S0-CVO-947

5TH EDITION

Maternity and Pediatric Nursing

5TH EDITION

Maternity and Pediatric Nursing

Susan Scott Ricci, APRN, MSN, MEd, CNE
Nursing Faculty
University of Central Florida
Orlando, Florida
Former Nursing Program Director and Faculty
Lake Sumter State College
Leesburg, Florida

Terri Kyle, DNP, APRN, CPNP, CNE
Professor of Nursing
RN to BSN, MSN Coordinator
AdventHealth University
Orlando, Florida

Susan Carman, MSN, MBA
Professor of Nursing
Most Recently, Edison Community College
Fort Myers, Florida

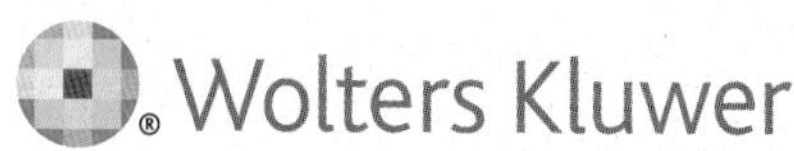

Philadelphia • Baltimore • New York • London
Buenos Aires • Hong Kong • Sydney • Tokyo

Vice President and Publisher: Julie K. Stegman
Director of Product Development: Jennifer K. Forestieri
Acquisitions Editor: Jodi Rhomberg
Development Editor: Devika Kishore
Editorial Coordinator: Erin E. Hernandez
Marketing Manager: Brittany Clements
Senior Production Project Manager: Catherine Ott
Art Director, Illustration: Jennifer Clements
Manager, Graphic Arts & Design: Stephen Druding
Manufacturing Coordinator: Margie Orzech
Prepress Vendor: S4Carlisle Publishing Services

Fifth Edition

Copyright © 2025 Wolters Kluwer.
Copyright © 2021, 2017 Wolters Kluwer. Copyright © 2013, 2009 Wolters Kluwer Health | Lippincott Williams & Wilkins. All rights reserved. This book is protected by copyright. No part of this book may be reproduced or transmitted in any form or by any means, including as photocopies or scanned-in or other electronic copies, or utilized by any information storage and retrieval system without written permission from the copyright owner, except for brief quotations embodied in critical articles and reviews. Materials appearing in this book prepared by individuals as part of their official duties as U.S. government employees are not covered by the above-mentioned copyright. To request permission, please contact Wolters Kluwer at Two Commerce Square, 2001 Market Street, Philadelphia, PA 19103, via email at permissions@lww.com, or via our website at shop.lww.com (products and services).

9 8 7 6 5 4 3 2 1

Printed in Mexico

Library of Congress Cataloging-in-Publication Data available upon request from publisher.

ISBN-13: 978-1-975220-41-9

Library of Congress Control Number: 2024915668

This work is provided "as is," and the publisher disclaims any and all warranties, express or implied, including any warranties as to accuracy, comprehensiveness, or currency of the content of this work.

This work is no substitute for individual patient assessment based upon healthcare professionals' examination of each patient and consideration of, among other things, age, weight, gender, current or prior medical conditions, medication history, laboratory data and other factors unique to the patient. The publisher does not provide medical advice or guidance and this work is merely a reference tool. Healthcare professionals, and not the publisher, are solely responsible for the use of this work including all medical judgments and for any resulting diagnosis and treatments.

Given continuous, rapid advances in medical science and health information, independent professional verification of medical diagnoses, indications, appropriate pharmaceutical selections and dosages, and treatment options should be made and healthcare professionals should consult a variety of sources. When prescribing medication, healthcare professionals are advised to consult the product information sheet (the manufacturer's package insert) accompanying each drug to verify, among other things, conditions of use, warnings and side effects and identify any changes in dosage schedule or contraindications, particularly if the medication to be administered is new, infrequently used or has a narrow therapeutic range. To the maximum extent permitted under applicable law, no responsibility is assumed by the publisher for any injury and/or damage to persons or property, as a matter of products liability, negligence law or otherwise, or from any reference to or use by any person of this work.

shop.lww.com

QUADM0824

This book is dedicated to the love of my life, my husband, Glenn, who fortifies me and encourages me in all my endeavors. Appreciate your support, encouragement, and expertise in editing. You are my rock and I am so blessed to have you at my side. And also to my children, Brian and Jennifer, and my grandchildren—Alyssa, Leyton, Sandon, Peyton, Wyatt, Michael, Rylan, Brody, Veda, and Reese—who bring me life's greatest joys. You make it all worthwhile.

—SUSAN SCOTT RICCI

This text is dedicated to all of the children and families I have been so honored to care for as a pediatric nurse and pediatric nurse practitioner. Thank you to my forever supportive husband, John, my amazing and delightful children, Christian and Caitlin, and the loves of my life: granddaughters Sophia and Chloe.

—TERRI KYLE

This book is dedicated to all the children out there and the wonderful nurses who care for them. They inspire me to become a better nurse, educator, and person. It is the major impact nurses have on the health of children and their families that drives me to find the best methods of teaching clinical judgment; our children deserve only the best pediatric nurses, with thorough education and training. This book is also dedicated to my loving and supportive family. My husband, Chris, without whom I could not have reached this accomplishment. My four beautiful girls, Grace, Ella, Lily, and Maya, who have allowed me to learn firsthand about growth and development and who truly amaze me each and every day. My parents, Lene and Kishor Patel, who always taught me I could do whatever I put my mind to. To Terri Kyle, thank you for this opportunity, your endless support, and your incredible vision.

—SUSAN CARMAN

ABOUT THE AUTHORS

SUSAN SCOTT RICCI

Susan Scott Ricci earned a diploma in nursing from the Washington Hospital Center School of Nursing with a BSN and an MSN from the Catholic University of America located in Washington, DC, as well as an MEd in Counseling from the University of Southern Mississippi. She is licensed as a women's health nurse practitioner (APRN) by the University of Florida. She recently renewed her national certification as a certified nurse educator (CNE). She has worked in numerous women's health care settings including labor and birth, postpartum, prenatal, and family planning ambulatory care clinics. Susan has spent more than 30 years in practice and in nursing education teaching in LPN, ADN, and BSN programs. She is involved in several professional nursing organizations and holds memberships in Sigma Theta Tau International Honor Society of Nursing, Association of Women's Health, Obstetric and Neonatal Nurses (AWHONN), American Nurses Association (ANA), National Association of OB/GYN Nurses, Who's Who in Professional Nursing, American Nurses Association, and the Florida Council of Maternal–Child Nurses.

With Susan's wealth of practical and educational experience, it is essential to concentrate on evidence-based nursing practice and reduce the amount of "nice to know" information that is presented to students. As an educator, she recognizes the tendency for nursing educators to want to "cover the world" when teaching, rather than focusing on the facts that students need to know for safe practice. With this mission in mind, Susan has directed her energy to the birth of these essential facts in this textbook.

She recognizes that nursing school instructional time is reduced, as the world of health care is expanding exponentially. Therefore, with the valuable instructional time allotted, she has recognized the urgent need to present pertinent facts as concisely as possible to promote application of knowledge within nursing practice.

TERRI KYLE

Terri Kyle earned a Bachelor of Science in Nursing from the University of North Carolina at Chapel Hill and a Master of Science in Nursing from Emory University in Atlanta, Georgia. Terri received her Doctorate of Nursing Practice in Educational Leadership from American Sentinel University. She is a certified pediatric nurse practitioner and certified nurse educator. Practicing pediatric nursing for over 40 years, Terri has had the opportunity to serve children and their families in a variety of diverse settings.

She has experience in inpatient pediatrics in pediatric and neonatal intensive care units, newborn nursery, specialized pediatric units, and community hospitals. She has worked as a pediatric nurse practitioner in pediatric specialty clinics and primary care. She has been involved in teaching nursing for over 32 years with experience in both undergraduate and graduate nursing education. Terri delights in providing innovative leadership to nursing educators and their students. She is a fellow in the National Association of Pediatric Nurse Practitioners and a member of Sigma Theta Tau International Honor Society of Nursing, the National League for Nursing, and the Society of Pediatric Nurses.

SUSAN CARMAN

Susan Carman earned a Bachelor of Science in Nursing from the University of Wisconsin–Madison and a Master of Science in Nursing and Master in Business Administration from the University of Colorado–Denver. As a pediatric nurse for over 25 years, Susan has had the opportunity to care for children in a variety of diverse settings and in many of the major children's hospitals throughout the United States. She also has provided volunteer nursing care in a variety of settings including the Dominican Republic and India. She has been involved in teaching nursing for the past 20 years and enjoys watching students transform into competent nurses with strong clinical judgment.

REVIEWERS

Barbara Caton, RN, MSN, CNE
Department Chair and Associate Professor of Nursing
Missouri State University
West Plains, Missouri

Mary Cimador, RN, MSN
Professor of Nursing
Community College of Allegheny County
Pittsburgh, Pennsylvania

Terri Enslein, EdD, MSN, RNC-OB, CNE
Associate Dean of Graduate Programs
Xavier University
Cincinnati, Ohio

Diane Hare, ADN, BSN, MSN, RN
Instructor of Allied Health
Lamar State College
Port Arthur, Texas

Jessica Huber, PhD, MSN, RN, CCRN, CPN
Assistant Professor of Nursing
Carlow University
Pittsburgh, Pennsylvania

Rebecca Logan, PhD, RN
Associate Professor of Nursing
Berry College
Mount Berry, Georgia

Jessica Marcus, DNP, RNC, WHNP-BC, CNE
Clinical Assistant Professor
Georgia State University
Atlanta, Georgia

Maureen Murt, MSN, RN, CCE
Associate Professor of Nursing
Bucks County Community College
Newtown, Pennsylvania

Sherry Obert, BSN, MSN
Professor of Nursing
Allegany College of Maryland
Everett, Pennsylvania

Sara Rippie, MS, AHN-BC, RNC-OB
Assistant Professor of Nursing
St. Catherine University
St. Paul, Minnesota

Rebecca Shabo, RN, PhD
Assistant Director of Accreditation and Assessment
Kennesaw State University
Kennesaw, Georgia

Tara Smith, MSN, RN
Assistant Professor of Nursing
Westmoreland County Community College
Youngwood, Pennsylvania

Alicia Stone, PhD, RN, FNP, CCES
Assistant Professor of Nursing
Molloy University
Rockville Centre, New York

Lisa Wallace, DNP, RNC-OB, NE-BC
Assistant Professor of Nursing
Morehead State University
Morehead, Kentucky

Donna Williams-Newman, PhD, DNP, MSN RN
Associate Professor of Nursing
Nova Southeastern University
Fort Lauderdale, Florida

PREFACE

Many nursing curricula combine and teach maternity and pediatrics in tandem. This can be viewed as a *natural fit* of two content areas that belong together. Nursing education in general is founded upon the principle of mastering simpler concepts first and incorporating those concepts into the student's knowledge base. The student is then able to progress to problem solving in more complex situations. In today's education climate with reduced class time devoted to specialty courses, it is particularly important for nursing educators to focus on key concepts, rather than attempting to cover everything within a specific topic.

The intent of *Maternity and Pediatric Nursing* is to provide the nurse the basis needed for sound nursing care of women and children. The content in the book will enable the reader to guide women and children toward higher levels of wellness throughout the life cycle. In addition, the focus of the textbook will allow the reader to anticipate, identify, and address common problems and provide timely, evidence-based interventions to reduce long-term sequelae.

This textbook is designed as a practical approach to understanding the health of women and children. The main objective is to help the student build a strong knowledge base and assist with the development of critical thinking skills and clinical reasoning. Women in our society are becoming empowered to make informed and responsible choices regarding their health and that of their children, but to do so they need the encouragement and support of nurses who care for them. This textbook focuses on women and children throughout their lifespan, covering a broad scope of topics with emphasis placed upon common issues. Maternity nursing content coverage is comprehensive yet presented in a concise and straightforward manner. The pediatric nursing content presents the important differences when caring for children compared with caring for adults. Utilizing the nursing process, a concept-based approach to the care of children and their families provides relevant information in a concise and nonredundant manner.

Since women's health has expanded to include care throughout their lifespan, the emphasis of this textbook is on promoting and maintaining their health. The focus of this fifth edition has now expanded to the global outreach of various cultures and traditions that nurses will encounter in their daily practice settings. Nurses are key players in the global community who improve the lives of mothers and infants. Safe nursing practice requires skills and knowledge, with application of sound evidence-based clinical judgment. It is vital for nurses to understand their clients to help promote an optimal outcome to all women and their families. Childbirth today has returned to a more natural practice that honors the normal process of birth. Several chapters focus on physiologic births and the nurse's role to accomplish this. With these imperatives in mind, the chapters present an overview of common health conditions encountered by many women and how to care for them. The new content presented can be used as a framework in caring for clients from diverse backgrounds, histories, and cultures.

The focus when caring for children is also to maintain and promote their health, as well as provide developmentally appropriate care whether the child is well or ill. Restoration of a child's health when an illness is experienced is paramount for timely accomplishment of suitable growth and development. Nurses are in a prime position for influencing children's health, not only through the direct care they provide to children but also through the connections they make with caregivers and their ability to educate families to best care for their children. Focusing on conceptual learning, students may develop complex critical thinking leading to the ability to clinically reason within various health care environments. This approach is supported by many of the book's features, such as the reoccurring features: Unfolding Case Studies, Clinical Reasoning Alerts, and Thinking About Development.

ORGANIZATION

Each chapter of *Maternity and Pediatric Nursing* focuses on a different aspect of maternity and/or pediatric nursing care. The book is divided into 11 units, beginning with general concepts related to maternity and pediatric nursing care, progressing from women's health, pregnancy and birth, through to child health promotion and nursing management of alterations in children's health.

Unit I: Introduction to Maternity and Pediatric Nursing

Unit I helps build a foundation for the student beginning the study of the care of women, infants, and children. This unit explores contemporary issues and trends in maternity and pediatric nursing. Perspectives on female health and pediatric nursing, core concepts of maternal and pediatric nursing, including family-centered and atraumatic care, and communication, and community-based nursing are addressed.

Unit II: Women's Health Throughout the Lifespan

Unit II introduces the student to selected female health topics, including structure and function of the reproductive system, common reproductive concerns, sexually transmitted infections, problems of the breast, and benign disorders and cancers of the female reproductive tract. This unit encourages the student to assist female patients in maintaining their quality of life, reducing their risk of disease, and becoming active partners with their health care professional.

Unit III: Pregnancy

Unit III addresses topics related to normal pregnancy, including fetal development, genetics, and maternal adaptation to pregnancy. Nursing management during normal pregnancy is addressed, encouraging application of basic knowledge to nursing practice. Nursing management includes maternal and fetal assessment throughout pregnancy, interventions to promote self-care and minimize common discomforts, and patient education.

Unit IV: Labor and Birth

Unit IV begins with an explanation of the normal labor and birth process, including maternal and fetal adaptations. This is followed by content focusing on the nurse's role during normal labor and birth, which includes maternal and fetal assessment, pharmacologic and nonpharmacologic comfort measures and pain management, and specific nursing interventions during each stage of labor and birth.

Unit V: Postpartum Period

Unit V focuses on maternal adaptation during the normal postpartum period. Both physiologic and psychological aspects are explored. Paternal adaptation is also considered. This unit also presents related nursing management, including assessment of physical and emotional status, promoting comfort, assisting with elimination, counseling about sexuality and contraception, promoting nutrition, promoting family adaptation, and preparing for discharge.

Unit VI: The Newborn

Unit VI covers physiologic and behavioral adaptations of the normal newborn. It also delves into nursing management of the normal newborn, including immediate assessment and specific interventions as well as ongoing assessment, physical examination, and specific interventions during the early newborn period.

Unit VII: Childbearing at Risk

Unit VII shifts the focus to at-risk pregnancy, childbirth, and postpartum care. Preexisting conditions of the woman, pregnancy-related complications, at-risk labor, emergencies associated with labor and birth, and medical conditions and complications affecting the postpartum woman are all covered. Treatment and nursing management are presented for each medical condition. This organization allows the student to build on a solid foundation of normal material when studying the at-risk content.

Unit VIII: The Newborn at Risk

Unit VIII continues to center on at-risk content. Issues of the newborn with birthweight variations, gestational age variations, congenital conditions, and acquired disorders are explored. Treatment and nursing management are presented for each medical condition. This organization helps cement the student's understanding of the material.

Unit IX: Health Promotion of the Growing Child and Family

Unit IX provides information related to growth and development expectations of the well child from newborn through adolescence. Although not exhaustive in nature, this unit provides a broad knowledge base related to normal growth and development that the nurse can draw on in any situation. Common concerns related to growth and development and client/family education are included in each age-specific chapter.

Unit X: Foundations of Pediatric Nursing

Unit X covers broad concepts that provide the foundation for providing nursing care for children. Rather than reiterating all aspects of nursing care, the unit focuses on specific details needed to provide nursing care for children in general. The content remains focused upon differences in caring for children compared with adults. Topics covered in this unit include atraumatic care, anticipatory guidance, routine well-child care (including immunization and safety), health assessment, nursing care of the child in diverse settings, including the hospital and at home, concerns common to special needs children, pediatric variations in medication and intravenous fluid delivery and nutritional support, and pain management in children.

Unit XI: Nursing Care of the Child With a Health Disorder

Unit XI focuses on children's responses to health disorders. This unit provides comprehensive coverage of illnesses affecting children and is presented according to broad topics of disorders organized with a body systems approach. It also includes infectious, genetic, and mental health disorders as well as pediatric emergencies. Each chapter follows a similar format in order to facilitate presentation of the information as well as reduce repetition. The chapters begin with a nursing process overview for the particular broad topic, presenting differences in children and how the nursing process applies. The approach provides a general framework for addressing disorders within the chapter. Individual disorders are then addressed with attention to specifics related to pathophysiology, nursing assessment, nursing management, and special considerations. Common pediatric disorders are covered in greater depth than less common disorders. The format of the chapters allows for the building of a strong knowledge base and encourages critical thinking. Additionally, the format is nursing process driven and consistent from chapter to chapter, providing a practical and sensible presentation of the information.

RECURRING FEATURES

To provide the instructor and student with an exciting and user-friendly text, a number of recurring features have been developed.

Key Terms

A list of terms that are considered essential to the chapter's understanding is presented at the beginning of each chapter. Each key term appears in boldface, with the definition included in the text. Phonetic spellings are provided for terms that may be new or difficult to pronounce.

Learning Objectives

Learning Objectives included at the beginning of each chapter guide the student in understanding what is important and why, leading the student to prioritize information for learning. These valuable learning tools also provide opportunities for self-testing or instructor evaluation of student knowledge and ability.

Words of Wisdom

Each chapter opens with inspiring Words of Wisdom (WOW), which offer helpful, timely, and interesting thoughts. These WOW statements set the stage for each chapter and give the student valuable insight into nursing care of women, children, and their families.

Threaded Case Studies

Real-life scenarios present relevant information regarding women, children, and families that is intended to improve the student's clinical reasoning skills. Questions that are threaded throughout the chapter about the scenario provide an opportunity for the student to critically evaluate the appropriate course of action.

Clinical Reasoning Alert

The Clinical Reasoning Alert promotes critical thinking in the nursing process on information key to clinical reasoning.

Unfolding Patient Stories

Unfolding Patient Stories, written by the National League for Nursing, are an engaging way to begin meaningful conversations in the classroom. These vignettes feature patients from Wolters Kluwer's *vSim for Nursing | Health Assessment* (codeveloped with Laerdal Medical) and DocuCare products; however, each Unfolding Patient Story in the book stands alone, not requiring purchase of these products. For your convenience, a list of these case studies, along with their location in the book, appears in the "Cases That Unfold Across Chapters" section later in this front matter.

Evidence-Based Practice

The consistent promotion of evidence-based practice is a key feature of the text. Throughout the chapters, pivotal questions addressed by current research have been incorporated into Evidence-Based Practice displays, which discuss recent evidence-based research findings and provide recommendations for nurses.

Healthy People 2030

Throughout the textbook, relevant Healthy People 2030 objectives are outlined in box format. The nursing implications or guidance provided in the box serves as a road map for improving the health of women, mothers, and children. These objectives reflect the Healthy People 2030 objectives.

Atraumatic Care

These highlights, located throughout the pediatric sections of the book, provide tips for providing atraumatic care to children in particular situations in relation to the topic being discussed.

Thinking About Development

The content featured in these boxes in chapters related to the care of children will encourage the student to think critically about special developmental concerns relating to the topic being discussed.

Teaching Guidelines

An important tool for achieving health promotion and disease prevention is health education. Throughout the textbook, Teaching Guidelines raise awareness, provide timely and accurate information, and are designed to ensure the student's preparation for educating women, children, and their families about various issues.

Consider This!

In every chapter the student is asked to *Consider This!* These first-person narratives engage the student in real-life scenarios experienced by their clients. The personal accounts evoke empathy and help the student to perfect caregiving skills. Each box ends with an opportunity for further contemplation, encouraging the student to think critically about the scenario.

Take Note!

The *Take Note!* feature draws the student's attention to points of critical emphasis throughout the chapter. This feature is often used to stress vitally important information.

Drug Guides

Drug guide tables summarize information about commonly used medications. The actions, indications, and significant nursing implications presented assist the student in providing optimum care to women, children, and their families.

Common Laboratory and Diagnostic Tests

The Common Laboratory and Diagnostic Tests tables in many of the chapters provide the student with a general understanding of how a broad range of disorders is diagnosed. Rather than reading the information repeatedly throughout the narrative, the student is then able to refer to the table as needed.

Common Medical Treatments

The Common Medical Treatments tables in many of the nursing management chapters provide the student with a broad awareness of how a common group of disorders is treated either medically or surgically. The tables serve as a reference point for common medical treatments.

Clinical Judgment and the Nursing Process

The Clinical Judgment & Nursing Process boxes provide concrete examples of particular steps of the nursing process and are provided in numerous chapters. Found within the nursing process overview section of the chapter, they summarize issue- or system-related content and outline a guide for delivering care.

Comparison Charts

These charts compare two or more disorders or other easily confused concepts. They serve to provide an explanation that clarifies the concepts for the student.

Nursing Procedures

Step-by-step Nursing Procedures are presented in a clear, concise format to facilitate competent performance of relevant procedures as well as to clarify maternity and pediatric variations when appropriate.

Dosage Calculation Box

This box provides a dosage calculation example in each of the pediatric alteration/disorder chapters. Reiteration of the significance of accurate dosage calculation assists the student with mastery of this critical concept.

Concept Mastery Alerts

Concept Mastery Alerts clarify maternity and pediatric nursing concepts to improve the reader's understanding of potentially confusing topics as identified by Misconception Alerts in Lippincott's Adaptive Learning Powered by PrepU. Data from thousands of actual students using this program in courses across the United States identified common misconceptions for the authors to clarify in this new edition.

Tables, Boxes, Illustrations, and Photographs

Abundant tables and boxes summarize key content throughout the book. Additionally, beautiful illustrations and photographs help the student to visualize the content. These features allow the student to quickly and easily access information.

Key Concepts

At the end of each chapter, Key Concepts provide a quick review of essential chapter elements. These bulleted lists help the student focus on the important aspects of the chapter.

References

References used in the development of the text are provided at the end of each chapter. These listings enable the student to further explore topics of interest. Many online resources are provided as a means for the student to electronically explore relevant content material. These resources can be shared with women, children, and their families to enhance patient education and support.

Developing Clinical Judgment

This section located at the end of each chapter assists the student with the development of clinical judgment through:

- **Practicing for NCLEX**—these NCLEX-RN style questions (multiple choice, multiple response, fill in the blanks) test the student's ability to utilize critical thinking in the application of the nursing process to chapter material. The questions are styled similarly to the national licensing exam (NCLEX-RN). Next-Gen NCLEX-RN style questions are now included in most chapters.
- **Dosage calculation questions**—these applicable problems test the student's ability to accurately determine medication dosages particular to children.
- **Critical thinking exercises**—these exercises serve to stimulate the student to incorporate the current material with previously learned concepts and reach a satisfactory conclusion. The exercises encourage students to think critically, problem solve, and consider their own perspective on given topics.
- **Study activities**—these activities promote student participation in the learning process. This section encourages increased interaction/learning via clinical, online, and community activities.
- **Answers**—answers to the Developing Clinical Judgment questions are provided to instructors on thePoint®.

INCLUSIVE LANGUAGE

A note about the language used in this book: Wolters Kluwer recognizes that people have a diverse range of identities, and we are committed to using the most inclusive, nonbiased language possible in our products. In line with the principles of nursing, we strive not to define people by their diagnoses, but to recognize their personhood first and foremost, using as much as possible the language diverse groups use to define themselves, and including only information that is relevant to nursing care.

We strive to better address the unique perspectives, complex challenges, and lived experiences of diverse populations traditionally underrepresented in health literature. When describing or referencing populations discussed in research studies, we will adhere to the identities presented in those studies to maintain fidelity to the evidence presented by the study investigators. We follow best practices of language set forth by the *Publication Manual of the American Psychological Association*, 7th edition, but acknowledge that language evolves rapidly, and we anticipate continuing to modify our language in future editions of our products.

TEACHING–LEARNING PACKAGE

Instructor's Resources

Tools to assist you with teaching your course are available upon adoption of this text.

- The **E-Book** gives you access to the book's full text and images online.
- A **Test Generator** features hundreds of questions within a powerful tool to help the instructor create quizzes and tests.
- **PowerPoint presentations** with **Guided Lecture Notes** provide an easy way for you to integrate the textbook with our students' classroom experience, either via slide shows or handouts. Multiple choice and true/false questions are integrated into the presentations to promote class participation and allow you to use iClicker technology.
- An **Image Bank** lets you use the photographs and illustrations from this textbook in your PowerPoint slides or as you see fit in your course.
- **Case Studies** with related questions (and suggested answers) give students an opportunity to apply their knowledge to a client case similar to one they might encounter in practice.
- **Journal Articles**, updated for the new edition, offer access to current research available in Lippincott Williams & Wilkins journals.
- **Multimedia Resources** appeal to a variety of learning styles, including:
  - **Watch and Learn Videos** highlight growth and development, communicating with children, and providing nursing care to the child in the hospital.
  - **Concepts in Action Animations** bring physiologic and pathophysiologic concepts to life and enhance student comprehension.
- **Journal Articles** offer access to current research available in Lippincott Williams & Wilkins journals. Contact your sales representative or check out LWW.com/Nursing for more details and ordering information.

Lippincott® CoursePoint+

The same trusted solution, innovation, and unmatched support that you have come to expect from *Lippincott CoursePoint+* is now enhanced with more engaging learning tools and deeper analytics to help prepare students for practice. This powerfully integrated digital learning solution combines learning tools, case studies, virtual simulation, real-time data, and the most trusted nursing education content on the market to make curriculum-wide learning more efficient and to meet students where they're at in their learning. And now, it's easier than ever for instructors and students to use, giving them everything they need for course and curriculum success!

Lippincott CoursePoint+ includes:

- Engaging course content provides a variety of learning tools to engage students of all learning styles.
- A more personalized learning approach, including adaptive learning powered by PrepU, gives students the content and tools they need at the moment they need it, giving them data for more focused remediation and helping to boost their confidence.
- Varying levels of case studies, virtual simulation, and access to Lippincott Advisor help students learn the critical thinking and clinical judgment skills to help them become practice-ready nurses.
- Unparalleled reporting provides in-depth dashboards with several data points to track student progress and help identify strengths and weaknesses.
- Unmatched support includes training coaches, product trainers, and nursing education consultants to help educators and students implement CoursePoint with ease.

CONTENTS IN BRIEF

CONTENTS

CASES THAT UNFOLD ACROSS CHAPTERS

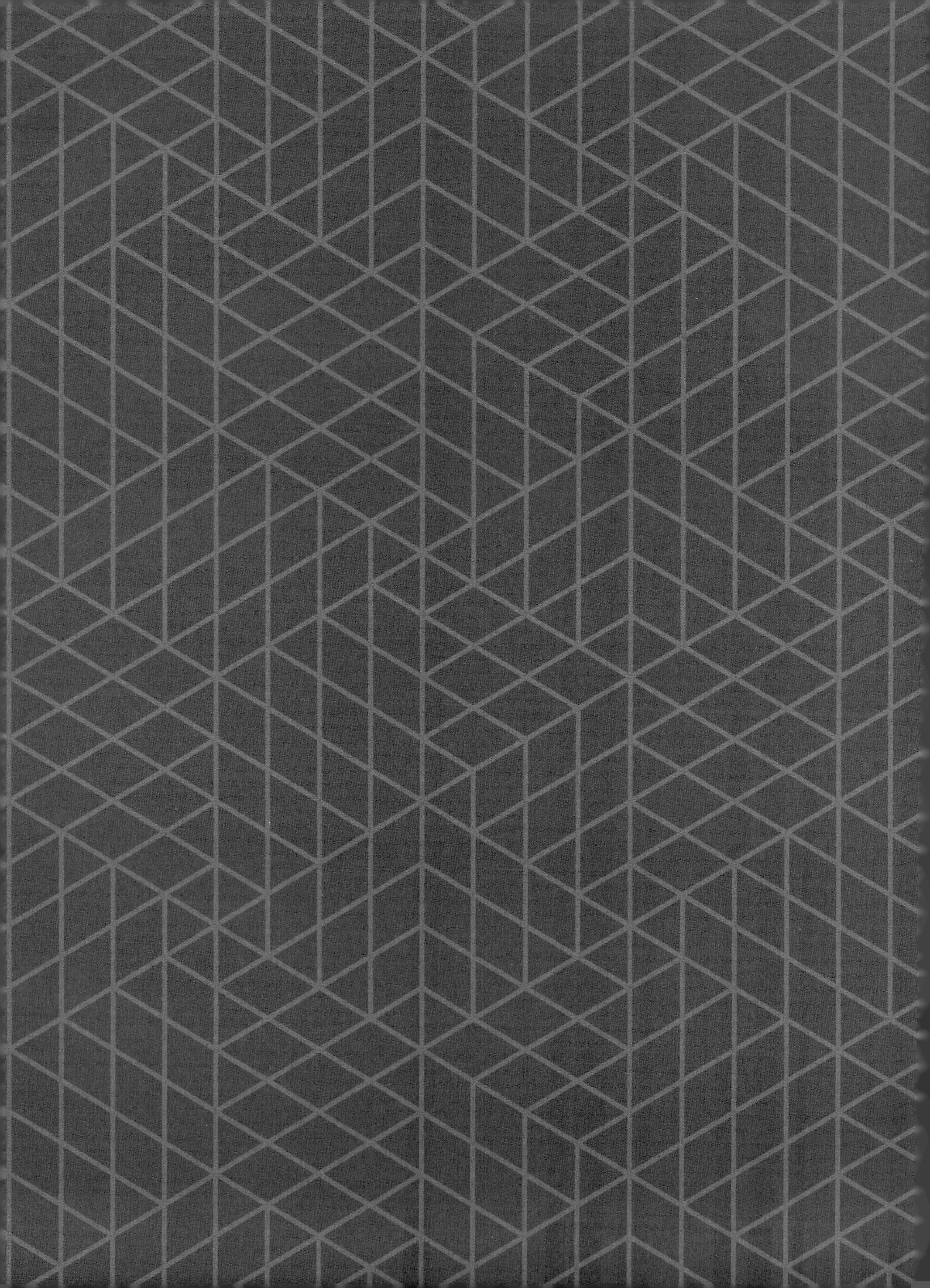

UNIT

I

Introduction to Maternity and Pediatric Nursing

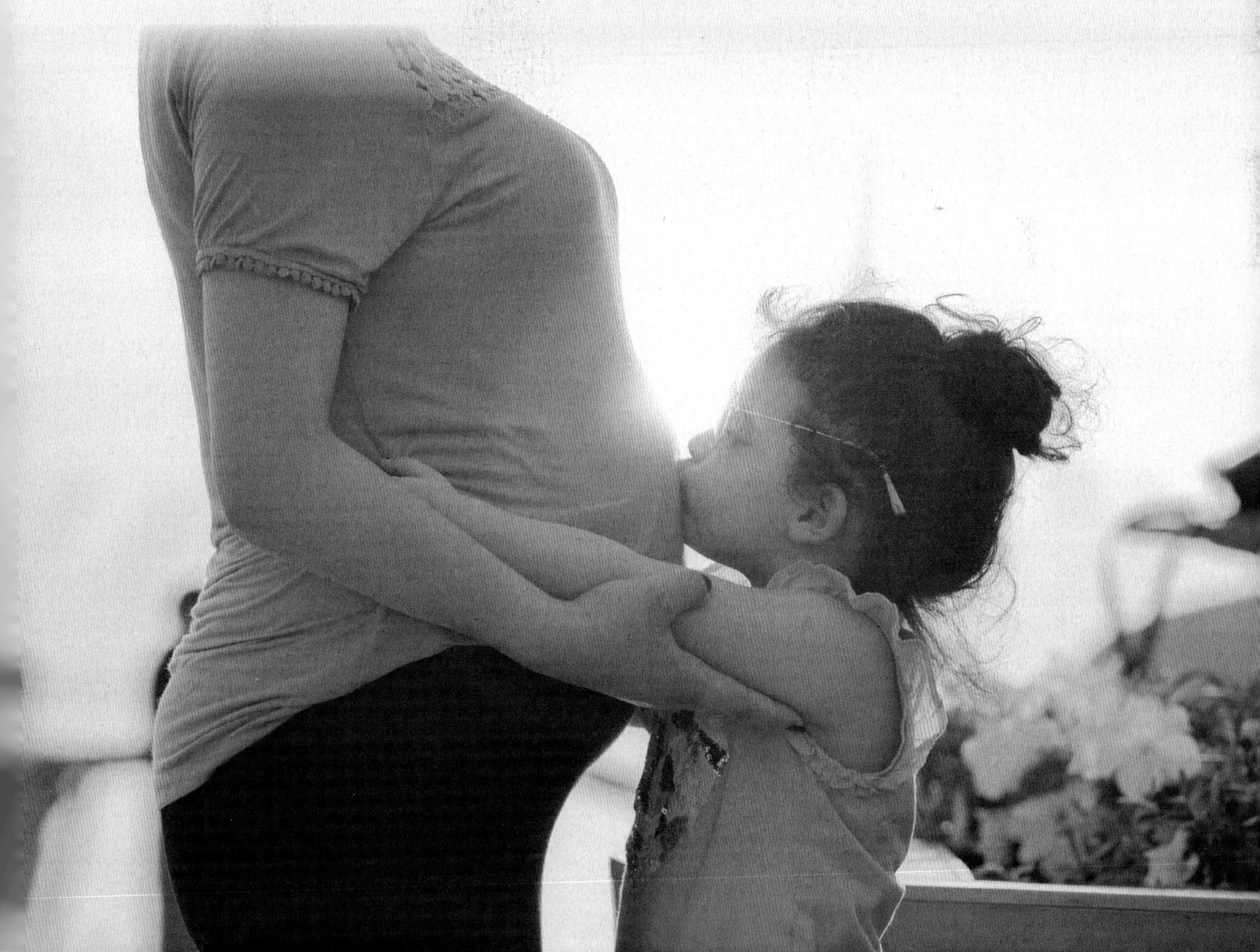

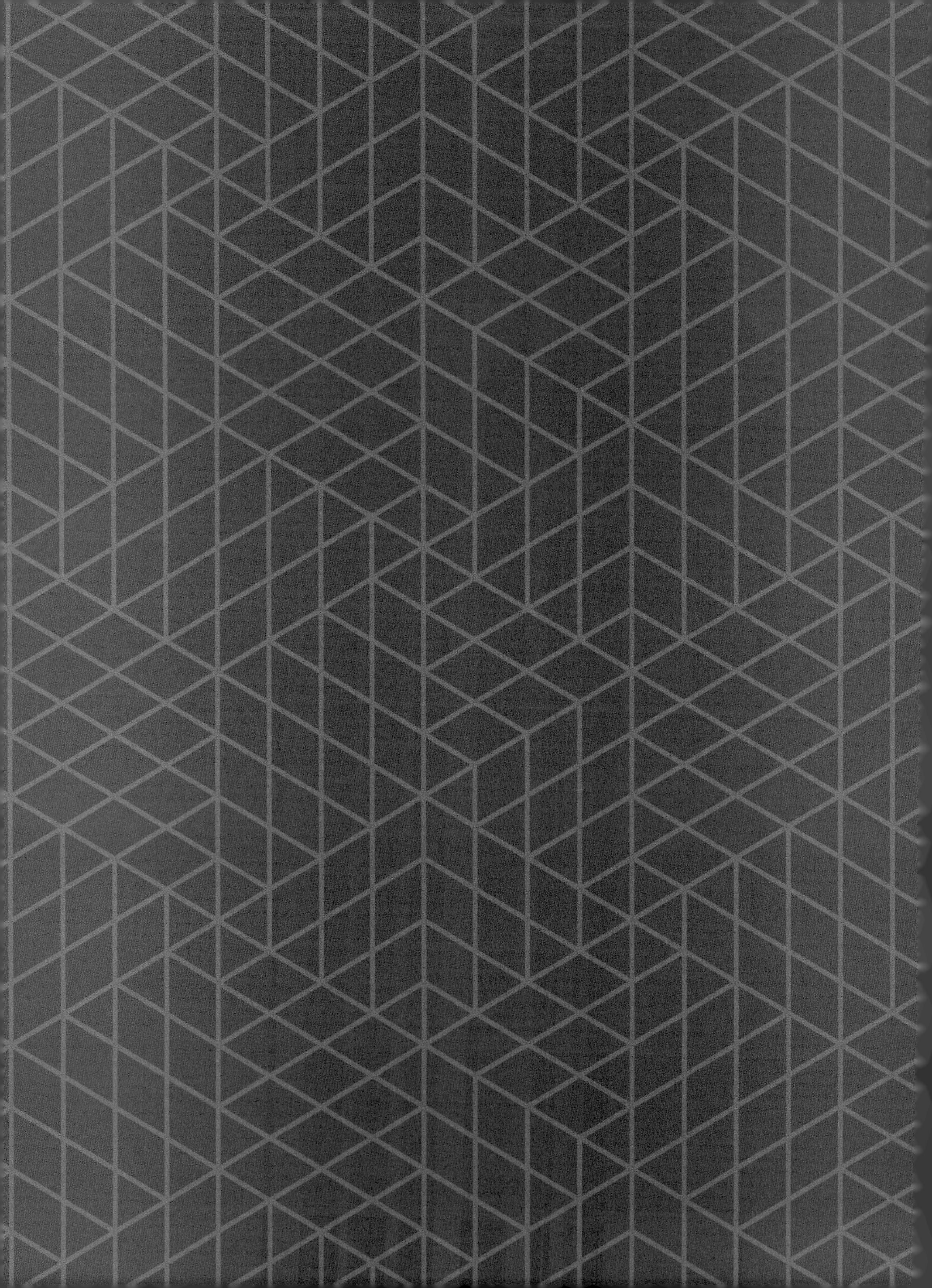

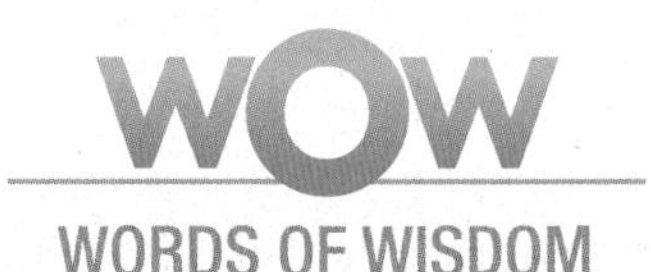

WORDS OF WISDOM

Being pregnant and giving birth is like crossing a narrow bridge: People can accompany you to the bridge, and they can greet you on the other side, but you walk that bridge alone. And the journey doesn't end there: Children are the future of a society and special gifts to the world. Changes in our society and world require us to be attentive to and value them and their health.

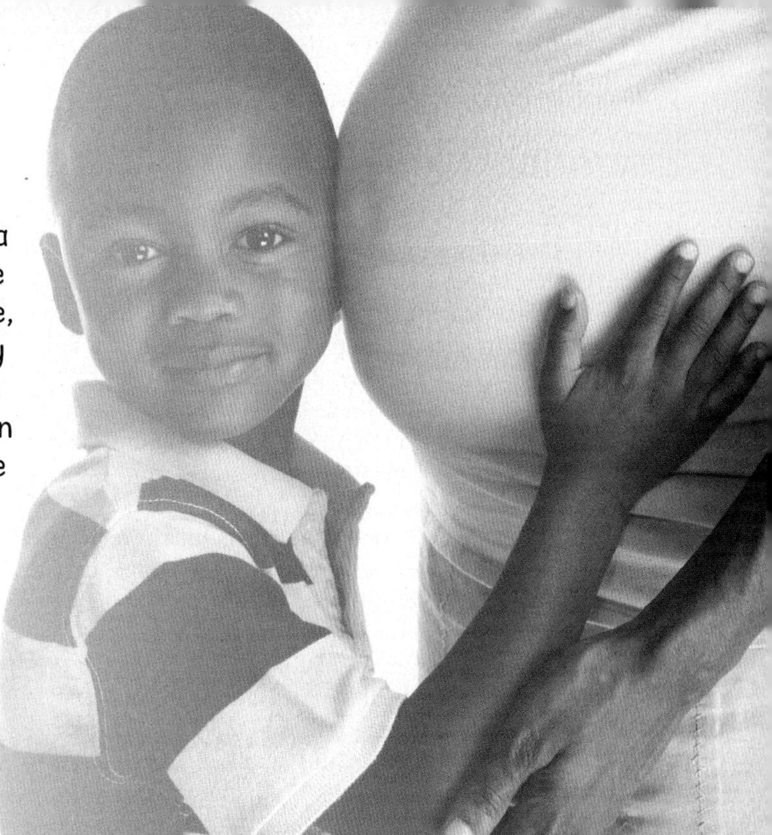

1

Perspectives on Maternal and Child Health Care

KEY TERMS

Affordable Care Act (ACA)
assent
certified nurse midwife (CNM)
childhood mortality rate
dissent
do-not-attempt-resuscitation (DNAR) orders
doula
emancipated minor
fetal mortality rate
infant mortality rate
maternal–fetal conflict
maternal mortality ratio
mature minor
morbidity
neonatal mortality rate

LEARNING OBJECTIVES

Upon completion of the chapter, you will be able to:

1. Analyze the key milestones in the history of maternal, newborn, and child health and health care.
2. Outline the evolution of maternal, newborn, and pediatric nursing.
3. Compare the past definitions of health and illness with the current definitions, as well as the measurements used to assess health and illness in children.
4. Identify the ethical and legal issues that may arise when caring for birthing parents, children, and families.

Sophia Greenly, a 38-year-old patient pregnant with her third child, comes to the prenatal clinic for a routine follow-up visit. Her parent, Betty, accompanies her because Sophia's husband is out of town. Sophia lives with her husband and two children, ages 4 and 9. She works part-time as a lunch aide in the local elementary school. What factors may play a role in influencing the health of Sophia and her family?

INTRODUCTION

A person's ability to lead a fulfilling life and to participate fully in society depends largely on their health status. This is especially true for people whose familial roles make them responsible for not only their own health but also that of others: their children and families. In many cases, this role is fulfilled by women. Thus, it is important to concentrate on the health of women, children, and families. Children are the future of our society. Their overall health has improved, and rates of death and illness in some areas have decreased but we still must focus on children's health both in the United States and globally. Habits and practices established in childhood have profound effects on health and illness throughout life. It is crucial to foster a society that cares about women, children, and families and promotes preventive and quality health care and positive lifestyle choices. Nurses play a major role in this task.

It should be noted in this textbook that the term "woman" is primarily written from the perspective of cisgender women, but other gender identities have been included where possible. We acknowledge that those assigned female at birth are not always women, and not all women may have been assigned female at birth. Nurses will care and must advocate for patients from a wide range of gender identities, racial or ethnic groups, religions, sexual orientations, age groups, socioeconomic statuses, and disability statuses.

Maternity care is an integrated care process, which consists of different services (prenatal, intranatal, and postnatal), involves different professionals, and covers extended time frames. Maternal and newborn nursing encompasses a wide scope of practice typically associated with childbearing. It includes care of the patient before pregnancy; care of the pregnant patient and fetus during pregnancy; care of the patient after pregnancy; and care of the newborn, usually during the first 6 weeks after birth. The overall goal of maternal and newborn nursing is to promote and maintain optimal health of the patient and their family. Providing quality maternity care includes patient satisfaction and achieving the best evidence-based outcomes with the fewest interventions. Child health nursing, commonly referred to as pediatric nursing, involves the care of the child from infancy through adolescence. In the United States, the number of children under age 18 years is approximately 72.5 million, accounting for 22% of the population (Federal Interagency Forum on Child and Family Statistics [FIFCFS], 2023). Since the 1960s, children have decreased as a percentage of the total U.S. population; the percentage is projected to slowly decline through 2050 (FIFCFS, 2023). The overall goal of pediatric nursing practice is to promote and assist the child in maintaining optimal levels of health while recognizing the influence of the family on the child's well-being. This goal involves health promotion and disease and injury prevention as well as assisting with care during illness. The common thread in both of these is the care of the family.

This chapter presents a general overview of the health care of women, children, and the legal and ethical issues involved in maternal and child health care. Nurses need to be knowledgeable about these concepts to ensure that they provide safe, professional care.

HISTORICAL DEVELOPMENT

The health care of women and children has changed over the years due in part to changes in childbirth methods, devastating epidemics, social trends in the United States, economic circumstances, physical environment, safety, exposure to violence, illicit substance misuse, changes in the health care system, and federal and state regulations. By reviewing historical events, nurses can gain a better understanding of the current and future status of maternal and child health and how maternal and pediatric nursing care has evolved.

The History of Maternal and Newborn Health and Health Care

Childbirth in colonial America was a difficult and dangerous experience. Death in childbirth was so common that many colonial women regarded pregnancy with dread. In addition to her anxieties about pregnancy, an expectant birthing parent was faced with the possible death of her newborn child.

Centuries ago, "granny midwives" handled the birthing process in most cases. Midwifery skills have traditionally been passed from one woman to another within families, grandparents to birthing parents to daughters, and also through apprenticeships with more experienced midwives. In the late 1800s and early 1900s, childbirth became very medicalized due to advances in pain relief, improved antiseptic and aseptic surgical procedures, and an increased belief in scientific medicine (Martucci, 2018).

During the early 1900s, university-trained primary providers attended about half the births in the United States. Midwives often cared for women who could not afford a doctor. Many women were attracted to hospitals because this showed affluence; additionally, hospitals could provide pain management, which was not available for home births. In the 1950s, natural childbirth practices advocating birth without medication and focusing on relaxation techniques were introduced (Handley-Cousins, 2021). These techniques opened the door to childbirth education classes and encouraged the nonbirthing parent's participation in the experience. Both partners could participate by taking an active role in pregnancy, childbirth, and parenting (Fig. 1.1).

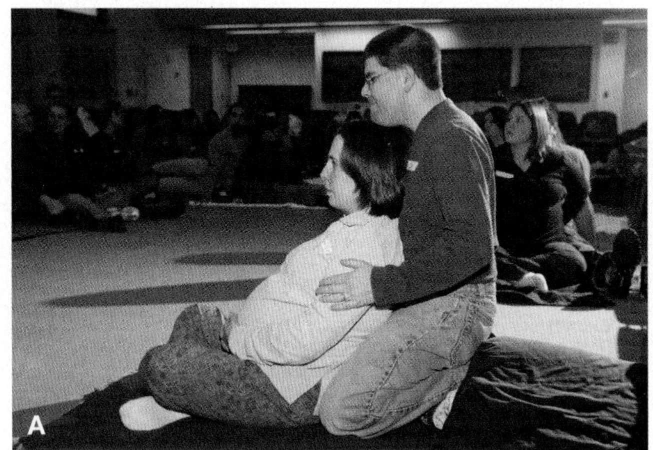

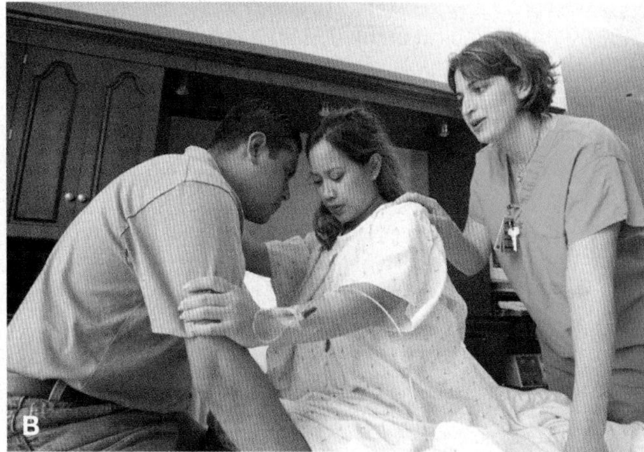

FIGURE 1.1 Today nonbirthing parents and partners are often encouraged to take an active role in the pregnancy and childbirth experience. **A.** A couple can participate together in childbirth education classes. (Photo by Gus Freedman.) **B.** Nonbirthing parents and partners can assist the birthing parent throughout their labor and delivery. (Photo by Joe Mitchell.)

Before World War II, American women moved from home to the hospital for childbirth in part because they were convinced the hospital setting would improve birth outcomes. Hospitals were the major employers of maternity nurses. Early ambulation and rooming-in induced changes in the focus of care for the growing numbers of birthing parents and infants. Maternity nurses' focus shifted away from carrying out tasks and performing procedures to teaching new parents about self- and infant care. Improved staffing patterns within hospitals meant longer hospital stays for the new parents, which allowed maternity nurses to spend more time with them for teaching purposes. Maternity nursing has changed dramatically since the baby boom era. The natural childbirth movement became a catalyst to bring about a change in nursing practice in postpartum nursing units.

Other changes that came later included breastfeeding and rooming-in to facilitate maternal–newborn bonding. Maternity nurses were then able to help the new birthing parents learn better how to care for their infants, to promote breastfeeding and bonding. The mid-1960s and early 1970s ushered in a consumer revolt that brought back home births, prepared childbirth, birth centers, a more humanizing maternity care focus, the nonbirthing parent's or partner's involvement in the birthing process, and nurse midwives—which had all but disappeared from the American health system (Martucci, 2018). Maternal–infant bonding became recognized as an essential part of postnatal care, and maternity nurses took a lead role in facilitating it. Box 1.1 shows a timeline of childbirth in America.

The History of Child Health and Child Health Care

In past centuries in the United States, the health of the country's population was overall poorer than it is today: Mortality rates were high, and life expectancy was short. When large numbers of people emigrated from Europe and immigrants settled in eastern U.S. cities, infectious diseases were rampant due to crowded living conditions, inadequate and unsafe food (e.g., contaminated milk), lack of childhood immunizations, and unsafe working conditions (including child labor). Devastating epidemics of smallpox, diphtheria, scarlet fever, and measles hit children the hardest. During this period, the prevalent view was that children were a commodity; their role was to increase the population and share in the work to be done. This view has changed over the years. Public schools were established, and the court system began viewing children as minors. The country began to pay more and more attention to the health of children.

As the end of the 19th century neared, doctors and scientists gained a better understanding of the root causes of illness. This knowledge helped fuel public health efforts, such as the campaign for a safe milk supply, which led to pasteurizing milk and to dispensing free milk in some cities (Maternal and Child Health Bureau [MCHB], Health Resources and Services Administration [HRSA], U.S. Department of Health and Human Services, n.d.). Compulsory vaccination programs began during this time. In the late 1800s, some states mandated smallpox vaccination as a condition of school attendance. These public health efforts led to a decrease in infant and child deaths (MCHB, HRSA, U.S. Department of Health and Human Services, n.d.).

In the late 19th and early 20th centuries, cities became healthier places to live due to urban public health improvements, such as sanitation services, treated municipal water, and improvements in hygiene (MCHB, HRSA, U.S. Department of Health and Human Services, n.d.). The threat of childhood diseases such as diphtheria, cholera, polio, and yellow fever began to take less of a toll on children (MCHB, HRSA, U.S. Department of Health and Human Services, n.d.). At the turn of the 20th century, researchers were achieving a new

BOX 1.1 Childbirth in the United States: A Timeline

1700s Society expected that women cared for women; men did not attend births because it was considered improper.
Women feared childbirth due to the risk of death; it was not generally viewed as joyous.
Female midwives attended most births at the woman's home.

1800s There was a shift from using midwives to doctors among middle-class women.
Puerperal (childbed) fever was occurring in epidemic proportions.
Louis Pasteur showed that streptococci were the major cause of puerperal fever that was killing birthing parents after delivery.
The first surgical birth (also called a cesarean delivery) was performed in Boston in 1894.
The x-ray was developed in 1895 and was used to assess pelvic size for birthing purposes.

1900s At the beginning of the decade, few women (<5%) gave birth in a hospital setting.
Twilight sleep (a heavy dose of narcotics and amnesiacs) was used on women during childbirth in the United States. Of all women who gave birth, 50% did so in hospitals by 1940 and 97% by 1960.
Nurseries were established because birthing parents could not care for their babies for several days after receiving chloroform gas.
In 1950, Sister Mary Stella introduced the idea of family-centered maternity care.
In 1933, Dr. Grantly Dick-Read wrote a book advocating natural childbirth entitled *Childbirth Without Fear*; he aimed to reduce the "fear–tension–pain" cycle women experienced during labor and birth.
In 1984, Dr. Fernand Lamaze wrote a book entitled *Painless Childbirth: The Lamaze Method*, which advocated distraction and relaxation techniques to minimize the perception of pain.
In the 1960s, the first birth control pills became available.
The 1970s and 1980s saw a growing trend to return to the "basics" of childbirth with nonmedicated, nonintervening care.
In the late 1900s, freestanding birthing centers were designed, and the number of home births began to increase.

2000s About one in three women undergoes a surgical birth.
Certified nurse midwives once again assist birthing parents with natural childbirth at home, in hospitals, or in freestanding facilities.
Childbirth classes of every flavor abound in most communities.

Feldhusen, A. E. (2000). The history of midwifery and childbirth in America: A time line. https://www.midwiferytoday.com/web-article/history-midwifery-childbirth-america-time-line/; Martucci, J. (2018). Beyond the nature/medicine in maternity care. *AMA Journal of Ethics, 20*(12), 1168–1174. https://doi.org/10.1001/amajethics.2018.1168

understanding of nutrition, sanitation, bacteriology, pharmacology, medication, and psychology. Penicillin, corticosteroids, and the increased number of vaccines developed during this time assisted with the fight against communicable diseases. Thus, by the end of the 20th century, unintentional injuries surpassed disease as the leading cause of death for children older than 1 year (Guyer et al., 2000).

By the end of the 1990s, technologic advances had significantly affected all aspects of health care. These trends led to increased survival rates in children. However, many children who survive illnesses that were previously considered fatal are left with chronic disabilities. For example, before the 1960s, extremely premature infants did not survive because of the immaturity of their lungs. The use of medications to foster lung development has increased survival rates in premature infants, but many of these children have chronic illnesses such as chronic lung disease (bronchopulmonary dysplasia), retinopathy of prematurity, cerebral palsy, and neurodevelopmental impairments (Mandy, 2022, 2023). Increased survival has resulted in a significant increase in chronic illness relative to acute illness as a cause of hospitalization and mortality (Mandy, 2023).

The beginning of the 21st century has brought tremendous improvements in technology and biomedicine. This has created a trend toward earlier diagnosis and treatment of disorders and diseases. Remarkable progress has been made linking genetics and pathophysiologic processes. Gene therapy holds the promise of correcting genetic disease before birth as research in this area continues to progress. In 2019, the U.S. Food and Drug Administration (FDA, 2019) approved an intravenous gene therapy construct for spinal muscle atrophy. In addition, many genetic defects are being identified early; thus, counseling and treatment may occur. Advancements in diagnostic technology and treatment methods continue to improve child health. For example, inhaled insulin, which is less invasive than an injection or pump, has been FDA approved for adults and is currently being studied for use in children ages 4 to 18 (U.S. National Library of Medicine, ClinicalTrials.gov, 2022).

In addition to improvements in technology and biomedicine in recent years, a number of national and international organizations devoted to protecting children's rights both in the United States and worldwide have been established. These organizations focus on events and circumstances that can negatively impact health: violence and abuse, child labor and soldiering, juvenile justice, child immigrants, orphaned children, and children who are abandoned or experiencing homelessness. A child whose rights are restored and upheld has an improved opportunity for growth, development, education, and health.

The gains in child health have been huge; unfortunately, these gains are not shared equally among all children. Certain health concerns, such as poor nutrition, obesity, lead poisoning, and asthma, affect children from families with lower incomes at higher rates and with greater severity than those from families with higher incomes (American Academy of Pediatrics, Council on Community Pediatrics, 2016, reaffirmed 2021). Unintentional injuries continue to be the leading cause of death in children older than 1 year, but children's health remains threatened by illnesses and other health-related conditions in the 21st century (Centers for Disease Control and Prevention [CDC]/National Center for Health Statistics, 2022). Obesity, environmental toxins, allergies, substance misuse, child abuse and neglect, and mental health problems are among the key issues that endanger children's health today.

Evolution of Maternal and Newborn Nursing

The evolution of maternity nursing is characterized by innovations that became common practice in later years. These innovations include fetal monitoring, birthing parent/baby care, and early postpartum discharge. The driving forces behind changes in care within the social context of the times were scientific and medical developments and families' desires for the best possible childbearing experience.

The childbirth process itself hasn't changed over the years, but many things associated with childbirth have, including the birthing parent's expectations for the birthing experience, pain management options, the economics of childbirth, the U.S. system of health care, and the technology used during pregnancy and birth. In many ways, childbirth practices in the United States have come full circle; for example, the demand for nurse midwives and doulas during childbirth has risen recently (Niles & Zephyrin, 2023). The concept of women helping other women during childbirth is not new; people who labored and gave birth at home were traditionally attended by relatives and midwives (Evidence-Based Practice 1.1). A **certified nurse midwife (CNM)** has postgraduate training in the care of normal pregnancy and childbirth and is certified by the American College of Nurse Midwives. A **doula** is a birth assistant who provides emotional, physical, and educational support to the pregnant person and their family during childbirth and the postpartum period. Many nurses working in labor and birth areas today are credentialed in their specialties so that they can provide optimal care to the birthing person and their newborn. Childbirth choices are often based on what works best for the birthing person, child, and family.

Evolution of Pediatric Nursing

In 1870, the first pediatric professorship for a physician was awarded in the United States to Abraham Jacobi,

EVIDENCE-BASED PRACTICE **1.1**

Women's Response to Continuous Labor Support

Historically and cross-culturally, women have been attended to and supported by other women during childbirth. Women historically help other women in labor by providing emotional support, comfort measures, information, and advocacy. According to the World Health Organization (WHO), a laboring person's companion can be any person from their family, from their work setting, or from their social network chosen by the laboring person to offer continuous support during labor and childbirth.

STUDY

A qualitative study was done to assess the effect of having a birth companion offering continuous support on the laboring woman's level of pain perception. It was a nonrandomized pretest–posttest control study with 54 participants (27 in each group). The experimental group was allowed a birth companion in the labor room, whereas the control group was not. Pain levels were assessed every 2 hours using a numeric pain rating scale in both groups.

Findings

Women receiving continuous intrapartum support indicated reduced pain experienced from the worst and severe levels to a moderate to mild level of pain in the subsequent posttest. Comparing the mean pain of both groups showed a statistically significant difference between the two groups within the group with continuous labor support. The study concluded that the presence of a birth companion for the laboring woman did reduce women's perception of pain.

Nursing Implications

Continuous support during labor may improve birth outcomes and pain perceptions for the birthing person. Based on findings from this research, women in labor clearly benefit from one-on-one support during labor. Nurses can use the information gained from this study to educate birthing people about the importance of having a support person during labor and birth. Nurses can also act as patient advocates in facilities where they work to foster an environment that encourages the use of support people during the intrapartum period. The focus of nursing needs to be individualized, supportive, and collaborative with the family during their childbearing experience. In short, nurses should place the needs of the birthing person and their family first in providing a continuum of care and encourage the provision of birth companions in labor rooms. These practices help the patient to have a less painful childbirth experience.

Preksha, Vahitha, S., Chanu, S. M., & Venkatesh, A. (2022). The effect of birth companion on the level of pain perception among primi-parturient admitted for labor. *Journal of Obstetrics and Gynecological Nursing, 10*(1), 8–13. https://indianjournals.com/ijor.aspx?target=ijor:tnnmcjogn&volume=10&issue=1&article=002

who is considered the founder of pediatrics. For the first time, the medical community realized the need to provide specialized training and education about children to health care providers. In the early 1900s, Lillian Wald established the Henry Street Settlement House in New York City; this was the start of public health nursing. This facility provided medical and other services to families with low income. These services included home nurse visits to teach birthing parents about health care.

During this time, health care personnel were trained to take care of children in hospitals, but parents of hospitalized children were discouraged from visiting to prevent the spread of infection. Restricting parents from being involved in their child's care was also thought to minimize emotional stress.

Nursing in public schools began in 1902 with the appointment of Lina Rogers as a full-time public school nurse in New York. A professional course in pediatric nursing was started in the early 1900s at Teachers' College of Columbia University.

In the 1960s, changes in the health care delivery system and shifts in the population's health status led to the development of the nurse practitioner role. Loretta Ford was the founder of the first nurse practitioner program. In response to rapid escalation of health care expenditures, the federal government instituted cost control systems in the 1970s. In addition, the considerable changes in the U.S. health care system in the 1980s affected pediatric nursing and child health care. The emphasis of care was on quality outcomes and cost containment. Some of these changes brought more advanced practice nurses into the field of pediatrics.

In the 1980s, the Division of Maternal–Child Health Nursing Practice of the American Nurses Association (ANA) developed maternal–child health standards to provide important guidelines for delivering nursing care.

In the 1990s, the Institute of Medicine published reports outlining the need to improve the quality and safety of the American health care system. This led to an increased focus on improving health care outcomes. As the health care environment continued to increase in complexity and patients hospitalized got sicker, programs were created for nurses to obtain a level of expertise and validate mastery of their skills and knowledge by passing a national standardized examination. Registered nurses and nurse practitioners can be certified in their specialty, such as pediatrics. These certifications show a commitment to lifelong learning and the ability to stay up to date in the rapidly changing health care environment. In recent years, pediatric nursing certifications have become increasingly specialized; for example, certifications are available in pediatric hematology/oncology nursing and in pediatric emergency nursing.

HEALTH STATUS OF WOMEN AND CHILDREN

At one time, health was defined simply as the absence of disease. Health was measured by monitoring the mortality and morbidity of a group. Over the past century, however, the focus on health has shifted to disease prevention, health promotion, and wellness. The definition of health is complex. The WHO (2023a) defines health as "a state of complete physical, mental, and social well-being, and not merely the absence of disease or infirmity."

In 1979, the U.S. Surgeon General's Healthy People initiative presented an agenda for the nation that identified the most significant preventable threats to health. With the series of updates that followed, including the present one, Healthy People 2030, the United States has a comprehensive health promotion and disease prevention agenda with specific goals and objectives for improving the quantity and quality of life in America. Overarching goals are to attain healthy, thriving lives and eliminate preventable disease, disability, injury, and premature death; achieve health equity, eliminate disparities, and attain health literacy to improve the health of all groups; create physical, economic, and social environments that promote good health and well-being for all; promote healthy development and behaviors across every stage of life; and engage leadership, the public, and key constituents to take action and develop policies that will improve the health and well-being of all (U.S. Department of Health and Human Services, n.d.). The principle behind this agenda is that setting national objectives and monitoring their progress can motivate action and change. The agenda incorporates input from public health and prevention experts; federal, state, and local governments; over 2,000 organizations; and the public to develop health objectives.

There are specific health topic areas, including women's and children's health topics, which serve as a method for evaluation of progress made in public health. These topic areas also serve as focal points to coordinate national health improvement efforts. For example, one objective under the physical activity topic is to increase the proportion of adolescents who meet current federal physical activity guidelines for aerobic physical activity and for muscle-strengthening activity (U.S. Department of Health and Human Services, n.d.). See the Healthy People 2030 features throughout the text for specific objectives, nursing implications, and guidance related to working toward achieving these objectives. Measuring health status is not always a simple process. For example, some people with chronic illnesses do not see themselves as "ill" if their disease is under control. A traditional method of measuring health is to examine mortality and morbidity data. This information is collected and analyzed to provide an objective description of the nation's health.

Mortality

Mortality is the incidence or number of people who have died over a specific period. This statistic is presented as a rate per 100,000 and is calculated from a sample of death certificates. The National Center for Health Statistics (NCHS), under the U.S. Department of Health and Human Services (USDHHS), collects, analyzes, and disseminates data on U.S. mortality rates. The CDC collects, stores, and shares their data collected through the Pregnancy Mortality Surveillance System (PMSS).

Maternal Mortality

A major predictor of a nation's overall health is maternal mortality, which recently has risen dramatically in the United States as compared to other high-income countries and globally (Brown & Small, 2024). The **maternal mortality ratio** is the annual number of female deaths from any cause related to or aggravated by pregnancy or its management (excluding inadvertent or incidental causes) during pregnancy and childbirth or within 42 days of termination of pregnancy, irrespective of the duration and site of the pregnancy. It is reported as a ratio of deaths per 100,000 live births for a specified year.

The death of a person during pregnancy, during birth, or postpartum is a tragedy for their family and for society as a whole. About 1,200 women die annually in the United States as a result of pregnancy or childbirth complications (Hoyert, 2023). In 2021, maternal mortality in the United States was 32.9 maternal deaths per 100,000 live births (Hoyert, 2023). Risk factors for maternal mortality include race and ethnicity: Black women have a maternal mortality rate more than double that of non-Hispanic White and Hispanic women (Brown & Small, 2024). Maternal age is also a risk factor as maternal mortality increases as maternal age increases (Hoyert, 2023).

The United States is highly advanced in terms of medicine and technology and has the highest per capita spending on health care in the world, but maternal mortality has steadily increased over the years. Increased maternal age, high body mass index (BMI), and comorbidities during pregnancy may contribute to the rise in maternal mortality (Brown & Small, 2024). It is estimated that 80% of maternal deaths are preventable. The leading causes of pregnancy-related death are mental health conditions, hemorrhage, and cardiovascular problems (Brown & Small, 2024). The striking difference in the pregnancy-related mortality ratio between Black women and women of other races is the largest disparity in the area of maternal health (Brown & Small, 2024). Researchers do not entirely understand what accounts for this disparity but believe it is related to social and structural rather than biologic determinants (Brown & Small, 2024). Lack of care during pregnancy is a major factor contributing to a poor outcome. Prenatal care prevents complications of pregnancy and supports the birth of healthy infants, but not all pregnant people receive the same quality and quantity of health care.

The CDC has called for more research and monitoring to understand and address racial disparities and for increased funding for prenatal and postpartum care. Research is needed to identify causes and to design initiatives to reduce health disparities, and the CDC is calling on Congress to expand programs to provide preconception and prenatal care to underserved people. Commitment from people, organizations, and the health care community as a whole will be needed to improve reproductive care for all.

Fetal Mortality

The terms "fetal death," "fetal demise," "stillbirth," and "stillborn" all refer to an intrauterine death of a fetus with no signs of life as demonstrated by the absence of breathing, heartbeat, definite movements of voluntary muscles, or lack of pulsation of the umbilical cord (Ross, 2023). The **fetal mortality rate**, or fetal death rate, refers to the spontaneous intrauterine death of a fetus at any time during pregnancy per 1,000 live births. Fetal deaths later in pregnancy than 20 weeks' gestation are also referred to as stillbirths; prior to 20 weeks, they are referred to as spontaneous abortion (Ross, 2023). Fetal mortality may be attributable to maternal factors (e.g., malnutrition, disease, preterm cervical dilation) or fetal factors (e.g., chromosomal abnormalities, poor placental attachment).

Fetal mortality is a major but often overlooked public health problem. The fetal mortality rate in the United States is 5.7 per 1,000 live births (Ross, 2023). Much of the public concern regarding reproductive loss has concentrated on infant mortality because less is known about fetal mortality. However, the impact of fetal mortality on families in the United States is considerable; moreover, it provides an overall picture of the quality of maternal health and prenatal care.

Neonatal and Infant Mortality

The **neonatal mortality rate** is the number of infant deaths occurring in the first 28 days of life per 1,000 live births. The neonatal mortality rate in the United States in 2021 was 3.49 per 1,000 live births; it has been declining since 1995 (Ely & Driscoll, 2023). The reliability of the neonatal mortality estimates depends on the accuracy and completeness of reporting and recording of births and deaths. Underreporting and misclassification are common, especially for deaths occurring early in life.

The perinatal mortality rate encompasses late fetal and early neonatal mortalities; it is also a useful health status indicator. In the United States, the perinatal mortality rate was 5.69 per 1,000 live births in 2019 (Zacharias, 2023). Prematurity, postterm, congenital malformations, multiple gestation pregnancy, and being of African ancestry are risk factors for increased perinatal and neonatal mortality (Zacharias, 2023).

The **infant mortality rate** refers to the number of deaths occurring in the first 12 months of life. It is also documented as the number of deaths of infants younger than 1 year of age per 1,000 live births. The infant mortality rate is used as an index of the general health of a country. Generally, this statistic is one of the more significant measures of children's health. The current infant mortality rate in the United States is 5.4 per 1,000 live births (CDC, 2024b) (Fig. 1.2).

The infant mortality rate varies greatly from state to state as well as among racial and ethnic groups. The United States has one of the highest gross national products in the world and is known for its technologic capabilities, but its infant mortality rate is much higher than (and in some cases double) that of most other nations with similar resources (Central Intelligence Agency, 2023). The main causes of early infant death in the United States include congenital malformations, short gestation, low birth weight, sudden infant death syndrome (SIDS), unintentional injuries, and maternal complications during pregnancy (Ely & Driscoll, 2023).

TAKE NOTE!

Non-Hispanic Black infants have consistently had higher infant mortality rates compared to other racial groups (CDC, 2024b).

Preterm births and low birth weight are key risk factors for infant death: The lower the birth weight, the higher the risk of infant mortality. The percentage of infants born preterm in the United States peaked in 2006; thus, the impact of preterm-related causes of infant death increased during this time. From 2007 to 2018, preterm birth rates declined each year, with the exception of 2015, until 2019 when they began to rise again. In 2021, preterm birth rates hit an all-time high (Hamilton et al., 2022). This trend will need to be closely monitored to understand what is contributing to the increase and what can be done to decrease the incidence of preterm birth.

After birth, other health promotion strategies can significantly improve an infant's health and chances of survival. Breastfeeding has been shown to reduce rates of infection in infants and to improve their long-term health. Human milk also reduces the risk for certain chronic diseases such as allergic conditions, celiac disease, and inflammatory bowel disease (IBD), as well as the risk of obesity and its complications (Meek, 2023). Emphasizing the importance of placing an infant on their

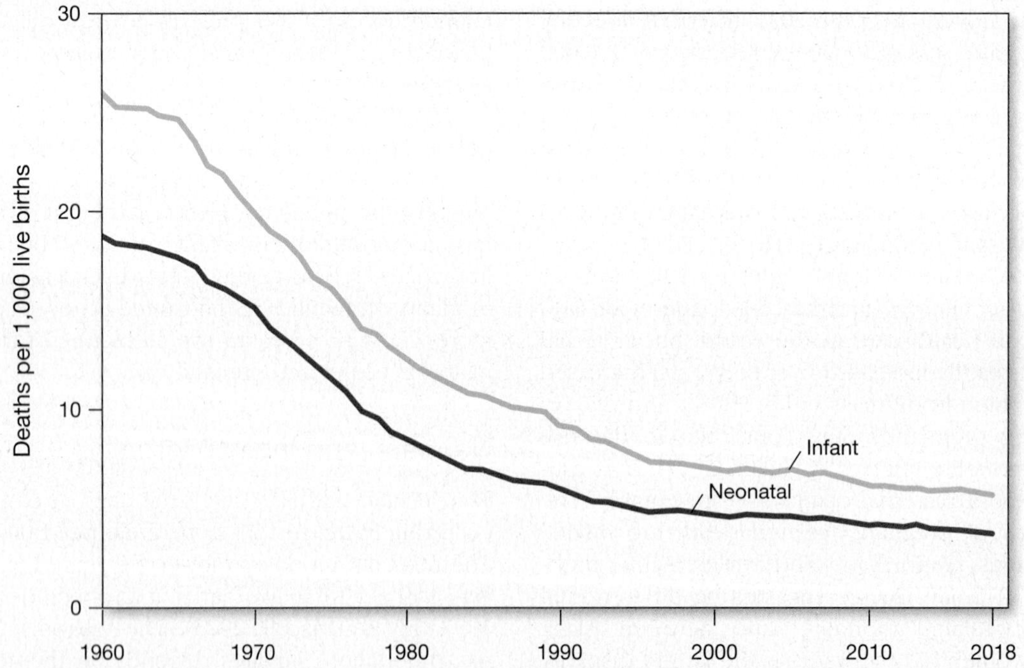

NOTE: Rates are infant (under 1 year) and neonatal (under 28 days) deaths per 1,000 live births in specified group.
SOURCE: NCHS, National Vital Statistics System, Mortality.

FIGURE 1.2 Infant and neonatal mortality from 1995 to 2020. (Data from Ely, D. M., & Driscoll, A. K. [2022]. Infant mortality in the United States, 2020: Data from the period linked birth/infant death file. *National Vital Statistics Reports*, *71*[5]. National Center for Health Statistics. https://dx.doi.org/10.15620/cdc:120700)

back to sleep will reduce the incidence of SIDS. In addition, parents and caregivers should not share a bed with an infant (Kellams, 2024). Encouraging pregnant people to join support groups to prevent postpartum depression and learn sound childrearing practices will improve the health of both the new parent and their infant.

Childhood Mortality

The **childhood mortality rate** is the number of deaths per 100,000 population in children 1 to 14 years of age. The childhood mortality rate in the United States has remained relatively steady however, disparities by sex, age, race, and ethnicity persist (America's Health Rankings, United Health Foundation, 2024). In 2020, the mortality rate for children between ages 1 and 4 years was 22.7 per 100,000, with the leading cause of death being unintentional injuries followed by congenital malformations, then homicide (CDC/National Center for Health Statistics, 2022). The mortality rate for children aged 5 to 14 years was 13.7 per 100,000, with the leading cause being unintentional injuries followed by cancer, then congenital malformations (CDC/National Center for Health Statistics, 2022). Other causes of childhood mortality include suicide, diseases of the heart, influenza, and pneumonia.

Even as research continues into the preventable nature of childhood injuries, unintentional injury, such as from motor vehicle collisions, fires, drowning, bicycle or pedestrian collisions, poisoning, and falls, remains a leading cause of mortality and morbidity in children (FIFCFS, 2023). These injuries have far-reaching consequences for children, families, and society in general. Risk factors associated with childhood injuries include young age, male sex, low socioeconomic status, parents who are unmarried or single, low maternal education level, poor housing, parental drug or alcohol misuse, and low level of support within the family. These deaths can often be prevented through education about the value of using car seats and seat belts; the dangers of driving under the influence of alcohol and other substances; and the importance of pedestrian and bicycle, fire, water, and home safety.

TAKE NOTE!

In the United States, Native American, Alaska Native, and Black children have the highest rates of death by unintentional injury (CDC, 2024a).

Morbidity

Morbidity is the measure of the prevalence of a specific illness in a population at a particular time. The rate is presented as a number per 1,000 population. Morbidity is often difficult to define and record because the definitions used vary widely. For example, morbidity may be defined as visits to the primary provider or diagnosis for hospital admission. Also, data may be difficult to obtain. Morbidity statistics are revised less frequently than mortality statistics because of the difficulty in defining or obtaining the information. The WHO (2023b) has identified four noncommunicable diseases that cause the most worldwide morbidities and mortalities—cardiovascular disease (CVD), cancers, chronic respiratory diseases, and diabetes.

Female Health Indicators

Disease can be of genetic origin but can also arise from poor personal habits. Only recently have researchers and the medical community focused on women's special health needs.

A better understanding of the extent of maternal morbidity is needed to help inform change that can safeguard the lives and well-being of girls and women. Globally, there is greater awareness of the plight of people who have complications associated with pregnancy or childbirth and who continue to experience long-term problems. Maternal health is a social and economic phenomenon, not just a clinical and biologic issue. The current goal should be to address health risks in all people before pregnancy so they enter pregnancy healthier, start prenatal care earlier, and are less likely to develop health conditions that lead to long-term morbidity. Every childbirth is unique, and the health care community must address inequalities that impact health outcomes, especially inequalities related to sexual and reproductive rights and gender.

The passage of the **Affordable Care Act (ACA)** and the publishing of Healthy People 2030 hold great promise for women's health. The emphasis on access to preventive health care aims to make a positive impact on the areas of deficiency. It is essential that women take advantage of the benefits, expansions, and improvements included in the law. Nurses have a critical role to play in understanding the ACA to make sure all women receive the health care they need and deserve.

The health status of all women across the United States must be improved. Far too many states fail to meet the Healthy People goals for satisfactory health status, and states are only slowly grappling with policy changes that can make improvements in women's health. Many states have made positive changes in their policies, but there is still a great distance to go. Much more needs to be done to improve access to health insurance and health care providers and services and to increase access to reproductive health services. Additionally, women often need help attaining the economic security that would greatly improve their health and the health of their families. Citizens can advocate for improvement in the health care system by writing a letter to their Congressional representatives demanding they implement health policies that promote all women's health.

Major Health Issues for Women

CARDIOVASCULAR DISEASE

CVD is the number one cause of death of women across racial and ethnic groups. In 2021, about 310,600 women died of CVD, which is approximately one in five female deaths and greater than 60 million women are living with some form of heart disease (CDC, 2024e). Initial presenting symptoms of myocardial infarction (MI) in males and females are often similar; however, females are more likely to present without chest pain than males, and MI is more likely to go unrecognized in females than in males (Pagidipati & Douglas, 2024).

Pregnancy places an increased workload on the heart, including increases in circulating blood volume, plasma volume, heart rate, and cardiac output. This is usually well tolerated by healthy people, but not by those with preexisting CVD who have inadequate cardiovascular reserve.

Nurses need to look beyond the textbook "crushing chest pain" symptom that heralds MI in males and recognize that a female patient may be experiencing MI in the absence of that symptom. Symptoms may be atypical; for example, patients may experience dyspnea rather than chest pain. Causes of heart disease also differ between males and females in several ways; causes for females include menopause (associated with a significant rise in coronary events); history of preeclampsia; diabetes, high cholesterol levels, and left ventricular hypertrophy; smoking, including second-hand smoke (which has a greater effect on females due to their smaller average body size); gestational hypertension; polycystic ovary syndrome; increasing maternal age; prepregnancy obesity; blood vessel inflammation; and repeated episodes of weight loss and gain (leading to increased coronary morbidity and mortality). In the United States, the leading cause of mortality in women is CVD (Office on Women's Health, 2023). Nurses have a major role in empowering patients to engage in a heart-healthy lifestyle to prevent CVD and to educate patients regarding the signs and symptoms of MI and the importance of seeking treatment early. Preconception counseling is necessary for all patients with preexisting CVD who may become pregnant to clearly define both maternal and fetal risks of pregnancy.

CANCER

Cancer is the second leading cause of death among women (Office on Women's Health, 2023). Breast, colon, endometrial, lung, cervical, skin, and ovarian cancers most often affect women. Approximately one third of cancer deaths are caused by smoking, obesity, minimal fruit and vegetable consumption, alcohol, and lack of exercise (WHO, 2023c). Although much attention is focused on cancers of the reproductive system, lung cancer is the most fatal cancer in women (CDC, 2024c). This is often the result of smoking and second-hand smoke. Lung cancer has no early symptoms, making early detection challenging.

Breast cancer occurs in one in every eight women in a lifetime (ACS, 2024). In 2024, approximately 310,720 new cases of invasive breast cancers were diagnosed among females in the United States. An estimated 42,250 women are expected to die from the disease in 2024 (ACS, 2024). Black women are more likely to die from breast cancer than women in any other racial group (ACS, 2024).

As of 2023, there are over 4 million breast cancer survivors in the United States (ACS, 2024). It is the most common malignancy in women, second only to lung cancer as a cause of cancer mortality in women (ACS, 2024). Although a family history of breast cancer, aging, and irregularities in the menstrual cycle at an early age are major risk factors, there are controllable risk factors such as higher body weight, not having children, not being physically active, not breastfeeding, oral contraceptive use, excessive alcohol consumption, a high-fat diet, and long-term use of hormone replacement therapy.

Breast cancer rates have dropped steadily for many years, possibly due to earlier detection through screening, increased awareness, and improvement in treatments (ACS, 2024). Early detection and timely treatment continue to offer the best chance for a cure, and reducing the overall risk of cancer by decreasing avoidable risk factors continues to be the best preventive plan.

PREGNANCY AND HEALTH ISSUES

Pregnant patients are by no means immune to any of the above health issues. Many start a pregnancy with health conditions that might include hypertension, higher body weight, CVD, diabetes, autoimmune diseases, anemia, asthma, sexually transmitted infections (STIs), depression, or cancer. Although many pregnant people are young and fairly healthy, the incidence of many chronic health issues in young people and childhood obesity is increasing secondary to the obesity epidemic in the United States. Over the last few decades, the incidence of obesity has risen to epidemic proportions worldwide, which has led to obesity in pregnancies. Obesity increases the risk of blood clots, surgical births, long labors, preterm birth, macrosomia, shoulder dystocia, stillbirths, gestational diabetes, congenital defects, preeclampsia, gestational hypertension, obstructive sleep apnea, and postpartum infections (ACOG, 2023a).

Women's health is a complex issue, and no single policy or law can be passed that will quickly change access, discrimination, or health insurance coverage or improve care for historically underserved populations.

Although progress in science and technology has helped reduce the incidence of and improve the survival rates for several diseases, women's health issues continue to have an impact on U.S. society. By eliminating or decreasing some of the risk factors and causes of prevalent diseases and illnesses, society and science could minimize certain chronic health problems.

Childhood Morbidity

As reported in a summary of health statistics for children, the vast majority of children are considered to be in excellent, very good, or good health, with only 2.6% reporting fair or poor health based on data collected via survey (CDC/National Center for Health Statistics, 2023a). Factors that may increase morbidity include homelessness, poverty, low birth weight, chronic health disorders, foreign-born adoption, attendance at day care centers, and other barriers to health care. For example, 16.1% of children live in poverty. These children have a higher incidence of disease; limited coordination of health services; and limited access to health care, except for visits to the emergency department (Creamer et al., 2022). The overall poverty rate in 2021 was 11.6%, marking the second increase in the past 5 years (Creamer et al., 2022). However, the poverty rate among Black and Hispanic Americans is 19.5% and 17.1%, respectively; these children are particularly at increased risk for illness (Creamer et al., 2022).

The most important aspect of morbidity is the degree of disability it produces, which is identified in children as the number of days missed from school or confined to bed. In 2022, 8.9% of school-age children (ages 5 to 17) missed 11 or more days of school because of injury or illness (CDC/National Center for Health Statistics, 2023b).

Common health problems in children include respiratory disorders, gastrointestinal disturbances that lead to malnutrition and dehydration, and injuries. In 2018, acute bronchitis, asthma, pneumonia, epilepsy/convulsions, and depressive disorders were the major causes of hospitalization in children 1 to 17 years of age (McDermott & Roemer, 2021). Inpatient hospital stays due to depressive disorders were twice as high for females as for males (McDermott & Roemer, 2021).

As more immunizations become available, common childhood communicable diseases affect fewer children. The tracking of the leading topics from Healthy People provides some positive information related to improving children's health. Improvements have occurred in child health, but morbidity and disability from some conditions, such as asthma, diabetes, attention deficit disorders, and obesity, have increased in recent decades. Also, disparities in health status among children in the United States reflect widening social inequalities.

One trend in the United States is the increasing number of children with mental health disorders and related emotional, social, or behavioral problems. It is estimated that one in five children in the United States have a mental, emotional, developmental, or behavioral disorder (Office of the Surgeon General, 2021). Recent research has found that depressive and anxiety symptoms increased during the COVID-19 pandemic (Office of the Surgeon General, 2021). These problems may limit the child's educational success and increase the risk for significant mental health problems later in life, emotional problems, use of firearms, reckless driving, risky sexual activity, and substance misuse during adolescence. Overall, these behavioral, social, and educational problems can interfere with children's social and academic development. Access to treatment is a concern in part because insurance may not reimburse for treating these problems.

> ***TAKE NOTE!***
>
> The U.S. Surgeon General issued an advisory to call the American people's attention to the increasing concerns regarding the mental health of the country's youth and the negative effects of social media on their mental health (Office of the Surgeon General, 2023).

Environmental and psychosocial factors are an area of concern in children. They include academic difficulties, complex psychiatric disorders, self-harm and harm to others, use of firearms, hostility at school, substance misuse, HIV/AIDS, and adverse effects of the media.

LEGAL AND ETHICAL ISSUES IN MATERNAL AND CHILD HEALTH CARE

Law and ethics are interrelated and affect all aspects of nursing. Every nurse is responsible for knowing current information regarding ethics and laws related to their practice. Numerous federal programs have had a major impact on women's and children's health (Table 1.1).

> ***TAKE NOTE!***
>
> As advocates for children, nurses support policies that protect children's rights and improve children's health care.

Parents and guardians generally make choices about their child's health and services. As the legal custodians of minor children, they have the responsibility to decide what is best for their children. Nurses caring for children and their families make the child's and family's needs a priority. Moral development (the ability to function in an ethical manner) and the legal requirements involved in working with women and children affect nurses on a daily basis. Maternity and pediatric nurses must function

TABLE 1.1 • Milestones in Federal Programs in Support of the Health of Women and Children

Date	Action	Impact
1909	First White House Conference on Care of Dependent Children (convened by President Theodore Roosevelt) Prevention of Infant Mortality Association formed	Addressed the poor working and living conditions of many children in the United States Aimed at improving the lives of children The Association played a major role in creating a new registration procedure for all infant births and deaths nationally.
1912/1913	U.S. Children's Bureau	Established the first governmental agency to oversee children's health and environmental conditions Purpose is to research and report all issues pertaining to all children's well-being; to assist state and local governments in preventing child abuse and neglect
1921	Maternity & Infancy (Sheppard–Towner) Act	Provided grants to states to establish maternal and child health divisions in state health departments
1930	White House Conference on Child Welfare Standards	Produced the Children's Charter, documenting the child's need for health, education, welfare, and protection
1935	The Social Security Act Introduction of vitamin K to newborns	Established federal–state partnership, Aid to Dependent Families and Children (ADFC), maternal–child health services, and child welfare services Led to the prevention of hemorrhagic disease in newborns
1935	Title V Maternal Child Health Block Grant	Provides funding for ensuring the health of U.S. birthing parents and children through grants to states Serves >2.5 million pregnant people, 4 million infants, and 30 million children annually
1938	Initiation of the March of Dimes	Through research, defeated polio and now improves lives through the prevention of birth defects, prematurity, and infant mortality
1946	National School Lunch Program	Provides nutritious, well-balanced lunches to children each day at school for free or at low cost Provides meal supplements for children in afterschool care and nutrition programs for children experiencing homelessness
1946	Centers for Disease Control and Prevention established	The CDC is globally recognized as a leading force in public health expertise.
1962	National Institute of Child Health and Human Development (NICHD)	Supports and performs research on child, maternal, adult, and family health issues
1964	Head Start developed	Head Start provides child development programs to pregnant people, families, and children from birth to age 5 with the overarching goal of increasing school readiness for children from families of low income.
1965	Medicaid Program under Title XIX of the Social Security Act; special programs such as the Child Health Assessment Program	Provided state block grants to reduce financial barriers to health care for people with low incomes and special services to pregnant people, young children, and people with disabilities
1966/1974	Women, Infants, and Children (WIC) program	Provided nutritional supplementation and education to families with low incomes; pregnant, postpartum, and lactating people; and infants and children up to age 5
1968	Expansion of National School Lunch Act	Provides year-round food for school-age children whose families have low income and children in day care and Head Start programs whose families have low income
1969	U.S. Children's Bureau moves to Office of Health, Education, & Welfare (HEW)	Established greater presence for the programs
1972	Head Start to serve children with disabilities	Congress mandated that at least 10% of the children enrolled in Head Start must have disabilities.

TABLE 1.1 • Milestones in Federal Programs in Support of the Health of Women and Children

Impact	Impact	Impact
1975	Education for All Handicapped Children Act (Public Law 94-142)	Established federally mandated special education in public schools
	Title XX Social Services	Provided block grants to day care, emergency shelters, counseling, family planning, and other services for children
1976	Improved Pregnancy Outcome Projects	Raised awareness of the importance of maternal health during pregnancy to reduce infant mortality
1976	The Supplemental Security Income (SSI) Disabled Children's Program	Provided cash to families with low income who have children with disabilities to help those families manage health care costs
1979	National health objectives for 1990	These early efforts resulted in Healthy People 2010 and 2020. Now 2030 is developed.
1981	Alcohol, Drug Abuse, & Mental Health block grants	Began funding services for children and adolescents with mental health issues
	Healthy Mothers, Healthy Babies Coalition	Raised public awareness of prenatal care, good nutrition, and avoidance of drugs, and promoted breastfeeding
1986	Education of Handicapped Act Amendments (Public Law 99-457)	Established federal funding for states to create statewide, comprehensive, coordinated, and multidisciplinary early-intervention services for infants and toddlers with disabilities
1990	Omnibus Budget Reconciliation Act	Extended Medicaid coverage to all children (6–18 years) of families with income below 133% of poverty level
1990	Bright Futures initiated	Provided a comprehensive set of child health supervision guidelines for health professionals, families, and communities; trained these groups to work toward optimal child health
1991	Healthy Start initiated	Community-based program that provides services to at-risk childbearing people from preconception to postpartum to help reduce infant mortality
1993	Family & Medical Leave Act (FMLA)	Allowed eligible employees to take up to 12 weeks of unpaid leave from their jobs every year to care for newborns or newly adopted children or children, parents, or spouses who have a serious health condition with assurance the employee can return to their previous job or a comparable job with the same conditions
1994	Back to Sleep Campaign	National campaign to prevent sudden infant death syndrome (SIDS) by placing infants on their backs to sleep
1995	Early Head Start Program	Federally funded community-based program for families with low incomes (infants, toddlers, and pregnant people) that focuses on child development
1997	Children's Health Insurance Program (CHIP) (formerly known as State Children's Health Insurance Program [SCHIP])	Offers federal assistance with state-based health insurance for families with low incomes that are not eligible for Medicaid but cannot afford private insurance
2000	Children's Health Act	Led to increased research and treatment of children's health issues such as autism, asthma, epilepsy, and oral health
2002	No Child Left Behind Act	Aimed at ensuring all children in all classrooms received research-based curricula, well-prepared teachers, and safe learning environments
2006	Combating Autism Act	Led to increased awareness of autism by increasing funding for research, surveillance, diagnosis, and treatment
2007	WIC Food Package revised	Designed to improve nutritional intake of WIC recipients by supporting and promoting long-term breastfeeding and adding fruits and vegetables, whole grains, soy-based foods, and a variety of culturally appropriate foods
2008	Newborn Screening Saving Lives Act	Provided increased funding for newborn screening grants and provided more education and outreach, coordination of follow-up care after screening, and evaluation of newborn screening programs

(continued)

TABLE 1.1 • Milestones in Federal Programs in Support of the Health of Women and Children (*continued*)

Date	Action	Impact
2009	Children's Health Insurance Program Reauthorization Act	Expanded the program to cover more children without insurance
2009	American Recovery and Reinvestment Act	Designated money to fund and expand programs such as Head Start, foster care, and the Supplemental Nutrition Assistance Program (Food Stamp Program) and to create new jobs and improve services such as community health centers and unemployment benefits during the economic recession
2010	Affordable Care Act (Patient Protection & Affordable Care Act); Health Care & Education Reconciliation Act	Increased coverage by expanding Medicaid, ended exclusion of preexisting conditions for children; holds insurance companies accountable by ending lifetime coverage limits, requiring insurance companies to publicly justify premium increases; decreases health care costs; increases choice and enhances quality of care for all Americans by covering all preventive care
2014	Birth to Five: Watch Me Thrive	A federal initiative program that promotes developmental and behavioral screening for children with the goal of improving early diagnosis and treatment of children with developmental delays
2018	Helping Ensure Access for Little Ones, Toddlers, and Hopeful Youth by Keeping Insurance Delivery Stable Act (HEALTHY KIDS Act)	Extended funding for CHIP through the 2027 National Conference
2018	Maternal, Infant, and Early Childhood Home Visiting (MIECHV) program	The Bipartisan Budget Control Act extended funding for 5 years for the MIECHV program (2018), which provides home visits to improve health and development outcomes for children who are at risk.

Adapted from Hoban, C. (2019). *Federal programs improve women and children's healthcare.* Emergency and Disaster Management Digest. Retrieved December 19, 2023, from https://edmdigest.com/preparedness/federal-programs-healthcare/; U.S. Department of Agriculture. (2024). *Special supplemental nutrition program for women, infants, and children (WIC).* Food and Nutrition Service. https://www.fns.usda.gov/wic; Health Resources & Services Administration. (2018). *Early periodic screening, diagnosis, and treatment.* Retrieved December 19, 2023, from https://mchb.hrsa.gov/maternal-child-health-initiatives/mchb-programs/early-periodic-screening-diagnosis-and-treatment; Association of Maternal & Child Health Programs. (2019). *Title V overview.* Retrieved December 19, 2023, from http://www.amchp.org/AboutTitleV/Pages/default.aspx; Yarrow, A. L. (2011). A history of federal child antipoverty and health policy in the United States since 1900. *Child Development Perspectives, 5*(1), 66–72. https://doi.org/10.1111/j.1750-8606.2010.00157.x; GovTrack.us. (2022). *H.R. 3921—115th Congress: HEALTHY KIDS Act.* Retrieved November 7, 2023, from https://www.govtrack.us/congress/bills/115/hr3921; Maternal and Child Health Bureau, Health Resources and Services Administration, U.S. Department of Health and Human Services. (n.d.). *MCH timeline.* Retrieved October 24, 2023, from https://mchb.hrsa.gov/about/timeline/index.asp; and U.S. Department of Health and Human Services. (2022a). *About the Affordable Care Act.* Retrieved November 7, 2023, from https://www.hhs.gov/healthcare/about-the-aca/index.html

within ethical and legal boundaries related to their care. They must understand their state's legal requirements for routine care, consent for treatment, hospitalization, and research.

Several areas are of particular importance to the health care of women and children. These include abortion, substance misuse, fetal therapy, maternal–fetal conflict, stem cell research, umbilical cord blood (UCB) banking, informed consent, patient rights, and confidentiality.

Abortion

Abortion has been a legal medical procedure in the United States for many decades, yet it continues to be hotly debated as a volatile legal, social, and political issue. It was the subject of contention even before *Roe v. Wade*, the 1973 Supreme Court decision that ruled the government cannot excessively restrict the right to an abortion. The Supreme Court ruled that, in consultation with a health care provider, a person has a constitutionally protected right to have an abortion during the early stages of pregnancy—that is, before viability—free from government interference. *Roe v. Wade* protected a person's right to choose to have an abortion, but it did not end the debate; in fact, it led to some of the more intense social and political clashes in U.S. society.

The Supreme Court's decision in June 2022 to overturn *Roe v. Wade* now gives the states the authority to set their own abortion policies. These state laws vary widely, and many tighten the restrictions on access to abortion. Abortion has been a health care option frequently needed by people impacted by structural inequalities of poverty and racism, LGBTQ+ people, people with disabilities, and people of color. Many people feel access to reproductive health care—including abortions—should be available without barriers or political interference. They believe people deserve the right to control their own body no matter how much money they have or where they live, two factors that greatly impact access with states controlling abortion rights. See Chapter 4 for further information regarding abortion.

The issue of abortion separates people into two groups that largely refer to themselves as "pro-choice" and "pro-life." The pro-choice group supports the right of anyone to make decisions about their reproductive functions based on their own moral and ethical beliefs. The pro-life group believes abortion is murder and that the fetus has a basic right to life. It is unlikely that the debate over the issue of abortion will come to a close for years to come.

Abortion is a complex issue, and the controversy is not only in the public arena. Many nurses struggle with a conflict between their personal convictions and their professional duties. However, nurses are expected to be supportive patient advocates and to maintain a nonjudgmental attitude under all circumstances, even when their personal and political views differ from those of their patients.

Nurses need to clarify their personal values and beliefs regarding abortion and must be committed to providing unbiased care before assuming responsibility for patients who might be in a position to consider abortion. The decision to care for or refuse to care for such patients affects staff unity, influences staffing decisions, and challenges the ethical concept of duty. The ability of nurses to care for their patients as individuals illustrates the nature of empowerment as nurses work to help patients meet their health care goals. Nurses are frequently the first point of contact for information about reproductive health for many patients. As more restrictions and state laws surrounding abortion change, potential barriers may prevent nurses from safely executing their responsibilities (Blitchok, 2022).

The ANA's Code of Ethics for Nurses upholds the nurse's right to refuse to care for a patient undergoing an abortion if the nurse ethically opposes the procedure. However, nurses must take care to balance the health care professionals' right to exercise their conscience with the patient's right to access a full range of health care services. Nurses who oppose abortion need to make their stance known to their managers before encountering patients seeking an abortion so that alternative staffing arrangements can be made. Open communication and acceptance of the personal beliefs of others can promote a comfortable working environment.

Substance Misuse

Engaging in substance misuse is harmful to anybody, but when it is done during pregnancy, substance misuse can cause preterm birth, placental abruption, poor weight gain, low birth weight, stillbirth, spontaneous abortion, a variety of behavioral and cognitive problems in exposed children, and fetal injury; thus, it has legal and ethical implications. Approximately 7% of pregnant women self report use of prescription opioids during the perinatal period (CDC, 2024d). Regular use of drugs can cause neonatal abstinence syndrome (NAS), in which the newborn goes through withdrawal symptoms after birth. Currently, NAS is diagnosed every 24 minutes in the United States (Anbalagan et al., 2024; CDC, 2024d). Many state laws require evidence of prenatal drug exposure to be reported, which may lead to charges of negligence and child endangerment against the pregnant person. It has been found that incarceration or threat of it has no effect on reducing the number of cases of alcohol or substance misuse. Laws that criminalize drug use during pregnancy usually deter pregnant people from seeking prenatal care that can provide them access to appropriate counseling, referral, and monitoring. Mandatory reporting may be critical for the health of the pregnant person and their infant, but many state policies may create or exacerbate barriers to a person's access to appropriate substance misuse disorder treatments while pregnant (Department of Justice, 2022).

The punitive approach to fetal injury raises ethical and legal questions about the degree of government control that is appropriate in the interests of child safety. All pregnant people and people who can become pregnant should be screened periodically for alcohol, tobacco, and prescription and illicit drug use. Nurses should employ a flexible approach to the care of patients who have a substance use disorder, and nurses should encourage the use of all available community resources. Nurses should take a calm, nonjudgmental approach to counseling patients about the risks of preconception, antepartum, and postpartum substance misuse (Prince & Ayers, 2022). Pregnant people with substance use disorder should be provided access to preventive, supportive, and recovery services that meet their special needs. The nurse can be instrumental in facilitating referrals to community programs for both pregnant and postpartum people; participation in these programs can help ensure their full recovery from substance misuse and better lives for themselves and their children.

Fetal Therapy

Fetal therapy is performed for the benefit of the fetus and newborn before separation of the fetus from the placenta at birth. The goal may be to achieve a cure or eliminate a genetic mutation to optimize maternal and fetal outcomes. Progress in prenatal diagnosis can lead to the diagnosis of severe fetal abnormalities that previously would have resulted in a fatal outcome or the development of severe disability despite optimal postnatal care. Maternal–fetal surgery or therapy was first performed over 30 years ago. Today, fetal surgery is a growing branch of maternal–fetal medicine that covers numerous surgical techniques that are used to treat birth defects in fetuses who are still in the pregnant uterus. Intrauterine therapy can now be offered in these selected cases and also in the treatment of fetal obstructive uropathy, intrauterine transfusions for fetal anemia, spina bifida repair, and stem cell transplantation. Intrauterine therapy is a procedure that involves opening the uterus during pregnancy, performing a surgery, and replacing the fetus in the uterus. Although the risks to the fetus and the pregnant person are both great, fetal therapy may be used to correct many different anatomic anomalies and improve the quality of life of the infant. This technology and therapy do demonstrate increasing efficacy; however, ethically speaking, there is tension between maternal and fetal interests (Rousseau et al., 2022). Some argue that medical technology should not interfere with nature and that this intervention should not take place. Others argue that surgical intervention improves the child's quality of life. For many people, technology is the subject of debate and intellectual discussion; however, for nurses, these procedures may be part of their daily work.

Nurses play an important supportive role in caring and advocating for patients and their families. As the use of technology grows, situations that test a nurse's belief system will surface more frequently. Encouraging open discussions to address emotional issues and differences of opinion among staff members is healthy and increases respect for differing points of view.

Maternal–Fetal Conflict

Advances in prenatal care have brought about a greater understanding of the special status of the fetus to the point that it is considered an individual in its own regard. Current ethical viewpoints range from absolute respect for maternal autonomy to gentle persuasion to overt interventions that override a woman's autonomy. In maternity nursing, the ethical principles of beneficence and autonomy provide the fundamental framework that guides the management of all pregnant people. Because the fetus also needs to be considered, autonomy can become a complex issue giving rise to what is sometimes called **maternal–fetal conflict**.

Fetal care becomes problematic when what is required to benefit one member of the dyad will cause unacceptable harm to the other. Even when a fetal condition poses no health threat to the pregnant person, caring for the fetal patient will always carry some degree of risk to the pregnant person without direct therapeutic benefit for them. The ethical principles of beneficence (be of benefit) and nonmaleficence (do no harm) can come into conflict.

Because the patients are biologically linked, both or neither must be treated alike. It would be unethical to recommend fetal therapy as if it were medically indicated for both patients. Still, given a recommendation for fetal therapy, pregnant people, in many cases, will consent to treatment that promotes fetal health. When a pregnant person refuses therapy, health care providers must remember that the ethical injunction against harming one patient in order to benefit another is absolute.

The use of court orders to force treatment on pregnant people raises many ethical concerns. Court orders force pregnant people to forfeit their autonomy in ways not required of competent nonpregnant people. There is an inconsistency in allowing competent adults to refuse therapy in all cases but pregnancy. The American College of Obstetricians and Gynecologists (ACOG, 2020) advocates counseling and education to allow the patient to make a thoughtful decision and condemns the use of coercion on a pregnant person because this violates the intent of the informed consent process. Faced with a continuing disagreement with a pregnant patient, a primary provider should turn to an institutional ethics committee. Resorting to the legal system is almost never justified.

Stem Cell Research

Stem cell science has expanded in the past few decades. Stem cells possess the unique ability to differentiate into many distinct cell types in the body. The goal of stem cell research is the relief of human suffering, which is good ethically. Benefits of stem cell research include providing therapies for Parkinson disease and diabetes, regenerating diseased body tissues, repairing spinal cord injuries, growing organs for transplant, and numerous other therapies.

The therapeutic needs of sick patients along with the potential benefits of therapy must be balanced with ensuring rigorous scientific standards and effective consent procedures related to stem cell research. The ethical concerns surrounding stem cell research vary depending on the origin of the stem cells. Adult stem cells can replace old cells by reproducing new ones such as blood and liver cells. Bone marrow transplants are examples of the use of adult stem cells in medical therapy. Embryonic stem cells are derived from the inner cell mass of an early embryo. Stem cells have been touted as a potential cure for everything from type 1 diabetes to stroke. Although they hold great promise, they are not without controversy due to some embryonic stem cells coming from discarded human embryos. The controversy is not about whether stem cells should be used; it is about the source of stem cells and how they are obtained (Okere & Minimah, 2022).

The process of obtaining embryonic stem cells results in the destruction of the embryo. Some people argue that the destruction of the human embryo constitutes the killing of a human being, and they reject this practice on moral or religious grounds. Views about when life begins and whether the early embryo is considered a person with moral status are at the heart of the ethical deliberations related to the use of embryonic stem cells. Everyone must decide how they feel about this issue for themselves on the basis of personal values and ethical background. Although the promise of stem cells for use in future therapies is exciting, years of intensive research remain due to current technical barriers (National Institute of Neurological Disorders and Stroke [NINDS], 2023).

Umbilical Cord Blood Banking

UCB is the blood remaining in the umbilical cord at birth; it can be collected at birth and be a source of stem cells for a person in need of a bone marrow transplant later in life or who has other conditions. The use of UCB as an alternative source of hematopoietic stem cells for the treatment of certain diseases has increased tremendously. These stem cells can be used to produce healthy new cells, replace damaged cells, and treat diseases such as genetic, hematologic, and malignant disorders (ACOG, 2023b). UCB provides a source of stem cells with a minimal collection process and immense benefits. UCB is a potentially vast source of primitive hematopoietic stem and progenitor cells available for clinical applications.

Private for-profit banks were initially developed to store cord blood stem cells from newborns for a fee for potential future use by the same child or a family member if they developed a disease later in life. Today, public nonprofit cord blood banks store stem cells for free that can be used by anyone needing them; this is similar to how public blood banks work. As the providers of umbilical cord tissue, these banks are a central component in both medical treatment and scientific research with stem cells. Although some people view the creation of umbilical cord banks as a successful practice, others view it as ethically risky.

Pregnant people should be aware that stem cells from UCB cannot currently be used to treat inborn errors of metabolism or other genetic diseases in the same person from whom they were collected because the UCB would have the same genetic mutation. UCB collected from a newborn who later develops childhood leukemia cannot be used to treat that leukemia for much the same reason.

The fact that private cord banks offer their services as "biologic insurance" to obtain informed consent from parents (by ensuring that the tissue will be made available if their child needs it in the future) raises the issue of whether the consent is freely given or given under coercion. Another consideration that must be made in relation to privately owned cord banks has to do with the ownership of the stored umbilical cord. Many primary providers own private blood banks. Conflicts between economic interests and moral principles cause dilemmas in the clinical practice of UCB storage and use, especially in regard to privately owned banks (Aliouche, 2022).

Both ACOG (2023b) and the American Academy of Pediatrics (AAP) (Shearer et al., 2017) have issued statements opposing the use of for-profit cord banks and criticizing their marketing tactics. They recommended that parents instead donate cord blood to public banks, which make it available for free to anyone who needs it. Globally, other organizations have done the same. Currently, it is recommended that delaying the clamping and cutting of the umbilical cord constitutes best practice. Therefore, cord blood stem cell collection should not alter the timing of umbilical cord clamping. Nurses providing prenatal care to pregnant people need increased awareness and knowledge about options for storage, or "banking," of cord blood and tissue in order to present information to expectant parents that is accurate, evidence based, and without bias.

Informed Consent

In the United States, clinicians have a clear ethical and legal responsibility to obtain informed consent for tests, treatments, and procedures. Most care given in a health care setting is covered by the initial consent for treatment signed when the person becomes a patient at that office or clinic, or by the consent to treatment signed upon admission to the hospital or other inpatient facility. Certain procedures, however, require a specific process of informed consent. Procedures that require informed consent include major and minor surgery; invasive procedures such as amniocentesis, internal fetal monitoring, lumbar puncture, or bone marrow aspiration; treatments placing the person at higher risk, such as chemotherapy or radiation therapy; procedures or treatments involving research; application of restraints; and photography involving the person.

Generally, only people over the age of majority (18 years of age) can legally provide consent for health care. Because children are minors, the process of consent involves obtaining written permission from a parent or legal guardian. In cases requiring a signature for consent, usually, the parent gives consent for the care of children younger than 18 years of age except in certain situations (see discussion that follows).

TAKE NOTE!

Never assume that the adult accompanying the child is the parent or legal guardian. Always clarify the relationship of the accompanying adult.

The informed consent process, which must be done before the procedure or specific care, addresses the legal and ethical requirement of informing the person about the procedure. It originates from the right of the child and family to direct their care and the ethical responsibility of health care providers to involve the child and family in health care decisions. Nurses have many roles in the informed consent process. Nurses should involve children and adolescents in the decision-making process to the extent possible, though the parent is still ultimately responsible for giving consent. The primary provider or advanced practitioner providing or performing the treatment and/or procedure is responsible for informing the child and family about the procedure and obtaining consent by providing a detailed description of the procedure or treatment, the potential risks and benefits, and alternative methods available.

The nurse's responsibility related to informed consent includes the following:

- Determining whether the patient, parents, or legal guardians understand what they are signing by asking them pertinent questions.
- Ensuring that the consent form is signed by the patient (or parents or legal guardians if the patient is a child).
- Serving as a witness to the signature process.

Box 1.2 describes the key elements of informed consent; keep in mind that laws vary from state to state. Nurses must become familiar with state laws as well as the policies and procedures of the health care agency. Treating children without obtaining proper informed consent violates their rights, and the primary provider and/or facility may be held liable for any damages (Olson & Middleman, 2022).

Special Situations Related to Informed Consent

There are special situations related to informed consent. If the parent is not available, then the person in charge (relative, babysitter, or teacher) may give consent for emergency treatment if that person has a signed form from the parent or legal guardian allowing them to do so. During an emergency situation, verbal consent via telephone may be obtained. Two witnesses must be listening simultaneously and will sign the consent form, indicating that consent was received via telephone. Health care providers can provide emergency treatment to a child without consent if they have made reasonable attempts to contact the child's parent or legal guardian (American Academy of Pediatrics et al., 2011, reaffirmed 2021). In urgent or emergent situations, appropriate medical care should never be delayed or withheld due to an inability to obtain consent (American Academy of Pediatrics et al., 2011, reaffirmed 2021). Certain federal laws, such as the Emergency Medical Treatment and Labor Act (EMTALA), require that every patient who presents at an emergency department is given a medical examination regardless of informed consent or reimbursement ability (American Academy of Pediatrics et al., 2011, reaffirmed 2021). Table 1.2 gives further information about other special situations.

BOX 1.2 Key Elements of Informed Consent

- The decision maker must be of legal age in that state, with full civil rights, and must be competent (have the ability to make the decision).
- Present information that is simple, concise, and appropriate to the decision maker's level of education and language.
- The decision must be voluntary and without coercion, force, or influence of duress.
- Have a witness to the process of informed consent.
- Have the witness sign the consent form.

Exceptions to Parental Consent Requirement

In some states, a **mature minor** may give consent to certain medical treatments. The health care provider must determine that the adolescent (usually over 14 years of age) is sufficiently mature and intelligent to make the decision for treatment. The provider also considers the complexity of the treatment, its risks and benefits, and whether the treatment is necessary or elective before obtaining consent from a mature minor (American Academy of Pediatrics et al., 2011, reaffirmed 2021).

State laws vary in relation to the definition of an emancipated minor and the types of treatment that may be obtained by an emancipated minor (without parental consent). The nurse must be familiar with the particular state's law. Emancipation may be considered in any of the following situations, depending on the state's laws:

- Membership in a branch of the armed services
- Marriage
- Court-determined emancipation
- Financial independence and living apart from parents
- Pregnancy
- Birthing parent younger than 18 years of age

The emancipated minor is considered to have the legal capacity of an adult and may make their own health care decisions (American Academy of Pediatrics et al., 2011, reaffirmed 2021).

Many states do not require the consent or notification of parents or legal guardians when providing specific care to minors. Depending on the state law, health care may be provided to minors for certain conditions in a confidential manner without including the parents. These types of care may include pregnancy counseling, prenatal care, contraception, testing for and treatment of STIs and communicable diseases (including HIV), substance misuse, and mental illness counseling and treatment (American Academy of Pediatrics et al., 2011, reaffirmed 2021; Guttmacher Institute, 2023). These exceptions allow minors to seek help in a confidential

TABLE 1.2 • Special Considerations Related to Informed Consent

Issue	Definition	Nursing Considerations
Child not living with biologic or adoptive parents	Child living: • In foster care • With potential adoptive parent(s) • With a relative	A legally appointed guardian must provide consent. Verify the guardian's authority and include documentation of the legally appointed guardian in the child's medical record.
Parental consent after divorce	The right to give consent for health care rests with the parent who has legal custody by divorce decree.	Determine if the parents have joint custody or if there is sole custody by one parent. The parent who only has physical custody may give consent for emergency care. Court involvement may be needed if there is joint legal custody and the parents disagree on care.
Consent for organ donation	For a minor to donate, their parents must be aware of the risks and benefits and must provide emotional support to the child, and there should be a close relationship between the donor and recipient if living-related donation is occurring.	Potential donors should be referred to a local organ procurement organization. Educate the family about policies related to organ donation. The legal guardian or parent must consent to organ donation.
Consent for medical experimentation	The requirements include consent of parents, assent of child, and a perceived benefit to the child.	Comply with all federal regulations if federal funds are received. Refer to the "Assent" section.

American Academy of Pediatrics, Committee on Hospital Care, Section on Surgery, & Section on Critical Care. (2010, reaffirmed 2019). Pediatric organ donation and transplantation. *Pediatrics, 125*(4), 822–828. https://doi.org/10.1542/peds.2010-0081; Office for Human Research Protection. (2016). *Children: Information on special protections for children as research subjects.* Retrieved June 12, 2024 from https://www.hhs.gov/ohrp/regulations-and-policy/guidance/special-protections-for-children/index.html

manner; they might otherwise avoid care if they were required to inform their parents or legal guardians. Again, laws vary by state, so the nurse must be knowledgeable about the laws in the state where they are licensed to practice.

Assent

Assent means agreeing to something. In pediatric health care, the term assent refers to the child's participation in the decision-making process about their health care (Katz et al., 2016, reaffirmed 2023). The age of assent depends on the child's developmental level, maturity, and psychological state. The AAP recommends that children and adolescents be involved in discussions about their health care and kept informed in an age-appropriate manner (Katz et al., 2016, reaffirmed 2023). As a child gets older, assent and its converse **dissent** (disagreeing with the treatment plan) should be given more serious consideration. The pediatric patient needs to be empowered by health care providers to the extent of their capabilities; as children mature and develop over time, they should become the primary decision maker regarding their own health care (Katz et al., 2016, reaffirmed 2023). The AAP recommends that if a provider asks the child's opinion about the direction of treatment or participation in research, then the child's view and desires should be seriously considered (Katz et al., 2016, reaffirmed 2023).

When obtaining assent, first help the child to understand their health condition, depending on the child's developmental level. Next, inform the child of the treatment planned and discuss what they should expect. Then determine what the child understands about the situation and make sure they are not being unduly influenced to make a decision one way or another. Lastly, ascertain the child's willingness to participate in the treatment or research (Katz et al., 2016, reaffirmed 2023). Assent is a process that should continue throughout the course of treatment or research protocol.

Dissent needs to be carefully considered and respected if it occurs. If the primary provider is not going to honor the patient's dissent, then the argument can be made that the provider should not ask for the patient's assent. In some cases, such as in those of significant morbidity or mortality, dissent may need to be overridden. These cases need to be looked at on an individual basis. If the decision is made to move forward with treatment despite the child's dissent, then this decision must be explained to the child in developmentally appropriate terms.

There has been an increased emphasis on including children in research studies. Children are not little adults; however, less than 50% of medications have labeling with specific pediatric information (Frattarelli et al., 2014, reaffirmed 2021). In research studies, investigators and institutional review boards (IRBs) are responsible for ensuring measures are taken to protect the children in the studies. The nurse caring for these children also has the responsibility to ensure protection at all stages of the research process. Nurses can become members of the IRB and can become familiar with studies that have been approved in their work setting to help ensure that their pediatric patients are protected.

TAKE NOTE!

Whenever possible, assent for participation should be obtained from the child.

Refusal of Medical Treatment

All patients have the right to refuse medical treatment, based on the American Hospital Association's Bill of Rights. Parental autonomy (the right to decide for or against medical treatment) is a fundamental constitutionally protected right but is not an absolute one. The general assumption is that parents act in the best interest of their children. Ideally, medical care without informed consent should be used only when the patient's life is in danger. In some cases, the patient may refuse medical treatment, or the parents may refuse medical treatment for their child. This refusal may arise when treatment conflicts with the parents' religious or cultural beliefs, and the nurse should be aware of some of these common beliefs. People of some religions, such as Christian Science, may prefer prayer or faith healing to allopathic medicine, and some Jehovah's Witnesses refuse blood product administration based on their religious beliefs. Muslims may refuse the use of any potentially addictive substances such as narcotics or medicines containing alcohol. Sometimes, common ground may be reached between the family's religious or cultural beliefs and the health care team's recommendations; adequate communication and education are essential in this situation.

TAKE NOTE!

Do not assume what a patient's beliefs are based on religious affiliation. Assess each patient's views on an individual basis.

In other cases, parents may refuse treatment if they perceive that their child's quality of life may be significantly impaired by the medical care that is offered. The health care team must appropriately educate the family and communicate with them, ensuring they can understand. The child and family should be informed of what to expect with certain tests or treatments. The health care team should make a clinical assessment of the child's and family's understanding of the situation and their reasons for refusing treatment. Active listening may allow the health care provider to address the concerns, fears, or reservations the family may have regarding their child's care.

Refusal of medical care may be considered a form of child neglect. If providing medical treatment may prevent substantial harm and suffering or save a child's life, providers and the judicial system strive to advocate for the child. The state has an overriding interest in the health and welfare of the child and can order that the medical treatment proceeds without signed informed consent; this is referred to as "parens patriae" (the state has a right and a duty to protect children). If the parents refuse treatment and the health care team feels the treatment is reasonable and warranted, the patient should be referred to the institution's ethics committee. If the issue remains unresolved, or if the case is complex, the judicial system may become involved (Katz et al., 2016, reaffirmed 2023). Nurses should document "informed refusal" just as they would informed consent and include assessment information of the patient's decisional capacity along with details regarding the reasons for refusal (Peterson, 2022).

Advance Directives

The Patient Self-Determination Act of 1990 established the concept of advance directives. Advance directives determine the patient's and family's wishes should life-sustaining care become necessary. An advance directive is a "living will" that describes the medical ambitions of the patient's end-of-life care. Parents are generally the surrogate decision makers for children; however, the AAP encourages health care providers to take into consideration the child's views when possible. If the child's interests are not served by prolonged survival, then the primary provider or advanced practitioner should educate the parents about the extent of the child's illness, diagnostic and therapeutic options, and potential for ongoing quality of life (Pozgar, 2020; Weise et al., 2017, reaffirmed 2023). After discussion with other family members, friends, and spiritual advisers, the parents may make the decision to forego life-sustaining medical treatment, either withdrawing treatment or deciding to withhold further treatment or opt not to resuscitate in the event of cardiopulmonary arrest (Weise et al., 2017, reaffirmed 2023).

Life-sustaining care may include antibiotics, chemotherapy, dialysis, ventilation, cardiopulmonary resuscitation (CPR), and artificial nutrition and hydration. Some families may choose to withdraw these treatments if they are already in place or to not begin them should the need arise. **Do-not-attempt-resuscitation (DNAR) orders** are in place for some patients, particularly people who are terminally ill. Some institutions have started using the term AND (Allow Natural Death). No matter what term is used, these orders should include specific instructions regarding the patient's and family's wishes (e.g., some families may desire oxygen but not chest compressions or code medications). When the child is hospitalized, the DNAR order must be documented in the primary provider's orders and updated according to the facility's policy. DNAR orders may also be in place in the home, but only a few states allow emergency medical services to honor a child's DNAR order in the home. Children with DNAR orders may also still be attending school. In that case, the health care professionals involved should meet with school officials (the board of education and its legal counsel) to discuss how the DNAR request can be upheld in the school setting. The health care provider should help educate school officials and staff about the child's condition, potential complications, and health care goals (Weise et al., 2017, reaffirmed 2023). They should work with the school and family on developing an individualized health care plan that will include what to do instead of CPR, such as comfort measures (Weise et al., 2017, reaffirmed 2023).

The Baby Doe regulations, which are an amendment to the U.S. Child Abuse Protection and Treatment Act, provide specific guidelines on how to treat extremely ill, premature, terminally ill, and/or disabled infants regardless of the parents' wishes (Butts & Rich, 2020; National Child Abuse and Neglect Training and Publications Project, 2014). These cases encompass complex ethical issues and are characterized by legal uncertainty. Therefore, providers must continue to work with parents of extremely sick or premature infants to ensure that they are accurately informed about their child's condition and the risks and benefits of treatment. Health care providers must also be aware of federal, state, and hospital policies regarding the care of newborns who are very ill, premature, and/or with disability. The nurse must be knowledgeable about the laws related to the health care of children in the state where they practice as well as the policies of their health care institution. The nurse must be sensitive to the various ethical situations in which they may become involved and should apply knowledge of laws as well as concepts of ethics to provide appropriate care.

Patient Rights

The American Hospital Association first established a Patient's Bill of Rights in 1972 as a way to promote the patient's value and dignity. This information is updated periodically. Most health care agencies and professional organizations have developed some type of document that addresses patient rights.

Ensuring that patient rights are upheld is a key aspect in the care of any patient. For the pregnant person, two patients must be considered—the pregnant person and their fetus. The American Foundation for Maternal and Child Health developed the Pregnant Patient's Bill of Rights to address specific concerns and situations involving the health and well-being of the pregnant person and their fetus. In addition, the USDHHS has issued laws related to protecting the welfare of newborns (the Baby Doe law). A child, due to their age and developmental level, may lack mature decision-making abilities. Many pediatric institutions have adopted a bill of rights for children's health care specific to that institution. This might include the following rights:

- To be called by name
- To receive compassionate health care in a careful, prompt, and courteous manner
- To know the names of all providers caring for the child
- To have basic needs met and usual schedules or routines honored
- To make choices whenever possible
- To be kept without food or drink only when necessary and for the shortest time possible
- To be unrestrained if able
- To access information contained in their records within a reasonable time frame
- To have parents or other important people present with the child
- To have personal privacy protected
- To receive care in a safe setting, free from verbal or physical abuse or harassment
- To have an interpreter for the child and family when needed
- To object noisily if desired
- To be educated honestly about the child's health care
- To be respected as a person (e.g., not having people talk about the child within earshot unless the child knows what is happening)
- For all health care providers to respect the child's confidentiality about their illness at all times (adapted from Society of Pediatric Nurses [SPN], 2021)

Confidentiality

With the establishment of the Health Insurance Portability and Accountability Act (HIPAA) of 1996, the confidentiality of health care information became required. The primary intent of the law is to maintain health insurance coverage for workers and their families when they change or lose jobs. Another aspect of the law requires the USDHHS to establish national standards for electronic transmission of patients' health information. Due to the increased use of electronic medical records (EMRs) and electronic billing, there is an increased possibility that personal health information might be inappropriately distributed. Patient confidentiality and privacy must be maintained in the same manner as it is with paper documentation. Nurses can ensure that privacy is maintained when using computerized documentation and EMRs by doing the following:

- Always maintain the security of personal log-in information; never share it with other health care providers or other people.

- Always log off when leaving the computer.
- Do not leave patient information visible on a monitor screen when the computer/monitor is unattended.
- Use safeguards such as encryption when using alternative means of communication such as e-mail.

HIPAA also addresses security and privacy issues involving a person's health information. The HIPAA Security Rule established national standards to protect electronic personal health information. The HIPAA Privacy Rule ensures proper protection of personal health information while allowing for the flow of health information needed to provide and promote high-quality care (U.S. Department of Health and Human Services, 2022b). As long as reasonable precautions have been taken to protect the patient's privacy, the privacy rule allows certain disclosures that assist in patient care. State privacy laws and professional practice standards also exist to protect personal health information, and care providers must follow whichever guidelines are more stringent. In the pediatric area, information is shared only with the legal parents or guardians or with other people as established in writing by the parents. This law, along with professional obligation, promotes the security and privacy of children's health information.

Exceptions to confidentiality exist. For example, all states require reporting of suspicion of physical or sexual child abuse and injuries caused by a weapon or criminal act. Abuse cases are reported to the child welfare authorities, and criminal acts to the police. If the minor is a threat to themselves, information may need to be disclosed to protect the child. The provider must also follow public health laws that require reporting certain infectious diseases to the local health department (e.g., tuberculosis, hepatitis, HIV, and other STIs). Finally, there is a duty to warn third parties when a specific threat is made to an identifiable person.

Providers must strike a balance between confidentiality and required disclosure. Even if disclosure is required, it is recommended that the provider discuss the issue with the child and, when possible, inform the minor of the limits to confidentiality and consent prior to the initiation of care (Middleman & Olson, 2023).

KEY CONCEPTS

- Healthy People 2030 presents a national set of health goals and objectives for adults and children; these goals focus on health promotion and disease prevention.
- One method to establish the aggregate health status of women, infants, and children is with statistical data, such as mortality and morbidity rates.
- The infant mortality rate is used as an index of the general health of a country. The infant mortality rate in the United States is higher when compared with other high-income countries. This high rate may be the result of the increase in low birth weight infants born in this country.
- Law and ethics are interrelated and affect all of nursing. Based on the American Hospital Association's Bill of Rights, all patients have the right to refuse medical treatment. Parents have the legal right to decide for or against medical treatment for their child. Minor children (under the age of 18 years) must have their parents or legal guardians provide consent for health care in most cases.
- In certain states, mature minors and emancipated minors may consent to their own health care, and certain health care may be provided to adolescents without parental notification. This includes contraception, pregnancy counseling, prenatal care, testing and treatment of STIs and communicable diseases (including HIV), substance misuse, and mental illness counseling and treatment.
- The nurse must be knowledgeable about the laws related to health care of women and children in the specific state of nursing practice and about the specific policies of the health care institution where they work.

REFERENCES AND RECOMMENDED READINGS

Aliouche, H. (2022). *Insight into umbilical cord blood banking*. *News-Medical*. https://www.news-medical.net/health/Insight-into-Umbilical-Cord-Blood-Banking.aspx

American Academy of Pediatrics, Committee on Hospital Care, Section on Surgery, & Section on Critical Care. (2010, reaffirmed 2019). Pediatric organ donation and transplantation. *Pediatrics*, *125*(4), 822–828. https://doi.org/10.1542/peds.2010-0081

American Academy of Pediatrics, Committee on Pediatric Emergency Medicine, & Committee on Bioethics. (2011, reaffirmed 2021). Consent for emergency medical services for children and adolescents. *Pediatrics*, *128*(2), 427–433. https://doi.org/10.1542/peds.2011-1166

American Academy of Pediatrics, Council on Community Pediatrics. (2016, reaffirmed 2021). Poverty and child health in the United States. *Pediatrics*, *137*(4), e20160339. https://doi.org/10.1542/peds.2016-0339

American Cancer Society. (2024). *Key statistics for breast cancer*. https://www.cancer.org/cancer/types/breast-cancer/about/how-common-is-breast-cancer.html

American College of Obstetricians and Gynecologists. (2020). *Opposition to criminalization of individuals during pregnancy and the postpartum period: Statement of policy*. https://www.acog.org/clinical-information/policy-and-position-statements/statements-of-policy/2020/opposition-criminalization-of-individuals-pregnancy-and-postpartum-period

American College of Obstetricians and Gynecologists. (2023a). *Obesity and pregnancy*. https://www.acog.org/womens-health/faqs/obesity-and-pregnancy

American College of Obstetricians and Gynecologists. (2023b). *Umbilical cord blood banking*. https://www.acog.org/clinical/clinical-guidance/committee-opinion/articles/2019/03/umbilical-cord-blood-banking

America's Health Rankings, United Health Foundation. (2024). *Child mortality in the United States*. Retrieved June 12, 2024 from https://www.americashealthrankings.org/explore/measures/child_mortality_a

Anbalagan, S., Falkowitz, D. M., & Mendez, M. D. (2024). *Neonatal abstinence syndrome*. In *StatPearls*. StatPearls Publishing. https://www.ncbi.nlm.nih.gov/books/NBK551498/

Association of Maternal & Child Health Programs. (2019). *Title V overview*. Retrieved December 19, 2023, from http://www.amchp.org/AboutTitleV/Pages/default.aspx

Blitchok, A. (2022). *Roe v. Wade overturned, what it means for healthcare*. Nursing Organization. https://nurse.org/articles/roe-v-wade-abortion-healthcare-impact/

Brown, H. L., & Small, M. J. (2024). Overview of maternal mortality. *UpToDate*. Retrieved April 9, 2024, from https://www.uptodate.com/contents/overview-of-maternal-mortality

Butts, J. B., & Rich, K. L. (2020). *Nursing ethics: Across the curriculum and into practice* (5th ed.). Jones & Bartlett Learning.

Centers for Disease Control and Prevention. (2024a) Child Passenger Safety:RiskFactors for Child Passengers. Retrieved June 12, 2024 from https://www.cdc.gov/child-passenger-safety/risk-factors/index.html

Centers for Disease Control and Prevention. (2024b). *Reproductive health; Infant mortality*. Retrieved June 12, 2024, from https://www.cdc.gov/maternal-infant-health/infant-mortality/

Centers for Disease Control and Prevention. (2024c). *Lung cancer statistics*. https://www.cdc.gov/lung-cancer/statistics/

Centers for Disease Control and Prevention. (2024d). *Data and statistics about opioid use during pregnancy*. https://www.cdc.gov/opioid-use-during-pregnancy/about/index.html

Centers for Disease Control and Prevention. (2024e). *Women and heart disease*. https://www.cdc.gov/heart-disease/about/women-and-heart-disease.html

Centers for Disease Control and Prevention/National Center for Health Statistics. (2022). *Child health*. Retrieved October 24, 2023, from https://www.cdc.gov/nchs/fastats/child-health.htm

Centers for Disease Control and Prevention/National Center for Health Statistics. (2023a). *Percentage of fair or poor health status for children under age 18 years, United States, 2019–2022*. National Health Interview Survey. Generated interactively October 25, 2023, from https://wwwn.cdc.gov/NHISDataQueryTool/SHS_child/index.html

Centers for Disease Control and Prevention /National Center for Health Statistics. (2023b). *Percentage of missing 11 or more school days due to illness, injury, or disability in the past 12 months for children aged 5–17 years, United States, 2019–2020*. National Health Interview Survey. Generated interactively, Retrieved October 25, 2023, from https://wwwn.cdc.gov/NHISDataQueryTool/SHS_child/index.html

Central Intelligence Agency. (2023). *The world factbook: Field listing—Infant mortality rate*. Retrieved April 9, 2024, from https://www.cia.gov/the-world-factbook/field/infant-mortality-rate

Creamer, J., Shrider, E. A., Burns, K., & Chen, F. (2022). *U.S. Census Bureau, current population reports, P60-277, poverty in the United States: 2021*. U.S. Government Publishing Office.

Department of Justice. (2022). *Substance use and pregnancy—Current state policies on mandatory reporting of substance use during pregnancy, and their implications*. https://bja.ojp.gov/library/publications/substance-use-and-pregnancy-part-1-current-state-policies-mandatory-reporting

Ely, D. M., & Driscoll, A. K. (2022). *Infant mortality in the United States, 2020: Data from the period linked birth/infant death file* (*National Vital Statistics Reports*, Volume *71*, *Issue* 5). *National Center for Health Statistics*. https://doi.org/10.15620/cdc:120700

Ely, D. M., & Driscoll, A. K. (2023). *Infant mortality in the United States, 2021: Data from the period linked birth/infant death file* (*National Vital Statistics Reports*, Volume *72*, Issue 11). National Center for Health Statistics. https://www.cdc.gov/nchs/data/nvsr/nvsr72/nvsr72-11.pdf

Federal Interagency Forum on Child and Family Statistics. (2023). *America's children: Key national indicators of well-being, 2023*. U.S. Government Printing Office. https://www.childstats.gov/pdf/ac2023/ac_23.pdf

Feldhusen, A. E. (2000). *The history of midwifery and childbirth in America: A time line*. https://www.midwiferytoday.com/web-article/history-midwifery-childbirth-america-time-line/

Frattarelli, D. A., Galinkin, J. L., Green, T. P., Johnson, T. D., Neville, K. A., Paul, I. M., Van Den Anker, J. N., & American Academy of Pediatrics Committee on Drugs. (2014, reaffirmed 2021). Policy statement: Off-label use of drugs in children. *Pediatrics*, *133*(3), 563–567. https://doi.org/10.1542/peds.2013-4060

GovTrack.us. (2022). *H.R. 3921—115th Congress: HEALTHY KIDS Act*. Retrieved November 7, 2023, from https://www.govtrack.us/congress/bills/115/hr3921

Guttmacher Institute. (2023). *An overview of consent to reproductive health services by young people*. Retrieved October 30, 2023, from https://www.guttmacher.org/state-policy/explore/overview-minors-consent-law

Guyer, B., Freedman, M. A., Strobino, D. M., & Sondik, E. J. (2000). Annual summary of vital statistics: Trends in the health of Americans during the 20th century. *Pediatrics*, *106*(6), 1307–1317. https://doi.org/10.1542/peds.106.6.1307

Hamilton, B. E., Martin, J. A., & Osterman, M. J. K. (2022). *Births: Provisional data for 2021* (*Vital Statistics Rapid Release*, No. 20). *National Center for Health Statistics*. https://dx.doi.org/10.15620/cdc:116027

Handley-Cousins, S. (2021). *A history of childbirth in America*. https://digpodcast.org/2021/08/15/a-history-of-childbirth-in-america/

Health Resources & Services Administration. (2018). *Early periodic screening, diagnosis, and treatment*. Retrieved December 19, 2023, from https://mchb.hrsa.gov/maternal-child-health-initiatives/mchb-programs/early-periodic-screening-diagnosis-and-treatment

Hoban, C. (2019). *Federal programs improve women and children's healthcare*. Emergency and Disaster Management Digest. Retrieved December 19, 2023, from https://edmdigest.com/preparedness/federal-programs-healthcare/

Hoyert, D. L. (2023). Maternal mortality rates in the United States, 2021. *NCHS Health E-Stats*. https://dx.doi.org/10.15620/cdc:124678

Katz, A. L., Webb, S. A., & Committee on Bioethics. (2016, reaffirmed 2023). Informed consent in decision-making in pediatric practice. *Pediatrics, 138*(2), e20161485. https://doi.org/10.1542/peds.2016-1485

Kellams, A. (2024). Breastfeeding: Parental education and support. *UpToDate*. Retrieved April 9, 2024, from https://www.uptodate.com/contents/breastfeeding-parental-education-and-support

Mandy, G. T. (2022). Preterm birth: Definitions of prematurity, epidemiology, and risk factors for infant mortality. *UpToDate*. Retrieved October 24, 2023, from https://www.uptodate.com/contents/preterm-birth-definitions-of-prematurity-epidemiology-and-risk-factors-for-infant-mortality

Mandy, G. T. (2023). Overview of the long-term complications of preterm birth. *UpToDate*. Retrieved October 24, 2023, from https://www.uptodate.com/contents/overview-of-the-long-term-complications-of-preterm-birth

Martucci, J. (2018). Beyond the nature/medicine divide in maternity care. *AMA Journal of Ethics, 20*(12), 1168–1174. https://doi.org/10.1001/amajethics.2018.1168

Maternal and Child Health Bureau, *Health Resources and Services Administration*, U.S. Department of Health and Human Services. (n.d.). *MCH timeline*. Retrieved October 24, 2023, from https://mchb.hrsa.gov/about-us/timeline

McDermott, K. W., & Roemer, M. (2021). *Most Frequent Principal Diagnoses for Inpatient Stays in U.S. Hospitals, 2018. HCUP Statistical Brief #277*. Agency for Healthcare Research and Quality. https://www.hcup-us.ahrq.gov/reports/statbriefs/sb277-TopReasons-Hospital-Stays-2018.pdf

Meek, J. Y. (2023). Infant benefits of breastfeeding. *UpToDate*. Retrieved October 24, 2023, from https://www.uptodate.com/contents/infant-benefits-of-breastfeeding

Middleman, A. B., & Olson, K. A. (2023). Confidentiality in adolescent health care. *UpToDate*. Retrieved October 31, 2023, from https://www.uptodate.com/contents/confidentiality-in-adolescent-health-care

National Child Abuse and Neglect Training and Publications Project. (2014). *The Child Abuse Prevention and Treatment Act: 40 years of safeguarding America's children*. U.S. Department of Health and Human Services, Children's Bureau.

National Institute of Neurological Disorders and Stroke. (2023), *Focus on stem cell research*. https://www.ninds.nih.gov/current-research/focus-tools-topics/focus-stem-cell-research

Niles, P. M., & Zephyrin, L. C. (2023). *How expanding the role of midwives in U.S. health care could help address the maternal health crisis*. https://www.commonwealthfund.org/publications/issue-briefs/2023/may/expanding-role-midwives-address-maternal-health-crisis

Office for Human Research Protection. (2016). *Children: Information on special protections for children as research subjects*. Retrieved June 12, 2024 from https://www.hhs.gov/ohrp/regulations-and-policy/guidance/special-protections-for-children/index.html

Office of the Surgeon General. (2021). *Protecting youth mental health: The U.S. Surgeon General's Advisory*. https://www.hhs.gov/sites/default/files/surgeon-general-youth-mental-health-advisory.pdf

Office of the Surgeon General. (2023). *Social media and youth mental health: The U.S. Surgeon General's Advisory*. https://www.hhs.gov/sites/default/files/sg-youth-mental-health-social-media-advisory.pdf

Office on Women's Health. (2023). *Disparities and the leading causes of death in women—National Women's Health Week 2023*. https://www.womenshealth.gov/node/1374#

Okere, Z. C., & Minimah, F. I. (2022). Moral views on the use of human embryonic stem cells. *International Journal of Research Publication and Reviews, 3*(1), 475–481. https://ijrpr.com/uploads/V3ISSUE1/IJRPR2340.pdf

Olson, K. A., & Middleman, A. B. (2022). Consent in adolescent health care. *UpToDate*. Retrieved October 30, 2023, from https://www.uptodate.com/contents/consent-in-adolescent-health-care

Pagidipati, N., & Douglas, P. S. (2024). Clinical features and diagnosis of coronary heart disease in women. *UpToDate*. Retrieved April 10, 2024, from https://www.uptodate.com/contents/clinical-features-and-diagnosis-of-coronary-heart-disease-in-women

Peterson, K. (2022). Informed refusal: A patient's right? *Nursing, 52*(9), 15–20. https://doi.org/10.1097/01.NURSE.0000853984.71390.98

Pozgar, G. D. (2020). *Legal and ethical issues for health professionals* (5th ed.). Jones & Bartlett Learning.

Preksha, Vahitha, S., Chanu, S. M., & Venkatesh, A. (2022). The effect of birth companion on the level of pain perception among primi-parturient admitted for labor. *Journal of Obstetrics and Gynecological Nursing, 10*(1), 8–13. https://indianjournals.com/ijor.aspx?target=ijor:tnnmcjogn&volume=10&issue=1&article=002

Prince, M. K., & Ayers, D. (2022). *Substance use in pregnancy*. In *StatPearls*. StatPearls Publishing. https://www.ncbi.nlm.nih.gov/books/NBK542330/

Ross, M. G. (2023). Evaluation of fetal death. *eMedicine*. https://emedicine.medscape.com/article/259165-overview

Rousseau, A. C., Riggan, K. A., Schenone, M. H., Whitford, K. J., Pittock, S. T., & Allyse, M. A. (2022). Ethical considerations of maternal-fetal surgery. *Journal of Perinatal Medicine, 50*(5), 519–527. https://doi.org/10.1515/jpm-2021-0476

Shearer, W. T., Lubin, B. H., Cairo, M. S., Section on Hematology/Oncology, & Section on Allergy and Immunology. (2017). Cord blood banking for potential future transplantation. *Pediatrics, 140*(5), e20172695. https://doi.org/10.1542/peds.2017-2695

Society of Pediatric Nurses. (2021). *SPN informational paper: Pediatric bill of rights*. https://www.pedsnurses.org/assets/docs/Informational-Papers/SPN%20Informational%20Paper-%20Pediatric%20Bill%20of%20Rights.pdf

U.S. Department of Agriculture. (2024). *Special supplemental nutrition program for women, infants, and children (WIC)*. Food and Nutrition Service. https://www.fns.usda.gov/wic

U.S. Department of Health and Human Services. (n.d.). Healthy People 2030 objectives. https://health.gov/healthypeople

U.S. Department of Health and Human Services. (2022a). *About the Affordable Care Act*. Retrieved November 7, 2023, from https://www.hhs.gov/healthcare/about-the-aca/index.html

U.S. Department of Health and Human Services. (2022b). *Summary of the HIPAA Privacy Rule*. Retrieved October 31, 2023, from https://www.hhs.gov/hipaa/for-professionals/privacy/laws-regulations/index.html

U.S. Food and Drug Administration. (2019). *FDA approves innovative gene therapy to treat pediatric patients with spinal muscular atrophy, a rare disease and leading genetic cause of infant mortality* [Press release]. https://www.fda.gov/news-events/press-announcements/fda-approves-innovative-gene-therapy-treat-pediatric-patients-spinal-muscular-atrophy-rare-disease

U.S. National Library of Medicine, ClinicalTrials.gov. (2022). *Afrezza® INHALE-1 study in pediatrics (INHALE-1)*. https://clinicaltrials.gov/ct2/show/NCT04974528

Weise, K. L., Okun, A. L., Carter, B. S., Christian, C. W., Committee on Bioethics, Section on Hospice and Palliative Medicine, & Committee on Child Abuse and Neglect. (2017, reaffirmed 2023). Policy statement: Guidance on forgoing life-sustaining medical treatment. *Pediatrics, 140*(3), e20171905. https://doi.org/10.1542/peds.2017-1905

World Health Organization. (2023a). *Constitution*. Retrieved October 24, 2023, from https://www.who.int/about/governance/constitution

World Health Organization. (2023b). *Noncommunicable disease—Key facts*. Retrieved November 12, 2023, from https://www.who.int/news-room/fact-sheets/detail/noncommunicable-diseases#

World Health Organization. (2023c). *Cancer—Key facts*. https://www.who.int/news-room/fact-sheets/detail/cancer

Yarrow, A. L. (2011). A history of federal child antipoverty and health policy in the United States since 1900. *Child Development Perspectives, 5*(1), 66–72. https://doi.org/10.1111/j.1750-8606.2010.00157.x

Zacharias, N. (2023). Perinatal mortality. *UpToDate*. Retrieved April 9, 2024, from https://www.uptodate.com/contents/perinatal-mortality

DEVELOPING CLINICAL JUDGMENT

PRACTICING FOR NCLEX

1. The nurse is preparing a presentation for a local women's group on women's health problems. What will the nurse include as the top cause of mortality for women in the United States?
  a. Breast cancer
  b. Childbirth complications
  c. Injury resulting from violence
  d. Heart disease

2. The nurse is developing strategies to increase the number of people in the community who receive prenatal care. Which factor would most likely be responsible for a pregnant person's failure to receive adequate prenatal care in the United States?
  a. Belief that it is not necessary for a normal pregnancy
  b. Use of denial to cope with pregnancy
  c. Lack of health insurance to cover expenses
  d. Distrust of traditional medical practices

3. When caring for an adolescent, in which instance must the nurse share information with the parents, no matter in which state care is provided?
  a. Pregnancy counseling
  b. Depression
  c. Contraception
  d. Tuberculosis

4. The nurse is developing a community outreach program to help reduce childhood mortality. Which topic(s) are essential to include? Select all that apply.
  a. HIV routes of transmission
  b. Treatment options for congenital anomalies
  c. Appropriate restraints in motor vehicles
  d. Low birth weight prevention strategies
  e. Proper bicycle helmet fit
  f. Water safety

5. The school nurse is planning a screening program. What items should be included to address issues related to the "new morbidity"?
  a. Academic difficulties, violence, and other mental health issues
  b. The number of children with chronic illness at the school
  c. Statistics related to health insurance coverage for the children
  d. HIV infection, asthma, and respiratory allergy testing

CRITICAL THINKING EXERCISES

1. As a nurse working in a federally funded low-income clinic offering women's health services, you are becoming increasingly frustrated with the number of "no-shows," or appointments missed, in your maternity clinic. Some patients come for their initial prenatal intake appointment and never come back. You realize that some patients forget their appointments, but most don't call to notify you. Many of the patients are high risk and are therefore jeopardizing their health and the health of their future child.
  a. What changes might be helpful to address this situation?
  b. Outline what you might say at your next staff meeting to address the issue of patients making one clinic visit and then never returning.
  c. What strategies might you use to improve attendance and notification?
  d. Describe what cultural and customer service techniques might be needed.

2. At your next staff meeting, you have been asked to present material to your nursing unit discussing special situations related to the informed consent of children. Describe the topics that you should address.

3. A 12-year-old is to undergo research treatment for a serious illness. Explain the concept of assent as it relates to this situation.

STUDY ACTIVITIES

1. Research a current policy, bill, or issue being debated on the community, state, or national level that pertains to the health and welfare of women or children. Summarize the major facts and supporting and opposing arguments, and prepare an oral report on your findings.

2. Within your clinical group, debate the following question: Should access to health care be a right or a privilege?

3. Visit a local community health center that offers services to a culturally diverse population of women and children. Interview the staff about any barriers to health care that they have identified. Investigate what the staff members have done to minimize those barriers.

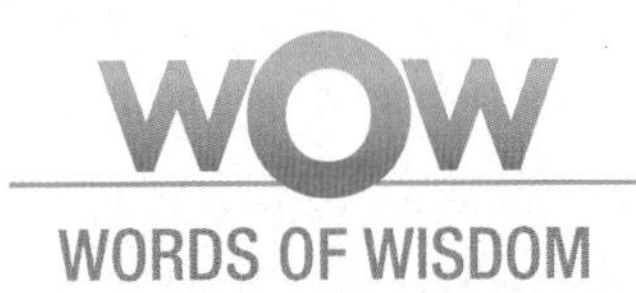

WORDS OF WISDOM

To recognize diversity in others and respect it, we must first have some awareness of who we are.

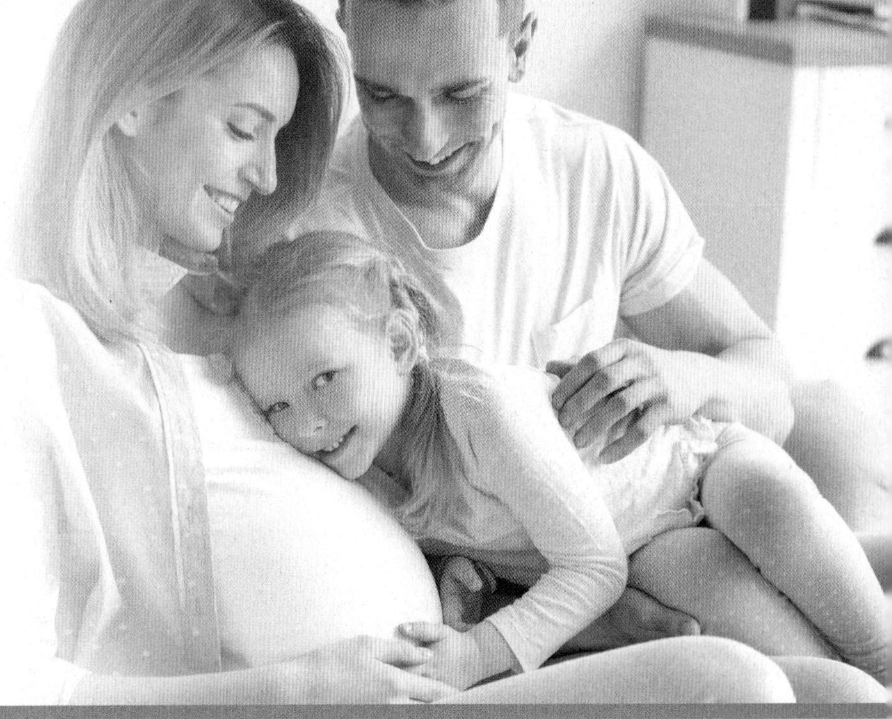

2 Caring for Women and Children

LEARNING OBJECTIVES

Upon completion of the chapter, you will be able to:

1. Identify the core concepts associated with the nursing management of women, children, and families.
2. Examine the major components and key elements of family-centered care.
3. Determine examples of cultural considerations relevant to providing nursing care.
4. Demonstrate the ability to use excellent therapeutic communication skills when interacting with women, children, and families.
5. Apply the process of health teaching as it relates to women, children, and families.
6. Assess the factors that affect maternal and child health.
7. Differentiate the structures, roles, and functions of the family and how they affect the health of women and children.
8. Evaluate how society and culture can influence the health of women, children, and families.
9. Examine access and barriers to health care and its effect on women, children, and family's health.
10. Discuss community and its effects on a child's health.
11. Examine the sources of violence and how exposure to violence affects children.
12. Describe the impact of poverty and social determinants of health on women and children.

KEY TERMS

atraumatic care
cultural humility
discipline
evidence-based practice
family-centered care
family structure
nonverbal communication
personal health literacy
resilience
verbal communication

Maria was home a few days after giving birth to her first child. She had just changed her newborn son and placed him on his stomach for a nap when the community health nurse arrived for a postpartum visit. Because the nurse didn't speak Spanish and Maria didn't speak English, a great deal of gesturing followed. After examining Maria, the nurse then picked up her son and placed him on his back in the crib. How might the nurse have prepared for this home visit? What message did the nurse convey in changing the newborn's position?

INTRODUCTION

Now more than ever, nurses contribute to nearly every health care experience. Historically, people were born at home, cared for when ill at home, and then died at home surrounded by loved ones. Today, these events from birth to death, and every health care emergency in between, will likely involve the presence of a nurse. Involvement of a knowledgeable, supportive, comforting nurse often leads to a positive health care experience. Skilled nursing practice depends on a solid base of knowledge and clinical expertise provided in a caring, holistic manner. Nurses, using their knowledge and passion, help meet the health care needs of their patients throughout the lifespan, whether the patient is a pregnant person, a fetus, a partner, a child, or the parents or family members of a child. Nurses fill a variety of roles in helping patients live healthier lives by providing direct care, emotional support, comfort, information, advice, advocacy, support, and counseling.

This chapter describes the core concepts of maternal and child health nursing and discusses the factors affecting maternal and child health. Nurses need to be knowledgeable about these concepts and factors affecting maternal and child health to ensure that they provide professional, effective care that leads to positive health outcomes.

CORE CONCEPTS OF MATERNAL AND CHILD HEALTH NURSING

Maternal and child health nursing focuses on providing evidence-based care to the patient within the context of the family. This care involves the implementation of an interdisciplinary plan in a collaborative manner to ensure continuity of care that is cost effective, quality oriented, and outcome focused. Nurses can provide this care by focusing on the family, using evidence-based practice (EBP), working collaboratively, providing atraumatic therapeutic care, communicating effectively, providing education, utilizing a continuum of care strategy, providing preventive care, and providing culturally congruent nursing care.

Family-Centered Care

Family-centered care and family-centered maternity care refer to the collaborative partnership among the patient, family, and caregivers to determine goals, share information, offer support, and formulate plans for health care. It is generally understood to be an approach in which patients and their families are considered integral components of the health care decision-making and delivery processes. It is based on mutual trust and collaboration among patients, children, families, and the health care professional. It is a partnership approach between families and their caregivers that recognizes the strength and integrity of the family. The following are the basic principles of family-centered maternity care:

- Childbirth is considered a normal, healthy event that affects the entire family.
- Care must be individualized and respectful.
- Continuous support during labor benefits the birthing parent and family.
- Efforts toward collaborative decision making among the patient and their health care providers is important.
- Education is based on current evidence-based knowledge.
- Birthing parents and newborns should stay together with skin-to-skin contact (Katz, n.d.).

The philosophy of family-centered care recognizes the family as the constant. The health and functioning of the family affect the health of the patient and other members of the family. Family members support one another well beyond the health care provider's brief time with them, such as during the childbearing process or during a child's illness.

Family-centered care requires sensitivity to the patient's and family's beliefs and culture. This involves listening to the family's needs and a shift of the nurse's authoritarian role to empower the family to make their own decisions within the context of a supportive environment. The concept of family-centered care shifts control and power out of the hands of those who give care into the hands of those who receive it.

With family-centered care, support and respect for the uniqueness and diversity of families are essential, along with encouragement and enhancement of the family's strengths and competencies. It is important to create opportunities for families to demonstrate their abilities and skills. Families also can acquire new abilities and skills to maintain a sense of control and empowerment in meeting the needs of the patient. Family-centered care promotes greater family self-determination, decision-making abilities, control, and self-efficacy, thereby enhancing the patient's and family's sense of empowerment. When implementing family-centered care, nurses seek caregiver input. These suggestions and advice are incorporated into the patient's plan of care as the nurse counsels and teaches the family appropriate health care interventions. Today, as nurses partner with various experts to provide high-quality and cost-effective care, one expert partnership that nurses can make is with the patient's family.

The impact of family-centered care can be seen in the models of care delivery for women and children. From the 1980s to the present, there has been increased access to care for all women (regardless of their ability to pay) and hospital redesigns (labor, delivery, and recovery [LDR] rooms and labor, delivery, recovery, and postpartum [LDRP] spaces) aimed at keeping families together during the childbirth experience and to minimize interruptions in breastfeeding dyads (Feldhusen, 2000). This impact can also be seen in the care of children. For example, rooming-in and liberal visiting policies allow parents and other family members to participate in the child's care (Fig. 2.1).

Family-centered care works well in all arenas of health care, from preventive care to long-term care. Using a family-centered approach is associated with positive outcomes, such as decreased anxiety, improved pain management, shorter recovery times, and enhanced confidence and problem-solving skills. Communication between the health care team and the family is also improved, leading to greater satisfaction for both health care providers and patients. It is important for nurses to remain neutral to all they hear and see in order to enhance trust and maintain open communication lines with all family members. Nurses need to remember that patients are experts of their own health; thus, nurses should work within patients' framework when planning health promotion interventions.

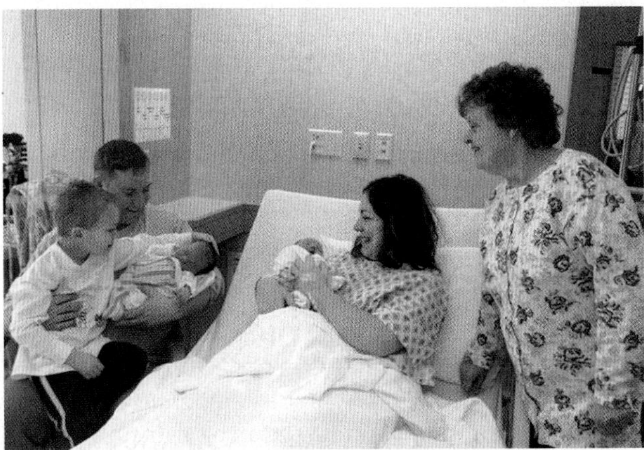

FIGURE 2.1 Providing an opportunity for the parent to interact with the child is an important component of family-centered nursing care.

Evidence-Based Care

Evidence-based practice (EBP) is a problem-solving approach to making nursing clinical decisions based on the most current research findings in holistic, high-quality nursing care (ANA, 2023). Nurses use EBP to identify, critically appraise, and then apply the best available evidence in making decisions about the care of patients. EBP involves the collection, interpretation, and integration of validated research-derived evidence from a variety of resources, such as research findings, internal evidence from outcome management or process improvement processes, and patient preferences. Nurses are challenged to integrate the best available scientific evidence into practice to achieve the best outcomes consistent with the aims of health care—to improve the experience of care, to improve the health of parents and infants, and to reduce the costs of health care. Nurses must have a clear concept of the rationale and principles behind the research to ensure correct implementation in clinical practice. It is important that nurses develop the skills and knowledge necessary to ask pertinent clinical questions, search for current best evidence, analyze the evidence, integrate the evidence into practice when appropriate, and evaluate outcomes. EBP may lead to a decrease in variations in care while at the same time increasing quality and improving health care.

Scientific research findings help nurses stay current not only in their clinical specialties but also in their choice of the most effective interventions. Many of the professional organizations, such as the Association of Women's Health, Obstetric and Neonatal Nurses (AWHONN), American Academy of Pediatrics (AAP), American Nurses Association (ANA), and National League for Nursing (NLN), have developed evidence-based clinical practice guidelines for the safest and most effective delivery of family-centered nursing care. Nurses should be diligent in seeking out these evidence-based guidelines to ensure excellence in their daily practice.

Collaborative Care

The nurse is a collaborator, care coordinator, and consultant. Collaborating with the interdisciplinary health care team, the nurse integrates the patient's, child's, and family's needs into a coordinated plan of care. In the role of consultant, the pediatric nurse ensures that the child's and family's needs are met through activities such as support group facilitation or working with the school nurse to plan the child's care. Collaboration in nursing involves enhanced communication and teamwork; when incorporated into nursing care, collaboration leads to increased nurse satisfaction, efficient and effective patient care, increased staff communication, and increased feelings of support (American Association of Critical Care Nurses [AACN], n.d.; Ferramosca et al., 2023). Nurses must embrace interprofessional collaborative care. Modern health care focuses on an interdisciplinary plan of care designed to meet a patient's physical, developmental, educational, spiritual, and psychosocial needs.

Atraumatic Care

Children undergo a wide range of interventions, many of which can be traumatic, stressful, and painful. The various settings where the child receives care can be scary and overwhelming to the child and family. The child and family interact with various health care personnel, which leads to an increased potential for anxiety. A major component of the child health nursing philosophy is the importance of providing atraumatic care. **Atraumatic care** refers to the therapeutic delivery of care that minimizes or eliminates the psychological and physical distress experienced by children and their families in the health care system (Wong, 1995). The key principles of atraumatic care include the following:

- Preventing or minimizing physical stressors
- Preventing or minimizing separation of the child from the family
- Promoting a sense of control

Nurses must be alert for any situation that has the potential for causing distress and should be able to identify potential stressors. Pediatric nurses should minimize separation of the child from the family, should decrease the child's exposure to stressful situations, and should strive to prevent or minimize pain and injury. The importance of providing atraumatic care to children is integrated throughout this text and discussed in detail in Chapter 30.

Communication

Communication is a way of conveying messages to various people using a common system of symbols, signs, or behaviors. Infants start their first communication soon after birth when they cry to convey the message of discomfort or hunger. Effective therapeutic communication with women, children, and families is essential to the provision of quality atraumatic nursing care. Effective patient- and family-centered communication increases satisfaction with nursing care and aids in improving knowledge and health care skills (Betancourt et al., 2023). The significance of communication revolves around its effectiveness and the climate in which communication occurs. Trust, respect, and empathy are three factors needed to create and foster effective therapeutic communication between people. (See Chapter 30 for specifics on effective communication when working with children.)

Verbal Communication

Communicating through the use of words, either written or spoken, is termed **verbal communication**. Nurses use verbal communication throughout the day when interacting with patients. Good verbal communication skills are necessary when performing nursing assessments and providing child/family teaching. General guidelines for appropriate verbal communication include the following:

- Use open-ended questions that do not restrict the patient's answers.
- Redirect the conversation to maintain focus.
- Use reflection to clarify the patient's feelings.
- Paraphrase the patient's feelings to demonstrate empathy.
- Acknowledge emotions.
- Demonstrate active listening by using the patient's own words.

When working with families, remember that most parents are laypeople, so avoid using medical jargon. The abbreviations and shortened terms that health care providers use sometimes without thinking may sound scary or foreign to children and parents. When medical terminology is necessary, provide a definition using developmentally appropriate language.

Nonverbal Communication

Nonverbal communication, or body language, includes attending to others and active listening. The nurse should listen to the other person's verbal communication from the beginning of the interaction. When parents and children feel they are being heard, trust and rapport are established. Guidelines for appropriate nonverbal communication include the following:

- Relax; maintain an open posture, with the arms uncrossed.
- Sit opposite the person and lean forward slightly.
- Maintain eye contact.
- Nod your head to demonstrate interest.
- Note the person's posture, eye contact, and facial expressions.

TAKE NOTE!

People of all ages desire to be listened to without interruption.

Active listening is critical to the communication process. Listening may uncover fears or concerns that the nurse may not have discovered through questioning.

Paying attention while someone talks is a powerful communication tool. By not listening, the nurse may miss critical information and the person may be reluctant to share further. When interacting with a child and their family, determine whether the messages sent by the child's or family member's verbal and nonverbal communication are congruent.

Recall Maria, who recently was discharged from the hospital with her newborn son. How did the nurse communicate with Maria? Did the nurse's actions during the visit promote the development of trust between Maria and the nurse? What might have been done differently to foster trust?

Communicating Across Cultures

Because nurses work with diverse populations, knowing the best way to respect cultural differences is a must. Understanding and respecting the patient's and family's culture helps foster good communication and improves child and family education about health care. Culture is shaped by many factors, such as religion, spirituality, race, ethnicity, geography, income, education, sexual orientation, and gender identity or expression (Betancourt et al., 2023). These factors are intertwined and affect the patient's and family's communication styles, health status, and health beliefs. It is important to be aware of a person's background, lifestyle, and health care practices to meet their information needs.

Learning about the practices of various cultures is just the beginning; the nurse must assess each family's individual beliefs and practices, not generalize. The best way to assess the family's cultural practices is to ask and then listen. Determine the language spoken at home and observe the use of eye contact and other physical contact. Demonstrate a caring, nonjudgmental attitude and sensitivity to the patient's and family's unique background.

WORKING WITH AN INTERPRETER

Attempting to communicate with a family who does not speak the nurse's language can be frustrating. In this situation, trained interpreters are an invaluable aid and an essential component of patient and family education. Whether working with an interpreter in person or over the phone/computer, it is important to coordinate efforts so that both the family and the interpreter understand the information to be communicated. Working as a team, the nurse questions or informs and the interpreter conveys the information completely and accurately. Well-trained translators can also help prevent cultural missteps and can help guide the health care provider to provide information in a culturally congruent manner; therefore, the use of untrained translators, such as family members or bilingual hospital employees, is not appropriate (AAP, 2021; Betancourt et al., 2023). Box 2.1 presents tips for working with an interpreter to maximize teaching efforts.

On the second visit to Maria's home, the nurse brought a Spanish-speaking interpreter who explained the reason for the "back to sleep" position and demonstrated to Maria several other useful positions for feeding and holding. Maria was smiling when the nurse left and asking when she would be back. What made the difference in their relationship the second visit? What interventions demonstrate culturally congruent care?

BOX 2.1 Tips on Working With an Interpreter

- **Help the interpreter prepare and understand what needs to be done ahead of time.** A few minutes of preparation may save a lot of time and help communication flow more smoothly in the long run.
- **The interpreter is the "communication bridge," not the "content expert."** The nurse's presence at teaching sessions is vital.
- **Ensure enough time is allotted.** It may take longer to say something in some languages than it does in English; therefore, plan for more time than you normally would.
- **Speak slowly and clearly.** Avoid jargon. Use short sentences and be concise. Avoid interrupting the interpreter.
- **Pause every few sentences so the interpreter can translate your information.** After 30 seconds of speaking, stop and let the interpreter express the information.
- **Talk directly to the child and family, not the interpreter.** This demonstrates that the information is coming from you and facilitates communication between you and the child and family. This also helps to limit side conversations that may occur between the interpreter and the child and family.
- **Give the family and the interpreter a break.** Keep sessions short; sessions that last >20 or 30 minutes are too long for attention spans and concentration.
- **Express the information in two or three different ways if needed.** There may be cultural barriers as well as language and dialect differences that interfere with understanding. Interpreters may know the correct communication protocols for the family.
- **Ask the interpreter to help ensure the family can read and understand translated written materials.** The interpreter can also help answer questions and evaluate learning.
- **Avoid side conversations during sessions.** These can be uncomfortable for the family and jeopardize child and family–provider relationships and trust.
- **Just because someone speaks another language doesn't mean they will make an effective interpreter.** An interpreter who has no medical background or training may not understand or interpret correctly, no matter how fluent they are.
- **Children should not be used as interpreters.** Doing so can affect family relationships, proper understanding, and adherence to health care.

Based on Levetown, M., & American Academy of Pediatrics Committee on Bioethics. (2008, reaffirmed 2017). Communicating with children and families: From everyday interactions to skill in conveying distressing information. *Pediatrics, 121*(5), e1441–e1460. https://doi.org/10.1542/peds.2008-0565; Betancourt, J. R., Green, A. R., & Carrillo, J. E. (2023). The patient's culture and effective communication. *UpToDate.* https://www.uptodate.com/contents/the-patients-culture-and-effective-communication

COMMUNICATING WITH PATIENTS WITH HEARING LOSS AND THEIR FAMILIES

Hearing loss is a common chronic disability and an invisible one. Around 432 million people worldwide have disabling hearing loss, and 34 million of these are children (World Health Organization [WHO], 2023). Health care providers are under a duty to provide auxiliary aids and services to establish effective communication with their patients. Providing assistance to people with hearing loss in health care settings is critically important because without assistance through auxiliary aids and services, health care can be difficult to access for people with hearing loss (National Association of the Deaf [NAD], 2023).

Pregnant people with hearing loss, their children, or their parents may be neglected due to a lack of understanding of how best to care for people with different communication needs. Nurses have a key role in exchanging information and taking the time to understand their needs in order to act as an advocate and improve communication with people with hearing loss.

When working with people with hearing loss, determine the method of communication used: lip reading, American Sign Language (ASL), another method, or some combination. If the nurse is not proficient in ASL and the patient or family uses it, then an ASL interpreter must be available if another adult family member is not present for translation. According to federal law (Americans with Disabilities Act), Deaf patients and Deaf family members must be given the opportunity to communicate effectively with health care providers (NAD, 2023).

Education

Illness and hospitalization are two situations that increase the need for assistance and education. Due to shortened hospital stays and decreased admissions, providing patient and family education is a key role for nurses. Many times, teaching begins in the primary care setting and then continues in the community setting, especially the home. In the community-based setting, patient education is often focused on assisting the patient and family to achieve independence.

Regardless of the type of setting, nurses are in a unique position to help patients and families manage their own health care needs. Patients and families need to be knowledgeable about areas such as their condition, the health care management plan, and when and how to contact health care providers. With the limited time available in all health care arenas, nurses must focus on teaching goals and begin teaching at the earliest opportunity.

Patient education occurs when nurses share information, knowledge, and skills with patients and families, allowing them to take responsibility for their health care, make informed decisions about treatment plans, and cope effectively with their illness and symptoms.

When thorough and structured education begins in the hospital setting, it can carry over into the home setting, which can decrease the likelihood of hospital readmission.

Steps of Patient and Family Education

The steps of patient and family education are similar to the steps of the nursing process. The nurse must assess the patient, develop a plan, implement services needed, perform follow-up evaluation, and, finally, document education. Once the nurse achieves a level of comfort and experience with each of these steps, they all blend together into one harmonious whole that becomes an everyday part of nursing practice. Patient education begins with the first patient encounter and proceeds through discharge and beyond. Reassessment after each step or change in the process is critical to ensuring success.

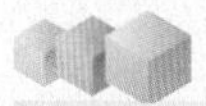
Concept Mastery Alert

When a patient is given a diagnosis that will have a significant impact on a family's life, it is important for the nurse to allow the family time to take in the information about the diagnosis. When communicating with parents about a child's diagnosis, the nurse should provide small amounts of information at a time to allow the parents time to absorb it.

ASSESSING TEACHING AND LEARNING NEEDS

Excellent nursing care begins with a thorough assessment of the patient. In the same way, patient and family education begins with a learning needs assessment that includes the patient's and family's learning needs, learning styles and preferences, and potential barriers to learning. Based on the results of the assessment, an individualized plan can be developed to reduce the time and effort required for teaching while maximizing learning for the patient and family. Although actual nursing care in pediatrics is given to the child, the educational process is targeted toward both the child (when developmentally appropriate) and the adult members of the family. Therefore, it is advisable to conduct a learning needs assessment on both the adult caregivers and the child, when appropriate. Box 2.2 describes the components of a learning needs assessment. This is also a good time to establish rapport with the family, demonstrating your interest in them and your confidence in their ability to learn.

Share the assessment with all members of the interdisciplinary team so that the entire team can support the patient's and family's learning. Although assessment generally takes place during the first or second meeting with the patient and family, it should also occur with each encounter to check for any changes that may occur.

BOX 2.2 Components of Learning Needs Assessment

Assess

- Learner characteristics: Find out more about the patient and family's life and how the patient's illness has affected it. Learn more about the patient and family's social, cultural, and spiritual values.
- Learner needs and readiness: Find out about what they want and need to know and what they know already, readiness and willingness to learn, motivation to learn and emotional concerns, and capacity to learn such as physical or cognitive abilities, including the ability to read and their developmental level.
- Learning style: Determine how the patient and family learn best, as well as preferred learning methods and modalities, such as audio, video, written, or modeling.
- Learning barriers: Identify cultural or language barriers, cognitive or physical disabilities, presence of pain, and status of the patient's support network.

Malcolm Knowles outlined core learning principles to consider when teaching adults (Culatta, 2023; Knowles et al., 2015). He found that instruction for adults needs to focus more on the process than on the content. Box 2.3 lists adult learner-centered principles.

In addition to determining the language spoken in the home and use of eye and physical contact, investigate the following during the assessment:

- Who is the person caring for the child at home?
- Who is the authority figure in the family?
- What is the social support structure?
- Are there any special dietary needs and concerns?
- Are any alternative and complementary health practices used?
- Are any special clothes or other items used to help maintain health?
- What religious beliefs, ceremonies, and spiritual practices are important to the family?

This information will help the nurse direct patient education and adapt their teaching style to meet the learning needs for each individual family. Learning needs can then be negotiated with the family and met based on the assessment. Considerations when teaching families of various backgrounds might include confusion regarding the use of the imperial versus the metric scale, a family's tendency to prepare formulas and medicines using a "handful" or "pinch" of ingredients rather than specific measurements such as a measuring cup or syringe, access to refrigeration for liquid antibiotics, and breastfeeding practices.

BOX 2.3 Specific Learning Principles Related to Adults

- **Adults are self-directed.** Adults value independence and want to learn on their own terms. The most helpful teaching strategies include such concepts as role-playing, demonstration, and self-evaluation. Using this model, nurses can partner with families to ensure that education is interactive and adopt the role of facilitator rather than lecturer.
- **Adults are problem focused and task oriented.** Adults learn best when they perceive there is a gap in their knowledge base and want information and skills to fill the gap. Providing a reason to learn can motivate families that appear slow to adhere to care and education for the patient.
- **Adults are goal oriented.** Adults learn best at a time when learning meets an immediate need. Presenting information in an organized, sequential, and timely manner can often help families understand the importance of learning a particular piece of information or task.
- **Adults value past experiences and beliefs.** Adults bring an accumulated wealth of experiences to each health care encounter; this provides a rich base for new learning. Education should take into account a wide range of backgrounds. Appreciating and using individual differences during teaching encounters can help improve adherence and reduce resistance to educational goals.

Knowles, M. S., Holton III, E. F., & Swanson, R. A. (2015). *The adult learner: The definitive classic in adult education and human resource development* (8th ed.). Routledge.

LITERACY ISSUES

A major barrier to understanding information is the inability to read. Adequate literacy skills benefit patient and family education, yet many people in the United States today have low literacy. In the United States, more than 54% of adults aged 16 to 74 years read at or below the level of the average sixth grader (Rothwell, 2020).

Even people with adequate literacy skills may have difficulty reading, understanding, and applying information to health care situations (Fig. 2.2). **Personal health literacy** is the ability to read, understand, and use health care information and services to make appropriate health care decisions and successfully navigate the health care system (Centers for Disease Control and Prevention [CDC], 2022a). In addition to the ability to read and understand health care information, personal health literacy includes listening; displaying oral, analytic, and decision-making skills; and using electronic technology. Applying these skills to health care situations allows the patient and family to use the information available to make well-informed health care decisions. The inability to comprehend health care information is an enormous problem for many Americans today; about 45% of all American adults have low health literacy (Betancourt et al., 2023).

Organizational health literacy refers to the ability of an organization to equitably empower a person to find, read, process, understand, and use health care information and services to make appropriate health care decisions (CDC, 2022a). Practices that improve personal and organizational health literacy have the potential to

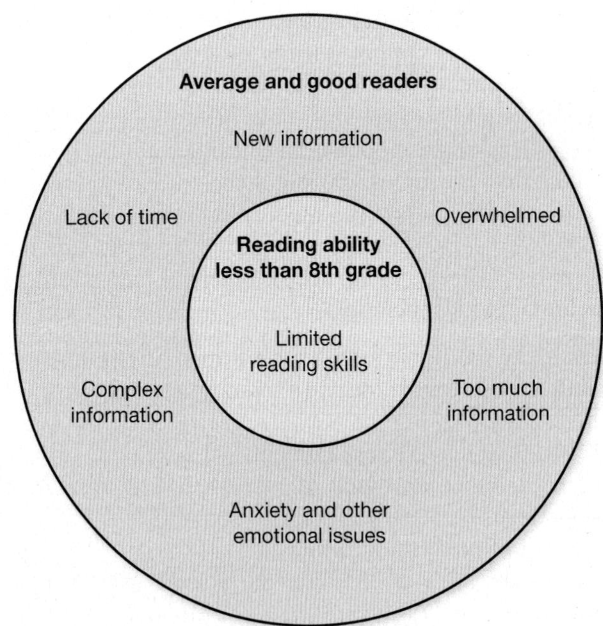

FIGURE 2.2 Factors contributing to poor health literacy.

decrease health disparities and improve health equity. Research has shown that health literacy leads to improved health outcomes, increased patient satisfaction, increased use of preventive health care, fewer dosing errors, decreased unneeded emergency department visits, and decreased hospital readmissions (Health Resources and Service Administration [HRSA], 2022).

TAKE NOTE!

Health literacy is a central focus of Healthy People 2030. One of the overarching goals is to "eliminate health disparities, achieve health equity, and attain health literacy to improve the health and well-being of all" (U.S. Department of Health and Human Services, n.d.).

Medical information is becoming increasingly complex, while the amount of time nurses are allotted to spend with patients is decreasing. Also, when unfamiliar information is introduced or when a person is experiencing emotional distress, reading ability and understanding are further reduced. Therefore, all health care providers should use universal literacy precautions and focus on providing easy-to-understand information during every patient encounter.

TAKE NOTE!

Federal programs, such as the Affordable Care Act of 2010 (ACA), the Department of Health and Human Services' National Action Plan to Improve Health Literacy, and the Plain Writing Act of 2010, have been developed to improve health literacy (CDC, 2022b; Koh et al., 2012).

Low literacy and health literacy are difficult to recognize; appearance, verbal ability, employment status, and educational level cannot reliably indicate a person's literacy or health literacy. People with low literacy may go to great lengths to hide this. Low health literacy affects all segments of the population, but older adults, people with limited resources, people from underrepresented groups, people who are medically underserved, and people who speak English as a second language are at a higher risk (Hickey et al., 2018). Potential indications of low literacy skills include:

- Difficulty filling out registration forms, questionnaires, and consent forms; forms are incomplete, incorrect, or inaccurate.
- Frequently missed appointments
- Nonadherence and lack of follow-up with treatment regimens
- History of medication errors
- Responses such as "I forgot my glasses" or "I'll read this when I get home"
- Inability to answer common questions about their treatment or medications
- Avoiding asking questions for fear of looking "stupid" (Center for Health Care Strategies, 2024)

Nurses need to provide understandable and accessible information to all patients, regardless of their literacy or education level. This includes avoiding medical jargon, breaking down information or instructions into small concrete steps, limiting the focus of a visit to three key points or tasks, and assessing for comprehension. In addition, printed information should be written at or below a fifth- to sixth-grade reading level with plenty of visual aids or pictures (Wittenberg et al., 2018).

Planning Education

Once the assessment is completed, plan mutually agreed-upon, achievable, individualized learning goals and objectives. It is important that both the teacher and the learner believe the goals can be accomplished. Finding common ground and building a bridge between the patient's and family's concerns and what the health care team believes they need to know is a critical part of an education plan. This is also an excellent time to consider which patient education materials and resources can be used to maximize learning and retention. No single teaching method will suit every patient and family. The nurse should individualize educational methods to meet the learning needs and abilities of the person they are teaching. Ensuring instructional methods are chosen based on educational outcomes is a key to success.

Research has shown that 40% to 80% of verbal information given during an office visit is forgotten immediately, and almost half of what is retained is incorrect (Brega et al., 2015; Krontoft, 2021). Verbal instruction continues to be an important component of patient education, but it is not always effective and should be used along with other teaching methods. Using multiple teaching strategies, such as using videos, dolls, play therapy, or computer-based instruction along with written material, at an appropriate reading level for the general population, for future reference is beneficial. Visual aids such as pictures and illustrations are helpful and can assist those with low literacy.

Planning patient and family education should involve input from the entire interdisciplinary team when appropriate. Through effective communication and collaboration, team members can work together to empower the patient and family to become knowledgeable and skillful caregivers. Leaving behind the traditional path of teacher-centered education and providing family-centered education instead require thought and skill.

Practical Interventions to Enhance Learning

The assessed needs and planned learning objectives lead to good teaching interventions. Evaluate these interventions frequently to ensure that the child and family are learning and meeting agreed-upon goals. Table 2.1 presents six techniques that can help improve learning.

Experts, including the American Medical Association and the Agency for Healthcare Research and Quality (AHRQ), recommend practicing universal literacy precautions, which means delivering care as if everyone has low health literacy (AHRQ, 2010, reviewed 2020).

Nurses are in an excellent position to create a "blame-free" environment and offer help. It is entirely appropriate to say to the patient or family member, "Many people have a problem reading and remembering the information on this teaching sheet (booklet, manual). Is this ever a problem for you?"

Several steps that the nurses can take to enhance learning include:

- Draw pictures or use medical illustrations.
- Use videos.
- Color-code medications or the steps of a procedure.
- Record an audiotape.
- Repeat verbal information often and organize it into small groups.
- Teach another family member who can reinforce the learning.

Evaluating Learning

Teaching, even when done well, does not necessarily mean that learning has occurred. Evaluation of learning is critical to ensure that the patient and family have actually learned what was taught. In a health care setting, perform an evaluation with each educational encounter and adjust goals and interventions accordingly. The nurse, along with the rest of the interdisciplinary team, is responsible for patient and family learning. Help ensure understanding by asking for feedback and offering an opportunity for questions. Also, assessing for signs of confusion, such as increased anxiety, can help evaluate learning. If the patient or family has not learned the information, the health care team ensures that teaching strategies are adjusted so that the patient or family does learn it.

The ultimate goal of education is a change in behavior on the part of the patient and family; this change can occur in their level of knowledge, skill, or both.

Evaluation can occur in several different ways, depending on the topic and the method of teaching. The patient or family may:

- demonstrate a skill, often referred to as *return demonstration*. Learning can quickly and easily be identified using this method.

TABLE 2.1 • Six Techniques to Improve Learning

Technique	Explanation
Slow down and repeat information often.	Since most of the education in a health care setting is done verbally, repeat important information at least four or five times.
Speak in conversational style using plain, nonmedical language.	When writing directions, write only several words, bullet points, or phrases. Use common, informal language containing one or two syllables whenever possible.
Group information and teach it in small amounts using logical steps.	This is especially important when there are large amounts of complex information for the family to learn. Teach for 10–15 minutes, give the learner a break, and return later to teach again.
Prioritize information and teach "survival skills" first.	Due to time constraints and multiple demands on the part of staff, coupled with the rapid turnaround times of health care encounters for patients, there never seems to be enough time to teach. Nurses must provide the patient and family with the necessary information to meet their immediate needs. This may include information about the following: • The child's medical condition • Treatment information • Why the information is important • Possible problems, adverse effects, or concerns • What to do if problems arise • Who to contact for further help, information, or supplies
Use visuals, such as pictures, videos, and models.	Use visual resources to enhance and reinforce learning when available. Drawing simple pictures and charts or using alternative methods such as color-coding often allows learning to occur for families who are having difficulty grasping information or concepts.
Teach using an interactive, "hands-on" approach.	When the learner uses hands-on practice or participates in care, learning occurs more quickly and easily. Learning first on a doll or model can ease anxiety and bolster self-confidence before actually doing care or procedures on themselves or the child.
Teach using demonstration, return demonstration, and teach back, tell back.	Show the learner how to do something, have them show you what they learned to do, and have the learner state in their own words what they know or have learned to do.

- repeat back or teach back the information using their own words.
- answer open-ended questions. Open-ended questions provide an opportunity to assess for missing or incorrect information. Open-ended questions are those that cannot be answered with a simple "yes" or "no."

Another option to evaluate learning is to provide a "pretend" scenario for the patient or family, mentally placing them in their own home. Have them verbalize all the steps needed to care for their child, from routine care to handling an emergency situation. They will need to convey information accurately and completely as they walk through the steps necessary to provide care for their child independently at home.

Documenting Education for the Child and Family

Documenting patient care and education on the medical record is part of every nurse's professional practice and serves four main purposes. First and foremost, the child's medical record serves as a communication tool that the entire interdisciplinary team can use to keep track of what the patient and family have learned already and what learning still needs to occur. Second, it serves to testify to the education the patient and family received if and when legal matters arise. Third, it verifies standards set by The Joint Commission, Centers for Medicare & Medicaid Services (CMS), and other accrediting bodies that hold health care providers accountable for patient and family education activities. Finally, it informs third-party payers of goods and services provided for reimbursement purposes.

Documentation of patient and family education is imperative. It is the only way to ensure that the family's educational plan and objectives have been completed and that the family is ready for discharge. Documentation of patient and family education should include the following topics:

- The learning needs assessment
- Information on the patient's medical condition and plan of care
- Goals of patient education and the dates those goals are met
- Teaching method used and how it was received by the patient and family
- Medications, including drug–drug and drug–food interactions
- Modified diets and nutritional needs
- Safe use of medical equipment
- Follow-up care and community resources discussed

Patient and family education plays an essential role in promoting safe self-management practice. To ensure that patients and their families attain the required abilities, patient and family education needs to be competency based. When developing and applying a competency-based education lesson/program, the nurse must identify essential competencies to be taught, optimal teaching methods, best method to evaluate achievement, and documentation of evidence of learning taken place (Rivers et al., 2019).

The Continuum of Care Emphasis

A "continuum of care" strategy provides more efficient and effective services. This continuum extends from acute care settings such as hospitals to outpatient settings such as ambulatory care clinics, primary care offices, rehabilitative units, community care settings, long-term facilities, homes, and even schools. For example, the hospital stay is now integrated into a continuum that allows the patient to complete therapy at home, school, or other community settings while reentering the hospital for short periods for specific treatments or illnesses. Nurses play a primary role in providing better follow-up and smoother transitions from one setting to the next.

As a result of recently improved diagnosis methods and treatments, nurses will care for patients at all stages along the health–illness continuum. For example, at one time, people with congenital heart disease did not live long enough to become pregnant. However, with the help of new surgical techniques to correct the defect, many patients survive and become pregnant, progressing through their pregnancies without significant problems. Moreover, the pediatric nurse now cares for children who have survived once-fatal situations, are living well beyond the usual life expectancy for a specific illness, or are functioning and attending school with chronic disabilities. While positive and exciting, these advances and trends pose new challenges for the health care community. For example, as care for premature newborns improves and survival rates have increased, so too has the incidence of long-term chronic conditions, such as respiratory airway dysfunction or developmental delays. As a result, pediatric nurses must learn to care for children who are well in addition to those who are occasionally ill and those with chronic, sometimes disabling, conditions.

Preventive Care

The concept of prevention is a key part of maternal and pediatric nursing. Health screenings, well-child checkups, routine physical examinations, immunizations, prenatal/postpartum care, and treatment of common acute illnesses are essential to good health. Anticipatory guidance is vital during each health contact with women, children, and families. Education of the family includes everything from keeping the home safe to preventing illness. It is the responsibility of all nurses to incorporate health promotion and disease prevention activities into their professional roles. Applying scientific principles to prevent disease and disability is basic to nursing practice. All health professionals have a special role in health promotion, health protection, and disease prevention. Much of nursing involves prevention, early identification, and prompt treatment of health problems and monitoring for emerging threats that might lead to health problems. This care often involves advocacy for services to meet the patient's needs.

Culturally Congruent Nursing Care

The United States contains an ever-changing mix of numerous, diverse cultural groups of people who arrive daily from countries around the world. The United States has more immigrants than any other nation; the foreign-born population currently makes up about one in seven residents (American Immigration Council, 2021). It is projected that over the next four decades, the United States will experience a dramatic increase in racial and ethnic diversity, and beginning around 2030, immigration will account for more than half of population growth (Vespa et al., 2018, revised 2020). The population of people identifying as two or more races is expected to more than double; the Asian population is expected to double; the Hispanic population is expected to nearly double; and all other racial groups will see an increase, with the exception of non-Hispanic White people, who are expected to decline in number (Vespa et al., 2018, revised 2020).

This growing diversity has significant implications for the health care system. Nurses are tasked with providing optimal health care that meets the needs of women and children and their families from varied cultures and ethnic groups. In addition to displaying competence in technical skills, nurses must also become knowledgeable in caring for patients from varied cultural, ethnic, and racial backgrounds. Adapting to different cultural beliefs and practices requires flexibility and acceptance of others' viewpoints. Nurses must listen to patients and learn about their beliefs about health and wellness. To provide culturally appropriate care to diverse populations, nurses need to know, understand, and respect culturally influenced health behaviors.

The goal is for the nurse to view culture as a point of congruence rather than a potential source of conflict. The nurse needs to combine cultural respect with **cultural humility**. This is an ongoing process that includes self-reflection of one's own biases, a continued willingness to learn from others, and a desire to honor each person's individual beliefs, customs, and values. By combining cultural respect and knowledge with cultural humility, the nurse will be able to provide more effective care to women and children and their families. This cultural awareness allows nurses to care for the whole patient and to improve the quality of care and health outcomes.

The relationship of culture to health care can become obscured by the use of broad group titles. In reality, there are many distinct cultural groups, and within a group, there may be many subcultures. It is crucial that the nurse remembers that diversity exists within cultures and that this is as important as the diversity among different cultures. Every person is a unique individual with their own beliefs, values, and history. The nurse needs to assess each patient and family and ask questions to understand their unique beliefs and values.

CONSIDER THIS!

Our medical mission took a team of nurse practitioners into the rural mountains of Guatemala to offer medical services to people there. One day, a distraught parent brought her 10-year-old daughter to the mission clinic, asking me if there was anything I could do about her daughter's right wrist. She had sustained a wrist fracture a year ago, and it had not healed properly. As I looked at the girl's malformed wrist, I asked if it had been splinted to help with alignment, knowing that it likely had not. The interpreter then explained that this young girl would never marry and have children because of this injury. I was puzzled at the interpreter's prediction of this girl's future. It was later explained to me that if the girl couldn't make tortillas from corn meal for her husband because of her wrist disability, she would be considered unworthy of becoming someone's wife and thus would probably live with her parents the rest of her life.

I reminded myself during the week of the medical mission not to impose my cultural values on the women for whom I was caring and to accept their cultural mores without judgment. These silent self-reminders helped me remain open to learning about our patients' lifestyles and customs.

Thoughts: What must the young girl be feeling at the age of 10, being rejected for a disability that isn't her fault? What might have happened if I had imposed my value system on this patient? How effective would I have been in helping her if she didn't feel accepted? This incident ripped my heart out, for this young girl may be deprived of a fulfilling family life based on a wrist disability. To me, it feels like this is just another example of female suppression that happens all over the world—such a tragedy. And yet, it is a part of the patient's culture, which we as nurses should respect to provide optimal care.

Barriers to Cultural Humility

Illness is culturally shaped in the sense that how we perceive, experience, and cope with disease is based upon our explanations of sickness. When a health care provider lacks knowledge of a patients' cultural practices and beliefs or when the provider's beliefs differ from the patient's, the provider may be unprepared to respond when the patient makes health care decisions the provider does not expect. System-related barriers can occur if agencies that have not been designed for cultural diversity want all patient to conform to their established rules and regulations and attempt to fit everyone into the same mold.

Complementary and Alternative Medicine

The federal government formed the National Center for Complementary and Alternative Medicine (NCCAM) to conduct and support research and provide education and information on complementary and alternative medicine (CAM) to health care providers and the public.

The use of CAM is not unique to a specific ethnic or cultural group; interest in CAM therapies continues to grow nationwide and will affect care of many patients. People of various socioeconomic statuses and education levels and from all regions use CAM. It is a multibillion-dollar industry (Adams-Leander, 2022). Overall, CAM use is more common among women than men (Stussman et al., 2020). In the United States, approximately 37% of adults and approximately 12% of children are using some form of CAM (Nahin et al., 2024). Pregnant people and people in labor commonly use CAM to help manage symptoms and improve pain.

Types of CAM and Integrative Medicine

Complementary medicine is used together with conventional medicine, such as using aromatherapy to reduce discomfort after surgery or to reduce pain during a procedure or during early labor. Alternative medicine is used in place of conventional medicine, such as eating a special natural diet to control nausea and vomiting or taking herbal medicines to treat cancer instead of undergoing surgery, chemotherapy, or radiation that has been recommended by a conventional doctor. Integrative medicine combines mainstream medical therapies with CAM therapies for which there is some scientific evidence of safety and effectiveness (Adams-Leander, 2022).

Integrative health includes acupuncture, reflexology, therapeutic touch, meditation, yoga, massage, herbal therapies, nutritional supplements, homeopathy, naturopathic medicine, and many more modalities used for the promotion of health and well-being.

The philosophy of integrative medicine focuses on treating the whole person, not just the disease, as it combines conventional Western medicine with complementary treatments. The goal is to treat the mind, body, and spirit all at the same time. In science, treatment is never determined by the results of a single study but rather by the collective weight of the evidence. Medicine rests on a foundation that begins with good clinical observations, case reports, and careful interpretations. Replication of a particular approach's results by other scientists establishes whether those clinical observations are important and perhaps applicable; this attempt at replication is the hallmark of valid science. Health care providers need to be aware of the evidence that supports or does not support certain complementary practices in order to provide information and guidance to their patients (Bao et al., 2023). The nurse should avoid judgment and encourage the patient or family to research all evidence-based approaches that support healthy outcomes. Table 2.2 describes select CAM therapies and treatments.

Nursing Implications of CAM

Many people integrate CAM into their health care. Nurses play a significant role in communicating with patients about their CAM utilization. Because of heightened interest in CAM and its widening use, anecdotal efficacy, and growing supporting research-based evidence, nurses must be sensitive to patients' interest and knowledgeable enough to answer many of the questions patients ask and

TABLE 2.2 • Selected Complementary and Alternative Therapies

Therapy	Description
Aromatherapy	Use of essential oils to stimulate the sense of smell for balancing mind, body, and spirit
Homeopathy	Based on the theory of "like treats like"; helps restore the body's natural balance
Acupressure	Restoration of balance by pressing an appropriate point so self-healing capacities can take over
Feng shui (pronounced fung shway)	The Chinese art of placement. Objects are positioned in the environment to induce harmony with chi.
Guided imagery	Use of consciously chosen positive and healing images along with deep relaxation to reduce stress and to help people cope
Reflexology	Use of deep massage on identified points of the foot or hand to scan and rebalance body parts that correspond with each point
Therapeutic touch	Balancing of energy by centering, invoking an intention to heal, and moving the hands from the head to the feet several inches from the skin
Herbal medicine	The therapeutic use of plants for healing and treating diseases and conditions
Spiritual healing	Praying, chanting, presence, laying on of hands, rituals, and meditation to assist in healing
Chiropractic therapy	Aimed at removing irritants to the nervous system to restore proper function—spinal manipulation done for musculoskeletal complaints
Massage therapy	Therapeutic stroking or kneading of the body to decrease pain, produce relaxation, and/or to improve circulation to that body part

Adapted from National Center for Complementary and Integrative Health. (2021). *Complementary, alternative, or integrative health: What's in a name?* https://www.nccih.nih.gov/health/complementary-alternative-or-integrative-health-whats-in-a-name

to guide them in a safe, objective, and supportive way (Adams-Leander, 2022). Nurses have a unique opportunity to provide services that facilitate wholeness. They need to understand all aspects of CAM, including costs, patient knowledge, and drug interactions, if they are to promote holistic strategies for patients and families.

Many patients who use CAM do not reveal this fact to their health care providers. Therefore, one of the nurse's most important roles during the assessment phase of the nursing process is to encourage patients to communicate their use of these therapies to eliminate the possibility of harmful interactions and contraindications with other prescribed medical therapies. When assessing patients, ask specific questions about any nonprescription medications they may be taking, including vitamins, minerals, or herbs. Patients should also be asked about any therapies they are taking that have not been ordered by their primary health care providers.

When caring for patients and their families who practice CAM, nurses need to:

- be culturally sensitive to nontraditional treatments.
- acknowledge and respect different beliefs, attitudes, and lifestyles.
- keep an open mind, remembering that standard medical treatments do not work for all patients.
- accept CAM and integrate it if it brings comfort without harm.
- provide accurate information, not unsubstantiated opinions.
- advise patients on how they can best monitor their conditions using CAM.
- discourage practices only if they are harmful to the patient's health.
- instruct the patient to weigh the risks and benefits of CAM use.
- avoid confrontation when asking patients about CAM.
- be reflective, nonjudgmental, and open minded about CAM.

Many pregnant people suffer from nausea and vomiting in early pregnancy. The use of CAM is widespread to alleviate these symptoms. Ginger lollipops or tea, Sea-Bands, peppermint, acupuncture or acupressure, and vitamin B_6 are frequently used to manage morning sickness with varying results (National Center for Complementary and Integrative Health [NCCIH], 2021b). Although these may not cause any ill effects during pregnancy, most substances ingested cross the placenta and have the potential to reach the fetus. Therefore, nurses should stress to all pregnant patients that they should discuss all remedies with their care providers.

People at risk for osteoporosis may seek alternative therapies. Some of the alternative therapies for osteoporosis include soy isoflavones and red clover (NCCIH, 2021b). In addition, menopausal people may seek CAM therapies for hot flashes. Despite anecdotes suggesting effectiveness, many of these modalities have not undergone scientific testing and thus could place the patient at risk.

If patients are considering the use of or are using CAM therapies, suggest they check with their health care providers before taking any substance, even if it is natural. Offer patients the following instructions:

- Keep in mind that natural does not necessarily mean safe.
- Seek medical care when you are ill.
- Always inform your health care provider if you are taking herbs or other therapies.
- Be sure that any product package contains a list of all ingredients and the amounts of each.
- Be aware that frequent or continual use of large doses of a CAM preparation is not advisable, and harm may result if therapies are mixed (e.g., vitamin E, garlic, and aspirin all have anticoagulant properties).

All nurses, especially nurses working in the community, must educate themselves about the pros and cons of CAM and be prepared to discuss and help their patients understand information about CAM. Understanding and respecting diverse cultures and patients' use of and interest in CAM will enable nurses to provide the best treatment options for patients and their families receiving community-based care.

The Nursing Process

The maternal and pediatric nurse performs all of these tasks using the framework of the nursing process. The nursing process is used to care for patients and their families during health promotion, maintenance, restoration, and rehabilitation. It is a problem-solving method based on the scientific method that allows nursing care to be planned and implemented in a thorough, organized manner to ensure quality and consistency of care. The nursing process is applicable to all health care settings and consists of five steps: assessment, nursing analysis (diagnosis), outcome identification and planning, implementation, and outcome evaluation.

1. Assessment. Assessment involves collecting data about the patient and family and performing physical assessment during community-based health services, at admission to an acute care setting, at periodic times during the patient's hospitalization or care, and during home care visits.
2. Nursing analysis. The nurse analyzes the data collected during assessment to make clinical judgments about the patient's health and developmental status. From this analysis, the nurse develops a list of patient issues, concerns, problems, opportunities, or nursing analyses, which differ from medical diagnoses in that they are issues the nurse can address within their

scope of practice. The actual or potential health problems that result from this clinical judgment process suggest health promotion and health patterns that pediatric nurses can manage.

3. Planning and expected outcomes. The next step in the process involves developing a plan of care that incorporate goals or expected outcomes that improve the patient's dysfunctional health patterns, promote appropriate health patterns, or provide for optimal developmental outcomes. The plan of care includes the specific nursing actions that assist in obtaining the outcomes.
4. Implementation. These interventions are implemented, adapted to the child's developmental level and family status, and modified if the patient's response indicates the need. The plan of care incorporates the family in addition to the patient.
5. Evaluation. The process is continually evaluated and updated during the partnership with the patient and their family.

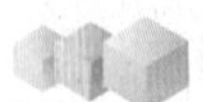
Concept Mastery Alert

Assessment

When prioritizing care for children who witnessed a traumatic incident, the nurse must remember that assessment is the first step in the nursing process.

Standardized care plans for specific nursing analyses/patient issues or concerns and critical pathways for case management are often used in various maternal and pediatric settings. In general, care plans and critical pathways are becoming more evidence based, using a combination of research, group consensus, and past health care decisions to identify the most effective interventions for the patient and family. Evidence-based care planning systems or tools can help bring EBP to the point of care. These templates can help improve the quality of patient care. The nurse is responsible for individualizing these standardized care plans based on the data collected during the assessment of the patient and family and for evaluating the patient's and family's response to the nursing interventions.

Standards of Care and Performance

In any role, the professional nurse is held accountable for nursing actions that adhere to the standards of care. A standard of care is a minimally accepted action expected of a person of a certain skill or knowledge level and reflects what a reasonable and prudent person would do in a similar situation. Professional standards from regulatory agencies, state or federal laws, nurse practice acts, and other specialty groups regulate nursing practice in general.

The ANA, the National Association of Pediatric Nurse Practitioners (NAPNAP), and the Society of Pediatric Nurses (SPN) (2015) have formulated specific standards of care and professional performance for pediatric clinical nursing practice. Standards of practice include assessment, diagnosis/analysis, outcome identification, planning, implementation, and evaluation (refer to "The Nursing Process" section for a description of these standards). Standards of professional performance include ethics, education, EBP and research, quality of practice, communication, leadership, collaboration, professional practice evaluation, resource utilization, environmental health, and advocacy.

The AWHONN updated their *Standards for Professional Nursing Practice in the Care of Women and Newborns* in 2019. These standards include assessment, diagnosis/analysis, outcomes, planning, implementation, evaluation (refer to "The Nursing Process" section for a description of these standards), ethics, culturally congruent practice, communication, collaboration, leadership, education, EBP and research, quality of practice, professional practice evaluation, resource utilization, and environmental health.

These standards are tools that determine whether care constitutes adequate, effective, and acceptable nursing practice. They also serve as guides and legal measures for this special area of practice. These standards promote consistency in practice, provide important guidelines for care planning, assist with the development of outcome criteria, and ensure quality nursing care. The ANA–SPN standards specify what is adequate and effective for general pediatric nursing and promote consistency in practice.

Based on the Institute of Medicine's competencies for nursing, Quality and Safety Education for Nurses (QSEN) initiatives were developed to be integrated into nursing education. Nurses need to understand these initiatives or competencies and utilize them to continue to improve the quality and safety of their nursing practice.

FACTORS AFFECTING MATERNAL AND CHILD HEALTH

From conception, children are shaped by a myriad of factors, such as genetics and the environment. As members of a family, they are also members of a specific community, culture, and society. As they learn and grow, they are affected by multiple complex and ever-changing influences around them. For example, dramatic demographic changes in the United States have led to shifts in communities of color. Globalization has led to an international focus on health. In addition, access to health care and the types of health care available have changed due to modifications in health care delivery and financing. Furthermore, health care delivery in the United States is affected by factors such as immigration, poverty, natural disasters, literacy, violence, and homelessness. The factors affecting maternal and child health discussed in this section include genetics, health status and lifestyle, family, culture, spirituality and religion, community, U.S. society, and global society.

These factors may affect the person positively, by promoting healthy growth and development, or negatively, by increasing the person's health risks. Nurses, especially those working with women and children, need to understand how these influences affect the quality of nursing care and health outcomes. They must examine the impact of these variables to gain the knowledge and skills needed to plan effective care, thereby achieving the best possible outcomes for women, children, and families.

Genetics

Genetics, the study of heredity and its variations, is a field that has applications to all stages of life and all types of diseases. Heredity is the process of transmitting genetic characteristics from parent to offspring. The child's biologic traits, including sex, physical characteristics, some behavioral traits, and the presence of certain diseases or illnesses, are directly linked to genetic inheritance.

Sex

The child's sex is established when the sex chromosomes join. A child's sex can influence many aspects, such as physical characteristics and personal attributes. In addition to the development of male or female genitalia, body development, and hair distribution, some diseases or illnesses can be sex related. For example, scoliosis is more prevalent in those assigned female at birth, and color-vision deficiency is more common in those assigned male at birth. The survival rate of premature infants is correlated with sex; premature females have a higher survival rate than premature males (Mandy, 2022).

Physical Characteristics

Race is the categorization of people based on the perception that physical traits are shared among people of particular heritage or from a particular place. These traits include features such as skin color, bone structure, or blood type. Some physical characteristics may be common among people of a particular race but may be considered an identifying characteristic of a disorder if identified in someone of a different race. For example, epicanthal folds (the vertical folds of skin that partially or completely cover the inner canthi of the eye) are expected in children of Asian descent but may also occur with genetic conditions, such as Down syndrome. In addition, specific malformations and diseases have higher prevalence among people of specific groups. For example, sickle cell anemia occurs more often in African, African American, and Mediterranean population groups, and Tay-Sachs disease is seen most often in people of Ashkenazi Jewish or French-Canadian descent (Sutton & Meng, 2023; Vichinsky, 2022). It is important to note, however, that these disorders can occur in people of any ancestry (Sutton & Meng, 2023; Vichinsky, 2022).

Public awareness is important in educating couples at genetic risk for a particular disease about the benefits of screening programs and proactively seeking preconception genetic counseling to consider options that could include preimplantation genetic diagnosis (the use of in vitro fertilization technology to screen for unaffected embryos). Preimplantation genetic diagnosis was developed as an alternative to prenatal diagnosis for people with a family history of genetic disease or people wishing to avoid passing on to their offspring a known genetic mutation, such as BRCA1 or BRCA2 (Breast Cancer Organization, 2023). Racial and ethnic disparities in the utilization of genetic testing services may reflect a lack of awareness and knowledge about genetic testing (Hong et al., 2023). By educating patients at genetic risk about genetic counseling, nurses can assist patients in gaining awareness that will empower them to make informed reproductive decisions for their families.

Behavioral Traits

Temperament is innate qualities that determine the manner in which a child interacts with their environment. Research supports that hundreds of genes strongly influence temperament (Cloninger et al., 2019). The way a child experiences a particular event will be influenced by their temperament, and the child's temperament will influence the responses of others, including the parents, to the child. Early on, infants demonstrate differences in their behaviors in response to stimuli. These responses are an integral part of the infant's developing personality and individuality. Knowing a child's temperament can help parents and caregivers understand and accept the characteristics of the child without feeling responsible for having caused them.

It is important to recognize that there is a wide range of temperaments within normal development. If the definition of temperament is too narrow, certain behaviors may be mislabeled as development delays or concerns. Children's temperaments are commonly categorized into groups: even-tempered, challenging, and slow to warm up. Various temperaments exist that are a combination of these groups (Bogues & Levine, 2023). Even-tempered children have regular biologic functions, predictable behavior, and positive attitudes toward new experiences. Challenging children have irregular biologic functions, are highly active and intense, react to new experiences by withdrawing, and are frustrated easily. Children in the slow-to-warm-up category are cautious and less active and have more irregular reactions; they react to new experiences with mild but passive resistance and need extra time to adjust to new situations. Many children will exhibit a mix of these temperaments.

There may be friction in a family if parents' and children's temperaments conflict (e.g., a challenging 2-year-old with slow-to-warm-up parents). If parents want and expect their child to be predictable but that is not the child's style, those parents may perceive the child to have problems; this conflict may then affect the child's health. The key is not to label the child but to recognize the strengths and challenges of each type of temperament. Knowing a child's temperament can help parents anticipate and understand a child's characteristics and behaviors and allow them to adjust their parenting styles.

Genetically Linked Diseases

New technologies in molecular biology and biochemistry have led to better understanding of the mechanisms involved in hereditary transmission, including those associated with genetic disorders. These advances are now leading to better diagnostic tests and management options.

Reproductive genetic testing, counseling, and other genetic services can be valuable components in the reproductive health care of childbearing people and their families.

Two major areas of study in genetics that are important to pediatrics are cytogenetics and the Human Genome Project. Cytogenetics is the study of genetics at the chromosome level. Since the genetic code was deciphered, much has been learned about the chromosomal structure shared by all human organisms. Chromosomal anomalies, such as trisomies 21, 18, and 13, occur in 0.6% of all live births and negatively affect fetal viability (Breilyn & Levy, 2023). Anomalies are even more common in cases of spontaneous abortions and stillbirths. The Human Genome Project was an international research effort involving the localization, isolation, and characterization of human genes and investigation of the function of the gene products and their interaction with one another. It was considered a highly ambitious and successful international research collaboration. Completion of this project provided scientists with greatly enhanced information about how DNA shapes species development and genetic diseases to aid in developing new ways to identify, treat, cure, or even prevent them. Chapters 10 and 49 offer more detailed discussion of genetics.

Health Status and Lifestyle

A person's general health status and specific lifestyle influence their health. Health status may be a factor soon after birth. Societal shifts including a greater focus on education and careers have resulted in a trend toward delayed childbearing in the United States (Morris, 2023). This delayed timing has contributed to an increased incidence of multiple births due to the increased use of in vitro fertilization and other assisted reproductive technologies (Qian et al., 2023). Potential complications of multiple births include prematurity and intrauterine growth restriction, which may lead to chronic health problems in the child. There is a higher rate of chronic health problems among babies born prematurely or who suffered other in utero complications, such as intrauterine growth restriction (Mandy, 2023). Children with chronic health conditions may also have developmental delays, especially in acquiring skills related to cognition, communication, adaptation, social functioning, and motor functioning. Thus, a child's beginning health status may affect their long-term health and development.

> ***TAKE NOTE!***
>
> The lifestyle of the parents basically is the lifestyle of the children. For instance, parents who are physically inactive and eat less nutritious foods will likely have children who do the same; unhealthy habits are associated with health problems such as diabetes, obesity, and early heart disease that are showing up earlier in children and adolescents. It is important for parents to serve as role models for their children, modeling a nutritious diet and physical activity (through sports, hobbies, or other activities).

Developmental Level and Disease Distribution

The way a child develops is the result of genetics and the environment within the context of a variety of biopsychosocial forces. Biologic influences include genetics, in utero exposure to teratogens, postpartum illnesses, exposure to hazardous substances, and maturation. Chapters 25 through 29 discuss the factors affecting the growth and development for each age group.

Developmental level has a major impact on a person's health status. In general, the distribution of diseases or illnesses varies with age. For example, adolescents who become pregnant are at a higher risk for certain complications, such as anemia, hypertension, preterm labor, cephalopelvic disproportion, and postpartum hemorrhage. Pregnant adolescents also experience higher rates of intimate partner violence and substance use disorder. Moreover, substance misuse can contribute to low birth weight, intrauterine growth restriction, preterm births, stillbirth, newborn addiction, and sepsis (CDC, 2022f). People who become pregnant after age 35 are at risk for hypertension, dystocia, and postpartum hemorrhage; they are also more likely to have a preexisting condition that could complicate the pregnancy. Moreover, their fetuses are at higher risk for chromosomal abnormalities.

Certain communicable diseases are more commonly associated with certain age groups. Roseola, which is a viral illness resulting in high fevers and rash, is most often seen in infants 7 to 13 months old. Scarlet fever, which is an infection from group A streptococci, is a disease that primarily affects children older than 3 years (CDC, 2022g; Tremblay & Brady, 2023). The physiologic immaturity of an infant's body system increases the risk of infection. Ingestion of toxic substances and the risk of poisoning are major health concerns for toddlers as they become more mobile and inquisitive. Because preschool- and school-aged children are generally very active, they are more prone to injury and accidents. Adolescents are establishing their identity, which may lead them to separate from family values and traditions for a period of time and attempt to conform to their peers' behaviors and expectations. This may contribute to risk-taking behaviors, resulting in injuries or other situations that may impair their health.

Nutrition

Nutrition provides the body with the calories and nutrients to sustain life, promote growth, maintain health, and prevent illness. Adequate nutrition is beneficial for the developing child; conversely, nutritional deprivation can seriously interfere with brain development and other functions. Nutritional requirements change over the child's life and have a great influence on the child's physical growth and intellectual development. Good nutrition provides the essentials required to maintain health and prevent illness (Fig. 2.3). Chapters 3 through 7 discuss the specific nutritional requirements and the impact of deficiencies for each developmental stage.

Nutritional deficiencies, such as iron deficiency anemia, or excesses, such as those that can lead to childhood obesity, are still common problems in the United States. Some factors contributing to poor nutrition include inadequate food intake, nutritionally unsound social and cultural food practices, the easy accessibility of processed and nutritionally inadequate foods, lack of nutrition education in homes and schools, and the presence of illness that interferes with ingestion, digestion, and absorption of food. In a growing child, inadequate nutrition is associated with delayed development, increased susceptibility to childhood illnesses and infections, increased risk for morbidity and mortality, delayed development, and stunted physical growth (Buchanan & Marquez, 2023a). Childhood obesity places the child at a higher risk for adult obesity and for certain diseases, such as type 2 diabetes and cardiovascular disease at an earlier age (Buchanan & Marquez, 2023b).

A pregnant person needs additional calories to support fetal growth and development as well as to support their own needs, and an adequate intake of folic acid is important to prevent neural tube defects. Discussion of nutrition and its effects on health status is integrated throughout this text.

Lifestyle Choices

Lifestyle choices that affect a person's health include patterns of eating; amount and type of exercise; use of tobacco, drugs, or alcohol; and methods of coping with stress. A

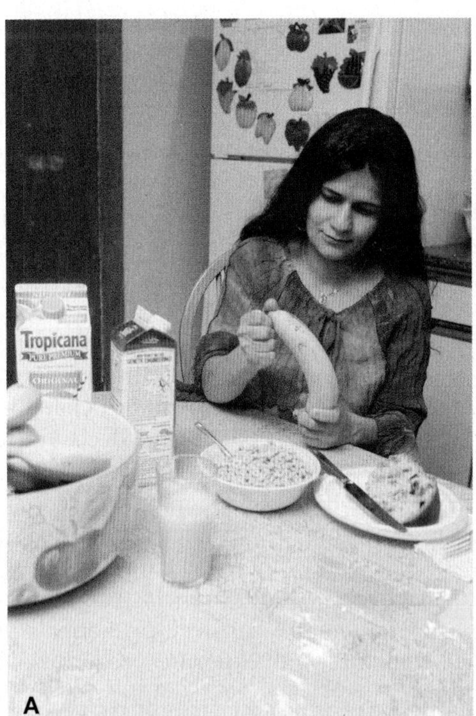

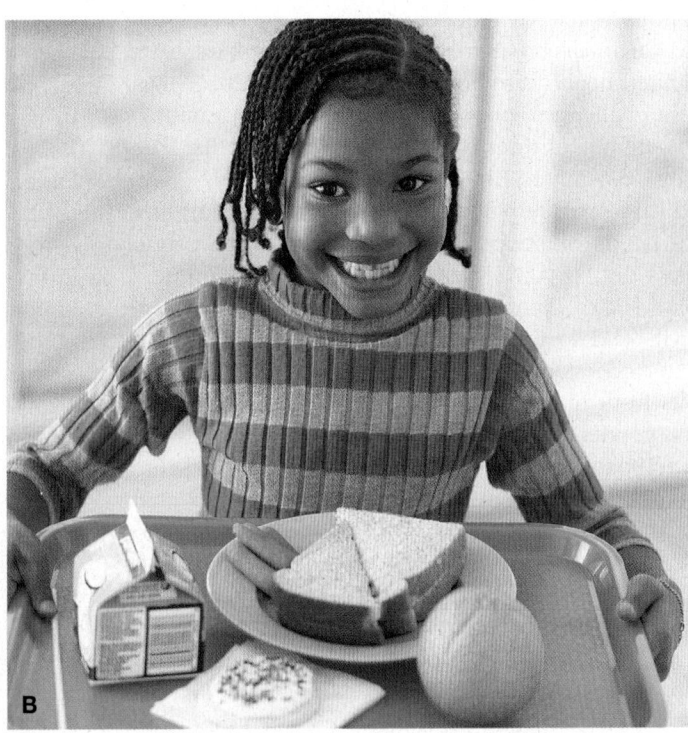

FIGURE 2.3 **A.** A pregnant patient eating a healthy meal to ensure adequate nutrition. **B.** The dietary habits established early in life can have a long-lasting impact on the child's health and quality of life.

person's lifestyle contributes to their wellness and health problems. Children take on their parents' lifestyle. Parents who are not physically active and who eat foods with inadequate nutrition commonly have children with the same habits; those habits can contribute to diabetes and early heart disease. Once thought of as adult problems, these conditions are being diagnosed more frequently in children and adolescents today (Drozdz et al., 2021). Parents should self-evaluate their own dietary and activity habits and make changes to support their own health and then strive to encourage healthy eating habits and an appropriate level of physical activity in the child's life through sports, hobbies such as dancing, and family activities.

Gender and Sexual Identity

In addition to the specific biologic and physical traits related to the child's sex, there are also social factors related to their gender. The child often develops specific gender attitudes and behaviors that are aligned with their culture. Interactions with family members and peers as well as activities and societal values affect how children perceive their and others' genders. A child is assigned a sex at birth, and in many cases, this is congruent with their gender identity. However, sex and gender do not always match, and the child may be transgender or gender diverse (Forcier & Olson-Kennedy, 2023).

Sexual identity can also have an impact on a child's overall health and development. People who are lesbian, gay, bisexual, transgender, queer, intersex, asexual, or of other minoritized gender or sexual identities (LGBTQ+) disproportionately experience challenges in health care due to factors such as discrimination, social pressure, and limited health care access (Bass & Nagy, 2022). Due to these challenges, people in the LGBTQ+ community experience higher rates of depression, tobacco use, and sexually transmitted infections (Bass & Nagy, 2022). Health care providers need to learn and understand the special needs of people of diverse sexual and gender identities and provide them with culturally congruent, compassionate, comprehensive, and high-quality care. This will lead to improved health outcomes. Providers need to understand and use respectful terminology for patients from minoritized sexual and gender communities, use gender-neutral language and language that aligns with each patient's identified pronouns, and understand, assess, and treat patients for the unique risks and challenges they may face, as appropriate. See Box 2.4 for commonly used terms related to gender identity. This list is not all inclusive, and the exact terms a health care provider uses are secondary to the importance of being sensitive and aware of each person's identity. One way to do this is to use the terms that align with each individual patient's identity. Strong parental and social support are essential to healthy development for children who are LGBTQ+.

BOX 2.4 Gender Identity Terms

- Binary: The person identifies as a man or woman.
- Nonbinary: The person's gender identity does not fit into the categories of man or woman.
- Cisgender/cis: The person's gender identity aligns with their sex assigned at birth.
- Transgender/trans: The person's gender identity is different from their sex assigned at birth.
- Agender: The person does not identify as any gender.
- Genderqueer: The person's gender identity is not binary.
- Gender-expansive: The person has a more flexible gender identity beyond the binary.
- Gender transition: The process of bringing oneself and one's body in alignment with one's gender identity.
- Gender dysphoria: Distress or discomfort experienced due to the lack of alignment between one's assigned sex at birth and one's gender identity.
- Bigender: The person's identity includes two genders or is moving between two genders.
- Affirmed gender: A person's true gender, which may or may not align with their sex assigned at birth.
- Genderfluid: Moving among genders and not adhering to one fixed gender.

Adapted from Bass, B., & Nagy, H. (2022). Cultural competence in the care of LGBTQ patients. In: *StatPearls* [Internet]. StatPearls Publishing. https://www.ncbi.nlm.nih.gov/books/NBK563176/; Parent, Families and Friends of Lesbians and Gays. (2023). *LGBTQ+ Glossary.* Retrieved October 8, 2023, from https://pflag.org/glossary/

Environmental Exposure

Environmental pollutants are not only hazardous to the ecosystem, but they can also lead to various health problems that affect the human population worldwide, irrespective of sex, gender, race, or age. Some environmental exposures can jeopardize health. In utero, poor nutrition or exposure to the pregnant parent's use of alcohol, tobacco, or drugs or infections can affect the fetus. Nurses caring for pregnant patients should be aware of the risks to the fetus posed by certain drugs, chemicals, and dietary agents, as well as maternal illnesses. These agents, known as *teratogens*, may be linked to birth defects in children. However, not all drugs or agents are associated with fetal effects, and research is ongoing to identify the correlations between teratogens and other variables.

The environment continues to affect a child's health after birth. Exposure to air pollution, tobacco, and water or food contaminants can impair a child's health status. Safety hazards in the home or community can contribute to falls, burns, drowning, or other accidents. Exposure to secondhand smoke and other pollutants, such as from radiation or chemicals, is also a health hazard for children. Because children are smaller than adults and still developing, environmental exposures can cause them additional health problems. For example, due to young children's rapidly developing nervous system, they are more sensitive than adults to the effects of lead. Lead exposure is a common preventable poisoning in children, especially among children less than 6 years of age (Sample, 2024). Sources include lead paint, pottery and ceramics, imported toys, lead-contaminated dust, and lead contained in soil and water. Lead exposure can result in developmental and behavioral problems ranging from inattentiveness and hyperactivity to permanent brain damage and death, depending on the level of exposure.

TAKE NOTE!

Thirdhand smoke refers to residual tobacco smoke and carcinogens that remain after a cigarette is extinguished. These toxins cling to the hair and clothes of the person smoking and can be present on any surface in the house, such as carpet and cushions. Children are particularly susceptible to thirdhand smoke since they breathe near, crawl on, touch, and may put their mouths on contaminated surfaces (Samet & Sockrider, 2022).

Stress, Coping, and Adverse Childhood Experiences

Children are exposed to various situations and events that can produce stress. These events can contribute to common problems associated with growth and development, such as entering a new classroom, learning a new skill, or being teased by a classmate. However, they can also be associated with exposure to or experience with poverty, illness, divorce, violence, suicide, substance use, mental illness, or other potential sources of trauma. These experiences are referred to as *adverse childhood experiences* (ACEs). Exposure to ACEs in childhood leads to an increased risk for chronic health problems, mental illness, and substance use in adulthood (CDC, 2024d). ACEs are preventable, and health care providers can help families and communities create safe, stable environments with nurturing healthy relationships for children.

TAKE NOTE!

People assigned female at birth and non-Hispanic American Indians and Alaska Natives were found to have a higher risk for experiencing one or more ACEs (CDC, 2024e).

Stressors such as war, terrorism, school violence, pandemics, climate change, displacement, and natural disasters can have a significant impact on the well-being of women, children, and families. Exposure to traumatic events and violence may have long-term effects on a person's psychosocial development and status. Exposure to stress is not limited to disasters or traumatic events, however. Stress can also include areas such as inadequate finances, family crises such as divorce, inadequate support systems, illness, or violence. Similar to disasters and traumatic events, the effects of these stressors can dramatically affect the health status of an adult, child, or family.

Some adults and children can adapt and respond to the stress, while others have more difficulty. **Resilience** refers to the ability to adapt and cope with significant adverse events or stresses and to recover and function successfully with positive outcomes.

Various internal and external protective factors promote resiliency. Internal factors include the person's ability to take control and be proactive; to be responsible for their own decisions; to understand and accept their own limits and abilities; and to be goal directed, knowing when to continue or when to stop. External factors include caring relationships with a family member; a positive, safe learning environment at school (including membership in clubs and social organizations); and positive influences in the community (see the discussion earlier in this chapter under violence in the home providing examples of protective factors and violence). Promoting the development of resiliency in children aids in the achievement of positive developmental and health outcomes (Gartland et al., 2019).

Access to Health Care

The health care system, including the delivery and financing of this system, continues to change and evolve. Health insurance coverage is a critical factor in making health care affordable and accessible. In the United States, changes in the health care system result from pressures from many directions. These changes reflect shifts in social and economic realities and the results of the biomedical and technologic progress over the past several decades. The effects are felt by everyone who seeks health care in any form. Access to health care is negatively affected by the lack of health insurance. People without health insurance typically cannot afford to seek health care for maintenance and prevention interventions. People who work full time may not earn enough money to afford health insurance or medical care, and people who work part time do not typically receive benefits, such as health insurance. Women are less likely than men to be uninsured due to the expansion of ACA, but they often have inadequate access to care, receive a lower standard of care, and have poorer outcomes (Kaiser Family Foundation, 2020).

Families without insurance may delay care for their children and are less likely to have a usual place of care for their children (Federal Interagency Forum on Child and Family Statistics [FIFCFS], 2023). The percentage of children without health insurance for 12 months has declined since 2010 and is currently at 4% to 5% (FIFCFS, 2023). This decrease is largely attributed to the expansion of Medicaid and the Child's Health Insurance Program

(CHIP, which was created as the State Children's Health Insurance Program [SCHIP] through legislation passed in 1997) (Mykyta et al., 2022). Medicaid is a joint federal and state program that provides health insurance to families with lower incomes. It is state administered, and each state has its own set of guidelines. The purpose of CHIP is to help insure children whose families are ineligible for Medicaid but cannot afford private health insurance. This program is also funded jointly by the federal and state governments but administered by individual states.

Insurance coverage for 36% of children comes from Medicaid or CHIP, while over 60% of children are covered by private insurance or employer-based health insurance (Mykyta et al., 2022). In recent years, Medicaid and CHIP have focused on increasing enrollment by increasing outreach, simplifying enrollment procedures, and retaining eligible enrollees. Legislation such as the Children's Health Insurance Program Reauthorization Act of 2009 (CHIPRA) and the ACA have helped support this effort. Medicaid and CHIP provide a good base of coverage for children from families with lower incomes, but eligibility for parents is much more limited. These programs rely on adequate state and federal funding. Therefore, the continued success of these programs depends on future legislation. Changes in employer-based and private health insurance will continue to challenge the nation in ensuring adequate health care for all children.

Barriers to Health Care

Women are major consumers of health care services, in many cases arranging not only their own care but also that of family members. See Evidence-Based Practice 2.1. Even with the federal and state programs available to assist woman, children, and families, there remain barriers to appropriate, cost-effective, coordinated, and timely health care.

FINANCES

Financial barriers are one of the most important factors limiting access to care. Childbirth is the leading reason for hospitalization in the United States. For both private insurers and Medicaid, hospital maternity and newborn charges exceed those for any other condition. In U.S. hospitals, vaginal and cesarean births are costly. Many people have limited or no health insurance and cannot afford to pay for maternity care. Compared with people from other ethnic groups, African American women tend to be younger when they give birth, are more likely to have a surgical birth, experience more preterm births, stay longer in the hospital, and incur higher Medicaid costs. Black women experience a higher rate of adverse pregnancy outcomes than do White women (CDC, 2023e). Racial disparities in adverse pregnancy outcomes represent not only potential preventable human suffering but also avoidable economic costs. Although Medicaid

EVIDENCE-BASED PRACTICE 2.1

Strategies to reduce stigma and discrimination in sexual and reproductive health care settings: A mixed-methods systematic review

BACKGROUND

Sexual and reproductive health and rights are important to achieve positive health outcomes, but they remain out of reach for many worldwide. Both manifest in broader society involving privilege, power, and disadvantages. Stigma and discrimination within health care organizations cause health inequalities and an imbalance of power within society. People who are stigmatized may receive substandard care and delay or forgo seeking health care in the future. Eliminating both stigma and discrimination from health care settings is vital to the attainment of reproductive justice and respectful care for all people. This study aimed to address this health care injustice and offer recommendations for interventions to promote respectful, person-centered care for all.

STUDY

Quantitative, qualitative, and mixed-methods studies that focused on strategies to reduce stigma and discrimination in sexual and reproductive community settings were included. This was a mixed-methods systematic review of 8,262 articles screened, with 12 articles from 10 studies meeting the inclusion criteria. Six articles contributed qualitative evidence, and the remainder provided quantitative evidence. Findings were consistent with previous systematic reviews on strategies to address stigma and discrimination in maternity care.

Findings

Many interventions were identified to address stigma and discrimination within community settings. They included improving health care providers' awareness of their behaviors and educating them about health conditions and consequences of their behaviors to improve empathy in clinical encounters. Policy reform may create environments that foster safe, respectful, and inclusive care without creating barriers.

Nursing Implications

Perceptions and experiences of stigma and discrimination are well documented globally, but critical problems remain in understanding them and taking action to bring about changes that will address them. More research is needed to develop strategies to address the problems of stigma and discrimination of marginalized people in health care settings. The findings from this review have important implications for policy and practice. Nurses need to evaluate how they offer reproductive care to patients and their families and how improvement in health care providers' behaviors can be made. All nurses need to reexamine their practice to make sure that it is respectful, safe, family centered, and of high quality, regardless of the practice setting.

Bohren, M. A., Corona, M. V., Odiase, O. J., Wilson, A. N., Sudhinaraset, M., Diamond-Smith, N., Berryman, J., Tuncalp, O., & Afulani, P. A. (2022). Strategies to reduce stigma and discrimination in sexual and reproductive healthcare settings: A mixed-methods systematic review. *PLOS Global Public Health*. https://doi.org/10.1371/journal.pgph.0000582

covers more than 40% of U.S. births overall and 65% of births to Black birthing parents, expanding and enhancing the coverage is needed to address the disparities that comprise a Black maternal health crisis (Center on Budget and Policy Priorities, 2021). Moreover, the paperwork and enrollment process for health insurance can be so overwhelming that many people do not register.

In 2021, 29% of children were living in families with lower incomes and 15.3% were living below the federal poverty threshold (Shrider & Creamer, 2023; Wildsmith & Alvira-Hammond, 2023). Many children and families do not have health insurance, do not have enough insurance to cover the services they need, or cannot pay for services. Nurses need to assess for financial barriers to health care and be aware of resources available to help families overcome these barriers.

SOCIOCULTURAL BARRIERS

Lack of transportation and the need for both parents to work also pose barriers to seeking health care. It can be difficult to attend all recommended prenatal health care visits or well-child visits, especially if the patient has other small children who must be taken along on the visit. These challenges can reduce the adherence to scheduled appointments and follow-up. Knowledge barriers (e.g., lack of understanding of the importance of prenatal care or preventive health care), language barriers (e.g., speaking a different language than the health care providers do), or spiritual barriers (e.g., religious beliefs discouraging some forms of treatment) also exist.

CONSIDER THIS!

I was a 17-year-old pregnant migrant worker needing prenatal care. I didn't speak much English, so when I saw the receptionist I pointed to my "big belly" and asked for services. All the receptionist seemed interested in was a social security number and health insurance card—neither of which I had. She proceeded to ask me personal questions concerning who the father was and commented on how young I looked. The receptionist then demanded in a loud voice that I sit down and wait for an answer from someone in the back, but I never actually saw her contact anyone. It felt like all eyes were on me while I found an empty seat in the waiting room. After sitting there quietly for over an hour without any attention or answer, I left.

Thoughts: Why did this patient leave before receiving any health care service? What must they have been feeling during the long wait? Would you come back to this clinic again? Why or why not?

Family

The family is considered the basic social unit. The U.S. Census Bureau (2023) defines a *family* as a group of two or more people related by birth, marriage, or adoption and living together. Traditional definitions of family emphasize the legal ties or genetic relationships of people living in the same household with specific roles. Given the diversity of families in today's society, some believe that family should be defined as whatever the child says it is (Fig. 2.4) (Patterson, 1995).

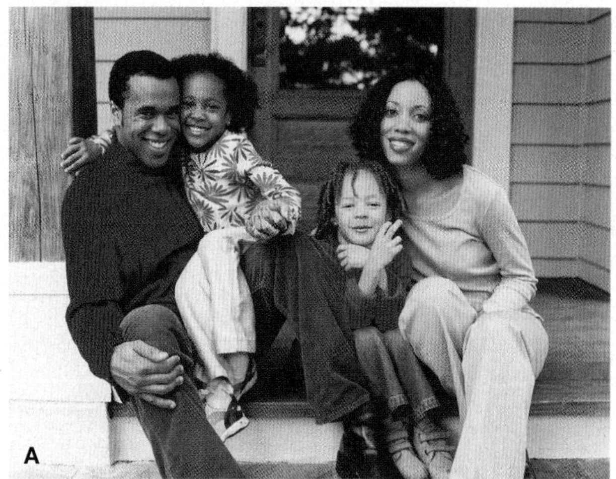

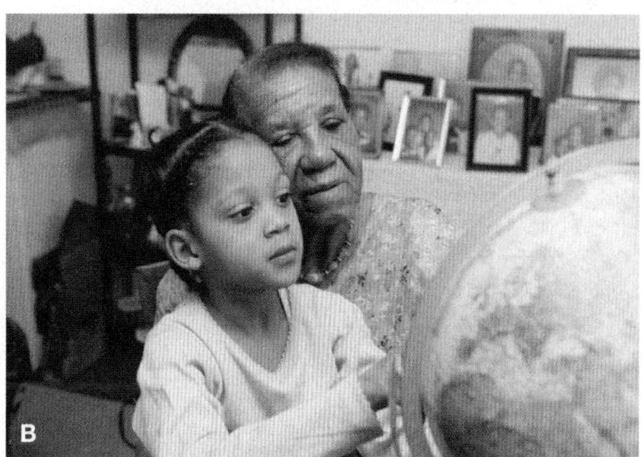

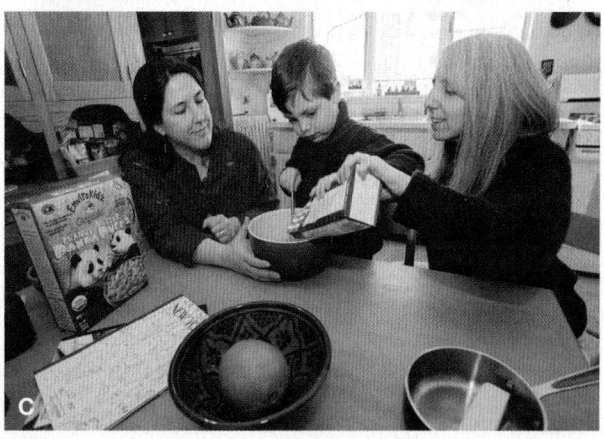

FIGURE 2.4 **A**. Nurses must recognize family dynamics when providing health care. There are many different family structures that influence the patient's needs. The traditional nuclear family is composed of two parents and their biologic or adopted children. **B**. The extended family includes the nuclear family plus other family members, such as grandparents, aunts, uncles, and cousins. **C**. In gay and lesbian families, people of the same sex or gender share a committed relationship with or without children.

The family greatly influences the development and health of its members. For example, children learn health care activities, health beliefs, and health values from their family. The family's structure, the roles assumed by family members, and social changes that affect the family's life can influence the parent's and child's health status. Families are unique; each one has different views and requires distinct methods for support.

Various theories and models have been generated to explain the concept of family. They have influenced the definition of family, the understanding of the structure and function of the family, and the way family coping and adaptation are assessed. Table 2.3 summarizes some of the major theories related to family.

Family Structure

Family structure is the composition of people who interact with one another on a regular, recurring basis in socially sanctioned ways. It describes how the family unit is organized, which often influences the relationships among the members of the family. Family members

TABLE 2.3 • Summary of Major Theories Related to Family

Theory	Description	Key Components
Friedman's structural functional theory (1998)	Emphasizes the social system of family, such as the organization or structure of the family and how the structure relates to the function	Identified five functions of families: 1. Affective function: meeting the love and belonging needs of each member 2. Socialization and social placement function: teaching children how to function and assume adult roles in society 3. Reproductive role: continuing the family and society in general 4. Economic function: ensuring the family has necessary resources with appropriate allocation 5. Health care function: involving the provision of physical care to keep family healthy
Duvall's developmental theory (1977)	Emphasizes the developmental stages that all families go through, beginning with marriage; the longitudinal career of the family is also known as the family life cycle	Described eight chronologic stages with specific predictable tasks that each family completes: 1. Marriage: beginning of family 2. Childbearing stage 3. Family with preschool children 4. Family with school-aged children 5. Family with adolescents 6. Family with young adults 7. Middle-aged parents 8. Family in later years
Von Bertalanffy: general system theory applied to families (1968)	Emphasizes the family as a system with interdependent, interacting parts that endure over time to ensure the survival, continuity, and growth of its components; the family is not the sum of its parts but is characterized by wholeness and unity	Used to define how families interact with and are influenced by family and society and how to analyze the interrelationships of the members and the impact that change affecting one member will have on other members
Family stress theory	Addresses the way families respond to stress and how the family copes with the stress as a group as well as how each individual member copes	Described stress as elements occurring internally within the family (e.g., values, beliefs, structure) that the family can control or change or externally from outside the family (e.g., culture of the surrounding community, genetics, the family's current time or place) over which the family has no control Described mobilization of family resources resulting in either a positive response of constructive coping or a negative response of a crisis Identified the main determinant of adequate coping based on the meaning of the stressful event to the family and its individual members
Resiliency model of family stress and family adjustment, and adaptation response model	Addresses the way families adapt to stress and can rebound from adversity	Identified the elements of risks and protective factors that aid a family in achieving positive outcomes

Adapted from Friedman, M. M. (1998). *Family nursing: Theory and practice* (4th ed.). Appleton & Lange; Duvall, E. (1977). *Marriage and family development* (5th ed.). J. B. Lippincott; Von Bertalanffy, L. (1968). *General systems theory.* Penguin Press; Boss, P. (2001). *Family stress management: A contextual approach* (2nd ed.). Sage Publications, Inc.; and Patterson, J. (2002). Integrating family resilience and family stress theory. *Journal of Marriage and Family, 64*(2), 349–360. https://doi.org/10.1111/j.1741-3737.2002.00349.x

can be gained or lost through events, such as divorce, marriage, birth, adoption, death, abandonment, and incarceration. All of these events alter the family structure, and roles are then redefined or redistributed.

The traditional nuclear family is no longer considered the dominant family structure in the United States. From 1960 to 2022, the percentage of children who were living with two parents decreased from 88% to 65% (FIFCFS, 2023; U.S. Census Bureau, 2016). Table 2.4 lists some of the family structures the nurse may encounter. Nurses working with children need to understand the child's family structure and any changes that are occurring within it so they can help the family maintain or achieve optimal health and well-being.

Families face complex challenges in nurturing, developing, and socializing their members. Family structure changes such as divorce, blending families, adoption, or foster care can have wide-ranging and lifelong effects. Some situations may require astute assessment and

TABLE 2.4 • Types of Family Structures

Structure	Description	Specific Issues
Nuclear family	Two parents living in the same household with their children	May include biologic or adopted children Once considered the traditional family structure; now decreased due to trends in divorce rates or increases in alternative structures
Binuclear family	Structure in which a child is a member of two nuclear families due to joint custody; parenting is considered a joint venture	Always better for the child when their interests are put above the parents' needs and desires
Single-parent family	One parent responsible for care of children	May encounter several challenges because of economic, social, and personal restraints; one person as household manager, caregiver, and financial provider
Commuter family	Adults in the family living and working apart for professional or financial reasons, often leaving the daily care of children to one parent	Similar to single-parent family
Blended family	Adults with children from previous marriages and/or from the new marriage	May lead to family conflict due to different expectations for the child and adults; may have different views and practices related to child care and health
Extended family	May include grandparents, cousins, aunts, uncles, and other family members	Need to determine decision maker as well as primary caregiver of the children Extended families may be more involved in the child's life in some cultures than in others
LGBTQ+ family	Family in which some of its members are gay, lesbian, transgender, bisexual, queer, or nonbinary, with or without children	May face prejudice and discrimination
Communal family	Group of people living together to raise children and manage household, unrelated by blood or marriage	May face prejudice and discrimination Need to determine the decision maker and caregiver of children
Foster family	A temporary family for children who are placed away from their parents to ensure their emotional and physical well-being	May include foster family's children and other foster children in the home Foster children more likely to have unmet health needs and chronic health problems because they may have been living in a variety of settings
Grandparents-as-parents families	Grandparents raising their grandchildren if parents are unable to do so	May increase the risk for physical, financial, and emotional stress on older adults May lead to confusion and emotional stress for child if parents are in and out of the child's life
Adolescent families	Young parents still mastering the developmental tasks of their own childhoods	Greater risk for health problems during pregnancy and for delivery of premature infants, leading to risk of subsequent health and developmental problems Probably still need support from their families related to financial, emotional, and school issues

proactive intervention to minimize the risk to the child and family.

DIVORCED FAMILY

Divorce is a common reason why family structure changes. Today, just under 40% of marriages end in divorce, and many of the affected families include children (Fortin & Downes, 2023). Divorce can have a great impact on the child, sometimes with chronic and devastating results. Changes may have been occurring in the family for years, and children may have been exposed to turmoil, violence, or changes in structure before the actual divorce. Children may feel scared and confused by the threat divorce poses to their security. The initial response of children to divorce depends on their age as well as their developmental level, their temperament, and the circumstances surrounding the divorce. Problems for children are often most apparent in the first couple of years immediately following the divorce. Children may feel anger, anxiety, guilt, and depression, and they may exhibit nonadherence; however, most children show effective adjustment a few years after divorce (Fortin & Downes, 2023). Children in divorced families may experience long-term distress and are two to three times more likely to require psychological help than children whose parents remained married (Fortin & Downes, 2023).

Parents need to understand the impact divorce can have on their children so they can place the children's interest in the forefront. By appropriately supporting the child and utilizing the strengths of the child and family, parents can help their children constructively adjust to divorce. Parents can use the suggestions in Box 2.5 to help reduce tension and conflict, thereby minimizing the impact of separation and divorce on their children. Health care providers can offer support, guidance, and resources to help make the strain of divorce easier on the entire family.

BOX 2.5 Recommendations for Divorcing Parents

1. Tell your children about the divorce and the reasons for the divorce in terms they can understand. Be sure you and your spouse are both present when telling the children; tell all the children at the same time.
2. Reassure your children that the divorce is not their fault. Repeat this as often as possible and as necessary.
3. Inform the children well in advance of anyone moving out of the house (except when abuse is present or there are concerns for immediate safety).
4. Clearly inform the children about the family structure after the divorce, such as who will live with whom and where; also discuss visitation clearly and honestly.
5. Do not expect your children to be or act like adults. Seek support from other adults in your life.
6. Do not discuss money or finances with your children.
7. Minimize unpredictable schedules and maintain routines, rules, and discipline. Be consistent in this area.
8. Never force or allow your children to take sides.
9. Avoid belittling your former spouse when the children can hear. However, do not lie to cover up for irresponsible behavior by the other parent.
10. Never put your children in the middle between you and your ex-spouse.
11. Keep each parent involved in the child's life. Write letters, emails, phone calls, and text messages to continue communication. This shows the child they remain important to you even when they are with the other parent.
12. Communicate directly with the other parent. Avoid making the child your messenger.
13. Allow and assist the child to express their feelings about the divorce and offer support.

Adapted from Kemp, G., Smith, M., & Segal, J. (2022). *Children and divorce.* https://www.helpguide.org/articles/parenting-family/children-and-divorce.htm; Fortin, K., & Downes, A. H. (2023). Section 5: Psychosocial issues. In K. J. Marcdante, R. M. Kleigman, & A. M. Schuh (Eds.), *Nelson essentials of pediatrics* (9th ed., pp. 79–100). Elsevier.

SINGLE-PARENT FAMILIES

Single-parent families result from a variety of situations: divorce or separation, death of a partner, an unmarried person raising their own child, adoption, and so on. Approximately 27% of children younger than age 18 live with one parent, with 22% living with the female parent only and 5% living with the male parent only (FIFCFS, 2023).

The nurse should be aware of multiple factors that can affect the health of children in a single-parent family. Life in a single-parent household may include unique stressors for both the adult and the children. The single parent may feel overwhelmed if they have no one to share the day-to-day responsibilities of care of the children, maintaining a job, and keeping up with the home and finances. These issues may be compounded by other pressures, such as custody problems, limited time to spend with children, continuing conflicts between parents who are separated or divorced, or changes in relationships with extended family members.

Communication and support are essential to the optimal functioning of the single-parent family. The parent and children need to be able to express their feelings and work through any problems together. Single parents must often individually provide greater support for their children than a parent in a household with more than one adult does. Even though single parents may feel alone, they need to ensure they treat their children as children and not a substitute for a partner; they must receive support and comfort from sources who aren't their children. Community resources can be helpful. "Parents Without Partners," for instance, is an international organization that has more than 200 chapters in the United States and Canada.

BLENDED FAMILIES

Though it is increasingly common, creating a blended family (parents and stepchildren) can be stressful for the parents and children alike. Although it can create new structure and stability and reduce the financial stress of single parenthood, making the transition to a blended family takes time. Children may feel jealous of a stepparent or worry they are being disloyal to the parent who is not in this new relationship. There may be competition or rivalry among stepchildren. The child may fear that a stepparent is interfering with the child's relationship with their parent or taking away the child's source of love, affection, and attention.

Mutual respect and open, honest communication among all people involved are essential, and this should include the parent(s) outside the new parent–stepparent relationship when possible. Responsibilities for parenting, including decisions about expectations, limits, and discipline, must be shared. The continued role of the child's parents and stepparents in the child's life are important to address.

ADOPTED FAMILIES

Adoption is the process of a nonbiologic parent or parents creating a legal relationship with a child. Adoption can occur domestically (through an agency or intermediary such as an attorney in the family's own area or country), or the family may choose to adopt a child from another country. The child may be of a different culture, race, or ethnicity than the parents (Fig. 2.5). Most children in need of adoption in the United States and overseas are not infants (Schulte, 2023). Recent trends in adoption include an increase in transcultural adoptions, adoptions by same-sex parents, and single-parent adoptions along with increases in adoption of children with disabilities and increased openness in the adoption process (Schulte, 2023).

The amount of contact between the child and the birthing parent can vary greatly. In a closed adoption, there is no contact among the adoptive parents, the adopted child, and the birthing parent. In an open adoption, there is as much contact among the people as desired. Regardless of whether the adoption is closed or open, families with adopted children may be faced with unique issues. The children may have been exposed to poverty, neglect, infectious diseases, and lack of adequate food, clothing, shelter, and nurturing. These factors contribute to higher risk for medical problems, physical growth and development delays or abnormalities, and behavioral, cognitive, and emotional problems. The adoptive parents may know about these problems, but in other situations, little if any history may be available.

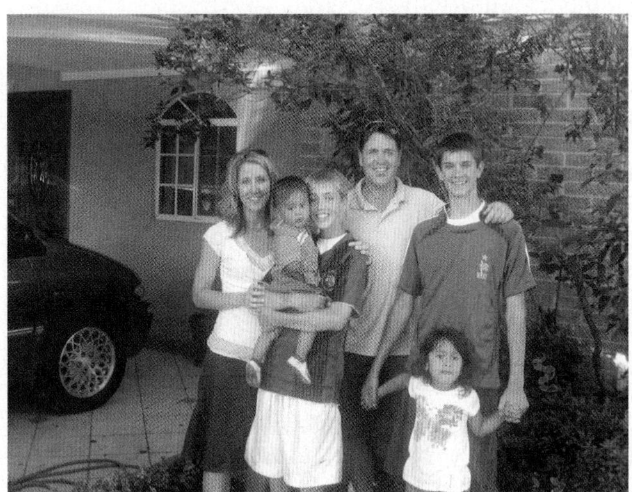

FIGURE 2.5 An adoptive family with children from a culture different from the parents'.

Differences in culture, ethnicity, or race can influence the adopted child's sense of identity (Jones et al., 2012, reaffirmed 2017). Children from underrepresented groups may be subjected to racism or bigotry. Extended family members may not accept the child as part of the family. Parents need to emphasize that the adopted child is their child and is as much a part of the family as any other member. Parents need to openly recognize differences that exist between them and their child. They should encourage and assist the child in learning about the child's racial–ethnic history and heritage and their ethnic origin culture as part of their socialization process (Jones et al., 2012, reaffirmed 2017). People who were adopted may feel a need to identify their biologic parents. People adopted from other countries may travel to the country of their birth, and people adopted domestically may search for biologic relatives. Although these actions are indicative of healthy emotional growth, it may upset the adoptive parents, who may feel rejected.

> ***TAKE NOTE!***
>
> People who are adopted as adolescents typically experience unique challenges adjusting to adoption because of the added complexity of identity issues people in this age group typically experience (Jones et al., 2012, reaffirmed 2017).

Clear, open, honest communication and discussion are essential to promoting a healthy, strong relationship. Support, guidance, and open communication are key for all parties involved. Open acknowledgment of the adoptive relationship helps to nurture trust, security, and a child's self-esteem as they learn to understand what it means to be part of a family through adoption (Jones et al., 2012, reaffirmed 2017).

The pediatric nurse needs to be sensitive, understanding, and supportive when interacting with adopted children and their families. When discussing the topic of adoption, the nurse should use positive language. This includes saying "birth parent" when referring to a biologic parent instead of "natural parent" or "real parent" and using the term "parent" when talking about an adoptive parent (Jones et al., 2012, reaffirmed 2017). Also, it is inappropriate to refer to the child as the "adopted child" and to other children in the family as "natural children" (Jones et al., 2012, reaffirmed 2017). When discussing adoption, the nurse should use phrases such as "make an adoption plan" instead of "give away" or "give up for adoption" (Schulte, 2023). The nurse also needs to provide reassurance and understanding regarding missing health information and provide appropriate resources and referrals to resources that are knowledgeable about adoption and sensitive to the issues that may arise.

FOSTER CARE FAMILIES

In foster care, a child is cared for in an alternative living situation apart from their parents or legal guardians. The child may be placed in this living situation because of difficulties related to their original living situation, such as abuse, neglect, abandonment, or the parents' inability to meet the child's needs due to illness, substance use disorder, or death. The child may be sent to live with relatives (kinship care) or foster parents, who are nonrelatives who provide protection and shelter in a state-approved foster home.

As of 2020, there were about 407,493 children in the United States living in some form of foster care (U.S. Department of Health and Human Services et al., 2021). There has been a decline in the number of children in foster care over the past several years, and about 45% of children in foster care live in nonrelative homes (U.S. Department of Health and Human Services et al., 2021). In 2020, 48% of children who left foster care were reunified with their parents, 6% went to live with other relatives, and 25% were adopted (U.S. Department of Health and Human Services et al., 2021). The goal of foster care is to temporarily protect the child's safety and health until the child can return home to their family or be adopted. Children may remain in foster care for several years or longer and may be moved from one foster family to another.

Many children who are placed in foster care have been the victims of abuse or neglect. Children in foster care are more likely to exhibit a wide range of medical, emotional, behavioral, educational, or developmental problems (Fortin & Downes, 2023). They may experience one or more of the following:

- Unmet health care needs
- Significant mental health problems, such as depression, social problems, anxiety, and posttraumatic stress disorder due to trauma, loss, and unpredictability
- Behavioral problems such as substance use disorder, legal problems, and self-destructive behaviors
- Interruptions in developmental stages and developmental delays
- Educational difficulties due to frequent moves and gaps in education
- Self-blame and feelings of guilt
- Feelings of being unwanted
- Feelings of helplessness and powerlessness
- Insecurity about the future
- Ambivalent feelings related to foster parents and/or feelings of being disloyal to birth parents (Fortin & Downes, 2023)

Individual attention to the child in foster care is essential. A multidisciplinary approach to care that includes the birth parents (when possible), the foster parents, the child, health care professionals, and support services is important to meet the child's needs for growth and development. Nurses play a key role in advocating for the child.

Family Roles and Functions

Regardless of the structure of the family, the role of the family in caring for the child includes not only providing physical and emotional care but also imparting the rules and expected behaviors of society through teaching and discipline techniques. The expected behaviors depend on the family's culture, values, and beliefs and the child's developmental stage and physical and cognitive abilities. Roles and functions are further defined by each family's own traditions and values and the family's standards for interaction within and outside the family. For instance, some families may value privacy more than others.

CAREGIVER–CHILD INTERACTION

The caregiver–child interaction is critical to the young child's survival and healthy development (WHO, 2012). Responsive caregiving is essential for positive socioemotional development in children. Most often, the primary caregivers are the parents. Ideally, parents nurture their children and provide them with an environment in which they can become competent, productive, self-directed members of society. For young children in particular, growth, health, and their personhood itself depend on the ability of the adults in their life to understand and respond to them.

Parental Roles

Parenting is an enormous responsibility and takes a lot of time as well as physical and mental energy. Parental roles are vast and numerous. Typical parental roles include nurturer/caregiver, financial provider, decision maker, schedule manager, financial manager, problem solver, counselor, teacher, behavior support and manager, and health manager.

CHANGES IN PARENTAL ROLES OVER TIME

Parental roles evolve due to societal and economic changes as well as individual family changes. In the past in the United States, the role of provider was most often assigned to the father. Today, however, with many more women in the workforce and more households with two parents working, both parents are often the providers as well as the nurturers to the children. Technologic innovations have provided parents with opportunities to work at home, allowing some parents to simultaneously fulfill the provider role and the nurturer and health manager roles. Fathers are taking on greater responsibilities related to household management and child care. Additionally, a significant number of children are being raised by their grandparents (Joshi & Lebrun-Harris, 2022). Moreover, as Baby Boomers age, Generation X and Millennial parents may find themselves caring for both their children and their own parents.

Being a parent is a highly challenging job. However, there is no definitive manual that teaches people how to be successful at it. Nurses must encourage involvement of both parents in two-parent families by inviting them both to the maternity suite, learning their names, directing questions at them, and listening to their answers. By ensuring parents feel involved and important from the first signs of pregnancy, during childbirth, and afterward, the building blocks of family well-being can be laid and will contribute to improved cognitive and socioemotional development of their children.

PARENTING STYLES

Following on the psychologist Diana Baumrind's work in the 1960s, in the 1980s, Eleanor Maccoby and John Martin conducted further research that led to the conceptualization of four major parenting styles common in U.S. society: authoritarian, authoritative, permissive, and uninvolved, rejecting, or neglecting (Baumrind, 1966; Cherry, 2022). The styles are defined by the amount of support and control the parents exert over the child. Many parents use more than one parenting style and are characterized somewhere in between styles instead of adhering strictly to just one. Also, some parents may change parenting styles as the child ages and matures. Nurses need to recognize different parenting styles and provide support to parents by discussing the effects of different parenting models and teaching parenting skills.

Authoritarian

The authoritarian parent expects obedience from the child and discourages the child from questioning the family's rules. The parent provides low support and high control over the child. The rules and standards set forth by the parents are strictly enforced and firm. The parents expect the child to accept the family's beliefs and values and demand respect for these beliefs. The parents are the ultimate authority and allow little, if any, participation by the child in making decisions. Behavior that does not adhere to the family's rules and standards is punished. This parenting style is associated with children who are obedient and proficient but who may also experience negative effects on self-esteem, happiness, and social skills as well as increased aggression and defiance (Cherry, 2022).

Authoritative

The authoritative or democratic parent shows some respect for the child's opinions. Although parents still have the ultimate authority and expect the child to adhere to the rules, authoritative parents allow children to be different and believe that each child is a unique individual. They exhibit warmth, and they consistently, fairly, and firmly enforce the family's rules and standards without emphasizing punishment. This type of parenting is associated with increased independence, happiness, and self-confidence that helps children become socially responsible adults (Cherry, 2022).

Permissive

Permissive or laissez-faire parents have little control over their children's behavior. Rules or standards may be inconsistent, unclear, or nonexistent. Permissive parents allow their children to determine their own standards and rules for behavior. Discipline can be lax, inconsistent, or absent. Parents can be warm, cool, or uninvolved. There are more negative than positive effects associated with this style of parenting. Negative effects include impulsivity, low happiness, poor school performance, problems with authority, and lack of responsibility and independence (Cherry, 2022).

Uninvolved, Rejecting, or Neglecting

Uninvolved parents are indifferent. They do not provide rules or standards. The child's basic needs are often met, but the parents are disconnected from the child's life. In some cases, the parents may neglect or reject the child. They can be cold and uninterested in meeting the child's needs. They minimize their interactions and time with the children. This type of parenting is associated with negative effects, such as disinterest in school, disinterest in the future, and limited emotional and self-control (Cherry, 2022). This type of parenting may also lead to issues with trust, low self-esteem, and less competency than the child's peers (Cherry, 2022).

Discipline

Much of parenting involves increasing desirable behavior and decreasing or eliminating undesirable behavior through a process generally known as **discipline**. There are various opinions in U.S. society about the best or most effective methods of discipline. Each child and family are unique. Discipline that works with one child or within one family may not work for another family. Discipline should focus on the development of the child and should preserve their self-esteem and dignity. It should be based on age-appropriate expectations with clear, consistent guidelines and should offer meaningful choices when possible. Discipline involves teaching and is ongoing, not something that is done only when the child misbehaves.

The AAP focuses on the importance of teaching good behavior rather than punishing bad behavior and on teaching the child to manage or regulate their behavior (Sege et al., 2018). Effective discipline relies on understanding a child's normal growth and development. Nurses can assist families by educating them on their child's development and on effective discipline techniques. Teaching Guidelines 2.1 provides some tips to help a child learn acceptable behavior as they grow.

POSITIVE REINFORCEMENT

Attention from parents is a powerful form of positive reinforcement and can help increase desirable behaviors. The key is to focus on the child's appropriate behaviors rather than emphasize the inappropriate ones. Immediate, consistent, and frequent feedback is crucial. This feedback can be in the form of smiles, praise, special attention, or rewards, such as extra privileges or a special token or activity. Providing the feedback immediately is important so that the child learns to associate the feedback with the appropriate behavior; this reinforces the behavior.

EXTINCTION

Another form of discipline is extinction, which focuses on reducing or eliminating the positive reinforcement for inappropriate behavior. Examples include ignoring a toddler's temper tantrums, withholding or removing privileges, and requiring a "time-out." Withholding or removing privileges such as the use of a TV, music device, computer, or phone is most effective for older children and adolescents. The adolescent may be grounded for a short time or not allowed to drive the car. To be effective, the privilege being withheld or removed must be something that the child values.

Time-out is an extinction discipline method that is most effective with toddlers, preschoolers, and early school-aged children. It involves removing the child from the problem area and placing them in a neutral, nonthreatening, safe area where no interaction occurs between the child and the parents or others for a specifically determined period of time (Fig. 2.6).

TEACHING GUIDELINES 2.1 Teaching to Promote Effective Discipline

- Set clear, consistent, and developmentally appropriate expected behaviors; offer choices whenever possible.
- Maintain consistency in responding to behaviors; provide encouragement and affection.
- Role-model appropriate behaviors.
- Provide an age-appropriate explanation of the consequence if the child demonstrates unacceptable behavior.
- Always administer the consequence soon after the unacceptable behavior.
- Keep the consequence appropriate to the age of the child and the situation.
- Stay calm but firm without showing anger when administering the consequence.
- Always praise the child for displaying appropriate behavior (positive reinforcement).
- Set up the environment to assist the child in accomplishing the appropriate behavior; remove temptations that may lead to inappropriate behavior.
- Reinforce that the child's behavior was undesirable but the child themselves is not bad.

TAKE NOTE!

The amount of time a child spends in time-out is typically 1 minute per year of age; around the age of 3, the parent may allow the child to dictate the length of time they spend in time-out, such as by saying, "Come back when you feel ready and calm." This allows the child to learn self-management skills (AAP, 2018).

PUNISHMENT

Discipline is often confused with punishment, but punishment involves a negative or unpleasant experience or consequence for doing or not doing something.

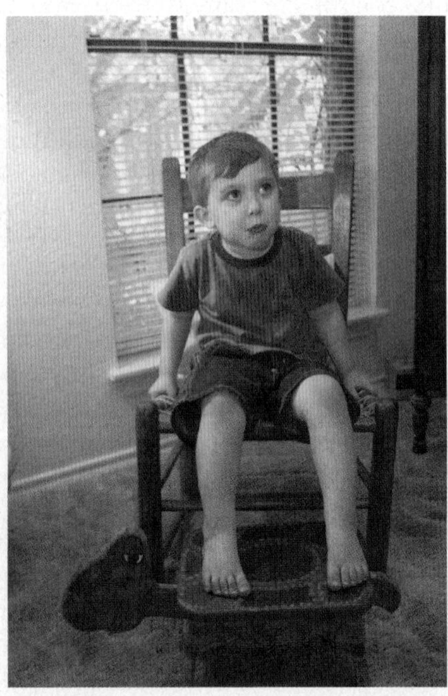

FIGURE 2.6 Although they might not like it, quiet solitude helps the child develop inner control.

Punishment may be verbal or corporal. Verbal punishment commonly takes the form of reprimands or scolding (the use of disapproving statements). The statements are intended to change or eliminate the inappropriate behavior. Verbal reprimands can be effective in the short term if they are used sparingly and are focused on the child's specific behavior. If verbal reprimands are used frequently and indiscriminately, they lose their effectiveness, can provoke anxiety in the child, and encourage the child to ignore the parent.

Corporal punishment involves the use of physical pain as a means to decrease inappropriate behavior. The most common form of corporal punishment is spanking (the use of an open hand to the buttocks or an extremity with the intention of modifying behavior without causing injury) (Sege et al., 2018). Recent research shows that the use of corporal punishment is declining, with only 50% of parents reporting ever spanking their child (Sege et al., 2018).

Initially, spanking may be effective in dissuading a particular behavior because of its sudden and shocking nature. However, over time, it loses its effectiveness because its shock value declines. Spanking may stop the undesirable behavior; however, it increases the risk of physical injury, especially for infants and young children, and may lead to altered caregiver–child relationships (Sege et al., 2018). Because the effects of spanking diminish, the intensity of the spanking must be increased to achieve the same effects. It is important for parents to understand the consequences of its use.

Various studies have linked spanking in childhood with subsequent aggressive behavior in childhood and persistent anger in adulthood (Sege et al., 2018). Because of the negative consequences of spanking and because it has been shown to be no more effective than other methods for managing inappropriate behavior, the AAP recommends parents use methods other than spanking to respond to inappropriate behavior (Sege et al., 2018).

Culture

Culture is the view of the world and implementation of a set of traditions and practices used by a specific social group that passes those traditions to subsequent generations. Culture plays a critical role in shaping a person or family, including their health and health practices. Culture is a complex phenomenon involving the integration of many components such as beliefs, values, language, time, personal space, and view of the world, all of which shape a person's actions and behavior. People learn these patterns of cultural behaviors from their family and community through a process called enculturation, which involves acquiring knowledge and internalizing values.

Culture is learned first in the family, then in school, the community, and other social organizations. Culture influences every aspect of development and is reflected in childbearing and child-rearing beliefs and practices designed to promote adaptation to the social group's expectations. Typically, a child begins to understand their culture at approximately 5 years of age (Andrews, 2020).

Nurses must be able to incorporate cultural knowledge into their interventions so that they can care effectively for culturally diverse adults, children, and families. They must be aware of the wide range of cultural traditions, values, and ethics that exist in the United States. All nurses must establish knowledge about a patient's culture so that health care interventions can be adapted to meet the needs of the patient. The nurse should know about various culture-based health practices and how they may affect children, as well as about the demographics of the local population.

The goal is for the nurse to view culture as a point of congruence rather than a potential source of conflict. The nurse needs to combine cultural respect with cultural humility. This is an ongoing process that includes self-reflection on one's own biases, a continued willingness to learn from others, and a desire to honor each person's personal beliefs, customs, and values. By combining cultural respect and knowledge with cultural humility, the nurse will be able to provide more effective care to children and their families.

The relationship of culture to health care can become obscured by the use of broad group titles. In reality, there are many distinct cultural groups, and within a group, there may be many subcultures. It is crucial that the nurse remembers that diversity exists within cultures, and this is as important as the diversity among different cultures. Every patient is a unique person with their own beliefs, values, and history. The nurse needs to assess each adult, child, and family and ask questions to understand their unique beliefs and values.

Cultural Health Practices

Health practices are often the result of health beliefs derived from a person's culture. For example, does the adult, child, or family view health and illness as the result of natural forces, supernatural forces, or the imbalance of forces? Many cultures have remedies that people may use or consider before they seek professional health care. Families may go to complementary or alternative medicine practitioners who they believe can cure certain illnesses.

If culturally influenced complementary or alternative care practices are compatible with the health regimen and support appropriate health practices, these practices do no harm; in fact, they can be beneficial to the patient and family. However, these practices should not contribute to a delay in beneficial treatment or create other problems.

TAKE NOTE!

Nurses can help to shape a person's lifelong perceptions of health and health services. An understanding of how the adult's, child's, and family's culture affects their health practices gives the nurse an opportunity to incorporate appropriate and beneficial health practices into the family's cultural milieu, providing sources of strength rather than areas of conflict.

Changing Cultural Demographics

Although in the United States, the proportion of children is decreasing in relationship to the adult population, the racial, ethnic, and cultural diversity among children is significantly increasing (FIFCFS, 2021). Thus, the diversity among children entering the health care system in the United States is increasing. In 2022, approximately 49% of the population identified as White non-Hispanic, 26% as Hispanic, 14% as Black non-Hispanic, 6% as Asian, and 6% as non-Hispanic, all other races (FIFCFS, 2023). It is projected that by 2050, 31% of the U.S. population of children will be identified as Hispanic, 39% as White non-Hispanic, 14% as Black non-Hispanic, 7% as Asian, and 9% as non-Hispanic, all other races (FIFCFS, 2023). In addition, the increasing number of relationships between people from different backgrounds is producing an increasing number of children whose heritage represents more than one cultural group.

Immigration

Employment and economic opportunities, expanded human rights, educational opportunities, and other types of freedoms and opportunities encourage many people from other countries to move to the United States. Approximately one in four children in the United States are immigrants or members of an immigrant family (Children's Defense Fund, 2023). This includes both children born outside the United States and those with at least one foreign-born parent. Some communities welcome newcomers, but others do not.

Immigration can affect the health, educational, and social services provided in the United States. Immigration is a factor in access to care and the types of care that need to be offered. There are higher rates of poverty, lack of health insurance coverage, and low educational attainment among families who have immigrated as compared to their nonimmigrant counterparts (Kaiser Family Foundation, 2022). Immigration can impose unique stresses on women, children, and families, including:

- Depression, grief, or anxiety associated with leaving their country of origin and pressure for acculturation
- Separation from family and other support systems
- Language barriers
- Differences in social, professional, and economic status between their country of origin and the United States
- Traumatic events, such as war, that may have occurred in their country of origin (Linton et al., 2019)

The inability to speak English can hinder educational attainment, economic opportunities, and the ability to join the societal mainstream. Fourteen percent of children born in immigrant families have difficulty speaking English, and 16% of children in immigrant families live in a linguistically isolated home (i.e., no person aged 14 years or older speaks English "very well") (Kids Count Data Center, 2022a, 2022b). Parents who do not speak English may have trouble accessing health care and health insurance, enrolling their children in school, becoming involved in school activities, and accessing work or higher paying jobs.

Women and children from other countries may arrive in the United States with significant health problems. They may present with diseases that are more common in their countries of origin and rarely seen in the United States, such as malaria. Their health status may be compromised due to the lack of at-birth and early childhood screenings, which may manifest in problems such as inborn errors of metabolism, lack of preventive care, no immunizations, and no dental care. Due to financial, language, cultural, and other types of barriers that immigrant families sometimes face, children may not receive necessary preventive care or receive care for minor conditions until the condition becomes more serious. Stressors, such as those associated with relocation, separation, and traumatic events, also can have a negative impact on psychological and physical health.

Spirituality and Religion

Spirituality is a belief in something greater than oneself and a faith that affirms life positively. It is a major influence in many people's lives, providing meaning or purpose to life and a foundation for and source of love, relationships, and service. Spirituality is considered a universal human phenomenon with an assumption of the wholeness of people and their connectedness to a higher being. During life-changing events and crises, such as a serious illness or the birth of a child with a congenital defect, families often turn to spirituality for hope, comfort, and relief.

The word "religion" is often used interchangeably with spirituality in U.S. society. However, "spirituality" can describe a more private and individual belief, while "religion" is an organized way of sharing beliefs and practicing worship. Of Americans, 81% report believing in God (Jones, 2022). Therefore, spirituality and religion are an important focus when working with women, children, and their families. A person's reaction to health and illness may be affected by these beliefs. Different religions may present illness as a punishment for sin or wrongdoing, a curse, or a test of strength (Andrews, 2020).

People appreciate the recognition of and respect for their beliefs. Therefore, identifying the individual's and family's religious beliefs and customs is important. People may adhere to special dietary restrictions, rituals such as baptism or Holy Communion, the use of amulets or icons, or practices related to death and dying that can be incorporated into the plan of care. Using open-ended questions and observing for the use of religious articles during assessment can provide clues to a patient's or family's beliefs and practices. Visits from spiritual leaders may also be noted.

TAKE NOTE!

Never make assumptions about a family's religious or spiritual affiliation. Although they may belong to a particular religion, family members may not adhere to all of its beliefs or participate in all aspects of the religion. Be alert for clues that provide insight into their specific beliefs.

Community

Community encompasses a broad range of concepts, from the nation where a person lives, to a particular neighborhood or group. The surrounding community affects many aspects of a person's health and general welfare. The quality of life within a community has a great influence on a person's ability to develop and become a functional member of society. Community influences include the school, which is a community in itself, and peer groups. The support and assistance offered to women, children, and families from other areas of the community, such as school programs and community centers, can improve the person's overall health and well-being.

Schools and Other Community Centers

Children today start school at an earlier age, spend more time in childcare settings, and are involved in various community centers and activities. By age 3 or 4, many children are in a preschool setting for several hours a day. Some children spend more awake time in school and childcare settings than in their family home. Thus, schools and childcare settings have become major influences on children.

School also provides a means of socialization. School rules about attendance and authority relationships and the system of sanctions and rewards based on achievement help to teach children behavioral expectations they will need for future employment and relationships in the adult world. Although the primary role of schools has always been academic education, today, schools are performing more health-related functions. Schools play an important role in promoting healthy behaviors and educating children about proper exercise, nutrition, safety, sex, drugs, and mental health.

Academic success is linked to healthy behaviors. Academic success is a good indicator of childhood well-being and is a predictor of adult health outcomes (CDC, 2022d). Academic failure is linked to higher risk behaviors, such as substance use, eating a diet with low nutritional value, and physical inactivity (CDC, 2022d). School health programs have positive impacts on health outcomes and health risk behaviors along with educational outcomes (CDC, 2022d).

Because many families have two parents who both work, many children are enrolled in childcare and afterschool programs. Thus, the socialization process begins earlier and involves a larger percentage of the child's waking hours (Fig. 2.7).

Afterschool hours are a critical time during which children may participate in higher risk behaviors if they are not provided with supervised, structured activity through which they can learn and grow. Community centers and afterschool programs can provide an opportunity for children to learn new skills, have new experiences, and develop relationships with caring adults in a safe and supportive environment.

Peer Groups

A child's friends can have a major influence on their growth and development. Peer group relationships often begin early and are a large part of the child's world, particularly for school-aged children and adolescents. This influence starts in playgroups in preschool or elementary school. The child is confronted with a variety of values and belief systems from interactions with their friends. To be accepted, the child must conform to the specific values and beliefs of the group. When these values and beliefs differ from those of the adults in the child's world,

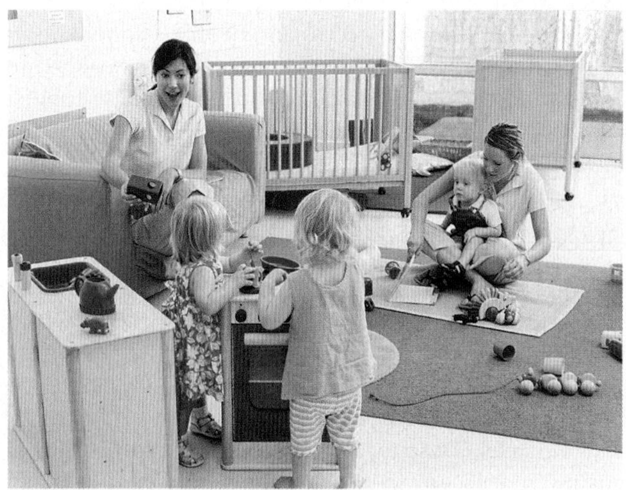

FIGURE 2.7 Day care centers provide socialization and support for young children.

conflicts can occur, possibly distancing children from the adults and strengthening their sense of belonging to the peer group.

When the child's friends are successful in school or other activities, the growth and development of the child continues in a healthy and positive way. When these groups demonstrate healthy behaviors, the influence is positive; however, peer groups can also exert negative influences on the child. Thus, it is vital to identify the important peer groups in a child's life and the positive or negative behaviors exhibited within these groups.

Society

Society has a major impact on the health of women, children, and families. Major societal factors that influence women's and children's health include social roles, social determinants of health, the media, and the expanding global nature of society. Each of these areas may influence a person's self-concept, the community where they live, their choice of lifestyle, and their health. Nurses need to assess these areas and their influence on the woman, child, and family so that individualized strategies can be designed and implemented to enhance the positive effects and minimize the negative effects on the woman's, child's, and family's health.

Social Roles

Societal norms often prescribe specific patterns of behaviors: Certain behaviors are permitted, and others are prohibited. These patterns influence social roles and can be an important factor in the development of self-concept. A person's self-concept can strongly influence their health.

Social Determinants of Health

Social determinants of health are conditions in the environment where people live, work, learn, and play that affect their health, well-being, and quality of life. Examples include education access and quality, economic stability, neighborhood and built environments, health care access and quality, and social and community context (Healthy People 2030 et al., n.d.).

Socioeconomic Status and Economic Stability

An important influence on children is the family's socioeconomic status (relative position in society), which takes into account the family's economic, occupational, and educational levels. Children are raised differently based on their parents' educational levels, occupations, and incomes. Despite advances and improvements in quality and access to health care, disparities in health status among socioeconomic classes have continued (AHRQ, 2021). Income inequality is an important factor in explaining this variation. Parents with lower incomes may need to work longer hours to provide basic necessities and have little time or money to enrich the child's life with outside resources or to promote healthy lifestyle choices. However, families in this situation may have stronger family relationships if they need to rely on the broader family network to meet some of their physical and emotional needs.

Low socioeconomic status can have an adverse influence on children's health. Some families may not be able to afford health insurance or health care. Meals may be unbalanced or irregular. The family's house or apartment may be overcrowded and may have poor sanitation or lead paint. Some families may not understand the importance of preventive care or may not be able to afford it, and as a result, the children may be inadequately immunized against communicable diseases or lack preventive care. Studies have documented that children who come from low socioeconomic backgrounds are more likely to suffer negative physical and mental health outcomes, such as depression, behavioral problems, substance misuse, and injuries (Bitsko et al., 2022). Basic financial stability enhances the general health and well-being of children; thus, an important negative influence on children's health is poverty. Children living in poverty are more likely to have poor health, complete fewer years of school, experience violent crimes, and become adults with lower incomes (FIFCFS, 2023).

The poverty threshold is based on the family's size and income and is used to determine whether a family is living in poverty (Table 2.5). According to the U.S. Census Bureau in 2022, the official poverty rate was 11.5%. (Shrider & Creamer, 2023). Overall, 12.4% of children younger than age 18 were living in poverty (Shrider & Creamer, 2023). According to the Children's Defense Fund (2023), 11.1 million American children live in poverty, with 5.5 million living in extreme poverty. The rate of poverty is closely tied to the overall health of the economy. In times of recession, a rise in the number of

TABLE 2.5 • 2023 U.S. Poverty Guidelines

Size of Family Unit	48 Contiguous States and Washington, D.C.	Alaska	Hawaii
1	$13,580	$18,210	$16,770
2	$19,720	$24,640	$22,680
3	$24,860	$31,070	$28,590
4	$30,000	$37,500	$34,500
5	$35,140	$43,930	$40,410

Data from U.S. Department of Health and Human Services. (2023). *HHS poverty guidelines for 2023.* Retrieved December 17, 2023, from https://aspe.hhs.gov/topics/poverty-economic-mobility/poverty-guidelines

people living below the federal poverty threshold usually occurs.

Family structure is an important factor associated with poverty rates for children. The poverty rate for married-couple families is lower than that for families headed by a single parent. Of the families living below the poverty level, 24.7% were female householder families with no spouse present, 11.6% were male householder families with no spouse present, and 5.4% were headed by married couples (Shrider & Creamer, 2023). Educational level is another important factor: As education increases, unemployment declines and annual income rises. However, a chronic physical or emotional problem in any wage earner may lead to unemployment, and this can cause the family to experience an economic decline.

The effects of poverty on children's health can be wide ranging. The family may be able to afford only inadequate housing or a house or an apartment in a neighborhood with unsanitary conditions, toxins, or violence. These families may also experience homelessness.

Neighborhoods, Built Environments, and Homelessness

The neighborhood and environment where a child lives, plays, and learns is an important determinant of their health. Refer to the content discussed under the "Community" section earlier in the chapter. Housing is a critical social determinant of health in children. During the 2020 to 2021 school year, approximately 1.1 million children who were enrolled in school did not have housing. In other words, one in 45 children enrolled in public school were without a home (Children's Defense Fund, 2023). It is impossible to measure homelessness with 100% accuracy. Therefore, looking at trends is important to demonstrate whether progress is being made. Recent data suggest that homelessness among families is increasing (Children's Defense Fund, 2023).

Homelessness occurs across geographic regions. The principal causes of homelessness are poverty and lack of affordable housing. Other causes include cutbacks in public welfare programs; mental health issues; traumatic events, such as unemployment, illness, or accidents; and personal crises, such as divorce, domestic violence, and substance use disorder. Children may be forced out of their houses or choose to run away because they have been abused or neglected, lived in foster homes, or were placed in residential treatment or juvenile detention centers.

The basic need for stable shelter goes unmet for children experiencing homelessness. This is not conducive to appropriate growth and development in children. These children are more likely to have behavioral and emotional problems, be diagnosed with a mental illness, be victims of physical and sexual abuse, and suffer educational disabilities. They also have a higher incidence of acute and chronic health problems such as increased rates of asthma; ear infections; gastrointestinal disorders, such as diarrhea; speech problems; mental health problems such as anxiety, depression, and withdrawal; violence and victimization; substance use disorder, pregnancy; and sexually transmitted diseases. They may be exposed to environmental hazards in homeless shelters or overcrowded housing, or they may experience exposure to the elements, lack of sanitary facilities, and an increased risk of injuries. An unbalanced diet may place children without homes at risk for nutritional deficits, which can lead to delayed growth and development. Adolescents without homes often engage in high-risk behaviors such as drug use or unprotected sex with multiple partners, so they are more likely to need emergency care, experience depression, contract sexually transmitted diseases, or become pregnant (AAP, 2013, reaffirmed 2022).

Children experiencing homelessness may have limited access to health care services, especially preventive care such as immunizations, dental care, and well-child services. Lack of immunizations can lead to delayed enrollment in school, and education is vital to help break the cycle of homelessness. Families may need to use their money for food and shelter instead of health care. If they do seek health care, they may need to use an emergency department or a free clinic rather than a consistent family care provider. They may access care sporadically, which is not conducive to the ongoing health needs of a growing child. The family may not be able to follow up with care because they cannot afford it, lack health insurance, or do not have transportation to the clinic or pharmacy.

Some children experiencing homelessness do not go to school or go to various schools because the family moves from place to place. The stress the family experiences creates an environment that is not conducive to learning. As a result, children may present with learning problems, socialization issues, or other behavioral issues.

Media

Children are inundated with various forms of media via television, mobile phones and tablets, video and computer games, social media, the internet, movies, magazines, books, and newspapers (Fig. 2.8). Media has become a major factor in children's lives, with TV remaining the dominant medium (AAP & Council on Communications and Media, 2016b, reaffirmed 2022b). Media can have both positive and negative effects on the development of children; those effects largely depend on the content to which they are exposed (AAP & Council on Communications and Media, 2016b, reaffirmed 2022b; Chassiakos et al., 2016). Positive effects include exposure to early learning, new knowledge and information

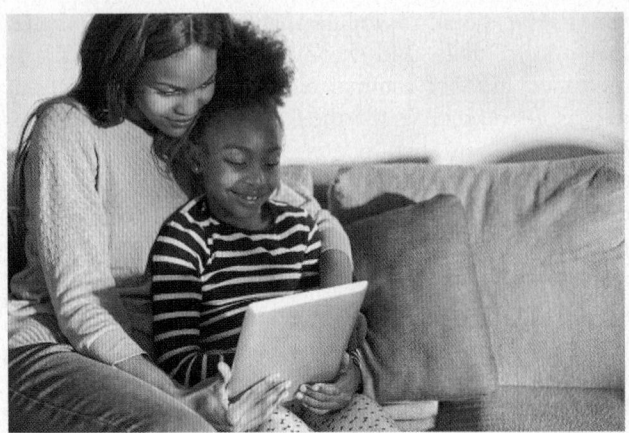

FIGURE 2.8 Computer games can be fun and educational, but the child should be monitored while using the computer and other forms of media to minimize negative effects.

including health promotion messages, increased awareness of current events and issues, and increased social contact and support (AAP & Council on Communications and Media, 2016b, reaffirmed 2022b; Chassiakos et al., 2016). The media can be a positive influence, such as when it offers educational programming or public service messages on the negative effects of substance use and misuse, smoking, or gang involvement. Public broadcasting networks often offer valuable programming. However, media can have adverse health effects on sleep, attention, learning, activity, and mental health (AAP & Council on Communications and Media, 2016b, reaffirmed 2022b; Chassiakos et al., 2016). The media's influence stem not only from content but also from total viewing time. For example, excessive TV viewing has been linked to obesity, poor cognitive skills, and irregular sleep patterns. Overuse of computer or video games may lead to poor school performance.

Increased support and connection from social media used in moderation has been found to be beneficial to a child's mental health (AAP & Council on Communications and Media, 2016b, reaffirmed 2022b). Increased risk of depression has been found with both high and low social media usage (AAP & Council on Communications and Media, 2016b, reaffirmed 2022b). The images and information found in social media are not always in the best interests of children. Children may identify with and mimic people or characters who engage in risk-taking behaviors or lifestyles.

Evidence is clear that media exposure can contribute to many risks and health problems, such as excessive caloric intake, physical inactivity, smoking, early initiation of sexual behaviors, and underage drinking (AAP & Council on Communications and Media, 2016b, reaffirmed 2022b; Chassiakos et al., 2016). Research has established a strong link between media violence and violent, aggressive behavior (Chassiakos et al., 2016). If an image or type of behavior is portrayed as the norm, children may view this as acceptable behavior without examining the potential health risks or other long-term consequences. For example, when thinness is overvalued in the media, this can contribute to some children developing unhealthy dieting or other behaviors to develop that body type. For the child who has a body type that does not match the ones they see valued in media, depression or self-esteem issues may develop.

Overall, the images and messages children view every day will affect their behavior and, possibly, their health, and pediatric nurses should take this into account when working with children and their families.

A media history is helpful and important information to obtain. The nurse is encouraged to ask questions regarding media use, such as the amount of recreational screen time a child engages in and if the child has a television or internet-connected device in their bedroom (Chassiakos et al., 2016). The AAP recommends families develop a family media plan. This allows a family to develop and individualize family rules and guidelines surrounding media use. The AAP Family Media Use Plan can be accessed at www.healthychildren.org/MediaUsePlan (AAP & Council on Communications and Media, 2016b, reaffirmed 2022b; Chassiakos et al., 2016). It is important for parents to set limits and to know what their children are viewing, regardless of the device.

TAKE NOTE!

The AAP discourages the use of media, with the exception of video chatting, in children younger than 18 months. In children aged 18 to 24 months, media should be limited to educational programming with adult interaction during the media viewing and no more than 1 hour a day of media for children aged 2 to 5 years. For children older than 5 years of age, the recommendation includes 2 hours or less of sedentary screen time daily and no screens during meals or 1 hour before bed (AAP & Council on Communications and Media, 2016a, reaffirmed 2022a; 2016b, reaffirmed 2022b; Chassiakos et al., 2016).

Widespread access to the internet has fostered a connection to other areas of the world that would not have been possible in previous years. Children are no longer limited to their immediate surroundings, and they have access to a wealth of information. The internet can be a valuable resource for parents and children to access information, learn new things, and communicate with friends and family. However, the child's health and safety can be threatened online by sexual predators, pornography, violence, and bigotry. Parents need to be alert to these hazards and set up safety guidelines (Teaching Guidelines 2.2).

TEACHING GUIDELINES 2.2 Teaching to Promote Safe Internet Use

- Develop a family media use plan.
- Determine a time limit for your child's daily or weekly digital media use, and maintain consistency in enforcing this time limit.
- Ensure that the use of the internet does not replace or interfere with homework, sleep, physical activity, friends, or household or school activities.
- Tell your child *never* to share personal information with anyone online unless you know the person and the child has your permission to do so.
- Urge your child *never* to share their password with anyone, even friends.
- Review internet sites with your child, and explain which sites are appropriate. Use the safety and parental controls offered by your internet service provider.
- Avoid placing the computer or having digital media in the child's room. Instead, place the computer and encourage digital media use in a public area of your home, such as the den or kitchen, so that you can monitor your child's use.
- Discuss with your child the need for safety while using the internet. Explain potential hazards in terms the child can understand.
- Advise your child to immediately close any sites or stop any communications that make them confused or uncomfortable. Tell your child *never* to arrange any face-to-face meetings with people they meet online. Urge your child to tell you if someone suggests such a meeting.
- Teach the child *never* to open email from any unknown senders.
- Be aware of digital media use policies in your child's school.

Global Society

The world is connected in many ways. Many people are able to travel from one nation to another easily, new products are distributed globally every day, people immigrate to new countries at increasing levels, and the internet makes worldwide communication simple. The United Nations Children's Fund (UNICEF, 2022) and the WHO lead the world in addressing global children's issues. Every year, about 5.2 million children younger than 5 years of age and 500,000 children aged 5 to 9 years die around the world (WHO, 2020). Thousands of children born in resource-limited countries are moving to resource-abundant countries such as the United States as refugees, immigrants, or international adoptees. These children become part of this nation.

Nurses need to be aware of the impact of worldwide events, such as natural and human-made disasters, on children. Families can be displaced by events such as hurricanes or wars, placing them at increased risk for problems, such as infectious diseases, malnutrition, and psychological trauma.

Young children bear the brunt of the global burden of disease, but progress has been made in reducing mortality in children younger than 5 years (WHO, 2020). The UNICEF and the WHO have identified major problems affecting child growth and development and survival:

- Preterm birth complications and birth asphyxia
- Acute respiratory infections, such as pneumonia
- Malnutrition, including micronutrient deficiency
- Diarrhea related to lack of clean water and sanitation
- Vaccine-preventable diseases such as measles
- Malaria
- Poor health care of pregnant and nursing people (WHO, 2020)

UNICEF and the WHO work to eradicate these conditions to improve the health of children around the world.

Society as a whole and families have concerns over world threats to safety. Disasters such as terrorist attacks, mass shootings, and extreme weather events can have a significant impact on the well-being of women and children. These stressors put women, children, and families at risk for experiencing mental health difficulties. Children who have experienced traumatic events are at risk for issues, such as posttraumatic stress disorder, behavioral problems, depression, anxiety, sleep disturbances, restlessness, irritability, aggression, abnormal eating patterns, physiologic responses such as gastrointestinal symptoms, decline in academic performance, social isolation, and safety and security concerns (Fortin & Downes, 2023; UNICEF, 2022). Children's coping abilities may be reduced, and they may experience alterations in growth and development. Children's reactions depend on age and developmental level and are highly influenced by the emotional state of their caregivers. Nurses must be aware of the effects of world threats on women, children, and families so that they can assess for alterations and intervene to promote security and stability.

Violence

Per the chief of the United Nations, the longest, deadliest pandemic in the world may be violence against women and girls (United Nations, 2022). A partner or family member kills a woman, often in her own home, every 11 minutes (United Nations, 2022). Millions of women and girls worldwide suffer some form of gender-based violence, be it domestic violence, female genital mutilation/cutting, dowry-related killing, human trafficking, sexual violence, and other manifestations of abuse. The United Nations defines *violence* against women as "any act of gender-based violence that results in physical, sexual, or mental harm or suffering to women, including threats of such acts, coercion, or arbitrary deprivation of liberty" (WHO, 2024). Violence can occur in any setting and can involve anyone. One in three women in the world report having experienced physical and/or sexual violence at some point in their lifetime (WHO, 2024). Violence affects people of all ages, ethnicities, races, educational levels, and socioeconomic levels. Pregnancy is often a time when physical abuse starts or escalates, resulting in poorer outcomes for the birthing parent and the baby.

Nurses are typically the first health care providers whom victims of violence encounter when they are injured. Nurses serve their patients best not by trying to rescue them, but by helping them build on their strengths and providing support, thereby empowering the patients to help themselves. All nurses need to include a screening tool like "RADAR" (Box 2.6) in every patient visit (Families and Communities Together, 2016; U.S. Prevention Services Task Force [USPSTF], 2018).

VIOLENCE IN THE HOME

Violence in the home environment, known as *domestic violence*, affects many lives in the United States. It is estimated that one in three women will experience rape, physical violence, or stalking by an intimate partner in their lifetime, with many women experiencing their first episode during adolescence (Weil, 2023). Domestic violence includes intimate partner violence and violence between family members. Refer to Chapter 9 for further information on violence and abuse, including gender-based violence and intimate partner violence.

Children exposed to family violence are more likely to be a victim or perpetrator of violence in adulthood (Franchek-Roa, 2022). The Federal Child Abuse Prevention and Treatment Act (CAPTA) defines *child abuse and neglect* as any recent act or failure to act on the part of a parent or caregiver that results in death, serious physical or emotional harm, or sexual abuse or exploitation, or an act or failure to act that presents an imminent risk of serious harm to a child (U.S. Department of Health and Human Services, 2014).

In 2020, approximately 618,000 cases of child maltreatment occurred in the United States (U.S. Department of Health and Human Services et al., 2022). Of the number of children identified as being maltreated, 76.1% were victims of neglect, 16.5% were victims of physical abuse, and 9.4% were victims of sexual abuse (U.S. Department of Health and Human Services et al., 2022). Approximately 1,750 children died from abuse and neglect in 2020; 68% of those children were younger than 3 years of age (U.S. Department of Health and Human Services et al., 2022).

BOX 2.6 RADAR

R—Routinely screen every patient for abuse.
A—Ask direct questions.
D—Document your findings.
A—Assess for your patient's safety before they leave the medical setting.
R—Review options and make referrals.

Families and Communities Together. (2016). *RADAR: A domestic violence intervention.* https://www.factoc.org/radar-a-domestic-violence-intervention/

TAKE NOTE!

American Indian, Alaska Native, and African American children experience higher rates of abuse and neglect according to the U.S. Department of Health and Human Services, Administration for Children and Families, Administration on Children, Youth and Families, and Children's Bureau (2022). The incidence of child abuse and neglect is five times higher for children from families with low socioeconomic status (CDC, 2022c).

Children who are exposed to stressors such as domestic violence or who are victims of childhood abuse or neglect are at high risk for short- and long-term problems. These problems manifest differently based on the child's age and developmental ability. The younger the child and the longer the exposure, the more serious the problems. Short-term problems include sleep disturbances, headaches, stomachaches, depression, asthma, fear of harm, inability to experience empathy or guilt, habitual lying, low frustration tolerance, poor judgment, shame, fear about the future, enuresis, and aggressive behaviors, such as increased peer aggression and bullying, decreased social competencies, withdrawal, avoidance attachment, developmental regression, fears, anxiety, and learning problems. Long-term problems may include poor school performance, truancy, absenteeism, and difficulty with adult relationships and tasks. There is a strong correlation between the number of exposures to ACEs and negative behaviors and health concerns such as early initiation of smoking, sexual activity, illicit drug use, adolescent pregnancy, obesity, depression, and suicide attempts (Bradford, 2020).

TAKE NOTE!

Witnessing and being exposed to violence in childhood result in a higher tolerance for and greater use of violence as an adult (Franchek-Roa, 2022).

Due to the potential impact of violence on children and families, it is important to perform a thorough assessment to identify violence in the family (Box 2.7). The nurse should provide referrals to shelters and child advocacy centers and intervene to assist children who are exposed to or victims of violence.

BOX **2.7** **Assessing for Violence**

Questions for the Parent

- Do you ever feel afraid in your home?
- What happens when you and (partner's name) argue?
- Do arguments ever become physical (hitting, kicking, pushing, throwing, or punching/breaking objects)?
- Has (partner's name) ever threatened you with a weapon (e.g., gun, knife)?
- Have you ever felt trapped or like a prisoner in your own home? Does your partner ever lock you in/out of the house or take your car keys?
- Have your children ever seen or heard violence in the home?
- Have the police ever been involved due to violence in your home?
- Is the violence ever directed at the children? Does (partner's name) ever hit, kick, push, or yell at your child when they are angry?
- How do you and (partner's name) discipline the children?

Questions for the Child

- What happens when Mommy and Daddy (or appropriate partner names) argue or fight? Is there any hitting, pushing, and so forth?
- How do you feel when Mommy and Daddy (or appropriate partner names) fight?
- What happens to you when you get in trouble?
- If hitting or other physical forms of discipline occur, ask:
- What does (name of person) hit you with? Where on your body? Does it ever leave a mark or bruise?
- Who hits or kicks you? How often does it happen?

Not all children who are exposed to violence suffer negative consequences. Studies have identified protective factors that can help buffer children from the effects of violence and reduce the risk that the child will develop violent behaviors in the future (CDC, 2022e). Examples of protective factors include the following:

- Feelings of connectedness or a secure attachment to a nonviolent parent or caregiver
- Strong commitment to school and academic performance
- Involvement in social activities
- Social and community support
- Positive sibling and peer relationships
- Ability to discuss problems with parents or a supportive adult
- Consistent presence of a parent at least once during the day, such as in the morning on awakening, when getting home from school, at dinnertime, or when going to bed
- Positive view of self
- Strong cultural and/or spiritual identity

Interventions need to focus on reducing children's exposure to violence and fostering protective factors.

YOUTH VIOLENCE

Youth violence is "the intentional use of physical force or power to threaten or harm others by young people ages 10 to 24" (CDC, 2023a). A young person can be involved with youth violence as a victim, offender, or witness. Youth violence affects the community as well as the child and family. Studies have shown that youth violence is associated with a disruption in social services, negative impact on school attendance, an increase in health care costs, and a decline in property values (CDC, 2024a). Research continues to show that children exposed to violence suffer serious consequences, such as problems with development, behavior, economic health of all community residents, and physical and mental health issues, which last a lifetime (CDC, 2023a).

VIOLENT CRIMES

Violent crimes include murder, rape, robbery, and aggravated assault. Statistics from the CDC (2023a) show that for people aged 10 to 24 years:

- More than 800 are treated in emergency departments for injuries due to physical violence.
- Homicide is the third leading cause of death for all people in this age group and is the leading cause of death for non-Hispanic Black or African American young people.

SUICIDE

Suicide is a serious public health problem affecting people today. In the United States, it is one of the leading causes of death, and in people aged 10 to 14 years and 20 to 34 years, it is the second leading cause of death (CDC, 2023c). Many more people think about or attempt suicide every year than die from suicide (CDC, 2023c).

TAKE NOTE!

There are variations in suicide rates among populations: Non-Hispanic Native Americans, Alaska Natives, and non-Hispanic White people have the highest rates of suicide (CDC, 2023c).

SCHOOL VIOLENCE

In recent years, due to several high-profile cases of school shootings, much attention has been directed at school violence and concern for student safety. Statistically, however, less than 2% of school-aged homicides occur on the way to or from school, at school events, or during school hours (CDC, 2021b). Although students are less likely to be victims of crime at school, some schools continue to have violence problems, highlighting the importance of school violence prevention (CDC, 2024b). In 2019, the CDC conducted a nationwide survey of high school students about risk behavior and found that approximately 8% of the students reported that they had been involved in a physical altercation on school property, while 7%

reported being injured or threatened by a person with a weapon on school grounds (CDC, 2021a).

Much of school violence involves bullying, which is defined as repeated negative actions that are clearly malicious and unwarranted by one or more people directed at a victim. It has been estimated that one in five students in the ninth and 10th grades in the United States are a target of bullying (CDC, 2021a). Many cases of bullying go unreported; however, bullying can have long-lasting traumatic effects, such as depression, low self-esteem, anxiety, academic problems, sleep problems, and violence later in adolescence and adulthood (CDC, 2021a). School nurses need to be aware of bullying and offer support, guidance, and intervention to students and staff.

Safe schools are essential for proper learning, growth and development, development of healthy relationships, and overall health of children. Violence in schools has a negative effect not only on students but also on the school and the entire community. The continued coordination among schools, law enforcement, social services, and mental health systems and the development of effective programs will help to reduce these risk behaviors.

KEY CONCEPTS

- Core concepts of maternal and pediatric nursing include family-centered care, EBP, collaborative care, atraumatic therapeutic care, communication, education, continuum of care strategy, preventive care, and culturally congruent care.
- Family-centered care recognizes the concept of the family as the constant. The health and functioning ability of the family influences and impacts the health of the patient and other members of the family. Family-centered care recognizes and respects family strengths and individuality, encourages referrals for family support, and facilitates collaboration.
- It is important that nurses develop the skills and knowledge necessary to ask pertinent clinical questions, search for current best evidence, analyze the evidence, integrate the evidence into practice when appropriate, and evaluate outcomes.
- Open, honest lines of communication are essential for nurses. The use of an interpreter may be necessary to ensure effective communication with patients and their families. Maintaining confidentiality and privacy is key.
- A family's knowledge related to the patient's health or illness is vitally important. Nurses play a major role in educating women, children, and their families. For children, teaching is provided based on their developmental level.
- The family is considered the basic social unit. The family greatly influences the development and health of its members. Members learn health care activities, health beliefs, and health values from their family.
- Social roles are often an important factor in the development of one's self-concept, which can have a very positive influence on health or present various limitations and problems, possibly resulting in a negative influence on health.
- Culture influences every aspect of development and is reflected in childbearing and child-rearing beliefs and practices designed to promote adaptation to the social group's expectations.
- Spirituality, a major influence for many people, provides meaning and purpose to life and is a foundation for and a source of love, relationships, and service. Spiritual and religious beliefs and views can provide strength and support to women, children, and their families during times of stress and illness.
- Other factors impacting the health of women and children include genetics, global society, health status and lifestyles, access to health care, and improved diagnosis and treatment. Barriers to health care can result from lack of finances; sociocultural barriers, including lack of transportation, the need for both parents to work, high health insurance premiums, and discrimination; language differences; and health care delivery system barriers, including inconvenient clinic hours and unsupportive or judgmental attitudes by health care workers.

Unfolding Patient Stories: Fatime Sanogo Part 1

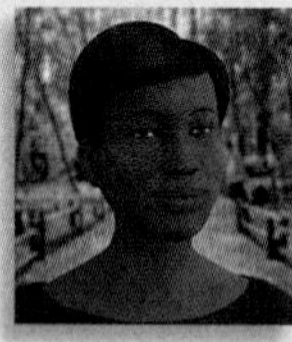

Fatime Sanogo, a 23-year-old, is being seen by the nurse in the prenatal clinic. The nurse learns that this is her first pregnancy, she is Muslim, and she recently moved to the United States from Mali, West Africa, with her husband. What cultural factors are important for the nurse to assess that guide culturally humble care during Fatime's pregnancy and preparation for delivery? (Fatime Sanogo's story continues in Chapter 14.)

Care for Fatime and other patients in a realistic virtual environment: ***vSim** for Nursing* **(thepoint.lww.com/vSimMaternity).** Practice documenting these patients' care in DocuCare **(thepoint.lww.com/DocuCareEHR).**

REFERENCES AND RECOMMENDED READINGS

Adams-Leander, S. (2022). Public health nursing in the community. In C. Rector & M. J. Stanley (Eds.), *Community and public health nursing: Promoting the public's health* (10th ed., pp. 94–119). Wolters Kluwer Health.

Agency for Healthcare Research and Quality. (2010, reviewed 2020). *AHRQ health literacy universal precautions toolkit.* https://www.ahrq.gov/health-literacy/improve/precautions/index.html

Agency for Healthcare Research and Quality. (2021).*Disparities in healthcare. 2021 National Healthcare Quality and Disparities Report.* https://www.ncbi.nlm.nih.gov/books/NBK578532/

American Academy of Pediatrics. (2013, reaffirmed 2022). Policy statement: Providing care for children and adolescents facing homelessness and housing insecurity. *Pediatrics, 131*(6), 1206–1210. https://doi.org/10.1542/peds.2013-0645

American Academy of Pediatrics. (2018). *What's the best way to discipline my child?* HealthyChildren. http://www.healthychildren.org/english/family-life/family-dynamics/communication-discipline/pages/disciplining-your-child.aspx

American Academy of Pediatrics. (2021). *Addressing low health literacy and limited English proficiency.* https://www.aap.org/en/practice-management/providing-patient--and-family-centered-care/addressing-low-health-literacy-and-limited-english-proficiency/

American Academy of Pediatrics, & Council on Communications and Media. (2016a, reaffirmed 2022a). Policy statement: Media and young minds. *Pediatrics, 138*(5). https://doi.org/10.1542/peds.2016-2591

American Academy of Pediatrics, & Council on Communications and Media. (2016b, reaffirmed 2022b). Policy statement: Media use in school-aged children and adolescents. *Pediatrics, 138*(5), e20162592. https://doi.org/10.1542/peds.2016-2592

American Association of Critical Care Nurses. (n.d.). *True collaboration.* Retrieved November 19, 2023, from https://www.aacn.org/nursing-excellence/healthy-work-environments/true-collaboration

American Immigration Council. (2021). *Fact sheet: Immigrants in the United States.* https://www.americanimmigrationcouncil.org/research/immigrants-in-the-united-states#

American Nurses Association. (2023). *What is evidence-based practice in nursing?* https://www.nursingworld.org/content-hub/resources/workplace/evidence-based-practice-in-nursing/

American Nurses Association, National Association of Pediatric Nurse Practitioners, & Society of Pediatric Nurses. (2015). *Pediatric nursing: Scope and standards of practice* (2nd ed.). American Nurses Publishing.

Andrews, M. M. (2020). Transcultural perspectives in nursing care of children. In M. M. Andrews, J. S. Boyle, & J. W. Collins (Eds.), *Transcultural concepts in nursing care* (8th ed., pp. 172–208). Wolters Kluwer.

Bao, T., Greenlee, H., Lopez, A. M., Kadro, Z., Lopez, G., & Carlson, L. E. (2023). How to make evidence-based integrative medicine a part of everyday oncology practice. *American Society of Clinical Oncology Educational Book, 43*, e389830. https://doi.org/10.1200/EDBK_389830

Bass, B., & Nagy, H. (2022). Cultural competence in the care of LGBTQ patients. In *StatPearls* [Internet]. StatPearls Publishing. https://www.ncbi.nlm.nih.gov/books/NBK563176/

Baumrind, D. (1966). Effects of authoritative parental control on child behavior. *Child Development, 37*(4), 887–907. https://doi.org/10.2307/1126611

Betancourt, J. R., Green, A. R., & Carrillo, J. E. (2023). The patient's culture and effective communication. *UpToDate.* https://www.uptodate.com/contents/the-patients-culture-and-effective-communication

Bitsko, R. H., Claussen, A. H., Lichstein, J., Black, L. I., Jones, S. E., Danielson, M. L., Hoenig, J. M., Jack, S. P. D., Brody, D. J., Gyawali, S., Maenner, M. J., Warner, M., Holland, K. M., Ruth Perou, R., Crosby, A. E., Blumberg, S. J., Shelli Avenevoli, S., Kaminski, J. W., & Ghandour, R. M. (2022). Mental health surveillance among children—United States, 2013–2019. *MMWR Supplements, 71*(2), 1–42. https://doi.org/10.15585/mmwr.su7102a1

Bogues, L., & Levine, D. A. (2023). Section 2: Growth and development. Chapter 7: Normal development. In K. J. Marcdante, R. M. Kleigman, & A. M. Schuh (Eds.), *Nelson essentials of pediatrics* (9th ed., pp. 14–16). Elsevier.

Bohren, M. A., Corona, M. V., Odiase, O. J., Wilson, A. N., Sudhinaraset, M., Diamond-Smith, N., Berryman, J., Tuncalp, O., & Afulani, P. A. (2022). Strategies to reduce stigma and discrimination in sexual and reproductive healthcare settings: A mixed-methods systematic review. *PLOS Global Public Health.* https://doi.org/10.1371/journal.pgph.0000582

Boss, P. (2001). *Family stress management: A contextual approach* (2nd ed.). Sage Publications, Inc.

Bradford, K. (2020). Reducing the effects of adverse childhood experiences. *LegisBrief, 28*(29). https://www.ncsl.org/research/health/reducing-the-effects-of-adverse-childhood-experiences.aspx#:~:text=The%20more%20ACEs%20a%20child,depression%2C%20substance%20misuse%20and%20suicide

Breast Cancer Organization. (2023). *How BRCA and other gene mutations work.* https://www.breastcancer.org/genetic-testing/brca

Brega, A. G., Barnard, J., Mabachi, N. M., Weiss, B. D., DeWalt, D. A., Brach, C., Cifuentes, M., Albright, K., West, D. R. (2015). *AHRQ health literacy universal precautions toolkit* (2nd ed.). Agency for Healthcare Research and Quality. Retrieved February 4, 2020, from https://www.ahrq.gov/sites/default/files/publications/files/healthlittoolkit2_4.pdf

Breilyn, M. S., & Levy, P. A. (2023). Section 9: Human genetics and dysmorphology. Chapter 49: Chromosomal disorders. In K. J. Marcdante, R. M. Kleigman, & A. M. Schuh (Eds.), *Nelson essentials of pediatrics* (9th ed., pp. 189–192). Elsevier.

Buchanan, A. O., & Marquez, M. L. (2023a). Section 6: Pediatric nutrition and nutritional disorders. Chapter 30: Pediatric undernutrition. In K. J. Marcdante, R. M. Kleigman, & A. M. Schuh (Eds.), *Nelson essentials of pediatrics* (9th ed., pp. 114–118). Elsevier.

Buchanan, A. O., & Marquez, M. L. (2023b). Section 6: Pediatric nutrition and nutritional disorders. Chapter 29: Obesity. In K. J. Marcdante, R. M. Kleigman, & A. M. Schuh (Eds.), *Nelson essentials of pediatrics* (9th ed., pp. 109–114). Elsevier.

Center for Health Care Strategies. (2024). Health Literacy Fact Sheets: Identifying Limited Health Literacy. https://www.chcs.org/media/2-Identifying-Limited-Health-Literacy_2024.pdf

Center on Budget and Policy Priorities. (2021). *Closing the coverage gap would improve Black maternal health.* https://www.cbpp.org/research/health/closing-the-coverage-gap-would-improve-black-maternal-health

Centers for Disease Control and Prevention (CDC). (2024e, April 9). About Adverse Childhood Experiences. https://www.cdc.gov/aces/about/index.htmll

Centers for Disease Control and Prevention. (2021b). *Preventing bullying*. https://www.cdc.gov/violenceprevention/pdf/yv/Bullying-factsheet_508_1.pdf

Centers for Disease Control and Prevention. (2021c, September 2). *Key findings: School-associated violent death study*. https://www.cdc.gov/violenceprevention/youthviolence/schoolviolence/SAVD.html

Centers for Disease Control and Prevention. (2022a). *What is health literacy?* https://www.cdc.gov/healthliteracy/learn/index.html

Centers for Disease Control and Prevention. (2022b). *CDC's health literacy action plan*. https://www.cdc.gov/healthliteracy/planact/cdcplan.html

Centers for Disease Control and Prevention. (2022c). *Preventing child abuse & neglect*. https://www.cdc.gov/violenceprevention/pdf/can/CAN-factsheet_2022.pdf

Centers for Disease Control and Prevention. (2022d, August 19). *Health and academics*. https://www.cdc.gov/healthyschools/health_and_academics/index.htm

Centers for Disease Control and Prevention. (2022e, April 6). *Child abuse and neglect prevention: Risk and protective factors*. https://www.cdc.gov/violenceprevention/childabuseandneglect/riskprotectivefactors.html

Centers for Disease Control and Prevention. (2022g, June 27). *Scarlet fever*. https://www.cdc.gov/groupastrep/diseases-hcp/scarlet-fever.html

Centers for Disease Control and Prevention. (2023a). *Preventing youth violence*. Retrieved December 5, 2023, from https://www.cdc.gov/youth-violence/prevention/index.html

Centers for Disease Control and Prevention. (2023c). *Facts about suicide*. https://www.cdc.gov/suicide/facts/index.html

Centers for Disease Control and Prevention. (2023e). *Working together to reduce Black maternal mortality*. https://www.cdc.gov/healthequity/features/maternal-mortality/

Centers for Disease Control and Prevention. (2024a). *About Youth Violence*. https://www.cdc.gov/youth-violence/about/index.html

Centers for Disease Control and Prevention. (2024b, April 19). *About school violence*. https://www.cdc.gov/youth-violence/about/about-school-violence.html

Centers for Disease Control and Prevention. (2024c, May 15). *Substance use during pregnancy*. https://www.cdc.gov/maternal-infant-health/pregnancy-substance-abuse/

Centers for Disease Control and Prevention. (2024d, April 24). *Preventing adverse childhood experiences*. https://www.cdc.gov/aces/prevention/index.html

Chassiakos, Y. R., Radesky, J., Christakis, D., Moreno, M. A., Cross, C., & Council on Communications and Media. (2016). Technical report: Children and adolescents and digital media. *Pediatrics, 138*(5), e20162593. https://doi.org/10.1542/peds.2016-2593

Cherry, K. (2022). *Why parenting styles matter when raising children*. https://www.verywellmind.com/parenting-styles-2795072

Children's Defense Fund. (2023). *The state of America's children*. https://www.childrensdefense.org/the-state-of-americas-children/

Cloninger, C. R., Cloninger, K. M., Zwir, I., & Keltikangas-Järvinen, L. (2019). The complex genetics and biology of human temperament: A review of traditional concepts in relation to new molecular findings. *Translational Psychiatry, 9*(1), 290. https://doi.org/10.1038/s41398-019-0621-4

Culatta, R. (2023). *Andragogy (Malcolm Knowles)*. Retrieved December 18, 2023, from https://www.instructionaldesign.org/theories/andragogy/

Drozdz, D., Alvarez-Pitti, J., Wójcik, M., Borghi, C., Gabbianelli, R., Mazur, A., Herceg-Čavrak, V., Lopez-Valcarcel, B. G., Brzeziński, M., Lurbe, E., & Wühl, E. (2021). Obesity and cardiometabolic risk factors: From childhood to adulthood. *Nutrients, 13*(11), 4176. https://doi.org/10.3390/nu13114176

Duvall, E. (1977). *Marriage and family development* (5th ed.). J. B. Lippincott

Families and Communities Together. (2016). *RADAR: A domestic violence intervention*. https://www.factoc.org/radar-a-domestic-violence-intervention/

Federal Interagency Forum on Child and Family Statistics. (2021). *America's children: Key national indicators of well-being, 2021*. U.S. Government Printing Office. https://www.childstats.gov/pdf/ac2021/ac_21.pdf

Federal Interagency Forum on Child and Family Statistics. (2023). *America's children: Key national indicators of well-being, 2023*. U.S. Government Printing Office. https://www.childstats.gov/pdf/ac2023/ac_23.pdf

Feldhusen, A. E. (2000). *The history of midwifery and childbirth in America: A time line*. https://www.midwiferytoday.com/web-article/history-midwifery-childbirth-america-time-line/

Ferramosca, F. M. P., De Maria, M., Ivziku, D., Raffaele, B., Lommi, M., Tolentino Diaz, M. Y., Montini, G., Porcelli, B., De Benedictis, A., Tartaglini, D., & Gualandi, R. (2023). Nurses' organization of work and its relation to workload in medical surgical units: A cross-sectional observational multi-center study. *Healthcare (Basel, Switzerland), 11*(2), 156. https://doi.org/10.3390/healthcare11020156

Forcier, M., & Olson-Kennedy, J. (2023). Gender development and clinical presentation of gender diversity in children and adolescents. *UpToDate*. Retrieved December 10, 2023, from https://www.uptodate.com/contents/gender-development-and-clinical-presentation-of-gender-diversity-in-children-and-adolescents

Fortin, K., & Downes, A. H. (2023). Section 5: Psychosocial issues. In K. J. Marcdante, R. M. Kleigman, & Abigail M. Schuh (Eds.), *Nelson essentials of pediatrics* (9th ed., pp. 79–100). Elsevier.

Franchek-Roa, K. M. (2022). Intimate partner violence: Childhood exposure. *UpToDate*. Retrieved December 4, 2023, from https://www.uptodate.com/contents/intimate-partner-violence-childhood-exposure

Friedman, M. M. (1998). *Family nursing: Theory and practice* (4th ed.). Appleton & Lange.

Gartland, D., Riggs, E., Muyeen, S., Giallo, R., Afifi, T. O., MacMillan, H., Herrman, H., Bulford, E., & Brown, S. J. (2019). What factors are associated with resilient outcomes in children exposed to social adversity? A systematic review. *BMJ Open, 9*(4). e024870. https://doi.org/10.1136/bmjopen-2018-024870

Health Resources and Services Administration. (2022). *Addressing health literacy*. Retrieved January 27, 2019, from https://www.hrsa.gov/about/organization/bureaus/ohe/health-literacy

Healthy People 2030, U.S. Department of Health and Human Services, & Office of Disease Prevention and Health

Promotion. (n.d.). *Social determinants of health* https://health.gov/healthypeople/objectives-and-data/social-determinants-health

Hickey, K. T., Masterson Creber, R. M., Reading, M., Sciacca, R. R., Riga, T. C., Frulla, A. P., & Casida, J. M. (2018). Low health literacy: Implications for managing cardiac patients in practice. *The Nurse Practitioner*, *43*(8), 49–55. https://doi.org/10.1097/01.NPR.0000541468.54290.49

Hong, Y.-R., Yadav, S., Wang, R., Vadaparampil, S., Bian, J., George, T. J., & Braithwaite, D. (2023). Genetic testing for cancer risk and perceived importance of genetic information among US population by race and ethnicity: A cross-sectional study. *Journal of Racial and Ethnic Health Disparities*, *11*, 392–394. https://doi.org/10.1007/s40615-023-01526-4

Jones, J. M. (2022). *Belief in god in U.S. dips to 81%, a new low.* Retrieved December 8, 2023, from https://news.gallup.com/poll/393737/belief-god-dips-new-low.aspx

Jones, V. F., Schulte, E. E., & Committee on Early Childhood and Council on Foster Care, Adoption, and Kinship Care. (2012, reaffirmed 2017). The pediatrician's role in supporting adoptive families. *Pediatrics*, *130*(4):e1040–e1049. https://doi.org/10.1542/peds.2012–2261

Joshi, D. S., & Lebrun-Harris, L. A. (2022). Child health status and health care use in grandparent—Versus parent-led households. *Pediatrics*, *150*(3), e2021055291. https://doi.org/10.1542/peds.2021-055291

Kaiser Family Foundation. (2020). *Women's health insurance coverage*. https://www.kff.org/womens-health-policy/fact-sheet/womens-health-insurance-coverage-fact-sheet/

Kaiser Family Foundation. (2022). *Key facts on health coverage of immigrants.* https://www.kff.org/racial-equity-and-health-policy/fact-sheet/key-facts-on-health-coverage-of-immigrants/

Katz, B. (n.d.). *ICEA position paper: Family-centered maternity care.* https://icea.org/wp-content/uploads/2018/02/ICEA-Position-Paper-Family-Centered-Maternity-Care.pdf

Kemp, G., Smith, M., & Segal, J. (2022). *Children and divorce.* https://www.helpguide.org/articles/parenting-family/children-and-divorce.htm

Kids Count Data Center. (2022a). *Children who have difficulty speaking English by family nativity in United States.* Retrieved December 6, 2023, from https://datacenter.kidscount.org/data/tables/128-children-who-have-difficulty-speaking-english-by-family-nativity?loc=1#detailed/1/any/false/1729,870/78,79/470,471

Kids Count Data Center. (2022b). *Children living in linguistically isolated households by family nativity in United States.* Retrieved December 6, 2023, from https://datacenter.aecf.org/data/tables/129-children-living-in-linguistically-isolated-households-by-family-nativity#detailed/1/any/false/1095,2048,1729,37,871,870,573,869,36,868/78,79/472,473

Knowles, M. S., Holton III, E. F., & Swanson, R. A. (2015). *The adult learner: The definitive classic in adult education and human resource development* (8th ed.). Routledge.

Koh, H. K., Berwick, D. M., Clancy, C. M., Baur, C., Brach, C., Harris, L. M., & Zerhusen, E. G. (2012). New federal policy initiatives to boost health literacy can help the nation move beyond the cycle of costly "crisis care." *Health Affairs*, *31*(2), 434–443. https://doi.org/10.1377/hlthaff.2011.1169

Krontoft, A. (2021). How do patients prefer to receive patient education material about treatment, diagnosis and procedures? *Open Journal of Nursing*, *11*, 809–827. https://doi.org/10.4236/ojn.2021.1110068

Levetown, M., & American Academy of Pediatrics Committee on Bioethics. (2008, reaffirmed 2017). Communicating with children and families: From everyday interactions to skill in conveying distressing information. *Pediatrics*, *121*(5), e1441–e1460. https://doi.org/10.1542/peds.2008-0565

Linton, J. M., Green, A., & Council on Community Pediatrics. (2019). Providing care for children in immigrant families. *Pediatrics*, *144*(3), e20192077. https://doi.org/10.1542/peds.2019-2077

Mandy, G. T. (2022). Preterm birth: Definitions of prematurity, epidemiology, and risk factors for infant mortality. *UpToDate.* Retrieved November 28, 2023, from https://www.uptodate.com/contents/preterm-birth-definitions-of-prematurity-epidemiology-and-risk-factors-for-infant-mortality

Mandy, G. T. (2023). Overview of the long-term complications of preterm birth. *UpToDate.* Retrieved December 8, 2023, from https://www.uptodate.com/contents/overview-of-the-long-term-complications-of-preterm-birth

Morris, M. E. (2023). Advancing maternal age: Infertility evaluation and management. *UpToDate.* Retrieved on December 15, 2023, from https://www.uptodate.com/contents/advancing-maternal-age-infertility-evaluation-and-management

Mykyta, L., Keisler-Starkey, K., & Bunch, L. (2022). *More children were covered by Medicaid and CHIP in 2021.* United States Census Bureau. https://www.census.gov/library/stories/2022/09/uninsured-rate-of-children-declines.html

Nahin, R. L., Rhee, A., & Stussman, B. (2024). Use of complementary health approaches overall and for pain management by US adults. *JAMA*, *331*(7), 613–615. https://www.nccih.nih.gov/research/national-health-interview-survey-2022

National Association of the Deaf. (2023). *Position statement on health care access for deaf patients.* https://www.nad.org/about-us/position-statements/position-statement-on-health-care-access-for-deaf-patients/

National Center for Complementary and Integrative Health. (2021a). *Complementary, alternative, or integrative health: What's in a name?* https://www.nccih.nih.gov/health/complementary-alternative-or-integrative-health-whats-in-a-name

National Center for Complementary and Integrative Health. (2021b). *Women's health and complementary approaches.* https://www.nccih.nih.gov/health/womens-health-and-complementary-approaches

Patterson, J. (1995). Promoting resilience in families experiencing stress. *Pediatric Clinics of North America*, *42*(1), 47–63. https://doi.org/10.1016/S0031-3955(16)38907-6

Patterson, J. (2002). Integrating family resilience and family stress theory. *Journal of Marriage and Family*, *64*(2), 349–360. https://doi.org/10.1111/j.1741-3737.2002.00349.x

Qian, L., Wu, W., Jiang, J., & Wu, Y. (2023). The epidemiology of multiple pregnancy and perinatal outcome with the aid of machine learning-based forecasting models [Abstract]. *Soft Computing.* https://doi.org/10.1007/s00500-023-08745-1

Rivers, C., Gibson, S., Contreras, E., Livingston, T., & Hanson, P. (2019). Competency-based education: An evolutionary higher education business model. *Journal of Competency-Based Education*, *4*, e01179. https://doi.org/10.1002/cbe2.1179

Rothwell, J. (2020). *Assessing the economic gains of eradicating illiteracy nationally and regionally in the United States.* Gallup. https://www.barbarabush.org/wp-content/uploads/2020/09/BBFoundation_GainsFromEradicatingIlliteracy_9_8.pdf

Samet, J. M., & Sockrider, M. (2022). Control of secondhand smoke exposure. *UpToDate.* Retrieved December 10, 2023, from https://www.uptodate.com/contents/control-of-secondhand-smoke-exposure

Sample, J.A. (2024). Childhood lead poisoning: Clinical manifestations and diagnosis. *UpToDate.* Retrieved on June 24, 2024 from https://www.uptodate.com/contents/childhood-lead-poisoning-clinical-manifestations-and-diagnosis

Schulte, E. E. (2023). Adoption. *UpToDate.* Retrieved November 29, 2023, from https://www.uptodate.com/contents/adoption

Sege, R. D., Siegel, B. S., Council on Child Abuse and Neglect, & Committee on Psychosocial Aspects of child and Family Health. (2018). Effective discipline to raise healthy children. *Pediatrics*, 2018, *142*(6), Article 20183112. https://doi.org/10.1542/peds.2018-3112

Shrider, E. A., & Creamer, J. (2023). *Poverty in the United States: 2022: Current population reports*, 60–280. U.S. Government Publishing Office. https://www.census.gov/content/dam/Census/library/publications/2023/demo/p60-280.pdf

Stussman, B. J., Nahin, R. R., Barnes, P. M., & Ward, B. W. (2020). U.S. physician recommendations to their patients about the use of complementary health approaches. *Journal of Alternative and Complementary Medicine*, *26*(1), 25–33. https://doi.org/10.1089/acm.2019.0303

Sutton, V. R., & Meng, L. (2023). Gene test interpretation: HEXA (Tay–Sachs disease gene). *UpToDate.* Retrieved November 29, 2023 from https://www.uptodate.com/contents/gene-test-interpretation-hexa-tay-sachs-disease-gene

Tremblay, C., & Brady, M. T. (2023). Roseola infantum (exanthem subitum). *UpToDate.* Retrieved December 10, 2023, from https://www.uptodate.com/contents/roseola-infantum-exanthem-subitum

United Nations. (2022). Women and girls deserve to live without violence in 'safety, dignity and freedom.' *UN News.* https://news.un.org/en/story/2022/03/1114472

United Nations Children's Fund. (2022). *Mental health and psychosocial support in emergencies.* https://www.unicef.org/protection/mental-health-psychosocial-support-in-emergencies

U.S. Census Bureau. (2016). *The majority of children live with two parents, Census Bureau Reports.* https://www.census.gov/newsroom/archives/2016-pr/cb16-192.html

U.S. Census Bureau. (2023). *Subject definitions.* Retrieved November 29, 2023, from https://www.census.gov/programs-surveys/cps/technical-documentation/subject-definitions.html#family

U.S. Department of Health and Human Services. (n.d.). *Healthy People 2030.* https://health.gov/healthypeople

U.S. Department of Health and Human Services. (2014). *What is child abuse or neglect? What is the definition of child abuse and neglect?* https://www.hhs.gov/answers/programs-for-families-and-children/what-is-child-abuse/index.html

U.S. Department of Health and Human Services. (2023). *HHS poverty guidelines for 2023.* Retrieved December 17, 2023, from https://aspe.hhs.gov/topics/poverty-economic-mobility/poverty-guidelines

U.S. Department of Health and Human Services, Administration for Children and Families, Administration on Children, Youth and Families, & Children's Bureau. (2021). *The AFCARS report.* https://www.acf.hhs.gov/sites/default/files/documents/cb/afcarsreport28.pdf

U.S. Department of Health and Human Services, Administration for Children and Families, Administration on Children, Youth and Families, & Children's Bureau. (2022). *Child Maltreatment 2020.* https://www.acf.hhs.gov/cb/data-research/child-maltreatment

U.S. Prevention Services Task Force. (2018). *Intimate partner violence, elder abuse, and abuse of vulnerable adults: Screening.* https://www.uspreventiveservicestaskforce.org/uspstf/recommendation/intimate-partner-violence-and-abuse-of-elderly-and-vulnerable-adults-screening

Vespa, J., Medina, L., & Armstrong, D. M. (2018, revised 2020). *Demographic turning points for the United States: Population projections for 2020 to 2060: Population estimates and projections: Current population reports.* https://www.census.gov/content/dam/Census/library/publications/2020/demo/p25-1144.pdf

Vichinsky, E. P. (2022). Diagnosis of sickle cell disorders. *UpToDate.* Retrieved November 29, 2023 from https://www.uptodate.com/contents/diagnosis-of-sickle-cell-disorders

Von Bertalanffy, L. (1968). *General systems theory.* Penguin Press.

Weil, A. (2023). Intimate partner violence: Epidemiology and health consequences. *UpToDate.* Retrieved December 4, 2023 from https://www.uptodate.com/contents/intimate-partner-violence-epidemiology-and-health-consequences

Wildsmith, E., & Alvira-Hammond, M. (2023). *Data on families with low incomes across America can inform two-generation approaches.* Child Trends. https://doi.org/10.56417/1147h453i

Wittenberg, E., Ferrell, B., Kanter, E., & Buller, H. (2018). Nurse communication challenges with health literacy support. *Clinical Journal of Oncology Nursing, 22*(1), 53–61. https://doi.org/10.1188/18.CJON.53-61

Wong, D. (1995). *Whaley & Wong's nursing care of infants and children* (5th ed.). Mosby.

World Health Organization. (2012). *Care for child development: Participant manual.* https://www.unicef.org/media/91176/file/3-CCD-Participant-Manual.pdf

World Health Organization. (2020). *Children: Improving survival and well-being.* https://www.who.int/en/news-room/fact-sheets/detail/children-reducing-mortality

World Health Organization. (2023). *Deafness and hearing loss.* https://www.who.int/news-room/fact-sheets/detail/deafness-and-hearing-loss

World Health Organization. (2024). *Violence against women.* https://www.who.int/news-room/fact-sheets/detail/violence-against-women

DEVELOPING CLINICAL JUDGMENT

PRACTICING FOR NCLEX

1. The nurse is teaching a group of students about children's health status factors related to immigration. Which statement by a student would indicate the need for additional teaching?
   a. "The children of immigrants have better access to preventive care."
   b. "The children of immigrants may have limited involvement in activities due to language barriers."
   c. "The children of immigrants may lack adequate support systems."
   d. "The children of immigrants face increased stressors due to relocation."

2. The nurse is working with a group of adolescents who have been exposed to violence in their homes. Which examples would the nurse identify as protective factors that will help buffer the adolescents from the effects of violence? Select all that apply.
   a. Participating in a mentorship program
   b. Limiting involvement in social activities to help at home
   c. Limiting communication with parents
   d. Committing to school work
   e. Joining the school's student government

3. When planning education for a patient and their family, what is the first step the nurse should take?
   a. Decide which procedures and medications the patient will be discharged on.
   b. Determine the patient's and family's learning needs and styles.
   c. Ask the family if they have ever performed this type of procedure.
   d. Tell the patient and family what the goals of the teaching session are.

4. The clinic nurse is concerned about the patient's health literacy level and their ability to understand the instructions given. Which of the following can the nurse employ to increase the patient's understanding of the instructions?
   a. Draw pictures of the procedure and write down the steps to it.
   b. Instruct the patient to call the nurse if they have questions.
   c. Discuss the instructions with an older adult family member in addition to the patient.
   d. Question the patient about their reading level and educational level.

5. The nurse is preparing a class for a group of students about homelessness. Which factors contribute to homelessness? Select all that apply.
   a. Decrease in the number of people living in poverty
   b. Rises in unemployment
   c. Exposure to abuse or neglect
   d. Cutbacks in public welfare programs
   e. Development of community crisis centers

CRITICAL THINKING EXERCISES

1. A 3-year-old girl from Saudi Arabia has become seriously ill while on a visit to the United States. It is projected that she will require a lengthy hospitalization. Describe the steps the nurse should take to communicate with and provide extensive health care teaching to this child's family.

2. Vanessa Walters brings her 3-year-old son, Tyler, for a well-child visit. Vanessa states, "Tyler is a handful. He always seems to be misbehaving. I just don't know what to do." How should the nurse respond, and what suggestions might be helpful?

3. You have been asked by the local school district to speak to a group of middle school students about internet safety. Describe the topics that you should address.

STUDY ACTIVITIES

1. Discuss with fellow students the different types of family structures. Include information about your own family structure. Compare and contrast the roles assumed by each member in the different structures.

2. Create a culture diary or journal for use in clinical practice. Record observations made while caring for children and families of cultural or ethnic backgrounds different from your own. Include the preferences that the children and families had relating to food, health care, decision making for the family, view of children, and general health practices.

3. Perform a "spiritual inventory" on yourself. Identify your beliefs about higher authority, life after death, purpose in life, and your thoughts about people who have different beliefs.

4. Search the internet for websites that provide information about violence and its impact on children's health.

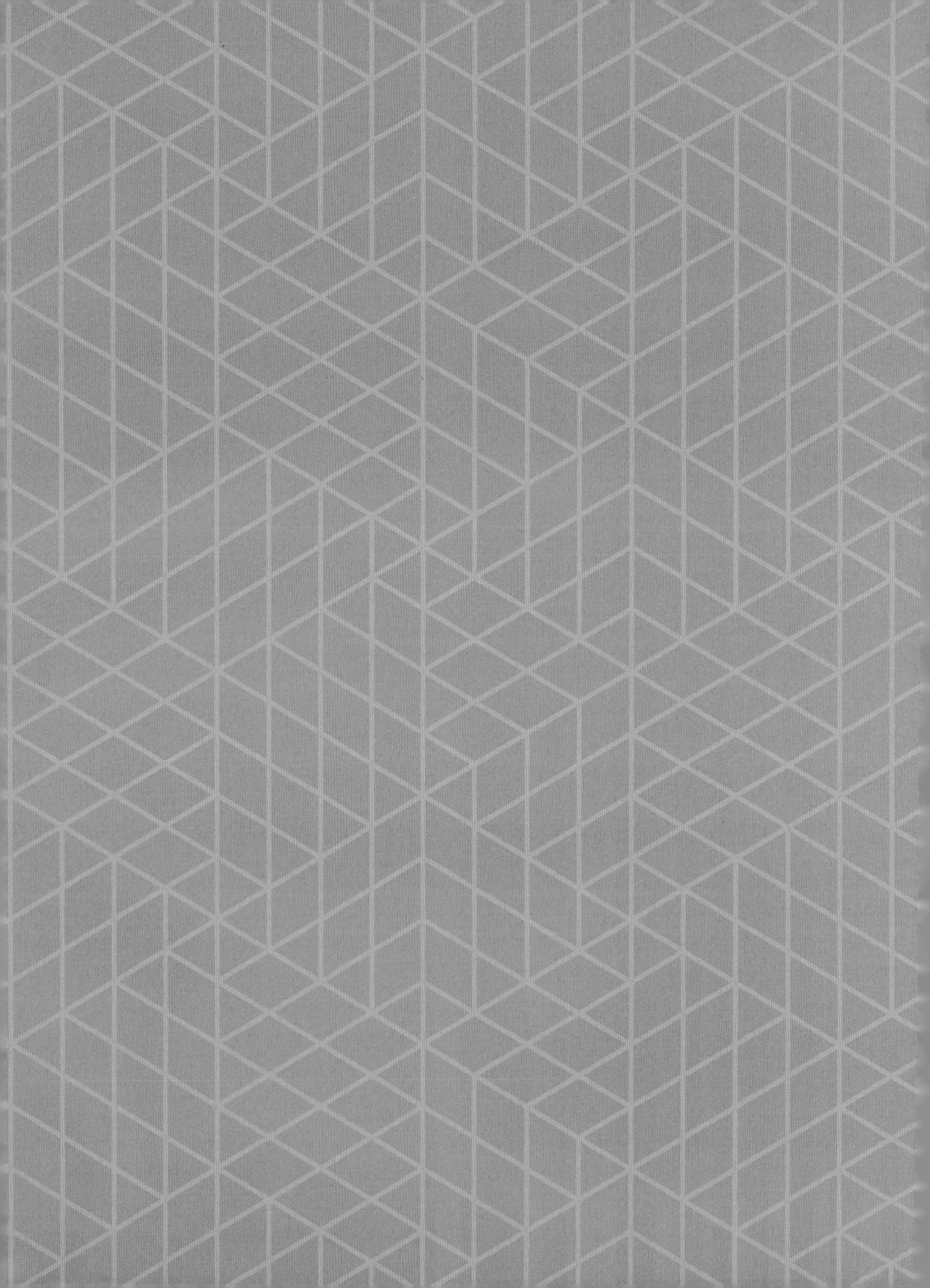

UNIT

II

Women's Health Throughout the Lifespan

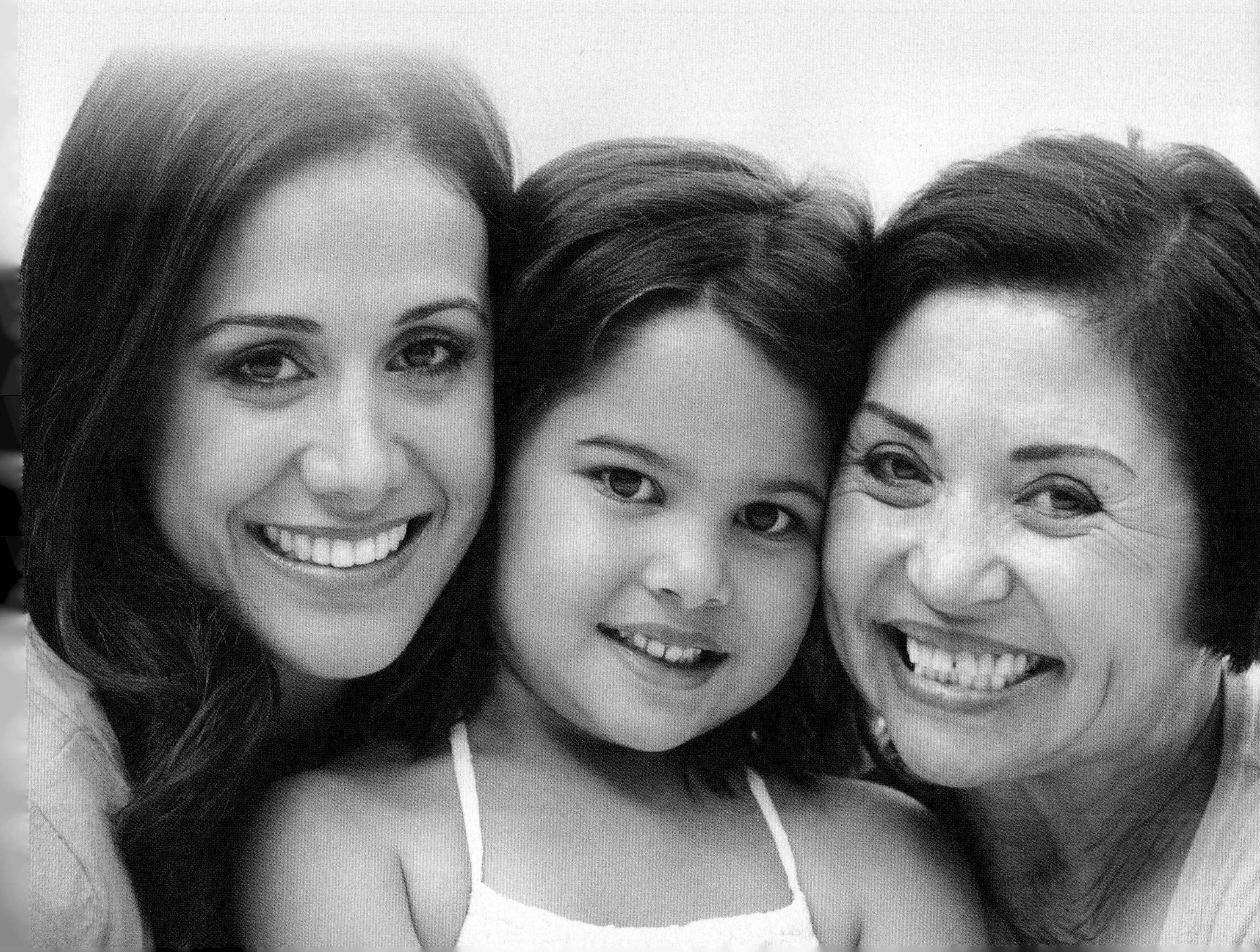

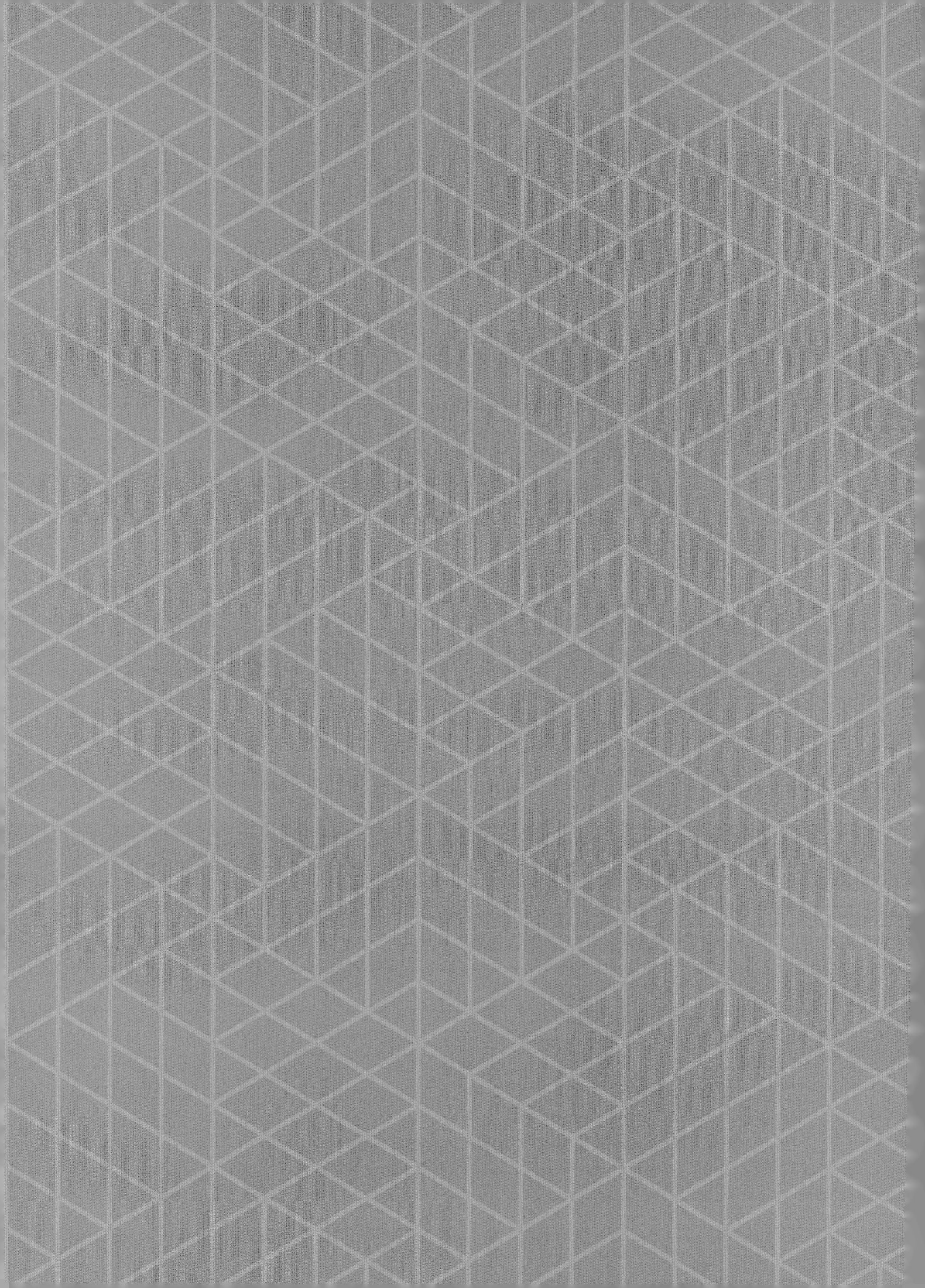

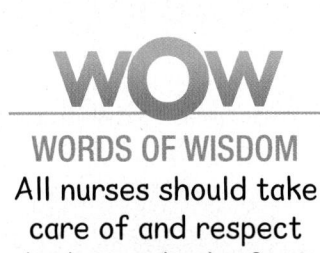

WORDS OF WISDOM

All nurses should take care of and respect the human body, for it is a wondrous precision machine.

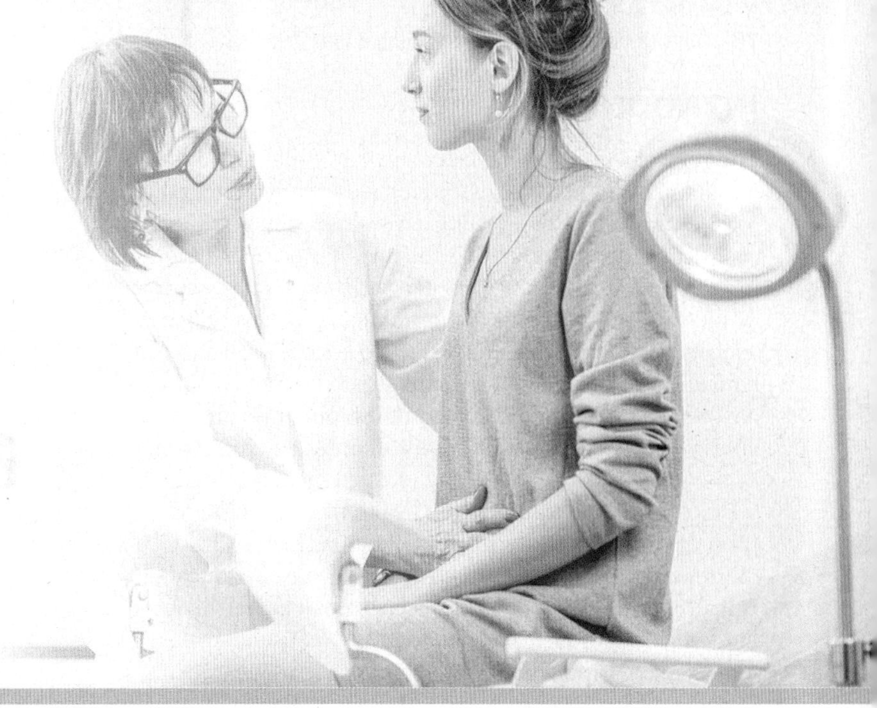

3 Anatomy and Physiology of the Female Reproductive System

LEARNING OBJECTIVES

Upon completion of the chapter, you will be able to:

1. Differentiate the structures and functions of the major external and internal female genital organs.
2. Outline the phases of the menstrual cycle, the dominant hormones involved, and the changes taking place in each phase.

KEY TERMS

breasts
cervix
endometrium (en'dō-mē'trē-ŭm)
estrogen
fallopian tubes (fă-lō'pē-ăn)
follicle-stimulating hormone (FSH)
luteinizing hormone (LH) (lū'tē-in-ī'zing)
menarche (men-ahr'kē)
menstruation (men'strū-ā'shŭn)
ovaries
ovulation (ov'yū-lā'shŭn)
progesterone (prŏ-jes'tĕr-ōn)
uterus
vagina
vulva

Linda, 52, started menstruating when she was 12 years old. Her menstrual periods have always been regular, but now she is experiencing irregular, heavier, and longer ones. She wonders if there is something wrong or if this is normal.

INTRODUCTION

The reproductive system is a collection of internal and external organs in both males and females that work together for the purpose of procreating. Scientists argue that the reproductive system is among the most important systems in the entire body since it plays a vital role in the survival of the human species. Without the ability to reproduce, a species dies. The female reproductive system produces the female reproductive cells (the eggs or ova) and contains an organ (**uterus**) in which the development of the fetus takes place. Nurses need to have a thorough understanding of the anatomy and physiology of the female reproductive system to be able to assess the health of these systems, to promote their health, to care for conditions that might affect the reproductive organs, and to provide patient education concerning the reproductive system. This chapter reviews the female reproductive system and the menstrual cycle as it relates to reproduction.

FEMALE REPRODUCTIVE ANATOMY AND PHYSIOLOGY

The female reproductive system is composed of both external and internal reproductive organs. It consists of the paired ovaries and oviducts, the uterus, the vagina, the external genitalia, and the mammary glands. All of these structures have evolved for the important functions of ovulation, fertilization of an ovum by a sperm, support of the developing embryo and fetus, and the birth and care of a newborn.

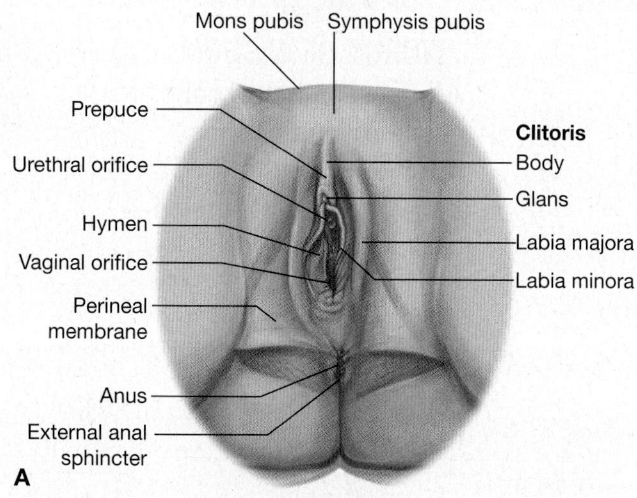

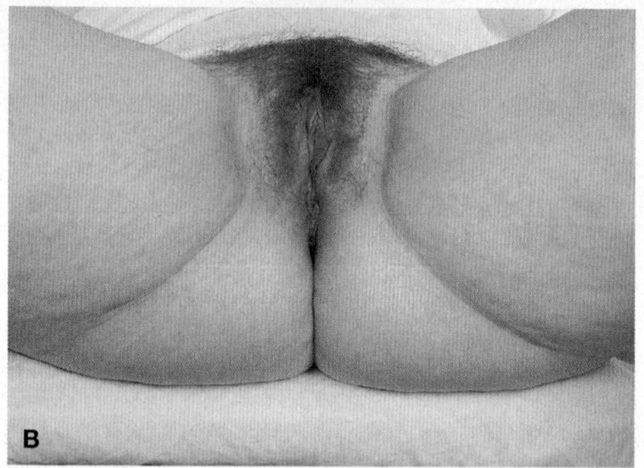

FIGURE 3.1 **A.** The external female reproductive organs. **B.** Normal appearance of external structures. (Photo by B. Proud.)

External Female Reproductive Organs

The external female reproductive organs are collectively called the **vulva** (which means "covering" in Latin). It encompasses the mons pubis, both sets of labia (majora and minora), the head of the clitoris and its prepuce, the structures within the vestibule, the opening of the urethra, the opening of the vagina, and the perineum (Fig. 3.1). The vulva serves to protect the urethral and vaginal openings, and this area, particularly the clitoris, is highly sensitive to touch to increase the female's pleasure during sexual arousal (Nath, 2023).

Mons Pubis

The mons pubis is the elevated, rounded, fleshy prominence made up of fatty tissue that overlays the symphysis pubis. The skin of this fatty tissue is covered with coarse, curly pubic hair after puberty. The mons pubis protects the symphysis pubis during sexual intercourse.

Labia

The labia majora (large lips), which are relatively large and fleshy, are comparable to the scrotum in males. The labia majora contain sweat and sebaceous (oil-secreting) glands; after puberty, they are covered with hair. Their function is to protect the vaginal opening and provide cushioning during sexual activity. The labia minora (small lips) are the delicate hairless inner folds of skin; they can be very small or up to 2 in wide. They lie just inside the labia majora and surround the openings to the vagina and urethra. The labia minora grow down from the anterior inner part of the labia majora on each side. These lips surround the vaginal opening and extend upward to form protection around both the clitoris and urethra. They are highly vascular and abundant in nerve supply. They lubricate the vulva, swell in response to stimulation, and are highly sensitive.

Clitoris and Prepuce

The clitoris is a small, cylindrical mass of erectile tissue and nerves. It is highly sensitive during arousal and stimulation and is analogous to the head of the penis. Unlike the penis, however, the function of the clitoris is purely erogenous. Most of the components of the clitoris are buried under the skin and connective tissue of the vulva. It is located at the anterior junction of the labia minora.

There are folds above and below the clitoris. The joining of the folds above the clitoris forms the prepuce, a hoodlike covering over the clitoris; the junction below the clitoris forms the frenulum.

TAKE NOTE!

The hoodlike covering over the clitoris is the site for female genital mutilation or cutting, which is a cultural ritual still practiced in some countries, including the United States. It is internationally recognized as a human rights violation against women.

A rich supply of blood vessels gives the clitoris a pink color. Like the penis, the clitoris is sensitive to touch, stimulation, and temperature and can become erect. For its small size, 9 to 11 cm, it has a generous blood and nerve supply. There are more free nerve endings of sensory reception located on the clitoris than on any other part of the body, and it is therefore unsurprisingly the most erotically sensitive part of the genitalia for most females. Its function is sexual stimulation and is found in people assigned female at birth.

TAKE NOTE!

The word clitoris is from the Greek word for "key"; in ancient times, the clitoris was thought to be the key to female sexuality.

Vestibule

The vestibule is an oval area enclosed by the two labia minora laterally. It is inside the labia minora and outside of the hymen and is perforated by six openings. Opening into the vestibule are the urethra from the urinary bladder, the vagina, and two sets of glands. The opening to the vagina is called the introitus, and the half-moon-shaped area behind the opening is called the fourchette. Through tiny ducts beside the introitus, Bartholin glands, when stimulated, secrete mucus that supplies lubrication for intercourse. Skene glands are located on either side of the opening to the urethra. They secrete a small amount of mucus, which is believed to be antimicrobial, to keep the opening moist and lubricated for the passage of urine (Nguyen & Duong, 2023).

The vaginal opening is surrounded by the hymen. The hymen is a tough, elastic, perforated, mucosa-covered tissue across the vaginal introitus. Without a history of penetration, the hymen may completely cover the opening, but it usually encircles the opening like a tight ring. Because the degree of tightness varies among people, the hymen may tear at the first attempt at intercourse, or it may be so soft and pliable that no tearing occurs. The hymen may also tear during exercise or insertion of a tampon or diaphragm. In a female who has a history of penetration, the hymen usually appears as small tags of tissue surrounding the vaginal opening, but the presence or absence of the hymen can neither confirm nor rule out sexual experience (Mishori et al., 2019).

TAKE NOTE!

Heavy physical exertion, use of tampons, or injury to the area can alter the appearance of the hymen in females who have not been sexually active.

Perineum

The perineum is the most posterior part of the external female reproductive organs. This external region is located between the vulva and the anus. It is made up of skin, muscle, and fascia. The perineum can become lacerated or incised (episiotomy) during childbirth and may need to be repaired with sutures. Incising the perineum area to provide more space for the presenting part is called an episiotomy. See Chapter 14 for further information.

Internal Female Reproductive Organs

The internal female reproductive organs consist of the vagina, uterus, fallopian tubes, and ovaries (Fig. 3.2). These structures develop and function according to specific hormonal influences that affect fertility and childbearing.

Vagina

The **vagina** is a highly muscular and distensible canal situated in front of the rectum and behind the bladder. It is a tubular, fibromuscular organ lined with mucous membrane that lies in a series of transverse folds called rugae. The rugae allow for extreme dilation of the canal during labor and birth. The vagina is a canal that connects the external genitals (vulva) to the cervix. It receives the penis and the sperm ejaculated during sexual intercourse, and it serves as an exit passageway for menstrual blood and for the fetus during childbirth. The front and back walls normally touch each other so that there is no space in the vagina except when it is opened (e.g., during a pelvic examination or intercourse). In the adult, the vaginal cavity is 3 to 4 in long. Muscles that control its diameter surround the lower third of the vagina. The upper two thirds of the vagina lie above these muscles and can be stretched easily. During the female reproductive years, the mucosal lining of the vagina has a corrugated appearance and is resistant to bacterial colonization. Before puberty and after menopause (if the person is not taking estrogen), the mucosa is smooth due to lower levels of estrogen. Genitourinary syndrome of menopause

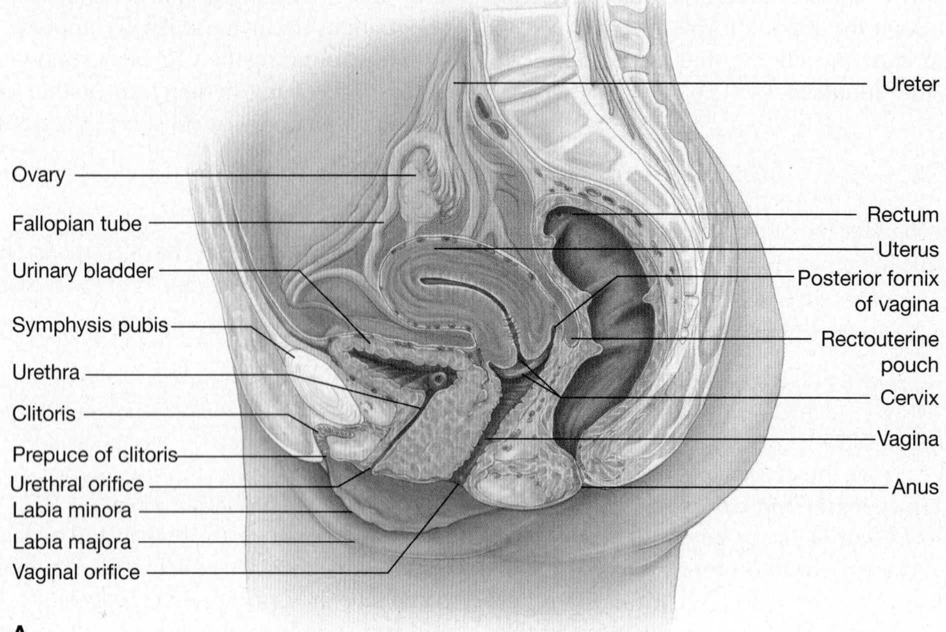

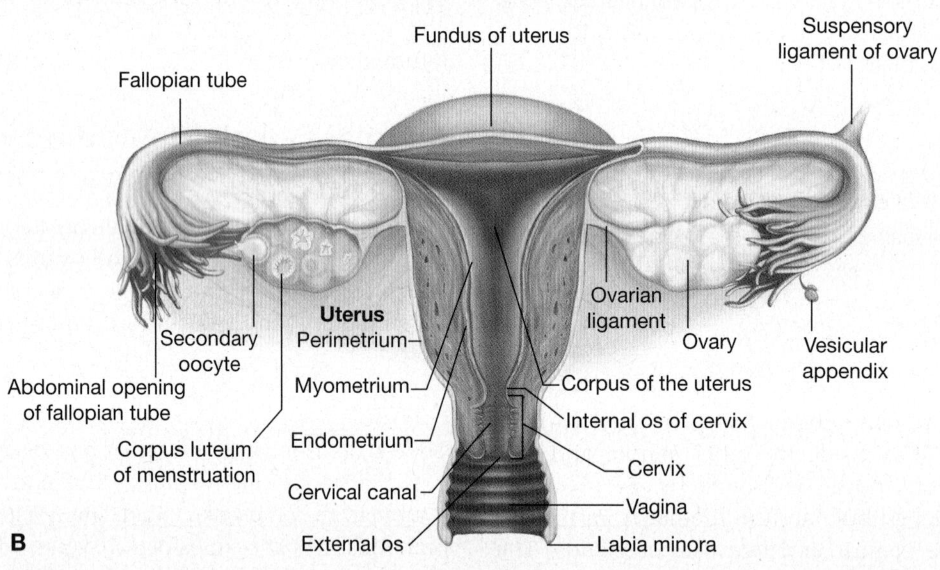

FIGURE 3.2 The internal female reproductive organs. **A.** Lateral view. **B.** Anterior view. (Reprinted with permission from Anatomical Chart Company. [2001]. *Atlas of human anatomy*. Springhouse.)

(GSM) occurs when estrogen is reduced and can have adverse effects on the health and quality of life in midlife. This syndrome includes genital dryness, burning and irritation, lack of vaginal lubrication, urinary symptoms of urgency, dysuria, dyspareunia, and recurrent urinary tract infections. Physical changes may include labial atrophy, vaginal dryness, and clitoral atrophy (Agency for Healthcare Research and Quality [AHRQ], 2023).

The vagina has an acidic environment, which protects it against ascending infections. Antibiotic therapy, douching, perineal hygiene sprays, and deodorants upset the acid balance within the vaginal environment and can predispose females to infections.

Uterus

The uterus is an inverted, pear-shaped muscular organ at the top of the vagina. It lies behind the bladder and in front of the rectum and is anchored in position by eight ligaments, though it is not firmly attached or adherent to any part of the skeleton. A full bladder tilts the uterus backward; a distended rectum tilts it forward. The uterus alters its position by gravity or with change of posture, and it is the size and shape of an inverted pear. It is the site of menstruation, receiving a fertilized ovum, development of the fetus during pregnancy, and contracting to help in the expulsion of the fetus and placenta. Before the first pregnancy, it measures approximately 3 in long, 2 in wide, and 1 in thick. After a pregnancy, the uterus remains larger than before the pregnancy. After menopause, it becomes smaller and atrophies.

The uterine wall is relatively thick and composed of three layers: the endometrium (innermost layer), the myometrium (muscular middle layer), and the perimetrium (outer serosal layer that covers the body of the uterus). The **endometrium** is the mucosal layer that lines the uterine cavity in nonpregnant people. It varies in thickness from 0.5 to 5 mm and has an abundant supply of glands and blood vessels. It is the primary target tissue for the hormone estrogen (Yu et al., 2022). The myometrium makes up the major portion of the uterus and is composed of smooth muscle linked by connective tissue with numerous elastic fibers. During pregnancy, the upper myometrium undergoes marked hypertrophy, but there is limited change in the cervical muscle content.

Anatomic subdivisions of the uterus include the convex portion above the uterine tubes (the fundus); the central portion (the corpus or body) between the fundus and the cervix; and the cervix, or neck, which opens into the vagina.

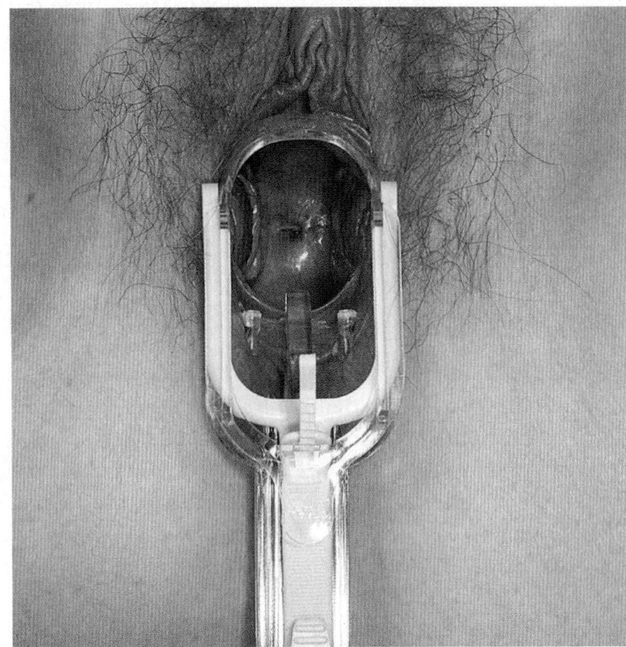

FIGURE 3.3 Appearance of normal cervix. Note. This is the cervix of a multipara female. (Photo by B. Proud.)

CERVIX

The **cervix**, the lower part of the uterus, is sometimes called the neck of the uterus. It opens into the vagina and has a channel that allows sperm to enter the uterus and menstrual discharge to exit. It is composed of fibrous connective tissue. During a pelvic examination, the part of the cervix that protrudes into the upper end of the vagina can be visualized. Like the vagina, this part of the cervix is covered by mucosa, which is smooth, firm, and doughnut shaped, with a visible central opening called the external os (Fig. 3.3). Before childbirth, the external cervical os is a small, regular, oval opening. After childbirth, the opening is converted into a transverse slit that resembles lips (Fig. 3.4). Except during menstruation or ovulation, the cervix is usually a good barrier against bacteria. The cervix has an alkaline environment, which protects the sperm from the acidic environment in the vagina.

The canal or channel of the cervix is lined with mucus-secreting glands. This mucus is thick and impenetrable to sperm until just before the ovaries release an egg (ovulation). At ovulation, the consistency of the mucus changes so that sperm can swim through it, allowing fertilization. At the same time, the mucus-secreting glands of the cervix actually become able to store live sperm for 2 or 3 days. These sperm can later move up through the corpus and into the fallopian tubes to fertilize the egg; thus, intercourse 1 or 2 days before ovulation can lead to pregnancy. Because ovulation is not always consistent, pregnancy can occur at varying times after the last menstrual period. During pregnancy, the cervix is the vital mechanical barrier that resists compressive and tensile loads generated from a growing fetus. The channel in the cervix is too narrow for the fetus to pass through during pregnancy, but during labor, it stretches to let the newborn through.

CORPUS

The corpus, or the main body of the uterus, is a highly muscular organ that enlarges to hold the fetus during pregnancy. The inner lining of the corpus (endometrium) undergoes cyclic changes as a result of the changing levels of hormones secreted by the ovaries; it is thickest during the part of the menstrual cycle in which a fertilized egg would be expected to enter the uterus and is thinnest just after menstruation. If fertilization does not take place during this cycle, most of the endometrium is shed and bleeding occurs, resulting in the monthly period. If fertilization does take place, the embryo attaches to the wall of the uterus, where it becomes embedded in the endometrium (about 1 week after fertilization); this process is called implantation. Implantation is the usual

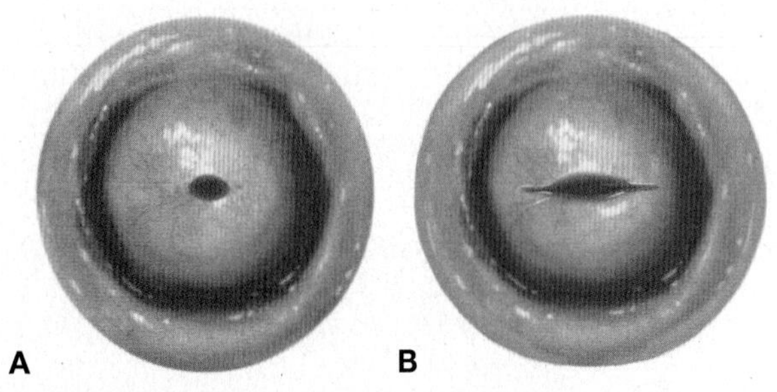

FIGURE 3.4 **A.** Nulliparous cervical os. **B.** Parous cervical os.

marker for the start of a pregnancy. Events that occur during the first week of conception include fertilization, mitotic cleavage of the blastomere, morula formation, blastocyst formation, and, finally, implantation of the blastocyst (Khan & Ackerman, 2023). Menstruation then ceases during the 40 weeks (280 days) of pregnancy. During labor, the muscular walls of the corpus contract to push the baby through the cervix and into the vagina.

Fallopian Tubes

The **fallopian tubes**, also known as oviducts, are hollow, cylindrical structures that extend 2 to 3 in from the upper edges of the uterus toward the ovaries. Each tube is about 7 to 10 cm long (4 in) and approximately 0.7 cm in diameter. The end of each tube flares into a funnel shape, providing a large opening for the egg to fall into when it is released from the ovary. Cilia (beating, hairlike extensions on cells) line the fallopian tube and the muscles in the tube's wall. The fallopian tubes convey the ovum from the ovary to the uterus and sperm from the uterus toward the ovary. This movement is accomplished via ciliary action and peristaltic contraction. If sperm are present in the fallopian tube as a result of sexual intercourse or artificial insemination, fertilization of the ovum can occur in the distal portion of the tube. If the egg is fertilized, it will divide over a period of 4 days while it moves slowly down the fallopian tube and into the uterus, where it implants into the uterine lining.

Ovaries

The **ovaries** are a set of paired glands resembling unshelled almonds that are the organs of gamete production in the female. They are set in the pelvic cavity below and to either side of the umbilicus. They are usually pearl colored, oblong, and have a lumpy surface. They are homologous to the testes. Each mature ovary is about 3.5 cm long, 2 cm wide, and 1 cm thick (Gibson & Mahdy, 2023). The ovaries are not attached to the fallopian tubes but are suspended nearby from several ligaments, which help hold them in position. The development and the release of the ovum and the secretion of the female hormones **estrogen** and **progesterone** are the two primary functions of the ovary. The ovaries link the reproductive system to the body's system of endocrine glands, as they produce the ova (eggs) and secrete estrogen and progesterone cyclically. After an ovum matures, it passes into the fallopian tubes.

Breasts

The two mammary glands, or **breasts**, are accessory organs of the female reproductive system that are specialized to secrete milk following pregnancy. They overlie the pectoralis major muscles and extend from the second to the sixth ribs and from the sternum to the axilla. Each breast has a nipple located near the tip, which is surrounded by a circular area of pigmented skin called the areola. Each breast is composed of approximately nine lobes (the number can range between 4 and 18), which contain glands (alveolar) and a duct (lactiferous) that leads to the nipple and opens to the outside (Fig. 3.5). Fibrous connective tissue and bands along with adipose tissue are dispersed between the lobes, which help support the weight of the breasts and give the breasts shape (Harigopal & Singh, 2022).

During pregnancy, placental estrogen and progesterone stimulate the development of the mammary glands. Because of this hormonal activity, the breasts may double in size during pregnancy in preparation for milk production. At the same time, glandular tissue replaces the adipose tissue of the breasts.

Following childbirth and the expulsion of the placenta, levels of placental hormones (progesterone and lactogen) fall rapidly, and the action of prolactin (milk-producing hormone) is no longer inhibited. Prolactin stimulates the production of milk within a few days after childbirth, but in the interim, dark yellow fluid called colostrum is secreted. Colostrum contains more minerals and protein but less sugar and fat than mature breast milk. Colostrum secretion may continue

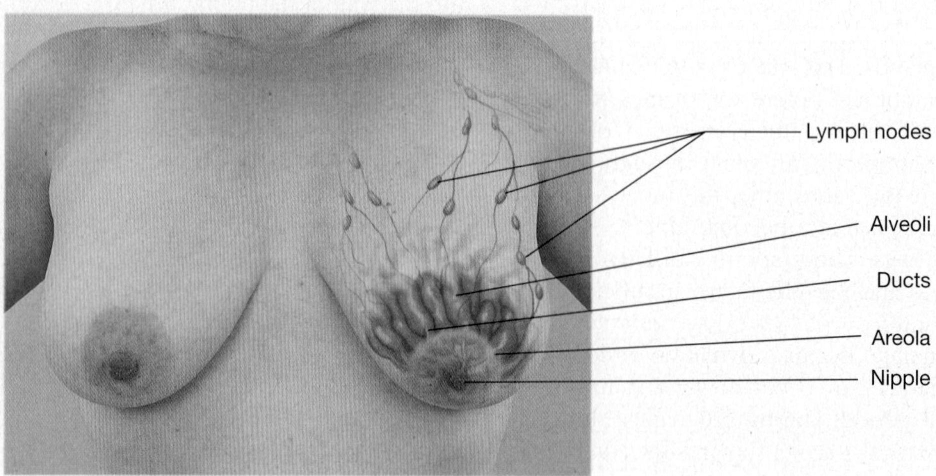

FIGURE 3.5 Anatomy of the breasts. (Photo by B. Proud.)

for approximately a week after childbirth, with gradual conversion to mature milk. Colostrum is rich in maternal antibodies, especially immunoglobulin A (IgA), which offers protection for the newborn against enteric pathogens.

Female Sexual Response

Sexual arousal is a physiologic response to internal and external stimuli and is mediated by both the central and peripheral nervous systems. The sexual response in females is governed primarily by the nervous system rather than by hormones. It is characterized by changes in sensation, tissue contractility, vasocongestion, and lubrication. The sexual cycle is usually thought of as having five phases: desire, excitement, plateau, orgasm, and resolution:

1. *Desire:* Starts with a desire for sexual intimacy, also known as *libido.*
2. *Excitement:* Females have a heightened sexual awareness. During sexual arousal, the brain coordinates a patterned sexual response cycle consisting of increased heart rate, respiratory rate, blood pressure, and general level of excitement (Sexual Medicine Society of North America [SMSNA], 2021). With sexual stimulation, tissues in the clitoris and breasts and around the vaginal orifice fill with blood and the erectile tissues swell. At the same time, the vagina begins to expand and elongate to accommodate the penis. As part of the whole vasocongestive reaction, the labia majora and minora swell and darken. As sexual stimulation intensifies, the vestibular glands secrete mucus to moisten and lubricate the tissues to facilitate insertion of the penis. Hormones play an integral role in the female sexual response as well. Adequate estrogen and testosterone must be available for the brain to sense incoming arousal stimuli. Research indicates that estrogen preserves the vascular function of female sex organs and affects genital sensation. It is also believed to promote blood flow to these areas during stimulation. Recent research findings also suggest that testosterone therapy improves sexual desire, arousal, and satisfaction in females (Shifren, 2022).
3. *Plateau:* The heart rate, blood pressure, level of muscle tension, and respiration rate all increase. During this phase, the penile erection intensifies and the vagina constricts around the penis. Continued stimulation of the clitoris and penis with movement leads to the next phase of the sexual response, the *orgasmic phase.*
4. *Orgasm:* The shortest phase of the sexual response is the orgasm. Orgasm is an intense sensation of pleasure achieved by stimulation of erogenous zones. Females experience rhythmic contractions of the pelvic muscles and vaginal walls. Typically, the person feels warm and relaxed after an orgasm. Within a short time after orgasm, the two physiologic mechanisms that created the sexual response, vasocongestion and muscle contraction, rapidly dissipate. The orgasmic experience varies from person to person and from time to time in the same person. Females do not have a refractory period after each orgasm and can therefore experience multiple orgasms. Clitoral sexual response and the female orgasm are not affected by aging.
5. *Resolution:* At the completion of the sexual episode, the brain and body return to an unaroused state, which is termed *sexual resolution.* During this phase, the heart rate, blood pressure, and respirations slow; the muscles relax. Frequently, fatigue sets in for both people.

THE FEMALE REPRODUCTIVE CYCLE

The female reproductive cycle functions to produce gametes and reproductive hormones. It is a complex process that encompasses an intricate series of chemical secretions and reactions to produce the ultimate potential for fertility and birth. The female reproductive cycle is a general term that includes the ovarian cycle, the endometrial (uterine) cycle, and the hormonal changes that regulate them. The endometrium, ovaries, pituitary gland, and hypothalamus are all involved in the cyclic changes that help prepare the body for fertilization. Absence of fertilization results in **menstruation**, the monthly shedding of the uterine lining. Menstruation marks the beginning and end of the monthly cycle. Menopause is the naturally occurring cessation of menstrual cycles.

The menstrual cycle results from a functional hypothalamic–pituitary–ovarian axis and a precise sequencing of hormones that lead to ovulation. The ovarian cycle, during which ovulation occurs, and the endometrial cycle, during which menstruation occurs, are divided at midcycle by ovulation. **Ovulation** occurs when the ovum is released from its follicle; after leaving the ovary, the ovum enters the fallopian tube and journeys toward the uterus. If a sperm cell fertilizes the ovum during its journey, pregnancy occurs (Fig. 3.6).

Menstrual Cycle Hormones

The menstrual cycle involves a complex interaction of hormones. The predominant hormones include gonadotropin-releasing hormone (GnRH), follicle-stimulating hormone (FSH), luteinizing hormone (LH), estrogen, progesterone, and prostaglandins. Box 3.1 summarizes menstrual cycle hormones.

Gonadotropin-Releasing Hormone

GnRH is secreted from the hypothalamus in a pulsatile manner throughout the reproductive cycle. It pulsates slowly during the follicular phase and increases during the luteal phase. GnRH causes the pituitary gland to induce the release of FSH and LH to assist with ovulation.

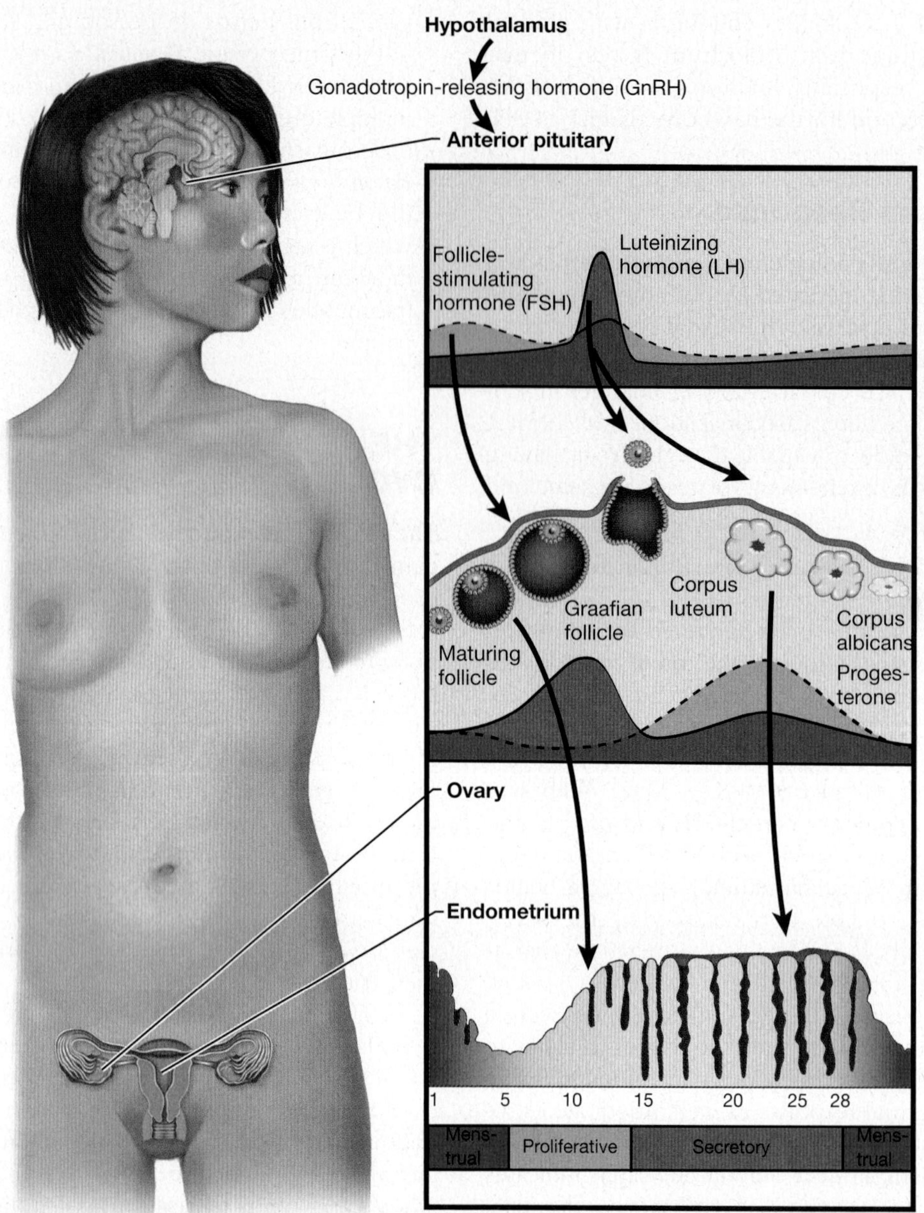

FIGURE 3.6 Menstrual cycle summary based on a 28-day (average) menstrual cycle.

BOX 3.1 Summary of Menstrual Cycle Hormones

- LH rises and stimulates the follicle to produce estrogen.
- As estrogen is produced by the follicle, estrogen levels rise, inhibiting the output of LH.
- Ovulation occurs after an LH surge damages the estrogen-producing cells, resulting in a decline in estrogen.
- The LH surge results in establishment of the corpus luteum, which produces estrogen and progesterone.
- Estrogen and progesterone levels rise, suppressing LH output.
- Lack of LH promotes degeneration of the corpus luteum.
- Cessation of the corpus luteum means a decline in estrogen and progesterone output.
- The decline of the ovarian hormones ends their negative effect on the secretion of LH.
- LH is secreted, and the menstrual cycle begins again.

LH, luteinizing hormone.

Follicle-Stimulating Hormone

FSH is secreted by the anterior pituitary gland and is primarily responsible for the release and maturation of the ovarian follicle. FSH secretion is highest and most important during the first week of the follicular phase of the reproductive cycle.

Luteinizing Hormone

LH is produced and secreted by the anterior pituitary gland and is required for both the final maturation of preovulatory follicles and luteinization of the ruptured follicle. LH stimulates ovulation and the formation of corpus luteum. As a result, estrogen production declines and progesterone secretion continues. Thus, estrogen levels fall a day before ovulation, and progesterone levels begin to rise.

Estrogen

Estrogen is a steroid hormone associated with the development of female sexual characteristics. Estrogen is secreted by the ovaries and is crucial for the development and maturation of the follicle. Estrogen is predominant at the end of the proliferative phase, directly preceding ovulation. After ovulation, estrogen levels drop sharply as progesterone dominates. In the endometrial cycle, estrogen induces proliferation of the endometrial glands. Estrogen also causes the uterus to increase in size and weight because of increased glycogen, amino acids, electrolytes, and water. Blood supply is expanded as well.

Progesterone

Progesterone is secreted by the corpus luteum, a temporary endocrine gland that is produced after ovulation during the second half of the menstrual cycle. Progesterone levels increase just before ovulation and peak 5 to 7 days after ovulation. During the luteal phase, progesterone induces swelling and increased secretion of the endometrium, which prepares it for the potential of pregnancy after ovulation. This hormone is often called the hormone of pregnancy because of its calming effect (reduces uterine contractions) on the uterus, allowing pregnancy to be maintained.

Prostaglandins

Prostaglandins are hormonelike primary mediators of the body's inflammatory processes and are essential for the normal physiologic function of the female reproductive system. They are a closely related group of oxygenated fatty acids that are produced by the endometrium with a variety of effects throughout the body. Prostaglandins increase during follicular maturation and play a key role in ovulation by freeing the ovum inside the graafian follicle. Large amounts of prostaglandins are found in menstrual blood. Current research suggests that the pathogenesis of menstrual cramps and pain is due to prostaglandin F2a (PGF2a), a potent myometrial stimulant and vasoconstrictor, in the secretory endometrium (Barcikowska et al., 2020). Elevated PGF levels are found in the endometrial fluid of females with dysmenorrhea (painful menses), and this correlates with their degree of pain (Barcikowska et al., 2020).

Ovarian Cycle

The ovarian cycle is a set of predictable changes in the female's oocytes and ovarian follicles. The series of events are associated with a developing oocyte (ovum or egg) within the ovaries. Whereas males manufacture sperm daily, often into advanced age, females are born with a single lifetime supply of ova that are released from the ovaries gradually throughout the childbearing years. In the female ovary, 600,000 to 1,000,000 oocytes are present at birth and by puberty this number has decreased in half (Park et al., 2022). Typically, a female ovulates one oocyte per month over an approximately 40-year reproductive lifespan. This accounts for the loss of 400 to 500 follicles. By age 50, follicular supply will be nearly zero, and most females will have reached menopause (Park et al., 2022). The ovarian cycle begins when the follicular cells (ovum and surrounding cells) swell and the maturation process starts. The maturing follicle at this stage is called a graafian follicle. The ovary raises many follicles monthly, but usually only one follicle matures to reach ovulation. The ovarian cycle consists of three phases: the follicular phase, ovulation, and the luteal phase.

Follicular Phase

This phase is so named because it is when the follicles in the ovary grow and form a mature egg. The goal of this phase is to produce an ovum for fertilization. This phase starts on day 1 of the menstrual cycle and continues until ovulation, approximately 10 to 14 days later. Increasing levels of estrogen secreted from the maturing follicular cells and the continued growth of the dominant follicle cell induce proliferation of the endometrium and myometrium. This thickening of the uterine lining supports an implanted ovum if pregnancy occurs. If no egg has been fertilized by male sperm, the top layers of the endometrium sluff off and menstrual bleeding occurs.

Prompted by the hypothalamus, the pituitary gland releases **follicle-stimulating hormone (FSH)**, which stimulates the ovary to produce immature follicles. Each follicle houses an immature oocyte or egg. The follicle that is targeted to mature fully will soon rupture and expel a mature oocyte in the process of ovulation. A surge in **luteinizing hormone (LH)** from the anterior pituitary gland is responsible for affecting the final development and subsequent rupture of the mature follicle. The follicular phase ends the day before the LH surge occurs (Welt, 2023).

Ovulation

Ovulation is the physiologic process defined by the release of an oocyte from the ovary into the fallopian tube where it has the potential to become fertilized by a sperm. At ovulation, a mature follicle ruptures in response to a surge of LH from the pituitary gland, releasing a mature oocyte. The LH surge is the trigger that sets in motion and coordinates both the final stages of oocyte maturation and follicular rupture. No one single event causes ovulation. This occurs approximately on day 14 in a 28-day cycle. When ovulation occurs, there is a drop in estrogen. Typically, ovulation takes place approximately 36 hours after the LH surge (Welt, 2023). The distal ends of the fallopian tubes become active near the time of ovulation and create currents that help carry the ovum into the uterus. The lifespan of the ovum is only about 24 hours; unless it meets a sperm on its journey within that time, it will die.

During ovulation, the cervix produces thin, clear, stretchy, slippery mucus that is designed to capture the sperm, nourish it, and help the sperm travel up through the cervix to meet the ovum for fertilization. Ovulation symptoms also include vaginal spotting, an increase in vaginal discharge, giving the person a "feeling of wetness," increased libido leading to more desire to be intimate, a slight rise in basal body temperature, and lower abdominal cramping.

The one constant, whether a menstrual cycle is 28 days or 120 days, is that ovulation takes place at least 14 days before menstruation (Holesh et al., 2023). Research finds that ovulation occurs more often from the right ovary; oocytes from the right ovary have a better chance for pregnancy than those from the left ovary (Fukuda et al., 2022).

TAKE NOTE!

Over 40% of females may feel a pain on one side of the abdomen around the time the egg is released (Brott & Le, 2023). This midcycle pain is called mittelschmerz.

CONSIDER THIS!

We had been married for 2 years when my husband and I decided to start a family. I began thinking back to my high school biology class and tried to remember about ovulation and what to look for. I also used the internet to find the answers I was seeking. As I was reading, it all started to come into place. During ovulation, cervical mucus increases and the ovulating person experiences a wet sensation for several days midcycle. The mucus also becomes stretchable during this time. In addition, body temperature rises slightly and then falls if no conception takes place. Armed with this knowledge, I began to check my temperature daily before arising and began to monitor the consistency of my cervical mucus. I figured that monitoring these two signs of ovulation could help me discover the best time to conceive. After 6 months of trying without results, I wondered what I was doing wrong. Did I really understand my body's reproductive activity?

Thoughts: What additional suggestions might the nurse offer this person in their journey to conception? What community resources might be available to assist this couple? How does knowledge of the reproductive system help nurses care for people who are trying to become pregnant?

Luteal Phase

The luteal phase begins at ovulation and lasts until the menstrual phase of the next cycle. It typically occurs on days 15 through 28 of a 28-day cycle. After the follicle ruptures as it releases the egg, it closes and forms a corpus luteum. The corpus luteum secretes increasing amounts of the hormone progesterone, which interacts with the endometrium to prepare it for implantation. At the beginning of the luteal phase, progesterone induces the endometrial glands to secrete glycogen, mucus, and other substances. These glands become tortuous and have large lumens due to increased secretory activity. The progesterone secreted by the corpus luteum causes the temperature of the body to rise slightly until the start of the next period. A significant increase in temperature, usually 0.5°F to 1°F (0.28°C–0.56°C), is generally seen within a day or two after ovulation has occurred; the temperature remains elevated until 3 days before the onset of the next menstruation. If the basal body temperature elevation does not decrease, it could be an early sign of pregnancy (Steward & Raja, 2023). This rise in temperature can be plotted on a graph and gives an indication of when ovulation has occurred. In the absence of fertilization, the corpus luteum begins to degenerate and consequently ovarian hormone levels decrease. As estrogen and progesterone levels decrease, the endometrium undergoes involution. FSH and LH are generally at their lowest levels during the luteal phase and highest during the follicular phase.

Endometrial (Uterine) Cycle

The endometrial (uterine) cycle occurs in response to cyclic hormonal changes. The four phases of the endometrial cycle are the proliferative phase, secretory phase, ischemic phase, and menstrual phase.

Proliferative Phase

The proliferative phase of the endometrial cycle corresponds to the follicular phase of the ovarian cycle. It starts with enlargement of the endometrial glands in response to dramatically increasing amounts of estrogen. The blood vessels become dilated, and the endometrium gradually increases in thickness in preparation for implantation of the fertilized ovum (Welt, 2023). Cervical mucus becomes thin, clear, stretchy, and more alkaline, making it more favorable to sperm to enhance the opportunity for fertilization. The proliferative phase starts on about day 5 of the menstrual cycle and lasts until the time of ovulation. This phase depends on estrogen stimulation resulting from ovarian follicles, and this phase coincides with the follicular phase of the ovarian cycle.

Secretory Phase

The secretory phase begins at ovulation to about 3 days before the next menstrual period. Under the influence of progesterone released by the corpus luteum after ovulation, the endometrium becomes thickened and more vascular (growth of the spiral arteries) and glandular (secretion of more glycogen and lipids). These dramatic changes are all in preparation for implantation if it is to occur. This phase typically lasts from day 15 (after ovulation) to day 28 and coincides with the luteal phase of the ovarian cycle. In the absence of fertilization by day 23 of the menstrual cycle, the corpus luteum begins to degenerate and consequently ovarian hormone levels decrease. As estrogen and progesterone levels decrease, the endometrium undergoes involution.

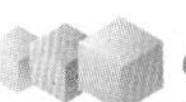
Concept Mastery Alert

Proliferative Versus Secretory Phases of the Uterine Cycle

During the proliferative phase, the ovarian follicles are producing increased amounts of estrogen, and the endometrium prepares for possible fertilization with pronounced growth. The secretory phase begins at the time of ovulation. If the ovum is not fertilized, then the corpus luteum degenerates and hormone levels fall, ultimately resulting in menstruation.

Ischemic Phase

If fertilization does not occur, the ischemic phase begins. Estrogen and progesterone levels drop sharply during this phase as the corpus luteum starts to degenerate. Changes in the endometrium occur with spasm of the arterioles, resulting in ischemia of the basal layer. The ischemia leads to shedding of the endometrium down to the basal layer, and menstrual flow begins.

Menstrual Phase

The menstrual phase begins as the spiral arteries rupture secondary to ischemia, releasing blood into the uterus, and the sloughing of the endometrial lining begins. If fertilization does not take place, the corpus luteum degenerates. As a result, both estrogen and progesterone levels fall, and the thickened endometrial lining sloughs away from the uterine wall and passes out through the vagina. The beginning of the menstrual flow marks the end of one menstrual cycle and the start of a new one. Menstruation is a term derived from the Latin word *mensis*, meaning "month." It is the normal, predictable physiologic process that typically occurs monthly. The normal number of days of menstrual bleeding is defined as less than or equal to 8 days. The amount of menstrual flow varies and is subjective. Normal volume is considered menstrual blood loss that does not disrupt physical, social, and emotional quality of life but can be quantified as less than or equal to 80 mL in volume per cycle (Welt, 2023).

Menstruation has many effects on menstruating people, including emotional and self-image changes. Menarche is defined as the first period of a female adolescent. In the United States, the average age at **menarche** is 12.4 years with a range between 10 and 16 and varies by race and ethnicity (Biro & Chan, 2023; Lacroix et al., 2023). Genetics is an important factor in determining the age at which menarche starts, but general health, nutritional status, socioeconomic conditions, exercise, and family environment are also important (Biro & Chan, 2023; Lacroix et al., 2023).

Pubertal events preceding the first menses have an orderly progression: thelarche, the development of breast buds; adrenarche, the appearance of pubic and then axillary hair followed by a growth spurt; and menarche (occurring about 2 years after the start of breast development). In healthy pubertal females, the menstrual period varies in flow heaviness and may remain irregular in occurrence for up to 2 years following menarche. After that time, the regular menstrual cycle should be established. Normal, regular menstrual cycles vary in frequency and blood loss (Welt, 2023).

Think back to Linda, who was introduced at the beginning of the chapter. What questions might need to be asked to assess her condition? What laboratory work might be anticipated to validate her heavier flow?

Although menstruation is a normal process, various cultures have taken a wide variety of attitudes toward it, seeing it as everything from a sacred time to an unclean time. Cultural beliefs surrounding menstrual-related matters have considerable implications for symptom expression and treatment-seeking behavior. Recent research findings imply the need for education and improved access to period products to help adolescents manage menstrual symptoms and increase awareness of the benefit of treating them (Schmitt et al., 2022). Given that menstrual-related information comes from familial, societal, and cultural sources, negative attitudes toward monthly cycles can be formed in young, impressionable females. Many adolescents lack adequate education about menstruation. Nurses, through formal instruction or casual one-on-one discussions, can open doors to many conversations with young patients to help shape good menstrual attitudes and a more positive image of this natural physiologic process.

TAKE NOTE!

Knowledge about menstruation has increased significantly, and attitudes have changed. What was once discussed only behind closed doors is discussed openly today.

Perimenopause and Menopause

Perimenopause or menopausal transition and menopause are biologic markers of the transition from young adulthood to middle age. Perimenopause is the period between the onset of irregular menstrual cycles and the last menstrual period. Neither of these is a symptom or disease but rather a natural maturing of the reproductive system.

Menopause is a universal and irreversible part of the overall aging process involving the female reproductive system after menstruation ends. This naturally occurring phase in every female body marks the end of childbearing capacity. The average age of natural menopause—defined as 1 year without a menstrual period—is 51.4 years old, with a typical range somewhere between 47 and 55 years; however, this varies among different people and populations (Casper, 2023; Endocrine Society, 2022).

See Chapter 4 for more information about menopausal transition and menopause.

Recall Linda, who was experiencing changes in her menstrual patterns. Which hormones might be changing, and which systems might they affect? What approach should the nurse take to enlighten Linda about what is happening in her body?

KEY CONCEPTS

- The female reproductive system produces the female reproductive cells (the eggs or ova) and contains an organ (uterus) where the fetus develops.
- The internal female reproductive organs consist of the vagina, the uterus, the fallopian tubes, and the ovaries. The external female reproductive organs make up the vulva. These include the mons pubis, the labia majora and minora, the clitoris and prepuce, structures within the vestibule, and the perineum.
- The breasts are accessory organs of the female reproductive system that are specialized to secrete milk following pregnancy.
- The main function of the reproductive cycle is to stimulate growth of a follicle to release an egg and prepare a site for implantation if fertilization occurs.
- Menstruation, the monthly shedding of the uterine lining, marks the beginning and end of the cycle if fertilization does not occur.
- The ovarian cycle is the series of events associated with a developing oocyte (ovum or egg) within the ovaries.
- At ovulation, a mature follicle ruptures in response to a surge of LH, releasing a mature oocyte (ovum).
- The endometrial cycle is divided into four phases: the follicular or proliferative phase, the luteal or secretory phase, the ischemic phase, and the menstrual phase.
- The menstrual cycle involves a complex interaction of hormones. The predominant hormones are GnRH, FSH, LH, estrogen, progesterone, and prostaglandins.

REFERENCES AND RECOMMENDED READINGS

Agency for Healthcare Research and Quality. (2023). *Genitourinary syndrome of menopause.* https://effectivehealthcare.ahrq.gov/products/genitourinary-syndrome/protocol

Barcikowska, Z., Rajkowska-Labon, E., Grzybowska, M. E., Hansdorfer-Korzon, R., & Zorena, K. (2020). Inflammatory markers in dysmenorrhea and therapeutic options. *International Journal of Environmental Research and Public Health, 17*(4), 1191. https://doi.org/10.3390/ijerph17041191

Biro, F. M., & Chan, Y. M. (2023). Normal puberty. *UpToDate.* Retrieved March 4, 2024, from https://www.uptodate.com/contents/normal-puberty

Brott, N. R., & Le, J. K. (2023). Mittelschmerz. *StatPearls.* https://www.ncbi.nlm.nih.gov/books/NBK549822/

Casper, R. F. (2023). Clinical manifestations and diagnosis of menopause. *UpToDate.* Retrieved March 3, 2024, from https://www.uptodate.com/contents/clinical-manifestations-and-diagnosis-of-menopause

Endocrine Society. (2022). *Menopause.* https://www.endocrine.org/patient-engagement/endocrine-library/menopause

Fukuda, M., Fukuda, K., Mason, S., Tatsumi, K., Shimizu, T., Akahori, T., Matsumoto, T., Tahara, M., & Andersen, C. Y. (2022). Ovulation patterns affect the offspring sex ratios and change with the women's age. *Reproductive health, 19*(1), 159. https://doi.org/10.1186/s12978-022-01462-2

Gibson, E., & Mahdy, H. (2023). Anatomy, abdomen and pelvis, ovary. *StatPearls.* https://www.ncbi.nlm.nih.gov/books/NBK545187/

Harigopal, M., & Singh, K. (2022). Breast development and morphology. *UpToDate.* Retrieved February 29, 2024, from https://www.uptodate.com/contents/breast-development-and-morphology

Holesh, J. E., Bass, A. N., & Lord, M. (2023). Physiology, ovulation. *StatPearls.* https://www.ncbi.nlm.nih.gov/books/NBK441996/

Khan, Y. S., & Ackerman, K. M. (2023). Embryology, week 1. *StatPearls.* https://www.ncbi.nlm.nih.gov/books/NBK554562/

Lacroix, A. E., Gondal, H., Shumway, K. R., & Langaker, M. D. (2023). Physiology, menarche. *StatPearls.* https://www.ncbi.nlm.nih.gov/books/NBK470216/

Mishori, R., Ferdowsian, H., Naimer, K., Volpellier, M., & McHale, T. (2019). The little tissue that couldn't—Dispelling myths about the Hymen's role in determining sexual history and assault. *Reproductive Health, 16*(1), 74. https://doi.org/10.1186/s12978-019-0731-8

Nath, J. (2023). Altered reproductive function. In J. Nath (Ed.), *Applied pathophysiology* (4th ed., pp. 344–369). Wolters Kluwer.

Nguyen, J. D., & Duong, H. (2023). Anatomy, abdomen and pelvis: Female external genitalia. *StatPearls.* https://www.ncbi.nlm.nih.gov/books/NBK547703/

Park, C. J., Oh, J. E., Feng, J., Cho, Y. M., Qiao, H., & Ko, C. (2022). Lifetime changes of the oocyte pool: Contributing factors with a focus on ovulatory inflammation. *Clinical and Experimental Reproductive Medicine, 49*(1), 16–25. https://doi.org/10.5653/cerm.2021.04917

Schmitt, M. L., Booth, K., & Sommer, M. (2022). A policy for addressing menstrual equity in schools: A case study from New York city, U.S.A. *Frontiers in Reproductive Health*, *3*, 725805. https://doi.org/10.3389/frph.2021.725805

Sexual Medicine Society of North America. (2021). *An overview of the sexual response cycle*. https://www.smsna.org/news/smsna/an-overview-of-the-sexual-response-cycle

Shifren, J. L. (2022). Overview of sexual dysfunction in females: Epidemiology, risk factors, and evaluation. *UpToDate*. https://www.uptodate.com/contents/overview-of-sexual-dysfunction-in-females-epidemiology-risk-factors-and-evaluation

Steward, K., & Raja, A. (2023). Physiology, ovulation and basal body temperature. *StatPearls*. https://pubmed.ncbi.nlm.nih.gov/31536292/

Welt, C. K. (2023). Normal menstrual cycle. *UpToDate*. Retrieved February 29, 2024, from https://www.uptodate.com/contents/normal-menstrual-cycle

Yu, K., Huang, Z. Y., Xu, X. L., Li, J., Fu, X. W., & Deng, S. L. (2022). Estrogen receptor function: Impact on the human endometrium. *Frontiers in Endocrinology*, *13*, 827724. https://pubmed.ncbi.nlm.nih.gov/35295981/

DEVELOPING CLINICAL JUDGMENT

PRACTICING FOR NCLEX

1. The predominant anterior pituitary hormone that orchestrates the menstrual cycle is
   a. thyroid-stimulating hormone (TSH).
   b. follicle-stimulating hormone (FSH).
   c. corticotropin-releasing hormone (CRH).
   d. gonadotropin-releasing hormone (GnRH).
2. Which glands are located on either side of the female urethra and secrete mucus to keep the opening moist and lubricated for urination?
   a. Cowper
   b. Bartholin
   c. Skene
   d. Seminal
3. What event occurs during the proliferative phase of the menstrual cycle?
   a. Menstrual flow starts.
   b. Endometrium thickens.
   c. Ovulation occurs.
   d. Progesterone secretion peaks.
4. Which hormone is produced in high levels to prepare the endometrium for implantation just after ovulation by the corpus luteum?
   a. Estrogen
   b. Prostaglandins
   c. Prolactin
   d. Progesterone
5. The nurse is preparing to teach a class regarding the most common vasomotor symptoms experienced during menopause and possible modalities of treatment available. Which are common vasomotor symptoms?
   a. Chronic fatigue and confusion
   b. Forgetfulness and irritability
   c. Night sweats and hot flashes
   d. Decrease in sexual response and appetite

CRITICAL THINKING EXERCISE

1. The school nurse was asked to speak to a 10th-grade biology class about menstruation. The teacher felt that the students did not understand this monthly event and wanted the nurse to dispel some myths about it. After the nurse explains the factors influencing the menses, one girl asks, "Could someone get pregnant if she has sex during her period?"
   a. How should the nurse respond to this question?
   b. What factor regarding the menstrual cycle was not clarified?
   c. What additional topics might this question lead to that might be discussed?

STUDY ACTIVITIES

1. Should sex education be taught in public schools, and if so, what topics should be addressed? Debate the pros and cons of teaching this and outline which topics should be covered.
2. Respond to the following as a topic sentence: "When I was growing up, talking about sexual matters with my parents was _____ because ______. Now the situation is ______."
3. List the predominant hormones and their functions in the menstrual cycle.
4. The ovarian cycle describes the series of events associated with the development of the ____________ within the ovaries.

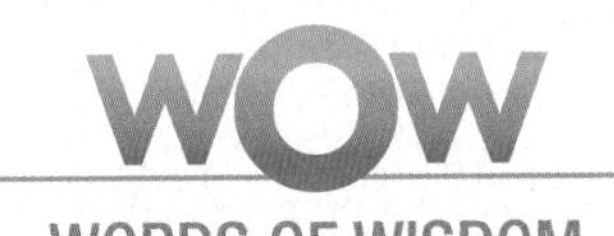

WORDS OF WISDOM

When female patients bare their souls, nurses must respond without judgment.

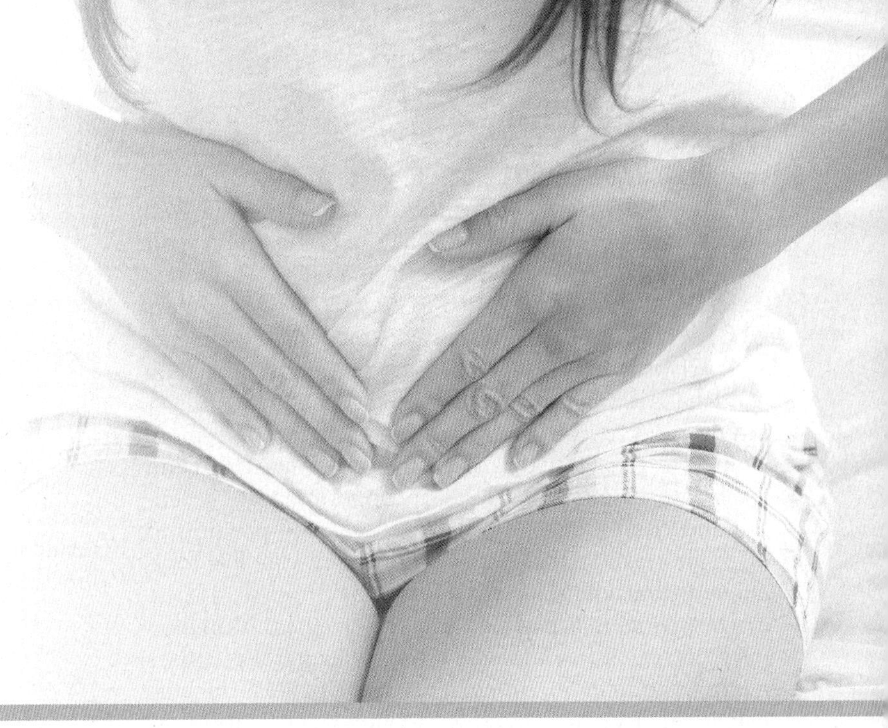

4

Common Gynecologic Issues

KEY TERMS

abnormal uterine bleeding (AUB)
abortion
amenorrhea (ā-men′ŏ-rē′ă)
basal body temperature (BBT)
cervical cap
cervical mucus ovulation method
coitus interruptus (kō′i-tŭs in-tĕr-rŭ-p′tŭs)
condoms
contraception (kon′tră-sep′shŭ-n)
contraceptive sponge
Depo-Provera
diaphragm
dysmenorrhea (dis-men′ōr-ē′ ă)
dyspareunia (dis′păr-ū′nē-ă)
emergency contraception (EC)
endometriosis (en′dō-mē-trē-ō′sis)
fertility awareness
implant
infertility
intrauterine devices (IUDs)
lactational amenorrhea method (LAM)
menopausal transition
oral contraceptives (OCs)
osteoporosis (os′tē-ō-pŏr-ō′sis)
premenstrual disorders (PMD)
sexual abstinence
standard days method (SDM)
sterilization
symptothermal method
transdermal patch
tubal ligation
vaginal ring
vasectomy (vas-ek′tŏ-mē)

LEARNING OBJECTIVES

Upon completion of the chapter, you will be able to:

1. Examine common gynecologic concerns in terms of symptoms, diagnostic tests, and appropriate interventions.
2. Evaluate risk factors and outline appropriate patient education needed in common gynecologic disorders.
3. Delineate the nursing management needed for patients experiencing common gynecologic disorders.
4. Analyze the physiologic and psychological aspects of menopausal transition.
5. Compare and contrast the various contraceptive methods available and their overall effectiveness.
6. Explore the challenges associated with induced abortion in our society today.

Izzy, a 27-year-old patient, presents to her health care provider complaining of progressive severe pelvic pain associated with her monthly periods. She has to take off work and "dope up" with pills to endure the pain. In addition, she has been trying to conceive for over a year without any results.

INTRODUCTION

Good health throughout the life cycle begins with the individual. People today can expect to live well into their 80s and need to be proactive in maintaining their own quality of life. Patients must take steps to reduce their risk of disease and need to become active partners with their health care professionals to identify problems early when treatment may be most successful (Teaching Guidelines 4.1). Nurses can assist patients in maintaining their quality of life by helping them become more attuned to their bodies and their bodies' clues and can use the assessment period as an opportunity for teaching and counseling. Nurses are in a prime position to offer information that provides patients with the tools needed to maintain healthy lifestyles and assist in altering behaviors that may cause harm or illness. Common reproductive issues addressed in this chapter that nurses might encounter in caring for female patients include menstrual disorders, infertility, contraception, abortion, and the menopausal transition.

MENSTRUAL CONCERNS

Menstrual patterns can be an indicator of overall health and self-perception of well-being. Many people sail through their monthly menstrual cycles with little or no concerns. With few symptoms to worry about, their menses are like clockwork, starting and stopping at nearly the same times every month. For others, the menstrual cycle causes physical and emotional symptoms that initiate visits to their health care providers for consultation. The following menstruation-related conditions will be discussed in this section: amenorrhea, dysmenorrhea, abnormal uterine bleeding (AUB), premenstrual syndrome (PMS), premenstrual dysphoric disorder (PMDD), menopausal transition and menopause, and endometriosis.

TEACHING GUIDELINES 4.1 Tips for Being an Active Partner in Managing Your Health

- Become an informed consumer. Read, ask, and search.
- Know family history and know factors that put you at high risk for different disorders.
- Maintain a healthy lifestyle and let moderation be your guide.
- Complete preventive screenings, exams, and immunizations as recommended.
- Schedule regular medical checkups and screenings for early detection.
- Ask your health care provider for a full explanation of any treatment.
- Seek a second medical opinion if you feel you need more information.
- Know when to seek medical care by being aware of disease symptoms.
- Take control of your own health and don't let it take control of you!

Amenorrhea

Amenorrhea simply means the absence of menses. It is a symptom, not a diagnosis. Amenorrhea is normal in prepubertal, pregnant, postpartum, and postmenopausal females. It usually indicates a dysfunction somewhere in the hypothalamic–pituitary–ovarian–uterine axis to induce cyclic changes in the endometrium that normally result in menses. All of these parts of the body must function properly and in harmony for a menstrual cycle to occur. Amenorrhea is categorized as either primary or secondary. Primary amenorrhea is defined as the failure to reach menarche in females of reproductive age. Of females living in the United States, 98% menstruate by age 15 (Lacroix et al., 2023). Studies over the past 30 years suggest that pubertal development, and hence menarche, continues to begin earlier in Americans than it did decades ago (Biro & Chan, 2023). Once menarche has occurred, cycles may take up to 2 years to become regular, ovulatory cycles. Secondary amenorrhea is the absence of regular menses for three cycles or irregular menses for 6 months in those who have previously menstruated regularly and are not pregnant, breastfeeding, or menopausal.

Nurses need to consider the causes of amenorrhea as due to one of many factors including ovarian failure, polycystic ovarian syndrome, congenital absence of the uterus and vagina, gonadotropin-releasing hormone (GnRH) deficiency, elevated follicle-stimulating hormone (FSH) levels, or constitutional delay of puberty. Outflow area problems are obstructive in nature and can be found on physical exam, while ovarian, pituitary, and central nervous system problems involve disruptions in the hypothalamic–pituitary–ovarian–uterine axis that controls the neuroendocrine processes required for a normal menstrual cycle and are generally found through laboratory analysis (Gasner & Rehman, 2023).

Etiology

Primary amenorrhea is typically caused by a genetic or anatomic abnormality; common causes include:

- Congenital abnormalities of the reproductive system
- Turner syndrome—defective development of the gonads (ovary or testes)
- Müllerian agenesis (absence of vagina, sometimes with the absence of uterus)
- Physiologic delay of puberty
- Isolated GnRH deficiency
- Transverse vaginal septum

- Stress from a major life event
- Excessive exercise
- Weight loss/eating disorders (anorexia nervosa)
- Polycystic ovary syndrome (PCOS)
- Hypothyroidism
- Imperforate hymen
- Chronic illness—diabetes, thyroid disease, depression
- Pregnancy
- Ovarian or adrenal tumors (Welt & Barbieri, 2023a)

Causes of secondary amenorrhea can include:

- Pregnancy
- Intrauterine adhesions (Asherman syndrome)
- Functional hypothalamus amenorrhea (functional hypothalamic GnRH deficiency) may be related to eating disorders, stress, or excessive exercise
- Systemic diseases such as type 1 diabetes mellitus and celiac disease
- Pituitary, ovarian, or adrenal tumors
- Hyperprolactinemia
- Postpartum pituitary necrosis (Sheehan syndrome)
- Hyperthyroid or hypothyroid conditions
- PCOS
- Primary ovarian insufficiency (premature ovarian failure) (Welt & Barbieri, 2023b)

Therapeutic Management

Therapeutic intervention depends on the cause of the amenorrhea. The treatment of primary and secondary amenorrhea focuses on the correction of the underlying issue, interventions to achieve fertility if wanted, and treatment to prevent complications of the disease such as estrogen replacement therapy to stimulate the development of secondary sexual characteristics if they are absent or to prevent osteoporosis (Welt & Barbieri, 2022a, 2022b). Treatment modalities may include surgery and medications, but specific treatment type is based on the underlying cause of the primary or secondary amenorrhea.

Nursing Assessment

Nursing assessment for the patient experiencing amenorrhea includes a thorough health history, physical examination, and laboratory and diagnostic tests of selected hormone levels to help identify any underlying causes.

HEALTH HISTORY AND PHYSICAL EXAMINATION

A thorough history and physical examination are needed to determine the etiology. The history should include questions about the patient's menstrual onset and patterns; eating and exercise habits; presence of psychosocial stressors; body weight changes; past illnesses; hospitalizations and surgeries; obstetric history; use of prescription and over-the-counter drugs; recent or past lifestyle changes; and history of present illness with an assessment of any bodily changes.

The physical examination should begin with an overall assessment of the patient's nutritional status and general health. A sensitive and gentle approach to the pelvic examination is critical, especially in young patients. Height, weight, and body mass index (BMI) should be taken, along with vital signs. Hypothermia, bradycardia, hypotension, and reduced subcutaneous fat may be observed in patients with anorexia nervosa. Facial hair and acne might be evidence of androgen excess secondary to a tumor. The presence or absence of axillary and pubic hair may indicate adrenal and ovarian hyposecretion or delayed puberty. A general physical examination may uncover unexpected findings that are indirectly related to amenorrhea. For example, a low hairline and webbed neck may indicate the presence of Turner syndrome (Welt & Barbieri, 2022a). Examination of the breasts also deserves careful attention because breast development is a reliable indicator of estrogen production. The sexual maturity rating scale developed by Tanner in 1962 is used to describe breast development and should be noted to describe breast development. The Tanner stages include:

- Stage I—Papilla elevation only (tip of the nipple is raised)
- Stage II—Breast buds palpable and areolae enlarge at approximately 11 years old.
- Stage III—Elevation of breast contour; areolae enlarge at approximately 12 years old.
- Stage IV—Areolae forms a secondary mound on the breast at approximately 13 years old.
- Stage V—Adult breast contour; areola recesses to breast contour (Tanner, 1962).

Information gained from the history and physical exam can clearly exclude certain diagnostic possibilities, but first impressions can be deceiving and lead to errors in judgment. A methodical, systematic approach to identify the etiology of amenorrhea is best.

LABORATORY AND DIAGNOSTIC TESTS

Common laboratory tests that might be ordered to determine the cause of amenorrhea include:

- Karyotype (might be positive for Turner syndrome)
- Pelvic and/or vaginal ultrasound to assess the presence and development of ovaries, uterus, and cervix
- Quantitative human chorionic gonadotropin (hCG) test to rule out pregnancy
- Thyroid function studies to determine thyroid disorder
- Prolactin level (an elevated level might indicate a pituitary tumor)
- FSH level (an elevated level might indicate ovarian failure)

- Luteinizing hormone (LH) level (an elevated level might indicate gonadal dysfunction)
- 17-Ketosteroids (an elevated level might indicate an adrenal tumor, PCOS) (Pagana et al., 2023; Welt & Barbieri, 2022a, 2022b)

Nursing Management

Counseling and education are primary interventions and appropriate nursing roles. Address the diverse causes of amenorrhea, the relationship to sexual identity, possible infertility, and the possibility of a tumor or a life-threatening disease. Evidence is mounting that loss of menstrual regularity is a risk factor for later development of osteoporosis and hip fractures, so treatment to restore regular menstrual cycles is essential (Behary & Comninos, 2022). In addition, inform the patient about the purpose of each diagnostic test, how it is performed, and when the results will be available to discuss. Listening sensitively, interviewing, and presenting treatment options are paramount to gain the patient's cooperation and understanding.

Nutritional counseling is also vital in managing this disorder, especially if the patient has findings suggestive of an eating disorder. The relationship between eating disorders and menstrual dysfunction has been identified in research studies. It has been found that menstrual irregularity is experienced by over 50% of females with an eating disorder (MacNeil, 2022). Careful evaluation of menstrual status is warranted for all female patients with eating disorders. Although not all causes can be addressed by making lifestyle changes, emphasize maintaining a healthy lifestyle for the best possible outcomes (Teaching Guidelines 4.2).

TEACHING GUIDELINES 4.2 Tips for Maintaining a Healthy Lifestyle

- Balance energy expenditure with energy intake to maintain the ideal weight range.
- Modify diet to maintain healthy BMI (18.5–24.9 kg/m^2).
- Avoid excessive use of alcohol and mood-altering or sedative drugs.
- Avoid cigarette smoking, which accelerates bone loss.
- Identify areas of emotional stress and seek assistance to resolve them.
- Consume adequate fiber to promote bowel regularity.
- Balance work, recreation, and rest to reduce anxiety and stress in life.
- Maintain a positive outlook regarding any diagnoses and prognoses.
- Participate in ongoing care and screenings to monitor any medical conditions.
- Maintain bone density through:
  - Calcium intake (1,200 mg daily)
  - Vitamin D intake (800 IU/daily)
  - Weight-bearing exercise (30 minutes or more daily)
  - Hormone therapy (HT) for low-risk patients

Centers for Disease Control and Prevention. (2022a). *Promoting health for adults*. https://www.cdc.gov/chronicdisease/resources/publications/factsheets/promoting-health-for-adults.htm; Rosen, H. N., & Lewiecki, E. M. (2024). Overview of the management of low bone mass and osteoporosis in postmenopausal women. *UpToDate*. Retrieved March 10, 2024, from https://www.uptodate.com/contents/overview-of-the-management-of-low-bone-mass-and-osteoporosis-in-postmenopausal-women

Dysmenorrhea

Dysmenorrhea refers to painful menstruation and is a highly prevalent problem among menstruating people. This condition has also been termed *cyclic perimenstrual pain*. Usually, pain starts 1 to 2 days before the start of bleeding and diminishes over the next 12 to 72 hours (Smith & Kaunitz, 2023b). The term *dysmenorrhea* is derived from the Greek words *dys*, meaning "difficult, painful, or abnormal," and *rrhea*, meaning "flow." Based on the results of surveys, it is estimated that it may impact 50% to 90% of menstruating people (Smith & Kaunitz, 2023b). It is a significant cause of absenteeism at work and school and has adverse effects on quality of life (Smith & Kaunitz, 2023b). Risk factors associated with dysmenorrhea include younger age, smoking, and stress (Smith & Kaunitz, 2023b). Uterine contractions occur during all periods, but in some people, these cramps can be frequent and very intense. Dysmenorrhea is a symptom, not a full diagnosis. It is classified as primary (spasmodic) or secondary (congestive) (Smith & Kaunitz, 2023b).

Etiology

Primary dysmenorrhea refers to painful menstrual bleeding in the absence of any identified underlying pelvic pathology. It is caused by increased prostaglandin production by the endometrium in an ovulatory cycle. This hormone causes contraction of the uterus, and levels tend to be higher in people with severe menstrual pain than in people who experience mild or no menstrual pain. Dysmenorrhea is caused by the activation of prostaglandins released at the beginning of menses from endometrial shedding, and this results in increased rhythmic uterine contractions from vasoconstriction of the small vessels of the uterine wall (Smith & Kaunitz, 2023b). This condition usually begins within a few years of the onset of ovulatory cycles at menarche.

Secondary dysmenorrhea is painful menstruation due to pelvic or uterine pathology. It typically begins after years of relatively less painful periods. It may be caused by endometriosis, pelvic adhesions, adenomyosis, fibroids, pelvic inflammatory disease (PID), an intrauterine system (IUS), cervical stenosis, or congenital uterine or vaginal abnormalities. Adenomyosis involves the ingrowth of tissue similar to that of the endometrium into the uterine musculature. Endometriosis involves ectopic implantation of tissue similar to that of the endometrium in other parts of the pelvis and throughout the body. It is most commonly diagnosed in the third or fourth decade of life and affects approximately 10% of females of reproductive age (American College of Obstetricians and Gynecologists [ACOG], 2021a). Endometriosis is a significant cause of secondary dysmenorrhea and is associated with pain beyond menstruation, dyspareunia, low back pain, heavy or irregular bleeding, chronic fatigue, and infertility (Schenken, 2024). The most effective treatment involves removing the underlying pathology, but there is no cure.

Think back to Izzy from the chapter opener. Is her pelvic pain complaint a common one?

Therapeutic Management

The goal of treatment is to provide adequate pain relief and to build coping strategies to allow the patient to perform their usual activities. Treatment is supportive and should be guided by individual needs to include patient education and reassurance (Smith & Kaunitz, 2023a). First-line treatment measures usually include nonsteroidal anti-inflammatory drugs (NSAIDs) and hormonal contraceptives. See Table 4.1 for select first-tier treatment options. Hormonal treatment is often associated with unwanted side effects and recurrence of symptoms when stopped. Severe dysmenorrhea can be distressing, adversely affecting social and occupational activities. For some, satisfactory pain relief is difficult to achieve, and they increasingly seek alternative options. Complementary therapies such as massage therapy, acupuncture (needles used to stimulate certain points of the body to balance the flow of energy within the body), and acupressure (the use of fingers and hands to stimulate acupoints to maintain the balance of energy) are gaining popularity as different ways to cope with the cyclic discomfort. If treatments are not effective after 3 to 6 months, further testing is warranted to focus treatment

TABLE 4.1 • Select Tier 1 Treatment Options for Dysmenorrhea

Therapy Options	Dosage	Comments
Nonsteroidal anti-inflammatory agents (NSAIDs)		NSAIDs prevent prostaglandin synthesis, reducing cramping.
Ibuprofen (Advil, Motrin, Midol)	400–800 mg every 4–6 hours (not to exceed 2,400 mg/day)	Take with meals. Do not take with aspirin.
Naproxen (Anaprox, Naprelan, Naprosyn, Aleve)	250–550 mg every 6–8 hours (not to exceed 1,250–1,375 mg/day)	Avoid alcohol. Watch for signs of GI bleeding. Same as above Both ibuprofen and naproxen available without a prescription
Fenamates such as mefenamic acid	Initial dose 500 mg then 250 mg every 6 hours (not to exceed 1,000 mg/day)	Same as above May have slightly better efficacy than ibuprofen or naproxen (Smith & Kaunitz, 2023a)
Acetic acids such as diclofenac	Initial dose 75–100 mg then 50 mg TID	Same as above Available by prescription
Hormonal contraceptives		Decrease prostaglandin synthesis. Choice of method determined by patient preferences and desired clinical result
Combined estrogen–progestin products	Variable based on the product chosen; available as oral pills, transdermal patches, or vaginal ring	Cause thinning of the endometrium over time therefore resulting in decreased blood flow and uterine contractions
Progestin-only options	Variable based on the product chosen; available as oral pills, implant, injection, or intrauterine device (IUD)	Cause atrophy of the endometrium over time May lead to irregular bleeding Option for patients for whom estrogen is contraindicated

GI, gastrointestinal; TID, three times a day.

Adapted from Smith, R. P., & Kaunitz, A. M. (2023a). Dysmenorrhea in adult females: Treatment. *UpToDate*. Retrieved March 6, 2024, from https://www.uptodate.com/contents/dysmenorrhea-in-adult-females-treatment; Nagy, H., Carlson, K., & Khan, M. A. B. (2023). Dysmenorrhea. *StatPearls* [Internet]. https://www.ncbi.nlm.nih.gov/books/NBK560834

on the underlying cause. Second-tier treatment options include the use of transcutaneous electrical nerve stimulation. GnRH analog has been shown to be effective in treating dysmenorrhea from endometriosis but is not considered a long-term treatment due to its high cost and adverse effects (Smith & Kaunitz, 2023a). Other second-tier treatments include diagnostic laparoscopy and endometrial ablation (Smith & Kaunitz, 2023a).

Nursing Assessment

As with any gynecologic complaint, a thorough focused history and physical examination are necessary to make the diagnosis of primary or secondary dysmenorrhea. With primary dysmenorrhea, the history usually reveals the typical cramping pain with menstruation, and the physical examination is completely normal. With secondary dysmenorrhea, the history discloses cramping pain with a pelvic abnormality or an underlying issue, occurrence later in life with symptoms worsening over time, infertility, heavy menstrual flow, irregular cycles, and little response to NSAIDs, oral contraceptives (OCs), or both (Smith & Kaunitz, 2023b).

HEALTH HISTORY AND CLINICAL MANIFESTATIONS

Note the past medical history, including any chronic illnesses and family history of gynecologic concerns. Determine medication and substance use, such as prescription medications, contraceptives, anabolic steroids, tobacco, cannabis, cocaine, or other recreational drugs. A detailed sexual history is essential to assess for inflammation and scarring (adhesions) secondary to PID. A history of PID and sexually transmitted infections (STIs) can result in secondary dysmenorrhea (Smith & Kaunitz, 2023b).

During the initial interview, the nurse might ask some of the following questions to assess the patient's history of dysmenorrhea:

- At what age did your menstrual cycles start?
- When was the first day of your last menstrual cycle?
- Have your cycles always been painful, or did the pain start recently?
- When in your cycle do you experience the pain?
- How would you describe the pain you feel?
- Are you sexually active?
- How many days does your cycle last from the start to when it completely stops?
- What impact does your cycle have on your physical and social activities?
- Was the flow of your last menstrual cycle a normal amount for you?
- Do your cycles tend to be heavy or last longer than 5 days?
- Are your cycles generally regular and predictable?
- What have you done to relieve your discomfort? Is it effective?
- Has there been a progression of symptom severity?
- Do you have any other symptoms, such as nausea, diarrhea, headache, general malaise, or chronic fatigue? (Smith & Kaunitz, 2023b)

Assess for clinical manifestations of dysmenorrhea. Those who are affected experience sharp, intermittent spasms of pain, usually in the suprapubic area. Pain may radiate to the back of the legs or the lower back. Pain usually develops within hours of the start of menstruation and peaks as the flow becomes heaviest during the first day or two of the cycle (Smith & Kaunitz, 2023b).

PHYSICAL EXAMINATION

The physical examination performed by the health care provider centers on the bimanual pelvic examination. This examination is done during the nonmenstrual phase of the cycle. Explain to the patient how it is to be performed, especially if it is their first pelvic examination. Prepare the patient in the examining room by offering them a cover gown to put on and covering their lap with a privacy sheet on the examination table. Remain in the examining room throughout the examination to assist the health care provider with any procedures or specimens and to offer the patient reassurance.

LABORATORY AND DIAGNOSTIC TESTS

Common diagnostic tests that may be ordered to determine the cause of dysmenorrhea can include:

- Complete blood count to rule out anemia
- Urinalysis to rule out a bladder infection
- Pregnancy test (hCG level) to rule out pregnancy
- Cervical culture to exclude STI
- Erythrocyte sedimentation rate to detect an inflammatory process
- Stool guaiac test to exclude gastrointestinal bleeding or disorders
- Pelvic and/or vaginal ultrasound to detect pelvic masses or cysts
- Diagnostic laparoscopy and/or laparotomy (rarely required) to visualize pathology that may account for the symptoms (Pagana et al., 2023; Smith & Kaunitz, 2023b)

> What diagnostic tests might be ordered to diagnose Izzy's pelvic pain?

Nursing Management

Educating the patient about the normal events of the menstrual cycle and the etiology of their pain is paramount in achieving a successful outcome. Although dysmenorrhea itself is not life-threatening, it can have a profound negative impact on a person's day-to-day life. The nurse should keep this in mind and not minimize this condition.

Explaining the normal menstrual cycle will teach the patient the correct terms to use so they can communicate their symptoms more accurately; this will also help dispel myths. Provide the patient with monthly graphs, charts, or apps to record menses, the onset of pain, the timing of medication, relief afforded, and coping strategies used. This involves the patient in their care and provides objective information so therapy can be modified if necessary. Educate patients about the associated risk factors for dysmenorrhea such as stress or anxiety, disruption of social networks, small familial predisposition, nulliparity, and smoking (Smith & Kaunitz, 2023b).

The nurse should explain in detail the dosing regimen and the side effects of the medication therapy selected. Commonly prescribed drugs include NSAIDs such as ibuprofen (Motrin, Advil) or naproxen (Naprosyn). The primary goal of NSAID therapy for dysmenorrhea is to preempt the production of prostaglandins; thus, starting the medication prophylactically and using sufficient doses to maximally suppress prostaglandin production are essential. If pain relief is not achieved in two to four cycles, a low-dose combination OC may be initiated. Patient education and counseling should include information about how to take pills, side effects, and danger signs to watch for.

The positive role of exercise in decreasing the symptoms of dysmenorrhea is supported by evidence, but further study into the type, duration, and frequency is needed (Smith & Kaunitz, 2023a). Nonmedical approaches such as behavioral interventions (biofeedback, hypnosis, relaxation), massage therapy, yoga, acupuncture, acupressure, and dietary or herbal supplements may be used in an effort to relieve the pain of dysmenorrhea. The data on the effectiveness of such interventions remain limited (Smith & Kaunitz, 2023a). Encourage the patient to apply a heating pad or warm compress to alleviate menstrual cramps. Additional lifestyle changes that the patient can make to restore some sense of control and active participation in their care are listed in Teaching Guidelines 4.3.

TEACHING GUIDELINES 4.3 Tips for Managing Dysmenorrhea

- Exercise to increase endorphins and suppress prostaglandin release.
- Eat a balanced diet rich in vitamins and minerals.
- Increase water consumption to serve as a natural diuretic; limit caffeine.
- Increase fiber intake with fruits and vegetables to prevent constipation.
- Use heating pads or warm baths to increase comfort.
- Take warm showers to promote relaxation.
- Sip on warm beverages, such as decaffeinated green tea.
- Keep legs elevated while lying down or lie on your side with knees bent.
- Use stress management techniques to reduce emotional stress.
- Practice relaxation techniques to enhance the ability to cope with pain.
- Stop smoking and decrease alcohol use which causes vasoconstriction.

Adapted from Smith, R. P., & Kaunitz, A. M. (2023a). Dysmenorrhea in adult females: Treatment. *UpToDate*. Retrieved March 6, 2024, from https://www.uptodate.com/contents/dysmenorrhea-in-adult-females-treatment

Abnormal Uterine Bleeding

Disturbances of menstrual bleeding manifest in a wide range of presentations. **Abnormal uterine bleeding (AUB)** is the umbrella term used to describe any deviation from normal menstruation or from a normal menstrual cycle pattern. It is further defined as a change in volume, regularity, or timing that has presented for 6 months or longer. It can occur in people of any age, with a prevalence of up to 25% among females of reproductive age (Price, 2022). The key characteristics are that regularity, frequency, volume or heaviness of flow, and duration of flow are abnormal, but each of these may exhibit considerable variability.

AUB is a disorder that occurs most frequently in females at the beginning and end of their reproductive years. It is common and somewhat debilitating in females of reproductive age. AUB is defined as painless endometrial bleeding that is prolonged, excessive, and irregular, and not attributed to any identified underlying structural or systemic disease. The International Federation of Gynecology and Obstetrics (FIGO) recommends the use of the term "AUB" to describe any aberration of menstrual volume, regulation, duration, and/or frequency in a female who isn't pregnant (Munro et al., 2018). FIGO also recommends discarding such terminology as "menorrhagia," "metrorrhagia," and "dysfunctional uterine bleeding," as they are controversial, confusing, and poorly defined. In addition, symptoms of AUB are too often overlooked by parents, patients, and health care workers. Consequently, they are underrecognized, underreported, and usually undertreated (Kaunitz, 2024a; Munro et al., 2018). AUB is frequently associated with anovulatory cycles, which are common for the first year after menarche and associated with immaturity of the hypothalamic–pituitary–ovarian axis. It also occurs later in life as people approach menopause and experience irregular menstrual cycles.

The pathophysiology of AUB can be related to changes in the structure of the uterus from conditions such as polyps or hyperplasia, changes in clotting pathways such as coagulopathies, or a hormone disturbance such as ovulatory or endocrine disorders that lead to alterations in menstruation (Davis & Sparzak, 2023). If the bleeding is heavy enough and frequent enough, anemia can result.

Etiology

The most common causes of AUB can be classified using the PALM-COEIN acronym, which categorizes potential causes of AUB:

- PALM (structural)
  - Polyp
  - Adenomyosis
  - Leiomyoma
  - Malignancy and hyperplasia
- COEIN (other)
  - Coagulopathy
  - Ovulatory dysfunction
  - Endometrial
  - Iatrogenic
  - Not yet classified (Kaunitz, 2024a)

Therapeutic Management

Treatment of AUB depends on the cause of the bleeding, the age and health status of the patient, and whether they desire future fertility. When known, the underlying cause of the disorder is treated. Otherwise, the goal of treatment is to normalize the bleeding, correct anemia, prevent or diagnose early cancer, and restore quality of life. Once malignancy and pelvic pathology have been ruled out, medical treatment is an effective first-line therapeutic option. In cases of chronic AUB, complications of anemia, infertility, and endometrial cancer may occur (Davis & Sparzak, 2023).

Management of AUB might include medical care with pharmacotherapy. Drug categories used in the treatment of AUB include:

- *Estrogens*: cause vasospasm of the uterine arteries to decrease bleeding
- *Progestins*: used to stabilize an estrogen-primed endometrium
- *OCs*: regulate the cycle and suppress the endometrium
- *NSAIDs:* inhibit prostaglandins in ovulatory menstrual cycles
- *Levonorgestrel intrauterine devices (IUDs)*: suppress endometrial growth
- *Androgens*: create a high-androgen/low-estrogen environment that inhibits endometrial growth
- *Antifibrinolytic drugs*: (tranexamic acid) prevent fibrin degradation to reduce bleeding
- *Iron replacement therapy*: replenishes iron stores lost during heavy bleeding

If the patient does not respond to medical therapy, surgical intervention might include dilation and curettage (D&C), endometrial ablation, uterine artery embolization, or hysterectomy. Surgery should only be considered for patients for whom medical treatment has failed, cannot be tolerated, or is contraindicated (Kaunitz, 2024b). Endometrial ablation is an alternative to hysterectomy, but both would only be for the patient who no longer desires fertility as both procedures can cause infertility. Techniques used for ablation include laser, electrosurgery excision procedure, freezing, heated fluid infusion, or thermal balloon ablation. Most patients will have reduced menstrual flow following endometrial ablation, and up to half will stop having periods. Younger patients are less likely than older patients to respond to endometrial ablation. Hysterectomy is the definitive treatment for uterine bleeding; however, it brings a risk of perioperative complications.

Nursing Assessment

A thorough history should be taken to differentiate between AUB and other conditions that might cause vaginal bleeding, such as pregnancy and pregnancy-related conditions (abruptio placentae, ectopic pregnancy, abortion, or placenta previa); systemic conditions such as Cushing disease, blood dyscrasias, liver disease, renal disease, or thyroid disease; and genital tract pathology such as infections, tumors, or trauma. Review of medications should include the use of contraceptives, postmenopausal HT, tamoxifen, corticosteroids, phenytoin, antipsychotic drugs, antibiotics, medications that can cause hyperprolactinemia (such as metoclopramide), and anticoagulants (Kaunitz, 2024a).

Assess for clinical manifestations of AUB, which commonly include vaginal bleeding between periods, irregular menstrual cycles (usually less than 24 days between cycles), infertility, mood swings, hot flashes, vaginal tenderness, variable menstrual flow ranging from scanty to profuse, obesity, acne, stress, anorexia, thyroid disease, and diabetes. Signs of polycystic ovary syndrome might be present because it is associated with unopposed estrogen stimulation, elevated androgen levels, obesity, and insulin resistance or elevated insulin levels, and it is a common cause of anovulation (Endocrine Society, 2023).

Measure orthostatic blood pressure and orthostatic pulse; a drop in pressure or pulse rate may occur with anemia. With the nurse assisting, the health care provider performs a pelvic examination to identify any structural abnormalities.

Common diagnostic/lab tests that may be ordered to determine the cause of AUB include:

- Complete blood count to detect anemia
- Prothrombin time to detect blood dyscrasias
- Pregnancy test to rule out a spontaneous abortion or ectopic pregnancy

- Thyroid-stimulating hormone level to screen for hypothyroidism
- Transvaginal ultrasound to measure endometrium
- Pelvic ultrasound to view any structural abnormalities
- Endometrial biopsy to check for intrauterine pathology
- D&C for diagnostic evaluation

Nursing Management

Educate the patient about normal menstrual cycles and the possible reasons for their abnormal pattern. Inform the patient about treatment options. Do not simply encourage them to "live with it." Instruct the patient about any prescribed medications and potential side effects. For example, if high-dose estrogens are prescribed, the patient may experience nausea. Teach them to take antiemetics as prescribed and encourage them to eat small, frequent meals to alleviate nausea. Adequate follow-up and evaluation are essential for patients who do not respond to medical management. See Clinical Judgment & Nursing Process 4.1: Overview of a Patient With Abnormal Uterine Bleeding.

TAKE NOTE!

Chronic anovulation can result in infertility and the long-term problem of hyperandrogenism. Severe anemia can also result secondary to prolonged or heavy menses. Depression and embarrassment may be secondary to the irregular and heavy bleeding. Endometrial cancer is associated with prolonged buildup of the endometrial lining and most commonly presents with abnormal uterine bleeding (ACOG, 2023b).

CLINICAL JUDGMENT & NURSING PROCESS 4.1 Overview of a Patient With Abnormal Uterine Bleeding

Stacy, a 52-year-old patient with obesity, comes to her gynecologist with a complaint of heavy erratic bleeding. Her periods were fairly regular until about 4 months ago, and since that time, they have been unpredictable, excessive, and prolonged. Stacy reports she is tired all the time, can't sleep, and feels "out of sorts" and anxious. She is fearful she has cancer.

NURSING ANALYSIS: Fear related to current signs and symptoms possibly indicating a life-threatening condition

OUTCOME IDENTIFICATION AND EVALUATION

The patient will acknowledge their fears as evidenced by statements made that fear and anxiety have been lessened after explanation of diagnosis.

INTERVENTIONS: *Reducing Fear and Anxiety*

- Distinguish between anxiety and fear *to determine appropriate interventions.*
- Check complete blood count and assess for possible anemia secondary to excessive bleeding *to determine if fatigue is contributing to anxiety and fear.* Fatigue occurs because the oxygen-carrying capacity of the blood is reduced.
- Reassure patient that symptoms can be managed *to help address current concerns.*
- Provide patient with factual information and explain what to expect *to assist patient with identifying fears and help them cope with their condition.*
- Provide symptom management *to reduce concerns associated with the cause of bleeding.*
- Teach patient about early manifestations of fear and anxiety *to aid in prompt recognition and to minimize the escalation of anxiety.*
- Assess patient's use of coping strategies in the past and reinforce use of effective ones *to help control anxiety and fear.*
- Instruct patient in relaxation methods, such as deep breathing exercises and imagery, *to provide them with additional methods for controlling anxiety and fear.*

NURSING ANALYSIS: Lack of knowledge related to perimenopausal transition and its management

OUTCOME IDENTIFICATION AND EVALUATION

The patient will demonstrate understanding of their symptoms as evidenced by making health-promoting lifestyle choices, verbalizing appropriate health care practices, adhering to measures, and complying with therapy.

INTERVENTIONS: *Providing Patient Education*

- Assess patient's understanding of menopausal transition and its treatment *to provide a baseline for teaching and developing a plan of care.*
- Review instructions about prescribed procedures and recommendations for self-care, frequently obtaining feedback from the patient *to validate adequate understanding of information.*
- Outline the link between anovulatory cycles and excessive buildup of uterine lining during menopausal transition *to assist patient in understanding the etiology of their bleeding.*
- Provide written material with pictures *to promote learning and help patient visualize what is occurring with their body during menopausal transition.*
- Inform patient about the availability of community resources, and make appropriate referrals as needed *to provide additional education and support.*
- Document details of teaching and learning *to allow for continuity of care and further education if needed.*

Premenstrual Disorders

Premenstrual disorders (PMD) is an umbrella category that includes PMS and PMDD. Premenstrual syndrome (PMS) describes a constellation of recurrent physical, emotional, and behavioral symptoms that occur during the luteal phase or the last half of the menstrual cycle and resolve with the onset of menstruation. A majority of females in their reproductive years experience a variety of premenstrual symptoms that can alter their behavior and well-being. Females have between 400 and 500 menstrual cycles over their reproductive years, and since premenstrual distress symptoms peak during 4 to 7 days prior to menses, consistently symptomatic people may spend up to 10 years of their lives in a state of compromised physical functioning and/or psychological well-being; thus, it constitutes a major health problem. The ACOG defines PMS as at least one emotional or physical symptom that causes severe distress and interferes with some aspect of the person's life either socially or at work or in the home (Yonkers & Casper, 2022). It is thought the symptoms are related to the interaction between hormonal events and central neurotransmitter function, most notably serotonin (Yonkers & Casper, 2024).

As defined by the American Psychiatric Association, PMDD is a more severe variant of PMS (Yonkers & Casper, 2022). Experts compare the difference between PMS and PMDD to the difference between a mild tension headache and a migraine. Risk factors identified that predispose to PMS and PMDD are lower education, cigarette smoking, an anxiety disorder, a family history of PMDD, and stressful or traumatic life events (Yonkers & Casper, 2024).

Therapeutic Management

Treatment of PMS is often frustrating for both patients and health care providers. Clinical outcomes can be expected to improve as a result of recent consensus on the diagnostic criteria for PMS and PMDD, data from clinical trials, and the availability of evidence-based clinical guidelines.

The management of PMS or PMDD requires a multidimensional approach because these conditions are not likely to have a single cause, and they appear to affect multiple systems within the body; therefore, they are not likely to be amenable to treatment with a single therapy. A clear diagnosis of either one needs to be established before treatment is considered (Casper & Yonkers, 2022). To reduce the negative impact of PMDs on a person's life, education along with reassurance and anticipatory guidance are needed for patients to feel they have some control over this condition.

TAKE NOTE!

Because there are no diagnostic tests that can reliably determine the existence of PMS or PMDD, the patient must decide that they need help for these symptoms. They must embrace multiple therapies and become an active participant in their treatment plan to find the best level of symptom relief.

Therapeutic interventions for PMS and PMDD address the symptoms since the exact causes of this condition are still unknown. Treatments may include vitamin supplements, dietary changes, exercise, lifestyle changes, and medications (Box 4.1). Pharmacotherapies (particularly selective serotonin reuptake inhibitors [SSRIs] and serotonin–norepinephrine reuptake inhibitors [SNRIs]) represent the first-line treatment for the mood and behavioral symptoms of PMDD. Unlike the approach to the treatment of depression, antidepressants need not be given daily, but may be effective when used cyclically, only in the luteal phase, or even limited to the duration of the symptoms.

COMPLEMENTARY AND ALTERNATIVE THERAPIES

No single treatment is universally recognized as effective, and many patients often turn to therapeutic approaches outside of conventional medicine. Many people use dietary supplements and herbal remedies for their menstrual health and bleeding disorders, though there has been little research to demonstrate their efficacy (Casper & Yonkers, 2022). Alternative treatments for treating PMDD may include vitex agnus castus (chaste tree berry), primrose oil, cognitive behavioral therapy, and relaxation therapies, such as yoga (Casper & Yonkers, 2022). Although research has not conclusively validated the efficacy of these alternative therapies, it is important for the nurse to be aware of the alternative products that patients may choose to use and to base recommendations on evidence-based practice.

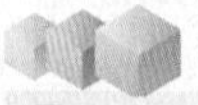

Concept Mastery Alert

Treatments for Premenstrual Syndrome

Possible treatment options for PMS include reduction of caffeine intake, vitamin and mineral supplements, diuretic therapy, and NSAIDs. Medication therapy that has been found to be helpful for patients with PMS includes antidepressants and anxiolytics.

BOX 4.1 Treatment Options for PMS and PMDD

- Lifestyle changes
  - Reduce stress.
  - Exercise three to five times a week.
  - Eat a balanced diet and increase water intake.
  - Decrease caffeine intake.
  - Stop smoking and limit the intake of alcohol.
  - Attend a PMS or female health support group.
- Medications
  - NSAIDs taken a week prior to menses
  - OCs (low dose)
  - Selective serotonin reuptake inhibitors (SSRIs)
  - GnRH agonists

GnRH, gonadotropin-releasing hormone; NSAIDs, nonsteroidal anti-inflammatory drugs; OC, oral contraceptive; PMDD, premenstrual dysphoric disorder; PMS, premenstrual syndrome.

Casper, R. F., & Yonkers, K. A. (2022). Treatment of premenstrual syndrome and premenstrual dysphoric disorder. *UpToDate*. Retrieved March 7, 2024, from https://www.uptodate.com/contents/treatment-of-premenstrual-syndrome-and-premenstrual-dysphoric-disorder; Gudipally, P. R., & Sharma, G. K. (2023). Premenstrual syndrome. *StatPearls* [Internet]. https://pubmed.ncbi.nlm.nih.gov/32809533/

Nursing Assessment

Although the description of symptoms about what constitutes PMS and PMDD varies, the physical and psychological symptoms are real. The extent to which the symptoms debilitate or incapacitate a person is highly variable.

More than 150 symptoms are assigned to PMS, but the most prominent and consistently described are irritability; increased appetite and food cravings; mood swings; depression; sleep disturbances; headache; fatigue; bloating; edema of the face, abdominal area, and extremities; difficulty concentrating; breast tenderness; anxiety/tension; hot flashes (in people who are not postpartum, perimenopausal, or menopausal); and decreased interest in activities (Yonkers & Casper, 2022). To establish the diagnosis of PMS, elicit a description of cyclic symptoms occurring before the patient's menstrual period. The patient should chart their daily symptoms for two cycles. These data will help demonstrate symptoms clustering around the luteal phase of ovulation with resolution after bleeding starts. Ask the patient to bring this list of symptoms to the next appointment. Gather information regarding the effect these symptoms have on daily life and if they interfere with the patient's ability to function.

In PMDD, the main symptoms of internal tension, anger, or irritability are more prominent (Yonkers & Casper, 2022). These symptoms must have occurred in most menstrual cycles over the past year and must cause significant distress and interfere with usual daily activities (Yonkers & Casper, 2022).

Nursing Management

Educate the patient about the management of PMS or PMDD. Advise them that lifestyle changes often result in significant symptom improvement without pharmacotherapy. Encourage patients to eat a balanced diet that includes nutrient-rich foods to avoid hypoglycemia and associated mood swings. Encourage all patients to participate in aerobic exercise three times a week to promote a sense of well-being, decrease fatigue, and reduce stress. NSAIDs may be useful for painful physical symptoms, and spironolactone (Aldactone) may help with bloating and water retention. Herbs such as vitex agnus castus (chaste tree berry) and evening primrose, as well as SAM-e (*S*-adenosylmethionine; a dietary supplement used to enhance mood), may be recommended; though not harmful unless the patient has a contraindication, not all herbs have enough clinical or research evidence to document their efficacy. Nutritional treatments include a diet low in salt, alcohol, caffeine, and sugar; furthermore, deep-fried foods should be avoided. A diet rich in vegetables, fruits, and fiber is recommended (Siminiuc & Turcanu, 2023).

Explain to the patient the relationship between cyclic estrogen fluctuation and changes in serotonin levels and how the different management strategies help maintain serotonin levels, thus improving mood symptoms. It is important to rule out other conditions that might cause erratic or dysphoric behavior. If the initial treatment regimen does not work, explain to the patient that they should return for further testing. Behavioral counseling and stress management might help patients regain control during these stressful periods. Reassuring them that support and help are available through many community resources and support groups can be instrumental in their acceptance of this monthly disorder. Nurses can be a calming force for many people experiencing PMS or PMDD. A holistic approach, including lifestyle modifications, pharmacotherapy, herbal therapies, acupuncture, and cognitive behavioral therapy, is most beneficial for symptom reduction, improvement in daily functioning, and quality of life.

> *TAKE NOTE!*
>
> Adolescent and adult females who experience more extensive emotional symptoms with PMS should be evaluated for PMDD because they may require antidepressant therapy.

MENOPAUSAL TRANSITION AND MENOPAUSE

Midlife is a critical time for female patients because it encompasses both chronologic aging and menopause. This is a time of pronounced changes in body composition, cardiovascular health, mood, sleep, cognition, and overall functioning. More than 1.3 million people in the United States experience menopause annually (Peacock et al., 2023). The term **menopausal transition** refers to the transition from the female reproductive phase of life to the final menstrual period. This period is also referred to as *perimenopause*. The transition may begin between the ages of 45 and 55, with the average age being 47 years, and can last 7 to 14 years in some people (Casper, 2023; National Institute on Aging, 2021a). Menopause is a natural process that occurs in all female lives as part of normal aging. *Meno* is derived from the Greek word for "month," and *pause* is derived from the Greek word for "pause" or "halt." Menopause is the technical term for a point in time at which menses and fertility cease (Casper, 2023). People call it many things: The change of life. The end of fertility. The beginning of freedom. Whatever people call it, menopause is a unique and personal experience for every person who experiences it. The average age of natural menopause, defined as 1 year without a menstrual period, is 51.4 years (Casper, 2023). The average age of natural menopause has remained constant for the last several 100 years despite improvements in nutrition and health care. With current female life expectancy at 84 years, this event comes in roughly the middle of a female adult's life. Many people go through the menopausal transition with few or no symptoms, while some have significant or even disabling symptoms.

TAKE NOTE!

Humans are virtually the only species to outlive their reproductive capacities.

Menopause signals the end of an era for many people. Menopause does not happen in isolation. Midlife is often experienced as a time of change and reflection. Change happens in many arenas; children are leaving or returning home, employment pressures intensify as career moves or decisions are required, older adult parents require more care or the death of a parent may have a major impact, and partners are retrenching or undergoing their own midlife changes. Females must negotiate all these changes in addition to menopause. Managing this stress can be challenging for many as they make this transition.

A female is born with approximately 1 million follicles in an ovary; by puberty, about 250,000 to 400,000 remain (Peacock et al., 2023). The absolute number of ova in the ovary is a major determinant of fertility. Over the course of premenopausal life, there is a steady decline in the number of immature ova (Coney, 2023). No one understands this depletion, but it does not occur in isolation. Maturing ova are surrounded by follicles that produce two major hormones: estrogen, in the form of estradiol, and progesterone. The cyclic maturation of the ovum is directed by the hypothalamus. The hypothalamus triggers a cascade of neurohormones, which act through the pituitary and the ovaries as a pulse generator for reproduction. This hypothalamic–pituitary–ovarian–uterine axis begins to break down in response to a decrease in estrogen, resulting from the absence of ovulation; therefore, endometrial development may not occur, leading to irregular menstrual cycles (Peacock et al., 2023). The final act in this process is amenorrhea.

Hormone changes during menopausal transition and menopause can lead to stress, fatigue, and tense emotions (Silver, 2023). With its dramatic decline in estrogen, menopausal transition and menopause affect not only the reproductive organs but also other body systems:

- Brain and central nervous system: hot flashes, irritability, disturbed sleep, mood, and cognitive changes (such as forgetfulness and brain fog), depression, and anxiety
- Cardiovascular: lower levels of high-density lipoprotein (HDL) and increased risk of cardiovascular disease (CVD)
- Skeletal: rapid loss of bone density that increases the risk of osteoporosis; joint aches and pains
- Breasts: breast pain and tenderness
- Genitourinary: vaginal dryness, stress incontinence, cystitis, irregular menstrual cycles
- Gastrointestinal: less absorption of calcium from food, increasing the risk for fractures
- Integumentary: dry, thin skin and decreased collagen levels; increased aging; and wrinkling skin
- Body shape: gain fat mass and lose lean muscle; more abdominal fat; waist size that swells relative to hips

Several therapies can be considered to help manage these complaints. Choosing an appropriate treatment approach for the management of these symptoms requires careful assessment of the risk-to-benefit ratio of each evidence-based management option as well as individual patient preference.

Therapeutic Management

Menopausal transition should be managed individually. The Women's Health Initiative showed adverse effects of menopausal hormone therapy (MHT) in females over 60 or with more than 10 years since menopause (Martin & Barbieri, 2022). Years later, there remains widespread uncertainty as to how to advise menopausal patients and when and how to prescribe MHT. The Agency for Healthcare Research and Quality (AHRQ) concluded recently that people taking MHT for primary prevention of chronic conditions do experience some benefits, but also an increased risk of harm (Gartlehner et al., 2022).

Recent research has found that people taking MHT between the ages of 50 and 59 with less than 10 years since the initiation of menopause did not have an increased risk of coronary artery disease (CAD) (Martin & Barbieri, 2022). Menopause predisposes people to osteoporosis due to declining estrogen levels. There is considerable evidence that estrogen or MHT reduces the risk of postmenopausal osteoporotic fracture of both the spine and hip along with reducing modifiable risk factors through dietary and lifestyle changes. For patients with osteoporosis, lifelong management is required. New therapy guidelines from the North American Menopause Society now state that MHT's effectiveness in treating vasomotor, genitourinary syndrome, and use for bone loss prevention should be considered (Carr, 2022). The 2022 recommendations state that for healthy people under 60 with less than 10 years since menopause onset, the benefits of MHT outweigh the risks ("The 2022 Hormone Therapy Position Statement of The North American Menopause Society" Advisory Panel, 2022).

A number of treatment options are available, but factors in the patient's history should be the driving force when determining therapy. Patients need to educate themselves about the latest research findings and collaborate with their health care providers on the right menopause therapy. Individualized therapy needs to be reevaluated to ensure that it continues to maximize benefits and minimize risks as the patient ages.

Many people consider nonhormonal therapies such as bisphosphonates and selective estrogen receptor modulators (SERMs). Consider weight-bearing exercises, calcium, vitamin D, smoking cessation, and avoidance of alcohol to treat or prevent osteoporosis. Regular breast examinations and mammograms are essential. Local estrogen creams can be used for vaginal atrophy. Many people consider herbal therapies such as black cohosh for symptoms, though their efficacy is not well established (Loprinzi & Casper, 2023).

Although numerous symptoms have been attributed to menopause, some of them are more closely related to the aging process than to estrogen deficiency. A few of the more common menopausal conditions and their management are discussed next.

Managing Hot Flashes and Night Sweats

Hot flashes during menopause are distressing and result in poor quality of life. When they happen at night, they are termed night sweats. These occurrences negatively affect sleep. Hot flashes and night sweats are classic signs of estrogen deficiency and the predominant complaint during perimenopause and menopause (Casper, 2023). A hot flash is a transient and sudden sensation of warmth that spreads over the body, particularly the neck, face, and chest. Hot flashes are caused by vasomotor instability. This instability causes inappropriate peripheral vasodilation of superficial blood vessels, which gives the sensation of heat. Nearly 80% of menopausal people experience them (Casper, 2023). Hot flashes are an early and acute sign of estrogen deficiency. These flashes can be mild or extreme, can last as long as 4 minutes, and may occur as frequently as every hour to several times per week. On average, patients experience hot flashes for a period of 6 months to 2 years, but the symptoms may last up to 10 years or more. Severe vasomotor symptoms can have a significant and detrimental effect on quality of life. Factors that trigger vasomotor symptoms are individualized but commonly include caffeine and alcohol consumption, smoking, intake of hot drinks and spicy foods, hot environment, stress, and anxiety (Endocrine Society, 2022a).

Many options are available for treating hot flashes. Treatment must be based on symptom severity, the patient's medical history, and the patient's values and concerns. Although the gold standard in the treatment of hot flashes is estrogen, this is not recommended for all patients who have high-risk factors in their history.

TRADITIONAL THERAPIES FOR THE MANAGEMENT OF HOT FLASHES

The following are traditional therapies for the management of hot flashes:

- MHT unless contraindicated
- Tissue selective estrogen complexes (TSECs)—a combination of a SERM (such as bazedoxifene) and a conjugated estrogen
- SSRIs and SNRIs such as venlafaxine (Effexor), paroxetine (Paxil), and escitalopram (Lexapro)
- Antiepileptics such as gabapentin
- Other medications including oxybutynin and gabapentin
- Neurokinin 3 receptor (NK3R) antagonists (fezolinetant) (Loprinzi & Casper, 2023)

TAKE NOTE!

Bioidentical hormones, which are derived from soy and plant abstracts and are the same molecular structure as hormones in our bodies, have gained in popularity. Current recommendations in the literature advise against the use of this approach until there is evidence to support its safety and efficacy (Martin & Barbieri, 2022).

COMPLEMENTARY AND ALTERNATIVE THERAPIES FOR MANAGEMENT OF HOT FLASHES

Nurses can play a major role in assisting menopausal patients by educating and counseling them about the multitude of options available for disease prevention and treatments for symptoms during this time of change. Menopause should be an opportunity for patients to strive for healthy, long lives, and nurses can help to make this opportunity a reality. Nonhormonal therapies that are not recommended for vasomotor symptoms include paced respiration, supplements/herbal remedies, cooling techniques, avoiding triggers, exercise, yoga, mindfulness-based intervention, relaxation, soy, cannabinoids, acupuncture, and clonidine ("The 2023 Nonhormone Therapy Position Statement of The North American Menopause Society" Advisory Panel, 2023).

Many patients choose complementary and alternative medicine (CAM) treatments for managing menopausal symptoms such as cognitive behavioral therapy, hypnosis, stress management and relaxation techniques, mindfulness techniques, aromatherapy, phytoestrogens, and herbal medicines. Evidence supporting the efficacy and safety of most CAM remedies for the relief of hot flashes is limited (Loprinzi & Casper, 2023). Because of their natural origin, patients sometimes believe CAM treatments are safer. The interest in phytoestrogens came about because of the low prevalence of hot flashes in Asian patients, which was attributed to their diet being rich in phytoestrogens. Inconsistent evidence on the efficacy of plant-based therapies (phytoestrogens and herbal remedies such as black cohosh) along with paced respiration, weight loss, and exercise is available in the literature (Loprinzi & Casper, 2023). Evidence is lacking for acupuncture, exercise, evening primrose oil, flaxseed, ginseng, dongquai, wild yam, and progesterone creams (Loprinzi & Casper, 2023).

Although research thus far has been skeptical about efficacy, many patients report easing of symptoms with CAM treatments, and use has skyrocketed. Although patients may experience some benefits from their use, evidence of the efficacy of CAM treatments in menopause is largely anecdotal. Small, preliminary clinical trials might demonstrate the safety of some of the nonpharmacologic products. Nurses should be aware of CAM practices and the purported action of these agents as well as any adverse effects or drug interactions in order to help guide patients to effective and safe care practices.

The following are lifestyle changes and CAM therapies for the treatment of hot flashes:

- Lower room temperature; use fans, carry a portable fan.
- Wear clothing in layers for easy removal.
- Limit caffeine and alcohol intake.
- Use a cold washcloth on the back of your neck during a hot flash.
- Stop smoking.
- Avoid hot drinks and spicy food.
- Maintain a healthy weight.
- Keep a diary to identify triggers of hot flashes.
- Try mind–body practices such as relaxation techniques, deep breathing, and meditation (National Institute on Aging, 2021b).

Managing Genitourinary Syndrome

Genitourinary syndrome of menopause describes the multiple changes that occur in female external genitalia, bladder and urethra, pelvic floor tissues, and libido. These chronic genitourinary changes are the result of reduced estrogen levels and aging. These changes include the ovaries and uterus reducing in size, the vagina shortening and becoming narrower, loss of bone mass, and loss of muscle tone leading to pelvic floor weakening (Habeeb, 2022). Physiologically, this syndrome manifests with symptoms of vaginal dryness, irritation, and itching; decreased lubrication during intercourse; dysuria; and urinary frequency and urgency (Bachmann & Pinkerton, 2023a). Menopausal transition and menopause can be a physically and emotionally challenging time. In addition to the psychological burden of leaving behind the reproductive phase of life and the stigma of an aging body, sexual difficulties resulting from urogenital changes plague many patients but are frequently not addressed. Sexual desire is affected by endocrine and psychosocial factors. Menopausal hormonal changes are relevant to the causes of sexual dysfunction during reproductive aging. The frequency of sexual intercourse declines as people enter midlife. While partner availability and function may play a role, menopausal symptoms, such as vaginal dryness, are also present (Bachmann & Pinkerton, 2023a).

Vaginal atrophy occurs during menopause because of declining estrogen levels. These changes include thinning of the vaginal walls, an increase in pH, irritation, increased susceptibility to infection, **dyspareunia** (difficult or painful sexual intercourse), loss of lubrication with intercourse, vaginal dryness, and a decrease in sexual desire related to these changes. Decreased estrogen levels can also influence female sexual function as well. Delayed clitoral reaction, decreased vaginal lubrication, diminished circulatory response during sexual stimulation, and reduced contractions during orgasm have all been linked to low estrogen levels. Genitourinary syndrome symptoms are caused by estrogen deficiency and are progressive, worsening over time. Despite the high prevalence of symptoms, many people do not seek treatment for these issues due to embarrassment; cultural, religious, or societal beliefs; believing it is a normal consequence of the aging process; lack of awareness of safe and effective treatment options; and health care providers failing to assess patients for these symptoms (Bachman & Pinkerton, 2023a).

Genitourinary syndrome of menopause causes multiple changes in genitourinary tissues and does not improve with time after menopause. Management of these changes might include the use of vaginal moisturizers and lubricants (Astroglide), estrogen vaginal tablets (Vagifem), Premarin cream, or Estring (an estrogen-releasing vaginal ring that lasts for months) (Bachman & Pinkerton, 2023b). A positive outlook on sexuality and a supportive partner are also needed to make the sexual experience enjoyable and fulfilling. Nurses are in a unique position to sensitively discuss symptoms and can advise, educate, and provide information that can improve the sexual health and quality of life in menopausal patients by offering them choices about managing them. It is essential that nurses recognize the chronic nature of this syndrome and the need for clinical intervention.

TAKE NOTE!

Sexual health is an important aspect of the human experience. By keeping an open mind, listening to patients, and providing evidence-based treatment options, the nurse can help improve the quality of life for menopausal people.

Preventing and Managing Osteoporosis

Menopause predisposes patients to osteoporosis due to declining estrogen levels. This results in a decrease in bone mineral density and an increase in fractures.

Osteoporosis has been recognized as a significant worldwide public health problem. As the world's population ages, both in the United States and internationally, the prevalence of osteoporosis is expected to increase significantly. **Osteoporosis** is the state of diminished bone density in which bones become structurally weaker over time. This disorder is a progressive, systemic skeletal disease characterized by low bone mass and microarchitectural deterioration of bone tissue with a consequent increase in bone fragility.

According to recent information from the Bone Health and Osteoporosis Foundation (BHOF, 2022a), osteoporosis is a major medical problem that affects millions of people worldwide. It affects one in two females and one in four males over the age of 50. By 2040, it is predicted that osteoporosis will be responsible for over 3.2 million fractures annually at a cost of over $95 billion in medical expenses (BHOF, 2022a). Osteoporosis continues to be underdiagnosed and undertreated because it is often not recognized until the first fracture occurs.

Patients are greatly affected by osteoporosis after menopause. Bone mass declines to such an extent that fractures can occur with minimal trauma. Bone loss begins in the third or fourth decade of a female's life and accelerates rapidly after menopause (Endocrine Society, 2022b). It is a "silent" disease because bone loss occurs without the person being aware of it (Endocrine Society, 2022b). This condition puts many patients into long-term care with a resulting loss of independence. Figure 4.1 shows the skeletal changes associated with osteoporosis.

Most patients with osteoporosis do not know they have the disease until they sustain a fracture, usually of the wrist or hip. Risk factors for osteoporosis-related fractures include:

- Advancing age
- Weight less than 57.6 kg (127 lbs)
- Family history of osteoporosis or hip fracture
- Long-term use of steroids (longer than 3 months)
- Thyroid replacement drugs
- Smoking
- Low calcium and vitamin D intake
- Excessive consumption of alcohol
- Personal history of nontraumatic fracture (Yu, 2024)

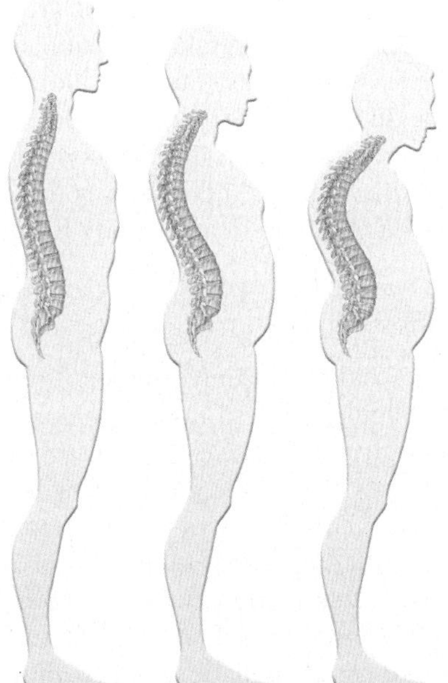

FIGURE 4.1 Skeletal changes associated with osteoporosis. (Reprinted with permission from Evans, R. J., Evans, M. K., & Brown, Y. M. R. [2014]. *Canadian maternity, newborn & women's health nursing: Comprehensive care across the life span* [2nd ed.]. Wolters Kluwer.)

Currently, no method exists for directly measuring bone mass. Instead, a bone mass density (BMD) measurement is obtained using dual-energy x-ray absorptiometry (DEXA). BMD is a two-dimensional measurement of the average content of mineral in a section of bone. BMD evaluations are made at the hip, femoral neck, and spine. There is a significant relationship between BMD and fracture: as BMD is reduced, the risk of fracture increases (BHOF, 2022b). Screening tests to measure bone density are not good predictors for young people who might be at risk for developing this condition. DEXA is a screening test that calculates the mineral content of the bone at the spine and hip. It is highly accurate, fast, and relatively inexpensive. The DEXA scan is the gold standard radiologic method for identifying osteoporosis through measuring BMD (BHOF, 2022b).

Fractures in older people often lead to functional decline, reduced quality of life, disability, chronic pain, and an increased risk of mortality. Hip fractures are the most devastating of the fragility fractures secondary to osteoporosis. A number of medical, social, and economic consequences follow a hip fracture. The concern surrounding osteoporosis is not the rate of fracture alone but also the potential for lifelong disability secondary to fracture.

Early identification and intervention are needed to reduce the burden of osteoporotic fractures. Care for a patient with osteoporosis or osteopenia (bone loss that hasn't reached the extent of that of osteoporosis) includes assessment of fracture risk, evaluation of secondary causes, and selection of the appropriate treatment plan. The best management for this painful, crippling, and potentially fatal disease is prevention.

People can modify many risk factors by doing the following:

- Engage in daily weight-bearing exercise, such as walking, to increase osteoblast activity.
- Adequate intake of vitamin D—800 IU daily
- Adequate intake of calcium—1,200 mg/daily
- Remove indoor and outdoor falling hazards.
- Avoid smoking and excessive alcohol (more than two drinks per day).
- Discuss bone health with a health care provider (Rosen & Lewiecki, 2024).

Medications that can help prevent and manage osteoporosis include:

- Bisphosphonates (Actonel, Fosamax, or Boniva)
- SERMs (raloxifene [Evista])
- Calcium and vitamin D supplements
- Romosozumab (Evenity) (bone builder)
- MHT
- Parathyroid hormone (Forteo) (Rosen & Lewiecki, 2024)

Preventing and Managing CVD

Over the last decade, CVD has become the leading cause of death worldwide. It is largely driven by modifiable risk factors, such as smoking, drinking alcohol, lack of physical activity, high levels of stress, and diets high in fat and sodium (CDC, 2024). One in five females die from heart disease, making it the leading cause of death in females (CDC, 2024). Many health care providers still think of CVD as a "man's disease," so they ignore symptoms in female patients and delay treatment. Awareness campaigns, such as the Heart Truth and the Red Dress symbol, appear to have improved recognition of CVD risk in female patients. Further, female-specific guidelines have been developed to prevent and reduce CVD. Though the current understanding of the role of MHT on CVD risk remains controversial and not clear, studies suggest that the use of MHT in early menopause does not seem to be associated with an increased risk of CVD compared to MHT taken by older menopausal patients (Martin & Rosenson, 2023).

For the first half of a female's life, estrogen seems to be a protective substance for the cardiovascular system by smoothing, relaxing, and dilating blood vessels. It even helps boost HDL and lower low-density lipoprotein (LDL) levels, helping keep the arteries clean from plaque accumulation. But when estrogen levels plummet with age and menopause, the incidence of CVD increases dramatically. Females are more likely to have atypical cardiovascular symptoms when compared to males. This may lead to a delayed or misdiagnosis of CVD and suboptimal treatment. These symptoms may include:

- A—Angina (chest pain)
- B—Breathlessness
- C—Chronic fatigue
- D—Dizziness
- E—Edema of hands and feet
- F—Fluttering of the heart
- G—Gastric upset
- H—Heavy pain in back and shoulders

Menopause is not the only factor that increases a female's risk for CVD. Lifestyle and medical history factors such as the following play a major role:

- Smoking
- Obesity
- High-fat diet
- Sedentary lifestyle
- High cholesterol levels
- Family history of CVD
- Hypertension
- Apple-shaped body
- Diabetes

Two of the major risk factors for coronary heart disease are hypertension and dyslipidemia. Both are modifiable and can be prevented by lifestyle changes and if needed, controlled by medication. This is why prevention is essential. In addition, patients who experience early menopause lose the protection afforded by endogenous estrogen to the cardiac system and are at greater risk for more extensive atherosclerosis.

The nurse is often a patient's first and most consistent point of contact within the health care system. Nurses who work in primary care settings can identify patients at risk for CVD, counsel them about their risk factors, and encourage and initiate primary and secondary prevention strategies. Nurses, particularly those caring for patients during their reproductive years, are uniquely positioned to provide education and support for long-term cardiovascular health for all patients. Raising awareness of heart disease in females is an essential role for nurses. The good news is that CVD is largely preventable. Because CVD is a chronic disease that develops over time, primary prevention lifestyle modification interventions are most effective if initiated before the development of overt disease. The gold standard of treatment and risk reduction for all females, regardless of their risk category, is adhering to a healthy lifestyle, including diet, exercise, adequate sleep, stress reduction, decreased alcohol intake, weight reduction, and smoking cessation. Stressing the importance of lifestyle modifications must begin early in life and should be reinforced from the beginning of a young person's reproductive years through menopause. Education is the cornerstone to reducing CVD risk and death among female patients.

Nursing Assessment

Menopausal transition is a universal and irreversible part of the overall aging process involving the reproductive system. Although not a disease state, menopausal transition does place females at greater risk for the development of many conditions of aging. Nurses can help the patient become aware of their risk for menopausal diseases as well as strategies to prevent them. The nurse can be instrumental in assessing risk factors and planning interventions in collaboration with the patient. These might include:

- Screening for osteoporosis, CVD, and cancer risk
- Assessment of blood pressure to identify hypertension

- Blood cholesterol test to identify hyperlipidemia risk
- Mammogram to find a cancerous lesion
- Pap smear to identify cervical cancer
- Pelvic examination to identify endometrial cancer or masses
- Digital rectal examination to assess for colon cancer
- Bone density testing as a baseline at menopause to identify osteopenia (low bone mass), which might lead to osteoporosis
- Assessing lifestyle to plan strategies to prevent chronic conditions:
  - Dietary intake of fat, cholesterol, and sodium
  - Weight management
  - Calcium intake
  - Use of tobacco, alcohol, and caffeine
  - Amount and type of daily exercise routines

Nursing Management

There is no "magic bullet" in managing menopause. Nurses can counsel patients about their risks and help them prevent disease and debilitating conditions with specific health maintenance education. Patients should make their own decisions, but the nurse should make sure they are armed with the facts to do so intelligently. Nurses can offer a thorough explanation of the menopausal process, including the latest research findings, to help patients understand and make decisions about this inevitable event.

If the patient decides to use MHT to control menopausal symptoms after being thoroughly educated, they will need frequent reassessment. There are no hard-and-fast rules that apply to meeting a person's individual needs. The nurse can provide realistic expectations of the therapy to reduce anxiety and concerns.

It is also useful to emphasize the value of friends to gain support and share information and resources. Often just talking about emotional difficulties such as the death of a parent or problematic relationships helps solve problems. It also shows the patient that their emotional responses are valid.

Living a healthy lifestyle is vital to health and longevity, and it is important to keep these on the patient's agenda when discussing menopause (American Heart Association [AHA], 2023). Evidence-based interventions include lifestyle modifications, risk management therapies, and preventive drug interventions, such as:

- Participate actively in maintaining health.
- Stay current on health screenings and vaccinations.
- Exercise regularly to prevent CVD and osteoporosis.
- Ensure adequate calcium intake (or use calcium supplements) and eat appropriately to prevent osteoporosis.
- Stop smoking to prevent lung and heart diseases.
- Reduce caffeine and alcohol intake to prevent osteoporosis.
- Monitor blood pressure, lipids, and diabetes (drug therapy management).
- Reduce dietary intake of fat, cholesterol, and sodium to prevent CVD.
- Maintain a healthy weight for body frame.
- Establish good sleep habits to feel energized throughout the day.
- Perform breast self-examinations for breast awareness.
- Control stress to prevent depression (Peacock et al., 2023).

These life approaches may be low-tech, but they can stave off menopause-related complications such as CVD, osteoporosis, and depression. These tips for healthy living work well, and the patient needs to be motivated to stick with them.

Endometriosis

Endometriosis is a complex syndrome characterized by an estrogen-dominant chronic inflammatory process that affects primarily pelvic tissues, including the ovaries. It is caused when tissue similar to that of the endometrium implants outside of the uterus, most commonly throughout the abdominal cavity including the bowel, bladder, ovary, uterosacral ligaments, diaphragm, and pleural cavity. Although it is a benign process, it can cause dysmenorrhea, dyspareunia, infertility, and chronic pelvic pain (WHO, 2023a). It is one of the most common gynecologic diseases affecting up to 10% of the adult female population globally (WHO, 2023a). Endometriosis tissue is commonly found attached to the ovaries, fallopian tubes, the outer surface of the uterus, the bowels, the area between the vagina and the rectum (rectovaginal septum), and the pelvic side wall (Fig. 4.2) though lesions have been found in locations as far from the uterus as the brain. The places where the tissue attaches are called implants or lesions. These lesions create their own blood supply and respond to hormones released during the menstrual cycle in the same way as the endometrial lining within the uterus.

At the beginning of the menstrual cycle, when the lining of the uterus is shed and menstrual bleeding begins, endometriosis implants swell and bleed as well. In short, the person with endometriosis experiences several "mini-periods" throughout their abdomen, wherever this endometriosis tissue exists. In addition to cyclic bleeding outside the uterus, pelvic pain that can be debilitating, scarring, and adhesion formation occur throughout the pelvis. Symptoms begin as early as adolescence and may settle after menopause.

Think back to Izzy, with her progressive pelvic pain and infertility concerns. After a pelvic examination, her health care provider suspects she has endometriosis.

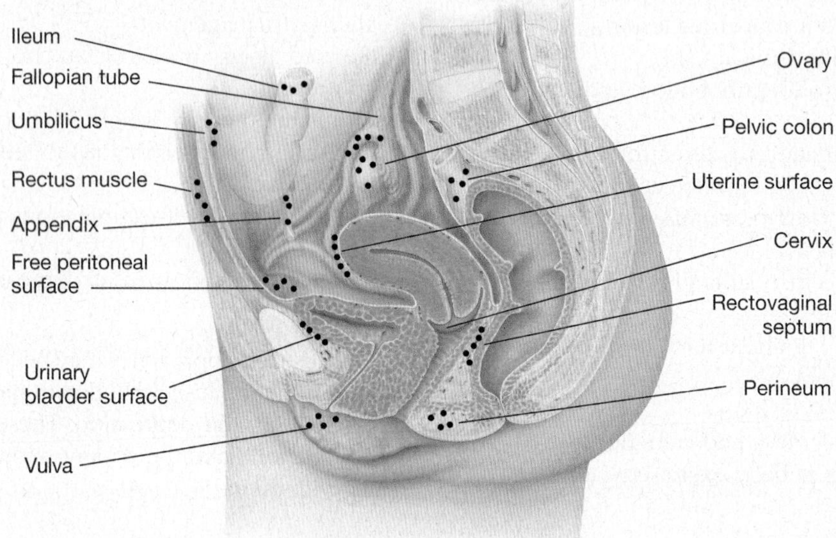

FIGURE 4.2 Common sites of endometriosis formation. (Reprinted with permission from Stewart, J. G. [2017]. *Anatomical Chart Company atlas of pathophysiology* [4th ed.]. Wolters Kluwer.)

Etiology and Risk Factors

It is not currently known why endometriosis tissue implants and grows in other parts of the body. Despite some progress, critical gaps remain in understanding the epidemiology of this condition. Several theories exist, but to date, none has been scientifically proven. However, several factors tend to be correlated with a diagnosis of endometriosis:

- Tall height
- Lower BMI
- Family history of endometriosis in a first-degree relative
- Short menstrual cycle (<27 days apart)
- Heavy menstrual flow
- Late menopause
- Obstruction of menstrual flow
- Young age of menarche (younger than 11 to 13 years of age)
- No pregnancies (nulliparity) (Schenken, 2024)

Therapeutic Management

Therapeutic management of the patient with endometriosis falls into three categories: pain relief, hormonal suppression, and surgery. The plan must take into consideration the following factors: severity of symptoms, desire for fertility, degree of the disease, and the patient's therapy goals. Currently, a definitive diagnosis of endometriosis is only possible via laparoscopy and visualization of the lesions; to date, no imaging modality can prove the presence of lesions. Treatment of endometriosis involves surgery to remove the lesions. Ovarian suppressive agents (OCs, progestins, long-acting GnRH analogs, and androgenic agents like danazol) can manage symptoms. Many people with endometriosis do not experience adequate pain relief from existing medical or surgical treatments (Mechsner, 2022). The gold standard for endometriosis treatment is laparoscopic excision surgery while pain-relieving drugs and hormone suppressants can address symptoms. Alternative therapies may be used, including heat application, acupuncture, exercise, stress-reducing therapies (such as meditation), yoga, and turmeric. Alternative therapies allow the patient to self-manage their pain and give them control, but efficacy data are limited and more research is warranted (Li et al., 2023). Because endometriosis has no cure and surgery with an endometriosis specialist is not widely accessible, surgery with a general gynecologist may only control symptoms temporarily. Patients with endometriosis frequently experience only short-term relief. Endometriosis-associated pelvic pain can be managed by suppression of ovulatory menses and estrogen production, cyclooxygenase inhibitors, and surgical removal of pelvic lesions. Many pain relief and hormonal suppression therapies have significant adverse effects and limits on the duration of therapy (Table 4.2).

Nursing Assessment

Nurses encounter patients with endometriosis in a variety of settings: community health settings, schools, clinics, day surgical centers, and hospitals. Health care professionals must not trivialize or dismiss the concerns of these patients, because early recognition is essential to improve long-term quality of life and preserve fertility. The diversity of presenting symptoms and a high rate

TABLE 4.2 • Treatment Options for Endometriosis

Therapy Options	Comment
Surgical Intervention	
Conservative surgery	Laparoscopic surgery. Removal of implants/lesions using laser, cautery, or small surgical instruments for excision. This intervention may reduce pain and allow pregnancy to occur in the future but may need to be repeated.
Definitive surgery	Abdominal hysterectomy with or without bilateral salpingo-oophorectomy. Will eliminate bleeding but will leave a patient unable to become pregnant in the future. Pain may not resolve if extrauterine lesions are not completely removed.
Medication Therapy	
NSAIDs	First-line treatment to reduce pain; taken early when premenstrual symptoms are first felt. Limited data demonstrating efficacy
Combined estrogen/progestin contraceptives	Suppresses ovarian function and cyclic hormonal response of the endometriosis tissue
Progestins	Inhibits endometrial tissue growth
Gonadotropin-releasing hormone analogs (GnRH-a)	Suppresses endometriosis symptoms by creating a temporary pseudomenopause

NSAIDs, nonsteroidal anti-inflammatory drugs.

Schenken, R. S. (2023). Endometriosis: Treatment of pelvic pain. *UpToDate.* Retrieved March 6, 2024, from https://www.uptodate.com/contents/endometriosis-treatment-of-pelvic-pain

of misdiagnosis contribute to patients with endometriosis falling through the cracks and not being diagnosed promptly.

HEALTH HISTORY

Endometriosis may be difficult to diagnose because its symptoms mimic those of other pelvic and gastrointestinal disorders, and the severity of the symptoms does not always reflect the extent of the disease. Obtain a health history to determine risk factors and elicit a description of signs and symptoms. Endometriosis can be asymptomatic, but it can also be a severe and debilitating condition. It is chronic and progressive. Ask specifically about menarche, history of menstrual problems, details of pregnancies, and difficulties with conception. Assess the patient for clinical manifestations, which include:

- Chronic pelvic pain
- Infertility
- Back pain
- Pain before and during menstrual periods
- Pain during or after sexual intercourse
- Painful urination
- Chronic fatigue
- Painful bowel movements
- Diarrhea or constipation
- Hypermenorrhea (heavy menses)
- Pelvic adhesions
- Blood in urine
- Irregular and more frequent menses (Schenken, 2024)

Classic symptoms seen in endometriosis are pelvic pain, infertility, or ovarian mass (Schenken, 2024). Endometriosis occurs in 25% to 50% of females with infertility and up to 70% of females with chronic pelvic pain (Hornstein et al., 2024; Schenken, 2024).

What are the most common symptoms experienced by people with endometriosis? Is Izzy's profile typical? As a nurse, what would be your role in Izzy's continued workup?

PHYSICAL EXAMINATION AND LABORATORY AND DIAGNOSTIC TESTS

The pelvic examination typically correlates with the extent of the endometriosis growth. The usual finding is nonspecific pelvic tenderness. The hallmark finding is the presence of tender nodular masses on the uterosacral ligaments, the posterior uterus, or the posterior cul-de-sac. A skilled endometriosis specialist may be able to identify suspected adhesions with a pelvic exam, but the only definitive diagnosis is the one made during surgery and with biopsy (Schenken, 2024).

After a thorough history and a pelvic examination, the health care provider may suspect endometriosis, but the only certain method of diagnosing it is by seeing it. Pelvic or transvaginal ultrasound is used to assess pelvic organ structures and rule out any cysts or fibroids. However, a laparoscopy is needed to diagnose endometriosis. Laparoscopy is the direct visualization of the internal organs with a lighted instrument inserted through an abdominal incision. A tissue biopsy of the suspected implant taken at the same time and examined microscopically confirms the diagnosis. Endometriosis can be treated during laparoscopy by removing the suspected tissue.

Nurses can play a role by offering a thorough explanation of the condition and explaining why tests are needed to diagnose endometriosis. The nurse can set up appointments for imaging studies and laparoscopy.

Nursing Management

In addition to the interventions outlined previously, the nurse should encourage the patient to adopt healthy lifestyle habits with respect to diet, exercise, sleep, and stress management. Referrals to support groups and internet resources (Box 4.2) can help the patient understand this condition and cope with chronic pain. Dealing with the symptoms and complications of endometriosis can be distressing. A number of organizations provide information about the diagnosis and treatment of endometriosis and offer support to patients and their families. Nurses are uniquely situated to improve patient outcomes by assisting patients in making informed treatment decisions. A prompt diagnosis ensures the best possible outcomes for this chronic disease.

INFERTILITY

The desire to have children can be powerful and widespread, but for many, that desire can also be unfulfilled. **Infertility** is defined as a disease characterized by the inability to conceive a child after 1 year of regular sexual intercourse unprotected by contraception. Infertility impacts approximately one in six people globally at least once in their lifetime (WHO, 2023c). Secondary infertility is the inability to conceive after a previous pregnancy. Many people take the ability to conceive and produce a child for granted, but infertility affects more than 48 million couples and 186 million individuals globally (Dourou et al., 2023). Infertility is a widespread problem that has an emotional, social, and economic impact on individuals and couples. It affects relationships, leads to tension and anger between partners, and can result in severe sexual dysfunction and breakdown of the relationship. Nurses must recognize infertility and understand its causes and treatment options so they can help patients and families understand the possibilities as well as the limitations of current therapies. Nurses have a central role in providing support through these stressful treatments. Patients and families will frequently confide in a nurse and can gain great benefit from a sympathetic and sensible discussion. Patients wish to be treated with respect and dignity and given appropriate information and support. Patients deserve to have their distress recognized, to feel cared for, and to have confidence in health care providers in situations in which outcomes are uncertain. Prevention of infertility through education should also be incorporated into any patient–nurse interaction.

BOX 4.2 Organizations and Web Resources to Assist the Patient With Endometriosis

- American College of Obstetricians and Gynecologists
  http://www.acog.org
- American Society of Reproductive Medicine
  http://www.asrm.org
- Endometriosis Association
  http://www.endometriosisassn.org
- Endometriosis Foundation of America
  http://www.endofound.org
- National Institutes of Health (U.S. Department of Health and Human Services)
  https://www.nichd.nih.gov/health/topics/endometriosis

> After completing several diagnostic tests, the doctor strongly suspects Izzy has endometriosis. She asks you about her chances of becoming pregnant and becoming pain free. What treatment options would you explain to Izzy? What information can you give about her future childbearing ability?

Cultural Considerations

Infertility is not only a physiologic problem, but it is one that can initiate a life crisis that is experienced with psychological, familial, social, and cultural consequences. Cross-culturally, the expectation for couples to reproduce is an accepted norm, and the inability to conceive may be considered a violation of this cultural norm. In this context, infertility represents a crisis for the individual and/or the couple. The manner in which different cultures, ethnic groups, and religious groups perceive and manage infertility may be very different. For example, many African Americans believe that assisted reproductive techniques are unnatural and that they remove the spiritual or divine nature of creation from conception. For this reason, they may seek spiritual rather than medical assistance when trying to conceive. Those belonging to Hispanic cultures may believe that children validate the marriage, so families are often large. Like African Americans, Hispanic people are often spiritual and may consider infertility a test of faith, leading them to seek spiritual counseling. Disappointing one's spouse can often be of concern to African American females, while avoiding the stigmatization of infertility can be a top concern to Asian American females. African Americans and Asian Americans alike may find themselves living with partner tensions, criticism from relatives, and stigmatization from the community. Many people of color do not reveal their infertility experiences, which often leaves them feeling alone in this process experiencing feelings of depression, anxiety, and grief (American Psychological Association, 2022).

Religion often influences cultural factors and, for this reason, may also be considered when pursuing treatment for infertility. In the Orthodox Jewish religion, procreation is considered to be a "mitzvah," a religious good deed. However, Orthodox Jews do accept the use of contraceptives to prevent conception when it is not desired. Conservative and Reform Jews put no restrictions on contraception and a lesser demand on procreation. Roman Catholics have a restrictive view of the use of assisted reproductive technologies since in their view, procreation cannot be separated from the relationship between parents. Thus, God wants human life to begin through the "conjugal act" and not artificially. Most religious teachings speak to the significance of procreation, so infertility can impact the self and relational identities of the couple wishing to become parents. Nurses must be cognizant of the patient's cultural and religious background and how it may dictate which, if any, reproductive treatment options are chosen. Nurses need to include this awareness in their counseling of couples dealing with infertility.

CONSIDER THIS!

We had been married for 3 years and wanted to start a family, but much to our dismay, nothing happened after a year of trying. I had some irregular periods and was finally diagnosed with endometriosis and put on Clomid for three cycles. After that time without achieving a pregnancy, I went to a fertility expert. The doctor lasered the misplaced endometriosis tissue, sent carbon dioxide through my tubes to make sure they were patent, and put me back on Clomid, but still we had no luck. Finally, 2 years later, we considered in vitro fertilization (IVF) and prayed we could find the money for the procedure. By then I felt I was a failure as a woman. We then decided that it was more important for us to be parents than it was for me to be pregnant, so we considered adoption. We tried for another year without any results.

We went to the adoption agency to fill out the paperwork for the process to begin. Our blood was taken and we waited for an hour, wondering the whole time why it was taking so long for the results. The nurse finally appeared and handed a piece of paper to me with the word "positive" written on it. I started to cry tears of joy because I was pregnant and our long journey of infertility was finally ending.

Thoughts: For many people, the dream of having a child is not easily realized. Infertility can affect self-esteem, disrupt relationships, and result in depression. This couple experienced many years of frustration in trying to have a family. What help can be offered to couples during this time? What can be said to comfort the patient who feels they are a failure?

Etiology and Risk Factors

Reproduction requires the interaction of the female and the male reproductive tracts, which involves (1) the release of a normal preovulatory oocyte, (2) the production of adequate spermatozoa, (3) the normal transport of the gametes to the ampullary portion of the fallopian tube (where fertilization takes place), and (4) the subsequent transport of the cleaving embryo into the endometrial cavity for implantation and development (Nath, 2023).

Multiple known and unknown factors affect fertility. Female-factor infertility is detected in about 50% of cases, male-factor infertility in about 26% of cases, and 28% fall into a category of combined (both male and female factors) or are considered unexplained (Kuohung & Hornstein, 2023b). In females, ovarian dysfunction and tubal damage are the primary contributing factors to infertility (Kuohung & Hornstein, 2023b).

Risk factors and causes for female infertility include:

- Overweight or underweight (can disrupt hormone function)
- Scarred fallopian tubes from infections
- Uterine fibroids
- Tubal blockages
- Oligoovulation and anovulation
- Luteal phase defect
- Cervical stenosis
- Reduced oocyte quality
- Chromosomal abnormalities
- Congenital anomalies of the uterus
- Immune system disorders
- Chronic illnesses such as diabetes, celiac disease
- STIs
- Ectopic pregnancy
- Increased age
- Endometriosis
- Turner syndrome
- Eating disorders
- History of PID
- Smoking and heavy alcohol consumption
- Daily vigorous exercise
- Multiple miscarriages
- Environmental toxins
- Menstrual abnormalities
- Exposure to chemotherapeutic agents (Hornstein et al., 2022; Kuohung & Hornstein, 2023c)

Risk factors and causes for male infertility include:

- Exposure to toxic substances (lead, mercury, x-rays, chemotherapy)
- Cigarette smoke
- Diabetes
- Heavy alcohol consumption
- Use of certain prescription drugs such as cimetidine
- Exposure of the genitals to high temperatures (hot tubs or saunas)
- Use of anabolic steroids
- Pituitary or testicular cancers
- Low levels of sperm
- Obesity associated with decreased sperm quality
- Kleinfelter syndrome
- Frequent long-distance cycling
- STIs
- Undescended testicles (cryptorchidism)
- Mumps after puberty (Anawalt, 2020; WHO, 2023b)

Therapeutic Management

As noted earlier, the main causes of infertility are female factor (e.g., ovarian dysfunction, tubal damage, endometriosis), male factor (e.g., low or absent numbers of motile sperm in the ejaculate, erectile dysfunction), or unexplained (CDC, 2023a). The test results are presented to the couple and different treatment options are suggested. The majority of infertility cases are treated with drugs or surgery. Treatment options include lifestyle changes, such as weight loss and smoking cessation; taking clomiphene to promote ovulation; hormone injections to promote ovulation; intrauterine insemination; and IVF. Various ovulation enhancement drugs and timed intercourse might be used for ovulation problems. The patient should understand a drug's benefits and side effects before consenting to take it. Depending on the type of drug used and the dosage, some may experience multiple pregnancies. If the female reproductive organs are damaged, surgery can be done to repair them. Still, other couples might opt for the hi-tech approaches of artificial insemination (Fig. 4.3), IVF (Fig. 4.4), embryo transfer, and egg donation, or they may contract for a gestational carrier or surrogate (Ho, 2023). Table 4.3 lists selected treatment options for infertility.

Nursing Assessment

Couples dealing with infertility may be under tremendous pressure and often keep the problem a secret, considering it to be personal. Individuals and couples are often beset by feelings of inadequacy and guilt, and many are subject to pressures from both family and friends. As the problem becomes more chronic, they may begin to blame one another, with consequent marital discord. Seeking help is often a difficult step, and it may take a lot of courage to discuss something about which they feel embarrassed or upset. The nurse working in this specialty setting must be aware of the conflict and problems couples experience and must be sensitive to their needs.

A full medical history should be taken from both partners, along with a physical examination. The data needed for the infertility evaluation are sensitive and of a personal nature, so the nurse must use professional interviewing skills.

Infertility has numerous causes and contributing factors, so it is important to use the process of elimination, determining what problems do not exist to better comprehend the problems that may exist. At the first visit, a plan of investigation is outlined and a complete health history is taken. This first visit forces many couples to confront the reality that a desired pregnancy may not occur naturally. Alleviate some of the anxiety associated with diagnostic testing by explaining the timing and reasons for each test.

Assessing Male Factors

The initial screening evaluation for the male partner should include a reproductive history and a semen analysis. This is the cornerstone of male infertility evaluation. From the male perspective, three things must happen for conception to take place: the number of sperm must be adequate, those sperm must be healthy and mature, and the sperm must be able to penetrate and fertilize the egg. Normal males have more than 15 million sperm per milliliter with greater than 40% motility (Anawalt, 2022). The patient should abstain from sexual activity for 2 to 5 days before giving the sample. For a semen examination, the patient is asked to produce a specimen by ejaculating into a specimen container and delivering it to the laboratory for analysis within 1 hour. When the specimen is brought to the laboratory, it is analyzed for volume, viscosity, number of sperm, sperm viability, motility, and sperm shape.

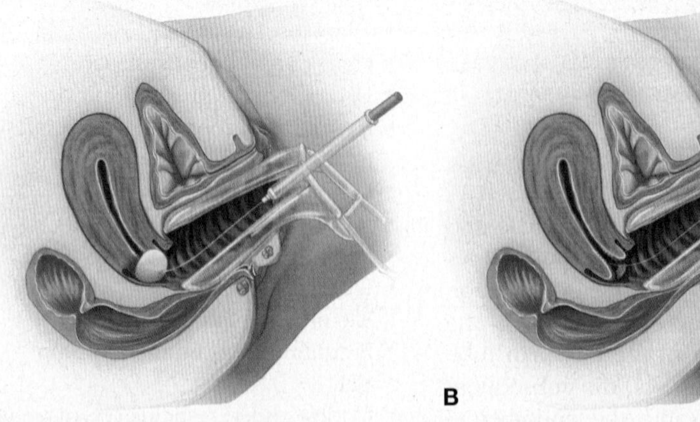

FIGURE 4.3 Artificial insemination. Sperm are deposited next to the cervix (**A**) or injected directly into the uterine cavity (**B**).

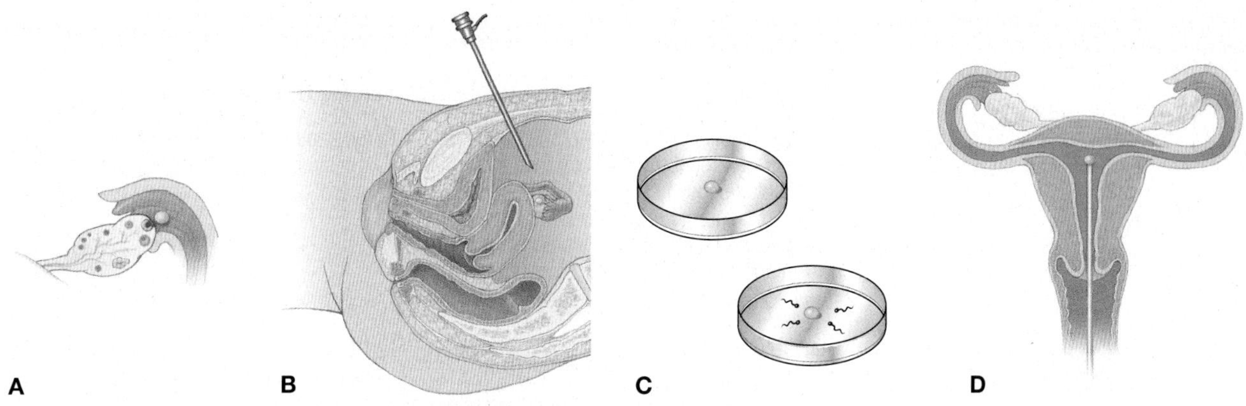

FIGURE 4.4 Steps involved in in vitro fertilization. **A.** Ovulation. **B.** Capture of the ova (done here intra-abdominally). **C.** Fertilization of ova and growth in culture medium. **D.** Insertion of fertilized ova into the uterus.

TABLE **4.3** • Selected Treatment Options for Infertility

Procedure	Comments	Nursing Considerations
Fertility Drugs		
Clomiphene citrate (Clomid)	A selective estrogen receptor modulator (SERM) used to induce ovulation. Clomid is limited to less than 12 cycles and after 3–6 unsuccessful cycles further evaluation is warranted.	Nurse can advise the couple to have intercourse every other day for 1 week starting after day 5 of medication.
Aromatase inhibitors (letrozole–currently not FDA approved for this use; Casper & Mitwally, 2022)	Blocks estrogen biosynthesis to induce ovulation	Same as above Drug of choice for people with PCOS Lower chance of multiple gestation
Gonadotropin therapy	Induces ovulation by direct stimulation of ovarian follicle	Same as above Higher chance of multiple gestation
Artificial insemination	The insertion of a prepared semen sample into the cervical os or intrauterine cavity Enables sperm to be deposited closer to improve chances of conception Husband's or donor sperm can be used.	Nurse needs to advise the couple that the procedure might need to be repeated if not successful the first time.
Assisted Reproductive Technologies		
In vitro fertilization (IVF)	Oocytes are fertilized in the lab and transferred to the uterus. Usually indicated for tubal obstruction, endometriosis, pelvic adhesions, and low sperm counts	Nurse advises patient to take medication to stimulate ovulation so the mature ovum can be retrieved by needle aspiration.
Gamete intrafallopian transfer (GIFT)	Oocytes and sperm are combined and immediately placed in the fallopian tube so fertilization can occur naturally. Requires laparoscopy and general anesthesia, which increases the risk	Nurse needs to inform couple of risks and have consent signed.
Intracytoplasmic sperm injection (ICSI)	One sperm is injected into the cytoplasm of the oocyte to fertilize it. Indicated for male-factor infertility	Nurse needs to inform the male that sperm will be aspirated by a needle through the skin into the epididymis.
Donor oocytes or sperm	Eggs or sperm are retrieved from a donor, and the eggs are inseminated; resulting embryos are transferred via IVF. Recommended for people older than 40 years and those with poor-quality eggs	Nurse needs to support couple in their ethical/religious discussions prior to deciding.

(*continued*)

TABLE 4.3 • Selected Treatment Options for Infertility (*continued*)

Procedure	Comments	Nursing Considerations
Preimplantation genetic diagnosis (PGD)	Used to identify genetic defects in embryos created through IVF before pregnancy This is done specifically when one or both genetic parents have a known genetic abnormality and testing is performed on an embryo to see if it also carries a genetic abnormality.	Nurse should inform couple about this option and support them until the test results return.
Gestational carrier (surrogacy)	Laboratory fertilization takes place, and embryos are transferred to the uterus of another female, who will carry the pregnancy or intrauterine insemination can be done with the male sperm. Medical legal issues have resulted over the "true ownership" of the resulting infant.	Nurse should encourage an open discussion regarding implications of this method with the couple.

FDA, U.S. Food and Drug Administration; IVF, in vitro fertilization; PCOS, polycystic ovary syndrome.

Kuohung, W., & Hornstein, M. D. (2023d). Female infertility: Treatments. *UpToDate.* Retrieved March 12, 2024, from https://www.uptodate.com/contents/female-infertility-treatments; Casper, R. F., & Mitwally, M. F. M. (2022). Ovulation induction with letrozole. *UpToDate.* Retrieved March 12, 2024, from https://www.uptodate.com/contents/ovulation-induction-with-letrozole; Seli, E., & Arici, A. (2023). Ovulation induction with clomiphene citrate. *UpToDate.* Retrieved March 12, 2024, from https://www.uptodate.com/contents/ovulation-induction-with-clomiphene-citrate; Salem, W. (2023). Assisted reproductive technology: Pregnancy and maternal outcomes. *UpToDate.* Retrieved March 12, 2024, from https://www.uptodate.com/contents/assisted-reproductive-technology-pregnancy-and-maternal-outcomes

The physical examination routinely includes:

- A general exam for overall health, assessing for signs of endocrine problems, such as a thyroid disorder or Cushing disease
- Assessment for appropriate male sexual characteristics, such as body hair distribution, development of the Adam's apple, and muscle development
- Examination of the penis, scrotum, testicles, epididymis, prostate, and vas deferens for abnormalities (e.g., nodules, irregularities, varicocele)
- Assessment for abnormal development of external genitalia (e.g., small testicles, micropenis) (Anawalt, 2022)

Assessing Female Factors

The initial assessment of the female should include a thorough history of factors associated with ovulation and the pelvic organs. The history should include duration of infertility, along with sexual, menstrual, and gynecologic history. The physical examination routinely includes:

- A general exam for overall health, assessing for signs of potential causes of infertility such as endocrine problems (e.g., a thyroid disorder or androgen excess such as hirsutism)
- Assessment for appropriate female secondary sexual characteristics
- Examination for uterine enlargement or tenderness
- Assessment for normal development of external genitalia (Kuohung & Hornstein, 2023a)

Diagnostic tests to determine female infertility may include:

- Assessment of ovarian function
- Urinary LH level
- Assessment of pelvic organs
- Papanicolaou (Pap) smear to rule out cervical cancer or inflammation
- Cervical culture to rule out any STIs
- Ultrasound to assess pelvic structures
- Hysterosalpingography (HSG) to visualize structural defects and tubal occlusion (Kuohung & Hornstein, 2023a)

Laboratory and Diagnostic Testing

The diagnostic procedures that should be done during an infertility workup should be guided by the couple's history. They generally proceed from less to more invasive tests.

HOME OVULATION PREDICTOR KITS

Home ovulation predictor kits contain monoclonal antibodies specific for LH and use an enzyme-linked immunosorbent assay (ELISA) test to determine the amount of LH present in the urine. A significant color change from baseline indicates the LH surge and presumably the most fertile day of the month.

CLOMIPHENE CITRATE CHALLENGE TEST

The clomiphene citrate challenge test is used to assess ovarian reserve (ability of eggs to become fertilized).

FSH levels are drawn on cycle day 3 and on cycle day 10 after the patient has taken 100 mg of clomiphene citrate on cycle days 5 through 9. If the FSH level is greater than 15, the result is considered abnormal and the likelihood of conception with their own eggs is low (Kuohung & Hornstein, 2023a).

HYSTEROSALPINGOGRAPHY

HSG is the gold standard in assessing patency (being open and unobstructed) of the fallopian tubes. Fallopian tube obstruction is among the most common causes of female-factor infertility. Ultrasonography and magnetic resonance imaging (MRI) are used in this assessment. In hysterosalpingography, 3 to 10 mL of an opaque oil-based contrast medium is slowly injected through a catheter into the endocervical canal so that the uterus and tubes can be visualized during fluoroscopy and radiography. If the fallopian tubes are patent, the dye will ascend upward to distend the uterus and the tubes and will spill out into the peritoneal cavity (Fig. 4.5) (Mayer & Deedwania, 2023).

LAPAROSCOPY

Laparoscopy offers direct visualization of the female pelvic anatomy to diagnose tubal and peritoneal abnormalities that may be interfering with fertility. A laparoscopy is usually performed early in the menstrual cycle. It is not part of the routine infertility evaluation. It is used when abnormalities are found on the ultrasound or the hysterosalpingogram or when endometriosis is suspected. Because of the added risks of surgery, the need for anesthesia, and operative costs, it is only used when clearly indicated. During the procedure, an endoscope is inserted through a small incision in the anterior abdominal wall. Visualization of the peritoneal cavity in patient with female infertility may reveal endometriosis, pelvic adhesions, tubal occlusion, fibroids, or polycystic ovaries (Arab, 2022).

Nursing Management

Nurses play an important role in the care of people with infertility. They are pivotal educators about preventive health care. A number of potentially modifiable risk factors are associated with the development of impaired fertility in females, and patients need to be aware of these risks to institute change. The nurse is most effective when they offer care and treatment in a professional manner and regard the patient and couple as valued and respected people. The nurse must be respectful of and mindful that many people may seek spiritual help for their infertility issues in addition to traditional medical modalities. Throughout the entire process, the nurse's role is to provide information, anticipatory guidance, stress management, and counseling. The couple's emotional distress is often high, and the nurse must be able to recognize that anxiety and provide emotional support. The nurse may need to refer couples to a reproductive endocrinologist or surgeon, depending on the problem identified.

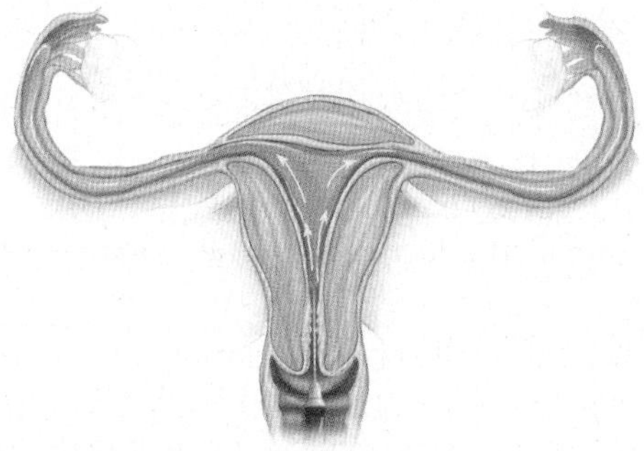

FIGURE 4.5 Insertion of a dye for a hysterosalpingogram. The contrast dye outlines the uterus and fallopian tubes on an x-ray to demonstrate patency.

There is no absolute way to prevent infertility per se because so many factors are involved in conception. Nurses can be instrumental in educating people about the factors that contribute to infertility. The nurse can also outline the risks and benefits of treatments so that the couple can make an informed decision. As couples struggle with infertility, they frequently turn to nurses for empathy, counseling, and support. By understanding the struggles and lived experiences of people experiencing infertility, the nurse can tailor their approach to better meet the couple's needs so that the pregnancy and birth experience is healing, transformative, and positive.

With advances in genetics and reproductive medicine also come a myriad of ethical, social, and cultural issues that will affect the couple's decisions. With this in mind, provide an opportunity for the couple to make informed decisions in a nondirective, nonjudgmental environment. It is important to encourage couples to remain optimistic throughout investigation and treatment.

Finances and insurance coverage often dictate the choice of treatment. Help couples decipher their insurance coverage and help them weigh the costs of various procedures by explaining what each will provide in terms of their infertility problems. Assisting them in making a priority list of diagnostic tests and potential treatment options will help the couple plan a financial strategy.

Many couples dealing with infertility are not prepared for the emotional roller coaster of grief and loss that accompanies infertility treatments. Financial concerns and coping as a couple are two major areas of stress when treatment is undertaken. During the course of what may be months or even years of infertility care, it is essential to develop a holistic approach to nursing care. Stress management and anxiety reduction need to be addressed, and referral to a peer support group such as RESOLVE might be in order (Box 4.3).

BOX 4.3 Organizations and Web Resources to Assist the Patient With Infertility

- RESOLVE: a nationwide network of chapters dedicated to providing education, advocacy, and support for people facing infertility. They provide a helpline, medical referral services, and a member-to-member contact system (http://www.resolve.org).
- American Society of Reproductive Medicine (ASRM): provides fact sheets and other resources on infertility, treatments, insurance, and other issues (http://www.asrm.org).
- International Counsel on Infertility (INCIID): provides information about infertility, support forums, and a directory of infertility specialists (http://www.inciid.org).
- American Fertility Association: offers education, referrals, research, support, and advocacy for couples dealing with infertility (http://www.americaninfertility.org).
- Office on Women's Health—Infertility health topic: (https://www.womenshealth.gov/a-z-topics/infertility).
- International Consumer Support for Infertility: an international network engaged in advocacy on behalf of couples faced with infertility via fact sheets and information (icsicommunity.org).

HEALTHY PEOPLE 2030

Objective	Nursing Significance
Increase the proportion of pregnancies that are intended.	Would reduce the number of unplanned pregnancies and females not finishing their education. This would in turn reduce the number of single parents on state financial assistance.
Reduce pregnancies among adolescent females.	Awareness of contraceptive methods and accessibility brings about better compliance and prevention of unintended pregnancies.
Increase the proportion of female adolescents who receive formal instruction on reproductive health topics before they are 18 years old.	Accessibility of reproductive resources can offer pregnancy prevention and preventive education.
Increase the proportion of females in need of publicly supported contraceptive services and supplies who receive those services and supplies.	Would increase accessibility to contraception and prevent unintended pregnancies.

Healthy People Objectives retrieved from http://www.healthypeople.gov

CONTRACEPTION

The terms "**contraception**," "family planning," and "birth control" are used interchangeably when referring to the intentional prevention of pregnancy through the use of various devices, agents, drugs, sexual practices, and surgical procedures. This allows people control over their reproductive health and active participation in family planning. Among females in their reproductive years in the United States who do not want to become pregnant, 90% use some form of contraception. Therefore, nurses will often encounter patients using some type of contraception (Britton et al., 2020). See the Healthy People 2030 box.

In addition to unplanned pregnancies, some contraceptives help prevent transmission of STIs and human immunodeficiency virus (HIV). The CDC (2023c) states that about 36,000 people in the United States received an HIV diagnosis every year. Much of this suffering could be prevented by access to and consistent use of safe, efficient, appropriate, modern contraception for everyone who wants it, as well as proper education regarding benefits and instructions for use (see Evidence-Based Practice 4.1). See Chapter 5 for more information on STIs.

Types of Contraceptive Methods

Contraceptive methods can be divided into four types: behavioral methods, barrier methods, hormonal methods, and permanent methods. Patients must decide which method is appropriate for them to meet their changing contraceptive needs throughout their life cycles. Nurses can educate and assist patients during this selection process. This part of the chapter will outline the most common birth control methods available.

In an era when many people wish to delay pregnancy and avoid STIs, choices can be difficult. Numerous methods of contraception are available today, and many more will be offered in the near future. The ideal contraceptive method for many people would have the following characteristics: ease of use, safety, effectiveness, minimal side effects, widely available, acceptable to all cultures and religions, be nonhormonal, and be immediately reversible. The best birth control method is one that is used consistently with minimal adverse effects (Kaunitz, 2023a). Currently, no contraceptive method offers everything. Box 4.4 outlines the contraceptive methods available today. Table 4.4 provides a detailed summary of each type, including information on failure rates, advantages, disadvantages, STI protection, and danger signs.

Contraceptive methods can be grouped according to their estimated effectiveness in preventing pregnancy as follows:

- Most effective methods: male and female sterilization, intrauterine contraception, and implant
- Very effective methods: injectable contraceptive, contraceptive patch, ring, pills, and diaphragm
- Less effective methods: external (male) and internal (female) condoms, cervical cap, sponge, spermicide, and fertility awareness (ACOG, 2023a)

EVIDENCE-BASED PRACTICE 4.1

Telehealth for Female Preventive Services

BACKGROUND

While telehealth has been around for decades, it has made leaps and bounds in recent years as patients and providers have embraced it. Patients now have access to high-quality care from the comfort of their homes. With the COVID-19 pandemic that forced many people to become homebound for long periods of time, the use of telehealth has increased substantially to meet many health care needs. The objective of this study was to evaluate the effectiveness, use, and implementation of telehealth for female preventive services for reproductive health needs and interpersonal violence as compared to in-person care. It also evaluated patient preferences.

STUDY

Searches of 5,704 articles that addressed telehealth interventions were independently reviewed for inclusion in the study using predefined criteria. Sixteen were included in this study.

Findings

Based on 16 studies, outcomes of telehealth compared with face-to-face care were similar for adolescent and adult females presenting for contraceptive care or receiving services for screening, assessment, or intervention for interpersonal violence. The COVID-19 pandemic increased telehealth utilization. Barriers to telehealth interventions included limited internet access, low digital literacy, and confidentiality concerns.

Nursing Implications

The study demonstrated evidence, though limited due to the low number of studies included in the final analysis, that telehealth interventions for contraceptive care and interpersonal violence services result in equivalent patient-reported outcomes as face-to-face care. Telehealth is a viable alternative and resource for patients in need of reproductive care services who face barriers to health care. Nurses can suggest this modality of care to patients experiencing access issues such as limited transportation, babysitting issues, and time restraints.

Cantor, A. G., Nelson, H. D., Pappas, M., Atchison, C., Hatch, B., Huguet, N., Flynn, B., & McDonagh, M. (2022). *Telehealth for women's preventive services.* Comparative effectiveness Review No. 256. Agency for Healthcare Research and Quality. https://doi.org/10.23970/AHRQEPCCER256

BOX 4.4 Outline of Contraceptive Methods

Reversible Methods

- Behavioral
  - Abstinence
  - Fertility awareness–based methods (FAMs)
  - Withdrawal (coitus interruptus)
  - Lactational amenorrhea method (LAM)
- Barrier
  - Condom (male and female)
  - Diaphragm
  - Cervical cap
  - Sponge
- Hormonal
  - Oral contraceptive (OC)
  - Injectable contraceptive
  - Transdermal patch
  - Vaginal ring
  - Implantable contraceptive
  - Intrauterine contraceptive
  - Emergency contraceptive

Permanent Methods

- Tubal ligation for females
- Vasectomy for males

Sexual Abstinence

Sexual abstinence (not having intercourse) is one of the least expensive forms of contraception and has been used for thousands of years to avoid unintended pregnancy. Pregnancy cannot occur if sperm is kept out of the vagina. It also reduces the risk of contracting HIV/AIDS and other STIs, unless body fluids are exchanged through oral sex; however, some infections, like herpes and human papillomavirus (HPV), can still be passed by skin-to-skin contact. Dental dams can be used to prevent transmission, however. There are many pleasurable options for sex play without intercourse ("outercourse"), such as kissing, masturbation, erotic massage, sexual fantasy, sex toys such as vibrators, and oral sex.

Many people have strong feelings about abstinence based on religious and moral beliefs. There are many reasons to choose abstinence. For some, it is a way of life, while for others it is a temporary choice. Some people choose sexual abstinence because they want to:

- Wait to have sex until they are older.
- Wait to have sex for a long-term relationship.
- Avoid pregnancy or STIs.
- Relieve feelings of depression or anxiety.
- Follow religious or cultural expectations.

Fertility Awareness–Based Methods

Fertility awareness methods (FAMs) are based on identifying fertile days in the female cycle and avoiding sexual intercourse during that time. FAMs use physical signs and symptoms that change with hormone fluctuations throughout the menstrual cycle to predict female fertility. Ovulation occurs on 1 day during each menstrual cycle, and the several days preceding ovulation are when intercourse is most likely to result in pregnancy. Collectively, the potentially fertile days up to and including the day of ovulation are called the "fertile window," which is approximately 6 days. Awareness of fertility is a better fertility-producing method than a contraceptive method. The unifying theme of FAMs is that a person can reduce their chance of pregnancy by abstaining from coitus or using

TABLE 4.4 • Summary of Contraceptive Methods

Type	Description	Failure Rate	Pros	Cons	STI Protection	Danger Signs	Comments
Nothing/chance	No birth control method used	85%					
Fertility awareness–based methods	Refrain from sex during fertile period	23%	No side effects; acceptable to most religious groups	High failure rate with incorrect use	None	None	Requires high level of couple commitment
Withdrawal (coitus interruptus)	Male withdraws before ejaculation.	22%	Involves no devices and is always available	Requires considerable self-control by the male	None	None	Places female in trusting and dependent role
Lactational amenorrhea method (LAM)	Uses lactational infertility for protection from pregnancy	0.45%–7.5% chance of pregnancy in first 6 months	No cost; not coitus linked	Temporary method; effective for only 6 months after giving birth	None	None	Person must breastfeed infant on demand without supplementation for 6 months.
Male condom	Thin sheath placed over an erect penis, blocking sperm	13%	Widely available; low cost; physiologically safe	Decreased sensation; interferes with sexual spontaneity; breakage risk	Provides protection against STIs	Latex allergy	Couple must be instructed on proper use of condom.
Female condom	Polyurethane sheath inserted vaginally to block sperm	21%	Use controlled by female; eliminates postcoital drainage of semen	Expensive for frequent use; cumbersome; noisy during sex act; for single use only	Provides protection against STIs	Allergy to polyurethane	Couple must be instructed on proper use of condom.
Diaphragm with spermicide	Shallow latex cup with spring mechanism in its rim to hold it in place in the vagina	17%	Nonhormonal; considered medically safe; provides some protection against cervical cancer	Requires accurate fitting by health care professional; increase in UTIs	None	Allergy to latex, rubber, polyurethane, or spermicide Report symptoms of toxic shock syndrome May become dislodged in female superior position	Patient must be taught to insert and remove the diaphragm correctly.
Cervical cap with spermicide	Soft cup-shaped latex device that fits over base of the cervix	17%–23%	No use of hormones; provides continuous protection while in place	Requires accurate fitting by health care professional; odor may occur if left in too long	None	Irritation, allergic reaction; abnormal Pap test; risk of toxic shock syndrome	Instructions on insertion and removal must be understood by patient.

Sponge with spermicide	Disk-shaped polyurethane device containing a spermicide that is activated by wetting it with water	14% if nulliparous 27% if multiparous	Offers immediate and continuous protection for 24 hours; OTC	Can fall out of vagina with voiding; is not form fitting in the vagina	None	Irritation, allergic reactions; toxic shock syndrome can occur if the sponge is left in too long.	Caution patient not to leave sponge in beyond 24 hours.
Oral contraceptives (combination)	A pill that suppresses ovulation by combined action of estrogen and progestin	7%	Easy to use; high rate of effectiveness; protection against ovarian and endometrial cancer	User must remember to take pill daily; possible undesirable side effects; high cost for some people; prescription needed	None	Dizziness, nausea, mood changes, high blood pressure, blood clots, heart attacks, strokes	Each patient must be assessed thoroughly to make sure they are not a smoker and do not have a history of thromboembolic disease.
Oral contraceptives (progestin-only mini-pills)	A pill containing only progestin that thickens cervical mucus to prevent sperm from penetrating	7%	No estrogen-related side effects; may be used by lactating patient; may be used by patient with a history of thrombophlebitis	Must be taken with meticulous accuracy; may cause irregular bleeding; less effective than combination pills	None	Irregular bleeding, weight gain, increased incidence of ectopic pregnancy	Patients should be screened for history of functional ovarian cysts, previous ectopic pregnancy, and hyperlipidemia prior to giving prescription.
Patch (Ortho Evra)	Transdermal patch that releases estrogen and progestin into circulation	7%	Easy system to remember; very effective	May cause skin irritation where it is placed; may fall off and not be noticed and thus provide no protection	None	Less effective in people weighing more than 200 lb	Instruct patient to apply patch every week for 3 weeks and then not to wear one during week 4.
Ring (NuvaRing)	Vaginal contraceptive ring about 2 in in diameter that is inserted into the vagina; releases estrogen and progestin	7%	Easy system to remember; very effective	May cause a vaginal discharge; can be expelled without noticing and not offer protection	None	Similar to oral contraceptives	Instruct patient to use a backup method if ring is expelled and remains out for more than 3 hours.
Depo-Provera injection	An injectable progestin that inhibits ovulation	4%	Long duration of action (3 months); highly effective; estrogen free; may be used by smokers; can be used by lactating people	Menstrual irregularities; return visit needed every 12 weeks; weight gain, headaches, depression; return to fertility delayed up to 12 months	None	If depression is a problem, this method may increase the depression.	Inform patient that fertility is delayed after stopping the injections.

(*continued*)

TABLE 4.4 • Summary of Contraceptive Methods (*continued*)

Type	Description	Failure Rate	Pros	Cons	STI Protection	Danger Signs	Comments
Implant (Nexplanon)	A time-release implant (one rod) of levonorgestrel for 3 years	0.1%	Long duration of action; low dose of hormones; reversible; estrogen free	Irregular bleeding; weight gain; breast tenderness; headaches; difficulty in removal	None	If bleeding is heavy, anemia may occur.	Before insertion, assess patient to make sure they are aware that this method will produce about 3 years of infertility.
Intrauterine contraception device or system (IUD or IUS)	A T-shaped device inserted into the uterus that releases copper, progesterone, or levonorgestrel	0.1%–0.8%	It is immediately and highly effective; allows for sexual spontaneity; can be used during lactation; return to fertility not impaired; requires no active compliance by the user after insertion	Insertion requires a skilled professional; menstrual irregularities; prolonged amenorrhea; can be unknowingly expelled; may increase the risk of pelvic infection; user must regularly check string for placement; no protection against STIs; delay of fertility after discontinuing for possibly 6–12 months	None	Cramps, bleeding, pelvic inflammatory disease; infertility; perforation of the uterus	Instruct patient how to locate string to check monthly for placement.
Postcoital emergency contraceptives (ECs)	Combination of levonorgestrel-only pills; combined estrogen and progestin pills; or the copper IUS inserted within 72 hours after unprotected intercourse	2.2%	Provides a last chance to prevent a pregnancy	Risk of ectopic pregnancy if EC fails	None	Nausea, vomiting, abdominal pain, fatigue, headache	Inform patient that ECs do not interrupt an established pregnancy, and the sooner they are taken, the more effective they are.
Permanent Sterilization							
Male	Sealing, tying, or cutting the vas deferens	0.15%	One-time decision provides permanent sterility; short recovery time; low long-term risks	Procedures are difficult to reverse; initial cost may be high; chance of regret; some pain/discomfort after procedures	None for both	Postoperative complications: pain, bleeding, infection	Counsel both as to permanence of procedure and urge them to think it through prior to signing consent.
Female	Fallopian tubes are blocked to prevent conception.	0.5%					

OTC, over the counter; STIs, sexually transmitted infections; UTIs, urinary tract infections.

Adapted from Paradise, S. L., Landis, C. A., & Klein, D. A. (2022). Evidence-based contraception: Common questions and answers. *American Family Physician.* https://www.aafp.org/dam/AAFP/documents/journals/afp/Paradise.pdf; American College of Obstetricians and Gynecologists. (2023a). *Effectiveness of birth control methods.* https://www.acog.org/womens-health/infographics/effectiveness-of-birth-control-methods; Centers for Disease Control and Prevention. (2023b). *Contraception.* https://www.cdc.gov/reproductivehealth/contraception/index.htm; Sonalkar, S., & Mody, S. K. (2023). Contraception: Postpartum counseling and methods. *UpToDate.* Retrieved March 15, 2024, from https://www.uptodate.com/contents/contraception-postpartum-counseling-and-methods

barrier methods during times of fertility. These methods require couples to take an active role in preventing pregnancy through their sexual behaviors, and menstrual cycles need to be regular for it to be effective. Couples agree to practice certain techniques, use calculations, and be observant of the fertile and the nonfertile periods in a monthly menstrual cycle. Using these methods for birth control requires a strong commitment from both partners. The normal physiologic changes caused by hormonal fluctuations during the menstrual cycle can be observed and charted. This information can then be used to avoid or promote pregnancy. Many apps are currently available and easily downloaded to mobile devices. Some are geared toward enhancing fertility while others are designed for contraception. FAMs rely on the following assumptions:

- A single ovum is released from the ovary 14 days before the next menstrual period. It lives approximately 24 hours.
- People using this method must have regular menstrual cycles for it to be effective.
- Sperm can live up to 5 days after intercourse. The fertile period during the menstrual cycle is thus approximately 6 days before and 1 day after ovulation. Because body changes start to occur before ovulation, the person can become aware of them and not have intercourse on these days or use another method to prevent pregnancy.
- The exact time of ovulation cannot be determined, so 2 to 3 days may be added to the beginning and end to avoid pregnancy.

Techniques used to determine fertility include the cervical mucus ovulation method, the basal body temperature (BBT) method, the symptothermal method, standard days method (SDM), and 2-day method (Jennings, 2023). FAMs are moderately effective but are unforgiving if not carried out as prescribed. FAMs can be used in combination with coital abstinence or barrier methods during fertile days if pregnancy is not desired.

CERVICAL MUCUS OVULATION METHOD

Cervical mucus is a jellylike vaginal discharge that comes from the cervix. The **cervical mucus ovulation method** is used to assess the character of the cervical mucus to help determine fertile days. Cervical mucus changes in consistency during the menstrual cycle and plays a vital role in the fertilization of the egg. In the days preceding ovulation, fertile cervical mucus helps draw sperm up and into the fallopian tubes, where fertilization usually takes place. It also helps maintain the survival of sperm. As ovulation approaches, the mucus becomes more abundant, clear, slippery, and smooth; it can be stretched between two fingers without breaking. Under the influence of estrogen, this mucus looks like egg whites. It is called *spinnbarkeit* mucus (Fig. 4.6). After ovulation, the cervical mucus becomes thick and dry under the influence of progesterone.

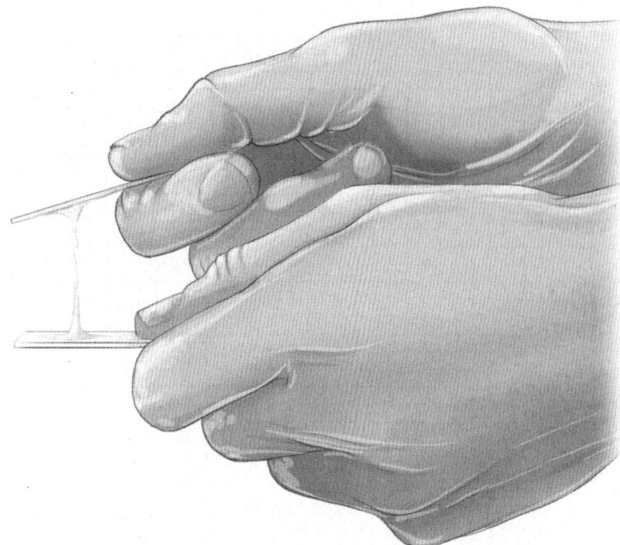

FIGURE 4.6 Spinnbarkeit mucus is cervical mucus that can stretch a distance before breaking.

This method works because the person becomes aware of the body changes that accompany ovulation. When they notice these changes, they abstain from sexual intercourse or use another method to prevent pregnancy. Each person's fertile time of the month is unique and thus must be individually assessed and determined.

BASAL BODY TEMPERATURE METHOD

The **basal body temperature (BBT)** refers to the lowest temperature reached on awakening. The person takes their temperature orally before rising and records it on a chart. Preovulation temperatures are suppressed by estrogen, while postovulation temperatures are increased under the influence of heat-inducing progesterone. Temperatures typically rise within a day or two after ovulation and remain elevated for approximately 2 weeks (at which point bleeding usually begins). If using this method by itself, the person should avoid unprotected intercourse until the BBT has been elevated for 3 days. Nurses should instruct patients using the BBT method that it is important to keep in mind that illness and any drugs, including alcohol, can raise body temperature and give a false reading. Other FAMs should be used along with BBT for better results (Fig. 4.7).

SYMPTOTHERMAL METHOD

The **symptothermal method** relies on a combination of techniques to recognize ovulation, including BBT, cervical mucus changes, alterations in the position and firmness of the cervix, and other symptoms of ovulation, such as increased libido, *mittelschmerz* (midcycle, lower abdominal pain at ovulation), pelvic fullness or tenderness, and breast tenderness (Jennings, 2023). Combining all these predictors increases the awareness of when ovulation occurs and increases the effectiveness of this method. A home predictor test for ovulation is also

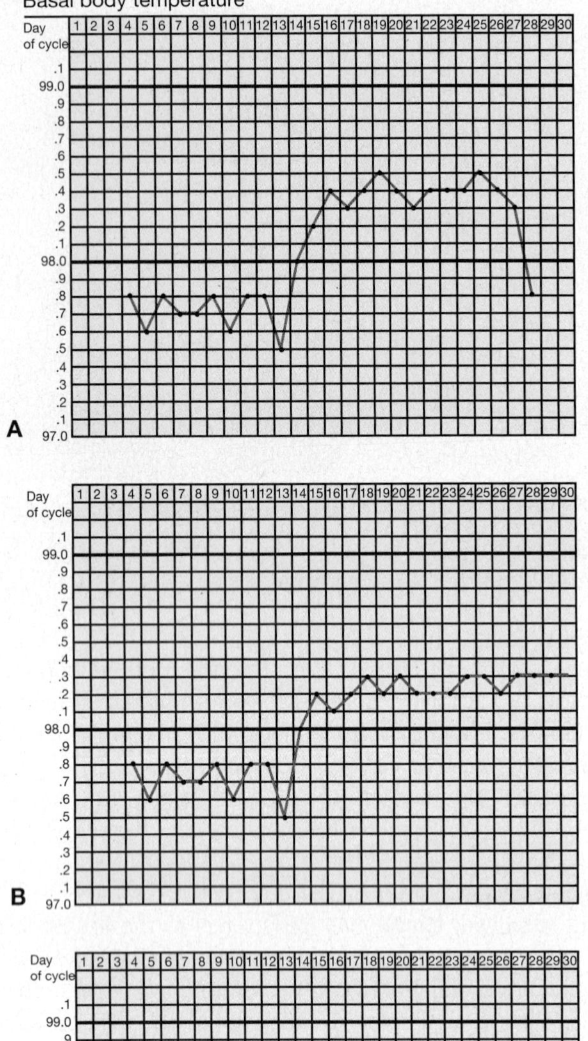

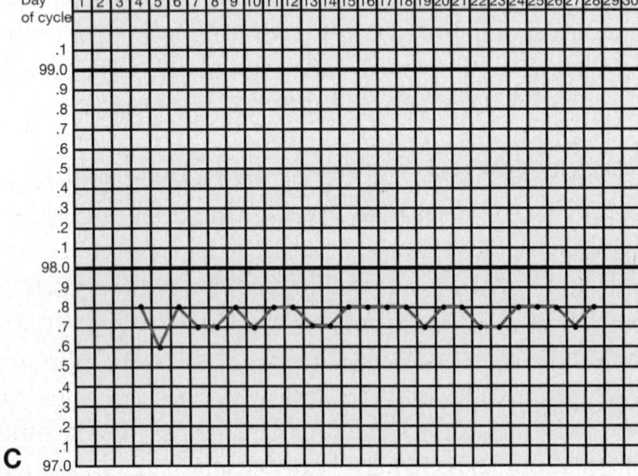

FIGURE 4.7 Basal body temperature graph. **A.** The female's temperature dips slightly at midpoint in the menstrual cycle, then rises sharply, an indication of ovulation. Toward the end of the cycle (the 24th day), the temperature begins to decline, indicating that progesterone levels are falling and that they did not conceive. **B.** The female's temperature rises at the midpoint in the cycle and remains at that elevated level past the time of the normal menstrual flow, suggesting that pregnancy has occurred. **C.** There is no preovulatory dip and no rise of temperature anywhere during the cycle. This is the typical pattern of a female who does not ovulate.

available in most pharmacies. It measures LH levels to pinpoint the day before or the day of ovulation. These tests are widely used for fertility and infertility regimens.

THE SDM AND THE 2-DAY METHOD

The **standard days method (SDM)** and the 2-day method are both natural methods of contraception developed by Georgetown University Medical Center's Institute for Reproductive Health. Both methods provide simple, clear instructions for identifying fertile days. People with menstrual cycles between 26 and 32 days long can use the SDM to prevent pregnancy by avoiding unprotected intercourse on days 8 through 19 of their cycles. SDM identifies the 12-day "fertile window" of the menstrual cycle. These 12 days take into account the lifespan of the egg (about 24 hours) and the viability of the sperm (about 5 days) as well as the variation in the actual timing of ovulation from one cycle to another. To help keep track of the days to avoid unprotected intercourse, a string of 32 color-coded string of beads called CycleBeads can be used, with each bead representing a day of the menstrual cycle. Starting with the red bead, which represents the first day of the menstrual period, the person moves a small rubber ring one bead each day. The brown beads are the days when pregnancy is unlikely, and the white beads represent fertile days (Jennings, 2023). This method has been used in underdeveloped countries for people with limited educational resources (Fig. 4.8).

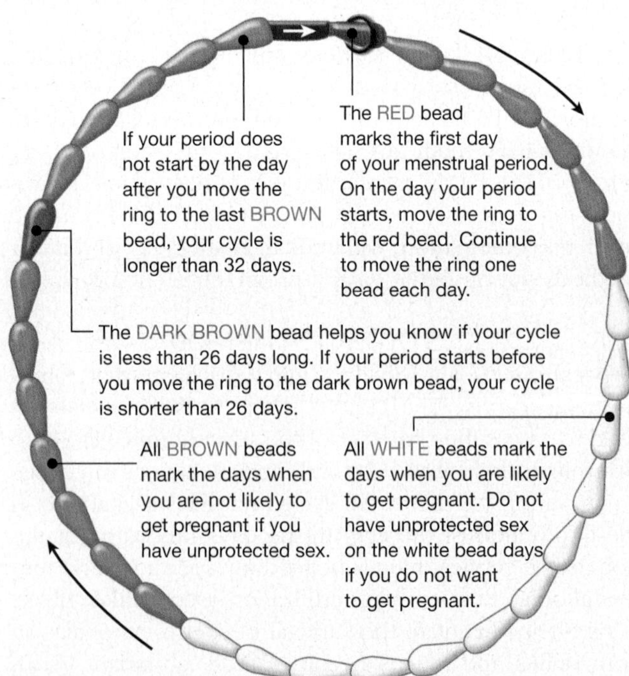

FIGURE 4.8 CycleBeads help people to remember to use the standard days method.

With the 2-day method, a person observes the presence or absence of cervical secretions by examining toilet paper or underwear or by monitoring their physical sensations. Every day, the person asks two simple questions: "Did I note any secretions yesterday?" and "Did I note any secretions today?" If the answer to either question is yes, they consider themselves fertile and avoid unprotected intercourse. If the answers are no, they have a low risk of becoming pregnant from unprotected intercourse on that day (Jennings, 2023).

Withdrawal (Coitus Interruptus)

In **coitus interruptus**, also known as withdrawal, a male partner controls their ejaculation during sexual intercourse and ejaculates outside the vagina. It is better known colloquially as "pulling out." It is one of the oldest and most widely used means of preventing pregnancy in the world and one of the least effective methods for preventing pregnancy. The problem with this method is that the first few drops of the true ejaculate contain the greatest concentration of sperm, and if some pre-ejaculatory fluid escapes from the urethra before orgasm, conception may result. This method requires that the female partner rely solely on the cooperation and judgment of the male partner. Nurses might discuss the use of emergency contraceptives with this couple or the use of a more effective method of contraception.

Lactational Amenorrhea Method

The **lactational amenorrhea method (LAM)** is an effective temporary method of contraception used by breastfeeding parents. It relies on physiologic changes associated with breastfeeding for contraception. Continuous breastfeeding can usually postpone ovulation and thus prevent pregnancy. Breastfeeding stimulates the hormone prolactin, which is necessary for milk production, and it also inhibits the release of another hormone, gonadotropin, which is necessary for ovulation.

Breastfeeding as a contraceptive method can be fairly effective for up to 6 months after giving birth if:

- The person has not had menses since giving birth.
- It has been less than 6 months since delivery.
- The person is fully or nearly fully breastfeeding (breastfeeding at least every 4 to 6 hours) (CDC, 2023b).

Barrier Methods

Barrier contraceptives are physical or chemical devices that prevent pregnancy by preventing the sperm from reaching the ovum. Mechanical barriers include condoms, diaphragms, cervical caps, and sponges. These devices are placed over the penis or cervix to physically obstruct the passage of sperm through the cervix. Chemical barriers called spermicides may be used along with mechanical barrier devices. They come in creams, jellies, foam, suppositories, and vaginal films. They chemically destroy the sperm in the vagina. Condoms are a barrier method that not only provides a physical barrier for sperm but also protects against STIs. Barrier methods may contain latex; therefore, a person with a latex allergy needs to be aware of which products are safe for them to use.

CONDOMS

Condoms are barrier methods of contraceptives made for both males and females. The external condom is made from latex or polyurethane (synthetic) or natural membrane and may be coated with spermicide. External condoms are available in many colors, textures, sizes, shapes, and thicknesses. When used correctly, the external condom is put on over an erect penis before it enters the vagina and is worn throughout sexual intercourse (Fig. 4.9). It serves as a barrier to pregnancy by trapping seminal fluid and sperm after orgasm and offers protection against STIs. Natural condoms may not prevent against STIs (CDC, 2023b). Condoms are not perfect barriers, however, because breakage and slippage can occur. If this happens, emergency postcoital contraception may need to be sought to prevent a pregnancy.

The internal condom is a polyurethane or nitrile pouch inserted into the vagina to catch the male ejaculate. It consists of an outer and inner ring that is inserted vaginally and held in place by the pubic bone. Some people complain that the female condom is cumbersome to use and makes noise during intercourse. Female condoms are readily available, are inexpensive, and can be carried inconspicuously. The female condom was the first female-controlled method that offered protection against pregnancy and some STIs.

VAGINAL DIAPHRAGM

The **diaphragm** is a nonhormonal method that is a reusable soft silicone dome device surrounded by a metal spring. Used in conjunction with a spermicidal jelly or cream, it is inserted into the vagina to cover the cervix (Fig. 4.10). The diaphragm may be inserted up to 2 hours before intercourse and must be left in place for at least 6 hours afterward. Diaphragms are available in a single one-size-fits-most (commercially named Caya) or multisize styles. The failure rate is similar between the single and multisize diaphragms (Bartz, 2023). Both are only available by prescription. The multisize diaphragm

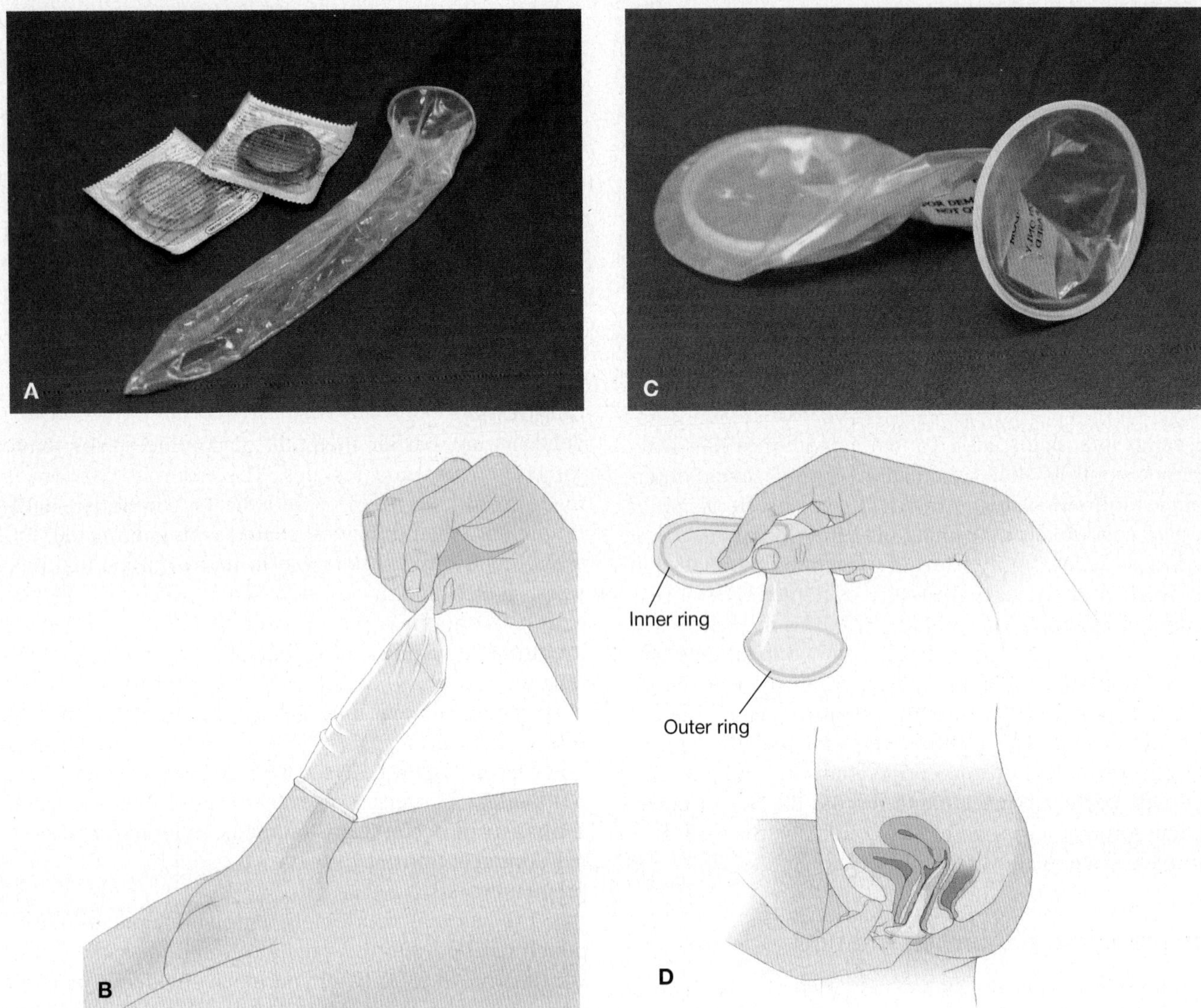

FIGURE 4.9 **A.** External condom. **B.** Applying a male condom. Leaving space at the tip helps to ensure the condom will not break with ejaculation. **C.** The internal condom. **D.** Insertion technique.

requires professional fitting by a health care provider (Bartz, 2023). Patients may need to be refitted with a different-sized diaphragm after pregnancy, abdominal or pelvic surgery, or weight loss or gain of 10 lb or more. As a general rule, diaphragms should be replaced every 2 years (Bartz, 2023).

Diaphragms require motivation at every sexual act and some skill to use. They are not effective unless used correctly. Patients need to receive thorough instructions about diaphragm use and should practice putting one in and taking it out before they leave the health care office (Fig. 4.11). Diaphragm care includes not using oil-based lubricants or powders on the diaphragm, washing it with soap and water, and storing it in a clean and dry container (Bartz, 2023).

CERVICAL CAP

The **cervical cap** is smaller than the diaphragm and covers only the cervix; it is held in place by suction. It is nonhormonal, shaped like a sailor's hat, and prevents sperm from entering the cervix. Caps are made from silicone and are used with spermicide (Fig. 4.12). The FemCap is the only cervical cap device currently available in the United States and comes in three sizes: small, medium, and large (Bartz, 2023). The cap may be inserted up to 6 hours before intercourse and provides protection for 48 hours. The cap must be kept in the vagina for 6 hours after the final act of intercourse and should be replaced every year of use. A refitting may also be necessary after pregnancy, abortion, or weight changes. Failure rates are higher after birthing a baby as the cervix is larger and the

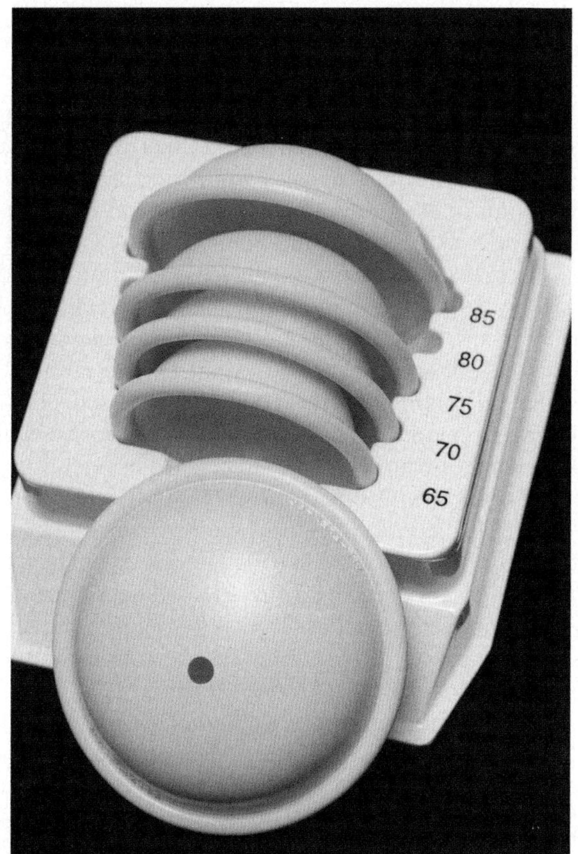

FIGURE 4.10 Sample diaphragm used for measuring.

cervical cap does not fit as well (Bartz, 2023). The dome of the cap is filled about one third full with spermicide. Spermicide should not be applied to the rim because it might interfere with the seal that must form around the cervix. The cap is available online, but it is preferred to see a health care professional to get fitted and receive teaching regarding proper insertion and removal (Bartz, 2023). Contraindications to the use of a cervical cap include cervical cancer, recent urinary tract infection, latex allergy, pelvic organ prolapse, and history of toxic shock syndrome (TSS). Using the cervical cap during menstruation is not recommended (Bartz, 2023). Cervical cap care is similar to diaphragm care discussed earlier.

CONTRACEPTIVE SPONGE

The **contraceptive sponge** is a round, nonhormonal, nonprescription device that includes both a barrier and a spermicide (commercially known as Today Sponge). Most are generally about 2 in in diameter and have a ring for easy removal.

It is a soft concave device that prevents pregnancy by covering the cervix and releasing spermicide. The sponge, made of polyurethane saturated with 1 g of nonoxynol-9, releases 125 mg of the spermicide over

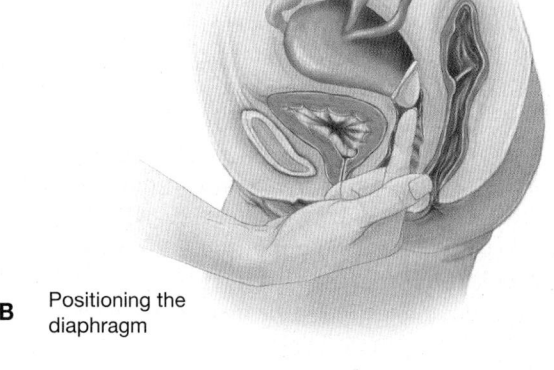

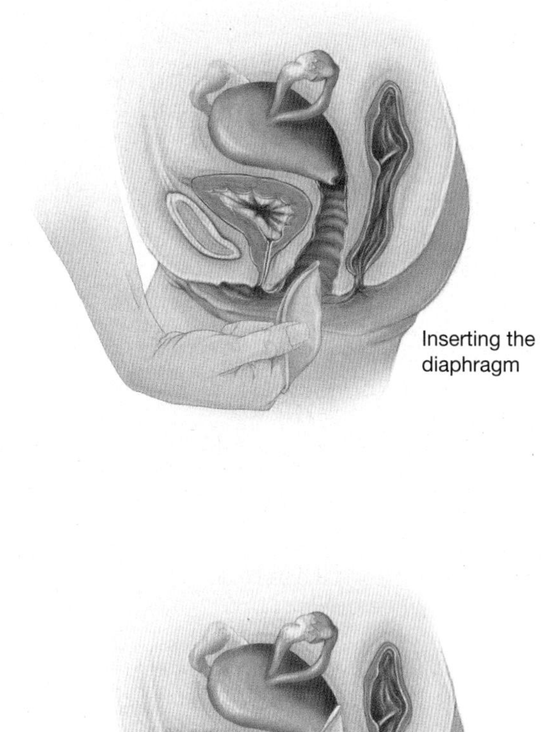

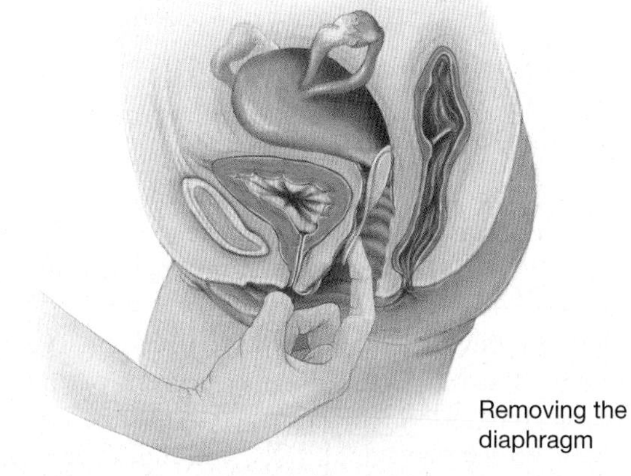

FIGURE 4.11 Application of a diaphragm. **A.** To insert, fold the diaphragm in half, separate the labia with one hand, then insert upward and back into the vagina. **B.** To position, make certain the diaphragm securely covers the cervix. **C.** To remove, hook a finger over the top of the rim and bring the diaphragm down and out.

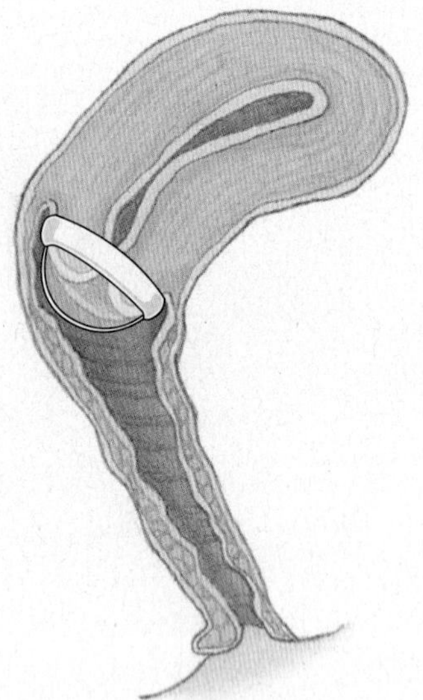

FIGURE 4.12 A cervical cap is placed over the cervix and used with a spermicidal jelly, the same as a diaphragm.

24 hours of use. Unlike the diaphragm, the sponge can be used for more than one coital act within 24 hours without the insertion of additional spermicide, and it does not require fitting from a health care provider and is available over the counter (Bartz, 2023). While it is less effective than several other methods and does not offer protection against STIs, the sponge achieved a wide following among people who appreciated the spontaneity with which it could be used and its easy availability.

To use the sponge, the user first wets it with water, squeezes it until it is thoroughly wet and foamy, and then inserts it into the vagina with a finger, using a cord loop attachment. It can be inserted up to 24 hours before intercourse and should be left in place for at least 6 hours following intercourse. The sponge provides protection for up to 12 hours, but should not be left in for more than 30 hours after insertion (Bartz, 2023).

Hormonal Methods

Several options are available for long-term but reversible protection against pregnancy. These methods of contraception work by altering the hormones within the female body. They rely on estrogen and progestin or progestin alone to prevent ovulation. When used consistently, these methods are a reliable way to prevent pregnancy. Hormonal methods include **oral contraceptives (OCs)** injectables, implants, vaginal rings, and transdermal patches.

ORAL CONTRACEPTIVES

As early as 1937, scientists recognized that the injection of progesterone inhibited ovulation in rabbits and provided contraception. The first hormonal pill, called *Enovid*, was approved by the U.S. Food and Drug Administration (FDA) in May 1960. It contained high levels of estrogen to prevent ovulation. Since that time, it has evolved through gradual lowering of estrogen and is now combined with many different progestins.

Development of hormonal oral contraception marked a revolutionary step in social change that has improved the lives of people and families worldwide. Since the first OC was introduced, hormonal contraception has undergone various stages of advancement. Today, OC regimens are safer and more tolerable with equal or improved efficacy than that of the early formulations. Incremental decreases in the estrogen dosage helped alleviate some of the unwanted side effects of the pill (Roe et al., 2023). Oral contraception is the most commonly prescribed type of contraception in the United States, with approximately 25% of females who are on contraception using it as their method of choice (Cooper et al., 2022) (Fig. 4.13).

The FDA recently approved the first over-the-counter birth control pill (Opill), allowing Americans to buy this progestin-only contraceptive medication without a prescription. This approval may reduce barriers to contraceptive access by allowing people to obtain an oral contraceptive without the need to first see a health care provider (FDA, 2023).

Although most commonly prescribed for contraception, OCs have long been used in the management of a wide range of conditions and have many health benefits, such as:

- Reduced incidence of ovarian and endometrial cancer
- Treatment of symptoms of endometriosis
- Decreased incidence of acne and hirsutism
- Decreased incidence of ectopic pregnancy
- Decreased incidence of pelvic pain
- Reduced incidence of benign cystic breast disease
- Decreased perimenopausal symptoms
- Improved bone density
- Improvement in asthmatic symptoms
- Decreased risk for rheumatoid arthritis
- Increased menstrual cycle regularity
- Lower incidence of colorectal cancer
- Decreased number of pregnancy-related deaths by preventing pregnancy

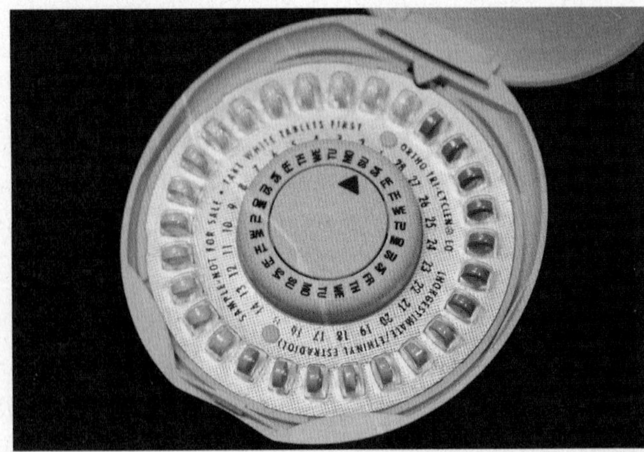

FIGURE 4.13 Oral contraceptive.

- Reduced iron-deficiency anemia due to heavy menstrual bleeding
- Reduced incidence of dysmenorrhea (Allen, 2023; Schuiling & Likis, 2022)

OCs work primarily by suppressing ovulation by adding estrogen and progesterone to the body, thus mimicking pregnancy. This hormonal level stifles GnRH, which in turn suppresses FSH and LH and thus inhibits ovulation. Cervical mucus also thickens, which hinders sperm transport into the uterus. Implantation is inhibited by suppression of the maturation of the endometrium and alterations of uterine secretions (Allen, 2023).

The combination pills are prescribed as monophasic pills, which deliver fixed dosages of estrogen and progestin, or as multiphasic ones. Multiphasic pills (e.g., biphasic and triphasic OCs) alter the amount of progestin and estrogen within each cycle. To maintain adequate hormonal levels for contraception and enhance adherence to the regimen, OCs should be taken at the same time daily.

OCs that contain progestin are sometimes called mini-pills. Progestin-only pills (POPs) have both advantages and disadvantages when compared to combined pills. The pill-taking regimen is simple and fixed; no pill color changes or days without pill-taking occur. These pills are appropriate for people who cannot or should not take estrogen in combined OCs, for example, a person older than 35 years who smokes cigarettes. These OCs work primarily by thickening the cervical mucus to prevent penetration of the sperm and make the endometrium unfavorable for implantation. POPs must be taken at a certain time every 24 hours. Breakthrough bleeding and a higher risk of pregnancy have made these OCs less popular than combination OCs.

Extended-cycle or continuous-use OC regimens have been used for the management of menstrual disorders and endometriosis and are attracting wider attention. Surveys asking people about their willingness to reduce their menstrual cycles from 12 to 4 annually were returned with a resounding "yes." Research has confirmed that the extended use of active OC pills carries the same safety profile as the conventional 28-day regimens (Allen, 2023). OCs taken in continuous or in extended cycles offer benefits with regard to PMS and PMDD, reduced menstrual bleeding, symptoms related to endometriosis, dysmenorrhea, and management of symptoms during perimenopause (Allen, 2023). The extended regimen consists of 84 consecutive days of active combination pills followed by 7 days of placebos (Allen, 2023). The user has four withdrawal-bleeding episodes a year. Continuous cycle OCs provide more hormonal exposure on a yearly basis (365 days) (Allen, 2023). There is no physiologic requirement for cyclic hormonal withdrawal bleeds while taking these OCs (Allen, 2023).

The balance between the benefits and the risks of OCs must be determined for each patient when they are being assessed for this type of contraceptive. It is a highly effective contraceptive when taken properly but can aggravate many medical conditions, especially in those who smoke. Comparison Chart 4.1 lists the advantages

COMPARISON CHART 4.1 Advantages and Disadvantages of Oral Contraceptives

Advantages	Disadvantages
Regulate and shorten the menstrual cycle	Offer no protection against STIs
Decrease severe cramping and bleeding	
Reduce anemia Reduce premenstrual dysphoric disorder	Modest risk for venous thrombosis and pulmonary emboli
Reduce ovarian, endometrial, and colorectal cancer risk	
Decrease benign breast disease Reduces iron-deficiency anemia	Associated with increased risk for myocardial infarction, stroke, and hypertension
Improve acne and reduce the incidence of menstrual headaches	May increase the risk of depression May increase the risk for cervical cancer if taken >5 years
Minimize perimenopausal symptoms	User must remember to take pill daily.
Decrease incidence of rheumatoid arthritis	High, ongoing cost for some patients
Improve PMS symptoms	
Protect against loss of bone density and reduce the risk of osteoporosis	

Newhouse, R. (2022). Contraception. In K. D. Schuiling & F. E. Likis (Eds.), *Gynecologic health care* (4th ed., pp. 235–266). Jones & Bartlett Learning; Allen, R. H. (2023). Combined estrogen-progestin oral contraceptives: Patient selection, counseling, and use. *UpToDate.* Retrieved March 14, 2024, from https://www.uptodate.com/contents/combined-estrogen-progestin-oral-contraceptives-patient-selection-counseling-and-use

and disadvantages of OCs. A thorough history and pelvic examination, including a Pap smear, are not required before the medication is prescribed, but a regular medical follow-up is advised. Patients should also be counseled that the effectiveness of OCs is decreased when taking antibiotics; thus, an alternative or secondary method should be used during this period to prevent pregnancy.

Nurses need to provide OC users with a great deal of education before they leave the health care facility. They need to be able to identify early signs and symptoms that might indicate a problem.

> **TAKE NOTE!**
>
> The mnemonic "ACHES" can help people remember the early warning signs of oral, transdermal, or vaginal ring contraceptive complications that necessitate a return to the health care provider (Box 4.5).

INJECTABLE CONTRACEPTION

Injectable contraception includes progestin-only and a combination of estrogen and progestin agents that provide safe and highly effective birth control for up to 3 months. Injectable agents are widely available and play an important role in family planning worldwide. They offer a discrete, convenient, reversible, and noncoital-dependent method of birth control. Recent research finds that allowing self-administration of injectable contraceptives can lead to improved contraceptive continuation rates compared to provider administration (Kaunitz, 2023b).

Depo-Provera (depot medroxyprogesterone acetate [DMPA]) is the trade name for a 3-month injectable of a progesterone-only contraceptive that works at the hypothalamic/pituitary level to stop the hormonal cycle. Depo-Provera works by suppressing ovulation and the production of FSH and LH by the pituitary gland, increasing the viscosity of cervical mucus and causing endometrial atrophy. It is available in two strengths: 150 mg/1 mL for intramuscular injection and 104 mg/0.65 mL for subcutaneous injection. It acts like other progestin-only products to prevent pregnancy for 3 months at a time (Fig. 4.14). The primary side effects of Depo-Provera are menstrual cycle disturbances such as unscheduled bleeding or amenorrhea, weight gain, headache, and loss of bone mineral density (Kaunitz, 2023c). It should also be noted that cycles may not be restored fully for up to 9 months following the last Depo-Provera injection.

Concerns have been raised about Depo-Provera's impact on bone mineral density, and substantial controversy has surrounded this issue (Kaunitz, 2023c). Evidence prompted the manufacturer and the FDA to issue a warning about the long-term use (over 2 years) of Depo-Provera and bone loss (Newhouse, 2022). Some experts have called for the removal of this warning as the overall belief from professional organizations including ACOG and the CDC is the advantages of Depo-Provera outweigh the risk of skeletal harm (Kaunitz, 2023c). Recent studies have shown that premenopausal and young females using Depo-Provera for up to 5 years saw a reversal in the decline in their bone mineral density after the use of Depo-Provera was stopped (Kaunitz, 2023c).

TRANSDERMAL PATCHES

The **transdermal patch** is a 2-in square adhesive that contains ethinyl estradiol and norelgestromin or estradiol and levonorgestrel (LNG). These substances are absorbed through the skin when placed on the lower abdomen, upper outer arm, buttocks, or upper torso (avoiding the breasts). The patch is applied weekly for 3 weeks followed by a patch-free week when withdrawal bleeding occurs. The patch delivers continuous levels of progesterone and estrogen. Transdermal absorption allows the drug to enter the bloodstream directly, avoiding rapid inactivation in the liver known as first-pass metabolism. This delivery method allows for a lower total

BOX 4.5 Early Signs of Combined Complications for Users of Oral Contraceptives, Combined Transdermal Contraceptives (Patch), Combined Vaginal Ring Contraceptives

- A = Abdominal pain may indicate liver problems or ectopic pregnancy.
- C = Chest pain or shortness of breath may indicate a pulmonary embolus or myocardial infarction.
- H = Headaches may indicate hypertension or impending stroke.
- E = Eye problems may indicate hypertension or a possible clot in the eye.
- S = Severe leg pain may indicate a thromboembolic event.

Adapted from Department of Health and Environmental Control. (2021). *Warning signs & cautions (ACHES)*. Retrieved March 14, 2024, from https://scdhec.gov/sites/default/files/Library/ML-005064.pdf

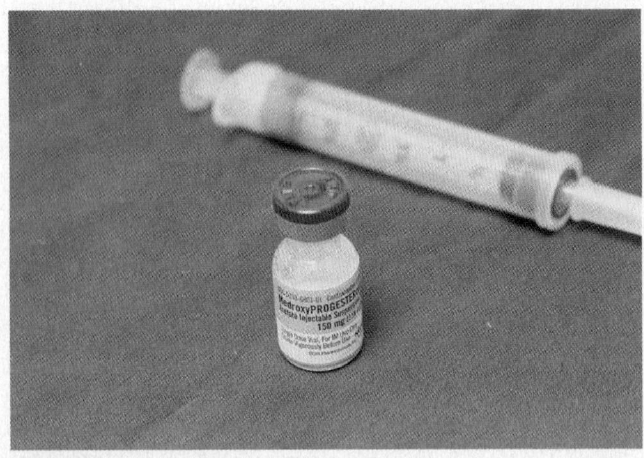

FIGURE 4.14 Injectable contraceptive.

hormone dose when compared to that of oral products that are metabolized in the liver. Because estrogen and progesterone are metabolized by liver enzymes, avoiding first-pass metabolism was thought to reduce adverse effects. However, recent evidence suggests that the risk of venous thrombosis and embolism is increased with the patch but still lower than the risk of venous thromboembolism during pregnancy (Burkman, 2022). Additional studies are underway to understand the clinical significance of these findings, but in the interim, nurses need to focus on ongoing risk assessment and should be prepared to discuss current research findings with patients.

Adherence to the regimen of combination contraceptive patch use has been shown to be significantly greater than adherence with OCs. In addition, research suggests that people with obesity (BMI >30 kg/m^2) should be advised of the potentially decreased effectiveness of the patch and increased incidence of venous thromboembolism (Burkman, 2022). The patch provides combination HT with a side effect profile similar to that of OCs (Fig. 4.15).

VAGINAL RINGS

The contraceptive **vaginal ring**, commercially known as the NuvaRing, EluRyng, Haloette, and EnilloRing, is a flexible, soft, transparent ring that contains both estrogen and progesterone. It is inserted by the user for a 3-week period of continuous use followed by a ring-free week to allow withdrawal bleeding (Fig. 4.16). Ethinyl estradiol and etonogestrel are rapidly absorbed through the vaginal epithelium and result in a steady serum concentration. Because the hormones are released directly into the vagina, a lower daily dose of hormones is required in comparison with OC doses. Studies have demonstrated that the efficacy, safety, and adverse effects of the ring are equivalent to those of OCs (Kerns & Darney, 2023). Patients report being highly satisfied with the vaginal ring due to ease of use, low doses of hormones, and once a month administration (Kerns & Darney, 2023).

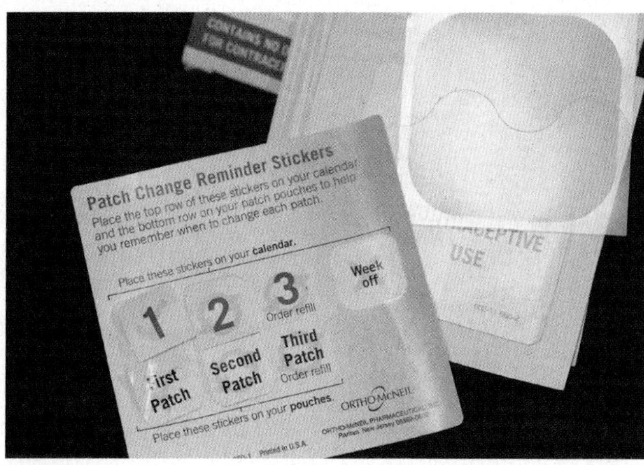

FIGURE 4.15 Transdermal patch.

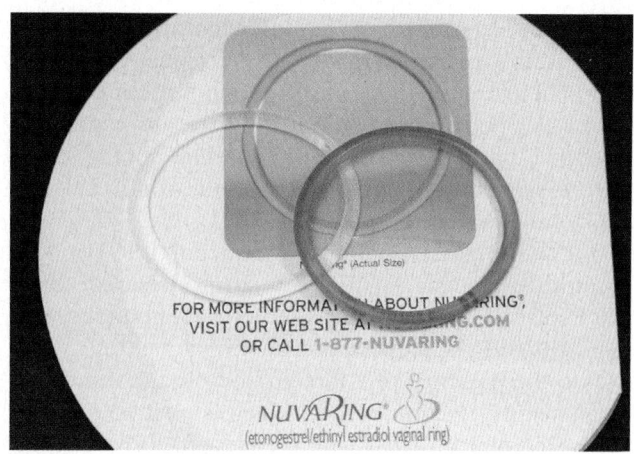

FIGURE 4.16 Vaginal ring.

The ring provides effective cycle control as well as symptom relief for people with endometriosis-related pain (Kerns & Darney, 2023). Reported problems associated with the use of vaginal rings are rare but include ring expulsion, interference with coitus, and vaginal discomfort due to feeling the ring (Kerns & Darney, 2023). The ring can be inserted by the patient and does not have to be fitted. The patient compresses the ring and inserts it into the vagina, behind the pubic bone, as far back as possible, but precise placement is not critical. The hormones are absorbed through the vaginal mucosa. It is left in place for 3 weeks and then removed and discarded. Recent data support continuous ring use in people desiring fewer days of withdrawal bleeding (Kerns & Darney, 2023). Patients need to be counseled regarding the timely insertion of the ring and what to do in case of accidental expulsion.

LONG-ACTING REVERSIBLE CONTRACEPTIVES

Long-acting reversible contraceptives (LARCs) include the subdural single-rod contraceptive implant (commercially known as Nexplanon) and IUSs or intrauterine contraceptives, commonly referred to as **intrauterine devices (IUDs)**. LARCs are highly effective because they are forgettable methods of contraception. The **implant** is a subdermal time-release method that delivers synthetic progestin that inhibits ovulation. Once in place, it delivers 3 years of continuous, highly effective contraception. Like POPs, implants act by inhibiting ovulation and thickening cervical mucus, so sperm cannot penetrate. Nexplanon is 4-cm long and 2 mm in diameter, and it contains 68 mg of progestin. It is one of the most effective contraceptive methods (Darney, 2024). The side effects are also similar to those of POPs—irregular bleeding, headaches, weight gain, acne, increased appetite, breast tenderness, and depression. Fertility is restored quickly after it is removed. Implants require a minor surgical procedure for both insertion and removal. The implants do not offer any protection against STIs.

Hormonal side effects are not exclusive to implants but tend to be a problem with all hormonal contraceptives. Therefore, with the implant, preinsertion counseling by the nurse is essential to prepare the patient for any such side effects. Expert counseling should cover the one side effect most likely to cause discontinuation—initial irregular bleeding (Darney, 2024).

IUDs are classified as either hormonal (LNG) or nonhormonal (copper). An IUD is a small T-shaped object that is placed inside the uterus to provide contraception (Fig. 4.17). IUDs prevent pregnancy in multiple ways. Due to the presence of a foreign body in the uterus, an inflammatory reaction occurs, which is toxic to ova and sperm and inhibits implantation (Madden, 2023). The implants contain either copper or progesterone to enhance their effectiveness. One or two attached strings protrude into the vagina so that the user can check its placement.

Four T-shaped IUDs are currently available in the United States, including the copper ParaGard-TCu-380A and LNG-releasing intrauterine systems (LNG-IUSs). The LNG-IUSs are available in three different formulations: LNG-52 mg marketed as Mirena and Liletta, LNG-19.5 mg marketed as *Kyleena*, and LNG-13.5 mg marketed as *Skyla*. The ParaGard-TCu-380A is approved for 10 years of use and is nonhormonal. Its mechanism of action is based on the release of copper ions, which alone are spermicidal. Additionally, the device causes an inflammatory action leading to a hostile uterine environment. The ParaGard-TCu-380A is also approved for use as emergency contraception (EC) (Madden, 2023). Mirena and Liletta are approved for 8 years of use, *Kyleena* is approved for 5 years, and Skyla for 3 years (Madden, 2023). These three devices release a low dose of progestin causing thinning of the endometrium and thickening of cervical mucus, which inhibits sperm entry into the upper genital tract. Their use results in a major reduction in menstrual flow and dysmenorrhea. The use of LNG-52 mg (Mirena and Liletta) has been approved by the FDA for the treatment of heavy menstrual bleeding (Madden, 2023).

The IUDs provide a safe, highly effective, long-lasting, reversible method of contraception. Expanding access to IUDs is an effective measure to reduce the rate of unintended pregnancy in the United States. Nurses should consider including them in their discussion to appropriate candidates, including patients who are nulliparous, adolescent, immediately postpartum, or postabortion; those who desire EC; and those who want an alternative to permanent sterilization. IUD insertion can take place on any day of the menstrual cycle if the absence of pregnancy is confirmed (Bartz & Pocius, 2023). Pain and irregular bleeding patterns are the most common side effects (Madden, 2023). Complications with IUDs are uncommon (Madden, 2023).

EMERGENCY CONTRACEPTION

Using an emergency contraceptive provides a second chance to prevent an unintended pregnancy. **Emergency contraception (EC)** reduces the risk of pregnancy after unprotected intercourse or contraceptive failure such as condom breakage but before pregnancy is established (Fig. 4.18). It is used within 72 to 120 hours of unprotected intercourse to prevent pregnancy. The sooner ECs are taken, the more effective they are. They reduce the risk of pregnancy for a single act of unprotected sex by almost 95% (WHO, 2021). The methods currently available in the United States are highly effective and include ulipristal acetate (UPA), an oral progesterone receptor agonist–antagonist (Ella); LNG, an oral progestin (Plan B One-Step); the copper intrauterine device (Cu-IUD); LNG-52 mg IUD; and combined oral contraceptives (Yuzpe method) (Turok, 2023).

Access to ECs has been controversial for minors. Prior to 2013, the pills were available by prescription only, and even when approved for nonprescription status, access was restricted based on age. In 2013, several judicial courts and the FDA ruled in favor of nonprescription access to EC by all people regardless of age, and it is now sold over the counter. The only contraindication to the use of any of the EC methods is a known pregnancy as defined as implantation.

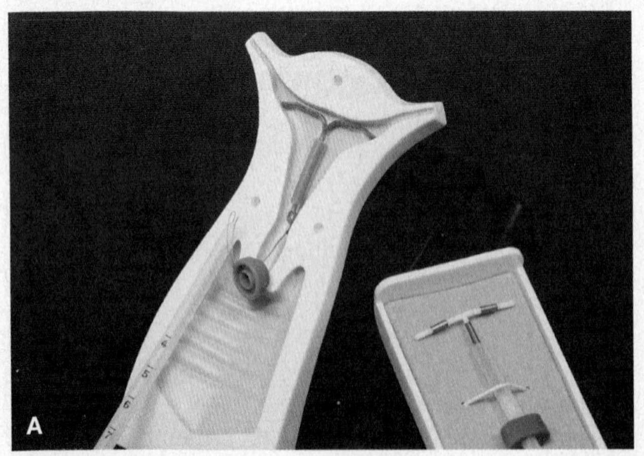

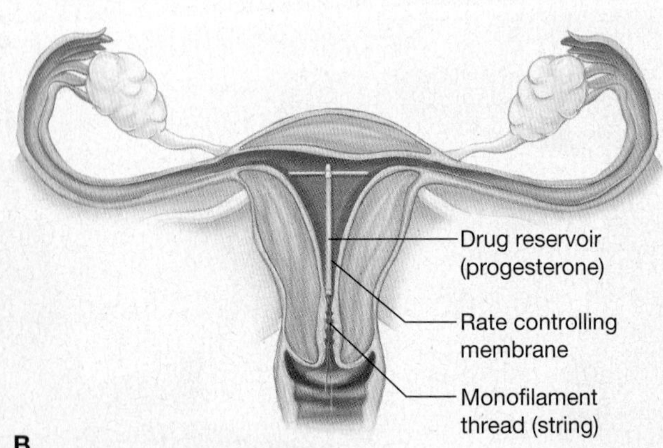

FIGURE 4.17 A. Intrauterine contraceptive. **B.** An intrauterine device (IUD) in place in the uterus.

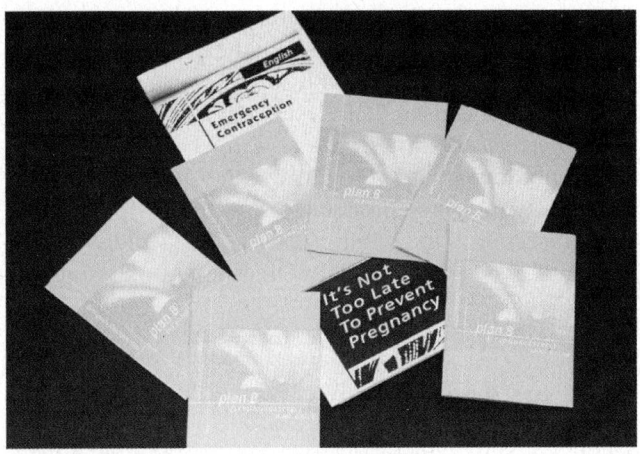

FIGURE 4.18 Emergency contraceptive kit.

Although access to EC has increased with nonprescription status and approval of Plan B One-Step and Ella as a single-dose pill without age restrictions, many barriers remain in public awareness, and unintended pregnancies continue to rise. Because of the lack of awareness of EC and the politics surrounding it, EC is not used as widely as would be warranted by the incidence of unprotected coitus. Contraceptive care is an essential health service, but inequalities exist in marginalized groups. Many people from marginalized groups report bias, discrimination, and poor health outcomes. Nurses need to educate their patients to bring about increased awareness of this second-chance method and use approaches to care that mitigate bias and discrimination (Loder & Solomon, 2022). Table 4.5 lists recommended oral medication and intrauterine regimens.

Prime points to stress concerning ECs are:

- ECs do not offer any protection against STIs or future pregnancies.
- ECs may cause the next menses to be early or late, so evaluation for pregnancy is needed if menses does not occur within 3 weeks after EC use.
- Report any heavy bleeding accompanied by severe abdominal pain to the health care provider immediately.
- ECs are contraindicated if pregnant (Turok, 2023).

TAKE NOTE!

Contrary to popular belief, ECs do not induce abortion and are not related to mifepristone or RU-486, the so-called abortion pill approved by the FDA in 2000. Mifepristone chemically induces abortion by blocking the body's progesterone receptors, which are necessary for pregnancy maintenance. ECs simply prevent embryo creation and uterine implantation from occurring in the first place. There is no evidence that ECs have any effect on an already implanted ovum.

Sterilization

Sterilization is a permanent, safe, and highly effective method of contraception for those who are certain they do not want any or any more children. Vasectomy is the only highly reliable form of male contraception.

TABLE **4.5** • Emergency Postcoital Contraception Options

Product	Dosage (within 72 hours)	Comments
Combined estrogen and progestin pills (Yuzpe regimen)	OCs are taken in various formulations to prevent conception.	Interfere with the cascade of events that result in ovulation and fertilization; significant risk of nausea and vomiting; decreased effectiveness in people with obesity
Plan B One-Step; My Way; Next Choice	1.5-mg pill taken	Can cause nausea and vomiting; decreased effectiveness in people with obesity
Ulipristal acetate (Ella or ellaOne)	Single 30-mg tablet	Can cause nausea and vomiting; decreased effectiveness in people with obesity
Levonorgestrel 52 mg IUD (Mirena and Liletta)	Inserted within 5 days after unprotected sexual episode	Can be left in for long-term contraception (8 years); most effective; not affected by BMI
Copper-bearing IUD (ParaGard-TCu-380A)	Inserted within 5 days after unprotected sexual episode	Can be left in for long-term contraception (10 years); most effective; not affected by BMI

BMI, body mass index; IUD, intrauterine device; OC, oral contraceptive.

Paradise, S. L., Landis, C. A., & Klein, D. A. (2022). Evidence-based contraception: Common questions and answers. *American Family Physician.* https://www.aafp.org/dam/AAFP/documents/journals/afp/Paradise.pdf; Turok, D. (2023). Emergency contraception. *UpToDate.* Retrieved March 15, 2024, from https://www.uptodate.com/contents/emergency-contraception

Sterilization refers to surgical procedures intended to render the person infertile. Laparoscopic, abdominal, and hysteroscopic methods of female sterilization are available in the United States, with many of these procedures performed outside the hospital. Sterilization is the world's most common method of family planning (Braaten & Dutton, 2024). More females than males undergo surgical sterilization. According to Sung and Abramovitz (2024), approximately 30% of females undergo female sterilization in comparison with 17% of males in the United States. Sterilization should be considered a permanent end to fertility because reversal surgery is difficult, expensive, and sometimes unsuccessful. Because these methods are intended to be irreversible, all couples should be appropriately counseled about the permanency of sterilization and the availability of highly effective, long-acting, reversible methods of contraception before this decision is made.

TUBAL LIGATION

Tubal ligation, the sterilization procedure for females, can be performed postpartum, after an abortion, or as an interval procedure unrelated to pregnancy. Mini-laparotomies and laparoscopies are the two most common techniques. In the laparoscopy procedure, the abdomen is filled with carbon dioxide gas so that the abdominal wall balloons away from the tubes to provide a view of the fallopian tubes. They are grasped and sealed with a cauterizing instrument or with rings, bands, or clips, or cut and tied (Fig. 4.19).

VASECTOMY

Male sterilization is accomplished with a minor surgical procedure known as a **vasectomy**. This is the fourth most common contraceptive method in the United States behind condoms, birth control pills, and tubal ligations (Stormont & Deibert, 2022). It is usually performed under local anesthesia in a urologist's office, and most patients can return to work and normal activities in a day or two. The procedure involves making a small incision into the scrotum and cutting the vas deferens, which carries sperm from the testes to the penis (Fig. 4.20). Complications from vasectomy are rare and minor in nature. Immediate risks include infection, hematoma, and pain. After vasectomy, semen no longer contains sperm. This is not immediate, though, and the patient must submit semen specimens for analysis around 3 months after a vasectomy and again another 1 to 2 months after that until two specimens show that no sperm is present (Viera, 2023).

Nursing Assessment

When assessing which contraceptive method might meet the patient's needs, the nurse might ask:

- Do your religious beliefs interfere with any methods?
- Will this method interfere with your sexual pleasure?
- Are you aware of the various methods currently available?
- Is cost a major consideration, or does your insurance cover it?
- Does your partner influence which method you choose?
- Are you in a stable, monogamous relationship?
- Have you heard anything that troubles you about any of the methods?
- How comfortable are you touching your own body?
- What are your future plans for having children?

Although deciding on a contraceptive is a personal decision, nurses can assist in this process by performing a complete health history and physical examination and by educating the patient or couple about necessary laboratory and diagnostic testing. Areas of focus during the nursing assessment are:

- Medical history: smoking status, cancer of the reproductive tract, diabetes mellitus, migraines, hypertension, thromboembolic disorder, allergies, risk factors for CVD

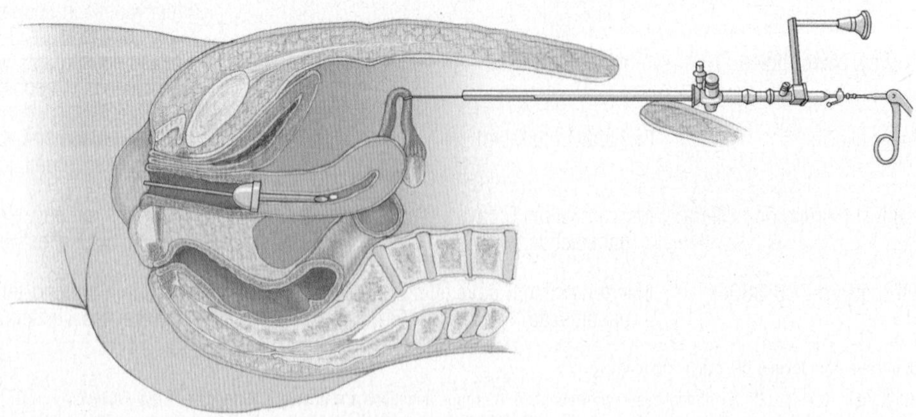

FIGURE 4.19 Laparoscopy for tubal sterilization.

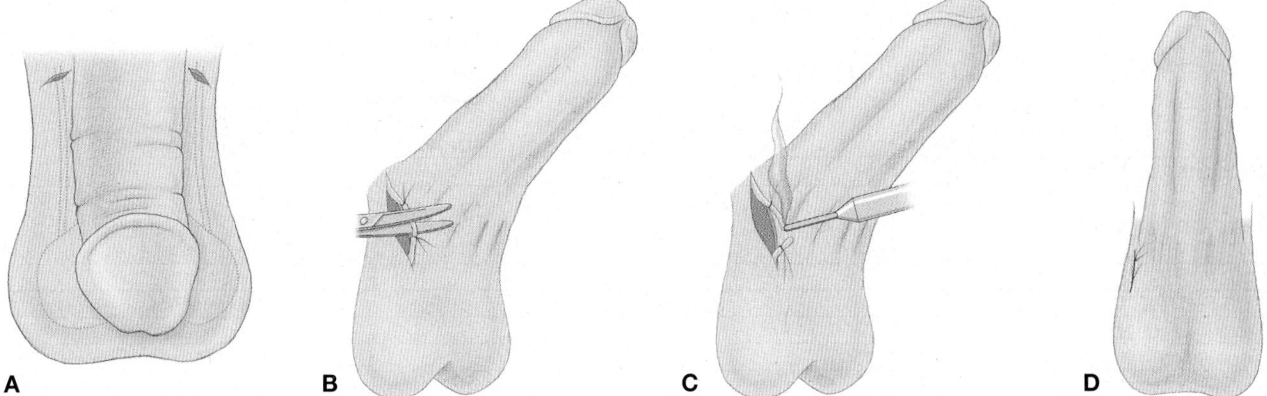

FIGURE 4.20 Vasectomy. **A.** Site of vasectomy incisions. **B.** The vas deferens is cut with surgical scissors. **C.** Cut ends of the vas deferens are cauterized to ensure blockage of the passage of sperm. **D.** Final skin suture.

- Family history: cancer, CVD, hypertension, stroke, diabetes
- Obstetrics and gynecology (OB/GYN) history: menstrual disorders, current contraceptive, previous STIs, PID, vaginitis, sexual activity
- Personal history: use of tampons and female hygiene products, plans for childbearing, comfort with touching oneself, number of sexual partners and their involvement in the decision
- Physical examination: height, weight, blood pressure, breast examination, thyroid palpation, pelvic examination
- Diagnostic testing: urinalysis, complete blood count, Pap smear, wet mount to check for STIs, HIV/AIDS tests, lipid profile, glucose level

Figure 4.21 shows an example of a family planning flow record that can be used during the assessment. After collecting the assessment data, consider the medical factors to help decide if the patient is a candidate for all methods or whether some should be eliminated. For example, if they report multiple sex partners and a history of pelvic infections, they would not be a good candidate for an IUD. Barrier methods (male or female condoms) of contraception might be recommended to this patient instead to offer protection against STIs.

Nursing Management

The choice of a contraceptive method is a personal one involving many factors. In making contraceptive choices, people must balance their sexual lives, their reproductive goals, and each partner's health and safety. Facilitate this process by establishing a trusting relationship with the patient and by providing unbiased, accurate information about all methods available. As a nurse, honestly reflect on your feelings about contraceptives while allowing the patient's feelings to be paramount. Be aware of the practical issues involved in contraceptive use, and avoid making assumptions, making decisions on the patient's behalf, and making judgments about them and their situation. To do so, it is important to keep up to date on the latest methods available and convey this information to patients. Encourage patients to take control of their lives by sharing information that allows them to plan their futures, encourages shared decision making, and focuses on patient preferences.

If a contraceptive is to be effective, the patient must understand how it works, must be able to use it correctly and consistently, and must be comfortable and confident with it. If a patient cannot adhere to taking a pill daily, consider a method used once a week (transdermal patches), once every 3 weeks (transvaginal ring), or once every 3 months (Depo-Provera injection). Another option may be a LARC that lasts several years and may reduce menstrual flow significantly (if hormonal).

Regardless of which method is chosen, the patient's needs should be paramount in the discussion. The nurse can educate patients about which methods are available and their advantages and disadvantages, efficacy, costs, and safety. Knowledge of contraceptive effectiveness is crucial to making an informed choice. The patient or couple must comprehend the pros and cons of the contraceptive methods being considered. Choice may be influenced by understanding the likelihood of pregnancy with each method and factors that influence effectiveness. Counseling can help patients and couples choose a contraceptive method that is efficacious and fits their preferences and lifestyle (see Evidence-based Practice 4.1).

The following guidelines are helpful in counseling and educating the patient or couple about contraceptives:

- Encourage the patient to discuss preferences regarding contraceptives.
- Provide patient education. The patient must become an informed user before the method is chosen. Education should be targeted to the patient's level so it is understood. Provide step-by-step teaching and

FAMILY PLANNING FLOW (VISIT) RECORD

Name:__________
ID #:__________
Date of Birth:__________

	Date:		Date:	
Current Method				
Reason for Visit				
LMP				
SUBJECTIVE DATA	**Pt.**	**Comments**	**Pt.**	**Comments**
Severe headaches				
Depression				
Visual abnormalities				
Dyspnea/chest pain				
Breast changes				
SBE				
Abdominal pain				
Nausea and vomiting				
Dysuria/frequency				
Menstrual irregularities				
Vaginal discharge/infections				
Leg pain				
Surgery, injury, infections, or serious illness since last visit				
Allergic reaction				
Pregnancy plans				
Other				
OBJECTIVE DATA	**Weight**	**B.P.**	**Weight**	**B.P.**
Other				
Lab				
ASSESSMENT Check here if assessment continues on progress notes	**O**		**O**	
PLAN Type of contraceptive given				
COUNSELING/EDUCATION				
Next appointment				
SIGNATURE/TITLE				
SIGNATURE/TITLE				

O = normal ✓= abnormal

FIGURE 4.21 Family planning flow (visit) record. LMP, last menstrual period.

an opportunity to practice certain methods (cervical caps, diaphragms, vaginal rings, and condoms) (see Teaching Guidelines 4.4 and Figure 4.22).
- Discuss contraindications for all selected contraceptives.
- Consider the patient's cultural and religious beliefs when providing care.
- Address myths and misperceptions about the methods under consideration in your initial discussion of contraceptives.

It is also important to clear up common misconceptions about contraception and pregnancy. Resolving misconceptions will permit new learning to take hold and a better patient response to whichever methods are explored and ultimately selected. Some common misconceptions include:

- Breastfeeding protects against pregnancy.
- Pregnancy can be avoided if the male partner "pulls out" before ejaculating.

TEACHING GUIDELINES 4.4 Tips for the Use of Cervical Caps, Diaphragms, Vaginal Rings, and Condoms

Cervical Cap Insertion/Removal Technique

- It is important to be involved in the fitting process.
- To insert the cap, pinch the sides together, compress the cap dome, insert it into the vagina, and place it over the cervix.
- Use one finger to feel around the entire circumference to make sure there are no gaps between the cap rim and the cervix.
- After a minute or two, pinch the dome and tug gently to check for evidence of suction. The cap should resist the tug and not slide off easily.
- To remove the cap, press the index finger against the rim and tip the cap slightly to break the suction. Gently pull out the cap.
- The patient should practice inserting and removing the cervical cap three times to validate their proficiency with this device.

Patient Education and Counseling Regarding the Cervical Cap

- Fill the dome of the cap up about one third full with spermicide cream or jelly. Place about one-quarter teaspoon along the rim. Turn the cap over and over and add one-quarter teaspoon of spermicide in the groove between the dome and the brim.
- Wait approximately 30 minutes after insertion before engaging in sexual intercourse to be sure that a seal has formed between the rim and the cervix.
- Leave the cervical cap in place for a minimum of 6 hours after sexual intercourse. It can be left in place for up to 48 hours without additional spermicide being added.
- Do not use during menses.
- Replace the cervical cap after each year of use.
- Inspect the cervical cap prior to insertion for cracks, holes, or tears.
- After using the cervical cap, wash it with soap and water, dry it thoroughly, and store in its container.

Diaphragm Insertion/Removal Technique

- Always empty the bladder prior to inserting the diaphragm.
- Inspect the diaphragm for holes or tears by holding it up to a light source, or fill it with water and check for a leak.
- Place approximately a tablespoon of spermicidal jelly or cream in the dome and around the rim of the diaphragm.
- The diaphragm should be inserted within 1 hour before intercourse.
- Select the position that is most comfortable for insertion:
  - Squatting
  - Leg up, raising the nondominant leg up on a low stool
  - Reclining position, lying on back in bed
  - Sitting forward on the edge of a chair
- Hold the diaphragm between the thumb and fingers and compress it to form a "figure eight" shape.
- Insert the diaphragm into the vagina, directing it downward as far as it will go.
- Tuck the front rim of the diaphragm behind the pubic bone so that the rubber hugs the front wall of the vagina.
- Feel for the cervix through the diaphragm to make sure it is properly placed.
- To remove the diaphragm, insert the finger up and over the top side and move slightly to the side, breaking the suction.
- Pull the diaphragm down and out of the vagina.

(*continued*)

TEACHING GUIDELINES 4.4 Tips for the Use of Cervical Caps, Diaphragms, Vaginal Rings, and Condoms (*continued*)

Patient Education and Counseling Regarding the Diaphragm

- Avoid the use of oil-based products, such as baby oil, because they may weaken the rubber.
- Wash the diaphragm with soap and water after use and dry thoroughly.
- Place the diaphragm back into the storage case.
- The diaphragm may need to be refitted after weight loss or gain or childbirth.
- Diaphragms should not be used by people with latex, silicone, or spermicidal sensitivity allergies.

Vaginal Ring Insertion/Removal Technique and Counseling

- Each ring is used for one menstrual cycle, which consists of 3 weeks of continuous use followed by a ring-free week to allow for menses.
- No fitting is necessary; one size fits all.
- The ring is compressed and inserted into the vagina, behind the pubic bone, as far back as possible.
- Precision placement is not essential.
- Backup contraception is needed for 7 days if the ring is expelled for more than 3 hours during the 3-week period of continuous use.
- The vaginal ring is left in place for 3 weeks then removed and discarded.

External (Male) Condom Insertion/Removal Technique and Counseling

- Always keep the condom in its original package until ready to use.
- Store in a cool, dry place.
- Spermicidal condoms should be used if available.
- Check the expiration date before using.
- Use a new condom for each sexual act.
- Condom is placed over the erect penis prior to insertion.
- Place condom on the head of the penis and unroll it down the shaft.
- Leave a half inch of empty space at the end to collect ejaculate.
- Avoid use of oil-based products because they may cause breakage.
- After intercourse, remove the condom while the penis is still erect.
- Discard condom after use.

Internal (Female) Condom Insertion/Removal Technique and Counseling

- Practice wearing and inserting prior to first use with sexual intercourse.
- Condom can be inserted before intercourse.
- Condom is intended for one-time use.
- It can be purchased over the counter; one size fits all.
- Avoid wearing rings to prevent tears; long fingernails can also cause tears.
- Spermicidal lubricant can be used if desired.
- Insert the inner ring high in the vagina against the cervix.
- Place the outer ring on the outside of the vagina.
- Make sure the erect penis is placed inside the female condom.
- Remove the condom after intercourse. Avoid spilling the ejaculate.

Education and Counseling of Patients Using Injectable Contraceptives

- Consume a diet high in calcium and vitamin D to prevent bone mineral loss.
- Know the conditions that need to be reported to the health care provider:
  - Significant headaches
  - Abnormal uterine bleeding
  - Depression
  - Severe abdominal pain
  - Any infection occurring at the injection site

Adapted from Bartz, D. A. (2023). Pericoital (on demand) contraception: Diaphragm, cervical cap, spermicides, and sponge. *UpToDate*. Retrieved March 14, 2024, from https://www.uptodate.com/contents/pericoital-contraception-diaphragm-cervical-cap-spermicides-and-sponge

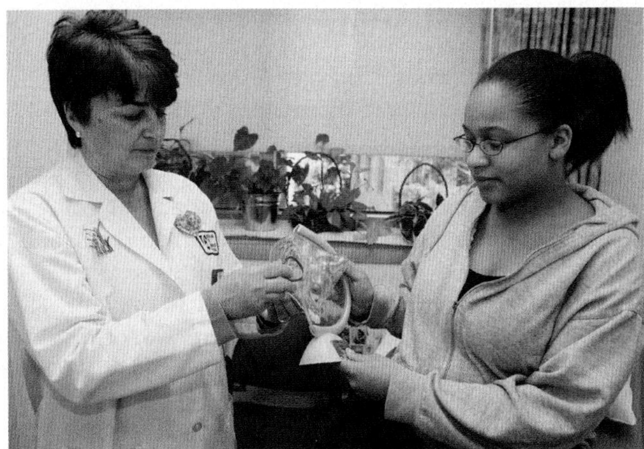

FIGURE 4.22 The nurse demonstrates insertion of a vaginal ring during patient education.

- Pregnancy cannot occur during menses.
- Douching after sex will prevent pregnancy.
- Pregnancy will not happen during the first sexual experience.
- Taking birth control pills protects against STIs.
- The female is too old to get pregnant.
- If female orgasm is not reached, conception is not likely.
- Irregular menstruation prevents pregnancy.

When discussing in detail each method of contraception, focus on specific information for each method outlined. Include information such as how this particular method works to prevent pregnancy under normal circumstances of use; the potential noncontraceptive benefits; advantages and disadvantages of all methods; the cost involved for each particular method; danger signs that need to be reported to the health care provider; and the required frequency of office visits needed for the particular method.

In addition, outline factors that place the patient at risk for method failure. Contraceptives can fail for any of many reasons. Use Table 4.6 to provide patient education concerning a few of the reasons for contraceptive failure. Help patients who have chosen abstinence or FAMs define the sexual activities in which they do or do not want to participate. This helps them set sexual limits or boundaries. Help them develop communication and negotiation skills that will allow them to be successful. Supporting, encouraging, and respecting a patient's or couple's choice of abstinence is vital for nurses.

After patients have chosen a method of contraception, it is important to complete the following:

- Emphasize that a second method to use as a backup is always needed.
- Provide both oral and written instructions on the method chosen.
- Discuss the need for STI protection if not using a barrier method.
- Inform the patient about the availability of ECs.

Steady progress in contraception research has been achieved over the past several years. Hormonal and nonhormonal contraceptives have improved female lives by reducing different health conditions that contribute to morbidity. However, the contraceptives available today are not suitable for all users, and the need to expand contraceptive choices still exists. It is hoped that the introduction of newer methods in the

TABLE 4.6 • Contraceptive Problems and Educational Needs

Contraceptive Failure Problem	Patient Education Needed
Not following instructions for use of contraceptive correctly	Take pill the same time every day. Use condoms properly and check the condition before using. Make sure the diaphragm or cervical cap covers the cervix completely. Check IUD for placement monthly.
Inconsistent use of contraceptive	Contraceptives must be used regularly to achieve maximum effectiveness. All it takes is one unprotected act of sexual intercourse to become pregnant. During use, 2%–5% of condoms will break or tear.
Condom broke during sex	Check expiration date. Store condoms properly. Use only a water-based lubricant. Watch for tears caused by long fingernails. Use spermicides to decrease possibility of pregnancy.Seek emergency postcoital conception.
Use of antibiotics or other herbs taken with OCs	Use alternative methods during the antibiotic therapy, plus seven additional days. Implement on day 1 of taking antibiotics.
Belief that you can't get pregnant during menses or that it is safe "just this one time"	It may be possible to become pregnant on almost any day of the menstrual cycle.

IUD, intrauterine device; OC, oral contraceptive.

near future with additional health benefits will continue to help people and couples meet their family planning needs.

There is no "best" method of contraception, and the choice depends on multiple factors including the patient's overall health, age, frequency of sexual activity, number of sexual partners, desire for future fertility, family history of certain diseases, possible side effects, and comfort in using the method. A clear understanding of the available contraceptive methods allows the nurse to counsel patients about the various methods that are most consistent with their health status, lifestyles, and comfort levels to ensure the highest levels of success.

PREGNANCY TERMINATION OR ABORTION

Pregnancy termination, also referred to as abortion, sits at the intersection of issues such as public health, human rights, reproductive justice, and bodily autonomy. It has remained controversial for decades. **Abortion** is defined in a variety of ways in medical and legal literature but at its basic level is the expulsion or extraction of an embryo or fetus before it is viable (Shakhatreh et al., 2022). Abortion can be a medical or surgical procedure. Both are safe. The purpose of abortion is to terminate a pregnancy. One in four females will end a pregnancy by abortion at some time in their reproductive lives (Ajmal et al., 2023). Globally, more than one fifth of all known pregnancies end in abortion (Ajmal et al., 2023). The practice of abortion was legal in the United States until the Supreme Court overturned *Roe versus Wade*, a decision that had affirmed the constitutional right to abortion, through its ruling in the *Dobbs versus Jackson Women's Health Organization* case in 2022. Abortion policies are now left up to individual states.

Debate has continued over how and when abortions are provided. Every state has laws regulating some aspects of abortion, and many have passed restrictions such as parental consent or notification requirements, mandated counseling and waiting periods, and limits on funding for abortion. Each state addresses these matters independently, and the laws that are passed or enforced are legislative decisions and a function of the political system.

It is imperative that nurses honor all patients' rights to self-determination, autonomy, respect, and privacy. As uncertainty about abortion access within the various states unfolds, it is important for nurses to provide patients that desire abortion with accurate information about regulations within their state and disregard their personal viewpoints regarding abortion (NPWH, 2022).

Procedural Abortion

Two types of procedural abortion are available: uterine aspiration or dilation and evacuation (D&E). Method selection is based on gestational age. It is an ambulatory procedure done under local anesthesia. The cervix is dilated prior to surgery and then the products of conception are removed by suction evacuation. The uterus may gently be scraped by curettage to make sure that it is empty. The entire procedure lasts about 10 minutes. The overall risk of complications is less than 1% for surgical termination (Shih & Wallace, 2023). The major risks and complications in the first trimester are infection, retained tissue or hemorrhage, uterine perforation, retained products of conception, infection, pelvic pain, low-grade fever, or cervical tear (Sajadi-Ernazarova & Martinez, 2023). For patients whose blood is Rh-negative, RhoGAM is indicated prior to the start of either medical or surgical termination.

Medication Abortion

Medication abortions account for the majority (54%) of all abortions in the United States (Guttmacher Institute, 2022). The most common regimen in the United States involves the use of two different medications, mifepristone and misoprostol. Mifepristone blocks progesterone, which is essential to the development of pregnancy. Misoprostol, taken 24 to 48 hours later, works to empty the uterus by causing cramping and bleeding. A follow-up visit is scheduled later to confirm the pregnancy was terminated via ultrasound or blood test. Medication abortion is a safe and effective method to terminate a pregnancy but does carry about a 2% risk of complications, which is higher than procedural abortions (Sajadi-Ernazarova & Martinez, 2023; Shih & Wallace, 2023). Complications of medical abortions include incomplete expulsion of uterine contents, failed abortion, infection, and hemorrhage (Sajadi-Ernazarova & Martinez, 2023).

The assessment of the patient with an unintended pregnancy should be performed with cautious sensitivity. It is essential to explore the patient's feelings about pregnancy before congratulating or consoling them. The encounter should be guided by the feelings of the patient, not by the assumptions and values of the nurse.

Abortion can be an emotional, deeply personal issue. Considerate and sensitive communication is key in dealing with cases of termination of pregnancy. Provide support and accurate information. If you feel unable to actively participate in the care of a patient undergoing an abortion for personal, religious, or ethical reasons, you still have the professional responsibility to ensure that the patient receives the nursing care and help they require. This may necessitate a transfer to another area or a staffing reassignment. Nurses must keep in mind that all patients have the right to have access to unbiased, factual information about available reproductive health choices, whether they seek to end or start a pregnancy, from which they can then make informed decisions about their own reproductive health.

KEY CONCEPTS

- Establishing good health habits and avoiding risky behaviors early in life will prevent chronic conditions later in life.
- PMS has more than 150 symptoms, and at least two different syndromes are recognized—PMS and PMDD.
- Endometriosis is a condition in which tissue similar to that of the endometrium is located outside the uterine cavity.
- Infertility is a widespread problem that has an emotional, social, and economic impact on couples.
- Hormonal methods include OCs, injectables, implants, vaginal rings, and transdermal patches.
- Recent studies have shown that the extension of active extended-cycle OC pills carries the same safety profile as the conventional 28-day regimens.
- The IUDs available in the United States include the copper ParaGard-TCu-380A and the LNG-IUSs. The LNG-IUSs are available in three different formulations: LNG-52 mg (Mirena and Liletta), LNG-19.5 mg (Kyleena), and LNG-13.5 mg (Skyla).
- With a dramatic decline in estrogen levels, menopause affects not only the reproductive organs but also other body systems.
- Most people with osteoporosis do not know they have the disease until they sustain a fracture, usually of the wrist or hip.
- Nurses should aim to have a holistic approach to the sexual health of patients from menarche through menopause.

Unfolding Patient Stories: Carla Hernandez • Part 1

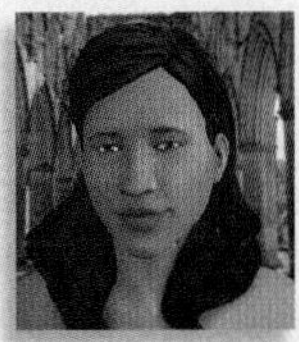

Carla Hernandez is a 32-year-old in her second pregnancy. She is at 39 5/7 weeks' gestation when her partner brings her to the hospital. She and her partner tell the nurse that after delivery of the baby, they want to discuss options for preventing a future pregnancy. What information can the nurse prepare to help them make an informed decision? What questions asked by the nurse can help guide the discussion toward methods that correspond with their beliefs and values? (Carla Hernandez's story continues in Chapter 14.)

Care for Carla and other patients in a realistic virtual environment: ***vSim** for Nursing* (**thepoint.lww.com/vSimMaternity**). Practice documenting these patients' care in DocuCare (**thepoint.lww.com/DocuCareEHR**).

REFERENCES AND RECOMMENDED READINGS

Ajmal, M., Sunder, M., & Akinbinu, R. (2023). Abortion. *StatPearls* [Internet]. https://www.ncbi.nlm.nih.gov/books/NBK518961/

Allen, R. H. (2023). Combined estrogen-progestin oral contraceptives: Patient selection, counseling, and use. *UpToDate*. Retrieved March 14, 2024, from https://www.uptodate.com/contents/combined-estrogen-progestin-oral-contraceptives-patient-selection-counseling-and-use

American College of Obstetricians and Gynecologists. (2021a). *Endometriosis*. https://www.acog.org/womens-health/faqs/endometriosis

American College of Obstetricians and Gynecologists. (2023a). *Effectiveness of birth control methods*. https://www.acog.org/womens-health/infographics/effectiveness-of-birth-control-methods

American College of Obstetricians and Gynecologists. (2023b). *Endometrial cancer*. https://www.acog.org/womens-health/faqs/endometrial-cancer#

American Heart Association. (2023). *Heart-healthy lifestyle linked to a longer life, free of chronic health conditions*. https://newsroom.heart.org/news/heart-healthy-lifestyle-linked-to-a-longer-life-free-of-chronic-health-conditions

American Psychological Association. (2022). *Infertility and BIPOC (Black, Indigenous & People of Color) women*. https://www.apa.org/pi/women/committee/infertility-bipoc

Anawalt, B. D. (2020). Causes of male infertility. *UpToDate*. Retrieved March 12, 2024, from https://www.uptodate.com/contents/causes-of-male-infertility

Anawalt, B. D. (2022). Approach to the male with infertility. *UpToDate*. Retrieved March 12, 2024, from https://www.uptodate.com/contents/approach-to-the-male-with-infertility

Arab, W. (2022). Diagnostic laparoscopy for unexplained subfertility: A comprehensive review. *JBRA Assisted Reproduction, 26*(1), 145–152. https://doi.org/10.5935/1518-0557.20210084

Bachmann, G., & Pinkerton, J. V. (2023a). Genitourinary syndrome of menopause (vulvovaginal atrophy): Clinical manifestations and diagnosis. *UpToDate*. Retrieved March 10, 2024, from https://www.uptodate.com/contents/genitourinary-syndrome-of-menopause-vulvovaginal-atrophy-clinical-manifestations-and-diagnosis

Bachmann, G., & Pinkerton, J. V. (2023b). Genitourinary syndrome of menopause (vulvovaginal atrophy): Treatment. *UpToDate*. Retrieved March 10, 2024, from https://www.uptodate.com/contents/genitourinary-syndrome-of-menopause-vulvovaginal-atrophy-treatment

Bartz, D. A. (2023). Pericoital (on demand) contraception: Diaphragm, cervical cap, spermicides, and sponge. *UpToDate*. Retrieved March 14, 2024, from https://www.uptodate.com/contents/pericoital-contraception-diaphragm-cervical-cap-spermicides-and-sponge

Bartz, D. A., & Pocius, K. D. (2023). Intrauterine contraception: Insertion and removal. *UpToDate*. Retrieved March 15, 2024, from https://www.uptodate.com/contents/intrauterine-contraception-insertion-and-removal

Behary, P., & Comninos, A. N. (2022). Bone perspectives in functional hypothalamic amenorrhoea: An update and future avenues. *Frontiers in Endocrinology*, 13. https://doi.org/10.3389/fendo.2022.923791

Biro, F. M., & Chan, Y. M. (2023). Normal puberty. *UpToDate*. Retrieved March 4, 2024, from https://www.uptodate.com/contents/normal-puberty

Bone Health and Osteoporosis Foundation. (2022a). *Facts about bone health*. https://www.bonehealthpolicyinstitute.org/bone-facts

Bone Health and Osteoporosis Foundation. (2022b). *Evaluation of bone health/bone density testing*. https://www.bonehealthandosteoporosis.org/patients/diagnosis-information/bone-density-examtesting/

Braaten, K. P., & Dutton, C. (2024). Overview of female permanent contraception. *UpToDate*. Retrieved March 15, 2024, from https://www.uptodate.com/contents/overview-of-female-permanent-contraception

Britton, L. E., Alspaugh, A., Greene, M. Z., & McLemore, M. R. (2020). CE: An evidence-based update on contraception. *The American Journal of Nursing*, *120*(2), 22–33. https://doi.org/10.1097/01.NAJ.0000654304.29632.a7

Burkman, R. T. (2022). Contraception: Transdermal contraceptive patches. *UpToDate*. Retrieved March 14, 2024, from https://www.uptodate.com/contents/contraception-transdermal-contraceptive-patches#:~:text=The%20transdermal%20contraceptive%20patches%20are,can%20safely%20use%20this%20method

Cantor, A. G., Nelson, H. D., Pappas, M., Atchison, C., Hatch, B., Huguet, N., Flynn, B., & McDonagh, M. (2022). *Telehealth for women's preventive services*. Comparative Effectiveness Review No. 256. Agency for Healthcare Research and Quality. https://doi.org/10.23970/AHRQEPCCER256

Carr, L. (2022). New hormone therapy guidelines from the North American Menopause Society. *Contemporary OB/GYN*. https://www.contemporaryobgyn.net/view/new-hormone-therapy-guidelines-from-the-north-american-menopause-society

Casper, R. F. (2023). Clinical manifestations and diagnosis of menopause. *UpToDate*. Retrieved March 9, 2024, from https://www.uptodate.com/contents/clinical-manifestations-and-diagnosis-of-menopause

Casper, R. F., & Mitwally, M. F. M. (2022). Ovulation induction with letrozole. *UpToDate*. Retrieved March 12, 2024, from https://www.uptodate.com/contents/ovulation-induction-with-letrozole

Casper, R. F., & Yonkers, K. A. (2022). Treatment of premenstrual syndrome and premenstrual dysphoric disorder. *UpToDate*. Retrieved March 7, 2024, from https://www.uptodate.com/contents/treatment-of-premenstrual-syndrome-and-premenstrual-dysphoric-disorder

Centers for Disease Control and Prevention. (2022a). *Promoting health for adults*. https://www.cdc.gov/chronicdisease/resources/publications/factsheets/promoting-health-for-adults.htm

Centers for Disease Control and Prevention. (2023a). *Infertility FAQs*. https://www.cdc.gov/reproductivehealth/infertility/index.htm

Centers for Disease Control and Prevention. (2023b). *Contraception*. https://www.cdc.gov/reproductivehealth/contraception/

Centers for Disease Control and Prevention. (2023c). *HIV basics: Basic statistics*. https://www.cdc.gov/hiv/basics/statistics.html

Centers for Disease Control and Prevention. (2024). *Lower your risk for the number 1 killer of women*. https://www.cdc.gov/healthequity/features/heartdisease/index.html

Coney, P. (2023). Menopause. *eMedicine*. https://emedicine.medscape.com/article/264088-overview

Cooper, D. B., Patel, P., & Mahdy, H. (2022). Oral contraceptive pills. *StatPearls* [Internet]. https://www.ncbi.nlm.nih.gov/books/NBK430882/

Darney, P. D. (2024). Contraception: Etonogestrel implant. *UpToDate*. Retrieved March 15, 2024, from https://www.uptodate.com/contents/contraception-etonogestrel-implant

Davis, E., & Sparzak, P. B. (2023). Abnormal uterine bleeding. *StatPearls* [Internet]. https://www.ncbi.nlm.nih.gov/books/NBK532913/

Department of Health and Environmental Control. (2021). Warning signs and cautions (ACHES). Retrieved March 14, 2024, from https://scdhec.gov/sites/default/files/Library/ML-005064.pdf

Dourou, P., Gourounti, K., Lykeridou, A., Gaitanou, K., Petrogiannis, N., & Sarantaki, A. (2023). Quality of life among couples with a fertility related diagnosis. *Clinics and practice*, *13*(1), 251–263. https://doi.org/10.3390/clinpract13010023

Endocrine Society. (2022a). *Menopause: Hot flashes*. https://www.endocrine.org/patient-engagement/endocrine-library/menopause

Endocrine Society. (2022b). *Osteoporosis*. https://www.endocrine.org/patient-engagement/endocrine-library/osteoporosis

Endocrine Society. (2023). *Obesity appears to increase the risk of developing polycystic ovary syndrome*. https://www.endocrine.org/news-and-advocacy/news-room/2023/endo-2023-press-amiri

Gartlehner, G., Patel, S. V., Reddy, S., Rains, C., Coker-Schwimmer, M., & Kahwati, L. (2022). Hormone therapy for the primary prevention of chronic conditions in postmenopausal persons: An evidence review for the U.S. preventive services task force. *Evidence Synthesis* No. 222. Agency for Healthcare Research and Quality. https://www.ncbi.nlm.nih.gov/books/NBK586478/pdf/Bookshelf_NBK586478.pdf

Gasner, A., & Rehman, A. (2023). Primary amenorrhea. *StatPearls* [Internet]. https://www.ncbi.nlm.nih.gov/books/NBK554469/

Gudipally, P. R., & Sharma, G. K. (2023). Premenstrual syndrome. *StatPearls* [Internet]. https://pubmed.ncbi.nlm.nih.gov/32809533/

Guttmacher Institute. (2022). *Medication abortion now accounts for more than half of all US abortions*. https://www.guttmacher.org/article/2022/02/medication-abortion-now-accounts-more-half-all-us-abortions

Habeeb, S. (2022). HRT in menopause & role of nurse. *Journal of Physical Medicine Rehabilitation Studies & Reports*, *4*(2). https://www.onlinescientificresearch.com/articles/hrt-in-menopause-amp-role-of-nurse.pdf

Ho, J. (2023). In vitro fertilization: Overview of clinical issues and questions. *UpToDate*. Retrieved March 12, 2024, from https://www.uptodate.com/contents/in-vitro-fertilization-overview-of-clinical-issues-and-questions

Hornstein, M. D., Gibbons, W. E., & Schenken, R. S. (2022). Natural fertility and impact of lifestyle factors. *UpToDate*. Retrieved March 11, 2024, from https://www.uptodate.com/contents/natural-fertility-and-impact-of-lifestyle-factors

Hornstein, M. D., Gibbons, W. E., & Young, S. L. (2024). Endometriosis: Treatment of infertility in females. *UpToDate*. Retrieved March 11, 2024, from https://www.uptodate.com/contents/endometriosis-treatment-of-infertility-in-females

Jennings, V. (2023). Fertility awareness-based methods of pregnancy prevention. *UpToDate*. Retrieved March 12, 2024, from https://www.uptodate.com/contents/fertility-awareness-based-methods-of-pregnancy-prevention

Kaunitz, A. M. (2023a). Patient education: Hormonal methods of birth control (beyond the basics). *UpToDate*. Retrieved March 12, 2024, from https://www.uptodate.com/contents/hormonal-methods-of-birth-control-beyond-the-basics

Kaunitz, A. M. (2023b). Depot medroxyprogesterone acetate (DMPA): Formulations, patient selection and drug administration. *UpToDate*. Retrieved March 14, 2024, from https://www.uptodate.com/contents/depot-medroxyprogesterone-acetate-dmpa-formulations-patient-selection-and-drug-administration

Kaunitz, A. M. (2023c). Depot medroxyprogesterone acetate (DMPA): Efficacy, side effects, metabolic impact, and benefits. *UpToDate*. Retrieved March 14, 2024, from https://www.uptodate.com/contents/depot-medroxyprogesterone-acetate-dmpa-efficacy-side-effects-metabolic-impact-and-benefits

Kaunitz, A. M. (2024a). Abnormal uterine bleeding in nonpregnant reproductive-age patients: Terminology, evaluation, and approach to diagnosis. *UpToDate*. Retrieved March 7, 2024, from https://www.uptodate.com/contents/abnormal-uterine-bleeding-in-nonpregnant-reproductive-age-patients-terminology-evaluation-and-approach-to-diagnosis

Kaunitz, A. M. (2024b). Abnormal uterine bleeding in nonpregnant reproductive-age patients: Management. *UpToDate*. Retrieved March 7, 2024, from, https://www.uptodate.com/contents/abnormal-uterine-bleeding-in-nonpregnant-reproductive-age-patients-management

Kerns, J., & Darney, P. D. (2023). Contraception: Hormonal contraceptive vaginal rings. *UpToDate*. Retrieved March 14, 2024, from https://www.uptodate.com/contents/contraception-hormonal-contraceptive-vaginal-rings

Kuohung, W., & Hornstein, M. D. (2023a). Female infertility: Evaluation. *UpToDate*. Retrieved March 12, 2024, from https://www.uptodate.com/contents/evaluation-of-female-infertility

Kuohung, W., & Hornstein, M. D. (2023b). Overview of infertility. *UpToDate*. Retrieved March 11, 2024, from https://www.uptodate.com/contents/overview-of-infertility

Kuohung, W., & Hornstein, M. D. (2023c). Female infertility: Causes. *UpToDate*. Retrieved March 12, 2024, from https://www.uptodate.com/contents/female-infertility-causes

Kuohung, W., & Hornstein, M. D. (2023d). Female infertility: Treatments. *UpToDate*. Retrieved March 12, 2024, from https://www.uptodate.com/contents/female-infertility-treatments

Lacroix, A. E., Gondal, H., Shumway, K. R., & Langaker, M. D. (2023). Physiology, menarche. *StatPearls* [Internet]. https://www.ncbi.nlm.nih.gov/books/NBK470216/

Li, L., Lou, K., Chu, A., O'Brien, E., Molina, A., & Riley, K. (2023). Complementary therapy for endometriosis related pelvic pain. *Journal of Endometriosis and Pelvic Pain Disorders, 15*(1):34–43. https://doi.org/10.1177/22840265231159704

Loder, C., & Solomon, L. M. (2022). Improving contraceptive care for marginalized populations. *Contemporary OB/GYN, 67*(9), 10–13. https://www.contemporaryobgyn.net/view/improving-contraceptive-care-for-marginalized-populations

Loprinzi, C. L., & Casper, R. F. (2023). Menopausal hot flashes. *UpToDate*. Retrieved March 10, 2024, from https://www.uptodate.com/contents/menopausal-hot-flashes

MacNeil, B. A. (2022). Examining predictors of menstrual irregularity among women receiving outpatient treatment for an eating disorder: Psychiatric diagnosis, age of onset, physical, and psychological symptoms. *Psychiatry Research Communications, 2*(2), 100049. https://www.sciencedirect.com/science/article/pii/S2772598722000307

Madden, T. (2023). Intrauterine contraception: Background and device types. *UpToDate*. Retrieved March 15, 2024, from https://www.uptodate.com/contents/intrauterine-contraception-background-and-device-types#:~:text=The%20intrauterine%20device%20(IUD)%20is,as%20effective%20as%20surgical%20sterilization

Martin, K. A., & Barbieri, R. L. (2022). Menopausal hormone therapy: Benefits and risks. *UpToDate*. Retrieved March 10, 2024, from https://www.uptodate.com/contents/menopausal-hormone-therapy-benefits-and-risks

Martin, K. A., & Rosenson, R. S. (2023). Menopausal hormone therapy and cardiovascular risk. *UpToDate*. Retrieved March 11, 2024, from https://www.uptodate.com/contents/menopausal-hormone-therapy-and-cardiovascular-risk

Mayer, C., & Deedwania, P. (2023). Hysterosalpingogram. *StatPearls* [Internet]. https://www.ncbi.nlm.nih.gov/books/NBK572146/

Mechsner, S. (2022). Endometriosis, an ongoing pain-step-by-step treatment. *Journal of Clinical Medicine, 11*(2), 467. https://doi.org/10.3390/jcm11020467

Munro, M. G., Critchley, H. O. D., Fraser, I. S., & Federation of Gynecology and Obstetrics. (2018). The two FIGO systems for normal and abnormal uterine bleeding symptoms and classification of causes of abnormal uterine bleeding in the reproductive years: 2018 revisions. *International Journal of Genecology and Obstetrics, 143*, 393–408. https://doi.org/10.1002/ijgo.12666

Nagy, H., Carlson, K., & Khan, M. A. B. (2023). Dysmenorrhea. *StatPearls* [Internet]. https://www.ncbi.nlm.nih.gov/books/NBK560834

Nath, J. (2023). Altered reproductive function. In J. Nath (Ed.), *Applied pathophysiology* (4th ed., pp. 344–369). Wolters Kluwer.

National Institute on Aging. (2021a). *What is menopause?* https://www.nia.nih.gov/health/what-menopause#transition

National Institute on Aging. (2021b). *Hot flashes: What can I do?* https://www.nia.nih.gov/health/menopause/hot-flashes-what-can-i-do#lifestyle

Newhouse, R. (2022). Contraception. In K. D. Schuiling & F. E. Likis (Eds.), *Gynecologic health care* (4th ed., pp. 235–266). Jones & Bartlett Learning.

Nurse Practitioners in Women's Health. (2022). *NPWH position statement: Access to safe abortion care*. https://cdn.ymaws.com/npwh.org/resource/resmgr/positionstatement/Updated_Abortion_Care.pdf

Pagana, K. D., Pagana, T. J., & Pagana, T. N. (2023). *Mosby's diagnostic and laboratory test reference* (16th ed.). Elsevier.

Paradise, S. L., Landis, C. A., & Klein, D. A. (2022). Evidence-based contraception: Common questions and answers. *American Family Physician*. https://www.aafp.org/dam/AAFP/documents/journals/afp/Paradise.pdf

Peacock, K., Carlson, K., & Ketvertis, K. M. (2023). Menopause. *StatPearls* [Internet]. https://www.ncbi.nlm.nih.gov/books/NBK507826/

Price, T. M. (2022). Abnormal uterine bleeding. *eMedicine*. https://emedicine.medscape.com/article/257007-overview

Roe, A. H., Bartz, D. A., & Douglas, P. S. (2023). Combined estrogen-progestin contraception: Side effects and health concerns. *UpToDate*. https://www.uptodate.com/contents/combined-estrogen-progestin-contraception-side-effects-and-health-concerns

Rosen, H. N., & Lewiecki, E. M. (2024). Overview of the management of low bone mass and osteoporosis in postmenopausal women. *UpToDate*. Retrieved March 10, 2024, from https://www.uptodate.com/contents/overview-of-the-management-of-low-bone-mass-and-osteoporosis-in-postmenopausal-women

Sajadi-Ernazarova, K. R., & Martinez, C. L. (2023). Abortion complications. *StatPearls* [Internet]. https://www.ncbi.nlm.nih.gov/books/NBK430793/

Salem, W. (2023). Assisted reproductive technology: Pregnancy and maternal outcomes. *UpToDate*. Retrieved March 12, 2024, from https://www.uptodate.com/contents/assisted-reproductive-technology-pregnancy-and-maternal-outcomes

Schenken, R. S. (2023). Endometriosis: Treatment of pelvic pain. *UpToDate*. Retrieved March 6, 2024, from https://www.uptodate.com/contents/endometriosis-treatment-of-pelvic-pain

Schenken, R. S. (2024). Endometriosis: Clinical features, evaluation, and diagnosis. *UpToDate*. Retrieved on March 6, 2024, from https://www.uptodate.com/contents/endometriosis-clinical-features-evaluation-and-diagnosis

Schuiling, K. D., & Likis, F. E. (2022). *Gynecologic health care* (4th ed.). Jones & Bartlett Learning.

Seli, E., & Arici, A. (2023). Ovulation induction with clomiphene citrate. *UpToDate*. Retrieved March 12, 2024, from https://www.uptodate.com/contents/ovulation-induction-with-clomiphene-citrate

Shakhatreh, H. J. M., Salih, A. J., Aldrou, K. K. A. R., Alazzam, F. A. F., & Issa, M. S. B. (2022). Medico-legal aspects of abortion: Updates of the literature. *Medical Archives (Sarajevo, Bosnia and Herzegovina)*, *76*(5), 373–376. https://doi.org/10.5455/medarh.2022.76.373-376

Shih, G., & Wallace, R. (2023). First-trimester pregnancy termination: Uterine aspiration. *UpToDate*. Retrieved March 15, 2024, from https://www.uptodate.com/contents/first-trimester-pregnancy-termination-uterine-aspiration/print

Silver, N. E. (2023). Mood changes during perimenopause are real. Here's what to know. *American College of Obstetricians and Gynecologists*. https://www.acog.org/womens-health/experts-and-stories/the-latest/mood-changes-during-perimenopause-are-real-heres-what-to-know

Siminiuc, R., & Turcanu, D. (2023). Impact of nutritional diet therapy on premenstrual syndrome. *Frontiers in Nutrition*, *10*, 1079417. https://doi.org/10.3389/fnut.2023.1079417

Smith, R. P., & Kaunitz, A. M. (2023a). Dysmenorrhea in adult females: Treatment. *UpToDate*. Retrieved March 6, 2024, from https://www.uptodate.com/contents/dysmenorrhea-in-adult-females-treatment

Smith, R. P., & Kaunitz, A. M. (2023b). Dysmenorrhea in adult females: Clinical features and diagnosis. *UpToDate*. Retrieved March 6, 2024, from https://www.uptodate.com/contents/dysmenorrhea-in-adult-females-clinical-features-and-diagnosis

Sonalkar, S., & Mody, S. K. (2023). Contraception: Postpartum counseling and methods. *UpToDate*. Retrieved March 15, 2024, from https://www.uptodate.com/contents/contraception-postpartum-counseling-and-methods

Stormont, G., & Deibert, C. M. (2022). Vasectomy. *StatPearls* [Internet]. https://www.ncbi.nlm.nih.gov/books/NBK549904/

Sung, S., & Abramovitz, A. (2024) Tubal ligation. *StatPearls* [Internet]. https://www.ncbi.nlm.nih.gov/books/NBK549873/

Tanner, J. M. (1962). *Growth at adolescence*. Blackwell Scientific Publications.

"The 2022 Hormone Therapy Position Statement of The North American Menopause Society" Advisory Panel. (2022). The 2022 hormone therapy position statement of the North American Menopause Society. *Menopause*, *29*(7), 767–794. https://doi.org/10.1097/GME.0000000000002028

"The 2023 Nonhormone Therapy Position Statement of The North American Menopause Society" Advisory Panel. (2023). The 2023 nonhormone therapy position statement of the North American Menopause Society. *Menopause*, *30*(6), 573–590. https://doi.org/10.1097/GME.0000000000002200

Turok, D. (2023). Emergency contraception. *UpToDate*. Retrieved March 15, 2024, from https://www.uptodate.com/contents/emergency-contraception

U.S. Department of Health and Human Services. (n.d.). *Healthy people 2030*. https://health.gov/healthypeople

U.S. Food & Drug Administration. (2023). *FDA approves first nonprescription daily oral contraceptive*. https://www.fda.gov/news-events/press-announcements/fda-approves-first-nonprescription-daily-oral-contraceptive

Viera, A. J. (2023). Vasectomy. *UpToDate*. Retrieved March 15, 2024, from https://www.uptodate.com/contents/vasectomy

Welt, C. K., & Barbieri, R. L. (2022a). Evaluation and management of primary amenorrhea. *UpToDate*. Retrieved March 5, 2024, from https://www.uptodate.com/contents/evaluation-and-management-of-primary-amenorrhea?topicRef=7402&source=see_link

Welt, C. K., & Barbieri, R. L. (2022b). Evaluation and management of secondary amenorrhea. *UpToDate*. Retrieved March 5, 2024, from https://www.uptodate.com/contents/evaluation-and-management-of-secondary-amenorrhea?source=related_link

Welt, C. K., & Barbieri, R. L. (2023a). Causes of primary amenorrhea. *UpToDate*. Retrieved March 5, 2024, from https://www.uptodate.com/contents/causes-of-primary-amenorrhea

Welt, C. K., & Barbieri, R. L. (2023b). Epidemiology and causes of secondary amenorrhea. *UpToDate*. Retrieved March 5, 2024, from https://www.uptodate.com/contents/epidemiology-and-causes-of-secondary-amenorrhea

World Health Organization. (2021). *Emergency contraception*. https://www.who.int/news-room/fact-sheets/detail/emergency-contraception

World Health Organization. (2023a). *Endometriosis*. https://www.who.int/news-room/fact-sheets/detail/endometriosis

World Health Organization. (2023b). *Infertility*. https://www.who.int/news-room/fact-sheets/detail/infertility

World Health Organization. (2023c). 1 in 6 people globally affected by infertility: WHO. https://www.who.int/news/item/04-04-2023-1-in-6-people-globally-affected-by-infertility

Yonkers, K. A., & Casper, R. F. (2022). Clinical manifestations and diagnosis of premenstrual syndrome and premenstrual dysphoric disorder. *UpToDate*. Retrieved March 7, 2024, from https://www.uptodate.com/contents/clinical-manifestations-and-diagnosis-of-premenstrual-syndrome-and-premenstrual-dysphoric-disorder

Yonkers, K. A., & Casper, R. F. (2024). Epidemiology and pathogenesis of premenstrual syndrome and premenstrual dysphoric disorder. *UpToDate*. Retrieved March 7, 2024, from https://www.uptodate.com/contents/epidemiology-and-pathogenesis-of-premenstrual-syndrome-and-premenstrual-dysphoric-disorder

Yu, E. W. (2024). Screening for osteoporosis in postmenopausal women and men. *UpToDate*. Retrieved March 10, 2024, from https://www.uptodate.com/contents/screening-for-osteoporosis-in-postmenopausal-women-and-men

DEVELOPING CLINICAL JUDGMENT

PRACTICING FOR NCLEX

1. The nurse is teaching a couple about infertility and they ask, "After how many months of trying to conceive would we then be considered infertile?" Which is the appropriate response by the nurse?
   a. "6 months"
   b. "12 months"
   c. "18 months"
   d. "24 months"

2. The nurse is caring for a couple in the clinic. They report that the condom broke while they were having sexual intercourse last night. What would the nurse advise to prevent pregnancy?
   a. "Inject a spermicidal agent into the vagina immediately."
   b. "Obtain emergency contraceptives and take them immediately."
   c. "Douche with a solution of vinegar and hot water tonight."
   d. "Take a strong laxative now and again at bedtime."

3. The nurse is working with a postmenopausal patient. Which measure would the nurse recommend to the patient to help prevent osteoporosis?
   a. Supplementing with iron
   b. Sleeping 8 hours nightly
   c. Eating lean meats only
   d. Weight-bearing exercise

4. The nurse is teaching a female patient about oral contraceptives. Which activity does the nurse teach will increase the risk of cardiovascular disease (CVD) when combined with OCs?
   a. Eating a high-fiber diet
   b. Smoking cigarettes
   c. Taking daily multivitamins
   d. Drinking alcohol

5. The nurse is preparing to teach a class to a group of middle-aged people regarding the most common vasomotor symptoms experienced during menopause. Which is an example of a vasomotor symptom experienced by people in menopause?
   a. Weight gain
   b. Decreased bone density
   c. Hot flashes
   d. Heart disease

6. A group of people is taking a class on female health promotion. What does the nurse teach that throughout life is the most proactive activity to promote female health?
   a. Consistent exercise
   b. Socialization with friends
   c. Quality quiet time with themselves
   d. Consuming water

7. A female patient is discussing contraception options with the nurse. Which comment by the patient would indicate that a diaphragm is not the best contraceptive device for them?
   a. "My partner says it is my job to keep from getting pregnant."
   b. "I have a hard time remembering to take my vitamins daily."
   c. "Hormones cause cancer and I don't want to take them."
   d. "I am not comfortable touching myself down there."

8. A nurse educator has taught a group of nursing students about menstrual abnormalities. Which response by the students demonstrates an understanding of the most common cause of menstrual abnormality in a reproductive-age female?
   a. "Ectopic pregnancy"
   b. "Coagulopathy"
   c. "Carcinoma"
   d. "Anovulation"

CRITICAL THINKING EXERCISE

1. Ms. London, age 25, comes to your family planning clinic requesting to have an IUD inserted because "birth control pills give you cancer." In reviewing her history, you note she has been into the STI clinic three times in the past year with vaginal infections and was hospitalized for PID last month. When you question her about her sexual history, she reports having sex with multiple partners and not always using protection.
   a. Is an IUD the most appropriate method for this patient? Why or why not?
   b. What myths/misperceptions will you address in your counseling session?
   c. Outline the safer sex discussion you plan to have with her.

STUDY ACTIVITIES

1. Develop a teaching plan for an adolescent with PMS and dysmenorrhea.

2. Arrange to shadow a nurse working in family planning for the morning. What questions does the nurse ask to ascertain the kind of family planning

method that is right for each patient? What teaching goes along with each method? What follow-up care is needed? Share your findings with your classmates during a clinical conference.

3. Access the internet and locate three resources for couples experiencing infertility to consult that provide support and resources.

4. Sterilization is the most prevalent method of contraception used by married couples in the United States. Contact a local urologist and gynecologist to learn about the procedure involved and the cost of male and female sterilization. Which procedure poses less risk to the person and costs less?

5. Take a field trip to a local drugstore to check out the variety and costs of male and female condoms. How many different brands did you find? What was the range of costs?

6. What are the noncontraceptive benefits of combined oral contraceptives? Select all that apply.
   a. Protection against ovarian cancer
   b. Protection against endometrial cancer
   c. Protection against breast cancer
   d. Reduction in incidence of ectopic pregnancy
   e. Prevention of functional ovarian cysts
   f. Reduction in the risk of deep venous thrombosis
   g. Reduction in the risk of colorectal cancer

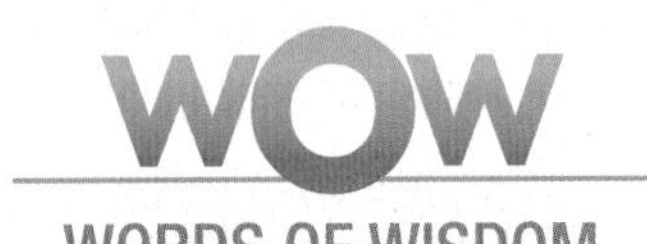

WORDS OF WISDOM

Unconditional self-acceptance in patients is the core to reducing risky behavior and fostering peace of mind.

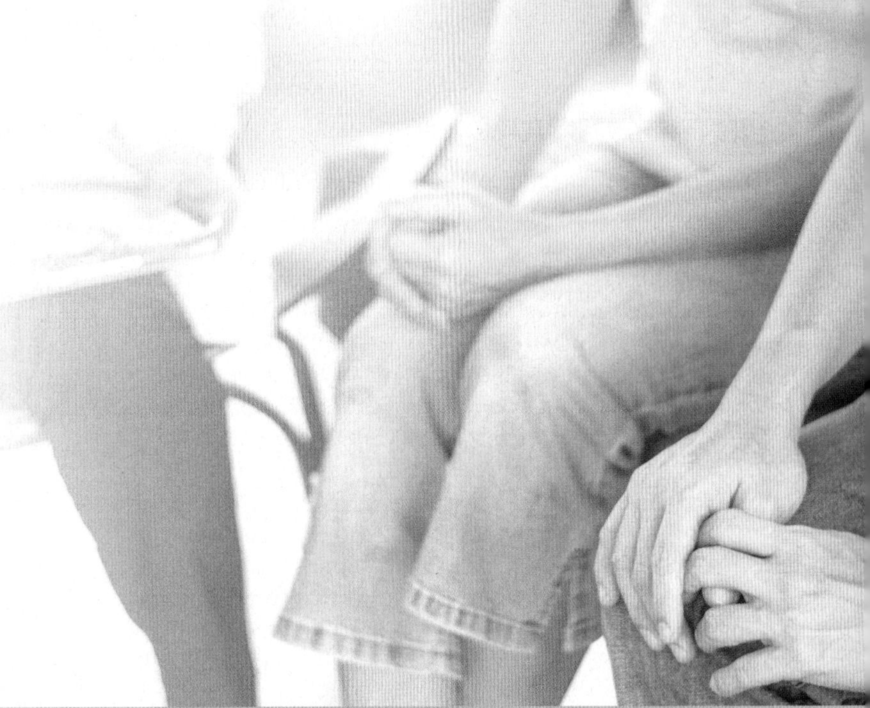

5

Sexually Transmitted Infections

LEARNING OBJECTIVES

Upon completion of the chapter, you will be able to:

1. Examine the cultural and psychological components of sexually transmitted infections (STIs).
2. Analyze the pathology, spread, control, and prevention of STIs.
3. Relate the risk factors, and outline patient education appropriate to common STIs.
4. Outline the nursing management needed for patients with STIs characterized by vaginal discharge, cervicitis, and genital ulcers.
5. Determine the long-term sequelae that pelvic inflammatory disease (PID) can cause and prevention measures.
6. Design a teaching plan to educate patients about vaccine-preventable STIs.
7. Summarize household measures to prevent the spread of ectoparasitic infections among family members.
8. Formulate a teaching presentation for youth about human immunodeficiency virus (HIV), including transmission, clinical signs and symptoms, treatment, and prevention.
9. Describe how the nurse can play a role in the prevention of STIs.

KEY TERMS

acquired immunodeficiency syndrome (AIDS)
bacterial vaginosis (bak-tēr'ē-ăl vaj'i-nō'sis)
chlamydia (kla-mid'ē-ă)
ectoparasites
genital herpes
genital/vulvovaginal candidiasis (kan'di-dī'ă-sis)
gonorrhea
human immunodeficiency virus (HIV)
human papillomavirus (HPV)
pelvic inflammatory disease (PID)
sexually transmitted infection (STI)
syphilis
trichomoniasis (trik'ō-mō-nī'ă-sis)

Sandy, a 19-year-old, couldn't imagine what these "things" were that appeared "down there" in her genital area last week. She was too embarrassed to tell anyone, so she stopped by the college health service today to find out what they were.

INTRODUCTION

Sexually transmitted infections (STIs) are infections of the reproductive tract caused by microorganisms transmitted through vaginal, anal, or oral sexual intercourse (Centers for Disease Control and Prevention [CDC], 2023c). STIs are a significant health challenge globally, which pose a serious threat not only to female sexual health but also to the general health and well-being of millions of people worldwide (see Box 5.1 for STI classification). According to the World Health Organization (WHO), every day worldwide, 1 million new cases of STIs are acquired (WHO, 2023b). In the United States, one in five people have an STI on any given day (CDC, 2022d). STIs constitute an epidemic of tremendous magnitude. An estimated 1.2 million people in the United States currently live with human immunodeficiency virus (HIV), an incurable STI, and approximately 36,000 Americans become infected with HIV annually (CDC, 2023b). About 13% of them (one in seven) are unaware they are infected, and they account for 40% of new HIV infections (Kaiser Family Foundation [KFF], 2022). The incidence of STIs continues to rise and costs the United States over $16 billion annually (CDC, 2022d).

STIs present a greater risk and cause more complications among young people and females than among males (CDC, 2022d). Due to anatomic differences, females are more susceptible than males to acquire a STI. After only a single exposure, females are twice as likely as males to acquire infections from pathogens that cause gonorrhea, chlamydial infection, hepatitis B, and syphilis. STIs contribute to cervical cancer, infertility, ectopic pregnancy, chronic pelvic pain, and death. Certain infections can be transmitted in utero to the fetus or during childbirth to the newborn (Table 5.1).

Psychological distress is commonly associated with STIs; people may feel shame, anxiety, embarrassment, isolation, fear of rejection, and depression after being diagnosed with an STI (Singh & Singh, 2021). The patient may be afraid or embarrassed to tell their partner and ask them to seek treatment. In some instances, females may be afraid that telling their partner may place them in danger of escalating abuse. The nurse can empathize with the patient's feelings and suggest specific ways of talking with partners that will help decrease anxiety and assist in efforts to control infection. It is important for the nurse to be aware of the specific context of female vulnerability to STIs and identify any barriers to care. To maximize the impact of behavioral interventions and risk reduction programs, the nurse must adjust for social and cultural differences within all diverse populations. Based on the findings of numerous studies, the U.S. Preventive Services Task Force (USPSTF) recommends behavioral counseling for sexually active adolescents and high-risk adults to reduce their risk (USPSTF, 2020). Nurses play a crucial role in supporting patients from diverse cultures within sexual health services and as trusted health care providers in a range of settings. Preventing, identifying, and managing STIs are vital components of offering good health care.

Additional information on STIs during pregnancy can be found in Chapter 20.

BOX 5.1 CDC Classifications of STIs

- Infections characterized by vaginal discharge
  - Vulvovaginal candidiasis
  - Trichomoniasis
  - Bacterial vaginosis
- Infections characterized by cervicitis
  - Chlamydia
  - Gonorrhea
- Infections characterized by genital ulcers
  - Genital herpes simplex
  - Syphilis
- Vaccine-preventable STIs
  - Hepatitis A
  - Hepatitis B
  - Hepatitis C
  - Human papillomavirus
- Ectoparasitic infections
  - Pediculosis pubis
  - Scabies

CDC, Centers for Disease Control and Prevention; STI, sexually transmitted infection.

Centers for Disease Control and Prevention. (2023c). *Sexually transmitted diseases (STDs): CDC fact sheets.* https://www.cdc.gov/std/healthcomm/fact_sheets.htm

MARGINALIZED POPULATIONS

Marginalized populations continue to face severe disparities in all reportable STIs, but Black females are the group most affected (Dall, 2023). Gonorrhea rates among Black females are higher than for any other racial or ethnic group and seven times higher than for White females (Cohn & Harrison, 2022). There is a higher prevalence of STIs among transgender and non-binary people than the general population (Rietmeijer, 2024). It is imperative that the health care team work together to improve access to effective STI prevention and treatment services in local communities for those who need it the most. By adopting a multicultural approach to the control of STIs, nurses can address specific cultural attitudes and behaviors that may impact exposure to STIs and intervene to reduce them.

The lesbian, gay, bisexual, transgender, queer, intersex, and asexual (LGBTQIA+) community comprises a significant, growing patient population that faces a unique set of health care challenges that must be addressed by the health care system and nurses who work within it. This community has experienced historic oppression and discrimination, leading many to withdraw from seeking needed health care and refrain from disclosing their LGBTQIA+ identities. This has resulted in delayed treatment and poor outcomes.

TABLE 5.1 • Maternal and Fetal Effects From STIs

STI	Maternal Effects	Fetal Effects
Candidiasis	Resistant to treatment during pregnancy; uncomfortable localized genital itching and discharge	Can acquire thrush in the mouth during birthing process if birthing parent infected
Trichomoniasis	Has been implicated in causing PROM and preterm births	Risk of prematurity and low birth weight
Bacterial vaginosis	Increases risk for spontaneous abortion, PROM, chorioamnionitis, postpartum endometritis, and preterm labor	Risk of low birth weight and neonatal sepsis
Chlamydia	Postpartum endometritis, PROM, and preterm birth	Conjunctivitis, which can lead to blindness, low birth weight, neonatal sepsis, and pneumonitis
Gonorrhea	Chorioamnionitis, spontaneous abortion, preterm birth, PROM, IUGR, and postpartum sepsis	Pharyngeal and eye infection (*gonococcal ophthalmia*), which can cause blindness
Genital herpes	Spontaneous abortion, intrauterine infection, preterm labor, PROM, and IUGR	Contamination during birth, newborn can develop skin or mouth sores, birth anomalies, neurologic impairment, and transplacental infection
Syphilis	Spontaneous abortion, preterm birth, and stillbirth	Congenital syphilis, leading to multisystem organ failure and structural damage as well as intellectual disability
Human papillomavirus	May cause dystocia if large wartlike genital lesions	May develop warts in throat, uncommon but life-threatening
Hepatitis B	May cause preterm birth; can be transmitted to fetus if active in last trimester	Can become chronic carrier of hepatitis B, which may lead to liver cancer or cirrhosis
Human immunodeficiency virus	Fatigue, nausea, and weight loss	Transmission can occur transplacentally, during childbirth or through breast milk.

IUGR, intrauterine growth restriction; PROM, premature rupture of membranes; STI, sexually transmitted infection.

Centers for Disease Control and Prevention. (2023). *STDs during pregnancy: CDC detailed fact sheet.* https://www.cdc.gov/std/pregnancy/stdfact-pregnancy-detailed.htm#details; Centers for Disease Control and Prevention. (2023c). *Sexually transmitted diseases (STDs): CDC fact sheets.* https://www.cdc.gov/std/healthcomm/fact_sheets.htm

Living in a country that allows the free practice of various religions and lifestyles, nurses must be able to understand the needs and practices of each person, while being careful to not cast judgment or impose personal opinions of their worldview. Therapeutic communication is an essential component of the nurse–patient relationship and must be cultivated in the ongoing effort toward providing culturally competent care.

Nursing Assessment

When caring for patients from marginalized populations, nurses need to assess the sexual history, behavior, and STI risk through open dialogue and a nonjudgmental approach. Assessment will be directed by the person's anatomy and sexual behaviors.

Nursing Management

Nurses cannot ignore the glaring racial and cultural disparities present in rates of STIs. Nurses must be receptive to the health care concerns of all patients, understand their cumulative experiences, and be responsive to each person's specific needs. Nurses must adopt strategies that can help to bridge the gap in achieving equity in reproductive and sexual health for all people. To truly maximize the impact of behavioral interventions and risk reduction programs, nurses must adjust for social and cultural differences within any diverse population group for which they care.

ADOLESCENTS

STIs occur disproportionately among adolescents. An estimated 46% of all STIs occur among people aged 15 to 24 years (CDC, 2022d). In the United States, all states allow minors to consent for their own STI services. No state requires parental consent for STI care. Of high school students in 2021, 30% report having been sexually active, with nearly half of these students not using a condom during their last sexual encounter (CDC, 2023e). These data reinforce existing recommendations for sexual health education and STI prevention targeting adolescents before they become sexually active. See Healthy People 2030 box.

HEALTHY PEOPLE 2030

STI Objectives	Nursing Significance
Increase the proportion of adolescents who get formal sex education before age 18 years. Reduce the proportion of adolescents and young adults with genital herpes. Increase the proportion of adolescents who get recommended doses of the HPV vaccine.	Educate adolescents that abstinence is the only way to completely avoid contracting STIs. Encourage adolescents to postpone initiation of sexual intercourse for as long as possible. For teens who have already had sexual intercourse, encourage abstinence at this point. Encourage adolescents to minimize their lifetime number of sexual partners. Encourage adolescents to always use condoms if participating in any sexual act. Educate about the HPV vaccine and encourage patients to receive recommended vaccinations.

HPV, human papillomavirus; STI, sexually transmitted infection.
Healthy People Objectives retrieved from http://www.healthypeople.gov

Risk Factors

Because of biologic and behavioral factors, adolescents are at a particularly high risk for acquiring STIs and for the serious, long-term, potentially life-altering sequelae that can develop from undiagnosed, untreated infections. During adolescence and young adulthood, female columnar epithelial cells are especially sensitive to invasion by sexually transmitted organisms, such as chlamydia and gonococci (the organism that causes gonorrhea). These cells extend out over the vaginal surface of the cervix, where they are unprotected by cervical mucus; with age, they recede to a more protected location.

Behaviorally, adolescents and young adults tend to think they are invincible and deny the risks of their behaviors. This risky behavior may expose them to STIs, including HIV/acquired immunodeficiency syndrome (AIDS). Adolescents frequently have unprotected intercourse, engage in partnerships of limited durations, and face many obstacles that prevent them from using the health care system. High-risk factors in adolescents include sexual activity in early to middle adolescence, alcohol and substance use, males having sex with males, living in a detention center, having a mood disorder, adverse childhood experiences (such as maltreatment or sexual abuse), and having multiple or new sexual partners or a partner with multiple partners and not using condoms (Fortenberry, 2023). Inexperience with condoms can also lead to more condom accidents, such as breakage caused by storage in a hot environment, opening packages with teeth, using long fingernails to put condoms on, slippage if the wrong size condom is used, or failure to hold the condom while withdrawing.

Furthermore, some adolescents are unwilling to disclose their sexual activity. If symptoms of an STI develop, they may misperceive them as normal, consequently delaying medical treatment. Untreated STIs can cause pelvic inflammatory disease (PID), which can lead to infertility, adverse pregnancy outcomes, and anogenital and cervical cancers. In addition, the presence of other STIs increases the likelihood of both transmitting and acquiring HIV, since a break in the skin can make it easier for the virus to enter the body (CDC, 2022e).

Nursing Assessment

Many health care providers fail to assess adolescent sexual behavior and STI risks, to screen for infection without symptoms during clinic visits, or to counsel adolescents on STI risk reduction. Nurses need to remember that they play a key role in the detection, prevention, and treatment of STIs in adolescents. All 50 states in the United States recognize chlamydia, gonorrhea, syphilis, chancroid, and HIV as notifiable conditions (CDC, 2024a). This means that federal law mandates health care providers to report new cases of these infections to public health authorities. Reporting STIs allows for their incidence to be monitored and tracked. Specific STIs seen in females and adolescents are discussed further.

Nursing Management

Prevention of STIs among adolescents is critical. Health care providers have a unique opportunity to provide counseling and education to their patients. Adolescents are less willing to be open to nurses and less likely to return for care if they are uncertain about confidentiality. Nurses working with adolescents need to convey their willingness to discuss sexual habits, and any interactions with patients need to be direct and nonjudgmental.

Nurses can provide effective guidance and promote sexual health so that primary or repeat infections can be avoided. Adolescents bear disproportionate burdens when it comes to STIs, so education is needed to help them protect their reproductive futures. Specific actions to take include:

- Encourage the patient to complete antibiotic prescriptions (specific management for each type of STI is discussed further).
- Adapt the style and content of any message to the patient's developmental level.
- Identify risk factors and risk behaviors, and guide the patient in developing specific individualized actions of prevention.
- Teach adolescents about their sexual development to foster understanding of their bodily changes, the role of hormones, and the emotions they are experiencing.
- Encourage adolescents to postpone initiation of sexual intercourse for as long as possible, but if they choose to have sexual intercourse, explain the necessity of using barrier methods, such as male external or female internal condoms (Teaching Guidelines 5.1). For adolescents who have already had sexual intercourse, the clinician can encourage abstinence at this point. If adolescents are sexually active, they should be directed to teen clinics, and contraceptive options should be explained. In areas where specialized teen clinics are not available, nurses should feel comfortable discussing sexuality, safety, and contraception with teens. Encourage adolescents to minimize their lifetime number of sexual partners, to use barrier methods consistently and correctly, and to be aware of the connection between drug and alcohol use and the incorrect use of barrier methods. Table 5.2 discusses barriers to condom use and means to overcome them.

Think back to Sandy, who was introduced at the beginning of the chapter. How should the nurse handle Sandy's anxious state? What specific questions should the nurse ask Sandy to determine the source of the possible infection in her genital area?

TEACHING GUIDELINES 5.1 Proper External Condom Use

- Use latex or polyurethane condoms to create a mechanical barrier for sexually transmitted infections and pregnancy.
- Use a new condom with each act of sexual intercourse. Never reuse a condom.
- Handle condoms with care to prevent damage from sharp objects such as fingernails and teeth.
- Ensure condom has been stored in a cool, dry place away from direct sunlight. Do not store condoms in a wallet or automobile or anywhere they would be exposed to extreme temperatures.
- Check the expiration date on the condom package.
- Open the condom wrapper carefully. Don't use teeth or scissors that could tear or puncture the condom inside.
- Do not use a condom if it appears brittle, sticky, or discolored. These are signs of aging.
- Put condom on before any genital contact because sperm is present in pre-ejaculate fluid.
- Put condom on when penis is erect. Ensure it is placed so it will readily unroll.
- Hold the tip of the condom while unrolling. Ensure there is a space at the tip for semen to collect, but make sure no air is trapped in the tip. Pinch the air out of the top tip.
- Ensure adequate lubrication during intercourse. If external lubricants are used, use only water-based lubricants such as K-Y Jelly with latex condoms. Oil-based or petroleum-based lubricants, such as body lotion, massage oil, or cooking oil, can weaken latex condoms.
- Polyurethane condoms are more expensive and thinner than latex condoms. They also have a looser fit, but are just as effective as latex. However, polyurethane breaks more often when compared with latex condoms. They are not compatible with all the different kinds of lubricants (water, silicone, silicone hybrid, and oil), so checking each lubricant brand for compatibility is wise.
- Withdraw while penis is still erect, and hold condom firmly against base of penis.

Proper Internal Condom Use

- Do not use an external condom with an internal condom.
- The thick inner ring with the closed end goes into the vagina (similar to inserting a tampon); the thin outer ring remains outside the body.
- Ensure condom is not twisted, that penis does not slip between the condom and vaginal wall, and the outer ring does not get pushed into the vagina.

Adapted from Centers for Disease Control and Prevention. (2022f). *Condom effectiveness: Male (external) condom use.* https://www.cdc.gov/condomeffectiveness/external-condom-use.html; and Centers for Disease Control and Prevention. (2022c). *Condom effectiveness: Female (internal) condom use*. https://www.cdc.gov/condomeffectiveness/internal-condom-use.html?CDC_AA_refVal=https%3A%2F%2Fwww.cdc.gov%2Fcondomeffectiveness%2FFemale-condom-use.html

TABLE 5.2 • Guidelines: Barriers to Condom Use and Means to Overcome Them

Perceived Barrier	Intervention Strategy
Decreases sexual pleasure (sensation) Note: Often perceived by those who have never used a condom	• Encourage patient to try. • Put a drop of water-based lubricant or saliva inside the tip of the condom or on the glans of the penis before putting on the condom. • Try a thinner latex condom or a different brand or more lubrication.
Decreases spontaneity of sexual activity	• Incorporate condom use into foreplay. • Remind patient that peace of mind may enhance pleasure for self and partner.
Embarrassing, juvenile, "unmanly"	• Remind patient that it is "manly" to protect themselves and others.
Poor fit (too small or too big, slips off, uncomfortable)	• Smaller and larger condoms are available.
Requires prompt withdrawal after ejaculation	• Reinforce the protective nature of prompt withdrawal and suggest substituting other postcoital sexual activities.
Fear of breakage may lead to less vigorous sexual activity.	• With prolonged intercourse, lubricant wears off and the condom begins to rub. Have a water-soluble lubricant available to reapply.
Nonpenetrative sexual activity	• Condoms have been advocated for use during fellatio; unlubricated condoms may prove best for this purpose due to the taste of the lubricant. • Other barriers, such as dental dams or an unlubricated condom, can be cut down the middle to form a barrier; these have been advocated for use during certain forms of nonpenetrative sexual activity (e.g., cunnilingus and anolingual sex).
Allergy to latex	• Polyurethane external and internal condoms are available. • A natural skin condom can be used together with a latex condom to protect the person from contact with latex.

Copyright © All rights reserved. Public Health Agency of Canada. [2008]. *Updates to the Canadian guidelines on sexually transmitted infections.* Reproduced and Adapted with permission from the Minister of Health, 2024. https://publications.gc.ca/collections/collection_2008/phac-aspc/HP40-1-2008E.pdf

INFECTIONS CHARACTERIZED BY VAGINAL DISCHARGE

"Vaginitis" is a generic term that means inflammation and infection of the vagina. Vaginitis has many causes, but more often than not, the cause is infection by one of three organisms:

- *Candida*, a fungus
- *Trichomonas*, a protozoan
- *Gardnerella*, a bacterium

The complex balance of microbiologic organisms in the vagina is a key element in the maintenance of health. Subtle shifts in the vaginal environment may allow organisms with pathologic potential to proliferate, causing infectious symptoms.

The nurse's role in managing vaginitis is one of primary prevention and education to limit recurrences of these infections. In addition to assessing patients for the common signs and symptoms and risk factors, primary prevention begins with changing the sexual behaviors that place them at risk for infection.

Genital/Vulvovaginal Candidiasis

Genital/vulvovaginal candidiasis (VVC) is one of the most common causes of vaginal discharge. It is also referred to as yeast, monilia, and fungal infection. It is not considered an STI because *Candida* is a normal constituent in the vagina and becomes pathologic only when the vaginal environment becomes altered. An estimated 75% of females will have at least one episode of VVC, and about 40% to 45% will have two or more episodes in their lifetimes (CDC, 2021).

Therapeutic Management

Treatment of candidiasis is indicated in patients with symptoms and a positive diagnostic test and includes one of the following medications:

- Miconazole (Monistat) vaginal cream or suppository (available over the counter [OTC])
- Clotrimazole (Gyne-Lotrimin) vaginal tablet or cream (available OTC)
- Tioconazole (Monistat-1 or Vagistat-1) vaginal tablet or cream (available OTC), single dose
- Terconazole vaginal ointment
- Butoconazole (Gynazole-1) vaginal cream, single dose
- Fluconazole (Diflucan) 150 mg oral tablet typically given as a single dose but second dose may be needed (Sobel, 2023)
- Ibrexafungerp (Brexafemme) 150 mg oral tablet, two tablets given twice in 1 day; used in nonpregnant patients who cannot use fluconazole

Most of the above medications are used intravaginally in the form of a cream, tablet, or suppositories for 3 to 7 days. If fluconazole (Diflucan) is prescribed, a 150-mg oral tablet is taken as a single dose.

Topical azole preparations are effective in the treatment of VVC, relieving symptoms and producing negative cultures in 80% to 90% of patients who complete therapy (CDC, 2021). If VVC is not treated effectively during pregnancy, the newborn can develop an oral infection known as thrush during the birth process; that infection must be treated with a local azole preparation after birth.

Nursing Assessment

Assess the patient's health history for predisposing factors for VVC, which include:

- Pregnancy
- Use of oral contraceptives with high estrogen content
- Use of broad-spectrum antibiotics
- Diabetes mellitus
- Obesity
- Use of steroid and immunosuppressive drugs
- HIV infection
- Wearing tight, restrictive clothes and nylon underpants
- Trauma to vaginal mucosa from chemical irritants or douching

Assess the patient for clinical manifestations of VVC. Typical symptoms, which can worsen just before menses, include:

- Pruritus
- Vaginal discharge (thick, white, curdlike)
- Vaginal soreness
- Vulvar burning
- Erythema in the vulvovaginal area
- Dyspareunia
- External dysuria

Figure 5.1 shows the typical appearance of VVC.

Speculum examination will reveal white plaques on the vaginal walls. The vaginal pH remains within normal range. Definitive diagnosis is made by a wet smear, which reveals the filamentous hyphae and spores characteristic of a fungus when viewed under a microscope.

Nursing Management

Teach the following preventive measures to patients with frequent VVC infections:

- Avoid douching to prevent altering the vaginal environment.
- Use condoms to avoid spreading the organism.
- Urinate with knees spread wide apart.
- Avoid tights, nylon underpants, and tight clothes that hold heat and moisture.

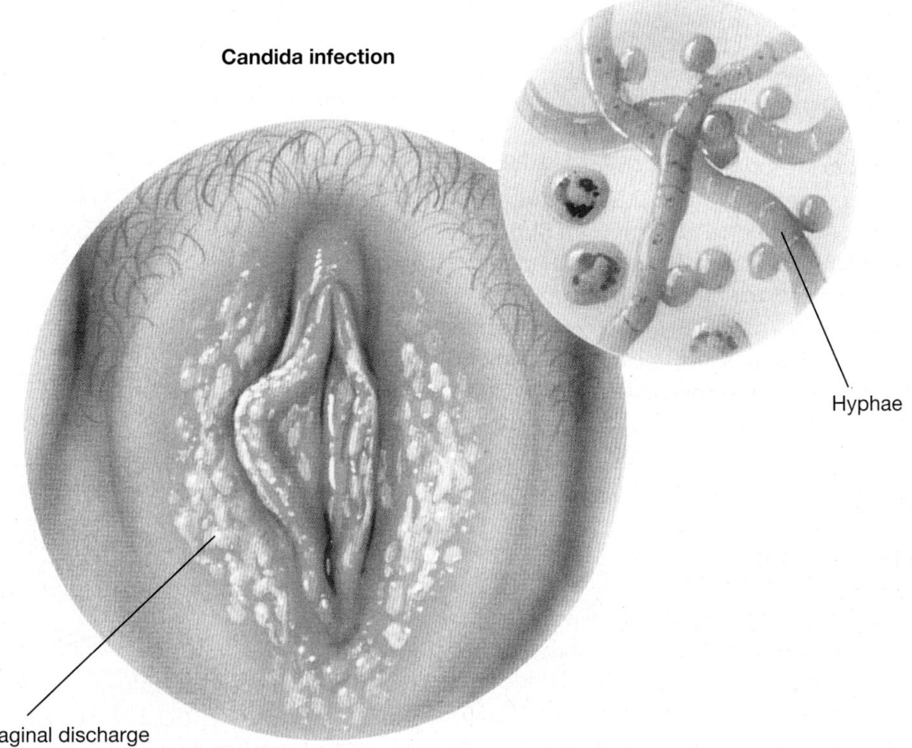

FIGURE 5.1 Vulvovaginal candidiasis. (Reprinted with permission from Stewart, J. G. [2017]. *Anatomical Chart Company atlas of pathophysiology* [4th ed.]. Wolters Kluwer.)

- Wipe from front to back after using the toilet.
- Wash with hypoallergenic or mild, unscented bar soaps; avoid using liquid soaps or body washes.
- Avoid powders, bubble baths, and perfumed vaginal sprays.
- Wear clean cotton underpants.
- Wash and dry the vulvar area gently after baths or showers.
- Limit the number of sexual partners, and use condoms for safer sex.
- Change out of wet bathing suits as soon as possible.
- Become familiar with the signs and symptoms of vaginitis.
- Reduce dietary intake of simple sugars and soda.
- Wash underwear in unscented laundry detergent and hot water.
- Dry underwear in a hot dryer to kill the yeast that clings to the fabric.
- Practice good body hygiene.
- Avoid the use of superabsorbent tampons (use pads instead).

Trichomoniasis

Trichomoniasis is a flagellated protozoan that is a common parasite found in all sexes. *Trichomonas vaginalis* is an ovoid, single-cell protozoan parasite that can be observed under the microscope making a jerky swaying motion. It is mainly sexually transmitted, but it can also live on damp/wet surfaces and poorly cleaned/maintained hot tubs, drains, towels, and bathing suits. Infection is more common in females than in males, and older females are more likely than younger females to become infected (CDC, 2022g). In the United States, an estimated 2 million people have the infection, but only about 30% develop any symptoms (CDC, 2022g). The female patient may be markedly symptomatic or without symptoms. Males are often without symptoms. Although this infection is localized, there is increasing evidence of preterm birth, premature rupture of membranes, low-birth-weight infants, PID, and infertility in people with this type of vaginitis (Sobel & Mitchell, 2023a). The high prevalence of this infection worldwide and frequency of coinfection with other STIs make trichomoniasis a compelling public health concern. Notably, infection with trichomoniasis doubles the risk of HIV susceptibility (Sobel & Mitchell, 2023a). Although an STI, trichomoniasis is not nationally reportable.

Therapeutic Management

A single 2-g dose of oral metronidazole (Flagyl), tinidazole (Tindamax), or secnidazole for both partners is a common treatment for this infection. Multidose therapy, consisting of 500 mg twice a day for 5 to 7 days, is also available and is the preferred treatment in females when using metronidazole (Sobel &Mitchell, 2023b). Sex partners of females with trichomoniasis should be treated to avoid recurrence of infection.

Nursing Assessment

Assess the patient for clinical manifestations of trichomoniasis, which include:

- A heavy yellow/green or grayish frothy or bubbly discharge
- Vaginal pruritus and vulvar soreness
- Lower abdominal pain
- Dyspareunia
- A cervix that may bleed on contact
- Dysuria
- Vaginal odor described as foul
- Vaginal or vulvar erythema
- Petechiae on the cervix (also called "strawberry cervix")

Figure 5.2 shows the typical appearance of trichomoniasis.

The diagnosis is confirmed via nucleic acid amplification tests (NAATs), which are highly accurate with sensitivity and specificity near 100% (Sobel & Mitchell, 2023a). Evaluation of vaginal pH and microscopy, where a motile flagellated trichomonad is visualized under the microscope, are also available options, which are faster and more convenient but also less accurate. A vaginal pH of greater than 4.5 is a typical finding (Sobel &Mitchell, 2023a).

Nursing Management

Patient education plays an important role in management as does partner notification and treatment. Instruct patients to avoid sex until they and their sex partners are cured (i.e., when therapy has been completed and both partners are symptom-free). In addition, it is important to provide information regarding infection cause and transmission, effects on reproductive organs and future fertility, and the need for partner notification and treatment. Follow-up testing is not indicated if symptoms resolve with treatment.

> **TAKE NOTE!**
>
> For patients receiving oral nitroimidazoles, antibiotics such as metronidazole and avoiding alcohol consumption have been recommended in the past by the manufacturer. Current data do not support this; therefore, in practice, patients may not be advised to abstain from alcohol during treatment (Sobel, 2024).

Bacterial Vaginosis

Bacterial vaginosis (BV) is a common condition that results from a shift in the balance of the vaginal microflora. It is the most prevalent cause of vaginal discharge or malodor, but up to 50% to 70% of those infected are without

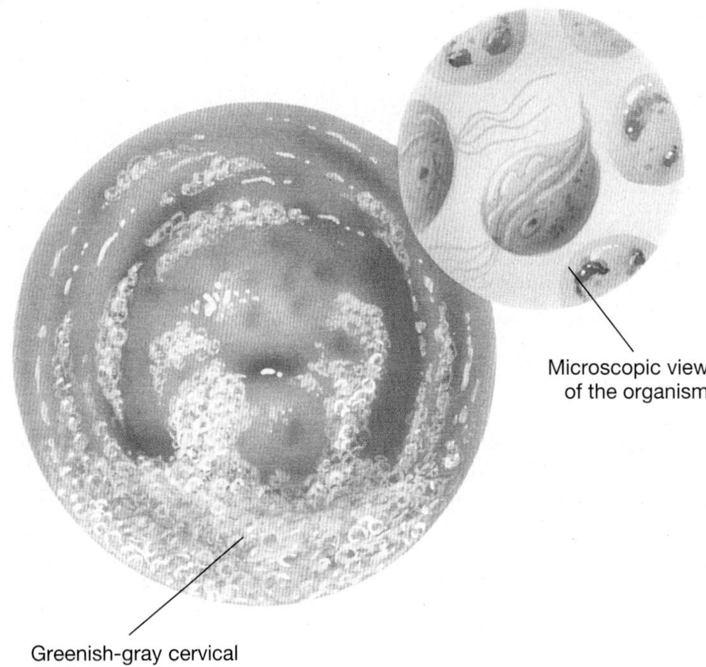

FIGURE 5.2 Trichomoniasis. (Reprinted with permission from Stewart, J. G. [2017]. *Anatomical Chart Company atlas of pathophysiology* [4th ed.]. Wolters Kluwer.)

symptoms (Sobel & Mitchell, 2023c). BV is a sexually transmitted infection characterized by alterations in vaginal flora in which lactobacilli in the vagina are replaced with high concentrations of anaerobic bacteria. BV was named so because bacteria are the etiologic agents and an associated inflammatory response is lacking. The bacterial imbalance is associated with sexual contact but is not usually spread through sex. The cause of the microbial alteration is not fully understood but is associated with having new or multiple sex partners, douching, and not using condoms (CDC, 2022h). Research suggests that BV is associated with preterm labor, high risk of contracting HIV and other STIs, low birth weight, endometritis, and PID (CDC, 2022h).

Therapeutic Management

Treatment is indicated for patients with confirmed BV who are symptomatic or are having a gynecologic procedure involving the vagina (Sobel, 2024). Treatment for BV typically includes oral or vaginal metronidazole (Flagyl) or clindamycin (Cleocin) cream. Treatment of the male sex partner is not indicated; however, it can spread between female sex partners (CDC, 2022h). Therefore, female sex partners need to be counseled on the signs and symptoms of BV and advised to seek treatment if symptoms develop (Sobel, 2024).

Nursing Assessment

Assess the patient for clinical manifestations of BV. Primary symptoms are a thin, white/grayish homogeneous vaginal discharge, pain, itching and burning in the vagina, burning when urinating, itching around the outside of the vagina, and a characteristic "stale fish" odor, often recognized only after sexual intercourse. Figure 5.3 shows the typical appearance of BV.

To diagnose BV, three of the following four criteria must be met:

- Thin, white/grayish vaginal discharge that adheres to the vaginal mucosa
- Vaginal pH higher than 4.5
- Positive "whiff test" (secretion is mixed with a drop of 10% potassium hydroxide on a slide, producing a characteristic stale fishy odor)
- The presence of clue cells on wet-mount examination (Sobel & Mitchell, 2023c)

Nursing Management

The nurse's role is one of primary prevention and education to limit recurrences of these infections. Since BV is similar to several other conditions (chlamydia, gonorrhea, genitourinary syndrome of menopause, trichomoniasis), it is essential that symptomatic people see their health care providers for an accurate diagnosis and treatment. Nurses need to reinforce the importance of following medication instructions and finishing the entire course of antibiotics prescribed. In addition to assessing patients for common signs, symptoms, and risk factors, the nurse can help patients avoid vaginitis or prevent a recurrence by teaching them about behaviors that place them at risk, such as recent antibiotic use, douching,

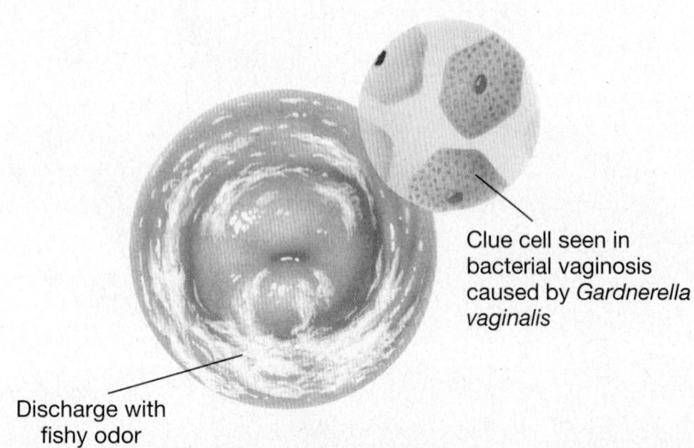

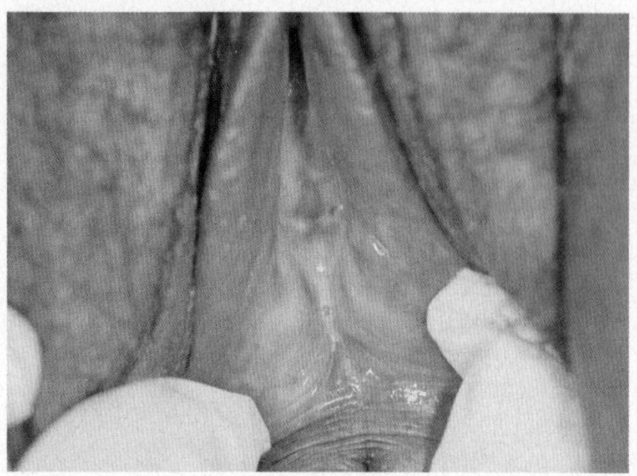

FIGURE 5.3 Bacterial vaginosis. (Left: Reprinted with permission from Stewart, J. G. [2017]. *Anatomical Chart Company atlas of pathophysiology* [4th ed.]. Wolters Kluwer. Right: Photograph reprinted with permission from Sweet, R. L., & Gibbs, R. S. [2005]. *Atlas of infectious diseases of the female genital tract*. Lippincott Williams & Wilkins.)

sexual activity with multiple partners, and not using condoms, and ways to minimize these risks.

INFECTIONS CHARACTERIZED BY CERVICITIS

"Cervicitis" is a catchall term that implies the presence of inflammation or infection of the cervix. It is used to describe everything from symptomless erosions to an inflamed cervix that bleeds on contact and produces quantities of purulent discharge containing organisms not ordinarily found in the vagina. Cervicitis is usually caused by gonorrhea or chlamydia, as well as almost any pathogenic bacterial agent and a number of viruses. The highest incidence is in young females aged 15 to 24 years and in HIV-positive females (Iqbal & Willis, 2023). The treatment of cervicitis involves the appropriate therapy for the specific organism that has caused it. Nurses should institute the ABC (abstinence, being monogamous, condom use) strategy when educating patients about engaging in prevention behaviors (Iqbal & Willis, 2023).

Chlamydia

Chlamydia *trachomatis* is the bacterium that causes chlamydia, which is the most commonly reported bacterial STI in the United States and globally (Hsu, 2023a). It is an intracellular parasite that cannot produce its own energy and depends on the host for survival. It is often difficult to detect, and this can pose problems for female patients due to the long-term consequences of untreated infection.

The highest rates of infection are among those ages 14 to 24 years (Hsu, 2023a). The most common risk factors associated with chlamydia are young age, history of a previous chlamydia infection, new sexual partner or multiple sexual partners in the past 3 months, lack of use of barrier contraception, disadvantaged socioeconomic conditions, and being a Black female (Hsu, 2023a). Infection without symptoms is common among both males and females (Hsu, 2022). Many cases go undiagnosed, unreported, and untreated.

Females with chlamydia who are left undiagnosed and untreated can develop cervicitis; urethritis; PID, which leads to infertility; chronic pelvic pain; and ectopic pregnancies (Hsu, 2022). Moreover, lack of treatment provides more opportunity for the infection to be transmitted to sexual partners. When untreated in pregnancy, chlamydia is associated with premature rupture of membranes, preterm labor, and low-birth-weight newborns (Hsu, 2022). Newborns born to infected birthing parents may develop ophthalmia neonatorum, which is an acute mucopurulent conjunctivitis occurring in the first month of birth. It is essentially an infection acquired during vaginal delivery. The most frequent infectious agents involved are *C. trachomatis* and *Neisseria gonorrhoeae* (Ochoa & Mendez, 2023). The CDC recommends yearly testing for chlamydia of all sexually active or pregnant females ages 25 and younger, as well as older or pregnant females with risk factors for chlamydial infections (CDC, 2022i).

Therapeutic Management

The diagnosis is generally based on NAATs on the cervical or vaginal swabs and urine samples. Antibiotics are usually used to treat the patient and their sexual partners and prevent reinfection. The CDC treatment options for chlamydia include doxycycline (preferred treatment) 100 mg orally twice a day for 7 days or azithromycin (Zithromax) 1 g orally in a single dose if doxycycline is contraindicated (Hsu, 2023b). Pregnant patients who are diagnosed with chlamydia should be treated with azithromycin as doxycycline is avoided during pregnancy (Hsu, 2023b). Retesting in 3 months to identify reinfection is suggested (CDC, 2022a). All patients positive for chlamydia should be tested and treated for other STIs.

Nursing Assessment

Assess the health history for significant risk factors for chlamydia, which may include:

- Being younger than 24 years of age
- Having multiple sex partners
- Having a new sex partner
- Engaging in unprotected vaginal, anal, or oral sex
- Using oral contraceptives
- Being HIV-positive
- Being pregnant
- Having a history of another STI (Hsu, 2023a)

Assess the patient for clinical manifestations of chlamydia. Recognize that the majority of females are without symptoms (Hsu, 2022). If the patient is symptomatic, clinical manifestations include:

- Mucopurulent vaginal discharge
- Urethritis
- Bartholinitis
- Endometritis
- Salpingitis
- Dysfunctional uterine bleeding

Gonorrhea

Gonorrhea is a serious and potentially severe bacterial infection that can occur in the genitals, rectum, or throat. It is the second most commonly reported infection in the United States (Bash & Connelly, 2023). The cause of gonorrhea is an aerobic Gram-negative intracellular diplococcus, *N. gonorrhoeae*. The site of infection is the columnar epithelium of the endocervix. Gonorrhea is almost exclusively transmitted by sexual activity. In pregnant patients, gonorrhea is associated with chorioamnionitis, premature labor, spontaneous abortion, premature rupture of membranes, and low-birth-weight or small-for-gestational-age infants (Ghanem, 2023). It can also be transmitted to the newborn in the form of ophthalmia neonatorum during vaginal births by direct contact with gonococcal organisms in the cervix. Ophthalmia neonatorum is highly contagious and, if untreated, leads to blindness in the newborn (Ochoa & Mendez, 2023). Gonorrhea increases the risk of PID, infertility, ectopic pregnancy, chronic pelvic pain, along with other STIs and HIV acquisition and transmission (Ghanem, 2023). It can be difficult to cure due to antibiotic resistance (Ghanem, 2023). Infection without symptoms is common among females, which is a major factor in the spread of gonorrhea (Ghanem, 2023).

The CDC recommends yearly testing for gonorrhea of all sexually active or pregnant females ages 25 and younger, as well as older or pregnant females with risk factors for gonococcal infections (CDC, 2022i). Pregnant patients should be screened during the first trimester and again in the third trimester if they are at high risk for STIs. Nucleic acid hybridization tests (GenProbe) are used for diagnosis (Seña & Cohen, 2023).

Therapeutic Management

Gonorrhea can currently be cured with the right treatment. The treatment of choice for uncomplicated gonococcal infections is a single intramuscular high dose of ceftriaxone (Rocephin) 500 mg for pregnant and nonpregnant females weighing less than 150 kg (CDC, 2022a). If chlamydia has not been ruled out, proper treatment for chlamydia should be started (Seña & Cohen, 2023). Retesting in 3 months to identify reinfection is suggested (CDC, 2022a). To prevent gonococcal ophthalmia neonatorum, which can result in corneal ulceration and in turn permanent blindness, a prophylactic agent (erythromycin ointment or azithromycin solution) should be instilled into the eyes of all newborns (Ochoa & Mendez, 2023).

Nursing Assessment

Assess the patient's health history for risk factors, which may include low education level, low socioeconomic status, single status, inconsistent use of barrier contraceptives, age under 25 years, being of an underrepresented ethnic population, substance misuse, history of previous gonorrhea, having a new sex partner, and having multiple sex partners (Bash & Connelly, 2023). Assessment involves taking a health history that includes a comprehensive sexual history. Ask about the number of sex partners and the use of safer sex techniques. Review previous and current symptoms. Assess the patient for clinical manifestations of gonorrhea, keeping in mind that 70% of females infected with gonorrhea are totally symptom-free (Ghanem, 2023). If symptoms are present, they might include:

- Mucopurulent vaginal discharge
- Dysuria
- Dyspareunia
- Abnormal vaginal bleeding
- Bartholin abscess
- Abdominal or pelvic pain

Sometimes a local gonorrheal infection is self-limiting (there is no further spread), but usually the organism ascends upward through the endocervical canal to the endometrium of the uterus, further on to the fallopian tubes, and out into the peritoneal cavity. When the peritoneum and the ovaries become involved, the condition is known as PID (discussed later in this chapter).

If gonorrhea remains untreated, it can enter the bloodstream and produce a disseminated gonococcal infection. This severe form of infection can invade the joints (arthritis), the heart (endocarditis), the brain (meningitis), and the liver (toxic hepatitis). Figure 5.4 shows the typical appearance of gonorrhea.

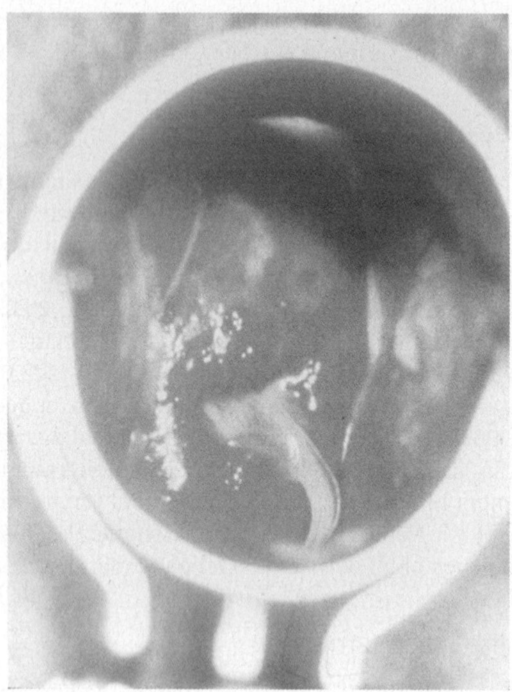

FIGURE 5.4 Gonorrhea. (Reprinted with permission from Gorbach, S. L., Bartlett, J. G., & Blacklow, N. R. [Eds.]. [2004]. *Infectious diseases* [3rd ed.]. Lippincott Williams & Wilkins.)

Nursing Management of Chlamydia and Gonorrhea

Sexual health is an important part of a person's physical and mental health, and nurses have a professional obligation to address it. Be particularly sensitive when addressing STIs because patients are often embarrassed, guilty or angry, or even fearful of outcomes related to telling partners about the diagnosis. There is still a social stigma attached to STIs, so patients need to be reassured about confidentiality.

The nurse's knowledge about chlamydia and gonorrhea should include treatment strategies, referral sources, and preventive measures. The nurse should be skilled at patient education and counseling and be comfortable talking with and advising patients diagnosed with these infections. Of utmost importance is the willingness to listen and show interest and respect in a nonjudgmental manner. Provide education about risk factors for these infections. Emphasize the importance of seeking treatment, adhering to prescribed treatment regimens, and informing sex partners. Discuss the importance of completing medication course and receiving any recommended follow-up testing.

In addition to meeting the health needs of patients with chlamydia and gonorrhea, the nurse is responsible for educating the public about these infections. This information should include high-risk behaviors associated with these infections, signs and symptoms, and the treatment modalities available. Stress that both of these STIs can lead to infertility and long-term sequelae. Although many prevention programs are available, improvements can be made in raising awareness about chlamydia and gonorrhea, increasing screening coverage, and enhancing partner services. In addition, nurses can focus their efforts on reaching disproportionately affected groups. See Healthy People 2030 box.

INFECTIONS CHARACTERIZED BY GENITAL LESIONS

In the United States, the majority of young, sexually active patients who have genital ulcers have genital herpes, syphilis, or chancroid. The frequency of each condition differs by geographic area and patient population; however, herpes simplex virus (HSV) is the most prevalent cause, followed by syphilis (Tuddenham & Ghanem, 2023). More than one of these diseases can be present in a patient who has genital ulcers. All three of these diseases have been associated with an increased risk of HIV infection (Tuddenham & Ghanem, 2023). Not all genital ulcers are caused by STIs.

HEALTHY PEOPLE 2030

STI Objectives	Nursing Significance
Increase the proportion of sexually active adolescent and young females who get screened for chlamydia.	Provide confidential care to all young females. Assess for sexual behaviors and STI risks during clinic visits; take every opportunity to educate on risks of STIs and risk reduction. Encourage all sexually active females under 25 years of age to be tested for chlamydia.
Reduce pelvic inflammatory disease in adolescent and young females.	Provide an open, nonjudgmental environment so patients will report symptoms and seek treatment earlier. Encourage patients to minimize their lifetime number of sexual partners. Educate about the importance of correct and consistent condom use with every sexual act.

STI, sexually transmitted infection.
Healthy People Objectives retrieved from http://www.healthypeople.gov

Genital Herpes

Genital herpes is a recurrent, lifelong viral infection that has the potential for transmission throughout the lifespan. It is characterized by painful, recurrent outbreaks of genital and anal lesions. Once a person is infected with herpes, they remain infected for life. Genital HSV infections are common, with over 572,000 new cases estimated annually (CDC, 2022j). Infection during pregnancy is common, and the most devastating consequence of maternal genital herpes is neonatal herpes disease, which ranges from 3 to 30 per 100,000 births in the United States and has a high mortality rate (Riley & Wald, 2022). The risk of neonatal infection is highest with a primary genital HSV infection acquired near the time of delivery and significantly reduced in patients with a recurrent HSV infection (Riley & Wald, 2022).

Genital herpes infects females twice as much as males in part due to prolonged contact with semen during vaginal intercourse (WHO, 2023a). Two serotypes of HSV have been identified: HSV-1 and HSV-2. HSV-1 is associated mainly with oral herpes (commonly called cold sores and fever blisters), and HSV-2 is mainly associated with genital herpes; both types can cause outbreaks in either location. Most HSV-1 infections are acquired during childhood.

HSV is transmitted by contact of mucous membranes or breaks in the skin with visible or nonvisible lesions. Most genital herpes infections are transmitted by people unaware that they have an infection. Many have mild or unrecognized infections but still shed the herpes virus intermittently. HSV is transmitted primarily by direct contact with an infected person who is shedding the virus. Kissing, sexual contact (including oral sex), and vaginal delivery are means of transmission.

Having sex with an infected partner places a person at risk for contracting HSV. After the primary outbreak, the virus remains dormant in the nerve cells for a lifetime, resulting in periodic recurrent outbreaks. Immunocompromised females have more frequent and more severe recurrent outbreaks than other hosts. A genital herpes infection during pregnancy may lead to a spontaneous abortion or preterm labor (CDC, 2022j). Transmission to the neonate usually occurs during delivery due to direct contact with the virus shed from an infected site (Riley & Ward, 2022).

Living with genital herpes can be difficult due to the erratic, recurrent nature of the infection, the location of the lesions, the unknown causes of the recurrences, and the lack of a cure. Upon diagnosis, patients have important concerns related not to the physical nature of the disease but to the social consequences, including transmission and the impact on their sex lives. Furthermore, the stigma associated with this infection may affect the person's feelings about themselves and their interactions with partners. Potential psychosocial consequences may include emotional distress, isolation, fear of rejection by a partner, depression, fear of transmission of the disease, and altered perceptions of self-esteem (Devine et al., 2022).

Therapeutic Management

No cure exists, but antiviral drug therapy helps reduce or suppress symptoms, shedding, and recurrent episodes. Advances in treatment with acyclovir (Zovirax) 400 mg orally three times daily for 7 to 10 days, famciclovir (Famvir) 250 mg orally three times daily for 7 to 10 days, or valacyclovir (Valtrex) 1 g orally twice daily for 7 to 10 days have resulted in an improved quality of life for those infected with HSV (Albrecht, 2024). Oral antiviral therapy may be used in patients with recurrent infections to reduce recurrences, improve symptoms, and decrease the risk of transmission (Albrecht, 2024). The natural course of the disease is for recurrences to be less frequent over time.

Nursing Assessment

Assess the patient for clinical manifestations of HSV. Clinical manifestations can be divided into the primary episode and recurrent infections. The first or primary episode is usually the most severe with a prolonged period of viral shedding. Primary HSV is a systemic disease characterized by multiple painful vesicular lesions, mucopurulent discharge, superinfection with candida, fever, chills, malaise, dysuria, headache, genital irritation, inguinal tenderness, and lymphadenopathy. The lesions in the primary herpes episode are frequently located on the vulva, vagina, and perineal areas. The vesicles will open and weep and finally crust over, dry, and disappear without scar formation (Fig. 5.5). This viral shedding process usually takes up to 2 weeks to complete.

Recurrent infection episodes may occur five to eight times per year and are usually much milder with fewer lesions and shorter in duration than the primary one. Tingling, itching, pain, unilateral genital lesions, and a more rapid resolution of lesions are characteristics of recurrent infections. Recurrent herpes is a localized disease characterized by typical HSV lesions at the site of initial viral entry. Recurrent herpes lesions are fewer in number, less painful, and resolve more rapidly (Albrecht, 2022).

Diagnosis of HSV is often based on clinical signs and symptoms, and the preferred diagnostic tests include viral culture or polymerase chain reaction (PCR) (Albrecht, 2022). All patients should be tested for all common STIs, especially if they have new sexual partners.

Syphilis

Syphilis is a systemic, curable bacterial infection caused by the spirochete *Treponema pallidum*. It is often thought to be a disease of the past, largely eradicated in modern

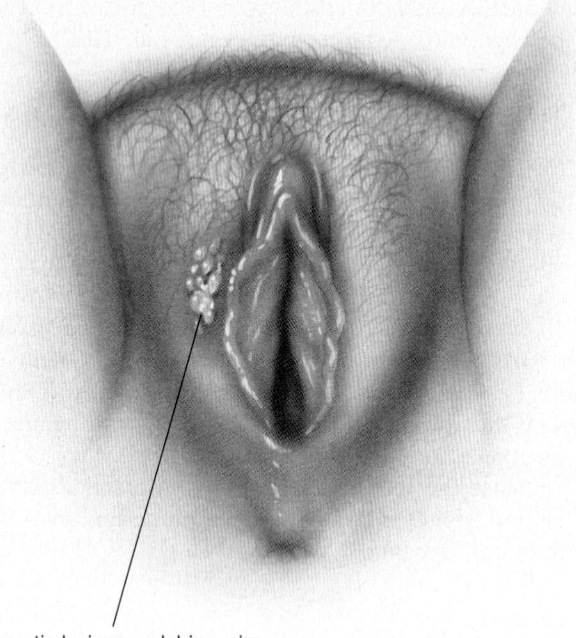

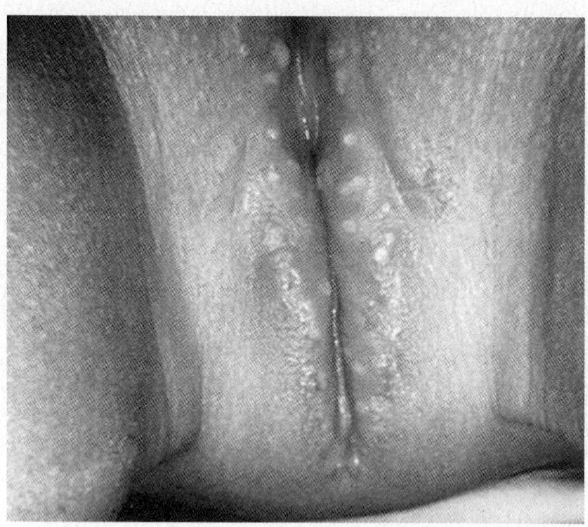

FIGURE 5.5 Genital herpes simplex. (Illustration provided by Anatomical Chart Co. Photograph courtesy of Stephen Ludwig, MD.)

America, but its incidence has been increasing since the year 2000 (Hicks & Clement, 2023a). It is a serious systemic disease that can lead to disability and death if untreated. Syphilis has a complex life cycle during which episodes of active clinical disease are punctuated with periods of latency. The syphilis spirochete rapidly penetrates intact mucous membranes or microscopic lesions in the skin and within hours enters the lymphatic system and bloodstream to produce a systemic infection long before the appearance of a primary lesion. The site of entry may be vaginal, rectal, or oral (Hicks & Clement, 2023a). The syphilis spirochete can cross the placenta. Congenital syphilis can occur when an infected birthing parent directly infects the fetus through transplacental transmission or during delivery due to direct contact with a lesion (Norwitz & Hicks, 2024). Maternal infection consequences for the newborn include spontaneous abortion, low birth weight, prematurity, stillbirth, and multisystem problems of the bones, liver, pancreas, intestine, kidney, and spleen (Arrieta, 2023). All pregnant patients should be screened for syphilis infection at the first prenatal visit, with repeat testing at 28 weeks and before delivery for high-risk patients (CDC, 2022i). Screen patients without symptoms who are considered high risk (CDC, 2022i).

Therapeutic Management

Fortunately, an effective treatment is available for syphilis. An injection of penicillin G can cure primary, secondary, or early latent syphilis. Preparation, dosage, and treatment length depend on the disease stage (CDC, 2024b). For late latent syphilis, three doses of penicillin at weekly intervals are needed. Pregnant people should be treated with the same regimen for whichever stage they present with. Other medications, such as doxycycline, are available if the patient is allergic to penicillin.

Patients should be reevaluated at 6 and 12 months after treatment for primary or secondary syphilis with additional serologic testing. Patients with latent syphilis should be followed up with clinically and serologically at 6, 12, and 24 months (Hicks & Clement, 2023c).

 *Concept Mastery Alert*

Syphilis Transmission in Pregnancy

Syphilis easily crosses the placenta of a pregnant person and is devastating to the developing fetus. Syphilis can affect the fetus's bone, brain, heart, lungs, and abdominal organs.

Nursing Assessment

Syphilis has many nonspecific signs and symptoms that may be overlooked by the health care provider or may simply be indistinguishable from other more common diseases. Regrettably, undiagnosed and untreated syphilis may lead to life-threatening complications such as hepatitis, cardiovascular issues, and central nervous system damage (Hicks & Clement, 2023a). Assess the patient for any clinical manifestations of syphilis. If untreated, syphilis is a lifelong infection progressing in orderly staging. The five stages of syphilis infection are (1) primary, (2) secondary, (3) early latent, (4) late latent, and (5) tertiary. The primary, secondary, and early latent stages are considered the most infectious.

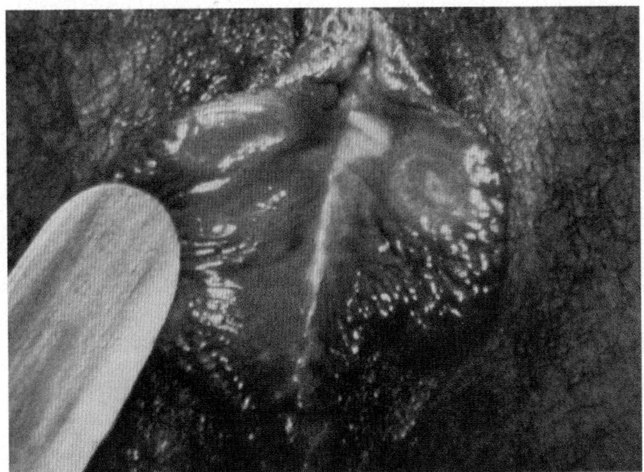

FIGURE 5.6 Chancre of primary syphilis. (Reprinted with permission from Sweet, R. L., & Gibbs, R. S. [2005]. *Atlas of infectious diseases of the female genital tract*. Lippincott Williams & Wilkins.)

HEALTHY PEOPLE 2030

STI Objectives	Nursing Significance
STI-03 Reduce the syphilis rate in females.	Provide confidential care to all young females. Assess for sexual behaviors and STI risks during clinic visits; take every opportunity to educate on risks of STIs and risk reduction. Encourage people to minimize their lifetime number of sexual partners. Educate about the importance of correct and consistent condom use.

STI, sexually transmitted infection.
Healthy People Objectives retrieved from http://www.healthypeople.gov

Primary syphilis presents as a chancre (painless ulcer) at the site of bacterial entry that will disappear within 3 to 6 weeks without intervention (Fig. 5.6). Motile spirochetes are present on dark-field examination of the ulcer exudate. In addition, painless bilateral adenopathy is present during this highly infectious period. The patient is highly infectious whenever chancres are present. If left untreated, the infection progresses to the secondary stage.

Secondary syphilis appears 2 to 6 months after the initial exposure and is manifested by flulike symptoms and a maculopapular rash of the trunk, palms, and soles. Alopecia and adenopathy are both common during this stage. In addition to rashes, secondary syphilis may present with symptoms of fever, sore throat, weight loss, myalgias, and fatigue (Hicks & Clement, 2023a). The secondary stage of syphilis lasts about 2 years. Once the secondary stage subsides, the latency periods (early and late) begin. These stages are characterized by the absence of any clinical manifestations of disease, though the serology is positive. This stage can last as long as 20 years. If not treated, *tertiary* or *late syphilis* occurs, with life-threatening cardiovascular syphilis, gumma syphilis, and central nervous system syphilis that slowly destroys the heart, along with inflammation of the aorta, eyes, brain, central nervous system, and skin (Hicks & Clements, 2023a).

Serologic testing for syphilis is evaluated by using both nontreponemal and treponemal tests. Nontreponemal tests measure immunoglobulin M (IgM) and immunoglobulin G (IgG). Although these tests are less specific, they are commonly used for primary screening because they are rapid to perform and inexpensive. The most commonly used nontreponemal tests are the rapid plasma regain (RPR) and the Venereal Disease Research Laboratory (VDRL) tests. Treponemal tests detect treponema-specific immunoglobulin A (IgA), IgM, and IgG antibodies, giving these tests greater accuracy. The preferred treponemal test is the *T. pallidum* enzyme immunoassay (TP-EIA) (Hicks & Clement, 2023b).

A presumptive diagnosis can be made by using two serologic tests:

- Nontreponemal tests (VDRL and RPR)
- Treponemal tests (fluorescent treponemal antibody absorption [FTA-ABS] and *T. pallidum* particle agglutination [TP-PA])

Dark-field microscopic examinations and direct fluorescent antibody tests of lesion exudate or tissue are the definitive methods for diagnosing early syphilis (CDC, 2024b).

Nursing Management of Herpes and Syphilis

Genital ulcers from either herpes or syphilis can be devastating, and the nurse can be instrumental in helping patients through this difficult time. Therapeutic management also includes counseling regarding the natural history of the disease, the risk of sexual and perinatal transmission, current treatment regimens, and the use of methods to prevent further spread. Referral to a support group may be helpful. Address the psychosocial aspects of these STIs with patients by discussing appropriate coping skills, acceptance of the lifelong nature of the condition (herpes), and options for treatment and rehabilitation. Teaching Guidelines 5.2 highlights appropriate teaching points for the patient with genital ulcers. Encourage all patients to inform their current sex partners that they have an STI and to inform future partners before initiating a sexual relationship. Finally, many experts recommend a sympathetic, nonjudgmental approach. See Healthy People 2030 box.

TEACHING GUIDELINES **5.2** Caring for Genital Ulcers

- Abstain from intercourse during the prodromal period and when lesions are present.
- Wash hands with soap and water after touching lesions to avoid autoinoculation.
- Use comfort measures such as wearing non-constricting clothes, wearing cotton underwear, urinating in water if urination is painful, taking lukewarm sitz baths, and air-drying lesions with a hair dryer on low heat.
- Apply cool compresses to the area.
- Avoid extremes of temperature such as ice packs or hot pads to the genital area as well as application of steroid creams, sprays, or gels.
- Use condoms with all new or noninfected partners.
- Inform health care professionals of your condition.

PELVIC INFLAMMATORY DISEASE

Pelvic inflammatory disease (PID) is a spectrum of inflammatory disorders usually caused by an ascending polymicrobial infection of the genital tract from chlamydia or gonorrhea (Fig. 5.7). It refers to an inflammatory state of the upper female genital tract and nearby structures. It encompasses a broad category of diseases, including endometritis, salpingitis, salpingo-oophoritis, tubo-ovarian abscess, and pelvic peritonitis. In the United States, about 4% of females 18 to 44 years of age report having PID (Ross, 2023a). Long-term complications of PID are ectopic pregnancies, infertility, and chronic pelvic pain (Jennings & Krywko, 2023). All sexually active females are at risk for PID, but common risk factors include age younger than 25 years, multiple sexual partners, insertion of an intrauterine device (IUD) within the past 3 weeks, history of STIs in the patient or their partner, lack of barrier contraceptive use, and a previous episode of PID (Ross, 2023a). Because of the seriousness of the complications of PID, an accurate diagnosis is critical.

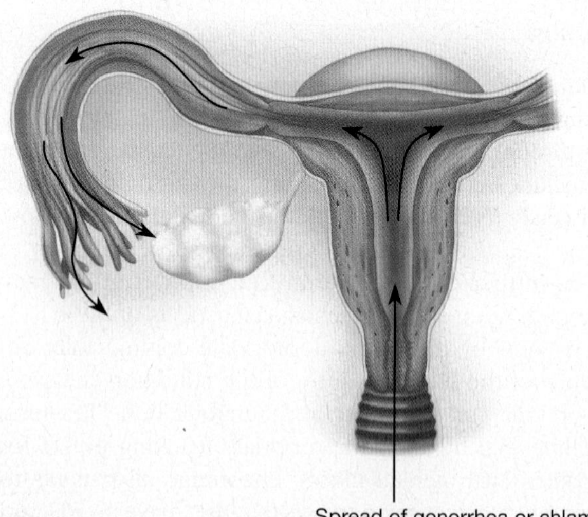

FIGURE 5.7 Pelvic inflammatory disease. Chlamydia or gonorrhea spreads up the vagina into the uterus and then to the fallopian tubes and ovaries.

Therapeutic Management

Broad-spectrum antibiotic therapy is generally required to cover chlamydia, gonorrhea, or any anaerobic infection. The current CDC recommendation is ceftriaxone 1 g intravenously once daily, plus doxycycline 100 mg orally every 12 hours, plus metronidazole 500 mg orally or intravenously every 12 hours; cefoxitin 2 g intravenously every 6 hours plus doxycycline 100 mg orally or intravenously every 12 hours; or cefotetan 2 g intravenously every 12 hours plus doxycycline 100 mg orally or intravenously every 12 hours (Wiesenfeld, 2024). Treatment will be outpatient or hospital based.

The decision to hospitalize a patient is based on clinical judgment and the severity of the symptoms (e.g., severely ill with high fever, a tubo-ovarian abscess is suspected, the patient is immunocompromised or presents with protracted vomiting). Treatment then includes intravenous antibiotics, increased oral fluids to improve hydration, bed rest, and pain management. Follow-up is needed to validate that the infectious process has disappeared to prevent the development of chronic pelvic pain.

Nursing Assessment

Nursing assessment of the patient with PID involves a complete health history and assessment of clinical manifestations, physical examination, and laboratory and diagnostic testing. The diagnosis of PID provides an opportunity to educate adolescent and young females about prevention of STIs, including abstinence, consistent use of barrier methods of protection, immunizations, and the importance of receiving periodic screening for STIs and HIV.

Health History

Explore the patient's current and past medical and sexual health history for risk factors for PID, which may include:

- Adolescence or young adulthood
- Having multiple sex partners
- History of PID or STI
- Having intercourse with a partner who has untreated urethritis
- Recent insertion of an IUD
- Lack of consistent condom use
- Lack of contraceptive use (Ross, 2023b)

Physical Examination and Laboratory and Diagnostic Tests

Assess the patient for clinical manifestations of PID, keeping in mind that, because of the wide variety of clinical manifestations of PID, clinical diagnosis can be challenging. Inspect the patient for presence of fever or vaginal discharge. Palpate the abdomen, noting tenderness over the uterus or ovaries. No single test is highly specific or sensitive for the disease. To reduce the risk of missed diagnosis, the CDC has established criteria for the diagnosis of PID. A presumptive clinical diagnosis is made in sexually active females with lower abdominal tenderness, adnexal tenderness, and cervical motion tenderness determined from a pelvic exam. Additional supportive criteria that support a diagnosis of PID are:

- Abnormal cervical or vaginal mucopurulent discharge
- Oral temperature higher than 101°F (38.3°C)
- *N. gonorrhoeae* or *C. trachomatis* infection documented (causative bacterial organism)
- Abundant white blood cells on saline vaginal smear
- Elevated erythrocyte sedimentation rate (inflammatory process)
- Elevated C-reactive protein level (inflammatory process) (CDC, 2022k)

Nursing Management

If the patient with PID is hospitalized, maintain hydration via intravenous fluids if necessary and administer analgesics as needed for pain. Semi-Fowler positioning facilitates pelvic drainage. A key element to treatment of PID is education to prevent recurrence. Depending on the clinical setting (hospital or community clinic) where the nurse encounters the patient diagnosed with PID, a risk assessment should be done to ascertain what interventions are appropriate to prevent recurrence. To gain the patient's cooperation, explain the various diagnostic tests needed. Discuss the implications of PID and the risk factors for the infection; their sexual partner should be included if possible. Sexual counseling should include practicing safer sex, limiting the number of sexual partners, using barrier contraceptives consistently, considering another contraceptive method if using an IUD with multiple sexual partners, and completing the course of antibiotics as prescribed. Explain the serious sequelae that may occur if the condition is not treated or if the patient does not adhere to the treatment plan. Ask the patient to have their partner go for evaluation and treatment to prevent a repeat infection. Provide nonjudgmental support while stressing the importance of barrier contraceptive methods and follow-up care. Teaching Guidelines 5.3 provides further information related to PID prevention.

TEACHING GUIDELINES 5.3 Preventing Pelvic Inflammatory Disease

- Advise sexually active patients to insist their partners use condoms.
- Discourage routine vaginal douching, as this may lead to bacterial overgrowth.
- Encourage regular sexually transmitted infection (STI) screenings.
- Emphasize the importance of having each sexual partner receive antibiotic treatment if diagnosed with an STI.

Human Papillomavirus

Human papillomavirus (HPV) is the most common STI in the United States and is responsible for anogenital warts and several cancers including cervical, vaginal, vulvar, oropharyngeal, and anal cancers (CDC, 2022l). HPV is so common that nearly 80% of all sexually active people will get at least one type of HPV at some point in their lives (Office on Women's Health, 2022). Genital warts or condylomata (Greek for "warts") are caused by HPV. Conservative estimates suggest that in the United States, approximately 20 million people have productive HPV infection, and 5.5 million Americans acquire it annually (Palefsky, 2022). Strong evidence has established that HPV is linked to cervical cancer, which is the fourth most common female cancer in the world (Palefsky, 2022; WHO, 2024). Every year in the United States, almost 14,000 people are diagnosed with cervical cancer and over 4,000 die from this disease (American Cancer Society [ACS], 2024). More than 200 types of HPV can infect the genital tract, of which at least 14 are cancer causing.

Therapeutic Management

There is currently no medical treatment or cure for HPV. Instead, therapeutic management focuses heavily on prevention through the use of the HPV vaccine, education, and treatment of lesions and warts caused by HPV.

In the United States, 9-valent vaccine is used. The CDC's Advisory Committee on Immunization Practices (ACIP) has recommended the vaccine for routine administration to 11- and 12-year-old children. The ACIP also endorses the use of an HPV vaccine for children as young as age 9 and recommends that females between 11 and 26 years of age receive the vaccination series. Children who start the vaccine series before their 15th birthday need only two doses to be fully protected. After the age of 15, three doses are needed to be fully protected. Researchers are now investigating whether a single dose might be effective (Palefsky, 2022;

National Cancer Institute [NCI], 2023). All HPV vaccines are prophylactic and designed primarily for cervical cancer prevention. The vaccine can protect against about 90% of cervical, vulvar, vaginal, penile, and anal cancers (Liao et al., 2022). Prophylactic HPV vaccines are relatively safe, well tolerated, and highly efficacious in preventing persistent infections and cervical diseases associated with HPV vaccine types among young females. See Evidence-Based Practice 5.1 regarding the HPV vaccine's effectiveness in preventing cervical cancer.

If the female patient does not receive primary prevention with the vaccine, then secondary prevention would focus on education about the importance of receiving regular Pap smears and, for female patients over 30 years of age, including an HPV test to determine whether they have a latent high-risk virus that could lead to precancerous cervical changes. Genital warts are typically diagnosed visually. Finally, treatment options for precancerous cervical lesions or genital warts caused by HPV are numerous and may include:

- Topical trichloroacetic acid (TCA) 80% to 90%
- Liquid nitrogen cryotherapy ablation
- Topical imiquimod 5% cream (Aldara)
- Topical podophyllin 0.15% to 0.5%
- Topical sinecatechins 15% ointment
- Topical isotretinoin
- Laser carbon dioxide vaporization
- Electrocauterization
- Patient-applied podofilox 0.5% solution or gel
- Simple surgical excision (Leslie et al., 2023)

The goal of treating genital warts is to remove the warts and induce wart-free periods for the patient. Treatment of genital warts should be guided by the preference of the patient and available resources. No single treatment has been found to be ideal for all patients, and most treatment modalities appear to have comparable efficacy. Because genital warts can proliferate and become friable during pregnancy, they should be removed using a local agent. A cesarean birth is not indicated solely to prevent transmission of HPV infection to the newborn unless the pelvic outlet is obstructed by warts (Zhu et al., 2022).

Nursing Assessment

Nursing assessment of the patient with HPV involves a complete health history and assessment of clinical manifestations, physical examination, and laboratory and diagnostic testing. A patient with HPV lesions may have symptoms such as profuse, irritating vaginal discharge, itching, dyspareunia, or bleeding after intercourse. They may also report "bumps" on their labia. Physical inspection of the external genitalia is important whenever HPV lesions are suspected or seen.

HEALTH HISTORY, PHYSICAL EXAMINATION, AND LABORATORY AND DIAGNOSTIC TESTS

Assess the patient's health history for risk factors for HPV, which include sexually active, multiple sex partners, new sex partner, and age 15 to 25 years (Palefsky, 2022).

Assess the patient for clinical manifestations of HPV. Most HPV infections are without symptoms, unrecognized, or subclinical. Visible genital warts are usually caused by HPV types 6 or 11. In addition to the external genitalia, genital warts can occur on the cervix and in the vagina, urethra, anus, and mouth. Depending on the size

EVIDENCE-BASED PRACTICE 5.1

Targeted Interventions to Encourage the Uptake of Cervical Screening

BACKGROUND

Human papillomaviruses (HPVs) are sexually transmitted infections (STIs), and they are common in young people. Usually, they are cleared by the immune system, but when high-risk types HPV 16 and 18 (which cause most cervical cancers worldwide) persist, cervical cancer can develop. Preventive vaccination triggers the production of antibodies, which protects against future HPV infections. Cervical screening detects the presence of HPV or abnormal cells.

STUDY

Comprehensive literature searches identified 2,597 studies; of these, 70 studies with a total of 257,899 female subjects met the inclusion criteria. The purpose of the review was to assess the effectiveness of invitational and educational interventions, lay worker involvement, or counseling and risk factor assessment to increase cervical cancer screenings.

Findings

There was moderate-certainty evidence to support the use of invitation letters to increase the number of people having cervical cancer screenings. The promotion of cervical screening by lay health workers to populations of ethnic minorities may increase the number of cervical screenings, but not conclusively. Education by a health promotion nurse to encourage cervical screenings may increase uptake of screenings.

Nursing Implications

Based on the findings from this study, nurses should utilize invitation letters, lay health workers, and education to encourage and increase cervical screenings. Primary prevention strategies for cervical cancer need to focus on reducing HPV infections by getting the HPV vaccine and increased cervical screenings.

Staley, H., Shiraz, A., Shreeve, N., Bryant, A., Martin-Hirsh, P. P. L., & Gajjar, K. (2021). Interventions targeted at women to encourage the uptake of cervical screening. *Cochrane Database of Systematic Reviews, 9*(9), CD002834. https://doi.org/10.1002/14651858.CD002834.pub3

and location, genital warts can be painful, friable (easily pulverized or crumbled), and pruritic (itching), although most are typically without symptoms (Fig. 5.8).

Clinically, visible warts are diagnosed by inspection. The warts are fleshy papules with a warty, granular surface. Lesions can grow large during pregnancy, affecting urination, defecation, mobility, and descent of the fetus (Ardekani et al., 2022). Large lesions, which may resemble cauliflowers, exist in coalesced clusters and bleed easily.

Pap smears are now performed every 3 to 5 years for low-risk females starting at the age of 21. This current standard of care, calling for less frequent cervical cancer screening than in the past, makes it critical for patients to understand when they are to have them and follow through to get them. These regular Pap smears will detect the cellular changes associated with HPV. The Food and Drug Administration (FDA) has approved an HPV test as a follow-up for patients who have an ambiguous Pap test. In addition, this HPV test may be a helpful addition to the Pap test for general screening of people aged 30 and over. The HPV test is a diagnostic test that can determine the specific HPV strain, which is useful in discriminating between low-risk and high-risk HPV types. A specimen for testing can be obtained with a fluid-phase collection system such as Thin Prep. The HPV test can identify 13 of the high-risk types of HPV associated with the development of cervical cancer and can detect high-risk types of HPV even before there are any conclusive visible changes to the cervical cells. If the test is positive for the high-risk types of HPV, the patient should be referred for colposcopy, which is a visual examination of the cervix using magnification and simple staining solutions such as acetic acid and Lugol's solution. It is sometimes accompanied by a biopsy to confirm a cervical abnormality (Cooper & Dunton, 2023).

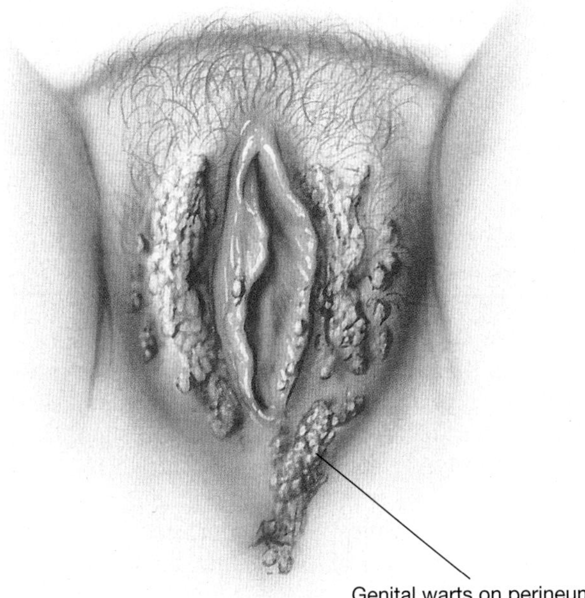

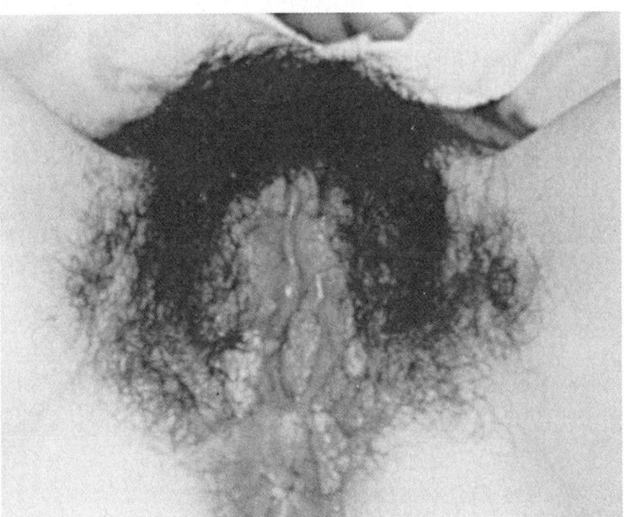

FIGURE 5.8 Genital warts. (Reprinted with permission from Gorbach, S. L., Bartlett, J. G., & Blacklow, N. R. [Eds.]. [2004]. *Infectious diseases* [3rd ed.]. Lippincott Williams & Wilkins.)

Upon physical examination, it is determined that Sandy has genital warts. The nurse finds out that Sandy engaged in high-risk behavior with a stranger she "hooked up" with recently at school. She couldn't imagine that he would give her an STI because "he looked so clean-cut." She wonders how she could possibly have genital warts. What information should be given to Sandy about STIs in general? What specific information about HPV should be stressed?

Nursing Management

Key nursing roles are teaching about prevention of HPV infection and promotion of vaccines and screening tests in order to reduce the morbidity and mortality associated with cervical cancer caused by HPV infection. Teach all patients that the only way to prevent HPV is to refrain from any genital contact with another person. Although the effect of condoms in preventing HPV infection is unknown, latex condom use has been associated with a lower rate of cervical cancer (NCI, 2024). Teach patients about the link between HPV and cervical cancer. Explain that in most cases, there are no signs or symptoms of infection with HPV. Strongly encourage all females between the ages of 9 and 26 (and in the case of young patients between 9 and 18, also their parents) to consider receiving the vaccine against HPV. For females 27 through 45 years, it is recommended that a shared clinical decision be made with their health care provider based on their risk profile. For all female patients, promote the importance of obtaining regular Pap smears and for female patients over age 30, suggest an HPV test to rule out the presence of a latent high-risk strain of HPV.

Education and counseling are important aspects of managing female patients who have genital warts. Teach the patient that:

- Even after genital warts are removed, HPV may remain, and viral shedding may continue.
- The likelihood of transmission to future partners and the duration of infectivity after treatment for genital warts are unknown.
- The recurrence of genital warts within the first few months after treatment is common and usually indicates recurrence rather than reinfection (Carusi, 2023).

In the absence of major national health policy mandates, a multilevel, multifaceted approach will be needed to achieve high rates of HPV vaccination in the United States. Nurses must focus on the education of their patients regarding indications of HPV vaccination and work on approaches to communicating most effectively with parents about the safety and benefits of vaccination and the risks associated with not vaccinating their children.

Sandy is being treated for HPV and is anxious for her "things" to disappear and never return. What education is needed to prevent further transmission from Sandy to any future sexual partners?

TAKE NOTE!

Sexually active females, particularly those with multiple partners, are at risk for contracting hepatitis A, B, and C through sexual contact. Proper use of barrier protection and following immunization recommendations (available for hepatitis A and B) will help prevent hepatitis. There is no current vaccine for hepatitis C. Recommended screening for hepatitis B includes females at risk and all pregnant people at their first prenatal visit and retesting near delivery for high-risk patients. Hepatitis C screening is recommended for all females 18 years of age and older once in their lifetime (CDC, 2022i).

ECTOPARASITIC INFECTIONS

Ectoparasites are parasites that live on the outside of the body (host). They are a common cause of skin rash and pruritus throughout the world, affecting people of all ages, races, and socioeconomic groups. Overcrowding, weakened immune systems, global traveling, immigration, delayed diagnosis and treatment, and poor public education contribute to the prevalence of ectoparasites in both industrial and nonindustrial nations. These infections include infestations of scabies and pubic lice. Because these parasites are easily passed from one person to another during sexual intimacy, patients should be assessed for them when receiving care for other STIs.

Scabies is a highly contagious intensely pruritic dermatitis caused by a mite. The worldwide prevalence has been estimated at about 200 million cases annually (Gilson & Crane, 2023). In general, transmission occurs by direct skin-to-skin contact, sexual contact, and overcrowded living conditions. Intense itching occurs weeks after the initial infection, especially at night. The female mite burrows under the skin and deposits eggs, which hatch. The lesions start as a small papule that reddens, erodes, and sometimes crusts. Presumptive diagnosis may be made based on history and clinical findings such as appearance of linear burrows in the webs between the fingers, on the elbows, and in the axillae, buttocks, and the genitalia (Goldstein & Goldstein, 2022). Aggressive infestation can occur in immunodeficient, debilitated, or malnourished people, but healthy people do not usually suffer sequelae. Scabies treatment includes topical administration of a scabicidal agent (e.g., permethrin, crotamiton, or ivermectin), as well as an antibiotic if a secondary infection is present.

Lice are blood-sucking insects that can be found on people's heads, bodies, or pubic areas. Patients with pediculosis pubis (pubic louse) usually seek treatment because of the pruritus, because of a rash brought on by skin irritation from scratching, or because they notice lice or nits in their pubic hair, axillary hair, abdominal and thigh hair, and sometimes in the eyebrows, eyelashes, and beards. Infestation is usually without symptoms until after a week or so, when bites cause pruritus and secondary infections from scratching. Diagnosis is based on history and the presence of nits (small, shiny, yellow/white, oval, dewdroplike eggs) affixed to hair shafts or lice (a tan to grayish, short, wingless insect that appears crablike) (Fig. 5.9) (Bragg & Willis, 2023).

Treatment has two aspects: medication and environmental control measures. Medications used include topical antilouse agents such as permethrin or pyrethrin shampoos, malathion, spinosad, or ivermectin. Bedding and clothing should be washed in hot water and dried using a hot setting on the dryer or dry cleaning or sealing clothes in plastic bags for 2 weeks to decontaminate them. Sexual partners should also be treated, as well as family members who live in close contact with the infected person.

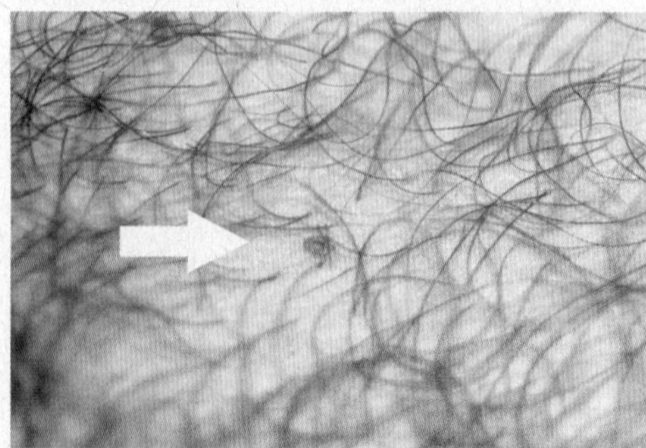

FIGURE 5.9 Pubic lice. A small brown living crab louse is seen at the base of hairs (arrow). (Reprinted with permission from Goodheart, H., & Gonzalez, M. [2015]. *Goodheart's photoguide of common pediatric and adult skin disorders* [4th ed.]. Lippincott Williams & Wilkins.)

TEACHING GUIDELINES 5.4 Treating and Minimizing the Spread of Scabies and Pubic Lice

- Use the medication according to the manufacturer's instructions.
- Retreat as directed.
- Remove nits with a fine-toothed nit comb.
- Practice safer sex. Avoid sexual contact until both people are successfully treated.
- Wash hands on a regular basis, especially after handling raw foods or feces.
- Do not share any personal items with others or accept items from others.
- Treat objects, clothing, and bedding and wash them in hot water.

Nursing care of a patient infested with lice or scabies involves a three-tiered approach: eradicating the infestation with medication, removing the nits, and preventing spread or recurrence by managing the environment. The CDC recommends regimens using pyrethrins and permethrins. Frequently, a combination of malathion or ivermectin is also added. Nurses should provide education about these products (Teaching Guidelines 5.4). The nurse can follow these same guidelines to prevent the health care facility from becoming infested.

HUMAN IMMUNODEFICIENCY VIRUS

The first diagnosis of AIDS occurred in the United States in 1981. Females were rarely impacted in the early 1980s, but as years passed, they became a hard-hit group. Globally, half of all of those living with HIV are female (The Well Project, 2023). In the United States, one in five females receive a diagnosis of HIV infection (The Well Project, 2023). Black females and transgender people are affected by HIV to a much greater degree than other groups (The Well Project, 2023).

Human immunodeficiency virus (HIV) targets the immune system and weakens the body's defense systems against infections and some types of cancer. Many advances have been made in the prevention of HIV transmission and management of HIV/AIDS. One of the most important discoveries has been antiretroviral treatment, which can halt the replication of the virus and ease symptoms, turning AIDS into a manageable chronic condition instead of a rapid terminal illness.

Acquired immunodeficiency syndrome (AIDS) is a breakdown in the immune function caused by HIV, a retrovirus. A sufficient quantity of viruses must be transferred to infect a person. The virus cannot live long outside the human body; it cannot be transmitted via tears or sweat. The HIV infection is associated with continued activation of immune system and is the driving force behind CD4 T-cell depletion and progression to AIDS. The infected person develops opportunistic infections or malignancies that become fatal. The progression from HIV to AIDS timeline is individualized and depends on treatment and adherence to treatment protocols. HIV infection is acquired through:

- Sexual intercourse
- Exposure to infected blood
- Perinatal transmission

Females are particularly vulnerable to heterosexual transmission of HIV as a result of substantial mucosal exposure to seminal fluids. Heterosexual intercourse is the most commonly reported risk factor in females (Aberg & Cespedes, 2024).

An infected birthing parent can transmit HIV infection to their newborn before or during birth and through breastfeeding. Most cases of birthing parent-to-child HIV transmission, the cause of the majority of pediatric-acquired infections worldwide, occur late in pregnancy or during delivery. The efficacy of the use of combination antiretroviral therapy (ART) during pregnancy has decreased the HIV transmission from birthing parent to fetus to less than 1% (Aberg & Cespedes, 2024). Screening for HIV is recommended in all females aged 13 to 64 years, all females who seek evaluation and treatment for an STI, and all pregnant people at first prenatal appointment and retest during the third trimester if at high risk (CDC, 2022i).

Clinical Manifestations

HIV infection undergoes three distinct phases: acute seroconversion, chronic HIV without AIDS (without symptoms), and then progression to AIDS. When a person is initially infected with HIV, they go through an acute primary infection period for about 3 weeks. The HIV viral load drops rapidly because the host's immune system works well to fight this initial infection. The onset of the acute primary infection occurs 2 to 6 weeks after exposure. Symptoms include fever, pharyngitis, rash, and myalgia. Most people do not associate this flulike condition with HIV infection. After initial exposure, there is a period of 3 to 12 months before seroconversion. The person is considered infectious during this time.

After the acute phase, the infected person is without symptoms, but the HIV virus begins to replicate. Even though there are no symptoms, the immune system runs down. A normal person has a CD4 T-cell count of 450 to 1,200 cells/μL. When the CD4 T-cell count reaches 200 or less, the person is considered to have AIDS. The immune system begins a constant battle to fight this viral invasion, but over time, it falls behind. A viral reservoir occurs in T cells that can store various stages of the virus. The onset and severity of the disease correlate directly with the viral load; the more HIV virus that is present, the worse the person will feel. As profound immunosuppression begins to occur, opportunistic infections will occur, qualifying the person for the diagnosis of AIDS.

Diagnosis

There are three kinds of HIV tests to diagnose HIV: nucleic acid tests, antibody tests, and antigen/antibody tests. These tests are designed to detect antigens, antibodies, or RNA. In addition, several point-of-care or rapid antibody tests along with self-tests are available. Two categories of screening methods currently used include rapid HIV tests and confirmatory tests. The rapid tests allow for screening at the point of care and quick results. A positive result is followed up with laboratory-based test.

Rapid point-of-service HIV tests are becoming powerful screening tools in various health care settings because they offer the opportunity to not only screen for HIV but also to educate the person regarding risk factors and discuss their test results all in one clinical visit. Most use a fingerstick drop of blood or a swab of saliva taken from the mouth. Results are typically ready within 10 to 20 minutes. If the confirmation test (Western blot [WB] or immunofluorescent assay [IFA]) is positive, the person is infected with HIV and can transmit the virus to others.

Therapeutic Management

The goals of ART include:

- Decrease the HIV viral load below the level of detection.
- Restore the body's ability to fight off pathogens.
- Prevent HIV transmission to others.
- Improve the patient's quality of life.
- Reduce HIV morbidity and mortality (Gillespie, 2023).

Pregnant people will adhere to their prescribed ART during pregnancy and delivery. The infant will receive HIV medications for 2 to 6 weeks after birth to decrease the risk of transmission (CDC, 2023a).

Dramatic new treatment advances with antiretroviral medications have turned a disease that used to be a death sentence into a chronic, manageable one for people who live in countries where ART is available. Despite these advances in treatment, however, only a minority of HIV-positive people in the United States who take antiretroviral medications are receiving the full benefits because they are not adhering to the prescribed regimens. Successful ART requires nearly perfect adherence to a complex medication regimen; less-than-perfect adherence leads to drug resistance.

Adherence is difficult because of the complexity of the regimen and the lifelong duration of treatment. A typical antiretroviral regimen may consist of daily oral medications. Adherence is made even more difficult because of the unpleasant side effects, such as nausea and diarrhea. People in early pregnancy already experience these, and the antiretroviral medication only exacerbates them.

Preexposure prophylaxis (PrEP) is a medication taken to prevent HIV. PrEP is taken by people who are HIV-negative because it reduces the risk of acquiring HIV from sex by approximately 99% and from injection drug use by 74% (CDC, 2022b). It is only effective if taken as prescribed and consistently. Although PrEP medications are very effective preventive measures, only 25% of people at high risk for acquiring HIV take them (Johns Hopkins Bloomberg School of Public Health, 2023). High costs and side effects (nausea, vomiting, and diarrhea) are the main reasons this population does not take PrEP medications (Johns Hopkins Bloomberg School of Public Health, 2023).

Nursing Management

Nurses can play a major role in caring for the HIV-positive patient by helping them accept the possibility of a shortened lifespan, cope with others' reactions to a stigmatizing illness, and develop strategies to maintain their physical and emotional health. Educate the patient about changes they can make in their behavior to prevent spreading HIV to others, and refer them to appropriate community resources such as HIV medical care services, substance misuse services, mental health services, and social services. See Clinical Judgment & Nursing Process 5.1.

Promoting Adherence to Medication Regimen

The goal of ART is to suppress viral replication so that the viral load becomes undetectable by diagnostic tests. This is done to preserve immune function and delay disease progression, but it is a challenge because of the side effects of nausea and vomiting, diarrhea, altered taste, anorexia, flatulence, constipation, headaches, anemia, and fatigue. Although not everyone experiences all of the side effects, the majority do have some of them.

Adherence to medication regimens is crucial for treatment success. The nurse should identify the barriers to adherence in order to help the patient overcome them. Some of the common barriers exist because the patient:

- Has poor patient–provider relationships
- Fears revealing their HIV status by being seen taking medication
- Lacks access to social services (food, housing, transportation)
- Lacks physical and emotional support from friends/family
- Has not adjusted emotionally to the HIV diagnosis
- Fears telling their family about the diagnosis
- Has few financial resources to afford therapy
- Does not understand the dosing regimen or schedule
- Experiences unpleasant side effects frequently
- Feels anxious or depressed (Aberg & Cespedes, 2024; The Foundation for AIDS Research, 2023)

CLINICAL JUDGMENT & NURSING PROCESS 5.1 Overview of the Patient Who Is HIV-Positive

A 28-year-old Black person is living with HIV. They acquired HIV through unprotected sexual contact. They have been inconsistent in taking antiretroviral medications and present today stating they are tired and do not feel well.

NURSING ANALYSIS: Infection risk related to positive HIV status and inconsistent adherence to antiretroviral therapy regimen

OUTCOME IDENTIFICATION AND EVALUATION

The patient will remain free of opportunistic infections as evidenced by temperature within acceptable parameters and absence of signs and symptoms of opportunistic infections.

INTERVENTIONS: *Minimizing the Risk of Opportunistic Infections*

- Assess CD4 count and viral loads *to determine disease progression* (CD4 counts 500/L and viral loads >10,000 copies/L = increased risk of opportunistic infections).
- Assess complete blood count *to identify presence of infection* (>10,000 cells/μL may indicate infection).
- Assess oral cavity and mucous membranes for painful white patches in mouth *to evaluate for possible fungal infection.*
- Teach patient to monitor for general signs and symptoms of infections, such as fever, weakness, and fatigue, *to ensure early identification.*
- Provide information explaining the importance of avoiding people with infections when possible *to minimize the risk of exposure to infections.*
- Teach importance of keeping appointments so the CD4 count and viral load can be monitored *to alert the health care provider about changes in immune system status.*
- Instruct them to reduce their exposure to infections via:
  - Meticulous hand hygiene
  - Thorough cooking of meats, eggs, and vegetables
  - Wearing shoes at all times, especially when outdoors
- Encourage a balance of rest with activity throughout the day *to prevent overexertion.*
- Stress the importance of maintaining prescribed antiretroviral drug therapies *to prevent disease progression and resistance.*
- If necessary, refer to a nutritionist to help them understand what constitutes a well-balanced diet with supplements *to promote health and reduce the risk of infection.*

NURSING ANALYSIS: Lack of knowledge related to HIV infection and possible complications

OUTCOME IDENTIFICATION AND EVALUATION

The patient will demonstrate increased understanding of HIV infection as evidenced by verbalizing appropriate health care practices and adhering to therapy to reduce the risk of further exposure and disease progression.

INTERVENTIONS: *Providing Patient Education*

- Assess their understanding of HIV and its treatment *to provide a baseline for teaching.*
- Establish trust and be honest with them; encourage them to talk about fears and the impact of the disease *to provide an outlet for their concerns.* Encourage them to discuss reasons for nonadherence to therapy.
- Provide a nonjudgmental, accessible, confidential, and culturally sensitive approach *to promote the patient's self-esteem and allow them to feel like a priority.*
- Explain measures, including safer sex practices and birth control options, *to prevent disease transmission*; determine their willingness to practice safer sex to protect others *to determine further teaching needs.*
- Discuss the signs and symptoms of disease progression and potential opportunistic infections *to promote early detection for prompt intervention.*
- Outline with the patient the availability of community resources and make appropriate referrals as needed *to provide additional education and support.*
- Monitor for signs of loneliness, depression, and social isolation *to open up a conversation.*
- Encourage the patient to keep scheduled appointments *to ensure follow-up and allow early detection of potential problems.*

HIV, human immunodeficiency virus.

Educate the patient about the prescribed medication therapy and stress that it is important to take the regimen as prescribed. Offer suggestions about how to cope with anorexia, nausea, vomiting, and diarrhea by:

- Separating the intake of food and fluids
- Eating dry crackers upon arising
- Eating six small meals daily
- Using high-protein supplements (Boost, Ensure) to provide quick and easy protein and calories
- Eating "comfort foods," which may appeal when other foods do not

Stress the importance of taking the prescribed ARTs by explaining that they help prevent replication of the retroviruses and subsequent progression of the disease and also decrease the risk of perinatal transmission of HIV. In addition, provide written materials describing diet, exercise, medications, and signs and symptoms of complications and opportunistic infections. Reinforce this information at each visit.

Preventing Human Immunodeficiency Virus Infection

The core of HIV prevention is to reduce each person's high-risk sexual behaviors. However, it is important to recognize that not all patients have the economic and social power to make all their own life choices. Nurses must address the factors that will give patients more control over their lives by providing anticipatory guidance, giving ample opportunities to practice negotiation techniques and refusal skills in a safe environment, and encouraging the use of condoms to protect against this deadly virus. Prevention is the key to decreasing HIV infection.

Nurses need to routinely take a sexual and injection use history for all of their patients in an open and nonjudgmental manner. They should be informed that acquisition of HIV can be prevented with medication (USPSTF, 2023). Reviewing high-risk behaviors and that consistent use of condoms decreases their risk is important, along with frequent follow-up with their prescriber. See Healthy People 2030 box.

Providing Care During Pregnancy and Childbirth

Voluntary counseling and HIV testing should be offered to all pregnant people as early in the pregnancy as possible to identify people living with HIV so that treatment can be initiated early. Once a pregnant person is identified as living with HIV, they should be informed about the risk of perinatal transmission.

HEALTHY PEOPLE 2030

STI Objectives	Nursing Significance
Reduce the number of new HIV infections.	• Discourage intravenous illicit drug use. • Educate sexually active females about the risks of HIV transmission. • Encourage proper and consistent condom use with all sexual activity.
Increase knowledge of HIV status.	• Encourage sexually active females to seek appropriate reproductive health care and screening.
Reduce the rate of birthing parent-to-child HIV transmission.	• For pregnant people, encourage HIV testing to determine status. • Encourage the HIV-positive pregnant person to comply with HIV treatment as prescribed.

HIV, human immunodeficiency virus; STI, sexually transmitted infection.
Healthy People Objectives retrieved from http://www.healthypeople.gov

In addition, the patient needs instructions on ways to enhance their immune system by following these guidelines during pregnancy:

- getting adequate sleep each night (7 to 9 hours)
- avoiding infections (e.g., staying out of crowds, practicing good hand hygiene)
- decreasing stress
- consuming adequate protein and vitamins
- increasing fluid intake to 2 L daily to stay hydrated
- planning rest periods throughout the day to prevent fatigue

As previously stated, despite the dramatic reduction in perinatal transmission, some infants will be born infected with HIV. The birth of each infected infant is a missed prevention opportunity. To minimize perinatal HIV transmission, identify HIV infection in female patients, preferably before pregnancy; provide information about disease prevention; and encourage patients living with HIV to follow the prescribed drug therapy.

Providing Appropriate Referrals

The person with HIV may have difficulty coping with the normal activities of daily living because they have less energy and decreased physical endurance. They may be overwhelmed by the financial burdens of medical and drug therapies, the emotional responses to a life-threatening condition, and, if pregnant, concern about their infant's future. A case management approach is needed to deal with the complexity of their needs during this time. Be an empathetic listener and make appropriate referrals for nutritional services, counseling, homemaker services, spiritual care, and local support groups. Many community-based organizations have developed programs to address the numerous issues regarding HIV/AIDS. The national AIDS hotline (1-800-342-AIDS) is a good resource.

PREVENTING SEXUALLY TRANSMITTED INFECTIONS

Education about safer sex practices—and the resulting increase in the use of condoms—can play a vital role in reducing STI rates all over the world. Clearly, knowledge and prevention are the best defenses against STIs. The prevention and control of STIs are based on the following guidelines:

1. Education and counseling of people at risk about safer sexual behavior
2. Recommending immunizations that prevent hepatitis B and HPV preexposure
3. Educating people that condoms offer protection and reduce risk of transmission
4. Identifying infected people without symptoms and symptomatic people unlikely to seek diagnosis and treatment

5. Effectively diagnosing and treating infected people
6. Evaluating, treating, and counseling sex partners of people who are infected with STIs
7. Encouraging a reduction in the number of sex partners people may have
8. Encouraging people to get tested for STIs if engaging in unprotected sexual acts
9. Informing people to be knowledgeable about the sexual practices of partner (Rietmeijer, 2024)

Nurses play an integral role in identifying and preventing STIs. They have a unique opportunity to educate the public about this serious public health issue by communicating the methods of transmission and symptoms associated with each condition, tracking the most up-to-date CDC treatment guidelines, and offering patients strategic preventive measures to reduce the spread of STIs. Nurses have a huge role to play to ensure all people are well educated about STIs by informing them how these infections are transmitted, symptoms, risk factors, potential for adverse effects, screening, and treatment recommendations. Armed with this knowledge, people can make fully informed decisions about accepting screening and adhering to treatment and follow-up advice.

Challenges to prevention of STIs include lack of resources and difficulty in changing the behaviors that contribute to their spread. Regardless of the challenging factors involved, nurses must continue to educate and meet the needs of all patients to promote their sexual health. Successful treatment and prevention of STIs is impossible without education. Successful teaching approaches include giving clear, accurate messages that are age-appropriate and culturally sensitive.

Primary prevention strategies include educating all patients, especially adolescents, regarding the risk of early sexual activity, the number of sexual partners, and STIs. Sexual abstinence is ideal but often not practiced; therefore, the use of barrier contraception (condoms) should be encouraged (see Teaching Guidelines 5.1).

Secondary prevention involves the need for screening examinations for all sexually active people, regardless of age. Many female patients with STIs are without symptoms, so regular screening examinations are paramount for early detection. Understanding the relationship between poor socioeconomic conditions and poor patterns of sexual and reproductive self-care is significant in disease prevention and health promotion strategies.

Every successful form of prevention requires a change in behavior. The nursing role in teaching and rendering quality health care is invaluable evidence that the key to reducing the spread of STIs is through behavioral change. Nurses working in these specialty areas have a responsibility to educate themselves, their patients, their families, and the community about STIs and to provide compassionate and supportive care to patients. Some strategies nurses can use to prevent the spread of STIs are detailed in Box 5.2.

BOX 5.2 Selected Nursing Strategies to Prevent the Spread of STIs

- Provide basic information about STI transmission.
- Outline safer sexual behaviors for people at risk for STIs.
- Refer patients to appropriate community resources to reduce risk.
- Screen people with STIs without symptoms.
- Identify barriers to STI testing and remove them.
- Offer preexposure immunizations for vaccine-preventable STIs.
- Respond honestly about testing results and options available.
- Counsel and treat sexual partners of people with STIs.
- Educate school administrators, parents, and teens about STIs.
- Support youth development activities to reduce sexual risk-taking.
- Promote the use of barrier methods (condoms, diaphragms) to prevent the spread of STIs.
- Assist patients in gaining skills in negotiating safer sex.
- Discuss reducing the number of sexual partners to reduce risk.

STI, sexually transmitted infection.

CONSIDER THIS!

I was thinking of my carefree college days, when the most important thing was having an active sorority life and meeting guys. I had been raised by strict parents and was never allowed to date while growing up. Since I attended an out-of-state college, I figured that my parents' outdated advice and rules no longer applied. Abruptly, my thoughts of the past were interrupted by the HIV counselor asking about my feelings concerning my positive diagnosis. What was there to say at this point? I had a lot of fun in college but never dreamed it would haunt me for the rest of my life, which was possibly going to be shortened considerably now. I only wish I could turn back time and listen to my parents' advice, which somehow doesn't seem so outdated now.

Thoughts: All of us have thought back on our lives to better times and wondered how our lives would have changed if we had made better choices or gone down another path. We only have one chance to make good, sound decisions at times. What would you have changed in your life if given a second chance? Can you still make a change for the better now?

KEY CONCEPTS

- Avoiding risky sexual behaviors may preserve fertility and prevent chronic conditions later in life.
- The most reliable way to avoid transmission of STIs is to abstain from sexual intercourse (i.e., oral, vaginal, or anal sex) or to be in a long-term, mutually monogamous relationship with an uninfected partner.
- Barrier methods of contraception are recommended because they increase protection from contact with urethral discharge, mucosal secretions, and lesions of the cervix or penis.
- The high rate of transmission of STIs without symptoms calls for teaching high-risk people the nature of transmission and how to recognize infections.

- Nurses should practice good hand hygiene and follow standard precautions to protect themselves and their patients from STIs.
- Nurses are in an important position to promote the sexual health of all people. Nurses should make their patients and the community aware of the perinatal implications and lifelong sequelae of STIs.

REFERENCES AND RECOMMENDED READINGS

Aberg, J. A., & Cespedes, M. S. (2024). HIV and women. *UpToDate.* Retrieved March 21, 2024, from https://www.uptodate.com/contents/hiv-and-women

Albrecht, M. A. (2022). Epidemiology, clinical manifestations, and diagnosis of genital herpes simplex virus infection. *UpToDate.* Retrieved March 19, 2024, from https://www.uptodate.com/contents/epidemiology-clinical-manifestations-and-diagnosis-of-genital-herpes-simplex-virus-infection

Albrecht, M. A. (2024). Treatment of genital herpes simplex virus infection. *UpToDate.* Retrieved March 19, 2024, from https://www.uptodate.com/contents/treatment-of-genital-herpes-simplex-virus-infection

American Cancer Society. (2024). *Key statistics for cervical cancer.* https://www.cancer.org/cancer/cervical-cancer/about/key-statistics.html

Ardekani, A., Taherifard, E., Mollalo, A., Hemadi, E., Roshanshad, A., Fereidooni, R., Rouholamin, S., Rezaeinejad, M., Farid-Mojtahedi, M., Razavi, M., & Rostami, A. (2022). Human papillomavirus infection during pregnancy and childhood: A comprehensive review. *Microorganisms, 10*(10), 1932. https://doi.org/10.3390/microorganisms10101932

Arrieta, A. C. (2023). Congenital syphilis: Clinical manifestations, evaluation, and diagnosis. *UpToDate.* https://www.uptodate.com/contents/congenital-syphilis-clinical-manifestations-evaluation-and-diagnosis

Bash, M. C., & Connelly, M. (2023). Epidemiology and pathogenesis of *Neisseria gonorrhoeae* infection. *UpToDate.* Retrieved March 19, 2024, from https://www.uptodate.com/contents/epidemiology-and-pathogenesis-of-neisseria-gonorrhoeae-infection

Bragg, B. N., & Willis, C. (2023). Pediculosis. In *StatPearls.* StatPearls Publishing. https://www.ncbi.nlm.nih.gov/books/NBK470343/

Carusi, D. A. (2023). Condylomata acuminata (anogenital warts): Treatment of vulvar and vaginal warts. *UpToDate.* Retrieved March 21, 2024, from https://www.uptodate.com/contents/condylomata-acuminata-anogenital-warts-treatment-of-vulvar-and-vaginal-warts

Centers for Disease Control and Prevention. (2021). *Vulvovaginal candidiasis (VVC).* https://www.cdc.gov/std/treatment-guidelines/candidiasis.htm

Centers for Disease Control and Prevention. (2022a). *STI treatment guidelines, 2021: Gonococcal infections among adolescents and adults.* https://www.cdc.gov/std/treatment-guidelines/gonorrhea-adults.htm

Centers for Disease Control and Prevention. (2022b). *Pre-exposure prophylaxis (PrEP).* https://www.cdc.gov/hiv/risk/prep/index.html

Centers for Disease Control and Prevention. (2022c). *Condom effectiveness: Female (internal) condom use.* https://www.cdc.gov/condomeffectiveness/internal-condom-use.html?CDC_AA_refVal=https%3A%2F%2Fwww.cdc.gov%2Fcondomeffectiveness%2FFemale-condom-use.html

Centers for Disease Control and Prevention. (2022d). *Incidence, prevalence, and cost of sexually transmitted infections in the United States.* https://www.cdc.gov/nchhstp/newsroom/fact-sheets/std/STI-Incidence-Prevalence-Cost-Factsheet.html

Centers for Disease Control and Prevention. (2022e). *STDs and HIV—CDC basic fact sheet.* https://www.cdc.gov/std/hiv/stdfact-std-hiv.htm

Centers for Disease Control and Prevention. (2022f). *Condom effectiveness: Male (external) condom use.* https://www.cdc.gov/condomeffectiveness/external-condom-use.html

Centers for Disease Control and Prevention. (2022g). *Trichomoniasis—CDC basic fact sheet.* https://www.cdc.gov/std/trichomonas/stdfact-trichomoniasis.htm

Centers for Disease Control and Prevention. (2022h). *Bacterial vaginosis—CDC basic fact sheet.* https://www.cdc.gov/std/bv/stdfact-bacterial-vaginosis.htm

Centers for Disease Control and Prevention. (2022i). *Screening recommendations and considerations referenced in treatment guidelines and original sources.* https://www.cdc.gov/std/treatment-guidelines/screening-recommendations.htm

Centers for Disease Control and Prevention. (2022j). *Genital herpes—CDC basic fact sheet.* https://www.cdc.gov/std/herpes/stdfact-herpes.htm

Centers for Disease Control and Prevention. (2022k). *Sexually transmitted infections treatment guidelines, 2021: Pelvic inflammatory disease (PID).* https://www.cdc.gov/std/treatment-guidelines/pid.htm

Centers for Disease Control and Prevention. (2022l). *Human Papillomavirus (HPV): Genital HPV infection—Basic fact sheet.* https://www.cdc.gov/std/hpv/stdfact-hpv.htm

Centers for Disease Control and Prevention. (2023a). *HIV and perinatal transmission: Preventing perinatal HIV transmission.* https://www.cdc.gov/hiv/group/pregnant-people/transmission.html

Centers for Disease Control and Prevention. (2023b). *HIV basics: Basic statistics.* https://www.cdc.gov/hiv/basics/statistics.html

Centers for Disease Control and Prevention. (2023c). *Sexually transmitted diseases (STDs): CDC fact sheets.* https://www.cdc.gov/std/healthcomm/fact_sheets.htm

Centers for Disease Control and Prevention. (2023d). *STDs during pregnancy: CDC detailed fact sheet.* https://www.cdc.gov/std/pregnancy/stdfact-pregnancy-detailed.htm#details

Centers for Disease Control and Prevention. (2023e). *Youth risk behavior survey: Data summary & trends report: 2011–2021.* https://www.cdc.gov/healthyyouth/data/yrbs/pdf/YRBS_Data-Summary-Trends_Report2023_508.pdf

Centers for Disease Control and Prevention. (2024a). Sexually transmitted infections surveillance, 2022*: National Notifiable Diseases Surveillance System (NNDSS).* https://www.cdc.gov/std/statistics/2022/nndss.htm

Centers for Disease Control and Prevention. (2024b). *Sexually transmitted infections treatment guidelines, 2021: Syphilis.* https://www.cdc.gov/std/treatment-guidelines/syphilis.htm

Cohn, T., & Harrison, C. V. (2022). A systematic review exploring racial disparities, social determinants of health, and sexually transmitted infections in Black women. *Nursing for Women's Health, 26*(2), 128–142. https://doi.org/10.1016/j.nwh.2022.01.006

Cooper, D. B., & Dunton, C. J. (2023). Colposcopy. In *StatPearls*. StatPearls Publishing. https://www.ncbi.nlm.nih.gov/books/NBK564514/

Dall, C. (2023). *Sexually transmitted infections continue to climb in US*. https://www.cidrap.umn.edu/sexually-transmitted-infections/sexually-transmitted-infections-continue-climb-us#

Devine, A., Xiong, X., Gottlieb, S. L., Mello, M. B., Fairley, C. K., & Ong, J. J. (2022). Health-related quality of life in individuals with genital herpes: A systematic review. *Health and Quality of Life Outcomes, 20*(1), 25. https://doi.org/10.1186/s12955-022-01934-w

Fortenberry, J. D. (2023). Sexually transmitted infections: Issues specific to adolescents. *UpToDate*. Retrieved January 26, 2024, from https://www.uptodate.com/contents/sexually-transmitted-infections-issues-specific-to-adolescents

Ghanem, K. G. (2023). Clinical manifestations and diagnosis of *Neisseria gonorrhoeae* infection in adults and adolescents. *UpToDate*. Retrieved March 19, 2024, from https://www.uptodate.com/contents/clinical-manifestations-and-diagnosis-of-neisseria-gonorrhoeae-infection-in-adults-and-adolescents

Gillespie, S. L. (2023). The adolescent with HIV infection. *UpToDate*. https://www.uptodate.com/contents/the-adolescent-with-hiv-infection

Gilson, R. L., & Crane, J. S. (2023). Scabies. In *StatPearls*. StatPearls Publishing. https://www.ncbi.nlm.nih.gov/books/NBK544306/

Goldstein, B. G., & Goldstein, A. O. (2022). Scabies: Epidemiology, clinical features, and diagnosis. *UpToDate*. Retrieved March 20, 2024, from https://www.uptodate.com/contents/scabies-epidemiology-clinical-features-and-diagnosis

Hicks, C. B., & Clement, M. (2023a). Syphilis: Epidemiology, pathophysiology, and clinical manifestations in patients without HIV. *UpToDate*. Retrieved March 20, 2024, from https://www.uptodate.com/contents/syphilis-epidemiology-pathophysiology-and-clinical-manifestations-in-patients-without-hiv

Hicks, C. B., & Clement, M. (2023b). Syphilis: Screening and diagnostic testing. *UpToDate*. Retrieved March 20, 2024, from https://www.uptodate.com/contents/syphilis-screening-and-diagnostic-testing

Hicks, C. B., & Clement, M. (2023c). Syphilis: Treatment and monitoring. *UpToDate*. Retrieved March 20, 2024, from https://www.uptodate.com/contents/syphilis-treatment-and-monitoring

Hsu, K. (2022). Clinical manifestations and diagnosis of *Chlamydia trachomatis* infections. *UpToDate*. Retrieved March 19, 2024, from https://www.uptodate.com/contents/clinical-manifestations-and-diagnosis-of-chlamydia-trachomatis-infections

Hsu, K. (2023a). Epidemiology of *Chlamydia trachomatis* infections. *UpToDate*. Retrieved March 19, 2024, from https://www.uptodate.com/contents/epidemiology-of-chlamydia-trachomatis-infections

Hsu, K. (2023b). Treatment of *Chlamydia trachomatis* infection in adults and adolescents. *UpToDate*. Retrieved March 19, 2024, from https://www.uptodate.com/contents/treatment-of-chlamydia-trachomatis-infection-in-adults-and-adolescents

Iqbal, U., & Willis, C. (2023). Cervicitis. In *StatPearls*. StatPearls Publishing. https://www.ncbi.nlm.nih.gov/books/NBK562193/

Jennings, L. K., & Krywko, D. M. (2023). Pelvic inflammatory disease. In *StatPearls*. StatPearls Publishing. https://www.ncbi.nlm.nih.gov/books/NBK499959/

Johns Hopkins Bloomberg School of Public Health. (2023). *Study suggests side-effects and costs are biggest issues for users of HIV pre-exposure prophylaxis*. https://publichealth.jhu.edu/2023/study-suggests-side-effects-and-costs-are-biggest-issues-for-users-of-hiv-pre-exposure-prophylaxis

Kaiser Family Foundation. (2022). *HIV testing in the United States*. https://www.kff.org/hivaids/fact-sheet/hiv-testing-in-the-united-states/

Leslie, S. W., Sajjad, H., & Kumar, S. (2023). Genital warts. In *StatPearls*. StatPearls Publishing. https://www.ncbi.nlm.nih.gov/books/NBK441884/

Liao, C. I., Francoeur, A. A., Kapp, D. S., Caesar, M. A. P., Huh, W. K., & Chan, J. K. (2022). Trends in human papillomavirus-associated cancers, demographic characteristics, and vaccinations in the US, 2001–2017. *JAMA Network Open, 5*(3), e222530. https://jamanetwork.com/journals/jamanetworkopen/fullarticle/2790165

National Cancer Institute. (2023). *Human papillomavirus (HPV) vaccines*. https://www.cancer.gov/about-cancer/causes-prevention/risk/infectious-agents/hpv-vaccine-fact-sheet

National Cancer Institute. (2024). *Cervical cancer prevention (PDQ®)—Health professional version*. https://www.cancer.gov/types/cervical/hp/cervical-prevention-pdq#

Norwitz, E. R., & Hicks, C. B. (2024). Syphilis in pregnancy. *UpToDate*. Retrieved March 20, 2024, from https://www.uptodate.com/contents/syphilis-in-pregnancy

Ochoa, K. J. C., & Mendez, M. D. (2023). Ophthalmia neonatorum. In *StatPearls*. StatPearls Publishing. https://www.ncbi.nlm.nih.gov/books/NBK551572/

Office on Women's Health. (2022). *Human papillomavirus*. https://www.womenshealth.gov/a-z-topics/human-papillomavirus

Palefsky, J. M. (2022). Human papillomavirus infections: Epidemiology and disease associations. *UpToDate*. Retrieved March 19, 2024, from https://www.uptodate.com/contents/human-papillomavirus-infections-epidemiology-and-disease-associations

Rietmeijer, K. (2024). Prevention of sexually transmitted infections. *UpToDate*. Retrieved March 18, 2024, from https://www.uptodate.com/contents/prevention-of-sexually-transmitted-infections

Riley, L. E. & Wald, A. (2022). Genital herpes simplex virus infection and pregnancy. *UpToDate*. Retrieved March 19, 2024, from https://www.uptodate.com/contents/genital-herpes-simplex-virus-infection-and-pregnancy

Ross, J. (2023a). Pelvic inflammatory disease: Pathogenesis, microbiology, and risk factors. *UpToDate*. Retrieved March 19, 2024, from https://www.uptodate.com/contents/pelvic-inflammatory-disease-pathogenesis-microbiology-and-risk-factors

Ross, J. (2023b). Pelvic inflammatory disease: Clinical manifestations and diagnosis. *UpToDate*. Retrieved March 19, 2024, from https://www.uptodate.com/contents/pelvic-inflammatory-disease-clinical-manifestations-and-diagnosis

Seña, A. C., & Cohen, M. S. (2023). Treatment of uncomplicated gonorrhea (*Neisseria gonorrhoeae* infection) in adults and adolescents. *UpToDate*. Retrieved March 19, 2024, from https://www.uptodate.com/contents/treatment-of-uncomplicated-gonorrhea-neisseria-gonorrhoeae-infection-in-adults-and-adolescents

Singh, S., & Singh, S. K. (2021). Psychological health and well-being in patients with sexually transmitted infections: A prospective cross-sectional study. *Indian Journal of Sexually Transmitted Diseases and AIDS, 42*(2), 125–131. https://doi.org/10.4103/ijstd.IJSTD_77_19

Sobel, J. D. (2023). Candida vulvovaginitis in adults: Treatment of acute infection. *UpToDate*. Retrieved March 19, 2024, from https://www.uptodate.com/contents/candida-vulvovaginitis-in-adults-treatment-of-acute-infection

Sobel, J. D. (2024). Bacterial vaginosis: Initial treatment. *UpToDate*. Retrieved March 19, 2024, from https://www.uptodate.com/contents/bacterial-vaginosis-initial-treatment

Sobel, J. D., & Mitchell, C. (2023a). Trichomoniasis: Clinical manifestations and diagnosis. *UpToDate*. Retrieved March 19, 2024, from https://www.uptodate.com/contents/trichomoniasis-clinical-manifestations-and-diagnosis

Sobel, J. D., & Mitchell, C. (2023b). Trichomoniasis: Treatment. *UpToDate*. Retrieved March 19, 2024, from https://www.uptodate.com/contents/trichomoniasis-treatment

Sobel, J. D., & Mitchell, C. (2023c). Bacterial vaginosis: Clinical manifestations and diagnosis. *UpToDate*. Retrieved March 19, 2024, from https://www.uptodate.com/contents/bacterial-vaginosis-clinical-manifestations-and-diagnosis

Staley, H., Shiraz, A., Shreeve, N., Bryant, A., Martin-Hirsh, P. P. L., & Gajjar, K. (2021). Interventions targeted at women to encourage the uptake of cervical screening. *Cochrane Database of Systematic Reviews, 9*(9), CD002834. https://doi.org/10.1002/14651858.CD002834.pub3

The Expert Working Group on the Canadian Guidelines for Sexually Transmitted Infections. (2008). *Canadian guidelines on sexually transmitted infections*. Public Health Agency of Canada.

The Foundation for AIDS Research. (2023). *Understanding the barriers to HIV care*. https://www.amfar.org/news/understanding-the-barriers-to-hiv-care/

The Well Project. (2023). *Women and HIV*. https://www.thewellproject.org/hiv-information/women-and-hiv

Tuddenham, S., & Ghanem, K. G. (2023). Approach to the patient with genital ulcers. *UpToDate*. https://www.uptodate.com/contents/approach-to-the-patient-with-genital-ulcers

U.S. Department of Health and Human Services. (n.d.). *Healthy People 2030*. https://health.gov/healthypeople

U.S. Preventive Services Task Force. (2020). *Sexually transmitted infections: Behavioral counseling*. https://www.uspreventiveservicestaskforce.org/uspstf/recommendation/sexually-transmitted-infections-behavioral-counseling

U.S. Preventive Services Task Force. (2023). *Prevention of acquisition of HIV: Preexposure prophylaxis*. https://uspreventiveservicestaskforce.org/uspstf/recommendation/prevention-of-human-immunodeficiency-virus-hiv-infection-pre-exposure-prophylaxis

Wiesenfeld, H. C. (2024). Pelvic inflammatory disease: Treatment in adults and adolescents. *UpToDate*. Retrieved March 19, 2024, from https://www.uptodate.com/contents/pelvic-inflammatory-disease-treatment-in-adults-and-adolescents

World Health Organization. (2023a). *Herpes simplex virus*. https://www.who.int/news-room/fact-sheets/detail/herpes-simplex-virus

World Health Organization. (2023b). *Sexually transmitted infections (STIs)*. https://www.who.int/news-room/fact-sheets/detail/sexually-transmitted-infections-(stis)

World Health Organization. (2024). *Cervical cancer*. https://www.who.int/news-room/fact-sheets/detail/cervical-cancer

Zhu, P., Qi, R. Q., Yang, Y., Huo, W., Zhang, Y., He, L., Wang, G., Xu, J., Zhang, F., Yang, R., Tu, P., Ma, L., Liu, Q., Li, Y., Gu, H., Cheng, B., Chen, X., Chen, A., Xiao, S., … Gao, X. H. (2022). Clinical guideline for the diagnosis and treatment of cutaneous warts (2022). *Journal of Evidence-Based Medicine, 15*(3), 284–301. https://doi.org/10.1111/jebm.12494

DEVELOPING CLINICAL JUDGMENT

PRACTICING FOR NCLEX

1. The nurse working in an internal medicine clinic recognizes their primary role related to STIs is
   a. case reporting of partners.
   b. detection and education.
   c. sexual counseling.
   d. diagnosis and treatment.
2. A 16-year-old comes to the clinic for routine care and is diagnosed with gonorrhea. The patient asks the nurse why she needs treatment for this since she has no symptoms. The nurse should explain that possible complications of lack of treatment could result in
   a. infertility, birth defects, and miscarriage.
   b. the need for future births by cesarean section.
   c. skin rashes and hearing loss.
   d. disseminated systemic infections.
3. The nurse is teaching a class to a group about contraceptive methods. Which method offers protection against STIs?
   a. Oral contraceptives
   b. Withdrawal
   c. Latex condom
   d. IUD
4. The nurse is teaching a patient about HIV transmission. Which example given by the patient of how the virus *cannot* be transmitted demonstrates understanding?
   a. Shaking hands
   b. Sharing drug needles
   c. Sexual intercourse
   d. Breastfeeding
5. The nurse is caring for a female patient in the clinic recently diagnosed with HPV. Upon assessment, the nurse is likely to note which finding?
   a. Profuse, pus-filled vaginal discharge
   b. Clusters of genital warts
   c. Single painless ulcer
   d. Multiple vesicles on genitalia
6. The nurse is discharging a female patient with PID. The discharge teaching plan for the patient should reinforce which potentially life-threatening complication?
   a. Involuntary infertility
   b. Chronic pelvic pain
   c. Depression
   d. Ectopic pregnancy
7. The nurse is working with a patient with a possible diagnosis of primary syphilis. Upon examination, the nurse may observe which finding on the external genitalia that would support this diagnosis?
   a. A highly variable skin rash
   b. A yellow-green vaginal discharge
   c. A nontender, indurated ulcer
   d. A localized gumma formation

CRITICAL THINKING EXERCISES

1. Sally, age 17, comes to the clinic saying she is in pain and has some "crud" between her legs. The nurse takes her into the examining room and questions her about her symptoms. Sally states she had numerous genital bumps that had been filled with fluid, then ruptured and turned into ulcers with crusts. In addition, she has pain on urination and overall body pain. Sally says she had unprotected sex with several males when she was drunk at a party a few weeks back, but she thought they were "clean."
   a. What STI would the nurse suspect?
   b. The nurse should give immediate consideration to which of Sally's complaints?
   c. What should be the goal of the nurse in teaching Sally about STIs?

STUDY ACTIVITIES

1. Go to the CDC website and select a specific STI of interest. Educate yourself about one specific STI thoroughly, and share your expertise with your clinical group.
2. Contact your local health department and request current statistics regarding three STIs. Ask them to compare the current number of cases reported to last year's report. Has the number of STIs increased or decreased? What may be some of the reasons for the change in the number of cases reported?
3. Request permission to attend a local STI clinic to shadow a nurse for a few hours. Describe the nurse's counseling role with patients and what specific information is emphasized to patients.
4. Two common STIs that appear together and are commonly treated together regardless of identification of the secondary one are ________________ and ______________________.
5. Genital warts can be treated with which therapies? Select all that apply.
   a. Penicillin
   b. Podophyllin
   c. Imiquimod
   d. Cryotherapy
   e. ART
   f. Acyclovir

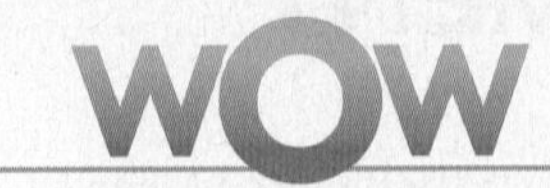

WORDS OF WISDOM

Focus on reducing fear, anxiety, pain, and loneliness in all patients diagnosed with a breast disorder.

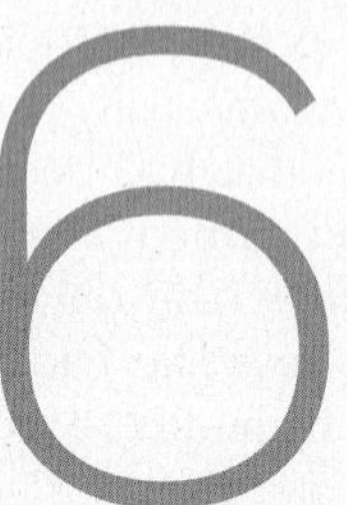

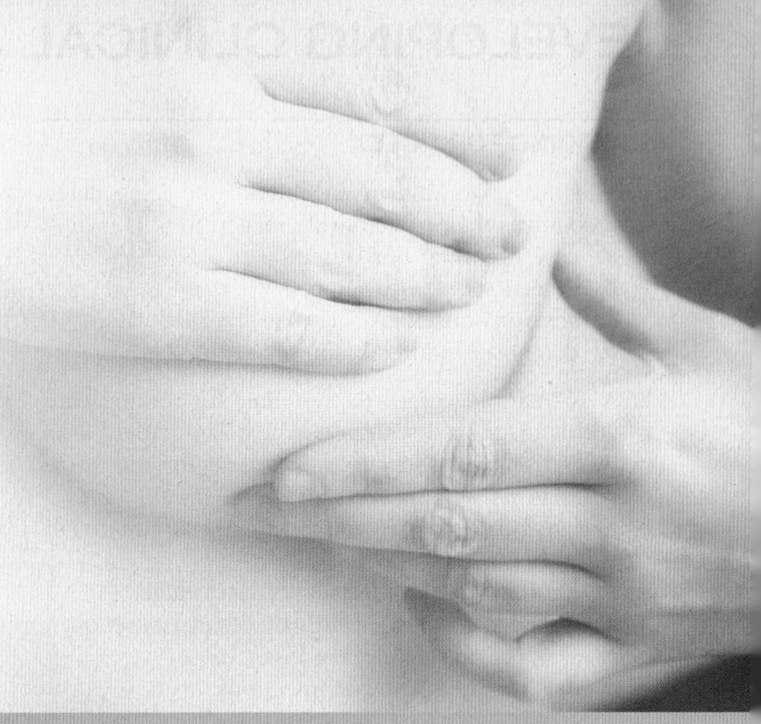

Disorders of the Breasts

LEARNING OBJECTIVES

Upon completion of the chapter, you will be able to:

1. Identify the incidence, risk factors, screening methods, and treatment modalities for benign breast conditions.
2. Analyze the incidence, risk factors, treatment modalities, and nursing considerations related to breast cancer.
3. Appraise reasons behind breast augmentation including the potential benefits and risks.
4. Outline preventive strategies for breast cancer through lifestyle changes and health screening.
5. Develop an educational plan to teach breast self-awareness to a group of high-risk patients.

Nancy hasn't been able to sleep well since she felt the lump in her left breast over a month ago, just after her 60th birthday. She knows she is at high risk because her mother died of breast cancer, but she can't bring herself to have it checked out.

KEY TERMS

benign breast disorder
breast augmentation (awg'men-tā'shŭn)
breast cancer
breast-conserving surgery
breast self-awareness
carcinoma
chemotherapy
duct ectasia (dŭkt ek-tā'zē-ă)
endocrine therapy
fibroadenomas (fī'brō-ad-ē-nō'măz)
mammography
modified radical mastectomy
nonproliferative epithelial lesions
simple (total) mastectomy

INTRODUCTION

The breasts, or mammary glands, are modified sweat glands lying over the pectoralis major muscles of the anterior chest wall. Physiologically, the breast is an organ specialized for milk formation to nourish offspring. Each breast extends approximately from the second to the seventh rib. The female breasts are closely linked to societal views of womanhood in American culture. The female breasts are seen as physical markers for transitions from one stage of life to another, and although the primary function of the breasts is lactation, they are often perceived as elements of a person's physical attractiveness and sexuality.

This chapter discusses assessments, screening procedures, and management of specific benign and malignant breast disorders. Nurses play a key role in helping patients maintain breast health by providing education and screening. A good working knowledge of early detection techniques, diagnosis, and treatment options is essential.

BENIGN BREAST DISORDERS

A **benign breast disorder** is any noncancerous breast abnormality. Benign breast disorders represent a wide range of conditions that come to clinical attention via imaging abnormalities or are discovered as palpable lesions upon examination. Benign breast disorders are a common complaint among patients from puberty to menopause. Though not life-threatening, benign disorders can cause pain and discomfort, and they account for a large number of visits to primary care providers. As the breasts are constantly undergoing changes due to hormonal influences, there is a lot of confusion in differentiating between normal and pathologic findings. Fully understanding benign breast disorders should enable the nurse to appropriately evaluate symptoms, determine which breast findings require treatment, and identify patients who are at increased risk for breast cancer.

Depending on the type of benign breast disorder, treatment may or may not be necessary. Although these disorders are benign, the emotional trauma patients experience can be severe. Fear, anxiety, disbelief, helplessness, and depression are just a few of the feelings a patient may have when they discover a lump in their breast. Many people believe that all lumps are cancerous, but in reality, approximately 90% of the lumps discovered are benign and need no treatment (Sabel, 2023a). Patience, support, and education are essential components of nursing care.

Some of the more commonly encountered benign breast disorders in females include nonproliferative epithelial lesions, such as breast cysts and fibrocystic changes of the breasts, and proliferative lesions atypia, such as fibroadenomas. Although these breast disorders are considered benign, fibrocystic changes of the breasts may carry a cancer risk depending on the type of atypical cells found, with prolific masses and hyperplastic changes occurring within the breasts. Generally speaking, fibrocystic changes and fibroadenomas carry little risk for cancer (Sabel, 2023b).

TAKE NOTE!

Nonlactational mastitis is a benign breast disorder that can be caused by *duct ectasia*, which occurs when the milk ducts become congested with secretions and debris, resulting in periductal inflammation. Patients with these types of abscesses present with greenish nipple discharge, nipple retraction, and noncyclical pain. Treatment is mainly supportive, including warm compresses, keeping the area clean, and wearing a supportive bra to help with discomfort; however, in some instances, antibiotics may be prescribed, or surgery may be warranted to remove the duct (Hamwi & Winters, 2023).

Nonproliferative Epithelial Lesions

Nonproliferative epithelial lesions are a type of benign breast lesions that include breast cysts (most common) and fibrocystic changes (Sabel, 2023b). It is estimated that 50% of all females will experience a noncancerous lump at some point in their life, with about 25% of these lumps being a breast cyst (Sabel, 2023b). Fibrocystic changes are caused by an overgrowth of fibrous tissues in the connective tissues supporting the breasts. This is frequently accompanied by the presence of fluid-filled cysts, which contribute to the lumpy feeling the patient may notice. Pain and tenderness occur that fluctuate with the menstrual cycle. Nonproliferative lesions are not associated with an increased risk of breast cancer (Sabel, 2023b).

Fibrocystic breast changes are most common between the ages of 30 and 50. The condition is rare in postmenopausal people not taking hormone replacement therapy (HRT) (Malherbe et al., 2023).

Therapeutic Management

Management of the symptoms of fibrocystic breast changes begins with self-care. For some patients, diet and lifestyle changes help reduce discomfort. Other options include wearing a supportive bra, taking over-the-counter pain relievers, applying warm or cool compresses, and limiting the consumption of salt and fat (Malherbe et al., 2023). Some people report that avoiding caffeine in coffee, tea, and soft drinks has improved their symptoms, although current research available does not show a clear link (American Cancer Society, 2022a). In severe cases, drugs including bromocriptine (a dopamine receptor agonist that lowers prolactin levels), tamoxifen (which blocks the effects of estrogen), or danazol (a synthetic male hormone) can be used to reduce the influence of estrogen on breast tissue. However, several undesirable side effects, including masculinization, have been documented. Aspiration or surgical removal of breast lumps will reduce pain and swelling by removing space-occupying masses, but they may recur.

Nursing Assessment

Nursing assessment consists of a health history, which should include issues having to do with the onset; frequency; quality and quantity of any pain, discharge, or masses; medications taken; physical activity; family history; reproductive history; any associated symptoms; physical examination of the breasts; and laboratory and diagnostic tests.

HEALTH HISTORY

Ask the patient about common clinical manifestations, which include lumpy, tender breasts and a feeling of fullness, particularly during the week before menses. Changes in breast tissue produce pain by nerve irritation from edema in connective tissue and by fibrosis from nerve pinching. The pain is cyclic and frequently dissipates after the onset of menses. The pain is described as a dull, aching feeling of fullness. Masses or nodularity usually appear in both breasts and are often found in the upper outer quadrants. Some patients also experience spontaneous clear to yellow nipple discharge when the breast is squeezed or manipulated.

PHYSICAL EXAMINATION

It is best to examine a patient's breast a week after menses, when swelling has subsided. Observe the breasts for fibrosis or thickening of the normal breast tissues, which occurs in the early stages. When performing a breast exam, the health care provider palpates the breasts using the pads of the middle three fingers. Techniques used are varied and based on provider preference, but a key approach is to follow a consistent pattern to prevent missing any areas (Henderson et al., 2023). Cysts form in the later stages and feel like multiple, smooth, well-delineated tiny pebbles or bumpy oatmeal under the skin (Fig. 6.1). On physical examination of the breasts, a few characteristics might be helpful in differentiating a cyst from a cancerous lesion. Cancerous lesions are typically fixed and painless and may cause skin retraction (pulling). Cysts tend to be mobile and tender and do not cause skin retraction in the surrounding tissue.

LABORATORY AND DIAGNOSTIC TESTS

Mammography can be helpful in distinguishing fibrocystic changes from breast cancer. Ultrasound is a useful adjunct to mammography for breast evaluation because it helps differentiate a cystic mass from a solid one. Ultrasound produces images of the breasts by sending sound waves through a gel applied to the breasts. Fine-needle aspiration biopsy can also be done to differentiate a solid tumor, cyst, or malignancy. A fine-needle aspiration biopsy uses a thin needle guided by ultrasound to the mass. In a method called stereotactic needle biopsy, a computer maps the exact location of the mass using mammograms taken from two angles, and the map is used to guide the needle.

Nursing Management

A nurse caring for a patient with fibrocystic breast changes can teach the patient about the condition, provide tips for self-care (Teaching Guidelines 6.1), suggest lifestyle changes, and demonstrate how to perform breast self-awareness to monitor the changes. Clinical Judgment & Nursing Process 6.1 presents a plan of care for a patient with fibrocystic breast changes.

TEACHING GUIDELINES 6.1 Relieving Symptoms of Fibrocystic Breast Changes

- Wear an extra supportive, well-made bra to prevent undue strain on the ligaments of the breasts to reduce discomfort.
- Take oral contraceptives as recommended by a health care practitioner to stabilize the monthly hormonal levels.
- Eat a low-fat diet rich in fruits, vegetables, and grains to maintain a healthy nutritional lifestyle and ideal weight.
- Consider taking supplemental vitamins E and D and evening primrose oil.
- Apply heat or cool packs to the breasts to help reduce pain.
- Take diuretics as recommended by a health care practitioner to counteract fluid retention and swelling of the breasts.
- Reduce salt intake to reduce fluid retention and swelling in the breasts.
- Take over-the-counter medications, such as acetylsalicylic acid (Aspirin) or ibuprofen (Motrin, Advil, Nuprin), to reduce inflammation and discomfort.
- Use thiamine and vitamin E therapy. This has been found helpful for some people, but research has failed to demonstrate a direct benefit from either therapy.
- Take medications as prescribed (e.g., bromocriptine, tamoxifen, or danazol).
- Discuss the possibility of aspiration or surgical removal of breast lumps with a health care practitioner.
- Restrict use of alcohol.

Malherbe, K., Khan, M., & Fatima, S. (2023). Fibrocystic breast disease. *StatPearls*. https://www.ncbi.nlm.nih.gov/books/NBK551609/; Shabanian, S., Rozbeh, A., Mohammadi, B., Ahmadi, A., & Arjmand, M.-H. (2023). The association between vitamin D deficiency and fibrocystic breast disorder. *Current Molecular Medicine, 24*(7), 899–905. https://doi.org/10.2174/1566524023666230623155659

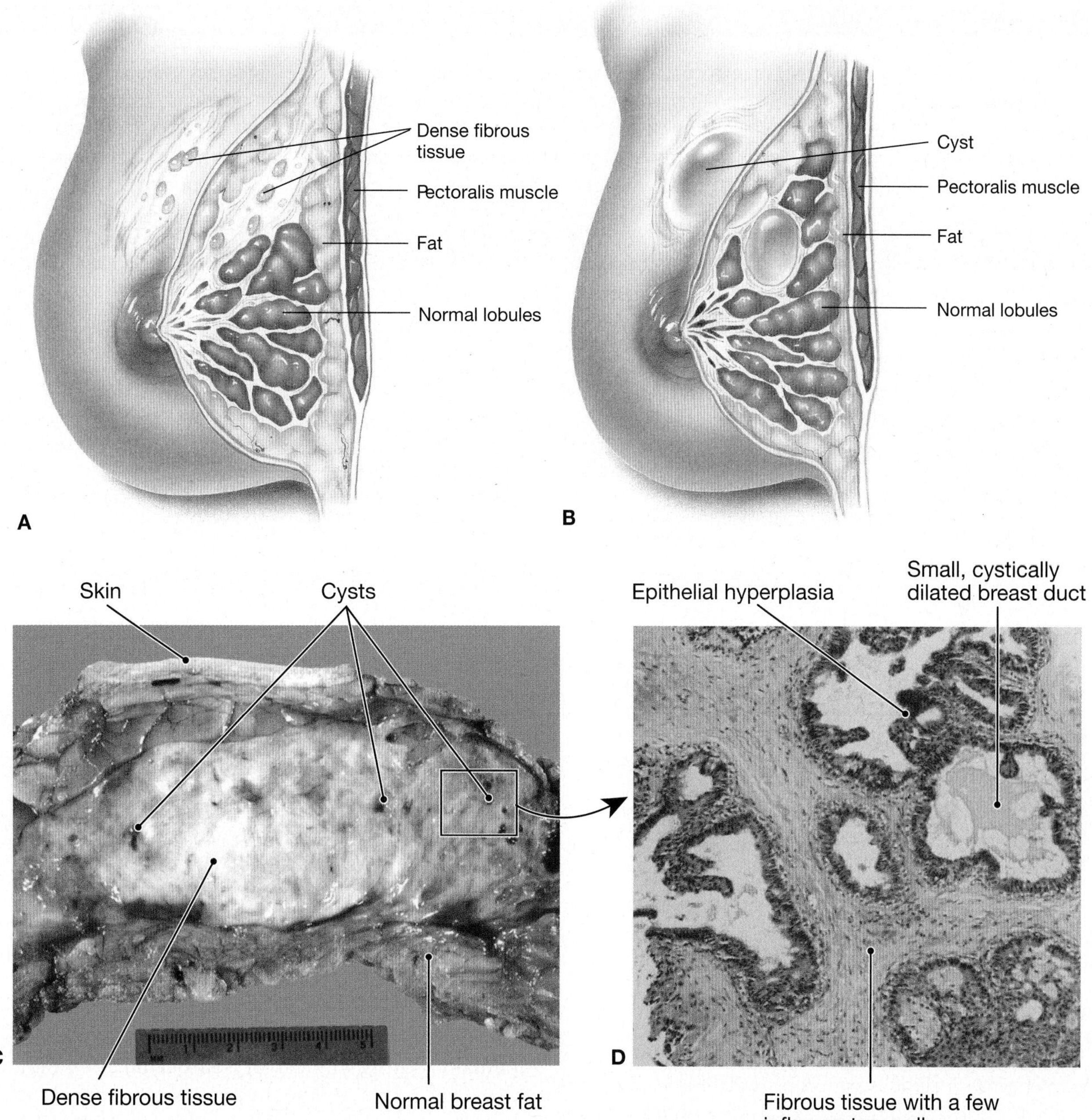

FIGURE 6.1 **A.** Fibrocystic breast changes. **B.** Breast cysts. **C.** This gross study shows that most of the abnormal tissue is fibrous. Cysts are relatively inconspicuous in this example. **D.** The microscopic study shows dense fibrous tissue containing dilated ducts lined by hyperplastic epithelium. (**A, B,** reprinted with permission from Stewart, J. G. [2017]. *Anatomical Chart Company atlas of pathophysiology* [4th ed.]. Lippincott Williams & Wilkins. **C, D,** reprinted with permission from McConnell, T. H. [2014]. *The nature of disease pathology for the health professions* [2nd ed.]. Lippincott Williams & Wilkins.)

Fibroadenomas

Fibroadenomas, also classified as proliferative lesions without atypia (cell abnormalities), are the most common benign tumor type of the breasts and account for up to half of all breast biopsies (Sabel, 2023b). They are the most common mass in females ages 15 to 35 years but can be found in females of any age (Breast Cancer Organization, 2022a; Sabel, 2023b). They are considered hyperplastic lesions associated with an aberration of normal development and involution rather than a neoplasm. Fibroadenomas can be stimulated by hormones, particularly estrogen, as they seem to grow during pregnancy and get smaller during menopause (Ajmal et al., 2023). They are composed of both fibrous and glandular tissue that feels round or oval, firm, rubbery, and smooth, and they are mobile and may be tender. They are usually unilateral but may present in both breasts (Sabel, 2023b). Giant fibroadenomas are frequently larger than 10 cm, and excision is recommended (Sabel, 2023b). Simple fibroadenomas are rarely associated with an increased risk of cancer (Sabel, 2023b).

CLINICAL JUDGMENT & NURSING PROCESS 6.1 Overview of the Patient With Fibrocystic Breast Changes

Sheree Rollins is a 37-year-old patient who comes to the clinic for her routine checkup. During the examination, she says, "Sometimes my breasts feel so heavy, and they ache a lot. I noticed a couple of lumpy areas in my breast last week just before I got my period. Is this normal? Now they feel like they're almost gone. Should I be worried?" The clinical breast examination reveals two small (pea-sized), mobile, slightly tender nodules in each breast bilaterally. No skin retraction noted. Previous mammogram revealed fibrocystic breast changes.

NURSING ANALYSIS: Pain related to changes in breast tissue

OUTCOME IDENTIFICATION AND EVALUATION

The patient will demonstrate a decrease in breast pain as evidenced by a pain rating of 1 or 2 on a pain rating scale of 0 to 10 and statements that pain is lessened.

INTERVENTIONS: *Relieving Pain*

- Ask the patient to rate her pain using a numeric pain rating scale *to establish a baseline.*
- Discuss with the patient any measures used to relieve pain *to determine effectiveness of the measures.*
- Encourage use of a supportive bra *to aid in reducing discomfort.*
- Instruct the patient in use of over-the-counter analgesics *to promote pain relief.*
- Advise the patient to apply warm compresses or allow warm water from the shower to flow over her breasts *to promote vasodilation and subsequent pain relief.*
- Tell the patient to reduce her intake of salt *to reduce risk of fluid retention and swelling leading to increased pain.*

NURSING ANALYSIS: Lack of knowledge related to fibrocystic breast changes and appropriate care measures

OUTCOME IDENTIFICATION AND EVALUATION

The patient will verbalize understanding of condition as evidenced by statements about the cause of breast changes and appropriate choices for lifestyle changes and demonstration of self-care measures.

INTERVENTIONS: *Providing Patient Education*

- Assess the patient's knowledge of fibrocystic breast changes *to establish a baseline for teaching.*
- Explain the role of monthly hormonal level changes, and describe the signs and symptoms *to promote understanding of this condition.*
- Teach the patient how to perform breast self-awareness after her menstrual period *to monitor for changes.*
- Encourage the patient to report any changes promptly *to ensure early detection of problems.*
- Suggest the patient speak with her primary care provider about the use of oral contraceptives *to help stabilize monthly hormonal levels.*
- Review lifestyle choices, such as eating a low-fat diet rich in fruits, vegetables, and grains, and adhering to screening recommendations *to promote health.*
- Discuss measures for pain relief *to minimize discomfort associated with breast changes.*

Therapeutic Management

Treatment may include a period of "watchful waiting" because many fibroadenomas stop growing or shrink on their own without any treatment. Other growths may need to be surgically removed if they do not regress or if they remain unchanged. Cryoablation (cryotherapy), an alternative to surgery, can also be used to remove a tumor. In this procedure, extremely cold gas is piped into the tumor using ultrasound guidance. The tumor freezes and dies. The current trend is toward a more conservative approach to treatment after careful evaluation and continued monitoring.

Nursing Assessment

Ask the patient about clinical manifestations of fibroadenomas. These lumps are felt as firm, rubbery, round, well-circumscribed, freely mobile nodules that might or might not be tender when palpated.

Breast fibroadenomas are usually detected incidentally during clinical or self-examinations and are usually located in the upper outer quadrant of the breast; more than one may be present (Fig. 6.2). Several other breast lesions have similar characteristics, so every patient with a breast mass should be evaluated to exclude cancer. A clinical breast examination by a health care provider is critical. In addition, diagnostic studies include imaging studies (mammography, ultrasound, or both) and some form of biopsy, most often a fine-needle aspiration, core needle biopsy, or stereotactic needle biopsy. The core needle biopsy removes a small cylinder of tissue from the breast mass, more than the fine-needle aspiration biopsy. If additional tissue needs to be evaluated, the advanced breast biopsy instrument (ABBI) is used. This instrument removes a larger cylinder of tissue for examination by using a rotating circular knife.

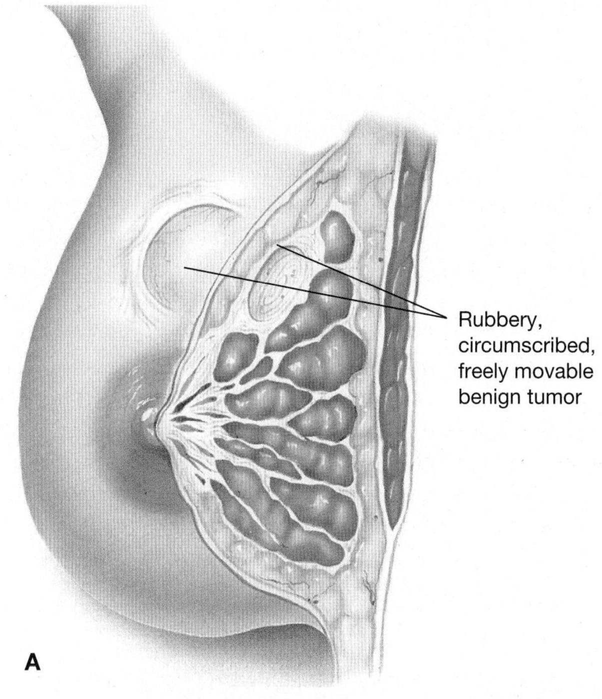

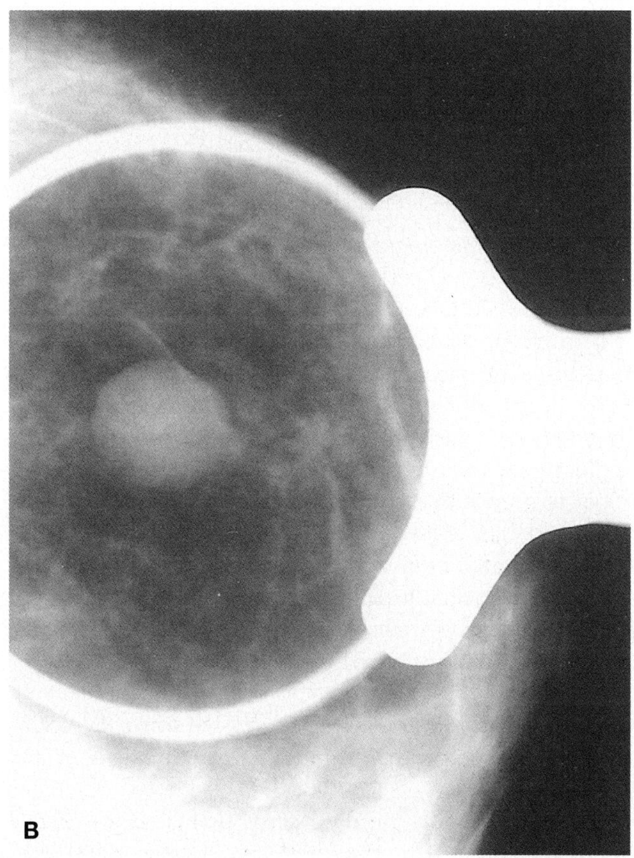

FIGURE 6.2 **A.** Fibroadenoma. (Reprinted with permission from Stewart, J. G. [2017]. *Anatomical Chart Company atlas of pathophysiology* [4th ed.]. Lippincott Williams & Wilkins.) **B.** Spot compression view of a smoothly marginated mass proven to represent a fibroadenoma. Ultrasonography demonstrated a solid mass.

Nursing Management

The nurse should urge the patient to return for revaluation in 6 months, practice breast self-awareness, and return annually for a clinical breast examination if recommended by their provider. Patients with high breast density are at a higher risk for future breast cancer (American Cancer Society [ACS], 2023a). Patients with low breast density are at a low risk, regardless of their benign pathologic diagnosis. Dense breast tissue also makes it harder for radiologists to visualize cancerous lesions on mammograms (ACS, 2023a). This is all the more reason for patients to have close monitoring over time.

MALIGNANT BREAST DISORDERS

Breast cancer is a neoplastic disease in which normal body cells mutate and grow out of control and create a malignant mass or tumor (Breast Cancer Organization, 2023a). It is the second most common cancer in females in the United States and the second leading cause of cancer deaths (lung cancer is first) among American females (ACS, 2024; CDC, 2023). See the Healthy People 2030 box below. Breast cancer accounts for one of every three cancers diagnosed in the United States (ACS, 2024).

It is estimated that about 310,700 new cases of invasive breast cancer will be diagnosed in females in the United States in 2024 (National Cancer Institute [NCI], 2024a). Black females have a higher rate of mortality from breast cancer than people in any other racial or ethnic group (ACS, 2024). Breast cancer can also affect males, but only 1% of all people diagnosed with breast cancer annually are male (NCI, 2024a).

The cause of breast cancer, while not well understood, is thought to be a complex interaction between environmental, genetic, and hormonal factors. Breast cancer is a progressive rather than a systemic disease, meaning that most cancers grow from a small size with

HEALTHY PEOPLE 2030

Objective	Nursing Significance
Reduce the female breast cancer death rate.	• Educate patients regarding risk factors, screening recommendations, and lifestyle modifications to decrease risk of breast cancer. • Support and encourage patients to maintain a healthy weight in adulthood, especially in the postmenopausal years.

Healthy People Objectives retrieved from http://www.healthypeople.gov

low metastatic potential to a larger size and greater metastatic potential. Tumor stage, size, and lymph node involvement are major predictors of metastatic potential and prognosis (Min et al., 2021).

CONSIDER THIS!

It was pouring down rain and I was driving alone along dark wet streets to my 8 a.m. appointment for a breast ultrasound. I recently had my annual mammogram, and the radiologist thought he saw something suspicious on my right breast. I was on my way to find out if his suspicions were right, and I couldn't keep focused on the road ahead. For the past few days, I had been so anxious, fearing the worst. I was playing it out in my mind, what I would do if...? What changes would I make in my life, and how would I react when told? I have been through such personal turmoil since that doctor announced he wanted "more tests."

Thoughts: This person is worrying and is emotionally devastated before they even have a conclusive diagnosis. Is this a typical reaction to a breast disorder? Why do patients sometimes fear the worst? Many patients use denial to mask their feelings and hope the doctor made a mistake or misread the mammogram. How would you react if you or a family member, friend, or significant other were confronted with a breast disorder?

Pathophysiology

Cancer is not just one disease but rather a group of diseases that result from unregulated cell growth. Without regulation, cells divide and grow uncontrollably until they eventually form a tumor. Extensive research has determined that all cancer is the result of changes in DNA or chromosome structure that cause the mutation of specific genes. Most genetic mutations that cause cancer are acquired sporadically, which means they occur by chance and are not necessarily due to inherited mutations, while 5% to 10% of breast cancers are hereditary (Breast Cancer Organization, 2024a). Cancer development is thought to be clonal in nature, which means that each cell is derived from another cell. If one cell develops a mutation, any daughter cell derived from that cell will have that same mutation, and this process continues until a malignant tumor forms.

Breast cancer starts in the epithelial cells that line the mammary ducts within the breast. The growth rate depends on hormonal influences, mainly that of estrogen and progesterone. The two major categories of breast cancer are noninvasive and invasive. Noninvasive (in situ) breast cancers are those that have not extended beyond the duct, lobule, or other point of origin into the surrounding breast tissue. Conversely, invasive (infiltrating) breast cancers have extended into the surrounding breast tissue with the potential to metastasize. Breast cancer metastasizes widely and to almost all organs of the body, but primarily to the bone, lungs, lymph nodes, liver, and brain. The first sites of metastases are usually local or regional, involving the chest wall or axillary supraclavicular lymph nodes or bone (Lee, 2024).

Invasive Ductal Carcinoma

By far the most common breast cancer is invasive or infiltrating ductal carcinoma (IDC), which represents 70% to 80% of all cases (Joe, 2023). **Carcinoma** is a malignant tumor that occurs in epithelial tissue; it tends to infiltrate and give rise to metastases. It spreads rapidly to axillary and other lymph nodes, even while small. IDC may take various histologic forms—well differentiated (Grade 1); slower growing, moderately differentiated (Grade 2); and poorly differentiated (Grade 3) and more aggressive (Bleiweiss, 2022). This common type of breast cancer starts in the ducts, breaks through the duct wall, and invades the fatty breast tissue.

Invasive Lobular Carcinoma

Invasive lobular carcinoma (ILC) is the second most common type of breast cancer. Invasive or infiltrating lobular carcinomas originate in the terminal lobular units of breast ducts and account for 8% of all cases of breast cancer (Joe, 2023). The peak incidence is in females in their early 60s (Trotter, 2022). It presents as an area of ill-defined thickening rather than a palpable mass.

Other Invasive Carcinomas

Several other histologic types account for the remaining invasive breast cancers seen. Several examples are discussed here. Tubular carcinoma accounts for less than 2% of invasive breast cancers. These tumors are often small, metastases are rare, and the prognosis is favorable (Bleiweiss, 2022). Mucinous or colloid carcinoma accounts for 1% to 2% of invasive breast cancers. It is more common in older patients, is characterized by the presence of large pools of mucus interspersed with small islands of tumor cells, and has a favorable prognosis (Bleiweiss, 2022). Medullary carcinoma accounts for 1% to 10% of invasive breast cancers. It occurs more frequently in younger females and grows into large tumor masses (Bleiweiss, 2022). Inflammatory breast cancer accounts for 1% to 5% of breast cancers; often presents with skin edema, redness, and warmth; and is an aggressive form. Typically, the patient is seen with advanced disease (Merajver, 2022). Paget disease accounts for 1% of breast cancers, originates in the nipple, and typically occurs with invasive ductal carcinoma or ducal carcinoma in situ (Trotter, 2022).

Staging of Breast Cancer

Cancer staging is the process of determining how much cancer is in the body and its location. The American Joint Committee on Cancer (AJCC) and the International

Union for Cancer Control classification system for tumors, nodes, and metastases (TNM) is used and was last updated in 2018 (Joe, 2023). This update incorporates biologic markers such as grade, estrogen receptor (ER) status, progesterone receptor status, and *HER2* (human epidermal growth factor receptor 2, a gene that can be a factor in developing breast cancer) status, along with tumor size, lymph node involvement, and evidence of metastasis (Burnstein, 2022). Additional test results, such as Oncotype DX, Mammaprint, and Prosigna, may be included to further assist in staging and treatment plan (ACS, 2021a, 2021b). Staging of breast cancer is more complex than that for some other cancers. As a general, rule the lower the number in staging, the less the cancer has spread; a higher number indicates the cancer has spread more. Tumor staging helps determine the probability that the tumor has metastasized to decide on an appropriate course of therapy and assess the patient's prognosis. The overall 5-year survival rate for a patient with stage I breast cancer is 99.6%; for a patient with stage II, it is about 86.7% (NCI, 2022a). The outlook is significantly decreased (about 32%) for patients with cancer that has metastasized (NCI, 2022a).

There is no completely accurate way to know whether the cancer has micro-metastasized to distant organs, but certain tests can help determine if the cancer has spread. A bone scan can be performed to assess the bones, and magnetic resonance imaging (MRI) can be used to detect metastases to the liver, abdominal cavity, lungs, or brain.

Risk Factors

Breast cancer is thought to develop in response to a number of related factors: aging; sex (99% of cases occur in females); delayed childbearing or nulliparity; never breastfeeding a child; genetic influences; *BRCA1* and *BRCA2* genetic mutations; history of receiving ionizing radiation to the chest, especially during puberty or young adulthood; high breast density on a mammogram; postmenopausal obesity; family history of cancer; hormonal factors such as early menarche younger than 12 years, late menopause older than 55 years, or first term pregnancy after 30 year old; HRT with estrogen plus progestin; recent use of oral contraceptives; physical inactivity; White race; and ingestion of two drinks or more of alcohol each day (NCI, 2022b; Trotter, 2022).

Since 1970, the number of new cases of breast cancer has gradually risen each year by about 1% (NCI, 2022a). This slight increase in incidence might be explained in a variety of ways. Better detection and screening tools are available, which have identified more cases; people are living to older ages when their risk increases; and lifestyle changes in Americans (such as having their first pregnancy at an older age and having fewer children) might have produced the higher numbers. Age is a significant risk factor. Because rates of breast cancer increase with age, estimates of risk at specific ages are more meaningful than estimates of lifetime risk. The estimated chances of a female being diagnosed with breast cancer between the ages of 30 and 70 are detailed in Table 6.1.

Risk factors for breast cancer can be divided into those that cannot be changed (nonmodifiable risk factors) and those that can be changed (modifiable risk factors). Nonmodifiable risk factors (NCI, 2024b) include:

- Sex (female)
- Aging (older than 50 years old)
- Genetic mutations (*BRCA1* and *BRCA2* genes)
- Personal history of ovarian or colon cancer
- Increased breast density on mammography
- Family history of breast cancer
- Personal history of breast cancer
- Race and ethnicity
- Previous abnormal breast biopsy (atypical hyperplasia)
- Exposure to chest radiation (radiation damages DNA)
- Previous breast radiation
- Early menarche (younger than 12 years old) or late onset of menopause (older than 55 years old), which represents increased estrogen exposure over the lifetime

Modifiable risk factors related to lifestyle choices (ACS, 2022b; NCI, 2024b) include:

- Not having children at all or not having children until after age 30; this increases the risk of breast cancer by not reducing the number of menstrual cycles.
- Postmenopausal use of estrogens and progestins, long-term use of menopausal hormone therapy (MHT)
- Not breastfeeding for up to a year after pregnancy; increase in the risk of breast cancer may be because it does not reduce the total number of lifetime menstrual cycles.
- Alcohol consumption; the risk increases with increased amounts of drinking.
- Smoking; exposure to carcinogenic agents found in cigarettes

TABLE 6.1 • Estimated Risk of Breast Cancer at Specific Ages

Age 30	1 out of 204
Age 40	1 out of 65
Age 50	1 out of 42
Age 60	1 out of 28
Age 70	1 out of 24

National Cancer Institute. (2020). *Breast cancer risk in American Women.* https://www.cancer.gov/types/breast/risk-fact-sheet

- Obesity after menopause; fat cells produce and store estrogen, so more fat cells create higher estrogen levels.
- Sedentary lifestyle and lack of physical exercise increase body fat, which houses estrogen.

Breast cancer incidence rates are higher in non-Hispanic White women compared with Black women; however, Black women are more likely to be diagnosed with an advanced stage cancer and are more likely to die from breast cancer (ACS, 2022c). The gap is due in part to social factors and inequalities in social determinants of health, including less access to high-quality treatment, higher prevalence of comorbidities such as obesity, and inadequate health insurance (ACS, 2022c). Some studies have also found genetic differences in the type of cancers that develop in people of African ancestry; for example, Black women are more likely to be diagnosed with aggressive, more difficult-to-treat breast cancer such as inflammatory breast cancer (Giaquinto et al., 2022).

The presence of risk factors, especially several of them, calls for careful ongoing monitoring and evaluation to promote early detection. Even though risk factors are important considerations, many patients with newly diagnosed breast cancer have no known risk factors. Although routine mammography and breast self-awareness are prudent for high-risk patients, these precautions may become lifesavers for early detection of cancerous lesions.

Screening for breast cancer begins with a routine history and physical exam. Nurses should take every opportunity to educate and emphasize the goal of breast cancer screening: Early detection reduces mortality. Screening may also include practicing breast self-awareness, clinical breast exams (varies by provider and based on risk status of the patient), and mammography.

Diagnosis

Many studies can be performed to make an accurate diagnosis of a malignant breast lump. Diagnostic tests include:

- Diagnostic mammography or digital mammography to determine breast density
- Magnetic resonance mammography (MRM) or breast MRI
- Ultrasound
- Fine-needle aspiration
- Stereotactic, ultrasound, or MRI-guided needle biopsy
- Sentinel lymph node biopsy
- Hormone receptor status
- HER2/neu genetic marker (Trotter, 2022)

Mammography

Mammography has become an accepted screening procedure that is sanctioned by most cancer organizations and is paid for annually by most health insurance agencies. Mammography can provide a diagnosis while screening for preclinical disease to prevent adverse outcomes, improve survival, and avoid intensive treatment. Mammography involves taking x-ray pictures of a bare breast while it is compressed between two plastic plates. This can identify and characterize a breast mass and detect an early malignancy. Radiologists are now required to report the density of breast tissue within their mammography report as people with dense breasts have a higher risk of breast cancer compared to those with less dense breasts (ACS, 2023a). Dense breasts can make cancer challenging to detect on a mammogram, leading to missed or underdiagnosed cancers (ACS, 2023a). It remains the gold standard screening method for females at average risk for breast cancer. It is relatively inexpensive, requires only a low dose of radiation, and reliably identifies malignant tumors, including those that are too small to feel. See the Healthy People 2030 box. It can also be used to investigate breast lumps and other symptoms. A screening mammogram typically consists of four views, two per breast (Fig. 6.3). Digital tomosynthesis, or 3D mammography, has been shown to detect more cancer and have fewer false positives (Slanetz & Lee, 2024). In the United States, 3D ultrasounds are available in most settings but may not be covered by all health plans.

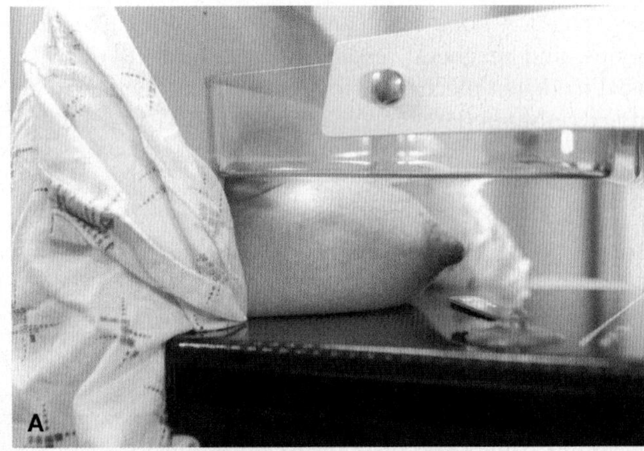

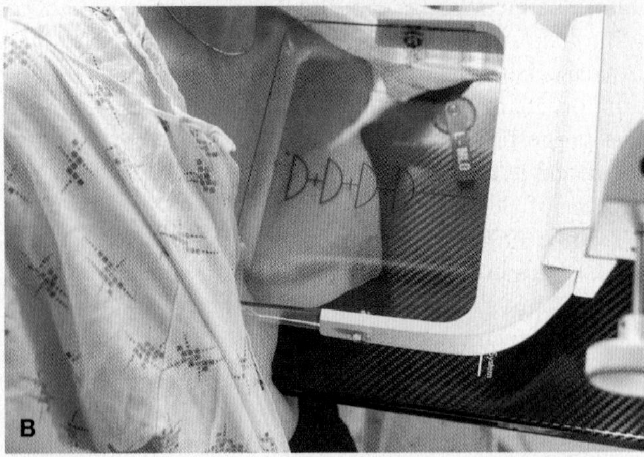

FIGURE 6.3 Mammography. **A.** A top-to-bottom view of the breast. **B.** A side view of the breast.

HEALTHY PEOPLE 2030

Objective	Nursing Significance
Increase the proportion of females who get screened for breast cancer.	• Educate patients using the latest evidence-based research to help them make informed decisions on when to begin mammogram screening based on their age, overall health status, and family history of cancer. • Encourage and support patients to get the proper screening by explaining the procedure and answering any questions or concerns to help increase adherence to recommendations.

Healthy People Objectives retrieved from http://www.healthypeople.gov

TEACHING GUIDELINES 6.2 Preparing for a Screening Mammogram

- Schedule the procedure just after menses when breasts are less tender.
- Do not use deodorant or powder on the day of the procedure, because they can appear on the x-ray film as calcium spots.
- Acetaminophen (Tylenol) or acetylsalicylic acid (aspirin) can relieve any discomfort after the procedure.
- Remove all jewelry from around the neck because the metal can cause distortions on the film image.
- Select a facility that is accredited by the American College of Radiology to ensure appropriate credentialed staff.

A diagnostic mammogram is performed when a patient has suspicious clinical findings on a breast examination or an abnormality has been found on a screening mammogram. A diagnostic mammogram uses additional views of the affected breast as well as magnification views. Diagnostic mammography provides the radiologist with additional detail to render a more specific diagnosis. Currently, digital mammography is being used to diagnose breast lesions.

Most patients find the 10-minute mammography procedure uncomfortable but not painful. Teaching Guidelines 6.2 offers tips for a patient to follow before they undergo this procedure.

Recommendations for mammogram screening vary among different professional societies such as the U.S. Preventive Services Task Force (USPSTF), the ACS, and the American College of Obstetricians and Gynecologists (ACOG). This conflicting information can be confusing to people trying to make decisions about breast cancer screening. Nurses can present the latest evidence-based research to help patients make informed decisions based on their age, overall health status, and family history of cancer (see Table 6.2 for a helpful outline). Because they contradict one another, there isn't any clear direction from the authoritative organizations; each patient and their health care provider should make the best choice for the patient. The associated risk is delay in detecting a breast lesion early when it could be treated earlier.

TABLE 6.2 • Mammogram Screening Recommendations for People at Average Risk of Developing Breast Cancer

U.S. Preventive Services Task Force (USPSTF)	Recommendations updated in 2023 include biennial screening mammography for females starting at age 40. In addition, the USPSTF concluded that the current evidence is insufficient and further research is needed to determine if patients with dense breasts should have additional screening via breast ultrasound or magnetic resonance imaging (MRI) and to assess the benefits and harms of screening mammography in patients 75 years and older.
American Cancer Society (ACS)	The ACS still recommends annual mammograms for females starting at age 45–54 and then biennially starting at age 55. For females aged 40–44, the decision is individualized and should be discussed with their provider.
American College of Obstetricians and Gynecologists (ACOG)	In 2021, ACOG reaffirmed their recommendation that screening mammograms be offered annually or biennially to females starting at age 40, initiated at ages 40–49 if the patient desires after counseling, and recommended by age 50 if the patient has not already started.

Barsouk, A., Saginala, K., Aluru, J. S., Rawla, P., & Barsouk, A. (2022). US cancer screening recommendations: Developments and the impact of COVID-19. *Medical Sciences, 10*(1), 16. https://doi.org/10.3390/medsci10010016; American Cancer Society. (2023b). *American Cancer Society recommendations for the early detection of breast cancer.* https://www.cancer.org/cancer/breast-cancer/screening-tests-and-early-detection/american-cancer-society-recommendations-for-the-early-detection-of-breast-cancer.html; U.S. Preventive Services Task Force. (2023). *Task force issues draft recommendation statement on screening for breast cancer.* https://www.uspreventiveservicestaskforce.org/uspstf/sites/default/files/file/supporting_documents/breast-cancer-screening-draft-rec-bulletin.pdf; American College of Obstetricians and Gynecologists. (2021). *Breast cancer risk assessment and screening in average-risk women.* https://www.acog.org/clinical/clinical-guidance/practice-bulletin/articles/2017/07/breast-cancer-risk-assessment-and-screening-in-average-risk-women; and Elmore, J. G., & Lee, C. I. (2024). Screening for breast cancer: Strategies and recommendations. *UpToDate.* Retrieved April 25, 2024, from https://www.uptodate.com/contents/screening-for-breast-cancer-strategies-and-recommendations

Magnetic Resonance Mammography

MRI of the breast or MRM of the breast uses a powerful magnetic field, radio waves, and a computer to produce detailed three-dimensional images of the breast structures. It allows for earlier detection because it can detect smaller lesions and provide finer detail. MRM has high sensitivity (71% to 100%) but is a costly tool (10 to 15 times more than a mammogram or ultrasound) (Slanetz, 2024). Contrast infusion is used to evaluate the rate at which the dye initially enters the breast tissue. The basis of the high sensitivity of MRM is the tumor angiogenesis (vessel growth) that accompanies a majority of breast cancers, even early ones. Currently, MRM is used for screening patients with a significantly high risk for breast cancer as it has a higher sensitivity than mammography or ultrasound in detecting breast cancer in high-risk populations (Slanetz, 2024). It may also be used in cases of inconclusive findings using other traditional methods such as mammography or ultrasound (Slanetz, 2024).

Fine-Needle Aspiration Biopsy or Core Biopsy

Fine-needle aspiration biopsy is done to identify a solid tumor, cyst, or malignancy. It is a simple office procedure that can be performed with or without anesthesia. A small (23- to 27-gauge) needle connected to a 10-mL or larger syringe is inserted into the breast mass, and suction is applied to withdraw the contents. The aspirate is then sent to the cytology laboratory to be evaluated for abnormal cells.

A core needle biopsy is much like a fine-needle biopsy except that a larger needle is used to withdraw small cylinders or cores of tissue from the abnormal area of the breast. It takes longer than the fine-needle biopsy, but more tissue is sampled to be tested.

Stereotactic Needle-Guided Biopsy

Stereotactic needle-guided biopsy is used to target and identify mammographically detected nonpalpable lesions in the breast. This procedure is less expensive than an excisional biopsy. The procedure takes place in a specially equipped room and generally takes about an hour. The patient is required to lie prone and must be able to remain still for approximately 20 minutes while the biopsy is taken. When proper placement of the breast mass is confirmed by digital mammograms, the breast is locally anesthetized and a spring-loaded biopsy gun is used to obtain two or three core biopsy tissue samples. After the procedure is finished, the biopsy area is cleaned and a sterile dressing is applied.

Sentinel Lymph Node Biopsy

With a sentinel lymph node biopsy, the clinician can determine whether breast cancer has spread to the axillary lymph nodes without having to do a traditional axillary lymph node dissection. Experience has shown that the lymph ducts of the breast typically drain to one lymph node before draining through the rest of the lymph nodes under the arm. The first lymph node is called the sentinel lymph node. If the sentinel node is negative, then there is a good chance the cancer has not spread outside of the breast (Breast Cancer Organization, 2022b). This procedure can be performed under local anesthesia. A radioactive blue dye is injected 2 hours before the biopsy to identify the afferent sentinel lymph node. The surgeon usually removes one to three nodes and sends them to the pathologist to determine whether cancer cells are present. The sentinel lymph node biopsy is usually performed before a lumpectomy to make sure the cancer has not spread. Removing only the sentinel lymph node can allow people with breast cancer to avoid many of the side effects (lymphedema) associated with a traditional axillary lymph node dissection. This procedure is associated with less morbidity compared to the axillary lymph node dissection, which results in more accurate staging, better axillary tumor control, and improved survival.

Hormone Receptor Status

Normal breast epithelium has hormone receptors and responds specifically to the stimulatory effects of estrogen and progesterone. Most breast cancers retain ERs, and for those tumors, estrogen will retain proliferative control over the malignant cells. It is therefore useful to know the hormone receptor status of the cancer to predict which patients will respond to hormone manipulation. Hormone receptor status reveals whether the tumor is stimulated to grow by estrogen and/or progesterone. Eighty percent of breast cancers in females tend to be ER-positive (have cancer cells that grow in response to estrogen), while 65% are both ER-positive and PR-positive (progesterone receptor) (Breast Cancer Organization, 2023d). To determine hormone receptor status, a sample of breast cancer tissue obtained during a biopsy or a tumor removed surgically during a lumpectomy or mastectomy is examined by a cytologist.

Therapeutic Management

People diagnosed with breast cancer have many treatments available to them. Generally, treatments fall into two categories: local and systemic. Local treatments are surgery and radiation therapy. Effective systemic treatments include chemotherapy, hormonal therapy, and immunotherapy.

Treatment plans are based on multiple factors, with the primary factors being the stage and grade of the cancer, the number of cancerous axillary lymph nodes, the presence of certain biomarkers such as hormone receptor status, and the patient's overall health and preferences (NCI, 2022c). These factors along with current medical advice will help guide the patient and health care provider, using shared decision making, to develop the best treatment plan for the patient. A combination of surgical options and adjunctive therapy is often recommended.

Another consideration in making decisions about a treatment plan is genetic testing for *BRCA1* and *BRCA2* genetic mutations. This genetic testing became available in 1995 and can identify people who have a significantly increased risk for breast cancer, ovarian cancer, and contralateral breast cancer; people with *BRCA1* and *BRCA2* mutations have up to a 72% lifetime risk of breast cancer by the age of 70 and up to a 50% risk of ovarian cancer within 20 years (Petrucelli et al., 2022). Most cases of breast and ovarian cancers are sporadic in nature rather than resulting from genetic inheritance (Peshkin & Isaacs, 2023). DNA (from a blood or saliva sample) is needed for mutation testing. The sample is sent to a laboratory for analysis. Testing positive for a *BRCA1* or *BRCA2* mutation can significantly alter health care decisions. The clinical importance of genetic testing of *BRCA1* and *BRCA2* in breast, ovarian, prostate, and pancreatic cancers is widely recognized, but there may be additional cancers linked to this genetic mutation. Knowing the risk posed by a *BRCA* mutation can help patients and their health care teams determine the prognosis and ultimately treatment. Some patients may choose to have a preventive mastectomy.

Surgical Options

The primary goal of breast cancer surgery is to successfully remove the breast cancer from the patient. A secondary and important goal is to reconstruct the removed tissue so as to allow the patient to feel whole from a psychological perspective. People with locally advanced breast cancer may undergo neoadjuvant chemotherapy or radiotherapy to shrink the tumor before surgical removal is attempted (Chalasani, 2023). The surgical options depend on the type and extent of cancer. The choices are typically either breast-conserving surgery (lumpectomy typically with radiation) or mastectomy with or without reconstruction. Research has shown that the survival rates in people with early-stage breast cancer who have undergone breast-conserving surgery followed by radiation are improved as compared to those who have had mastectomies (Ji et al., 2022). However, lumpectomy may not be an option for some patients, including those:

- Who are diagnosed with inflammatory breast cancer
- Who have two or more cancer sites that cannot be removed through one incision
- Whose surgery will not result in a clean margin of tissue
- Who have active connective tissue conditions (lupus or scleroderma) that make body tissues especially sensitive to the side effects of radiation
- Who have had previous radiation to the affected breast
- Who have a large tumor relative to breast size (Sabel, 2023c)

These decisions are made jointly between the patient and their surgeon. If mastectomy is chosen, because of either tumor characteristics or patient preference, then discussion needs to include breast reconstruction and regional lymph node biopsy versus sentinel lymph node biopsy. The mastectomy techniques are a simple mastectomy with sentinel node biopsy or a radical mastectomy with regional node biopsy. Removal of numerous lymph nodes places the patient at high risk for lymphedema.

BREAST-CONSERVING SURGERY

Breast-conserving surgery, the least invasive procedure, is the wide local excision (or lumpectomy) of the tumor along with a 1-cm margin of normal tissue. A lumpectomy is often used for early-stage localized tumors. The goal of breast-conserving surgery is to remove the suspicious mass along with tissue free of malignant cells to prevent recurrence. The results are less drastic and emotionally less scarring than having a mastectomy to the patient. Patients undergoing breast-conserving therapy may receive radiation after lumpectomy with the goal of eradicating residual microscopic cancer cells to limit locoregional recurrence. In patients who do not require adjuvant chemotherapy, radiation therapy typically begins 2 to 4 weeks after surgery to allow healing of the lumpectomy incision site. Radiation is administered to the entire breast at daily doses over a period of several weeks and has been found to increase survival rates over mastectomy without radiation (Kunkler et al., 2023).

A sentinel lymph node biopsy may also be performed since the lymph nodes draining the breast are located primarily in the axilla. Theoretically, if breast cancer is to metastasize to other parts of the body, it will probably do so via the lymphatic system. If malignant cells are found in the nodes, more aggressive systemic treatment may be needed.

MASTECTOMY

A **simple (total) mastectomy** is the removal of all breast tissue, the nipple, the areola, and the underlying fascia of the pectoral muscle. The axillary nodes and pectoral muscles are spared. A sentinel lymph node dissection may be performed (Breast Cancer Organization, 2023b). This procedure would be used for a large tumor or multiple tumors that have not metastasized to adjacent structures or the lymph system.

A **modified radical mastectomy** involves removal of breast tissue, underlying fascia of the pectoralis muscle, and a few positive axillary nodes (usually about 10). Other surgical techniques include a skin-sparing mastectomy (most of the skin over the breast is left intact) and a nipple-areolar-sparing mastectomy (Kwong & Sabel, 2022). In conjunction with the mastectomy, lymph node surgery (removal of underarm nodes) may need to be done to reduce the risk of distant metastasis and improve a patient's chance of long-term survival. For patients with a positive sentinel node biopsy, 10 to 20 underarm lymph nodes may need to be removed. Complications associated with axillary lymph node surgery include nerve damage during surgery, causing temporary numbness down the upper aspect of the arm; seroma formation (fluid buildup) followed by wound infection; restrictions in arm mobility (some patients need physiotherapy); and lymphedema (swelling related to the lymph glands). In many patients, lymphedema can be avoided or minimized by:

- Avoiding using the affected arm for drawing blood, inserting intravenous lines, or measuring blood pressure (can cause trauma and possible infection)
- Self-monitoring lymphedema and seeking medical care immediately if the affected arm swells
- Keeping weight under control, as higher body weight can worsen lymphedema
- Taking steps to reduce the risk of injury or infection to the arm including good skin hygiene and nail care
- Avoiding sunburn and exposure to excessive heat from saunas and hot tubs
- Engaging in aerobic exercise and weight-lifting to reduce the severity of lymphedema
- Avoiding wearing clothes that restrict lymphatic fluid flow to and from the arm
- Wearing a well-fitted compression sleeve to promote drainage return (Mehrara, 2022)

People having mastectomies must decide whether to have further surgery to reconstruct the breast. If the patient decides to have reconstructive surgery, it is ideally performed immediately after the mastectomy. The patient must also determine whether they want the surgeon to use saline implants or natural tissue from the patient's abdomen (transverse rectus abdominis muscle (TRAM) flap method) or back (latissimus dorsi (LAT) flap method).

If reconstructive surgery is desired, the ultimate decision regarding the method will be determined by the patient's anatomy (e.g., sufficient fat and muscle to permit natural reconstruction) and overall health status. Both procedures require a prolonged recovery period.

Some patients opt for no reconstruction, and many of them choose to wear breast prostheses. Some prostheses are worn in the bra cup and others fit against the skin or into special pockets in their clothing.

Whether to have reconstructive surgery is an individual and complex decision. Each patient must be presented with all of the options and then allowed to decide. The nurse can play an important role here by presenting the facts to the patient so that they can make an intelligent decision to meet their unique situation. Breast reconstruction surgery can help restore the look and feel of the breast after a mastectomy. Performed by a plastic surgeon, breast reconstruction can be done immediately after the mastectomy or at a later date. Breast reconstruction can be done with breast implants (filled with saline or silicone gel); natural tissue flaps (using skin fat and muscle from the patient's own body); or a combination of both. Side effects or complications include risk of rupture, hardening of the tissues around the implant, infection, and pain. Nurses need to educate the patient about these potential problems and make sure they understand before consenting to breast reconstruction. See Figure 6.4 for examples of postmastectomy and reconstruction.

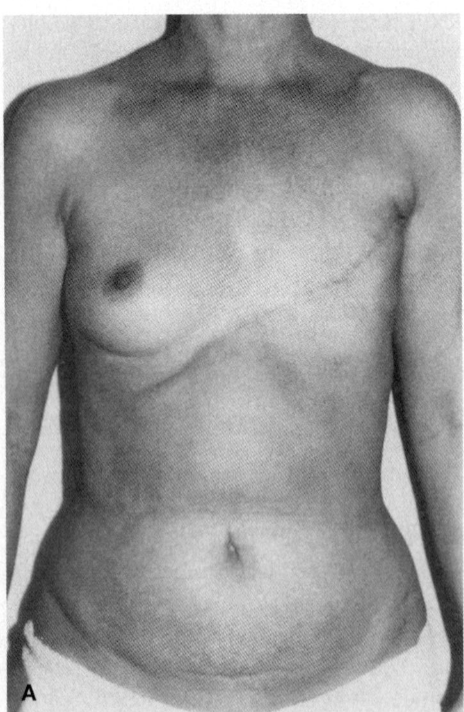

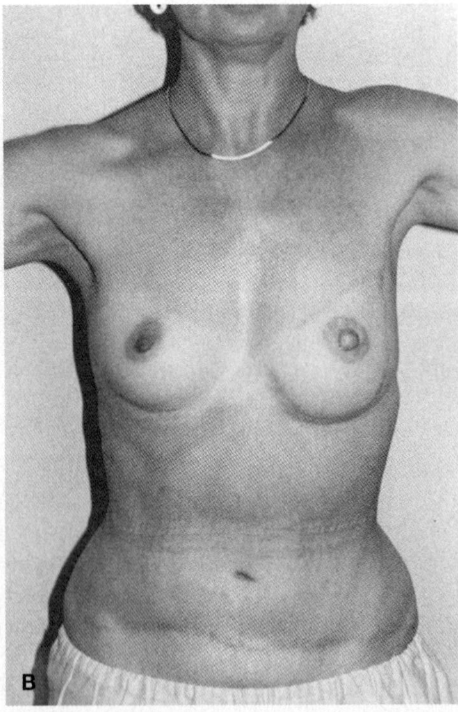

FIGURE 6.4 Before (**A**) and after (**B**) photos of postmastectomy and reconstruction.

BREAST AUGMENTATION

Breast augmentation is a surgical procedure by which the breast size is enhanced. It is a common surgical procedure with patients undergoing it with implants for a variety of reasons ranging from aesthetic to reconstructive surgery following a mastectomy. Saline-filled or silicone gel-filled implants are used in cosmetic enhancement and reconstructive surgeries, but both have an outer silicone shell. The exact anatomic placement of breast implants can vary, but the location is typically subglandular (over the pectoral muscle) or subpectoral (under the muscle). Breast implants are not lifetime devices, but most are guaranteed for approximately 10 years in case of rupture. Breast augmentation with implants is not without risks. Potential complications include capsular contracture, rippling, implant rupture, asymmetry, breast pain, infection, or hematoma. Capsular contraction occurs when scar tissue forms, contracts, and hardens around the implant. Rippling most often occurs when wrinkles form in the implant or as a complication of contracture (U.S. Food & Drug Administration, 2023).

Breast examination in patients with reconstructive surgery is done exactly the same way as for natural breasts. Breasts with implants in place usually feel firmer than normal breast tissue on palpation due to the formation of a fibrotic band or capsule around the implant. If implants are used, press firmly inward at the edges of the implant to feel the ribs beneath it.

Adjunctive Therapy

Adjunctive therapy is supportive or additional therapy that is recommended after surgery. Adjunctive therapies include local therapy such as radiation therapy and systemic therapies using chemotherapy, hormonal therapy, and immunotherapy.

RADIATION THERAPY

Radiation therapy (also called radiotherapy) uses high-energy rays to destroy cancer cells that might have been left behind in the breast, chest wall, or underarm area after a tumor has been removed surgically. Radiation therapy damages all cells, both healthy cells and cancer cells, but its effect on cancer cells is greater (DePolo, 2024c). Traditionally, serial radiation doses were given 5 days a week to the tumor site for 5 to 7 weeks postoperatively, but advances in technology have led to overall shorter treatment durations (Taghian, 2024). Each treatment takes only a few minutes and is typically painless, but the dose is cumulative; therefore, over time, local irritation or discomfort may occur. The goal of adjuvant radiation therapy is to eradicate residual microscopic cancer cells in order to reduce the risk of recurrence and to improve survival (Taghian, 2024).

Side effects of radiation therapy include redness; swelling; skin changes in the treated area such as sunburnlike appearance, itching, soreness, or burning; and breast pain and fatigue (DePolo, 2024a). Changes to the breast tissue and skin usually resolve in about 6 to 12 months in most patients (DePolo, 2024a). This type of therapy can be given with external beam radiation, which delivers a carefully focused dose of radiation from a machine outside the body, or internal radiation, or with brachytherapy, in which tiny pellets that contain radioactive material are placed into the tumor.

High-dose brachytherapy is used only after a lumpectomy (DePolo, 2024b). A balloon catheter is used to insert radioactive seeds into the breast after the tumor has been removed surgically. The seeds deliver a concentrated dose directly to the operative site; this is important because most cancer recurrences in the breast occur at or near the lumpectomy site (DePolo, 2024b). This allows a high dose of radiation to be delivered to a small target volume with a minimal dose to the surrounding normal tissue. This procedure takes a few days as opposed to the 3 to 7 weeks that traditional radiation therapy takes; it also eliminates the need to delay radiation therapy to allow for wound healing. Brachytherapy is an option used after breast-conserving surgery in selected patients as an alternative to whole breast irradiation (DePolo, 2024b). Side effects of brachytherapy include redness or discharge around catheters, fever, and infection. Daily cleansing of the catheter insertion site with a mild soap and application of an antibiotic ointment will minimize the risk of infection.

Newer types of radiation therapy include intraoperative radiation therapy (radiation therapy delivered during the surgery to remove the tumor) and proton therapy (which uses protons instead of x-rays to treat the cancer) (DePolo, 2024c). Research is ongoing to evaluate new types and the impact of all of these advances in radiation therapy.

CHEMOTHERAPY

Chemotherapy refers to the use of drugs that are toxic to all cells and interfere with a cell's ability to reproduce. They are particularly effective against malignant cells but affect all rapidly dividing cells, especially those of the skin, the hair follicles, the mouth, the gastrointestinal tract, and the bone marrow. Breast cancer is a systemic disease in which micro-metastases may already be present in other organs by the time the breast cancer is diagnosed. Chemotherapeutic agents perform a systemic "sweep" of the body to reduce the chances that distant tumors will start growing. Chemotherapy can be given before surgery (referred to as neoadjuvant chemotherapy) or after surgery (referred to as adjuvant chemotherapy).

Chemotherapy may be indicated for patients who are premenopausal, with positive lymph nodes, or with cancer of an aggressive type (DePolo, 2024d). Chemotherapy is prescribed in regimens and cycles, with each period of treatment followed by a rest period. Treatment typically lasts 3 to 6 months, depending on the dose and medications used and the patient's health status.

Different classes of drugs affect different aspects of cell division and are used in combinations or "cocktails." There are many chemotherapeutic agents that can be used to treat breast cancer, and the medication used will be based on individual factors of each patient.

Side effects of chemotherapy depend on the agents used, the intensity of dosage, the dosage schedule, the type and extent of cancer, and the patient's physical and emotional status. Nurses need to remain updated on new treatments and the side-effect profiles and recognize that each patient will have individual reactions. This knowledge is vital in providing evidence-based, personalized care for patients receiving these treatments. However, typical side effects include nausea and vomiting, diarrhea or constipation, hair loss, weight loss, stomatitis, fatigue, and immunosuppression. The most serious is bone marrow suppression (myelosuppression). This causes an increased risk of infection, bleeding, and a reduced red blood cell count, which can lead to anemia. Treatment of the side effects can generally be addressed through appropriate support medications such as antinausea drugs. In addition, growth-stimulating factors, such as epoetin alfa (Procrit) and filgrastim (Neupogen), help keep blood counts from dropping too low. Counts that are too low can stop or delay the use of chemotherapy.

HORMONAL THERAPY

One of estrogen's normal functions is to stimulate the growth and division of healthy cells in the breasts. However, in people with hormone receptor-positive breast cancer, this normal function contributes to the growth and division of cancer cells.

The objective of **endocrine therapy** is to block or counter the effect of estrogen. Approximately two out of three females with breast cancer have hormone-sensitive disease (ER-positive and/or progesterone receptor-positive), and adjuvant hormone therapy plays an essential role in reducing the risk of recurrence and improving survival (ACS, 2023c). Hormone therapy acts by preventing the body from producing estrogen or by eliminating the hormone receptors on cells, making it impossible for estrogen to properly attach itself to breast cell tissue to grow (NCI, 2022d). Several different drug classes are used to interfere or block ERs. They include selective estrogen receptor modulators (SERMs), ER down regulators, aromatase inhibitors, and luteinizing hormone–releasing hormone agonists (NCI, 2022d). Many patients with ER-positive breast cancer take a hormonelike medication—known as a SERM antiestrogenic agent—daily for up to 5 to 10 years after initial treatment. Certain areas in the female body (breasts, uterus, ovaries, skin, vagina, and brain) contain specialized hormone receptors that allow estrogen to enter the cell and stimulate it to divide. SERMs enter these same receptors, and estrogen cannot attach; this therefore turns off the signal for growth inside the cell (Breast Cancer Organization, 2022c). A commonly used SERM is tamoxifen. Although it works well in preventing the further spread of cancer, it is also associated with increased incidence of endometrial cancer, deep vein thrombosis, stroke, cataracts, and liver problems (Breast Cancer Organization, 2022c). Common side effects include hot flashes, depression, loss of libido, vaginal discharge, nausea, mood swings, dry skin, constipation, thinning hair, and fatigue (Breast Cancer Organization, 2022c).

Another class of endocrine agents, aromatase inhibitors, works by inhibiting the conversion of androgens to estrogens. Aromatase inhibitors include letrozole (Femara, 2.5 mg daily), exemestane (Aromasin, 25 mg daily), and anastrozole (Arimidex, 1 mg daily for 5 years), all of which are taken orally. These are usually given to patients with breast cancer who are postmenopausal or whose ovaries no longer produce estrogen because the drugs block the conversion of androgens into estrogens (Breast Cancer Organization, 2023c). Research is ongoing to study the effects of aromatase inhibitors in premenopausal patients given ovarian suppression medication (Breast Cancer Organization, 2023c). Side effects include joint pain or stiffness, heart problems, osteoporosis, and broken bones (Breast Cancer Organization, 2023c).

IMMUNOTHERAPY

Immunotherapy, used as an adjunct to surgery, represents an attempt to stimulate the body's natural defenses to recognize and attack cancer cells. It uses the immune system to identify, target, and attack cancer cells. Pembrolizumab (Keytruda), Trastuzumab emtansine (Kadcyla), trastuzumab (Herceptin), and pertuzumab (Perjeta) are a few immunotherapy options (Breast Cancer Organization, 2024b). Immunotherapy is a relatively new treatment with less extensive research than that for other treatment modalities (Breast Cancer Organization, 2024b). However, immunotherapy treatment has the potential to improve outcomes for patients with breast cancer.

Concept Mastery Alert

Tamoxifen Versus Trastuzumab in Breast Cancer Treatment

Tamoxifen is a SERM used to prevent the further spread of breast cancer in patients with ER-positive breast cancer. Trastuzumab is a monoclonal antibody used in the treatment of breast cancer and is considered immunotherapy.

Nursing Process for the Patient With Breast Cancer

When a patient is diagnosed with breast cancer, they face treatment that may alter their body shape, may make them feel unwell, and may not carry a certainty of cure. Nurses can support patients from the time of diagnosis, through the treatments, and through follow-up after the surgical and adjunctive treatments have been completed. Allowing patients the time to ask questions and to discuss any necessary preparations for treatment is critical. As our understanding of breast disorders keeps improving, treatments continue to change.

Although the goal of treatment remains improved survival, increasing emphasis is being focused on prevention. Breast cancer prevention measures focus on evaluating and reducing risk factors. Approaches for reducing breast cancer risk include lifestyle modifications (diet and physical exercise); maintaining a healthy weight; consuming less meat; eating more fruit, vegetables, and whole grains; limiting alcohol; quitting smoking, chemoprevention (SERMs and aromatase inhibitors); and prophylactic surgery (bilateral salpingo-oophorectomy and bilateral prophylactic mastectomy) for patients at high risk (Breast Cancer Research Foundation, 2022). Nurses can have an impact on early detection of breast disorders, treatment, and symptom management. A nurse who is involved in the patient's treatment plan from the beginning can effectively offer support throughout the whole experience.

Teamwork is important in breast screening and caring for patients with breast disorders. Treatment is often fragmented between the hospital and community treatment centers, and this can be emotionally traumatic for the patient and their family. The advances being made in the diagnosis and treatment of breast disorders mean that guidelines are constantly changing, requiring all health care providers to keep up to date. Informed nurses can provide support, information, and most importantly, continuity of care for the patient undergoing treatment for a breast problem.

The nurse plays a particularly important role in providing psychological support and self-care teaching to patients with breast cancer. Nurses can influence both physical and emotional recovery, which are both important aspects of care that help in improving the patient's quality of life and the ability to survive. The nurse's role should extend beyond helping patients; spreading the word in the community about screening and prevention is a big part of the ongoing fight against cancer. The community should see nurses as both educators and valued sources of credible information. This role will help improve clinical outcomes while achieving high levels of patient satisfaction.

Remember Nancy from the chapter opener. Is this a typical response for someone discovering a lump in their breast? Nancy confides her discovery of the lump and her worries to you. What advice would you give her?

Assessment

Early breast cancer has no symptoms. The earliest sign of breast cancer is often an abnormality seen on a screening mammogram before the patient or the health care provider feels it. A healthy, asymptomatic presentation is typical. However, symptoms may include a lump in the breast that is usually nontender, fixed, and hard with irregular borders. In the patient presenting with a breast disorder, take a thorough history of the problem and explore risk factors for breast cancer. Assess the patient for clinical manifestations of breast cancer, such as changes in breast appearance and contour which become apparent with advancing breast cancer (ACS, 2022d). These changes include:

- Continued and persistent changes in the breast
- A lump or thickening in one breast
- Breast or nipple pain
- Unusual breast swelling or asymmetry
- Skin dimpling that looks like an orange peel
- A lump or swelling in the axilla or near collarbone
- Changes in skin color or texture (red, dry, flaking, or thickened)
- Nipple retraction, tenderness, or discharge

The recommendations available from professional societies on whether or not to perform a clinical breast exam on people at average risk is conflicting. It will be very important to assess the patient for risk factors and to discuss the option of a clinical breast exam. In cases where the patient has a complaint or concern about their breast health, the advanced practice provider should perform an exam. For patients with no complaints and average risk, ACOG recommends the practitioner offer a clinical breast exam every 3 to 5 years to patients 25 to 39 years of age and every year to patients 40 years of age or older (ACOG, 2021). The ACS currently does not recommend a clinical breast exam in people at average risk, while the USPSTF states there is currently insufficient evidence to recommend for or against regular clinical breast exam (ACOG, 2021; ACS, 2023b). Helpful characteristics in evaluating palpable breast masses are described in Table 6.3. If a lump can be palpated, the cancer has been there for quite some time.

Be cognizant of the impact that breast cancer has on a person's emotional state, coping ability, and quality of life. Patients may experience sadness, vulnerability, loss of control, alteration of body image and integrity, anger, the illness's impact on relationships,

TABLE 6.3 • Characteristics of Benign Versus Malignant Breast Masses

Benign Breast Masses Are Described as	Malignant Breast Masses Are Described as
• Frequently painful • Firm, rubbery mass • Bilateral masses • Induced nipple discharge • Regular margins (clearly delineated) • No skin dimpling • No nipple retraction • Mobile, not affixed to the chest wall • No bloody discharge	• Hard on palpation • Painless • Irregularly shaped (poorly delineated) • Immobile, fixed to the chest wall • Skin dimpling • Nipple retraction • Unilateral mass • Bloody, serosanguineous, or serous nipple discharge • Spontaneous nipple discharge

fear of mortality, the need to reprioritize their life, and guilt as a result of having breast cancer. Closely monitor patients for their psychosocial adjustment to diagnosis and treatment and be able to identify those who need further psychological intervention. By giving practical advice, the nurse can help the patient adjust to their altered body image and accept the changes in their life.

Because family members play a significant role in supporting patients through breast cancer diagnosis and treatment, assess the emotional distress of family members during the course of treatment, and if needed, make a referral for psychological counseling. By identifying interpersonal strain, negative psychosocial side effects of cancer treatment can be minimized.

Nursing Analysis

Appropriate nursing analyses for a patient with a diagnosis of breast cancer might include:

- Altered body image related to:
  - Loss of body part (breast)
  - Loss of femininity
  - Loss of hair due to chemotherapy
- Fear related to:
  - Diagnosis of cancer
  - Prognosis of disease
- Knowledge deficiency related to:
  - Cancer treatment options
  - Reconstructive surgery decisions
  - Breast self-awareness

Nursing Interventions

Offer information, support, and perioperative care to patients diagnosed with breast cancer who are undergoing treatment. See Evidence-Based Practice 6.1. Implement health promotion and disease prevention strategies to minimize the risk for developing breast cancer and to promote optimal outcomes.

Remember Nancy, who discovered a breast lump? You offer to go with her to the doctor. After a full examination and several diagnostic tests, the results come back positive for breast cancer. What treatment options does Nancy have, and what factors need to be considered in selecting those options?

EVIDENCE-BASED PRACTICE 6.1

Specialist Breast Care Nurses for Supportive Care of Patients With Breast Cancer.

BACKGROUND

Breast cancer is one of the most feared conditions that impact numerous people globally. Survival rates have improved tremendously in the last few decades due to treatment advances, better screening methods, and a multiprofessional management approach. Supportive breast care nurses can meet patients when they are diagnosed and provide information, emotional support, and patient advocacy and assist them to navigate through the health care pathway toward recovery.

STUDY

Nine randomized controlled studies with a total of 1,469 participants were included. The studies compared a specialist breast care nurse intervention with usual care. The evidence from all of the studies was summarized and analyzed; special attention was paid to the consistency of the results.

Findings

The evidence suggests that psychosocial interventions carried out by specially trained breast care nurses for patients with a primary diagnosis of breast cancer can improve their quality of life and reduce their rates of depression, anxiety, distress, and physical symptoms. Telephone follow-up interventions by the nurses were equally effective in demonstrating high levels of satisfaction by the study participants.

Nursing Implications

People going through the emotional journey of breast cancer treatment are positively impacted by interventions from nurses educated with extensive breast cancer knowledge who address their multifactorial needs. After diagnosis, patients with breast cancer are at high risk to experience psychological distress and may have decreased health-related quality of life. Patients with breast cancer need support from nurses who can provide anticipatory guidance for them throughout this experience. This can be a new role for nurses as part of the multidisciplinary health care team to improve the quality-of-life outcomes for patients with breast cancer.

Brown, T., Cruickshank, S., & Noblet, M. (2021). Specialist breast care nurses for support of women with breast cancer. *Cochrane Database of Systematic Reviews, 2021*(2), CD005634. https://doi.org/10.1002/14651858.CD005634.pub3

Providing Patient Education

Help the patient and their partner and/or family members prioritize the voluminous amount of information given to them so that they can make informed decisions. Explain all treatment options in detail so the patient and their family understand them. By preparing an individualized packet of information and reviewing it with the patient and their family, the nurse can help the patient understand their specific type of cancer, the diagnostic studies and treatment options they may choose, and the goals of treatment. For example, nurses play an important role in educating patients about the use of endocrine therapies, observing patients' experiences with treatment, and communicating those observations to their primary health care providers to make dosage adjustments, in addition to contributing to the knowledge base of endocrine therapy in the treatment of breast cancer.

Providing information is a central role of the nurse in caring for the patient with a diagnosis of breast cancer. This information can be given via telephone counseling, one-to-one contact, and pamphlets. Telephone counseling with patients and their partners and families may be an effective method to improve symptom management and quality of life.

Providing Emotional Support

Many people perceive their breasts as intrinsic to their femininity, self-esteem, and sexuality, and the possibility of losing a breast can provoke extreme tension (Webb et al., 2019). Considering the huge role psychological factors play in people's overall well-being, it is important that a comprehensive treatment regimen include appropriate levels of screening and support to address the psychological needs of the patient diagnosed with breast cancer. Nurses need to address the physical, emotional, and spiritual needs of the patient for whom they are caring as well as the needs of the patient's family. Nurses should identify the patient's personal coping style, which has an impact on how the patient experiences and copes with distress after a diagnosis.

The diagnosis of cancer affects all aspects of life for a patient and their family. The threatening nature of the disease and feelings of uncertainty about the future can lead to anxiety and stress. Address the patient's need for:

- Information about diagnosis and treatment
- Physical care while undergoing treatments
- Contact with supportive people
- Education about disease, options, and prevention measures
- Discussion and support by a caring, competent nurse

Reassure the patient and their family in regard to the concerns they have about the diagnosis of breast cancer. They may need reassurance that the diagnosis does not necessarily mean imminent death, a decrease in attractiveness, or diminished sexuality. Encourage the patient to express their fears and worries. Be available to listen and address the patient's concerns in an open manner to help their recovery. All aspects of care must include sensitivity to the patient's personal efforts to cope and heal. Some patients will become involved in organizations or charities that support cancer research; they may participate in breast cancer walks to raise awareness or become a volunteer to help others. Each patient copes in their own personal manner, and all of these efforts can be positive motivators for the patient's own healing.

To help patients cope with the diagnosis of breast cancer, the ACS created a program called Reach to Recovery (RTR). Specially trained survivors of breast cancer give patients and their families opportunities to express their feelings, verbalize their fears, and get answers. Most importantly, RTR volunteers offer understanding, support, and hope through face-to-face visits or by telephone; they are proof that people can survive breast cancer and live productive lives. National contact information is 1-800-277-2345, and it is easy to join online at reach.cancer.org.

Providing Postoperative Care

For the patient who has had surgery to remove a malignant breast lump or an entire breast, excellent postoperative nursing care is crucial. Tell the patient what to expect in terms of symptoms and when they usually occur during treatment and after surgery. This allows the patient to anticipate these symptoms and proactively employ management strategies to improve the experience. Postoperative care includes immediate postoperative care, pain management, care of the affected arm, wound care, mobility care, respiratory care, emotional care, referrals, and educational needs.

IMMEDIATE POSTOPERATIVE CARE

Assess the patient's respiratory status by auscultating the lungs and observing the breathing pattern. Assess circulation; note vital signs, monitor urinary output, skin color, and skin temperature. Observe the patient's neurologic status by evaluating the level of alertness and orientation. Monitor the wound for amount and color of drainage. Monitor the intravenous lines for patency, correct fluid, and rate. Assess the drainage tube for amount, color, and consistency of drainage.

PAIN MANAGEMENT

Provide analgesics as needed. Reassure the patient that their pain will be controlled. Teach the patient how to communicate their pain intensity on a scale of 0 to 10, with 10 being the worst pain imaginable. Assess the patient's pain level frequently and anticipate pain before assisting the patient in ambulating.

AFFECTED ARM CARE

Elevate the affected arm on a pillow to promote lymph drainage. Make sure no treatments are performed on the affected arm, including laboratory draws, intravenous lines, blood pressures, and so on. Place a sign above the bed to warn others not to touch the affected arm.

WOUND CARE

Observe the wound often and empty drainage reservoirs as needed. Tell the patient to report any evidence of infection early, such as fever, chills, or any area of redness or inflammation along the incision line. Also tell the patient to report any increase in drainage, foul odor, or separation at the incision site.

MOBILITY CARE

Perform active range-of-motion and arm exercises as ordered. Encourage self-care activities for successful rehabilitation. Perform dressing and drainage care; explain the care during the procedure.

Respiratory Care

Assist with turning, coughing, and deep breathing every 2 hours. Explain that this helps to expand collapsed alveoli in the lungs, promotes faster clearance of inhalation agents from the body, and prevents postoperative pneumonia and atelectasis.

EMOTIONAL CARE AND REFERRALS

Encourage the patient to participate in their care. Assess the patient's coping strategies preoperatively. Explain possible body image concerns after discharge. Promote the ACS websites, which provide the latest cancer therapy news. Encourage the patient to attend local support groups for breast cancer survivors, such as RTR.

EDUCATIONAL NEEDS

Provide follow-up information about adjunctive therapy. Explain that radiation therapy may start postoperatively within weeks. Discuss chemotherapy, its side effects and cycles, home care during treatment, and future monitoring strategies. Explain hormonal therapy, including anti-estrogens or aromatase inhibitors. Teach progressive arm exercises to minimize lymphedema. Explain that ongoing surveillance is needed to detect recurrence of cancer or a new primary site and that the patient will typically see the health care provider every 6 months.

Nancy underwent a mastectomy with radiation and chemotherapy. What follow-up care is needed? How can the nurse assist Nancy in coping with her uncertain future? What community resources might help her?

IMPLEMENTING HEALTH PROMOTION AND DISEASE PREVENTION STRATEGIES

Combining extensive clinical knowledge of breast cancer with an understanding of the support needs of patients, nurses play an essential role in making positive impacts on patients' lives. Many advances in treating breast cancer have been made, and nurses can serve as the first line of communication for questions throughout the entire journey from diagnosis through treatment.

Prior to any diagnosis of breast cancer, nurses can help guide patients toward breast cancer prevention through screenings, lifestyle changes, and health care practices to decrease their risks. In the fight against cancer, nurses often assume a variety of roles, such as educator, counselor, advocate, and role model. Nurses can offer education about:

- Prevention
- Early detection
- Screening
- Dispelling myths and fears
- Breast self-awareness technique
- Individual risk status and strategies for risk reduction

It is important to be knowledgeable about the most current evidence-based practices and cognizant of how the media presents this information. Offer prevention strategies within the context of the patient's life. Factors such as lifestyle choices, economic status, and multiple roles need to be taken into consideration when counseling patients. Advocate for healthy lifestyles and making sound choices to prevent cancer. Nurses, like all health care providers, should offer guidance from a comprehensive perspective that acknowledges the unique needs of each person. Provide patients with information about detection and risk factors, inform them about the new ACS screening guidelines, instruct them on breast self-awareness, and outline dietary changes that might reduce the risk of breast cancer.

Awareness is the first step toward a change in habits. Raising the level of awareness about breast cancer is of paramount importance, and nurses can play an important role in health promotion, disease prevention, and education.

Breast Cancer Screening

Finding breast cancer early and receiving early treatment are essential to decreasing mortality (ACS, 2023b). The ACS (2023b) and ACOG (2021) have issued breast cancer screening guidelines that offer specific guidance for the person at average risk and greater clarification of the role of breast examinations; these guidelines will be discussed below. Screening guidelines are revised about every few years to include new scientific findings and developments.

Patients are exposed to multiple sources of cancer prevention information, and much of it may not be sound. Discuss the benefits, risks, and potential limitations of breast self-examination (BSE), clinical breast exam, and mammography with each patient and tailor the information to their specific risk factors (ACS, 2023b). Based on the new guidelines, make clinical judgments as to the appropriateness of recommending BSE, and reevaluate the need to teach the procedure to all patients; the focus might instead be on encouraging regular mammograms (depending, of course, on the patient's individual risk factors).

Breast Self-Awareness

BSE is a technique that enables a person to detect changes in their breasts. BSEs, once thought essential for early breast cancer detection, are now considered optional. Instead, breast self-awareness is stressed. **Breast self-awareness** refers to a person being familiar with the normal consistency of both breasts and the underlying tissue. This emphasis is now on awareness of breast changes, not just discovery of cancer. Research has shown that BSE plays a small role in detecting breast cancer compared with self-awareness (ACOG, 2021). However, doing BSE is one way for a person to know how their breasts normally feel so that they can notice any changes that do occur (National Breast Cancer Foundation, 2024).

> *TAKE NOTE!*
>
> BSE is no longer recommended for average-risk people due to the lack of evidence demonstrating its benefit. Most people discover a lump or changes during normal activities of daily living (ADLs) such as dressing and bathing, and there is risk of harm from false positives (ACOG, 2021; ACS, 2023b).

If appropriate, there are two steps in conducting a BSE: visual inspection and tactile palpation. The visual part should be done in three separate positions: with the arms up behind the head, with the arms down at the sides, and bending forward. Instruct the patient to look for:

- Changes in shape, size, contour, or symmetry
- Skin discoloration or dimpling, bumps/lumps
- Sores or scaly skin
- Discharge or puckering of the nipple

In the second part, the tactile examination, the patient should feel the breasts in one of three specific patterns: spiral, pie-shaped wedges, or a vertical strip (up and down). When using any of the three patterns, the patient should use a circular rubbing motion (in dime-sized circles) without lifting the fingers. They should check not only the breasts but also between the breast and the axilla, the axilla itself, and the area above the breast up to the clavicle and across the shoulder. The pads of the three middle fingers on the right hand are used to assess the left breast; the pads of the three middle fingers on the left hand are used to assess the right breast. Instruct the patient to use three different degrees of pressure:

- Light (move the skin without moving the tissue underneath)
- Medium (midway into the tissue)
- Hard (down to the ribs)

Nutrition and Physical Activity

As discussed previously, nutrition and physical activity play a critical role in all health promotion and disease prevention. Cancer is considered to be a chronic disease that may be influenced at many stages by nutrition and physical activity. These factors may affect prevention, progression, and treatment of the disease. Increasingly, research suggests there is a connection between diet and physical activity and cancer mortality and that reducing alcohol intake, increasing fruit and vegetable intake in the diet, decreasing saturated fat intake and red meat, and increasing levels of physical activity lead to a decrease in cancer mortality in both pre- and postmenopausal women (Jia et al., 2022). Being overweight or having obesity is a risk factor for breast cancer in postmenopausal people (Pati et al., 2023). Evidence has shown that obesity as measured by body mass index (BMI) 30 kg/m^2 or greater is linked to poorer breast cancer outcomes and greater mortality risks because increased adipose tissue synthesizes more estrogen (particularly in postmenopausal people), subsequently promoting carcinogenesis (Devericks et al., 2022). There is a complex reciprocal relationship among adipose fat, immune cells, and tumor growth that appears to promote breast cancer development in people with obesity (Nunez-Ruiz et al., 2022). Dozens of studies demonstrate that people who are overweight (BMI $>$ 25 kg/m^2) or have obesity (BMI $>$ 30 kg/m^2) at the time of breast cancer diagnosis are at an increased risk of cancer recurrence and death compared with people with a BMI lower than 25 kg/m^2, and some evidence suggests that patients who gain weight after a breast cancer diagnosis may also be at increased risk of poor outcomes (Pati et al., 2023). Some research suggests the Mediterranean diet, which is high in fruits, vegetables, and high-fiber carbohydrates and low in animal fat, seems to offer some protection against breast cancer while facilitating weight control; however, there is currently insufficient data to support its recommendation for these purposes (Jia et al., 2022).

The ACS made the following recommendations to reduce the risk for developing breast cancer:

- Engaging in 150 to 300 minutes of moderate exercise and 75 to 150 minutes of vigorous physical activity each week

- Consuming foods high in nutrients and a variety of fruits and whole grains
- Not smoking or using any tobacco products
- Staying at a healthy weight and avoiding weight gain in adult life
- Limiting intake of processed foods and refined sugar
- Consuming a wide variety of plant-based foods to increase fiber intake
- Limiting consumption of red and processed meats and sugary drinks
- Limiting intake of fatty foods, particularly those of animal origin (Rock et al., 2020)

Research has shown that phytochemicals can help prevent bladder, breast, esophagus, lung, and skin cancers (Waldron, 2022). This area of research provides hope for people seeking to prevent breast cancer as well as those recovering from it. Although the mechanism is not clear, certain foods demonstrate anticancer properties and boost the immune system. Phytochemical-rich foods include:

- Blueberries
- Strawberries
- Raspberries
- Watermelon
- Bell peppers
- Tomato
- Cherries
- Peaches
- Plums
- Spinach
- Kale (Waldron, 2022)

Adopt a holistic approach when addressing the nutritional needs of patients with breast cancer. Incorporate nutritional assessment into the general overall assessment of all patients. Culturally sensitive nutritional assessment tools need to be developed and used to enhance this process. Providing examples of appropriate foods associated with the patient's current dietary habits, relating current health status to nutritional intake, and placing proposed modifications within a realistic personal framework may increase the patient's willingness to incorporate needed changes in their nutritional behavior. Be able to interpret research results and stay up to date on nutritional influences so that you can transmit this key information to the public.

KEY CONCEPTS

- Many patients believe that all lumps are cancerous, but actually more than 90% of lumps discovered are benign and need no treatment.
- The most commonly encountered benign breast disorders in females include nonproliferative epithelial lesions, such as breast cysts and fibrocystic changes of the breasts, and proliferative lesions atypia, such as fibroadenomas.
- Fibroadenomas are common benign solid breast tumors that can be stimulated by external estrogen, progesterone, lactation, and pregnancy.
- Breast cancer is the second most common cancer in females and the second leading cause of cancer deaths (lung cancer is first) among American females.
- Breast cancer metastasizes widely and to almost all organs of the body but primarily to the bone, lungs, lymph nodes, liver, and brain.
- The cause of breast cancer, while not well understood, is thought to be a complex interaction among environmental, genetic, and hormonal factors.
- Breast cancer treatments fall into two categories: local and systemic. Local treatments are surgery and radiation therapy. Effective systemic treatments include chemotherapy, hormonal therapy, and immunotherapy.
- Patients often perceive their breasts as intrinsic to their femininity, self-esteem, and/or sexuality, and the risk of losing a breast can provoke extreme tension (Webb et al., 2019).
- Nurses can influence both physical and emotional recovery, which are both important aspects of care that help in improving the patient's quality of life and the ability to survive.
- Health promotion measures that will reduce the risk of breast cancer include breastfeeding, daily exercise, avoiding alcohol, and maintaining a healthy BMI (18.5 to 24.9 kg/m^2).
- The common ways to screen for breast cancer in people who are at average risk include mammography and practicing breast self-awareness to get to know one's own breasts to be better able to identify any abnormal lesions.
- Providing up-to-date information and emotional support are central roles of the nurse in caring for the patient with a diagnosis of breast cancer.

REFERENCES AND RECOMMENDED READINGS

Ajmal, M., Khan, M., & Van Fossen, K. (2023). Breast fibroadenoma. *StatPearls*. https://www.ncbi.nlm.nih.gov/books/NBK535345/

American Cancer Society. (2021a). *Breast cancer stages*. https://www.cancer.org/cancer/types/breast-cancer/understanding-a-breast-cancer-diagnosis/stages-of-breast-cancer.html

American Cancer Society. (2021b). *Breast cancer gene expression tests*. https://www.cancer.org/content/dam/CRC/PDF/Public/8580.00.pdf

American Cancer Society. (2022a). *Non-cancerous breast conditions: Fibrocystic changes in the breast*. https://www.cancer.org/cancer/breast-cancer/non-cancerous-breast-conditions/fibrosis-and-simple-cysts-in-the-breast.html

American Cancer Society. (2022b). *Lifestyle-related breast cancer risk factors*. https://www.cancer.org/cancer/breast-cancer/risk-and-prevention/lifestyle-related-breast-cancer-risk-factors.html

American Cancer Society. (2022c). *More Black women die from breast cancer than any other cancer*. https://www.cancer.org/latest-news/facts-and-figures-african-american-black-people-2022-2024.html

American Cancer Society. (2022d). *Breast cancer signs and symptoms*. https://www.cancer.org/cancer/breast-cancer/screening-tests-and-early-detection/breast-cancer-signs-and-symptoms.html

American Cancer Society. (2023a). *Breast density and your mammogram report*. https://www.cancer.org/cancer/breast-cancer/screening-tests-and-early-detection/mammograms/breast-density-and-your-mammogram-report.html

American Cancer Society. (2023b). *American Cancer Society recommendations for the early detection of breast cancer*. https://www.cancer.org/cancer/breast-cancer/screening-tests-and-early-detection/american-cancer-society-recommendations-for-the-early-detection-of-breast-cancer.html

American Cancer Society. (2023c). *Hormone therapy for breast cancer*. https://www.cancer.org/cancer/types/breast-cancer/treatment/hormone-therapy-for-breast-cancer.html

American Cancer Society. (2024). *Key statistics for breast cancer*. https://www.cancer.org/cancer/breast-cancer/about/how-common-is-breast-cancer.html

American College of Obstetricians and Gynecologists. (2021). *Breast cancer risk assessment and screening in average-risk women*. https://www.acog.org/clinical/clinical-guidance/practice-bulletin/articles/2017/07/breast-cancer-risk-assessment-and-screening-in-average-risk-women

Barsouk, A., Saginala, K., Aluru, J. S., Rawla, P., & Barsouk, A. (2022). US cancer screening recommendations: Developments and the impact of COVID-19. *Medical Sciences, 10*(1), 16. https://doi.org/10.3390/medsci10010016

Bleiweiss, I. J. (2022). Pathology of breast cancer. *UpToDate*. Retrieved April 23, 2024, from https://www.uptodate.com/contents/pathology-of-breast-cancer

Breast Cancer Organization. (2022a). *Fibroadenomas of the breast: Causes, symptoms, and treatment*. https://www.breastcancer.org/benign-breast-conditions/fibroadenoma

Breast Cancer Organization. (2022b). *Sentinel lymph node dissection*. https://www.breastcancer.org/treatment/surgery/lymph-node-removal/sentinel-node-dissection

Breast Cancer Organization. (2022c). *Tamoxifen*. https://www.breastcancer.org/treatment/hormonal-therapy/tamoxifen

Breast Cancer Organization. (2023a). *About breast cancer*. https://www.breastcancer.org/about-breast-cancer

Breast Cancer Organization. (2023b). *Types of mastectomy*. https://www.breastcancer.org/treatment/surgery/mastectomy/types#section-modified-radical-mastectomy

Breast Cancer Organization. (2023c). *Aromatase inhibitors*. https://www.breastcancer.org/treatment/hormonal-therapy/aromatase-inhibitors

Breast Cancer Organization. (2023d). *Hormone receptor status*. https://www.breastcancer.org/pathology-report/hormone-receptor-status

Breast Cancer Organization. (2024a). *Genetics*. https://www.breastcancer.org/risk/risk-factors/genetics

Breast Cancer Organization. (2024b). *Immunotherapy*. https://www.breastcancer.org/treatment/immunotherapy

Breast Cancer Research Foundation. (2022). *Ten ways to reduce breast cancer risk and improve overall health*. https://www.bcrf.org/blog/breast-cancer-prevention-breast-cancer-risk-reduction/

Brown, T., Cruickshank, S., & Noblet, M. (2021). Specialist breast care nurses for support of women with breast cancer. *Cochrane Database of Systematic Reviews, 2021*(2), CD005634. https://doi.org//10.1002/14651858.CD005634.pub3

Burnstein, H. J. (2022). Tumor, node, metastasis (TNM) staging classification for breast cancer. *UpToDate*. Retrieved on April 23, 2024, from https://www.uptodate.com/contents/tumor-node-metastasis-tnm-staging-classification-for-breast-cancer

Centers for Disease Control and Prevention. (2023). *Breast cancer statistics*. https://www.cdc.gov/cancer/breast/statistics/index.htm

Chalasani, P. (2023). Breast cancer treatment & management. *eMedicine*. https://emedicine.medscape.com/article/1947145-treatment

DePolo, J. (2024a). *Breast radiation side effects*. Breast Cancer Organization. https://www.breastcancer.org/treatment/radiation-therapy/side-effects

DePolo, J. (2024b). *Brachytherapy or internal radiation*. Breast Cancer Organization. https://www.breastcancer.org/treatment/radiation-therapy/internal

DePolo, J. (2024c). *Radiation therapy*. Breast Cancer Organization. https://www.breastcancer.org/treatment/radiation-therapy

DePolo, J. (2024d). *Chemotherapy for breast cancer*. Breast Cancer Organization. https://www.breastcancer.org/treatment/chemotherapy

Devericks, E. N., Carson, M. S., McCullough, L. E., Coleman, M. F., & Hursting, S. D. (2022). The obesity-breast cancer link: A multidisciplinary perspective. *Cancer and Metastasis Reviews*, 41(3), 607–625. https://doi.org/10.1007/s10555-022-10043-5

Elmore, J. G., & Lee, C. I. (2024). Screening for breast cancer: Strategies and recommendations. *UpToDate*. Retrieved April 25, 2024, from https://www.uptodate.com/contents/screening-for-breast-cancer-strategies-and-recommendations

Giaquinto, A. N., Miller, K. D., Tossas, K. Y., Winn, R. A., Jemal, A., & Siegel, R. L. (2022). Cancer statistics for African American/Black People 2022. *CA: A Cancer Journal for Clinicians, 72*(3), 202–229. https://doi.org/10.3322/caac.21718

Hamwi, M. W., & Winters, R. (2023). Mammary duct ectasia. *StatPearls*. https://www.ncbi.nlm.nih.gov/books/NBK557665/

Henderson, J. A., Duffee, D., & Ferguson, T. (2023). Breast examination techniques. *StatPearls*. https://www.ncbi.nlm.nih.gov/books/NBK459179/

Ji, J., Yuan, S., He, J., Liu, H., Yang, L., & He, X. (2022). Breast-conserving therapy is associated with better survival than mastectomy in early-stage breast cancer: A propensity score analysis. *Cancer Medicine, 11*, 1646–1658. https://doi.org/10.1002/cam4.4510

Jia, T., Liu, Y., Fan, Y., Wang, L., & Jiang, E. (2022). Association of healthy diet and physical activity with breast cancer: Lifestyle interventions and oncology education. *Frontiers in Public Health, 10*, 797794. https://doi.org/10.3389/fpubh.2022.797794

Joe, B. N. (2023). Clinical features, diagnosis, and staging of newly diagnosed breast cancer. *UpToDate*. Retrieved April 23, 2024, from https://www.uptodate.com/contents/clinical-features-diagnosis-and-staging-of-newly-diagnosed-breast-cancer

Kunkler, I. H., Williams, L. J., Jack, W. J. L., Cameron, D. A., & Dixon, J. M. (2023). Breast-conserving surgery with or without irradiation in early breast cancer. *New England Journal of Medicine, 388*(7), 585–594. https://doi.org/10.1056/nejmoa2207586

Kwong, A., & Sabel, M. S. (2022). Mastectomy. *UpToDate*. Retrieved April 25, 2024, from https://www.uptodate.com/contents/mastectomy

Lee, V. (2024). *Metastatic breast cancer?* Breast Cancer Organization. https://www.breastcancer.org/types/metastatic#section-what-is-metastatic-breast-cancer

Malherbe, K., Khan, M., & Fatima, S. (2023). Fibrocystic breast disease. *StatPearls*. https://www.ncbi.nlm.nih.gov/books/NBK551609/

Mehrara, B. (2022). Clinical staging and conservative management of peripheral lymphedema. *UpToDate*. Retrieved on April 25, 2024, from https://www.uptodate.com/contents/clinical-staging-and-conservative-management-of-peripheral-lymphedema

Merajver, S. D. (2022). Inflammatory breast cancer: Pathology and molecular pathogenesis. *UpToDate*. Retrieved on April 23, 2024, from https://www.uptodate.com/contents/inflammatory-breast-cancer-pathology-and-molecular-pathogenesis

Min, S. K., Lee, S. K., Woo, J., Jung, S. M., Ryu, J. M., Yu, J., Lee, J. E., Kim, S. W., Chae, B. J., & Nam, S. J. (2021). Relation between tumor size and lymph node metastasis according to subtypes of breast cancer. *Journal of Breast Cancer*, *24*(1), 75–84. https://doi.org/10.4048/jbc.2021.24.e4

National Breast Cancer Foundation. (2024). *Breast self-exam*. https://www.nationalbreastcancer.org/breast-self-exam/

National Cancer Institute. (2020). *Breast cancer risk in American women*. https://www.cancer.gov/types/breast/risk-fact-sheet

National Cancer Institute. (2022a). *Cancer stat facts: Female breast cancer*. https://seer.cancer.gov/statfacts/html/breast.html

National Cancer Institute. (2022b). *Who is at risk?* https://www.cancer.gov/types/breast/hp/breast-prevention-pdq#_558

National Cancer Institute. (2022c). *Treatment option overview*. https://www.cancer.gov/types/breast/patient/breast-treatment-pdq#_185

National Cancer Institute. (2022d). *Hormone therapy for breast cancer*. https://www.cancer.gov/types/breast/breast-hormone-therapy-fact-sheet

National Cancer Institute. (2024a). *General information about breast cancer*. https://www.cancer.gov/types/breast/hp/breast-treatment-pdq#_1

National Cancer Institute. (2024b). *Breast Cancer Prevention (PDQ)—Health Professional Version: Overview*. https://www.cancer.gov/types/breast/hp/breast-prevention-pdq#_1

Nunez-Ruiz, A., Sanchez-Brena, F., Lopez-Pacheco, C., Acevedo-Dominguez, N. A., & Soldevilia, G. (2022). Obesity modulates the immune macroenvironment associated with breast cancer development. *PLoS One*, *17*(4), e0266827. https://doi.org/10.1371/journal.pone.0266827

Pati, S., Irfan, W., Jameel, A., Ahmed, S., & Shahid, R. K. (2023). Obesity and cancer: A current overview of epidemiology, pathogenesis, outcomes, and management. *Cancers*, *15*(2), 485. https://doi.org/10.3390/cancers15020485

Peshkin, B. N., & Isaacs, C. (2023). Overview of hereditary breast and ovarian cancer syndromes. *UpToDate*. Retrieved April 25, 2024, from https://www.uptodate.com/contents/overview-of-hereditary-breast-and-ovarian-cancer-syndromes

Petrucelli, N., Daly, M. B., & Pal, T. (2022). BRCA1 and BRCA2-associated hereditary breast and ovarian cancer. *Gene Reviews*. https://www.ncbi.nlm.nih.gov/books/NBK1247/

Rock, C. L., Thomson, C., Gansler, T., Gapstur, S. M., McCullough, M. L., Patel, A. V., Andrews, K. S., Bandera, E. V., Spees, C. K., Robien, K., Hartman, S., Sullivan, K., Grant, B. L., Hamilton, K. K., Kushi, L. H., Caan, B. J., Kibbe, D., Black, J. D., Wiedt, T. L., McMahon, C., . . . & Doyle, C. (2020). American Cancer Society guideline for diet and physical activity for cancer prevention. *CA: A Cancer Journal for Clinicians*, *70*, 245–271. https://doi.org/10.3322/caac.21591

Sabel, M. S. (2023a). Clinical manifestations, differential diagnosis, and clinical evaluation of a palpable breast mass. *UpToDate*. Retrieved on April 8, 2024, from https://www.uptodate.com/contents/clinical-manifestations-differential-diagnosis-and-clinical-evaluation-of-a-palpable-breast-mass

Sabel, M. S. (2023b). Overview of benign breast diseases. *UpToDate*. Retrieved on April 8, 2024, from https://www.uptodate.com/contents/overview-of-benign-breast-diseases

Sabel, M. S. (2023c). Breast-conserving therapy. *UpToDate*. Retrieved on April 8, 2024, from https://www.uptodate.com/contents/breast-conserving-therapy

Shabanian, S., Rozbeh, A., Mohammadi, B., Ahmadi, A., & Arjmand, M.-H. (2023). The association between vitamin D deficiency and fibrocystic breast disorder. *Current Molecular Medicine*, *24*(7), 899–905. https://doi.org/10.2174/1566524023666230623155659

Slanetz, P. J. (2024). MRI of the breast and emerging technologies. *UpToDate*. Retrieved April 25, 2024, from https://www.uptodate.com/contents/mri-of-the-breast-and-emerging-technologies

Slanetz, P. J., & Lee, C. I. (2024). Breast imaging for cancer screening: Mammography and ultrasonography. *UpToDate*. Retrieved on April 24, 2024, from https://www.uptodate.com/contents/breast-imaging-for-cancer-screening-mammography-and-ultrasonography

Taghian, A. (2024). Adjuvant radiation therapy for women with newly diagnosed, non-metastatic breast cancer. *UpToDate*. Retrieved April 26, 2024, from https://www.uptodate.com/contents/adjuvant-radiation-therapy-for-women-with-newly-diagnosed-non-metastatic-breast-cancer/print

Trotter, K. J. (2022). Breast conditions. In K. D. Schuiling & F. E. Likis (Eds.), *Gynecologic health care* (4th ed., pp. 337–352). Jones & Bartlett Learning.

U.S. Department of Health and Human Services. (n.d.). *Healthy People 2030*. https://health.gov/healthypeople

U.S. Food & Drug Administration. (2023). *Risks and complications of breast implants*. https://www.fda.gov/medical-devices/breast-implants/risks-and-complications-breast-implants

U.S. Preventive Services Task Force. (2023). *Task force issues draft recommendation statement on screening for breast cancer*. https://www.uspreventiveservicestaskforce.org/uspstf/sites/default/files/file/supporting_documents/breast-cancer-screening-draft-rec-bulletin.pdf

Waldron, K. (2022). *Food for thought: Nutrition and cancer*. Rutgers Cancer Institute of New Jersey. https://www.cinj.org/food-thought-nutrition-and-cancer

Webb, C., Jacox, N., & Temple-Oberle, C. (2019). The making of breasts: Navigating the symbolism of breasts in women facing cancer. *Plastic Surgery*, *27*(1), 49–53. https://doi.org/10.1177/2292550318800500

DEVELOPING CLINICAL JUDGMENT

PRACTICING FOR NCLEX

1. The nurse is educating a group of patients regarding breast self-awareness. These patients will learn that breast self-awareness involves
   a. palpation of cervical lymph nodes.
   b. firm squeezing of both nipples.
   c. visualizing both breasts for any changes.
   d. a mammogram to evaluate breast tissue.
2. The nurse is educating a group of patients regarding breast cancer. Which of the following will the nurse explain is the strongest risk factor for breast cancer?
   a. Advancing age and being female
   b. High number of children
   c. Genetic mutations in *BRCA1* and *BRCA2* genes
   d. Family history of colon cancer
3. The nurse is caring for a patient with breast cancer who will begin adjuvant chemotherapy. The nurse will explain the most serious potential adverse reaction from chemotherapy is
   a. thrombocytopenia.
   b. deep vein thrombosis.
   c. alopecia.
   d. myelosuppression.
4. A patient comes to the clinic with complaints of painful fibrocystic breast changes. What suggestion can the nurse provide that would be helpful for this patient?
   a. Increase their caffeine intake.
   b. Take a mild analgesic when needed.
   c. Reduce their intake of leafy vegetables.
   d. Wear a loose-fitting bra without support.
5. The nurse is caring for a patient who has had a mastectomy. Upon discharge, the nurse should refer the patient to which organization for assistance and support?
   a. National Organization for Women (NOW)
   b. Food and Drug Administration (FDA)
   c. March of Dimes Foundation (MDF)
   d. RTR
6. A 25-year-old patient presents with a breast mass without symptoms. Which statement is true concerning the patient's diagnosis and treatment?
   a. All breast masses should be considered premalignant.
   b. The breast mass should be surgically removed immediately.
   c. Ultrasound is typically used to determine the diagnosis.
   d. Since it is without symptoms, only reassurance is needed now.

CRITICAL THINKING EXERCISES

1. Mrs. Gordon, 48 years, presents to the women's community clinic where you work as a nurse. She is upset and crying. She tells you that she found lumps in her breast: "I know that it's cancer and I will die." When you ask her about her problem, she says she does not check her breasts monthly and hasn't had a mammogram for years because "they're too expensive." She also describes the intermittent pain she experiences.
   a. What specific questions would you ask this patient to get a clearer picture?
   b. What education is needed for this patient regarding breast health?
   c. What community referrals are needed to meet this patient's future needs?
2. Ms. Davis, 51 years, stops in at the urgent care facility with an anxious look on her face. She tells the nurse practitioner that she has green discharge coming from her right breast and discomfort intermittently. She can't understand how this would happen since she hasn't previously had any nipple discharge or pain.
   a. What benign breast condition might the nurse practitioner suspect based on her description?
   b. What specific information should the nurse practitioner give Ms. Davis about duct ectasia?
   c. The typical treatment of this benign breast condition would include what?

STUDY ACTIVITIES

1. Discuss with a group of patients what their breasts symbolize to them and to society. Do they symbolize something different to each one?
2. When a person experiences a breast disorder, what feelings might they be experiencing and how can a nurse help them sort out those feelings?
3. Interview a patient who has fibrocystic breast changes and find out how they manage this condition. Which interventions work and which don't seem to help?

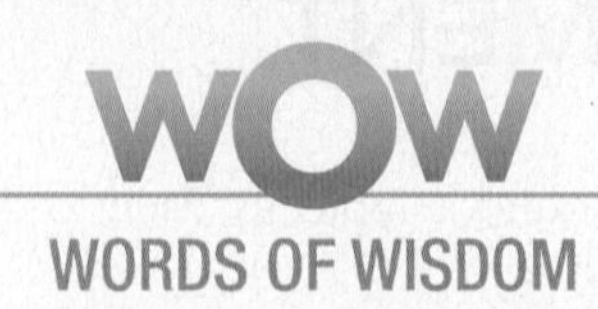

WORDS OF WISDOM

People can influence the aging process by making wise lifestyle choices early on.

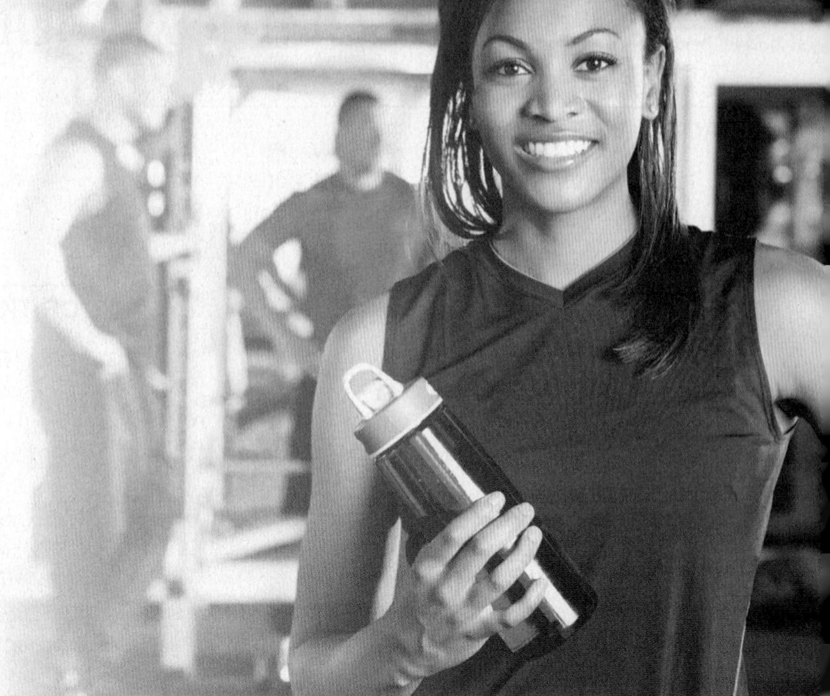

7

Benign Disorders of the Female Reproductive Tract

KEY TERMS

Bartholin cysts

cystocele (sis'tō-sēl)

enterocele (en'tĕr-o-sēl)

ovarian cyst

pelvic floor muscle exercises (Kegel exercises)

pelvic organ prolapse (POP)

pessary

polycystic ovary syndrome (PCOS)

polyps

rectocele (rek'tō-sēl)

urinary incontinence (UI)

urogenital fistulas

uterine fibroids

uterine prolapse

LEARNING OBJECTIVES

Upon completion of the chapter, you will be able to:

1. Characterize the major pelvic relaxation disorders in terms of etiology, management, and nursing interventions.
2. Evaluate urinary incontinence (UI) in terms of pathology, clinical manifestations, treatment options, and effect on quality of life.
3. Compare the various benign growths in terms of their symptoms and management.
4. Analyze the emotional impact of polycystic ovary syndrome (PCOS) and the nurse's role as a counselor, educator, and advocate.

Liz, a 26-year-old patient with a higher body weight, presented to the clinic with hirsutism and facial acne and told the nurse that she was concerned about her irregular menstrual periods. She also said that recently the hair on top of her head seemed to be falling out. What diagnostic tests might the nurse anticipate with this patient? How can the nurse prepare Liz for them?

INTRODUCTION

The incidence of several benign pelvic disorders increases as females age. For instance, people may experience pelvic floor disorders related to pelvic relaxation or UI. These disorders generally develop after years of wear and tear on the muscles and tissues that support the pelvic floor. This can result from childbearing, chronic coughing, straining, surgery, or simply aging. In addition to pelvic floor disorders, females may experience various benign neoplasms of the reproductive tract, such as cervical polyps, uterine leiomyomas (fibroids), ovarian cysts, genital fistulas, and Bartholin cysts. This chapter provides an overview of various pelvic floor disorders and benign neoplasms, discussing the assessment, treatment, and prevention strategies for each.

PELVIC FLOOR DISORDERS

Pelvic floor disorders include UI, pelvic organ prolapse (POP), fecal incontinence, and other sensory and emptying abnormalities. These are widely prevalent and largely undertreated.

Researchers report that nearly one quarter of all females and more than one third of older females in the United States have at least one symptom of a pelvic floor disorder (Kenne et al., 2022). According to recent studies, the frequency of pelvic floor disorders increases with age (Kenne et al., 2022). Determining the actual incidence of pelvic floor disorders is difficult as the array of symptoms and conditions spans over many disciplines, and it is unknown how many people do not seek treatment (Grimes & Stratton, 2023; Rogers & Fashokun, 2022). Pelvic floor disorders can cause significant physical and psychological morbidity and can diminish a person's social interactions, emotional well-being, and overall quality of life. Because these disorders increase with age, the problem grows worse as our population ages. Studies show there is a lack of knowledge among females of all ages about pelvic floor disorders, including the risk factors and treatment options (Fante et al., 2019).

The term "pelvic floor" refers to the group of muscles that form a sling or hammock across the pelvis. Together with their surrounding tissues, these muscles hold the pelvic organs (uterus, bladder, and bowel) in place so they can function correctly. These disorders occur as a result of weakness of the connective tissue and muscular support of pelvic organs due to factors including pregnancy and vaginal childbirth, which are the main factors (American College of Obstetricians and Gynecologists [ACOG], 2021a). Additional factors include menopause; aging; obesity (body mass index [BMI] greater than 30 kg/m^2); lifting; chronic cough from smoking, asthma, or other conditions; and straining at defecation secondary to constipation (ACOG, 2021a). The female anatomy is susceptible to the development of pelvic floor disorders because of its vertical structure placement. The bony pelvis has an exaggerated lumbar spinal curve and a downward tilt to it. The bladder rests on the symphysis and the posterior organs rest on the sacrum and coccyx. The pelvis holds the organs, but a person's erect posture causes a funneling effect and constant downward pressure.

Pelvic Organ Prolapse

Pelvic organ prolapse (POP) (from the Latin *prolapsus*, "a slipping forth") refers to the abnormal descent or herniation of the pelvic organs from their original attachment sites or their normal position in the pelvis. POP occurs when structures of the pelvis shift and protrude into or outside the vaginal canal. This disorder affects a person's micturition, defecation, and sexual activity. The Egyptians were the first to describe prolapse of the genital organs. In 400 B.C., Hippocrates made reference to placing a pomegranate half into the vagina to treat organ prolapse. POP, a disorder exclusive to females, can affect a person's daily activities and quality of life (Ghanbari et al., 2022). It is difficult to determine the incidence of POP because the disorder is often without symptoms and many people do not seek treatment. Studies have shown a correlation between increased parity, increased age, and a higher incidence of POP (Aboseif & Liu, 2022). Each year, over 300,000 people undergo surgery to repair the prolapse (Culligan et al., 2022). This number is expected to increase by 50% by the year 2050 as the older adult population continues to grow (Culligan et al., 2022).

The prevalence of obesity (BMI greater than 30 kg/m^2) is increasing globally and causing significant health care problems. Obesity is associated with a high prevalence of pelvic floor disorders. Obesity can also aggravate symptoms of POP, fecal incontinence, sexual dysfunction, and stress UI and increase the risk of endometrial polyps and symptomatic fibroids. Weight reduction enhances reproductive outcomes, diminishes symptoms of UI, improves sexual dysfunction, and reduces morbidity following gynecologic surgery.

The treatment and diagnosis of POP are challenging and problematic.

Types of POP

The four most common types of pelvic or genital prolapse are cystocele, rectocele, enterocele, and uterine prolapse (Fig. 7.1):

- **Cystocele** occurs when the bladder drops into the vagina.
- **Rectocele** occurs when the rectum sags and bulges into the vagina.
- **Enterocele** occurs when the small intestine bulges into the vagina.
- **Uterine prolapse** occurs when the uterus drops into the vagina. Multiparous people are at particular risk

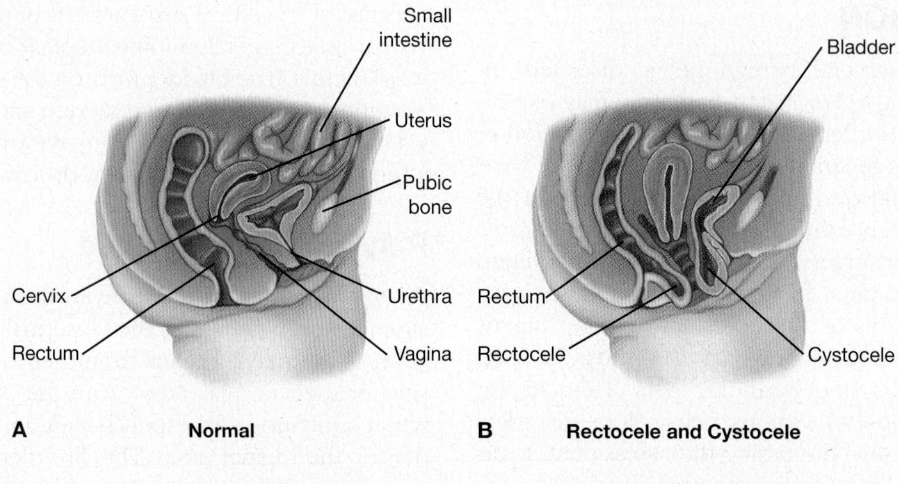

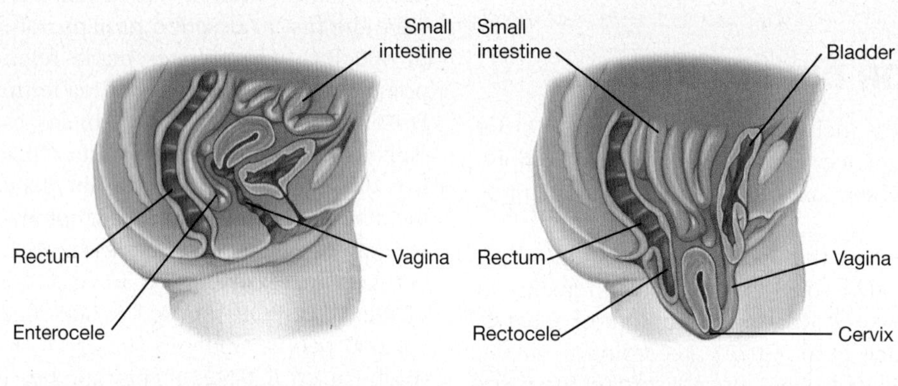

FIGURE 7.1 Types of pelvic prolapses. **A.** Normal. **B.** Rectocele and cystocele. **C.** Enterocele. **D.** Uterine prolapse.

for uterine prolapse. The extent of uterine prolapse is classified in terms of stages:

- *Stage 0:* No descent of pelvic structure during straining
- *Stage I:* The prolapsed descending organ is more than 1 cm above the hymenal ring.
- *Stage II:* The prolapsed organ is less than 1 cm above or below the hymenal ring.
- *Stage III:* The prolapsed organ extends over 1 cm (but no more than 2 cm) below the hymenal ring.
- *Stage IV:* The vagina is completely everted or the prolapsed organ is more than 2 cm below the hymenal ring (Fashokun & Rogers, 2023).

Etiology

Anatomic support of the pelvic organs is mainly provided by the levator ani muscle complex and the connective tissue attachments of the pelvic organ fascia. Dysfunction of one or both of these components can lead to loss of support and eventually POP. Many risk factors for POP have been suggested, but the true cause is likely multifactorial. Causes might include:

- Multiparity: weakening of pelvic support related to childbirth trauma; instrumental childbirth
- Increasing age: atrophy of supporting tissues with aging
- Menopause: decline of estrogen levels
- Obesity
- Reproductive surgery, including hysterectomy
- Family history of POP
- Connective tissue disorders
- Increased abdominal pressure secondary to:
  - Lifting of children or heavy objects
  - Straining due to chronic constipation
  - Respiratory problems or chronic coughing (Rogers & Fashokun, 2022)

Therapeutic Management

Treatment options for POP depend on the symptoms and their effect on the patient's quality of life. Important considerations when deciding on nonsurgical or surgical options include the severity of symptoms; the patient's preferences, health status, age, and suitability for surgery; and the presence of other pelvic conditions (urinary or fecal incontinence). Conservative measures such as pelvic floor muscle exercises (PFMEs) supplemented by lifestyle interventions such as weight loss, and avoidance of straining (reducing lifting heavy weights, treatment of chronic cough and constipation) are recommended as first-line management.

When surgery is being considered, the nature of the procedure and the likely outcome must be fully explained and discussed with the patient and, if they have one and wish to include them, their partner. In addition to PFMEs and surgery, treatment options for POP may include estrogen replacement therapy, dietary and lifestyle modifications, weight loss, and/or the use of a pessary (a removable device placed into the vagina to support pelvic organs).

PELVIC FLOOR MUSCLE EXERCISES

Pelvic floor muscle exercises (PFME), previously termed Kegel exercises, strengthen the pelvic floor muscles to support the inner organs, prevent further prolapse, and provide urethral support to prevent urine leakage and suppress urgency. They are generally accepted as first-line treatment for stress and urge UI and are also widely used for anal incontinence. Prior to starting this therapy, contributing lifestyle factors must be addressed and possibly modified—weight loss, avoiding constipation, reducing consumption of alcohol and sodas, and smoking cessation. PFME was first introduced in 1936. Since then, a wealth of research has supported the benefits of PFMEs in treating both UI and POP (Lukacz, 2024a). The purpose of pelvic floor exercises is to increase the muscle volume, which will result in a stronger muscular contraction. The goal of PFME is to teach patients how to prevent urine loss by occluding the urethra using active contraction of pelvic floor muscles. PFMEs might limit the progression of mild prolapse and alleviate mild prolapse symptoms, including low back pain and pelvic pressure. They will not, however, help severe uterine prolapse (see Evidence-Based Practice 7.1).

HORMONE REPLACEMENT THERAPY

Hormone replacement therapy, or HRT (orally, transdermally, low-dose vaginal ring, or vaginal cream), may improve the tone, natural thickness, and vascularity of the supporting tissue in perimenopausal and menopausal patients by increasing blood perfusion and the elasticity of the vaginal wall. Currently, no data exist supporting the use of systemic or topical estrogen as a primary treatment of POP (Rogers & Fashokun, 2022). There have been some promising results, but data are insufficient to advise its use as a routine treatment (Rogers & Fashokun, 2022). HRT has many benefits as well as risks. It is essential that the benefits are weighed against the risks to the patient before this therapy is initiated.

DIETARY AND LIFESTYLE MODIFICATIONS

Dietary and lifestyle modifications may help prevent pelvic relaxation and chronic problems later in life. Specific lifestyle changes would include avoiding constipation, bladder irritants, heavy lifting, high-impact exercise, weight loss, and smoking cessation. Dietary habits can exacerbate the prolapse by causing constipation and

EVIDENCE-BASED PRACTICE 7.1

Pelvic Floor Muscle Training for Urinary Incontinence With or Without Biofeedback or Electrostimulation in Women: A Systematic Review

BACKGROUND

Involuntary leakage of urine (urinary incontinence [UI]) affects women of all ages. It is considered a health, social, and hygienic problem. Some women leak urine during exercise or when they cough or sneeze (stress UI). This may occur as a result of weakness of the pelvic floor muscles due to factors such as damage during childbirth. Other women leak urine before going to the toilet when there is a sudden and compelling need to pass urine (urgency UI). This may be caused by an involuntary contraction of the bladder muscle. Mixed UI is the combination of both stress and urgency UI. Pelvic floor muscle training (PFMT) is a first-line treatment that involves muscle-clenching exercises to strengthen the pelvic floor muscles. This study was done to determine the effectiveness of PFMT with or without biofeedback or electrostimulation in reducing UI in women.

STUDY

Following a systematic literature review, 15 randomized control studies were selected with a total of 2,441 women analyzed for UI. Participants in the study had stress, urge, or mixed UI.

Findings

The results of this systemic review show that PFMT was effective in reducing UI and improving muscle contraction with or without biofeedback or electrostimulation. Participants experienced a significant decline in depressive symptoms and improvement in their quality of life as UI was reduced.

Nursing Implications

Overall, according to this study, there is sufficient evidence to support the widespread recommendation that PFMT should be included in a first-line conservative management program for patients with stress, urge, or mixed UI. Previous studies have validated that pelvic floor exercises do help in bringing tone to the muscles that control micturition. Nurses can continue to instruct female patients with UI to perform PFMT daily to improve their urinary control and their quality of life.

Adapted from Alouini, S., Memic, S., & Couillandre, A. (2022). Pelvic floor muscle training for urinary incontinence with or without biofeedback or electrostimulation in women: A systematic review. *International Journal of Environmental Research and Public Health, 19*(5), 2789. https://doi.org/10.3390/ijerph19052789

consequently chronic straining. The stools of a constipated person are hard and dry, and typically they must strain while bearing down to defecate. This straining to pass a hard stool increases intra-abdominal pressure, which over time causes the pelvic organs to prolapse. Dietary modifications can help establish regular bowel movements without discomfort and eliminate flatus and bloating. A weight loss regimen might also need to be instituted if the person is overweight.

PESSARIES

A vaginal **pessary** is a synthetic support device inserted in the vagina to provide support to the bladder and other pelvic organs as a corrective measure for UI and/or POP (Fig. 7.2). Almost all pessaries are made of medical-grade silicone, which provides many advantages. Silicone pessaries are pliable and have a long shelf life; lack odor and secretion absorption; are biologically inert, nonallergenic, and noncarcinogenic; and they can be boiled or autoclaved for sterilization. Although many types and shapes are available, the most commonly used pessary is a firm ring that presses against the wall of the vagina and urethra to help decrease leakage and support a prolapsed vagina or uterus (Clemons, 2024). Pessaries are a low-risk treatment option with the advantage of being cost-effective and minimally invasive. They also provide immediate relief of symptoms.

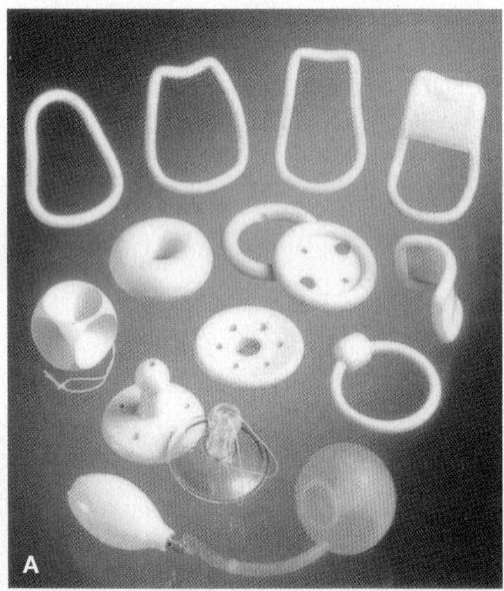

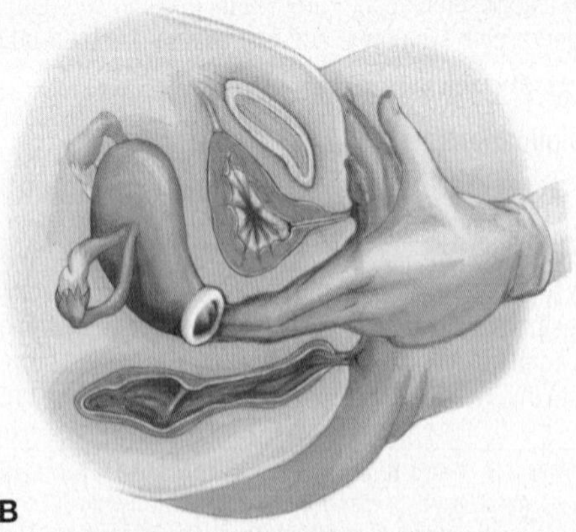

FIGURE 7.2 Examples of pessaries. **A.** Various shapes and sizes of pessaries available. **B.** Insertion of one type of pessary.

Indications for pessary use include uterine prolapse or cystocele, especially among older patients for whom surgery is contraindicated; younger patients with prolapse who plan to have additional children; and patients with marked prolapse who prefer to use a pessary rather than undergo surgery (Clemons, 2024). Many patients use pessaries for only a short period of time and become free of symptoms. Long-term use can lead to pressure necrosis and the development of fistulas in some patients; in this situation, other methods of support should be explored. Pessaries are fitted by trial and error; the patient often needs to try several sizes or styles. The largest pessary that the patient can wear comfortably is generally the most effective. The patient should be instructed to report any discomfort or difficulty with urination or defecation while wearing the pessary and also to attend follow-up care appointments to check positioning.

Nurses need to be aware of the personal isolation, embarrassment, and social and cultural implications that POP and UI may cause as well as the subjective experiences of using a pessary. With appropriate support, vaginal pessaries can provide people with the freedom to lead active, engaged social lives.

SURGICAL INTERVENTIONS

There are two types of surgical interventions for POP: reconstructive, which is the most common, and obliterative (ACOG, 2022). Obliterative surgery is used for patients who have comorbidities that put them at high risk for requiring an extensive surgery and for patients who do not plan to have vaginal sexual intercourse in the future, as the procedure removes or closes off all or part of the vaginal canal (Jelovsek, 2024). The goal of reconstructive surgery is to correct specific defects to restore normal anatomy and to preserve function. There are many different types of surgery approaches for POP, including vaginal or abdominal with or without grafts (Rogers & Fashokun, 2022). However, surgery is not an option for all patients. Patients who have POP without symptoms; plan to give birth to more children; are at high risk of suffering recurrent prolapse after a surgical repair; or have a BMI greater than 40 kg/m^2, chronic obstructive pulmonary disease, or medical conditions in which general anesthesia would be risky are not good candidates for surgical repair. Noninvasive treatment strategies should be discussed with such patients (Jelovsek, 2024).

Nursing Assessment

Nursing assessment for patients with POP includes a thorough health history, a physical examination, and several laboratory and diagnostic tests.

HEALTH HISTORY AND CLINICAL MANIFESTATIONS

A history and general assessment of the patient is important to exclude pathology and evaluate various factors that may influence choice and success of management. Evaluation of systems such as bowel, urinary and sexual function, coexistent morbidities, medical and surgical history, any physical or mental impairment, and lifestyle are important, particularly in older patients. The patient's social circumstances and support systems, desire for treatment, and expectations will have implications on the management options.

The cause of prolapse is multifactorial. Assessment of risk factors in the patient's history will assist the health care provider in the diagnosis and treatment of POP. The history should include questions about:

- Obstetrical history (number of pregnancies, weight of newborns, pregnancy spacing)
- Age
- Menopausal status
- Weight history (loss or gain)
- Constipation (frequency and chronicity)
- Chronic respiratory conditions (e.g., chronic coughing)
- Work history (e.g., physical labor or light office work)
- Connective tissue disorders or congenital abnormalities
- Family history (family member with POP)
- UI
- Previous pelvic surgeries (Rogers & Fashokun, 2022)

Assess for clinical manifestations of POP. POP is often without symptoms, but when symptoms do occur, they are often related to the site and type of prolapse. Symptoms common to all types of prolapse are a feeling of dragging, a lump in the vagina, or something "coming down." People with POP can present either with one symptom, such as vaginal bulging or pelvic pressure, or with several complaints, including multiple bladder, bowel, and pelvic symptoms. Symptoms associated with POP are summarized in Box 7.1.

Patients present with varying degrees of uterine descent. Uterine prolapse, due to the weakening of its surrounding support structures, is the most troubling type of pelvic relaxation because it is often associated with concomitant defects of the vagina in the anterior, posterior, and lateral compartments that can result in urinary and fecal incontinence, leading to sexual dysfunction and a poor body image (Chen & Thompson, 2022).

BOX 7.1 Symptoms Associated With Pelvic Organ Prolapse

- Vaginal bulge or pressure
- Stress incontinence
- Frequency (diurnal and nocturnal)
- Urgency and urge incontinence
- Hesitancy
- Feeling of pelvic pressure
- Poor or prolonged stream
- Feeling of incomplete emptying
- Symptoms worsening throughout the day
- Difficulty with defecation
- Incontinence of flatus or liquid or solid stool
- Urgency of defecation
- Feeling of incomplete evacuation
- Rectal protrusion or prolapse after defecation
- Lack of satisfaction or orgasm
- Incontinence during sexual activity
- Pain in the vagina or perineum
- Low back pain after long periods of standing
- Difficulty in walking due to a protrusion from the vagina
- Difficulty inserting or keeping a tampon in place

Adapted from American College of Obstetricians and Gynecologists. (2021a). *Pelvic support problems.* https://www.acog.org/womens-health/faqs/pelvic-support-problems; and Rogers, R. G., & Fashokun, T. B. (2022). Pelvic organ prolapse in females: Epidemiology, risk factors, clinical manifestations, and management. *UpToDate.* Retrieved April 30, 2024, from https://www.uptodate.com/contents/pelvic-organ-prolapse-in-females-epidemiology-risk-factors-clinical-manifestations-and-management

PHYSICAL EXAMINATION

The pelvic examination performed by the health care provider includes an external genital inspection to visualize any obvious protrusion of the uterus, bladder, urethra, or vaginal wall occurring at the vaginal opening. Usually, the patient is asked to perform the Valsalva maneuver (bearing down) while the examiner notes which organ prolapses first and the degree to which it occurs. Any urine leakage during the examination is important to note. The patient is asked to contract the pubococcygeal muscles (PFME); the health care provider inserts two fingers into the vagina to assess the strength and symmetry of the contraction. Because pelvic or genital organ prolapse can cause urinary symptoms such as incontinence, bladder function should be assessed by determining postvoid residual with a catheter. If the patient has more than 100 mL of retained urine, they should be referred for further urodynamic evaluation and testing.

LABORATORY AND DIAGNOSTIC TESTS

Common laboratory tests that may be ordered to determine the cause of POP include a urinalysis to rule out a bacterial infection, urine culture to identify the specific organism if present, visualization of urine loss during the pelvic examination, and measurement of postvoid urine volume.

Nursing Management

Help the patient understand the nature of the condition, the treatment options, and the likely outcomes. Nursing considerations might include:

- Describe normal anatomy and causes of pelvic prolapse.
- Assess how this condition has affected the patient's life.
- Outline the options with the advantages and disadvantages of each.
- Allow the patient to make the decision that is right for them.
- Provide education.
- Schedule preoperative activities needed for surgery.
- Reassure the patient that there is a solution for their symptoms.
- Provide community education about genital prolapse.

Clinical Judgment & Nursing Process 7.1 provides an overview of care for a patient with POP.

PROMOTE PREVENTION STRATEGIES

Researchers are studying ways to prevent POP, but a nurse needs to first understand its incidence, risk factors, prevalence, clinical implications, and treatment options

CLINICAL JUDGMENT & NURSING PROCESS 7.1 Overview of a Patient With Pelvic Organ Prolapse (POP)

Katherine, a 62-year-old multiparous patient, came to her gynecologist with complaints of a chronic dragging or heavy painful feeling in her pelvis, lower backache, constipation, and urine leakage. Her symptoms increase when she stands for long periods. She has not had menstrual cycles for at least a decade. She tells you, "I'm not taking any of those menopausal hormones." She also states that she is self-conscious and embarrassed about her urine leakage and restricts her outside activities.

NURSING ANALYSIS: Altered body image related to relaxation of pelvic support and elimination difficulties

OUTCOME IDENTIFICATION AND EVALUATION

The patient will report improved body image after management of POP and improved urinary control.

INTERVENTIONS: *Providing Pain Management*

- Obtain a thorough history including ongoing embarrassing experiences, methods of urine control used, what worked, what didn't, any changes in sexual practices related to this, and the effect of this condition on activities of daily living *to provide a baseline and enable a systematic approach to address it.*
- Assess the frequency, severity, precipitating factors, and aggravating/alleviating factors *to identify characteristics of the patient's abnormal urinary patterns to plan appropriate interventions.*
- Educate the patient about any medications prescribed (correct dosage, route, side effects, and precautions) *to increase the patient's understanding of the therapy and promote adherence.*
- Assess problematic elimination patterns *to identify underlying factors from which to plan appropriate prevention strategies.*
- Encourage the patient to increase fluids and fiber in the diet and increase physical activity daily *to promote peristalsis.*
- Assist the patient with establishing regular toileting patterns by setting aside time daily for bowel elimination *to promote regular bowel function and evacuation.*
- Urge the patient to avoid the routine use of laxatives *to reduce the risk of compounding constipation.*

NURSING ANALYSIS: Knowledge deficiency related to causes of structural disorders and treatment options

OUTCOME IDENTIFICATION AND EVALUATION

The patient will demonstrate an understanding of the current condition and treatments as evidenced by identifying treatment options, making health-promoting lifestyle choices, verbalizing appropriate health care practices, and adhering to the treatment plan.

INTERVENTIONS: *Providing Patient Education*

- Assess the patient's understanding of POP and its treatment options *to provide a baseline for teaching.*
- Review information provided about surgical procedures and recommendations for a healthy lifestyle, obtaining feedback frequently, *to validate the patient's understanding of instructions.*
- Discuss association between uterine, bladder, and rectal prolapse and symptoms *to help the patient understand the etiology of their symptoms and pain.*
- Have the patient verbalize and discuss information related to diagnosis, surgical procedure, preoperative routine, and postoperative regimen *to ensure adequate understanding and provide time for correcting or clarifying any misinformation or misconceptions.*
- Provide written material with pictures *to promote learning and help the patient visualize what has occurred to their body secondary to aging, weight gain, childbirth, and gravity.*
- Discuss pros and cons of hormone replacement therapy, osteoporosis prevention, and cardiovascular events common in postmenopausal people *to promote informed decision making by the patient about available menopausal therapies.*
- Inform the patient about the availability of community resources and make appropriate referrals as needed *to provide additional education and support.*
- Document details of teaching and learning *to allow for continuity of care and further education if needed.*

to be an effective caregiver for the patient. The nurse's understanding will not only improve their ability to treat this growing patient population but will also help in developing preventive strategies to address the patient's suffering from this condition.

Approaches include lifestyle changes that reduce modifiable risk factors, such as losing weight, avoiding heavy lifting, stopping smoking to prevent chronic coughing, and choosing foods with high fiber to prevent constipation. Explore with the patient what factors in their lifestyle might be modified to reduce their risk of developing POP (primary prevention) or to improve their quality of life after receiving treatment (secondary prevention).

ENCOURAGE PELVIC FLOOR MUSCLE TRAINING

Encourage the patient to perform PFMEs daily (Teaching Guidelines 7.1). Discuss current research findings and educate the patient about estrogen therapy, allowing the patient to make their own informed decision about whether to use hormones.

ENCOURAGE DIETARY AND LIFESTYLE MODIFICATIONS

Instruct patients to increase dietary fiber and fluids to prevent constipation. A high-fiber diet with an increase in fluid intake alleviates constipation by increasing stool bulk and stimulating peristalsis. It is accomplished by replacing refined, low-fiber foods with high-fiber foods. The recommended intake of fiber is 20 to 35 g/day (Wald, 2022). In addition to increasing the amount of fiber in the patient's diet, encourage them to drink eight 8-oz glasses of fluid daily and to engage in regular low-impact aerobic exercise, which promotes muscle tone and stimulates peristalsis.

Educate the patient about other lifestyle changes that will assist with prolapse, such as:

- Achieve a healthy BMI (18.5 to 24.9 kg/m^2) to reduce intra-abdominal pressure and strain on pelvic organs, including pressure on the bladder.
- Wear a girdle or abdominal support to support the muscles surrounding the pelvic organs.
- Avoid lifting heavy objects to reduce the risk of increasing intra-abdominal pressure, which can push the pelvic organs downward.
- Avoid high-impact aerobics, jogging, or jumping repeatedly to minimize the risk of increasing intra-abdominal pressure, which places downward pressure on the organs.
- Give up smoking to minimize the risk for a chronic "smoker's cough," which increases intra-abdominal pressure and forces the pelvic organs downward.

TEACHING GUIDELINES 7.1 Performing Pelvic Floor Exercises

- Squeeze the muscles in your rectum as if you are trying to prevent passing flatus.
- Stop and start urinary flow to help identify the pubococcygeus muscle.
- Tighten the pubococcygeus muscle for a count of three and then relax it.
- Contract and relax the pubococcygeus muscle rapidly 10 times.
- Try to bring up the entire pelvic floor and bear down 10 times.
- Repeat pelvic floor muscle exercises at least five times daily.

PROVIDE TEACHING FOR PESSARY USE

Educate the patient about pessary use. Discuss complications as part of the instruction. Although the pessary is a safe device, it is still a foreign body in the vagina. Because of this, the most common side effects of the pessary are increased vaginal discharge, bleeding, erosions, and odor (Clemons, 2023). Vaginal discharge and odors can be reduced by using a pH-lowering product, such as Trimo-San gel, inserted vaginally (Clemons, 2023). Low-dose vaginal estrogen cream can also be used to help reduce vaginal discharge, odor, erosion, and bleeding (Clemons, 2023).

The patient must be capable of managing the use of the pessary, either alone or with the help of their health care provider or caregiver. The most common recommendations for pessary care include removing the pessary every 1 to 2 weeks, leaving it out of the vagina for one night; cleaning it with soap and water; using a lubricant for insertion; and having regular follow-up examinations every 6 to 12 months after an initial period of adjustment.

Besides cleaning, the patient must properly reinsert the device into their vaginal cavity, and they must also be willing to participate in all aspects of care of the pessary for this treatment option to be successful. Any patient who chooses this option must be instructed in the care of their pessary so that they feel comfortable with all aspects of it before leaving the health care facility. Health care visits should allow adequate time for the patient to share their concerns, anxieties, and fears surrounding the transition to life with a pessary.

PROVIDE PERIOPERATIVE CARE

Prepare the patient for surgery by reinforcing the risks and benefits of surgery and describing the postoperative course. Explain that a Foley catheter will be in place for up to 1 week and that the patient might not be able to urinate due to the swelling after the catheter has been removed. Provide home care instructions for the Foley catheter. The patient should cleanse the perineal area daily with mild soap and water, especially around where the catheter enters the urinary meatus. If the patient is provided with a leg bag to be worn during waking hours, instruct them to empty it frequently and keep it below the level of the bladder to prevent backflow. The same principles are applied to the primary Foley bag when emptying it.

During the recovery period for several weeks, instruct the patient to avoid activities that cause an increase in abdominal pressure, such as straining, sneezing, and coughing. In addition, advise the patient to avoid lifting anything heavy or straining to push anything. Explain to the patient that stool softeners and gentle laxatives might be prescribed to prevent constipation and straining with bowel movements. Avoiding vaginal intercourse will be recommended until the operative area is healed in 6 weeks.

Urinary Incontinence

Urinary incontinence (UI) is the involuntary leakage of urine (Lukacz, 2024b). This disorder affects over 20 million females in the United States, and at least 50% of all females over the age of 50 experience some form of UI (McKinney et al., 2022). The psychosocial costs and morbidities are difficult to quantify. Embarrassment and depression are common. Despite the considerable impact of incontinence on quality of life, many people are unlikely to bring up the subject of their lack of bladder control and few seek help or treatment for incontinence concerns. There are several possible explanations for why patients do not talk about their bladder control issues. The patient may:

- Believe UI is inevitable and not amenable to treatment
- Feel UI is a "normal" part of aging
- Believe UI is part of being "female." Females tend to accept urinary symptoms such as UI more than males do.
- Feel embarrassed and try to deny that it is a real problem
- Think that the only treatment option is surgical intervention
- Consider UI a hygiene problem and not a medical condition

TAKE NOTE!

Incontinence is preventable, treatable, and often curable. However, many people believe that loss of bladder function is a normal and expected part of aging.

Incontinence can have far-reaching effects. Some people experience anxiety, depression, social isolation, embarrassment, insomnia, fear, feelings of uncleanliness, worry, vulnerability, shame, limits in the ability to travel far from home or have social engagements, and disruptions in self-esteem and dignity. UI can cause the person to stop working, traveling, socializing, and enjoying sexual relationships. In addition, incontinence can create a tremendous burden for caregivers and is a common reason for admission to a long-term care facility. People often try to cope with UI through lifestyle modifications such as wearing protective pads, avoiding certain activities, emptying the bladder frequently, and modifying diet and fluid intake. People who experience UI are often distressed by the social implications and many go to great efforts to hide their symptoms. In some cultures, UI is abhorred to the point at which the person may be shunned by their community. A sense of control, normality, and self-esteem are central issues in living with UI. Generally, with time and a worsening of symptoms, a person will pursue medical evaluation and treatment (ACOG, 2021b).

The types of UI are defined based on their presenting symptoms and signs. The three most common types of incontinence are urgency UI (overactive bladder caused by detrusor muscle contractions resulting in a strong urge to urinate and leaking urine), stress incontinence (inadequate urinary sphincter function resulting in leaking urine during exertion), and mixed incontinence (involves both stress and urge incontinence) (ACOG, 2021b; Tran & Puckett, 2023). Comparison Chart 7.1 details these types of UI.

COMPARISON CHART 7.1 Urge Incontinence Versus Stress Incontinence

	Urge Incontinence	Stress Incontinence
Description	Precipitous loss of urine, preceded by a strong urge to void, with increased bladder pressure and detrusor contraction	Accidental leakage of urine that occurs with increased pressure on the bladder from coughing, sneezing, laughing, or physical exertion
Etiology	Causes might be neurologic, idiopathic, or infectious	Develops commonly in females in their 40s and 50s, usually as the result of weakened muscles and ligaments in the pelvis following childbirth
Signs and symptoms	Urgency, frequency, nocturia, and a large amount of urine loss	Involuntary loss of a small amount of urine in response to physical activity that raises intra-abdominal pressure

Pathophysiology and Etiology

Urinary continence requires several factors, including effective functioning of the bladder, adequate pelvic floor muscles, neural control from the brain, and integrity of the neural connections that facilitate voluntary control. The bladder neck and proximal urethra function as a sphincter. During urination, the sphincter relaxes and the bladder empties. The ability to control urination requires the integrated function of numerous components of the lower urinary tract, which must be structurally sound and functioning normally.

Incontinence can develop if the bladder muscles become overactive due to weakened sphincter muscles, if the bladder muscles become too weak to contract properly, or if signals from the nervous system to the urinary structures are interrupted. A major factor in females that contributes to urinary continence is the estrogen level because this hormone helps maintain bladder sphincter tone. In perimenopausal or menopausal people, incontinence can be a problem as estrogen levels begin to decline and genitourinary changes occur. In simple terms, the bladder is the reservoir, the urethra is the seal, and the levator ani muscle is the gate that holds pressure against the outflow of urine by supporting the urethra and bladder from below. When any of these three structures is not functioning normally, incontinence occurs. Weakened pelvic floor muscles also prevent complete closure of the urethra, resulting in urine leakage during physical stress. This problem is not limited to older patients; UI has been documented in people as young as 20 years of age (Tran & Puckett, 2023).

Contributing factors in UI include:

- Fluid intake, especially alcohol, carbonated drinks, and caffeinated beverages
- Constipation: alters the position of the pelvic organs and puts pressure on the bladder
- Habitual "preventive" emptying: may result in training the bladder to hold only small amounts of urine
- Urinary tract infection
- Menopause and depletion of estrogen
- Chronic diseases such as stroke, multiple sclerosis, or diabetes
- Smoking: nicotine increases detrusor muscle contractions.
- Advancing age: age-related anatomic changes result in less pelvic support.
- Pregnancy and childbirth: damage to pelvic structures during childbirth
- Obesity: increases abdominal pressure (ACOG, 2021b; Lukacz, 2024b)

Therapeutic Management

Treatment options depend on the type of UI. In general, the least invasive procedure with the fewest risks is the first choice for treatment. Surgery is used only if other methods have failed. There is a widespread belief that UI is an inevitable problem of getting older and that little or nothing can be done to relieve symptoms or reverse it. However, nothing is further from the truth, and attitudes must change so that people will feel comfortable seeking help for what can be an embarrassing condition.

For many patients with urge incontinence, simple reassurance and lifestyle interventions might help. The promotion of a healthy weight can help reduce incontinence related to obesity. See additional contributing factors above. However, if more than simple lifestyle measures are needed, effective treatments might include:

- Bladder training to establish normal voiding intervals (every 3 to 5 hours)
- PFMEs to strengthen the pelvic floor musculature (see Evidence-Based Practice 7.1)
- A pessary to support pelvic structures that have weakened
- Topical vaginal estrogen for peri- or postmenopausal patients (Lukacz, 2024a)

For patients with stress incontinence, treatment is not always a cure, but it can minimize the impact of this condition on the patient's quality of life. Some treatment options for stress incontinence might include:

- Weight loss if indicated
- Avoidance of constipation
- Smoking cessation
- PFMEs to strengthen the pelvic floor
- Pessaries
- Weighted vaginal cones to improve the tone of pelvic floor muscles
- Periurethral injection (injecting a bulking agent [collagen] to form a bulge that brings the urethral walls closer together to achieve a better closure)
- Medications such as duloxetine (Cymbalta, Yentreve) to increase urethral sphincter contractions during the storage phase of the urination cycle (not routinely used due to adverse effects) (Lukacz, 2024a)
- Estrogen replacement therapy to improve bladder sphincter tone
- Surgery to correct genital prolapse and improve urethral and bladder tone

CONSIDER THIS!

Life can be complicated and embarrassing at times when we least expect it. I met a man in church who seemed interested in me, and he asked me out for coffee after Sunday services. I have been alone for 10 years, and this prospect seemed exciting to me. We talked for hours over coffee and seemed to have a great deal in common, especially since both of us had lost our spouses to cancer. He asked me to go square dancing with him since that was an activity we both had enjoyed in the past with our spouses. I hadn't been out or physically active for ages and didn't realize how my body had changed with age.

It was during the first dance that I noticed a wet sensation between my legs, which I was unable to control. I managed to continue on and pretend that all was fine, but then realized what many of my friends were talking about—stress incontinence. Not being able to control one's urine is very embarrassing and it complicates your life, but I made up my mind that it wasn't going to control me.

Thoughts: Gravity and childbirth take a toll on the female reproductive organs by pushing them downward. This person is not going to let stress incontinence curtail their outside activity, which demonstrates a good attitude. What can be done to mitigate the person's embarrassment and lack of control? Were there any preventive strategies they could have used at an earlier age?

Nursing Assessment

The assessment of the patient experiencing UI includes a history, physical examination, laboratory tests, and possibly urodynamic testing. The onset, frequency, severity, and pattern of incontinence should be determined, as well as any associated symptoms such as frequency, dysuria, urgency, and nocturia. Incontinence may be quantified by asking the patient if they wear a pad and how often the pad is changed. A review of the patient's current medications, including over-the-counter medications, should be included in the history.

A complete physical examination should be carried out by the health care provider; it should include a neurologic assessment and pelvic and rectal examinations. The presence of associated POP should be noted because it can contribute to the patient's voiding problems and may have an impact on diagnosis and treatment. A rectal examination is done to evaluate sphincter tone and perineal sensation. A "cough stress test" can be performed by asking the patient to cough with a full bladder and subsequently observing for leakage of urine from the urethra. This can also help in assessing the patient's ability to control voiding.

A urinalysis is performed to look for hematuria, pyuria, glucosuria, or proteinuria. A urine culture is done if there is pyuria or bacteriuria. Postvoid residual should be measured either with pelvic ultrasound or directly with a catheter. If the residual exceeds the limit set, urodynamic testing is then used to diagnose the incontinence.

Nursing Management

Incontinence can be devastating and can cause psychosocial concerns and isolation. Nurses can encourage patients with troublesome symptoms to seek help. Discuss the treatment options with the patient, including benefits and potential outcomes, and encourage them to select the continence treatment best for their lifestyle. Provide education about good bladder habits and strategies to reduce the incidence or severity of incontinence (Teaching Guidelines 7.2). Provide support and encouragement to ensure adherence to the guidelines. Remember that aging can increase the risk of incontinence, but incontinence is not an inevitable part of aging. Review the anatomy and physiology of the urinary system and offer simple explanations to help the patient cope with urinary alterations. Therapeutic listening is important. Be aware of the courage it takes for a patient to disclose an embarrassing condition.

TEACHING GUIDELINES 7.2 Managing Urinary Incontinence

- Avoid drinking too much fluid (i.e., 2 L total daily limit).
- Reduce intake of fluids and foods that are bladder irritants and precipitate urgency, such as chocolate, caffeine, carbonated beverages such as sodas, alcohol, artificial sweetener, citrus fruits, and tomatoes.
- Increase fiber and fluids in your diet to reduce constipation.
- Control blood glucose levels to prevent polyuria.
- Treat chronic cough.
- Remove any barriers that delay you from reaching the toilet.
- Practice good perineal hygiene by using mild soap and water. Wipe from front to back to prevent urinary tract infections.
- Become aware of adverse drug effects.
- Take your medications as prescribed.
- Continue to do pelvic floor muscle exercises.

American College of Obstetricians and Gynecologists. (2021b). *Urinary incontinence.* https://www.acog.org/womens-health/faqs/urinary-incontinence; and Tran, L. N., & Puckett, Y. (2023). Urinary incontinence. *StatPearls*. In StatPearls Publishing. https://www.ncbi.nlm.nih.gov/books/NBK559095/

TAKE NOTE!

Simple diet and lifestyle alterations combined with a proper pelvic floor muscle strengthening program can often produce significant improvements for patients of all ages.

BENIGN GROWTHS

The most common benign growths of the reproductive tract include cervical, endocervical, and endometrial polyps; uterine fibroids (leiomyomas); genital fistulas; Bartholin cysts; and ovarian cysts.

Polyps

Polyps are small, usually benign mucous membrane growths. The incidence of malignancy in cervical polyps is less than 1.5% (Alkilani & Apodaca-Ramos, 2023).

Malignancy is more common in postmenopausal people over the age of 40 (Alkilani & Apodaca-Ramos, 2023). The cause of polyp growth is not well understood, but theories point to infection, chronic inflammation, an abnormal local response to increased levels of estrogen, or local congestion of the cervical vasculature as potential causes (Alkilani & Apodaca-Ramos, 2023). Single or multiple polyps might occur. They are most common in multiparous, premenopausal people (Alkilani & Apodaca-Ramos, 2023). Polyps can appear anywhere but are most common at or near the cervical os and in the uterus (Fig. 7.3).

Endometrial polyps are benign tumors or localized overgrowths of the endometrium. They can be a single lesion or multiple lesions and are friable and easily bleed on contact. These polyps can occur at any age, but the peak incidence is in females 40 to 49 years of age (Mansour & Chowdhury, 2023). The polyps are typically benign, but some females, including those who are postmenopausal or who are taking tamoxifen, are at an increased risk for malignancy (Stewart, 2024a). Endometrial polyps are one of the more common causes of abnormal genital bleeding in females (Stewart, 2024a).

Therapeutic Management

The management of cervical polyps depends mostly on their clinical characteristics. Treatment of polyps usually consists of simple removal with small forceps done on an outpatient basis and then cauterized or lasered to prevent bleeding and polyp recurrence. The polyp base can be removed by laser vaporization. Because many polyps are infected, an antibiotic may be ordered after removal as a preventive measure or to treat early signs of infection.

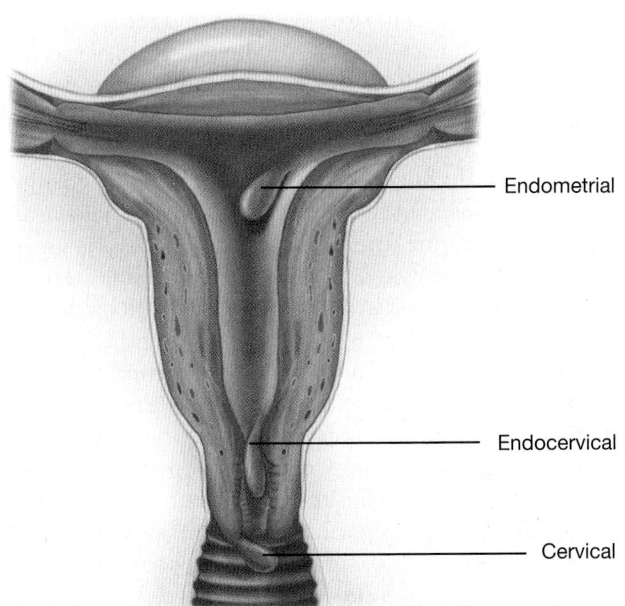

FIGURE 7.3 Cervical, endocervical, and endometrial polyps.

Although polyps are rarely cancerous, a specimen should be sent after surgery to a pathology laboratory to exclude malignancy. A cervical biopsy typically reveals mildly atypical cells and signs of infection. Polyps rarely return after they are removed. Regularly scheduled Pap smears are suggested for patients with cervical polyps to detect any future abnormal growths that may be malignant.

Nursing Assessment

Nursing assessment for a patient with polyps includes assisting with the physical examination and preparing the collected specimen to be sent to the cytologist.

CLINICAL MANIFESTATIONS

Assess for clinical manifestations of polyps. Cervical and endocervical polyps are often without symptoms, but they can produce mild symptoms such as abnormal vaginal bleeding (after intercourse, between menses) or discharge. The most common clinical manifestation of endometrial polyps is irregular, acyclic bleeding.

PHYSICAL EXAMINATION AND LABORATORY AND DIAGNOSTIC STUDIES

Typically, cervical polyps are diagnosed when the cervix is visualized through a speculum during the patient's annual gynecologic examination (Alkilani & Apodaca-Ramos, 2023). Endometrial polyps are not detected on physical examination but rather with ultrasound or hysteroscopy (introduction of a small camera through the cervix to visualize the uterine cavity).

Nursing Management

Nursing management of polyps involves explaining the condition and the rationale for removal and giving follow-up care instructions. The nurse also assists the health care provider with the removal procedure. Every excised polyp should be sent to the lab for a histologic assessment to rule out malignancy.

Uterine Fibroids

Uterine fibroids, also known as myomas or leiomyomas, are benign tumors composed of smooth muscle and fibrous connective tissue in the uterus. They are the most common pelvic tumors in females, with the highest incidence during reproductive years (Stewart & Laughlin-Tommaso, 2024). They can vary in size from that of a pea to larger than a grapefruit. Unlike cancerous tumors, fibroids usually grow more slowly, responding to present estrogen levels, and their cells do not break away and invade other parts of the body. Fibroids are

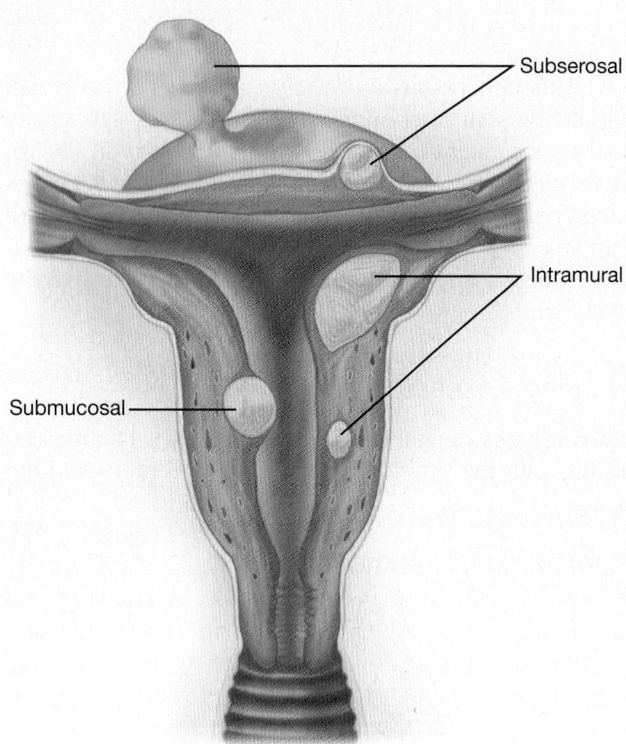

FIGURE 7.4 Submucosal, intramural, and subserosal fibroids.

classified according to their position in the uterus and on the uterine layer most involved (Fig. 7.4):

- *Subserosal fibroids:* lie underneath the outermost peritoneal layer of the uterus and grow outside the uterus. They are attached to the uterus by a stalk or peduncle.
- *Intramural fibroids:* grow within the wall of the uterus and are the most common type
- *Submucosal fibroids:* grow from immediately below the inner uterine surface (endometrium) into the uterine cavity
- *Cervical fibroids:* located in the cervix rather than in the uterine cavity (Stewart & Laughlin-Tommaso, 2024)

Fibroids are estrogen dependent and thus grow rapidly during the childbearing years when estrogen is plentiful, but they shrink during menopause when estrogen levels decline. It is believed that these benign tumors develop in up to 70% to 80% of females by age 50, but many are small and without symptoms (Mutch & Biest, 2023). It is difficult to be precise because fibroids may cause no symptoms, so many people do not know they have them.

Fibroids are the most common indication for hysterectomy in the United States (Barjon & Mikhail, 2023). The peak incidence occurs around 35 to 45 years of age, and they are more prevalent in Black women than in White women (Stewart & Laughlin-Tommaso, 2024).

Etiology

Although the cause of fibroids is unknown, several predisposing factors have been identified, including:

- Genetic predisposition
- African ancestry
- Hypertension
- Early menarche
- Vitamin D deficiencies
- Alcohol consumption
- Smoking
- Chronic stress
- Nulliparity
- Diabetes
- Obesity (Stewart & Laughlin-Tommaso, 2024)

Therapeutic Management

Treatment depends on the size of the fibroids and the patient's symptoms, which can include heavy or painful menses, a feeling of "fullness" or pressure in the lower pelvis, urinating frequently, constipation, pain during sexual intercourse, lower back pain, and infertility (Stewart & Laughlin-Tommaso, 2024). Several treatment options exist, ranging from watchful waiting to surgery.

MEDICAL MANAGEMENT

The goals of medical therapy are to reduce symptoms and/or the tumor size. This can be accomplished with pain medications to treat mild or occasional pain from fibroids; birth control pills, a progestin-releasing intrauterine device, or tranexamic acid (a nonhormonal medication) to control heavy menses; gonadotropin-releasing hormone (GnRH) antagonists, such as elagolix, relugolix, and linzagolix; or GnRH agonists such as leuprolide, nafarelin, or goserelin to stop ovulation and the production of estrogen (Stewart, 2024b). All these therapies produce regression and reduce the size of the tumors without surgery, but long-term therapy is expensive and not well tolerated by most patients. The side effects of GnRH medications include hot flashes, headaches, mood changes, vaginal dryness, musculoskeletal malaise, bone loss, and depression. Uterine artery embolization (UAE) is an option in which polyvinyl alcohol pellets are injected into selected blood vessels via a catheter to block circulation to the fibroid, causing it to shrink and producing symptom resolution. The procedure is carried out by an interventional radiologist who makes a tiny incision in the groin, introduces a fine catheter into the main artery leading to the uterus, and injects tiny particles of plastic or gelatin sponge into the artery that supplies blood to the fibroid. These particles stop the flow of blood, causing the fibroid to shrink or disappear completely over time. UAE has short-term advantages over surgery, such as lower risk of major complications and faster recovery time, but there is a higher reintervention rate after 2 years (van der Kooij & Hehenkamp, 2024). The decision to offer UAE should be based on the patient's needs and desires, including their plans for childbearing; the patient should be educated about treatment alternatives and their success rates, limitations, and side effects (Stewart, 2024b; van der Kooij & Hehenkamp, 2024).

Magnetic resonance-guided focused ultrasound (MRgFUS) creates coagulative necrosis, which destroys fibroids by using high-intensity ultrasound that directs focused ultrasound waves through the skin. This procedure is performed on an outpatient basis with sedation and no incisions. It is usually recommended for patients with large fibroids. Overall, this option has been shown to be effective and safe for decreasing fibroid size and/or volume but is time consuming and expensive and has a higher rate of reintervention than UAE (Stewart, 2024b). Case studies have documented successful pregnancy outcomes following MRgFUS (Stewart, 2024b).

SURGICAL MANAGEMENT

For patients with large fibroids or severe uterine bleeding, surgery is preferred over medical treatment. Surgical management might involve myomectomy, laser surgery, or hysterectomy.

Myomectomy. Myomectomy involves removing the fibroid alone and leaves the healthy areas of the uterus intact to preserve fertility. A myomectomy is performed via laparoscopy, through an abdominal incision or via the vagina. The advantage is that only the fibroid is removed; fertility is not jeopardized because this procedure leaves the uterine muscle walls intact. Myomectomy relieves symptoms but does not affect the underlying process; thus, fibroids grow back and further treatment will be needed in the future.

Hysterectomy. A hysterectomy is the surgical removal of the uterus. It is the most effective treatment for symptomatic fibroids with no recurrence. After a cesarean delivery, it is the most frequently performed surgical procedure for females in the United States (Walters & Ferrando, 2024). Common conditions associated with hysterectomies are pelvic relaxation, fibroids, endometriosis, and uterine prolapse (Pillarisetty & Mahdy, 2023). A hysterectomy to remove fibroids eliminates both the symptoms and the risk of recurrence, but it also terminates the patient's ability to bear children. Several types of hysterectomy surgeries are available: vaginal hysterectomy, laparoscopically assisted vaginal hysterectomy, and abdominal hysterectomy.

In a vaginal hysterectomy, the uterus is removed through an incision in the posterior vagina. Advantages include a shorter hospital stay and recovery time and no abdominal scars. Disadvantages include a limited operating space and poor visualization of other pelvic organs.

In a laparoscopically assisted vaginal hysterectomy, the uterus is removed through a laparoscope, through which structures within the abdomen and pelvis are visualized. Small incisions are made in the abdominal wall to permit the laparoscope to enter the surgical site. Advantages include a better surgical field, less pain, lower cost, and a shorter recovery time. Disadvantages include potential injury to the bladder and the inability to remove enlarged uteruses and scar tissue.

In an abdominal hysterectomy, the uterus and other pelvic organs are removed through an incision in the abdomen. This procedure allows the surgeon to visualize all pelvic organs and is typically used when a malignancy is suspected or the patient has a very large uterus. Disadvantages include the need for general anesthesia, a longer hospital stay and recovery period, more pain, higher cost, and a visible scar on the abdomen.

Complications of hysterectomy vary based on the route of surgery and technique. Possible complications include infection, bladder injury, venous thromboembolism, genitourinary and gastrointestinal injuries, and hemorrhage (Pillarisetty & Mahdy, 2023). With astute nursing observations and assessments, these complications can be reduced or minimized. A summary of treatment options for uterine fibroids is presented in Table 7.1.

Nursing Assessment

Nursing assessment for the patient with uterine fibroids includes a thorough health history, physical examination, and laboratory and diagnostic studies.

HEALTH HISTORY AND CLINICAL MANIFESTATIONS

The history should include questions about the patient's menstrual cycle, including alterations in the menstrual pattern (e.g., pain or pressure, aggravating and alleviating factors), history of infertility, and any history of spontaneous abortion, which might indicate a space-occupying uterine lesion. Ask if any female relatives have had fibroids because there is a familial predisposition. Assess for clinical manifestations of uterine fibroids. Symptoms of fibroids depend on the size and location and may include:

- Chronic pelvic pain
- Changes in menstrual cycle
- Low back pain
- Iron-deficiency anemia secondary to bleeding
- Constipation
- Infertility (with large tumors)
- Dysmenorrhea
- Miscarriage
- Sciatica
- Dyspareunia
- Urinary frequency, urgency, incontinence
- Irregular vaginal bleeding (menorrhagia)
- Feeling of heaviness in the pelvic region (United States Food & Drug Administration, 2023; Stewart & Laughlin-Tommaso, 2024)

TABLE 7.1 • Summary of Treatment Options for Uterine Fibroids

Method	Advantages	Disadvantages
Hormones	Noninvasive Reduces the size of fibroids Symptom improvement	Serious side effects with long-term use Fibroids regrow when meds stopped
Uterine artery embolization	Minimally invasive Dramatic decrease in symptoms Future fertility possible	Procedure frequently painful Requires radiation and contrast dye Permanently implanted material Possible negative fertility impact
Myomectomy	Performed as minor surgery Uterus is preserved.	Requires general anesthesia New growth of fibroids occurs.
Hysterectomy	Complete removal of fibroids Immediate symptom relief	Requires general anesthesia Major surgery with associated risks Fertility not preserved
Magnetic resonance-focused ultrasound	Noninvasive treatment with a short recovery time; rapid resolution of symptoms	Typically used for large fibroids and can be expensive

PHYSICAL EXAMINATION AND LABORATORY AND DIAGNOSTIC STUDIES

The bimanual examination performed by the health care provider typically shows an enlarged, irregular uterus. The uterus may be palpable abdominally if the fibroid is very large. Ultrasound may be used to confirm the diagnosis.

Nursing Management

The level of support that nurses can provide patients with fibroids depends on the type of treatment offered and the patient's choice. Nurses should be able to explain any current treatment options and the implications of a diagnosis of fibroids. Many patients have not yet heard of fibroids and need reassurance that they are both common and benign. If medication is prescribed, it is essential to explain the possible side effects and why medication can only be taken for a limited duration. If surgery is selected, verbal and written information about it and the aftercare should be addressed (Box 7.2).

A patient undergoing a hysterectomy for the treatment of fibroids often needs special care and can benefit from presurgical and postsurgical support provided by nurses. Personalized nursing, tailored to the individual patient's needs, enhances the patient's coping strategies and alleviates different adverse psychological sequelae following gynecologic surgery. Patients may experience a variety of psychological adjustment difficulties related to changes in self-image, self-esteem, loss of femininity or identity, and sexual dysfunction. The incidence of postsurgical problems can be reduced greatly with proper patient-centered perioperative nursing care.

BOX 7.2 Nursing Interventions for a Patient Undergoing a Hysterectomy

Preoperative Care

- Instruct the patient and their family about the procedure and postoperative care.
- Provide interventions to reduce anxiety (due to perceived threats to the patient's self-concept and role functioning) and fear of alteration in body image, complications, and pain. Prepare the patient so that they know what to expect throughout the perioperative experience. Explain postoperative pain management procedures that will be used. Identify the high-risk patient early to reduce their stress.
- Teach turning, deep breathing, and coughing before surgery to prevent postoperative atelectasis and respiratory complications such as pneumonia.
- Encourage the patient to discuss their feelings. Some people attach great importance to their reproductive capability, and the loss of the uterus could evoke grieving.
- Complete all preoperative orders in a timely manner to allow for rest.

Postoperative Care

- Provide comfort measures.
- Administer analgesics promptly or use a patient-controlled anesthesia pump.
- Administer antiemetics to control nausea and vomiting per order.
- Change the patient's linens and gown frequently to promote hygiene.
- Change the patient's position frequently and use pillows for support to promote comfort and pain management.
- Assess the incision, the dressing, and vaginal bleeding and report if bleeding is excessive (soaking perineal pad within an hour).
- Monitor elimination and provide increased fluids and fiber to prevent constipation and straining.
- Encourage ambulation and active range-of-motion exercises when in bed to prevent thrombophlebitis and venous stasis.
- Monitor vital signs to detect early complications.
- Be comfortable discussing sexual concerns with the patient.

BOX 7.2 **Nursing Interventions for a Patient Undergoing a Hysterectomy**

Discharge Planning

- Advise the patient to reduce their activity level to avoid fatigue, which might inhibit healing.
- Advise the patient to rest when they are tired and when ready, to increase their activity level slowly.
- Educate the patient on the need for pelvic rest (nothing in the vagina) for 6 weeks.
- Instruct the patient to avoid heavy lifting or straining for about 6 weeks to prevent an increase in intra-abdominal pressure, which could weaken the sutures.
- Teach the patient the signs and symptoms of infection.
- Advise the patient to take showers instead of tub baths to reduce the risk of infection.
- Encourage the patient to eat a healthy diet with increased intake of fluids to prevent dehydration and fluid and electrolyte imbalance.
- Instruct the patient to change their perineal pad frequently to prevent infection.
- Explain and schedule follow-up care appointments as needed.
- Provide information about community resources for support and help.

Urogenital Fistulas

Urogenital fistulas are abnormal communications between the female genital tract and the urinary system or rectum. In the United States and other resource-abundant countries, these are uncommon and typically result as a complication after a hysterectomy (Garely & Mann, 2022). In resource-limited countries, approximately 3 million females (both adults and children) worldwide are affected, mostly in Africa and South Asia (Medlen & Barbier, 2023). A fistula can result from a congenital anomaly, surgical complications, Bartholin gland abscesses, radiation, or malignancy, but the majority of fistulas that occur in resource-limited countries are related to obstetric trauma, typically from a long obstructed labor and female genital mutilation/cutting, which makes delivery more difficult (United Nations Population Fund, 2023a). During normal labor, the bladder is displaced upward into the abdomen, and the anterior vaginal wall, the base of the bladder, and the urethra are compressed between the fetal head and the posterior pubis. When labor is obstructed or prolonged, this unrelieved compression causes ischemia, which causes pressure necrosis and subsequent fistula formation. The direct consequences of this damage include UI and fecal incontinence if the rectum is involved.

Common types of fistulas include:

- *Vesicovaginal:* communication between the bladder and genital tract
- *Urethrovaginal:* communication between the urethra and the vagina
- *Rectovaginal:* communication between the rectum or sigmoid colon and the vagina

Despite being internationally recognized as a human rights violation, 230 million people alive today have undergone female genital mutilation/cutting; if current rates persist, an estimated 68 million more will be cut by 2030 (United Nations Population Fund, 2023b). Because of immigration, health care providers in the United States are increasingly confronted with the range of negative urogynecologic effects that result from this practice. Nurses need to have a deeper understanding of related history, cultural beliefs, medical complications, and methods of surgical reconstruction to provide culturally congruent care to patients who have undergone female genital mutilation/cutting. This cultural practice will be addressed in detail in Chapter 9.

Therapeutic Management

The best management for fistulas is preventing the complication during a hysterectomy or recognizing and repairing the injury during the primary surgery (Garely & Mann, 2022). Many small fistulas will heal with stent placement, but large fistulas often require surgical repair; surgery may be postponed until the edema or inflammation in the surrounding tissues has dissipated.

Nursing Assessment

The history should include questions about any changes in the patient's urinary and bowel patterns. Assess for common signs and symptoms of fistulas, which are related to the type of fistula. If the opening involves the rectum, feces and flatus will leak through the vagina. If it involves the bladder, urine will leak from the vagina. Depending on the location and size of the fistula, the patient may or may not experience discomfort. The health care provider can detect these abnormal openings through inspection and palpation during the pelvic examination. Diagnostic or laboratory tests are generally not ordered once this condition is found.

Nursing Management

Provide guidance and support. Offer information to help the patient learn about their condition and with appropriate intervention, to improve their quality of life. Begin by making sure the patient understands their anatomy and why they are having such symptoms. Provide a thorough explanation of the treatment options so that the patient can make an informed decision. Be sensitive to the patient's feeling of shame and fear about their incontinence; these feelings may be why the patient delayed seeking treatment. Address all of the patient's needs, both physical and emotional.

Bartholin Cysts

The Bartholin glands are two mucus-secreting glandular pea-sized structures with duct openings located bilaterally at the base of the labia minora near the opening of the vagina. They provide lubrication during sexual arousal. Normally, these glands cannot be felt or seen unless they are infected. **Bartholin cysts** are swollen, fluid-filled, saclike structures that result when one of the ducts of the Bartholin gland becomes blocked. The cyst may become infected, and an abscess may develop in the gland. Bartholin cysts and abscesses account for about 2% of gynecologic visits each year (Chen, 2023).

Therapeutic Management

Treatment can be conservative or surgical depending on the symptoms, the size of the cyst, and whether it is infected or not. Small cysts without symptoms do not require treatment. Sitz baths along with analgesics are used to reduce discomfort. Antibiotics are prescribed if the gland is infected. The aim of treatment for a larger cyst or abscess is to create a fistulous tract from the dilated duct to the outside vulva by incision and drainage. However, cysts or abscesses tend to return if this option is used.

Other treatment options beyond incision and drainage include placement of a Word catheter with a balloon tip (performed in the office and preferred first choice) or a small loop of plastic tubing secured in place to prevent closure and to allow drainage (referred to as marsupialization and performed in an operating room) (Lee & Wittler, 2023). Both procedures are safe and effective alternatives to surgery (Lee & Wittler, 2023). Treatment for a pregnant patient with a Bartholin cyst depends on the severity of the symptoms and whether an infection is present. Surgery may be delayed until after the patient gives birth if there are no symptoms.

Nursing Assessment

Nursing assessment for the patient with a Bartholin cyst includes a thorough health history, physical examination, and laboratory and diagnostic tests.

HEALTH HISTORY

The history should include questions about the patient's sexual practices and protective measures used. Assess for common signs and symptoms of Bartholin cysts. The patient may be without symptoms if the cyst is small (less than 5 cm) and not infected. If infection is present, symptoms include varying degrees of pain, especially when walking or sitting; unilateral edema; redness around the gland; and dyspareunia. Extensive inflammation may cause systemic symptoms. Abscess formation occurs when the cystic fluid becomes infected. An abscess usually develops rapidly over a 2- to 3-day period and may spontaneously rupture. A history of sudden relief of pain following profuse discharge is highly suggestive of spontaneous rupture (Quinn, 2022).

PHYSICAL EXAMINATION AND LABORATORY AND DIAGNOSTIC STUDIES

The diagnosis of Bartholin cysts or abscesses is primarily made during a physical examination when a protruding tender labial mass is located. In postmenopausal people, there is an increased risk of malignancy; however, Bartholin gland carcinoma is overall rare (Chen, 2023). Cultures of the purulent abscess fluid and of the cervix should be obtained for aerobic bacteria and *Neisseria gonorrhoeae* and *Chlamydia trachomatis* to rule out a sexually transmitted infection (Chen, 2023).

Nursing Management

Nurses must be aware of and knowledgeable about vulvar cysts and treatment options. The patient may be aware of a vulvar cyst secondary to the pain or may be unaware of it if it is without symptoms. A Bartholin cyst may be an incidental finding during a routine pelvic examination. Explain the cause of the cyst and assist with cultures if needed. Provide reassurance and support.

Ovarian Cysts

An **ovarian cyst** is a fluid-filled sac that forms on the ovary (Fig. 7.5). These common growths are often without symptoms and discovered incidentally during an ultrasound or routine pelvic exam (Mobeen & Apostol, 2022). Ovarian cysts occur in 20% of females within their lifetime (Mobeen & Apostol, 2022). When the cysts grow large and exert pressure on surrounding structures, people often seek medical help.

Types of Ovarian Cysts

The most common benign ovarian cysts are follicular cysts, corpus luteum (lutein) cysts, and theca-lutein cysts. Although PCOS includes the term "cyst," the "cysts" that form are actually follicles. However, the condition will be discussed here.

FOLLICULAR CYSTS

Small follicular cysts are commonly found in the ovaries of prepubertal females and those of reproductive age, and in most cases, they are of no clinical significance. They are usually self-limiting and resolve spontaneously. Follicular cysts are caused by the failure of the ovarian follicle to rupture at the time of ovulation. Follicular cysts seldom grow larger than 5 cm in diameter; most regress and require no treatment. They can occur at any age and are rare after menopause. They are detected by vaginal ultrasound.

CORPUS LUTEUM (LUTEIN) CYSTS

A corpus luteum cyst forms when the corpus luteum becomes cystic or hemorrhagic and fails to degenerate after 14 days. They typically grow to 3 cm in size. These cysts

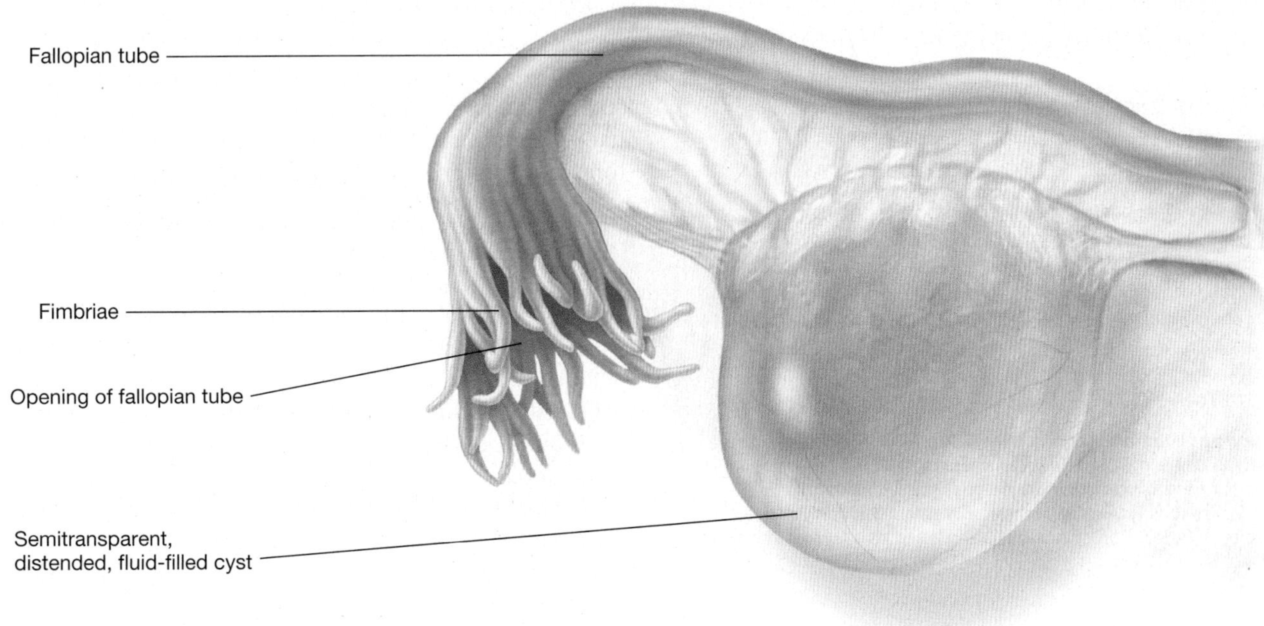

FIGURE 7.5 Ovarian cyst. (Reprinted with permission from Stewart, J. G. [2017]. *Anatomical Chart Company atlas of pathophysiology* [4th ed.]. Wolters Kluwer.)

might cause pain and delay the next menstrual period. A pelvic ultrasound helps to make this diagnosis. Typically, these cysts appear after ovulation and resolve without intervention.

POLYCYSTIC OVARY SYNDROME

Polycystic ovary syndrome (PCOS) is one of the more common endocrine conditions in females of reproductive age; it affects 6% to 10% of this population (Azziz, 2023). It is a heterogeneous condition that involves elevated male sex hormones (androgens), failure of the ovary to release eggs (ovulation), and ovarian enlargement with cyst formation (WHO, 2023). In PCOS, the follicles have a cystlike appearance. With normal functioning, the egg would mature and the follicle would release it, but with PCOS, the eggs never mature and ovulation does not occur. It is a multifaceted disorder, and central to its pathogenesis are hyperandrogenemia, genetics, and hyperinsulinemia, which are targets for treatment. Current science implicates insulin resistance as the major cause of this disorder (Zhao et al., 2023). It is associated with obesity, impaired glucose tolerance, obstructive sleep apnea, infertility, type 2 diabetes, cardiovascular risk, depression, endometrial cancer, nonalcoholic fatty liver disease, metabolic syndrome, and dyslipidemia (Rasquin et al., 2022). People with PCOS have a higher risk of pregnancy and birth complications such as gestational diabetes, gestational hypertension, preeclampsia, preterm birth, labor induction, large for gestational age infants, and a higher cesarean delivery rate (Bahri Khomami et al., 2022). In the United States, PCOS is the most common cause of infertility (Pinkerton, 2023).

Therapeutic Management

Diagnosis is based on the presence of at least two of the following criteria: hyperandrogenism (evidenced by testosterone excess, hirsutism); ovarian dysfunction (anovulation); and the detection of specific polycystic ovarian morphology (Rasquin et al., 2022). Treatment is centered on the clinical manifestations and should be initiated early to prevent or limit long-term complications. Oral contraceptives, antidiabetic agents, and statins are some of the common therapies used to address the symptoms of this complex hormonal condition. Weight loss and surgery may also be beneficial as nondrug options.

Treatment of ovarian cysts focuses on differentiating a benign cyst from a solid ovarian malignancy. Transvaginal ultrasound is useful in distinguishing fluid-filled cysts from solid masses. Laparoscopy may be needed to remove the cyst if it is large and pressing on surrounding structures. Oral contraceptives are often prescribed to suppress gonadotropin levels, which may help resolve the cysts. Pain medication is also prescribed if needed.

Medical management of PCOS is aimed at the treatment of metabolic derangements, anovulation, hirsutism, and menstrual irregularity. This includes both drug and nondrug therapy, along with lifestyle modifications. Goals of therapy focus on reducing the production and circulating levels of androgens, protecting the endometrium against the effects of unopposed estrogens, supporting lifestyle changes to achieve a healthy BMI (18.5 to 24.9 kg/m^2), lowering the risk of cardiovascular disease, avoiding the effects of hyperinsulinemia on the risk of cardiovascular disease and diabetes, and inducing ovulation to achieve pregnancy if desired. Treatment modalities for PCOS are highlighted in Box 7.3.

BOX 7.3 Treatment Modalities for Polycystic Ovary Syndrome

- Oral contraceptives to treat menstrual irregularities, hirsutism, and acne
- Mechanical hair removal (shaving, waxing, plucking, or electrolysis) to treat hirsutism
- Glucophage (metformin), which improves insulin uptake by fat and muscle cells, to treat hyperinsulinemia; also improves menstrual cycles and abnormal waist-to-hip ratios
- Ovulation induction agents (Clomid) to treat infertility
- Lifestyle changes (e.g., weight loss, exercise, balanced low-fat diet)
- Referral to support groups to help improve emotional state and build self-esteem

Adapted from Barbieri, R. L., & Ehrmann, D. A. (2022b). Treatment of polycystic ovary syndrome in adults. *UpToDate*. Retrieved May 1, 2024, from https://www.uptodate.com/contents/treatment-of-polycystic-ovary-syndrome-in-adults; Rasquin, L. I., Anastasopoulou, C., & Mayrin, J. V. (2022). Polycystic ovarian disease. In *StatPearls*. StatPearls Publishing. https://www.ncbi.nlm.nih.gov/books/NBK459251/

Nursing Assessment

Nursing assessment for the patient with PCOS includes a thorough health history, physical examination, and laboratory and diagnostic tests.

HEALTH HISTORY

The history should include questions about the patient's symptoms, including onset, location, frequency, quality, intensity, and aggravating and alleviating factors of their discomfort. Note the last menstrual period and whether or not the patient's cycles are regular. Ask about their overall general health and any changes recently noticed, such as a change in abdominal girth without a concomitant weight gain. Assess for common signs and symptoms of ovarian cysts. Findings might include:

- Hirsutism (face and chin, upper lip, areola, lower abdomen, and perineum)
- Alopecia (female pattern baldness)
- Menstrual irregularity and infertility (oligomenorrhea or amenorrhea, anovulation)
- Polycystic ovaries (12 or more follicles on ovaries)
- Obesity (occurs in more than 50% of people with PCOS)
- Metabolic syndrome (elevated cholesterol, triglycerides, and low-density lipoprotein; risk of cardiovascular disease)
- Psychological impact (depression, frustration, anxiety, eating disorders; see Evidence-Based Practice 7.2)
- Acne (face and shoulders) (Barbieri & Ehrmann, 2022a)

PHYSICAL EXAMINATION AND LABORATORY AND DIAGNOSTIC STUDIES

The physical examination includes inspection, auscultation, and palpation of the abdomen because large ovarian masses may cause visible changes in the abdomen. A complete pelvic examination by an advanced health care provider is performed to assess the location, size, shape, texture, mobility, and tenderness of any palpable mass.

EVIDENCE-BASED PRACTICE 7.2

Psychosocial Interventions for Patients With Polycystic Ovary Syndrome: A Systematic Review of Randomized Controlled Trials

BACKGROUND

Polycystic ovary syndrome (PCOS) is a common endocrine disorder affecting women of reproductive age across their lifespan; worldwide, the prevalence of this disorder is up to 20% in this population. Insulin resistance and hyperandrogenism play essential roles in its development. Prior research studies have suggested that PCOS can be associated with mood and psychiatric disorders due to the multifactorial nature and distressing signs and symptoms of this condition.

STUDY

The objective of this study was to evaluate the effects of psychosocial interventions aimed at improving depression, anxiety, quality of life, and other psychological conditions in women living with PCOS. The literature search included seven studies, with an average sample size of 83 participants. Interventions from these studies included a total of 579 participants. The psychosocial interventions used were cognitive behavioral therapy, acceptance and commitment therapy, mindfulness-based stress reduction, and lifestyle modifications.

Findings

Within the intervention groups, significant positive impacts were observed for depression, anxiety, quality of life, self-esteem, body image, and perceived stress. These findings demonstrate proof of concept that psychosocial interventions improve PCOS-related mental health issues.

Nursing Implications

Based on this study, it is important for nurses to understand that PCOS is associated with an increased risk of diagnosis of depression and anxiety, low self-esteem, poor body image, and quality of life issues. The high prevalence rate of these psychological disorders in this population suggests that the initial evaluation of all patients with PCOS should also include an assessment of their mental health. Psychological support by nurses should take on an important role in the management of the person with PCOS. This does not suggest that medical treatment of PCOS is not required, but a thorough cooperation between medical treatment and psychological support would improve the situation of patients with PCOS. The physical and psychosocial aspects of the management of PCOS go hand in hand. Meeting physical management goals (e.g., weight loss, reduction in hyperandrogenism manifestations) can lessen some of the distressing psychosocial effects and enhance self-esteem.

Adapted from Phimphasone-Brady, P., Palmer, B., Vela, A., Johnson, R. L., Harnke, B., Hoffecker, L., Coons, H. L., & Epperson, N. (2022). Psychosocial interventions for women with polycystic ovary syndrome: A systematic review of randomized controlled trials. *F & S Reviews*, *3*(1), 42–56. https://doi.org/10.1016/j.xfnr.2021.11.004

Diagnostic tests include a pregnancy test to rule out ectopic pregnancy. Gonorrhea and chlamydia testing is warranted if an ovarian abscess is suspected. An ultrasound may be ordered to differentiate between functional or simple ovarian cysts and a solid tumor. Additional tests may be performed depending on the findings.

Remember Liz, the patient with irregular menses, facial hair, and acne? Her glucose level is elevated, multiple cysts were felt on her ovaries during the pelvic examination, and laboratory tests found elevated lipid and lipoprotein levels. What education should the nurse provide Liz regarding her PCOS diagnosis? What medications might be prescribed to address her abnormal laboratory values?

Nursing Management

Nursing care should include education about the condition, treatment options, diagnostic test arrangements, and referral for surgery if needed. Provide support and reassurance during the diagnostic period to allay anxiety in the patient and their family. Reassure the patient that the majority of ovarian cysts are benign, but continue to stress the importance of follow-up care. Listen to the patient's concerns about their appearance, infertility, and facial hair growth. Offer suggestions to help the patient feel better about themselves and their health.

Nurses can have a positive impact on patients with PCOS through counseling and education. Provide support for patients dealing with negative self-image secondary to the physical manifestations of PCOS. Through education, help the patient understand the syndrome and its associated risk factors to prevent long-term health problems. Encourage the patient to make positive lifestyle changes. Make community referrals to local support groups to help the patient build their coping skills.

Liz returns to the clinic a month later for a revaluation of her PCOS. She has been taking metformin to reduce her insulin resistance, has followed her exercise regimen, reduced her caloric intake to lose weight, but she is still concerned about her facial hair and acne. What interventions might be helpful to address this problem? What medication might also be prescribed to regularize her menses and relieve the hirsutism?

KEY CONCEPTS

- Pelvic floor disorders such as POP and urinary and fecal incontinence are prevalent conditions in aging females. They cause significant physical and psychological morbidity, negatively affecting people's social interactions, emotional well-being, and overall quality of life.
- The four most common types of genital prolapse are cystocele, rectocele, enterocele, and uterine prolapse.
- The purpose of PFMEs is to increase the muscle volume, which will result in a stronger muscular contraction. These exercises might limit the progression of mild prolapse and alleviate mild prolapse symptoms, including low back pain and pelvic pressure.
- UI is the involuntary loss of urine sufficient enough to be a social or hygiene problem. It affects approximately 20 million females in the United States.
- The three most common types of incontinence are urge incontinence (overactive bladder caused by detrusor muscle contractions), stress incontinence (inadequate urinary sphincter function), and mixed incontinence (involves both stress and urge incontinence).
- The most common benign growths of the reproductive tract include cervical, endocervical, and endometrial polyps; uterine fibroids (leiomyomas); genital fistulas; Bartholin cysts; and ovarian cysts.
- PCOS involves the presence of multiple inactive follicles within the ovary that interfere with ovarian function. Hyperandrogenism, insulin resistance, and chronic anovulation characterize PCOS. Careful attention should be given to this condition because people with it are at increased risk for long-term health problems such as cardiovascular disease, obesity, metabolic syndrome, stroke, obstructive sleep apnea, liver damage, depression, anxiety, dyslipidemia, infertility, type 2 diabetes, and cancer (endometrial).

REFERENCES AND RECOMMENDED READINGS

Aboseif, C., & Liu, P. (2022). Pelvic organ prolapse. In *StatPearls*. StatPearls Publishing. https://www.ncbi.nlm.nih.gov/books/NBK563229/

Alkilani, Y. G., & Apodaca-Ramos, I. (2023). Cervical polyps. In *StatPearls*. StatPearls Publishing. https://www.ncbi.nlm.nih.gov/books/NBK562185/#

Alouini, S., Memic, S., & Couillandre, A. (2022). Pelvic floor muscle training for urinary incontinence with or without biofeedback or electrostimulation in women: A systematic review. *International Journal of Environmental Research and Public Health*, *19*(5), 2789. https://doi.org/10.3390/ijerph19052789

American College of Obstetricians and Gynecologists. (2021a). *Pelvic support problems*. https://www.acog.org/womens-health/faqs/pelvic-support-problems

American College of Obstetricians and Gynecologists. (2021b). *Urinary incontinence*. https://www.acog.org/womens-health/faqs/urinary-incontinence

American College of Obstetricians and Gynecologists. (2022). *Surgery for pelvic organ prolapse*. https://www.acog.org/womens-health/faqs/surgery-for-pelvic-organ-prolapse

Azziz, R. (2023). Epidemiology, phenotype, and genetics of the polycystic ovary syndrome in adults. *UpToDate*. Retrieved

May 1, 2024, from https://www.uptodate.com/contents/epidemiology-phenotype-and-genetics-of-the-polycystic-ovary-syndrome-in-adults

Bahri Khomami, M., Teede, H. J., Joham, A. E., Moran, L. J., Piltonen, T. T., & Boyle, J. A. (2022). Clinical management of pregnancy in women with polycystic ovary syndrome: An expert opinion. *Clinical Endocrinology*, *97*, 227–236. https://doi.org/10.1111/cen.14723

Barbieri, R. L., & Ehrmann, D. A. (2022a). Clinical manifestations of polycystic ovary syndrome in adults. *UpToDate*. Retrieved May 1, 2024, from https://www.uptodate.com/contents/clinical-manifestations-of-polycystic-ovary-syndrome-in-adults

Barbieri, R. L., & Ehrmann, D. A. (2022b). Treatment of polycystic ovary syndrome in adults. *UpToDate*. Retrieved May 1, 2024, from https://www.uptodate.com/contents/treatment-of-polycystic-ovary-syndrome-in-adults

Barjon, K., & Mikhail, L. N. (2023). Uterine leiomyomata. In *StatPearls*. StatPearls Publishing. https://www.ncbi.nlm.nih.gov/books/NBK546680/

Chen, C. J., & Thompson, H. (2022). Uterine prolapse. In *StatPearls*. StatPearls Publishing. https://www.ncbi.nlm.nih.gov/books/NBK564429/

Chen, K. T. (2023). Bartholin gland masses. *UpToDate*. Retrieved May 1, 2024, from https://www.uptodate.com/contents/bartholin-gland-masses

Clemons, J. L. (2023). Vaginal pessaries: Insertion and fitting, management, and complications. *UpToDate*. Retrieved April 30, 2024, from https://www.uptodate.com/contents/vaginal-pessaries-insertion-and-fitting-management-and-complications

Clemons, J. L. (2024). Vaginal pessaries: Indications, devices, and approach to selection. *UpToDate*. Retrieved April 30, 2024, from https://www.uptodate.com/contents/vaginal-pessaries-indications-devices-and-approach-to-selection

Culligan, P. J., Saiz, C. M., & Rosenblatt, P. L. (2022). Contemporary use and techniques of laparoscopic sacrocolpopexy with or without robotic assistance for pelvic organ prolapse. *Obstetrics & Gynecology*, *139*(5), 922–932. https://pubmed.ncbi.nlm.nih.gov/35576354/

Fante, J. F., Silva, T. D., Mateus-Vasconcelos, E. C. L., Ferreira, C. H. J., & Brito, L. G. O. (2019). Do women have adequate knowledge about pelvic floor dysfunctions? A systematic review. *Revista brasileira de ginecologia e obstetricia (RBGO)*, *41*(8), 508–519. https://doi.org/10.1055/s-0039-1695002

Fashokun, T. B., & Rogers, R. G. (2023). Pelvic organ prolapse in women: Diagnostic evaluation. *UpToDate*. Retrieved April 30, 2024, from https://www.uptodate.com/contents/pelvic-organ-prolapse-in-women-diagnostic-evaluation

Garely, A. D., & Mann, W. J., Jr. (2022). Urogenital tract fistulas in females. *UpToDate*. Retrieved May 1, 2024, from https://www.uptodate.com/contents/urogenital-tract-fistulas-in-females

Ghanbari, Z., Ghaemi, M., Shafiee, A., Jelodarian, P., Hosseini, R. S., Pouyamoghaddam, S., & Montazeri, A. (2022). Quality of life following pelvic organ prolapse treatments in women: A systematic review and meta-analysis. *Journal of Clinical Medicine*, *11*(23), 7166. https://doi.org/10.3390/jcm11237166

Grimes, W. R., & Stratton, M. (2023). Pelvic floor dysfunction. In *StatPearls*. StatPearls Publishing. https://www.ncbi.nlm.nih.gov/books/NBK559246/

Jelovsek, J. E. (2024). Pelvic organ prolapse in women: Choosing a primary surgical procedure. *UpToDate*. Retrieved April 30, 2024, from https://www.uptodate.com/contents/pelvic-organ-prolapse-in-women-choosing-a-primary-surgical-procedure

Kenne, K. A., Wendt, L., & Jackson, J. B. (2022). Prevalence of pelvic floor disorders in adult women being seen in a primary care setting and associated risk factors. *Scientific Reports*, *12*, 9878. https://doi.org/10.1038/s41598-022-13501-w

Lee, W. A., & Wittler, M. (2023). Bartholin gland cyst. In *StatPearls*. StatPearls Publishing. https://www.ncbi.nlm.nih.gov/books/NBK532271

Lukacz, E. S. (2024a). Female urinary incontinence: Treatment. *UpToDate*. Retrieved April 30, 2024, from https://www.uptodate.com/contents/female-urinary-incontinence-treatment

Lukacz, E. S. (2024b). Female urinary incontinence: Evaluation. *UpToDate*. Retrieved April 30, 2024, from https://www.uptodate.com/contents/female-urinary-incontinence-evaluation

Mansour, T., & Chowdhury, Y. S. (2023). Endometrial polyp. In *StatPearls*. StatPearls Publishing. https://www.ncbi.nlm.nih.gov/books/NBK557824/

McKinney, J. L., Keyser, L. E., Pulliam, S. J., & Ferzandi, T. R. (2022). Female urinary incontinence evidence-based treatment pathway: An infographic for shared decision-making. *Journal of Women's Health*, *31*(3). https://doi.org/10.1089/jwh.2021.0266

Medlen, H., & Barbier, H. (2023). Vesicovaginal fistula. In *StatPearls*. StatPearls Publishing. https://www.ncbi.nlm.nih.gov/books/NBK564389/

Mobeen, S., & Apostol, R. (2022). Ovarian cyst. In *StatPearls*. StatPearls Publishing. https://www.ncbi.nlm.nih.gov/books/NBK560541/

Mutch, D. G., & Biest, S. W. (2023). Uterine fibroids. *Merck Manual*. https://www.merckmanuals.com/professional/gynecology-and-obstetrics/uterine-fibroids/uterine-fibroids

Phimphasone-Brady, P., Palmer, B., Vela, A., Johnson, R. L., Harnke, B., Hoffecker, L., Coons, H. L., & Epperson, N. (2022). Psychosocial interventions for women with polycystic ovary syndrome: A systematic review of randomized controlled trials. *F & S Reviews*, *3*(1), 42–56. https://doi.org/10.1016/j.xfnr.2021.11.004

Pillarisetty, L. S., & Mahdy, H. (2023). Vaginal hysterectomy. In *StatPearls*. StatPearls Publishing. https://www.ncbi.nlm.nih.gov/books/NBK554482/

Pinkerton, J. V. (2023). Polycystic ovary syndrome (PCOS). *Merck Manual*. https://www.merckmanuals.com/professional/gynecology-and-obstetrics/menstrual-abnormalities/polycystic-ovary-syndrome-pcos

Quinn, A. (2022). Bartholin gland diseases clinical presentation. *eMedicine*. https://emedicine.medscape.com/article/777112-clinical

Rasquin, L. I., Anastasopoulou, C., & Mayrin, J. V. (2022). Polycystic ovarian disease. In *StatPearls*. StatPearls Publishing. https://www.ncbi.nlm.nih.gov/books/NBK459251/

Rogers, R. G., & Fashokun, T. B. (2022). Pelvic organ prolapse in females: Epidemiology, risk factors, clinical manifestations, and management. *UpToDate*. Retrieved April 30, 2024, from https://www.uptodate.com/contents/pelvic-organ-prolapse-in-females-epidemiology-risk-factors-clinical-manifestations-and-management

Stewart, E. A. (2024a). Endometrial polyps. *UpToDate*. Retrieved April 30, 2024, from https://www.uptodate.com/contents/endometrial-polyps

Stewart, E. A. (2024b). Uterine fibroids (leiomyomas): Treatment overview. *UpToDate*. https://www.uptodate.com/contents/uterine-fibroids-leiomyomas-treatment-overview

Stewart, E. A., & Laughlin-Tommaso, S. K. (2024). Uterine fibroids (leiomyomas): Epidemiology, clinical features, diagnosis, and natural history. *UpToDate*. Retrieved April 30, 2024, from https://www.uptodate.com/contents/uterine-fibroids-leiomyomas-epidemiology-clinical-features-diagnosis-and-natural-history

Tran, L. N., & Puckett, Y. (2023). Urinary incontinence. In *StatPearls*. StatPearls Publishing. https://www.ncbi.nlm.nih.gov/books/NBK559095/

United Nations Population Fund. (2023a). *Obstetric fistula*. https://esaro.unfpa.org/en/topics/obstetric-fistula

United Nations Population Fund. (2023b). *Female genital mutilation*. https://www.unfpa.org/female-genital-mutilation

United States Food & Drug Administration. (2023). *Uterine fibroids*. https://www.fda.gov/consumers/womens-health-topics/uterine-fibroids

van der Kooij, S. M., & Hehenkamp, W. J. K. (2024). Uterine fibroids (leiomyomas): Treatment with uterine artery embolization. *UpToDate*. Retrieved May 1, 2024, from https://www.uptodate.com/contents/uterine-fibroids-leiomyomas-treatment-with-uterine-artery-embolization

Wald, A. (2022). Patient education: High-fiber diet (beyond the basics). *UpToDate*. Retrieved April 30, 2024, from https://www.uptodate.com/contents/high-fiber-diet-beyond-the-basics

Walters, M. D., & Ferrando, C. (2024). Hysterectomy (benign indications): Patient-important issues and surgical complications. *UpToDate*. Retrieved May 1, 2024, from https://www.uptodate.com/contents/hysterectomy-benign-indications-patient-important-issues-and-surgical-complications

World Health Organization. (2023). *Polycystic ovary syndrome*. https://www.who.int/news-room/fact-sheets/detail/polycystic-ovary-syndrome

Zhao, H., Zhang, J., Cheng, X., Nie, X., & He, B. (2023). Insulin resistance in polycystic ovary syndrome across various tissues: An updated review of pathogenesis, evaluation, and treatment. *Journal of Ovarian Research*, *16*(1), 9. https://doi.org/10.1186/s13048-022-01091-0

DEVELOPING CLINICAL JUDGMENT

PRACTICING FOR NCLEX

1. The nurse is interviewing a patient with uterine fibroids. What subjective data would you expect to find in their history?
   a. Cyclic migraine headaches
   b. Urinary tract infections
   c. Chronic pelvic pain
   d. Chronic constipation

2. The nurse is caring for a patient in the clinic with POP. The nurse explains which conservative treatment options are available for this patient?
   a. Pessaries and PFMEs
   b. External pelvic fixation devices
   c. Weight gain and yoga
   d. Firm panty-and-girdle garments

3. The nurse is teaching a group of postmenopausal patients about changes that occur with aging. Which dietary and lifestyle modification might the nurse recommend to help prevent pelvic relaxation?
   a. Eat a high-fiber diet to avoid constipation and straining.
   b. Avoid sitting for long periods; get up and walk around frequently.
   c. Limit the amount of exercise to prevent overdeveloping muscles.
   d. Space children a year apart to reduce wear and tear on the uterus.

4. The nurse is caring for a patient with PCOS. The nurse understands that this patient is at an increased risk for developing which long-term health problem?
   a. Osteoporosis
   b. Lupus
   c. Type 2 diabetes
   d. Migraine headaches

5. The nurse is teaching a patient about medications taken for uterine fibroids. The nurse explains side effects experienced by patients taking GnRH agonists for the treatment of fibroids closely resemble those of
   a. anorexia nervosa.
   b. osteoarthritis.
   c. depression.
   d. menopause.

6. The nurse is obtaining a health history of a 65-year-old female patient seen in the clinic. Which clinical manifestation described by the patient would the nurse suspect is related to POP?
   a. Chronic abdominal pain
   b. Heavy feeling or dragging in the vagina
   c. Uterine cramping and backache
   d. Weight gain and edema of ankles

CRITICAL THINKING EXERCISE

1. Faith, a 42-year-old multiparous woman, presents to the women's health clinic complaining of pelvic pain, heavy menstrual bleeding, and vaginal discharge. She says she has been having these problems for several months. Upon examination, her uterus is enlarged and irregular in shape. Her blood studies reveal anemia.
   a. What condition might Faith have based on her symptoms?
   b. What treatment options are available to address this condition?
   c. What educational interventions should the nurse discuss with Faith?

STUDY ACTIVITIES

1. Prepare an educational session to teach patients how to do PFMEs to prevent stress incontinence and pelvic floor relaxation.

2. In a small group, discuss the personal, social, and sexual issues that might affect a patient with POP. How might these issues affect their socialization? How might a support group help?

3. List the symptoms that a patient with uterine fibroids might have. Discuss how these symptoms might mimic a more frightening condition and why the patient might delay seeking treatment.

4. A bladder that herniates into the vagina is a ________________.

5. A rectum that herniates into the vagina is a ________________.

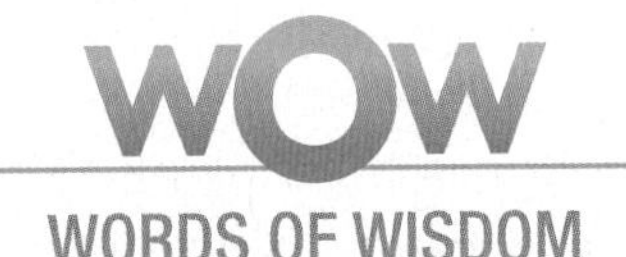

WORDS OF WISDOM

The word "cancer" can strike fear into anyone who hears it. But when it involves a reproductive organ, this fear is often magnified.

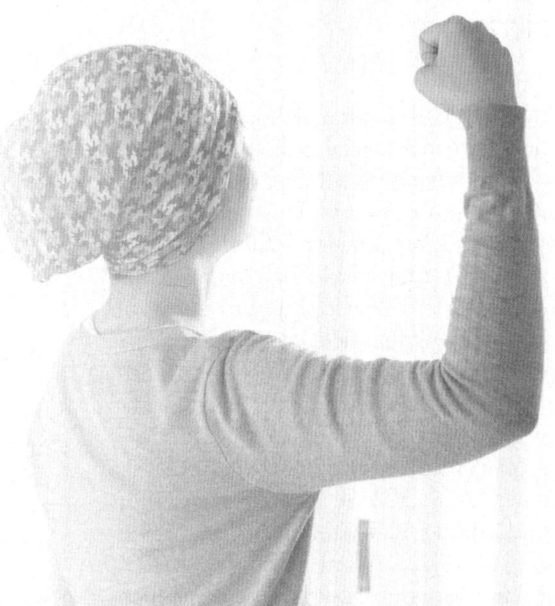

8

Cancers of the Female Reproductive Tract

LEARNING OBJECTIVES

Upon completion of the chapter, you will be able to:

1. Analyze the national and global statistics related to reproductive cancer rates in females.
2. Plan, implement, and evaluate using the nursing process for patients with cancer of the reproductive tract.
3. Describe the assessment, collaborative care, and nursing management of patients with a diagnosis of ovarian cancer.
4. Identify the clinical manifestations, diagnostic procedures, and treatment options for patients with endometrial cancer.
5. Examine lifestyle changes and health screenings that reduce the risk of or prevent cervical cancers.
6. Outline the nursing and collaborative management needed for a patient diagnosed with vaginal cancer.
7. Appraise the psychological distress felt by patients diagnosed with any reproductive cancer and resources available to those patients.

Carmella is a 58-year-old woman who has obesity (body mass index [BMI] greater than 30 kg/m^2). She presents to her woman's health care provider with vaginal bleeding. She has been through menopause and wonders why she is having a period again. Her history includes infertility and hypertension. Three years ago, she had a mastectomy for breast cancer, and she has been taking tamoxifen (Nolvadex) to prevent recurrent breast cancer since her surgery. What risk factors in Carmella's history might predispose her to a reproductive tract cancer? What additional information is needed to make a diagnosis?

KEY TERMS

cervical cancer

cervical dysplasia (ser'vĭ-kăl dis-pl-ā'zē-ă)

colposcopy (kol-pos'kŏ-pē)

endometrial cancer (en'dō-mē'trē-ăl kan'ser)

human papillomavirus (hyū'măn pap'i-lō'mă-vĭ'rŭs)

ovarian cancer

Papanicolaou (Pap) test (pa-pă-ni'kō-low test)

vaginal cancer

vulvar cancer

INTRODUCTION

Cancer is a major public health problem globally and the second leading cause of death for females in the United States, surpassed only by cardiovascular disease (Centers for Disease Control and Prevention [CDC],/National Center for Health Statistics, 2024a). Cardiovascular disease is and should continue to be a major focus of efforts in female health. However, this should not overshadow the fact that many females are developing and dying of cancer; breast cancer is one of the most common cancers and the second leading cause of cancer death (American Cancer Society [ACS], 2023a; National Cancer Institute [NCI], 2020). Females have a one-in-three lifetime risk of developing cancer and a one-in-six lifetime risk of dying from cancer (ACS, 2024a). There is a higher cancer mortality rate among Black females than White females (Giaquinto et al., 2022). Racial, ethnic, socioeconomic, and geographic disparities in cancer occurrence and outcomes stem from historical and structural racism and discriminatory practices that place barriers to cancer prevention, early detection, and treatments. Despite significant advancements in cancer outcomes and treatment options, disparities still exist (Collins, 2024). The ACS (2023b) estimated that in 2023, there would be about 948,000 new cases of cancer diagnosed in females and about 288,000 cancer deaths in females in the United States.

Nurses need to focus their energies on screening, education, and early detection to reduce these numbers. Because cancer risk is strongly associated with lifestyle and behavior, screening programs are of particular importance for early detection. There is evidence that prevention and early detection have reduced cancer mortality rates and prevented reproductive cancers (CDC, 2023a).

This chapter begins with a nursing process overview of the care of patients with reproductive cancer. It then describes selected cancers of the reproductive system: ovarian, endometrial, cervical, vaginal, and vulvar cancers. The chapter discusses the nurse's role through diagnosis, intervention, and follow-up care. Cancer management requires a multidisciplinary approach, including specialists in surgical, medical, and radiation oncology. The nurse can provide guidance and support to the patient who has cancer.

Nursing Process Overview for Patients With Cancer of the Reproductive Tract

The word "cancer" is associated with fear and dread. These feelings may worsen when the cancer involves a person's reproductive tract. The diagnosis of reproductive tract cancer can have a profound impact on a person's sexuality because it affects the parts of the body associated with these functions. The loss of the reproductive body part as well as the possible loss of childbearing ability can have a significant effect on patients and their partners. Nurses need to remember this when counseling patients and their partners about cancer treatment and side effects as well as potential changes in the patient's body image and sexuality.

When a person is first diagnosed with a reproductive tract cancer, two primary needs arise: information and emotional support. When the diagnosis is made, the patient typically has many questions, such as "What is going to happen to me?" "How will this change my life?" and "Will I survive?" Nurses can play a major role in helping patients find the answers to their questions and directing them to the resources they need. A few reliable sources of general cancer information and support are the National Cancer Institute, Cancer Support Community Hotline, Patient Advocacy Foundation, Cancer Care, and the ACS. They can be reached via the internet or by phone.

The nurse also plays a key role in offering emotional support, determining appropriate sources of support, and helping the patient use effective coping strategies. A recent research study found that peer social support, which is support from people who have been diagnosed and treated for cancer, increased psychological empowerment for women and therefore improved coping, self-efficacy, and knowledge (Ziegler et al., 2022). Implications for nurses working with patients following a cancer diagnosis include assessing patients' definitions and availability of support; respecting varied needs for informational support; providing a supportive clinical environment; educating clinicians, family, and friends regarding unsupportive responses within the cultural context; and validating patients' control and balancing of support needs. Patients without a social support network may need a social work referral or may need to be guided toward support groups to receive the emotional support they need. The care provided by nurses to patients undergoing treatment and recovery is invaluable in maintaining their quality of life and managing the unpleasant side effects that many patients experience.

In addition, patients with cancer have a strong need for hope. Cancer is a debilitating and feared disease, so providing psychological, social, and emotional support is inherent to professional nursing roles. Strategies for inspiring hope may include active listening, touch, presence, and helping patients overcome communication barriers. A cancer diagnosis does not determine how strong a person is, but rather can show them they have the courage to face cancer, the tenacity, and the strength to battle it. Often it is not what nurses say or do, but just their presence that counts. The ability for patients to depend on a trusted nurse during this difficult time in their lives is something that can have a profound effect on their emotional state and energy levels during their recovery process.

Assessment

Assessment of a patient with cancer of the reproductive tract involves a thorough history and physical examination. In addition, various laboratory and diagnostic tests may be done to evaluate for a malignancy.

Health History and Physical Examination

Interview the patient carefully to determine any current or past factors that might increase their risk of cancer, such as early menarche, late menopause, sexually transmitted infections (STIs), use of hormonal agents, or infertility. Find out if the patient has a family history of cancer. Be thorough in obtaining the patient's past medical history, especially their reproductive, obstetric, and gynecologic history. Ask about their lifestyle and behaviors, including higher risk behaviors such as engaging in unprotected sexual intercourse or sexual intercourse with multiple partners. Find out if the patient has had routine or recommended screening procedures.

Ask if the patient has had any symptoms, such as abnormal vaginal bleeding or discharge or vaginal discomfort. Often the symptoms of cancer are vague and nonspecific, and the patient may attribute them to another problem, such as aging, stress, or a less nutritious diet.

Perform a complete physical examination, including a review of body systems. A pelvic examination will be performed by an advanced practitioner. Observe for lesions or masses in the perineal area. Note any masses when palpating the abdomen or whether any are noted by the practitioner during the pelvic examination.

Laboratory and Diagnostic Testing

Some of the laboratory and diagnostic tests used to help diagnose cancer of the reproductive tract are discussed in Common Laboratory and Diagnostic Tests 8.1.

Nursing Analyses and Related Interventions

Upon completion of a thorough assessment, the nurse might identify several nursing analyses, including:

- Knowledge deficiency
- Altered body image perception
- Acute anxiety
- Fear
- Pain

Nursing goals, interventions, and evaluation for patients with reproductive tract cancer are based on the nursing analyses. Clinical Judgment & Nursing Process 8.1 may be used as a guide in planning nursing care for patients with reproductive tract cancer. It should be individualized based on the patient's symptoms and needs.

COMMON LABORATORY AND DIAGNOSTIC TESTS 8.1

Test	Explanation	Indications	Nursing Implications
Pap test	Cervical cytology screening to diagnose cervical cancers	Aids in detecting abnormal cells of the cervix (from squamocolumnar junction of the cervix; most cervical cancers arise here.)	• Encourage all sexually active females to receive a pelvic examination, including a Pap test if they have a high-risk profile, to promote early detection of cervical cancer.
Transvaginal ultrasound	Screening for pelvic pathology to assist in diagnosing endometrial cancers	Allows measurement of endometrial thickness to determine if endometrial biopsy is needed for postmenopausal bleeding	• Review the risk factors for the development of endometrial cancer and the reason for this screening test. • Assist in preparing the patient for this examination.
Cancer antigen 125 (CA-125)	A protein found in the blood at higher levels in about 80% of people with ovarian cancer[a]; tumor marker for ovarian and other cancers	Elevation of marker suggests malignancy but is not specific to ovarian cancer.	• Review risk factors for ovarian cancer and explain that a series of diagnostic tests may be performed (transvaginal ultrasound, computed tomography (CT) scan, CA-125) to assist in the diagnosis and treatment plan. • Elevated marker levels are not specific to ovarian cancer; they can be elevated in other types of cancer.

[a]Gandhi, T., Zubair, M., & Bhatt, H. (2023). Cancer antigen 125. In *StatPearls*. StatPearls Publishing. https://www.ncbi.nlm.nih.gov/books/NBK562245/

CLINICAL JUDGMENT & NURSING PROCESS 8.1 Overview of a Patient With a Reproductive Tract Cancer

Molly, a 28-year-old, comes to the free health clinic complaining of a thin, watery vaginal discharge and spotting after sex. Molly says they have had multiple sex partners since the age of 15. They had an abnormal Pap smear "a while back" but didn't return to the clinic for follow-up. Cervical cancer is suspected.

NURSING ANALYSIS: Acute anxiety related to uncertainty of diagnosis, possible diagnosis of cancer, and eventual outcome as evidenced by patient's report of signs and symptoms and statements of being worried and not knowing what they would do

OUTCOME IDENTIFICATION AND EVALUATION

The patient will demonstrate measures to cope with anxiety as evidenced by statements acknowledging anxiety, use of positive coping strategies, and verbalization that anxiety has decreased.

INTERVENTIONS: *Reducing Anxiety*

- Encourage patient to express their feelings and concerns *to reduce anxiety and to determine appropriate interventions.*
- Assess the meaning of the diagnosis to the patient, clarify misconceptions, and provide reliable, realistic information *to enhance their understanding of their condition, subsequently reducing their anxiety.*
- Assess patient's psychological status *to determine the degree of emotional distress related to diagnosis and treatment options.*
- Identify and address verbalized concerns, providing information about what to expect *to decrease uncertainty about the unknown.*
- Assess the patient's use of coping mechanisms in the past and their effectiveness *to foster the use of positive strategies.*
- Teach patient about early signs of anxiety and help them recognize those signs (e.g., fast heartbeat, sweating, or feeling flushed) *to minimize escalation of anxiety.*
- Provide positive reinforcement that the patient's condition can be managed *to relieve their anxiety.*

NURSING ANALYSIS: Knowledge deficiency related to diagnosis, prevention strategies, disease course, and treatment as evidenced by patient's statements about hoping nothing is wrong, lack of follow-up for a previous abnormal Pap test, and higher risk behaviors

OUTCOME IDENTIFICATION AND EVALUATION

The patient will demonstrate an understanding of diagnosis as evidenced by making health-promoting lifestyle choices, verbalizing appropriate health care practices, describing the condition once diagnosed, and adhering to measures associated with therapy.

INTERVENTIONS: *Providing Patient Teaching*

- Assess patient's current knowledge about the diagnosis and proposed therapeutic regimen *to establish a baseline from which to develop a teaching plan.*
- Review contributing factors associated with the development of reproductive tract cancer, including lifestyle behaviors, *to foster an understanding of the etiology of cervical cancer.*
- Review information about treatments and procedures and recommendations for a healthy lifestyle, obtaining feedback frequently *to validate an adequate understanding of instructions.*
- Discuss strategies, including using condoms and limiting the number of sexual partners, *to reduce the risk of transmission of STIs*, including HPV, which is associated with cervical cancer.
- Encourage patient to obtain prompt treatment of any vaginal or cervical infections *to minimize the risk for cervical cancer.*
- Urge the patient to have an annual Pap smear and/or HPV test *to allow screening and early detection.*
- Describe the treatment measures used *to provide patient with knowledge of what may be necessary.*
- Provide written material with pictures *to allow for patient review and to help them visualize what is occurring in their body.*
- Inform patient about available community resources and make appropriate referrals as needed *to provide additional education and support.*
- Document details of teaching and learning *to allow for continuity of care and further education if needed.*

NURSING ANALYSIS: Altered body image perception related to suspected reproductive tract cancer and impact on patient's sexuality and sense of self as evidenced by statement of being worried about not being the same

OUTCOME IDENTIFICATION AND EVALUATION

The patient will verbalize or demonstrate a positive self-esteem in relation to body image as evidenced by positive statements about self, sexuality, and participation in activities with others.

INTERVENTIONS: *Promoting Healthy Body Image*

- Assess patient's use of self-criticism *to determine patient's current state of coping and adjustment.*
- Determine if the patient's change in body image has contributed *to social isolation to provide a direction for care.*
- Provide opportunities for the patient to explore their feelings related to issues of sexuality, including past behaviors that may have placed them at risk, *to minimize feelings of guilt about their condition.*
- Acknowledge the patient's feelings about possible changes in their body and sexuality and their illness *to foster trust and allow patient to ventilate feelings and concerns.*
- Facilitate contact with other patients with the same type of cancer *to promote sharing of feelings and decrease feelings of isolation.*
- Initiate referrals for counseling and community support groups as necessary *to assist patient in gaining a positive image of themselves.*

Nurses have traditionally served as advocates in the health care arena and should continue to be on the forefront of health education and diagnosis, acting as leaders in the fight against cancer. The public needs to know that not only are these deaths preventable, but many of the cancers themselves are preventable. Nurses need to work to improve the availability and quality of cancer-screening services, making them accessible to patients from underserved and socioeconomically disadvantaged communities. Through the unified effort of health care providers, health policy experts, government agencies, health insurance companies, the media, educational institutions, and patients themselves, along with consistency and continuity, nurses can offer quality care to all patients with cancer.

Educating to Prevent Cancer

Between 30% and 50% of all cancers are preventable by avoiding risk factors and implementing existing evidence-based prevention strategies (World Health Organization [WHO], 2023). Nurses need to provide patients with information to help prevent disease and enhance quality of life. Educate patients about the importance of consistent and timely screenings to identify cancer early. Emphasize the importance of having an annual pelvic examination. Also stress the need for follow-up screenings as recommended. Provide patients with information if further diagnostic testing is required. Nurses also play a key role in promoting cancer awareness, prevention, and control. Advocate improving the availability of cancer-screening services and work to provide public education about risk factors for cancer.

Nurses can be instrumental in helping patients identify and change behaviors that put them at risk for various reproductive tract cancers (Teaching Guidelines 8.1). Do not limit your interventions to providing preventive education only; inform patients about the consequences of doing nothing about their conditions and what the long-term outcomes might be without treatment. For example, stress the importance of visiting a health care provider if certain signs and symptoms appear:

- Blood in a bowel movement
- Unusual vaginal discharge or chronic vulvar itching
- Persistent abdominal bloating or constipation
- Irregular vaginal bleeding
- Urinary frequency
- Pelvic pain or pressure
- Persistent low backache not related to standing
- Itching, burning, pain, or discolored vulvar lesions
- Bleeding after menopause
- Unexplained significant weight loss
- A lump anywhere on your body
- Pain or bleeding after sexual intercourse

Teaching the Patient About Their Diagnosis

Provide information about tests that may be required to confirm or rule out the diagnosis. Review with the patient what they have been told about their diagnosis and their understanding of their condition. It is not unusual for the patient to hear the diagnosis and then become overwhelmed by the thought of cancer, blocking out whatever is said after that. Answer any questions the patient may have. Go slowly and repeat the information as necessary. Use written materials to explain and reinforce the teaching. Provide information about the condition and recommended therapies. For example, if a patient is undergoing surgery, discuss postoperative issues such as incision care, pain, and activity level. Instruct the patient on health maintenance activities after treatment, and inform the patient and their family about available support resources.

Providing Emotional Support

Once the diagnosis is made, provide the patient and their family with emotional support. Validate the patient's feelings and provide realistic hope, using a nonjudgmental approach and therapeutic communication skills during all interactions. Nurses can be invaluable

TEACHING GUIDELINES 8.1 Reducing Your Risk for Cancer

- Do not smoke.
- Drink alcohol only in moderation (no more than one drink daily).
- Be physically active daily.
- Receive the human papillomavirus (HPV) vaccine.
- Eat a healthy diet.
- Avoid long-term sun and ultraviolet radiation exposure.
- Avoid using tanning beds.
- Stay current with immunizations.
- Use a condom with every sexual encounter.
- Reach and maintain a healthy weight.
- Take preventive medicines if needed.
- Get recommended screening tests:
  - Body mass index (BMI)
  - Mammogram as recommended by provider
  - Pap smears every 1–3 years if sexually active, starting at age 21
  - Cholesterol checked annually starting at age 45
  - Blood pressure checked at least every 2 years
  - Diabetes test if hypertensive or hypercholesterolemia
  - Check for STIs if sexually active.

National Cancer Institute. (2022). *Cancer prevention overview (PDQ®)—Health professional version.* https://www.cancer.gov/about-cancer/causes-prevention/hp-prevention-overview-pdq; https://www.cdc.gov/ovarian-cancer/prevention/; and Colditz, G. A. (2022). Overview of cancer prevention. *UpToDate.* https://www.uptodate.com/contents/overview-of-cancer-prevention

when assisting patients who are coping with the uncertainty of their future by providing positive communication and support. Nurses need to focus on the physical, psychosocial, and economic concerns from diagnosis through treatment and if applicable, until the end of life for all of the patients for whom they care. Individualize the care based on the patient's cultural traditions and beliefs as explained in the following section.

Ensuring Cultural Humility

Demonstrating cultural humility with cancer care can improve outcomes and decrease disparities in care. If nurses are to meet the needs of diverse populations, they must be culturally sensitive, appreciative of differing health beliefs and practices, and flexible in the way they approach health care. It is nurses who must adapt, expand, and learn. Cultural humility encourages developing an attitude of *not knowing* the patient's culture and learning about it from the patient.

Nurses have the opportunity to learn about diverse cultures, religions, and faith traditions that support patients and families during their cancer journeys and while facing a serious life-limiting illness. Nursing care practices should embrace all patients with whom they come in contact, and by having a better understanding of diverse groups, nurses can build trust in patients seeking oncology care needs that range from detection to diagnosis to treatment and possibly through palliative and end-of-life care.

Be aware of the patient's cultural background, religion, migration history, degree of acculturation, living conditions, educational level, and legal status, because each of these factors can affect the patient's understanding of their diagnosis and the eventual outcome. A person's reaction to a cancer diagnosis and their decisions about treatment are influenced by their cultural values and how their community views cancer. A diagnosis of cancer carries deep physical, psychosocial, and cultural implications. Sensitive cross-cultural communication and cultural congruency are vital for all nurses to deliver equal care to all patients with cancer. Nurses need to understand health care disparities and the influence of those disparities on health outcomes. Patients with cancer reflect demographic variations across the United States, representing differences in culture, religion, socioeconomic status, race, and lifestyle. Nurses need to relinquish the role of expert to the patient, and instead become the student of the patient, explicitly expressing that the patient is a capable and full partner in the therapeutic alliance. Nurses need to realize the importance of recognizing diversity and applying cultural humility for successful outcomes. In some cultures, sharing news of a serious illness like cancer is considered disrespectful and impolite, or even inhumane or unnecessarily cruel. Out of respect for aging family members, some people may withhold discussions of serious illness to avoid causing unnecessary anxieties. There may be a reluctance to tell the truth or to have open communication, as this can be viewed as impolite. The patient may have a preference for family-centered decision-making styles (Mori et al., 2023). Integrate this knowledge into your care to ensure a culturally competent approach.

> **TAKE NOTE!**
> When a diagnosis of cancer is made, assessing a person's strengths and weaknesses from a cultural perspective will help the nurse provide culturally congruent care.

Because American society is increasingly multilingual, multicultural, and multireligious, learning about patients' values and cultural beliefs is critical. Be willing to learn about patient preferences; doing so promotes caring and cultural humility.

OVARIAN CANCER

Ovarian cancer is a malignant neoplastic growth of the ovary (Fig. 8.1). It is the second most common gynecologic cancer among females and is the deadliest because it is often diagnosed during later stages (CDC, 2024b). A female's lifetime risk of getting ovarian cancer is about one in 87, and their lifetime risk of dying from invasive ovarian cancer is about one in 130 (ACS, 2024b). Ovarian cancer rates are highest in older people, with about 50% of those diagnosed being over 63 years of age (ACS, 2024b). The incidence is higher among White women than among Black women (ACS, 2024b).

The most important variable influencing the prognosis is the extent of the disease. About 20% of people with ovarian cancer receive their diagnosis when the disease is in the early stages (ACS, 2020a). The relative survival rate is about 89% when it is diagnosed in stage 1, 71% when diagnosed in stage II, but only about 40% and 20% when discovered in stages III and IV, respectively (Carlson, 2024). Survival depends on the stage of the tumor, grade of differentiation, gross findings at surgery, amount of residual tumor after surgery, and effectiveness of any adjunct treatment postoperatively. Many patients with ovarian cancer will experience recurrence despite best efforts to eradicate the cancer through surgery, radiation, or chemotherapy to eliminate residual tumor cells. The likelihood of cure in the event of recurrence is low (Duska, 2023).

Pathophysiology

Ovarian cancer, the cause of which is unknown, can originate from different cell types. About 95% of ovarian cancers are thought to originate in the ovarian epithelium (Chen & Berek, 2024a). New insights now propose

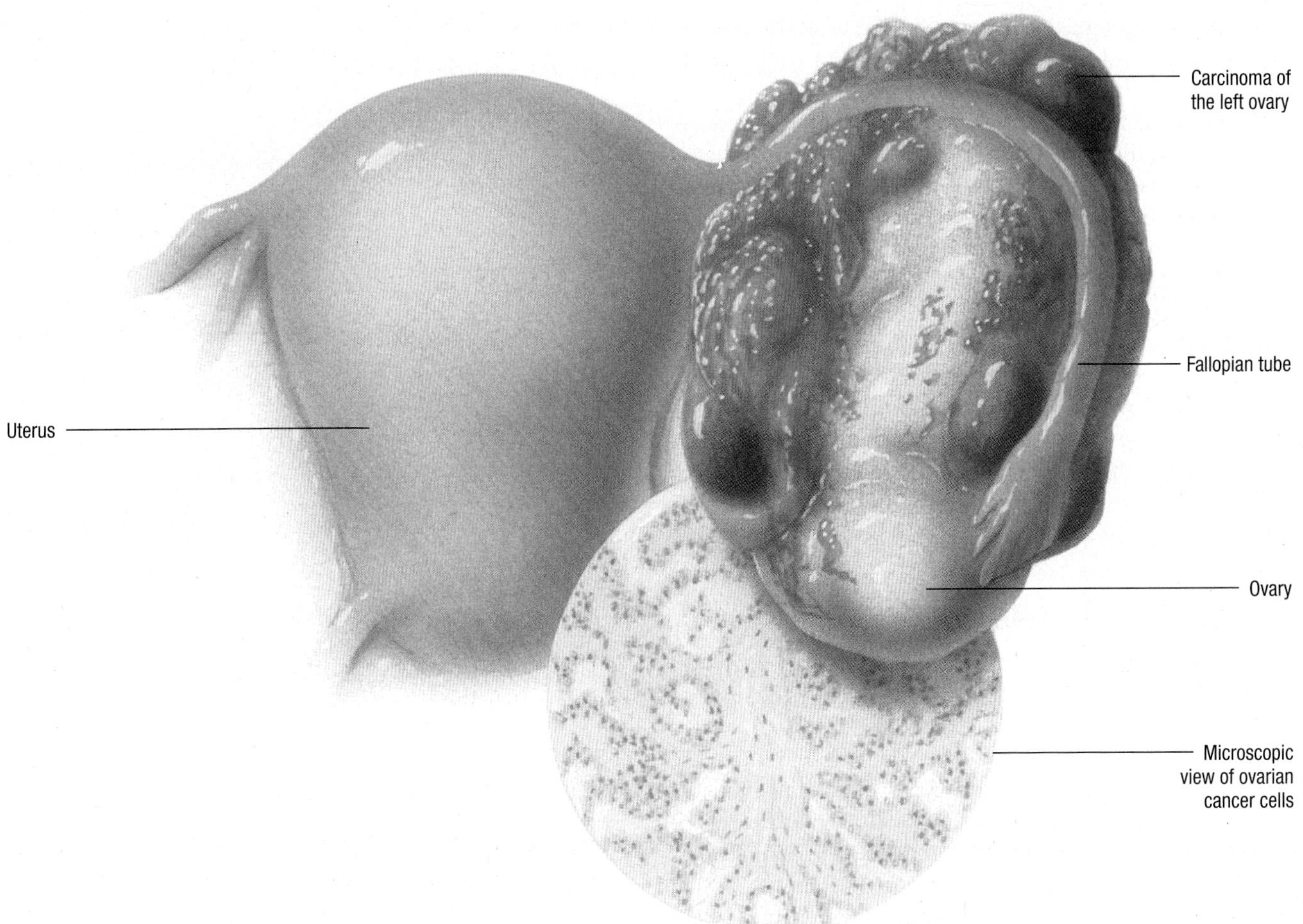

FIGURE 8.1 Ovarian cancer. (Reprinted with permission from Stewart, J. G. [2017]. *Anatomical Chart Company atlas of pathophysiology* [4th ed.]. Wolters Kluwer.)

a pivotal role for the fallopian tube during ovarian cancer pathogenesis. Increasing evidence suggests that serous ovarian cancer, the most common subtype of epithelial ovarian cancer, originates from the fimbriated distal end of the fallopian tube, while the ovary gets involved at a later stage. These represent 75% of all epithelial ovarian cancers (Chen & Berek, 2024a). Based on this finding, a postreproductive salpingectomy deserves consideration as a prophylactic intervention that may confer protection against an often-deadly disease (Green, 2022).

Tumors usually present as solid masses that have spread beyond the ovary and seeded into the peritoneum prior to diagnosis. A thorough understanding of the true pathogenesis of this cancer's origin could lead to the development of new and more effective therapies as well as novel biomarkers in early detection.

Screening and Diagnosis

Patients with ovarian cancer are typically diagnosed at a late stage, because of its vague early symptoms and lack of reliable screening tools, when the cancer has spread into the peritoneal cavity and complete surgical removal is challenging. Late discovery of ovarian cancer is common primarily because there is still no adequate screening test. The U.S. Preventive Services Task Force (USPSTF, 2018), along with the American College of Obstetricians and Gynecologists (ACOG) and the American Medical Association (AMA), recently reviewed the evidence for ovarian cancer screening and did not recommend screening for people at average risk because they found that such screening does not reduce ovarian cancer deaths. However, people with increased risk related to *BRCA1/2* gene mutations or a family history of ovarian cancer should be considered for genetic counseling to further evaluate their risk (USPSTF, 2018).

Two genes, *BRCA1* and *BRCA2*, are linked with hereditary breast and ovarian cancers. Blood tests can be performed to assess DNA in white blood cells to detect mutations in the *BRCA* genes. These genetic markers do not predict whether the person will develop cancer. Rather, they provide information regarding the risk of developing cancer: A patient who is BRCA-positive may have up to a 70% chance of developing breast cancer and up to a 40% chance of developing ovarian cancer (Petrucelli et al., 2023).

Specific clinical guidelines for ovarian cancer screening have not been developed, so the disease is often not diagnosed until it has metastasized. The USPSTF recommends against routine screening for ovarian cancer with serum CA-125, a transvaginal ultrasound, or a bimanual pelvic exam because these have not been shown to reduce mortality, and they are associated with a high rate of false positives (Carlson, 2024). CA-125 is a biologic tumor marker associated with ovarian cancer. Although its levels are elevated in many people with ovarian cancer, CA-125 is not specific for this cancer, and the levels may be elevated with other malignancies too (pancreatic, liver, colon, breast, and lung cancers). Despite the discovery that CA-125 and other serum markers increase before the clinical onset of ovarian cancer, it has proven surprisingly difficult to devise a successful screening program for patients with ovarian cancer without symptoms. Currently, due to its low specificity and low positive predictive value, it does not serve as a reliable screening tool alone (Carlson, 2024).

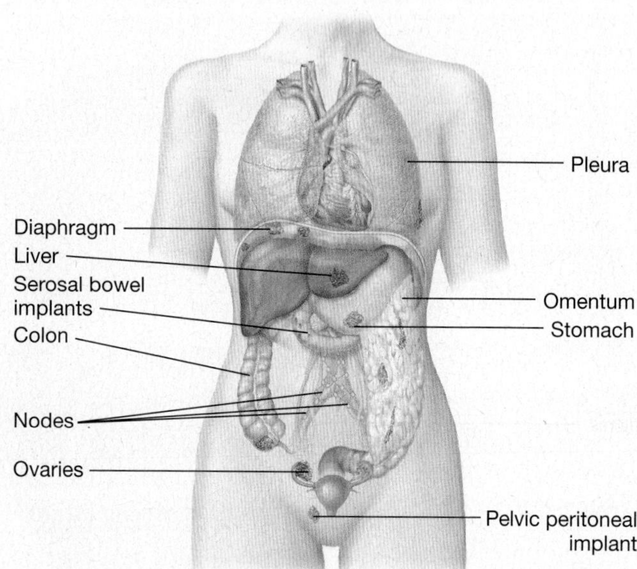

FIGURE 8.2 Common metastatic sites for ovarian cancer. (Reprinted with permission from Stewart, J. G. [2017]. *Anatomical Chart Company atlas of pathophysiology* [4th ed.]. Wolters Kluwer.)

Therapeutic Management

Treatment options for ovarian cancer vary depending on the stage and severity of the disease. Cancer staging is the extent to which the cancer has spread from the site of origin. Usually, a laparoscopy (abdominal exploration with an endoscope) is performed for diagnosis and staging, as well as evaluation for therapy. Staging is done using the 2017 8th Edition American Joint Committee on Cancer (AJCC) and the International Federation of Gynecology and Obstetrics (FIGO) Tumor, Node, Metastasis (TNM) classification system (Salani & Cosgrove, 2024). In general terms, in stage I, the cancer is limited to the ovaries. In stage II, the growth involves one or both ovaries, with pelvic extension. Stage III cancer involves one or both ovaries and other organs or structures inside the abdominal cavity and outside the pelvis; it may or may not have spread to the lymph nodes. In stage IV, the cancer has metastasized to distant sites (Salani & Cosgrove, 2024). Figure 8.2 shows the likely metastatic sites for ovarian cancer.

Surgical intervention remains the mainstay of the management of ovarian cancer. The management approach for most patients with ovarian cancer includes surgical staging, cytoreduction or debulking surgery, and adjuvant chemotherapy (Chen & Berek, 2024a). Because most patients are diagnosed with advanced-stage ovarian cancer, aggressive management involving debulking or cytoreductive surgery is commonly performed. This surgery involves resecting all visible tumors from the peritoneum, taking peritoneal biopsies, sampling lymph nodes, and removing all reproductive organs and the omentum. This aggressive surgery has been shown to increase the chance that chemotherapy will result in improved long-term survival rates (Chen & Berek, 2024a).

Chemotherapy is recommended for all stages of ovarian cancer, either before or after surgical intervention. Intraperitoneal chemotherapy, combined with surgery, has produced encouraging results for overall survival at acceptable morbidity and mortality rates. The landscape of maintenance drug therapy to prevent reoccurrence is evolving, with the FDA approving a few medications with promising results. Despite all of these therapies, virtually the only agreement about treatment for advanced disease is that surgery and chemotherapy both play a role, and current treatment and ability to detect cancer in its early stages are both ineffective in far too many patients (Arora et al., 2023).

Nursing Assessment

Ovarian cancers are considered the worst of all the gynecologic malignancies, primarily because they develop slowly and remain silent without symptoms until the cancer is far advanced. It has been described as the "overlooked disease" or "silent killer" because patients and health care providers often ignore or rationalize early symptoms. For example, patients may attribute gastrointestinal problems to stress and midlife changes. However, these vague complaints may precede more obvious symptoms by months. The most common early symptoms include abdominal bloating, early satiety, difficulty eating, vague abdominal or pelvic pain, and urinary frequency or urgency. Additional symptoms include fatigue, anorexia, nausea, dyspepsia, dyspareunia, constipation, menstrual irregularities, and back pain (Goff, 2024).

TAKE NOTE!

A symptom index has been created to help health care providers evaluate patients for early symptoms of ovarian cancer. This index requires further study to validate its use. It is not recommended for clinical use at this time (Goff, 2024).

Obtain a thorough history of the patient's symptoms, including their onset, duration, and frequency. Review the patient's history for risk factors such as:

- Nulliparity or childbirth later in life
- Obesity (BMI greater than 30 kg/m^2)
- Smoking
- Family history of ovarian, breast, or colorectal cancer
- Genetics: Eastern European or Ashkenazi Jewish descent
- Positive *BRCA1* and *BRCA2* mutations
- Personal history of breast cancer
- Hormone replacement therapy (HRT) for more than 10 years
- Fertility treatment (CDC, 2023b; National Ovarian Cancer Coalition [NOCC], 2023)

Perform a complete physical examination. Inspect the abdomen, noting any distention or bloating. Palpate the abdomen. Be alert for a mass or pain on palpation. Anticipate further testing to confirm the diagnosis.

Nursing Management

The complexities of ovarian cancer make a multidisciplinary approach necessary for optimal management. With the subtle nature and high risk of recurrence and mortality of this condition, most patients find it an emotionally exhausting and devastating experience. The presence of hope is essential for patients at the time of the diagnosis; they want to believe in being cured and able to continue life as usual with loved ones, friends, and relatives. Still, the newly received cancer diagnosis makes patients oscillate between hope and hopelessness, between positive expectations of getting cured and frightening feelings of the disease taking command. Nurses are invaluable resources in inspiring patients to find hope in life when diagnosed with cancer. Nursing management needs to focus on measures to promote early detection, educate the patient about the disease and its treatments, and provide emotional support. Nurses should show a positive attitude that communicates understanding and reassurance.

Promoting Early Detection

Nurses need to ensure that patients are aware of the risk factors for ovarian cancer. Urge patients not to dismiss seemingly innocuous symptoms as "just a part of aging." Encourage patients to describe such nonspecific complaints at health visits.

Assess the patient's family and personal history for risk factors and encourage genetic testing for patients with affected family members. Outline screening guidelines for patients with hereditary cancer syndrome and inform patients at high risk about the appropriate screening strategies.

Urge patients to have yearly bimanual pelvic examinations and a transvaginal ultrasound to allow identification of ovarian masses in their early stages. After menopause, a mass on an ovary is not a cyst; physiologic cysts can arise only from a follicle that has not ruptured or from the cystic degeneration of the corpus luteum. Ovarian cancer is not always silent and may manifest with several vague gastrointestinal symptoms. Although screening the general population is not recommended, nurses need to know what factors place patients at high risk and listen carefully to patient's complaints to detect this type of cancer before it becomes advanced.

TAKE NOTE!

A small ovarian "cyst" found on ultrasound in a postmenopausal patient without symptoms should arouse suspicion. Any mass or ovary palpated in a postmenopausal patient should be considered cancerous until proven otherwise (Matalliotakis et al., 2023).

Educating the Patient

Education is a major focus of nursing care. This teaching involves risk reduction and health promotion. Teach the patient about risk reduction strategies; for instance, pregnancy, use of oral contraceptives, and breastfeeding reduce the risk of ovarian cancer. Review the lifetime risks related to *BRCA1* and *BRCA2* genes and the options available should the patient test positive for these genes. Help promote community awareness of ovarian cancer by educating the public about risk-reducing behaviors. See research on primary prevention of reproductive cancer.

Instruct the patient about the importance of healthy lifestyles. Stress the importance of maintaining a healthy BMI (18.5 to 24.9 kg/m^2) to reduce risk. Encourage patients to eat a low-fat diet. Factors associated with a reduced risk of ovarian cancer include the use of oral contraceptives for 5 or more years, giving birth, breastfeeding, bilateral tubal ligation, removal of the ovaries, and hysterectomy (CDC, 2023c).

For the patient who is diagnosed with ovarian cancer, describe in simple terms the tests, treatment modalities, and follow-up needed. For example, if the patient will be having surgery, the nurse needs to provide thorough teaching about what to expect before, during, and after surgery. Outline the treatment options and the implications of choices. Assist the patient and their family in deciphering the large amount of information related to staging, tests, and treatments. Teach the patient about additional treatment measures, such as radiation therapy or chemotherapy, including how to handle the common adverse effects of treatment.

Supporting the Patient and Family

The diagnosis of ovarian cancer, like any cancer, can be overwhelming. In addition, the treatments and their effects can be highly stressful, both physically and emotionally. Provide one-to-one support for patients facing treatment for ovarian cancer. Ovarian cancer involves the reproductive system, which can have a direct impact on the patient's view of themselves. Encourage open discussion of sexuality and the impact of cancer. Listen and support the patient and their family as they try to cope with this disease. By being aware of patients' individual needs and different coping strategies, nurses can improve support for patients in this vulnerable situation. Encourage the use of appropriate coping strategies to allow for the best quality of life. Try to restore hope to patients with ovarian cancer, and stress treatment adherence. Nurses should not forget about the family caregivers who need help with managing emotions about prognosis, balancing their own and the patient's needs, work, and decision-making when there is uncertainty. If appropriate, encourage participation in clinical trials to offer hope for all patients. Continue to offer support to the patient and their family members as they experience sadness and grief.

CONSIDER THIS!

I felt I was a lucky woman because I had been in remission from breast cancer for 12 years, and I had been given the gift of life to share with my beloved family. Recently, I became ill with stomach problems like pain, indigestion, bloating, and nausea. My doctor treated me for gastric reflux disease, but the symptoms persisted. I was then referred to a gastroenterologist, a urologist, and then a gynecologist, who did an ultrasound, which was negative. I received reassurance from all three that there was nothing wrong with me. As time went by, I experienced more pain, more symptoms, and increased frustration. Six months after seeing all three specialists, a repeat ultrasound revealed I had ovarian cancer, and I needed surgery as soon as possible. I underwent a complete hysterectomy, and my surgeon found I was in stage III. Since then, I have undergone chemotherapy and participated in a clinical cancer study that was not successful for me. Now I am facing the fact that I am going to die soon.

Thoughts: This woman has tried everything to save her life, but time has run out for her with advanced ovarian cancer. People diagnosed with breast cancer are at a significant risk for developing ovarian cancer later in life. Of the string of doctors she saw, why did no one order more extensive testing, given her history of breast cancer? We are often haunted with the question: If health care providers had made different choices, would patients be faced with advanced diagnoses? We will never know.

ENDOMETRIAL CANCER

Endometrial cancer (also known as uterine cancer) is a malignant neoplastic growth of the uterine lining. It is the most common gynecologic malignancy in the United States and the second most common cancer globally (Chen & Berek, 2024b, 2024c). The ACS (2024c) estimates that about 67,880 new cases will be diagnosed in people in 2024 and that approximately 13,250 of these people will die. Postmenopausal people are affected the most. Incidence peaks between 60 and 70 years, but as people age, the risk of endometrial cancer increases (ACS, 2024c). It is more common in Black females than White females (ACS, 2024c). Approximately 90% of endometrial malignancies are carcinomas of the endometrium (Chen & Berek, 2024c). Because endometrial cancer is usually diagnosed in the early stages, it has a better prognosis than cervical or ovarian cancer (Chen & Berek, 2024b).

The incidence and prevalence of endometrial cancer are rising along with the global obesity epidemic, which is considered a major underlying cause (Crosbie et al., 2022). Additional risk factors include eating a high-fat diet, being physically inactive, chronic anovulation, type 2 diabetes, hypertension, polycystic ovary syndrome, long-term use of unopposed estrogens for HRT after menopause, use of tamoxifen, personal history of breast or ovarian cancer, and family history of endometrial cancer (Chen & Berek, 2024c). Protection against endometrial cancer includes increased parity, daily physical activity, use of combined oral contraceptives, increased age at last childbirth, and breastfeeding (Chen & Berek, 2024c).

Pathophysiology

Endometrial cancer appears to begin with endometrial proliferation that is hormonally stimulated by either endogenous or exogenous unopposed estrogen resulting in endometrial hyperplasia (Mahdy et al., 2022). Atypical premalignant lesions (referred to as endometrial hyperplasia neoplasia) change to endometrioid cancer (Mahdy et al., 2022). The majority of endometrial cancers are endometrioid adenocarcinoma; are low grade, meaning they are generally confined to the uterus and generally have a good prognosis; and account for 80% to 90% of endometrioid cancers (Creasman, 2022; Mahdy et al., 2022). Although metastatic spread is uncommon, it can be seen upon presentation or can be a recurrence of a primary tumor after initial treatment (Campos & Cohn, 2024a).

Early tumor growth is characterized by friable and spontaneous bleeding. Later tumor growth is characterized by myometrial invasion and growth toward the cervix (Fig. 8.3).

Remember Carmella, the woman with postmenopausal bleeding? In postmenopausal people, any bleeding is abnormal and warrants further assessment. What diagnostic testing would the nurse anticipate to determine the diagnosis? What would be the nurse's role during this testing?

Screening and Diagnosis

There is no specific screening test currently available to detect endometrial cancer. Screening for endometrial cancer is not routinely done because it is not practical or

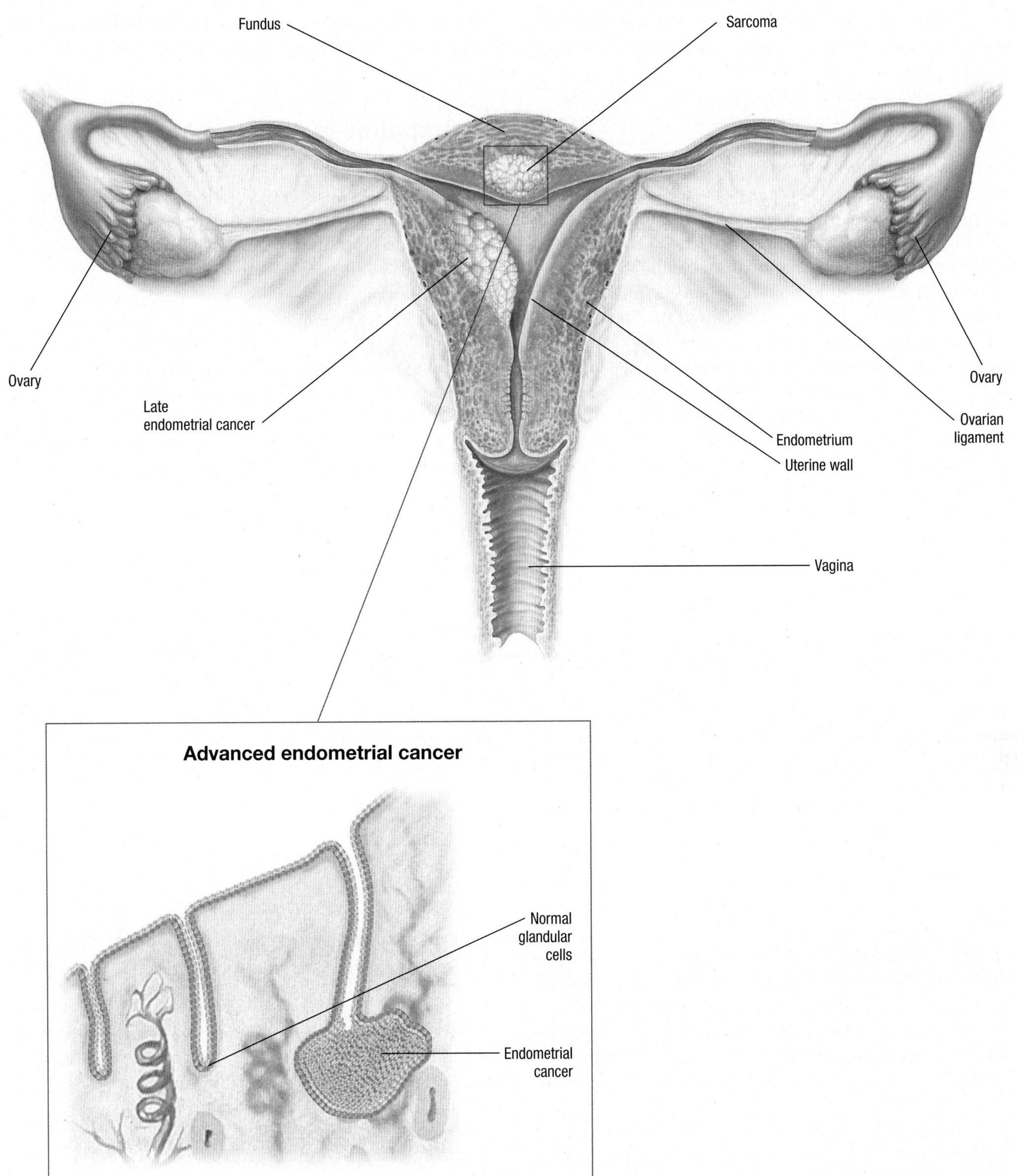

FIGURE 8.3 Progression of endometrial cancer. (Reprinted with permission from Stewart, J. G. [2017]. *Anatomical Chart Company atlas of pathophysiology* [4th ed.]. Wolters Kluwer.)

cost effective. The ACS (2020b) recommends patients be informed about the risks and symptoms of endometrial cancer at the onset of menopause and strongly encouraged to report any unexpected bleeding or spotting to the health care provider. A pelvic examination is frequently normal in the early stages of the disease. Changes in the size, shape, or consistency of the uterus or its surrounding support structures may exist when the disease is more advanced. Among all patients, 75% to 90% will present with early symptoms, typically abnormal bleeding, while the cancer remains only in the uterus; effective therapy results in high survival rates (Chen & Berek, 2024b).

During the past few decades, the role of ultrasound in the evaluation of postmenopausal bleeding has changed markedly, from little or no role to a major role today. Transvaginal ultrasound can be used to evaluate the endometrial cavity and measure the thickness of the endometrial lining. It can be used to detect endometrial hyperplasia. Numerous studies have shown that ultrasound is at least as sensitive as endometrial biopsy for endometrial cancer and that ultrasound can reliably exclude cancer without the need for biopsy in some patients with postmenopausal bleeding. The depth of myometrium is an important diagnostic factor. In particular, numerous studies have shown that people with an endometrial thickness of 4 mm or less have an extremely low likelihood of endometrial cancer and thus do not need to undergo an endometrial biopsy, though a follow-up scan could be offered (Saccardi et al., 2022). Ultrasound can also help in the selection of an appropriate biopsy technique. In a patient with postmenopausal bleeding and a thick endometrium, a sonohysterogram can determine whether the endometrium is diffusely thick or has focal areas of thickening. With diffuse thickening, an endometrial biopsy is appropriate. When one or more focal areas of thickening are present, hysteroscopic biopsy is likely to be the better choice.

Endometrial biopsy is an office procedure that is used after a suspicious transvaginal ultrasound has been done in the diagnosis of endometrial cancer in a patient with postmenopausal bleeding. The biopsy is obtained through an endometrial suction catheter that is inserted through the cervix into the uterine cavity and a tissue sample is taken. The sensitivity and specificity of the biopsy procedure tend to be in the range of 90% or higher for the detection of endometrial cancer or other pathologies (Chen & Berek, 2024b).

As indicated earlier, staging is the process of looking at all of the information the doctors have learned about the tumor to determine how much the cancer may have spread. Endometrial cancer classification has progressed over time. The FIGO has divided endometrial cancer into two categories: aggressive and less aggressive tumors. These categories are further subdivided into molecular subtypes (Huvila & McAlpine, 2023). This categorization helps improve both predictive and prognostic information (Huvila & McAlpine, 2023). The stage of endometrial cancer is the most important factor in choosing a treatment plan. It can spread locally to other parts of the uterus or regionally to nearby lymph nodes. The regional lymph nodes are found in the pelvis and farther away along the aorta. Finally, the cancer can spread (metastasize) to distant lymph nodes or organs such as the lung, liver, bone, brain, and others.

In stage I, the tumor is confined to the corpus and ovary. In stage II, it has spread to the connective tissue of the cervix, but not outside the uterus. In stage III, it has spread locally and regionally. In stage IV, it has invaded the bladder mucosa and bowel mucosa, lymph nodes, with distant metastases to the lungs, liver, and bone (Cohn, 2024).

Therapeutic Management

Typically, the stage of the disease directs treatment. It usually involves surgery with adjunct therapy based on pathologic findings. Surgery most often involves the removal of the uterus (hysterectomy) and the fallopian tubes and ovaries (salpingo-oophorectomy). Removal of the fallopian tubes and ovaries is recommended because tumor cells spread early to the ovaries, and any dormant cancer cells could be stimulated to grow by ovarian estrogen. In more advanced cancers, radiation and chemotherapy are used as adjuncts to surgery. Routine surveillance intervals for follow-up may be necessary since the majority of recurrences occur in the first 3 years after diagnosis (Campos & Cohn, 2024b).

Nursing Assessment

Obtain a thorough history from the patient, ascertaining their primary complaint. Most commonly, the major initial symptom of endometrial cancer is abnormal and painless vaginal bleeding. Obtain a menstrual history and inquire if the patient is taking any hormones. Also ascertain if they have a personal or family history of breast, ovarian, or colon cancer. These key pieces of information will assist in identifying patients at high risk for endometrial cancer.

TAKE NOTE!

Any episode of bright red bleeding that occurs after menopause should be investigated. Abnormal uterine bleeding is rarely the result of uterine malignancy in a young person, but in the postmenopausal person, it should be regarded with suspicion.

Also review the patient's history for any risk factors, including:

- Obesity (BMI greater than 30 kg/m^2)
- Diabetes mellitus
- Hypertension
- History of pelvic radiation
- Polycystic ovary syndrome
- Early menarche (before 12 years old)
- Use of prolonged exogenous unopposed estrogen with an intact uterus
- Endometrial hyperplasia
- Personal history of breast, colon, or ovarian cancer
- Late onset of menopause (after age 55)
- Tamoxifen use
- Lynch syndrome (Chen & Berek, 2024c)

Assess the patient for additional manifestations, such as dyspareunia, low back pain, purulent genital discharge, dysuria, pelvic pain, weight loss, and a change in bladder and bowel habits. These may suggest an advanced disease.

Perform a physical examination or assist with a pelvic examination as appropriate. Observe for vaginal discharge. Note any changes in the size, shape, or consistency of the uterus or surrounding structures or patient reports of pain during examination. Anticipate the need for transvaginal ultrasound to identify endometrial hyperplasia (usually greater than 4 mm) and endometrial biopsy if needed to identify malignant cells.

Nursing Management

Ensure that the patient understands all of the treatment options. Address any concerns the patient expresses, including questions about sexuality. Ensure that follow-up appointments are scheduled appropriately. Refer the patient to a support group. Offer the patient and family explanations and emotional support throughout the experience.

Educate the patient about preventive measures or follow-up care if they have been treated for cancer. Education may be the most important tool currently available for the early detection of endometrial cancer. Many risk factors for endometrial cancer are modifiable or treatable, including obesity (BMI greater than 30 kg/m^2), hypertension, and diabetes. Educating patients about risk factors and ways to decrease the risks is essential so that patients can learn about their own risk profiles and can become partners in the fight against this gynecologic cancer (Teaching Guidelines 8.2).

Carmella's endometrial biopsy indicates endometrial adenocarcinoma. Her health care provider recommends surgery and adjuvant radiation therapy. How long will Carmella need to follow up after surgery? What lifestyle changes will the nurse need to stress with Carmella?

TEACHING GUIDELINES 8.2 Preventive and Follow-Up Measures for Endometrial Cancer

- Visit health care practitioner for early evaluation of any abnormal bleeding after menopause.
- Maintain a low-fat, healthy diet throughout life.
- Engage in regular physical activity.
- Manage weight and maintain a healthy BMI (18.5–24.9 kg/m^2) to discourage hyperestrogenic states, which predispose patients to endometrial hyperplasia.
- Pregnancy serves as a protective factor by reducing estrogen. Breastfeed your baby if possible.
- Use combination estrogen and progestin pills for contraception.
- Be aware of risk factors for endometrial cancer and make modifications as needed.
- Report any of the following symptoms immediately:
  - Bleeding or spotting after sexual intercourse
  - Bleeding that lasts longer than a week
  - Reappearance of bleeding after 6 months or more of no menses
- After cancer therapy, schedule follow-up appointments for the next few years.
- After cancer therapy, frequently communicate with your health care provider concerning your status.
- After surgery, maintain a healthy BMI (18.5–24.9 kg/m^2).

CERVICAL CANCER

Cervical cancer is a malignancy located in the uterine cervix. The majority of cervical cancers are caused by the human papillomavirus (HPV). HPV is detected in 99.7% of cervical cancers (Frumovitz, 2024). Other HPV-related cancers include oropharyngeal, anal, penile, vaginal, and vulvar cancers. HPV is transmitted through vaginal intercourse, anal and oral sex, and other intimate skin-to-skin contact (CDC, 2022c). Cervical cancer is the third most common female gynecologic malignancy in the United States after cancers of the endometrium and the ovary (Frumovitz, 2024). The ACS (2024d) estimates that about 13,800 cases of invasive cervical cancer will be diagnosed in the United States in 2024 and approximately 4,360 patients will die. Worldwide, cervical cancer is the fourth most frequently diagnosed cancer in females, with over 660,000 new cases diagnosed annually, but it develops over time and is one of the most preventable types of cancer (WHO, 2024). Over the past 50 years, there has been a significant decrease in the incidence and mortality of cervical cancer (Frumovitz, 2024). However, in recent years, there has been an increase in the annual incidence of cervical cancer in females 30 to 44 years of age, and the incidence of advanced-stage cervical cancer is rising in the United States among White and Black women (Frumovitz, 2024; Thomas, 2022). This emphasizes the continued importance of access to routine health care and recommended screenings and immunizations (Frumovitz, 2024; Thomas, 2022). The 5-year survival rate for all stages of cervical cancer is about 67% (ACS, 2024e). Cervical cancer remains a disease of socioeconomic disparity. Barriers to screening and prevention of cervical cancer include lack of health insurance, procrastination, the person's fear of finding out that they have cancer and embarrassment about having a Papanicolaou (Pap) test. The incidence and mortality rates of cervical cancer have decreased noticeably in the past several decades, with most of the reduction attributed to the Pap and HPV screening tests, which detect cervical cancer and some precancerous lesions. The **Papanicolaou (Pap) test** (also known as a Pap smear) is a procedure used to obtain cells from the cervix for cytology screening. Cervical cancer is one of the most treatable cancers when detected at an early stage (Guimarães et al., 2022). See the Healthy People 2030 box. Cervical cancer tends to occur in midlife. Most cases are found in people younger than age 50, with the highest incidence in people aged 35 to 44 years (ACS, 2024d). It rarely develops in people younger than age 20 (ACS, 2024d). Many older people do not realize that the risk of developing cervical cancer is still present as they age (ACS, 2024d).

HEALTHY PEOPLE 2030

Objectives	Nursing Significance
Increase the proportion of females who get screened for cervical cancer. Reduce infections of HPV types prevented by the vaccine in young adults. Increase the proportion of adolescents who get recommended doses of the HPV vaccine.	• Will help improve mortality rates and quality of life and reduce health care costs related to the treatment of malignancies • Will reflect the importance of promoting evidence-based screening for cervical cancer by lowering mortality rates • Will help to promote screening and early detection. Regular Pap tests decrease cervix cancer incidence and mortality tremendously. Many patients diagnosed with invasive cervical cancer have never had a Pap test or haven't had one recently. • Educate patients about the importance of cervical cancer screening and assist if resources are needed. • Will raise awareness of cancer screening and prevention on local and national levels to improve and promote the health of all females • Educate patients about the HPV immunization recommendations and assist if resources are needed. • Will reduce the number of new cancer cases, as well as the illness, disability, and death caused by cancer

Healthy People Objectives retrieved from http://www.healthypeople.gov

Pathophysiology

HPV types 16 and 18 cause 75% of cervical cancer cases (Fowler et al., 2023). Cervical cancer starts with gradual abnormal changes in the cellular lining or surface of the cervix. Typically, these changes occur in the squamous–columnar junction of the cervix, as the majority of cervical cancer is squamous cell carcinoma (SCC) (ACS, 2024f). Here, cylindrical secretory epithelial cells (columnar) meet the protective flat epithelial cells (squamous) from the outer cervix and vagina in what is termed the transformation zone. Adenocarcinoma, which results from the glandular mucus-producing cells, accounts for the majority of the remaining cases of cervical cancer (ACS, 2024f). Figure 8.4 shows the pathophysiology of cervical cancer.

Human papillomavirus (HPV) occurs in the majority of sexually active females. Most people who have HPV are without symptoms and therefore do not realize they have the virus. The vast majority of squamous cervical cancers contain HPV DNA, and the virus is now accepted as a major causative factor in the development of cervical cancer and its precursor, **cervical dysplasia** (disordered growth of abnormal cells). However, only a small proportion of HPV infections actually progress to cancer; 90% of such infections clear on their own, demonstrating that other factors must be involved in the process of carcinogenesis (Boardman, 2022).

Screening and Diagnosis

Screening for cervical cancer is effective because the presence of a precursor lesion, cervical intraepithelial neoplasia, helps determine whether further tests are needed. Lesions start as dysplasia and progress in a predictable fashion over a long period, allowing ample opportunity for intervention at a precancerous stage. Progression from low-grade to high-grade dysplasia takes an average of 9 years, and progression from high-grade dysplasia to invasive cancer takes up to 2 years. Three main factors have been postulated to influence the progression of low-grade dysplasia to high-grade dysplasia. These include the type and duration of viral infection, with high-risk HPV type and persistent infection predicting a higher risk for progression; host conditions that compromise immunity, such as multiparity or poor nutritional status; and environmental factors such as smoking, oral contraceptive use, or vitamin deficiencies. In addition, various gynecologic factors, including history of STI, age of first intercourse, and number of sexual partners, significantly increase the risk for cervical cancer (Boardman, 2022).

Widespread use of the Pap test (cervical cytology), HPV test, or a combination of the two (cotesting) is credited with saving thousands of lives and decreasing deaths from cervical cancer. Routine Pap smears and HPV testing for all sexually active females has been one of the primary screening methods for early detection of cervical irregularities related to HPV and is crucial for the prevention of cervical cancer.

Despite its outstanding record of success as a screening tool for cervical cancer (it detects approximately 95%

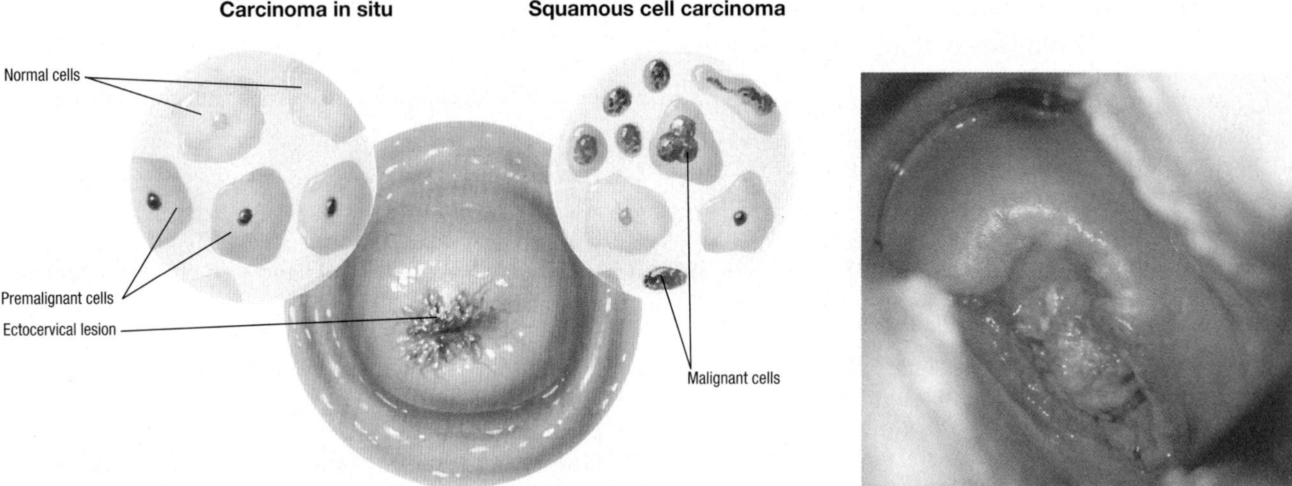

FIGURE 8.4 Cervical cancer. (Reprinted with permission from Stewart, J. G. [2017]. *Anatomical Chart Company atlas of pathophysiology* [4th ed.]. Wolters Kluwer.)

of early cancer changes), the conventional Pap smear has a 20% to 30% false-negative rate (NCI, 2024a). Many technologies have been developed to improve the sensitivity and specificity of Pap testing, including:

- *ThinPrep:* In this liquid-based technique, the cervical specimen is placed into a vial of preservative solution rather than on a glass slide.
- *ThinPrep Imaging System:* An algorithm-based decision-making technology identifies slides that should be rescreened by cytopathologists by selecting samples that exceed a certain threshold for the likelihood of abnormal cells (Feldman & Crum, 2023).

The high rate of false-negative results may also be due to other factors, including errors in sampling the cervix, in preparing the slide, and in patient preparation. Although cytology-based nationwide cervical screening has been helpful in identifying abnormal cervical cells, the sensitivity of cytology for the detection of high-grade precursor lesions is limited. Additionally, adenocarcinoma and its precursors are often missed by cytology. The current insight that infection with HPV is the causative agent of cervical cancer and its precursors has led to the development of molecular tests for the detection of HPV. Strong evidence now supports the use of HPV testing in the prevention of cervical cancer. It is evident that HPV can be detected in urine-based testing and menstrual blood sampling; these might eventually become helpful tools in cervical cancer screening and HPV surveillance efforts (Feldman & Crum, 2023). Nurses need to keep up to date on the latest research developments as well as the strengths and weaknesses of various screening methods.

Although professional medical organizations disagree as to the recommended frequency of screening and the age at which screening for cervical cancer should begin, ACOG (2021) recommends that cervical cancer screening begin at age 21 years (regardless of sexual history), since females younger than age 21 are at very low risk of cancer. In addition, ACOG advises Pap smears every 3 years for females between ages 21 and 29 years; females between ages 30 and 65 years can choose to have a Pap test and HPV test (cotesting) every 5 years, a Pap test alone every 3 years, or an HPV test along every 5 years. Cervical cancer screening can be stopped after age 65 in patients who have an adequate screening history. Patients who have had a hysterectomy should stop screening. Patients who have received the HPV vaccine should be screened according to the same guidelines as those who have not been vaccinated. In addition, patients must have a clear understanding of the results of Pap smear testing and follow-up guidelines. Patients at higher risk should continue to have annual Pap smears throughout their lives.

Pap smear results are classified using the Bethesda system, which provides a uniform diagnostic terminology that allows clear communication between the laboratory and the health care provider. The information provided by the laboratory is divided into categories: specimen type, specimen adequacy, general categorization of cytologic findings, and interpretation or result (Wang et al., 2023). The main categories under interpretation/results include negative for intraepithelial lesion or malignancy, non-neoplastic findings, organism, epithelial cell abnormalities, and other malignant neoplasms (Crum et al., 2022). If a patient has an abnormal screening result, the health care provider will provide follow-up recommendations regarding further testing or necessary treatment, taking into consideration the patient's previous screening results, any previous treatment for cervical cell changes, and personal health factors (NCI, 2023a).

Therapeutic Management

Treatment for abnormal Pap smears depends on the severity of the results and the health history of the patient. Therapeutic choices all involve destroying as many affected cells as possible. With the introduction of multimodality therapy for cervical cancer, many patients will be long-term survivors in need of comprehensive surveillance care. Obesity (BMI greater than 30 kg/m^2) and smoking are significant comorbidities that may complicate care in cervical cancer survivors. Nurses can focus their interventions on modifying these risk factors to increase the quality of life for cervical cancer survivors. Box 8.1 describes treatment options.

Colposcopy is a microscopic examination of the lower genital tract using a magnifying instrument called a colposcope. Specific patterns of cells that correlate well with certain histologic findings can be visualized.

BOX 8.1 Treatment Options for Cervical Cancer

- *Cryotherapy*—destroys abnormal cervical tissue by freezing with liquid nitrogen, Freon, or nitrous oxide. It is used for early in-situ lesions or cervical dysplasia. Healing takes up to 6 weeks, and the patient may experience a profuse, watery vaginal discharge for 3–4 weeks.
- *Cone biopsy or conization*—removes a cone-shaped section of cervical tissue usually for stage Ia1 lesions. The base of the cone is formed by the ectocervix (outer part of the cervix) and the point or apex of the cone is from the endocervical canal. The transformation zone is contained within the cone sample. The cone biopsy is also a treatment and can be used to completely remove any precancers and very early cancers. Two methods are commonly used for cone biopsies.
- *LEEP* (loop electrosurgical excision procedure) or LLETZ (large loop excision of the transformation zone)—the abnormal cervical tissue is removed with a wire that is heated by an electrical current. For this procedure, a local anesthetic is used. It is performed in the health care provider's office in approximately 10 minutes. Mild cramping and bleeding may persist for several weeks after the procedure.
- *Cold knife cone biopsy*—a surgical scalpel or a laser is used instead of a heated wire to remove tissue. This procedure requires general anesthesia and is done in a hospital setting. After the procedure, cramping and bleeding may persist for a few weeks.
- Laser therapy—destroys diseased cervical tissue by using a focused beam of high-energy light to vaporize it (burn it off). After the procedure, the patient may experience a watery brown discharge for a few weeks. Very effective in destroying precancers and preventing them from developing into cancers
- Hysterectomy—removes the uterus and cervix surgically. Radical hysterectomy also includes tissues next to the uterus.
- Radical trachelectomy—removes the cervix and upper part of the vagina but not the body of the uterus, therefore maintaining the patient's ability to bear children
- Radiation therapy—delivered by internal radium applications to the cervix or external radiation therapy that includes lymphatics of the pelvis
- Chemoradiation—weekly chemotherapeutic drug therapy concurrent with radiation

American Cancer Society. (2024g). *Treatment options for cervical cancer, by stage.* https://www.cancer.org/cancer/cervical-cancer/treating/by-stage.html; American Cancer Society. (2020c). *Surgery for cervical cancer.* https://www.cancer.org/cancer/types/cervical-cancer/treating/surgery.html

Nursing Assessment

Obtain a thorough history and physical examination of the patient. Investigate their history for risk factors such as:

- Early age at first intercourse
- Lower socioeconomic status
- Higher risk sexual partner
- Unprotected sexual intercourse
- Family history of cervical cancer (first-degree female relative)
- Sexual intercourse with uncircumcised males
- History of STIs such as genital herpes or chlamydia
- Multiple sex partners
- Cigarette smoking
- History of vulvar or vaginal squamous intraepithelial neoplasia
- Immunosuppression with HIV infection
- Oral contraceptive use
- Moderate dysplasia found on Pap smear within the past 5 years
- HPV infection (Frumovitz, 2024)

Question the patient about any signs and symptoms. Clinically, the first sign is abnormal vaginal bleeding, usually after sexual intercourse. Also be alert for reports of vaginal discomfort, malodorous discharge, and dysuria. In some cases, the patient is without symptoms, with detection occurring at an annual gynecologic examination and Pap test.

Perform a physical examination. Inspect the perineal area for vaginal discharge or genital warts. Perform or assist with a pelvic examination, including the collection of a Pap smear as indicated (Nursing Procedure 8.1).

TAKE NOTE!

Suspect advanced cervical cancer in patients with pelvic, back, or leg pain, weight loss, anorexia, weakness and fatigue, and fractures.

Prepare the patient for further diagnostic testing if indicated, such as a colposcopy. In a colposcopy, the patient is placed in the lithotomy position and their cervix is cleansed with acetic acid solution. Acetic acid makes abnormal cells appear white, which is referred to as "acetowhite." These white areas are then biopsied and sent to the pathologist for assessment. Although this test is not painful, it has minor side effects (minor bleeding, cramping, and a risk of an infection developing after the biopsy). It can be performed safely in the clinic or office setting, though patients may be apprehensive or anxious about it because it is done to identify and confirm potential abnormal cell growth. Some health care providers request that the patient premedicate with a mild analgesic such as ibuprofen prior to undergoing the procedure.

NURSING PROCEDURE 8.1 Assisting With Collection of a Pap Smear

Purpose: To Obtain Cells From the Cervix for Cervical Cytology Screening

1. Explain the procedure to the patient (Fig. A).
2. Instruct patient to empty their bladder.
3. Wash hands thoroughly.
4. Assemble equipment, maintaining sterility of equipment (Fig. B).
5. Position patient on stirrups or foot pedals so that their knees fall outward.
6. Drape patient with a sheet for privacy, covering the abdomen but leaving the perineal area exposed.
7. Open packages as needed.
8. Encourage patient to relax.
9. Provide support to patient as the practitioner obtains a sample by spreading the labia; inserting the speculum; inserting the cytobrush and swabbing the endocervix; or inserting the plastic spatula and swabbing the cervix (Figs. C–H).

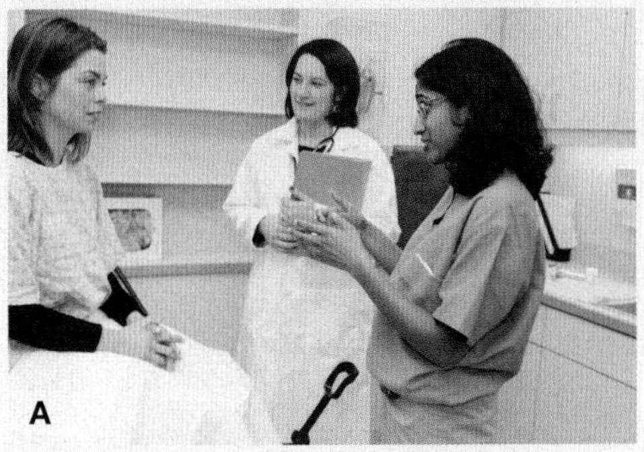
A

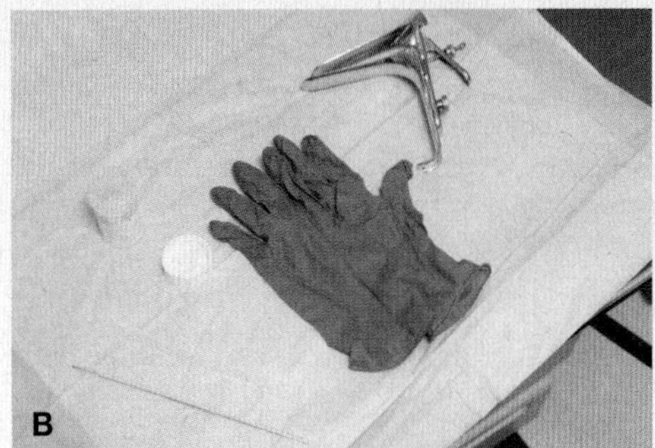
B

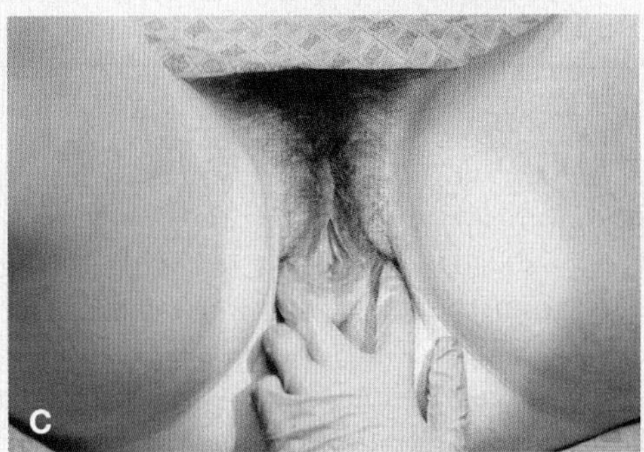
C

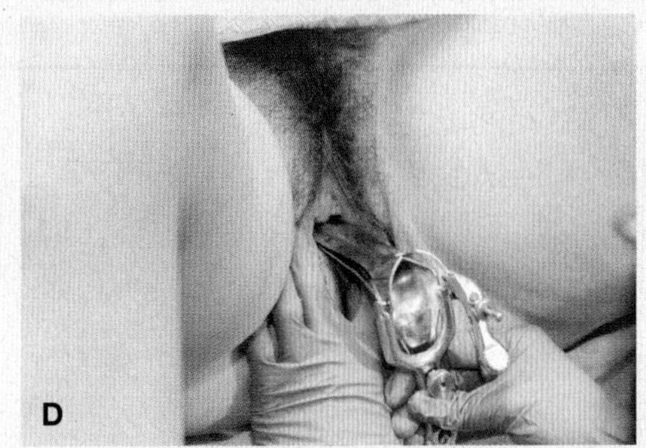
D

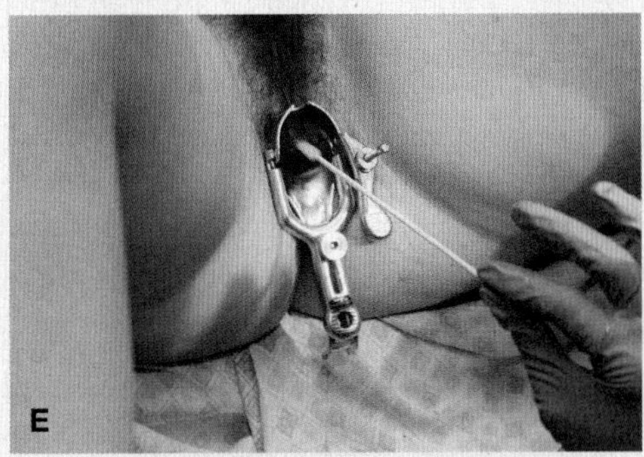
E

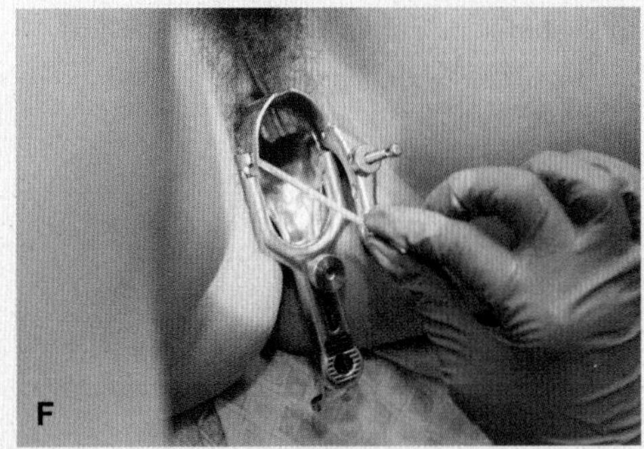
F

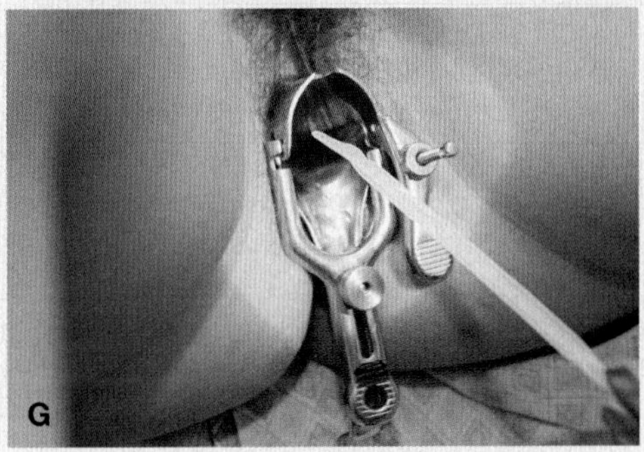
G

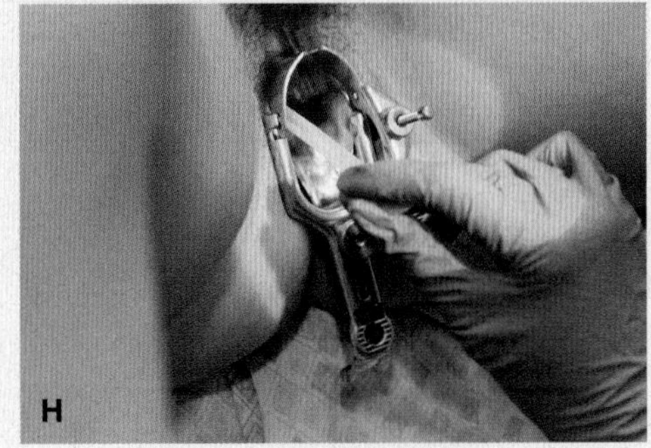
H

(*continued*)

NURSING PROCEDURE 8.1 Assisting With Collection of a Pap Smear (*continued*)

10. Transfer the specimen to a container (Fig. I) or a slide. If a slide is used, spray the fixative on the slide holding the spray container about 6 in away from the slide.
11. Place sterile lubricant on the practitioner's fingertip when indicated for the bimanual examination.
12. Wash hands thoroughly.
13. Label specimen according to facility policy.
14. Rinse reusable instruments and dispose of waste appropriately (Fig. J).
15. Wash hands thoroughly.
16. Assist the patient up after the exam is completed.

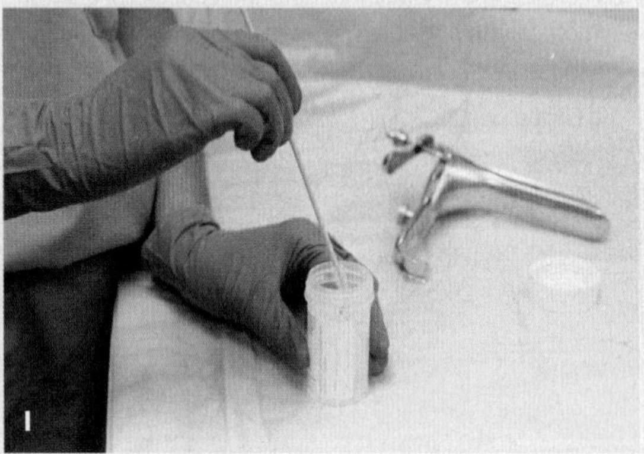
I

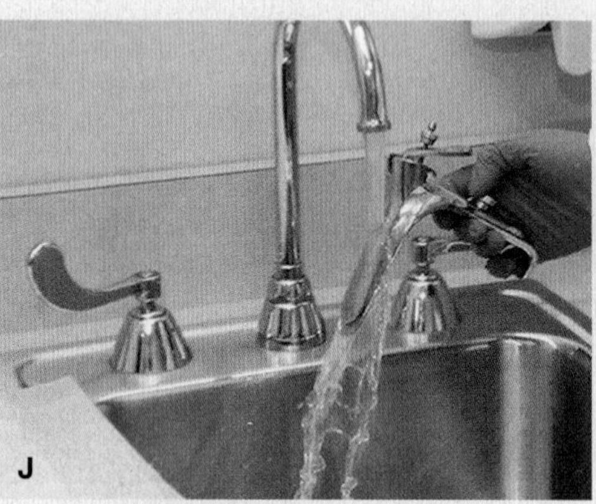
J

Adapted from Kamal, M. (2022). Pap smear collection and preparation: Key points. *CytoJournal, 19*, 24. https://dx.doi.org/10.25259/CMAS_03_05_2021; Feldman, S., & Crum, C. P. (2023). Cervical cancer screening tests: Techniques for cervical cytology and human papillomavirus testing. *UpToDate*. Retrieved May 5, 2024, from https://www.uptodate.com/contents/cervical-cancer-screening-tests-techniques-for-cervical-cytology-and-human-papillomavirus-testing

Nursing Management

The nurse's role involves primary prevention by educating patients about risk factors and ways to prevent cervical cancer.

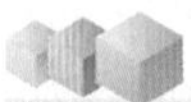
Concept Mastery Alert

Cervical Cancer Prevention

The key points to remember in cervical cancer prevention education are smoking cessation, limiting alcohol consumption, encouraging teens to refrain from early sexual activity, and having multiple partners.

Gardasil 9 is the vaccine currently approved by the U.S. Food and Drug Administration to protect children and adults from HPV from the ages of 9 to 45 years. The vaccines prevent infection from the nine strains of HPV responsible for most penile and cervical cancers. The vaccine is highly effective in preventing persistent HPV infection and has the potential to prevent more than 90% of HPV-attributable cancers (CDC, 2024d). The vaccine is administered by intramuscular injection, and the recommended schedule is a two-dose or three-dose series, depending on the person's age. The need to use two versus three injections will be determined by the health care provider. Usually, the younger the person is (9 to 14 years), the fewer injections needed. The vaccine protects against infection with these types of HPV for about 10 years. It is not known if the protection lasts longer. The vaccines do not treat or protect anyone already infected with HPV (CDC, 2024d). Barriers to receiving this vaccine are related to the belief the vaccine is not proven to be safe or effective, lack of knowledge and awareness of HPV and vaccination schedule, and parental feelings that their child is too young for the vaccine (Zhu et al., 2023). Nurses need to increase parental awareness, provide access, address psychological barriers to the HPV vaccine, and utilize evidence-based interventions to increase the usage of this effective vaccine to prevent cancers. This vaccine is not a substitute for routine cervical cancer screening, and vaccinated patients should have Pap smears as recommended. See Evidence-Based Practice 8.1.

Focus primary prevention education on the following:

- Identify high-risk behaviors in patients and teach them how to reduce such behaviors.
- Take steps to prevent STIs.
- Practice sexual abstinence.
- Avoid early sexual activity.
- Avoid long-term use of oral contraceptives.
- Faithfully use barrier methods of contraception.
- Avoid active and passive exposure to smoking.
- Receive the HPV vaccine.
- Instruct patients on the importance of screening for cervical cancer by having Pap smears, HPV tests, or a combination test.

EVIDENCE-BASED PRACTICE 8.1

Clinical Communication Strategies Associated With Increased Uptake of the Human Papillomavirus (HPV) Vaccine: A Systematic Review

BACKGROUND

HPV causes about 35,000 cancer cases annually in the United States. A very effective (nearly 100%) vaccine for HPV (Gardasil 9) can prevent those cancers, but there is low public acceptance of administering it in children. Only about half of adolescents have received Gardasil 9; parental concerns and lack of trust seem to play a role in the low acceptance of it. The purpose of this study was to determine specific communication strategies for promoting uptake of the HPV in children and adults.

STUDY

Database searches retrieved 106 related studies; of these, 46 met the inclusion criteria for this review that contained conversations with adolescents and parents. Quality assessment was performed with all studies included and each study was scored.

Findings

It was found that robust, direct communication about the HPV vaccine to the adolescent and/or parents (as compared to a more casual approach) was a workable strategy to gain acceptance of the vaccine. Although parental confidence in the HPV vaccine remains a challenge despite a favorable safety profile, effective, strong health recommendations with a presumptive style and communication on the part of the health care provider or nurse yielded positive results and acceptance of the vaccine.

Nursing Implications

Nurses are on the frontlines of providing vaccinations and encouraging adolescents and their parents to receive them for their own protection against a variety of cancers. Nurses need to understand the factors that influence hesitancy, acceptance, and demand for adolescent vaccination in different settings. A strong recommendation with a presumptive style positively affected vaccination rates and therefore should be considered an evidence-based practice. It is hoped that using this approach will reduce the incidence of HPV-associated cancers in the United States.

Constable, C., Ferguson, K., Nicholson, J., & Quinn, G. P. (2022). Clinician communication strategies associated with increased uptake of the human papillomavirus (HPV) vaccine: A systematic review. *Cancer, 72*(6), 561–569. https://doi.org/10.3322/caac.21753

TAKE NOTE!

The patient does not need to do any special preparation before a Pap test. It is not necessary to avoid intercourse, tampon use, douching, or vaginal gel lubricants 48 hours prior to the Pap test. The patient may be asked to schedule the test during a time they are not menstruating, but if they end up menstruating on the day of the test, it can still be performed. Cytologic results using liquid-based Pap tests do not appear to be affected by the presence of blood (Feldman & Crum, 2023).

Nurses also can advocate for patients by making sure that the Pap smear is sent to an accredited laboratory for interpretation. Doing so reduces the risk of false-negative results. The identification and treatment of early precancerous lesions is critical to the prevention of cervical cancer.

Secondary prevention focuses on reducing or limiting the area of cervical dysplasia. Explain in detail all procedures that might be needed. Encourage the patient who has undergone any cervical treatment to allow the pelvic area to rest for approximately 1 month. Discuss this rest period with the patient and their partner to gain cooperation. Outline alternatives to vaginal intercourse, such as cuddling, holding hands, and kissing. Remind the patient about any follow-up procedures that are needed, and assist them with scheduling if necessary.

Tertiary prevention focuses on minimizing disability or the spread of cervical cancer. It involves the diagnosis and treatment of confirmed cases of cancer. Treatment is typically through surgery, radiotherapy, and, frequently, chemotherapy. Palliative care is provided to patients when the disease has already reached an incurable stage. Knowing that the patient and their family have been told about her prognosis, the nurse is in a position to support them when the impact of the diagnosis is realized.

Throughout the process, provide emotional support to the patient and their family. During the decision-making process, the patient may be overwhelmed by the diagnosis and all the information being presented. Refer the patient and their family to appropriate community resources and support groups as indicated. It is crucial for all patients to be given correct information regarding safe sexual practices, informed about the preventive role of the HPV vaccination, and educated about the role of the Pap test as a secondary screening measure for cervical cancer. The emotional needs of the patient diagnosed with cancer can best be met by a warm, friendly personality; an attitude of empathy rather than sympathy; and skilled communication. Nurses across all settings are in a powerful position to be advocates for safe health care practices of patients through education at personal, community, and national levels.

VAGINAL CANCER

Vaginal cancer is an uncommon malignant tissue growth arising in the vagina. Primary vaginal cancer is rare, as most tumors in the vagina spread from another primary site. It only accounts for 1% to 2% of reproductive cancers (Kaltenecker et al., 2023). About 75% of vaginal cancers are caused by HPV (NCI, 2023b). The incidence increases with age, with 50% of cases in people over 70 years of age and the average age of diagnosis being 67 years (Kaltenecker et al., 2023). The prognosis of vaginal cancer depends largely on the stage of the disease and the type of tumor. The 5-year survival rate for stage I vaginal cancer is 87%; for stage II and more advanced cancers, it is 57% (Kaltenecker et al., 2023). Vaginal cancer can be effectively treated, and when found early, it is often curable.

Pathophysiology

The etiology of vaginal cancer has not been identified. Malignant diseases of the vagina are either primary vaginal cancers or metastatic forms from adjacent or distant organs. About 80% to 90% of vaginal cancers are metastatic, primarily from the cervix and endometrium (Kaltenecker et al., 2023). These cancers invade the vagina directly. Cancers from distant sites that metastasize to the vagina through the blood or lymphatic system are typically from the colon, kidneys, skin (melanoma), or breast.

SCCs that begin in the epithelial lining of the vagina account for about 90% of vaginal cancers (Kaltenecker et al., 2023). SCCs develop slowly over a period of years, commonly in the upper third of the vagina. They tend to spread early by directly invading the bladder and rectal walls. They also metastasize through blood and lymphatics. The remaining 5% to 10% are adenocarcinomas, which differ from SCC by an increase in pulmonary metastases and supraclavicular and pelvic node involvement (NCI, 2024b).

Therapeutic Management

Treatment of vaginal cancer depends on the type of cells involved and the stage of the disease. If the cancer is localized, radiation, wide local incision, laser surgery, or all may be used. If the cancer has spread, radical surgery such as a hysterectomy, or removal of the upper vagina with dissection of the pelvic nodes in addition to radiation therapy, might be needed.

Nursing Assessment

Begin the history and physical examination by reviewing for risk factors. Although direct risk factors for the initial development of vaginal cancer have not been identified, associated risk factors include advancing age; HPV infection; exposure to diethylstilbestrol (DES) in utero; and history of hysterectomy due to benign, premalignant, or malignant disease (NCI, 2024b).

Question the patient about any symptoms. Most people with vaginal cancer are without symptoms. Those with symptoms have painless vaginal bleeding (often after sexual intercourse), abnormal vaginal bleeding outside of their menstrual cycle, dyspareunia, dysuria, constipation, a mass in the vaginal wall that can be palpated, and pelvic pain (NCI, 2024b). During the physical examination, observe for any obvious vaginal discharge or genital warts or changes in the appearance of the vaginal mucosa. Anticipate colposcopy with a biopsy of suspicious lesions to confirm the diagnosis.

Nursing Management

Nursing management for this cancer is similar to that for other reproductive tract cancers, with an emphasis on sexuality counseling and referral to local support groups. Patients undergoing radical surgery need intensive counseling about the nature of the surgery, risks, potential complications, changes in physical appearance and physiologic function, and sexuality alterations. Nurses should focus their care on patient education, patient pain and symptom management, communication with the patient and their family, and coordination of care across all settings.

VULVAR CANCER

Vulvar cancer is a rare but aggressive gynecologic malignancy. It is an abnormal neoplastic growth on the external female genitalia including the clitoris, vaginal lips, and opening to the vagina (Fig. 8.5). Vulvar cancer accounts for approximately 6% of all female genital malignancies. In the United States, females have a one-in-333 chance of developing vulvar cancer at some point in their lifetimes (ACS, 2024h). When detected early, it is highly curable. Typically, vulvar cancer is diagnosed at an early stage. It presents as a visible cancer that can be seen by the patient as an abnormal lesion or growth in their genital region (Berek & Karam, 2024).

Vulvar cancer is found most commonly in postmenopausal people in their mid-60s to mid-70s, with the average age of diagnosis being 68 years of age (Berek & Karam, 2024). The overall 5-year survival rate if localized is 87.5%, but it drops to 52.5% when the lymph nodes have been invaded (Capria et al., 2023).

Pathophysiology

Vulvar cancer can be classified into two groups according to predisposing factors. The first type is associated with HPV infection and occurs mostly in younger people. The second group is not HPV associated and occurs in older people without cancerous disorders. Seventy-five percent or more of vulvar tumors are SCCs (Berek & Karam, 2024). This type of cancer forms slowly over several years and is usually preceded by precancerous changes. These precancerous changes are termed vulvar intraepithelial neoplasia (VIN). The two major types of

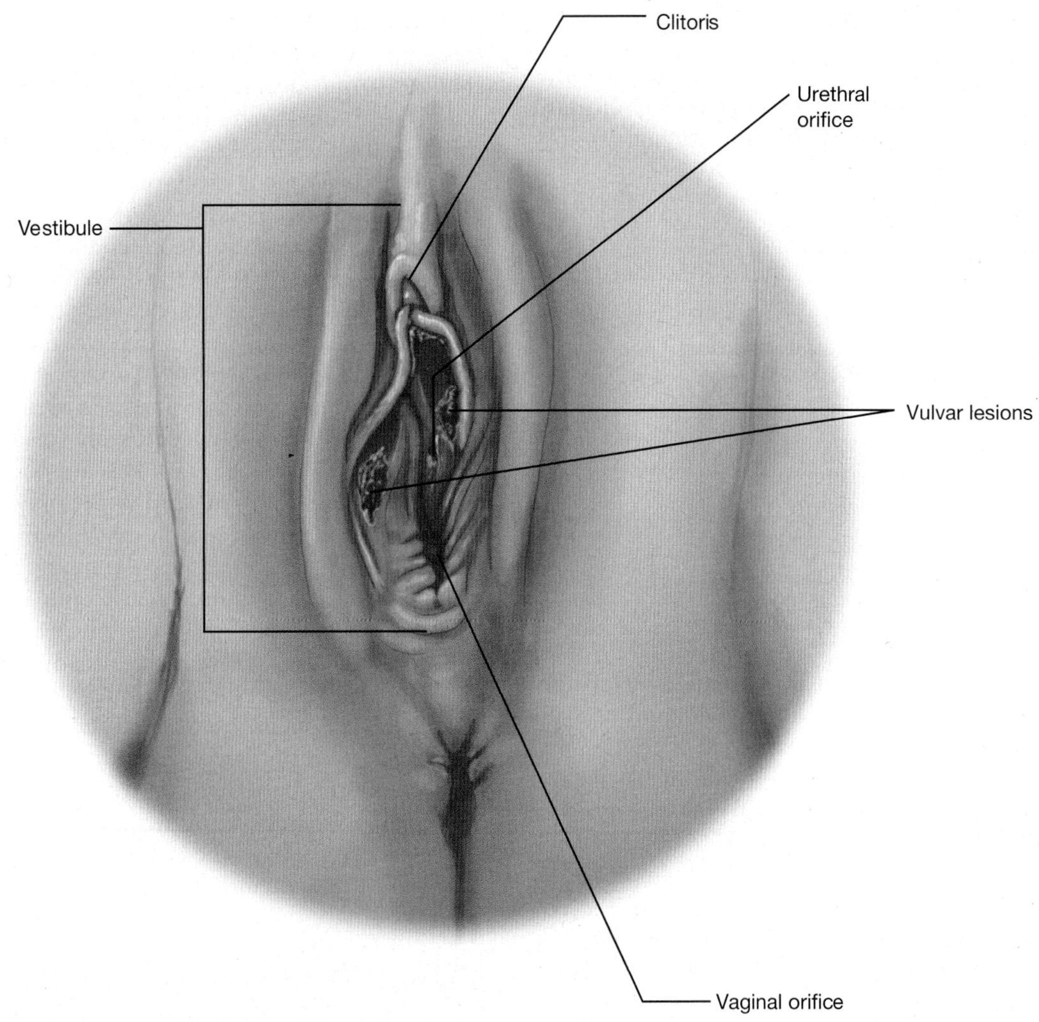

FIGURE 8.5 Vulvar cancer. (Redrawn with permission from Stewart JG. [2017]. *Anatomical Chart Company Atlas of Pathophysiology*, 4th ed. Wolters Kluwer.)

VIN are classic (undifferentiated) and simplex (differentiated). Classic VIN, the more common one, is associated with HPV infection (genital warts due to types 16, 18, and 33) and is typically found in younger patients (Berek & Karam, 2024). In contrast to classic VIN, simplex VIN usually occurs in postmenopausal people and is associated not with HPV but instead with vulvar dystrophies such as lichen sclerosus (Berek & Karam, 2024).

Screening and Diagnosis

Annual vulvar examination is the most effective way to prevent vulvar cancer. Careful inspection of the vulva during routine annual gynecologic examinations remains the most productive diagnostic technique. Liberal use of biopsies of any suspicious vulvar lesion is usually necessary to make the diagnosis and to guide treatment. However, many people do not seek health care evaluation for months or years after noticing an abnormal lump or lesion. Leading presenting complaints of patients with vulvar cancer include vulvar pruritus, vulvar bleeding or pain, and painful urination (Berek & Karam, 2024). The diagnosis of vulvar cancer is made by a biopsy of the suspicious lesion, which is usually found on the labia majora.

TAKE NOTE!

Vulvar pruritus or a lump is present in the majority of patients with vulvar cancer. Lumps should be biopsied even if the patient is without symptoms.

Therapeutic Management

Treatment varies depending on the extent of the disease. Surgery is the standard therapy with adjuvant radiation therapy or chemotherapy depending on the cancer stage. Larger lesions may need more extensive surgery and skin grafting. The traditional treatment of radical vulvectomy has been mostly replaced with more limited surgery with a more local excision to minimize morbidity (NCI, 2024c).

Nursing Assessment

Typically, no single specific clinical symptom heralds this disease, so diagnosis is often delayed significantly. Therefore, it is important to review the patient's history for risk factors such as:

- Exposure to HPV type 16
- Age over 50 years
- HIV infection
- VIN
- Lichen sclerosus (a patchy skin disorder)
- Multiple sex partners
- Smoking
- Metabolic syndrome
- Family history of breast cancer or cervical cancer (especially a first-degree relative)
- Immune suppression
- Hypertension
- Diabetes mellitus
- Obesity (Bucchi et al., 2022)

In most cases, the patient reports persistent vulvar itching, burning, and edema that do not improve with the use of creams or ointments. A history of condyloma, gonorrhea, and herpes simplex are some of the factors for greater risk for VIN. Diagnosis of vulvar carcinoma is often delayed. Patients neglect to seek treatment for an average of 6 months from the onset of symptoms. In addition, a delay in diagnosis often occurs after the patient presents to their primary provider. In many cases, a biopsy of the lesion is not performed until the problem fails to respond to numerous topical therapies. During the physical examination, observe for any masses or thickening of the vulvar area. A vulvar lump or mass is most often noted. The vulvar lesion is usually raised and may be fleshy, ulcerated, leukoplakic (looking like white patches), or warty. The cancer can appear anywhere on the vulva, often on the labia majora (Berek & Karam, 2024). Less commonly, the patient may present with vulvar bleeding, discharge, dysuria, and pain.

Nursing Management

Patients with vulvar cancer must clearly understand the disease, treatment options, and prognosis. To accomplish this, provide information and establish effective communication with the patient and their family. Act as an educator and advocate.

Teach the patient about healthy lifestyle behaviors, such as smoking cessation, and measures to reduce risk factors. For example, instruct the patient how to examine their genital area, urging them to do so monthly between menstrual periods. Tell the patient to look for any changes in appearance (e.g., whitened or reddened patches of skin); changes in feel (e.g., areas of the vulva becoming itchy or painful); or the development of lumps, moles (e.g., changes in size, shape, or color), freckles, cuts, or sores on the vulva. Instruct the patient to report these changes to the health care provider immediately (ACS, 2020d). Also encourage the patient to get regular pelvic checkups by their health care provider (ACS, 2020d).

Teach the patient about preventive measures to prevent HPV infection. Educate them about the use of barrier methods of birth control (e.g., condoms) to reduce the risk of contracting HIV, herpes simplex virus, and HPV. Other prevention measures include delaying first sexual intercourse, avoiding sexual intercourse with multiple partners, and getting the HPV vaccine available for adolescent males and for females between 9 and 26 years old.

For the patient diagnosed with vulvar cancer, provide information and support. Discuss potential changes in sexuality if radical surgery is performed. Encourage them to communicate openly with their partner. Refer the patient to appropriate community resources and support groups. All nurses may come in contact with people in their clinical practices who have the potential to become patients with cancer, already have suspicious signs or symptoms of cancer, are already undergoing cancer treatment, or are patients with terminal cancer. The nurse should be involved with all aspects of cancer, from diagnosis through palliative care. Each nurse has an obligation to keep informed of current developments in the cancer field to function effectively and be able to educate the patient and their family.

KEY CONCEPTS

- Females have a one-in-three lifetime risk of developing cancer and a one-in-six risk of dying from cancer (ACS, 2024a).
- The nurse plays a key role in offering emotional support, determining appropriate sources of support, and helping the patient use effective coping strategies when facing a diagnosis of cancer of the reproductive tract.
- Ovarian cancer is the second most common gynecologic cancer among females and is the deadliest because it is often diagnosed during later stages (CDC, 2024b).
- Ovarian cancer has been described as the “overlooked disease” or “silent killer” because patients and health care practitioners often ignore or rationalize early symptoms. It is typically diagnosed in advanced stages.
- Unopposed endogenous and exogenous estrogens, obesity (BMI greater than 30 kg/m^2), menopause after the age of 55, and diabetes are etiologic risk factors associated with the development of endometrial cancer.
- The ACS recommends that patients be informed about the risks and symptoms of endometrial cancer

at the onset of menopause and strongly encouraged to report any unexpected bleeding or spotting to their health care providers.

- Malignant diseases of the vagina are either primary vaginal cancers or metastatic forms from adjacent or distant organs. Vaginal cancer tumors can be effectively treated and when found early, are often curable.
- Cervical cancer incidence and mortality rates have decreased noticeably in the past several decades, with most of the reduction attributed to the Pap and HPV screening tests, which detect cervical cancer and precancerous lesions.
- The nurse's role involves primary prevention of cervical cancer through education of patients regarding risk factors and preventive vaccines to avoid cervical cancer.
- The majority of diagnosed vaginal cancers are metastatic, primarily from the cervix and endometrium. These cancers invade the vagina directly.
- Diagnosis of vulvar cancer is often delayed significantly because there is no single specific clinical symptom that heralds it. The most common presentation is persistent vulvar itching that does not improve with the application of creams or ointments.

REFERENCES AND RECOMMENDED READINGS

American Cancer Society. (2020a). *Can ovarian cancer be found early?* https://www.cancer.org/cancer/types/ovarian-cancer/detection-diagnosis-staging/detection.html

American Cancer Society. (2020b). *Can endometrial cancer be found early?* https://www.cancer.org/cancer/endometrial-cancer/detection-diagnosis-staging/detection.html

American Cancer Society. (2020c). *Surgery for cervical cancer.* https://www.cancer.org/cancer/types/cervical-cancer/treating/surgery.html

American Cancer Society. (2020d). *Can vulvar cancer be prevented?* https://www.cancer.org/cancer/types/vulvar-cancer/causes-risks-prevention/prevention.html

American Cancer Society. (2023a). *Cancer facts for women.* https://www.cancer.org/healthy/cancer-facts/cancer-facts-for-women.html

American Cancer Society. (2023b). *Cancer facts & figures 2023.* https://www.cancer.org/content/dam/cancer-org/research/cancer-facts-and-statistics/annual-cancer-facts-and-figures/2023/2023-cancer-facts-and-figures.pdf

American Cancer Society. (2024a). *Lifetime risk of developing or dying from cancer.* https://www.cancer.org/cancer/risk-prevention/understanding-cancer-risk/lifetime-probability-of-developing-or-dying-from-cancer.html

American Cancer Society. (2024b). *Key statistics for ovarian cancer.* https://www.cancer.org/cancer/types/ovarian-cancer/about/key-statistics.html

American Cancer Society. (2024c). *Key statistics for endometrial cancer.* https://www.cancer.org/cancer/endometrial-cancer/about/key-statistics.html

American Cancer Society. (2024d). *Key statistics for cervical cancer.* https://www.cancer.org/cancer/cervical-cancer/about/key-statistics.html

American Cancer Society. (2024e). *Survival rates for cervical cancer.* https://www.cancer.org/cancer/types/cervical-cancer/detection-diagnosis-staging/survival.html

American Cancer Society. (2024f). *What is cervical cancer?* https://www.cancer.org/cancer/types/cervical-cancer/about/what-is-cervical-cancer.html

American Cancer Society. (2024g). *Treatment options for cervical cancer, by stage.* https://www.cancer.org/cancer/cervical-cancer/treating/by-stage.html

American Cancer Society. (2024h). *Key statistics for vulvar cancer.* https://www.cancer.org/cancer/vulvar-cancer/about/key-statistics.html

American College of Obstetricians and Gynecologists. (2021). *Cervical cancer screening.* https://www.acog.org/-/media/project/acog/acogorg/womens-health/files/infographics/cervical-cancer-screening.pdf

Arora, T., Mullangi, S., & Lekkala, M. R. (2023). Ovarian cancer. In *StatPearls.* StatPearls Publishing. https://www.ncbi.nlm.nih.gov/books/NBK567760/

Berek, J. S., & Karam, A. (2024). Vulvar cancer: Epidemiology, diagnosis, histopathology, and treatment. *UpToDate.* Retrieved May 6, 2024, from https://www.uptodate.com/contents/vulvar-cancer-epidemiology-diagnosis-histopathology-and-treatment

Boardman, C. H. (2022). Cervical cancer. *eMedicine.* https://emedicine.medscape.com/article/253513-overview#a3

Bucchi, L., Pizzato, M., Rosso, S., & Ferretti, S. (2022). New insights into the epidemiology of vulvar cancer: Systematic literature review for an update of incidence and risk factors. *Cancers, 14*(2), 389. https://doi.org/10.3390/cancers14020389

Campos, S. M., & Cohn, D. E. (2024a). Initial treatment of metastatic endometrial cancer. *UpToDate.* Retrieved May 4, 2024, from https://www.uptodate.com/contents/initial-treatment-of-metastatic-endometrial-cancer

Campos, S. M., & Cohn, D. E. (2024b). Management of locoregional recurrence of endometrial cancer. *UpToDate.* Retrieved May 4, 2024, from https://www.uptodate.com/contents/management-of-locoregional-recurrence-of-endometrial-cancer

Capria, A., Tahir, N., & Fatehi, M. (2023). Vulvar cancer. In *StatPearls.* StatPearls Publishing. https://www.ncbi.nlm.nih.gov/books/NBK567798/

Carlson, K. J. (2024). Screening for ovarian cancer. *UpToDate.* Retrieved May 3, 2024, from https://www.uptodate.com/contents/screening-for-ovarian-cancer

Centers for Disease Control and Prevention (CDC)/National Center for Health Statistics. (2024a). Women's Health, https://www.cdc.gov/nchs/fastats/womens-health.htm

Centers for Disease Control and Prevention. (2024b). *Ovarian cancer statistics.* https://www.cdc.gov/ovarian-cancer/statistics/

Centers for Disease Control and Prevention. (2024c). *About Genital HPV infection—https://www.cdc.gov/sti/about/about-genital-hpv-infection.html*

Centers for Disease Control and Prevention. (2024d). *HPV vaccination. https://www.cdc.gov/hpv/vaccines/*

Centers for Disease Control and Prevention. (2023a). *Preventing cancer.* https://www.cdc.gov/cancer/prevention/

Centers for Disease Control and Prevention. (2023b). *Ovarian cancer risk factors.* https://www.cdc.gov/ovarian-cancer/risk-factors/

Centers for Disease Control and Prevention. (2023c). *Reducing risk for ovarian cancer.* https://www.cdc.gov/ovarian-cancer/prevention/

Centers for Disease Control and Prevention. (2023d). *Healthy choices.* https://www.cdc.gov/cancer/prevention/healthy-choices.html

Chen, L. M., & Berek, J. S. (2024a). Overview of epithelial carcinoma of the ovary, fallopian tube, and peritoneum. *UpToDate.* Retrieved May 3, 2024, from https://www.uptodate.com/contents/overview-of-epithelial-carcinoma-of-the-ovary-fallopian-tube-and-peritoneum

Chen, L. M., & Berek, J. S. (2024b). Endometrial carcinoma: Clinical features, diagnosis, prognosis, and screening. *UpToDate.* Retrieved May 3, 2024, from https://www.uptodate.com/contents/endometrial-carcinoma-clinical-features-diagnosis-prognosis-and-screening

Chen, L. M., & Berek, J. S. (2024c). Endometrial carcinoma: Epidemiology, risk factors, and prevention. *UpToDate.* Retrieved May 3, 2024, from https://www.uptodate.com/contents/endometrial-carcinoma-epidemiology-risk-factors-and-prevention

Cohn, D. E. (2024). Endometrial carcinoma: Staging and surgical treatment. *UpToDate.* Retrieved May 3, 2024, from https://www.uptodate.com/contents/endometrial-carcinoma-staging-and-surgical-treatment

Colditz, G. A. (2022). Overview of cancer prevention. *UpToDate.* Retrieved May 2, 2024, from https://www.uptodate.com/contents/overview-of-cancer-prevention

Collins, S. (2024). *2024—First year the US expects more than 2M new cases of cancer.* https://www.cancer.org/research/acs-research-news/facts-and-figures-2024.html

Constable, C., Ferguson, K., Nicholson, J., & Quinn, G. P. (2022). Clinician communication strategies associated with increased uptake of the human papillomavirus (HPV) vaccine: A systematic review. *CA: A Cancer Journal for Clinicians, 72*(6), 561–569. https://doi.org/10.3322/caac.21753

Creasman, W. T. (2022). Endometrial carcinoma. *eMedicine.* https://emedicine.medscape.com/article/254083-overview#a3

Crosbie, E. J., Kitson, S. J., McAlpine, J. N., Mukhopadhyay, A., Powell, M. E., & Singh, N. (2022). Endometrial cancer. *The Lancet, 399*(10333), 1412–1428. https://doi.org/10.1016/S0140-6736(22)00323-3

Crum, C. P., Huh, W. K., & Einstein, M. H. (2022). Cervical cancer screening: The cytology and human papillomavirus report. *UpToDate.* Retrieved May 5, 2024, from https://www.uptodate.com/contents/cervical-cancer-screening-the-cytology-and-human-papillomavirus-report

Duska, L. R. (2023). Approach to survivors of epithelial ovarian, fallopian tube, or peritoneal carcinoma. *UpToDate.* Retrieved May 3, 2024, from https://www.uptodate.com/contents/approach-to-survivors-of-epithelial-ovarian-fallopian-tube-or-peritoneal-carcinoma

Feldman, S., & Crum, C. P. (2023). Cervical cancer screening tests: Techniques for cervical cytology and human papillomavirus testing. *UpToDate.* Retrieved May 5, 2024, from https://www.uptodate.com/contents/cervical-cancer-screening-tests-techniques-for-cervical-cytology-and-human-papillomavirus-testing

Fowler, J. R., Maani, E. V., Dunton, C. J., Gasalberti, D. P., & Jack, B. W. (2023). Cervical cancer. *In StatPearls.* StatPearls Publishing. https://www.ncbi.nlm.nih.gov/books/NBK431093/

Frumovitz, M. (2024). Invasive cervical cancer: Epidemiology, risk factors, clinical manifestations, and diagnosis. *UpToDate.* Retrieved May 4, 2024, from https://www.uptodate.com/contents/invasive-cervical-cancer-epidemiology-risk-factors-clinical-manifestations-and-diagnosis

Gandhi, T., Zubair, M., & Bhatt, H. (2023). Cancer antigen 125. In *StatPearls.* StatPearls Publishing. https://www.ncbi.nlm.nih.gov/books/NBK562245/

Giaquinto, A. N., Miller, K. D., Tossas, K. Y., Winn, R. A., Jemal, A., & Siegel, R. L. (2022). Cancer statistics for African American/Black people 2022. *CA: A Cancer Journal for Clinicians, 72*(3), 202–229. https://doi.org/10.3322/caac.21718

Goff, B. (2024). Early detection of epithelial ovarian cancer: Role of symptom recognition. *UpToDate.* Retrieved May 5, 2024, from https://www.uptodate.com/contents/early-detection-of-epithelial-ovarian-cancer-role-of-symptom-recognition

Green, A. E. (2022). Ovarian cancer. *eMedicine.* https://emedicine.medscape.com/article/255771-overview#a3

Guimarães, Y. M., Godoy, L. R., Longatto-Filho, A., & Reis, R. D. (2022). Management of early-stage cervical cancer: A literature review. *Cancers, 14*(3), 575. https://doi.org/10.3390/cancers14030575

Huvila, J., & McAlpine, J. N. (2023). Endometrial cancer: Pathology and classification. *UpToDate.* Retrieved May 5, 2024, from https://www.uptodate.com/contents/endometrial-cancer-pathology-and-classification

Kaltenecker, B., Dunton, C. J., & Tikaria, R. (2023). Vaginal cancer. In *StatPearls.* StatPearls Publishing. https://www.ncbi.nlm.nih.gov/books/NBK559126/

Kamal, M. (2022). Pap smear collection and preparation: Key points. *CytoJournal, 19,* 24. https://dx.doi.org/10.25259/CMAS_03_05_2021

Mahdy, H., Casey, M. J., & Crotzer, D. (2022). Endometrial cancer. In *StatPearls.* StatPearls Publishing. https://www.ncbi.nlm.nih.gov/books/NBK525981/

Matalliotakis, M., Matalliotaki, C., Krithinakis, K., Laliotis, A., Kapetanios, G., Tsakiridis, I., & Kalogiannidis, I. (2023). Anatomic distribution of benign ovarian tumors in perimenopausal and postmenopausal women. *Cureus, 15*(1), e34059. https://doi.org/10.7759/cureus.34059

Mori, M., Lin, C.-P., Cheng, S.-Y., Suh, S.-Y., Takenouchi, S., Ng, R., Chan, H., Kim, S. H., Chen, P.-J., Yuen, K.-K., Fujimori, M., Yamaguchi, T., Hamano, J., Kizawa, Y., Morita, T., & Martina, D. (2023). Communication in cancer care in Asia: A narrative review. *JCO Global Oncology, 9.* https://doi.org/10.1200/go.22.00266

National Cancer Institute. (2020). *Cancer statistics.* https://www.cancer.gov/about-cancer/understanding/statistics

National Cancer Institute. (2022). *Cancer prevention overview (PDQ®)—Health professional version.* https://www.cancer.gov/about-cancer/causes-prevention/hp-prevention-overview-pdq

National Cancer Institute. (2023a). *HPV and Pap test results: Next steps after an abnormal cervical cancer screening test.* https://www.cancer.gov/types/cervical/screening/abnormal-hpv-pap-test-results

National Cancer Institute. (2023b). *HPV and cancer.* https://www.cancer.gov/about-cancer/causes-prevention/risk/infectious-agents/hpv-and-cancer#

National Cancer Institute. (2024a). *Cervical cancer screening (PDQ®)—Health professional version.* https://www.cancer.gov/types/cervical/hp/cervical-screening-pdq#_54

National Cancer Institute. (2024b). *Vaginal cancer treatment (PDQ®)—Health professional version.* https://www.cancer.gov/types/vaginal/hp/vaginal-treatment-pdq#_116

National Cancer Institute. (2024c). *Vulvar cancer treatment (PDQ®)—Health professional version.* https://www.cancer.gov/types/vulvar/hp/vulvar-treatment-pdq#_67

National Ovarian Cancer Coalition. (2023). *Ovarian cancer risk factors: What are the risk factors for ovarian cancer?* https://ovarian.org/about-ovarian-cancer/whos-at-risk/

Petrucelli, N., Daily, M. B., & Pal, T. (2023). BRCA1- and BRCA2-associated hereditary breast and ovarian cancer. In: *GeneReviews*. University of Washington. https://www.ncbi.nlm.nih.gov/books/NBK1247/pdf/Bookshelf_NBK1247.pdf

Saccardi, C., Spagnol, G., Bonaldo, G., Marchetti, M., Tozzi, R., & Noventa, M. (2022). New light on endometrial thickness as a risk factor of cancer: What do clinicians need to know? *Cancer Management and Research, 14*, 1331–1340. https://doi.org/10.2147/CMAR.S294074

Salani, R., & Cosgrove, C. M. (2024). Epithelial carcinoma of the ovary, fallopian tube, and peritoneum: Surgical staging. *UpToDate*. Retrieved May 3, 2024, from https://www.uptodate.com/contents/epithelial-carcinoma-of-the-ovary-fallopian-tube-and-peritoneum-surgical-staging

Thomas, N. (2022). Advanced stage cervical cancer is rising in White and Black women in the US. *CNN Health*. https://www.cnn.com/2022/08/22/health/advanced-cervical-cancer-us-rise/index.html

U.S. Department of Health and Human Services. (n.d.). *Healthy People 2030*. https://health.gov/healthypeople

U.S. Preventive Services Task Force. (2018). *Final recommendation statement: Screening for ovarian cancer*. https://www.uspreventiveservicestaskforce.org/uspstf/announcements/final-recommendation-statement-screening-ovarian-cancer-0

Wang, T., Zhang, H., Liu, Y., & Zhao, C. (2023). Updates in cervical cancer screening guidelines, the Bethesda System for reporting cervical cytology, and clinical management recommendations. *Journal of Clinical and Translational Pathology, 3*(2), 75–83. https://www.xiahepublishing.com/2771-165X/JCTP-2023-00004

World Health Organization. (2023). *Cancer*. https://www.who.int/health-topics/cancer#tab=tab_1

World Health Organization. (2024). *Cervical cancer: Key facts*. https://www.who.int/news-room/fact-sheets/detail/cervical-cancer

Zhu, X., Jacobson, R. M., MacLaughlin, K. L., Sauver, J. St., Griffin, J. M., & Finney Rutten, L. J. (2023). Parent-reported barriers and parental beliefs associated with intentions to obtain HPV vaccination for children in a primary care patient population in Minnesota, USA. *Journal of Community Health, 48*(4), 678–686. https://doi.org/10.1007/s10900-023-01205-9

Ziegler, E., Hill, J., Lieske, B., Klein, J., von dem Knesebeck, O., & Kofahl, C. (2022). Empowerment in cancer patients: Does peer support make a difference? A systematic review. *Psycho-Oncology, 31*(5), 683–704. https://doi.org/10.1002/pon.5869

DEVELOPING CLINICAL JUDGMENT

PRACTICING FOR NCLEX

1. The nurse is working with a local women's group to increase awareness regarding gynecologic cancers. The nurse states ovarian cancer often is not diagnosed early because

a. the disease progresses slowly.
b. the early stages produce vague symptoms.
c. the disease is usually diagnosed only at autopsy.
d. patients do not follow up on acute pelvic pain.

2. A 60-year-old female patient is seen in the clinic by the nurse. The patient reports that she has started spotting again. Which action would the nurse take?

a. Instruct the patient to keep a menstrual diary for the next few months.
b. Tell her not to worry since this is a common but not serious event.
c. Have her start warm-water douches to promote healing.
d. Anticipate that the doctor will assess her endometrium thickness.

3. The nurse is caring for a patient recently diagnosed with reproductive cancer. Which of the following would the nurse identify as the priority psychosocial need for this patient?

a. Research findings
b. Hand-holding
c. Cheerfulness
d. Offering of hope

4. The nurse is teaching a group of patients about screening and early detection of cervical cancer. The nurse would include which procedure as the most effective?

a. Fecal occult blood test
b. CA-125 blood test
c. Pap smear and HPV test
d. Sigmoidoscopy

5. The nursing instructor is teaching a group of students about reproductive tract cancers. The nursing instructor determines that the teaching was successful when the students identify which as the deadliest type of female reproductive cancer?

a. Vulvar
b. Ovarian
c. Endometrial
d. Cervical

6. The nurse is attempting to reassure a female patient with obesity (BMI greater than 30 kg/m^2) about the discovery of an ovarian cyst after a pelvic exam. Which statement is accurate?

a. Frequently seen in polycystic kidney disease
b. Always painful and need to be removed surgically
c. A precursor to ovarian carcinoma
d. May be a syndrome that includes hypertension and diabetes

7. The nurse is educating a group of patients regarding cancers of the reproductive tract. Which response by the group would demonstrate learning has occurred?

a. Vitamin B_{12} deficiency is a risk factor for vulvar cancer.
b. Epstein–Barr virus is a risk factor for vulvar cancer.
c. Human papillomavirus is a risk factor for vulvar cancer.
d. Adenovirus is a risk factor for vulvar cancer.

CRITICAL THINKING EXERCISES

1. A 27-year-old sexually active White woman visits the Health Department family planning clinic and requests information about the various available methods of contraception. In taking her history, the nurse learns that she started having sex at age 15 and has had multiple sex partners since then. She smokes two packs of cigarettes daily. Because she has been unemployed for a few months, her health insurance policy has lapsed. She has never previously obtained any gynecologic care.

a. Based on her history, which risk factors for cervical cancer are present?
b. What recommendations would you make for her and why?
c. What are this patient's educational needs concerning health maintenance?

2. A 65-year-old nulliparous woman presents to the gynecologic oncology clinic after her health care provider palpated an adnexal mass on her right ovary. In taking her history, the nurse learns that she had experienced mild abdominal bloating and weight loss for the past several months but felt fine otherwise. She was diagnosed with breast cancer 15 years ago and was treated with a lumpectomy and radiation.

3. A transvaginal ultrasound reveals a complex mass in the right adnexa. She undergoes a total abdominal hysterectomy, bilateral salpingo-oophorectomy, and lymph node biopsy. Pathology confirms a diagnosis of stage III ovarian cancer with abdominal metastasis and positive lymph nodes.

a. Is this patient's profile typical for a person with this diagnosis?
b. What in her history might have increased her risk for ovarian cancer?
c. What can the nurse do to increase awareness of this cancer for all female patients?

STUDY ACTIVITIES

1. During your surgical clinical rotation, interview a female patient undergoing surgery for cancer of the reproductive organs. Ask the patient to recall the symptoms that brought them to the health care provider. Ask what thoughts, feelings, and emotions went through the patient's mind before and after the diagnosis. Finally, ask the patient how this experience will change their life in the future.
2. Visit an oncology and radiology treatment center to find out about the various treatment modalities available for reproductive cancers. Contrast the various treatment methods and report your findings to your class.
3. Visit a website related to reproductive tract cancers and explore a topic of interest concerning those cancers. How correct and current is the content? What is its level? Share your assessment with your classmates.
4. Taking oral contraceptives provides protection against ________________ cancer.
5. Two genes, *BRCA1* and *BRCA2*, are linked with hereditary ______________ and ______________ cancers.

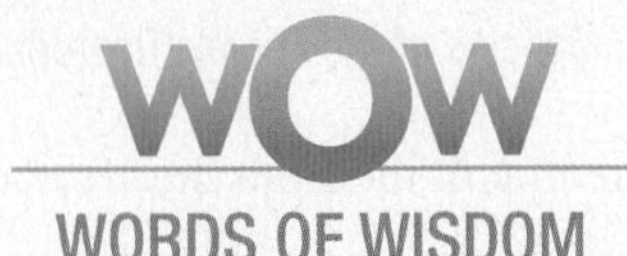

WORDS OF WISDOM

After being traumatized, a person is not defined by their past but by the strength they used to overcome it.

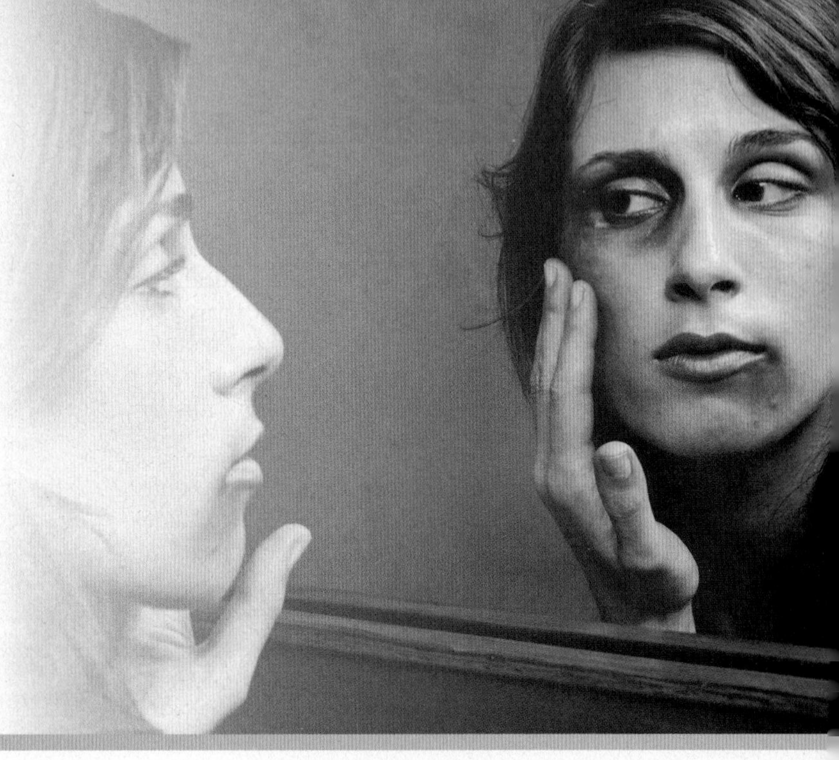

9

Violence and Abuse

LEARNING OBJECTIVES

Upon completion of the chapter, you will be able to:

1. Examine the incidence of violence against women.
2. Outline the role of the nurse who cares for women who have been abused.
3. Characterize the cycle of violence and appropriate interventions.
4. Evaluate the various myths and facts about violence.
5. Select the resources available to women experiencing abuse.
6. Analyze the dynamics of rape and sexual abuse.

KEY TERMS

cycle of violence
female genital mutilation/cutting (FGM/C)
human trafficking
incest
intimate partner violence (IPV)
posttraumatic stress disorder (PTSD)
rape
sexual abuse
statutory rape

Dorothy came to the prenatal clinic with a complaint of recurring headaches. She had been in twice this week already but insisted she be seen today and started to cry. When the nurse called her into the examination room, Dorothy's cell phone rang. She hurried to answer it and told the person on the other end that she was at the store. When the nurse asked if she was afraid at home, Dorothy answered "at times." What cues did the nurse pick up on to ask that question? How frequent is this problem among women?

INTRODUCTION

Violence against women is an international epidemic of global concern that is compounded by other crises such as wars, poor family relations, climate-related natural disasters, food insecurity, and human rights violations. Violence against women is devastating to families and to the local communities and nations in which they live. Globally, the World Health Organization (WHO) estimates that one in three women has been subjected to physical and/or sexual intimate partner violence (IPV) or nonpartner sexual violence in their lifetime (WHO, 2024a). Forms of violence against women include assault, rape, sexual enslavement, torture, verbal abuse, mutilation, and murder. Violence against women is a pervasive human rights issue. The United Nations defines violence against women as "any act of gender-based violence that results in or is likely to result in physical, sexual, or mental harm or suffering to women, including threats of such acts, coercion, or arbitrary deprivation of liberty whether occurring in public or private life" (WHO, 2024a).

Gender-based violence is a major global public health and human rights problem that often goes unrecognized and unreported. It is a common source of physical, psychological, and emotional morbidity. It occurs in all countries, irrespective of social, economic, religious, or cultural status. No segment of society is immune to this problem, which is related to the unequal power relations between men and women in many societies. The causes are multidimensional and are social, economic, cultural, political, and religious. Each form of abuse begets interrelated kinds of violence, and the "cycle of abuse" is often continued from exposed children into their adult relationships, and finally to the care of the older adults.

Pregnancy is a time of unique vulnerability to IPV because of changes in a woman's physical, social, emotional, and economic needs during this period. Although the true prevalence of violence during pregnancy is unclear, research suggests it is substantial and often continues into the postpartum period. Recent research found that homicide was a leading cause of death during pregnancy and the postpartum period in the United States, exceeding all other leading causes of maternal mortality (Wallace et al., 2021). Pregnancy was associated with a very high risk for Black women and for women younger than 24 years old across racial and ethnic subgroups (Wallace et al., 2021). The evidence suggests that the people closest to pregnant women are committing violence against women in their own homes; in most cases, a firearm is involved (Wallace et al., 2021). All pregnant women should be screened for violence at each visit and be provided with interventions and referrals to services if needed (Wallace et al., 2021).

Additionally, female-perpetrated violence against male partners receives little attention. Although women are victims of violence more frequently than men are, the prevalence of violence against men nonetheless represents a significant public health concern. In the United States, over 10 million adults experience violence against them annually (Huecker et al., 2023). One out of every nine men have experienced rape, physical violence, psychological aggression, and/or stalking by an intimate partner in their lifetimes (Huecker et al., 2023).

Although women can be violent toward their partners, including men, the overwhelming majority of partner violence consists of men committing violence against women. Nearly one in four women and one in 26 men in the United States have been raped (CDC, 2024b). Over 50% of assailants are acquaintances, family members, or romantic partners of the victims (Weil, 2023). The Federal Bureau of Investigation (FBI) expanded their definition of rape in 2018; they define it as "penetration, no matter how slight, of the vagina or anus with any body part or object, or oral penetration by a sex organ of another person without the consent of the victim" (FBI, 2018).

Gathering data about the prevalence, incidence, and nature of gender-based violence is complex for a variety of reasons. Many survivors do not report their experience of violence or may do so years later. Many times, survivors do not report their experience to law enforcement, health care providers, or other entities that track data (The White House, 2023). The National Intimate Partner and Sexual Violence Survey (NISVS) report indicates that 41% of women in the United States will experience some form of physical violence during their lifetime (The White House, 2023). Nearly half of all women murdered in the United States are killed by a past or present intimate partner (AbiNader et al., 2023).

Nurses play a major role in assessing women who have suffered some type of violence. Nurses have a central ethic of caring and an agenda of early intervention and health promotion for their patients to improve their health status and well-being. Often, after a person is victimized, they will have physical ailments that will prompt them to visit a health care setting. A visit to a health care agency is an ideal time for people to be assessed for violence. Because nurses are often viewed as trustworthy and sensitive about personal subjects, people often feel comfortable confiding in them and discussing these issues with them. As a professional nurse, the act of screening women seen in every health care setting is often the first step for a victim to feel that a better future is possible. Nurses have a responsibility to recognize and respond to signs of domestic and sexual abuse in order to address health inequalities, safeguard women, and ultimately save lives.

TAKE NOTE!

Nurses will encounter violence and sexual abuse no matter what health care setting they work in. Nurses must be ready to ask the right questions and to act on the answers because such action could be lifesaving.

This chapter addresses several types of gender-based violence: IPV, sexual violence, female genital mutilation/cutting (FGM/C), and human trafficking. All of these types of violence against women have devastating and costly consequences for all of society.

INTIMATE PARTNER VIOLENCE

Intimate partner violence (IPV) is actual or threatened physical or sexual violence or psychological/emotional abuse. Abuse often begins as emotional and then progresses to physical. Research suggests that physical violence in intimate relationships is accompanied by sexual abuse the majority of the time (Weil, 2023). Intimate partners include people who are currently in dating, cohabitating, or marital relationships, or those who have been in such relationships in the past. Some of the common terms used to describe IPV are domestic abuse, spouse abuse, domestic violence, gender-based violence, and rape. IPV affects a distressingly high percentage of the population and has physical, psychological, social, and economic consequences.

Because a nurse may be the first health care provider to assess and identify the signs of IPV, a nurse can have a profound impact on a person's decision to seek help. Nurses need to recognize and understand the intense volatility and danger of the patient's situation and communicate that they believe the patient. Therefore, it is important for nurses to be able to identify abuse, recognize *red flags* (behaviors that serve as warning signs that a person may become abusive or violent), and aid the victim. IPV can leave significant psychological scars, and a well-trained nurse can have a positive impact on the victim's mental and emotional health.

Incidence

Many IPV episodes go unreported; therefore, epidemiologic data are only estimates (Weil, 2024). Overall, lifetime, and 1-year estimates for sexual violence, stalking, and IPV are alarmingly high for adult Americans, with IPV alone affecting millions of people each year (CDC, 2024a). It is estimated that each year 5.7 million women experience IPV (The White House, 2023). Data from crime reports find that one in five homicide victims is killed by their intimate partner (CDC, 2024a).

Women are at risk for violence at nearly every stage of their lives. No woman is ever completely safe from the risk of IPV.

IPV is pervasive and crosses all boundaries of sexual orientation, race, and class. Violence within intimate relationships may go unreported for fear of harassment or ridicule. The medical community's efforts to address IPV must include members of the lesbian, gay, bisexual, transgender, queer, intersex, and asexual (LGBTQIA+) population. Recent studies show that IPV in the LGBTQIA+ community occurs at a rate equal to or higher than that in the heterosexual community (Weil, 2024). The role of the nurse as an advocate for these patients is critical.

The Violence Against Women Act was last reauthorized in March 2022 by Congress for 5 years, being updated to include coverage of same-sex partners and survivors from the LGBTQIA+ population, with additional funding for community services (The White House, 2022).

Background

Violence is pervasive in American society. In the past, the U.S. legal and judicial systems considered intervention into family disputes wrong and a violation of the family's right to privacy. IPV was often tolerated and sometimes even considered socially acceptable. Laws have changed to protect survivors and punish abusers. Healthy People 2030 shows there are violence prevention objectives.

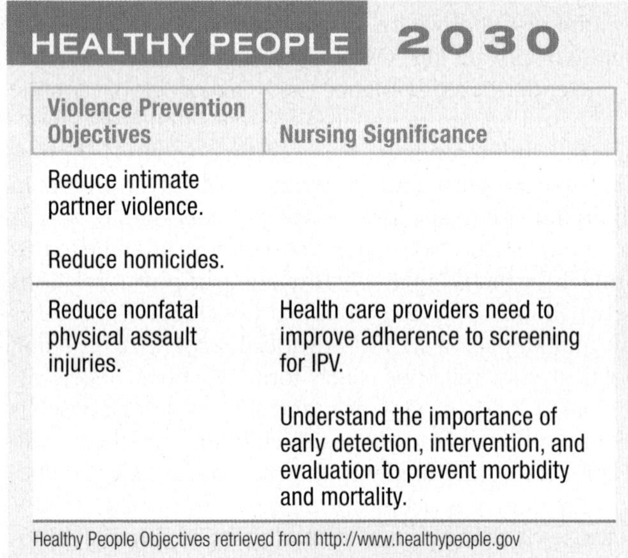

HEALTHY PEOPLE 2030

Violence Prevention Objectives	Nursing Significance
Reduce intimate partner violence. Reduce homicides.	
Reduce nonfatal physical assault injuries.	Health care providers need to improve adherence to screening for IPV. Understand the importance of early detection, intervention, and evaluation to prevent morbidity and mortality.

Healthy People Objectives retrieved from http://www.healthypeople.gov

Characteristics of Intimate Partner Violence

Although more research is needed in this area, studies have found certain risk factors that are associated with the occurrence of IPV. These risk factors can be divided into four different categories: individual factors, relationship factors, community factors, and societal factors. Specific risk factors within each category are listed in Table 9.1. Risk factors for perpetration include exposure to violence during childhood, unresolved posttraumatic stress disorder (PTSD), recent job loss/instability, and substance use disorder (Weil, 2024).

Generation-to-Generation Continuation of Violence

Violence is a learned behavior that, without intervention, can be self-perpetuating. It is a cyclical health problem.

TABLE 9.1 • Risk Factors for Committing Intimate Partner Violence (IPV)

Individual Factors (Victim)	Relationship Factors	Community Factors	Societal Factors
Young age (<24)	Marital dissatisfaction	High rates of crime	Social norms supportive of violence
Nontraditional gender expression	Reproductive coercion	High rates of violence	Exposure to war or political violence
Prior history of IPV	Adherence to traditional gender expectations	Delinquent peers	Traditional gender expectations
Depression or chronic mental illness	Dominance or control by one partner	Social norms supportive of violence	
Low academic achievement	Martial conflict	Low social support	
Witnessing or experiencing violence as a child	Poor family relationships	Poverty	
Low income and/or unemployment			
Refugee or asylum seeking			
Member of underrepresented group			

World Health Organization. (2022b). *Intimate partner violence*. https://apps.who.int/violence-info/intimate-partner-violence/; and Weil, A. (2024). Intimate partner violence: Epidemiology and health consequences. *UpToDate*. Retrieved May 7, 2024, from https://www.uptodate.com/contents/intimate-partner-violence-epidemiology-and-health-consequences

The long-term effects of violence on victims and children who witness it can be profound. Children who witness one parent abuse another are more likely to become abusers themselves because they see abuse as an integral part of a close relationship. Thus, an abusive relationship between parents can perpetuate future abusive relationships. The psychological consequences are huge, stemming from the paradox of the victim being abused by a member of the family with whom they expect to have a supportive, loving, and respectful relationship. Research has found that children who witness IPV are at risk for developing aggression, conduct disorders, impulsivity, anxiety, thoughts of violent events, disrupted sleep pattern, depression, low self-esteem, problems in school such as increased absenteeism, high-risk sexual behavior during adolescence, and substance use disorder later in life (Franchek-Roa, 2022).

Childhood maltreatment is a major health problem associated with a wide range of physical conditions, and it leads to high rates of psychiatric morbidity and social problems in adulthood. Consequences of violence extend far beyond the physical and mental suffering of victims and their families and have an impact on schools, neighborhoods, businesses, and the legal and health care systems. Women who were physically or sexually abused as children have an increased risk of victimization and poor sexual health practices such as having multiple sexual partners at the same time and having unprotected sex. They also have higher rates of mental health conditions like depression, anxiety, PTSD, and low self-esteem as adults (Willie et al., 2021).

In many cases when a parent is abused, the children are abused as well. Approximately one in seven children is abused annually in the United States; this is likely an underestimate (CDC, 2022a). The lifetime economic cost to society of childhood maltreatment is estimated to be $600 billion (CDC, 2022a). Young children who live with family violence represent a disempowered group because developmentally they have relatively limited verbal skills, emotional literacy, and high dependence on others for care.

The Cycle of Violence

In an abusive relationship, the **cycle of violence**, also referred to as the power and control wheel (Fig. 9.1), is composed of four distinct phases: the tension-building phase, the physically abusive incident, the reconciliation

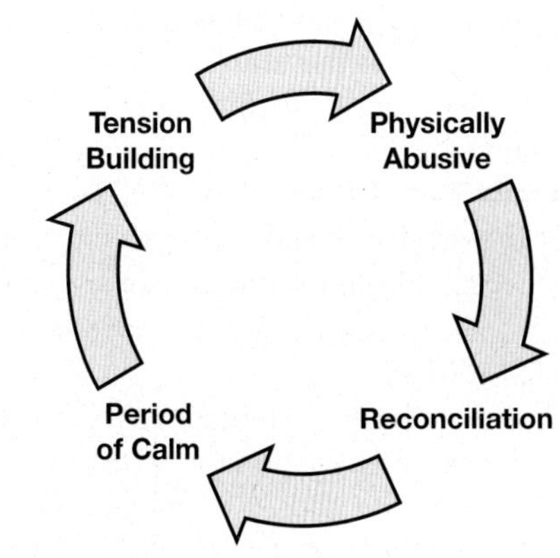

FIGURE 9.1 The cycle of violence.

(or honeymoon) phase, and the period of calm (Connections for Abused Women and Their Children [CAWC], 2023). The cyclical behavior begins with a time of tension-building arguments, progresses to violence, then settles into a making-up or reconciliation period, and then finally the calm stage. This cycle of violence increases in frequency and severity as it is repeated over and over again. The cycle can cover long or short periods of time. The calm phase gradually shortens and eventually disappears altogether. Abuse in relationships typically becomes accelerated and thus more dangerous over time. The abuser no longer feels the need to apologize and indulge in a reconciliation phase as the victim becomes increasingly disempowered in the relationship.

PHASE 1: TENSION BUILDING

During the first—and usually the longest—phase of the cycle, tension escalates between the partners. Excessive drinking, jealousy, or other factors might lead to name-calling, hostility, and friction. The victim might sense that the abuser is reacting to them more negatively, that they are on edge and react heatedly to any trivial frustration. A victim will often accept their abuser's building anger as legitimately directed toward them. The victim internalizes what they perceive as their responsibility to keep the situation from exploding. In their mind, if they do the job well, the abuser and the situation will remain calm. If the abuser's behavior escalates, the victim feels that the resulting violence is their own fault.

PHASE 2: PHYSICALLY ABUSIVE PHASE

The second phase of the cycle is the explosion of violence. The abuser may reach an emotional peak. They may physically assault or murder the victim. After a physically violent episode, many victims characterize themselves as lucky that the abuse was not worse, no matter how severe their injuries were. They often deny the seriousness of their injuries and may refuse to seek medical treatment.

PHASE 3: RECONCILIATION

The third phase of the cycle is a period of loving and contrite behavior on the part of the abuser. They express that they are sorry for the pain caused to the victim. They promise to make up for the abusive behavior, that they can control the violence, and that they will never hurt the victim again. The victim often wants to believe that the abuser really can change. Many victims feel responsible, at least in part, for the abuser's violent actions, and they may feel responsible for the abuser's well-being.

PHASE 4: CALM PHASE

During the fourth phase, justifications or explanations are discussed by both the victim and abuser to excuse or minimize the abuse. The abuser might put the blame on outside forces—work, stress, illness, having a bad day, or alcohol. The abuser may show remorse, promise it will not happen again, and may appear to be more understanding of the victim's needs. Refer to Box 9.1.

BOX 9.1 Cycle of Violence

- *Phase 1—Tension building:* Verbal or minor physical abuse occurs. Almost any subject, such as housekeeping or money, may trigger the buildup of tension. There is a breakdown of communication. The victim may attempt to calm the abuser. The victim may feel like they are "walking on eggshells" around the abuser.
- *Phase 2—Incident of violence:* Characterized by uncontrollable discharge of tension. Violence is rarely triggered by the victim's behavior; they are abused no matter how they respond. The start of the episode is unpredictable and beyond the victim's control.
- *Phase 3—Reconciliation:* First, the abuser expresses shame over the behavior. The abuser may try to minimize the abuse and blame it on the partner. The abuser may become loving, kind, and apologetic and express guilt. The abuser may work on making the victim feel responsible. This loving behavior strengthens the bond between partners and may convince the victim, once again, that leaving the relationship is not necessary.
- *Phase 4—Calm:* The abuser may continue to be attentive toward the victim, and abusive behaviors may be minimized. Both partners feel the relationship has returned to normal and they may feel close to each other. Even if the abuser claims they want to make things right, there is often an underlying tone of dismissal. The abuser may gaslight the victim to manipulate their behavior to gain control and power over them again.

Connections for Abused Women and their Children. (2023). *What is the cycle of abuse?* https://www.cawc.org/news/what-is-the-cycle-of-abuse/; PsychCentral. (2022). *The 4 stages of the cycle of abuse: From tension to calm and back.* https://psychcentral.com/health/cycle-of-abuse; and Ricee, S. (2022). *Cycle of abuse: An overview and its effects on victims.* Diversity for Social Impact. https://diversity.social/cycle-of-abuse/#0-what-is-the-cycle-of-abuse-and-what-it-means-for-the-victims

Types of Abuse

Abusers may use whatever it takes to control a situation—from emotional abuse and humiliation to physical assault. They often subject their victims to emotional, physical, financial, and sexual abuse. Some people remain in abusive relationships because they believe they deserve the abuse. Others feel they have no means of escape, and often an attempt to escape can be fatal for the victim.

Emotional Abuse

Emotional abuse includes:

- Promising, swearing, or threatening to harm the victim
- Forcing the victim to perform degrading or humiliating acts
- Threatening to harm children, pets, or close friends
- Humiliating the victim by name-calling and insults
- Threatening to leave the victim and their children
- Isolating the victim from family and friends
- Ridiculing or making fun of the victim

- Giving the victim the silent treatment
- Destroying the victim's valued possessions
- Controlling the victim's every move

Physical Abuse

Physical abuse includes:

- Hitting or grabbing the victim so hard that it leaves marks
- Throwing things at the victim
- Slapping, spitting at, biting, burning, pushing, choking, or shoving the victim
- Kicking or punching the victim, or slamming the victim against things
- Attacking the victim with weapons such as a knife, gun, rope, or electrical cord
- Controlling access to health care for injury

Financial Abuse

Financial abuse includes:

- Preventing the victim from getting a job
- Refusing to provide money for expenses
- Controlling how all money is spent
- Failing to contribute financially

Sexual Abuse

Sexual abuse includes:

- Forcing the victim to have vaginal, oral, or anal intercourse against their will
- Biting the victim's breasts or genitals
- Taking nonconsensual photos or videos of an undressed or nude victim
- Shoving objects into the victim's vagina or anus
- Forcing the victim to do something sexual that they find degrading or humiliating (OVW, 2023)

Myths and Facts About IPV

Table 9.2 lists many of the myths about IPV. Health care providers should take steps to dispel these myths.

Abuse Profiles

Victims

Victims often will not describe themselves as abused. The woman who is being abused often feels terrified, trapped, helpless, and alone. She reacts to any expression of anger or threat by avoidance and withdrawal behavior. Some women believe that the abuse is caused by a personality flaw or inadequacy in themselves (e.g., inability to keep the partner happy). Their partners reinforce and exploit these feelings of failure. After the

TABLE 9.2 • Common Myths and Facts About Intimate Partner Violence

Myths	Facts
Physical abuse occurs only among people of lower socioeconomic status.	Violence occurs in all socioeconomic classes.
Substance use disorder causes violence.	Violence is a learned behavior and can be changed. While substance use does not cause violence, the presence of drugs and alcohol can make a bad problem worse.
Violence happens to only a small percentage of women.	One in three women will be victims of violence in their lifetime (Weil, 2024).
Intimate partner violence (IPV) is typically a one-time, isolated occurrence and is always physical.	IPV is a pattern of coercion and control that one person exerts over another. It is repeated using a number of tactics, including intimidation, threats, economic deprivation, isolation, sexual abuse, and physical injury. The various forms of abuse utilized by abusers help them maintain power and control over their victims.
Women can easily choose to leave an abusive relationship.	Women often stay in abusive relationships because they feel they have no options. Frequently, leaving presents the greatest risk to the woman's life.
Only men with mental health problems commit violence against women.	No research supports this. Abuse and violence is a choice made by the abuser. Abusers often seem normal and do not appear to suffer from personality disorders or other forms of mental illness.
Pregnant women are protected from abuse by their partners.	IPV often begins or increases during pregnancy (Weil, 2024).
Women provoke their partners to abuse them, and abuse takes place because the abuser loses control and is angry.	Abuse and violence are a deliberate choice by the abuser to gain power and control.
IPV is rare in same-sex relationships.	People identifying as LGBTQIA+ experience IPV at rates similar to or higher than those in the straight population.

Rhodes, L. R. (2023). Addressing intimate partner violence with LGBTQ+ clients. *Counseling Today.* https://ctarchive.counseling.org/2023/06/addressing-intimate-partner-violence-with-lgbtq-clients/; Domestic Violence Action Center. (n.d.). *Common myths about domestic violence.* https://domesticviolenceactioncenter.org/common-myths/; Filipovic, J. (2023). *14 Misconceptions about domestic violence.* https://www.domesticshelters.org/articles/domestic-violence-op-ed-column/14-misconceptions-about-domestic-violence; and Smith, M., & Segal, J. (2023). *Domestic violence and abuse.* Help Guide Organization. https://www.helpguide.org/articles/abuse/domestic-violence-and-abuse.htm

abuser repeatedly tells the victim that they are "bad," some victims begin to believe it. Many victims were abused as children and may have poor health outcomes, PTSD, depression, low educational achievement, limited employment opportunities, or substance or alcohol use disorder (CDC, 2022a).

Abusers

Abusers come from all walks of life and often feel insecure, powerless, and helpless; feelings that are not in line with the image of strength they would like to project. The abuser expresses their inner feelings of low self-esteem and desire for power through acts of violence or aggression toward others (Kippert, 2023).

Violence typically occurs at home and is usually directed toward the intimate partner or the children who live there. Abusers refuse to share power and choose violence to control their victims. They often exhibit childlike aggression or antisocial behaviors. They may fail to accept responsibility or may blame others for their own problems. They might also have a history of substance use disorder; childhood physical or sexual abuse; trouble with the justice system; few close relationships or social isolation; a sensitivity to criticism; a tendency to hold grudges; involvement in power struggles; feelings of being misunderstood, mistreated, or victimized; an inability to admit fault; untreated mental illness; obsessive or extreme jealousy; low self-esteem; PTSD; controlling behaviors; generally violent behavior; erratic employment history; and/or financial problems (Kippert, 2023).

Violence Against Pregnant Women

Many think of pregnancy as a time of celebration and planning for the unborn child's future, but in an abusive relationship, it can be a time of escalating violence. The strongest predictor of abuse during pregnancy is prior abuse. Violence against pregnant people is more prevalent than diseases routinely investigated during prenatal care, such as gestational diabetes (Huecker et al., 2023). Pregnant people are more likely to die from homicide, which is linked to IPV, than from any pregnancy-related health issues (Wallace et al., 2021).

Women are at a higher risk for violence during pregnancy, and having children does not protect a person from IPV. On the contrary, IPV appears to last longer if the victim has children, and this also seems to be the case even after the partnership has come to an end. Pregnancy represents a dangerous time for people who become victims of IPV, given the potential for adverse outcomes for both the victim and their infant (Agarwal et al., 2023). Pregnant people are vulnerable during this time, and abusers can take advantage of this vulnerability. Abuse during pregnancy poses special risks and dynamics. Commonly found risk factors leading to violence during this time include:

- Pregnant person with low self-esteem
- History of IPV before pregnancy for the person or their partner
- Having less than a high school education
- Low income
- Unemployment
- Lack of social support from family and friends
- Economic stress
- Partner with substance use disorder
- Lack of community resources (Agarwal et al., 2023)

Abuse during pregnancy threatens the well-being of the pregnant person and fetus. Physical violence may involve injuries to the head, face, neck, thorax, breasts, and abdomen. The mental health consequences are also significant. Several studies have confirmed the relationship between abuse and poor mental health, especially depression and PTSD, negative self-image, increased distress, fearfulness, anxiousness, and stress (Agarwal et al., 2023; D'Angelo et al., 2022). For the childbearing person, many of these conditions most often manifest during the postpartum period.

TAKE NOTE!

Frequently, the fear of harm to their unborn child will motivate a pregnant person to try to escape an abusive relationship.

Additional adverse outcomes to the pregnant person and fetus include:

- Stillbirth
- Smoking and substance misuse
- Preterm labor
- Low-birth-weight infants (Guo et al., 2023; Huecker et al., 2023)

Dorothy, whom you met at the beginning of the chapter, has been frequenting the clinic with vague somatic complaints in recent weeks and admits she is sometimes afraid at home. She tells the nurse her partner doesn't want her to work, though he is only sporadically employed at low-paying jobs. What cues in her assessment might indicate abuse? What physical signs might the nurse observe?

Signs of abuse can emerge during pregnancy and may include poor attendance at prenatal visits, unrealistic fears, weight fluctuations, difficulty with pelvic examinations, and nonadherence to treatment.

Uncovering abuse in pregnant patients requires a consistent and direct approach to every patient by the nurse. Multiple assessments may enhance reporting by enabling the nurse to establish trust and rapport with the patient and identify changes in their behavior. Once abuse is discovered in a pregnant person, interventions should include safety planning, emotional support and counseling, referral to community services, ongoing prenatal care, and follow-up to avoid adverse health outcomes (Agarwal et al., 2023).

Violence Against Older People

Elder abuse is an umbrella term that may include physical, sexual, or emotional abuse; financial exploitation; and neglect, abandonment, or self-neglect of the vulnerable older person by a caregiver where there is an expectation of trust. Older women can experience the same forms of violence as younger women do, but the intersections of ageism and sexism, as well as factors such as illness, disability, isolation, widowhood, dependency, and mental impairment, increase the risk of violence against them (Huecker et al., 2023). Additional risk factors that may contribute to elder abuse include low income, depression, external family stressors or conflict such as caregiver burnout, poor physical health related to chronic health challenges, and cognitive impairment such as dementia or Alzheimer disease (Halphen, 2023). In 90% of cases, the abuser is someone the victim knows, usually a family member (Halphen, 2023). All 50 states have laws requiring health care providers to report elder or vulnerable person abuse. It is estimated that 3% to 10% of older people experience abuse, but many cases go unreported (Huecker et al., 2023). Research suggests that older females are abused at a higher rate than males and that the older a person is, the more likely they are to be abused (Halphen, 2023). Elder abuse is expected to increase as the population ages (WHO, 2022a). Although an injury may bring the older patient into the health care system, the physical and emotional sequelae of IPV may be more subtle and may include depression, insomnia, chronic pain, difficulty trusting others, low self-esteem, thoughts of suicide, substance abuse, anger issues, atypical chest pain, or other kinds of somatic symptoms. Accurate detection and assessment of misuse in older patients are essential duties of all nurses. Bruises, grip marks, and lacerations are just some of the potential indications of elder abuse. Nurses have frequent contact with older victims of abuse, giving nurses the opportunity to play a significant role in detecting, reporting, and intervening in such cases. As part of a thorough screening, nurses should determine what the patient has done to attempt to resolve the abuse and the effectiveness of those strategies. Actions taken by the patient prior to revealing the abuse issue to the nurse might have included passive acceptance, calling law enforcement, counseling, or other measures. In addition, taking time to establish rapport with older patients builds a sense of trust, safety, and openness. Nurses must listen carefully and nonjudgmentally. Judging or criticizing the victim for their decisions might create the impression that they deserve the abuse or that they are to blame. Finally, nurses should attempt to stay current in their knowledge of referral resources to assist the older person experiencing abuse. Some of these resources include housing, transportation, medical services, employment, social services, and local support groups. A coordinated and comprehensive response to IPV is essential to reduce its sequelae.

Nursing Management of IPV Victims

Nurses encounter thousands of abuse victims each year in their practice settings, but many victims slip through the cracks. As practicing universal violence assessment has increased in recent years, nurses need to be aware of not only how to screen for violence but also how to respond in a way that is helpful, sincere, nonjudgmental, and legally adequate. This will require nurses to move beyond a description of violence toward a response that is action oriented and evidence based, which includes safety planning and referrals. There are many things nurses can do to help victims. Early recognition and intervention can significantly reduce the morbidity and mortality associated with IPV. To stop the cycle of violence, nurses need to know how to assess for and identify IPV and implement appropriate actions.

Assessment

Routine screening for IPV is the first way to detect abuse. See Evidence-Based Practice 9.1. The nurse should build rapport by listening, showing an interest in the concerns of the patient, and creating an atmosphere of openness. Communicating support through a nonjudgmental attitude and telling the patient that no one deserves to be abused are the first steps toward establishing trust and rapport. Rather than overlooking abused patients, especially women, as "chronic complainers," astute nurses need to be vigilant for subtle clues of abuse. Learning how to assess for abuse is critical. Some basic assessment guidelines follow.

SCREEN FOR ABUSE DURING EVERY HEALTH CARE VISIT

Screening for violence takes only a few minutes and can have an enormously positive effect on the outcome for the abused person. Any woman could be a victim; no single sign marks a woman as an abuse victim, but the following clues may be helpful:

- Injuries—bruises on the upper arm, chest, and abdomen, scars from blunt trauma, minor lacerations, or weapon wounds on the face, head, and neck
- Injury sequelae—headaches, hearing loss from ruptured ear drums, joint pain, sinus infections, teeth marks, clumps of hair missing, dental trauma, pelvic pain, and breast or genital injuries

- Reported history of injury that is not consistent with the actual presenting problem
- Mental health problems—depression, anxiety or panic disorder, substance use disorder, eating disorders, suicidal ideation or suicide attempts, and PTSD
- Frequent urgent care or emergency room visits
- Nonadherence to medication regimen
- Inappropriate affect—avoids eye contact or is hostile
- Delay in seeking medical attention and patterns of repeated injury
- Missed appointments or late initiation of prenatal care
- Potential abuser's behavior at the health care visit: appears overly solicitous or overprotective, is unwilling to leave the patient alone with the health care provider, answers questions for the patient, and attempts to control the situation (Weil, 2022)

Most of the professional societies recommend screening all women for IPV regardless of setting; a recommended frequency is not given, but all clinicians should be alert to IPV during every health care encounter (Weil, 2022).

ISOLATE PATIENT IMMEDIATELY FROM ABUSER

If abuse is detected, immediately isolate the patient to provide privacy and prevent potential retaliation from the abuser. Asking about abuse in front of the perpetrator may trigger an abusive episode during the interview or at home. Ways to ensure the patient's safety include taking the victim to an area away from the abuser to ask questions. The assessment can take place anywhere that is private and away from the abuser, for example, an x-ray area, ultrasound room, elevator, restroom, or laboratory.

If abuse is detected, the nurse can do the following to enhance the nurse–patient relationship:

- Educate the patient about the connection between the violence and their symptoms.
- Help the patient acknowledge what has happened to them and begin to deal with the situation.
- Offer the patient referrals so they can get the help that will allow them to begin to heal.

Dorothy returns to the prenatal clinic a month later with anemia, inadequate weight gain, bruises on her face and neck, and second-trimester bleeding. This time she is accompanied by her partner, who stays close to Dorothy. What questions should the nurse ask to assess the situation? Where is the appropriate location to ask these questions? What legal responsibilities does the nurse have concerning their observations?

EVIDENCE-BASED PRACTICE 9.1

Intimate Partner Violence Screening and Referral Outcomes Among Transgender Patients in a Primary Care Setting

BACKGROUND

Transgender people, whose gender identity does not align with the sex assigned to them at birth, experience intimate partner violence (IPV) at higher rates than people in the cisgender population in the United States. IPV is a significant yet preventable public health problem that globally affects millions of people annually. According to recent statistics, transgender people are especially vulnerable to IPV. Screening for IPV is a standard of care recommended by the United States Preventive Services Task Force (USPSTF) and other professional organizations; however, they provide no clear guidance on screening or referral of transgender patients. Health care settings are a critical access point for IPV services, but many transgender patients face several barriers to accessing health care and negative experiences with health care providers. Nurses are in an advantageous position to screen these patients for IPV as they are able to build rapport with them.

The purpose of this study was to determine the effectiveness of routine IPV screening of transgender patients using an existing screening program and identify factors associated with referral and engagement in the care of transgender patients.

STUDY

A referral cascade was developed for 1,947 transgender patients, of whom 227 screened positive for IPV. Patients were included in the analysis regardless of their social, medical, or surgical transition status. Four IPV screening areas were used: isolation, sexual, coercive, and physical. Based on the screening results, referrals were made within the next 3 months, but many did not seek assistance.

Findings

The results of this study emphasized the feasibility and utility of universal routine IPV screening among transgender patients, who are currently excluded from national screening guidelines despite experiencing higher rates of IPV. Given the higher IPV rates in transgender aggregates when compared to cisgender communities, IPV screenings should be utilized at every health care encounter to identify and link transgender survivors with needed community services.

Nursing Implications

Health care encounters present a great opportunity for nurses to screen all patients for IPV. Nurses can build therapeutic rapport with their patients over the course of their health care visits, resulting in a trusting relationship. Based on the findings, it is important to screen for IPV at each health care visit and provide appropriate referrals for transgender patients in the primary care setting. It is essential for nurses to serve as advocates for all patients suffering from IPV by supporting them in their decisions and making necessary referrals. This universal action will help to ensure the benefits of IPV screening are applied equally for all people.

Adapted from Das, K. J. H., Peitzmeier, S., Berrahou, I. K., & Potter, J. (2022). Intimate partner violence (IPV) screening and referral outcomes among transgender patients in a primary care setting. *Journal of Interpersonal Violence, 37*(13–14). https://doi.org/10.1177/0886260521997460

ASK QUESTIONS ABOUT ABUSE

Violence against women is often unseen, unknown, and hidden in families. Questions to screen for abuse should be routine and handled just like any other questions. Many nurses feel uncomfortable asking questions of this nature, but broaching the subject is important, even if the answer comes later. Opening up the possibility for patients to express themselves about their experience of abuse to a nurse sends out a clear message that violence should never be tolerated or kept hidden; it also conveys the message that nurses care about the patient's experiences and want to offer a best practice initial response. Just knowing that someone else knows about the abuse may offer the victim some relief and may help them disclose it.

Ask difficult questions in an empathetic and nonthreatening manner and remain nonjudgmental in all responses and interactions. Choose the type of question that makes you most comfortable. Direct and indirect questions produce the same results. "Does your partner hit you?" or "Have you ever been or are you now in an abusive relationship?" are direct questions. If that approach feels uncomfortable, try indirect statements that imply questions to the patient: "We see many women with injuries or complaints like yours and often they are being abused, so I now ask every patient if this is what is happening to them;" or "Many women in our community experience abuse from their partners; therefore, we have now made it routine to ask every patient if this is happening in their life." With either approach, nurses need to maintain a nonjudgmental acceptance of whatever answers the patient offers.

Many screening tools are available, but no single screening tool is well established (Boyland & Berishaj, 2022; Weil, 2022). Lengthy tools have been evaluated in the literature but are not as realistic to use with every patient encounter in busy health care settings (Weil, 2022). Various short question models are available, and some advise that a single question such as "Do you feel safe in your relationship?" when asked routinely in a nonjudgmental way will increase the detection of IPV (Weil, 2022). The SAVE model is a recommended screening tool for all patients to screen for sexual violence (see Box 9.2).

ASSESS IMMEDIATE SAFETY

It is essential to assist the woman by assessing her safety and the safety of her children, if she has any. To do this, speak to the woman alone and ask her:

- Does she feel safe going home after her meeting with you?
- Does she need an immediate place of safety for herself or her children?
- Does she have a plan of escape if she becomes at risk for her safety?
- Does she need to consider an alternative exit from this building?
- Who are the people she could contact for help or support?

BOX 9.2 SAVE Model

SCREEN All of Your Patients for Sexual Violence by Asking

- Have you been touched sexually against your will or without consent?
- Do you feel you have control over your sexual relationships and will be listened to if you say "no" to having sex?
- Has anyone forced you to engage in sexual activities?

ASK Direct Questions in a Nonjudgmental Way

- Begin by normalizing the topic with the patient.
- Make continuous eye contact with the patient.
- Stay calm; avoid emotional reactions to what the patient tells you.
- Never blame the patient, even if they blame themselves.
- Do not dismiss or minimize what the patient tells you, even if they do.
- Wait for each answer patiently. Do not rush to the next question.
- Do not use formal, technical, or medical language.
- Avoid using leading questions; be direct and to the point.
- Use a nonthreatening, accepting approach.

VALIDATE the Patient by Telling Them

- You believe their story.
- You do not blame them for what happened.
- They are not alone.
- It is brave of them to tell you this.
- Help is available for them.
- Talking with you is a hopeful sign and a first big step.

EVALUATE, Educate, and Refer This Patient by Asking Them

- What type of violence was it?
- Are they now in any danger?
- How are they feeling now?
- Do they know that there are consequences to violence?
- Is the patient aware of community resources available to help them?

Adapted with permission from Florida Council Against Sexual Violence. (2012). *How to screen your patients for sexual assault: A guide for healthcare professionals.* https://www.yumpu.com/en/document/read/44966841/view-full-booklet-florida-council-against-sexual-violence

The Danger Assessment Tool (Box 9.3) helps women and health care providers assess the potential for homicidal behavior in an ongoing abusive relationship. It is based on research that showed several risk factors for abuse. It has proven validity and reliability, and it is recommended that health care providers perform this assessment on every patient who screens positively for IPV (Boyland & Berishaj, 2022; Garcia-Vergara et al., 2022). There are different versions available for specific groups such as immigrant women, Indigenous women, and women in same-sex relationships (Garcia-Vergara et al., 2022). It is free and available to the public.

DOCUMENT AND REPORT YOUR FINDINGS

If the interview reveals a history of abuse, accurate documentation is critical because this evidence may support the patient's case in court. Documentation must include details about the frequency and severity of abuse; the location, extent, and outcome of injuries; and any treatments or interventions. When documenting, use direct quotes and be specific: "He choked me." Describe any visible injuries and use a body map (outline of a patient's body) to show where the injuries are. Obtain photos (with informed consent) or document their refusal if the patient

BOX 9.3 Danger Assessment

Several risk factors have been associated with increased risk of homicides (murders) of women and men in violent relationships. We cannot predict what will happen in your case, but we would like you to be aware of the danger of homicide in situations of abuse and for you to see how many of the risk factors apply to your situation.

Using the calendar, please mark the approximate dates during the past year when you were abused by your partner or ex-partner. Write on that date how bad the incident was according to the following scale:

1. Slapping, pushing; no injuries and/or lasting pain
2. Punching, kicking; bruises, cuts, and/or continuing pain
3. "Beating up"; severe contusions, burns, broken bones
4. Threat to use weapon; head injury, internal injury, permanent injury, miscarriage or choking* (use a © in the date to indicate choking/strangulation/cut off your breathing- example 4©)
5. Use of weapon; wounds from weapon

(If **any** of the descriptions for the higher number apply, use the higher number.)

Mark **Yes** or **No** for each of the following. ("He" refers to your husband, partner, ex-husband, ex-partner, or whoever is currently physically hurting you.)

_____1. Has the physical violence increased in severity or frequency over the past year?
_____2. Does he own a gun?
_____3. Have you left him after living together during the past year?
3a. (If you have never lived with him, check here:___)
_____4. Is he unemployed?
_____5. Has he ever used a weapon against you or threatened you with a lethal weapon? (If yes, was the weapon a gun? check here:___)
_____6. Does he threaten to kill you?
_____7. Has he avoided being arrested for domestic violence?
_____8. Do you have a child that is not his?
_____9. Has he ever forced you to have sex when you did not wish to do so?
_____10. Does he ever try to choke/strangle you or cut off your breathing?
_____10a. (If yes, has he done it more than once, or did it make you pass out or black out or make you dizzy? check here:_______)
_____11. Does he use illegal drugs? By drugs, I mean "uppers" or amphetamines, "meth", speed, angel dust, cocaine, "crack", street drugs or mixtures.
_____12. Is he an alcoholic or problem drinker?
_____13. Does he control most or all of your daily activities? For instance, does he tell you who you can be friends with, when you can see your family, how much money you can use, or when you can take the car? (If he tries, but you do not let him, check here:_______)
_____14. Is he violently and constantly jealous of you? (For instance, does he say: "If I can't have you, no one can.")
_____15. Have you ever been beaten by him while you were pregnant? (If you have never been pregnant by him, check here:_____)
_____16. Has he ever threatened or tried to commit suicide?
_____17. Does he threaten to harm your children?
_____18. Do you believe he is capable of killing you?
_____19. Does he follow or spy on you, leave threatening notes or messages, destroy your property, or call you when you don't want him to?
_____20. Have you ever threatened or tried to commit suicide?
_____ Total "Yes" Answers

Thank you. Please talk to your nurse, advocate, or counselor about what the Danger Assessment means in your situation.

[a]Men are not the only perpetrators of violence. Alter your language to match the gender identities of the victim and abuser.

Jacquelyn C. Campbell, Ph.D., R.N. Copyright © 2003; update 2019. Retrieved July 5, 2024, from www.dangerassessment.com.

Campbell, J. C., Webster, D. W., & Glass, N. (2009). The danger assessment: Validation of a lethality risk assessment instrument for intimate partner femicide. *Journal of Interpersonal Violence, 24*(4), 653–674. https://doi.org/10.1177/0886260508317180

declines photos. Pictures or diagrams can be helpful. Figure 9.2 shows a sample documentation form for IPV.

Laws in many states require health care providers to alert the police to any injuries that involve knives, firearms, or other deadly weapons or that present life-threatening emergencies. If the assessment reveals suspicion or actual indication of abuse, the nurse can explain to the patient that they are required by law to report it.

Nursing Analysis

When violence is suspected or validated, the nurse needs to formulate nursing analyses based on the completed assessment. Possible nursing analyses related to violence against women might include:

- Knowledge deficiency related to understanding the cycle of violence and availability of resources
- Anxiety related to threat to self-concept, situational crisis of abuse
- Low self-esteem related to negative family interactions
- Powerlessness related to a lifestyle of helplessness
- Altered individual and family coping related to abusive patterns

Interventions

The response of nurses to people who are being abused can have a profound effect on their willingness to open up or seek help. Some responses to assist successful communication in these circumstances could include:

- *Listening*—"I hear and understand what you are saying." Being listened to can be an empowering experience for a person who has been abused.
- *Communicating belief*—"That must have been frightening for you."
- *Validating the decision to disclose*—"It must have been difficult for you to talk about this today."
- *Emphasizing the unacceptability of this violence*—"You don't deserve to be treated this way."

If abuse is identified, nurses can undertake interventions that can increase the patient's safety and improve their health. The goal of intervention is to enable the victim to gain control of their life. Provide sensitive, predictable care in an accepting setting. Offer step-by-step explanations of procedures. Provide educational materials about violence. Allow the victim to actively participate in their care and have control over all health care decisions. Pace your nursing interventions and allow the patient to take the lead. Communicate support through a nonjudgmental attitude. Carefully document all of your assessment findings and nursing interventions.

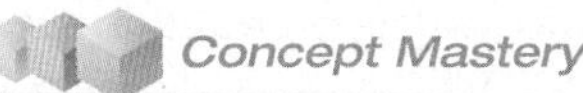
Concept Mastery Alert

Priorities in Intimate Partner Violence Interventions

Although it is important that a person in an abusive situation is safe, it is also important for them to regain a sense of control in their life. A lack of control is what can prevent the person from escaping an abusive situation.

Domestic Violence Screening/Documentation Form

DV Screen
☐ DV + (Positive)
☐ DV? (Suspected)

Date ____________ Patient ID# ____________
Patient Name ____________
Provider Name ____________
Patient Pregnant? ☐ Yes ☐ No

Assess Patient Safety

☐ Yes ☐ No Is abuser here now?
☐ Yes ☐ No Is patient afraid of their partner?
☐ Yes ☐ No Is patient afraid to go home?
☐ Yes ☐ No Has physical violence increased in severity?
☐ Yes ☐ No Has partner physically abused children?
☐ Yes ☐ No Have children witnessed violence in the home?
☐ Yes ☐ No Threats of homicide?
By whom? ____________
☐ Yes ☐ No Threats of suicide?
By whom? ____________
☐ Yes ☐ No Is there a gun in the home?
☐ Yes ☐ No Alcohol or substance abuse?
☐ Yes ☐ No Was safety plan discussed?

Referrals

☐ Hotline number given
☐ Legal referral made
☐ Shelter number given
☐ In-house referral made
Describe: ____________
☐ Other referral made
Describe: ____________

Reporting

☐ Law enforcement report made
☐ Child Protective Services report made
☐ Adult Protective Services report made

Photographs

☐ Yes ☐ No Consent to be photographed?
☐ Yes ☐ No Photographs taken?
Attach photographs and consent form

FIGURE 9.2 Intimate partner violence documentation form. (Reprinted with permission from Cassidy, K. [1999]. How to assess and intervene in domestic violence situations. *Home Healthcare Nurse*, *17*[10], 644–672. https://doi.org/10.1097/00004045-199910000-00008, Copyright © 1999, with permission from Lippincott Williams & Wilkins.)

A public health approach to violence prevention requires input from and coordination across sectors, including those of health, education, social services, justice, and policy. The goal of public health is to improve the health of the entire community or society. Depending on when in the cycle of violence the nurse encounters a patient experiencing abuse, goals may fall into three groups:

- *Primary prevention*—aimed at breaking the abuse cycle through community educational initiatives by nurses, primary providers, law enforcement, teachers, and clergy
- *Secondary prevention*—focuses on screening high-risk people and dealing with victims and abusers in the early stages with the goal of preventing the progression of abuse
- *Tertiary prevention*—geared toward helping adults and children experiencing severe abuse recover and become productive members of society and rehabilitating abusers to stop the cycle of violence; these activities are typically long-term and expensive.

EMPOWER is a mnemonic device to help remember an empowerment framework for providing sensitive nursing interventions to people experiencing abuse (Box 9.4). Specific nursing interventions for the person experiencing abuse include educating them about community services, providing emotional support, and offering a safety plan.

BOX 9.4 EMPOWER When Caring for People Who Have Been Abused

- **E** Empathetic listening
- **M** Making time to ensure accurate and appropriate documentation of findings
- Documentation should include:
  - A clear quoted statement about the abuse in the patient's own words
  - Accurate descriptions of injuries and the history of them
  - Information on the first, the worst, and the most recent abusive incident
  - Photos of the injuries (with the patient's consent)
- **P** Providing information and education about the cycle of violence and that it will escalate:
  - Educate about abuse and its health effects.
  - Help the patient understand that they are not alone.
  - Offer appropriate community support and referrals.
  - Display posters and brochures to foster awareness of this public health problem.
- **O** Offering choices and options
- **W** Working with domestic abuse specialists
- **E** Encouraging planning for safety, the most important aspect of the intervention. Ensure that the patient has resources and a plan of action to carry out if and when they decide to leave.
- **R** Referring the patient to local services and support groups

Adapted with permission from Boyland, C. M., & Berishaj, K. A. (2022). Intimate partner violence. In K. D. Schuiling & F. E. Likis (Eds.), *Gynecologic health care* (4th ed., pp. 303–325). Jones & Bartlett Learning.

EDUCATE THE PATIENT ABOUT COMMUNITY SERVICES

A wide range of support services are available to meet the needs of survivors of violence. Nurses should be prepared to help the patient take advantage of these opportunities. Services will vary by community but might include psychological counseling, legal advice, social services, crisis services, support groups, hotlines, housing, vocational training, and other community-based referrals.

Give the patient information about shelters or services even if they initially reject it. Give the patient the national domestic violence hotline number: (800) 799-7233 or website: www.thehotline.org.

PROVIDE EMOTIONAL SUPPORT

Providing reassurance and support to a person experiencing abuse is essential if the violence is to end. The physical, psychological, and emotional effects of IPV on survivors and their children can be severe and long lasting. Nurses in all clinical settings can help victims feel a sense of personal power and provide them with a safe and supportive environment. Appropriate action can help survivors express their thoughts and feelings in constructive ways, manage stress, and move on with their lives. Appropriate interventions include:

- Strengthen the person's sense of control over their life by:
  - Teaching coping strategies to manage stress
  - Assisting with activities of daily living to improve their lifestyle
  - Allowing them to make as many decisions as they can
  - Educating them about the symptoms of PTSD and their basis
- Encourage the person to establish realistic goals for themselves by:
  - Teaching problem-solving skills
  - Encouraging social activities to connect with other people
- Provide support and allow the person to grieve for their losses by:
  - Listening to and clarifying their reactions to the traumatic event
  - Discussing shock, disbelief, anger, depression, and acceptance
- Explain to the person that:
  - Abuse is never OK. They didn't ask for it, and they don't deserve it.
  - They are not alone, and help is available.
  - Abuse is a crime, and they are a victim.
  - Alcohol, drugs, money problems, depression, and jealousy do not cause violence, but these things can give the abuser an excuse for abusing the victim.
  - The actions of the abuser are not the victim's fault.
  - Their history of abuse is believed.
  - Making a decision to leave an abusive relationship can be hard and dangerous and takes time.

OFFER A SAFETY PLAN

The choice to leave must belong to the victim. Nurses cannot choose a life for the victim; they can only offer choices. Leaving is a process, not an event. Victims may try to leave their abusers as many as seven or eight times before succeeding. Frequently, the final attempt to leave results in the death of the victim. People planning to leave an abusive relationship should have a safety plan (Teaching Guidelines 9.1).

Nurses need to remember that their role is that of a guide, not a savior. A person will make the best decision they see fit at that moment in time. A nurse may be the person's most effective resource in a stress-filled environment. Just allowing the person to talk may be the most valuable intervention. The impact of the nurse's presence and support will stay with the person, no matter what decision they make. Nurses must remember that significant underlying factors in violence against women by men are inequality between men and women and the lesser status of women compared to men in many societies. These factors contribute to disrespect for women and place them at higher risk. Violence against women remains a worldwide public health problem of epidemic proportions, and nurses need to understand their roles in identifying and responding to it appropriately.

TEACHING GUIDELINES 9.1 Safety Plan for Leaving an Abusive Relationship

- When leaving an abusive relationship, prepare an emergency kit with the following items:
  - Driver's license or photo ID
  - Social Security number or green card/work permit
  - Birth certificates for you and any children
  - Phone numbers for social services, domestic violence shelter, or women's shelter
  - The deed or lease to your home or apartment
  - Any court papers or orders
  - Prescription medications
  - A change of clothing for you and your children
  - Pay stubs, check book, credit cards, and cash
  - Health insurance cards
  - Car keys
  - Money
- Back the car in the driveway and keep the tank full.
- Memorize important phone numbers.
- If you need to leave a domestic violence situation immediately, turn to authorities for assistance in gathering this material.
- Any 24-hour health care facility can be a safety net.
- Develop a plan for leaving, including where you will go. Rehearse it and share the plan with a trusted family member or friend.

Boyland, C. M., & Berishaj, K. A. (2022). Intimate partner violence. In K. D. Schuiling & F. E. Likis (Eds.), *Gynecologic health care* (4th ed., pp. 303–325). Jones & Bartlett Learning; and Healthy Alternatives to Violent Environments. (2022). *Safety planning*. https://www.havenstan.org/safety-planing

SEXUAL VIOLENCE

Sexual violence exacerbates inequalities of gender, race, ethnicity, class, age, sexuality, ability status, citizenship status, and nationality. It is both a public health problem and a human rights violation. Sexual violence includes IPV, human trafficking, incest, FGM/C, forced prostitution, bondage, exploitation, neglect, infanticide, and sexual assault. It occurs worldwide; impacts every community; and affects people of all genders, sexual orientations, and ages. Over 50% of women over a lifetime have experienced sexual violence involving physical contact (CDC, 2022b). Once every 2 minutes, 30 times an hour, 1,871 times a day in the United States, a perpetrator rapes a girl or woman. One in four women and one in 26 men have been the victim of an attempted or completed rape during their lifetimes (Basile et al., 2022). Nine out of 10 victims of rape are women (Rape, Abuse, & Incest National Network [RAINN], 2023a). Over the course of their lives, women may be the victims of more than one type of violence. Women aged 12 to 24 years are at the highest risk of sexual assault and rape (Melmer, 2023).

Sexual violence can have a variety of devastating short- and long-term effects. Victims of sexual violence can experience psychological, physical, and cognitive symptoms that affect them daily. These can include pelvic pain, genital injuries, headaches, STIs, pregnancy, anxiety, fear, sleep disturbances, substance misuse, depression, sexual health problems, PTSD, and suicidal ideation and attempts (Basile et al., 2022; CDC, 2022b). A traumatic experience not only damages a person's sense of safety in the world, but it also has the potential to reduce their self-esteem and ability to continue their education, to earn money and be productive, to have children, and if they have children, to nurture and protect them. A study found that women who have been sexually assaulted may exhibit lower functioning as they age as sexual assaults have been linked to structural alterations in brain regions (Thurston et al., 2022). This may increase the risk for dementia, strokes, and other brain disorders (Thurston et al., 2022).

Sexual Abuse

Sexual abuse occurs when someone forces another person to have sexual contact of any kind (vaginal, oral, or anal) without their consent. It includes sexual slavery, nonconsensual pornography, child abuse, and sexual assault. Twenty-six percent of females and 5% of males have been sexually abused by adulthood (Melmer, 2023). At every age in the lifespan, females are more likely to be sexually abused by a nonbirthing parent, brother, family member, neighbor, boyfriend, husband, partner, or ex-partner than by a stranger or anonymous assailant. Sexual abuse is not subject to economic or cultural barriers. Marriage does not constitute a tacit agreement for a spouse to inflict one's demands on the other without permission.

Childhood sexual abuse is any type of sexual exploitation that involves a child younger than 18 years old. Sexual abuse involves engaging a child in a sexual activity that they do not fully understand, cannot give informed consent to engage in, and are forced, manipulated, or coerced into participating in (Nienow, 2023). It might include disrobing, nudity, masturbation, fondling, digital penetration, forced performance of sexual acts on the perpetrator, and intercourse. It is estimated that one in four girls and one in 13 boys in the United States are likely to experience sexual abuse (Nienow, 2023). Child sexual abuse is a silent epidemic; it is estimated that fewer than half of all sexual assaults are reported (Melmer, 2023). Childhood sexual abuse has a lifelong impact on its survivors. There is strong evidence that sexual assault in childhood or adolescence can lead to long-term issues such as depression, anxiety, thoughts of suicide, PTSD, poor body image, low self-esteem, unhealthy behaviors such as drug and alcohol use, self-mutilation, and risky sexual behaviors (Whealin & Barnett, 2022). Women who were sexually abused during childhood are at a heightened risk for repeat abuse. This may be because the early abuse lowers their self-esteem and their ability to protect themselves and set firm boundaries. Childhood sexual abuse is a trauma that influences the way victims form relationships, deal with adversity, cope with daily problems, relate to their children and peers, protect their health, and live. See Evidence-Based Practice 9.2 for research regarding childhood maltreatment. Studies have shown that the more victimization a person experiences, the more likely it is that they will be victimized later in life (Rowe et al., 2022).

Interventions for sexually abused children or adults should include referral for mental health counseling. Follow-up for any medical problems (e.g., genitourinary complaints) should be arranged with the victim's primary provider. If the community has an abuse referral center, refer the victim there for follow-up care according to local protocol.

The medical consequences of sexual abuse require the prophylaxis and treatment of STIs, emergency contraception, and treatment of any injuries that resulted from the abuse. Victims with postassault bleeding require an

EVIDENCE-BASED PRACTICE 9.2

Sexual, Physical, and Emotional Maltreatment in Childhood Are Differentially Associated With Sexual and Physical Revictimization in Adulthood

BACKGROUND

Worldwide, it is estimated that half of all children are victims of sexual, physical, and/or emotional maltreatment annually. Experiencing maltreatment as a child is linked to a variety of negative outcomes including lower educational achievement, poorer mental health, and a lower overall quality of life. Current research suggests that maltreatment in childhood increases the risk of later revictimization. The purpose of this study was to examine if the risk of revictimization in adulthood is associated with specific maltreatment types such as sexual, physical, or emotional and which parent is more likely to be the perpetrator (birthing parent vs. nonbirthing parent).

STUDY

Participants in this study included 720 adult women recruited through the online platform Prolific Academic. All participants participated in two online sessions 2 weeks apart hosted by Prolific Academic. Statistical analyses were conducted to examine the relationships between revictimization and childhood maltreatment variables.

Findings

It was found that childhood maltreatment has a negative, often lifelong, effect on functioning and increases the risk for sexual or physical revictimization throughout adulthood. Childhood sexual maltreatment was significantly associated with revictimization. In addition, there was greater sexual revictimization risk as an adult in girls who had experienced emotional and physical nonbirthing parent–perpetrated maltreatment during childhood compared with girls who had experienced birthing parent–perpetrated maltreatment during childhood. In women who experience sexual attraction to more than one gender, the study found that birthing parent–perpetrated maltreatment was significantly associated with revictimization.

Nursing Implications

Knowledge of this study's findings will assist the nurse in identifying adult patients who were maltreated as children and are now at increased risk of being revictimized as an adult. Nurses should take a thorough history of each patient's childhood to determine if any maltreatment occurred. With sexually abused adults, nurses have the opportunity to assist adult survivors. The most important aspect of working with survivors is a caring, reliable nurse who creates a therapeutic environment. Many empowerment support strategies can be used to help the survivor. These results have important implications for identifying girls at the highest risk for revictimization early in life and providing them with targeted support and education to prevent revictimization in adulthood. Nurses must be knowledgeable of the potential vulnerabilities of adults who have experienced maltreatment as a child and protect them.

Adapted from Rowe, J., Chananna, J., Cunningham, S., & Harkness, K. L. (2022). Sexual, physical, and emotional maltreatment in childhood are differentially associated with sexual and physical revictimization in adulthood. *Journal of Interpersonal Violence, 38*, 3806–3830. https://doi.org/10.1177/08862605221111411

emergent evaluation and may need emergency treatment by a gynecologist for repair of genital injury. The psychosocial aspects of sexual abuse must also be addressed because appropriate therapeutic follow-up is essential to the victim's future emotional well-being.

Incest

Incest is defined as sexual activity between people so closely related that marriage between them is legally or culturally prohibited. It remains a major taboo in contemporary society. The exact incidence of childhood incest victimization is unknown. Such sexual abuse is not only a crime but also a symptom of acute and irreversible family dysfunction. Childhood incest abuse involves any kind of sexual exploitation between a child and another person that violates the social taboos of family roles; children cannot yet understand these activities and cannot give informed consent. Survivors of incest are often tricked, coerced, or manipulated. All adults appear powerful to children. Perpetrators might threaten victims so that they are afraid to disclose the abuse or might tell them the abuse is their fault. Often these threats serve to silence victims.

Incestuous relationships in the home endanger not only the child's intellectual and moral development but also the health of the child. Many children do not ask for help because they do not want to expose the "secret." For this reason, only the most obvious effects are statistically visible: serious injuries, internal damage, STIs, and pregnancy.

Whether an incest victim endured an isolated incident of abuse or ongoing assaults over an extended period, recovery can be painful and difficult. The recovery process begins with an admission of abuse and the recognition that help and services are needed. Resources for incest victims include books, self-help groups, workshops, therapy programs, and possibly legal remedies. In addition to listening to and believing incest victims, nurses need to search for ways to prevent future generations from enduring such abuse and from continuing the cycle of abuse in their own family and relationships. Every nurse bears the ethical and legal responsibility of being a mandated reporter of child sexual abuse. Nurses have the ability and the responsibility to function within an interdisciplinary system responsible for the assessment and ongoing treatment of families in which incest has been committed. Nurses can fulfill their roles as advocates for children while at the same time adding necessary referrals to social services and legal authorities. Forming this partnership with the social service and judicial communities will help protect the child from future abuse and ensure the child a safe environment in which to grow and develop. Nurses must educate society about incest and work toward preventing abuse and aiding survivors and their families in healing.

CONSIDER THIS!

At 53 years old, I stood and looked at myself in the mirror. The image staring back at me was one of a frightened, middle-aged, cowardly woman hiding her past. I had been sexually abused by my father for many years as a child and never told anyone. My mother knew of the abuse but felt helpless to make it stop. I married right out of high school to escape and felt I lived a "happy normal life" with my husband and three children. My children have left home and live far away, and my husband recently died of a sudden heart attack. I am now experiencing dreams and thoughts about my past abuse and feeling afraid again.

Thoughts: This woman suppressed her abusive past for most of her life and now her painful experience has surfaced. What can be done to reach out to her at this point? Did her health care providers miss the "red flags" that are common to women with a history of childhood sexual abuse all those years?

Rape

Rape is an expression of violence, not a sexual act. Rape distorts one of the most intimate forms of human interaction. It is not an act of lust or an overzealous release of passion; it is a violent, aggressive assault on the victim's body and integrity (Clifton, 2022). It may or may not include the use of a weapon. **Statutory rape** is sexual activity between an adult and a person under the age of 18 and is considered to have occurred even if the underage person was willing because someone who is underage is not legally considered capable of giving consent. Enforcement of laws, education, and community empowerment are all needed to prevent rape.

Some people believe strangers are more likely than known people to rape or assault women, or they may believe that perpetrators are more likely to rape women who are provocatively dressed. They may believe rapists are sex-starved people seeking sexual gratification. These myths are destructive beliefs about sexual aggression (i.e., its scope, causes, context, and consequences) that serve to deny, downplay, and justify sexually aggressive behavior. These myths serve to blame victims and exonerate perpetrators. Such myths and the actual facts are presented in Table 9.3.

Acquaintance Rape

In acquaintance rape, a person the victim knows socially penetrates the victim without their consent. For example, rape committed by a coworker, teacher, spouse's friend, or boss is considered acquaintance rape. Date rape, or rape that occurs within a dating relationship without the consent of one of the participants, is a form of acquaintance rape. Acquaintance and date rapes account for 80% to 90% of rapes that occur on college campuses (Wiemann & Miller, 2022).

TABLE 9.3 • Common Myths and Facts About Rape

Myths	Facts
People who are raped get over it quickly.	It can take many years to recover emotionally and physically from rape.
Most rape victims tell someone about it.	The majority of victims never tell anyone about it. In fact, almost two thirds of victims never report it to the police.
Once the rape is over, a survivor can again feel safe in their life.	The victim often feels vulnerable, betrayed, and insecure afterward.
Women who feel guilty after having sex then lie and say they were raped.	Few victims lie about rape. It is very traumatizing to be a victim. Coming forward with a rape allegation is often retraumatizing and detrimental to the victim's life.
Women who drink or take drugs deserve it if they get raped.	No one is ever to blame for being sexually assaulted. The responsibility for that crime lies with the perpetrator.
It is not rape if the victim is the perpetrator's girlfriend or wife.	Rape is always rape. If the other person doesn't consent, regardless of the relationship between victim and perpetrator, it is rape and is illegal.
When it comes to sex, men can be aroused to "a point of no return."	Men are physically able to stop at any point during sexual activity. Rape is not an act of impulsive, uncontrolled passion; it is a premeditated act of violence. A person has a right to end a sexual encounter at any moment.
Women who wear certain clothes, drink alcohol, or who are sex workers are "asking for it."	No victim invites sexual assault regardless of their clothing, lifestyle choices, or decision to be a sex worker.
Women have rape fantasies and want to be raped.	Reality and fantasy are different. Rape is always an act of violence on the part of the perpetrator, not sexual expression.
Only attractive women are raped.	Anyone can be raped, and since rape is an act of violence, attractiveness is not a relevant factor.
It is only rape if the victim is physically forced into sex and receives visible injuries.	During a rape, the victim may not be able to move or speak. Victims may or may not have injuries that aren't visible, but it doesn't mean they weren't assaulted. Rapists frequently use weapons or verbal threats to take control of the victim. Rapists may also use coercion or other nonviolent tactics during rape.

Rape Crisis Organization. (2022). *Myths vs facts.* https://rapecrisis.org.uk/get-informed/about-sexual-violence/myths-vs-realities/;
Tilton, E. C. R. (2022). Rape myths, catastrophe, and credibility. *Episteme.* https://www.cambridge.org/core/journals/episteme/article/rape-myths-catastrophe-and-credibility/9ED6425DB68E14C76B5EA28DF98F9551

Rapes are physically and emotionally devastating for the victims. Survivors of both acquaintance rape and rape committed by strangers report similar levels of depression, anxiety, complications in subsequent relationships, and difficulty attaining sexual satisfaction. Despite the violation and reality of physical and emotional trauma, victims of acquaintance rape often do not identify their experience as sexual assault. Many do not report the rape because they may have feelings of guilt (especially if drinking or drug use were involved), be confused if the act was consensual or forced, and feel it is only rape if the perpetrator is a stranger (Wiemann & Miller, 2022). Due to these feelings and the fact that eight out of 10 sexual assaults occur by someone the victims know, the Rape, Abuse, & Incest National Network suggests avoiding the potentially confusing labeling of rape as "date rape" or "acquaintance rape" and instead plainly naming the crime: rape (RAINN, 2023b).

A rapist might use alcohol or other drugs to sedate their victim (though rape does not always involve drugs). In 1996, the U.S. federal government passed a law making it a felony to give an unsuspecting person a "spiked substance" with the intent of raping them. Rape drugs are also known as "club drugs" because they are often used at venues such as nightclubs, fraternity parties, and all-night raves. The most common is Rohypnol (also known as "roofies," "forget pills," "mind erasers," or the "drop drug"). It comes in the form of a liquid or pill that quickly dissolves in liquid with no odor, taste, or color. This drug is 10 times as strong as diazepam (Valium). The effects can be felt within 30 minutes and produce memory loss for up to 8 hours. Gamma hydroxybutyrate (GHB; colloquially known as "liquid ecstasy" or "easy lay") is a liquid depressant that produces euphoria, an out-of-body high, sleepiness, increased sex drive, and memory loss. GHB takes effect in about 15 minutes and can last 3 to 4 hours. It comes in a white powder or liquid and may cause unconsciousness, depression, and coma. The third rape drug, ketamine (known as "special K," "vitamin K," or "super acid"), acts on the central nervous system very quickly to separate perception and sensation. Combining alcohol with these drugs can make the effects even stronger and in some cases fatal (Office on Women's Health, 2021). Rape drugs are dangerous, and people must be taught their use is unacceptable and harmful; in the meantime, there are a variety of ways people can protect themselves against rape drugs (Teaching Guidelines 9.2).

Rape Recovery

Recovery for rape survivors is an individual process with variable timing for healing. It may take weeks, months, or years to heal from their traumatic experiences. Some people never heal or get professional counseling, but most develop ways to cope. It may be challenging, but sharing their story can help victims in the healing process. Identifying people in their life who believe and support them is another helpful step toward healing. Rape is viewed as a situational crisis that the survivor is unprepared to handle because it is an unforeseen event.

A significant proportion of those who are raped also experience symptoms of **posttraumatic stress disorder (PTSD)**. PTSD develops when an event outside the range of normal human experience occurs that produces marked distress in the person. Symptoms of PTSD are divided into four groups:

1. Intrusion (reexperiencing the trauma, including nightmares, flashbacks, and recurrent thoughts)
2. Avoidance (avoiding trauma-related stimuli, social withdrawal, emotional numbing)
3. Hyperarousal (increased emotional arousal, exaggerated startle response, irritability)
4. Cognitive and mood symptoms (negative thoughts, depression, excessive guilt, and self-blame) (Sareen, 2022)

Not every victim of rape develops full-blown or even minor PTSD. Symptoms usually begin within 3 months of the incident but occasionally may only emerge years later. They must last more than a month to be considered PTSD. The condition varies from person to person. Some people recover within months, while others have symptoms for much longer.

TEACHING GUIDELINES 9.2 Protecting Oneself Against Spiked Substances

While society must work to shift to educate people not to harm each other, those who may be harmed must continue to be taught how to protect themselves. Tips to avoid getting drugged include:

- Pour your own drinks.
- Stick with your friends at parties and ask for help if you start feeling odd.
- Leave your cell phone on so your location can be traced.
- Be vigilant if you are drinking with strangers.
- Don't leave a party with someone you don't know.
- Never leave a drink of any kind unattended.
- Don't accept a drink from someone else.
- Only accept drinks from a bartender or in a closed container.
- If a drink is left unattended, pour it out, and don't drink it.
- Don't drink anything that tastes or smells strange.
- Don't drink beverages served from a punch bowl.
- If you think someone drugged you, call 911.

Office on Women's Health. (2021). *Date rape drugs*. https://www.womenshealth.gov/a-z-topics/date-rape-drugs

Nursing Care of Rape Victims

Health care providers, along with sexual assault nurse examiners (SANEs), can make a difference in the lives of survivors by understanding the facts, the effects this violence can have on mental and physical health, where to find information for themselves and their patients, and how to properly care for a survivor. A SANE is a registered nurse specially trained to conduct sexual assault evidentiary examinations for rape victims. In addition to the collection of forensic evidence, they may provide access to crisis intervention, STI testing, and emergency contraception.

Rape survivors undergo profound and complex trauma. The survivor should be provided with a safe and comfortable environment for a forensic examination. Nursing care of the rape survivor should focus on providing supportive care, collecting and documenting evidence, assessing for STIs, preventing pregnancy, and assessing for PTSD. Once initial treatment and evidence collection have been completed, follow-up care should include counseling, medical treatment, and crisis intervention. There is mounting evidence that early intervention and immediate counseling can accelerate a rape survivor's recovery (Buchanan, 2023). Clinical Judgment & Nursing Process 9.1 highlights a sample plan of care for a victim of rape.

TAKE NOTE!

Many rape survivors seek treatment in the hospital emergency department if no rape crisis center is available. Unfortunately, many emergency department doctors and nurses have little training in how to treat rape survivors or in collecting evidence. To make matters worse, if survivors have to wait for hours in public waiting rooms, they may leave the hospital, never receiving treatment or supplying the evidence needed to arrest and convict their assailants if they decide to take legal action.

CLINICAL JUDGMENT & NURSING PROCESS 9.1 Overview of the Patient Who Is a Victim of Rape

Lucy, a 20-year-old college junior, was admitted to the emergency room after police found her when a passerby called 911 to report an assault. She stated, "I was raped at a fraternity party a few hours ago. The stranger found me when I was walking back to my dorm room." Assessment reveals the following: numerous cuts and bruises of varying sizes on her face, arms, and legs; lip swollen and cut; right eye swollen and bruised; jacket and shirt ripped and bloodied; hair matted with grass and debris; vital signs within acceptable parameters; patient tearful, clutching her clothing, and trembling; perineal bruising and tearing.

NURSING ANALYSIS: Acute psychological trauma related to recent sexual assault

OUTCOME IDENTIFICATION AND EVALUATION

Patient will demonstrate adequate coping skills related to the effects of rape as evidenced by her ability to discuss the event, verbalize her feelings and fears, and exhibit appropriate actions to return to her precrisis level of functioning.

INTERVENTIONS: *Promoting Adequate Coping Skills*

- Stay with the patient *to promote feelings of safety.*
- Explain the procedures to be completed based on the facility's policy *to help alleviate patient's fear of the unknown.*
- Assist with physical examination for specimen collection *to obtain evidence for legal proceedings.*
- Administer prophylactic medication as ordered *to prevent pregnancy and STIs.*
- Provide care to wounds as ordered *to prevent infection.*
- Assist patient with hygiene measures as necessary *to promote self-esteem.*
- Allow patient to describe the events as much as possible *to encourage ventilation of feelings about the incident*; engage in active listening and offer nonjudgmental support *to facilitate coping and demonstrate understanding of the patient's situation and feelings.*
- Help the patient identify positive coping skills and personal strengths used in the past *to aid in effective decision making.*
- Assist patient in developing additional coping strategies and teach patient relaxation techniques *to help deal with the current crisis and anxiety.*
- Contact the rape counselor in the facility *to help the patient deal with the crisis.*
- Arrange for follow-up visit with the rape counselor *to provide continued care and to promote continuity of care.*
- Encourage the patient to contact a close friend, partner, or family member *to accompany her home to provide support.*
- Provide the patient with the telephone number of a counseling service or community support groups *to help her cope and obtain ongoing support.*
- Provide written instructions related to follow-up appointments, care, and testing *to ensure adequate understanding.*

PROVIDING SUPPORTIVE CARE

Establishing a therapeutic and trusting relationship will help the survivor describe their experience. Take the victim to a secure, isolated area away from family, friends, and other patients and staff so they can be open and honest when asked about the assault. Provide a change of clothes, access to a shower and toiletries, and a private waiting area for family and friends.

COLLECTING AND DOCUMENTING EVIDENCE

The victim should be instructed to bring all clothing, especially undergarments, worn at the time of the assault to the medical facility. The victim should not shower or bathe before presenting for care. Typically, a SANE will collect the evidence from the victim.

ASSESSING FOR SEXUALLY TRANSMITTED INFECTIONS

As part of the assessment, a pelvic examination will be done on females to collect vaginal secretions to rule out any STIs. This examination can be emotionally stressful for many patients and should be carried out gently and sensitively, explaining every step of the process to minimize further emotional trauma.

PREVENTING PREGNANCY

An essential element in the care of rape survivors involves offering them pregnancy prevention. After unprotected intercourse, including rape, pregnancy can be prevented by using an emergency contraceptive pill, sometimes called postcoital contraception or the "morning-after pill." Emergency contraceptive pills involve high doses of the same oral contraceptives that millions of people take every day. The emergency regimen consists of one dose taken within 72 to 120 hours of the unprotected intercourse. Emergency contraception works by preventing ovulation, fertilization, or implantation. Emergency contraception is most effective if it is taken within 12 hours of the rape; it becomes less effective with every 12 hours of delay thereafter.

ASSESSING FOR PTSD

Nurses can begin to assess the extent to which a survivor is suffering from PTSD by asking the following questions:

- To assess the presence of intrusive thoughts:
  - Do upsetting thoughts and nightmares of the trauma bother you?
  - Do you feel as though you are actually reliving the trauma?

- Does it upset you to be exposed to anything that reminds you of that event?
- To assess the presence of avoidance reactions:
  - Do you find yourself trying to avoid thinking or talking about the trauma?
  - Do you stay away from situations, people, or places that remind you of the event?
  - Do you have trouble recalling exactly what happened?
  - Do you feel emotionally numb, detached, negative beliefs about yourself and the world around you, and/or a persistent negative state?
- To assess the presence of physical symptoms:
  - Are you having trouble sleeping?
  - Have you demonstrated reckless or self-destructive behavior?
  - Do you have feelings of needing to protect yourself at all times?
  - Have you felt irritable or experienced outbursts of anger?
  - Do you have problems concentrating?
  - Do you have an extreme startle response? (Anxiety & Depression Association of America [ADAA], 2023).

With a growing body of knowledge about rape-related PTSD, help is available through most rape crisis and trauma centers. Support groups have been established where survivors can meet regularly to share experiences to help relieve the symptoms of PTSD. For some survivors, medication prescribed along with therapy is the best combination to relieve the pain. Just as in the treatment of any other illness, at the first opportunity, the victim should be encouraged to talk about the traumatic experience. This provides a chance to receive needed support and comfort, as well as an opportunity to begin processing the experience. In order to have a better understanding of the aftermath of criminal victimization such as sexual assault, nurses must begin to accept the reality that crime can happen to anyone regardless of the precautions that are taken to prevent it. Nurses must also understand that a victim's life is often turned upside down when they become a victim of crime. In order to help victims trust society again and regain a sense of balance and self-worth, nurses must educate all those who come in contact with victims and survivors to be sensitive to their needs.

Female Genital Cutting

Violence affects women and girls throughout the world and crosses cultural and economic boundaries. One major indicator of gender inequality is **female genital mutilation/cutting (FGM/C)**, sometimes called female circumcision. Like other forms of gender-based violence, FGM/C is pervasive and cannot be eradicated solely through laws criminalizing it. Universal awareness of this practice and consciousness raising must occur. This practice threatens the rights of young girls to health, life, self-determination, bodily integrity, and freedom from violence (American College of Nurse Midwives, 2022). FGM/C is often correlated with child marriage, forced sexual experience, and health complications throughout the lifespan. FGM/C involves any injury of the external female genitalia for cultural or nontherapeutic reasons. It confers severe health consequences for girls and women. The international community views this practice as a human rights violation, and it is considered an extreme form of discrimination against women. This practice is a grave form of violence and torture against women and girls. It violates the fundamental sexual and reproductive health rights of its victims (WHO, 2024b). The category of FGM/C is determined by the surgical removal of a portion or portions of the genitalia of female infants, girls, and women. See Box 9.5 for the major types of FGM/C procedures classified by the WHO. FGM/C is a worldwide practice that affects millions of women and girls. According to the WHO (2024b), 230 million women are victims of FGM/C. It is practiced routinely in over 25 countries, including countries in Africa, the Middle East, Asia, Eastern Europe, and Latin America. Prevalence in Sudan and Egypt has been estimated to be as high as 88% to 90% (United Nations Population Fund, 2024). The exact origins of FGM/C are not known. Although FGM/C may be interwoven into a particular culture, it is not mandated by any religion. All the reasons FGM/C is practiced appear to be cultural, traditional, and not rooted in any religious texts (WHO, 2024b). In some cultures, it is associated with feminine beauty and often signifies a rite of passage from childhood to adulthood.

FGM/C is performed for supposed reasons including decreasing a woman's sexual desires and ensuring her chastity until marriage, preserving fertility, ensuring

BOX 9.5 Four Major Types of Female Genital Cutting Procedures

- *Type I:* Excision of the prepuce with excision of part or the entire clitoris
- *Type II:* Excision of the clitoris and part or all of the labia minora with or without removal of labia majora
- *Type III (Infibulation):* Excision of all or part of the external genitalia and stitching/narrowing of the vaginal opening (narrows the vaginal opening by creating a covering seal)
- *Type IV:* All other harmful procedures on the genitals such as pricking, piercing, or incision of the clitoris or labia
  - Stretching of the clitoris and/or labia
  - Cauterizing by burning the clitoris and surrounding tissues
  - Scraping or cutting the vaginal orifice
  - Introduction of a corrosive substance into the vagina
  - Placing herbs into the vagina to narrow it

World Health Organization. (2024b). *Female genital mutilation.* https://www.who.int/news-room/fact-sheets/detail/female-genital-mutilation

marriageability, improving hygiene, and enhancing sexual pleasure for males (Nour, 2024). However, this practice has no health benefits and leads to a range of serious health complications. Notable complications include physical, psychological, social, and sexual harms to people who undergo this procedure. Complications vary, depending on the type of cutting and the way it was performed. It is frequently performed without anesthesia under nonsterile conditions. Cutting tools can be anything from razor blades to knives to pieces of glass or tin can lids. Complications can include infertility, dysmenorrhea, dyspareunia, sexual dysfunction, infection, hemorrhage after the procedure, vaginal stenosis, chronic vaginitis, pelvic inflammatory disease, urinary complications such as urinary retention and chronic urinary tract infections, and difficulty in giving birth (Nour, 2024). The most common long-term complication is the formation of inclusion clitoral dermoid cysts and labial fusion. These can become as large as a grapefruit and can lead to difficulty in walking and sitting, sometimes causing psychological distress from the deformity. The psychological effects include anxiety, flashbacks, depression, PTSD, and physical complaints such as headaches and pain that have no other physiologic cause (United Nations Population Fund, 2024).

TAKE NOTE!

From a Western perspective, FGM/C may be hard to comprehend. However, many females who have undergone FGM/C may not consider it to be mutilation and may not understand that females in other regions do not have this done. Health care providers need to understand this and be sensitive to their patients' experiences, taking a nonjudgmental approach when discussing FGM/C (Nour, 2024).

Since FGM/C has no health benefits and often leaves women with lifelong physical and emotional trauma, there is a human rights justification to end the practice. The U.S. government opposes FGM/C, and it is against the law to perform it on a child under 18 (U.S. Citizenship and Immigration Services, 2024). International pressure to end FGM/C has been mounting since 1997, when the WHO, United Nations Children's Fund (UNICEF), and United Nations Population Fund (UNFPA) issued a joint statement to call on governments to ban the practice. In 2008, the WHO passed a resolution on the elimination of FGM/C (Schadewald, 2022; WHO, 2024b; United Nations Children's Fund, 2024).

Nursing Care of the Patient Who Has Experienced FGM/C

As immigration to the United States increases, nurses are increasingly likely to encounter patients affected by FGM/C and its complications. The psychological pressure and trauma of living within two cultures and feeling different may weigh heavily on the patient in a new setting where FGM/C is foreign and banned. Nurses need updated education regarding women who have undergone FGM/C so that appropriate care for this population can be provided for this very sensitive health care problem. Well-informed nurses represent the best opportunity to provide culturally sensitive care to this population. Nurses are in a unique position to contact and educate patients who have been cut or are at risk for FGM/C. To advocate for these patients, a thorough understanding of the practice of FGM/C, its cultural significance, physical implications, and psychosocial effects is needed.

Helping patients who have had an FGM/C procedure requires good communication skills and often an interpreter since many may not speak the nurse's language. Nurses are educated to provide comprehensive, culturally sensitive care regardless of the patient's circumstances. Nurses must keep in mind that FGM/C is considered normal in many cultures and, for the patient, to not have it done may be unthinkable. Nurses have the opportunity to educate patients by providing accurate information and positive health care experiences. Make sure that you are comfortable with and aware of your own feelings about this practice before dealing with patients. Some guidelines include:

- Let the patient know you are concerned and interested and want to help.
- Speak clearly and slowly, using simple, accurate terms.
- Use the term or name for this practice that the recipient uses, not "female genital cutting" or "mutilation."
- Use pictures and diagrams to help the patient understand what you are saying.
- Be patient in allowing the patient to answer questions.
- Include male family members in any education, as they are influential in this practice.
- Repeat back your understanding of the patient's statements.
- Always look and talk directly to the patient, not the interpreter.
- Do not express judgment of the practice.
- Use trauma-sensitive language.
- Ensure the patient's privacy throughout the examination.
- Maintain respect for older people who have experienced FGM/C.
- Encourage the patient to express themselves freely.
- Maintain strict confidentiality.
- Provide culturally attuned care to all patients.

In short, FGM/C is a form of violence against women, and it is only through the education and empowerment of women that the practice can be reduced or eliminated.

This practice often defines a woman within her culture and becomes a part of her identity; nurses must understand this to be able to assist women who have undergone FGM/C. Nurses are in a unique position to contact and educate women who have been cut or are at risk for mutilation. Only through intense education will the next generation of girls be saved from this practice.

Human Trafficking

Human trafficking is a global crime in which people are traded and exploited for profit. The United Nations defines **human trafficking** as "the recruitment, transportation, transfer, harboring, or receipt of persons by means of threat or use of force, or other forms of coercion, abduction, fraud, or deception for the purpose of exploitation" (United Nations Office on Drugs and Crime [UNODC], 2023). Victims of trafficking can be any age, any sex or gender, and from anywhere in the world. Globally, one in three victims is a child (UNODC, 2023). Human trafficking is a global phenomenon to which no country is immune.

In the United States, forced labor is predominantly found in these sectors:

- Private-sector industries (63%)
- State-imposed forced labor (14%)
- Commercial sexual exploitation (23%) (Tracy & Macias-Konstantopoulos, 2023)

Human trafficking responds to and is driven by demand, and this demand persists at the expense of many vulnerable women and girls. Consider this scenario: A girl who was just 14 years old was held captive in a tiny trailer room, where she was forced to have sex with as many as 30 men a day. On her nightstand was a teddy bear that reminded her of her childhood in Mexico from where people abducted her and forced her into sexual slavery.

This scenario describes human trafficking, the enslavement of humans for profit. Within U.S. borders, thousands of foreign nationals and U.S. citizens, many of them children, are forced or coerced into sex work or various forms of labor every year (Polaris Project Organization, 2024a, 2024b). Human trafficking is both a global problem and a domestic problem. The United States is a major receiver of trafficked people. It wasn't made illegal in the United States until 2000. Any person is at risk for human trafficking, but people in certain populations have a higher vulnerability (Toney-Butler et al., 2023).

Women and children are the primary victims of human trafficking, many in the sex trade and others through forced-labor domestic servitude (Toney-Butler et al., 2023). This includes young people, particularly girls 12 to 16 years old. Risk of being a victim of human trafficking is increased by poverty; increased psychiatric complexity; being a member of a historically marginalized community; living in a rural location; low education level; disability; inadequate family support or protection; history of running away from home; identification as LGBTQIA+; recent migration; being a survivor of child abuse, sexual abuse, or IPV; and exposure to violence in the community or gang violence (Toney-Butler et al., 2023; Tracy & Macias-Konstantopoulos, 2023).

Trafficking people is hugely profitable: One estimate places global profits at approximately $150 billion annually (Toney-Butler et al., 2023). Some believe trafficking surpasses the market value of drug dealing (Toney-Butler et al., 2023). The United States is a profitable destination country for traffickers, and these profits contribute to the development of organized criminal enterprises worldwide. To help combat human trafficking, the Victims of Trafficking and Violence Protection Act of 2000 (U.S. Department of Justice, 2023) established the three Ps: protection, prevention, and prosecution.

Victims of human trafficking are exposed to serious and numerous health risks such as violence, rape, torture, physical injuries such as cigarette burns and bruises or fractures, PTSD, pregnancy, HIV/AIDS, STIs, cervical cancer, hazardous work environments, dehydration and malnourishment, and alcohol and substance use disorder (Toney-Butler et al., 2023; Tracy & Macias-Konstantopoulos, 2023). Health care is one of the most pressing needs of these victims. No nurse is immune to encountering a trafficking victim, and nurses need to be prepared to respond appropriately. Respect and openness are the bedrock of a nurse's interactions with victims to make them feel safer to talk. Nurses should be aware of the warning signs and recognize victims who require further investigation. Nurses and other health care providers who encounter victims of trafficking often do not realize they are being trafficked, and opportunities to intervene are lost. The challenge for nurses is identifying and helping victims because most victims fear the consequences they will face if they disclose their circumstances. Although no one sign can demonstrate with certainty when someone is being trafficked, clinicians should be aware of certain indicators. It is important to be alert for trafficking victims in any setting and to recognize cues (Box 9.6).

Nursing interventions in the care of trafficking victims include:

- Building trust as the top priority
- Knowing the at-risk groups for trafficking in the community
- Observing the relationship between the patient and the accompanying person
- Taking the time to listen and develop a rapport
- Screening in a private place to ensure confidentiality and safety
- Reassuring the potential victim
- Providing one-on-one interactions
- Thoroughly examining all injuries, even if they seem unintentional

BOX 9.6 Identifying Victims of Human Trafficking

Look beneath the surface and ask yourself: Is this person…
- A female or a child in poor health?
- Foreign-born and not an English speaker?
- Not registered in local schools?
- Displaying closed body language; e.g., avoiding eye contact?
- Nervous, fearful, withdrawn, submissive, or depressed?
- Dressed in ill-fitting clothing?
- Giving the appearance of being coached on what to say?
- In possession of few personal belongings?
- Experiencing problems with their jaw or neck?
- Displaying signs of neglect, malnourishment, or physical abuse?
- Presenting with debris in their vagina or rectum?
- Vague about their address or where they live?
- "Marked" with tattoos on their neck or other types of branding?
- Lacking immigration documents?
- Lacking control of money, identification, or passport?
- Refusing to change into a gown and/or cooperate with a physical exam?
- Giving an inconsistent explanation of injury?
- Exhibiting behavior that doesn't align with injury or complaint?
- Refusing treatment that takes place during a follow-up appointment?
- Reluctant to give any information about self, injury, home, or work?
- Fearful of authority figure or "sponsor" if present? ("Sponsor" might not leave victim alone with health care provider.)
- Living with the employer?

Sample questions to ask the potential victim of human trafficking:
- Can you leave your job or situation if you wish?
- Can you come and go as you please?
- Have you been threatened if you try to leave?
- Has anyone threatened your family with harm if you leave?
- What are your working and living conditions?
- Do you have to ask permission to go to the bathroom, eat, or sleep?
- Is there a lock on your door so you cannot get out?
- What brought you to the United States? Is your situation now in line with those plans?
- Are you free to leave your current work or home situation?
- Who has your immigration papers? Why don't you have them?
- Are you paid for the work you do?
- Are there times you feel afraid?
- How can your situation be changed?

U.S. Department of Homeland Security. (2023). *Identifying a victim.* https://www.dhs.gov/blue-campaign/identify-victim; Morris, G. (2022). How nurses can recognize and report human trafficking. *Nurse Journal.* https://nursejournal.org/articles/how-nurses-recognize-and-report-human-trafficking/; Association of Women's Health, Obstetric and Neonatal Nurses. (2022). Position statement: Human trafficking. *Journal of Obstetric, Gynecologic, & Neonatal Nursing, 51*(6), E1–E3. https://www.jognn.org/article/S0884-2175(22)00321-5/fulltext

- Assessing hydration, nutrition, and hygiene
- Not relying on the patient's interpreter if English isn't spoken
- Specifically asking about the patient's safety
- Offering paraphrased stories to clarify and therapeutically reflect the patient's statements
- Staying calm and on an even keel
- Understanding the risk these victims are taking by disclosing their plight
- Documenting your suspicion in your notes
- Calling the human trafficking hotline for guidance at 1-866-US-TIPLINE

Human trafficking is a violation of human rights. It is an unconscionable attack on the dignity of vulnerable people. Nurses are one of the few groups of professionals likely to interact with trafficked victims while they are still in captivity. They have the opportunity to screen, identify, intervene, and rescue these victims. Nurses are well positioned to identify and assist trafficked individuals as well as those who may be at risk for exploitation. If you suspect a trafficking situation, notify local law enforcement and a regional social service organization that has experience in dealing with trafficking victims. It is imperative to reach out to these victims and stop the cycle of abuse by following through on your suspicions. Nurses can also reach out within their communities to bring about awareness through community education about human trafficking to increase pressure on the government to take action to stop it.

Across the world, in communities both large and small, individual stories of suffering and injustice make up the ugly mosaic of human trafficking. No matter the impetus, nurses are not defenseless in the fight against human trafficking. Rather, they are a powerful part of the solution.

Trauma-Informed Care

Every patient is a potential trauma survivor. Nurses should approach all patient encounters with trauma-informed care (TIC) (Tracy & Macias-Konstantopoulos, 2023). Trauma includes any experience that causes an intense psychological or physical reaction. Trauma has no boundaries and can impact anyone. Traumatic events can include IPV, sexual assault, childhood abuse, discrimination, adverse childbirth experience, natural disasters, wars, separation from family, or any other harmful experiences (Nurse Practitioners in Women's Health [NPWH], 2022). Trauma can have a powerful influence on a person's health and well-being. Aggregates exposed to discrimination at individual and systemic levels include those from underrepresented groups, LGBTQIA+ people, people with disabilities, people with higher body weight, and people living in poverty. Inequalities place people in these groups at increased risk of exposure to trauma.

Trauma survivors may suffer an array of symptoms including depression, mood swings, fearfulness, anxiety, agitation, irritability, insomnia, poor concentration levels, anger outbursts, flashbacks, poor trusting ability, and an overall disconnectedness (NPWH, 2022). Traumatized people experience difficulties accessing medical care, following through with treatment plans, and feeling safe when receiving care.

TIC is an essential ingredient of evidence-based treatment, so nurses should be utilizing it when caring for their patients. This approach to providing health care recognizes that trauma impacts a person's life (Tracy & Macias-Konstantopoulos, 2023). Nurses need to recognize that many patient experiences or nursing interventions have the potential to retraumatize a trauma victim (NPWH, 2022). Key components in implementing TIC are to avoid reinjury by developing settings that ensure the patient's physical and emotional safety; empower the patient and emphasize survivor strengths and resilience; aid empowerment, healing, and recovery; and promote the development of survivorship skills (Tracy & Macias-Konstantopoulos, 2023). Examples of ways the nurse can incorporate TIC include obtaining permission from the patient prior to touching them and allowing the patient to remain clothed until the physical exam is performed and then providing appropriate cover during the exam when possible (Tracy & Macias-Konstantopoulos, 2023).

SUMMARY

The causes of violence against women are complex. Previously, violence against women was largely invisible and was even considered natural and trivial. Many people did not consider intimate or community violence against women to be a human rights violation. Raising awareness and developing evidence-based programs, practices, and policies to prevent IPV and sexual assault are essential in stopping violent behavior before it starts. Many women will experience some type of violence in their lives, and it can have a debilitating effect on their health and future relationships. Nurses have the skills, professional experience, and perspective to be an important part of comprehensive violence prevention efforts in communities. Violence frequently leaves a legacy of pain to future generations. Nurses can empower women and encourage them and provide resources to assist them in taking control of their lives. When women live in peace and security, free from violence, they have an enormous potential to contribute to their own communities and to the national and global society. Nurses can play an important role in working toward reducing violence in the community, but they must first become informed. Nurses must insist that health care agencies that employ them accept this responsibility and work together to reach out to those being abused. The time is ripe for nurses to act and ensure serious inroads are made in improving the health and well-being of all women across the world.

Violence against women is not normal, legal, or acceptable, and it should never be tolerated or justified. It can and must be stopped by the entire world community. Early education and prevention provide the best hope for creating healthy futures and fostering a global society without violence. As a global society, nurses have the opportunity and responsibility to address violence to effectively intervene within families, schools, and communities to inject resiliency, help, and healing.

KEY CONCEPTS

- Violence against women is a major public health and social problem because it violates a woman's human rights and causes numerous mental and physical health sequelae.
- Every woman has the potential to become a victim of violence.
- There are Healthy People 2030 objectives that focus on reducing the rate of physical and sexual assaults.
- Abuse may be emotional, physical, or sexual in nature, or it may be a combination of all of these.
- The cycle of violence includes four phases: tension building, incidence of violence, honeymoon/reconciliation, and period of calm.
- Pregnancy can precipitate violence toward the pregnant person or escalate it.
- Many people experience PTSD after being sexually assaulted. PTSD can inhibit a survivor from adapting or coping in a healthy manner.
- FGM/C is practiced worldwide, and nurses in the United States need to become knowledgeable about it and place no judgment on people who have undergone the practice.
- Human trafficking is a violation of human rights, and nurses who suspect it should report it to stop the cycle of abuse against vulnerable people.
- The nurse's role in dealing with survivors of violence is to establish rapport; open up lines of communication; apply the nursing process to assess and screen all patients in all settings; and implement and intervene as appropriate.

Unfolding Patient Stories: Brenda Patton • Part 1

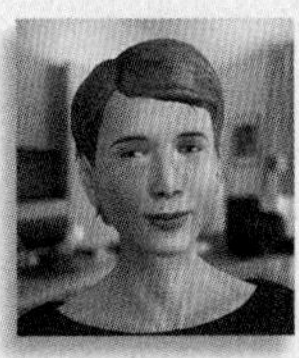

Brenda Patton is 18 years old and pregnant with her first child. When her live-in boyfriend accompanies her to a prenatal visit, the nurse notices that Brenda seems nervous around him. Brenda also has some bruises on her arm. Explain what the nurse should do if she suspects IPV. What counseling and resource information should the nurse provide to Brenda in this situation? (Brenda Patton's story continues in Chapter 10.)

Care for Brenda and other patients in a realistic virtual environment: ***vSim** for Nursing* (thepoint.lww.com/vSimMaternity). Practice documenting these patients' care in DocuCare (**thepoint.lww.com/DocuCareEHR**).

REFERENCES AND RECOMMENDED READINGS

AbiNader, M. A., Graham, L. M., & Kafka, J. M. (2023). Examining intimate partner violence-related fatalities: Past lessons and future directions using U.S. National Data. *Journal of Family Violence, 38*, 1–12. Advance online publication. https://doi.org/10.1007/s10896-022-00487-2

Agarwal, S., Prasad, R., Mantri, S., Chandrakar, R., Gupta, S., Babhulkar, V., Srivastav, S., Jaiswal, A., & Wanjari, M. B. (2023). A comprehensive review of intimate partner violence during pregnancy and its adverse effects on maternal and fetal health. *Cureus, 15*(5), e39262. https://doi.org/10.7759/cureus.39262

American College of Nurse Midwives. (2022). *Position statement: Female genital cutting*. https://www.midwife.org/acnm/files/acnmlibrarydata/uploadfilename/000000000068/2022_ps_female-genital-cutting.pdf

Anxiety & Depression Association of America. (2023). *Screening for posttraumatic stress disorder (PTSD)*. https://adaa.org/screening-posttraumatic-stress-disorder-ptsd

Association of Women's Health, Obstetric and Neonatal Nurses. (2022). Position statement: Human trafficking. *Journal of Obstetric, Gynecologic, & Neonatal Nursing, 51*(6), E1–E3. https://www.jognn.org/article/S0884-2175(22)00321-5/fulltext

Basile, K. C., Smith, S. G., Kresnow, M., Khatiwada, S., & Leemis, R. W. (2022). *The National Intimate Partner and Sexual Violence Survey: 2016/2017 report on sexual violence*. National Center for Injury Prevention and Control, Centers for Disease Control and Prevention. https://www.cdc.gov/violenceprevention/pdf/nisvs/nisvsReportonSexualViolence.pdf

Boyland, C. M., & Berishaj, K. A. (2022). Intimate partner violence. In K. D. Schuiling & F. E. Likis (Eds.), *Gynecologic health care* (4th ed., pp. 303–325). Jones & Bartlett Learning.

Buchanan, J. A. (2023). Patient education: Care after sexual assault (beyond the basics). *UpToDate*. Retrieved May 9, 2024, from https://www.uptodate.com/contents/care-after-sexual-assault-beyond-the-basics

Campbell, J. C., Webster, D. W., & Glass, N. (2009). The danger assessment: Validation of a lethality risk assessment instrument for intimate partner femicide. *Journal of Interpersonal Violence, 24*(4), 653–674. https://doi.org/10.1177/0886260508317180

Centers for Disease Control and Prevention. (2022a). *Preventing child abuse and neglect*. https://www.cdc.gov/child-abuse-neglect/prevention/index.html

Centers for Disease Control and Prevention. (2022b). *Preventing sexual violence*. https://www.cdc.gov/sexual-violence/prevention/index.html

Centers for Disease Control and Prevention. (2024a). *Fast facts: About intimate partner violence*. https://www.cdc.gov/intimate-partner-violence/about/

Centers for Disease Control and Prevention. (2024b). *About sexual violence*. https://www.cdc.gov/sexual-violence/about/index.html

Clifton, E. G. (2022). Medical examination of the sexual assault victim. *MSD Manual*. https://www.msdmanuals.com/professional/gynecology-and-obstetrics/domestic-violence-and-sexual-assault/medical-examination-of-the-sexual-assault-victim?mredirectid=2116

Connections for Abused Women and their Children. (2023). *What is the cycle of abuse?* https://www.cawc.org/news/what-is-the-cycle-of-abuse/

D'Angelo, D. V., Bombard, J. M., Lee, R. D., Kortsmit, K., Kapaya, M., & Fasula, A. (2022). Prevalence of experiencing physical, emotional, and sexual violence by a current intimate partner during pregnancy: Population-based estimates from the pregnancy risk assessment monitoring system. *Journal of Family Violence, 38*, 117–126. https://doi.org/10.1007/s10896-022-00356-y

Das, K. J. H., Peitzmeier, S., Berrahou, I. K., & Potter, J. (2022). Intimate partner violence (IPV) screening and referral outcomes among transgender patients in a primary care setting. *Journal of Interpersonal Violence, 37*(13–14). https://doi.org/10.1177/0886260521997460

Domestic Violence Action Center. (n.d.). *Common myths about domestic violence*. https://domesticviolenceactioncenter.org/common-myths/

Federal Bureau of Investigation. (2018). *Crime in the United States: Rape*. https://ucr.fbi.gov/crime-in-the-u.s/2018/crime-in-the-u.s.-2018/topic-pages/rape

Filipovic, J. (2023). *14 Misconceptions about domestic violence*. https://www.domesticshelters.org/articles/domestic-violence-op-ed-column/14-misconceptions-about-domestic-violence

Florida Council Against Sexual Violence. (2012). *How to screen your patients for sexual assault: A guide for health care professionals*. https://www.yumpu.com/en/document/read/44966841/view-full-booklet-florida-council-against-sexual-violence

Franchek-Roa, K. M. (2022). Intimate partner violence: Childhood exposure. *UpToDate*. Retrieved May 8, 2024, from https://www.uptodate.com/contents/intimate-partner-violence-childhood-exposure

Garcia-Vergara, E., Almeda, N., Fernández-Navarro, F., & Becerra-Alonso, D. (2022). Risk assessment instruments for intimate partner femicide: A systematic review. *Frontiers in Psychology, 13*, 896901. https://doi.org/10.3389/fpsyg.2022.896901

Guo, C., Wan, M., Wang, Y., Wang, P., Tousey-Pfarrer, M., Liu, H., Yu, L., Jian, L., Zhang, M., Yang, Z., Ge, F., & Zhang, J. (2023). Associations between intimate partner violence and adverse birth outcomes during pregnancy: A systematic review and meta-analysis. *Frontiers in Medicine, 10*. https://doi.org/10.3389/fmed.2023.1140787

Halphen, J. M. (2023). Elder abuse, self-neglect, and related phenomena. *UpToDate*. Retrieved May 8, 2023, from https://www.uptodate.com/contents/elder-abuse-self-neglect-and-related-phenomena

Healthy Alternatives to Violent Environments. (2022). *Safety planning*. https://www.havenstan.org/safety-planing

Huecker, M. R., King, K. C., Jordan, G. A., & Smock, W. (2023). Domestic violence. *StatPearls*. https://www.ncbi.nlm.nih.gov/books/NBK499891/

Kippert, A. (2023). *Profile of an abuser*. Domestic Shelters Organization. https://www.domesticshelters.org/articles/identifying-abuse/profile-of-an-abuser

Melmer, M. N. (2023). Child sexual abuse and neglect. *StatPearls*. https://www.statpearls.com/ArticleLibrary/viewarticle/19407

Morris, G. (2022). How nurses can recognize and report human trafficking. *Nurse Journal*. https://nursejournal.org/articles/how-nurses-recognize-and-report-human-trafficking/

Nienow, S. (2023). *Preventing child sexual abuse: What parents need to know*. American Academy of Pediatrics. https://

www.healthychildren.org/English/safety-prevention/at-home/Pages/Sexual-Abuse.aspx

Nour, N. M. (2024). Female genital cutting. *UpToDate*. Retrieved May 9, 2024, from https://www.uptodate.com/contents/female-genital-cutting

Nurse Practitioners in Women's Health. (2022). *Position statement: Trauma-informed care*. https://sigma.nursingrepository.org/server/api/core/bitstreams/97f98c62-6cd3-4923-a32b-ca79c6d0df1a/content

Office on Women's Health. (2021). *Date rape drugs*. https://www.womenshealth.gov/a-z-topics/date-rape-drugs

Office on Violence Against Women. (2023). *Domestic violence*. U.S. Department of Justice. https://www.justice.gov/ovw/domestic-violence

Polaris Project Organization. (2024a). *Understanding human trafficking*. https://polarisproject.org/understanding-human-trafficking/

Polaris Project Organization. (2024b). *Myths, facts, and statistics*. https://polarisproject.org/myths-facts-and-statistics/

Rape, Abuse, & Incest National Network. (2023a). *Scope of the problem: Statistics*. https://www.rainn.org/statistics/scope-problem

Rape, Abuse, & Incest National Network. (2023b). *Key terms and phrases*. https://www.rainn.org/articles/key-terms-and-phrases

Rape Crisis Organization. (2022). *Myths vs facts*. https://rapecrisis.org.uk/get-informed/about-sexual-violence/myths-vs-realities/

Rhodes, L. R. (2023). Addressing intimate partner violence with LGBTQ+ clients. *Counseling Today*. https://ctarchive.counseling.org/2023/06/addressing-intimate-partner-violence-with-lgbtq-clients/

Ricee, S. (2022). *Cycle of abuse: An overview and its effects on victims*. Diversity for Social Impact. https://diversity.social/cycle-of-abuse/#0-what-is-the-cycle-of-abuse-and-what-it-means-for-the-victims

Rowe, J., Chananna, J., Cunningham, S., & Harkness, K. L. (2022). Sexual, physical, and emotional maltreatment in childhood are differentially associated with sexual and physical revictimization in adulthood. *Journal of Interpersonal Violence*, *38*, 3806–3830. https://doi.org/10.1177/08862605221111411

Sareen, J. (2022). Posttraumatic stress disorder in adults: Epidemiology, pathophysiology, clinical features, assessment, and diagnosis. *UpToDate*. Retrieved May 9, 2024, from https://www.uptodate.com/contents/posttraumatic-stress-disorder-in-adults-epidemiology-pathophysiology-clinical-features-assessment-and-diagnosis

Schadewald, D. (2022). Perinatal considerations for women who have experienced type 3 female genital cutting/infibulation. *Women's Healthcare*, *10*(5), 37–42. https://doi.org/10.51256/WHC102237

Smith, M., & Segal, J. (2023). *Domestic violence and abuse*. Help Guide Organization. https://www.helpguide.org/articles/abuse/domestic-violence-and-abuse.htm

The White House. (2022). *Fact sheet: Reauthorization of the Violence Against Women Act (VAWA)*. https://www.whitehouse.gov/briefing-room/statements-releases/2022/03/16/fact-sheet-reauthorization-of-the-violence-against-women-act-vawa/

The White House. (2023). *U.S. National Plan to End Gender-Based Violence: Strategies for action*. https://www.whitehouse.gov/wp-content/uploads/2023/05/National-Plan-to-End-GBV.pdf

Thurston, R. C., Jakubowski, K. P., Wu, M., Aizenstein, H. J., Chang, Y., Derby, C. A., Koenen, K. C., Barinas-Mitchell, E., & Maki, P. M. (2022). Sexual assault and white matter hyperintensities among midlife women. *Brain Imaging and Behavior*, *16*(2), 773–780. https://doi.org/10.1007/s11682-021-00536-2

Tilton, E. C. R. (2022). Rape myths, catastrophe, and credibility. *Episteme*. https://www.cambridge.org/core/journals/episteme/article/rape-myths-catastrophe-and-credibility/9ED6425DB68E14C76B5EA28DF98F9551

Toney-Butler, T. J., Ladd, M., & Mittel, O. (2023). Human trafficking. *StatPearls*. https://www.ncbi.nlm.nih.gov/books/NBK430910/

Tracy, E. E., & Macias-Konstantopoulos, W. (2023). Human trafficking: Identification and evaluation in the health care setting. *UpToDate*. Retrieved May 10, 2024, from https://www.uptodate.com/contents/human-trafficking-identification-and-evaluation-in-the-health-care-setting

United Nations Children's Fund. (2024). *Female genital mutilation (FGM)*. https://data.unicef.org/topic/child-protection/female-genital-mutilation/

United Nations Office on Drugs and Crime. (2023). *Human trafficking FAQs*. https://www.unodc.org/unodc/en/human-trafficking/faqs.html

United Nations Population Fund. (2024). *Female genital mutilation (FGM) frequently asked questions*. https://www.unfpa.org/resources/female-genital-mutilation-fgm-frequently-asked-questions#whatisfgm

U.S. Citizenship and Immigration Services. (2024). *Female genital mutilation or cutting (FGM/C)*. https://www.uscis.gov/FGMC

U.S. Department of Health and Human Services. (n.d.). *Healthy People 2030 objectives*. https://health.gov/healthypeople

U.S. Department of Homeland Security. (2023). *Identifying a victim*. https://www.dhs.gov/blue-campaign/identify-victim

U.S. Department of Justice. (2023). *Key legislation*. https://www.justice.gov/humantrafficking/key-legislation#:

Wallace, M., Gillispie-Bell, V., Cruz, K., Davis, K., & Vilda, D. (2021). Homicide during pregnancy and the postpartum period in the United States, 2018-2019. *Obstetrics and Gynecology*, *138*(5), 762–769. https://doi.org/10.1097/AOG.0000000000004567

Whealin, J., & Barnett, E. (2022). *Child sexual abuse*. National Center for PTSD. https://www.ptsd.va.gov/professional/treat/type/sexual_abuse_child.asp

Weil, A. (2022). Intimate partner violence: Diagnosis and screening. *UpToDate*. Retrieved May 7, 2024, from https://www.uptodate.com/contents/intimate-partner-violence-diagnosis-and-screening

Weil, A. (2023). Intimate partner violence: Epidemiology and health consequences. *UpToDate*. Retrieved May 7, 2024, from https://www.uptodate.com/contents/intimate-partner-violence-epidemiology-and-health-consequences

Wiemann, C. M., & Miller, E. (2022). Date rape: Identification and management. *UpToDate*. Retrieved May 9, 2024, from https://www.uptodate.com/contents/date-rape-identification-and-management

Willie, T. C., Kershaw, T., & Sullivan, T. P. (2021). The impact of adverse childhood events on the sexual and mental health of women experiencing intimate partner violence. *Journal of*

Interpersonal Violence, 36(11–12), 5145–5166. https://doi.org/10.1177/0886260518802852

World Health Organization. (2022a). *Abuse of older people.* https://www.who.int/news-room/fact-sheets/detail/abuse-of-older-people

World Health Organization. (2022b). *Intimate partner violence.* https://apps.who.int/violence-info/intimate-partner-violence/

World Health Organization. (2024a). *Violence against women.* https://www.who.int/news-room/fact-sheets/detail/violence-against-women

World Health Organization. (2024b). *Female genital mutilation.* https://www.who.int/news-room/fact-sheets/detail/female-genital-mutilation

DEVELOPING CLINICAL JUDGMENT

PRACTICING FOR NCLEX

1. The nurse is working at a women's shelter. The primary goal of intervention in working with abused women is to
   a. set up an appointment with a mental health counselor for the victim.
   b. convince them to set up safety plans to use when they leave.
   c. help them develop courage and financial support to leave their abusers.
   d. empower them and improve their self-esteem to gain control of their lives.
2. The nurse is providing community education to a group of women. The nurse explains that the first phase of the abuse cycle is characterized by
   a. the victim provoking the abuser to bring about abuse.
   b. tension building and verbal or minor battery.
   c. a honeymoon period that lulls the victim into forgetting.
   d. an acute episode of physical abuse.
3. The nurse is teaching nursing students about caring for women who experience IPV. The nurse helps the students understand that women recovering from abusive relationships need to learn ways to improve their
   a. educational level by getting college degrees.
   b. earning power so they can move to better neighborhoods.
   c. self-esteem and communication skills to increase assertiveness.
   d. relationship skills so they will be better prepared to deal with their partners.
4. The nurse is caring for a woman who is the victim of violence in her home. Which statement might empower this woman to take action?
   a. "You don't deserve to be treated this way."
   b. "Your children deserve to grow up in a two-parent family."
   c. "Try to figure out what you do to trigger his abuse and stop it."
   d. "Give your partner more time to come to his senses about this."
5. Nurses play an important role in screening and assessment of any patient abuse or violence. Which statement is correct?
   a. Most patients are extremely reluctant to come forth with private matters.
   b. Any IPV questions should be asked in the presence of both partners.
   c. To invite disclosure, assure the woman that you won't document her statements.
   d. The best statement to make to the person experiencing abuse is, "You don't deserve this."
6. The nurse is caring for a patient whose history prompts suspicion of IPV. What should the nurse do if this patient chooses not to disclose information about her abusive relationship during the interview?
   a. Confront the victim with the physical evidence and telltale signs of abuse.
   b. Contact family members to tell you about the abusive relationship.
   c. Call the local police department to inquire about domestic disturbance calls.
   d. Respect the patient's right of self-determination and provide her with resources.
7. The nurse is caring for a new patient at the clinic. Which patient behavior would raise a "red flag" to the nurse that the patient may be a human trafficking victim?
   a. Looks nurse straight in the eyes when responding to questions
   b. Appears calm and cooperative during examination
   c. Acts like it is "no big deal," even with concerning injuries
   d. Changes into examination gown quickly without hesitation

CRITICAL THINKING EXERCISES

1. Mrs. Bennett has three children under the age of 5 and is 6 months pregnant with her fourth child. She has made repeated unscheduled visits to your clinic with vague somatic complaints regarding the children as well as herself but has missed several scheduled prenatal appointments. On occasion, she has worn sunglasses to cover bruises around her eyes. As a nurse, you sense there is something else bothering her, but she doesn't seem to want to discuss it with you. She appears sad and the children cling to her.
   a. Outline your conversation when you broach the subject of abuse with this patient.
   b. What is your role as a nurse in caring for a family in which you suspect abuse is occurring?
   c. What ethical and legal considerations are important in planning care for this family?

STUDY ACTIVITIES

1. Visit the *National Domestic Violence Hotline* website for victims of violence. Discuss what you discovered on this site and your reactions to it.
2. Research the statistics about violence against women in your state. Are law enforcement and community interventions reducing the incidence of sexual assault and intimate partner violence?

3. Attend a college dorm orientation at a local college to hear about measures in place to protect women's safety on campus. Find out the number of sexual assaults reported and what strategies the college uses to reduce this number.

4. Volunteer to spend a weekend evening at the local sheriff's department 911 hotline desk to observe the number and nature of calls received reporting intimate partner violence. Interview the dispatch operator about the frequency and trends of these calls.

5. Identify three community resources that could be useful to a victim of violence. Identify their sources of funding and the services they provide.

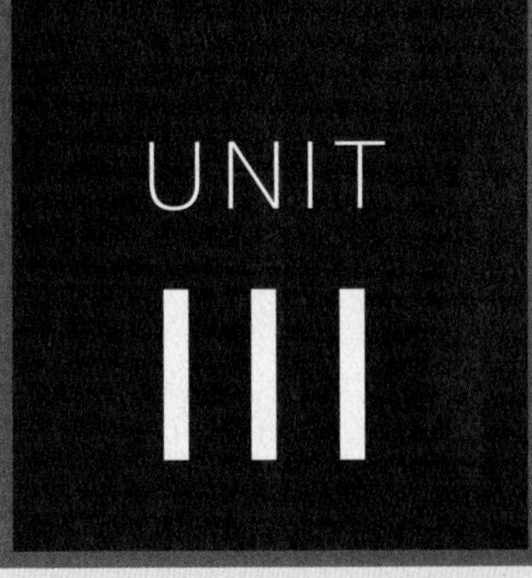

UNIT III

Pregnancy

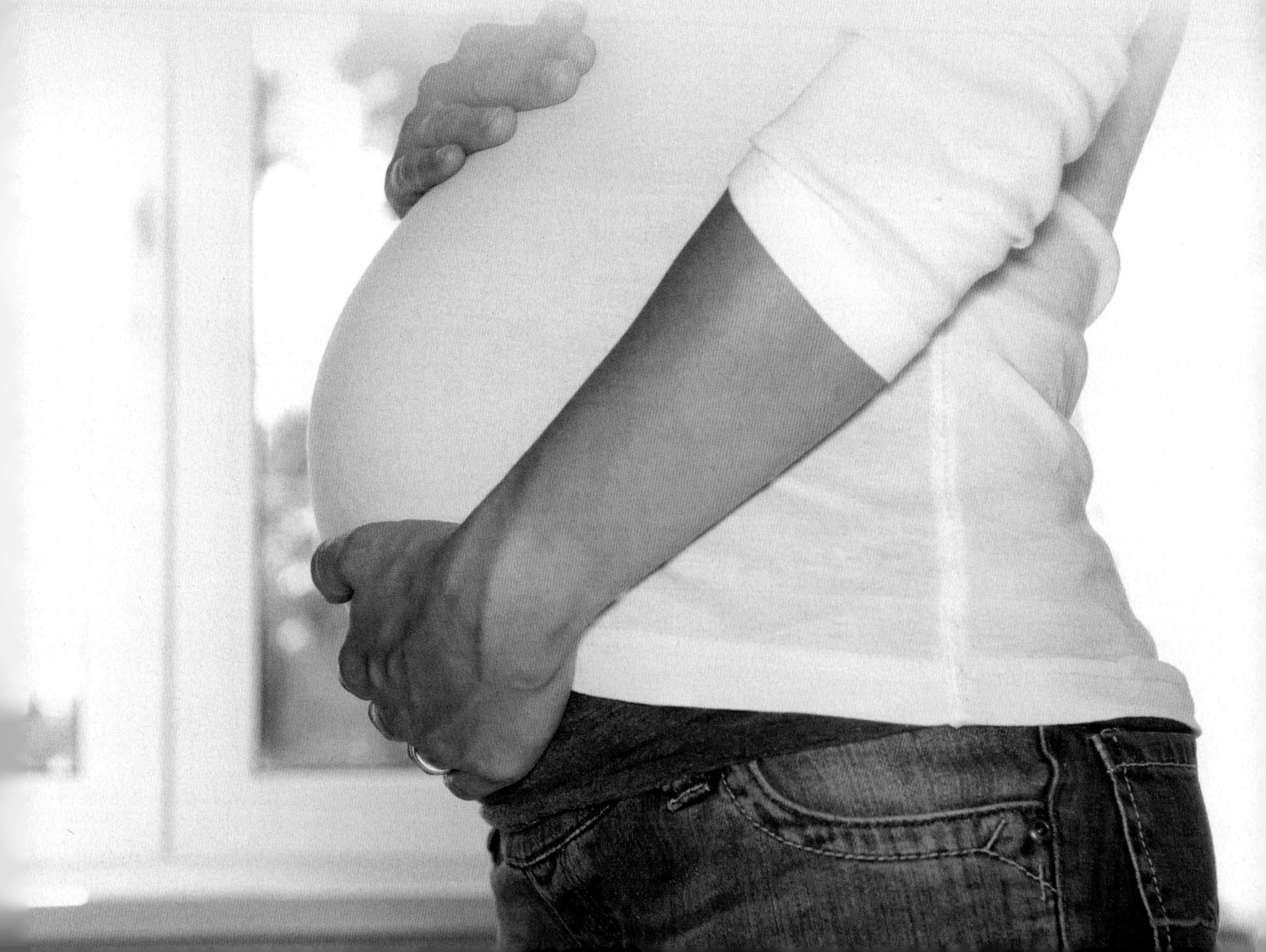

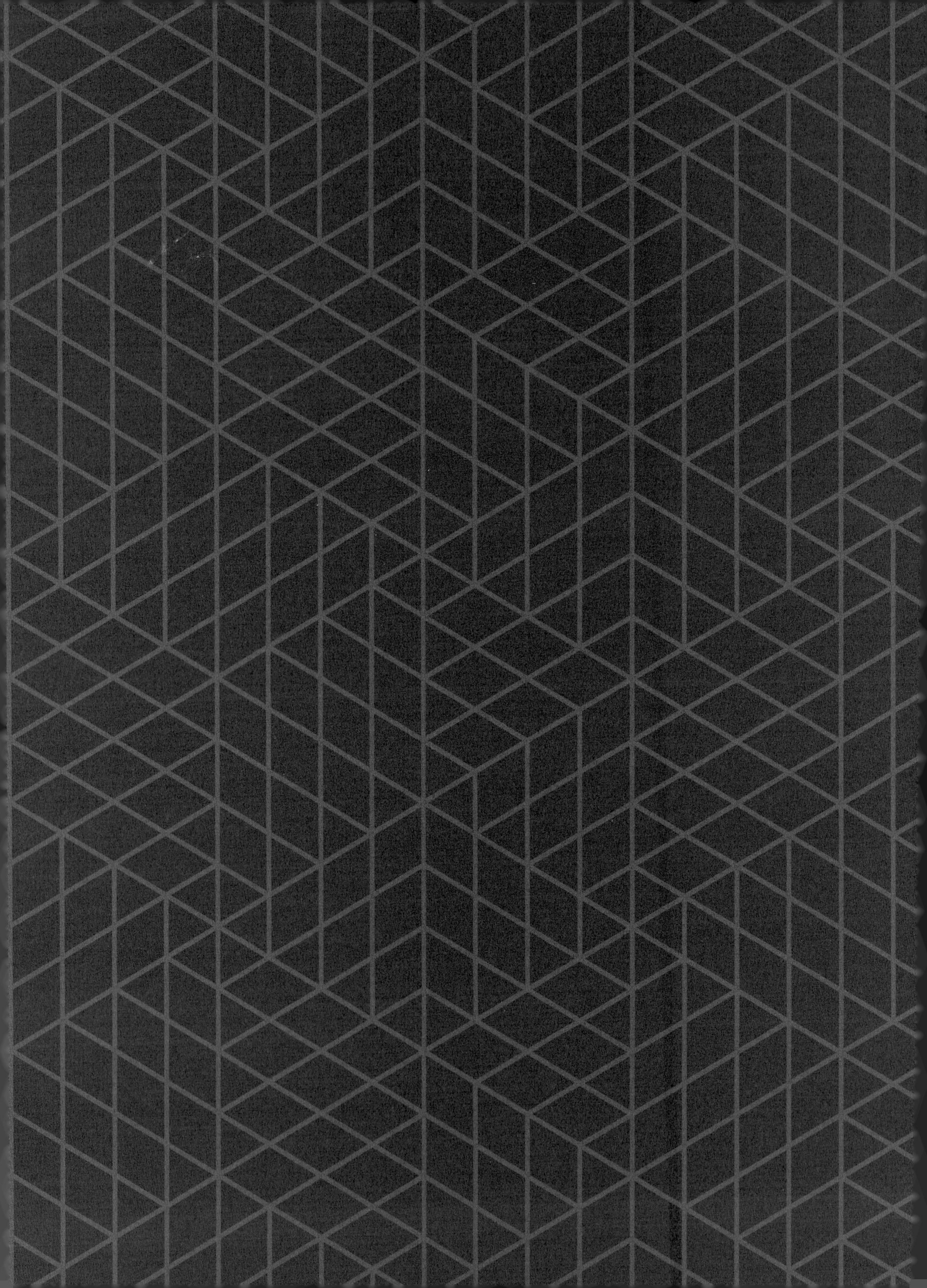

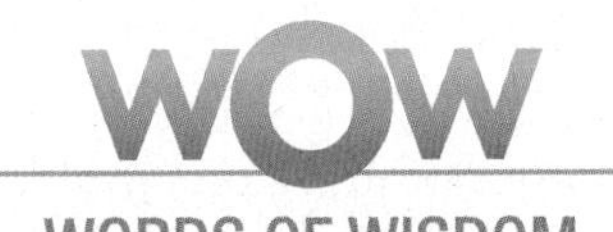

WORDS OF WISDOM

Being a nurse without awe is like food without spice. Nurses only have to witness the miracle of life to find their lost awe.

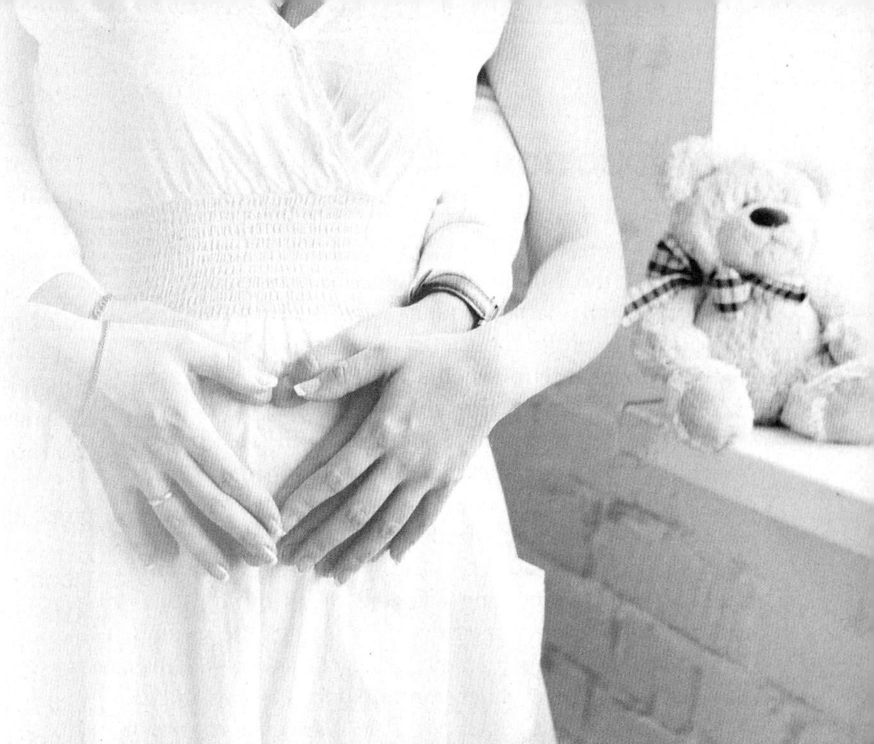

10 Fetal Development and Genetics

KEY TERMS

allele (ă-lēl')
blastocyst
embryonic stage
fertilization
fetal stage
genes
genetic counseling
genetics
genomics
genotype
heterozygous (het'ĕr-ō-zī'gŭs)
homozygous (hō'mō-zī'gŭs)
implantation
karyotype (kar'ē-ō-tīp)
morula
phenotype
placenta
preembryonic stage
teratogen (ter'ă-tō-jen)
trophoblast (trof'ō-blast)
umbilical cord
zygote (zī'gōt)

LEARNING OBJECTIVES

Upon completion of the chapter, you will be able to:

1. Describe the process of fertilization, implantation, and cell differentiation.
2. Outline normal fetal development from conception through birth.
3. Examine the functions of the placenta, umbilical cord, and amniotic fluid.
4. Analyze examples of ethical and legal issues surrounding genetic testing.
5. Compare the various inheritance patterns, including nontraditional patterns of inheritance.
6. Explain the role of the nurse in genetic counseling and genetic-related activities.

Robert and Kate have just received the news that Kate's pregnancy test was positive. It had been a long and anxious 3 years of trying to start a family. Although both are elated about the prospect of becoming parents, they are also concerned about the possibility of a genetic problem because Kate is 41 years old. What might be the first step in looking into their concerns? As a nurse, what might raise concerns for you?

INTRODUCTION

Pregnancy is a dynamic and precisely coordinated process involving systemic and local changes in the female body that support the supply of nutrients and oxygen to the fetus for growth and subsequent lactation. Human reproduction is one of the most intimate spheres of a person's life. Conception occurs when a healthy ovum is released from the ovary, passes into an open fallopian tube, and starts its journey downward. Sperm from the male is deposited into the vagina and swims approximately 7 in to meet the ovum at the outermost portion of the fallopian tube, the area where fertilization takes place. Fertilization takes about 24 hours to complete. The zygote forms as a result of sperm combining with the ovum during fertilization. When one spermatozoon penetrates the ovum's thick outer membrane, a new living cell is formed that is unlike the cells of either parent. Soon, the two nuclei will fuse, bringing together about 25,000 genes to guide human development.

Nurses caring for the childbearing family need to have a basic understanding of conception and prenatal development so they can identify problems or variations and can initiate appropriate interventions should any problems occur. This chapter presents an overview of fetal development beginning with conception. It also discusses hereditary influences on fetal development and the nurse's role in genetic counseling.

FETAL DEVELOPMENT

Fetal development during pregnancy is measured by the number of weeks after fertilization. An average human pregnancy lasts for about 280 days or 40 weeks from the date of the last menstrual period (LMP). Traditionally, it has been calculated as 10 lunar months or 9 months by the modern calendar. Fertilization of the egg by the sperm, however, usually occurs (considering an average menstrual cycle of 28 days) 14 days after the last period. Thus, the average actual duration of a human pregnancy (gestation period) is 280 days minus 14 days for 266 days.

The three stages of fetal development during pregnancy are as follows:

1. *Preembryonic stage*—fertilization through the 2nd week
2. *Embryonic stage*—end of the 2nd week through the 8th week
3. *Fetal stage*—end of the 8th week until birth

Fetal circulation is a significant aspect of fetal development that spans all three stages.

Preembryonic Stage

The **preembryonic stage** begins with fertilization, also called *conception*. **Fertilization** is the union of ovum and sperm, which is the starting point of pregnancy. Development during this stage takes place in an organized fashion that is cephalocaudal, proximal to distal, and general to specific. Fertilization requires a timely interaction between the release of the mature ovum at ovulation and the ejaculation of enough healthy, mobile sperm to survive the hostile vaginal environment through which they must travel to meet the ovum. All things considered, the act of conception is difficult at best. To say that it occurs when the sperm unites with the ovum is overly simplistic because this union requires an intricate interplay between hormonal preparation and overcoming an overwhelming number of natural barriers. A human being is truly an amazing outcome of this elaborate process.

Prior to fertilization, the ovum and the spermatozoon undergo the process of meiosis. The primary oocyte completes its first meiotic division before ovulation. The secondary oocyte begins its second meiotic division just before ovulation. Primary and secondary spermatocytes undergo meiotic division while still in the testes. Gametogenesis is the process by which gametes (ovum or sperm cells) are produced to initiate the development of a new person. The gametes must have a haploid number of chromosomes (a single set, i.e., 23) so when they come together to form the **zygote**, the normal human diploid number of chromosomes (combination of two sets, i.e., 46) is established (Fig. 10.1).

Although each milliliter of ejaculated semen contains more than 200 million sperm, only one is able to enter the ovum to fertilize it. All others are blocked by the clear protein layer called the **zona pellucida**. The zona pellucida disappears in about 5 days. Once the sperm reaches the plasma membrane, the ovum resumes meiosis and forms a nucleus with half the number of chromosomes (23). When the nucleus from the ovum and the nucleus of the sperm make contact, they lose their respective nuclear membranes and combine their maternal and paternal chromosomes. Because each nucleus contains a haploid number of chromosomes (23), this union restores the diploid number (46). The resulting zygote begins the process of a new life.

The genetic information from both ovum and sperm establishes the unique physical characteristics of the person. Sex determination is also determined at fertilization and depends on whether the ovum is fertilized by a Y-bearing sperm or an X-bearing sperm. Approximately 50% of sperm cells carry the XX chromosome while the other 50% carry XY. An XX zygote will become a female and an XY zygote will become a male (Fig. 10.2). That is why it is scientifically correct to say that the sex of the infant is determined by the nonbirthing parent and not by the birthing parent (Schnebly, 2021).

Fertilization takes place in the outer third of the ampulla of the fallopian tube. When the ovum is fertilized by the sperm, a great deal of activity immediately takes place. Mitosis, or *cleavage*, occurs as the zygote is slowly transported into the uterine cavity by tubal muscular movements (Fig. 10.3). After a series of four cleavages, the 16 cells appear as a solid ball of cells or a **morula**, meaning "little mulberry." The morula continues to divide and transforms into a blastocyst as it moves further

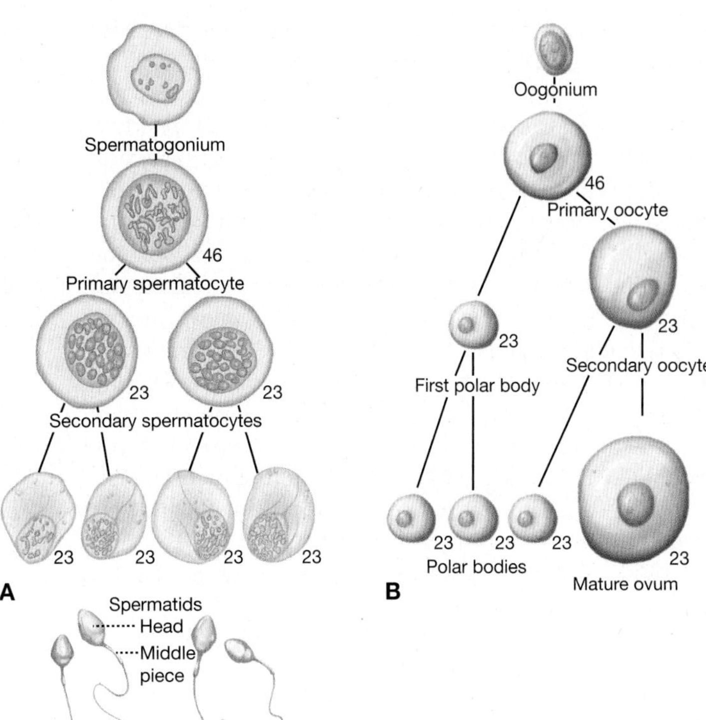

FIGURE 10.1 The formation of gametes by the process of meiosis is known as gametogenesis. **A.** Spermatogenesis. One spermatogonium gives rise to four spermatozoa. **B.** Oogenesis. From each oogonium, one mature ovum and three abortive cells are produced. The chromosomes are reduced to one half the number characteristic for the general body cells of the species. In humans, the number in the body cells is 46, and the number in the mature spermatozoon and secondary oocyte is 23.

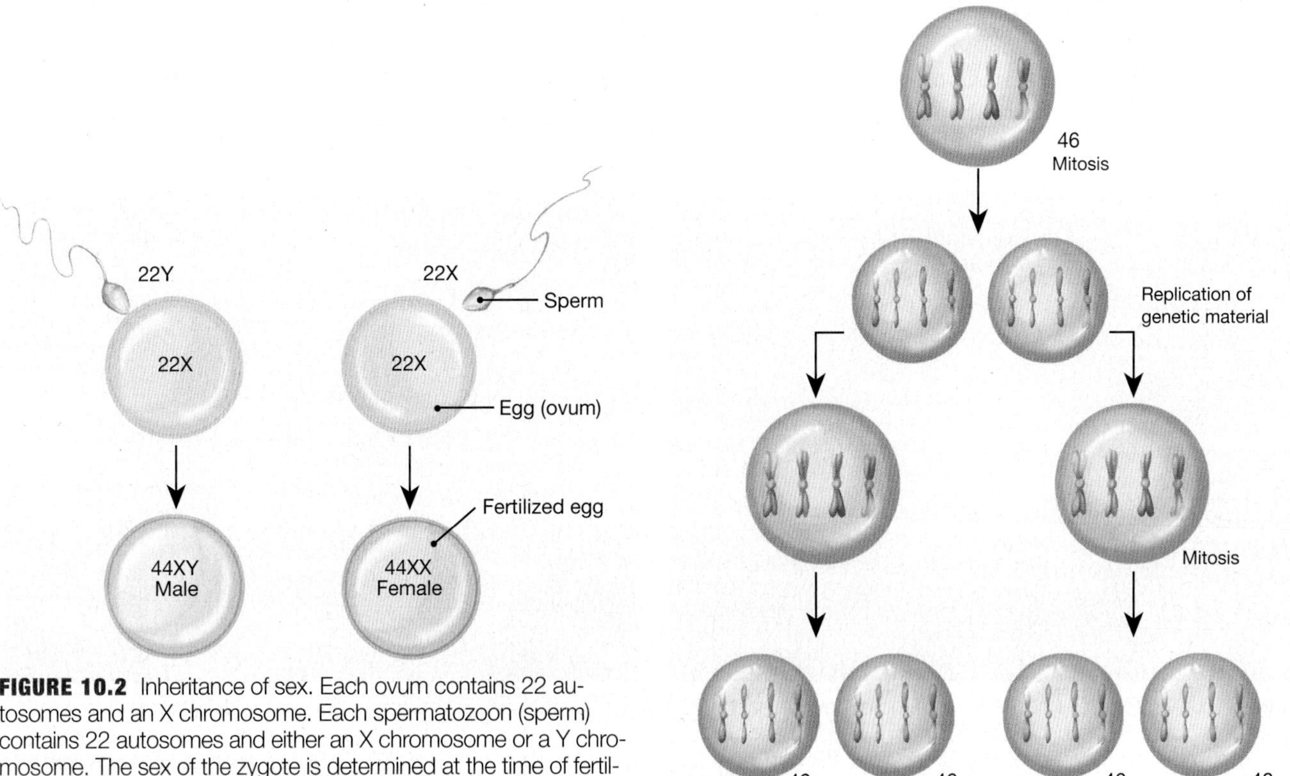

FIGURE 10.2 Inheritance of sex. Each ovum contains 22 autosomes and an X chromosome. Each spermatozoon (sperm) contains 22 autosomes and either an X chromosome or a Y chromosome. The sex of the zygote is determined at the time of fertilization by the combination of the sex chromosomes of the sperm (either X or Y) and the ovum (X).

FIGURE 10.3 Mitosis of the stoma cells.

into the uterus. The morula reaches the uterine cavity about 72 hours after fertilization (Bastauros, 2023).

Multiple fetuses can also occur at the time of fertilization when more than one ovum is fertilized. Identical twins (also called monozygotic twins) occur when one fertilized egg splits and develops into two (or occasionally more) fetuses. The fetuses usually share one placenta. Identical twins have the same genes, so they generally look alike and are of the same sex. Fraternal twins (also called dizygotic twins) develop when two separate eggs are fertilized by two different sperm. Each twin usually has its own placenta. Fraternal twins (like other siblings) share about 50% of their genes, so they can be different sexes. They generally do not look any more alike than siblings born from different pregnancies. Fraternal twins are more common than identical twins (see Chapter 19 for further details).

With additional cell division, the morula divides into specialized cells that will later form fetal structures. Within the morula, an off-center, fluid-filled space appears, transforming it into the hollow ball of cells called a **blastocyst** (Fig. 10.4). The inner surface of the blastocyst will form the embryo and amnion. The outer layer of cells surrounding the blastocyst cavity is called a **trophoblast**. Eventually, the trophoblast develops into one of the embryonic membranes, the chorion, and helps to form the placenta.

Currently, the developing blastocyst needs more food and oxygen to keep growing. The trophoblast attaches itself to the surface of the endometrium for further nourishment. Normally, implantation occurs in the upper uterus (fundus), where a rich blood supply is available. This area also contains strong muscular fibers, which clamp down on blood vessels after the placenta separates from the inner wall of the uterus. Additionally, the lining is thickest here so the placenta cannot attach so strongly that it remains attached after birth. The process of attachment and placental formation is termed **implantation**. Figure 10.5 shows the process of fertilization and implantation.

Concurrent with the development of the trophoblast and implantation, further differentiation of the inner cell mass occurs. Some of the cells become the embryo itself, and others give rise to the membranes that surround and protect it. The three embryonic layers of cells formed are:

1. *Ectoderm*—forms the central nervous system, special senses, skin, and glands
2. *Mesoderm*—forms the skeletal, urinary, circulatory, and reproductive organs
3. *Endoderm*—forms the respiratory system, liver, pancreas, and digestive system

These three layers are formed at the same time as the embryonic membranes, and all tissues, organs, and organ systems develop from these three primary germ cell layers (Muhr et al., 2023). Box 10.1 summarizes preembryonic development.

Despite the intense and dramatic activities going on internally to create a human life, many pregnant people are unaware that they have become pregnant at all. Several weeks will pass before even one of the presumptive signs of pregnancy—missing the first menstrual period—will take place.

Embryonic Stage

The **embryonic stage** of development begins at Day 15 after conception and continues through week 8. Basic structures of all major body organs and the main external

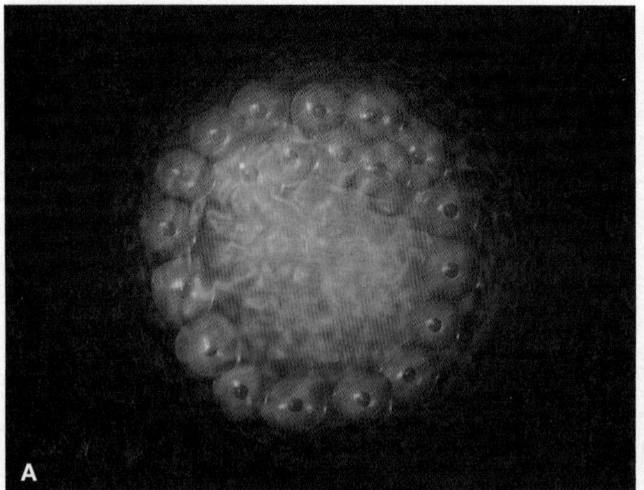

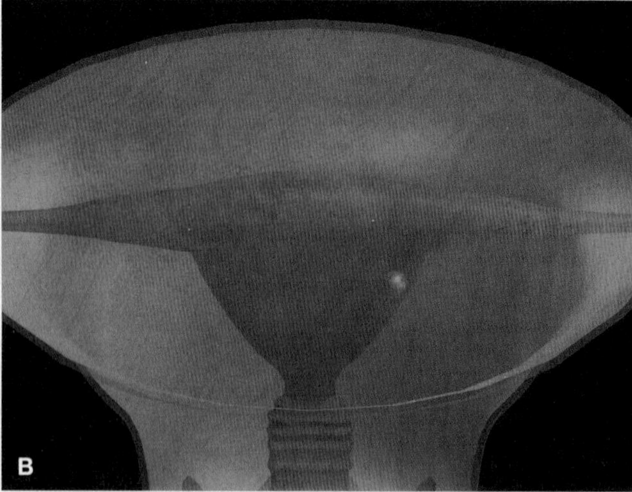

FIGURE 10.4 A. Fertilized human egg (zygote) having reached the blastocyst stage. The zygote contains 20 to 30 eggs and a fluid-filled blastocele is beginning to form. **B.** Implantation. Stylized image showing a frontal view of a uterus with a blastocyst about to implant into the endometrium of the uterus. (Reprinted with permission from LifeART: 3D Super Anatomy 6. Copyright © 2024 Lippincott Williams & Wilkins. All rights reserved.)

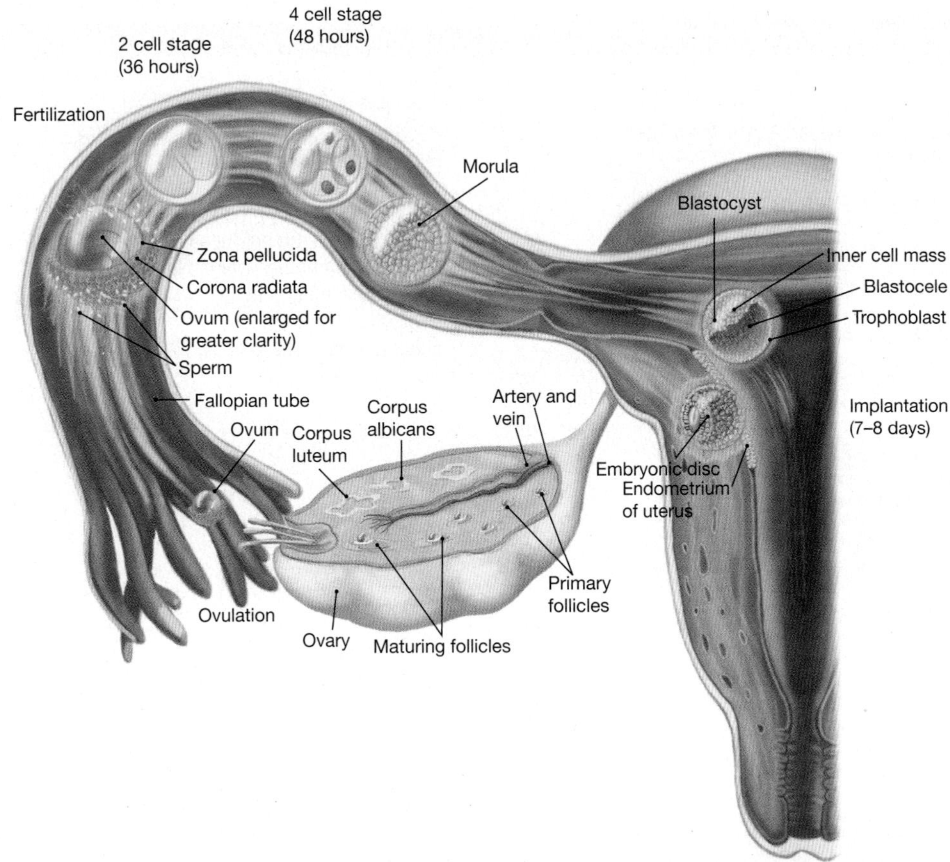

FIGURE 10.5 Fertilization and tubal transport of the zygote. From fertilization to implantation, the zygote travels through the fallopian tube, experiencing rapid mitotic division (cleavage). During the journey toward the uterus, the zygote evolves through several stages, including morula and blastocyst.

features are completed during this time period, including internal organs. Table 10.1 and Figure 10.6 summarize embryonic development.

The embryonic membranes (Fig. 10.7) begin to form around the time of implantation. The chorion consists of trophoblast cells and a mesodermal lining. The chorion has fingerlike projections called *chorionic villi* on its surface. The amnion originates from the ectoderm germ layer during the early stages of embryonic development. It is a thin protective membrane that contains amniotic fluid. Alongside of the amnion, a yolk sac develops as a second cavity about Day 8 or 9 after conception. The yolk sac aids in transferring maternal nutrients and oxygen to the embryo during the 2nd and 3rd weeks' gestation when development of the uteroplacental circulation is underway. As the pregnancy progresses, the yolk sac atrophies and is incorporated into the umbilical cord. As the embryo grows, the amnion expands until it touches the chorion. These two fetal membranes form the fluid-filled amniotic sac, or bag of waters, that protects the floating embryo. Both membranes contribute to inflammatory homeostasis, which allows for normal gestation progression (Truong et al., 2023).

Amniotic fluid surrounds the embryo and increases in volume as the pregnancy progresses, reaching approximately a liter at term. Amniotic fluid is derived from two sources: fluid transported from the maternal blood across the amnion and fetal urine. Its volume changes constantly as the fetus swallows and voids. Sufficient amounts of amniotic fluid help maintain a constant body temperature for the fetus, permit symmetric growth and development, cushion the fetus from trauma, allow the umbilical cord to be relatively free from compression,

BOX 10.1 Summary of Preembryonic Development

- Fertilization takes place in ampulla of the fallopian tube.
- Union of sperm and ovum forms a *zygote* (46 chromosomes).
- Cleavage cell division continues to form a *morula* (mass of 16 cells).
- The inner cell mass is called a *blastocyst*, which forms the embryo and amnion.
- The outer cell mass is called a *trophoblast*, which forms the placenta and chorion.
- Implantation occurs 7 to 10 days after conception in the endometrium.

TABLE 10.1 • Embryonic and Fetal Development

WEEK 3
Neural tube forms, which later becomes the spinal cord.
Beginning development of the heart
Beginning development of the gastrointestinal tract

WEEK 4
Neural tube closes.
Four chambers of heart formed
Brain differentiates.
Limb buds grow and develop.
Diaphragm and lungs begin to form.
Stomach, pancreas, liver, urinary tract, and genitalia begin to form.

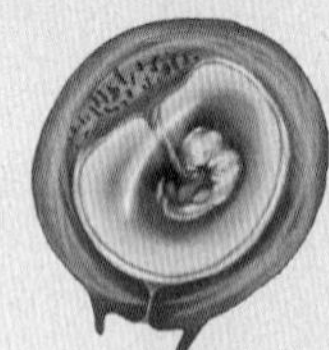
4 weeks

WEEK 5
Heart now beats at a regular rhythm.
Beginning structures of eyes and face
Some cranial nerves are visible.
Muscles innervated

WEEK 6
Fetal circulation established
Liver produces red blood cells.
Further development of the brain
Primitive skeleton forms.
Central nervous system forms.
Brain waves detectable

WEEK 7
Straightening of trunk, characteristic C shape
Beginning of ear development
Nipples and hair follicles form.
Elbows and toes visible
Legs move
Diaphragm formed
Mouth with lips and early tooth buds

WEEK 8
Rotation of intestines
Facial features continue to develop.
Heart development completes.
Resembles a human being
Penis, urethra, scrotum (male) or clitoris and labia (female) begin to form.
Placenta is working.
Eyelids form and grow but are sealed shut.
Organogenesis is complete.

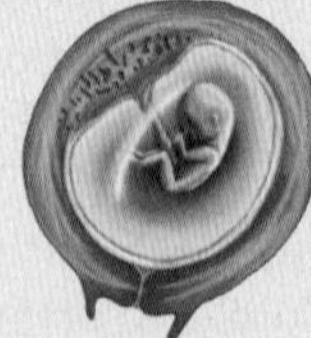
8 weeks

WEEKS 9–12
Sexual differentiation continues.
Buds for all 20 temporary teeth laid down
Digestive system shows activity.
Head makes up nearly half the fetus size.
Face and neck are well formed.
Urogenital tract completes development.
Red blood cells are produced in the liver.
Urine begins to be produced and excreted.
Fetal sex can be determined by week 12.
Limbs are long and thin.
Digits are well formed.
Fetus moves, kicks, and swallows.

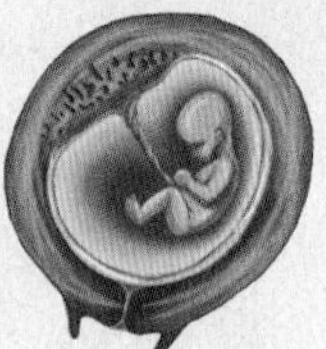
12 weeks

WEEKS 13–16
Fetal skin is almost transparent.
Bones become harder.
Fetus makes active movement.
Sucking motions are made with the mouth.
Amniotic fluid is swallowed.
External genitalia are recognizable.
Fingernails and toenails present
Formation of pinna
Weight quadruples.
Fetal movement (also known as *quickening*) detected by pregnant person

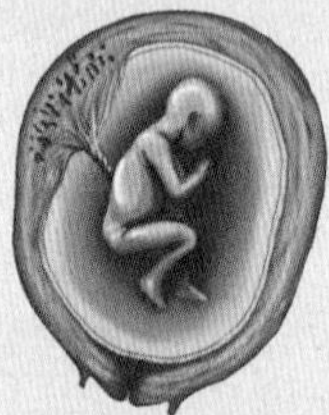
16 weeks

WEEKS 17–20
Rapid brain growth occurs.
Fetal heart tones can be heard with stethoscope.
A fine hair called *lanugo* develops on the head.
Kidneys continue to secrete urine into the amniotic fluid.
Vernix caseosa, a white greasy film, covers the fetus.
Eyebrows and head hair appear.
Brown fat deposited to help maintain temperature
Nails are present on both fingers and toes.
Muscles are well developed.

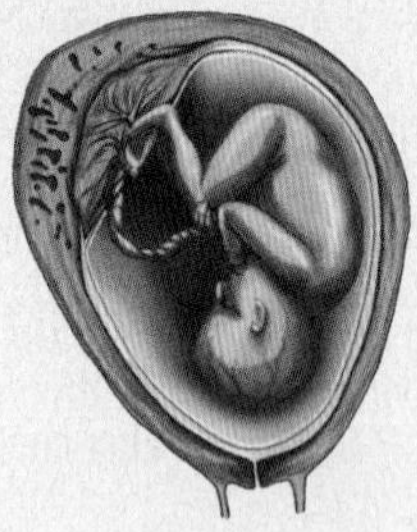
20 weeks

TABLE **10.1** • Embryonic and Fetal Development

WEEKS 21–24
Eyebrows and eyelashes are well formed.
Fetus has a hand grasp and startle reflex.
Alveoli forming in lungs
Skin is translucent and red.
Eyelids remain sealed.
Lungs begin to produce *surfactant.*

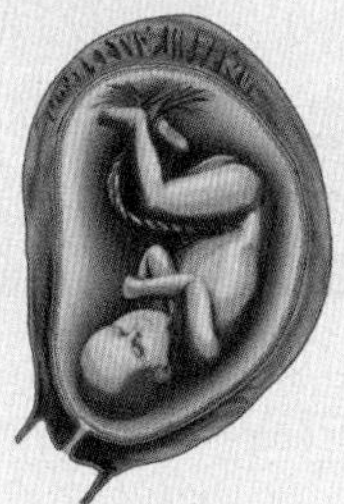

25 weeks

WEEKS 25–28
Fetus reaches a length of 15 in.
Brow formation
Rapid brain development
Eyelids open and close.
Nervous system controls some functions.
Fingerprints are set.
Subcutaneous fat is visible under the skin.
Blood formation shifts from spleen to bone marrow.
Fetus usually assumes head-down position.
Fetus responds to light and sound.
Fetus can open and shut eyes and suck thumb.

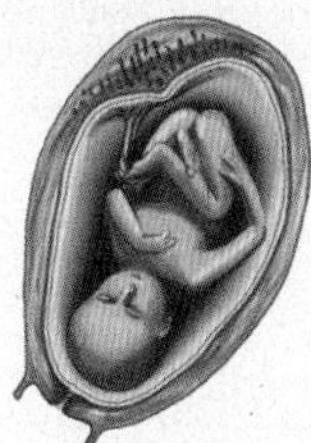

28 weeks

WEEKS 29–32
Rapid increase in the amount of body fat
Increased central nervous system control over body functions
Rhythmic breathing movements occur.
Lungs are not fully mature.
Pupillary light reflex is present.
Fetus stores iron, calcium, and phosphorus.

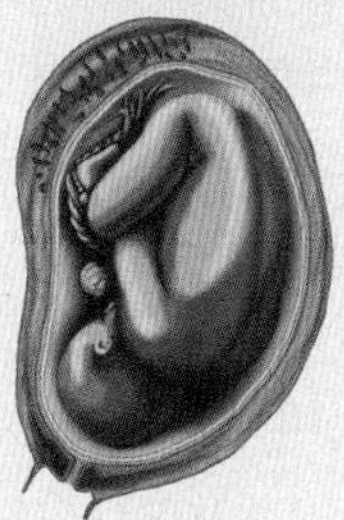

32 weeks

WEEKS 33–39
Testes are in scrotum of male fetus.
Lanugo begins to disappear.
Has strong hand grasp reflex
Increase in body fat
Earlobes formed and firm
Fingernails reach the end of fingertips.
Small breast buds are present on both sexes.
Pregnant person supplies fetus with antibodies against disease.
Fetus is considered full term at 39 weeks.
Fetus fills uterus and moves to a head-down position.

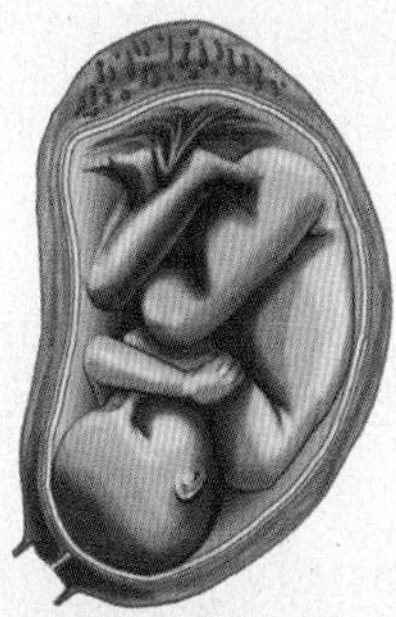

37 weeks

Adapted from Donovan, M. F., & Cascella, M. (2022). Embryology, weeks 6–8. *StatPearls.* https://www.ncbi.nlm.nih.gov/books/NBK563181/; Cunningham, F. G., Leveno, K. J., Dashe, J. S., Hoffman, B. L., Spong, C. Y., & Casey, B. M. (2022). Embryogenesis and fetal development. In F. G. Cunningham, K. J. Leveno, J. S. Dashe, B. L. Hoffman, C. Y., Spong, & B. M. Casey (Eds.), *William's obstetrics* (26th ed.). McGraw-Hill.

and promote fetal movement to enhance musculoskeletal development. Amniotic fluid is composed of 98% water and 2% organic matter. It is slightly alkaline and contains albumin, urea, uric acid, creatinine, bilirubin, lecithin, sphingomyelin, epithelial cells, vernix, and fine hair called lanugo that floats in it. Amniotic fluid is essential for fetal growth and development, especially fetal lung development.

The volume of amniotic fluid is important in determining fetal well-being. It gradually fluctuates throughout the pregnancy. The rate of change of amniotic fluid volume depends on the gestational age. During the fetal stage, the increase is 10 mL/week, and it increases to 50 to 60 mL/week at 19 to 25 weeks' gestation. The volume is at a maximum at 34 weeks' gestation before it undergoes a gradual decrease by term. Alterations in amniotic fluid volume can be associated with problems in the fetus. Too little amniotic fluid, termed *oligohydramnios*, is associated with complications such as uteroplacental insufficiency, umbilical cord compression, meconium aspiration, fetal deformation, and pulmonary hypoplasia (Beloosesky & Ross, 2022). Too much amniotic fluid,

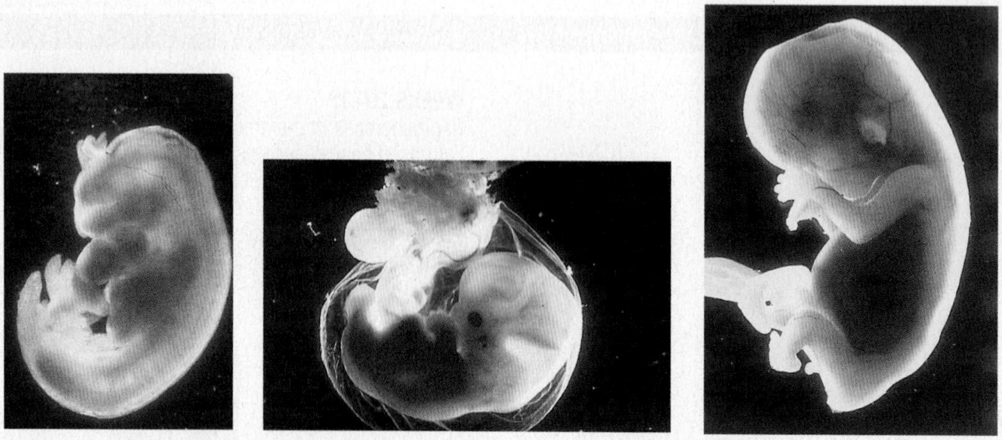

FIGURE 10.6 Embryonic development. **A.** Four-week embryo. **B.** Five-week embryo. **C.** Six-week embryo.

termed *polyhydramnios*, is associated with complications such as premature rupture of membranes, preterm labor and birth, macrosomia, umbilical cord prolapse, maternal respiratory compromise, prolonged second stage of labor, and postpartum uterine atony (Beloosesky & Ross, 2024) (see Chapter 19 for further information).

While the placenta is developing (end of the 2nd week), the **umbilical cord** is also formed from the amnion. It is the lifeline from the pregnant person to the growing embryo. It contains one large umbilical vein and two small umbilical arteries; the former carries oxygenated blood to the fetus and the latter transport deoxygenated blood with waste products from the fetus to the placenta. Wharton jelly (a specialized connective tissue) surrounds these three blood vessels in the umbilical cord to prevent compression, which would cut off fetal blood and nutrient supply. At term, the average umbilical cord is 50 to 60 cm (20 to 24 in) long and about 2 cm (1 in) wide (Heil & Bordoni, 2023).

The precursor cells of the placenta—the trophoblasts—first appear 4 days after fertilization as the outer layer of cells of the blastocyst. These early blastocyst

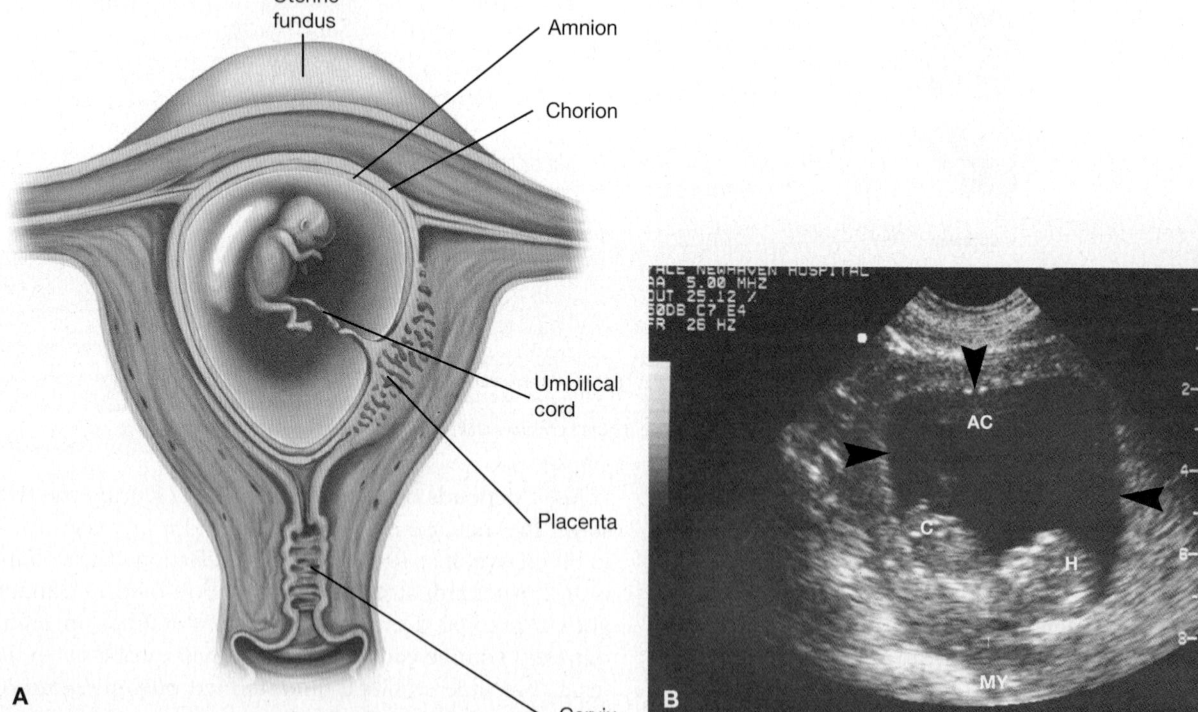

FIGURE 10.7 A. The embryo is floating in amniotic fluid, surrounded by the protective fetal membranes (amnion and chorion). **B.** Longitudinal sonogram of a pregnant uterus at 11 weeks showing the intrauterine gestational sac (*black arrowheads*) and the amniotic cavity (AC) filled with amniotic fluid; the fetus is seen in longitudinal section with the head (H) and coccyx (C) well displayed. The myometrium (MY) of the uterus can be identified. (Figure B courtesy of L. Scoutt.)

trophoblasts differentiate into all the cells that form the placenta. When fully developed, the placenta serves as the interface between the pregnant person and the developing fetus. Most commonly, the placenta develops at the uterine fundus. As early as 3 days after conception, the trophoblasts make human chorionic gonadotropin (hCG), a hormone that ensures the endometrium will be receptive to the implanting embryo. During the next few weeks, the placenta begins to make hormones that control the basic physiology of the pregnant person in such a way that the fetus is supplied with the nutrients and oxygen needed for growth.

The **placenta** is the least understood human organ and arguably one of the most important. It is a highly complex endocrine organ that controls the selective exchange of gas, nutrients, and waste between the maternal and fetal circulation. It is a transient fetal organ and unnecessary once birth takes place. As the placenta develops, it brings oxygen and nutrients to the growing fetus and moves waste away from it. It also protects the fetus from immune attack by the pregnant person's body and induces them to eat more, thereby bringing more food to the placenta. Near the time of delivery, it produces hormones that ready fetal organs for life outside the uterus. The placenta allows the developing fetus to rely on the maternal circulation to fulfill its bioenergetic needs while growing undisturbed in the protected environment of the uterus (Kapilia & Chaudhry, 2023).

Theoretically, at no time during pregnancy does the maternal blood mix with fetal blood because there is no direct contact between their blood; layers of fetal tissue always separate the maternal blood and the fetal blood. These fetal tissues are called the *placental barrier.* Materials can be interchanged only through diffusion. The maternal uterine arteries deliver the nutrients to the placenta, which in turn provides nutrients to the developing fetus; the pregnant person's uterine veins carry fetal waste products away. The structure of the placenta is usually completed by week 12.

The placenta is not only a transfer organ but a hormone factory as well. Placental hormones have profound effects on maternal metabolism, initially building up energy reserves and then releasing these to support fetal growth in later pregnancy and lactation postnatally. Several hormones are produced that are necessary for normal pregnancy including hCG, human chorionic somatomammotropin (hCS), progesterone, estrogen, and glucocorticoids (Roberts & Myatt, 2023).

The placenta acts as a pass-through between the pregnant person and fetus, not a barrier. Almost everything the person ingests (food, alcohol, and drugs) passes through to the developing conceptus. This is why it is so important to advise pregnant people not to use unprescribed drugs, alcohol, and tobacco, because they can be harmful to the fetus. Although prescription drug use is common during pregnancy (nine in 10 pregnant people take medicine during pregnancy), the human teratogenic risks are undetermined for many prescription medications because of a scarcity of data from pregnant humans (CDC, 2023a). This lack of data poses the risk that these medications may turn out to be harmful for the fetus if taken during pregnancy (CDC, 2023a). Pregnant people must check with their health care providers whether their prescribed drugs are safe for use during pregnancy.

During the embryonic stage, the fetus grows rapidly as all organs and structures are forming. During this critical period of differentiation, the growing embryo is most susceptible to damage from external sources, including teratogens (substances that cause birth defects, such as alcohol and drugs), infections (such as rubella or cytomegalovirus), radiation, and nutritional deficiencies.

Teratogens

A **teratogen** is any substance, organism, physical agent, or deficiency state present during gestation that is capable of inducing abnormal postnatal structure or function by interfering with normal embryonic and fetal development. Teratogens may produce physical or functional defects in the human embryo or fetus after the pregnant person has been exposed to that substance. Teratogens affect the fetus or embryo in a number of ways, causing physical deformities, problems in the behavioral or emotional development of the child, and decreased intellectual quotient (IQ) in the child. Additionally, teratogens may also affect pregnancies and cause complications such as preterm labors and spontaneous abortions. Susceptibility to teratogenic agents is dependent on the timing of the exposure and the developmental stage of the embryo or fetus. Teratogens are classified into four types: physical agents, metabolic conditions, infection, and drugs or chemical agents.

Select harmful teratogens to fetuses include the following:

- *Ionizing radiation*—leads to abnormal brain development, mental impairment, and leukemia
- *Organic mercury*—leads to damage of the neural system, mental impairment, behavioral and cognitive problems, and blindness
- *Lead exposure*—can cause spontaneous abortion, delayed fetal development, increased risk of fetal death, or abnormal mental or physical development
- *Toxoplasma*—leads to spontaneous abortion or stillbirth, underdeveloped fetal brain, blindness, and seizures
- *Syphilis bacteria*—can cause fetal death, spontaneous abortion, liver and spleen enlargement, and congenital syphilis
- *Rubella virus*—leads to abnormal brain development
- *Cytomegalovirus*—leads to underdevelopment of the fetal brain, blindness, deafness, jaundice, and liver and spleen dysfunction

- *Varicella zoster*—leads to underdeveloped limbs and brain or eye malformations
- *Herpes virus*—causes fetal death, microcephaly, herpetic pneumonia, and meningoencephalitis
- *Maternal conditions*—obesity, diabetes, hypothyroidism, hyperthyroidism, and phenylketonuria (PKU)
- *Medications*—antiepileptic drugs (cognitive defects, structural malformations); vitamin A in large doses (thymic and cardiac anomalies); anticoagulants (fetal skeletal abnormalities); and certain antimicrobials such as tetracycline (liver necrosis, bone and teeth defects) (Tsamantioti & Hashmi, 2024)

TAKE NOTE!

In 2015, the USFDA implemented the Pregnancy and Lactation Labeling Rule to improve drug safety categorization and to assist health care providers when counseling pregnant patients on medication use (Tsamantioti & Hashmi, 2024).

Fetal Stage

The average pregnancy lasts 280 days from the first day of the LMP. The **fetal stage** is the time from the end of the 8th week until birth. It is the longest period of prenatal development. During this stage, the embryo is mature enough to be called a fetus. Although all major systems are present in their basic form, dramatic growth and refinement of all organ systems take place during the fetal period (see Table 10.1). Figure 10.8 depicts a 12- to 15-week-old fetus.

Fetal Circulation

In contrast to the adult, who is surrounded by air, the developing fetus is surrounded by amniotic fluid. The fetus relies on the maternal circulation for nutrients and for respiration, including oxygen supply and carbon dioxide removal. The fetal heart begins developing approximately 22 days after conception. In the fetus, gas exchange occurs at the placenta with an oxygenation saturation of approximately 70% to 80% (Remien & Majmundar, 2023). Fetal circulation differs from adult circulation due to the presence of certain vessels and shunts. These shunts will close after birth and most of these vessels will be seen as remnants in adult circulation. The function of these shunts is to direct oxygen-rich venous blood to the systemic circulation and to ensure that oxygen-depleted venous blood bypasses the underdeveloped pulmonary circulation. Prostaglandins from the placenta keep the shunts open during fetal life.

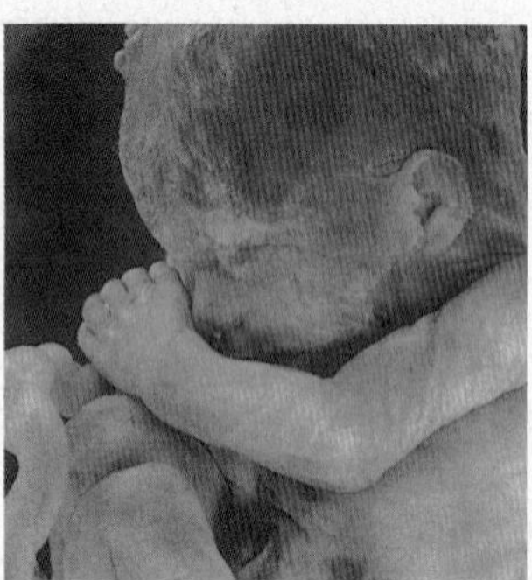

FIGURE 10.8 Fetal development: 12- to 15-week fetus.

Three shunts are present during fetal life:

1. *Ductus venosus*—connects the umbilical vein to the inferior vena cava
2. *Ductus arteriosus*—connects the main pulmonary artery to the aorta
3. *Foramen ovale*—anatomic opening between the right and left atria

TAKE NOTE!

Fetal circulation functions to carry highly oxygenated blood to vital areas (e.g., heart, brain) while first shunting it away from less important ones (e.g., lungs, liver). The placenta essentially takes over the functions of the lungs and liver during fetal life. As a result, large volumes of oxygenated blood are not needed.

Refer to Chapter 17 for additional information regarding fetal transition after birth.

GENETICS

Every species has a particular series of inherited characteristics, which determines a developmental plan and distinguishes one species from another. Different variations between members of the same species are the result of genetic, epigenetic, or environmental factors. **Genetics** refers to the study of heredity—its transmission and characteristic variation. **Genomics**, a relatively new science, is the study of all genes of a person and includes interactions among genes as well as interactions between genes and the environment. Genomics plays a role in complex conditions such as heart disease and diabetes. Another emerging area of research is that of pharmacogenomics, the study of genetic and genomic influences on pharmacodynamics and pharmacotherapeutics. While pharmacogenetics describes genetic variations between people and their influence on the efficacy and side effects of drugs, pharmacogenomics examines interactions of drugs with the entire genome. The main goal of both fields is the individual prediction of desirable and undesirable drug effects. A person's genetics influences wellness and health issues throughout that person's life cycle.

According to the Centers for Disease Control and Prevention (CDC, 2023b), birth defects and genetic disorders occur in one in 33 infants born in the United States and cause one in five infant deaths. Globally, an estimated 8 million newborns are born with a birth defect every year (WHO, 2023). Traditionally, genetics has been associated with making decisions about childbearing and caring for children with genetic disorders. Currently, genetic and technologic advances are expanding our understanding of how genetic changes affect human diseases such as diabetes, cancer, Alzheimer disease, and other multifactorial diseases that are prevalent in adults. Today's genetic technologies are not yet a crystal ball for seeing a child's future, but scientists are closer to routinely glimpsing the genetic blueprints of a fetus just months after sperm meets egg. Genomic reconstruction can reveal future disease risk and genetic traits in the first trimester of pregnancy. Newborn screening is perhaps the most widely used application of genetics in perinatal and neonatal care. Our ability to diagnose genetic conditions is more advanced than our ability to cure or treat the disorders. However, accurate diagnosis has led to improved treatment and outcomes for those affected with these disorders.

TAKE NOTE!

Genetic science has the potential to revolutionize health care with regard to national screening programs, predisposition testing, detection of genetic disorders, and pharmacogenetics.

Genetics has been a part of perinatal care for decades. Rapid development and implementation of advanced genetics technology in prenatal settings includes the ability to screen for and diagnose a broader range of diseases and conditions of the fetus in early gestational ages. Ultrasounds and maternal serum screening have become routine elements of prenatal care. Preconception carrier screening for conditions such as Tay–Sachs disease has been in place among high-risk populations such as those of Ashkenazi Jewish, French–Canadian, or Cajun descent. Amniocentesis is used as a diagnostic test that may confirm a genetic anomaly in a developing fetus, but it is an invasive technique. A fetal nuchal translucency test, seen on ultrasound, may suggest the presence of trisomy 21 or Down syndrome if increased nuchal thickness is found between 11 and 13 weeks' gestation. Modern technology makes it possible to screen for and diagnose conditions prior to birth, such as open neural tube defects, chromosomal aneuploidies (e.g., trisomies 13, 18, and 21), congenital defects, as well as single-gene inheritable disorders (e.g., cystic fibrosis, Huntington disease, Duchenne muscular dystrophy, and hemophilia).

Testing for genetic diseases before they cause symptoms, making a diagnosis in a person who has disease symptoms, and seeking treatment as early as possible can help people make informed decisions about managing their health care. In many cases, health insurance plans will cover the costs of genetic testing when it is recommended by the health care provider. However, patients must check their individual plans because different health insurance providers have different policies about which tests are covered.

Advances in genetics and genomics have profound implications for health care; the growing importance and relevance of genetics for nursing practice is apparent. Today, nurses are required to have basic skills and knowledge in genetics, genetic testing, and genetic counseling so they can assume these roles and provide information and support to patients and their families. Roles for maternity nurses in genetic health care have expanded significantly as genetics education and counseling have become a standard of care. Today, nurses may provide preconception counseling for patients at risk for the transmission of a genetic disorder. In addition, they may provide prenatal care for patients with genetically linked disorders that require specialized care or may participate in screening infants for birth defects and genetic disorders. Nurses employed in prenatal care settings need to have accurate information they can provide to patients so they understand the benefits and limitations of screening. Timely presentation of information and identification of available resources will help nurses minimize a patient's confusion and provide support as they proceed with pregnancy screening. Nurses at all levels should participate in risk assessments for genetic conditions and disorders, explaining genetic risk and genetic testing, and supporting informed health decisions and opportunities for early intervention. Nurses have a social and professional responsibility to ensure they provide current accurate information to patients and their families amid rapidly developing technology. This is especially true for nurses who value and support well-informed decision making that is patient and family centered.

Genomics is relevant to all health care providers across the health care continuum. In the future, as the era of personalized health care moves forward, nurses will be responsible for ensuring that the scientific principles, ethical standards, and professional accountability of genetics and genomics practice are integrated into nursing practice. Nurses are increasingly doing this as they gain the necessary knowledge and skills. The strength of the nursing voice in genetics and genomic research will be the link to the bedside and the commitment to ensure that new knowledge is translated into competent, safe, effective, and evidence-based patient care. For further information suitable for patient education, nurses may want to visit the CDC's web page on genomics.

Advances in Genetics and Genetic Technology

Human Genome Project

The publication of the first sequence of the human genome was a result of the Human Genome Project (HGP), regarded as one of the most ambitious and successful international research collaborations in modern biology. It was started in 1990 by the Department of Energy and the National Institutes of Health (NIH) and was completed in May 2003. The goals of the HGP were to map, sequence, and determine the function of the human genome, which led to advances in the field of genetics and genetic testing (National Human Genome Research Institute, 2023). A person's **genome** represents their genetic blueprint, which determines **genotype** (the gene pairs inherited from parents; the specific genetic makeup) and **phenotype** (observed outward characteristics of a person). A person's genetic profile can help guide decisions made regarding prevention, diagnosing, and treating disease. This is a profound shift in thinking from genetics that only addressed rare disorders to the use of genetic information in all aspects of health care.

Genetic Testing, Diagnosis, and Therapy

Recent advances in genetic knowledge and technology have affected all areas of health, including testing, diagnosis, and treatment. Approximately 80% of rare diseases have a genetic origin, making them amenable to gene therapy (Kruse et al., 2022). These advances have increased the number of health interventions that can be undertaken with regard to genetic disorders. For example, genetic prenatal testing that determines the risk of certain disorders is available (Evidence-Based Practice 10.1). Genetic testing can now also diagnose presymptomatic conditions in children and adults.

Gene therapy is a technique to prevent, treat, or cure a medical condition. It works by adding new copies of a broken gene, replacing a defective or missing gene with a healthy version of that gene. Nearly 50 years after the concept was first proposed, gene therapy is now considered a promising treatment option for multiple human diseases. It can be used to replace or repair defective or missing genes with normal ones. Gene therapy may be used for a variety of disorders, including cystic fibrosis, blindness, neuromuscular diseases, immunodeficiency disorders, melanoma, diabetes, human immunodeficiency virus (HIV), and hepatitis (Flomenberg & Daniel, 2024). Both inherited genetic conditions (hemophilia and sickle cell disease) and acquired disorders (leukemia) have been treated with gene therapy (National Human Genome Research Institute, 2024).

Current and potential applications of advances in genetic technology in health care include rapid and more specific diagnosis of disease with hundreds of genetic

EVIDENCE-BASED PRACTICE 10.1

Prenatal Genetic Screening and Diagnostic Testing: Assessing Patient's Knowledge, Clinical Experiences, and Utilized Resources in Comparison to Provider's Perceptions

BACKGROUND

Prenatal genetic testing focuses on identifying people at risk for giving birth to infants with chromosomal abnormalities. Despite the explosion of genetic services and research, there remains a deficit in understanding of these services when patients consider screening tests. Prenatal genetic screening and testing are common now, but patients must be well-informed if they are to understand the results and implications of the test's findings on the health of their newborn. The objective of this survey study was to evaluate patients' knowledge, clinical resources, and utilized resources about genetic screening and diagnostic tests.

STUDY

Patient and provider surveys were used to gather data. Five hundred were completed, but only 441 were analyzed. Among providers, only 66 of 229 responded to the online surveys. The questionnaire focused on general genetics-related knowledge and health implications. Many patients reported that they needed to access web links to help improve their understanding. The conversations between patients and providers in the health care office fell short of offering an understandable explanation of the tests to the patients.

Findings

Patients reported that conversations with their health care providers and nurses about prenatal screening and testing helped them with gaining knowledge about the purpose and results of the tests. Many patients reported that, although information was provided, there remained a deficit in their understanding the applications of these services.

Nursing Implications

Based on this study's findings, patients considering prenatal genetic diagnostic testing could benefit from patient–provider discussions in the office setting to improve patient knowledge and understanding. Inadequate understanding of the implications of prenatal testing and genetic services can impact decision making, especially in the context of prenatal care. Nurses should take a lead role in offering that support to these families to assist them through this challenging time in their lives. Nurses should provide current, comprehensive, and accurate prenatal testing information to prenatal patients to help in their decisions as to whether to undergo prenatal genetic testing or not. Based on their genetic risk profile, referral to a genetic counselor might be in order. Nurses have a responsibility to be knowledgeable about available genetic tests so they can assist their patients to become informed consumers of genetic-based health care.

Adapted from Delgado, A., Schulkin, J., & Macri, C. J. (2022). Prenatal genetic screening and diagnostic testing: Assessing patient's knowledge, clinical experiences, and utilized resources in comparison to provider's perceptions. *American Journal of Perinatology Reports, 12*(1), 27–32. https://doi.org/10.1055/s-0041-1742236

tests available in research or clinical practice; earlier detection of genetic predisposition to disease; less emphasis on treating the symptoms of a disease and more emphasis on looking at the fundamental causes of the disease; new classes of drugs; avoidance of environmental conditions that may trigger disease; and augmentation or replacement of defective genes through gene therapy. This genetic knowledge and technology, along with the commercialization of this knowledge, is changing both professional and parental understanding of genetic disorders. Current reproductive applications, however, remain restricted to mostly the prevention of transmitting an at-risk gene or genes and do not include full treatments or cures. As such, the scientific and ethical issues associated with reproductive applications will continue to affect decision making of at-risk people.

Ethical, Legal, and Social Issues of Genetic Technology

The potential benefits of these discoveries are vast, but so is the potential for misuse. These advances challenge all health care providers to consider the many ethical, legal, and social ramifications of genetics in human lives. In the near future, individualized risk profiling based on a person's unique genetic makeup will be used to tailor prevention, treatment, and ongoing management of health conditions. This profiling will raise issues associated with patient privacy and confidentiality related to workplace discrimination and access to health insurance. Issues of autonomy are equally problematic as society considers how to address the injustices that will inevitably surface when disease risk can be determined years before the disease occurs. People are currently protected from genetic discrimination by health insurers and employers through the Genetic Information Nondiscrimination Act of 2008, but this does not extend to providers of life, disability, or long-term care insurance (Scott & Lee, 2020a). Nurses will play an important role in developing policies and providing direction and support in this arena, and to do so, they will need a basic understanding of genetics, including inheritance and inheritance patterns.

Inheritance

DNA and Genetic Information

The nucleus within the cell is the controlling factor in all cellular activities because it contains chromosomes, long continuous strands of DNA that carry genetic information. Each chromosome is made up of genes. **Genes** are individual units of heredity of all traits and are organized into long segments of DNA that occupy a specific location on a chromosome and determine a particular characteristic in an organism.

Genotypes and Alleles

The genotype—the specific genetic makeup of a person, usually in the form of DNA—is the internally coded inheritable information. It refers to the particular **allele**, which is one of two or more alternative versions of a gene at a given position or locus on a chromosome that imparts the same characteristic of that gene. For instance, each human has a gene that controls height, but the variations of these genes, or alleles, code for a specific height. As another example, a gene that controls eye color may have an allele that can produce blue eyes or an allele that produces brown eyes. The genotype, together with environmental variation that influences the person, determines the phenotype. A human inherits two genes, one from each parent. Therefore, one allele comes from each biologic parent. These alleles may be the same for the characteristic (**homozygous**) or different (**heterozygous**). For example, WW stands for homozygous dominant; ww stands for homozygous recessive. Heterozygous would be indicated as Ww. If the two alleles differ, such as Ww, the dominant one will usually be expressed in the phenotype of the person.

Chromosomes

Human beings typically have 46 chromosomes. This includes 22 pairs of nonsex chromosomes, or autosomes, and one pair of sex chromosomes (two X chromosomes in females, and an X chromosome and a Y chromosome in males). Offspring receive one chromosome of each of the 23 pairs from each parent.

The pictorial analysis of the number, form, and size of a person's chromosomes is termed the **karyotype**. This analysis commonly uses white blood cells and fetal cells in amniotic fluid and is often used in prenatal testing to diagnose or predict genetic diseases. The chromosomes are numbered from the largest to the smallest, 1 to 22, and the sex chromosomes are designated by the letter X or Y. A female karyotype is designated as 46, XX and a male karyotype is designated as 46, XY. Figure 10.9 illustrates an example of a karyotyping pattern.

Genetic Mutations

A genetic **mutation** is a permanent change in a DNA sequence that changes the function of the gene. Regulation and expression of the thousands of human genes are complex processes and are the result of many intricate interactions within each cell.

Mutations occur throughout the natural world and are a major fuel of evolution. Genetic mutations can be inherited, spontaneous, or acquired. Inherited mutations are passed on from parent to child in the egg and sperm; then, they are passed on to all cells in that child's body when the body cells reproduce. A spontaneous mutation

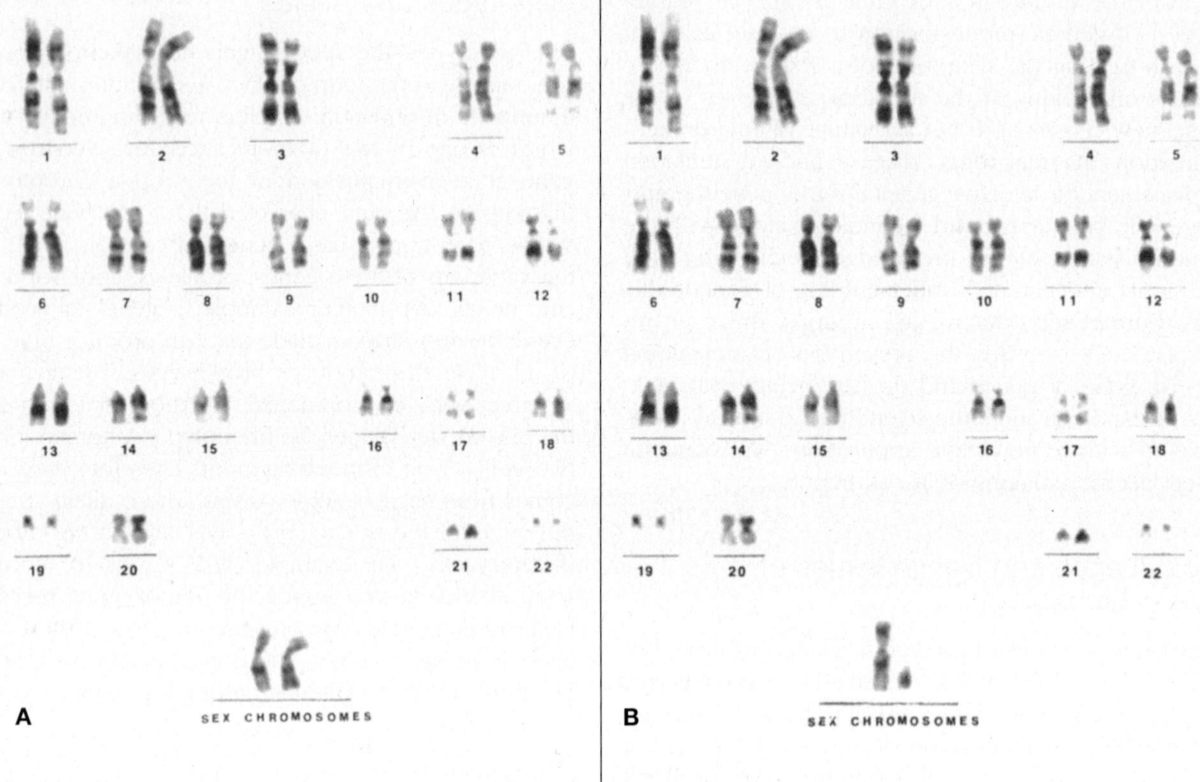

FIGURE 10.9 Karyotype pattern. **A.** Normal female karyotype. **B.** Normal male karyotype.

can occur in individual eggs or sperm at the time of conception. A person who has the new spontaneous mutation has the risk of passing it on to their offspring. Acquired mutations occur in body cells other than egg or sperm. They involve changes in DNA that take place after conception during a person's lifetime. Acquired mutations are passed on when they reproduce to daughter cells. These changes can be caused by environmental exposures (USFDA, 2022). Some genetic mutations have no significant effect, while others can have a tremendous impact on the health of the person. For example, cystic fibrosis is a disease caused by an inherited mutation and Marfan syndrome is a disease caused by an acquired mutation. Other genetic disorders such as cancer, sickle cell disease, PKU, and hemophilia can also result from mutations.

Patterns of Inheritance for Genetic Disorders

Patterns of inheritance demonstrate how a genetic disorder can be passed on to offspring. A genetic disorder is a disease caused by an abnormality in a person's genetic material or genome. Diagnosis of a genetic disorder is usually based on clinical signs and symptoms or on laboratory confirmation of the presence of an altered gene associated with the disorder. Accurate diagnosis can be aided by recognition of the pattern of inheritance within a family. The pattern of inheritance is also vital to understand when teaching and counseling families about the risks in future pregnancies.

Mendelian or Monogenic Laws of Inheritance

Principles of inheritance of single-gene disorders are the same that govern the inheritance of other traits, such as eye and hair color. These are known as Mendel's laws of inheritance, named for Gregor Mendel, an Austrian naturalist who conducted genetic research. These patterns occur because a single gene is defective and the disorders that result are referred to as monogenic or, sometimes, mendelian disorders. If the defect occurs on the autosome, the genetic disorder is termed autosomal; if the defect is on the X chromosome, the genetic disorder is termed X linked. The defect also can be classified as dominant or recessive. Monogenic disorders include autosomal dominant, autosomal recessive, X-linked dominant, and X-linked recessive. Not all single-gene disorders follow typical mendelian inheritance, as the pattern of inheritance can be complicated by other genes, epigenetic changes, or environmental factors. These nontraditional inheritance patterns are discussed in the following sections (Raby, 2021).

AUTOSOMAL DOMINANT INHERITANCE

Autosomal dominant inheritance occurs when a single gene in the heterozygous state is capable of producing the phenotype. In these instances, the abnormal or mutant gene overshadows the normal gene and the person will demonstrate signs and symptoms of the disorder. The affected person usually has one affected parent. However, there can be varying degrees of presentation, termed variable expression, among individuals in a family. For example, a parent with a mild form of the disorder could have a child with a more severe form. In some autosomal dominant disorders, there may be no history of an affected family member. This can be due to the child presenting a new mutation or the result of incomplete or reduced penetrance, which means that a person with the genetic mutation does not develop phenotypic features of the disorder. Incomplete or reduced penetrance may result from a combination of genetic, environmental, and lifestyle factors; age; and sex.

Offspring of an affected parent will have a 50% chance of inheriting two normal genes (thus, being disorder free) and a 50% chance of inheriting one normal and one abnormal gene (thus, inheriting the disorder) (Scott & Lee, 2020b) (Fig. 10.10). Females and males are equally affected by autosomal dominant disorders. Affected males can pass these disorders on their male offspring (Scott & Lee, 2020b). This male-to-male transmission is important in distinguishing autosomal dominant inheritance from X-linked inheritance. Common types of genetic disorders that follow the autosomal dominant pattern of inheritance include achondroplasia, neurofibromatosis, Huntington disease, Marfan syndrome, and osteogenesis imperfecta type 1 (Breilyn & Levy, 2023).

AUTOSOMAL RECESSIVE INHERITANCE

Autosomal recessive inheritance occurs when two copies of the mutant or abnormal gene in the homozygous state are necessary to produce the phenotype. In other words, two abnormal genes are needed (one from each parent) for the person to demonstrate signs and symptoms of the disorder. Both parents of the affected person must be heterozygous carriers of the gene (clinically normal but carry the gene). Offspring of two carriers of the abnormal gene have a 25% chance of inheriting two normal genes; a 50% chance of inheriting one normal gene and one abnormal gene (becoming a carrier); and a 25% chance of inheriting two abnormal genes (and, thus, the inheriting the disorder) (Scott & Lee, 2020b) (Fig. 10.11). Affected people are usually present in only one generation of the family; females and males are equally affected. Male-to-male transmission is possible (Scott & Lee, 2020b). The chance that any two parents will both be carriers of the mutant gene is increased if the couple is consanguineous (having a common ancestor) (Scott & Lee, 2020b). Common types of genetic disorders that follow the autosomal recessive inheritance pattern include cystic fibrosis (a disease involving generalized dysfunction of the exocrine glands); galactosemia (an inborn error of metabolism in which the body is unable to metabolize galactose to glucose); PKU (an inborn error of metabolism involving a deficiency in a liver enzyme that leads to the

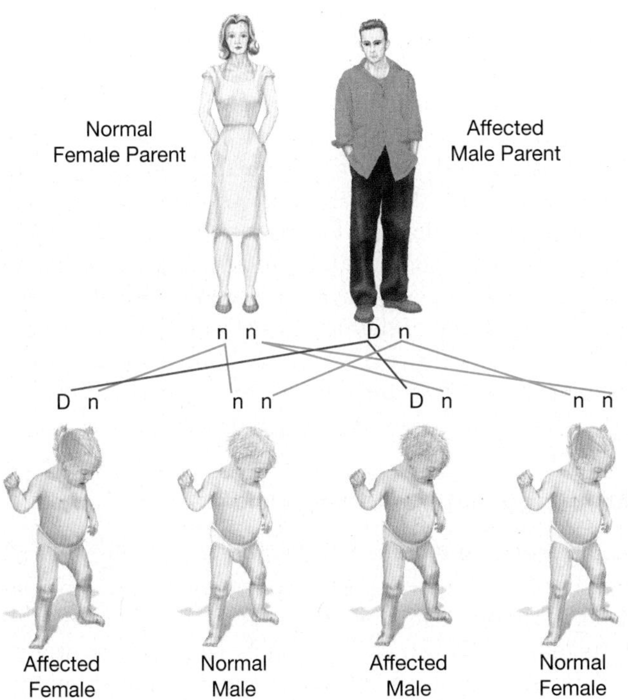

FIGURE 10.10 Autosomal dominant inheritance.

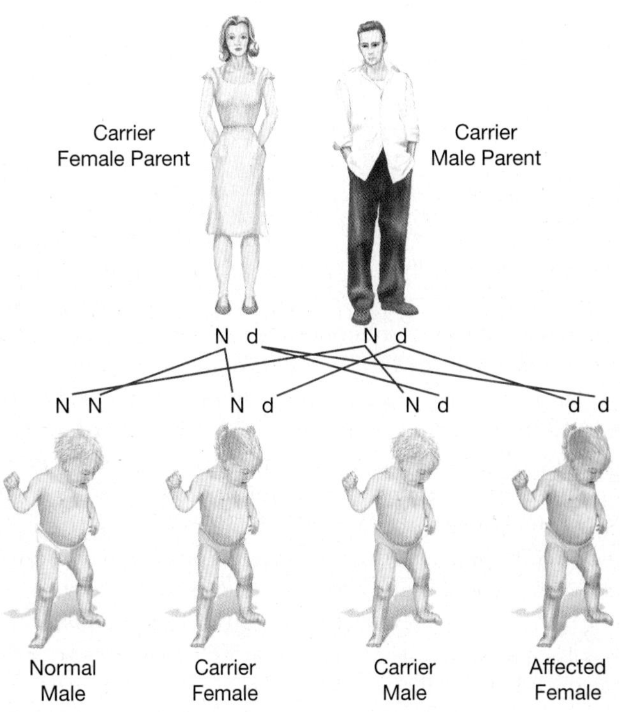

FIGURE 10.11 Autosomal recessive inheritance.

inability to process the essential amino acid phenylalanine); Tay–Sachs disease (an inborn error of metabolism caused by insufficient activity of the enzyme hexosaminidase A, which is necessary for the breakdown of certain fatty substances in the brain and nerve cells); and sickle cell disease (a disease in which the red blood cells carry an ineffective type of hemoglobin instead of the normal adult hemoglobin) (Breilyn & Levy, 2023).

X-LINKED INHERITANCE

X-linked inheritance is associated with altered genes present on the X chromosome. X-linked inheritance disorders differ from autosomal disorders. If a male inherits an X-linked altered gene, they will express the condition. Because a male has only one X chromosome, all the genes on the X chromosome will be expressed (the Y chromosome carries no normal allele to compensate for the altered gene). Because females inherit two X chromosomes, they can be either heterozygous or homozygous for any allele. Therefore, X-linked disorders in females are expressed similarly to autosomal disorders.

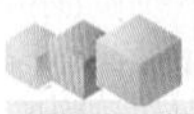

Concept Mastery Alert

Male Children in Pattern of Inheritance of Duchenne Muscular Dystrophy

The gene for Duchenne muscular dystrophy is X-linked, which means that a male child who inherits this gene will be affected by, but will not be a carrier of, this disease. A female child will not be affected by the disease.

TAKE NOTE!

The distinction between X-linked recessive and X-linked dominant inheritance is not clear; some experts believe a distinction should not even be made. This is because it is possible for females with uneven X-inactivation to demonstrate clinical features of X-linked conditions (Raby, 2021).

X-linked inheritance disorders can be either recessive or dominant, but most demonstrate a recessive pattern of inheritance (Breilyn & Levy, 2023). In the X-linked recessive pattern of inheritance, there are more affected males than females because all the genes on a male's X chromosome will be expressed since a male has only one X chromosome (Raby, 2021). On the other hand, a female will usually need two abnormal X chromosomes to exhibit the disease and one normal and one abnormal X chromosome to be a carrier of the disease. There is no male-to-male transmission (since no X chromosome from the male is transmitted to male offspring), but any male who is affected will have carrier female offspring. If a female is a carrier, there is a 50% chance that their male children will be affected and a 50% chance that their female children will be carriers (Breilyn & Levy, 2023) (Fig. 10.12). Common types of genetic disorders

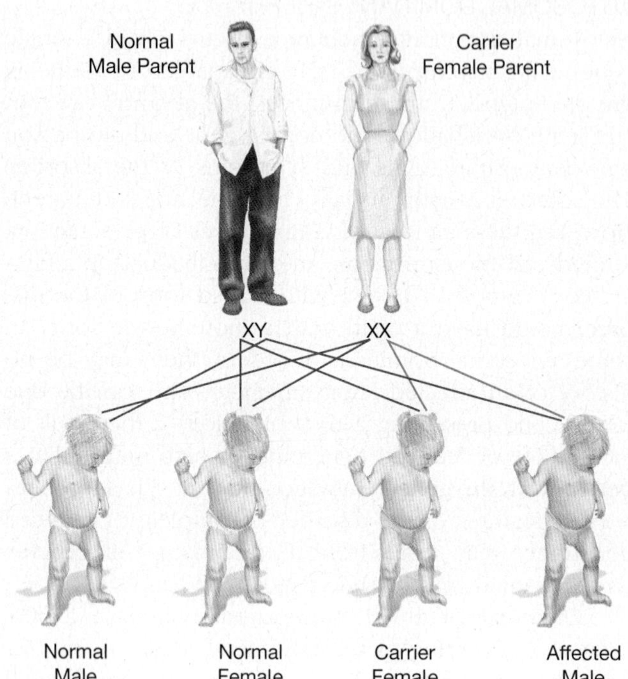

FIGURE 10.12 X-linked recessive inheritance.

that follow X-linked recessive inheritance patterns include hemophilia (a genetic disorder involving a deficiency of one of the coagulation factors in the blood); color blindness; and Duchenne muscular dystrophy (a disorder involving progressive muscular weakness and wasting) (Breilyn & Levy, 2023).

X-linked dominant inherited disorders are not very common (Breilyn & Levy, 2023). X-linked dominant inheritance occurs when a male has an abnormal X chromosome or a female has one abnormal X chromosome. All the female offspring and none of the male offspring of an affected male have the condition, while both male and female offspring of an affected female have a 50% chance of inheriting and presenting with the condition (Raby, 2021) (Fig. 10.13). Males are more severely affected than females. Many X-linked dominant disorders have lethal results in males (Raby, 2021). In females, even though the gene is dominant, having a second normal X gene offsets the effects of the dominant gene to some extent, resulting in decreased severity of the disorder. X-linked dominant disorders are rare; an example is hypophosphatemic (vitamin D-resistant) rickets (Raby, 2021).

Multifactorial Inheritance

Multifactorial inheritance disorders are thought to be caused by multiple genetic (polygenic) and environmental factors. Many of the common congenital malformations, such as cleft lip, cleft palate, spina bifida, pyloric stenosis, clubfoot, developmental hip dysplasia, and cardiac defects, are attributed to multifactorial inheritance (Scott & Lee, 2020b). A combination of genes

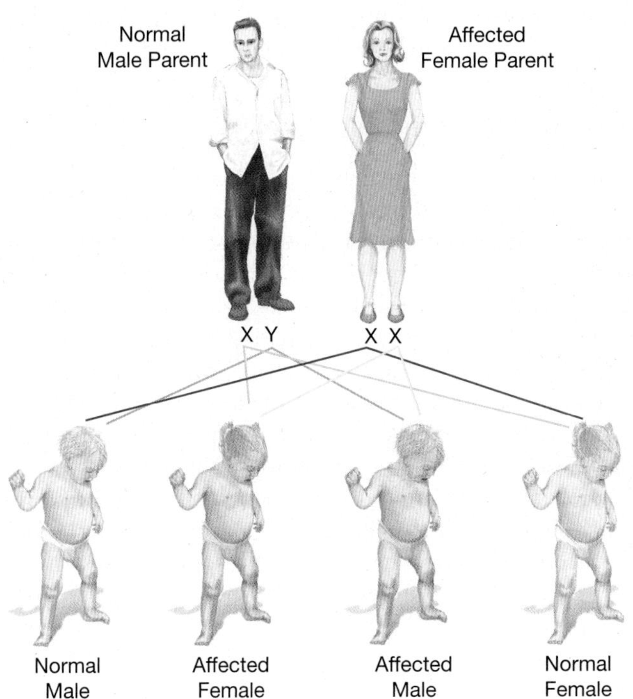

FIGURE 10.13 X-linked dominant inheritance.

from both parents, along with unknown environmental factors, produces the trait or condition. A person may inherit a predisposition to a particular anomaly or disease. The anomalies or diseases vary in severity, and often a sex bias is present. For example, pyloric stenosis is seen more often in males, while developmental hip dysplasia is much more likely to occur in females. Multifactorial conditions tend to run in families, but the pattern of inheritance is not as predictable as with single-gene disorders. The chance of recurrence is also less than in single-gene disorders, but the degree of risk is related to the number of genes in common with the affected person. The closer the degree of relationship, the more genes a person has in common with the affected family member, resulting in a higher chance that the person's offspring will have a similar defect. In multifactorial inheritance, the likelihood that both identical twins will be affected is not 100%, indicating that there are nongenetic factors involved.

Nontraditional Inheritance Patterns

Molecular studies have revealed that some genetic disorders are inherited in ways that do not follow the typical patterns of dominant, recessive, X-linked, or multifactorial inheritance. Examples of nontraditional inheritance patterns include mitochondrial inheritance and genomic imprinting. As the science of molecular genetics advances and we learn more about inheritance patterns, other nontraditional patterns of inheritance may be discovered or may be found to be relatively common.

MITOCHONDRIAL INHERITANCE

Certain diseases result from mutations in the mitochondrial DNA. Mitochondria (the part of the cell responsible for energy production) are inherited almost exclusively from the female parent. Therefore, mitochondrial inheritance is usually passed from the female to the offspring, regardless of the offspring's sex (thereby differentiating mitochondrial inheritance from X-linked recessive inheritance). These mutations are often deletions and abnormalities and are often seen in one or more organs, such as the brain, eye, and skeletal muscle. They are often associated with energy deficits in cells with high energy requirements, such as nerve and muscle cells. These disorders tend to be progressive, and the age of onset can vary from infancy to adulthood. There is an extreme amount of variability in symptoms within a family. Examples of disorders that follow mitochondrial inheritance include Kearns–Sayre syndrome (a neuromuscular disorder) and Leber hereditary optic neuropathy (which causes progressive visual impairment) (Scott & Lee, 2020b).

GENETIC IMPRINTING

Another nontraditional inheritance pattern results from a process called genetic imprinting. Genetic imprinting plays a critical role in fetal growth and development and placental functioning. It is a phenomenon by which the expression of a gene is determined by its parental origin. In genomic imprinting, both the maternal and paternal alleles are present, but only one is expressed; the other is inactive. Genetic imprinting does not alter the genetic sequence itself, but affects the phenotype observed. In these cases, the altered genes in a certain region of the genome have very different expressions depending on whether they were inherited from the male or female parent. Several human syndromes are known to be associated with defects in gene imprinting. Disorders that result from a disruption of imprinting usually involve a growth phenotype and include varying degrees of developmental problems. Common examples include Prader–Willi syndrome (a condition resulting in severe hypotonia and hyperphagia, leading to obesity and intellectual disability), Angelman syndrome (a neurodevelopmental disorder associated with intellectual disability, jerky movements, and seizures), and Beckwith–Wiedemann syndrome (characterized by somatic overgrowth, congenital malformations, and a predisposition to embryonic neoplasia) (Scott & Lee, 2020b).

Chromosomal Abnormalities

In some instances of genetic disorders, the abnormality occurs due to problems with the chromosomes. Chromosomal abnormalities do not follow straightforward patterns of inheritance. Although some chromosomal disorders can be inherited, most others occur due to random events during the formation of reproductive cells or in early fetal development.

Sperm and egg cells each have 23 unpaired chromosomes. When they unite during conception, they form a fertilized egg with 46 chromosomes. Sometimes, before pregnancy begins, an error occurs during the process of cell division, leaving an egg or sperm with too many or too few chromosomes. If this egg or sperm cell joins with a normal egg or sperm cell, the resulting embryo has a chromosomal abnormality. Chromosomal abnormalities can also occur due to an error in the structure of the chromosome. Small pieces of the chromosome may be deleted, duplicated, inverted, misplaced, or exchanged with part of another chromosome.

Most chromosomal abnormalities occur due to an error in the egg or sperm. Therefore, the abnormality is present in every cell of the body. Some abnormalities can happen after fertilization, during mitotic cell division, and result in mosaicism. Mosaicism, or the mosaic form, is when the chromosomal abnormalities do not show up in every cell; only some cells or tissues carry the abnormality. In mosaic forms of the disorder, symptoms are usually less severe than they would be if all the cells were abnormal.

Chromosomal abnormalities occur in about 1% to 2% of live births (Bacino & Lee, 2020). There is a much higher frequency of chromosomal abnormalities in spontaneous abortions and stillbirths (Bacino & Lee, 2020). Congenital anomalies and intellectual disability are often associated with chromosomal abnormalities (Bacino & Lee, 2020). These abnormalities occur on autosomal or nonsex chromosomes as well as sex chromosomes and can result from abnormalities of either chromosome number or chromosome structure.

Numeric Abnormalities

Chromosomal abnormalities of number often result from nondisjunction or failure of the chromosome pair to separate during cell division, meiosis, or mitosis. Few chromosomal numeric abnormalities are compatible with full-term development, and most result in spontaneous abortion.

Some numeric abnormalities do support development to term because the chromosome on which the abnormality is present carries relatively few genes (such as chromosome 13, 18, 21, or X). Two common abnormalities of chromosome number are monosomies and trisomies. In **monosomies**, there is only one copy of a particular chromosome instead of the usual pair (an entire single chromosome is missing). In these cases, all fetuses spontaneously abort in early pregnancy. Survival is seen only in mosaic forms of these disorders. In **trisomies**, there are three of a particular chromosome instead of the usual two (an entire single chromosome is added). Trisomies may be present in every cell or may present in the mosaic form. The most common trisomies include trisomy 21 (Down syndrome), trisomy 18, and trisomy 13.

Structural Abnormalities

Chromosomal abnormalities of structure usually occur when a portion of one or more chromosomes is broken or lost, and during the repair process, the broken ends are rejoined incorrectly. Structural abnormalities usually lead to too much or too little genetic material. Altered chromosome structure can take on several forms. Deletions occur when a portion of the chromosome is missing, resulting in a loss of that chromosomal material. Duplications are seen when a portion of the chromosome is duplicated and an extra chromosomal segment is present. Clinical findings vary depending on how much chromosomal material is involved. Inversions occur when a portion of the chromosome breaks off at two points and is turned upside down and reattached; therefore, the genetic material is inverted. With inversion, there is no loss or gain of chromosomal material, and carriers are phenotypically normal. However, they are at increased risk for miscarriage and having chromosomally abnormal offspring (Bacino & Lee, 2020). Ring chromosomes are seen when a portion of a chromosome has broken off in two places and has formed a circle or ring.

The most clinically significant structural abnormality is a translocation. This occurs when part of one chromosome is transferred to another chromosome and an abnormal rearrangement is present.

Structural abnormalities can be balanced or unbalanced. Balanced abnormalities involve the rearrangement of genetic material with neither an overall gain nor loss. People who inherit a balanced structural abnormality are usually phenotypically normal but are at a higher risk for miscarriages and chromosomally abnormal offspring. Examples of structural rearrangements that can be balanced include inversions, translocations, and ring chromosomes. Unbalanced structural abnormalities are similar to numeric abnormalities because genetic material is either gained or lost. Unbalanced structural abnormalities can encompass several genes and result in severe clinical consequences.

Sex Chromosome Abnormalities

Chromosomal abnormalities can also involve sex chromosomes. These cases are usually less severe in their clinical effects than autosomal chromosomal abnormalities. Sex chromosome abnormalities are sex specific and involve a missing or extra sex chromosome (Bacino & Lee, 2020). They affect sexual development and may cause infertility, growth abnormalities, and possibly behavioral and learning problems (Bacino, 2023). Many affected people lead essentially normal lives. Examples are Turner syndrome (in females) and Klinefelter syndrome (in males).

Genetic Evaluation and Counseling

Genetic counseling is a communication and educational process in which the influence of genetics on health is explained, along with information regarding a specific genetic disorder, its transmission, its inheritance, and options available in testing, management, and family planning (Raby & Kohlmann, 2024). A person should be referred for genetic counseling for any of a variety of reasons. Box 10.2 lists those who may benefit from genetic counseling. In many instances, geneticists and genetic counselors provide information to families regarding genetic diseases. However, an experienced family physician, pediatrician, or nurse who has received special training in genetics may also provide the information.

A genetic consultation involves evaluation of a person or a family. Its purposes are to confirm, diagnose, or rule out genetic conditions; to identify medical management issues; to calculate and communicate genetic risks to a family; to discuss ethical and legal issues; and to provide and arrange psychosocial support. Genetic counselors serve as educators and resource people for other health care providers and the general public.

The ideal time for genetic counseling is before conception. Preconception counseling gives people the chance to identify and reduce potential pregnancy risks, plan for known risks, and establish early prenatal care. Unfortunately, some people may delay seeking prenatal care until their second or third trimesters after the crucial time of organogenesis. Therefore, it is important that preconception counseling be offered to all patients as they seek health care throughout their childbearing years, especially if they are contemplating pregnancy. This requires health care providers to take a proactive role.

CONSIDER THIS!

As I waited for the genetic counselor to come into the room, my mind was filled with numerous fears and questions. What does an inconclusive amniocentesis really mean? What if this pregnancy produced an abnormal baby? How would I cope parenting a child with disabilities? If only I had gone to the midwife sooner when I thought I was pregnant, but I was still in denial. Why did I not stop drinking and smoking when I found out I was pregnant? If only I had started to take my folic acid pills when prescribed. Why didn't I research my family's history to know of any hidden genetic conditions? What about my sister who has a child with Down syndrome? What was I thinking? I guess I could play the "what if" game forever and never come up with answers. Is it too late to do anything about this? I am 37 years old and alone. I started to pray silently when the counselor opened the door.

Thoughts: This patient is reviewing the past few weeks, looking for answers to their greatest fears. Inconclusive screenings can introduce emotional torment for many patients as they wait for validating results. Are these common thoughts and fears for many people facing potential genetic disorders? What supportive interventions might the nurse offer?

BOX 10.2 Those Who May Benefit From Genetic Counseling

- Maternal age of 35 years or older when the baby is born
- Paternal age of 40 years or older
- Previous child, parents, or close relatives with an inherited disease, congenital anomalies, metabolic disorders, developmental disorders, or chromosomal abnormalities
- Consanguinity or incest
- Pregnancy screening abnormality, including alpha-fetoprotein, triple/quadruple screen, amniocentesis, or ultrasound
- Stillborn with congenital anomalies
- Two or more pregnancy losses
- Teratogen exposure or risk
- Concerns about genetic defects that occur frequently in their ethnic or racial group (for instance, those of African descent are most at risk for having a child with sickle cell anemia)
- Abnormal newborn screening
- Couples with a family history of X-linked disorders
- Carriers of autosomal recessive or dominant diseases
- Child born with one or more major malformations in a major organ system
- Child with abnormalities of growth
- Child with developmental delay, intellectual disability, blindness, or deafness

Data from Lee, B. (2020). Integration of genetics into pediatric practice. In R. M. Kleigman, J. W. St. Geme III, N. J. Blum, S. S. Shah, R. C. Tasker, K. M. Wilson, & R. E. Behrman (Eds.), *Nelson textbook of pediatrics* (21st ed., pp. 3789–3820). Elsevier.

Genetic screening and counseling can raise serious ethical and moral issues for a couple. The results of prenatal genetic testing can lead to the decision to terminate a pregnancy, even if the results are not conclusive but indicate a strong possibility that the child will have an abnormality. The severity of the abnormality may not be known, and some may find the decision to terminate unethical. Another difficult situation that provides an example of the ethical and moral issues surrounding genetic screening and counseling involves disorders that affect offspring of only one sex. A female may find they are a carrier of a gene for a disorder for which there is no prenatal screening test available. In these instances, the pregnant person may decide to terminate any pregnancy where the fetus is the affected sex, even though there is a 50% chance that the child will not inherit the disorder. In these situations, the choice is the patient's, and information and support must be provided in a nondirective, nonjudgmental manner.

Genetic counseling is particularly important if a congenital anomaly or genetic disease has been diagnosed prenatally or if a child is born with a life-threatening congenital anomaly or genetic disease. In these instances, families need information urgently so they can make immediate decisions. If a diagnosis with genetic implications is made later in life, if a person with a family history of a genetic disorder or a previous child with a genetic disorder is planning a family, or if there is suspected teratogen exposure, urgency of information is not such an issue. In these situations, the family needs time to ponder all their options. This may involve several meetings over a longer period of time.

Genetic counseling involves extensive information gathering regarding birth history, past medical history, and current health status as well as a family history of congenital anomalies, intellectual disability, genetic diseases, reproductive history, general health, and causes of death. A detailed family history is imperative and, in most instances, will include the development of a pedigree, which is like a family tree (Fig. 10.14). Information is ideally gathered on three generations, but if the family history is complicated, information from more distant relatives may be needed. Families receiving genetic counseling may benefit from being told in advance that this information will be necessary; they may need to discuss these sensitive, private issues with family members to obtain the needed facts. When necessary, medical records may be requested for family members, especially those who have a genetic disorder, to help ensure accuracy of the information. Sometimes a pedigree may reveal confidential information not known by all family members, such as an adoption, a child conceived through in vitro fertilization, or a partner not being the biologic parent of a baby. Therefore, maintaining confidentiality is extremely important. After careful analysis of the data obtained, referral to a genetic counselor when indicated is appropriate.

Medical genetic knowledge has increased dramatically during the past few decades. This has greatly expanded the role of the genetic counselor. Not only is it possible to detect specific diseases with genetic mutations, but it is also possible to test for a genetic predisposition to various diseases or conditions and certain physical characteristics. This leads to complex ethical, moral, and social issues. Maintaining patient privacy and confidentiality and administering care in a nondiscriminatory manner are essential while maintaining sensitivity to cultural differences. It is essential to respect patient autonomy and present information in a nondirective, nonjudgmental manner.

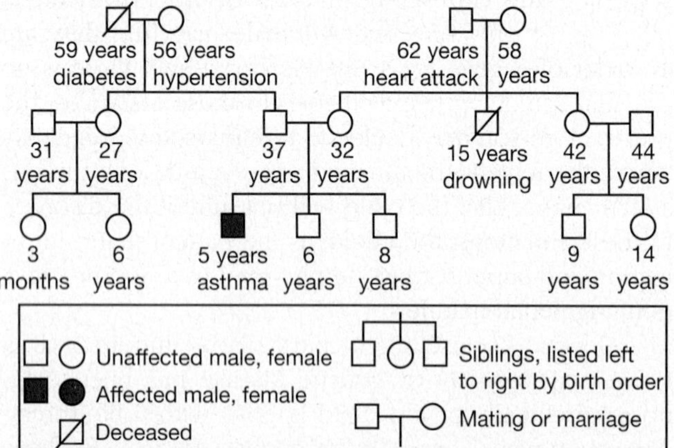

FIGURE 10.14 A pedigree is a diagram made using symbols that demonstrates the links between family members and focuses on medical and health information for each relative.

NURSING ROLES AND RESPONSIBILITIES

Nurses are at the forefront of patient care and will participate fully in genetic-based and genomic-based activities. The nurse is likely to interact with the patient in a variety of ways related to genetics: taking a family history, scheduling genetic testing, explaining the purposes of all screening and diagnostic tests, answering questions, providing information and psychosocial support to people and families, and addressing concerns raised by family members. Nurses are often the first health care providers to encounter patients with preconception and prenatal issues. Genetic counseling is more than providing the patient with information. It is a form of communication that facilitates decisions on choosing a course of action that are made solely by the patient. Nurses play an important role in beginning the preconception counseling process and referring patients and their partners for further genetic testing when indicated.

An accurate and thorough family history is an essential part of preconception counseling. Nurses in any practice setting can obtain a patient's history during the initial encounter. At a basic level, all nurses should be able to take a family medical history to help identify those at risk for genetic conditions, and then initiate a referral when appropriate. Box 10.3 presents examples of focused assessment questions that can be used. Based on the information gathered during the history, the nurse must decide whether a referral to a genetic specialist is necessary or whether further evaluation is needed. Families identified with genetic issues need unique clinical care including management of acute illnesses, screening for long-term complications, discussion of the etiology of the condition, connections to social supports, clarification of the recurrence risks, and prenatal testing and treatment options. Prenatal testing to assess for genetic risks and defects might be used to identify genetic disorders. Refer to Chapter 12 for additional information.

> Remember Robert and Kate? Based on the information gathered from their genetic history, they were referred to a genetic specialist. What prenatal tests might be ordered to assess their risk for genetic disorders? What would be the nurse's role related to genetic counseling?

Talking with family members who have recently been diagnosed with genetic disorders or who have had a child born with congenital anomalies can be difficult.

BOX 10.3 Focused Health Assessment: Genetic History

- What was the cause and age of death for family members who died at an early age?
- Does any consanguinity exist between relatives?
- Do any serious illnesses or chronic conditions exist? If so, what was the age of onset?
- Do any female family members have a history of miscarriages, stillbirths, or diabetes?
- Do any female members have a history of alcohol or drug use during pregnancy?
- What were the ages of female members during childbearing, especially if older than 35 years?
- Do any family members have intellectual disabilities or developmental delays?
- Do any family members have known or suspected metabolic disorders such as phenylketonuria?
- What is the age of both parents presently during this pregnancy?
- Do any family members have an affective disorder such as bipolar disorder?
- Have any close relatives been diagnosed with any type of cancer?
- What is your racial and ethnic background (to explore as related to certain disorders)?
- Do any family members have a known or suspected chromosomal disorder?
- Do any family members have a progressive neurologic disorder?

Raby, B. A., & Kohlmann, W. (2024). Genetic counseling: Family history interpretation and risk assessment. *UpToDate*. https://www.uptodate.com/contents/genetic-counseling-family-history-interpretation-and-risk-assessment; Centers for Disease Control and Prevention. (2023c). *Family health history and planning for pregnancy*. https://www.cdc.gov/genomics/famhistory/famhist_plan_pregnancy.htm

Many times, the nurse may be the one who has first contact with these parents and will be the one to provide follow-up care. Genetic disorders are significant, life-changing, and possibly life-threatening situations. Genetic information is highly technical, and the field is undergoing significant technologic advances. Nurses need an understanding of who will benefit from genetic counseling and must be able to discuss the role of the genetic counselor with families. The goal is to ensure that families at risk are aware that genetic counseling is available before they attempt to have another baby.

Based on the results of their genetic tests, Robert and Kate are placed at moderate risk for having an infant with an autosomal recessive genetic disorder. The couple asks the nurse what all of this means. What information should the nurse provide about concepts of probability and disorder susceptibility for this couple? How can the nurse help this couple to make knowledgeable decisions concerning their reproductive future?

Nurses play an essential role in providing emotional support to the family through this challenging time. Genetics permeates all aspects of health care. Nurses who have an understanding of genetics and genomics will possess the foundation to provide high-quality, evidence-based care especially with follow-up counseling after the couple or family has been to the genetic specialist.

TAKE NOTE!

Nurses need to be actively engaged with patients and their families and help them consider the facts, values, and context in which they are making decisions. Nurses need to be open and honest with families as they discuss these sensitive and emotional choices.

Nurses should provide ongoing support and education for patients and their families. This includes coping with the disease burden, helping patients and families adapt to a condition in the family, and ensuring adequate understanding of the genetic risks and the available prenatal diagnostic and reproductive choices. The nurse is in an ideal position to help families review what has been discussed during the genetic counseling sessions and to answer any additional questions they might have. Referral to appropriate agencies, support groups, and resources, such as a social worker, clergy, or an ethicist, is another key role when caring for families with suspected or diagnosed genetic disorders. In short, nurses need to be equipped to integrate genetics and genomics into their practice to improve patient care for all families encountered.

KEY CONCEPTS

- Fertilization, which takes place in the outer third of the ampulla of the fallopian tube, leads to the formation of a zygote. The zygote undergoes cleavage, eventually implanting in the endometrium about 7 to 10 days after conception.
- Three embryonic layers of cells are formed: the ectoderm, which forms the central nervous system, special senses, skin, and glands; the mesoderm, which forms the skeletal, urinary, circulatory, and reproductive systems; and the endoderm, which forms the respiratory system, liver, pancreas, and digestive system.
- Amniotic fluid surrounds the embryo and increases in volume as the pregnancy progresses, reaching approximately a liter by term.
- At no time during pregnancy is there any direct connection between the blood of the fetus and the blood of the pregnant person, so there is no mixing of blood.
- The placenta protects the fetus from immune attack by the pregnant person's body, removes waste

products from the fetus, induces the pregnant person to eat more and thereby bring more food to the placenta, and, near the time of delivery, produces hormones that mature fetal organs in preparation for life outside the uterus.

- The purpose of fetal circulation is to carry highly oxygenated blood to vital areas (heart and brain) while first shunting it away from less vital ones (lungs and liver).
- Humans have 46 paired chromosomes that are found in all cells of the body, except the ovum and sperm cells, which have just 23 chromosomes. Each person has a unique genetic constitution, or genotype.
- Research from the HGP has provided a better understanding of the genetic contribution to disease.
- Genetic disorders can result from abnormalities in patterns of inheritance or chromosomal abnormalities involving chromosomal number or structure.
- Autosomal dominant inheritance occurs when a single gene in the heterozygous state is capable of producing the phenotype. Autosomal recessive inheritance occurs when two copies of the mutant or abnormal gene in the homozygous state are necessary to produce the phenotype. X-linked inheritance disorders are those associated with altered genes present on the X chromosome. They can be dominant or recessive.
- In some instances of genetic disorders, a chromosomal abnormality occurs. Chromosomal abnormalities do not follow straightforward patterns of inheritance. These abnormalities occur on autosomal as well as sex chromosomes and can result from changes in the number of chromosomes or changes in the structure of the chromosomes.
- Genetic counseling involves evaluation of a person or a family. Its purpose is to confirm, diagnose, or rule out genetic conditions; identify medical management issues; calculate and communicate genetic risks to a family; discuss ethical and legal issues; and assist in providing and arranging psychosocial support.
- Legal, ethical, and social issues that can arise related to genetic testing include the privacy and confidentiality of genetic information, who should have access to personal genetic information, psychological impact and stigmatization due to individual genetic differences, use of genetic information in reproductive decision making and reproductive rights, and whether testing is to be performed if no cure is available.
- Preconception screening and counseling can raise serious ethical and moral issues for people. The results of prenatal genetic testing can lead to the decision to terminate a pregnancy.
- Nurses play an important role in beginning the preconception counseling process and referring patients for further genetic information when indicated. Many times, the nurse is the one who has first contact with these patients and will be the one to provide follow-up care.
- Nurses need to have a solid understanding of who will benefit from genetic counseling and must be able to discuss the role of the genetic counselor with families, ensuring that families at risk are aware that genetic counseling is available before they attempt to have another baby.
- Nurses play an essential role in providing emotional support and referrals to appropriate agencies, support groups, and resources when caring for families with suspected or diagnosed genetic disorders. Nurses can assist patients with their decision making by referring them to a social worker, a chaplain, or an ethicist.

Unfolding Patient Stories: Brenda Patton • Part 2

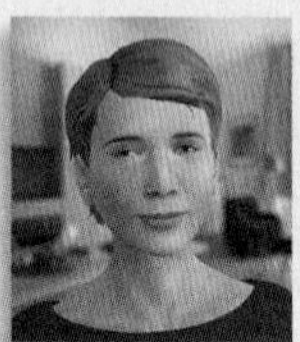

Recall from Chapter 9 Brenda Patton. She is 18 years old at 24 weeks' gestation with her first child. During each prenatal visit, what questions would the nurse ask to evaluate fetal well-being? What factors can interfere with normal growth and development of the fetus? Describe the assessments the nurse performs to monitor fetal growth and development.

Care for Brenda and other patients in a realistic virtual environment: ***vSim** for Nursing* (thepoint.lww.com/vSimMaternity). Practice documenting these patients' care in DocuCare (thepoint.lww.com/DocuCareEHR).

REFERENCES AND RECOMMENDED READINGS

Bacino, C. A. (2023). Sex chromosome abnormalities. *UpToDate*. Retrieved April 1, 2024, from https://www.uptodate.com/contents/sex-chromosome-abnormalities

Bacino, C. A., & Lee, B. (2020). Cytogenetics. In R. M. Kleigman, J. W. St. Geme III, N. J. Blum, S. S. Shah, R. C. Tasker, K. M. Wilson, & R. E. Behrman (Eds.), *Nelson textbook of pediatrics* (21st ed., pp. 3903–3999). Elsevier.

Bastauros, H. (2023). *Human reproduction: A clinical approach*. https://iastate.pressbooks.pub/humanreproduction/chapter/cleavage-stage/

Beloosesky, R., & Ross, M. G. (2022). Oligohydramnios: Etiology, diagnosis, and management in singleton gestations. *UpToDate*. Retrieved April 1, 2024, from https://www.uptodate.com/contents/oligohydramnios-etiology-diagnosis-and-management-in-singleton-gestations

Beloosesky, R., & Ross, M. G. (2024). Polyhydramnios: Etiology, diagnosis, and management in singleton gestations. *UpToDate*. Retrieved April 1, 2024, from https://www.uptodate.com/contents/polyhydramnios-etiology-diagnosis-and-management-in-singleton-gestations

Breilyn, M. S., & Levy, P. A. (2023). Human genetics and dysmorphology. In K. J. Marcdante, R. M. Kleigman, & A. M. Schuh (Eds.), *Nelson essentials of pediatrics* (9th ed., pp. 177–199). Elsevier.

Centers for Disease Control and Prevention. (2023a). *Medicine and pregnancy.* https://www.cdc.gov/pregnancy/meds/treatingfortwo/index.html

Centers for Disease Control and Prevention. (2023b). *Birth defects: Data & statistics on birth defects.* https://www.cdc.gov/ncbddd/birthdefects/data.html

Centers for Disease Control and Prevention. (2023c). *Family health history and planning for pregnancy.* https://www.cdc.gov/genomics/famhistory/famhist_plan_pregnancy.htm

Cunningham, F. G., Leveno, K. J., Dashe, J. S., Hoffman, B. L., Spong, C. Y., & Casey, B. M. (2022). Embryogenesis and fetal development. In F. G. Cunningham, K. J. Leveno, J. S. Dashe, B. L. Hoffman, C. Y., Spong, & B. M. Casey (Eds.), *William's obstetrics* (26th ed.). McGraw-Hill.

Delgado, A., Schulkin, J., & Macri, C. J. (2022). Prenatal genetic screening and diagnostic testing: Assessing patient's knowledge, clinical experiences, and utilized resources in comparison to provider's perceptions. *American Journal of Perinatology Reports, 12*(1), 27–32. https://doi.org/10.1055/s-0041-1742236

Donovan, M. F., & Cascella, M. (2022). Embryology, weeks 6–8. *StatPearls.* https://www.ncbi.nlm.nih.gov/books/NBK563181/

Flomenberg, P., & Daniel, R. (2024). Overview of gene therapy, gene editing, and gene silencing. *UpToDate.* Retrieved April 1, 2024, from https://www.uptodate.com/contents/overview-of-gene-therapy-gene-editing-and-gene-silencing

Heil, J. R., & Bordoni, B. (2023). Embryology, umbilical cord. *StatPearls.* https://www.ncbi.nlm.nih.gov/books/NBK557490/

Kapilia, V., & Chaudhry, K. (2023). Physiology, placenta. *StatPearls.* https://www.ncbi.nlm.nih.gov/books/NBK538332/

Kruse, J., Mueller, R., Aghdassi, A. A., Lerch, M. M., & Salloch, S. (2022). Genetic testing for rare diseases: A systematic review of ethical aspects. *Frontiers in Genetics*, 12, 701988. https://doi.org/10.3389/fgene.2021.701988

Lee, B. (2020). Integration of genetics into pediatric practice. In R. M. Kleigman, J. W. St. Geme III, N. J. Blum, S. S. Shah, R. C. Tasker, K. M. Wilson, & R. E. Behrman (Eds.), *Nelson textbook of pediatrics* (21st ed., pp. 3789–3820). Elsevier.

Muhr, J., Arbor, T. C., & Ackerman, K. M. (2023). Embryology, gastrulation. *StatPearls.* https://www.ncbi.nlm.nih.gov/books/NBK554394/#:

National Human Genome Research Institute. (2023). *The human genome project.* https://www.genome.gov/human-genome-project

National Human Genome Research Institute. (2024). *Gene therapy.* https://www.genome.gov/genetics-glossary/Gene-Therapy#

Raby, B. A. (2021). Inheritance patterns of monogenic disorders (Mendelian and non-Mendelian). *UpToDate.* Retrieved May 26, 2023, from https://www.uptodate.com/contents/inheritance-patterns-of-monogenic-disorders-mendelian-and-non-mendelian

Raby, B. A., & Kohlmann, W. (2024). Genetic counseling: Family history interpretation and risk assessment. *UpToDate.* Retrieved April 1, 2024, from https://www.uptodate.com/contents/genetic-counseling-family-history-interpretation-and-risk-assessment

Remien, K., & Majmundar, S. H. (2023). Physiology, fetal circulation. *StatPearls.* https://www.ncbi.nlm.nih.gov/books/NBK539710/

Roberts, V., & Myatt, L. (2023). Placental development and physiology. *UpToDate.* Retrieved April 2, 2024, from https://www.uptodate.com/contents/placental-development-and-physiology

Schnebly, A. R. (2021). Sex determination in humans. *Embryo Project Encyclopedia.* https://embryo.asu.edu/pages/sex-determination-humans

Scott, D. A., & Lee, B. (2020a). The genetic approach in pediatric medicine. In R. M. Kleigman, J. W. St. Geme III, N. J. Blum, S. S. Shah, R. C. Tasker, K. M. Wilson, & R. E. Behrman (Eds.), *Nelson textbook of pediatrics* (21st ed., pp. 3821–3837). Elsevier.

Scott, D. A., & Lee, B. (2020b). Patterns of genetic transmission. In R. M. Kleigman, J. W. St. Geme III, N. J. Blum, S. S. Shah, R. C. Tasker, K. M. Wilson, & R. E. Behrman (Eds.), *Nelson textbook of pediatrics* (21st ed., pp. 3862–3902). Elsevier.

Truong, N., Richardson, L., & Menon, R. (2023). The role of fetal membranes during gestation, at term, and preterm labor: Fetal membranes role during pregnancy. *Placenta and Reproductive Medicine*, *2*, 1–8. https://doi.org/10.54844/prm.2022.0296

Tsamantioti, E. S., & Hashmi, M. F. (2024). Teratogenic medications. *StatPearls.* https://www.ncbi.nlm.nih.gov/books/NBK553086/

U.S. Food & Drug Administration. (2022). *How gene therapy can cure or treat diseases.* https://www.fda.gov/consumers/consumer-updates/how-gene-therapy-can-cure-or-treat-diseases

World Health Organization. (2023). *World Birth Defects Day: Many birth defects, one voice.* https://www.who.int/southeastasia/news/detail/02-03-2023-world-birth-defects-day-many-birth-defects-one-voice

DEVELOPING CLINICAL JUDGMENT

PRACTICING FOR NCLEX

1. The nurse educator is teaching a group of students about fertilization. The nurse determines that the teaching was successful when the group identifies which as the usual site of fertilization?
   a. Fundus of the uterus
   b. Endometrium of the uterus
   c. Upper portion of fallopian tube
   d. Follicular tissue of the ovary
2. The nurse is counseling a couple in which one person is affected by an autosomal dominant disorder. They express concerns about the risk of transmitting the disorder. What is the best response by the nurse regarding the risk that their baby may have the disease?
   a. "You have a one-in-four (25%) chance."
   b. "The risk is 12.5%, or a one-in-eight chance."
   c. "The chance is 100%."
   d. "Your risk is 50%, or a one-in-two chance.
3. The nurse is performing a preconception assessment. What does the nurse determine is the first step in assessing a couple's risk for their offspring having a genetic disorder?
   a. Observing the patient and family over time
   b. Conducting extensive psychological testing
   c. Obtaining a thorough family health history
   d. Completing an extensive exclusionary list
4. The nurse working in a women's health clinic determines that genetic counseling may be appropriate for a person (Select any three):
   a. who just had their first miscarriage at 10 weeks.
   b. who is 30 years old and planning to conceive.
   c. whose history reveals a close relative with fragile X syndrome.
   d. who is 18 weeks pregnant and whose triple screen came back normal.
   e. who reports a history of three miscarriages.
   f. who reports their first-born child had a cleft lip.

CRITICAL THINKING EXERCISE

1. Mr. and Mrs. Martin wish to start a family, but they cannot agree on something important: Mr. Martin wants his wife to be tested for cystic fibrosis (CF) to see if she is a carrier. Mr. Martin had a brother with CF and watched his parents struggle with the hardship and the expense of caring for him, and he does not want to experience it in his own life. Mr. Martin has found out he is a CF carrier. Mrs. Martin does not want to have the test because she figures that once a baby is in their arms, they will be glad, no matter what.
   a. What information and education should this couple consider before deciding whether to have the test?
   b. How can you assist this couple in their decision-making process?
   c. What is your role in this situation if you don't agree with their decision?

STUDY ACTIVITIES

1. Obtain the video *Miracle of Life* or any current childbirth video, which shows conception and fetal development. What are your impressions? Is the title of this video appropriate?
2. Select websites related to genetics and pregnancy and explore the topic of genetics. Critique the information presented. Is it understandable to a layperson? What specifically did you learn? Share your findings with your classmates during a discussion group.
3. Draw your own family pedigree, identifying inheritance patterns. Share it with your family to validate its accuracy. What did you discover about your family's past health?
4. Select one of the various prenatal screening tests (alpha-fetoprotein, amniocentesis, or fetal nuchal translucency) and research it in depth. Role-play with another nursing student how you would explain its purpose, the procedure, and potential findings to an expectant couple at risk for a fetal abnormality.

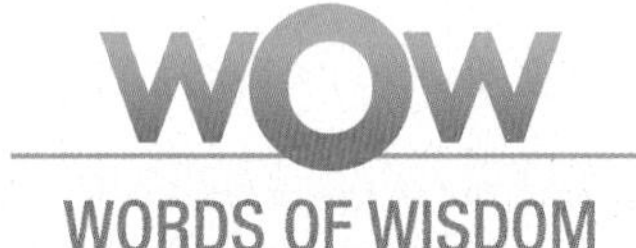

WORDS OF WISDOM

When a person discovers they are pregnant, they must remember to protect and nourish the fetus by making wise choices.

11

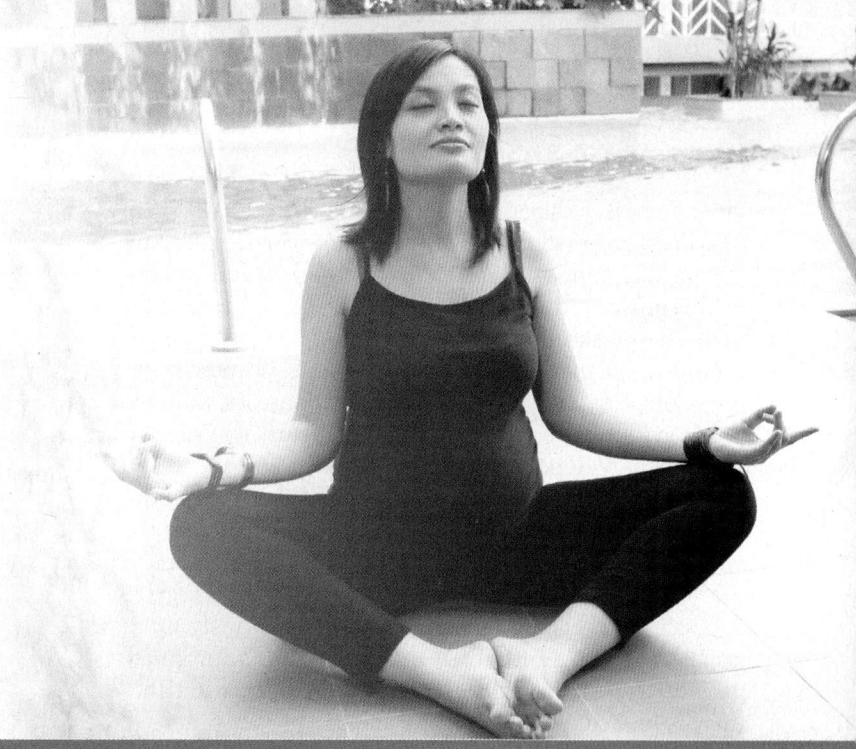

Maternal Adaptation During Pregnancy

LEARNING OBJECTIVES

Upon completion of the chapter, you will be able to:

1. Differentiate between subjective (presumptive), objective (probable), and diagnostic (positive) signs of pregnancy.
2. Describe maternal physiologic changes that occur during pregnancy.
3. Summarize the nutritional needs of the pregnant person and their fetus.
4. Characterize the emotional and psychological changes that occur during pregnancy.

KEY TERMS

ballottement (bal-ot-mōn[h]')
Braxton Hicks contractions
Chadwick sign
dietary reference intakes (DRIs)
Goodell sign
Hegar sign
linea nigra
physiologic anemia of pregnancy
pica
quickening
trimester

Marva, age 17, appeared at the health department clinic complaining that they had a stomach virus and needed to be seen right away. When the nurse asked Marva additional questions about the illness, Marva reported that they had been sick to their stomach and "exhausted" for days. They had stopped eating to avoid any more nausea and vomiting.

INTRODUCTION

Pregnancy is a dynamic and precisely coordinated process involving systemic and local changes in the pregnant person that support the supply of nutrients and oxygen to the growing fetus in utero and in subsequent lactation. The person's body goes through immense changes during pregnancy that impact all organs in their body. Pregnancy involves a coordinated response of multiple organ systems to support the growing fetus. The success of pregnancy depends on (1) fertilization and successful implantation of the developing embryo into the endometrium; (2) development and function of the placenta, which sustains the pregnancy and meets the demands of the fetus; (3) adaptation of the maternal physiology to support the pregnant person and fetus and satisfy nutritional, metabolic, and physical demands; (4) appropriate growth and functional development of organs and homeostatic systems in the fetus; and (5) proper timing of birth so that the fetus is mature enough to survive outside the uterus (Pascual & Langaker, 2023).

A pregnancy is divided into three **trimesters** of 13 weeks each. Within each trimester, numerous adaptations take place that facilitate the growth of the fetus. The most obvious are physical changes to accommodate the growing fetus, but pregnant people also undergo psychological changes as they prepare to give birth. A thorough understanding of these numerous changes and adaptations is essential for all nurses caring for people who are pregnant.

What additional information is necessary to complete the assessment of Marva, the 17-year-old, with nausea and vomiting? What diagnostic tests might be done to confirm the nurse's suspicion that Marva is pregnant?

SIGNS AND SYMPTOMS OF PREGNANCY

Traditionally, signs and symptoms of pregnancy have been grouped into the following categories: presumptive, probable, and positive (Box 11.1). The only signs that can determine a pregnancy with 100% accuracy are positive signs.

Presumptive Signs

Presumptive, or subjective, signs are those signs that the pregnant person can perceive. The most obvious presumptive sign of pregnancy is the absence of menstruation. Skipping a period is not a reliable sign of pregnancy by itself, but if it is accompanied by consistent nausea, fatigue, breast tenderness, and urinary frequency, the person may be pregnant.

Presumptive changes can be caused by conditions other than pregnancy. For example, amenorrhea can be caused by early menopause, endocrine dysfunction, malnutrition, anemia, diabetes mellitus, long-distance running, cancer, or stress. Nausea and vomiting can be caused by gastrointestinal disorders, food poisoning, acute infections, or eating disorders. Fatigue could be caused by anemia, stress, or viral infections. Breast tenderness may result from chronic cystic mastitis, premenstrual changes, or the use of oral contraceptives. Urinary frequency could have a variety of causes other than pregnancy, such as infection, cystocele, structural disorders, pelvic tumors, or emotional tension.

Probable Signs

Physical Signs

Probable signs of pregnancy are those that can be detected on physical examination by a health care provider. Common probable signs of pregnancy include softening of the lower uterine segment or isthmus (**Hegar sign**), softening of the cervix (**Goodell sign**), and a bluish-purple coloration of the vaginal mucosa and cervix (**Chadwick sign**). Other probable signs include changes in the

BOX **11.1** Signs and Symptoms of Pregnancy

Presumptive (Time of Occurrence)	Probable (Time of Occurrence)	Positive (Time of Occurrence)
Amenorrhea Breast enlargement and tenderness Nausea and vomiting Urinary frequency without dysuria Excessive fatigue Fetal movements known as **quickening** (18–20 weeks)	Braxton Hicks contractions (16–28 weeks) Positive pregnancy test (4–12 weeks) Hyperpigmentation of the skin Increased abdominal girth from uterine enlargement Ballottement (16–28 weeks) Goodell sign (5 weeks) Chadwick sign (6–8 weeks) Hegar sign (about 16 weeks) Palpable fetal outline	Ultrasound verification of embryo or fetus outline Fetal movement felt by experienced clinician (20 weeks) Auscultation of fetal heart tones Fetal heart rate seen on ultrasound (5–6 weeks)

Adapted from Adams, E. D. (2022). Anatomic and physiologic adaptations of normal pregnancy. In K. D. Schuiling & F. E. Likis (Eds.), *Gynecologic health care* (4th ed., pp. 677–682). Jones & Bartlett Learning.

CONSIDER THIS!

Jim and I decided to start our family, so I stopped taking the pill 3 months ago. One morning when I got out of bed to take the dog out, I felt queasy and lightheaded. I hoped I was not coming down with the flu. By the end of the week, I was feeling really tired and started taking naps in the afternoon. In addition, I seemed to be going to the bathroom frequently, despite not drinking much fluid. When my breasts started to tingle and ache, I decided to make an appointment with my doctor to see what illness I had contracted.

After listening to my list of physical complaints, the office nurse asked me if I might be pregnant. My eyes opened wide; I had somehow missed the link between my symptoms and pregnancy. I started to think about when my last period was, and it had been 2 months ago. The office nurse ran a pregnancy test, and much to my surprise, it was positive!

Thoughts: *Many people stop contraceptives in an attempt to achieve pregnancy but miss the early signs of pregnancy. This patient was experiencing several signs of early pregnancy—urinary frequency, fatigue, morning nausea, and breast tenderness. What advice can the nurse give this patient to ease these symptoms? What additional education related to pregnancy would be appropriate at this time?*

shape and size of the uterus, abdominal enlargement, Braxton Hicks contractions, and **ballottement** (the examiner pushes against the patient's cervix during a pelvic examination and feels a rebound from the floating fetus).

Pregnancy Tests

Along with these physical signs, pregnancy tests are also considered a probable sign of pregnancy. Several pregnancy tests are available. These tests vary in sensitivity, specificity, and accuracy and are influenced by the length of gestation, specimen concentration, presence of blood, the presence of some drugs, and user technique. Serum and urine tests for pregnancy measure the presence of human chorionic gonadotropin (hCG), which is a glycoprotein and the earliest biochemical marker for pregnancy. Many pregnancy tests are based on the recognition of hCG or a beta subunit of hCG. An hCG level lower than 5 mIU/mL is considered negative for pregnancy; anything higher than 25 mIU/mL is considered positive for pregnancy. hCG levels in normal pregnancy usually double every 29 to 53 hours during the first 30 days after implantation and peak around 8 to 10 weeks' gestation (Bastian & Brown, 2023). The hCG doubling time has been used as a marker by clinicians to differentiate normal from abnormal gestations. Low levels are associated with an ectopic pregnancy, and higher-than-normal levels may indicate a multiple-gestation pregnancy (Bastian & Brown, 2023).

In-home pregnancy testing became available in the United States in late 1977. In-home testing appealed to the general public because of convenience, cost, and confidentiality. In-home tests are highly accurate, but it is recommended that a positive test be confirmed via Doppler of fetal heart sounds, ultrasound, physical examination, or serum pregnancy test (Bastian & Brown 2023). Some in-home tests can detect 97% of pregnancies as early as one day after a missed menses if done properly, but others will detect only 50% to 60% of pregnancies on the first day of missed menses (Bastian & Brown, 2023). A major concern with home pregnancy tests is the possibility of a false negative when the test is performed too early and the hCG level has not risen high enough to be detected by the test. It is recommended that if absence of menses continues, the person should retest for pregnancy in 1 week (Bastian & Brown, 2023). The limitations of these tests must be understood so that pregnancy detection is not significantly delayed. Early pregnancy detection allows for the commencement of prenatal care, potential medication changes, and lifestyle changes to promote a healthy pregnancy.

TAKE NOTE!

This elevation of hCG corresponds to the morning sickness period of approximately 6 to 12 weeks during early pregnancy.

Although probable signs suggest pregnancy and are more reliable than presumptive signs, they still are not 100% reliable in confirming a pregnancy. For example, uterine tumors, polyps, infection, and pelvic congestion can cause changes to uterine shape, size, and consistency. And although pregnancy tests are used to establish the diagnosis of pregnancy when the physical signs are still inconclusive, they are not completely reliable, because conditions other than pregnancy (e.g., ovarian cancer, choriocarcinoma, hydatidiform mole) can also elevate hCG levels.

Positive Signs

Usually within 2 weeks after missed menses, enough subjective symptoms are present so that a person can be reasonably sure that they are pregnant. However, an experienced health care provider can confirm the person's suspicions by identifying positive signs of pregnancy that can be directly attributed to the fetus. The positive signs of pregnancy confirm that a fetus is growing in the uterus. Visualizing the fetus by ultrasound, palpating for fetal movements, and hearing a fetal heartbeat are all signs that make the pregnancy a certainty.

If the pregnancy test is positive, the clinical visit should include an estimation of gestational age so that appropriate counseling can be provided. In addition, patients should receive information about the normal signs and symptoms of early pregnancy and should be instructed to report any concerns to the health care provider for further evaluation. Once pregnancy has been confirmed, the health care provider will set up a schedule of prenatal visits to assess the patient and the fetus throughout the entire pregnancy. Assessment and education begin at the first prenatal visit and continue throughout the pregnancy (see Chapter 12).

Remember Marva, who thought they had a stomach virus? Their pregnancy test was positive. During the assessment, Marva acknowledged missing two menstrual periods and being sexually active with their boyfriend without using protection. What is the nurse's role at this point in caring for Marva? What instructions might be given to Marva while they wait for their first prenatal visit?

PHYSIOLOGIC ADAPTATIONS DURING PREGNANCY

Every system of a person's body changes during pregnancy to accommodate the needs of the growing fetus, and these changes occur with startling speed. The physical changes of pregnancy can be uncomfortable, though every person reacts uniquely.

Reproductive System Adaptations

Immense changes occur throughout the person's body during pregnancy to accommodate the growing fetus. Many have a protective role for maternal homeostasis and are essential in meeting the demands of both the pregnant person and the fetus. Many adaptations are reversible after the person gives birth, but some persist for life.

Uterus

In pregnancy, there is a decrease in uterine vascular and muscle tone and a rise in blood flow. The uterus grows at a steady and predictable rate during pregnancy. Normally pear-shaped, the uterus expands more in length than width and exits the pelvis by 12 weeks' gestation. During the first few months of pregnancy, estrogen stimulates uterine growth, and the uterus undergoes a tremendous increase in size, weight, length, width, depth, volume, and overall capacity. The weight of the uterus increases from 70 g (1 oz) to about 1,100 g (2.2 lb) at term; its capacity increases from 10 to 5,000 mL (Pascual & Langaker, 2023). The uterine walls thin to 1.5 cm (0.59 in) or less; the shape changes from an inverted pear shape that is solid to a soft, hollow globe (Records & Clark, 2024).

Uterine growth occurs as a result of both hyperplasia and hypertrophy of the myometrial cells, which do not increase much in number but do increase in size. In early pregnancy, uterine growth is due to hyperplasia of uterine smooth muscle cells within the myometrium; however, the major component of myometrial growth occurs after mid-gestation due to smooth muscle cell hypertrophy caused by mechanical stretch of uterine tissue by the growing fetus (Adams, 2022). Blood vessels elongate, enlarge, dilate, and sprout new branches to support and nourish the growing muscle tissue, and the increase in uterine weight is accompanied by a large increase in uterine blood flow, which is necessary to perfuse the uterine muscle and accommodate the growing fetus. As pregnancy progresses, 80% to 90% of uterine blood flow goes to the placenta with the remainder distributed between the endometrium and myometrium. During pregnancy, the diameter of the main uterine artery approximately doubles in size to accommodate the increased blood volume needed to supply the placenta (Chaudhry & Chaudhry, 2023).

Uterine contractility is enhanced as well. Spontaneous, irregular, and painless contractions, called **Braxton Hicks contractions**, begin during the first trimester. These contractions continue throughout pregnancy, becoming especially noticeable during the last month, when they function to thin out or efface the cervix before birth (see Chapter 12, for more information).

The lower portion of the uterus (the isthmus) does not undergo hypertrophy and becomes increasingly thinner as pregnancy progresses, thereby forming the lower uterine segment. Changes in the lower uterus occurring during the first 6 to 8 weeks' gestation indicate some of the typical findings, including a positive Hegar sign. This softening and compressibility of the lower uterine segment results in exaggerated uterine anteflexion during the early months of pregnancy (Reports & Clark, 2024).

The uterus remains in the pelvic cavity for the first 3 months of pregnancy, after which it progressively ascends into the abdomen (Fig. 11.1). As the uterus grows, it presses on the urinary bladder and causes the increased frequency of urination experienced during early pregnancy. In addition, the heavy gravid uterus in the last trimester can fall back against the inferior vena cava in the supine position, resulting in vena cava compression, which reduces venous return and decreases cardiac output and blood pressure, increasing orthostatic stress. This occurs when the pregnant person changes their position from recumbent to sitting to standing. This acute hemodynamic change, termed *supine hypotensive syndrome*, causes the person to experience symptoms of weakness, lightheadedness, nausea, dizziness, or syncope (Fig. 11.2). These changes are reversed when the person is in the side-lying position, which displaces the uterus to the left and off the vena cava.

The uterus becomes ovoid as length increases over width. By 20 weeks' gestation, the fundus, or top of the uterus, is at the level of the umbilicus and measures 20 cm. A monthly measurement of the height of the top of the uterus in centimeters, which corresponds to the number of gestational weeks, is commonly used to date the pregnancy.

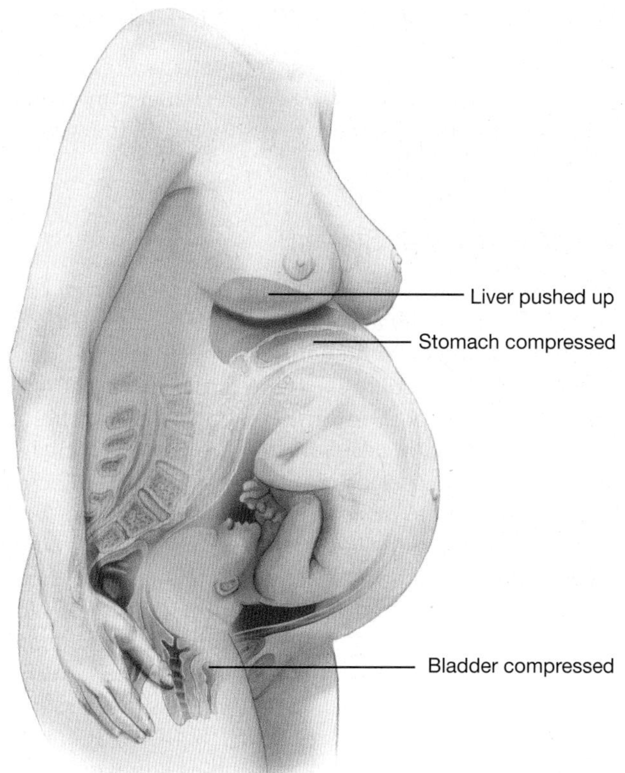

FIGURE 11.1 The growing uterus in the abdomen.

TAKE NOTE!

Fundal height can usually be correlated with gestational weeks most accurately between 18 and 32 weeks. Obesity, hydramnios, and uterine fibroids interfere with the accuracy of this correlation.

The fundus reaches its highest level, at the xiphoid process, at approximately 36 weeks. Between 38 and 40 weeks, fundal height drops as the fetus begins to descend and engage into the pelvis. Because it pushes against the diaphragm, many pregnant people experience shortness of breath. By 40 weeks, the fetal head begins to descend and engage in the pelvis, which is termed *lightening*. For the person who is pregnant for the first time, lightening usually occurs approximately 2 weeks before the onset of labor; for the person who is experiencing a second or subsequent pregnancy, it usually occurs at the onset of labor. Although breathing becomes easier because of this descent, the pressure on the urinary bladder now increases and the person now experiences urinary frequency again, as they had in the first trimester of pregnancy.

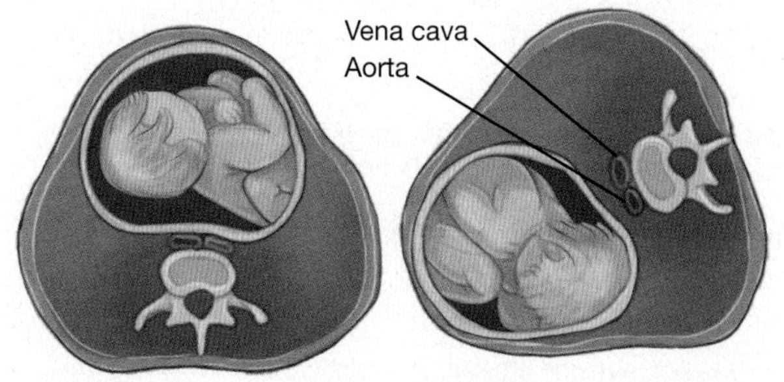

FIGURE 11.2 Supine hypotensive syndrome.

Cervix

Between weeks 6 and 8 of pregnancy, the cervix begins to soften (Goodell sign) due to vasocongestion and the influence of estrogen. Along with the softening, the endocervical glands increase in size and number and produce more cervical mucus. Under the influence of progesterone, a thick mucus plug is formed that blocks the cervical os and protects the opening from bacterial invasion. At about the same time, increased vascularization of the cervix causes Chadwick sign, a cyanosis or bluish-purple discoloration. Cervical ripening (softening, effacement, and increased distensibility) begins about 4 weeks before birth. The connective tissues of the cervix undergo biochemical modifications in preparation for labor that result in changes to its elasticity and strength. The cervix begins to soften and thin (referred to as cervical ripening) due to increasing estrogen and changes in the solubility of collagen (Adams, 2022).

Vagina

During pregnancy, vascularity increases because of the influences of estrogen, resulting in pelvic congestion and hypertrophy of the vagina in preparation for the distention needed for birth. The vaginal mucosa thickens, the connective tissue begins to loosen, the smooth muscle begins to hypertrophy, and the vaginal vault begins to lengthen in preparation for expansion during birth (Adams, 2022). Most people experience an increase in a whitish/yellowish vaginal discharge, called leukorrhea, during the second trimester of pregnancy. Vaginal pH increases, leading to an increased risk for candidiasis (Adams, 2022). Candidiasis is a benign fungal condition that is uncomfortable for the person and can be transmitted from an infected person to their newborn at birth. Neonates develop an oral infection known as thrush, which presents as white patches on the mucous membranes of their mouths. It is self-limiting and is treated with local antifungal agents.

Ovaries

The increased blood supply to the ovaries causes them to enlarge until approximately the 12th to 14th week of gestation. The ovaries are not palpable after that time because the uterus fills the pelvic cavity. Ovulation ceases during pregnancy because of the elevated levels of estrogen and progesterone, which block secretion of follicle-stimulating hormone (FSH) and luteinizing hormone (LH) from the anterior pituitary. The ovaries are active in hormone production to support the pregnancy until about weeks 6 to 7, when the corpus luteum regresses and the placenta takes over the major production of progesterone.

Breasts

The breasts increase in fullness, become tender, and grow larger throughout pregnancy under the influence of estrogen and progesterone. The breasts become highly vascular, and veins become visible under the skin. The nipples become larger and more erect. Both the nipples and the areola become deeply pigmented, and tubercles of Montgomery (sebaceous glands) become prominent. These sebaceous glands keep the nipples lubricated for breastfeeding.

The tremendous growth of and the thinning of the skin on the breasts may lead to striae (stretch marks) in many pregnant people (Adams, 2022). Initially, they appear as pink to purple lines on the skin, but they eventually fade to a silver color. Although they become less conspicuous in time, they never completely disappear.

Creamy, yellowish breast fluid called colostrum can be expressed from the breast, if squeezed, by the third trimester. This fluid provides nourishment for the breastfeeding newborn during the first few days of life before breast milk comes in (see Chapters 15 and 16, for more information). Table 11.1 summarizes reproductive system adaptations.

General Body System Adaptations

In addition to changes in the reproductive system, the pregnant person also experiences changes in virtually every other body system in response to the growing fetus.

Gastrointestinal System

The gastrointestinal (GI) system begins in the oral cavity and ends at the rectum. The secretory and absorptive functions of the GI system are not much affected during pregnancy, but motility is. There is displacement of the intra-abdominal portion of the esophagus into the thorax, in addition to relaxation of the lower esophageal sphincter and a decrease in gastric tone due to increasing progesterone. This leads to dyspepsia (Adams, 2022). During pregnancy, the gums become hyperemic, swollen, and friable and tend to bleed easily. This change is influenced by estrogen and increased proliferation of blood vessels and circulation to the mouth. Taste perception often changes during pregnancy, but the cause is unknown (Bianco, 2023). In addition, the saliva produced in the mouth becomes more acidic. Some people report excessive salivation, termed *ptyalism* or *sialorrhea*, which may be caused by the decrease in unconscious swallowing by the person when nauseated in early gestation. It can include massive volumes of produced saliva, up to 2 L daily. Many people experiencing this issue need to use cups, tissues, and other measures to dispose of excessive saliva. Ptyalism typically resolves spontaneously during the second trimester, although it sometimes endures throughout the pregnancy. Some people get temporary relief from gum chewing, frequent sips of

TABLE 11.1 • Summary of Reproductive System Adaptations

Reproductive Organ	Adaptations
Uterus	Size increases to 20 times that of nonpregnant size. Capacity increases by about 500 times to accommodate the developing fetus. Increased strength and elasticity allow uterus to contract and expel fetus during birth.
Cervix	Increases in mass, water content, and vascularization Changes from a relatively rigid to a soft, distensible structure that allows the fetus to be expelled Under the influence of progesterone, a thick mucus plug is formed, which blocks the cervical os and protects the developing fetus from bacterial invasion.
Vagina	Increased vascularity because of estrogen influences, results in pelvic congestion and hypertrophy. Increased thickness of mucosa, along with an increase in vaginal secretions, helps prevent bacterial infections.
Ovaries	Increased blood supply to the ovaries causes them to enlarge until approximately the 12th to 14th week of gestation. They actively produce hormones to support the pregnancy until weeks 6–7 when the placenta takes over the production of progesterone.
Breasts	Breast changes begin soon after conception; they increase in size and areolar pigmentation. The tubercles of Montgomery enlarge and become more prominent, and the nipples become more erect. The blood vessels become more prominent, and blood flow to the breast doubles.

water, sucking on hard candies, or antiemetics, but no definitive treatment for this condition exists (Bianco, 2023). Dental plaque, calculus, and debris deposits increase during pregnancy and are all associated with periodontal disease, which includes gingivitis and periodontitis. An increased production of female hormones during pregnancy contributes to the development of gingivitis and periodontitis because both vascular permeability and possible tissue edema are increased. Periodontal disease may be a risk factor for negative pregnancy outcomes; however, current research remains inconclusive at this time (Robinson & Norwitz, 2024; Wilder & Moretti, 2023).

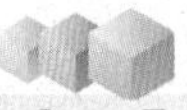
Concept Mastery Alert

Gum Fragility in Pregnancy

Bleeding of gums during pregnancy results from increased estrogen levels that cause blood vessel proliferation. This then leads to increased blood vessels in the gums and an increased chance of bleeding.

Smooth muscle relaxation and decreased peristalsis occur related to the influence of progesterone. Elevated progesterone levels cause smooth muscle relaxation, which results in delayed gastric emptying and decreased peristalsis. The transition time of food throughout the GI tract may be much slower, resulting in more water than normal being reabsorbed, leading to bloating and constipation. Constipation can also result from low-fiber food choices, reduced fluid intake, the use of iron supplements, decreased activity levels, and intestinal displacement secondary to a growing uterus. Constipation, increased venous pressure, and the pressure of the gravid uterus contribute to the formation of hemorrhoids.

The slowed gastric emptying combined with relaxation of the cardiac sphincter allows reflux, which causes heartburn. Acid indigestion or heartburn (pyrosis) seems to be a universal problem for pregnant people. It is caused by regurgitation of the stomach contents into the upper esophagus and may be associated with the generalized relaxation of the entire digestive system. Over-the-counter antacids will usually relieve the symptoms, but they should be taken only with the health care provider's knowledge and as directed.

The formation of gallstones is more likely to occur in pregnant patients compared with nonpregnant patients (Brooks, 2024). The emptying time of the gallbladder is prolonged secondary to the smooth muscle relaxation from progesterone. Cholelithiasis (gallstone disease) during the perinatal and postpartum period has an incidence of approximately 12% (Rampersad et al., 2022). Hypercholesterolemia can follow, increasing the risk of gallstone formation. Other risk factors for gallstone formation during pregnancy include higher weight during prepregnancy (body mass index [BMI] greater than 30 kg/m^2) and multiparity (Brooks, 2024). Laparoscopic cholecystectomy is a safe procedure in all trimesters of pregnancy if removal of the gallbladder is warranted (Brooks, 2024).

Nausea and vomiting, better known as morning sickness, can plague up to 90% of pregnant people (Smith et al., 2024). This condition is usually self-limiting, but the symptoms can be distressing and interfere with work, social activities, and sleep. Symptoms usually start about 6 weeks into the pregnancy and subside by 20 weeks but may sometimes continue into the third trimester. Although it occurs most often in the morning, the nauseated feeling can last all day in some people. The highest incidence of morning sickness occurs between 6 and 12 weeks. The physiologic basis for morning sickness is still debatable and likely has several causes. It has been linked to high levels of hCG, high levels of circulating estrogen and progesterone, increased gastric acidity and gastroesophageal reflux, genetic factors, and lowered tone and motility of the digestive tract (Smith et al., 2023).

Cardiovascular System

Cardiovascular changes occur early during pregnancy to meet the demands of the enlarging uterus and the placenta for more blood and more oxygen. The changes include an increase in heart rate, an increase in cardiac output, reduced total peripheral resistance, increased blood volume, reduced systemic vascular resistance and blood pressure, and increased plasma volume (Valente & Economy, 2024). Perhaps the most striking cardiac alteration occurring during pregnancy is the increase in blood volume.

BLOOD VOLUME

Blood volume increases by approximately 1,100 to 1,600 mL, or about 30% to 50% above nonpregnant levels, peaks by the 30th to 34th week of gestation, and remains more or less constant thereafter (Adams, 2022). The increase is made up of 75% plasma plus a smaller amount of increased red blood cell (RBC) volume (Adams, 2022). It is not clear how this occurs, but retention of sodium seems to be involved. It begins at weeks 10 to 12, peaks at weeks 32 to 34, and decreases slightly by week 40.

TAKE NOTE!

The rise in blood volume correlates directly with fetal weight, supporting the concept of the placenta as an arteriovenous shunt in the maternal vascular compartment.

This increase in blood volume is needed to provide adequate hydration of fetal and maternal tissues, to supply blood flow to perfuse the enlarging uterus, and to provide a reserve to compensate for blood loss at birth and during the postpartum period. The maternal blood volume expansion occurs at a larger proportion than the increase in RBC mass, which results in physiologic anemia and hemodilution. This dilution of RBCs is termed **physiologic anemia of pregnancy**. This is reflected in a lowered hematocrit and hemoglobin. These changes are considered a normal adaptation of pregnancy (Gandhi & Gupta, 2023). This increase is also necessary to meet the increased metabolic needs of the pregnant person and to meet the need for increased perfusion of other organs, especially the person's kidneys since they are excreting waste products for both themselves and the fetus.

CARDIAC OUTPUT AND HEART RATE

Cardiac output, the product of stroke volume and heart rate, is a measure of the functional capacity of the heart. It increases by 30% to 40% over the nonpregnant rate, typically peaks at 20 to 24 weeks' gestation, and declines slightly later in the third trimester as the pregnancy approaches 40 weeks' gestation (Valente & Economy, 2024). The increase in cardiac output is associated with an increase in venous return and greater right ventricular output, especially when the pregnant person is lying in the left lateral position, particularly after 20 weeks (Valente & Economy, 2024). Conversely, if the pregnant person is lying in the supine position, the uterus can compress the inferior cava and significantly reduce cardiac output and venous return to the heart and can lead to dizziness, lightheadedness, and tachycardia (Valente & Economy, 2024). Heart rate increases by 10 to 30 beats/min; this persists to term (Valente & Economy, 2024). There is slight hypertrophy or enlargement of the heart during pregnancy. This is probably to accommodate the increase in blood volume and cardiac output. The heart works harder and pumps more blood to supply the oxygen needs of the fetus, as well as those of the pregnant person. Both heart rate and venous return are increased in pregnancy, contributing to the increase in cardiac output seen throughout gestation. A person with preexisting heart disease may have symptoms and begin to decompensate during the time the blood volume peaks. Close monitoring is warranted during 28 to 35 weeks' gestation.

BLOOD PRESSURE

Blood pressure, especially the diastolic pressure, declines slightly during pregnancy as a result of peripheral vasodilation caused by progesterone. It usually reaches a low-point mid-pregnancy and thereafter increases to prepregnancy levels until term. During the first trimester, blood pressure typically remains at the prepregnancy level. During the second trimester, the blood pressure decreases 5 to 10 mm Hg and thereafter returns to first-trimester levels. This decrease in blood pressure begins at about 7 weeks' gestation and persists until 32 weeks' gestation, when it begins to rise to prepregnancy levels. A BMI higher than 25 kg/m^2 typically drives the blood pressure higher throughout pregnancy (Knight, 2023). Any significant rise in blood pressure during pregnancy should be investigated to rule out gestational hypertension.

BLOOD COMPONENTS

The number of RBCs also increases throughout pregnancy to a level that is 20% to 30% higher than nonpregnant values, depending on the amount of iron available. This increase is necessary to transport the additional oxygen required during pregnancy. Although there is an increase in RBCs, there is a greater increase in the plasma volume as a result of hormonal factors and sodium and water retention. Because the plasma increase exceeds the increase of RBC production, normal hemoglobin and hematocrit values decrease, resulting in physiologic anemia of pregnancy. Changes in RBC volume are mainly due to increased circulating erythropoietin, which increases by 50%, resulting in accelerated RBC production (Valente & Economy, 2024).

Iron requirements during pregnancy increase because of the demands of the growing fetus and the increase in maternal blood volume. The fetal tissues prevail over the pregnant person's tissues with respect to use of iron stores. With the accelerated production of RBCs, iron is necessary for hemoglobin formation, the oxygen-carrying component of RBCs.

> **TAKE NOTE!**
>
> Many people enter pregnancy with insufficient iron stores and thus need supplementation to meet the extra demands of pregnancy.

Both fibrin and plasma fibrinogen levels increase along with various blood clotting factors. These factors make pregnancy a hypercoagulable state. These changes, coupled with venous stasis secondary to venous pooling, which occurs during late pregnancy after long periods of standing in the upright position with the pressure exerted by the uterus on the large pelvic veins, contribute to slowed venous return, pooling, and dependent edema. These factors also increase the person's risk for venous thrombosis. Refer to Chapter 22, for further information on venous thromboembolic conditions.

Respiratory System

Pregnancy puts less stress on the respiratory system than on the cardiovascular system, but adaptations to this system do take place during pregnancy. The primary changes occur in lung volume and ventilation. Oxygen consumption reflects the uptick of maternal metabolism by increasing between 20% and 30% by the time full term is reached. During pregnancy, the amount of space available to house the lungs decreases as the uterus puts pressure on the diaphragm and causes it to shift upward by 4 cm above its usual position. The growing uterus does change the size and shape of the thoracic cavity, but diaphragmatic excursion increases, chest circumference increases by 2 to 3 in, and the transverse diameter increases by an inch, allowing a larger tidal volume, as evidenced by deeper breathing. Tidal volume, or the volume of air inhaled, increases by 30% to 40% as the pregnancy progresses (Pascual & Langaker, 2023). This increase results in maternal hyperventilation and hypocapnia. As a result of these changes, the person's breathing becomes more diaphragmatic than abdominal. Sixty percent to 75% of pregnant people experience dyspnea during the latter part of pregnancy (Weinberger, 2024). Concomitant with the increase in tidal volume is a 30% increase in maternal oxygen consumption due to the increased oxygen requirements of the developing fetus, placenta, and maternal organs (Adams, 2022).

Because of these various changes, pregnant people with asthma, pneumonia, or other respiratory pathology are at risk for further compromise and more susceptible to early decompensation (Adams, 2022).

A pregnant person breathes faster and more deeply because they and the fetus need more oxygen. Oxygen consumption increases during pregnancy even as airway resistance and lung compliance remain unchanged. Changes in the structures of the respiratory system take place to prepare the body for the enlarging uterus and increased lung volume (Kepley et al., 2023). As muscles and cartilage in the thoracic region relax, the chest broadens with a conversion from abdominal breathing to thoracic breathing. This leads to a 50% increase in air volume per minute. All of these structural alterations are temporary and revert back to their prepregnant state at the end of the pregnancy.

Increased vascularity of the respiratory tract is influenced by increased estrogen levels, leading to congestion. Rising levels of sex hormones and heightened sensitivity to allergens may influence the nasal mucosa, precipitating epistaxis (nosebleed) and rhinitis. This congestion gives rise to nasal and sinus stuffiness (Weinberger, 2024).

Renal/Urinary System

The renal and urinary systems undergo dramatic changes in response to pregnancy. The kidneys must adapt to an increase in blood volume and increased maternal and fetal waste. Hormonal changes during pregnancy allow for increased blood flow to the kidneys. The renal system must handle the effects of increased maternal intravascular and extracellular volume and metabolic waste products, as well as excretion of fetal wastes. The predominant structural change in the renal system during pregnancy is dilation of the renal pelvis and uterus. Changes in renal structure occur as a result of the hormonal influences of estrogen and progesterone, pressure from an enlarging uterus, and an increase in maternal blood volume. Dilation of the kidneys and ureters increases the potential for urinary stasis and infection. Like the heart, the kidneys work harder throughout the pregnancy. Changes in kidney function occur to accommodate a heavier workload while maintaining a stable electrolyte balance and blood pressure. As more blood flows to the kidneys, the glomerular filtration rate (GFR) increases, leading to an increase in urine flow and volume, substances delivered to the kidneys, and filtration and excretion of protein, amino acids, and glucose (Thadhani & Maynard, 2024).

Anatomically, the kidneys enlarge during pregnancy. Each kidney increases in length, by approximately 1 to 1.5 cm, and weight as a result of hormonal effects that cause increased tone and decreased motility of the smooth muscle. The renal pelvis becomes dilated. The ureters (especially the right ureter) elongate, widen, and become more curved above the pelvic rim by the second trimester (Thadhani & Maynard, 2024). Progesterone is thought to cause both of these changes because of its relaxing influence on smooth muscle.

Blood flow to the kidneys increases by 50% to 80% as a result of the increase in cardiac output and relaxin, which causes a decrease in both efferent and afferent resistance. This in turn leads to an increase in the GFR by as much as 50% starting during the second trimester, resulting in hyperfiltration (Pascual & Langaker, 2023). This elevation continues until birth. This change has important clinical implications for medication use because drugs excreted through the kidneys may require higher doses and more frequent administration for therapeutic blood levels during pregnancy (Pinheiro & Stika, 2020). Further research on pregnancy-specific dosing guidelines is needed (Pinheiro & Stika, 2020).

The activity of the kidneys normally increases when a person lies down and decreases upon standing. This difference is amplified during pregnancy, which is one reason a pregnant person feels the need to urinate frequently while trying to sleep. Late in the pregnancy, the increase in kidney activity is even greater when the person lies on their side rather than their back. Lying on either side relieves the pressure that the enlarged uterus puts on the vena cava carrying blood from the legs. Subsequently, venous return to the heart increases, leading to increased cardiac output. Increased cardiac output results in increased renal perfusion and glomerular filtration. As a rule, all the physiologic changes maximize by the end of the second trimester and then start to return to the prepregnant level. However, changes in this anatomy can take 4 to 6 weeks postpartum to subside, and urinary incontinence may last even longer (Thadhani & Maynard, 2024).

Musculoskeletal System

The musculoskeletal system undergoes significant changes during pregnancy and childbirth. Pregnancy represents a window of opportunity to adopt an active, healthy lifestyle, but it also places a person at risk for musculoskeletal disorders, impairments, and other discomforts. Weight gain, the enlargement of the uterus, and a shift in the body's center of gravity can contribute to several musculoskeletal problems. Changes in the musculoskeletal system are progressive, resulting from the influence of hormones, fetal growth, and maternal weight gain. Pregnancy is characterized by changes in posture and gait. The ligaments that hold the sacroiliac joints and the pubis symphysis in place begin to soften and stretch, and the articulations between the joints widen and become more movable (Bermas, 2023). The relaxation of the joints peaks by the beginning of the third trimester. These changes increase the size of the pelvic cavity and make delivery easier.

The postural changes of pregnancy—an increased swayback and an upper spine extension to compensate for the enlarging abdomen—coupled with the loosening of the sacroiliac joints may result in lower back pain. The person's center of gravity shifts forward, requiring a realignment of the spinal curvatures. Factors thought to contribute to these postural changes include the alteration to the center of gravity that come with pregnancy, the influence of the pregnancy-related hormone relaxin on the pelvic joints, and the increasing weight and position of the growing fetus.

An increase in the normal lumbosacral curve (lordosis) occurs, and a compensatory curvature in the cervicodorsal area develops to assist the person in maintaining their balance (Fig. 11.3). In addition, relaxation and increased mobility of joints occur because of the hormones progesterone and relaxin, which lead to the characteristic "waddle" gait that pregnant people demonstrate as they near term. Increased weight gain can add to this discomfort by accentuating the lumbar and dorsal curves. Common issues include low back pain, disk disease, pelvic girdle and hip pain, leg and foot pain/cramps, and hand and wrist pain (Bermas, 2023).

Integumentary System

The integumentary system includes the skin, hair, nails, and sebaceous and sweat glands. There are a variety of integumentary changes that are associated with pregnancy, including changes in pigment, vascular supply, connective skin tissue, hair growth, nail structure, and gland functions. Almost all pregnant people will show signs of hyperpigmentation during pregnancy, typically localized and mild (Pomeranz, 2023). The skin of pregnant people undergoes hyperpigmentation primarily resulting from elevated estrogen, progesterone, and melanocyte-stimulating hormone levels. These changes are mainly seen on the nipples, areola, umbilicus, perineum, and axilla. Although many integumentary changes disappear after giving birth, some only fade. Many pregnant people express concerns about stretch marks, changes in skin color, and hair loss. Little is known about how to avoid these changes.

Complexion changes are not unusual. Increased pigmentation that appears on the breasts and genitalia also develops on the face, forming what is known as the "mask of pregnancy," which is also called *facial melasma*. This occurs in up to 75% of pregnant people (Pomeranz,

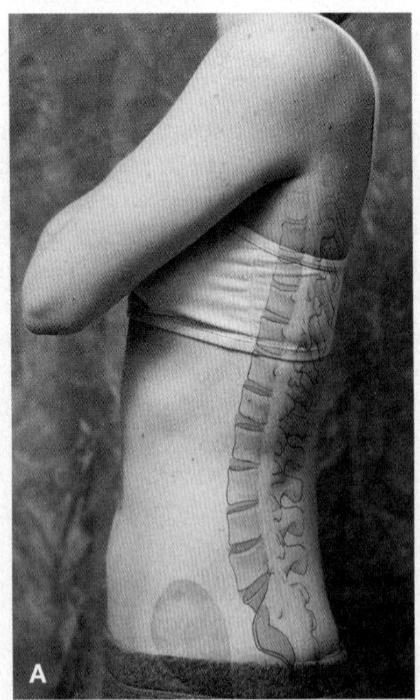

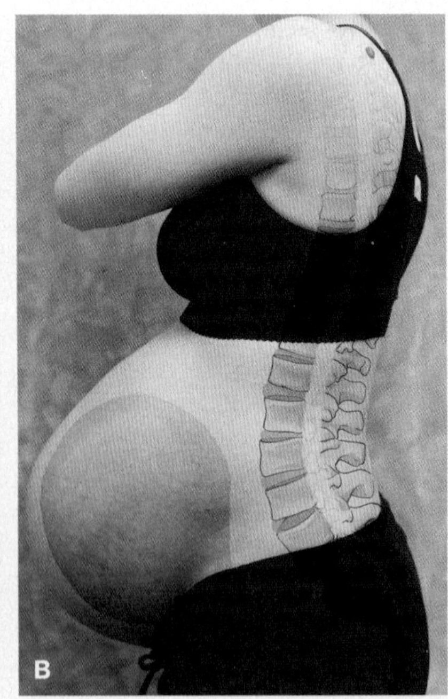

FIGURE 11.3 Postural changes during **(A)** the first trimester and **(B)** the third trimester.

2023). There is a genetic predisposition toward melasma, which is exacerbated by sun exposure and tends to recur in subsequent pregnancies. This blotchy, brownish pigment covers the forehead and cheeks in dark-haired people. Most facial pigmentation fades as hormone levels subside toward the end of the pregnancy, but some may linger. The skin in the middle of the abdomen may develop a pigmented line called the **linea nigra**, which extends from the umbilicus to the pubic area (Fig. 11.4).

Striae gravidarum, or stretch marks, are irregular reddish streaks that appear most often on the abdomen, breasts, and thighs, but also on the lower back, buttocks, and upper arms. Striae are most prominent by 6 to 7 months (Pomeranz, 2023). The exact cause is not well understood, but striae are thought to result from many contributing factors, such as genetics, hormone changes, reduced connective tissue strength resulting from elevated adrenal steroid levels, tension on the skin, and stretching of the structures secondary from fetal growth (Pomeranz, 2023). Striae are more common in younger people, people with a family history, those carrying larger infants, or those with a higher BMI (Pomeranz, 2023). Several creams and lotions, such as cocoa butter and olive oil, have been touted as preventing striae gravidarum, but current research does not validate these claims (Pomeranz, 2023). Over time, many striae improve in appearance and fade to a light silver color but do not disappear.

VASCULAR-RELATED SKIN CHANGES

Vascular changes during pregnancy manifest in the integumentary system include varicosities of the legs, vulva, and perineum. Varicose veins are commonly the result of distention, instability, and poor circulation secondary to prolonged standing or sitting and the heavy gravid uterus placing pressure on the pelvic veins, preventing complete venous return. Interventions to reduce the risk of developing varicosities include the following:

- Elevating both legs when sitting or lying down
- Avoiding prolonged standing or sitting; changing position frequently
- Resting in the left lateral position
- Walking daily for exercise
- Avoiding tight clothing or knee-high hosiery
- Wearing support hose if varicosities are a preexisting condition to pregnancy

Another skin manifestation, believed to be secondary to vascular changes and high estrogen levels, is the appearance of small blood vessels called *vascular spiders*. These may appear on the neck, thorax, face, and arms. They are especially obvious in White people and typically disappear after childbirth. Palmar erythema is a well-delineated pinkish area on the palmar surface of the hands. This integumentary change is also related to elevated estrogen levels and other factors that cause vascular changes, such as vascular distention, instability, and proliferation of blood vessels (Pomeranz, 2023).

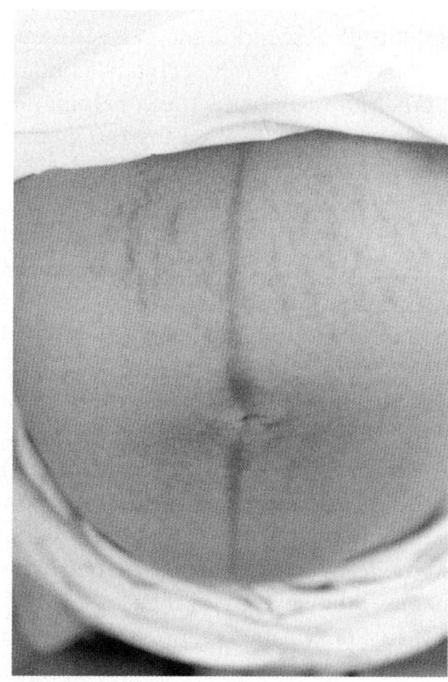

FIGURE 11.4 Linea nigra.

HAIR AND NAILS

Some people also notice a decrease in hair growth during pregnancy. The hair follicles normally undergo a growing and resting phase. The resting phase is followed by a loss of hair; the hairs are then replaced by new ones. During pregnancy, fewer hair follicles go into the resting phase. After delivery, the body catches up with subsequent hair loss for several months. Nails typically grow faster during pregnancy. Pregnant people may experience increased brittleness, distal separation of the nail bed, whitish discoloration, and transverse grooves on the nails; however, most of these conditions resolve in the postpartum period (Pomeranz, 2023).

Endocrine System

The endocrine system undergoes many changes during pregnancy, because hormonal changes are essential in meeting the needs of the growing fetus. Hormonal changes play a major role in controlling the supplies of maternal glucose, amino acids, and lipids to the fetus. Although estrogen and progesterone are the main hormones involved in pregnancy changes, other endocrine glands and hormones also change during pregnancy.

THYROID GLAND

Multiple organs undergo physiologic changes during pregnancy, and the thyroid is no exception. The thyroid gland enlarges slightly and becomes more active during pregnancy as a result of increased vascularity and hyperplasia. Increased gland activity results in an increase in thyroid hormone secretion starting during the first trimester; levels taper off within a few weeks after birth and return to normal limits. Maternal thyroid hormone is transferred to the fetus beginning soon after conception and is critical for fetal brain development, neurogenesis, and organizational processes prior to 20 weeks when fetal thyroid production is low. However, even after the fetal thyroid is producing increasing amounts of hormone, much of the thyroxin (T_4) needed for development continues to be provided by the birthing parent. Low maternal thyroid levels with thyroid insufficiency, hypothyroidism, or low or inadequate iodine intake may compromise fetal neurologic development and places the fetus at higher risk of fetal hypothyroidism (Pande & Anjankar, 2023). With an increase in the secretion of thyroid hormones, the basal metabolic rate (the amount of oxygen consumed by the body over a unit of time in milliliters per minute) progressively increases by 20% to 25% (Records & Clark, 2024).

PITUITARY GLAND

During pregnancy, major endocrine and metabolic alterations occur due to the physiologic hormonal secretion from the placenta. The pituitary gland adapts to these changes, and all secretory axes are affected. During pregnancy, the pituitary gland enlarges and grows in size mainly because of an increase in blood supply. It returns to normal size after birth.

The anterior lobe of the pituitary is glandular tissue and produces multiple hormones. The release of these hormones is regulated by releasing and inhibiting hormones produced by the hypothalamus. Some of these anterior pituitary hormones induce other glands to secrete their hormones. The increase in blood levels of the hormones produced by the final target glands (e.g., the ovary or thyroid) inhibits the release of anterior pituitary hormones.

FSH and LH secretion are inhibited during pregnancy, probably as a result of hCG produced by the placenta and corpus luteum, as well as increased secretion of prolactin by the anterior pituitary gland. These hormone levels remain decreased until after delivery. Thyroid-stimulating hormone (TSH) levels are reduced during the first trimester but usually return to normal for the remainder of the pregnancy.

Growth hormone (GH) is an anabolic hormone that promotes protein synthesis. It stimulates most body cells to grow in size and divide, facilitating the use of fats for fuel and conserving glucose. During pregnancy, there is a decrease in the number of GH-producing cells and a corresponding decrease in GH blood levels. The action of human chorionic somatomammotropin (hCS), formerly known as human placental lactogen (hPL), is thought to decrease the need for and use of GH. During pregnancy, prolactin is secreted in pulses and increases 10-fold to promote breast development and the lactation process. High levels of progesterone secreted by the placenta inhibit the direct influence of prolactin on the breast during pregnancy, thus suppressing lactation. At birth, when the placenta is expelled and progesterone levels drop, lactogenesis can begin. Prolactin, released from the anterior pituitary gland in response to suckling by the newborn, is the major hormonal signal responsible for stimulation in the breasts (Al-Chalabi et al., 2023).

Melanocyte-stimulating hormone (MSH), another anterior pituitary hormone, increases during pregnancy. For many years, its increase was thought to be responsible for many of the skin changes of pregnancy, particularly changes in skin pigmentation (e.g., darkening of the areola, melasma, and linea nigra). However, it is currently thought that these skin changes are due to estrogen (and possibly progesterone), as well as the increase in MSH.

The two hormones, oxytocin and antidiuretic hormone (ADH), released by the posterior pituitary are actually synthesized in the hypothalamus. They migrate along the nerve fibers to the posterior pituitary and are stored until stimulated to be released into the general circulation. Oxytocin is released by the posterior pituitary gland, and its production gradually increases as the fetus matures (Adams, 2022). Oxytocin is responsible for uterine contractions, both before and after delivery. The muscle layers of the uterus (myometrium) become more sensitive to oxytocin near term. Toward the end of a term pregnancy, levels of progesterone decline and contractions that were previously suppressed by progesterone begin to occur more frequently, with stronger intensity. This change in the hormonal levels is believed to be one of the initiators of labor.

Oxytocin is responsible for stimulating the uterine contractions that bring about delivery. Contractions lead to cervical thinning and dilation. They also exert pressure, helping the fetus to descend in the pelvis for eventual delivery. After delivery, oxytocin secretion continues, causing the myometrium to contract and helping to constrict the uterine blood vessels, decreasing the amount of vaginal bleeding after delivery. Oxytocin is also responsible for milk ejection during breastfeeding. Stimulation of the breasts through sucking or touching stimulates the secretion of oxytocin from the posterior pituitary gland. Oxytocin causes contraction of the myoepithelial cells in the lactating mammary gland and allows for milk "let down."

Cramping pain and discomfort occur following childbirth as the uterus contracts and returns to its prepregnant size. These postpartum pains are caused by involuntary contractions and usually last for a few days after childbirth. They are more evident in people who have previously had a baby. Breastfeeding signals the release of oxytocin, which stimulates the uterus to contract and can increase the severity of these after-birth pains.

ADH, also known as vasopressin, functions to inhibit or prevent the formation of urine via vasoconstriction, which results in increased blood pressure and hypervolemia. Overall, the release of ADH is unchanged in pregnancy (Reports & Clark, 2024).

PANCREAS

The pancreas is both an exocrine organ, supplying digestive enzymes and buffers, and an endocrine organ. The endocrine pancreas consists of the islets of Langerhans, which are groups of cells scattered throughout, each containing four cell types. One of these types is the beta cell, which produces insulin. Insulin lowers blood glucose by increasing the rate of glucose uptake and utilization by most body cells. The growing fetus needs significant amounts of glucose, amino acids, and lipids. Even during early pregnancy, the fetus makes demands on the maternal glucose stores. Ideally, hormonal changes of pregnancy help meet fetal needs without putting the pregnant person's metabolism out of balance.

A person's insulin secretion works on a supply versus demand mode. As the demand to meet the needs of pregnancy increases, more insulin is secreted. Maternal insulin does not cross the placenta, so the fetus must produce its own supply to maintain glucose control (Box 11.2).

BOX 11.2 Pregnancy, Insulin, and Glucose

- During early pregnancy, maternal glucose levels decrease because of the heavy fetal demand for glucose. The fetus is also drawing amino acids and lipids from the pregnant person, decreasing the person's ability to synthesize glucose. Maternal glucose is diverted across the placenta to assist the growing embryo/fetus during early pregnancy, and thus levels decline in the pregnant person. As a result, maternal glucose concentrations decline to a level that would be considered "hypoglycemic" in a nonpregnant person.
- During early pregnancy, there is also a decrease in maternal insulin production and insulin levels. The pancreas is responsible for the production of insulin, which facilitates entry of glucose into cells. Although glucose and other nutrients easily cross the placenta to the fetus, insulin does not. Therefore, the fetus must produce its own insulin to facilitate the entry of glucose into its own cells.
- After the first trimester, hPL from the placenta and steroids (cortisol) from the adrenal cortex act against insulin. hPL acts as an antagonist against maternal insulin, and thus more insulin must be secreted to counteract the increasing levels of hPL and cortisol during the last half of pregnancy.
- Human chorionic somatomammotropin (also known as human placental lactogen), placental GH, glucocorticoids, estrogen, and progesterone are also thought to cause insulin resistance. As a result, glucose is less likely to enter the pregnant person's cells and is more likely to cross over the placenta to the fetus.

Adapted from Records, K., & Clark, A. (2024). Physiology of pregnancy. In B. J. Baker, J. Janke, & AWHONN (Eds.), *Core curriculum for maternal-newborn nursing* (6th ed., Chapt. 8). Elsevier; Tal, R., & Taylor, H. S. (2021). Endocrinology of pregnancy. In K. R. Feingold, B. Anawalt, M. R. Blackman, A. Boyce, G. Chrousos, E. Corpas, W. W. de Herder, K. Dhatariya, K. Dungan, J. Hofland, S. Kalra, G. Kaltsas, N. Kapoor, C. Koch, P. Kopp, M. Korbonits, C. S. Kovacs, W. Kuohung, B. Laferrère, ... D. P. Wilson (Eds.), *Endotext*. https://www.ncbi.nlm.nih.gov/books/NBK278962/; Pascual, Z. N., & Langaker, M. D. (2023). Physiology, pregnancy. In *StatPearls*. StatPearls Publishing. https://www.ncbi.nlm.nih.gov/books/NBK559304/

Maternal glucose metabolism during pregnancy differs from the nongravid state to allow the pregnant person to meet their own and the growing fetus's energy needs. During the first half of pregnancy, much of the maternal glucose is diverted to the growing fetus, and thus the pregnant person's glucose levels are low. Hormonal antagonists, including hCS, increase during the second half of pregnancy. Therefore, the pregnant person must produce more insulin to overcome the resistance by these hormones. Insulin resistance (the inability of insulin to increase glucose uptake and utilization) in pregnancy is consequent to the physiologic adaptation necessary to provide glucose to the growing fetus.

If the pregnant person has normal beta cells of the islets of Langerhans, there is usually no problem meeting the demands for extra insulin. However, if the person has inadequate numbers of beta cells, they may be unable to produce enough insulin and will develop glucose intolerance during pregnancy. If the person has glucose intolerance, they are not able to meet the increasing demands and their blood glucose level increases.

ADRENAL GLANDS

During pregnancy, there is an increase in hormone production by the adrenal glands. Pregnancy does not cause much change in the size of the adrenal glands themselves, but there are changes in some secretions and activity. One of the key changes is the marked increase in cortisol secretion, which regulates carbohydrate and protein metabolism and is helpful in times of stress. Although pregnancy is considered a normal condition, it is a time of stress for a person's body. The rate of secretion of cortisol by maternal adrenals is not increased during pregnancy, but the rate of clearance is decreased. Cortisol level increases in response to increased estrogen levels and the placenta's release of corticotropin-releasing hormone during the second and third trimesters (Nana & Williamson, 2022). The majority (80% to 90%) of cortisol is deactivated to cortisone by a placental enzyme to protect the fetus (Nana & Williamson, 2022).

The amount of aldosterone, also secreted by the adrenal glands, is increased during pregnancy. It normally regulates absorption of sodium from the distal tubules of the kidney. During pregnancy, progesterone allows salt to be wasted (or lost) in the urine. Aldosterone is a key regulator of electrolyte and water homeostasis and plays a central role in blood pressure regulation. Hormonal changes during pregnancy, among them increased progesterone and aldosterone production, lead to the required plasma volume expansion of the maternal body as an accommodation mechanism for fetus growth.

PROSTAGLANDIN SECRETION DURING PREGNANCY

Prostaglandins are not protein or steroid hormones; they act as chemical mediators, or local hormones. Although hormones circulate in the blood to influence distant tissues, prostaglandins act locally on adjacent cells. Both the fetal membranes of the amniotic sac—the amnion and chorion—are believed to be involved in the production of prostaglandins. Various maternal and fetal tissues, as well as the amniotic fluid itself, are considered to be sources of prostaglandins, but details about their composition and sources are limited. It is widely believed that prostaglandins play a part in softening the cervix and initiating or maintaining labor, but the exact mechanism is unclear. What is theorized is that increased production of prostaglandins occurs, which facilitates uterine contractions, promotes cervical ripening, and increases myometrial sensitivity to oxytocin that is needed for the labor process (Norwitz, 2024). Along with oxytocin, the influence of prostaglandins on the uterine myometrium predominates to promote uterine contractile activity.

PLACENTAL SECRETION

The placenta is an organ that serves to prevent the direct exchange between the blood of the fetus and the blood of the pregnant person. The placenta is not only a transfer organ but also a factory. It is capable of synthesizing enzymes and proteins and manufactures fats and carbohydrates that serve as a source of stored energy. The placenta also functions as an endocrine gland, manufacturing and secreting hormones. The placenta has a feature possessed by no other endocrine organ—the ability to form protein and steroid hormones. Very early during pregnancy, the placenta begins to produce the following hormones:

- hCG
- hPL
- Relaxin
- Progesterone
- Estrogen

Table 11.2 summarizes the role of these hormones.

Immune System

The immune system is made up of organs and specialized cells with the primary purpose of defending the body from foreign substances (antigens) that may cause tissue injury or disease. The mechanisms of innate and adaptive immunity work cooperatively to prevent, control, and eradicate foreign antigens in the body.

TABLE 11.2 • Placental Hormones

Hormone	Description
Human chorionic gonadotropin (hCG)	• Responsible for maintaining the maternal corpus luteum, which secretes progesterone and estrogens with synthesis occurring before implantation • Production by fetal trophoblast cells until the placenta is developed sufficiently to take over that function • Basis for early pregnancy tests because it appears in the maternal bloodstream soon after implantation (as early as day 8 after conception) • Production peaks between 8 and 10 weeks and then gradually declines
Human chorionic somatomammotropin (hCS; originally known as human placental lactogen [hPL])	• Preparation of mammary glands for lactation and involved in the process of making glucose available for fetal growth by altering maternal carbohydrate, fat, and protein metabolism • Antagonist of insulin because it decreases tissue sensitivity or alters the ability to use insulin • Increase in the amount of circulating free fatty acids for maternal metabolic needs and decrease in maternal metabolism of glucose to facilitate fetal growth
Relaxin	• Secretion by the placenta as well as the corpus luteum during pregnancy • Thought to act synergistically with progesterone to maintain pregnancy • Increase in flexibility of the pubic symphysis, permitting the pelvis to expand during delivery • Dilation of the cervix, making it easier for the fetus to enter the vaginal canal; thought to suppress the release of oxytocin by the hypothalamus, thus delaying the onset of labor contractions
Progesterone	• Produced by the corpus luteum during the first few weeks of pregnancy and then by the placenta until term • Often called the "hormone of pregnancy" because of the critical role it plays in supporting the endometrium of the uterus • Supports the endometrium to provide an environment conducive to fetal survival • Maintains the endometrium, inhibits uterine contractility, suppresses maternal immune response, and assists in the development of the breasts for lactation
Estrogen	• Promotes enlargement of the genitals, uterus, and breasts and increases vascularity, causing vasodilatation • Relaxation of pelvic ligaments and joints • Associated with hyperpigmentation, vascular changes in the skin, increased activity of the salivary glands, and hyperemia of the gums and nasal mucous membranes • Aids in developing the ductal system of the breasts in preparation for lactation

Adapted from Kapila, V., & Chaudhry, K. (2024). Physiology, placenta. In *StatPearls*. StatPearls Publishing. https://www.ncbi.nlm.nih.gov/books/NBK538332/; Records, K., & Clark, A. (2024). Physiology of pregnancy. In B. J. Baker, J. Janke, & AWHONN (Eds.), *Core curriculum for maternal-newborn nursing* (6th ed., Chap. 8). Elsevier.

A general enhancement of innate immunity (inflammatory response and phagocytosis) and suppression of adaptive immunity (protective response to a specific foreign antigen) take place during pregnancy. These immunologic alterations help prevent the pregnant person's immune system from rejecting the fetus (foreign body), increase their risk of developing certain infections such as urinary tract infections, and influence the course of chronic disorders such as autoimmune diseases. Some chronic conditions worsen (diabetes), while others seem to stabilize (asthma) during pregnancy; but this is individualized and not predictable. In general, immune function in pregnant people is similar to immune function in nonpregnant females. Table 11.3 summarizes the general body systems' adaptations to pregnancy.

Marva returns for their first prenatal appointment and tells the nurse that their whole body is "out of sorts." Marva is overwhelmed and feels bad. Outline the bodily changes Marva can expect each trimester to help them understand the adaptations taking place. What guidance can the nurse give Marva to help them understand the changes of pregnancy?

CHANGING NUTRITIONAL NEEDS OF PREGNANCY

The reproductive period is a critical time because it becomes a determinant of lifetime risk of chronic diseases for both the pregnant person and the fetus. Consuming

TABLE 11.3 • Summary of General Body System Adaptations

System	Adaptation
Gastrointestinal system	*Mouth and pharynx:* Gums become hyperemic, swollen, and friable and tend to bleed easily. Saliva production increases. *Esophagus:* Decreased lower esophageal sphincter pressure and tone, which increases the risk of developing heartburn *Stomach:* Decreased tone and mobility with delayed gastric emptying time, which increases the risk of gastroesophageal reflux and vomiting *Intestines:* Decreased intestinal tone motility with increased transit time, which increases risk of constipation and flatulence *Gallbladder:* Decreased tone and motility, which may increase risk of gallstone formation
Cardiovascular system	*Blood volume:* Marked increase in plasma and RBCs compared to nonpregnant values. Causes hemodilution, which is reflected in a lower hematocrit and hemoglobin levels. *Cardiac output and heart rate:* Cardiac output increases from 30% to 40% over the nonpregnant rate. The increase in cardiac output is associated with an increase in venous return and greater right ventricular output, especially in the left lateral position. Heart rate increases by 10–30 beats/min and this increase will persist to term. *Blood pressure:* Blood pressure decreases to reach its lowest point by mid-pregnancy; it then gradually returns to nonpregnant baseline values by term. *Blood components:* The number of RBCs increases throughout pregnancy to a level 25% higher than nonpregnant values. Both fibrin and plasma fibrinogen levels increase, along with various blood clotting factors. These factors make pregnancy a hypercoagulable state.
Respiratory system	Enlargement of the uterus shifts the diaphragm up to 4 cm above its usual position. As muscles and cartilage in the thoracic region relax, the chest broadens with conversion from abdominal breathing to thoracic breathing. This leads to a 30%–40% increase in air volume per minute. Tidal volume, or the volume of air inhaled, increases gradually by 30%–40% as the pregnancy progresses.
Renal/urinary system	The renal pelvis becomes dilated. The ureters (especially the right ureter) elongate, widen, and become more curved above the pelvic rim. Bladder tone decreases and bladder capacity doubles by term. Glomerular filtration rate increases by 50% during pregnancy. Blood flow to the kidneys increases by 50%–80% as a result of the increase in cardiac output.
Musculoskeletal system	Distention of the abdomen with growth of the fetus tilts the pelvis forward, shifting the center of gravity. The pregnant person's body compensates by developing an increased curvature (lordosis) of the spine. Relaxation and increased mobility of joints occur because of the hormones progesterone and relaxin, which lead to the characteristic "waddle gait" that pregnant people demonstrate toward term.

(*continued*)

TABLE 11.3 • Summary of General Body System Adaptations (*continued*)

System	Adaptation
Integumentary system	Hyperpigmentation of the skin is the most common alteration during pregnancy. The most common areas include the areola, genital skin, axilla, inner aspects of the thighs, and linea nigra. Striae gravidarum, or stretch marks, are irregular reddish streaks that may appear on the abdomen, breasts, and buttocks in about half of pregnant people. The skin in the middle of the abdomen may develop a pigmented line called the linea nigra, which extends from the umbilicus to the pubic area. Melasma ("mask of pregnancy") occurs in up to 75% of pregnant people. It is characterized by irregular, blotchy areas of pigmentation on the face, most commonly on the cheeks, chin, and nose.
Endocrine system	Controls the integrity and duration of gestation by maintaining the corpus luteum via hCG secretion; production of estrogen, progesterone, hPL, and other hormones and growth factors via the placenta; release of oxytocin (by the posterior pituitary gland), prolactin (by the anterior pituitary), and relaxin (by the ovary, uterus, and placenta)
Immune system	A general enhancement of innate immunity (inflammatory response and phagocytosis) and suppression of adaptive immunity (protective response to a specific foreign antigen) take place during pregnancy. These immunologic alterations help prevent the pregnant person's immune system from rejecting the fetus (foreign body), increase their risk of developing certain infections, and influence the course of chronic disorders such as autoimmune diseases.

Adapted from Valente, A. M., & Economy, K. (2024). Maternal adaptations to pregnancy: Cardiovascular and hemodynamic changes. *UpToDate*. Retrieved May 22, 2024, from https://www.uptodate.com/contents/maternal-adaptations-to-pregnancy-cardiovascular-and-hemodynamic-changes; and Pascual, Z. N., & Langaker, M. D. (2023). Physiology, pregnancy. In *StatPearls*. StatPearls Publishing. https://www.ncbi.nlm.nih.gov/books/NBK559304/

a healthy diet before and during pregnancy improves outcomes for both the pregnant person and the child. Maternal body weight and diet quality, even prepregnancy, can affect the uterine environment, birth weight, and the infant's subsequent health into adulthood. Healthy eating during pregnancy enables optimal gestational weight gain and reduces complications, both of which are associated with positive birth outcomes. During pregnancy, maternal nutritional needs change to meet the demands of the pregnancy. Healthy eating can help ensure that adequate nutrients are available for both the pregnant person and the fetus.

Nutritional intake during pregnancy has a direct effect on fetal well-being and birth outcome. Inadequate or excessive nutritional intake may contribute to preterm birth, congenital anomalies, miscarriage, gestational diabetes, small-for-gestational-age newborns, hypertensive disorders, and neurocognitive developmental issues (Garner, 2024).

Since the requirements for so many nutrients increase during pregnancy, pregnant people may need to take a vitamin and mineral supplement daily. Prenatal vitamins are prescribed routinely, almost universally in the United States, as a safeguard against less-than-optimal diets. Iron and folic acid need to be supplemented because their increased requirements during pregnancy are usually too great to be met through diet alone. Iron and folic acid are needed to form new blood cells for the expanded maternal blood volume and to prevent anemia. Iron is essential for fetal growth and brain development and in the prevention of maternal anemia. An increase in folic acid is essential before pregnancy and in the early weeks of pregnancy to prevent neural tube defects in the fetus. For most pregnant people, supplements of 27 mg of ferrous iron and 400 to 800 mcg of folic acid per day are recommended as **dietary reference intakes (DRIs)**, which are reference values of estimates of nutrient intakes (Garner, 2023; Office of Disease Prevention and Health Promotion [ODPHP], 2023). People with previous histories of fetuses with neural tube defects are often prescribed higher doses of folic acid.

There is an abundance of conflicting advice about nutrition during pregnancy and what is good or bad to eat. Overall, the following guidelines are helpful:

- Increase consumption of fruits and vegetables, taking up half the plate with these.
- Consume dairy, including fat-free or low-fat milk, yogurt, and cheese.
- Consume protein-rich foods.
- Choose whole grains in place of refined grains.
- Limit consumption of added sugars, saturated fats, and sodium.
- Read and check nutritional labels to make healthy choices.
- Follow food safety tips to avoid foodborne illnesses.
- Choose foods high in fiber to prevent constipation.
- Do not consume any alcoholic beverages.
- Limit caffeine to less than 200 to 300 mg/day.
- Eat at least 8 to 12 oz of lower methylmercury fish weekly, with one of them being an oily fish.
- Consume 2.3 L (76 oz) of water daily (Garner, 2024; U.S. Department of Agriculture & U.S. Department of Health and Human Services, 2020).

In the months before conception, food choices are key. The foods and vitamins consumed can ensure that the pregnant person and their fetus will have the nutrients that are essential for the very start of pregnancy.

While most people recognize the importance of healthy eating during pregnancy, some find it challenging to achieve. Many people say they have little time and energy to devote to meal planning and preparation. Another barrier to healthy eating is conflicting messages from various sources, resulting in a lack of clear, reliable, and relevant information. Moreover, many people restrict calories in an effort to control their weight, putting them at greater risk of inadequate nutrient intake.

Nutritional Requirements During Pregnancy

Pregnancy is a time of intense fetal growth and development, as well as maternal physiologic changes. Good nutrition during pregnancy promotes these processes, while under- or overnutrition is associated with poor pregnancy, maternal, and pediatric outcomes. Optimal maternal health via good nutritional practices during pregnancy reduces the risk of suboptimal fetal development.

The Food and Nutrition Board of the National Research Council has made recommendations for nutrient intake for people living in the United States. These DRIs are more comprehensive than previous nutrient guidelines issued by the Food and Nutrition Board. They have replaced previous recommendations because they are not limited to preventing deficiency diseases. Rather, the DRIs incorporate current concepts about the role of nutrients and food components in reducing the risk of chronic disease, developmental disorders, and other related problems. The DRIs can be used to plan and assess diets for healthy people (National Academies of Sciences, Engineering, and Medicine [NASEM], 2023).

These dietary recommendations also include information for people who are pregnant or lactating, because growing fetal and maternal tissues require increased quantities of essential dietary components. For example, current DRIs suggest an increase in the pregnant person's intake of protein from 46 to 71 g/day during the second and third trimesters, iron from 18 to 27 mg/day, and folic acid from 400 to 800 mcg/day, along with an increase in the second and third trimesters, respectively, of 340 to 450 calories/day over the recommended intake of 1,800 to 2,200 calories/day for nonpregnant females (Table 11.4) (Garner, 2024; ODPHP, 2023).

TAKE NOTE!

Good food sources of folic acid include dark green vegetables such as broccoli, romaine lettuce, and spinach; baked beans; black-eyed peas; citrus fruits; peanuts; and liver.

Food Concerns During Pregnancy

ARTIFICIAL SWEETENERS

Artificial sweeteners or intense sweeteners are sugar substitutes that are used as an alternative to table sugar. They are many times sweeter than natural sugar and contain no calories. The U.S. Food and Drug Administration (FDA)

TABLE **11.4** • Dietary Recommendations for the Pregnant and Lactating Person

Nutrient	Nonpregnant Female	Pregnant Person	Lactating Person
Calories	1,800–2,200	2,200–2,400 (2nd trimester) 2,400–2,600 (3rd trimester)	2,200–2,400
Protein	56 g	71 g	71 g
Vitamin A	900 mcg	750–770 mcg	1,200–1,300 mcg
Vitamin C	90 mg	80–85 mg	115–120 mg
Vitamin D	600 IU	600 IU	600 IU
Folate	400 mcg	600 mcg	500 mcg
Calcium	1,000 mg	1,000–1,300 mg	1,000–1,300 mg
Iodine		220 mcg	290 mcg
Iron	8 mg	27 mg	9–10 mg
Zinc	11 mg	11–12 mg	12–13 mg

U.S. Department of Agriculture & U.S. Department of Health and Human Services. (2020). *Dietary guidelines for Americans, 2020–2025* (9th ed). https://www.dietaryguidelines.gov

has stated the following nonnutritive sweeteners are safe to use during pregnancy: acesulfame potassium (Sunett, Sweet One), advantame, aspartame (NutraSweet, Equal), neotame (Newtame), saccharin (Sweet Low), luo han guo (Siraitia grosvenorii Swingle) fruit extract, lower than 95% purity steviol glycosides (e.g., Stevia, Truvia, SweetLeaf), sucralose (e.g., Splenda), or stevioside (Garner, 2023). Studies on short- and long-term effects are limited, but no data have shown that ingestion of nonnutritive sweeteners leads to increased risk of congenital anomalies (Garner, 2023). Recent evidence has linked nonnutritive sweeteners with higher newborn birth weights, low increase in preterm birth, altered childhood preference for sweet taste, and increased rates of higher weight (BMI greater than 30 kg/m^2) in childhood (Garner, 2023). Overall, artificial sweeteners should be used minimally.

FISH, SHELLFISH, AND LEVELS OF MERCURY

Fish and shellfish are an important part of a healthy diet because they contain high-quality protein, are low in saturated fat, and contain omega-3 fatty acids. However, nearly all fish and shellfish contain traces of mercury, and some contain higher levels of mercury that may harm a developing fetus's central nervous system if ingested by the pregnant person in large amounts. Human exposure to mercury primarily occurs through the consumption of fish contaminated through atmospheric mercury releases. Once airborne, rainfall transfers mercury particles into waterways, where it is converted to the neurotoxic methylmercury form through a microbial process. Plankton absorbs methylmercury, which is then consumed by small fish. As the larger predatory fish consume these smaller fish, methylmercury bioaccumulates up the food chain and can reach humans. Mercury exposure in pregnancy has been associated with both pregnancy complications and developmental problems in infants. Apart from the environmental exposures, mercury exposure is likely to arise from predatory fish consumption. All pregnant people should avoid these potential problems to minimize any risk.

All fish contain methylmercury, regardless of the size or geographic location of the waters from which the fish is caught, although these factors can influence the amounts of methylmercury present. With this in mind, the FDA and the Environmental Protection Agency (EPA) advise people who may become pregnant, pregnant people, and those who are breastfeeding to:

- avoid consumption of fish with moderate to high mercury levels for 6 to 12 months prior to conception and throughout pregnancy.
- avoid eating shark, swordfish, king mackerel, marlin, orange roughy, bigeye tuna, and tilefish because they are high in mercury levels.
- eat 8 to 12 oz (two average meals) weekly of fish known to have low mercury levels, such as shrimp, white albacore tuna (limit to 6 oz/week), salmon, lobster, sole, tilapia, cod, haddock, pollock, and catfish.
- check local advisories about the safety of fish caught by family and friends in local lakes, rivers, and coastal areas (American College of Obstetricians and Gynecologists [ACOG], 2023; U.S. Food and Drug Administration [FDA] & U.S. Environmental Protection Agency, 2021).

See Evidence-Based Practice 11.1.

EVIDENCE-BASED PRACTICE **11.1**

Vitamin D: Before, During, and After Pregnancy: Effect on Neonates and Children

BACKGROUND

A global prevalence of vitamin D deficiency exists, with a growing concern of the potential adverse effects on pregnant people and their offspring. Vitamin D enhances bone health in the body and functions as a regulator of calcium and phosphate metabolism. Deficiency during pregnancy may lead to hypocalcemia and nutritional rickets in newborn. Supplementation with vitamin D can reduce maternal and newborn complications. The purpose of this study was to review observational and interventional studies to see the influence of vitamin D deficiency on fertility, pregnancy, and offspring outcomes.

STUDY

Numerous studies were reviewed internationally to provide an overview of the effects of vitamin D supplementation on various aspects of health before, during, and after pregnancy. Systematic reviews, meta-analyses, and review articles were included in the analysis.

Findings

Supplementation with vitamin D and achievement of optimal levels of vitamin D reduced maternal–fetal and newborn complications, such as preeclampsia, gestational diabetes, preterm births, low birth weights, infertility, and lower bone mass in infants and children. These findings validated the roles of vitamin D deficiency and the consequences of intervention from preconception through infancy.

Nursing Implications

These findings suggest a positive impact of vitamin D supplementation on several birth outcomes, such as onset of preeclampsia, preterm births, low birth weight, gestational diabetes, and positive changes in the bone mass of the newborn. A balanced diet is necessary for a healthy pregnancy, but a majority of people do not consume one that provides all the micronutrients needed to support a healthy pregnancy. Nurses can be instrumental in offering advice to patients on vitamin D supplementation and good nutrition to improve pregnancy outcomes.

Adapted from Mansur, J. L., Oliveri, B., Giacoia, E., Fusaro, D., & Constanzo, P. R. (2022). Vitamin D: Before, during and after pregnancy: Effects on neonates and children. *Nutrients, 14*(9), 1900. https://doi.org/10.3390/nu14091900

LISTERIOSIS AND PREGNANCY

Another food issue concern for pregnant people is consumption of food contaminated with the Gram-positive bacillus *Listeria monocytogenes*. *Listeria* is a type of bacteria found in soil, groundwater, animals, and sometimes on plants. It is commonly found in processed and prepared foods and in raw or unpasteurized milk, and it causes listeriosis. Listeriosis is associated with high morbidity and mortality. Although *Listeria* is all around our environment, most *Listeria* infections in people result from eating contaminated foods. Pregnant people are 10 times as likely to get listeriosis as compared to healthy, nonpregnant adults (Gelfand et al., 2022a). Listeriosis during pregnancy usually presents as an unremarkable flulike febrile illness in the pregnant person but can be fatal for the fetus and newborn. Reliable laboratory testing for early diagnosis is lacking. Listeriosis can be passed to an unborn baby through the placenta even if the pregnant person is not showing signs of illness. This can lead to miscarriage, preterm labor, neonatal sepsis, meningitis, and neonatal mortality (Gelfand et al., 2022a). Pregnant people with known or suspected listeriosis should be treated with ampicillin IV or amoxicillin orally for 7 days (Gelfand et al., 2022b). Appropriate preventive treatment should be initiated to avoid complications. Advice for pregnant people to avoid listeriosis include the following:

- Wash hands frequently during food preparation.
- Refrigerate all perishable foods within 2 hours to prevent harmful bacteria from proliferating.
- Avoid getting fluid from hot dog packages on other foods, utensils, and food preparation surfaces, and wash hands after handling hot dogs, luncheon meats, and deli meats.
- Do not eat soft cheeses such as feta, Brie, Camembert, and blue-veined cheeses.
- It is safe to eat hard cheeses and semi-soft cheeses such as mozzarella, pasteurized processed cheese slices and spreads, cream cheese, and cottage cheese.
- Do not eat refrigerated pâté or meat spreads.
- It is safe to eat canned or shelf-stable pâté and meat spreads.
- Do not eat refrigerated smoked seafood, unless it is an ingredient in a cooked dish such as a casserole. Examples of refrigerated smoked seafood include salmon, trout, whitefish, cod, tuna, and mackerel and are most often labeled as "nova-style," "lox," "kippered," "smoked," or "jerky." These refrigerated smoked fish are found in the refrigerated section or sold at delicatessens and deli counters of grocery stores.
- It is safe to eat canned fish such as salmon and tuna or shelf-stable smoked seafood.
- Do not drink raw (unpasteurized) milk or eat foods that contain unpasteurized milk.
- Use all refrigerated perishable items that are precooked or ready-to-eat as soon as possible.
- Use a refrigerator thermometer to make sure that the refrigerator always stays at 40°F (about 4°C) or below and the freezer stays at 0°F (−18°C).
- Do not eat salads made in the store such as ham salad, chicken salad, egg salad, tuna salad, or seafood salad.
- Check expiration and "use by" dates, and throw out foods that are outdated.
- Thaw or marinate foods in the refrigerator, never on the kitchen counter.
- Avoid hot dogs and deli meats unless they are reheated until steaming hot.
- Thoroughly wash all fruits and vegetables even if you are peeling them.
- Do not eat raw or lightly cooked sprouts of any kind.
- Clean your refrigerator regularly (Gelfand et al., 2022b; U.S. FDA, 2018).

Maternal Weight Gain

The amount of weight a person gains during pregnancy is not as important as what they eat. A person can lose extra weight after a pregnancy, but they can never make up for poor nutritional status during the pregnancy. Earlier guidelines recommended weight gain that would be optimal for the infant, but new guidelines also consider the well-being of the pregnant person (Table 11.5).

Weight gain during pregnancy reflects increased maternal stores as well as those of the developing fetus and placenta. The National Academies of Sciences, Engineering, and Medicine (previously the Institute of Medicine) has made weight gain recommendations for a

TABLE 11.5 • Normal Distribution of Weight Gain During Pregnancy

Component	Weight
Infant birth weight	7–8 lb (3.2–3.6 kg)
Blood volume increase	3–4 lb (1.4–1.8 kg)
Uterus	2 lb (0.9 kg)
Increase in breast tissue	1–3 lb (0.45–1.4 kg)
Placenta	1.5 lb (0.7 kg)
Maternal fluid volume	2–3 lb (0.9–1.4 kg)
Maternal fat tissue	6–8 lb (2.7–3.6 kg)
Amniotic fluid	2 lb (0.9 kg)
Approximate total weight gain	24.5–31.5 lb (11.1–14.3 kg)

Adapted from Poston, L. (2024). Gestational weight gain. *UpToDate.* Retrieved May 24, 2024, from https://www.uptodate.com/contents/gestational-weight-gain

BOX 11.3 Body Mass Index

Body mass index (BMI) provides an estimate of total body fat and is considered a good method to assess overweight and higher weight in people. BMI is a weight-to-height ratio calculation that can be determined by dividing a person's weight in kilograms by the height in meters squared. BMI can also be calculated by weight in pounds divided by the height in inches squared, multiplied by 704.5.

The Centers for Disease Control and Prevention (CDC, 2024) categorizes BMI as follows:

- Underweight: lower than 18.5
- Normal: 18.5–24.9
- Overweight: 25–29.9
- Obesity: 30–39.9

Use this example to calculate BMI:
Mary is 5 ft 5 in tall and weighs 150 lb.

1. Convert weight into kilograms: 150 ÷ 2.2 lb/kg = 68.18 kg
2. Convert height into meters:
   a. 5 ft 5 in = 65 in ÷ 2.54 cm/in = 165.1 cm
   b. 165.1 cm ÷ 100 cm = 1.65 m
3. Then square the height in meters: 1.65 × 1.65 = 2.72
4. Calculate BMI: 68.18 kg ÷ 2.72 = 25

Adapted from Centers for Disease Control and Prevention. (2024). *Weight gain during pregnancy.* https://www.cdc.gov/maternal-infant-health/pregnancy-weight

person pregnant with one fetus based on BMI (Box 11.3) (CDC, 2024; Poston, 2024) as follows:

- BMI less than 18.5: total weight gain range 28 to 40 lb
- BMI 18.5 to 24.9: total weight gain range 25 to 35 lb
- BMI 25 to 29.9: total weight gain range 15 to 25 lb
- BMI 30 or higher: total weight gain range 11 to 20 lb

A person who has a low BMI before pregnancy or who has a low maternal weight gain pattern should be monitored carefully because they are at risk of preterm birth and of giving birth to a low-birth-weight infant (lighter than 2,500 g or 5.5 lb) (Poston, 2024). Frequently, people with a low BMI need advice on what to eat to add weight. They should be encouraged to eat high-calorie snacks such as nuts, peanut butter, milkshakes, cheese, fruit, yogurt, and ice cream. Any person who has a prepregnancy BMI less than 18.5 should be encouraged to reach a healthy BMI before pregnancy. They should be offered referral to a nutritionist, and the health care provider should consider the presence of an eating disorder (Poston, 2024).

Excessive gestational weight gain is a global epidemic. People who start a pregnancy at a higher weight (BMI of 25 to 29.9) run the risk of having a high-birth-weight infant with resulting cephalopelvic disproportion and a potential surgical birth (Poston, 2024). Around 30% to 50% of females in the United States have a higher weight (BMI greater than 25 kg/m^2) and are at risk for numerous adverse pregnancy outcomes such as early pregnancy loss, gestational diabetes and hypertension, preterm birth, and preeclampsia, in addition to surgical birth (Poston, 2024; Ramsey & Schenken, 2024). When maternal obesity is present, the fetus is at an increased risk for congenital anomalies; fetal, neonatal, and infant death; preterm birth; large for gestational age; having higher weight in childhood; and neurodevelopmental and psychiatric disorders such as autism spectrum disorder, attention-deficit disorder, anxiety, and depression (Ramsey & Schenken, 2024). Dieting during pregnancy is never recommended, even for people with higher weight. Severe restriction of caloric intake is associated with a decrease in birth weight. Because of the expansion of maternal blood volume and the development of fetal and placental tissues, some weight gain is essential for a healthy pregnancy. The best way to assess whether a pregnant person is consuming enough calories is to follow their pattern of weight gain. All pregnant people should aim for a steady rate of weight gain throughout pregnancy. If they are gaining in a steady, gradual manner, then they are taking in enough calories. However, consuming an adequate number of calories does not guarantee the nutrient intake is also sufficient. It is critical to evaluate both the quantity and the quality of the foods eaten.

During the first trimester, for people whose prepregnancy BMI is healthy (18.5 to 24.9 kg/m^2), weight gain should be about 3.5 to 5 lb. For people with a lower BMI (less than 18.5 kg/m^2), weight gain should be at least 5 lb. For people who have a higher BMI (25 kg/m^2), weight gain should be about 2 lb. Much of the weight gained during the first trimester is caused by growth of the uterus and expansion of the blood volume.

During the second and third trimesters, the following pattern is recommended: For people whose prepregnancy BMI is healthy (18.5 to 24.9 kg/m^2), weight gain should be about 1 lb per week. For people with a lower BMI (less than 18.5 kg/m^2), weight gain should be slightly more than 1 lb per week. For people who have a higher BMI (greater than 25 kg/m^2), weight gain should be about 0.5 to 0.6 lb per week (ACOG, 2013, reaffirmed 2023).

Nutrition Promotion

Through education, nurses can play an important role in ensuring adequate nutrition for pregnant people. During the initial prenatal visit, health care providers conduct a thorough assessment of a patient's typical dietary practices and address any conditions that may cause inadequate nutrition, such as nausea, vomiting, or lack of access to adequate food. Assess and reinforce dietary information at every prenatal visit to promote good nutrition. A normal pregnancy and a well-balanced diet generally provide most of the recommended nutrients, except iron and folate, both of which must be supplemented in the form of prenatal vitamins (Teaching Guidelines 11.1).

TEACHING GUIDELINES 11.1 Teaching to Promote Optimal Nutrition During Pregnancy

- Follow a healthy dietary pattern and select a variety of foods from each group (vegetables of all types, whole fruits, grains [at least half whole grains], dairy, protein-rich food, and plant-based oils).
- Gain between 11 and 40 lb in a gradual and steady manner depending on prepregnancy BMI as follows:
  - BMI less than 18.5: total weight gain range 28 to 40 lb
  - BMI 18.5 to 24.0: total weight gain range 25 to 35 lb
  - BMI 25 to 29: total weight gain range 15 to 25 lb
  - BMI 30 or higher: total weight gain range 11 to 20 lb
- Take prenatal vitamins and mineral supplementations daily.
- Avoid weight reduction diets during pregnancy.
- Do not skip meals; eat three meals with one or two snacks daily.
- Limit the intake of sugary beverages and added sugars and saturated fats.
- Limit caffeine to 200 to 300 mg/day.
- Avoid consuming any alcohol.
- Do not restrict the use of salt unless instructed to do so by your health care provider.
- Practice safe food handling.
- Engage in reasonable physical activity for 150 minutes each week.

Adapted from Garner, C. D. (2024). Nutrition in pregnancy: Dietary requirements and supplements. *UpToDate.* Retrieved May 23, 2024, from https://www.uptodate.com/contents/nutrition-in-pregnancy-dietary-requirements-and-supplements; and U.S. Department of Agriculture & U.S. Department of Health and Human Services. (2020). *Dietary guidelines for Americans, 2020–2025* (9th ed). https://www.dietaryguidelines.gov

Special Nutritional Considerations

Many factors play an important role in shaping a person's food habits, and these factors must be taken into account if nutritional counseling is to be realistic and appropriate. Nurses need to be aware of these factors to ensure individualized teaching and care.

Cultural Variations and Restrictions

Food is important to every cultural group. It is often part of celebrations and rituals. The nurse needs to adapt nutritional guidelines to meet each person's nutritional needs within their cultural framework and preferences. Food choices and variations for different cultures might include foods with which the health care provider is unfamiliar, and they must understand the nutritional content of each patient's individual diet preferences.

Lactose Intolerance

Food plays an essential role in normal cellular processes and is required for survival of all living organisms. In some people with allergies and food intolerances, it can trigger or worsen certain disease states. The best source of calcium is milk and dairy products, but for those with lactose intolerance, adaptations are necessary. People with lactose intolerance lack an enzyme (lactase) that is needed for the breakdown of lactose into its component simple sugars, glucose, and galactose. Without adequate lactase, lactose passes through the small intestine undigested and causes abdominal discomfort, gas, and diarrhea. Lactose intolerance is more common among females of African, Asian, and South American descent (Malik & Panuganti, 2023).

Additional or substitute sources of calcium and vitamin D may be necessary. Encourage the patient who is intolerant to lactose to drink and eat lactose-free dairy products or calcium-enriched orange juice or soy milk.

Vegetarians

People choose a vegetarian diet for various reasons, including environmental, animal rights, philosophical, religious, and health beliefs. Vegetarians choose not to eat meat, poultry, and fish. Their diets consist mostly of plant-based foods, such as legumes, vegetables, whole grains, nuts, and seeds. Vegetarian diets vary based on which animal proteins a person avoids and fall into groups defined by the types of foods they eat. Lacto-ovo-vegetarians omit red meat, fish, and poultry but eat eggs, milk, and dairy products in addition to plant-based foods. Lacto vegetarians consume milk and dairy products along with plant-based foods; they omit eggs, meat, fish, and poultry. Vegans eliminate all foods originating from animals, including eggs, milk, and milk products, and eat only plant-based foods (Garner, 2023).

The concern with any form of vegetarianism, especially during pregnancy, is that the diet may be inadequate in nutrients. Other risks of vegetarian eating patterns during pregnancy may include low-birth-weight or small-for-gestational-age infant; iron-deficiency anemia; and low vitamin D, E, and choline (Garner, 2023). Certain diets can become so restrictive that the person does not gain weight during pregnancy or consistently does not eat enough from one or more of the food groups. Generally, the more restrictive the diet is, the greater the chance of nutrient deficiencies.

Well-balanced vegetarian diets in general provide adequate caloric and nutrient intake and are considered safe during pregnancy and lactation (Garner, 2023). It is important to assess each patient and consider their specific diet restrictions to determine risks for nutrient deficiencies. Pregnant vegetarians must pay special attention to their intake of protein, iron, calcium, vitamin D, and vitamin B_{12}. Suggestions include:

- *For protein:* Substitute soy foods, beans, lentils, nuts, grains, and seeds.
- *For iron:* Eat a variety of meat alternatives along with vitamin C–rich foods.
- *For calcium:* Substitute soy, calcium-fortified orange juice, kale, broccoli, and tofu.
- *For vitamin D:* Consume fortified milk and fish and fortified cereal, and take a prenatal vitamin.
- *For vitamin B_{12}:* Eat fortified soy foods and cereals, and take a B_{12} supplement.

Pica

Pica is a term used to describe the intense craving for and eating of nonfood items over a period of time of at least 1 month. Many people experience unusual food cravings during their pregnancy. Having cravings during pregnancy is perfectly normal. Sometimes, however, a pregnant person craves substances that have no nutritional value and can even be dangerous to themselves and the fetus. Pica is the compulsive ingestion of nonfood substances. Pica is derived from the Latin term for magpie, a bird that is known to consume a variety of nonfood substances. Unlike the bird, however, pregnant people who develop pica typically have one or two specific cravings.

Many factors have been implicated in the etiology of pica, but the exact cause of pica is not known. Many theories have been advanced to explain it, but none has been proven scientifically. The incidence of pica is difficult to determine since it is underreported. It is more common in pregnant people than any other demographic group (Young & Cox, 2023). Common substances ingested include dirt; clay; raw starch such as cornstarch, laundry starch, or flour; and ice or freezer frost (Young & Cox, 2023). Other pica cravings include paper, toilet paper, charcoal, baby powder, chalk, coffee grounds, paint chips, and ashes (Young & Cox, 2023).

The three main substances consumed by pregnant people with pica are soil or clay (geophagia), ice (pagophagia), and laundry starch (amylophagia). Nutritional and clinical implications include the following:

- *Soil and clay:* replaces nutritive sources and causes iron-deficiency anemia and low gestational weight gain; produces constipation; can contain toxic substances and cause parasitic infection or hypokalemia
- *Ice:* can cause iron-deficiency anemia, tooth fractures, jaw pain, freezer burn injuries, and low gestational weight gain
- *Laundry starch:* replaces iron-rich foods; leads to iron deficiencies, abdominal discomfort, poor glucose control, and excessive weight gain (Young & Cox, 2023).

Secrecy surrounding pica makes research and diagnosis difficult because some people do not view their behavior as anything unusual, harmful, or worth reporting. Because of the clinical implications, pica should be discussed with all pregnant people as a preventive measure. The topic can be part of a general discussion of cravings, and the nurse should stress the harmful effects of consuming nonfood items.

A nonjudgmental, understanding, and culturally supportive environment can facilitate reporting of pica by the patient. Suspect pica when the patient exhibits anemia though their dietary intake is appropriate. Ask about their usual dietary intake, and include questions about the ingestion of nonfood substances. Consider the potential negative outcomes for the pregnant person and their fetus, and take appropriate action. The nurse's focus should be to change potentially harmful eating habits and to be supportive to the patient in making the change.

PSYCHOSOCIAL ADAPTATIONS DURING PREGNANCY

Pregnancy is a unique time in a person's life. It marks a period of emotional, physical, and relational changes that are shaped by each person's individual circumstances. The transition to parenthood is characterized by physiologic, psychological, and social changes. It is a time of dramatic alterations in the person's body and appearance, as well as a time of change in their social status. All of these changes occur simultaneously. Concurrent with the physiologic changes within the person's body systems are psychosocial changes within the pregnant person and their family members as they face significant role and lifestyle changes. Nurses should inquire at every prenatal visit about the person's emotional well-being to assess their psychosocial adjustments throughout the pregnancy.

Maternal Emotional Responses

Parenthood holds special significance for many people. Women are socialized to seek fulfillment and satisfaction in the role of the "ever-bountiful, ever-giving, self-sacrificing mother." Pregnancy and transitioning to parenthood are critical experiences in a person's life, stirring a whole range of powerful emotions. Many people describe pregnancy as a moody time in their lives. People of any culture, age, income, or educational level can develop perinatal mood and anxiety disorders. Significant symptoms of depression or anxiety occur in approximately 15% to 20% of pregnant and postpartum people (Postpartum Support International, 2023). Given the high expectations typically applied to new parenthood, many pregnant people experience various emotions throughout their pregnancy. The person's approach to these emotions is influenced by their emotional makeup, their sociologic and cultural background, their acceptance or rejection of the pregnancy, if the pregnancy was planned, if they have a partner, and their support network. Pregnant people impacted by adverse childhoods and social determinants, such as economic insecurity, violence, lack of access to high-quality health care, language barriers, safe housing and neighborhoods, few job skills, few job opportunities, and food insecurity, are at increased risk for perinatal mood and anxiety disorders. Nurses should be highly aware of symptoms of depression and anxiety during the perinatal period and understand the diagnostic criteria and screening methods used to identify both (Association of Women's Health, Obstetric and Neonatal Nurses, 2022). Nurses can also initiate effective interventions to ensure the safety of the birthing parent and infant and make appropriate community referrals for treatment.

Despite the wide-ranging emotions associated with pregnancy, many pregnant people experience similar responses. These responses commonly include ambivalence, introversion, acceptance, mood swings, and changes in body image.

Ambivalence

The realization of a pregnancy can lead to fluctuating responses, possibly at opposite ends of the spectrum. For example, regardless of whether the pregnancy was planned or not, the person may feel proud and excited by the news, while at the same time fearful and anxious of the implications. These reactions are influenced by several factors, including the way the person was raised, their current family situation, the quality of the relationship with their partner, and their hopes for the future. Some people may express concerns over the timing of the pregnancy, wishing that goals and life objectives had been met before the pregnancy. Other people may question how a newborn or infant will affect their careers or their relationships with friends and family. These feelings can cause conflict and confusion about the pregnancy.

Ambivalence, or having conflicting feelings at the same time, is a universal feeling and is considered normal when preparing for a lifestyle change and new role. Pregnant people commonly experience ambivalence during the first trimester. Usually, ambivalence evolves into acceptance by the second trimester, when fetal movement is felt. The pregnant person's personality, their ability to adapt to changing circumstances, and the reactions of their partner will affect the person's adjustment to being pregnant and their acceptance of impending parenthood.

Introversion

Introversion, or focusing on oneself, is common during the early part of pregnancy. The person may withdraw and become increasingly preoccupied with themselves and their fetus. As a result, they may participate less with the outside world, and they may appear passive to their family and friends.

This introspective behavior is a normal psychological adaptation for most pregnant people. Introversion seems to heighten during the first and third trimesters, when the person's focus is on behaviors that will ensure a safe and health pregnancy outcome. Patients, partners, and families need to be aware of this behavior and should be informed about measures to maintain and support the focus on the family.

Acceptance

During the second trimester, the physical changes of the growing fetus, including an enlarging abdomen and fetal movement, bring a sense of reality and validity to the pregnancy. There are many tangible signs that someone separate from themselves is present. The pregnant person feels fetal movement and may hear the heartbeat. They may see the fetal image on an ultrasound screen and feel distinct parts, recognizing independent sleep and wake patterns.

Many people will verbalize positive feelings about the pregnancy and will conceptualize the fetus as a person. The pregnant person may accept their new body image and talk about the new life within. Generating a discussion about the person's feelings and offering support and validation at prenatal visits are important.

Mood Swings

Emotional lability is characteristic throughout most pregnancies. One moment a person can feel great joy, and within a short time, they can feel shock and disbelief. Frequently, pregnant people will start to cry without any apparent cause. Some people feel as though they are riding an "emotional roller coaster." These extremes in emotion can make it difficult for partners and family members to communicate with the pregnant person without placing blame on themselves for their mood changes. Clear explanations about how common mood swings are during pregnancy are essential.

Change in Body Image

The way in which pregnancy affects a person's body image varies greatly from person to person. Some people feel as if they have never been more beautiful, while others spend their pregnancy feeling unhappy with their appearance and uncomfortable. For some people, pregnancy is a relief from worrying about weight, while for others it exacerbates fears of weight gain. Changes in body image are normal but can be stressful for the pregnant person. Offering a thorough explanation and initiating discussion of the expected bodily changes may help the family to cope with them.

Becoming a Parent

Reva Rubin (1984) identified maternal tasks that a woman must accomplish to incorporate the maternal role into her personality. Accomplishing these tasks helps the expectant parent develop their self-concept as a parent and form a mutually gratifying relationship with the infant. These tasks are listed in Box 11.4.

Pregnancy and Sexuality

Sexuality is an important part of health and well-being. It is a lifelong biopsychosocial concept that is affected by attitudes, behaviors, and society. Sexual behavior modifies as pregnancy progresses, influenced by biologic, psychological, and social factors. The way a pregnant person feels and experiences their body during pregnancy can affect their sexuality. The person's changing shape, emotional status, fetal activity, changes in breast size, pressure on the bladder, and other discomforts of pregnancy result in increased physical and emotional demands. These can produce stress on the sexual relationship between the pregnant person and their partner. As the changes of pregnancy ensue, many partners become confused, anxious, and fearful of how the relationship may be affected.

The sexual desire of pregnant people may change throughout the pregnancy. During the first trimester, the person may be less interested in sex because of fatigue, nausea, and fear of disturbing the early embryonic development. During the second trimester, their interest may increase because of the stability of the pregnancy. During the third trimester, their enlarging physical size may produce discomfort during sexual activity.

Theoretical complications of sex during pregnancy include preterm labor, infectious complications, release of oxytocin during orgasm, and direct action of prostaglandins in semen; however, there is insufficient evidence to recommend against sexual intercourse in a healthy pregnancy (Lockwood & Magriples, 2024). Abstinence is usually only recommended for people with pregnancy complications, such as vaginal bleeding or preterm cervical dilation or who are at risk for preterm labor or for antepartum hemorrhage because of placenta previa (Lockwood & Magriples, 2024).

A person's sexual health is intimately linked to their own self-image. Sexual positions to increase comfort as the pregnancy progresses as well as alternative noncoital modes of sexual expression, such as cuddling, caressing, and holding, should be discussed. Giving permission to talk about and then normalizing sexuality can help enhance the sexual experience during pregnancy and ultimately the couple's relationship. If avenues of communication are open regarding sexuality during pregnancy, any fears and myths the couple may have can be dispelled.

BOX 11.4 Rubin's Maternal Tasks

- Ensuring safe passage throughout pregnancy and birth
  - Primary focus of the pregnant person's attention
  - First trimester: person focuses on themselves, not on the fetus
  - Second trimester: person develops attachment of great value to the fetus
  - Third trimester: person has concern for themselves and the fetus as a unit
  - Participation in positive self-care activities related to diet, exercise, and overall well-being
- Seeking acceptance of infant by others
  - First trimester: acceptance of pregnancy by themselves and others
  - Second trimester: family needs to relate to the fetus as member
  - Third trimester: unconditional acceptance without rejection
- Seeking acceptance of self in maternal role to infant ("binding in")
  - First trimester: pregnant person accepts idea of pregnancy, but not of infant
  - Second trimester: with sensation of fetal movement (quickening), person acknowledges fetus as a separate entity within them
  - Third trimester: person longs to hold infant and becomes tired of being pregnant
- Learning to give of oneself
  - First trimester: identifies what must be given up to assume new role
  - Second trimester: identifies with infant and learns how to delay own desires
  - Third trimester: questions their ability to become a good parent to infant

Rubin, R. (1984). *Maternal identity and the maternal experience.* Springer.

Pregnancy and the Partner

Nursing care related to childbirth has expanded from a narrow emphasis on the physical health needs of the pregnant person and infant to a broader focus on family-related social and emotional needs. One prominent feature of this family-centered approach is the recent movement toward promoting the bond between the birthing parent and the infant. But to achieve a truly family-centered practice, nursing must make a comparable commitment to understanding and meeting the needs of the partner in the emerging family.

Reactions to pregnancy and to the psychological and physical changes by the pregnant person's partner vary greatly. Some enjoy taking on a nurturing role, while others experience alienation and may seek comfort or companionship elsewhere. Some male partners may view pregnancy as proof of their masculinity and assume a dominant role, while others see their role as minimal, leaving the pregnancy up to the pregnant person entirely. Each expectant partner reacts uniquely.

Emotionally and psychologically, an expectant partner may undergo fewer visible changes than the pregnant person, but changes do occur and may remain unexpressed and unappreciated. Partners often play a key role in pregnancy and childbirth preparedness in terms of economic and emotional support. Expectant partners also experience a multitude of adjustments and concerns. Physically, they may gain weight around the middle and experience nausea and other GI disturbances—a reaction termed *couvade syndrome* that is a sympathetic response to their partner's pregnancy. They may also experience ambivalence during early pregnancy, with extremes of emotions (e.g., pride and joy vs. an overwhelming sense of impending responsibility).

During the second trimester of pregnancy, partners often go through acceptance of the role as caregiver and support person. They come to accept the reality of the fetus when movement is felt, and they experience confusion when dealing with the pregnant person's mood swings and introspection. During the third trimester, the expectant partner prepares for the reality of this new role and negotiates what the role will be during the labor and birthing process. Many express concerns about being the primary support person during labor and birth and worry how they will react when faced with their loved one in pain. Expectant partners share many of the same anxieties as their pregnant partners. However, it is uncommon for them to reveal these anxieties to the pregnant partner or health care providers. Often, how the expectant partner responds during the third trimester depends on the state of the marriage or partnership. When the marriage or partnership is struggling, the impending increase in responsibility toward the end of pregnancy may drive the expectant partner further away. It may manifest as working late, staying out late with friends, or beginning new or superficial relationships. In the stable partnership, the expectant partner who may have been struggling to find their place in the pregnancy now finds concrete tasks to do—for example, painting the nursery, assembling the car seat, or attending childbirth classes.

Pregnancy and Siblings

A sibling's reaction to pregnancy is age dependent. Some children might express excitement and anticipation, while others might have negative reactions. A young toddler might regress in toilet training or ask to drink from a bottle again. An older school-aged child may ignore the new addition to the family and engage in outside activities to avoid the new member. The introduction of an infant into the family can be the beginning of sibling rivalry, which results from the child's fear of change in the security of the relationship with their parents. Preparation of the siblings for the anticipated birth is imperative and must be designed according to the age and life experiences of the sibling at home. Constant reinforcement of love and caring will help reduce the older child's fear of change and worry about being replaced by the new family member.

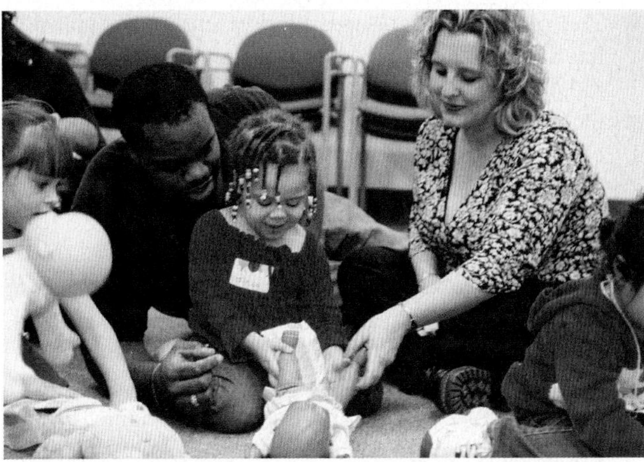

FIGURE 11.5 Parents preparing sibling for the birth of a new baby.

If possible, parents should include siblings in preparation for the birth of the new baby to help them feel as if they have an important role to play (Fig. 11.5). Get the older sibling involved by allowing them to choose a present or clothes for the new baby, help choose a name for the new baby or decide where to put baby supplies and toys, and give them opportunities to care for the new baby in small ways. Parents must also continue to focus on the older sibling, provide one-on-one time with the older child after the birth, and discuss with the child how they may be feeling to help reduce regressive or aggressive behavior toward the newborn.

Pregnancy is an extremely busy time, not only in terms of the bodily changes taking place but tasks that must be done such as choosing health care providers, preparing for the new family member in a matter of months, and making lifestyle modifications to promote the best possible pregnancy outcome. We will explore this more in Chapter 12.

KEY CONCEPTS

- Pregnancy is a normal life event that involves considerable physical, psychosocial, emotional, and relationship adjustments.
- The signs and symptoms of pregnancy have been grouped into those that are subjective (presumptive) and experienced by the pregnant person themselves; those that are objective (probable) and observed by the health care provider; and those that are the positive (diagnostic) signs.
- Physiologically, almost every system of a person's body changes during pregnancy with startling rapidity to accommodate the needs of the growing fetus. A majority of these changes are influenced by hormonal changes.

- The placenta is a unique kind of endocrine gland; it has a feature possessed by no other endocrine organ—the ability to form protein and steroid hormones.
- Occurring in conjunction with the physiologic changes in the person's body systems are psychosocial changes occurring within the pregnant person and their family members, as they face significant role and lifestyle changes.
- Commonly experienced emotional responses to pregnancy in the pregnant person include ambivalence, introversion, acceptance, mood swings, and changes in body image.
- Reactions of expectant partners to pregnancy and to the physical and psychological changes in the pregnant person vary greatly.
- Sibling reactions to pregnancy are age dependent. The introduction of a new infant to the family may be the beginning of sibling rivalry, which results from the child's fear of change in security of their relationships with their parents. Therefore, preparation of the siblings for the anticipated birth is imperative.

REFERENCES AND RECOMMENDED READINGS

Adams, E. D. (2022). Anatomic and physiologic adaptations of normal pregnancy. In K. D. Schuiling & F. E. Likis (Eds.), *Gynecologic health care* (4th ed., pp. 677–682). Jones & Bartlett Learning.

Al-Chalabi, M., Bass, A. N., & Alsalman, I. (2023). Physiology, prolactin. In *StatPearls*. StatPearls Publishing. https://www.ncbi.nlm.nih.gov/books/NBK507829/

American College of Obstetricians and Gynecologists (2013, reaffirmed 2023). Weight gain during pregnancy. Committee opinion no. 548. *Obstetrics and Gynecology*, *121*, 210–212.

American College of Obstetricians and Gynecologists. (2023). *Nutrition during pregnancy*. https://www.acog.org/womens-health/faqs/nutrition-during-pregnancy

Association of Women's Health, Obstetric and Neonatal Nurses. (2022). AWHONN position statement: Perinatal mood and anxiety disorders. *JOGNN*, *51*(4), E1–E4. https://doi.org/10.1016/j.jogn.2022.03.007

Bastian, L. A., & Brown, H. L. (2023). Clinical manifestations and diagnosis of early pregnancy. *UpToDate*. Retrieved May 13, 2024, from https://www.uptodate.com/contents/clinical-manifestations-and-diagnosis-of-early-pregnancy

Bermas, B. L. (2023). Maternal adaptations to pregnancy: Musculoskeletal changes and pain. *UpToDate*. Retrieved May 22, 2024, from https://www.uptodate.com/contents/maternal-adaptations-to-pregnancy-musculoskeletal-changes-and-pain

Bianco, A. (2023). Maternal adaptations to pregnancy: Gastrointestinal tract. *UpToDate*. Retrieved May 21, 2024, from https://www.uptodate.com/contents/maternal-adaptations-to-pregnancy-gastrointestinal-tract

Brooks, D. C. (2024). Gallstones diseases in pregnancy. *UpToDate*. Retrieved May 21, 2024, from https://www.uptodate.com/contents/gallstone-diseases-in-pregnancy

Centers for Disease Control and Prevention. (2024). *Weight gain during pregnancy*. https://www.cdc.gov/maternal-infant-health/pregnancy-weight

Chaudhry, R., & Chaudhry, K. (2023). Anatomy, abdomen and pelvis: Uterine arteries. In *StatPearls*. StatPearls Publishing. https://www.ncbi.nlm.nih.gov/books/NBK482267/

Gandhi, M. H., & Gupta, V. (2023). Physiology, maternal blood. In *StatPearls*. StatPearls Publishing. https://www.ncbi.nlm.nih.gov/books/NBK557783/

Garner, C. D. (2023). Nutrition in pregnancy: Assessment and counseling. *UpToDate*. Retrieved May 23, 2024, from https://www.uptodate.com/contents/nutrition-in-pregnancy-assessment-and-counseling

Garner, C. D. (2024). Nutrition in pregnancy: Dietary requirements and supplements. *UpToDate*. Retrieved May 23, 2024, from https://www.uptodate.com/contents/nutrition-in-pregnancy-dietary-requirements-and-supplements

Gelfand, M. S., Swamy, G. K., & Thompson, J. L. (2022a). Clinical manifestations and diagnosis of *Listeria monocytogenes* infection. *UpToDate*. Retrieved May 24, 2024, from https://www.uptodate.com/contents/clinical-manifestations-and-diagnosis-of-listeria-monocytogenes-infection

Gelfand, M. S., Thompson, J. L., & Swamy, G. K. (2022b). Treatment and prevention of *Listeria monocytogenes* infection. *UpToDate*. Retrieved May 24, 2024, from https://www.uptodate.com/contents/treatment-and-prevention-of-listeria-monocytogenes-infection

Kapila, V., & Chaudhry, K. (2024). Physiology, placenta. In *StatPearls*. StatPearls Publishing. https://www.ncbi.nlm.nih.gov/books/NBK538332/

Kepley, J. M., Bates, K., & Mohiuddin, S. S. (2023). Physiology, maternal changes. In *StatPearls*. StatPearls Publishing. https://www.ncbi.nlm.nih.gov/books/NBK539766/

Knight, J. (2023). Pregnancy 1: Effects on hematological and cardiovascular systems. *Nursing Times*, *119*(9). https://www.nursingtimes.net/clinical-archive/womens-health/pregnancy-1-effects-on-haematological-and-cardiovascular-systems-29-08-2023/

Lockwood, C. J., & Magriples, U. (2024). Prenatal care: Patient education, health promotion, and safety of commonly used drugs. *UpToDate*. Retrieved May 24, 2024, from https://www.uptodate.com/contents/prenatal-care-patient-education-health-promotion-and-safety-of-commonly-used-drugs

Malik, T. F., & Panuganti, K. K. (2023). Lactose intolerance. In *StatPearls*. StatPearls Publishing. https://www.ncbi.nlm.nih.gov/books/NBK532285/

Mansur, J. L., Oliveri, B., Giacoia, E., Fusaro, D., & Constanzo, P. R. (2022). Vitamin D: Before, during and after pregnancy: Effects on neonates and children. *Nutrients*, *14*(9), 1900. https://doi.org/10.3390/nu14091900

Nana, M., & Williamson, C. (2022). Pituitary and adrenal disorders of pregnancy. In K. R. Feingold, B. Anawalt, M. R. Blackman, A. Boyce, G. Chrousos, E. Corpas, W. W. de Herder, K. Dhatariya, K. Dungan, J. Hofland, S. Kalra, G. Kaltsas, N. Kapoor, C. Koch, P. Kopp, M. Korbonits, C. S. Kovacs, W. Kuohung, B. Laferrère, … D. P. Wilson (Eds.), *Endotext*. https://www.ncbi.nlm.nih.gov/books/NBK279043/

National Academies of Sciences, Engineering, and Medicine. (2023). *Dietary reference intakes for energy*. https://nap.nationalacademies.org/catalog/26818/dietary-reference-intakes-for-energy

Norwitz, E. R. (2024). Physiology of parturition at term. *UpToDate*. Retrieved May 23, 2024, from https://www.uptodate.com/contents/physiology-of-parturition-at-term

Office of Disease Prevention and Health Promotion. (2023). *Eat healthy during pregnancy: Quick tips*. https://health.gov/myhealthfinder/pregnancy/nutrition-and-physical-activity/eat-healthy-during-pregnancy-quick-tips

Pande, A., & Anjankar, A. (2023). A narrative review on the effect of maternal hypothyroidism on fetal development. *Cureus, 15*(2), e34824. https://doi.org/10.7759/cureus.34824

Pascual, Z. N., & Langaker, M. D. (2023). Physiology, pregnancy. In *StatPearls*. StatPearls Publishing. https://www.ncbi.nlm.nih.gov/books/NBK559304/

Pinheiro, E. A., & Stika, C. S. (2020). Drugs in pregnancy: Pharmacologic and physiologic changes that affect clinical care. *Seminars in Perinatology, 44*(3), 151221. https://doi.org/10.1016/j.semperi.2020.151221

Pomeranz, M. K. (2023). Maternal adaptations to pregnancy: Skin and related structures. *UpToDate*. Retrieved May 22, 2024, from https://www.uptodate.com/contents/maternal-adaptations-to-pregnancy-skin-and-related-structures

Poston, L. (2024). Gestational weight gain. *UpToDate*. Retrieved May 24, 2024, from https://www.uptodate.com/contents/gestational-weight-gain

Postpartum Support International. (2023). *Perinatal mental health disorders*. https://www.postpartum.net/learn-more/

Rampersad, F. S., Chan, A., Persaud, S., Maharaj, P., & Maharaj, R. (2022). Choledocholithiasis in pregnancy: A case report. *Cureus, 14*(2), e22610. https://www.ncbi.nlm.nih.gov/pmc/articles/PMC8958046/

Ramsey, P. S., & Schenken, R. S. (2024). Obesity in pregnancy: Complications and maternal management. *UpToDate*. Retrieved May 24, 2024, from https://www.uptodate.com/contents/obesity-in-pregnancy-complications-and-maternal-management

Records, K., & Clark, A. (2024). Physiology of pregnancy. In B. J. Baker, J. Janke, & AWHONN (Eds.), *Core curriculum for maternal-newborn nursing* (6th ed., Chap. 8). Elsevier.

Robinson, J. N., & Norwitz, E. R. (2024). Spontaneous preterm birth: Overview of risk factors and prognosis. *UpToDate*. Retrieved May 21, 2024, from https://www.uptodate.com/contents/spontaneous-preterm-birth-overview-of-risk-factors-and-prognosis

Rubin, R. (1984). *Maternal identify and maternal experience*. Springer Publishers.

Smith, J. A., Fox, K. A., & Clark, S. M. (2023). Nausea and vomiting of pregnancy: Treatment and outcome. *UpToDate*. https://www.uptodate.com/contents/nausea-and-vomiting-of-pregnancy-treatment-and-outcome

Smith, J. A., Fox, K. A., & Clark, S. M. (2024). Nausea and vomiting of pregnancy: Clinical findings and evaluation. *UpToDate*. Retrieved May 21, 2024, from https://www.uptodate.com/contents/nausea-and-vomiting-of-pregnancy-clinical-findings-and-evaluation

Tal, R., & Taylor, H. S. (2021). Endocrinology of pregnancy. In K. R. Feingold, B. Anawalt, M. R. Blackman, A. Boyce, G. Chrousos, E. Corpas, W. W. de Herder, K. Dhatariya, K. Dungan, J. Hofland, S. Kalra, G. Kaltsas, N. Kapoor, C. Koch, P. Kopp, M. Korbonits, C. S. Kovacs, W. Kuohung, B. Laferrère, … D. P. Wilson (Eds.), *Endotext*. https://www.ncbi.nlm.nih.gov/books/NBK278962/

Thadhani, R. I., & Maynard, S. E. (2024). Maternal adaptations to pregnancy: Renal and urinary tract physiology. *UpToDate*. Retrieved May 22, 2024, from https://www.uptodate.com/contents/maternal-adaptations-to-pregnancy-renal-and-urinary-tract-physiology

U.S. Department of Agriculture & U.S. Department of Health and Human Services. (2020). *Dietary guidelines for Americans, 2020–2025* (9th ed.). https://www.dietaryguidelines.gov

U.S. Food and Drug Administration. (2018). *Listeria from food safety for moms to be*. https://www.fda.gov/food/health-educators/listeria-food-safety-moms-be

U.S. Food and Drug Administration & U.S. Environmental Protection Agency. (2021). *Advice about eating fish*. https://www.fda.gov/food/consumers/advice-about-eating-fish

Valente, A. M., & Economy, K. (2024). Maternal adaptations to pregnancy: Cardiovascular and hemodynamic changes. *UpToDate*. Retrieved May 22, 2024, from https://www.uptodate.com/contents/maternal-adaptations-to-pregnancy-cardiovascular-and-hemodynamic-changes

Weinberger, S. E. (2024). Maternal adaptations to pregnancy: Dyspnea and other physiologic respiratory changes. *UpToDate*. Retrieved May 22, 2024, from https://www.uptodate.com/contents/maternal-adaptations-to-pregnancy-dyspnea-and-other-physiologic-respiratory-changes

Wilder, R. S., & Moretti, A. (2023). Overview of gingivitis and periodontitis in adults. *UpToDate*. Retrieved May 21, 2024, from https://www.uptodate.com/contents/overview-of-gingivitis-and-periodontitis-in-adults

Young, S. L., & Cox, J. T. (2023). Pica in pregnancy. *UpToDate*. Retrieved May 24, 2024, from https://www.uptodate.com/contents/pica-in-pregnancy

DEVELOPING CLINICAL JUDGMENT

PRACTICING FOR NCLEX

1. The nurse is teaching nursing students about care of the pregnant person. The nursing students demonstrate understanding when they explain that which factor would change during a pregnancy if the hormone progesterone were reduced or withdrawn?
   a. The person's gums would become red and swollen and would bleed easily.
   b. The uterus would contract more, and peristalsis would increase.
   c. Morning sickness would increase and would be prolonged.
   d. The secretion of prolactin by the pituitary gland would be inhibited.
2. A 26-year-old female is seen in the clinic. She states her last menstrual period was 6 weeks ago. Which additional signs or symptoms would be presumptive for pregnancy? Select all that apply.
   a. Restlessness
   b. Elevated mood
   c. Urinary frequency
   d. Low backache
   e. Breast tenderness
   f. Nausea
3. The nurse is obtaining a blood test for pregnancy. The patient asks which hormone the test measures. What is the correct response by the nurse?
   a. Human chorionic gonadotropin (hCG)
   b. Human placental lactogen (hPL)
   c. Follicle-stimulating hormone (FSH)
   d. Luteinizing hormone (LH)
4. The nurse is teaching a prenatal class. The nurse explains that during pregnancy, the pregnant person should reduce or avoid which foods?
   a. Refrigerated Brie
   b. Fresh washed apples
   c. Whole grain toast
   d. Shrimp cocktail
5. A patient is seen in your clinic and has just received a diagnosis of pregnancy. The nurse is not surprised when the patient expresses which feeling?
   a. Acceptance
   b. Depression
   c. Jealousy
   d. Ambivalence
6. Reva Rubin identified four major tasks that a pregnant person undertakes to form a mutually gratifying relationship with their infant. What is "binding in?"
   a. Ensuring safe passage through pregnancy, labor, and birth
   b. Seeking acceptance of this infant by others
   c. Seeking acceptance of self as parent to the infant
   d. Learning to give of oneself on behalf of the infant
7. A pregnant patient close to term comes to the clinic for an examination. The patient complains about experiencing shortness of breath. The nurse knows that this may be caused by:
   a. the fetus needing more oxygen due to its larger size.
   b. the fundus of the uterus pushing the diaphragm upward.
   c. the patient experiencing an allergic reaction because of high histamine levels.
   d. the oxygen partial pressure concentration becoming lower during the third trimester.

CRITICAL THINKING EXERCISES

1. When interviewing a patient at their first prenatal visit, the nurse asks about the patient's feelings. The patient replies, "I am frightened and confused. I do not know whether I want to be pregnant or not. Being pregnant means changing our whole life, and now having somebody to care for all the time. I am not sure I would be a good parent. Plus, I'm a bit afraid of all the changes that will happen to my body. Is this normal? Am I OK?"
   a. How should the nurse answer this question?
   b. What specific information is needed to support the patient during this pregnancy?
2. Sally, age 23, is 9 weeks pregnant. At her clinic visit she says, "I am so tired I can barely make it home from work. Then once I am home, I do not have the energy to make dinner." She says she is so sick in the morning that she is frequently late to work and spends much of the day in the bathroom. Sally's current lab work is within normal limits.
   a. What explanation can the nurse offer Sally about her discomforts?
   b. What interventions can the nurse offer to Sally?
3. Bringing a new infant into the family affects the siblings. What strategies can a nurse discuss when a pregnant person asks how to deal with this?

STUDY ACTIVITIES

1. Go to your local health department's maternity clinic and interview several patients regarding about their feelings and the bodily changes that have taken place since becoming pregnant. Based on your findings, place them into the appropriate trimesters of pregnancy.
2. Search the internet for information about the psychological changes that occur during pregnancy. Share the information from the websites you find with your clinical group.
3. During pregnancy, the plasma volume increases by 75%, but the RBC volume increases by a much smaller amount. This disproportion manifests as ________________.
4. When a pregnant person in their third trimester lies on their back and experiences dizziness and lightheadedness, the underlying cause of this is ________________.

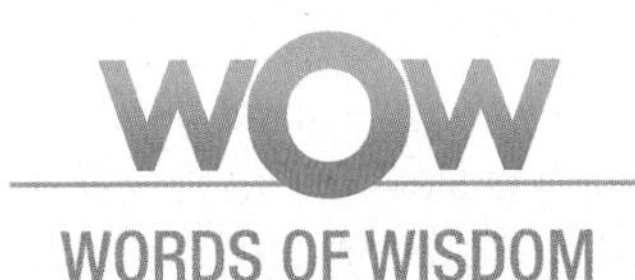

WORDS OF WISDOM

The secret of human touch is simple: showing a sincere liking and interest in people. Nurses need to use touch often.

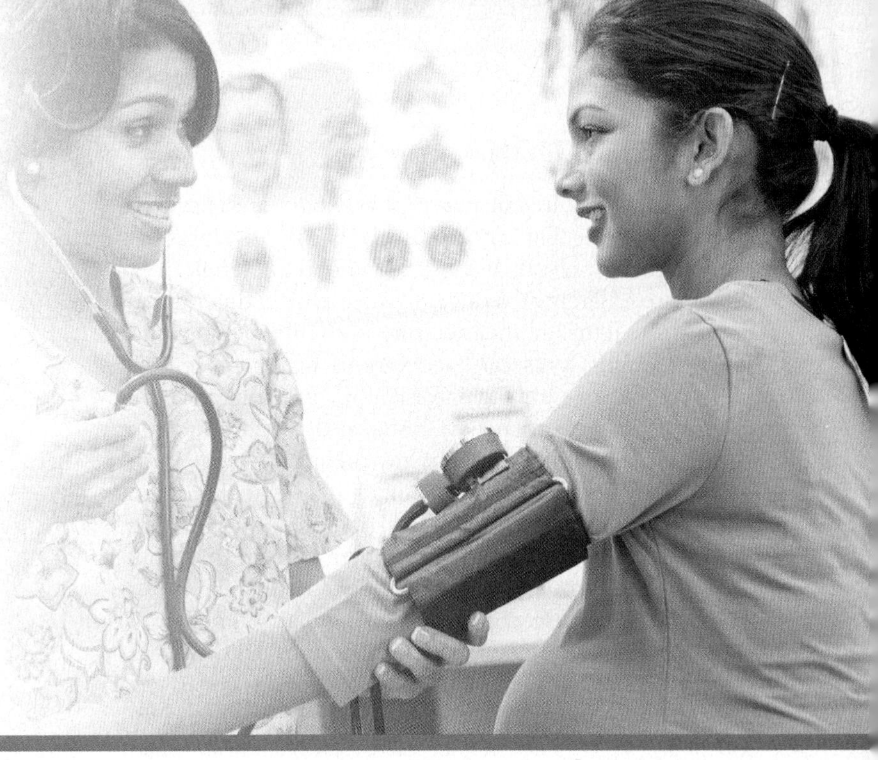

12 Nursing Management During Pregnancy

LEARNING OBJECTIVES

Upon completion of the chapter, you will be able to:

1. Relate the information typically collected at the initial prenatal visit.
2. Prepare an appropriate reproductive life plan based on a risk profile.
3. Select the assessments completed at follow-up prenatal visits.
4. Evaluate the tests used to assess maternal and fetal well-being, including nursing management for each.
5. Outline appropriate nursing management to promote maternal self-care and to minimize the common discomforts of pregnancy.
6. Examine the key components of perinatal education.

KEY TERMS

alpha-fetoprotein (al'fă-fē'tō-prō'tēn)
amniocentesis (am'nē-ō-sen-tē'sis)
biophysical profile (BPP)
chorionic villus sampling (CVS) (kō'rē-on'ik vil'ŭs)
gravida
high-risk pregnancy
linea nigra (lin'ē-ă nī'gră)
natural childbirth
para
perinatal education
preconception care

Linda and her husband Rob are eager to start a family within the next year. They are stable in their careers and feel financially secure. They decide to investigate a new nurse–midwife practice associated with the local hospital, and they go for a preconception appointment. They leave their appointment overwhelmed with all the information they were given about having a healthy pregnancy.

INTRODUCTION

Pregnancy is a time of many physiologic and psychological changes that can positively or negatively affect the pregnant person, their fetus, and their family. For the approximately 9 months during which the person carries the fetus in their uterus, both the person and the developing fetus can face various health risks. Misconceptions, inadequate information, and unanswered questions about pregnancy, birth, and parenthood are common. The ultimate goal of any pregnancy is the birth of a healthy newborn while maintaining the health of the birthing parent, and nurses play a major role in helping the pregnant person and their partner achieve this goal. Ongoing assessment and education are essential.

This chapter describes the nursing management and care required during pregnancy. It begins with a brief discussion of preconception care and then describes the assessment of the patient at the first prenatal visit and on follow-up visits. The chapter discusses tests commonly used to assess maternal and fetal well-being, including specific nursing management related to each test. The chapter also identifies important strategies to minimize the common discomforts of pregnancy and promote self-care. Finally, the chapter discusses perinatal education, including childbirth education, birthing options, health care provider options, preparation for breastfeeding or bottle-feeding, and final preparation for labor and birth.

PRECONCEPTION AND INTERCONCEPTION CARE

Ideally, people thinking about having children should schedule visits with the health care provider for preconception counseling to ensure that they are in the best possible state of health before pregnancy. **Preconception care** is the promotion of the health and well-being of a person and their partner before pregnancy. The goal of preconception care is to identify and modify biomedical, behavioral, and social risks to the person's health or pregnancy outcome through prevention and management interventions. The interconception period is the time between pregnancies when the person can improve their health status, especially if the prior pregnancy experience had a poor outcome or adverse events occurred (Centers for Disease Control and Prevention [CDC], 2024a). These interventions focus on risk factors that can be modified and/or eliminated prior to conception to optimize birth outcomes (Khekade et al., 2023).

Preconception and interconception care are both advocated throughout the world as tools for improving perinatal outcomes. Preconception and interconception care should occur any time a health care provider sees a person who can become pregnant. Primary nursing care for all people of childbearing potential should include a routine assessment of the person's reproductive goals and planning. People who could potentially become pregnant should be assessed for preconception or interconception risks and educated about the importance of maternal health in ensuring healthy pregnancies. People may be motivated to address modified health risks by learning about the way their present health will affect a future pregnancy. For people not intending a pregnancy soon, preconception care should focus on contraception counseling and optimizing overall health that may be aggravated by pregnancy if it occurs (Khekade et al., 2023). Personal and family history, physical examination, laboratory screening, reproductive planning, nutrition, supplements, weight, exercise, vaccinations, and injury prevention should be reviewed in all patients. Encourage folic acid 400 to 800 mcg per day depending on risk profile, as well as proper diet and exercise. Patients should receive the influenza vaccine if planning pregnancy during flu season; the rubella and varicella vaccines if there is no evidence of immunity to these viruses; and tetanus/diphtheria/pertussis if lacking adult vaccination. Offer specific interventions to reduce morbidity and mortality for both the baby and the birthing parent who has been identified with chronic diseases or exposed to teratogens or illicit substances. Several interventions have been proven to effectively improve pregnancy outcomes when provided as preconception care. Research suggests that events occurring in the uterine decidua even before a person knows they are pregnant may have a significant impact on pregnancy complications and the outcome of pregnancy (Tong et al., 2022). Decidualization is the process during which the endometrial stromal cells differentiate into decidual cells and secrete molecules essential for a successful pregnancy. Failure of adequate decidualization in terms of hormones, immunology, and biochemistry may lead to preeclampsia, preterm labor, and miscarriage (Tong et al., 2022). New insights reveal that the early embryo is extremely sensitive to signals from gametes, trophoblastic tissue, and periconception maternal lifestyles. Also, environmental factors, such as exposure to pollutants prior to and after conception, have an enormous impact on the developing embryo and cause long-term health problems (Rani & Dhok, 2023). The fetus is susceptible to environmental contaminants in its developing phase in early pregnancy and is impacted negatively by their effects. There is a growing body of evidence that environmental factors, such as exposure to heavy metals like mercury, lead, or cadmium, during embryonic development, can cause irreversible alteration in epigenetic markers. This can lead to negative pregnancy outcomes, such as stillbirth, preterm birth, and low birth weight, and can induce various diseases, including cardiovascular, neurologic, and metabolic disorders, and cognitive defects later in life (Rani & Dhok, 2023). With this in mind, shifting the focus on the preconception and interconception periods and the early stages of pregnancy can have significant benefits to the health of both the birthing parent and the infant. The overall aim should be to effectively provide counseling, education, and risk assessment before pregnancy to prevent poor perinatal outcomes (Fowler et al., 2023).

The CDC (2006) offers 10 guidelines for preconception care, and the American College of Obstetricians and Gynecologists (ACOG) and the American Society of Reproductive Medicine (ASRM) offer recommendations and conclusions related to prepregnancy care. See Box 12.1.

Risk Factors for Adverse Pregnancy Outcomes

Preconception and interconception care are just as important as prenatal care in reducing adverse pregnancy outcomes, such as maternal and infant mortality, preterm births, and low-birth-weight infants. Adverse pregnancy outcomes constitute a major public health challenge; 10.38% of infants are born preterm, with 9.5% of White infants and 14.5% of Black infants born preterm; 8.6% of infants are born with low birth weight, with 7% of White infants and 14.75% of Black infants born with low birth weight (Osterman et al., 2024). Starting a pregnancy with overweight (body mass index [BMI] >25 kg/m^2) or obesity (BMI >30 kg/m^2) and gaining more weight than recommended during the pregnancy increase a person's risk for late fetal death, complications during childbirth, delivery by cesarean birth, and instrument use during a vaginal delivery (Reed et al., 2023). Risk factors for these adverse pregnancy outcomes are prevalent among people who can become pregnant as demonstrated by the following statistics:

- 5.4% of people smoke during pregnancy, which can lead to fetal addiction to nicotine (Kipling et al., 2021).

BOX 12.1 Guidelines for Preconception/Interconception Care

- **Recommendation 1.** Individual responsibility across the lifespan: Each person and couple should be encouraged to have a reproductive life plan.
- **Recommendation 2.** Consumer awareness: Increase public awareness of the importance of preconception health behaviors and preconception care services by using information and tools appropriate across various ages; literacy, including health literacy; and cultural/linguistic contexts.
- **Recommendation 3.** Preventive visits: As a part of primary care visits, provide risk assessment and educational and health promotion counseling to all people who can become pregnant to reduce reproductive risks and improve pregnancy outcomes.
- **Recommendation 4.** Interventions for identified risks: Increase the proportion of patients who receive interventions as a follow-up to preconception risk screening, focusing on high-priority interventions (i.e., those with evidence of effectiveness and greatest potential impact).
- **Recommendation 5.** Interconception care: Use the interconception period to provide additional intensive interventions to patients who have had a previous pregnancy that ended in an adverse outcome (i.e., infant death, fetal loss, birth defects, low birth weight, or preterm birth).
- **Recommendation 6.** Prepregnancy checkup: Offer, as a component of maternity care, one prepregnancy visit for couples and people planning pregnancy.
- **Recommendation 7.** Health insurance coverage for patients with low incomes: Increase public and private health insurance coverage for patients with low incomes to improve access to preventive health and preconception and interconception care.
- **Recommendation 8.** Public health programs and strategies: Integrate components of preconception health into existing local public health and related programs, including emphasis on interconception interventions for patients with previous adverse outcomes.
- **Recommendation 9.** Research: Increase the evidence base and promote the use of the evidence to improve preconception health.
- **Recommendation 10.** Monitoring improvements: Maximize public health surveillance and related research mechanisms to monitor preconception health.

American College of Obstetricians and Gynecologists (ACOG) and the American Society of Reproductive Medicine (ASRM) Recommendations and Conclusions

- Any encounter with a person who can become pregnant should include counsel about wellness and healthy habits. This may help improve reproductive and pregnancy outcomes if and when they choose to reproduce.
- Ask "Would you like to become pregnant in the next year?"
- The goal is to reduce the risk of adverse health effects for the patient, fetus, and neonate by addressing modifiable risk factors and providing education about healthy pregnancy.
- Encourage patients to seek medical care before attempting to become pregnant or as soon as they believe they are pregnant.
- Ensure chronic medical conditions, such as diabetes and hypertension, are optimally managed before pregnancy.
- Review with the patient all prescription and nonprescription medications, including nutritional supplements and herbal products.
- Offer prepregnancy patients the same genetic screening recommended for pregnant patients.
- Assess immunization status annually for tetanus toxoid, reduced diphtheria toxoid, and acellular pertussis (Tdap); measles, mumps, and rubella; hepatitis B; and varicella. Recommend the annual influenza vaccination.
- Assess the need for screening for sexually transmitted infections.
- Counsel regarding potential exposure to infectious diseases, such as Zika, and travel restrictions and appropriate waiting time before attempting pregnancy.
- Assess alcohol, nicotine, and drug use, including prescription opioids.
- Screen for intimate partner violence.
- Encourage prepregnancy folic acid supplementation.
- Screen the patient's diet and vitamin supplements to confirm they are meeting their recommended daily allowances for calcium, iron, vitamin A, vitamin B, vitamin D, and vitamin B_{12}.
- Encourage the patient to attain a healthy body mass index (BMI, 18.5–24.9 kg/m^2).

Adapted from Centers for Disease Control and Prevention. (2006). *Recommendations to improve preconception health and health care—United States.* https://www.cdc.gov/mmwr/preview/mmwrhtml/rr5506a1.htm; and American College of Obstetricians and Gynecologists. (2019, reaffirmed 2020). Prepregnancy counseling. ACOG Committee Opinion No. 762. *Obstetrics & Gynecology, 133*, e78–e89. https://www.acog.org/clinical/clinical-guidance/committee-opinion/articles/2019/01/prepregnancy-counseling

- 13.5% of people consume alcohol during pregnancy, which can lead to fetal alcohol spectrum disorder (Gosdin et al., 2022).
- More than 50% of pregnant people are overweight or have obesity, which may increase their risk of developing hypertension, diabetes, and thromboembolic disease and may increase the need for cesarean birth (Paredes et al., 2021).

All these factors pose risks to pregnancy and could be addressed with early interventions if the patient seeks preconception health care. Specific recognized risk factors for adverse pregnancy outcomes that fall into one or more of these categories are listed in Box 12.2.

The period of greatest environmental sensitivity and consequent risk for the developing embryo is between days 17 and 56 after conception. The first prenatal visit, which is usually a month or later after a missed menstrual period, may occur too late to affect reproductive outcomes associated with abnormal organogenesis secondary to poor lifestyle choices. In some cases, such as with unplanned pregnancies, a person may delay seeking health care because they deny that they are pregnant. Thus, commonly used prevention practices may begin too late to avert the morbidity and mortality associated with congenital anomalies and low birth weight. A more global preventive strategy is needed to reduce the high rates of pregnancy complications in all populations. Securing international-level political priority for maternal and newborn care remains critical to accomplishing the goal of better health for all families. All people or couples should take on the responsibility of developing their reproductive life plan and share it with their health care providers at office visits. A reproductive life plan is an individualized plan of reproduction with goals based on personal beliefs and values. Its purpose is to reflect future intentions regarding pregnancy and take appropriate actions to optimize health status beforehand (Gregory, 2023).

What is the purpose of couples like Linda and Rob going for preconception counseling? What are the goals of preconception care for this couple? What psychological support can be offered by the nurse to this couple at this stage?

BOX 12.2 Risk Factors for Adverse Pregnancy Outcomes

- **Isotretinoins:** Use of isotretinoins (e.g., Accutane) in pregnancy to treat acne significantly increases the risk of serious birth defects, such as cleft palate, congenital heart defects, hearing loss, and microcephaly.
- **Alcohol misuse:** No time during pregnancy is safe to drink alcohol, and harm can occur early, before a patient has realized that they are or might be pregnant. Fetal alcohol syndrome and other alcohol-related birth defects can be prevented if the person ceases intake of alcohol before conception.
- **Antiepileptic drugs:** Certain antiepileptic drugs are known teratogens (e.g., valproic acid). Recommendations suggest that before conception, patients who are on a regimen of these drugs and who are contemplating pregnancy should be prescribed lower dosages of these drugs or change to antiepileptic medicines that are proven to have low fetal risks.
- **Diabetes (preconception):** The increase in the prevalence of birth defects among infants of birthing parents with type 1 and type 2 diabetes is substantially reduced through proper management of diabetes.
- **Folic acid deficiency:** Daily use of vitamin supplements containing folic acid (400 mcg) has been demonstrated to reduce the occurrence of neural tube defects by two thirds.
- **Hepatitis B:** Vaccination is recommended for all people who are at risk for acquiring hepatitis B virus (HBV) infection. Preventing HBV infection in people who can become pregnant prevents transmission of infection to infants and eliminates the risk to the person of HBV infection and sequelae, including hepatic failure, liver carcinoma, cirrhosis, and death.
- **HIV/AIDS:** If HIV infection is identified before conception, timely antiretroviral treatment can be administered, and patients (or couples) can be given additional information that can help prevent parent-to-child transmission.
- **Rubella seronegativity:** Rubella vaccination provides protective seropositivity and prevents congenital rubella syndrome.
- **Obesity:** Adverse perinatal outcomes associated with maternal obesity (body mass index [BMI] > 30 kg/m^2) include preeclampsia, gestational diabetes, cesarean birth, and stillbirth. Appropriate weight loss and nutritional intake before pregnancy reduce these risks.
- **Sexually transmitted infections (STIs): Chlamydia trachomatis** and **Neisseria gonorrhoeae** have been strongly associated with ectopic pregnancy, infertility, and chronic pelvic pain. STIs during pregnancy might result in fetal death or substantial physical and developmental disabilities, including intellectual disability and blindness. Early screening and treatment prevent these adverse outcomes.
- **Smoking:** Preterm birth, stillbirth, low birth weight, and other adverse perinatal outcomes associated with maternal smoking in pregnancy can be prevented if the person stops smoking before or during early pregnancy. Cessation of smoking is recommended before pregnancy.
- **Hypertension:** Maternal hypertension places infants at risk for preterm birth, low birth weight, eclampsia, and stroke. The pregnant person is more prone to complications including preeclampsia, placental abruption, and gestational diabetes. Early identification and treatment of hypertension will reduce these risks.

Centers for Disease Control and Prevention. (2024b). *Pregnancy complications.* https://www.cdc.gov/maternal-infant-health/pregnancy-complications/; Centers for Disease Control and Prevention. (2024c). *Alcohol and pregnancy.* https://www.cdc.gov/alcohol-pregnancy/about/index.html; Office on Women's Health. (2022). *Pregnancy complications.* https://www.womenshealth.gov/pregnancy/youre-pregnant-now-what/pregnancy-complications; McElrath, T., & Gerard, E. (2024). Management of epilepsy during preconception, pregnancy, and the postpartum period. *UpToDate.* Retrieved May 25, 2024, from https://www.uptodate.com/contents/management-of-epilepsy-during-preconception-pregnancy-and-the-postpartum-period; Owen, C. (2024). Oral isotretinoin therapy for acne vulgaris. *UpToDate.* Retrieved May 25, 2024, from https://www.uptodate.com/contents/oral-isotretinoin-therapy-for-acne-vulgaris

Nursing Management

In the United States, rates of maternal mortality, unintended pregnancies, low birth weight, and preterm infants continue to rise, making the need for preconception care a priority for all nurses. Traditionally, people have thought that preconception care is a single visit made before getting pregnant; however, the maximum benefits are obtained when the person and their partner receive preconception and interconception care throughout the reproductive years. The nurse's role is vital in identifying risk factors and encouraging healthier behaviors that potentially improve maternal and perinatal outcomes. Preconception care involves obtaining a complete health history and physical examination of the person and their partner. Key areas include:

- Immunization status of the patient
- Underlying medical conditions, such as cardiovascular, metabolic conditions, and respiratory problems or genetic disorders
- Reproductive health data, such as pelvic examinations, use of contraceptives, and sexually transmitted infections (STIs)
- Sexuality and sexual practices, such as safer sex practices and body image issues
- Nutrition history and present status, including BMI
- Lifestyle practices, including occupation and recreational activities
- Determining genetic disorders and carrier status
- Psychosocial issues such as levels of stress and exposure to abuse and violence
- Medication and drug use, including use of tobacco, alcohol, over-the-counter (OTC) and prescription medications, and illicit drugs
- Support system, including family, friends, and community (Fowler et al., 2023)

Figure 12.1 gives a sample preconception screening tool.

This information provides a foundation for planning health promotion activities and education. For example, to have a positive impact on the pregnancy:

- Ensure that the patient's immunizations are up to date.
- Create a reproductive life plan to address and outline reproductive needs.
- Take a thorough history of both partners to identify any medical or genetic conditions that need treatment, screening, or a referral to specialists.
- Identify history of STIs and high-risk sexual practices so they can be modified and determine the need for screening for STIs.
- Complete a dietary history combined with nutritional counseling.
- Gather information regarding exercise and lifestyle practices to encourage daily exercise for well-being and weight maintenance.
- Stress the importance of taking folic acid to prevent neural tube defects.
- Encourage the patient to achieve a healthy BMI (18.5 to 25.9 kg/m^2) before a pregnancy.
- Identify work environment and any needed changes to promote health.
- Address substance use issues, including smoking and drugs.
- Identify victims of violence and assist them to get help.
- Manage chronic conditions such as diabetes and asthma.
- Educate the patient or couple about environmental hazards, including metals and herbs.
- Offer genetic counseling to identify carriers.
- Suggest the availability of support systems, if needed (Phillippi & Sanders, 2022).

Nurses can act as advocates and educators, creating healthy, supportive communities for people and their partners in the childbearing phases of their lives. It is important to enter into a collaborative partnership with the patient and their partner, enabling them to examine their own health and its influence on the health of their future baby. Provide information to allow the patient and their partner to make an informed decision about having a baby, but keep in mind that this decision rests solely with the patient or couple.

TAKE NOTE!

Because all people who can become pregnant, from menarche to menopause, benefit from preventive care, preconception and interconception care should be an integral part of that continuum (Health Resources & Services Administration [HRSA], 2024; Women's Preventive Services Initiative [WPSI], 2024).

Linda and Rob decide to change several aspects of their lifestyle and nutritional habits before conceiving a baby based on advice from the nurse midwife. They both want to lose weight, stop smoking, and increase their intake of fruits and vegetables. How will these lifestyle and dietary changes benefit Linda's future pregnancy? What other areas might need to be brought up to date to prepare for a future pregnancy?

THE FIRST PRENATAL VISIT

The focus of prenatal care is to reduce the risk of adverse health effects for the pregnant person, fetus, and newborn by addressing modifiable risk factors and providing education about having a healthy pregnancy. Once a pregnancy is suspected and, in some cases, tentatively confirmed by a home pregnancy test, the person should

FIGO
International Federation of Gynecology and Obstetrics
the Global Voice for Women's Health

FIGO Preconception Checklist for women desiring pregnancy

This checklist is designed for girls/women* to complete together with their healthcare professional to assess their health status before getting pregnant and provide a basis for their healthcare professional to give advice on the best possible way to prepare for conception.

Date of birth: ☐ Blood type: ☐

Has your mother/father/siblings had health problems such as hypertension, diabetes, thrombosis, genetic diseases or others? Yes ☐ No ☐ Don't know ☐

Nutrition

For assessment, use the FIGO Nutrition Checklist for pre-pregnancy/early pregnant women (https://survey.figo.org/c/kuxayx3e)

Weight: ☐ kg, Height: ☐ m², BMI: ☐ kg/m²

If your BMI is higher than 30kg/m² or lower than 18.5 kg/m², refer to a dietician.

Supplementation

a) Start taking folic acid at least 3 months before conception:

- **0.4 mg per day** if you are at low risk of neural tube defects (NDTs)
- **4–5 mg per day** if you are at increased risk of NTDs (e.g. BMI higher than 30, NTD history in a previous child, epilepsy, anticonvulsant use, type 2 diabetes)

b) Start taking multiple micronutrients

c) Your hemoglobin levels should be checked and anemia corrected if necessary

d) Your calcium and vitamin D levels should be checked and any deficiency corrected if necessary

Lifestyle variables

a) Do you smoke tobacco? Yes ☐ No ☐

If you have replied YES, you should stop smoking before trying to get pregnant. If you smoke regularly, you may need to be assessed in more detail by an expert

b) Do you consume alcoholic drinks? Yes ☐ No ☐

If you have replied YES, you should avoid drinking alcohol when trying to get pregnant. If you consume alcohol regularly, you may need to be assessed in more detail by an expert

c) Do you use substances/illicit drugs? Yes ☐ No ☐

If you have replied YES, and your use is occasional you should stop. If you use regularly, you may need to be assessed in more detail by an expert

d) Do you think you are exposed to any toxic environmental chemicals? Yes ☐ No ☐ Don't know ☐

If you have replied YES, you should be given specific advice on how to avoid/reduce exposure

e) Do you practice regular physical activity? Yes ☐ No ☐

Please remember that moderate physical activity of at least 30 minutes a day, 5 days a week, for a minimum of 150 minutes of moderate exercise per week is usually recommended before and during pregnancy

Vaccines

a) Measles–Mumps–Rubella Yes ☐ No ☐ Don't know ☐
b) Hepatitis B Yes ☐ No ☐ Don't know ☐
c) Human Papilloma Viruses Yes ☐ No ☐ Don't know ☐
d) Meningococcal (ACWY and B) Yes ☐ No ☐ Don't know ☐
e) Varicella Yes ☐ No ☐ Don't know ☐
f) Tetanus, Diphtheria and Pertussis Yes ☐ No ☐ Don't know ☐
g) Influenza Yes ☐ No ☐ Don't know ☐

If you have replied NO, you should consider vaccination to prevent complications for yourself and your baby

Interpregnancy intervals

a) How many previous pregnancies have you had? 1 2 3 4 or more ☐
b) When? Dates ☐
c) Did you have complications during any pregnancy and/or delivery? Yes ☐ No ☐

If you have replied YES, please specify in more detail ☐

(Please remember that a time lapse of 12 to 24 months between one pregnancy and another is likely the optimal interval to minimize complications for your baby and yourself)

*Within our documents, we often use the terms 'woman', 'girl' and 'women and girls'. We recognise that not all people who require access to gynaecological and obstetric services identify as a woman or girl. All individuals, regardless of gender identity, must be provided with access to appropriate, inclusive and sensitive services and care

This document is based on "FIGO Preconception Checklist: Preconception care for mother and baby". *Int J Gynecol Obstet* 2024; 165:2. FIGO, Benedetto C, Borella F, Divakar H et al.

FIGO is the world's largest alliance of national societies of obstetrics and gynaecology dedicated to the health and wellbeing of women, girls and newborns.

FIGURE 12.1 Sample preconception screening tool. DES, diethylstilbestrol, HPV, human papillomavirus. (Modified with permission from Benedetto, C., Borella, F., Divakar, H., O'Riordan, S. L., Mazzoli, M., Hanson, M., O'Reilly, S., Jacobsson, B., Conry, J. A., McAuliffe, F. M., & FIGO Committee on Well Woman Healthcare, FIGO Committee on the Impact of Pregnancy on Long-Term Health. [2024]. FIGO preconception checklist: Preconception care for mother and baby. *International Journal of Gynaecology and Obstetrics*, *165*, 1–8. https://doi.org/10.1002/ijgo.15446. Copyright © 2024 The Authors. *International Journal of Gynecology and Obstetrics* published by John Wiley & Sons Ltd on behalf of *International Federation of Gynecology and Obstetrics*.)

seek prenatal care to promote a healthy outcome. Although the most opportune window (preconception) for improving pregnancy outcomes may be missed, appropriate nursing management starting at conception and continuing throughout the pregnancy can have a positive impact on the health of pregnant people and their unborn children.

The assessment process begins at this initial prenatal visit and continues throughout the pregnancy. The initial visit is an ideal time to screen for factors that might place the patient and their fetus at risk for problems such as preterm delivery. The initial visit is also an optimal time to begin educating the patient about changes that will affect their life. Researchers found that a delayed initiation of prenatal care was associated with increased rates of neonatal intensive care unit (NICU) admissions (Sarker et al., 2019). Overall, there is evidence of the benefits of prenatal care, but the components have not been extensively evaluated. However, the opportunity to improve maternal health and reduce adverse newborn outcomes is lost when prenatal care is not sought (Lockwood & Magriples, 2024a).

Prenatal care can be delivered in one of the two methods: either individually or in a group format termed *centering*. The first method is the traditional model whereby a pregnant person sees their health care provider at specified interims throughout the pregnancy and all visits occur on a one-to-one basis. The centering pregnancy model of group prenatal care involves groups of up to a dozen people in similar gestational ages meeting with their health care provider for 10 sessions of approximately 1.5 to 2 hours each. Researchers are exploring if the centering group method produces better perinatal outcomes than traditional individually delivered prenatal care due to increased patient–provider interaction, increased social support, and greater sense of community (Magriples, 2023). See Evidence-Based Practice 12.1.

Gestational diabetes is a common complication of pregnancy. The overall gestational diabetes rate has been increasing over the past 10 years in the United States and currently is approximately 8.3 per 100 births (CDC, 2024d).

Gestational diabetes results in short- and long-term complications for both the birthing parent and the fetus. There is an increased risk of preeclampsia, large for gestational age newborn, and the development of type 2 diabetes later in life (Durnwald, 2023).

It is estimated that approximately 30% of females aged 18 to 44 years have some degree of abnormal glucose metabolism (Durnwald, 2023). Therefore, early

Pre-existing medical conditions

a) Did/do you have high blood glucose levels/diabetes?	Yes ☐ No ☐ Don't know ☐
b) Did/do you have a congenital or acquired endocrine disorder?	Yes ☐ No ☐ Don't know ☐
c) Did/do you have high blood cholesterol levels?	Yes ☐ No ☐ Don't know ☐
d) Did/do you have high blood pressure?	Yes ☐ No ☐ Don't know ☐
e) Have you had a thromboembolic/thrombotic event?	Yes ☐ No ☐ Don't know ☐
f) Do you have congenital or acquired thrombophilia?	Yes ☐ No ☐ Don't know ☐
g) Do you have congenital or acquired heart disease?	Yes ☐ No ☐ Don't know ☐
h) Have you had a heart attack/stroke?	Yes ☐ No ☐ Don't know ☐
i) Did/do you have congenital or acquired lung disease?	Yes ☐ No ☐ Don't know ☐
j) Did/do you have congenital or acquired kidney disease?	Yes ☐ No ☐ Don't know ☐
k) Do you have recurrent urinary tract infections?	Yes ☐ No ☐ Don't know ☐
l) Did/do you have congenital or acquired liver and/or bowel disease?	Yes ☐ No ☐ Don't know ☐
m) Did/do you have congenital or acquired neurological disease?	Yes ☐ No ☐ Don't know ☐
n) Did/do you suffer from depression, or any other mental disorder?	Yes ☐ No ☐ Don't know ☐
o) Did/do you suffer from eating disorders (anorexia, bulimia)?	Yes ☐ No ☐ Don't know ☐
p) Did/do you have an autoimmune disease?	Yes ☐ No ☐ Don't know ☐
q) Did/do you have anemia or any other blood disorder?	Yes ☐ No ☐ Don't know ☐
r) Did/do you have a sexually transmitted infection?	Yes ☐ No ☐ Don't know ☐
s) Did/do you have cancer?	Yes ☐ No ☐ Don't know ☐
t) Did/do you have any other known congenital or acquired disease?	Yes ☐ No ☐ Don't know ☐
u) Do you take specific medications regularly?	Yes ☐ No ☐ Don't know ☐

If you have replied YES to any of the above questions you may need to be assessed in more detail

This document is based on "FIGO Preconception Checklist: Preconception care for mother and baby". *Int J Gynecol Obstet* 2024; 165:2. FIGO, Benedetto C, Borella F, Divakar H et al.

FIGO is the world's largest alliance of national societies of obstetrics and gynaecology dedicated to the health and wellbeing of women, girls and newborns.

FIGURE 12.1 *(continued)*

pregnancy screening of hemoglobin A1C may be performed (Durnwald, 2023). Also, the ACOG and the American Diabetes Association (ADA) recommend targeted screening for people at increased risk of type 2 diabetes; this includes people with gestational diabetes in a previous pregnancy; a BMI higher than 25 kg/m^2; and one or more additional risk factors including a first-degree relative with diabetes, being of a higher risk race or ethnicity, history of cardiovascular disease or hypertension, elevated high-density lipoprotein and/or triglycerides,

EVIDENCE-BASED PRACTICE 12.1

Psychosocial Outcomes of Group Prenatal Care

BACKGROUND

Group prenatal care offers its attendees education, collaboration with other pregnant peers, and group discussions. Prior research found that participating in group prenatal care was associated with a reduced risk of preterm labor and low-birth-weight infants, increased pregnancy knowledge, and less stress. *CenteringPregnancy*, an evidence-based model of group prenatal care, has demonstrated improved health outcomes when compared to individual prenatal care, including a reduction in the risk of preterm and low birth weights, a decrease in neonatal intensive care unit admissions, a reduction in the rates of fetal death, an increase in rates of breastfeeding, an increase in the likelihood of vaginal versus surgical birth, and an increase in the use of postpartum family planning. Another worthy area of focus is depression, which impacts up to 12% of pregnant people. The purpose of this study was to assess factors in group prenatal care that might reduce the risk of depression when compared to traditional individual prenatal care.

STUDY

This quasi-experimental study recruited participants on their first prenatal visit. Of the 129 total participants, 54 were placed in the centering (group) prenatal care cohort and 75 in the individual prenatal care cohort. Depression pre- and post-tests were administered and compared in both cohorts.

Findings

This research confirmed the superior effects of group prenatal care compared to traditional prenatal care regarding increased pregnancy knowledge among participants but failed to show statistically significant differences in depression scores between the two cohorts. Participants in the group prenatal care cohort expressed very positive feelings and felt supported throughout their pregnancy by the group's members.

Nursing Implications

This study supports the group prenatal model to change health behaviors in pregnant people and help them become more confident in their pregnancy and postpartum decisions. The additional education given to the prenatal group cohort produced positive pregnancy and postpartum outcomes. Nurses can encourage participation in group prenatal care, if offered, by educating the pregnant patient about the positive aspects related to it.

Adapted from Boothe, E., Olenderek, M., Noyola, M. C., Rushing, J., Allred, E., & Kaplan, S. (2022). Psychosocial outcomes of group prenatal care. *Journal of Public Health, 30,* 1373–1380. https://doi.org/10.1007/s10389-020-01441-6

EVIDENCE-BASED PRACTICE 12.2

The Prevention of Gestational Diabetes Mellitus (the Role of Lifestyle): A Meta-Analysis

BACKGROUND

Gestational diabetes is a common complication of pregnancy and has adverse consequences on both the fetus and the pregnant person. Complications include excessive fetal growth, impaired glucose metabolism, cardiovascular disease, and hypertension. The current treatment modalities include physical activity, dietary modifications, insulin administration, or oral hypoglycemic agents. The role of maternal lifestyle brings up several barriers that may lead to poor glycemic control. This study reviewed the role of lifestyle in the prevention of gestational diabetes through diet and exercise.

STUDY

Several databases were searched; 66 studies were screened, and 19 studies were selected. In the current review, 6 studies assessed the effects of diet, and 13 studies pertained to exercise. A comparison of three diets—Dietary Approach to Stop Hypertension (DASH), the Mediterranean diet, and Alternate Healthy Eating Index (aHEI)—were included.

Findings

This meta-analysis showed that diet alone was effective in preventing gestational diabetes mellitus, although exercise was not, if introduced in the second trimester. Of the three different diets studied, the aHEI was superior when compared to the DASH or Mediterranean diet. Exercise was effective in the first trimester, but not during the second one. Moderate exercise before or in early pregnancy was effective in reducing gestational diabetes.

Nursing Implications

It is clear that consistent lifestyle modifications both prenatally and continued into pregnancy can prevent the development of gestational diabetes. Nurses can recommend specific dietary modifications to some patients and moderate exercises to all patients to enhance positive outcomes of their pregnancies and the prevention of short- and long-term complications.

Adapted from Altemani, A. H., & Alzaheb, R. A. (2022). The prevention of gestational diabetes mellitus (The role of lifestyle): A meta-analysis. *Diabetology & Metabolic Syndrome, 14*, 83. https://doi.org/10.1186/s13098-022-00854-5

polycystic ovary syndrome (PCOS), physical inactivity, HIV infection, or age over 35 years (Durnwald, 2023). Screening, diagnosis, and classification have been established and offer the potential to stop the cycle of diabetes and obesity (BMI >30 kg/m^2) caused by hyperglycemia in pregnancy. Normoglycemia is the goal in all aspects of pregnancy and offers the benefits of decreased short- and long-term complications of diabetes. See Evidence-Based Practice 12.2. Refer to Chapter 20 for more information on diabetes in pregnancy.

Counseling and education of the pregnant person and their partner are critical to ensure healthy outcomes for the pregnant person and infant. Pregnant people and their partners frequently have questions, misinformation, or misconceptions about what to eat, weight gain, physical discomforts, drug and alcohol use, sexuality, and the birthing process. The nurse needs to allow time to answer questions and provide anticipatory guidance during the pregnancy and to make appropriate community referrals to meet the needs of these patients. To address these issues and foster the overall well-being of pregnant people and their fetuses, specific national health goals have been established (see the Healthy People 2030 box).

Comprehensive Health History

During the initial visit, the patient should feel supported by a skilled, knowledgeable, and well-prepared nurse. A comprehensive health history is obtained, including age, menstrual history, prior obstetric history, past medical and surgical history, psychological screening, family history, genetic screening, dietary habits, lifestyle and health practices, medication or drug use, and history of exposure to STIs. The focus of prenatal care includes risk assessment, health promotion and education, and therapeutic interventions (Lockwood & Magriples, 2023). Often, the use of a prenatal history form (Fig. 12.2) is the best way to document the data collected.

HEALTHY PEOPLE 2030

Objective	Nursing Significance
Increase the proportion of pregnant people who receive early and adequate prenatal care.	Will contribute to reduced rates of perinatal illness, disability, and death by helping identify possible risk factors and implementing measures to lessen these factors that contribute to poor outcomes
Increase the proportion of people who can become pregnant who have optimal red blood cell folate concentrations.	Risk of maternal and infant mortality and pregnancy-related complications can be reduced by educating patients to take folic acid prenatally and throughout pregnancy to reduce the risk of neural tube birth defects; will enhance healthy birth outcomes and early identification and treatment of health.
Increase the proportion of people delivering a live birth who had a healthy weight prior to pregnancy.	Will reduce the risks associated with overweight (body mass index [BMI] >25 kg/m^2) and/or obesity (BMI >30 kg/m^2) for better perinatal outcomes for birthing parent and infant

Healthy People Objectives retrieved from http://www.healthypeople.gov

MNRS Maternal/Newborn Record System™

Health History Summary

Page 1 of 2

To order call: 1.800.245.4080 Re-order No. 5700N

Patient's Name ______

ID. No. ______

Demographic Data

Date of Birth ______ Age ______ Language ☐ English ☐ ______ Interpreter ☐ None ☐ ______

Religion ☐ N/A ☐ ______ Race/Ethnicity ______

Marital Status S M SEP D W Father of Baby's Name ______

Education	Occupation	Full	Part	Self	Unemp	Work Tel No	Home Tel No
Patient		☐	☐	☐	☐		
Father of Baby		☐	☐	☐	☐		

Allergy/Sensitivity

☐ **None** ☐ **Latex** ☐ **Food**

☐ Other ______

Primary/Referring Physician

Menstrual History

Menarche	Interval	Length	Abnormalities ☐ **None**
yrs	days	days	

LMP ___/___/___ Certain ☐ Yes ☐ No Normal ☐ Yes ☐ No

Positive Pregnancy Test ___/___/___ ☐ Blood ☐ Urine

EDD By Dates ___/___/___ By Ultrasound ___/___/___ Date of Ultrasound ___/___/___

Pregnancy History

Gravida	Full Term	Premature	Spontaneous Ab	Induced Ab	Ectopic	Multiple Births	Live

No	Month/ Year	Infant Sex	Weight at Birth	Wks Gest	Hours In Labor	Type of Delivery	Anesthesia	Comments/Complications
1								
2								
3								
4								
5								
6								
7								

Medical History

Check and detail positive findings below. Use reference numbers.

Obstetric (Patient)

1. Anemia ☐
2. Fetal/Neonatal Death or Anomaly ☐
3. Gestational Diabetes ☐
4. Hemorrhage ☐
5. Hyperemesis ☐
6. Incompetent Cervix ☐
7. Intrauterine Growth Retardation ☐
8. Isoimmunization ☐
9. Polyhydramnios ☐
10. Postpartum Depression ☐
11. Pregnancy Induced Hypertension ☐
12. Preterm Labor or Birth ☐
13. PROM-Chorioamnionitis ☐
14. Rhogam Given ☐
15. RH Neg ☐

Gynecologic

16. Contraceptive Use ☐
17. Abnormal PAP ☐
18. Fibroids ☐
19. GYN Surgery ☐

Gynecologic (Cont'd.) (Patient)

20. Infertility ☐
21. In Utero Exposure to DES ☐
22. Uterine/Cervical Anomaly ☐

Sexually Transmitted Diseases

23. Chlamydia ☐
24. Gonorrhea ☐
25. Herpes (HSV) ☐
26. Syphilis ☐

Vaginal/Genital Infections

27. Trichomonas ☐
28. Condylomata ☐
29. Candidiasis ☐

Other Infections

30. Toxoplasmosis ☐
31. Group B Streptococcus ☐
32. Rubella or immunization ☐
33. Varicella or immunization ☐
34. Cytomegalovirus (CMV) ☐
35. AIDS (HIV) ☐
36. Hepatitis (type ______) ☐ or immunization (type ______)

FIGURE 12.2 Sample prenatal history form. DES, diethylstilbestrol, GYN, gynecology. (Reprinted with permission. Copyright Briggs Healthcare.)

MNRS Maternal/Newborn Record System™

Health History Summary

Page 2 of 2

To order call: 1.800.245.4080 Re-order No. 5700N

Patient's Name ______

ID. No. ______

Check and detail positive findings below. Use reference numbers.

Cardiovascular (Patient / Family)

37. Myocardial Infarction ☐ ☐
38. Heart Disease ☐ ☐
39. Rheumatic Fever ☐
40. Valve Disease ☐
41. Chronic Hypertension ☐ ☐
42. Disease of the Aorta ☐ ☐
43. Varicosities Thrombophlebitis ☐ ☐
44. Previous Pulmonary Embolism ☐
45. Blood Disorders ☐ ☐
46. Anemia/ Hemoglobinopathy ☐ ☐
47. Blood Transfusions ☐
48. Other ☐

Pulmonary

49. Asthma ☐
50. Tuberculosis ☐ ☐
51. Chronic Obstructive Pulmonary Disease ☐ ☐

Endocrine

52. Diabetes ☐ ☐
53. Thyroid Dysfunction ☐ ☐
54. Maternal PKU ☐
55. Endocrinopathy ☐ ☐
56. **Gastrointestinal** ☐
57. **Liver Disease** ☐

Renal Disease (Patient / Family)

58. Cystitis ☐
59. Pyelonephritis ☐
60. Asymptomatic Bacteriuria ☐
61. Chronic Renal Disease ☐ ☐
62. Autoimmune Disease ☐ ☐
63. Cancer ☐ ☐

Neurologic Disease

64. Cerebrovascular Accident ☐ ☐
65. Seizure Disorder ☐ ☐
66. Migraine Headaches ☐ ☐
67. Degenerative Disease ☐ ☐
68. Other ______ ☐

Psychiatric/Surgical

69. Psychiatric Disease/ Mental Illness ☐ ☐
70. Physical Abuse or Neglect ☐ ☐
71. Emotional Abuse or Neglect ☐ ☐
72. Addiction (Drug, Alcohol, Nicotine) ☐ ☐
73. Other ______ ☐
74. Major Accidents ☐
75. Surgery ☐
76. Anesthetic Complications ☐
77. Non-Surgical Hospitalization ☐
78. **No Known Disease/Problems** ______ ☐

Genetic History

(Patient / Father of Baby / Family)

79. Age 35 or older (female) 50 or older (male) ☐ ☐
80. Cerebral Palsy ☐ ☐ ☐
81. Cleft Lip/Palate ☐ ☐ ☐
82. Congenital Anomalies ☐ ☐ ☐
83. Congenital Heart Disease ☐ ☐ ☐
84. Consanguinity ☐ ☐ ☐
85. Cystic Fibrosis ☐ ☐ ☐
86. Down's Syndrome ☐ ☐ ☐
87. Hemophilia ☐ ☐ ☐
88. Huntington's Chorea ☐ ☐ ☐
89. Mental Retardation ☐ ☐ ☐
90. Muscular Dystrophy ☐ ☐ ☐
91. Neural Tube Defect ☐ ☐ ☐
92. Sickle Cell Disease or Trait ☐ ☐ ☐
93. Tay-Sachs Disease ☐ ☐ ☐
94. Test for Fragile X ☐ ☐ ☐
95. Thalassemia A or B ☐ ☐ ☐
96. Other ______ ☐ ☐ ☐
97. Other ______ ☐ ☐ ☐
98. Other ______ ☐ ☐ ☐

Historical Risk Status

☐ **No Risk Factors Noted**

☐ **At Risk (Identify)**

Signature

FIGURE 12.2 *(continued)*

The initial health history typically includes questions about three major areas: the reason for seeking care; the patient's past medical, surgical, and personal history, including that of the family and the patient's partner; and the patient's reproductive history. During the history-taking process, the nurse and patient establish the foundation of a trusting relationship and jointly develop a plan of care for the pregnancy. They tailor this plan to the patient's lifestyle as much as possible and focus primarily on education for overall wellness during the pregnancy. The ultimate goal for the first prenatal visit is to collect baseline data about the patient and their partner and their needs, to estimate gestational age of the pregnancy, to screen for potential teratogenic medications, and to detect any risk factors that need to be addressed to facilitate a healthy pregnancy (Phillippi & Sanders, 2022).

Reason for Seeking Care

The patient commonly comes for prenatal care based on the suspicion that they are pregnant. The patient may report that they have missed their menstrual period or have had a positive result on a home pregnancy test. Ask the patient for the date of their last normal menstrual period (LMP). Also ask about any presumptive or probable signs of pregnancy that the patient might be experiencing. Typically, a urine or blood test to check for evidence of human chorionic gonadotropin (hCG) is done to confirm the pregnancy.

Past History

Ask about the patient's past medical and surgical history. This information is important because conditions that the patient experienced in the past (e.g., urinary tract infections) may recur or be exacerbated during pregnancy. Also, chronic illnesses, such as diabetes or heart disease, can increase the risk for complications during pregnancy for the patient and their fetus. Ask about any history of allergies to medications, foods, or environmental substances. Ask about any mental health problems, such as depression or anxiety. Gather similar information about the patient's family and partner.

The patient's personal history is also important. Ask about their occupation, possible exposure to teratogens, exercise and activity level, recreational patterns (including the use of substances such as alcohol, tobacco, and drugs), use of alternative and complementary therapies, sleep patterns, nutritional habits, and general lifestyle. Each of these may have an impact on the outcome of the pregnancy. For example, if the patient smokes during pregnancy, nicotine in the cigarettes causes vasoconstriction in the patient, leading to reduced placental perfusion. As a result, the newborn may be small for gestational age. The newborn will also go through nicotine withdrawal soon after birth. In addition, no safe level of alcohol ingestion in pregnancy has been determined. Many fetuses exposed to heavy alcohol levels during pregnancy develop fetal alcohol spectrum disorder, a collection of deformities and disabilities.

Reproductive History

The patient's reproductive history includes a menstrual, obstetric, and gynecologic history. Typically, this history begins with a description of the patient's menstrual cycle, including their age at menarche, number of days in their cycle, typical flow characteristics, and any discomfort experienced. The use of contraception is also important, including when the patient last used it.

Establishing an accurate due date is one of the most important assessments for a pregnant person, one that has both social and medical significance. For patients and their families, this estimated date of delivery (EDD) represents the long-awaited birthday of their child and is a timeframe around which many economic and social activities are planned. This endpoint date provides guidance for the timing of specific maternal and fetal testing throughout pregnancy, gauges fetal growth parameters, and provides well-established timelines for specific interventions in the management of prenatal complications, such as preterm labor management.

Ask the patient the date of their LMP to determine the EDD. Several methods may be used to estimate the date of birth. Nagele's rule can be used to establish the EDD (Box 12.3). An alternative way is to add 7 days and then add 9 months = year where needed. This date has a margin of error of plus or minus 2 weeks.

Because of the normal variations in people's menstrual cycles, differences in the normal length of gestation among groups based on ancestry, and errors in dating methods, there is no such thing as an exact due date. In general, a birth 2 weeks before or 2 weeks after the EDD is considered normal. Nagele's rule is less accurate if the person's menstrual cycles are irregular, if they conceive while breastfeeding, if they conceive before their regular menstrual cycle is reestablished after childbirth, or if they

BOX 12.3 Nagele's Rule for Calculating the Estimated Due Date (EDD)

1. Use the first day of the last normal menstrual period.	10/14/23
2. Subtract 3 from the number of months.	7/14/23
3. Add 7 to the number of days.	7/21/23
4. Adjust the year by adding 1 year.	7/21/24
5. Estimated due date (+ or − 2 weeks) = July 21, 2024.	

ovulate even when experiencing amenorrhea. If the person starts prenatal care late, a second trimester fetal head circumference measurement via ultrasound can also be used to predict EDD or a transvaginal ultrasound can identify an intrauterine pregnancy about 4 weeks after the LMP (Edwards & Itzhak, 2023).

A gestational or birth calculator or wheel can also be used to calculate the due date (Fig. 12.3). Some practitioners use ultrasound to more accurately determine the gestational age and date of the pregnancy. Ultrasound is typically the most accurate method of dating a pregnancy.

Typically, an obstetric history provides information about the patient's past pregnancies, including any problems encountered during the pregnancy, labor, birth, and postpartum. Such information can provide clues to problems that might develop in the current pregnancy. Some common terms used to describe and document an obstetric history include gravid, **gravida**, gravida I (primigravida), gravida II (secundigravida), multigravida, and **para** (Table 12.1).

Other systems may be used to document a patient's obstetric history. These systems often break down the category of para more specifically (Box 12.4).

Information about the patient's gynecologic history is important. Ask about any reproductive tract surgeries the patient has undergone. For example, surgery on the uterus may affect its ability to contract effectively during labor. A history of tubal pregnancy increases the person's risk for another tubal pregnancy. Also ask about safer sex practices and any history of STIs.

Physical Examination

The next step in the assessment process is the physical examination, which detects any physical problems that may affect the pregnancy outcome. The initial physical examination provides the baseline for evaluating changes during future visits.

Preparation

Instruct the patient to undress and put on a gown. Also ask them to empty their bladder, and when doing so, to collect a urine specimen. Typically, this specimen is a clean-catch urine specimen that is sent to the laboratory for a urinalysis to detect possible urinary tract infections.

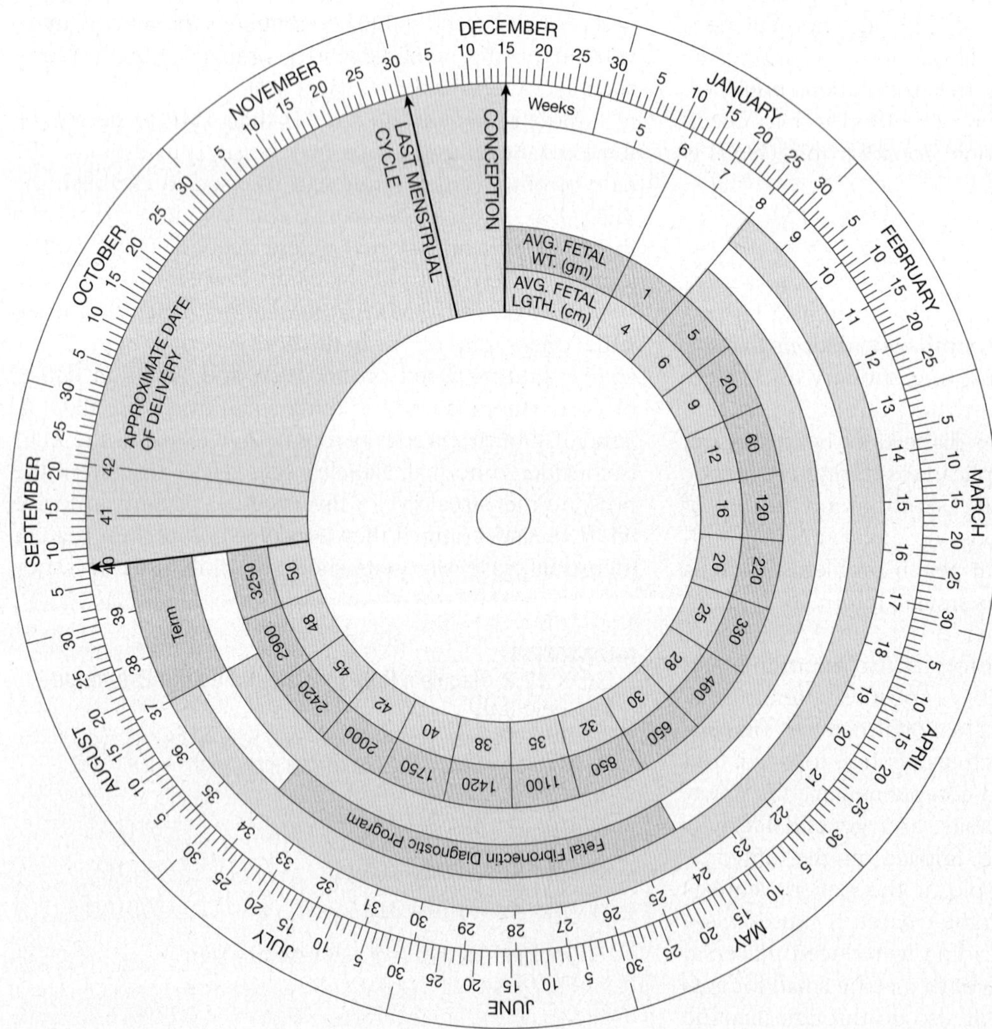

FIGURE 12.3 Estimated date of delivery (EDD) using a birth wheel. The first day of the person's last normal menstrual period was October 1. Using the birth wheel, their EDD would be approximately July 8 of the following year. AFP, alpha-fetoprotein; CVS, chorionic villus sampling.

TABLE **12.1** • Pregnancy Terms

Term	Definition
Gravid	The state of being pregnant
Gravida/gravidity	The total number of times a person has been pregnant, regardless of whether the pregnancy resulted in a termination or if multiple infants were born from a pregnancy
Nulligravida	A person who has never experienced pregnancy
Primigravida	A person pregnant for the first time
Secundigravida	A person pregnant for the second time
Multigravida	A person pregnant for at least the third time
Para	The number of times a person has given birth to a fetus of at least 20 gestational weeks (viable or not), counting multiple births as one birth event
Parity	Refers to the number of pregnancies, not the number of fetuses, carried to the point of viability, regardless of the outcome
Nullipara (para 0)	A person who has not produced a viable offspring
Primipara	A person who has given birth once after a pregnancy of at least 20 weeks, commonly referred to as a "primip" in clinical practice
Multipara	A person who has had two or more pregnancies of at least 20 weeks' gestation resulting in viable offspring, commonly referred to as a "multip"

Begin the physical examination by obtaining vital signs. Also measure the patient's height and weight. Abnormalities such as an elevated blood pressure may suggest pregestational hypertension, requiring further evaluation. Abnormalities in pulse rate and respiration require further investigation for possible cardiac or respiratory disease. If the patient weighs less than 100 lb or more than 200 lb or there has been a sudden weight gain, report these findings to the primary care provider; medical treatment or nutritional counseling may be necessary.

BOX **12.4** **Obstetric History Terms: GTPAL or TPAL**

G, gravida; T, term births; P, preterm births; A, abortions; L, living children

- G—the current pregnancy to be included in count
- T—the number of term gestations delivering between 38 and 42 weeks
- P—the number of preterm pregnancies ending >20 weeks or viability but before completion of 37 weeks
- A—the number of pregnancies ending before 20 weeks or viability
- L—the number of children currently living

Consider this example:
Mary is pregnant for the fourth time. She had one abortion at 8 weeks' gestation. She has a daughter who was born at 40 weeks' gestation and a son born at 34 weeks. Mary's obstetric history would be documented as follows:

- Using the gravida/para method: gravida 4, para 2
- Using the TPAL method: 1112 (T = 1 [daughter born at 40 weeks]; P = 1 [son born at 34 weeks]; A = 1 [abortion at 8 weeks]; L = 2 [two living children])

Head-to-Toe Assessment

A complete head-to-toe assessment is usually performed by the health care provider. Every body system is assessed. Some of the major areas are discussed here. Throughout the assessment, be sure to drape the patient appropriately to ensure privacy and prevent chilling.

HEAD AND NECK

Assess the head and neck area for any previous injuries and sequelae. Evaluate for any limitations in range of motion. Palpate for any enlarged lymph nodes or swelling. Note any edema of the nasal mucosa or hypertrophy of gingival tissue in the mouth; these are typical responses to increased estrogen levels in pregnancy. Palpate the thyroid gland for enlargement. Slight enlargement is normal, but marked enlargement may indicate hyperthyroidism, requiring further investigation.

CHEST

Auscultate heart sounds, noting any abnormalities. A soft systolic murmur caused by the increase in blood volume may be noted. Anticipate an increase in heart rate by 10 to 15 beats/min (bpm) (starting between 14 and 20 weeks of pregnancy) secondary to increases in cardiac output and blood volume. The body adapts to the increase in blood volume with peripheral dilation to maintain blood pressure. Progesterone causes peripheral dilation.

Auscultate the chest for breath sounds, which should be clear. Also note symmetry of chest movement and thoracic breathing patterns. Estrogen promotes relaxation of the ligaments and joints of the ribs with a resulting increase in the anteroposterior chest diameter. Expect a slight increase in respiratory rate to accommodate the increase in tidal volume and oxygen consumption.

Inspect and palpate the breasts and nipples for symmetry and color. Increases in estrogen and progesterone and blood supply make the breasts feel full and more nodular with increased sensitivity to touch. Blood vessels become more visible, and there is an increase in breast size. Striae gravidarum (stretch marks) may be visible in patients with large breasts. Darker pigmentation of the nipple and areola is present, along with enlargement of Montgomery glands. Colostrum (yellowish secretion that precedes mature breast milk) is excreted typically in the third trimester.

TAKE NOTE!

Use this opportunity to reinforce and teach breast self-awareness if the person has a high-risk history.

ABDOMEN

The appearance of the abdomen depends on the number of weeks of gestation. The abdomen enlarges progressively as the fetus grows. Inspect the abdomen for striae, scars, shape, and size. Inspection may reveal striae gravidarum and the **linea nigra**, a thin brownish black pigmented line running from the umbilicus to the symphysis pubis, depending on the duration of the pregnancy. Palpate the abdomen, which should be rounded and nontender. A decrease in muscle tone may be noted due to the influence of progesterone.

Typically, the height of the fundus is measured when the uterus arises out of the pelvis to evaluate fetal growth. At 12 weeks' gestation, the fundus can be palpated at the symphysis pubis. At 16 weeks' gestation, the fundus is midway between the symphysis and the umbilicus. At 20 weeks, the fundus can be palpated at the umbilicus and measures approximately 20 cm from the symphysis pubis. By 36 weeks, the fundus is just below the xiphoid process and measures approximately 36 cm.

EXTREMITIES

Inspect and palpate both legs for dependent edema, pulses, and varicose veins. If edema is present in early pregnancy, further evaluation may be needed to rule out gestational hypertension. During the third trimester, dependent edema is a normal finding. Ask the patient if they have any pain in their calf that increases when they ambulate. This might indicate a deep vein thrombosis (DVT). High levels of estrogen during pregnancy place the patient at higher risk for DVT.

Pelvic Examination

The pelvic examination provides information about the internal and external reproductive organs. In addition, it aids in assessing some of the presumptive and probable signs of pregnancy and allows for the determination of pelvic adequacy. During the pelvic examination, remain in the examining room to assist the health care provider with any specimen collection, fixation, and labeling. Also provide comfort and emotional support for the patient, who might be anxious. Throughout the examination, explain what is happening and why, and answer any questions as necessary.

EXTERNAL GENITALIA

After the patient is placed in the lithotomy position and draped appropriately, the external genitalia are inspected visually. They should be free from lesions, discharge, hematomas, varicosities, and inflammation upon inspection. A culture for STIs may be collected at this time.

INTERNAL GENITALIA

Next, the internal genitalia are examined via a speculum. The cervix should be smooth, long, thick, and closed. Because of increased pelvic congestion, the cervix will be softened (Goodell sign), the uterine isthmus will be softened (Hegar sign), and there will be a bluish coloration of the cervix and vaginal mucosa (Chadwick sign).

The uterus is typically pear shaped and mobile with a smooth surface. It will undergo cell hypertrophy and hyperplasia so that it enlarges throughout the pregnancy to accommodate the growing fetus.

During the pelvic examination, a Papanicolaou (Pap) smear may be obtained. Additional cultures, such as for gonorrhea and chlamydia screening, may also be obtained. Ensure that all specimens obtained are labeled correctly and sent to the laboratory for evaluation. A rectal examination is done last to assess for lesions, masses, prolapse, or hemorrhoids.

Once the examination of the internal genitalia is completed and the speculum is removed, a bimanual examination is performed to estimate the size of the uterus to confirm dates and to palpate the ovaries. The ovaries should be small and nontender without masses. At the conclusion of the bimanual examination, the health care provider reinserts the index finger into the vagina and the middle finger into the rectum to assess the strength and regularity of the posterior vaginal wall.

PELVIC SIZE, SHAPE, AND MEASUREMENTS

The size and shape of the patient's pelvis can affect their ability to deliver vaginally. Pelvic shape is typically classified as one of the four types: gynecoid, android, anthropoid, and platypelloid. Refer to Chapter 13 for an in-depth discussion of pelvic size and shape.

Taking internal pelvic measurements determines the actual diameters of the inlet and outlet through which the fetus will pass. This is extremely important if the patient has never given birth vaginally. Taking pelvic measurements is unnecessary for the patient who has given birth vaginally before (unless they have experienced some type of trauma to the area) because vaginal delivery demonstrates that the pelvis is adequate for the passage of the fetus.

Three measurements are assessed: diagonal conjugate, true conjugate, and ischial tuberosity (Fig. 12.4). The diagonal conjugate is the distance between the anterior surface of the sacral prominence and the anterior surface of the inferior margin of the symphysis pubis (Siccardi et al., 2023). This measurement, usually 12.5 cm or greater, represents the anteroposterior diameter of the pelvic inlet through which the fetal head passes first. The diagonal conjugate is the most useful measurement for estimating pelvic size because a misfit with the fetal head occurs if it is too small.

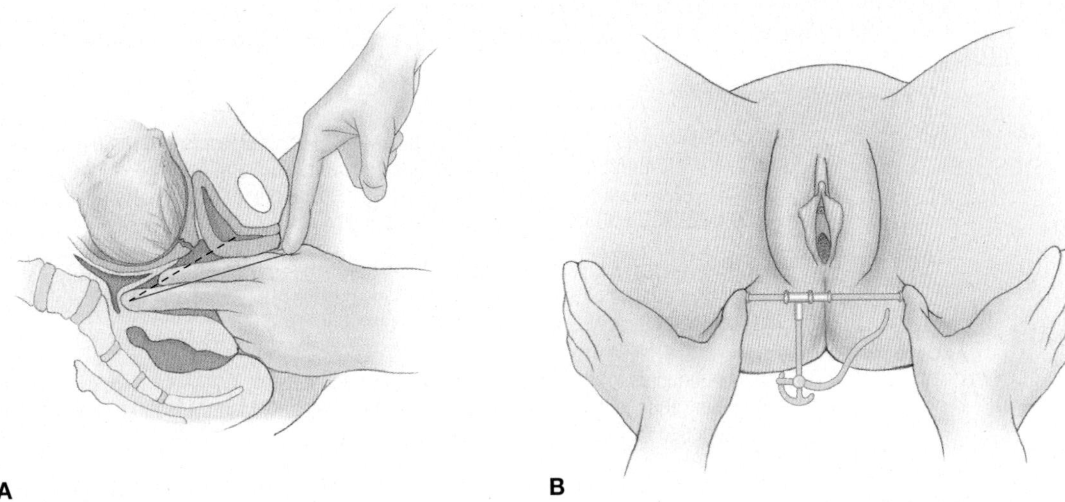

FIGURE 12.4 Pelvic measurements. **A.** Diagonal conjugate (solid line) and true conjugate (dotted line). **B.** Ischial tuberosity diameter.

The true conjugate, also called the *obstetric conjugate*, is the measurement from the anterior surface of the sacral prominence to the posterior surface of the inferior margin of the symphysis pubis. This diameter cannot be measured directly; rather, it is estimated by subtracting 1 to 2 cm from the diagonal conjugate measurement. The average true conjugate diameter is 11 cm (Siccardi et al., 2023). This measurement is important because it is the smallest front-to-back diameter through which the fetal head must pass when moving through the pelvic inlet.

The ischial tuberosity diameter is the transverse diameter of the pelvic outlet. This measurement is made outside the pelvis at the lowest aspect of the ischial tuberosities. A diameter of 10.5 cm or more is considered adequate for passage of the fetal head (Siccardi et al., 2023).

Laboratory Tests

A series of tests is generally ordered during the initial visit so that baseline data can be obtained, allowing for early detection and prompt intervention if any problems occur. Tests that are generally conducted for all pregnant patients include urinalysis and blood studies. The urine is analyzed for albumin, glucose, ketones, and bacteria casts. Blood studies usually include a complete blood count (CBC) (hemoglobin, hematocrit, red and white blood cell counts, and platelets), blood typing and Rh factor, glucose screening for high-risk patients, a rubella titer, hepatitis B surface antibody antigen, HIV, venereal disease research laboratory (VDRL) or rapid plasma reagin (RPR) tests, and cervical smears to detect STIs (Common Laboratory and Diagnostic Tests 12.1). In addition, most offices and clinics have ultrasound equipment available to validate an intrauterine pregnancy and assess early fetal growth.

The need for additional laboratory studies is determined by a patient's history, physical examination findings, current health status, and risk factors identified in the initial interview. Additional tests can be offered (e.g., screening for genetic diseases, blood lead screening, rubeola), but ultimately the patient and their partner make the decision about undergoing them. Educate the patient and their partner about the tests, including the rationale. In addition, support the patient and their partner in their decision-making process, regardless of whether you agree with the couple's decisions. The couple's decisions about their health care are based on the ethical principle of autonomy, which allows a person the right to make decisions about their own body.

Remember Linda and Rob, the couple who want to start a family? Ten months after the preconception appointment, Linda calls to make a first prenatal appointment. What key areas will be addressed at this first prenatal visit? What interventions might be suggested for Linda to implement in order to ensure a healthy newborn? What emotional support might Linda need during her first trimester of pregnancy?

FOLLOW-UP VISITS

Continuous prenatal care is important for a successful pregnancy outcome. The recommended follow-up visit schedule for a healthy pregnant person is:

- Every 4 weeks up to 28 weeks (7 months)
- Every 2 weeks from 29 to 36 weeks
- Every week from 37 weeks to birth

At each subsequent prenatal visit, the following assessments are completed:

- Weight and blood pressure, which are compared with baseline values

COMMON LABORATORY AND DIAGNOSIS TESTS 12.1

Test	Explanation
Complete blood cell count (CBC)	Evaluates hemoglobin (12–14 g) and hematocrit (42% ± 5%) levels and red blood cell count (4.2–5.4 million/mm^3) to detect the presence of anemia; identifies white blood cell level (5,000–10,000 mm^{-3}), which, if elevated, may indicate an infection; determines platelet count (150,000–450,000 mL^3) to assess clotting ability
Blood typing	Determines patient's blood type and Rh status to rule out any blood-incompatibility issues early; Rh-negative birthing parent would likely receive anti-D immune globulin (at 28 weeks' gestation) and possibly again within 72 hours after childbirth
Rubella titer	Detects antibodies for the virus that causes German measles; if titer is ≤1:8, the patient is not immune; requires immunization after birth, and the patient is advised to avoid people with undiagnosed rashes
Hepatitis B	Determines if the patient has hepatitis B by detecting the presence of hepatitis antibody surface antigen (HbsAg) in their blood
HIV testing	Detects HIV antibodies and, if positive, requires more specific testing, counseling, and treatment during pregnancy with antiretroviral medications to prevent transmission to fetus
Sexually transmitted infection (STI) screening: venereal disease research laboratory (VDRL) or rapid plasma reagin (RPR) serologic tests or by cervical smears, cultures, or visual identification of suspicious lesions	Detects STIs (such as syphilis, herpes, human papillomavirus [HPV], hepatitis C virus [HCV], chlamydia, and gonorrhea) so that treatment can be initiated early to prevent transmission to fetus
Cervical smears	Detects abnormalities such as cervical cancer (Pap test) or infections such as gonorrhea, chlamydia, or group B *Streptococcus* so that treatment can be initiated if positive

Centers for Disease Control and Prevention. (2024e). *Recommended clinical timeline for screening for syphilis, HIV, HCV, HBV, chlamydia, and gonorrhea.* https://www.cdc.gov/nchhstp/pregnancy/screening/clinician-timeline.html; and Lockwood, C. J., & Magriples, U. (2024a). Prenatal care: Initial assessment. *UpToDate.* Retrieved May 26, 2024, from https://www.uptodate.com/contents/prenatal-care-initial-assessment

- Urine testing for protein, glucose, ketones, and nitrites
- Fundal height measurement to assess fetal growth
- Assessment for quickening/fetal movement to determine fetal well-being
- Assessment of fetal heart rate (should be 110 to 160 bpm)

At each follow-up visit, answer questions, provide anticipatory guidance and education, review nutritional guidelines, and evaluate the patient for adherence to prenatal vitamin therapy. Throughout the pregnancy, encourage the patient's partner to participate if possible.

Follow-Up Visit Intervals and Assessments

Up to 28 weeks' gestation, follow-up visits involve assessment of the patient's blood pressure and weight. The urine is tested for protein and glucose. Fundal height and fetal heart rate are assessed at every office visit.

There is no universal consensus about the best procedure for screening and diagnosing gestational diabetes (Durnwald, 2023). All strategies involve an oral glucose test, but there remains disagreement about how many grams of glucose (50, 75, or 100 g) the patient should ingest and how long afterward their blood sample should be drawn. A recent release of *Standards of Medical Care in Diabetes—2023* by the ADA concluded that there was insufficient evidence to determine which assessment test is the best method to use to identify people who have gestational diabetes. Screening for gestational diabetes is best done between 24 and 28 weeks' gestation, unless screening is warranted in the first trimester for high-risk reasons (obesity [BMI >30 kg/m^2]; older age; family history of diabetes; history of gestational diabetes; or the patient being of Hispanic, Native American, Alaska Native, Native Hawaiian, South or East Asian, or Pacific Islander descent) (Durnwald, 2023). Because insulin resistance increases as pregnancy advances, testing at this gestational point yields a higher rate of abnormal test results. There are two commonly used screening approaches for gestational diabetes: one-step and two-step. In the *one-step method*, in a fasting patient, a blood glucose level is obtained using a 75-g oral glucose load followed by a 2-hour plasma glucose determination. If the result is elevated, then a positive gestational diabetes diagnosis is made. The *two-step method* starts with a 1-hour glucose challenge test in a nonfasting patient after consuming a 50-g glucose drink. Blood is drawn 1 hour later. Patients with an elevated glucose level move to step two, which measures blood glucose at 1, 2, and 3 hours after consuming a 100-g glucose drink to a fasting patient. Gestational diabetes is diagnosed if at least two of the values are elevated (ADA, 2023; Durnwald, 2023).

During this time, review the common discomforts of pregnancy, evaluate any patient complaints, and answer questions. Reinforce the importance of good nutrition and use of prenatal vitamins, along with daily exercise.

Between 29 and 36 weeks' gestation, all the assessments of previous visits are completed, along with assessment for edema. Special attention is focused on the presence and location of edema during the last trimester. Pregnant people commonly experience dependent edema of the lower extremities from constriction of blood vessels secondary to the heavy gravid uterus. Periorbital edema around the eyes, edema of the hands, and pretibial edema (edema on the front, or shin part of the leg) are abnormal and could be signs of gestational hypertension. Inspecting and palpating both extremities, listening for complaints about rings becoming too tight on the fingers, and observing for swelling around the eyes are important assessments. Abnormal findings in any of these areas need to be reported.

If the pregnant person is Rh negative, their antibody titer is evaluated at this time to test for Rh incompatibility. *Rh incompatibility* refers to the discordant pairing of maternal and fetal Rh types; it can result in Rh sensitization and hemolytic disease of the neonate (Moise, 2023). Anti-D immune globulin is given if indicated. Anti-D immune globulin is used to prevent the development of antibodies to Rh-positive red cells whenever fetal cells are known or suspected of entering the maternal circulation, such as after a spontaneous abortion or amniocentesis. It is also recommended at 28 weeks' gestation and following birth if the infant is D positive (Moise, 2024). The patient is also evaluated for risk of preterm labor. At each visit, ask if the patient is experiencing any common signs or symptoms of preterm labor (e.g., uterine contractions, dull backache, feeling of pressure in the pelvic area or thighs, increased vaginal discharge, menstrual-like cramps, vaginal bleeding). If the patient has had a previous preterm birth, they are at risk for another, and close monitoring is warranted. An initial preterm labor evaluation if the patient reports signs and symptoms of preterm labor includes review of prenatal record for risk factors, evaluation of reported symptoms (uterine contractions, vital signs, fetal heart rate, pelvic examination for cervical dilation and effacement assessment, and status of fetal membranes), and a urine culture to diagnose asymptomatic bacteriuria. A cervical dilation of over 3 cm supports the diagnosis of preterm labor (Lockwood, 2024). If positive for preterm labor, the patient may be requested to rest and medications to stop contractions may be in order.

Counsel the patient about choosing a health care provider for the newborn if they have not selected one yet. Along with completion of a breast assessment, the nurse should discuss and educate the patient about the choice of breastfeeding versus bottle-feeding. The American Academy of Pediatrics (AAP) does encourage all birthing parents to breastfeed their offspring, but the decision to do so is ultimately the birthing parent's. The nurse can refer the patient to the Nursing Mothers and La Leche League websites for further information to assist them in making that decision. Reinforce the importance of daily fetal movement monitoring as an indicator of fetal well-being. Reevaluate hemoglobin and hematocrit levels to assess for anemia.

Between 37 and 40 weeks' gestation, the same assessments are done as for the previous weeks. In addition, screening for group B *Streptococcus*, gonorrhea, and chlamydia is done. Fetal presentation and position (via Leopold maneuvers) are assessed. Review the signs and symptoms of labor and forward a copy of the prenatal record to the hospital labor department for future reference. Review the patient's desire for family planning after birth as well as their decision to breastfeed or bottle feed. Remind the patient that an infant car seat is required by law and must be used to drive the newborn home from the hospital or birthing center.

Fundal Height Measurement

Fundal height is the distance (in centimeters) measured with a tape measure from the top of the pubic bone to the top of the uterus (fundus) with the patient lying on their back with their knees slightly flexed (Fig. 12.5). Measurement in this way is termed the *McDonald method*. Fundal height typically increases as the pregnancy progresses; it reflects fetal growth and provides a gross estimate of the duration of the pregnancy.

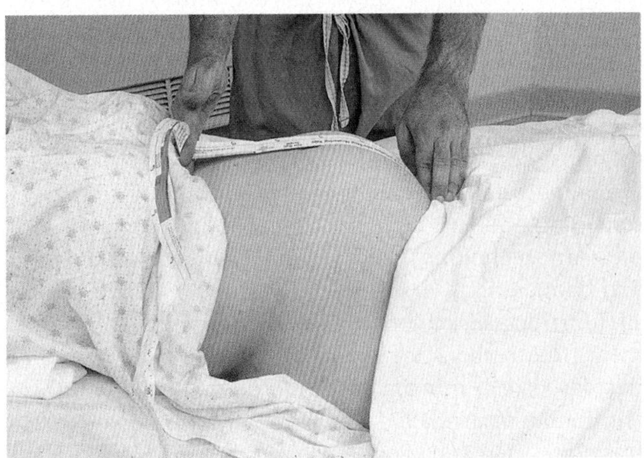

FIGURE 12.5 Fundal height measurement.

Between 12 and 14 weeks' gestation, the fundus can be palpated above the symphysis pubis. The fundus reaches the level of the umbilicus at approximately 20 weeks and measures 20 cm. Fundal measurement should approximately equal the number of weeks of gestation until week 36. For example, a fundal height of 24 cm suggests a fetus at 24 weeks' gestation. After 36 weeks, the fundal height then drops due to lightening and may no longer correspond with the week of gestation.

It is expected that the fundal height will increase progressively throughout the pregnancy, reflecting fetal growth. However, if the growth curve flattens or stays stable, it may indicate the presence of fetal growth restriction (FGR). If the fundal height measurement is greater than expected from the weeks of gestational age, further evaluation is warranted if a multifetal gestation has not been diagnosed or hydramnios has not been ruled out (Adams & Schuiling, 2022).

Fetal Movement Determination

Fetal movements felt by the patient during the pregnancy are a sign that the fetus is growing in size and strength. Perception of fetal movement typically begins in the second trimester, between the 16th and 22nd weeks of pregnancy and occurs earlier in multiparous people than in nulliparous people (Fretts, 2024). The pregnant person's first perception of fetal movement, termed "quickening," is commonly described as a gentle fluttering. This perceived fetal movement is most often related to trunk and limb motion and rollovers, or flips. Maternal perception of fetal movement is an important screening method for fetal well-being, because decreased fetal movement is associated with a range of pregnancy pathologies and poor pregnancy outcomes. Decreased fetal movement may indicate hypoxemia. If compromised, the fetus decreases its oxygen requirements by decreasing activity. Reduced fetal movement is a warning sign of fetal impairment or risk and warrants further evaluation (Huecker et al., 2023).

Fetal movement counting is a method used by the pregnant person to quantify their fetus's movement. However, the optimal number of movements and the ideal duration of counting them remain controversial. Many variations for determining fetal movement, also called *fetal movement counts*, have been developed, but the most common method is described as follows. Determining fetal movement is a noninvasive method of screening and can be easily taught to all pregnant people. Any technique used requires patient participation and cooperation.

Instruct the patient about how to count fetal movements, the reasons for doing so, and the significance of decreased fetal movements. Urge the patient to perform the counts in a relaxed environment and a comfortable position, such as semi-Fowler or side lying. Provide the patient with detailed information concerning fetal movement counts, and stress the need for consistency in monitoring (at approximately the same time each day) and the importance of informing the health care provider promptly of any reduced movements. Providing patients with "fetal kick count" charts to record movement helps promote adherence to instructions. No values for fetal movement have been established that indicate fetal well-being, so the patient needs to be aware of a decrease in the number of movements when last assessed. The most common method used is "Count to 10," with which a pregnant person focuses their attention on the fetus's movement and records how long it takes to document 10 movements. If it takes longer than 2 hours, the person should contact the health care provider for further evaluation. Fetal kick counting in current prenatal care appears to be underutilized, and nurses need to educate patients about this assessment in their pregnancy care.

Fetal Heart Rate Measurement

Fetal heart rate measurement is integral to fetal surveillance throughout the pregnancy. Auscultating the fetal heart rate with a handheld Doppler at each prenatal visit helps confirm that the intrauterine environment is still supportive to the growing fetus. The purpose of assessing fetal heart rate is to determine the rate and rhythm. The normal fetal heart rate range is 110 to 160 bpm. Nursing Procedure 12.1 lists the steps for measuring fetal heart rate.

Teaching About the Danger Signs During Pregnancy

It is important to educate the patient about danger signs during pregnancy that require further evaluation. Explain that the patient should contact their health care provider immediately if they experience any of the following:

- *During the first trimester:* spotting or bleeding (miscarriage), painful urination (infection), severe persistent vomiting, weight loss, reduced appetite, (hyperemesis gravidarum), fever higher than 100°F (37.7°C; indicative of infection), dizziness or fainting, headache that gets worse over time, and lower abdominal pain with dizziness and accompanied by shoulder pain and vaginal bleeding (indicative of ruptured ectopic pregnancy)
- *During the second trimester:* regular uterine contractions, back pain, increased vaginal discharge (preterm labor); pain in calf, often increased with foot flexion (indicative of DVT); sudden gush or leakage of fluid from vagina (prelabor rupture of membranes); and absence of fetal movement for more than 12 hours (indicative of possible fetal distress or demise)
- *During the third trimester:* sudden weight gain; periorbital or facial edema, severe upper abdominal

NURSING PROCEDURE 12.1 Measuring Fetal Heart Rate

Purpose: To Assess Fetal Well-Being

1. Assist the patient onto the examining table and have them lie down.
2. Cover the patient with a sheet to ensure privacy and then expose their abdomen.
3. Palpate the abdomen to determine the fetal lie, position, and presentation.
4. Locate the back of the fetus (the ideal position to hear the heart rate).
5. Apply lubricant gel to the abdomen in the area where the back has been located.
6. Turn on the handheld Doppler device, and place it on the spot over the fetal back.
7. Listen for the sound of the amplified heart rate, moving the device slightly from side to side as necessary to obtain the loudest sound. Assess the patient's pulse rate and compare it to the amplified sound. If the rates appear the same, reposition the Doppler device.
8. Once the fetal heart rate has been identified, count the number of beats in 1 minute and record the results.
9. Remove the Doppler device and wipe off any remaining gel from the patient's abdomen and the device.
10. Record the heart rate on the patient's medical record; normal range is 110–160 bpm.
11. Provide information to the patient regarding fetal well-being based on findings.

pain, or headache with visual changes and extreme swelling of face or hands (indicative of gestational hypertension and/or preeclampsia); a decrease in fetal daily movement for more than 24 hours (indicative of fetal hypoxia and possible demise); and late pregnancy bleeding (indicative of placenta previa, abruptio placentae, or placenta accreta)

Any of the first- and second-trimester warning signs and symptoms can also be present in the last trimester (Adams & Schuiling, 2022; Office on Women's Health, 2022).

Early Contractions

One of the warning signs that should be emphasized is early contractions, which can lead to preterm birth. The pregnant person should not confuse these early preterm contractions with Braxton Hicks contractions, which are not true labor pains, because they go away when walking around or resting. They also often go away when the pregnant person goes to sleep. Braxton Hicks contractions are usually felt in the abdomen rather than in the lower back as with true preterm labor contractions. Signs of preterm labor that a person may experience include contractions every 10 minutes or more frequently; change in vaginal discharge; pelvic pressure and cramping; low, dull backache radiating to the abdomen and menstrual-like cramps; and diarrhea (Adams & Schuiling, 2022).

All pregnant people need to be able to recognize early signs of contractions to prevent preterm labor, which is a major public health problem in the United States. Approximately 10% of all live births in the United States occur before 37 weeks, and almost 3% occur at less than 34 weeks (Mandy, 2022). Preterm births among non-Hispanic Black people are higher (14%) when compared to non-Hispanic White (9.1%) or Hispanic (9.7%) people (Mandy, 2022). These preterm infants (born earlier than 37 weeks' gestation) can suffer lifelong health consequences, such as intellectual disability, chronic lung disease, cerebral palsy, seizure disorders, anxiety, depression, autism spectrum disorders, attention-deficit/hyperactivity disorder (ADHD), and vision and hearing loss (Suman & Luther, 2023). Preterm labor can happen to any pregnant person at any time. In many cases, it can be stopped with medications if it is recognized early, before significant cervical dilation has taken place. If the person experiences menstrual-like cramps occurring every 10 minutes accompanied by a low, dull backache, they should stop what they are doing and lie down on their left side for 1 hour and drink two or three glasses of water. If the symptoms worsen or do not subside after 1 hour, they should contact their health care provider.

ASSESSMENT OF FETAL WELL-BEING

During the antepartum period, several tests are routinely performed to monitor fetal well-being and to detect possible problems. When a high-risk pregnancy is identified, additional antepartum testing can be initiated to promote positive maternal, fetal, and neonatal outcomes. **High-risk pregnancy** is a broad term that includes pregnancies that are complicated by maternal or fetal conditions (coincidental with or unique to pregnancy) or by social or demographic factors that jeopardize the health status of the birthing parent and put the fetus at risk for adverse outcomes or a complicated birth (Lockwood & Magriples,

2023). Additional antepartum fetal testing or interventions will be based on specific causes of the pregnancy complication.

Ultrasonography

Since its introduction in the late 1950s, ultrasonography has become a useful diagnostic tool in obstetrics. Diagnostic ultrasound is employed in a variety of circumstances during pregnancy, such as concerns regarding fetal growth and after maternal complications. Real-time scanners can produce a continuous picture of the fetus on a monitor screen. A transducer that emits high-frequency sound waves is placed on the pregnant person's abdomen and moved to visualize the fetus (Fig. 12.6). The fetal heartbeat and any malformations in the fetus can be assessed, and measurements can be made accurately from the picture on the monitor screen.

Obstetric ultrasound is a standard component of prenatal care used to identify pregnancy complications and establish an accurate gestational age in order to improve pregnancy outcomes. Because the ultrasound procedure is noninvasive, it is a safe practice for low-risk patients and an accurate and cost-effective tool. It provides important information about fetal activity, growth, and gestational age; assesses fetal well-being; and determines the need for invasive intrauterine tests. If a single screening is performed, the optimal time is between 18 and 20 weeks' gestation (Shipp, 2023).

There are no hard-and-fast rules as to the number of ultrasounds a person should have during their pregnancy. A low-risk patient does not necessarily require any, but most practices do them as part of the prenatal care routine. A transvaginal ultrasound may be performed in the first trimester to confirm pregnancy, exclude ectopic (in which a fertilized egg implants somewhere other than the main cavity of the uterus) or molar (hydatidiform mole, a benign tumor that develops in the uterus) pregnancies, and confirm cardiac pulsation. A second abdominal scan may be performed at about 18 to 20 weeks to look for congenital malformations, exclude multifetal pregnancies, and verify dates and growth. A third abdominal scan may be done at around 32 to 36 weeks to evaluate fetal size and amniotic fluid volume, assess fetal growth, and verify placental position (Shipp, 2023). An ultrasound is used to confirm placental location during amniocentesis and to provide visualization during chorionic villus sampling (CVS). An ultrasound is also ordered whenever an abnormality is suspected.

During the past several years, ultrasound technology has advanced significantly. Now available for pregnant patients is three-/four-dimensional (3D/4D) ultrasound imaging. Unlike traditional 2D imaging, which takes a look at the developing fetus from one angle (thus creating the "flat" image), 3D imaging takes a view of the fetus from three different angles. A software then takes these three images and merges them to produce a 3D image. Because the fourth dimension is time and movement, with 4D, parents are able to watch the live movements of their fetus in 3D.

Nursing management during the ultrasound procedure focuses on educating the patient about the ultrasound test and reassuring them that they will not experience any sensation from the sound waves during the test. No special patient preparation is needed before performing the ultrasound, although in early pregnancy, the patient may need to have a full bladder. Inform the patient that they may experience some discomfort from the pressure on the full bladder during the scan, but it will last only a short time. Tell the patient that the conducting gel used on the abdomen during the scan may feel cold initially.

Doppler Flow Studies

Doppler ultrasonography is the use of sound waves to examine the flow of blood in blood vessels. Comprehensive assessment of fetal well-being involves monitoring of fetal growth, placental function, central venous pressure, and cardiac function. Primary indications

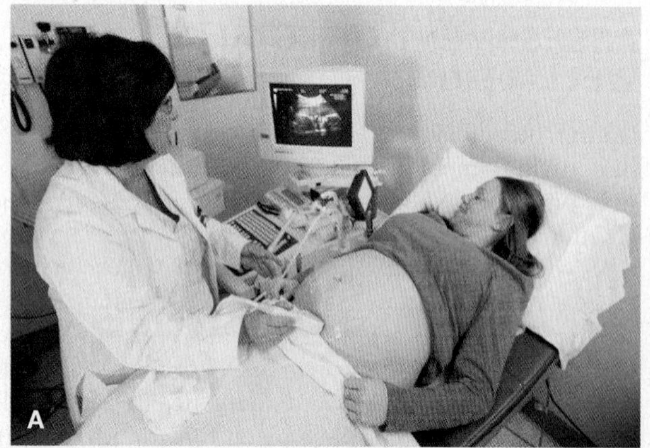

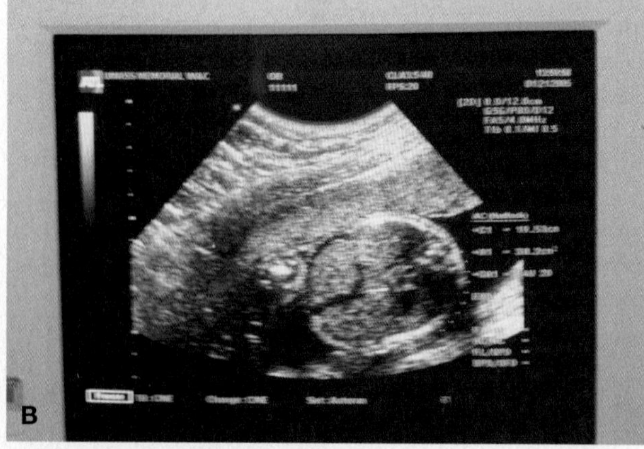

FIGURE 12.6 Ultrasound. **A.** Ultrasound device being applied to patient's abdomen. **B.** View of monitor.

for the use of Doppler ultrasonography include FGR, pregnancy-induced hypertension, preeclampsia, abnormalities of fetal heart rate or arrhythmias, and suspicion of cardiac defects (Faber et al., 2021). Doppler flow studies can be used to measure the velocity of blood flow via ultrasound. Doppler flow studies can detect fetal compromise in high-risk pregnancies. The test is noninvasive and has no contraindications. The images produced help to identify abnormalities in diastolic flow within the umbilical vessels. The velocity of the fetal red blood cells can be determined by measuring the change in the frequency of the sound wave reflected off the cells. Thus, Doppler flow studies can detect the movement of red blood cells in vessels to investigate fetal hemodynamics to use these findings for fetal surveillance. Placental defects are related to the etiology of preeclampsia, FGR, and newborns who are small for gestational age. In pregnancies complicated by hypertension or FGR, diastolic blood flow may be absent or even reversed (Faber et al., 2021). Doppler flow studies can also be used to evaluate the blood flow through other fetal blood vessels, such as the aorta and those in the brain. Research continues to determine the indications for Doppler flow studies to improve pregnancy outcomes. Nursing care of the patient undergoing Doppler flow studies is similar to that described for an ultrasound.

Alpha-Fetoprotein Analysis

Alpha-fetoprotein (AFP) is a glycoprotein produced initially by the yolk sac and fetal gut, and later predominantly by the fetal liver. In a fetus, the serum AFP level increases until approximately 14 to 15 weeks and then falls progressively by 32 weeks' gestation. In normal pregnancies, AFP from fetal serum enters the amniotic fluid (in microgram quantities) through fetal urination, fetal gastrointestinal (GI) secretions, and transudation across fetal membranes (amnion and placenta). If a developmental defect is present, such as failure of the neural tube to close, more AFP escapes into amniotic fluid from the fetus. AFP then enters the maternal circulation by crossing the placenta, and the level in maternal serum can be measured. The optimal time for AFP screening is 16 to 18 weeks' gestation, but it is frequently offered between the 15th and 20th weeks of gestation (Dukhovny & Wilkins-Haug, 2024).

In the past, this biomarker screening test had been recommended for all pregnant people along with other prenatal screening tests depending on the risk profile. Currently, all pregnant patients should be offered a second-trimester ultrasound for fetal structure defects between 18 and 22 weeks' gestation. With the availability of high-quality ultrasound technology, the midtrimester ultrasound has gradually replaced measuring maternal serum AFP (MSAFP) levels as a screening method because it appears to detect more neural tube defects than low MSAFP alone (Dukhovny & Wilkins-Haug, 2024). Therefore, if ultrasound screening is performed, MSAFP screening may not be necessary unless optimal images cannot be obtained (Dukhovny & Wilkins-Haug, 2024).

Correct information about gestational dating, maternal weight, race, number of fetuses, and presence of maternal diabetes is necessary to ensure the accuracy of this screening test (Dukhovny & Wilkins-Haug, 2024). If incorrect maternal information is submitted or the blood specimen is not drawn during the appropriate time frame, false-positive results may occur; this could cause the patient anxiety. Subsequently, further testing might be ordered based on an inaccurate interpretation, resulting in additional financial and emotional costs to the patient.

Increased levels of MSAFP may indicate conditions such as neural tube defect, multiple gestation, omphalocele, gastroschisis, renal abnormalities, and threatened miscarriage (Fischbach et al., 2022). Lower than expected MSAFP levels are seen when fetal gestational age is overestimated or in cases of fetal death, hydatidiform mole, increased maternal weight, and fetal trisomy 21 (Down syndrome) or trisomy 18 (Edward syndrome) (Adigun et al., 2024).

Measurement of MSAFP is minimally invasive, requiring only a venipuncture for a blood sample. AFP has now been combined with other biomarker screening tests (triple, quad, or penta screens) to determine the risk of neural tube defects and Down syndrome.

Nursing management for AFP testing consists of preparing the patient for this screening test by gathering accurate information about the date of their LMP, weight, race, and gestational dating. Accurately determining the window of 16 to 18 weeks' gestation will help ensure that the test results are correct. Also explain that the test involves obtaining a blood specimen.

Marker Screening Tests

Using maternal serum is an effective, noninvasive method for identifying fetal risk for aneuploidy (trisomies 13, 18, and 21) and neural tube defects. Prenatal screening for Down syndrome in the early second trimester with multiple maternal serum markers has been available for more than 15 years. Abnormalities in maternal serum marker levels and fetal measurements obtained during the first-trimester screening can be markers not only for certain chromosomal disorders and anomalies in the fetus but also for specific pregnancy complications. Pregnancy-associated plasma protein A (PAPP-A) is a complex, high-molecular-weight glycoprotein and is a key regulator of insulin-like growth factor essential for normal fetal development. In maternal blood, this protein increases with gestational age. It is routinely used for Down syndrome screening in the first trimester. A low maternal serum PAPP-A at 11 to 13 weeks' gestation is associated with the placenta not working as it should and can indicate stillbirth, preterm birth, preeclampsia, and chromosomal abnormalities (Gordon & Langaker, 2023; Livrinova et al., 2019).

Multiple blood screening tests may be used to determine the risk of open neural tube defects and Down syndrome: the triple-marker screen measures three hormones (AFP, hCG, and unconjugated estriol), while the quad screen includes the triple screening tests with the addition of a fourth marker, inhibin A (glycoprotein secreted by the placenta). The quad screen is used to enhance the accuracy of screening for Down syndrome in pregnant people younger than 35 years of age. High inhibin A levels indicate the possibility of Down syndrome (Gordon & Langaker, 2023). The penta screen includes AFP, hCG, unconjugated estrogen, dimeric inhibin A (DIA), and hyperglycosylated hCG (h-hCG). These biomarkers are merely screening tests and identify patients who need further definitive procedures (i.e., ultrasound, amniocentesis, and genetic counseling) to make a diagnosis of neural tube defects (anencephaly, spina bifida, and encephalocele) or Down syndrome in the fetus. Most screening tests are performed between 15 and 22 weeks' gestation (16 to 18 weeks is ideal), except for the cell-free fetal DNA (cffDNA) test, which can be performed around 9 to 10 weeks' gestation. The cffDNA test offers clinical benefits over existing prenatal screening tests by detecting the presence of trisomy 21 with high sensitivity and specificity at an earlier time frame (Messerlian et al., 2022).

Accurate test interpretation and risk determination are dependent on accurate pregnancy dating and reporting of relevant maternal characteristics. This is why it is so important, if an abnormal test result is reported, for nurses to confirm pregnancy dating and report any significant maternal factors relevant to test accuracy. In addition, nurses have a prominent role in providing education about the tests to the pregnant person and their partner. Prenatal screening has become standard in prenatal care. However, for many people, it remains confusing, emotionally charged, and filled with uncertain risks. Offer a thorough explanation of the test, reinforcing the information given by the health care professional. Provide a description of the risks and benefits of performing these screens, emphasizing that these tests are for screening purposes only. Remind the patient or couple that a definitive diagnosis is not made without further tests, such as an amniocentesis. Answer any questions about these prenatal screening tests and respect the patient's decision if they choose not to have them done. Many people may choose not to know because they would not consider having an abortion, regardless of the test results. Prenatal tests are expanding rapidly and will continue to provide families with more reproductive choices but at the same time may introduce ethical challenges.

Nuchal Translucency Screening

The nuchal area is a normal, fluid-filled subcutaneous space at the back of the fetal neck. Nuchal translucency screening (ultrasound) is done in the first trimester between 11 and 14 weeks. This allows for early detection and diagnosis of some fetal chromosomal and structural abnormalities. Over the years, it has become clear that increased nuchal translucency is a marker for chromosomal abnormalities and is also associated with a wide spectrum of structural anomalies (particularly cardiac anomalies), genetic syndromes, and high risk of spontaneous abortion and fetal death (Simpson, 2024). Increased nuchal translucency is associated with chromosomal abnormalities, such as trisomies 21, 18, and 13. Infants with trisomies tend to have more collagen and elastic connective tissue, allowing for accumulation. See Chapter 10 for more information.

Amniocentesis

Amniocentesis involves a transabdominal puncture of the amniotic sac to obtain a sample of amniotic fluid for analysis. It is an invasive procedure. The fluid contains fetal cells that are examined to detect chromosomal abnormalities and several hereditary metabolic defects in the fetus before birth. In addition, amniocentesis is used to confirm a fetal abnormality when other screening tests detect a possible problem.

Amniocentesis is typically performed in the second trimester, usually between 15 and 20 weeks' gestation. At this age, the amount of fluid is adequate (~150 mL), and the ratio of viable to nonviable cells is the greatest. More than 40 different chromosomal abnormalities as well as inborn errors of metabolism, intrauterine infections, degrees of hemolytic anemia, blood or platelet type, hemoglobinopathy, and neural tube defects can be diagnosed with amniocentesis (Ghidini, 2024). It can replace a genetic probability with a diagnostic certainty, allowing the patient and their partner to make an informed decision about the option of therapeutic abortion.

Amniocentesis can be performed in any of the three trimesters of pregnancy. An early amniocentesis (performed between weeks 11 and 14) is done to detect genetic anomalies. However, early amniocentesis has been associated with a high risk of spontaneous miscarriage and postprocedural amniotic fluid leakage compared with transabdominal chorionic villus screening (Jindal et al., 2023).

Table 12.2 lists amniotic fluid analysis findings and their implications.

Procedure

Amniocentesis is performed after an ultrasound examination identifies an adequate pocket of amniotic fluid free of fetal parts, the umbilical cord, or the placenta

TABLE 12.2 • Amniotic Fluid Analysis and Implications

Test Component	Normal Findings	Fetal Implications of Abnormal Findings
Color	Clear with white flecks of vernix caseosa in a mature fetus	Blood of maternal origin is usually harmless. "Port wine" fluid may indicate abruptio placentae. Fetal blood may indicate damage to the fetal, placental, or umbilical cord vessels. Changes in color are associated with fetal distress.
Bilirubin	Absent at term	High levels indicate hemolytic disease of the neonate in isoimmunized pregnancy and are associated with impending fetal death.
Meconium	Absent (except in breech presentation)	Presence indicates fetal hypotension, hypoxia, or distress.
Creatinine	>2 mg/dL in a mature fetus	Decrease may indicate immature fetus (<37 weeks).
Lecithin-to-sphingomyelin ratio (L/S ratio)	>2 generally indicates fetal pulmonary maturity	A ratio of <2 indicates pulmonary immaturity and subsequent respiratory distress syndrome.
Phosphatidylglycerol (PG)	Present	Absence indicates pulmonary immaturity.
Glucose	<45 mg/dL	Excessive increases at term or near term indicate hypertrophied fetal pancreas and subsequent neonatal hypoglycemia.
Alpha-fetoprotein (AFP)	Variable, depending on gestation age and laboratory technique; highest concentration	Inappropriate increases indicate neural tube defects such as spina bifida or anencephaly, multiple gestations, impending fetal death, abdominal wall defects, teratomas, Rh sensitization, or fetal distress; decreased AFP is associated with trisomy 21.
Bacteria	Absent	Presence indicates chorioamnionitis.
Chromosomes	Normal karyotype	Abnormal karyotype may indicate fetal sex and chromosomal disorders.
Acetylcholinesterase	Absent	Presence may indicate neural tube defects, exomphalos, or other serious malformations.

Jindal, A., Sharma, M., Karena, Z. V., & Chaudhary, C. (2023). Amniocentesis. In *StatPearls*. StatPearls Publishing. https://www.ncbi.nlm.nih.gov/books/NBK559247/; and Fischbach, F. T., Fischbach, M. A., & Stout, K. (2022). *A manual of laboratory and diagnostic tests* (11th ed.). Wolters Kluwer.

(Fig. 12.7). The health care provider inserts a long pudendal or spinal needle, a 22-gauge, 5-in needle, into the amniotic cavity and aspirates amniotic fluid, which is placed in an amber or foil-covered test tube to protect it from light. When the desired amount of fluid has been withdrawn, the needle is removed and slight pressure is applied to the site. If there is no evidence of bleeding, a sterile bandage is applied to the needle site. The specimens are then sent to the laboratory immediately for the cytologist to evaluate.

Examining a sample of fetal cells directly produces a definitive diagnosis rather than a "best guess" diagnosis based on indirect screening tests. It is an invaluable diagnostic tool, but the risks include lower abdominal discomfort and cramping, leakage of amniotic fluid, chorioamniotic separation, direct or indirect fetal injury, maternal or fetal infection (low incidence), and fetal loss (Ghidini, 2024; Jindal et al., 2023). Obtaining the test results may take up to 3 weeks. Rather than undergoing invasive testing such as amniocentesis, pregnant people today are more often choosing noninvasive prenatal testing despite those tests not being 100% correct. Patients

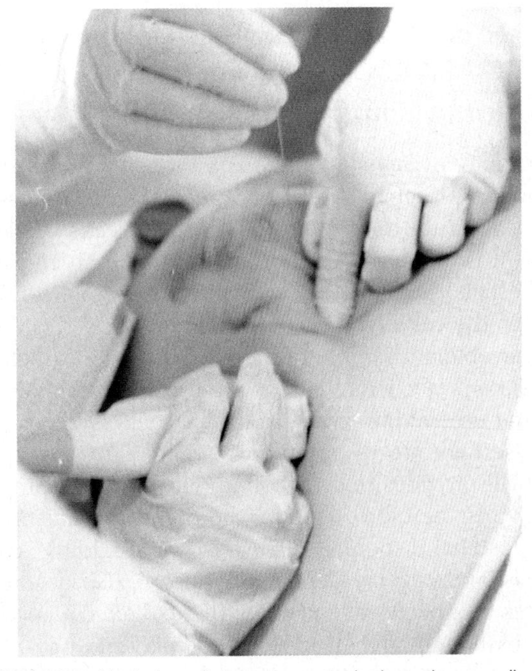

FIGURE 12.7 Technique for amniocentesis: inserting needle.

who receive reassuring results from noninvasive testing and normal ultrasound findings seem satisfied to forgo invasive procedures over the risk of procedure-related pregnancy loss. The number of invasive procedures has declined since the availability of noninvasive prenatal testing, and it is predicted that they will replace the more invasive procedures in the future (Ghidini, 2024).

Nursing Management

When preparing the patient for an amniocentesis, explain the procedure and its potential complications, and encourage the patient to empty their bladder just before the procedure to avoid the risk of bladder puncture. Inform the patient that a 20-minute electronic fetal monitoring strip is usually obtained to evaluate fetal well-being and obtain a baseline to compare after the procedure is completed. Obtain and record maternal vital signs.

After the procedure, assist the patient into a position of comfort and administer anti-D immune globulin if the patient is Rh negative to prevent potential sensitization to fetal blood if ordered. Assess maternal vital signs and fetal heart rate every 15 minutes for an hour after the procedure. Observe the puncture site for bleeding or drainage. Instruct the patient to rest after returning home and remind them to report fever, leaking amniotic fluid, vaginal bleeding, or uterine contractions or any changes in fetal activity (increased or decreased) to the health care provider.

When the test results come back, be available to offer support, especially if a fetal abnormality is found. Also prepare the patient and their partner for the need for genetic counseling. Trained genetic counselors can provide accurate medical information and help couples interpret the results of the amniocentesis so they can make the decisions that are right for them as a family.

Chorionic Villus Sampling

Chorionic villus sampling (CVS) is a procedure performed to biopsy placental tissue for prenatal genetic testing, generally in the first trimester after 10 weeks (Ghidini, 2023). It is an invasive procedure in which an 18-gauge needlestick is inserted either transabdominally or through the cervix with ultrasound guidance. This test is used to obtain a sample of the chorionic villi, which are fingerlike projections that cover the embryo and anchor it to the uterine lining before the placenta is developed. Because they are of embryonic origin, sampling chorionic villi provides information about the developing fetus. CVS is, therefore, used for the prenatal evaluation of chromosomal disorders, such as Down syndrome, cystic fibrosis, and enzyme deficiencies. It can also determine the sex of the fetus and identify sex-linked disorders, such as hemophilia, sickle cell anemia, and Tay–Sachs disease (Jones & Montero, 2022).

There has been an impetus to develop earlier prenatal diagnostic procedures so that couples can make an early decision to terminate the pregnancy if an anomaly is confirmed. Early prenatal diagnosis by CVS has been proposed as an alternative to routine amniocentesis, which is done later in the pregnancy to minimize procedural risks. In addition, the results of CVS testing are available sooner than those of amniocentesis.

Procedure

CVS is generally performed 10 to 13 weeks after the LMP. Earlier, chorionic villi may not be sufficiently developed for adequate tissue sampling and the risk of limb defects is increased (Ghidini, 2023). First, an ultrasound is done to confirm gestational age and viability. Then, under continuous ultrasound guidance, CVS is performed using either a transcervical or transabdominal approach. With the transcervical approach, the patient is placed in the lithotomy position and a sterile catheter is introduced through the cervix and inserted into the placenta, where a sample of chorionic villi is aspirated. This approach requires the patient to have a full bladder to push the uterus and placenta into a position that is more accessible to the catheter. A full bladder also helps in better visualization of the structures. With the transabdominal approach, an 18-gauge spinal needle is inserted through the abdominal wall into the placental tissue and a sample of chorionic villi is aspirated. Regardless of the approach used, the sample is sent to the cytogenetics laboratory for analysis.

Potential complications of CVS include postprocedural vaginal bleeding and cramping (most common), spontaneous abortion, limb abnormalities, rupture of membranes (rare), infection (rare), and fetal–maternal hemorrhage (Ghidini, 2023). The pregnancy loss and procedure-related miscarriage rates after CVS are similar to those of amniocentesis (Ghidini, 2023). In addition, patients who are Rh negative should receive anti-D immune globulin to avoid isoimmunization (Moise, 2023).

Nursing Management

Explain to the patient that the procedure will last about 15 minutes. An ultrasound will be done first to locate the embryo, and a baseline set of vital signs will be taken before starting. Make sure the patient is informed of the risks related to the procedure, including their incidence. If a transabdominal CVS procedure is planned, advise the patient to fill their bladder by drinking increased amounts of water. Inform them that a needle will be inserted through their abdominal wall and samples will be collected. Once the samples are collected, the needle will be withdrawn, and the samples will be sent to the genetics laboratory for evaluation.

For transcervical CVS, inform the patient that a speculum will be placed into the vagina under ultrasound guidance. Then, the vagina will be cleaned, and a small catheter inserted through the cervix. The samples obtained through the catheter are then sent to a laboratory.

After either procedure, assist the patient into a position of comfort and clean any excess lubricant or secretions from the area. Instruct the patient about signs to watch for and report, such as fever, cramping, and vaginal bleeding. Urge them not to engage in any strenuous activity for the next 48 hours. Assess the fetal heart rate for changes and administer anti-D immune globulin to an unsensitized Rh-negative patient after the procedure.

Nonstress Test

The nonstress test (NST) is used to test fetal well-being before the onset of labor. It is the most common method of prenatal testing used in practice today. The NST provides an indirect measurement of uteroplacental function and identifies fetuses at risk for hypoxemia or death (Miller, 2023). Unlike the fetal movement counting done by the pregnant person alone, this procedure requires specialized equipment and trained personnel. The basis for the NST is that the normal fetus produces characteristic fetal heart rate patterns in response to fetal movements. In the healthy fetus, there is an acceleration of the fetal heart rate with fetal movement. The NST is used from 32 weeks' gestation until delivery for surveillance of high-risk pregnancies in which the fetus is at risk for hypoxia or demise (Umana & Siccardi, 2023). The NST is a noninvasive test that requires no initiation of contractions. It is quick to perform, and there are no known side effects.

Procedure

Before the procedure, the patient eats a meal to stimulate fetal activity. Then the patient is placed in the left lateral recumbent position to avoid supine hypotension syndrome. An external electronic fetal monitoring device is applied to the patient's abdomen. The device consists of two belts, each with a sensor. One of the sensors records uterine activity, while the second sensor records fetal heart rate. The patient is handed an "event marker" with a button that they push every time they perceive fetal movement. When the button is pushed, the fetal monitor strip is marked to identify that fetal movement has occurred. The procedure usually lasts 20 to 30 minutes.

Nursing Management

Prior to the NST, explain the testing procedure and have the patient empty their bladder. Position the patient in a semi-Fowler position and apply the two external monitor belts. Document the date and time the test is started, patient information, the reason for the test, and the maternal vital signs. Obtain a baseline fetal monitor strip over 15 to 30 minutes.

During the test, observe for signs of fetal activity with a concurrent acceleration of the fetal heart rate. Interpret the NST as reactive or nonreactive. A reactive NST includes at least two fetal heart rate accelerations from the baseline of at least 15 bpm for at least 15 seconds within the 20-minute recording period. If the test does not meet these criteria after 40 minutes, it is considered nonreactive. A nonreactive NST is characterized by the absence of two fetal heart rate accelerations using the 15-by-15 criterion in a 20-minute time frame. A nonreactive test may be a sign of interrupted fetal oxygenation, but other causes include fetal immaturity, fetal sleeping, maternal smoking, fetal cardiac or neurologic anomalies, sepsis, or maternal ingestion of drugs with cardiac effects (Miller, 2023). More than half of nonreactive NSTs may be false positives; therefore, further evaluation is warranted, such as repeating the test, performing vibroacoustic stimulation, or performing another test, such as a biophysical profile (BPP) or a contraction stress test (Miller, 2023).

After the NST procedure, assist the patient off the table, provide them with fluids, and allow them to use the restroom. Typically, the health care provider discusses the results with the patient at this time. Provide teaching about signs and symptoms to report. If serial NSTs are being done, schedule the next testing session.

Biophysical Profile

A **biophysical profile (BPP)** uses a real-time ultrasound and NST to allow assessment of various parameters of fetal well-being that are sensitive to hypoxia. A BPP includes ultrasound monitoring of fetal movements, fetal tone, and fetal breathing as well as ultrasound assessment of amniotic fluid volume with or without assessment of the fetal heart rate. A BPP is performed in an effort to identify fetuses at risk of poor pregnancy outcome so that additional assessments of well-being may be performed or labor may be induced or a cesarean birth performed to expedite birth. The primary objectives of the BPP are to reduce stillbirth and to detect hypoxia early enough to allow delivery in time to avoid permanent fetal damage resulting from fetal asphyxia. These parameters, together with the NST, constitute the BPP. Each parameter is controlled by a different structure in the fetal brain: fetal tone by the cortex, fetal movements by the cortex and motor nuclei, fetal breathing movements by the centers close to the fourth ventricle, and the NST by the posterior hypothalamus and medulla. The amniotic fluid is the result of fetal urine volume. Some clinicians do not perform an NST unless other parameters of the profile are abnormal, as a normal BPP without NST has the same high predictive value as a normal BPP accompanied by a reactive NST (Manning, 2023). The BPP is based on the concept that a fetus who experiences hypoxia loses certain behavioral parameters in the reverse order in which they were acquired during fetal development (normal order of development: tone at 8 weeks, movement at 9 weeks, breathing at 20 weeks, and fetal heart rate reactivity at 24 weeks).

Scoring and Interpretation

The BPP is a scored test with five components, each worth two points if present. A total score of 10 is possible if the NST is used (without the NST, the total score possible is 8). Thirty minutes are allotted for testing, though less than 10 minutes are usually needed. The following criteria must be met to obtain a score of 2; anything less is scored as 0 (Manning, 2023).

- *Body movements:* three or more discrete limb or trunk movements
- *Fetal tone:* one or more instances of full extension and flexion of a limb or trunk
- *Fetal breathing:* one or more fetal breathing movements of more than 30 seconds
- *Amniotic fluid volume:* one or more pockets of fluid measuring more than 2 cm
- *NST:* normal NST = 2 points; abnormal NST = 0 points

Interpretation of the BPP score can be complicated, depending on several fetal and maternal variables. Because it is indicated as a result of a nonreassuring finding from previous fetal surveillance tests, this test can be used to quantify the interpretation, and intervention can be initiated if appropriate. A maximum score of 10 can be achieved, and the test is complete once all of the variables have been observed. For the test to be judged abnormal and a score of zero awarded for the absence of fetal movement, fetal tone, or fetal breathing movements, a period of not less than 30 minutes must have elapsed. Because of the excellent sensitivity of fetal NST for fetal acidemia, it has been proposed that this acute marker alone may be used for fetal assessment in combination with the amniotic fluid volume assessment, a chronic marker. This combination, also known as the *modified BPP*, has been shown to have excellent false-negative rates that compare with those of the complete BPP.

One of the important factors is the amniotic fluid volume, taken in conjunction with the results of the NST. Amniotic fluid volume evaluation is standard in the surveillance of fetal well-being, especially in high-risk pregnancies. Amniotic fluid is largely composed of fetal urine. As placental function decreases, perfusion of fetal organs, such as kidneys, decreases, and this can lead to a reduction of amniotic fluid. If oligohydramnios or decreased amniotic fluid is present, the potential exists for antepartum or intrapartum fetal compromise (Manning, 2023).

Overall, a score of 8 to 10 is considered normal if the amniotic fluid volume is adequate. A score of 6 or below is suspicious, possibly indicating a compromised fetus; further investigation of fetal well-being is needed.

Because the BPP is an ultrasonographic assessment of fetal behavior, it requires more extensive equipment and more highly trained personnel than other testing modalities. The cost is much greater than those of less sophisticated tests. It permits conservative therapy and prevents premature or unnecessary intervention. There is a lower incidence of false negatives using a BPP test than using the NST alone (Sapoval et al., 2023).

Nursing Management

Nursing care focuses primarily on offering the patient support and answering their questions. Expect to complete the NST before scheduling the BPP and explain why further testing might be needed. Tell the patient that the ultrasound will be done in the diagnostic imaging department.

NURSING MANAGEMENT FOR THE COMMON DISCOMFORTS OF PREGNANCY

Most people experience common discomforts during pregnancy and ask a nurse's advice about ways to minimize them. However, other people will not bring up their concerns unless asked. Therefore, the nurse needs to address the common discomforts that occur in each trimester at each prenatal visit and provide realistic measures to help the patient deal with them (Teaching Guidelines 12.1). Clinical Judgment & Nursing Process 12.1 applies the nursing process to the care of a patient experiencing some discomforts of pregnancy.

First-Trimester Discomforts

During the first 3 months of pregnancy, the person's body undergoes numerous changes. Some people experience many discomforts, but others have few. These discomforts are caused by the changes taking place within the body, and they pass as the pregnancy progresses.

Urinary Frequency or Incontinence

Urinary frequency or incontinence is common in the first trimester because the growing uterus compresses the bladder. This is also a common complaint during the third trimester, especially when the fetal head settles into the pelvis. However, the discomfort tends to improve in the second trimester, when the uterus becomes an abdominal organ and moves away from the bladder region.

After infection and gestational diabetes have been ruled out as causative factors of increased urinary frequency, suggest that the patient decrease their fluid intake 2 to 3 hours before bedtime and limit their intake of caffeinated beverages. Increased voiding is normal, but encourage the patient to report any pain or burning during urination. Also explain that increased urinary frequency may subside as they enter their second trimester,

CLINICAL JUDGMENT & NURSING PROCESS 12.1 Overview of the Patient Experiencing Common Discomforts of Pregnancy

Alicia, a 32-year-old, G1 P0, at 10 weeks' gestation, comes to the clinic for a visit. During the interview, she tells you, "I'm running to the bathroom to urinate it seems like all the time, and I'm so nauseous that I'm having trouble eating." She denies any burning or pain on urination. Vital signs are within acceptable limits.

NURSING ANALYSIS: Altered urinary elimination related to frequency secondary to physiologic changes of pregnancy

OUTCOME IDENTIFICATION AND EVALUATION

The patient will report a decrease in urinary complaints as evidenced by a decrease in the number of times she uses the bathroom to void, reports that she feels her bladder is empty after voiding, and use of pelvic floor muscle exercises.

INTERVENTIONS: *Promoting Normal Urinary Elimination Patterns*

- Assess patient's usual bladder elimination patterns *to establish a baseline for comparison.*
- Obtain a urine specimen for analysis *to rule out infection or glucosuria.*
- Review with patient the physiologic basis for the increased frequency during pregnancy; inform patient that frequency should abate during the second trimester and that it most likely will return during her third trimester. *This will promote understanding of the problem.*
- Encourage the patient to empty her bladder when first feeling a sensation of fullness *to minimize the risk of urinary retention.*
- Suggest patient to avoid caffeinated drinks, *which can stimulate the need to void.*
- Encourage patient to drink adequate amounts of fluid throughout the day; however, have patient reduce her fluid intake before bedtime *to reduce nighttime urination.*
- Urge patient to keep perineal area clean and dry *to prevent irritation and excoriation from any leakage.*
- Instruct patient on pelvic floor muscle exercises *to increase perineal muscle tone and control over leakage.*
- Teach patient about the signs and symptoms of urinary tract infection and urge her to report them should they occur *to ensure early detection and prompt intervention.*

NURSING ANALYSIS: Undernutrition risk related to nausea and vomiting

OUTCOME IDENTIFICATION AND EVALUATION

The patient will ingest adequate amounts of nutrients for maternal and fetal well-being as evidenced by acceptable weight gain pattern and statements indicating an increase in food intake with a decrease in the number of episodes of nausea and vomiting.

INTERVENTIONS: *Promoting Adequate Nutrition*

- Obtain weight and compare to baseline *to determine the effects of nausea and vomiting on nutritional intake.*
- Review patient's typical dietary intake over 24 hours *to determine nutritional intake and patterns so that suggestions can be individualized.*
- Encourage patient to eat five or six small frequent meals throughout the day *to prevent her stomach from becoming empty.*
- Suggest that she munch on dry crackers, toast, cereal, or cheese, or drink a small amount of lemonade before arising *to minimize nausea.*
- Encourage patient to arise slowly from bed in the morning and avoid sudden movements *to reduce stimulation of the vomiting center.*
- Advise patient to drink fluids between meals rather than with meals *to avoid overdistention of the abdomen and subsequent increase in abdominal pressure.*
- Encourage her to increase her intake of foods high in vitamin B_6 such as meat, poultry, bananas, fish, green leafy vegetables, peanuts, raisins, walnuts, and whole grains, as tolerated, *to ensure adequate nutrient intake.*
- Advise the patient to avoid greasy, fried, or highly spiced foods and to avoid strong odors, including foods such as cabbage, *to minimize gastrointestinal upset.*
- Encourage the patient to avoid wearing tight or restrictive clothes *to minimize pressure on the expanding abdomen.*
- Arrange for consultation with nutritionist as necessary *to assist with diet planning.*

only to recur in the third trimester. Teach the patient to perform pelvic floor muscle training exercises, to increase support of the uterus, bladder, small intestine, and rectum throughout the day; this will help strengthen perineal muscle tone, thereby enhancing urinary control and decreasing the possibility of incontinence.

Fatigue

Fatigue plagues all pregnant people, primarily in the first and third trimesters (the highest energy levels typically occur during the second trimester), even if they get their normal amount of sleep at night. First-trimester fatigue is most often related to the many physical changes (e.g., increased oxygen consumption, increased levels of progesterone and relaxin, increased metabolic demands) and psychosocial changes (e.g., mood swings, multiple role demands) of pregnancy. Third-trimester fatigue can be caused by sleep disturbances from increased weight (many people cannot find comfortable sleeping positions due to the enlarging abdomen), physical discomforts such as heartburn, and insomnia due to mood swings, multiple role anxiety, and a decrease in exercise.

TEACHING GUIDELINES 12.1 Managing the Discomforts of Pregnancy

Urinary Frequency or Incontinence

- Try pelvic floor muscle exercises to increase control over leakage.
- Empty bladder when a full sensation is first felt.
- Avoid caffeinated drinks, which stimulate voiding.
- Reduce fluid intake after dinner to reduce nighttime urination.

Fatigue

- Attempt to get a full night's sleep without interruptions.
- Eat a healthy balanced diet.
- Schedule a nap in the early afternoon daily.
- When feeling tired, pause and rest.

Nausea and Vomiting

- Avoid an empty stomach at all times.
- Eat dry crackers/toast in bed before arising.
- Eat five to six small meals throughout the day.
- Avoid brushing teeth immediately after eating to avoid gag reflex.
- Acupressure wristbands can be worn daily.
- Prepare bland foods and avoid spicy or hot foods.
- Drink fluids between meals rather than with meals.
- Avoid greasy, fried foods or ones with a strong odor, such as cabbage or Brussels sprouts.

Backache

- Avoid standing or sitting in one position for long periods.
- Apply heating pad (low setting) to the small of back.
- Support lower back with pillows when sitting.
- Use proper body mechanics for lifting anything.
- Avoid excessive bending, lifting, or walking without rest periods.
- Wear supportive low-heeled shoes; avoid high heels.
- Stand with shoulders back to maintain correct posture.

Leg Cramps

- Elevate legs above heart level frequently throughout the day.
- If a cramp occurs, straighten both legs and flex feet up toward the body.
- Ask health care provider about taking additional calcium supplements, which may reduce leg spasms.

Varicosities

- Walk daily to improve circulation to extremities.
- Elevate both legs above heart level while resting.
- Avoid standing in one position for long periods of time.
- Don't wear constrictive stockings and socks.
- Don't cross the legs when sitting for long periods.
- Wear support stockings to promote better circulation.

Hemorrhoids

- Establish a regular time for daily bowel elimination.
- Avoid constipation and straining during defecation.
- Prevent straining by drinking plenty of fluids and eating fiber-rich foods and exercising daily.
- Use warm sitz baths and cool witch hazel compresses for comfort.

Constipation

- Increase intake of foods high in fiber and drink at least eight 8-oz glasses of fluid daily.
- Ingest prunes or prune juice, which are natural laxatives.
- Consume warm liquids (e.g., tea) upon rising to stimulate peristalsis.
- Exercise each day (brisk walking) to promote movement through the intestine.
- Reduce the amount of cheese consumed.

Heartburn/Indigestion

- Avoid spicy or greasy foods and eat small frequent meals.
- Sleep on several pillows so that your head is elevated 30 degrees.
- Stop smoking and avoid caffeinated drinks to reduce stimulation.
- Avoid lying down for at least 3 hours after meals.
- Try drinking sips of water to reduce burning sensation.
- Avoid foods that trigger symptoms—fried foods, citrus, soda, chocolate.
- Take antacids sparingly if burning sensation is severe.

Braxton Hicks Contractions

- Keep in mind that these contractions are a normal sensation. Try changing your position or engaging in mild exercise to help reduce the sensation.
- Drink more fluids if possible.

Once anemia, infection, and blood dyscrasias have been ruled out as contributing to the patient's fatigue, advise them to arrange work, child care, and other demands in their life to permit additional rest periods. Work with the patient to devise a realistic schedule for rest. Using pillows for support in the left-side–lying position relieves pressure on major blood vessels that supply oxygen and nutrients to the fetus when resting (Fig. 12.8). Also recommend the use of relaxation techniques, providing instructions as necessary, and suggest the patient increase their daily exercise level.

Nausea and Vomiting

It is estimated that up to 90% of pregnant people experience nausea and vomiting (Smith et al., 2024). The

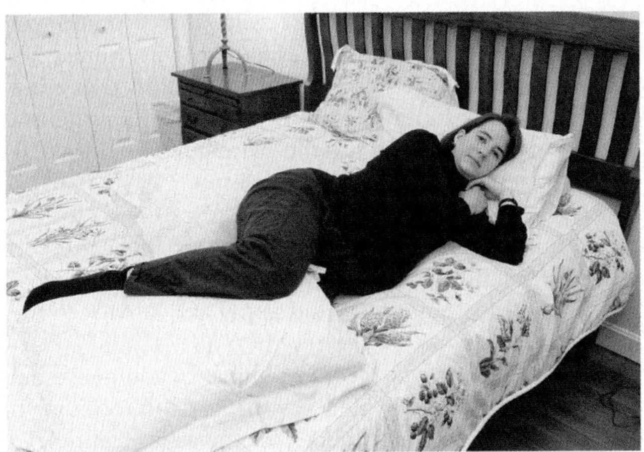

FIGURE 12.8 Using pillows for support in the side-lying position.

problem is generally time-limited, with the onset about the fifth week after the LMP, a peak at 8 to 12 weeks, and resolution by 16 to 18 weeks. Despite popular use of the term *morning sickness*, nausea and vomiting of pregnancy persists throughout the day in the majority (80%) of affected people (Smith et al., 2024). The physiologic changes that cause nausea and vomiting are unknown, but research suggests that unusually high levels of estrogen, progesterone, and hCG, along with abnormal GI motility and a vitamin B_6 or zinc deficiency, may be contributing factors (Smith et al., 2024). In summary, the etiology of nausea and vomiting in pregnancy is physiologic; thus, assessment of the condition focuses on severity, and the management is largely supportive.

Nausea and vomiting of pregnancy can take a physical and psychological toll on the pregnant person and may have an adverse effect on their partner, family members, and even coworkers. People tend to minimize the burden it places on the pregnant person, as it is considered a normal part of pregnancy; thus, it may not be considered worthy of evaluation, diagnosis, management, and emotional support. As a result, it may not be taken seriously because it is so common and time-limited, leading some pregnant people to feel frustrated and feel guilty that they are even complaining about their symptoms. Nurses need to pick up on this, address it, and provide support for the pregnant person.

The goal of treatment is to improve symptoms while minimizing risks to the pregnant person and fetus. Treatment management ranges from simple dietary modifications to drug therapy. To help alleviate nausea and vomiting, advise the patient to eat small, frequent meals that are bland and low in fat (five or six times a day) to prevent their stomach from becoming completely empty. Other helpful suggestions include eating dry crackers, Cheerios, or cheese or drinking lemonade before getting out of bed in the morning and increasing their intake of foods high in vitamin B_6, such as meat, poultry, bananas, fish, green leafy vegetables, peanuts, raisins, walnuts, and whole grains, or making sure they are receiving enough vitamin B_6 by taking their prescribed prenatal vitamins.

Some people find ginger is effective in reducing mild-to-moderate nausea and vomiting during pregnancy. Vitamin B_6 (pyridoxine), taken 10 to 25 mg orally every 6 to 8 hours, is an OTC medication that can improve nausea (Smith et al., 2023). The U.S. Food and Drug Administration (FDA) has approved doxylamine succinate 10 mg per pyridoxine hydrochloride 10 mg (Diclegis) as a medication to specifically treat morning sickness in pregnancy if vitamin B_6 alone does not work. It is considered safe to take two tablets at bedtime during pregnancy and, if that is not sufficient, to add one tablet in the morning and one in mid-afternoon (Smith et al., 2023).

Other pharmacotherapies that might be considered may include diphenhydramine (e.g., Benadryl), dimenhydrinate (e.g., Dramamine), meclizine (e.g., Antivert), prochlorperazine (e.g., Compazine), promethazine (e.g., Phenergan), or ondansetron (e.g., Zofran).

Other helpful tips to deal with nausea and vomiting include:

- Get out of bed in the morning slowly.
- Avoid sudden movements.
- Eat before or as soon as you feel hungry to avoid an empty stomach.
- Avoid triggers that stimulate or exacerbate nausea—strong food odors.
- Eat a high-protein snack before getting out of bed in the morning and snacks during the night to prevent an empty stomach.
- Take ginger (up to 1 g in divided doses daily; 250-mg capsules QID), which increases tone and peristalsis in the GI tract.
- Open a window to remove odors of food being cooked.
- Eat more protein than carbohydrates and take in more liquids than solids.
- Limit intake of fluids or soups during meals (drink them between meals).
- Avoid fried foods and foods cooked with grease, oils, or fatty meats, because they tend to upset the stomach.
- Increase periods of rest.
- Suck on popsicles throughout the day.
- Avoid highly seasoned foods such as those cooked with garlic, onions, peppers, and chili.
- Drink a small amount of caffeine-free carbonated beverage (ginger ale) if nauseated.
- Trying acupressure using a wristband has been FDA approved for nausea.
- Avoid wearing tight or restricting clothes, which might place increased pressure on the expanding abdomen.
- Avoid stress (Phillippi & Sanders, 2022; Smith et al., 2023).

Breast Tenderness

Breast tenderness is often the first symptom of pregnancy, occurring as early as a week or 2 after conception. As a result of increased estrogen and progesterone levels, which cause the fat layer of breasts to thicken and the number of milk ducts and glands to increase during the first trimester, many pregnant people experience breast tenderness. Offering a thorough explanation to the patient about the reasons for the breast discomfort is important. Wearing a larger, properly fitting bra with good support and wide straps, even while sleeping, can help alleviate this discomfort (Phillippi & Sanders, 2022).

Constipation

Constipation affects up to 40% of pregnancies (Bianco, 2023). Increasing levels of progesterone during pregnancy lead to decreased contractility of the GI tract, slowed movement of substances through the colon, and a resulting increase in water absorption. All of these factors lead to constipation. Lack of exercise or too little fiber or fluids in the diet can also promote constipation. In addition, the large bowel is mechanically compressed by the enlarging uterus, adding to this discomfort. The iron and calcium in prenatal vitamins can also contribute to constipation during the first and third trimesters.

Explain how pregnancy exacerbates the symptoms of constipation and offer the following suggestions:

- Eat fresh or dried fruit daily.
- Eat more raw fruits and vegetables, including their skins.
- Eat whole-grain cereals and breads such as raisin bran or bran flakes.
- Participate in physical activity every day.
- Engage in pelvic floor exercises, stretching exercises, and yoga daily.
- Eat meals at regular intervals.
- Establish a time of day to defecate and elevate feet on a stool to avoid straining.
- Drink six to eight glasses of water daily.
- Decrease intake of refined carbohydrates.
- Drink warm fluids upon arising to stimulate bowel motility.
- Decrease consumption of sugary sodas.
- Avoid eating large amounts of cheese.

If the abovementioned suggestions are ineffective, suggest that the patient use a bulk-forming laxative, such as Metamucil (Lockwood & Magriples, 2024b).

Nasal Stuffiness, Bleeding Gums, and Epistaxis (Nosebleeds)

Increased levels of estrogen cause edema of the mucous membranes of the nasal and oral cavities. Advise the pregnant patient to drink extra water for hydration of the mucous membranes or to use a cool mist humidifier in their bedroom at night. If they need to blow their nose to relieve nasal stuffiness, advise them to blow gently, one nostril at a time. Advise the patient to avoid the use of nasal decongestants and sprays.

If a nosebleed occurs, advise the patient to loosen the clothing around their neck, sit with their head tilted forward, pinch their nostrils with their thumb and forefinger for 10 to 15 minutes, and apply an ice pack to the bridge of their nose.

If the patient has bleeding gums, encourage them to practice good oral hygiene by using a soft toothbrush and flossing daily. Warm saline mouthwashes can relieve discomfort. If the gum problem persists, instruct the patient to see their dentist.

Cravings

Food craving refers to an intense desire to consume a specific food. Commonly reported cravings include fast food; pickles; pizza; starchy carbohydrates; dairy, such as ice cream; chocolate; and other sweets (Blau et al., 2020). Pregnant people commonly have food cravings (Blau et al., 2020). Desires for certain foods and beverages are likely to begin during the first trimester but do not appear to reflect any physiologic need. Foods with a high sodium or sugar content are often the ones craved. At times, some pregnant people crave nonfood substances, such as clay, cornstarch, laundry detergent, baking soda, soap, paint chips, dirt, ice, or wax. As explained in Chapter 11, this craving for nonfood substances, termed "pica," may indicate a severe dietary deficiency of minerals or vitamins; pica may have cultural roots or psychological factors, such as stress (Nasser et al., 2023).

Leukorrhea

Vaginal discharge, also known as *leukorrhea*, in a person who can become pregnant typically consists of 1 to 4 mL in 24 hours; this amount is considered normal. It is usually transparent, mucous like, and whitish yellow (Adams, 2022). Increased vaginal discharge begins during the first trimester of pregnancy. The physiologic changes behind leukorrhea arise from the high levels of estrogen, which cause increased vascularity and hypertrophy of cervical glands as well as vaginal cells (Adams, 2022; Sim et al., 2020). The result is progressively increasing vaginal secretions throughout pregnancy.

Advise the patient to keep the perineal area clean and dry, washing the area with mild soap and water during their daily shower. Also recommend that the patient avoid wearing pantyhose and other tight-fitting nylon clothes that prevent air from circulating to the genital area. Encourage the use of cotton underwear and suggest wearing a nightgown rather than pajamas to allow for increased airflow. Also instruct the patient to avoid douching and tampon use.

Second-Trimester Discomforts

A sense of well-being typically characterizes the second trimester for most pregnant people. By this time, the fatigue, nausea, and vomiting have subsided, and the uncomfortable changes of the third trimester are a few months away. Not every pregnant person experiences the same discomforts during this time, so nursing assessments and interventions must be individualized.

Backache

Musculoskeletal pain is a common occurrence during pregnancy and the postpartum period. It is most prevalent during the second half of pregnancy. Up to 60% of people report having back pain at some point during pregnancy (Bermas, 2023). This can seriously impact a person's quality of life and have socioeconomic impacts from lost days at work. The pain can be lumbar or sacroiliac. The pain may also be present only at night. Back pain is thought to be due to multiple factors, which include shifting of the center of gravity caused by the enlarging uterus, increased joint laxity due to an increase in relaxin, stretching of the ligaments (which are pain-sensitive structures), and pregnancy-related circulatory changes.

Treatment includes heat and ice, acetaminophen, massage, proper posturing, good support shoes, and a good exercise program for strength and conditioning. Pregnant people may also relieve back pain by placing one foot on a stool when standing for long periods of time and placing a pillow between the legs when lying down (Bermas, 2023). After ruling out other potential causes such as uterine contractions, urinary tract infection, ulcers, or musculoskeletal back disorders, the following instructions may be helpful:

- Maintain correct posture with head up and shoulders back.
- Wear low-heeled shoes with good arch support.
- Get daily exercise to strengthen back muscles.
- Sit in chairs that offer good back support.
- Avoid lifting heavy objects and bending from the waist.
- Attempt to be active daily to help strengthen back muscles.
- Move feet when turning around to avoid twisting spine.
- Try swimming or aquatic therapy to relieve joint and muscle pressure.
- Consider investing in a firm mattress for better back support.
- When standing for long periods, place one foot on a stool or box.
- Use good body mechanics when lifting objects.
- Sleep on the left side with a pillow between the legs for support.
- When sitting, use foot supports and pillows behind the back.
- Try pelvic tilt or rocking exercises to strengthen the back (Bermas, 2023).

The pelvic tilt or pelvic rock is used to alleviate pressure on the lower back during pregnancy by stretching the core lower back muscles. It can be done sitting, standing, or on all fours. To do it on all fours, the hands are positioned directly under the shoulders and the knees under the hips. The back should be in a neutral position, with the head and neck aligned with the straight back. The person then presses up with the lower back and holds this position for a few seconds, then relaxes to a neutral position. This exercise helps strengthen the abdominal muscles and relieves lumbar lordosis (Bermas, 2023).

Leg Cramps

During pregnancy, up to 50% of people can be affected by leg cramps, typically in the last 3 months of pregnancy, especially at night (Bordoni et al., 2023). Leg cramps occur primarily in the second and third trimesters and could be related to the pressure of the gravid uterus on pelvic nerves and blood vessels. Along with lack of exercise, diet can also be a contributing factor if the pregnant person is not consuming enough of certain minerals, such as calcium and magnesium.

Encourage the patient to gently stretch the muscle by dorsiflexing the foot up toward the body. Wrapping a warm, moist towel around the leg muscle can also help the muscle relax. Advise the patient to avoid stretching their legs, pointing their toes, and walking excessively. Stress the importance of wearing low-heeled shoes and support hose and arising slowly from a sitting position. If the leg cramps are due to deficiencies in minerals, the condition can be remedied by eating more foods rich in these nutrients. Also instruct the patient on calf-stretching exercises: have them stand 3 ft from the wall and lean toward it, resting their lower arms against it while keeping their heels on the floor. This may help reduce cramping if it is done before going to bed.

Elevating the legs throughout the day will help relieve pressure and minimize strain. Instruct the patient to avoid standing in one spot for a prolonged period or crossing their legs. If the patient must stand for prolonged periods, suggest that they change their position at least every 2 hours by walking or sitting to reduce the risk of leg cramps. Encourage the patient to drink eight 8-oz glasses of fluid throughout the day to ensure adequate hydration. Taking daily walks can also help reduce leg cramping because ambulation improves circulation to the muscles.

Varicosities of the Vulva and Legs

Varicose veins are abnormally enlarged superficial veins due to vasodilation caused by progesterone's effects on the vessel walls and valves. Approximately 50% of pregnant people experience varicose veins in their lower extremities (Pomeranz, 2023). Varicosities of the vulva and legs are associated with the increased venous stasis caused by the pressure of the gravid uterus on pelvic vessels. Progesterone relaxes the vein walls, making it difficult for blood to return to the heart from the extremities; pooling can result. Genetic predisposition, inactivity, obesity, and poor muscle tone are also contributing factors.

Supportive therapy of leg varicosities includes leg elevation, sleeping on the left side, compression hosiery, and avoiding long periods of standing or sitting. Exercise may prevent varicose veins if started early in the pregnancy. Encourage the patient to wear support hose that have gradient pressure in them and teach the patient how to apply them properly. Advise the patient to elevate their legs above their heart while lying on their back for 10 minutes before they get out of bed in the morning, thus promoting venous return before the patient applies the hose. Instruct the patient to avoid crossing their legs and avoid wearing knee-high stockings. These cause constriction of leg vessels and muscles and contribute to venous stasis. Also encourage the patient to elevate both the legs above the level of the heart for 5 to 10 minutes at least twice a day (Fig. 12.9), to wear low-heeled shoes, and to avoid long periods of standing or sitting, frequently changing their position. If the patient has vulvar varicosities, suggest that they apply ice packs to the area when they are lying down.

Hemorrhoids

Hemorrhoids are varicosities of the rectum and may be external (outside the anal sphincter) or internal (above the sphincter) (Wedro, 2023). They occur as a result of progesterone-induced vasodilation and from pressure of the enlarged uterus on the lower intestine and rectum. Hemorrhoids are more common in people with constipation, obesity (BMI >30 kg/m^2), a low-fiber diet, poor fluid intake or poor dietary habits, a habit of smoking, a sedentary lifestyle, or a previous history of natural childbirth and hemorrhoids. It is estimated they occur in about 40% of pregnant and postpartum people (Buzinskiene et al., 2022).

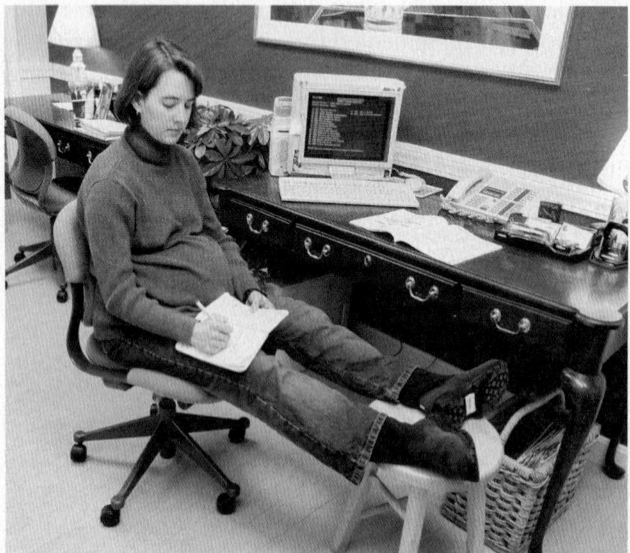

FIGURE 12.9 Pregnant person elevating their legs while working.

Instruct the patient in measures to prevent constipation, including increasing fiber intake and drinking at least 2 L of fluid per day. Recommend the use of topical anesthetics (e.g., Preparation H, Anusol, witch hazel compresses such as Tucks) to reduce pain, itching, and swelling, if permitted by the health care provider. Teach the patient about local comfort measures, such as warm sitz baths, witch hazel compresses, or cold compresses. To minimize the patient's risk of straining while defecating, suggest that they elevate their feet on a stool. Also encourage the patient to avoid prolonged sitting on the toilet (Buzinskiene et al., 2022).

Flatulence With Bloating

Flatulence and gas pain are another result of decreased GI motility. The physiologic changes that result in constipation (reduced GI motility and dilation secondary to progesterone's influence) may also result in increased flatulence. As the enlarging uterus compresses the bowel, it delays the passage of food through the intestines, thus allowing more time for gas to be formed by bacteria in the colon. The patient usually reports increased passage of rectal gas, abdominal bloating, or belching. Instruct the patient to avoid gas-forming foods, such as beans, cabbage, and onions, as well as foods that have a high content of white sugar. Adding more fiber to the diet, increasing fluid intake, eating and drinking slowly, avoiding carbonated beverages, and increasing physical exercise are also helpful in reducing flatus. In addition, wearing clothing that is loose around the abdomen, breathing deeply and slowly, and reducing the amount of swallowed air (if chewing gum) will reduce gas buildup. The knee–chest position may also help with discomfort from unexpelled gas. Consuming six smaller meals a day will help avoid digestive system overload. Taking a brisk walk after meals will help mobilize gas for expulsion. Reducing the intake of cheese and eating mints can also help reduce flatulence during pregnancy.

Third-Trimester Discomforts

As people enter the third trimester, many experience a return of the first-trimester discomforts of fatigue, urinary frequency, leukorrhea, and constipation. These discomforts are secondary to the enlarging uterus compressing adjacent structures, increasing hormone levels, and the metabolic demands of the fetus. In addition to these discomforts, many people experience shortness of breath, heartburn, indigestion, swelling, and Braxton Hicks contractions.

Shortness of Breath and Dyspnea

Dyspnea, or shortness of breath, is a common complaint in pregnant people during the first and third trimesters. Physiologic and hemodynamic changes can result in significant dyspnea in such cases. In some people, dyspnea in normal daily activities can be a sign of heart and lung disease and may be associated with poor perinatal and cardiac outcomes in which early detection can prevent adverse events. The increasing growth of the uterus prevents complete lung expansion late in pregnancy. As the uterus enlarges upward in the second and third trimesters, the expansion of the diaphragm is limited. Dyspnea can occur when the patient lies on their back and the pressure of the gravid uterus against the vena cava reduces venous return to the heart. Sixty percent to 75% of pregnant people experience periodic dyspnea (Weinberger, 2024).

Reassure the patient that dyspnea is normal and will improve when the fetus drops into the pelvis (lightening). Instruct the patient to adjust their body position to allow for maximum expansion of the chest and to avoid large meals, which increase abdominal pressure. Raising the head of the bed on blocks or placing pillows behind the back can be helpful too. Under normal circumstances, resting with the head elevated while taking slow, deep breaths reduces shortness of breath. In addition, emphasize that lying on the left side will displace the uterus off the vena cava and improve breathing. Having the patient periodically stand up and stretch their arms above their head and take a deep breath is helpful with relieving dyspnea. Also advise the patient to avoid exercise that precipitates dyspnea, to rest after exercise, and to avoid overheating in warm climates. If the patient still smokes, encourage them to stop.

Heartburn and Indigestion

Heartburn, also termed *gastroesophageal reflux*, is common during pregnancy. Heartburn and indigestion result when high progesterone levels cause relaxation of the cardiac sphincter, allowing food and digestive juices to flow backward from the stomach into the esophagus. Irritation of the esophageal lining occurs, causing the burning sensation known as *heartburn*. It occurs in 40% to 85% of people at some point during pregnancy with an increased frequency seen in the third trimester (Bianco, 2023). The pain may radiate to the neck and throat. It worsens when the person lies down, bends over after eating, or wears tight clothes. In addition, the stomach is displaced upward and compressed by the large uterus in the third trimester, thus limiting the stomach's capacity to empty quickly. Food sits, causing heartburn and indigestion.

Review the patient's usual dietary intake and suggest that they limit or avoid gas-producing or fatty foods and large meals. Instruct the patient to pay attention to the timing of the discomfort. Usually, it is heartburn when the pain occurs 30 to 45 minutes after a meal. Encourage the patient to maintain proper posture and remain in the sitting position for 1 to 3 hours after eating to prevent reflux of gastric acids into the esophagus by gravity. Urge the patient to consume small, frequent meals and eat slowly, chewing food thoroughly to prevent excessive swallowing of air, which can lead to increased gastric pressure. Instruct the patient to avoid foods that act as triggers, such as caffeinated drinks; greasy, gas-forming foods; citrus; spiced foods; chocolate; coffee; alcohol; and spearmint or peppermint. These items stimulate the release of gastric digestive acids, which may cause reflux into the esophagus. The patient should avoid late night or large meals and gum chewing. Finally, elevating the head of the bed by 10 to 30 degrees may help.

Dependent Edema

Edema, a term for swelling or puffiness, of the lower legs is common during pregnancy. Total body fluids increase by 6 to 8 L during pregnancy, most of which is extracellular. Swelling is the result of increased capillary permeability caused by elevated hormone levels and increased blood volume. Sodium and water are retained, and thirst increases. Edema occurs most often in dependent areas such as the legs and feet throughout the day due to gravity after walking, standing, and sitting in a chair for a long period of time or at the end of the day; it improves after a night's sleep. Warm weather or prolonged standing or sitting may increase edema. Appropriate suggestions to minimize dependent edema include:

- Elevate your feet and legs above the level of the heart periodically throughout the day.
- Wear compression stockings when standing or sitting for long periods.
- Change position frequently throughout the day.
- Walk at a sensible pace to help contract leg muscles to promote venous return.
- When taking a long car ride, stop to walk around every 2 hours.
- When standing, rock from the ball of the foot to the toes to stimulate circulation.
- Lie on your left side to keep the gravid uterus off the vena cava to return blood to the heart.
- Avoid foods high in sodium, such as lunch meats, potato chips, and bacon.
- Avoid wearing knee-high stockings.
- Drink six to eight glasses of water daily (Lockwood & Magriples, 2024b; Sterns, 2023).

CLINICAL REASONING ALERT

Generalized edema, especially if present on the face, accompanied by a sudden and rapid increase in weight (>5 lb/week [2.3 kg/week]) can signal preeclampsia and warrants further evaluation (August & Sibai, 2024).

Braxton Hicks Contractions

Braxton Hicks contractions are irregular, painless contractions that occur without cervical dilation. Typically, they intensify in the third trimester in preparation for labor. In reality, they have been present since early in the pregnancy but may have gone unnoticed. They are thought to increase the tone of uterine muscles for labor purposes (Raines & Cooper, 2023).

CONSIDER THIS!

One has to wonder sometimes why pregnant people go through what they do. During my first pregnancy, I was sick for the first 2 months. I would experience waves of nausea from the moment I got out of bed until midmorning. Needless to say, I wasn't the happiest. After the third month, my life seemed to settle down, and I was beginning to think that being pregnant wasn't too bad after all. For the moment, I was fooled. Then, during my last 2 months, another wave of discomfort struck—heartburn and constipation—a double whammy! I now feared eating anything that might trigger acid indigestion and also might remain in my body too long. I literally had to become the "fiber queen" to combat these two challenges. However, my suffering was well worth our bright-eyed baby girl in the end.

Thoughts: Despite the various discomforts associated with pregnancy, most people probably wouldn't change the end result. Do most pregnant people experience these discomforts? What suggestions could be made to reduce them?

Reassure the patient that these contractions are normal. Instruct the patient on how to differentiate between Braxton Hicks and labor contractions. Explain that true labor contractions usually grow longer, stronger, and closer together and occur at regular intervals. Walking usually strengthens true labor contractions, while Braxton Hicks contractions tend to decrease in intensity and taper off. Advise the patient to keep themselves well hydrated and to rest in a left-side–lying position to help relieve the discomfort. Suggest that the patient use breathing techniques to ease the discomfort.

NURSING MANAGEMENT TO PROMOTE SELF-CARE

Pregnancy is a natural event for many people and should be considered a time of health, not illness. Health promotion and maintenance activities are essential to promoting an optimal outcome for the pregnant person and their fetus. Pregnant people commonly have many questions about the changes occurring during pregnancy: how these changes affect usual routines, such as working, traveling, exercising, or engaging in sexual activity; how the changes influence typical self-care activities, such as bathing, perineal care, or dental care; and whether these changes are signs of a problem.

TAKE NOTE!

Patients may have heard stories about or been told by many others what to do and what not to do during pregnancy, leading to many misconceptions and much misinformation.

Nurses can play a major role in providing anticipatory guidance and teaching to foster the patient's responsibility for self-care, helping to clarify misconceptions and correct any misinformation. Educating the patient to identify threats to safety posed by their lifestyle or environment and proposing ways to modify them to avoid a negative outcome are important. Counseling should also include healthy ways to prepare food, advice to avoid medications unless they are prescribed for the patient, and advice on identifying teratogens within the patient's environment or at work and how to reduce the risk from exposure. The pregnant patient can better care for themselves and the fetus if their concerns are anticipated and identified by the nurse and are incorporated into teaching sessions at each prenatal visit.

Personal Hygiene

Hygiene is a necessity for the maintenance of good health. Cleansing the skin removes dirt, bacteria, sweat, dead skin cells, and body secretions. Counsel patients to wash their hands and under their fingernails frequently throughout the day in order to lower the bacterial count on both. During pregnancy, a person's sebaceous (sweat) glands become more active under the influence of hormones, and sweating is more profuse. This increase may make it necessary to use a stronger deodorant and shower more frequently. The cervical and vaginal glands also produce more secretions during pregnancy. Frequent showering helps keep the area dry and promotes better hygiene. Encourage the use of cotton underwear to allow greater air circulation. Taking a tub bath in early pregnancy is permitted, but closer to term, when the person's center of gravity shifts, it is safer to shower to prevent the risk of slipping.

Hot Tubs and Saunas

Caution pregnant people to avoid using hot tubs, saunas, whirlpools, and tanning beds during pregnancy. The heat may cause fetal tachycardia as well as raise the maternal temperature. Exposure to bacteria in hot tubs that have not been cleaned sufficiently is another reason to avoid them during pregnancy.

Perineal Care

The glands in the cervical and vaginal areas become more active during pregnancy secondary to hormonal influences. This increase in activity will produce more vaginal secretions, especially in the last trimester. Advise pregnant people to shower frequently and wear all-cotton underwear to minimize the effects of these secretions. Caution pregnant people not to douche, because douching can increase the risk of infection, and not to wear panty liners, which block air circulation and promote moisture. Explain that they should also avoid perfumed soaps, lotions, perineal sprays, and harsh laundry detergents to help prevent irritation and potential infection.

Dental Care

Oral health is integral to systemic health and has profound effects during pregnancy. It is essential in general health and well-being to maintain overall quality of life. Physiologic changes that occur in pregnant people, however, can adversely affect oral health. Elevations in estrogen and progesterone enhance the inflammatory response and consequently alter gingival tissue. During pregnancy, the incidence of gingivitis and periodontitis increases (Butera et al., 2023). Pregnancy is a time when a person can be receptive to health messaging. It is a time when nurses can help patients understand that good oral health and regular dental care are important to a healthy pregnancy and can decrease the risk of dental caries in their children. When people see oral health as a priority for themselves, they are more likely to place a high priority on their children's oral health.

Periodontal disease is a contributing factor to systemic conditions, such as heart disease, respiratory diseases, diabetes mellitus, and adverse pregnancy outcomes (preterm births, low-birth-weight infants, gestational diabetes, and preeclampsia) (Butera et al., 2023). Research has established that elevated levels of estrogen and progesterone during pregnancy cause people to be more sensitive to the effects of bacterial dental plaque, which can cause gingivitis, an oral infection characterized by swollen and bleeding gums (Butera et al., 2023).

Nurses should assess all pregnant patients' oral health status by taking oral health histories; checking their mouths for swollen or bleeding gums, untreated dental decay, mucosal lesions, and signs of infection; and documenting findings in the prenatal record. Oral health care and dental interventions should be completed before conception to prevent adverse pregnancy outcomes.

Additional guidelines that the nurse should stress regarding maintaining dental health include:

- Seek professional dental care before conception or during the first trimester for assessment and care and every 6 months for regular checkups throughout the pregnancy.
- Be reassured that dental x-rays and typical medications used in dental procedures are safe for the fetus.
- Be reassured that oral health care is safe during pregnancy in any trimester.
- Obtain treatment for dental pain and infection promptly during pregnancy.
- Brush twice daily for 2 minutes, especially before bed, with fluoridated toothpaste and rinse well. Use a soft-bristled toothbrush and be sure to brush at the gum line to remove food debris and plaque to keep gums healthy.
- Floss teeth daily with dental floss, and rinse well afterward with plain water.
- Eat healthy foods, especially those high in vitamins A, C, and D and calcium.
- Avoid sugary snacks.
- Do not smoke.
- Chew sugar-free gum for 10 minutes after a meal if brushing is not possible.
- After vomiting, rinse your mouth immediately with baking soda (1 tsp) and warm water (1 c) to neutralize the acid (March of Dimes, 2023).

Breast Care

Breast care during pregnancy helps to avoid problems during breastfeeding. Because the breasts enlarge significantly and become heavier throughout pregnancy, stress the need to wear a firm, supportive bra with wide straps to balance the weight of the breasts. Instruct the patient to anticipate buying a larger sized bra about halfway through their pregnancy because of the increasing size of the breasts. The nipples and areola may also double in size and darken. This darkening helps the newborn zero in on the nipple when feeding. Advise the patient to avoid using soap on the nipple area because it can be drying. Encourage the patient to rinse the nipple area with plain water while bathing to keep it clean. The Montgomery glands (located in the areolar part of the nipple) secrete a lubricating substance that keeps the nipples moist and discourages the growth of bacteria, so there is no need to use alcohol or other antiseptics on the nipples.

If the patient has chosen to breastfeed, nipple preparation is unnecessary unless their nipples are inverted and do not become erect when stimulated. During the last trimester, nipples may leak colostrum. Use breast pads inside the bra to soak up any leaks.

Clothing

Many clothes are loose fitting and layered, so the patient may not need to buy an entirely new wardrobe to accommodate their pregnancy. Some pregnant people may continue to wear tight clothes. Point out that loose clothing may be more comfortable for the patient and their expanding waistline.

Advise pregnant patients to avoid wearing constricting clothes and girdles that compress the growing abdomen. Urge the patient to avoid knee-high pantyhose, which might impede lower extremity circulation and increase the risk of developing DVT. Low-heeled shoes will minimize pelvic tilt and possible backache. Wearing layered clothing that can be removed as the temperatures fluctuate may be more comfortable, especially toward term, when the patient may feel overheated.

Exercise

Regular physical exercise improves cardiovascular health, helps maintain a healthy BMI (18.5 to 24.9 kg/m^2) and avoid medical comorbidities associated with higher body weight, and improves longevity. A physically inactive lifestyle is associated with an increase in chronic diseases, such as cardiovascular disease, type 2 diabetes, osteoporosis, and cancer. The proportion of pregnant people who are overweight (BMI >25 kg/m^2) or have obesity (BMI >30 kg/m^2) is increasing globally, so exercise is essential to reduce these risks and promote a healthy pregnancy. Exercise is well tolerated by a healthy person during pregnancy (Fig. 12.10). It promotes a feeling of well-being; improves circulation; helps reduce constipation, bloating, and swelling; may help prevent or treat gestational diabetes; reduces the risk of developing hypertensive disorders of pregnancy; promotes muscle tone, strength, and endurance; increases likelihood of vaginal birth; increases energy level; improves posture; helps sleep and promotes relaxation and rest; and relieves pregnancy-related musculoskeletal discomforts, such as lower back discomfort and lumbopelvic and pelvic girdle pain (Artal, 2024). However, the duration and difficulty of exercise should be modified throughout pregnancy because of a decrease in performance efficiency with gestational age. At least 30 minutes of moderate-intense physical activity daily (ideally 150 minutes per week) is recommended (Cooper & Yang, 2023). Some pregnant people continue to push themselves to maintain their prior level of exercise, but most find that as their shape changes and their abdominal area enlarges, they must modify their exercise routines. Modification also helps to reduce the risk of injury caused by laxity of the joints and connective tissue due to the hormonal effects. Exercise during pregnancy is contraindicated in people with preterm labor, placenta previa, incompetent cervix, second- or third-trimester bleeding, preterm premature rupture of membranes, significant heart or lung disease, preeclampsia, or severe anemia (Cooper & Yang, 2023). It is believed that pregnancy is a unique time for behavior modification and that healthy behaviors maintained or adopted during pregnancy may improve the person's health for the rest of their life. Exercise helps the person to avoid gaining excess weight during pregnancy.

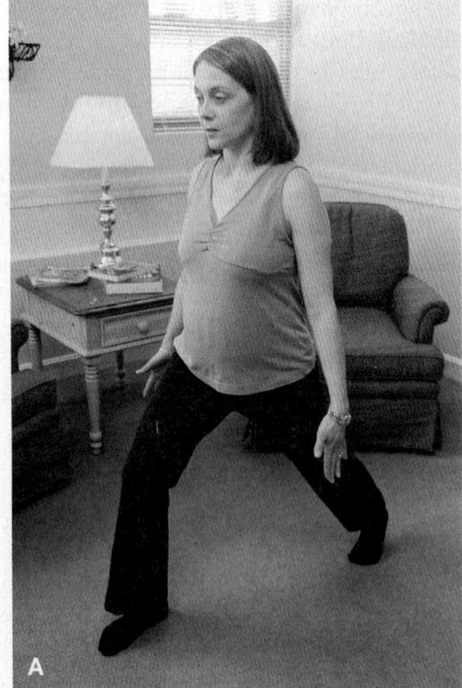

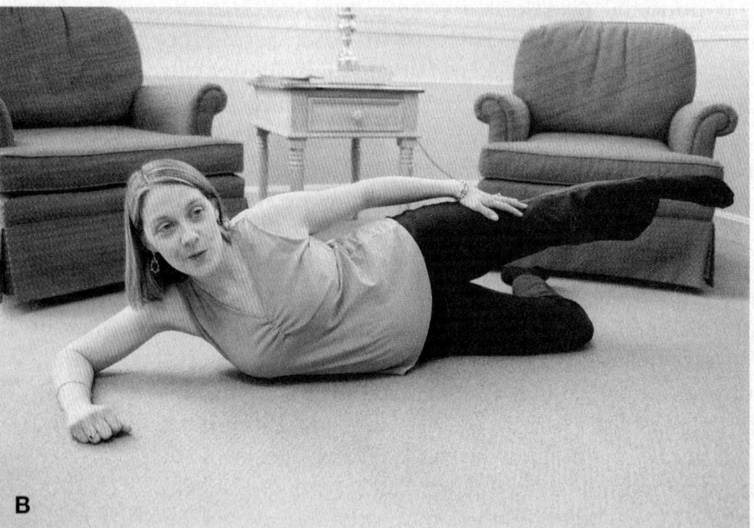

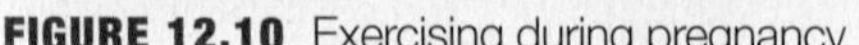

FIGURE 12.10 Exercising during pregnancy.

Teaching Guidelines 12.2 highlights recommendations for exercise during pregnancy.

Sleep and Rest

Getting enough sleep helps a person feel better and promotes optimal performance levels during the day. The body releases its greatest concentration of growth hormone during sleep, helping the body repair damaged tissue and grow. Also, with the increased metabolic demands during pregnancy, fatigue is a constant challenge to many pregnant people, especially during the first and third trimesters. Chronic sleep deprivation lowers the body's immune system and appears to be linked to gestational diabetes mellitus; poor sleep appears to be a risk factor for preterm birth, low birth weight, painful labor, surgical delivery, and depression (Pacheco & Callender, 2023). The following tips can help promote adequate sleep:

- Stay on a regular schedule by going to bed and waking up at the same times.
- Eat regular meals at regular times to keep external body cues consistent.
- Take time to unwind and relax before bedtime.
- Prioritize sleep—it is one of the healthiest things for the body.
- Establish a bedtime routine or pattern and follow it.
- Avoid any electronic screen use for at least 1 hour prior to bedtime.
- Create a proper sleep environment by reducing the light and lowering the room temperature.
- Go to bed when you feel tired; if sleep does not occur, read a book until you are sleepy.
- Avoid naps late in the day.
- Reduce caffeine intake later in the day; avoid caffeine after noon.
- Limit fluid intake after dinner to minimize trips to the bathroom.
- Exercise daily to improve circulation and well-being.
- Use a modified Sims position to improve circulation in the lower extremities; use pillows to help with comfort (under the knees and abdomen and behind the back).
- Avoid lying on your back after the fourth month, which may compromise circulation to the uterus.
- Keep anxieties and worries out of the bedroom. Set aside a specific area in the home or time of day for them (Lockwood & Magriples, 2024b).

TEACHING GUIDELINES 12.2 Promoting Exercise During Pregnancy

- Consume liquids before, during, and after exercising.
- Consult with your health care provider before you start a new exercise routine.
- Avoid exercising in hot, humid weather or when you have a fever.
- Stop exercising and notify your health care provider if you experience vaginal bleeding, dizziness, syncope, chest pain, headache, muscle weakness that affects balance, calf pain or swelling, uterine contractions, decreased fetal movement, or fluid leaking from the vagina.
- Exercise three or four times each week, not sporadically.
- Engage in brisk walking, swimming, biking, or low-impact aerobics; these are considered ideal activities.
- Avoid getting overheated during exercise.
- Wear comfortable exercise footwear that gives strong ankle and arch support.
- Contact sports should be avoided during pregnancy.
- Include relaxation and stretching before and after your exercise program.
- Reduce the intensity of workouts in late pregnancy.
- Avoid jerky, bouncy, or high-impact movements.
- Avoid lying flat (supine) after the fourth month because of hypotensive effect.
- Use pelvic tilt and pelvic rocking to relieve backache.
- Start with 5–10 minutes of stretching exercises.
- Rise slowly following an exercise session to avoid dizziness.
- Avoid activities such as skiing, surfing, scuba diving, and ice hockey.
- Never exercise to the point of exhaustion.

Cooper, D. B., & Yang, L. (2023). Pregnancy and exercise. In *StatPearls*. StatPearls Publishing. https://www.ncbi.nlm.nih.gov/books/NBK430821/; Artal, R. (2024). Exercise during pregnancy and the postpartum period. *UpToDate.* Retrieved May 28, 2024, from https://www.uptodate.com/contents/exercise-during-pregnancy-and-the-postpartum-period

Sexual Activity and Sexuality

Sexuality is a central aspect of human existence, present throughout all phases of the life cycle, and an important part of health and well-being. Pregnancy is characterized by intense biologic, psychological, and social changes. These changes have direct and indirect, conscious and unconscious effects on a person's sexuality. The person experiences dramatic alterations in their physiology, appearance, body, and relationships. Contraindications to sexual intercourse during pregnancy include unexplained vaginal bleeding, placenta previa, ruptured membranes, preterm cervical dilatation/effacement, and preterm contractions (Lockwood & Magriples, 2024b). A person's sexual responses during pregnancy vary widely.

Common symptoms and discomforts of pregnancy such as fatigue, nausea, vomiting, breast soreness, urinary frequency, changing shape, and fetal activity may reduce the person's desire for sexual intimacy. However, many pregnant people report enhanced sexual desire due to increasing levels of estrogen, resulting in an increase in pelvic congestion and lubrication that may heighten orgasm. Usually, sexual satisfaction does not change in pregnancy compared with the prepregnancy patterns despite a decline in sexual activity during the third trimester. A discussion of expected changes in sexuality should be routinely done in order to improve the patient's or couple's perception of possible sexual modifications induced by pregnancy. It is clear that despite some difficulties related to sexual activity during pregnancy, its need and importance are recognized for both participants.

TAKE NOTE!

Fluctuations in sexual desire are normal and a highly individualized response throughout pregnancy.

Often, pregnant people ask whether sexual intercourse is allowed during pregnancy or whether there are specific times when they should refrain from having sex. This is a good opportunity to educate patients about sexual behavior during pregnancy and also to ask about their expectations and individual experience related to sexuality and possible changes. It is also a good time for nurses to address the impact of the changes associated with pregnancy on sexual desire and behavior. People may enjoy sexual activity more because there is no fear of pregnancy and no need to disrupt spontaneity by using birth control.

If applicable to your patient, inform the patient or couple that engaging in sexual activity, including vaginal penetration, will not injure the fetus. Suggest that certain positions may be more comfortable (e.g., the pregnant person on top or side lying) than others, especially during the later stages of pregnancy. Some of the physical changes in pregnancy, which can affect a couple's relationship, for example, halitosis that can result from dehydration, can still be alleviated, in this case with extra fluids and better oral hygiene. Pregnant people can have breast tenderness and skin changes that can cause them to feel less attractive to the partner during pregnancy. In addition, they can be worried about increases in vaginal discharge and need to know what is expected and what can be a sign of infection. Nurses should make patients feel comfortable talking about their fears, encouraging them to find acceptance of their changing bodies.

Employment

Globally, most people work throughout their pregnancies for reasons such as career fulfillment, career advancement, financial necessity, keeping health insurance coverage, and saving leave time for the postpartum period. Fifty-six percent of pregnant people in the United States worked full time during their first pregnancy (Fowler & Culpepper, 2024). For the most part, people can continue working until giving birth if they have no complications during pregnancy and the workplace does not present any special hazards. Hazardous occupations include health care workers, daycare providers and teachers, construction crews, manufacturing workers, service workers and flight attendants, firefighters and law enforcement, and farm and greenhouse workers (National Institute for Occupational Safety and Health [NIOSH], 2024). Jobs requiring strenuous work such as heavy lifting, climbing, carrying heavy objects, and standing for prolonged periods place a pregnant person at risk for complications, such as miscarriage or preterm birth, if modifications are not instituted (NIOSH, 2024).

Assess for environmental and occupational factors that place the pregnant person and their fetus at risk for injury. Interview the patient about their employment environment. Ask about possible exposure to teratogens (substances with the potential to alter the fetus permanently in form or function) and the physical demands of employment: Is the patient exposed to temperature extremes? Do they need to stand for prolonged periods in a fixed position? A description of the work environment is important in providing anticipatory guidance to the patient.

Because of the numerous physiologic and psychosocial changes that people experience during their pregnancies, the employer may need to make special accommodations to reduce the pregnant person's risk of hazardous exposures and heavy workloads. The employer may need to provide adequate coverage so that the person can take rest breaks, remove the person from any areas where they might be exposed to toxic substances, and avoid work assignments that require heavy lifting, hard physical labor, continuous standing, or constant moving. Some recommendations for working while pregnant are provided in Teaching Guidelines 12.3.

Travel

Pregnancy does not curtail a person's ability to travel in a car or in a plane. However, the pregnant person should follow a few safety guidelines to minimize the risk to themselves and their fetuses. According to ACOG (2023a), pregnant people can travel safely throughout pregnancy, although mid-pregnancy (14 to 28 weeks) is perhaps the best time to travel because there is the least chance of complications. Pregnant people considering international travel should evaluate the problems that could occur during the journey as well as the quality of medical care available at the destination.

A person in the third trimester should be advised to defer international travel because of concerns about access to medical care in case of problems such as

TEACHING GUIDELINES 12.3 Teaching for the Pregnant Person Who Is Working

- Plan to take rest periods throughout the day and be sure there is a place available for you to rest, preferably in the side-lying position, with a restroom readily available.
- Avoid jobs that require strenuous workloads; if this is not possible, then request a modification of work duties (lighter tasks) to reduce your workload.
- Change your position from standing to sitting or vice versa at least every 2–3 hours.
- Ensure that you are allowed time off without penalty, if necessary, to ensure a healthy outcome for you and your fetus.
- Make sure the work environment is free of toxic substances.
- Ensure the work environment is smoke free so passive smoke inhalation is not a concern.
- Minimize stooping, bending, squatting, and heavy lifting.
- Reduce or avoid lifting heavy objects from the floor, lifting heavy objects while reaching or bending, and lifting or reaching overhead.

Adapted from National Institute for Occupational Safety and Health. (2024). *About physical job demands and reproductive health.* https://www.cdc.gov/niosh/reproductive-health/prevention/physical-demands.html

hypertension, Zika virus and malaria infection from mosquito bites, phlebitis, or premature labor. Some airlines will allow travel until 36 weeks' gestation, but always check before booking (CDC, 2022). Pregnant people should be advised to consult with their health care providers before making any travel decisions.

TAKE NOTE!

Clinical manifestations that indicate the need for immediate medical attention while traveling are vaginal bleeding, pelvic or abdominal pain or cramps, contractions, symptoms of preeclampsia (generalized swelling, severe headache, nausea and vomiting, and vision changes), ruptured membranes, hypertension, excessive leg swelling or pain, and dehydration (CDC, 2022; Ram et al., 2023).

Advise pregnant patients to be aware of the potential for injuries and traumas related to traveling and teach them ways to prevent these from occurring. Teaching Guidelines 12.4 offers tips for safe travel on planes and to foreign areas.

When traveling by car, the major risk is a collision. Motor vehicle crashes account for more than 50% of all traumas during pregnancy and a large percentage of fetal deaths occurring during these crashes (Krywko et al., 2022). The impact and momentum can lead to traumatic separation of the placenta from the wall of the uterus. Shock and massive hemorrhage might result. Tips that nurses can offer to promote safety during ground travel include:

- Always wear a three-point seat belt, no matter how short the trip, to prevent ejection or serious injury from collision.
- Apply a nonpadded shoulder strap properly; it should cross between the breasts and over the upper

TEACHING GUIDELINES 12.4 Promoting Safe Travel on Planes and During International Travel

- Bring along a copy of the prenatal record if your travel will be prolonged in case there is a medical emergency away from home.
- Before leaving home, find hospitals or clinics that provide obstetric care near where you will be staying.
- Understand your health insurance plan and coverage for travel.
- Travel with at least one companion at all times for personal safety.
- Check with your health care provider before receiving any immunizations necessary for foreign travel; some may be harmful to the fetus.
- Depending on which country you are visiting, avoid fresh fruit, vegetables, and local water.
- Avoid any milk that is not pasteurized.
- Depending on the country you are visiting, consume only bottled water to prevent microbial diarrhea.
- Avoid destinations with extremely hot weather and high altitudes.
- Eat only meat that is well cooked to avoid exposure to toxoplasmosis.
- Request an aisle seat and walk about the airplane every 2 hours.
- While sitting on long flights, practice calf-tensing exercises to improve circulation to the lower extremities.
- Be aware of typical problems encountered by pregnant travelers, such as fatigue, heartburn, indigestion, constipation, vaginal discharge, leg cramps, urinary frequency, and hemorrhoids.
- Always wear support hose while flying to prevent the development of blood clots.
- Drink plenty of water to keep well hydrated throughout the flight.
- Postpone travel if risks outweigh benefits.

American College of Obstetricians and Gynecologists. (2023a). *Travel during pregnancy.* https://www.acog.org/womens-health/faqs/travel-during-pregnancy; and Centers for Disease Control and Prevention. (2022). *Pregnant travelers.* https://wwwnc.cdc.gov/travel/page/pregnant-travelers

abdomen, above the uterus; the lap portion should sit on your hip bones, below your belly (Fig. 12.11).

- If no seat belts are available (buses or vans), ride in the back seat of the vehicle.
- Leave the airbag operational. Move the seat as far back from the dashboard as possible to minimize impact on the abdomen.
- Never use a cellular phone while driving to prevent distraction.
- As much as possible, avoid sharp turns and sudden braking while driving.
- Adjust your seatbelt to be comfortable; leave as much space between it and the abdomen as possible.
- Plan driving breaks to stretch legs, use the restroom, and refresh.
- Stay hydrated and well fed to keep blood glucose level stable.
- Avoid driving at night on unfamiliar or rural roads.
- Avoid driving when fatigued and in the first and third trimesters.
- Avoid late night driving when visibility might be compromised.
- Direct a tilting steering wheel away from the abdomen (ACOG, 2023a).

Immunizations and Medications

Vaccines are among the greatest primary prevention public health achievements of the 21st century, credited with significant reduction of morbidity and mortality from many diseases caused by bacteria and viruses. Ideally, patients should receive all childhood immunizations before conception to protect the fetus from any risk of congenital anomalies. If the patient comes for a preconception visit, review the adult immunization schedule such as measles, mumps, and rubella (MMR) (given 1 month or more before pregnancy); varicella (3 months before pregnancy); tetanus, diphtheria, and pertussis (Tdap); flu; COVID-19 (recommended before, during, and after pregnancy); pneumonia; certain types of meningitis; and hepatitis A and B (Yawetz, 2024).

The risk to a developing fetus from vaccination of the pregnant person is primarily theoretical. However, no evidence exists of risk from vaccinating pregnant people with inactivated virus or bacterial vaccines or toxoids (Yawetz, 2024). Routine immunizations are not usually indicated during pregnancy; if performed, the theoretical risks of vaccination must be weighed against the risks of the disease to the pregnant person and fetus (Yawetz, 2024).

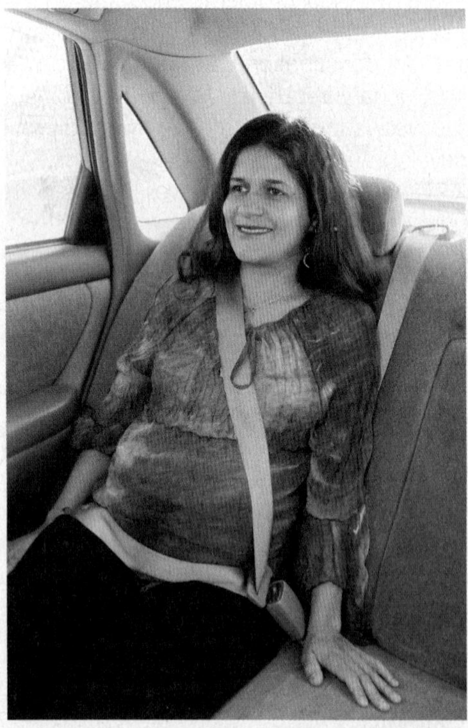

FIGURE 12.11 Proper application of a seat belt during pregnancy.

TAKE NOTE!

Advise pregnant patients to avoid live virus vaccines (MMR and varicella). Advise female patients to avoid becoming pregnant within 28 days after receiving the MMR vaccination or 3 months after receiving varicella vaccination because of the theoretical risk of transmission to the fetus (Yawetz, 2024).

The CDC guidelines for vaccine administration are outlined in Box 12.5.

BOX 12.5 CDC Guidelines for Vaccine Administration During Pregnancy

Vaccines That Should Be Considered Unless Contraindicated

- Hepatitis B
- Influenza (inactivated) injection
- Tetanus, diphtheria, and pertussis (Tdap)
- Respiratory syncytial virus (RSV)
- COVID-19

Vaccines to Avoid During Pregnancy

- Influenza (live, attenuated vaccine) nasal spray
- Human papillomavirus (HPV)
- Measles
- Mumps
- Rubella
- Varicella
- BCG (tuberculosis)
- RZV (recombinant zoster vaccine)
- Typhoid`

Yawetz, S. (2024). Immunizations during pregnancy. *UpToDate.* Retrieved May 28, 2024, from https://www.uptodate.com/contents/immunizations-during-pregnancy; and Immunize.org & ACOG. (2023). *Vaccinations needed during pregnancy.* https://www.immunize.org/catg.d/p4040.pdf

About 80% of people in the United States take at least one OTC or prescription medication while they are pregnant (U.S. Food & Drug Administration [USFDA], 2023a). Not all medicines are safe to take during pregnancy, since they have not been tested on pregnant people.

Pregnant people use a wide variety of both prescription and OTC medications for both pregnancy-related conditions and conditions unrelated to pregnancy conditions. Emphasize to the patient that they should always ask a health care professional before taking any medicines, herbs, or vitamins (USFDA, 2023a). Little is known about the effects of taking most medications during pregnancy. Less than 10% of medications approved by the FDA since 1980 have enough information to determine their risk for birth defects (CDC, 2024f). Based on this lack of evidence, it is best for pregnant people to not take any medications during their pregnancy. At the very least, encourage them to discuss with the health care provider their current medications and any herbal remedies they take so that they can learn about any potential risks should they continue to take them during pregnancy. In general, if the patient is taking medicine for seizures, high blood pressure, or asthma, the benefits of continuing the medicine during pregnancy outweigh the risks to the fetus. The safety profile of some medications may change according to the gestational age of the fetus. Embryogenesis is completed by the end of the first trimester, when all fetal organs are complete. Thus, avoiding fetal drug exposure in the first 12 weeks of gestation is crucial (Lockwood & Magriples, 2024b).

The FDA has developed a system of ranking drugs that appears on drug labels and package inserts. These risk categories are summarized in Box 12.6. Always advise patients to check with their health care providers for guidance.

BOX 12.6 FDA Pregnancy Risk Classification of Drugs

- The "Pregnancy" subsection of each drug's information will provide information relevant to the use of the drug in pregnant people, such as dosing and potential risks to the developing fetus, and will require information about whether there is a registry that collects and maintains data on how pregnant people are affected when they use the drug or biologic product. Information in drug labeling about the existence of any pregnancy registries has been previously recommended, but not required until now. This subsection includes labor and birth.
- The "Lactation" subsection will provide information about using the drug while breastfeeding, such as the amount of drug in human milk and potential effects on the breastfed child.
- The "Females and Males of Reproductive Potential" subsection will include information about pregnancy testing, contraception, and infertility as it relates to the drug. This information has been included in labeling, but there was no consistent placement for it until now.

Leek, J. C., & Arif, H. (2023). Pregnancy medications. In *StatPearls*. StatPearls Publishing. https://www.ncbi.nlm.nih.gov/books/NBK507858/

A common concern of many pregnant people involves the use of OTC medications and herbal agents. Although OTC medications may seem harmless and herbal medications are commonly thought of as "natural" alternatives to other medicines, they can be just as potent as some prescription medications. A major concern about herbal medicine is the lack of consistent potency in the active ingredients in any given batch of product, making it difficult to know the exact strength by reading the label. Also, many herbs contain chemicals that cross the placenta and may cause harm to the fetus.

Nurses are often asked about the safety of OTC medicines and herbal agents. Unfortunately, many drugs have not been evaluated in controlled studies, and it is difficult to make general recommendations for these products. Therefore, encourage pregnant patients to check with their health care providers before taking anything. Questions about the use of OTC and herbal products are part of the initial prenatal interview.

NURSING CARE TO PREPARE THE PATIENT AND THEIR PARTNER FOR LABOR, BIRTH, AND PARENTHOOD

Pregnancy and birth are unique to every person. Individual people and families hold different expectations during childbearing based on their knowledge, experiences, belief systems, culture, and social and family backgrounds. These differences should be understood and respected by the nurse, and care for them adapted to meet the individual needs of the pregnant person and families. Knowing a pregnant person's needs, values, cultural background, preferences, and expectations during childbirth helps nurses provide high-quality care to them. Childbirth today is a different experience from childbirth in past generations. In the past, pregnant people were literally "put to sleep" with anesthetics, and they woke up with a baby. Most birthing people never remembered the details and had a passive role in childbirth as the primary provider delivered the newborn. In the 1950s, consumers began to insist on taking a more active role in their health care, and couples desired to be together during the extraordinary event of childbirth. Compared to the past, there is a stronger push for partners of pregnant people to play a greater role in the pregnancy and childbirth today. Partners want to be seen as individuals who are part of the childbirth experience. If they are left out, they tend to feel helpless; this can result in a feeling of panic and anxiety that can put support for the birthing person at risk. Perinatal nurses need to make sure that partners are invited to be involved and that they feel vital in the childbirth experience.

Health beliefs related to pregnancy and childbirth exist in various cultures. A pregnant person's perception of their own status is critical to their decision-making process, because their personal behaviors can significantly alter their pregnancy-related risks. Pregnant people come from diverse cultures and hold a number of beliefs related to diet, behavior related to prenatal care, and the use of herbs during pregnancy and after birth. Nurses need to be aware of these cultural beliefs so as to incorporate these into their practices while respectfully discouraging the use of those posing any health risks. To move forward as a profession, nursing must address inequities and unconscious biases so nurses can deliver culturally responsive care that is respectful for every patient (Johnson, 2022).

Childbirth education began because people demanded to become more involved in their birthing experience rather than simply turning control over to a health care provider. Nurses played a pivotal role in bringing about this change by providing information and supporting patients and their families, fostering a more active role in preparing for the upcoming birth.

Traditional childbirth education classes focused on developing and practicing techniques for use in managing pain and facilitating the progress of labor. Today, the focus of this education has broadened. The term used to describe this broad range of topics is **perinatal education**. Subjects commonly addressed in perinatal education include:

- Anatomy and physiology of birth
- Fetal growth and development
- Prenatal maternal exercise
- Physiologic and emotional changes during pregnancy
- Sex during pregnancy
- Infant growth and development
- Nutrition and healthy eating habits during pregnancy
- Teratogens and their impact on the fetus
- Signs and symptoms of labor
- Right to respectful nursing care
- Preparation for labor and birth (for parents, siblings, and other family members)
- Options for birth
- Ways the partner can be supportive during labor and birth
- A variety of comfort measures including techniques for relaxing and ways to cope during labor
- Pain management approaches for labor
- Complications of labor and birth and ways to prevent and manage them
- Positions for birth
- Infant nutrition, including preparation for breastfeeding
- Infant care, including safety, cardiopulmonary resuscitation, and first aid
- Family planning, including contraception (Prabhu, 2024)

Childbirth Education Classes

Childbirth education classes teach pregnant people and their support people about pregnancy, birth, and parenting. The classes are offered in local communities or online and are usually taught by certified childbirth educators. The major focus is to provide pregnant people with confidence in their own ability to give birth, to increase their knowledge and support needed to make decisions about the childbirth process that is congruent with their values and preferences, to foster their comfort as labor progresses by using learned techniques, and to see that they are supported by family, friends, and professionals (Prabhu, 2024). Many childbirth classes support the concept of **natural childbirth** (a birth without pain-relieving medications) so that the pregnant person can be in control throughout the experience as much as they choose. The classes differ in their approach to specific comfort techniques and breathing patterns. The three most common childbirth methods are the Lamaze (psychoprophylactic) method, the Bradley (partner-coached childbirth) method, and the Dick-Read (natural childbirth) method.

Lamaze Method

Lamaze is a psychoprophylactic ("mind prevention") method of preparing for labor and birth that promotes the use of specific breathing and relaxation techniques. Dr. Fernand Lamaze, a French obstetrician, popularized this method of childbirth preparation in the 1960s. Lamaze believed that conquering fear through knowledge and preparation, along with conditioning to diminish the pain reflex, was important (Prabhu, 2024). Lamaze felt strongly that all pregnant people have the right to deliver their babies with minimal or no medication while maintaining their dignity, minimizing their pain, maximizing their self-esteem, and enjoying the miracle of birth.

Contemporary Lamaze classes continue with the philosophy that birth is normal and natural, and breathing is one of many comfort strategies taught (Prabhu, 2024). The breathing techniques are used in labor to enhance relaxation and to reduce the birthing person's perception of pain. The goal is for pregnant people to become aware of their own comfortable rate of breathing in order to maintain relaxation and adequate oxygenation of the fetus. The following breathing techniques are an effective attention-focusing strategy to reduce pain:

- *Paced breathing* involves breathing techniques used to decrease stress responses and, therefore, decrease pain. This type of breathing implies self-regulation by the birthing person. The person starts off by taking a cleansing breath at the onset and end of each contraction. This cleansing breath symbolizes freeing the person's mind from worries and concerns. This breath enhances oxygenation and puts the person in a relaxed state.

- *Slow-paced breathing* is associated with relaxation and should be half the normal breathing rate (6 to 9 breaths per minute). This type of breathing is the most relaxed pattern and is recommended throughout labor. Abdominal or chest breathing may be used. It is generally best to breathe in through the nose and breathe out either through the nose or through the mouth, whichever is more comfortable for the person.
- *Modified-paced breathing* can be used for increased work or stress during labor to increase alertness or focus attention or when slow-paced breathing is no longer effective in keeping the person relaxed. The person's respiratory rate increases, but it does not exceed twice their normal rate. Modified-paced breathing is a quiet upper chest breath that is increased or decreased according to the intensity of the contraction. The inhalation and the exhalation are equal. This breathing technique should be practiced during pregnancy for optimal use during labor.
- *Patterned-paced breathing* is similar to modified-paced breathing but with a rhythmic pattern. It uses a variety of patterns, with an emphasis on the exhalation breath at regular intervals. Different patterns can be used, such as 4/1, 6/1, and 4/1. A 4/1 rhythm is four upper chest breaths followed by an exhalation (a sighing out of air, like blowing out a candle). Random patterns can be chosen for use as long as the basic principles of rate and relaxation are met.

Pregnant people and their support people practice these breathing patterns typically during the last few months of the pregnancy until they feel comfortable using them. Focal points (visual fixation on a designated object), effleurage (light abdominal massage by the birthing person or support person), massage, and imagery (journey of the mind to a relaxing place) are also added to aid in relaxation. Breathing is only one of many comfort strategies taught. Birthing people are now encouraged to work with their labor, find comfort within their contractions, push when they feel the urge to push, and not let the labor control their bodies (Prabhu, 2024). From the nurse's perspective, encourage the patient to breathe at a level of comfort that allows them to cope. Always remain quiet during the patient's periods of imagery and focal point visualization to avoid breaking their concentration.

Bradley (Partner-Coached) Method

The Bradley method uses various exercises and slow, controlled abdominal breathing to accomplish relaxation. Dr. Robert Bradley, a Denver-based obstetrician, advocated a completely unmedicated labor and birth experience. In 1965, Bradley wrote *Husband-Coached Childbirth*, which advocated for the active participation of the partner as labor coach.

A pregnant person is conditioned to work in harmony with their body using breath control and deep abdominopelvic breathing to promote general body relaxation during labor. This method stresses that childbirth is a joyful, natural process and emphasizes the partner's involvement during pregnancy, labor, birth, and the early newborn period. Thus, the training techniques are directed toward the coach, not the birthing person. The coach is educated in massage and comfort techniques to use on the birthing person throughout the labor and birth process.

Dick-Read Method

In 1944, Grantly Dick-Read, a British obstetrician, wrote *Childbirth Without Fear.* He believed that the attitude of a person toward their birthing process had a considerable influence on the ease of the person's labor, and he believed that fear is the primary pain-producing agent in an otherwise normal labor. He proposed that fear builds a state of tension, creating an antagonistic effect on the laboring muscles of the uterus, which results in pain. A private, undisturbed, and dark environment, where the birthing person can feel safe, can promote the release of oxytocin, the hormone responsible for uterine contractions thought to promote the release of the pain-relieving hormones endorphins. When this is not achieved, people can experience fear–tension–pain syndrome, impeding labor progress and causing increased levels of pain (Prabhu, 2024). Dick-Read sought to interrupt the circular pattern of fear, tension, and pain during the labor and birthing process.

Dick-Read believed that prenatal instruction was essential for pain relief and that emotional factors during labor interfered with the normal labor progression. The pregnant person achieves relaxation and reduces pain by arming themselves with the knowledge of normal childbirth and using abdominal breathing during contractions.

HYPNOBIRTHING METHOD

HypnoBirthing is a spinoff of the Dick-Read method with self-hypnosis added. It was created by hypnotherapist Marie Mongan and detailed in her 1989 book, *HypnoBirthing—A Celebration of Life*. With the aid of hypnosis, the birthing person can bring their body into a state of deep relaxation and allow their muscles to work in a way that is supportive of childbirth. This method is based on the power of suggestion, relaxation, breathing, meditation, and body toning. The birthing person can use positive suggestions and visualizations to relax their body, guide their thoughts, and control their breathing.

Nursing Management and Childbirth Education

Childbirth education is less about methods than about mastery. The overall aim of any method is to promote an internal locus of control that will enable each birthing person to yield their body to the process of birth. As the person gains success and tangible benefits from the exercises they are taught, they begin to reframe their beliefs and gain practical knowledge, and the impetus will be there for the person to engage in the conscious use of the techniques (Fig. 12.12). Nurses play a key role in supporting and encouraging each birthing person's and support person's use of the techniques taught in childbirth education classes.

Every birthing person's labor is unique, and it is important for nurses not to generalize or stereotype their patients. The most effective support a nurse can offer a person using prepared childbirth methods is encouragement and presence. These nursing measures must be adapted to each patient throughout the labor process. Offering encouraging phrases such as "great job" or "you can do it" helps reinforce their efforts and at the same time empowers them to continue. Using eye contact to engage the birthing person's total attention is important if they appear overwhelmed or appear to lose control during the transition phase of labor.

Nurses play a significant role in enhancing the birthing person and support person's relationship by respecting the involvement of the partner and demonstrating concern for their needs throughout labor. Offering to stay with the birthing person to give the partner a break periodically allows them to meet their needs while at the same time still actively participating. Offer anticipatory guidance to the birthing person and their partner and assist during critical times in labor. Demonstrate many of the coping techniques to the partner and praise their successful use to increase self-esteem. Focus on strengths and the positive elements of the labor experience. Congratulating both the patient and the support person for a job well done is paramount.

Throughout the labor experience, demonstrate personal warmth and project a friendly attitude. Frequently, a nurse's touch may help prevent a crisis by reassuring the patient they are doing well.

Options for Birth Settings and Care Providers

From the moment a person discovers they are pregnant, numerous decisions await them—where the infant will be born, which birth setting is best, and who will assist with the birth. The majority of pregnant people are well and healthy and can consider the full range of birth settings—hospital, birth center, or home setting—and care providers. They should be given information about each to ensure the most informed decision.

Birth Settings

HOSPITALS

Hospitals are the most common site for birth in the United States. If the pregnant person has a serious medical condition or is at high risk for developing one, they will probably need to plan to give birth in a hospital setting under the care of an obstetrician. Giving birth in a hospital is advantageous for several reasons. Hospitals are best equipped to diagnose and treat birthing people and newborns with complications, trained personnel are available if necessary, and no transportation is needed if a complication should arise during labor or birth. Disadvantages include the clinical atmosphere, strict policies and restrictions that might limit who can be with the birthing person, and the medical model of care.

Within the hospital setting, however, choices do exist regarding birth environments. The conventional delivery room resembles an operating room, where the health care professional delivers the newborn from the birthing person, who is positioned in stirrups. The patient is then

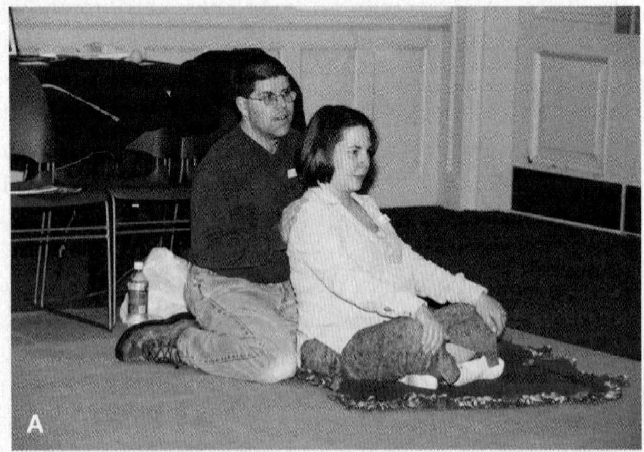

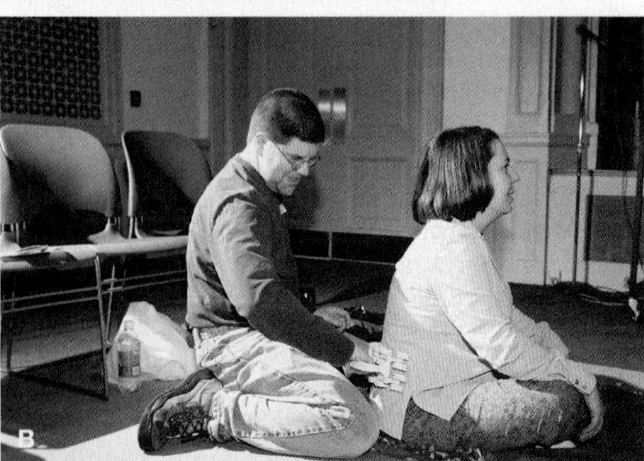

FIGURE 12.12 A couple practicing the techniques taught in a childbirth education class. **A.** Practicing breathing techniques to use during labor. **B.** Partner practicing applying sacral pressure.

transferred to the recovery area on a stretcher and then again to the postpartum unit. The birthing suite is the other option within the hospital setting. In the birthing suite, the birthing person and their partner or support person remain in one place for labor, birth, and recovery. The birthing suite is a private room decorated to look as home-like as possible. For example, the bed converts to allow for various birthing positions, and there may be a rocking chair or an easy chair for the birthing person's partner. Despite the homey atmosphere, the room is still equipped with emergency resuscitative obstetric equipment and electronic fetal monitors in case they are needed quickly (Fig. 12.13A). Such settings provide a more personal childbirth experience in a less formal and intimidating atmosphere compared to the traditional delivery room.

FREESTANDING BIRTH CENTERS

A freestanding birth center offers birthing people a comfortable setting where they can receive maternity care with appropriate levels of intervention. A freestanding birth center (Fig. 12.13B) can be a good choice for a person who wants more personalized care than that of a hospital, but does not feel comfortable with a home birth. In contrast to the institutional environment in hospitals, most freestanding birth centers have a home-like atmosphere, and many are located in converted homes. Some are located on hospital property and are affiliated with the hospitals. Birth centers are designed to provide maternity care to birthing people judged to be at low risk for obstetric complications. People are allowed and encouraged to give birth in the position most comfortable for them. Care in birth centers is often provided by midwives and is more relaxed, with no routine intravenous lines, fetal monitoring, and restrictive protocols. A disadvantage of the birth center is the need to transport the birthing person to a hospital quickly if an emergency arises because emergency equipment is not readily available. Research shows that in low-risk pregnancies, maternal outcomes are better and neonatal outcomes are the same or better in birth centers when compared to hospital care (Alliman et al., 2022). Personal preferences, risk status, and available birth setting options should be considered in a person's or couple's decision making regarding whether to use a freestanding birth center (Alliman et al., 2022).

> **TAKE NOTE!**
>
> A recent study showed that people giving birth at a community birth center experienced reduced racial and ethnic disparities and reduced experiences of discrimination when compared to a hospital-based system (Almanza et al., 2021).

HOME BIRTHS

Home births in the United States comprise approximately 1.5% of all births, which is the highest percentage since 1990 when home birth recording first started (Declercq & Stotland, 2024). Most people who choose a home birth believe that birth is a natural process that requires little medical intervention and express a desire for freedom and personal control in the birth process (Declercq & Stotland, 2024). Research has shown that people believe that planned home births increase comfort and convenience, increase freedom of choice and control over the birth process, limit newborn and birthing parent separation, are associated with reduced rates of medical interventions, and facilitate family involvement in a relaxed, peaceful atmosphere (Declercq & Stotland, 2024).

The safety of home births is a topic of ongoing debate in the United States. The ACOG states that hospitals and accredited birth centers are the safest settings for birth; however, they recognize that each pregnant person has the right to make their own decision regarding delivery (ACOG, 2023b). The ACOG considers planned home birth to be safe as long as the birthing person and

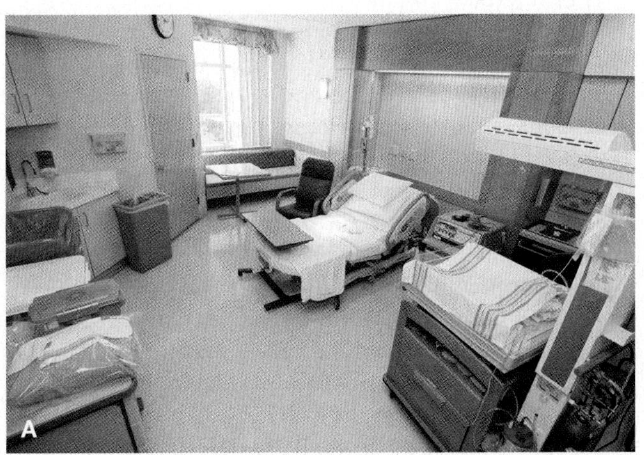

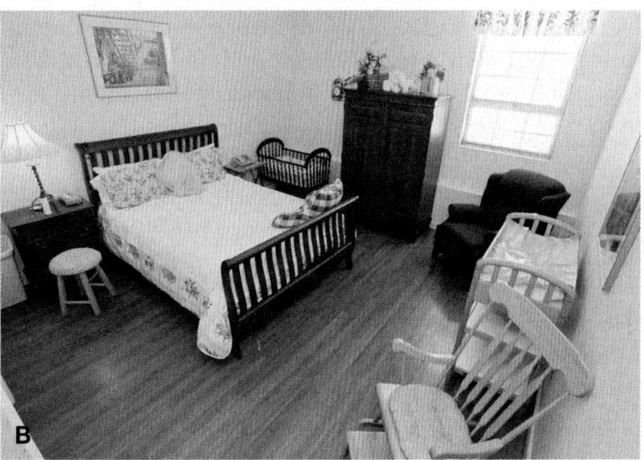

FIGURE 12.13 **A.** Birthing suite in hospital setting. **B.** Childbirth room in birthing center.

the pregnancy meet certain criteria, such as a low-risk pregnancy, singleton fetus, cephalic fetus at term, and no prior cesarean birth (ACOG, 2023b). Home births can be safe if there are qualified, experienced attendants and an emergency transfer system in place in case of complications. Many pregnant people choose the home setting out of a strong desire to control birth and to give birth surrounded by family members. Most home birth caregivers are midwives who have provided continuous care to the birthing person throughout the pregnancy. Disadvantages include the need to transport the person to the hospital during or after labor if a problem arises and the limited pain management available in the home setting.

Care Providers

While most pregnant people in the United States still receive pregnancy care from an obstetrician, an increasing number are choosing midwives for their care. The difference is a matter of degrees. Obstetricians must finish a 4-year residency in obstetrics and gynecology in addition to medical school. Certified nurse midwives are registered nurses who have graduated from a nurse midwifery education program accredited by the Accreditation Commission for Midwifery Education (ACME) and have passed a national certification examination to receive the professional designation of certified nurse midwife. As of 2010, a graduate degree is required for entry into midwifery practice in the United States. Midwives usually care for people with low-risk pregnancies in a variety of settings. They are able to write prescriptions and provide prenatal care, childbirth care, postpartum care, newborn care, and well-woman care throughout the lifespan. Family practice doctors also provide maternity, woman's care, and well-baby care. Many deliver their patients' newborns in hospitals or birthing centers. Obstetricians can handle high-risk pregnancies and delivery emergencies, can administer or order pain-relief drugs, and are assisted by support staff in the hospital setting. Midwives work in hospitals, birthing centers, and home settings to deliver care. They believe in normalizing birth and tolerating wide variations of what is considered normal during labor, which leads to fewer interventions applied during the process. Certified nurse midwives attend approximately 10.3% of total U.S. births (American College of Nurse-Midwives, 2022). Midwives do handle high-risk and emergency births, but because many are not always predictable, they typically have an obstetrician as backup when they do occur to assist them.

In addition to the pregnant person's primary health care provider, some people hire a doula to be with them during the childbearing process. "Doula" is a Greek word that means "woman's servant." A doula is a layperson trained to provide birthing people and their families with encouragement, emotional and physical support, and information through late pregnancy, labor, birth, and postpartum. Doulas provide birthing people with continuous support throughout labor but do not perform any clinical procedures.

Preparation for Breastfeeding or Bottle-Feeding

Pregnant people are faced with a decision about which method of feeding to choose. Educate the pregnant patient about the advantages and disadvantages of each method, allowing the patient and their partner to make an informed decision about the best method for their situation. Providing the patient and their partner with this information will increase the likelihood of a successful experience, regardless of the method of feeding chosen. As part of health promotion and evidence-based interventions, nurses should be encouraging and educating all pregnant patients about breastfeeding while respecting each patient's ultimate decision.

Breastfeeding

Substantial scientific evidence documents the health benefits of breastfeeding for newborns. The AAP, the American Academy of Family Physicians, the ACOG, and the World Health Organization recommend that infants be breastfed exclusively until the age of 6 months and then continue to be breastfed for a year and/or for as long as it is mutually desired, with appropriate solid foods introduced (Meek, 2024). In addition, a lack of breastfeeding contributes to a negative impact on the health care system by increasing the number of patient visits, the number of hospital admissions, and health care costs.

Human milk provides an ideal balance of nutrients for newborns (Meek, 2024). Breastfeeding is advantageous for the following reasons:

- Human milk is digestible and economical and requires no preparation.
- Bonding between the breastfeeding parent and child is promoted.
- Cost is less than purchasing formula.
- Ovulation is suppressed (however, this is not a reliable birth control method).
- It reduces the risk of ovarian, breast, and endometrial cancer.
- It reduces the risk of maternal cardiovascular disease and type 2 diabetes.
- Oxytocin is released to promote more rapid uterine involution with less bleeding.
- Sucking helps to develop the muscles in the infant's jaw.
- The immunologic properties of human milk help prevent infections in the baby.
- It reduces the risks of the baby developing otitis media, respiratory disease, gastroenteritis and diarrhea,

urinary tract infections, neonatal sepsis, sudden unexpected infant death (SUID), allergic conditions, celiac disease, inflammatory bowel disease, childhood obesity (BMI >30 kg/m^2), type 1 and type 2 diabetes, and leukemia and lymphoma.
- Absorption of lactose and minerals in the newborn is improved.
- The composition of human milk adapts to meet the infant's changing needs as they grow.
- Human milk offers neurobehavioral benefits for the infant and appears to have an analgesic effect (Meek, 2024; Perez-Escamilla & Segura-Perez, 2024).

Some people assume that lactation and breastfeeding are so natural that they should just happen on their own accord, but this is not the case. Learning to breastfeed takes practice, requires support from the partner, and requires dedication and patience on the part of the breastfeeding person; it may be necessary to work closely with a lactation consultant to be successful and comfortable when breastfeeding. Figure 12.14 shows the different positions that may be used for breastfeeding. Nurses can encourage breastfeeding for all birthing parents, except those who are HIV positive and are untreated or who do not have sustained viral suppression, who have human T-lymphotropic retrovirus (HTLV) I or HTLV II infection, who use illicit drugs, or who have suspected or confirmed Ebola virus (Kellams, 2024a). Nurses can also advise new parents who breastfeed their infants that once breastfeeding is well established (usually within the first 2 to 4 weeks), a pacifier can be offered (Kellams, 2024b).

Breastfeeding has some uncomfortable side effects for the breastfeeding parent, including breast discomfort, sore nipples, nipple blebs or milk blisters, mastitis, engorgement, breast abscess, *Candida* infection, milk stasis, and flat or inverted nipples (Spencer, 2024). The most common cause of nipple pain is an improper latch, and such discomfort is usually piercing, immediate, and short-lived, typically occurring as soon as the baby starts nursing and gradually subsiding during the feeding. Some people feel breastfeeding is inconvenient or embarrassing, limits other activities, limits partner involvement, increases their dependency by being tied to the infant all the time, and restricts their use of alcohol or drugs. Nurses can help breastfeeding parents cope with their fear of dependency and feelings of obligation by emphasizing the positive aspects of breastfeeding and encouraging bonding experiences. Nurses can be instrumental in helping parents prepare and continue to breastfeed after they return to work.

PREPARATION FOR BREASTFEEDING

Nipple preparation is not necessary during the prenatal period unless the nipples are inverted and do not become erect when stimulated. Assess for this by placing the forefinger and thumb above and below the areola and compressing behind the nipple. If it flattens or inverts, enlist assistance from lactation experts during the first stages of breastfeeding (Kellams, 2024b). Early recognition and assistance is the key to success (Kellams, 2024b). Encourage the patient to request a certified lactation specialist (CLS) at the hospital, if giving birth there. Lactation specialists are health care providers who specialize in the clinical management of breastfeeding. Some run their own breastfeeding support groups as well. In addition, suggest that the patient attends a breastfeeding support group (e.g., La Leche League), provide them with sources of information about infant feeding, and suggest they read a good reference book about lactation. All of these activities will help in the patient's decision-making process and will be invaluable to them should they choose to breastfeed their newborn. Breastfeeding parents returning to work can pump their breasts and store the milk in the freezer for future use.

Bottle-Feeding

Once the placenta no longer provides nutrition, a newborn's survival depends on the ability to consume nutrients.

Bottle-feeding an infant is not just a matter of "open, pour, and feed." Parents need information on the types of formulas, preparation and storage of formula, equipment, and feeding positions. It is recommended that normal full-term infants receive conventional cow's milk-based formulas; the primary provider should direct this choice. If the infant has a reaction (diarrhea, vomiting, abdominal pain, excessive gas) to the first formula, another formula should be tried. Sometimes a soy-based formula is substituted. In terms of preparation of formula and its use, the following guidelines should be stressed:

- Obtain adequate equipment (six 4-oz bottles, eight 8-oz bottles, and nipples).
- Consistency is important. Stay with a nipple that is comfortable to the infant.
- Frequently assess nipples for any loose pieces of rubber at the opening.
- Correct formula preparation is critical to the health and development of the infant. Formula is available in three forms: ready-to-feed, liquid concentrate, and powder.
- Read the formula label thoroughly before mixing.
- Using the formula before the "use by" date is important to guarantee the nutrient content and quality of the formula.
- All feeding items should be cleaned after every use.
- Correct formula dilution is important to avoid fluid imbalances. For ready-to-use formula, use as is without dilution. For concentrated formulas, dilute with equal parts of water. For powdered formulas, follow the instructions on the infant formula container. Always measure water first, then the powder.

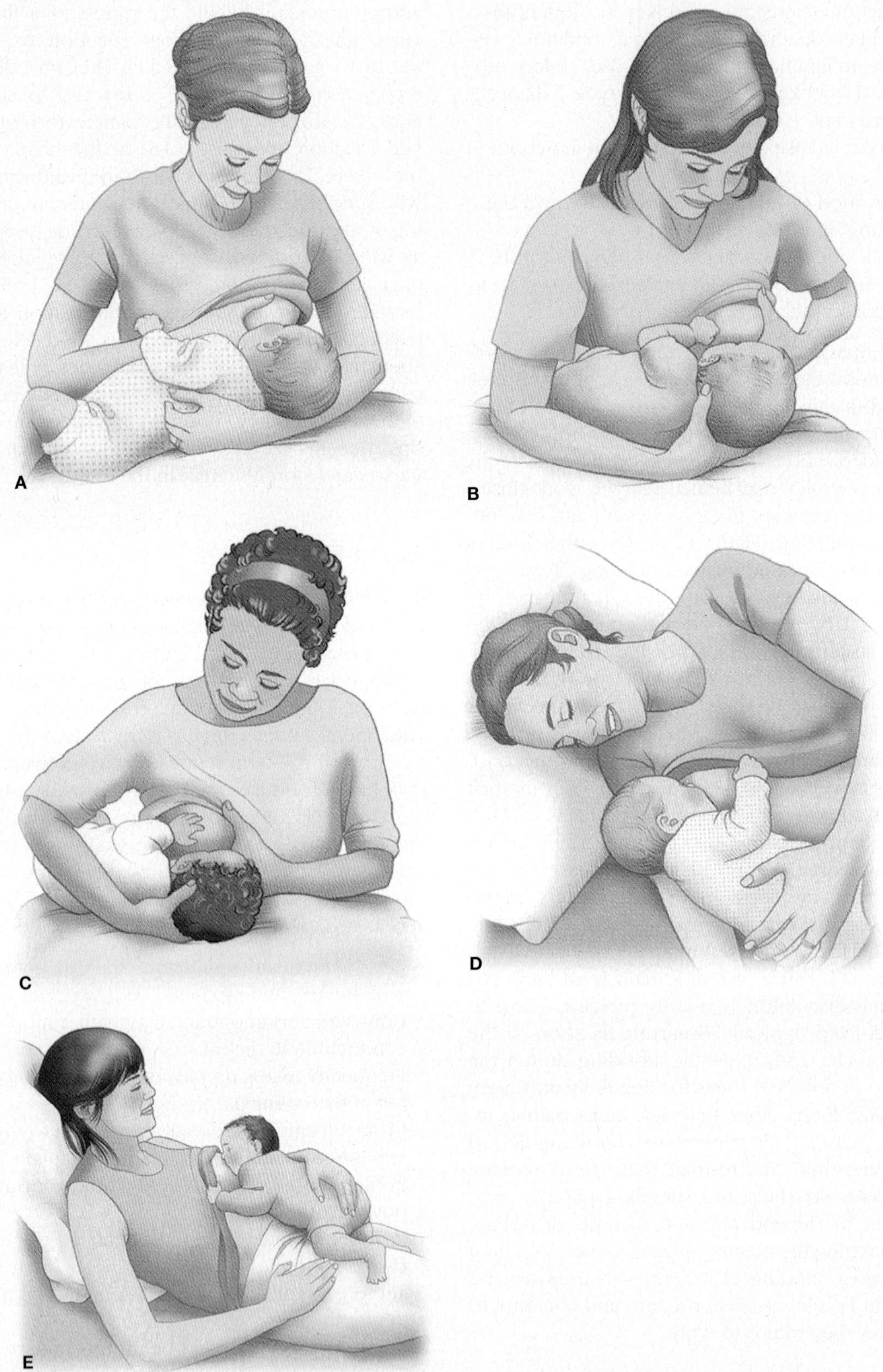

FIGURE 12.14 Positions for breastfeeding. **A.** Cradle hold—infant's head is held in the breastfeeding parent's forearm to nurse. **B.** Cross cradle or transitional hold—infant is held along the opposite arm from the breast. **C.** Clutch or football hold—infant is held on breastfeeding parent's side hip almost under the parent's arm. **D.** Side-lying position—infant lies parallel to breastfeeding parent's side-lying position to nurse. **E.** Prone or laid-back position—infant lies stomach to stomach on top of breastfeeding parent to nurse. (From U.S. Department of Health and Human Services, Office on Women's Health. [2021]. *Getting a good latch.* https://www.womenshealth.gov/breastfeeding/learning-breastfeed/getting-good-latch#4)

- If the water supply is safe, sterilization is not necessary.
- If the water supply is questionable, water should be boiled for 5 minutes before use, or bottled water should be used.
- Bottles and nipples should be washed and sanitized in hot, sudsy water using a bottlebrush.
- Formula can be served at room temperature.
- Formula should not be heated in a microwave oven, because it is heated unevenly.
- Formula can be prepared 24 hours ahead of time and stored in the refrigerator. If it is not stored in the refrigerator, use it within 2 hours of preparation.
- If the baby is less than 2 months of age, was born premature, or has a weakened immune system, discuss with your health care provider the need for extra precautions (CDC, 2023; USFDA, 2023b).

Teach the birthing parent and other caregivers to feed the infant in a semi-upright position using the cradle hold in the arms. This position allows for face-to-face contact between the infant and the caregiver. Advise the caregiver to hold the bottle so that the nipple is kept full of formula to prevent excessive air swallowing. Instruct the caregiver to feed the infant every 3 to 4 hours and adapt the feeding times to the infant's needs. Frequent burping of the infant (every ounce) helps prevent gas from building up in the stomach. Caution the caregiver not to prop the bottle; doing so can cause choking.

Bottle-feeding should mirror breastfeeding as closely as possible. While nutrition is important, so are the emotional and interactive components of feeding. Encourage the caregiver to cuddle the infant closely and position the infant so that their head is in a comfortable position. Also encourage communication with the infant during feedings. Nurses should know the different types of formulas available to provide advice to parents who have made the informed choice not to breastfeed or to stop breastfeeding.

TAKE NOTE!

Warn the caregiver about the danger of putting the infant to bed with a bottle. This can lead to "baby bottle tooth decay" (nursing caries) because sugars in the formula stay in contact with the infant's developing teeth for prolonged periods.

Final Preparation for Labor and Birth

The nurse has played a supportive and education role for the pregnant person or couple throughout the pregnancy and now needs to assist in preparing them for their "big event" by making sure they have made informed decisions and completed the following checklist:

- Attended childbirth preparation classes and practiced breathing techniques
- Selected a birth setting and made arrangements there
- Chose one or more people for continuous labor support
- Know what to expect during labor and birth; wrote out a birth plan
- Toured the birthing facility
- Packed a suitcase to take to the birthing facility when labor starts
- Made arrangements to have siblings and/or pets taken care of during labor
- Been instructed regarding signs and symptoms of labor and what to do
- Know what to do if membranes rupture prior to going into labor
- Know how to reach the health care provider when labor starts
- Communicated their needs and desires concerning pain management
- Discussed the possibility of a cesarean birth if complications occur
- Discussed possible names for the newborn
- Selected a feeding method (breast or bottle) with which they feel comfortable
- Made a decision regarding circumcision if the baby is male
- Purchased an infant safety car seat in which to bring their newborn home
- Decided on a pediatrician
- Have items needed to prepare for the newborn's homecoming:
  - Infant clothes in several sizes
  - Nursing bras
  - Infant crib with spaces between the slats that are 2 in or less apart
  - Diapers (cloth or disposable)
  - Feeding supplies (bottles and nipples if bottle-feeding)
  - Infant thermometer
- Selected a family planning method to use after the birth (Prabhu, 2024)

At each prenatal visit, the nurse has had the opportunity to discuss and reinforce the importance of being prepared for the birth of the child with the parents. It is now up to the parents to use the nurse's guidance and put it into action to be ready for the upcoming birth.

All nurses have the responsibility to impart their knowledge to all birthing people and their families—and that starts with teaching themselves first. The evidence is clear that birthing people have better outcomes when nurses intervene only when needed in the childbirth process. Nurses need to personalize their care to every patient based on that patient's needs, desires, and state of health. Nurses must focus on teaching patients and their families to understand the value of birth and its long-lasting effects on the family. In addition, nurses must provide information about birth settings that are safe, whether in the hospital, birth center, or at home. Any birth setting should provide continuous support in labor, allow the birthing person the freedom to move and assume positions of choice, offer nourishment of the person's body and spirit, use nonpharmacologic pain-relief modalities whenever possible, and ensure seamless, collaborative teamwork.

KEY CONCEPTS

- Preconception and interconception care include promotion of the health and well-being of a person and their partner before and between pregnancies. The goal of preconception and interconception care is to identify and modify any areas such as health problems, lifestyle habits, or social concerns that might unfavorably affect pregnancy.
- A thorough history and physical examination are performed on the initial prenatal visit.
- A primary aspect of nursing management during the antepartum period is counseling and educating the pregnant person and their partner to promote healthy outcomes for all involved.
- Nagele's rule can be used to establish the estimated date of birth. Using this rule, subtract 3 months from the month of the LMP, add 7 days to the first day of the LMP, then correct the year by adding 1 to it. This date is within plus or minus 2 weeks (the margin of error).
- Continuous prenatal care is important for a successful outcome. The recommended schedule is every 4 weeks up to 28 weeks (7 months), every 2 weeks from 29 to 36 weeks, and every week from 37 weeks to birth.
- The height of the fundus is measured when the uterus arises out of the pelvis to evaluate fetal growth.
- The fundus reaches the level of the umbilicus at approximately 20 weeks and measures 20 cm. The fundal measurement should approximately equal the number of weeks of gestation until week 36.
- At each visit, the patient is asked whether they are having any common signs or symptoms of preterm labor, which might include uterine contractions, dull backache, pressure in the pelvic area or thighs, increased vaginal discharge, menstrual-like cramps, and vaginal bleeding.
- Prenatal screening has become standard in prenatal care to detect neural tube defects and genetic abnormalities.
- The nurse should matter-of-factly address common discomforts that occur in each trimester at all prenatal visits and should provide realistic measures to help the patient deal with them effectively.
- The pregnant patient can better care for themselves and the fetus if their concerns are anticipated by the nurse and incorporated into guidance sessions at each prenatal visit.
- Iron and folic acid need to be supplemented because their increased requirements during pregnancy are usually too great to be met through diet alone.
- Throughout pregnancy, a well-balanced diet is critical for a healthy baby.
- Perinatal education has broadened its focus to include preparation for pregnancy and family adaptation to the new parenting roles. Childbirth education began because of increasing pressure from consumers who wanted to become more involved in their birthing experience.
- Common childbirth education methods are Lamaze (psychoprophylactic), Bradley (partner-coached childbirth), Dick-Read (natural childbirth), and HypnoBirthing (hypnosis).
- Most pregnant people in the United States are well and healthy and can consider the full range of birth settings: hospital, birth center, or home.
- All pregnant people need to be able to recognize early signs of contractions to prevent preterm labor.

Unfolding Patient Stories: Amelia Sung • Part 1

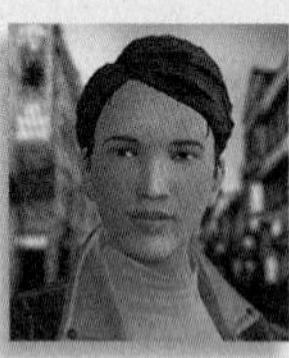

Amelia Sung is 36 years old and 8 weeks' pregnant with her second child. She tells the nurse that she is considering an amniocentesis due to her age. What information would the nurse include when providing education on amniocentesis? (Amelia Sung's story continues in Chapter 20.)

Care for Amelia and other patients in a realistic virtual environment: ***vSim** for Nursing* (**thepoint.lww.com/vSimMaternity**). Practice documenting these patients' care in DocuCare (**thepoint.lww.com/DocuCareEHR**).

REFERENCES AND RECOMMENDED READINGS

Adams, E. D. (2022). Anatomic and physiologic adaptations of normal pregnancy. In K. D. Schuiling & F. E. Likis (Eds.), *Gynecologic health care* (4th ed., pp. 677–682). Jones & Bartlett Learning.

Adams, E. D., & Schuiling, K. D. (2022). Common complications of pregnancy. In K. D. Schuiling & F. E. Likis (Eds.), *Gynecologic health care* (4th ed., pp. 697–712). Jones & Bartlett Learning.

Adigun, O. O., Yarrarapu, S. N. S., Zubair, M., & Khetarpal, S. (2024). Alpha-fetoprotein analysis. In *StatPearls*. StatPearls Publishing. https://www.ncbi.nlm.nih.gov/books/NBK430750/

Alliman, J., Bauer, K., & Williams, T. (2022). Freestanding birth centers: An evidence-based option for birth. *Journal of Perinatal Education, 31*(1), 8–13. https://doi.org/10.1891/JPE-2021-0024

Almanza, J. I., Karbeah, J. M., Tessier, K. M., Neerland, C., Stoll, K., Hardeman, R. R., & Vedam, S. (2021). The impact of culturally-centered care on peripartum experiences of autonomy and respect in community birth centers: A comparative study. *Maternal and Child Health Journal, 26*, 895–904. https://doi.org/10.1007/s10995-021-03245-w

Altemani, A. H., & Alzaheb, R. A. (2022). The prevention of gestational diabetes mellitus (The role of lifestyle): A meta-analysis. *Diabetology & Metabolic Syndrome, 14*, 83. https://doi.org/10.1186/s13098-022-00854-5

American College of Nurse-Midwives. (2022). *Fact sheet: Essential facts about midwives.* https://www.midwife.org/acnm/files/cclibraryfiles/filename/000000008273/EssentialFactsAboutMidwives_Final_2022.pdf

American College of Obstetricians and Gynecologists. (2019, reaffirmed 2020). Prepregnancy counseling. ACOG Committee Opinion No. 762. *Obstetrics & Gynecology, 133*, e78–e89. https://www.acog.org/clinical/clinical-guidance/committee-opinion/articles/2019/01/prepregnancy-counseling

American College of Obstetricians and Gynecologists. (2023a). *Travel during pregnancy.* https://www.acog.org/womens-health/faqs/travel-during-pregnancy

American College of Obstetricians and Gynecologists. (2023b). *Committee on Obstetric Practice: Planned home birth.* https://www.acog.org/clinical/clinical-guidance/committee-opinion/articles/2017/04/planned-home-birth

American Diabetes Association. (2023). *Classification and diagnosis of diabetes: Standards of care in diabetes—2023.* https://diabetesjournals.org/care/article/46/Supplement_1/S19/148056/2-Classification-and-Diagnosis-of-Diabetes

Artal, R. (2024). Exercise during pregnancy and the postpartum period. *UpToDate.* Retrieved May 28, 2024, from https://www.uptodate.com/contents/exercise-during-pregnancy-and-the-postpartum-period

August, P., & Sibai, B. M. (2024). Preeclampsia: Clinical features and diagnosis. *UpToDate.* Retrieved May 28, 2024, from https://www.uptodate.com/contents/preeclampsia-clinical-features-and-diagnosis

Bermas, B. L. (2023). Maternal adaptations to pregnancy: Musculoskeletal changes and pain. *UpToDate.* Retrieved May 27, 2024, from https://www.uptodate.com/contents/maternal-adaptations-to-pregnancy-musculoskeletal-changes-and-pain

Bianco, A. (2023). Maternal adaptations to pregnancy: Gastrointestinal tract. *UpToDate.* Retrieved May 27, 2024, from https://www.uptodate.com/contents/maternal-adaptations-to-pregnancy-gastrointestinal-tract

Blau, L. E., Lipsky, L. M., Dempster, K. W., Eisenberg Colman, M. H., Siega-Riz, A. M., Faith, M. S., & Nansel, T. R. (2020). Women's experience and understanding of food cravings in pregnancy: A qualitative study in women receiving prenatal Care at the University of North Carolina-Chapel Hill. *Journal of the Academy of Nutrition and Dietetics, 120*(5), 815–824. https://doi.org/10.1016/j.jand.2019.09.020

Boothe, E., Olenderek, M., Noyola, M. C., Rushing, J., Allred, E., & Kaplan, S. (2022). Psychosocial outcomes of group prenatal care. *Journal of Public Health, 30*, 1373–1380. https://doi.org/10.1007/s10389-020-01441-6

Bordoni, B., Sugumar, K., & Varacallo, M. (2023). Muscle cramps. In *StatPearls*. StatPearls Publishing. https://www.ncbi.nlm.nih.gov/books/NBK499895/

Butera, A., Maiorani, C., Morandini, A., Trombini, J., Simonini, M., Ogliari, C., & Scribante, A. (2023). Periodontitis in pregnant women: A possible link to adverse pregnancy outcomes. *Healthcare (Basel, Switzerland), 11*(10), 1372. https://doi.org/10.3390/healthcare11101372

Buzinskiene, D., Sabonyte-Balsaitiene, Z., & Poskus, T. (2022). Perianal diseases in pregnancy and after childbirth: Frequency, risk factors, impact on women's quality of life and treatment methods. *Frontiers in Surgery, 9*, 788823. https://doi.org/10.3389/fsurg.2022.788823

Centers for Disease Control and Prevention. (2006). *Recommendations to improve preconception health and health care—United States.* https://www.cdc.gov/mmwr/preview/mmwrhtml/rr5506a1.htm

Centers for Disease Control and Prevention. (2022). *Pregnant travelers.* https://wwwnc.cdc.gov/travel/page/pregnant-travelers

Centers for Disease Control and Prevention. (2023). *Infant formula preparation and storage.* https://www.cdc.gov/nutrition/infantandtoddlernutrition/formula-feeding/infant-formula-preparation-and-storage.html

Centers for Disease Control and Prevention. (2024a). *About planning for pregnancy.* https://www.cdc.gov/pregnancy/about/index.html

Centers for Disease Control and Prevention. (2024b). *Pregnancy complications.* https://www.cdc.gov/maternal-infant-health/pregnancy-complications/

Centers for Disease Control and Prevention. (2024c). *Alcohol and pregnancy.* https://www.cdc.gov/alcohol-pregnancy/about/index.html

Centers for Disease Control and Prevention. (2024d). QuickStats: Percentage of mothers with gestational diabetes, by maternal age—National Vital Statistics System, United States, 2016 and 2021. *MMWR Morbidity and Mortality Weekly Report 2023, 72*, 16. http://dx.doi.org/10.15585/mmwr.mm7201a4

Centers for Disease Control and Prevention. (2024e). *Screening and testing for HIV, viral hepatitis, STD & tuberculosis in pregnancy.* https://www.cdc.gov/pregnancy-hiv-std-tb-hepatitis/php/screening/

Centers for Disease Control and Prevention. (2024f). *Medicine and pregnancy: An overview.* https://www.cdc.gov/medicine-and-pregnancy/about/index.html

Cooper, D. B., & Yang, L. (2023). Pregnancy and exercise. In *StatPearls*. StatPearls Publishing. https://www.ncbi.nlm.nih.gov/books/NBK430821/

Declercq, E., & Stotland, N. E. (2024). Planned home birth. *UpToDate.* Retrieved May 29, 2024, from https://www.uptodate.com/contents/planned-home-birth

Dukhovny, S., & Wilkins-Haug, L. (2024). Neural tube defects: Overview of prenatal screening, evaluation, and pregnancy management. *UpToDate*. Retrieved May 27, 2024, from https://www.uptodate.com/contents/neural-tube-defects-overview-of-prenatal-screening-evaluation-and-pregnancy-management

Durnwald, C. (2023). Gestational diabetes mellitus: Screening, diagnosis, and prevention. *UpToDate*. Retrieved May 26, 2024, from https://www.uptodate.com/contents/gestational-diabetes-mellitus-screening-diagnosis-and-prevention

Edwards, K. I., & Itzhak, P. (2023). Estimated date of delivery. In *StatPearls*. StatPearls Publishing. https://www.ncbi.nlm.nih.gov/books/NBK536986/

Faber, R., Heling, K. S., Steiner, H., & Gembruch, U. (2021). Doppler ultrasound in pregnancy—Quality requirements of DEGUM and clinical application (part 2). *European Journal of Ultrasound, 42*(5), 541–550. https://doi.org/10.1055/a-1452-9898

Fischbach, F. T., Fischbach, M. A., & Stout, K. (2022). *A manual of laboratory and diagnostic tests* (11th ed.). Wolters Kluwer.

Fowler, J. R., & Culpepper, L. (2024). Working during pregnancy. *UpToDate*. Retrieved May 28, 2024, from https://www.uptodate.com/contents/working-during-pregnancy

Fowler, J. R., Jenkins, S. M., & Jack, B. W. (2023). Preconception counseling. In *StatPearls*. StatPearls Publishing. https://www.ncbi.nlm.nih.gov/books/NBK441880/

Fretts, R. C. (2024). Decreased fetal movement: Diagnosis, evaluation, and management. *UpToDate*. Retrieved May 26, 2024, https://www.uptodate.com/contents/decreased-fetal-movement-diagnosis-evaluation-and-management

Ghidini, A. (2023). Patient education: Chorionic villus sampling. *UpToDate*. Retrieved May 27, 2024, from https://www.uptodate.com/contents/chorionic-villus-sampling-beyond-the-basics

Ghidini, A. (2024). Diagnostic amniocentesis. *UpToDate*. Retrieved May 27, 2024, from https://www.uptodate.com/contents/diagnostic-amniocentesis

Gordon, S., & Langaker, M. D. (2023). Prenatal genetic screening. In *StatPearls*. StatPearls Publishing. https://www.ncbi.nlm.nih.gov/books/NBK557702/

Gosdin, L. K., Deputy, N. P., Kim, S. Y., Dang, E. P., & Denny, C. H. (2022). Alcohol consumption and binge drinking during pregnancy among adults aged 18–49 years—United States, 2018–2020. *MMWR Morbidity and Mortality Weekly Report, 71*, 10–13. http://dx.doi.org/10.15585/mmwr.mm7101a2

Gregory, K. D. (2023). *Reproductive life planning: A tool to shape your future*. https://www.acog.org/womens-health/experts-and-stories/the-latest/reproductive-life-planning-a-tool-to-shape-your-future

Health Resources & Services Administration. (2024). *Women's preventive services guidelines*. https://www.hrsa.gov/womens-guidelines

Huecker, B. R., Jamil, R. T., & Thistle, J. (2023). Fetal movement. In *StatPearls*. StatPearls Publishing. https://www.ncbi.nlm.nih.gov/books/NBK470566/

Immunize.org & ACOG. (2023). *Vaccinations needed during pregnancy*. https://www.immunize.org/catg.d/p4040.pdf

Jindal, A., Sharma, M., Karena, Z. V., & Chaudhary, C. (2023). Amniocentesis. In *StatPearls*. StatPearls Publishing. https://www.ncbi.nlm.nih.gov/books/NBK559247/

Johnson, C. (2022). Maternity care: How to address bias and increase cultural humility. *Kaiser Permanente*. https://www.kpihp.org/blog/maternity-care-how-to-address-bias-and-increase-cultural-humility/

Jones, T. M., & Montero, F. J. (2022). Chorionic villus sampling. In *StatPearls*. StatPearls Publishing. https://pubmed.ncbi.nlm.nih.gov/33085448/

Kellams, A. (2024a). Breastfeeding: Parental education and support. *UpToDate*. Retrieved May 29, 2024, from https://www.uptodate.com/contents/breastfeeding-parental-education-and-support

Kellams, A. (2024b). Initiation of breastfeeding. *UpToDate*. Retrieved May 29, 2024, from https://www.uptodate.com/contents/initiation-of-breastfeeding

Khekade, H., Potdukhe, A., Taksande, A. B., Wanjari, M. B., & Yelne, S. (2023). Preconception care: A strategic intervention for the prevention of neonatal and birth disorders. *Cureus, 15*(6), e41141. https://doi.org/10.7759/cureus.41141

Kipling, L., Bombard, J., Wang, X., & Cox, S. (2021). Cigarette smoking among pregnant women during the perinatal period: Prevalence and health care provider inquiries—Pregnancy Risk Assessment Monitoring System, United States, 2021. *MMWR Morbidity and Mortality Weekly Report, 73*, 393–398. http://dx.doi.org/10.15585/mmwr.mm7317a2

Krywko, D. M., Toy, F. K., Mahan, M. E., & Kiel, J. (2022). Pregnancy trauma. In *StatPearls*. StatPearls Publishing. https://www.ncbi.nlm.nih.gov/books/NBK430926/

Leek, J. C., & Arif, H. (2023). Pregnancy medications. In *StatPearls*. StatPearls Publishing. https://www.ncbi.nlm.nih.gov/books/NBK507858/

Livrinova, V., Petrov, I., Samardziski, I., Jovanovska, V., Boshku, A. A., Todorovska, I., Dabeski, D., & Shabani, A. (2019). Clinical importance of low level of PAPP-A in first trimester of pregnancy—An obstetrical dilemma in chromosomally normal fetus. *Open Access Macedonian Journal of Medical Sciences, 7*(9), 1475–1479. https://www.ncbi.nlm.nih.gov/pmc/articles/PMC6542385/

Lockwood, C. J. (2024). Preterm labor: Clinical findings, diagnostic evaluation, and initial treatment. *UpToDate*. Retrieved May 26, 2024, from https://www.uptodate.com/contents/preterm-labor-clinical-findings-diagnostic-evaluation-and-initial-treatment

Lockwood, C. J., & Magriples, U. (2023). Prenatal care: Second and third trimesters. *UpToDate*. Retrieved May 26, 2024, from https://www.uptodate.com/contents/prenatal-care-second-and-third-trimesters

Lockwood, C. J., & Magriples, U. (2024a). Prenatal care: Initial assessment. *UpToDate*. Retrieved May 26, 2024, from https://www.uptodate.com/contents/prenatal-care-initial-assessment

Lockwood, C. J., & Magriples, U. (2024b). Prenatal care: Patient education, health promotion, and safety of commonly used drugs. *UpToDate*. Retrieved May 27, 2024, from https://www.uptodate.com/contents/prenatal-care-patient-education-health-promotion-and-safety-of-commonly-used-drugs

Magriples, U. (2023). Group prenatal care. *UpToDate*. Retrieved May 26, 2024, from https://www.uptodate.com/contents/group-prenatal-care

Mandy, G. T. (2022). Preterm birth: Definitions of prematurity, epidemiology, and risk factors for infant mortality. *UpToDate*. Retrieved May 26, 2024, https://www.uptodate.com/contents/preterm-birth-definitions-of-prematurity-epidemiology-and-risk-factors-for-infant-mortality

Manning, F. A. (2023). Biophysical profile test for antepartum fetal assessment. *UpToDate*. Retrieved May 27, 2024, from https://www.uptodate.com/contents/biophysical-profile-test-for-antepartum-fetal-assessment

March of Dimes. (2023). *Dental health during pregnancy.* https://www.marchofdimes.org/find-support/topics/pregnancy/dental-health-during-pregnancy

McElrath, T., & Gerard, E. (2024). Management of epilepsy during preconception, pregnancy, and the postpartum period. *UpToDate.* Retrieved May 25, 2024, from https://www.uptodate.com/contents/management-of-epilepsy-during-preconception-pregnancy-and-the-postpartum-period

Meek, J. Y. (2024). Infant benefits of breastfeeding. *UpToDate.* Retrieved May 29, 2024, from https://www.uptodate.com/contents/infant-benefits-of-breastfeeding

Messerlian, G. M., Halliday, J. V., & Palomaki, G. E. (2022). Down syndrome: Overview of prenatal screening. *UpToDate.* Retrieved May 26, 2024, from https://www.uptodate.com/contents/down-syndrome-overview-of-prenatal-screening

Miller, D. A. (2023). Nonstress test and contraction stress test. *UpToDate.* Retrieved May 27, 2024, from https://www.uptodate.com/contents/nonstress-test-and-contraction-stress-test

Moise, K. J. (2023). RhD alloimmunization in pregnancy: Overview. *UpToDate.* Retrieved May 26, 2024, from https://www.uptodate.com/contents/rhd-alloimmunization-in-pregnancy-overview

Moise, K. J. (2024). RhD alloimmunization: Prevention in pregnant and postpartum patients. *UpToDate.* Retrieved May 26, 2024, from https://www.uptodate.com/contents/rhd-alloimmunization-prevention-in-pregnant-and-postpartum-patients

Nasser, Y. A., Muco, E., & Alsaad, A. J. (2023). Pica. In *StatPearls.* StatPearls Publishing. https://www.ncbi.nlm.nih.gov/books/NBK532242/

National Institute for Occupational Safety and Health. (2024). *About physical job demands and reproductive health.* https://www.cdc.gov/niosh/reproductive-health/prevention/physical-demands.html

Office on Women's Health. (2022). *Pregnancy complications.* https://www.womenshealth.gov/pregnancy/youre-pregnant-now-what/pregnancy-complications

Osterman, M. J. K., Hamilton, B. E., Martin, J. A., Driscoll, A. K., & Valenzuela, C. P. (2024). Births: Final data for 2022. *National Vital Statistics Reports, 73*(2). National Center for Health Statistics. https://dx.doi.org/10.15620/cdc:145588

Owen, C. (2024). Oral isotretinoin therapy for acne vulgaris. *UpToDate.* Retrieved May 25, 2024, from https://www.uptodate.com/contents/oral-isotretinoin-therapy-for-acne-vulgaris

Pacheco, D., & Callender, E. (2023). Pregnancy and sleep. *Sleep Foundation.* https://www.sleepfoundation.org/pregnancy

Paredes, C., Hsu, R. C., Tong, A., & Johnson, J. R. (2021). Obesity and pregnancy. *NeoReviews, 22*(2), e78–e87. https://doi.org/10.1542/neo.22-2-e78

Perez-Escamilla, R., & Segura-Perez, S. (2024). Maternal and economic benefits of breastfeeding. *UpToDate.* Retrieved May 29, 2024, from https://www.uptodate.com/contents/maternal-and-economic-benefits-of-breastfeeding

Phillippi, J. C., & Sanders, B. (2022). Overview of prenatal care. In K. D. Schuiling & F. E. Likis (Eds.), *Gynecologic health care* (4th ed., pp. 683–696). Jones & Bartlett Learning.

Pomeranz, M. K. (2023). Maternal adaptations to pregnancy: Skin and related structures. *UpToDate.* Retrieved May 28, 2024, from https://www.uptodate.com/contents/maternal-adaptations-to-pregnancy-skin-and-related-structures

Prabhu, M. (2024). Preparation for childbirth. *UpToDate.* Retrieved May 28, 2024, from https://www.uptodate.com/contents/preparation-for-childbirth

Raines, D. A., & Cooper, D. B. (2023). Braxton hicks contractions. In *StatPearls.* StatPearls Publishing. https://www.ncbi.nlm.nih.gov/books/NBK470546/

Ram, S., Ram, H. S., Neuhof, B., Shlezinger, R., Rosenthal, Y. S., Chodick, G., & Yogev, Y. (2023). Air travel during pregnancy and the risk of venous thrombosis. *American Journal of Obstetrics & Gynecology,* 5(1), 100751. https://doi.org/10.1016/j.ajogmf.2022.100751

Rani, P., & Dhok, A. (2023). Effects of pollution on pregnancy and infants. *Cureus, 15*(1), e33906. https://doi.org/10.7759/cureus.33906

Reed, J., Case, S., & Rijhsinghani, A. (2023). Maternal obesity: Perinatal implications. *SAGE Open Medicine, 11,* 20503121231176128. https://doi.org/10.1177/20503121231176128

Sapoval, J., Singh, V., & Carter, R. E. (2023). Ultrasound biophysical profile. In *StatPearls.* StatPearls Publishing. https://www.ncbi.nlm.nih.gov/books/NBK539866/

Sarker, M. R., Skeith, A. E., Bacheller, H., Caughey, A. B., & Valent, A. M. (2019). 344: Impact of delayed initiation of prenatal care on neonatal outcomes. *American Journal of Obstetrics & Gynecology, 220*(1), S240. https://doi.org/10.1016/j.ajog.2018.11.365

Shipp, T. D. (2023). Overview of ultrasound examination in obstetrics and gynecology. *UpToDate.* Retrieved May 26, 2024, from https://www.uptodate.com/contents/overview-of-ultrasound-examination-in-obstetrics-and-gynecology

Siccardi, M. A., Imonugo, O., Arbor, T. C., & Valle, C. (2023). Anatomy, abdomen and pelvis, pelvic inlet. In *StatPearls.* StatPearls Publishing. https://www.ncbi.nlm.nih.gov/books/NBK519068

Sim, M., Logan, S., & Goh, L. H. (2020). Vaginal discharge: Evaluation and management in primary care. *Singapore Medical Journal, 61*(6), 297–301. https://doi.org/10.11622/smedj.2020088

Simpson, L. L. (2024). Enlarged nuchal translucency and cystic hygroma. *UpToDate.* Retrieved May 27, 2024, from https://www.uptodate.com/contents/enlarged-nuchal-translucency-and-cystic-hygroma

Smith, J. A., Fox, K. A., & Clark, S. (2023). Nausea and vomiting of pregnancy: Treatment and outcome. *UpToDate.* Retrieved May 27, 2024, from https://www.uptodate.com/contents/nausea-and-vomiting-of-pregnancy-treatment-and-outcome

Smith, J. A., Fox, K. A., & Clark, S. (2024). Nausea and vomiting of pregnancy: Clinical findings and evaluation. *UpToDate.* Retrieved May 27, 2024, from https://www.uptodate.com/contents/nausea-and-vomiting-of-pregnancy-clinical-findings-and-evaluation

Spencer, J. (2024). Common problems of breastfeeding and weaning. *UpToDate.* Retrieved May 29, 2024, from https://www.uptodate.com/contents/common-problems-of-breastfeeding-and-weaning

Sterns, R. H. (2023). Patient education: Edema (swelling) (Beyond the basics). *UpToDate.* https://www.uptodate.com/contents/edema-swelling-beyond-the-basics

Suman, V., & Luther, E. E. (2023). Preterm labor. In *StatPearls.* StatPearls Publishing. https://www.ncbi.nlm.nih.gov/books/NBK536939/

Tong, J., Lv, S., Yang, J., Li, H., Li, W., & Zhang, C. (2022). Decidualization and related pregnancy complications. *Maternal-Fetal Medicine, 4*(1), 24–35. https://doi.org/10.1097/FM9.0000000000000135

Umana, O. D., & Siccardi, M. A. (2023). Prenatal non-stress test. In *StatPearls.* StatPearls Publishing. https://www.ncbi.nlm.nih.gov/books/NBK537123/

U.S. Department of Health and Human Services. (n.d.). *Healthy People 2030*. https://health.gov/healthypeople

U.S. Department of Health and Human Services, Office on Women's Health. (2021). *Getting a good latch*. https://www.womenshealth.gov/breastfeeding/learning-breastfeed/getting-good-latch#4

U.S. Food & Drug Administration. (2023a). *Medicine and pregnancy*. https://www.fda.gov/consumers/free-publications-women/medicine-and-pregnancy

U.S. Food & Drug Administration. (2023b). *Infant formula: Safety do's and don'ts*. https://www.fda.gov/consumers/consumer-updates/infant-formula-safety-dos-and-donts

Wedro, B. (2023). Hemorrhoids (Piles). *MedicineNet*. https://www.medicinenet.com/hemorrhoids_piles/article.htm

Weinberger, S. E. (2024). Maternal adaptations to pregnancy: Dyspnea and other physiologic respiratory changes. *UpToDate*. Retrieved May 28, 2024, from https://www.uptodate.com/contents/maternal-adaptations-to-pregnancy-dyspnea-and-other-physiologic-respiratory-changes

Women's Preventive Services Initiative. (2024). *2024 Recommendations for women's preventive health care: A well-woman chart*. https://www.womenspreventivehealth.org/wp-content/uploads/FINAL_2024-Well-Woman-Chart-English.pdf

Yawetz, S. (2024). Immunizations during pregnancy. *UpToDate*. Retrieved May 28, 2024, from https://www.uptodate.com/contents/immunizations-during-pregnancy

DEVELOPING CLINICAL JUDGMENT

PRACTICING FOR NCLEX

1. The nurse is working with a nursing student. When discussing assessment of fetal well-being, the nurse would explain that which biophysical profile finding indicates poor oxygenation to the fetus?
- **a.** Two pockets of amniotic fluid
- **b.** Well-flexed arms and legs
- **c.** Decrease in fetal movement
- **d.** Fetal breathing movements noted

2. The nurse teaches the pregnant patient how to perform pelvic floor muscle exercises as a way to accomplish which action?
- **a.** Prevent perineal lacerations
- **b.** Stimulate labor contractions
- **c.** Increase pelvic muscle tone
- **d.** Lose pregnancy weight quickly

3. During a clinic visit, a pregnant patient at 30 weeks' gestation tells the nurse, "I've had some mild cramps that are pretty irregular. What does this mean?" The cramps are probably
- **a.** the beginning of labor in the very early stages.
- **b.** an ominous finding indicating that the patient is about to have a miscarriage.
- **c.** related to overhydration of the patient.
- **d.** Braxton Hicks contractions, which occur throughout pregnancy.

4. The nurse is preparing her teaching plan for a patient who has just had their pregnancy confirmed. Which information should be included in it? Select all that apply.
- **a.** Prevent constipation by taking a daily laxative.
- **b.** Balance your dietary intake by increasing your calories by 300 daily.
- **c.** Continue your daily walking routine just as you did before this pregnancy.
- **d.** Tetanus and MMR vaccines will be given to you now.
- **e.** Avoid tub baths now that you are pregnant to prevent vaginal infections.
- **f.** Sexual activity is permitted as long as your membranes are intact.
- **g.** Increase your consumption of milk to meet your iron needs.

5. A pregnant patient's LMP was on August 10. Using Nagele's rule, the nurse calculates that the patient's EDD will be when?
- **a.** June 23
- **b.** July 10
- **c.** July 30
- **d.** May 17

6. The nurse is teaching a group of pregnant people about breastfeeding. Which statement about breastfeeding made by a member of the group is not true?
- **a.** Breastfed infants experience more infections and allergies.
- **b.** Human milk is perfectly suited to the infant's nutritional needs.
- **c.** Human milk contains maternal antibodies to stimulate the infant's immunity.
- **d.** Breastfeeding enhances paternal bonding and attachment.

7. Practicing good oral hygiene is important for all people throughout pregnancy. As a nurse providing anticipatory guidance for pregnant patients, what condition can result from periodontal disease if good dental care is not practiced?
- **a.** Post-term pregnancy
- **b.** Large for gestational age infant
- **c.** Advanced reproductive cancer
- **d.** Preterm or low-birth-weight infant

8. The nurse is caring for a patient in their first trimester of pregnancy. What anticipatory guidance regarding sexual activity during pregnancy will be included in patient education? Select all that apply.
- **a.** Sexual activity is contraindicated throughout pregnancy.
- **b.** Most people don't desire intimacy after the first trimester.
- **c.** Sexual activity may continue up until the end of the second trimester.
- **d.** Sexual intercourse is prohibited if a history of preterm labor exists.
- **e.** Pregnant people's sexual desire may change throughout the pregnancy.
- **f.** Couples can try a variety of positions during intercourse for comfort during pregnancy.

9. The nurse is doing a first prenatal visit assessment on a newly pregnant patient. Which would be considered risk factors for psychological well-being during the patient's pregnancy? Select all that apply.
- **a.** Limited support system and network of friends and family
- **b.** Introverted personality at any point in the pregnancy
- **c.** Ambivalence any time during the pregnancy
- **d.** High levels of stress due to family discord
- **e.** History of previous high-risk pregnancy with complications
- **f.** Depression prior to pregnancy and on medication

CRITICAL THINKING EXERCISES

1. Mary Jones comes to the Women's Health Center, where you work as a nurse. She is in her first trimester of pregnancy and tells you her main complaints are nausea and fatigue, to the point that she wants to sleep most of the time and eats one meal daily. She appears pale and tired. Her mucous membranes are pale. She reports that she gets 8 to 9 hours of sleep each night but still can't seem to stay awake and alert at work. She tells you she knows that she is not eating as she should, but she isn't hungry. Her hemoglobin and hematocrit are low.
   a. What subjective and objective data do you have to make your assessment?
   b. What is your impression of this patient?
   c. What nursing interventions would be appropriate for this patient?
   d. How will you evaluate the effectiveness of your interventions?

2. Monica, a 16-year-old high school student, is here for her first prenatal visit. Her LMP was 2 months ago, and she states she has been "sick ever since." She is 5 ft, 6 in tall and weighs 110 lb. In completing her dietary assessment, the nurse asks about her intake of milk and dairy products. Monica reports that she doesn't like "that stuff" and doesn't want to put on too much weight because it "might ruin my figure."
   a. In addition to the routine obstetric assessments, which additional ones might be warranted for this patient?
   b. What dietary instruction should be provided to this patient based on her history?
   c. What follow-up monitoring should be included in subsequent prenatal visits?

3. Devon, a 27-year-old patient in their last trimester of pregnancy (34 weeks), complains to the clinic nurse that they are constipated and feel miserable most of the time. Devon reports that they have started taking laxatives, but the laxatives don't help much. When questioned about their dietary habits, Devon replies that they eat beans and rice and drink tea with most meals. Devon says they have tried to limit their fluid intake so they don't have to go to the bathroom so often.
   a. What additional information would the nurse need to assess Devon's complaint?
   b. What interventions would be appropriate for Devon?
   c. What adaptations will Devon need to make to alleviate their constipation?

STUDY ACTIVITIES

1. Visit a freestanding birth center and compare it to a traditional hospital setting in terms of restrictions, type of pain management available, and costs.

2. Arrange to shadow a nurse midwife for a day to see their role in working with the childbearing family.

3. Request permission to attend a childbirth education class in your local area and help a person without a partner practice the paced breathing exercises. Present the information you learned and think about how you can apply it while taking care of a patient during labor.

4. A layperson with a specialized education and experience in assisting birthing people during labor is a ____________________.

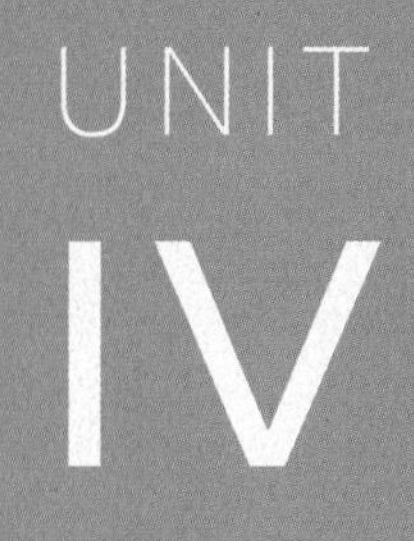

UNIT IV

Labor and Birth

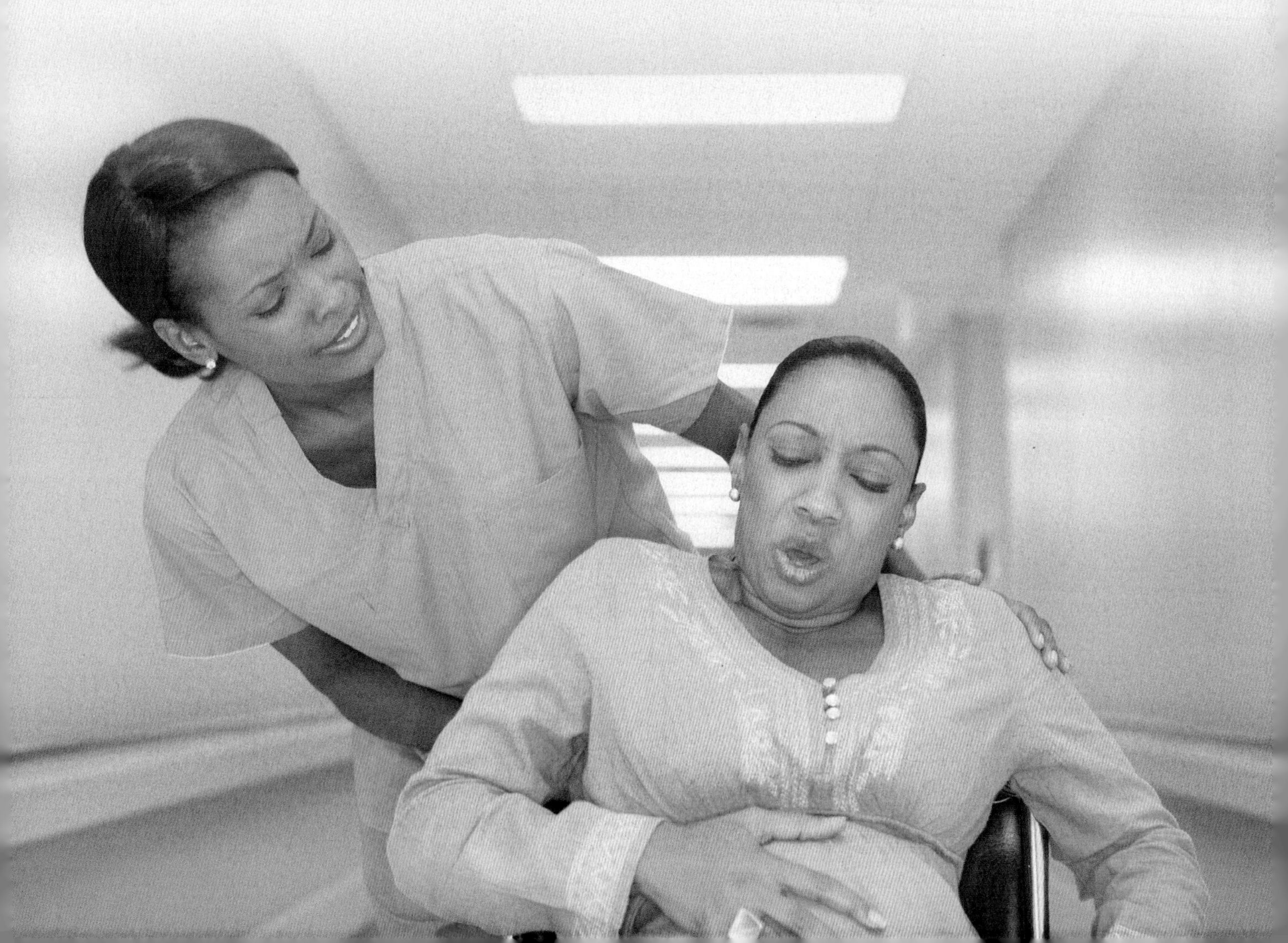

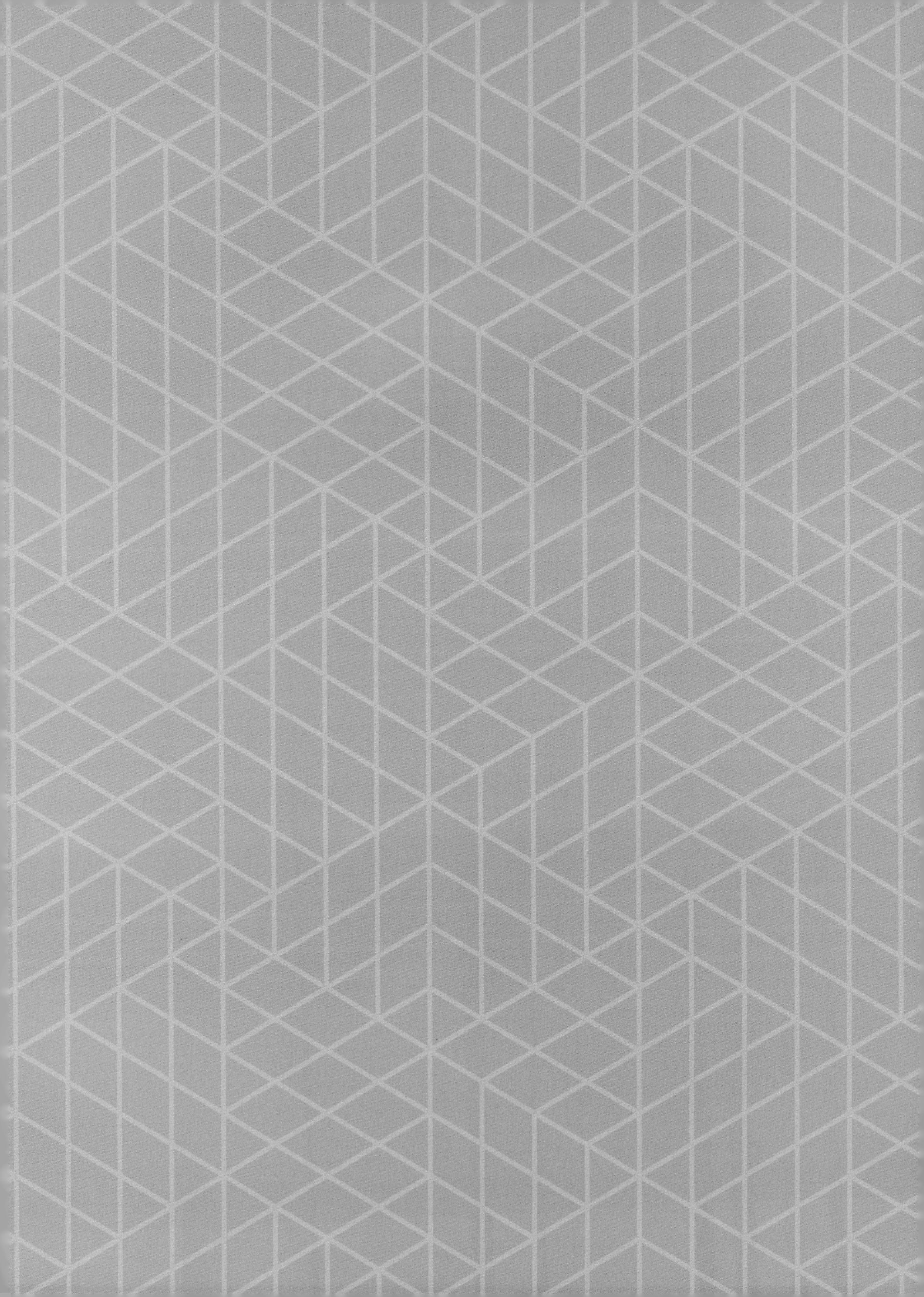

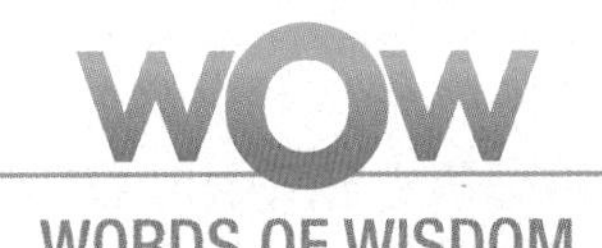

WORDS OF WISDOM

Intense physical and emotional support promotes a positive and memorable birthing experience.

13

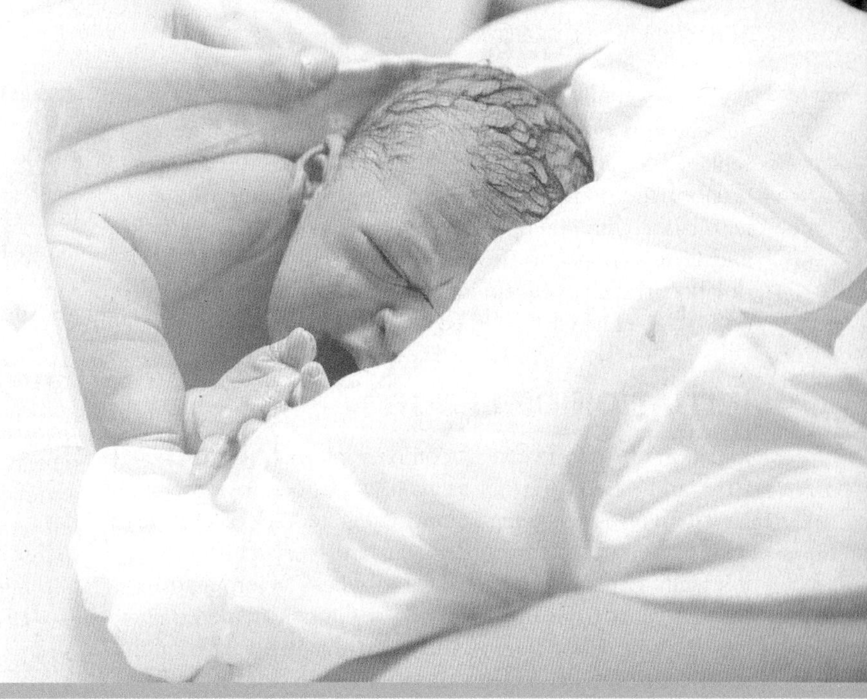

Labor and Birth Process

LEARNING OBJECTIVES

Upon completion of the chapter, you will be able to:

1. Identify premonitory signs of labor.
2. Compare and contrast true versus false labor.
3. Categorize the critical factors affecting labor and birth.
4. Analyze the cardinal movements of labor.
5. Evaluate the maternal and fetal responses to labor and birth.
6. Examine the concept of pain as it relates to the person in labor.
7. Classify the stages of labor and the critical events in each stage.
8. Characterize the normal physiologic/psychological changes occurring during all stages of labor.

KEY TERMS

attitude
dilation
doula
duration
effacement
engagement
frequency
intensity
lie
lightening
molding
position
presentation
station

Kathy and Chuck have been eagerly awaiting the birth of their first child for what seems to them an eternity. When Kathy finally feels contractions in her abdomen, she and Chuck rush to the birthing center. After the obstetric nurse finishes a complete history and physical assessment, she informs Kathy and her husband that she must have experienced "false labor" and that they should return home until she starts true labor.

INTRODUCTION

Experiencing childbirth is one of the most significant events in a person's life. Labor is the process by which the birth canal is prepared to allow the fetus to pass from the uterine cavity to the outside world. The process of labor and birth involves more than the birth of a newborn. Numerous physiologic and psychological events occur, which ultimately result in the birth of a newborn and the creation or expansion of the family. This chapter describes labor and birth as a process. It addresses the initiation of labor, the premonitory signs of labor, including true and false labor, critical factors affecting labor and birth, maternal and fetal response to the laboring process, and the stages of labor. The chapter also identifies critical factors related to each stage of labor: the "10 Ps of labor."

INITIATION OF LABOR

Initiation of labor involves a complex interplay of maternal, fetal, and genetic factors as well as endocrine signaling. Labor involves a sequential and integrated set of changes within the myometrium, decidua, and cervix that occur gradually over a period of days to weeks in order to expel the fetus from the uterus. It is difficult to determine exactly why labor begins and what initiates it. Although several theories have been proposed to explain the onset and maintenance of labor, none of these has been scientifically proved. It is widely believed that labor is influenced by a cascade of events, including uterine stretch from the fetus and amniotic fluid volume, progesterone withdrawal to estrogen dominance, increased oxytocin sensitivity, and increased release of prostaglandins (Norwitz, 2024).

One theory suggests that labor is initiated by a change in the estrogen-to-progesterone ratio. During the last trimester of pregnancy, estrogen levels increase and progesterone levels decrease. This change leads to an increase in the number of myometrium gap junctions. Gap junctions are proteins that connect cell membranes and facilitate the coordination of uterine contractions and myometrial stretching. At term, it is likely that a cascade of events happens that removes calming uterine mechanisms and ushers in factors that promote uterine contractions. Prostaglandins, oxytocin, cytokines, and other peptides play a regulating role in labor, birth, breastfeeding, and attachment (Norwitz, 2024). It is preferred to allow labor to begin on its own and not through induction via medications—so these hormones and other peptides can carry out their roles as nature intended.

Although physiologic evidence for the role of oxytocin in the initiation of labor is inconclusive, the number of oxytocin receptors in the uterus increases at the end of pregnancy. This creates an increased sensitivity to oxytocin. Estrogen, the levels of which are also rising, increases myometrial sensitivity to oxytocin. With the increasing levels of oxytocin in the maternal blood in conjunction with increasing fetal cortisol levels that synthesize prostaglandins, uterine contractions are initiated. Oxytocin also aids in stimulating prostaglandin synthesis through receptors in the decidua. Prostaglandins lead to additional contractions, cervical softening, gap junction induction, and myometrial sensitization, thereby leading to a progressive cervical **dilation** (the opening or enlargement of the external cervical os). Uterine contractions have two main functions: to dilate the cervix and to push the fetus through the birth canal (Ehsanipoor & Satin, 2023).

PREMONITORY SIGNS OF LABOR

Before the onset of labor, a pregnant person's body undergoes several changes in preparation for the birth of the newborn. The changes that occur often lead to characteristic signs and symptoms that suggest that labor is near. These premonitory signs and symptoms can vary, and not everyone experiences every one of them.

Braxton Hicks Contractions

Braxton Hicks contractions, which may have been experienced throughout the pregnancy, may become stronger and more frequent. Braxton Hicks contractions are typically felt as a tightening or pulling sensation of the top of the uterus. They occur primarily in the abdomen and groin and gradually spread downward before relaxing. In contrast, true labor contractions are more commonly felt in the lower back. These contractions aid in moving the cervix from a posterior position to an anterior position. They also help in ripening and softening the cervix. However, the contractions are irregular and can be decreased by walking, voiding, eating, increasing fluid intake, or changing position.

Braxton Hicks contractions usually last about 30 seconds but can persist for as long as 2 minutes. As birth draws near and the uterus becomes more sensitive to oxytocin, the frequency and intensity of these contractions increase. However, if the contractions last longer than 30 seconds and occur more often than four to six times an hour, advise the patient to contact their health care provider so that she can be evaluated for possible preterm labor, especially if less than 38 weeks pregnant.

TAKE NOTE!

An infant born between 34 0/7 and 36 6/7 weeks' gestation is identified as "late preterm" and experiences many of the same health issues as other preterm birth infants (Barfield & Lee, 2023).

Lightening

Lightening occurs when the fetal presenting part begins to descend into the true pelvis. The uterus lowers and moves into a more anterior position. The shape of the abdomen changes as a result of the change in the uterus. With this descent, breathing becomes easier and there is a decrease in gastric reflux. However, the patient may complain of increased pelvic pressure, leg cramping, dependent edema in the lower legs, and low back discomfort. There may be an increase in vaginal discharge and more frequent urination. In primiparas, lightening can occur 2 weeks or more before labor begins; among multiparas, it may not occur until labor starts (American Pregnancy Association, 2024).

Increased Energy Level

Some people report a sudden increase in energy before labor. This is sometimes referred to as nesting because many people will focus this energy on childbirth preparation by cleaning, cooking, preparing the nursery, and spending extra time with other children in the household. The increased energy level usually occurs 24 to 48 hours before the onset of labor (American Pregnancy Association, 2024).

Bloody Show

At the onset of labor or before, the mucus plug that fills the cervical canal during pregnancy is expelled as a result of cervical softening and increased pressure of the presenting part. These ruptured cervical capillaries release a small amount of blood that mixes with mucus, resulting in the pink-tinged secretions known as bloody show.

Cervical Changes

The rigid cervix of pregnancy must become distensible to expel the fetus. Before labor begins, cervical softening and possible cervical dilation with descent of the presenting part into the pelvis occur. These changes can occur 1 month to 1 hour before actual labor begins.

As labor approaches, the cervix changes from an elongated structure to a shortened, thinned segment. Cervical collagen fibers undergo enzymatic rearrangement into smaller, more flexible fibers that facilitate water absorption, leading to a softer, more stretchable cervix. These changes occur secondary to the effects of prostaglandins and pressure from Braxton Hicks contractions. The ripening and softening of the cervix are essential for effacement and dilation, which reflect the enhanced collagen breakdown that was previously inhibited by progesterone. Cervical stretch receptors send signals to the hypothalamus, which in turn stimulates the release of oxytocin to progressively increase contractions (Evbuomwan & Chowdhury, 2023).

Spontaneous Rupture of Membranes

Rupture of membranes with loss of amniotic fluid prior to the onset of labor is termed prelabor rupture of membranes (PROM). The rupture of membranes can result in either a sudden gush or a steady leakage of amniotic fluid. Although much of the amniotic fluid is lost when the rupture occurs, a continuous supply is produced to ensure protection of the fetus until birth.

After the amniotic sac has ruptured, the barrier to infection is gone and an ascending infection is possible. In addition, there is a danger of cord prolapse if engagement has not occurred with the sudden release of fluid and pressure with rupture. Due to the possibility of these complications, advise patients to notify their health care providers and go in for an evaluation.

CONSIDER THIS!

I always pictured myself as a dignified woman and behaved in ways to demonstrate that, because this was the way I was raised. My mother and grandmother always stressed that you should look polished, dress well, and do nothing to embarrass yourself in public. I did a fairly good job of living up to their expectations until an incident occurred at the end of my first pregnancy. I recall I was overdue according to my dates and was miserable in the summer heat. I decided to go to the store for some ice cream. As I waddled down the grocery aisles, all of a sudden, my water broke and came pouring down my legs all over the floor. Not wanting to make a spectacle of myself and remembering what my mother always said about being dignified at all times in public, I quickly reached up onto the grocery shelf and "accidentally" knocked off a large jar of pickles right where my puddle was. As I walked hurriedly away from that mess without my ice cream, I heard on the store loudspeaker, "Clean-up on Aisle 13!"

Thoughts: We tend to live by what we are taught, and in this case, this woman felt the need to save face from her ruptured membranes. Many people experience ruptured membranes before the onset of labor, so it is not out of the ordinary for this to happen in public. What risks can occur when membranes rupture? What action should this woman take now to minimize these risks? How can the nurse validate this patient's feelings?

TRUE VERSUS FALSE LABOR

Not all contractions indicate labor. False labor is a condition occurring during the latter weeks of some pregnancies when irregular uterine contractions are felt, but the cervix is not affected. In contrast, true labor is characterized by contractions occurring at regular intervals that increase in frequency, duration, and intensity. True labor contractions bring about progressive cervical dilation and effacement. Table 13.1 summarizes the differences between true and false labor. False labor, prodromal labor, and Braxton Hicks contractions are all names for contractions that do not contribute in a measurable way toward the goal of birth. Distinguishing between true and false labor is an essential nursing assessment skill and one that develops with experience.

Many people fear being sent home from the hospital with false labor. Everyone feels anxious when they feel contractions, but they should be informed that labor could be a long process, especially if it is the first pregnancy. Encourage your patients to think of false labor or prelabor signs as positive because they are part of the entire labor continuum. Describe early contractions as a phase of preparatory activity by the body in advance of active labor. With first pregnancies, the cervix can take up to about 20 hours to dilate completely (Hutchison et al., 2023).

Remember Kathy and Chuck, the anxious couple who came to the hospital too early? Kathy felt sure she was in labor and is now confused. What explanations and anticipatory guidance should be offered to this couple? What term describes her contractions?

STAGES OF LABOR

Labor is typically divided into these stages: dilation, expulsive, placental, and restorative. Table 13.2 summarizes the major events of each stage.

TABLE 13.1 • Differences Between True and False Labor

Parameters	True Labor	False Labor
Contraction timing	Regular, becoming closer together, usually 4–6 minutes apart, lasting 30–60 seconds	Irregular, not occurring close together
Contraction strength	Become stronger with time; vaginal pressure is usually felt.	Frequently weak, not getting stronger with time or alternating (a strong one followed by weaker ones)
Contraction discomfort	Start in the back and radiates around toward the front of the abdomen	Usually felt in the front of the abdomen
Any change in activity	Contractions continue no matter what positional change is made.	Contractions may stop or slow down with walking or making a position change.
Stay or go?	Stay home until contractions are 5 minutes apart, last 45–60 seconds, and are strong enough so that a conversation during one is not possible—then go to the hospital or birthing center.	Drink fluids and walk around to see if there is any change in the intensity of the contractions; if the contractions diminish in intensity after either or both, stay home.

Aubin, S. L. (2023). Clinical course of normal labor. In G. Posner, A. Black, G. Jones, & J. Dy, *Oxorn-Foote human labor and birth* (7th ed.). McGraw Hill; Lothian, J. (2024). Normal childbirth. In B. J. Baker, J. Janke, & Association of Women's Health, Obstetric, and Neonatal Nurses, *Core curriculum for maternal-newborn nursing* (6th ed.). Elsevier.

TABLE 13.2 • Stages and Phases of Labor

	First Stage	Second Stage	Third Stage	Fourth Stage
Description	From 0 to 10 cm dilation; consists of three phases	From complete dilation (10 cm) to birth of the newborn; may last up to 3 hours	Separation and delivery of the placenta; usually takes 5–10 minutes, but may take up to 30 minutes	1–4 hours after the birth of the newborn; time of maternal physiologic adjustment
Phases	**Latent phase** (0–6 cm dilation) • Cervical dilation from 0 to 6 cm • Cervical effacement from 0% to 40% • Nullipara can last up to 20 hours; multipara, can last up to 14 hours. • Contraction frequency every 5–10 minutes • Contraction duration 30–45 seconds • Contraction intensity mild to palpation **Active phase** (6–10 cm dilation) • Cervical dilation from 6 to 10 cm • Cervical effacement from 40% to 100% • Nullipara, lasts up to 6 hours; multipara, lasts up to 4 hours • Contraction frequency every 2–5 minutes • Contraction duration 45–60 seconds • Contraction intensity moderate to palpation	**Pelvic phase** (period of fetal descent) **Perineal phase** (period of active pushing) • Nullipara, lasts up to 3 hours; multipara, lasts up to 2 hours • Contraction frequency every 2–3 minutes or less • Contraction duration 60–90 seconds • Contraction intensity strong by palpation • Strong urge to push during the later perineal phase	**Placental separation:** detaching from uterine wall **Placental expulsion:** coming outside the vaginal opening	

Aubin, S. L. (2023). Clinical course of normal labor. In G. Posner, A. Black, G. Jones, & J. Dy, *Oxorn-Foote human labor and birth* (7th ed.). McGraw Hill; Cunningham, F. G., Leveno, K. J., Dashe, J. S., Hoffman, B. L., Spong, C. Y., & Casey, B. M. (2022b). Normal labor. In F. G. Cunningham, K. J. Leveno, J. S. Dashe, B. L. Hoffman, C. Y. Spong, & B. M. Casey (Eds.), *William's obstetrics* (26th ed.). McGraw-Hill.

The first stage, dilation, is the longest; it begins with the first true contraction and ends with full dilation (opening) of the cervix. Because this stage lasts so long, it is divided into two phases, latent and active, each corresponding to the progressive dilation of the cervix. Previously, there were thought to be three phases—latent, active, and transitional—but the transitional stage is no longer used (American College of Obstetricians and Gynecologists [ACOG], 2021).

The second stage, the expulsive stage, begins when the cervix is completely dilated and ends with the birth of the newborn. The expulsive stage can last from minutes to hours. The contractions typically occur every 2 to 3 minutes, lasting 60 to 90 seconds, and are strong by palpation. The laboring person is usually intent on the work of pushing during this stage.

The third stage, placental expulsion, starts after the newborn is born and ends with the separation and birth of the placenta. Continued uterine contractions typically cause the placenta to be expelled within 5 to 30 minutes. If the newborn is stable, bonding of the infant and birthing parent takes place during this stage through touching, holding, and skin-to-skin contact.

The fourth stage, the restorative stage or immediate postpartum period, lasts from 1 to 4 hours after birth. This period is when the birthing parent's body begins to stabilize after the hard work of labor and the loss of the products of conception. The fourth stage is often not recognized as a true stage of labor, but it is a critical period for maternal physiologic transition as well as new family attachment. Close monitoring of both the birthing parent and newborn is done during this stage (Hutchison et al., 2023).

First Stage

During the first stage of labor, the fundamental change underlying the process is progressive dilation of the cervix. Cervical dilation is gauged subjectively by vaginal examination and is expressed in centimeters. The first stage ends when the cervix is dilated to 10 cm in diameter and is large enough to permit the passage of a fetal head of average size. The fetal membranes usually rupture during the first stage, but they may have burst earlier or may even remain intact until birth. For the primigravida, the first stage of labor can last up to 20 hours without being considered prolonged. However, this time can vary widely; for the multiparous person, it can last up to 14 hours (ACOG, 2021).

During the first stage of labor, patients usually perceive the visceral pain of diffuse abdominal cramping and uterine contractions. Pain during the first stage of labor is primarily a result of the dilation of the cervix and lower uterine segment and the distention (stretching) of these structures during contractions. The first stage is divided into two phases: latent and active.

Latent Phase

The latent phase gives rise to the familiar signs and symptoms of labor. This phase begins with the start of regular contractions and ends when rapid cervical dilation begins. During the latent phase, the cervix dilates slowly to approximately 6 cm. Sedation can increase the duration of this phase.

Contractions usually occur every 5 to 10 minutes, last 30 to 45 seconds, and are described as mild by palpation by the nurse. Assessment of intensity is evaluated by pressing down on the fundus during a contraction to see if it can be dented with the nurse's fingers. The ability to indent the fundus at the peak of the contraction would typically indicate a mild contraction. Effacement of the cervix is from 0% to 40%. Many people remain talkative during this period, perceiving their contractions to be similar to menstrual cramps. They may remain at home during this phase, contacting their health care provider about the onset of labor.

During this phase, patients are often apprehensive but excited about the start of labor after the long gestational period.

Think back to the couple who were sent home from the hospital birthing center. Three days later, Kathy awakens with a wet sensation and intense discomfort in her back spreading around to her abdomen. She decides to go for a walk, but her contractions don't diminish. Instead, her contractions continue to occur every few minutes and grow stronger in intensity. She and Chuck decide to go back to the hospital birthing center. Was there a difference in the location of Kathy's discomfort this time? What changes will the admission nurse find in Kathy if this is true labor?

Active Phase

The active phase of labor encompasses the time from an increase in the rate of cervical dilation (end of latent phase of labor) until the completion of cervical dilation. Cervical dilation begins to occur more rapidly and predictably until it reaches 10 cm and cervical dilation and effacement are complete. Active labor with more rapid cervical dilation generally dilates at a rate of 1.2 to 1.5 cm per hour (Ehsanipoor & Satin, 2023). The fetus descends farther in the pelvis. Contractions become more frequent (every 2 to 5 minutes) and increase in duration (45 to 60 seconds). The laboring person's discomfort intensifies (moderate to strong by palpation). They become more intense and inwardly focused, absorbed in the serious work of labor. They limit interactions with those in the room. If they have attended childbirth education classes, they will begin to use the relaxation and paced breathing techniques that they learned to cope with the contractions.

In assessing Kathy, the nurse finds she is 4 cm dilated and 50% effaced with ruptured membranes. In what stage and phase of labor would this assessment finding place Kathy?

Second Stage

The second stage of labor begins with complete cervical dilation (10 cm) and effacement and ends with the birth of the newborn. This stage is usually much shorter than the first stage but may extend for many hours. Although the previous stage of labor primarily involved the thinning and opening of the cervix, this stage involves moving the fetus through the birth canal and out of the body. The cardinal movements of labor occur during the early phase of passive descent in the second stage of labor.

Contractions occur every 2 to 3 minutes, last 60 to 90 seconds, and are described as strong by palpation. Parity, delayed pushing, use of epidural analgesia, maternal body mass index, birth weight, pelvis shape, occiput posterior position, and fetal station at complete dilation all have been shown to affect the length of the second stage of labor. A longer duration of the second stage of labor is associated with adverse maternal outcomes, such as higher rates of puerperal infection, and the fetus can suffer acidemia, shoulder dystocia, bony fractures, nerve palsies, scalp hematomas, and anoxic brain injuries. Similarly, a host of traumatic complications can start to develop, such as uterine rupture or hemorrhage, vaginal laceration, cervical laceration, third- and fourth-degree perineal lacerations, amniotic fluid embolism, and death (Hutchison et al., 2023). During this expulsive stage, the laboring person usually feels more in control and less irritable and agitated. They are focused on the work of pushing. The maternal urge to push is generally felt when there is direct contact of the fetus to the pelvic floor. Stretch receptors in the wall of the vagina, rectum, and perineum communicate the pressure of the fetus descending in the birth canal that, along with increased abdominal pressure, causes the overwhelming urge to push described by laboring people (Aubin, 2023).

Pushing

During the second stage of labor, active pushing is the time in which the laboring person feels rectal pressure by the fetal presenting part and physiologically feels the urge to push. The patient receiving neuraxial analgesia (i.e., epidural or spinal) should receive the least amount possible to maintain pain control and still allow the laboring person to feel the sensation to push (Toledano & Leffert, 2024).

In the second stage of labor, the perineum bulges, and there is an increase in bloody show. The fetal head becomes apparent at the vaginal opening but disappears between contractions. When the top of the head no longer regresses between contractions, it is said to have crowned. The fetus rotates as it maneuvers out. Today, evidence demonstrates labor progresses more slowly than was previously thought. In nulliparous people without neuraxial analgesia, the second stage averages 0.6 hour, while in those with neuraxial analgesia the average length is 1 hour (Ehsanipoor & Satin, 2023). Many patients may need a little more time to labor and give birth vaginally avoiding surgical birth (Fig. 13.1).

SPONTANEOUS PUSHING VERSUS DIRECTED PUSHING

There are two ways of conducting the second stage of labor: *spontaneous pushing* (following the birthing parent's spontaneous urge) and *directed pushing* (pushing directed by the caregiver). Spontaneous pushing represents a natural way of managing the second stage of labor. Evidence is mounting that the management of the second stage, particularly pushing, is a modifiable risk factor in long-term perinatal outcomes (Cunningham et al., 2022b).

In the second stage, the adoption of a physiologic, patient-directed approach to bearing down is advocated. Delayed pushing may result in increased neonatal morbidity and place the birthing parent at increased risk for postpartum hemorrhage and other complications (ACOG, 2024). The American College of Obstetricians and Gynecologists (2024) advises open-glottis pushing to begin when cervical dilatation is complete. Using an open-glottis method (involuntary pushing with expiratory grunting and vocalization) to push supports the birthing parent's involuntary bearing-down efforts (Oppenheimer & Black, 2023). Laboring down (promotion of passive descent) is an alternative strategy for second-stage management in patients with epidurals. Using this approach, the fetus descends with delay in initiation of pushing efforts. Labor nurses need to develop an evidence-based approach that acknowledges and reinforces the patient's innate ability to give birth and refrain from trying to direct pushing behaviors (Association of Women's Health, Obstetric, and Neonatal Nurses [AWHONN], 2023) (see Evidence-Based Practice 13.1).

Third Stage

The ideal placement for the newborn immediately following the birth is on the birthing parent's abdomen or chest, in skin-to-skin contact, which promotes a positive transition from intrauterine to extrauterine life. While the birthing parent is getting to know the newborn, the third stage of labor occurs. Lasting from 5 to 30 minutes, it begins with the birth of the newborn and ends with the separation and delivery of the placenta. The uterus is continuing to contract strongly, and the uterine surface area has decreased, resulting in a shearing force leading to placental separation (the first phase of the third stage). Expulsion of the placenta follows. The average blood loss during a spontaneous vaginal delivery is less than 500 mL (Funai & Norwitz, 2024).

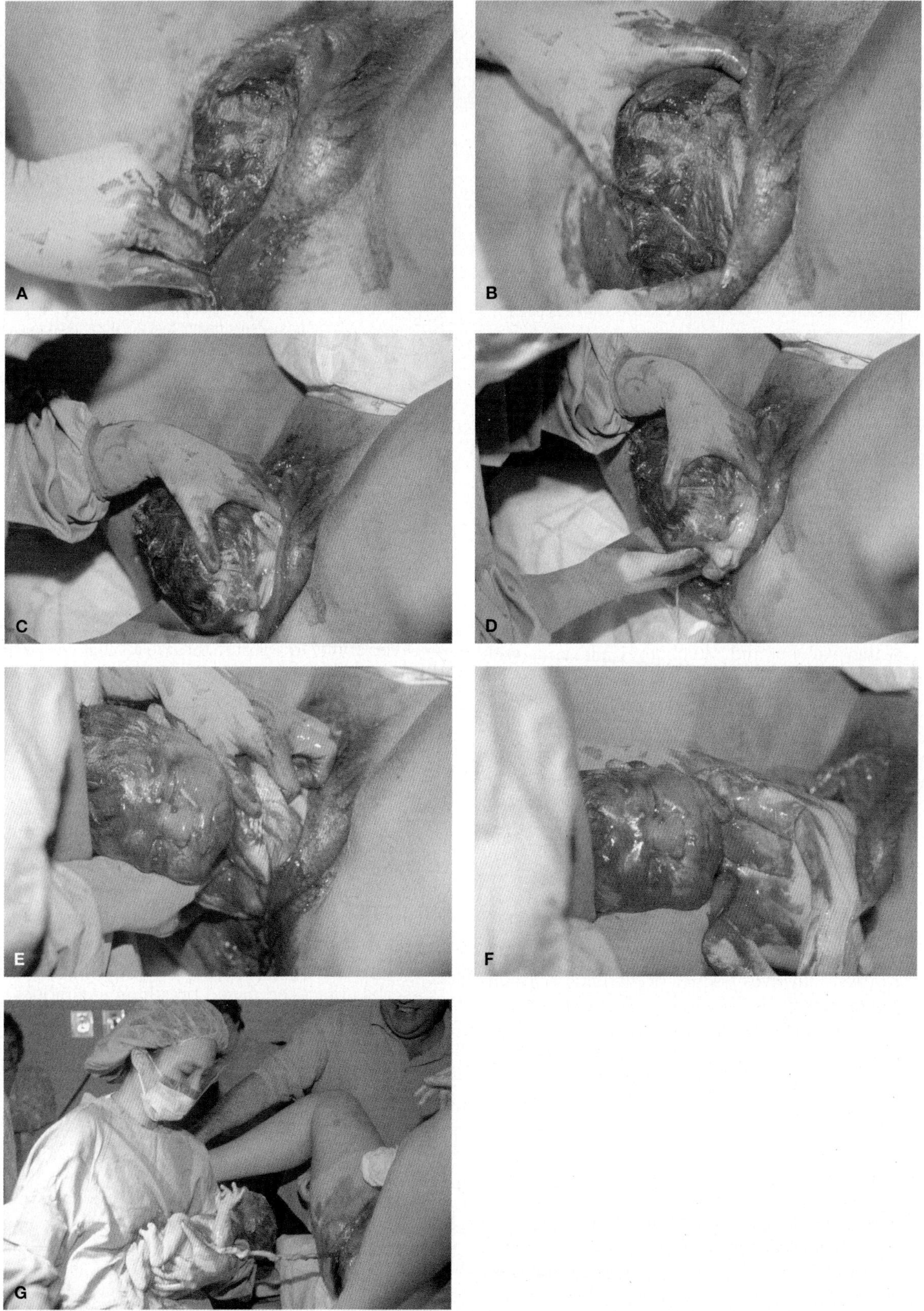

FIGURE 13.1 Birth sequence from crowning through the birth of the newborn. **A.** Early crowning of the fetal head. Notice the bulging of the perineum. **B.** Late crowning. Notice that the fetal head is appearing face down. This is the normal OA position. **C.** As the head extends, you can see that the occiput is to the laboring person's right side–ROA position. **D.** The cardinal movement of extension. **E.** The shoulders are born. Notice how the head has turned to line up with the shoulders—the cardinal movement of external rotation. **F.** The body easily follows the shoulders. **G.** The newborn is held for the first time. ROA, right occiput anterior. (Photo by B. Proud.)

EVIDENCE-BASED PRACTICE **13.1**

Postpartum Urinary Incontinence and Birth Outcomes as a Result of Pushing Technique: A Systematic Review and Meta-Analysis

BACKGROUND

Pregnancy and childbirth are contributing factors to pelvic floor dysfunction and lead to urinary incontinence in about 30% of females who give birth. Spontaneous pushing during labor involves natural inhalation within a time frame of less than 10 seconds. Direct pushing involves consistent strong abdominal pressure and bearing down longer than 10 seconds. The purpose of the study was to determine if the pushing technique used by laboring patients in the second stage of labor contributes to postpartum urinary incontinence and poor birth outcomes.

STUDY

There were 742 studies screened overall, with 17 meeting the eligibility criteria. There were 4,606 nulliparas in the spontaneous pushing group and 2,282 nulliparas in the direct pushing group.

Findings

Analysis of the studies' results revealed that spontaneous pushing statistically reduced urinary incontinence compared with directed pushing. Repeated strong abdominal pressure can lead to bladder neck descent, which can cause postpartum urinary incontinence. Maternal spontaneous pushing in a recumbent position lengthened the duration of the second stage of labor. In short, laboring in an upright position using spontaneous pushing can reduce the likelihood of postpartum urinary incontinence.

Nursing Implications

Based on this study's findings, nurses should discourage directed pushing when laboring patients do not feel a natural urge to push and support them to follow their own expulsive urges for better perinatal outcomes. This will hopefully preserve the pelvic floor muscles and prevent postpartum urinary incontinence.

Adapted from Shinozaki, K., Suto, M., Ota, E., Eto, H., & Horiuchi, S. (2022). Postpartum urinary incontinence and birth outcomes as a result of the pushing technique: A systematic review and meta-analysis. *International Urogynecology Journal, 33*(6), 1435–1449. https://doi.org/10.1007/s00192-021-05058-5

Fourth Stage

The fourth stage begins with the completion of the expulsion of the placenta and membranes and ends with the initial physiologic adjustment and stabilization of the birthing parent (a few hours after birth). This stage initiates the postpartum period (Paudel et al., 2023). The birthing parent usually feels a sense of peace and excitement, is wide awake, and is initially talkative. The attachment process begins with inspecting the newborn and desiring to cuddle and breastfeed them.

PHYSIOLOGIC RESPONSES TO LABOR

The labor process involves a series of rhythmic, involuntary, uterine muscle contractions. The contractions bring about effacement and dilation of the cervix. After a period of time, the infant is born (Norwitz, 2024). During this process, the postpartum person and fetus make several physiologic adaptations.

Maternal Responses

As childbirth progresses, numerous physiologic responses occur that assist the laboring person to adapt to the labor process. The labor process stresses several body systems, which react through numerous compensatory mechanisms. Maternal physiologic responses include:

- Slight increase in heart rate, 30% to 40% increase in cardiac output, and increased blood pressure
- Increase in white blood cell count to 20,000 cells/mm^3
- Increase in respiratory rate, hyperventilation
- Decrease in gastric motility, gastric emptying, and food absorption (Lothian, 2024)

The ability to adapt to the stress of labor is influenced by the pregnant person's psychological state. Among the many factors that affect coping ability are:

- Previous birth experiences and their outcomes (complications and previous birth outcomes)
- Current pregnancy experience (planned vs. unplanned, discomforts experienced, age, risk status of pregnancy)
- Cultural considerations (values and beliefs about health status)
- Support system (presence and support of a valued partner during labor)
- Childbirth preparation (attended childbirth classes and has practiced paced breathing techniques)
- Expectations of the birthing experience (viewed as a meaningful or stressful event)
- Anxiety level (excessive anxiety may interfere with labor progress) (Hurst & Baker, 2024)

Fetal Responses

Although the focus during labor may be on assessing the birthing parent's adaptations, several physiologic adaptations occur in the fetus as well. The fetus is experiencing labor along with the birthing parent. If the fetus is healthy, the stress of labor usually has no adverse effects. The nurse needs to be alert to any abnormalities in the fetus's adaptation to labor. Fetal responses to labor include:

- Periodic fetal heart rate accelerations and slight decelerations related to fetal movement, fundal pressure, and uterine contractions

- Decrease in circulation and perfusion to the fetus secondary to uterine contractions (a healthy fetus is able to compensate for this drop)
- Mild decrease in oxygenation with contractions (Cypher, 2024)

TAKE NOTE!

Respiratory changes during labor help prepare the fetus for extrauterine respiration immediately after birth.

FACTORS AFFECTING THE LABOR PROCESS

Traditionally, the critical factors that affect the process of labor and birth are outlined as the "five Ps:"

1. Passageway (birth canal)
2. Passenger (fetus and placenta)
3. Powers (contractions)
4. Position (maternal)
5. Psychological response

These critical factors are commonly accepted and discussed by health care providers. However, five additional "Ps" can also affect the labor process:

1. Philosophy (low tech, high touch)
2. Partners (support caregivers)
3. Patience (natural timing)
4. Patient preparation (childbirth knowledge base)
5. Pain management (comfort measures)

These five additional Ps are helpful in planning care for the laboring patient and their family. These patient-focused factors are an attempt to foster labor that can be managed through the use of high touch, patience, support, knowledge, and pain management.

Passageway

The birth passageway is the route through which the fetus must travel to be born vaginally. Compared to other primates, childbirth is remarkably difficult in humans because the head of the neonate is large relative to the birth-relevant dimensions of the maternal pelvis. The passageway consists of the maternal pelvis and soft tissues. Of the two, however, the maternal bony pelvis is more important because it is relatively unyielding (except for the coccyx). Typically, the pelvis is assessed and measured during the first trimester, often at the first visit to the health care provider, to identify any abnormalities that might hinder a successful vaginal birth. As the pregnancy progresses, the hormones relaxin and estrogen cause the connective tissues to become more relaxed and elastic and cause the joints to become more flexible to prepare the laboring person's pelvis for birth. Additionally, the soft tissues usually yield to the forces of labor.

Bony Pelvis

The main purpose of the pelvic bones is to transfer the weight of the upper body onto the lower limbs while standing or walking. It also protects the organs within it—the bladder, urethra, rectum, and uterus (Burgess & Lui, 2023). The maternal bony pelvis can be divided into true and false portions. The false (or greater) pelvis is composed of the upper flared parts of the two iliac bones with their concavities and the wings of the base of the sacrum. The false pelvis is divided from the true pelvis by an imaginary line drawn from the sacral prominence at the back to the superior aspect of the symphysis pubis at the front of the pelvis. This imaginary line is called the linea terminalis. The false pelvis lies above this imaginary line; the true pelvis lies below it (Fig. 13.2). The true pelvis is the bony passageway through which

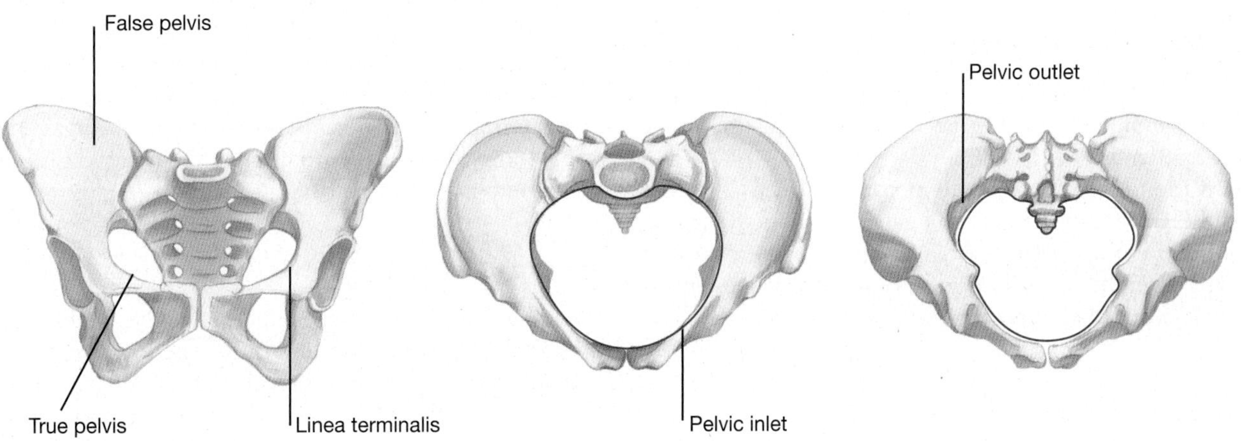

FIGURE 13.2 The bony pelvis.

the fetus must travel. It is made up of three planes: the inlet, the mid-pelvis (cavity), and the outlet.

PELVIC INLET

The pelvic inlet, or upper pelvic narrow, is oval in shape and forms the entrance toward the birth canal. It allows entrance to the true pelvis. It is bounded by the sacral prominence in the back, the ilium on the sides, and the superior aspect of the symphysis pubis in the front (Siccardi et al., 2023). The pelvic inlet is wider in the transverse aspect (sideways) than it is from front to back.

MID-PELVIS

The mid-pelvis (cavity) occupies the space between the inlet and outlet. It is through this snug, curved space that the fetus must travel to reach the outside. As the fetus passes through this small area, their chest is compressed, causing lung fluid and mucus to be expelled. This expulsion removes the space-occupying fluid so that air can enter the lungs with the newborn's first breath.

PELVIC OUTLET

The pelvic outlet defines the lower margin of the true pelvis and is bound by the ischial tuberosities, the lower rim of the symphysis pubis, and the tip of the coccyx. In comparison with the pelvic inlet, the outlet is wider from front to back. For the fetus to pass through the pelvis, the outlet must be large enough. To ensure the adequacy of the pelvic outlet for vaginal birth, the following pelvic measurements are assessed:

- Diagonal conjugate of the inlet (distance between the anterior surface of the sacral prominence and the anterior surface of the inferior margin of the symphysis pubis)
- Transverse or ischial tuberosity diameter of the outlet (distance at the medial and lowest aspect of the ischial tuberosities, at the level of the anus; a known hand span or clenched-fist measurement is generally used to obtain this measurement)
- True or obstetric conjugate (distance estimated from the measurement of the diagonal conjugate; 1.5 cm is subtracted from the diagonal conjugate measurement) (Eggleton & Cunha, 2023)

For more information about pelvic measurements, see Chapter 12.

If the diagonal conjugate measures at least 11.5 cm and the true or obstetric conjugate measures 10 cm or more (1.5 cm less than the diagonal conjugate or about 10 cm), then the pelvis is large enough for a vaginal birth of what would be considered a normal-sized newborn.

Pelvic Shape

In addition to size, the shape of the female pelvis may be a determining factor for a vaginal birth. The pelvis is divided into four main shapes, defined by the anterior–posterior and transverse diameters: gynecoid, anthropoid, android, and platypelloid (Fig. 13.3). These four labeled pelvic shapes were first classified and described in the 1930s by Caldwell and Moloy; however, they have recently been called into question. Today, it is believed that many pelvic shapes exist that lead to uncomplicated births and good outcomes for parents and newborns. There is a call to move away from labeling pelvic types (VanSickle et al., 2022).

An important principle is that most pelvises are not purely defined but occur in nature as mixed types. Many females have a combination of these four basic pelvis types, with no two pelvises shaped exactly the same. Regardless of the pelvic shape, the newborn can be born vaginally if size and positioning remain compatible. The narrowest part of the fetus attempts to align itself with the narrowest pelvic dimension (e.g., biparietal to interspinous diameters, which means the fetus generally tends to rotate to the amplest portion of the pelvis).

Soft Tissues

The soft tissues of the passageway consist of the cervix, the pelvic floor muscles, and the vagina. Through **effacement**, the cervix effaces (thins) to allow the presenting fetal part to descend into the vagina.

> **TAKE NOTE!**
>
> The process of cervical effacement and dilation is analogous to that of pulling a turtleneck sweater over your head.

The pelvic floor muscles help the fetus rotate anteriorly as it passes through the birth canal. The soft tissues of the vagina expand to accommodate the fetus during birth.

Passenger

The fetus (with placenta) is the passenger. The fetal head (size and presence of molding), fetal attitude (degree of body flexion), fetal lie (relationship of body parts), fetal presentation (first body part), fetal position (relationship to maternal pelvis), fetal station, and fetal engagement are all important factors that have an impact on the ultimate outcome in the birthing process.

Fetal Head

The fetal head is the largest fetal structure, making it an important factor in labor and birth. There is considerable variation in the size and diameter of the fetal skull.

Compared with an adult's head, the fetal head is large in proportion to the rest of the body. The bones that make up the face and cranial base are fused and

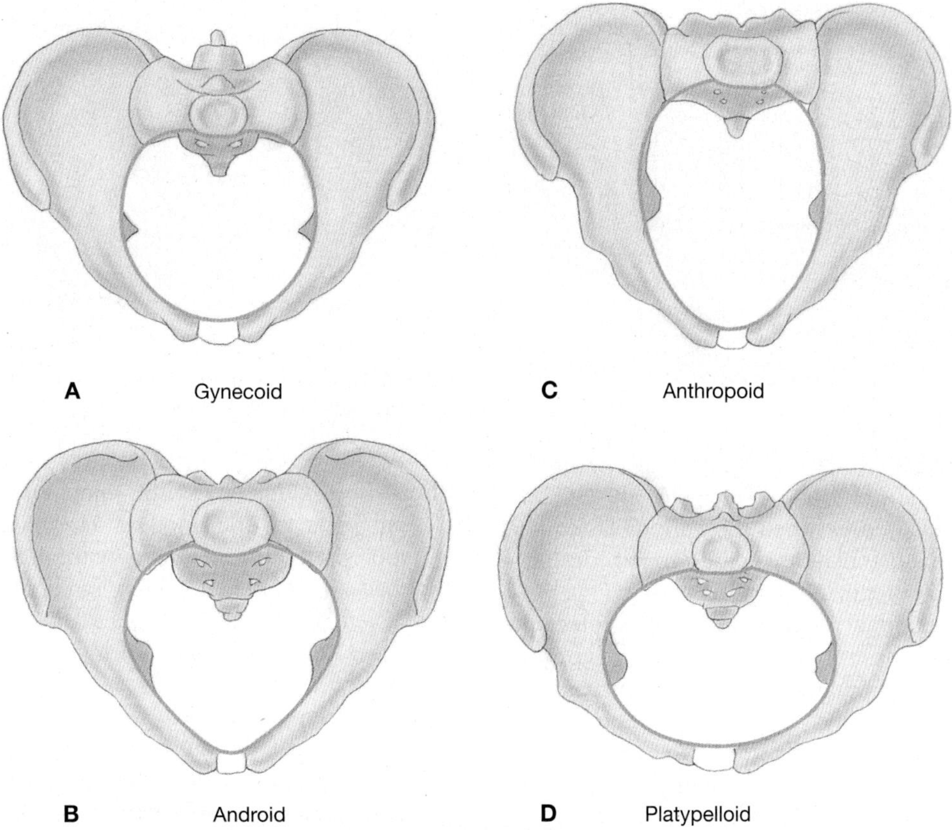

FIGURE 13.3 Pelvic shapes. **A.** Gynecoid. **B.** Android. **C.** Anthropoid. **D.** Platypelloid.

essentially fixed. However, the five bones that make up the rest of the cranium (two frontal bones, two parietal bones, and the occipital bone) are not fused; rather, they are soft and pliable, with gaps between the plates of bone. These gaps, membranous spaces between the cranial bones, are called sutures, and the intersections of these sutures are called fontanelles. Sutures are important because they allow the cranial bones to overlap in order for the head to adjust in shape (elongate) when pressure is exerted on it by uterine contractions or the maternal bony pelvis. Some diameters shorten, while others lengthen as the head is molded during the labor and birthing process (Moura et al., 2021). After birth, the sutures close as the bones grow and the brain reaches its full growth.

A newborn may occasionally endure minor physical injury during the childbirth process involving structural or tissue impairment. Most are temporary and self-limiting with full recovery. The changed (elongated) shape of the fetal skull at birth as a result of overlapping of the cranial bones is known as **molding**. Along with molding, fluid can also collect in the scalp (caput succedaneum) or blood can collect beneath the scalp (cephalohematoma), further distorting the shape and appearance of the fetal head. Refer to Chapter 24 for additional information.

TAKE NOTE!

Parents may become concerned about the distortion of the newborn's head. However, reassurance that the oblong shape is only temporary is usually all that is needed to reduce their anxiety.

Sutures also play a role in helping to identify the position of the fetal head during a vaginal examination. Figure 13.4 shows a fetal skull. During a pelvic examination, palpation of these sutures by the examiner reveals the position of the fetal head and the degree of rotation that has occurred.

The anterior and posterior fontanelles are also useful in helping to identify the position of the fetal head. They allow for molding and are important when evaluating the newborn. The anterior fontanelle is the famous "soft spot" of the newborn's head and is the largest of all fontanelles. It is a diamond-shaped space that measures from 1 to 4 cm. The posterior fontanelle corresponds to the anterior one but is located at the back of the fetal head; it is triangular, measuring about 1 cm at its widest diameter (Smith, 2022).

The diameter of the fetal skull is an important consideration during the labor and birth process. Fetal skull

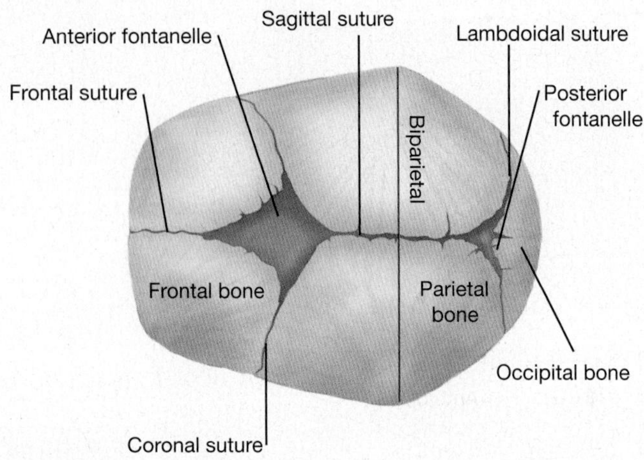

FIGURE 13.4 Fetal skull.

diameters are measured between the various landmarks of the skull. Diameters include occipitofrontal, occipitomental, suboccipitobregmatic, and biparietal (Fig. 13.5). The two most important diameters that can affect the birth process are the suboccipitobregmatic (approximately 9.5 cm at term) and the biparietal (approximately 9.25 cm at term) diameters. The suboccipitobregmatic diameter, measured from the base of the occiput to the center of the anterior fontanelle, identifies the smallest anteroposterior diameter of the fetal skull. The biparietal diameter measures the largest transverse diameter of the fetal skull—the distance between the two parietal bones. In a cephalic (head first) presentation, occurring in most term births, if the fetus presents in a flexed position in which the chin is resting on the chest, the optimal or smallest fetal skull dimensions for a vaginal birth are present (Cunningham et al., 2022b). If the fetal head is not fully flexed at birth, the anteroposterior diameter increases. This increase in dimension might prevent the fetal skull from entering the maternal pelvis.

Fetal Attitude

Fetal attitude is another important consideration related to the passenger. Fetal **attitude** refers to the posturing

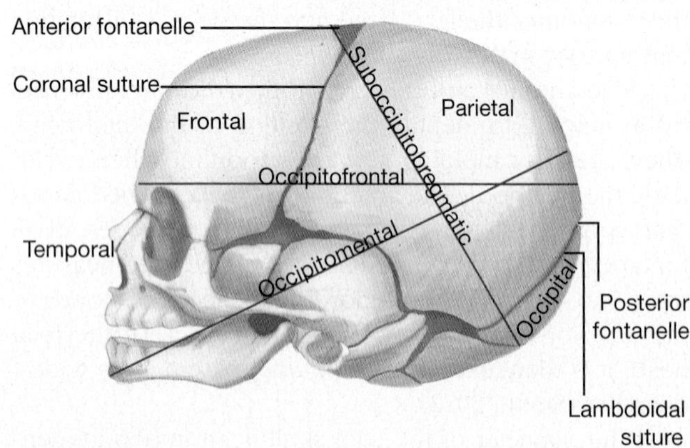

FIGURE 13.5 Fetal skull diameters.

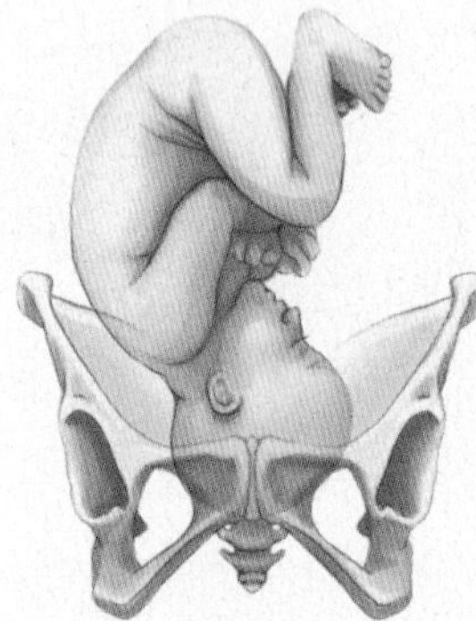

FIGURE 13.6 Fetal attitude: full flexion. Note that the smallest diameter presents to the pelvis.

(flexion or extension) of the joints and the relationship of fetal parts to one another. The most common fetal attitude when labor begins is with all joints flexed—the fetal back is rounded, the chin is on the chest, the thighs are flexed on the abdomen, and the legs are flexed at the knees (Fig. 13.6). This normal fetal position is most favorable for vaginal birth, presenting the smallest fetal skull diameters to the pelvis.

When the fetus presents to the pelvis with abnormal attitudes (no flexion or extension), the nonflexed position can increase the diameter of the presenting part as it passes through the pelvis, increasing the difficulty of birth. An attitude of extension tends to present larger fetal skull diameters, which may make birth difficult.

Fetal Lie

Fetal **lie** refers to the relationship of the long axis (spine) of the fetus to the long axis (spine) of the laboring person. There are three possible lies: longitudinal (the most common), transverse (Fig. 13.7), and oblique.

A longitudinal lie, considered ideal for labor and delivery, occurs when the long axis of the fetus is parallel to that of the laboring person (fetal spine to maternal spine side-by-side). A transverse lie occurs when the long axis of the fetus is perpendicular to the long axis of the birthing parent (fetal spine lies across the maternal abdomen and crosses the birthing parent's spine). In an oblique lie, the fetal long axis is at an angle to the bony inlet, and no palpable fetal part is presenting. This lie is usually transitory and occurs during fetal conversion between other lies. A fetus in a transverse or oblique lie position cannot be delivered vaginally (Cunningham et al., 2022c).

Fetal Presentation

Fetal **presentation** refers to the body part of the fetus that enters the pelvic inlet first (the "presenting part"). This is the fetal part that lies over the inlet of the pelvis or the cervical os. Knowing which fetal part is coming first at birth is critical for planning and initiating appropriate interventions.

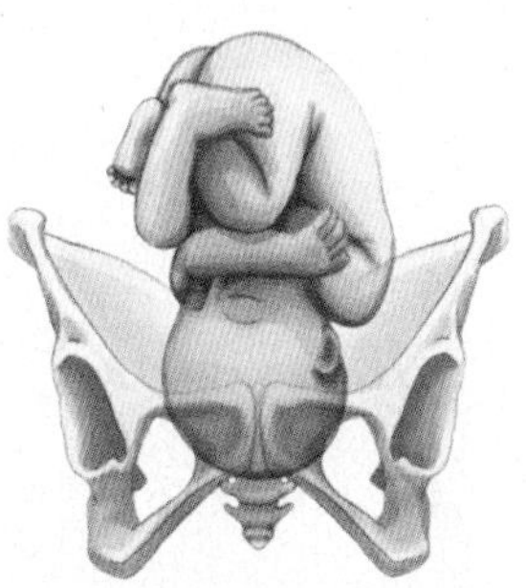

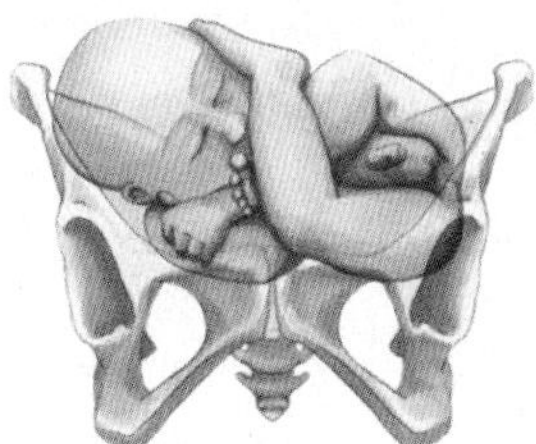

FIGURE 13.7 Fetal lie. **A.** Fetal long axis (spine) runs parallel to the laboring person's spine. **B.** Fetal long axis (spine) runs transverse or perpendicular to that of the laboring person's spine.

The three main fetal presentations are cephalic (head first), breech (pelvis first), and shoulder (scapula first). The majority of term newborns (95% to 96%) are born in a cephalic presentation; breech presentations account for 3% to 4% of term births and shoulder presentations for approximately 1% (Mohammed & El-Chaâr, 2023).

In a cephalic presentation, the presenting part is usually the occipital portion of the fetal head (Fig. 13.8). This presentation is also referred to as a vertex presentation. Variations in a vertex presentation include the military, brow, and facial presentations.

BREECH PRESENTATION

In early pregnancy, fetuses have a variable lie within the uterus. As the pregnancy approaches the final weeks, the majority of singleton pregnancies have a longitudinal lie and the fetus enters the pelvis in a cephalic presentation. Breech presentation occurs when the fetal buttocks or feet enter the maternal pelvis first and the fetal skull enters last. This abnormal presentation occurs in 2% to 3% of singleton term births and poses several challenges at birth (Cunningham et al., 2022b). Primarily, the largest part of the fetus (skull) is born last and may become stuck in the pelvis. In addition, the umbilical cord can become compressed between the fetal skull and the maternal pelvis after the fetal chest is born because the head is the last to exit. Moreover, unlike the hard fetal skull, the buttocks are soft and are not as effective as a cervical dilator during labor compared with a cephalic presentation. Finally, there is the possibility of trauma to the head as a result of the lack of opportunity for molding.

The types of breech presentations are determined by the positioning of the fetal legs (Fig. 13.9). In a frank breech (50% to 70%), the buttocks present first with both legs extended up toward the face. In a full or complete breech (5% to 10%), the fetus sits cross-legged above the cervix. In a footling or incomplete breech (10% to 40%), one or both legs are presenting. Breech presentations are associated with prematurity, previous history of breech birth, placenta previa, multiparity, contracted maternal pelvis, uterine abnormalities (fibroids), extreme volumes of amniotic fluid, and some congenital anomalies such as hydrocephaly (Hofmeyr, 2023). A frank breech can result in a vaginal birth, but complete, footling, and incomplete breech presentations generally necessitate a cesarean birth.

SHOULDER PRESENTATION

A shoulder presentation occurs when the fetus is in a transverse lie with the shoulder as the presenting part. Conditions associated with shoulder dystocia include placenta previa, prematurity, high parity, premature rupture of membranes, multiple gestation, or fetal anomalies. A cesarean birth is usually necessary unless the fetus is very small (<800 g) (Cunningham et al., 2022c).

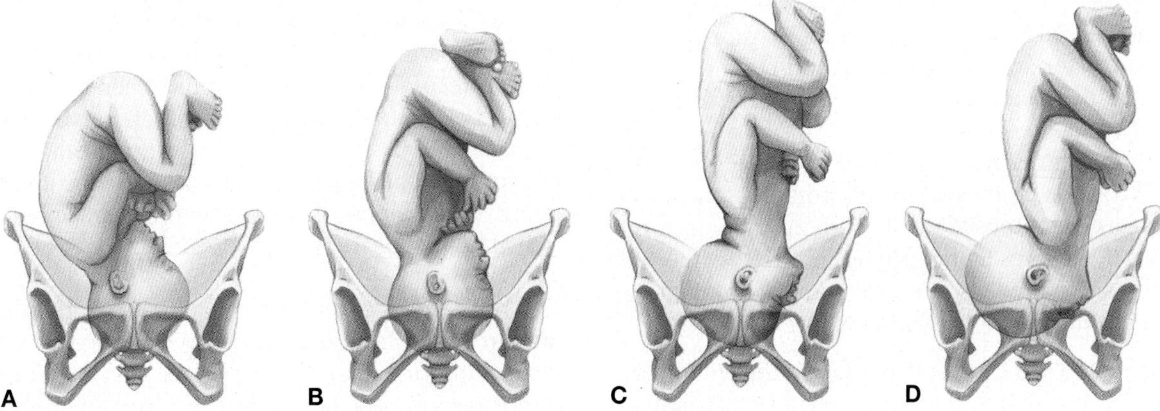

FIGURE 13.8 Fetal presentation: cephalic presentations. **A.** Vertex. **B.** Military. **C.** Brow. **D.** Face.

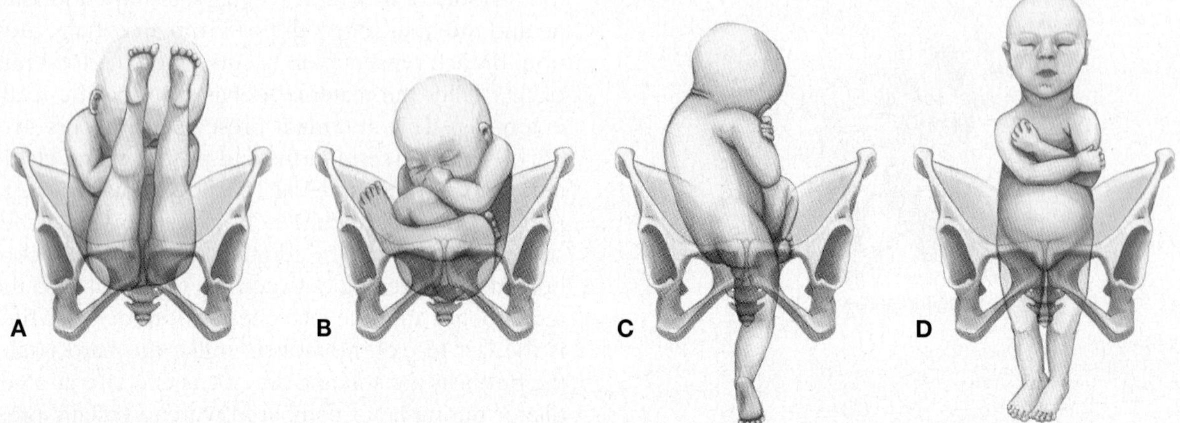

FIGURE 13.9 Breech presentations. **A.** Frank breech. **B.** Complete breech. **C.** Single footling breech. **D.** Double footling breech.

Fetal Position

Fetal **position** describes the relationship of a given point on the presenting part of the fetus to a designated point of the maternal pelvis (Garber & Dy, 2023). The landmark fetal presenting parts include the occipital bone (O), which designates a vertex presentation; the chin (mentum [M]), which designates a face presentation; the buttocks (sacrum [S]), which designate a breech presentation; and the scapula (acromion process [A]), which designates a shoulder presentation.

In addition, the maternal pelvis is divided into four quadrants: right anterior, left anterior, right posterior, and left posterior. These quadrants designate whether the presenting part is directed toward the front, back, left, or right side of the pelvis. Fetal position is determined first by identifying the presenting part and then the maternal quadrant the presenting part is facing (Fig. 13.10). Position is indicated by a three-letter abbreviation as follows:

- The first letter defines whether the presenting part is tilted toward the left (L) or the right (R) side of the maternal pelvis.
- The second letter represents the particular presenting part of the fetus: O for occiput, S for sacrum, M for mentum, A for acromion process, and D for dorsal (refers to the fetal back) when denoting the fetal position in shoulder presentations.
- The third letter defines the location of the presenting part in relation to the anterior (A) portion of the maternal pelvis or the posterior (P) portion of the maternal pelvis. If the presenting part is directed to the side of the maternal pelvis, the fetal presentation is designated as transverse (T) (Garber & Dy, 2023).

For example, if the occiput is facing the left anterior quadrant of the pelvis, then the position is termed left occiput anterior and is recorded as LOA.

TAKE NOTE!

LOA is currently the most common (and most favorable) fetal position for birthing, followed by right occiput anterior (ROA). The positioning of the fetus allows the fetal head to contour to the diameters of the maternal pelvis. LOA and ROA are optimal positions for vaginal birth.

An occiput posterior position may lead to a long and difficult birth, and other positions may or may not be compatible with vaginal birth.

Fetal Station

Fetal **station** refers to the relationship of the presenting part to the level of the maternal pelvic ischial spines. Fetal station is measured in centimeters and is referred to as a minus or plus, depending on its location above or below the ischial spines. Typically, the ischial spines are the narrowest part of the pelvis and are the natural measuring point for the birth progress.

Zero (0) station is designated when the presenting part is at the level of the maternal ischial spines. When the presenting part is above the ischial spines, the distance is recorded as minus stations. When the presenting part is below the ischial spines, the distance is recorded as plus stations. For instance, if the presenting part is above the ischial spines by 1 cm, it is documented as being a −1 station; if the presenting part is below the ischial spines by 1 cm, it is documented as being a +1 station.

Assessment of fetal head station is based on the distal part of the fetal skull and is a vital determination in monitoring progression in labor. An easy way to understand this concept is to think in terms of meeting the goal, which is birth. If the fetus is descending downward

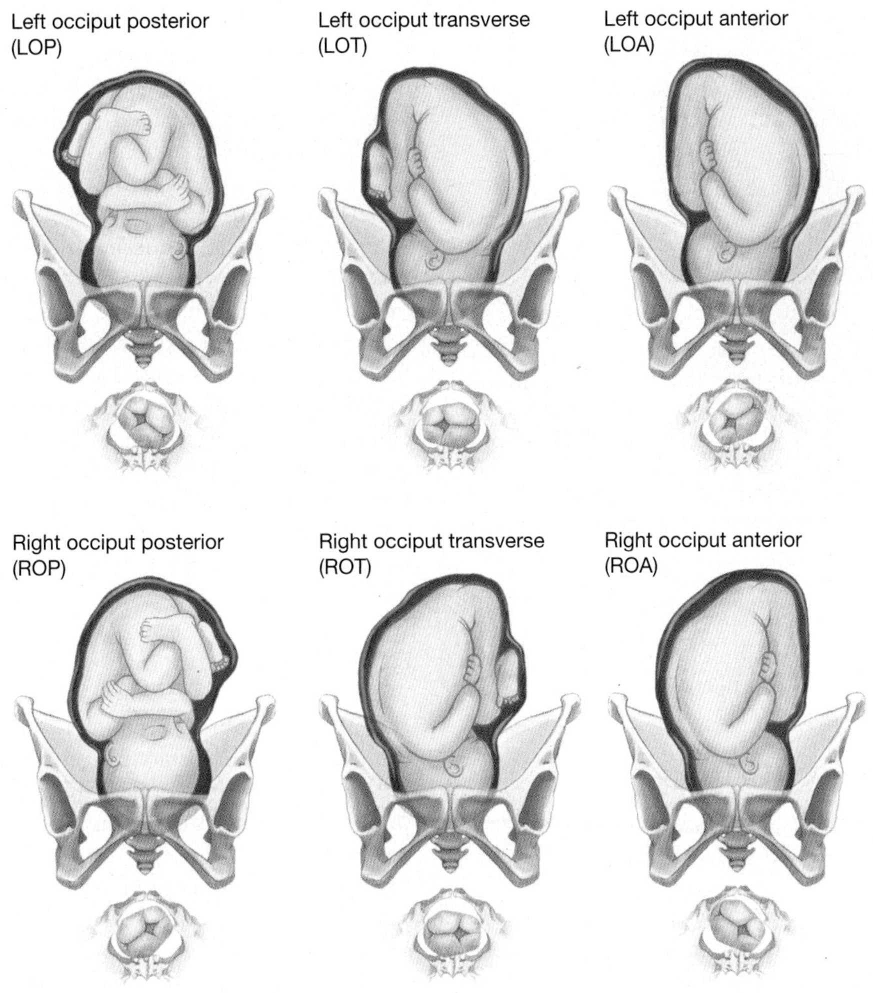

FIGURE 13.10 Examples of fetal positions in a vertex presentation. The lie is longitudinal for each illustration. The attitude is one of flexion. Notice that the view of the top illustration is seen when facing the pregnant person. The bottom view is that seen with the person in a dorsal recumbent position.

(past the ischial spines) and moving toward meeting the goal of birth, then the station is positive and the centimeter numbers grow bigger from +1 to +4. If the fetus is not descending past the ischial spines, then the station is negative and the centimeter numbers grow from −1 to −4. The farther away the presenting part from the outside, the larger the negative number (−4 cm). The closer the presenting part of the fetus is to the outside, the larger the positive number (+4 cm). Figure 13.11 shows stations of the presenting part.

Fetal Engagement

Fetal **engagement** signifies the entrance of the largest diameter of the fetal presenting part (usually the fetal head) into the smallest diameter of the maternal pelvis (Posner, 2023). The fetus is said to be engaged in the pelvis when the presenting part reaches 0 station. Engagement is determined by pelvic examination.

The largest diameter of the fetal head is the biparietal diameter. It extends from one parietal prominence to the other. It is an important factor in the navigation through the maternal pelvis. Engagement typically occurs in primigravidas 2 weeks before term, while multiparas may experience engagement several weeks before the onset of labor or not until labor begins.

> **TAKE NOTE!**
>
> The term *floating* is used when engagement has not occurred because the presenting part is freely movable above the pelvic inlet.

Cardinal Movements of Labor

The fetus goes through many positional changes as it travels through the passageway. These positional changes are known as the cardinal movements of labor. They are deliberate, specific, and precise movements that allow the smallest diameter of the fetal head to pass through a corresponding diameter of the laboring person's pelvic structure. Although cardinal movements are

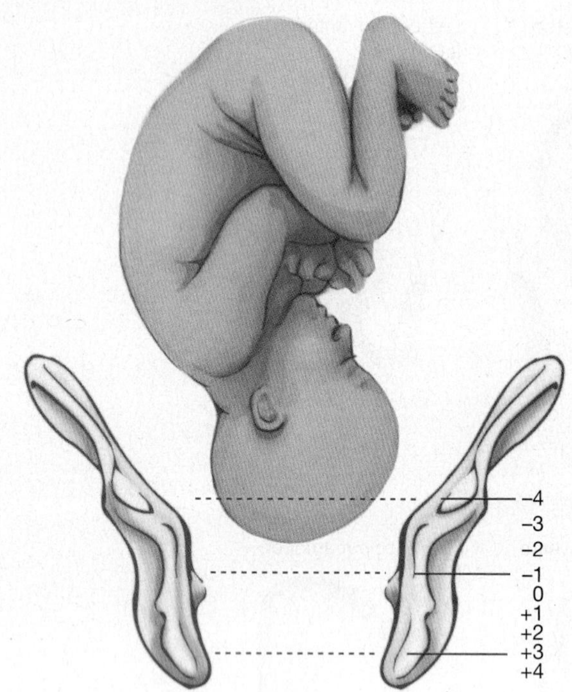

FIGURE 13.11 Fetal stations.

conceptualized as separate and sequential, the movements are typically concurrent (Fig. 13.12).

ENGAGEMENT

Engagement occurs when the greatest transverse diameter of the head in the vertex (biparietal diameter) passes through the pelvic inlet (usually 0 station). The head usually enters the pelvis with the sagittal suture aligned in the transverse diameter.

DESCENT

Descent is the downward movement of the fetal head until it is within the pelvic inlet. Descent occurs intermittently with contractions and is brought about by one or more of the following forces:

- Pressure of the amniotic fluid
- Direct pressure of the fundus on the fetus's buttocks or head (depending on which part is located in the top of the uterus)
- Contractions of the abdominal muscles (second stage)
- Extension and straightening of the fetal body

Descent occurs throughout labor, ending with birth. During this time, the laboring person experiences discomfort, but she is unable to isolate this particular fetal movement from her overall discomfort.

FLEXION

Flexion occurs as the vertex meets resistance from the cervix, the walls of the pelvis, or the pelvic floor. As a result, the chin is brought into contact with the fetal thorax and the presenting diameter is changed from occipitofrontal to suboccipitobregmatic (9.5 cm), which achieves the smallest fetal skull diameter presenting to the maternal pelvic dimensions.

INTERNAL ROTATION

After engagement, as the head descends, the lower portion of the head (usually the occiput) meets resistance from one side of the pelvic floor. As a result, the head rotates about 45 degrees anteriorly to the midline under the symphysis. This movement is known as *internal rotation*. Internal rotation brings the anteroposterior diameter of the head in line with the anteroposterior diameter of the pelvic outlet. It aligns the long axis of the fetal head with the long axis of the maternal pelvis. The widest portion of the maternal pelvis is the anteroposterior diameter, and thus the fetus must rotate to accommodate the pelvis.

EXTENSION

With further descent and full flexion of the head, the nucha (the base of the occiput) becomes impinged under the symphysis. Resistance from the pelvic floor causes the fetal head to extend so that it can pass under the pubic arch. *Extension* occurs after internal rotation is complete. The head emerges through extension under the symphysis pubis along with the shoulders. The anterior fontanelle, brow, nose, mouth, and chin are born successively.

EXTERNAL ROTATION (RESTITUTION)

After the head is born and is free of resistance, it untwists, causing the occiput to move about 45 degrees back to its original left or right position (restitution). The sagittal suture has now resumed its normal right-angle relationship to the transverse (bisacromial) diameter of the shoulders (i.e., the head realigns with the position of the back in the birth canal). *External rotation* of the fetal head allows the shoulders to rotate internally to fit the maternal pelvis.

EXPULSION

Expulsion of the rest of the body occurs more smoothly after the birth of the head and the anterior and posterior shoulders. Expulsion begins when the fetal head enters the birth canal and ends with the birth. Manual control of the fetus expulsion and perineal support by the health care provider reduces the risk of perineal injury to the laboring person (Garber & Dy, 2023). See Figure 13.4 for an image of a fetal skull.

Recent research findings have challenged the number of cardinal movements and suggest they be reduced to four, not seven. It is proposed that engagement, descent, and expulsion be excluded from the rotational movements because they are all part of the fetal

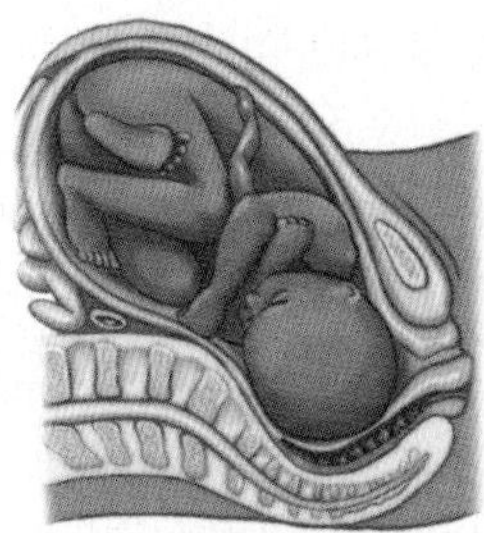

Engagement, descent, flexion

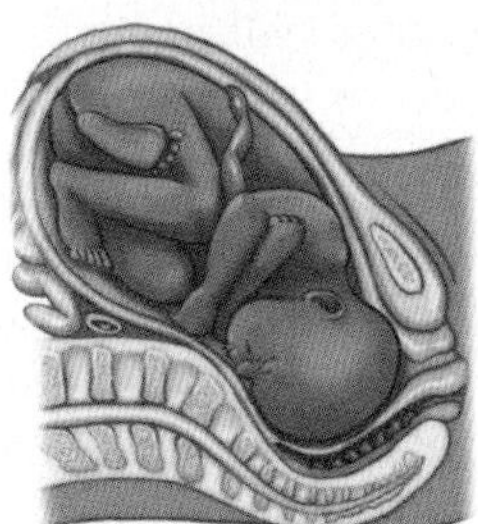

Internal rotation

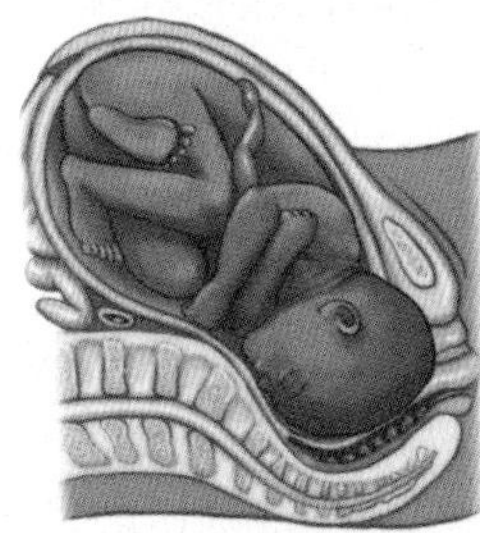

Extension beginning (rotation complete)

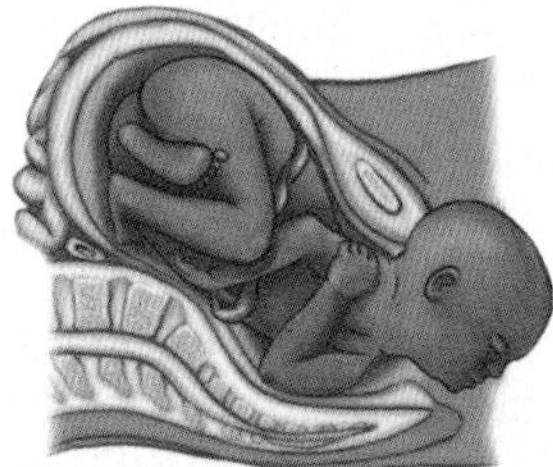

Extension complete

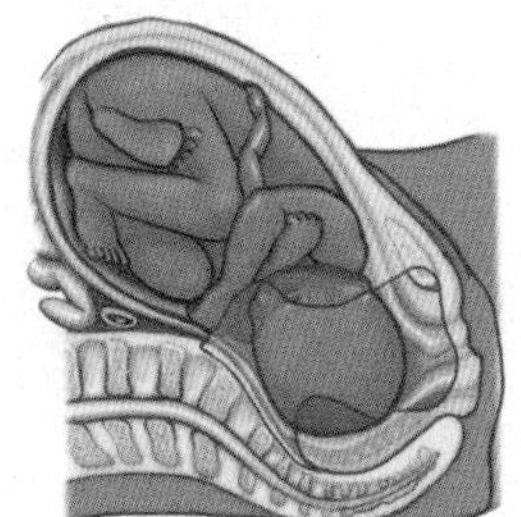

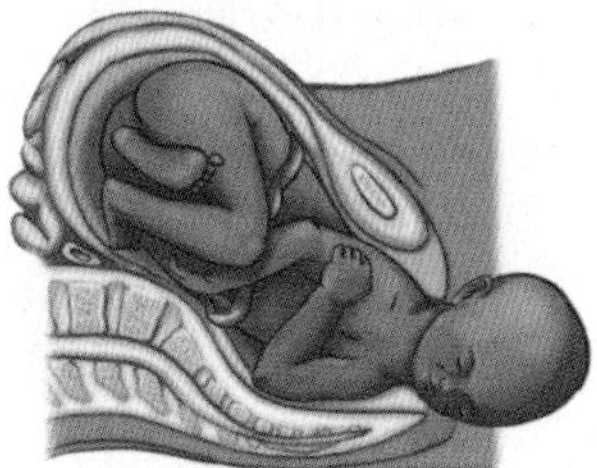

External rotation (restitution)

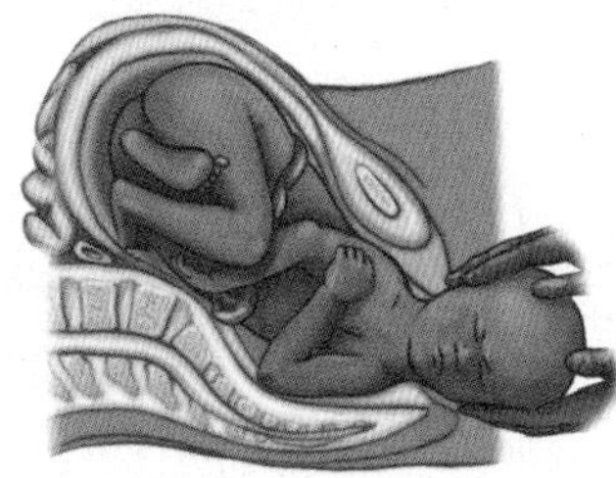

External rotation (shoulder rotation)

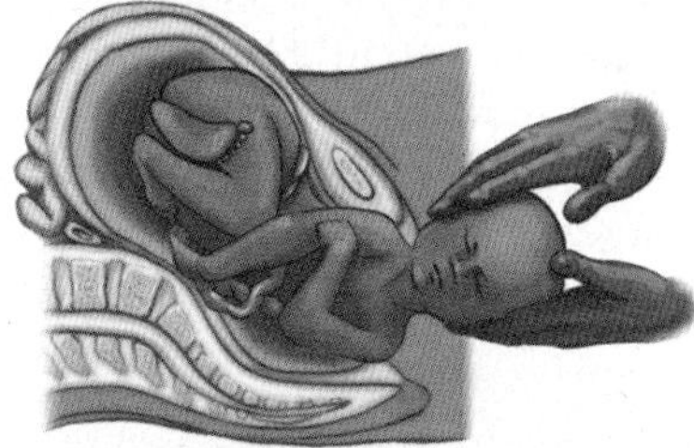

Expulsion

FIGURE 13.12 Cardinal movements of labor.

descent process. This research was gathered using the results of clinical examinations and ultrasounds (Iversen et al., 2021).

Powers

The primary stimulus powering labor is uterine contraction. Contractions cause complete dilation and effacement of the cervix during the first stage of labor. The secondary powers in labor involve the use of intra-abdominal pressure (voluntary muscle contractions) exerted by the laboring patient as they push and bears down during the second stage of labor.

Uterine Contractions

Uterine contractions are involuntary and therefore cannot be controlled by the person experiencing them, regardless of whether they are spontaneous or induced. Uterine contractions are rhythmic and intermittent, with a period of relaxation between contractions. This pause allows the person and the uterine muscles to rest. In addition, this pause restores blood flow to the uterus and placenta, which is temporarily reduced during each uterine contraction.

Uterine contractions are responsible for thinning and dilating the cervix, then thrusting the presenting part

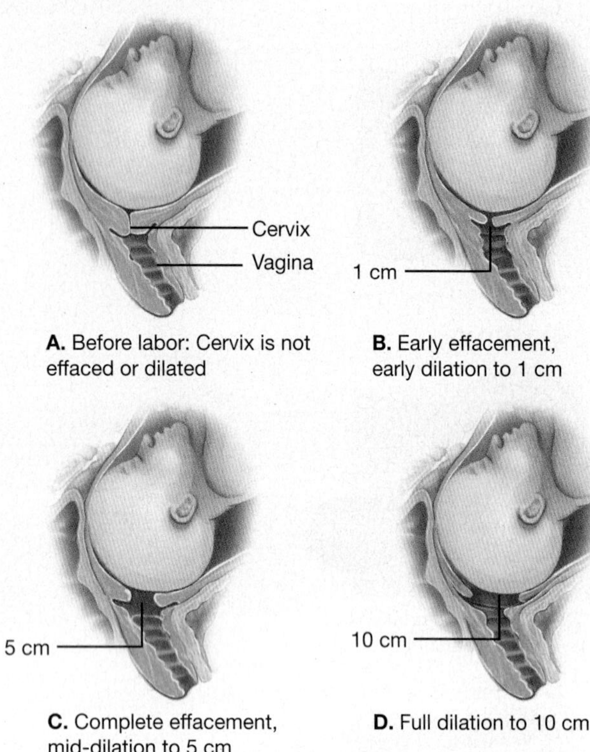

FIGURE 13.13 Cervical effacement and dilation. Cervical dilation is expressed in centimeters. **A.** Shows cervix not effaced or dilated. **B.** 50% effaced. **C.** 100% effaced. **D.** Fully dilated at 10 cm.

toward the lower uterine segment. The cervical canal reduces in length from 2 cm to a paper-thin entity and is described in terms of percentages from 0% to 100%. In primigravidas, effacement typically starts before the onset of labor and usually begins before dilation; in multiparas, however, neither effacement nor dilation may start until labor ensues (Fig. 13.13). On clinical examination, the following may be assessed:

- Cervical canal 2 cm in length is described as 0% effaced.
- Cervical canal 1 cm in length is described as 50% effaced.
- Cervical canal 0 cm in length is described as 100% effaced.

Dilation is dependent on the pressure of the presenting part and the contraction and retraction of the uterus. The diameter of the cervical os increases from less than 1 cm to approximately 10 cm to allow for birth. When the cervix is fully dilated, it is no longer palpable on vaginal examination. Descriptions may include:

- External cervical os closed: 0 cm dilated
- External cervical os half open: 5 cm dilated
- External cervical os fully open: 10 cm dilated

During early labor, uterine contractions are described as mild, they last about 30 seconds, and they occur about every 5 to 7 minutes. As labor progresses, contractions last longer (60 seconds), occur more frequently (2 to 3 minutes apart), and are described as being moderate to high in intensity. Each contraction has three phases: increment (buildup of the contraction), acme (peak or highest intensity), and decrement (descent or relaxation of the uterine muscle fibers) (see Figure 13.14).

Uterine contractions are monitored and assessed according to three parameters: frequency, duration, and intensity.

1. **Frequency** refers to how often the contractions occur and is measured from the beginning of one contraction to the beginning of the next contraction.
2. **Duration** refers to how long a contraction lasts and is measured from the beginning of one contraction to the end of that same contraction.
3. **Intensity** refers to the strength of the contraction determined by manual palpation or measured by an internal intrauterine pressure catheter. The catheter is positioned in the uterine cavity through the cervix after the membranes have ruptured. It reports intensity by measuring the pressure of the amniotic fluid inside the uterus in millimeters of mercury. It is not recommended for routine use in low-risk laboring patients due to the potential risk of infection and injury

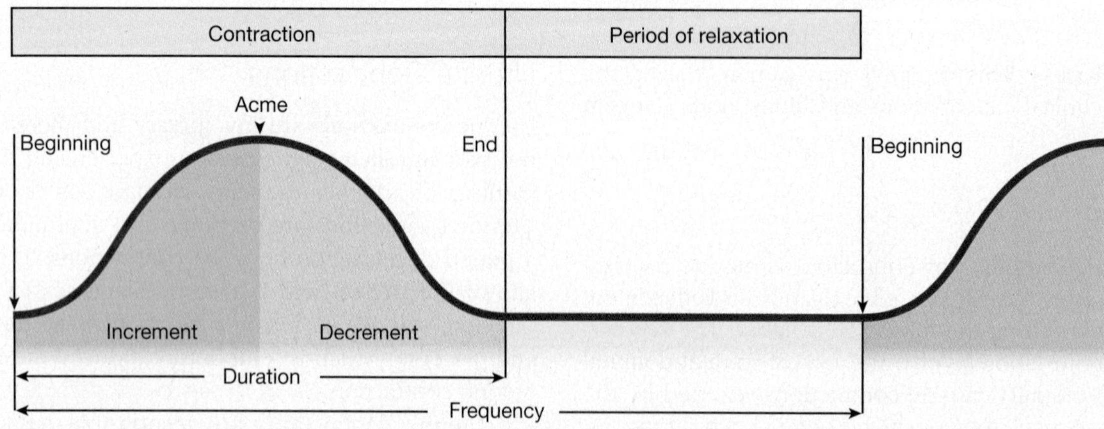

FIGURE 13.14 The three phases of a uterine contraction.

to the placenta or fetus. In a recent study using noninvasive technology, it was found that using a multichannel electromyogram that acquires a uterine signal and maternal and fetal electrocardiograms gave more accurate results than those of an external Doppler and fetal scalp electrode monitor. Therefore, the multichannel electromyogram can be used to help differentiate between term, preterm, and imminent delivery labors based on the detected uterine electrical activity (Zhang et al., 2022).

Intra-Abdominal Pressure

Increased intra-abdominal pressure (voluntary muscle contractions) occurs during stage 2 of labor and is achieved by pushing. This pressure compresses the uterus and adds to the power of the expulsion forces of the uterine contractions (Cunningham et al., 2022a). Coordination of these forces in unison promotes birth of the fetus and expulsion of the fetal membranes and placenta from the uterus. Interference with these forces (such as when a patient is highly sedated or extremely anxious) can compromise the effectiveness of these powers.

Position (Maternal)

Maternal positioning impacts the biomechanics of and physiologic adaptations to labor. Birth positions are usually described as upright, lateral, or supine. Positioning for normal labor and birth has evolved. Until about 250 years ago, women were depicted in art and described in essays as sitting upright with flexed hips, squatting, or less commonly standing or kneeling during the childbirth process. These positions maintain flexion at the hip joint and somewhat straighten the pelvis. In upright positions, the maternal pelvis is at its widest and the pull of gravity aids in the fetal head descent. Flexible sacrum position is an upright position in which the laboring person's weight is taken off the sacrum, allowing the pelvic outlet to expand and promoting flexibility of the sacroiliac joints (Badi et al., 2022). In the past 250 years, dorsal and dorsal lithotomy positions evolved for unclear reasons ascribed to Western medicine. Childbirth medicalization has reduced the opportunity for a laboring person to be in a spontaneous position of choice in favor of a recumbent one. Medical historians posit that the evolution was for convenience after administration of anesthesia and to facilitate forceps usage, vacuum-assisted births, episiotomies, and fetal monitoring. Studies have shown that other positions such as squatting, side-lying, or being on hands and knees have many benefits, including easing pain, hastening birth, and producing better maternal and fetal outcomes (Irvin et al., 2022).

Maternal positioning during labor has only recently been the subject of well-controlled research. Scientific evidence has shown that nonmoving, back-lying positions during labor are not healthy. Supine positions are linked to greater fetal heart rate abnormalities and fewer spontaneous vaginal deliveries than upright or side-lying positions (Familiari et al., 2023; Satone & Tayade, 2023). In an upright position, gravity can help in bringing the fetus down, and there is less risk of compressing the maternal aorta which supplies oxygen to the fetus.

Although many labor and birthing facilities claim that all laboring patients are allowed to adopt any position of comfort during their laboring experience, many patients still spend their time on their backs during labor and birth. Patients should be encouraged to assume any position of comfort for them. In a recent randomized controlled study, the use of a birth ball placed between the laboring person's legs during labor decreased the length of labor and increased the rate of vaginal births. Use of the birth ball was associated with a significantly lower incidence of cesarean births. The birth ball can be a potentially successful nursing intervention to help progress labor and support vaginal birth, along with position changes, for patients laboring under epidural analgesia. The use of the birth ball was found to be effective for pain management, correct fetal presentation, and reduction in the duration of labor (Jha et al., 2023; Martinez et al., 2022).

TAKE NOTE!

If the only furniture provided is a bed, this is what the laboring patient will use. Furnishing rooms with comfortable chairs, beanbag chairs, and other birth props allows them to choose from a variety of positions and to be free to move around during labor.

Changing positions and moving around during labor and birth offer several benefits. Maternal position can influence pelvic size and contours. Changing position and walking affect the pelvis joints, which may facilitate fetal descent and rotation. Assuming an upright position to give birth reduces the risk of aorta compression, which allows a better oxygen supply to the uterus and fetus. Squatting enlarges the pelvic inlet and outlet diameters, and a kneeling position removes pressure on the maternal vena cava and helps rotate the fetus from a posterior position to an anterior one to facilitate birth (Jyoti et al., 2022). The use of any upright or lateral position compared to supine or lithotomy positions may:

- Reduce the length of the first stage of labor.
- Reduce the duration of the second stage of labor.
- Reduce the number of assisted deliveries (vacuum and forceps).
- Reduce episiotomies and perineal tears.
- Contribute to fewer abnormal fetal heart rate patterns.
- Increase comfort and reduce requests for pain medication.

- Enhance a sense of control by the laboring person.
- Alter the shape and size of the pelvis, which assists in descent.
- Assist gravity to move the fetus downward (Oppenheimer & Black, 2023).

Using the research available can promote better outcomes, heightened professionalism, and evidence-based practice in childbearing practices. Current guidelines discourage from lying supine or semisupine during labor and encourage them to adapt to any other position that they find comfortable since lying on the back is associated with longer labor, increase in surgical births, increased pain, and a higher incidence of fetal heart rate abnormalities (AWHONN, 2022; National Institute for Health and Care Excellence, 2023). Nurses need to encourage upright positioning and freedom of movement throughout labor to achieve the best outcomes (see Evidence-Based Practice 13.2).

Psychological Response

Childbearing can be one of the most life-altering experiences for a person. The experience of childbirth goes beyond the physiologic aspects: It can influence their self-confidence; ability to bond with the newborn; self-esteem; future childbirth decisions; and their view of life, relationships, and children. Their state of mind (psyche) throughout the entire process is critical to bringing about a positive outcome for them and their family. Research finds that maternal anxiety, distress, and fear are associated with an increase in surgical births, prolonged labor, and use of epidural analgesia (Sanni et al., 2022). Nurses need to understand and tune into the patient's perceptions and expectations of childbirth to promote a positive experience and outcome. Factors promoting a positive birth experience include:

- Clear information about procedures
- Support; not being alone
- Sense of mastery, self-confidence
- Trust in staff assisting with labor and delivery
- Sense of empowerment in body
- Increased awareness of the laboring process
- Involvement and support of partner
- Positive reaction to the pregnancy
- Personal control over breathing
- Preparation for the childbirth experience (AWHONN, 2022)

Having a strong sense of self and meaningful support from others can often help people manage labor well. Feeling safe and secure typically promotes a sense of control and the ability to withstand the challenges of the childbearing experience. Anxiety and fear, however, decrease a person's ability to cope with the discomfort of labor. Maternal catecholamines secreted in response to anxiety and fear can inhibit uterine blood flow and placental perfusion (Rakers et al., 2020). In contrast, relaxation can augment the natural process of labor (Kaple & Patil, 2023). Preparing mentally for childbirth is important so that the laboring person can work with, rather than against, the natural forces of labor.

EVIDENCE-BASED PRACTICE **13.2**

Evaluating the Effects of Maternal Positions in Childbirth: An Overview of Cochrane Systematic Reviews

BACKGROUND

The mechanisms of childbirth positions are associated with pelvic dimensions, intrauterine pressure, fetal head molding, and progression of fetal descent through the maternal birth canal. In the United States, laboring people generally recline in a recumbent position to make it easier for nurses to monitor fetal progress and perform vaginal exams. However, recumbent positions result in supine hypotension, diminishing uterine activity, and a reduction in the dimensions of the pelvic outlet. The purpose of this overview was to provide a summary of the effects of maternal positioning on duration of labor and birth, as well as operative birth.

STUDY

An electronic search for studies was conducted within the Cochrane database. Three systematic reviews were included in this overview, which included 65 trials with a total of 18,697 participants.

Findings

In the first stage of labor, upright positions were significantly associated with a shorter duration of labor and fewer surgical births. In the second stage of labor, the upright position was associated with a shorter duration of labor and a reduction in the number of assisted births, but not a reduction in surgical births.

Nursing Implications

Based on the results of this study, nurses should actively encourage laboring patients to walk around, stand, sit, kneel, or squat to allow gravity to speed the cervix to dilate. Ambulation can reduce the duration of labor, need for analgesia, and improve maternal comfort. Encouraging an upright position improves frequency, strength, and length of contractions; decreases the use of oxytocin to augment labor; and improves the oxygen supply to the fetus. Gravity can improve the descent of the fetus and an upright position is also beneficial to maternal cardiac output, which promotes better fetal circulation. Nurses can inform all low-risk laboring patients about the benefits of assuming upright positions or their free choice of position, which provides comfort for the patient during the first stage of labor, and support them in their choices.

Adapted from Kibuka, M., Price, A., Onakpoya, I., Tierney, S., & Clarke, M. (2021). Evaluating the effects of maternal positions in childbirth: An overview of Cochrane systematic reviews. *European Journal of Midwifery, 5*, 57. https://doi.org/10.18332/ejm/142781

Philosophy

Not everyone views childbirth in the same way. A philosophical continuum exists that extends from viewing labor as a disease process to a normal process. One end of the spectrum assumes laboring people cannot manage the birth experience adequately and therefore need constant expert monitoring and management. The other philosophy assumes that they are capable and reasonable people who can actively participate in their birth experience.

The health care system in the United States today seems to lean toward the former philosophy, applying technologic interventions to most birthing parents who enter the hospital system. Giving birth in a hospital in the 21st century has become "intervention intensive." It is designed to start, continue, and end labor with extensive medical management, rather than allowing the normal process of birth to unfold. The increase in surgical births has resulted in a decline in quality and respect for some patients. Advances in medical care have improved the safety of patients with high-risk pregnancies. However, the routine use of intravenous therapy, electronic fetal monitoring, uterine augmentation, and epidural anesthesia has not improved birth outcomes for all patients (Sabetghadam et al., 2022). Perhaps supporting a physiologic approach to childbirth using fewer unnecessary medical interventions is the way to improve birth outcomes in the United States.

During the 1970s, family-centered maternity care was developed in response to the consumer reaction to the depersonalization of birth. The hope was to shift the philosophy from "medicalization" to physiologic childbirth. The term "physiologic" is more appropriate today to denote the low-tech, high-touch approach requested by many childbearing people who view childbirth as a normal process. Physiologic childbirth is an approach to care that supports the body's ability to perform processes during childbirth while considering the laboring person's philosophy, values, and preferences during this life event.

Certified nurse midwives (CNMs) are champions of physiologic birthing, and their participation in the childbirth process is associated with fewer unnecessary interventions when compared to obstetricians. CNMs subscribe to a normal birth process during which the patient uses their own instincts and bodily signs during labor. Use of midwives is linked to fewer surgical births, lower preterm birth rates, lower episiotomy rates, higher breastfeeding rates, and a more positive childbirth experience (Niles & Zephyrin, 2023). Midwives encourage movement throughout labor and let nature take its course. In short, midwives empower laboring people within the birthing environment (Morningstar, 2022). No matter what philosophy is held, it is ideal if everyone involved in the particular birth process—from the health care provider to the laboring person—shares the same philosophy toward the birth process.

Partners

Laboring people desire support and attentive care during labor and birth. Caregivers can convey emotional support by offering their continued presence and words of encouragement. Throughout the world, few people are left to labor totally alone; emotional, physical, and/or spiritual support during labor is the norm for most cultures. A caring partner can use massage, light touch, acupressure, hand-holding, stroking, and relaxation; can help the person in labor communicate their wishes to the staff; and can provide a continuous, reassuring presence, all of which bring some degree of comfort. Partners need emotional and informational support from nurses to be actively involved and play an important, supportive role for the birthing parent (ACOG, 2023; Schmitt et al., 2022). Although the presence of the significant other at the birth provides special emotional support, a partner can be anyone who is present to support the laboring person throughout the experience. For many laboring people, the essential ingredients for a safe and satisfying birth include a sense of empowerment and success in coping with or transcending the experience in addition to having solid, positive encouragement from a support companion.

Worldwide, women usually support other women in childbirth. **Doula** is a Greek word meaning woman servant or caregiver. It now commonly refers to a woman who offers emotional and practical support to a birthing parent or couple before, during, and after childbirth. A doula believes in "mothering the mother," and clinical support remains the job of the midwife or medical staff (International Doula Institute, 2024). The continuous presence of a trained female support person reduces the need for medication for pain relief, the use of vacuum or forceps delivery, and the need for cesarean births. Continuous support has also been associated with a slight reduction in the length of labor. The doula, who is an experienced labor companion, provides the laboring patient and their partner with emotional and physical support and information throughout the entire labor and birth experience.

Research finds that nursing care during labor decreases the likelihood of negative evaluations of the childbirth experience, spontaneous vaginal births, feelings of tenseness during labor, and finding labor worse than expected. Evidence also notes less perineal trauma, reduced difficulty in parenting the newborn, and reduced likelihood of early cessation of breastfeeding. Continuous support by nurses includes reassurance, encouragement, praise, advocacy, nurturing, and explanation of the labor progress (Kiti et al., 2022).

Nursing care of patients during labor should incorporate finding a way to connect with them and to understand what they are experiencing (knowing); spending time with them (presence); protecting them and preserving their dignity (doing for); providing information and explanations in a clear methodical manner (enabling); and ensuring a safe childbirth experience. Given the many benefits of intrapartum support, laboring patients should always have the option to receive partner support, whether from nurses, doulas, significant others, or family. Whoever the support partner is, they should provide the laboring person with continuous presence and hands-on comfort and encouragement. The overall objective of providing support for patients during childbirth is to create a positive experience for them while preserving their physical and psychological health (AWHONN, 2022).

Patience

The birth process takes time. If more time were allowed for labor to progress naturally without intervention, the cesarean birth rate would most likely be reduced. In one study, continuous support provided by midwives during labor reduced the duration of labor and the number of cesarean births; this model of support should be available to all patients (AWHONN, 2022). The literature suggests that delaying interventions can give a patient enough time to progress in labor and reduce the need for surgical intervention (ACOG, 2021).

Healthy People 2030 includes one goal related to cesarean births in the United States, "MICH-06: Reduce cesarean births among low-risk women with no prior births" (U.S. Department of Health and Human Services, n.d.). We are a long way from achieving this and other goals; in the United States, the cesarean birth rate ranges from 24.1% to 35.8% depending on the state (Centers for Disease Control and Prevention, 2022). Cesarean birth rate is associated with increased morbidity and mortality for both birthing parent and infant as well as increased inpatient length of stay and health care costs (Angolile et al., 2023).

It is difficult to predict how labor will progress and therefore equally difficult to determine how long an person's labor will last. There is no way to estimate the likely strength and frequency of uterine contractions, the extent to which the cervix will soften and dilate, and how much the fetal head will need to mold to fit through the birth canal. It is not known beforehand whether the complex fetal rotations needed for an efficient labor will properly take place. All of these factors are unknown when labor starts.

Patient Preparation: Prenatal Education

Basic prenatal education can help patients manage the labor process and feel in control of their birthing experience. The literature indicates that if a pregnant person is prepared before the labor and birth experience, the labor is more likely to remain natural without the need for medical intervention. An increasing body of evidence also indicates that the well-prepared patient with good labor support is less likely to need analgesia or anesthesia and is less likely to require cesarean birth (Lothian, 2022).

Prenatal education teaches the pregnant person about the childbirth experience and increases their sense of control. They are then able to work as an active participant during the labor and birth experience (Gallant, 2023). The research also suggests that prenatal preparation may affect intra- and postpartum psychosocial outcomes (Vanderlaan et al., 2022). Special consideration of each patient's culture, age, cognitive skills, access to health information, and health literacy all impact their understanding of the content presented. Nurses play an essential role in providing evidence-based education throughout the prenatal period.

TAKE NOTE!

Learning about labor and birth allows pregnant people and couples to express their needs and preferences ahead of time, enhance their confidence, and improve communication between themselves and the staff.

Pain Management

The perception of pain can be influenced by a number of factors—past experiences of pain, culture and beliefs, stoicism, and anxiety and depression. To manage a patient's plan, nurses need to understand what it is and provide support to the laboring patient to enable them to deal with the pain and challenges of labor. Labor and birth, though a normal physiologic process, can produce significant pain. Pain during labor is a nearly universal experience. Controlling the uterine discomfort without harming the fetus or labor process is the major focus of pain management during childbirth. Many options exist if and when the patient might decide to use them (Petruska, 2022). Pain is a subjective experience involving a complex interaction of physiologic, spiritual, psychosocial, cultural, and environmental influences. Cultural values and learned behaviors influence perception and response to pain, as do anxiety and fear, both of which tend to heighten the sense of pain. Patients in labor need to feel in control and have input in the decision-making regarding the pain management process during labor (Grant & Reale, 2024). The challenge for care providers is to find the right combination of pain management methods to keep the discomfort manageable while minimizing the negative effect on the fetus, the normal physiology of labor, maternal–infant bonding, breastfeeding, and a laboring patient's perception of the labor itself (Lothian, 2024). Chapter 14 presents a full discussion of pain management during labor and birth.

KEY CONCEPTS

- Labor is a complex, multifaceted interaction between the birthing parent and fetus. Thus, it is difficult to determine exactly why labor begins and what initiates it.
- Before the onset of labor, the pregnant body undergoes several changes in preparation for the birth of the newborn, often leading to characteristic signs and symptoms that suggest labor is near. These changes include cervical changes, lightening, increased energy level, bloody show, Braxton Hicks contractions, and spontaneous rupture of membranes.
- False labor is a condition seen during the latter weeks of some pregnancies in which irregular uterine contractions are felt, but the cervix is not affected.
- Labor is typically divided into stages that are unequal in length.
- During the first stage, the fundamental change underlying the process is progressive dilation of the cervix. It is further divided into two phases: latent phase and active phase.
- The second stage of labor is from complete cervical dilation (10 cm) and effacement through the birth of the infant.
- The third stage is that of separation and birth of the placenta. It consists of two phases: placental separation and placental expulsion.
- The fourth stage begins after the birth of the placenta and membranes and ends with the initial physiologic adjustment and stabilization of the birthing parent (1 to 4 hours).
- As the patient experiences and progresses through childbirth, numerous physiologic responses occur that assist their adaptation to the laboring process.
- The critical factors in labor and birth are designated as the 10 Ps: passageway (birth canal), passenger (fetus and placenta), powers (contractions), position (maternal), psychological response, philosophy (low tech, high touch), partners (support caregivers), patience (natural timing), patient preparation (childbirth knowledge base), and pain management (comfort measures).
- The size and shape of the female pelvis are determining factors for a vaginal birth. The female pelvis is classified according to four main shapes: gynecoid, anthropoid, android, and platypelloid, but these classifications have recently been questioned for validity.
- The diameters of the fetal skull vary considerably, with some diameters shortening and others lengthening as the head is molded during the labor and birth process.
- The labor process is comprised of a series of rhythmic, involuntary, usually quite uncomfortable uterine muscle contractions that bring about a shortening (effacement) and opening (dilation) of the cervix, and a bursting of the fetal membranes. Important parameters of uterine contractions are frequency, duration, and intensity.
- Laboring patients should change positions frequently, assuming a desired position while avoiding supine positioning.
- Mentally preparing pregnant and laboring people for childbirth is important to enable them to work with the natural forces of labor and not against them.
- Pain during labor is a nearly universal experience. Having a strong sense of self and meaningful support from others can often help patients manage labor well and reduce the sensation of pain.

REFERENCES AND RECOMMENDED READINGS

American College of Obstetricians and Gynecologists. (2021). *ACOG Committee Opinion No. 766: Approaches to limit intervention during labor and birth.* (Reaffirmed, 2021). https://www.acog.org/clinical/clinical-guidance/committee-opinion/articles/2019/02/approaches-to-limit-intervention-during-labor-and-birth

American College of Obstetricians and Gynecologists. (2023). *A partner's guide to pregnancy.* https://www.acog.org/womens-health/faqs/a-partners-guide-to-pregnancy

American College of Obstetricians and Gynecologists. (2024). First and second stage labor management: ACOG clinical practice guideline no. 8. *Obstetrics and Gynecology, 143*(1), 144–162. https://doi.org/10.1097/AOG.0000000000005447

American Pregnancy Association. (2024). *Signs of labor.* https://americanpregnancy.org/healthy-pregnancy/labor-and-birth/signs-of-labor/

Angolile, C. M., Max, B. L., Mushemba, J., & Mashauri, H. L. (2023). Global increased cesarean section rates and public health implications: A call to action. *Health Science Reports, 6*(5), e1274. https://doi.org/10.1002/hsr2.1274

Association of Women's Health, Obstetric and Neonatal Nurses. (2022). Evidence-based clinical practice guideline: Labor support for intended vaginal birth. *Journal of Obstetric, Gynecologic, and Neonatal Nursing, 51*(6), S1-S42. https://doi.org/10.1016/j.jogn.2022.04.006

Aubin, S. L. (2023). Clinical course of normal labor. In G. Posner, A. Black, G. Jones, & J. Dy, *Oxorn-Foote human labor and birth* (7th ed.), McGraw Hill.

Badi, M. B., Abebe, S. M., Weldetsadic, M. A., Christensson, K., & Lindgren, H. (2022). Effect of flexible sacrum position on maternal and neonatal outcomes in public health facilities, Amhara Regional State, Ethiopia: A quasi-experimental study. *International Journal of Environmental Research and Public Health, 19*(15), 9637. https://doi.org/10.3390/ijerph19159637

Barfield, W. D., & Lee, K. G. (2023). Late preterm infants. *UpToDate.* Retrieved March 5, 2024, from https://www.uptodate.com/contents/late-preterm-infants

Burgess, M. D., & Lui, F. (2023). Anatomy, bony pelvis and lower limb: Pelvic bones. *StatPearls.* https://www.ncbi.nlm.nih.gov/books/NBK551580/

Centers for Disease Control and Prevention. (2022). *Cesarean delivery rate by state.* https://www.cdc.gov/nchs/pressroom/sosmap/cesarean_births/cesareans.htm

Cunningham, F. G., Leveno, K. J., Dashe, J. S., Hoffman, B. L., Spong, C. Y., & Casey, B. M. (2022a). Physiology of labor. In F. G. Cunningham, K. J. Leveno, J. S. Dashe, B. L. Hoffman, C. Y. Spong, & B. M. Casey (Eds.), *William's obstetrics* (26th ed.). McGraw-Hill.

Cunningham, F. G., Leveno, K. J., Dashe, J. S., Hoffman, B. L., Spong, C. Y., & Casey, B. M. (2022b). Normal labor. In F. G. Cunningham, K. J. Leveno, J. S. Dashe, B. L. Hoffman, C. Y. Spong, & B. M. Casey (Eds.), *William's obstetrics* (26th ed.). McGraw-Hill.

Cunningham, F. G., Leveno, K. J., Dashe, J. S., Hoffman, B. L., Spong, C. Y., & Casey, B. M. (2022c). Abnormal labor. In F. G. Cunningham, K. J. Leveno, J. S. Dashe, B. L. Hoffman, C. Y., Spong & B. M. Casey (Eds.), *William's obstetrics* (26th ed.). McGraw-Hill.

Cypher, R. L. (2024). Intrapartum fetal assessment. In B. J. Baker, J. Janke, & Association of Women's Health, Obstetric and Neonatal Nurses, *Core curriculum for maternal-newborn nursing* (6th ed.). Elsevier.

Eggleton, J. S., & Cunha, B. (2023). Anatomy, abdomen and pelvis, pelvic outlet. *StatPearls*. https://www.ncbi.nlm.nih.gov/books/NBK557602/

Ehsanipoor, R. M., & Satin, A. J. (2023). Labor: Overview of normal and abnormal progression. *UpToDate*. Retrieved March 4, 2024, from https://www.uptodate.com/contents/labor-overview-of-normal-and-abnormal-progression

Evbuomwan, O., & Chowdhury, Y. S. (2023). Physiology, cervical dilation. *StatPearls*. https://www.ncbi.nlm.nih.gov/books/NBK557582/

Familiari, A., Neri, C., Passananti, E., Marco, G. D., Felici, F., Ranieri, E., Flacco, M. E., & Lanzone, A. (2023). Maternal position during the second stage of labor and maternal-neonatal outcomes in nulliparous women: A retrospective cohort study. *AJOG Global Reports*, *3*(1), 100160. https://doi.org/10.1016/j.xagr.2023.100160

Funai, E. F., & Norwitz, E. R. (2024). Labor and delivery: Management of the normal third stage after vaginal birth. *UpToDate*. Retrieved February 29, 2024, from https://www.uptodate.com/contents/labor-and-delivery-management-of-the-normal-third-stage-after-vaginal-birth

Gallant, C. (2023). Obstetric anesthesia and analgesia. In G. Posner, A. Black, G. Jones, & J. Dy, *Oxorn-Foote human labor and birth* (7th ed.). McGraw Hill.

Garber, A., & Dy, J. (2023). Normal mechanisms of labor. In G. Posner, A. Black, G. Jones, & J. Dy, *Oxorn-Foote human labor and birth* (7th ed.). McGraw Hill.

Grant, G. J., & Reale, S. (2024). Pharmacologic management of pain during labor and delivery. *UpToDate*. Retrieved March 5, 2024, from https://www.uptodate.com/contents/pharmacologic-management-of-pain-during-labor-and-delivery

Hofmeyr, G. J. (2023). Overview of breech presentation. *UpToDate*. Retrieved March 5, 2024, from https://www.uptodate.com/contents/overview-of-breech-presentation

Hurst, H. M., & Baker, B. (2024). Essential forces and factors. In B. J. Baker, J. Janke, & Association of Women's Health, Obstetric and Neonatal Nurses, *Core curriculum for maternal-newborn nursing* (6th ed.). Elsevier.

Hutchison, J., Mahdy, H., & Hutchison, J. (2023). Stages of labor. *StatPearls*. https://www.ncbi.nlm.nih.gov/books/NBK544290/

International Doula Institute. (2024). *What is a doula?* https://internationaldoulainstitute.com/what-is-a-doula/

Irvin, L., De Leo, A., & Davison, C. (2022). Stand and deliver: An integrative review of the evidence around birthing upright. *British Journal of Midwifery*, *30*(3). https://www.britishjournalofmidwifery.com/content/literature-review/stand-and-deliver-an-integrative-review-of-the-evidence-around-birthing-upright

Iversen, J. K., Kahrs, B. H., & Eggebø, T. M. (2021). There are 4, not 7 cardinal movements in labor. *American Journal of Obstetrics & Gynecology*, *3*(6), 100436. https://doi.org/10.1016/j.ajogmf.2021.100436

Jha, S., Vyas, H., Nebhinani, M., Singh, P., & Deviga, T. (2023). The effect of birthing ball exercises on labor pain and labor outcome among primigravid parturient mothers at a tertiary care hospital. *Cureus*, *15*(3), e36088. https://doi.org/10.7759/cureus.36088

Jyoti, R., Sharma, M., & Pareek, S. (2022). The effects and outcomes of different maternal positions on the second stage of labor. *Journal of Health Sciences*, *10*(2), 21–24. https://doi.org/10.4103/mjhs.mjhs_49_21

Kaple, G. S., & Patil, S. (2023). Effectiveness of Jacobson relaxation and Lamaze breathing techniques in the management of pain and stress during labor: An experimental study. *Cureus*, *15*(1), e33212. https://doi.org/10.7759/cureus.33212

Kibuka, M., Price, A., Onakpoya, I., Tierney, S., & Clarke, M. (2021). Evaluating the effects of maternal positions in childbirth: An overview of Cochrane systematic reviews. *European Journal of Midwifery*, *5*, 57. https://doi.org/10.18332/ejm/142781

Kiti, G., Prata, N., & Afulani, P. A. (2022). Continuous labor support and person-centered maternity care: A cross-sectional study with women in rural Kenya. *Maternal and Child Health Journal*, *26*, 205–216. https://doi.org/10.1007/s10995-021-03259-4

Lothian, J. (2024). Normal childbirth. In B. J. Baker, J. Janke, & Association of Women's Health, Obstetric, and Neonatal Nurses, *Core curriculum for maternal-newborn nursing* (6th ed.). Elsevier.

Lothian, J. A. (2022). Preparation for childbirth. *UpToDate*. Retrieved March 6, 2024, from https://www.uptodate.com/contents/preparation-for-childbirth

Martinez, E. E., Serrano, M. O., Barrios, N. E. C., Gordon, G. P., Cornejo, S. V., & Garcia, Z. G. (2022). Birth ball for pain management and its effects in natural childbirth. *Alerta*, *5*(1), 57–63. https://doi.org/10.5377/alerta.v5i1.11223

Mohammed, R., & El-Chaâr, D. (2023). Abnormal cephalic presentations. In G. Posner, A. Black, G. Jones, & J. Dy, *Oxorn-Foote human labor and birth* (7th ed.). McGraw Hill.

Morningstar, S. (2022). Birth beyond medicalization. Midwifery Today, 142. https://www.midwiferytoday.com/mt-articles/birth-beyond-medicalization/

Moura, R., Borges, M., Vila Pouca, M. C. P., Oliveira, D. A., Parente, M. P . L., Kimmich, N., Mascarenhas, T., & Natal, R. M. (2021). A numerical study on fetal head molding during labor. *International Journal of Numerical Methods in Biomedical Engineering*, *37*, e3411. https://doi.org/10.1002/cnm.3411

National Institute for Health and Care Excellence. (2023). *Intrapartum care: NICE guideline [NG235]*. https://www.nice.org.uk/guidance/ng235

Niles, P. M., & Zephyrin, L. C. (2023). *How expanding the role of midwives in U.S. health care could help address the maternal health crisis*. The Commonwealth Fund. https://www

.commonwealthfund.org/publications/issue-briefs/2023/may/expanding-role-midwives-address-maternal-health-crisis

Norwitz, E. R. (2024). Physiology of parturition at term. *UpToDate*. Retrieved February 29, 2024, from https://www.uptodate.com/contents/physiology-of-parturition-at-term

Oppenheimer, L., & Black, A. (2023). The second stage of labor. In G. Posner, A. Black, G. Jones, & J. Dy, *Oxorn-Foote human labor and birth* (7th ed.). McGraw Hill.

Paudel, A. K., Chhetri, M. R., Baniya, A., Chhetri, M., & Gurung, A. (2023). Factors associated with postpartum care during the fourth stage of labor in Nepal: A hospital-based cross-sectional study. *Journal of Social, Behavioral, and Health Sciences, 17*(1), 67–79. https://doi.org/10.5590/JSBHS.2023.17.1.06

Petruska, S. E. (2022). *Making sense of childbirth pain relief options*. https://www.acog.org/womens-health/experts-and-stories/the-latest/making-sense-of-childbirth-pain-relief-options

Posner, G. (2023). Engagement, synclitism, asynclitism. In G. Posner, A. Black, G. Jones, & J. Dy, *Oxorn-Foote human labor and birth* (7th ed.). McGraw Hill.

Rakers, F., Rupprecht, S., Dreiling, M., Bergmeier, C., Witte, O. W., & Schwab, M. (2020). Transfer of maternal psychosocial stress to the fetus. *Neuroscience & Biobehavioral Reviews, 117*, 185–197. https://doi.org/10.1016/j.neubiorev.2017.02.019

Sabetghadam, S., Keramat, A., Goli, S., Malary, M., & Chamani, S. R. (2022). Assessment of medicalization of pregnancy and childbirth in low-risk pregnancies: A cross-sectional study. *International Journal of Community Based Nursing and Midwifery, 10*(1), 64–73. https://doi.org/10.30476/IJCBNM.2021.90292.1686

Sanni, K. R., Eeva, E., Noora, S. M., Laura, K. S., Linnea, K., & Hasse, K. (2022). The influence of maternal psychological distress on the mode of birth and duration of labor: Findings from the Finn Brain Birth Cohort Study. *Archives of Women's Mental Health. 25*, 463–472. https://doi.org/10.1007/s00737-022-01212-0

Satone, P. D., & Tayade, S. (2023). Alternative birthing positions compared to the conventional position in the second stage of labor: A review. *Cureus, 15*(4), e37943. https://doi.org/10.7759/cureus.37943

Schmitt, N., Striebich, S., Meyer, G., Berg, A., & Ayerle, G. M. (2022). The partner's experiences of childbirth in countries with a highly developed clinical setting: A scoping review. *BMC Pregnancy and Childbirth, 22*, 742. https://doi.org/10.1186/s12884-022-05014-1

Shinozaki, K., Suto, M., Ota, E., Eto, H., & Horiuchi, S. (2022). Postpartum urinary incontinence and birth outcomes as a result of the pushing technique: A systematic review and meta-analysis. *International Urogynecology Journal, 33*(6), 1435–1449. https://doi.org/10.1007/s00192-021-05058-5

Siccardi, M. A., Imonugo, O., Arbor, T. C., & Valle, C. (2023). Anatomy, abdomen and pelvis, pelvic inlet. *StatPearls*. https://www.ncbi.nlm.nih.gov/books/NBK519068/

Smith, D. (2022). The newborn infant. In M. Bunik, W. W. Hay, M. J. Levin, & M. J. Abzug (Eds.), *Current diagnosis & treatment: Pediatrics* (26th ed.). McGraw-Hill.

Toledano, R. D., & Leffert, L. (2024). Neuraxial analgesia for labor and delivery (including instrumental delivery). *UpToDate*. Retrieved March 6, 2024, from https://www.uptodate.com/contents/neuraxial-analgesia-for-labor-and-delivery-including-instrumental-delivery

U.S. Department of Health and Human Services. (n.d.).*Reduce cesarean births among low-risk women with no prior births—MICH-06*. https://health.gov/healthypeople/objectives-and-data/browse-objectives/pregnancy-and-childbirth/reduce-cesarean-births-among-low-risk-women-no-prior-births-mich-06

Vanderlaan, J., Gatlin, T., & Shen, J. (2022). Outcomes of childbirth education in PRAMS, phase 8. *Maternal and Child Health Journal, 27*, 82–91. https://doi.org/10.1007/s10995-022-03494-3

VanSickle, C., Liese, K. L., & Rutherford, J. N. (2022). Textbook typologies: Challenging the myth of the perfect obstetric pelvis. *The Anatomical Record, 305*, 753–1031. https://anatomypubs.onlinelibrary.wiley.com/doi/epdf/10.1002/ar.24880

Zhang, Y., Hao, D., Yang, L, Zhou, X., Ye-Lin, Y., & Yang, Y. (2022). Assessment of features between multichannel electrohysterogram for differentiation of labors. *Sensors, 22*(9), 3352. https://doi.org/10.3390/s22093352

DEVELOPING CLINICAL JUDGMENT

PRACTICING FOR NCLEX

1. The nurse is determining the frequency of contractions. Which period of time will the nurse measure?
   - a. Start of one contraction to the start of the next contraction
   - b. Beginning of one contraction to the end of the same contraction
   - c. Peak of one contraction to the peak of the next contraction
   - d. End of one contraction to the beginning of the next contraction
2. Which fetal lie is most conducive to a spontaneous vaginal birth?
   - a. Transverse
   - b. Longitudinal
   - c. Perpendicular
   - d. Oblique
3. The nurse is caring for a laboring person. Which observation would suggest that placental separation is occurring?
   - a. Uterus stops contracting altogether.
   - b. Umbilical cord pulsations stop.
   - c. Uterine shape changes to globular.
   - d. Maternal blood pressure drops.
4. The nurse is explaining the difference between true versus false labor to her childbirth class. Which participant response indicates an understanding of what the major difference between them is?
   - a. Discomfort level is greater with false labor.
   - b. Progressive cervical changes occur in true labor.
   - c. There is a feeling of nausea with false labor.
   - d. There is more fetal movement with true labor.
5. The nurse is teaching an antepartum patient about labor. What does the nurse teach the patient is the most intense time during labor?
   - a. Latent phase
   - b. Active phase
   - c. Membranes breaking
   - d. Placental expulsion phase
6. A laboring patient is admitted to the labor and birth suite at 4-cm dilation. Which stage of labor does the nurse determine the patient is in?
   - a. Latent
   - b. Active
   - c. Late
   - d. Early
7. A patient has arrived at the hospital because they think they are in labor. Which assessment would indicate that the patient is in true labor?
   - a. Contractions are irregular, not close together.
   - b. Many of the contractions are weak-feeling.
   - c. Cervix is 4 cm dilated, 90% effaced.
   - d. Contractions last 30 seconds every 5 to 10 minutes.
8. Which of the following are cardinal movements of labor? Select all that apply.
   - a. Extension and rotation
   - b. Descent and engagement
   - c. Presentation and position
   - d. Attitude and lie
   - e. Flexion and expulsion
9. Several patients have completed a childbirth education series. Which participant statement indicates how physiologic preparation for labor would be demonstrated?
   - a. "I will feel a decrease in the Braxton Hicks contractions."
   - b. "My appetite will increase, and I will gain weight."
   - c. "My belly will look lower when lightening occurs."
   - d. "Movements by my baby will increase in frequency."
10. The nurse is caring for a patient in active labor. Which maternal position will the nurse advocate for? Select three.
    - a. Dorsal lithotomy with stirrups
    - b. Sitting on the birthing ball
    - c. Supine to ensure patient comfort
    - d. Nonsupine position of comfort
    - e. Patient up on hands and knees

CRITICAL THINKING EXERCISES

1. Cindy, a 20-year-old primipara, calls the birthing center where you work as a nurse and reports that she thinks she is in labor because she feels labor pains. Her due date is this week. The midwives have been giving her prenatal care throughout this pregnancy.
   - a. What additional information do you need to respond appropriately?
   - b. What suggestions and recommendations would you make to her?
   - c. What instructions need to be given to guide her decision-making process?
   - d. About what other premonitory signs of labor might the nurse ask?
   - e. What manifestations would be found if Cindy is experiencing true labor?

2. You are assigned to lead a community education class for women in the third trimester of pregnancy to prepare them for the upcoming birth. Prepare an outline of topics that should be addressed.

STUDY ACTIVITIES

3. During clinical postconference, share with the other nursing students how the critical forces of labor influenced the length of labor and the birthing process for a laboring patient assigned to you.

4. Interview a patient on the mother–baby unit who has given birth within the past few hours. Ask them to describe their experience and examine psychological factors that may have influenced their laboring process.

5. On the following illustration, identify the parameters of uterine contractions by marking an "X" where the nurse would measure the duration of the contraction.

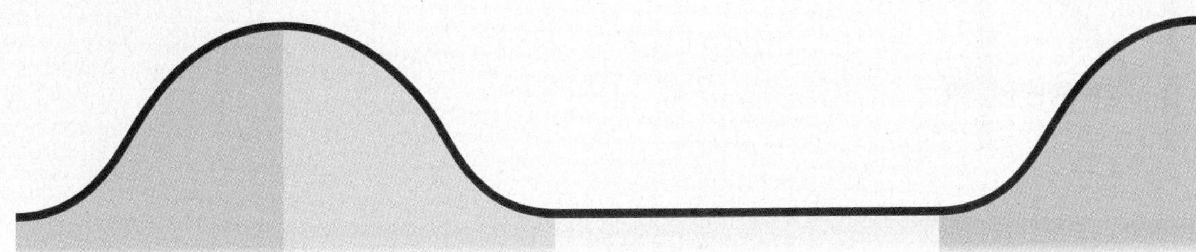

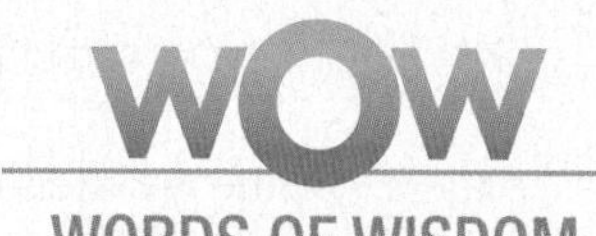

WORDS OF WISDOM

Wise nurses are not always silent, but they know when to be during the miracle of birth.

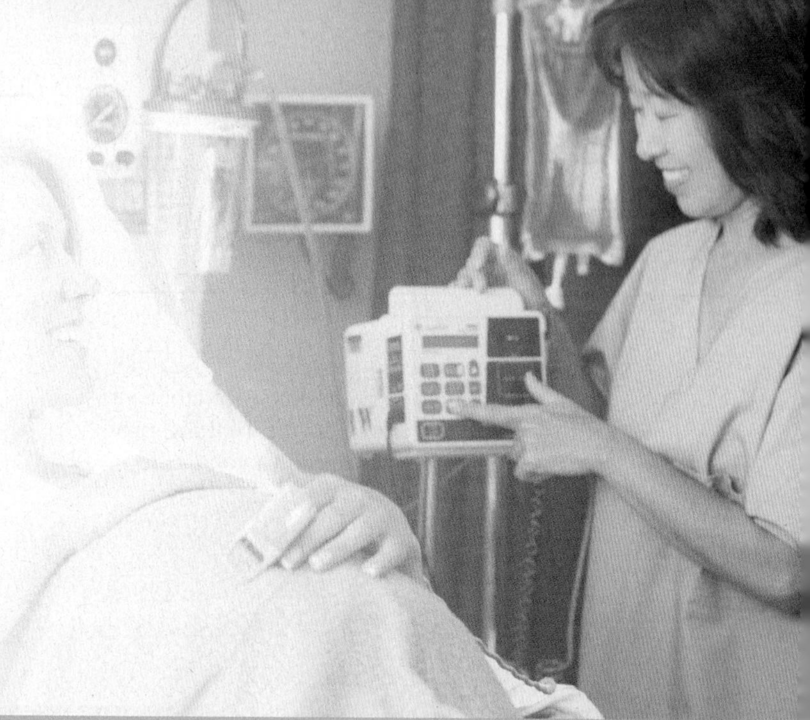

14

Nursing Management During Labor and Birth

KEY TERMS

accelerations
artifact
baseline fetal heart rate
baseline variability
crowning
deceleration
electronic fetal monitoring (EFM)
episiotomy (e-piz'ē-ot'ŏ-mē)
Leopold maneuvers
neuraxial (nū-rak'sē-ăl) analgesia/anesthesia
periodic baseline changes

LEARNING OBJECTIVES

Upon completion of the chapter, you will be able to:

1. Examine the measures used to evaluate maternal status during labor and birth.
2. Discuss the advantages and disadvantages of external and internal fetal monitoring, including the appropriate use for each.
3. Choose appropriate nursing interventions to address the categories of fetal heart rate patterns.
4. Outline the nurse's role in fetal assessment.
5. Appraise the various comfort promotion and pain relief strategies used during labor and birth.
6. Summarize the assessment data collected upon admission to the perinatal unit.
7. Relate the ongoing assessments involved in each stage of labor and birth.
8. Analyze the nurse's role throughout the labor and birth process.

Sheila was admitted in active labor to the labor and birth unit. She has progressed to 8 cm dilated and is becoming increasingly more uncomfortable. She is using a patterned-paced breathing now but is thrashing around in the hospital bed.

INTRODUCTION

The laboring and birthing process is a life-changing event. Childbirth is the culmination of a human pregnancy with the emergence of a newborn from the birthing parent's uterus. Nurses need to be respectful, available, nurturing, encouraging, supportive, and professional in dealing with all patients. Just the nurse's presence in the room can be comforting and reassuring to the laboring patient. Nursing management for labor and birth involves assessment, comfort measures, emotional support, information and instruction, advocacy, and support for the partner. Providing the highest quality in maternity care is dependent on nurses valuing the childbirth experience and recognizing it as a life-changing experience for laboring patients and their families; caring nurse practice encompasses technical skills and caring behaviors; giving care that protects, promotes, and supports physiologic childbirth; providing optimal, evidence-based care; and recognizing health disparity and cultural diversity in all patients cared for to improve their childbirth experience across time, settings, and disciplines. One of the components for evidence-based care and patient-centered care is patients' preferences to guide care for themselves during the birthing process. In a recent study, participants' needs and expectations during labor and birth were assessed. Several themes emerged—thoughtful and effective communication, anticipation of needs, trustworthiness, respect, presence of a companion, efforts made to relieve pain, instruction and advocacy, and emotional helpfulness (Wanyenze et al., 2022). In addition, labor companionship increased spontaneous vaginal births, shortened labor duration, and increased overall satisfaction with the childbirth experience (Dubey et al., 2023). It is important that nurses identify the expectations and needs of patients in their care to empower them to fully participate in their childbirth experience.

In most cases, nurses are the first health care providers that patients and their families encounter, making the initial assessment an excellent opportunity for building equitable care that addresses diversity and inclusion to make everyone feel welcome and accepted. Nurses bring their own personal experiences, biases, and beliefs about race, sexual orientation, ethnicity, and gender identity into the clinical setting. They must look closely at how their views may impact their ability to care for diverse patients. During the assessment process, nurses can learn about each patient's uniqueness and convey the message of caring through inclusion (Park, 2022).

The health of birthing parents and their infants is of critical importance, both as a reflection of the current health status of a large segment of our population and as a predictor of the health of the next generation. This chapter provides information about nursing management during labor and birth. First, the essentials for in-depth assessment of maternal and fetal status during labor and birth are discussed. This is followed by a thorough description of the major methods of promoting comfort and providing pain management during the labor and birth process. The chapter concludes by putting all the information together with a discussion of the nursing care specific to each stage of labor, including the necessary data to be obtained with the admission assessment, methods to evaluate labor progress during the first stage of labor, and key nursing measures that focus on maternal and fetal assessments and pain relief for all stages of labor.

MATERNAL ASSESSMENT DURING LABOR AND BIRTH

During labor and birth, various techniques are used to assess maternal status. These techniques provide an ongoing source of data to determine the laboring person's response and their progress during labor:

- Assess maternal vital signs, including temperature, blood pressure, pulse, respiration, and pain, which are primary components of the physical examination and ongoing assessment.
- Also review the prenatal record to identify risk factors that may contribute to a decrease in uteroplacental circulation during labor.
- Determine the integrity of membranes via a vaginal examination, nitrazine test, or AmniSure rupture of membrane (ROM) test.
- If there is no vaginal bleeding upon admission, a vaginal examination or ultrasound assessment is performed to assess cervical dilation, after which it is monitored periodically as necessary to identify progress.
- Evaluate maternal pain and the effectiveness of pain management strategies at regular intervals during labor and birth (Lothian, 2024).

Vaginal Examination

Vaginal examinations form a part of the care for patients in labor to assess the progress of labor. However, these examinations are highly invasive and can be distressing or painful for many patients. Nurses need to ensure that there is a clear indication to perform them, and that the exam will provide information that will aid in the patient's care. Prior to performing a vaginal exam, a full explanation should be given to the laboring patient and their birth companion. The patient's privacy and dignity should be maintained during the exam. A full explanation of the nurse's findings should be given to the patient and birth partner with details of how the findings may impact the plan of care for the labor. It is important that the examination be done with sensitivity and gentleness (Moncrief et al., 2022).

TAKE NOTE!

A vaginal examination is an assessment skill that takes time and experience to develop; only by doing it frequently in clinical practice can the practitioner's skill level improve.

The purpose of performing a vaginal examination is to assess the amount of cervical dilation, the percentage of cervical effacement, and the fetal membrane status and to gather information on presentation, position, station, degree of fetal head flexion, and presence of fetal skull swelling or molding (Fig. 14.1). Prepare the patient by informing them about the procedure, what information will be obtained from it, how they can assist with the procedure, how it will be performed, and who will be performing it.

The patient is typically in a semi-recumbent or supine position during the vaginal examination. The vaginal examination is performed gently with concern for the patient's comfort. If it is the initial vaginal examination to check for membrane status, water is used as a lubricant.

After donning sterile gloves, the examiner inserts their index and middle fingers into the vaginal introitus. Next, the cervix is palpated to assess dilation, effacement, and position (e.g., posterior or anterior). If the cervix is open to any degree, the presenting fetal part, fetal position, station, and presence of molding can be assessed. In addition, the membranes can be evaluated and described as intact, bulging, or ruptured.

At the conclusion of the vaginal examination, the findings are discussed with the patient and their labor partner to bring them up to date about labor progress. In addition, the findings are documented either electronically or in writing and reported to the primary health care provider in charge of the patient's care.

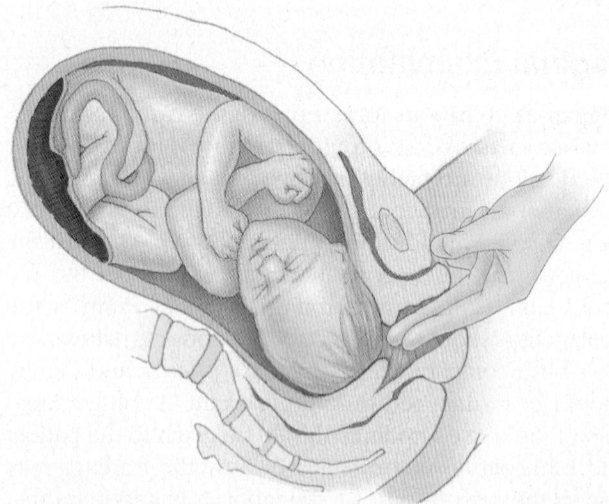

FIGURE 14.1 Vaginal examination to determine cervical dilation and effacement.

Cervical Dilation and Effacement

During the first stage of labor, the cervix opens and thins to allow descent of the fetus into the birth canal. The amount of cervical dilation (opening) and the degree of cervical effacement (thinning) are key areas assessed during the vaginal examination as the cervix is palpated with the gloved index finger. Although this finding is somewhat subjective, experienced examiners typically come up with similar findings. The width of the cervical opening determines dilation, and the length of the cervix assesses effacement. Effacement and dilation are used to assess cervical changes as follows:

- Effacement:
  - 0%: Cervical canal is 2 cm long.
  - 50%: Cervical canal is 1 cm long.
  - 100%: Cervical canal is obliterated.
- Dilation:
  - 0 cm: External cervical os is closed.
  - 5 cm: External cervical os is halfway dilated.
  - 10 cm: External os is fully dilated and ready for birth passage.

The information yielded by this examination serves as a basis for determining which stage of labor the patient is in and what their ongoing care should be.

Fetal Descent and Presenting Part

In addition to cervical dilation and effacement findings, the vaginal examination or ultrasound can also determine fetal descent (station) and presenting part. During the vaginal examination, the gloved index finger is used to palpate the fetal skull (if vertex presentation) through the opened cervix or the buttocks in the case of a breech presentation. Station is assessed in relation to the maternal ischial spines and the presenting fetal part. These spines are not sharp protrusions but rather blunted prominences at the midpelvis. The ischial spines serve as landmarks and have been designated as 0 station. If the presenting part is palpated higher than the maternal ischial spines, a negative number is assigned; if the presenting fetal part is felt below the maternal ischial spines, a positive number is assigned, denoting how many centimeters below 0 station (see Chapter 13 for a more detailed discussion).

Progressive fetal descent (−5 to +4) is the expected norm during labor—moving downward from the negative stations to 0 station to the positive stations in a timely manner. If progressive fetal descent does not occur, a disproportion between the maternal pelvis and the fetus might exist and needs to be investigated.

Rupture of Membranes

The integrity of the membranes can be determined during the vaginal examination or a bedside test kit such as AmniSure ROM, which detects the presence of amniotic fluid in vaginal secretions. Typically, if intact, the membranes will be felt as a soft bulge that is more prominent during a contraction. If the membranes have ruptured, the patient may have reported a sudden gush of fluid. Membrane rupture may also occur as a slow trickle of fluid. When membranes rupture, the priority focus should be on assessing fetal heart rate (FHR) first to identify a deceleration, which might indicate cord compression secondary to cord prolapse. If the membranes are ruptured when the patient comes to the hospital, the health care provider should ascertain when this occurred. Prolonged ruptured membranes increase the risk of infection because of ascending vaginal pathologic organisms for both birthing parent and fetus. Signs of intrauterine infection to be alert for include maternal fever, fetal and maternal tachycardia, foul odor of vaginal discharge, and an increase in white blood cell count.

The fetal membranes usually rupture during the first stage of labor. To confirm if they have ruptured, a sample of fluid is taken from the vagina via a nitrazine yellow dye swab to determine the fluid's pH. Vaginal fluid is acidic, while amniotic fluid is alkaline and turns a nitrazine swab blue. Sometimes, however, false-positive results can occur, especially in patients experiencing a large amount of bloody show because blood is alkaline. The membranes are most likely intact if the nitrazine swab remains yellow to olive green with pH between 5 and 6. The membranes are probably ruptured if the nitrazine swab turns a blue-green to deep blue with pH ranging from 6.5 to 7.5. Another assessment of the integrity of the membranes would be to visually confirm if there is amniotic fluid draining from the cervix or pooling in the vagina. A third way to assess membrane integrity would be to use an ultrasound to assess amniotic fluid volume (Duff, 2023). Many bedside tests are available (Actim, AmniSure, ROM Plus) to determine a change in vaginal pH or the presence of amniotic components such as insulinlike growth factor–binding protein 1 (a gene that may predict placental dysfunction, gestational diabetes, and preterm labor) or alpha-fetoprotein (AFP) in the vaginal fluid. In the AmniSure ROM bedside test, a swab from the collection kit is placed in the vagina for 1 minute to become saturated with fluid and then rotated in a solvent vial. The swab is read within 5 to 10 minutes. Negative means membranes have not ruptured; positive suggests it is likely that the membranes have ruptured (Qiagen, 2024; UNC Health/McLendon Clinical Laboratories, 2023). These tests determining membrane rupture should be part of an overall clinical assessment, and health care providers should not rely exclusively on one test (Nichols et al., 2022).

Assessing Uterine Contractions

The primary power of labor is uterine contractions, which are involuntary. Uterine contractions increase intrauterine pressure, causing tension on the cervix. This tension leads to cervical dilation and thinning, which in turn eventually forces the fetus through the birth canal. Normal uterine contractions have a contraction (systole) and a relaxation (diastole) phase. The contraction resembles a wave, moving downward to the cervix and upward to the fundus of the uterus. Each contraction starts with a building up (increment), gradually reaching an acme (peak intensity), and then a letting down (decrement). Each contraction is followed by an interval of rest, which ends when the next contraction begins. At the acme (peak) of the contraction, the entire uterus is contracting with the greatest intensity in the fundal area. The relaxation phase follows and occurs simultaneously throughout the uterus.

Uterine contractions during labor are monitored by palpation of the uterine fundus and by electronic monitoring. Assessment of the contractions includes frequency, duration, intensity, and uterine resting tone (see Chapter 13 for a more detailed discussion). Resting uterine tone is 10 to 15 mm Hg during labor. In the first stage of labor, contractions demonstrate an intensity of 25 to 50 mm Hg. During active labor, the intensity usually reaches as high as 80 to 100 mm Hg (Das et al., 2020).

To palpate the fundus for contraction intensity, place the pads of your fingers on the fundus and describe how it feels: like the tip of the nose (mild), like the chin (moderate), or like the forehead (strong). Palpation of intensity is a subjective judgment of the indentability of the uterine wall; a descriptive term is assigned (mild, moderate, or strong) (Fig. 14.2).

TAKE NOTE!

Frequent clinical experience is needed to gain accuracy in assessing the intensity of uterine contractions.

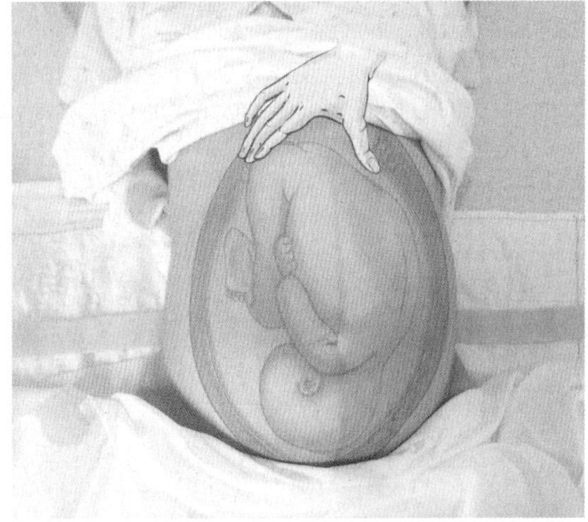

FIGURE 14.2 Nurse palpating the patient's fundus during a contraction.

The second method used to assess the intensity of uterine contractions is electronic monitoring, either external or internal. Both methods provide a reasonable measurement of the intensity of uterine contractions. Although the external fetal monitor is sometimes used to estimate the intensity of uterine contractions, it is not as accurate an assessment tool.

Performing Leopold Maneuvers

Leopold maneuvers are a method for determining the presentation, position, and lie of the fetus using four specific steps. This method involves inspection and palpation of the maternal abdomen as a screening assessment for malpresentation. The flat palmar surfaces of the nurse's hands with the fingers together palpate the uterus. A longitudinal lie is expected, and the presentation can be cephalic, breech, or shoulder. Each maneuver answers a question:

- *Maneuver 1*: What fetal part (head or buttocks) is located in the fundus (top of the uterus)?
- *Maneuver 2*: On which maternal side is the fetal back located? (Fetal heart tones are best auscultated through the back of the fetus.)
- *Maneuver 3*: What is the presenting part?
- *Maneuver 4*: Is the fetal head flexed and engaged in the pelvis?

Leopold maneuvers are described in Nursing Procedure 14.1.

FETAL ASSESSMENT DURING LABOR AND BIRTH

A fetal assessment identifies well-being or signs that indicate compromise. The character of the amniotic fluid is assessed, but the fetal assessment focuses primarily on determining the FHR pattern. Umbilical cord blood

NURSING PROCEDURE 14.1 Performing Leopold Maneuvers

Purpose: To Determine Fetal Presentation, Position, and Lie

1. Place the patient in the supine position and stand beside them.
2. Perform the first maneuver to determine presentation.
   a. Facing the patient's head, place both hands on the abdomen to determine fetal position in the uterine fundus.
   b. Feel for the buttocks, which will feel soft and irregular (indicates vertex presentation); feel for the head, which will feel hard, smooth, and round (indicates a breech presentation).

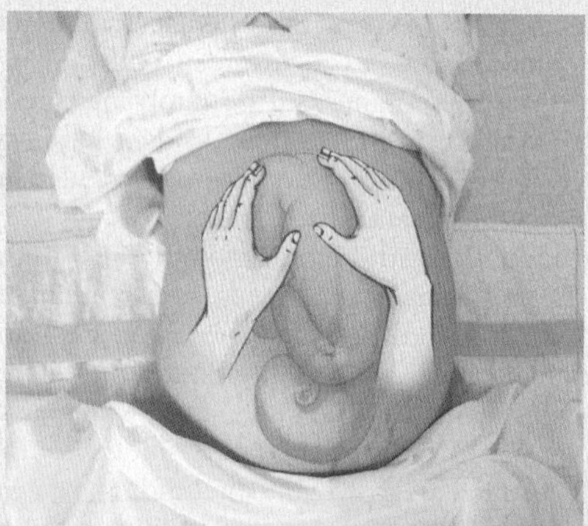

3. Complete the second maneuver to determine position.
   a. While still facing the patient, move hands down the lateral sides of the abdomen to palpate on which side the back is located (feels hard and smooth).
   b. Continue to palpate to determine on which side the limbs are located (irregular nodules with kicking and movement).

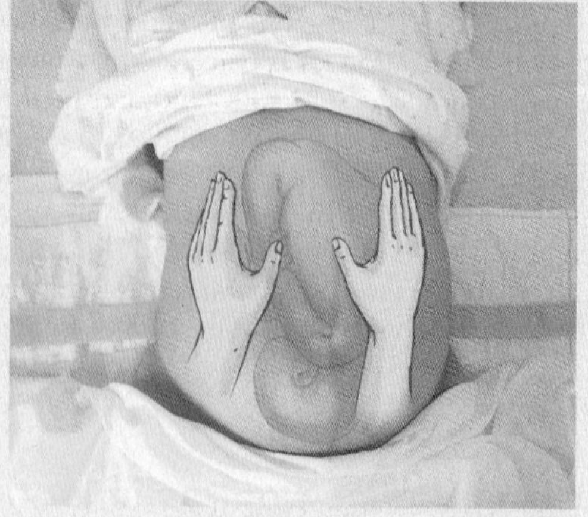

NURSING PROCEDURE 14.1 Performing Leopold Maneuvers

4. Perform the third maneuver to confirm presentation.
   a. Move hands down the sides of the abdomen to grasp the lower uterine segment and palpate the area just above the symphysis pubis.
   b. Place thumb and fingers of one hand apart and grasp the presenting part by bringing fingers together.
   c. Feel for the presenting part. If the presenting part is the head, it will be round, firm, and ballottable; if it is the buttocks, it will feel soft and irregular.

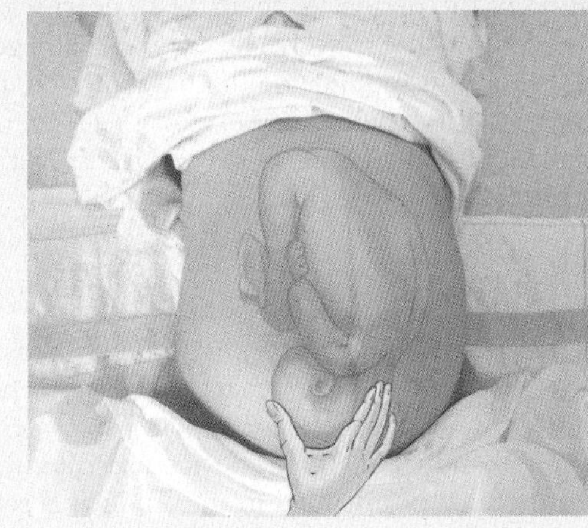

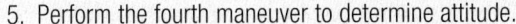

5. Perform the fourth maneuver to determine attitude.
   a. Turn to face the patient's feet and use the tips of the first three fingers of each hand to palpate the abdomen.
   b. Move fingers toward each other while applying downward pressure in the direction of the symphysis pubis. If you palpate a hard area on the side opposite the fetal back, the fetus is in flexion because you have palpated the chin. If the hard area is on the same side as the back, the fetus is in extension because the area palpated is the occiput.

Also, note how your hands move. If the hands move together easily, the fetal head is not descended into the patient's pelvic inlet. If the hands do not move together and stop because of resistance, the fetal head is engaged into the patient's pelvic inlet (Superville & Siccardi, 2023).

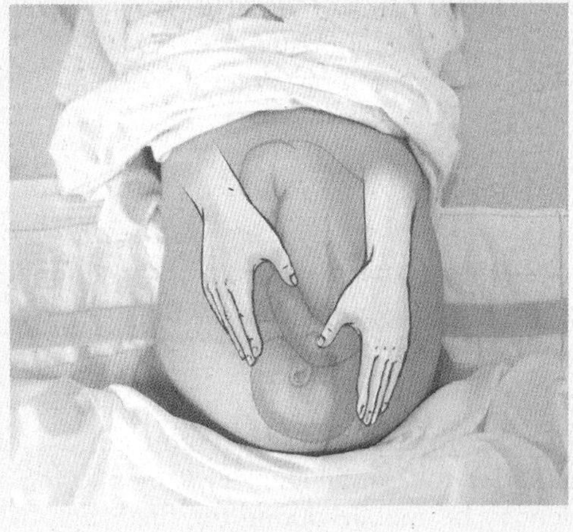

analysis and fetal scalp stimulation are additional assessments performed as necessary in the case of questionable FHR patterns.

Analysis of Amniotic Fluid

Amniotic fluid is composed of 98% water and electrolytes, with 2% being peptides, carbohydrates, lipids, and hormones (Fitzsimmons & Bajaj, 2023). Amniotic fluid should be clear when the membranes rupture. Rupturing of membranes is either spontaneous or artificial by means of an amniotomy, during which a disposable plastic hook (an Amnihook) is used to perforate the amniotic sac. Cloudy or foul-smelling amniotic fluid indicates infection. Green fluid may indicate that the fetus has passed meconium secondary to transient hypoxia, prolonged pregnancy, cord compression, intrauterine growth restriction (IUGR), maternal hypertension, diabetes, or chorioamnionitis; however, it is considered a normal occurrence if the fetus is in a breech presentation (Skelly et al., 2023). If it is determined that meconium-stained amniotic fluid is due to fetal hypoxia, the maternity and pediatric teams work together to prevent meconium aspiration syndrome, which can lead to respiratory distress. This would necessitate suctioning after the head is born before the infant takes a breath and perhaps direct tracheal suctioning after birth if the Apgar score is low. In some cases, an amnioinfusion (introduction of warmed, sterile normal saline or Ringer's lactate solution into the uterus) is used to dilute moderate to heavy meconium released in utero to assist in preventing meconium aspiration syndrome.

Analysis of the FHR

Monitoring of the FHR throughout labor and birth is important to ensure fetal well-being to optimize neonatal outcomes. Analysis of the FHR is one of the primary evaluation tools used to determine fetal oxygen status indirectly. FHR assessment can be done intermittently using a fetoscope (a modified stethoscope attached to a headpiece) or a Doppler (ultrasound) device, or continuously with an electronic fetal monitor applied externally or internally. The object of FHR monitoring is to reduce mortality and morbidity by ensuring that all fetal hypoxic insults are identified in time to allow removal or alteration of the reason for them, or to enable a safe birth of the fetus before irreversible asphyxia damage occurs. The areas assessed include the baseline rate, presence of accelerations, periodic or episodic decelerations, baseline variability, and trends of FHR patterns over time (Gibb & Arulkumaran, 2024).

Intermittent FHR Monitoring

Intermittent auscultation is a primary method of fetal surveillance in labor. It is the practice of using a handheld Doppler or fetoscope for periodic assessment of the FHR. The handheld Doppler device uses ultrasound waves that bounce off the fetal heart, producing echoes or clicks that reflect the rate of the fetal heart (Fig. 14.3). Intermittent auscultation of the FHR is an acceptable option for low-risk laboring patients (Cypher, 2024). Intermittent FHR auscultation promotes physiologic births.

TAKE NOTE!

Doppler devices to detect FHRs are relatively low in cost and are used in hospitals and in home births and birthing centers routinely. Many nurses use them in their work settings.

The nurse listens to FHR for short periods of time at regular intervals. Intermittent FHR monitoring allows the patient to be mobile during the first stage of labor. They are free to move around and change position at will since they are not attached to a stationary electronic fetal monitor. However, intermittent monitoring does not provide a continuous FHR recording and does not document how the fetus responds to the stress of labor (unless listening is done during the contraction). The best way to assess fetal well-being would be to start listening to the FHR at the end of the contraction (not after one) so that late decelerations could be detected. However, the pressure of the device during a contraction is uncomfortable and can distract the patient from using paced breathing patterns.

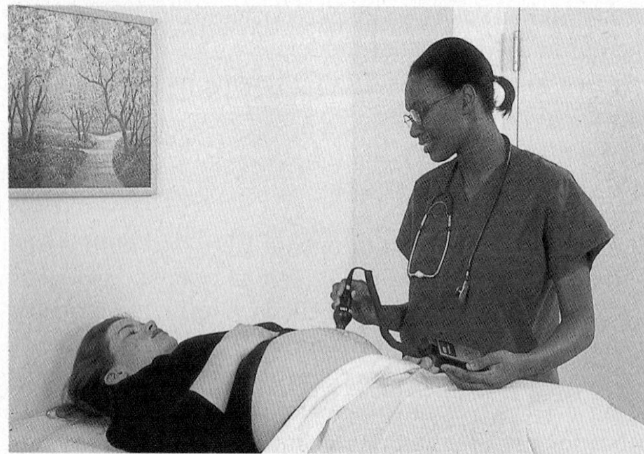

FIGURE 14.3 Nurse using a handheld Doppler to obtain a fetal heart rate.

Intermittent FHR auscultation can be used to detect FHR baseline and rhythm and changes from baseline. However, it cannot detect variability and types of decelerations as **electronic fetal monitoring (EFM)** can. Research finds no differences between continuous fetal monitoring (cardiotocography) versus intermittent fetal monitoring as they relate to Apgar scores, cord blood gases, rates of low-oxygen brain damage, admission to the neonatal intensive care unit (NICU), or perinatal death rates (Miller, 2022). During intermittent auscultation to establish a baseline, the FHR is assessed for a full minute after a contraction. From then on, unless there is a problem, listening for 30 seconds and multiplying the value by two is sufficient. If the patient experiences a change in condition during labor (such as ruptured membranes or onset of bleeding), auscultation assessments should be more frequent. After periods of ambulation, a vaginal examination, administration of pain medication, or other clinically important events, the FHR should be checked.

The FHR is heard most clearly at the fetal back. In a cephalic presentation, the FHR is best heard in the lower quadrant of the maternal abdomen. In a breech presentation, it is heard at or above the level of the maternal umbilicus (Fig. 14.4). As labor progresses, the FHR location will change accordingly as the fetus descends into the maternal pelvis for the birthing process. To ensure that the maternal heart rate is not confused with the FHR, palpate the patient's radial pulse simultaneously while the FHR is being auscultated through the abdomen.

For low-risk laboring patients, the FHR and contraction characteristics should be assessed every 15 to 30 minutes in active labor and every 5 to 15 minutes while pushing, as well as before and after any digital vaginal examinations, membrane rupture, medication administered, and ambulation to the restroom (Cypher, 2024).

Nursing Procedure 12.1 lists detailed steps for using a Doppler device to assess FHR. In brief, a small amount of water-soluble gel is applied to the abdomen or ultrasound device before auscultation with the Doppler device to promote sound wave transmission. Usually, the FHR is best heard in the lower abdominal quadrants; if the FHR is not found quickly, it may help locate the fetal back by performing Leopold maneuvers.

Although the intermittent method of FHR assessment allows the patient to move during labor, the information obtained doesn't provide a complete picture of the well-being of the fetus from moment to moment. This leads to the question of what the fetal status is during the times that are not assessed. For patients who are

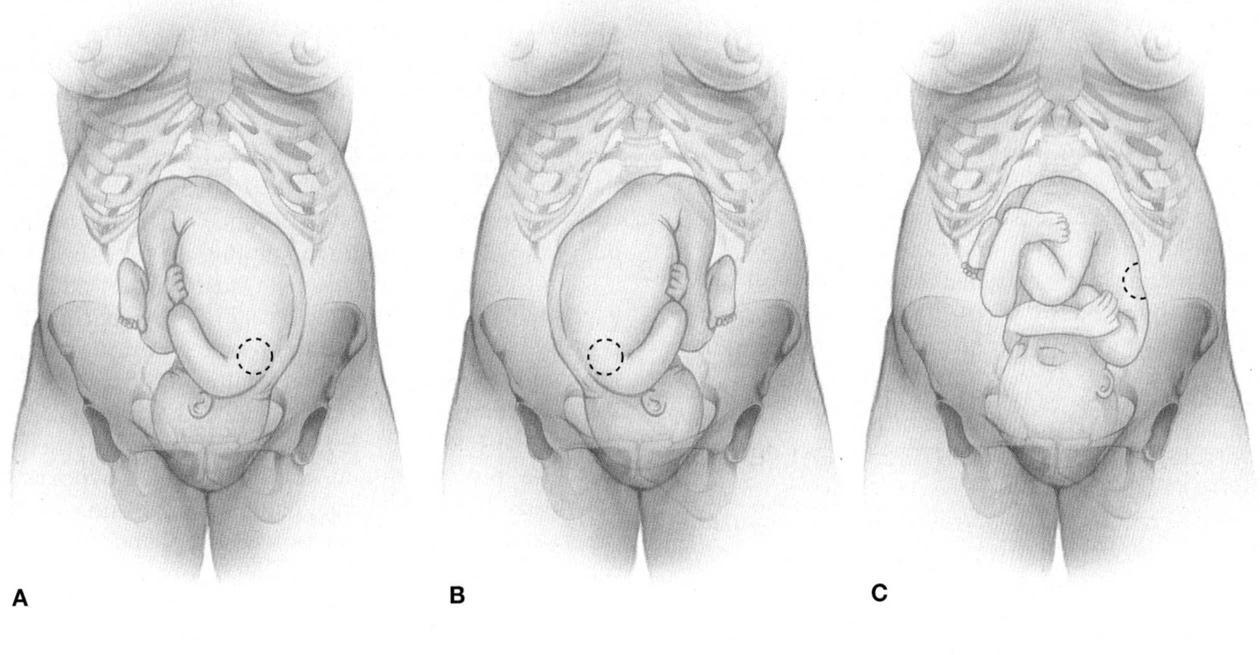

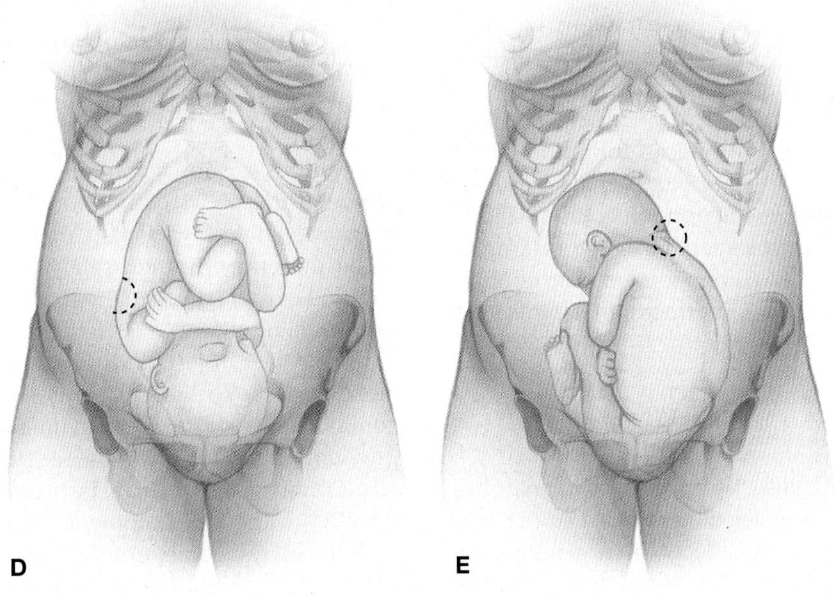

FIGURE 14.4 Locations for auscultating fetal heart rate based on fetal position. **A.** Left occiput anterior (LOA). **B.** Right occiput anterior (ROA). **C.** Left occiput posterior (LOP). **D.** Right occiput posterior (ROP). **E.** Left sacral anterior (LSA).

considered at low risk for complications, these periods without assessment are not a problem. However, for the undiagnosed high-risk patient, it might prove ominous.

GUIDELINES FOR ASSESSING FHR

National professional organizations have provided general guidelines for the frequency of assessments based on existing evidence. The American College of Obstetricians and Gynecologists (ACOG) and the Association of Women's Health, Obstetric and Neonatal Nurses (AWHONN) have published guidelines designed to assist clinicians in caring for laboring patients. Their recommendations are supported by large, controlled studies. They recommend the following guidelines for assessing FHR:

- Initial 10- to 20-minute continuous FHR assessment upon entry into labor and birth area
- Completion of a prenatal and labor risk assessment on all patients
- Intermittent auscultation every 30 minutes during active labor for a low-risk patient and every 15 minutes for a high-risk patient
- During the second stage of labor, every 15 minutes for the low-risk patient and every 5 minutes for the high-risk patient and during the pushing stage
- Avoid routine use of oxygen supplementation in patients with normal oxygen saturation for category II or III fetal heart tracings for the purpose of fetal intrauterine resuscitation (ACOG, 2023; Cypher, 2024).

EVIDENCE-BASED RESULTS: INTERMITTENT VERSUS ELECTRONIC MONITORING

In several randomized controlled studies comparing intermittent auscultation with electronic monitoring in both low- and high-risk patients, no difference in intrapartum fetal death or improved maternal well-being was found, but an increase in surgical births occurred with electronic monitoring when compared to intermittent Doppler monitoring (Miller, 2022). There is insufficient evidence to indicate specific situations in which continuous electronic FHR monitoring might result in better outcomes when compared to intermittent assessment. However, in pregnancies involving an increased risk of maternal or fetal compromise (abruption or unexplained vaginal bleeding, chorioamnionitis or sepsis, diabetes mellitus, growth restriction, meconium-stained amniotic fluid, previous cesarean birth, preeclampsia, postterm pregnancy), it is recommended that continuous EFM be used rather than intermittent fetal auscultation (Miller, 2022).

Continuous EFM

EFM detects the fetal pulse by sensing and analyzing tissue movements via Doppler ultrasound. The machine uses a transducer that is capable of both sending and receiving ultrasound waves. The waves travel through the ultrasound gel, then body tissues, and are eventually reflected by any tissue. The fast reflections are analyzed and software in the machine determines the FHR. EFM is the recommended method of intrapartum fetal surveillance for high-risk pregnancies. Despite mixed evidence regarding the ability of EFM to affect neonatal mortality, continuous cardiotocography (CTG) remains the predominant method of fetal monitoring today (Kauffmann & Silberman, 2023).

EFM is not a substitute for appropriate, professional nursing care and support of patients in labor. The indications for offering patients continuous fetal monitoring in labor are documented in the National Institute for Health and Care Excellence (NICE) guidelines. These include patients receiving oxytocin infusions; patients who have epidural analgesia; and when there are a variety of problems related to a compromise in either fetal or maternal health like prolonged ROM (longer than 24 hours), moderate hypertension (higher than 150/100 mm Hg), confirmed delay in the first or second stage of labor, and the presence of meconium (NICE, 2022).

EFM uses a machine to produce a continuous tracing of the FHR. When the monitoring device is in place, a sound is produced with each heartbeat. In addition, a graphic record of the FHR pattern is produced. The primary objective of EFM is to provide information about fetal oxygenation and prevent fetal injury that could result from impaired fetal oxygenation during labor. The purpose of EFM is to detect FHR changes early before they are prolonged and profound. Fetal hypoxia is demonstrated in a heart rate pattern change and is by far the most common etiology of fetal injury and death that can be prevented with optimal fetal surveillance during labor and early interventions (Miller, 2022).

With EFM, there is a continuous record of the FHR; no gaps exist as they do with intermittent auscultation. The concept of hearing and evaluating every beat of the fetus's heart to allow for early intervention seems logical. However, using continuous monitoring can limit maternal movement and encourages the laboring patient to lie in the supine position, which reduces placental perfusion.

Various groups within the medical community have criticized the use of continuous fetal monitoring for all pregnant patients, especially those at low risk. Concerns about the efficiency and safety of routine EFM in labor have led expert panels in the United States to recommend that such monitoring be limited to high-risk pregnancies. However, its use in low-risk pregnancies continues globally. Despite the criticisms, EFM remains the most common method for determining fetal health status by providing a moment-to-moment printout of FHR status.

Continuous EFM can be performed externally (indirectly) with the equipment attached to the maternal abdominal wall or internally (directly) with the equipment attached to the fetus. Both methods provide a continuous printout of the FHR, but they differ in their specificity. The efficacy of EFM depends on the accurate interpretation of the tracings, not necessarily which method (external or internal) is used.

CONTINUOUS EXTERNAL MONITORING

In external or indirect monitoring, two ultrasound transducers, each of which is attached to a belt, are applied around the laboring patient's abdomen. They are similar to the handheld Doppler device. One transducer is called a tocotransducer, a pressure-sensitive device that is applied against the uterine fundus. It detects changes in uterine pressure and converts the pressure registered into an electronic signal that is recorded in the electronic health record or can be printed on graph paper (Cypher, 2024). The tocotransducer is placed over the uterine fundus in the area of greatest contractility to monitor uterine contractions. The other ultrasound transducer records the baseline FHR, long-term variability, accelerations, and decelerations. It is positioned on the maternal abdomen in the midline between the umbilicus and the symphysis pubis. The diaphragm of the ultrasound transducer is moved to either side of the abdomen to obtain a stronger sound and is then attached to the second elastic belt (Fig. 14.5).

Continuous data are provided on the FHR. External monitoring can be used while the membranes are still intact, and the cervix is not yet dilated but also can be used with ruptured membranes and a dilating cervix. It is not invasive and can detect relative changes in abdominal pressure between uterine resting tone and contractions. External monitoring also measures the approximate duration and frequency of contractions, providing a permanent record of FHR (Cypher, 2024).

However, external monitoring can restrict the birthing parent's movements. It also cannot detect short-term variability. Signal disruptions can occur due to maternal obesity, fetal malpresentation, and fetal movement as well as by artifact. The term **artifact** is used to describe irregular variations or absence of the FHR on the fetal monitor record that result from mechanical limitations of the monitor or electrical interference. Loss of signal or confusion between the maternal heart rate and FHR is common in the second stage of labor. For instance, the monitor may pick up transmissions from radios used by drivers on nearby roads and translate them into a signal. Additionally, gaps in the monitor strip can occur periodically without explanation. These challenges are heightened in laboring patients with obesity as signals can be lost in layers of adipose tissue.

New technology has been developed that shows promise in solving current clinical and technologic challenges. For example, the noninvasive fetal electrocardiogram obtains data from the maternal abdomen and provides real-time visualization of the FHR. The wireless device is placed on the maternal abdomen like an adhesive patch. It is unaffected by maternal obesity and allows full ambulation and mobility during labor. The ability to "set and forget" the monitor will free up the nurse to focus on the patient and not the technology. Remote fetal monitoring is associated with high patient satisfaction and time reduction (Nir et al., 2024).

CONTINUOUS INTERNAL MONITORING

Continuous internal monitoring is usually indicated for laboring patients or fetuses considered to be at high risk. Possible conditions might include multiple gestation, decreased fetal movement, abnormal FHR on auscultation, IUGR, maternal fever, preeclampsia, dysfunctional labor, preterm birth, or medical conditions such as diabetes or hypertension. It involves the placement of a spiral electrode into the fetal presenting part, usually the parietal bone on the head, to assess FHR, and a pressure transducer placed internally within the uterus to record uterine contractions (Fig. 14.6). The fetal spiral electrode is considered the most accurate method of detecting fetal heart characteristics and patterns because it involves receiving a signal directly from the fetus (Ross & Beall, 2023). An intrauterine electrode may also be placed at the same time but is not required as the external tocotransducer

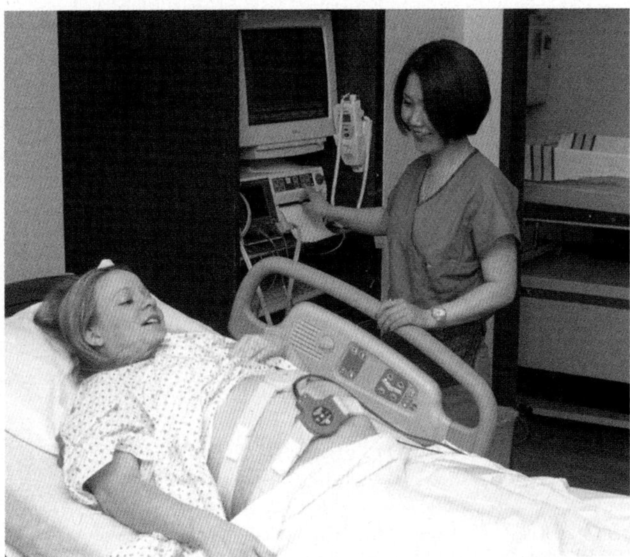

FIGURE 14.5 Continuous external electronic fetal monitoring device applied to the patient in labor.

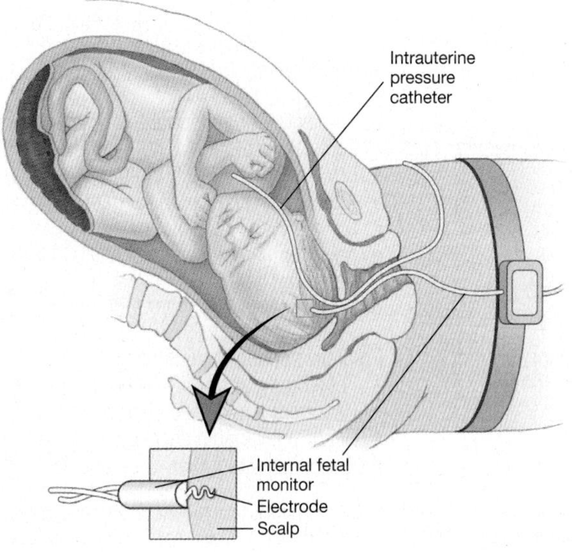

FIGURE 14.6 Continuous internal electronic fetal monitoring.

may still be used. Both the FHR and the duration and interval of uterine contractions are recorded. This method permits accurate evaluation of baseline heart rate and changes in rate and pattern.

Four specific criteria must be met for this type of monitoring to be used:

- Ruptured membranes
- Cervical dilation of at least 2 cm
- Presenting fetal part low enough to allow placement of the scalp electrode
- Skilled practitioner available to insert the spiral electrode (Ross & Beall, 2023)

Compared with external monitoring, continuous internal monitoring can accurately detect both short-term (moment-to-moment) changes and variability (fluctuations within the baseline) and FHR dysrhythmias. The application of artificial intelligence computer programs to the fetal electrocardiogram signal processing has led to better FHR pattern interpretations (Miller, 2022). In addition, maternal position changes and movement do not interfere with the quality of the tracing.

Determining FHR Patterns

Due to the rising costs of litigation related to birth asphyxia of the newborn and increasing complexity of obstetric populations, it has become mandatory that all nurses responsible for the care of patients in labor are trained adequately in interpretation and documentation of electronic tracings, as well as the guidelines for interventions based on the assessment of the tracing and overall clinical situation. Assessment parameters of the FHR include baseline FHR and variability, presence of accelerations, periodic or episodic decelerations, and changes or trends of FHR patterns over time.

The nurse must be able to interpret the various parameters to determine if the FHR pattern is:

- *Category I*—Strongly predictive of normal fetal acid–base status at the time of observation and needs no intervention
- *Category II*—Not predictive of abnormal fetal acid–base status but does require evaluation and continued monitoring
- *Category III*—Predictive of abnormal fetal acid–base status at the time of observation and requires prompt evaluation and interventions, changing maternal position, discontinuing labor augmentation medication, or treating maternal hypotension (Cypher, 2024). Table 14.1 summarizes these categories.

BASELINE FHR

Baseline fetal heart rate refers to the average FHR that occurs during a 10-minute segment that excludes periodic or episodic rate changes, such as tachycardia or bradycardia. It is assessed when the laboring person has no contractions, and the fetus is not experiencing episodic FHR changes. The normal baseline FHR ranges between 110 and 160 beats per minute (bpm) (Cypher, 2024). The

TABLE 14.1 • Interpreting Fetal Heart Rate Patterns

Category I: normal	Predictive of normal fetal acid–base status and do not require intervention • Baseline rate (110–160 bpm) • Baseline variability moderate • Present or absent accelerations • Present or absent early decelerations • No late or variable decelerations • Can be monitored with intermittent auscultation during labor
Category II: indeterminate	Not predictive of abnormal fetal acid–base status, but require evaluation and continued surveillance • Fetal tachycardia (>160 bpm) present • Bradycardia (<110 bpm) not accompanied by absent baseline variability • Absent baseline variability not accompanied by recurrent decelerations • Minimal or marked variability • Recurrent late decelerations with moderate baseline variability • Recurrent variable decelerations accompanied by minimal or moderate baseline variability, overshoots, or shoulders • Prolonged decelerations >2 minutes but <10 minutes
Category III: abnormal	Predictive of abnormal fetus acid–base status and require intervention • Fetal bradycardia (<110 bpm) • Recurrent late decelerations • Recurrent variable decelerations—declining or absent • Sinusoidal pattern (smooth, undulating baseline)

Association of Women's Health, Obstetric, and Neonatal Nurses. (2022). Antepartum and intrapartum fetal heart monitoring: Clinical competencies and education guide (7th ed.). *Journal of Obstetric, Gynecologic, and Neonatal Nursing, 51*(3), E1–E9. https://doi.org/10.1016/j.jogn.2022.01.004; Miller, D. A. (2022). Intrapartum fetal heart monitoring: Overview. *UpToDate.* Retrieved March 7, 2024, from https://www.uptodate.com/contents/intrapartum-fetal-heart-rate-monitoring-overview

normal baseline FHR can be obtained by auscultation, ultrasound, or Doppler or by a continuous internal direct fetal electrode.

Fetal bradycardia occurs when the FHR is below 110 bpm and lasts 10 minutes or longer (Macones, 2023). Causes of fetal bradycardia might include fetal hypoxia, placental abruption, cord prolapse, prolonged umbilical cord compression, maternal hypoglycemia, hypothermia, and maternal hypotension (Cypher, 2024). Bradycardia may be benign if it is an isolated event, but it is considered an ominous sign when accompanied by a decrease in baseline variability and late decelerations.

Fetal tachycardia is a baseline FHR greater than 160 bpm that lasts for 10 minutes or longer (Macones, 2023). It can represent an early compensatory response to asphyxia. Other causes of fetal tachycardia include fetal hypoxia, maternal fever, maternal dehydration, amnionitis, drugs (e.g., cocaine, amphetamines, nicotine), maternal hyperthyroidism, maternal anxiety, fetal anemia, prematurity, fetal infection, chronic hypoxemia, congenital anomalies, fetal heart failure, and fetal dysrhythmia. Fetal tachycardia is considered an ominous sign (predictive of fetal acidemia) if it is accompanied by a decrease in variability and late decelerations (Cypher, 2024).

BASELINE VARIABILITY

Baseline variability is defined as irregular fluctuations in the baseline FHR, which is measured as the amplitude of the peak to trough in beats per minute. It is categorized as absent, minimal, moderate, and marked (Cypher, 2024). It represents the interplay between the parasympathetic and sympathetic nervous systems. The constant interplay (push-and-pull effect) on the FHR from the parasympathetic and sympathetic systems produces a moment-to-moment change in the FHR. Because variability is in essence the combined result of autonomic nervous system branch function, its presence implies that both branches are working and receiving adequate oxygen (Miller, 2022). Thus, variability is one of the most important characteristics of the FHR because moderate levels indicate a well-oxygenated fetus, whereas reduced levels are associated with a compromised fetus. Variability is described in four categories as follows:

- Fluctuation range undetectable
- Fluctuation range observed at fewer than 5 bpm
- Fluctuation ranges from 6 to 25 bpm
- Fluctuation ranges more than 25 bpm

Absent or minimal variability is typically caused by fetal acidemia secondary to uteroplacental insufficiency, cord compression, a preterm fetus, maternal hypotension, uterine hyperstimulation, abruptio placentae, or a fetal dysrhythmia. Interventions to improve uteroplacental blood flow and perfusion through the umbilical cord include lateral positioning of the birthing parent, increasing the intravenous (IV) fluid rate to improve maternal

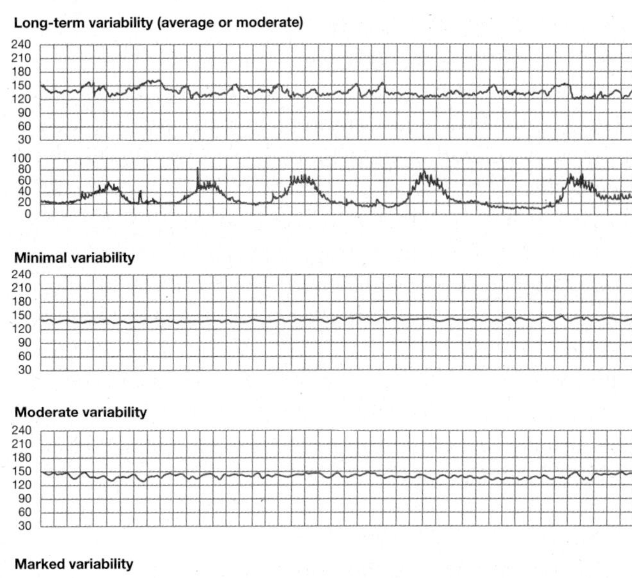

FIGURE 14.7 Examples of fetal monitoring strips.

circulation, administering oxygen at 8 to 10 L/min by mask, considering internal fetal monitoring, documenting findings, and reporting to the health care provider. Preparation for a surgical birth may be necessary if no changes occur after attempting the interventions.

Moderate viability indicates that the autonomic nervous system and central nervous system (CNS) of the fetus are well developed and well oxygenated. It is considered a good sign of fetal well-being and correlates with the absence of significant metabolic acidosis (Fig. 14.7). Marked variability occurs when there are more than 25 beats of fluctuation in the FHR baseline (Cypher, 2024). It may occur with labor induction and assisted vaginal deliveries; it is associated with an increased risk for fetal acidosis (Loussert et al., 2023).

FHR variability is an important clinical indicator that is predictive of fetal acid–base balance and cerebral tissue perfusion. It is influenced by fetal oxygenation status, cardiac output, and drug effects (Cypher, 2024). As the CNS is desensitized by hypoxia and acidosis, FHR decreases until a smooth baseline pattern appears. Loss of variability may be associated with a poor outcome.

TAKE NOTE!

External EFM cannot assess variability accurately. Therefore, if external monitoring shows a baseline that is smoothing out, use of an internal spiral electrode should be considered to gain a more accurate picture of the fetal health status.

PERIODIC BASELINE CHANGES

Periodic baseline changes are temporary, recurrent changes made in response to a stimulus such as a contraction. The FHR can demonstrate patterns of acceleration or deceleration in response to most stimuli. Fetal **accelerations** are transitory abrupt increases in the FHR above the baseline that last less than 30 seconds from onset to peak. They are associated with sympathetic nervous stimulation. They are visually apparent, with elevations of FHR of more than 15 bpm above the baseline, and their duration is longer than 15 seconds but less than 2 minutes (Funai & Norwitz, 2023). They are generally considered reassuring and require no interventions. Accelerations denote fetal movement and fetal well-being and are the basis for nonstress testing.

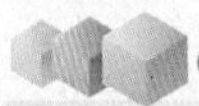

Concept Mastery Alert

Responding to FHR Distress During Labor

During possible fetal distress that involves lack of variability, late decelerations, and fetal tachycardia, simply changing the laboring patient's position is inadequate. The nurse should notify the health care provider immediately regarding the situation.

A **deceleration** is a transient fall in FHR caused by stimulation of the parasympathetic nervous system. Decelerations are described by their shape and association to a uterine contraction. They are classified as early, late, and variable only (Fig. 14.8).

Early decelerations are visually apparent, usually symmetrical, and characterized by a gradual decrease in the FHR in which the nadir (lowest point) occurs at the peak of the contraction. They rarely decrease more than 30 to 40 bpm below the baseline. Typically, the onset, nadir, and recovery of the deceleration occur at the same time as the onset, peak, and recovery of the contraction. They are most often seen during the active stage of any normal labor, during pushing, crowning, or vacuum extraction. They are thought to be a result of fetal head compression that results in a reflex vagal response with a resultant slowing of the FHR during uterine contractions. Early decelerations are not indicative of fetal distress and do not require intervention.

Late decelerations are visually apparent, usually symmetrical, transitory decreases in FHR that occur after the peak of the contraction. They have a gradual waveform and can be recurrent, occurring with each contraction over a period of time. The FHR does not return to baseline levels until well after the contraction has ended. Delayed timing of the deceleration occurs with the nadir of the uterine contraction. Late decelerations are associated with uteroplacental insufficiency, which occurs when blood flow within the intervillous space is decreased to the extent that fetal hypoxia or myocardial depression exists (Miller, 2022). Conditions that may decrease uteroplacental perfusion with resultant decelerations include maternal hypotension, gestational hypertension, placental aging secondary to diabetes and postmaturity, hyperstimulation via oxytocin infusion, maternal smoking, anemia, and cardiac disease. They imply some degree of fetal hypoxia. Recurrent or intermittent late decelerations are always category II (indeterminate) or category III (abnormal) regardless of depth of deceleration. Acute episodes with moderate variability are more likely to be correctable, while chronic episodes with loss of variability are less likely to be correctable (Macones, 2023). Box 14.1 highlights interventions for category III decelerations.

Variable decelerations present as visually apparent abrupt decreases in FHR below baseline and have

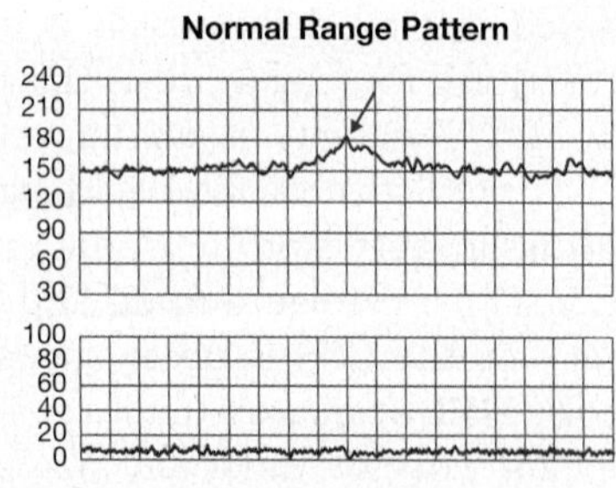

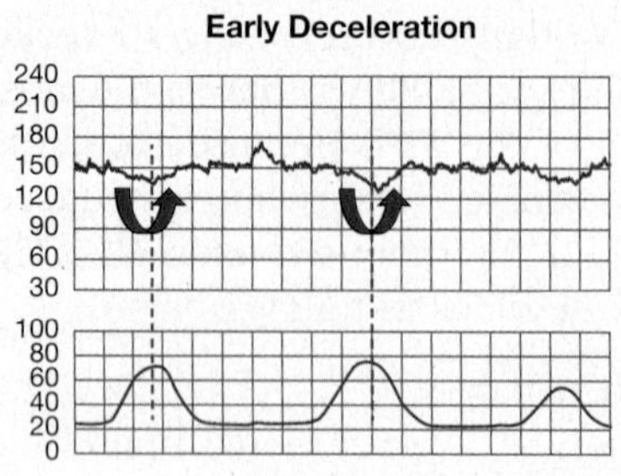

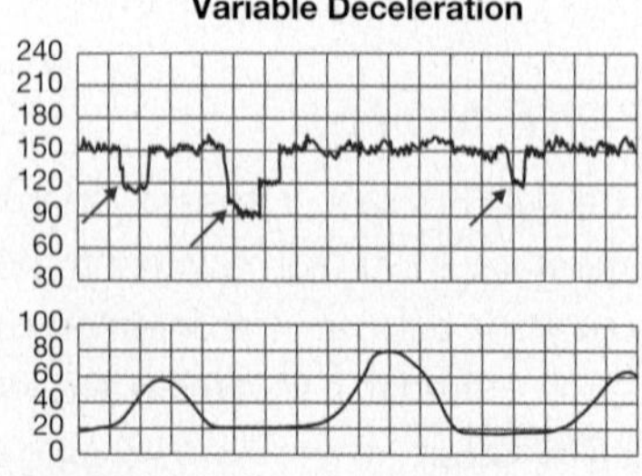

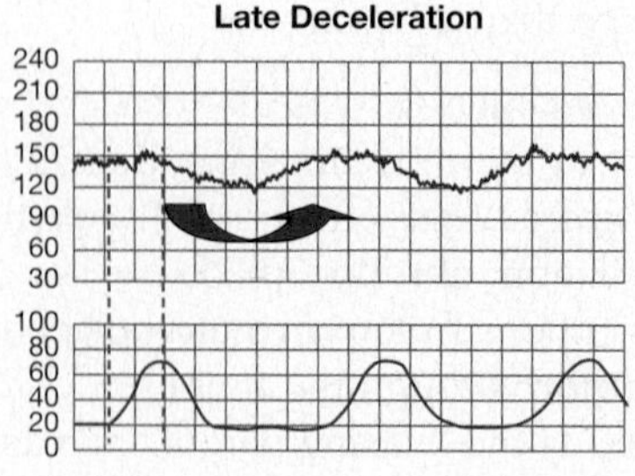

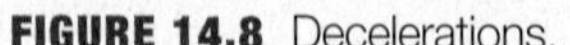

FIGURE 14.8 Decelerations.

BOX 14.1 Interventions for Category III Patterns

- Notify the health care provider about the pattern and obtain further orders, making sure to document all interventions and their effects on the FHR pattern.
- Discontinue oxytocin or other uterotonic agent as dictated by the facility's protocol if it is being administered.
- Turn the patient on their left or right lateral, knee–chest, or hands and knees to increase placental perfusion or relieve cord compression.
- Administer oxygen via nonrebreather face mask to increase fetal oxygenation.
- Increase the IV fluid rate to improve intravascular volume and correct maternal hypotension.
- Assess the patient for any underlying contributing causes.
- Provide reassurance that interventions are to effect pattern change.
- Modify pushing in the second stage of labor to improve fetal oxygenation.
- Document all interventions and any changes in FHR patterns.
- Prepare for an expeditious surgical birth if the pattern is not corrected in 30 minutes.

FHR, fetal heart rate; IV, intravenous.

Association of Women's Health, Obstetric, and Neonatal Nurses. (2022a). Antepartum and intrapartum fetal heart monitoring: Clinical competencies and education guide (7th ed.). *Journal of Obstetric, Gynecologic, and Neonatal Nursing, 51*(3), E1–E9. https://doi.org/10.1016/j.jogn.2022.01.004; Gibb, D., & Arulkumaran, S. (2024). *Fetal monitoring in practice* (5th ed.). Churchill Livingstone.

an unpredictable shape on the FHR baseline, possibly demonstrating no consistent relationship to uterine contractions. The shape of variable decelerations may be of a U, V, or W, or they may not resemble other patterns (Aubin & El-Chaâr, 2023). Variable decelerations usually occur abruptly with quick deceleration. They are the most common deceleration pattern found in the laboring patient and are usually transient and correctable (Aubin & El-Chaâr, 2023). Variable decelerations are associated with cord compression. However, they are classified either as category II or III depending on the accompanying change in baseline variability (Macones, 2023; Miller, 2022). The pattern of variable deceleration consistently related to the contractions with a slow return to FHR baseline warrants further monitoring and evaluation.

Prolonged decelerations are abrupt FHR declines of at least 15 bpm that last longer than 2 minutes but less than 10 minutes (Miller, 2022). The rate usually drops to less than 90 bpm. The causes of prolonged decelerations are similar to those of variable or late decelerations, but fetal hypoxia lasts longer (Miller, 2022).

A *sinusoidal pattern* has a smooth, sine wavelike undulating pattern in the FHR baseline, lasts for more than 20 minutes, and demonstrates a cycle frequency of 3 to 5 bpm that persists for more than 20 minutes. A true sinusoidal FHR pattern is rare (Miller, 2022). Historically, it is believed that the sinusoidal pattern results from fetal anemia, but a number of other fetal issues can also be the cause. A sinusoidal pattern indicates the fetus is in marked jeopardy and delivery is generally indicated (Cypher, 2024).

Other Fetal Assessment Methods

In situations suggesting the possibility of fetal compromise, such as category II or III FHR patterns, further ancillary testing such as umbilical cord blood analysis and fetal scalp stimulation may be used to validate the FHR findings and assist in planning interventions.

Umbilical Cord Blood Analysis

Neonatal and childhood mortality and morbidity are often attributed to fetal acidosis as indicated by a low cord pH at birth. Umbilical cord blood acid–base analysis drawn at birth provides an objective method of evaluating a newborn's condition, identifying the presence of intrapartum hypoxia and acidemia. This test is considered a good indicator of fetal oxygenation and acid–base condition at birth (Olofsson, 2023). The normal mean pH value range is 7.2 to 7.3. Metabolic acidosis in the fetus is indicated by pH of 7.0 or less and base deficit of 12.0 mmol/L or more.

Fetal Scalp Stimulation

An indirect method used to evaluate fetal oxygenation and acid–base balance to identify fetal hypoxia is fetal scalp stimulation. Fetal scalp stimulation is accomplished by placing a gloved finger on the fetal scalp and applying firm pressure. An expected healthy response is an acceleration of 15 bpm above the baseline heart rate that lasts at least 15 seconds. An absence of acceleration is considered abnormal (Aubin & El-Chaâr, 2023). Vibroacoustic stimulation should demonstrate the same response. An electronic artificial larynx is applied 1 cm from or directly on the patient's lower abdomen and turned on for 3 to 5 seconds to produce sound and vibration (Cunningham et al., 2022a).

Nurses play an essential role in the evaluation of maternal and fetal status during labor, continued surveillance, initiation of corrective measures when indicated, and reevaluation. A vital attribute of nursing surveillance is that it is a systematic process for assessment, intervention, and evaluation.

PROMOTING COMFORT AND PROVIDING PAIN MANAGEMENT DURING LABOR

Pain during labor is a universal experience, though the intensity of the pain may vary. Labor pain is unique to every person based on various contributing physiologic, emotional, social, and cultural factors. Although labor and childbirth are viewed as natural processes, both can produce significant pain and discomfort. The physical causes of pain during labor include cervical stretching; hypoxia of the uterine muscle due to a decrease in perfusion during contractions; pressure on the urethra, bladder, and rectum; and distention of the pelvic floor muscles (Funai & Norwitz, 2023).

Pain during labor is a physiologic phenomenon. The etiology of pain during the first stage of labor is associated with ischemia of the uterus during contractions. In the second stage, pain is caused by the stretching of the vagina and perineum and compression of the pelvic structures. Pain perception can be influenced by previous experiences with pain, fatigue, pain anticipation, genetics, positive or negative support system, health care provider's presence and encouragement, labor and birth environment, cultural expectations, and level of emotional stress and anxiety. Pain perception during labor changes in intensity and nature as labor progresses, and this is associated with behavioral changes in the laboring patient. Continuous labor support with the presence of a partner, doula, or nursing staff has been found to offer many advantages for the laboring patient, including a reduced need for oxytocin, shorter duration of labor, reduced need for medication, and a decrease in surgical births (National Partnership for Women & Families, 2024).

The techniques used to manage the pain of labor vary according to geography and culture. The need for culturally appropriate care is central to the World Health Organization (WHO) strategy to improve maternal outcomes and reduce morbidity and mortality (2022a). Some patients may request that their birthing parents, not their husbands, attend their births; partners do not actively participate in the birthing process. Some laboring patients may remain quiet during labor and birth and not complain of pain because outwardly expressing pain is not appropriate in their cultures. Never interpret quietness as freedom from pain. The concept of pain and pain expression during labor has different meanings for people of different cultures. Several points for the nurse to consider when caring for culturally diverse patients include using a qualified interpreter to communicate about pain as needed, offering and supporting culturally acceptable forms of pain relief, and assessing for pain frequently (Kennedy & Devane-Johnson, 2024).

Immigrating to a new country is a stressful process of readjustment and change. Effective verbal communication and understanding nonverbal social cues are invaluable when providing care to diverse cultures. Regardless of culture, childbearing families present to the labor and birth suites with the same needs and desires. Give all families the same respect and sense of welcome. Make sure they have a high-quality birth experience; uphold their religious, ethnic, and cultural values; and integrate them into their own care.

Today, there are many safe nonpharmacologic and pharmacologic choices for the management of pain during labor and birth, which may be used separately or in combination with one another. Pharmacologic approaches are directed at eliminating the physical sensation of labor pain, while nonpharmacologic approaches are largely directed at prevention of suffering.

Nurses are in an ideal position to provide childbearing patients with balanced, clear, concise information about effective nonpharmacologic and pharmacologic measures to relieve pain. Pain management standards issued by The Joint Commission mandate that pain be assessed in all patients admitted to a health care facility. Attention to the pain that occurs during labor and childbirth should be a priority of care for nurses and the medical team (Zuarez-Easton et al., 2023). Thus, it is important for nurses to be knowledgeable about the most recent scientific research on labor pain relief modalities, to make sure that accurate and unbiased information about effective pain relief measures is available to laboring patients, to be sure that the patient determines what is an acceptable labor pain level for them, and to allow the patient the choice of pain relief method.

Nonpharmacologic Measures

Nonpharmacologic measures may include continuous labor support, hydrotherapy, hypnosis, ambulation and maternal position changes, transcutaneous electrical nerve stimulation (TENS), acupuncture and acupressure, attention focusing and imagery, therapeutic touch, massage, breathing techniques, laboring in a shower or bathtub, and effleurage. Most of these methods are based on the *gate control theory of pain*, which proposes that local physical stimulation can interfere with pain stimuli by closing a hypothetical gate in the spinal cord, thus blocking pain signals from reaching the brain (Zuarez-Easton et al., 2023). It has long been a standard of care for labor nurses to first provide or encourage a variety of nonpharmacologic measures before moving to the pharmacologic interventions. Educating patients on what to expect with labor pain can help reduce their anxiety and their sense of loss of control.

Nonpharmacologic measures are usually simple, safe, and inexpensive to use. Many of these measures are taught in childbirth classes, and pregnant people should be encouraged to try a variety of methods prior to the real labor. Many of the measures need to be practiced for best results and coordinated with the partner or coach. The nurse provides support and encouragement for the patient and their partner using nonpharmacologic methods. Although patients cannot consciously direct the labor contractions, they can control how they respond to them, thereby enhancing their feelings of control. See Evidence-Based Practice 14.1 for more information.

EVIDENCE-BASED PRACTICE **14.1**

A Cross-Sectional Survey of Labor Pain Control and Patient Satisfaction

BACKGROUND

The pain experienced during labor can be intense, with body tension, anxiety, and fear increasing it. The pain experienced during childbirth is mostly a physiologic symptom, but psychological factors contribute to the perception of pain as well. Appropriate analgesia is essential because pain increases the level of circulating catecholamines, which reduce the perfusion to the uterus. The purpose of this study was to evaluate labor pain intensity before and after using pharmacologic and nonpharmacologic interventions and to evaluate patient satisfaction of labor pain management.

STUDY

The multicenter study was conducted using an interview questionnaire on the patient's second day postpartum. A total of 500 participants from different hospitals were surveyed regarding their pain relief method used and their satisfaction with its effectiveness. They were divided into two groups according to the method used during labor: pharmacologic and nonpharmacologic. Pharmacologic methods reported were parenteral opioids, inhalation of nitrous oxide, and regional methods. Nonpharmacologic methods included water immersion, physical activity (walking, moving), a birthing ball, massages, or transcutaneous electrical nerve stimulation (TENS) units.

Findings

The use of both pharmacologic and nonpharmacologic methods resulted in a significant reduction in pain. Water immersion (shower or bathtub) and epidural anesthesia proved to be the most effective pain relievers. The use of TENS units proved to be the least effective in relieving pain. Epidural anesthesia was the most effective method used overall, but its use was not correlated with maternal satisfaction. Maternal satisfaction was most influenced by the positive response of staff to the patient's pain, receiving education on available pain relief methods, and the ability to choose one's own method of pain relief.

Nursing Implications

Nurses need to have a basic understanding of pain relief methods so that they can advise patients during childbirth. Laboring patients want to use strategies to break the fear–tension–pain cycle and work effectively with the pain. Nurses working with laboring patients can suggest a variety of methods along with support and encouragement, such as finding comfortable positions, immersion in water, and self-help techniques to assist each patient through their labor process.

Adapted from Pietrzak, J., Medrzycka-Dabrowska, W., Tomaszek, L., & Grzybowska, M. E. (2022). A cross-sectional survey of labor pain control and women's satisfaction. *International Journal of Environmental Research and Public Health, 19*(3), 1741. https://doi.org/10.3390/ijerph19031741

Continuous Labor Support

Childbirth is a life-changing experience and can create lifelong memories. Nurses need to be familiar with diverse needs during childbirth, which include emotional, physical, and informational needs. Continuous labor support involves offering a sustained presence to the laboring patient by providing emotional support, comfort measures, advocacy, information about labor progress, advice on coping techniques, and support for the partner. It is a nonpharmacologic, evidence-based strategy associated with reduced cesarean rates. The evidence reveals that having a companion present throughout the childbirth process may improve birth outcomes and result in less use of interventions (Hurst & Baker, 2024). The family, midwife, nurse, doula, or anyone else close to the laboring person can provide this continuous presence. A support person can assist the patient with ambulating, repositioning, and using breathing techniques. A support person can also aid with the use of acupressure, massage, music therapy, or therapeutic touch. During the natural course of childbirth, a laboring patient's functional ability is limited secondary to pain, and they often have trouble making decisions. The support person can help make them based on their knowledge of the birth plan and personal wishes. Good interpersonal relationships can reduce fear associated with childbirth and subsequently contribute to a satisfactory birth experience.

Research has supported the value of continuous labor support versus intermittent support in terms of fewer operative deliveries, cesarean births, and requests for pain medication. Continuous labor support has been shown to have beneficial effects on the birthing parent and the newborn primarily due to the reduction in anxiety during the laboring experience. Most participants expressed greater satisfaction with their childbirth experience if they had continuous support during labor. Therefore, companionship throughout childbirth is recommended as a component of respectful maternity care (WHO, 2018).

TAKE NOTE!

The human presence is of immeasurable value to make the laboring patient feel secure.

Hydrotherapy

Laboring or giving birth in water is an ancient tradition. Hydrotherapy is the external use of any form of water for health promotion. It is a nonpharmacologic measure that may involve showering or soaking in a regular tub or whirlpool bath. When showering is the selected method of hydrotherapy, the laboring person stands or sits in a shower chair in a warm shower and allows the water to gently glide over their abdomen and back. If a tub or whirlpool is chosen, they are immersed in warm water for relaxation and relief of discomfort. The warmth and buoyancy of the water can impart a sense of well-being (Reviriego-Rodrigo et al., 2023). Warm water immersion reduces pain perception, relaxes the patient's muscles, and alleviates stress and tension. The water's buoyancy facilitates the finding of comfortable positions, which aids in labor progression and the rotation of the fetus (Mellado-García et al., 2024). Recent research findings reported that participants who used hydrotherapy during labor had significantly reduced surgical birth rates, a shorter second stage of labor, reduced analgesic requirements, and a lower incidence of perineal trauma. The research concluded that hydrotherapy during labor significantly aids the labor process, minimizes the use of analgesic medications, allows for various birth positions that can increase the diameter of the true pelvis, reduces the risk of perineal trauma, offers fast- and short-acting pain and anxiety relief, and should be considered a safe and effective birthing aid (Ergin et al., 2023).

A wide range of hydrotherapy options are available, from ordinary bathtubs to whirlpool baths and showers, combined with low lighting and music. Many hospitals provide showers and whirlpool baths for laboring patients for pain relief. However, hydrotherapy is more commonly practiced in birthing centers managed by midwives. The recommendation for initiating hydrotherapy is that the patient be in active labor (more than 6 cm dilated) to prevent the slowing of labor contractions secondary to muscular relaxation. Their membranes can be intact or ruptured. Patients are encouraged to stay in the bath or shower as long as they feel they are comfortable. The water temperature should not exceed body temperature.

Hydrotherapy is an effective pain management option for many patients. Those who are experiencing a healthy pregnancy can be offered this option. The potential risks associated with hydrotherapy include hyperthermia, umbilical cord avulsion, hypothermia, changes in maternal heart rate, fetal tachycardia, and unplanned underwater birth. The benefits include reducing pain, relieving anxiety, and promoting a sense of control during labor (Reviriego-Rodrigo et al., 2023).

Ambulation and Position Changes

Positioning during labor is influenced by cultural factors, obstetric practices, place of childbirth, technology, and the preferences of the laboring person and health care providers. Ambulation and position changes during labor are another extremely useful comfort measure. Historically, a variety of positions have been used during labor; the recumbent position was rarely used until during the first half of the 20th century. The medical profession has favored recumbent positions during labor but without evidence to demonstrate their appropriateness. Recent evidence indicates that upright positions may shorten the second stage of labor, reduce the episiotomy rate, and decrease abnormal FHR patterns needing intervention, but demonstrated increased rate of second-degree perineal trauma (Zang et al., 2021). Patients should be encouraged to use whatever position they find most comfortable in the first stage of labor (Spinning Babies, 2024).

Changing position frequently (every 30 minutes or so)—sitting, walking, kneeling, standing, lying down, getting on hands and knees, and using a birthing ball—helps relieve pain (Fig. 14.9). Position changes may also help speed labor by adding the benefits of gravity and changing the shape of the pelvis. Research has found that the position that the laboring patient assumes and the frequency of position changes have a profound effect on uterine activity and efficiency. Allowing the patient to obtain a position of comfort frequently facilitates a favorable fetal rotation by altering the alignment of the presenting part with the pelvis. As the laboring person continues to change position based on comfort, the optimal presentation is afforded. Supine positions should be avoided since they may interfere with labor progress and can cause compression of the vena cava and decrease blood return to the heart.

Swaying from side to side, rocking, or other rhythmic movements may also be comforting. If labor is progressing slowly, ambulating may speed it up again. Upright positions such as walking, kneeling forward, or doing a lunge on the birthing ball give most people a greater sense of control and active movement than just lying down. Table 14.2 highlights some of the more common positions that can be used during labor and birth.

Acupuncture and Acupressure

Acupuncture and acupressure can be used to relieve pain during labor. Although controlled research studies of these methods are limited, there is adequate evidence that both are useful in relieving pain associated with labor and birth (Smith et al., 2020). However, both methods require a trained, certified clinician, and such a person is not available in many birth facilities.

Acupuncture involves stimulating key trigger points with needles. This form of Chinese medicine has been practiced for approximately 2,500 years. Classical Chinese teaching holds that throughout the body there are meridians or channels of energy (*qi*) that when in balance regulate body functions. Pain reflects an imbalance or obstruction of the flow of energy. The purpose of acupuncture is to restore balance, thus diminishing pain (Van Hal et al., 2023). Stimulating the trigger points causes the release of endorphins, reducing the perception of pain.

Acupressure involves the application of a firm finger, thumb, knuckles, or massage used on similar points to those used in acupuncture to reduce the pain sensation. The amount of pressure is important. The intensity

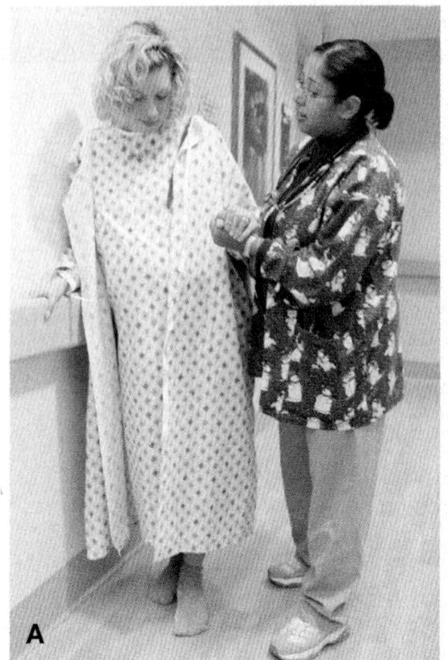

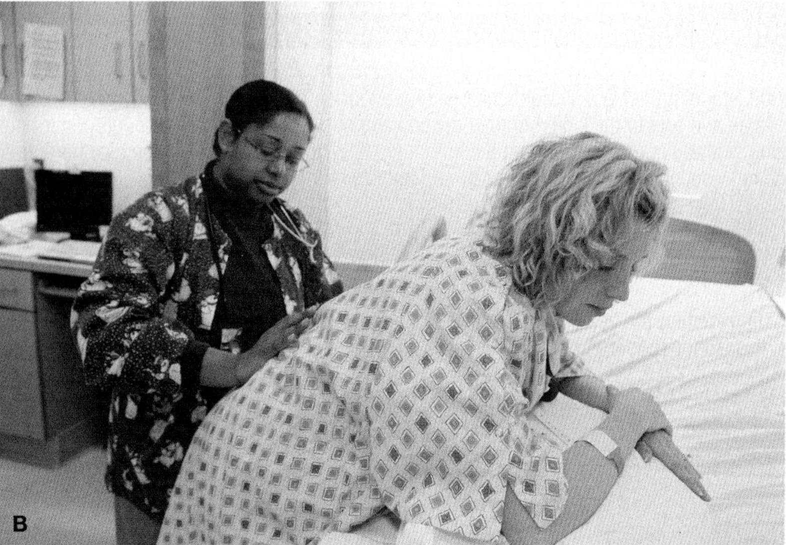

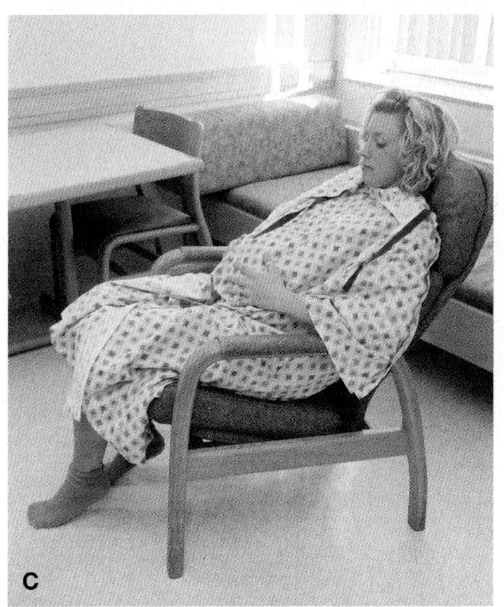

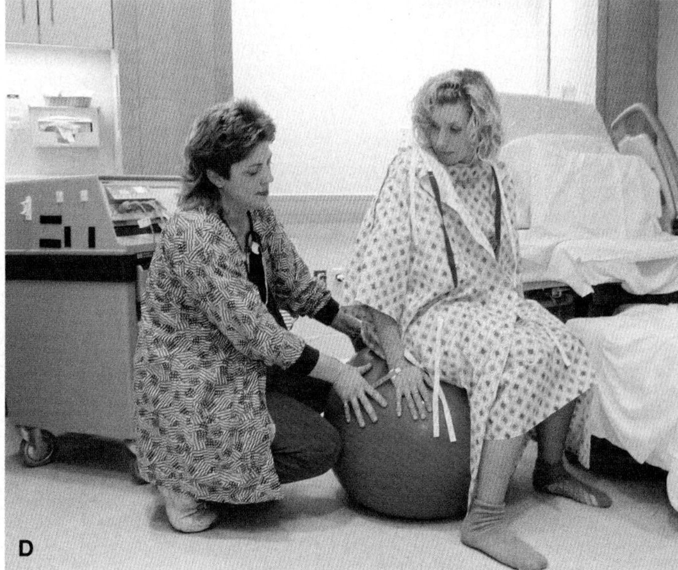

FIGURE 14.9 Various positions for use during labor. **A.** Ambulation. **B.** Leaning forward. **C.** Sitting in a chair. **D.** Using a birthing ball.

Table 14.2 • Common Positions for Use During Labor and Birth

Standing	• Takes advantage of gravity during and between contractions • Makes contractions feel less painful and be more productive • Helps fetus line up with angle of maternal pelvis • Helps increase urge to push in second stage of labor
Walking	• Has the same advantages as standing • Causes changes in the pelvic joints, helping the fetus move through the birth canal
Standing and leaning forward on partner, bed, or birthing ball	• Has the same advantages as standing • Is a good position for a backrub • May feel more restful than standing • Can be used with electronic fetal monitor
Slow dancing (standing with the laboring person's arms around partner's neck, head resting on the partner's chest or shoulder, with the partner's hands rubbing the laboring person's lower back; sway to music and breathe in rhythm if it helps)	• Has the same advantages as walking • Back pressure helps relieve back pain. • Rhythm and music help laboring person relax and provide comfort.

(*continued*)

Table 14.2 • Common Positions for Use During Labor and Birth (*continued*)

Position	Advantages
The lunge (standing facing a straight chair with one foot on the seat with knee and foot to the side; bending raised knee and hip, and lunging sideways repeatedly during a contraction, holding each lunge for 5 seconds; partner holds chair and helps with balance)	• Widens one side of the pelvis (the side toward lunge) • Encourages rotation of the baby • Can also be done in a kneeling position
Sitting upright	• Helps promote rest • Has more gravity advantage than lying down • Can be used with electronic fetal monitor
Semi-sitting (setting the head of the bed at a 45-degree angle with pillows used for support)	• Has the same advantages as sitting upright • Is an easy position if on a bed
Sitting on toilet or commode	• Has the same advantages as sitting upright • May help relax the perineum for effective bearing down
Rocking in a chair	• Has the same advantages as sitting upright • May help speed labor (rocking movement)
Sitting, leaning forward with support	• Has the same advantages as sitting upright • Is a good position for a backrub
On all fours, on hands and knees	• Helps relieve backache • Assists rotation of baby in posterior position • Allows for pelvic rocking and body movement • Relieves pressure on hemorrhoids • Allows for vaginal examinations • Is sometimes preferred as a pushing position by people with back labor pain
Kneeling, leaning forward with support on a chair seat, the raised head of the bed, or on a birthing ball	• Has the same advantages as all-fours position • Puts less strain on wrists and hands
Side-lying	• Is a good position for resting and convenient for many kinds of medical interventions • Helps lower elevated blood pressure • May promote progress of labor when alternated with walking • Is useful in slowing a rapid second stage • Avoids vena cava syndrome • May offer increased control of pushing efforts • Takes pressure off hemorrhoids • Facilitates relaxation between contractions
Squatting	• May relieve backache • Takes advantage of gravity • Requires less bearing-down effort • Widens pelvic outlet by approximately 28% • Pressure is evenly distributed to the perineum, reducing the need for episiotomy. • May help fetus turn and move down in a difficult birth • Helps if the person feels no urge to push • Allows freedom to shift weight for comfort • Offers an advantage when pushing, since upper trunk presses on the top of the uterus
Supported squat (leaning back against partner, who supports the laboring person under the arms and takes the entire laboring person's weight, standing up between contractions)	• Requires great strength in partner • Lengthens trunk, allowing more room for fetus to maneuver into position • Lets gravity help
Dangle (partner sitting high on bed or counter with feet supported on chairs or footrests and thighs spread; laboring person leaning back between partner's legs, placing flexed arms over partner's thighs; partner gripping laboring person's sides with their thighs; laboring person lowering themselves and allowing partner to support their full weight; standing up between contractions)	• Has the same advantages of a supported squat • Requires less physical strength from the partner

Lothian, J. (2024). Normal childbirth. In B. J. Baker, J. Janke, & Association of Women's Health, Obstetric and Neonatal Nurses, *Core curriculum for maternal-newborn nursing* (6th ed.). Elsevier; Jyoti, R., Sharma, M., & Pareek, S. (2022). The effects and outcomes of different maternal positions on the second stage of labor. *Journal of Health Sciences*, *10*(2), 21–24. https://doi.org/10.4103/mjhs.mjhs_49_21; Spinning Babies. (2024). *Maternal positioning*. https://www.spinningbabies.com/about/maternal-positioning/

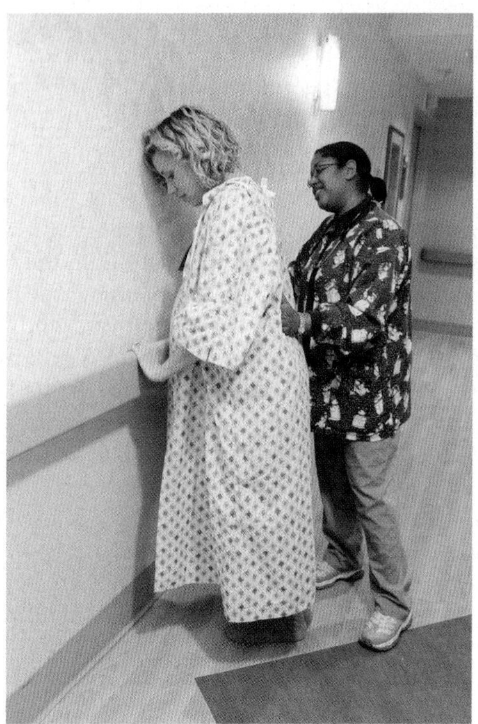

FIGURE 14.10 Nurse massaging the patient's back during a contraction while they ambulate during labor.

of the pressure is determined by the needs of the person. Holding and squeezing the hand of a person in labor may trigger the point most commonly used for both techniques. Some acupressure points are found along the spine, neck, shoulder, toes, and soles of the feet. Pressure along the side of the spine can help relieve back pain during labor (Fig. 14.10; Kirca & Gul, 2022). A recent study found that acupuncture and acupressure may indeed reduce labor pain, increase maternal satisfaction with pain management, and reduce use of pharmacologic management. However, there is a need for further research (Kirca & Gul, 2022).

Application of Heat and Cold

Superficial applications of heat or cold in various forms are popular with laboring people. They are easy to use, inexpensive, require no prior practice, and have minimal negative side effects when used properly. Heat causes vasodilation, improves blood supply, and according to gate control theory stops pain signals from reaching the brain (Goswami et al., 2022). Apply heat to the person's back, lower abdomen, groin, or perineum using a hot water bottle, heated rice-filled sock, warm compress (washcloth soaked in warm water and wrung out), electric heating pad, or warm blanket. A warm bath or shower is also useful. In addition to being used for pain relief, heat is used to relieve chills or trembling, decrease joint stiffness, reduce muscle spasm, and increase connective tissue extensibility.

Cold therapy, or cryotherapy, eases pain during the active phase of labor and may decrease labor time, without affecting perineal laceration, FHR, or Apgar score (Mascarenhas et al., 2019). Apply cold to the back or lower abdomen during dilation. Forms of cold include a bag or surgical glove filled with ice, a frozen gel pack, camper's "ice," a hollow, plastic rolling pin or bottle filled with ice, a washcloth dipped in cold water, soda cans chilled in ice, and even a frozen bag of vegetables. "Instant" cold packs, often available in hospitals, usually are not cold enough to effectively relieve labor pain. People who routinely feel cold usually need to feel warm before they can comfortably tolerate using a cold pack. Chilled soda cans and rolling pins filled with ice give the added benefit of mechanical pressure when rolled on the low back.

With appropriate safety precautions, heat and cold therapy offer comfort and relief, and their use should be dictated by the desires and responses of the laboring patient.

Attention Focusing and Imagery

Visualization or guided imagery uses many of the senses and the mind to focus on stimuli. It involves dwelling on a positive mental image to reduce stress and improve a person's sense of well-being. It stimulates the body's relaxation response. The laboring person can focus on tactile stimuli such as touch, massage, or stroking. They may focus on auditory stimuli such as music, humming, or verbal encouragement. Visual stimuli might be any object in the room, or they can imagine the beach, a mountaintop, a happy memory, or even the contractions of the uterine muscle pulling the cervix open and the fetus pressing downward to open the cervix. Some people focus on a particular mental activity such as a song, a chant, counting backward, or a religious verse. Breathing, relaxation, positive thinking, and positive visualization work well for people in labor. The use of these techniques keeps the sensory input perceived during the contraction from reaching the pain center in the cortex of the brain (West, 2022).

Effleurage and Massage

Effleurage is a light, stroking, superficial touch using slow, long, or continuous strokes on the abdomen, in rhythm with breathing during contractions. It is used as a relaxation and distraction technique from discomfort. External fetal monitor belts may interfere with the ability to accomplish this.

Effleurage and massage use the sense of touch to promote relaxation and pain relief. Massage works as a form of pain relief by increasing the production of endorphins in the body. Endorphins reduce the transmission of signals between nerve cells and thus lower the perception of pain. Because touch receptors go to the brain faster than pain receptors, massage—anywhere on the body—can block the pain message to the brain. In addition, light touch has been found to release endorphins and induce a relaxed state. In addition, touching and massage distract the laboring person from discomfort. Massage involves manipulation of the body's soft tissues. It is commonly used to help relax tense muscles and to soothe and calm the person. Massage may help relieve pain by assisting with relaxation, inhibiting sensory transmission in the pain pathways, or improving blood flow and oxygenation of tissues. Research indicates the use of massage leads to decreased pain during the first stage of labor and no ill effects have been demonstrated (Caughey & Tilden, 2023).

Breathing Techniques

Conscious use of breath by the person has the power to profoundly influence their labor and how they engage with it. The first action anyone takes in any situation is a breath. The breath affects the lungs, immediately cueing the nervous system. The nervous system responds by sending messages, which impact the entire psychophysiologic system. Messages sent from the nervous system affect us physically, emotionally, and mentally. If we alter how we breathe, we alter the constellation of messages and reactions in our entire mind–body experience. It reduces the duration of labor and brings pain relief (Amru et al., 2021; Issac et al., 2023).

Breathing techniques are effective in producing relaxation and pain relief using distraction. If the person is concentrating on slow-paced rhythmic breathing, they are not likely to fully focus on contraction pain. Breathing techniques are often taught in childbirth education classes (see Chapter 12 for additional information).

Controlled breathing helps reduce the pain experienced by using stimulus–response conditioning. The person selects a focal point within their environment to stare at during the first sign of a contraction. This focus creates a visual stimulus that goes directly to the brain. The person takes a deep cleansing breath, which is followed by rhythmic breathing. Verbal commands from their partner supply an ongoing auditory stimulus to their brain. Benefits of practicing patterned breathing include breathing that:

- Becomes an automatic response to pain
- Increases relaxation and can be used to deal with life's everyday stresses
- Is calming during labor
- Provides a sense of well-being and a measure of control
- Brings purpose to each contraction, making them more productive
- Helps form a visual focus to accompany conscious breathing
- Provides more oxygen for the laboring person and fetus (Terreri, 2023)

Many couples learn patterned-paced breathing during their childbirth education classes. Three levels may be taught, each beginning and ending with a cleansing breath or sigh after each contraction. In the first pattern, also known as slow-paced breathing, the laboring person inhales slowly through their nose and exhales through pursed lips. The breathing rate is typically 6 to 9 breaths per minute. In the second pattern, the laboring person inhales and exhales through their mouth at a rate of 4 breaths every 5 seconds. The rate can be accelerated to 2 breaths per second to assist them to relax. The third pattern is similar to the second pattern except that the breathing is punctuated every few breaths by a forceful exhalation through pursed lips. All breaths are kept equal and rhythmic and can increase as contractions increase in intensity (American Pregnancy Association, 2024).

Many childbirth educators do not recommend specific breathing techniques or try to teach parents to breathe the "right" way during labor and birth. Laboring people are encouraged to find breathing styles that enhance their relaxation and use them. There are numerous benefits to controlled and rhythmic breathing in childbirth (outlined previously), and many people choose these techniques to manage discomfort during labor.

Pharmacologic Measures

The goal for all laboring patients is the provision of adequate comfort and analgesia in labor and safety for them and the newborn. With varying degrees of success, generations of women have sought ways to relieve the pain of childbirth. Childbirth is a natural phenomenon, but it is painful. Pharmacologic pain relief during labor includes systemic analgesia and regional or local anesthesia. There have been dramatic changes in pharmacologic pain management options over the years. Methods have evolved from biting down on a stick to cope with pain, experiencing "twilight sleep" and not remembering what happened, to a more complex pharmacologic approach such as epidural/intrathecal analgesia. Systemic analgesia and regional analgesia/anesthesia have become less common, while newer neuraxial analgesia/anesthesia techniques involving minimal motor blockade have become more popular. **Neuraxial analgesia/anesthesia** is the administration of analgesic (opioids) or anesthetic (capable of producing a loss of sensation in an area of the body) agents, either continuously or intermittently, into the epidural or intrathecal space to relieve pain. Low-dose and ultra-low-dose epidural analgesia, spinal analgesia, and combined spinal–epidural (CSE) analgesia have replaced the traditional epidural for labor. Neuraxial analgesia does not interfere with the progress or outcome of labor. There is no need to withhold neuraxial analgesia until the active stage of labor; it can be initiated at any stage (Toledano & Leffert, 2023). This shift in pain management techniques allows the laboring person to be an active participant in labor.

TAKE NOTE!

Regardless of which approach is used during labor, the patient has the right to choose the methods of pain control that will best suit them and meet their needs.

Neuraxial Analgesia

Neuraxial analgesia involves the use of local anesthetic agents with or without added opioids to bring about pain relief or numbness through the drug's effects on the spinal cord and nerve roots. Approximately 70% of laboring people in the United States receive neuraxial analgesia for pain relief during labor (Grant & Reale, 2024). The routes of neuraxial analgesia for pain relief during active labor and birth include epidural block, CSE, and intrathecal (spinal) analgesia/anesthesia. The major advantage of these types of pain management techniques is that the patient can participate in the birthing process and still have good pain control.

EPIDURAL ANALGESIA

Lumbar epidurals provide an effective labor analgesic that has become very popular with laboring people. Epidural analgesia is used to obtain a partial or complete loss of pain sensation below T10 level of the spinal cord (Cunningham et al., 2022b). People requesting epidural analgesia in labor will do so when they feel they need pain relief, and for some, it might be quite early in their labor. Epidural analgesia for labor and birth involves the injection of a local anesthetic agent (e.g., lidocaine or bupivacaine) and an opioid analgesic agent (e.g., morphine or fentanyl) into the lumbar epidural space. A small catheter is then passed through the epidural needle to provide continuous access to the epidural space for maintenance of analgesia throughout labor and birth (Fig. 14.11). Epidural analgesia can increase the duration of the second stage of labor and may increase the rate of instrument-assisted vaginal deliveries as well as that of oxytocin administration (Cunningham et al., 2022b). The addition of opioids, such as fentanyl or morphine, to the local anesthetic helps decrease the amount of motor block obtained.

An epidural involves the injection of a drug into the epidural space, which is located outside the dura mater between the dura and the spinal canal. The epidural space is typically entered through the third and fourth lumbar vertebrae with a needle, and a catheter is threaded into the epidural space. An epidural can be used for both vaginal and cesarean births. It has evolved from a regional block producing total loss of sensation to analgesia with minimal blockade. The effectiveness of epidural analgesia depends on the technique and medications used. Theoretically, epidural local anesthetics could block all labor pain if used in large volumes and

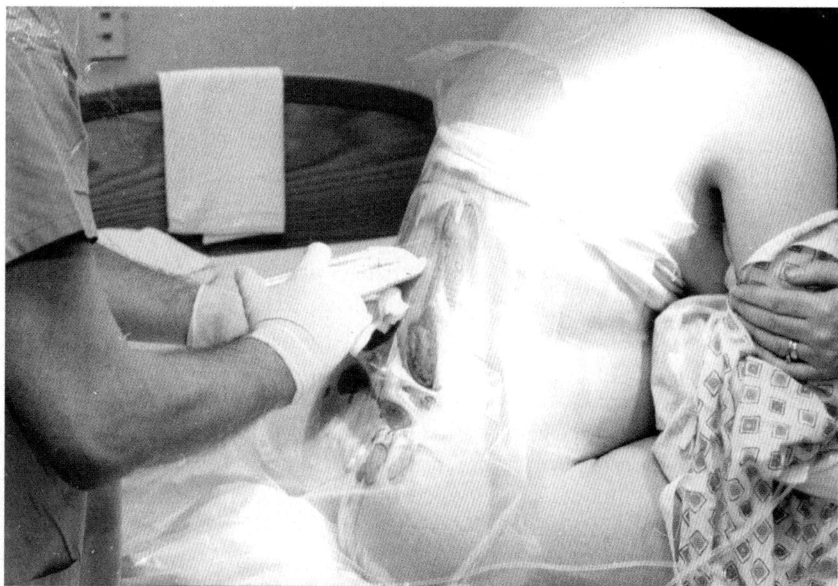

A

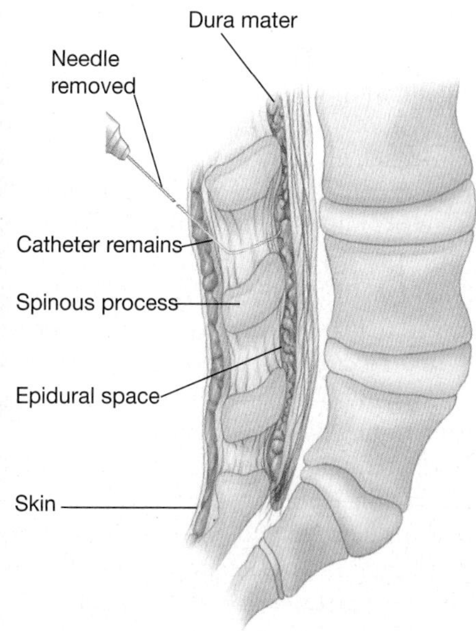

B

FIGURE 14.11 Epidural catheter insertion. **A.** A needle is inserted into the epidural space. **B.** A catheter is threaded into the epidural space; the needle is then removed. The catheter allows medication to be administered intermittently or continuously to relieve pain during labor and childbirth.

high concentrations. However, pain relief is balanced against other goals such as walking during the first stage of labor, pushing effectively in the second stage, and minimizing maternal and fetal side effects. Before the insertion procedure, the patient should be counseled on the risks and benefits. An epidural is contraindicated for patients with uncorrected hypovolemia, coagulopathy defects, sepsis, or infection at the intended puncture site, and increased intracranial pressure (Gallant, 2023; Toledano & Leffert, 2023).

Complications include nausea and vomiting, hypotension, fever (which affects one in five people), pruritus (if opioids are used), intravascular injection, maternal fever, urinary retention, allergic reaction, and respiratory depression. Effects on the fetus during labor include fetal distress secondary to maternal hypotension (Grant & Reale, 2024). Ensuring that the patient avoids a supine position and maintains a lateral position after an epidural catheter has been placed will help minimize hypotension.

PATIENT-CONTROLLED EPIDURAL ANALGESIA

Patient-controlled epidural analgesia (PCEA) involves the use of an indwelling epidural catheter with an infusion of medication and a programmed pump that allows the patient to control the dosing. This method allows the patient to have a sense of control over the pain and reach their own individually acceptable analgesia level. When compared with traditional epidural analgesia, PCEA provides equivalent analgesia with lower anesthetic use, lower rates of supplementation, and higher patient satisfaction.

With PCEA, the patient uses a handheld device connected to an analgesic agent that is attached to an epidural catheter. When they push the button, a bolus dose of agent is administered via the catheter to reduce pain. This method allows the patient to manage their pain at will without having to ask a staff member to provide pain relief. Evidence supports the use of PCEA, which appears to result in greater maternal satisfaction and lower overall medication use (Gallant, 2023).

SPINAL (INTRATHECAL) ANALGESIA/ANESTHESIA

The spinal (intrathecal) pain management technique involves injection of an anesthetic agent with or without opioids into the subarachnoid space to provide pain relief during labor or cesarean birth. The subarachnoid space is a fluid-filled area located between the dura mater and the spinal cord. Spinal anesthesia is frequently used for elective and emergent cesarean births. The contraindications are similar to those for an epidural block. Adverse reactions for the patient include hypotension and spinal headache.

The subarachnoid injection of opioids alone or in combination, a technique termed "intrathecal narcotics," has been used for laboring patients successfully for decades. A narcotic is injected into the subarachnoid space, providing rapid pain relief while still maintaining motor function and sensation. Morphine is a commonly used opioid due to its long duration of action (Champagne et al., 2023). Compared with epidural blocks, intrathecal narcotics are easy to administer, require a smaller volume of medication, produce excellent muscular relaxation, provide rapid-onset pain relief, are less likely to cause newborn respiratory depression, and do not cause motor blockade. The most frequent side effects of spinal analgesia are pruritus, hypotension, and prolonged decelerations (Ahmadi et al., 2022). Although pain relief is rapid with this technique, it is limited by the narcotic's duration of action, which may be only a few hours and not last through the labor.

COMBINED SPINAL–EPIDURAL ANALGESIA

Another epidural technique is CSE analgesia. This technique involves inserting the epidural needle into the epidural space and subsequently inserting a small-gauge spinal needle through the epidural needle into the subarachnoid space. An opioid without a local anesthetic is injected into this space. The spinal needle is then removed, and an epidural catheter is inserted for later use.

CSE is advantageous because of its rapid onset of pain relief (within 3 to 5 minutes) that can last up to 3 hours. It also allows the patient's motor function to remain active. Their ability to bear down during the second stage of labor is preserved because the pushing reflex is not lost, and their motor power remains intact. The CSE technique provides greater flexibility and reliability for labor than either spinal or epidural analgesia alone (Ituk & Wong, 2023). When compared with traditional epidural or spinal analgesia, which often keeps the patient lying in bed, CSE allows them to ambulate ("walking epidural").

Ambulating during labor provides several benefits; it may help to control pain better, shorten the first stage of labor, increase the intensity of the contractions, and decrease the possibility of an operative vaginal or cesarean birth. Although patients can walk with CSE, they often choose not to because of sedation and fatigue. Often health care providers do not encourage or assist them with ambulating for fear of injury. Nurses need to evaluate for ambulation safety including no postural hypotension and normal leg strength by demonstrating a partial knee bend while standing. Always assist with ambulation. As compared with epidural analgesia, CSE analgesia is associated with increased pruritis and fetal bradycardia (Toledano & Leffert, 2023). In addition, CSE analgesia had a faster onset of pain relief, yet there is an increased incidence of early FHR changes and maternal hypotension (Van de Velde, 2022).

Complications include maternal hypotension, intravascular injection, inadvertent intrathecal blockade, postdural puncture headache, pruritus, inadequate or failed block, maternal fever, and pruritus. Hypotension and associated FHR changes are managed with maternal positioning (semi-Fowler position), IV hydration, and supplemental oxygen (Grant, 2023).

Regional Analgesia/Anesthesia

Regional pain relief may also be achieved via local infiltration or pudendal block. These methods are used during birth for episiotomies (surgical incisions into the perineum to facilitate birth). Similar to neuraxial analgesia/anesthesia, regional analgesia/anesthesia provides pain relief without loss of consciousness.

LOCAL INFILTRATION

Local infiltration involves the injection of a local anesthetic, such as lidocaine, into the superficial perineal nerves to numb the perineal area. This technique is done by the primary provider or midwife just before performing an episiotomy or before suturing a laceration. Local infiltration does not alter the pain of uterine contractions, but it does numb the immediate area of the episiotomy or laceration. Local infiltration does not cause side effects for the patient or their newborn.

PUDENDAL NERVE BLOCK

The pudendal nerve block provides long-lasting perineal analgesia. A pudendal nerve block refers to the injection of a local anesthetic agent (e.g., bupivacaine, ropivacaine) into the pudendal nerves near each ischial spine. It provides pain relief in the lower vagina, vulva, and perineum (Fig. 14.12).

A pudendal block is used for the second stage of labor, an episiotomy, or an operative vaginal birth with outlet forceps or vacuum extractor. Pain impulses are transmitted through the pudendal nerve primarily in the second stage of labor; therefore, the pudendal nerve block is used to target this pain center (Beke, 2022). It must be administered about 15 minutes before it would be needed to ensure its full effect. A transvaginal approach is generally used to inject an anesthetic agent at or near the pudendal nerve branch. Neither maternal nor fetal complications are common.

General Anesthesia

Obstetric guidelines recommend neuraxial anesthesia for cesarean births in most patients. General anesthesia is typically reserved for emergency cesarean births when there is not enough time to provide spinal or epidural anesthesia or if the patient has a contraindication to the use of regional anesthesia. It can be started quickly and causes a rapid loss of consciousness. General anesthesia can be administered by IV injection, inhalation of anesthetic agents, or both. Commonly, thiopental, a short-acting barbiturate, or propofol is given IV to produce unconsciousness. This is followed by administration of a muscle relaxant. After the patient is intubated, nitrous oxide and oxygen are administered. A volatile halogenated agent may also be administered to produce amnesia (Nixon & Leffert, 2023).

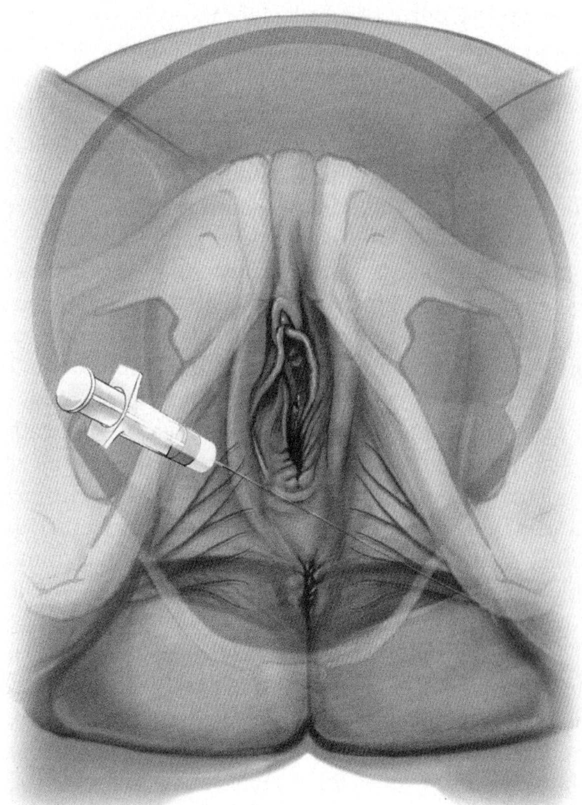

FIGURE 14.12 Pudendal nerve block.

All anesthetic agents cross the placenta and affect the fetus. The primary complication with general anesthesia is fetal depression, along with uterine relaxation and potential maternal vomiting and aspiration. General anesthesia complications are usually due to maternal aspiration or the inability to intubate the patient.

Although the anesthesiologist or nurse anesthetist administers the various general anesthesia agents, the nurse needs to be knowledgeable about the pharmacologic aspects of the drugs used and must be aware of airway management. Ensure that the patient is not taking anything by mouth (NPO) and has a patent IV line. In addition, there might be an order to administer a nonparticulate (clear) oral antacid or a proton pump inhibitor to reduce gastric acidity. Assist with placement of a wedge under the patient's right hip to displace the gravid uterus and prevent vena cava compression in the supine position. Once the newborn has been removed from the uterus, assist the perinatal team in providing supportive care.

Systemic Analgesia

Systemic analgesia involves the use of one or more drugs administered orally, intramuscularly, or IV; they become distributed throughout the body via the circulatory system. Depending on which administration method is used, the therapeutic effect of pain relief can occur within minutes and last for several hours. The most important complication associated with the use of this class of drugs is respiratory depression. Therefore, patients given these drugs require careful monitoring. Opioids given close to the time of birth can cause CNS depression in the newborn, necessitating the administration of naloxone (Narcan) to reverse the depressant effects of the opioids.

Systemic analgesics are typically administered parenterally, usually through an existing IV line. Nearly all medications given during labor cross the placenta and have a depressant effect on the fetus; therefore, it is important for the patient to receive the least amount of systemic medication that relieves their discomfort so that it does not cause any harm to the fetus (Grant & Reale, 2024). Historically opioids have been administered by nurses, but currently there has been increasing use of patient-controlled IV analgesia. With this system, the patient is given a button connected to a computerized pump on the IV line. When the patient desires analgesia, they press the button, and the pump delivers a preset amount of medication. This system provides the patient with a sense of control over their own pain management and active participation in the childbirth process. Drug Guide 14.1 highlights some of the major drugs used for systemic analgesia.

OPIOIDS

Opioids are morphinelike medications that are most effective for the relief of moderate to severe pain. Opioids typically are administered IV. All opioids are lipophilic and cross the placental barrier. Opioids may be associated with maternal and newborn CNS and respiratory depression (Gallant, 2023). To reduce the incidence of newborn depression, birth should occur within 1 hour or after 4 hours of administration to prevent neonatal respiratory depression.

OPIOID ANTAGONISTS

Opioid antagonists such as naloxone (Narcan) are given to reverse the effects of the CNS depression, including respiratory depression, caused by opioids. Given epidurally, opioid antagonists may also be used to reverse the side effects of neuraxial opioids such as pruritus, nausea, and vomiting, without significantly decreasing analgesia (Choi et al., 2020).

ANTIEMETICS

The antiemetic group of medications is used in combination with an opioid to decrease nausea and vomiting and lessen anxiety. These adjunct drugs potentiate the effectiveness of the opioid so that a lesser dose can be given. They may also be used to increase sedation.

BENZODIAZEPINES

Benzodiazepines are used for minor tranquilizing and sedative effects. They can be administered to calm a patient who feels out of control, thereby enabling them to relax enough so that they can participate effectively during the labor process rather than fighting against it.

Inhaled Analgesics

Inhaled nitrous oxide is a colorless, odorless gas that offers a safe and effective means of labor analgesia for many laboring patients. Nitrous oxide is known by most people as "laughing gas." The onset of action is approximately 30 to 60 seconds, so it should be administered 30 seconds before contraction onset (Grant & Reale, 2024). For labor pain, half nitrous oxide gas (50%) is mixed with half oxygen (50%) and inhaled through a mask or mouthpiece (Hill & Granlund, 2023). Self-administration of nitrous oxide is empowering for patients, giving them a sense of control. It is eliminated quickly via the lungs and does not cause respiratory depression in newborns. Potential side effects of nitrous oxide include nausea and vomiting, which are more common, dizziness, and dysphoria, although these are rare. It does not affect uterine contractile activity, progression of labor, or mode of delivery (Grant & Reale, 2024).

CONSIDER THIS!

When I was expecting my first child, I was determined to put my best foot forward and do everything right. I was an experienced obstetrics nurse, and in my mind doing everything right was expected behavior. I was already 2 weeks past my calculated due date, and I was becoming increasingly worried. That particular day I went to work with a backache but felt no contractions.

I managed to finish my 12-hour shift but felt completely wiped out. As I walked to my car outside the hospital, my water broke, and I felt the warm fluid run down my legs. I went back inside to be admitted for this much-awaited event.

Although I had helped so many women go through their childbirth experiences, I was now the one in the bed and not standing alongside it. My husband and I had practiced our breathing techniques to cope with the discomfort of labor, but this "discomfort" in my mind was more than I could tolerate. So, despite my best intentions of doing everything "right," within an hour, I begged for a painkiller to ease the pain. While the medication took the edge off my pain, I still felt every contraction and truly now appreciate the meaning of the word "labor." Although I wanted to use natural childbirth without any medication, I know that I was a full participant in my son's birthing experience, and that is what "doing everything right" was for me!

Thoughts: Doing what is "right" varies for each person, and as nurses, we need to support whatever that is. Having a positive outcome from the childbirth experience is the goal; the means it takes to achieve it are less important. How can nurses support patients in making their personal choices to achieve a healthy outcome? Is anyone a "failure" if they ask for pain medication to tolerate labor? How can nurses help patients overcome any stigma of using pharmacologic analgesia?

DRUG GUIDE 14.1

COMMON AGENTS USED FOR SYSTEMIC ANALGESIA

Type—Action	Drug	Comments
Opioids—Decrease the transmission of pain impulses by binding to receptor site pathways that transmit the pain signals to the brain	Morphine	Given IV or via epidural Rapidly crosses the placenta, causes a decrease in FHR variability Can cause maternal and neonatal CNS depression Decreases uterine contractions
	Butorphanol (Stadol)	Given IV Is rapidly transferred across the placenta Causes neonatal respiratory depression
	Nalbuphine (Nubain)	Given IV Causes less maternal nausea and vomiting Causes decreased FHR variability, fetal bradycardia, and respiratory depression
	Remifentanil (Ultiva)	Given via IV bolus or patient-controlled analgesia or epidurally Has rapid onset and is ultra-short-acting opioid Rapidly crosses placenta Can cause maternal and newborn respiratory depression
	Fentanyl (Sublimaze)	Given IV via patient-controlled analgesia, or via epidural Can cause maternal hypotension, maternal and fetal respiratory depression Rapidly crosses placenta
Antiemetics	Hydroxyzine (Vistaril)	Given IM Cannot be given IV Does not relieve pain but reduces anxiety and potentiates opioid analgesic effects Used to decrease nausea and vomiting
	Promethazine (Phenergan)	Recommended to be given IM secondary to risk of tissue damage with IV administration Used for antiemetic effect when combined with opioids Causes sedation, reduces apprehension May be given with morphine sulfate for sleep during prolonged latent phase May contribute to maternal hypotension and neonatal depression
	Prochlorperazine (Compazine)	Given IV or IM Frequently given with morphine sulfate for sleep during prolonged latent phase Counteracts nausea caused by opioids
Benzodiazepines	Diazepam (Valium)	Given IV Enhances pain relief of opioid and causes sedation May be used to stop eclamptic seizures Decreases nausea and vomiting Can cause newborn depression; therefore, lowest possible dose should be used.
	Midazolam (Versed)	Given IV Not used for analgesic but amnesia effect Used as adjunct for anesthesia Excreted in breast milk

CNS, central nervous system; FHR, fetal heart rate; IM, intramuscular; IV, intravenous.

Gallant, C. (2023). Obstetric anesthesia and analgesia. In G. Posner, A. Black, G. Jones, & J. Dy, *Oxorn-Foote human labor and birth* (7th ed.). McGraw Hill; Gill, P., Henning, J. M., Carlson, K., Van Hook, J. W., & Haddad, L. M. (2023). Abnormal labor (nursing). *StatPearls.* https://www.ncbi.nlm.nih.gov/books/NBK568801/; Grant, G. J., & Reale, S. (2024). Pharmacologic management of pain during labor and delivery. *UpToDate*. Retrieved March 9, 2024, from https://www.uptodate.com/contents/pharmacologic-management-of-pain-during-labor-and-delivery; UpToDate, Inc. (2024). *Lexi-comp® (Version 8.1.0)* [Mobile app]. Wolters Kluwer. https://apps.apple.com/us/app/lexicomp/id313401238

NURSING CARE DURING LABOR AND BIRTH

Childbirth, a physiologic process that is fundamental to human existence, can be one of the most significant cultural, psychological, spiritual, and behavioral events in a childbearing person's life. Although the act of giving birth is a universal phenomenon, it is a unique experience for each person. Continuous evaluation and appropriate intervention for patients during labor are essential to promoting a positive outcome for the family.

Care will vary at the different stages of labor, but what is essential is that an effective partnership with the patient is established, built upon successful communication and mutual trust. The nurse's role in childbirth is to ensure a safe environment for the patient and their newborn. Nurses begin evaluating the laboring patient and fetus during the admission procedures at the health care agency and continue to do so throughout labor. It is critical to provide anticipatory guidance and explain each procedure (fetal monitoring, IV therapy, and medications given and their expected reactions) and what will happen next. This will prepare the patient for the upcoming physical and emotional challenges, thereby helping reduce their anxiety. Acknowledging members of their support system (e.g., family, doula, or partner) helps allay their fears and concerns, thereby assisting them in carrying out their supportive role. Knowing how and when to evaluate a patient during the various stages of labor is essential for all labor and birth nurses to ensure a positive maternal experience and a healthy newborn.

A major focus of care for the patient during labor and birth is assisting them with maintaining control over their pain, emotions, and actions while being an active participant. Nurses can help and support patients' active involvement in their childbirth experience by allowing time for discussion, offering companionship and mere presence, listening to worries and concerns, paying attention to emotional needs, and offering information to explain what is happening in each stage of labor.

Nursing Management During the First Stage of Labor

Depending on how far advanced the patient's labor is when they arrive at the facility, the nurse will determine assessment parameters of maternal–fetal status and plan care accordingly. The nurse will provide high-touch, low-tech supportive nursing care during the first stage of labor when admitting the patient and orienting them to the labor and birth suite. The nurse is usually the primary gatekeeper of observations, interventions, treatments, and often the management of labor in the inpatient perinatal setting. Nursing care during this stage will include taking an admission history (reviewing the prenatal record); checking the results of routine laboratory tests and any special diagnostic tests such as chorionic villi sampling, amniocentesis, genetic studies, and biophysical profile done during pregnancy; asking the patient about their childbirth preparation (birth plan, classes taken, coping skills); and completing a physical assessment of the patient to establish baseline values for future comparison.

Key nursing interventions include the following:

- Identifying the estimated date of birth from the patient and the prenatal chart
- Validating the patient's prenatal history to determine fetal risk status
- Determining fundal height to validate dates and fetal growth
- Performing Leopold maneuvers to determine fetal position, lie, and presentation
- Checking FHR
- Performing a vaginal examination as appropriate to evaluate effacement and dilation progress
- Instructing the patient and their partner about monitoring techniques and equipment
- Assessing fetal response and FHR to contractions and recovery time
- Interpreting fetal monitoring strips
- Checking FHR baseline for accelerations, variability, and decelerations
- Repositioning the patient to obtain an optimal FHR pattern
- Recognizing FHR problems and initiating corrective measures
- Checking amniotic fluid for meconium staining, odor, and amount
- Comforting the patient throughout the testing period and labor
- Documenting times of notification for team members if problems arise
- Knowing appropriate interventions when abnormal FHR patterns present
- Recognizing and intervening appropriately in the different stages of labor
- Assessing the current level of maternal fatigue and emotional stress in each stage
- Supporting the patient's decisions regarding intervention or avoidance of intervention
- Assessing the patient's support system and coping status frequently (Lothian, 2024)

In addition to these interventions to promote optimal outcomes for the laboring patient and fetus, the nurse must document care accurately and in a timely fashion. Accurate and timely documentation helps decrease professional liability exposure, minimize the risk of preventable injuries to patients and infants during labor and birth, and preserve families (Hankey, 2023). Guidelines for recording care include documenting:

- All care rendered to prove standards were met
- Conversations with all providers including notification times
- Nursing interventions before and after notifying the provider
- Use of the chain of command and response at each level
- All flow sheets and forms to validate care given
- All education given to the patient and the response to it

- Facts, not personal opinions
- Detailed descriptions of any adverse outcome
- Initial nursing assessment, all encounters, and discharge plan
- All telephone conversations (Hankey, 2023)

Assessing the Patient Upon Admission

The nurse usually first encounters the patient either by phone or in person. The nurse should ascertain whether they are in true or false labor and whether they should be admitted or sent home. Upon admission to the labor and birth suite, the highest priorities include assessing FHR, assessing cervical dilation and effacement, and determining whether membranes have ruptured or are intact. These assessment data will guide the critical thinking in planning care for the patient.

If the initial contact is by phone, establish a therapeutic relationship with the patient. Speaking in a calm and caring tone facilitates this. Nurses providing a telephone triage service need to have sufficient clinical experience and have clear lines of responsibility to enable sound decision making. When completing a phone assessment, include questions about:

- Estimated date of birth to determine if term or preterm
- Fetal movement (frequency in the past few days)
- Other premonitory signs of labor experienced
- Parity, gravida, and previous childbirth experiences
- Time from start of labor to birth in previous labors
- Characteristics of contractions, including frequency, duration, and intensity
- Appearance of any vaginal bloody show
- Membrane status (ruptured or intact)
- Presence of supportive adult in household or if they are alone (Long & McMullen, 2019)

When speaking with the patient over the telephone, review the signs and symptoms that denote true versus false labor, and suggest various positions they can assume to provide comfort and increase placental perfusion. Also suggest walking, massage, and taking a warm shower to promote relaxation. Outline what foods and fluids are appropriate for oral intake in early labor. Throughout the phone call, listen to the patient's concerns and answer any questions clearly.

Reducing the risk of liability exposure and avoiding preventable injuries to patients and fetuses during labor and birth can be accomplished by adhering to two basic tenets of clinical practice: (1) use applicable evidence or published standards and guidelines as the foundation of care, and (2) whenever a clinical choice is presented, choose patient safety (The Joint Commission, 2022). With these two tenets in mind, advise the patient on the phone to contact their health care provider for further instructions or to come to the facility to be evaluated, since ruling out true labor and possible maternal–fetal complications cannot be done accurately over the phone. Additional nursing responsibilities associated with a phone assessment include the following:

- Consulting the patient's prenatal record for parity status, estimated date of birth, and untoward events
- Calling the health care provider to inform them of the patient's status
- Preparing for admission to the perinatal unit to ensure adequate staff assignment
- Notifying the admissions office of a pending admission

If the nurse's first encounter with the patient is in person, an assessment is completed to determine whether they should be admitted to the perinatal unit or sent home until their labor advances. Recent research findings suggest that patients admitted before active labor and with less than 80% cervical effacement are more likely to have their labor augmented with oxytocin and give birth via cesarean section when compared with patients admitted in active labor (Gjaerum et al., 2022). Nurses need to make careful assessment of labor progression *prior* to labor admission to decrease early admissions and to improve labor safety and birth outcomes.

An admission assessment includes maternal health history, physical assessment, fetal assessment, laboratory studies, and assessment of psychological status. Usually, the facility has a form that can be used throughout labor and birth to document assessment findings (Fig. 14.13).

MATERNAL HEALTH HISTORY AND CULTURAL ASSESSMENT

A maternal health history should include typical biographical data such as the patient's name and age and the name of the delivering health care provider. Other information that is collected includes reason for admission, such as labor, cesarean birth, or observation for a complication; the prenatal record data, including the estimated date of birth, a history of the current pregnancy, and the results of any laboratory and diagnostic tests, such as blood type, Rh status, and group B streptococcal (GBS) status; past pregnancy and obstetric history; past health history and family history; prenatal education; list of medications; risk factors such as diabetes, hypertension, and use of tobacco, alcohol, or illicit drugs; pain management plan; history of potential domestic violence; history of previous preterm births; allergies; time of last food ingestion; method chosen for infant feeding; and name of birth attendants and pediatrician.

Ascertaining this information is important so that an individualized plan of care can be developed for the patient. If, for example, the due date is still 2 months away, it is important to establish this information so interventions can be initiated to arrest the labor immediately or

ADMISSION ASSESSMENT OBSTETRICS

▲ PATIENT IDENTIFICATION ▲

ADMISSION DATA

Date	Time	Via ☐ Ambulatory ☐ Wheelchair ☐ Stretcher					
Grav.	Term	Pre-term	Ab.	Living	EDC	LMP	GA

Prev. adm. date ______ Reason ______
Obstetrician ______ Pediatrician ______
Ht.____ Wt. ____ Wt. gain ______
Allergies (meds/food) ☐ None ______ ☐ Hx latex sensitivity
BP ______ T ______ P ______ R ______
FHR ______ Vag exam ______

Reason for Admission

☐ Labor / SROM ☐ Induction ______
☐ Primary C/S ______ ☐ Repeat C/S
☐ Observation ______
☐ OB / Medical complication ______

Onset of labor: ☐ Not in labor
Date ______ Time ______
Membranes: ☐ Intact
☐ Ruptured / Date ______ Time ______
☐ Clear ☐ Meconium ☐ Bloody ☐ Foul
Vaginal bleeding: ☐ None
☐ Normal show ☐ ______

Current Pregnancy Labs ☐ NPC

☐ POL ☐ PPROM ☐ Cerclage
☐ PIH ☐ Chr. HTN ☐ Other ______
☐ Diabetes ______ Diet ______
☐ Insulin ______
☐ Amniocentesis ______ Results ______
Bld type / RH____ Date Rhogam____
Antibody screen ☐ Neg ☐ Pos
Rubella ☐ Non-immune ☐ Immune
Diabetic screen ☐ Normal ☐ Abnormal
Recent exposure to chick pox ☐
Current meds: ______

	Pos	Neg	Tested
Hepatitis B	☐	☐	☐ No
HIV	☐	☐	☐ No
Group B strep	☐	☐	☐ No
GC	☐	☐	☐ No
Chlamydia	☐	☐	☐ No
RPR	☐	☐	☐ No

Previous OB History

☐ POL ☐ Multiple gestation
☐ Prev C/S type ______ Reason ______
☐ PIH ☐ Chronic HTN ☐ Diabetes ______
☐ Stillbirth/demise ☐ Neodeath ☐ Anomalies
☐ Precipitous labor (<3 H) ☐ Macrosomia
☐ PP Hemorrhage
☐ Hx Transfusion reaction ☐ Yes ☐ No
☐ Other ______

Latest risk assessment ☐ None
1. ______ 3. ______
2. ______ 4. ______

Date ______
Signature ______ Time ______

NEUROLOGICAL

☐ WNL
Variance: ☐ HA
☐ Scotoma / visual changes
Reflexes ☐ < 2 + ☐ > 2 +
☐ Clonus___ bts
☐ Numbness ☐ Tingling
☐ Hx Seizures
☐ ______

RESPIRATORY

☐ WNL
Variance: ☐ Hx Asthma ☐ URI
Respirations: ☐ < 12 ☐ > 24
Effort: ☐ SOB
☐ Shallow ☐ Labored
Auscultation:
☐ Diminished ☐ Crackles
☐ Wheezes ☐ Rhonchi

	No	Yes
Cough for greater than 2 weeks?	☐	☐
Is the cough productive?	☐	☐
Blood in the sputum?	☐	☐
Experiencing any fever or night sweats?	☐	☐
Ever had TB in the past?	☐	☐
Recent exposure to TB?	☐	☐
Weight loss in last 3 weeks?	☐	☐

If the patient answers yes to any three of the above questions implement policy and procedure # 5725-0704.

GASTROINTESTINAL

☐ WNL
Variance: ☐ Heartburn
☐ Epigastric pain Nausea
☐ Vomiting ☐ Diarrhea
☐ Constipation ☐ Pain
☐ Wt. Gain < 2lbs / month**
☐ Recent change in appetite of < 50% of usual intake for > 5 days
☐ ______

INTEGUMENTARY

☐ WNL
Variance: ☐ Rash ☐ Lacerations
☐ Abrasion ☐ Swelling
☐ Urticaria ☐ Bruising
☐ Diaphoretic/hot
☐ Clammy/cold
☐ Scars
☐ ______

FETAL ASSESSMENT

☐ WNL
Variance:
☐ NRFS
FHR ☐ < 110 ☐ > 160
LTV ☐ Absent ☐ Minimal
☐ Increased
STV Absent
Decelerations: ______
☐ Decreased fetal movement
☐ IUGR
☐ ______

CARDIOVASCULAR

☐ WNL
Variance:
☐ MVP
Heart rate: ☐ < 60 ☐ > 100
B/P: Systolic: ☐ < 90 ☐ > 140
Diastolic: ☐ < 50 ☐ > 90
☐ Edema ______
☐ Chest pain / palpitations
☐ ______

MUSCULOSKELETAL

☐ WNL
Variance:
☐ Numbness ☐ Tingling
☐ Paralysis ☐ Deformity
☐ Scoliosis
☐ ______

GENITOURINARY

☐ WNL
Variance: ☐ Albumin ______
Output: ☐ < 30 cc/Hr.
☐ UTI ☐ Rx ☐ Frequency
☐ Dysuria ☐ Hematuria
☐ CVA Tenderness
☐ Hx STD ______
☐ Vag. discharge ______
☐ Rash ☐ Blisters
☐ Warts ☐ Lesions
☐ ______

EARS, NOSE, THROAT, AND EYES

☐ WNL
Variance:
☐ Sore throat ☐ Eyeglasses
☐ Runny nose ☐ Contact lenses
☐ Nasal congestion
☐ ______

PSYCHOSOCIAL

☐ WNL
Variance: ☐ Hx depression
☐ Yes ☐ No
☐ Emotional behavioral care
Affect: ☐ Flat ☐ Anxious
☐ Uncooperative ☐ Combative
Living will ☐ Yes ☐ No
☐ On chart
Healthcare surrogate ☐ Yes ☐ No
☐ On chart
Are you being hurt, hit, frightened by anyone at home or in your life? ☐ Yes ☐ No
Religious preference ______

Tobacco use	☐ Denies	☐ Yes	Amt ______
Alcohol use	☐ Denies	☐ Yes	Amt ______
Drug use	☐ Denies	☐ Yes	Amt type ______
Primary language	☐ English	☐ Spanish	☐ ______

PAIN ASSESSMENT

1. Do you have any ongoing pain problems? ☐ No ☐ Yes
2. Do you have any pain now? ☐ No ☐ Yes
3. If any of the above questions are answered yes, the patient has a positive pain screening.
4. *Patient to be given pain management education material. Complete pain / symptom assessment on flowsheet.*
5. *Please proceed to complete pain assessment.*

FIGURE 14.13 Sample documentation form used for admission to the perinatal unit. (Used with permission. Briggs Corporation, 2001.)

notify the intensive perinatal team to be available. In addition, if the patient has diabetes, it is critical to monitor their glucose levels during labor, to prepare for a surgical birth if dystocia of labor occurs, and to alert the newborn nursery of potential hypoglycemia in the newborn after birth. By collecting important information about each patient they care for, nurses can help improve the outcomes for all concerned.

Be sure to observe the patient's emotions, support system, verbal interaction, cultural background and language spoken, body language and posture, perceptual acuity, and energy level. This psychosocial information provides cues about their emotional state, culture, and communication systems. For example, if the patient arrives at the labor and birth suite extremely anxious, alone, and unable to communicate in English, how can the nurse meet their needs and plan their care appropriately? It is only by assessing each patient physically and psychosocially that the nurse can make astute decisions regarding proper care. In this case, an interpreter would be needed to assist in the communication process between the staff and the patient to initiate proper care.

It is important to acknowledge and try to understand the perspectives and needs of patients with cultural backgrounds different from that of the nurse. Attitudes toward childbirth are heavily influenced by the culture in which the person has been raised. As a result, within every society, specific attitudes and values shape the person's childbearing behaviors. Be aware of what these are. When carrying out a cultural assessment during the admission process, ask questions (Box 14.2) to help plan culturally competent care during labor and birth.

BOX 14.2 Questions for Providing Culturally Competent Care/Practicing Cultural Humility During Labor and Birth

- Where were you born? How long have you lived in the United States?
- What languages do you speak and read?
- Who are your major support people?
- What are your religious practices?
- How do you view childbearing?
- Are there any special precautions or restrictions that are important?
- Is birth considered a private or a social experience?
- How would you like to manage your labor discomfort?
- Who will provide your labor support?

American College of Obstetricians and Gynecologists. (2021b). *Effective patient–physician communication, committee opinion number 587 (reaffirmed 2021).* https://www.acog.org/clinical/clinical-guidance/committee-opinion/articles/2014/02/effective-patient-physician-communication; Kennedy, M. B., & Devane-Johnson, S. (2024). Perinatal diversity. In B. J. Baker, J. Janke, & Association of Women's Health, Obstetric and Neonatal Nurses, *Core curriculum for maternal-newborn nursing* (6th ed.). Elsevier.

PHYSICAL EXAMINATION

The physical examination typically includes a generalized assessment of the patient's body systems, including hydration status, vital signs, auscultation of heart and lung sounds, and measurement of height and weight. The physical examination also includes the following assessments:

1. Pain level and coping behaviors demonstrated
2. Uterine activity, including contraction frequency, duration, and intensity
3. Fetal status, including heart rate, position, and station
4. Cervical dilation and degree of effacement
5. Status of membranes (intact or ruptured)
6. Assessing vital signs: temperature, pulse, respirations, and blood pressure
7. Performing Leopold maneuvers to determine fetal lie
8. Fundal height measurement
9. Ability to ambulate safely

These assessment parameters form a baseline against which the nurse can compare all future values throughout labor. The findings should be similar to those of the patient's prepregnancy and pregnancy findings except for their pulse rate, which might be elevated secondary to their anxious state with beginning labor.

LABORATORY STUDIES

Upon admission, laboratory studies are typically done to establish a baseline. Although the exact tests may vary among facilities, they usually include a urinalysis via clean-catch urine specimen and complete blood count. Blood typing and Rh factor analysis may be necessary if the results of these are unknown or unavailable. In addition, if the following test results are not included in the maternal prenatal history, it may be necessary to perform them at this time. They include syphilis screening, hepatitis B surface antigen (HbsAg) screening, GBS, human immune deficiency virus (HIV) testing, and possible drug screening if the history is positive.

GBS is a Gram-positive organism that colonizes in the female genital tract and rectum and is present in 10% to 25% of all healthy females (Cunningham et al., 2022c). These people are carriers without any symptoms but can cause GBS disease of the newborn through vertical transmission during labor and horizontal transmission after birth. The mortality rate of infected newborns varies according to time of onset (early or late). Risk factors for GBS include maternal intrapartum fever, preterm birth, prolonged ruptured membranes (longer than 12 to 18 hours), previous birth of an infected newborn, and GBS bacteriuria in the present pregnancy.

ACOG and the American Academy of Pediatrics (AAP) recommend following the published guidelines advising universal screening via vaginal–rectal cultures of pregnant patients at 36 to 37 6/7 weeks' gestation for GBS and intrapartum antibiotic therapy for GBS carriers

(ACOG, 2022). These guidelines reaffirm the major prevention strategy—universal antenatal GBS screening and intrapartum antibiotic prophylaxis for culture-positive and high-risk patients. Also included are new recommendations for laboratory methods for identification of GBS colonization during pregnancy, algorithms for screening and intrapartum prophylaxis for patients with preterm labor and premature ROM, updated prophylaxis recommendations for patients with a penicillin allergy, and a revised algorithm for the care of newborn infants (ACOG, 2022). Maternal infections associated with GBS include acute chorioamnionitis, endometritis, and urinary tract infection. Neonatal clinical manifestations include pneumonia and sepsis. Identified GBS carriers receive IV antibiotic prophylaxis (penicillin G or ampicillin) at the onset of labor or ruptured membranes.

The ACOG, Centers for Disease Control and Prevention (CDC), AWHONN, and the U.S. Preventive Services Task Force recommend that all pregnant people have a screening test for HIV antibodies at their first prenatal visit, again during the third trimester if engaging in high-risk behaviors, and upon admission to the labor and birth area. The CDC estimates that approximately 36,000 people acquire HIV in the United States each year (CDC, 2023).

If their HIV status is not documented, the patient being admitted to the labor and birth suite should have rapid HIV testing done. To reduce perinatal transmission, patients who are HIV positive are given a combination of antiretroviral drugs. To further reduce the risk of perinatal transmission, ACOG and the U.S. Public Health Service recommend that patients who are infected with HIV and have plasma viral loads of more than 1,000 copies/mL be counseled regarding the benefits of elective cesarean birth (ACOG, 2024). In the absence of any medical intervention, the rate of vertical transmission of HIV to the fetus is 15% to 45% (WHO, 2024). About 3,500 people infected with HIV give birth annually in the United States and with the use of antiretroviral regimens, the transmission rate is reduced to less than 1% (Panel on Treatment of HIV During Pregnancy and Prevention of Perinatal Transmission, 2024).

Additional interventions to reduce the transmission risk would include avoiding use of a scalp electrode for fetal monitoring or doing a scalp blood sampling for fetal pH, delaying amniotomy, encouraging formula feeding after birth, and avoiding invasive procedures such as using forceps or vacuum-assisted devices. The nurse stresses the importance of all interventions and the goal to reduce transmission of HIV to the newborn.

Continuous Assessment During the First Stage of Labor

After the admission assessment is complete and the laboring patient and their support person have been oriented to the room, equipment, and procedures, assessment continues for changes that would indicate that labor is progressing as expected. Assess the patient's knowledge, experience, and expectations of labor. During the active phase of labor, vital signs are assessed every 30 minutes. Temperature is taken every 4 hours throughout the first stage of labor and every 2 hours after membranes have ruptured to detect an elevation indicating an ascending infection.

Vaginal examinations are performed periodically to track labor progress. This assessment information is shared with the patient to reinforce that they are making progress toward the goal of birth. Uterine contractions are monitored for frequency, duration, and intensity every 30 to 60 minutes during the latent phase, and every 15 to 30 minutes during the active phase. Note the changes in the character of the contractions as labor progresses and inform the patient of their progress. Continually determine the patient's level of pain and ability to cope and use relaxation techniques effectively.

When the fetal membranes rupture, spontaneously or artificially, assess the FHR and check the amniotic fluid for color, odor, and amount. Assess the FHR intermittently or continuously via electronic monitoring. During the latent phase of labor, assess the FHR every 30 to 60 minutes; in the active phase, assess the FHR at least every 15 to 30 minutes. Also, be sure to assess the FHR before ambulation, before any procedure, and before administering analgesia or anesthesia to the laboring person. The continuous monitoring of the FHR provides the nurse with insight into fetal well-being. Table 14.3 summarizes assessments for the first stage of labor.

Remember Sheila from the chapter-opening scenario? What is the nurse's role with Sheila in active labor? What additional comfort measures can the labor nurse offer Sheila?

Nursing Interventions

Nursing interventions during the admission process should include:

- Asking about the patient's expectations of the birthing process
- Providing information about labor, birth, pain management options, and relaxation techniques
- Presenting information about fetal monitoring equipment and the procedures needed
- Monitoring FHR and identifying patterns that need further intervention
- Monitoring the patient's vital signs to obtain a baseline for later comparison
- Reassuring the patient that their labor progress will be monitored closely, and nursing care will focus on ensuring fetal and maternal well-being throughout

TABLE 14.3 • Summary of Assessments During the First Stage of Labor

Assessments[a]	Latent Phase (0–6 cm)	Active Phase (6–10 cm)
Vital signs (BP, pulse, respirations)	Every 30–60 minutes	Every 15–30 minutes
Temperature	Every 4 hours; more frequently if membranes are ruptured	Every 4 hours; more frequently if membranes are ruptured
Contractions (frequency, duration, intensity)	Every 30–60 minutes by palpation or continuously if EFM	Every 15–30 minutes by palpation or continuously if EFM
Fetal heart rate	Every hour by Doppler or continuously by EFM	Every 15–30 minutes by Doppler or continuously by EFM
Vaginal examination	Initially on admission to determine phase and as needed based on maternal cues to document labor progression	As needed to monitor labor progression
Behavior/psychosocial	With every patient encounter: talkative, excited, anxious	With every patient encounter: self-absorbed in labor; intense and quiet now

BP, blood pressure; EFM, electronic fetal monitoring.
[a]The frequency of assessments is dictated by the health status of the patient and fetus and can be altered if either one of their conditions changes.
Funai, E. F., & Norwitz, E. R. (2023). Labor and delivery: Management of the normal first stage. *UpToDate.* Retrieved March 7, 2024, from https://www.uptodate.com/contents/labor-and-delivery-management-of-the-normal-first-stage; Lothian, J. (2024). Normal childbirth. In B. J. Baker, J. Janke, & Association of Women's Health, Obstetric and Neonatal Nurses, *Core curriculum for maternal-newborn nursing* (6th ed.). Elsevier.

As the patient progresses through the first stage of labor, nursing interventions include:

- Encouraging the support partner to participate
- Keeping the patient and partner up to date on the progress of the labor
- Orienting the patient and partner to the labor and birth unit and explaining all the birthing procedures
- Providing clear fluids (e.g., ice chips) as needed or requested
- Maintaining the patient's parenteral fluid intake at the prescribed rate if they have an IV
- Initiating or encouraging comfort measures, such as backrubs, cool cloths to the forehead, frequent position changes, ambulation, showers, slow dancing, leaning over a birth ball, side-lying, or counterpressure on lower back (Teaching Guidelines 14.1)
- Encouraging the partner's involvement with breathing techniques
- Assisting the patient and partner with focusing on breathing techniques
- Informing the patient that the discomfort will be intermittent and of limited duration; urging them to

TEACHING GUIDELINES 14.1 Positioning During the First Stage of Labor

- Walking with support from the partner (adds the force of gravity to contractions to promote fetal descent)
- Slow-dancing position with the partner holding the laboring person (adds the force of gravity to contractions and promotes support from and active participation of the partner)
- Side-lying with pillows between the knees for comfort (offers a restful position and improves oxygen flow to the uterus)
- Semi-sitting in bed or on a couch leaning against the partner (reduces back pain because fetus falls forward, away from the sacrum)
- Sitting in a chair with one foot on the floor and one on the chair (changes pelvic shape)
- Leaning forward by straddling a chair, a table, or a bed or kneeling over a birth ball (reduces back pain, adds the force of gravity to promote descent; possible pain relief if partner can apply sacral pressure)
- Encourage any position of comfort the laboring person chooses to labor in and give birth.
- Sitting in a rocking chair or on a birth ball and shifting weight back and forth (provides comfort because rocking motion is soothing; uses the force of gravity to help fetal descent)
- Lunge by rocking weight back and forth with foot up on chair during contraction (uses force of gravity by being upright; enhances rotation of fetus through rocking)
- Laboring people should be allowed to position themselves in whatever position they find most comfortable.
- Open knee–chest position (helps relieve back discomfort) (Dekker, 2022a; Spinning Babies, 2024)

rest between contractions to preserve their strength; and encouraging them to use distracting activities to lessen the focus on contractions
- Changing bed linens and gown as needed
- Keeping the perineal area clean and dry
- Supporting the patient's decisions about pain management
- Monitoring maternal vital signs frequently and reporting any abnormal values
- Ensuring that the patient takes deep cleansing breaths before and after each contraction to enhance gas exchange and oxygen to the fetus
- Educating the patient and partner about the need for rest and helping them plan strategies to conserve strength
- Monitoring FHR for baseline, accelerations, variability, and decelerations
- Checking on bladder status and encouraging voiding at least every 2 hours to facilitate birth
- Repositioning the patient as needed to obtain optimal heart rate pattern
- Communicating requests from the patient to appropriate personnel
- Respecting the patient's sense of privacy by covering them when appropriate
- Offering human presence by being present with the patient, not leaving them alone for long periods
- Being patient with the natural labor pattern to allow time for change
- Encouraging maternal movement throughout labor to increase the patient's level of comfort
- Dimming the lights in the room when pushing and requesting softened voices be used to maintain a calm and centered ambiance
- Reporting any deviations from normal to the health care professional so that interventions can be initiated early to be effective (ACOG, 2021a; Lothian, 2024)

See Clinical Judgment & Nursing Process Box 14.1.

Nursing Management During the Second Stage of Labor

Management of the second stage of labor often follows tradition-based routines rather than evidence-based practices. Current scientific evidence for management of the second stage of labor supports the practices of delayed pushing, spontaneous (nondirected) pushing, and maternal choice of positions (Funai & Norwitz, 2024). To be able to help patients through the second stage of labor requires the nurse to have a comprehensive understanding of physiology, be aware of the latest evidence-based research, and apply it to practice (Gimovsky & Berghella, 2022). A kind word, a squeeze of their hand, and a pat on their back can have a lasting impact and encouragement on the laboring patient.

Nursing care during the second stage of labor focuses on supporting the patient and their partner in making active decisions about their care and labor management, implementing strategies to prolong the early passive phase of fetal descent, supporting involuntary bearing-down efforts, providing instruction and assistance, and using maternal positions that can enhance descent and reduce pain (Jyoti et al., 2022). People in the past gave birth unaided by following their bodies' signals to birth their babies, so the role of the nurse should be to support the patient in their choice of pushing method and to encourage confidence in their instinct of when and how to push.

In the absence of any complications, nurses should not be controlling this stage of labor but rather empowering them to achieve a satisfying experience. The primary rationale for directing people to push is to shorten the second stage of labor. Common practice in many labor units is still to coach patients to use closed glottis pushing with every contraction, starting at 10 cm of dilation, a practice that is not supported by research. Research suggests that directed pushing during the second stage may be accompanied by a decline in fetal pH and may cause maternal muscle and nerve damage if done too early (Pouca et al., 2022). Shortening the phase of active pushing and lengthening the early phase of passive descent can be achieved by encouraging the patients not to push until they have a strong desire to do so and until the descent and rotation of the fetal head are well advanced. Effective pushing can be achieved by assisting the patient with assuming a more upright or squatting position. Supporting spontaneous pushing and encouraging patients to choose their own method of pushing should be accepted as best clinical practice.

Perineal lacerations or tears can occur during the second stage when the fetal head emerges through the vaginal introitus. The extent of the laceration is defined by depth: a first-degree laceration extends through the skin; a second-degree laceration extends through the muscles of the perineal body; a third-degree laceration continues through the anal sphincter muscle; and a fourth-degree laceration also involves the anterior rectal wall. Risk factors for perineal lacerations include advancing gestational age, Asian race, increased fetal weight, malpresentation, midline episiotomy, nulliparity, and operative vaginal delivery. Special attention needs to be paid to third- and fourth-degree lacerations to prevent fecal incontinence. Risks for third- or fourth-degree lacerations include forceps or vacuum deliveries, large fetus, and midline episiotomy (Ramar & Grimes, 2023). The primary care provider should repair any lacerations during the third stage of labor.

An **episiotomy** is an incision made in the perineum to enlarge the vaginal outlet and theoretically to shorten the second stage of labor. Alternative measures such as

CLINICAL JUDGMENT & NURSING PROCESS 14.1 Overview of a Patient in the Active Phase of the First Stage of Labor

Candice, a 23-year-old gravida 1, para 0 (G1P0), is admitted to the labor and birth suite at 39 weeks' gestation having contractions of moderate intensity every 5 to 6 minutes. A vaginal examination reveals that her cervix is 80% effaced and 5 cm dilated. The presenting part (vertex) is at 0 station and her membranes ruptured spontaneously 4 hours ago at home. She is admitted and an intravenous (IV) line is started for hydration and vascular access. An external fetal monitor is applied. Fetal heart rate (FHR) is 140 bpm and regular. Her partner is present at her bedside. Candice is now in the active phase of the first stage of labor, and her assessment findings are as follows: cervix dilated 7 cm, 80% effaced; moderate to strong contractions occurring regularly every 3 to 5 minutes lasting 45 to 60 seconds; at 0 station on pelvic examination; FHR auscultated loudest below umbilicus at 140 bpm; vaginal show—pink or bloody vaginal mucus; currently apprehensive, inwardly focused, with increased dependency; voicing concern about ability to cope with pain; limited ability to follow directions.

NURSING ANALYSIS: Anxiety related to labor and birth process and fear of the unknown related to patient's first experience

OUTCOME IDENTIFICATION AND EVALUATION

The patient will remain calm and in control as evidenced by ability to make decisions and use positive coping strategies.

INTERVENTIONS: Promoting Positive Coping Strategies

- Provide instruction regarding the labor process *to allay anxiety.*
- Orient the patient to the physical environment and equipment as necessary *to keep them informed of events.*
- Encourage verbalization of feelings and concerns *to reduce anxiety.*
- Listen attentively to the patient and their partner *to demonstrate interest and concern.*
- Inform the patient and their partner of standard procedures and processes *to ensure adequate understanding of events and procedures.*
- Frequently update patient of progress and labor status *to provide positive reinforcement for actions.*
- Reinforce relaxation techniques and provide instruction if needed *to aid in coping.*
- Encourage participation of the partner in the coaching role; role model *to facilitate partner participation in labor process to provide support and encouragement to the patient.*
- Provide a presence and remain with the patient as much as possible *to provide comfort and support.*

NURSING ANALYSIS: Acute pain related to uterine contractions and stretching of the cervix and birth canal

OUTCOME IDENTIFICATION AND EVALUATION

The patient will maintain a tolerable level of pain and discomfort as evidenced by statements of pain relief, pain rating of 2 or less on a pain rating scale, and absence of adverse effects in patient and fetus from analgesia or anesthesia.

INTERVENTIONS: *Providing Pain Relief*

- Monitor vital signs, observe for signs of pain, and have patient rate pain on a scale of 0 to 10 *to provide baseline for comparison.*
- Encourage patient to void every 1 to 2 hours *to decrease pressure from a full bladder.*
- Assist patient in changing positions frequently *to increase comfort and promote labor progress.*
- Encourage use of distraction *to reduce focus on contraction pain.*
- Suggest pelvic rocking, massage, or back counterpressure *to reduce pain.*
- Assist with use of relaxation and breathing techniques *to promote relaxation.*
- Use touch appropriately (backrub) when desired by the patient *to promote comfort.*
- Integrate use of nonpharmacologic measures for pain relief, such as warm water, birthing ball, or other techniques *to facilitate pain relief.*
- Administer pharmacologic agents as ordered when requested *to control pain.*
- Provide reassurance and encouragement between contractions *to foster self-esteem and continued participation in the labor process.*

NURSING ANALYSIS: Infection risk related to multiple vaginal examinations following rupture of membranes and tissue trauma

OUTCOME IDENTIFICATION AND EVALUATION

The patient will remain free of infection as evidenced by the absence of signs and symptoms of infection, vital signs and FHR within acceptable parameters, lab test results within normal limits, and clear amniotic fluid without odor.

INTERVENTIONS: *Preventing Infection*

- Monitor vital signs (every 2 hours after rupture of membranes) and FHR frequently as per protocol *to allow for early detection of problems*; report fetal tachycardia (early sign of maternal infection) *to ensure prompt treatment.*
- Provide frequent perineal care and pad changes *to maintain good perineal hygiene.*
- Change linens and patient's gown as needed *to maintain cleanliness.*
- Ensure that vaginal examinations are performed only when needed *to prevent introducing pathogens into the vaginal vault.*
- Monitor lab test results such as white blood cell count *to assess for elevations indicating infection.*
- Encourage the patient to empty her bladder at least every 2 hours *to not impede fetal descent.*
- Use aseptic technique for all invasive procedures *to prevent infection transmission.*
- Carry out good handwashing techniques before and after procedures and use standard precautions as appropriate *to minimize risk of infection transmission.*
- Document amniotic fluid characteristics like color and odor *to establish baseline for comparison.*

warm compresses and continual massage with oil have been successful in stretching the perineal area to prevent cutting it. Certified nurse midwives can cut and repair episiotomies, but they frequently use alternative measures if possible.

TAKE NOTE!

Restrictive use of episiotomy has been recommended by the ACOG and the WHO given the risks of the procedure, unclear benefits of routine use, and lack of defining criteria for its use (Berkowitz & Foust-Wright, 2023).

The midline episiotomy has been the most commonly used one in the United States because it can be easily repaired and causes the least amount of pain. The application of warmed compresses or intrapartum perineal massage during the pushing phase is associated with a decrease in trauma to the perineal area and reduced need for an episiotomy (Dekker, 2022b). Routine episiotomy has declined since liberal usage has been discouraged by ACOG and WHO except to avoid several maternal lacerations or to expedite difficult births. Anal sphincter laceration rates with spontaneous vaginal delivery have decreased, likely reflecting the decreased usage of episiotomy. The decline in operative vaginal delivery corresponds with a sharp increase in cesarean births, which may indicate that health care providers are favoring cesarean births for difficult births (Bernstein & Coggin-Carr, 2024). Figure 14.14 shows episiotomy locations.

Continuous Assessment During the Second Stage of Labor

Assessment is continuous during the second stage of labor. Hospital policies dictate the specific type and timing of assessments, as well as the way in which they are documented. Assessment involves identifying the signs typical of the second stage of labor, including:

- Increase in apprehension or irritability
- Spontaneous ROM
- Sudden appearance of sweat on upper lip
- Increase in blood-tinged show
- Low grunting sounds from the patient
- Complaints of rectal and perineal pressure
- Beginning of involuntary bearing-down efforts

Other ongoing assessments include the contraction frequency, duration, and intensity; maternal vital signs every 5 to 15 minutes; fetal response to labor as indicated by FHR monitor strips; amniotic fluid for color, odor, and amount when membranes are ruptured; and the coping status of the patient and their partner (Table 14.4).

Assessment also focuses on determining the progress of labor. Associated signs include bulging of the perineum, labial separation, advancing and retreating of the newborn's head during and between bearing-down efforts, and **crowning** (fetal head is visible at vaginal opening; Fig. 14.15).

A vaginal examination is completed to determine if it is appropriate for the patient to push. Pushing is appropriate if the cervix has fully dilated to 10 cm and the patient feels the urge to do so.

Nursing Interventions

Nursing interventions during this stage focus on motivating the patient, assisting them with positioning, encouraging them to put all their efforts to pushing this newborn to the outside world, and giving feedback on their progress. If the patient is pushing without progress, suggest that they keep their eyes open during the contractions and look toward where the newborn is coming out. Changing positions frequently will also help them

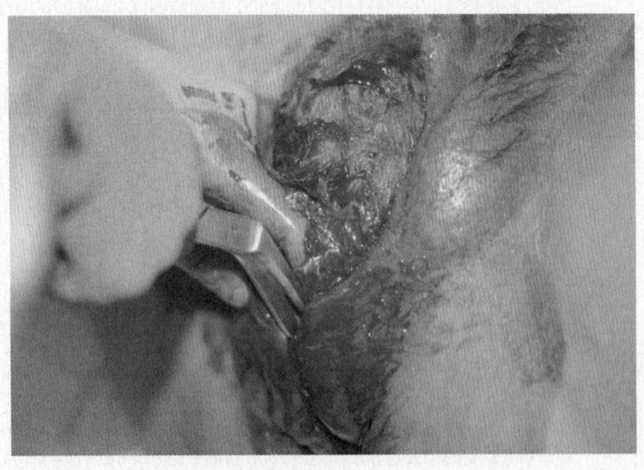

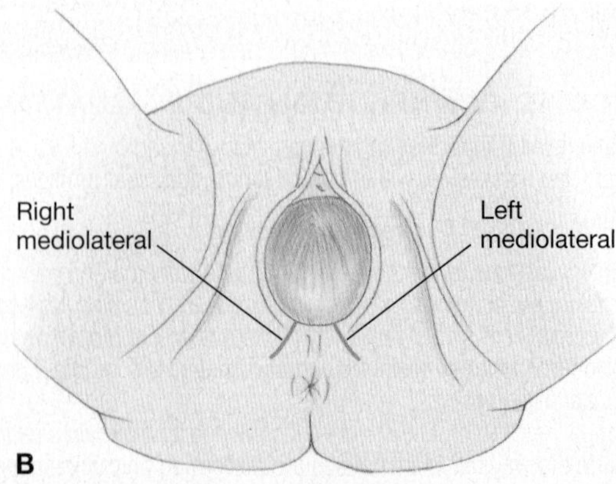

FIGURE 14.14 Location of an episiotomy. **A.** Midline episiotomy. **B.** Right and left mediolateral episiotomies.

TABLE 14.4 • Summary of Assessments During the Second, Third, and Fourth Stages of Labor

Assessments[a]	Second Stage of Labor (Birth of Neonate)	Third Stage of Labor (Placenta Expulsion)	Fourth Stage of Labor (Recovery)
Vital signs (BP, pulse, respirations)	Every 5–15 minutes	Every 15 minutes	Every 15 minutes
Fetal heart rate	Every 5–15 minutes by Doppler or continuously by EFM	Apgar scoring at 1 and 5 minutes	Newborn—complete head-to-toe assessment; vital signs every 15 minutes until stable
Contractions/uterus	Palpate every one	Observe for placental separation	Palpating for firmness and position every 15 minutes for first hour
Bearing down/ pushing	Assist with every effort	None	None
Vaginal discharge	Observe for signs of descent—bulging of perineum, crowning.	Assess bleeding after expulsion	Assess every 15 minutes with fundus firmness
Behavior/ psychosocial	Observe every 15 minutes: co-operative, focus is on work of pushing newborn out.	Observe every 15 minutes: often feelings of relief after hearing newborn crying; calmer.	Observe every 15 minutes: usually excited, talkative, awake; needs to hold newborn, be close, and inspect body.

BP, blood pressure; EFM, electronic fetal monitoring.
[a]The frequency of assessments is dictated by the health status of the person in labor and fetus and can be altered if either one of their conditions changes.Gimovsky, A. C., & Berghella, V. (2022). Evidence-based labor management: Second stage of labor (part 4). *American Journal of Obstetrics & Gynecology: Maternal Fetal Medicine*, *4*(2), 100548. https://doi.org/10.1016/j.ajogmf.2021.100548; Lothian, J. (2024). Normal childbirth. In B. J. Baker, J. Janke, & Association of Women's Health, Obstetric and Neonatal Nurses, *Core curriculum for maternal-newborn nursing* (6th ed.). Elsevier.

make progress. Positioning a mirror so the patient can visualize the birthing process and how successful their pushing efforts are can help motivate them.

During the second stage of labor, an ideal position would be one that opens the pelvic outlet as wide as possible, provides a smooth pathway for the fetus to descend through the birth canal, takes advantage of gravity to assist the fetus to descend, and gives them a sense of being safe and in control of the labor process (Jyoti et al., 2022). Some suggestions for positions in the second stage include:

- Lithotomy with feet up in stirrups: Most convenient position for caregivers, though evidence does not support this position physiologically
- Semi-sitting with pillows underneath knees, arms, and back
- Lateral/side-lying with curved back and upper leg supported by partner
- Sitting on birthing stool: Opens pelvis, enhances the pull of gravity, and helps with pushing
- Squatting/supported squatting: Gives the laboring person a sense of control
- Using a peanut ball between the legs to widen the pelvic diameter
- Kneeling with hands on bed and knees comfortably apart

Other important nursing interventions during the second stage include:

- Providing continuous comfort measures such as mouth care, encouraging position changes, changing bed linen and underpads, and providing a quiet, focused environment

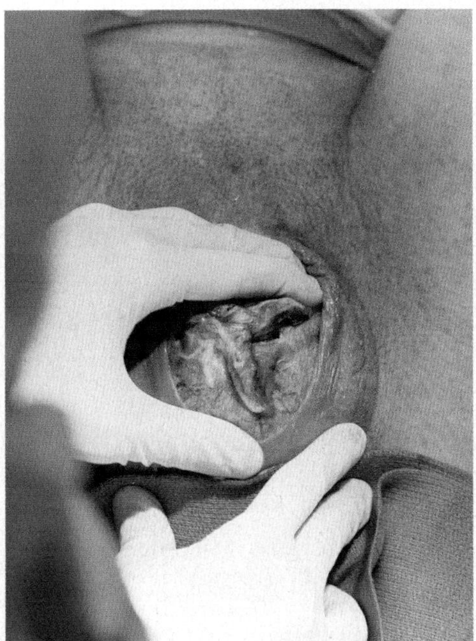

FIGURE 14.15 Crowning.

- Instructing the patient on the following bearing-down positions and techniques:
  - Pushing only when they feel an urge to do so
  - Delaying pushing for up to 90 minutes after complete dilation
  - Using abdominal muscles when bearing down
  - Using short pushes of 6 to 7 seconds
  - Focusing attention on the perineal area to visualize the newborn
  - Relaxing and conserving energy between contractions
  - Pushing several times with each contraction
  - Pushing with an open glottis and slight exhalation (Lothian, 2024)
- Continuing to monitor contractions and FHR patterns to identify problems
- Providing brief, explicit directions throughout this stage
- Continuing to provide psychosocial support by reassuring and coaching
- Facilitating the upright position to encourage the fetus to descend
- Continuing to assess blood pressure, pulse, respirations, uterine contractions, bearing-down efforts, FHR, and coping status of the patient and their partner
- Providing pain management if needed
- Providing a continuous nursing presence
- Offering praise for the patient's efforts
- Preparing for and assisting with delivery by:
  - Notifying the health care provider of the estimated time frame for birth
  - Preparing the delivery bed and positioning the patient
  - Preparing the perineal area according to the facility's protocol
  - Offering a mirror and adjusting it so the patient can watch the birth
  - Explaining all procedures and equipment to the patient and their partner
  - Setting up delivery instruments needed while maintaining sterility
  - Using standard precautions during the birthing process to avoid body fluid splashes
  - Recording the time of birth, time of placenta, and type of birth
  - Receiving the newborn and transporting them to a warming environment, or covering the newborn with a warmed blanket on their abdomen
  - Providing initial care and assessment of the newborn (see the "Birth" section that follows)

Sheila is completely dilated now and experiencing the urge to push. How can the nurse help Sheila with her pushing efforts? What additional interventions can the labor nurse offer Sheila now? In addition to encouraging Sheila to rest between pushing and offering praise for her efforts, what is the nurse's role during the birthing process?

BIRTH

The second stage of labor ends with the birth of the newborn. The maternal position for birth varies from the standard lithotomy position to side-lying to squatting to standing or kneeling depending on the birthing location, the patient's preference, and standard protocols. Once the patient is positioned for birth, cleanse the vulva and perineal areas. The primary health care provider then takes charge after donning protective eyewear, masks, gowns, and gloves and performing hand hygiene.

Once the fetal head has emerged, the primary care provider explores the fetal neck to see if the umbilical cord is wrapped around it. If it is, the cord is slipped over the head to facilitate delivery. As soon as the head emerges, the health care provider suctions the newborn's mouth first (because the newborn is an obligate nose breather) and then the nares with a bulb syringe to prevent aspiration of mucus, amniotic fluid, or meconium (Fig. 14.16). The umbilical cord is double-clamped and cut between the clamps by the birth attendant or the patient's partner if desired. With the first cries of the newborn, the second stage of labor ends. For care of the patient undergoing a surgical birth, see Chapter 21.

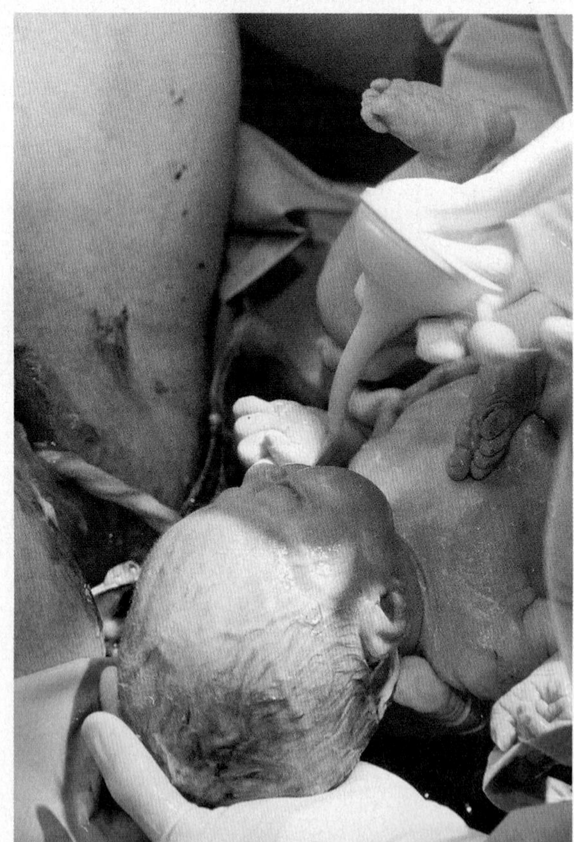

FIGURE 14.16 Suctioning the newborn immediately after birth.

IMMEDIATE CARE OF THE NEWBORN

Once birth takes place, the newborn is placed under a radiant warmer, dried, assessed, wrapped in warmed blankets, and placed on the birthing parent's abdomen for warmth and closeness. In some health care facilities, the newborn is placed on the birthing parent's abdomen immediately after birth and covered with a warmed blanket without being dried or assessed. In either scenario, the stability of the newborn dictates the location of aftercare. The nurse can also assist the patient with breastfeeding their newborn for the first time. All nurses that assist in the childbirth should be trained in the neonatal resuscitation guidelines, the use of equipment needed to carry it out, and the Apgar scoring system for evaluating the newborn (WHO, 2022b).

Assessment of the newborn begins at the moment of birth and continues until the newborn is discharged. Drying the newborn and providing warmth to prevent heat loss by evaporation is essential to help support thermoregulation and provide stimulation. Placing the newborn under a radiant heat source and putting on a cap will further reduce heat loss after drying.

Assess the newborn by assigning an Apgar (appearance, pulse, grimace, activity, and respiration) score at 1 and 5 minutes. The Apgar score assesses five parameters—(1) heart rate (absent, slow, or fast), (2) respiratory effort (absent, weak cry, or good strong yell), (3) muscle tone (limp, or lively and active), (4) response to irritation stimulus, and (5) color—that evaluate a newborn's cardiorespiratory adaptation after birth. The parameters are arranged from the most important (heart rate) to the least important (color). The newborn is assigned a score of 0 to 2 in each of the five parameters. The purpose of the Apgar assessment is to evaluate the physiologic status of the newborn; see Chapter 18 for additional information on Apgar scoring.

Secure two identification bands on the newborn's wrist and ankle that match the band on the birthing parent's wrist to ensure the newborn's identity. This identification process is completed in the birthing suite before anyone leaves the room. Some health care agencies also take an early photo of the newborn for identification in the event of abduction (National Center for Missing and Exploited Children [NCMEC], 2024).

Other types of newborn security systems can also be used to prevent abduction. Some systems have sensors that are attached to the newborn's identification bracelet or cord clamp. An alarm is set off if the bracelet or clamp activates receivers near exits. Others have an alarm that is activated when the sensor is removed from the newborn (Fig. 14.17). Even with the use of electronic sensors, the parents, nursing staff, and security personnel are responsible for prevention strategies and ensuring the safety and protection of all newborns (NCMEC, 2024). Nurses can help prevent newborn abduction by educating parents about abduction risks, using identically numbered bands on the baby and parents, instructing parents to keep their newborn in their direct line of vision within their hospital room at all times, taking color photographs of the infant, wearing color photograph ID badges themselves, discouraging parents and families from publishing birth notices in the public media with the birthing parent's name and address, controlling access to the nursery or postpartum unit with locked doors, and utilizing infant security tags or abduction alarm systems (NCMEC, 2024).

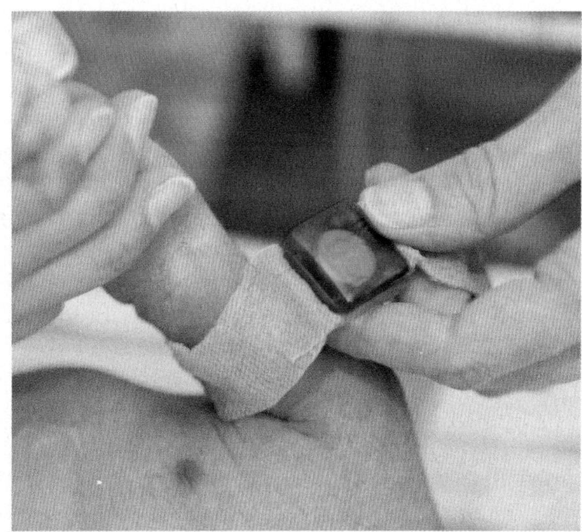

FIGURE 14.17 An example of a security sensor applied to a newborn's arm.

> Sheila gave birth to a healthy 7-lb, 7-oz baby girl. She is eager to hold and nurse her newborn. What is the initial care of the newborn? How can the nurse meet the needs of both the newborn and Sheila, who is exhausted but eager to bond with her newborn?

Nursing Management During the Third Stage of Labor

During the third stage of labor, strong uterine contractions continue at regular intervals under the continuing influence of oxytocin. The uterine muscle fibers shorten, or retract, with each contraction, leading to a gradual decrease in the size of the uterus, which helps shear the placenta away from its attachment site. The third stage is complete when the placenta is delivered. Nursing care during the third stage of labor primarily focuses on immediate newborn care and assessment and observing for signs of placental separation, being available to assist with the delivery of the placenta, recording the time of expulsion, and inspecting the placenta for intactness.

The nurse should also be assessing the laboring patient by palpating the uterus before and after placental expulsion.

Three hormones play important roles in the third stage. During this stage, the patient experiences peak levels of oxytocin and endorphins, while the high adrenaline levels that occurred during the second stage of labor to aid with pushing begin falling. The hormone oxytocin causes uterine contractions and helps the patient to enact instinctive nurturing behaviors such as holding the newborn close to their body and cuddling the baby.

Skin-to-skin contact immediately after birth and the newborn's first attempt at breastfeeding further augment maternal oxytocin levels, strengthening the uterine contractions that will help the placenta separate and the uterus contract to prevent hemorrhage. Endorphins, the body's natural opiates, produce an altered state of consciousness and aid in blocking out pain. In addition, the drop in adrenaline level from the second stage, which had kept the birthing parent and baby alert at first contact, causes most patients to shiver and feel cold shortly after giving birth.

TAKE NOTE!

A crucial role for nurses during the third stage of labor is to protect the natural hormonal process by ensuring unhurried and uninterrupted contact between birthing parent and newborn after birth, providing warmed blankets to prevent shivering, and allowing skin-to-skin contact with initial breastfeeding.

Continuing Assessment During the Third Stage of Labor

Assessment during the third stage of labor includes:

- Monitoring placental separation by looking for the following signs:
  - Firmly contracting uterus
  - Change in uterine shape from discoid to globular ovoid
  - Sudden gush of dark blood from vaginal opening
  - Lengthening of umbilical cord protruding from vagina
  - Examining placenta and fetal membranes for intactness the second time (the health care provider assesses the placenta for intactness the first time) (Fig. 14.18)
- Assessing for any perineal trauma, such as the following, before allowing the birth attendant to leave:
  - Firm fundus with bright red blood trickling: laceration
  - Boggy fundus with red blood flowing: uterine atony
  - Boggy fundus with dark blood and clots: retained placenta
  - Inspecting the perineum for condition of episiotomy if performed
  - Assessing for perineal lacerations and ensuring repair by birth attendant

Nursing Interventions

Interventions during the third stage of labor include:

- Describing the process of placental separation to the patient and support partner
- Instructing the patient to push when signs of separation are apparent
- Administering an oxytocic agent if ordered and indicated after placental expulsion (Berghella, 2023)
- Providing support and information about episiotomy or laceration if applicable
- Explaining what assessments will be carried out over the next hour and offering positive reinforcement for actions
- Cleaning and assisting the patient into a comfortable position after birth, making sure to lift both legs out of stirrups (if used) simultaneously to prevent strain
- Monitoring maternal physical status by assessing:

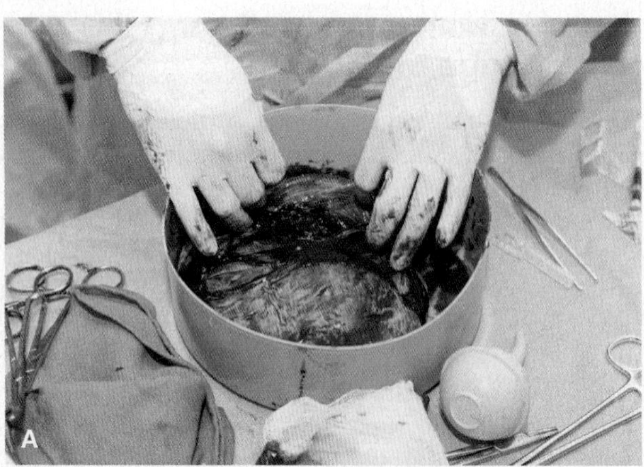

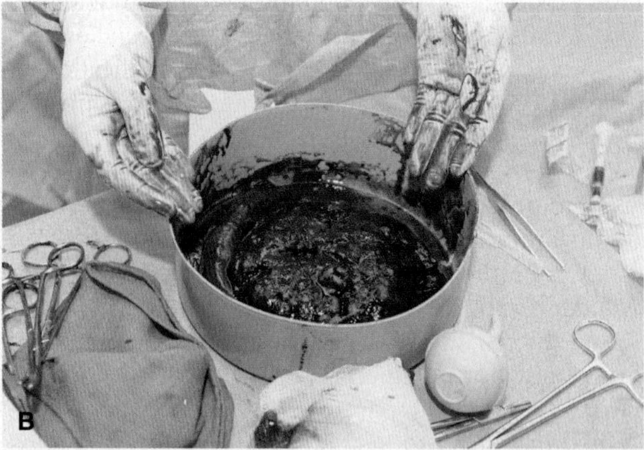

FIGURE 14.18 Placenta. **A.** Fetal side. **B.** Maternal side.

- Vaginal bleeding: amount, consistency, and color
- Vital signs: blood pressure, pulse, and respirations taken every 15 minutes
- Uterine fundus, which should be firm, in the midline, and at the level of the umbilicus

- Providing warmth by replacing warmed blankets over the patient
- Applying an ice pack to the perineal area to provide comfort to episiotomy if indicated
- Assessing the patient's knowledge of breastfeeding to determine educational needs
- Educating the patient about latching on, positioning, infant sucking and swallowing
- Repositioning the birthing bed to serve as a recovery bed if applicable
- Assisting with transfer to the recovery area if applicable
- Ascertaining any needs
- Recording all birthing statistics and securing primary caregiver's signature
- Documenting birthing event in the birth book (official record of the facility that outlines every birth event), detailing any deviations

Nursing Management During the Fourth Stage of Labor

The fourth stage of labor begins after the placenta is expelled and lasts up to 4 hours after birth, during which time recovery takes place. This recovery period may take place in the same room where the patient gave birth, in a separate recovery area, or in the postpartum room. During this stage, the patient's body is beginning to undergo the many physiologic and psychological changes that occur after birth. The focus of nursing management during the fourth stage of labor involves frequent close observation for hemorrhage, provision of comfort measures, and promotion of family attachment.

Assessment

Assessments during the fourth stage center on the patient's vital signs, status of the uterine fundus and perineal area, comfort level, lochia amount, and bladder status. During the first hour after birth, vital signs are taken every 15 minutes, then every 30 minutes for the next hour if needed. The patient's blood pressure should remain stable and within normal range after giving birth. A decrease may indicate uterine hemorrhage; an elevation might suggest preeclampsia.

The pulse is usually typically slower (60 to 70 bpm) than during labor. This may be associated with a decrease in blood volume following placental separation. An elevated pulse rate may be an early sign of blood loss. The blood pressure usually returns to its prepregnancy level and therefore is not a reliable early indicator of shock. Fever is indicative of dehydration (less than 100.4°F or 38°C) or infection (above 101°F [38.33°C]), which may involve the genitourinary tract. Respiratory rate is usually between 16 and 24 breaths per minute and regular. Respirations should be unlabored unless there is an underlying preexisting respiratory condition.

Assess fundal height, position, and firmness every 15 minutes during the first hour following birth. The fundus needs to remain firm to prevent excessive postpartum bleeding. The fundus should be firm (feels like the size and consistency of a grapefruit), located in the midline and below the umbilicus. If it is not firm (boggy), gently massage it until it is firm (see Nursing Procedure 22.1 for more information). Once firmness is obtained, stop massaging. Assess vaginal discharge (lochia) every 15 minutes for the first hour and every 30 minutes for the next hour. Palpate the fundus at the same time to ascertain its firmness and help estimate the amount of vaginal discharge.

TAKE NOTE!

If the fundus is displaced to the right of the midline, suspect a full bladder as the cause.

The vagina and perineal areas are quite stretched and edematous following a vaginal birth. Assess the perineum including the episiotomy if present for possible hematoma formation. Suspect a hematoma if the patient reports excruciating pain or cannot void or if a mass is noted in the perineal area. Also assess for hemorrhoids, which can cause discomfort.

Assess the patient's comfort level frequently to determine the need for analgesia. Ask the patient to rate their pain on a scale of 1 to 10; it should be less than 3. If it is higher, further evaluation is needed to make sure there aren't any deviations contributing to the discomfort.

Palpate the bladder for fullness, since many patients receiving an epidural block experience limited sensation in the bladder region. Voiding should produce large amounts of urine (diuresis) each time. Palpating the bladder after each voiding helps in assessing it and ensuring complete emptying. A full bladder will displace the uterus to either side of the midline and potentiate uterine hemorrhage secondary to bogginess.

Nursing Interventions

Nursing interventions during the fourth stage might include:

- Providing support and information to the patient regarding episiotomy repair and related pain relief and self-care measures
- Applying an ice pack to the perineum to promote comfort and reduce swelling

- Assisting with hygiene and perineal care; teaching the patient how to use the perineal bottle after each pad change and voiding; helping the patient into a new gown
- Monitoring for return of sensation and ability to void (if regional anesthesia was used)
- Encouraging the patient to void by ambulating to the bathroom, listening to running water, or pouring warm water over the perineal area with the peri bottle
- Monitoring vital signs and fundal and lochia status every 15 minutes and documenting them
- Assessing for postpartum hemorrhage and urinary retention via uterine palpation
- Promoting comfort by offering analgesia for afterpains and warm blankets to reduce chilling
- Offering fluids and nourishment if desired
- Encouraging parent–infant attachment by providing privacy for the family
- Being knowledgeable about and sensitive to typical cultural practices after birth
- Assisting and encouraging the patient to nurse, if they choose, during the recovery period to promote uterine firmness (the release of oxytocin from the posterior pituitary gland stimulates uterine contractions)
- Teaching the patient how to assess the fundus for firmness periodically and to massage it if it is boggy
- Describing the lochia flow and normal parameters to observe for postpartum
- Teaching safety techniques to prevent newborn abduction
- Demonstrating the use of the portable sitz bath as a comfort measure for the perineum if the patient had a laceration or an episiotomy repair
- Explaining comfort and hygiene measures and when to use them
- Assisting with ambulation when getting out of bed for the first time
- Providing information about the routine on the mother–baby unit or nursery during the stay
- Observing for signs of early parent–infant attachment: fingertip touch to palm touch to enfolding of the infant (Berens, 2024; Lothian, 2024)

The nurse's role in labor and birth is a privileged one, supporting patients during one of their most vulnerable times—childbirth. The nurse's focus during this time should be on supporting, protecting, advocating for, and empowering patients. Nurses plan and provide excellence in care of people in childbirth with their agreement and input. They provide informational support, which allows the patient to realize their aspirations and goals by making decisions through informed choice. Nurses make a long-term difference in the lives of childbearing people with small things they do for their patients that can make a big difference.

KEY CONCEPTS

- A nurse provides physical and emotional support during the labor and birth process to assist a patient in achieving their goals.
- When a laboring person is admitted to the labor and birth area, the admitting nurse must assess and evaluate the risk status of the pregnancy and initiate appropriate interventions to provide optimal care for the patient.
- Completing an admission assessment includes taking a maternal health history; performing a physical assessment on the patient and fetus, including their emotional and psychosocial status; and obtaining the necessary laboratory studies.
- The nurse's role in fetal assessment for labor and birth includes determining fetal well-being and interpreting signs and symptoms of possible compromise. Determining the FHR pattern and assessing amniotic fluid characteristics are key.
- FHR can be assessed intermittently or continuously. Although the intermittent method allows the patient to move around during labor, the information obtained intermittently does not provide a complete picture of fetal well-being from moment to moment.
- Assessment parameters of the FHR are classified as baseline rate, baseline variability, and periodic changes in the rate (accelerations and decelerations).
- The nurse monitoring the laboring patient needs to be knowledgeable about which category the FHR pattern is in so that appropriate interventions can be instituted.
- For a category III FHR pattern, the nurse should notify the health care provider about the pattern and obtain further orders, making sure to document all interventions and their effects on the FHR pattern.
- In addition to interpreting assessment findings and initiating appropriate inventions for the laboring patient, accurate and timely documentation must be carried out continuously.
- Today, laboring patients have many safe nonpharmacologic and pharmacologic choices for the management of pain during childbirth. They may be used individually or in combination to complement one another.
- Nursing management for the patient during labor and birth includes comfort measures, emotional support, information and instruction, advocacy, and support for the partner.
- Nursing care during the first stage of labor includes taking an admission history (reviewing the prenatal record), checking the results of routine laboratory work and special tests done during pregnancy, asking the patient about their childbirth preparation

(birth plan, classes taken, coping skills), and completing a physical assessment of the patient to establish baseline values for future comparison.

- Nursing care during the second stage of labor focuses on supporting the patient and their partner in making decisions about the patient's care and labor management, implementing strategies to prolong the early passive phase of fetal descent, supporting involuntary bearing-down efforts, providing support and assistance, and encouraging the use of maternal positions that can enhance descent and reduce the pain.
- Nursing care during the third stage of labor primarily focuses on immediate newborn care and assessment and being available to assist with the delivery of the placenta and inspecting it for intactness.
- The focus of nursing management during the fourth stage of labor involves frequently observing the patient for hemorrhage, providing comfort measures, and promoting family attachment.

Unfolding Patient Stories: Fatime Sanogo • Part 2

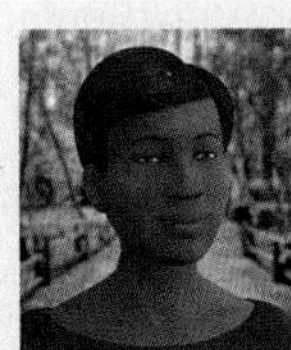

Recall Fatime Sanogo, the primiparous 23-year-old you met in Chapter 2. Fatime is now at 41 4/7 weeks' gestation and admitted to the hospital for induction of labor. What physical findings should be present before labor is induced? What nursing assessments are performed and what nursing interventions are implemented to safely manage induction of labor with an oxytocin infusion? What assessment data should be documented when artificial ROM is performed?

Care for Fatime and other patients in a realistic virtual environment: ***vSim** for Nursing* (**thepoint.lww.com/vSimMaternity**). Practice documenting these patients' care in DocuCare (**thepoint.lww.com/DocuCareEHR**).

Unfolding Patient Stories: Carla Hernandez • Part 2

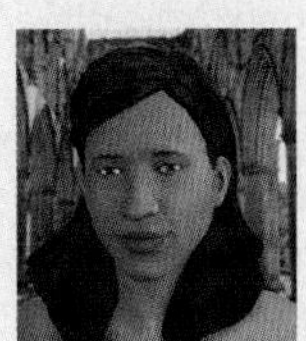

Recall Carla Hernandez from Chapter 4. She is at 39 5/7 weeks' gestation when her husband brings her to the hospital. How does the nurse determine that she is in active labor? If she is in active labor, how will the nurse monitor the progress of labor? What nursing assessments are done to identify the signs of potential complications during labor? What questions would the nurse ask Carla to identify symptoms of potential complications of labor? What nursing interventions can assist the couple's ability to cope with pain and stress experienced during labor?

Care for Carla and other patients in a realistic virtual environment: ***vSim** for Nursing* (**thepoint.lww.com/vSimMaternity**). Practice documenting these patients' care in DocuCare (**thepoint.lww.com/DocuCareEHR**).

REFERENCES AND RECOMMENDED READINGS

Ahmadi, S., Farahani, K., Aklamli, M., Ahmadi, K., & Beheshti, N. (2022). Spinal anesthesia in labor on maternal and neonatal outcomes: A retrospective cross-sectional study. *Journal of Obstetrics, Gynecology and Cancer Research, 7*(3), 186–191. https://doi.org/10.30699/jogcr.7.3.186

American College of Obstetricians and Gynecologists. (2021a). *Approaches to limit intervention during labor and birth, committee opinion number 766 (reaffirmed 2021).* https://www.acog.org/clinical/clinical-guidance/committee-opinion/articles/2019/02/approaches-to-limit-intervention-during-labor-and-birth

American College of Obstetricians and Gynecologists. (2021b). *Effective patient–physician communication, committee opinion number 587 (reaffirmed 2021).* https://www.acog.org/clinical/clinical-guidance/committee-opinion/articles/2014/02/effective-patient-physician-communication

American College of Obstetricians and Gynecologists. (2022). *Prevention of group B streptococcal early-onset disease in newborns, committee opinion number 797 (reaffirmed 2022).* https://www.acog.org/clinical/clinical-guidance/committee-opinion/articles/2020/02/prevention-of-group-b-streptococcal-early-onset-disease-in-newborns

American College of Obstetricians and Gynecologists. (2023). *Oxygen supplementation in the setting of category II or III fetal heart tracings, practice advisory (reaffirmed 2023).* https://www.acog.org/clinical/clinical-guidance/practice-advisory/articles/2022/01/oxygen-supplementation-in-the-setting-of-category-ii-or-iii-fetal-heart-tracings

American College of Obstetricians and Gynecologists. (2024). *Labor and delivery management of women with human immunodeficiency virus infection, committee opinion number 791 (reaffirmed 2024).* https://www.acog.org/clinical/clinical-guidance/committee-opinion/articles/2018/09/labor-and-delivery-management-of-women-with-human-immunodeficiency-virus-infection

American Pregnancy Association. (2024). *Patterned breathing during labor.* https://americanpregnancy.org/healthy-pregnancy/labor-and-birth/patterned-breathing/

Amru, D. E., Umiyah, A., Yastirin, P. A., Susanti, N. Y., & Ningsih, D. A. (2021). Effect of deep breathing techniques on intensity of labor pain in the active phase. *The International Journal of Social Sciences World, 3*(2), 359–364. https://doi.org/10.5281/zenodo.5808532

Association of Women's Health, Obstetric, and Neonatal Nurses. (2022). Antepartum and intrapartum fetal heart monitoring: Clinical competencies and education guide (7th ed.). *Journal of Obstetric, Gynecologic, and Neonatal Nursing, 51*(3), E1–E9. https://doi.org/10.1016/j.jogn.2022.01.004

Aubin, S. L., & El-Chaâr, D. (2023). Fetal surveillance during labor. In G. Posner, A. Black, G. Jones, & J. Dy, *Oxorn-Foote human labor and birth* (7th ed.). McGraw Hill

Beke, A. (2022). Effect of new peripudendal block (PPB) in the second stage of labor on perineal relaxation and on the reduction of episiotomy rate: A randomized control trial. *Obstetrics and Gynecology International, 2022*, 9352540. https://doi.org/10.1155/2022/9352540

Berens, P. (2024). Overview of the postpartum period: Normal physiology and routine maternal care. *UpToDate.* Retrieved March 9, 2024, from https://www.uptodate.com/contents/overview-of-the-postpartum-period-normal-physiology-and-routine-maternal-care

Berghella, V. (2023). Management of the third stage of labor: Prophylactic pharmacotherapy to minimize hemorrhage. *UpToDate.* https://www.uptodate.com/contents/management-of-the-third-stage-of-labor-prophylactic-pharmacotherapy-to-minimize-hemorrhage

Berkowitz, L. R., & Foust-Wright, C. E. (2023). Approach to episiotomy. *UpToDate.* Retrieved March 9, 2024, from https://www.uptodate.com/contents/approach-to-episiotomy

Bernstein, I. M., & Coggin-Carr, D. (2024). Assisted (operative) vaginal birth. *UpToDate.* Retrieved March 9, 2024, from https://www.uptodate.com/contents/assisted-operative-vaginal-birth

Caughey, A. B., & Tilden, E. (2023). Nonpharmacologic approaches to management of labor pain. *UpToDate.* Retrieved March 9, 2024, from https://www.uptodate.com/contents/nonpharmacologic-approaches-to-management-of-labor-pain

Centers for Disease Control and Prevention. (2023). *HIV basic statistics.* https://www.cdc.gov/hiv/basics/statistics.html

Champagne, K., Fecek, C., & Goldstein, S. (2023). Spinal opioids in anesthetic practice. *StatPearls.* https://www.ncbi.nlm.nih.gov/books/NBK564409/

Choi, J. H., Lee, J., Choi, J. H., & Bishop, M. J. (2020). Epidural naloxone reduces pruritus and nausea without affecting analgesia by epidural morphine in bupivacaine. *Canadian Journal of Anaesthesia, 47*(1), 33–37. https://doi.org/10.1007/BF03020728

Cunningham, F. G., Leveno, K. J., Dashe, J. S., Hoffman, B. L., Spong, C. Y., & Casey, B. M. (2022a). Intrapartum assessment. In F. G. Cunningham, K. J. Leveno, J. S. Dashe, B. L. Hoffman, C. Y. Spong, & B, M. Casey, *William's obstetrics* (26th ed.). McGraw Hill.

Cunningham, F. G., Leveno, K. J., Dashe, J. S., Hoffman, B. L., Spong, C. Y., & Casey, B. M. (2022b). Obstetrical analgesia and anesthesia. In F. G. Cunningham, K. J. Leveno, J. S. Dashe, B. L. Hoffman, C. Y. Spong, & B, M. Casey, *William's obstetrics* (26th ed.). McGraw Hill.

Cunningham, F. G., Leveno, K. J., Dashe, J. S., Hoffman, B. L., Spong, C. Y., & Casey, B. M. (2022c). Infectious diseases. In F. G. Cunningham, K. J. Leveno, J. S. Dashe, B. L. Hoffman, C. Y. Spong, & B. M. Casey, *William's obstetrics* (26th ed.). McGraw Hill.

Cypher, R. L. (2024). Intrapartum fetal assessment. In B. J. Baker, J. Janke, &Association of Women's Health, Obstetric and Neonatal Nurses, *Core curriculum for maternal-newborn nursing* (6th ed.). Elsevier.

Das, S., Obaidullah, S. K., Santosh, K. C., Roy, K., & Kumar, C. (2020). Cardiotocograph-based labor stage classification from uterine contraction pressure during ante-partum and intra-partum period: A fuzzy theoretic approach. *Health Information Science and Systems, 8*(1), 16. https://doi.org/10.1007/s13755-020-00107-7

Dekker, R. (2022a). *The evidence on: Birthing positions.* Evidence-Based Birth. https://evidencebasedbirth.com/evidence-birthing-positions/

Dekker, R. (2022b). *The evidence on perineal massage during labor with Dr. Rebecca Dekker.* Evidence-Based Birth. https://evidencebasedbirth.com/the-evidence-on-perineal-massage-during-labor-with-dr-rebecca-dekker/

Dubey, K. K., Sharma, N., Chawla, D., Khaduja, R., & Jain, S. (2023). Impact of birth companionship on maternal and fetal outcomes in primigravida women in a government tertiary care center. *Cureus, 15,* e38497. https://doi.org/10.7759/cureus.38497

Duff, P. (2023). Preterm prelabor rupture of membranes: Clinical manifestations and diagnosis. *UpToDate.* Retrieved March 7, 2024, from https://www.uptodate.com/contents/preterm-prelabor-rupture-of-membranes-clinical-manifestations-and-diagnosis

Ergin, A., Aşci, Ö., Bal, M. D., Öztürk, G. G., & Karaçam, Z. (2023). The use of hydrotherapy in the first stage of labor: A systematic review and meta-analysis. *International Journal of Nursing Practice, 30,* e13192. https://doi.org/10.1111/ijn.13192

Fitzsimmons, E. D., & Bajaj, T. (2023). *Embryology, amniotic fluid.* StatPearls. https://www.ncbi.nlm.nih.gov/books/NBK541089/

Funai, E. F., & Norwitz, E. R. (2023). Labor and delivery: Management of the normal first stage. *UpToDate.* Retrieved March 7, 2024, from https://www.uptodate.com/contents/labor-and-delivery-management-of-the-normal-first-stage

Funai, E. F., & Norwitz, E. R. (2024). Labor and delivery: Management of the normal second stage. *UpToDate.* Retrieved March 7, 2024, from https://www.uptodate.com/contents/labor-and-delivery-management-of-the-normal-second-stage

Gallant, C. (2023). Obstetric anesthesia and analgesia. In G. Posner, A. Black, G. Jones, & J. Dy, *Oxorn-Foote human labor and birth* (7th ed.). McGraw Hill.

Gjaerum, R., Johansen, I. H., Oian, P., Bernitz, S., & Dalbye, R. (2022). Associations between cervical dilatation on admission and mode of delivery, a cohort study of Norwegian nulliparous women. *Sexual and Reproductive Health, 31,* 100691. https://doi.org/10.1016/j.srhc.2021.100691

Gibb, D., & Arulkumaran, S. (2024). *Fetal monitoring in practice* (5th ed.). Churchill Livingstone.

Gill, P., Henning, J. M., Carlson, K., Van Hook, J. W., & Haddad, L. M. (2023). Abnormal labor (nursing). *StatPearls.* https://www.ncbi.nlm.nih.gov/books/NBK568801/

Gimovsky, A. C., & Berghella, V. (2022). Evidence-based labor management: Second stage of labor (part 4). *American Journal of Obstetrics & Gynecology: Maternal Fetal Medicine, 4*(2), 100548. https://doi.org/10.1016/j.ajogmf.2021.100548

Goswami, S., Jelly, P., Sharma, D. K., Negi, R., & Sharma, R. (2022). The effect of heat therapy on pain intensity, duration of labor during first stage among primiparous women and Apgar scores: A systematic review and meta-analysis. *European Journal of Midwifery, 6*(66). https://doi.org/10.18332/ejm/156487

Grant, G. J. (2023). Adverse effects of neuraxial analgesia and anesthesia for obstetrics. *UpToDate.* Retrieved March 9, 2024, from https://www.uptodate.com/contents/adverse-effects-of-neuraxial-analgesia-and-anesthesia-for-obstetrics

Grant, G. J., & Reale, S. (2024). Pharmacologic management of pain during labor and delivery. *UpToDate.* Retrieved March 9, 2024, from https://www.uptodate.com/contents/pharmacologic-management-of-pain-during-labor-and-delivery

Hankey, L. (2023). Proper documentation protects patients and your license. American Nurse. https://www.myamericannurse.com/proper-documentation-protects-patients-and-your-license/

Hill, N. E., & Granlund, B. (2023). Anesthesia for labor, delivery, and cesarean section in high-risk heart disease. *StatPearls.* https://www.ncbi.nlm.nih.gov/books/NBK574578/

Hurst, H. M., & Baker, B. (2024). Essential forces and factors. In B. J. Baker, J. Janke, &Association of Women's Health, Obstetric and Neonatal Nurses, *Core curriculum for maternal-newborn nursing* (6th ed.). Elsevier.

Issac, A., Nayak, S. G., T, P., Balakrishnan, D., Halemani, K., Mishra, P., P, I., VR, V., Jacob, J., & Stephen, S. (2023). Effectiveness of breathing exercise on the duration of labor: A systematic review and meta-analysis. *Journal of Global Health, 13*, 04023. https://doi.org/10.7189/jogh.13.04023

Ituk, U., & Wong, C. A. (2023). Epidural and combined spinal–epidural anesthesia: Techniques. *UpToDate*. Retrieved March 9, 2024, from https://www.uptodate.com/contents/epidural-and-combined-spinal-epidural-anesthesia-techniques

Jyoti, R., Sharma, M., & Pareek, S. (2022). The effects and outcomes of different maternal positions on the second stage of labor. *Journal of Health Sciences, 10*(2), 21–24. https://doi.org/10.4103/mjhs.mjhs_49_21

Kauffmann, T., & Silberman, M. (2023). Fetal monitoring. *StatPearls*. https://www.ncbi.nlm.nih.gov/books/NBK589699/

Kennedy, M. B., & Devane-Johnson, S. (2024). Perinatal diversity. In B. J. Baker, J. Janke, & Association of Women's Health, Obstetric and Neonatal Nurses, *Core curriculum for maternal-newborn nursing* (6th ed.). Elsevier.

Kirca, A. S., & Gul, D. K. (2022). Effects of acupressure and shower applied in the delivery on the intensity of labor pain and postpartum comfort. *European Journal of Obstetrics & Gynecology and Reproductive Biology, 273*, 98–104. https://doi.org/10.1016/j.ejogrb.2022.04.018

Long, V. E., & McMullen, P. C. (Eds.). (2019). *Telephone triage for obstetrics and gynecology* (3rd ed.). Wolters Kluwer Health.

Lothian, J. (2024). Normal childbirth. In B. J. Baker, J. Janke, & Association of Women's Health, Obstetric and Neonatal Nurses, *Core curriculum for maternal-newborn nursing* (6th ed.). Elsevier.

Loussert, L., Berveiller, P., Magadoux, A., Allouche, M., Vayssiere, C., Garabedian, C, & Guerby, P. (2023). Association between marked fetal heart rate variability and neonatal acidosis: A prospective cohort study. *British Journal of Obstetrics and Gynecology, 130*(4), 407–414. https://doi.org/10.1111/1471-0528.17345

Macones, G. (2023). Intrapartum category I, II, and III fetal heart rate tracings: Management. *UpToDate*. Retrieved March 7, 2024, from https://www.uptodate.com/contents/intrapartum-category-i-ii-and-iii-fetal-heart-rate-tracings-management

Mascarenhas, V. H., Lima, T. R., Silva, F. M., Negreiros, F. S., Santos, J. D., Moura, M. A., Gouveia, M. T., & Jorge, H. M. (2019). Scientific evidence on non-pharmacological methods for relief of labor pain. *Acta Paulista de Enfermagem, 32*(3), 350–357. https://doi.org/10.1590/1982-0194201900048

Mellado-García, E., Díaz-Rodríguez, L., Cortés-Martín, J., Sánchez-García, J. C., Piqueras-Sola, B., Higuero Macías, J. C., & Rodríguez-Blanque, R. (2024). Systematic reviews and synthesis without meta-analysis on hydrotherapy for pain control in labor. *Healthcare, 12*, 373. https://doi.org/10.3390/healthcare12030373

Miller, D. A. (2022). Intrapartum fetal heart rate monitoring: Overview. *UpToDate*. Retrieved March 7, 2024, from https://www.uptodate.com/contents/intrapartum-fetal-heart-rate-monitoring-overview

Moncrief, G., Gyte, G. M. L., Dahlen, H. G., Thomson, G., Singata-Madliki, M., Clegg, A., & Downe, S. (2022). Routine vaginal examinations compared to other methods for assessing progress of labour to improve outcomes for women and babies at term. *Cochrane Database of Systematic Reviews*. https://doi.org/10.1002/14651858.CD010088.pub3

National Center for Missing and Exploited Children. (2024). *Infant abductions*. https://www.missingkids.org/theissues/infantabductions#overview

National Institute for Health and Care Excellence. (2022). *Fetal monitoring in labour, NICE guideline [NG229]*. https://www.nice.org.uk/guidance/indevelopment/gid-ng10174

National Partnership for Women & Families. (2024). *What does research say about labor support?* https://nationalpartnership.org/childbirthconnection/giving-birth/labor-support/research-evidence/

Nichols, J. H., Ali, M., Anetor, J. I., Chen, L. S., Chen, Y., Collins, S., Das, S., Devaraj, S., Fu, L., Karon, B. S., Kary, H., Nerenz, R. D., Rai, A. J., Shajani-Yi, Z., Thakur, V., Wang, S., Yu, H. Y. E., & Zamora, L. E. (2022). AACC guidance document on the use of point-of-care testing in fertility and reproduction. *Journal of Applied Laboratory Medicine, 7*(5), 1202–1236. https://doi.org/10.1093/jalm/jfac042

Nir, O., Gur, D., Galler, E., Axelrod, M., Farhi, A., Barkai, G., Weisz, B., Sivan, E., Shali, S. M., & Tsur, A. (2024). Integrating technologies to provide comprehensive remote fetal surveillance: A prospective pilot study. *International Journal of Gynecology and Obstetrics, 64*(2), 662–667. https://doi.org/10.1002/ijgo.15018

Nixon, H., & Leffert, L. (2023). Anesthesia for cesarean delivery. *UpToDate*. Retrieved March 9, 2024, from https://www.uptodate.com/contents/anesthesia-for-cesarean-delivery

Olofsson, P. (2023). Umbilical cord pH, blood gases, and lactate at birth: normal values, interpretation, and clinical utility. *American Journal of Obstetrics & Gynecology, 228*(5), S1222–S1240. https://doi.org/10.1016/j.ajog.2022.07.001

Panel on Treatment of HIV During Pregnancy and Prevention of Perinatal Transmission. (2024). *Recommendations for the use of antiretroviral drugs during pregnancy and interventions to reduce perinatal HIV transmission in the United States*. https://clinicalinfo.hiv.gov/en/guidelines/perinatal

Park, M. (2022). Asking difficult questions. *American Nurse, 17*(10), 12–17. https://www.myamericannurse.com/asking-difficult-questions/

Pietrzak, J., Medrzycka-Dabrowska, W., Tomaszek, L., & Grzybowska, M. E. (2022). A cross-sectional survey of labor pain control and women's satisfaction. *International Journal of Environmental Research and Public Health, 19*(3), 1741. https://doi.org/10.3390/ijerph19031741

Pouca, M. C. P., Ferreira, J. P. S., Parente, M. P. L., Jorge, R. M. N., & Ashton-Miller, J. A. (2022). On the management of maternal pushing during the second stage of labor: A biomechanical study considering passive tissue fatigue damage accumulation. *American Journal of Obstetrics and Gynecology, 227*(2), 267.e1–267.e20. https://doi.org/10.1016/j.ajog.2022.01.023

Qiagen. (2024). *Amnisure ROM test training video [video]*. https://www.qiagen.com/us/clp/amnisure-rom-test-training-video

Ramar, C. N., & Grimes, W. R. (2023). Perineal lacerations. *StatPearls*. https://www.ncbi.nlm.nih.gov/books/NBK559068/

Reviriego-Rodrigo, E., Ibargoyen-Roteta, N., Carreguí-Vilar, S., Mediavilla-Serrano, L., Uceira-Rey, S., Iglesias-Casás, S., Martín-Casado, A., Toledo-Chávarri, A., Ares-Mateos, G., Montero-Carcaboso, S., Castelló-Zamora, B., Burgos-Alonso, N., Moreno-Rodríguez, A., Hernández-Tejada, N., & Koetsenruyter, C. (2023). Experiences of water immersion during childbirth: a qualitative thematic synthesis.

BMC Pregnancy and Childbirth, *23*(1), 395. https://doi.org/10.1186/s12884-023-05690-7

Ross, M. G., & Beall, M. H. (2023). *Scalp lead placement*. Medscape. https://emedicine.medscape.com/article/1998111-overview

Skelly, C. L., Zulfiqar, H., & Sankararaman, S. (2023). Meconium. *StatPearls*. https://www.ncbi.nlm.nih.gov/books/NBK542240/

Smith, C. A., Collins, C. T., Levett, K. M., Armour, M., Dahlen, H. G., Tan, A. L., & Mesgarpour, B. (2020). Acupuncture or acupressure for pain management during labour. *Cochrane Database of Systematic Reviews*, *2*(2), CD009232. https://doi.org/10.1002/14651858.CD009232.pub2

Spinning Babies. (2024). *Maternal positioning*. https://www.spinningbabies.com/about/maternal-positioning/

Superville, S. S., & Siccardi, M. A. (2023). Leopold maneuvers. *StatPearls*. https://www.ncbi.nlm.nih.gov/books/NBK560814/

Terreri, C. (2023). *Benefits of breathing during pregnancy & birth*. https://www.lamaze.org/Giving-Birth-with-Confidence/GBWC-Post/benefits-of-breathing-during-pregnancy-birth

The Joint Commission. (2022). *New requirements for the advanced certification in perinatal care*. https://www.jointcommission.org/-/media/tjc/documents/standards/prepublications/effective-2023/acpc_prepub_jan2023.pdf

Toledano, R. D., & Leffert, L. (2023). Neuraxial analgesia for labor and delivery (including instrumental delivery). *UpToDate*. Retrieved March 9, 2024, from https://www.uptodate.com/contents/neuraxial-analgesia-for-labor-and-delivery-including-instrumented-delivery

UNC Health/McLendon Clinical Laboratories. (2023). *Amnisure ROM test*. https://www.uncmedicalcenter.org/mclendon-clinical-laboratories/available-tests/amnisure-rom-test/

UpToDate, Inc. (2024). *Lexi-comp® (Version 8.1.0)* [Mobile app]. Wolters Kluwer. https://apps.apple.com/us/app/lexicomp/id313401238

Van de Velde, M. (2022). Combined spinal–epidural analgesia for labor. In R. Fernando, P. Sultan, & S. Phillips (Eds.), *Quick hits in obstetric anesthesia*. Springer Nature. https://doi.org/10.1007/978-3-030-72487-0_2

Van Hal, M., Dydyk, A. M., & Green, M. S. (2023). Acupuncture. *StatPearls*. https://www.ncbi.nlm.nih.gov/books/NBK532287/

Wanyenze, E. W., Byamugisha, J. K., Tumwesigye, N. M., Muwanguzi, P. A., & Nalwadda, G. K. (2022). A qualitative exploratory interview study on birth companion support actions for women during childbirth. *BMC Pregnancy and Childbirth*, *22*(1), https://doi.org/10.1186/s12884-022-04398-4

West, M. (2022). What to know about guided imagery. *Medical News Today*. https://www.medicalnewstoday.com/articles/guided-imagery

World Health Organization. (2018). *WHO recommendations: Intrapartum care for a positive childbirth experience*. https://www.ncbi.nlm.nih.gov/books/NBK513805/

World Health Organization. (2022a). *WHO recommendations on maternal and newborn care for a positive postnatal experience*. https://www.ncbi.nlm.nih.gov/books/NBK579653/

World Health Organization. (2022b). *Early essential newborn care: Clinical practice guide (2nd ed.)*. https://www.who.int/tools/essential-newborn-care-course

World Health Organization. (2024). *Mother-to-child transmission of HIV*. https://www.who.int/teams/global-hiv-hepatitis-and-stis-programmes/hiv/prevention/mother-to-child-transmission-of-hiv

Zang, Y., Lu, H., Zhang, H., Huang, J., Zhao, Y., & Ren, L. (2021). Benefits and risks of upright positions during the second stage of labour: An overview of systematic reviews. *International Journal of Nursing Studies*, *114*, 103812. https://doi.org/10.1016/j.ijnurstu.2020.103812

Zuarez-Easton, S., Erez, O., Zafran, N., Carmeli, J., Garmi, G., & Salim, R. (2023). Pharmacological and non-pharmacological options for pain relief during labor: an expert review. *American Journal of Obstetrics and Gynecology*, *228*(5), S1246–S1259. https://doi.org/10.1016/j.ajog.2023.03.003

DEVELOPING CLINICAL JUDGMENT

PRACTICING FOR NCLEX

1. The nurse is caring for a patient in labor who is fully dilated. Which instruction would be most effective to encourage effective pushing?

a. "Hold your breath and push through the entire contraction."
b. "Use chest breathing with the contraction."
c. "Pant and blow during each contraction."
d. "Wait until you feel the urge to push."

2. During the fourth stage of labor, the nurse assesses the patient at frequent intervals after giving childbirth. What assessment data would cause the nurse the most concern?

a. Moderate amount of dark red lochia drainage on peripad
b. Uterine fundus palpated to the right of the umbilicus
c. An oral temperature reading of 100.6°F (38.11°C)
d. Perineal area bruised and edematous beneath the patient's ice pack

3. The nurse is caring for a laboring patient. What should the nurse take into consideration when managing the patient's pain?

a. Make sure the agents given do not prolong labor.
b. Know that all pain relief measures are similar.
c. Support the patient's decisions and requests.
d. Do not recommend nonpharmacologic methods.

4. The nurse is caring for a patient during the active phase of labor without continuous EFM. How often should the nurse intermittently assess FHR?

a. 15- to 30-minute intervals
b. 5- to 10-minute intervals
c. 45- to 60-minute intervals
d. 60- to 75-minute intervals

5. The nurse notes the presence of transient fetal accelerations on the fetal monitoring strip. Which intervention would be most appropriate?

a. Reposition the patient on the left side.
b. Begin 100% oxygen via face mask.
c. Document this as indicating a normal pattern.
d. Call the health care provider immediately.

6. The nurse is caring for a patient in the second stage of labor. Which assessment indicates the end of the second stage?

a. The cervix is fully dilated and effaced.
b. The placenta is detached and expelled.
c. The fetus is born and on the patient's chest.
d. The patient may request pain medication.

7. The nurse is assisting a patient in a physiologic birth. Which practice would *not* be included?

a. Early induction of labor before 39 weeks' gestation
b. Freedom of movement for the laboring patient
c. Continuous presence and support throughout labor
d. Encouraging spontaneous pushing when urge *is* felt

CRITICAL THINKING EXERCISES

1. A 20-year-old primigravida at term comes to the birthing center in active labor (dilation 7 cm and 80% effaced, −1 station) with ruptured membranes. She states she wants an "all-natural" birth without medication. Her partner is with her and appears anxious but supportive. Upon the admission assessment, this patient's prenatal history is unremarkable; vital signs are within normal limits; FHR via Doppler ranges between 140 and 144 bpm and is regular.

a. Based on your assessment data and the patient's request not to have medication, what nonpharmacologic interventions could you offer her?
b. What positions might be suggested to facilitate fetal descent?

2. Several hours later, the patient complains of nausea and turns to her partner and angrily tells them to not touch her and to go away.

a. What assessment needs to be done to determine what is happening?
b. What explanation can you offer the patient's partner regarding the patient's change in behavior?

STUDY ACTIVITIES

1. Share experiences within a postclinical conference group regarding the pain management interventions of the patients to which you were assigned. Compare and evaluate the effectiveness of different methods used, maternal behavior observed, and neonatal outcome in terms of Apgar scores.

2. On the fetal heart monitor, the nurse notices an elevation of the fetal baseline with the onset of contractions. This elevation would describe ____________.

3. Compare and contrast a local birthing center to a community hospital's birthing suite in terms of the pain management techniques and fetal monitoring used.

4. Select a childbirth website for expectant parents and critique the information provided in terms of its educational level and amount of advertising.

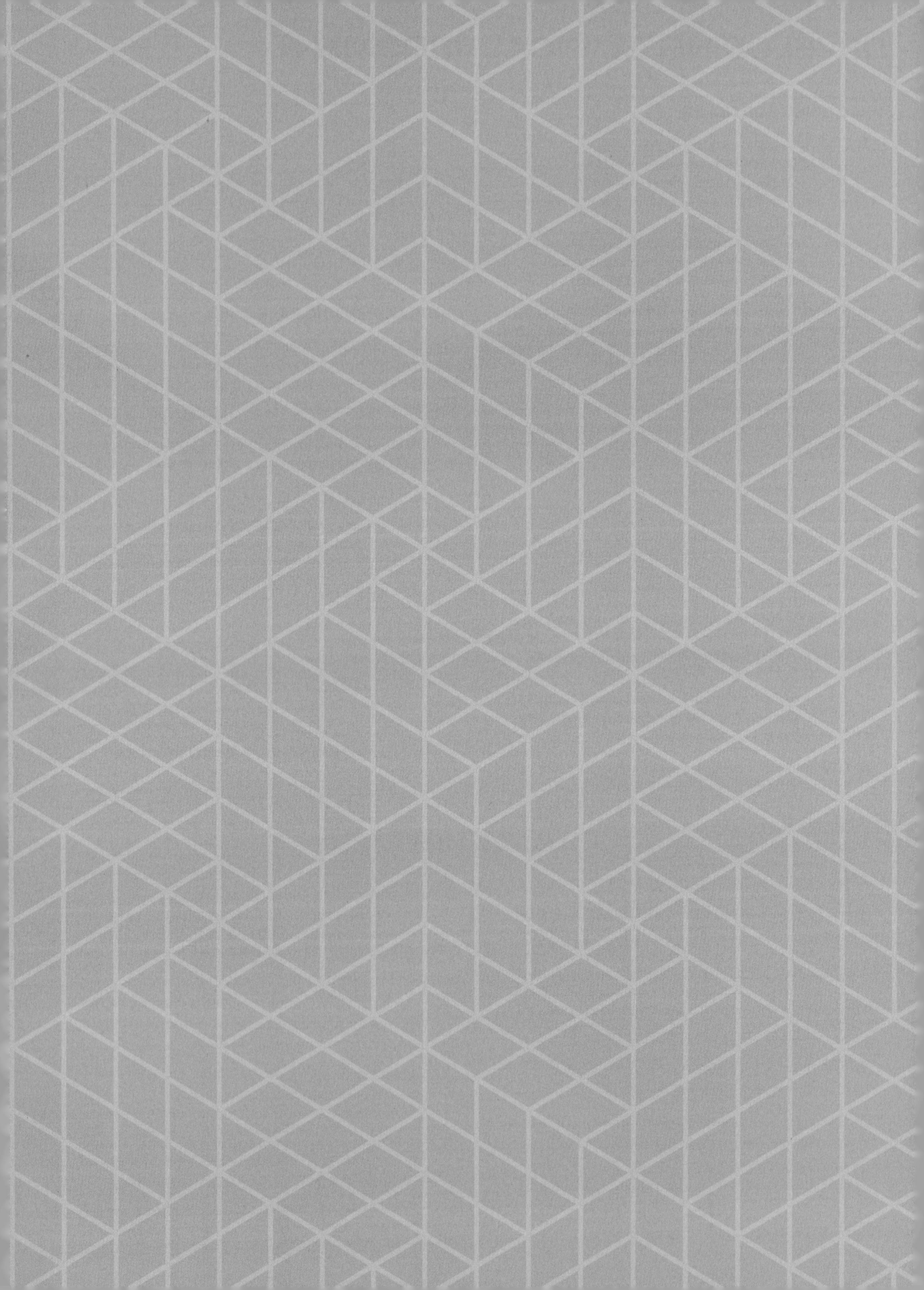

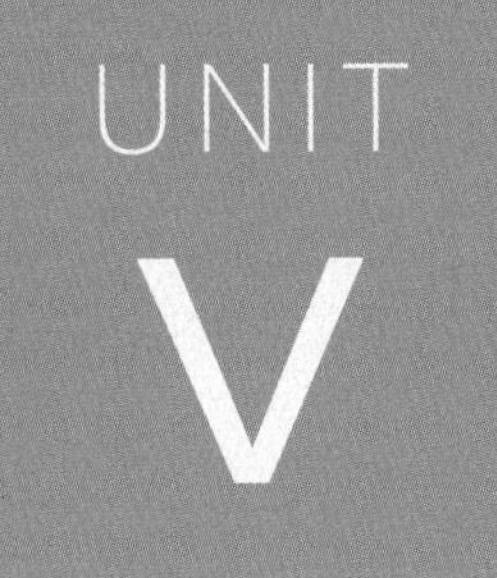

Postpartum Period

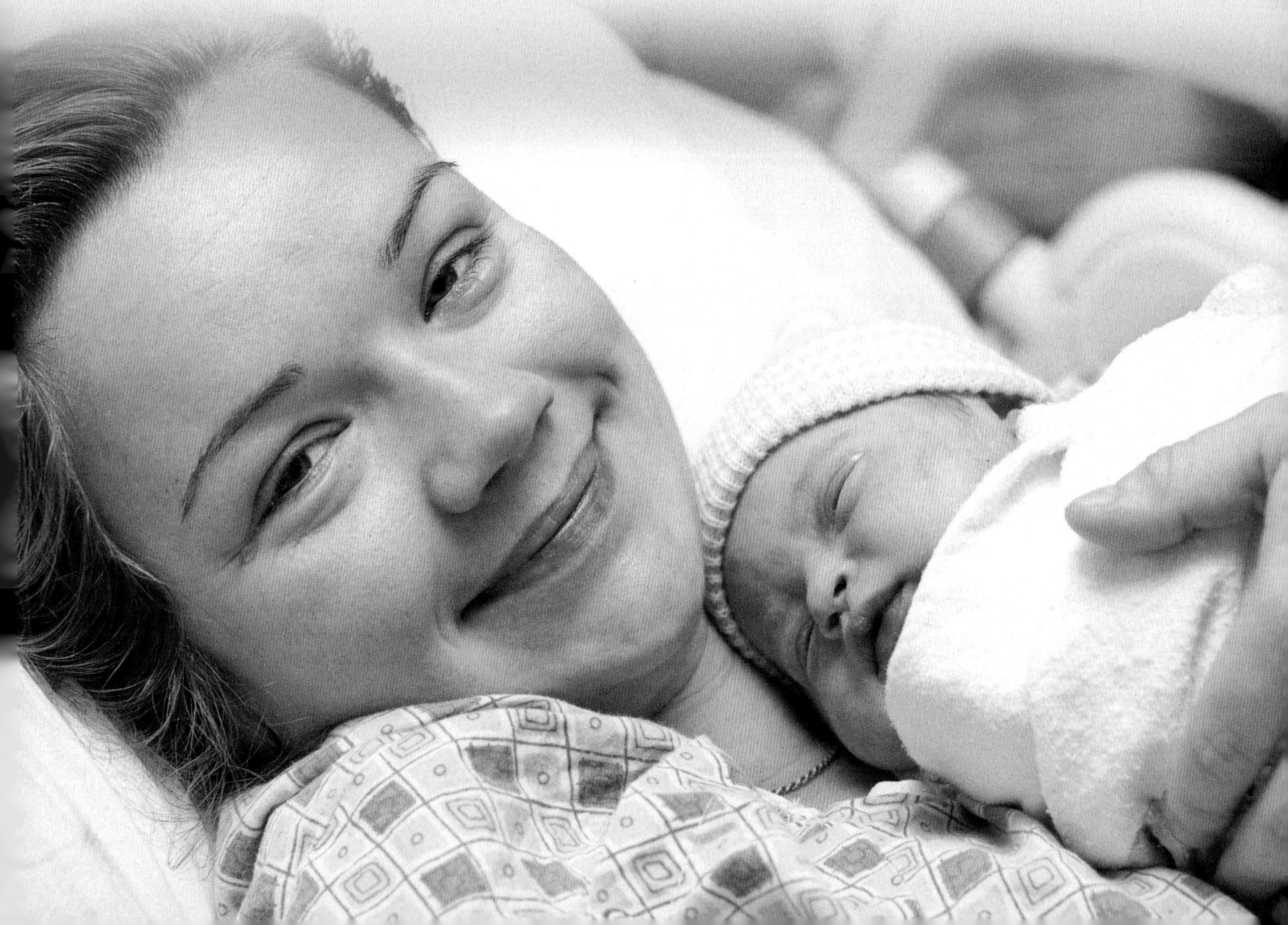

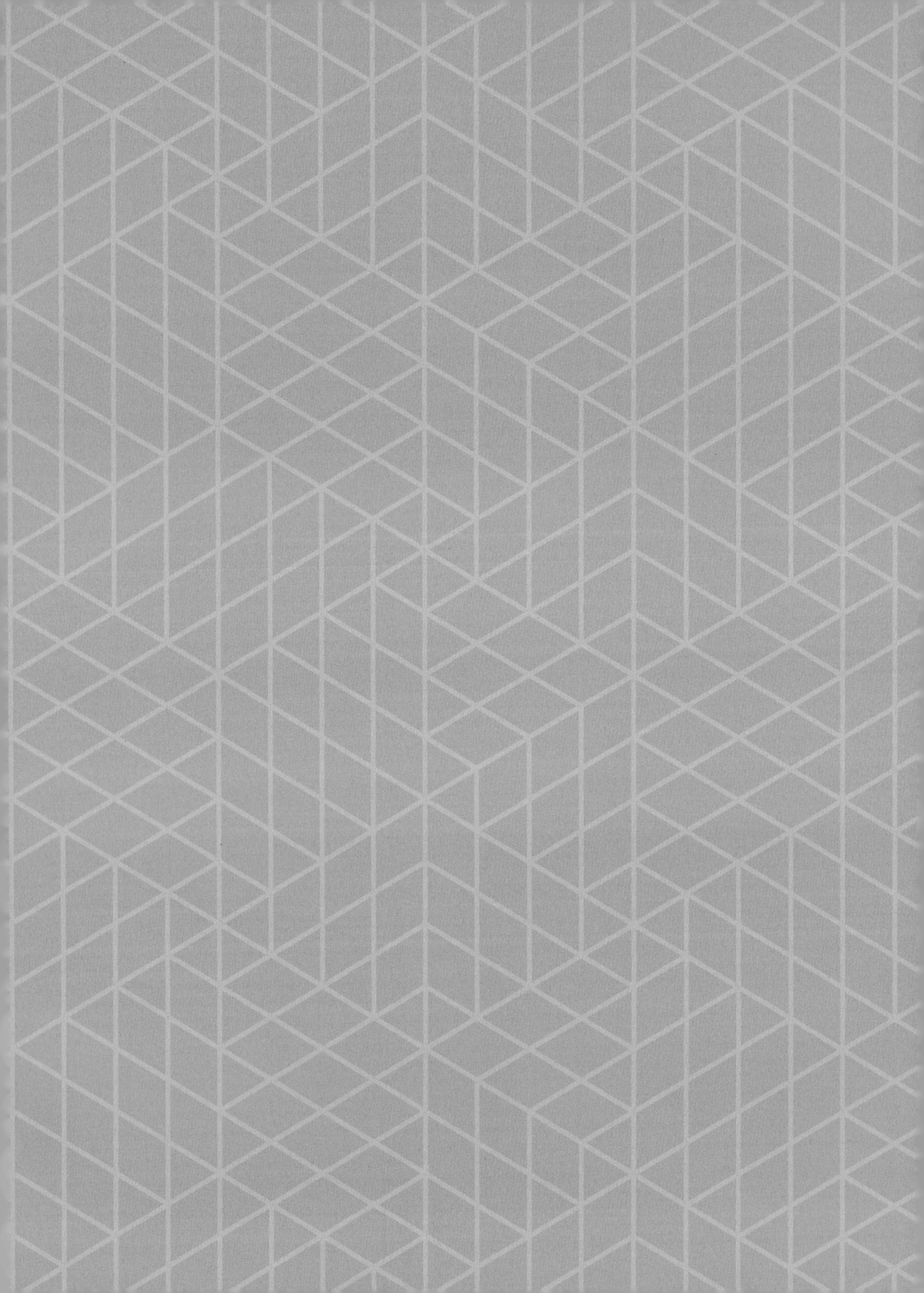

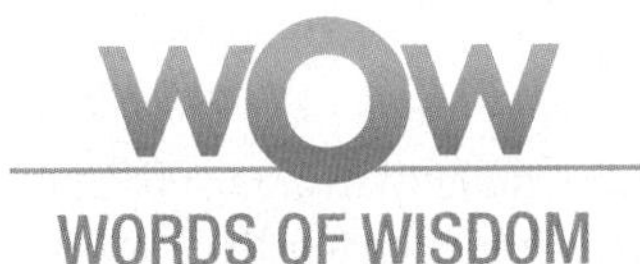

WORDS OF WISDOM

A new parent's expectations may be seen through rose-colored glasses, and at times their fantasy is better than the reality.

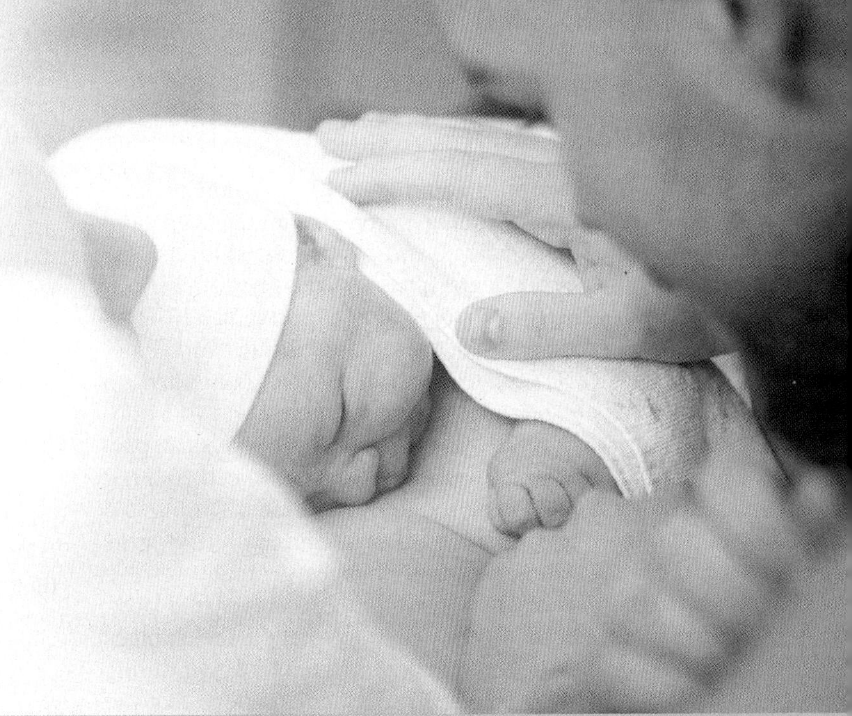

15

Postpartum Adaptations

LEARNING OBJECTIVES

Upon completion of the chapter, you will be able to:

1. Examine the systemic physiologic changes occurring in the birthing parent after childbirth.
2. Integrate dimensions of postpartum care with consideration of culture.
3. Determine the psychological changes that occur in patients in the postpartum period.
4. Plan postpartum nursing care with interventions to foster parent–infant bonding.
5. Assess the phases of parental role adjustment and accompanying behaviors.
6. Analyze the psychological adaptations occurring in the birthing parent's partner after childbirth.

KEY TERMS

attachment
engorgement
engrossment (en-grōs'ment)
involution (in'vō-lū'shŭn)
lactation
letting-go phase
lochia (lō'kē-ă)
puerperium (pyū-er-pē'rē-ŭm)
taking-hold phase
taking-in phase
uterine atony (yū'tĕr-in at'ŏ-nē)

Betsy had been home 3 days when she called the obstetrics unit where she had given birth and asked to speak to the lactation consultant. She reported pain in both breasts. Her nipples were tender due to frequent breastfeeding, and she described her breasts as heavy, hard, and swollen.

INTRODUCTION

The **puerperium** (postpartum period) is a critical transitional time for a birthing parent, their newborn, and their family on physiologic and psychological levels. The postpartum period begins after the delivery of the placenta and is currently thought to last approximately 6 to 8 weeks. The American College of Obstetricians and Gynecologists (ACOG) suggests the duration be extended up to 12 weeks to provide "[patient]-centered and individualized care that includes the assessments of physical, psychological, and social well-being" (ObG Project, 2022). It is also frequently called the fourth trimester. During this period, the birthing parent's body begins to return to its prepregnant state, and these changes generally resolve by the sixth week after giving birth. However, the postpartum period can also be defined to include the changes in all aspects of the birthing parent's life that occur during the first year after a child is born. Some believe that the postpartum adjustment period lasts well into the first year, making the fourth trimester the longest. Keeping this in mind, the true postpartum period may last longer as the birthing parent's body returns to its prepregnant state, as they psychologically adjust to the changes in their life, and as they take on the role of a new parent.

Nurses caring for childbearing families should consider all aspects of culture, including communication, space, and family roles. Beliefs, traditions, values, and culture are all reflected in practices transferred from one society to another. Communication encompasses an understanding of not only a person's language and loudness of speech but also the meaning of touch and gestures. The concept of personal space and the dimensions of comfort zones differ from culture to culture. Touching, placing patients in proximity to others, and taking away personal possessions can reduce a patient's personal security and heighten their anxiety. Nurses must be sensitive to how people respond when being touched and should refrain from touching if the patient's response indicates it is unwelcome. Cultural norms also have an impact on family roles, expectations, and behaviors associated with a member's position in the family. For example, culture may influence whether a male partner actively participates in pregnancy and childbirth. Maternity health care professionals in the United States expect partners to be involved, but this role expectation may conflict with that of many of the diverse groups living in the United States. Some groups may view the birthing experience as a woman's affair, so male partners and family members may be disengaged from the pregnancy and childbirth. The need for increased engagement of men in maternal health is one aspect of promoting gender equity. Cultural differences and prejudices can be a source of conflict; therefore, nurses must provide culturally competent care to avoid these (Yava et al., 2023). There is evidence of improvement in maternal health outcomes when male partners are actively involved in maternity care. One barrier that keeps men from participating in reproductive health includes an unfriendly atmosphere in centers from the staff toward them, which makes them feel marginalized (Roudsari et al., 2023). Nurses must be professional in interacting with all patients and their partners in a welcoming manner.

Our major role as nurses is to provide safe and evidence-based care to promote optimal birth outcomes for all birthing parents, regardless of their backgrounds. Nurses need to remember that there is more than one way to provide this care. Traditional postpartum practices are still dominant in many cultural groups. Nurses must educate birthing parents and provide strategies to help them integrate their beliefs into contemporary practices. Resources and opportunities are not equally accessible across all races, ages, languages, socioeconomic statuses, sexual orientations, and gender identities. Research finds that people of color face health disparities in health status and health outcomes (Boufides, 2022). Nurses are important cultural brokers as they welcome birthing parents and their families into obstetric units, where nurses share with those families one of the most intimate experiences of their lives (Garcia-Izquierdo & Montalt, 2022).

This chapter describes the major physiologic and psychological changes that occur in a birthing parent after childbirth. Various systemic adaptations take place throughout the person's body. In addition, the birthing parent and the family adjust to the new addition psychologically. The birth of a child changes the family structure and the roles of the family members. The adaptations are dynamic and continue to evolve as physical changes occur and new roles emerge.

MATERNAL PHYSIOLOGIC ADAPTATIONS

During pregnancy, the birthing parent's entire body changes to accommodate the needs of the growing fetus. After birth, the person's body once again undergoes significant changes as all body systems return to the prepregnant state. The World Health Organization (WHO) has made several recommendations on maternity care for a positive postnatal experience, including:

- Frequent assessment of vaginal bleeding, uterine tone, fundal height, and vital signs should be done during the first 24 hours after childbirth.
- After 24 hours after birth, the patient's well-being should be evaluated along with urinary status, bowel function, healing of perineal area, if necessary, pain assessment and perineal hygiene, breast status, uterine tenderness, and lochia amount.
- Birthing parents should be counseled and supported to practice good positioning and attachment of the infant to the breast for breastfeeding.

- Patients should be screened for postpartum depression and anxiety and given appropriate referrals if necessary.
- Comprehensive information about contraceptives should be offered to all birthing patients (2022).

Reproductive System Adaptations

The reproductive system goes through tremendous adaptations to return to the prepregnancy state. All organs and tissues of the reproductive system are involved. The female reproductive system is unique in its capacity to remodel itself throughout the person's reproductive life. The events after birth, with the shedding of the placenta and subsequent uterine involution, involve substantial tissue destruction and subsequent repair and remodeling. For example, the person's menstrual cycle, interrupted during pregnancy, will begin to return several weeks after childbirth if the person is not breastfeeding. Ovulation can return any time, so breastfeeding should not be considered a safe contraceptive and other methods should be used to prevent pregnancy. The uterus, which has undergone tremendous expansion during pregnancy to accommodate progressive fetal growth, will return to its prepregnant size over several weeks. The birthing parent's breasts have grown to prepare for lactation and do not return to their prepregnant size as the uterus does.

Uterine Involution

The uterus returns to its normal size through a gradual process of **involution**, which involves retrogressive changes that return it to its nonpregnant size and condition. A major indicator in the process of normal uterine involution is demonstrated in the decreasing height of the uterine fundus. Involution involves three retrogressive processes:

1. Contraction of muscle fibers to reduce those previously stretched during pregnancy
2. Catabolism, which shrinks enlarged individual myometrial cells
3. Regeneration of uterine epithelium from the lower layer of the decidua after the upper layers have been sloughed off and shed during lochial discharge (Chauhan & Tadi, 2022)

The uterus, which weighs approximately 1,000 g (2.2 lb) soon after birth, undergoes physiologic involution as it returns to its nonpregnant state. Approximately 1 week after birth, the uterus shrinks in size by 50% and weighs about 500 g (1 lb); at the end of 6 weeks, it weighs approximately 50 g, about the weight it was before the pregnancy (Chauhan & Tadi, 2022) (Fig. 15.1). During the first 12 hours postpartum, the fundus of the uterus is located at the level of the umbilicus. Over the first few days after birth, the uterus typically descends from the level of the umbilicus at a rate of 1 cm (one fingerbreadth) per day. By 3 days, the fundus lies two to three fingerbreadths below the umbilicus (or slightly higher in multiparous people). By the end of 10 days, the fundus usually cannot be palpated because it has descended into the true pelvis.

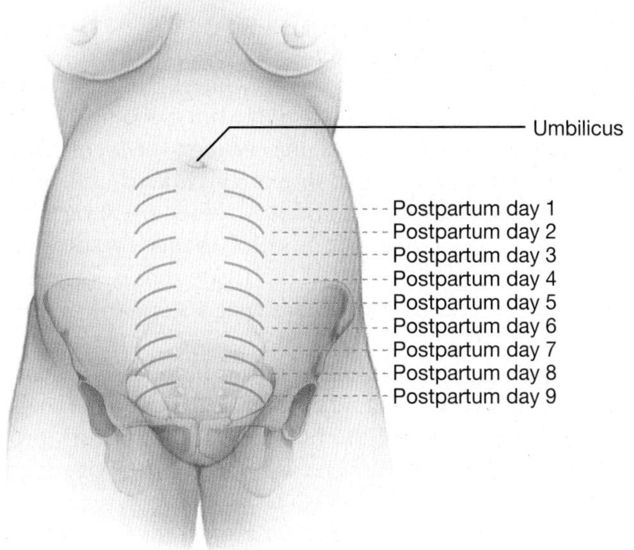

FIGURE 15.1 Uterine involution.

If these retrogressive changes do not occur as a result of retained placental fragments or infection, then subinvolution of the uterus typically results (delayed or absent involution). Subinvolution is generally responsive to early diagnosis and treatment. Appropriate uterine involution is noted by a midline, firm uterine fundus upon palpation. Factors that facilitate uterine involution include complete expulsion of amniotic membranes and placenta at birth, a complication-free labor and birth process, breastfeeding, and early ambulation. **Uterine atony** refers to a soft boggy uterus and inhibits involution of the blood vessels at the placental site. Factors leading to uterine atony and inhibited involution include prolonged labor, rapid delivery, incomplete expulsion of amniotic membranes and placenta, intra-amniotic infection, overdistention of uterine muscles (such as by multiple gestation, hydramnios, or a large singleton fetus), a full bladder (which displaces the uterus and interferes with contractions), oxytocin administration, medications relaxing uterine muscles (e.g., halogenated anesthetics, magnesium sulfate, nitroglycerin, terbutaline), and grand multiparity (Kansky & Isaacs, 2021).

LOCHIA

The process of involution and restoration of the endometrium is reflected in the characteristics of the lochia. **Lochia** is the vaginal discharge that occurs after birth and continues for approximately 4 to 8 weeks. The total volume of lochia secretion is 200 to 500 mL, which is discharged over approximately a month (Berens, 2024).

It results from involution, during which the superficial layer of the decidua basalis becomes necrotic and is sloughed off. Immediately after childbirth, lochia is bright red and consists mainly of blood, fibrinous products, decidual cells, and red and white blood cells. The lochia from the uterus is alkaline but becomes acidic as it passes through the vagina. Patterns of lochia flow vary in amount and duration among patients and pregnancies. Each day, the amount of bleeding should be less and the color lighter. The color changes result from the changing composition of the tissue that is sloughed and expelled during the endometrial restoration process (Berens, 2024).

Patients who have had cesarean births tend to have less flow because the uterine debris is removed manually along with delivery of the placenta by the primary provider. Lochia is present after a surgical birth with most patients experiencing it for up to 6 weeks.

Lochia passes through three stages:

- *Lochia rubra* is a deep-red mixture of mucus, tissue debris, and blood that occurs for the first 3 to 4 days after birth. As uterine bleeding subsides, it becomes paler and more serous.
- *Lochia serosa* is the second stage. It is pinkish brown and is expelled 3 to 10 days postpartum. Lochia serosa primarily contains leukocytes, decidual tissue, red blood cells, and serous fluid.
- *Lochia alba* is the final stage. The discharge is creamy white or light brown and consists of leukocytes, decidual tissue, and reduced fluid content. It occurs from days 10 to 14 but can last 3 to 6 weeks postpartum in some patients and still be considered normal (Lopez-Gonzalez & Kopparapu, 2023).

Lochia at any stage should have a fleshy smell; an offensive odor usually indicates an infection, such as endometritis.

TAKE NOTE!

A danger sign is the reappearance of bright-red blood after lochia rubra has stopped. Reevaluation by a health care provider is essential if this occurs.

AFTERPAINS

Part of the involution process involves uterine contractions. Immediately after birth and delivery of the placenta, the uterus begins to contract, constricting the intramyometrial vessels and impeding blood flow; this is the primary mechanism preventing hemorrhage from the placental site. Deficient uterine contractions may result in uterine atony, which can lead to an early postpartum hemorrhage (Berens, 2024). These painful uterine contractions are often called *afterpains*. All birthing people experience afterpains, but they are more acute in multiparous and breastfeeding people secondary to repeated stretching of the uterine muscles from multiple pregnancies or stimulation during breastfeeding with oxytocin released from the pituitary gland. Primiparous people typically experience mild afterpains because the uterus is able to maintain a contracted state. Both breastfeeding and administration of exogenous oxytocin cause powerful and painful uterine contractions. Afterpains usually respond to oral analgesics such as ibuprofen and acetaminophen (Wisner, 2022).

TAKE NOTE!

Afterpains are usually stronger during breastfeeding because oxytocin released by the sucking reflex strengthens the contractions. Mild analgesics can reduce this discomfort.

Cervix

Immediately after a vaginal birth, the cervix extends into the vagina and remains partly dilated, bruised, and edematous. The cervix typically returns to its prepregnant state by week 6 of the postpartum period. The cervix gradually closes but never regains its prepregnant appearance. Immediately after childbirth, the cervix is shapeless and edematous and is easily distensible for several days. The internal cervical os gradually closes and returns to normal by 2 weeks, while the external os widens and never appears the same after childbirth. The external cervical os is no longer shaped like a circle, but instead appears as a jagged slitlike opening (Fig. 15.2) (Cunningham et al., 2022a).

Vagina

Shortly after birth, the vaginal mucosa is edematous, relaxed, and thin with few rugae. As ovarian function returns and estrogen production resumes, the mucosa thickens and rugae return in approximately 3 weeks. The vagina gapes at the opening and is generally lax.

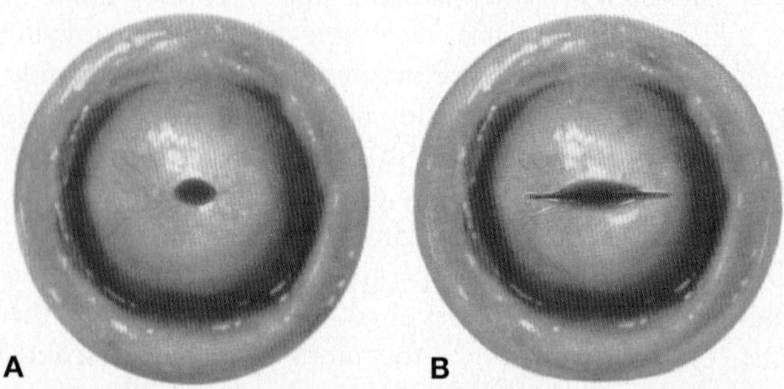

FIGURE 15.2 Appearance of the cervical os. **A.** Before the first pregnancy. **B.** After pregnancy.

It returns to its approximate prepregnant size by 6 to 8 weeks postpartum but will always remain a bit larger than it had been before pregnancy.

Normal mucus production and thickening of the vaginal mucosa usually return with ovulation. The vagina gradually decreases in size and regains tone over several weeks. By 3 to 4 weeks, the edema and vascularity have decreased. The vaginal epithelium is generally restored by 6 to 8 weeks postpartum. Vaginal tone then continues to improve over time, but never reaches its same prepregnancy condition (Karsnitz & Wilhite, 2022). Localized dryness and coital discomfort (dyspareunia) plague many patients until menstruation returns. Water-soluble lubricants can reduce discomfort during intercourse.

Perineum

The perineum stretches during childbirth to allow passage of the newborn, but many birthing people sustain some degree of perineal trauma during childbirth, which can be painful postpartum. The muscle tone may or may not return to normal, depending on the extent of injury to muscle, nerve, and connecting tissues (Berens, 2024). The perineum is often edematous and bruised for the first day or two after birth. About 53% to 89% of women will experience some form of perineal laceration during childbirth. The most common risk factors include nulliparity, delivering a large fetus, instrumental vaginal delivery, midline episiotomy, malpresentation, and advancing gestational age (Ramar & Grimes, 2023). If the birth involved an episiotomy or laceration, complete healing may take as long as 4 to 6 months in the absence of complications at the site, such as hematoma or infection. Perineal lacerations may extend into the anus and cause considerable discomfort for the birthing person when they are attempting to defecate or ambulate. The presence of swollen hemorrhoids may also heighten discomfort.

Supportive tissues of the pelvic floor are stretched during the childbirth process, and restoring their tone may take up to 6 months. Pelvic relaxation can occur in any patient experiencing a vaginal birth. Pelvic floor dysfunction is one of the most common complications of childbirth following a vaginal birth, and it can have a significant impact on the person's quality of life as they age. Nurses should identify risk factors that contribute to pelvic floor muscle dysfunction in the postpartum period and encourage all people who have given birth to practice pelvic floor muscle training (PFMT) exercises to improve pelvic floor muscle tone, strengthen the perineal muscles, and promote healing (see Evidence-Based Practice 15.1).

TAKE NOTE!

Failure to maintain and restore perineal muscular tone can lead to urinary incontinence later in life for many people who have given birth.

EVIDENCE-BASED PRACTICE 15.1

The Influence of Obstetric Factors on the Occurrence of Pelvic Floor Dysfunction in People in the Early Postpartum Period

BACKGROUND

Pelvic floor muscle dysfunction describes a weakening of the support structures of the pelvic floor muscles, which causes a relaxation that can result in stress urinary and fecal incontinence, sexual dysfunction, and pelvic organ prolapse. All of these disorders can seriously impact a person's quality of life. Up to 40% of females experience pelvic floor muscle dysfunction; this rate is increasing and poses a public health threat. The timely identification of risk factors and postpartum rehabilitation are needed. The purpose of the study was to analyze the effect of obstetric factors on the development of pelvic floor muscle dysfunction in the early postpartum period and address them.

STUDY

Clinical data from 300 participants were retrospectively analyzed. The participants had all experienced first, singleton pregnancies and were between the ages of 22 and 42 years. There were 46 people with pelvic organ prolapse and 82 people with stress urinary incontinence confirmed at 6 to 8 weeks after childbirth. Statistical Product and Service Solutions (SPSS) was used for the statistical analysis.

Findings

Obstetric factors such as age, mode of delivery, prolonged second stage of labor, large fetal size, and perineal tears increased the risk of experiencing pelvic floor muscle dysfunction disorders. It is important that these risk factors be identified early and addressed promptly to promote recovery of the pelvic floor muscle function.

Nursing Implications

The accumulation of evidence from this study and other literature shows that impairment of pelvic floor tissue, which maintains the normal position of the rectum, bladder, and other reproductive organs can lead to pelvic organ prolapse, stress urinary and fecal incontinence, sexual dysfunction, and ultimately a lowered quality of life. In order to prevent postpartum pelvic floor dysfunction disorders, nurses need to identify risk factors for each patient and try to minimize damage to the pelvic floor muscles and fascia during the childbirth experience. Nurses can address these potential conditions with all postpartum patients to encourage the use of pelvic floor muscle training to improve or prevent symptoms of urinary incontinence, sexual dysfunction, pelvic organ prolapse, and lowered quality of life as they age.

Adapted from Yang, F., & Liao, H. (2022). The influence of obstetric factors on the occurrence of pelvic floor dysfunction in women in the early postpartum period. *International Journal of General Medicine*, *15*, 3353–3361. https://doi.org/10.2147/IJGM.S355913

Cardiovascular System Adaptations

Childbirth alters the patient's hemodynamics and can lead to cardiovascular instability during the immediate postpartum period. The cardiovascular system undergoes dramatic changes after birth. During pregnancy, the heart is displaced slightly upward and to the left. This reverses as the uterus undergoes involution. Cardiac output remains high for the first few days postpartum and then gradually declines to nonpregnant values within 3 months of birth.

Blood volume, which increases substantially during pregnancy, drops rapidly after birth and returns to normal within 4 weeks postpartum. The decrease in both cardiac output and blood volume reflects the birth-related blood loss (an average of 500 mL with a vaginal birth and 1,000 mL with a cesarean birth). The cardiac output decreases to prelabor values 24 to 72 hours postpartum, rapidly falls over the next 2 weeks, and usually returns to nonpregnant levels within 6 to 8 weeks postpartum. Blood plasma volume is further reduced through diuresis, which occurs over the first 2 weeks postpartum (Chauhan & Tadi, 2022). Despite the decrease in blood volume, the hematocrit level remains relatively stable and may even increase, reflecting the predominant loss of plasma. Thus, an acute decrease in hematocrit is not an expected finding and may indicate hemorrhage.

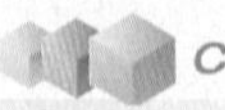
Concept Mastery Alert

Prioritizing Postpartum Vital Signs

It is not uncommon for patients to have a temperature elevation up to 100.4°F (38°C) in the first 24 hours postpartum due to mild dehydration. There may also be a slight decrease in blood pressure. The nurse should be most concerned about a blood pressure elevation because preeclampsia may occur during the early postpartum period.

Pulse and Blood Pressure

The increase in cardiac output and stroke volume during pregnancy begins to diminish after birth once the placenta has been delivered. This decrease in cardiac output is reflected in relative bradycardia for up to the first 2 weeks postpartum. Gradually, cardiac output returns to prepregnant levels within 14 days after childbirth (Ferraro, 2024).

Tachycardia (heart rate above 100 bpm) in the postpartum patient warrants further investigation. It may indicate hypovolemia, dehydration, or hemorrhage. However, because of the increased blood volume during pregnancy, a considerable loss of blood may be well tolerated and not cause a compensatory cardiovascular response such as tachycardia. In most instances of postpartum hemorrhage, blood pressure and cardiac output remain increased because of the compensatory increase in heart rate. Thus, a decrease in blood pressure and cardiac output are not expected changes during the postpartum period. Early identification is essential to ensure prompt intervention.

Blood pressure falls mostly in the first 2 days, increases after childbirth, and then returns to prepregnancy levels by 16 weeks (Chauhan & Tadi, 2022). A significant increase accompanied by headache might indicate preeclampsia and requires further investigation. Decreased blood pressure may suggest an infection or a uterine hemorrhage.

Coagulation

Normal physiologic changes of pregnancy, including alterations in hemostasis that favor coagulation, reduced fibrinolysis, and pooling and stasis of blood in the lower limbs, place the birthing person at risk for blood clots. These changes, which usually return to prepregnant levels after 3 weeks postpartum, are important for minimizing blood loss during childbirth. Risk factors for thromboembolus include a personal history of thrombosis, anemia, cesarean delivery, postpartum hemorrhage, multifetal gestation, higher body weight, preeclampsia, and postpartum infection (Cunningham et al., 2022b).

Clotting factors that increase during pregnancy tend to remain elevated during the early postpartum period. Giving birth stimulates this hypercoagulability state further. As a result, these coagulation factors remain elevated for 2 to 3 weeks postpartum. Compared with nonpregnant females, there is up to a 60-fold increase in the risk of developing venous thromboembolism for people in a postpartum period (Blondon & Skeith, 2022). This hypercoagulable state, combined with vessel damage during birth and immobility, places the patient at risk for thromboembolism (blood clots) in the lower extremities and the lungs.

Blood Cellular Components

Red blood cell production ceases early in the puerperium, causing mean hemoglobin and hematocrit levels to decrease slightly in the first 24 hours. During the next 2 weeks, both levels rise slowly. The white blood count, which increases in labor, remains elevated for the first 4 to 6 days after birth but then falls to 6,000 to 10,000/mm^3. This white blood cell elevation can complicate a diagnosis of infection in the immediate postpartum period.

Urinary System Adaptations

Pregnancy and birth can have profound effects on the urinary system. During pregnancy, the glomerular filtration rate and renal plasma flow increase significantly.

Both usually return to normal by 6 weeks after birth. There is a gradual return of bladder tone and normal size and function of the bladder, ureters, and renal pelvis, all of which were dilated during pregnancy.

Many people have difficulty feeling the sensation to void after giving birth if they received an anesthetic block during labor (which inhibits neural functioning of the bladder) or if they received oxytocin to induce or augment labor (antidiuretic effect). These patients will be at risk for incomplete emptying, bladder distention, difficulty voiding, and urinary retention. In addition, urination may be impeded by:

- Generalized swelling and bruising of the perineum and tissues surrounding the urinary meatus nulliparity
- First and second stages of labor longer than 11 to 12 hours
- Prolonged second stage of labor
- Vacuum-assisted or instrumental delivery
- Perineal lacerations
- Episiotomy
- Large fetal birth weight
- Cesarean delivery (for failure to progress in labor)
- Intermittent catheterization
- Decreased bladder tone as a result of regional anesthesia (Mohr et al., 2022)

Difficulty voiding can lead to urinary retention, bladder distention, and ultimately urinary tract infection. Urinary retention and bladder distention can cause displacement of the uterus from the midline to the right and can inhibit the uterus from contracting properly, which increases the risk of postpartum hemorrhage. Urinary retention is a major cause of uterine atony, which allows excessive bleeding. Frequent voiding of small amounts (less than 150 mL) suggests urinary retention with overflow, and catheterization may be necessary to empty the bladder to restore tone.

During pregnancy, the blood volume is increased, and relative extracellular sodium and water retention occur. After birth, this process is physiologically reversed (Cunningham et al., 2022a). Levels of atrial natriuretic peptide (ANP) increase by 1.5 times. This increased ANP level promotes urinary sodium excretion by inhibiting the actions of aldosterone, angiotensin II, and vasopressin. The result is significant diuresis in the 2 weeks following childbirth. Urine output may be as high as 3,000 mL/day (Chauhan & Tadi, 2022).

CONSIDER THIS!

Have you ever felt embarrassed when you were unable to complete a task that has always been simple for you? I had a beautiful baby boy after only 6 hours of labor. My epidural worked well, and I actually felt very little discomfort throughout my labor. Because it was in the middle of the night when they brought me to my postpartum room, I felt a few hours of sleep would be all I needed to be back to normal. During an assessment early the next morning, the nurse found my uterus had shifted to the right from my midline, and I was instructed to empty my bladder. I didn't understand why the nurse was concerned about where my uterus was located, and besides, I didn't feel any sensation of a full bladder. But I did get up anyway and tried to comply. Despite all the nurse's tricks of running the faucet for sound effects, in addition to having warm water poured over my thighs via the peribottle, I was unable to urinate. How could I not accomplish such a simple task?

Thoughts: Birthing patients who receive regional anesthesia frequently experience reduced sensation to their perineal area and do not feel a full bladder. The nursing assessment revealed a displaced uterus secondary to a full bladder. What additional "tricks" can be used to assist this patient in voiding? What explanation should be offered regarding why they are having difficulty urinating?

Gastrointestinal System Adaptations

The gastrointestinal system quickly returns to normal after birth because the gravid uterus is no longer filling the abdominal cavity and producing pressure on the abdominal organs. Progesterone levels, which caused relaxation of smooth muscle during pregnancy and diminished bowel tone, are also declining.

Regardless of the type of delivery, most patients experience decreased bowel tone and sluggish bowels for several days after birth. Decreased peristalsis occurs in response to analgesics, surgery, diminished intra-abdominal pressure, a low-fiber diet, insufficient fluid intake, and diminished muscle tone. In addition, patients with episiotomies, perineal lacerations, or hemorrhoids may fear pain or damage to the perineum with the first bowel movement and may attempt to delay it. Subsequently, constipation is a common problem during the postpartum period. A stool softener can be prescribed for this reason.

Most patients are hungry and thirsty after childbirth, commonly related to nothing-by-mouth (NPO) restrictions and the energy expended during labor. Many freestanding birth centers and some hospitals allow patients to eat food and drink fluids during labor. A recent Cochrane review did not find any evidence of harm resulting from eating and drinking during labor. Several professional organizations, including the WHO, the American College of Nurse-Midwives (ACNM), the National Institute for Health and Care Excellence (NICE), and the Society of Obstetricians and Gynecologists of Canada (SOGC), recommend that those at low risk for complications eat and drink as they desire during labor to replenish their energy levels (Dekker, 2022).

TAKE NOTE!

The WHO, ACNM, NICE, and SOGC recommend that people at low risk for complications eat and drink as they desire during labor to replenish their energy levels.

Musculoskeletal System Adaptations

The effects of pregnancy on the muscles and joints vary widely. Musculoskeletal changes associated with pregnancy, such as increased ligament laxity, weight gain, change in the center of gravity, and carpal tunnel syndrome, revert during the postpartum period. During pregnancy, the hormones relaxin, estrogen, and progesterone relax the joints. After birth, levels of these hormones decline, resulting in a return of all joints to their prepregnant state (Karsnitz & Wilhite, 2022). The exception is the patient's feet; parous people may note a flattening of the arch and a permanent increase in shoe size (Segal et al., 2013).

Birthing people commonly experience fatigue and activity intolerance and have a distorted body image for weeks after birth secondary to declining relaxin and progesterone levels, which cause hip and joint pain that interferes with ambulation and exercise. Good body mechanics and correct positioning are important during this time to prevent low back pain and injury to the joints. Within 6 to 8 weeks after delivery, joints are completely stabilized and return to normal.

During pregnancy, stretching of the abdominal wall muscles occurs to accommodate the enlarging uterus. This stretching leads to a loss in muscle tone and possibly separation of the longitudinal muscles (rectus abdominis muscles) of the abdomen. Separation of the rectus abdominis muscles, called diastasis recti, is more common in people who have poor abdominal muscle tone before pregnancy. After birth, muscle tone is diminished, and the abdominal muscles are soft and flabby. Specific exercises are necessary to help the patient regain muscle tone. Fortunately, diastasis responds well to exercise, and abdominal muscle tone can be improved (see Chapter 16 for more information about exercises to improve muscle tone).

TAKE NOTE!

If rectus muscle tone is not regained through exercise, support may not be adequate during future pregnancies.

Integumentary System Adaptations

Another system that experiences lasting effects of pregnancy is the integumentary system. As estrogen and progesterone levels decrease, the darkened pigmentation on the abdomen (linea nigra), face (melasma), and nipples gradually fades. Some people experience hair loss during pregnancy and the postpartum periods. Approximately 90% of hairs are growing at any one time, with the other 10% entering a resting phase. Because of the high estrogen levels present during pregnancy, an increased number of hairs go into the resting phase, which is part of the normal hair loss cycle. The most common period for hair loss is within 3 months after birth when estrogen returns to normal levels and more hairs are allowed to fall out. This hair loss is usually temporary, and regrowth generally returns to normal levels 6 to 15 months following delivery (Berens, 2024).

Striae gravidarum (stretch marks) often develop during pregnancy on the breasts, abdomen, buttocks, thighs, and hips. During pregnancy, dermal stretching leads to dermal scarring (Oakley & Patel, 2023). Approximately 43% to 88% of pregnant people have stretch marks (Oakley & Patel, 2023). Eventually, these stretch marks gradually fade to silvery lines though they do not disappear completely. Although many products on the market claim to make stretch marks disappear, their effectiveness is highly questionable.

The profuse diaphoresis (sweating) that is common during the early postpartum period is one of the most noticeable adaptations in the integumentary system. Many people who are postpartum will wake up drenched with perspiration during the puerperium. This postpartum diaphoresis is a mechanism to reduce the amount of fluids retained during pregnancy and restore prepregnant body fluid levels. It can be profuse at times. It is common, especially at night during the first week after birth. Reassure the patient that this is normal and encourage them to change their night clothes to prevent chilling.

Respiratory System Adaptations

Respirations usually remain within the normal adult range of 16 to 24 breaths/min. As the abdominal organs resume their nonpregnant positions, the diaphragm returns to its usual position. Anatomic changes in the thoracic cavity and rib cage caused by increasing uterine growth resolve quickly. As a result, discomforts such as shortness of breath and rib aches are relieved. Tidal volume, minute volume, vital capacity, and functional residual capacity return to prepregnant values, typically within 1 to 3 weeks of birth (Kodali & Segal, 2023).

Endocrine System Adaptations

With the delivery of the placenta, there is rapid clearance of placenta hormones. Levels of circulating estrogen and progesterone drop quickly with delivery of the placenta. Progesterone is returned to the prepregnancy level within 48 hours, and estrogen by 1 to 2 weeks (Karsnitz & Wilhite, 2022). Human chorionic gonadotropin (hCG) hormone levels decline rapidly after birth (Berens, 2024).

Luteinizing hormone (LH) and follicle-stimulating hormone (FSH) are low for about 2 weeks postpartum; they gradually return to normal levels (Karsnitz & Wilhite, 2022). Lactation interferes with the return of LH and FSH to prepregnancy levels. Prolactin levels decline within 2 weeks for a person who is not breastfeeding but remain elevated for a lactating person. Prolactin maintains continuous and effective lactation. The ovarian response to FSH and LH is inhibited in the presence of high prolactin (Chauhan & Tadi, 2022). Prolactin inhibits gonadotropin-releasing hormone (GnRH) secretion from the hypothalamus, thereby suppressing ovulation. People who practice exclusive breastfeeding may not ovulate for 6 months, but the onset of ovulation and return of menstruation are variable (Berens, 2024).

Weight Loss After Childbirth

Excessive weight gain and postpartum weight retention can increase the risk of obesity. Postpartum obesity is a clinical and public health concern because it can become a lifelong health issue if not addressed after childbirth. Breastfeeding has been shown to have many health benefits for both parent and infant; however, evidence of its effectiveness in postpartum weight loss is mixed. Lactation is usually not sufficient for the parent to return to the prepregnancy weight. Postpartum patients should be guided to engage in physical activity within 4 to 6 weeks after childbirth or as soon as they feel comfortable. They should gradually increase the intensity and duration over time (ACOG, 2022).

The rate and amount of weight loss in the postpartum period seem to be determined by the same factors that determine weight loss at any point in a person's life, including existing weight, body mass index (BMI), diet, age, and activity level (Liu et al., 2022). Thus, there is a benefit from overall lifestyle interventions on weight loss in postpartum patients, which include exercise plus dietary changes to achieve any weight reduction goals (see Evidence-Based Practice 15.2).

Sexual Health

Childbirth is an important period in a birthing person's life. Postpartum adaptations affect their physical well-being, mood, relationship, and sexual health. Sexuality is a central aspect of being human that is present throughout one's life. Hormones, physical and psychological changes, parenting roles, infant care, breastfeeding, insomnia, fatigue, customs, beliefs, and traditions are all factors that influence sexual functioning in the postpartum period. Caring for a newborn while attempting to maintain a romantic relationship is challenging. The sexual problems people have in the postpartum period typically relate to sexual drive, inability to reach orgasm, arousal, exhaustion, insomnia, reduced frequency

EVIDENCE-BASED PRACTICE 15.2

Effects of a Lifestyle Intervention on Postpartum Weight Retention Among People With Elevated Weight

BACKGROUND

Pregnancy and postpartum periods are critical times that may predispose women to gain weight. People experience significant weight gain during pregnancy and need to lose it after childbirth. Excessive weight gain during pregnancy is a known predictor of postpartum weight retention. Postpartum weight retention contributes to the development of obesity in midlife and postmenopausal periods. Overweight and obesity comprise a global public health problem and a major risk factor for diabetes, cancer, dyslipidemia, hypertension, and cardiovascular disease. The purpose of this study was to examine the impact of a pregnancy and postpartum behavioral lifestyle intervention versus standard care on postpartum weight retention.

STUDY

This randomized controlled study enrolled 219 White and Black participants (107 in the standard care group and 112 in the intervention group). Starting in early pregnancy and continuing until 6 months postpartum, the intervention group received two in-depth counseling sessions, telephone counseling, behavioral podcasts, and support on social media. Lifestyle interventions focused on physical activity, diet, and weight gain counseling. The participants receiving standard care were encouraged to attend prenatal visits. Multiple logistic regression models were applied to assess the effect of behavioral lifestyle intervention on weight outcomes.

Findings

The combined pregnancy and postpartum behavioral lifestyle intervention group participants experienced significantly reduced postpartum weight retention outcomes at 6 and 12 months after giving birth when compared to the standard group participants. Findings from this study suggest that continuing lifestyle interventions after childbirth positively contributes to postpartum weight loss.

Nursing Implications

The postpartum period is a challenging and stressful time for the person who has given birth. Many feel overwhelmed and exhausted due to sleep deprivation, hormonal changes, high demands of the infant, lack of time, and adaptation to the new parenting role. Postpartum weight retention has important public health implications as it has a significant impact on long-term weight and future health risks. Nurses should identify patients who are overweight or obese during pregnancy who will be at high risk of retaining their postpartum weight and provide them instructions on healthy lifestyle activities that would assist in weight loss. Patients look to nurses for direction about their health, eating, and appropriate weight ranges. Interventions by nurses might tip the scales for improved health in all patients' futures.

Adapted from Liu, J., Wilcox, S., Hutto, B., Turner-McGrievy, G., & Wingard, E. (2022). Effects of a lifestyle intervention on postpartum weight retention among women with elevated weight. *Obesity: A Research Journal, 30*(7), 1370–1379. https://doi.org/10.1002/oby.23449

of sexual activity, and uncomfortable intercourse due to lack of natural lubrication (Delgado-Perez et al., 2022; Rahmani et al., 2023). Based on research findings, people who identify as women tend to speak with female friends who are parents, rather than health care providers, about resuming sexual activity after childbirth (O'Malley et al., 2022). Nurses need to provide patients with opportunities to express, identify, and resolve their sexual problems, contributing to enhancing health and quality of life. Nurses can provide anticipatory guidance and counseling to patients and their partners about sexual problems they may experience during the postpartum period as well as their causes and possible solutions. Moreover, supporting patients as they navigate postpartum sexuality changes may help ease their concerns and enhance their sexual well-being.

Lactation

Lactation is the secretion of milk by the breasts. It is thought to be brought about by the interaction of progesterone, estrogen, prolactin, and oxytocin. Breast milk typically appears within 4 to 5 days after childbirth.

Think back to Betsy, the woman experiencing painful changes in her breasts. What might Betsy be describing? Why has the condition of her breasts changed compared with when she was in the hospital?

Breastfeeding

Breastfeeding is a dynamic process that requires coupling between periodic motions of the infant's jaws, undulation of the tongue, and breast milk ejection reflex. All mechanisms must be coordinated to be successful. All major health organizations recommend breastfeeding. The American Academy of Pediatrics (AAP) recommends exclusive breastfeeding for 6 months followed by the introduction of appropriate complementary foods and continued breastfeeding for 2 years and beyond (Meek et al., 2022). This recommendation is considered the standard of care today and is consistent with similar guidelines from the National Association of Pediatric Nurse Practitioners (2019), and the American Academy of Family Physicians (AAFP, 2024). Nurses have an important role in promoting, supporting, and protecting breastfeeding. They must have the necessary knowledge and skills to provide breastfeeding education to all birthing parents. Proper positioning, latching-on, sucking, and swallowing are the foundation for successful breastfeeding. Although breastfeeding is recommended by international and national organizations, the nurse must respect and support all patients in either of the infant feeding methods chosen.

During pregnancy, the breasts increase in size and functional ability in preparation for breastfeeding. Estrogen stimulates growth of the milk collection (ductal) system, while progesterone stimulates growth of the milk production system. Within the first month of gestation, the ducts of the mammary glands grow branches, forming more lobules and alveoli. These structural changes make the breasts larger, more tender, and heavy. The glandular cells fill with secretions, blood vessels increase in number, and the amounts of connective tissue and fat cells increase (Pillay & Davis, 2023).

Prolactin from the anterior pituitary gland, secreted in increasing levels throughout pregnancy, triggers the synthesis and secretion of milk after the person gives birth. During pregnancy, prolactin, estrogen, and progesterone cause the synthesis and secretion of *colostrum*, which contains protein and carbohydrates but no milk fat. It is only after birth takes place, when the high levels of estrogen and progesterone are abruptly withdrawn, that prolactin is able to stimulate the glandular cells to secrete milk instead of colostrum. This takes place within 4 to 5 days after giving birth.

Oxytocin acts so that milk can be ejected from the alveoli to the nipple. Therefore, sucking by the newborn will release milk. A decrease in the quality of stimulation causes a decrease in prolactin surges and thus a decrease in milk production. Prolactin levels increase in response to nipple stimulation during feedings. Prolactin and oxytocin result in milk production if stimulated by sucking (Pillay & Davis, 2023) (Fig. 15.3). If the stimulus (sucking) is not present, as with a birthing parent who is not breastfeeding, breast engorgement and milk production will subside within days postpartum.

Skin-to-skin contact during the first hour following birth is the gold standard to initiate breastfeeding if the birthing parent decides this is the method of feeding for their newborn. A newborn's instinct is to seek nourishment after birth. A newborn moves on their parent's abdomen up to their breast instinctively. Researchers term this movement the *breast crawl* that helps initiate breastfeeding immediately after childbirth. This instinct occurs when a newborn, left undisturbed and skin-to-skin on the birthing parent's trunk following birth, moves toward their parent's breast for the purpose of locating and self-attaching for the first feeding. From there, the newborn uses leg and arm movements to propel toward the breast. Upon reaching the sternum, the newborn will bounce their head up and down and side to side. As the newborn approaches the nipple, the mouth opens and after several attempts, latch-on and suckling take place. Research has found that the early initiation of breastfeeding is linked to a higher likelihood of breastfeeding success as well as a longer duration. It is also associated with a reduced long-term risk of chronic diseases such as hypertension, diabetes, cardiovascular disease, metabolic syndrome, and ovarian and breast cancers in

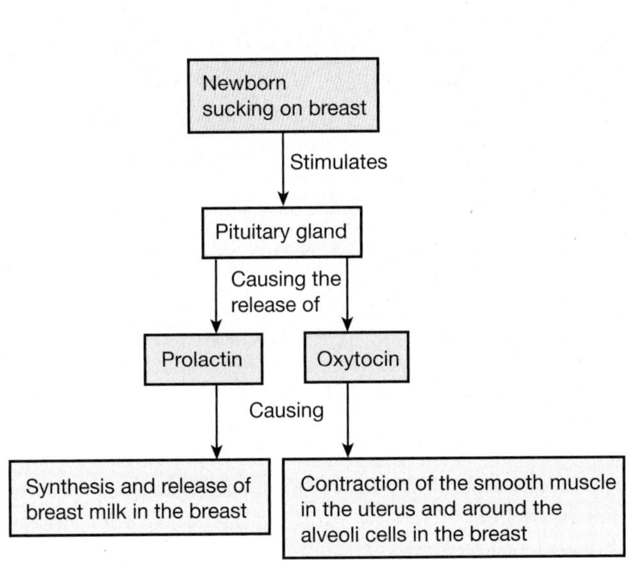

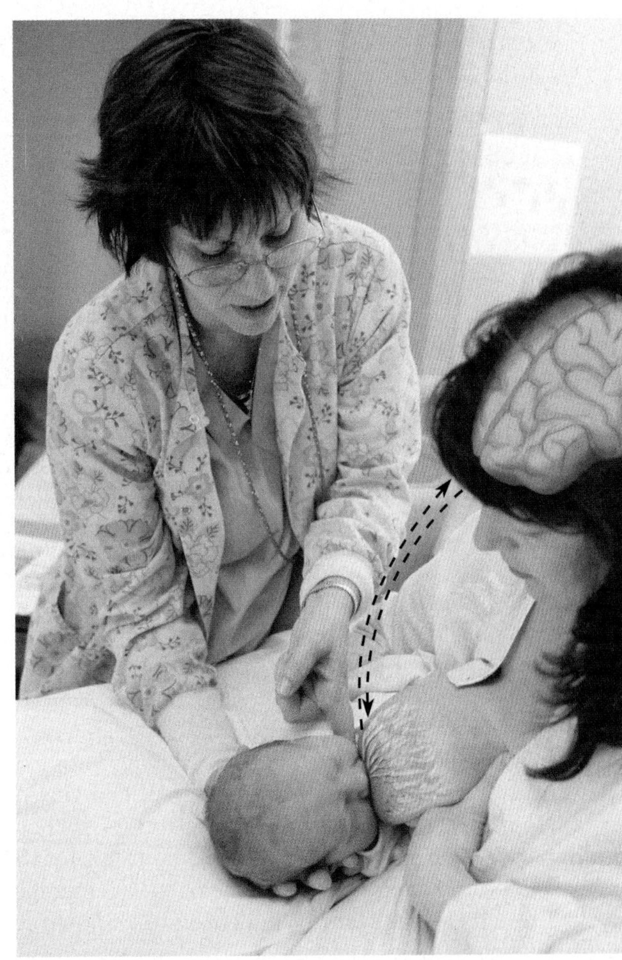

FIGURE 15.3 Physiology of lactation.

the birthing parent (Wang et al., 2022). Newborns have senses and skills that enable early initiation of feeding at the breast. Nurses can help facilitate the breast crawl as a continuation of the birthing process. Nurses have a responsibility to promote the health of their childbearing families and provide evidence-based care. Encouraging the use of the breast crawl can be the first step in health promotion for every newborn.

Breast milk production can be summarized as follows:

- Prolactin levels increase at term with a decrease in estrogen and progesterone levels.
- Estrogen and progesterone levels decrease after the placenta is delivered.
- Prolactin is released from the anterior pituitary gland and initiates milk production.
- Oxytocin is released from the posterior pituitary gland to promote milk let-down.
- Infant sucking at each feeding provides continuous stimulus for prolactin and oxytocin release (Pillay & Davis, 2023).

Typically, during the first 2 days after birth, the breasts are soft and nontender. The birthing parent may also report a tingling sensation in both breasts, which is the "let-down reflex" that occurs immediately before or during breastfeeding. After this time, breast changes depend on whether the person is breastfeeding or taking measures to prevent lactation.

Engorgement is a postnatal physiologic painful condition in which distention and swelling of the breast tissue occur as a result of an increase in blood and lymph supply as a precursor to lactation (Fig. 15.4). Breasts increase in vascularity and swell in response to prolactin 2 to 3 days after birth (Baker, 2024). Engorgement can occur from a delayed start to breastfeeding, poor breast attachment, overabundant milk supply, or infrequent feeding (United Nations International Children's Emergency Fund [UNICEF], 2022). If engorged, the breasts will be hard and tender to touch. They are temporarily full, tender, and uncomfortable until the milk supply is ready. Frequent emptying of the breasts helps minimize discomfort and resolve engorgement. Standing in a warm shower or applying warm compresses immediately before feedings will help to soften the breasts and nipples in order to allow the newborn to latch on more easily (Baker, 2024).

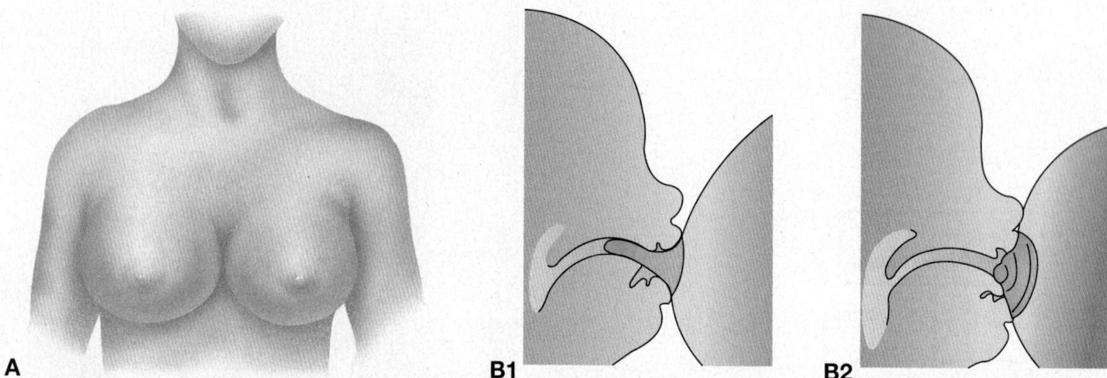

FIGURE 15.4 **A.** Image of engorged breasts. Note swelling and inflammation of both breasts. **B.** Breast engorgement can disrupt breastfeeding: (1) When sucking at a normal breast, the infant's lips compress the areola and fit neatly against the sides of the nipple. The infant also has adequate room to breathe. (2) When a breast is engorged, however, the infant has difficulty grasping the nipple and breathing ability is compromised. (**A**, reprinted with permission from Willis, L. M. [2016]. *Health assessment made incredibly visual!* [3rd ed.]. Wolters Kluwer. **B**, Reprinted with permission from Silbert-Flagg, J. [2022]. *Maternal and child health nursing* [9th ed.]. Wolters Kluwer.)

Treatments to reduce the pain of breast engorgement include heat or cold applications, cabbage leaf compresses, changing positions each breastfeeding period, standing in a warm shower, nursing or expressing milk every 2 hours, making sure that the infant is latching properly, breast massages, and breast pumping (La Leche League International, 2024). Anti-inflammatory agents, even those in nonprescription medications, can also be taken for the breast discomfort and swelling resulting from engorgement. These measures will also enhance the let-down reflex. Between feedings, applying cold compresses to the breasts helps reduce swelling. To maintain milk supply, the breasts need to be stimulated by a nursing infant, a breast pump, or manual expression of the milk (Fig. 15.5).

> Remember Betsy, who experienced breast discomfort? The lactation consultant explains that Betsy was experiencing normal breast engorgement and offered several suggestions to help her. What relief measures might be suggested? What reassurance can be given to Betsy at this time?

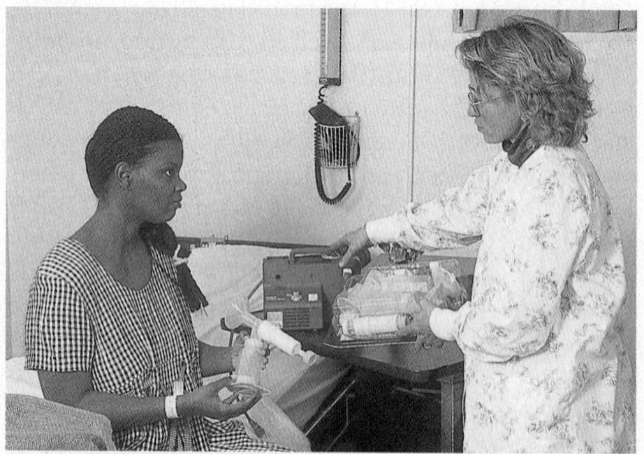

FIGURE 15.5 Nurse instructs the new breastfeeding parent about the use of a breast pump. (Photo by B. Proud.)

SUPPRESSING LACTATION

Various pharmacologic and nonpharmacologic interventions have been used to suppress lactation after childbirth and relieve associated symptoms; however, many of these medications carry significant risk and therefore are not recommended (Berens, 2024). Current research does not support the use of any medication for lactation suppression (Berens, 2024). It is estimated that more than 30% of birthing parents in the United States do not breastfeed their infants, and a larger proportion discontinues breastfeeding within 2 weeks of childbirth. Sixty percent of birthing parents do not breastfeed in the recommended time span due to issues with latching, cultural norms, lack of family/community support, and unsupportive work setting policies (CDC, 2023a). Although physiologic cessation of lactation eventually occurs in the absence of physical stimulus such as infant suckling, a large number of people in the postpartum period experience moderate to severe milk leakage and discomfort before lactation ceases. People who do not breastfeed experience engorgement and breast pain that typically subside within 2 to 3 days (Baker, 2024).

Ovulation and Return of Menstruation

Changing hormone levels constantly interact with one another to produce bodily changes. Four major hormones are influential during the postpartum period: estrogen, progesterone, prolactin, and oxytocin. Estrogen plays a major role during pregnancy, but levels drop profoundly at birth and reach their lowest level a week into the postpartum period. Progesterone quiets the uterus to prevent a preterm birth during pregnancy, and its increasing levels during pregnancy prevent lactation from starting before birth takes place. As with estrogen, progesterone levels decrease dramatically after birth and return to the prepregnant state within 48 hours after childbirth (Karsnitz & Wilhite, 2022).

During the postpartum period, oxytocin stimulates the uterus to contract during the breastfeeding session and for as long as 20 minutes after each feeding. Oxytocin also acts on the breast by eliciting the milk let-down reflex during breastfeeding. Prolactin is also associated with the breastfeeding process by stimulating milk production. The levels of prolactin fluctuate in proportion to nipple stimulation. Prolactin levels decrease in nonlactating patients, reaching prepregnant levels by the third postpartum week.

The timing of first menses and ovulation after birth differs between birthing parents who are breastfeeding and those who are not breastfeeding. For nonlactating people, menstruation may resume as early as 7 to 9 weeks after giving birth, but the majority take up to 3 months. The first cycle may be anovulatory (Berens, 2024). The return of menses in the lactating woman depends on breastfeeding frequency and duration. It can return any time after childbirth, depending on whether the person is exclusively breastfeeding or supplementing with formula. This underscores the importance of starting postpartum contraception in a timely manner.

TAKE NOTE!

Ovulation may occur before menstruation. Therefore, breastfeeding is not a totally reliable method of contraception unless the birthing parent exclusively breastfeeds, has had no menstrual period since giving birth, and has an infant younger than 6 months (Durbin, 2022).

Betsy tries several of the measures the lactation consultant suggested to relieve her breast discomfort but is still having heaviness and pain. She feels discouraged and tells the nurse that she is thinking of reducing her breastfeeding and using the formula to feed her newborn. What should Betsy consider when deciding if this is a good choice for her and her baby? Why or why not? What interventions will help Betsy get through this difficult time?

CULTURAL CONSIDERATIONS FOR THE POSTPARTUM PERIOD

People vary in their postpartum beliefs, practices, and customs. Nurses practice in an increasingly multicultural society. Therefore, they must be open, respectful, nonjudgmental, and willing to learn about culturally diverse populations. Although childbirth and the postpartum period are unique experiences for each birthing parent, how the person perceives and makes meaning of them is culturally defined. An estimated 60% of maternal deaths occur in the postpartum period, and 45% happen within the first 24 hours after childbirth in low- to middle-income countries (Clark-Deelder et al., 2023). This is a very vulnerable time period, and birthing parents in all countries need close monitoring and prompt management to reduce the risk of morbidity and mortality. Birthing parents of Latin American descent traditionally have a 40-day resting period called "cuarentena" with family (Grigsby, 2023). Birthing parents in other countries (e.g., Mexico, China, Japan, Korea, and many eastern European countries) have similar rest periods during which they stay home for several weeks after childbirth (Major, 2020).

Balance of Hot and Cold

Some cultures have specific beliefs about confinement and the balance of hot and cold after childbirth. In the United States, childbearing and recovery are typically viewed as healthy states, and birthing parents receive little formal support for both their recovery and infant care. In China, childbearing and postpartum are traditionally viewed as states that disturb the normal health balance between yin and yang. In order to restore balance in health, postpartum people engage in practices for a month related to the parental role, do not exercise, sleep long hours, stay indoors, allow the infant to be cared for by nannies or a grandmother, maintain body warmth by wearing warm clothes, consume six meals daily, limit use of electronics, and consume certain foods (Daxue Consulting, 2022). Although this confinement period is sometimes viewed as restrictive and isolating, it is well received by many. Recently, postpartum confinement practices have changed considerably and have been modified by many Singaporean women living in the United States (Tan et al., 2022). Nurses need to be aware of and familiar with the practice of confinement after childbirth for patients they may care for who participate in it.

Many cultures believe good health requires the balancing of hot and cold substances. Because childbirth involves the loss of blood, which is considered hot, the postpartum period is considered cold, so the birthing parent must balance that with the intake of hot food. Foods consumed should be hot in nature, and cold foods, such as fruits and vegetables, should be avoided. Western practices frequently use cold packs or sitz baths to reduce perineal swelling and discomfort. These practices are not acceptable to birthing parents of many cultures and can be viewed as harmful. For example, Vietnamese people traditionally view the postpartum period as a cold state (duong) and protect themselves with warmth. Cultural practices include warm water for hygiene and stimulation of lactation, consuming warm foods, and staying indoors.

Postpartum Cultural Beliefs

With increasing multiculturalism in the United States, understanding various cultures' views of the postnatal period as it relates to their recovery and well-being after childbirth is important for all nurses. Postpartum nurses need to understand these diverse cultural beliefs and provide creative strategies for encouraging hygiene (sponge baths, perineal care), exercise, and balanced nutrition while remaining respectful of the cultural significance of different practices. The best approach is to ask each birthing parent to describe what cultural practices are important to them and plan accordingly.

PSYCHOLOGICAL ADAPTATIONS

The process of becoming a parent requires extensive psychological, social, and physical work. Birthing parents experience heightened vulnerability and face tremendous challenges as they make this transition. Nurses have a remarkable opportunity to help birthing parents learn, gain confidence, and experience growth as they assume this new identity.

The transition to parenthood, while an exciting time to celebrate the life of a new child, causes parents to face new challenges such as physical exhaustion, role overload, and less time for themselves and each other. The arrival of an infant can be a joyful event, but it brings about changes in self-concepts, social roles, and the daily routines of parents. As the parenting role takes priority above all else, birthing parents often neglect their own needs. This may leave them exhausted, distressed, and struggling with too many new tasks and responsibilities (Bogdan et al., 2022). Birthing parents' and their partners' experiences of pregnancy are necessarily different, and this difference continues after childbirth as they both adjust to their new parenting roles. Many people struggle to adapt to parenthood.

Parenting involves caring for infants physically and emotionally to foster the growth and development of responsible, caring people. A substantial body of research finds no biologically based differences between birthing parents and their partners in sensitivity to infants, capacity to provide care, or acquisition of parenting skills. The birthing parent may experience postpartum depression, which is traditionally seen as a female condition, but their partners also are affected. Studies show that about one in 10 partners develops postpartum depression and about one in nine birthing parents will also develop depression. Partner postpartum depression is less discussed. Many partners deny it and do not seek help, thinking they will sort it out on their own. They may feel sad, tired, and overwhelmed. These are similar feelings as the birthing parent. They are also likely to engage in avoidance or escapist behaviors by spending more time away from home. Postpartum depression in partners can go undiagnosed and untreated (Sheppard, 2023). Nurses need to learn more about partner depression and reach out to partners to provide care to them as well by including them in the whole pregnancy and birthing experience from the beginning (AAP, 2023; Ruggeri, 2022). Early parent–infant contact after birth improves attachment behaviors.

Parental Attachment Behaviors

The postpartum period is a unique time distinguished by the inseparable relationship parents have with the newborn. To enable an attachment to be built, closeness of this family unit is essential. **Attachment** is the formation of a relationship between a parent and a newborn through a process of physical and emotional interactions. When a parent is sensitive and responsive to their infant's needs, they are seen as a secure attachment figure and a safe haven for the infant. Attachment between a birthing parent and their newborn has lifelong implications (Li, 2024). This attachment has the potential to affect both child development and parenting. The bond between a parent and the newborn is one of strength, power, and potential. Attachment begins before birth, during the prenatal period when acceptance and nurturing of the growing fetus takes place. It continues after giving birth as parents learn to recognize the newborn's cues, adapt to the newborn's behaviors and responses, and meet the newborn's needs.

Several factors take place during the early postpartum period that can have a large influence on the attachment and bonding that occur during this time. Oxytocin plays an essential role in the chemistry aspect of bonding (Kohlhoff et al., 2022). Early and sustained contact between newborns and their parents is vital for initiating this relationship.

Nurses play a crucial role in assisting the attachment process by promoting early parent–newborn interactions. In addition, nurses can facilitate skin-to-skin contact (kangaroo care) by placing the infant onto the bare chests of birthing parents and their partners to enhance parent–newborn attachment. This activity will enable them to get close to their newborn, experience an intense feeling of connectedness, and evoke feelings of being nurturing parents. Encouraging breastfeeding is another way to foster attachment between birthing parents and their newborns. Finally, nurses can encourage nurturing activities and contact such as touching, talking, singing, comforting, changing diapers, and feeding—in short, participating in routine newborn care.

The process of attachment is complex and influenced by many factors including environmental circumstances, the newborn's health status, and the quality of nursing care. The nurse must be able to recognize positive or impaired attachment behaviors between the birthing parent and their infant and create a plan of care to improve family dynamics. Nurses need to minimize parent–newborn separation by promoting parent–newborn interactions through kangaroo care, breastfeeding, and participation in their newborn care. Nurses who provide positive psychosocial support and clear communication with parents will help support the attachment process within family units. Encouraging consistently warm and nurturing infant care will enhance secure attachment behaviors.

The Birthing Parent's Psychological Adaptations

Childbirth can be a joyous period in a person's life and involves the sometimes-spiritual experience of giving life to another being. For many, this is life changing and throughout history has been anticipated with excitement and joy, often considered a blessing. However, childbirth and child-rearing can also be stressful, exhausting, financially challenging, and emotionally demanding.

Mood Disorders

Many people consider childbirth a time of happiness and well-being, but it is common for birthing parents to experience changes in their mood during this time. This may include being fatigued, irritable, and worried, and frequently these feelings become severe enough to require medical intervention. Perinatal mood disorders are one of the most common complications to occur during the postpartum period, impairing caregiving skills. In the postpartum period, mood disorders can be divided into two distinct types: postpartum baby blues and postpartum major depression (with or without psychosis). These disorders, however, have not been clearly demarcated, and it is a matter of much debate whether they are discrete disorders or a single disorder that ranges along a continuum of severity. Birthing parents who experience baby blues are at an increased risk for developing postpartum depression or psychosis (Balaram & Marwaha, 2023).

Fifty percent (or more) of people who have recently given birth suffer from the short-lived postpartum mood disorder colloquially called the baby blues, which are characterized by mild depressive symptoms, anxiety, crying, irritability, mood swings, loss of appetite, trouble sleeping, tearfulness (often for no discernible reason), increased sensitivity, and fatigue (CDC, 2023b). These symptoms typically peak on postpartum days 4 and 5, may last hours to days, and usually resolve by day 10. If these symptoms persist beyond 2 weeks, a depressive disorder may be occurring. Although these symptoms may be distressing, they do not reflect psychopathology, and they typically do not affect the parent's ability to function and care for their child. For additional information, see Chapter 22.

Phases of the Birthing Parent's Adaptation to Parenthood

Parenthood is a highly anticipated and frequently a positive event for many people. Becoming a parent is an important transition that adds new roles and responsibilities to daily life. It is a time of great change and heightened vulnerability, and a person faces tremendous challenges as they undergo this transition. Parenthood is often portrayed as idealized, romanticized, and joyful. However, a large proportion of birthing parents do not feel this way and instead experience postnatal psychological distress. Society has constructed many ideal images of parenthood, creating sometimes unrealistic standards for birthing parents to live up to, frequently setting them up for disappointment. Most people are able to experience this mismatch between their ideal and actual selves and adapt with minimal disruption. However, many birthing parents do not adapt well, and this period may result in a crisis if adaptation is not achieved (Simsek et al., 2022). It is paramount that nurses give care, support, and education to patients from the moment they decide to become pregnant throughout the pregnancy cycle and beyond to assist in the adaptation to parenthood. The birthing parent experiences a variety of responses as they adjust to a new family member and to postpartum discomforts, changes in their body image, and the reality of change in their life. In the early 1960s, Reva Rubin first identified three phases that a birthing parent goes through to adjust to their new role—taking in, taking hold, and letting go. Rubin's maternal role framework can be used to monitor the patient's progress as they "try on" this new role as a parent. The absence of these processes or the inability to progress through the phases satisfactorily may impede the appropriate development of the parental role. Parental role attainment is an interactional and developmental process occurring over time in which the birthing parent becomes attached to their infant, acquires competence in their caregiving tasks, and feels a sense of harmony (Frese & Nguyen, 2022). Although Rubin's maternal role development theories are of value, some of her observations regarding the length of each phase may not be completely relevant for the contemporary birthing parent of the 21st century. Today, many parents know their infant's sex, have "seen" their fetus in utero through four-dimensional ultrasound, and have a working knowledge of childbirth and child care. They are less passive than in years past and progress through the phases of attaining their new role at a much faster pace than Rubin expected in her research. Still, Rubin's three-phase framework is timeless for assessing and monitoring expected role behaviors when planning care and appropriate interventions.

TAKING-IN PHASE

The **taking-in phase** is the time immediately after birth when the birthing parent needs sleep, depends on others to meet their needs, and relives the events surrounding the birth process. This phase is characterized by dependent behavior. During the first 24 to 48 hours after giving birth, birthing parents often assume a passive role in meeting their own basic needs for food, fluids, and rest, allowing the nurse to make decisions for them concerning activities and care. They spend time recounting their labor experience to others. Such actions help the parent integrate the birth experience into reality; the pregnancy is over, and the newborn is now a unique individual, separate from the birthing parent. When interacting with the newborn, new birthing parents spend time claiming the newborn and touching them, commonly identifying specific features in the newborn, such as "he has my nose" or "her fingers are long like her father's." This is not an optimal time to instruct infant care to the birthing parent (Fig. 15.6).

TAKE NOTE!

The taking-in phase typically lasts 1 to 2 days and may be the only phase observed by nurses in the hospital setting because of the shortened postpartum stays that are the norm today.

TAKING-HOLD PHASE

The **taking-hold phase**, the second phase of maternal adaptation, is characterized by dependent and independent birthing parent behavior. This phase typically starts on the second to third day postpartum and may last several weeks.

As the patient regains control over their bodily functions during the next few days, they will be taking hold and becoming preoccupied with the present. They will be particularly concerned about their health, the infant's condition, and their ability to care for the infant. The birthing parent demonstrates increased autonomy and mastery of their own body's functioning, and a desire to take charge with support and help from others. They will show independence by caring for themselves and learning to care for their newborn, but they still require assurance that they are doing well as a parent. The birthing parent expresses a strong interest in caring for the infant by themselves. This is a good time to teach infant care to the birthing parent.

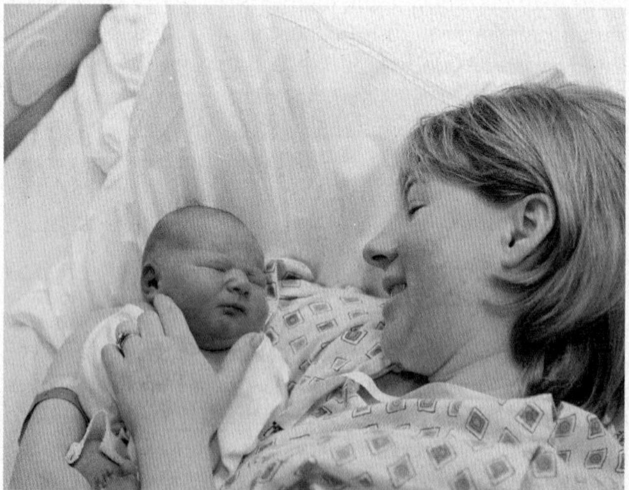

FIGURE 15.6 Parent bonding with newborn during the taking-in phase.

LETTING-GO PHASE

In the **letting-go phase**, the third phase of maternal adaptation, the birthing parent reestablishes relationships with other people. They adapt to parenthood in their new role. They assume the responsibility and care of the newborn with a bit more confidence (Rubin, 1984). The focus of this phase is to move forward by assuming the parental role and to separate themselves from the symbiotic relationship that they and their newborn had during pregnancy. The birthing parent establishes a lifestyle that includes the infant. The birthing parent relinquishes the fantasy infant and accepts the real one.

Nurses have recognized the importance of the process of what is traditionally called becoming a mother (BAM) to maternal–infant nursing since Rubin's report on maternal role attainment (MRA). Birthing parents' perceptions of their competence and/or confidence in parenting and their expressions of love for their infants are affected by age, relationship with their parenting partner, socioeconomic status, birth experience, stress, available support, personality traits, self-concept, child-rearing attitudes, role strain, health status, preparation during pregnancy, relationships with their own parents, depression, and anxiety. Infant variables identified as influencing MRA/BAM include appearance, responsiveness, temperament, and health status. More current research has led to renaming the four stages a birthing parent progresses through in establishing their new identity in BAM because some believe BAM encompasses the transformation the birthing parent experiences better than MRA does:

1. Commitment, attachment to the unborn baby, and preparation for delivery and parenthood during pregnancy
2. Acquaintance/attachment to the infant, learning to care for the infant, and physical restoration during the first 2 to 6 weeks following birth
3. Moving toward a new normal
4. Achievement of a parental identity through redefining self to incorporate parenthood (around 4 months); the birthing parent feels self-confident and competent in their parenting and expresses love for and pleasure in interacting with their infant (Hwang et al., 2022).

The birthing parent's work in the first stage is to make a commitment to the pregnancy and to the safe birth and care of their unborn child. This commitment is associated with a positive adaptation to parenthood. During the second stage while the birthing parent is placing the infant in their family context and learning how to care for the infant, their attachment and attitude toward their infant and their self-confidence and/or sense of competence in parenting consistently indicate an interdependence of these two variables. The nursing care provided during the first two stages is especially important in assisting birthing parents as they begin to parent. Follow-up is needed as parents move toward a new normal, and recognizing a transformation of themselves can continue to reinforce their capabilities (Hwang et al., 2022).

To foster MRA, three specific interventions for nurses were identified in a review of the literature (McCarter et al., 2022). First, instructions about infant care and the infant's capabilities are more effective if they are specifically focused on that particular parent's infant. Second, birthing parents prefer live classes rather than videos so they can ask questions. In short, interactive nurse–patient relationships are associated with positive growth in the parental role. Third, identifying barriers that reduce skin-to-skin periods of parent-to-infant contact during the postpartum hospital stay and intervening to reduce them have implications for both MRA and breastfeeding success, if the birthing parent has chosen this method. Providing times for skin-to-skin contact has a positive impact on the long-term health of both the birthing parent and baby. Nurses who interact with patients long-term during pregnancy, childbirth, and well-child care help build parental competence. Pregnancy, birth, and becoming a parent collectively represent a critical period of physical and emotional upheaval in a birthing person's life. The need for a holistic care approach that supports the emotional and physical health of the dyad is imperative.

Rubin's maternal role framework is far from the only maternal adaptation theory used, especially in recent years. Another theorist, Ramona Mercer, has added to the MRA literature by describing four stages of acquisition birthing parents go through—anticipatory, formal, informal, and personal. The primary process involves the birthing parent bonding with their infant, acquiring competency in caregiving tasks, and finally deriving pleasure in their new role (Mercer, 2004). However, all "transition to motherhood" theories describe the birthing parent in a prescribed role—that of being a "mother" and in a way, a predetermined type of mother. In that sense, transition to motherhood theory is baby centered. New theories need to be developed that are patient centered and conceptualize the birthing parent as an embodied self who is powerful in their own life. Nurses have a vital role to play throughout the entire process to assist the parent in attaining a parental identity.

Partner Psychological Adaptations

For partners, whether they are spouses, significant others, life partners, or friends, becoming a parent or simply sharing in the childbirth experience can be a perplexing time as well as a time of great change. Becoming a new parent can be scary. This transition is influenced by many factors, including participation in childbirth, relationships with significant others, competence in child care, the family role organization, the individual's cultural background, and the method of infant feeding.

Nurses can play a key role in supporting a partner's transition to parenthood by keeping partners informed about birth and postpartum routines, reporting on their newborn's health status, and reviewing infant development. They can also contribute by creating a participative space for new partners during the postpartum period. This can be achieved, for example, by helping partners take on the new role by supporting and promoting their degree of involvement in the process. They can also be encouraged to actively participate in caring for and maintaining contact with the newborns.

TAKE NOTE!

Most research findings stress the importance of early contact between the partner and the newborn as well as participation in infant care activities to foster the relationship (Steen, 2022).

Infants have a powerful effect on their parents and others, who become intensely involved with them (Fig. 15.7). The partner's developing bond with the newborn—a time of intense absorption, preoccupation, and interest—is called **engrossment**.

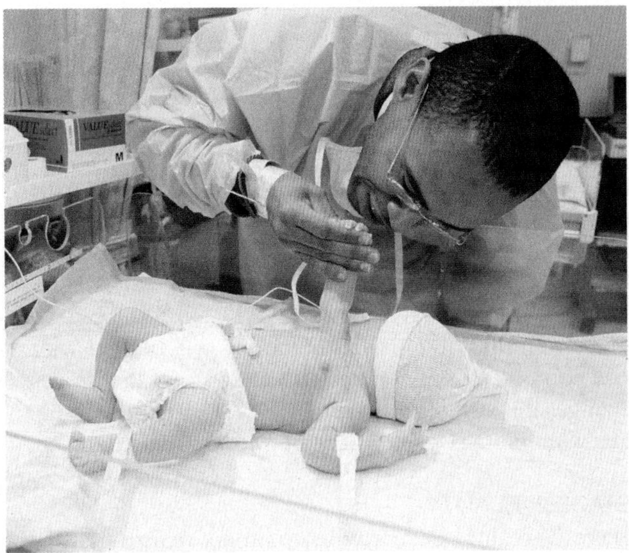

FIGURE 15.7 Engrossment of the new parent and their newborn.

Engrossment

Engrossment is characterized by seven behaviors:

1. Visual awareness of the newborn—the partner perceives the newborn as beautiful.
2. Tactile awareness of the newborn—the partner has a desire to touch or hold the newborn and considers this activity pleasurable.
3. Perception of the newborn as perfect—the partner does not "see" any imperfections.
4. Strong attraction to the newborn—the partner focuses all their attention on the newborn when in the room.
5. Awareness of distinct features of the newborn—the partner can distinguish the newborn from others in the nursery.
6. Extreme elation—the partner feels "high" after the birth of the child.
7. Increased sense of self-esteem—the partner feels proud, "bigger," more mature, and older after the birth of the child (Sears et al., 2022).

Frequently, partners are portrayed as well-meaning but bumbling when caring for newborns. However, they have their own unique way of relating to their newborns and can become just as nurturing—even if they did not give birth to the newborn. A partner's nurturing responses may be less automatic and slower to unfold, but they are capable of a strong bonding attachment to their newborns. Encouraging partners to express their feelings by seeing, touching, and holding the newborn and by cuddling, talking to, and feeding them will help cement this new relationship. Reinforcement of this engrossing behavior helps partners make a positive attachment during this critical period to engage early to build a bond that will serve them well throughout life. Investing in both the infant and their partner early will pay off in later years; infants benefit greatly from having parents with a happy relationship (Sears et al., 2022).

Three-Stage Role Development Process

Similar to birthing parents, partners also go through a predictable three-stage process during the first 3 weeks as they too "try on" their roles as parents. The three stages are expectations, reality, and transition to mastery (Sears et al., 2022).

STAGE 1: EXPECTATIONS

New partners pass through stage 1 (expectations) with preconceptions about what home life will be like with a newborn. Many partners may be unaware of the dramatic changes that can occur when this newborn comes home to live with them. For some, it is an eye-opening experience.

STAGE 2: REALITY

Stage 2 (reality) occurs when partners realize that their expectations in stage 1 are not in line with reality. Their feelings change from elation to sadness, ambivalence, jealousy, and frustration. Many wish to be more involved in the newborn's care and yet do not feel prepared to do so. Some find parenting fun but at the same time do not feel fully prepared to take on that role.

A partner's stress, irritability, and frustration in the days, weeks, and months after the birth of the child can turn into depression, just like that experienced by the birthing parent. Unfortunately, partners rarely discuss their feelings or ask for help, especially during a time when they are supposed to be the "strong one" for the parent who gave birth. Depression in partners can lead to conflicts between the couple, reckless or violent behavior, irritability, substance misuse, interference with infant bonding leading to emotional detachment, feelings of inadequacy, withdrawn parental interactions with the newborn, poor job performance, and substance misuse (Rodriguez, 2023).

Risk factors for partner postpartum depression include previous history of depression, financial problems, a poor relationship with the birthing parent, and an unplanned pregnancy. Symptoms of depression appear 1 to 3 weeks after birth and can include feelings of high stress, anxiety, discouragement, fatigue, headaches, and resentment toward the infant and the attention they are getting. Partners experiencing these symptoms should understand that it is not a sign of weakness, and professional help can be helpful.

STAGE 3: TRANSITION TO MASTERY

In stage 3 (transition to mastery), the partner makes a conscious decision to take control and be at the center of the newborn's life regardless of preparedness. This adjustment period is similar to that of the birthing parent's letting-go phase when they incorporate the newest member into the family.

KEY CONCEPTS

- The puerperium period refers to the first 6 weeks after delivery. During this period, the birthing parent experiences many physiologic and psychological adaptations to return them to the prepregnant state.
- Involution involves three processes: contraction of muscle fibers to reduce stretched ones, catabolism (which reduces enlarged, individual cells), and regeneration of uterine epithelium from the lower layer of the decidua after the upper layers have been sloughed off and shed in lochia.
- Lochia passes through three stages: lochia rubra, lochia serosa, and lochia alba during the postpartum period.
- The birthing parent's blood plasma volume decreases rapidly after birth and returns to normal within 4 weeks postpartum.

- Reva Rubin identified three phases the birthing parent goes through to adjust to their new role: the taking-in, taking-hold, and letting-go phases.
- The transition to parenthood for a partner is influenced by many factors, including participation in childbirth, relationships with significant others, competence in child care, the family role organization, the cultural background, and the method of infant feeding.
- Partners of those who have given birth also go through a predictable three-stage process during the first 3 weeks as they too "try on" their roles as partners. The three stages include expectations, reality, and transition to mastery.

REFERENCES AND RECOMMENDED READINGS

American Academy of Family Physicians. (2024). *Advocate for breastfeeding.* https://www.aafp.org/family-physician/patient-care/prevention-wellness/birth-control-pregnancy-childbirth/breastfeeding.html

American Academy of Pediatrics. (2023). *Perinatal depression in partners: Can both parents get the "baby blues?"* https://www.healthychildren.org/English/ages-stages/prenatal/delivery-beyond/Pages/dads-can-get-postpartum-depression-too.aspx#

American College of Obstetricians and Gynecologists. (2022). *Exercise after pregnancy.* https://www.acog.org/womens-health/faqs/exercise-after-pregnancy

Baker, B. (2024). Physical and psychological changes after childbirth. In B. J. Baker, J. Janke, & The Association of Women's Health, Obstetric and Neonatal Nurses (Eds.), *Core curriculum for maternal-newborn nursing* (6th ed.). Elsevier.

Balaram, K., & Marwaha, R. (2023). Postpartum blues. *StatPearls.* https://www.ncbi.nlm.nih.gov/books/NBK554546/

Berens, P. (2024). Overview of the postpartum period: Normal physiology and routine maternal care. *UpToDate.* Retrieved April 14, 2024, from https://www.uptodate.com/contents/overview-of-the-postpartum-period-normal-physiology-and-routine-maternal-care

Blondon, M., & Skeith, L. (2022). Preventing postpartum venous thromboembolism in 2022: A narrative review. *Frontiers in Cardiovascular Medicine, 9,* 886416. https://doi.org/10.3389/fcvm.2022.886416

Bogdan, I., Turliuc, M. N., & Candel, O. S. (2022). Transition to parenthood and marital satisfaction: A meta-analysis. *Frontiers in Psychology, 13,* 901362. https://doi.org/10.3389/fpsyg.2022.901362

Boufides, C. H. (2022). Despite being crucial to reducing health disparities, culturally-relevant health care programs remain poorly funded. *The Network for Public Health Law.* https://www.networkforphl.org/news-insights/despite-being-crucial-to-reducing-health-disparities-culturally-relevant-health-care-programs-remain-poorly-funded/

Centers for Disease Control and Prevention. (2023a). *Breastfeeding: Facts.* https://www.cdc.gov/breastfeeding/data/facts.html

Centers for Disease Control and Prevention. (2023b). *Depression during and after pregnancy.* https://www.cdc.gov/reproductivehealth/features/maternal-depression/

Chauhan, G., & Tadi, P. (2022). Physiology, postpartum changes. *StatPearls.* https://www.ncbi.nlm.nih.gov/books/NBK555904/

Clarke-Deelder, E., Opondo, K., Achieng, E., Garg, L., Han, D., Henry, J., Guha, M., Lightbourne, A., Makin, J., Miller, N., Otieno, B., Borovac-Pinheiro, A., Suarez-Rebling, D., Menzies, N. A., Burke, T., Oguttu, M., McConnell, M., & Cohen, J. (2023). Quality of care for postpartum hemorrhage: A direct observation study in referral hospitals in Kenya. *PLOS Global Public Health, 3*(3), e0001670. https://doi.org/10.1371/journal.pgph.0001670

Cunningham, F. G., Leveno, K. J., Dashe, J. S., Hoffman, B. L., Spong, C. Y., & Casey, B. M. (2022a). The puerperium. In F. G. Cunningham, K. J. Leveno, J. S. Dashe, B. L. Hoffman, C. Y. Spong, & B. M. Casey (Eds.), *William's obstetrics* (26th ed.). McGraw Hill.

Cunningham, F. G., Leveno, K. J., Dashe, J. S., Hoffman, B. L., Spong, C. Y., & Casey, B. M. (2022b). Thromboembolic disorders. In F. G. Cunningham, K. J. Leveno, J. S. Dashe, B. L. Hoffman, C. Y. Spong, & B. M. Casey (Eds.), *William's obstetrics* (26th ed.). McGraw Hill.

Daxue Consulting. (2022). *The endless steps of Chinese postpartum traditions: Confinement.* https://daxueconsulting.com/chinese-postpartum-traditions/

Dekker, R. (2022). *Evidence on: Eating and drinking during labor.* https://evidencebasedbirth.com/evidence-eating-drinking-labor/

Delgado-Perez, E., Rodriguez-Costa, I., Vergara-Perez, F., Blanco-Morales, M., & Torres-Lacomba, M. (2022). Recovering sexuality after childbirth. What strategies do women adopt? A qualitative study. *International Journal of Environmental Research and Public Health, 19*(2), 950. https://www.ncbi.nlm.nih.gov/pmc/articles/PMC8775547/

Durbin, K. (2022). *Lactational amenorrhea: Fertility, birth control and breastfeeding.* https://www.llli.org/lactational-amenorrhea-fertility-birth-control-and-breastfeeding/

Ferraro, L. M. (2024). Postpartum care. In M. O'Connell, J. A. Smith, & L. M. Borgelt (Eds.), *Women's health across the lifespan* (3rd ed.). McGraw Hill.

Frese, B. J., & Nguyen, M. H. T. (2022). The evolution of maternal role attainment: A theory analysis. *Advances in Nursing Science, 45*(4), 323–334. https://pubmed.ncbi.nlm.nih.gov/35533316/

Garcia-Izquierdo, I., & Montalt, V. (2022). Cultural competence and the role of the patient's mother tongue: A exploratory study of health professionals' perceptions. *Societies, 12*(2), 53. https://doi.org/10.3390/soc12020053

Grigsby, L. L. (2023). *What other cultures can teach the US about postpartum rituals.* Parents. https://www.parents.com/pregnancy/giving-birth/what-the-u-s-can-learn-about-the-time-after-birth-from-cultures-around-the-world/

Hwang, W. Y., Choi, S. Y., & An, H. J. (2022). Concept analysis of transition to motherhood: A methodological study. *Korean Journal of Women's Health Nursing, 28*(1), 8–17. https://doi.org/10.4069/kjwhn.2022.01.04

Kansky, C., & Isaacs, C. (2021). *Normal and abnormal puerperium.* https://emedicine.medscape.com/article/260187-overview#a1

Karsnitz, D. B., & Wilhite, K. (2022). Overview of postpartum care. In K. D. Schuiling & F. E. Likis (Eds.), *Gynecologic health care* (4th ed., pp. 1706–1747). Jones & Bartlett Learning.

Kodali, B. S., & Segal, S. (2023). Maternal physiological changes during pregnancy, labor, and the postpartum period. In S. Segal & B. S. Kodali (Eds.), *Datta's obstetric anesthesia handbook* (pp. 1–17). Springer. https://doi.org/10.1007/978-3-031-41893-8_1

Kohlhoff, J., Karlov, L., Dadds, M., Barnett, B., Silove, D., & Eapen, V. (2022). The contributions of maternal oxytocin and maternal sensitivity to infant attachment security. *Attachment & Human Development, 24*(4), 525–540. https://doi.org/10.1080/14616734.2021.2018472

La Leche League International. (2024). *Engorgement.* https://www.llli.org/breastfeeding-info/engorgement/

Li, P. (2024). *Attachment theory by Bowlby & Ainsworth.* https://www.parentingforbrain.com/what-is-attachment-parenting-attachment-theory/

Liu, J., Wilcox, S., Hutto, B., Turner-McGrievy, G., & Wingard, E. (2022). Effects of a lifestyle intervention on postpartum weight retention among women with elevated weight. *Obesity: A Research Journal, 30*(7), 1370–1379. https://doi.org/10.1002/oby.23449

Lopez-Gonzalez, D. M., & Kopparapu, A. K. (2023). Postpartum care of the new mother. *StatPearls.* https://www.ncbi.nlm.nih.gov/books/NBK565875/

Major, M. (2020). *What postpartum care looks like around the world, and why the U.S. is missing the mark.* https://www.healthline.com/health/pregnancy/what-post-childbirth-care-looks-like-around-the-world-and-why-the-u-s-is-missing-the-mark#Readiness

McCarter, D., Law, A. A., Cabullo, H., & Pinto, K. (2022). Scoping review of postpartum discharge education provided by nurses. *Journal of Obstetric, Gynecologic, & Neonatal Nursing, 51*(4), 377–387. https://doi.org/10.1016/j.jogn.2022.03.002

Meek, J. Y., Noble, L., & Section on Breastfeeding. (2022). Policy statement: Breastfeeding and the use of human milk. *Pediatrics, 150*(1), e2022057988. https://doi.org/10.1542/peds.2022-057988

Mercer, R. T. (2004). Becoming a mother versus maternal role attainment. *Journal of Nursing Scholarship, 36*(3), 226–232. https://doi.org/10.1111/j.1547-5069.2004.04042.x

Mohr, S., Raio, L., Gobrecht-Keller, U., Imboden, S., Mueller, M. D., & Kuhn, A. (2022). Postpartum urinary retention: What are the sequelae? A long-term study and review of the literature. *International Urogynecology Journal, 33*(6), 1601–1608. https://doi.org/10.1007/s00192-021-05074-5

National Association of Pediatric Nurse Practitioners, Breastfeeding Education Special Interest Group, Busch, D. W., Silbert-Flagg, J., Ryngaert, M., & Scott, A. (2019). NAPNAP position statement on breastfeeding. *Journal of Pediatric Health Care, 33,* A6–A10 https://doi.org/10.1016/j.pedhc.2018.08.011

O'Malley, D., Smith, V., & Higgins, A. (2022). Sexual health issues postpartum—A mixed methods study of women's help-seeking behavior after the birth of their first baby. *Midwifery, 104,* 103196. https://doi.org/10.1016/j.midw.2021.103196

Oakley, A. M., & Patel, B. C. (2023). Stretch marks. *StatPearls.* https://www.ncbi.nlm.nih.gov/books/NBK436005/

ObG Project. (2022). *ACOG redefines the postpartum visit—The 'fourth Trimester.'* https://www.obgproject.com/2022/04/25/acog-revises-redefines-postpartum-visit/

Pillay, J., & Davis, T. J. (2023). Physiology, lactation. *StatPearls.* https://www.ncbi.nlm.nih.gov/books/NBK499981/

Rahmani, A., Fallahi, A., Allahqoli, L., Grylka-Baeschlin, S., & Alkatout, I. (2023). How do new mothers describe their postpartum sexual quality of life? A qualitative study. *BMC Women's Health, 23*(1). https://doi.org/10.1186/s12905-023-02619-2

Ramar, C. N., & Grimes, W. R. (2023). Perineal lacerations. *StatPearls.* https://www.ncbi.nlm.nih.gov/books/NBK559068/

Rodriguez, A. (2023). Dads develop postpartum depression, too, and it can impact their child's mental health. *USA Today.* https://www.usatoday.com/story/news/health/2023/08/19/postpartum-depression-affects-dads-too-can-put-child-at-risk/70603530007/

Roudsari, R. L., Sharifi, F., & Goudarzi, F. (2023). Barriers to the participation of men in reproductive health care: A systematic review and meta-synthesis. *BMC Public Health, 23*(1), 818. https://doi.org/10.1186/s12889-023-15692-x

Rubin, R. (1984). *Maternal identity and the maternal experience.* Springer.

Ruggeri, A. (2022). *Male postnatal depression: Why men struggle in silence.* https://www.bbc.com/worklife/article/20220601-male-postnatal-depression-why-men-struggle-in-silence

Sears, W., Sears, M., Sears, R. W., & Sears, J. (2022). *The Sears baby book: Everything you need to know about your baby from birth to age two* (4th ed.). Hachette Book Group.

Segal, N. A., Boyer, E. R., Teran-Yengle, P., Glass, N. A., Hillstrom, H. J., & Yack, H. J. (2013). Pregnancy leads to lasting changes in foot structure. *American Journal of Physical Medicine & Rehabilitation, 92*(3), 232–240. https://doi.org/10.1097/PHM.0b013e31827443a9

Sheppard, S. (2023). *How postpartum depression affects dads.* https://www.verywellmind.com/what-is-male-postpartum-depression-5188022

Simsek, A., Balkan, E., & Caliskan, E. (2022). Determination of mothers' thoughts and adaptation behaviors regarding the infant: A descriptive study. *Pediatrics & Neonatology, 63*(3), 276–282. https://doi.org/10.1016/j.pedneo.2021.12.009

Steen, M. (2022). Why is newborn baby skin-to-skin contact with dads and non-birthing parents important? Here's what the science says. *The Conversation,* https://theconversation.com/why-is-newborn-baby-skin-to-skin-contact-with-dads-and-non-birthing-parents-important-heres-what-the-science-says-188927

Tan, M. L., Ng, K. L., Loh, L. W. L., Haugan, G., Wang, W., & He, H. G. (2022). A descriptive qualitative study exploring the postpartum confinement experiences among first-time mothers from the three major ethnic groups in Singapore. *Midwifery, 114,* 103463. https://doi.org/10.1016/j.midw.2022.103463

United Nations International Children's Emergency Fund. (2022). *Five common breastfeeding problems.* https://www.unicef.org/parenting/food-nutrition/5-common-breastfeeding-problems

Wang, Y. X., Arvizu, M., Rich-Edwards, J. W., Manson, J. E., Wang, L., & Missmer, S. A. (2022). Breastfeeding duration and subsequent risk of mortality among US women: A prospective cohort study. *The Lancet, 54,* 101693. https://doi.org/10.1016/j.eclinm.2022.101693

Wisner, K. (2022). Postpartum pain management. *MCN, The American Journal of Maternal/Child Nursing, 47*(1), 52. https://doi.org/10.1097/NMC.0000000000000774

Yang, F., & Liao, H. (2022). The influence of obstetric factors on the occurrence of pelvic floor dysfunction in women in the early postpartum period. *International Journal of General Medicine, 15,* 3353–3361. https://doi.org/10.2147/IJGM.S355913

Yava, A., Tosun, B., Papp, K., Tóthová, V., Şahin, E., Yılmaz, E., Dirgar, E., Hellerová, V., Tricas-Sauras, S., Prosen, M., Ličen, S., Karnjuš, I., Tamayo, M., & Leyva-Moral, J. M. (2023). Developing the better and effective nursing education for improving transcultural nursing skills cultural competence and cultural sensitivity assessment tool (BENEFITS-CCCSAT). *BMC Nursing, 22*(1), 331. https://doi.org/10.1186/s12912-023-01476-6

DEVELOPING CLINICAL JUDGMENT

PRACTICING FOR NCLEX

1. Postpartum breast engorgement occurs 48 to 72 hours after giving birth. What physiologic change influences breast engorgement?
   a. An increase in blood and lymph supply to the breasts
   b. An increase in estrogen and progesterone levels
   c. A dramatic increase in colostrum production
   d. Fluid retention in the breasts due to the intravenous fluids given during labor

2. In the taking-in maternal role phase described by Rubin, the nurse would expect the birthing parent's behavior to be characterized in what way?
   a. Gaining self-confidence
   b. Adjusting to their new relationships
   c. Being passive and dependent
   d. Resuming control over their life

3. The nurse is explaining to a postpartum patient 48 hours after childbirth that the afterpains they are experiencing can be the result of which factor?
   a. Abdominal cramping as a sign of endometriosis
   b. A small infant weighing less than 8 lb
   c. Pregnancies that were too closely spaced
   d. Contractions of the uterus after birth

4. The nurse would expect a postpartum patient to experience lochia in which sequence?
   a. Rubra, alba, serosa
   b. Rubra, serosa, alba
   c. Serosa, alba, rubra
   d. Alba, rubra, serosa

5. The nurse is assessing a patient who gave birth to their first child 5 days ago. What findings would the nurse expect?
   a. Cream-colored lochia; uterus above the umbilicus
   b. Bright-red lochia with clots; uterus two fingerbreadths below umbilicus
   c. Light pink or brown lochia; uterus four to five fingerbreadths below umbilicus
   d. Yellow, mucousy lochia; uterus at the level of the umbilicus

6. Prioritize the postpartum patient's needs 4 hours after giving birth by placing a number 1, 2, 3, or 4 in the blank before each need.
   a. ________ Learn how to hold and cuddle the infant.
   b. ________ Watch a baby bath demonstration given by the nurse.
   c. ________ Sleep and rest without being disturbed for a few hours.
   d. ________ Interaction time (first 30 minutes) with the infant to facilitate bonding.

7. Immediately after childbirth in the recovery area, the nurse observes the patient's partner's fascination and interest in the new child. What is this behavior termed?
   a. Attachment
   b. Engrossment
   c. Bonding
   d. Temperament

8. The nurse provided instructions to a postpartum patient about postpartum blues. Which statement by the patient indicates understanding?
   a. "I will need to take medication daily to treat the anxiety and sadness."
   b. "I will call the OB support line only if I start to hear voices."
   c. "I will contact my doctor if I become dizzy and felt nauseated."
   d. "I will feel like laughing 1 minute and crying the next minute."

CRITICAL THINKING EXERCISES

1. A new nurse assigned to the postpartum unit comments on the oncoming shift that a 25-year-old primipara seems lazy and shows no initiative in taking care of themselves or their baby. The nurse reported that this patient talks excessively about their labor and birth experience and seems preoccupied with their own needs, not their newborn's care. The nurse wonders if something is wrong with this patient because they seem so self-centered and have to be directed to do everything.
   a. Is there something to be concerned about in this patient's behavior? Why or why not?
   b. What maternal role phase is being described by the nurse?
   c. What role can the nurse play to support the patient through this phase?

2. A primipara gave birth to a healthy baby yesterday. Their partner seemed elated at the birth, calling their friends and family on their cell phone minutes after the birth. The partner praised the birthing parent for their efforts. Today, when the nurse walked into their room, the partner seemed anxious around the infant and called for the nurse whenever the baby cried or needed a diaper change. The partner seemed standoffish when asked to hold the infant and spent time talking to other people in the waiting room, leaving the birthing parent alone in the room.
   a. Would you consider this behavior to be normal at this time?
   b. What might the partner be feeling at this time?
   c. How can the nurse help this new parent adjust to their new role?

STUDY ACTIVITIES

1. Find an internet resource that discusses general postpartum care for new parents who might have questions after discharge. Evaluate the website's information as to how credible, accurate, and current the information is.
2. Prepare a teaching plan for new birthing parents, outlining the various physiologic changes that will take place after discharge.
3. The term that describes the return of the uterus to its prepregnant state is ___________.
4. A deviated fundus to the right side of the abdomen would indicate a ____________.

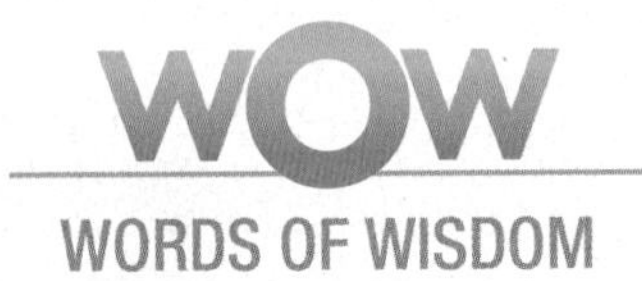

WORDS OF WISDOM

Parenting is an intimate, interactive, and continuous lifelong process.

16

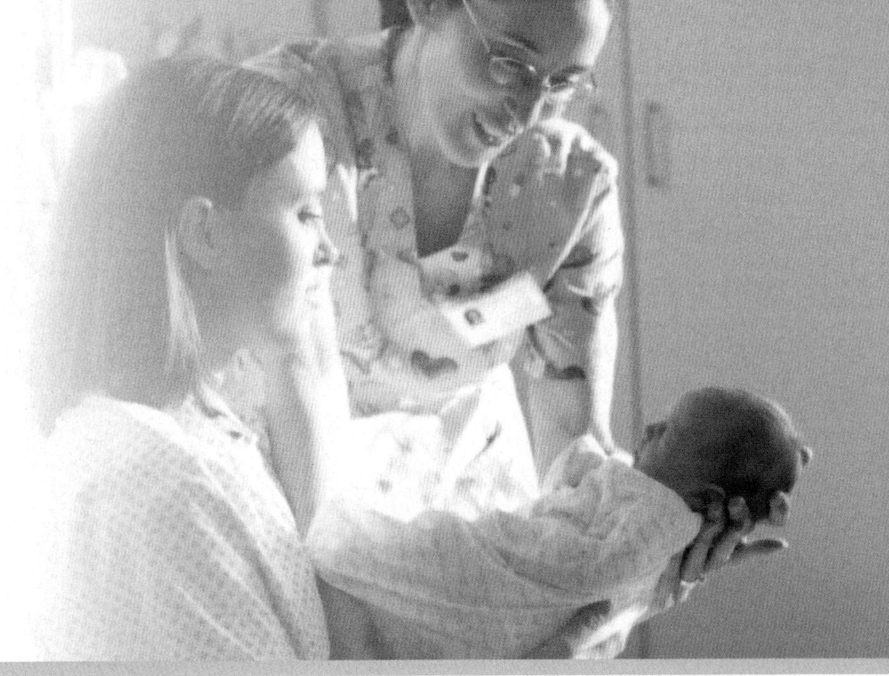

Nursing Management During the Postpartum Period

LEARNING OBJECTIVES

Upon completion of the chapter, you will be able to:

1. Characterize the normal physiologic and psychological adaptations to the postpartum period.
2. Determine the parameters that need to be assessed during the postpartum period.
3. Compare and contrast bonding to the attachment process.
4. Select behaviors that enhance or inhibit the attachment process.
5. Outline nursing management for the birthing parent and their family during the postpartum period.
6. Examine the role of the nurse in promoting successful breastfeeding.
7. Plan areas of health education needed for discharge planning, home care, and follow-up.

KEY TERMS

attachment
bonding
en face position (on[h] fas pŏ-zish′ŏn)
pelvic floor muscle exercises
peribottle
postpartum blues
sitz bath

Raina, a 24-year-old primipara, has just been admitted to the postpartum unit. Her husband sits at the bedside but doesn't seem to outwardly provide her any physical or emotional support after Raina's lengthy labor and difficult birth.

INTRODUCTION

Parenthood can be special, but the postpartum period is a time of major adjustments and adaptations not just for the birthing parent but for all members of the family. It is during this time that parenting starts and a relationship with the newborn begins. A positive, loving relationship between parents and the newborn promotes the emotional well-being of all. This relationship endures and has profound effects on the child's growth and development.

TAKE NOTE!

Parenting is a skill that is often learned by trial and error with varying degrees of success. Successful parenting, a continuous and complex interactive process, requires parents to learn new skills and integrate the new member into the family.

Once the infant is born, each system in the birthing parent's body takes several weeks to return to its nonpregnant state. The physiologic changes that take place during the postpartum period are dramatic. Nurses should be aware of these changes and should be able to make observations and assessments to validate normal occurrences and detect any deviations.

This chapter describes the nursing care of the birthing person and their family during the postpartum period. (See Chapter 21 for a detailed discussion of the postpartum care of the patient undergoing a surgical birth.) Nursing care during the postpartum period focuses on assessing the patient's ability to adapt to the physiologic and psychological changes occurring at this time (see Chapter 15 for a detailed discussion of these adaptations). This chapter outlines physical assessment parameters for new birthing parents and newborns. It also focuses on bonding and attachment behaviors; nurses need to be aware of these behaviors so they can perform appropriate interventions as needed. Family members are also assessed to determine how well they are making the transition to this new stage.

Based on the assessment findings, the nurse plans and implements care to address the family's needs. Steps to address physiologic needs such as comfort, self-care, nutrition, and contraception are described. Ways to help the birthing parent and their family adapt to the birth of the newborn are also discussed (Fig. 16.1). Because of today's shortened hospital stays, the nurse may be able to focus only on priority needs and may need to arrange for follow-up in the home to ensure that all the family's needs are met.

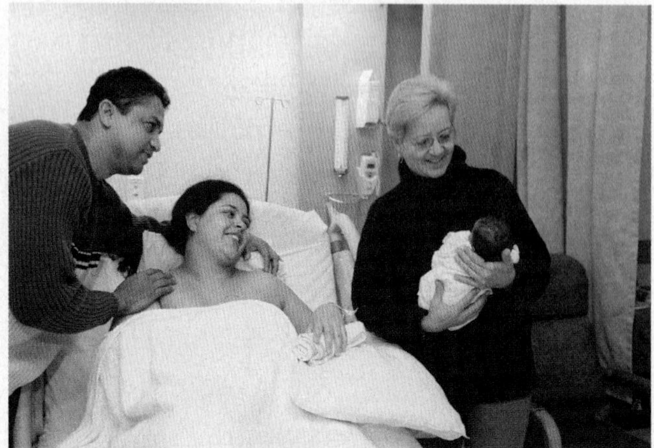

FIGURE 16.1 Parents and grandmother interacting with the newborn.

SOCIAL SUPPORT AND CULTURAL CONSIDERATIONS

The postpartum period is a critical stage in which a series of changes in the patient occurs, which impact them at the physical, psychological, and social levels. In addition to physical assessment and care of the patient in the postpartum period, strong social support is vital to help them integrate the baby into the family. A key to providing effective postpartum care is to understand the patient in their social and cultural context so that all care provided demonstrates cultural humility and is sensitive. In today's mobile society, extended families may live far away and may be unable to help care for the new family. As a result, many new parents turn to health care providers for information as well as physical and emotional support during this adjustment period. Nurses can be an invaluable resource by serving as mentors, teaching about self-care measures and baby care basics, and providing emotional support. Nurses can support the new parent by offering physical care, emotional support, information, and practical help. The nurse's support and care through this critical time can increase the new parents' confidence, giving them a sense of accomplishment in their parenting skills. One important intervention during the postpartum period is the promotion of breastfeeding.

As in all nursing care, nurses should provide care using cultural humility during the postpartum period. The nurse should engage in ongoing cultural self-assessment and address any stereotypes that perpetuate prejudice or discrimination against any patient. The postpartum period is noted for traditional practices related to rest, healing, and consumption of food and drink. In many cultures, birthing parents and grandparents have a great deal of influence over new parents, so nurses need to be aware of the patient's culture and help them integrate their beliefs and practices into contemporary health care practice. New parents may need guidance in areas of physical warmth, massage, hygiene, and physical activity where cultural practices may vary (LER Team, 2022). Providing culturally humble and competent nursing care during the postpartum period requires time, open-mindedness, and patience. It is vital that nurses know the cultural preferences of the patient they serve since we live in a multicultural society. Cultural practices and rituals are important for family-building. Allow the patient and their family to educate you about their cultural practices. Listen with an open mind and be willing to learn something new (LER Team, 2022). The global migration of diverse populations presents nurses with the challenge of providing care to unprecedented numbers of patients and their families with health care beliefs and practices that differ from their own. Sensitivity cannot be assumed; it needs to be nurtured and developed. The skill set needed by nurses to provide culturally humble care to postpartum patients and their families includes understanding their beliefs, experiences, and family environment; facilitating their language through appropriate use of interpreters so that the information provided can be understood; and compassionately respecting patients and their human rights. For instance, many cultures value traditions and the involvement of elders in the extended family. For example, Chinese females are traditionally cared for by other female family members for a month following childbirth, and they must follow rigid rules related to tradition. Many modern Chinese birthing parents want to abandon some of those rules and will seek the support of their health care provider in explaining to family members why they feel those rules are unnecessary (Zhang & Hanser, 2023). This can create tension among family members. To promote positive outcomes, the nurse should be sensitive to the patient's and family's culture, religion, and influences based on heritage and ethnicity. It is important to understand, respect, and support patients of all cultures and their practices around childbirth (see "Providing Optimal Cultural Care" in the "Nursing Interventions" section).

Remember the couple introduced at the beginning of the chapter? When the postpartum nurse comes to examine Raina, her husband quickly leaves the room and returns a short time later after the examination is complete. How do you interpret his behavior toward his wife? What might you communicate to this couple?

NURSING ASSESSMENT IN THE POSTPARTUM PERIOD

Many adaptations and adjustments must be made to accommodate the new family member. Nurses need to carry out a thorough assessment of the patient's discomfort and attempt to implement both preventive and therapeutic measures to reduce any discomfort to improve the patient's quality of life in one of the more complex phases of their life (Wisner, 2022). The nurse's focus is on assisting families to maximize their adjustment, surveillance for maladaptation, education, consultation, and collaboration as needed. Comprehensive nursing assessment begins within an hour after the patient gives birth and continues through discharge.

TAKE NOTE!

Nurses need a firm grasp of expected findings to be able to recognize unexpected findings and intervene appropriately.

This postpartum assessment includes vital signs and physical and psychosocial assessments. It also includes assessing the parents and other family members, such as siblings and grandparents, for attachment and bonding with the newborn. Although the exact protocol may vary among facilities, postpartum assessment is typically performed as follows:

- During the first hour: every 15 minutes
- During the second hour: every 30 minutes
- During the first 24 hours: every 4 hours
- After 24 hours: Follow the institution's protocol (Baker, 2024).

During each assessment, keep in mind risk factors that may lead to complications such as infection or hemorrhage during the recovery period (Box 16.1). Early identification is critical to ensure prompt intervention.

The postpartum period is a time of transition for the birthing parent. The end of the pregnancy and childbirth initiates physiologic changes as many body systems return to their nonpregnant states. Nurses need to be aware of

BOX **16.1** Factors Increasing a Birthing Person's Risk for Postpartum Complications

Risk Factors for Postpartum Infection

- Operative procedure (forceps, cesarean birth, vacuum extraction)
- History of diabetes, including gestational-onset diabetes
- Prolonged labor (more than 24 hours)
- Use of indwelling urinary catheter
- Anemia (hemoglobin <10.5 mg/dL)
- Multiple vaginal examinations during labor
- Prolonged rupture of membranes (>24 hours)
- Manual extraction of placenta
- Compromised immune system (HIV-positive)

Risk Factors for Postpartum Hemorrhage

- Precipitous labor (less than 3 hours)
- Uterine atony
- Placenta previa or abruptio placenta
- Labor induction or augmentation
- Operative procedures (vacuum extraction, forceps, cesarean birth)
- Retained placental fragments
- Prolonged third stage of labor (more than 30 minutes)
- Multiparity, more than three births closely spaced
- Uterine overdistention (large infant, twins, hydramnios)
- Obesity

Boushra, M., & Rahman, O. (2023). Postpartum infection. *StatPearls*. https://www.ncbi.nlm.nih.gov/books/NBK560804/; Smith, J. R., Talavera, F., & Rivlin, M. E. (2022). *Postpartum hemorrhage*. Medscape. https://emedicine.medscape.com/article/275038-overview#a7

the normal physiologic and psychological changes that take place in patients' bodies and minds in order to provide comprehensive care during the postpartum period. In addition to patient and family teaching, one of the most significant responsibilities of the postpartum nurse is to recognize potential complications after childbirth.

As with any assessment, always review the patient's medical records for information about their pregnancy, labor, and birth. Note any preexisting conditions, any complications that occurred during pregnancy, labor, birth, and immediately afterward, and any treatments provided.

Postpartum assessment of the birthing parent typically includes vital signs, pain level, epidural site inspection for infection, and a systematic head-to-toe review of body systems. The acronym BUBBLE-EE—*b*reasts, *u*terus, *b*ladder, *b*owels, *l*ochia, *e*pisiotomy/perineum/epidural site, *e*xtremities, and *e*motional status—can be used as a guide for this head-to-toe review.

While assessing the patient and their family during the postpartum period, be alert for danger signs (Box 16.2). Notify the primary health care provider immediately if any are noted.

Vital Signs Assessment

Obtain vital signs and compare them with the previous values, noting and reporting any deviations. Vital sign changes can be an early indicator of complications.

Temperature

Use a consistent measurement technique (oral, axillary, or tympanic) to get the most accurate readings. Typically, the birthing parent's temperature during the first 24 hours postpartum is within the normal range or a low-grade elevation up to 99°F (37.2°C). This elevation may be the result of dehydration, sweating, or diaphoresis. The rise in temperature can also be attributed to the systemic absorption of metabolites accumulated due to muscle contractions. Temperature should be normal after 24 hours with the replacement of fluids lost during labor and birth (Chauhan & Tadi, 2023).

BOX 16.2 Postpartum Danger Signs

- Fever > 100.4°F (38°C)
- Foul-smelling lochia or an unexpected change in color or amount
- Large blood clots or bleeding that saturates a peripad in an hour
- Severe headaches or blurred vision that do not go away
- Visual changes, such as blurred vision or spots, or headaches
- Calf pain with dorsiflexion of the foot
- Sudden weight gain
- Feeling faint, dizzy, or weak
- Rapid heart rate
- Swelling, redness, or discharge at the episiotomy, epidural, or abdominal sites
- Dysuria, burning, or incomplete emptying of the bladder
- Shortness of breath or difficulty breathing without exertion
- Depression or extreme mood swings

Ogunyemi, D. (2024b). *Three conditions to watch for after childbirth.* https://www.acog.org/womens-health/experts-and-stories/the-latest/3-conditions-to-watch-for-after-childbirth

Pulse

The patient's pulse rate may be elevated for a few hours after a temperature above 99°F (37.2°C) at any time, or an abnormal temperature after the first 24 hours may indicate infection and must be reported. Abnormal temperature readings warrant continued monitoring until an infection can be ruled out through cultures or blood studies. An elevated temperature can identify sepsis, which results in significant morbidity and mortality worldwide. To improve the outcome, it is essential that nurses be vigilant in obtaining accurate values and monitoring childbirth due to the labor pain experienced, which usually normalizes by the next day (Chauhan & Tadi, 2023). Pulse rates of 60 to 80 beats/min (bpm) are normal during the first week after birth, yet in the first few days, the pulse may be as low as 40 to 60 bpm (Baker, 2024). This pulse rate is called puerperal bradycardia. Tachycardia in the postpartum patient can suggest anxiety, excitement, fatigue, pain, excessive blood loss or delayed hemorrhage, infection, or underlying cardiac problems. Any pulse rate higher than 100 bpm warrants further investigation to rule out complications (Baker, 2024).

Respirations

Respiratory rates in the postpartum patient should be within the normal range of 12 to 20 breaths/min at rest. Pulmonary function typically returns to the prepregnant state after childbirth when the diaphragm descends and the organs revert to their normal positions. Any change in respiratory rate out of the normal range might indicate pulmonary edema, atelectasis (a side effect of epidural anesthesia), or pulmonary embolism (PE) and must be reported. Lungs should be clear on auscultation.

Blood Pressure

Assess the patient's blood pressure (BP) and compare it with their usual range. Report any deviation from this range. Immediately after childbirth, the BP should remain the same as during labor. An increase in BP could indicate gestational hypertension, while a decrease could indicate dehydration, shock, orthostatic hypotension, or a side effect of epidural anesthesia. In the patient with preeclampsia, BP usually gradually returns to normal levels following childbirth. Postpartum onset of preeclampsia may occur from 2 days to 6 weeks following birth, and investigation is necessary if the BP is higher than 140/90 mm Hg (August & Sibai, 2024). BP may also vary based on the patient's position, so assess BP with the patient in the same position every time. Be alert for orthostatic hypotension, which can occur when the patient moves rapidly from a lying or sitting position to a standing one.

Pain

Pain, the fifth vital sign, is assessed along with the other four parameters. Question the patient about the type of pain, its location, and severity. Have the patient rate the pain using a numeric scale from 0 to 10 points. Nursing care should focus on providing comfort measures to ease pain, which might include perineal care, a clean gown, mouth care, providing warm blankets, ensuring adequate fluid intake to facilitate healing, repositioning frequently, and encouraging rest between assessments.

Many postpartum orders will have the nurse premedicate the patient routinely for afterbirth pains rather than waiting for the patient to experience them first. The goal of pain management is to have the patient's pain scale rating maintained between 0 and 2 points at all times, especially after breastfeeding. This can be accomplished by assessing the patient's pain level frequently and preventing pain by administering analgesics. If the patient has severe pain in the perineal region despite the use of physical comfort measures, check for a hematoma by inspecting and palpating the area. If one is found, notify the health care provider immediately.

Physical Examination

Physical examination of the postpartum patient focuses on assessing the breasts, uterus, bladder, bowels, lochia, episiotomy/perineum and epidural site, and extremities.

Breasts

Inspect the breasts for size, contour, asymmetry, engorgement, or erythema. Check the nipples for cracks, redness, fissures, or bleeding, and note whether they are erect, flat, or inverted. Flat or inverted nipples can make breastfeeding challenging for both parent and infant. Cracked, blistered, fissured, bruised, or bleeding nipples in the breastfeeding person are generally indications that the baby is improperly positioned on the breast. Palpate the breasts lightly to ascertain if they are soft, filling, or engorged, and document your findings. For parents who are not breastfeeding, use a gentle, light touch to avoid breast stimulation, which would exacerbate engorgement.

Lactogenesis (the onset of milk secretion) is initially triggered by the delivery of the placenta, which results in falling levels of estrogen and progesterone with the continued presence of prolactin. If the parent is not breastfeeding, the prolactin levels fall and return to normal levels within 2 to 3 weeks. As milk starts to come in, the breasts become firmer; this is charted as "filling." Engorged breasts are hard, tender, and taut. Ask the patient if they are having any nipple discomfort. Palpate the breasts for any nodules, masses, or areas of warmth, which may indicate a plugged duct that may progress to mastitis if not treated promptly. Any discharge from the nipple should be described and documented if it is not colostrum (creamy yellow) or foremilk (bluish white). Over the first week, the breast milk matures and contains all necessary nutrients in the neonatal period. The breast milk continues to change throughout the breastfeeding period to meet the changing demands of the growing infant.

Uterus

Assess the fundus (top portion of the uterus) to determine the degree of uterine involution. If possible, have the patient empty their bladder before assessing the fundus and auscultate their bowel sounds prior to uterine palpation. If the patient has had a cesarean birth and has a patient-controlled anesthesia (PCA) pump, instruct them to self-medicate prior to fundal assessment to decrease their discomfort.

Using a two-handed approach with the patient in the supine position with their knees flexed slightly and the bed in a flat position or as low as possible, palpate the abdomen gently, feeling for the top of the uterus while the other hand is placed on the lower segment of the uterus to stabilize it (Fig. 16.2).

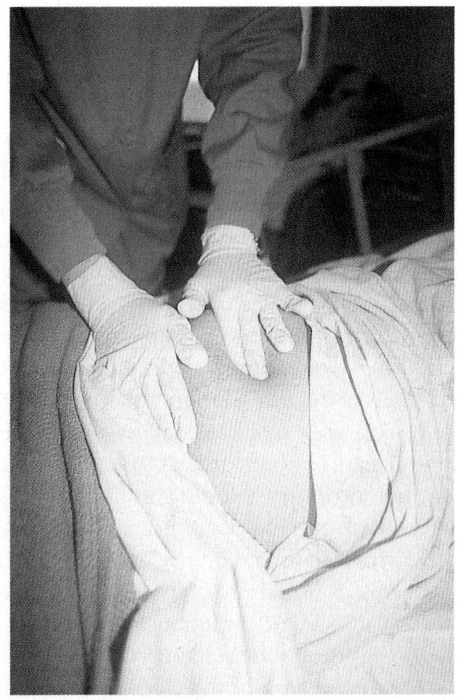

FIGURE 16.2 Palpating the fundus.

The fundus should be midline and should feel firm. A boggy or relaxed uterus is a sign of uterine atony (loss of muscle tone in the uterus). This can be the result of bladder distention, which displaces the uterus upward and to the right, or retained placental fragments. Either situation predisposes the patient to hemorrhage.

Once the fundus is located, place your index finger on the fundus and count the number of fingerbreadths between the fundus and the umbilicus (one fingerbreadth is approximately equal to 1 cm). One to two hours after birth, the fundus is typically between the umbilicus and the symphysis pubis. Approximately 6 to 12 hours after birth, the fundus is usually at the level of the umbilicus. If the fundal height is above the umbilicus, which would be an unexpected finding, investigate this immediately to prevent excessive bleeding. Frequently, the patient's bladder is full, thus displacing the uterus up and to either side of the midline. Ask the patient to empty their bladder, and reassess the uterus again.

Normally, the fundus progresses downward at a rate of 1 cm per day after childbirth and should be nonpalpable by 10 to 14 days postpartum. By Day 14, the uterus has descended below the rim of the symphysis pubis and is no longer palpable (Baker, 2024). On the first postpartum day, the top of the fundus is located 1 cm below the umbilicus and is recorded as u/1. Similarly, on the second postpartum day, the fundus would be 2 cm below the umbilicus and should be recorded as u/2, and so on. Health care agencies differ according to how fundal heights are charted, so follow their protocols for this. If the fundus is not firm, gently massage the uterus using a circular motion until it becomes firm.

Bladder

Considerable diuresis—as much as 3,000 mL/day—begins within 12 hours after childbirth and continues for several days, up to 2 weeks (Chauhan & Tadi, 2023). A single voiding may be 500 mL or more. However, many postpartum people do not sense the need to void even if their bladder is full. In this situation, the bladder can become distended and displace the uterus upward and to the side, which prevents the uterine muscles from contracting properly and can lead to excessive bleeding. Postpartum urinary retention is defined as the inability to empty the bladder within 6 hours after a vaginal birth. Urinary retention as a result of decreased bladder tone and emptying can lead to urinary tract infections and postpartum hemorrhage. Voiding should be encouraged and monitored to prevent asymptomatic urinary retention with overflow. It is imperative that nurses monitor patients for signs of urinary tract infections, including fever, urinary frequency and/or urgency, difficult or painful urination, and tenderness over the costovertebral angle (Berens, 2023). Patients who received regional anesthesia during labor are at risk for urinary tract infections due to continuous urinary catheterization to prevent urinary retention during labor, which is thought to delay fetal descent. They also experience difficulty voiding and loss of sensation and must wait until it returns to feel a full bladder, which might be several hours after childbirth.

Assess for voiding problems by asking the patient the following questions:

- Have you (voided, urinated, gone to the bathroom) yet?
- Have you noticed any burning or discomfort with urination?
- Do you have any difficulty passing your urine?
- Do you feel that your bladder is empty when you finish urinating?
- Do you have any signs of infection, such as urgency, frequency, or pain?
- Are you able to control the flow of urine by squeezing your muscles?
- Have you noticed any leakage of urine when you cough, laugh, or sneeze?

Assess the bladder for distention and adequate emptying after efforts to void. Palpate the area over the symphysis pubis. If empty, the bladder is not palpable. Palpation of a rounded mass suggests bladder distention. Also percuss the area; a full bladder is dull to percussion. If the bladder is full, lochia drainage will be more than normal because the uterus cannot contract to suppress the bleeding.

TAKE NOTE!

Note the location and condition of the fundus; a full bladder tends to displace the uterus up and to the right.

After the patient voids, palpate and percuss the area again to determine adequate emptying of the bladder. If the bladder remains distended, the patient may be retaining urine in their bladder, and measures to initiate voiding should be instituted. Be alert for signs of infection, including infrequent or insufficient voiding, discomfort, burning, urgency, or foul-smelling urine (Berens, 2023). Document all urine output.

Bowels

Constipation is one of the most common gastrointestinal symptoms in postpartum people. The etiology of postpartum constipation is multifactorial. Local pelvic floor trauma; taking pain medications; lack of dietary fiber, fluids, and infant care all contribute to constipation. Spontaneous bowel movements may not occur for 1 to 3 days after giving birth because of a decrease in muscle tone in the intestines as a result of elevated progesterone levels. About 2 to 3 days following childbirth, usual bowel elimination returns (Baker, 2024). Often birthing parents are hesitant to have a bowel movement due to pain in the perineal area resulting from an episiotomy, lacerations, or hemorrhoids. Some are fearful that they may "rip their stitches" should they strain. Nurses should reassure their patients that stool softeners and/or laxatives to treat constipation have been prescribed for them to reduce discomfort.

Inspect the patient's abdomen for distention, auscultate for bowel sounds in all four quadrants prior to palpating the uterine fundus, and palpate for tenderness. The abdomen is typically soft, nontender, and nondistended. Bowel sounds are present in all four quadrants. Ask the patient if they have had a bowel movement or have passed gas since giving birth, because constipation is common during the postpartum period, and many patients do not offer this information unless asked about it. Normal assessment findings are active bowel sounds, passing gas, and a nondistended abdomen.

Lochia

Assess lochia in terms of amount, color, odor, and change with activity and time. To assess how much a patient is bleeding, ask them how many perineal pads they have used in the past 1 to 2 hours and how much drainage was on each pad. For example, did they saturate the pad completely, or was only half of the pad covered with drainage? Ask about the color of the drainage, odor, and the presence of any clots. Lochia has a definite musky scent, with an odor similar to that of menstrual flow without any large clots (fist size). Foul-smelling lochia suggests an infection, and large clots suggest poor uterine involution, necessitating additional intervention.

To determine the amount of lochia, observe the amount of lochia saturation on the perineal pad and relate it to time (Fig. 16.3). Also, take into consideration the specific type of peripad used, because some are more absorbent than others. Lochia flow will increase when the patient gets out of bed (lochia pools in the vagina and the uterus while the patient is lying down) and when they breastfeed (oxytocin release causes uterine contractions). If there are concerns with the volume of lochia, it is recommended to measure the volume of lochia by accurately weighing the peripad (Baker, 2024). A patient who saturates a perineal pad within 30 to 60 minutes is bleeding much more than one who saturates a pad in 2 hours.

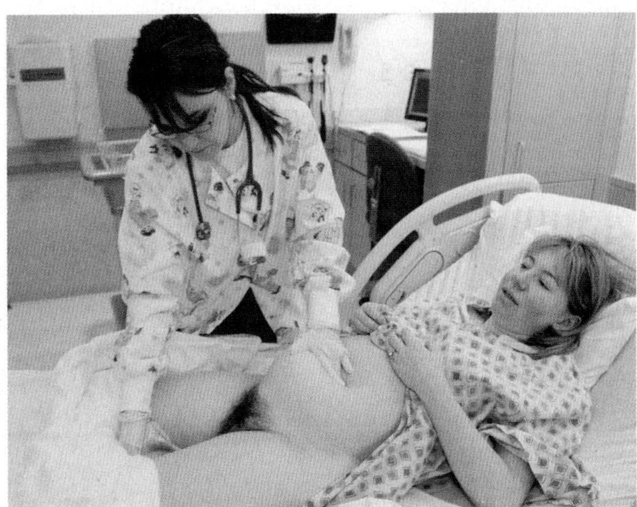

FIGURE 16.3 Assessing lochia.

The total volume of lochial discharge varies based on parity, but the amount decreases daily. Check under the patient by turning them to either side to make sure additional blood is not hidden and not absorbed on the perineal pad. This is also a good time to assess for the presence and condition of hemorrhoids since the nurse is visually inspecting the perineum.

Report any abnormal findings, such as heavy, bright red lochia with large tissue fragments or a foul odor. If excessive bleeding occurs, the first step would be to massage the boggy fundus until it is firm to reduce the flow of blood. Document all findings.

Patients who had cesarean births will have less lochia discharge than those who had vaginal births, but stages and color changes remain the same. Although the patient's abdomen will be tender after surgery, the nurse must palpate the fundus and assess the lochia to make sure they are within the normal range and that there is no excessive bleeding.

Anticipatory guidance to give the patient at discharge should include information about lochia and the expected changes. Urge the patient to notify their health care provider if lochia rubra returns after the serosa and alba transitions have taken place. This is abnormal and may indicate subinvolution or that the patient is too active and needs to rest more. Lochia is an excellent medium for bacterial growth. Explain to the patient that frequent changing of perineal pads, continued use of their peribottle for rinsing the perineal area, and hand hygiene before and after pad changes are important infection control measures.

Episiotomy/Perineum and Epidural Site

If the patient has an episiotomy, which is no longer routinely done, to assess the episiotomy and perineal area, position the patient on their side with their top leg flexed upward at the knee and drawn up toward their waist. If necessary, use a penlight to provide adequate lighting during the assessment. Wearing gloves and standing at the patient's side with their back to you, gently lift the upper buttock to expose the perineum and anus (Fig. 16.4). Inspect the episiotomy for irritation, ecchymosis, tenderness, or hematomas. Assess for hemorrhoids and their condition.

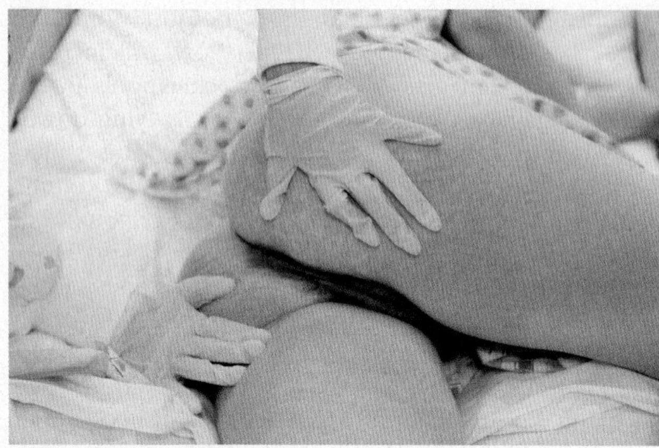

FIGURE 16.4 Inspecting the perineum.

During the early postpartum period, the perineal tissue surrounding the episiotomy is typically edematous and slightly bruised. The normal episiotomy site should not have redness, discharge, or edema. The majority of healing takes place within the first 2 weeks (Baker, 2024).

Lacerations to the perineal area sustained during the birthing process that were identified and repaired also need to be assessed to determine their healing status. Lacerations are classified based on severity and tissue involvement:

- *First-degree laceration:* involves only skin and superficial structures above muscle
- *Second-degree laceration:* extends through perineal muscles
- *Third-degree laceration:* extends through the anal sphincter muscle
- *Fourth-degree laceration:* continues through anterior rectal wall (Cunningham et al., 2022)

Assess the episiotomy and any lacerations at least every 8 hours to detect hematomas or signs of infection. Large areas of swollen, bluish skin with complaints of severe pain in the perineal area indicate pelvic or vulvar hematomas. Redness, swelling, increasing discomfort, or purulent drainage may indicate infection. Both findings need to be reported immediately.

A white line running the length of the episiotomy is a sign of infection, as is swelling or discharge. Severe, intractable pain, perineal discoloration, and ecchymosis indicate a perineal hematoma, a potentially dangerous condition. Report any unusual findings. Ice can be applied to relieve discomfort and reduce edema; sitz baths also can promote comfort and perineal healing (see "Promoting Comfort" in the "Nursing Interventions" section).

If the patient has had an epidural during labor, assessment of the epidural wound site is important as well as checking for any side effects of the medication injected such as itching, nausea and vomiting, or urinary retention. Visual inspection of the epidural site and an accurate documentation of intake and output are essential.

Extremities

Pregnancy is associated with an increased risk of venous thromboembolism (VTE), which includes PE and deep vein thrombosis (DVT). During pregnancy, the state of hypercoagulability protects the birthing parent against excessive blood loss during childbirth and placental separation. However, this hypercoagulable state can increase the risk of thromboembolic disorders during pregnancy and postpartum. Pregnant people have a five-fold higher risk of VTE when compared to nonpregnant people, and it becomes a 30- to 60-fold increase in the postpartum period. DVT events are more common during pregnancy while PE events are more likely to occur during the postpartum period. History of prior VTE, cigarette smoking, hypertension, or thrombophilia; advanced maternal age; obesity (BMI > 30kg/m^2); multiple gestation; multiparity; preeclampsia; premature or prolonged labor; and operative deliveries further increase the risk of VTE (Couto & Junior, 2022). The effective prevention and management of VTE is paramount to prevent a clot from dislodging and traveling to the lungs (Kalaitzopoulos et al., 2022).

While inspecting the patient's extremities, also determine the degree of sensory and motor function return (recovery from anesthesia) by asking the patient if they feel sensation in various areas the nurse touches and also by observing the patient's ambulation stability.

Psychosocial Assessment

Psychosocial assessment of the postpartum patient focuses on the emotional status, bonding, and attachment.

Emotional Status

Assess the patient's emotional status by observing how they interact with their family, the patient's level of independence, energy levels, eye contact with their infant (within a cultural context), posture and comfort level while holding the newborn, and sleep and rest patterns. Be alert for mood swings, irritability, or crying episodes.

> Remember Raina and her quiet husband? The postpartum nurse informs Raina that her doctor, Dr. Nancy Schultz, has been called away for emergency surgery and won't be available the rest of the day. The nurse explains that Dr. Robert Nappo will be making rounds for her. Raina and her husband become upset. What should the nurse have confirmed with the couple? Is culturally competent care being provided to this couple?

Bonding and Attachment

Nurses can be instrumental in promoting attachment by assessing attachment behaviors (positive and negative) and intervening appropriately if needed. Nurses must be able to identify any family discord that might interfere with the attachment process. Remember, however, that people from different cultures may behave differently from what is expected in one's own culture. For example, some parents may handle their newborns less often and use cradle boards to carry them. Some delay breastfeeding until their milk comes in, discarding colostrum in the first few days (Gutierrez, 2022). Do not assume that a behavior different from that of your own culture is wrong.

Meeting the newborn for the first time after birth can be an exhilarating experience for parents. Although parents may have spent many hours dreaming of their unborn baby and how they will look, it is not until after birth that they meet face to face. They need to get to know one another and to develop feelings for one another.

Bonding is the close emotional attraction to a newborn by the parents that develops during the first 30 to 60 minutes after birth. It is unidirectional, from parent to infant. It is thought that optimal bonding of the parents to a newborn requires a period of close contact within the first few minutes to a few hours after birth. Bonding is a continuation of the relationship that began during pregnancy (Sears & Sears, 2020a). It is affected by a multitude of factors, including the parents' socioeconomic status, family history, role models, support systems, cultural factors, and birth experiences. The birthing parent initiates bonding when they caress their infant and exhibit certain behaviors typical of a parent tending to their child. The infant's responses to this, such as body and eye movements, are a necessary part of the process. During this initial period, the infant is in a quiet, alert state, looking directly at the person holding them.

TAKE NOTE!

The length of time necessary for bonding depends on the health of the infant and birthing parent as well as the circumstances surrounding the labor and birth. It is completely normal to take a few days, a few weeks, or several months to feel that special bond (Ogunyemi, 2024a).

Attachment is the development of strong affection between an infant and a significant other (e.g., parent, sibling, or caregiver). This attachment is reciprocal; both the significant other and the newborn exhibit attachment behaviors. The attachment relationship formed between the infant and primary caregiver influences the child's view of the world and future relationships (United Nations International Children's Emergency Fund [UNICEF], n.d.). This tie between two people is psychological rather than biologic, and it does not occur overnight. The process of attachment follows a progressive or developmental course that changes over time. Attachment is an individualized and multifactorial process that differs based on the health of the infant, the birthing parent, environmental circumstances, and the quality of care the infant receives. The newborn responds to the significant other by cooing, grasping, smiling, and crying. Nurses can assess for attachment behaviors by observing the interaction between the newborn and the person holding them (American Family Physician [AFP], 2024). It occurs through mutually satisfying experiences. Maternal attachment begins during pregnancy as the result of fetal movement and maternal fantasies about the infant and continues through the birth and postpartum periods. Attachment behaviors include seeking; physical caregiving behaviors; emotional attentiveness to the infant's needs; staying close to, touching, kissing, cuddling, and choosing the ***en face* position** (face to face) while holding or feeding the newborn; expressing pride in the newborn; and exchanging gratifying experiences with the infant. All infants require a culture of warmth, responsiveness, and a protective environment from their primary caregiver for appropriate growth and development (Stoodley et al., 2022). In a high-risk pregnancy, the attachment process may be complicated by premature birth (lack of time to develop a relationship with the unborn baby) and by parental stress due to fetal and/or maternal vulnerability.

Bonding is a vital component of the attachment process and is necessary in establishing parent–infant attachment and a healthy, loving relationship. During this early period of acquaintance, birthing parents touch their infants in a characteristic manner. Birthing parents visually and physically "explore" their infants, initially using their fingertips on the infant's face and extremities and progressing to massaging and stroking the infant with their fingers. This is followed by palm contact on the trunk. Eventually, birthing parents draw their infant toward them and hold the infant (Fig. 16.5).

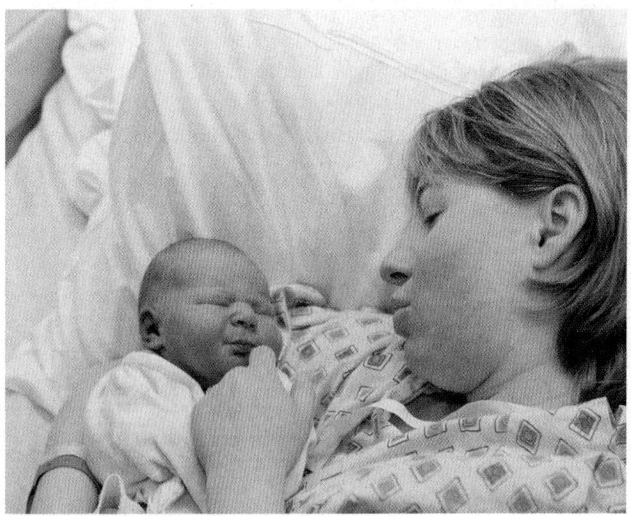

FIGURE 16.5 *En face* position.

Generally, research on attachment has found that the process is similar for partners as for birthing parents, but the pace may be different. Like birthing parents, partners manifest attachment behaviors during pregnancy. Partners develop emotional ties with their infants in a variety of ways. They seek and maintain closeness with the infant and can recognize the characteristics of the infant. Another study further described partner attachment as a permanent, cyclical concept characterized by changes in response to the child's developmental stage. When children have a secure, supportive, and sensitive relationship with the birthing parent's partner, they are generally better adjusted than those who have a nonsupportive relationship. It is important for nurses to support and enable partners to have skin-to-skin contact with their newborns to enhance the bonding and attachments between them. Studies confirm the positive impacts of skin-to-skin contact in terms of exploring, touching, caring, and enhancing the partner–neonate attachment (Dong et al., 2022).

Attachment is a process; it does not occur instantaneously, even though many parents believe in a romanticized version of attachment, which happens right after birth. A delay in the attachment process can occur if a birthing parent's physical and emotional states are adversely affected by exhaustion, pain, and the absence of a support system; if they have an infant in a neonatal intensive care unit (NICU) and are separated from them; or if they have a traumatic birth experience, substance use disorder, anesthesia, or an unwanted outcome such as an ill infant (AFP, 2024).

TAKE NOTE!

Touch is a basic instinctual interaction between a parent and their infant and has a vital role in the infant's early development. Attachment is established, in part, through sensory processes. Parents provide a variety of tactile stimulation while addressing their infant's daily care routines (Ogunyemi, 2024a).

The developmental task for the infant is learning to differentiate between trust and mistrust. If the parent or caregiver is consistently responsive to the infant's care, meeting the baby's physical and psychological needs, the infant will likely learn to trust the caregiver, view the world as a safe place, and grow up to be secure, self-reliant, trusting, cooperative, and helpful. However, if the infant's needs are not met, the child is more likely to face developmental delays, neglect, and child abuse (Sears & Sears, 2020a).

Factors associated with the health care facility or birthing unit can also hinder attachment. These include:

- Separation of infant and parents immediately after birth and for long periods during the day
- Policies that discourage unwrapping and exploring the infant
- Intensive care environment, restrictive visiting policies
- Staff indifference or lack of support for parents' caregiving attempts and abilities

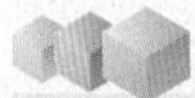
Concept Mastery Alert

Grief After Delivery of a Child With Special Needs

It is important for parents to visit the child in the special care nursery, but the priority is to assist them in dealing with the grief that can accompany giving birth to a child with a disability. The parents may first need to mourn the loss of what they pictured as the "perfect child."

CRITICAL ATTRIBUTES OF ATTACHMENT

The terms "bonding" and "attachment" are often used interchangeably, even though they involve different time frames and interactions. Attachment stages include proximity, reciprocity, and commitment.

Proximity refers to the physical and psychological experience of the parents being close to their infant. This attribute has three dimensions:

1. *Contact:* The sensory experiences of touching, holding, and gazing at the infant are part of proximity-seeking behavior.
2. *Emotional state:* The emotional state emerges from the affective experience of the new parents toward their infant and the parental role.
3. *Individualization:* Parents are aware of the need to differentiate the infant's needs from themselves and to recognize and respond to them appropriately, making the attachment process also, in a way, one of detachment.

Reciprocity is the process by which the infant's abilities and behaviors elicit parental response. Reciprocity is described by two dimensions: complementary behavior and sensitivity. Complementary behavior involves taking turns and stopping when the other is not interested or becomes tired. An infant can coo and stare at the parent to elicit a similar parental response to complement their behavior. Parents who are sensitive and responsive to their infant's cues will promote their development and growth. Parents who become skilled at recognizing the ways their infant communicates will respond appropriately by smiling, vocalizing, touching, and kissing.

Commitment refers to the enduring nature of the relationship. The components of this are twofold: centrality and parent role exploration. In centrality, parents place the infant at the center of their lives. They acknowledge and accept their responsibility to promote the infant's safety, growth, and development. Parent role exploration is the parents' ability to find their own way and integrate the parental identity into themselves (Sears & Sears, 2020a).

POSITIVE AND NEGATIVE ATTACHMENT BEHAVIORS

Positive bonding behaviors include maintaining close physical contact; making eye-to-eye contact; speaking in soft, high-pitched tones; and touching and exploring the infant. Table 16.1 highlights typical positive and negative attachment behaviors.

NURSING INTERVENTIONS

In terms of postpartum hospital stays today, "less is more." If the patient had a vaginal delivery, they may be discharged within 24 to 48 hours or sooner. If they had a cesarean birth, they may remain hospitalized for up to 72 hours. These shortened lengths of stay leave little time for nurses to prepare the patient and their family for the many changes that will occur when the patient returns home (see Clinical Judgment & Nursing Process 16.1). Research shows that birthing parents feel unprepared, uninformed, and unsupported during the postpartum period as they struggle with physical and emotional issues, infant caregiving, breastfeeding concerns, and lifestyle adjustments. Being discharged from the hospital before they're ready can place the patient at risk of not being able to meet their own needs and also place their newborn at risk. International organizations have provided the following key criteria to improve readiness for discharge: undergoing an assessment of patient and infant physiological stability; having knowledge on self-care and infant care; the availability of support at home; and the availability of professional care following discharge (H. Smith et al., 2022). Nurses need to focus on pain and discomfort, immunizations, nutrition, activity and exercise, infant care, lactation instruction, discharge teaching, sexuality and contraception, and follow-up with the limited time they have with their patients.

TAKE NOTE!

Always adhere to standard precautions when providing direct care to reduce the risk of disease transmission.

Providing Optimal Cultural Care

Because the population of the United States is diverse, nurses must be prepared to care for childbearing families from various cultures. In many cultures, birthing parents and their families are cared for and nurtured by their communities for weeks and even months after the birth of a new family member. Cultural humility helps nurses explore cultural competency as a process rather than an outcome. Overall, culturally humble care for all childbearing families includes understanding traditional cultural beliefs; involvement and support by family members; respect; presence of a significant other; breastfeeding and healthy eating; observing the principles of hot and cold; avoidance of postnatal sexual intercourse; encouragement; empowerment; the importance of spiritual dimensions; avoidance of evil spirits; and the hope that nurses will anticipate the needs of the birthing parent and infant (Srivastava, 2023). To provide appropriate nursing care, the nurse should determine, never assume, the patient's preferences before intervening through clear communication.

Nurses need to remember that childbearing practices and beliefs vary from culture to culture. Cultural practices may include dietary restrictions; certain clothes; taboos; activities for maintaining mental health; and the use of silence, prayer, or meditation. Restoring health may involve taking folk medicines or conferring with a tribal healer. A language barrier might interfere with communication between patients and health providers, possibly leading to them feeling reluctant to use health services in the future—especially when the language barrier is followed by a lack

TABLE 16.1 • Positive and Negative Attachment Behaviors

	Positive Behaviors	Negative Behaviors
Infant	Smiles; is alert; demonstrates strong grasp reflex to hold parent's finger; sucks well, feeds easily; enjoys being held close; makes eye-to-eye contact; follows parent's face; appears facially appealing; is consolable when crying	Feeds poorly, regurgitates often; cries for long periods, colicky and inconsolable; shows flat affect, rarely smiles even when prompted; resists holding and closeness; sleeps with eyes closed most of the time; stiffens body when held; is unresponsive to parents; doesn't pay attention to parents' faces
Parent	Makes direct eye contact; assumes *en face* position when holding infant; claims infant as a family member, pointing out common features; expresses pride in the infant; assigns meaning to infant's actions; smiles and gazes at infant; touches infant, progressing from fingertips to holding; names infant; requests to be close to infant as much as allowed; speaks positively about infant	Expresses disappointment or displeasure in the infant; fails to "explore" infant visually or physically; fails to claim infant as part of the family; avoids caring for the infant; finds excuses not to hold infant close; has negative self-concept; appears uninterested in having an infant in the room; frequently asks to have infant taken back to nursery to be cared for; assigns negative attributes to infant and calls infant inappropriate, negative names

Ogunyemi, D. (2024a). *Bonding with your newborn: What to know if you don't feel connected right away.* https://www.acog.org/womens-health/experts-and-stories/the-latest/bonding-with-your-newborn-heres-what-to-know-if-you-dont-feel-connected-right-away; Sears, W., & Sears, M. (2020a). *Bonding with baby.* https://www.askdrsears.com/topics/pregnancy-childbirth/tenth-month-post-partum/bonding-with-your-newborn/bonding-with-baby/; United Nations International Children's Emergency Fund. (n.d.). *What you need to know about parent-child attachment.* https://www.unicef.org/parenting/child-care/what-you-need-know-about-parent-child-attachment

CLINICAL JUDGMENT & NURSING PROCESS 16.1 Overview of the Postpartum Patient

A 26-year-old G2P2 is a patient on the postpartum unit after giving birth to a term 8-lb, 12-oz baby boy yesterday. The night nurse reports that the patient has an episiotomy, complains of a pain rating of 7 points on a scale of 1 to 10, is having difficulty breastfeeding, and had heavy lochia most of the night. The nurse also reports that the patient seems focused on their own needs and not on those of the infant. Assessment this morning reveals the following:

B: **Breasts** are soft with colostrum leaking; nipples cracked
U: **Uterus** is 1 cm below the umbilicus; deviated to the right
B: **Bladder** is palpable; patient states they haven't been up to void yet.
B: **Bowels** have not moved; bowel sounds present; passing flatus
L: **Lochia** is moderate; peripad soaked from night accumulation
E: **Episiotomy** site intact; swollen, bruised; hemorrhoids present
E: **Extremities** have no edema over the tibia; no warmth or tenderness in the calf
E: **Emotional status** is distressed as a result of discomfort and fatigue.

NURSING ANALYSIS: Altered tissue integrity related to episiotomy

OUTCOME IDENTIFICATION AND EVALUATION

The patient will remain free of infection without any signs and symptoms of infection and exhibit evidence of progressive healing as demonstrated by clean, dry, decreased/absent edema, and an intact episiotomy site.

INTERVENTIONS: *Promoting Tissue Integrity*

- Monitor episiotomy site for redness, edema, warmth, or discharge *to identify infection.*
- Assess vital signs at least every 4 hours *to identify changes suggesting infection.*
- Apply ice pack to the episiotomy site *to reduce swelling.*
- Instruct patient on the use of sitz bath *to promote healing, hygiene, and comfort.*
- Encourage frequent perineal care and peripad changes *to prevent infection.*
- Recommend ambulation *to improve circulation and promote healing.*
- Instruct patient on positioning *to relieve pressure on the perineal area.*
- Demonstrate the use of anesthetic sprays *to numb the perineal area.*

NURSING ANALYSIS: Acute pain related to episiotomy, sore nipples, and hemorrhoids

OUTCOME IDENTIFICATION AND EVALUATION

The patient will experience a decrease in pain as evidenced by reporting that their pain has diminished to a tolerable level and rating it as 2 points or less.

INTERVENTIONS: *Providing Pain Relief*

- Thoroughly inspect the perineum *to rule out hematoma as the cause of pain.*
- Administer analgesic medication as ordered and as needed *to promote comfort.*
- Carry out comfort measures to episiotomy as outlined earlier *to reduce pain.*
- Explain discomforts and reassure the patient that they are time limited *to assist in coping with pain.*
- Apply witch hazel pads to swollen hemorrhoids *to induce shrinkage and reduce pain.*
- Suggest frequent use of sitz bath *to reduce hemorrhoid pain.*
- Administer stool softener and laxative *to prevent straining with the first bowel movement.*
- Observe positioning and latching-on technique while breastfeeding. Offer suggestions based on observations *to correct positioning/latching on to minimize trauma to the breast.*
- Suggest air-drying of nipples after breastfeeding and use of plain water *to prevent nipple cracking.*
- Teach relaxation techniques when breastfeeding *to reduce anxiety and discomfort.*

NURSING ANALYSIS: Risk for coping impairment related to mood alteration and pain

OUTCOME IDENTIFICATION AND EVALUATION

The patient will cope with mood alterations, as evidenced by positive statements about the newborn and participation in newborn care.

INTERVENTIONS: *Promoting Effective Coping*

- Provide a supportive, nurturing environment and encourage the patient to vent their feelings and frustrations *to relieve anxiety.*
- Provide opportunities for the patient to rest and sleep *to combat fatigue.*
- Encourage the patient to eat a well-balanced diet *to increase their energy level.*

CLINICAL JUDGMENT & NURSING PROCESS 16.1 Overview of the Postpartum Patient

- Provide reassurance and explanations that mood alterations are common after birth secondary to waning hormones after pregnancy *to increase the patient's knowledge.*
- Allow the patient relief from newborn care *to afford the opportunity for self-care.*
- Discuss with the partner the expected behavior from patient and how additional support and help are needed during this stressful time *to promote partner's participation in care.*
- Make appropriate community referrals for parent–infant support *to ensure continuity of care.*
- Encourage frequent skin-to-skin contact and closeness between parent and infant *to facilitate bonding and attachment behaviors.*
- Encourage patient to participate in infant care and provide instructions as needed *to foster a sense of independence and self-esteem.*
- Offer praise and reinforcement of positive parent–infant interactions *to enhance self-confidence in care.*

of cultural sensitivity by the health care provider. Thus, honoring the culture and language of birthing parents is a key component of health equity (Feuerstein, 2022). Providing culturally competent care within our global community is challenging for all nurses because they must remember that a person's culture cannot be easily summarized in a reference book but rather is best learned and appreciated through life experiences.

Raina and her husband, who are Muslims, are upset at the thought of having a male doctor care for Raina; they want her to have a same-sex care provider. What should the nurse do in this situation?

Promoting Comfort

The postpartum patient may have discomfort and pain from a variety of sources, such as an episiotomy, perineal lacerations, backache as a result of the epidural, pain from a full bladder, an edematous perineum, inflamed hemorrhoids, engorged breasts, afterbirth pains secondary to uterine contractions in breastfeeding and multiparous patients, and sore nipples if breastfeeding. Relieving the underlying problem is the first step in pain management. Using shared decision making can help the health care team provide nonpharmacologic and pharmacologic measures to manage the birthing parent's discomfort (Wisner, 2022).

Applications of Cold and Heat

COLD

An ice pack is commonly the first measure used after a vaginal birth to relieve perineal discomfort from edema, an episiotomy, or a laceration. An ice pack can minimize edema, reduce inflammation, decrease capillary permeability, and reduce nerve conduction to the site. It is applied during the fourth stage of labor and can be used for the first 24 hours to reduce perineal edema and to prevent hematoma formation, thus reducing pain and promoting healing. Ice packs are wrapped in a disposable covering or clean washcloth and are applied to the perineal area. Usually, the ice pack is applied intermittently for 20 minutes and removed for 10 minutes. Many commercially prepared ice packs are available, but a surgical glove filled with crushed ice and covered with a wash cloth can also be used if the birthing parent is not allergic to latex. Ensure that the ice pack is changed frequently to promote good hygiene and to allow for periodic assessments.

HEAT

The **peribottle** is a plastic squeeze bottle filled with warm tap water that is sprayed over the perineal area after each voiding and before applying a new perineal pad. Usually, the peribottle is introduced to the patient when they are assisted to the bathroom to freshen up and void for the first time—in most instances, once vital signs are stable after the first hour. Provide the patient with instructions on how and when to use the peribottle. Reinforce this practice each time the patient changes their pad, voids, or defecates, making sure that they understand how to direct the flow of water from front to back. The patient can take the peribottle home and use it over the next several weeks until lochia discharge stops. The peribottle can be used by people who had either vaginal or cesarean births to provide comfort and hygiene to the perineal area.

Within the first 24 hours, a **sitz bath** with room-temperature water may be prescribed and substituted for the ice pack to reduce local swelling, promote muscle relaxation, and promote comfort for an episiotomy, perineal trauma and other wounds, inflammation, hemorrhoids, and anorectal infections (Choudhari et al., 2022). The change from cold to room-temperature therapy enhances vascular circulation and healing. Before using a sitz bath, the patient should cleanse the perineum with a peribottle or take a shower using a mild soap.

Hydrotherapy is the external use of any form of water for health promotion or treatment with varying temperatures, duration, and application sites. Most health care agencies use plastic disposable sitz baths that patients can take home. The plastic sitz bath consists of a basin that fits on the commode; a bag filled with warm water is hung on a hook and connected via a tube onto the front of the basin (Fig. 16.6). Teaching Guidelines 16.1 highlights the steps in using a sitz bath.

Advise the patient to use the sitz bath several times daily to provide hygiene and comfort to the perineal area. Encourage them to continue this measure after discharge. Some facilities have hygienic sitz baths called Suri-Gators in the bathroom that spray an antiseptic, water, or both onto the perineum. The patient sits on the toilet with their legs apart so that the nozzle spray reaches their perineal area.

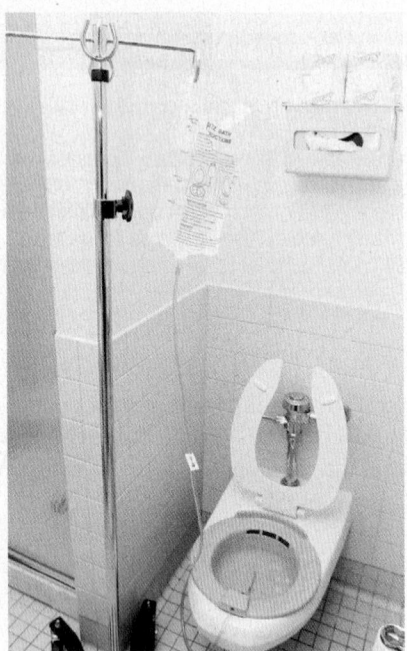

FIGURE 16.6 Sitz bath setup.

Keep in mind that tremendous hemodynamic changes are taking place within the patient during this early postpartum period, and their safety must be a priority. Fatigue, blood loss, the effects of medications, and lack of food may cause the patient to feel weak when they stand up.

TEACHING GUIDELINES 16.1 Using a Sitz Bath

1. Close the clamp on tubing before filling the bag with water to prevent leakage.
2. Fill sitz bath basin and plastic bag with room-temperature water (comfortable to touch).
3. Place the filled basin on the toilet with the seat raised and the overflow opening facing toward the back of the toilet.
4. Hang the filled plastic bag on a hook close to the toilet or an intravenous (IV) pole.
5. Attach the tubing to the opening on the basin.
6. Sit on the basin positioned on the toilet seat and release the clamp to allow warm water to irrigate the perineum.
7. Remain sitting on the basin for approximately 15 to 20 minutes.
8. Stand up and pat the perineum area dry. Apply a clean peripad.
9. Tip the basin to remove any remaining water and flush the toilet.
10. Wash the basin with warm water and soap, and dry it in the sink.
11. Store the basin and tubing in a clean, dry area until the next use.
12. Wash hands with soap and water.

Assisting the patient to the bathroom to instruct them on how to use the peribottle and sitz bath is necessary to ensure the patient's safety. Many birthing parents become lightheaded or dizzy when they get out of bed and need direct physical assistance. Staying in the patient's room, ensuring that the emergency call light is readily available, and being available if needed during this early period will ensure safety and prevent accidents and falls.

Topical Preparations

Several treatments may be applied topically for temporary relief of perineal pain and discomfort. One such treatment is a local anesthetic spray such as benzocaine topical. These agents numb the perineal area and are used after cleansing the area with water via the peribottle and/or a sitz bath.

Postpartum patients are predisposed to hemorrhoid development due to pressure during vaginal birth, constipation, relaxation of the smooth muscles in vein walls, and impaired blood return, all related to increased pressure from the heavy gravid uterus. Nonpharmacologic measures to reduce hemorrhoid discomfort include ice packs, ice sitz baths, and application of cool witch hazel pads. The pads are placed at the rectal area, between the hemorrhoids and the perineal pad. These pads cool the area, help relieve swelling, and minimize itching. Pharmacologic methods used to reduce hemorrhoid pain include local anesthetics (dibucaine) or steroids (hydrocortisone acetate); stool softeners help to prevent constipation. To reduce the discomfort of hemorrhoids and prevent or correct constipation, the patient should consume large amounts of water and eat high-fiber foods and fruits, perform frequent ambulation, utilize proper toileting habits, and avoid straining during defecation (Sujawaty et al., 2023).

In the breastfeeding person, nipple pain is a common issue and often leads to early weaning (Douglas, 2022). Nipple pain is difficult to treat, though a wide variety of topical creams, ointments, and gels are available to do so. This group includes beeswax, glycerin-based products, petrolatum, lanolin, and hydrogel products. Many people find these products comforting, though research does not support the manufacturer's claims that lanolin or hydrogel sheets provide healing benefits for nipple damage (Douglas, 2022). Lanolin does not need to be removed before breastfeeding. Hydrogel, beeswax, glycerin-based products, and petrolatum all need to be removed before breastfeeding. These products should be avoided in order to limit infant exposure because the process of removal may increase nipple irritation. Applying expressed breast milk to nipples and allowing them to dry has been suggested to reduce nipple pain. Usually, the pain is due to an incorrect latch and/or removal of the nursing infant from the breast. Early assistance with breastfeeding to ensure correct positioning can help prevent nipple trauma.

Analgesics

Analgesics such as acetaminophen and oral nonsteroidal anti-inflammatory drugs (NSAIDs) such as ibuprofen or naproxen are prescribed to relieve mild postpartum discomfort. For moderate to severe pain, a narcotic analgesic such as codeine or oxycodone in conjunction with aspirin or acetaminophen may be prescribed. Instruct the patient about the adverse effects of any medication prescribed. Common adverse effects of oral analgesics include dizziness, lightheadedness, nausea and vomiting, constipation, and sedation (UpToDate, Inc., 2024).

Also inform the patient that the drugs are secreted in breast milk. Nearly all medications that the patient takes are passed into their breast milk; however, mild analgesics (e.g., acetaminophen or ibuprofen) are considered relatively safe for breastfeeding people (Etzel & Ambizas, 2022). Administering a mild analgesic approximately an hour before breastfeeding will usually relieve afterpains and/or perineal discomfort.

Assisting With Elimination

The bladder is edematous, hypotonic, and congested immediately postpartum. Consequently, bladder distention, incomplete emptying, and the inability to void are common. A full bladder interferes with uterine contraction and may lead to hemorrhage because it will displace the uterus out of the midline. Encourage the patient to void. Often, assisting them in assuming the normal voiding position on the commode facilitates this. If the patient has difficulty voiding, pouring warm water over the perineal area, hearing the sound of running tap water, blowing bubbles through a straw, taking a warm shower, drinking fluids, providing them with privacy, or placing their hand in a basin of warm water may stimulate voiding. If these actions do not stimulate urination within 4 to 6 hours after giving birth, catheterization may be needed. Palpate the bladder for distention and ask the patient if they are voiding in small amounts (less than 100 mL) frequently (retention with overflow). If catheterization is necessary, use a sterile technique to reduce the risk of infection.

Constipation is one of the most common postpartum problems. Decreased bowel motility during labor, high iron content in prenatal vitamins, postpartum fluid loss, and the adverse effects of pain medications and/or anesthesia may predispose the postpartum patient to constipation. In addition, the patient may fear that bowel movements will cause pain or injury, especially if they had an episiotomy or a laceration that was repaired with sutures.

The choice of treatments for postpartum constipation remains a challenge. Usually, a stool softener, such as docusate, with or without a laxative might be helpful if the patient has difficulty with bowel elimination. Other measures, such as ambulating and increasing fluid and fiber intake, may also help. Nutritional instruction might include increasing fruits and vegetables in the diet; drinking plenty of fluids (8 to 12 c daily) to keep the stool soft; drinking small amounts of prune juice and/or hot liquids to stimulate peristalsis; eating high-fiber foods such as bran cereals, whole grains, dried fruits, fresh fruits, and raw vegetables; and walking daily.

Promoting Activity, Rest, and Exercise

The postpartum period is an ideal time for nurses to promote the importance of physical fitness, help birthing parents incorporate exercise into their lifestyles, and encourage them to overcome barriers to exercise. The lifestyle changes that occur postpartum may affect a birthing person's health for decades. Early ambulation is encouraged to reduce the risk of thromboembolism and to improve strengthening.

Many changes occur postpartum, and caring for a newborn alters parental eating and sleeping habits, work schedules, and time allocation. Postpartum fatigue is common during the early days after childbirth, and it may continue for weeks or months. Having adequate sleep is critical for new parents because shorter sleep time, a high percentage of sleep disturbances, and greater fatigue are associated with depressive symptoms in postpartum people and their partners (Pacheco & Snyder, 2024). Working partners with newborns experience fatigue during early parenthood and are unable to recover due to interrupted and poor sleep patterns. This sleep deficit can compromise their work safety and can also have long-term adverse effects for years, which include increased psychological stress, increased risk for mood disorders, and reduced quality of life and life satisfaction (Divine et al., 2022). The sleep deficit also affects parents' relationships with significant others and their ability to fulfill household and childcare responsibilities. Be sure that parents recognize their need for rest and sleep and are realistic about their expectations. Some suggestions include:

- Nap when the infant is sleeping because getting uninterrupted sleep at night is difficult.
- Reduce participation in outside activities, and limit the number of visitors.
- Determine the infant's sleep–wake cycles and attempt to increase wakeful periods during the day so the baby sleeps for longer periods at night.
- Eat a balanced diet to promote healing and to increase energy levels.
- Share household tasks to conserve energy.
- Ask other family members to provide infant care during the night periodically so that parents can get an uninterrupted night of sleep if they are not breastfeeding.
- Review the family's daily routine, and try to "cluster" activities to conserve energy and promote rest.

The demands of parenthood may reduce or prevent exercise in even the most committed person. A targeted exercise program and proper body mechanics can help new parents deal with the physical challenges of parenthood. Emphasize the benefits of a regular exercise program, which include:

- Helps the person lose pregnancy weight
- Increases overall postpartum well-being
- Reduces the risk of postpartum depression
- Maintains cardiovascular fitness
- Reduces mental fatigue (Mannarino & Jo, 2023)

Overweight and obesity constitute an epidemic in the United States. Obesity is a risk factor for numerous conditions, including diabetes, hypertension, high cholesterol, stroke, heart disease, cancer, and arthritis. Although the average gestational weight gain is small (approximately 25 to 35 lb), excess weight gain and not losing weight after pregnancy are important predictors of long-term obesity. The postpartum period is a vulnerable time for excessive weight retention, particularly for the increasing number of birthing parents who have a higher body weight at the start of pregnancy and subsequently find it difficult to lose the additional weight gained during pregnancy.

The postpartum person may face some obstacles to exercising, including physical changes (ligament laxity), competing demands (newborn care), lack of information about weight retention (inactivity equates to weight gain), and stress incontinence (leaking of urine during activity).

A healthy person with an uncomplicated vaginal birth can resume light exercise in the immediate postpartum period. Advise the person to start slowly and increase the level of exercise over a period of several weeks as tolerated. Infant strollers and carriers may be an option for some people, allowing them to walk with their newborns for exercise. Jogging strollers can be used later when the infant is 6 to 12 months old and can hold their head up. Also, exercise videos and home exercise equipment allow the parent to work out while the newborn naps.

Exercising after giving birth promotes feelings of well-being and restores muscle tone lost during pregnancy. Routine exercise should be resumed gradually, beginning with pelvic floor muscle exercises on the first postpartum day and by the second week, progressing to abdominal, buttock, and thigh-toning exercises. Walking is an excellent form of early exercise as long as the person avoids jarring and bouncing movements because joints do not stabilize until 6 to 8 weeks postpartum. Exercising too much too soon can cause the person to bleed more, and their lochia may return to bright red. If this occurs, instruct the person to stop exercising and rest by lying down until the bleeding slows. This increase in bleeding should be a warning to the person that they are overextending themselves and need to slow down their exercise routine.

Recommended exercises for the first few weeks postpartum include abdominal breathing, head lifts, modified sit-ups, double knee roll, and pelvic tilt (Teaching Guidelines 16.2). The number of exercises and their duration is gradually increased as the person gains strength.

TEACHING GUIDELINES 16.2 Postpartum Exercises

Abdominal Breathing

1. While lying on a flat surface (floor or bed), take a deep breath through your nose, and expand your abdominal muscles (they will rise up from your midsection).
2. Slowly exhale and tighten your abdominal muscles for 3 to 5 seconds.
3. Repeat this several times.

Head Lift

1. Lie on a flat surface with knees flexed and feet flat on the surface.
2. Lift your head off the flat surface, tuck it onto your chest, and hold for 3 to 5 seconds.
3. Relax your head and return to the starting position.
4. Repeat this several times.

Modified Sit-Ups

1. Lie on a flat surface and raise your head and shoulders 6 to 8 in so that your outstretched hands reach your knees.
2. Keep your waist on the flat surface.
3. Slowly return to the starting position.
4. Repeat, increasing in frequency as your comfort level allows.

Double Knee Roll

1. Lie on a flat surface with your knees bent.
2. While keeping your shoulders flat, slowly roll your knees to your right side to touch the flat surface (floor or bed).
3. Roll your knees back over your body to the left side until they touch the opposite side of the flat surface.
4. Return to the starting position on your back and rest.
5. Repeat this exercise several times.

Pelvic Tilt

1. Lie on your back on a flat surface with your knees bent and your arms at your side.
2. Slowly contract your abdominal muscles while lifting your pelvis up toward the ceiling.
3. Hold for 3 to 5 seconds and slowly return to your starting position.
4. Repeat several times.

Remember that there are different cultural attitudes toward exercise. Some cultures expect postpartum people to observe a specific period of bed rest or activity restriction; it would be inappropriate to recommend active exercise during the early postpartum period to a person from such a culture (Srivastava, 2023).

Preventing Stress Incontinence

Urinary incontinence is a condition in which a person experiences involuntary leakage of urine. Of all parous people, up to 50% develop some degree of pelvic prolapse in their lifetime that is associated with stress incontinence (Nygaard et al., 2021). Stress incontinence causes reduced quality of life and withdrawal from fitness and exercise activities typically. Research suggests that having a vaginal delivery results in direct pelvic muscle trauma and disruption of fascial supports as well as damage to the levator ani muscle and pudendal nerve injury. The National Institute for Health and Care Excellence recommends offering instruction for exercising the pelvic floor muscles to all birthing parents during their first pregnancy and again after having a vaginal birth (Okeahialam et al., 2022). Nurses can suggest these exercises as a first-line intervention in the prevention of urinary incontinence postpartum (Okeahialam et al., 2022). The more vaginal deliveries a person has had, the more likely they are to have stress incontinence. Stress incontinence can occur with any activity that causes an increase in intra-abdominal pressure. Postpartum people might consider low-impact activities such as walking, biking, swimming, or low-impact aerobics so they can resume physical activity while strengthening the pelvic floor.

Suggestions to prevent stress incontinence include modifications to lifestyle:

- Start a regular program of pelvic floor muscle training exercises after childbirth.
- Increase physical activity daily.
- Practice bladder retraining to lengthen the amount of time between voidings (scheduled voiding).
- Lose weight if necessary; obesity is associated with stress incontinence.
- Limit the intake of alcohol and caffeinated food and beverages, which irritate the bladder and increase urinary incontinence symptoms.
- Maintain fluid intake of 64 oz per day.
- Avoid constipation (Lukacz, 2022).

Pelvic floor muscle exercises help strengthen the pelvic floor muscles if done properly and regularly (Brubaker, 2023). These pelvic floor muscle-strengthening exercises were originally developed by Dr. Arnold Kegel in the 1940s as a method of controlling incontinence after childbirth. The principle behind these exercises is that strengthening the muscles of the pelvic floor improves urethral sphincter function.

While providing postpartum care, instruct patients about the primary prevention of stress incontinence by discussing the value and purpose of pelvic floor muscle exercises. Approach the subject sensitively, avoiding the term *incontinent*. The terms *leakage, loss of urine*, or *bladder control issues* are more acceptable to most patients.

Patients can perform pelvic floor muscle exercises by doing ten 10-second contractions whenever they change diapers, talk on the phone, or watch TV (at least three sets daily). Teach the patient to perform pelvic floor muscle exercises properly; help them identify the correct muscles by trying to stop and start the flow of urine when sitting on the toilet (Teaching Guidelines 16.3). Pelvic floor muscle exercises can be done without anyone knowing.

Assisting With Self-Care Measures

Demonstrate and discuss with the patient ways to prevent infection during the postpartum period. Because they may experience lochia drainage for as long as a month after childbirth, describe practices to promote well-being and healing. These measures include:

- Frequently change perineal pads, applying and removing them from front to back to prevent spreading contamination from the rectal area to the genital area.
- Avoid using tampons after giving birth to decrease the risk of infection.

TEACHING GUIDELINES 16.3 Performing Pelvic Floor Muscle Training Exercises

1. Identify the correct pelvic floor muscles by contracting them to stop the flow of urine while sitting on the toilet.
2. Repeat this contraction several times to become familiar with it.
3. Start the exercises by emptying the bladder.
4. Tighten the pelvic floor muscles and hold for 10 seconds.
5. Relax the muscles completely for 10 seconds.
6. Perform 10 exercises at least three times daily. Progressively increase the number you perform.
7. Perform the exercises in different positions, such as standing, lying, and sitting.
8. Keep breathing during the exercises.
9. Don't contract your abdominal, thigh, leg, or buttock muscles during these exercises.
10. Relax while doing pelvic floor muscle training exercises, and concentrate on isolating the right muscles.
11. Attempt to tighten your pelvic muscles before sneezing, jumping, or laughing.
12. Remember that you can perform these exercises anywhere without anyone noticing.

- Shower once or twice daily using a mild soap. Avoid using soap on nipples.
- Use a sitz bath after every bowel movement to cleanse the rectal area and relieve enlarged hemorrhoids.
- Begin pelvic floor muscle exercises to increase urinary tone and perineal circulation.
- Use the peribottle filled with warm water after urinating and before applying a new perineal pad.
- Avoid tub baths for 4 to 6 weeks until joints and balance are restored to prevent falls.
- Wash your hands before changing perineal pads, after disposing of soiled pads, and after voiding (Karsnitz & Wilhite, 2022).

To reduce the risk of infection at the episiotomy site, reinforce proper perineal care with the patient, showing them how to rinse their perineum with the peribottle after they void or defecate. Stress the importance of always patting gently from front to back and washing their hands thoroughly before and after perineal care. For hemorrhoids, have the patient apply witch hazel–soaked pads, ice packs to relieve swelling, or hemorrhoidal cream or ointment if ordered.

Ensuring Safety

One safety concern during the postpartum period is orthostatic hypotension. When the patient rapidly moves from a lying or sitting position to a standing one, their BP can suddenly drop, causing their pulse rate to increase. The patient may become dizzy and faint. Be aware of this problem and initiate the following safeguards:

- Check BP first before ambulating the patient.
- Check for low hemoglobin and hematocrit on lab work before ambulating the patient.
- Elevate the head of the bed for a few minutes before ambulating the patient.
- Have the patient sit on the side of the bed for a few moments before getting up.
- Help the patient to stand up, and stay with them.
- Ambulate alongside the patient and provide support if needed.
- Frequently ask the patient how their head feels.
- Stay close by to assist if the patient feels lightheaded.

Additional topics to address orthostatic hypotension that may concern infant safety include instructing the patient to place the newborn back in the crib on their back if the patient is feeling sleepy to prevent a fall. If the patient falls asleep while holding the infant, they might drop the baby. Also, instruct patients to keep the door to the room closed when their infant is in the room with them. They should check the identification of anyone who enters their room or who wants to take the infant out of the room. This will prevent infant abduction.

Counseling About Sexuality and Contraception

Pregnancy and childbirth are special periods in a person's life that involve significant physical, hormonal, psychological, social, and cultural changes that may influence their own sexuality as well as the health of a couple's sexual relationship. This is often a time period filled with excitement, changes, and challenges. Birthing parents often face changes in their own sexuality in their adjustment to parenthood. Sexuality is an important part of many people's lives. Birthing parents often want to get back to "normal" as soon as possible after giving birth, but sexual relationships cannot be isolated from the psychological and psychosocial adjustments that people and their partners go through surrounding childbirth.

Childbirth is a significant life transition that has a measurable impact on postpartum people's sexual function. There are physical, psychological, and contextual factors that contribute to the change in many people's sex lives after experiencing childbirth. Postpartum people may hesitate to resume sexual relations for a number of reasons. Many postpartum people have fatigue, weakness, loss of sexual desire, perception of decreased attractiveness, change in body appearance, vaginal bleeding, perineal discomfort, hemorrhoids, sore breasts, decreased vaginal lubrication resulting from low estrogen levels, and dyspareunia. Fatigue, the physical demands made by the infant, and the stress of new roles and responsibilities may stress people's emotional reserves. New parents may not get much privacy or rest, both of which are necessary for sexual pleasure. Parenthood requires adapting to new situations, including sexual relations. Typically, sexual activity progressively resumes over months after giving birth, but previous levels of sexual function and frequency will tend not to normalize until 6 months postpartum (Delgado-Perez et al., 2022).

Partners of the birthing parent may feel they now have a secondary role within the family, and they may not understand the birthing parent's daily routine. The delicate nature of postpartum sexuality makes it a difficult topic of discussion. These issues, combined with the birthing parent's typical increased investment in the parenting role, can strain a sexual relationship.

Although people are reluctant to ask, they often want to know when they can safely resume sexual intercourse after childbirth. Typically, sexual intercourse can be resumed once bright red bleeding has stopped and the perineum is healed from an episiotomy or lacerations. This is usually by the third to the sixth week postpartum. However, there is no set, prescribed time at which to resume sexual intercourse after childbirth. There is no scientific basis for the traditional recommendation to delay sexual activity until the 6-week postpartum checkup. Each person must set their own time frame when they feel it is appropriate to resume sexual intercourse. Despite fears and myths about sexual activity during pregnancy, maintaining sexual interactions throughout pregnancy and the postpartum period can promote sexual health and well-being and a greater depth of intimacy.

Postpartum sexual health and sexual problems are common; they may receive little attention from health care providers during the postpartum period, but they need to be addressed. A healthy sex life is a cornerstone of a person's overall health; thus, this topic should be explored with both birthing parents and their partners. Sex after childbirth may take time and effort, and intimacy can take many forms (Ruddy, 2023). When counseling people about sexuality, determine what knowledge and concerns they have about their sexual relationship. Emphasize that fluctuations in sexual interest are normal. Reassure the breastfeeding person that they may notice a let-down reflex during orgasm and find their breasts sensitive when touched by their partner. Also inform people about how to prevent discomfort. Precoital vaginal lubrication may be impaired during the postpartum period, especially in people who are breastfeeding. Use of water-based gel lubricants can help. Pelvic floor muscle training exercises, in addition to preventing stress incontinence, can enhance sensation.

Initiation of contraception during the postpartum period is important to prevent unintended pregnancy and short birth intervals, which can lead to negative health outcomes for the birthing parent and infant. Contraceptive options should be included in the discussions with birthing parents and partners so that they can make an informed decision before resuming sexual activity. Many people are overwhelmed with the amount of new information given to them during their brief hospitalization, so many are not ready for a lengthy discussion about contraceptives. Presenting a brief overview of the options, along with literature, may be appropriate. It may be suitable to ask them to think about contraceptive needs and preferences and advise them to use a barrier method (condom with spermicidal gel or foam) until they choose another form of contraception. This advice is especially important if the follow-up appointment will not occur for 4 to 6 weeks after childbirth because many people will resume sexual activity before this time. Some postpartum people ovulate before their menstrual period returns and thus need contraceptive protection to prevent another pregnancy.

Use of hormonal contraceptives in breastfeeding people raises questions about the effect on milk production and the risk to the breastfeeding person. Progestin-only contraceptives are the hormonal contraceptives of choice because they appear to have no effect on the quality or quantity of milk. Combined estrogen–progestin contraceptive pills are not ideal during lactation because they reduce the quantity and quality of milk and may increase the risk of DVT in the already hypercoagulable postpartum period. If used, they should not be started until after 6 weeks postpartum and after lactation is well established (National Institute of Child Health and Human Development, 2023).

Open and effective communication is necessary for effective contraceptive counseling so that information is clearly understood. Provide clear, consistent information appropriate to each person's language, culture, and educational level. This will help patients and partners select the best contraceptive method. Research supports that postpartum education about contraception leads to more contraception use and fewer unplanned pregnancies and that both short-term and multiple-contact interventions had effects. The use of contraceptives was highest when contraceptive counseling was provided prenatally and again in the postpartum period (Sonalkar & Mody, 2023).

Promoting Postpartum Nutrition

During postpartum, it is critical for postpartum people to develop healthy eating patterns to adequately support breastfeeding, optimize weight, and become good role models to their children. The postpartum period can be a stressful one for myriad reasons, such as fatigue, the physical stress of pregnancy and birth, and the nonstop work required to take care of the newborn and to meet the needs of other family members. As a result, the new parent may ignore their own nutritional needs. Whether they are breastfeeding or bottle-feeding, encourage the postpartum patient to take good care of themselves and eat a healthy diet so that the nutrients lost during pregnancy can be replaced and they can return to a healthy weight. In general, nutrition recommendations for the postpartum person include:

- Eat a wide variety of foods with high nutrient density.
- Minimize or avoid processed foods.
- Make sure all foods are well cooked to prevent bacterial ingestion.
- Avoid high-fat fast foods.
- Eat protein-rich foods, such as soups and stews made with bone broth.
- Eat plenty of fruit and vegetables—select a variety of colors.
- Incorporate whole grains into diet such as oatmeal, quinoa, brown rice, and farro.
- Drink plenty of fluids daily.
- Avoid fad weight reduction diets and harmful substances such as alcohol.
- Avoid excessive intake of fat, salt, sugar, and caffeine.
- Eat the recommended daily servings from each food group (Box 16.3) (Gouza, 2023).

Nutrition for the Breastfeeding Person

The breastfeeding person's nutritional needs are higher than they were during pregnancy. The person's diet and

BOX 16.3 Recommendations for Nutrition During the Postpartum Period

Recommendations for the Lactating Person From the *MyPlate* Food Guide

- Follow the MyPlate recommendations for the nonlactating person, increasing daily calories by 400.
- Choose a variety of fruits and vegetables.
- For grains, make at least ½ of them whole grains.
- Drink or eat low-fat or fat-free dairy milk or yogurt.
- Protein sources may include lean meats, poultry, seafood, beans, peas, lentils, nuts, and eggs (United States Department of Agriculture, n.d.-a).

General Dietary Guidelines for Americans From the *MyPlate* Food Guide for the Nonlactating Person

- Fruits: Make half of your plate fruits and vegetables.
- Vegetables: Eat red, orange, and dark green vegetables.
- Milk: Switch to skim milk or 1%.
- Breads, grains, and cereals should be whole grains.
- Meat, poultry, fish, and eggs: Eat seafood twice a week and beans, which are high in fiber.
- Eat the right amount of calories for you; enjoy your food, but eat less.
- Be physically active with activities you enjoy.
- Fats, oils, and sweets: Cut back.
- Use food labels to help you make better choices.

United States Department of Agriculture. (n.d.-b). *What is my plate?* https://www.myplate.gov/eat-healthy/what-is-myplate

nutritional status influence the quantity and quality of breast milk. To meet the needs for breast milk production, nutritional needs increase as follows:

- *Calories:* +400 kcal/day for the first 6 months, then +380 kcal/day thereafter
- *Calcium:* 1,000 mg daily (adolescent females 1,300 mg daily); for example, consuming four or more servings of milk
- *Iodine:* 290 mcg daily; for example, if using salt, make sure it is iodized, and increase intake of kale and cruciferous vegetables
- *Omega-3 fatty acids*: 200 to 300 mg daily; for example, two servings of low-mercury fish weekly
- *Fluid:* It is recommended to drink when thirsty; keep a bottle of healthy liquid nearby (Butte & Stuebe, 2024).

Some foods eaten by the breastfeeding person may affect the flavor of the breast milk or cause gastrointestinal problems for the infant. Not all infants are affected by the same foods. It is suggested that the parent identify the food item that may be causing a problem for the infant and reduce or eliminate their intake of it.

Nutritional needs for breastfeeding parents are based on the nutritional content of breast milk and the energy expended to produce it. If the intake of calories exceeds the energy expended, weight gain occurs. The highest incidence of obesity in females occurs during the childbearing years. Patients need to be made aware that weight gained during the reproductive years will have a negative impact on health with age. Nurses can assist patients in their postpartum weight management program by assessing their readiness to change to lose their pregnancy weight gain; assessing their breastfeeding status, dietary intake, and activity levels; and assessing them for stress and depressive symptoms, which might hinder weight loss. The goal of nursing care is to promote the physical well-being of parent and infant and support the growing relationship between them. Good nutrition for the parent can enhance this goal during the postnatal period (Said et al., 2022).

TAKE NOTE!

During a birthing parent's brief stay in a health care facility, they may demonstrate a healthy appetite and eat well. Nutritional problems usually start at home when the person needs to make their own food selections and prepare their own meals. This is a crucial area to address during follow-up.

Supporting Parental Choice of Infant Feeding Method

Both national and international health care organizations have released position statements in support of breastfeeding, and nurses should be encouraging it as part of evidence-based practice (Zimlich, 2022). See the Healthy People 2030 box. Although there is considerable evidence that breastfeeding has numerous health benefits for both parent and infant, many parents choose to feed their infants formula for the first year of life. Nurses must be able to deliver sound, evidence-based information to help the new parent choose the best way to feed their infant and must support the parent in their decision. Many factors affect a person's choice of feeding method, such as culture, employment demands, support from significant others and family, and knowledge base. Although breastfeeding is encouraged, be sure that people have the information they need to make informed decisions. Encouraging breastfeeding to improve the child's health is an important message for nurses to impart to new parents (Evidence-Based Practice 16.1). However, the patient's autonomy is paramount, and nurses must support and respect the patient's choice.

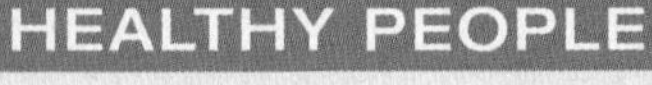

Objective	Nursing Significance
Increase the proportion of infants who are breastfed exclusively through 6 months.	• Educate parents about the benefits of breastfeeding. • Support and encourage parents in their attempts to initiate breastfeeding.

Healthy People Objectives retrieved from http://www.healthypeople.gov

EVIDENCE-BASED PRACTICE **16.1**

Breastfeeding Duration and Subsequent Risk of Mortality in the United States: A Prospective Cohort Study

BACKGROUND

According to the American Academy of Pediatrics (AAP), World Health Organization (WHO), and CDC, there is sufficient evidence that breastfeeding provides the best nutrition for newborns and should be done for the first 6 months postpartum continuing into the first year or more as solid foods are introduced to the infant. The short- and long-term benefits of breastfeeding are well supported by evidence showing reduced incidences of childhood illnesses in those breastfed as infants. Breastfeeding has also been associated with a reduced risk of long-term, chronic maternal diseases such as hypertension, endometriosis, diabetes, cardiovascular disease, metabolic syndrome, and ovarian and breast cancers. The purpose of this study was to investigate the potential interaction between breastfeeding duration and lifestyle factors on mortality risk across the reproductive lifespan.

STUDY

This study included 166,708 women taken from two large prospective cohorts who experienced at least one pregnancy during their reproductive lifespan. Participants reported their lifetime breastfeeding duration in three follow-up questionnaires. Descriptive analysis was conducted for baseline characteristics according to breastfeeding duration by standardizing to participants' age distribution.

Findings

It was found that a longer lifetime total breastfeeding duration was associated with a modestly lower risk of mortality. This inverse relationship appeared to be independent of parity and persisted during the average duration of breastfeeding per infant.

Nursing Implications

These results strengthen and refine the evidence of lifelong benefits of breastfeeding. This study provides valuable insight into the relationship between breastfeeding duration and lower maternal mortality in later life. The longer lifetime breastfeeding duration was associated with a lower risk of mortality in the breastfeeding person. Those who breastfed for a total of 18 to 24 months experienced the lowest risk. Efforts to promote continued breastfeeding throughout a child's first year of life by nurses is a worthwhile endeavor to improve the overall health of children and their parents. Additionally, the rates of childhood obesity would be lowered. Nurses can impart this study's findings to postpartum patients or prenatally to provide patients with information as they decide on infant nutrition.

Adapted from Wang, Y. X., Arvizu, M., Rich-Edwards, J. W., Manson, J. E., Wang, L., Missmer, S. A., & Chavarro, J. E. (2022). Breastfeeding duration and subsequent risk of mortality among US women: A prospective cohort study. *eClinicalMedicine, 54*. https://doi.org/10.1016/j.eclinm.2022.101693

People Who Should Not Breastfeed

Breastfeeding is the optimal way to feed infants, benefiting both the breastfeeding parent and the infant. However, certain people should not breastfeed, including those:

- Who are taking illicit drugs such as opioids, cocaine, or phencyclidine (PCP) as their metabolites enter the breast milk and may be harmful to the infant. (Note that people who are stable on methadone treatment may breastfeed.)
- With human immunodeficiency virus (HIV) infection who are not on antiretroviral therapy and achieving viral suppression: There is an increased risk of HIV transmission to the newborn.
- With active herpes infections on their breast (They should not breastfeed from the affected breast.)
- Whose newborn has galactosemia
- With mpox or brucellosis infection
- With active tuberculosis or varicella infection (though expressed breast milk may be fed to the infant) (Centers for Disease Control and Prevention [CDC], 2023a)

Providing Assistance With Breastfeeding and Bottle-Feeding

First-time parents often have many questions about feeding, and even people who have had experience with feeding may have questions. Regardless of whether the postpartum patient is breastfeeding or bottle-feeding their newborn, they can benefit from instruction.

PROVIDING ASSISTANCE WITH BREASTFEEDING

The American Academy of Pediatrics (Meek et al., 2022) recommends breastfeeding for all full-term newborns. Exclusive breastfeeding is sufficient to support optimal growth and development for approximately the first 6 months after birth. Breastfeeding should be continued for at least the first year of life and beyond for as long as mutually desired by parent and child. Educating a parent about breastfeeding will increase the likelihood of a successful breastfeeding experience.

At birth, all newborns should be quickly dried, assessed, and if stable, placed immediately in uninterrupted skin-to-skin contact (kangaroo care) with the birthing parent. This is good practice regardless of whether the infant will be breastfed or bottle-fed. Numerous benefits of kangaroo care have been reported related to both the physiologic (thermoregulation, cardiorespiratory stability) and behavioral (sleep, breastfeeding duration, and degree of exclusivity) domains as an effective therapy to relieve procedural pain and improve neurodevelopment. In addition, kangaroo care provides the newborn with optimal physiologic stability, relief of stress, greater weight gain, warmth, and opportunities for the first breastfeeding (Canadas et al., 2022).

The benefits of breastfeeding for infants are clear (see Chapter 18). To promote breastfeeding, the Baby-Friendly Hospital Initiative, an international program of the World

Health Organization (WHO) and the UNICEF, was started in 1991. This global health promotion initiative was put forth to improve maternal–infant health by improving rates of exclusive breastfeeding. The initial guidelines have been revised to reflect more evidence-based practice. As part of this program, the hospital or birth center should take the following 10 steps to provide "an optimal environment for the promotion, protection, and support of breastfeeding":

1. Have a written breastfeeding policy that is communicated to all staff.
2. Ensure that staff have sufficient knowledge, competence, and skills to support breastfeeding.
3. Discuss the importance and management of breastfeeding with pregnant people and their families.
4. Facilitate immediate and uninterrupted skin-to-skin contact, and support birthing parents in initiating breastfeeding as soon as possible after birth.
5. Support birthing parents in initiating and maintaining breastfeeding, and manage common difficulties.
6. Demonstrate to all birthing parents how to initiate and maintain breastfeeding.
7. Encourage breastfeeding on demand.
8. Counsel birthing parents on the use and risks of feeding bottles, teats, and pacifiers.
9. Establish breastfeeding support groups and refer birthing parents to them.
10. Enable birthing parents and their infants to remain together and to practice rooming-in 24 hours a day (Baby-Friendly USA, 2024).

The nurse is responsible for protecting, promoting, and supporting breastfeeding when appropriate. For the person who chooses to breastfeed their infant, the nurse or lactation consultant will need to spend time instructing them about how to do so successfully. Many people have the impression that breastfeeding is simple. The first few days of life are a critical period to facilitate breastfeeding, but a person may experience some difficulty in breastfeeding their newborn despite it being a natural process. Nurses can assist birthing parents in smoothing out this transition. Assist and provide one-to-one instruction to breastfeeding parents, especially first-time breastfeeding parents, to ensure correct technique. Suggestions are highlighted in Teaching Guidelines 16.4.

TAKE NOTE!

Some newborns "latch on and catch on" right away, and others take more time and patience. Inform new parents about this to reduce their frustration and uncertainty about their ability to breastfeed.

Tell birthing parents that they need to believe in themselves and their ability to accomplish this task. They

TEACHING GUIDELINES 16.4 Breastfeeding Suggestions

1. Explain that breastfeeding is a learned skill for both parties.
2. Offer a thorough explanation of the actions involved.
3. Instruct the parent to wash their hands before starting.
4. Inform the parent that their afterpains will increase during breastfeeding.
5. Make sure the parent is comfortable (pain free) and not hungry.
6. Tell the parent to start the feeding with an awake and alert infant showing hunger signs.
7. Assist the parent in positioning themselves correctly for comfort.
8. Urge the parent to relax to encourage the let-down reflex.
9. Guide the parent's hand to form a "C" to access the breast with the thumb on top and the other four fingers under the breast.

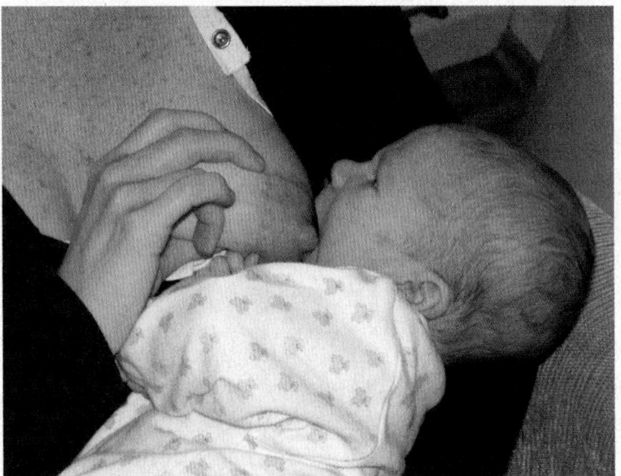

10. Have the parent lightly tickle the infant's upper lip with their nipple to stimulate the infant to open the mouth wide.
11. Aid the parent in helping the infant latch on by bringing the infant rapidly to the breast with a wide-open mouth.
12. Show the parent how to check that the newborn's mouth position is correct, and tell them to listen for a sucking noise.
13. Demonstrate correct removal from the breast, using their finger to break the suction.
14. Instruct the parent on how to burp the infant before changing from one breast to another.
15. Show them different positions, such as cradle and football holds and side-lying positions (see Chapter 18).

TEACHING GUIDELINES **16.4** Breastfeeding Suggestions

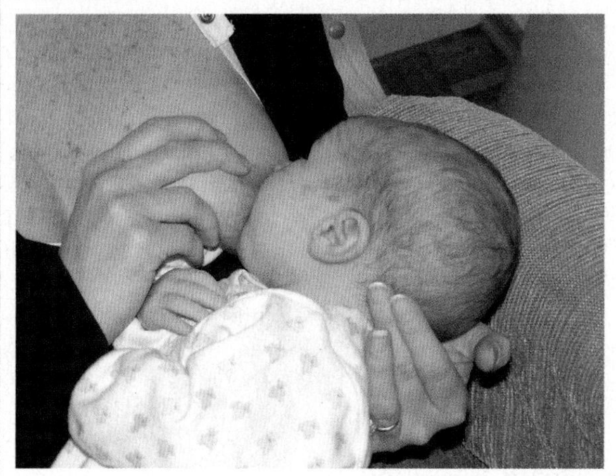

16. Reinforce and praise the parent for their efforts.
17. Allow ample time to answer questions and address concerns.
18. Refer the parent to support groups and community resources.

should not panic if breastfeeding does not go smoothly at first; it takes time and practice. Additional suggestions to help parents relax and feel more comfortable breastfeeding, especially when they return home, include:

- Select a quiet corner or room where you won't be disturbed.
- Use a rocking chair to soothe both you and your infant.
- Take long, slow deep breaths to relax before nursing.
- Drink water while breastfeeding to replenish body fluids.
- Listen to soothing music while breastfeeding.
- Cuddle and caress the infant while feeding.
- Set out extra cloth diapers within reach to use as burping cloths.
- Allow sufficient time to enjoy each other in an unhurried atmosphere.
- Involve other family members in all aspects of the infant's care from the start.
- Contact a local La Leche League or a nursing parents' group for continued guidance and support.

Because obesity in the United States is increasing, it is important for nurses to be knowledgeable about how it impacts breastfeeding and ways to support the birthing parent who has a higher body weight. Research shows that breastfeeding parents who have a body mass index (BMI) over 30 are less likely to initiate lactation, have difficulties with latching, have delayed lactogenesis, experience mechanical challenges, and are prone to early cessation of breastfeeding. Having skin-to-skin contact with their newborns can help these parents decrease breastfeeding disparities. Prevention of obesity is essential during pregnancy, as maternal obesity is associated with an increased risk for childhood obesity (Ramsey & Schenken, 2024). Obesity rates are highest among African American women, who also have the lowest rate of breastfeeding initiation and shortest duration when compared with women of other demographic groups. Improving rates of breastfeeding within Black communities could significantly improve the health of Black birthing parents and infants (Cleaves, 2020). Women who are of higher body weight have lowered prolactin responses to an infant sucking, thus milk production may be inhibited.

Nurses can assist in managing lactation challenges related to body weight by keeping the parent and newborn together to facilitate early and frequent sucking to trigger prolactin and oxytocin production, which will help negate the obesity-related blunting of the prolactin response. Suggesting a sandwich technique to insert the parent's breast into the newborn's mouth to elicit sucking might be helpful for the birthing parent with large breasts. In the sandwich technique, the parent is taught to grasp their breast by making a "C" with her thumb and index finger. The thumb stabilizes the top of the breast while the remaining four fingers support the breast from below. Massaging or pumping the breast may soften and extend the nipple for easier infant latch-on. In short, nurses can make a difference by observing lactation, assessing infant hydration and satisfaction, and reassuring the parent about their breastfeeding capacity.

PROVIDING ASSISTANCE WITH BOTTLE-FEEDING

If the parent has chosen to bottle feed the newborn, the nurse should respect and support this decision. Discuss with parents what type of formula they will use. Commercial formulas are classified as cow's milk-based, soy protein-based, or specialized or therapeutic formulas for infants with protein allergies. Commercial formulas can also be purchased in various forms: powdered (must be mixed with water), condensed liquid (must be diluted with equal amounts of water), ready to use (poured directly into bottles), and prepackaged (ready to use in disposable bottles).

Breast milk is a dynamic fluid with compositional changes occurring throughout the period of lactation that reflects the growth rate and developmental needs of the infant. Infant formula, in contrast, has a static composition intended to meet the nutritional requirements of infants from birth to 12 months of age. The formula ingredients are carbohydrates, oils and fats, protein, minerals, and vitamins (Patel & Rouster, 2023). Nurses need to bring this information to the attention of parents who choose to formula-feed their infants that changes may be needed in different stages of growth to meet the nutritional needs of the infant.

Newborns need about 110 to 135 cal/kg/day. Infant formulas supply about 20 kcal/oz (Patel & Rouster, 2023). Therefore, explain to parents that a newborn will need 2 to 4 oz to feel satisfied at each feeding. Until about 4 months of age, most bottle-fed infants need six feedings a day. After this time, the number of feedings declines to accommodate other foods in the diet, such as fruits, cereals, and vegetables (Langley-Evans, 2022). For more information on newborn nutrition and bottle-feeding, see Chapter 18.

When teaching a parent about bottle-feeding, provide the following guidelines:

- Wash hands with hot, soapy water, and dry using a clean or disposable cloth.
- Make sure all bottles, nipples, and other utensils are clean.
- Make feeding a relaxing time, a time to provide both food and comfort to the newborn.
- Use the feeding period to promote bonding by smiling, singing, making eye contact, and talking to the infant.
- Powdered formula mixes more easily and the lumps dissolve faster if you use room-temperature water.
- Store any formula prepared in advance in the refrigerator to keep bacteria from growing.
- Do not microwave formula; the microwave won't heat it evenly, causing hot spots.
- Always hold the newborn when feeding; never prop the bottle.
- Use a comfortable position when feeding the newborn. Place the newborn in the dominant arm, which is supported by a pillow. Alternately, have the newborn in a semi-upright position supported in the crook of your arm. This position reduces choking and the flow of milk into the middle ear.
- Tilt the bottle so that the nipple and the neck of the bottle are always filled with formula. This prevents the infant from taking in too much air.
- Stimulate the sucking reflex by touching the nipple to the infant's lips.
- Avoid placing any cereal or food in the bottle.
- Do not put the infant to bed with a bottle—it can cause tooth decay.
- Refrigerate any powdered formula that has been combined with tap water.
- Discard any formula not taken; do not keep it for future feedings.
- Burp the infant frequently, and place the baby on their back for sleeping.
- Avoid adding anything to the bottle to encourage fullness, such as cereal.
- Do not force feed at any time; monitor the infant's intake at each feeding.
- Do not dilute the powder formula to save money. This can lead to water intoxication.
- Prepared formula should be discarded within 1 hour after feeding an infant (CDC, 2021).

Teaching About Breast Care

Breasts and nipples do not need special care unless there are specific problems. Regardless of whether the parent is breastfeeding their newborn, urge them to wear a supportive, snug bra 24 hours a day to support enlarged breasts and promote comfort. A person who is breastfeeding should wear a supportive bra throughout the lactation period. A person who is not breastfeeding should wear it until engorgement ceases and then should wear a less restrictive one. The bra should fit snugly while still allowing the person to breathe without restriction. All postpartum people should use plain water to clean their breasts, especially the nipple area; soap has a drying effect on skin and should be avoided.

Assessing the Breasts

Instruct the patient on how to examine their breasts daily. Daily assessment includes the milk supply (breasts will feel full as they are filling), the condition of the nipples (red, bruised, fissured, or bleeding), and the success of breastfeeding. The fullness of the breasts may progress to engorgement in the breastfeeding person if feedings are delayed or breastfeeding is ineffective. Palpating both breasts will help identify whether the breasts are soft, filling, or engorged. A similar assessment of the breasts should be completed on the nonlactating postpartum person to identify any problems, such as engorgement or mastitis.

Alleviating Breast Engorgement

Breast engorgement usually occurs during the first week postpartum. It is a common response of the breasts to the sudden change in hormones and the presence of an increased amount of milk. Reassure the patient that this condition is temporary and usually resolves within 72 hours.

ALLEVIATING BREAST ENGORGEMENT IN THE BREASTFEEDING PATIENT

If the patient is breastfeeding, encourage frequent feedings at least every 2 to 3 hours, using manual expression just before feeding to soften the areola so the newborn can latch on more effectively. To help milk flow more easily, the breast can be gently massaged before feeding or expressing. Advise the patient to allow the newborn to feed on the first breast until it softens before switching to the other side (La Leche League International, 2022). See Chapter 18 for more information on alleviating breast engorgement and other common breastfeeding concerns.

ALLEVIATING BREAST ENGORGEMENT AND SUPPRESSING LACTATION IN THE BOTTLE-FEEDING PATIENT

If the patient is bottle-feeding, explain that breast engorgement is a self-limiting phenomenon that disappears as increasing estrogen levels suppress milk formation (i.e., lactation suppression). Encourage the patient to use ice packs, to wear a snug, supportive bra 24 hours a day, and to take mild analgesics such as acetaminophen. Encourage them to avoid any stimulation to the breasts that might foster milk production, such as warm showers or pumping or massaging the breasts. Medication is no longer given to hasten lactation suppression because these agents have limited effectiveness and adverse side effects. Teaching Guidelines 16.5 provides tips on lactation suppression.

Promoting Family Adjustment and Well-Being

The postpartum period involves extraordinary physiologic, psychological, and sociocultural changes in the life of a birthing parent and their family. Adapting to the role of a parent is not an easy process. The postpartum period is a "getting-to-know-you" time when parents begin to integrate the newborn into their lives as they reconcile the fantasy child with the real one. This can be a challenging period for families. Nurses play a major role in assisting families with adapting to the changes, promoting a smooth transition into parenthood. Appropriate and timely interventions can help parents adjust to the role changes and promote attachment to the newborn (Fig. 16.7).

For people who already have children, the addition of a new member may cause role conflict and challenges. The nurse should provide anticipatory guidance about siblings' potential responses to the new baby, increased emotional tension, child development, and meeting the multiple needs of the expanding family. Although the multiparous person has had experience with newborns, do not assume that their knowledge is current and accurate, especially if some time has elapsed since their previous child was born. Reinforcing information is important for all families.

TEACHING GUIDELINES 16.5 Suppressing Lactation

1. Wear a supportive, snugly fitting bra 24 hours daily, but not one that binds the breasts too tightly or interferes with breathing.
2. Suppression may take 5 to 7 days to accomplish.
3. Take mild analgesics to reduce breast discomfort.
4. Let shower water flow over your back rather than your breasts.
5. Avoid any breast stimulation in the form of sucking or massage.
6. Drink to quench your thirst. Restricting your fluid intake will not dry up your milk.
7. Reduce your salt intake to decrease fluid retention.
8. Use ice packs or cool compresses inside the bra to decrease local pain and swelling; change them every 30 minutes (Cross, 2023).

Promoting Parental Roles

Parents' roles develop and grow when they interact with the newborn (see Chapter 15 for information on parental adaptation). The pleasure they derive from this interaction stimulates and reinforces this behavior. With repeated, continued contact with the newborn, parents learn to recognize cues and understand the newborn's behavior. This positive interaction contributes to family harmony.

Nurses need to know the stages parents go through as they make their new parenting roles fit into their life experience. Assess the parents for attachment behaviors (normal and deviant), adjustment to the new parental role, family member adjustment, social support system, and educational needs. To promote parental role adaptation and parent–newborn attachment, provide the following nursing interventions:

- Provide as many opportunities as possible for parents to interact with their newborn. Encourage parents to explore, hold, and provide care for their newborn. Praise them for their efforts.
- Model behaviors by holding the newborn close, calling the newborn's name, and speaking positively.
- Speak directly to the newborn in a calm voice while pointing out the newborn's positive features to the parents.
- Evaluate the family's strengths, weaknesses, and readiness for parenting.
- Assess for risk factors such as lack of social support and the presence of stressors.
- Observe the effect of culture on family interaction to determine healthy family dynamics.
- Monitor parental attachment behaviors to determine whether alterations require referral. Positive behaviors include holding the newborn closely or in an *en face* position, talking to or admiring the newborn, or demonstrating closeness. Negative behaviors include avoiding contact with the newborn, calling them derogatory names, or showing a lack of interest in caring for them (see Table 16.1).
- Monitor the parents' coping behaviors to determine alterations that need intervention. Positive coping behaviors include positive conversations between the partners, both parents wanting to be involved with newborn care, and lack of arguments between the parents. Negative behaviors include not visiting, limited conversations or periods of silence, and heated arguments or conflict.
- Identify the support systems available to the new family and encourage them to ask for help. Ask direct questions about home or community support. Make referrals to community resources to meet the family's needs.
- Arrange for community home visits in high-risk families to provide positive reinforcement of parenting skills and nurturing behaviors with the newborn.

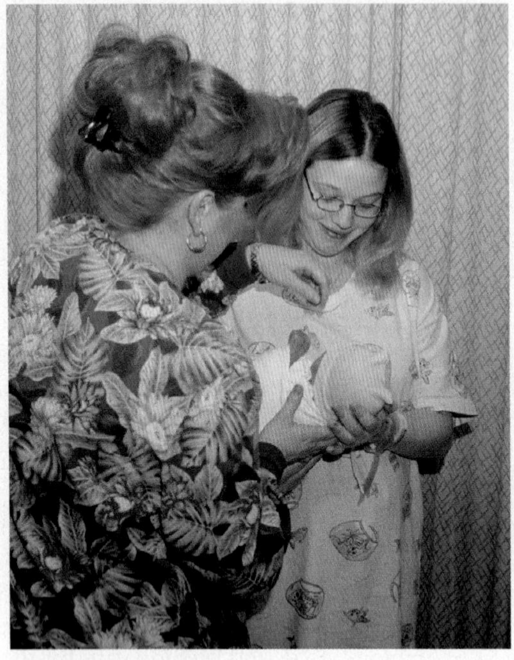

A

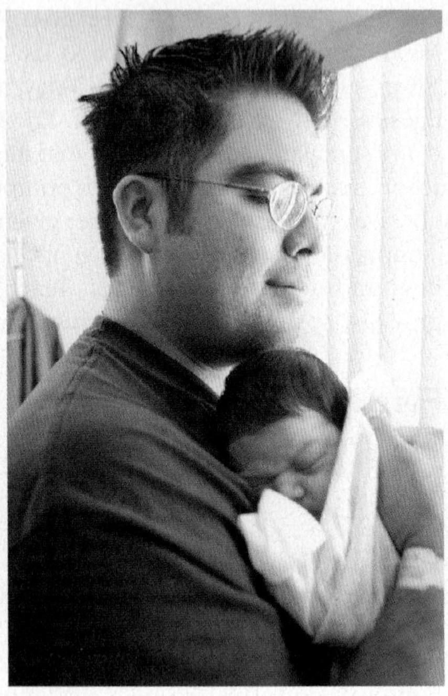

B

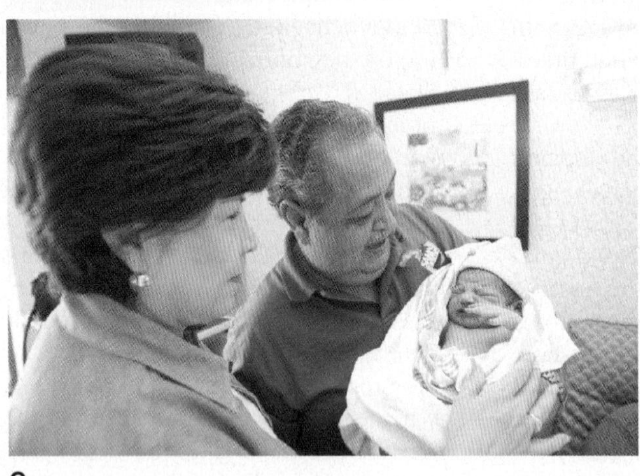

C

FIGURE 16.7 Examples of family members carrying out roles to promote adjustment and well-being. **A.** An aunt admiring the newest member of the family. **B.** A nonbirthing parent holding the newborn closely on his chest. **C.** Grandparents welcoming the newest member to the family circle.

- Provide anticipatory guidance about the following before discharge to reduce the new parents' frustration:
  - Newborn sleep–wake cycles (they may be reversed)
  - Variations in newborn appearance and developmental milestones (growth spurts)
  - How to interpret crying cues (hunger, wetness, discomfort) and what to do about them
  - Sensory enrichment and stimulation (colorful mobile)
  - Signs and symptoms of illness and how to assess for fever
  - Important phone numbers, follow-up care, and needed immunizations
  - Physical and emotional changes associated with the postpartum period
  - Need to integrate siblings into care of the newborn; stress that sibling rivalry is normal and offer ways to reduce it.
  - Ways for parents and partners to make time together

In addition, nurses can help partners feel more competent in assuming their parental role by teaching and providing information (Fig. 16.8). Education can dispel any unrealistic expectations they may have, helping them cope more successfully with the demands of parenthood, thereby fostering a nurturing family relationship.

Explaining Sibling Roles

Sibling adjustment is an important part of family adaptation. It can be overwhelming to a young child to have another family member introduced into their small, stable world. Although most parents try to prepare their

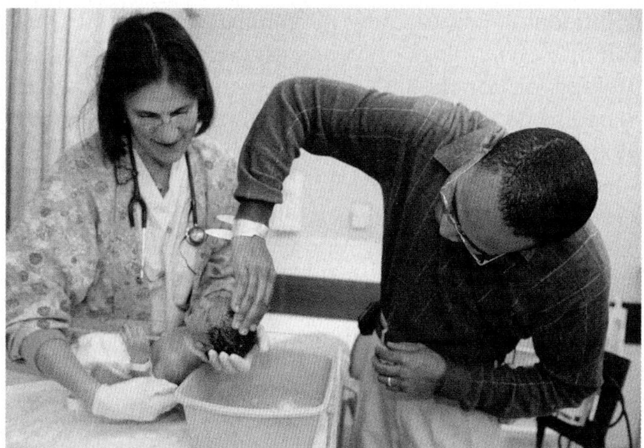

FIGURE 16.8 Nurse encouraging the partner of the birthing parent to participate in newborn care.

children for the arrival of a new sibling, many young children experience stress. They may view the new infant as competition, or fear that they will receive less of the parents' affection. All siblings need extra attention from their parents and reassurance that they are loved and important. Anticipatory guidance by nurses can help families navigate these sibling adjustments. Many parents need reassurance that sibling rivalry is normal. Suggest the following to help parents minimize sibling rivalry:

- Expect and tolerate some regression (thumb sucking, bedwetting).
- Explain childbirth in an appropriate way for the child's age.
- Encourage discussion about the new infant during relaxed family times.
- Encourage the sibling(s) to participate in decisions, such as the baby's name and toys to buy.
- Take the sibling on a tour of the maternity suite.
- Buy a T-shirt that says, "I'm the big (brother or sister)."
- Spend "special time" with the child.
- Read with the child. Some suggested titles include *Who? A Celebration of Babies* (Harris, 2018); *Poppy's Best Babies* (Eaddy, 2018); and *The New Small Person* (Child, 2015).
- Plan time for each child throughout the day.
- Role-play safe handling of a newborn using a doll. Give the preschooler or school-age child a doll to care for.
- Encourage older children to verbalize emotions about the newborn.
- Purchase a gift that the child can give to the newborn.
- Purchase a gift that can be given to the child by the newborn.
- Arrange for the child to come to the hospital to see the newborn (Fig. 16.9).
- Move the sibling from their crib to a youth bed months in advance of the birth of the newborn.
- Arrange a lot of outdoor time for the older child.
- Ignore "smallies"; address "biggies"—expect the older child to work out smaller problems.

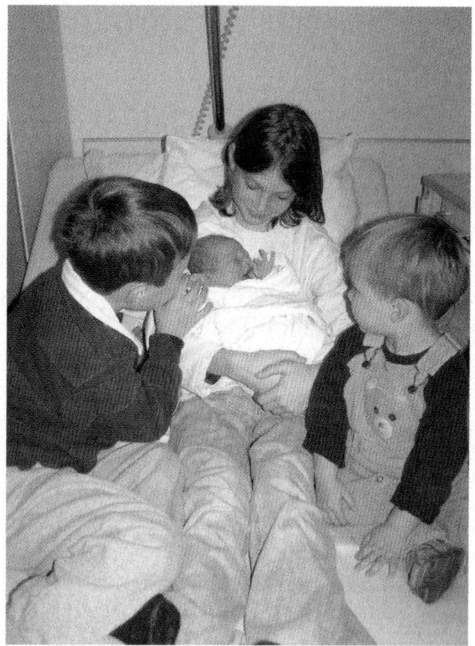

FIGURE 16.9 Sibling visitation.

- Show the older sibling photos of the baby growing. Let them pat the baby beneath the bulge, talk to the baby, and feel the baby kick.
- Help the older sibling feel important by giving them the title of "helper."
- Encourage grandparents to pay attention to the older child when visiting.
- Tell the older sibling that their friends come and go, but siblings are forever.
- Encourage "Do unto others as you would have them do unto you."
- Stay positive! (Sears & Sears, 2020b).

CONSIDER THIS!

Katie and Molly have been excited about having a new baby sister ever since they were told about their birthing parent's pregnancy. The 6-year-old twins are eagerly looking out the front window, waiting for their parents to bring their new sister, Jessica, home. The girls are big enough to help their birthing parent care for their new sibling, and for the past few months, they have been fixing up the new nursery and selecting baby clothes. They practiced diapering their dolls—their mother was specific about not using any powder or lotion on Jessica's bottom—and holding them correctly to feed them bottles. Finally, their mother arrives home from the hospital with Jessica in her arms.

The girls notice that their mother is protective of Jessica and watches them carefully when they care for her. They fight over the opportunity to hold her or feed her. What is special to both of them is the time they spend alone with their parents. Although a new family member has been added, the twins still feel special and loved by their parents.

Thoughts: Bringing a new baby into an established family can cause conflict and jealousy. What preparation did the older siblings have before Jessica arrived? Why is it important for parents to spend time with each sibling separately?

Discussing Grandparents' Role

Grandparents can be a source of support and comfort to the postpartum family if effective communication skills are used and roles are defined. The grandparents' role and involvement will depend on how close they live to the family, their willingness to become involved, and cultural expectations of their role. Just as parents and siblings go through developmental changes, so too do grandparents. These changes can have a positive or negative effect on the relationship.

Newborn care, feeding, and child-rearing practices have changed since the grandparents raised the parents. New parents may lack parenting skills but nonetheless want their parents' support without criticism. If a grandparent assumes a "take-charge approach," this may not be welcomed by new parents who are testing their own parenting roles, and family conflict may ensue. However, many grandparents respect their adult children's wishes for autonomy and remain "resource people" for them when requested.

> **TAKE NOTE!**
> Grandparents' involvement can enrich the lives of the entire family if accepted in the right context and dose by the family.

Nurses can assist in the grandparents' role transition by assessing their communication skills, role expectations, and support skills during the prenatal period. Find out whether the grandparents are included in the new parent's social support network and whether their support is wanted or helpful. If they are and it is, encourage grandparents to learn about the parenting, feeding, and child-rearing skills birthing parents and partners have learned in childbirth classes. This information is commonly found in "grandparenting" classes, which introduce new parenting concepts and bring the grandparents up to date on today's childbirth practices.

Teaching About the Postpartum Blues

The postpartum period is typically a happy yet stressful time because the birth of an infant is accompanied by enormous physical, social, and emotional changes. A sharp fall in hormones can be a predictor of mood changes in the postpartum period. **Postpartum blues** is a phase of emotional lability characterized by crying episodes, irritability, anxiety, confusion, and sleep disorders. Symptoms usually arise within 7 to 10 days after childbirth (Karsnitz & Wilhite, 2022). See Chapter 15 for a more thorough discussion of postpartum blues. Although postpartum blues is usually benign and self-limited, these mood changes can be frightening to the patient. It is prudent to ask the new parent about having pleasure and interest in things or feeling predominately down, depressed, or hopeless. Once postpartum blues are determined to be the likely cause of the mood symptoms, the nurse can offer anticipatory guidance that these mood swings are commonly experienced and usually resolve spontaneously within a week, offering reassurance. Postpartum blues is typically mild and transient with a short duration (Balaram & Marwaha, 2023). Patients should be counseled to seek further evaluation if these moods do not resolve within 2 weeks as postpartum depression may be developing.

> **TAKE NOTE!**
> Postpartum blues have been regarded as brief, benign, and without clinical significance, but research indicates an increased incidence of postpartum depression at 1 to 2 months following childbirth in birthing parents who experienced postpartum blues (Balaram & Marwaha, 2023).

Postpartum blues require no formal treatment other than support and reassurance because they do not usually interfere with the person's ability to function and care for their infant. Nurses can ease a postpartum patient's distress by encouraging them to vent their feelings and by demonstrating patience and understanding with the patient and their family. Suggest that getting outside help with housework and infant care might help the patient feel less overwhelmed until the blues ease. Provide telephone numbers they can call when they feel down during the day. Making patients aware of this disorder while they are pregnant will increase their knowledge about this mood disturbance, which may lessen their embarrassment and increase their willingness to ask for and accept help if it does occur.

The postpartum person is also at risk for postpartum depression and postpartum psychosis; these conditions are discussed in Chapter 22.

Preparing for Discharge

The WHO (2022) recommends that the length of stay in the health care facility should be individualized for each birthing parent and baby but should be at least 24 hours after birth; discharge from the hospital should not happen too early. Discharge can be considered if the following criteria are met:

- Birthing parent is afebrile, and vital signs are within normal range.
- Lochia is of appropriate amount and color for stage of recovery.
- The birthing parent's bleeding is controlled.

- The infant is feeding well.
- The birthing parent is voiding without documented difficulty.
- Hemoglobin and hematocrit values are within the normal range.
- Uterine fundus is firm; urinary output is adequate.
- ABO blood groups and RhD status are known and if indicated, anti-D immunoglobulin has been administered.
- Surgical wounds are healing, and no signs of infection are present.
- The birthing parent is able to ambulate without difficulty.
- Food and fluids are taken without difficulty.
- Self-care and infant care are understood and demonstrated.
- Family or other support system is available to care for both.
- The birthing parent is aware of possible complications (WHO, 2022).

Providing Immunizations

Prior to discharge, check all postpartum patients' immunity status for rubella and give a subcutaneous injection of rubella vaccine if they are not serologically immune (titer less than 1:8). Be sure that the patient signs a consent form to receive the vaccine. The rubella vaccine should not be given to any patient who is immunocompromised, and the immune status of their close contacts needs to be determined before any vaccine is administered to the patient to prevent a more virulent case of the vaccine-preventable illness or potential death. With the recent increase in the number of instances of pertussis in infants younger than 3 months of age, the Centers for Disease Control and Prevention (CDC, 2023b) is also recommending vaccination with (Tdap) (combination of diphtheria, pertussis, and tetanus vaccines) for the birthing parent during their postpartum stay. If it is flu season, the inactivated influenza vaccines are recommended to be administered. Breastfeeding parents can be vaccinated because the live, attenuated rubella virus is not communicable. Inform all patients receiving immunization about adverse effects (rash, joint symptoms, and a low-grade fever 5 to 21 days later) and the need to avoid pregnancy for at least 28 days after being vaccinated because of the risk of teratogenic effects (CDC, 2023b).

Rh Status

Each person's blood is one of four major types: A, B, AB, or O. Blood types are determined by the types of antigens on the red blood cells. Antigens are proteins on the surface of blood cells that can cause a response from the immune system. Approximately 15% of the U.S. population has Rh-negative blood (Salem & Singer, 2022). If the birthing parent is Rh-negative, check the Rh status of the newborn. Verify that the birthing parent is Rh-negative and has not been sensitized, that their indirect Coombs test (antibody screen) is negative, and that the newborn is Rh-positive. People who are Rh-negative and have given birth to an infant who is Rh-positive should receive an injection of Rh immunoglobulin within 72 hours after birth to prevent a sensitization reaction in the Rh-negative patient who received Rh-positive blood cells during the birthing process. Administering RhoGAM prevents initial isoimmunization in Rh-negative birthing parents by destroying fetal erythrocytes in the maternal system before maternal antibodies can develop and maternal memory cells become sensitized. This is a classic passive immunization technique. The usual protocol for the Rh-negative patient is to receive two doses of RhoGAM, one at 28 weeks' gestation and the second dose within 72 hours after childbirth. The standard dose of RhoGAM is 300 mcg given intramuscularly, which prevents the development of antibodies for an exposure of up to 15 mL of fetal red blood cells (UpToDate, Inc., 2024). A signed consent form is needed after a thorough explanation is provided about the procedure, including its purpose, possible adverse effects, and effects on future pregnancies.

RhoGAM contains actual Rh antibodies produced by people who have become sensitized. It is, therefore, a blood product. Each dose contains enough anti-D to suppress the immune response of 15 mL of Rh-positive red blood cells (Yoham & Casadesus, 2023). Jehovah's Witnesses and other people who belong to religions prohibiting the use of blood products should decide based on their conscience and possibly consultation with ecclesiastical leaders about the use of RhoGAM. Nurses need to respect whatever the patient's decision is.

Ensuring Follow-Up Care

New parents and their families need to be attended to over an extended period of time by nurses knowledgeable about postpartum patient care, infant feeding (both breastfeeding and bottle-feeding), infant care, and nutrition. Although continuous nursing care stops on discharge from the hospital or birthing center, extended episodic nursing care needs to be provided at home. Some of the challenges faced by families after discharge are described in Box 16.4.

Many postpartum patients are reluctant to "cut the cord" after their brief stay in the health care facility and need expanded community services. Birthing parents who are discharged too early from the hospital run the risk of uterine subinvolution, discomfort at

BOX 16.4 Challenges Facing Families After Discharge

- Lack of role models for breastfeeding and infant care
- Lack of support from the birthing parent's own birthing parent if they did not breastfeed
- Increased mobility of society, which means that extended family may live far away and cannot help care for the newborn and support the new family
- Nonsupportive, overwhelmed, and fatigued partner
- Feelings of isolation and limited community ties for birthing parents who work full-time
- Shortened hospital stays; parents may be overwhelmed by all the information they are given in the brief hospital stay.
- Prenatal classes usually focus on the birth itself rather than on skills needed to care for themselves and the newborn during the postpartum period.
- Limited access to education and support systems for families from diverse cultures

Ruderman, R. S., Dahl, E. C., Williams, B. R., Davis, K., Feinglass, J. M., Grobman, W. A., Kominiarek, M. A., & Yee1, L. M. (2021). Provider perspectives on barriers and facilitators to postpartum care for low-income individuals. *Women's Health Reports, 2*(1), 254–262. https://doi.org/10.1089/whr.2021.0009

an episiotomy or cesarean site, infection, fatigue, and maladjustment to their new role. Postpartum nursing care should include a range of family-focused care, including telephone calls, outpatient clinics, and home visits. Typically, public health nurses, community and home health nurses, and the health care provider's office staff will provide postpartum care after hospital discharge.

PROVIDING TELEPHONE FOLLOW-UP

Telephone follow-up typically occurs during the first week after discharge to check on how things are going at home. Calls can be made by perinatal nurses within the agency as part of follow-up care or by the local health department nurses. One disadvantage of a phone call assessment is that the nurse cannot see the patient and thus must rely on the patient's or the family's observations. The experienced nurse needs to be able to recognize distress and give appropriate advice and referral information if needed.

PROVIDING OUTPATIENT FOLLOW-UP

For patients with established health care providers such as private pediatricians and obstetricians, visits to the office are arranged soon after discharge. For the patient with an uncomplicated vaginal birth, an office visit is usually scheduled for 4 to 6 weeks after childbirth. A patient who had a cesarean birth is typically seen within 2 weeks after hospital discharge. Hospital discharge orders will specify when these visits should be made. Newborn examinations and further diagnostic laboratory studies are scheduled within the first week.

TAKE NOTE!

The hospital stay of the birthing parent and their healthy term newborn should be long enough to allow identification of early problems and to ensure that the family is able and prepared to care for the infant at home (WHO, 2022).

Outpatient clinics are available in many communities. If family members run into a problem, the local clinic is available to provide assessment and treatment. Clinic visits can replace or supplement home visits. Although these clinics are open during daytime hours only and the staff members are unfamiliar with the family, they can be a valuable resource for the new family with a problem or concern.

PROVIDING HOME VISIT FOLLOW-UP

Reduction in the postpartum lengths of stay has been advocated within the context of reducing health care system costs. Early discharge in combination with home visit follow-up programs has shown safe outcomes for both the parent and the infant. Home visits are usually made within the first week after discharge to assess the parent and newborn. During the home visit, the nurse assesses for and manages common physical and psychosocial problems. In addition, home nurses can help new parents adjust to the changes in their lives. Postpartum home visits usually include:

- *Maternal assessment:* general well-being, vital signs, breast health and care, abdominal and musculoskeletal status, voiding status, fundus and lochia status, psychological and coping status, family relationships, proper feeding technique, environmental safety check, newborn care knowledge, and health teaching needed (Fig. 16.10).
- *Infant assessment:* physical examination, general appearance, vital signs, home safety check, child development status, and education needed to improve parental skills

The home care nurse must be prepared to support and educate the birthing parent and their family in the following areas:

- Breastfeeding or bottle-feeding technique and procedures
- Appropriate parenting behavior and problem solving
- Maternal/newborn physical, psychosocial, and cultural–environmental needs
- Emotional needs of the new family
- Warning signs of problems and how to prevent or eliminate them
- Sexuality issues, including contraceptive use
- Immunization needs for both birthing parent and infant
- Family dynamics for a smooth transition
- Links to health care providers and community resources

MNRS Maternal/Newborn Record System™

Maternal Assessment

Page 1 of 2

To order call: 1.800.245.4080 Re-order No. 5842N

PATIENT IDENTIFICATION

Record No. ____

Name ____

Home address ____ STREET

CITY STATE ZIP

Date MO / DAY / YR Time Begin: ____ Date of Delivery MO / DAY / YR
Time End: ____

Medication Allergy ☐ None Identify ____

Significant Health History ☐ None Identify ____

PHYSICAL

TEMP.	PULSE	RESP.	BP /

Breasts ☐ Nursing ☐ Non-nursing

Color ☐ Normal ☐ Reddened

Condition ☐ Soft ☐ Firm ☐ Engorged ☐ Blocked Ducts

Secretion ☐ Colostrum ☐ Milk ☐ Other ____

Support Bra ☐ No ☐ Yes, Fit ☐ Appropriate ☐ Inappropriate

Nipples (If nursing) ☐ Erect ☐ Flat ☐ Inverted

Condition ☐ Intact ☐ Bruised ☐ Blistered ☐ Fissured ☐ Bleeding ☐ Scabbed

Care ☐ Water Only ☐ Soap ☐ Air Dry ☐ Topical Agent (type/frequency) ____ ☐ Other ____

Self-exam ☐ Accurate ☐ Inaccurate/Instructed

Abdomen

Diastasis Recti ☐ Absent ☐ Present ____ cm ☐ Exercise Taught

Incision ☐ None

Type ☐ Transverse ☐ Vertical ☐ Umbilical

Closure ☐ Staples ☐ Sutures ☐ Steri-strips

Condition ☐ Approximated ☐ Open ____ cm ☐ Redness ____ ☐ Swelling ____ ☐ Discharge ____ ☐ Other ____

Reproductive Tract

Uterus ☐ Firm ☐ Firm with Massage ☐ Boggy
Height ____ ☐ Midline ☐ Displaced L R
☐ Non Tender ☐ Tender ☐ with touch ☐ constant

Lochia ☐ Rubra ☐ Serosa ☐ Alba
☐ Clots (describe) ____
☐ Fleshy odor ☐ Foul odor
Pads Type ____ Number/Day ____
Saturation % 0 25 50 75 100

Perineum ☐ Intact ☐ Laceration
☐ Episiotomy Type ____ Extension ____ °

Condition ☐ Redness ____ ☐ Edema ____ ☐ Eccymosis ____ ☐ Discharge ____ ☐ Approximation ____

Care ☐ Front to Back Cleansing ☐ Peri-bottle ☐ Soap/Water ☐ Ice ☐ Sitz Bath ☐ warm ☐ cool ☐ Topical Agent (type/frequency) ____ ☐ Other ____

Elimination

Urinary Tract

Voiding Pattern ☐ Normal ☐ Incontinence ☐ Bladder Distention ☐ Catheter (type) ____

Signs of Infection ☐ None/Reviewed ☐ Urgency ☐ Frequency ☐ Dysuria ☐ CVA tenderness L R

Gastrointestinal Tract

Bowel Pattern ☐ Normal ☐ No BM ☐ Constipation ☐ Diarrhea ☐ Meds/Treatments (type, frequency, effect) ____

Hemorrhoids ☐ No ☐ Yes (describe) ____ ☐ Meds/Treatments (type, frequency, effect) ____

Lower Extremities

Edema ☐ None ☐ Pedal ☐ Ankle ☐ Pretibial ☐ Thigh ☐ Pitting (describe) ____

Signs of Thrombophlebitis ☐ None

	L	R		L	R
Homan's Sign	☐	☐	Redness	☐	☐
Pain	☐	☐	Warmth	☐	☐
Swelling	☐	☐			

Pain

	Level (0-10)	Type	Managed	Problematic
☐ Abdominal Incision	____	____	☐	☐
☐ Back	____	____	☐	☐
☐ Breasts	____	____	☐	☐
☐ Headache	____	____	☐	☐
☐ Hemorrhoid	____	____	☐	☐
☐ Nipple	____	____	☐	☐
☐ Perineum	____	____	☐	☐
☐ Uterine Cramping	____	____	☐	☐
☐ Other ____			☐	☐

Analgesic ☐ No ☐ Yes (type/dose/frequency) ____

Reportable Danger Signs ☐ Aware ☐ Unaware/Instructed

TESTS ☐ None ☐ Urinalysis ☐ CBC ☐ ____

IDENTIFIED NEEDS

Signature ____

Form 5842N Rev. 11/13 BRIGGS, Des Moines, IA (800) 245.4080 www.BriggsCorp.com
Copyright © 1998, Professional Nurse Associates, Inc. All rights reserved. Printed in U.S.A.

BRiGGS Healthcare® MATERNAL ASSESSMENT

FIGURE 16.10 Sample postpartum maternal home visit assessment form.(Used with permission. Copyright Briggs Corporation. Professional Nurse Associates. https://www.briggshealthcare.com/assets/itemdownloads/5842N.pdf.)

MNRS Maternal/Newborn Record System™

Maternal Assessment

Page 2 of 2

To order call: 1.800.245.4080 Re-order No. 5842N

PATIENT IDENTIFICATION

Record No. ____

Name ____

Home address ____ STREET

CITY STATE ZIP

ACTIVITIES OF DAILY LIVING - 24 HOUR HISTORY

Date MO / DAY / YR

Nutrition

Appetite ☐ Good ☐ Fair ☐ Poor

Usual Pattern ☐ Yes ☐ No ____

Special Diet ☐ No ☐ Yes ____

Food Intolerance/Allergy ☐ No ☐ Yes ____

Vitamin/Mineral Supplement ☐ No ☐ Yes ____

Fluid Intake (type/amount) ____ Alcohol ☐ No ☐ Yes (type/amount) ____

BREAKFAST	LUNCH	DINNER	SNACKS

General Hygiene ☐ Adequate ☐ Inadequate (describe) ____

Sleep/Activity

Amount of sleep

Night, uninterrupted ____ hrs

Naps ☐ No ☐ Yes ____ hrs

Fatigue ☐ none ☐ minimal ☐ moderate ☐ exhausted

Activities

Limitations ☐ None Identify ____

☐ Self Care ☐ Infant Care

	Appropriate	Inappropriate/Instructed
Stair Climbing	☐	☐
Lifting	☐	☐
Household Tasks	☐	☐
Outside Home	☐	☐

Other ____

Exercise

☐ None

	Accurate	Inaccurate/Instructed
Kegel	☐	☐
Postpartum	☐	☐

Other ____

PSYCHOLOGICAL

Review of Labor and Birth

Missing Pieces ☐ No ☐ Yes

Unmet Expectations ☐ No ☐ Yes

Unresolved Feelings ☐ No ☐ Yes

Pertinent Data ____

Postpartum Timetable (Key on reverse side)

☐ Taking In ☐ Taking Hold ☐ Letting Go

Emotional Status ☐ Happy ☐ Ambivalent ☐ Anxious ☐ Angry ☐ Sad ☐ Other ____

Postpartum-Depression (Key on reverse side)

☐ 0 ☐ 1 ☐ 2 ☐ 3 ☐ 4

☐ Signs/Symptoms Reviewed

General Comments (body image, role changes, concerns) ____

SEXUALITY

	Aware	Unaware/ Instructed
Relationship with Partner		
Adjustment	☐	☐
Expressions of Affection	☐	☐
Resuming Intercourse		
Timing (lack of lochia, comfort)	☐	☐
Vaginal Dryness	☐	☐
Milk Ejection (if lactating)	☐	☐
Position Variation	☐	☐
Libidinal Changes	☐	☐
Return of Menses	☐	☐

Contraceptive Method

☐ None ☐ Undecided/Aware of Options

☐ Natural Family Planning

☐ Cervical Cap

☐ Condom

☐ Diaphragm

☐ Hormones ☐ Pill ☐ Injection ☐ Implant

☐ IUD

☐ Spermicide

☐ Sterilization ☐ Female ☐ Male

☐ Other ____

Accurate use ☐ Yes ☐ No/Instructed

IDENTIFIED NEEDS ____

Signature ____

Form 5842N BRIGGS, Des Moines, IA (800) 245.4080 www.BriggsCorp.com

Copyright © 1998, Professional Nurse Associates, Inc. All rights reserved. Printed in U.S.A.

BRIGGS Healthcare® MATERNAL ASSESSMENT

FIGURE 16.10 *(continued)*

Postpartum Timetable

Taking In	Passive, dependent Concerned with own needs Hesitant about making decisions
Taking Hold	Strives for independence Initiates care of self and infant Anxious about mothering ability Mood swings
Letting Go	Begins to achieve interdependence Adapting to the reality of parenthood Accepts baby as a separate person Resumes role in family and society

Postpartum Depression Key

0	=	None	• No feelings of sadness, guilt, irritation • No periods of tearfulness • Able to make decisions and work toward goals with enthusiasm • Good appetite • No difficulty falling asleep/staying asleep
1	=	Blues	• Occasional feelings of sadness, guilt, irritation, restlessness • Occasional periods of tearfulness • Delayed decision making • Extra effort necessary to initiate activity
2	=	Moderate Depression	• Regular feelings of sadness, guilt, inadequacy • Cries easily • Difficulty concentrating, making decisions • Must push self very hard to do necessary activities • Lack of interest in pleasurable activities • Decreased appetite • Difficulty getting to sleep/staying asleep • Inability to cope
3	=	Severe Depression	• Intense feelings of sadness, guilt, inadequacy • Uncontrollable crying or inability to cry • Inability to make decisions or do any productive work • Severe insomnia, exhaustion • Thoughts of harming self or infant
4	=	Psychoses	• Delusions, hallucinations, disorganized behavior • Thoughts or verbalizations of suicide, infanticide

MATERNAL ASSESSMENT

FIGURE 16.10 *(continued)*

KEY CONCEPTS

- The transitional adjustment period between birth and parenthood includes education about baby care basics, the role of the new family, emotional support, breastfeeding or bottle-feeding support, and maternal mentoring.
- Sensitivity to how childbearing practices and beliefs vary for multicultural families and how best to provide appropriate nursing care to meet their needs are important during the postpartum period.
- A thorough postpartum assessment is key to preventing complications as is frequent hand hygiene by the nurse, especially between handling birthing parents and infants.
- The postpartum assessment that uses the acronym BUBBLE-EE (breasts, uterus, bowel, bladder, lochia, episiotomy/perineum/epidural site, extremities, and emotions) is a helpful guide in performing a systematic head-to-toe postpartum assessment.
- Lochia is assessed according to its amount, color, and change with activity and time. It proceeds from lochia rubra to serosa to alba.
- Because of shortened agency stays, nurses must use this brief time with the patient to address areas of comfort, elimination, activity, rest and exercise, self-care, sexuality and contraception, nutrition, family adaptation, discharge, and follow-up.
- The AAP advocates breastfeeding for all full-term newborns, maintaining that breast milk should ideally be the sole nutrient for the first 6 months and continued with foods until 12 months of life or longer.
- Successful parenting is a continuous and complex interactive process that requires the acquisition of new skills and the integration of the new member into the existing family unit.
- Bonding is a vital component of the attachment process and is necessary for establishing parent–infant attachment and a healthy, loving relationship; attachment behaviors include seeking and maintaining proximity to and exchanging gratifying experiences with the infant.
- Nurses can be instrumental in facilitating attachment by first understanding attachment behaviors (positive and negative) of newborns and parents and intervening appropriately to promote and enhance attachment.
- New parents and their families need to be attended to over an extended period of time by nurses knowledgeable about birthing parent care, newborn feeding (breastfeeding and bottle-feeding), newborn care, and nutrition.

REFERENCES AND RECOMMENDED READINGS

American College of Obstetrics and Gynecology. (2022). *Postpartum pain management.* https://www.acog.org/womens-health/faqs/postpartum-pain-management

American Family Physician. (2024). *Collections: Choosing wisely: 309: Don't separate mothers and their newborns at birth unless medically necessary.* https://www.aafp.org/pubs/afp/collections/choosing-wisely/309.html

August, P., & Sibai, B. M. (2024). Preeclampsia: Clinical features and diagnosis. *UpToDate.* Retrieved April 20, 2024, from https://www.uptodate.com/contents/preeclampsia-clinical-features-and-diagnosis

Baby-Friendly USA. (2024). *The ten steps to successful breastfeeding.* https://www.babyfriendlyusa.org/for-facilities/practice-guidelines/10-steps-and-international-code/

Baker, B. (2024). Physical and psychological changes after childbirth. In B. J. Baker, J. Janke, & Association of Women's Health, Obstetric and Neonatal Nurses (Eds.), *Core curriculum for maternal-newborn nursing* (6th ed.). Elsevier.

Balaram, K., & Marwaha, R. (2023). Postpartum blues. *StatPearls.* https://www.ncbi.nlm.nih.gov/books/NBK554546/

Berens, P. (2023). Overview of the postpartum period: Disorders and complications. *UpToDate.* Retrieved April 20, 2024, from https://www.uptodate.com/contents/overview-of-the-postpartum-period-disorders-and-complications

Boushra, M., & Rahman, O. (2023). Postpartum infection. *StatPearls.* https://www.ncbi.nlm.nih.gov/books/NBK560804/

Brubaker, L. (2023). Patient education: Pelvic floor muscle exercises (beyond the basics). *UpToDate.* Retrieved April 23, 2024, from https://www.uptodate.com/contents/pelvic-floor-muscle-exercises-beyond-the-basics/print

Butte, N. F., & Stuebe, A. (2024). Patient education: Health and nutrition during breastfeeding (beyond the basics). *UpToDate.* Retrieved April 26, 2024, from https://www.uptodate.com/contents/health-and-nutrition-during-breastfeeding-beyond-the-basics

Canadas, D. C., Carreno, T. P., Borja, C. S., & Perales, A. B. (2022). Benefits of kangaroo mother care on the physiological stress parameters of preterm infants and mothers in neonatal intensive care. *International Journal of Environmental Research and Public Health, 19*(12), 7183. https://doi.org/10.3390/ijerph19127183

Centers for Disease Control and Prevention. (2021). *Feeding from a bottle.* https://www.cdc.gov/nutrition/infantandtoddlernutrition/bottle-feeding/index.html

Centers for Disease Control and Prevention. (2023a). *Contraindications to breastfeeding or feeding expressed breast milk to infants.* https://www.cdc.gov/breastfeeding/breastfeeding-special-circumstances/contraindications-to-breastfeeding.html

Centers for Disease Control and Prevention. (2023b). *Vaccines during and after pregnancy.* https://www.cdc.gov/vaccines/pregnancy/vacc-during-after.html

Chauhan, G., & Tadi, P. (2023). Physiology, postpartum changes. *StatPearls.* https://www.ncbi.nlm.nih.gov/books/NBK555904/

Child, L. (2015). *The new small person* (1st U.S. ed.). Candlewick Press.

Choudhari, R. G., Tayade, S. A., Venurkar, S. V., & Deshpande, V. P. (2022). A review of episiotomy and modalities for relief of episiotomy pain. *Cureus, 14*(11), e31620. https://www.cureus.com/articles/110319-a-review-of-episiotomy-and-modalities-for-relief-of-episiotomy-pain

Cleaves, E. (2020). *Improving Black maternal and infant health requires breastfeeding support*. https://accesshealthnews.com/improving-black-maternal-and-infant-health-requires-breastfeeding-support/

Couto, E., & Junior, R. P. (2022). Prophylaxis for deep venous thrombosis during pregnancy, delivery, and postpartum. In: R. A. Moreira de Sa & E. B. de Fonseca (Eds.), *Perinatology*. Springer. https://doi.org/10.1007/978-3-030-83434-0_29

Cross, L. (2023). *Nursing guidelines: Breastfeeding support and promotion*. https://www.rch.org.au/rchcpg/hospital_clinical_guideline_index/Breastfeeding_support_and_promotion/

Cunningham, F. G., Leveno, K. J., Dashe, J. S., Hoffman, B. L., Spong, C. Y., & Casey, B. M. (2022). Vaginal delivery. In F. G. Cunningham, K. J. Leveno, J. S. Dashe, B. L. Hoffman, C. Y. Spong, & B. M. Casey, *William's obstetrics* (26th ed.). McGraw Hill.

Delgado-Perez, E., Rodriguez-Costa, I., Vergara-Perez, F., Blanco-Morales, M., & Torres-Lacomba, M. (2022). Recovering sexuality after childbirth. What strategies do women adopt? A qualitative study. *International Journal of Environmental Research and Public Health, 19*(2), 950. https://doi.org/10.3390/ijerph19020950

Divine, A., Blanchard, C., Benoit, C., Downs, D. S., & Rhodes, R. E. (2022). The influence of sleep and movement on mental health and life satisfaction during the transition to parenthood. *Sleep Health, 8*(5), 475–483. https://doi.org/10.1016/j.sleh.2022.06.013

Dong, Q., Steen, M., Wepa, D., & Eden, A. (2022). Exploratory study of fathers providing Kangaroo care in a neonatal intensive care unit. *Journal of Clinical Nursing, 00*, 1–12. https://onlinelibrary.wiley.com/doi/full/10.1111/jocn.16405

Douglas, P. (2022). Re-thinking lactation-related nipple pain and damage. *Women's Health, 18*, 17455057221087865. https://doi.org/10.1177/17455057221087865

Eaddy, S., & Bonnet, R. (2018). *Poppy's best babies*. Charlesbridge.

Etzel, J. V., & Ambizas, E. M. (2022). Breastfeeding and medication safety. *U.S. Pharmacist, 47*(7), 29–33. https://www.uspharmacist.com/article/breastfeeding-and-medication-safety

Feuerstein, K. (2022). *Caring for Black birthing families requires cultural responsiveness*. https://accesshealthnews.com/caring-for-black-birthing-families-requires-cultural-responsiveness/

Gouza, M. (2023). *Postpartum nutrition: A guide to healthy eating after giving birth*. https://www.nutrisense.io/blog/postpartum-nutrition-eat-healthy-after-giving-birth

Gutierrez, V. B. (2022). Culture and breastfeeding support. *British Journal of Midwifery, 30*(12). https://www.britishjournalofmidwifery.com/content/comment/culture-and-breastfeeding-support/

Harris, R. H., & Rosenberg, N. (2018). *Who?: A celebration of babies*. Abrams Appleseed.

Kalaitzopoulos, D. R., Panagopoulos, A., Samant, S., Ghalib, N., Kadillari, J., Daniilidis, A., Samartzis, N., Makadia, J., & Palaiodimos, L. (2022). Management of venous thromboembolism in pregnancy. *Thrombosis Research, 211*, 106–113. https://doi.org/10.1016/j.thromres.2022.02.002

Karsnitz, D. B., & Wilhite, K. (2022). Overview of postpartum care. In K. D. Schuiling & F. E. Likis (Eds.), *Gynecologic health care* (4th ed., pp. 1706–1747), Jones & Bartlett Learning.

La Leche League International. (2022). *Breast engorgement*. https://www.lllc.ca/breast-engorgement

Langley-Evans, S. C. (2022). Complementary feeding: Should baby be leading the way? *Journal of Human Nutrition and Dietetics, 35*(2), 247–249. https://doi.org/10.1111/jhn.12988

LER Team. (2022). *Cultural considerations: How postpartum traditions affect lactation*. https://www.lactationtraining.com/resources/blog/entry/cultural-considerations-how-postpartum-traditions-affect-lactation-1

Lukacz, E. S. (2022). Patient education: Urinary incontinence treatments for women (beyond the basics). *UpToDate*. Retrieved April 23, 2024, from https://www.uptodate.com/contents/urinary-incontinence-treatments-for-women-beyond-the-basics

Mannarino, M., & Jo, S. (2023). *Postpartum exercise: Your guide to working out after pregnancy*. https://www.forbes.com/health/family/postpartum-exercise-guide/

Meek, J. Y., Noble, L., & Section on Breastfeeding. (2022). Policy statement: Breastfeeding and the use of human milk. *Pediatrics, 150*(1), e2022057988. https://doi.org/10.1542/peds.2022-057988

National Institute of Child Health and Human Development. (2023). Contraceptives, oral, combined. *Drugs and Lactation Database (LactMed®)*. https://www.ncbi.nlm.nih.gov/books/NBK501295/

Nygaard, I. E., Wolpern, A., Bardsley, T., Egger, M. J., & Shaw, J. M. (2021). Early postpartum physical activity and pelvic floor support and symptoms 1 year postpartum. *American Journal of Obstetrics and Gynecology, 224*(2), 193.e1–193.e19. https://doi.org/10.1016/j.ajog.2020.08.033

Ogunyemi, D. (2024a). *Bonding with your newborn: What to know if you don't feel connected right away*. https://www.acog.org/womens-health/experts-and-stories/the-latest/bonding-with-your-newborn-heres-what-to-know-if-you-dont-feel-connected-right-away

Ogunyemi, D. (2024b). *Three conditions to watch for after childbirth*. https://www.acog.org/womens-health/experts-and-stories/the-latest/3-conditions-to-watch-for-after-childbirth

Okeahialam, N. A., Dworzynski, K., Jacklin, P., & McClurg, D. (2022). Prevention and non-surgical management of pelvic floor dysfunction: Summary of NICE guidance. *British Medical Journal, 376*, n3049. https://doi.org/10.1136/bmj.n3049

Pacheco, D., & Snyder, C. (2024). *Sleep deprivation and postpartum depression*. https://www.sleepfoundation.org/pregnancy/sleep-deprivation-and-postpartum-depression

Patel, J. K., & Rouster, A. S. (2023). Infant nutrition requirements and options. *StatPearls*. https://www.ncbi.nlm.nih.gov/books/NBK560758/

Ramsey, P. S., & Schenken, R. S. (2024). Obesity in pregnancy: Complications and maternal management. *UpToDate*. Retrieved April 26, 2024, from https://www.uptodate.com/contents/obesity-in-pregnancy-complications-and-maternal-management

Ruddy, E. Z. (2023). *What to know about sex after birth*. https://www.parents.com/parenting/relationships/sex-and-marriage-after-baby/how-to-have-great-postpartum-sex/

Ruderman, R. S., Dahl, E. C., Williams, B. R., Davis, K., Feinglass, J. M., Grobman, W. A., Kominiarek, M. A., & Yee1, L. M. (2021). Provider perspectives on barriers and facilitators to postpartum care for low-income individuals. *Women's Health Reports, 2*(1), 254–262. https://doi.org/10.1089/whr.2021.0009

Said, S. A. E., Elbana, H. M., & Salama, A. M. (2022). Effect of educational guideline on nurses performance regarding postnatal care of mothers and neonates. *SAGE Open Nursing, 8*. https://doi.org/10.1177/23779608211070154

Salem, L., & Singer, K. R. (2022). *Rh incompatibility*. Medscape. https://emedicine.medscape.com/article/797150-overview#a6

Sears, W., & Sears, M. (2020a). *Bonding with baby*. https://www.askdrsears.com/topics/pregnancy-childbirth/tenth-month-post-partum/bonding-with-your-newborn/bonding-with-baby/

Sears, W., & Sears, M. (2020b). *Sibling rivalry: 20 tips to stop the friction*. https://www.askdrsears.com/topics/parenting/discipline-behavior/bothersome-behaviors/sibling-rivalry/20-tips-stop-quibbling/

Smith, H., Harvey, C., & Portela, A. (2022). Discharge preparation and readiness after birth: A scoping review of global policies, guidelines and literature. *BMC Pregnancy and Childbirth, 22*(281). https://doi.org/10.1186/s12884-022-04577-3

Smith, J. R., Talavera, F., & Rivlin, M. E. (2022). *Postpartum hemorrhage*. Medscape. https://emedicine.medscape.com/article/275038-overview#a7

Sonalkar, S., & Mody, S. K. (2023). Contraception: Postpartum counseling and methods. *UpToDate*. Retrieved April 24, 2024, from https://www.uptodate.com/contents/postpartum-contraception-counseling-and-methods

Srivastava, R. H. (2023). *The health care professional's guide to cultural competence* (2nd ed.). Elsevier.

Stoodley, C., McKellar, L., Ziaian, T., Steen, M., Fereday, J., & Gwilt, I. (2022). Midwives supporting the development of the mother-infant relationship from pregnancy to six weeks after birth: A scoping review. *BMC Psychology, 11*(71). https://doi.org/10.21203/rs.3.rs-1717447/v1

Sujawaty, S., Tompunuh, M., Sataruno, A., Gobel, N., Labari, R., & Daaliuwa, R. (2023). Midwifery care for mothers with hemorrhoids. *Jurnal Aisyah: Jurnal Ilmu Kesehatan, 8*(S1), 67–70. https://doi.org/10.30604/jika.v8iS1.1690

United Nations International Children's Emergency Fund. (n.d.). *What you need to know about parent-child attachment*. https://www.unicef.org/parenting/child-care/what-you-need-know-about-parent-child-attachment

United States Department of Agriculture. (n.d.-a). *Pregnancy and breastfeeding*. https://www.myplate.gov/life-stages/pregnancy-and-breastfeeding

United States Department of Agriculture. (n.d.-b). *What is my plate?* https://www.myplate.gov/eat-healthy/what-is-myplate

UpToDate, Inc. (2024). *UpToDate® Lexidrug™* (Version 8.2.0) [Mobile app]. Wolters Kluwer. https://apps.apple.com/us/app/lexicomp/id313401238

U.S. Department of Health and Human Services. (n.d.). *Healthy People 2030*. https://health.gov/healthypeople

Wang, Y. X., Arvizu, M., Rich-Edwards, J. W., Manson, J. E., Wang, L., Missmer, S. A., & Chavarro, J. E. (2022). Breastfeeding duration and subsequent risk of mortality among US women: A prospective cohort study. *eClinicalMedicine, 54*. https://doi.org/10.1016/j.eclinm.2022.101693

Wisner, K. (2022). Postpartum pain management. *MCN: The Journal of Maternal-Child Nursing, 47*(1), 52. https://doi.org/10.1097/NMC.0000000000000774

World Health Organization. (2022). *WHO recommendations on maternal and newborn care for a positive postnatal experience*. https://www.who.int/publications/i/item/9789240045989

Yoham, A. L, & Casadesus, D. (2023). Rho(D) immune globulin. *StatPearls*. https://www.ncbi.nlm.nih.gov/books/NBK557884/

Zhang, Y., & Hanser, A. (2023). Be the mother, not the daughter: Immigrant Chinese women, postpartum care knowledge, and mothering autonomy. *Sociology of Health & Illness, 45*(5), 1028–1045. https://doi.org/10.1111/1467-9566.13631

Zimlich, R. (2022). Breast may be best, but bottles do the job too. *Contemporary Pediatrics Journal, 39*(3). https://www.contemporarypediatrics.com/view/breast-may-be-best-but-bottles-do-the-job-too

DEVELOPING CLINICAL JUDGMENT

PRACTICING FOR NCLEX-RN

1. The nurse is assessing a postpartum patient. Which finding would lead the nurse to suspect postpartum blues?
   a. Panic attacks and suicidal thoughts
   b. Anger toward self and infant
   c. Periodic crying and insomnia
   d. Obsessive thoughts and hallucinations

2. The nurse is caring for a childbearing family. Which of these activities would best help the postpartum nurse to provide culturally sensitive care?
   a. Taking a transcultural course
   b. Caring for only families of the nurse's cultural origin
   c. Teaching Western beliefs to families from other parts of the world
   d. Being open to having the patient educate the nurse about their cultural practices

3. A postpartum patient is trying to lose weight. Which suggestion would be most appropriate to include in the teaching plan?
   a. Increase fluid intake and acid-producing foods.
   b. Avoid empty-calorie foods, breastfeed, and increase exercise.
   c. Start a high-protein, low-carbohydrate diet, and restrict fluids.
   d. Eat no snacks or carbohydrates after dinner.

4. The nurse has taught a group of breastfeeding patients about nutritional needs. The nurse determines that the teaching was successful when the patients state that they need to increase their intake of which nutrients?
   a. Carbohydrates and fiber
   b. Fats and vitamins
   c. Calories and protein
   d. Iron-rich foods and minerals

5. The nurse is caring for a postpartum patient. Which finding would lead the nurse to suspect that the patient is developing a complication?
   a. Fatigue and irritability
   b. Perineal discomfort and pink discharge
   c. Pulse rate of 60 bpm
   d. Swollen, tender, hot area on the breast

6. A nurse has been observing parents interacting with their newborn. Which assessment finding indicates positive bonding is occurring?
   a. Holding the infant close to the body
   b. Having visitors hold the infant
   c. Buying expensive infant clothes
   d. Requesting that the nurses care for the infant

7. The nurse is planning teaching for a family with a newborn and one older child. Which activity would the nurse include in the teaching plan to reduce sibling rivalry when the newborn is brought home?
   a. Punishing the older child for bedwetting behavior
   b. Sending the sibling to the grandparents' house
   c. Planning a daily "special time" for the older sibling
   d. Allowing the sibling to share a room with the infant

8. A patient is scheduled for the first postpartum home care visit. What is the major purpose of this visit?
   a. Identifying complications that require interventions
   b. Obtaining a blood specimen for phenylketonuria (PKU) testing
   c. Completing the official birth certificate
   d. Supporting the new parents in their parenting roles

9. The nurse is instructing the postpartum patient who plans to bottle feed their newborn about measures to prevent breast engorgement when they are discharged. Which measure should the nurse include in the teaching plan?
   a. Decrease fluid intake for the first week at home.
   b. Wear a tight-fitting supportive bra 24 hours daily.
   c. Take a diuretic to release the extra fluid in the breasts.
   d. Manually express the milk that is accumulating.

10. A new parent gave birth 12 hours ago. Because this is their first child, which goal planned by the nurse is most appropriate?
    a. Early discharge for the parent and newborn
    b. Rapid transition into the role of being a parent/caregiver
    c. Minimal need for expression of feelings now
    d. Effective education of both parents before discharge

CRITICAL THINKING EXERCISES

1. As a nurse working on a postpartum unit, you enter the room of a 22-year-old primipara and find them chatting on the phone while their newborn is crying loudly in the bassinet, which has been pushed into the bathroom. You pick up and comfort the newborn. While holding the baby, you ask the patient if they were aware the newborn was crying. The patient replies, "That's about all that

monkey does since she was born!" You hand the newborn to the patient and they place the newborn on the bed away from them and continue the phone conversation.

a. What is your nursing assessment of this encounter?
b. What nursing interventions would be appropriate?
c. What specific discharge interventions may be needed?

2. A 34-year-old single primipara left the hospital after a 36-hour stay with their newborn son. The patient lives alone in a one-bedroom walk-up apartment. As the postpartum home health nurse visiting them 2 days later, you find:
   - Tearful patient pacing the floor holding their crying son
   - Home cluttered and in disarray
   - Fundus firm and displaced to the right of midline
   - Moderate lochia rubra; episiotomy site clean, dry, and intact
   - Vital signs within normal range; pain rating less than 3 points on a scale of 1 to 10
   - Breasts engorged slightly; supportive bra on
   - Newborn assessment within normal limits
   - Distended bladder upon palpation; reporting urinary frequency

   a. Which of these assessment findings warrants further investigation?
   b. What interventions are appropriate at this time and why?
   c. What health teaching is needed before you leave this home?

3. The nurse walks into the room of a 24-year-old primigravida. The patient asks the nurse to hand them the bottle sitting on the bedside table, stating, "I'm going to finish it off because my baby only ate half of it 3 hours ago when I fed him."

   a. What response by the nurse would be appropriate at this time?
   b. What action should the nurse take?
   c. What health teaching is needed for this new parent prior to discharge?

STUDY ACTIVITIES

1. Identify two questions that a nurse would ask a postpartum patient to assess for postpartum blues.
2. Find a website that offers advice to new parents about breastfeeding. Critique the site, the author's credentials, and the accuracy of the content.
3. Outline instructions you would give to a new parent on how to use their peribottle.
4. Breast tissue swelling secondary to vascular congestion after childbirth and preceding lactation describes ________________.
5. Listen to the postpartum story of one of your assigned patients and share it with your peers in class or as part of an online discussion.

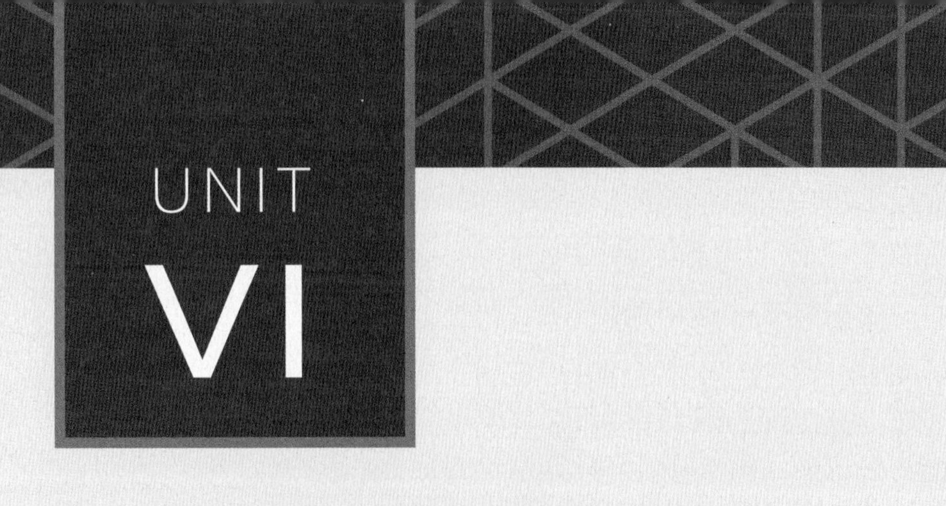

UNIT VI

The Newborn

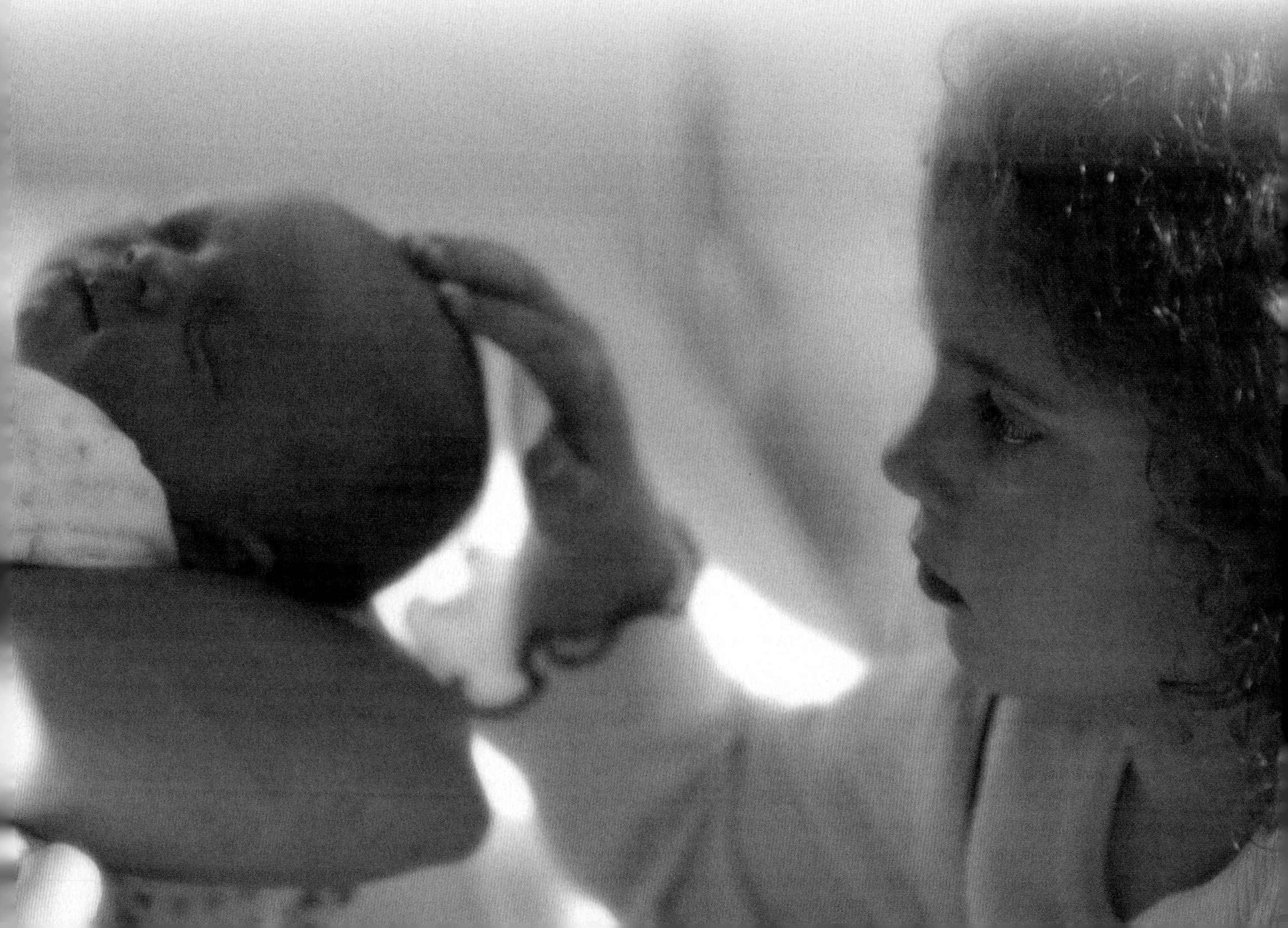

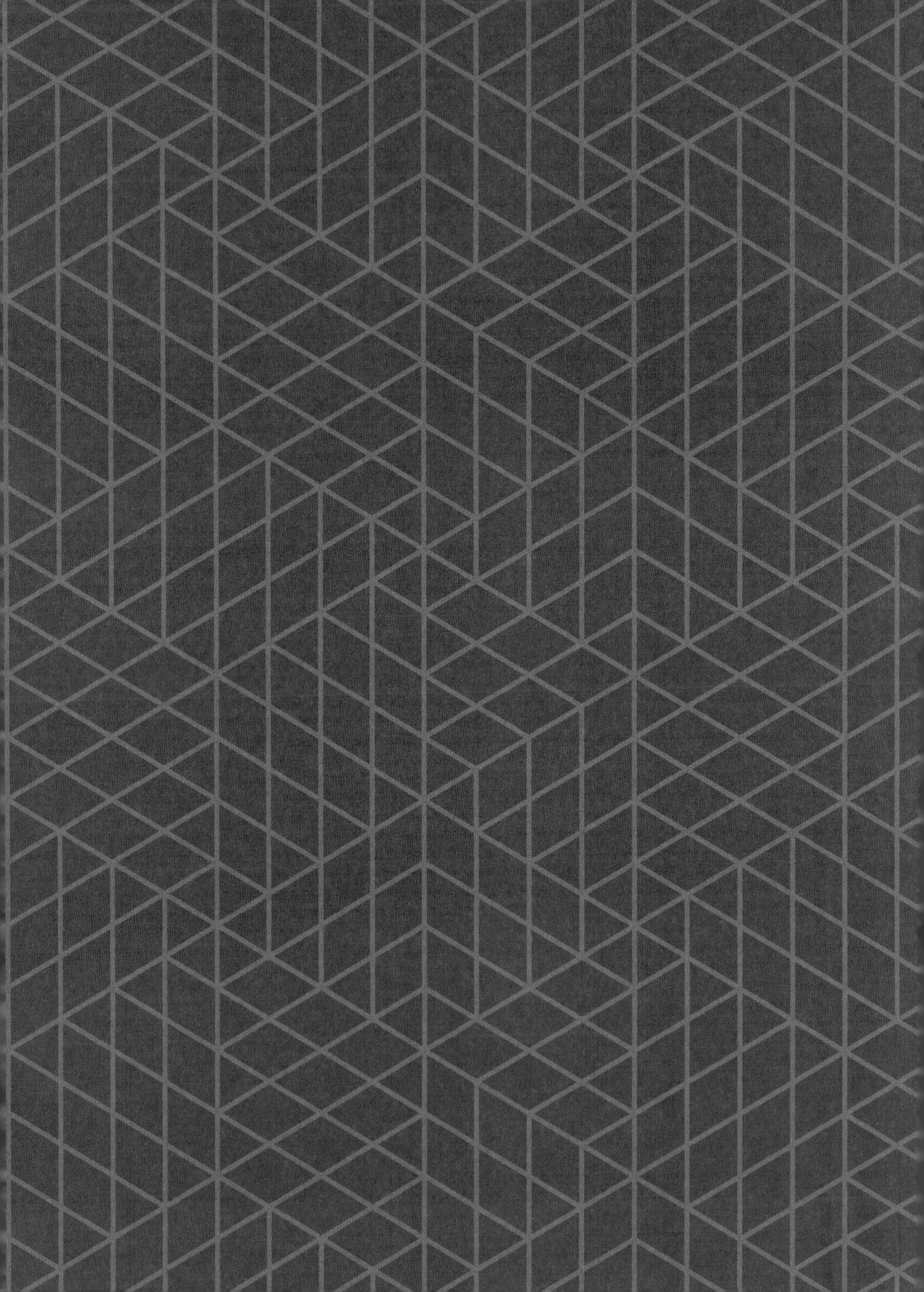

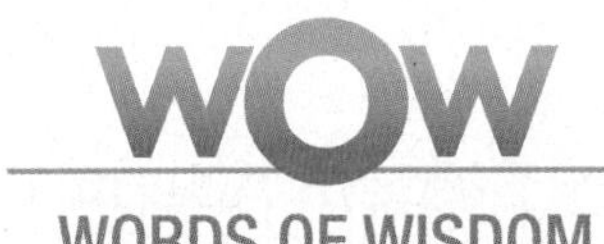

WORDS OF WISDOM

Newborns can't always be judged by their outer wrapping; rather, nurses should focus on the awesome gift inside.

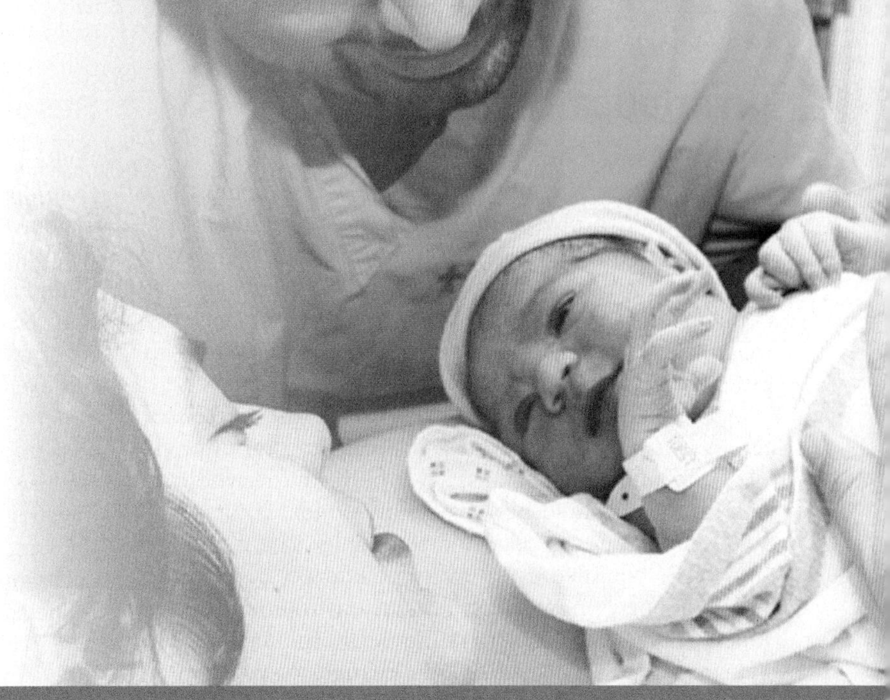

17

Newborn Transitioning

LEARNING OBJECTIVES

Upon completion of the chapter, you will be able to:

1. Examine the major physiologic changes that occur as the newborn transitions to extrauterine life.
2. Describe the cardiovascular changes that take place from fetal circulation to extrauterine circulation after birth.
3. Interpret the factors that influence the initiation of newborn respirations.
4. Relate characteristics that predispose newborns to heat loss after birth.
5. Distinguish primary immunoglobulins that help strengthen the newborn's immunologic system.
6. Determine the primary challenges faced by the newborn during the transition to extrauterine life.
7. Differentiate the behavioral patterns that newborns progress through after birth.
8. Assess the typical behavioral responses triggered by external stimuli of the newborn.

KEY TERMS

cold stress
jaundice (jawn'dis)
meconium (mē-kō'nē-ŭm)
neonatal period
neurobehavioral response
neutral thermal environment
periodic breathing
reflex
surfactant (sŭr-fak'tănt)
thermoregulation (thĕr'mō-reg'yū-lā'shŭn)

The Healthy Start home care nurse reviewed the patient's file in her car before she got out: 18-year-old primipara, 1 week postpartum with a term newborn girl weighing 7 lb. The new mother, **Maria,** greets the nurse at the door and lets her inside the house. After performing a postpartum assessment on Maria and an assessment of her newborn daughter, the nurse asked Maria if she has any questions or concerns. Maria's eyes well up with tears; she is worried that her daughter can't see.

INTRODUCTION

When a child is born, the exhaustion and stress of labor are over for the parents, but now the newborn must begin the work of physiologically and behaviorally adapting to the new environment. Birth is a relatively hypoxic event as newborns undergo a transition from the placenta as the organ of gas exchange to the lungs. Yet the majority of term newborns transition successfully, with little intervention (Fernandes, 2024).

The **neonatal period** is defined as the first 28 days of life. It is a period of the most dramatic and rapid physiologic changes in humans. After birth, the newborn is exposed to a whole new world of sounds, colors, outside temperatures, smells, and sensations. The newborn, previously confined to the warm, dark, wet intrauterine environment, is now thrust into an environment that is much brighter and cooler. As the newborn adapts to life after birth, numerous physiologic changes occur.

Awareness of the adaptations that are occurring forms the foundation for providing support to the newborn during this crucial time. Physiologic and behavioral changes occur quickly during this transition period. Being aware of any deviations from the norm is crucial to ensure early identification and prompt intervention.

This chapter describes the physiologic changes in the newborn's major body systems. It also discusses the behavioral adaptations, including behavioral patterns and the newborn's behavioral responses, which occur during this transition period.

PHYSIOLOGIC TRANSITIONING

At birth, the newborn has limited functional and structural adaptability. The first hour is often called the "golden hour of life," in recognition of the fact that the newborn's intrauterine to extrauterine transition is both dramatic and critical. The physiologic changes that characterize this transitional period are profound, unique, and unparalleled at any time else in life. This adaptation is complex and difficult but required for all humans. Maternal medical and fetal conditions can have a profound effect on the successful transition. The mechanics of birth require a change in the newborn for survival outside the uterus. Immediately at birth, respiratory gas exchange, along with circulatory modifications, must occur to sustain extrauterine life. During this time, as newborns strive to attain homeostasis, they also experience complex changes in major organ systems. The newborn's most dramatic and most rapid extrauterine transitions occur in four interdependent areas: the respiratory system, the circulatory system, thermoregulation, and their ability to stabilize their blood glucose levels. All four areas must make successful transitions for the newborn to adapt to extrauterine life.

Respiratory System Adaptations

Physiologic responsibility for gas exchange is transferred from the placenta to the newborn's lungs and pulmonary system at birth. The newborn's transition from fetal to neonatal life includes aeration of the lungs, establishment of pulmonary gas exchange, and changing the fetal circulation into the adult type. Lung aeration leads to the establishment of functional residual capacity, allowing pulmonary gas exchange to start. The first breath of life is a gasp that generates an increase in transpulmonary pressure and results in diaphragmatic descent. Hypercapnia, hypoxia, and acidosis resulting from normal labor become stimuli for initiating respirations. Inspiration of air and expansion of the lungs allow for an increase in tidal volume (amount of air brought into the lungs). **Surfactant** is a surface tension–reducing lipoprotein found in the newborn's lungs that prevents alveolar collapse at the end of expiration, prevents lung atelectasis, and loss of lung volume. It lines the alveoli to enhance aeration of gas-free lungs, thus reducing surface tension and lowering the pressure required to open the alveoli. Surfactant production starts at about 26 weeks' gestation and reaches maturity levels at approximately 35 weeks (Khawar & Marwaha, 2023). Normal lung function depends on surfactant, which permits a decrease in surface tension at end expiration (to prevent atelectasis) and an increase in surface tension during lung expansion (to facilitate elastic recoil on inspiration). Surfactant provides the lung stability needed for gas exchange. The newborn's first breath, in conjunction with the surfactant, overcomes the surface forces to permit aeration of the lungs. The chest wall of the newborn is floppy because of the high cartilage content and poorly developed musculature. Thus, accessory muscles that help in breathing are ineffective.

One of the most crucial adaptations that the newborn makes at birth is adjusting from a fluid-filled intrauterine environment to a gaseous extrauterine environment. During fetal life, the lungs are expanded with an ultrafiltrate of the amniotic fluid. During and after birth, this fluid must be removed and replaced with air. Passage through the birth canal allows intermittent compression of the thorax, which helps eliminate two thirds of the fluid in the lungs. Pulmonary capillaries and the lymphatics remove the remaining fluid.

If fluid is removed too slowly or incompletely (e.g., with decreased thoracic squeezing during birth or diminished respiratory effort), transient tachypnea (respiratory rate above 60 bpm) of the newborn occurs. Examples of situations involving decreased thoracic compression and diminished respiratory effort include cesarean birth and sedation in newborns. Research findings support the need for thoracic compression because the absence of the neonate's exposure to labor contractions in these situations is associated with an increased risk of transient tachypnea at term with oxygen supplementation being needed for a longer duration (Hooper & te Pas, 2022).

TAKE NOTE!

A neonate born by cesarean section does not have the same benefit of the birth canal squeeze as does the newborn born by vaginal birth. Closely observe the respirations of the newborn after cesarean births.

Lungs

Before the newborn's lungs can maintain respiratory function, the following certain events must occur:

- Initiation of respiratory movement
- Expansion of the lungs
- Establishment of functional residual capacity (ability to retain some air in the lungs on expiration)
- Increased pulmonary blood flow
- Redistribution of cardiac output (Rios et al., 2022)

Initial breathing is probably the result of a reflex triggered by pressure changes, noise, light, temperature changes, touching, compression of the fetal chest during the birthing process, and high carbon dioxide and low oxygen concentrations of the newborn's blood. Central chemoreceptors stimulated by hypoxia and hypercapnia further increase the respiratory drive.

Respirations

After respirations are established in the newborn, they are shallow and irregular, ranging from 30 to 60 breaths per minute, with short periods of apnea (less than 15 seconds). The newborn's respiratory rate varies according to their activity, the more active the newborn, the higher the respiratory rate on average. Signs of respiratory distress to observe for include central cyanosis, tachypnea, expiratory grunting, sternal retractions, and nasal flaring. Respirations should not be labored, and chest movements should be symmetric. In some instances, **periodic breathing** may occur, which is the cessation of breathing that lasts 5 to 10 seconds without changes in color or heart rate (Kondamudi et al., 2023). Periodic breathing may be observed in newborns within the first few days of life and requires close monitoring.

TAKE NOTE!

Apneic periods lasting more than 20 seconds or longer with cyanosis, pallor, and heart rate changes require further evaluation (Kondamudi et al., 2023).

Cardiovascular System Adaptations

It is important for the newborn, while taking their first breath, to shut down and rewire the intrauterine cardiovascular shunts present in their body. Not doing so can cause physiologic imbalances, such as not getting enough oxygen to the brain. During fetal life, the heart relies on certain unique structures that assist it in providing adequate perfusion of vital body parts. The umbilical vein carries oxygenated blood from the placenta to the fetus. The ductus venosus allows the majority of the umbilical vein blood to bypass the liver and merge with blood moving through the vena cava, bringing it to the heart sooner. The foramen ovale allows more than half the blood entering the right atrium to cross immediately to the left atrium, bypassing the pulmonary circulation. The ductus arteriosus connects the pulmonary artery to the aorta, which allows bypassing of the pulmonary circuit. Only a small portion of blood passes through the pulmonary circuit for the main purpose of perfusion of the structure, rather than for oxygenation. The fetus depends on the placenta to provide oxygen and nutrients and to remove waste products.

With the birth of the newborn and removal of the low-resistance placenta, there are major cardiovascular responses related to pressures, blood flow, and pulmonary circulation. At birth, the circulatory system must switch from fetal to newborn circulation and from placental to pulmonary gas exchange. Successful transition from fetal to postnatal circulation requires increased pulmonary blood flow, removal of the placenta, and closure of the intracardiac (foramen ovale) and extracardiac shunts (ductus venosus and ductus arteriosus). These changes are needed to increase left ventricular output (Fernandes, 2024). The physical forces of the contractions of labor and birth, mild asphyxia, increased intracranial pressure as a result of cord compression and uterine contractions, and the cold stress experienced immediately after birth lead to an increased release of catecholamines that is critical for the changes involved in the transition to extrauterine life. The increased levels of epinephrine and norepinephrine stimulate increased cardiac output and contractility, surfactant release, and promotion of pulmonary fluid clearance (Gupta & Paria, 2022).

Fetal to Neonatal Circulation Changes

At birth, multiple changes in circulation occur immediately as the fetus separates from the placenta (Fig. 17.1). All structures unique to fetal circulation are no longer needed and undergo changes into infant circulation. At birth, circulation alters in response to changes taking place in the lungs which now become the primary organs of respiration. When the umbilical cord is clamped, the first breath is taken, and the lungs begin to function. As a result, systemic vascular resistance increases and blood return to the heart via the inferior vena cava decreases. Concurrently, with these changes, there is a rapid decrease in pulmonary vascular resistance and an increase in pulmonary blood flow (Rios et al., 2022). The foramen ovale functionally closes with a decrease in pulmonary vascular resistance, which leads to a decrease in right-sided heart pressures. An increase in systemic pressure, after

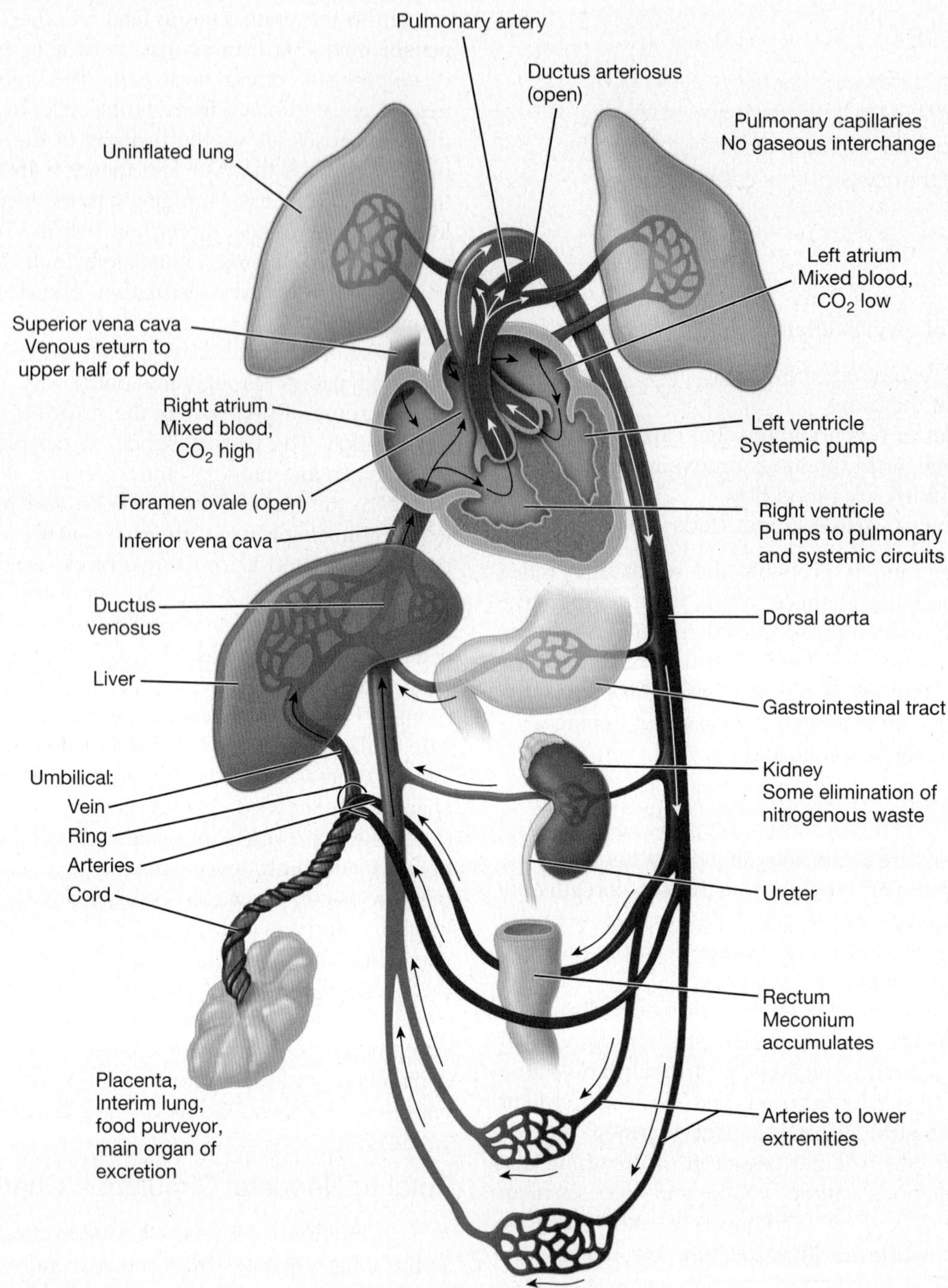

FIGURE 17.1 Cardiovascular adaptations of the newborn. Note the changes in oxygenation between (**A**) prenatal circulation and (**B**) postnatal (pulmonary) circulation.

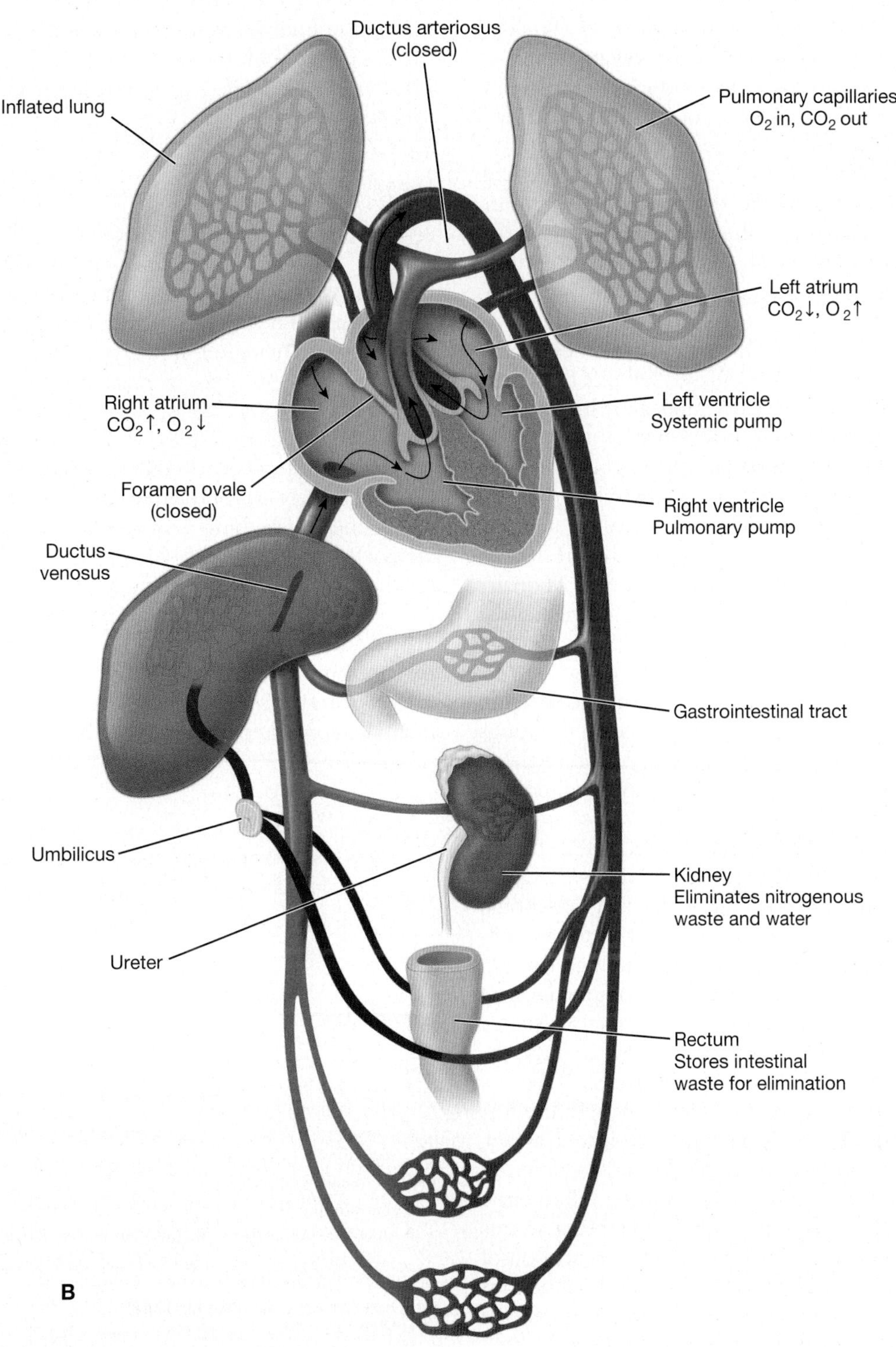

FIGURE 17.1 *(continued)*

clamping of the cord, leads to an increase in left-sided heart pressures. The ductus arteriosus, ductus venosus, and umbilical vessels that were vital during fetal life are no longer needed. Over a period of months, these fetal vessels form nonfunctional ligaments.

Before birth, the foramen ovale allowed most of the oxygenated blood entering the right atrium from the inferior vena cava to pass into the left atrium of the heart. With the newborn's first breath, air pushes into the lungs, triggering an increase in pulmonary blood flow and pulmonary venous return to the left side of the heart. As a result, the pressure in the left atrium becomes higher than in the right atrium. The increased left atrial pressure causes the foramen ovale to close, thus allowing the output from the right ventricle to flow entirely to the lungs. With closure of this fetal shunt, oxygenated blood is now separated from nonoxygenated blood. The subsequent increase in tissue oxygenation further promotes the increase in systemic blood pressure and continuing blood flow to the lungs. The foramen ovale normally closes functionally at birth when left atrial pressure increases and right atrial pressure decreases. Permanent anatomic closure, though, really occurs throughout the next several weeks.

During fetal life, the ductus arteriosus, connecting the aorta and the pulmonary artery, protected the lungs against circulatory overload by shunting blood (right to left) into the descending aorta, bypassing pulmonary circulation. Its patency during fetal life is promoted by continual production of prostaglandin E2 (PGE2) by the ductus arteriosus (Clyman, 2022). The ductus arteriosus becomes functionally closed within the first few hours after birth. Oxygen is the most important factor in controlling its closure. Closure depends on the high oxygen content of the aortic blood that results from aeration of the lungs at birth. At birth, pulmonary vascular resistance decreases, allowing pulmonary blood flow to increase and oxygen exchange to occur in the lungs. It occurs secondary to an increase in PO_2 coincident with the first breath and umbilical cord occlusion when it is clamped.

The ductus venosus shunted blood from the left umbilical vein to the inferior vena cava during intrauterine life. It closes within a few days after birth because this shunting is no longer needed as a result of activation of the liver. The activated liver now takes over the functions of the placenta (which was expelled at birth). The ductus venosus becomes a ligament in extrauterine life.

The two umbilical arteries and one umbilical vein begin to constrict at birth because, with placental expulsion, blood flow ceases. In addition, peripheral circulation increases. Thus, the vessels are no longer needed and they too become ligaments. Successful transition and closure of the three fetal shunts create a neonatal circulation by which deoxygenated blood returns to the heart through the inferior and superior vena cava. Deoxygenated blood enters the right atrium then into the right ventricle and travels through the pulmonary artery to the pulmonary vascular bed. Oxygenated blood returns through pulmonary veins to the left atrium, the left ventricle, and through the aorta to the systemic circulation (Rios et al., 2022). Box 17.1 provides a summary of fetal to neonatal circulation.

Heart Rate

As the transition from fetal to newborn circulation starts, massive rises in cortisol and catecholamines drive increases in cardiac output. During the first few minutes after birth, the newborn's heart rate is approximately 110 to 160 bpm. Thereafter, it begins to decrease to an average of 120 to 140 bpm, increasing with activity and decreasing with sleep (Vargo, 2025). The newborn is highly dependent on heart rate for maintenance of cardiac output and blood pressure. Although blood pressure is not taken routinely in the healthy term newborn, it is usually highest after birth and reaches a plateau within a week after birth. Cardiac defects may be identified in the newborn nursery by conducting a thorough and systematic physical assessment, including inspection, palpation, auscultation, and measurement of blood pressure and oxygen saturations. The ability of the nurse to identify irregular findings during physical assessment aids rapid identification and treatment.

TAKE NOTE!

Transient functional cardiac murmurs may be heard during the neonatal period as a result of the changing dynamics of the cardiovascular system at birth. Usually, they are benign (Vargo, 2025).

BOX 17.1 Summary of Fetal to Neonatal Circulation

- Clamping the umbilical cord after birth eliminates the placenta as a reservoir for blood.
- Onset of respirations causes a rise in PO_2 in the lungs and a decrease in pulmonary vascular resistance, *which...*
- Increases pulmonary blood flow and increases pressure in the left atrium, *which...*
- Decreases pressure in the right atrium of the heart, which causes closure of the foramen ovale (closes within minutes after birth secondary to a decreased pulmonary vascular resistance and increased left heart pressure).
- With an increase in oxygen levels after the first breath, an increase in systemic vascular resistance occurs, *which...*
- Decreases vena cava return, which reduces blood flow in the umbilical vein (constricts, becomes a ligament with functional closing)
- Closure of the ductus venosus (becomes a ligament) causes an increase in pressure in the aorta, which forces closure of the ductus arteriosus within 10 to 15 hours after birth.

Anthony, R., & McKinlay, C. J. D. (2022). Adaptation for life after birth: A review of neonatal physiology. *Anesthesia & Intensive Care Medicine, 24*(1), 1–9. https://doi.org/10.1016/j.mpaic.2022.11.002; and Chakkarapani, A. A., Roehr, C. C., Hooper, S. B., te Pas, A. B., & Samir Gupta, S. (2023). Transitional circulation and hemodynamic monitoring in newborn infants. *Pediatric Research.* https://doi.org/10.1038/s41390-022-02427-8

Cardiac murmurs arise from turbulent blood flow around structures of the heart. The fluctuations in both the heart rate and blood pressure tend to follow the changes in the newborn's behavioral state. An increase in activity, such as wakefulness, movement, or crying, corresponds to an increase in heart rate and blood pressure. In contrast, the compromised newborn demonstrates markedly less physiologic variability overall. Tachycardia may be found with volume depletion, cardiorespiratory disease, drug withdrawal, and hyperthyroidism. Bradycardia often occurs with apnea and is also associated with hypoxia.

Hematologic System Adaptations

Blood Volume

The blood volume of the newborn depends on the amount of blood transferred from the placenta at birth. Fetal blood volume is about 85 to 100 g or 30 mL/kg. Waiting to clamp the umbilical cord results in an increase of blood volume available to perfuse the lungs of the newborn after birth (Rabe et al., 2022). The current recommendation from the American College of Obstetrics and Gynecology (ACOG) and the American Academy of Pediatrics (AAP) is to delay cord clamping until 30 to 60 seconds after birth (Yamada et al., 2023). About 75% of blood available to transfer from the placenta to the infant is transferred within the first minute after birth (Funai & Norwitz, 2024). Clamping the cord in term infants in the recommended time frame provides the benefits of higher hemoglobin levels, preventing iron-deficiency anemia at 3 to 6 months of age, improved myelin brain volume to 12 months of age, and improved neurodevelopmental outcomes at 4 years of age(Funai & Norwitz, 2024; Rabe et al., 2022). Timing of cord clamping should not interfere with needed newborn resuscitation nor delay care when maternal or newborn safety is compromised (Funai & Norwitz, 2024).

Blood Components

Fetal red blood cell (RBC) development is independent from the birthing parent. The fetus has more RBCs per cubic millimeter than an adult, and they have a greater affinity for oxygen at a lower oxygen pressure than adult RBCs (Rios et al., 2022). After birth, the RBC count gradually increases as the cell size decreases, because the cells now live in an environment with much higher PO_2. A newborn's RBCs have a lifespan of 80 to 100 days, compared with 120 days in adults.

Hemoglobin levels are higher in newborns within the first few hours after birth. Levels peak at 4 to 6 hours, then slowly decrease over the next 12 to 18 hours and within the first few months of life. Hemoglobin initially declines as a result of a decrease in neonatal red cell mass (physiologic anemia of infancy). Leukocytosis (elevated white blood cells) is present as a result of birth trauma soon after birth. Fetal hemoglobin is gradually replaced by adult forms during infancy (Bahr & Ohls, 2022). The newborn's platelet count and aggregation ability are the same as those of adults.

The newborn's hematologic values are affected by the site of the blood sample (capillary blood has higher levels of hemoglobin and hematocrit compared with venous blood), placental transfusion (delayed cord clamping and normal shift of plasma to extravascular spaces, which causes higher levels of hemoglobin and hematocrit), and gestational age (increased age is associated with increased numbers of red cells and hemoglobin) (Bahr & Ohls, 2022). Table 17.1 lists expected newborn blood values.

Body Temperature Regulation

At birth, the fetus moves from a warm, moist intrauterine environment to the colder, drier extrauterine environment. Thermoregulation is an essential component to achieve for the stability and long-term positive outcomes for all newborns (Wood et al., 2022). Newborns are dependent on their environment for the maintenance of body temperature, much more so immediately after birth than later in life. One of the most important elements in a newborn's survival is obtaining a stable body temperature to promote an optimal transition to extrauterine life. On average, a newborn's temperature ranges from 97.9°F to 99.7°F (36.6°C to 37.6°C). Since newborns lose heat easily after birth, having skin-to-skin contact with their parents is recommended as the initial method for maintaining newborn body temperature. Skin-to-skin contact should be the first line of treatment for hypothermia and as a measure to establish successful breastfeeding immediately after birth. Research has shown that skin-to-skin care is effective for rewarming mildly hypothermic, low-risk term neonates (Kardum et al., 2022) (see Evidence-Based Practice 17.1).

Thermoregulation is the process of maintaining the balance between heat loss and heat production in order to maintain the body's core internal temperature (Sahni, 2022). It is a critical physiologic function that is

TABLE 17.1 • Expected Newborn Blood Values

Lab Data	Normal Range
Hemoglobin	15–24 g/dL
Hematocrit	44%–70%
Platelets	84,000–478,000/mm^3
Red blood cells	4.0–5.5 × 1,000,000/mm^3
White blood cells	9.1–34,000/mm^3

Data from American College of Clinical Pharmacy. (n.d.). *Reference values for common laboratory tests.* https://www.accp.com/docs/sap/Lab_Values_Table_PedSAP.pdf

EVIDENCE-BASED PRACTICE 17.1

Association Between Skin-to-Skin Contact Duration After Cesarean Section and Breastfeeding

BACKGROUND

Breastfeeding is important for maternal and infant health and has been recommended by most major professional maternal/neonatal associations worldwide. It can protect infants against infections and malocclusions. There is also evidence that breastfeeding can reduce the risk of the infant becoming overweight or developing obesity and diabetes. For people who are nursing, it can protect against breast cancer, ovarian cancer, and type 2 diabetes. Skin-to-skin contact immediately after birth stimulates the newborn's natural instinct to find and attach to the nipple and breastfeed. Immediate skin-to-skin contact is a beneficial practice that promotes positive breastfeeding outcomes. This study aimed to explore the association between skin-to-skin contact after cesarean sections in terms of breastfeeding outcomes and duration.

STUDY

The initial moments after birth are a sensitive period because this is the optimal time to establish effective breastfeeding. Frequently, the birthing parent and newborn are separated to place the newborn under radiant heat to prevent hypothermia. However, hypothermia can also be prevented by initiating skin-to-skin contact without separation. Skin-to-skin contact encourages newborns to move toward the nipples and latch effectively to breastfeed. A prospective study was conducted with 679 participants who had singleton pregnancies and delivered by cesarean section after 37 weeks' gestation using epidural or spinal anesthesia. The control group consisted of 136 participants who did not have skin-to-skin contact after their cesarean sections. There were 543 participants who had skin-to-skin contact and for whom early breastfeeding was initiated. Only 145 participants continued skin-to-skin contact after birth; the rest achieved lesser time spans.

Findings

This study demonstrated longer skin-to-skin duration after a cesarean section led to an increased rate of effective breastfeeding. The group that had 90 minutes of skin-to-skin time also had the highest rates of effective breastfeeding. Moreover, immediate skin-to-skin contact after childbirth is associated with higher rates of effective breastfeeding.

Nursing Implications

More attention should be paid to ensuring immediate skin-to-skin contact is practiced after surgical births to improve early breastfeeding initiation. To obtain the full benefits, longer durations of skin-to-skin contact periods should be encouraged. The initial moments after birth are a sensitive and critical period—this is the ideal time to start facilitating the newborn's nutritional behaviors and establish effective breastfeeding behaviors such as breast crawling and sucking.

The results of this prospective study found that maternal–infant skin-to-skin contact after birth increases the success rate and duration of breastfeeding, so it is a best practice for the postnatal care of newborns. The results of this study can be used by nurses in evidence-based decision making about ways to increase breastfeeding rates and hospital policies should be changed to enhance this practice.

Adapted from Juan, J., Zhang, X., Wang, X., Liu, J., Cao, Y., Tan, L., Gao, Y., Qui, Y., & Yang, H. (2022). Association between skin-to-skin contact duration after Cesarean section and breastfeeding. *Children*, *9*(11), 1742. https://doi.org/10.3390/children9111742

closely related to the transition and survival of the newborn. An appropriate thermal environment is essential for maintaining a normal body temperature. Compared with adults, newborns tolerate a narrower range of environmental temperatures and are extremely vulnerable to both underheating and overheating. Nurses play a key role in providing an appropriate environment to help newborns maintain thermal stability. Skilled nursing observation and proactive care are essential in preventing hypothermia in the newborn (Fig. 17.2).

Heat Loss

Newborns have several characteristics that predispose them to heat loss:

- Thin skin with blood vessels close to the surface
- Increased skin permeability to water
- Lack of shivering ability to produce heat until 3 months old
- Limited stores of metabolic substrates (glucose, glycogen, fat)
- Limited use of voluntary muscle activity or movement to produce heat
- Large surface area-to-body mass ratio, which promotes heat loss via conduction
- Lack of subcutaneous fat, which provides insulation
- More body water content
- Little ability to conserve heat by changing posture (fetal position) (Koop & Tadi, 2023)

Every newborn struggles to maintain body temperature from the moment of birth, when the newborn's wet body is exposed to the much cooler environment of the

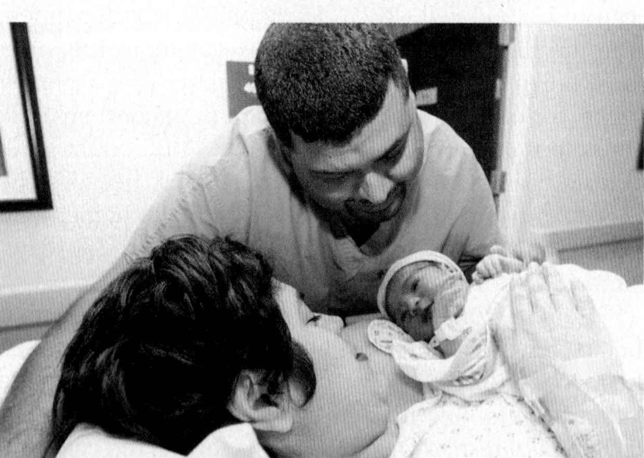

FIGURE 17.2 A couple looking at their newborn after birth. Note the newborn's hat and warm blanket to preserve body heat.

birthing room. The amniotic fluid covering the newborn cools as it evaporates rapidly in the low humidity and air conditioning of the room. The newborn's temperature may decrease 3°F to 5°F. within minutes after leaving the warmth of the uterus (99.6°F [37.5°C]). The skin of a newborn adjusts quickly to the challenging environmental conditions of extrauterine life. However, certain functions, for example, microcirculation, continue to develop beyond the neonatal period (Visscher & Narendran, 2022).

The transfer of heat depends on the temperature of the environment, air speed, and water vapor pressure or humidity. Heat exchange between the environment and the newborn involves the same mechanisms as those with any physical object and its environment. Heat can be lost by these four mechanisms: conduction, convection, evaporation, and radiation (Newnam & Tasket, 2024). Prevention of heat loss is a key nursing intervention (Fig. 17.3).

CONSIDER THIS!

When I look down at my little miracle of life in my arms, I can't help but beam with pride at this great accomplishment. She seems so vulnerable and defenseless and yet is equipped with everything she needs to survive at birth. When the nurse brought my daughter in for the first time after birth, I wanted to see and feel every part of her. Much to my dismay, she was wrapped up like a mummy in a blanket and she had a pink knit cap on her head. I asked the nurse why all the babies had to look like they were bound for the North Pole with all these layers on. Wasn't the nurse aware it was summertime and probably at least 85 degrees outside?

The nurse explained that newborns lose body heat easily and need to be kept warm until their temperature stabilizes. Even though I wanted to get up close and personal with my baby, I decided to keep the pink polar bear outfit on her.

Thoughts: Newborns may be born with "everything they need to survive" on the outside, but they still experience temperature instability and lose heat through radiation, evaporation, convection, and conduction. Because the newborn's head is the largest body part, a great deal of heat can be lost if a cap is not kept on the head. What guidance can be given to this mother before discharge to stabilize her daughter's temperature while at home? What simple examples can be used to demonstrate your point?

CONDUCTION

Conduction involves the transfer of heat from one object to another when the two objects are in direct contact with each other. Conduction refers to heat fluctuation between the newborn's body surface when in contact with other solid surfaces, such as a cold mattress, scale, or circumcision restraining board. Heat loss by conduction can also occur when touching a newborn with cold hands or when the newborn has direct contact with a colder object such as a metal scale or a cool mattress, blanket, or clothing.

CONVECTION

Convection involves the flow of heat from the body surface to cooler surrounding air or to air circulating over a body surface. Examples of convection-related heat loss would be a cool breeze that flows over the newborn, a cool room, cool corridors, or outside air currents.

EVAPORATION

Evaporation involves the loss of heat when a liquid is converted to vapor. Evaporative loss may be insensible (such as from skin and respiration) or sensible (such as from sweating). Insensible loss occurs, but the person is not aware of it. Sensible loss is objective and can be noticed. It depends on air speed and the absolute humidity of the air. For example, when the baby is born, the body is covered with amniotic fluid. The fluid evaporates into the air, leading to heat loss. Heat loss via evaporation also occurs when bathing a newborn.

RADIATION

Radiation involves the loss of body heat to cooler, solid surfaces that are in proximity but not in direct contact with the newborn. The amount of heat loss depends on the size of the cold surface area, the surface temperature of the newborn's body, and the temperature of the receiving surface area. For example, when a newborn is placed in a single-wall isolette next to a cold window, heat loss from radiation occurs. A newborn will become cold even though they are in a heated isolette.

To summarize, this is how each type of heat loss is likely to occur:

- Conductive heat loss: Placing newborns on a cold surface
- Convective heat loss: A flow of cooler ambient air carries heat away from newborn.
- Evaporative heat loss: Newborns are wet with amniotic fluid when born.
- Radiant heat loss: Bare skin of the newborn is exposed in an environment with cooler objects.

Overheating

The newborn is also prone to overheating. An overheated infant may have a flushed face and appear restless. Limited insulation and limited sweating ability can predispose any newborn to overheating. Control of body temperature is achieved via a complex negative feedback system that creates a balance between heat production, heat gain, and heat loss. The primary heat regulator is in the hypothalamus and the central nervous system (CNS). The immaturity of the newborn's CNS makes it

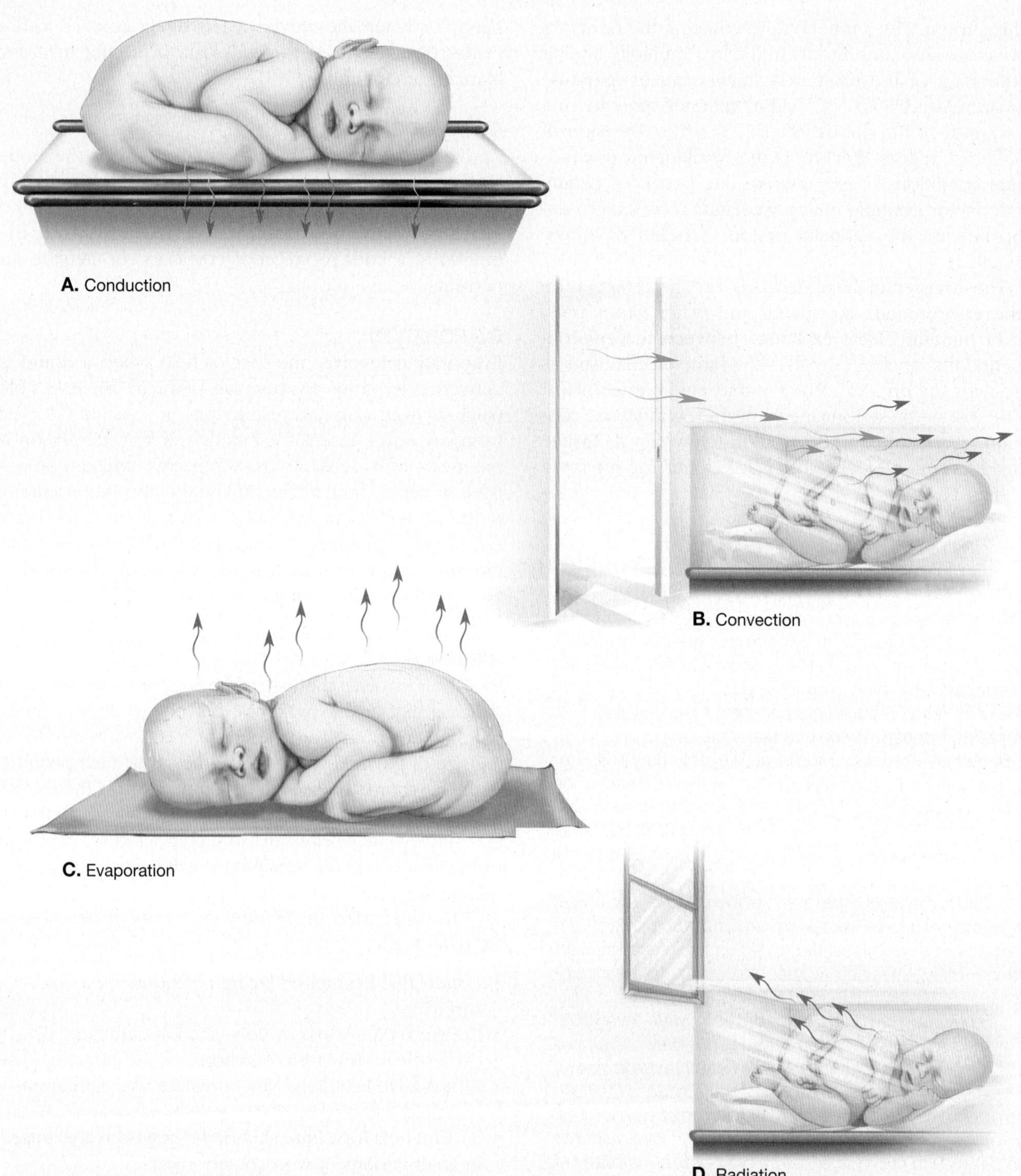

FIGURE 17.3 The four mechanisms of heat loss in the newborn. **A.** Conduction. **B.** Convection. **C.** Evaporation. **D.** Radiation.

difficult to create and maintain this balance. Therefore, the newborn can become overheated easily. For example, an isolette that is too warm or one that is left too close to a sunny window may lead to hyperthermia. Using too many layers of clothing and covering newborns with too many blankets can add to overheating. Although heat production can substantially increase in response to a cool environment, basal metabolic rate and the resultant heat produced cannot be reduced. Overheating increases fluid loss, the respiratory rate, and the metabolic rate considerably.

Thermoregulation

Humans can regulate body temperature within a narrow range. Newborns have a decreased ability to regulate body temperature, producing heat through nonshivering thermogenesis. Thermoregulation, the balance between heat loss and heat production, is related to the newborn's rate of metabolism and oxygen consumption. The newborn attempts to conserve heat and increase heat production by increasing the metabolic rate, oxidative glucose, fat, and protein metabolism, nonshivering thermogenesis of brown fat, muscular activity through movement, and peripheral vasoconstriction, and by assuming a fetal position to hold in heat and minimize exposed body surface area. If proper measures aren't taken to reduce heat loss immediately after birth, the newborn's temperature could drop 2°C to 4°C within the first 20 minutes of extrauterine life (Koop & Tadi, 2023).

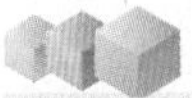 *Concept Mastery Alert*

Effects of Cold Stress in the Newborn's Brown Fat Metabolism

The newborn first experiences an increase in norepinephrine in response to a cold environment. This then influences the triglycerides to stimulate brown fat metabolism.

An environment in which body temperature is maintained without an increase in metabolic rate or oxygen use is called a **neutral thermal environment** (NTE). Within an NTE, the rates of oxygen consumption and metabolism are minimal, and internal body temperature is maintained because of thermal balance. In an NTE, a newborn maintains a normal body temperature while minimizing heat (energy) expenditure, water loss, and oxygen consumption. NTEs promote growth and stability and allow the newborn body to conserve energy for basic bodily functions. Newborns that experience thermal stability through an NTE demonstrate a decreased need for respiratory support, enhanced growth, decreased oxygen requirements, increased glucose stability, and reduced morbidities and mortalities associated with hyperthermia or hypothermia (Wood et al., 2022). Because newborns have difficulty maintaining body heat through shivering or other mechanisms, they need a higher environmental temperature to maintain an NTE. If the environmental temperature decreases, the newborn responds by consuming more oxygen. The respiratory rate increases (tachypnea) in response to the increased need for oxygen. As a result, the newborn's metabolic rate increases.

As noted earlier, the newborn's primary method of heat production is through nonshivering thermogenesis. This is a process in which brown fat (adipose tissue) is oxidized in response to cold exposure. Brown fat constitutes approximately 5% of body mass in the newborn and tends to reduce markedly in volume in adulthood (Hachemi & U-Din, 2023). Brown fat is a special kind of highly vascular fat that scientists once thought disappears by adulthood, but new research shows adults have brown fat as well (Hachemi & U-Din, 2023). Brown adipose tissue is a unique tissue that can convert chemical energy directly into heat when activated by the sympathetic nervous system. It is produced during the third trimester; it ordinarily is reduced by 3 to 5 weeks after birth and is vital for thermogenesis. The brown coloring is derived from the fat's rich supply of blood vessels and nerve endings. These fat deposits, which are capable of intense metabolic activity—and thus can generate a great deal of heat—are found between the scapulae, axillae, at the nape of the neck, in the mediastinum, and in areas surrounding the kidneys and adrenal glands. When the newborn experiences a cold environment, norepinephrine is released. This in turn stimulates brown fat metabolism by breaking down triglycerides. Cardiac output increases, increasing blood flow through the brown fat tissue. Subsequently, this blood becomes warmed as a result of the increased metabolic activity of the brown fat (Fig. 17.4).

Newborns can experience heat loss through all four mechanisms, ultimately resulting in cold stress. **Cold stress** is excessive heat loss that requires a newborn to use compensatory mechanisms (such as nonshivering thermogenesis and tachypnea) to maintain core body temperature (Bedwell & Holtzclaw, 2022). The consequences of cold stress can be quite severe. As the body temperature decreases, the newborn becomes less active, lethargic, hypotonic, and weaker. All newborns are at risk for cold stress, particularly within the first 12 hours of life. However, preterm newborns are at the greatest risk for cold stress and experience more profound effects than full-term newborns because they have fewer fat stores, poorer vasomotor responses, and less insulation to cope with a hypothermic event. Cold stress in the newborn can lead to hypoglycemia, metabolic acidosis, jaundice, and respiratory distress (Yitayew et al., 2020).

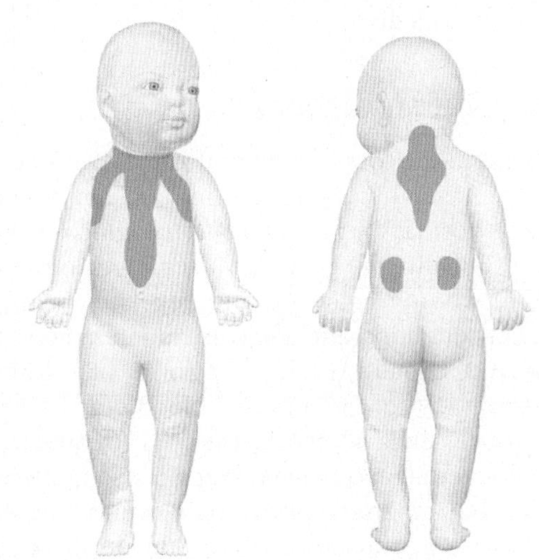

FIGURE 17.4 Areas of brown fat in a newborn.

> **TAKE NOTE!**
> Nurses must be aware of the thermoregulatory needs of the newborn and must ensure that these needs are met to provide the newborn with the best start possible. Maintenance of temperature stability should be focused on preventive measures.

These interventions allow the newborn to minimize their metabolic rate and oxygen consumption, thereby conserving vital energy stores required for optimum growth. By using preventive measures, competent assessments, and early interventions, cold stress and subsequent neonatal intensive care unit (NICU) admissions can be prevented.

Hepatic System Function

The liver has an essential role in the synthesis, degradation, and regulation of pathways involved in the metabolism of carbohydrates, proteins, lipids, trace elements, and vitamins. At birth, the newborn's liver slowly assumes the functions that the placenta handled during fetal life. Most enzymatic pathways are present in the newborn but are inactive at birth and generally become fully active at 3 months of age. These functions include blood coagulation, iron storage, carbohydrate metabolism, and conjugation of bilirubin, as discussed next. Glycogen reserves provide energy and may become depleted if the metabolic needs of the newborn increase, such as during cold or respiratory stress.

Iron Storage

Maturity, birth weight, and hemoglobin level determine the iron status of the newborn. As RBCs are destroyed after birth, their iron is released and stored by the liver until new RBCs need to be produced. If the maternal iron intake was adequate during pregnancy, sufficient iron has been stored in the newborn's liver for use during the first 6 months of age.

Carbohydrate Metabolism

Birth results in the loss of maternal glucose source. Glucose is an essential fuel for brain metabolism. When the placenta is lost at birth, the maternal glucose supply is cut off. Initially, the newborn's serum glucose levels decline. Newborns must learn to regulate their blood glucose concentration and adjust to an intermittent feeding schedule. Usually, a term newborn's blood glucose level is about 80% of the maternal blood glucose level at birth. Hypoglycemia is one of the most frequent problems encountered, and maintaining glucose homeostasis is one of the important physiologic events during the fetal-to-newborn transition. Major long-term sequelae may occur resulting in neurologic damage, seizures, developmental delays, and personality disorders. During the first 2 to 3 days hours of life, as normal neonates transition from intrauterine to extrauterine life, their plasma glucose levels are usually lower than later in life (Wernimont & Norris, 2022).

Glucose is the main source of energy for the first several hours after birth. With the newborn's increased energy needs after birth, the liver releases glucose from glycogen stores for the first 24 hours. Initiating early breastfeeding or bottle-feeding helps stabilize the newborn's blood glucose levels. Early feeding of all stable newborns will prevent hypoglycemia. No evidence supports universal invasive routine measurement of glucose in healthy term newborns. Selective screening of at-risk newborns is more appropriate (Rozance, 2023).

Bilirubin Conjugation

Before birth, bilirubin clearance is handled efficiently by the placenta and birthing parent's liver. After birth, the newborn's liver must assume full responsibility for bilirubin metabolism. Bilirubin is the yellow-to-orange bile pigment produced by the breakdown of RBCs.

Bilirubin normally circulates in plasma, is taken up by liver cells, and is changed to a water-soluble pigment that is excreted in the bile. This conjugated form of bilirubin is excreted from liver cells as a constituent of bile.

The principal source of bilirubin in the newborn is the hemolysis of erythrocytes. This is a normal occurrence after birth when fewer RBCs are needed to maintain extrauterine life. When RBCs die after approximately 80 days of life, the heme in their hemoglobin is converted to bilirubin. Bilirubin is released in an unconjugated form called indirect bilirubin, which is fat soluble. Enzymes, proteins, and different cells in the reticuloendothelial system and liver process the unconjugated bilirubin into conjugated bilirubin or direct bilirubin. This form is water soluble and now enters the gastrointestinal system via the bile and is eventually excreted through feces. The kidneys also excrete a small amount.

Newborns produce bilirubin at a rate of approximately 8 to 10 mg/kg/day. This is more than twice the production rate in adults, primarily because of relative polycythemia and increased RBC turnover. Bilirubin production typically declines to the adult level within 10 to 14 days after birth (Ansong-Assoku et al., 2023). In addition, the metabolic pathways of the liver are relatively immature and thus cannot conjugate bilirubin as quickly as needed.

Failure of the liver cells to break down and excrete bilirubin can cause an increased amount of bilirubin in the bloodstream, leading to jaundice. Bilirubin is toxic to the body and must be excreted. Blood tests ordered to determine bilirubin levels measure bilirubin in the serum. Total bilirubin is a combination of indirect (unconjugated) and direct (conjugated) bilirubin. When unconjugated bilirubin pigment is deposited in the skin and mucous membranes as a result of increased bilirubin levels, **jaundice**, also known as icterus, develops, with a yellowing of the skin, sclera, and mucous membranes. Visible jaundice as a result of increased blood bilirubin levels occurs in more than half of all healthy newborns; over 60% develop jaundice in the first week after birth. In the newborn, jaundice is not a disease, but a sign of elevated blood bilirubin level (Ansong-Assoku, 2023). It is typically mild, transient, self-limiting, and resolves without treatment. However, even in healthy term newborns, extremely elevated blood levels of bilirubin during the first week of life can cause bilirubin encephalopathy, a permanent and devastating form of brain damage (Qian et al., 2022). Jaundice in the newborn is discussed in more detail in Chapter 24.

Gastrointestinal System Adaptations

The full-term newborn has the capacity to swallow, digest, metabolize, and absorb food taken in soon after birth. At birth, the pH of the stomach contents is mildly acidic, reflecting the pH of the amniotic fluid. The once-sterile gut changes rapidly, depending on what feeding is received. Bowel sounds are normally heard shortly after birth but may be hypoactive on the first day.

Mucosal Barrier Protection

Humans start their development in a sterile intrauterine environment, but from the moment of birth, all epithelial surfaces in direct contact with the environment (skin, respiratory, gastrointestinal, and urogenital tract) are colonized by microorganisms. The intestinal mucosal barrier remains immature for 4 to 6 months following birth. An important adaptation of the gastrointestinal system is the development of this mucosal barrier to prevent the penetration of harmful substances (bacteria, toxins, and antigens) present within the intestinal lumen. At birth, the newborn must be prepared to deal with bacterial colonization of the gut. Colonization is dependent on oral intake. Nutrition, be it via breast milk or formula, plays a major role in early colonization patterns in the neonatal gut. It usually occurs within 24 hours of age and is required to produce vitamin K. A one-time vitamin K injection at birth is recommended to prevent low levels of vitamin K and bleeding (Centers for Disease Control and Prevention, 2023). After birth, environmental, oral, and cutaneous microbes from a parent will be mechanically transferred to the newborn by several processes including suckling, kissing, and caressing. Thus, the proximity of the birth canal and the anus, as well as parental expression of neonatal care, serves as effective methods of ensuring transmission of microbes from one generation to the next.

TAKE NOTE!

Human breast milk provides a passive mechanism to protect the newborn against the dangers of a deficient intestinal defense system. It contains antibodies, viable leukocytes, and many other substances that can interfere with bacterial colonization and prevent harmful penetration.

Stomach and Digestion

The newborn must rapidly adapt from receiving all nutrient and energy requirements via the placenta to obtaining them orally after birth. The physiologic capacity of the newborn stomach is considerably less than its anatomic capacity. There is a rapid gain in physiologic capacity during the first 4 days of life. After the first 4 days, the anatomic and physiologic capacities more closely approximate each other. The newborn stomach is capable of holding up to 30 mL of fluid (Mahe et al., 2022).

For bottle-fed newborns, small, frequent feedings set up a healthy eating pattern right from the start (breastfed newborns self-regulate how much they consume). Experts now advise adults that it is healthier to eat smaller amounts more often, and the same is true for babies and children. Coaxing an infant to take more milk leads to overfeeding. If feeling overfull at feedings becomes the norm for a young infant, this may lead to unhealthy eating habits that contribute to childhood and adult obesity later. Early-onset obesity is a precursor to a lifelong weight struggle and numerous comorbidities.

The cardiac sphincter and nervous control of the stomach are immature, which may lead to uncoordinated peristaltic activity and frequent regurgitation. Immaturity of the pharyngoesophageal sphincter and absence of lower esophageal peristaltic waves also contribute to the reflux of gastric contents. Avoiding overfeeding and stimulating frequent burping may minimize regurgitation. Most digestive enzymes are available at birth, allowing newborns to digest simple carbohydrates and protein. However, they have limited ability to digest complex carbohydrates and fats, because amylase and lipase levels are low at birth. As a result, newborns excrete a fair amount of lipids, resulting in fatty stools.

Adequate digestion and absorption are essential for newborn growth and development. Normally, term newborns lose 5% to 10% of their birth weight as a result of insufficient caloric intake within the first week after birth, shifting of intracellular water to extracellular space, and insensible water loss. To gain weight, the term newborn requires an intake of 108 kcal/kg/day from birth to 6 months of age. Understanding the role and importance of nutrition in early postnatal life on growth and development is vital, but how it links to later health has the potential of health benefits for all future generations. The first 1,000 days of life is the essential time when the foundations of newborn's long-term health are set. This is because the developing brain grows during this period (Likhar & Patil, 2022).

Bowel Elimination

The frequency, consistency, color, and type of stool passed by newborns vary widely. The evolution of a stool pattern begins with a newborn's first stool, which is **meconium**. Meconium is composed of amniotic fluid, shed mucosal cells, intestinal secretions, and blood. It is greenish black, has a tarry consistency, and is usually passed within 12 to 24 hours of birth. The first meconium stool passed is semi-sterile, but this changes rapidly with the ingestion of bacteria through feedings. After feedings are initiated, a transitional stool develops, which is greenish brown to yellowish brown, thinner in consistency, and seedy in appearance. If breastfed, the stools will resemble light mustard with seedlike particles. If formula-fed, the stools will be tan or yellow in color and firmer. The frequency of bowel movements varies widely from one infant to another.

TAKE NOTE!

Newborns who are fed early pass stools sooner, which helps reduce bilirubin buildup (La Leche League International, 2024).

The last development in the stool pattern is the milk stool. Its characteristics differ in breastfed and formula-fed newborns. The stools of the breastfed newborn are yellow-gold, loose, stringy to pasty in consistency, and typically sour-smelling. The stools of the formula-fed newborn vary depending on the type of formula ingested. They may be yellow, yellow-green, or greenish and loose, pasty, or formed in consistency, and they have an unpleasant odor.

Renal System Changes

A full complement of 1 million nephrons is present by 34 weeks' gestation. The glomeruli and nephrons are functionally immature at birth, resulting in a reduced glomerular filtration rate (GFR) and limited concentrating ability. A limited ability to concentrate urine and the reduced GFR make the newborn susceptible to both dehydration and fluid overload (Iacobelli & Guignard, 2022). Frequently, the newborn's kidneys are described as immature, but they can carry out their usual responsibilities and can handle the challenge of excretion and maintaining acid–base balance. Only when the newborn is faced with unexpected imbalances of water, electrolytes, or a disruption of acid–base status secondary to a preterm birth or illness does it lack the ability to handle the body's fluid homeostasis. A newborn infant's body mass is 75% water, the highest proportion of body water at any stage of a person's life. Most term newborns void immediately after birth, indicating adequate renal function. Although the newborn's kidneys can produce urine, they are limited in their ability to concentrate it until about 3 months of age, when the kidneys mature more. Until that time, a newborn voids frequently and the urine has a low specific gravity (1.001 to 1.020). About five to six voidings daily is average for most newborns; this indicates adequate fluid intake (Newnam & Tasket, 2024).

The renal cortex is relatively underdeveloped at birth and does not reach maturity until 12 to 18 months of age. The GFR is the amount of fluid filtered each minute by all the glomeruli of both kidneys and is one index of kidney function. At birth, the newborn's GFR is approximately 30% of normal adult values, reaching approximately 50% of normal adult values by age 1 month and full adult values by the first year of life (Guignard & Iacobelli, 2022). The low GFR and the limited excretion and conservation capability of the kidney affect the newborn's ability to excrete salt, water loads, and drugs.

TAKE NOTE!

The possibility of fluid overload is increased in newborns; keep this in mind when administering intravenous therapy to a newborn.

Immune System Adaptations

Essential to the newborn's survival is the ability to respond effectively to hostile environmental forces. The newborn's immune system begins working early in gestation, but many of the responses do not function adequately during the early neonatal period. The newborn is protected from certain infections, in part because of maternal antibodies circulating in their systems until about 6 months of age. Immunoglobulin G (IgG) crosses the placenta to the fetus while in utero. Newborns who are breastfed receive antibodies from the breast milk, including IgA, IgE, IgG, and IgM (Lawrence, 2022). The risk of acquiring an infection is great because a newborn's immune system is immature and is not able to respond for long periods of time to fight infections. The intrauterine environment usually protects the fetus from harmful microorganisms and the need for defensive immunologic responses. With exposure to a wide variety of microorganisms at birth, the newborn must develop a balance between host defenses and the hostile environmental organisms to ensure a safe transition to the outside world. Healthy infants begin to produce their own antibodies starting at 2 to 3 months of age.

Responses of the immune system serve three purposes: defense (protection from invading organisms), homeostasis (elimination of worn-out host cells), and surveillance (recognition and removal of enemy cells). The newborn's immune system response involves recognition of the pathogen or other foreign material followed by activation of mechanisms to react against and eliminate it. All immune responses primarily involve leukocytes (white blood cells).

The immune system's responses can be divided into two categories: natural and acquired immunity. These mechanisms are interrelated and interdependent; both are required for immunocompetency.

Natural Immunity

Natural immunity includes responses or mechanisms that do not require previous exposure to the microorganism or antigen to operate efficiently. Physical barriers (such as intact skin and mucous membranes), chemical barriers (such as gastric acids and digestive enzymes), and resident nonpathologic organisms make up the newborn's natural immune system. Natural immunity involves the most basic host defense responses: ingestion and killing of microorganisms by phagocytic cells.

Acquired Immunity

Acquired immunity involves two primary processes: (1) the development of circulating antibodies or immunoglobulins capable of targeting specific invading agents (antigens) for destruction and (2) formation of activated lymphocytes designed to destroy foreign invaders. Acquired immunity is absent until after the first invasion by a foreign organism or toxin.

Immunologic ability depends heavily on immunoglobulins such as IgG, IgM, and IgA. The newborn depends largely on these three immunoglobulins for defense against microorganisms associated with illness. Newborns remain susceptible to infections for months.

IgG is the major immunoglobulin and the most abundant, making up about 75% of all circulating antibodies (Kennelly, 2023). It is the only antibody that can pass through the placenta, thereby helping protect against neonatal infectious diseases and shaping the infant's gut bacteria and immunity. It is found in serum and interstitial fluid. It is the only class able to cross the placenta, with active placental transfer beginning at approximately 20 to 22 weeks' gestation. IgG produces antibodies against bacteria, bacterial toxins, and viral agents.

IgA is the most abundant immunoglobulin in the serum. IgA does not cross the placenta, and maximum levels are reached during childhood. This immunoglobulin is believed to protect mucous membranes from viruses and bacteria. IgA is predominantly found in the gastrointestinal and respiratory tracts, tears, saliva, colostrum, and breast milk.

TAKE NOTE!

A major source of IgA is human breast milk, so breastfeeding is believed to have significant immunologic advantages over formula feeding. Breast milk has high levels of IgA conferring passive immunity and contributing to the colonization of the infant gut microbiome (Ding et al., 2022).

IgM is found in blood and lymph fluid and is the first immunoglobulin to respond to infection. It does not cross the placenta, and levels are generally low at birth unless a congenital intrauterine infection is present. IgM offers a major source of protection from bloodborne infections. The predominant antibodies formed during neonatal or intrauterine infection are of this class.

Integumentary System Adaptations

The most important function of the skin is to provide a protective barrier between the body and the environment. It limits the loss of water, prevents absorption of harmful agents, protects thermoregulation and fat storage, and protects against physical trauma. The epidermal barrier begins to develop during midgestation and is fully formed by about 32 weeks' gestation. The newborn skin is critical to its transition from intrauterine to extrauterine environments and to the journey to self-sufficiency. The newborn's skin is a large organ, making up approximately 13% of body weight in contrast to 3% of body weight in an adult. It is sensitive, fragile, with a neutral pH on the surface, lower lipid content, thinner, and higher water content when compared with adults. Because of these characteristics, newborn skin is vulnerable to injury and infections, particularly in the preterm neonate (Visscher & Narendran, 2022). In a newborn, the risk of injury producing a break in the skin from the use of tapes and monitors and from handling is greater than for an adult. Improper handling of the newborn during daily skin care practices, such as bathing, can cause damage, prevent healing, and interfere with the normal maturation process.

Newborns vary greatly in appearance. Many of the variations are temporary and reflect the physiologic adaptations that the newborn is experiencing. Skin coloring varies, depending on the newborn's age, race, and ancestry; temperature; and whether they are crying. Skin color changes with both the environment and health status.

Neurologic System Adaptations

The nervous system is immature and continues to develop to achieve a full complement of cortical and brain stem cells by 1 year of age. The brain increases its size threefold during the first year of life. The nervous system consists of the brain, spinal cord, 12 cranial nerves, and a variety of spinal nerves that come from the spinal cord. Neurologic development follows cephalocaudal (head-to-toe) and proximal–distal (center-to-outside) patterns. Myelin develops early on in sensory impulse transmitters. Thus, the newborn has an acute sense of hearing, smell, and taste. The newborn's sensory capabilities include:

- *Hearing*—well developed at birth, responds to noise by turning to sound
- *Taste*—ability to distinguish between sweet and sour by 72 hours old
- *Smell*—ability to distinguish between birthing parent's breast milk and breast milk from others
- *Touch*—sensitivity to pain, responds to tactile stimuli
- *Vision*—incomplete at birth; maturation is dependent on nutrition and visual stimulation. Newborns can focus only on close objects (6 to 10 in away) with a visual acuity of 20/640 (Charlotte Lozier Institute, 2022). They demonstrate a preference for looking at faces.

Remember Maria, the new mother who is worried that her daughter can't see? What might the new mother notice about her daughter's behavior? What might be the new mother's expectations?

Congenital Reflexes

Primitive newborn reflexes are involuntary motor responses originating in the brainstem that facilitate infant survival. Most of these reflexes are integrated by 6 months of age as the brain matures and replaces them with voluntary motor activities (Kotagal, 2020). Successful adaptations demonstrated by the respiratory, circulatory, thermoregulatory, and musculoskeletal systems indirectly indicate the CNS's successful transition from fetal to extrauterine life, because the CNS plays a major role in all these adaptations. In the newborn, congenital reflexes are the hallmarks of maturity of the CNS, viability, and adaptation to extrauterine life.

The presence and strength of a reflex is an important indication of neurologic development and function. A **reflex** is an involuntary muscular response to a sensory stimulus. It is built into the nervous system and does not need the intervention of conscious thought to take effect. The physical assessment of the neurologic system of the newborn includes evaluating the major reflexes (gag, Babinski, Moro, and Galant) and minor ones (finger grasp, plantar grasp, rooting, sucking, head righting, stepping, and tonic neck).

To assess each reflex, the nurse progresses methodically, taking care to document each finding (Fanning, 2025). Many neonatal reflexes disappear with maturation, though some remain throughout adulthood. The arcs of these reflexes end at different levels of the spine and brain stem, reflecting the function of the cranial nerves and motor systems. The ways newborns blink, move their limbs, focus on a caregiver's face, turn toward sound, suck, swallow, and respond to the environment are all indications of their neurologic abilities. Defects or issues with the CNS are frequently not overt but may be revealed in abnormalities in tone, posture, alertness, or behavior (Kotagal, 2020). Damage to the nervous system (e.g., from birth trauma, perinatal hypoxia) during the birthing process can cause delays in the normal growth, development, and functioning of the newborn. Early identification may help to identify the cause and facilitate the start of early intervention to decrease long-term complications or permanent sequelae.

Newborn reflexes are assessed to evaluate neurologic function and development. Absent or abnormal reflexes in a newborn, persistence of a reflex past the age when it is normally lost, or redevelopment of an infantile reflex in an older child or adult may indicate neurologic pathology. (See Chapter 18 for a description of newborn reflex assessment.)

The nurse explains to Maria that all newborns are born with some degree of myopia (inability to see distances) and that 20/20 vision is not generally achieved until 5 to 7 years of age. What developmental information should the nurse discuss with Maria?

BEHAVIORAL ADAPTATIONS

In addition to adapting physiologically, the newborn adapts behaviorally. All newborns progress through a specific pattern of events after birth, regardless of their gestational age or the type of birth they experienced.

Behavioral Patterns

The newborn usually demonstrates a predictable pattern of behavior during the first several hours after birth, characterized by two periods of reactivity separated by a sleep phase. Behavioral adaptation is a defined progression of events triggered by stimuli from the extrauterine environment after birth.

First Period of Reactivity

The first period of reactivity begins at birth and may last from 30 minutes up to 2 hours. The newborn is alert and moving and may appear hungry. This period is characterized by myoclonic movements of the eyes, spontaneous Moro reflexes, sucking motions, chewing, rooting, and fine tremors of the extremities. Respiration and heart rate are elevated but gradually begin to slow as the next period begins.

This period of alertness allows parents to interact with their newborn and to enjoy close contact with their new baby (Fig. 17.5). The appearance of sucking and rooting behaviors provides a good opportunity for initiating breastfeeding. Many newborns latch on the nipple and suck well at this first experience.

Period of Decreased Responsiveness

At 30 to 120 minutes of age, the newborn enters the second stage of transition—that of the *sleep period* or a decrease in activity. This phase is referred to as a period of decreased responsiveness. Movements are less jerky and less frequent. Heart and respiratory rates decline as the newborn enters the sleep phase. The muscles become relaxed, and responsiveness to outside stimuli diminishes. During this phase, it is difficult to arouse or interact with the newborn. No interest in sucking is shown. This quiet time can be used for both parent and newborn to remain close and rest together after labor and the birthing experience.

Second Period of Reactivity

The second period of reactivity begins as the newborn awakens and shows an interest in environmental stimuli. This period typically lasts 2 to 8 hours (Newnam & Tasket, 2024). Heart and respiratory rates increase. Peristalsis also increases. Thus, it is not uncommon for the newborn to pass meconium or void during this period. In addition, motor activity and muscle tone increase in conjunction with an increase in muscular coordination (Fig. 17.6).

Interaction between the birthing parent and the newborn during this second period of reactivity is encouraged if the parent has rested and desires it. This period also provides a good opportunity for parents to examine their newborn and ask questions.

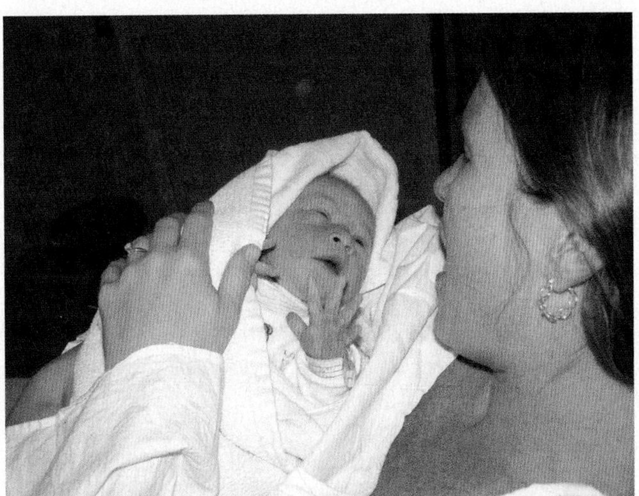

FIGURE 17.5 The first period of reactivity is an optimal time for interaction.

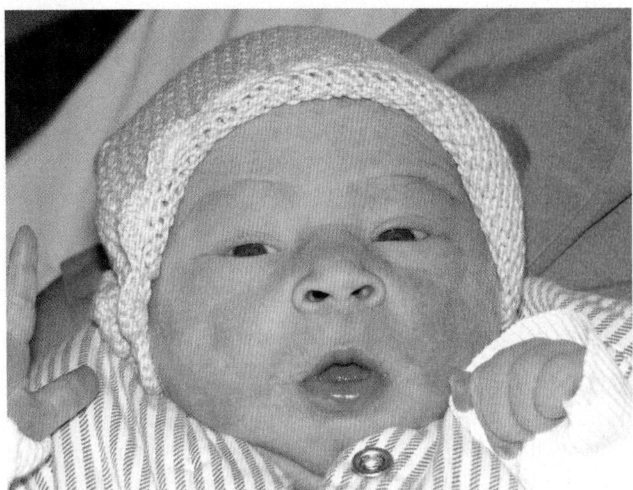

FIGURE 17.6 Newborn during the second period of reactivity. Note the newborn's wide-eyed interest.

TAKE NOTE!

Teaching about feeding, positioning for feeding, and diaper-changing techniques can be reinforced during the second period of reactivity.

Behavioral Responses

Newborn development reflects the dynamic relationship between endowment and the environment. Newborns demonstrate several predictable responses when interacting with their environments. How they react to the world around them is termed a **neurobehavioral response**. It comprises predictable periods that are probably triggered by external stimuli. Expected newborn behaviors include orientation, habituation, motor maturity, self-quieting ability, and social behaviors. Any deviation in behavioral responses requires further assessment, because it may indicate a complex neurobehavioral problem.

Orientation

The response of newborns to stimuli is called orientation. They become more alert when they sense a new stimulus in their environment. Orientation reflects newborn's response to auditory and visual stimuli, demonstrated by their movement of head and eyes to focus on that stimulus. Newborns prefer the human face and bright shiny objects. As the face or object comes into their line of vision, newborns respond by staring at the object intently. Newborns use this sensory capacity to become familiar with people and objects in their surroundings.

Remember Maria, who was concerned about her newborn daughter's vision? She told the nurse that her daughter did not show any interest in her pastel-colored homemade mobile she had hung across the room from her crib. What suggestions can the nurse make to Maria regarding the placement of the mobile and the types and colors of objects used to promote orientation in her daughter?

Habituation

Habituation is the newborn's ability to process and respond to visual and auditory stimuli. It is a measure of how well and appropriately an infant responds to the environment. Habituation is the ability to block out external stimuli after the newborn has become accustomed to the activity. During the first 24 hours after birth, newborns should increase their ability to habituate to environmental stimuli and sleep. Habituation provides a useful indicator of neurobehavioral intactness.

Motor Maturity

Motor maturity depends on gestational age and involves the evaluation of posture, tone, coordination, and movements. These activities enable newborns to control and coordinate movement. When stimulated, newborns with good motor organization demonstrate movements that are rhythmic and spontaneous. Bringing the hand up to the mouth is an example of good motor organization. As newborns adapt to their new environments, smoother movements should be observed. Such motor behavior is a good indicator of the newborn's ability to respond and adapt accordingly; it indicates that the CNS is processing stimuli appropriately.

Self-Quieting Ability

Self-quieting ability (also called self-soothing) refers to newborns' ability to quiet and comfort themselves. Newborns vary in their ability to console themselves or to be consoled. Consolability is how newborns can change from the crying state to an active alert, quiet alert, drowsy, or sleep state. They console themselves by hand-to-mouth movements and sucking, alerting to external stimuli, and motor activity.

Social Behaviors

Newborns begin extrauterine life already able to engage with the world using their sensory capabilities, and communicate with their environments through a complex repertoire of behaviors. Social behaviors include cuddling and snuggling into the arms of the parent when the newborn is held. Newborns are usually sensitive to being touched, cuddled, and held. Cuddliness is important to parents because they frequently gauge their ability to care for their newborn by the newborn's acceptance or positive response to their actions. This can be assessed by the degree to which the newborn nestles into the contours of the holder's arms. Most newborns cuddle, but some will resist. Assisting parents in assuming comforting behaviors (e.g., cooing while holding their newborn) and praising them for their efforts can help foster cuddling behaviors.

KEY CONCEPTS

- The neonatal period is defined as the first 28 days of life. As the newborn adapts to life after birth, numerous physiologic changes occur.
- At birth, the cardiopulmonary system must switch from fetal to neonatal circulation and from placental to pulmonary gas exchange.
- One of the most crucial adaptations that the newborn makes at birth is the adjustment of a fluid medium exchange from the placenta to the lungs and that of a gaseous environment.
- Neonatal RBCs have a lifespan of 80 to 100 days in comparison with the adult RBC lifespan of 120 days. This difference in RBC lifespan causes several adjustment problems.
- Thermoregulation is the maintenance of balance between heat loss and heat production. It is a critical physiologic function that is closely related to the transition and survival of the newborn.
- The newborn's primary method of heat production is through nonshivering thermogenesis, a process in which brown fat (adipose tissue) is oxidized in response to cold exposure. Brown fat is a special kind of highly vascular fat found in all humans.
- Heat loss in the newborn is the result of four mechanisms: conduction, convection, evaporation, and radiation.
- Responses of the immune system serve three purposes: defense (protection from invading organisms), homeostasis (elimination of worn-out host cells), and surveillance (recognition and removal of enemy cells).
- In the newborn, congenital reflexes are the hallmarks of maturity of the CNS, viability, and adaptation to extrauterine life.
- The newborn usually demonstrates a predictable pattern of behavior during the first several hours after birth, characterized by two periods of reactivity separated by a sleep phase.

REFERENCES AND RECOMMENDED READINGS

American College of Clinical Pharmacy. (n.d.). *Reference values for common laboratory tests.* https://www.accp.com/docs/sap/Lab_Values_Table_PedSAP.pdf

Ansong-Assoku, B., Shah, S. D., Adnan, M., & Ankola, P. A. (2023). Neonatal jaundice. *StatPearls*. https://www.ncbi.nlm.nih.gov/books/NBK532930/

Anthony, R., & McKinlay, C. J. D. (2022). Adaptation for life after birth: A review of neonatal physiology. *Anesthesia & Intensive Care Medicine, 24*(1), 1–9. https://doi.org/10.1016/j.mpaic.2022.11.002

Bahr, T. M., & Ohls, R. K. (2022). Developmental erythropoiesis. In R. A. Polin, S. H. Abman, D. H. Rowitch, W. E. Benitz, & W. W. Fox (Eds.), *Fetal and neonatal physiology* (6th ed., pp. 1104–1124.e5). Elsevier.

Bedwell, S., & Holtzclaw, B. J. (2022). Early interventions to achieve thermal balance in term neonates. *Nursing for Women's Health, 26*(5), 389–396. https://doi.org/10.1016/j.nwh.2022.07.006

Chakkarapani, A. A., Roehr, C. C., Hooper, S. B., te Pas, A. B., & Samir Gupta, S. (2023). Transitional circulation and hemodynamic monitoring in newborn infants. *Pediatric Research*. https://doi.org/10.1038/s41390-022-02427-8

Charlotte Lozier Institute. (2022). *The newborn senses: Sight and eye color*. https://lozierinstitute.org/dive-deeper/the-newborn-senses-sight-and-eye-color/

Centers for Disease Control and Prevention. (2023). *Vitamin K deficiency bleeding*. https://www.cdc.gov/ncbddd/vitamink/index.html

Clyman, R. I. (2022). Mechanisms regulating closure of the ductus arteriosus. In R. A. Polin, S. H. Abman, D. H. Rowitch, W. E. Benitz, & W. W. Fox (Eds.), *Fetal and neonatal physiology* (6th ed., pp. 553–564.e6). Elsevier.

Ding, L., Chen, X., Cheng, H., Zhang, T., & Li, Z. (2022). Advances in IgA glycosylation and its correlation with diseases. *Frontiers in Chemistry, 10*. https://www.frontiersin.org/articles/10.3389/fchem.2022.974854/full

Fanning, B. A. (2025). Neurologic assessment. In C. L. Witt & C. M. Wallman (Eds.), *Tappero & Honeyfield's physical assessment of the newborn* (7th ed.). Springer.

Fernandes, C. J. (2024). Physiologic transition from intrauterine to extrauterine life. *UpToDate*. Retrieved March 23, 2024, from https://www.uptodate.com/contents/physiologic-transition-from-intrauterine-to-extrauterine-life

Funai, E. F., & Norwtiz, E. R. (2024). Labor and delivery: Management of the normal third stage after vaginal birth. *UpToDate*. Retrieved March 22, 2024, from https://www.uptodate.com/contents/labor-and-delivery-management-of-the-normal-third-stage-after-vaginal-birth

Guignard, J.-P., & Iacobelli, S. (2022). Postnatal development of glomerular filtration rate in neonates. In R. A. Polin, S. H. Abman, D. H. Rowitch, W. E. Benitz, & W. W. Fox (Eds.), *Fetal and neonatal physiology* (6th ed., pp. 975–984.e2). Elsevier.

Gupta, A., & Paria, A. (2022). Transition from fetus to neonate. Surgery, 40(11), 685–690. https://doi.org/10.1016/j.mpsur.2022.10.001

Hachemi, I., & U-Din, M. (2023). Brown adipose tissue: Activation and metabolism in humans. *Endocrinology and Metabolism, 38*(2), 214–222. https://doi.org/10.3803/enm.2023.1659

Hooper, S. B., & te Pas, A. B. (2022). Physiology of neonatal resuscitation. In R. A. Polin, S. H. Abman, D. H. Rowitch, W. E. Benitz, & W. W. Fox (Eds.), *Fetal and neonatal physiology* (6th ed., pp. 1589–1605.e2). Elsevier.

Iacobelli, S., & Guignard, J.-P. (2022). Concentration and dilution of urine. In R. A. Polin, S. H. Abman, D. H. Rowitch, W. E. Benitz, & W. W. Fox (Eds.), *Fetal and neonatal physiology* (6th ed., pp. 1030–1047.e3). Elsevier.

Juan, J., Zhang, X., Wang, X., Liu, J., Cao, Y., Tan, L., Gao, Y., Qui, Y., & Yang, H. (2022). Association between skin-to-skin contact duration after cesarean section and breast-feeding. *Children, 9*(11), 1742. https://doi.org/10.3390/children9111742

Kardum, D., Bell, E. F., Grcic, B. F., & Muller, A. (2022). Duration of skin-to-skin care and rectal temperatures in late preterm and term infants. *BMC Pregnancy Childbirth, 22*, 655. https://doi.org/10.1186/s12884-022-04983-7

Kennelly, P. J. (2023). Plasma proteins & immunoglobulins. In P. J. Kennelly, K. M., Botham, O. P. McGuinness, V. M. Rodwell, & P. Weil (Eds.), Harper's illustrated biochemistry (32nd ed). McGraw Hill Education.

Khawar, H., & Marwaha, K. (2023). Surfactant. *StatPearls*. https://www.ncbi.nlm.nih.gov/books/NBK546600/

Kondamudi, N. P., Krata, L., & Wilt, A. S. (2023). Infant apnea. *StatPearls*. https://www.ncbi.nlm.nih.gov/books/NBK441969/

Kotagal, S. (2020). Neurologic examination of the newborn. *UpToDate*. Retrieved March 22, 2024, from https://www.uptodate.com/contents/neurologic-examination-of-the-newborn

La Leche League International. (2024). Breastfeeding info: Jaundice. https://llli.org/breastfeeding-info/jaundice/

Lawrence, R. M. (2022). Host-resistance factors and immunologic significance of human milk. In R. A. Lawrence (Ed.), *Breastfeeding* (9th ed., pp. 145–192). Elsevier.

Likhar, A., & Patil, M. S. (2022). Importance of maternal nutrition in the first 1,000 days of life and its effects on child development: A narrative review. *Cureus, 14*(10), e30083. https://doi.org/10.7759/cureus.30083

Mahe, M. M., Helmrath, M. A., & Shroyer, N. F. (2022). Organogenesis of the gastrointestinal tract. In R. A. Polin, S. H. Abman, D. H. Rowitch, W. E. Benitz, & W. W. Fox, *Fetal and neonatal physiology* (6th ed, pp. 845–854.e2). Elsevier.

Newnam, K. M., & Tasket, A. (2024). Transitional care of the newborn. In B. J. Baker, J. Janke, & AWHONN (Eds.), *Core curriculum for maternal-newborn nursing* (6th ed.). Elsevier.

Rios, D. R., El-Khuffash, A. F., & McNamara, P. J. (2022). Oxygen transport and delivery. In R. A. Polin, S. H. Abman, D. H. Rowitch, W. E. Benitz, & W. W. Fox (Eds.), *Fetal and neonatal physiology* (6th ed., pp. 684–696.e2). Elsevier.

Qian, S., Kumar, P., & Testai, F. D. (2022). Bilirubin encephalopathy. *Current Neurology and Neuroscience Reports, 22*(7), 343–353. https://doi.org/10.1007/s11910-022-01204-8

Rabe, H., Mercer, J., & Erickson-Owens, D. (2022). What does the evidence tell us? Revising optimal cord management at the time of birth. *European Journal of Pediatrics, 181*(5), 1797–1807. https://link.springer.com/article/10.1007/s00431-022-04395-x

Rozance, P. J. (2023). Pathogenesis, screening, and diagnosis of neonatal hypoglycemia. *UpToDate*. Retrieved March 22, 2024, from https://www.uptodate.com/contents/pathogenesis-screening-and-diagnosis-of-neonatal-hypoglycemia

Sahni, R. (2022). Temperature in newborn infants. In R. A. Polin, S. H. Abman, D. H. Rowitch, W. E. Benitz, & W. W. Fox (Eds.), *Fetal and neonatal physiology* (6th ed., pp. 423–445.e2). Elsevier.

Vargo, L. (2025). Cardiovascular assessment. In C. L. Witt & C. M. Wallman (Eds.), *Tappero & Honeyfield's physical assessment of the newborn* (7th ed.). Springer.

Visscher, M. O., & Narendran, V. (2022). Physiologic development of the skin. In R. A. Polin, S. H. Abman, D. H. Rowitch, W. E. Benitz, & W. W. Fox (Eds.), *Fetal and neonatal physiology* (6th ed., pp. 454–472.e4). Elsevier.

Wernimont, A. A., & Norris, A. W. (2022). Glucose metabolism in the fetus and newborn, and methods for its investigation. In R. A. Polin, S. H. Abman, D. H. Rowitch, W. E. Benitz, & W. W. Fox (Eds.), *Fetal and neonatal physiology* (6th ed., pp. 358–368.e3). Elsevier.

Wood, T., Johnson, M., Temples, T., & Bordelon, C. (2022). Thermoneutral environment for neonates: Back to the basics. *Neonatal Network, 41*(5), 289–296. https://pubmed.ncbi.nlm.nih.gov/36002281/

Yamada, N. K., Szyld, E., Strand, M. L., Finan, E., Illuzzi, J. L., Kamath-Rayne, B. D., Kapadia, V. S., Niermeyer, S., Schmölzer, G. M., Williams, A., Weiner, G. M., Wyckoff, M. H., Lee, H. C, American Heart Association, & American Academy of Pediatrics. (2023). 2023 American Heart Association and American Academy of Pediatrics focused update on neonatal resuscitation: An update to the American Heart Association Guidelines for cardiopulmonary resuscitation and emergency cardiovascular care. *Circulation, 149,* e157–e166. https://doi.org/10.1161/CIR.0000000000001181

Yitayew, Y. A., Aitaye, E., B., Lechissa, H. W., & Gebeyehu, L. O. (2020). Neonatal hypothermia and associated factors among newborns admitted in the neonatal intensive care unit of Dessie Referral Hospital, Amhara region, northeast Ethiopia. *International Journal of Pediatrics,* 3013427. https://doi.org/10.1155/2020/3013427

DEVELOPING CLINICAL JUDGMENT

PRACTICING FOR NCLEX-RN

1. When assessing the term newborn, the nurse observes: newborn is alert, heart and respiratory rates have stabilized, and meconium has been passed. Which period of early newborn transition does the nurse determine the infant is exhibiting?
   a. Initial period of reactivity
   b. Second period of reactivity
   c. Decreased responsiveness period
   d. Sleep period

2. A nurse observes a 3-day-old term newborn who is starting to appear mildly jaundiced. What might explain this condition?
   a. An elevated bilirubin level in the newborn
   b. Hemolytic disease of the newborn due to blood incompatibility
   c. Exposing the newborn to high levels of oxygen
   d. Overfeeding the newborn with too much glucose water

3. The nurse educator taught a group of nursing students about thermoregulation and appropriate measures to prevent heat loss by evaporation. Which student behavior indicates successful teaching?
   a. Transporting the newborn in an isolette
   b. Maintaining a warm room temperature
   c. Placing the newborn on a warmed surface
   d. Drying the newborn immediately after birth

4. After birth, the nurse would expect which fetal structure to close as a result of increases in the pressure gradients on the left side of the heart?
   a. Foramen ovale
   b. Ductus arteriosus
   c. Ductus venosus
   d. Umbilical vein

5. The nurse is caring for several newborns. Which newborn could be described as breathing normally?
   a. Newborn A is breathing deeply with a regular rhythm at a rate of 20 bpm.
   b. Newborn B is breathing diaphragmatically with sternal retractions at a rate of 70 bpm.
   c. Newborn C is breathing shallowly with 40-second periods of apnea and cyanosis.
   d. Newborn D is breathing shallowly at a rate of 36 bpm with short periods of apnea.

6. When assessing a term newborn (6 hours old), the nurse auscultates bowel sounds and documents recent passing of meconium. What do these findings indicate?
   a. Abnormal gastrointestinal newborn transition that requires reporting
   b. An intestinal anomaly that needs immediate surgery
   c. A patent anus with no bowel obstruction and normal peristalsis
   d. Malabsorption syndrome resulting in fatty stools

7. A nursing student asks the nursery nurse why they do not bathe the newborn immediately upon admission to the nursery observation area after birth. What does the nurse explain early bathing will increase the risk of?
   a. Jaundice
   b. Infection
   c. Hypothermia
   d. Anemia

8. Because the newborn's RBCs break down much sooner than those of an adult, what might result?
   a. Anemia
   b. Bruising
   c. Apnea
   d. Jaundice

9. The nurse performs a physical examination on a newborn 2 hours after birth. Which findings should be reported to the primary provider or nurse practitioner? Select all that apply.
   a. Respiratory rate of 50 breaths per minute
   b. Intermittent episodes of apnea lasting less than 10 seconds each
   c. Absent Moro reflex when startled
   d. Preauricular skin tag noted on the left ear
   e. White raised bumps noted on nose and face
   f. Yellow blanching of the skin when pressure is applied to the nose

CRITICAL THINKING EXERCISES

1. As the nurse manager, you have been orienting a new nurse in the nursery for the past few weeks. Although they have been demonstrating adequacy with most procedures, today you observe the new nurse bathing several newborns without covering them, weighing them on the scale without a cover, leaving the storage door open with the transporter nearby, and leaving the newborns' head covers and blankets off after showing them to family members through the nursery observation window.
   a. What is your impression of this behavior?
   b. What principles concerning thermoregulation need to be reinforced?
   c. How will you evaluate whether your instructions have been effective?

2. The most important adaptations for the newborn to make after birth are to establish respirations, make cardiovascular adjustments, and establish thermoregulation. Nursing care focuses on monitoring and supporting adjustments to extrauterine adaptation. Develop appropriate nursing interventions to help achieve the following newborn adaptations:

a. Respiratory adaptation
b. Safety, including prevention of infection
c. Thermoregulation

STUDY ACTIVITIES

1. While in the nursery clinical setting, identify the period of behavioral reactivity (first, inactivity, or second period) for two newborns born at different times. Share your findings during the post conference for that clinical day.
2. Dramatic changes occur in the cardiovascular system at birth. When the umbilical cord is clamped and the placenta is separated, there is a resultant increase in systemic blood pressure and changes to the three major fetal shunts (ductus venosus, foramen ovale, and ductus arteriosus) occur. Outline what happens to cause their functional closures during this period of transition.
3. Find two websites about the transition to extrauterine life that can be shared with other nursing students as well as nursery nurses. Critique the information presented in terms of how accurate and current it is.
4. The most common mechanism of heat loss in the newborn is ___________________.
5. The newborn creates heat in three ways—by shivering, through muscle activity, and through thermogenesis by the metabolism of brown adipose tissue. Which is the most effective?

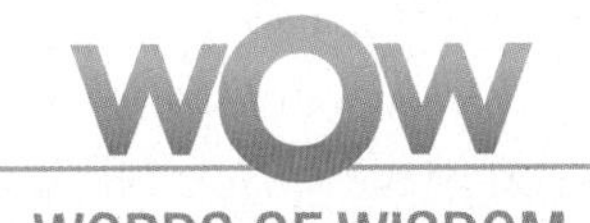

WORDS OF WISDOM

You can send a more powerful message with your actions and behavior than with words alone.

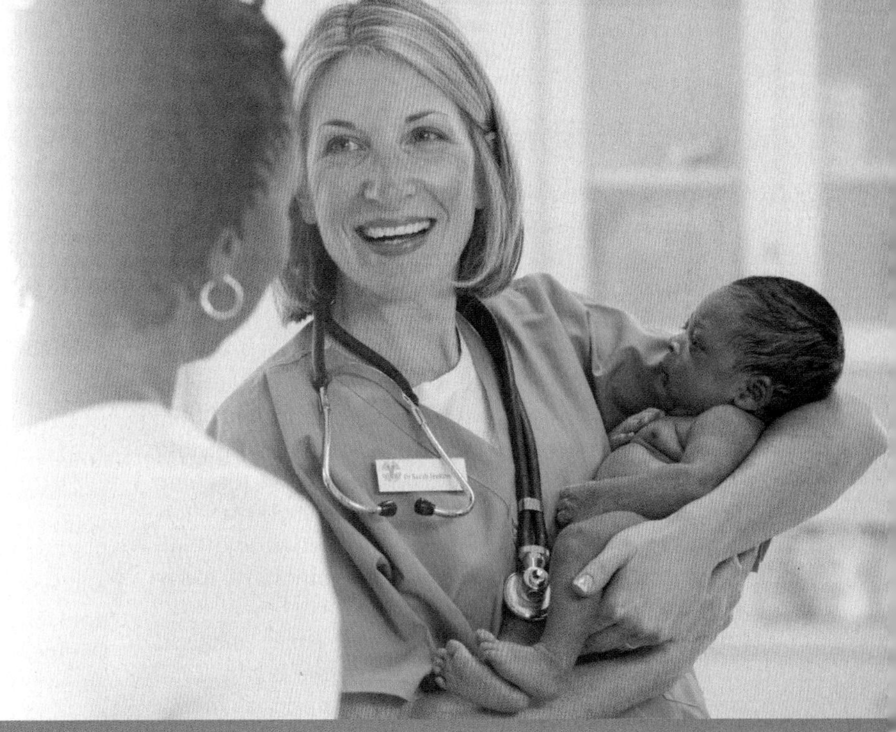

18 Nursing Management of the Newborn

KEY TERMS

acrocyanosis (ak'rō-sī-ă-nō'sis)
Apgar score (ap'gar skōr)
circumcision (ser'kŭm-sizh'ŭn)
congenital dermal melanocytosis (kŏn-jen'i-tăl dĕr'măl mel'ă-nō-sī tō'sis)
Epstein pearls
erythema toxicum neonatorum (er'i-thē'mă tok'si-kŭm nē'ō-nā-tōr-ŭm)
gestational age
harlequin syndrome
infant abduction
milia
molding
nevus flammeus (nē'vŭs flam'ē-ŭs)
nevus vasculosus (nē'vŭs vas'kyū-lō-sŭs)
ophthalmia neonatorum (of'thal'mē-ă nē'ō-nā-tōr-ŭm)
pseudomenstruation
stork bites
vernix caseosa (ver'niks kā'sē-ō'să)

LEARNING OBJECTIVES

Upon completion of the chapter, you will be able to:

1. Perform the assessments needed during the immediate newborn period.
2. Employ interventions that meet the immediate needs of the term newborn.
3. Demonstrate the components of a typical physical examination of a newborn.
4. Distinguish common variations that can be noted during a newborn's physical examination.
5. Plan for common interventions that are appropriate during the early newborn period.
6. Compare the importance of the newborn screening tests.
7. Characterize common concerns in the newborn and appropriate interventions.
8. Analyze the nurse's role in meeting the newborn's nutritional needs.
9. Outline discharge planning content and education needed for the family with a newborn.

Kelly, a 16-year-old first-time parent, calls the hospital maternity unit 3 days after being discharged home. She tells the nurse that her newborn son "looks yellow, like a canary" and "isn't nursing well." She wonders what is wrong.

INTRODUCTION

The birth of a newborn is an exciting time for a family. Immediately after the birth of a newborn, all parents are faced with the task of learning and understanding as much as possible about caring for this new family member, even if they already have other children. In their new or expanded role as parents, they will face many demands and challenges. For many, this is a wonderful, exciting time filled with many discoveries and much information.

Parents learn as they watch the nurse interacting with the newborn. Nurses play a major role in teaching the newborn's caregivers about normal newborn characteristics and about ways to foster optimal growth and development. This role is even more important today because of limited hospital stays.

The newborn has come from a dark, small, enclosed space in the birthing parent's uterus into the bright, cold, extrauterine environment. The newborn transitions from a warm, calm, and fluid environment to one in which physiologic adaptations must be made quickly in order to sustain extrauterine life successfully. Nurses can easily forget they are caring for a small human being who is experiencing their first taste of human interaction outside the uterus. The newborn period is an extremely important one.

It is also easy to overlook the intensity with which birthing parents, partners, and other visitors observe the actions of nurses as they care for the new family member. Nurses need to serve as a model for giving nurturing care to newborns. This chapter provides information about assessment and interventions in the period immediately following the birth of a newborn and during the early newborn period.

NURSING MANAGEMENT DURING THE IMMEDIATE NEWBORN PERIOD

The period of transition from intrauterine to extrauterine life occurs during the first several hours after birth. During this time, the newborn is undergoing numerous adaptations, many of which are occurring simultaneously (see Chapter 17 for more information on the newborn's adaptation). The neonate's temperature, respirations, and cardiovascular dynamics stabilize during this period. Close observation of the newborn's status is essential. Careful examination of the newborn at birth allows for detection of anomalies, birth injuries, and disorders that can compromise adaptation to extrauterine life. Problems that occur during this critical time can have a lifelong impact.

Resuscitating the Newborn

Newborns normally start to breathe without assistance and often cry after birth, stimulated by a change in pressure gradients and environmental temperature. The work of taking that first breath is primarily due to overcoming the surface tension of the walls of the terminal lung units at the gas–tissue interface. Subsequent breaths require less inspiratory pressure since there is an increase in functional capacity and air retained. By 1 minute of age, most newborns are breathing well.

Preparing for Newborn Delivery

The vast majority of newborns require only supportive care during initial resuscitation. Of the remaining infants, only about 5% to 7% of term newborns must have positive pressure ventilation (PPV) with a facemask to ventilate the lungs and begin spontaneous respiratory effort (Weiner & Zaichkin, 2022). An even smaller number will need further resuscitation involving tracheal intubation, chest compressions, or medication administration (Weiner & Zaichkin, 2022). The aim of neonatal resuscitation is to prevent neonatal death and adverse long-term neurodevelopmental sequelae associated with perinatal asphyxia. Anticipation, adequate preparation, accurate evaluation, and prompt initiation of support are critical for successful newborn resuscitation. Have all basic equipment immediately available and in working order. Ensure the equipment is evaluated daily, and document its condition and any needed repairs. Refer to Box 18.1 for basic equipment needed for newborn resuscitation.

Anticipating the potential need for more advanced resuscitation involves assessment of antepartum and intrapartum risk factors, knowing the anticipated gestation age, and determining the status of the amniotic fluid when the membranes ruptured.

Determining Need for and Providing Resuscitation Measures

Determine the newborn's risk status. Ask:

- Is this a full-term newborn?
- Is the infant's muscle tone good?
- Is the newborn breathing and crying?

BOX 18.1 Basic Equipment for Newborn Resuscitation

- A wall clock to document timing of activities and events
- A supply of disposable gloves in a variety of sizes for staff to use
- Naloxone (Narcan)
- Pulse oximeter
- A wall source or tank source of 100% oxygen with a flow meter
- A neonatal self-inflating ventilation bag with correctly sized face masks
- A selection of endotracheal tubes (2.5, 3.0, or 3.5 mm) with introducers
- A laryngoscope with a small, straight blade and spare batteries and bulbs
- Epinephrine
- Volume-expanding fluids

Weiner, G. M., & Zaichkin, J. (2021). *Textbook of neonatal resuscitation* (8th ed.). American Academy of Pediatrics.

When the answer to these questions is yes, the newborn does not need advanced resuscitative measures. All newborns need a clear airway and to be dried and warmed. Follow these steps, in this sequence, moving on to the next rapidly and only as needed:

1. Stabilize the infant: Dry the newborn thoroughly with a warm towel; provide warmth by placing them under a radiant heater to prevent rapid heat loss through evaporation. Position the head in a neutral position to open the airway, clear the airway with a bulb syringe or suction catheter, and stimulate the newborn to breathe by rubbing them with a dry towel. At times, handling and rubbing the newborn with a dry towel may be all that is needed to stimulate respirations.
2. Assess the infant's breathing: Provide PPV with an ambu-bag if the newborn is apneic or gasping.
3. Determine oxygen saturation: Place a pulse oximeter on the newborn's right hand.
4. Provide ongoing PPV if needed.
5. Assess the infant's heart rate (HR): If it is less than 100 when breathing on their own, or less than 60 and not improving with effective PPV, perform chest compressions using a 3:1 compression to ventilation ratio.
6. Reassess the newborn's HR: If the HR remains below 60 despite effective PPV and compressions, administer epinephrine (provide volume expansion if HR does not improve with epinephrine) (Fernandez, 2023).

The decision to progress from one set of actions to the next and the need for further resuscitative efforts are determined by the assessment of respirations, HR, and color. Serial clinical assessment of the response to interventions is fundamental to a successful resuscitation (Weiner & Zaichkin, 2021). To remember the steps used in resuscitation for all newborns regardless of gestational age, use the "ABC" mnemonic. Refer to Box 18.2 for additional information.

When the newborn requires more than drying, warming, positioning, suctioning, and stimulating, keep the parents informed of what is happening to their newborn and what is being done and why. Provide support through this initial crisis. Once the newborn has been stabilized, encourage bonding by having them stroke; touch; and, when appropriate, hold the newborn.

Maintaining Thermoregulation

Newborns have trouble regulating their temperature, especially during the first few hours after birth (see Chapter 17 for a complete discussion). Therefore, maintaining body temperature is crucial.

Assess body temperature frequently during the immediate newborn period. The infant's temperature should be taken every 30 minutes for the first 2 hours or until their temperature has stabilized and then every 8 hours until discharge or per hospital protocols. The newborn's temperature should remain stable for at least 12 hours before discharge (McKee-Garrett, 2023). Attach a thermistor probe (automatic sensor) to the newborn's skin to record body temperature on a monitoring device on the radiant warmer. Avoid placement of a skin temperature probe over a bony area or one with brown fat, because it does not give an accurate assessment of the whole-body temperature. The probe is taped to the newborn's abdomen, usually in one of the upper quadrants, which allows for position changes from supine to side-lying without having to readjust the probe (Bedwell & Holtzclaw, 2022). The other end of the thermistor probe is inserted into the radiant heat control panel. Temperature parameters are set on an alarm system connected to the heat panel that will sound if the newborn's temperature falls out of the set range. Check the probe connection periodically to make sure it remains secure. Remember the potential for heat loss in newborns, and perform all nursing interventions in a way that minimizes heat loss and prevents hypothermia.

Axillary temperature can also be used to assess the newborn's body temperature. Place the thermometer probe into the newborn's axillary area and place their arm over their chest to keep the thermometer in place and provide comfort to the newborn.

BOX 18.2 ABC for Newborn Resuscitation

ABC Newborn Resuscitation Protocol

- **Airway**
  - Place the infant's head in "sniffing" position, with the head tilted back and the chin tilted forward to open the airway.
  - Suction the infant's mouth, then nose.
- **Breathing**
  - Use positive pressure ventilation (PPV) for apnea, gasping, or pulse <100 bpm.
  - Form a seal around both the mouth and nose when giving breaths. Ventilate at a rate of one breath per 30 chest compressions.
  - Look for slight chest movement with each breath.
  - Auscultate for rising heart rate (HR), audible breath sounds.
- **Circulation**
  - Start compressions if the HR is <60 after 30 seconds of effective PPV.
  - Give rapid chest compressions, 90 per minute.
  - Maintain a compression to ventilation ratio of 3:1.
  - Compressions should be performed with two fingers at the center of the chest, or compress one third of the anterior–posterior diameter of the chest with thumbs.

Weiner, G. M., & Zaichkin, J. (2022). Updates for the neonatal resuscitation program and resuscitation guidelines. *NeoReviews, 23*(4), 238–249. https://doi.org/10.1542/neo.23-4-e238

Concept Mastery Alert

Use of a Radiant Heater in Preventing Newborn Heat Loss

A 1-day-old infant should have adequate thermoregulation to remain out of the radiant heater. The best way to prevent heat loss is to ensure that the infant does not come in contact with cold surfaces and has ongoing skin-to-skin contact with a parent.

Nursing interventions to help maintain body temperature include:

- Prewarm blankets and hats to reduce heat loss through conduction.
- Place the newborn under a temperature-controlled radiant warmer (Fig. 18.1).
- Dry the newborn immediately after birth to prevent heat loss through evaporation.
- Put a cap on the newborn's head after it is thoroughly dried after birth.
- Wrap the baby in warmed blankets to reduce heat loss via convection.
- Measure the newborn's axillary temperature soon after birth to establish a baseline.
- Use a warmed cover on the scale to weigh the unclothed newborn.
- Warm stethoscopes and hands before examining the infant or providing care.
- Delay the initial bath for 6 to 24 hours after birth when the infant demonstrates a stable temperature to prevent heat loss through evaporation.
- Encourage skin-to-skin contact with a parent, with both parent and infant covered with a warmed blanket, as soon as the newborn is stabilized to prevent body heat loss.
- Avoid placing newborns in drafts or near air vents to prevent heat loss through convection.
- Avoid placing cribs near cold outer walls to prevent heat loss through radiation.
- If oxygen is required, ensure it is heated and humidified (Bedwell & Holtzclaw, 2022; Tourneux et al., 2022).

Apgar Scoring

The **Apgar score**, introduced in 1952 by Dr. Virginia Apgar, is used worldwide to evaluate a newborn's physical condition at 1 and 5 minutes after birth (Newnam & Tasket, 2024). Endorsed by both the American College of Obstetricians and Gynecologists (ACOG) and the American Academy of Pediatrics (AAP), the Apgar score is the most commonly used assessment to quantify a newborn's status after birth (ACOG, 2021). An additional Apgar assessment is done at 10 minutes if the 5-minute score is less than 7 points. Rapidly determining a newborn's Apgar score immediately after birth provides an indication of success to the neonate's transition to extrauterine life and their ability to survive. Assessment of the newborn at 1 minute provides data about the newborn's initial adaptation to extrauterine life. Assessment at 5 minutes provides a clearer indication of the newborn's overall central nervous system status.

Five parameters are assessed with Apgar scoring. A quick way to remember the parameters of Apgar scoring is:

- A: appearance (color)
- P: pulse (HR)
- G: grimace (reflex irritability)
- A: activity (muscle tone)
- R: respiratory (respiratory effort)

Each parameter is assigned a score ranging from 0 to 2 points. A score of 0 points indicates an absent or poor response; a score of 2 points indicates a normal response (Table 18.1). A normal newborn's total score should be 8 to 10 points. If the Apgar score is 8 points or higher, no intervention is needed other than supporting normal respiratory efforts and maintaining thermoregulation. Scores of 4 to 7 points signify moderate difficulty with newborn transition, and scores of 0 to 3 points represent severe distress in adjusting to extrauterine life. The Apgar score is influenced by the newborn's physiologic

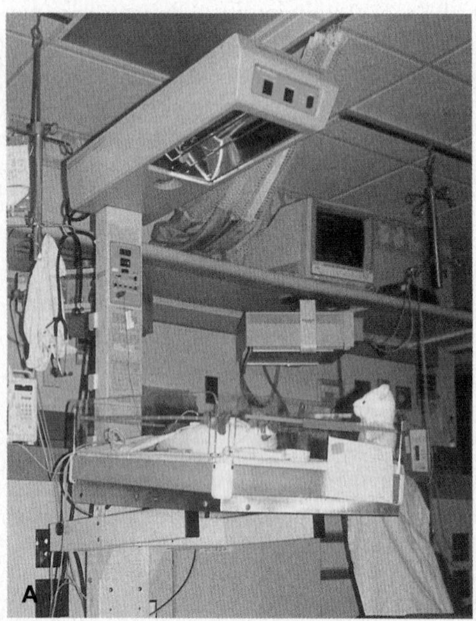

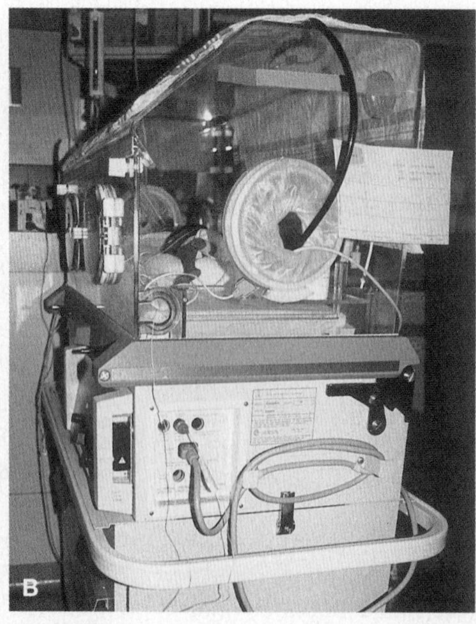

FIGURE 18.1 Maintaining thermoregulation. **A.** Radiant warmer. **B.** Isolette.

TABLE 18.1 • Apgar Scoring for Newborns

Parameter (Assessment Technique)	0 Point	1 Point	2 Points
Heart rate (auscultation of apical heart rate for 6 seconds, then multiply by 10)	Absent	Slow (<100 bpm)	>100 bpm
Respiratory effort (observation of the volume and vigor of the newborn's cry; auscultation of depth and rate of respirations)	Apneic	Slow, irregular, shallow	Regular respirations (usually 30–60 breaths/min), strong, good cry
Muscle tone (observation of the extent of flexion in the newborn's extremities and newborn's resistance when the extremities are pulled away from the body)	Limp, flaccid	Some flexion, limited resistance to extension	Tight flexion, good resistance to extension with quick return to flexed position after extension
Reflex irritability (flicking of the soles of the feet or suctioning of the nose with a bulb syringe)	No response	Grimace or frown when irritated	Sneeze, cough, or vigorous cry
Skin color (inspection of trunk and extremities with the appropriate color for race appearing within minutes after birth)	Cyanotic or pale	Appropriate body color; blue extremities (acrocyanosis)	Completely appropriate color (pink on both trunk and extremities)

Newnam, K. M., & Tasket, A. (2024). Transitional care of the newborn. In B. J. Baker, J. Janke, & Association of Women's Health, Obstetric and Neonatal Nurses, *Core curriculum for maternal-newborn nursing* (6th ed.). Elsevier; Weiner, G. M., & Zaichkin, J. (2021). *Textbook of neonatal resuscitation* (8th ed.). American Academy of Pediatrics.

maturity; birth weight; gestational age; the presence of congenital anomalies, neuromuscular disorders, or infection; labor management and birthing parent age; and sedation via medications.

Initial Newborn Assessment

An initial newborn assessment is completed shortly after birth to determine the newborn's overall health status (e.g., birth injury, respiratory status, heart murmur) and to identify apparent physical abnormalities (McKee-Garrett, 2023). Moreover, the results of the assessments must be relayed to the parents of the newborn.

During the initial newborn assessment, look for signs that might indicate a problem, including:

- Abnormal newborn size: small or large for gestational age
- Respiratory concerns:
  - Generalized cyanosis or pallor
  - Labored breathing, nasal flaring, chest retractions
  - Abnormal respiratory rate (tachypnea, more than 60 breaths/min; bradypnea, less than 25 breaths/min)
  - Grunting on exhalation
  - Abnormal breath sounds (rhonchi, crackles [rales], wheezing, and stridor)
  - Apneic episodes
- Abnormal HR (tachycardia, more than 160 bpm; bradycardia, less than 100 bpm)
- Flaccid body posture
- Bulging or sunken fontanelles on newborn's head
- Abdominal distention or hernias (Witt & Wallman, 2025)

If any of these findings is noted, medical intervention may be necessary.

Nursing Interventions

During the immediate newborn period, care focuses on helping the newborn make the transition to extrauterine life. In addition to maintaining thermoregulation, nursing interventions include maintaining airway patency, ensuring proper identification, and administering prescribed medications.

Maintaining Airway Patency

Routine suctioning of the mouth and airways is not required in all newborns. Immediately after birth, if fluids are blocking the airways, the newborn may be suctioned to remove fluids and mucus from the mouth and nose (Fig. 18.2). If suctioning with a bulb syringe is needed to remove large amounts of secretions from the nose and mouth, compress the bulb before placing it into the oral or nasal cavity. Typically, the newborn's mouth is suctioned first to remove debris, and then the nose is suctioned. Suctioning in this manner helps prevent aspiration of fluid into the lungs by an unexpected gasp. Release bulb compression slowly, making sure the tip is placed away from the mucous membranes to draw up the excess secretions. Remove the bulb syringe from the mouth or nose, and then, while holding the bulb syringe tip over an emesis basin lined with paper towel or tissue, compress the bulb to expel the secretions. Repeat the procedure until all secretions are removed;

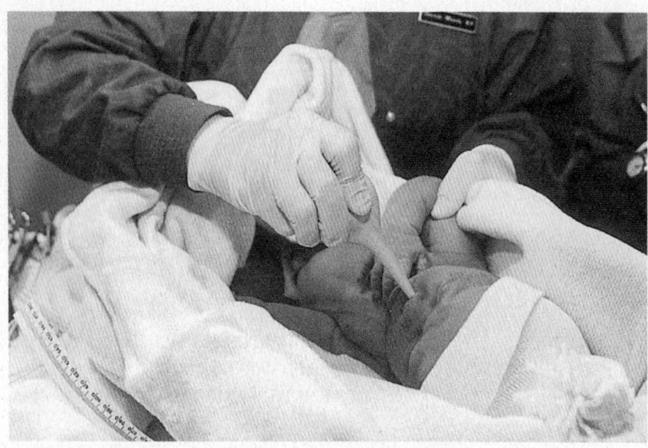

FIGURE 18.2 A newborn is suctioned by means of a bulb syringe to remove mucus from the mouth and nose. The head-down-and-to-the-side position facilitates drainage. Care is given with the infant under a radiant heat source. (Copyright Caroline Brown, RNC, MS, DEd.)

if appropriate, switch to using a towel to wipe away secretions per hospital policy.

> *TAKE NOTE!*
>
> Always keep a bulb syringe near the newborn when feeding them in case they develop sudden choking or a blockage in the nose. It may be lifesaving.

Ensuring Proper Identification

Recently, there has been an increase in possible challenges to health care security, ranging from terrorist attacks to active shooters to infant abductions. **Infant abduction** continues to be a threat in hospitals and health care organizations across the country. Abduction by nonfamily members of newborns from health care facilities has become a subject of concern for parents, parent–child care nurses, health care security and risk management administrators, law enforcement officials, and the National Center for Missing and Exploited Children (NCMEC). In cases of newborn abductions, 59% of the infants are taken from the birthing parent's room (Webster et al., 2021). The Joint Commission (2024) considers infant abduction or discharge to nonparents a sentinel event. Staff identification (ID) badges, training, video surveillance, access control, and tagging systems can help prevent a newborn from being abducted from the hospital. Proactive security measures must become everyone's responsibility to ensure the safety of all newborns and their families in all hospital settings. Infant abductions have been given security code names, such as "Code Pink," in many hospitals.

Before the newborn and their family leave the birthing area, be sure that hospital policy about ID has been followed. Typically, the birthing parent, the newborn, and the birthing parent's partner or support person of their choosing receive ID bracelets. The newborn commonly receives two ID bracelets, one on a wrist and the other on an ankle. The birthing parent receives a matching one, usually on their wrist. The ID bands usually include name, sex, date and time of birth, and ID number. The same ID number is on the bracelets of all family members.

These ID bracelets are provided for the safety of the newborn and must be secured before the birthing parent and newborn leave the birthing area. The ID bracelets are checked by all nurses to validate that the correct newborn is brought to the right birthing parent if they are separated for any period of time (Fig. 18.3). They also serve as the newborn's official ID and should be checked before initiating any procedure on that newborn and on discharge from the unit (Lee & Oh, 2023). Taking the newborn's picture within 2 hours after birth with a color camera or color video or digital image also helps prevent mix-ups and abduction. Many facilities use electronic devices that sound an alarm if a newborn is taken beyond a certain point on the unit or removed from the area.

It is critical not to allow anyone without ID to take an infant for any reason and to keep the infant within the sight of the parent or nursery staff at all times. Although infant abductions are rare, the safety and security of birthing parents and infants should remain a high priority for nurses. By being aware of the physical security of postpartum units, educating expectant parents on the methods used by potential abductors, and working with community resources, these incidents can be prevented.

Administering Prescribed Medications

During the immediate newborn period, infants are at risk for two conditions: vitamin K deficiency bleeding (VKDB) and ophthalmia neonatorum. Newborns are at risk for VKDB because they have not yet established an efficient gastrointestinal microbiome (for ongoing vitamin

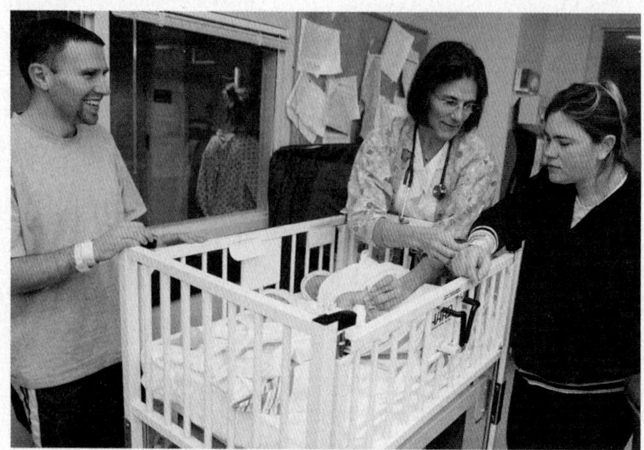

FIGURE 18.3 The nurse checks the newborn's identification band against the birthing parent's.

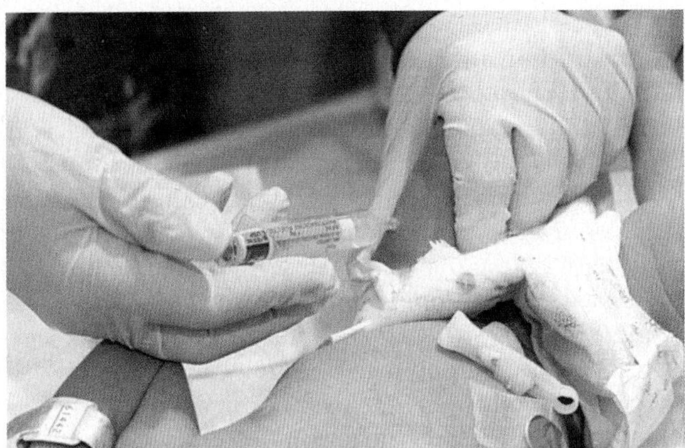

FIGURE 18.4 The nurse administers vitamin K intramuscularly to the newborn.

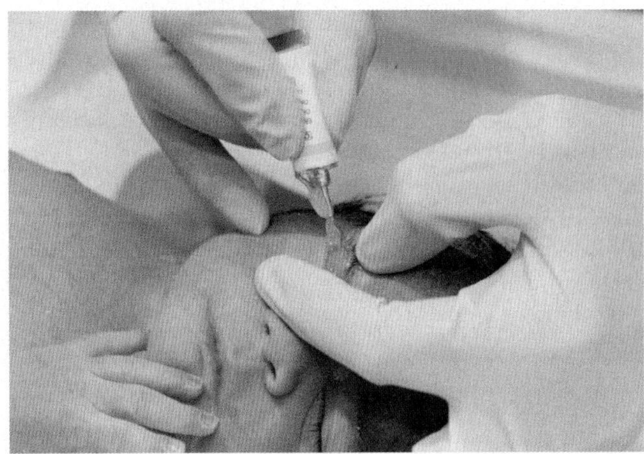

FIGURE 18.5 The nurse administers eye prophylaxis.

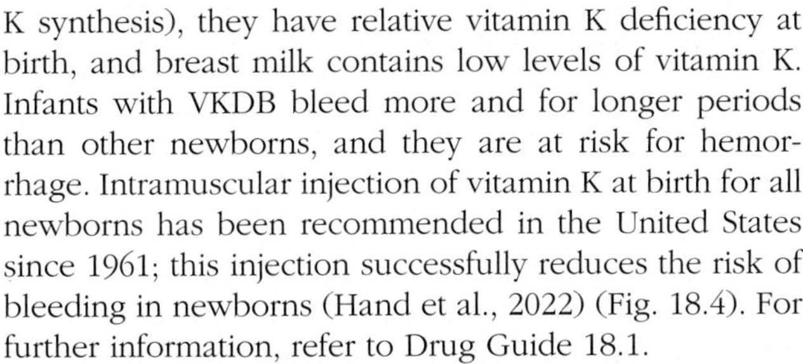

K synthesis), they have relative vitamin K deficiency at birth, and breast milk contains low levels of vitamin K. Infants with VKDB bleed more and for longer periods than other newborns, and they are at risk for hemorrhage. Intramuscular injection of vitamin K at birth for all newborns has been recommended in the United States since 1961; this injection successfully reduces the risk of bleeding in newborns (Hand et al., 2022) (Fig. 18.4). For further information, refer to Drug Guide 18.1.

Ophthalmia neonatorum is also called neonatal conjunctivitis. It may be caused by several different types of bacteria. Gonococcal causes of neonatal conjunctivitis can result in corneal perforation and blindness within 24 hours of age (Mukhopadhyay & Puopolo, 2023; U.S. Preventive Services Task Force [USPSTF], 2019). The USPSTF recommends that all newborns, regardless of birth method, receive prophylaxis for ophthalmia neonatorum within 1 hour of birth (2019). Erythromycin ophthalmic ointment is the only medication approved for use in the United States for prevention of ophthalmia neonatorum (USPSTF, 2019) (Fig. 18.5). For further information, refer to Drug Guide 18.1.

It is also recommended that **immunizations** begin at birth. The first dose of the hepatitis B vaccine is recommended to be given at birth. If the birthing parent is HbsAg-positive, then in addition to the hepatitis B vaccine, the newborn should receive hepatitis B immunoglobulin intramuscularly within 12 hours of birth. For infants born during October through March in most of the continental United States, assess the birthing parent's Respiratory Syncytial Virus (RSV) vaccination status. If the birthing parent was vaccinated fewer than 14 days prior to delivery, the newborn should receive the RSV immunization within 1 week of birth (Centers for Disease Control and Prevention [CDC], 2023a). Educate the parents about the risks and benefits for each vaccine and

DRUG GUIDE 18.1

DRUGS FOR THE NEWBORN

Drug	Action/Indication	Nursing Implications
Phytonadione (vitamin K [Aqua-MEPHYTON, Konakion, Mephyton])	Provides the newborn with vitamin K (necessary for production of adequate clotting factors II, VII, IX, and X by the liver) during the first week of birth until newborn can manufacture it Prevents vitamin K deficiency bleeding (VKDB) of the newborn	• Administer within 6 hours after birth. • Administer as an IM injection at a 90-degree angle into the outer middle third of the vastus lateralis muscle. • Use a 25-gauge, 5/8-in needle for injection. • Hold the leg firmly and inject the medication slowly. • Adhere to standard precautions. • Assess for bleeding at the injection site after administration.
Erythromycin ophthalmic ointment 0.5%	Provides bactericidal and bacteriostatic actions to prevent *Neisseria gonorrhoeae* and *Chlamydia trachomatis* conjunctivitis Prevents ophthalmia neonatorum	• Be alert for chemical conjunctivitis for 1–2 days. • Wear gloves, and open the infant's eyes by placing your thumb and finger above and below the eye. • Gently squeeze the tube or ampule to apply medication into the conjunctival sac from the inner canthus to the outer canthus of each eye. • Do not touch the tip to the eye. • Close the eye to make sure the medication permeates. • Wipe off excess ointment after 1 minute.

Hand, I., Noble, L., Abrams, S. A., & the Committee on Fetus and Newborn, Section on Breastfeeding, Committee on Nutrition. (2022). Vitamin K and the newborn infant. *Pediatrics, 149*(3), e2021056036. https://doi.org/10.1542/peds.2021-056036; UpToDate, Inc. (2024). *UpToDate® Lexidrug™* (Version 8.2.0) [Mobile app]. Wolters Kluwer. https://apps.apple.com/us/app/lexicomp/id313401238

possible adverse effects, obtain the parents' consent for vaccination, and provide them with the corresponding Vaccine Information Statement (VIS) (CDC, 2023b).

For vitamin K and erythromycin, educate parents about why the medications are recommended, what problems may arise if the treatment is not given, and possible adverse effects of the treatment. If eye ointment administration is delayed to allow the newborn time to visualize the parents and for them to bond, make sure the ointment is given as soon as feasible.

TAKE NOTE!

Ophthalmia neonatorum is a severe form of conjunctivitis gonococcal infection that is potentially a blinding condition in newborns.

NURSING MANAGEMENT DURING THE EARLY NEWBORN PERIOD

The early newborn period is a time of great adjustment for both the birthing parent and the newborn; they are adapting to many physiologic and psychological changes.

The nurse's role is to assist the birthing parent and their newborn through this dramatic transition period. The newborn needs continued health assessment, and the parent needs to be taught to care for the new baby. At discharge, the new parent may panic and feel insecure about their role as a primary caregiver. Nurses play a major role in promoting the newborn's transition by providing ongoing assessment and care and in promoting the birthing parent's confidence by serving as a role model and teaching about proper newborn care.

Assessment

The newborn requires ongoing assessment after leaving the birthing area to ensure that their transition to extrauterine life is progressing without problems. The nurse uses the data gathered during the initial assessment as a baseline for comparison.

Perinatal History

Pertinent birthing parent and fetal data are vital to formulate a plan of care for the birthing parent and their newborn. Historical information is obtained from the medical record and from interviewing the birthing parent. Review the parent's history because it provides pertinent information, such as the presence of certain risk factors that could affect the newborn. Keep in mind that a comprehensive patient history may not be available, especially if the birthing parent has had limited or no prenatal care. Historical information usually includes:

- Birthing parent's name, medical record number, blood type, serology result, rubella and hepatitis status, and history of substance use disorder.
- Other tests that are relevant to the newborn and care, such as human immunodeficiency virus (HIV) and group B streptococcus status.
- Intrapartum antibiotic therapy (type, dose, and duration).
- Birthing parent illness that can affect the pregnancy, evidence of chorioamnionitis, use of medications such as steroids.
- Prenatal care, including timing of first visit and subsequent visits.
- Risk for blood group incompatibility, including Rh status and blood type.
- Fetal distress or any category II or III fetal HR patterns during labor.
- Known inherited conditions such as sickle cell anemia and phenylketonuria (PKU).
- Birth weights of previous live-born children, along with identification of any newborn problems.
- Social history, including tobacco, alcohol, and recreational drug use.
- History of depression or domestic violence.
- Cultural factors, including primary language and educational level.
- Pregnancy complications associated with abnormal fetal growth, fetal anomalies, or abnormal results from tests of fetal well-being.
- Information on the progress of labor, birth, labor complications, duration of ruptured membranes, and presence of meconium in the amniotic fluid.
- Medications given during labor, at birth, and immediately after birth.
- Time and method of delivery, including presentation and the use of forceps or a vacuum extractor.
- Status of the newborn at birth, including Apgar scores at 1 and 5 minutes, the need for suctioning, weight, gestational age, vital signs, and umbilical cord status.
- Medications administered to the newborn.
- Postbirth birthing parent information, including placental findings, positive cultures, and presence of fever.

Newborn Physical Examination

The initial newborn physical examination, which may demonstrate subtle differences related to the newborn's age, is carried out within the first 24 hours after birth. For example, a newborn who is 30 minutes old has not yet completed the normal transition from intrauterine to extrauterine life, and, thus, variability may exist in vital signs and in respiratory, neurologic, gastrointestinal, skin, and cardiovascular systems. Therefore, a comprehensive examination should be delayed until after the newborn has completed the transition.

The physical examination should not be initiated if the newborn is crying or appears to be upset. Instead, it is best to postpone the assessment until the newborn is calm. In a quiet newborn, begin the examination with the least invasive and less noxious elements of the examination (auscultation of heart and lungs). Then, examine the areas most likely to irritate the newborn (e.g., examining the hips and eliciting the Moro reflex). A general visual assessment provides an enormous amount of information about the well-being of a newborn. Initial observation gives an impression of a healthy (stable) versus an ill newborn and a term versus a preterm newborn.

A typical physical examination of a newborn includes a general survey of skin color, posture, state of alertness, head size, overall behavioral state, respiratory status, biologic sex, and any obvious congenital anomalies. Check the overall appearance for anything unusual. Then, complete the examination in a systematic fashion.

Remember Kelly, who called the home health nurse and said her newborn son "looks like a canary?" What additional information is needed about the baby? What might be causing his yellow color?

ANTHROPOMETRIC MEASUREMENTS

Shortly after birth, after the biologic sex of the child is revealed, most parents want to know the weight of their newborn to report to their family and friends. Additional measurements, including length and head and chest circumference, are also taken and recorded. Abdominal measurements are not routinely obtained unless there is a suspicion of pathology that causes abdominal distention. The newborn's progress from that point onward will be validated based on these early measurements. These measurements will be compared with future serial measurements to determine growth patterns, which are plotted on growth charts to evaluate normalcy. Therefore, accuracy is paramount.

Length

The average length of most newborns is 50 cm (20 in), but it can range from 48 to 53 cm (19 to 21 in) (Newnam & Tasket, 2024). Measure length with the unclothed newborn lying on a warmed blanket placed on a flat surface with the knees held in an extended position. Because of the flexed position of the newborn after birth, it is necessary to extend the leg completely and hold it when measuring the length. Use a disposable tape measure or a built-in measurement board located on the side of some scales. Measure from the head to the soles of the feet—and record this measurement in the newborn's record (see Fig. 18.6).

Weight

Weight is affected by genetics, maternal age, size of the parents, the birthing parent's nutrition, the birthing parent's prenatal weight, gestational duration, pregnancy complications, cigarette use by the birthing parent, age of the birthing parent, substance misuse during pregnancy, and placental perfusion (Liu et al., 2022). The average full-term newborn birth weight ranges from 2,500 to 4,000 g (5 lb, 8 oz to 8 lb, 13 oz) (Newnam & Tasket, 2024). Newborns are weighed immediately after birth and then daily. Newborns usually lose 7% to 10% of their birth weight within the first 3 to 4 days of life due to loss of meconium, extracellular fluid, and limited food intake. The infant then gains weight, returning to the birth weight by 2 weeks of age (Caglar, 2022).

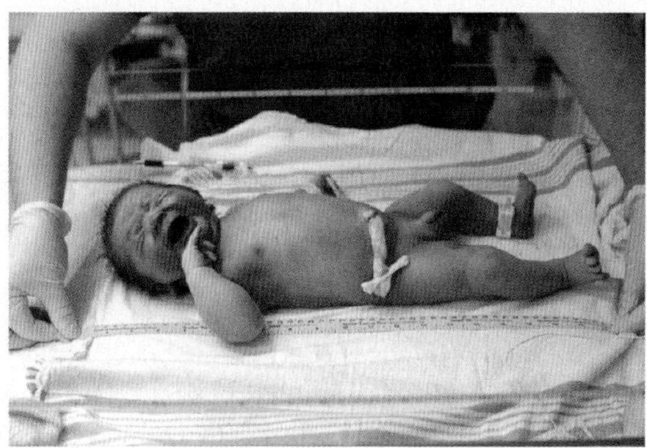

FIGURE 18.6 Measuring a newborn's length.

Newborns are weighed on admission to the nursery or are taken to a digital scale to be weighed and returned to the birthing parent's room. First, balance the scale if it is not balanced. Place a warmed protective cloth or paper as a barrier on the scale to prevent heat loss by conduction; recalibrate the scale to 0 after applying the barrier. Next, place the unclothed newborn in the center of the scale. Keep a hand above the newborn for safety (see Fig. 18.7).

Weight should be correlated with gestational age. A newborn who weighs more than the average might be large for gestational age (LGA) or an infant of a diabetic birthing parent. A newborn who weighs less than average might be small for gestation age (SGA), preterm, or have a genetic syndrome. It is important to identify the cause of the deviation in size and to monitor the newborn for complications common to that etiology.

Newborns are classified by their birth weight regardless of their gestational age as follows:

- Low birth weight (LBW): less than 2,500 g (less than 5.5 lb)
- Very low birth weight (VLBW): less than 1,500 g (less than 3.5 lb)

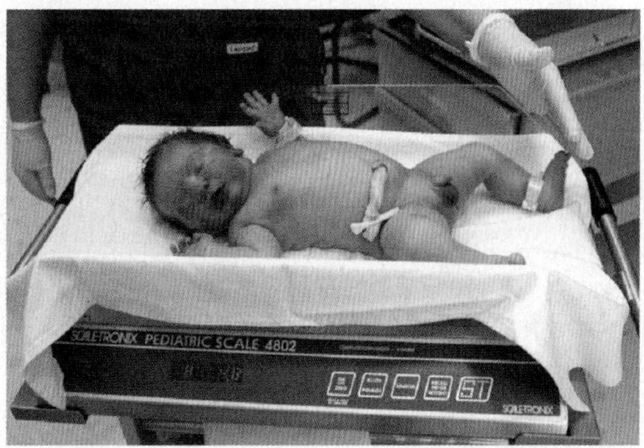

FIGURE 18.7 Weighing the newborn. Note how the nurse uses their hand to guard the newborn to prevent falling.

- Extremely low birth weight (ELBW): less than 1,000 g (less than 2.5 lb)
- Normal birth weight (NBW): between 2,500 and 4,000 g (5.5 to 8.8 lb)
- High birth weight (HBW): more than 4,000 kg (8.8 lb) (Smialek, 2024)

Head Circumference

The head circumference should be approximately one fourth of the newborn's length or about half the infant's body length plus 10 cm. The average newborn head circumference is 33 to 35.5 cm (13 to 14 in) (Newnam & Tasket, 2024). Measure the circumference at the head's widest diameter (the occipitofrontal circumference). Wrap a flexible or paper measuring tape snugly around the newborn's head and record the measurement (Fig. 18.8A). A small head circumference might indicate microcephaly or that the infant is SGA. A larger head circumference might indicate hydrocephalus or another cause of increased intracranial pressure. Both small and large head circumference need to be documented and reported for further investigation.

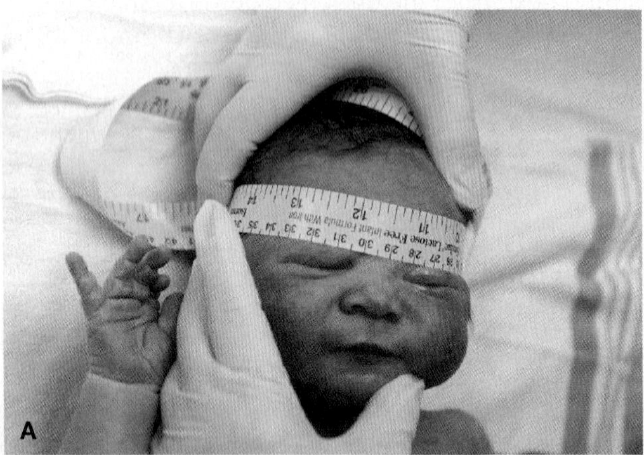

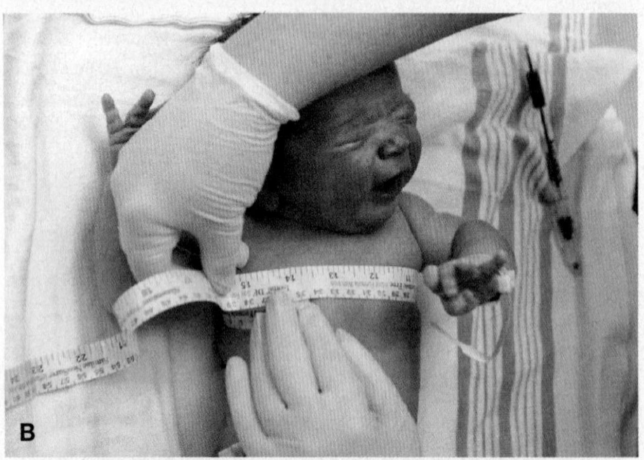

FIGURE 18.8 **A.** Measuring head circumference. **B.** Measuring chest circumference.

TAKE NOTE!

Head circumference may need to be remeasured at a later time if the shape of the head is altered from birth.

Chest Circumference

The average chest circumference is 30.5 to 33 cm (12 to 13 in). It is generally equal to or about 1 to 2 cm less than the head circumference (Newnam & Tasket, 2024). Measure the newborn's chest circumference by placing a flexible or paper tape measure around the unclothed newborn's chest just below the nipple line without pulling it taut (Fig. 18.8B).

TAKE NOTE!

The head and chest circumferences are usually equal by about 1 year of age.

VITAL SIGNS

HR and respiratory rate are assessed immediately after birth with Apgar scoring. Temperature, HR, and respiratory rate are assessed frequently within the first 4 hours of life and according to hospital policy. Following that, they should be assessed every 6 to 8 hours, strictly in accordance with the facility's policy (Newnam & Tasket, 2024). Vital signs are used for identifying a variety of complications and for ensuring the well-being of the newborn. In some health care agencies, the newborn's temperature is taken immediately after the Apgar score has been taken to allow for identification of hypothermia, which then requires a glucose check. However, nurses need to follow each facility's protocols on this assessment timing.

Take the newborn's temperature via the axillary method. In term newborns, the normal axillary temperature range should be maintained at 36.5°C to 37.5°C (97.7°F to 99.5°F) (Newnam & Tasket, 2024). Hold the thermometer or temperature probe in the midaxillary space according to manufacturer's directions and hospital protocol. Rectal temperatures are not taken because of the risk of perforation and infant distress (Kain & Mannix, 2023).

Following the immediate stabilization period after birth, count the apical pulse for one full minute. The average newborn HR is about 120 to 140 beats per minute (bpm). The HR may decrease to as low as 70 to 90 bpm when the infant is sleeping and may increase to 170 bpm or higher when the newborn is crying or very active (Vargo, 2025). Assess the newborn's respirations when they are quiet or sleeping. Place a stethoscope on the right side of the newborn's chest and count the breaths for one full minute to identify any irregularities. The typical neonatal respiratory rate is 30 to 60 breaths/min with symmetric chest movement (Fraser, 2025).

Blood pressure is not assessed as part of a newborn examination unless there is a clinical indication, such as suspected congenital heart or renal defect, or low Apgar score. If assessed, an oscillometer (Dinamap) is used. The typical range for a newborn weighing 3.5 kg is 50 to 80 mm Hg (systolic) and 30 to 55 mm Hg (diastolic) (Vargo, 2025). Blood pressure may be affected by activity level, behavioral state, and temperature. Refer to Table 18.2 for the expected newborn vital signs ranges.

SKIN

The newborn's skin is similar in structure to an adult's, but many of the functions are not fully developed. Observe the overall appearance of the skin, including color, texture, turgor, and integrity. The newborn's skin should be smooth and flexible, and the color should be consistent with racial background.

Skin Condition and Color

Check skin turgor by elevating a small area of skin over the chest or abdomen, and note how quickly it returns to its original position. In a well-hydrated newborn, the skin should return to its normal position immediately. Skin that remains "tented" after being pinched may indicate dehydration. A small amount of lanugo (fine downy hair) may be observed over the shoulders and on the sides of the face and upper back. There may be some cracking and peeling of the skin. The skin should be warm to the touch and intact.

The newborn's skin often appears blotchy or mottled, especially in the extremities. Persistent cyanosis of fingers, hands, toes, and feet with mottled blue or red discoloration and coldness is called **acrocyanosis** (Fig. 18.9). It is a typical finding in newborns during the first few weeks of life. In the first 12 to 24 hours of life circumoral cyanosis may be noted, yet it will not persist past 24 hours of age (Witt, 2025). Any change in color of the newborn skin needs further investigation.

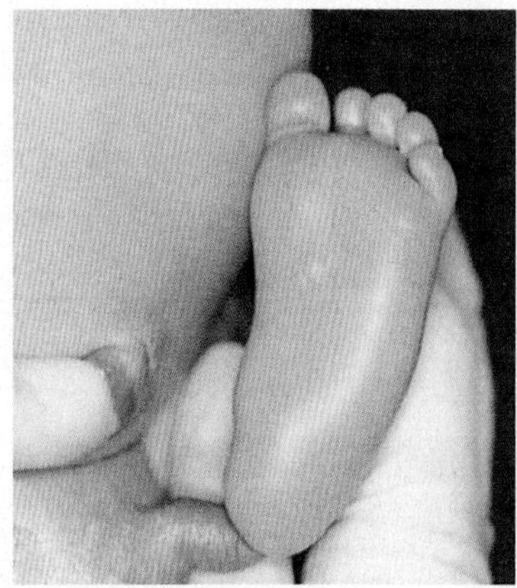

FIGURE 18.9 Acrocyanosis. This commonly appears on the feet and hands of babies shortly after birth. This infant is a 32-week-old newborn. (Reprinted with permission from Fletcher, M. [1998]. *Physical diagnosis in neonatology* [p. 115]. Lippincott-Raven Publishers.)

TABLE 18.2 • Newborn Vital Signs

Newborn Vital Signs	Ranges of Values
Temperature	36.5–37.5°C (97.7–99.5°F)
Heart rate (pulse)	120–140 bpm (as low as 70 with sleep, as high as 170+ with activity or crying)
Respirations	30–60 breaths/min at rest, increasing with crying
Blood pressure	50–80 mm Hg systolic, 30–55 mm Hg diastolic

Fraser, D. (2025). Chest and lung assessment. In C. L. Witt & C. M. Wallman (Eds.), *Tappero & Honeyfield's physical assessment of the newborn: A comprehensive approach to the art of physical examination* (7th ed.). Springer; Newnam, K. M., & Tasket, A. (2024). Transitional care of the newborn. In B. J. Baker, J. Janke, & Association of Women's Health, Obstetric and Neonatal Nurses, *Core curriculum for maternal-newborn nursing* (6th ed.). Elsevier; and Vargo, L. (2025). Cardiovascular assessment. In C. L. Witt & C. M. Wallman (Eds.), *Tappero & Honeyfield's physical assessment of the newborn: A comprehensive approach to the art of physical examination* (7th ed.). Springer.

Newborn Skin Variations

While assessing the skin, make note of any rashes, ecchymoses or petechiae, nevi, or dark pigmentation. Skin lesions can be congenital or transient; they may be a result of infection or may result from the mode of birth. If any of them are present, observe the anatomic location, arrangement, type, and color. Bruising may result from the use of devices such as a vacuum extractor during delivery. Petechiae may be the result of pressure on the skin during the birth process. Forceps marks may be observed over the cheeks and ears. A small puncture mark on the scalp may be seen if internal fetal scalp electrode monitoring was used during labor.

Common skin variations include vernix caseosa, stork bites or salmon patches, milia, congenital dermal melanocytosis, erythema toxicum neonatorum, harlequin syndrome, nevus flammeus, and nevus vasculosus (Fig. 18.10).

Vernix caseosa is a thick white substance that protects the skin of the fetus. It is formed by secretions from the fetus' oil glands and is found during the first 2 or 3 days after birth in body creases and the hair. It does not need to be removed because it will be absorbed into the skin.

Stork bites or salmon patches are superficial vascular areas found on the nape of the neck, on the eyelids, and between the eyes and the upper lip (Fig. 18.10A). The name comes from the marks on the back of the neck where, as myth goes, a stork picked up the baby. They are caused by a concentration of immature blood vessels and are most visible when the newborn is crying. They are considered a normal variant, and most fade and disappear completely within the first year.

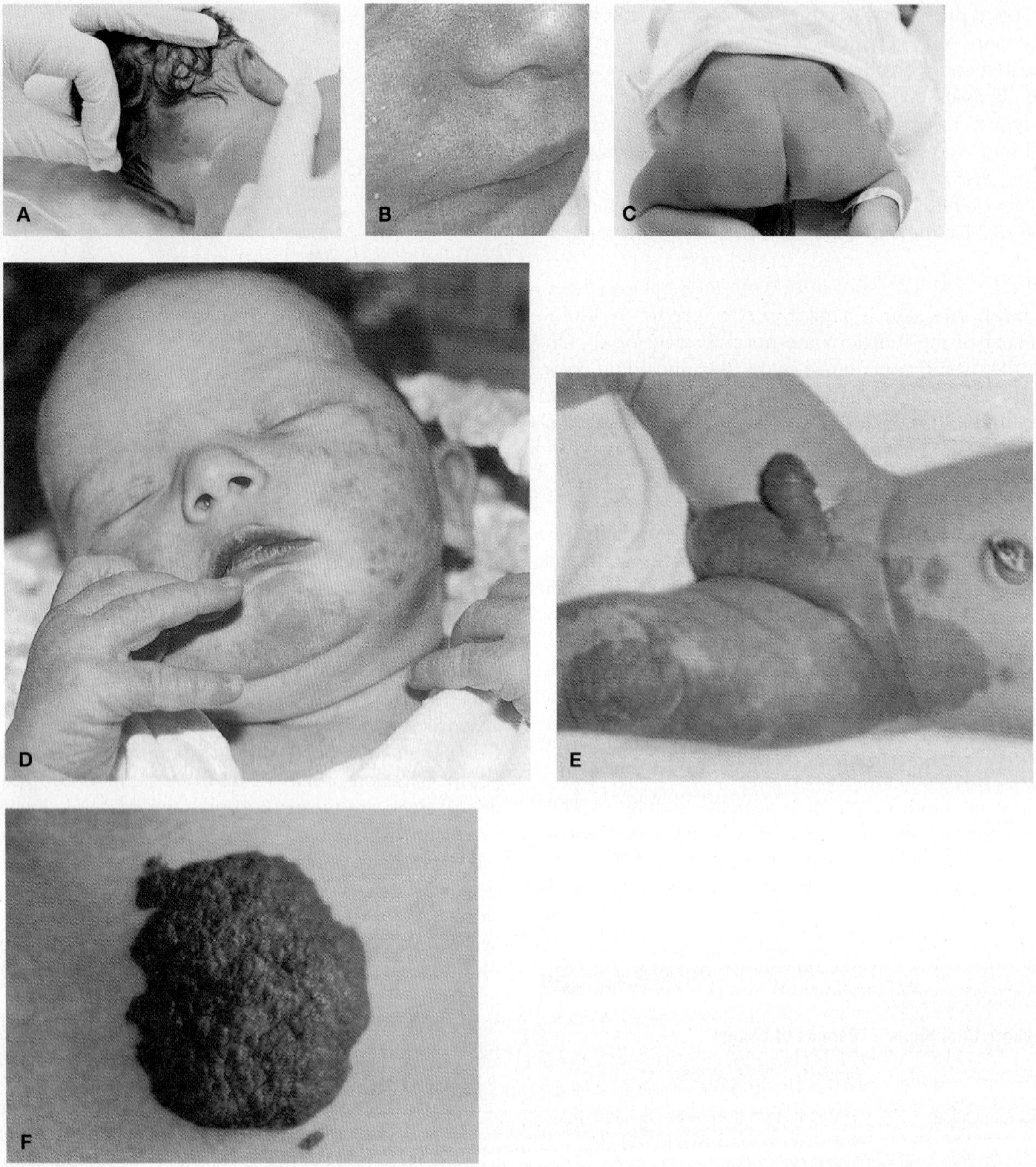

FIGURE 18.10 Common skin variations. **A.** Stork bite. **B.** Milia. **C.** Congenital dermal melanocytosis. **D.** Erythema toxicum. **E.** Nevus flammeus (port wine stain). **F.** Strawberry hemangioma.

Milia are multiple pearly white or pale yellow unopened sebaceous glands frequently found on a newborn's nose. They may also appear on the chin and forehead (Fig. 18.10B). They form from oil glands and disappear on their own within 2 to 4 weeks. When they occur in a newborn's mouth and gums, they are termed **Epstein pearls**. They occur on the palate in 65% to 80% of newborns and on the gingivae in 25% to 53% (Diaz de Ortiz & Mendez, 2023). Most lesions break spontaneously within the first few weeks of life.

Congenital dermal melanocytosis refers to benign blue or purple splotches that appear solitary on the lower back and buttocks of newborns but may occur as multiples over the legs and shoulders (Fig. 18.10C). They occur most often in Black, Asian, Hispanic, and Native American newborns but can develop in darker-skinned newborns of all races. The spots are caused by a concentration of pigmented cells; they usually fade spontaneously by 1 year and rarely persist after 6 years of life. Congenital dermal melanocytosis is usually benign and does not require treatment. The spots should not be confused with bruises caused by trauma (Chua & Pico, 2023).

Erythema toxicum neonatorum (newborn rash) is a benign, idiopathic, generalized, transient rash that occurs in 48% to 72% of all full-term newborns during the first week of life (Roques et al., 2023). It consists of small papules or pustules on the skin resembling fleabites. It is often mistaken for staphylococcal pustules. The rash is common on the face, chest, and back (Fig. 18.10D). One of the chief characteristics of this rash is its lack of pattern. It is caused by the newborn's eosinophils reacting to the environment as the immune system matures.

Harlequin syndrome refers to the dilation of blood vessels on only one side of the body, giving the newborn the appearance of wearing a clown suit. It gives a distinct midline demarcation, which is described as pale on the nondependent side and red on the opposite, dependent side. Harlequin syndrome occurs in about 10% of newborns, resolving by 3 weeks of age (Witt, 2025). It results from immature autonomic vasomotor control, with each episode lasting up to 30 minutes.

Nevus flammeus, also called a port wine stain, appears on the newborn's body; the head and neck areas are the most commonly affected (Fig. 18.10E). It is a capillary angioma located directly below the dermis. Nevus flammeus is flat with sharp demarcations. In light-skinned infants, the color is purple red; in dark-skinned infants it appears jet black in color (Witt, 2025). Nevus flammeus ranges in size from a few millimeters to large, occasionally involving as much as half the body surface. Port wine stains do not regress, but grow in proportion to the child's growth, becoming thicker and darker in color with age.

Nevus vasculosus, also called a strawberry mark or strawberry hemangioma, is a benign capillary hemangioma in the dermal and subdermal layers. It is raised, rough, dark red, and sharply demarcated (Fig. 18.10F). It is commonly found in the head region within a few weeks after birth and can increase in size or number. Nevus vasculosus affects about 4% to 5% of newborns (Chamli et al., 2023). This type of hemangioma may be subtle or even absent in the first few weeks of life, but they proliferate in the first few months.

HEAD

The newborn's head has five major bones—two frontal, one occipital, and two parietals. These bones are separated by connective tissue junctions termed cranial sutures. The bones are not yet fused, permitting slight movement for successful passage through the birth canal. Spaces between the bones are called fontanels, with the two commonly assessed being the anterior and posterior fontanels. The anterior fontanel is at the intersection of the coronal, metopic, and sagittal sutures; is diamond shaped; and is 0.6 to 4.7 cm in size. The posterior fontanel is triangular in shape; is 0.5 to 0.7 cm in size; and is located where the sagittal suture meets the lambdoidal suture, separating the occipital and parietal bones.

Inspect the infant's head for shape and anomalies. Palpate the cranium, noting overriding sutures and the size and flatness of the fontanels.

Variations in Head Size and Appearance

During inspection and palpation, be alert for common variations that may cause asymmetry. These include molding, caput succedaneum, and cephalhematoma.

Molding: this refers to elongated shaping of the fetal head to accommodate passage through the birth canal (Fig. 18.11). It typically resolves within a week after birth without intervention.

Caput succedaneum: localized edema on the scalp occurs from the pressure of the birth process. It presents as a poorly demarcated soft tissue swelling that crosses suture lines (Fig. 18.12A). The swelling will gradually dissipate in a few days without any treatment.

Cephalhematoma: this refers to benign localized subperiosteal collection of blood confined by one cranial bone. It is noted by a well-demarcated, often fluctuant swelling with no overlying skin discoloration (Fig. 18.12B). It resolves over several weeks.

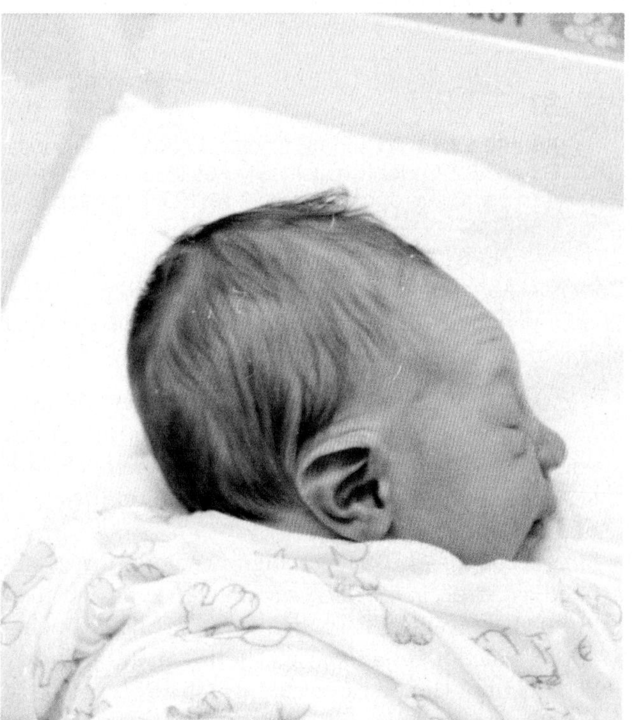

FIGURE 18.11 Molding of a newborn's head.

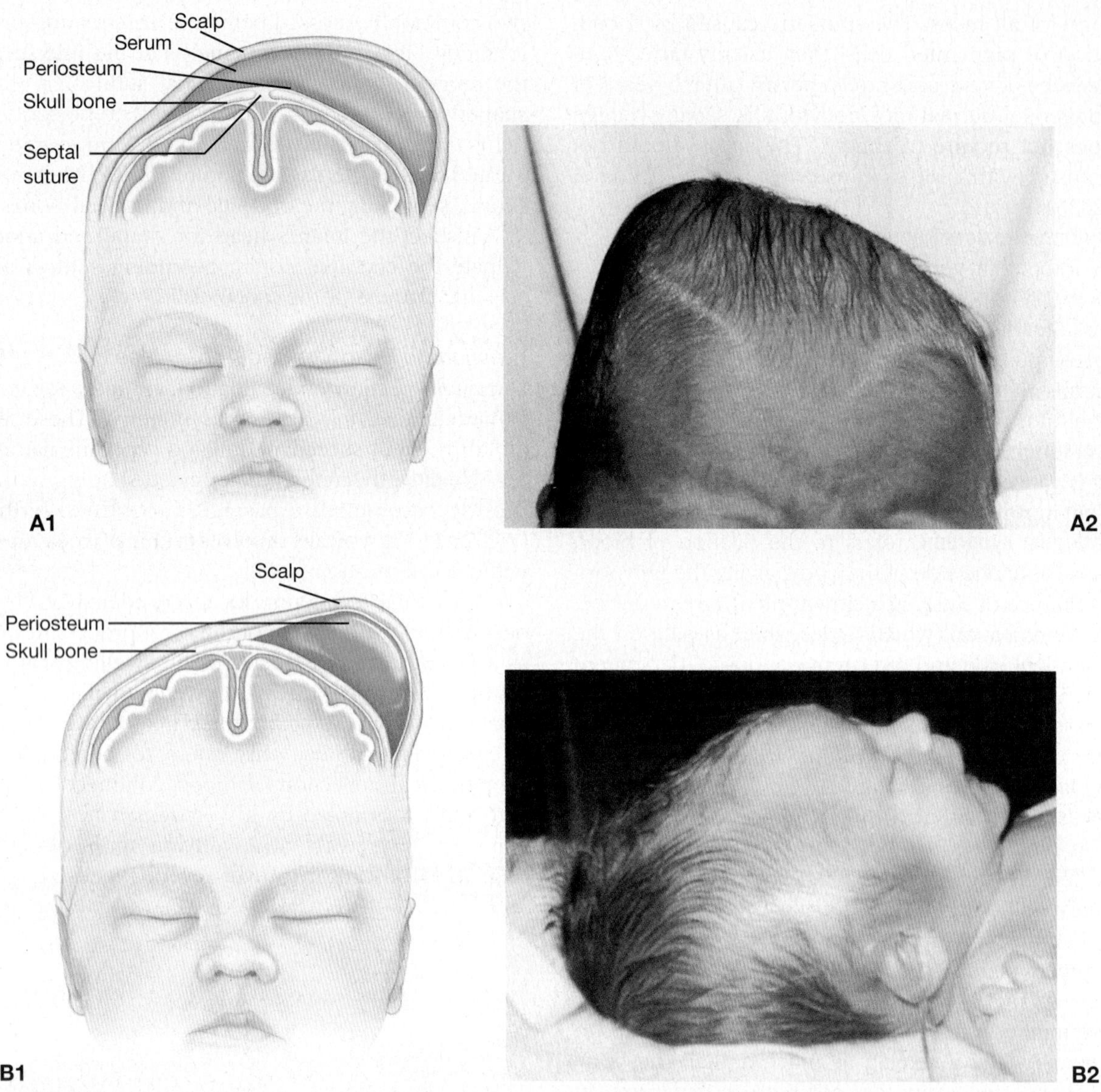

FIGURE 18.12 A1 and **A2.** Caput succedaneum involves the collection of serous fluid and often crosses the suture line. **B1** and **B2.** Cephalhematoma involves the collection of blood and does not cross the suture line. (**A2** and **B2**: Reprinted with permission from Fletcher, M. A. [1998]. *Physical diagnosis in neonatology* [p. 185]. Lippincott–Raven Publishers.)

Common Abnormalities in Head or Fontanel Size

Common abnormalities in head or fontanelle size that may indicate a problem include:

- *Microcephaly*—a congenital anomaly described as a head circumference more than two standard deviations below average or less than the 3rd percentile for gestational age (Johnson, 2025). It reflects failure of brain development.
- *Macrocephaly*—a usually benign condition that is defined as an occipitofrontal circumference greater than the 90th percentile despite weight and length being appropriate for gestational age (Johnson, 2025). It may be benign or can be associated with hydrocephalus or genetic conditions or syndromes.
- *Large anterior fontanel*—this occurs more often in Black infants. It is usually benign but may be associated with achondroplasia, congenital hypothyroidism, increased intracranial pressure, Down syndrome, or rickets (Lipsett et al., 2023).

FACE

Observe the newborn's face for fullness and symmetry. The face should have full cheeks and should be symmetric when the baby is resting and crying. If asymmetrical movement of the face occurs, facial nerve palsy may be present (see Chapter 24).

Eyes

Inspect the external eye structures, including the eyelids, lashes, conjunctiva, sclera, iris, and pupils, for position, color, size, and movement. There may be marked edema of the eyelids and subconjunctival hemorrhages due to pressure during birth. The eyes should be clear and symmetrically placed. Test the blink reflex by bringing an object close to the eye; the newborn should respond quickly by blinking. Also test the newborn's pupillary reflex: The pupils should be equal, round, and reactive to light bilaterally. Assess the newborn's gaze: They should be able to track objects to the midline. Movement may be uncoordinated during the first few weeks of life. Many newborns have transient strabismus (deviation or wandering of eyes independently) and searching nystagmus (involuntary repetitive eye movement), which is caused by immature muscular control. These are normal for the first 3 to 6 months of age.

Examine the internal eye structures. A red reflex (luminous red appearance seen on the retina) should be seen bilaterally with ophthalmoscopy. The red reflex normally shows no dullness or irregularities.

Chemical conjunctivitis commonly occurs within 24 hours of instillation of eye ointment after birth. There is lid edema with sterile discharge from both eyes. Usually, it resolves within 48 hours without treatment.

Ears

Inspect the ears for size, shape, skin condition, placement, and amount of cartilage. The ears should be soft and pliable and should recoil quickly and easily when folded and released. The ear pinnae should be aligned with the outer canthi of the eyes. Low-set ears and abnormally shaped ears are characteristic of many syndromes as well as genetic and renal system abnormalities. Findings of sinuses or preauricular skin tags should prompt further evaluation for possible renal abnormalities since both systems develop at the same time. An otoscopic examination is not typically done because the newborn's ear canals are filled with amniotic fluid and vernix caseosa, which would make visualization of the tympanic membrane difficult. To assess for hearing ability generally, observe the newborn's response to noises and conversations. The newborn typically turns toward sounds and startles with loud noises.

Nose

Inspect the nose for size, symmetry, position, and lesions. The newborn's nose is smaller and flatter than the adult's. Due to preferential nose breathing, sneezing is common, but there should be no actual drainage. The nose should have a midline placement, patent nares, and an intact septum. The nostrils should be of equal size and patent.

Mouth

Inspect the newborn's mouth, lips, and interior structures. The lips should be intact with symmetric movement and positioned in the midline; there should not be any lesions. Inspect the lips for appropriate color, moisture, and cracking. The lips should encircle the examiner's finger to form a vacuum.

Assess the inside of the mouth for alignment of the mandible, intact soft and hard palate, sucking pads inside the cheeks, a midline uvula, a free-moving tongue, and working gag, swallow, and sucking reflexes. The mucous membranes lining the oral cavity should be pink and moist with minimal saliva present. Normal variations might include Epstein pearls, erupted natal teeth that may need to be removed to prevent aspiration (Fig. 18.13), and thrush (white plaque inside the mouth caused by exposure to *Candida albicans* during birth), which cannot be wiped away with a cotton-tipped applicator.

NECK

Inspect the newborn's neck for movement and ability to support the head. The newborn's neck will appear almost nonexistent because it is so short. Creases are usually noted. The neck should move freely in all directions and should be capable of holding the head in a midline position. The newborn should have enough head control to be able to hold it up very briefly without support. Report any deviations such as restricted neck movement or absence of head control.

Also inspect the clavicles (collarbone), which should be straight and intact. Edema, crepitus, decreased or absent movement, and pain or tenderness on movement of the arm on the affected side may indicate clavicular fracture.

CHEST

Inspect the newborn's chest for size, shape, and symmetry. The newborn's chest should be barrel-shaped with equal anteroposterior and lateral diameters, symmetric, and 2 to 3 cm smaller than the head circumference. The xiphoid process may be prominent at birth, but it usually becomes less apparent when adipose tissue accumulates. Nipples may be engorged and may secrete a white discharge, dissipating within a few weeks. This discharge, which occurs regardless of sex, is a result of exposure to high levels of maternal estrogen while in utero. Some newborns may have extra nipples, called supernumerary nipples, which are generally benign. They are typically small, raised, pigmented areas vertical to the main nipple

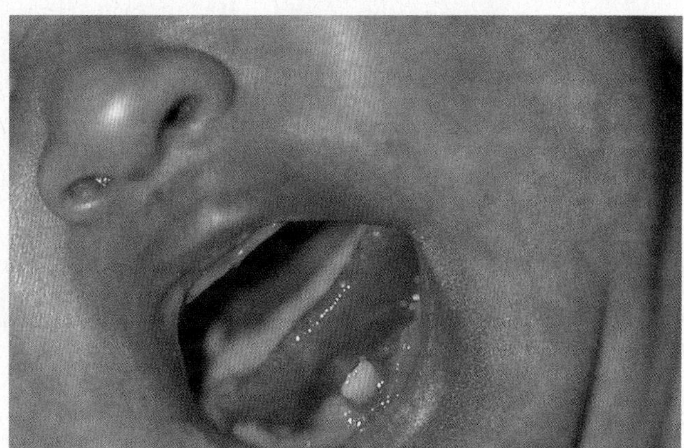

FIGURE 18.13 A natal tooth in a 16-day-old neonate. Natal teeth can be present at birth and are usually considered benign. No treatment is needed if they don't interfere with feeding.

line, 5 to 6 cm below the normal nipple. Supernumerary nipples may be unilateral or bilateral, and they may include an areola, nipple, or both.

Assess respirations by observing the rise and fall of the chest for one full minute. Respirations should be symmetric, slightly irregular, shallow, and unlabored at a rate of 30 to 60 breaths/min (Fraser, 2025). The newborn's respirations are predominantly diaphragmatic, but they are synchronous with abdominal movements after birth. Abnormalities include tachypnea, bradypnea, retractions, grunting, gasping, periods of apnea lasting longer than 20 seconds, and asymmetry or decreased chest expansion.

Auscultate the lungs bilaterally for equal breath sounds. Clear breath sounds should be heard with little difference between inspiration and expiration. Fine crackles can be heard on inspiration soon after birth as a result of amniotic fluid being cleared from the lungs. Abnormalities include diminished breath sounds, rhonchi and crackles, and sternal retractions. Some variations might exist early (Fraser, 2025).

The point of maximal impulse is a lateral of midclavicular line located at the fourth intercostal space. A displaced point of maximal impulse may indicate tension pneumothorax or cardiomegaly. Listen to the heart when the newborn is quiet or sleeping. Obtain an apical pulse by placing the stethoscope over the fourth intercostal space on the chest. Listen for a full minute, noting rate, rhythm, and abnormal sounds such as murmurs. In the typical newborn, the HR is 120 to 160 bpm with wide fluctuations with activity and sleep (Vargo, 2025). S1 and S2 heart sounds are accentuated at birth. Sinus arrhythmia is a normal finding. Murmurs are common during the 2 days of life while the peripheral vascular resistance is decreasing and the ductus arteriosus is not yet closed (Vargo, 2025). Also palpate the apical, femoral, and brachial pulses for presence and equality (Fig. 18.14).

ABDOMEN

Inspect the abdomen for shape and movement. Typically, the newborn's abdomen is protuberant but not distended. This contour is a result of the immaturity of the abdominal muscles. Abdominal movements are synchronous with respirations because newborns are abdominal breathers at times. Inspect the umbilical cord area for the presence of three blood vessels (two arteries and one vein). The umbilical vein is larger than the two umbilical arteries. Evidence of only a single umbilical artery is associated with renal and gastrointestinal anomalies. Also inspect the umbilical area for signs of bleeding, infection, inflammation, redness, swelling, purulent drainage or bleeding, erythema around the umbilicus, granuloma, or abnormal communication with the intra-abdominal organs. See Evidence-Based Practice 18.1.

Auscultate bowel sounds in all four quadrants, and then palpate the abdomen for consistency, masses, and tenderness. Perform auscultation and palpation systematically in a clockwise fashion until all four quadrants have been assessed. Palpate gently to feel the liver, the kidneys, and any masses. The liver edge is normally palpable 1 to 2 cm below the right costal margin. The kidneys are found at about 45 degrees lateral to and below both sides of the umbilicus, although the left may be more difficult to palpate (Bohara, 2025). Normal findings

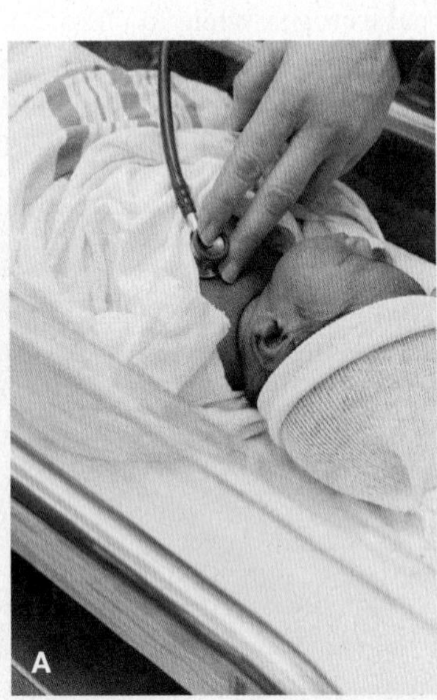

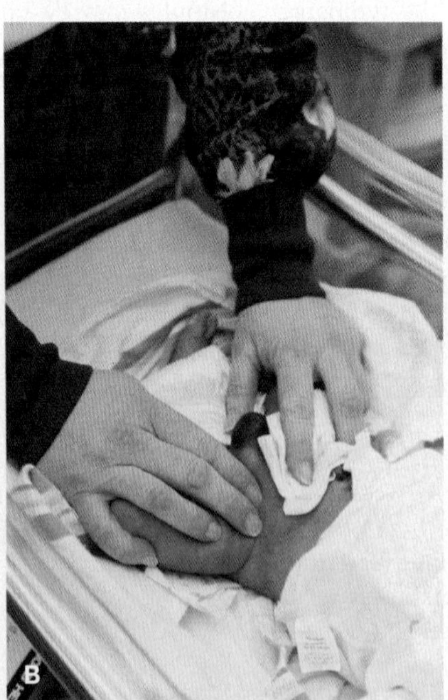

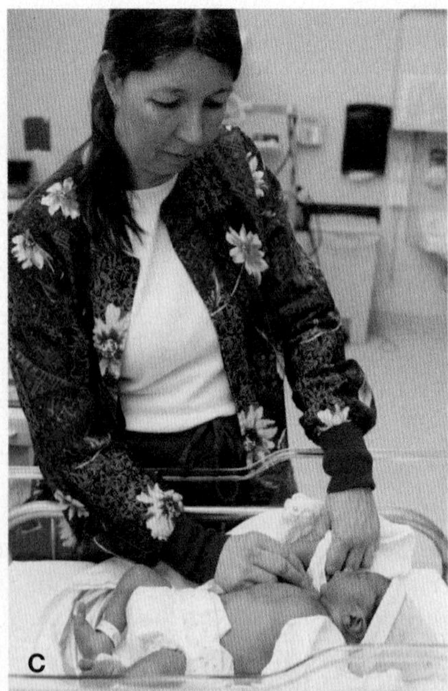

FIGURE 18.14 Assessing the newborn's pulses. **A.** Assessing the apical pulse. **B.** Palpating the femoral pulse. **C.** Palpating the brachial pulse.

EVIDENCE-BASED PRACTICE 18.1

What Is the Effect of Topical Breast Milk Application on Umbilical Cord Separation Among Healthy Babies in the Middle East?

BACKGROUND

Umbilical cord care practices are variable worldwide due to cultural traditions and global health practices. The WHO recommends dry cord care without the application of a topical substance in countries with low rates of neonatal mortality. Application of topical chlorhexidine is recommended in areas with higher infant mortality. Some studies found that the use of antiseptics prolonged the time of umbilical cord separation. Early cord detachment is preferred. The use of topical breast milk has been suggested as an effective umbilical cord care substance because it has antimicrobial healing properties and antiinflammatory effects. The purpose of this review was to evaluate the efficacy of topical application of human breast milk to reduce cord separation time.

STUDY

This literature review (three studies met the inclusion criteria) investigated the correlation between the topical application of breast milk on the umbilical cord and its separation among infants born in hospitals in the Middle East. One study included 400 infants using a simple random assignment technique, with 200 newborns placed in each of two groups. One group would use breast milk and the other group would utilize dry umbilical cord care. All newborns in the sample had their umbilical cords swabbed immediately after birth and then again in 3 days to determine the presence of infection. Another study with 174 infant participants compared the effects of chlorhexidine with those of breast milk used for umbilical cord care and timing of cord separation.

Findings

Comparing the results of all studies, it was found that breast milk was effective in shortening the separation time of the umbilical cord over dry cord care in two studies and just as effective in decreasing signs of infection when compared to chlorhexidine.

Nursing Implications

Umbilical cord care is an essential component of neonatal care. This review found a significant reduction in the time of the cord separation with the topical application of human breast milk compared to dry cord care. Optimal umbilical cord care has the potential to reduce neonatal morbidity and mortality. Nurses should instruct birthing parents to wash their hands before expressing their milk, apply several drops of breast milk to the umbilical stump, and allow it to dry. The human breast milk cord care regimen is safe, convenient, feasible, cost-effective, and noninvasive. This regimen should be considered as an alternative method in hospital settings.

Adapted from Awopileda, M. (2022). What is the effect of topical breast milk application on umbilical cord separation among healthy babies in the Middle East? *Vanderbilt Undergraduate Research Journal, 12*(1), 25–30. https://doi.org/10.15695/vurj.v12i1.5273

would include bowel sounds in all four quadrants and no masses or tenderness on palpation. Absent or hyperactive bowel sounds might indicate an intestinal obstruction, as might abdominal distention (Bohara, 2025).

GENITALIA AND ANUS

Inspect the anus in newborns for position and patency. Passage of meconium indicates patency. If meconium is not passed, a lubricated rectal thermometer can be inserted or a digital examination performed to determine patency. Abnormal findings would include anal fissures or fistulas and no meconium passed within 24 hours after birth.

Male

Inspect the penis and scrotum in the male. In the circumcised male newborn, the glans should be smooth, with the meatus centered at the tip of the penis. It will appear reddened until it heals. On the uncircumcised penis, the foreskin should cover the glans. Check the position of the urinary meatus; it should be in the midline at the glans's tip. If it is on the ventral surface of the penis, the condition is termed hypospadias; if it is on the dorsal surface of the penis, it is termed epispadias. In either case, circumcision should be avoided until further evaluation (Cavaliere, 2025).

Inspect the scrotum for size, symmetry, color, presence of rugae, and location of testes. The scrotum usually appears relatively large with well-formed rugae that should cover the scrotal sac. There should not be bulging, edema, or discoloration (Fig. 18.15A). Palpate the scrotum for evidence of the testes, which should be in the scrotal sac. The testes should feel firm and smooth and should be of equal size on both sides of the scrotal sac in the term newborn. Undescended testes (cryptorchidism) might be palpated in the inguinal canal in preterm infants; they can be unilateral or bilateral. In most infants, the testes descend by 3 month of age (Di Carlo & Crigger, 2025).

Female

In the female newborn, inspect the external genitalia. The urethral meatus is located below the clitoris in the midline. In contrast to the male genitalia, the female genitalia will be engorged; the labia majora and minora may both be edematous. The labia majora is large and covers the labia minora. The clitoris is large, and the hymen is thick. These findings are due to the maternal hormones estrogen and progesterone (Fig. 18.15B). A vaginal discharge composed of mucus mixed with blood may also be present during the first few weeks of life. This discharge, called **pseudomenstruation**, requires no treatment. Variations in female newborns may include a labial bulge, which might indicate an inguinal hernia; ambiguous genitalia; a rectovaginal fistula with feces present in the vagina; and an imperforate hymen.

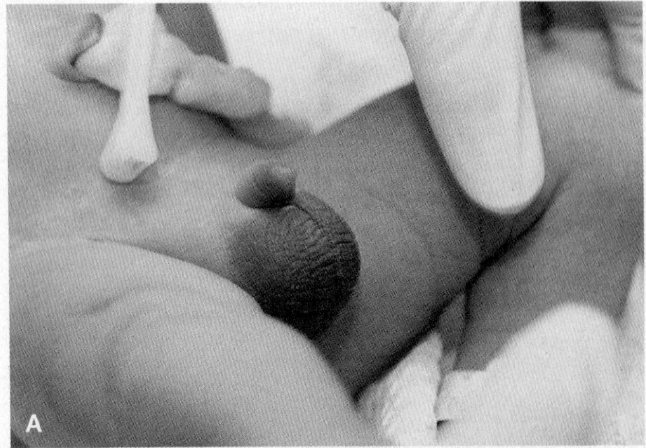

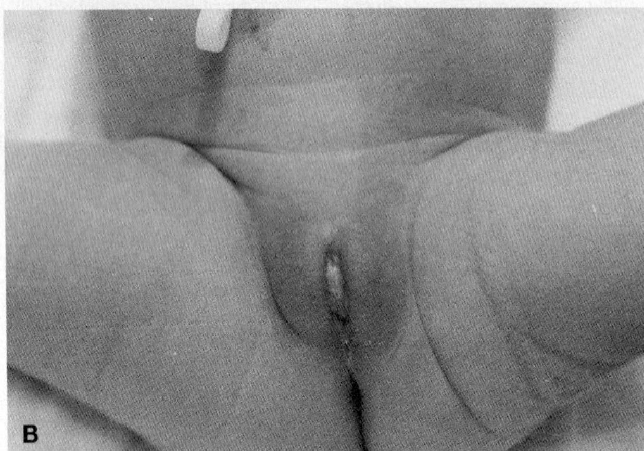

FIGURE 18.15 Newborn genitalia. **A.** Male genitalia. Note the darkened color of the scrotum. **B.** Female genitalia.

Difference in Sex Development

A difference in sex development (also termed intersex by some) occurs in 1 in 1,000 to 4,500 live births (Chan & Levitsky, 2023). It is an alteration in gonadal development resulting in the external genitalia not being what is typically expected. This biologic variance may result in genitalia that do not appear either male or female or in external genitalia that do not match the infant's internal gonads or biologic sex phenotype. The most common causes of differences in sex development include congenital adrenal hyperplasia, sex chromosome anomalies with X/XY mosaicism, and partial or complete androgen insensitivity syndrome in a person with an XY phenotype (Chan & Levitsky, 2022).

UPPER EXTREMITIES

Inspect the newborn's upper extremities for equality in appearance and movement. Inspect the hands for shape, presence of palmar creases, and number and position of fingers. The newborn's arms and hands should be symmetric and should spontaneously move through the range of motion without hesitation. An arm that hangs limp or does not move with the Moro reflex may indicate a brachial plexus injury. Each hand should have five digits. Note any extra digits (polydactyly) or fusing of two or more digits (syndactyly). Most newborns have three palmar creases on the hand. A single palmar crease is frequently associated with Down syndrome.

LOWER EXTREMITIES

Assess the lower extremities in the same manner. They should be of equal length with symmetric skinfolds. Perform the Ortolani and Barlow maneuvers to identify congenital hip dislocation, commonly termed developmental dysplasia of the hip. Nursing Procedure 18.1 highlights the steps for performing these maneuvers. Inspect and palpate the feet, noting movement and range of motion. An abnormal finding is clubfoot (see Chapter 24). Assess the toes, noting five on each foot and absence of polydactyly or syndactyly.

BACK

Inspect the back. Hold the infant in a prone position with your hand under the infant's chest and abdomen. The spine should appear straight and flat and should be easily flexed. Observe for the abnormal findings of a tuft of hair, a pilonidal dimple in the midline, a cyst, or a mass along the spine.

NEUROLOGIC STATUS

The newborn should be alert and not persistently lethargic. Note the quality of the infant's cry, which should be loud and lusty. The normal posture is hips abducted and partially flexed, with knees flexed. Arms are adducted and flexed at the elbow. Fists are often clenched, with fingers covering the thumb. To assess for muscle tone, suspend the newborn in a prone position with one hand under the chest and abdomen. Observe how the neck muscles hold the head. The neck extensors should be able to hold the head in line briefly. With the infant lying supine, pull the newborn from a supine position to a sitting one, noting the amount of head lag.

Newborn Reflexes

Assess the newborn's reflexes to evaluate neurologic function and development. Reflexes are present in all newborns; absent or abnormal reflexes in the newborn may indicate neurologic pathology. Reflexes commonly assessed in the newborn include sucking, Moro, stepping, tonic neck, rooting, Babinski, palmar grasp, and plantar grasp reflexes. Spinal reflexes tested include truncal incurvation (Galant reflex) and the anocutaneous reflex (anal wink).

The *sucking reflex* is elicited by gently stimulating the newborn's lips by touching them. The newborn will typically open the mouth and begin a sucking motion. Placing a gloved finger in the newborn's mouth will also elicit a sucking motion (Fig. 18.16A).

The *Moro reflex* occurs when the neonate is startled. To elicit this reflex, place the newborn on their back.

NURSING PROCEDURE 18.1 Performing Ortolani and Barlow Maneuvers

Purpose: To Detect Congenital Developmental Dysplasia of the Hip

Ortolani Maneuver

1. Place the newborn in the supine position, and flex the hips and knees to 90 degrees at the hip.
2. Place your fingers on the trochanter, and use the thumbs to grip the femur. Abduct the thighs and lift the femur forward.

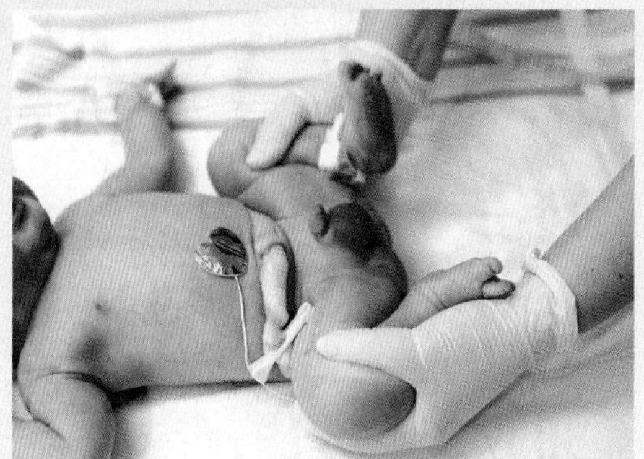

3. Listen for any sounds and feel for abnormalities during the maneuver. There should be no clunk felt. (This would indicate the femoral head is hitting the acetabulum as the head re-enters the area, suggesting developmental dysplasia of the hip [DDH]). A click or pop may be heard; this is considered benign.

Barlow Maneuver

4. Using the same positions of the newborn and the examiner's hands as those for the Ortolani maneuver, adduct the thighs while applying outward and downward pressure to the thighs.
5. Feel for a clunk as the femoral head slips out of the acetabulum (suggesting DDH). A click or pop may be heard; this is considered benign.

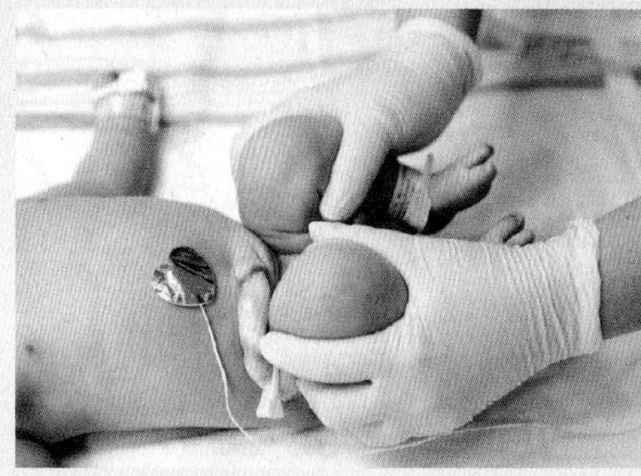

Tappero, E. P. (2025). Musculoskeletal system assessment. In C. L. Witt & C. M. Wallman (Eds.), *Tappero & Honeyfield's physical assessment of the newborn: A comprehensive approach to the art of physical examination* (7th ed.). Springer.

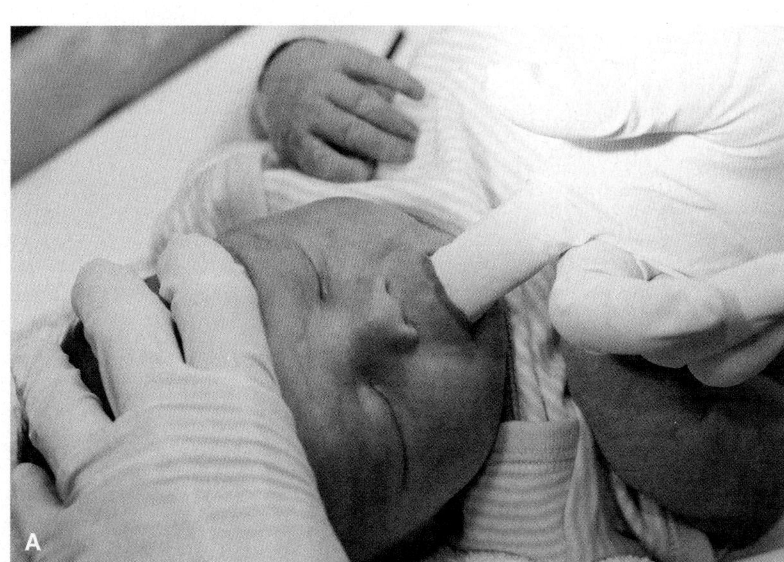

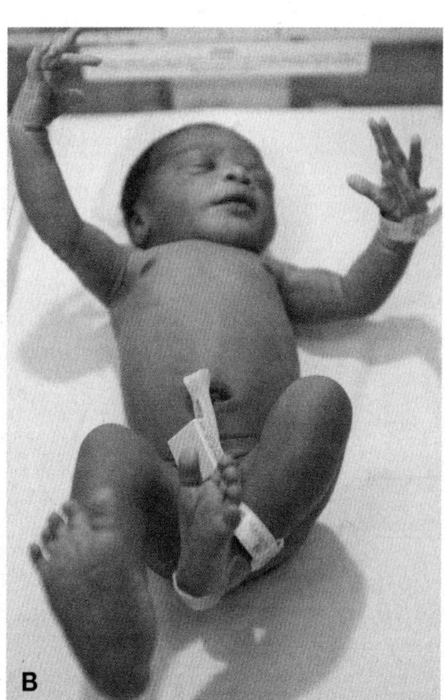

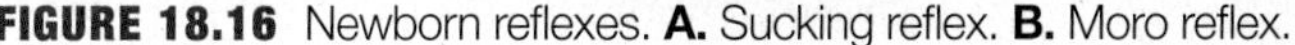

FIGURE 18.16 Newborn reflexes. **A.** Sucking reflex. **B.** Moro reflex.

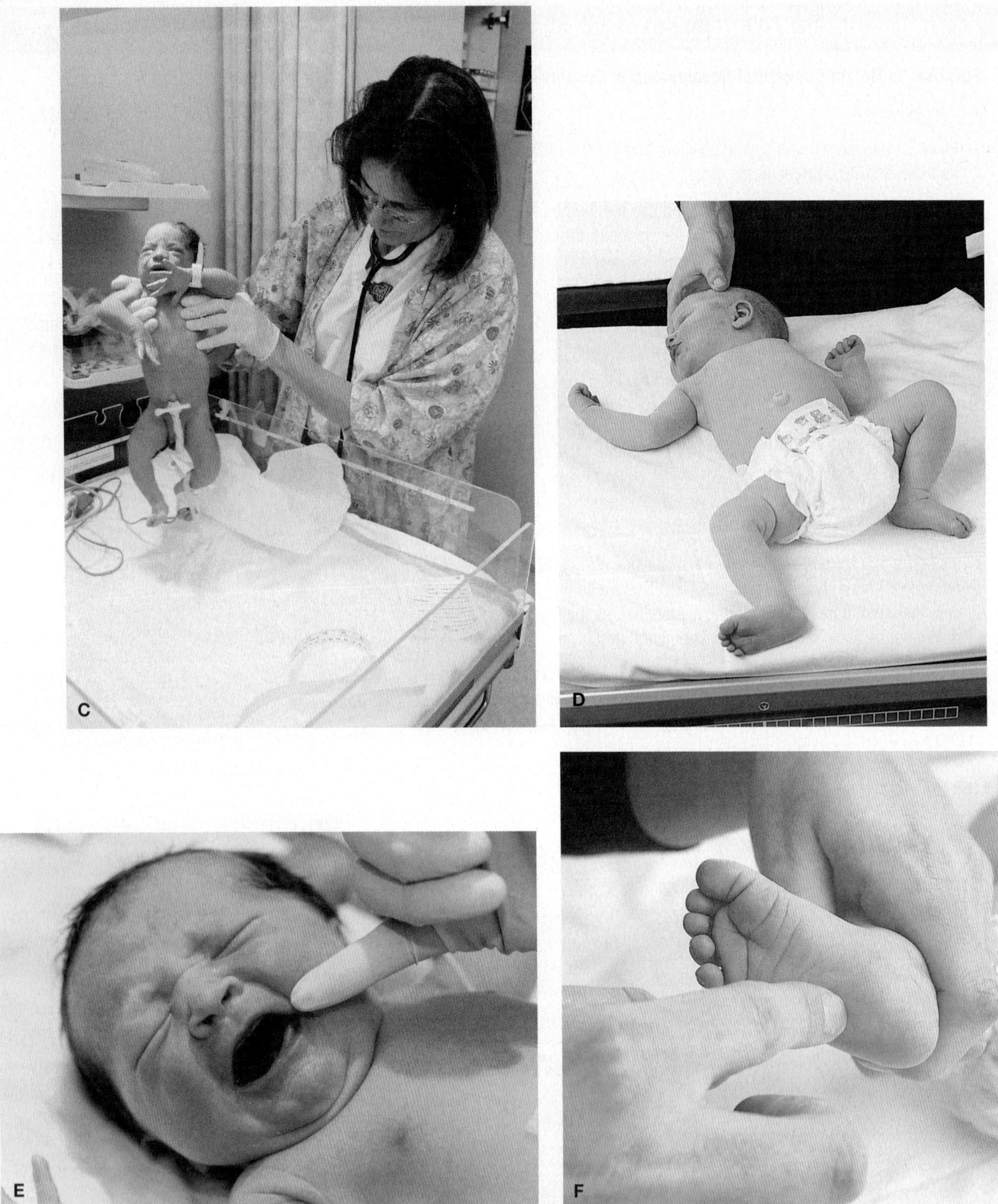

FIGURE 18.16 *(continued)* **C.** Stepping reflex. **D.** Tonic neck reflex. **E.** Rooting reflex. **F.** Babinski reflex.

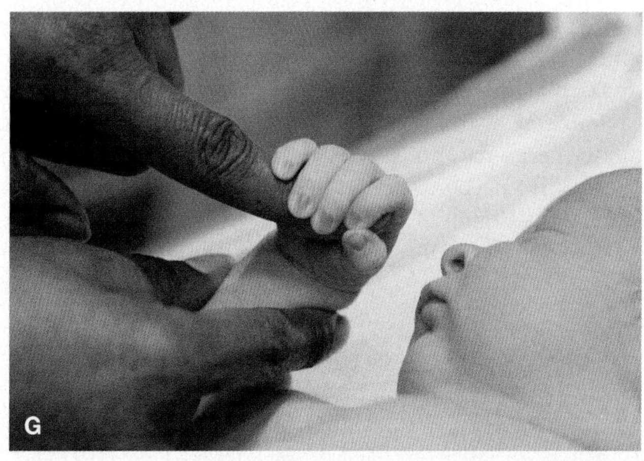

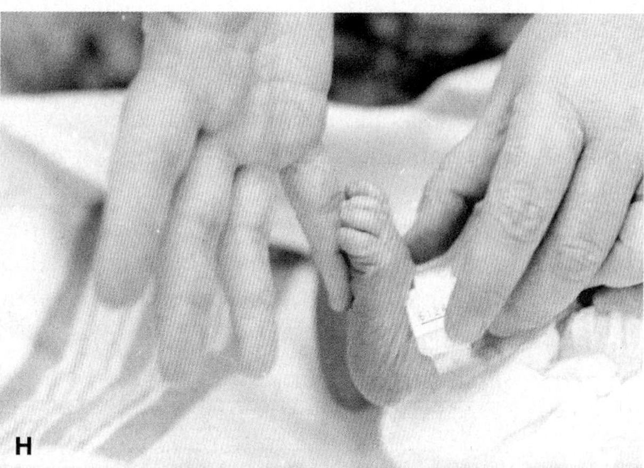

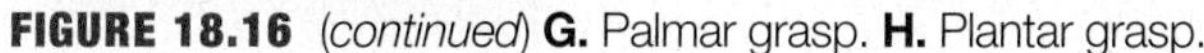

FIGURE 18.16 *(continued)* **G.** Palmar grasp. **H.** Plantar grasp.

Support the upper body weight of the supine newborn by the arms, using a lifting motion, without lifting the newborn off the surface. Then release the arms suddenly. The newborn will throw the arms outward and flex the knees; the arms then return to the chest. The fingers also spread to form a C shape. The newborn initially appears startled and then relaxes to a normal resting position (Fig. 18.16B).

Assess the *stepping reflex* by holding the newborn upright and inclined forward with the soles of the feet touching a flat surface. The baby should make a stepping or walking motion, alternating flexion and extension with the soles of the feet (Fig. 18.16C).

The *tonic neck reflex* resembles the stance of a fencer and is often called the fencing reflex. Test this reflex by having the newborn lie on the back. Turn the baby's head to one side. The arm toward which the baby is facing should extend straight away from the body with the hand partially open, whereas the arm on the side away from the face is flexed, and the fist is clenched tightly. Reversing the direction to which the face is turned reverses the position (Fig. 18.16D).

Elicit the *rooting reflex* by stroking the newborn's cheek. The newborn should turn toward the side that was stroked and should begin to make sucking movements (Fig. 18.16E).

Elicit the *Babinski reflex* by stroking the lateral sole of the newborn's foot from the heel toward and across the ball of the foot. The toes should fan out. A diminished response indicates a neurologic problem and needs follow-up (Fig. 18.16F).

The newborn exhibits two grasp reflexes: *palmar grasp* and *plantar grasp*. Elicit the palmar grasp reflex by placing a finger on the newborn's open palm. The baby's hand will close around the finger. Attempting to remove the finger causes the grip to tighten. Newborns have strong grasps and can almost be lifted from a flat surface if both hands are used. The grasp should be equal bilaterally (Fig. 18.16G). The plantar grasp is similar to the palmar grasp. Place a finger just below the newborn's toes. The toes typically curl over the finger (Fig. 18.16H).

Blinking, sneezing, gagging, and *coughing* are all protective reflexes and are elicited when an object or light is brought close to the eye (blinking); something irritating is swallowed or a bulb syringe is used for suctioning (gagging and coughing); or an irritant is brought close to the nose (sneezing).

The *truncal incurvation reflex* (*Galant reflex*) is present at birth and disappears in a few days to 4 weeks (Fig. 18.17). With the newborn in a prone position or held in ventral suspension, apply firm pressure and run a finger down either side of the spine. This stroking will cause the pelvis to flex toward the stimulated side. This indicates T2–S1 innervation. Lack of response may indicate a neurologic or spinal cord problem.

The *anocutaneous reflex* (*anal wink*) is elicited by stimulating the perianal skin close to the anus. The external sphincter will constrict (wink) immediately with stimulation. This indicates S4–S5 innervations (Fanning, 2025).

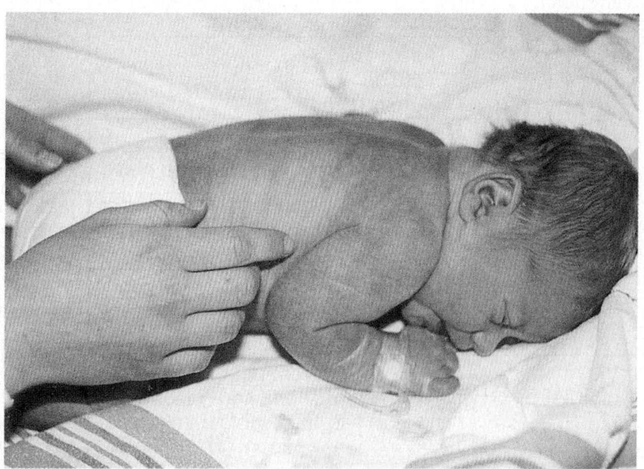

FIGURE 18.17 Trunk incurvation reflex. When the paravertebral area is stroked, the newborn flexes their trunk toward the stimulation. (Copyright Caroline Brown, RNC, MS, DEd.)

Gestational Age Assessment

To determine a newborn's **gestational age** (the stage of maturity), physical signs and neurologic characteristics are assessed. Typically, gestational age is determined by using a tool such as the Ballard gestational age assessment or Ballard Scale. A score is assigned to the various parameters, and the total score corresponds to a maturity rating in weeks of gestation (Fig. 18.18). This scoring system provides an objective estimate of gestational age by scoring the specific parameters of physical as well as neuromuscular maturity. Points are given for each assessment parameter, with a low score of −1 point or −2 points for extreme immaturity to 4 or 5 points for postmaturity. The scores from each section are added to correspond to a specific gestational age in weeks (from 20 to 44).

The physical maturity assessment section of the New Ballard Score evaluates six physical characteristics

NEUROMUSCULAR MATURITY

NEUROMUSCULAR MATURITY SIGN	SCORE −1	0	1	2	3	4	5	RECORD SCORE HERE
POSTURE								
SQUARE WINDOW (Wrist)	>90°	90°	60°	45°	30°	0°		
ARM RECOIL		180°	140°–180°	110°–140°	90°–110°	<90°		
POPLITEAL ANGLE	180°	160°	140°	120°	100°	90°	<90°	
SCARF SIGN								
HEEL TO EAR								
							TOTAL NEUROMUSCULAR MATURITY SCORE	

SCORE
Neuromuscular ___
Physical ___
Total ___

MATURITY RATING

Score	Weeks
−10	20
−5	22
0	24
5	26
10	28
15	30
20	32
25	34
30	36
35	38
40	40
45	42
50	44

PHYSICAL MATURITY

PHYSICAL MATURITY SIGN	SCORE −1	0	1	2	3	4	5	RECORD SCORE HERE
SKIN	sticky, friable, transparent	gelatinous, red, translucent	smooth, pink, visible veins	superficial peeling and/or rash, few veins	cracking pale areas, rare veins	parchment, deep cracking, no vessels	leathery, cracked, wrinkled	
LANUGO	–	sparse	abundant	thinning	bald areas	mostly bald		
PLANTAR SURFACE	heel-toe 40–50 mm: −1 <40 mm: −2	>50 mm no crease	faint red marks	anterior transverse crease only	creases ant. 2/3	creases over entire sole		
BREAST	impercep-tible	barely perceptible	flat areola no bud	stippled areola 1–2 mm bud	raised areola 3–4 mm bud	full areola 5–10 mm bud		
EYE–EAR	lids fused loosely: −1 tightly: −2	lids open pinna flat stays folded	sl. curved pinna; soft; slow recoil	well-curved pinna; soft but ready recoil	formed and firm instant recoil	thick cartilage, ear stiff		
GENITALS (Male)	scrotum flat, smooth	scrotum empty, faint rugae	testes in upper canal, rare rugae	testes descending, few rugae	testes down, good rugae	testes pendulous, deep rugae		
GENITALS (Female)	clitoris prominent and labia flat	prominent clitoris and small labia minora	prominent clitoris and enlarging minora	majora and minora equally prominent	majora large, minora small	majora cover clitoris and minora		
							TOTAL PHYSICAL MATURITY SCORE	

FIGURE 18.18 Gestational age assessment tool. (Adapted from [2014]. The new Ballard score. http://www.ballardscore.com.)

that differ depending on a newborn's gestational maturity. Newborns who are physically mature have higher scores than those who are not. The areas assessed on the physical maturity examination include:

- *Skin texture*—typically ranges from sticky and transparent to smooth with varying degrees of peeling and cracking, to parchment-like or leathery with significant cracking and wrinkling
- *Lanugo*—soft downy hair on the newborn's body, which is absent in preterm newborns; appears with maturity and then disappears again with postmaturity
- *Plantar creases*—creases on the soles of the feet, which range from absent to covering the entire foot, depending on maturity (the greater the number of creases, the greater the newborn's maturity)
- *Breast tissue*—the thickness and size of breast tissue and areola (the darkened ring around each nipple), which range from being imperceptible to full and budding
- *Eyes and ears*—eyelids can be fused or open, and ear cartilage and stiffness determine the degree of maturity (the greater the amount of ear cartilage with stiffness, the greater the newborn's maturity)
- *Genitals*—in males, evidence of testicular descent and appearance of scrotum (which can range from smooth to covered with rugae) determine maturity; in females, appearance and size of clitoris and labia determine maturity (a prominent clitoris with flat labia suggests prematurity, while a clitoris covered by labia suggests greater maturity)

The neuromuscular maturity section is typically completed within 24 hours after birth. Six activities or maneuvers with various body parts are evaluated to determine the newborn's degree of maturity:

1. *Posture*—How does the newborn hold their extremities in relation to the trunk? The greater the degree of flexion, the greater the maturity. For example, extension of the arms and legs is scored as 0 points, and full flexion of the arms and legs is scored as 4 points.
2. *Square window*—How far can the newborn's hands be flexed toward the wrist? The angle is measured and scored from more than 90 to 0 degrees to determine the maturity rating. As the angle decreases, the newborn's maturity increases. For example, an angle of more than 90 degrees is scored as −1 point, and an angle of 0 degrees is scored as 4 points.
3. *Arm recoil*—How far do the newborn's arms "spring back" to a flexed position? This measure evaluates the degree of arm flexion and the strength of recoil. The reaction of the arm is then scored from 0 to 4 points based on the degree of flexion as the arms are returned to their normal flexed position. The higher the points assigned, the greater the neuromuscular maturity (e.g., recoil less than a 90-degree angle is scored as 4 points).
4. *Popliteal angle*—How far will the newborn's knees extend? The angle created when the knee is extended is measured. An angle of less than 90 degrees indicates greater maturity. For example, an angle of 180 degrees is scored as −1 point, and an angle of less than 90 degrees is scored as 5 points.
5. *Scarf sign*—How far can the elbows be moved across the newborn's chest? An elbow that does not reach midline indicates greater maturity. For example, if the elbow reaches or nears the level of the opposite shoulder, this is scored as −1 point; if the elbow does not cross the proximate axillary line, it is scored as 4 points.
6. *Heel to ear*—How close can the newborn's feet be moved to the ears? This maneuver assesses hip flexibility; the lesser the flexibility, the greater the newborn's maturity. The heel-to-ear assessment is scored in the same manner as the scarf sign (Trotter, 2025).

After the scoring is completed, the 12 scores are totaled and then compared with standardized values to determine the appropriate gestational age in weeks. Scores range from very low for preterm newborns to very high for mature and postmature newborns.

TAKE NOTE!

Gestational age assessment is important because it allows the nurse to plot growth parameters and to anticipate problems related to prematurity, postmaturity, and growth abnormalities.

Typically, newborns are also classified according to their gestational age as:

- Term newborn subgroups:
  - *Early term*: 37 to 38 weeks 6 days
  - *Full term*: 39 to 40 weeks 6 days
  - *Late term*: 41 to 41 weeks 6 days (American College of Obstetricians and Gynecologists [ACOG], 2022)
- Preterm newborn subgroups:
  - *Extremely preterm*: fewer than 28 weeks
  - *Very preterm*: 28 to 32 weeks
  - *Moderate preterm*: 32 to 33 weeks 6 days
  - *Late preterm newborn* (near term): 34 to 36 weeks 6 days (Mandy, 2022)
- Post-term newborn: more than 42 completed weeks' gestation (ACOG, 2022)

Using the information about gestational age and then considering birth weight, newborns can also be classified as:

- *SGA*—birth weight less than the 10th percentile on standard growth charts
- *Appropriate for gestational age (AGA)*—birth weight between 10th and 90th percentiles

- LGA—birth weight more than the 90th percentile on standard growth charts (Trotter, 2025).

Table 18.3 summarizes the newborn assessment.

Nursing Interventions

Developing confidence in caring for a newborn can be challenging for new parents. It takes time and patience and a great deal of instruction provided by the nurse. "Showing and telling" parents about the newborn and all the procedures (e.g., feeding, bathing, changing, and handling) involved in daily care are key nursing interventions.

Providing General Newborn Care

Generally, newborn care involves bathing and hygiene, elimination and diaper area care, cord care, circumcision care, environmental safety measures, and prevention of infection. Nurses should teach these skills to parents and serve as role models for appropriate and consistent interaction with newborns. Demonstrating respect for the newborn and family helps foster a positive atmosphere to promote the newborn's growth and development.

BATHING AND HYGIENE

Immediately after birth, drying the newborn and removing blood may minimize the risk of infection caused by hepatitis B, herpes virus, and HIV, but the specific benefits of this practice remain unclear. Until the newborn has been thoroughly bathed, standard precautions should be used when handling the newborn. Newborns are bathed primarily for aesthetic reasons, and bathing is postponed until thermal and cardiorespiratory stability is ensured. The newborn's bath should be delayed until their temperature is stable. To prevent hypothermia and resultant hypoglycemia and to increase the likelihood of exclusive breastfeeding at discharge, delay the bath for at least

TABLE 18.3 • Newborn Assessment Summary

Assessment	Usual Findings	Variations and Common Problems
Anthropometric measurements	Head circumference: 33–37 cm (13–14 in) Chest circumference: 30–33 cm (12–13 in) Weight: 2,500–4,000 g (5.5–8.5 lb) Length: 45–55 cm (19–21 in)	SGA, LGA
Vital signs	Temperature: 97–99°F (36.5–37.5°C) Apical pulse: 110–160 bpm Respirations: 30–60 breaths/min	
Skin	Smooth, flexible, elastic skin turgor, well hydrated, warm	Jaundice, acrocyanosis, milia, dermal melanocytosis, stork bites
Head	Anterior and posterior fontanels soft and flat; overriding sutures are possible	Microcephaly, macrocephaly, enlarged fontanels
Face	Full cheeks with symmetric facial features	Facial nerve paralysis, nevus flammeus, nevus vasculosus
Nose	Small, placed in the midline, able to smell	Malformation or blockage
Mouth	Aligned in midline, symmetric, intact soft and hard palate	Epstein pearls, erupted precocious teeth, thrush
Neck	Short, creased, moves freely, infant holds head in midline	Restricted movement, clavicular fractures
Eyes	Clear and symmetrically placed on face; in line with ear pinnae	Chemical conjunctivitis, subconjunctival hemorrhage
Ears	Soft and pliable with quick recoil when folded and released	Low-set ears, hearing loss
Chest	Round, symmetric, smaller than head, evenly spaced nipples	Nipple engorgement, whitish discharge
Abdomen	Protuberant contour, soft, positive bowel sounds, three vessels in umbilical cord	Distended, only two vessels in umbilical cord
Genitals	Biologic male: smooth glans, meatus centered at tip of penis, testes may or may not be descended Biologic female: swollen female genitals as a result of birthing parent's estrogen	Edematous scrotum in males, vaginal discharge in females
Extremities and spine	Extremities symmetric with spontaneous, free movement	Hip subluxation, hair tuft or dimple on spine

bpm, beats per minute; LGA, large for gestation age; SGA, small for gestation age.

6 hours; ideally, wait until 24 hours of age for the first bath (Priyadarshi et al., 2022). Provide the parents with the opportunity to bathe their newborn while supported by the nurse. Follow hospital policies regarding the timing and procedures for newborn bathing and hygiene.

During the first bath, it is important for the nurse to wear gloves because of potential exposure to the birthing parent's blood on the newborn. Perform the bath quickly, drying the baby thoroughly to prevent heat loss by evaporation. After bathing, place the newborn under the radiant warmer and wrap them securely in blankets to prevent chilling. Check the baby's temperature within an hour to make sure it is within normal limits. If it is low, rewarm the infant slowly.

Other guidelines for bathing newborns are outlined in Teaching Guidelines 18.1.

ELIMINATION AND DIAPER AREA CARE

Check frequently to see whether a diaper change is needed, especially after feeding. Adhere to standard precautions when providing diaper area care. Cleanse the diaper area with clear water and mild soap (or use an unscented commercial baby wipe) at each diaper change. For females, teach the parents to clean from front to back. In the male uncircumcised newborn, do not force the foreskin back; it will retract normally over time.

Instruct parents to keep the top edge of the diaper folded down below the umbilical cord area to prevent irritation and to allow air to help dry the cord. For a male infant, point the penis down to prevent urine from wetting the top of the diaper, where the umbilicus is located. Choice of cloth or disposable diaper is the individual family's decision. Regardless of the type of diapers used, up to 10 diapers a day, or about 70 a week, will be needed.

Newborn elimination patterns are highly individualized. Usually, the urine is light amber in color. Soaking a minimum of six diapers a day indicates adequate hydration. Stools change in color, texture, and frequency without signaling a problem. Meconium is passed within the first 48 hours after birth; the stools appear thick, tarry, sticky, and dark green. Transitional stools (thin, brown to green, less sticky than meconium) typically appear by day 3 after initiation of feeding. The stool characteristics after transitional stool depend on whether the newborn is breastfed or bottle-fed. Breastfed newborns typically pass mustard-colored, soft, seedy stools. Formula-fed newborns pass yellow to brown, soft stools with a pasty consistency. As long as the newborn seems content, is eating normally, and shows no signs of illness, minor changes in bowel movements should not be a concern.

While performing diaper area care, parents should observe the area closely for irritation or rash. Tips for preventing or healing a diaper rash include:

- Change diapers frequently, especially after bowel movements.
- Apply a "barrier" cream, such as A&D ointment or Desitin, after cleaning with mild soap and water.
- Use dye- and fragrance-free detergents-to wash cloth diapers.
- Avoid the use of plastic pants because they tend to hold in moisture.
- Expose the newborn's bottom to air several times a day.
- Place the newborn's buttocks in warm water after they have had a diaper on all night.

TEACHING GUIDELINES **18.1** Bathing a Newborn

- Select a warm room with a flat surface at a comfortable working height.
- Before the bath, gather all supplies needed so they will be within reach.
- Never leave the newborn alone or unattended at any time during the bath.
- Undress the newborn down to shirt and diaper.
- Always support the newborn's head and neck when moving or positioning them.
- Place a blanket or towel underneath the newborn for warmth and comfort.
- In this order, progressing from the cleanest to the dirtiest areas:
  - Wipe eyes with plain water, using either cotton balls or a washcloth. Wipe from the inner corner of the eyes to the outer with separate wipes.
  - Wash the rest of the face, including ears, with plain water.
  - Using baby shampoo, gently wash the hair and rinse with water.
  - Pay special attention to body creases, and dry thoroughly.
  - Wash extremities, trunk, and back. Wash, rinse, dry, and cover.
  - Wash diaper area last, using soap and water, and dry; observe for rash.
- Put on a clean diaper and clean clothes on the newborn after the bath.
- Sponge bathe only (without submersion into the water) until the umbilical cord falls off and the navel area is healed completely (if circumcised, until that area has also healed, usually 1 to 2 weeks)

TAKE NOTE!

Advise parents that a rash that persists for more than 3 days may be fungal in origin and may require antifungal treatment. Encourage the parents to notify the health care provider.

With a moistened cloth, clean any milk spilled into the newborn's neck folds from breastfeeding or formula. The use of lotions, baby oil, and powders is not recommended. Oils and lotions can lead to skin irritation and rashes. If the parents want to use oils or lotions, have them apply a small amount onto their hands, away from the newborn (warming it), and then apply that lotion or oil sparingly. Powders should not be used because they can be inhaled, causing respiratory distress.

CORD CARE

The umbilical cord stump begins drying within hours after birth and is shriveled and blackened by the second or third day (Palazzi & Brandt, 2023). Within 7 to 10 days, it sloughs off and the umbilicus heals. During this transition, frequent assessments of the area are necessary to detect any bleeding or signs of infection. Cord bleeding is abnormal and may occur if the cord clamp is loosened. Any cord drainage is also abnormal; it may be caused by infection, which requires immediate treatment. Keeping the cord clean and dry and using only soap and water should be emphasized to caregivers.

To protect the cord area during each diaper change, keep the diaper folded below the cord to keep urine from soaking it and keep the cord stump clean and dry (Newnam & Tasket, 2024). Expect to remove the cord clamp approximately 24 hours after birth by using a cord-cutting clamp. However, if the cord is still moist, keep the clamp in place, and ensure a referral to home health care so that the home care nurse can remove it after discharge. Always adhere to agency policies regarding cord care; changes in policy may be necessary based on new research findings.

Many parents avoid contact with the cord site to make sure they don't "bother" it. Teach them how to care for the cord site when they go home to prevent complications (Teaching Guidelines 18.2).

CIRCUMCISION

Circumcision is one of the oldest and most common surgical procedures performed worldwide, but it remains controversial. It is performed for medical, religious, cultural, and social reasons. **Circumcision** is the surgical removal of all or part of the foreskin (prepuce) of the penis. It is often performed in the hospital before the newborn is discharged, but it may also be performed following discharge. The American Academy of Pediatrics (2022a) has determined that the benefits of circumcision (decreased urinary tract and sexually transmitted infection) outweigh the risks (bleeding, infection, and inappropriate foreskin cutting or healing). Circumcision is a personal decision for parents, and the nurse's major responsibility is to inform the parents of the risks and benefits of the procedure and to address concerns so that the parents can reach a fully informed decision.

There are three commonly used methods of circumcision: the Gomco clamp, the Hollister Plastibell device, and the Mogen clamp. During the circumcision procedure, part of the foreskin is removed by clamping and cutting with a scalpel (Gomco or Mogen clamp) or by using a Plastibell. The Plastibell is fitted over the glans, and the excess foreskin is pulled over the plastic ring. A suture is tied around the rim to apply pressure to the blood vessels, creating hemostasis. The excess foreskin is cut away. The plastic rim remains in place until healing occurs. The plastic ring typically loosens and falls off in approximately 1 week. Petroleum jelly should be applied to the circumcised area after the procedure is done with the Gomco or Mogen clamp (Schmitt, 2023a) (Fig. 18.19).

Research has found that newborns circumcised without analgesia experience pain and stress, indicated by changes in HR, blood pressure, oxygen saturation, and cortisol levels (Stockton, 2022). The AAP recommends that if parents decide to circumcise their newborn, pain relief must be provided. Analgesic methods may include EMLA cream (a topical mixture of local anesthetics, lidocaine, and prilocaine), ring block, a dorsal penile nerve block with buffered lidocaine, acetaminophen, skin-to-skin contact, a sucrose pacifier, and swaddling (Rossi et al., 2021).

TEACHING GUIDELINES 18.2 Umbilical Cord Care

- Observe for bleeding, redness, drainage, or foul odor from the cord stump, and report it to the newborn's primary care provider immediately.
- Avoid tub baths until the cord has fallen off and the area has healed.
- Expose the cord stump to the air as much as possible throughout the day.
- Fold diapers below the level of the cord to prevent contamination of the site and to promote air-drying of the cord.
- Observe the cord stump, which will change color from yellow to brown to black. This is normal.
- Never pull the cord or attempt to loosen it; it will fall off naturally.

TAKE NOTE!

The decision to circumcise the male newborn is often a social one, with the strongest factor being whether the newborn's parent is circumcised (Reeves & Mishtal, 2022).

Preoperative circumcision preparation should include confirmation of the following:

- Infant is at least 12 hours old.
- Infant has received standard vitamin K prophylaxis.
- Infant has voided normally at least once since birth.
- Infant has not eaten for at least an hour prior to the procedure.
- Written parental consent has been obtained.
- The infant has been correctly identified when brought to the procedure room.

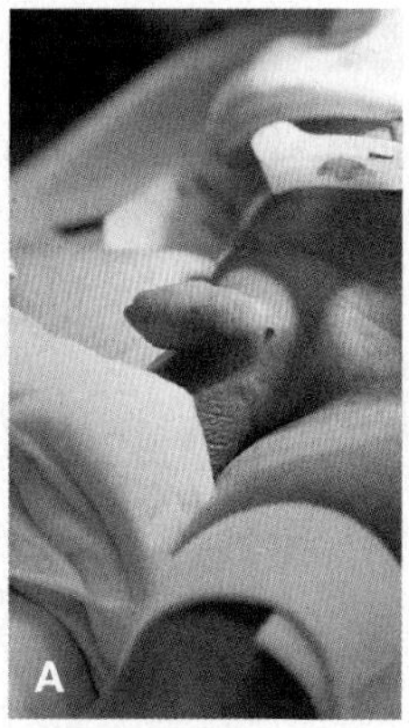
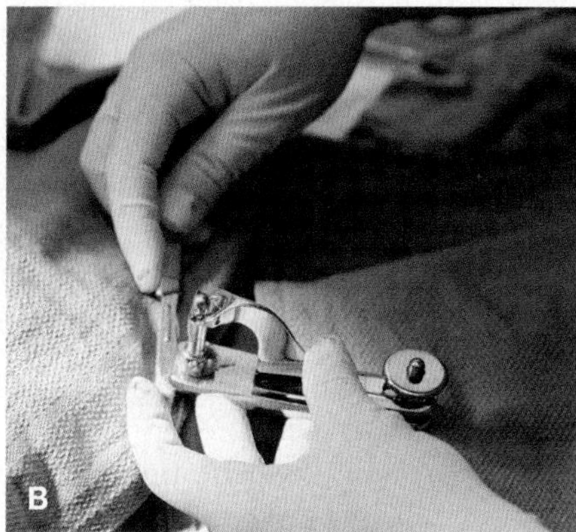
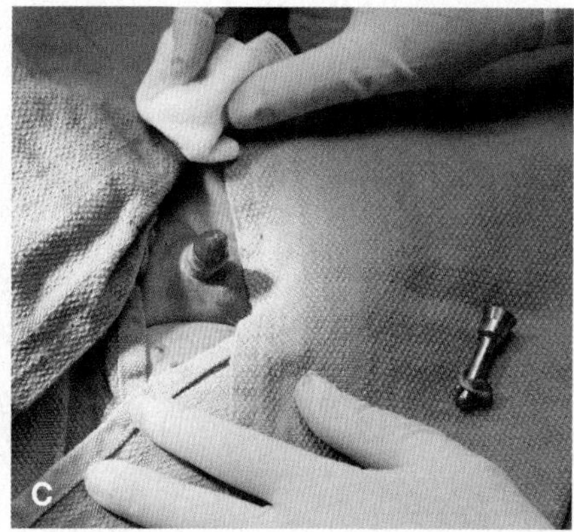

FIGURE 18.19 Circumcision. **A.** Before the procedure. **B.** Clamp applied and foreskin removed. **C.** Appearance after circumcision.

Immediately after circumcision, the tip of the penis is usually covered with petroleum jelly–coated gauze to keep the wound from sticking to the diaper. Continued care of this site includes:

- Assess for bleeding every 30 minutes for at least 2 hours.
- Document the first voiding to evaluate for urinary obstruction or edema.
- Squeeze soapy water over the area daily, and then rinse with warm water. Pat dry.
- Apply a small amount of petroleum jelly with every diaper change if the Plastibell was used; clean with mild soap and water if other techniques were used.
- Fasten the diaper loosely over the penis, avoiding placing the newborn on their abdomen to prevent friction.

If a Plastibell has been used, it will fall off by itself in about a week. Inform parents of this and advise them not to pull it off sooner. Also instruct the parents to check daily for any foul-smelling drainage, bleeding, or unusual swelling.

ENSURING SAFETY

Newborns are completely dependent on those around them to ensure their safety. Their safety must be ensured while in the health care facility and after they are discharged. Parental education is key, especially as the newborn grows, develops, and begins to respond to and explore their surroundings (Teaching Guidelines 18.3).

Car Safety

Every state requires the use of car seats for infants and children because motor vehicle crashes are still the leading cause of unintentional injury and death in children under age 5. The National Highway Traffic Safety Administration data shows that nearly half of deaths and injuries of infants occurred because they were not properly secured. When installed and used properly, child safety seats can prevent injuries and save lives (AAP, 2024c).

Make sure both parents understand the importance of safely transporting their newborn in a federally approved safety car seat every time the infant rides in a car. Do not release any newborn unless the parents have a car seat in place for the newborn's ride home (Fig. 18.20). If they cannot afford one, many community organizations will provide one for them. According to the AAP's policy statement on child passenger safety (AAP, 2024c), no one

TEACHING GUIDELINES 18.3 General Newborn Safety

- Have emergency telephone numbers readily available, such as those for emergency medical assistance and the poison control center.
- Keep small or sharp objects out of reach to prevent them from being aspirated.
- Do not leave the infant alone in any room without a portable intercom on.
- Always supervise the newborn in the tub; a newborn can drown in as little as 2 in of water.
- Make sure the crib or changing table is sturdy, without any loose hardware, and is painted with lead-free paint.
- Avoid placing the crib or changing table near blinds or curtain cords.
- Provide a smoke-free environment for all infants.
- Place all infants on their backs to sleep to prevent sudden unexplained infant death.
- Employ safe sleep strategies to reduce suffocation deaths of infants.
- Use car seats properly to reduce motor vehicle crash injuries and deaths.
- To prevent falls, do not leave the newborn alone on any elevated surface.
- Use sun shields on strollers and hats to avoid overexposing the newborn to the sun.
- To prevent infection, thoroughly wash your hands before preparing formula.
- Thoroughly investigate any infant care facility before using it.

Adapted from Centers for Disease Control and Prevention. (2024). *Infants & toddlers: Safety in the home & community*. https://www.cdc.gov/parents/infants/safety.html

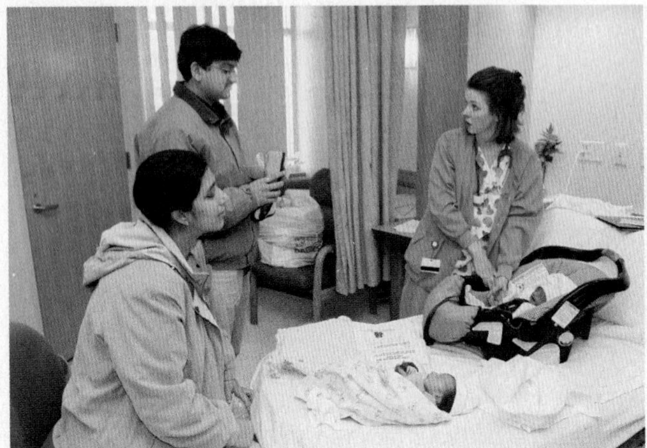

FIGURE 18.20 Newborn in a properly secured car seat.

car seat is considered to be the safest or the best; instead, consistent and proper use is the key to preventing injuries and deaths. Instruct parents in the following:

- Select a car seat that is appropriate for the child's size and weight.
- Caution caregivers against the placement of car seats on elevated or soft surfaces outside the car to prevent falling.
- All newborns discharged from the hospital should be brought home in rear-facing car safety seats secured in the back seat of the vehicle.
- Avoid using a rear-facing car seat in the front seat equipped with a passenger-side airbag.
- Never let an infant ride in the arms of an adult while in a moving vehicle.
- Use the car seat correctly every time the child is in the car.
- Use rear-facing car safety seats for most infants up to 2 years of age or until they reach the highest weight or height allowed by the manufacturer of the seat.
- Make sure the harness (most seats have a 3- to 5-point harness) is in the slots at or below the shoulders.

PREVENTING INFECTION

Nurses must adhere to infection control requirements within their health care facilities. The nurse plays a major role in preventing infection in the newborn environment. Ways to control infection are:

- Minimize exposure of newborns to organisms.
- Report understaffing at your facility as it can lead to nurses missing early signs of infection and thereby cause failure-to-rescue events.
- Wash your hands before and after providing care, and insist that all personnel wash their hands before handling any newborn.
- Visitors should be limited to those essential for the birthing parent's well-being and care.
- Do not allow ill staff or visitors to visit or handle newborns.
- Avoid sharing any infant supplies with another infant.
- Monitor the umbilical cord stump and circumcision site for signs of infection.
- Provide eye prophylaxis by instilling prescribed medication soon after birth (Nest 360 & United Nations International Children's Emergency Fund, n.d.).

Educate parents about appropriate home measures that will prevent infections, such as practicing good hand hygiene before and after diaper changes, keeping the newborn well hydrated, avoiding taking the infant into crowds (which may expose them to viruses), ensuring visitors also wash their hands, and keeping health care provider appointments for routine immunizations (Schmitt, 2023b).

Promoting Sleep

Although many parents feel their newborns need them every minute of the day, babies actually need to sleep much of the day at first. Usually, newborns sleep up to 15 hours daily. They sleep for 2 to 4 hours at a time but do not sleep through the night because their stomach capacity is too small to go long periods without nourishment.

> ***TAKE NOTE!***
>
> All newborns develop their own sleep patterns and cycles, but it may take several months before the newborn sleeps through the night. Frequently, newborns have their day and night hours reversed and tend to sleep more during the daytime and less during the night.

Parents should place the newborn on their back to sleep. Back sleeping reduces the risk of sudden unexplained infant death. Inform parent that the practice of "co-sleeping" (sharing a bed) is not safe as infants under 4 months of age who sleep in adult beds are more likely to suffocate than those who sleep in cribs (AAP, 2024b). Suffocation can occur when the infant gets entangled in bedding or caught under pillows, or slips between the bed and the wall or the headboard and mattress. The parent may accidentally roll against or on top of the baby. The safest place for a newborn to sleep is in a crib in the same room with the parents for up to a year, or at least 6 months, without any movable objects in the crib. Co-bedding is not recommended as it significantly raises the risk of infant injury or death and should not be done under any circumstances (AAP, 2024b).

Teach parents to use a crib that meets federal safety guidelines. To prevent suffocation, parents should not place fluffy bedding, quilts, sheepskins, stuffed animals, or pillows in the infant's crib. Teach parents not to allow window blind cords to hang loose in proximity to the crib. They should avoid exposing the infant to tobacco smoke, alcohol, and illicit drugs (AAP, 2024b). Recommendations for safe infant sleeping practices are an important aspect of education for new parents. It is important for nurses to assess families' cultural beliefs and their prior practices to fully understand how to make recommendations in a culturally sensitive manner. See the Healthy People 2030 box.

The AAP (2023) recommends the following to reduce the risk of sudden unexplained infant death (SUID):

- Always place the baby on their back to sleep for all sleep times, including naps; similarly, to avoid the newborn shifting to a tummy position, do not prop infants on their side when putting to sleep.
- Room share, not bed share—keep the baby's sleep area in the same room where the caregiver sleeps.
- Avoid infant exposure to tobacco smoke during pregnancy and after birth.
- Avoid wrapping the infant too tightly with a blanket, and stop when infant can roll over.
- Encourage breastfeeding as breastfed infants have a 50% lower risk of developing Sudden Infant Death Syndrome (SIDS).
- Keep the infant's sleep area in the same room where parents sleep for the first 6 months or, ideally, for the first year.
- Only bring the infant into the parents' bed to feed or comfort them.
- Allow supervised awake "tummy time" to counteract back sleeping on muscle development or development of a flattening of the head.
- If the infant falls asleep in the car seat, move them to a firm surface, laying them on their back.
- Use a firm sleep surface, free from soft objects, toys, blankets, and crib bumpers.
- Use a pacifier during infant sleep, but do not force its use.

HEALTHY PEOPLE 2030

Objective	Nursing Significance
Increase the proportion of infants who are put to sleep in a safe sleep environment. Increase the proportion of infants who are put to sleep on their backs.	• Teach parents about providing a safe sleep environment. • Educate parents about newborns sleeping on their back in a safe sleeping environment to prevent sudden unexplained infant death. • Encourage parents to provide "Tummy Time" while their infant is awake and alert to encourage appropriate development.

Healthy People Objectives retrieved from http://www.healthypeople.gov

Enhancing Bonding

Encourage and enhance parent–newborn interaction by involving both parents with the baby and demonstrating appropriate nurturing behaviors:

- Say "hello" and introduce yourself to the newborn.
- Ask the parents' permission to care for and hold the newborn. This helps parents realize they are responsible for their child and reminds nurses of their role.
- Show parents the power of a soothing voice to calm the newborn (Fig. 18.21).
- Provide care to the newborn in the least stressful way.
- Demonstrate ways to gently wake up the newborn for better feeding.
- Tell parents what you are doing, why you are doing it, and how they can duplicate what you are doing at home.
- Offer the opportunity for parents to perform care while you observe them. Support their efforts to soothe the newborn throughout the care process.
- Help parents interpret the communication cues the newborn uses.
- Point out the efforts the newborn is making to connect with the parents (e.g., alerting to the familiar voice, following the parents while they are speaking, quieting when held securely).

One of the most pleasurable aspects of newborn care is being close to them. Bonding begins soon after birth when parents cradle their newborn and gently stroke them with their fingers. Provide parents with opportunities for skin-to-skin contact with the newborn, holding the baby against their own skin when feeding or cradling. Many newborns respond positively to gentle

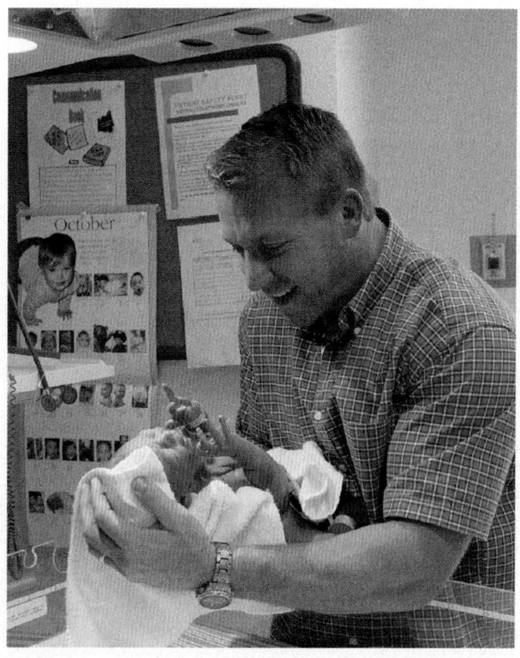

FIGURE 18.21 The new parent uses a soothing voice to calm the newborn.

massage. If necessary, recommend books and videos that cover the subject.

For newborns, crying is the only way to communicate something is wrong. Try to find out the reason why: Is the diaper wet? Is the room too hot or too cold? Is the baby uncomfortable (e.g., diaper rash or tight clothing)? Suggest the following ways in which parents can soothe an upset newborn:

- Try feeding or burping to relieve air or stomach gas.
- Lightly rub the newborn's back and speak softly to them.
- Let the infant suck on something, such as a pacifier, which is calming.
- Gently sway side to side, or rock back and forth in a rocking chair.
- Talk with the newborn while making eye contact.
- Take the newborn for a walk in a stroller or carriage to get fresh air.
- Change the baby's position from back to side or vice versa.
- Hold the crying infant close against your body and take calm, slow breaths.
- Place the infant across your lap on their belly and gently rub their back.
- Take a 5-minute walk with infant; then sit and hold them for another 5 minutes.
- Try singing, reciting poetry and nursery rhymes, or reading to the baby.
- Turn on a musical mobile above the newborn's head.
- Create "white noise," such as shushing, that drowns out other noises.
- Provide more physical contact by walking, rocking, or patting the newborn (AAP, 2022c).
- Swaddle the newborn to provide a sense of security and comfort. To do this:
    - Spread out a receiving blanket with one corner folded slightly.
    - Lay the newborn face up with the head at the folded corner.
    - Wrap the left corner over the baby's body and tuck it beneath the baby.
    - Bring the bottom corner over the baby's feet.
    - Wrap the right corner around the baby, leaving only the head exposed.
    - Arms can be released from the blanket to allow for self-comforting (Moon & Glassy, 2022).

Assisting With Screening Tests

Newborn screening has been among the most successful public health programs of the 21st century. The aim of screening is to identify newborns who appear healthy but could be at risk of having conditions with severe complications if left untreated. Newborn screening tests that are required in most states before discharge are used to check for certain genetic issues, inborn errors of metabolism, and hearing. Early identification and initiation of treatment can prevent significant complications and can minimize the negative effects of untreated disease.

GENETIC ISSUES AND INBORN ERRORS OF METABOLISM SCREENING

Each state mandates particular conditions that must be tested on the initial newborn screen. Common screening tests include sickle cell disease, congenital hypothyroidism, and inborn errors of metabolism such as PKU and galactosemia. Refer to Chapter 24 for additional information. Screening tests for genetic issues and inborn errors of metabolism require a few drops of blood taken from the newborn's heel (Fig. 18.22).

The trend toward early discharge of newborns can affect the timing of screening and the accuracy of some test results. For example, the newborn needs to ingest enough breast milk or formula to elevate phenylalanine levels for the screening test to identify PKU accurately, so newborn screening for PKU testing should not be performed before 24 to 48 hours of age. Be aware of which conditions your state routinely screens for at birth to ensure the parents are taught about the tests and the

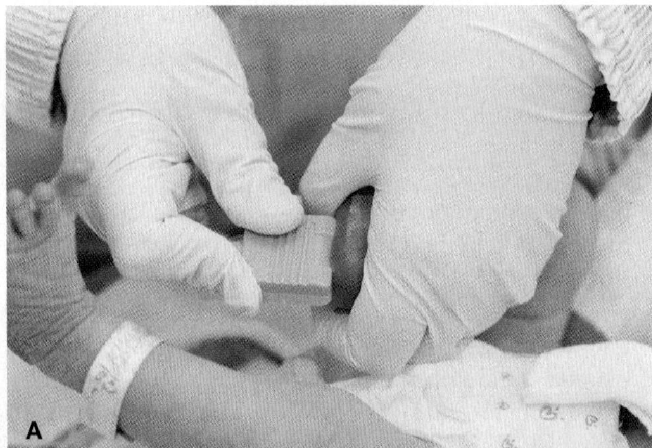

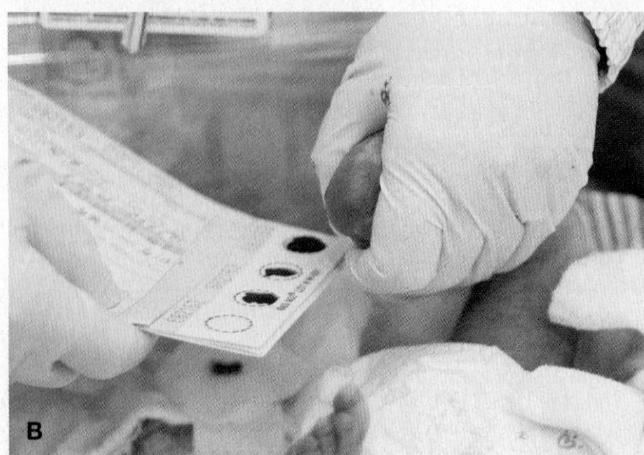

FIGURE 18.22 Screening for phenylketonuria (PKU). **A.** Performing a heel stick. **B.** Applying the blood specimen to the card for screening.

importance of early treatment. Also be familiar with the optimal time frame for screening and conditions that could affect the results. Ensure that a satisfactory specimen has been obtained at the appropriate time and that circumstances that could cause false results have been minimized. Refer to Table 18.4 for additional information regarding a selected few inborn errors of metabolism.

HEARING SCREENING

Unlike a physical deformity, hearing loss is not obviously clinically detectable at birth and thus remains difficult to assess. In the United States, among live births, approximately 1 to 3 of every 1,000 newborns have an atypical hearing threshold (AAP, 2024a). Congenital hearing loss may be inherited through a single gene, be a part of an associated syndrome, occur as a result of prenatal infection, or be a teratogenic effect of medications or toxins on the developing fetus (Smith & Gooi, 2023). Based on the AAP's recommendation to screen every newborn for hearing loss, each state has an Early Hearing Detection and Intervention program; most of them require an initial hearing screening prior to leaving the hospital (National Center for Hearing Assessment and Management, 2024). See the Healthy People 2030 box.

HEALTHY PEOPLE 2030

Objective	Nursing Significance
Increase the proportion of newborns who are screened for hearing loss no later than age 1 month. Increase the proportion of infants who did not pass the hearing screening test who get evaluated for hearing loss no later than age 3 months. Increase the proportion of infants with confirmed hearing loss who are enrolled for intervention services no later than age 6 months.	• Encourage appropriate hearing assessments. • Refer children who are diagnosed with a hearing deficit to appropriate local services.

Healthy People Objectives retrieved from http://www.healthypeople.gov

TABLE 18.4 • Select Conditions Screened for in the Newborn

Condition	Description	Clinical Picture/Effect If Not Treated	Treatment	Timing of Screening
Phenylketonuria (PKU)	Autosomal recessive inherited deficiency in one of the enzymes necessary for the metabolism of phenylalanine to tyrosine—essential amino acids found in most foods	Irritability, vomiting of protein feedings, and a musty odor to the skin or body secretions of the newborn; if not treated, cognitive impairment, motor retardation, seizures, microcephaly, and poor growth and development	Lifetime diet of foods low in phenylalanine (low protein) and monitoring of blood levels; special newborn formulas available: Phenex and Lofenalac	Universally screened for in the United States; testing is done 24–48 hours after protein feeding.
Congenital hypothyroidism	Deficiency of thyroid hormone necessary for normal brain growth, calorie metabolism, and development; may result from hypothyroidism in birthing parent	Increased risk in newborns with birth weight <2,000 g or >4,500 g, and those of Hispanic and Asian heritage; feeding problems, growth and breathing problems; if not treated, irreversible brain damage and intellectual disability before age 1	Lifelong thyroid replacement therapy	Testing (measures thyroxin [T_4] and thyroid stimulating hormone [TSH]) is done between days 4 and 6 of life.
Galactosemia	Absence of the enzyme needed for the conversion of the milk sugar galactose to glucose	Poor weight gain, vomiting, jaundice, mood changes, loss of eyesight, seizures, and intellectual disability; if untreated, galactose buildup causing permanent damage to the brain, eyes, and liver, and eventually death	Eliminate milk from diet; substitute soy milk. Breastfeeding not advised	First test done on discharge from the hospital with a follow-up test within 1 month
Sickle cell anemia	Recessively inherited abnormality in hemoglobin structure	Anemia developing shortly after birth; increased risk for infection, growth restriction, vaso-occlusive crisis	Maintenance of hydration and hemodilution, rest, electrolyte replacement, pain management, blood replacement, and antibiotics	Bloodspot obtained at same time of other newborn screening tests or prior to 3 months of age

Matern, D. (2023). Newborn screening for inborn errors of metabolism. *UpToDate*. Retrieved March 25, 2024, from https://www.uptodate.com/contents/newborn-screening-for-inborn-errors-of-metabolism

Review the hearing screen result with the family to facilitate tracking and follow-up (AAP, 2024a). The child with a positive screen for atypical hearing thresholds in one or both ears should be referred to an audiologist for diagnostic consultation and testing. Delays in identification and intervention may affect the child's language and cognitive development, as well as academic performance; detection before 3 months greatly improves outcomes. Early identification and intervention can prevent severe psychosocial, educational, and language development delays. Refer to Box 18.3 for additional information related to hearing screening methods.

PREVENTING HYPOGLYCEMIA

Hypoglycemia is the most common metabolic disturbance in the neonatal period. During the first 24 to 48 hours of life, as healthy newborns transition from intrauterine to extrauterine life, their plasma glucose levels are typically lower than later in life. Hypoglycemia affects as many as 40% of all full-term newborns. It is defined as a plasma glucose level of less than 30 mg/dL in the first 24 hours of life and less than 45 mg/dL after the first 24 hours (Cranmer, 2022). In newborns, blood glucose levels fall to a low point during the first few hours of life because the source of glucose from the birthing parent is removed when the umbilical cord is cut. This period of transition is usually smooth, but certain newborns are at greater risk for hypoglycemia: infants of birthing parents who have diabetes or high body weight; preterm newborns; newborns with fetal growth restriction (FGR); newborns born via cesarean section; and those with neonatal hypothermia, inadequate caloric intake, sepsis, asphyxia, hypothermia, polycythemia, glycogen storage disorders, or endocrine deficiencies (Chen et al., 2022).

Most newborns experience transient hypoglycemia and are asymptomatic. The symptoms, when present, are nonspecific and include jitteriness, sweating, hypothermia, irritability, lethargy, cyanosis, apnea, seizures, high-pitched or weak cry, hypothermia, and poor feeding. If hypoglycemia is prolonged or is left untreated, serious, long-term adverse neurologic sequelae such as learning disabilities and intellectual disabilities can occur (Cranmer, 2022).

Treatment of hypoglycemia in the newborn includes administration of a rapid-acting source of glucose such as dextrose gel, breastfeeding, or early formula feeding. In acute, severe cases, intravenous administration of glucose may be required. Continuous monitoring of glucose levels is not only prudent but mandatory in high-risk newborns. Although there is no specific means of preventing hypoglycemia in newborns except for early feeding, it is wise and cautious to monitor for symptoms and intervene as soon as symptoms are noted. Subsequently, early diagnosis and appropriate intervention are essential for all newborns.

Nursing care of the hypoglycemic newborn includes monitoring for signs of hypoglycemia or identifying high-risk newborns prone to this disorder based on their perinatal history, physical examination, body measurements, and gestational age. Glucose screening should be performed on at-risk infants and those with clinical signs compatible with hypoglycemia (Kain & Mannix, 2023).

BOX 18.3 Newborn Hearing Screening Methods

Newborn hearing screening is the standard of care in hospitals nationwide. A newborn's hearing can be screened in one of two ways: otoacoustic emission (OAE) or automated auditory brain stem response (AABR).

In OAE, a tiny microphone is placed in the infant's ear canal, and the sound waves produced by the newborn's inner ear are measured in response to certain tones or clicks presented through the earphone. Preset parameters in the equipment decide whether the OAEs are sufficient for the newborn to pass or whether a referral is necessary for further evaluation. The test may be done with the infant awake, but the best and quickest results are possible when the newborn is sleeping.

In AABR, an earphone is placed in the ear canal, or an earmuff is placed over the newborn's ear, and a soft, rapid tapping noise is presented. Electrodes placed around the newborn's head, neck, and shoulders record neural activity from the infant's brain stem in response to the tapping noises. The AABR tests how well the ear and the nerves leading to the brain work. The infant must be sleeping or quiet. Like OAEs, automated AABR screening is sensitive to more than mild degrees of hearing loss, but a "pass" does not guarantee normal hearing.

Vohr, B. R. (2023). Screening the newborn for hearing loss. *UpToDate*. Retrieved April 13, 2024, from https://www.uptodate.com/contents/screening-the-newborn-for-hearing-loss

Promoting Nutrition

Several physiologic changes dictate the type and method of feeding throughout the newborn's first year. Some of these changes include:

- Stomach capacity is limited at birth. The emptying time is short (2 to 3 hours) and peristalsis is rapid. Therefore, small, frequent feedings are needed at first, with amounts progressively increasing with maturity.
- The immune system is immature at birth, so the baby is at high risk for food allergies during the first 4 to 6 months of life. Introducing solid foods prior to this time increases the risk of developing food allergies.
- Pancreatic enzymes and bile to assist in digestion of fat and starch are in limited supply until about 3 to 6 months of age. Infants cannot digest cereal prior to this time.
- The kidneys are immature and unable to concentrate urine until about 4 to 6 weeks of age. Excess protein and mineral intake can place a strain on kidney function and can lead to dehydration. Infants need to consume more water per unit of body weight than adults do as a result of their high body weight from water.

NEWBORN NUTRITIONAL NEEDS

Once the placenta no longer provides nutrition, a newborn's survival depends on its ability to take in nutrients. As newborns grow, their energy and nutrient requirements change to meet their body's changing needs. During infancy, energy, protein, vitamin, and mineral requirements per pound of body weight are higher than at any other time of life. These high levels are needed to fuel the rapid growth and development during this stage of life. Generally, an infant's birth weight doubles in the first 4 to 6 months of life and triples within the first year.

A newborn's caloric needs range from 110 to 120 cal/kg body weight. Breast milk and formulas contain approximately 20 cal/oz, so the caloric needs of young infants can be met if several feedings are given throughout the day. Most full-term infants need a basic formula if the parent chooses not to breastfeed. These formulas are modeled after breast milk, which contains 20 cal/oz. There is no evidence to recommend one brand over the other since all of them are nutritionally interchangeable. All formulas are classified based on three parameters: caloric density, carbohydrate source, and protein composition (Table 18.5).

Fluid requirements for the newborn and infant range from 100 to 150 mL/kg daily. This requirement can be met through breastfeeding or bottle-feeding. Additional water supplementation is not necessary. Adequate carbohydrates, fats, protein, and vitamins are achieved through consumption of breast milk or formula. The AAP recommends that iron-fortified formula be used for all infants who are not breastfed from birth to 1 year of age. The breastfed infant draws on iron reserves for the first 6 months and then needs iron-rich foods or supplementation added at 6 months of age (Paulley & Duff, 2022). The AAP has also recommended that all infants (breastfed and bottle-fed) receive a daily supplement of 400 IU of vitamin D, starting within the first few days of life to prevent rickets and vitamin D deficiency (Porto & Abu-Alreesh, 2022).

Cultural beliefs can also influence feeding practices of newborns, which can impact an infant's nutritional status. Examples may include beliefs in avoidance of colostrum, human milk alone being insufficient, newborns needing solid foods as early as 2 weeks of age, different perceptions of what constitutes appropriate weight, and encouragement of prolonged bottle-feeding beyond 2 years of age. Nurses need to be open to learning various cultural feeding practices and utilize a sensitive approach to breastfeeding and nutritional guidance with parents (AAP, 2024d).

SUPPORTING THE CHOICE OF FEEDING METHOD

The benefits of breastfeeding are significant and well documented. Numerous health-related professional

TABLE 18.5 • Comparison of Breast Milk With Selected Formula Composition

Type	Brand Names	Calories per Ounce	Carbohydrate Source	Protein Source	Indications
Breast milk	None	20	Lactose	Human milk	Preferred for all infants
Term formula	Enfamil; Similac; Carnation Good Start	20	Lactose	Cow's milk	Appropriate for all term infants
Term formula with DHA and ARA	Enfamil Lipil; Good Start DHA and ARA; Similac Advance	20	Lactose	Cow's milk	Marketed to promote good vision and brain development; to make them more like breast milk
Preterm formula	Enfamil 24 Premature; Preemie SMA 24	24	Lactose	Cow's milk	Usually given to preterm infants <34 weeks' gestation
Soy formula	Enfamil Prosobee; Good Start Soy	20	Corn-based	Soy	For infants with galactosemia
Hypoallergenic formula	Similac Alimentum; Enfamil Nutramigen; Enfamil Pregestimil	20	Corn or sucrose	Extensively hydrolyzed	For infants with a milk protein allergy
Nonallergenic formula	Neocate; Nutramigen AA	20	Corn or sucrose	Amino acids	For infants with a milk protein allergy
Antireflux formula	Enfamil AR; Similac Sensitive RS	20	Lactose thickened with rice starch	Cow's milk	For infants with gastric reflux disorder

ARA, arachidonic acid; DHA, docosahexaenoic acid.

U.S. Food & Drug Administration. (2022). *Questions & answers for consumers concerning infant formula.* https://www.fda.gov/food/people-risk-foodborne-illness/questions-answers-consumers-concerning-infant-formula

organizations promote breastfeeding because of the health benefits for both the birthing parent and infant. Nurses should encourage and advocate breastfeeding for their patients and provide support for the family throughout their breastfeeding experiences. Parents typically decide about the method of feeding well before the infant is born. Prenatal and childbirth classes present information about breastfeeding versus bottle-feeding and allow the parents to make up their minds about which method is best for them. The decision to bottle-feed, rather than breastfeed, is influenced by various factors, including socioeconomic status, culture, sexual objectification, fear of a negative community reaction, lack of social support (especially from the partner), lack of self-efficacy, free formula provided by government programs, and lack of prenatal education and support for breastfeeding (Roberts et al., 2023). Nurses can provide evidence-based information to assist parents in making their decision. Regardless of which method is chosen, the nurse needs to respect and support parents' decisions.

FEEDING THE NEWBORN

The newborn can be fed at any time during the transition period if assessments are normal and a desire is demonstrated. Before the newborn can be fed, determine their ability to suck and swallow. Clear any mucus in the nares or mouth with a bulb syringe before initiating feeding. Auscultate bowel sounds, check for abdominal distention, and inspect the anus for patency. If these parameters are within normal limits, newborn feeding may be started. Most newborns should be fed on demand, and they should feed when they awaken. When they go home, parents are encouraged to feed their newborns every 2 to 4 hours during the day and only when the newborn awakens during the night for the first few days after birth.

Parents often have many questions about feeding. Generally, newborns should be fed on demand whenever they seem hungry. Most newborns will give clues about their hunger status by crying, placing their fingers or fist in their mouth, rooting around, and sucking.

Newborns differ in their feeding needs and preferences, but most breastfed newborns need to be fed every 2 to 3 hours, usually nursing for 10 to 20 minutes on each breast. The length of feedings is up to the parent and newborn. Encourage the parent to respond to cues from their infant and not feed according to a standard or preset schedule.

Formula-fed newborns usually feed every 3 to 4 hours, finishing a bottle in 30 minutes or less. In the first few days, the newborn has the capacity to take only about ½ oz of formula per feeding, increasing to 1 to 2 ounces per feeding after that (Jain & Bunik, 2024). If the newborn seems satisfied, wets six to 10 diapers daily, produces several stools a day, sleeps well, and is gaining weight regularly, then they are probably receiving sufficient breast milk or formula.

Newborns swallow air during feedings, which causes discomfort and fussiness. Parents can prevent this by burping them frequently throughout the feeding. Tips regarding burping include:

- *Over shoulder:* Hold the newborn upright with their head on the parent's shoulder (Fig. 18.23A). Support

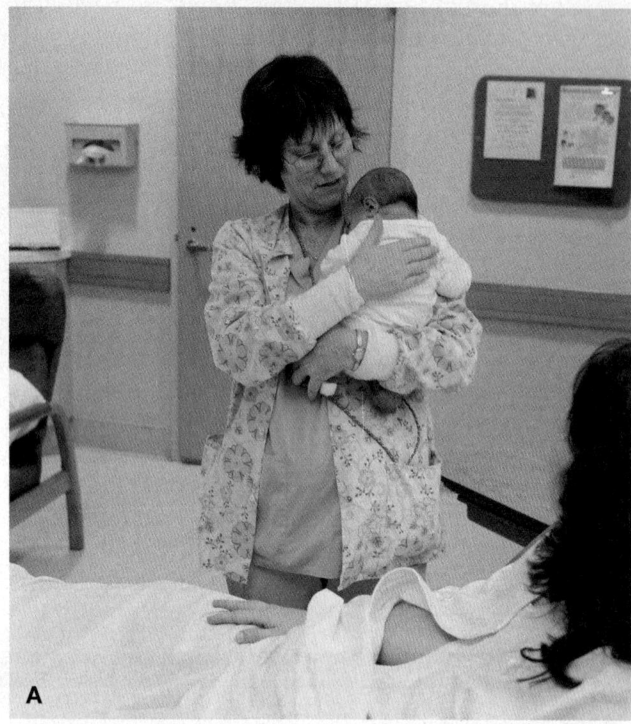

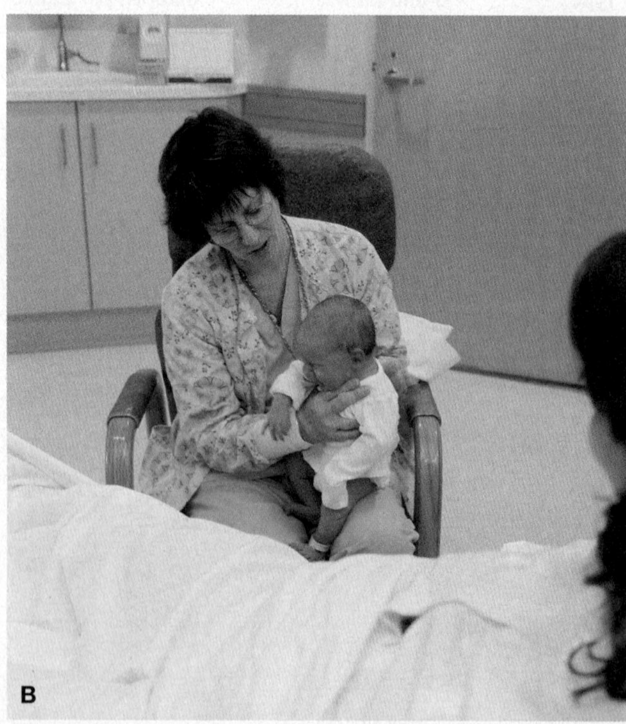

FIGURE 18.23 The nurse demonstrates **(A)** holding the newborn upright over the shoulder and **(B)** sitting the newborn upright, supporting the neck and chin.

the head and neck while the parent gently pats or rubs the newborn's back.

- *Sitting on lap*: Sit the newborn on the parent's lap, with the newborn facing away from the parent or to the side. Place the palm of the parent's hand flat against the newborn's chest and support their chin and jaw. Gently rub the newborn's back with the other hand (Fig. 18.23B).
- *Face-down on lap:* Lay the newborn on the parent's lap, with the baby's back facing up. Support the newborn's head in the crook of the parent's arm, and gently pat or rub the back (UNICEF, n.d.).

TAKE NOTE!

It is the upright position, not the strength of the patting or rubbing, that allows the newborn to release air accumulated in the stomach.

Stress to parents that feeding time is more than an opportunity to get nutrients into their newborn; it is also a time for closeness and sharing. Feedings are as much for the baby's emotional pleasure as their physical well-being. Encourage parents to maintain eye contact with the newborn during the feeding, hold the newborn comfortably close to them, and talk softly during the feeding to promote closeness and security.

BREASTFEEDING

Breast milk is universally recognized as the optimal form of nourishment for infants during the first 6 months to a year of life. There is consensus in the medical community that breastfeeding is ideal for all newborns. The AAP (Meek et al., 2022), the National Association of Pediatric Nurse Practitioners (NAPNAP, 2019), and the American Academy of Family Physicians (2024) recommend breastfeeding exclusively for the first 6 months of life, continuing it in conjunction with other food at least until the newborn's first birthday. Box 18.4 highlights the advantages of breastfeeding for the birthing parent and newborn. In addition, breastfeeding is associated with a lower incidence of necrotizing enterocolitis and SUID and then later in life, acute otitis media, type 2 diabetes, asthma, and higher weight (Meek et al., 2022). Parents should continue to breastfeed during mild illnesses such as colds or flu. However, in the United States, people with HIV and galactosemia are advised not to breastfeed.

The composition of breast milk changes over time from colostrum to transitional milk and, finally, to mature milk. Colostrum is a thick, yellowish substance secreted during the first few days after birth. It is composed of the macronutrients carbohydrates, protein, and fat. It is rich in immunoglobulins A, which help protect the newborn against infections. Colostrum helps to establish a healthy gut microbiome by coating the intestines (Duale et al., 2022). See the Healthy People 2030 box.

BOX 18.4 Advantages of Breastfeeding

Advantages for the Newborn

- Contributes to the development of a strong immune system
- Stimulates growth of positive bacteria in the digestive tract
- Reduces incidence of stomach upset, diarrhea, and colic
- Begins the immunization process at birth by providing passive immunity
- Promotes optimal parent–infant bonding
- Reduces the risk of newborn constipation
- Promotes greater developmental gains in preterm infants
- Provides easily tolerated and digestible food that is sterile; at proper temperature; and readily available with no artificial colorings, flavorings, or preservatives
- Is less likely to result in overfeeding, leading to unhealthy weight gain
- Promotes better tooth and jaw development as a result of sucking hard
- Provides protection against food allergies
- Lowers health care costs due to fewer illnesses
- Is associated with avoidance of type 1 diabetes and heart disease

Advantages for the Breastfeeding Parent

- Can facilitate postpartum weight loss by burning extra calories
- Stimulates uterine contractions to control bleeding
- Lowers risk for ovarian and endometrial cancers
- Facilitates bonding with the newborn infant
- Lowers risk of type 2 diabetes
- Breast milk, unlike formula, is free
- Reduces risk of postpartum depression
- Promotes uterine involution as a result of release of oxytocin
- Lowers the risk of breast cancer and osteoporosis
- Affords some protection against conception, although it is not a reliable contraceptive method

Campbell, S. H. (2022). *Lactation: A foundational strategy for health promotion.* Jones & Bartlett Learning; Meek, J. Y., Noble, L., & Section on Breastfeeding. (2022). Policy statement: Breastfeeding and the use of human milk. *Pediatrics, 150*(1), e2022057988. https://doi.org/10.1542/peds.2022-057988

Transitional milk occurs between colostrum and mature milk and contains all the nutrients in colostrum, but it is thinner and less yellow than colostrum. This transitional milk is replaced by true or mature milk around day 10 after birth. Mature milk appears bluish and is not as thick as colostrum. It provides 20 cal/oz and contains:

- *Protein*—Although the content is lower than formula, it is ideal for supporting growth and development for the newborn. The majority of the protein is whey, which is easy to digest.
- *Fat*—Approximately 58% of total calories are fat, but they are easy to digest. Essential fatty acid content is high, as is the level of cholesterol, which helps develop enzyme systems capable of handling cholesterol later in life. The fat content of human milk is necessary for continued brain growth in the infant.
- *Carbohydrate*—Approximately 40% of total calories are in the form of lactose, which stimulates the growth of natural defense bacteria in the gastrointestinal system and promotes calcium absorption.

- *Water*—Water, the major nutrient in breast milk, makes up 85% to 95% of the total volume. Total milk volume varies with the age of the infant and demand.
- *Minerals*—Breast milk contains calcium, phosphorus, chlorine, potassium, and sodium, with trace amounts of iron, copper, and manganese. Iron absorption is about 50%, compared with about 4% for iron-fortified formulas.
- *Vitamins*—All vitamins are present in breast milk; vitamin D is the lowest in amount.
- *Enzymes*—Lipase and amylase are found in breast milk to assist with digestion (Duale et al., 2022).

HEALTHY PEOPLE 2030

Objective	Nursing Significance
Increase the proportion of infants who are breastfed exclusively through 6 months.	• Educate parents about the benefits of breastfeeding. • Support and encourage parents in their attempts to initiate breastfeeding.

Healthy People Objectives retrieved from http://www.healthypeople.gov

Breastfeeding Assistance

Breastfeeding can be initiated immediately after birth. If the newborn is healthy and stable, wipe the newborn from head to toe with a dry cloth, and place them skin to skin on the birthing parent's abdomen. Then cover the newborn and parent with another warmed blanket to hold in the warmth. Immediate parent–newborn contact takes advantage of the newborn's natural alertness after a vaginal birth and fosters bonding. This immediate contact also reduces bleeding in the birthing parent, stabilizes the newborn's temperature and blood glucose level, helps regulate the newborn's heartbeat and breathing, encourages bonding, and reduces stress (Magge, 2022).

Left alone on the birthing parent's abdomen, a healthy newborn scoots upward, pushing with the feet, pulling with the arms, and bobbing the head until finding and latching onto the parent's nipple. A newborn's sense of smell is highly developed, which also helps in finding the nipple. As the newborn moves to the nipple, the birthing parent produces high levels of oxytocin, which contracts the uterus, thereby minimizing bleeding. Oxytocin also causes the breasts to release colostrum when the newborn sucks on the nipple. Colostrum is rich in antibodies and thus provides the newborn with the "first immunization" against infection.

Keys to successful breastfeeding include:

- Initiating breastfeeding within the first hour of life if the newborn is stable
- Placing the newborn on the birthing parent's chest or abdomen immediately after birth
- Following the newborn's feeding schedule—eight to 12 times in 24 hours
- Providing unrestricted periods of breastfeeding
- Offering no supplement unless medically indicated
- Having a lactation consultant observe a feeding session
- Avoiding artificial nipples and pacifiers except during a painful procedure
- Increasing fluid intake to encourage greater milk production
- Feeding from both breasts over each 24-hour period
- Relaxing the parent's shoulders and bringing the infant to the breast, rather than breast to the infant
- Having the breastfeeding parent hold the infant close during breastfeeding, tummy to tummy, nose to nipple
- Holding the infant close helps to build a secure and loving relationship
- Watching for indicators of sufficient intake from infant:
  - Six to 10 wet diapers daily
  - Waking up hungry eight to 12 times in 24 hours
  - Acting content and falling asleep after feeding
- Keeping the infant warm throughout breastfeeding experience
- Keeping the newborn with the birthing parent throughout the hospital stay
- Availability of the nurse or lactation consultant to guide and support the breastfeeding parent while on the postpartum unit (Campbell, 2022).

Help position the newborn so that latching on is effective and not painful for the breastfeeding parent. It may be helpful to place pillows or a folded blanket under the parent's head or roll them to one side and tuck the newborn next to them. Assess both the parent and the newborn during this initial session to determine needs for assistance and education. One tool used frequently in this assessment is the LATCH scoring tool (Divya et al., 2022). The LATCH scoring tool is a breastfeeding charting system that provides a systematic method for gathering information about individual breastfeeding sessions. The system assigns a numerical score of 0, 1, or 2 to five key components of breastfeeding. Each letter of the acronym "LATCH" denotes an area of assessment: "L" is for how well the infant latches onto the breast; "A" is for audible swallowing noted; "T" is for the breastfeeding parent's nipple type; "C" is for the parent's breast/nipple level of comfort; and "H" is for the holding position and amount of help the parent needs to hold their infant to the breast. The system is visually represented in the same form as the Apgar scoring grid, and the numbers are handled in the same way. With the LATCH system, the nurse can assess parent and infant variables, define areas of needed intervention, and determine priorities in providing patient care and teaching (Table 18.6). The higher the score, the greater the chance of successful breastfeeding and the lesser the nursing intervention needed by the parent and baby.

Breastfeeding Positioning

The parent and infant must be in comfortable positions to ensure breastfeeding success. The four most common

TABLE 18.6 • The Latch Scoring Tool

Parameters	0 Point	1 Point	2 Points
L: Latch	Sleepy infant, no sustained latch achieved	Must hold nipple in infant's mouth to sustain latch and suck; must stimulate infant to continue to suck	Grasps nipple; tongue down; lips flanged; rhythmic sucking
A: Audible swallowing	None	A few observed with stimulation	Spontaneous and intermittent both <24 hours old and afterward
T: Type of nipple	Inverted (drawn inward into breast tissue)	Flat (not protruding)	Everted or protruding out after stimulation
C: Comfort of nipple	Engorged, cracked bleeding; blisters or bruises; severe discomfort	Filling; reddened, small blisters or bruises; mild to moderate discomfort	Soft, nontender
H: Hold (positioning)	Nurse must hold infant to breast	Minimal assistance; help with positioning, then breastfeeding parent takes over	No assistance needed by nurse

Divya, R., Taksande, A., Balaji, M. K., & Sweetline, C. (2022). Efficacy of counseling in improving LATCH score and successful breastfeeding: A hospital-based prospective cohort study. *Journal of Clinical and Diagnostic Research*, *16*(8), 1. https://doi.org/10.7860/JCDR/2022/56968.16685; American Academy of Pediatrics. (2022b). *Ensuring proper latch on while breastfeeding*. https://www.healthychildren.org/English/ages-stages/baby/breastfeeding/Pages/Ensuring-Proper-Latch-On.aspx?gclid

positions for breastfeeding are the football, cross cradle, across-the-lap, and side-lying holds. With experimentation, each breastfeeding parent can decide which positions feel most comfortable for them (Fig. 18.24).

- In the *football hold*, the breastfeeding parent holds the infant's back and shoulders in their palm and tucks the infant under their arm. Remind the parent to keep the infant's ear, shoulder, and hip in a straight line.

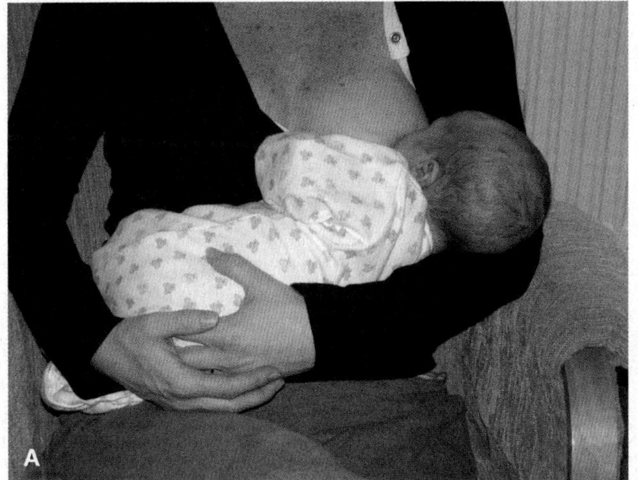

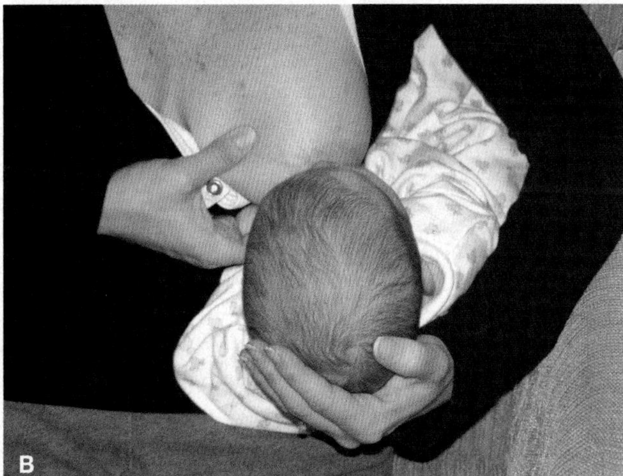

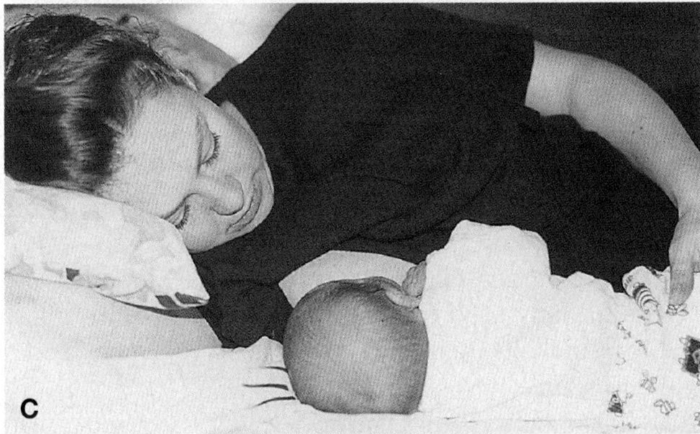

FIGURE 18.24 Breastfeeding positions. **A.** Cradling position. **B.** Football hold position. **C.** Side-lying position.

The parent supports the breast with their hand and brings it to the infant's lips to latch on. The parent continues to support the breast until the infant begins to nurse. This position allows the parent to see the infant's mouth as they guide the infant to the nipple. This is a good choice for birthing parents who have had cesarean births because it avoids pressure on the incision.

- The *cross-cradling position* is the one most commonly used. The breastfeeding parent holds the baby in the crook of their arm, with the infant facing the parent. The parent supports the breast with their opposite hand.
- In the *across-the-lap position*, the breastfeeding parent places a pillow across their lap, with the infant facing them. The parent supports the infant's back and shoulders with their palm and supports their breast from underneath. After the infant is in position, the infant is pulled forward to latch on.
- In the *side-lying position*, the breastfeeding parent lies on their side with a pillow supporting their back and another pillow supporting the newborn in the front. To start, the parent props themselves up on an elbow and supports the newborn with that arm while holding their breast with the opposite hand. Once nursing is started, the parent lies down in a comfortable position (La Leche League International [LLLI], 2024d).

To promote latching on, instruct the breastfeeding parent to make a C or a V shape with their fingers. In the C hold, the parent places their thumb well above the areola and the other four fingers below the areola and under the breast. In the V hold, the parent places their index finger above the areola and their other three fingers below the areola and under the breast. Either method can be used as long as the parent's hand is well away from the nipple so the infant can latch on.

Breastfeeding Education

Breastfeeding is not an innate skill in humans. Almost all birthing parents have the potential to breastfeed successfully, but many struggle to do so because of inadequate knowledge. Nursing Care Plan 18.1 outlines typical nursing analyses, outcomes, and interventions. For many parents and newborns, breastfeeding goes smoothly from the start, but for others it is a struggle. Nurses can help throughout the experience by not being judgmental and by demonstrating techniques and offering encouragement and praise for success. Correct positioning will enhance good attachment and will ensure effective milk transfer. Nurses should emphasize that the key to successful breastfeeding is correct positioning and latching on.

Prenatal and postnatal education by nurses regarding breastfeeding has been shown to have a significant effect on both the ability to breastfeed successfully and the duration of lactation (LeMoine et al., 2022). During the first few breastfeeding sessions, parents want to know how often they should be nursing, whether breastfeeding is going well, if the newborn is getting enough nourishment, and what problems may occur and how to cope with them. Education for the breastfeeding parent is highlighted in Teaching Guidelines 18.4.

TAKE NOTE!

Remember that the supply of milk is equal to the demand–the more sucking, the more milk.

Remember Kelly, who was concerned about jaundice in her newborn son? At her son's 2-week well-baby check-up at the clinic, his bilirubin level came back within normal limits. Kelly still felt he was not getting enough to eat and stated that she might switch to formula feeding her son. What information can the nurse present to promote and reinforce breastfeeding? Should the nurse make a referral to the lactation consultant?

Breast Milk Storage and Expression

If the breastfeeding parent becomes separated from the newborn for any reason (e.g., work, travel, or illness), they need instruction on how to express and store milk safely. Expressing milk can be done manually (hand compression of breast) or by using a breast pump. Manual or handheld pumps are inexpensive and can be used by parents who occasionally need an extra bottle if they are going out (Fig. 18.25A). Electric breast pumps are used for parents who experience a lengthy separation from their infants and need to pump their breasts regularly, for instance, while at the workplace (Fig. 18.25B).

To ensure the safety of expressed breast milk, instruct the breastfeeding parent as follows:

- Wash your hands before expressing milk or handling breast milk.
- Find a quiet, clean place to express milk.
- Use clean containers that have been washed in hot, soapy water to store expressed milk.
- Use sealed and chilled milk within 24 hours.
- All milk should be dated before storing.
- Discard any milk that has been refrigerated for more than 24 hours.
- Thaw frozen milk in refrigerator overnight and place in cup of warm water.
- Avoid boiling and microwaves to prevent loss of nutritional properties.
- Use any frozen expressed milk within 3 months.
- Discard any used milk; never refreeze it.
- Store milk in quantities to be used for each feeding (2 to 4 oz).
- Thaw milk in warm water before using (LLLI, 2024e).

TEACHING GUIDELINES 18.4 Breastfeeding

- Set aside a quiet place where you can be relaxed and won't be disturbed. Relaxation promotes milk letdown.
- Sit in a comfortable chair or rocking chair, or lie on a bed. Try to make each feeding calm, quiet, and leisurely. Avoid distractions.
- Listen to soothing music, and sip a nutritious drink during feedings.
- Initially, nurse the newborn every few hours to stimulate milk production. Remember that the supply of milk is equal to the demand—the more sucking, the more milk.
- Watch for signals from the infant to indicate that they are hungry, such as:
  - Nuzzling against the parent's breasts
  - Demonstrating the rooting reflex by making sucking motions
  - Placing fist or hands in mouth to suck on
  - Crying and squirming
  - Smacking the lips
- Stimulate the rooting reflex by touching the newborn's cheek to initiate sucking.
- Look for signs indicating that the newborn has latched on correctly: wide-open mouth with the nipple and much of the areola in the mouth, lips rolled outward, and tongue over lower gum, visible jaw movement drawing milk out, rhythmic sucking with an audible swallowing (soft "ka" or "ah" sound indicates the infant is swallowing milk).
- Hold the newborn closely, facing the breast, with the newborn's ear, shoulder, and hip in direct alignment.
- Nurse the infant on demand, not on a rigid schedule. Feed every 2 to 3 hours within a 24-hour period for a total of eight to 12 feedings.
- Alternate the breast you offer first; identify with a safety pin on the bra.
- Vary your position for each feeding to empty breasts and reduce soreness.
- Look for signs that the newborn is getting enough milk:
  - At least six wet diapers and two to five loose yellow stools daily
  - Steady weight gain after the first week of age
  - Pale yellow urine, not deep yellow or orange
  - Sleeping well, yet looks alert and healthy when awake
- Wake up the newborn if they have nursed less than 5 minutes by unwrapping them.
- Before removing the baby from the breast, break the infant's suction by inserting a finger.
- Burp the infant to release air when changing breasts and at the end of the breastfeeding session.
- Avoid supplemental formula feedings unless indicated for a medical reason. Do not take drugs or medications unless approved by the health care provider.
- Avoid drinking alcohol or caffeinated drinks, because they pass through milk.
- Do not smoke while breastfeeding; it increases the risk of SIDS.
- Always wash your hands before expressing or handling milk to store.
- Wear nursing bras and clothes that are easy to undo.

Campbell, S. H. (2022). *Lactation: A foundational strategy for health promotion*. Jones & Bartlett Learning; Meek, J. Y., Noble, L., & Section on Breastfeeding. (2022). Policy statement: Breastfeeding and the use of human milk. *Pediatrics*, *150*(1), e2022057988. https://doi.org/10.1542/peds.2022-057988

CLINICAL JUDGMENT & NURSING PROCESS 18.1 Overview of the Parent and Newborn Having Difficulty With Breastfeeding

Baby boy James, weight 7 lb, 4 oz, was born a few hours ago. His parent is a 19-year-old gravida 1, para 1. His Apgar scores were 9 points at both 1 and 5 minutes. Labor and birth were unremarkable, and James was admitted to the nursery for assessment. After stabilization, James was brought to his parent, who had said she wished to breastfeed. The postpartum nurse assisted the new parent with positioning and latching on and left the room for a few minutes. On returning, the parent was upset, James was crying, and she stated she wanted a bottle of formula to feed him since she didn't have milk and her nipples hurt.

Assessment reveals a young, inexperienced parent placed in an uncomfortable situation with limited knowledge of breastfeeding. Anxiety from the parent transferred to James, resulting in crying. The parent, apprehensive about breastfeeding, needs additional help.

NURSING ANALYSIS: Breastfeeding difficulty related to pain and limited skill

OUTCOME IDENTIFICATION AND EVALUATION

The parent will demonstrate understanding of breastfeeding skills, as evidenced by use of correct positioning and technique, and verbalization of appropriate information related to breastfeeding.

(continued)

CLINICAL JUDGMENT & NURSING PROCESS 18.1 Overview of the Parent and Newborn Having Difficulty With Breastfeeding (*continued*)

INTERVENTIONS: *Providing Education*

- Instruct the parent on proper positioning for breastfeeding; suggest use of football hold, side-lying position, modified cradle, and across-the-lap position *to ensure comfort and to promote ease in breastfeeding.*
- Review breast anatomy and milk letdown reflex *to enhance parent's understanding of lactation.*
- Observe newborn's ability to suck and latch on to the nipple *to assess whether newborn has adequate ability.*
- Monitor sucking and newborn swallowing for several minutes *to ensure adequate latching on and to assess intake.*
- Reinforce nipple care with water and exposure to air *to maintain nipple integrity.*

NURSING ANALYSIS: Acute anxiety related to breastfeeding ability and irritable, crying newborn

OUTCOME IDENTIFICATION AND EVALUATION

The parent will verbalize increased comfort with breastfeeding, as evidenced by positive statements related to breastfeeding and verbalization of desire to continue to breastfeed newborn.

INTERVENTIONS: *Reducing Anxiety*

- Ensure that the environment is calm and soothing without distractions *to promote maternal and newborn relaxation.*
- Show the parent correct latching-on technique *to promote breastfeeding.*
- Assist in calming newborn by holding and talking *to ensure the newborn is relaxed prior to latching on.*
- Reassure the parent she can be successful at breastfeeding *to enhance her self-esteem and confidence.*
- Encourage frequent trials and attempts *to enhance confidence.*
- Encourage the parent to verbalize her anxiety and fears *to reduce anxiety.*

NURSING ANALYSIS: Acute pain related to breastfeeding and incorrect latching-on technique

OUTCOME IDENTIFICATION AND EVALUATION

The parent will experience a decrease in pain during breastfeeding, as evidenced by statements of less nipple pain.

INTERVENTIONS: *Reducing Pain*

- Suggest several alternate positions for breastfeeding *to increase comfort.*
- Demonstrate how to break suction before removing infant from breast *to minimize trauma to nipple.*
- Inspect nipple area *to promote early identification of trauma.*
- Reinforce correct latching-on technique *to prevent nipple trauma.*
- Administer pain medication if indicated *to relieve pain.*
- Instruct about nipple care between feedings *to maintain nipple integrity.*

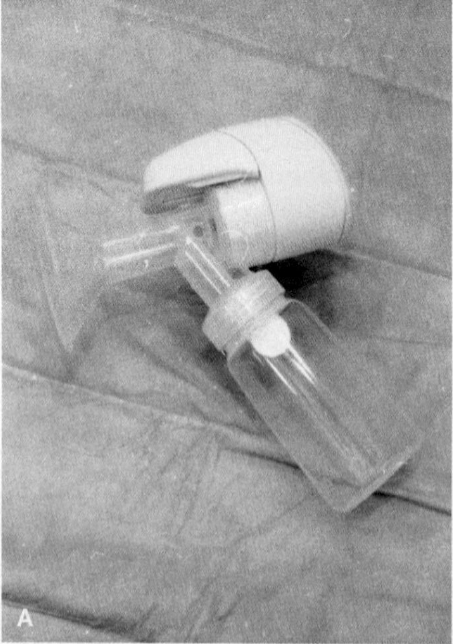

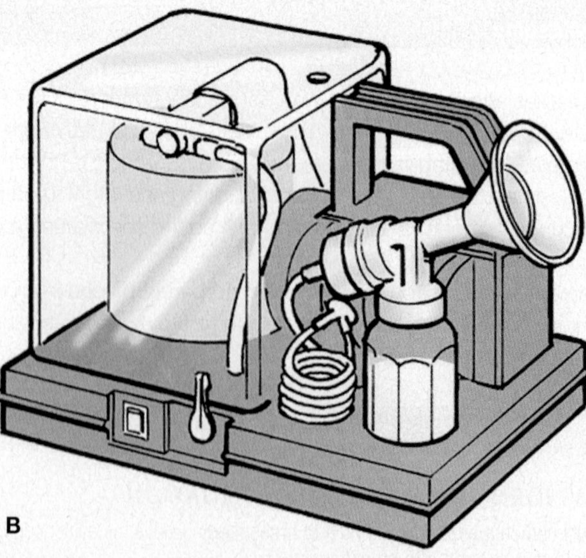

FIGURE 18.25 **A.** Handheld breast pump. **B.** Electric breast pump. (B. Reprinted with permission from Lippincott William & Wilkins. [2008]. *Lippincott nursing procedures* [5th ed.]. Wolters Kluwer.)

Common Breastfeeding Concerns

Breastfeeding parents may experience problems such as cracked nipples, engorgement (the painful overfilling of the breasts with milk), or mastitis (inflammation of the breast). Breastfeeding should not be painful for the parent. If they have sore, cracked nipples, the first step is to find the cause. Incorrect positioning or latching on, removing the infant from the breast without first breaking the suction, or wearing a bra that is too tight can cause cracked or sore nipples. Cracked nipples can increase the risk of mastitis because a break in the skin may allow *Staphylococcus aureus or* other organisms to enter the body.

Sore nipples are usually caused by improper infant attachment, which traumatizes the tissue. The nurse should review techniques for proper positioning and latching on. It is important to get this correct from the first feed to assist in the prevention of incorrect attachment and associated nipple trauma. Recommend the following to the breastfeeding parent:

- Use only warm water, not soap, to clean the nipples to prevent dryness.
- Express some milk before feeding to stimulate the milk ejection reflex.
- Avoid using breast pads with plastic liners, and change pads when they are wet.
- Wear a comfortable bra that is not too tight.
- Apply a few drops of breast milk to the nipples after feeding.
- Take systemic antiinflammatory drugs such as ibuprofen for discomfort.
- Rotate positions when feeding the infant to promote complete breast emptying.
- Leave the nursing bra flaps down after feeding to allow nipples to air-dry.
- Inspect the nipples daily for redness or cracks (LLLI, 2024a).

To ease nipple pain and trauma, reinforce appropriate latching-on techniques and remind the breastfeeding parent about the need to break the suction at the breast before removing the newborn from the breast. Additional measures may include applying cold compresses over the area and massaging breast milk onto the nipple after feeding.

Engorgement may occur as the milk comes in around day 3 or 4 after birth of the newborn. Explain to the parent that engorgement, although uncomfortable, is self-limited and will resolve as the newborn continues to nurse. The parent should continue to nurse during engorgement to avoid a plugged milk duct, which could lead to mastitis. Provide the following tips for relieving engorgement:

- Take warm to hot showers to encourage milk release.
- Express some milk manually before breastfeeding.
- Use a bag of frozen vegetables (such as peas) as a cold compress on sore breasts.
- Lie back to keep the breasts higher because fluids follow gravity.
- Wear a supportive nursing bra 24 hours a day to provide support.
- Feed the newborn in a variety of positions—sitting up and then lying down.
- Massage the breasts from under the axillary area down toward the nipple.
- Increase the frequency of feedings to at least every 2 hours.
- Keep infant with you to facilitate frequent breastfeeding.
- Apply warm compresses to the breasts prior to nursing.
- Stay relaxed while breastfeeding.
- Stand in a shower and let hot water hit the back to relax and release some milk.
- Use a breast pump if nursing or if manual expression is not effective.
- Remember that this condition is temporary and resolves quickly (LLLI, 2024b).

Mastitis, or inflammation of the breast, causes flu-like symptoms, chills, fever, and malaise. These symptoms may occur before the development of soreness, aching, swelling, and redness in the breast (usually the upper outer quadrant). This condition usually occurs in just one breast when a milk duct becomes blocked, causing inflammation, or through a cracked or damaged nipple, allowing bacteria to infect a portion of the breast. Treatment consists of rest, warm compresses, antibiotics, breast support, and continued breastfeeding (the infection will not pass into the breast milk). Explain to the parent that it is important to keep the milk flowing in the infected breast, whether it is through nursing or manual expression or with a breast pump (LLLI, 2024c).

FORMULA FEEDING

Despite the general acknowledgment that breastfeeding is the most desirable means of feeding infants, many parents choose formula feeding and need to be educated about this procedure. Formula-fed infants grow more rapidly than breastfed infants, not only in weight but also in length.

Formula feeding requires more than just opening, pouring, and feeding. Parents need information about the types of formula available, preparation and storage of formula, equipment, feeding positions, and the amount to feed the newborn. The parent also needs to know how to prevent lactation (see Chapter 16 for more information).

Commercially prepared formulas are regulated by the U.S. Food and Drug Administration (FDA), which sets minimum and maximum levels of nutrients. Formulas are manufactured by numerous manufacturers in the United States. Normal full-term infants usually receive conventional cow's milk-based formula, but the health care provider makes this decision. If the infant shows signs of a reaction or lactose intolerance, a switch to another formula type is recommended.

The general recommendation is for all infants to receive iron-fortified formula until the age of 1 year. The latest generation of infant formulas includes some fortification with docosahexaenoic acid (DHA) and arachidonic acid (ARA), two natural components of breast milk. Commercial formulas come in three forms: powder, concentrate, and easy-to-feed or ready-to-use. All are similar in terms of nutritional content but differ in expense. Powdered formula is the least expensive, with concentrated formula the next most expensive. Both must be mixed with water before using. Ready-to-feed formula is the most expensive; it can be opened and poured into a bottle and fed directly to the infant.

Parents need information about the equipment needed for formula feeding. Basic supplies are four to six 4-oz bottles, eight to 10 8-oz bottles, eight to 10 nipple units, a bottle brush, and a nipple brush. A key area of instruction is assessing for flow of formula through the nipple and checking for any nipple damage. When the bottle is filled and turned upside down, the flow from the nipple should be approximately one drop per second. If the parents are using bottles with disposable bags, instruct them to make sure they have a tight-fitting nipple to prevent leaks. Frequent observation of the flow rate from the nipple and the condition of the nipple will prevent choking and aspiration associated with too fast a rate of delivery. Ask the parents to fill a bottle with formula and then turn it upside down and observe the rate at which the formula drips from the bottle. If it is too fast (more than one drop per second), then the nipple should be replaced.

Correct formula preparation is critical to the newborn's health and development. Mistakes in dilution may result if the parents do not understand how to prepare the formula or make measurement errors. The safety of the water supply should be considered. The AAP states that municipal tap water is generally safe for mixing infant formula if there is not a current issue in the municipality (Abrams, 2024). If well water is used, parents should sterilize the water by boiling it or should use bottled water.

Opened cans of ready-made or concentrated formula should be covered and refrigerated after being prepared for the day (24 hours). Instruct parents to discard any unused portions after 48 hours.

TAKE NOTE!

Any formula left in the bottle after feeding should also be discarded because the infant's saliva has been mixed with it.

To warm refrigerated formula, advise the parents to place the bottle in a pan of hot water or an electric bottle warmer and test the temperature by letting a few drops fall on the inside of the wrist. If it is comfortably warm, it is the correct temperature.

Formula-Feeding Assistance

The process of feeding a newborn formula from a bottle should mirror breastfeeding as closely as possible. Although nutrition is important, so are the emotional and interactive components of feeding. Encourage parents to cuddle their newborn closely and position them so that the head is in a comfortable position, not too far back or turned, which makes swallowing difficult (Fig. 18.26). Also urge parents to communicate with the newborn during the feedings by talking and singing to them.

Although it may seem that bottle-feeding is not a difficult task, many new parents find it awkward. At first glance, holding an infant and a bottle appears simple enough, but both the position of the baby and the angle of the bottle must be correct.

Formula-Feeding Positions

Advise parents to feed their newborns in relaxed and quiet settings to create a sense of calm for themselves and the baby. Make sure that comfort is a priority for both parent and newborn. The parent can sit in a comfortable chair, using a pillow to support the arm in which they are holding the baby. The parent can cradle the newborn in a semi-upright position, supporting the newborn's head in the crook of the parent's arm. Holding the newborn close during feeding provides stimulation and helps prevent choking. Holding the newborn's head raised slightly will help prevent formula from washing backward into the eustachian tubes in the ears, which can lead to an ear infection.

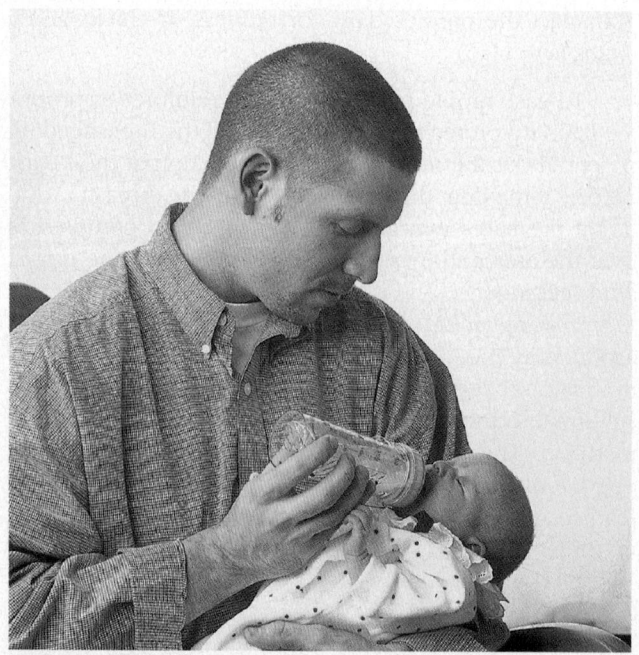

FIGURE 18.26 Parent holding a newborn securely while feeding.

Formula-Feeding Education

Parents require teaching about the correct preparation and storage of formula as well as the techniques for feeding; refer to Teaching Guidelines 18.5.

Proper positioning makes bottle-feeding easier and more enjoyable for both the parent and the newborn. As in breastfeeding, frequent burping is key. Advise parents to hold the bottle so formula fills the nipple, thus allowing less air to enter. Infants get fussy when they swallow air during feedings and need to be relieved of it every 2 to 3 oz.

Emphasize to parents that an electrolyte imbalance can occur in infants who are fed formula that has been incorrectly mixed. Mixing the formula with too *little* water (i.e., too thickly) can cause hypernatremia because the high concentration of sodium is too much for the baby's immature kidneys to handle. As a result, sodium is excreted along with water, leading to dehydration. Mixing the formula with too *much* water in an effort to save money can lead to failure to thrive, diminished nutrition, fluoride overdose, and lack of weight gain (Abrams, 2024).

TEACHING GUIDELINES **18.5** Formula Feeding

- Wash your hands with soap and water before preparing formula.
- Mix the formula and water amounts exactly as the label specifies.
- Always hold the newborn and bottle during feedings; never prop the bottle.
- Never freeze formula or warm it in the microwave.
- Place refrigerated formula in a pan of hot water for a few minutes to warm.
- Test the temperature of the formula by shaking a few drops on the wrist.
- Hold the bottle like a pencil, keeping it tipped to prevent air from entering. Position the bottle so that the nipple remains filled with milk.
- Burp the infant after every few ounces to allow air swallowed to escape.
- Move the nipple around in the infant's mouth to stimulate sucking.
- Always keep a bulb syringe close by to use if choking occurs.
- Avoid putting the infant to bed with a bottle to prevent "baby bottle tooth decay."
- Feed the newborn approximately every 3 to 4 hours.
- Use an iron-fortified formula for the first year.
- Prepare enough formula for the next 24 hours.
- Check nipples regularly and discard any that are sticky, cracked, or leaking.
- Store unmixed, open liquid formula in the refrigerator for up to 48 hours.
- Throw away any formula left in the bottle after each feeding (CDC, 2021).

Preparing for Discharge

Preparing the parents for discharge is an essential task for the nurse. Because of today's shorter hospital stays, the nurse must identify the major teaching topics that need to be covered. Nurses should assess the parents' baseline knowledge and learning needs and plan how to meet them. Using the following principles fosters a learner-centered approach:

- Make the environment conducive to learning. Promote comfort for the parents during this stressful time by using support and praise.
- Allow the parents to provide input about the content and the process of learning. What do they want and need to learn?
- Build the parents' self-esteem by confirming that their responses to the entire birthing process and aftercare are legitimate and that others have felt the same way.
- Ensure that what the parents learn is relevant to their day-to-day home situation.
- Encourage responsibility by reinforcing that their emotional and physical responses are within the normal range.
- Respect cultural beliefs and practices that are important to the family by taking into account their traditions and health beliefs regarding newborn care.

While in the hospital, birthing parents have ready access to support and hands-on instruction regarding feeding and newborn care. When the new parent is discharged, this close supervision and support by nurses should not end abruptly. Providing the new parents with the phone number of the postpartum unit will help them through this stressful transitional period. Giving the new family information and offering backup support via telephone will increase parenting success.

CONSIDER THIS!

I have always prided myself on being organized and in control in most situations, but survival at home after childbirth wasn't one of them. I left the hospital 24 hours after giving birth to my son because my doctor said I could. The postpartum nurse encouraged me to stay longer, but wanting to be in control and sleeping in my own bed again won out. I thought my baby would be sleeping while I sent out birth announcements to my friends and family—wrong! What happened instead was my son didn't sleep as I imagined and my nipples became sore after breastfeeding every few hours. I was weary and tired and wanted to sleep, but I couldn't. Somehow, I thought I would be getting a full night's sleep because I was up throughout the day, but that was a fantasy too. At 2 o'clock in the morning when you are up feeding your baby, you feel like you are the only one in the world up at that time and feel very much alone. My feelings of being organized and in control all the time have changed dramatically since I left the hospital. I have learned to yield to the important needs of my son and derive satisfaction from being able to bring comfort to him and to let go of my need for control.

Thoughts: It is interesting to see how a newborn changed this parent's need to organize and control their environment. What "tips of survival" could the nurse offer this patient to help in the transition to home with their newborn? How can friends and family help when parents arrive home from the hospital with their newborns?

ENSURING FOLLOW-UP CARE

Most newborns are scheduled for their first health follow-up appointment within 2 to 4 days after discharge so they can have additional laboratory work done as part of the newborn screening series, especially if they were discharged within 48 hours. After this first visit, the typical schedule of health care visits is as follows: 2 to 4 weeks of age and 2, 4, 6, 9, 12, 15, 18, and 24 months of age for checkups and vaccines or screenings as necessary. These appointments provide an opportunity for parents to ask questions and receive anticipatory guidance as the newborn grows and develops.

In addition to encouraging parents to keep follow-up appointments, advise parents to call the health care provider if they notice signs of illness in their newborn. They should know which over-the-counter medicines should be kept on hand. Review the following warning signs of illness with parents:

- Temperature of 100.4°F (38°C) or higher (AAP, 2021).
- Forceful, persistent vomiting, not just spitting up
- Refusal to take feedings
- Not moving or very weak
- Weak sucking or cannot suck for appropriate amount of time
- Two or more green, watery diarrheal stools
- Infrequent wet diapers and change in bowel movements from normal pattern
- Lethargy or excessive sleepiness
- Inconsolable crying and extreme fussiness
- Abdominal distention
- Difficult or labored breathing (Schmitt, 2024)

KEY CONCEPTS

- The period of transition from intrauterine to extrauterine life occurs during the first several hours after birth. It is a time of stabilization for the newborn's temperature, respiration, and cardiovascular dynamics.
- All newborns have the following resuscitation needs: being dry, warmth, position, suction, and stimulation.
- The newborn's bowel is sterile at birth. It usually takes about a week for the newborn to produce vitamin K in sufficient quantities to prevent VKDB.
- Nursing measures to maintain the newborn's body temperature include drying them immediately after birth to prevent heat loss through evaporation, wrapping them in prewarmed blankets, putting a hat on their head, and placing them under temperature-controlled radiant warmers.
- It is recommended that all newborns in the United States receive an instillation of a prophylactic agent (erythromycin or tetracycline ophthalmic ointment) in their eyes within an hour or two of being born.
- The specific components of a typical newborn examination include a general survey of the skin, including color; posture; state of alertness; head size; overall behavioral state; respiratory status; biologic sex; and any obvious congenital anomalies.
- Gestational age assessment is pertinent because it allows the nurse to plot growth parameters and to anticipate potential problems related to prematurity/postmaturity and growth abnormalities such as SGA/LGA.
- After the newborn has passed the transitional period and stabilized, the nurse needs to complete ongoing assessments, vital signs, weight and measurements, cord care, hygiene measures, newborn screening tests, and various other tasks until the newborn is discharged home from the birthing unit.
- Important topics about which to educate parents include environmental safety, newborn characteristics, feeding and bathing, circumcision and cord care, sleep and elimination patterns of newborns, safe infant car seats, holding and positioning, and follow-up care.
- Newborn screening tests consist of hearing and certain genetic issues and inborn errors of metabolism tests required in most states for newborns before discharge from the birth facility.
- The AAP, NAPNAP, and the American Association of Family Physicians recommend breastfeeding exclusively for the first 6 months of life and continuing along with other food at least until the first birthday.
- Parents who choose not to breastfeed need to know what types of formula are available, preparation and storage of formula, equipment, feeding positions, and how much to feed their infant.
- The newborn with hypoglycemia requires close monitoring for signs and symptoms of hypoglycemia if present. In addition, newborns at high risk need to be identified based on their perinatal history, physical examination, body measurements, and gestational age.

REFERENCES AND RECOMMENDED READINGS

Abrams, S. A. (2024). *How to safely prepare baby formula with water.* https://www.healthychildren.org/English/ages-stages/baby/formula-feeding/Pages/how-to-safely-prepare-formula-with-water.aspx

American Academy of Family Physicians. (2024). *Advocate for breastfeeding*. https://www.aafp.org/family-physician/patient-care/prevention-wellness/birth-control-pregnancy-childbirth/breastfeeding.html

American Academy of Pediatrics. (2021). *Fever in newborns: Treatment for babies who otherwise seem well*. https://www.healthychildren.org/English/news/Pages/Fever-in-Newborns.aspx

American Academy of Pediatrics. (2022a). *Circumcision: What you need to know*. https://doi.org/10.1542/peo_document019

American Academy of Pediatrics. (2022b). *Ensuring proper latch on while breastfeeding*. https://www.healthychildren.org/English/ages-stages/baby/breastfeeding/Pages/Ensuring-Proper-Latch-On.aspx?gclid

American Academy of Pediatrics. (2022c). *How to calm a fussy baby: Tips for parents & caregivers*. https://www.healthychildren.org/English/ages-stages/baby/crying-colic/Pages/Calming-A-Fussy-Baby.aspx

American Academy of Pediatrics. (2023). *Safe sleep*. https://www.aap.org/en/patient-care/safe-sleep/

American Academy of Pediatrics. (2024a). *American Academy of Pediatrics updates guidance on assessing hearing in infants, children and adolescents*. https://www.aap.org/en/news-room/news-releases/aap/2023/american-academy-of-pediatrics-updates-guidance-on-assessing-hearing-in-infants-children-and-adolescents/

American Academy of Pediatrics. (2024b). *American Academy of Pediatrics updates safe sleep recommendations: Back is best*. https://www.aap.org/en/news-room/news-releases/aap/2022/american-academy-of-pediatrics-updates-safe-sleep-recommendations-back-is-best/

American Academy of Pediatrics. (2024c). *Car seats: Information for families*. https://www.healthychildren.org/English/safety-prevention/on-the-go/Pages/Car-Safety-Seats-Information-for-Families.aspx

American Academy of Pediatrics. (2024d). *Newborn and infant nutrition*. https://www.aap.org/en/patient-care/newborn-and-infant-nutrition/

American College of Obstetricians and Gynecologists. (2021). *The Apgar score: Committee opinion 644 (reaffirmed 2021)*. https://www.acog.org/clinical/clinical-guidance/committee-opinion/articles/2015/10/the-apgar-score

American College of Obstetricians and Gynecologists. (2022). *Definition of term pregnancy: Committee opinion 579 (reaffirmed 2022)*. https://www.acog.org/clinical/clinical-guidance/committee-opinion/articles/2013/11/definition-of-term-pregnancy

Awopileda, M. (2022). What is the effect of topical breast milk application on umbilical cord separation among healthy babies in the Middle East? *Vanderbilt Undergraduate Research Journal, 12*(1), 25–30. https://doi.org/10.15695/vurj.v12i1.5273

Bedwell, S., & Holtzclaw, B. J. (2022). Early interventions to achieve thermal balance in term neonates. *Nursing for Women's Health*, 26(5),389-396. https://doi.org/10.1016/j.nwh.2022.07.006

Bohara, B. (2025). Abdominal assessment. In C. L. Witt & C. M. Wallman (Eds.), *Tappero & Honeyfield's physical assessment of the newborn: A comprehensive approach to the art of physical examination* (7th ed.). Springer.

Caglar, D. (2022). Evaluation of weight loss in infants six months of age and younger. *UpToDate*. Retrieved March 24, 2024, from https://www.uptodate.com/contents/evaluation-of-weight-loss-in-infants-six-months-of-age-and-younger

Campbell, S. H. (2022). *Lactation: A foundational strategy for health promotion*. Jones & Bartlett Learning.

Centers for Disease Control and Prevention. (2021). *Feeding from a bottle*. https://www.cdc.gov/nutrition/infantandtoddlernutrition/bottle-feeding/index.html

Centers for Disease Control and Prevention. (2023a). *Child and adolescent immunization schedule: Recommendations for ages 18 years or younger, United States, 2024*. https://www.cdc.gov/vaccines/schedules/hcp/imz/child-index.html

Centers for Disease Control and Prevention. (2023b). *Vaccine information statements (VISs)*. https://www.cdc.gov/vaccines/hcp/vis/

Centers for Disease Control and Prevention. (2024). *Infants & toddlers: Safety in the home & community*. https://www.cdc.gov/parents/infants/safety.html

Chamli, A., Aggarwal, P., Jamil, R., & Litaiem, N. (2023). Hemangioma. *StatPearls*. https://www.ncbi.nlm.nih.gov/books/NBK538232/

Chan, Y.-M., & Levitsky, L. L. (2022). Causes of differences of sex development. *UpToDate*. Retrieved April 11, 2024, from https://www.uptodate.com/contents/causes-of-differences-of-sex-development

Chan, Y.-M., & Levitsky, L. L. (2023). Evaluation of the infant with atypical genital appearance (difference of sex development). *UpToDate*. Retrieved April 11, 2024, from https://www.uptodate.com/contents/evaluation-of-the-infant-with-atypical-genital-appearance-difference-of-sex-development

Chen, Y. S., Ho, C. H., Lin, S. J., & Tsai, W. H. (2022). Identifying additional risk factors for early asymptomatic neonatal hypoglycemia in term and late preterm babies. *Pediatrics & Neonatology, 63*(6), 625–632. https://doi.org/10.1016/j.pedneo.2022.04.011

Chua, R. F., & Pico, J. (2023). Dermal melanocytosis. *StatPearls*. https://www.ncbi.nlm.nih.gov/books/NBK557408/

Cranmer, H. (2022). Neonatal hypoglycemia. *Medscape*. https://emedicine.medscape.com/article/802334-overview#a6

Diaz de Ortiz, L. E., & Mendez, M. D. (2023). Palatal and gingival cysts of the newborn. *StatPearls*. https://www.ncbi.nlm.nih.gov/books/NBK493177/

Di Carlo, H. N., & Crigger, C. B. (2025). Chapter 582: Disorders and anomalies of the scrotal contents. In R. M. Kliegman, J. W. St Geme, III, N. J. Blum, R. C. Tasker, K. M. Wilson, A. M. Schuh, C. L. Mack, & M. A Deardorff, *Nelson Textbook of Pediatrics* (22 ed.). Elsevier Health Sciences.

Divya, R., Taksande, A., Balaji, M. K., & Sweetline, C. (2022). Efficacy of counseling in improving LATCH score and successful breastfeeding: A hospital-based prospective cohort study. *Journal of Clinical and Diagnostic Research, 16*(8), p1. https://doi.org/10.7860/JCDR/2022/56968.16685

Duale, A., Singh, P., & Khodor, S. A. (2022). Breast milk: A meal worth having. *Frontiers in Nutrition, 8*, 800927. https://doi.org/10.3389/fnut.2021.800927

Fanning, B. A. (2025). Neurologic assessment. In C. L. Witt & C. M. Wallman (Eds.), *Tappero & Honeyfield's physical assessment of the newborn: A comprehensive approach to the art of physical examination* (7th ed.). Springer.

Fernandez, C. J. (2023). Neonatal resuscitation in the delivery room. *UpToDate*. Retrieved March 18, 2024, from https://www.uptodate.com/contents/neonatal-resuscitation-in-the-delivery-room

Fraser, D. (2025). Chest and lung assessment. In C. L. Witt & C. M. Wallman (Eds.), *Tappero & Honeyfield's physical assessment of the newborn: A comprehensive approach to the art of physical examination* (7th ed.). Springer.

Hand, I., Noble, L., Abrams, S. A., & the Committee on Fetus and Newborn, Section on Breastfeeding, Committee on Nutrition. (2022). Vitamin K and the newborn infant. *Pediatrics, 149*(3), e2021056036. https://doi.org/10.1542/peds.2021-056036

Jain, S., & Bunik, M. (2024). *How often and how much should your baby eat?* https://www.healthychildren.org/English/ages-stages/baby/feeding-nutrition/Pages/How-Often-and-How-Much-Should-Your-Baby-Eat.aspx#

Johnson, P. (2025). Head, eyes, ears, nose, mouth, and neck assessment. In C. L. Witt & C. M. Wallman (Eds.), *Tappero & Honeyfield's physical assessment of the newborn: A comprehensive approach to the art of physical examination* (7th ed.). Springer.

Kain, V., & Mannix, T. (2023). *Neonatal care for nurses and midwives: Principles for practice* (2nd ed.). Elsevier.

La Leche League International. (2024a). *Breastfeeding with sore nipples.* https://www.llli.org/breastfeeding-info/breastfeeding-sore-nipples/

La Leche League International. (2024b). *Engorgement.* https://www.llli.org/breastfeeding-info/engorgement/

La Leche League International. (2024c). *Mastitis and sore breasts.* https://www.llli.org/breastfeeding-info/mastitis/

La Leche League International. (2024d). *Positioning.* https://llli.org/breastfeeding-info/positioning/

La Leche League International. (2024e). *Storing human milk.* https://www.llli.org/breastfeeding-info/storingmilk/

Lee, H. K., & Oh, E. (2023). Care of the well newborn. In E. C. Eichenwald, A. R. Hansen, C. R. Martin, & A. R. Stark (Eds.), *Cloherty & Stark's manual of neonatal care* (9th ed.). Wolters Kluwer.

LeMoine, F. V., Witt, C., Howard, S., Chapple, A., Pam, L., & Sutton, E. F. (2022). Factors attributed to breastfeeding success in a tertiary obstetric hospital. *Women's Health Reports, 3*(1), 624–632. https://doi.org/10.1089/whr.2022.0045

Lipsett, B. J., Reddy, V., & Steanson, K. (2023). Anatomy, head and neck: Fontanelles. *StatPearls.* https://www.ncbi.nlm.nih.gov/books/NBK542197/

Liu, Z., Han, N., Su, T., Ji, Y., Bao, H., Zhou, S., Luo, S., Wang, H., Liu, J., & Wang, H.-J. (2022). Interpretable machine learning to identify important predictors of birth weight: A prospective cohort study. *Frontiers in Pediatrics, 10.* https://doi.org/10.3389/fped.2022.899954

Magge, H. (2022). *Kangaroo mother care may be the best 'medicine' in newborn care.* Bill & Melinda Gates Foundation. https://www.gatesfoundation.org/ideas/articles/kangaroo-mother-care-neonatal-skin-to-skin-contact

Mandy, G. T. (2022). Preterm birth: Definitions of prematurity, epidemiology, and risk factors for infant mortality. *UpToDate.* Retrieved March 18, 2024, from https://www.uptodate.com/contents/preterm-birth-definitions-of-prematurity-epidemiology-and-risk-factors-for-infant-mortality

Matern, D. (2023). Newborn screening for inborn errors of metabolism. *UpToDate.* Retrieved March 25, 2024, from https://www.uptodate.com/contents/newborn-screening-for-inborn-errors-of-metabolism

McKee-Garrett, T. M. (2023). Assessment of the newborn infant. *UpToDate.* https://www.uptodate.com/contents/assessment-of-the-newborn-infant

Meek, J. Y., Noble, L., & Section on Breastfeeding. (2022). Policy statement: Breastfeeding and the use of human milk. *Pediatrics, 150*(1), e2022057988. https://doi.org/10.1542/peds.2022-057988

Moon, R. Y., & Glassy, D. (2022). *Swaddling: Is it safe for your baby?* https://www.healthychildren.org/English/ages-stages/baby/diapers-clothing/Pages/Swaddling-Is-it-Safe.aspx

Mukhopadhyay, S., & Puopolo, K. M. (2023). Bacterial and fungal infections. In E. C. Eichenwald, A. R. Hansen, C. R. Martin, & A. R. Stark (Eds.), *Cloherty & Stark's manual of neonatal care* (9th ed.). Wolters Kluwer.

National Association of Pediatric Nurse Practitioners, Breastfeeding Education Special Interest Group, Busch, D. W., Silbert-Flagg, J., Ryngaert, M., & Scott, A. (2019). NAPNAP position statement on breastfeeding. *Journal of Pediatric Health Care, 33*, A6–A10 https://doi.org/10.1016/j.pedhc.2018.08.011

National Center for Hearing Assessment and Management. (2024). *State EHDI information.* https://www.infanthearing.org/states_home/

Nest 360, & United Nations International Children's Emergency Fund. (n.d.). *Infection prevention and control.* https://newborntoolkit.org/toolkit/infection-prevention-and-control/infection-prevention

Newnam, K. M., & Tasket, A. (2024). Transitional care of the newborn. In B. J. Baker, J. Janke, & Association of Women's Health, Obstetric and Neonatal Nurses, *Core curriculum for maternal-newborn nursing* (6th ed.). Elsevier.

Palazzi, D. L., & Brandt, M. L. (2023). Care of the umbilicus and management of umbilical disorders. *UpToDate.* https://www.uptodate.com/contents/care-of-the-umbilicus-and-management-of-umbilical-disorders

Paulley, L. M., & Duff, E. (2022). Iron deficiency in infants—What nurse practitioners need to know. *The Journal for Nurse Practitioners, 18*(6), 614–617. https://doi.org/10.1016/j.nurpra.2022.03.012

Porto, A., & Abu-Alreesh, S. (2022). *Vitamin D for babies, children & adolescents.* https://www.healthychildren.org/English/healthy-living/nutrition/Pages/vitamin-d-on-the-double.aspx

Priyadarshi, M., Balachander, B., Gupta, S., & Sankar, M. J. (2022). Timing of first bath in term healthy newborns: A systematic review. *Journal of Global Health, 12*, 12004. https://doi.org/10.7189/jogh.12.12004

Reeves, K. M., & Mishtal, J. (2022). Situating parents' circumcision decision-making within health research, knowledge, and experience. *SSM—Qualitative Research in Health, 2*, 100132. https://doi.org/10.1016/j.ssmqr.2022.100132

Roberts, D., Jackson, L., Davie, P., Zhao, C., Harrold, J. A., Fallon, V., & Silverio, S. A. (2023). Exploring the reasons why mothers do not breastfeed, to inform and enable better support. *Frontiers in Global Womens Health, 4.* https://doi.org/10.3389/fgwh.2023.1148719

Roques, E., Ward, R., & Mendez, M. D. (2023). Erythema toxicum. *StatPearls.* https://www.ncbi.nlm.nih.gov/books/NBK470222/

Rossi, S., Buonocore, G., & Bellieni, C. V. (2021). Management of pain in newborn circumcision: A systematic review. *European Journal of Pediatrics, 180*, 13–20. https://doi.org/10.1007/s00431-020-03758-6

Schmitt, B. (2023a). *Circumcision problems.* https://doi.org/10.1542/ppe_schmitt_045

Schmitt, B. (2023b). *Newborn—Taking care of baby.* https://doi.org/10.1542/ppe_schmitt_398

Schmitt, B. (2024). *Newborn illness—How to recognize*. https://www.healthychildren.org/English/tips-tools/symptom-checker/Pages/symptomviewer.aspx?symptom=Newborn+Illness+-+How+to+Recognize

Smialek, D. (2024). *Birth weight percentile calculator*. https://www.omnicalculator.com/health/birthweight-percentile#average-weight-of-newborn-baby

Smith, R. J. H., & Gooi, A. (2023). Hearing loss in children: Etiology. *UpToDate*. Retrieved April 13, 2024, from https://www.uptodate.com/contents/hearing-loss-in-children-etiology

Stockton, M. D. (2022). Nerve block, dorsal penile, neonatal. *Medscape*. https://emedicine.medscape.com/article/1355150-overview

Tappero, E. P. (2025). Musculoskeletal system assessment. In C. L. Witt & C. M. Wallman (Eds.), *Tappero & Honeyfield's physical assessment of the newborn: A comprehensive approach to the art of physical examination* (7th ed.). Springer.

The Joint Commission. (2024). *Sentinel event policy*. https://www.jointcommissioninternational.org/contact-us/sentinel-event-policy/

Tourneux, P., Thiriez, G., Renesme, L., Zores, C., Sizun, J., & Kuhn, P. (2022). Optimizing homeothermy in neonates: A systematic review and clinical guidelines from the French Neonatal Society. *Acta Pediatrica, 111*(8), 1490–1499. https://doi.org/10.1111/apa.16407

Trotter, C. W. (2025). Gestational age assessment. In C. L. Witt & C. M. Wallman (Eds.), *Tappero & Honeyfield's physical assessment of the newborn: A comprehensive approach to the art of physical examination* (7th ed.). Springer.

United Nations International Children's Emergency Fund. (n.d.). *Baby basics: How to burp your baby*. https://www.unicef.org/parenting/child-care/how-to-burp-baby

U.S. Department of Health and Human Services. (2020). *Healthy People 2030 infants*. https://health.gov/healthypeople/objectives-and-data/browse-objectives/infants

U.S. Food & Drug Administration. (2022). *Questions & answers for consumers concerning infant formula*. https://www.fda.gov/food/people-risk-foodborne-illness/questions-answers-consumers-concerning-infant-formula

U.S. Preventive Services Task Force. (2019). *Final recommendation statement: Ocular prophylaxis for gonococcal ophthalmia neonatorum: Preventive medication*. https://www.uspreventiveservicestaskforce.org/uspstf/recommendation/ocular-prophylaxis-for-gonococcal-ophthalmia-neonatorum-preventive-medication

Vargo, L. (2025). Cardiovascular assessment. In C. L. Witt & C. M. Wallman (Eds.), *Tappero & Honeyfield's physical assessment of the newborn: A comprehensive approach to the art of physical examination* (7th ed.). Springer.

Vohr, B. R. (2023). Screening the newborn for hearing loss. *UpToDate*. Retrieved April 13, 2024, from https://www.uptodate.com/contents/screening-the-newborn-for-hearing-loss

Webster, K., Stikes, R., Bunnell, L., & Petruska, S. (2021). Application of human factors methods to ensure appropriate infant identification and abduction prevention within the hospital setting. *Journal of Perinatal & Neonatal Nursing, 35*, 258–265. https://doi.org/10.1097/JPN.0000000000000554

Weiner, G. M., & Zaichkin, J. (2021). *Textbook of neonatal resuscitation* (8th ed.). American Academy of Pediatrics.

Weiner, G. M., & Zaichkin, J. (2022). Updates for the neonatal resuscitation program and resuscitation guidelines. *NeoReviews, 23*(4), 238–249. https://doi.org/10.1542/neo.23-4-e238

Witt, C. L. (2025). Skin assessment. In C. L. Witt & C. M. Wallman (Eds.), *Tappero & Honeyfield's physical assessment of the newborn: A comprehensive approach to the art of physical examination* (7th ed.). Springer.

Witt, C. L., & Wallman, C. M. (Eds.). (2025). *Tappero & Honeyfield's physical assessment of the newborn: A comprehensive approach to the art of physical examination* (7th ed.). Springer.

DEVELOPING CLINICAL JUDGMENT

PRACTICING FOR NCLEX

1. At birth, a newborn's assessment reveals the following: HR of 140 bpm, loud crying, some flexion of extremities, crying when bulb syringe is introduced into the nares, and a pink body with blue extremities. What would the nurse document the newborn's Apgar score as?
   a. 5 points
   b. 6 points
   c. 7 points
   d. 8 points

2. The nurse is caring for a newborn in the delivery room. What is the purpose of the nurse administering a dose of vitamin K intramuscularly?
   a. Promotes conjugation of bilirubin
   b. Prevents blood clotting
   c. Closes the foreman ovale
   d. Digests complex proteins

3. Shortly after delivery, a prophylactic agent is instilled in both eyes of the newborn. What condition does this prevent?
   a. Gonorrhea conjunctivitis
   b. Thrush and enterobacter
   c. *Staphylococcus* and syphilis
   d. Hepatitis B and herpes

4. The current recommendation is for all newborns be placed on their backs to sleep. The nurse will teach the parents that this position reduces the risk of what?
   a. Respiratory distress syndrome
   b. Bottle mouth syndrome
   c. SUID
   d. Gastrointestinal regurgitation syndrome

5. The nurse is teaching a new graduate about newborn vaccination. Which immunization will the nurse teach is given to newborns before hospital discharge?
   a. Pneumococcus
   b. Varicella
   c. Hepatitis A
   d. Hepatitis B

6. The nurse has completed the comprehensive assessment of a newborn. Which finding would the nurse document as abnormal when assessing the newborn's head?
   a. Two soft spots palpated between the cranial bones
   b. A spongy area of edema outlined on the head
   c. Head circumference 32 cm, chest 34 cm
   d. Asymmetry of the head with overriding bones

7. The nurse has completed assessment of a newborn. Which finding would be considered normal?
   a. Passage of meconium within the first 24 hours
   b. Respiratory rate of 80 breaths/min
   c. Yellow skin tones 10 hours after birth
   d. Bleeding from the umbilicus area

8. Which parameters are measured in determining an Apgar score? Select all that apply.
   a. Blood pressure
   b. Oxygen saturation
   c. Skin color
   d. Reflex irritability
   e. Alertness

CRITICAL THINKING EXERCISES

1. A birthing parent who delivered their first baby and is on the postpartum unit calls the nursery nurse into the room and expresses concern about how their daughter looks. The parent tells the nurse that the baby's head looks like a "banana" and is mushy to the touch and that she has "white spots" all over her nose. In addition, there appear to be "big bluish bruises" all over the baby's buttocks. The parent wants to know what is wrong with their baby and whether these problems will go away.
   a. How should the nurse respond to this parent's questions?
   b. What additional newborn instruction might be appropriate at this time?
   c. What reassurance can be given to this new parent regarding their daughter's appearance?

2. At approximately 12:30 a.m. on a Friday, a person enters a hospital through a busy emergency department. They are wearing a white uniform and a lab coat with a stethoscope around their neck. They identify themselves as a new nurse coming back to check on something they had left on the unit on an earlier shift. The person enters a postpartum patient's room containing a newborn, pushes the open crib down a hallway, and leaves through an exit. The security cameras aren't working. The infant isn't discovered missing until the 2 a.m. check by the nurse.
   a. What impact does an infant abduction have on the family and the hospital?
   b. What security measure was the weak link in the chain of security?
   c. What can hospitals do to prevent infant abduction?

STUDY ACTIVITIES

1. Obtain a set of vital signs (temperature, pulse, and respiration) of a newborn on admission to the nursery. Repeat this procedure and compare changes in the values several hours later. Discuss what changes in the vital signs you would expect during this transitional period.
2. Interview a new parent on the postpartum unit on their second day about the changes they have noticed in their newborn's appearance and behavior within the past 24 hours. Discuss your interview findings at post conference.
3. Demonstrate a newborn bath to a new parent in their room, using the principle of bathing from the cleanest to the dirtiest body part. Discuss the questions asked by the parent and their reaction to the demonstration in post conference.
4. Go to the La Leche League website. Review the information it provides on breastfeeding. How helpful would it be to a new parent?
5. Debate the risks and benefits of neonatal circumcision within your nursing group at post conference. Did either side present a stronger position? What is your opinion, and why?

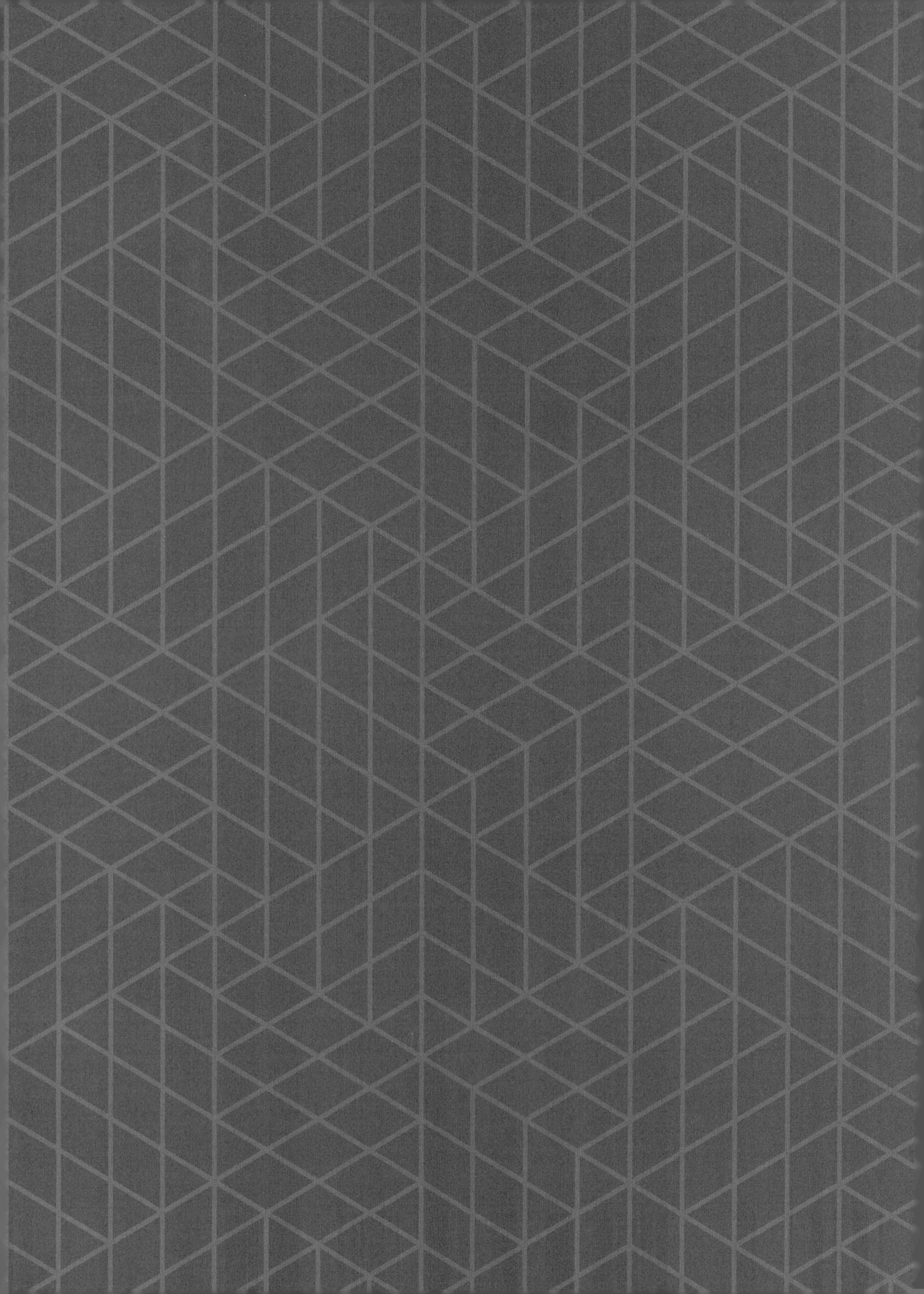

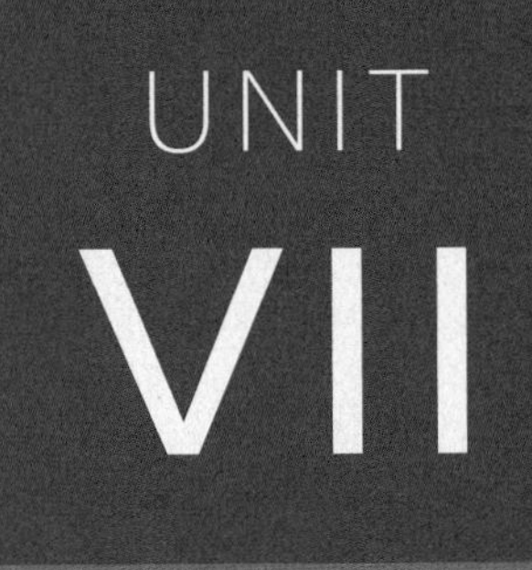

Childbearing at Risk

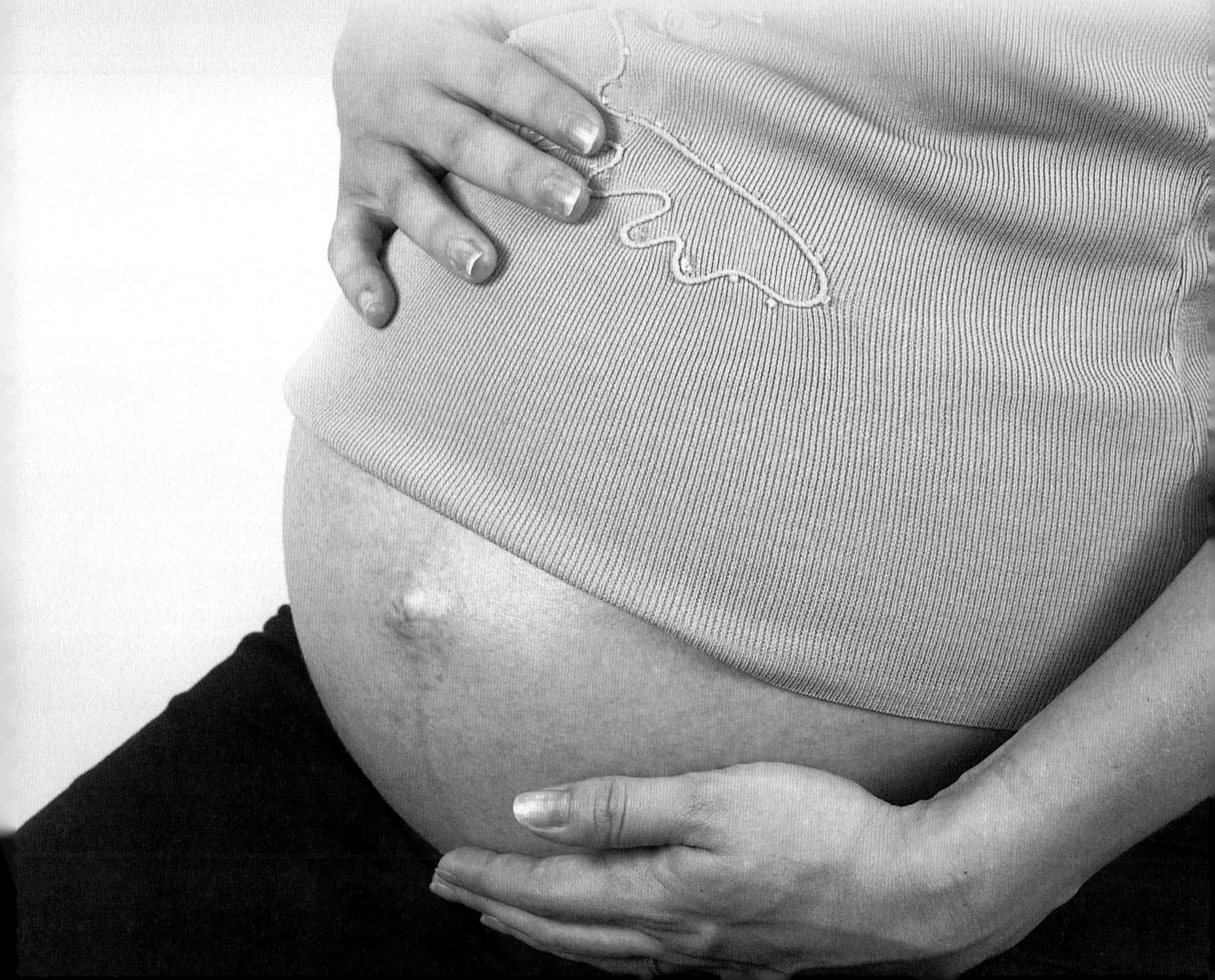

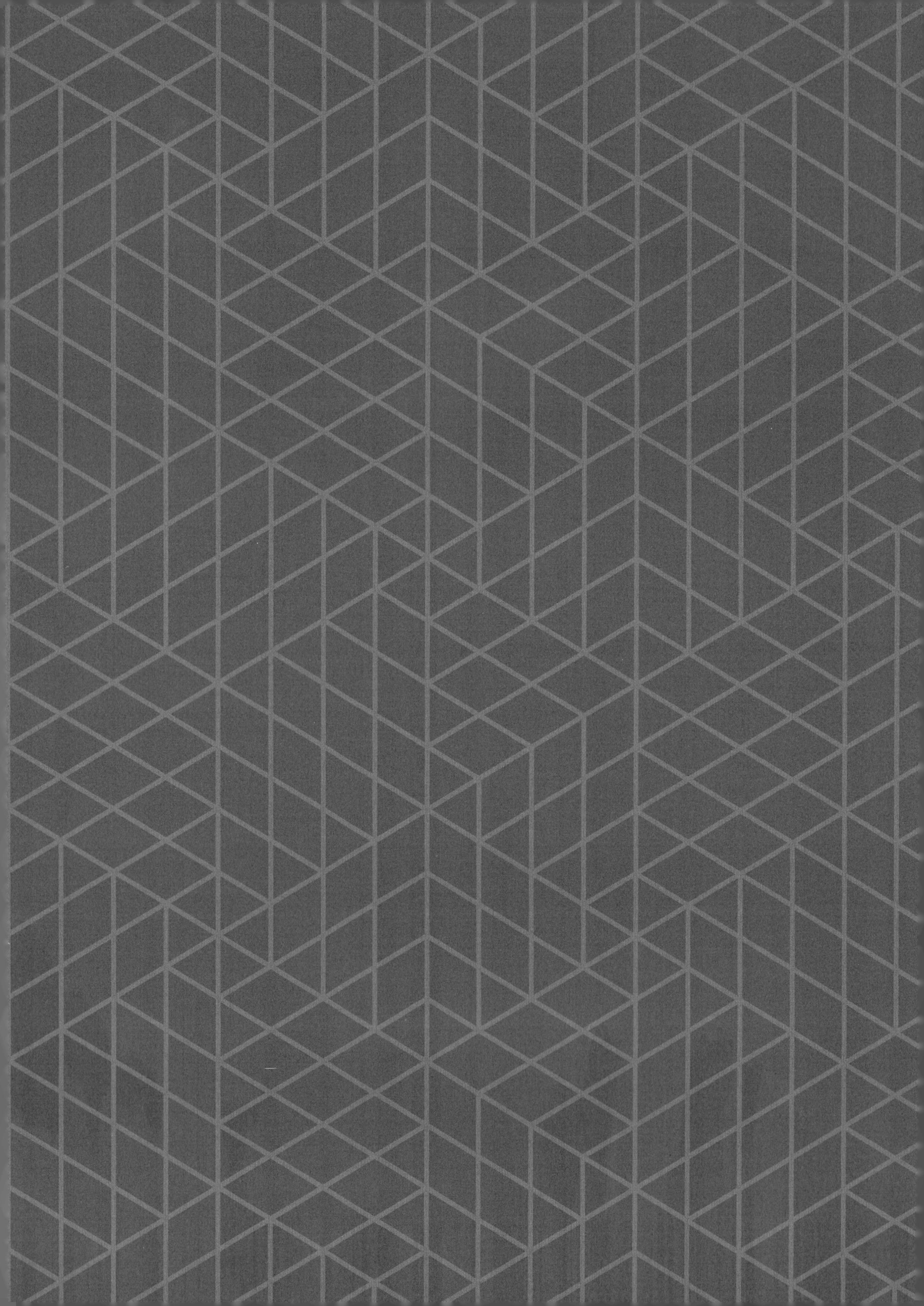

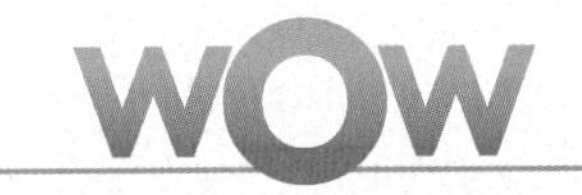

WORDS OF WISDOM

Detours and bumps along the road of life can be managed, but many cannot be entirely avoided.

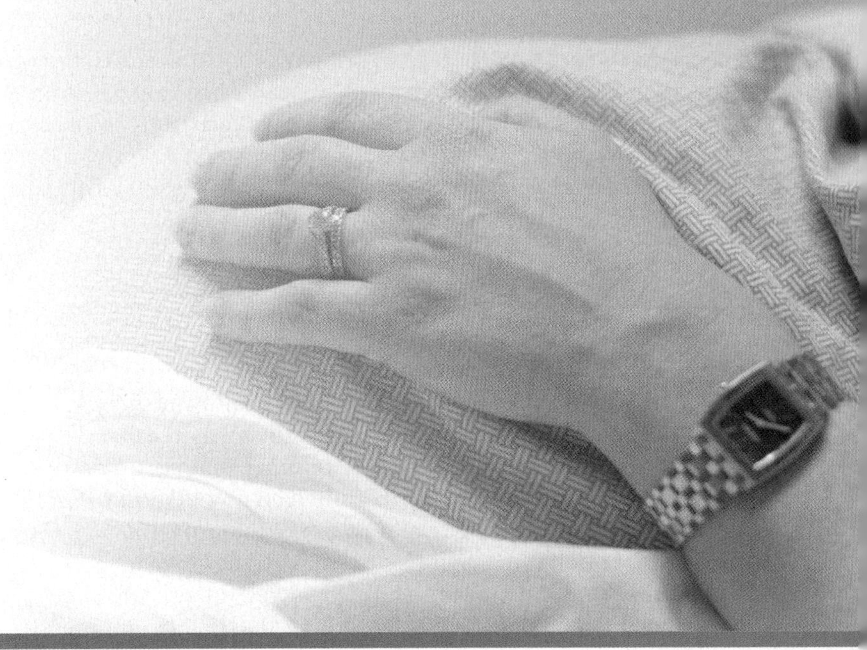

19

Nursing Management of Pregnancy at Risk: Pregnancy-Related Complications

KEY TERMS

abortion
eclampsia (ek-lamp'sē-ă)
ectopic pregnancy
gestational hypertension
gestational trophoblastic disease (GTD) (jes-tā'shŭn-ŭl trof'ō-blas'tik di-zēz)
high-risk pregnancy
hyperemesis gravidarum (hī'pĕr-em'ĕ-sis grav'i-dăr'ŭm)
multiple gestation
oligohydramnios (ol'i-gō-hī-dram'nē-os)
placenta accreta spectrum
placenta previa
placental abruption
polyhydramnios (pol'ē-hī-dram'nē-os)
preeclampsia
prelabor rupture of membranes (PROM)
preterm prelabor rupture of membranes (PPROM)

LEARNING OBJECTIVES

Upon completion of the chapter, you will be able to:

1. Compare and contrast a normal pregnancy to a high-risk one. Determine the common factors that might place a pregnancy at high risk.
2. Detect the causes of vaginal bleeding during early and late pregnancy.
3. Outline nursing assessment and management for the pregnant patient experiencing vaginal bleeding.
4. Identify current evidence-based guidelines used to effectively screen, diagnose, and manage placenta accreta spectrum disorders.
5. Develop plans of care for patients experiencing preeclampsia, eclampsia, and hemolysis, elevated liver enzymes, and low platelet count (HELLP) syndrome.
6. Describe Rh incompatibility and hemolytic disease of the newborn.
7. Examine the pathophysiology of imbalances in amniotic fluid and subsequent management.
8. Explore multiple gestation and possible complications for both the birthing parent and fetus.
9. Evaluate factors in a patient's prenatal history that place them at risk for prelabor rupture of membranes (PROM).
10. Formulate a teaching plan for maintaining the health of pregnant patients experiencing a high-risk pregnancy.

Helen, a 35-year-old G5P4, presents to the labor and birth suite with severe abdominal pain. She reports that the pain began suddenly about an hour ago while she was resting. She has had two prior cesarean births and thus far has had an uneventful past 32 weeks. Helen appears distressed and is moaning. What additional assessments do you need to do to care for Helen? What might be your immediate nursing action?

INTRODUCTION

Many people think of pregnancy as a natural process with a positive outcome—the birth of a healthy newborn. Unfortunately, conditions can occur that may result in negative outcomes for the fetus, birthing parent, or both. A **high-risk pregnancy** is one in which a condition exists that jeopardizes the health of the birthing parent, their fetus, or both. In a high-risk pregnancy, the birthing parent and fetus (or newborn) are at increased risk of morbidity or mortality prenatally, during the gestation, or postnatally.

Pregnant people who are considered to be at high risk have a higher morbidity and mortality compared with parents in the general population. The risk status of a pregnant person and their fetus can change during the pregnancy due to a number of problems occurring during labor, birth, or afterward, even in patients without any known previous prenatal risk. Preexisting chronic conditions are strongly linked to poor pregnancy outcomes (Myers, 2022). Examples of high-risk conditions include diabetes, hypertension, HIV infection, overweight or obesity, pregnancy history (preterm labor, fetal growth restriction, preeclampsia, still birth, or complications in a prior pregnancy), older or younger age, and multiple gestation (National Institute of Child Health and Human Development, 2022). Many obstetric complications and conditions are life-threatening emergencies with high morbidity and mortality rates. It is essential that these be identified early to ensure the best possible outcome for the birthing parent and infant.

The term "risk" may mean different things to different groups. For example, health care providers may focus on disease processes and treatments to prevent complications. Nurses may focus on nursing care and on the psychosocial impact on the patient and their family. Health insurance companies may focus on the economic issues related to the high-risk status. The birthing parent's attention may be focused on their own needs and those of their family. Together, working as a collaborative team, the goal of care is to ensure the best possible outcome for the patient, fetus, and family.

Risk assessment begins at the first prenatal visit and continues with each subsequent visit because factors may be identified in later visits that were not apparent during earlier visits. For example, as the nurse and patient develop a trusting relationship, previously unidentified or unsuspected factors (such as substance use disorder or intimate partner violence) may be revealed. Through education and support, the nurse can encourage the patient to inform the health care provider of these concerns, and necessary interventions or referrals can be made.

Various factors must be considered when determining a patient's risk for adverse pregnancy outcomes, and a comprehensive approach to high-risk pregnancy is needed. For example, prenatal stress and distress have been shown to have significant consequences for the birthing parent, child, and family. Pregnancy-specific stress such as depression, anxiety, and perceived stress may increase the risk for adverse birth outcomes and is associated with preterm births and intrauterine fetal growth restriction. Research results show screening for significant anxiety symptoms in the first and last terms can help prevent early births (Schetter et al., 2022). Another factor to be considered is race and ancestry: In the United States, severe maternal morbidity is consistently higher among Black, Latina, and Asian women when compared to White women, regardless of their age (Myers, 2022).

This chapter describes the major conditions directly related to pregnancy that can complicate a pregnancy, possibly affecting maternal and fetal outcomes. These include bleeding during pregnancy (spontaneous abortion, ectopic pregnancy, gestational trophoblastic disease [GTD], cervical insufficiency, placenta previa, placental abruption, and placenta accreta), hyperemesis gravidarum, gestational hypertension, HELLP syndrome, gestational diabetes, blood incompatibility, amniotic fluid imbalances (polyhydramnios and oligohydramnios), multiple gestation, and PROM. Chapter 20 addresses preexisting conditions that can complicate a patient's pregnancy as well as populations that are considered to be at high risk.

BLEEDING DURING PREGNANCY

Bleeding at any time during pregnancy is potentially life threatening. Every minute of every day, a person dies in pregnancy or childbirth. The biggest killer is obstetric hemorrhage, the successful treatment of which is a challenge worldwide. Management of obstetric hemorrhage involves early recognition, assessment, and resuscitation. Bleeding can occur early or late in the pregnancy and may result from numerous conditions. Bleeding is a common concern during the first trimester of pregnancy (Norwitz & Park, 2023). A transvaginal ultrasound is helpful in evaluating bleeding in early pregnancy to determine the cause (Norwitz & Park, 2023). Conditions commonly associated with early bleeding (first half of pregnancy) include spontaneous abortion, uterine fibroids, ectopic pregnancy, GTD, and cervical insufficiency. Conditions associated with late bleeding include placenta previa, placental abruption, and placenta accreta, which usually occur after the 20th week of gestation.

Spontaneous Abortion

Pregnancy is a significant event in a person's life and is often a time of great expectations. Therefore, experiencing a pregnancy loss can be not only a devasting experience but a very lonely one as the person is separated from their hopes and dreams. An **abortion** is the loss of an early pregnancy, usually before week 20 of gestation. Abortion can be spontaneous or induced. It is considered not only a major reproductive health matter but also a health risk factor for the patient's well-being. Spontaneous abortion, or miscarriage, is the most common complication of early pregnancy and can be both physically and emotionally painful (Prager et al., 2024). A spontaneous abortion refers to the loss of a fetus resulting from natural causes, that is, not elective or therapeutically induced by a procedure. Laypeople often use the term "miscarriage" to denote an abortion that has occurred spontaneously. A miscarriage can occur during very early pregnancy, and many people who miscarry may not even be aware that they are pregnant. The incidence of early pregnancy loss is as high as 31% in the first trimester (Prager et al., 2024). The frequency of spontaneous abortion increases further with advancing maternal age. The causes of spontaneous abortion are varied and often unknown. The terms threatened abortion, incomplete abortion, inevitable abortion, and missed abortion were historically used to categorize abortions. The terms are nonspecific and are no longer preferred for use.

While a miscarriage is a loss before the 20th week, a stillbirth is the loss of a fetus after the 20th week of development. Stillbirths are much less common than miscarriages, occurring in about six of every 1,000 pregnancies in the United States (Centers for Disease Control and Prevention [CDC], 2022).

A vaginal ultrasound may confirm an empty or partially filled amniotic sac. The provider may have human chorionic gonadotropin (hCG) levels drawn to determine pregnancy loss. In the first trimester, if the abortion is not complete and products of conception remain, cervical dilatation and suction curettage are implemented to reduce the risk of excessive bleeding and infection. An alternative is the administration of a prostaglandin analogue (misoprostol) to empty the uterus of retained tissue. In the second trimester, the patient is admitted to the hospital for an augmented labor and delivery. Nursing care would focus on the care of the laboring patient, with tremendous attention paid to providing emotional support to the patient and their family.

Nursing Assessment

When a pregnant person calls and reports vaginal bleeding, they must be seen as soon as possible by a health care professional to ascertain the etiology. Varying degrees of vaginal bleeding, low back pain, abdominal cramping, and passage of products of conception tissue may be reported. Ask the patient about the color of the vaginal bleeding (bright red is significant) and the amount—for example, question them about the frequency with which they are changing their peripads (saturation of one peripad hourly is significant) and the passage of any clots or tissue. Instruct the patient to save any tissue or clots that have passed and bring them to the health care facility. Also, obtain a description of any other signs and symptoms the patient may be experiencing, along with a description of their severity and duration. It is important to remain calm and listen to the patient's description.

When the patient arrives at the health care facility, assess their vital signs and observe the amount, color, and characteristics of the bleeding. Ask the patient to rate their current pain level, using an appropriate pain assessment tool. Also evaluate the amount and intensity of the patient's abdominal cramping or contractions, and assess the patient's level of understanding about what is happening to them.

Nursing Management

Nursing care for the patient with a spontaneous abortion focuses on providing continued monitoring and psychological support because the family is often experiencing acute loss and grief. An important component of this support is reassuring the patient that spontaneous abortions usually result from an abnormality and that their actions did not cause the abortion.

PROVIDING CONTINUED MONITORING

Continued monitoring and ongoing assessments are essential for the patient experiencing a spontaneous abortion. Monitor the amount of vaginal bleeding through pad counts and observe for passage of products of conception tissue. Assess for pain and provide appropriate pain management to address the cramping discomfort.

Assist in preparing the patient for procedures and treatments such as surgery to evacuate the uterus or medications such as misoprostol or prostaglandin E2 (PGE2). If the patient is Rh-negative and not sensitized, expect to administer RhoGAM within 72 hours after the abortion is complete. Drug Guide 19.1 provides more information about these medications.

DRUG GUIDE 19.1

MEDICATIONS RELATED TO ABORTIONS

Medication	Action/Indications	Nursing Implications
Misoprostol (Cytotec)	Stimulates uterine contractions to terminate a pregnancy and to evacuate the uterus after abortion to ensure passage of all the products of conception; taken 24–48 hours after mifepristone	• Monitor for side effects such as diarrhea, abdominal pain, nausea, vomiting, and dyspepsia. • Assess vaginal bleeding, and report any increased bleeding, pain, or fever. • Monitor for signs and symptoms of shock, such as tachycardia, hypotension, and anxiety.
Mifepristone (Korlym)	Acts as a progesterone antagonist, allowing prostaglandins to stimulate uterine contractions; causes the endometrium to slough; may be followed by administration of misoprostol within 48 hours	• Monitor for headache, vomiting, diarrhea, and heavy bleeding. • Anticipate administration of antiemetic prior to use to reduce nausea and vomiting. • Encourage the patient to use acetaminophen to reduce discomfort from cramping.
PGE2, dinoprostone (Prostin E2 suppository)	Stimulates uterine contractions, causing expulsion of uterine contents; expels uterine contents in fetal death or spontaneous abortion during the second trimester; effaces and dilates the cervix in pregnancy at term	• Bring the drug to room temperature prior to use. • Administer the suppository high in the vagina; it may be repeated every 3–5 hours. • Avoid contact with skin. • Use sterile technique to administer. • Keep the patient supine for 10 minutes after administering. • Explain the drug's purpose and expected response to the patient.
Rho(D) immunoglobulin (RhoGAM, Gamulin, HyperRho S/D, MICRhoGAM)	Suppresses immune response to prevent isoimmunization in nonsensitized Rh-negative patients exposed to Rh-positive blood after abortion, miscarriage, or pregnancy	• Administer intramuscularly in the deltoid area. • HyperRho mini-dose and MICRhoGAM for abortion up to 12 weeks gestation, RhoGAM after 12 weeks gestation • Educate the patient that they will need this after subsequent deliveries if the infants are Rh-positive; also check lab study results prior to administering the drug.

UpToDate, Inc. (2024). *UpToDate® Lexidrug*™ (Version 8.2.0) [Mobile app]. Wolters Kluwer. https://apps.apple.com/us/app/lexicomp/id313401238

PROVIDING SUPPORT

Pregnancy loss subjects parents to a multitude of emotions and may have significant consequences on their mental health. A patient's emotional reaction may vary depending on their desire for the pregnancy and their available support network. Provide both physical and emotional support. In addition, prepare the patient and their family for the assessment process and answer their questions.

Explaining some of the causes of spontaneous abortions can help the patient understand what is happening and may allay any possible fear or feelings of guilt that they did something to cause the pregnancy loss. Many patients experience an acute sense of loss and go through a grieving process with a spontaneous abortion. Providing sensitive listening, counseling, and anticipatory guidance to the patients and their family will allow them to verbalize their feelings and ask questions about future pregnancies.

The grieving period may last years after a pregnancy loss, with each person grieving in their own way. Encourage friends and family to be supportive, but give the family space and time to work through their loss. Referral to a community support group for parents who have experienced a loss can be helpful during this grief process. Sensitive, caring, and skilled nursing care for all patients experiencing a miscarriage will play an important role in their long-term emotional recovery.

Ectopic Pregnancy

The term "ectopic" is derived from the Greek word *ektopos,* meaning "out of place." Accordingly, an **ectopic pregnancy** is any pregnancy in which the fertilized ovum implants outside the main cavity of the uterus, including the fallopian tubes, cervix, ovary, and the abdominal cavity (Fig. 19.1). None of these anatomic sites can accommodate placental attachment or a growing embryo.

Ectopic pregnancies usually result from conditions that obstruct or slow the passage of the fertilized ovum through the fallopian tube to the uterus. This may be a physical blockage in the tube or failure of the tubal epithelium to move the zygote (the cell formed after the egg is fertilized) down the tube into the uterus. The most common extrauterine location for implantation is the fallopian tube, which accounts for 96% of all ectopic gestations (Tulandi, 2023c). The incidence increases with advancing maternal age.

The abnormally implanted embryo grows and draws its blood supply from the site of abnormal implantation. As the embryo enlarges, it creates the potential for organ rupture because only the uterine cavity is designed to expand and accommodate fetal development. Ectopic pregnancies carry high rates of morbidity and mortality

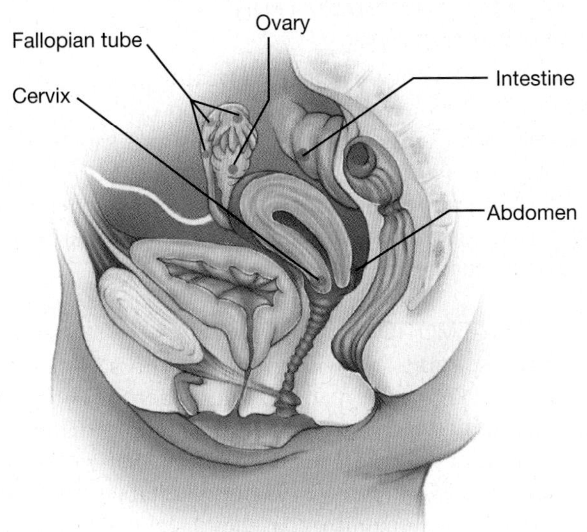

FIGURE 19.1 Possible sites for implantation with an ectopic pregnancy.

if not identified and treated promptly—they can lead to massive hemorrhage, infertility, or death.

Ectopic pregnancies occur in about 1.5% to 2% of pregnancies in the United States (Tulandi, 2023c). While the overall maternal mortality rate associated with ectopic pregnancy has decreased, the mortality rate is higher in Black people than in White people and also increases with advancing maternal age (Tulandi, 2023c). The discovery of ectopic pregnancies prior to rupture has increased dramatically in the past few decades as a result of improved diagnostic techniques such as the development of sensitive and specific radioimmunoassays for beta-hCG (levels will be low) and high-resolution ultrasonography allowing visualization of an extrauterine gestational sac (Tulandi, 2023b).

Ectopic pregnancy is a potentially life-threatening condition and involves pregnancy loss. With the growth of the embryo, rupture may occur, followed by hemorrhage. A ruptured ectopic pregnancy is a medical emergency; therefore, prediction of any tubal rupture before its occurrence is extremely important.

Therapeutic Management

In clinically stable patients who have been diagnosed with nonruptured ectopic pregnancies, intramuscular (IM) methotrexate administration or laparoscopic surgery are safe and effective treatments. In the hemodynamically stable patient with an early diagnosis, no signs of active bleeding in the peritoneal cavity, low beta-hCG levels, and a mass less than 4 cm in size, a single dose of methotrexate may be given. Medical management with methotrexate, though not approved by the U.S. Food and Drug Administration (FDA) for this purpose, has been endorsed by the American College of Obstetricians and Gynecologists (ACOG, 2022a). Methotrexate is a folic acid antagonist that inhibits cell division in the developing embryo. It typically has been used as a chemotherapeutic agent in the treatment of leukemia, lymphoma, and rheumatoid arthritis. Its results are similar to those of surgical therapy in terms of high success rate, low complication rate, and good reproductive potential (Tulandi, 2023a).

Surgical management for the unruptured fallopian tube might involve a linear salpingostomy to preserve the tube—an important consideration for the patient who wants to preserve future fertility. It may also be considered when medical treatment is considered unsuitable. With a ruptured ectopic pregnancy, surgery is necessary as a result of possible uncontrolled hemorrhage. A laparotomy with the removal of the tube (salpingectomy) may be necessary. With earlier diagnosis and medical management, the focus has changed from preventing maternal death to facilitating rapid recovery and preserving fertility.

Nursing Assessment

Nursing assessment focuses on determining the existence of an ectopic pregnancy and whether or not it has ruptured. A patient with a suspected ectopic pregnancy may have to undergo several diagnostic tests, some of which are invasive. Consider how the patient might feel during all of these tests, anticipate their questions, and offer them thorough explanations and reassurances.

HEALTH HISTORY AND PHYSICAL EXAMINATION

Determine risk factors for ectopic pregnancy including:

- Previous ectopic pregnancy
- History of pelvic inflammatory disease (PID), other genital infections, or endometriosis
- Infertility and assisted reproduction use
- Sterilization failure or intrauterine device use
- Cigarette smoking
- Routine vaginal douching
- In-utero exposure to diethylstilbestrol (DES)

Assess the patient thoroughly for signs and symptoms that may suggest an ectopic pregnancy. The onset of signs and symptoms varies, but they usually begin at about the seventh or eighth week of gestation. A missed menstrual period, adnexal fullness, and tenderness may indicate an unruptured tubal pregnancy. As the tube stretches, the pain increases. Pain may be unilateral, bilateral, or diffuse over the abdomen. Tubal rupture may be associated with an abrupt onset of severe pain. With more extensive, sufficient intra-abdominal bleeding, referred pain may be felt in the shoulder (Tulandi, 2023b).

> **TAKE NOTE!**
>
> The hallmark of ectopic pregnancy is abdominal pain with spotting within 6 to 8 weeks after a missed menstrual period. Many people have symptoms typical of early pregnancy, such as breast tenderness, nausea, fatigue, shoulder pain, and low back pain.

Nursing Management

Nursing care for the patient with an ectopic pregnancy focuses on pain management, providing medication, offering support, and providing education about treatment and follow-up. Administer analgesics as ordered to promote comfort and relieve discomfort from abdominal pain. Although the intensity of the pain can vary, patients often report a great deal of pain. With either medical or surgical treatment of ectopic pregnancy, ask the patient about their feelings and concerns related to future fertility, and provide teaching about the need to use contraceptives for at least three menstrual cycles to allow the reproductive tract to heal and the tissue to be repaired. If the patient has a spouse or partner, include them in this discussion to make sure both parties understand what has happened, what intervention is needed, and what the future holds regarding childbearing. Whether treated with medication or surgery, all Rh-negative nonsensitized patients are given Rh immunoglobulin (RhIG) to prevent isoimmunization in future pregnancies.

PROVIDING MEDICATION THERAPY

Prior to the patient receiving methotrexate to treat an unruptured ectopic pregnancy, counsel them about the risks; benefits; adverse effects; and possibility of failure of medical therapy, which would result in tubal rupture, necessitating surgery (ACOG, 2022a). Methotrexate is dosed based on the patient's body surface area and is usually given as a single-dose IM injection. As a chemotherapy agent, it should only be administered by people who have had education and training in the handling and administration of hazardous drugs.

Educate the patient about the potential adverse effects associated with methotrexate, including nausea, vomiting, stomatitis, diarrhea, gastric upset, increased abdominal pain, and dizziness. Instruct the patient to return on Days 4 and 7 for follow-up beta-hCG titers. After the beta-hCG level has decreased by more than 15%, it is then monitored weekly until it is nondetectable (Cunningham et al., 2022b). Outline the signs and symptoms of ectopic rupture (severe, sharp, stabbing, unilateral abdominal pain; vertigo/fainting; hypotension; and increased pulse), and advise the patient to seek medical help immediately if they occur.

PROVIDING PREOPERATIVE AND POSTOPERATIVE CARE

Prepare the patient physiologically and psychologically for surgery. Provide a clear explanation of the expected outcome. After surgery, closely assess and monitor the patient's vital signs and bleeding (peritoneal or vaginal) to identify hypovolemic shock. Assess the patient's pain, and provide nonpharmacologic comfort measures and prescribed analgesics to manage the pain.

PROVIDING EMOTIONAL SUPPORT

Emotional support following pregnancy loss is vital for the holistic care of the patient. The patient with an ectopic pregnancy requires support throughout diagnosis, treatment, and aftercare. A person's psychological reaction to an ectopic pregnancy is unpredictable. However, it is important to recognize that they have experienced a pregnancy loss in addition to undergoing treatment for a potentially life-threatening condition. The patient may find it difficult to comprehend what has happened to them because events occur so quickly. The patient may be confused, questioning why and how they had just started a pregnancy that now has ended abruptly. Bleeding during any pregnancy is traumatic because of the uncertainty of the outcome. Help the patient cope with this experience by encouraging the patient and their family to express their feelings and concerns openly and by validating that this is a loss of pregnancy and that it is OK to grieve over the loss. Although the patient may have physically recovered from an ectopic pregnancy, they may still experience significant emotional distress for a long time.

Provide emotional support, spiritual care, and information about community support groups (such as Resolve through Sharing) as the patient grieves for the loss of their unborn child and comes to terms with the medical complications of the situation. Acknowledge the patient's pregnancy and allow them to discuss their feelings about what the pregnancy means.

PREVENTING FUTURE ECTOPIC PREGNANCIES

Preventing ectopic pregnancies through screening and patient education is essential. Many can be prevented by avoiding conditions that might cause scarring of the fallopian tubes. In addition, a contributing factor to the development of ectopic pregnancy is a previous ectopic pregnancy. Therefore, educating the patient is crucial. Prevention education may include:

- Reduce risk factors such as sexual intercourse with multiple partners or intercourse without a condom.
- Avoid contracting sexually transmitted infections (STIs) that lead to PID.
- Use condoms to decrease the risk of infections that cause tubal scarring.
- Obtain early diagnosis and adequate treatment of STIs.

- If an intrauterine contraceptive system is chosen, recognize the signs of PID to reduce the risk of repeat ascending infections, which can be responsible for tubal scarring.
- Avoid smoking during childbearing years since a correlation with an increase in risk exists.
- Seek prenatal care early to confirm the location of the pregnancy.

Gestational Trophoblastic Disease

Gestational trophoblastic disease (GTD) is a spectrum of benign and malignant disorders that are created from abnormal trophoblastic tissue. The classification of GTD includes disorders of placental development (hydatidiform mole—complete and partial) and neoplasms of the trophoblast (choriocarcinoma, invasive mole, epithelioid trophoblastic tumor, and placental site trophoblastic tumor) (AlJulaih & Muzio, 2023). This discussion will focus on hydatidiform mole and choriocarcinoma.

GTD is a proliferation of trophoblastic tissue in pregnant or recently pregnant people. A common feature of all trophoblastic lesions is that they produce hCG, which serves as a clinical marker for the presence of persistent or progressive trophoblastic disease (Cunningham et al., 2022c). With GTD, there is abnormal hyperproliferation of trophoblastic cells that would normally develop into the placenta during pregnancy. Gestational tissue is present, but the pregnancy is not viable. The incidence is hard to determine due to uncommon diagnosis and inaccuracy of documentation of pregnancy loss, but it is thought to occur in about 110 to 120 per 100,000 pregnancies in the United States (National Cancer Institute, 2022).

Pathophysiology

The pathogenesis of GTD is unique because the maternal tumor arises from gestational rather than maternal tissue. Refer to Table 19.1 for an explanation of the pathophysiology of GTD.

Therapeutic Management

Molar pregnancy can be removed via surgical uterine evacuation (dilatation and curettage [D&C]) or a hysterectomy. Uterine evacuation preserves future childbearing ability. With either procedure, the risk of developing a gestational trophoblastic neoplasm is 15% to 20% (Berkowitz et al., 2022). Following surgery, serial measurements of beta hCG are taken until they become nondetectable. The patient should use a reliable contraceptive for at least 6 months (Cunningham et al., 2022c). Choriocarcinoma is treated with chemotherapy with an overall remission rate of around 90% (Cunningham et al., 2022c).

Nursing Assessment

The nurse plays a crucial role in identifying and bringing this condition to the attention of the health care provider based on sound knowledge of the typical clinical manifestations and astute prenatal assessments. Explore the patient's history for risk factors for molar pregnancy including extremes of maternal age, prior molar pregnancy, infertility, prior spontaneous abortion, and vitamin A deficiency (Berkowitz et al., 2023). The main risk factor for the development of choriocarcinoma is the history of complete hydatidiform mole (Berkowitz et al., 2022). Clinical manifestations of a molar pregnancy include vaginal bleeding, pelvic pressure or pain, enlarged uterus, preeclampsia, and hyperemesis gravidarum.

Typically, without symptoms, the first symptom of choriocarcinoma may be shortness of breath (80% of patients demonstrate metastasis to the lungs) (Berkowitz et al., 2022).

Nursing Management

Nursing care for the patient with GTD focuses on preparing them for a D&C, providing emotional support to deal with the loss and potential risks, and educating them

TABLE 19.1 • Pathophysiology of Gestational Trophoblastic Disease

Type	Incidence	Description	Development	Karyotype
Hydatidiform mole	80% of cases of GTD	Benign neoplasm of the chorion in which chorionic villi degenerate and become transparent vesicles	Complete mole: empty egg fertilized by sperm, embryo nonviable (dies) (Fig. 19.2) May transform into choriocarcinoma	46 all-paternal chromosomes
			Partial mole: Two sperm cells provide a double contribution by fertilizing the ovum.	Triploid (69 chromosomes)

GTD, gestational trophoblastic disease.

Source: Baergen, R. N. (2021). Gestational trophoblastic disease: Pathology. *UpToDate*. Retrieved April 28, 2024, from https://www.uptodate.com/contents/gestational-trophoblastic-disease-pathology; Berkowitz, R. S., Horowitz, N. S., & Elias, K. M. (2022). Gestational trophoblastic neoplasia: Epidemiology, clinical features, diagnosis, staging, and risk stratification. *UpToDate*. Retrieved April 28, 2024, from https://www.uptodate.com/contents/gestational-trophoblastic-neoplasia-epidemiology-clinical-features-diagnosis-staging-and-risk-stratification

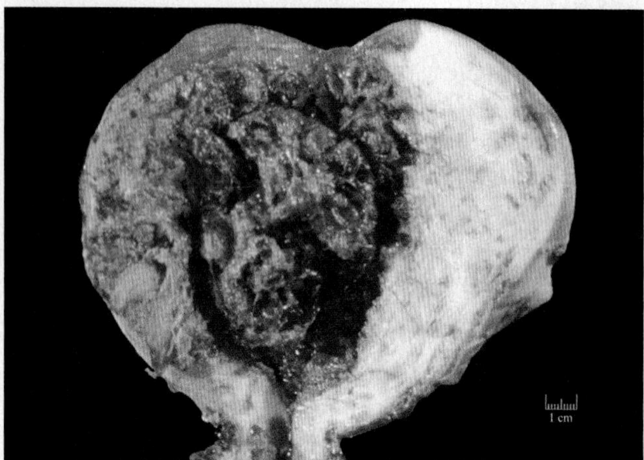

FIGURE 19.2 Complete hydatidiform mole as seen in a cutaway of a uterus. The chorionic villi degenerate and become filled with a viscid fluid, forming transparent vesicles. (Courtesy of Dr. Enrique Higa.)

about the risk that cancer may develop after a molar pregnancy and the strict adherence needed with the follow-up program. The patient must understand the need for the continued follow-up care regimen to improve their chances of future pregnancies and to ensure their continued quality of life.

PREPARING THE PATIENT

Upon diagnosis, the patient will need an immediate evacuation of the uterus. Perform preoperative care, preparing the patient physically and psychologically for the procedure.

PROVIDING EMOTIONAL SUPPORT

To aid the patient and their family in coping with the loss of the pregnancy and the possibility of a cancer diagnosis, use the following interventions:

- Listen to their concerns and fears.
- Allow them time to grieve for the pregnancy loss.
- Acknowledge their loss and sad feelings.
- Encourage them to express their grief; allow them to cry.
- Provide them with as much factual information as possible to help them make sense of what is happening.
- Enlist support from additional family and friends as appropriate and with the patient's permission.

EDUCATING THE PATIENT

After GTD is diagnosed, teach the patient about the condition and appropriate interventions that may be necessary to save their life. Explain each phase of treatment accurately and provide support for the patient and their family as they go through the grieving process.

As with any facet of health care, be aware of the latest research and new therapies. Inform the patient about follow-up care, which will probably involve close clinical surveillance for approximately 1 year, and reinforce its importance in monitoring the patient's condition. Tell the patient that serial serum beta-hCG levels are used to detect residual trophoblastic tissue. Continued high or increasing hCG titers are abnormal and need further evaluation.

Inform the patient about the possible use of chemotherapy, such as methotrexate, which may be started prophylactically. Strongly urge them to use a reliable contraceptive to prevent pregnancy for at least 1 year, because a pregnancy would interfere with tracking the serial beta-hCG levels used to identify a potential malignancy. Stress the need for the patient to adhere to the plan of therapy throughout this yearlong follow-up period.

CONSIDER THIS!

We had lived across the dorm hall from each other during nursing school but really did not get to know each other except for a casual hello in passing. When we graduated, Rose went to work in the emergency room (ER), and I worked in OB. We saw each other occasionally in the employee cafeteria, but a quick hello was all that we usually exchanged. I heard she married one of the paramedics who worked in the ER and was soon pregnant. I finally got to say more than hello when she was admitted to the OB unit bleeding during her fourth month of pregnancy. GTD was discovered instead of a normal pregnancy. I remember holding her in my arms as she wept. She was told she had a complete molar pregnancy after surgery, and she would need extensive follow-up for the next year. I lost track of her that summer as my life became busier. Around Thanksgiving time, I heard she had died from choriocarcinoma. I attended her funeral, finally, to get the time to say a final hello and good-bye, but this time with sadness and tears.

Thoughts: Rose was only 26 years old when she succumbed to this very virulent cancer. I think back and realize I missed knowing this brave young woman and wished that I had taken the time to say more than hello. Could her outcome have been different? Why wasn't it recognized earlier? I can only speculate regarding these questions. She lived a short but purposeful life, and hopefully continued research will change other women's outcomes in the future.

Cervical Insufficiency

Cervical insufficiency refers to painless cervical dilatation in the second trimester. Ultimately, an immature fetus will be expelled. It may result from cervical trauma or abnormal cervical development (possibly from in-utero DES exposure). Cervical insufficiency occurs more frequently in patients with Marfan syndrome and Ehlers–Danlos syndrome (Cunningham et al., 2022a). The exact etiology of cervical insufficiency is not known.

Therapeutic Management

Lifestyle changes such as bed rest, avoidance of coitus, and stopping working or exercise have not been well studied so are not universally recommended, though they may be beneficial to the patient with transvaginal ultrasound documentation of a shortened cervix (Berghella, 2024). A cervical cerclage may be placed during the second trimester, either transvaginally or transabdominally. Cervical cerclage involves using a heavy purse-string suture to secure and reinforce the internal os of the cervix (Fig. 19.3).

Nursing Assessment

Nursing assessment focuses on obtaining a thorough history to determine any risk factors that might have a bearing on the pregnancy, including previous cervical trauma, preterm labor, fetal loss in the second trimester, and previous surgeries or procedures involving the cervix. History may reveal a previous loss of pregnancy around 20 weeks.

Also be alert for complaints of vaginal discharge or pelvic pressure. With cervical insufficiency, the patient will often report a pink-tinged vaginal discharge or an increase in low pelvic pressure, cramping with vaginal bleeding, and loss of amniotic fluid. Cervical dilation also occurs. If this continues, rupture of the membranes, release of amniotic fluid, and uterine contractions occur, subsequently resulting in delivery of the fetus, often before it is viable.

TAKE NOTE!

The diagnosis of cervical insufficiency remains difficult in many circumstances. The cornerstone of diagnosis is a history of a pregnancy loss during the second or early third trimester associated with painless cervical dilation without evidence of uterine activity.

Nursing Management

Nursing management focuses on monitoring the patient closely for signs of preterm labor: backache, increase in vaginal discharge, rupture of membranes, and uterine contractions. Provide emotional support and education to allay any patient and family anxiety about the well-being of the fetus. Provide preoperative care and teaching as indicated if the patient will be undergoing cerclage. Teach the patient and their family about the signs and symptoms of preterm labor and the need to report any changes immediately. Also reinforce the need for activity restrictions (if appropriate) and continued regular follow-up. Continuing surveillance throughout the pregnancy is important to promote a positive outcome for the family. The nurse can play a pivotal role in identifying preterm labor through risk assessment, physical examination, and advocacy.

Placenta Previa

Placenta previa (meaning "afterbirth first") exists when the placenta is inserted wholly or partly into the lower uterine segment of the uterus, partially or completely covering the internal cervical opening. The source of bleeding is maternal and typically occurs during the last two trimesters of pregnancy. It poses a high risk of prenatal and postpartum hemorrhage as well as perinatal mortality. It is also associated with potentially serious consequences from abruption (separation) of the placenta and emergency cesarean birth. Placenta previa affects about 4 to 5 of every 1,000 live births (Lockwood & Russo-Stieglitz, 2024a).

The term placenta previa currently refers to the placenta covering the internal cervical os, while low-lying placenta refers to the placental edge being less than 2 cm from the internal os but does not cover it (Fig. 19.4). The exact cause of placenta previa is unknown.

Therapeutic Management

In the case of low-lying placenta without symptoms, transvaginal ultrasound and color Doppler are utilized to determine whether the placenta is migrating upward. To reduce the risk of bleeding, cervical examination is avoided. After 20 weeks' gestation, the patient should avoid strenuous activity and sexual activity leading to

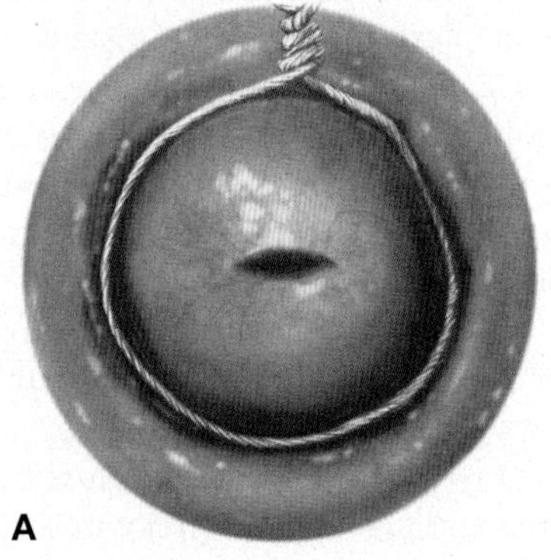

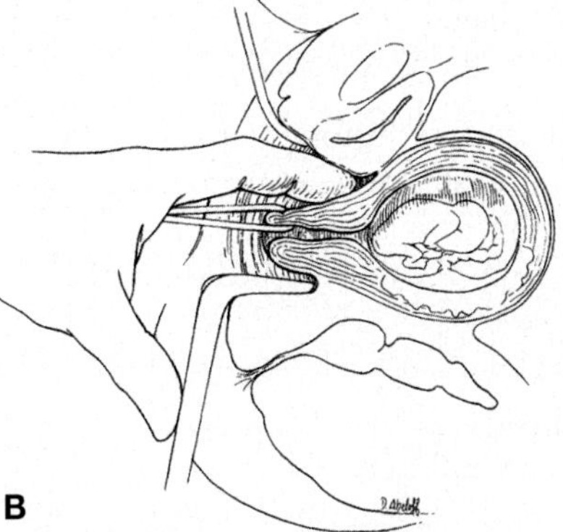

FIGURE 19.3 **A.** Cervical cerclage. **B.** Suturing the cervix for cervical insufficiency.

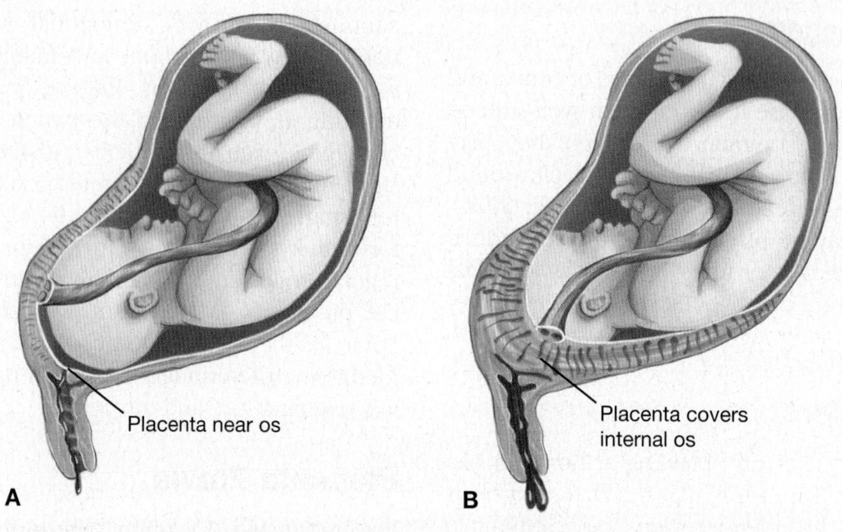

FIGURE 19.4 Classification of placenta previa. **A.** Low lying. **B.** Placenta previa.

orgasm. A patient with placenta previa who demonstrates active vaginal bleeding should be considered a potential obstetric emergency. The patient may be hospitalized for maternal and fetal assessment, fluid resuscitation and blood transfusion, and preparation for cesarean section if in active labor (Lockwood & Russo-Stieglitz, 2024b).

Nursing Assessment

Nursing assessment involves a thorough history including possible risk factors and a physical examination. Evaluate the patient's history for these risk factors:

- Previous placenta previa
- Previous cesarean birth
- Multiple gestation
- Increasing parity
- Increasing maternal age
- Previous uterine surgical procedure
- Infertility treatment
- Prior uterine artery embolization
- Endometriosis or abortion
- Maternal smoking or cocaine use
- Male fetus (Lockwood & Russo-Stieglitz, 2024a)

Assess for a previous or current history of painless vaginal bleeding. Determine if uterine contractions are occurring and auscultate the fetal rate to determine lack of distress. To validate the position of the placenta, a transvaginal ultrasound is done.

Nursing Management

Whether the care setting is in the patient's home or in the health care facility, the nurse focuses on monitoring the maternal–fetal status, including assessing for signs and symptoms of vaginal bleeding and fetal distress and providing support and education to the patient and their family, including providing information about the diagnostic studies and procedures that are performed. Monitor the patient's vital signs and uterine contractility frequently for changes. Have the patient rate their level of pain using an appropriate pain rating scale. With true placenta previa, a cesarean birth will be planned. Clinical Judgment & Nursing Process 19.1 discusses the nursing process for the patient with placenta previa.

> *TAKE NOTE!*
>
> Avoid doing vaginal examinations in the patient with placenta previa because they may disrupt the placenta and cause additional hemorrhage.

PROVIDING SUPPORT AND EDUCATION

Determine the patient's level of understanding about placenta previa and the associated procedures and treatment plan. Doing so is important to prevent confusion and gain the patient's cooperation. Provide information about the condition, and make sure that all related information is consistent with information from the health care provider. Explain all assessments and treatment measures as needed.

Act as a patient advocate in obtaining information for the family. Teach the patient how to perform and record daily fetal movements. This action serves two purposes: (1) It provides valuable information about the fetus and (2) it is an activity in which the patient can participate, thereby fostering some feeling of control over the situation.

If the patient may require prolonged hospitalization or home bed rest, assess the physical and emotional impact that this may have on them. Evaluate their coping mechanisms to help determine how well they will be able to adjust and adhere to the treatment plan. Allow the patient to verbalize their feelings and fears and provide emotional support. Also provide opportunities for distraction—educational videos, arts and crafts, video games, physical books, or audiobooks—and evaluate the patient's response.

In addition to the emotional impact of prolonged bed rest, thoroughly assess the patient's skin to prevent skin breakdown and to help alleviate their discomfort secondary to limited physical activity. Instruct the patient in appropriate skin care measures. Encourage them to eat a balanced diet with adequate fluid intake to ensure adequate nutrition and hydration and prevent complications associated with urinary and bowel elimination secondary to bed rest.

Teach the patient and their family about any signs and symptoms that should be reported immediately. In addition, prepare the patient for the possibility of a cesarean birth. The patient must notify their health care provider about any bleeding episodes or backaches (which may indicate preterm labor contractions) and must adhere to the prescribed bed rest regimen. To ensure adherence to the plan and a positive outcome, the patient needs to be aware of and understand the rationales for the ongoing observations.

CLINICAL JUDGMENT & NURSING PROCESS 19.1 Overview of the Patient With Placenta Previia

A 39-year-old G5P4 multigravida at 32 weeks' gestation was admitted to the labor and birth suite with sudden vaginal bleeding. She had no further active bleeding and did not complain of any abdominal discomfort or tenderness. She did complain of occasional "tightening" in her stomach. Her abdomen palpated soft. Fetal heart rates were in the 140s with accelerations with movement. She was placed on bed rest with bathroom privileges. Ultrasound identified a low-lying placenta with a viable, normal-growth fetus. She was diagnosed with placenta previa and admitted for observation and surveillance of fetal well-being. Her history revealed two previous cesarean births, smoking half a pack of cigarettes per day, and endometritis infection after the birth of her last newborn. Additional assessment findings included painless, bright red vaginal bleeding with initial bleeding ceasing spontaneously; irregular, mild, and sporadic uterine contractions; fetal heart rate and maternal vital signs within normal range; fetus in transverse lie; anxiety related to the outcome of pregnancy; and expression of feelings of helplessness.

NURSING ANALYSIS: Injury (fetal and maternal) risk related to threat to uteroplacental perfusion and hemorrhage

OUTCOME IDENTIFICATION AND EVALUATION

The patient will maintain adequate tissue perfusion as evidenced by stable vital signs, decreased blood loss, few or no uterine contractions, normal fetal heart rate patterns and variability, and positive fetal movement.

INTERVENTIONS: *Maintaining Adequate Tissue Perfusion*

- Establish intravenous (IV) access *to allow for the administration of fluids, blood, and medications as necessary.*
- Obtain type and cross-match for at least 2 units of blood products *to ensure availability should bleeding continue.*
- Obtain specimens as ordered for blood studies, such as complete blood count (CBC) and clotting studies, *to establish a baseline and use for future comparison.*
- Monitor output *to evaluate the adequacy of renal perfusion.*
- Administer IV fluid replacement therapy as ordered *to maintain blood pressure and blood volume.*
- Palpate for abdominal tenderness and rigidity *to determine bleeding and evidence of uterine contractions.*
- Institute bed rest *to reduce oxygen demands.*
- Assess for rupture of membranes *to evaluate for possible onset of labor.*
- Avoid vaginal examinations *to prevent further bleeding episodes.*
- Complete an Rh titer *to identify the need for RhIG.*
- Avoid nipple stimulation *to prevent uterine contractions.*
- Continuously monitor for contractions or PROM *to allow for prompt intervention.*
- Administer tocolytic agents as ordered *to stall preterm labor.*
- Monitor vital signs frequently *to identify possible hypovolemia and infection.*
- Assess frequently for active vaginal bleeding *to minimize the risk of hemorrhage.*
- Continuously monitor fetal heart rate with electronic fetal monitor *to evaluate fetal status.*
- Assist with fetal surveillance tests as ordered *to aid in determining fetal well-being.*
- Observe for abnormal fetal heart rate patterns, such as loss of variability, decelerations, and tachycardia, *to identify fetal distress.*
- Position the patient in a side-lying position with a wedge for support *to maximize placental perfusion.*
- Assess fetal movement *to evaluate for possible fetal hypoxia.*
- Teach the patient to monitor fetal movement *to evaluate fetal well-being.*
- Administer oxygen as ordered *to increase oxygenation to the pregnant person and fetus.*

(continued)

CLINICAL JUDGMENT & NURSING PROCESS 19.1 Overview of the Patient With Placenta Previa (*continued*)

NURSING ANALYSIS: Acute anxiety related to the threat to self and fetus, unknown future

OUTCOME IDENTIFICATION AND EVALUATION

The patient will experience a decrease in anxiety as evidenced by verbal reports of less anxiety, use of effective coping measures, and calm demeanor.

INTERVENTIONS: *Minimizing Anxiety*

- Provide factual information about diagnosis and treatment, and explain interventions and the rationale behind them *to provide the patient with an understanding of their condition.*
- Answer questions about health status honestly *to establish a trusting relationship.*
- Speak calmly to the patient and family members *to minimize environmental stress.*
- Encourage the use of past effective techniques for coping *to promote relaxation and feelings of control.*
- Acknowledge and facilitate the patient's spiritual needs *to promote effective coping.*
- Involve the patient and family in the decision-making process *to foster self-confidence and control over the situation.*
- Maintain a presence during stressful periods *to allay anxiety.*
- Use the sense of touch if appropriate *to convey caring and concern.*
- Encourage talking as a means *to release tension.*

PROM, prelabor rupture of membranes; RhIG, Rh immunoglobulin.

Placental Abruption

Placental abruption (also termed abruptio placentae) is the early separation of a normally implanted placenta after the 20th week of gestation prior to birth, which leads to hemorrhage. Abruption results from premature placental separation and rupture of maternal blood vessels in the decidua basalis, which leads to bleeding between the decidua and placenta. It is a significant cause of second- or third-trimester bleeding with a high mortality rate. It occurs in three to 10 per 1,000 births globally, with the United States being at the higher end (Ananth & Kinzler, 2023).

Maternal risks include obstetric hemorrhage, need for blood transfusions, emergency hysterectomy, disseminated intravascular coagulation (DIC), Sheehan syndrome or postpartum gland necrosis, and renal failure. The maternal mortality rate for placental abruption is 6% (Deering, 2023). The overall fetal mortality rate is about 119 per 1,000 births (Cunningham et al., 2022e). Placental abruption represents an emergency, with the main objective to extract the fetus quickly and to manage the maternal hemorrhage.

Pathophysiology

Abruption occurs when the maternal vessels tear away from the placenta and bleeding occurs between the uterine lining and the maternal side of the placenta. As the blood accumulates, it pushes the uterine wall and placenta apart. If the abruption continues, loss of placental function results in fetal hypoxia and possibly fetal death. The etiology of this condition is unknown; however, it has been proposed that abruption starts with degenerative changes in the small maternal blood vessels, resulting in blood clotting, degeneration of the decidua (uterine lining), and possible rupture of a vessel. Bleeding from the blood vessel forms a blood clot between the placenta and the uterine wall. Placental abruption also may be classified as partial or complete, depending on the degree of separation, or as concealed or apparent based on the type of bleeding (Fig. 19.5).

Remember Helen, the pregnant woman with severe abdominal pain? Electronic fetal monitoring revealed uterine hypertonicity with absent fetal heart sounds. Palpation of her abdomen revealed rigidity and extreme tenderness in all four quadrants. Her vital signs were as follows: temperature, afebrile; pulse, 94; respirations, 22; blood pressure, 130/90 mm Hg. What might you suspect as the cause of Helen's abdominal pain? What course of action would you anticipate for Helen?

Therapeutic Management

The onset of placental abruption is often unexpected, sudden, and intense, and it requires immediate treatment. Management of placental abruption is guided by fetal viability, severity of the abruption, and maternal status. Emergency measures include starting two large-bore intravenous (IV) lines with normal saline or lactated Ringer's solution to combat hypovolemia, obtaining blood specimens for evaluating hemodynamic status values and for typing and cross-matching, and frequently monitoring fetal and maternal well-being. After the severity of abruption is determined and appropriate blood and fluid replacement is given, cesarean birth is performed

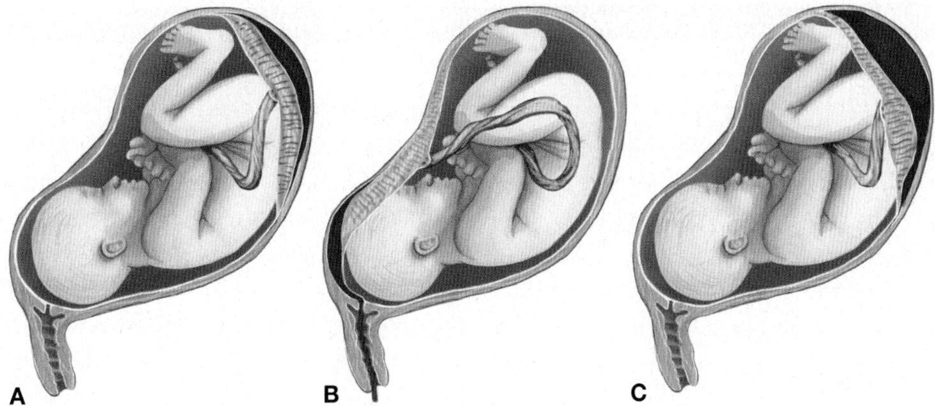

FIGURE 19.5 Classifications of placental abruption. **A.** Partial abruption with concealed hemorrhage. **B.** Partial abruption with apparent hemorrhage. **C.** Complete abruption with concealed hemorrhage.

immediately if fetal distress is evident. If the fetus is not in distress, close monitoring continues with birth planned at the earliest signs of fetal distress. Because of the possibility of fetal blood loss through the placenta, a neonatal intensive care team should be available during the birth process to assess and treat the newborn immediately for shock, blood loss, and hypoxia.

Placental abruption can result in uterine atony and the development of DIC (Box 19.1). Treatment of DIC involves fluid resuscitation with crystalloids, transfusion of blood products (packed red blood cells, fresh-frozen plasma, cryoprecipitate, platelets), and lyophilized human fibrinogen concentrate to restore appropriate coagulation (Belfort, 2023). Prompt identification and early intervention are essential for a patient with acute DIC associated with placental abruption to treat DIC and possibly save their life.

Nursing Assessment

Initial assessment should focus on maternal hemodynamic status and fetal well-being. The nurse plays a critical role in assessing the pregnant patient presenting with abdominal pain and/or experiencing vaginal bleeding, especially in a concealed hemorrhage, in which the extent of bleeding is not recognized. Rapid assessment is essential to ensure prompt, effective interventions to prevent maternal and fetal morbidity and mortality. Comparison Chart 19.1 compares placenta previa with placental abruption.

HEALTH HISTORY AND PHYSICAL EXAMINATION

Placental abruption produces a wide range of clinical effects, depending on the extent of placental separation and the amount of maternal blood loss. Begin the health

BOX 19.1 Disseminated Intravascular Coagulation

Disseminated intravascular coagulation (DIC) is a bleeding disorder characterized by an abnormal reduction in the elements involved in blood clotting resulting from their widespread intravascular clotting (Belfort, 2023). This disorder can occur secondary to placental abruption, amniotic fluid embolism, endotoxin sepsis after an abortion, retained dead fetus, posthemorrhagic shock, hydatidiform mole, HELLP syndrome, and gynecologic malignancies.

The clinical and pathologic manifestations of DIC can be described as a loss of balance between the clot-forming activity of thrombin and the clot-lysing activity of plasmin. Therefore, too much thrombin tips the balance toward the prothrombic state, and the patient develops clots. Alternately, too much clot lysis (fibrinolysis) results from plasmin formation, and the patient hemorrhages. Small clots form throughout the body, and eventually, the blood clotting factors are used up, rendering them unavailable to form clots at sites of tissue injury. Clot-dissolving mechanisms are also increased, resulting in potentially severe bleeding.

Complications of DIC include acute kidney failure, hepatic dysfunction, cardiac tamponade, gangrene and loss of digits, shock, and death (Levi & Schmaier, 2022). DIC is associated with high mortality and morbidity rates. No single laboratory test is sensitive or specific enough to diagnose DIC definitively, but it can be diagnosed by using a combination of multiple clinical and laboratory tests that reflect the pathophysiology of the syndrome.

Laboratory studies that assist in the diagnosis include:

- Decreased fibrinogen and platelets
- Prolonged PT and aPTT
- Positive D-dimer tests and fibrin (split) degradation products (objective evidence of the simultaneous formation of thrombin and plasmin) (Levi & Schmaier, 2022)

aPTT, activated partial thromboplastin time; HELLP, hemolysis, elevated liver enzymes, and low platelets; PT, prothrombin time.

Belfort, M. A. (2023). Disseminated intravascular coagulation (DIC) during pregnancy: Clinical findings, etiology, and diagnosis. *UpToDate*. Retrieved April 29, 2024, from https://www.uptodate.com/contents/disseminated-intravascular-coagulation-dic-during-pregnancy-clinical-findings-etiology-and-diagnosis; Levi, M. M., & Schmaier, A. H. (2022). Disseminated intravascular coagulation (DIC). *Medscape*. https://emedicine.medscape.com/article/199627-overview

COMPARISON CHART 19.1 Placenta Previa Versus Placental Abruption

Manifestation	Placenta Previa	Placental Abruption
Onset	Insidious	Sudden
Type of bleeding	Always visible; slight, then more profuse	Can be concealed or visible
Blood description	Bright red	Dark
Discomfort/pain	None (painless)	Constant; uterine tenderness on palpation
Uterine tone	Soft and relaxed	Firm to rigid
Fetal heart rate	Usually in the normal range	Fetal distress or absent
Fetal presentation	May be a breech or transverse lie; engagement is absent.	No relationship

history by assessing the patient for risk factors that may predispose them to placental abruption:

- Previous placental abruption
- Hypertension
- Uterine structural anomaly
- Cigarette use (synergistic with hypertension)
- Cocaine use
- Having been a small-for-gestational-age infant
- Sibling who experienced placental abruption
- Major fetal anomaly
- Fetal growth restriction
- Assistive reproductive technology use
- Asthma
- Subclinical hypothyroidism
- Previous cesarean birth
- Marginal placental cord insertion
- Short stature
- Grand multiparity (Ananth & Kinzler, 2023)

Placental abruption may also occur as a result of external trauma (Cunningham et al., 2022e).

Assess the patient for bleeding. As the placenta separates from the uterus, hemorrhage ensues. It can be apparent, appearing as vaginal bleeding, or it can be concealed. Quantify the amount of vaginal bleeding when present. Monitor the patient's perfusion status and level of consciousness, noting any signs or symptoms that may suggest shock.

TAKE NOTE!

Vital signs can be within the normal range, even with significant blood loss, because of increased intravascular volume in pregnancy. As a result, the patient can lose up to 30% to 40% of total blood volume without showing signs of shock (Smith, 2022).

Assess the patient for complaints of pain, including the type, onset, and location. Ask if they have had any contractions. Palpate the abdomen, noting any contractions, uterine tenderness, tenseness, or rigidity. Ask if the patient has noticed any changes in fetal movement and activity. Decreased fetal movement may be the presenting complaint, resulting from fetal jeopardy or fetal death (Cunningham et al., 2022d). Assess fetal heart rate and continue to monitor it electronically.

TAKE NOTE!

Classic manifestations of placental abruption include painful, dark red vaginal bleeding (port-wine color) because the bleeding comes from the clot that was formed behind the placenta; "knifelike" abdominal pain; uterine tenderness; contractions; and decreased fetal movement. Rapid assessment is essential to ensuring prompt, effective interventions to prevent maternal and fetal morbidity and mortality.

Nursing Management

The patient with placental abruption requires immediate care to provide the best outcome for both the birthing parent and fetus. Nursing care focuses on ensuring adequate tissue perfusion, monitoring fetal status, and providing education and support.

ENSURING ADEQUATE TISSUE PERFUSION

When the patient arrives at the facility, place them on strict bed rest and in a left lateral position to prevent pressure on the vena cava. This position provides uninterrupted perfusion to the fetus. Expect to administer oxygen therapy via nasal cannula to ensure adequate tissue perfusion. Monitor oxygen saturation levels via pulse oximetry to evaluate the effectiveness of interventions.

Obtain the patient's vital signs frequently, as often as every 15 minutes as indicated, depending on the patient's status and amount of blood loss. Observe for changes in vital signs suggesting hypovolemic shock and report them immediately. Also expect to insert an indwelling urinary (Foley) catheter to assess hourly urine output and initiate an IV infusion for fluid replacement using a large-bore catheter.

Assess fundal height for changes. An increase in size would indicate bleeding. Monitor the amount and characteristics of any vaginal bleeding as frequently as every 15 to 30 minutes. Be alert for signs and symptoms of DIC, such as bleeding gums, tachycardia, oozing from the IV insertion site, and petechiae, and administer blood products as ordered if DIC occurs.

Institute continuous electronic fetal monitoring. Assess uterine contractions, and report any increased uterine tenseness or rigidity. Also observe the tracing for tetanic uterine contractions or changes in fetal heart rate patterns suggesting that the fetus has been compromised.

PROVIDING SUPPORT AND EDUCATION

A patient diagnosed with placental abruption may be filled with a sense of heightened anxiety and apprehension for their own health as well as for the health of their fetus. Communicate empathy and understanding of the patient's experience, and provide emotional support throughout this potentially frightening time. Remain with the patient and their family, acknowledge their emotions and fears, and address their spiritual and cultural needs. Answer their questions about the status of their fetus openly and honestly, being sure to explain indicators of fetal well-being. Provide information about the various diagnostic tests, treatments, and procedures that may be done, including the possible need for a cesarean birth. Depending on the patient's status, extent of bleeding, and length of gestation, the fetus may not survive. If the fetus does survive, they most likely will require neonatal intensive care. Assist the patient and family in dealing with the loss or with the birth of a newborn in the neonatal intensive care unit.

Although placental abruption is not a preventable condition, patient education is important to help reduce the risk of a recurrence of this condition. Encourage the patient to avoid drinking alcohol, smoking, or using drugs during pregnancy. Urge them to seek early and continuous prenatal care and to receive prompt health care if any signs and symptoms occur in future pregnancies.

> Think back to Helen, the pregnant woman described at the beginning of the chapter. She was diagnosed with placental abruption and was prepared for an emergency cesarean birth. Upon exploration, there was almost a 75% abruption, with approximately 800 mL of concealed blood between the uterus and the placenta. In addition, she lost 500 mL during surgery. What factors in Helen's history may have placed her at increased risk for abruption? What assessments and interventions would be essential during her postpartum recovery secondary to her significant blood loss? What psychosocial interventions would be necessary due to her fetal loss?

Placenta Accreta Spectrum

Placenta accreta spectrum refers to a full range of accrete diagnoses, including placenta accreta (adherent placenta), as well as increta and percreta (invasive placentas). All three types entail trophoblast invasions of varying depths in which the placenta is anchored into the myometrium rather than the decidua. Consequently, the placenta does not separate at birth, and it must be manually removed. Placenta accreta disorders are potentially life-threatening obstetric hemorrhagic conditions that require a multidisciplinary approach to management. The incidence of placenta accreta has increased and seems to parallel the increasing rates of cesarean births or intrauterine procedures. Over the past 50 years, surgical births have risen globally by up to 30%, and at the same time, a 10-fold increase in the incidence of this spectrum has been reported (Morlando & Collins, 2022). **Placenta accreta spectrum** includes three conditions. *Accreta* is the most common (80%) and is a condition in which the placenta attaches itself too deeply into the wall of the uterus but does not penetrate the uterine muscle. *Placenta increta* occurs (15%) when the placenta invades the myometrium, and *placenta percreta* occurs (5%) when it has extended through the myometrium, uterine serosa, and adjacent tissue (Cunningham et al., 2022e). A common risk associated with placenta accreta when unsuspected at the time of birth is the possibility of hemorrhaging during manual attempts to detach the placenta (Silver, 2023). Placenta accreta occurs in as many as one in 272 pregnancies (ACOG, 2021a). The specific cause of placenta accreta is unknown, but it can be related to postoperative scar remodeling following previous cesarean births or uterine surgery, or it may be associated with preexisting uterine pathology (Silver, 2023).

Placenta accreta is typically diagnosed after birth when the placenta fails to normally separate from the uterine wall. Attempts to remove the adherent placenta manually may result in major hemorrhage, and maternal mortality with placenta accreta may be as high as 27% (Silver, 2023). A profuse hemorrhage may result because the uterus cannot contract to close off the open blood vessels. Care will depend on the severity of the bleeding and frequently necessitates a prompt hysterectomy. However, a recent study found that leaving the placenta in situ after delivery and using a high-intensity focused ultrasound shows promise as a fertility-preserving treatment. The ultrasound causes rapid heating of the tissue in the focal area and a coagulative necrosis of the area (Guan et al., 2022). Nurses need to be prepared to manage hemorrhage in this emergency situation and possibly to prepare the patient for a hysterectomy.

HYPEREMESIS GRAVIDARUM

Hyperemesis gravidarum is a severe form of nausea and intractable vomiting of pregnancy associated with significant costs and psychosocial impacts. It can be associated with acute starvation and may require hospitalization. Seventy to eighty percent of pregnant people experience nausea and vomiting during their pregnancies, but up to 3.6% of pregnancies in the United States are affected by this severe condition (Mares et al., 2022). The term "morning sickness" is often used to describe nausea and vomiting when symptoms are relatively mild. Such symptoms usually disappear after the first trimester. This mild form mostly affects the quality of life of the patient and their family, while the severe form—hyperemesis gravidarum—results in weight loss, anxiety and depression, work performance impairment, and consideration of termination of the current pregnancy or avoidance of future pregnancies (Smith & Fox, 2024).

Unlike morning sickness, hyperemesis gravidarum is a complication of pregnancy characterized by persistent, uncontrollable nausea and vomiting beginning by 5 to 6 weeks' gestation (Jennings & Mahdy, 2023). It results in dehydration, weight loss of more than 5% of prepregnancy body weight, ketosis, electrolyte imbalances, ketonuria, and nutritional deficiencies.

TAKE NOTE!

Every pregnant patient needs to be instructed to report any episodes of severe nausea and vomiting or episodes that extend beyond the first trimester.

Pathophysiology

Hyperemesis gravidarum is a multifactorial condition likely involving hormonal, gastrointestinal, and genetic factors. Elevated levels of hCG are present in all pregnant people during early pregnancy, usually declining after 12 weeks. This corresponds to the usual duration of morning sickness. In hyperemesis gravidarum, the hCG levels are often higher and extend beyond the first trimester. High estrogen levels during pregnancy may also be a contributing factor. Relaxed lower esophageal sphincter tone naturally occurring during pregnancy results in gastroesophageal reflux leading to nausea. Genetics may also play a role; family history of hyperemesis gravidarum results in increased risk (Jennings & Mahdy, 2023).

Therapeutic Management

Conservative management in the home is the first line of treatment for the patient with hyperemesis gravidarum. This usually focuses on dietary and lifestyle changes. If conservative management fails to alleviate the patient's symptoms and nausea and vomiting continue, hospitalization is necessary to reverse the effects of severe nausea and vomiting. Changing the patient's prenatal vitamin to folic acid only may help with nausea. Ginger supplements (250 mg) may be taken four times daily (Jennings & Mahdy, 2023).

Upon admission to the hospital, blood tests are ordered to assess the extent of the patient's dehydration, electrolyte imbalance, ketosis, and malnutrition. Fluid replacement is achieved with the use of normal saline, which aids in preventing hyponatremia, with vitamins (pyridoxine or vitamin B6) and electrolytes added. Oral food and fluids are withheld for the first 24 to 36 hours to allow the gastrointestinal tract to rest. Antiemetics may be administered rectally or intravenously to control the nausea and vomiting initially while the patient is nothing by mouth (NPO). Once the condition stabilizes and the patient is permitted oral intake, medications may be administered orally.

If the patient's condition does not improve after several days of bed rest, "gut rest," IV fluids, and antiemetics, total parenteral nutrition or feeding through a percutaneous endoscopic gastrostomy tube is instituted to prevent malnutrition. Administering antiemetics IV or IM is typically the second pillar of treatment for hyperemesis gravidarum. Refer to Drug Guide 19.2 for information about medications used to treat hyperemesis gravidarum.

DRUG GUIDE 19.2

MEDICATIONS USED FOR HYPEREMESIS GRAVIDARUM

Medication	Action/Indications	Nursing Implications
Promethazine (Phenergan)	Diminishes vestibular stimulation and acts on the chemoreceptor trigger zone (CTZ) Symptomatic relief of nausea, vomiting, and motion sickness	Be alert for urinary retention, dizziness, hypotension, and involuntary movements. Institute safety measures to prevent injury secondary to sedative effects. Offer hard candy and frequent rinsing of the mouth for dryness.
Pyridoxine and doxylamine (Diclegis)	Delayed-release medication containing a combination of an antihistamine and vitamin B6 Symptomatic relief of nausea and vomiting during pregnancy	Be alert for drowsiness, dizziness, headache, and irritability. Do not administer with any central nervous system depressants or sleeping medications. It must be taken daily, not as needed. It should be taken on an empty stomach with a full glass of water.
Ondansetron (Zofran)	Blocks serotonin release, which stimulates the vagal afferent nerves, thus stimulating the vomiting reflex	Monitor for possible side effects such as diarrhea, constipation, abdominal pain, headache, dizziness, drowsiness, and fatigue. Monitor liver function studies as ordered.
Pyridoxine (Vitamin B6)	Improves nausea with a good safety profile with minimal side effects	No major fetal malformations were found in the studies.

Jennings, L. K., & Mahdy, H. (2023). Hyperemesis gravidarum. *StatPearls*. https://www.ncbi.nlm.nih.gov/books/NBK532917/#article-27636.s2; UpToDate, Inc. (2024). *UpToDate® Lexidrug*™ (Version 8.2.0) [Mobile app]. Wolters Kluwer. https://apps.apple.com/us/app/lexicomp/id313401238

Few patients receive complete relief of symptoms from any one therapy. Complementary and alternative medicine therapies appeal to many patients as supplements to traditional ones. However, many of these therapies have not been rigorously studied and may or may not be useful. Acupressure to the *nei guan* acupoint on the wrist has been shown to help prevent nausea and vomiting (Nafiah et al., 2022).

Nursing Assessment

Nursing assessment of the patient with hyperemesis gravidarum requires a thorough history and physical examination to identify signs and symptoms associated with this disorder. The patient is extremely uncomfortable. They may experience many hours of lost work productivity and sleep, and hyperemesis may damage family relationships.

Health History and Physical Examination

Begin the history by asking about the onset, duration, and course of the patient's nausea and vomiting. Ask them about any medications or treatments they used and how effective they were in relieving the nausea and vomiting. Obtain a diet history from the patient, including a dietary recall for the past week. Note the patient's knowledge of nutrition and the need for appropriate nutritional intake. Be alert for patterns that may contribute to or trigger their distress. Also ask about any complaints of ptyalism (excessive salivation), anorexia, indigestion, abdominal pain, or distention, and about any blood or mucus in the patient's stool. Also note any complaints of weakness, fatigue, activity intolerance, dizziness, or sleep disturbances. Assess the patient's perception of the situation. Note any evidence of depression, anxiety, irritability, mood changes, and decreased ability to concentrate; all of these can add to the patient's emotional distress. Determine the people in the patient's support systems who are available to help.

Review the patient's history for possible risk factors, which are similar to the classic nausea and vomiting experienced during pregnancy:

- Prepregnancy history of nausea and vomiting with estrogen-containing products, migraine, or motion sickness
- Nausea and vomiting in previous pregnancies
- Nonuse of vitamins before 6 weeks' gestation or in the preconception period
- Molar pregnancy
- Acid reflux
- Multiple gestation (Smith & Fox, 2024)

Additionally, family history of hyperemesis gravidarum is a risk factor.

Weigh the patient and compare their weight with their weight before they began experiencing symptoms and to their prepregnancy weight to estimate the degree of loss. With hyperemesis, weight loss usually exceeds 5% of body mass. Inspect the mucous membranes for dryness and check skin turgor for lack of elasticity. Determine capillary refill (prolonged with dehydration). Assess blood pressure for changes, such as hypotension, which may suggest a fluid volume deficit.

The results of laboratory and diagnostic tests help determine the severity of the condition.

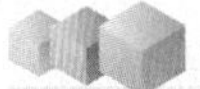
Concept Mastery Alert

Priority Interventions in Hyperemesis Gravidarum

Hyperemesis gravidarum is nausea and vomiting in early pregnancy that prevents the person from ingesting adequate nutrition. IV fluids may be required for rehydration, but the priority is to stop all intake of food and fluid for a period of time until vomiting has stopped.

Nursing Management

Nursing care of the patient with hyperemesis gravidarum focuses on promoting comfort by controlling the patient's nausea and vomiting and promoting adequate nutrition. In addition, the nurse plays a major role in supporting and educating the patient and their family.

Promoting Comfort and Nutrition

During the initial period, expect to withhold all oral food and fluids, maintaining NPO status to allow the gastrointestinal tract to rest. In addition, administer prescribed antiemetics to relieve the nausea and vomiting and IV fluids to replace fluid losses. Monitor the rate of infusion to prevent overload and assess the IV insertion site to prevent infiltration or infection. Also administer electrolyte replacement therapy as ordered to correct any imbalances, and periodically check serum electrolyte levels to evaluate the effectiveness of therapy.

Provide physical comfort measures such as hygiene measures and oral care. Pay special attention to the environment, making sure to keep the area free of pungent odors. As the patient's nausea and vomiting subside, gradually introduce oral fluids and foods in small amounts. Monitor intake and output and assess the patient's tolerance to the increase in intake.

Providing Support and Education

Patients with hyperemesis gravidarum are often fatigued physically and emotionally. Many are exhausted, frustrated, and anxious. Offer reassurance that all interventions are directed toward promoting positive pregnancy outcomes for both the patient and their fetus. Providing information about the expected plan of care may help alleviate the patient's anxiety. Listen to their concerns and feelings, answering all questions honestly. Educate the patient and their family about the condition and its treatment options (Teaching Guidelines 19.1).

TEACHING GUIDELINES 19.1 Teaching to Minimize Nausea and Vomiting

- Avoid noxious stimuli, such as strong flavors, perfumes, or strong odors like frying bacon, that might trigger nausea and vomiting.
- Avoid tight waistbands to minimize pressure on the abdomen.
- Eat small, frequent meals throughout the day.
- Separate fluids from solids by consuming fluids in between meals.
- Avoid lying down or reclining for at least 2 hours after eating.
- Use high-protein supplement drinks.
- Avoid foods high in fat.
- Increase your intake of carbonated beverages.
- Increase your exposure to fresh air to improve symptoms.
- Eat when you are hungry, regardless of normal mealtimes.
- Drink herbal teas containing peppermint or ginger.
- Avoid fatigue, and learn how to manage stress in life.
- Schedule daily rest periods to avoid becoming overtired.
- Eat foods that settle the stomach, such as dry crackers, toast, or soda.

Teach the patient about therapeutic lifestyle changes, such as avoiding stressors and fatigue that may trigger nausea and vomiting. Offer ongoing support and encouragement and promote active participation in care decisions, thereby empowering the patient and their family. Attempting to provide the patient with a sense of control may help them overcome the feeling that they have lost control. If necessary, refer the patient to a spiritual adviser or counselor. Also suggest possible local or national support groups that the patient may contact for additional information. Arrange for possible home care follow-up for the patient and reinforce discharge instructions to promote understanding. Timely counseling, balanced nutrition, pharmacotherapy, and emotional support are associated with favorable outcomes for the person with this condition. Collaborate with community resources to ensure continuity of care.

HYPERTENSIVE DISORDERS OF PREGNANCY

Hypertensive disorders of pregnancy, an umbrella term, include chronic hypertension, preeclampsia/eclampsia, preeclampsia superimposed on chronic hypertension, and gestational hypertension (Carson & Gibson, 2022). Hypertensive disorders complicate up to 16% of pregnancies and are the leading cause of maternal mortality in the United States (31.6% of maternal deaths) (Ford et al., 2022).

Hypertensive disorders of pregnancy comprise a spectrum of severity ranging from a mild elevation of blood pressure to severe preeclampsia and hemolysis. Recent data show that hypertensive disorders of pregnancy are associated with long-term cardiovascular risks, which include chronic hypertension, hypercholesterolemia, obesity, and diabetes following the pregnancy (Stuart et al., 2022).

Hypertension becomes more prevalent as age increases and weight increases (Bender, 2022). It results in frequent hospital admissions, maternal morbidity and mortality, and preterm births with concomitant neonatal morbidity and mortality. Regardless of its onset or subclassification, hypertension jeopardizes the well-being of the birthing parent as well as the fetus.

Although not accepted globally, specific hypertensive disorders of pregnancy are named based on the context in which the hypertension was first identified. The classification of hypertensive disorders in pregnancy currently consists of four categories: chronic hypertension, gestational hypertension, preeclampsia/eclampsia and HELLP syndrome, and chronic hypertension with superimposed preeclampsia (August & Sibai, 2023).

Chronic Hypertension

Chronic hypertension is defined as blood pressure exceeding 140/90 mm Hg before pregnancy or before 20 weeks' gestation. The latest clinical guidance from ACOG is to use 140/90 as the threshold for medical therapy for chronic hypertension in pregnancy rather than higher values to improve outcomes (2024). When hypertension is first identified during a patient's pregnancy and they are less than 20 weeks' gestation, blood pressure elevations usually represent chronic hypertension. Chronic hypertension occurs in up to 22% of females of childbearing age with the prevalence varying according to age, race, and body mass index (BMI) (Carson & Gibson, 2022). As the U.S. obesity rate rises, more people will start pregnancies with elevated blood pressures. About 20% to 25% of people with chronic hypertension develop preeclampsia during pregnancy (Carson & Gibson, 2022). Patients with chronic hypertension in pregnancy should be monitored for the development of worsening hypertension and/or the development of superimposed preeclampsia.

ACOG recommends antihypertensive therapy be initiated if chronic hypertension is detected with a blood pressure reading of 140/90 because of the long-term sequelae of stroke or acute renal failure (Ford et al., 2022). Patients with mild to moderate chronic hypertension do not require antihypertensive therapy during most of their pregnancy. Pharmacologic treatment of mild hypertension does not reduce the likelihood of developing preeclampsia later in gestation and increases the likelihood of intrauterine growth restriction. Nurses can play an important role in educating their patients with hypertension to help them understand potential complications and how simple changes in their lifestyles might be helpful in influencing the pregnancy outcome positively.

Gestational Hypertension

The gestational hypertension category is used in patients with nonproteinuric hypertension of pregnancy, in which the pathophysiologic disturbances of the preeclampsia syndrome do not develop before giving birth. Gestational hypertension is a temporary diagnosis for pregnant patients with hypertension who do not meet the criteria for preeclampsia (both hypertension and possibly proteinuria) or chronic hypertension (hypertension first detected before the 20th week of pregnancy).

Gestational hypertension is characterized by hypertension (higher than 140/90 mm Hg) in a previously normotensive patient without proteinuria after 20 weeks' gestation resolving by 12 weeks' postpartum (Melvin & Funai, 2024). Gestational hypertension is diagnosed when systolic blood pressure is over 140 mm Hg and/or diastolic pressure is over 90 mm Hg on at least two occasions at least 4 to 6 hours apart after the 20th week of gestation in patients known to be normotensive prior to this time and prior to pregnancy (Melvin & Funai, 2024). Gestational hypertension can be differentiated from chronic hypertension, which appears before the 20th week of gestation, or hypertension before the current pregnancy, which continues after the patient gives birth.

Preeclampsia/Eclampsia

Preeclampsia currently remains one of the leading causes of death and severe maternal morbidity worldwide. Normal physiologic adaptations to pregnancy are altered in the patient who develops preeclampsia. **Preeclampsia** can be described as new-onset hypertension accompanied by proteinuria and/or maternal organ dysfunction that targets the cardiovascular, hepatic, renal, and central nervous systems (CNS) (August & Sibai, 2024). Preeclampsia can present with severe features, or it may not. Each is associated with specific criteria. Comparison Chart 19.2 highlights these.

Pathophysiology

The progressive multisystem disorder preeclampsia results from abnormal placental plantation and a maternal vascular response (August & Sibai, 2024). The spiral arteries in the placenta fail to widen from thick-walled blood vessels to thinner, large-diameter saclike vessels with much larger diameters. This usual change in the spiral arteries permits the vessels to handle pregnancy's increased blood volume. In preeclampsia, this remodeling of the vessels either does not or only partially occurs, leading to decreased placental perfusion and hypoxia. Next, toxic substances are released due to placental ischemia, which cause endothelial cell dysfunction. Generalized vasospasm occurs, resulting in increased peripheral resistance, hypertension, and poor tissue perfusion in all organ systems (Dix, 2024).

Therapeutic Management

Current management of preeclampsia includes preconception counseling, perinatal blood pressure control and monitoring, prenatal aspirin therapy, betamethasone for

COMPARISON CHART 19.2 Preeclampsia Versus Eclampsia

	Preeclampsia Without Severe Features	Preeclampsia With Severe Features	Eclampsia
Blood pressure	≥140/90 mm Hg after 20 weeks' gestation	≥160/110 mm Hg on two occasions at least 6 hours apart while on bed rest	>160/110 mm Hg
Seizures/coma	No	No	Yes
Hyperreflexia	No	Yes	Yes
Other signs and symptoms		Headache Oliguria Blurred vision, scotomata (blind spots) Pulmonary edema Thrombocytopenia (platelet count <100,000 platelets/mm^3) Cerebral disturbances Persistent epigastric or right upper quadrant pain HELLP Progressive renal insufficiency	Severe headache Generalized edema Right upper quadrant or epigastric pain Visual disturbances Cerebral hemorrhage Renal failure HELLP

HELLP, hemolysis, elevated liver enzymes, and low platelets.

patients prior to 34 weeks' gestation, parenteral magnesium sulfate prophylaxis, and follow-up of postpartum blood pressures. Care of the patient with preeclampsia varies depending on the severity of their condition and its effects on the fetus. Typically, the patient is given conservative care if they are not experiencing severe features. However, if the condition progresses, the approach becomes more aggressive. After delivery of the fetus and placenta, blood pressure returns to normal within 4 weeks to 3 months (August & Sibai, 2024). According to recent studies, prevention of preeclampsia should be considered with daily low-dose aspirin (81 mg) from 12 weeks' gestation until delivery for patients with one or more high-risk factors (Wang et al., 2022) (see Evidence-Based Practice 19.1).

MANAGEMENT FOR PREECLAMPSIA WITHOUT SEVERE FEATURES

Conservative strategies for preeclampsia without severe features are used if the patient exhibits no signs of renal or hepatic dysfunction or coagulopathy. A patient with mild elevation in blood pressure may be placed on bed rest at home with instructions for blood pressure monitoring and fetal kick counts. Additionally, labs such as complete blood count (CBC), clotting studies, liver enzymes, and platelet levels will be periodically monitored. If home management fails to lower the blood pressure, admission to the hospital is warranted and the treatment strategy is individualized based on the severity of the condition and the gestational age at the time of diagnosis.

During hospitalization, the patient with preeclampsia without severe features is monitored closely for signs and symptoms of severe preeclampsia or impending eclampsia (e.g., persistent headache, hyperreflexia). Monitoring includes frequent blood pressure measurements and ongoing fetal surveillance. Expectant management (watchful waiting) usually continues until the pregnancy reaches at least 37 weeks' gestation, fetal lung maturity is documented, or complications develop that warrant immediate birth.

During labor, the focus is prevention of disease progression. Frequent blood pressure monitoring continues. A quiet environment is provided with continued close monitoring of neurologic status. An indwelling urinary catheter will allow for accurate measurement of urine output.

MANAGEMENT OF PREECLAMPSIA WITH SEVERE FEATURES

Before 37 weeks' gestation, expectant management may be appropriate unless the disease progresses and symptoms worsen. Preeclampsia with severe features may develop suddenly or within days and bring with it a blood pressure of more than 160/110 mm Hg, severe headache, visual symptoms, pulmonary edema, severe upper

EVIDENCE-BASED PRACTICE 19.1

Aspirin for the Prevention of Preeclampsia: A Systematic Review and Meta-Analysis of Randomized Controlled Studies

BACKGROUND

Preeclampsia is a pregnancy-specific disorder defined as a new onset of hypertension in pregnancy (>140/90) after the 20th week of gestation with the coexistence of either proteinuria (>300 mg/day) or maternal organ dysfunction. Organ dysfunction may include liver or renal insufficiency, neurologic or hematologic complications, uteroplacental dysfunction, or fetal growth restriction. The American College of Obstetricians and Gynecologists (ACOG) recommends that pregnant patients with any high-risk factors should receive low doses of aspirin (81 mg/day) to prevent preeclampsia starting between 12 and 16 weeks' gestation until childbirth. This systematic review was conducted to assess the use of aspirin to prevent preeclampsia.

STUDY

Hypertensive disorders are major causes of maternal and fetal complications worldwide, most notably preeclampsia. Aspirin has been a well-accepted therapy for the prevention of cardiovascular events. Therefore, it is hypothesized that aspirin, which is an antiplatelet agent, taken in early pregnancy may reduce pathologic coagulation and vasoconstriction in the placental circulation and promote placental growth, thus reducing the incidence of cardiovascular conditions in pregnant patients. A total of 1,241 articles were retrieved; of these, 39 were determined to be relevant and were used in the meta-analysis. Low-dose aspirin was given to patients at high risk for developing preeclampsia, and the treatment outcomes were compared to patients in the group not receiving aspirin in relation to preeclampsia prevention.

Findings

The systematic review found that aspirin was effective in preventing the occurrence of preeclampsia in pregnant patients at high risk if starting at 12 to 16 weeks' gestation. Aspirin is currently accepted for the prevention and treatment of preeclampsia.

Nursing Implications

Based on the findings of this review, nurses can be instrumental in identifying during early prenatal assessments those pregnant patients who are at high risk of developing preeclampsia so prophylactic, low-dose aspirin can be prescribed in early pregnancy if deemed appropriate by the health care provider. The nurse can provide instructions and rationales for the use and timing of this therapy to patients. Numerous studies and professional health organizations have recommended low-dose aspirin to prevent preeclampsia, so nurses can view this therapy as an evidence-based intervention to promote better outcomes for birthing parents and their infants.

Adapted from Wang, Y., Guo, X., Obore, N., Ding, H., Wu, C., & Yu, H. (2022). Aspirin for the prevention of preeclampsia: A systematic review and meta-analysis of randomized controlled studies. *Frontiers in Cardiovascular Medicine, 9*. https://doi.org/10.3389/fcvm.2022.936560

right quadrant or epigastric pain, impaired liver function, thrombocytopenia, and progressive renal insufficiency (August & Sibai, 2024). When severe features occur, immediate hospitalization is needed.

Preeclampsia with severe features is treated aggressively because hypertension poses a serious threat to the birthing parent and fetus. The goal of care is to stabilize the parent–fetus dyad and prepare for birth. Therapy focuses on controlling hypertension, preventing seizures, ensuring timely delivery, and preventing long-term morbidity and maternal, fetal, or newborn death (Norwitz, 2024). Intense maternal and fetal surveillance starts when the patient enters the hospital and continues throughout their stay.

Antihypertensive drugs are given to manage blood pressure, and magnesium sulfate is used to prevent seizure activity. Magnesium sulfate is given IV via an infusion pump. Refer to Drug Guide 19.3 for additional information. Decreased fetal heart rate variability may occur in response to magnesium sulfate. If at all possible, a vaginal delivery is preferable to a cesarean birth for better maternal outcomes and less risk associated

DRUG GUIDE 19.3

MEDICATIONS USED WITH PREECLAMPSIA AND ECLAMPSIA

Medication	Action/Indications	Nursing Implications
Magnesium sulfate	Blockage of neuromuscular transmission, vasodilation Prevention and treatment of eclamptic seizures	Administer loading dose of 4–6 g by intravenously (IV) in 100 mL of fluid administered over 15–30 minutes followed by a maintenance dose of 1–2 g as a continuous IV infusion. Monitor serum magnesium levels closely. Assess deep tendon reflexes (DTRs), and check for ankle clonus. Have calcium gluconate available in case of toxicity (give 10 mL of a 10% solution IV over 3 minutes). Monitor for signs and symptoms of toxicity, such as respiratory and central nervous system (CNS) depression, flushing, sweating, and hypotension. The drug should not be used longer than 5–7 days to avoid adverse fetal effects.
Hydralazine hydrochloride (Apresoline)	Vascular smooth muscle relaxant, thus improving perfusion to renal, uterine, and cerebral areas Reduction in blood pressure	Administer 5–10 mg by slow IV push every 20–40 minutes as needed. Use parenteral form immediately after opening the ampoule. Withdraw the drug slowly to prevent possible rebound hypertension. Monitor for adverse effects such as palpitations, headache, tachycardia, anorexia, nausea, vomiting, and diarrhea.
Labetalol hydrochloride (Normodyne)	α-1 and β blocker Reduction in blood pressure	Be aware that the drug lowers blood pressure without decreasing maternal heart rate or cardiac output. Administer an IV dose of 20 mg over 2 minutes. Increase subsequent doses by 20–40 mg given every 10–30 minutes (max dose 80 mg) or administer IV infusion of 0.5–2 mg/min until the desired blood pressure value is achieved. Monitor for possible adverse effects such as gastric pain, flatulence, constipation, dizziness, vertigo, and fatigue.
Nifedipine (Procardia)	Calcium channel blocker/dilation of coronary arteries, arterioles, and peripheral arterioles Reduction in blood pressure, stoppage of preterm labor	Administer 10 mg orally as the initial dose. After 20 minutes, if blood pressure (BP) remains elevated, give 10–20 mg; similarly, give a third dose. If BP remains elevated after three doses, another antihypertensive should be prescribed. Monitor for possible adverse effects such as dizziness, peripheral edema, angina, diarrhea, nasal congestions, and cough.
Sodium nitroprusside (Nitropress)	Rapid vasodilation (arterial and venous) Severe hypertension requiring rapid reduction in blood pressure	Administer via continuous IV infusion with a dose titrated according to BP levels. Wrap the IV infusion solution in foil or opaque material to protect it from light. Monitor for possible adverse effects, such as apprehension, restlessness, retrosternal pressure, palpitations, diaphoresis, and abdominal pain.
Furosemide (Lasix)	Diuretic action, inhibiting the reabsorption of sodium and chloride from the ascending loop of Henle Pulmonary edema (used only if the condition is present)	Administer via slow IV bolus at a dose of 20–40 mg. Monitor urine output hourly. Assess for possible adverse effects such as dizziness, vertigo, orthostatic hypotension, anorexia, vomiting, electrolyte imbalances, muscle cramps, and muscle spasms.

UpToDate, Inc. (2024). *UpToDate® Lexidrug*™ (Version 8.2.0) [Mobile app]. Wolters Kluwer. https://apps.apple.com/us/app/lexicomp/id313401238

with a surgical birth. PGE2 gel may be used to ripen the cervix. A cesarean birth may be performed if the patient is seriously ill. A pediatrician, neonatologist, and/or neonatal nurse practitioner should be available in the birthing room to care for the newborn. A newborn whose birthing parent received high doses of magnesium sulfate needs to be monitored for respiratory and neurologic depression (hypotonia, muscle weakness, loss of reflexes) and hypocalcemia (Numoto et al., 2021).

MANAGEMENT OF ECLAMPSIA

Eclampsia is the hallmark neurologic complication of preeclampsia, with the new onset of generalized, tonic–clonic seizure activity. Eclamptic seizures are a medical emergency and require immediate treatment to prevent mortality in both the birthing parent and fetus (Akre et al., 2022). Seizure management is provided, and magnesium sulfate may be continued. Magnesium sulfate is administered IV to prevent further seizures and continued for at least 24 hours after the patient's last seizure. After the patient's seizures are controlled, their stability is assessed. If they are stable, birth via induction or cesarean birth is performed (August & Sibai, 2023). If the patient's condition remains stable, they will be transferred to the postpartum unit for care. If they become unstable after giving birth, they may be transferred to the critical care unit for closer observation.

Nursing Assessment

Preventing complications related to preeclampsia requires the use of assessment, advocacy, and counseling skills. Assessment begins with the accurate measurement of the patient's blood pressure at each encounter. In addition, nurses need to assess for subjective complaints that may indicate the progression of the disease—visual changes, severe headaches, unusual bleeding or bruising, or right upper quadrant epigastric pain (August & Sibai, 2024). The significant signs of preeclampsia—proteinuria and hypertension—occur without the patient's awareness. Unfortunately, by the time symptoms are noticed, gestational hypertension can be severe.

> **TAKE NOTE!**
>
> The absolute blood pressure (a value that validates elevation) of 140/90 mm Hg should be obtained on two occasions 4 to 6 hours apart to be diagnostic of preeclampsia. Proteinuria is defined as 300 mg or more of urinary protein per 24 hours or more than 1+ protein by chemical reagent strip or dipstick of at least two random urine samples collected at least 4 to 6 hours apart with no evidence of urinary tract infection (UTI) (ACOG, 2024).

HEALTH HISTORY AND PHYSICAL EXAMINATION

Take a thorough history during the first prenatal visit to identify whether the patient is at risk for preeclampsia. Risk factors include:

- Primigravida status
- Age younger than 20 or older than 35
- Prepregnancy overweight or obesity
- History of preeclampsia in a previous pregnancy
- Prior pregnancy placental insufficiency
- History of diabetes, chronic hypertension or kidney disease, systemic lupus erythematosus, or antiphospholipid syndrome
- Assisted reproductive technology
- Multiple gestation
- Family history of preeclampsia (first-degree relative) (August & Sibai, 2024)

Patients at risk for preeclampsia require more frequent prenatal visits throughout their pregnancy, and they require teaching about problems so that they can report them promptly.

Blood pressure must be measured carefully and consistently. Obtain all measurements with the patient in the same position (recommended is on the right with the patient in a sitting position or lateral recumbent position with the arm at the level of the heart). Use the same technique (automated or manual) with appropriately calibrated devices (Dix, 2024). At each visit, also check a clean-catch urine specimen for protein using a dipstick. Monitor the fetus: At every prenatal visit, assess the fetal heart rate with a Doppler device.

> **TAKE NOTE!**
>
> Monitor the patient's weight frequently to identify sudden gains in a short time span. Nondependent edema in the face or hands may also occur (Carson & Gibson, 2022).

Various laboratory tests may be performed to evaluate the patient's status. These include a CBC, serum electrolytes, blood urea nitrogen (BUN), creatinine, and hepatic enzyme levels. If urine protein levels are 1 to 2+ or greater, a 24-hour urine collection is completed.

Nursing Management

Nursing care for the patient with preeclampsia focuses on close monitoring of blood pressure and ongoing assessment for evidence of disease progression. Throughout the patient's pregnancy, fetal surveillance is essential.

INTERVENING FOR PREECLAMPSIA WITHOUT SEVERE FEATURES

Typically, patients with preeclampsia without severe features and who are otherwise stable can be managed at home. Frequent monitoring to detect changes is necessary because preeclampsia can progress to eclampsia rapidly. Provide the patient with education about the disease process and blood pressure monitoring (see Teaching Guidelines 19.2). Instruct all patients to know the signs and symptoms of preeclampsia, and urge them to contact their health care provider for immediate evaluation should any occur. The home care nurse may make frequent visits and follow-up phone calls to assess the patient's condition, assist with scheduling periodic evaluations of the fetus (such as nonstress tests), and evaluate any changes that might suggest a worsening of the patient's condition.

Early detection and management of preeclampsia is associated with the greatest success in reducing the progression of this condition. As long as the patient carries out the guidelines of care as outlined by the health care provider and remains stable, home care can continue to maintain the pregnancy until the fetus is mature. If disease progression occurs, hospitalization is required. If hospitalized, the patient should be maintained in a quiet environment to minimize the risk of stimulation and to promote rest.

TEACHING GUIDELINES 19.2 Teaching for the Patient With Preeclampsia Without Severe Features

- Rest in a quiet environment to prevent cerebral disturbances.
- Drink eight to 10 glasses of water daily.
- Consume a balanced, high-protein diet including high-fiber foods.
- Obtain intermittent bed rest to improve circulation to the heart and uterus.
- Limit your physical activity to promote urination and subsequent decrease in blood pressure.
- Enlist the aid of your family so that you can obtain adequate rest time.
- Perform self-monitoring as instructed, including:
  - Taking your own blood pressure twice daily
  - Recording the number of fetal kicks daily
- Contact the home health nurse if any of the following occurs:
  - Increase in blood pressure
  - Burning or frequency when urinating
  - Decrease in fetal activity or movement
  - Headache (forehead or posterior neck region)
  - Dizziness or visual disturbances
  - Stomach pain, excessive heartburn, or epigastric pain
  - Decreased or infrequent urination
  - Contractions or low back pain
  - Easy or excessive bruising
  - Sudden onset of abdominal pain
  - Nausea and vomiting

INTERVENING FOR PREECLAMPSIA WITH SEVERE FEATURES

The patient with preeclampsia with severe features usually requires hospitalization. Keep the patient on complete bed rest in the left lateral lying position. Ensure that the room is dim and quiet to reduce stimulation. Give sedatives as ordered to encourage quiet bed rest. The patient is at risk for seizures if the condition progresses. Therefore, institute and maintain seizure precautions, such as padding the side rails and having oxygen, suction equipment, and a call button readily available to protect the patient from injury.

TAKE NOTE!

Preeclampsia increases the risk of placental abruption, preterm birth, intrauterine growth restriction, and fetal distress during childbirth. Always be prepared if you see symptoms of preeclampsia!

Closely monitor the patient's blood pressure. Administer antihypertensives as ordered to reduce blood pressure (Drug Guide 19.3). Assess the patient's vision and level of consciousness. Report any changes and any complaints of headache or visual disturbances. Recommend a high-protein diet with eight to 10 glasses of water daily. Monitor the patient's intake and output every hour, and administer fluid and electrolyte replacements as ordered. Assess the patient for signs and symptoms of pulmonary edema, such as crackles and wheezing heard on auscultation, dyspnea, decreased oxygen saturation levels, cough, neck vein distention, anxiety, and restlessness. The treatment of acute pulmonary edema is symptomatic and includes the administration of vasodilating agents and diuretics. The development of acute pulmonary edema in patients with hypertension during pregnancy is associated with high levels of IV fluid administration (Lim & Steinberg, 2022).

To achieve a safe outcome for the fetus, prepare the patient for possible testing to evaluate fetal status as preeclampsia progresses. Testing may include the nonstress test, serial ultrasounds to track fetal growth, and biophysical profile to evaluate ongoing fetal well-being (Carson & Gibson, 2022).

Administer parenteral magnesium sulfate as ordered to prevent seizures. Assess DTRs to evaluate the effectiveness of therapy. Patients with preeclampsia with severe features commonly present with hyperreflexia. Diminished or absent reflexes occur when the patient develops magnesium toxicity. Because magnesium is a potent neuromuscular blockade, the afferent and efferent nerve pathways do not relay messages properly and hyporeflexia develops. Nursing Procedure 19.1 highlights the steps for assessing the patellar reflex. The National Institute of Neurological Disorders and Stroke (NINDS) Muscle Stretch Reflex Scale grades reflexes from 0 to 4+. Grades 2+ and 3+ are considered normal, and grades 0

NURSING PROCEDURE 19.1 Assessing the Patellar Reflex

Purpose: To Evaluate for Nervous System Irritability Related to Preeclampsia

1. Place the patient in the supine position (or sitting upright with the legs dangling freely over the side of the bed or examination table).
2. If lying supine, have the patient flex their knee slightly.
3. Place a hand under the knee to support the leg and locate the patellar tendon. It should be midline just below the knee cap.
4. Using a reflex hammer or the side of your hand, strike the area of the patellar tendon firmly and quickly.
5. Note the movement of the leg and foot. A patellar reflex occurs when the leg and foot move (documented as 2+).
6. Repeat the procedure on the opposite leg.

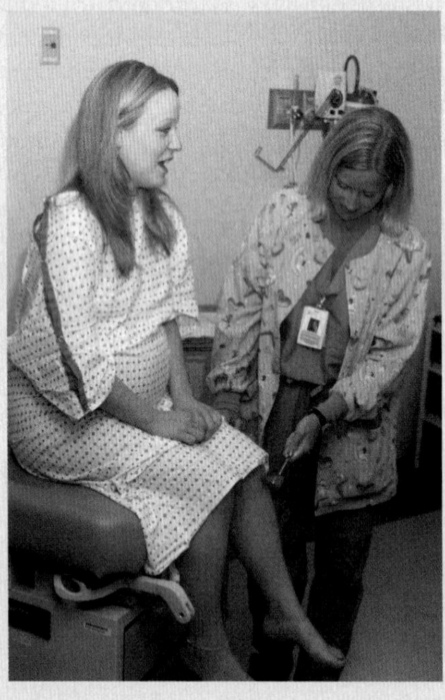

and 4 may indicate pathology (Table 19.2) (Zimmerman & Hubbard, 2023).

Clonus is the presence of rhythmic involuntary contractions, most often at the foot or ankle. Sustained clonus confirms CNS involvement. Nursing Procedure 19.2 highlights the steps when testing for ankle clonus.

CLINICAL REASONING ALERT!

In the patient receiving magnesium sulfate, toxicity is indicated by a respiratory rate of <12 breaths/min, absence of DTRs, and a decrease in urinary output (<30 mL/h).

TABLE 19.2 • Grading Deep Tendon Reflexes

Description of Finding	Grade
Reflex absent, none elicited	0
Hypoactive response, sluggish	1
Reflex in the lower half of the normal range	2
Reflex in the upper half of the normal range	3
Hyperactive, brisk, clonus present	4

Zimmerman, B., & Hubbard, J. B. (2023). Deep tendon reflexes. *StatPearls.* https://www.ncbi.nlm.nih.gov/books/NBK531502

NURSING PROCEDURE 19.2 Testing for Ankle Clonus

Purpose: To Evaluate for Nervous System Irritability Related to Preeclampsia

1. Place the patient in the supine position.
2. Have the patient slightly bend their knee, and place a hand under the knee to support it.
3. Dorsiflex the foot briskly and then quickly release it.

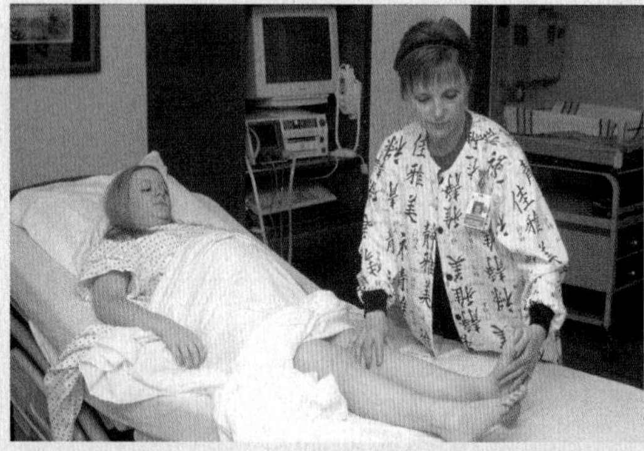

4. Watch for the foot to rebound smoothly against your hand. If the movement is smooth without any rapid contractions of the ankle or calf muscle, then clonus is not present; if the movement is jerky and rapid, clonus is present.
5. Repeat on the opposite side.

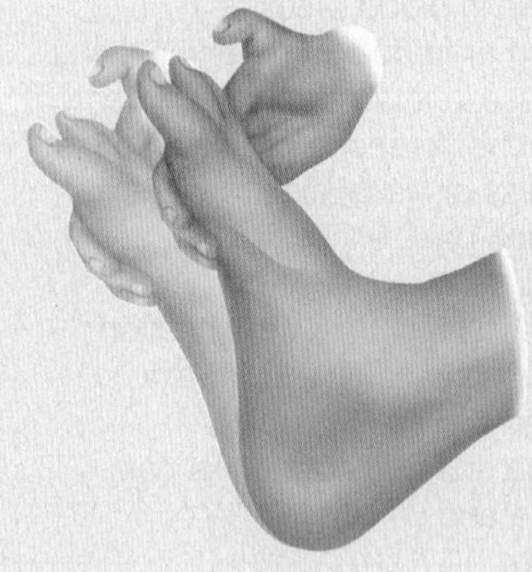

If signs and symptoms of magnesium toxicity develop, expect to administer calcium gluconate as the antidote.

Throughout the patient's stay, closely monitor them for signs and symptoms of labor. Perform continuous electronic fetal monitoring to assess fetal well-being. Note trends in baseline rate and presence or absence of accelerations or decelerations. Also observe for signs of fetal distress and report them immediately. Administer prescribed glucocorticoid treatment if ordered to enhance fetal lung maturity. Prepare for labor induction if the patient's condition warrants.

Keep the patient and family informed of the patient's condition and educate them about the course of treatment. Provide emotional support for the patient and family. Severe preeclampsia is frightening for the patient and their family, and most birthing parents are anxious about their own health as well as that of the fetus. To allay anxiety, use light touch to comfort and reassure the patient that the necessary actions are being taken. Actively listening to their concerns and fears and communicating them to the health care provider are important to keep the lines of communication open. Offering praise for small accomplishments can provide positive reinforcement for effective behaviors.

INTERVENING FOR ECLAMPSIA

The onset of seizure activity identifies eclampsia. Typically, eclamptic seizures are generalized and start with facial twitching. The body then becomes rigid in a state of tonic muscular contraction. The clonic phase of the seizure involves alternating contraction and relaxation of all body muscles. Respirations stop during seizure activity and resume shortly after it ends. Patient safety is the primary concern during eclamptic seizures. If possible, turn the patient to their side and remain with them. Make sure that the side rails are up and padded. Dim the lights and keep the room quiet.

Document the time and sequence of events as soon as possible. After the seizure activity has ceased, suction the nasopharynx as necessary and administer oxygen. Continue the magnesium sulfate infusion to prevent further seizures. Ensure continuous electronic fetal monitoring, evaluating fetal status for changes. Also assess the patient for uterine contractions. After the patient is stabilized, prepare them for the birthing process as soon as possible to reduce the risk of perinatal mortality.

PROVIDING FOLLOW-UP CARE

After the birth of the newborn, continue to monitor the patient for signs and symptoms of preeclampsia/eclampsia for at least 48 hours. Expect to continue to administer magnesium sulfate infusion for 24 hours to prevent seizure activity, and monitor serum magnesium levels for toxicity.

Assess vital signs at least every 4 hours, along with routine postpartum assessments: fundus, lochia, breasts, bladder, bowels, and the patient's emotional state. Monitor urine output closely. Diuresis is a positive sign that, along with a decrease in proteinuria, signals the resolution of the disease.

HELLP Syndrome

HELLP syndrome is an acronym for hemolysis, elevated liver enzymes, and low platelet count. It is a variant of the preeclampsia/eclampsia syndrome that occurs in 4% to 12% of patients with preeclampsia (Khan & Meirowitz, 2022). The onset is between 27 weeks' gestation and delivery and may also occur in the postpartum period. HELLP syndrome is characterized by abnormal vascular tone, vasospasm, and coagulation defects. People with HELLP syndrome are at increased risk for complications such as cerebral hemorrhage, retinal detachment, hematoma/liver rupture, DIC, placental abruption, eclampsia, acute renal failure, pulmonary edema, and maternal death (Khan & Meirowitz, 2022). It is a life-threatening obstetric complication considered by many to be a severe form of preeclampsia involving hemolysis, thrombocytopenia, and liver dysfunction. The recognition of HELLP syndrome, an aggressive multidisciplinary approach, and prompt transfer of these patients to obstetric centers with expertise in this field are required for the improvement of maternal–fetal prognosis.

Pathophysiology

Similar to preeclampsia, the essential phenomenon in HELLP's development is an abnormal trophoblastic invasion. Inadequate maternal immune tolerance may also play a role. Red blood cells become fragmented as they pass through small, damaged blood vessels, resulting in microangiopathic hemolytic anemia. Reduced blood flow to the liver secondary to obstruction from fibrin deposits leads to elevated liver enzymes. Endothelial damage and fibrin deposition in the liver lead to liver impairment, subsequent hyperbilirubinemia and jaundice, and possible hemorrhagic necrosis. Platelets aggregate at sites of vascular damage, with resultant thrombocytopenia (Khalid et al., 2023).

Therapeutic Management

Management focuses on the stabilization of blood pressure and assessment of fetal well-being to determine the optimal time for birth. The mainstay of treatment is lowering of high blood pressure with rapid-acting antihypertensive agents, prevention of convulsions or further seizures with magnesium sulfate, and administration of steroids to increase the preterm fetus's lung maturity. After 24 to 48 hours following steroid administration, the parental–fetal dyad is assessed to evaluate for delivery. If the birthing parent is unstable or fetal distress is present, immediate delivery of the fetus and placenta can be lifesaving for both the birthing parent and newborn (Khan & Meirowitz, 2022). The patient should be admitted or transferred to a tertiary center with a neonatal intensive care unit. Additional treatment includes correction of the coagulopathies that accompany HELLP syndrome.

Nursing Assessment

Nursing assessment of the patient with HELLP is similar to that for the patient with preeclampsia with severe features. Be alert for complaints of nausea (with or without vomiting), malaise, epigastric or right upper quadrant pain, headache, and changes in vision. Perform systematic assessments frequently as indicated by the patient's condition and response to therapy.

Nursing Management

Nursing care for the patient diagnosed with HELLP syndrome is the same as that for the patient with preeclampsia with severe features. If possible, the patient with HELLP syndrome should be transferred to a tertiary care center once they have been assessed and stabilized. Closely monitor the patient for changes and provide ongoing support throughout this experience.

BLOOD INCOMPATIBILITY

Blood incompatibility most commonly involves one of two issues: blood type or Rh factor. Blood type incompatibility, also known as ABO incompatibility, arises when a person with blood type O becomes pregnant with a fetus with a different blood type (type A, B, or AB). The pregnant person's serum contains naturally occurring anti-A and anti-B, which can cross the placenta and hemolyze fetal red blood cells. It is usually less severe than Rh incompatibility. One reason is that fetal red blood cells express less of the ABO blood group antigens when compared to adult levels. In addition, in contrast to the Rh antigens, the ABO blood group antigens are expressed by a variety of fetal (and adult) tissues, reducing the chances of anti-A and anti-B binding their target antigens on the fetal red blood cells. ABO incompatibility rarely causes significant hemolysis, and prenatal treatment is not warranted.

Rh isoimmunization occurs when a pregnant person's immune system creates antibodies against fetal Rh blood factors. Although the patient will exhibit no symptoms of Rh incompatibility, Rh antibodies adversely affect fetal health. Rh antibodies can cause fetal heart problems, breathing difficulties, jaundice, and a form of anemia known as hemolytic disease of the newborn. Rh sensitization occurs in approximately one in 1,000 births to Rh-negative birthing parents (Salem & Singer, 2022). Today, RH isoimmunization in pregnant people and hemolytic disease of the newborn are rarely seen, primarily because patients who are Rh-negative are given anti-D immune globulin prophylaxis (RhIG) in the third trimester of pregnancy and within 72 hours after childbirth if the newborn is Rh-positive.

Pathophysiology

Rhesus (Rh) incompatibility refers to the discordant pairing of maternal and fetal Rh types. This discordance becomes clinically significant if a birthing parent who is Rh-negative becomes sensitized to the D antigen and subsequently produces anti-D antibodies that can bind to and destroy Rh-positive red blood cells in the fetus (Sarwar & Sridhar, 2023).

Hemolysis associated with ABO incompatibility is limited to type O birthing parents with fetuses who have type A or B blood. In birthing parents with type A and B blood, naturally occurring antibodies are of the IgM class, which do not cross the placenta, while in type O birthing parents, the antibodies are predominantly IgG in nature. Because A and B antigens are widely expressed in a variety of tissues besides red blood cells, only a small portion of the antibodies crossing the placenta is available to bind to fetal red cells. The transplacental transport of the type O birthing parent's isoantibodies causes an immune reaction in the fetus (Whitehurst, 2020).

Rh Incompatibility (Hemolytic Disease of the Newborn or Alloimmune Hemolytic Disease of the Newborn)

Rh incompatibility is a condition that develops when a person with Rh-negative blood type is exposed to Rh-positive blood cells and subsequently develops circulating titers of Rh antibodies. People with an Rh-positive blood type have the D antigen present on their red cells, while people with an Rh-negative blood type do not. The presence or absence of the Rh antigen on the red blood cell membrane is genetically controlled.

In the United States, about 15% of the White population, 4% to 8% of the Black population, and 0.1% to 0.3% of the Asian population are Rh-negative. People otherwise are Rh-positive (Sarwar & Sridhar, 2023).

Rh incompatibility most commonly arises with exposure of a Rh-negative birthing parent to Rh-positive fetal blood during pregnancy or birth. Tiny amounts (0.1 mL) of fetal blood are transferred to the birthing parent during most pregnancies, but transplacental fetomaternal bleeding occurring with childbirth accounts for most cases of maternal D alloimmunization. Isoimmunization can also occur during an amniocentesis, ectopic pregnancy, placenta previa, placenta abruption, and in-utero fetal death, or due to small placental accidents (transplacental bleeds secondary to minor separation, trophoblastic disease, spontaneous abortion, or abdominal/pelvic trauma). After a significant exposure, alloimmunization or sensitization occurs. As a result, maternal antibodies are produced against the foreign Rh antigen (Moise, 2023).

Most firstborn infants with Rh-positive blood type are not affected because the short period from first exposure of Rh-positive fetal erythrocytes to the birth of the infant is insufficient to produce a significant maternal IgG antibody response. The risk and severity of alloimmune response increase with each subsequent pregnancy involving a fetus with Rh-positive blood. A second pregnancy with an Rh-positive fetus often produces an infant with mild anemia, while succeeding pregnancies produce infants with more serious hemolytic anemia.

Nursing Assessment

At the first prenatal visit, determine the patient's blood type and Rh status. Also obtain a thorough health history, noting any reports of previous events involving hemorrhage to delineate the risk for prior sensitization. When the patient's history reveals an Rh-negative birthing parent who may be pregnant with an Rh-positive fetus, prepare the patient for an antibody screen (indirect Coombs test) to determine whether they have developed isoimmunity to the Rh antigen. This test detects unexpected circulating antibodies in a pregnant person's serum, which could be harmful to the fetus.

Nursing Management

If the indirect Coombs test is negative (meaning no antibodies are present), then the patient is a candidate for RhIG. If the test is positive, RhIG is of no value because isoimmunization has occurred. In this case, the fetus is carefully monitored for hemolytic disease.

RhIG, which is pooled from human blood, helps destroy any fetal cells in the maternal circulation before sensitization occurs, thus inhibiting maternal antibody production. This provides temporary passive immunity, thereby preventing maternal sensitization (Yoham & Casadesus, 2023).

The incidence of isoimmunization has declined dramatically as a result of prenatal and postnatal RhIG administration after any event in which blood transfer may occur. The standard dose is 300 mcg, which is effective for 15 mL of fetal blood cells.

The current recommendation is for every Rh-negative nonimmunized pregnant person to receive RhIG at 28 weeks' gestation and again within 72 hours after giving birth. Other indications for receiving RhIG include:

- Ectopic pregnancy, abortion, miscarriage
- Chorionic villus sampling, amniocentesis, percutaneous umbilical sampling, fetal surgery
- Any bleeding during pregnancy
- Blunt trauma to the abdomen during pregnancy
- Manual fetal rotation for breech presentation (ACOG, 2022b)

Despite the availability of RhIG and laboratory tests to identify birthing parents and newborns at risk, isoimmunization remains a serious clinical reality that continues to contribute to perinatal and neonatal mortality. As patient advocates, nurses are in a unique position to make sure test results are brought to the health care provider's attention so appropriate interventions can be initiated. In addition, nurses must stay abreast of current literature and research regarding isoimmunization and its management. Stress to all patients who can become pregnant that early prenatal care can help identify and prevent this condition. Because Rh incompatibility is preventable with the use of RhIG, prevention remains the best treatment. Nurses can make a tremendous impact to ensure positive outcomes for the greatest possible number of pregnancies through education.

AMNIOTIC FLUID IMBALANCES

Amniotic fluid develops from several maternal and fetal structures, including the amnion, chorion, maternal blood, fetal lungs, gastrointestinal tract, kidneys, and skin. Any alteration in one or more of the various sources will alter the amount of amniotic fluid. Polyhydramnios and oligohydramnios are two imbalances associated with amniotic fluid.

Polyhydramnios

Polyhydramnios, also called hydramnios, is a condition in which there is an excessive volume of amniotic fluid (more than 2,000 mL) surrounding the fetus between 32 and 36 weeks' gestation. It occurs in approximately 1% to 2% of all pregnancies and is associated with maternal diabetes mellitus and fetal anomalies of development such as upper gastrointestinal obstruction or atresias, neural tube defects, and anterior abdominal wall defects, together with impaired swallowing in fetuses with chromosomal anomalies, such as trisomies 13 and 18 and anencephaly (Beloosesky & Ross, 2024). There is an increase in cesarean births for fetal labor intolerance, low 5-minute Apgar scores, increased neonatal birth weight, postpartum hemorrhage, cord prolapse, breech presentation, congenital anomalies, and newborn intensive care unit admissions for birthing parents with too much amniotic fluid at term (Beloosesky & Ross, 2024). Overall, it is associated with poorer fetal outcomes because of the increased incidence of preterm births, fetal malpresentation, and cord prolapse.

Therapeutic Management

Treatment may include close monitoring and frequent follow-up visits with the health care provider if the polyhydramnios is mild to moderate. In severe cases in which the birthing parent is in pain and experiencing shortness of breath, an amniocentesis or artificial rupture of the membranes is done to reduce the fluid and the pressure. Removal of fluid by amniocentesis is only transiently effective. A noninvasive treatment may involve the use of a prostaglandin synthesis inhibitor (indomethacin) to decrease amniotic fluid volume by decreasing fetal urinary output, but this may cause premature closure of the fetal ductus arteriosus and result in a transient decrease in fetal urine output (Hwang & Mahdy, 2023).

Nursing Assessment

Begin the assessment with a thorough history, staying alert to risk factors such as maternal diabetes or multiple gestations. Review the maternal history for information about possible fetal anomalies including fetal esophageal or intestinal atresia, neural tube defects, chromosomal deviations, fetal hydrops, CNS or cardiovascular anomalies, and hydrocephaly.

Polyhydramnios is initially suspected when uterine enlargement, maternal abdominal girth, and fundal height are larger than expected for the fetus's gestational age. Determine the gestational age of the fetus, and measure the patient's fundal height. With polyhydramnios, there is a discrepancy between fundal height and gestational age, or a rapid growth of the uterus is noted. Assess the patient for complaints of discomfort in their abdomen, such as being severely stretched and tight. Also note any reports of uterine contractions, which may result from overstretching of the uterus. Assess for shortness of breath resulting from pressure on the patient's diaphragm and inspect their lower extremities for edema, which results from increased pressure on the vena cava. Palpate the abdomen and obtain fetal heart rate. Often the fetal parts and heart rate are difficult to obtain because of the excess fluid present.

Prepare the patient for possible diagnostic testing to evaluate for the presence of possible fetal anomalies. An ultrasound is usually done to measure the pockets of amniotic fluid to estimate the total volume. In some cases, ultrasound is also helpful in finding the etiology of polyhydramnios, such as multiple pregnancy or a fetal structural anomaly.

Nursing Management

Nursing care of the patient with polyhydramnios focuses on ongoing assessment and monitoring for symptoms of abdominal pain, dyspnea, uterine contractions, and edema of the lower extremities. Explain to the patient and their family that this condition can cause the patient's uterus to become overdistended and may lead to preterm labor and PROM. Outline the signs and symptoms of both conditions, and instruct the patient to contact their health care provider if they occur. If a therapeutic amniocentesis is performed, assist the health care provider and monitor maternal and fetal status throughout for any changes.

Oligohydramnios

Oligohydramnios is a decreased amount of amniotic fluid expected for gestational age and is associated with poor pregnancy outcomes. The volume of amniotic fluid increases in a linear fashion until 34 to 36 weeks and then starts to decrease. It occurs in 2% to 10% of pregnancies at 4 to 42 weeks (Beloosesky & Ross, 2022). Oligohydramnios may result from any condition that prevents the fetus from making urine or blocks it from going into the amniotic sac. It is most common in the last trimester, but it can develop at any time in the pregnancy. About one in eight people whose pregnancies last 2 weeks past their expected due date develops oligohydramnios. This happens as amniotic fluid levels naturally decline. This condition puts the fetus at an increased risk of perinatal morbidity and mortality (Keilman & Shanks, 2022). Reduction in amniotic fluid reduces the ability of the fetus to move freely without the risk of cord compression, which increases the risk for fetal death and intrapartal hypoxia.

Therapeutic Management

Care for the patient with oligohydramnios can take place on an outpatient basis with serial ultrasounds and fetal surveillance through nonstress testing and biophysical profiles. As long as fetal well-being is demonstrated with frequent testing, no intervention is necessary. If fetal well-being is compromised, however, birth may be planned along with amnioinfusion (the transvaginal infusion of crystalloid fluid to compensate for the lost amniotic fluid). The fluid is introduced into the uterus through an intrauterine pressure catheter. The infusion is administered in a controlled fashion to prevent overdistention of the uterus. Amnioinfusion is thought to improve abnormal fetal heart rate patterns, decrease cesarean births, and possibly minimize the risk of neonatal meconium aspiration syndrome, but oral hydration of the birthing parent with up to 2 L of water may be an alternative to amnioinfusion to transiently increase amniotic fluid volume for up to 48 hours (Beloosesky & Ross, 2022).

Nursing Assessment

Though oligohydramnios can be idiopathic, there are multiple medical factors associated with it. Review the maternal and fetal histories for causes of oligohydramnios, including premature prelabor rupture of membranes, uteroplacental insufficiency (fetal growth restriction, preeclampsia, chronic abruption), and fetal anomalies.

Assess the patient for complaints of fluid leaking from the vagina. Leaking of amniotic fluid from the vagina occurs with rupture of the amniotic sac. Leaking in conjunction with a uterus that is small for expected dates of gestation also suggests oligohydramnios. However, the patient may not present with any symptoms. Typically, the reduced volume of amniotic fluid is identified on ultrasound.

Nursing Management

Nursing care of the patient with oligohydramnios involves continuous monitoring of fetal well-being during nonstress testing or during labor and birth by identifying category II and III patterns on the fetal monitor. Variable decelerations indicating cord compression are common. Changing the patient's position might be therapeutic in altering this fetal heart rate pattern. After the birth, evaluate the newborn for signs of postmaturity, congenital anomalies, and respiratory difficulty.

Continue to assess the patient's vital signs, contraction status, and fetal heart rate. Provide comfort measures such as changing the bed linens and the patient's bed clothes frequently because of the constant leakage of fluid from the vagina. Also provide frequent perineal care during the infusion.

MULTIPLE GESTATION

Multiple gestation is defined as a pregnancy with two or more fetuses. This includes twins, triplets, and higher order multiples such as quadruplets. The incidence of multiple gestations in the United States continues to increase because of the widespread use of fertility drugs, older age of people becoming pregnant, and the development of assisted reproductive technologies to treat infertility (Chasen, 2023).

In the United States, the overall prevalence of twins is about 3% of all live births, and about 70% are dizygotic (derived from two separate ova) (Gill et al., 2023). The increasing number of multiple gestations is a concern because birthing parents who are expecting more than one infant are at high risk for preterm labor, polyhydramnios, hyperemesis gravidarum, anemia, preeclampsia, and antepartum hemorrhage. Fetal/newborn risks or complications include prematurity, respiratory distress syndrome, birth asphyxia/perinatal depression, congenital anomalies (CNS, cardiovascular, and gastrointestinal defects), twin-to-twin transfusion syndrome (transfusion of blood from one twin [i.e., donor] to the other twin [i.e., recipient]), intrauterine growth restriction, and becoming conjoined twins (ACOG, 2021b).

Twins are either monozygotic (identical) or dizygotic (Fig. 19.6). Monozygotic twins develop when a single, fertilized ovum splits during the first 2 weeks after conception. Monozygotic twins are also called identical twins. Two sperm fertilizing two ova produce dizygotic twins, which are called fraternal twins. Separate amnions, chorions, and placentas are formed in dizygotic twins (fraternal). Triplets can be monozygotic, dizygotic, or trizygotic.

Therapeutic Management

When multiple gestation is confirmed, the patient is followed with serial ultrasounds to assess fetal growth patterns and development. Biophysical profiles along with nonstress tests are ordered to determine fetal well-being. Many patients are hospitalized in late pregnancy to prevent preterm labor and receive closer surveillance. During the intrapartum period, the patient is closely monitored with a perinatal team available to assist after birth. Operative delivery is frequently needed due to fetal malpresentation.

Nursing Assessment

Obtain a health history and perform a physical examination. Be alert for complaints of fatigue and severe nausea and vomiting. Assess the patient's abdomen and fundal height. Typically, with a multiple gestation, the uterus is larger than expected based on the estimated date of birth. Laboratory test results may reveal anemia. Prepare the patient for ultrasound, which typically confirms the diagnosis of a multiple gestation.

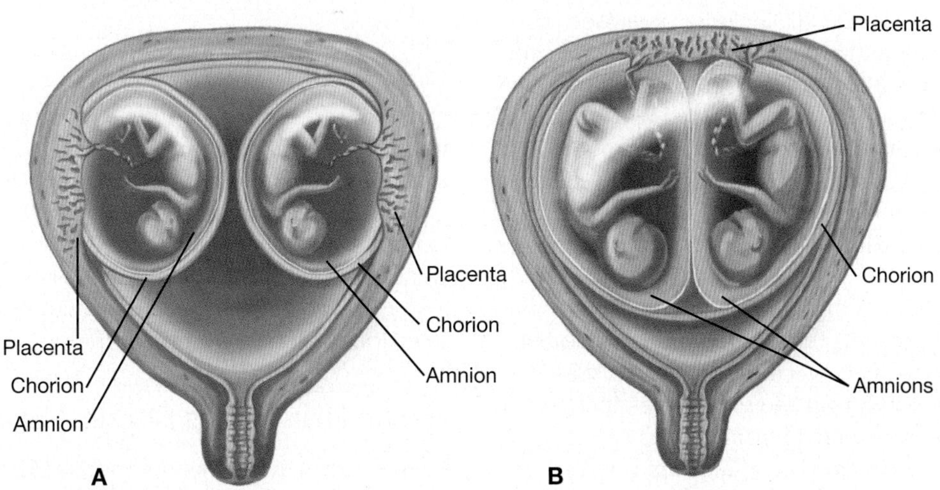

FIGURE 19.6 Multiple gestation with twins. **A.** Dizygotic twins; each fetus has its own placenta, amnion, and chorion. **B.** Monozygotic twins; the fetuses share one placenta, two amnions, and one chorion.

Nursing Management

During the prenatal period, provide education and support for the patient regarding nutrition, increased rest periods, and close observation for pregnancy complications such as anemia, excessive weight gain, proteinuria, edema, vaginal bleeding, and hypertension. Prevention of preterm labor is a major priority in caring for patients with a multifetal gestation. Instruct the patient to be alert for and immediately report any signs and symptoms of preterm labor, including contractions, uterine cramping, low backache, an increase in vaginal discharge, loss of mucus plug, pelvic pain, and pressure.

With the onset of labor, expect to monitor fetal heart rates continuously. Prepare the patient for an ultrasound to assess the presentation of each fetus to determine the best delivery approach. Ensure that extra nursing staff and the perinatal team are available for any birth or newborn complications.

After the babies are born, closely assess the birthing parent for hemorrhage by frequently assessing uterine involution. Palpate the uterine fundus and monitor the amount and characteristics of lochia.

Throughout the entire pregnancy, birth, and hospital stay, inform and support the patient and their family. Encourage them to ask questions and verbalize any fears and concerns.

PRELABOR RUPTURE OF MEMBRANES

Prelabor rupture of membranes (PROM) is the spontaneous rupture of the amniotic sac, sometimes called the bag of waters, before the onset of true labor. The exact cause of PROM is not known, but PROM may be associated with physiologic weakening of the amniotic membranes or with prelabor uterine contractions; it may also simply occur spontaneously (Dayal & Hong, 2023).

Complications of PROM include prolapsed cord, placental abruption, and preterm labor. High-risk factors associated with PROM include low socioeconomic status, multiple gestation, low BMI, tobacco use, history of preterm labor, placenta previa, placental abruption, UTI, vaginal bleeding at any time in pregnancy, illicit drug use, cerclage, and amniocentesis (Scorza, 2023). At term, it complicates approximately up to 8% of pregnancies (Scorza, 2023).

If prolonged (greater than 24 hours), the birthing parent's risk for infection (chorioamnionitis, endometritis, sepsis, and neonatal infections) increases and continues to increase the longer the time since the amniotic sac ruptured. The time interval from the rupture of membranes to the onset of regular contractions is termed the latent period. Fetal complications include intrauterine infection, umbilical cord compression, and placental abruption.

Patients with PROM present with leakage of fluid, vaginal discharge, vaginal bleeding, and pelvic pressure, but they are not having contractions. PROM is diagnosed by speculum vaginal examination of the cervix and vaginal cavity. Pooling of fluid in the vagina or leakage of fluid from the cervix, ferning of the dried fluid under microscopic examination, and alkalinity of the fluid as determined by nitrazine paper (pH indicator) confirm the diagnosis.

The terminology of PROM can be confusing. PROM is the rupture of the membranes prior to the onset of labor and is used appropriately when referring to a patient who is beyond 37 weeks' gestation, has presented with spontaneous rupture of the membranes, and is not in labor. A related term is **preterm prelabor rupture of membranes (PPROM)**, which is defined as the rupture of membranes prior to the onset of labor in a birthing parent who is *less* than 37 weeks' gestation. PPROM complicates 3% of all pregnancies yearly in the United States (Duff, 2024a).

Therapeutic Management

Treatment of PROM typically depends on the gestational age. Under no circumstances is an unsterile digital cervical examination done until the patient enters active labor to minimize infection exposure. If the fetal lungs are mature, induction of labor is initiated. PROM is not a lone indicator for surgical birth. If the fetal lungs are immature, expectant management is carried out with adequate hydration, reduced physical activity, pelvic rest, and close observation for possible infection, such as with frequent monitoring of vital signs and laboratory test results (e.g., white blood cell count). Corticosteroids may be given to enhance fetal lung maturity if lungs are immature, though this remains controversial. Recent studies have shown clear benefits of antibiotics in decreasing the incidence of chorioamnionitis and neonatal morbidity associated with PPROM (Duff, 2024b).

Nursing Assessment

Nursing assessment focuses on obtaining a complete health history and performing a physical examination to determine maternal and fetal status. An accurate assessment of the gestational age and knowledge of the maternal, fetal, and neonatal risks are essential to appropriate evaluation, counseling, and care for patients with PROM and PPROM. Nurses need to be aware that the risk of infection increases with the duration of PPROM.

Health History and Physical Examination

Review the maternal history for risk factors such as infection, increased uterine size (potential polyhydramnios, macrosomia, and multiple gestation), uterine and fetal anomalies, lower socioeconomic status, STIs, cervical insufficiency, vaginal bleeding, and cigarette smoking during pregnancy. Ask about any history or current symptoms of UTI (frequency, urgency, dysuria, or flank pain) or pelvic or vaginal infection (pain or vaginal discharge). Assess for symptoms of labor (cramping, pelvic pressure, or back pain). Also assess vital signs; fever or tachycardia may indicate the development of infection (Duff, 2024a).

Institute continuous electronic fetal heart rate monitoring to evaluate fetal well-being. Conduct a vaginal examination to ascertain the cervical status in PROM. If PPROM exists, a sterile speculum examination (during which the examiner inspects the cervix but does not palpate it) is done rather than a digital cervical examination because it may diminish latency (period of time from rupture of membranes to birth) and increase newborn morbidity (Duff, 2024a).

Observe the characteristics of the amniotic fluid. Note any evidence of meconium or a foul odor. When meconium is present in the amniotic fluid, it typically indicates fetal distress related to hypoxia. Meconium stains the fluid yellow to greenish brown, depending on the amount present. A foul odor of amniotic fluid indicates infection. Also observe the amount of fluid. A decreased amount of amniotic fluid reduces the cushioning effect, thereby making cord compression a possibility. Key assessments are summarized in Box 19.2.

BOX 19.2 Key Assessments With Prelabor Rupture of Membranes

For the patient with PROM, the following assessments are essential:

- Determining the date, time, and duration of membrane rupture by patient interview
- Ascertaining gestational age of the fetus based on the date of the birthing parent's last menstrual period, fundal height, and ultrasound dating
- Visualizing clear fluid pooled in the vaginal vault
- Questioning the patient about possible history of or recent UTI or vaginal infection that might have contributed to PROM
- Assessing for any associated labor symptoms, such as back pain or pelvic pressure
- Assisting with or performing diagnostic tests to validate leakage of fluid, such as nitrazine test, "ferning" on slide, and ultrasound; contamination of nitrazine tape with lubricant or insufficient fluid will render the assessment unreliable.
- Continually assessing for signs of infection including:
  - Elevation of maternal temperature and pulse rate
  - Abdominal/uterine tenderness
  - Fetal tachycardia >160 bpm
  - Elevated white blood cell count and C-reactive protein
  - Cloudy, foul-smelling amniotic fluid

PROM, prelabor rupture of membranes; UTI, urinary tract infection.

Dayal, S., & Hong, P. L. (2023). Premature rupture of membranes. *StatPearls*. https://www.ncbi.nlm.nih.gov/books/NBK532888/; Duff, P. (2024a). Preterm prelabor rupture of membranes: Clinical manifestations and diagnosis. *UpToDate*. Retrieved May 1, 2024, from https://www.uptodate.com/contents/preterm-prelabor-rupture-of-membranes-clinical-manifestations-and-diagnosis

Laboratory and Diagnostic Testing

To diagnose PROM or PPROM, several procedures may be used: the nitrazine test, fern test, or ultrasound. After the insertion of a sterile speculum, a sample of the fluid in the vaginal area is obtained. With a nitrazine test, the pH of the fluid is tested; amniotic fluid is more basic (7.0) than normal vaginal secretions (4.5). Nitrazine paper turns blue in the presence of amniotic fluid. However, false-positive results can occur if blood, urine, semen, or antiseptic chemicals are also present; all will increase the pH.

For the fern test, a sample of vaginal fluid is placed on a slide to be viewed directly under a microscope. Amniotic fluid will develop a fernlike pattern when it dries because of sodium chloride crystallization. If both of these tests are inconclusive, a transvaginal ultrasound can also be used to determine whether membranes have ruptured by demonstrating a decreased amount of amniotic fluid (oligohydramnios) in the uterus (Dayal & Hong, 2023).

Other laboratory and diagnostic tests that may be obtained are:

1. Urinalysis and urine culture for UTI or bacteriuria without symptoms
2. Cervical test or culture for chlamydia or gonorrhea
3. Vaginal culture for bacterial vaginosis and trichomoniasis
4. Vaginal introital/rectal culture for group B streptococcus

Nursing Management

Nursing care of the patient with PROM or PPROM focuses on preventing infection and identifying uterine contractions. The risk for infection is great because of the break in the amniotic fluid membrane and its proximity to vaginal bacteria. Therefore, maternal vital signs must be monitored closely. Be alert for a temperature elevation or an increase in pulse, which could indicate infection. Also monitor the fetal heart rate continuously, reporting any fetal tachycardia (which could indicate a maternal infection) or variable decelerations (suggesting cord compression). If variable decelerations are present, amnioinfusion may be used based on agency policy. Evaluate the results of laboratory tests such as a CBC. An elevation in white blood cells would suggest infection. Administer antibiotics if ordered.

Encourage the patient to verbalize their feelings and concerns. Educate them about the purpose of the protective membranes and the implications of early rupture. Keep them informed about planned interventions, including potential complications and required therapy. If the patient has a partner, include them in this encouragement and education. As appropriate, prepare the patient for induction or augmentation of labor as appropriate if they are near term.

If labor does not start within 48 hours, the patient with PPROM may be discharged home on expectant management, which may include:

- Antibiotics if cervicovaginal cultures are positive
- Activity restrictions
- Education about signs and symptoms of infection and when to call with problems or concerns (Teaching Guidelines 19.3)
- Frequent fetal testing for well-being
- Ultrasound every 3 to 4 weeks to assess amniotic fluid levels
- Possible corticosteroid treatment depending on gestational age
- Daily kick counts to assess fetal well-being

TEACHING GUIDELINES 19.3 Teaching for the Patient With PROM/PPROM

- Monitor your baby's activity by performing fetal kick counts daily.
- Check your temperature daily, and report any temperature increases to your health care provider.
- Watch for signs related to the beginning of labor. Report any tightening of the abdomen or contractions.
- Avoid any touching or manipulating of your breasts, which could stimulate labor.
- Do not insert anything into your vagina or vaginal area; do not use tampons and avoid vaginal intercourse.
- Do not swim in pools or in the ocean or sit in a hot tub or Jacuzzi.
- Take showers for daily hygiene needs; avoid sitting in a tub bath.
- Maintain any specific activity restrictions as recommended.
- Wash your hands thoroughly after using the bathroom, and make sure to wipe from front to back each time.
- Keep your perineal area clean and dry.
- Take your antibiotics as directed if your health care provider has prescribed them.
- Call your health care provider with changes in your condition, including fever, uterine tenderness, feeling like your heart is racing, and foul-smelling vaginal discharge (Baker & Hurst, 2024).

KEY CONCEPTS

- Identifying risk factors early on and throughout the pregnancy is important to ensure the best outcome for every pregnancy. Risk assessment should start with the first prenatal visit and continue with subsequent visits.
- The three most common causes of hemorrhage early in pregnancy (first half of pregnancy) are spontaneous abortion, ectopic pregnancy, and GTD.
- Ectopic pregnancies occur in about one in 40 pregnancies and have increased dramatically during the past few decades.
- Having a molar pregnancy results in the loss of the pregnancy and the possibility of developing choriocarcinoma, a chronic malignancy from the trophoblastic tissue.
- The classic clinical picture presentation for placenta previa is painless, bright red vaginal bleeding occurring during the third trimester.
- Treatment of placental abruption is designed to assess, control, and restore the amount of blood lost; to provide a positive outcome for both birthing parent and infant; and to prevent coagulation disorders.
- DIC can be described in simplest terms as a loss of balance between the clot-forming activity of thrombin and the clot-lysing activity of plasmin.
- Hyperemesis gravidarum is a complication of pregnancy characterized by persistent, uncontrollable nausea and vomiting in early pregnancy.
- Gestational hypertension is the leading cause of maternal death in the United States and the most common complication reported during pregnancy.
- HELLP is an acronym for hemolysis, elevated liver enzymes, and low platelet count.
- Rh incompatibility is a condition that develops when a birthing parent with Rh-negative blood is exposed to Rh-positive fetal blood cells and subsequently develops circulating titers of Rh antibodies.
- Polyhydramnios occurs in approximately 2% of all pregnancies and is associated with fetal anomalies of development.
- Nursing care for the patient with oligohydramnios involves continuous monitoring of fetal well-being during nonstress testing or during labor and birth by identifying category II and III patterns on the fetal monitor.
- The increasing number of multiple gestations is a concern because people who are pregnant with more than one infant are at high risk for preterm labor, hydramnios, hyperemesis gravidarum, anemia, preeclampsia, and antepartum hemorrhage.
- Nursing care related to PROM centers on infection prevention and identification of preterm labor contractions.
- Monitoring maternal vital signs for changes and the fetal heart rate once PPROM occurs is essential to increasing the chances of a good outcome.
- It is essential that nurses educate all pregnant patients about how to detect the early signs of PROM and what action is needed if it happens.

REFERENCES AND RECOMMENDED READINGS

Akre, S., Sharma, K., Chakole, S., & Wanjari, M. B. (2022). Eclampsia and its treatment modalities: A review article. *Cureus, 14*(9), e29080. https://doi.org/10.7759/cureus.29080

AlJulaih, G. H., & Muzio, M. R. (2023). Gestational trophoblastic neoplasia. *StatPearls*. https://www.ncbi.nlm.nih.gov/books/NBK562225/

American College of Obstetricians and Gynecologists. (2021a). *Placenta accreta spectrum (Reaffirmed)*. https://www.acog.org/clinical/clinical-guidance/obstetric-care-consensus/articles/2018/12/placenta-accreta-spectrum#

American College of Obstetricians and Gynecologists. (2021b). *Practice Bulletin 231: Multifetal gestations twin triplet and higher-order multifetal pregnancies*. https://www.acog.org/clinical/clinical-guidance/practice-bulletin/articles/2021/06/multifetal-gestations-twin-triplet-and-higher-order-multifetal-pregnancies

American College of Obstetricians and Gynecologists. (2022a). *Ectopic pregnancy*. https://www.acog.org/womens-health/faqs/ectopic-pregnancy

American College of Obstetricians and Gynecologists. (2022b). *The Rh factor: How it can affect your pregnancy*. https://www.acog.org/womens-health/faqs/the-rh-factor-how-it-can-affect-your-pregnancy

American College of Obstetricians and Gynecologists. (2024). *Clinical guidance for the integration of the findings of the chronic hypertension and pregnancy (CHAP) study (Reaffirmed)*. https://www.acog.org/clinical/clinical-guidance/practice-advisory/articles/2022/04/clinical-guidance-for-the-integration-of-the-findings-of-the-chronic-hypertension-and-pregnancy-chap-study

Ananth, C. V., & Kinzler, W. L. (2023). Acute placental abruption: Pathophysiology, clinical features, diagnosis, and consequences. *UpToDate*. Retrieved April 29, 2024, from https://www.uptodate.com/contents/acute-placental-abruption-pathophysiology-clinical-features-diagnosis-and-consequences

August, P., & Sibai, B. M. (2023). Hypertensive disorders in pregnancy: Approach to differential diagnosis. *UpToDate*. Retrieved April 28, 2024, from https://www.uptodate.com/contents/hypertensive-disorders-in-pregnancy-approach-to-differential-diagnosis

August, P., & Sibai, B. M. (2024). Preeclampsia: Clinical features and diagnosis. *UpToDate*. Retrieved April 28, 2024, from https://www.uptodate.com/contents/preeclampsia-clinical-features-and-diagnosis

Baergen, R. N. (2021). Gestational trophoblastic disease: Pathology. *UpToDate*. Retrieved April 28, 2024, from https://www.uptodate.com/contents/gestational-trophoblastic-disease-pathology

Baker, B., & Hurst, H. E. (2024). Labor and delivery at risk. In B. J. Baker, J. Janke, & Association of Women's Health, Obstetric and Neonatal Nurses, *Core curriculum for maternal-newborn nursing* (6th ed.). Elsevier.

Belfort, M. A. (2023). Disseminated intravascular coagulation (DIC) during pregnancy: Clinical findings, etiology, and diagnosis. *UpToDate*. Retrieved April 29, 2024, from https://www.uptodate.com/contents/disseminated-intravascular-coagulation-dic-during-pregnancy-clinical-findings-etiology-and-diagnosis

Beloosesky, R., & Ross, M. G. (2022). Oligohydramnios: Etiology, diagnosis, and management in singleton gestations. *UpToDate*. Retrieved May 1, 2024, from https://www.uptodate.com/contents/oligohydramnios-etiology-diagnosis-and-management-in-singleton-gestations

Beloosesky, R., & Ross, M. G. (2024). Polyhydramnios: Etiology, diagnosis, and management in singleton gestations. *UpToDate*. Retrieved May 1, 2024, from https://www.uptodate.com/contents/polyhydramnios-etiology-diagnosis-and-management-in-singleton-gestations

Bender, W. (2022). Deep dive into hypertensive disorders in pregnancy. *Contemporary OB/GYN, 67*(5), 16–20. https://www.contemporaryobgyn.net/view/deep-dive-into-hypertensive-disorders-in-pregnancy

Berghella, V. (2024). Cervical insufficiency. *UpToDate*. Retrieved April 28, 2024, from https://www.uptodate.com/contents/cervical-insufficiency

Berkowitz, R. S., Horowitz, N. S., & Elias, K. M. (2022). Gestational trophoblastic neoplasia: Epidemiology, clinical features, diagnosis, staging, and risk stratification. *UpToDate*. Retrieved April 28, 2024, from https://www.uptodate.com/contents/gestational-trophoblastic-neoplasia-epidemiology-clinical-features-diagnosis-staging-and-risk-stratification

Berkowitz, R. S., Horowitz, N. S., & Elias, K. M. (2023). Hydatidiform mole: Epidemiology, clinical features, and diagnosis. *UpToDate*. Retrieved April 28, 2024, from https://www.uptodate.com/contents/hydatidiform-mole-epidemiology-clinical-features-and-diagnosis

Carson, M. P., & Gibson, P. S. (2022). Hypertension and pregnancy. *Medscape*. https://emedicine.medscape.com/article/261435-overview

Centers for Disease Control and Prevention. (2022). *Stillbirth*. https://www.cdc.gov/ncbddd/stillbirth/index.html

Chasen, S. T. (2023). Twin pregnancy: Overview. *UpToDate*. Retrieved May 1, 2024, from https://www.uptodate.com/contents/twin-pregnancy-overview

Cunningham, F. G., Leveno, K. J., Dashe, J. S., Hoffman, B. L., Spong, C. Y., & Casey, B. M. (2022a). First- and second-trimester pregnancy loss. In F. G. Cunningham, K. J. Leveno, J. S. Dashe, B. L. Hoffman, C. Y. Spong, & B., M. Casey, *William's obstetrics* (26th ed.). McGraw-Hill.

Cunningham, F. G., Leveno, K. J., Dashe, J. S., Hoffman, B. L., Spong, C. Y., & Casey, B. M. (2022b). Ectopic pregnancy. In F. G. Cunningham, K. J. Leveno, J. S. Dashe, B. L. Hoffman, C. Y. Spong, & B., M. Casey, *William's obstetrics* (26th ed.). McGraw-Hill.

Cunningham, F. G., Leveno, K. J., Dashe, J. S., Hoffman, B. L., Spong, C. Y., & Casey, B. M. (2022c). Gestational trophoblastic disease. In F. G. Cunningham, K. J. Leveno, J. S. Dashe, B. L. Hoffman, C. Y. Spong, & B., M. Casey, *William's obstetrics* (26th ed.). McGraw-Hill.

Cunningham, F. G., Leveno, K. J., Dashe, J. S., Hoffman, B. L., Spong, C. Y., & Casey, B. M. (2022d). Antepartum fetal assessment. In F. G. Cunningham, K. J. Leveno, J. S. Dashe, B. L. Hoffman, C. Y. Spong, & B., M. Casey, *William's obstetrics* (26th ed.). McGraw-Hill.

Cunningham, F. G., Leveno, K. J., Dashe, J. S., Hoffman, B. L., Spong, C. Y., & Casey, B. M. (2022e). Hemorrhagic placental disorders. In F. G. Cunningham, K. J. Leveno, J. S. Dashe, B. L. Hoffman, C. Y. Spong, & B., M. Casey, *William's obstetrics* (26th ed.). McGraw-Hill.

Dayal, S., & Hong, P. L. (2023). Premature rupture of membranes. *StatPearls*. https://www.ncbi.nlm.nih.gov/books/NBK532888/

Deering, S. H. (2023). Abruptio placentae. *Medscape*. https://emedicine.medscape.com/article/252810-overview

Dix, D. (2024). Hypertensive disorders in pregnancy. In B. J. Baker, J. Janke, & Association of Women's Health, Obstetric and Neonatal Nurses, *Core curriculum for maternal-newborn nursing* (6th ed.). Elsevier.

Duff, P. (2024a). Preterm prelabor rupture of membranes: Clinical manifestations and diagnosis. *UpToDate*. Retrieved May 1, 2024, from https://www.uptodate.com/contents/preterm-prelabor-rupture-of-membranes-clinical-manifestations-and-diagnosis

Duff, P. (2024b). Preterm prelabor rupture of membranes: Management and outcome. *UpToDate*. Retrieved May 1, 2024, from https://www.uptodate.com/contents/preterm-prelabor-rupture-of-membranes-management-and-outcome

Ford, N. D., Cox, S., Ko, J. Y., Ouyang, L., Romero, L., Colarusso, T., Ferre, C. D., Kroelinger, C. D., Hayes, D. K., & Barfield, W. D. (2022). Hypertensive disorders in pregnancy and mortality at delivery hospitalization—United States, 2017–2019. *MMWR, Morbidity and Mortal Weekly Report*, *71*, 585–591. http://doi.org/10.15585/mmwr.mm7117a

Gill, P., Lende, M. N., & Van Hook, J. W. (2023). Twin births. *StatPearls*. https://pubmed.ncbi.nlm.nih.gov/29630252/

Guan, X., Huang, X., Ye, M., Huang, G., Xiao, X., & Chen, J. (2022). Treatment of placenta increta with high-intensity focused ultrasound ablation and leaving the placenta in situ: A multicenter comparative study. *Frontiers in Medicine*, *9*. https://doi.org/10.3389/fmed.2022.871528

Hwang, D. S., & Mahdy, H. (2023). Polyhydramnios. *StatPearls*. https://www.ncbi.nlm.nih.gov/books/NBK562140/

Jennings, L. K., & Mahdy, H. (2023). Hyperemesis gravidarum. *StatPearls*. https://www.ncbi.nlm.nih.gov/books/NBK532917/#article-27636.s2

Keilman, C., & Shanks, A. L. (2022). Oligohydramnios. *StatPearls*. https://www.ncbi.nlm.nih.gov/books/NBK562326/

Khalid, F., Mahendraker, N., & Tonismae, T. (2023). HELLP syndrome. *StatPearls*. https://www.ncbi.nlm.nih.gov/books/NBK560615/

Khan, H., & Meirowitz, M. B. (2022). HELLP syndrome. *Medscape*. https://emedicine.medscape.com/article/1394126-overview#a4

Levi, M. M., & Schmaier, A. H. (2022). Disseminated intravascular coagulation (DIC). *Medscape*. https://emedicine.medscape.com/article/199627-overview

Lim, K.-H., & Steinberg, G. (2022). Preeclampsia. *Medscape*. https://emedicine.medscape.com/article/1476919-overview#a1

Lockwood, C. J., & Russo-Stieglitz, K. (2024a). Placenta previa: Epidemiology, clinical features, diagnosis, morbidity and mortality. *UpToDate*. Retrieved April 28, 2024, from https://www.uptodate.com/contents/placenta-previa-epidemiology-clinical-features-diagnosis-morbidity-and-mortality

Lockwood, C. J., & Russo-Stieglitz, K. (2024b). Placenta previa: Management. *UpToDate*. Retrieved April 28, 2024, from https://www.uptodate.com/contents/placenta-previa-management

Mares, R., Morrow, A., Shumway, H., Zapata, I., Forstein, D., & Brooks, B. (2022). Assessment of management approaches for hyperemesis gravidarum and nausea and vomiting of pregnancy: a retrospective questionnaire analysis. *BMC Pregnancy and Childbirth*, *22*(1). https://doi.org/10.1186/s12884-022-04922-6

Melvin, L. M., & Funai, E. F. (2024). Gestational hypertension. *UpToDate*. Retrieved April 30, 2024, from https://www.uptodate.com/contents/gestational-hypertension

Moise, K. J. (2023). RhD alloimmunization in pregnancy: Overview. *UpToDate*. Retrieved April 30, 2024, from https://www.uptodate.com/contents/rhd-alloimmunization-in-pregnancy-overview

Morlando, M., & Collins, S. (2022). Placenta accreta spectrum disorders: Challenges, risks, and management strategies. *International Journal of Women's Health*, *12*, 1033–1045. https://doi.org/10.2147/IJWH.S224191

Myers, A. L. (2022). *Racial and ethnic disparities in maternal health*. https://www.bcbs.com/the-health-of-america/reports/racial-and-ethnic-disparities-maternal-health

Nafiah, M., Chieng, N., Zainuddin, W., Chew, A., Kalok, K., Abu, A., & Ng, M. (2022). Effect of acupressure at P6 on nausea and vomiting in women with hyperemesis gravidarum: A randomized controlled trial. *International Journal of Environmental Research and Public Health*, *19*(17), 10886. https://doi.org/10.3390/ijerph191710886

National Cancer Institute. (2022). *Gestational trophoblastic disease treatment (PDQ®)–Health professional version*. https://www.cancer.gov/types/gestational-trophoblastic/hp/gtd-treatment-pdq

National Institute of Child Health and Human Development. (2022). *Who is at increased risk of health problems during pregnancy?* https://www.nichd.nih.gov/health/topics/preconceptioncare/conditioninfo/risk

Norwitz, E. R. (2024). Preeclampsia: Antepartum management and timing of delivery. *UpToDate*. Retrieved April 29, 2024, from https://www.uptodate.com/contents/preeclampsia-antepartum-management-and-timing-of-delivery

Norwitz, E. R., & Park, J. S. (2023). Evaluation and differential diagnosis of vaginal bleeding before 20 weeks of gestation. *UpToDate*. Retrieved April 29, 2024, from https://www.uptodate.com/contents/overview-of-the-etiology-and-evaluation-of-vaginal-bleeding-in-pregnancy

Numoto, S., Kakita, H., Takeshita, S., Ueda, H., Kondo, T., Kurahashi, H., Wakatsuki, A., Yamada, Y., & Okumura, A. (2021). Effects of maternal magnesium sulfate treatment on newborns. *Pediatrics International*, *64*(1), e14747. https://doi.org.resource.ahu.edu/10.1111/ped.14747

Prager, S., Micks, E., & Dalton, V. K. (2024). Pregnancy loss (miscarriage): Terminology, risk factors, and etiology. *UpToDate*. Retrieved April 28, 2024, from https://www.uptodate.com/contents/pregnancy-loss-miscarriage-terminology-risk-factors-and-etiology

Salem, L., & Singer, K. R. (2022). Rh incompatibility. *Medscape*. https://emedicine.medscape.com/article/797150-overview#a6

Sarwar, A., & Sridhar, D. C. (2023). Rh hemolytic disease. *StatPearls*. https://www.ncbi.nlm.nih.gov/books/NBK560488/#article-28508.s5

Schetter, C. D., Rahal, D., Ponting, C., Julian, M., Ramos, I., Hobel, C. J., & Coussons-Read, M. (2022). Anxiety in pregnancy and length of gestation: Findings from the healthy babies before birth study. *Health Psychology*, *41*(12). https://doi.org/10.1037/hea0001210

Scorza, W. E. (2023). Prelabor rupture of membranes at term: management. *UpToDate*. Retrieved May 1, 2024, from https://www.uptodate.com/contents/prelabor-rupture-of-membranes-at-term-management

Sibai, B. M. (2023). HELLP syndrome (hemolysis, elevated liver enzymes, and low platelets). *UpToDate*. Retrieved May 1, 2024, from https://www.uptodate.com/contents/hellp-syndrome-hemolysis-elevated-liver-enzymes-and-low-platelets

Silver, R. M. (2023). Placenta accreta spectrum: Clinical features, diagnosis, and potential consequences. *UpToDate*. Retrieved April 29, 2024, from https://www.uptodate.com/contents/placenta-accreta-spectrum-clinical-features-diagnosis-and-potential-consequences

Smith, J. A., & Fox, K. A. (2024). Nausea and vomiting of pregnancy: Clinical findings and evaluation. *UpToDate*. Retrieved April 29, 2024, from https://www.uptodate.com/contents/nausea-and-vomiting-of-pregnancy-clinical-findings-and-evaluation

Smith, J. R. (2022). Postpartum hemorrhage. *Medscape*. https://emedicine.medscape.com/article/275038-overview#

Stuart, J. J., Tanz, L. J., Rimm, E. B., Spiegelman, D., Missmer, S. A., Mukamal, K. J., Rexrode, K. M., & Rich-Edwards, J. W. (2022). Cardiovascular risk factors mediate the long-term maternal risk associated with hypertensive disorders of pregnancy. *Journal of the American College of Cardiology*, *79*(19), 1901–1913. https://doi.org/10.1016/j.jacc.2022.03.335

Tulandi, T. (2023a). Ectopic pregnancy: Choosing a treatment. *UpToDate*. Retrieved April 28, 2024, from https://www.uptodate.com/contents/ectopic-pregnancy-choosing-a-treatment

Tulandi, T. (2023b). Ectopic pregnancy: Clinical manifestations and diagnosis. *UpToDate*. Retrieved April 28, 2024, from https://www.uptodate.com/contents/ectopic-pregnancy-clinical-manifestations-and-diagnosis

Tulandi, T. (2023c). Ectopic pregnancy: Epidemiology, risk factors, and anatomic sites. *UpToDate*. Retrieved April 28, 2024, from https://www.uptodate.com/contents/ectopic-pregnancy-epidemiology-risk-factors-and-anatomic-sites/

Wang, Y., Guo, X., Obore, N., Ding, H., Wu, C., & Yu, H. (2022). Aspirin for the prevention of preeclampsia: A systematic review and meta-analysis of randomized controlled studies. *Frontiers in Cardiovascular Medicine*, *9*. https://doi.org/10.3389/fcvm.2022.936560

Whitehurst, R. M. (2020). ABO incompatibility. In T. Gomella, F. G. Eyal, & F. Bany-Mohammed (Eds.), *Gomella's neonatology: Management, procedures, on-call problems, diseases, and drugs* (8th ed.). McGraw-Hill.

Yoham, A. L., & Casadesus, D. (2023). Rho(D) immune globulin. *StatPearls*. https://www.ncbi.nlm.nih.gov/books/NBK557884/

Zimmerman, B., & Hubbard, J. B. (2023). Deep tendon reflexes. *StatPearls*. https://www.ncbi.nlm.nih.gov/books/NBK531502/

DEVELOPING CLINICAL JUDGMENT

PRACTICING FOR NCLEX

1. The postpartum nurse is caring for several patients who delivered within the past 10 hours. Which patient should receive RhIG postpartum?
   a. Nonsensitized Rh-negative patient with an Rh-negative newborn
   b. Nonsensitized Rh-negative patient with an Rh-positive newborn
   c. Sensitized Rh-negative patient with an Rh-positive newborn
   d. Sensitized Rh-negative patient with an Rh-negative newborn
2. A patient is suspected of having placental abruption. Which finding would the nurse expect to assess as a classic symptom?
   a. Painless, bright red bleeding
   b. "Knifelike" abdominal pain
   c. Excessive nausea and vomiting
   d. Hypertension and headache
3. The nurse is preparing to administer RhIG to a newly delivered primipara who is Rh-negative. In addition to this situation, after which occurrence would Rh-negative birthing parents receive this medication?
   a. Therapeutic or spontaneous abortion
   b. Head injury from a car crash
   c. Blood transfusion after a hemorrhage
   d. Unsuccessful artificial insemination procedure
4. The nurse has taught a pregnant patient about hyperemesis gravidarum and how it differs from the typical nausea and vomiting of pregnancy. Which statement made by the patient indicates that the teaching was successful?
   a. "I can expect the nausea to last through my second trimester."
   b. "I should drink fluids with my meals instead of in between them."
   c. "I need to avoid strong odors, perfumes, or flavors."
   d. "I should lie down after I eat for about 2 hours."
5. A pregnant patient who is at approximately 12 weeks' gestation comes to the emergency department after calling their health care provider's office and reporting moderate vaginal bleeding. Assessment reveals cervical dilation and moderately strong abdominal cramps. The patient reports that they passed some tissue with the bleeding. The nurse interprets these findings to suggest which of the following?
   a. Placenta previa
   b. Spontaneous abortion
   c. Abruptio placentae
   d. Placenta accreta
6. The nurse will be administering magnesium sulfate to a patient with preeclampsia. The nurse explains to the patient that this drug is given for what?
   a. Reducing blood pressure
   b. Increasing the progress of labor
   c. Preventing seizures
   d. Lowering blood glucose levels
7. A patient is being discharged after receiving treatment for a hydatidiform molar pregnancy. The nurse should include which information in the discharge teaching?
   a. Do not become pregnant for at least a year; use contraceptives to prevent it.
   b. Have your blood pressure checked weekly in the clinic.
   c. RhIG must be given within the next month at the clinic.
   d. An amniocentesis can detect a recurrence of this disorder in the future.

CRITICAL THINKING EXERCISE

1. A 16-year-old primigravida presents to the maternity clinic complaining of continual nausea and vomiting for the past 3 days. The patient states they are approximately 15 weeks pregnant and have been unable to keep anything they eat down or take any fluids in without throwing up for the past 3 days. The patient reports they are dizzy and weak. Upon examination, they appear pale and anxious. Their mucous membranes are dry, skin turgor is poor, and lips are dry and cracked.
   a. What is your impression of this condition?
   b. What risk factors does the patient have?
   c. What intervention is appropriate for this patient?
2. A 39-year-old African American primigravida with higher body weight is diagnosed with gestational hypertension. The patient's history reveals that their sister developed preeclampsia during her pregnancy. When describing their diet to the nurse, the patient mentions that they tend to eat a lot of fast food.
   a. What risk factors does this patient have that increase their risk for gestational hypertension?
   b. When assessing this patient, what assessment findings would lead the nurse to suspect that the patient has developed severe preeclampsia?

STUDY ACTIVITIES

1. Ask a community health maternity nurse how the signs and symptoms of gestational hypertension (including preeclampsia and eclampsia) are taught and how effective efforts have been to reduce the incidence in the area.

2. Find a website designed to help parents who have suffered a pregnancy loss secondary to a spontaneous abortion. What is its audience level? Is the information up to date?

3. A pregnancy in which the blastocyst implants outside the uterus is a(n) __________________ pregnancy.

4. The most serious complication of hydatidiform mole is the development of __________________ afterward.

5. Discuss various activities a person with a multiple gestation could engage in to help pass the time when ordered to be on bed rest at home for 2 months.

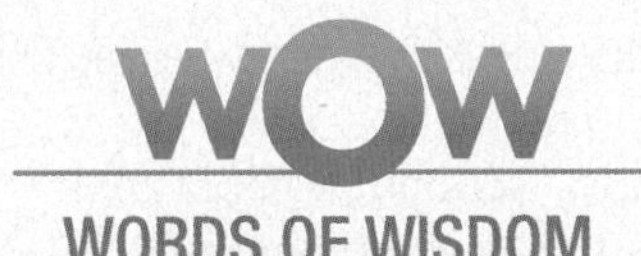

WORDS OF WISDOM

As the sun sets each day, nurses should make sure they have done something for others and should try to be understanding even under the most difficult of conditions.

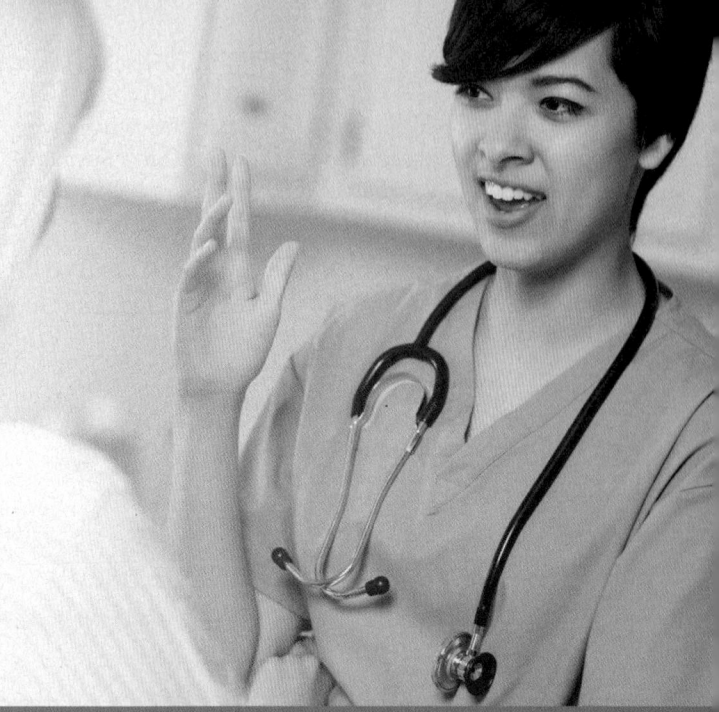

20 Nursing Management of the Pregnancy at Risk: Selected Health Conditions and Vulnerable Populations

KEY TERMS

acquired immunodeficiency syndrome (AIDS) (ă-kwīrd' im'yū-nō-dō-fish'en-sē sin'drōm)

adolescence

anemia

fibromyalgia (fi-bro-my-al-gi-a)

gestational diabetes mellitus

human immunodeficiency virus (HIV)

neonatal opioid withdrawal syndrome (NOWS)

perinatal drug misuse

pregestational diabetes

teratogen

LEARNING OBJECTIVES

Upon completion of the chapter, you will be able to:

1. Identify conditions present before pregnancy that can have negative effects on a pregnancy.
2. Examine how a condition present before pregnancy can affect the pregnant person physiologically and psychologically when they become pregnant.
3. Evaluate the nursing assessment and management for a pregnant person with diabetes from that of a pregnant person without diabetes.
4. Explore how congenital and acquired heart conditions can affect a pregnancy.
5. Design the nursing assessment and management of a pregnant person with cardiovascular disorders and respiratory conditions.
6. Differentiate the types of anemia affecting pregnant people in terms of prevention and management.
7. Relate the nursing care needed for the pregnant person with an autoimmune disorder.
8. Compare the most common infections that can jeopardize a pregnancy and propose possible preventive strategies.

9. Develop a plan of care for the pregnant person who is HIV-positive.
10. Outline the nurse's role in the prevention and management of adolescent pregnancy.
11. Determine the impact of pregnancy on a person over the age of 35.
12. Analyze the effects of substance misuse during pregnancy.

Rose, a 16-year-old who appears far along in her pregnancy, came into the clinic wheezing and having difficulty catching her breath. She had missed several previous prenatal visits but arrived at the clinic today in distress. Rose has a history of asthma since she was 5 years old. How might her current condition affect her pregnancy? Is this picture typical of a pregnant person with asthma?

INTRODUCTION

Pregnancy can be a special time in a person's life, but it can also be anxiety producing if it is accompanied by medical conditions that might complicate the pregnancy and jeopardize the fetal outcome. Ideally, the pregnant person is free of any conditions that can affect a pregnancy, but in reality, many people enter pregnancy with a multitude of health-related or psychosocial issues that can have a negative impact on the outcome. Currently, because of the obesity epidemic in the United States and people postponing their pregnancies until later in their lives, nurses will increasingly see more people with medical conditions that affect their pregnancies.

Many pregnant people express hope that their babies are born healthy. Nurses can play a major role in helping this become a reality by educating people about health promotion before they become pregnant. Conditions such as diabetes, cardiac and respiratory disorders, anemia, autoimmune disorders, and specific infections can frequently be controlled through close prenatal management so that the impact on pregnancy is minimized. Nurses can provide pregnancy prevention strategies when counseling adolescents. Meeting the developmental needs of pregnant adolescents is a challenge. Finally, lifestyle choices can place many people at risk during pregnancy, and nurses need to remain nonjudgmental when working with these populations. The use of alcohol, nicotine, and illicit substances during pregnancy is addressed in Healthy People 2030 as outlined in Healthy People 2030 box.

Chapter 19 described pregnancy-related conditions that place the pregnant person at risk. This chapter addresses common conditions that can have a negative impact on pregnancy and special populations at risk, outlining appropriate nursing assessment and management for each condition or situation. The unique skills of nurses, in conjunction with the other members of the health care team, can increase the potential for a positive outcome in many high-risk pregnancies.

DIABETES MELLITUS

Diabetes is a global public health concern with potential implications for the health of pregnant people with diabetes and their offspring. The prevalence of this condition in pregnancy has been increasing in relation to the global epidemic of obesity. Worldwide, one in seven pregnant people are diagnosed with gestational diabetes, which confers short- and long-term health risks for both the pregnant person and their child (Fuller et al., 2022). People in ethnic minority groups are affected more frequently than White European people (15% vs. 6%) (Fuller et al., 2022). Diabetes is a chronic disease characterized by a relative lack of insulin or the absence of the hormone that is necessary for glucose metabolism. The chronic hyperglycemia of diabetes is associated with long-term damage, dysfunction, and failure of the eyes, kidneys, nerves, heart, and blood vessels.

With diabetes, there is a deficiency of or resistance to insulin. This interferes with the body's ability to obtain essential nutrients for fuel and storage. Pregestational diabetes and gestational diabetes greatly affect the profound metabolic alterations during pregnancy that are necessary to support the growth and development of the fetus.

Diabetes is commonly classified based on disease etiology (Balasubramanyam, 2024). These groups include:

- **Pregestational diabetes**: Alteration in carbohydrate metabolism identified before conception
  - **Type 1 diabetes**: Absolute insulin deficiency due to autoimmune beta cell destruction
  - **Type 2 diabetes**: Insulin resistance or deficiency due to a progressive loss of beta cell insulin secretion frequently on the background of insulin resistance
- **Gestational diabetes mellitus**: Glucose intolerance with its onset during pregnancy usually diagnosed in the second or third trimester of pregnancy that was not clearly overt prior to gestation. Gestational diabetes

has become increasingly prevalent over the last three decades (Gregory & Ely, 2022).

Gestational diabetes is associated with neonatal complications such as macrosomia, hypoglycemia, birth trauma due to shoulder dystocia, and respiratory distress syndrome. Maternal complications include hypertension, preeclampsia, cesarean birth, and increased risk of developing diabetes mellitus (Rodriguez & Mahdy, 2023). Further specific issues related to the effects of diabetes on the pregnant person and fetus are provided in Table 20.1. During the past several decades, great strides have been made in improving the outcomes of pregnancy in people with diabetes, but this chronic metabolic disorder remains a high-risk condition during pregnancy. A favorable outcome requires commitment on the pregnant person's part to adhere to frequent prenatal visits, dietary restrictions, self-monitoring of blood glucose levels, frequent laboratory tests, intensive fetal surveillance, and perhaps hospitalization.

Pathophysiology

Pregnancy is characterized by a series of metabolic changes that promote accumulation of adipose tissue in early pregnancy followed by insulin resistance later in gestation. Maternal metabolism is directed toward supplying adequate nutrition for the fetus. In pregnancy, placental hormones cause insulin resistance at a level that tends to parallel the growth of the fetoplacental unit. As the placenta grows, more placental hormones are secreted. Human placental lactogen (hPL), progesterone, cortisol, prolactin, and growth hormone (somatotropin) increase in direct correlation with the growth of placental tissue, rising throughout the last 20 weeks of pregnancy and causing insulin resistance. Subsequently, insulin secretion increases to overcome the resistance of these two hormones. In the pregnant person without diabetes, the pancreas can respond to the demands for increased insulin production to maintain normal glucose levels throughout the pregnancy. However, the person with glucose intolerance or diabetes during pregnancy cannot cope with changes in metabolism resulting from insufficient insulin to meet needs during gestation (Fu & Retnakaran, 2022).

Reduced sensitivity to insulin in the liver, muscle, and adipose tissue, and a progressive decline in pancreatic beta cell function lead to impaired insulin secretion, eventually resulting in hyperglycemia (Sharma et al., 2022). With gestational diabetes, pancreatic beta cell dysfunction likely exists prior to pregnancy. This problem is then unmasked by the development of insulin resistance during pregnancy, which requires enhanced insulin production to maintain normal blood glucose ranges.

Therapeutic Management

Therapeutic care for the pregnant person with diabetes focuses on glycemic control, to decrease risk to both the pregnant person and the fetus.

TABLE 20.1 • Diabetes and Pregnancy: Effects on the Birthing Parent and Fetus

Effects on the Parent	Effects on the Fetus/Neonate
• Polyhydramnios due to fetal diuresis caused by hyperglycemia • Gestational hypertension of unknown etiology • Ketoacidosis due to uncontrolled hyperglycemia • Preterm labor secondary to premature membrane rupture • Stillbirth in pregnancies complicated by ketoacidosis and poor glucose control • Hypoglycemia as glucose is diverted to the fetus (occurring in the first trimester) • Urinary tract infections resulting from excess glucose in the urine (glucosuria), which promotes bacterial growth • Chronic monilial vaginitis due to glucosuria, which promotes the growth of yeast • Difficult labor, cesarean birth, postpartum hemorrhage secondary to an overdistended uterus to accommodate a macrosomic infant	• Cord prolapse secondary to polyhydramnios and abnormal fetal presentation • Congenital anomaly due to hyperglycemia in the first trimester (cardiac problems, neural tube defects, skeletal deformities, and genitourinary problems) • Macrosomia resulting from hyperinsulinemia stimulated by fetal hyperglycemia • Birth trauma due to the increased size of the fetus, which complicates the birthing process (shoulder dystocia) • Preterm birth secondary to polyhydramnios and an aging placenta, which places the fetus in jeopardy if the pregnancy continues • Fetal asphyxia secondary to fetal hyperglycemia and hyperinsulinemia • Intrauterine growth restriction secondary to maternal vascular impairment and decreased placental perfusion, which restricts growth • Perinatal death due to poor placental perfusion and hypoxia • Respiratory distress syndrome resulting from poor surfactant production secondary to hyperinsulinemia inhibiting the production of phospholipids, which make up surfactant • Polycythemia due to excessive red blood cell (RBC) production in response to hypoxia • Hyperbilirubinemia due to excessive RBC breakdown from hypoxia and an immature liver unable to break down bilirubin • Neonatal hypoglycemia resulting from ongoing hyperinsulinemia after the placenta is removed • Subsequent childhood obesity and carbohydrate intolerance

Cunningham, F. G., Leveno, K. J., Dashe, J. S., Hoffman, B. L., Spong, C. Y., & Casey, B. M. (2022d). Diabetes mellitus. In F. G. Cunningham, K. J. Leveno, J. S. Dashe, B. L. Hoffman, C. Y. Spong, & B., M. Casey, *William's obstetrics* (26th ed.). McGraw Hill.

Preconception Counseling for the Person With Pregestational Diabetes

Pregestational diabetes is a significant public health problem that increases the risk for structural birth defects affecting both maternal and neonatal pregnancy outcomes. People who have pregestational diabetes need comprehensive prenatal care. Achieving good metabolic control during the period prior to conception is essential to reducing congenital malformations that can occur in pregnancies complicated by diabetes. Preconception counseling is essential for the person with pregestational diabetes to ensure that the disease state is stable. The goals of preconception care involve a discussion of potential adverse outcomes and specifically are to:

- Integrate the person into the management of their diabetes.
- Achieve the lowest glycosylated hemoglobin A1c (HgbA1C) test results without excessive hypoglycemia.
- Ensure effective contraception until stable glycemia is achieved.
- Identify and evaluate long-term diabetic complications such as retinopathy, nephropathy, neuropathy, cardiovascular disease (CVD), and hypertension (Seely & Powe, 2024).

Care for the Pregnant Person With Diabetes

Lifestyle modification, nutritional changes, and encouragement of physical activities form the primary mode of therapy for diabetes during pregnancy. Therapeutic care of the pregnant person with diabetes mellitus focuses on tight glucose control. The recommendations include a fasting blood glucose level below 95 mg/dL with postprandial levels below 140 mg/dL at 1 hour and below 120 mg/dL at 2 hours (ElSayed et al., 2023). Such tight control has been advocated because it is associated with a reduction in macrosomia.

PHARMACOLOGIC THERAPY FOR DIABETES

The person with type 1 diabetes will need to continue insulin therapy throughout pregnancy. For the person with gestational diabetes, nutritional management and exercise may be all that are necessary. Pharmacologic therapy is considered if nutrition and exercise fail to maintain target glucose levels.

In uncontrolled gestational diabetes, in which target glycemic levels cannot be reached, insulin is also required. The Americans With Disabilities Act (ADA) affirms the use of insulin as the first-line pharmacotherapy for gestational diabetes when medication is necessary to control blood glucose levels (ElSayed et al., 2023). Insulin, which does not cross the placenta, has historically been the medication of choice for treating hyperglycemia in pregnancy. Combining intermediate- and short-acting insulin yields the best result for most patients. Two insulin doses are given daily with two thirds of the total insulin in the morning to cover the energy needs of the active day and one third at night. Insulin pump technology can also be used to regulate glucose levels. Generally, for the person with type 1 diabetes, insulin doses are reduced in the first trimester to prevent hypoglycemia resulting from increased insulin sensitivity as well as from nausea and vomiting. Short-acting insulins, which do not cross the placenta, may help reduce postprandial hyperglycemia and episodes of hypoglycemia between meals.

Some patients with diabetes cannot use insulin safely during pregnancy due to cost, language barriers, lack of comprehension, or cultural influences. Oral agents may be used as an alternative, after a discussion of risks. Metformin readily crosses the placenta and can cause neonatal hypoglycemia. It should not be used in pregnant people with hypertension or preeclampsia (ElSayed et al., 2023). Insulin therapy or oral hypoglycemic agents in addition to diet and exercise are major elements of achieving glycemic control (see Evidence-Based Practice 20.1).

After giving birth, the overt glycemic abnormalities of gestational diabetes usually resolve. This phenomenon suggests that diabetes is transient and that the consequences of gestational diabetes end with the birth of the infant. However, for the birthing parent, childbirth is not the end of the story. The diagnosis of gestational diabetes heralds future health risks. Knowledge of this "failed" stress test conveys new information about their future risk for type 2 diabetes, which warrants further screening and prevention efforts during the postpartum period and beyond.

Nursing Assessment

Nursing assessment begins at the first prenatal visit. A thorough history and physical examination in conjunction with specific laboratory and diagnostic testing aids in developing an individualized plan of care for the person with diabetes. Early screening, ideally before 13 weeks' gestation, is important to identify pregestational diabetes (Trout, 2019).

Health History and Physical Examination

For the person with pregestational diabetes, obtain a thorough history of the preexisting diabetic condition. Ask about the duration of the disease, management of glucose levels (insulin injections, insulin pump, or oral hypoglycemic agents), dietary adjustments, presence of vascular complications and current vascular status, current insulin regimen, and technique used for glucose testing. Review any information that they may have received as part of their preconception counseling and measures that were implemented during this time.

EVIDENCE-BASED PRACTICE 20.1

Effects of Resistance Exercise on Blood Glucose Level and Pregnancy Outcome in Patients With Gestational Diabetes Mellitus: A Randomized Controlled Study

BACKGROUND

Gestational diabetes accounts for about 90% to 95% of the total number of people with hyperglycemia during pregnancy and has increased by more than 30% in the last two decades. Adverse outcomes of this condition include preterm births, neonatal respiratory distress, fetal macrosomia, and increased risk of type 2 diabetes 5 to 10 years post childbirth for both the birthing parent and offspring. It is important to prevent these adverse outcomes to improve the health of parent and child. The purpose of this study was to investigate the effect of resistance exercise versus aerobic exercise on blood glucose level, insulin utilization rate, and pregnancy outcomes.

STUDY

Excessive gestational weight gain is associated with several adverse events and pathology during pregnancy for both the birthing parent and the fetus. Physical activity is an essential component for people with gestational diabetes. Exercise increases glucose uptake and increases insulin sensitivity, thus decreasing insulin resistance. Early intervention can positively impact pregnancy outcomes.

A randomized controlled trial included 100 pregnant people divided into an aerobic exercise group (51) and a resistance exercise group (49). Both groups received exercise intervention for 50 to 60 minutes, three times weekly, lasting for 6 weeks, in addition to their routine maternity care.

Findings

The resistance exercise group showed better postprandial blood glucose and exercise compliance than the aerobic exercise group. Resistance exercise is easier to perform, has better adherence, and is conducive to being carried out throughout pregnancy and postpartum.

Nursing Implications

The result of this study indicates that resistance and/or aerobic exercise throughout pregnancy can reduce the risk of adverse events and lower glucose levels. Resistance exercise is easier to perform, especially in late pregnancy because it can be carried out in a sitting position or lying down. Nurses should inform people about the benefits of exercise and provide literature and resources about specific exercises to engage in. Writing out a "prescription" for the type and amount of exercise may help people recognize the importance of this intervention and encourage them to do it. Encourage them to keep a daily log to track their regimen, and ask about it at every prenatal visit.

Adapted from Xie, Y., Zhao, H., Zhao, M., Huang, H., Liu, C., Huang, F., & Wu, J. (2022). Effects of resistance exercise on blood glucose level and pregnancy outcome in patients with gestational diabetes mellitus: A randomized controlled trial. *BMJ Open Diabetes Research and Care, 10*(2), e002622. https://doi.org/10.1136/bmjdrc-2021-002622

Be knowledgeable about the person's nutritional requirements and assess the adequacy and pattern of their dietary intake. Assess their blood glucose self-monitoring in terms of technique, frequency, and ability to adjust the insulin dose based on the changing patterns. Ask about the frequency of episodes of hypoglycemia or hyperglycemia to ascertain their ability to recognize and treat them. Continue to assess for signs and symptoms of hypoglycemia and hyperglycemia.

During antepartum visits, assess the patient's knowledge about their disease, including the signs and symptoms of hypoglycemia, hyperglycemia, and diabetic ketoacidosis; insulin administration techniques; and the impact of pregnancy on their chronic condition. If possible, have the person demonstrate their technique for blood glucose monitoring and insulin administration if appropriate. Exercise patience and understanding while frequently encouraging and reinforcing all verbal instructions with written material (Fig. 20.1).

Assess the risk for gestational diabetes at the first prenatal visit. Risk factors for gestational diabetes include:

- Overweight (body mass index [BMI] 25 to 29.9) or obesity (BMI ≥30)
- History of gestational diabetes or polyhydramnios in a previous pregnancy
- First-degree relative with diabetes
- Polycystic ovary syndrome
- Previous infant weighing more than 9 lb (4,000 g)
- Hypertension before pregnancy or in early pregnancy
- Hispanic, Native American, Pacific Islander, or African ancestry
- Signs and symptoms of glucose intolerance (polyuria, polyphagia, polydipsia, fatigue) (Rodriguez & Mahdy, 2023)

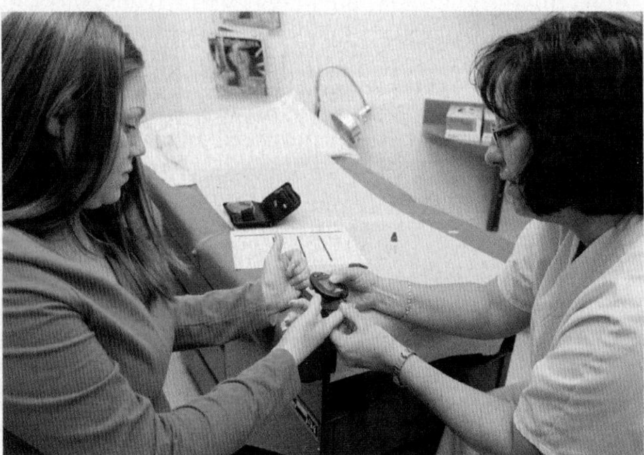

FIGURE 20.1 The nurse is demonstrating the technique for self-blood glucose monitoring with a pregnant patient who has diabetes.

People with clinical characteristics consistent with a high risk for gestational diabetes should undergo glucose testing as soon as feasible.

Also assess the person's psychosocial adaptation to their condition. This assessment is critical to gain cooperation for a change in regimen or the addition of a new regimen throughout pregnancy. Identify their support systems and note any financial constraints, because they will need intense monitoring and frequent fetal surveillance.

Laboratory and Diagnostic Testing

The diagnosis of preexisting previously undiagnosed diabetes may be made in early pregnancy. Screening for gestational diabetes routinely occurs at 24 to 28 weeks' gestation. Table 20.2 provides information on diagnosing and classifying hyperglycemia in pregnancy. People with pregestational diabetes and those diagnosed with gestational diabetes require ongoing maternal and fetal surveillance to promote the best outcome.

SURVEILLANCE

Maternal surveillance may include:

- Urine check for protein (may indicate the need for further evaluation for preeclampsia) and for nitrates and leukocyte esterase (may indicate a urinary tract infection)
- Urine check for ketones (may indicate the need for evaluation of eating habits)
- Kidney function evaluation every trimester for creatinine clearance and protein levels
- Eye examination in the first trimester to evaluate the retina for vascular changes
- HgbA1C every 4 to 8 weeks to monitor glucose trends (Zera & Brown, 2023)

Fetal surveillance may include ultrasound to provide information about fetal growth, activity, and amniotic fluid volume and to validate gestational age.

TABLE 20.2 • Recommendations for Diagnosing and Classifying Hyperglycemia in Pregnancy

When	Diagnosis	Test	Cutoff for Diagnosis
First prenatal visit	Overt (pregestational) diabetes	Fasting HgbA1C Random	126 mg/dL >7% 200 mg/dL
24–28 weeks	Gestational diabetes	Fasting	<92 mg/dL
		75 g OGTT–1 hour	<180 mg/dL
		75 g OGTT–2 hour	<153 mg/dL

HgbA1C, glycosylated hemoglobin; OGTT, oral glucose tolerance test.

American Diabetes Association. (2020a). Classification and diagnosis of diabetes: Standards of medical care in diabetes—2020. *Diabetes Care, 43*(Supplement 1), S14–S31. https://doi.org/10.2337/dc20-S002; and American Diabetes Association. (2020b). Glycemic targets: Standards of medical care in diabetes—2020. *Diabetes Care, 43*(Supplement 1), S66–S76. https://doi.org/10.2337/dc20-S006

Nursing Management

The ideal outcome of every pregnancy is a healthy newborn and birthing parent. Nurses can be pivotal in realizing this positive outcome for people with pregestational or gestational diabetes by implementing measures to minimize risks and complications. Since the person with diabetes is considered to be at high risk, prenatal visits occur more frequently (every 2 weeks up to 28 weeks and then twice a week until birth), providing the nurse with numerous opportunities for ongoing assessment, education, and counseling (Clinical Judgment & Nursing Process 20.1).

Providing Appropriate Nutrition

In addition to the nursing interventions provided earlier, the person with gestational diabetes needs nutritional counseling from the nurse or a registered dietitian. Nutritional management focuses on maintaining balanced glucose levels and providing enough energy and nutrients for the pregnant person and developing fetus while avoiding ketosis and minimizing the risk of hypoglycemia in people treated with insulin. For the patient to adopt and follow the nutritional plan, it must be in keeping with their present cultural dietary patterns and not radically different (Palmer, 2021). Nutrient-dense carbohydrates are a vital part of the diet, as they support glucose control, reduce free fatty acids, improve insulin action, and provide vascular benefits (Krewson, 2022). It is recommended to limit consumption of sugary beverages; read food labels; and include grains, oats, beans, vegetables, fruit, and dairy products in the diet. People who receive dietary advice and follow it have been shown to have better pregnancy outcomes than those who do not receive dietary advice (Helm et al., 2022).

Recommend three healthy meals per day using the Diabetes Plate Method. With this method, the pregnant person with diabetes should plan each meal based on a 9-in-diameter dinner plate half-filled with nonstarchy vegetables, quarter filled with lean protein, and quarter filled with complex carbohydrate foods, accompanied by water or other zero-calorie beverages. Snacks should be high in protein, fiber, and/or healthy fats (Diabetes Food Hub Team, 2020). For assistance with meal planning, refer patients to the American Diabetes Association's Diabetes Food Hub site (https://www.diabetesfoodhub.org/articles/tips-for-using-the-diabetes-food-hub-meal-planner-and-grocery-list.html) (Fig. 20.2).

CLINICAL JUDGMENT & NURSING PROCESS 20.1 Overview of the Pregnant Person With Type 1 Diabetes

Patty, a 30-year-old pregnant person with type 1 diabetes, presents to the maternity clinic for preconception care. She has had diabetes for 8 years and takes insulin twice daily by injection. She does blood glucose self-monitoring four times daily. She reports that her disease is fairly well controlled but says, "I'm worried about how my diabetes will affect a pregnancy and my baby. Will I need to make changes in my routine? Will my baby be normal?" She reports that she recently had a foot infection and needed to go to the emergency department because it led to an episode of ketoacidosis. She states that her last HgbA1C test results were abnormal.

NURSING ANALYSIS: Altered health maintenance: Maternal related to lack of knowledge regarding care in the diabetic condition in pregnancy as evidenced by questions about the effect on pregnancy, possible changes in regimen, and pregnancy outcome

OUTCOME IDENTIFICATION AND EVALUATION

The patient will demonstrate increased knowledge of type 1 diabetes and its effects on pregnancy as evidenced by proper techniques for blood glucose monitoring and insulin administration, the ability to modify insulin doses and dietary intake to achieve control, and verbalization of the need for glycemic control prior to pregnancy with blood glucose levels remaining within normal range.

INTERVENTIONS: *Providing Patient Teaching*

- Assess patient's knowledge of diabetes and pregnancy *to establish a baseline from which to develop an individualized teaching plan.*
- Review the underlying problems associated with diabetes and how pregnancy affects glucose control *to provide patient with a firm knowledge base for decision making.*
- Review signs and symptoms of hypoglycemia and hyperglycemia and prevention and management measures *to ensure patient can deal with them should they occur.*
- Provide written materials describing diabetes and care needed for control *to provide an opportunity for patient's review and promote retention of learning.*
- Observe patient administering insulin and self-glucose testing for technique and offer suggestions for improvement if needed *to ensure adequate self-care ability.*
- Discuss proper foot care *to prevent future infections.*
- Teach home treatment for symptomatic hypoglycemia *to minimize risk to patient and fetus.*
- Outline acute and chronic diabetic complications *to reinforce the importance of glucose control.*
- Discuss the use of contraceptives until blood glucose levels can be optimized before conception occurs *to promote the best possible health status before conception.*
- Explain the rationale for good glucose control and the importance of achieving excellent glycemic control before pregnancy *to promote a positive pregnancy outcome.*
- Review self-care practices (blood glucose monitoring and frequency of testing; insulin administration; adjustment of insulin dosages based on blood glucose levels) *to foster independence in self-care and feelings of control over the situation.*
- Refer patient for dietary counseling *to ensure optimal diet for glycemic control.*
- Outline obstetric management and fetal surveillance needed for pregnancy *to provide patient with information on what to expect.*
- Discuss strategies for maintaining optimal glycemic control during pregnancy *to minimize risks to patient and fetus.*

NURSING ANALYSIS: Acute anxiety related to the threat to self and fetus as evidenced by questions about the effect of the patient's condition on the baby and baby being healthy

OUTCOME IDENTIFICATION AND EVALUATION

The patient will openly express feelings related to diabetes and pregnancy as evidenced by statements of feeling better about their preexisting condition and pregnancy outlook, and statements of understanding related to future childbearing by linking good glucose control with positive outcomes for both the patient and offspring.

INTERVENTIONS: *Minimizing Anxiety*

- Review the need for a physical examination *to evaluate for any effects of diabetes on the patient's health status.*
- Explain the rationale for assessing patient's blood pressure, vision, and peripheral pulses at each visit *to provide information related to possible effects of diabetes on health status.*
- Identify any alterations in the present diabetic condition that need intervention *to aid in minimizing risks that may increase patient's anxiety level.*
- Review potential effects of diabetes on pregnancy *to promote patient understanding of risks and ways to control or minimize them.*
- Encourage active participation in decision making and planning pregnancy *to promote feelings of control over the situation and foster self-confidence.*
- Discuss feelings about future childbearing and managing pregnancy *to help reduce anxiety related to uncertainties.*
- Encourage patient to ask questions or voice concerns *to help decrease anxiety related to the unknown.*
- Emphasize the use of frequent and continued surveillance of patient and fetal status during pregnancy *to reduce the risk of complications and aid in alleviating anxieties related to the unknown.*
- Provide positive reinforcement for healthy behaviors and actions *to foster continued use and enhancement of self-esteem.*

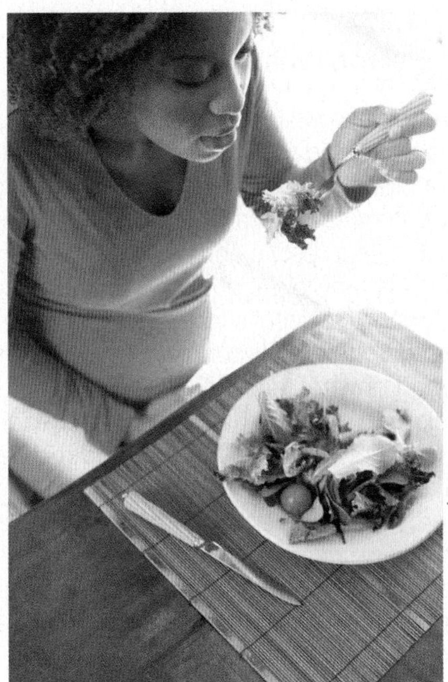

FIGURE 20.2 The pregnant patient with diabetes eating a nutritious meal to ensure adequate glucose control.

Promoting Physical Activity

Exercise is another important component of comprehensive prenatal care for the pregnant person with glucose intolerance. Regular exercise helps maintain glucose control by increasing the uptake of glucose into the cells and decreasing central body weight, hypertension, and dyslipidemia. This will ultimately decrease the person's insulin requirement. Regular physical activity has been proven to result in marked benefits for the birthing parent and fetus. Maternal benefits include improved cardiovascular function, limited pregnancy weight gain, decreased musculoskeletal discomfort, reduced incidence of muscle cramps and lower limb edema, mood stability, and reduction of gestational diabetes mellitus and gestational hypertension. Fetal benefits include decreased fat mass, improved stress tolerance, and advanced neurobehavioral maturation. Moderately intense exercise for 20 to 30 minutes on most days, or at least 150 minutes of moderately intense aerobic activity per week, is recommended (Onaade et al., 2021).

TAKE NOTE!

Nutrient requirements and recommendations for weight gain for the pregnant person with diabetes are the same as those for pregnant people without diabetes.

Promoting Optimal Glucose Control

At each visit, review blood glucose levels, including any laboratory tests and self-monitoring results. Ask the patient if they have had any episodes of hypoglycemia and what they did to alleviate them. Reinforce with the patient the need to perform blood glucose monitoring (usually four times a day, before meals and at bedtime) and to keep a record of the results. If appropriate, obtain a fingerstick blood glucose level to evaluate the accuracy of self-monitoring results. Also assess the patient's techniques for monitoring blood glucose levels and for administering insulin if ordered and offer support and guidance. If they are receiving insulin therapy, assist with any changes needed if glucose levels are not controlled. The goal is a fasting glucose level below 95 mg/dL and a 1-hour postprandial level below 140 mg/dL or a 2-hour postprandial level below 120 mg/dL (ElSayed et al., 2023). Obtain a urine specimen and check for glucose, protein, and ketones.

Preventing Complications

Assess the patient closely for signs and symptoms of complications at each visit. Anticipate possible complications and plan appropriate interventions or referrals. Check for blood pressure changes and evaluate for proteinuria when obtaining a urine specimen. These might suggest the development of preeclampsia. Measure the fundal height and review gestational age. Note any discrepancies between fundal height and gestational age or a sudden increase in uterine growth. These may suggest hydramnios.

Encourage the patient to perform daily fetal movement counts to monitor fetal well-being. Tell them specifically when to notify the health care provider. Also prepare the patient for the need for frequent laboratory and diagnostic testing to evaluate fetal status. Assist with serial ultrasounds to monitor fetal growth and with nonstress tests and biophysical profiles to assess fetal well-being.

CONSIDER THIS!

Scott and I had been busy all day setting up the new crib in our nursery, and we finally sat down to rest. I was due any day, and we had been putting this off until we had a long weekend to complete the task. I was excited to think about decorating my new daughter's room. I was sure that she would love it as much as I loved her already. A few days later, I barely noticed any fetal movement, but I thought that she must be as tired as I was by this point.

That night I went into labor and kept looking at the worried faces of the nurses and the midwife in attendance. I had been diagnosed with gestational diabetes a few months ago and had tried to follow the instructions regarding diet and exercise, but old habits are hard to change when you are 38 years old. I was finally told after a short time in the labor unit that they couldn't pick up a fetal heartbeat and an ultrasound was to be done; still no heartbeat was detected. Scott and I were finally told that our daughter was stillborn. All I could think about was that she would never get to see all the colors in the nursery.

Providing Patient Education and Counseling

The pregnant person with diabetes requires counseling and education about the need for strict glucose monitoring, diet and exercise, and signs and symptoms of complications. Encourage the patient and family to make any lifestyle changes needed to optimize the pregnancy outcome. At each visit, stress the importance of performing blood glucose screening and documenting the results. With proper instruction, the patient and family will be able to cope with all the changes in their body during pregnancy (Teaching Guidelines 20.1).

Instruct the patient about the benefits of breastfeeding related to blood glucose control. Breastfeeding helps normalize blood glucose level, so it should be encouraged. Also teach the person receiving insulin for diabetes that their insulin needs after birth will drastically decrease. People with gestational diabetes are at risk of developing type 2 diabetes and prediabetes in the postpartum period. Lactation is considered beneficial for maternal postpartum weight loss and control of glycemic metabolism, so it should be encouraged. Breastfeeding for more than 6 months reduces one's risk of recurrent gestational diabetes; a greater amount of breastfeeding in a lifetime decreases the risk of developing type 2 diabetes (Melov et al., 2022).

Review discussions about the timing of birth and the rationale. Counsel the patient about the possibility of cesarean birth for an infant who is large for gestational age (LGA). Inform the person who will be giving birth vaginally about the possible need for augmentation with oxytocin (Pitocin).

TAKE NOTE!

In the person with well-controlled diabetes, birth is typically not induced before term unless complications, such as preeclampsia or fetal compromise, arise. An early delivery date might be set for the person with poorly controlled diabetes or a large fetus who is having complications.

CARDIOVASCULAR DISEASE

Maternal heart disease has emerged as a major threat to cardiovascular health in pregnant people. Up to 4% of pregnant people may have cardiovascular complications despite a lack of previously diagnosed cardiac disease, and more than 25% of maternal deaths are attributed to CVD (American College of Obstetricians and Gynecologists [ACOG], 2022b). Pregnancy has profound effects on the cardiovascular system. These effects include increased cardiac output secondary to a 50% increase in intravascular volume, a decrease in blood pressure, and an increase in heart rate. Cardiac output is further

TEACHING GUIDELINES 20.1 Teaching for the Pregnant Person With Diabetes

- Be sure to keep your appointments for frequent prenatal visits and tests for fetal well-being.
- Perform blood glucose self-monitoring as directed, usually before each meal and at bedtime. Keep a record of your results and call your health care provider with any levels outside the established range. Bring your results to each prenatal visit.
- Perform daily fetal kick counts. Document them and report any decrease in activity.
- Drink eight to ten 8-oz glasses of water each day to prevent bladder infections and maintain hydration.
- Wear proper, well-fitted footwear when walking to prevent injury.
- Engage in a regular exercise program such as walking to aid in glucose control, but avoid exercising in temperature extremes.
- Consider breastfeeding your infant to lower your blood glucose levels.
- If you are taking insulin:
  - Administer the correct dose of insulin at the correct time every day.
  - Eat breakfast within 30 minutes after injecting regular insulin to prevent a reaction.
  - Plan meals at a fixed time and snacks to prevent extremes in glucose levels.
- Avoid simple sugars (cake, candy, cookies), which raise blood glucose levels.
- Know the signs and symptoms of hypoglycemia and the treatment needed:
  - Sweating, tremors, cold, clammy skin, headache
  - Feeling hungry, blurred vision, disorientation, irritability
  - Treatment: Drink 8 oz of milk and eat two crackers or take two glucose tablets.
  - Treatment: Carry "glucose boosters" (such as hard candies) to treat hypoglycemia.
- Know the signs and symptoms of hyperglycemia and the treatment needed:
  - Dry mouth, frequent urination, excessive thirst, rapid breathing
  - Feeling tired, flushed, hot skin, headache, drowsiness
  - Treatment: Notify your health care provider because hospitalization may be needed.
- Wear a diabetic identification bracelet at all times.
- Wash your hands frequently to prevent infections.
- Report any signs and symptoms of illness, infection, and dehydration to your health care provider, because these can affect blood glucose control.
- Remember, prevention is the best strategy for disease control!

affected in the third trimester by maternal positioning (Mohamad, 2022). The cardiovascular adaptations during pregnancy are well tolerated by the normal heart but may unveil undiagnosed underlying heart disease or tip the hemodynamic balance and lead to decompensation in those with existing heart disease. Pregnancy is a predictor of future cardiovascular health (Iftikhar & Biswas, 2023).

Congenital and Acquired Heart Disease

Congenital heart disease often involves structural defects that are present at birth but may not be discovered at that time (Table 20.3). Due to modern surgical techniques to correct these conditions, many people can complete a successful pregnancy at relatively low risk when appropriate counseling and optimal care are provided. Increasing numbers of people with complex congenital heart disease are reaching childbearing age. Complications such as growth restriction, preterm birth, newborn congenital heart defect, and fetal and neonatal mortality are more common among children of birthing parents with congenital heart disease (Waksmonski, 2023).

People with certain congenital conditions should avoid pregnancy. These include Fontan circulation for tetralogy of Fallot or transposition of the great arteries, bicuspid aortic valve stenosis with ascending aorta

TABLE 20.3 • Selected Heart Conditions Affecting Pregnancy

Condition	Description	Management
Congenital		
Atrial septal defect (ASD)	Congenital heart defect involving a communication or opening between the atria with left-to-right shunting due to greater left-sided pressure Arrhythmias present in some people	Treatment with atrioventricular nodal blocking agents and at times with electrical cardioversion
Ventricular septal defect (VSD)	Congenital heart defect involving an opening in the ventricular septum, permitting blood flow from the left to the right ventricle Complications include arrhythmias, heart failure, and pulmonary hypertension.	Rest with limited activity if symptomatic
Acquired		
Mitral valve prolapse	Very common in the general population, occurring most often in younger people Leaflets of the mitral valve prolapse into the left atrium during ventricular contraction The most common cause of mitral valve regurgitation if present during pregnancy Usually improvements in mitral valve function due to increased blood volume and decreased systemic vascular resistance of pregnancy; most people are able to tolerate pregnancy well.	Most people are without symptoms; diagnosis is made incidentally. Occasional palpitations, chest pain, or arrhythmias in some people, possibly requiring beta-blockers Usually, no special precautions are necessary during pregnancy.
Mitral valve stenosis	Most common chronic rheumatic valvular lesion in pregnancy Causes obstruction of blood flow from the atria to the ventricle, thereby decreasing ventricular filling and causing a fixed cardiac output Resultant pulmonary edema, pulmonary hypertension, and right ventricular failure In most pregnant people, this condition can be managed medically.	General symptomatic improvement with medical management involving diuretics, beta-blockers, and anticoagulant therapy Activity restriction, reduction in sodium, and potentially bed rest if the condition severe
Aortic stenosis	Narrowing of the opening of the aortic valve, leading to an obstruction to left ventricular ejection People with mild disease can tolerate hypervolemia of pregnancy; with progressive narrowing of the opening, cardiac output becomes fixed. Diagnosis can be confirmed with echocardiography. For most people, care can consist of medical therapy, bed rest, and close monitoring.	Diagnosis confirmed with echocardiography Pharmacologic treatment with beta-blockers and/or antiarrhythmic agents to reduce the risk of heart failure and/or dysrhythmias Bed rest/limited activity and close monitoring

(continued)

TABLE 20.3 • Selected Heart Conditions Affecting Pregnancy (*continued*)

Condition	Description	Management
Peripartum cardiomyopathy	Rare congestive cardiomyopathy that may arise during pregnancy Multiparity, age, multiple fetuses, hypertension, an infectious agent, autoimmune disease, or cocaine use may contribute to its presence. Development of heart failure in the last month of pregnancy or within 5 months of giving birth without any preexisting heart disease or any identifiable cause	Preload reduction with diuretic therapy Afterload reduction with vasodilators Improvement in contractility with inotropic agents Nonpharmacologic approaches include salt restriction and daily exercise such as walking or biking. The question of whether another pregnancy should be attempted is controversial due to the high risk of repeat complications.
Myocardial infarction (MI)	Rare during pregnancy, but incidence is expected to increase as people become pregnant later in life and the risk factors for coronary artery disease become more prevalent. Factors contributing to MI include family history, stress, smoking, age, obesity, multiple fetuses, hypercholesterolemia, and cocaine use. Increased plasma volume and cardiac output during pregnancy increase the cardiac workload as well as the myocardial oxygen demands; imbalance in supply and demand may contribute to myocardial ischemia.	Usual treatment modalities for any acute MI along with consideration for the fetus Anticoagulant therapy, rest, and lifestyle changes to preserve the health of both parties

Cunningham, F. G., Leveno, K. J., Dashe, J. S., Hoffman, B. L., Spong, C. Y., & Casey, B. M. (2022b). Cardiovascular disorders. In F. G. Cunningham, K. J. Leveno, J. S. Dashe, B. L. Hoffman, C. Y. Spong, & B., M. Casey, *William's obstetrics* (26th ed.). McGraw Hill; Mohamad, T. N. (2022). Cardiovascular disease and pregnancy. *Medscape.* https://emedicine.medscape.com/article/162004-overview; and Iftikhar, S. F., & Biswas, M. (2023). Cardiac disease in pregnancy. *StatPearls.* https://www.ncbi.nlm.nih.gov/books/NBK537261/

diameter greater than 50 mm, and Marfan syndrome with aorta dilation greater than 45 mm (Waksmonski, 2023).

Acquired heart diseases are conditions affecting the heart and its associated blood vessels that develop during a person's lifetime. Acquired heart diseases include chronic hypertension, coronary artery disease, coronary heart disease, rheumatic heart disease, diseases of the pulmonary vessels and the aorta, diseases of the tissues of the heart, and diseases of the heart valves. Chronic hypertension is discussed in Chapter 19. Contraindications to pregnancy for people with acquired heart disease include severe arterial pulmonary hypertension of any cause, severe mitral stenosis, and severe systemic ventricular systolic dysfunction (Waksmonski, 2023) (see Table 20.3).

Many people are postponing childbearing until their 30s and 40s. With advancing maternal age, underlying medical conditions such as hypertension, diabetes, and hypercholesterolemia contributing to ischemic heart disease become more common and increase the incidence of acquired heart disease complicating pregnancy. Coronary artery disease and myocardial infarction may result (Cunningham et al., 2022b).

A person's ability to function during pregnancy is often more important than what the particular cardiovascular condition is and can be classified by risk. The risk categories are based on how much the patient is limited during physical activity, normal breathing, and varying degrees of shortness of breath and/or chest pain:

- *Risk Class I*: No detectable increased risk of maternal mortality and no increase or a mild increase in morbidity; prepregnancy/pregnancy counseling suggested. Select conditions under this classification might include pulmonic stenosis, patent ductus arteriosus, and mitral valve prolapse.
- *Risk Class II*: Small increased risk of maternal mortality or moderate increase in morbidity; prepregnancy/pregnancy counseling and cardiac consult every trimester. Select conditions under this classification include atrial or ventricular septal defect, repaired tetralogy of Fallot defects, and most arrhythmias.
- *Risk Classes II and III*: Intermediate increased risk of maternal mortality or moderate to severe increase in morbidity; prepregnancy/pregnancy counseling with a cardiologist consult every trimester. Delivery at appropriate level hospital. Select conditions include mild left ventricular impairment or hypertrophic cardiomyopathy.
- *Risk Class III*: Significantly increased risk of maternal mortality or severe morbidity; prepregnancy/pregnancy counseling, cardiologist consult every other month, prenatal care, and delivery at the appropriate level hospital. Select conditions in this classification include moderate left ventricular impairment, mechanical valve, moderate mitral stenosis, and ventricular tachycardia.
- *Risk Class IV*: Pregnancy contraindicated. Extremely high risk of maternal mortality or severe morbidity. Cardiac team consult and follow-up monthly (Iftikhar & Biswas, 2023).

The classification may change as the pregnancy progresses, and the pregnant person's body must cope with the increasing stress on the cardiovascular system resulting from the numerous physiologic changes taking place. Typically, a person with class I or II cardiac disease can go through a pregnancy without major complications. A person with class III disease needs frequent visits with the cardiac care team throughout pregnancy. A person with class IV disease should typically be advised to avoid pregnancy (Waksmonski, 2023). People with cardiac disease may benefit from preconception counseling so that they know the risks before deciding to become pregnant. Maternal mortality varies directly with the functional class at pregnancy onset.

Pathophysiology

Numerous hemodynamic changes occur in all pregnant people. These normal physiologic changes can overstress the cardiovascular system, increasing the risk for problems. Increased cardiac workload and greater myocardial oxygen demand during pregnancy place additional stress on the cardiovascular system, resulting in increased risk for morbidity and mortality.

TAKE NOTE!

Uterine blood flow increases by at least 1 L/min, requiring the body to produce more blood during pregnancy. This results in a 25% increase in red blood cells (RBCs), a 50% expansion of plasma volume during pregnancy, and an overall hemodilution. In addition, the increase in total red blood cellular volume includes an increase in clotting factors and platelets, defining the hypercoagulable state of pregnancy (Cunningham et al., 2022a). These changes start as early as the second month of gestation.

Normal physiologic changes are important for a successful adaptation to pregnancy but create unique physiologic challenges for the patient with cardiac disease (Comparison Chart 20.1).

COMPARISON CHART 20.1 Cardiovascular Changes: Prepregnancy Versus Pregnancy

Measurement	Prepregnancy	Pregnancy
Heart rate	72 (±10 bpm)	+10%–20%
Cardiac output	4.3 (±0.9 L/min)	+30%–50%
Blood volume	5 L	+20%–50%
Stroke volume	73.3 (±9 mL)	+30%
Systemic vascular resistance	1,530 (±520 dyne/cm/sec)	−20%
Oxygen consumption	250 mL/min	+20%–30%

Cunningham, F. G., Leveno, K. J., Dashe, J. S., Hoffman, B. L., Spong, C. Y., & Casey, B. M. (2022a). Maternal physiology. In F. G. Cunningham, K. J. Leveno, J. S. Dashe, B. L. Hoffman, C. Y. Spong, & B., M. Casey, *William's obstetrics* (26th ed.). McGraw Hill; and Iftikhar, S. F., & Biswas, M. (2023). Cardiac disease in pregnancy. *StatPearls.* https://www.ncbi.nlm.nih.gov/books/NBK537261/

Therapeutic Management

Ideally, a person with a history of congenital or acquired heart disease should consult their health care provider and undergo a risk assessment before becoming pregnant. This risk assessment must consider the person's functional capacity, exercise tolerance, degree of cyanosis, medication needs, and history of arrhythmias. The impact of heart disease on a person's childbearing potential needs to be clearly explained, and providing information on how pregnancy may affect them and the fetus is important. This allows people to make an informed choice about whether they wish to accept the risks associated with pregnancy. When possible, any surgical procedures, such as valve replacement, should be done before pregnancy to improve fetal and maternal outcomes (Cunningham et al., 2022b).

If the patient presents for care after becoming pregnant, prenatal counseling focuses on the impact of the hemodynamic changes of pregnancy, the signs and symptoms of cardiac compromise, and dietary and lifestyle changes needed. More frequent prenatal visits (every 2 weeks until the last month and then weekly) are usually needed to ensure the health and safety of the pregnant person and fetus.

Nursing Assessment

Explore the patient's history. The key risk factors linked to CVD-related maternal morbidity and mortality include race/ethnicity (higher risk in non-Hispanic Black people vs. non-Hispanic White people), age (older than 40 years), hypertension, obesity (BMI ≥30), cigarette smoking, and hypercholesterolemia (American Heart Association, 2022). Frequent and thorough assessments are crucial during the antepartum period to ensure early detection of and prompt intervention for problems. Assess vital signs, noting any changes. Auscultate the apical heart rate and heart sounds, being especially alert for abnormalities, including rhythm irregularities or murmurs. Check the patient's weight and compare it with baseline and weights obtained on previous visits. Report any weight gain outside the expected parameters. Inspect the extremities for edema and note any pitting.

Question the patient about fetal activity and ask if they have noticed any changes. Report any changes such as a decrease in fetal movements. Ask the patient about any symptoms of preterm labor, such as low back pain, uterine contractions, increased pelvic pressure, and vaginal discharge, and report them immediately. Assess the fetal heart rate and review serial ultrasound results to monitor fetal growth.

Assess the patient's lifestyle and their ability to cope with the changes of pregnancy and its effect on cardiac status and ability to function. Evaluate the patient's understanding of their condition and what restrictions and lifestyle changes may be needed to provide the best outcome for them and their fetus. A healthy infant and birthing parent at the end of pregnancy is the ultimate goal. As the patient's pregnancy advances, expect their functional class to be revised based on their level of disability. Suggest realistic modifications.

The nurse plays a major role in recognizing the signs and symptoms of cardiac decompensation. Decompensation refers to the heart's inability to maintain adequate circulation. As a result, tissue perfusion in the pregnant person and the fetus is impaired. Common complaints of normal pregnancy, such as dyspnea, fatigue, palpitations, orthopnea, and pedal edema, mimic symptoms of worsening cardiac disease and create challenges when trying to evaluate pregnant people with cardiac disease.

TAKE NOTE!

Assessing the pregnant person with heart disease for cardiac decompensation is vital because their hemodynamic status impacts the health of the fetus.

Nursing Management

Nursing care for the pregnant person with heart disease focuses on assisting with measures to stabilize their hemodynamic status because a decrease in maternal blood pressure or volume will cause blood to be shunted away from the uterus, thus reducing placental perfusion. Pregnant people with cardiac disease also need assistance in reducing risks that would lead to complications or further cardiac compromise; therefore, education and counseling are critical. Collaboration between the cardiologist, obstetrician, perinatologist, and nurse is needed to promote the best possible outcome.

Drug therapy may be indicated for the pregnant person with a cardiac disorder. Possible drugs include diuretics such as furosemide to prevent heart failure, digitalis to increase contractility and decrease heart rates, antiarrhythmic agents (lidocaine), beta-blockers (labetalol), or calcium channel blockers (nifedipine) to treat hypertension, and anticoagulants (low-molecular-weight heparin). Warfarin (Coumadin) is not recommended because it crosses the placenta and may have teratogenic effects (UpToDate, Inc., 2024).

The U.S. Food and Drug Administration (FDA) is no longer using drug categories A, B, C, D, and X. The package inserts include three separate categories that provide information in a narrative format. The goal of this labeling is to provide information about the drug to the consumer. They now use specific subheadings under each of the three categories: pregnancy, lactation, and females and males of reproductive potential.

Encourage the patient to continue taking their cardiac medications as prescribed. Review the indications, actions, and potential side effects of the medications. Reinforce the importance of frequent prenatal visits and close medical supervision throughout the pregnancy.

Discuss the need to conserve energy. Help the patient prioritize household chores and child care to allow rest periods. Encourage the patient to rest in the side-lying position, which enhances placental perfusion.

Encourage the patient to eat nutritious foods and consume a high-fiber diet to prevent straining and constipation. Discuss limiting sodium intake if indicated to reduce fluid retention. Contact a dietitian to assist the patient in planning nutritionally appropriate meals.

Assist the patient in preparing for diagnostic tests to evaluate fetal well-being. Describe the tests that may be done, such as electrocardiogram (ECG), and explain the need for serial nonstress testing, usually beginning at approximately 32 weeks' gestation. Instruct the patient on how to monitor fetal activity and movements. Urge them to do this daily and report any changes in activity immediately.

Although the morbidity and mortality rates of pregnant people with cardiac disease have decreased greatly, hemodynamic changes during pregnancy (increased heart rate, stroke volume, cardiac output, and blood volume) have a profound effect, which may increase cardiac work and might exceed the functional capacity of the diseased heart. These changes may result in pulmonary hypertension, pulmonary edema, heart failure, or maternal death (Iftikhar & Biswas, 2023). Explain the signs and symptoms of these complications and review the signs and symptoms of cardiac decompensation, encouraging the patient to notify their health care provider if any occur.

Provide support and encouragement throughout the prenatal period. Assess the support systems available to the patient and family and encourage their use. If necessary, assist with referrals to community services for additional support.

ASTHMA

During pregnancy, the respiratory system is affected by hormonal changes, mechanical changes, and prior respiratory conditions. These changes can cause a patient with a history of compromised respiration to decompensate during pregnancy. Chronic respiratory conditions such as asthma can have a negative effect on the growing fetus when alterations in oxygenation occur in the pregnant person. The outcome of pregnancy in a person with asthma depends on the severity of the oxygen alteration as well as the degree and duration of hypoxia in the fetus.

Asthma

Worldwide, the prevalence of asthma among pregnant people is on the rise. Pregnancy leads to a worsening of asthma for about one third of people. Another third will remain unchanged, while the last third will see their symptoms improve (American Academy of Allergy Asthma & Immunology, 2023). Asthma affects up to 8% of pregnancies and is associated with an increased risk of preeclampsia, fetal growth restriction, preterm birth, low birth weight, and maternal and fetal mortality (Shebl & Chakraborty, 2023). As asthma severity increases, the risks also increase.

Remember Rose, the pregnant adolescent with asthma in acute distress described at the beginning of the chapter? What therapies might be offered to control her symptoms? Should she be treated differently than someone who is not pregnant? Why or why not?

Pathophysiology

Asthma is a chronic inflammatory response of the respiratory tract to various stimuli such as allergens (pollen and animal dander), irritants (cigarette smoke and chemicals), stress, infections (colds or flu), and physical exertion. The bronchioles constrict in response to these stimuli. Asthma is characterized by intermittently recurrent or persistent symptoms of bronchoconstriction, including breathlessness, wheezing, chest tightness, cough, and sputum production. In addition to bronchoconstriction, inflammation of the airways occurs and tenacious mucus is produced, limiting air movement and making ventilation difficult (Cunningham et al., 2022c).

The normal physiologic changes of pregnancy affect the respiratory system. Although the respiratory rate does not change, vital capacity and inspiratory capacity increase by 20% by late pregnancy. Diaphragmatic elevation and a decrease in functional lung residual capacity occur late in pregnancy, which may reduce the person's ability to inspire deeply to take in more oxygen. Both oxygen consumption and the metabolic rate increase, placing additional stress on the respiratory system (Cunningham et al., 2022c).

Therapeutic Management

The primary goal of asthma management during pregnancy is to maintain adequate oxygenation of the fetus by preventing hypoxic episodes in the parent. The management of asthma focuses on the prevention of airway inflammation to avoid airway hyperresponsiveness and an exacerbation of asthma symptoms. Treatment is the same as that of a person who is not pregnant (Shebl & Chakraborty, 2023). The mainstay of asthma control is avoidance of allergens or triggers. A stepwise approach is used to prevent and manage symptoms with inhaled corticosteroids and bronchodilators. When asthma symptoms worsen or are poorly controlled, treatment is stepped up to the next level.

Nursing Assessment

Obtain a thorough history of the patient's experience with asthma, including the usual therapy and control measures. Question the patient about asthma triggers and strategies used to reduce exposure to them. Review the patient's medication therapy regimen.

Note the patient's skin color (use the palms, soles, or mucosa to determine color in people with dark skin). Determine the heart rate, which may be elevated with an asthma exacerbation. Auscultate the lungs and assess respiratory and heart rates. Note the rate, rhythm, and depth of respirations, listening for a tight cough. Auscultate the lungs, which should be clear between episodes. During an acute exacerbation, wheezing and dyspnea may be noted (Lange-Vaidya, 2023). Assess the fetal heart rate.

CLINICAL REASONING ALERT!

Tachycardia, tachypnea, and a prolonged expiratory phase are indicators of the severity of an asthma exacerbation.

Nursing Management

Nursing management focuses on reinforcing asthma management with the patient. The asthma maintenance plan is individualized for each patient by the primary care provider or pulmonologist. Reinforce the importance of optimal asthma control. Observe the patient demonstrating the use of the inhaler to ensure its correct use. Offer resources such as smoking cessation programs and home environmental allergy controls. Ensure the pregnant patient understands concerning symptoms and who to contact in an emergency. Review potential perinatal complications with the patient to motivate them to adhere to the prescribed regimen.

Rose, the pregnant patient described earlier, is concerned about passing her asthma on to her baby. What should the nurse discuss with her?

HEMATOLOGIC CONDITIONS

Anemia, a reduction in RBC volume, is measured by hematocrit (Hct) or a decrease in the concentration of hemoglobin (Hgb) in the peripheral blood. This results in reduced capacity of the blood to carry oxygen to the vital organs of the pregnant person and the fetus. Anemia may be caused by nutrient deficiencies or a genetic hemoglobinopathy. Anemia during pregnancy is generally defined as an Hgb below 11 g/dL in the first and third trimesters, and below 10.5 g/dL in the second trimester (Auerbach & Landy, 2023).

Iron-Deficiency Anemia

In North and South America, about 19% of patients experience anemia during pregnancy; iron deficiency is the most common cause (Auerbach & Landy, 2023). Increased risk for iron deficiency during pregnancy is related to increased maternal blood volume, expanded maternal erythrocyte mass, and iron needs for fetal/placental growth and fetal erythrocyte production (Auerbach & Landy, 2023). A person who is pregnant often has insufficient iron stores to meet the demands of pregnancy. Iron-deficiency anemia accounts for most of the cases of anemia in pregnant people; it is usually related to an iron-deficient diet, gastrointestinal issues affecting absorption, or a short pregnancy interval (Auerbach & Landy, 2023).

Pregnant patients with iron-deficiency anemia are twice as likely to experience severe maternal morbidity and have an increased risk of preeclampsia, cesarean delivery, infection, and postpartum hemorrhage (Auerbach & Landy, 2023). Adequate iron is required for normal fetal brain development; maternal iron deficiency places the newborn at risk for neurodevelopmental sequelae (Auerbach & Landy, 2023).

Therapeutic Management

The goals of treatment for iron-deficiency anemia in pregnancy are to eliminate symptoms, correct the deficiency, and replenish iron stores. Screening for anemia with Hgb and Hct should occur at the first prenatal visit and again at 24 to 28 weeks' gestation. The first-line treatment is oral iron. The supplement ferrous sulfate may be given once or twice daily or on alternate days (which improves absorption and decreases side effects) (Auerbach & Landy, 2023).

Nursing Assessment

Review the patient's history for factors that may increase the risk for the development of iron-deficiency anemia, including poor nutrition, hemolysis, multiple gestation, limited intervals between pregnancies, and blood loss. Assess dietary intake as well as the quantity and timing of ingestion of substances that interfere with iron absorption, such as tea, coffee, chocolate, and high-fiber foods. Ask the patient if they have fatigue, weakness, malaise, anorexia, or symptoms of restless leg syndrome. Inspect the skin and mucous membranes, noting any pallor. Obtain vital signs and report any tachycardia.

> **TAKE NOTE!**
>
> Hgb and Hct decrease normally during pregnancy in response to an increase in blood plasma in comparison to RBCs. This hemodilution can lead to physiologic anemia of pregnancy, which does not indicate a decrease in oxygen-carrying capacity or true anemia.

Nursing Management

Nursing care of the person with iron-deficiency anemia focuses on encouraging adherence to iron drug therapy and providing dietary instruction about the intake of iron-rich foods. Stress the importance of taking prenatal vitamins, which contain 27 mg/day of iron, and (if prescribed) an iron supplement consistently. Encourage the patient to take the iron supplement with vitamin C–containing fluids such as orange juice, which will promote absorption, rather than milk, which can inhibit iron absorption. Taking iron on an empty stomach improves its absorption, but many people cannot tolerate the gastrointestinal discomfort it causes. In such cases, advise the patient to take it with meals. Instruct them about adverse effects, which are predominantly gastrointestinal and include abdominal pain, nausea, metallic taste, black stool, and constipation. Provide dietary counseling for increasing intake of iron-containing foods. Teaching Guidelines 20.2 highlights instructions for the pregnant person with iron-deficiency anemia.

TEACHING GUIDELINES 20.2 Teaching for the Person With Iron-Deficiency Anemia

- Take your prenatal vitamin daily; if you miss a dose, take it as soon as you remember.
- For best absorption, take iron supplements between meals and with orange juice.
- Be aware of the side effects of iron supplementation.
- Avoid taking iron supplements with coffee, tea, chocolate, and high-fiber foods.
- Eat foods rich in iron, such as:
  - Meats, green leafy vegetables, legumes, dried fruits, whole grains
  - Peanut butter, bean dip, whole-wheat fortified breads, and cereals
- For best iron absorption from foods, consume the food along with a food high in vitamin C.
- Increase your exercise, fluids, and high-fiber foods to reduce constipation.
- Plan frequent rest periods during the day.

Hemoglobinopathies

Sickle cell disease (SCD) and thalassemia are two hereditary hemoglobinopathies that result in anemia. SCD is an autosomal recessive inherited condition resulting in a defective hemoglobin molecule (hemoglobin S). The normal donut-shaped RBC is replaced with a rigid, sickle-shaped cell that has difficulty passing through small blood vessels, obstructing blood flow. The typical lifespan of sickled RBCs is approximately 15 days, compared to the 120-day lifespan of normal RBCs. Consequently, people with sickle cell anemia suffer from moderate to severe anemia. Beta thalassemia major is an autosomal recessive condition in which the beta chain of the hemoglobin molecule is defective, leading to hemolysis and resulting in significant anemia. It also results in hemochromatosis (excess iron deposition in the tissues and organs). People who have only one gene for SCD or thalassemia are carriers of the disease; carrier status has little effect on pregnancy.

TAKE NOTE!

Because of their association with iron overload, iron supplements are contraindicated in beta thalassemia major.

SCD during pregnancy is associated with more severe anemia and frequent vaso-occlusive crises resulting in increased perinatal morbidity and mortality including venous and arterial thromboembolism, infection, preeclampsia, eclampsia, cesarean birth, fetal growth restriction, low birth weight, and preterm birth (James & Oppong, 2023). It is recommended that low-dose aspirin be given after 12 weeks' gestation to prevent preeclampsia (ACOG et al., 2022). Hydroxyurea is routinely used for the management of SCD and may or may not be continued during pregnancy depending upon SCD severity. Prenatal vitamins should not contain iron, and higher doses of folic acid may be helpful. Analgesics will be needed during vaso-occlusive crises (James & Oppong, 2023).

The mainstay of treatment for beta thalassemia major is blood transfusion and ongoing iron chelation therapy. A person with beta thalassemia major is able to carry a fetus to term if they have a normal cardiac evaluation and have participated in chronic blood transfusion with iron chelation. The need for blood transfusions to maintain hemoglobin greater than 10 mg/dL will likely increase during pregnancy due to increased intravascular volume. Iron chelation is not advised during pregnancy due to its possible teratogenic effects (Benz & Angelucci, 2024).

Nursing Assessment

Early and continuous prenatal care of the patient with a hemoglobinopathy is needed to safeguard the fetus or newborn from potential complications. Explore the patient's health history for usual medications for SCD and a regular schedule of blood transfusions for beta thalassemia major. Ask the patient if they have fatigue, malaise, or dyspnea. Inspect the color of the skin and mucous membranes, noting any pallor. Assess hydration status. Note palpitations or tachycardia. Be alert for indicators of sickle cell vaso-occlusive crisis including leg, digit, or joint pain and chest or abdominal pain (Mangla et al., 2023). Monitor hemoglobin and ferritin levels frequently. Assess the fetal heart rate at each visit.

Nursing Management

Prenatal visits during the first and second trimesters should occur more frequently. Nurses should provide supportive care and expectant management throughout the pregnancy. In the presence of anemia, instruction to rest and to avoid infections is helpful. Urge the patient to drink eight to 10 glasses of fluid daily to prevent dehydration. Teach the patient about the need to avoid infections (including meticulous hand hygiene), cigarette smoking, alcohol consumption, and temperature extremes.

Predicting the clinical course of SCD or beta thalassemia during pregnancy is difficult. Outcomes have improved for pregnant people with hemoglobinopathy. Optimal management during pregnancy requires a multidisciplinary team and prompt, effective treatment of potential complications if they occur.

SELECTED MUSCULOSKELETAL AND AUTOIMMUNE DISORDERS

Musculoskeletal disorders often involve pain and are frequently treated with teratogenic medications. Autoimmune disorders are a group of more than 100 distinct diseases that emerge when the immune system launches an immune response against its own cells and tissues. It is thought that a genetic predisposition, environmental triggers, and hormones all contribute to disease development and activity. A greater number of autoimmune-related genes originate from the X chromosome, which creates a far greater possibility of mutations occurring (Angum et al., 2020). This places people with two X chromosomes at a greater risk for developing autoimmune diseases than those with only one. Of people affected by autoimmune diseases, approximately 80% are female. Previously, the general advice to people with autoimmune diseases was to avoid pregnancy because there was a high risk of maternal and fetal morbidity and mortality. However, it is now clear that these risks can generally be reduced by avoiding pregnancy when the diseases are active and continuing appropriate medication to reduce the chances of disease flare during pregnancy. At times considered an autoimmune disease, multiple sclerosis (MS) is likely an immune response to a viral trigger (Olek & Mowry, 2024). MS will be included in this discussion.

Pregnancies in people with an autoimmune disease may be considered high risk. At each prenatal visit, fetal well-being and growth must be assessed. Complications related to pregnancy with each disease are:

- Systemic lupus erythematosus (SLE): preeclampsia, eclampsia, preterm labor, unplanned cesarean delivery, fetal growth restriction (Bermas & Smith, 2023)
- Poorly controlled rheumatoid arthritis (RA): hypertensive disorders, fetal growth restriction, cesarean delivery (Bermas, 2023)
- Fibromyalgia: cesarean delivery (Koné et al., 2022)

The exception to complications in pregnancy is MS. Pregnancy seems to decrease MS relapses. Refer to Table 20.4 for an explanation of selected autoimmune and immune diseases and their therapeutic management and nursing implications.

TABLE 20.4 • Selected Musculoskeletal and Autoimmune Diseases

Disease and Explanation	Clinical Manifestations	Therapeutic Management	Nursing Implications
Musculoskeletal Diseases			
Multiple sclerosis—chronic inflammatory, demyelinating autoimmune disorder of the central nervous system	• Sensory loss in the face or limbs • Motor and gait disturbances • Balance issues, vertigo • Diplopia, vision loss • Bladder problems • Pain	Disease-modifying therapy (DMT) medications such as interferon and monoclonal antibodies	• In nonsevere cases of MS, DMTs should be stopped prior to conception. • Educate the patient to eat a balanced diet, avoid alcohol and smoking, take vitamin D and prenatal vitamins, and prioritize sleep hygiene.
Fibromyalgia—central pain sensitivity syndrome without joint damage	• Brain fog • Depression • Fatigue • Widespread musculoskeletal and other body pain	Pregabalin, duloxetine, and milnacipran	• Educate the patient about relaxation techniques, sleep hygiene, and the importance of exercise. • Duloxetine, milnacipran, and pregabalin cross the placenta. • If duloxetine or milnacipran are to be discontinued, they should be tapered rather than abruptly stopped.
Autoimmune Diseases			
Systemic lupus erythematosus (SLE)—chronic, relapsing autoimmune disease of the connective tissues affecting various organs (skin, joints, kidneys, serosal membranes)	• Swollen joints • Extreme fatigue • Oral ulcers • Fever • Skin rashes • Sensitivity to sunlight	Anti-inflammatory drugs and hydroxychloroquine (Plaquenil) are used to manage disease flares activated by estrogen, cigarette smoking, infections, stress, ultraviolet light exposure, or pregnancy.	• Recommend postponing conception until the disease has been stable or in remission for 6 months. • Assess for SLE signs and symptoms, urine for protein and specific gravity, and signs of infection. • Teach to monitor for flare symptoms and educate on energy conservation techniques.
Rheumatoid arthritis (RA)—joint inflammation (primarily synovial joints, tissues of the hands and feet) resulting in disability	• Painful joints • Loss of function • Joint deformity • Stiffness with inactivity • Decreased mobility	Anti-inflammatory drugs, glucocorticoids, DMT medications, methotrexate	• Educate to discontinue DMT drugs upon conception and methotrexate prior to conception. • Encourage physical activity within the limits of joint pain (swimming is excellent). • Advise about increased risk of disease flare in the postpartum period.

Bermas, B. L. (2023). Rheumatoid arthritis and pregnancy. *UpToDate*. Retrieved May 3, 2024, from https://www.uptodate.com/contents/rheumatoid-arthritis-and-pregnancy; Bermas, B. L., & Smith, N. A. (2023). Pregnancy in women with systemic lupus erythematosus. *UpToDate*. Retrieved May 3, 2024, from https://www.uptodate.com/contents/pregnancy-in-women-with-systemic-lupus-erythematosus; Bhargava, J., & Hurley, J. A. (2023). Fibromyalgia. *StatPearls*. https://www.ncbi.nlm.nih.gov/books/NBK540974/; Lee, M. J., Sullivan, C., & Graves, J. (2023). Multiple sclerosis: Pregnancy planning. *UpToDate*. Retrieved May 3, 2024, from https://www.uptodate.com/contents/multiple-sclerosis-pregnancy-planning; Olek, M. J., & Howard, J. (2024). Clinical presentation, course, and prognosis of multiple sclerosis in adults. *UpToDate*. Retrieved May 3, 2024, from https://www.uptodate.com/contents/clinical-presentation-course-and-prognosis-of-multiple-sclerosis-in-adults; UpToDate, Inc. (2024). *UpToDate® Lexidrug™* (Version 8.2.0) [Mobile app]. Wolters Kluwer. https://apps.apple.com/us/app/lexicomp/id313401238; and Wallace, D. J., & Gladman, D. D. (2023). Clinical manifestations and diagnosis of systemic lupus erythematosus in adults. *UpToDate*. Retrieved May 3, 2024, from https://www.uptodate.com/contents/clinical-manifestations-and-diagnosis-of-systemic-lupus-erythematosus-in-adults

INFECTIONS

A wide variety of infections can affect the progression of pregnancy, possibly negatively impacting the outcome. The effect of the infection depends on the timing and severity of the infection and the body systems involved. Common viral infections include cytomegalovirus (CMV), rubella, herpes simplex, hepatitis B, varicella, and parvovirus B19. Group B streptococcus (GBS), toxoplasmosis, and tuberculosis (TB) are common nonviral infections. Sexually transmitted infections (STIs) may be bacterial or viral. STIs are discussed in detail in Chapter 5. Refer to Table 20.5 for information relating to STIs during pregnancy.

TABLE 20.5 • Sexually Transmitted Infections (STIs) Affecting Pregnancy

Infection/Organism	Effect on Pregnancy and Fetus/Newborn	Implications
Herpes simplex virus (HSV)	Highest risk of transmission is with infection onset near the time of birth and vaginal birth with active lesions. Newborn infection may be localized or disseminated (high risk of mortality).	Antiviral agents during pregnancy may decrease the transmission rate. Avoid procedures causing a break in the infant's skin, such as artificial rupture of membranes, fetal scalp electrode, forceps, and vacuum extraction. Cesarean delivery indicated if active lesions noted at the time of birth
Syphilis (*Treponema pallidum*)	Maternal infection increases the risk of premature labor and birth. Newborn may be born with congenital syphilis, causing jaundice, rhinitis, anemia, fetal growth restriction, and central nervous system involvement.	All pregnant people should be screened for this STI and treated with benzathine penicillin G 2.4 million units IM to prevent placental transmission.
Gonorrhea (*Neisseria gonorrhea*)	Majority of people are without symptoms. It causes ophthalmia neonatorum in the newborn from birth through infected birth canal.	All pregnant people should be screened at the first prenatal visit with repeat screening in the third trimester. All newborns receive mandatory eye prophylaxis with erythromycin within the first hour of life. Birthing parent is treated with ceftriaxone (Rocephin) 125 mg IM in a single dose before going home.
Chlamydia (*Chlamydia trachomatis*)	Majority of people are without symptoms. Infection is associated with infertility and ectopic pregnancy, spontaneous abortions, preterm labor, premature rupture of membranes, low birth weight, stillbirth, and neonatal mortality. Infection is transmitted to the newborn through vaginal birth. Neonate may develop conjunctivitis or pneumonia.	All pregnant people should be screened at the first prenatal visit and treated with erythromycin.
Human papillomavirus (HPV)	Infection causes warts in the anogenital area, known as condylomata acuminata. These warts may grow large enough to block a vaginal birth. Fetal exposure to HPV during birth is associated with laryngeal papillomas.	Warts are treated with trichloroacetic acid, liquid nitrogen, or laser therapy under colposcopy. Two HPV vaccines have been FDA-approved and are licensed in the United States for people 9–45 years old, with recommended vaccination beginning at age 9. The vaccines are 95%–100% effective.
Trichomonas (*Trichomonas vaginalis*)	Infection produces itching and burning, dysuria, strawberry patches on the cervix, and vaginal discharge. Infection is associated with premature rupture of membranes and preterm birth.	Treatment is with a single 2-g dose of metronidazole (Flagyl).

FDA, U.S. Food and Drug Administration; IM, intramuscularly.

Cunningham, F. G., Leveno, K. J., Dashe, J. S., Hoffman, B. L., Spong, C. Y., & Casey, B. M. (2022e). Sexually transmitted infections. In F. G. Cunningham, K. J. Leveno, J. S. Dashe, B. L. Hoffman, C. Y. Spong, & B., M. Casey, *William's obstetrics* (26th ed.). McGraw Hill.

Cytomegalovirus

CMV is a member of the herpesvirus family and infects between 50% and 80% of the human population by age 40 (Cedeno-Mendoza, 2023). It is transmitted via body fluids such as saliva, urine, semen, vaginal fluids, blood, tears, and breast milk and can also pass through the placenta during pregnancy. Pregnant people acquire active disease primarily from sexual contact, blood transfusions, kissing, and contact with children in day care centers. CMV is typically without symptoms in most people, though it may cause influenzalike symptoms in some. Acute infection during pregnancy may lead to fetal growth restriction or an infant who is small for gestational age (SGA).

Prenatal screening for CMV infection is not routinely performed. In infants of previously seronegative birthing parents who acquire CMV infection during pregnancy, in utero fetal infection may occur. Between 10% and 15% of congenitally infected infants are acutely symptomatic at birth, displaying a blueberry muffin rash, central nervous system anomalies, jaundice, and hepatosplenomegaly (Fig. 20.3) (Plotogea et al., 2022). Congenital CMV infection often results in deafness and neurodevelopmental disabilities. There is no proven in utero treatment for infected fetuses (Plotogea et al., 2022).

Stressing the importance of good hand hygiene and the use of sound hygiene practices can help to reduce transmission of the virus. A few specific hygiene guidelines for pregnant people include:

- Wash hands frequently with soap and water and wear gloves, especially after diaper changes, feeding, wiping nose or drool, and handling children's toys.
- Do not share cups, plates, utensils, food, or toothbrushes.
- Do not share towels or washcloths.
- Avoid contact with tears and saliva when kissing a child.
- Do not put a child's pacifier in your mouth.
- Clean toys, countertops, and other surfaces that come in contact with children's urine or saliva.
- Practice safe sex, including limiting sexual partners and using condoms consistently.

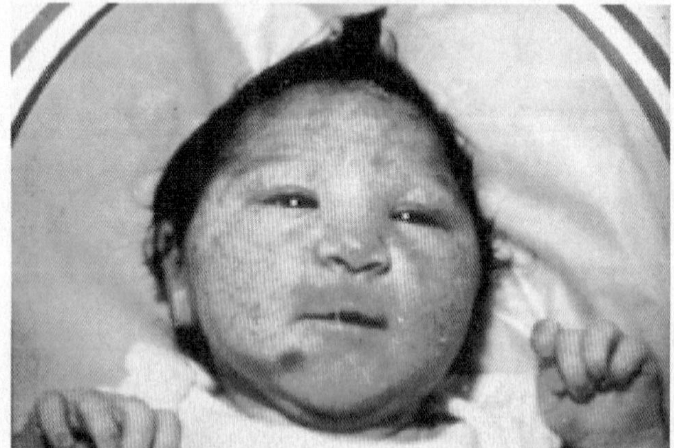

FIGURE 20.3 Clinical appearance of an infant with congenital cytomegalovirus with stigmata of disease, including petechial rash, microcephaly, jaundice, and abnormal posture of upper extremities secondary to central nervous system damage.

Rubella

Rubella, commonly called German measles, is a vaccine-preventable infection spread by droplets or through direct contact with a contaminated object (Edwards & Shetty, 2023). The risk of a pregnant person transmitting this virus through the placenta to the fetus increases with earlier exposure to the virus. The highest risk of transmission occurs when the pregnant person becomes infected within the first 10 weeks of gestation (Arrieta, 2023). Congenital rubella infection may result in spontaneous abortion or stillbirth. The newborn may have sensorineural hearing loss (most common); congenital cataracts or glaucoma; congenital heart defects; and later in life, developmental delay (Arrieta, 2023).

Education for primary prevention is the key. Ideally, everyone has been vaccinated and has adequate immunity against rubella. However, all patients are still screened at their first prenatal visits to determine their immune status. A rubella antibody titer of 1:8 or greater provides evidence of immunity. People who are not immune should be vaccinated during the immediate postpartum period so that they will be immune before becoming pregnant again (Riley, 2024).

Hepatitis B and C Virus

Hepatitis B virus (HBV) is one of the most prevalent chronic diseases in the world. Since 1998, rates of hepatitis B infection in pregnant people have increased by over 5% annually (Pressman & Ros, 2023). In the United States, the prevalence of chronic hepatitis B infection among pregnant people is approaching 1% (Asafo-Agyei & Samant, 2023). HBV can be transmitted through sexual contact, illicit drug use, and contaminated blood; sexual transmission accounts for most adult HBV infections. Hepatitis C virus (HCV) infection is becoming increasingly more prevalent during pregnancy, likely due to injectable drug use (Pressman & Ros, 2023). Both acute and chronic HBV and HCV infection may be vertically transmitted to the infant.

People with acute HBV and HCV infection may be completely without symptoms or may experience malaise, right upper quadrant abdominal pain, nausea, anorexia, jaundice, and dark urine (Asafo-Agyei & Samant, 2023; Feld, 2022). Both HBV and HCV may cause chronic infection, which is generally without symptoms. Maternal HBV and HCV infection increases the risk of preterm birth and neonatal death (Asafo-Agyei & Samant, 2023; Chen et al., 2023). Additionally, chronic HBV infection during pregnancy increases the risk for maternal death, fetal growth restriction, gestational hypertension, placental abruption, and preterm birth (Asafo-Agyei & Samant, 2023). With chronic HBV, if the hepatitis B surface antigen (HBsAg) is positive, the vertical transmission rate is 90% (Asafo-Agyei & Samant, 2023). The vertical transmission rate for HCV is almost 6% (with an increased rate of transmission for those also infected with HIV) (Goldman & O'Donovan, 2023).

Nursing Assessment

The ACOG (2023) recommends hepatitis B and hepatitis C screening at the first prenatal visit. HBsAg should also be evaluated.

Nursing Management

Pregnant people with a high viral load for hepatitis B may be treated with antivirals after 28 to 32 weeks of gestation to decrease the vertical transmission rate to 5% (Asafo-Agyei & Samant, 2023). People who are HBsAg-negative may be vaccinated safely during pregnancy, with the hepatitis B vaccine series given as two injections, 5 months apart. To decrease vertical transmission in people positive for hepatitis C, it is recommended to avoid cesarean birth if at all possible.

Patient education related to the prevention of HBV and HCV is essential. Teach the patient about safer sex practices, good hand hygiene techniques, and the use of standard precautions. All pregnant people should avoid injectable drug misuse.

Varicella Zoster Virus

Varicella zoster virus (VZV) is one of the eight herpes family viruses. It is the virus that causes both varicella (chickenpox) and herpes zoster (shingles). Primary VZV leads to varicella and establishes latency in the dorsal root ganglia. Reactivation of VZV causes herpes zoster. Herpes zoster can occur once the immune response against the virus wanes, usually with advancing age.

Due to prior immunity resulting from chickenpox in childhood or immunization series completion, pregnant people rarely develop varicella infection (Speer, 2023). When a seronegative person contracts varicella infection 2 to 5 days before delivery, the newborn fatality rate is 30% (Speer, 2023). If hospitalized, a seronegative pregnant person who is exposed to an active varicella infection 6 to 21 days before delivery must be isolated to prevent transmission to others. The newborn may stay in the birthing parent's room but should not be admitted to the nursery to prevent possible transmission to other infants.

If the birthing parent has signs and symptoms of varicella infection within 2 to 5 days of delivery, the newborn should receive varicella zoster immunoglobulin (Varizig) intramuscularly shortly after birth (Speer, 2023). Varicella infection can be prevented by appropriate immunization with the vaccine in people testing nonimmune to varicella. As a live vaccine, varicella immunization is contraindicated in pregnancy but should be given to seronegative people before or after pregnancy (Centers for Disease Control and Prevention [CDC], 2022a).

Parvovirus B19

Parvovirus B19 is a common, self-limiting, benign childhood virus that causes erythema infectiosum. It is estimated that 30% to 60% of adults have been infected previously with parvovirus (Riley & Fernandes, 2023). Parvovirus B19 is commonly called fifth disease and is transmitted by respiratory secretions or saliva, close person-to-person contact, and fomites (Jordan, 2023). Most infected people are without symptoms, though young children are most commonly infected and present with a slapped cheek appearance and lacy erythematous rash on the trunk and extremities (Riley & Fernandes, 2023). Infection usually results in lasting immunity. Fetal infection may be associated with a normal outcome; however, fetal death or fetal hydrops may occur (Riley & Fernandes, 2023).

Those most at risk for contracting parvovirus B19 infection are people in crowded environments, close household contacts of infected people, and day care workers and teachers (Jordan, 2023). Parvovirus B19 may be transmitted vertically via the placenta. The virus is toxic to fetal RBC precursors, resulting in fetal anemia. Fetal hydrops (abnormal accumulation of fluid in fetal serous cavities and tissues) then develops; this may spontaneously resolve or may quickly lead to fetal death (Riley & Fernandes, 2023). An immunization against parvovirus B19 does not exist. Advise pregnant patients to avoid contact with people known to be infected with the virus.

Group B Streptococcus

GBS is a gram-positive bacterium colonizing in the gastrointestinal and genitourinary tracts. GBS colonization is present in 10% to 30% of pregnant people (Morgan et al., 2023). GBS is transmitted to the newborn via vaginal labor and birth. GBS maternal colonization increases the risk for chorioamnionitis, endometritis, cesarean delivery, and postpartum wound infection. About 50% of colonized pregnant people transmit the infection to their infant, but only 1% to 2% of those infants develop GBS disease (Puopolo & Baker, 2023). GBS is the most common cause of sepsis and meningitis in newborns and is a frequent cause of newborn pneumonia (Morgan et al., 2023). Newborns with early-onset GBS infections usually present within 24 hours of birth (up to 6 days of age), while those with late-onset infection present between 7 and 89 days of age (Puopolo & Baker, 2023).

All pregnant people should be screened for GBS colonization with a rectovaginal culture at 35 to 37 weeks' gestation. Maternal intrapartum prophylaxis is necessary in GBS-positive people. A loading intravenous dose is followed by intermittent doses every 4 hours throughout labor. Penicillin G and ampicillin are the drugs of choice, with clindamycin being used in people who are allergic to penicillin. If the pregnant person's GBS status is unknown, intravenous antibiotics should be administered during labor for patients who present with preterm labor. Antibiotic prophylaxis should be initiated in patients with preterm labor or rupture of membranes longer than 18 hours, if the laboring person's temperature is greater than 100.4°F (38°C), or if there is history of invasive early-onset GBS infection in a sibling (Morgan et al., 2023).

Toxoplasmosis

Toxoplasmosis is an infection caused by the parasite *Toxoplasma gondii*; it infects more than 225,000 people in the United States annually (Hökelek, 2022). Cats are the definitive hosts of this parasite and shed it in their feces. It is transferred from hand to mouth after touching cat feces while changing the cat litter box or through gardening in contaminated soil. Consuming undercooked infected meat, such as pork, lamb, or venison; drinking contaminated water; and eating unwashed fruits and vegetables can also transmit this organism. Maternal infection is usually without symptoms (Petersen & Mandelbrot, 2024). Transplacental infection occurs in one infant per 10,000 live births each year in the United States (Guerina & Marquez, 2022).

Although 70% to 90% of infected newborns will be without symptoms, clinical manifestations occurring in 50% or more symptomatic cases of congenital toxoplasmosis include chorioretinitis, intracranial calcifications, hydrocephalus, abnormal cerebrospinal fluid, jaundice, thrombocytopenia, and anemia (Guerina & Marquez, 2022). Severity varies with gestational age (Petersen & Mandelbrot, 2024).

Maternal antibiotic administration may decrease the severity of effects on the fetus. It should be initiated at greater than 14 weeks' gestation to minimize teratogenic effects on the fetus. The treatment of choice is spiramycin in the first trimester (<14 weeks), and pyrimethamine–sulfadiazine when therapy is begun after 14 weeks of gestation (Petersen & Mandelbrot, 2024). Preventing infection in pregnant patients is key to avoiding infection in newborns (Teaching Guidelines 20.3).

TEACHING GUIDELINES 20.3 Teaching to Prevent Toxoplasmosis

- Avoid eating raw or undercooked meat, especially lamb or pork. Cook all meat to an internal temperature of 160°F (71°C) throughout.
- Clean cutting boards, work surfaces, and utensils with hot, soapy water after contact with raw meat or unwashed fruits and vegetables.
- Peel or thoroughly wash all raw fruits and vegetables before eating them.
- Wash hands thoroughly with warm water and soap after handling raw meat.
- Avoid feeding the cat raw or undercooked meats.
- Wash hands with soap and water after handling fruits and vegetables.
- Avoid emptying or cleaning the cat's litter box. Have someone else do it daily.
- Keep outdoor sandboxes covered to prevent cat feces contamination.
- Keep the cat indoors to prevent it from hunting and eating birds or rodents.
- Avoid uncooked eggs and unpasteurized milk.
- Avoid drinking unfiltered water in any setting.
- Avoid eating raw shellfish like oysters, clams, or mussels.
- Use a food thermometer to make sure it is cooked to a safe temperature.
- Wear gardening gloves when in contact with outdoor soil (Hökelek, 2022; Petersen & Mandelbrot, 2024).

Tuberculosis

TB is a disease that represents a global health hazard (Hui & Lao, 2022). It is caused by inhalation of *Mycobacterium tuberculosis*. In the United States, 2.5 cases occur per 100,000 people each year (CDC, 2024c). The most common site of infection is the pulmonary system, but extrapulmonary effects may also occur. Risk factors for TB include recent immigration, homelessness, overcrowded living situations, immunocompromised status, and injectable drug use.

When treated adequately, TB in pregnant people has outcomes equivalent to those in nonpregnant people, with neonatal and maternal morbidity also being reduced (Hui & Lao, 2022). Active TB infection increases the maternal risk of miscarriage, stillbirth, placenta previa, preeclampsia, eclampsia, preterm delivery, anemia, sepsis, cesarean delivery, and postpartum hemorrhage. Maternal TB increases the risk of fetal distress, low birth weight, fetal growth restriction, low Apgar scores, birth asphyxia, and congenital anomalies (Hui & Lao, 2022). The newborn is at risk of postnatally acquired TB if the birthing parent still has active TB at the time of birth. Therefore, prenatal diagnosis and effective treatment of the pregnant person are essential.

TB refers to an active TB infection resulting in signs and symptoms of the disease. These include fever, pleuritic pain, cough, fatigue, and arthralgia (Pozniak, 2024). Pregnant people who are at high risk for TB infection or who are demonstrating symptoms suggestive of TB should have a tuberculin skin test (TST) or interferon-γ release assay (IGRA). Both the TST and IGRA are positive in those with active TB but are not diagnostic of TB in the absence of a positive chest x-ray finding and sputum acid-fast bacilli culture (Friedman & Tanoue, 2024). The TST and IGRA are also positive in people with latent TB infection, but the person is without symptoms and is noninfectious (Pozniak, 2024).

Pregnant people should start treatment as soon as TB is identified. The multidrug treatment regimen lasts for 9 months. In the first 2 months, isoniazid (INH), rifampin, and ethambutol are given. The remaining 7 months of therapy include INH and rifampin. In addition, pyridoxine (vitamin B6) should be given to prevent peripheral neuropathy associated with INH treatment. Latent TB infection (without signs of disease) does not require treatment.

Adherence to multidrug therapy is critical to protect the patient and the fetus from the progression of TB. Provide education about the disease process, the mode of transmission, prevention, potential complications, and the importance of adhering to the treatment regimen.

Breastfeeding is not contraindicated during the time the birthing parent is on the medication regimen and should in fact be encouraged. If the birthing parent is untreated for TB at the time of childbirth, they should not breastfeed or be in direct contact with the newborn until at least 2 weeks after starting antitubercular medications (Friedman & Tanoue, 2024). Untreated lactating parents can be encouraged to pump their milk to feed their newborns until they can breastfeed directly (CDC, 2024a). Nurses should consult their hospital policies regarding parents with TB for additional guidance.

HIV Infection

The **human immunodeficiency virus (HIV)** infection is a chronic infection caused by the retrovirus HIV and is transmitted via blood and body fluids. The virus affects the T cells that express CD4 receptors causing immunodeficiency. Once infected, the person may remain without symptoms or develop an acute response, usually within 2 to 4 weeks but as long as 10 months (Sax, 2024). When symptomatic, acute HIV infection results in fever, diarrhea, headache, lymphadenopathy, myalgia/arthralgia, rash, sore throat, and weight loss (Sax, 2024). Without treatment, acute HIV infection progresses to chronic HIV infection. When the CD4-positive cell count falls below 200 cells/mm^3, **acquired immunodeficiency syndrome (AIDS)** occurs (HIVinfo.NIH.gov, 2023). With AIDS, certain opportunistic infections, particular cancers, neurocognitive decline, and eventual death occur. Though the incidence has been decreasing, each year nearly 7,000 females become infected with HIV (CDC, 2023). The majority become infected via heterosexual contact (Peterson & Kleeman, 2022). HIV during pregnancy places the fetus and newborn at risk for prematurity, fetal growth restriction, low birth weight, and infection.

Pathophysiology

HIV is an RNA retrovirus that is transmitted through infected blood and bodily secretions. The three recognized modes of HIV transmission are unprotected sexual intercourse with an infected partner, contact with infected blood or blood products, and perinatal (vertical) transmission. Once infected with HIV, the person develops antibodies that can be detected with an enzyme-linked immunosorbent assay (ELISA) and confirmed with the Western blot test about 3 weeks after infection. All pregnant people should be screened for HIV at the initial prenatal visit.

TAKE NOTE!

HIV is not transmitted by doorknobs, faucets, toilets, dirty dishes, mosquitoes, wet towels, coughing or sneezing, shaking hands, being hugged, or by any other indirect method.

Therapeutic Management

Pregnant people with HIV infection require antiretroviral therapy (ART). Combination ART has been shown to suppress the viral load, significantly decreasing the risk for perinatal transmission (Choudhary, 2022). The medications used to treat nonpregnant adults are also used in pregnant people with HIV infection: nucleoside reverse transcriptase inhibitors (NRTIs), protease inhibitors, integrase inhibitors, and non-NRTIs. A two- or three-drug regimen is used.

It is recommended that having a cesarean birth will reduce the risk of HIV infection (Hughes & Cu-Uvin, 2023). Efforts to reduce instrumentation, such as avoiding the use of an episiotomy, fetal scalp electrodes, and fetal scalp sampling, will also reduce the newborn's exposure to body fluids.

Nursing Assessment

Review the patient's history for risk factors such as higher risk sex practices, multiple sex partners, and injectable drug use. Ask about the presence of symptoms such as fever, diarrhea, headache, muscle or joint pain, rash, and sore throat. Perform a complete physical examination. Note lymphadenopathy if present. Obtain the patient's weight and determine if they have lost weight recently.

LABORATORY AND DIAGNOSTIC TESTING

Early screening allows for prompt confirmation of the HIV diagnosis and initiation of therapies to safeguard the patient's health. The American College of Obstetricians and Gynecologists (ACOG) (2024) recommends offering

HIV testing to pregnant patients at the initial visit. The recommended screening test is a combined antigen/antibody test. Subsequently, a nucleic acid test will determine the viral load. Those with HIV infection are often coinfected with HBV or HCV and should therefore be tested for those as well (Peterson & Kleeman, 2022).

TAKE NOTE!

Screening only people who are identified as high risk based on their histories is inadequate due to the prolonged latency period that can exist after exposure. Additionally, research indicating that treatment with antiretroviral agents could reduce vertical transmission from the infected person to the newborn has dramatically increased the importance of HIV infection screening in pregnancy.

Nursing Management

Pregnant patients are dealing with many issues at their first prenatal visit. The confirmation of pregnancy may be accompanied by feelings of joy, anxiety, depression, or other emotions. Understanding health education may be difficult in these circumstances. To expect patients to understand detailed explanations of HIV infection may be unrealistic. Determine the patient's readiness for this discussion. Identify the patient's individual needs for teaching, emotional support, and physical care, and approach education and counseling in a caring, sensitive manner. In addition to the importance of ongoing prenatal care, a well-balanced diet should be followed. Also address the following information:

- Infection control issues at home
- Safer sex precautions
- Stages of the HIV infectious process
- Symptoms of opportunistic infections
- Referrals to community support, counseling, and financial aid
- Patient's support system and potential caregiver
- Measures to reduce exposure to infections

Educate the patient about the importance of maintaining ART, and provide them with suggestions for dealing with medication side effects. ACOG (2022b) also recommends the discussion of preexposure prophylaxis (PrEP) medication with all sexually active patients, rather than providing this information to only those at high risk of acquiring HIV. Patients must be informed about PrEP to prevent HIV acquisition.

Be aware of the psychosocial sequelae of HIV/AIDS. The person with HIV infection may experience grief, fear, or anxiety about the future of themselves and their child. Along with the medications that are so important to health maintenance, address the patient's mental health needs, family dynamics, capacity to work, and social concerns, and provide appropriate support and guidance. Be aware of your personal beliefs and attitudes toward people with HIV infection. Incorporate this awareness in your actions as you help the patient face the reality of the diagnosis and treatment options. Empathy, understanding, caring, and assistance are key to helping the patient and their family.

PREPARING FOR LABOR, BIRTH, AND POSTPARTUM

Current evidence suggests that cesarean birth performed before the onset of labor and before the rupture of membranes in patients with a viral load greater than 1,000 copies/mL significantly reduces the rate of perinatal transmission. Cesarean section should be performed at 38 weeks' gestation and prior to rupture of membranes (Hughes & Cu-Uvin, 2023). For those with viral loads lower than 100 copies/mL, the method of delivery should be based on viral load, the duration of ruptured membranes, the progress of labor, and other pertinent clinical factors (Hughes & Cu-Uvin, 2023).

Prepare the patient physically and emotionally for the possibility of cesarean birth, and assist as necessary. Ensure that they understand the rationale for the surgical birth. For the patient without viral suppression and who did not take ART in the third trimester, breastfeeding is not recommended due to the increased risk of virus transmission to the newborn. Breastfeeding may be discussed with the provider as an option for birthing parents with viral suppression and who were maintained on ART throughout all of the third trimester (Hughes & Cu-Uvin, 2023).

After the birth of the newborn, the motivation for taking antiretroviral medications may be lower, thus affecting adherence to therapy. Encourage the patient to continue therapy for their own sake as well as that of the newborn. Nurses can make a difference in helping patients adhere to their complex drug regimens. Educate the patient with an HIV infection about self-care measures, including the proper method for disposing of perineal pads to reduce the risk of exposing others to infected body fluids. Finally, teach them the signs and symptoms of infection in newborns and infants, encouraging them to report any to the health care provider.

TAKE NOTE!

When providing direct care, *always* follow standard precautions.

VULNERABLE POPULATIONS

Risks for adverse pregnancy outcomes are dramatically increased for certain vulnerable populations: adolescents, people over the age of 35, people with obesity (BMI ≥30), and people who misuse substances. Although risks cannot be totally eliminated once pregnancy has begun, they can be reduced through appropriate and timely interventions. Every person's experience with pregnancy is unique and personal. Many people in these special population groups go through pregnancy feeling confusion, isolation, and desperately in need of help but not knowing where to go. Skilled nursing interventions are essential in promoting the best outcome for the patient and baby. Timely support and appropriate interventions during the perinatal period can have long-standing implications for the parent and their newborn, ultimately with the goal of stability and integration of the family as a unit.

Pregnant Adolescents

Adolescence lasts from the onset of puberty to the cessation of physical growth, roughly from 10 to 19 years of age. Adolescents are in between being children and being adults. They need to adjust to the physiologic changes their bodies are undergoing and establish a sexual identity during this time. They search for personal identity and desire freedom and independence of thought and action. It is also a time for building meaningful relationships with others (Fig. 20.4).

Adolescents have special needs when working to accomplish their developmental tasks and making a smooth transition to young adulthood. One of the biggest areas of need is sexual health. Sexuality is a natural aspect of being human, and sexual activity is a basic aspect of human development for young people. Adolescents' normal development includes an attitude of invulnerability and lack of planning for the future. In addition, adolescents often participate in sexual activity, sometimes in submission to peer pressure. They commonly lack the information, skills, and services necessary to make informed choices related to their sexual and reproductive health. As a result, unplanned pregnancies occur.

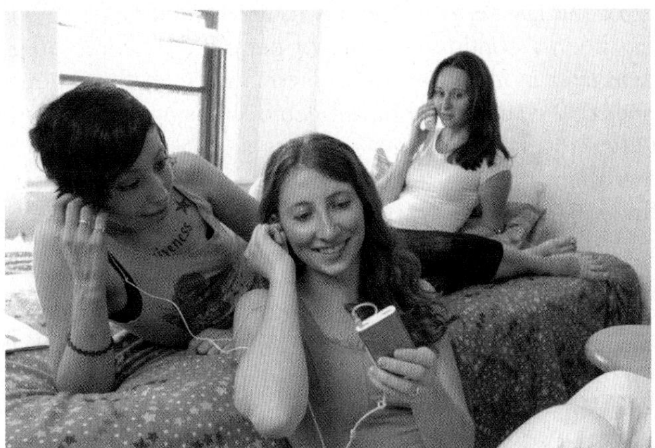

FIGURE 20.4 Adolescents sharing time together.

For the past three decades, pregnancy in adolescence has been decreasing and currently occurs at a rate of 16.7 per 1,000 live births (CDC, 2021). Currently, fewer high school students are having sexual intercourse, and more sexually active students are using some method of contraception (CDC, 2021). Adolescents need support from parents or other trusted adults, as well as access to youth-friendly reproductive health services. Pregnancy options including continuing with the pregnancy, pursuing adoption, or terminating the pregnancy should be discussed and appropriate referrals made (Berlan et al., 2022).

Health and Social Consequences

Adolescent parenthood can present a challenge. Health issues associated with adolescent pregnancy (particularly younger adolescents) include an increased risk for anemia, preeclampsia, instrumental delivery, preterm birth, low birth weight, fetal growth restriction, postpartum depression, and maternal and infant mortality compared with pregnant people aged 20 and older (Berlan et al., 2022; Chacko, 2023; Maheshwari et al., 2022). Improving adherence to prenatal care is critical for decreasing these risks for pregnant adolescents to improve outcomes for parents and infants. Adverse social outcomes include lower socioeconomic status, fewer years of education, and increased risk of intimate partner violence (Berlan et al., 2022). Children of adolescent birthing parents are at increased risk of mood and behavioral disorders, cognitive and learning problems, early sexual activity, and early parenthood (Chacko, 2023). Additionally, adolescent parents report an increased prevalence of alcohol ingestion and cigarette smoking (Prince & Ayers, 2023).

Recall Rose, the pregnant adolescent with asthma. What issues would be important for the nurse to discuss with her related to her pregnancy, her asthma, and her age?

Nursing Assessment

Assessment of the pregnant adolescent is the same as that for any pregnant person. Having an honest regard for adolescent patients requires getting to know them and being able to appreciate the important aspects of their lives. Doing so forms a basis for the nurse's clinical judgment and promotes care that takes into account the concerns and practical circumstances of the adolescent and family. Skillful practice includes knowing how and when to advise an adolescent and when to listen and refrain from giving advice.

Adolescent pregnancy is an area in which a nurse's moral convictions may influence the care that they provide to patients. Nurses need to examine their own beliefs about adolescent sexuality to identify personal assumptions. Putting aside one's moral convictions may be difficult, but it is necessary when working with pregnant adolescents. Giving advice insensitively and without context can be interpreted as "preaching," and the adolescent may be inclined to ignore the information. The nurse must be perceptive, flexible, and sensitive and must communicate in a manner that adolescents understand. Respecting adolescents as individuals helps to establish a therapeutic relationship (see the Healthy People 2030 box).

HEALTHY PEOPLE 2030

Objective	Nursing Significance
Reduce pregnancies among adolescents. Increase the proportion of adolescent females at risk for unintended pregnancy who use effective birth control.	• Provide education to adolescents about pregnancy prevention and safer sexual practices. • Teach adolescents about the personal and fetal risk of pregnancy during this period. • Provide confidential counseling to maintain the adolescent's privacy and trust.

Healthy People Objectives retrieved from http://www.healthypeople.gov

Nursing Management

For adolescents, as for adults, pregnancy can be a physically, emotionally, and socially stressful time. Nurses must support adolescents during the transition from childhood into adulthood, which is complicated by their emergence into parenthood. When caring for the pregnant adolescent:

- Assist the adolescent in identifying family and friends who want to be involved and provide support throughout the pregnancy.
- Help the adolescent identify the options for this pregnancy, such as abortion, self-parenting of the child, temporary foster care for the baby or themselves, or placement of the child for adoption.
- Explore with the adolescent if the pregnancy was planned or unintended (becoming aware of why they decided to have a child is necessary to help with the development of the adolescent and their ability to parent).
- Identify barriers to seeking prenatal care, such as lack of transportation, too many problems at home, financial concerns, the long wait for an appointment, and lack of sensitivity on the part of the health care system.
- Monitor maternal and fetal well-being throughout pregnancy and labor (Fig. 20.5).
- Stress that the patient's physical well-being is important for both themselves and their developing fetus, which depends on the patient for their own health-related needs.
- Emphasize the importance of attending prenatal education classes.
- Encourage the patient to set goals and work toward them.
- Assist them in returning to school and furthering their education.
- As appropriate, initiate a referral for career or job counseling.
- Assist with arrangements for care, including stress management and self-care.
- Provide appropriate teaching based on the adolescent's developmental level and emphasize the importance of continued prenatal and follow-up care.

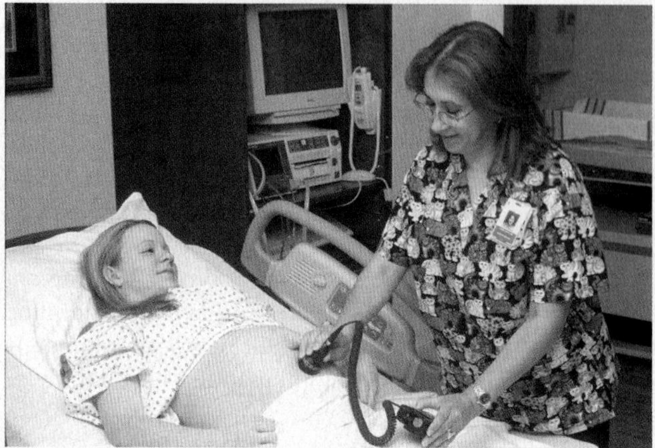

FIGURE 20.5 A pregnant adolescent receiving care during labor.

Nurses can play a major role in preventing adolescent pregnancies, perhaps by volunteering to talk to adolescent groups. Teaching Guidelines 20.4 highlights the key areas for teaching adolescents about pregnancy prevention.

The Pregnant Person of Advanced Maternal Age

Over the last several decades in the United States, there has been a continued trend for people to become pregnant later in life. Since 1990, pregnancy rates for patients under 30 years of age have been decreasing, while pregnancy rates for patients 30 years and older have been increasing (Fretts, 2023). Advanced maternal age is defined as pregnancy in a person 35 years of age or older. U.S. data from 2020 indicate patients of advanced maternal age account for 19% of all pregnancies and 11% of all first-time pregnancies (ACOG, 2022a). Pregnant women of advanced maternal age are at increased risk for gestational diabetes, preeclampsia, labor dystocia, cesarean delivery, preterm delivery, postpartum hemorrhage, neonatal low birth weight, and infant admission to the neonatal intensive care unit. The risks continue to

TEACHING GUIDELINES 20.4 Topics for Teaching Adolescents to Prevent Pregnancy

- High-risk behaviors that lead to pregnancy
- Absolute effectiveness of sexual abstinence
- Involvement in programs such as Teen Pregnancy Prevention (TPP) program, Personal Responsibility Education Program (PREP), or Sexual Risk Avoidance Education Programs
- Planning and goal setting to visualize futures in terms of career, college, travel, and education
- Choice of abstinence even after first becoming sexually active
- Discussions about sexuality with a wise adult, someone they respect who can help put things in perspective
- Protection against STIs and pregnancy if they choose to remain sexually active
- Empowerment to make choices that will shape their lives for years to come, including getting control of their own lives now
- Appropriate use of recreational time, such as sports, drama, volunteer work, music, jobs, religious or spiritual activities, and school clubs

American Academy of Pediatrics. (2023). *Considerations for providing adolescent care*. https://www.aap.org/en/patient-care/adolescent-sexual-health/adolescent-supportive-care/considerations-for-providing-adolescent-care/; and Congressional Research Service. (2022). *Federal teen pregnancy prevention programs*. https://crsreports.congress.gov/product/pdf/IF/IF10877

increase with each 5-year increment of advancing age. Additionally, people 35 years of age and older have a higher prevalence of chronic disorders such as diabetes mellitus, hypertension, and obesity (BMI ≥30), placing them at further risk (ACOG, 2022a).

Impact of Pregnancy on the Person of Advanced Maternal Age

Although maternal complications increase as a person ages, their pregnancy remains a physiologic, not a pathologic, process. In addition to the previously mentioned risks, data have shown that increased maternal age in a first pregnancy demonstrates further risk for premature rupture of membrane, retained placenta/placental fragments, severe perineal tear grade 3/4, placental abruption, chorioamnionitis, puerperal fever, maternal intensive care unit admission, and prolonged hospitalization (greater than 7 days after cesarean or greater than 5 days after vaginal delivery). Risks to the fetus include intrapartum intrauterine fetal death (IUFD), 5-min Apgar score below 7, birth asphyxia, congenital malformations, being LGA, meconium aspiration, jaundice, transient tachypnea of the newborn, brachial plexus injury, mechanical ventilation, seizures, hypoglycemia, sepsis, encephalopathy, and intracranial hemorrhage (Hochler et al., 2023). However, even though increased age implies increased complications, most people today who become pregnant after age 34 have healthy pregnancies and healthy newborns.

Nursing Assessment

Nursing assessment of pregnant people over age 35 is the same as that for any pregnant person. For a person of this age, a preconception visit is important to identify chronic health problems that might affect the pregnancy and also to address lifestyle issues that may take time to modify. Encourage the person of advanced maternal age to plan for the pregnancy by seeing their health care provider before getting pregnant to discuss preexisting medical conditions, medications, and lifestyle choices. Assess for risk factors such as cigarette smoking, poor nutrition, higher or lower body weight, alcohol use, or illicit drug use.

A preconception visit also provides the opportunity to educate the patient about risk factors and provide information on how to modify lifestyle habits to improve the pregnancy outcome. Assist the patient with lifestyle changes so that they can begin pregnancy in an optimal state of health. For example, if the patient is of higher weight, they may wish to discuss weight loss before becoming pregnant. Support them to stop drinking alcohol, start taking folic acid supplements, and stabilize any comorbidities they may have. If the patient smokes, encourage smoking cessation to reduce the effects of nicotine on themselves and the fetus.

Prepare the patient for laboratory and diagnostic testing to establish a baseline for future comparisons. The risk of having a baby with Down syndrome increases with age, especially over age 34. Amniocentesis is routinely offered to all older pregnant people to allow the early detection of numerous chromosomal abnormalities, including Down syndrome. Additionally, a quadruple blood test screen (alpha-fetoprotein [AFP], human chorionic gonadotropin [hCG], unconjugated estriol [UE], and inhibin A [placental hormone]) drawn between 15 and 20 weeks of pregnancy can be helpful in screening for Down syndrome and neural tube defects.

Nursing Management

During routine prenatal visits, the nurse can play a key role in promoting a healthy pregnancy. Consider social, genetic, and environmental factors that are unique to pregnant people of advanced maternal age and prepare to address these factors when providing care.

Assess the patient's knowledge about risk factors and measures to reduce them. Educate them about measures to promote a positive outcome. Encourage them to get early and regular prenatal care. Advise them to eat a variety of nutritious foods, especially fortified cereals, enriched grain products, and fresh fruits and vegetables; drink at least six to eight glasses of water daily; and take the prescribed vitamin containing 400 mcg of folic acid daily. Also stress the need for the patient to avoid alcohol intake during pregnancy, avoid exposure to second-hand smoke, and take no drugs unless they are prescribed. ACOG recommends the following as well:

- Daily intake of low-dose aspirin (81 mg/day) for the prevention of preeclampsia
- A first-trimester detailed fetal anatomic ultrasound
- An additional ultrasound for growth assessment one time in the third trimester (ACOG, 2022a)

Provide continued maternal and fetal surveillance throughout the pregnancy.

The Pregnant Person With Obesity

In the past two decades, the prevalence of pregnant people with obesity (BMI ≥30) has increased dramatically. Of all females aged 20 to 39 years, obesity demonstrates a near 40% prevalence rate. Data from live births in 2020 show that 26.7% of people were overweight (BMI 25 to 29.9) and 29.5% were obese when they became pregnant (Creanga et al., 2022). Higher body weight during pregnancy places the pregnant person and fetus at increased risk for complications. Maternal complications include miscarriage, gestational diabetes, gestational hypertension, preeclampsia, depression, anxiety, preterm birth, labor and delivery complications, cesarean delivery, venous thromboembolism, and postpartum hemorrhage (Creanga et al., 2022). Fetal complications include intrauterine fetal death, congenital anomalies, macrosomia, and being LGA (Creanga et al., 2022; Ramsey & Schenken, 2024).

Obesity is a medical condition in which adipose tissue as an active endocrine organ has dysregulatory effects on inflammatory, metabolic, and vascular pathways (Ramsey & Schenken, 2024). Preconception assessment and counseling are needed for people with higher weight and should include specific information about maternal and fetal risks of obesity in pregnancy, as well as encouragement to undertake a program that includes diet, exercise, and behavior modification to reduce weight prior to conception.

Pregnant people with obesity require individualized nursing care using a nonjudgmental approach. By lowering their body weight prior to pregnancy, insulin resistance, inflammation, and oxidative stress associated with obesity can be reduced, and adverse effects to the pregnant person or fetus can be minimized (Wei et al., 2022). Extra time may be needed to promote healthful practices, which should include dealing with issues of weight, diet, and exercise. Specialist dietary interventions and evidence-based guidelines for working with childbearing people must be seen as a public health priority by all nurses. This care must be done with honesty and respect for all of the patient's needs. There is an opportunity for health promotion aimed at disseminating information about the risks associated with higher body weight in pregnancy to people of childbearing age who may benefit from such information.

The Pregnant Person and Substance Misuse

Substance misuse in pregnancy is a significant public health problem causing increased morbidity in both the pregnant person and the fetus. The epidemic of substance misuse continues to pose a significant challenge around the globe. Drug misuse affects every social stratum, sex, and race, and pregnant people are no exception. **Perinatal drug misuse** includes the use of alcohol and other drugs by pregnant people. The incidence of substance misuse during pregnancy is highly variable because most pregnant people are reluctant to reveal the extent of their use. Illicit drugs used while pregnant include cannabis, heroin, opioids or psychotherapeutic drugs that were not prescribed by a health care provider, and cocaine.

Cannabis is the most widely used drug during pregnancy in the United States. It remains illegal at the federal level, but many states have legalized it for medicinal or recreational purposes (Substance Abuse and Mental Health Services Administration [SAMHSA], 2022). Between 5% and 15% people reported using cannabis while pregnant (Chang, 2024). In addition, more than 8% reported using alcohol and more than 15% reported smoking cigarettes during their pregnancy (Prince & Ayers, 2023). Cocaine and methamphetamine may also be used by pregnant people. Many pregnant people who use substances during pregnancy are polysubstance users, meaning they use more than one substance (CDC, 2022b).

Research shows that the use of tobacco, alcohol, illicit drugs, or misuse of prescription drugs by pregnant people can have serious health consequences for infants (National Institute on Drug Abuse [NIDA], 2020). Substance use can be viewed along a continuum between social recreational drug use and addiction. Substance misuse is prevalent and continues to remain undetected and underdiagnosed in many pregnant people. Substance misuse rarely starts during pregnancy. More often, people enter pregnancy already dependent on or misusing drugs. Many pregnant people with substance use disorder do not seek prenatal care for fear of legal proceedings or being reported to child protective services (SAMHSA, 2022).

The use of drugs, legal or not, increases the risk of medical complications in the pregnant person and poor birth outcomes in the newborn. The placenta acts as an active transport mechanism, not as a barrier, and substances pass from a pregnant person to the fetus through the placenta. Thus, along with the pregnant person, the fetus experiences substance use, misuse, and addiction. Additionally, fetal vulnerability to drugs is much greater because the fetus has not developed the enzymatic system needed to metabolize drugs (Prince & Ayers, 2023).

A nonjudgmental atmosphere and unbiased teaching to all pregnant people regardless of their choices or lifestyle is crucial. A caring, concerned manner is critical to helping these people feel safe and respond honestly to assessment questions.

Pregnancy can be a motivator for some who want to try treatment. The goal of therapy is to help the patient deal with pregnancy by developing a trusting relationship. Providing a full spectrum of medical, social, and emotional care is necessary.

Effects of Commonly Misused Substances

Substance misuse during pregnancy, particularly in the first trimester, has a negative effect on the health of the pregnant person and the growth and development of the fetus. The fetus experiences the same systemic effects as the pregnant person, but often more severely. The fetus cannot metabolize drugs as efficiently and will experience the effects long after the drugs have left the pregnant person's system. Substance misuse during pregnancy is associated with preeclampsia, preterm labor and delivery, premature rupture of membranes, spontaneous abortion, placental abruption, depressed Apgar scores, fetal growth restriction, meconium staining at birth, low birth weight, neurobehavioral abnormalities, and long-term childhood developmental consequences (Jansson, 2023). Refer to Table 20.6 for the effects of specific drugs.

TABLE 20.6 • Effects of Select Drugs on Pregnancy

Substance	Effect on Pregnancy
Alcohol	Spontaneous abortion, inadequate weight gain, IUGR, FASD (the leading cause of intellectual disability)
Caffeine	Vasoconstriction and mild diuresis in pregnant person; fetal stimulation, but teratogenic effects not documented via research
Nicotine	Vasoconstriction, reduced uteroplacental blood flow, decreased birth weight, spontaneous abortion, prematurity, placental abruption, fetal demise
Cocaine	Vasoconstriction, gestational hypertension, placental abruption, spontaneous abortion, central nervous system defects, IUGR
Cannabis	Anemia, inadequate weight gain, "amotivational syndrome," hyperactive startle reflex, newborn tremors, prematurity, IUGR
Opiates and narcotics	Maternal and fetal withdrawal, placental abruption, preterm labor, premature rupture of membranes, perinatal asphyxia, newborn sepsis and death, intellectual impairment, malnutrition
Sedatives	Central nervous system depression, newborn withdrawal, maternal seizures in labor, neonatal abstinence syndrome, delayed lung maturity

FASD, fetal alcohol spectrum disorder; IUGR, intrauterine growth restriction.

Centers for Disease Control and Prevention. (2022b). *Polysubstance use during pregnancy.* https://www.cdc.gov/pregnancy/polysubstance-use-in-pregnancy.html; Chang, G. (2024). Substance use during pregnancy: Overview of selected drugs. *UpToDate.* Retrieved May 7, 2024, from https://www.uptodate.com/contents/substance-use-during-pregnancy-overview-of-selected-drugs; and Prince, M. K., & Ayers, D. (2023). Substance use in pregnancy. *StatPearls.* https://www.ncbi.nlm.nih.gov/books/NBK542330/

CANNABIS

Cannabis is a preparation of the leaves and flowering tops of *Cannabis sativa*, the hemp plant, which contains a number of pharmacologically active agents. Tetrahydrocannabinol (THC) is the most active ingredient of cannabis. It is lipid soluble, so its distribution to the brain and fat occurs easily, and high fetal concentrations can be achieved with heavy exposure (Shukla & Doshi, 2023). Though the federal government continues to consider cannabis a Schedule I substance (having no medicinal uses and at high risk for misuse), several states have legalized it for adult recreational use or medicinal use (pain, nausea and vomiting, HIV/AIDS, cancer). Cannabis use increases the risk of preterm labor and delivery, decreased birth weight, and neonatal intensive care unit admission (Shukla & Doshi, 2023). Other newborn effects of in utero cannabis exposure are not yet known, as evidence thus far has been inconclusive or contradictory. Childhood effects include impulse control, attention, and problem-solving deficits, as well as lower global scholastic achievement (Shukla & Doshi, 2023). ACOG (2021c) advises cessation of cannabis use in pregnancy and lactation, even if it has been prescribed for medicinal purposes.

ALCOHOL

Alcohol misuse is a major public health issue in the United States. Alcohol is a **teratogen**, a substance known to be toxic to human development. The true rate of prenatal alcohol consumption is unknown. It is recognized that fetal alcohol spectrum disorder (FASD) is entirely preventable through alcohol abstinence. Theoretically, no parent would give a glass of wine, beer, or hard liquor to their newborn, but when they drink, the embryo or fetus is exposed to the same blood alcohol concentration as they are. Alcohol is a teratogen with irreversible central nervous effects on the newborn (Weitzman & Rojmahamongkol, 2022). Refer to Chapter 24 for further information about FASD. The preferred action taken to prevent alcohol consumption during pregnancy is abstinence, as no amount of alcohol consumption is considered safe during pregnancy. Damage to the fetus can occur at any stage of pregnancy, even before a person knows they are pregnant (ACOG, 2021b) (see the Healthy People 2030 box).

HEALTHY PEOPLE 2030

Objective	Nursing Significance
Increase abstinence from alcohol among pregnant people.	• Educate people in the preconception and prenatal periods to abstain from alcohol to avoid fetal effects. • Refer to self-help programs as needed.

Healthy People Objectives retrieved from http://www.healthypeople.gov

NICOTINE

Cigarette smoking during pregnancy is the biggest preventable cause of death and illness in pregnant people and infants and is associated with numerous obstetric, fetal, and developmental complications, as well as an increased risk of adverse health consequences in the adult offspring. Nicotine replacement therapy has been developed as a pharmacotherapy for smoking cessation and is considered to be a safer alternative to smoking during pregnancy. The safety of nicotine replacement therapy (transdermal patches and bupropion) use during pregnancy has been evaluated in a limited number of short-term human trials, but there is currently no information on the long-term effects of developmental nicotine exposure in humans. However, nicotine replacement therapies do help some people who smoke quit, so their use is considered safer than continued smoking (NIDA, 2022).

Nicotine is found in cigarettes and is another substance that is harmful to the pregnant person and their fetus. Nicotine, which causes vasoconstriction, transfers across the placenta and reduces blood flow to the fetus, contributing to fetal hypoxia. When compared with alcohol, cannabis, and other illicit drug use, tobacco use is less likely to decline as the pregnancy progresses (NIDA, 2022). Smoking is associated with adverse pregnancy outcomes. However, these adverse outcomes can be avoided if the person stops smoking before becoming pregnant.

Smoking increases the risk of spontaneous abortion; stillbirth; ectopic pregnancy; placental abruption; preterm labor and birth; preterm premature rupture of membranes; maternal hypertension; low birth weight; and increased signs of excitability, stress, and hypertonicity. Additionally, exposure to cigarette smoke significantly increases the risk of sudden unexplained infant death (SUID) (Rodriguez, 2023) (see the Healthy People 2030 box).

HEALTHY PEOPLE 2030

Objective	Nursing Significance
Increase abstinence from cigarette smoking among pregnant people.	• Educate pregnant people about the fetal effects of cigarette smoking. • Refer to the smoking cessation program. • Support the patient in their effort to quit smoking.

Healthy People Objectives retrieved from http://www.healthypeople.gov

CAFFEINE

Caffeine is a stimulant found in tea, coffee, soft drinks, chocolate, and energy drinks. About 90% of all adults worldwide consume caffeine daily (Bordeaux, 2023). During pregnancy, caffeine clearance from the blood slows down significantly. Evidence indicates maternal caffeine use is associated with growth restriction (low birth weight and shorter stature) (Gleason et al., 2022). Birth defects have not been linked to caffeine consumption, but maternal coffee consumption decreases iron absorption and may increase the risk of anemia during pregnancy.

All energy drinks surpass the FDA official soft drink concentration of caffeine limit, typically two to four times the amount seen in one serving of soda or tea. Adverse effects of energy drinks can even occur in healthy people, and pregnant people are considered an at-risk group, so they should avoid excessive caffeine intake, which has been linked to adverse reproductive outcomes, such as low birth weight. Evidence demonstrates consumption of energy drinks is associated with increased demand of the heart resulting in increased cardiac output, increased systolic and diastolic blood pressure, and QTc prolongation; anecdotal reports include atrial fibrillation, myocardial infarction, and sudden death (Somers & Svatikova, 2020). Health care providers recommend pregnant people exclude carbonated and energy drinks, as they contain large amounts of sugar, caffeine, colorants, and preservatives. Nurses should advise pregnant patients to drink water instead of soda or energy drinks.

COCAINE

Though cannabis, alcohol, and tobacco are used much more often by pregnant people, cocaine and stimulant use is on the rise (Chang & Rosenthal, 2024). Cocaine is sniffed into the mucous membranes of the nose, smoked, or injected. Because cocaine crosses the placenta as well as the fetal blood–brain barrier, it is thought that its primary mechanism for placental and fetal damage is vasoconstriction. Uteroplacental insufficiency may occur from reduced blood flow; this reduces placental perfusion. Adverse effects are related to dose and stage of pregnancy. In utero cocaine exposure increases the risk of preterm birth, low birth weight, shorter length for gestational age, and being SGA (Chang, 2024).

METHAMPHETAMINE

Methamphetamine is a powerful, highly addictive central nervous stimulant that alters the release and reuptake of neurotransmitters such as dopamine, serotonin, and norepinephrine. Approximately 2 million adults use it annually (Pew Charitable Trusts, 2024). A highly addictive stimulant, methamphetamine is smoked, injected, sniffed via the nasal mucosa, or taken orally. Maternal effects include an intense rush lasting 5 to 30 minutes, insomnia, acute anxiety, agitation, and psychotic or violent behavior (Yasaei & Saadabad, 2023). Signs of use include poor dental hygiene, injection track marks, unhealthy complexion, skin abscesses from skin picking, and pallor. Few studies have conclusively determined the fetal effects of maternal methamphetamine use, but it is known that it increases the risk for low birth weight, the newborn being SGA, and possibly childhood neurodevelopmental anomalies (ACOG, 2021a).

SEDATIVES

Sedatives relax the central nervous system and are used medically for inducing relaxation and sleep, relieving tension, and treating seizures. Sedatives easily cross the placenta and can cause birth defects and behavioral problems. Infants born to people who misuse sedatives during pregnancy may be physically dependent on the drugs themselves and are more prone to respiratory problems, vigorous sucking, vomiting, loose stools, hypertonicity, and poor weight gain (Jansson, 2023).

OPIOIDS AND NARCOTICS

Over the past decade, the United States has experienced an epidemic of prescription opioid misuse. Opioids and narcotics include opium, heroin, morphine, codeine, fentanyl, hydromorphone (Dilaudid), oxycodone (Percodan), meperidine (Demerol), and methadone. Opiates can be inhaled, injected, snorted, ingested, or used subcutaneously. These drugs are central nervous system depressants that soothe and lull. They may be prescribed medically for pain management, but all have a high potential for misuse. Most are capable of causing intense addiction in both the pregnant person and the newborn. Up to 2.7% of pregnancies are complicated by opioid misuse (Chang, 2024). Another concern is that maternal opiate overdose deaths have increased dramatically in recent years (Han et al., 2023).

Narcotic dependence is particularly problematic in pregnant people as the effects on the fetus can be severe (Seligman et al., 2023). Taking opiates or narcotics during pregnancy places the person at increased risk for preterm labor, fetal growth restriction, placental abruption, perinatal mortality, preterm rupture of membranes, and preeclampsia (Chang, 2024). Pain medications are the most commonly misused prescription drugs, while heroin is the most common illicitly used opioid. Heroin, which easily crosses the placenta, is derived from the seeds of the poppy plant and can be sniffed, smoked, or injected. The most common harmful effect of heroin and other opioids on newborns is withdrawal or **neonatal opioid withdrawal syndrome (NOWS)** (see Chapter 24).

Withdrawal from opiates during pregnancy is extremely dangerous for the fetus, so a prescribed oral methadone or buprenorphine maintenance program combined with psychotherapy is recommended for the pregnant person. This closely supervised treatment program reduces drug cravings, blocks the euphoric effects of narcotic drugs in order to reduce illicit drug use, and reduces withdrawal symptoms in the newborn. Useful therapies include self-help, 12-step groups, individual and group substance misuse counseling, and psychotherapy.

See the Healthy People 2030 box.

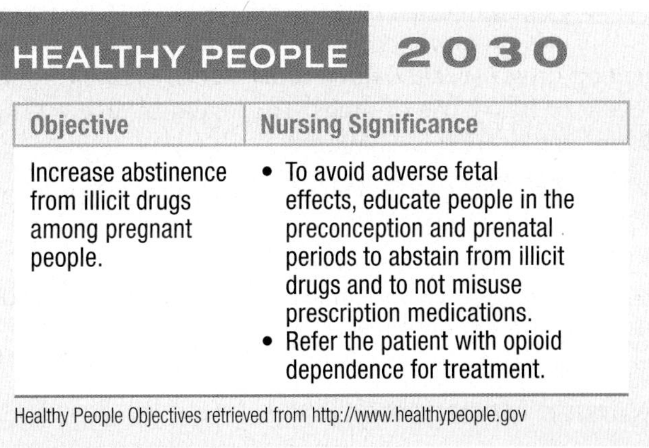

HEALTHY PEOPLE 2030

Objective	Nursing Significance
Increase abstinence from illicit drugs among pregnant people.	• To avoid adverse fetal effects, educate people in the preconception and prenatal periods to abstain from illicit drugs and to not misuse prescription medications. • Refer the patient with opioid dependence for treatment.

Healthy People Objectives retrieved from http://www.healthypeople.gov

Nursing Assessment

Routine screening and education of people of childbearing age remain the most important ways to reduce addiction in pregnancy. Complete a thorough history and physical examination to evaluate a patient for substance use and misuse. Substance misuse screening in pregnancy is done to detect the use of any substance known or suspected to exert a deleterious effect on the patient or their fetus. Routinely ask all people who can become pregnant about substance misuse, inform them of the risks involved, and advise them against continuing. Screening questionnaires are helpful in identifying potential use, may reduce the stigma of asking patients about substance misuse, and may result in a more accurate and consistent evaluation. The questions in Box 20.1 may be helpful in assessing a patient who is at risk for substance

BOX 20.1 Sample Questions for Assessing Substance Use

- Have you ever used recreational drugs? If so, when and what?
- Have you ever taken a prescription drug other than as intended?
- What are your feelings about drug use during pregnancy?
- How often do you smoke cigarettes? How many per day?
- How often do you drink alcohol?
- Have you ever felt guilty about drinking or drug use?

If the assessment reveals substance use, obtain additional information by using the CRAFFT questionnaire, which is a sensitive screening instrument for identifying substance misuse (CRAFFT):

- *C:* Have you ever ridden in a **c**ar driven by someone (including yourself) who was high or drunk?
- *R:* Do you drink or take drugs to **r**elax, improve your self-image, or fit in?
- *A:* Do you ever drink or take drugs while **a**lone?
- *F:* Do you have any close **f**riends who drink or take drugs?
- *F:* Does a close **f**amily member have a problem with alcohol or drugs?
- *T:* Have you ever gotten in **t**rouble from drinking or taking drugs?

National Institute on Drugs Abuse. (2023). *Screening and assessment tools chart.* https://nida.nih.gov/nidamed-medical-health-professionals/screening-tools-resources/chart-screening-tools; and Saxon, A. J. (2023). Screening for unhealthy use of alcohol and other drugs in primary care. *UpToDate.* Retrieved May 7, 2024, from https://www.uptodate.com/contents/screening-for-unhealthy-use-of-alcohol-and-other-drugs-in-primary-care

misuse during pregnancy. Using accepting terminology may encourage the patient to give honest answers without fear of reproach.

A urine toxicology screen may be helpful in determining drug use, although a urine screen identifies only recent or heavy use of drugs. The length of time a drug is present in urine is as follows:

- Cocaine: with 6 to 12 hours of use, up to 3 days after
- Opioids: 1 to 4 days after use
- Amphetamines: 1 to 3 days after use
- Cannabis: 1 week to 1 month after use but may yield false positives (Mukherji et al., 2023)

Nursing Management

If the patient's drug screen is positive, use this as an opportunity to discuss prenatal exposure to substances that may be harmful. The discussion may lead the nurse to refer the patient for a diagnostic assessment or identify an intervention such as counseling that may be helpful. Being nonjudgmental is a key to success; a patient is more apt to trust and reveal patterns of misuse if the nurse does not judge the patient and their choices.

A positive drug screen in a newborn may warrant an investigation by the state protection agency (according to state laws). If the newborn exhibits clinical manifestations of NOWS, institute measures to reduce stress and stimuli to promote the newborn's comfort (see Chapter 24 for a more in-depth discussion).

Be proactive, supportive, and accepting when caring for the patient. Assure people with substance use disorder that sharing information of a confidential nature with health care providers will not render them liable to criminal prosecution. Provide counseling and education, emphasizing the following:

- Effects of substance exposure on the fetus
- Interventions to improve parent–child attachment and improve parenting
- Psychosocial support if treatment is needed to reduce substance misuse
- Referral to outreach programs to improve access to treatment facilities
- Hazardous legal substances to avoid during pregnancy
- Follow-up of children born to parents with substance use disorder
- Dietary counseling to improve the pregnancy outcome for both parent and child
- Drug screening to identify all drugs a patient is using
- More frequent prenatal visits to monitor fetal well-being
- Maternal and fetal benefits of remaining drug free
- Cultural sensitivity
- Promotion of family involvement in a rehabilitation program
- Strengthening of individual and family coping skills
- Coping skills, support systems, and vocational assistance

There is nothing categorically different about addiction during pregnancy compared to addiction in general. Pregnant people with substance dependence issues are people who use drugs, get pregnant, and cannot stop using drugs. Substance misuse is a complex problem that requires sensitivity to each person's unique situation and contributing factors. Be sure to address individual psychological and sociocultural factors to help the patient regain control. Nurses must be aware of these people's unique needs and the related legal and ethical ramifications surrounding pregnancy. Treatment must combine different approaches and provide ongoing support for people learning to live drug free. Developing personal strengths, such as communication skills, assertiveness, and self-confidence, will help the patient to resist drug use. Encourage the use of appropriate coping skills. Enhancing self-esteem also helps provide a foundation to avoid drugs. Through therapeutic communication, nursing interventions, clinical assessment, and building trusting relationships, nurses can have a significant impact in managing patients with substance misuse.

KEY CONCEPTS

- Preconception counseling for the person with diabetes is helpful in promoting blood glucose control to prevent congenital anomalies.
- The classification system for diabetes is based on disease etiology and not pharmacology management;

the classification includes type 1 diabetes, type 2 diabetes, and gestational diabetes.

- The risk classification for heart disease during pregnancy helps determine how much risk the person has for morbidity and mortality.
- Chronic hypertension exists when the person has a blood pressure of 140/90 mm Hg or higher before pregnancy or before the 20th week of gestation or when hypertension persists for more than 12 weeks postpartum.
- Successful management of asthma in pregnancy involves the elimination of environmental triggers, drug therapy, and patient education.
- Ideally, people with hematologic conditions are screened before conception and are made aware of the risks to themselves and to a pregnancy.
- A wide variety of infections, such as CMV, rubella, herpes simplex, hepatitis B, varicella, parvovirus B19, and many STIs can affect a pregnancy, having negative impacts on its outcome.
- Cases of perinatal HIV transmission have decreased in the past several years in the United States, primarily because of the use of ART in pregnant people with HIV.
- ACOG recommends all pregnant people should be offered HIV antibody testing regardless of their risk of infection and that testing should be done during the initial prenatal evaluation.
- The nurse's role in caring for the pregnant adolescent is to assist in identifying the options for this pregnancy, including abortion, self-parenting of the child, temporary foster care for the baby or themselves, or placement for adoption.
- Pregnant people with substance use disorder commonly misuse several substances, making it difficult to ascribe a specific perinatal effect to any one substance. Societal attitudes regarding pregnant people and substance misuse may prohibit them from admitting the problem and seeking treatment.
- Substance misuse during pregnancy is associated with preterm labor, spontaneous abortion, low birth weight, central nervous system and fetal anomalies, and long-term childhood developmental consequences.

Unfolding Patient Stories: Amelia Sung • Part 2

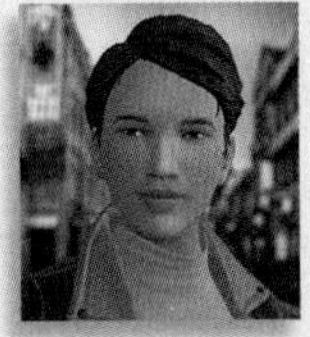

Think back to Amelia Sung, who, as you learned in Chapter 12, is 36 years old and gravida 2 para 1. She is diagnosed with gestational diabetes mellitus at 26 weeks. Explain the areas of education the nurse should provide regarding diabetes management. How does the nurse evaluate Amelia's understanding of the information provided and her ability to manage diabetes and maintain normal glucose levels?

Care for Amelia and other patients in a realistic virtual environment: ***vSim** for Nursing* (thepoint.lww.com/vSim-Maternity). Practice documenting these patients' care in DocuCare (thepoint.lww.com/DocuCareEHR).

- Nursing care for the person with substance misuse focuses on screening and preventing substance misuse to reduce the high incidence of obstetric and medical complications as well as the morbidity and mortality among passively addicted newborns.

REFERENCES AND RECOMMENDED READINGS

American Academy of Allergy Asthma & Immunology. (2023). *Asthma and pregnancy*. https://www.aaaai.org/Tools-for-the-Public/Conditions-Library/Asthma/Asthma-and-Pregnancy

American College of Obstetricians and Gynecologists. (2021a). *Methamphetamine abuse in women of reproductive age: Committee opinion #479 (Reaffirmed 2021)*. https://www.acog.org/clinical/clinical-guidance/committee-opinion/articles/2011/03/methamphetamine-abuse-in-women-of-reproductive-age

American College of Obstetricians and Gynecologists. (2021b). *Alcohol abuse and other substance use disorders: Ethical issues in obstetric and gynecologic practice: Committee opinion #633 (Reaffirmed 2021)*. https://www.acog.org/clinical/clinical-guidance/committee-opinion/articles/2015/06/alcohol-abuse-and-other-substance-use-disorders-ethical-issues-in-obstetric-and-gynecologic-practice

American College of Obstetricians and Gynecologists. (2021c). *Marijuana use during pregnancy and lactation: Committee opinion #637 (Reaffirmed 2021)*. https://www.acog.org/clinical/clinical-guidance/committee-opinion/articles/2017/10/marijuana-use-during-pregnancy-and-lactation

American College of Obstetricians and Gynecologists. (2022a). *Pregnancy at age 35 years or older: Committee on clinical census #11*. https://www.acog.org/clinical/clinical-guidance/obstetric-care-consensus/articles/2022/08/pregnancy-at-age-35-years-or-older

American College of Obstetricians and Gynecologists. (2022b). *Preexposure prophylaxis for the prevention of human immunodeficiency virus: Committee opinion # 595*. https://www.acog.org/clinical/clinical-guidance/practice-advisory/articles/2022/06/preexposure-prophylaxis-for-the-prevention-of-human-immunodeficiency-virus

American College of Obstetricians and Gynecologists. (2023). Viral hepatitis in pregnancy: ACOG practice guideline no. 6. *Obstetrics & Gynecology, 142*(3), 745–759. https://doi.org/10.1097/AOG.0000000000005300

American College of Obstetricians and Gynecologists, Eke, A. C., Gandhi, M., Kaimal, A. J., Moniz, M., & Shields, A. (2022). *Hemoglobinopathies in pregnancy: Practice bulletin no. 78 update*. https://www.acog.org/clinical/clinical-guidance/practice-advisory/articles/2022/08/hemoglobinopathies-in-pregnancy

American Diabetes Association. (2020a). Classification and diagnosis of diabetes: Standards of medical care in diabetes—2020. *Diabetes Care, 43*(Supplement_1), S14–S31. https://doi.org/10.2337/dc20-S002

American Diabetes Association. (2020b). Glycemic targets: Standards of medical care in diabetes—2020. *Diabetes Care, 43*(Supplement_1), S66–S76. https://doi.org/10.2337/dc20-S006

American Heart Association. (2022). *2022 Heart disease & stroke statistical update fact sheet: Females & cardiovascular diseases*. https://www.heart.org/-/media/PHD-Files-2/Science-News/2/2022-Heart-and-Stroke-Stat-Update/2022-Stat-Update-factsheet-Females-and-CVD.pdf

Angum, F., Khan, T., Kaler, J., Siddiqui, L., & Hussain, A. (2020). The prevalence of autoimmune disorders in women: A narrative review. *Cureus, 12*(5), e8094. https://doi.org/10.7759/cureus.8094

Arrieta, A. C. (2023). Congenital rubella. *UpToDate*. Retrieved May 4, 2024, from https://www.uptodate.com/contents/congenital-rubella

Asafo-Agyei, K. O., & Samant, H. (2023). Pregnancy and viral hepatitis. *StatPearls*. https://www.ncbi.nlm.nih.gov/books/NBK556026/

Auerbach, M., & Landy, H. J. (2023). Anemia in pregnancy. *UpToDate*. Retrieved May 3, 2024, from https://www.uptodate.com/contents/anemia-in-pregnancy

Balasubramanyam, A. (2024). Classification of diabetes mellitus and genetic diabetic syndromes. *UpToDate*. Retrieved April 2, 2024, from https://www.uptodate.com/contents/classification-of-diabetes-mellitus-and-genetic-diabetic-syndromes

Benz, E. J., & Angelucci, E. (2024). Management of thalassemia. *UpToDate*. Retrieved May 3, 2024, from https://www.uptodate.com/contents/management-of-thalassemia

Berlan, E. D., Menon, S., & Committee on Adolescence, 2021–2022. (2022). Options counseling for the pregnant adolescent patient. *Pediatrics, 150*(3), e2022058781. https://doi.org/10.1542/peds.2022-058781

Bermas, B. L. (2023). Rheumatoid arthritis and pregnancy. *UpToDate*. Retrieved May 3, 2024, from https://www.uptodate.com/contents/rheumatoid-arthritis-and-pregnancy

Bermas, B. L., & Smith, N. A. (2023). Pregnancy in women with systemic lupus erythematosus. *UpToDate*. Retrieved May 3, 2024, from https://www.uptodate.com/contents/pregnancy-in-women-with-systemic-lupus-erythematosus

Bhargava, J., & Hurley, J. A. (2023). Fibromyalgia. *StatPearls*. https://www.ncbi.nlm.nih.gov/books/NBK540974/

Bordeaux, B. (2023). Benefits and risks of caffeine and caffeinated beverages. *UpToDate*. Retrieved May 7, 2024, from https://www.uptodate.com/contents/benefits-and-risks-of-caffeine-and-caffeinated-beverages

Cedeno-Mendoza, R. (2023). Cytomegalovirus. *Medscape*. https://emedicine.medscape.com/article/215702-overview#a5

Centers for Disease Control and Prevention. (2021). *About teen pregnancy*. https://www.cdc.gov/reproductive-health/teen-pregnancy/

Centers for Disease Control and Prevention. (2022a). *Guidelines for vaccinating pregnant women*. https://www.cdc.gov/vaccines/pregnancy/hcp-toolkit/guidelines.html

Centers for Disease Control and Prevention.(2022b). *Polysubstance use during pregnancy*. https://www.cdc.gov/pregnancy/polysubstance-use-in-pregnancy.html

Centers for Disease Control and Prevention. (2023). Diagnoses of HIV infection in the United States and dependent areas, 2021. *HIV Surveillance Report 2023, 34*. https://www.cdc.gov/hiv/library/reports/hiv-surveillance/vol-34/index.html

Centers for Disease Control and Prevention. (2024a). *Contraindications to breastfeeding or feeding expressed breast milk to infants*. https://www.cdc.gov/breastfeeding-special-circumstances/hcp/contraindications/index.html

Centers for Disease Control and Prevention. (2024b). *HIV diagnoses, deaths, and prevalence*. https://www.cdc.gov/hiv-data/nhss/hiv-diagnoses-deaths-prevalence.html

Centers for Disease Control and Prevention. (2024c). *Tuberculosis (TB): Data and statistics*. https://www.cdc.gov/tb/statistics/default.htm

Chacko, M. R. (2023). Pregnancy in adolescents. *UpToDate*. Retrieved May 7, 2024, from https://www.uptodate.com/contents/pregnancy-in-adolescents

Chang, G. (2024). Substance use during pregnancy: Overview of selected drugs. *UpToDate*. Retrieved May 7, 2024, from https://www.uptodate.com/contents/substance-use-during-pregnancy-overview-of-selected-drugs

Chang, G., & Rosenthal, E. (2024). Substance use during pregnancy: Screening and prenatal care. *UpToDate*. Retrieved May 7, 2024, from https://www.uptodate.com/contents/substance-use-during-pregnancy-screening-and-prenatal-care

Chen, P., Johnson, L., Limketkai, B. N., Jusuf, E., Sun, J., Kim, B., Price, J. C., & Woreta, T. A. (2023). Trends in the prevalence of hepatitis C infection during pregnancy and maternal-infant outcomes in the US, 1998 to 2018. *JAMA Network Open, 6*(7), e2324770. https://doi.org/10.1001/jamanetworkopen.2023.24770

Choudhary, M. C. (2022). Antiretroviral therapy (ART) in pregnant people with HIV infection: Overview of HIV antiretroviral therapy in pregnancy. *Medscape*. https://emedicine.medscape.com/article/2042311-overview

Congressional Research Service. (2022). *Federal teen pregnancy prevention programs*. https://crsreports.congress.gov/product/pdf/IF/IF10877

Creanga, A. A., Catalano, P. M., & Bateman, B. T. (2022). Obesity in pregnancy. *New England Journal of Medicine, 387*(3), 248–259. https://doi.org/10.1056/nejmra1801040

Cunningham, F. G., Leveno, K. J., Dashe, J. S., Hoffman, B. L., Spong, C. Y., & Casey, B. M. (2022a). Maternal physiology. In F. G. Cunningham, K. J. Leveno, J. S. Dashe, B. L. Hoffman, C. Y. Spong, & B., M. Casey, *William's obstetrics* (26th ed.). McGraw Hill.

Cunningham, F. G., Leveno, K. J., Dashe, J. S., Hoffman, B. L., Spong, C. Y., & Casey, B. M. (2022b). Cardiovascular disorders. In F. G. Cunningham, K. J. Leveno, J. S. Dashe, B. L. Hoffman, C. Y. Spong, & B., M. Casey, *William's obstetrics* (26th ed.). McGraw Hill.

Cunningham, F. G., Leveno, K. J., Dashe, J. S., Hoffman, B. L., Spong, C. Y., & Casey, B. M. (2022c). Pulmonary disorders. In F. G. Cunningham, K. J. Leveno, J. S. Dashe, B. L. Hoffman, C. Y. Spong, & B., M. Casey, *William's obstetrics* (26th ed.). McGraw Hill.

Cunningham, F. G., Leveno, K. J., Dashe, J. S., Hoffman, B. L., Spong, C. Y., & Casey, B. M. (2022d). Diabetes mellitus. In F. G. Cunningham, K. J. Leveno, J. S. Dashe, B. L. Hoffman, C. Y. Spong, & B., M. Casey, *William's obstetrics* (26th ed.). McGraw Hill.

Cunningham, F. G., Leveno, K. J., Dashe, J. S., Hoffman, B. L., Spong, C. Y., & Casey, B. M. (2022e). Sexually transmitted infections. In F. G. Cunningham, K. J. Leveno, J. S. Dashe, B. L. Hoffman, C. Y. Spong, & B., M. Casey, *William's obstetrics* (26th ed.). McGraw Hill.

Diabetes Food Hub Team. (2020). *Create-your-plate: Simplify meal planning with the plate method*. https://www.diabetesfoodhub.org/articles/create-your-plate-simplify-meal-planning-with-the-plate-method.html

Edwards, M. S., & Shetty, A. (2023). Rubella. *UpToDate*. Retrieved May 4, 2024, from https://www.uptodate.com/contents/rubella

ElSayed, N. A., Aleppo, G., Aroda, V. R., Bannuru, R. R., Brown, F. M., Bruemmer, D., Collins, B. S., Hilliard, M. E., Isaacs, D., Johnson, E. L., Kahan, S., Khunti, K., Leon, J., Lyons, S. K.,

Perry, M. L., Prahalad, P., Pratley, R. E., Seley, J., Stanton, R. C., & Gabbay, R. A. (2023). 15. Management of diabetes in pregnancy: Standards of care in diabetes—2023. *Diabetes Care, 46*(Supplement_1), S254–S266. https://doi.org/10.2337/dc23-s015

Feld, J. J. (2022). Clinical manifestations, diagnosis, and treatment of acute hepatitis C virus infection in adults. *UpToDate*. Retrieved May 4, 2024, from https://www.uptodate.com/contents/clinical-manifestations-diagnosis-and-treatment-of-acute-hepatitis-c-virus-infection-in-adults

Fretts, R. C. (2023). Management of pregnancy in patients of advanced age. *UpToDate*. Retrieved May 7, 2024, from https://www.uptodate.com/contents/management-of-pregnancy-in-patients-of-advanced-age

Friedman, L. N., & Tanoue, L. T. (2024). Tuberculosis disease (active tuberculosis) in pregnancy. *UpToDate*. Retrieved May 5, 2024, from https://www.uptodate.com/contents/tuberculosis-disease-active-tuberculosis-in-pregnancy

Fu, J., & Retnakaran, R. (2022). The life course perspective of gestational diabetes: An opportunity for the prevention of diabetes and heart disease in women. *The Lancet, 45*, 101294. https://www.thelancet.com/journals/eclinm/article/PIIS2589-5370(22)00024-4/fulltext

Fuller, H., Moore, J. B., Iles, M. M., & Zulyniak, M. A. (2022). Ethnic-specific associations between dietary consumption and gestational diabetes mellitus incidence: A meta-analysis. *PLOS Global Public Health, 2*(5), e0000250. https://doi.org/10.1371/journal.pgph.0000250

Gleason, J. L., Sundaram, R., Mitro, S. D., Hinkle, S. N., Gilman, S. E., Zhang, C., Newman, R. B., Hunt, K. J., Skupski, D. W., Grobman, W. A., Nageotte, M., Robinson, M., Kannan, K., & Grantz, K. L. (2022). Association of maternal caffeine consumption during pregnancy with child growth. *JAMA Network Open, 5*(10), e2239609. https://doi.org/10.1001/jamanetworkopen.2022.39609

Goldman, E., & O'Donovan, D. J. (2023). Vertical transmission of hepatitis C virus. *UpToDate*. Retrieved May 4, 2024, from https://www.uptodate.com/contents/vertical-transmission-of-hepatitis-c-virus

Gregory, E. C. W., & Ely, D. M. (2022). Trends and characteristics in gestational diabetes: United States, 2016-2020. *National Vital Statistics Reports, 71*(3), https://www.cdc.gov/nchs/data/nvsr/nvsr71/nvsr71-03.pdf

Guerina, N. G., & Marquez, L. (2022). Congenital toxoplasmosis: Clinical features and diagnosis. *UpToDate*. Retrieved May 5, 2024, from https://www.uptodate.com/contents/congenital-toxoplasmosis-clinical-features-and-diagnosis

Han, B., Compton, W. M., Einstein, E. B., Elder, E., & Volkow, N. D. (2024). Pregnancy and postpartum drug overdose deaths in the US before and during the COVID-19 pandemic. *JAMA Psychiatry, 81*(3), 270–283. https://doi.org/10.1001/jamapsychiatry.2023.4523

Helm, M. M., Izuora, K., & Basu, A. (2022). Nutrition-education-based interventions in gestational diabetes: A scoping review of clinical trials. *International Journal of Environmental Research and Public Health, 19*(19), 12926. https://doi.org/10.3390/ijerph191912926

HIVinfo.NIH.gov. (2023). *HIV overview*. https://hivinfo.nih.gov/understanding-hiv/fact-sheets/hiv-and-aids-basics

Hochler, H., Lipschuetz, M., Suissa-Cohen, Y., Weiss, A., Sela, H. Y., Yagel, S., Rosenbloom, J. I., Grisaru-Granovsky, S., & Rottenstreich, M. (2023). The impact of advanced maternal age on pregnancy outcomes: A retrospective multicenter study. *Journal of Clinical Medicine, 12*(17), 5696. https://doi.org/10.3390/jcm12175696

Hökelek, M. (2022). Toxoplasmosis. *Medscape*. https://emedicine.medscape.com/article/229969-overview

Hughes, B. L., & Cu-Uvin, S. (2023). Intrapartum and postpartum management of pregnant women with HIV and infant prophylaxis in resource-rich settings. *UpToDate*. Retrieved May 5, 2024, from https://www.uptodate.com/contents/intrapartum-management-of-pregnant-women-with-hiv-and-infant-prophylaxis-in-resource-rich-settings

Hui, S. Y. A., & Lao, T. T. (2022). Tuberculosis in pregnancy. *Best Practice & Research Clinical Obstetrics & Gynecology, 85*(A), 34–44. https://doi.org/10.1016/j.bpobgyn.2022.07.006

Iftikhar, S. F., & Biswas, M. (2023). Cardiac disease in pregnancy. *StatPearls*. https://www.ncbi.nlm.nih.gov/books/NBK537261/

James, A. H., & Oppong, S. A. (2023). Sickle cell disease: Obstetric considerations. *UpToDate*. Retrieved May 3, 2024, from https://www.uptodate.com/contents/sickle-cell-disease-obstetric-considerations

Jansson, L. M. (2023). Neonatal abstinence syndrome (NAS): Clinical features and diagnosis. *UpToDate*. Retrieved July 18, 2024, from https://www.uptodate.com/contents/infants-with-prenatal-substance-use-exposure

Jordan, J. A. (2023). Virology, epidemiology, and pathogenesis of parvovirus B19 infection. *UpToDate*. Retrieved May 5, 2024, from https://www.uptodate.com/contents/virology-epidemiology-and-pathogenesis-of-parvovirus-b19-infection

Koné, M. C., Kambiré, N. A., Kouakou, K., & Ahoua, Y. (2022). Fibromyalgia of women who gave birth and pregnancy outcome parameters. *Open Journal of Epidemiology, 12*, 1–11. https://doi.org/10.4236/ojepi.2022.121001

Krewson, C. (2022). *How changes in diet can manage gestational diabetes*. https://www.contemporaryobgyn.net/view/how-changes-in-diet-can-manage-gestational-diabetes

Lange-Vaidya, N. (2023). Asthma in adolescents and adults: Evaluation and diagnosis. *UpToDate*. Retrieved May 3, 2024, from https://www.uptodate.com/contents/asthma-in-adolescents-and-adults-evaluation-and-diagnosis

Lee, M. J., Sullivan, C., & Graves, J. (2023). Multiple sclerosis: Pregnancy planning. *UpToDate*. Retrieved May 3, 2024, from https://www.uptodate.com/contents/multiple-sclerosis-pregnancy-planning

Maheshwari, M. V., Khalid, N., Patel, P. D., Alghareeb, R., & Hussain, A. (2022). Maternal and neonatal outcomes of adolescent pregnancy: A narrative review. *Cureus, 14*(6), e25921. https://doi.org/10.7759/cureus.25921

Mangla, A., Ehsan, M., Agarwal, N., Maruvada, S, & Doerr, C. (2023). Sickle cell anemia (nursing). *StatPearls*. https://www.ncbi.nlm.nih.gov/books/NBK568706/

Melov, S. J., White, L., Simmons, M., Kirby, A., Stulz, V., Padmanabhan, S., Alahakoon, T. I., Pasupathy, D., & Cheung, N. W. (2022). The BLIiNG study—Breastfeeding length and intensity in gestational diabetes and metabolic effects in a subsequent pregnancy: A cohort study. *Midwifery, 107*, 103262. https://doi.org/10.1016/j.midw.2022.103262

Mohamad, T. N. (2022). Cardiovascular disease and pregnancy. *Medscape*. https://emedicine.medscape.com/article/162004-overview

Morgan, J. A., Zafar, N., & Cooper, D. B. (2023). Group B streptococcus and pregnancy. *StatPearls*. https://www.ncbi.nlm.nih.gov/books/NBK482443/

Mukherji, P., Azhar, Y., & Sharma, S. (2023). Toxicology screening. *StatPearls*. https://www.ncbi.nlm.nih.gov/books/NBK499901/

National Institute on Drugs Abuse. (2020). *Substance use while pregnant and breastfeeding*. https://nida.nih.gov/publications/research-reports/substance-use-in-women/references

National Institute on Drugs Abuse. (2022). *What are the risks of smoking during pregnancy?* https://nida.nih.gov/publications/research-reports/tobacco-nicotine-e-cigarettes/what-are-risks-smoking-during-pregnancy

National Institute on Drugs Abuse. (2023). *Screening and assessment tools chart*. https://nida.nih.gov/nidamed-medical-health-professionals/screening-tools-resources/chart-screening-tools

Olek, M. J., & Howard, J. (2024). Clinical presentation, course, and prognosis of multiple sclerosis in adults. *UpToDate*. Retrieved May 3, 2024, from https://www.uptodate.com/contents/clinical-presentation-course-and-prognosis-of-multiple-sclerosis-in-adults

Olek, M. J., & Mowry, E. (2024). Pathogenesis and epidemiology of multiple sclerosis. *UpToDate*. Retrieved May 3, 2024, from https://www.uptodate.com/contents/pathogenesis-and-epidemiology-of-multiple-sclerosis

Onaade, O., Maples, J. M., Rand, B., Fortner, K. B., Zite, N. B., & Ehrlich, S. F. (2021). Physical activity for blood glucose control in gestational diabetes mellitus: Rationale and recommendations for translational behavioral interventions. *Clinical Diabetes and Endocrinology*, *7*, 7. https://doi.org/10.1186/s40842-021-00120-z

Palmer, S. (2021). Cultural humility in food & nutrition. *Today's Dietitian*, *23*(2), 24. https://www.todaysdietitian.com/newarchives/0221p24.shtml

Petersen, E., & Mandelbrot, L. (2024). Toxoplasmosis and pregnancy. *UpToDate*. Retrieved May 5, 2024, from https://www.uptodate.com/contents/toxoplasmosis-and-pregnancy

Peterson, A. T., & Kleeman, L. C. (2022). HIV in pregnancy. *Medscape*. https://emedicine.medscape.com/article/1385488-overview#a2

Pew Charitable Trusts. (2024). *Methamphetamine use, overdose deaths, and arrests soared from 2015 to 2019*. https://www.pewtrusts.org/en/research-and-analysis/articles/2022/08/16/methamphetamine-use-overdose-deaths-and-arrests-soared-from-2015-to-2019

Plotogea, M., Isam, A. J., Frincu, F., Zgura, A., Bacinschi, X., Sandru, F., Duta, S., Petca, R. C., & Edu, A. (2022). An overview of cytomegalovirus infection in pregnancy. *Diagnostics*, *12*(10), 2429. https://doi.org/10.3390/diagnostics12102429

Pozniak, A. (2024). Pulmonary tuberculosis: Clinical manifestations and complications. *UpToDate*. Retrieved May 5, 2024, from https://www.uptodate.com/contents/pulmonary-tuberculosis-clinical-manifestations-and-complications

Pressman, K., & Ros, S. (2023). Management of hepatitis B and C during pregnancy: Neonatal implications. *NeoReviews*, *24*(1), 24–30. https://doi.org/10.1542/neo.24-1-e24

Prince, M. K., & Ayers, D. (2023). Substance use in pregnancy. *StatPearls*. https://www.ncbi.nlm.nih.gov/books/NBK542330/

Puopolo, K. M., & Baker, C. J. (2023). Group B streptococcal infection in neonates and young infants. *UpToDate*. Retrieved May 5, 2024, from https://www.uptodate.com/contents/group-b-streptococcal-infection-in-neonates-and-young-infants

Ramsey, P. S., & Schenken, R. S. (2024). Obesity in pregnancy: Complications and maternal management. *UpToDate*. Retrieved May 7, 2024, from https://www.uptodate.com/contents/obesity-in-pregnancy-complications-and-maternal-management

Riley, L. E. (2024). Rubella in pregnancy. *UpToDate*. Retrieved May 4, 2024, from https://www.uptodate.com/contents/rubella-in-pregnancy

Riley, L. E., & Fernandes, C. J. (2023). Parvovirus B19 infection during pregnancy. *UpToDate*. Retrieved May 5, 2024, from https://www.uptodate.com/contents/parvovirus-b19-infection-during-pregnancy

Rodriguez, D. (2023). Cigarette and tobacco products in pregnancy: Impact on pregnancy and the neonate. *UpToDate*. Retrieved May 7, 2024, from https://www.uptodate.com/contents/cigarette-and-tobacco-products-in-pregnancy-impact-on-pregnancy-and-the-neonate

Rodriguez, Q., & Mahdy, H. (2023). Gestational diabetes. *StatPearls*. https://www.ncbi.nlm.nih.gov/books/NBK545196/

Sax, P. E. (2024). Acute and early HIV infection: Clinical manifestations and diagnosis. *UpToDate*. Retrieved May 5, 2024, from https://www.uptodate.com/contents/acute-and-early-hiv-infection-clinical-manifestations-and-diagnosis

Saxon, A. J. (2023). Screening for unhealthy use of alcohol and other drugs in primary care. *UpToDate*. Retrieved May 7, 2024, from https://www.uptodate.com/contents/screening-for-unhealthy-use-of-alcohol-and-other-drugs-in-primary-care

Seely, E. W., & Powe, C. E. (2024). Pregestational (preexisting) diabetes: Preconception counseling, evaluation, and management. *UpToDate*. Retrieved May 2, 2024, from https://www.uptodate.com/contents/pregestational-preexisting-diabetes-preconception-counseling-evaluation-and-management

Seligman, N.S., Rosenthal, E., & Berghella, V. (2023). Opioid use disorder: Overview of treatment during pregnancy. *UpToDate*. Retrieved May 7, 2024, from https://www.uptodate.com/contents/opioid-use-disorder-overview-of-treatment-during-pregnancy

Sharma, A. K., Singh, S., Singh, H., Mahajan, D., Kolli, P., Mandadapu, G., Kumar, B., Kumar, D., Kumar, S., & Jena, M. K. (2022). Deep insight of the pathophysiology of gestational diabetes mellitus. *Cells*, *11*(17), 2672. https://doi.org/10.3390/cells11172672

Shebl, E., & Chakraborty, R. K. (2023). Asthma in pregnancy. *StatPearls*. https://www.ncbi.nlm.nih.gov/books/NBK532283/

Shukla, S., & Doshi, H. (2023). Marijuana and maternal, perinatal, and neonatal outcomes. *StatPearls*. https://pubmed.ncbi.nlm.nih.gov/34033378/

Somers, K. R., & Svatikova, A. (2020). Cardiovascular and autonomic responses to energy drinks—Clinical implications. *Journal of Clinical Medicine*, *9*(2), 431. https://doi.org/10.3390/jcm9020431

Speer, M. E. (2023). Varicella-zoster infection in the newborn. *UpToDate*. Retrieved May 5, 2024, from https://www.uptodate.com/contents/varicella-zoster-infection-in-the-newborn

Substance Abuse and Mental Health Services Administration. (2022). *Marijuana and pregnancy*. https://www.samhsa.gov/marijuana/marijuana-pregnancy

Trout, K. K. (2019). Managing the sugar blues: Putting the latest gestational diabetes mellitus guidelines into practice. *Women's Healthcare: A clinical journal for NPs*, *7*(1), 37–43. https://www.npwomenshealthcare.com/wp-content/uploads/2019/04/WHNP_Q1Mar19_SugarBlues-1.pdf

UpToDate, Inc. (2024). *UpToDate® Lexidrug™* (Version 8.2.0) [Mobile app]. Wolters Kluwer. https://apps.apple.com/us/app/lexicomp/id313401238

U.S. Department of Health and Human Services. (2020). *Healthy People 2030: Objectives and data: Browse objectives by topic: Infants.* https://health.gov/healthypeople/objectives-and-data/browse-objectives/infants

Waksmonski, C. A. (2023). Pregnancy in women with congenital heart disease: General principles. *UpToDate.* Retrieved May 2, 2024, from https://www.uptodate.com/contents/pregnancy-in-women-with-congenital-heart-disease-general-principles

Wallace, D. J., & Gladman, D. D. (2023). Clinical manifestations and diagnosis of systemic lupus erythematosus in adults. *UpToDate.* Retrieved May 3, 2024, from https://www.uptodate.com/contents/clinical-manifestations-and-diagnosis-of-systemic-lupus-erythematosus-in-adults

Wei, W., Zhang, X., Zhou, B., Ge, B., Tian, J., & Chen, J. (2022). Effects of female obesity on conception, pregnancy and the health of offspring. *Frontiers in Endocrinology, 13*, 949228. https://doi.org/10.3389/fendo.2022.949228

Weitzman, C., & Rojmahamongkol, P. (2022). Fetal alcohol spectrum disorder: Clinical features and diagnosis. *UpToDate.* Retrieved May 2, 2024, from https://www.uptodate.com/contents/fetal-alcohol-spectrum-disorder-clinical-features-and-diagnosis

Xie, Y., Zhao, H., Zhao, M., Huang, H., Liu, C., Huang, F., & Wu, J. (2022). Effects of resistance exercise on blood glucose level and pregnancy outcome in patients with gestational diabetes mellitus: A randomized controlled trial. *BMJ Open Diabetes Research and Care, 10*(2), e002622. https://doi.org/10.1136/bmjdrc-2021-002622

Yasaei, R., & Saadabadi, A. (2023). Methamphetamine. *StatPearls.* https://www.ncbi.nlm.nih.gov/books/NBK535356/

Zera, C., & Brown, F. M. (2023). Pregestational (preexisting) diabetes mellitus: Antenatal glycemic control. *UpToDate.* Retrieved May 2, 2024, from https://www.uptodate.com/contents/pregestational-preexisting-diabetes-mellitus-antenatal-glycemic-control

DEVELOPING CLINICAL JUDGMENT

PRACTICING FOR NCLEX

1. The nurse is teaching a pregnant person about the pathophysiologic mechanisms associated with gestational diabetes. What should the nurse include in the teaching?
   a. Pregnancy fosters the development of carbohydrate cravings.
   b. There is progressive resistance to the effects of insulin.
   c. Hypoinsulinemia develops early in the first trimester.
   d. Glucose levels decrease to accommodate fetal growth.
2. The nurse is providing prenatal education to a pregnant person with asthma. Which action would be important for the nurse to take?
   a. Explain that the patient should avoid steroids during pregnancy.
   b. Demonstrate how the patient can assess their blood glucose levels.
   c. Teach correct administration of subcutaneous bronchodilators.
   d. Ensure the patient seeks treatment for any acute exacerbation.
3. Which condition would most likely cause a pregnant person with type 1 diabetes the greatest difficulty during pregnancy?
   a. Placenta previa
   b. Hyperemesis gravidarum
   c. Placental abruption
   d. Rh incompatibility
4. The nurse has provided preconceptual counseling about abstaining from alcohol ingestion when pregnant. What is the reason for this?
   a. Pregnant people often produce more alcohol dehydrogenase when drinking.
   b. Pregnant people typically become intoxicated more quickly than before pregnancy.
   c. Alcohol ingestion places the infant at risk for FASD.
   d. Weight gain throughout gestation will be a few pounds lower without alcohol.
5. The nurse is explaining HIV infection and transmission to a pregnant person. Which information would the nurse include?
   a. It primarily occurs when there is a large viral load in the blood.
   b. HIV is most commonly transmitted via sexual contact.
   c. It affects the majority of infants of birthing parents with HIV infection.
   d. Nurses are most frequently affected by needlesticks.
6. People with obesity have a greater risk of developing which condition during pregnancy?
   a. Type 1 diabetes
   b. Hypotension
   c. Low-birth-weight infant
   d. Gestational hypertension
7. The clinic nurse is following two pregnant patients. One is prescribed maintenance methadone, while the other is prescribed buprenorphine maintenance. These medications indicate that both patients have been using which drug?
   a. Alcohol
   b. Nicotine
   c. Opiates
   d. Cannabis

CRITICAL THINKING EXERCISES

1. A patient at 26 weeks' gestation came to the clinic to follow up on their previous 1-hour glucose screening. Their results had come back outside the accepted screening range, and a 3-hour glucose tolerance test (GTT) had been ordered. It resulted in three abnormal values, confirming a diagnosis of gestational diabetes. As the nurse in the prenatal clinic, you are seeing them for the first time.
   a. What additional information will you need to provide care for this patient?
   b. What education will they need to address this new diagnosis?
   c. How will you evaluate the effectiveness of your interventions?
2. A 14-year-old comes to the public health clinic with her parent. The parent tells you that the patient has been "out messing around and has gotten herself pregnant." The patient is crying quietly in the corner and avoids eye contact with you. The parent says their child "must be following in my footsteps" because she became pregnant when she was 15 years old. The patient's parent goes back out into the waiting room and leaves the patient with you.
   a. What is your first approach with the patient to gain her trust?
   b. List the patient's educational needs during this pregnancy.
   c. What prevention strategies are needed to prevent a second pregnancy?
3. A 27-year-old G3P2 is admitted to the labor and birth suite because of preterm rupture of membranes at an estimated 35 weeks' gestation. They have received no prenatal care and report this was an unplanned pregnancy. The patient appears distracted and very thin. They report that their two previous children have been in foster care since

birth because the child welfare authorities "didn't think I was an adequate parent." They deny any recent use of alcohol or drugs, but you smell alcohol on their breath. They had a spontaneous vaginal birth a few hours later, producing a 4-lb baby with Apgar scores of 8 at 1 minute and 9 at 5 minutes.

a. What aspects of this patient's history may lead the nurse to suspect that this infant may be at risk for FASD?

b. What additional screening or laboratory tests might validate your suspicion?

c. What physical and neurodevelopmental deficits might present later in life if the infant has FASD?

STUDY ACTIVITIES

1. In the maternity clinic or hospital setting, interview a pregnant person with a preexisting medical condition (e.g., diabetes, asthma, sickle cell anemia) and find out how this condition affects their life and this pregnancy, especially their lifestyle choices.

2. You have a close friend who you believe is misusing alcohol but denies it. The friend now admits to you that they think they are pregnant because they missed their period. What specific information and advice should you give your friend concerning alcohol use during pregnancy?

3. Should cannabis be legalized nationally in the United States? What impact might your view have on pregnant people and their offspring?

4. Outline a discussion you might have with a pregnant patient who is HIV-positive and doesn't see the need to take antiretroviral agents to prevent perinatal transmission.

5. The nurse is preparing a teaching session about breastfeeding for a group of pregnant people who have various infections listed below. The nurse would include people with which conditions? Select all that apply.

a. Hepatitis B

b. Parvovirus B19

c. Herpesvirus type 2

d. HIV-positive status

e. Cytomegalovirus

f. VZV

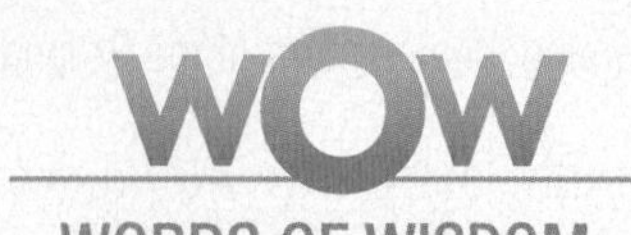

WORDS OF WISDOM

In the face of a crisis or a potentially bad outcome, add a mixture of warmth and serenity to your technical abilities.

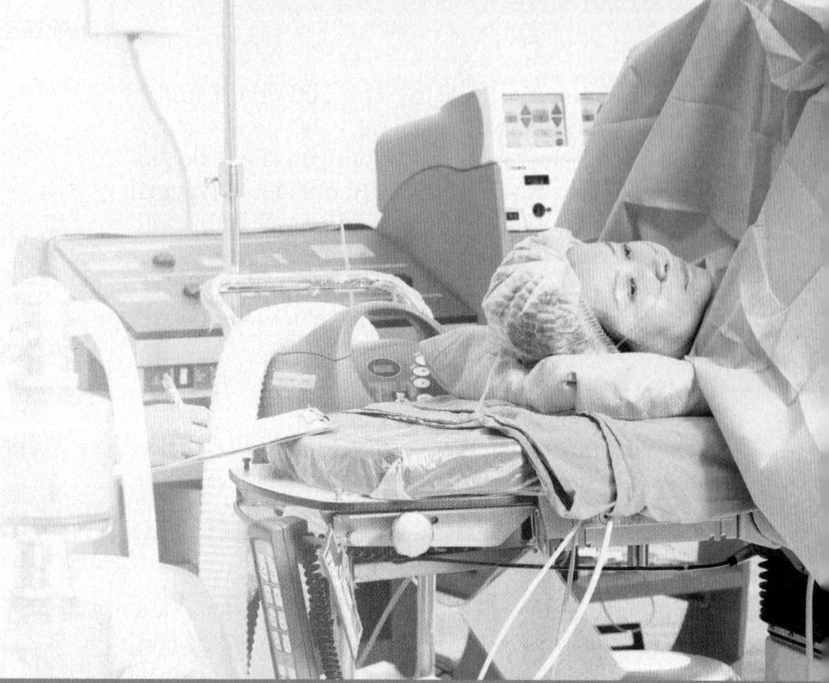

21

Nursing Management of Labor and Birth at Risk

KEY TERMS

arrest disorders
cesarean birth
dystocia (dis-tō'sē-ă)
forceps
hypertonic uterine dysfunction
hypotonic uterine dysfunction
labor induction
multiple gestation
perinatal loss
postterm pregnancy
precipitous labor (prē-sip'i-tŭs lā'bŏr)
preterm labor
protracted disorders
shoulder dystocia
tocolytic (tō'kō-lit'ik)
umbilical cord prolapse
vacuum extractor
vaginal birth after cesarean (VBAC)

LEARNING OBJECTIVES

Upon completion of the chapter, you will be able to:

1. Identify risk factors associated with dystocia.
2. Differentiate the major abnormalities or problems associated with dysfunctional labor patterns, giving examples of each problem.
3. Examine the nursing management for the patient with dysfunctional labor experiencing a problem with expulsive forces; fetal presentation, position, and development; the maternal bony pelvis or birth canal; or psychological maternal stress.
4. Devise a plan of care for the patient experiencing preterm labor.
5. Outline the nursing assessment and management of the patient experiencing a prolonged pregnancy.
6. Discuss the nursing management for the patient undergoing labor induction or augmentation.
7. Evaluate the key areas to be addressed when caring for a patient who undergoes a vaginal birth after cesarean (VBAC).
8. Assess obstetric emergencies that can complicate labor and birth, including appropriate management for each.
9. Discuss forceps-assisted and vacuum-assisted birth.
10. Summarize the plan of care for a patient who is to undergo a cesarean birth.

11. Identify risk factors associated with perinatal loss and the management of the family experiencing a stillbirth.
12. Outline the nontraditional family health care needs and the best practices of nursing care to address them.

Jennifer, a 29-year-old G1P0, is at 41 weeks' gestation. Her health care provider has recommended that she come in for induction. She is anxious about doing this since she has heard "horror stories" about the "hard, painful contractions" that can result. What can the nurse do to calm her fears?

INTRODUCTION

Pregnancy can be an exciting time, but the development of an unexpected problem can suddenly change circumstances dramatically. Consider the patient who has had a problem-free pregnancy and then suddenly develops a condition during labor, turning a routine situation into a possible crisis. Many complications occur with little or no warning and present challenges for the perinatal health care team as well as the family. Sadly, over 800 people die annually in the United States as a result of childbirth complications (Hoyert, 2022). The nurse plays a major role in identifying potential problems quickly and coordinating immediate intervention with the goal of achieving positive outcomes.

This chapter will address several conditions that can occur during labor and birth that may increase the risk of an adverse outcome for the pregnant person and/or fetus. It also describes birth-related procedures that may be necessary for the person who develops a condition that increases their risk or that may be needed to reduce their risk for developing a condition, thus promoting optimal maternal and fetal outcomes. Nursing management of the patient and family focuses on professional support and compassionate care. See the Healthy People 2030 box to learn more about actions to reduce maternal deaths.

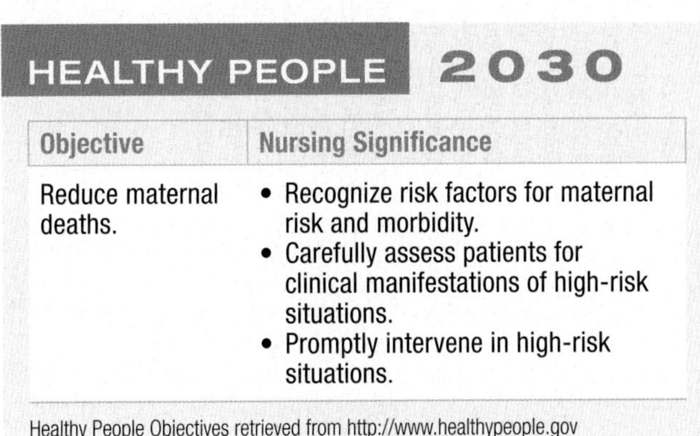

HEALTHY PEOPLE 2030

Objective	Nursing Significance
Reduce maternal deaths.	• Recognize risk factors for maternal risk and morbidity. • Carefully assess patients for clinical manifestations of high-risk situations. • Promptly intervene in high-risk situations.

Healthy People Objectives retrieved from http://www.healthypeople.gov

DYSTOCIA

Dystocia is the abnormal progression of labor typically caused by problems or abnormalities involving the expulsive forces; fetal presentation, position, and development; the maternal bony pelvis, or birth canal; and psychological maternal stress. It can be influenced by a number of maternal and fetal factors. Dystocia is characterized by a slow and abnormal progression of labor. It is a common complication of labor and accounts for about half of the unplanned cesarean births in low-risk nulliparous patients in the United States (Kissler & Hurt, 2022). Refer to Chapter 13 to review the progress of normal labor. Dystocia is a fatiguing factor for both the birthing parent and fetus and is associated with an increase in postpartum hemorrhage, infections, perineal lacerations, and anal sphincter injury. It frequently requires medical or surgical interventions, which increase the risk (Olsen & Karjane, 2022).

Early identification of and prompt interventions for dystocia are essential to minimize risk to the birthing parent and fetus. Admitting a pregnant person too early to the hospital while still in the early latent phase of labor may increase the diagnosis of dystocia and increase the risk of augmentation of labor and epidural analgesia. These two interventions may result in surgical birth. Adequate hydration, rest, emotional and physical support, and if needed, pharmacologic sedation can be encouraged as alternatives to early hospital admission. Patience is a critical factor.

The uterine contractions, the axis of engagement, the pelvic diameters, and the descending fetus should all work in unison to allow for a successful vaginal birth. Table 21.1 summarizes the diagnosis, therapeutic management, and nursing management of the common problems associated with dystocia.

Problems With the Expulsive Forces

When the expulsive forces of the uterus become dysfunctional, the uterus may either never fully relax (hypertonic contractions), placing the fetus in jeopardy, or

TABLE 21.1 • Diagnosis and Management of Common Problems Associated With Dystocia

	Description	Diagnosis	Therapeutic Management	Nursing Management
Problems With the Expulsive Forces				
Hypertonic uterine dysfunction	Occurring in the latent phase of the first stage of labor (cervical dilation of <4 cm); uncoordinated Force of contraction typically in the midsection of the uterus at the junction of the active upper and passive lower segments of the uterus rather than in the fundus Loss of downward pressure to push the presenting part against the cervix Patient commonly becomes discouraged due to lack of progress; also has increased pain secondary to uterine anoxia	Characteristic hypertonicity of the contractions and the lack of labor progress	Therapeutic rest with the use of sedatives to promote relaxation and stop the abnormal activity of the uterus Identification and intervention of any contributing factors Ruling out placental abruption (also associated with high resting tone and persistent pain) Onset of a normal labor pattern occurs in many people after a 4- to 6-hour rest period.	Institute bed rest and sedation to promote relaxation and reduce pain. Assist with measures to rule out fetopelvic disproportion and fetal malpresentation. Evaluate fetal tolerance to labor pattern, such as monitoring of FHR patterns. Assess for signs of maternal infection. Promote adequate hydration through IV therapy. Provide pain management via epidural or IV analgesics. Assist with amniotomy to augment labor. Explain to the patient and family about dysfunctional pattern. Plan for operative birth if normal labor pattern is not achieved.
Hypotonic uterine dysfunction	Often termed *secondary uterine inertia* because the labor begins normally and then the frequency and intensity of contractions decrease Possible contributing factors: overdistended uterus with multifetal pregnancy or large single fetus, too much pain medicine given too early in labor, fetal malposition, and regional anesthesia	Evaluation of the patient's labor to confirm they are having hypotonic active labor rather than a long latent phase Evaluation of maternal pelvis and fetal presentation and position to ensure that they are not contributing to the prolonged labor without noticeable progress	Identification of possible cause of inefficient uterine action (a malpositioned fetus, a too-small maternal pelvis, overdistention of the uterus with fluid, or a macrosomic fetus) Rupture of the amniotic sac (amniotomy) if all causes are ruled out Possible augmentation with oxytocin (Pitocin) to stimulate effective uterine contractions Cesarean birth if amniotomy and augmentation ineffective	Administer oxytocin as ordered once fetopelvic disproportion is ruled out. Assist with amniotomy if membranes are intact. Provide continuous electronic fetal monitoring. Monitor vital signs, contractions, and cervix continually. Assess for signs of maternal and fetal infection. Explain to the patient and family about dysfunctional pattern. Plan for surgical birth if normal labor pattern is not achieved or fetal distress occurs.
Precipitous labor	Abrupt onset of higher intensity contractions occurring in a shorter period of time instead of the more gradual increase in frequency, duration, and intensity that typifies most spontaneous labors	Identification based on the rapidity of progress through the stages of labor	Vaginal delivery if maternal pelvis is adequate	Closely monitor a patient with a previous history. Anticipate the use of scheduled induction to control labor rate. Administer pharmacologic agents, such as tocolytics, to slow labor. Stay in constant attendance to monitor progress.

Problems With the Fetal Presentation, Position, or Development				
Persistent occiput posterior position	Engagement of fetal head in the left or right occipito-transverse position with the occiput rotating posteriorly rather than into the more favorable occiput anterior position (fetus born facing upward instead of the normal downward position) Labor usually much longer and more uncomfortable (causing increased back pain during labor) if the fetus remains in this position Possible extensive caput succedaneum and molding from the sustained occiput posterior position	Leopold maneuvers and vaginal examination to determine position of the fetal head in conjunction with the patient's complaints of severe back pain (back of fetal head pressing on patient's sacrum and coccyx)	Labor to proceed, preparing the patient for a long labor (spontaneous resolution possible) Comfort measures and maternal positioning to help promote fetal head rotation	Assess for complaints of intense back pain in the first stage of labor. Anticipate possible use of forceps to rotate to anterior position at birth or manual rotation to anterior position at the end of the second stage. Assess for the prolonged second stage of labor with the arrest of descent (common with this malposition). Encourage maternal position changes to promote fetal head rotation: hands and knees and rocking pelvis back and forth; side-lying position; side lunges during contractions; sitting, kneeling, or standing while leaning forward; squatting position to give birth and enlarge pelvic outlet. Prepare for possible cesarean birth if rotation is not achieved. Administer agents as ordered for pain relief (effective pain relief crucial to help the patient tolerate the back discomfort). Apply low back counterpressure during contractions to ease the discomfort. Use other helpful measures to attempt to rotate the fetal head, including lateral abdominal stroking in the direction that the fetal head should rotate; assisting the patient into a hands-and-knees position (all fours); and squatting, pelvic rocking, stair climbing, assuming a side-lying position toward the side that the fetus should rotate, and side lunges. Provide measures to reduce anxiety. Continuously reinforce the patient's progress. Teach the patient about measures to facilitate fetal head rotation.
Face and brow presentation	Face presentation with complete extension of the fetal head Brow presentation: fetal head between full extension and full flexion so that the largest fetal skull diameter presents to the pelvis	Diagnosis only once labor is well established via vaginal examination; palpation of facial features as the presenting part rather than the fetal head	Vaginal birth possible with face presentation with an adequate maternal pelvis and fetal head rotation; cesarean birth if head rotates backward Cesarean birth for brow presentation unless head flexes	Assist with evaluating for fetopelvic disproportion. Anticipate cesarean birth if vertex position is not achieved. Explain fetal malposition to the patient and family. Provide close observation for any signs of fetal hypoxia as evidenced by late decelerations on the fetal monitor.

(*continued*)

TABLE 21.1 • Diagnosis and Management of Common Problems Associated With Dystocia (*continued*)

	Description	Diagnosis	Therapeutic Management	Nursing Management
Breech presentation	Fetal buttocks or breech, presenting first rather than the head 1. Frank breech: buttock as the presenting part, with hips flexed and legs and knees extended upward 2. Complete breech (or full breech): buttock as presenting part, with hips flexed and knees flexed in a “cannonball” position 3. Footling or incomplete breech: One or two feet as the presenting part, with one or both hips extended	Vaginal examination to determine breech presentation. Ideally, ultrasound to confirm a clinically suspected presentation and to identify any fetal anomalies	The optimal method of birth is controversial: cesarean birth by some providers unless the fetus is small, and the patient has a large pelvis; vaginal birth by others with each occurrence treated individually and labor monitored closely Regardless of the birth method selected, the risk for trauma is high. Breech vaginal births are not recommended by ACOG and come with a higher risk to the pregnant person and infant than a planned surgical birth. Vaginal delivery: fetus allowed to spontaneously deliver up to the umbilicus; then maneuvers to assist in the delivery of the remainder of the body, arms, and head; fetal membranes left intact as long as possible to act as a dilating wedge and to prevent cord prolapse; anesthesiologist and pediatrician present Cesarean birth: use of external cephalic version to reduce the chance of breech presentation at birth; attempted after the 35th week of gestation but before the start of labor (some fetuses spontaneously turn to a cephalic presentation on their own toward term, and some will return to the breech presentation if external cephalic version is attempted too early); variable success rates, with risk for fractured bones, ruptured viscera, placental abruption, fetomaternal hemorrhage, and umbilical cord entanglement Tocolytics to relax the uterus as well as other methods to facilitate external cephalic version at term Individual evaluation of each patient for all factors before any intervention is initiated	Assess for associated conditions such as placenta previa, hydramnios, fetal anomalies, and multifetal pregnancy. Arrange for an ultrasound to confirm fetal presentation. Assist with external cephalic version possible after 36 weeks and administer tocolytics to assist with external cephalic version. Anticipate trial labor for 4–6 hours to evaluate progress if the version is unsuccessful. Plan for cesarean birth if no progress is seen or fetal distress occurs. After external cephalic version, administer RhoGAM to the Rh-negative patient to prevent a sensitization reaction if trauma has occurred and the potential for mixing of blood exists.

Shoulder dystocia	Delivery of fetal head with neck not appearing; retraction of chin against the perineum; shoulders remaining wedged behind the birthing person's pubic bone, causing a difficult birth with potential for injury to both birthing person and baby If shoulders still above the brim at this stage, no advancement Newborn's chest trapped within the vaginal vault; chest unable to expand with respiration (although nose and mouth are outside) Risk of umbilical cord compression between the fetal body and the maternal pelvis	Emergency, often unexpected complication Diagnosis made when the newborn's head delivers without delivery of the neck and remaining body structures Primary risk factors, including suspected infant macrosomia (weight >4,500 g), maternal diabetes mellitus, excessive maternal weight gain, abnormal maternal pelvic anatomy, maternal obesity, postdated pregnancy, short stature, a history of previous shoulder dystocia, and use of epidural analgesia	If anticipated, preparatory tasks instituted: alerting of key personnel; education of patient and family regarding steps to be taken in the event of a difficult birth; emptying of patient's bladder to allow additional room for possible maneuvers needed for the birth McRoberts maneuver Suprapubic pressure (not fundal) (see Fig. 21.1) Combination of maneuvers effective in more than 50% of cases of shoulder dystocia Newborn resuscitation team readily available	Intervene immediately due to cord compression. Perform McRoberts maneuver and application of suprapubic pressure. Assist with positioning the patient in a squatting position, hands-and-knees position, or lateral recumbent position for birth to free shoulder. Anticipate cesarean birth if no success in dislodging shoulders. Clear room of unnecessary clutter to make room for additional personnel and equipment. After the birth, assess newborn for crepitus, deformity, Erb palsy, or bruising, which might suggest neurologic damage or a fracture.
Multiple pregnancy	More than one fetus, leading to uterine overdistention and possibly resulting in hypotonic contractions and abnormal presentations of the fetuses Fetal hypoxia during labor is a significant threat due to the placenta providing oxygen and nutrients to more than one fetus	Nearly all multiples are now diagnosed early by ultrasound. Most people go into labor before 37 weeks.	Admission to the facility with a specialized care unit if a patient goes into labor Spontaneous progression of labor if the patient has no complicating factors and the first fetus is in a longitudinal lie Separate monitoring of each FHR during labor and birth After the birth of the first fetus, clamping of cord and lie of the second twin assessed; possible external cephalic version necessary to assist in providing a longitudinal lie Second and subsequent fetuses at greater risk for birth-related complications, such as umbilical cord prolapse, malpresentation, and placental abruption Cesarean birth if risk factors are high.	Assess for hypotonic labor pattern due to overdistention. Evaluate for fetal presentation, maternal pelvic size, and gestational age to determine the mode of delivery. Ensure the presence of neonatal team for the birth of multiples. Anticipate the need for cesarean birth, which is common in multifetal pregnancy.

(*continued*)

TABLE 21.1 • Diagnosis and Management of Common Problems Associated With Dystocia (*continued*)

	Description	Diagnosis	Therapeutic Management	Nursing Management
Excessive fetal size and abnormalities	Macrosomia leading to fetopelvic disproportion (fetus unable to fit through the maternal pelvis to be born vaginally) Reduced contraction strength due to overdistention by a large fetus leading to a prolonged labor and the potential for birth injury and trauma Fetal abnormalities possibly interfering with fetal descent, leading to prolonged labor and difficult birth	A diagnosis of fetal macrosomia can be confirmed by measuring the birth weight after birth. Suspicion of macrosomia based on the findings of an ultrasound examination before the onset of labor (if suspected due to conditions such as maternal diabetes or obesity, estimation of fetal weight via ultrasound) Leopold maneuvers to estimate fetal weight and position on admission to labor and birth unit	Scheduled cesarean birth if diagnosis is made before the onset of labor to reduce the risk of injury to both the newborn and the patient If identified by Leopold maneuvers, possible trial of labor to evaluate progress; however, providers usually opt to proceed with a cesarean birth in a primigravida with a macrosomic fetus	Assess for the inability of the fetus to descend. Anticipate the need for vacuum- and forceps-assisted births (common). Plan for cesarean birth if maternal parameters are inadequate to give birth to a large fetus.
Problems With the Maternal Pelvis or Birth Canal				
	Contraction of one or more of the three planes of the pelvis Poorer prognosis for vaginal birth in people with android and platypelloid types of pelvis Contracted pelvis involving a reduction in one or more of the pelvic diameters interfering with progress of labor: inlet, midpelvis, and outlet contracture Obstruction in the birth canal, such as placenta previa that partially or completely obstructs the internal os of the cervix, fibroids in the lower uterine segment, a full bladder or rectum, an edematous cervix caused by premature bearing-down efforts, and human papillomavirus (HPV) warts	Shortest A-P diameter $<$10 cm or greatest transverse diameter $<$12 cm (approximation of A-P diameter via measurement of the diagonal conjugate, which in the contracted pelvis is $<$11.5 cm) X-ray pelvimetry to determine the smallest A-P diameter through which the fetal head must pass Interischial tuberous diameter of $<$8 cm possibly compromising outlet contracture (outlet and midpelvic contractures frequently occur together)	Focus on allowing natural forces of labor contractions to push the largest diameter (biparietal) of the fetal head beyond the obstruction or narrow passage. Possible forceps and vacuum extraction to assist navigation through this passageway	Assess for poor contractions, slow dilation, and prolonged labor. Evaluate bowel and bladder status to reduce soft tissue obstruction and allow increased pelvic space. Anticipate trial of labor; if no labor progression after an adequate trial, plan for cesarean birth.

Problems With Psychological Maternal Stress				
	Release of stress-related hormones (catecholamines, cortisol, epinephrine, beta-endorphin), which act on smooth muscle (uterus) and reduce uterine contractility Excessive release of catecholamines and other stress-related hormones not therapeutic Release also results in decreased uteroplacental perfusion and increased risk for poor newborn adjustment.	Ruling out of other possible causes of dystocia	Treatment dependent on patient's responses such as anxiety, fear, anger, frustration, or denial (highly variable due to patient's understanding of the condition itself, past experiences, previous coping mechanisms, and the amount of family and nursing support received) Appropriate medical or surgical interventions depending on the underlying condition	Provide comfortable environment, such as with dim lighting or music. Encourage partner to participate. Provide pain management to reduce anxiety and stress. Ensure continuous presence of staff to allay anxiety. Provide frequent updates concerning fetal status and progress. Provide ongoing encouragement to minimize the patient's stress, help to cope with labor, and promote a positive, timely outcome. Assist in relaxation and comfort measures to help their body work more effectively with the forces of labor. Engage the patient in conversation about their emotional well-being; offer anticipatory guidance and reassurance to increase self-esteem and ability to cope, decrease frustration, and encourage cooperation.

ACOG, American College of Obstetricians and Gynecologists; FHR, fetal heart rate; IV, intravenous.

Cunningham, F. G., Leveno, K. J., Dashe, J. S., Hoffman, B. L., Spong, C. Y., & Casey, B. M. (2022). Abnormal labor. In F. G. Cunningham, K. J. Leveno, J. S. Dashe, B. L. Hoffman, C. Y. Spong, & B. M. Casey, *William's obstetrics* (26th ed.). McGraw Hill; Dike, N. O., & Ibine, R. (2023). Hypotonic labor. *StatPearls.* https://www.ncbi.nlm.nih.gov/books/NBK564403/; Fischer, R., & Modena, A. B. (2022). Breech presentation. *Medscape.* https://emedicine.medscape.com/article/262159-overview; and Olsen, N. S., & Karjane, N. W. (2022). Abnormal labor. *Medscape.* https://emedicine.medscape.com/article/273053-overview

relax too much (hypotonic contractions), causing ineffective contractions. Additionally, the uterus may contract so frequently and with such intensity that a very rapid birth will take place (precipitous labor).

Hypertonic uterine dysfunction occurs when the uterus never fully relaxes between contractions. Subsequently, contractions are ineffectual, erratic, and poorly coordinated because they involve only a portion of the uterus and more than one uterine pacemaker is sending signals for contraction. Birthing people in this situation experience a prolonged latent phase, stay at 2 to 3 cm, and do not dilate as they should. Placental perfusion becomes compromised, thereby reducing oxygen to the fetus. Hypertonic contractions exhaust the birthing parent, who is experiencing frequent, intense, and painful contractions with little progression. This dysfunctional pattern occurs in early labor and affects nulliparous people more often than multiparous people (Simpson & O'Brien-Abel, 2021).

Hypotonic uterine dysfunction occurs during active labor (dilation more than 5 to 6 cm) when contractions become poor quality and lack sufficient intensity to dilate and efface the cervix. Factors associated with this abnormal labor pattern include overstretching of the uterus, a large fetus, multiple fetuses, hydramnios, multiple parity, bowel or bladder distention preventing descent, and excessive use of analgesia. Clinical manifestations of hypotonic uterine dysfunction include weak contractions that become milder, briefer, and more infrequent, and a uterine fundus that is not firm to palpation at the peak of each contraction (Dike & Ibine, 2023). The major risk with this complication is hemorrhage after giving birth because the uterus cannot contract effectively to compress blood vessels.

"Labor" refers to uterine contractions resulting in progressive dilation and effacement of the cervix accompanied by descent and expulsion of the fetus. "Abnormal labor," "dystocia," and "failure to progress" are imprecise terms used to describe a difficult labor pattern that deviates from that observed in the majority of people who have spontaneous vaginal deliveries. A better classification to characterize labor abnormalities is protracted disorders (i.e., slower-than-normal progress) or arrest disorders (i.e., complete cessation of progress).

Protracted disorders are a series of events including protracted active phase dilation (slower-than-normal rate of cervical dilation) and protracted descent (delayed descent of the fetal head in the active phase). A laboring person with a slower-than-normal rate of cervical dilation is said to have a protracted labor pattern disorder. Slow progress may be the result of cephalopelvic disproportion. Most people, however, benefit greatly from adequate hydration and some nutrition, emotional reassurance, and position changes; these people may go on and give birth vaginally.

Arrest disorders include secondary arrest of dilation (no progress in cervical dilation in over 2 hours), arrest of descent (fetal head does not descend for more than 1 hour in primiparas and more than 30 minutes in multiparas), and failure of descent (no descent). About 20% of labors involve either protracted or arrest disorders (Ehsanipoor & Satin, 2023).

Precipitous labor is labor that is completed in less than 3 hours from the start of contractions to birth. Not only can labor be too slow, but it can be abnormally rapid. The prevailing opinion has been that too rapid a labor can result in maternal injury and place the fetus at risk for traumatic or asphyxia insults. Precipitous labor occurs in up to 3% of labors in the United States (Chung et al., 2022). People experiencing precipitous labor typically have soft perineal tissues that stretch readily, permitting the fetus to pass through the pelvis quickly, or abnormally strong uterine contractions. Maternal risk factors include multiparity, chronic hypertension, and a low-birth-weight fetus. Maternal complications are rare if the maternal pelvis is adequate, and the soft tissues yield to a fast fetal descent. However, if the fetus delivers too fast, it does not allow the cervix to dilate and efface, which leads to cervical lacerations, postpartum hemorrhage, placental abruption, and the potential for uterine rupture. Erb or Duchenne palsy may occur in the neonate as a result of precipitous labor (Cunningham et al., 2022).

Precipitous labor is an anxiety-producing situation and frequently very painful with little rest between contractions. Continuous monitoring, frequent updates on labor progress, pain management, and reassurance about the patient's condition can assist their anxiety. Management includes the readiness of the health care team for this rapid birth.

Problems With Presentation, Position, and Development of the Fetus

Any presentation other than occiput anterior (head down and anterior facing) or a slight variation of the fetal position or size increases the probability of dystocia. These variations can affect the contractions or fetal descent through the maternal pelvis. Common problems involving the fetus include occiput posterior position, breech presentation, multifetal pregnancy, excessive size (macrosomia) as it relates to cephalopelvic disproportion, and structural anomalies.

Persistent occiput posterior is the most common malposition, occurring in up to 5% of laboring people (Argani & Satin, 2023). The reasons for this malposition are often unclear. This position presents slightly larger diameters to the maternal pelvis, thus slowing fetal descent. A fetal head that is poorly flexed may be responsible. In addition, poor uterine contractions may not push the fetal head down into the pelvic floor to the extent that the fetal occiput sinks into it rather than being pushed to rotate in an anterior direction. Risk factors for this malposition include nulliparity, obesity, previous occiput posterior birth, advanced maternal age, and small pelvic outlet (Argani & Satin, 2023).

Face and brow presentations are rare and are associated with fetal abnormalities (anencephaly, severe hydrocephalus), multiple nuchal cord, cephalopelvic disproportion, pelvic contractures or platypelloid pelvis, multiparity, placenta previa, polyhydramnios, previous cesarean birth, preterm birth, low birth weight, and macrosomia (Galerneau, 2023).

By 35 to 36 weeks' gestation, the majority of fetuses will spontaneously settle into the vertex presentation (head down toward the birth canal). In about 3% of patients, however, the fetus will remain in a breech presentation with the buttocks or feet presenting (Hofmeyr, 2023). There is less risk to the fetus and birthing person when the head is down at the time of birth. Breech presentation is frequently associated with multifetal or multiple pregnancies, grand multiparity (more than five births), pregnancy over age 35, placenta previa, hydramnios, preterm births, uterine malformations or fibroids, a scarred uterus, a female infant, laxity of maternal abdominal wall, and fetal anomalies such as hydrocephaly (Fischer & Modena, 2022). Infants in a breech presentation have an increased incidence of subtle fetal abnormalities and mild deformation, developmental dysplasia of the hip, and torticollis as compared with infants in the vertex position (Hofmeyr, 2023).

External cephalic version refers to a procedure in which the fetus is rotated from the breech to the cephalic presentation by manipulation through the pregnant person's abdominal wall at or near term. External cephalic version is successful in approximately 60% of patients, with a 40% reduction in cesarean delivery (Hofmeyr, 2023).

Shoulder dystocia is defined as the obstruction of fetal descent and birth by the axis of the fetal shoulders after the fetal head has been delivered. Shoulder dystocia is a fundamentally mechanical problem. It is virtually impossible to predict or prevent this problem. The incidence of shoulder dystocia is increasing due to increasing birth weight, with reports of it occurring in about one in every 200 (3%) vaginal births. It is an obstetric emergency that requires a coordinated team response, as there is no reliable way to predict it and thus decreases the rate at which adverse outcomes occur (Hill et al., 2020). It can be one of the most anxiety-provoking emergencies encountered during labor. Failure of the shoulders to deliver spontaneously places both the birthing person and the fetus at risk for injury. Fundal pressure and strong lateral traction or forced head rotation should all be avoided in the management of shoulder dystocia, as they are counterproductive and increase the risk of brachial plexus injury (Allen & Allen, 2023). Postpartum hemorrhage secondary to uterine atony, vaginal lacerations, anal tears, and uterine rupture are major complications to the birthing person. Transient Erb or Duchenne brachial plexus palsies and clavicular or humeral fractures are the most common fetal injuries encountered with shoulder dystocia. The occurrence of neonatal brachial plexus palsy in the United States is about 0.9 to 2.6 per 1,000 live births, with significant arm weakness occurring in 0.4 to 5 infants per 1,000 live births (Basit et al., 2023). Prompt recognition and appropriate management, such as with the McRoberts maneuver, can reduce the severity of injuries to the birthing person and newborn (Fig. 21.1).

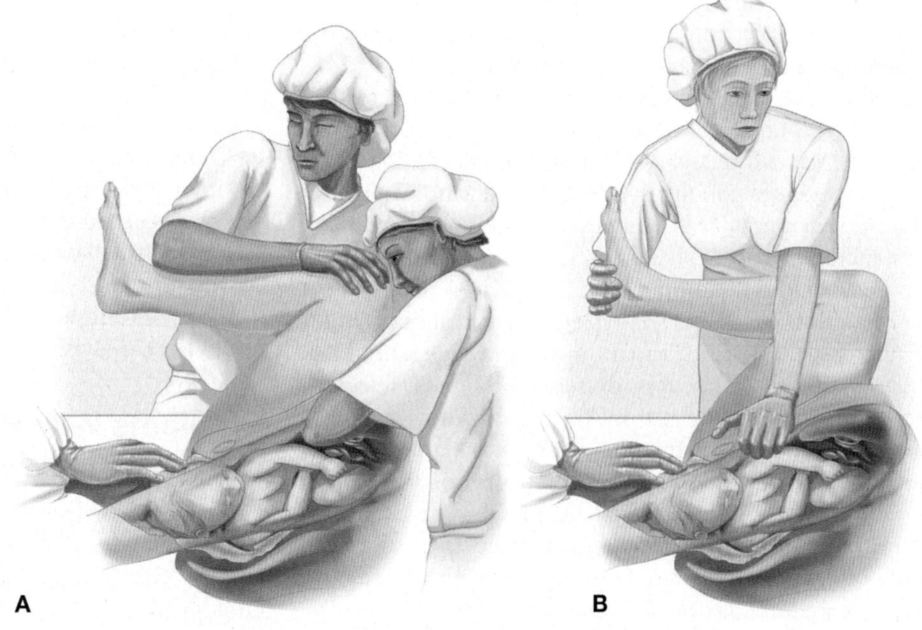

FIGURE 21.1 Maneuvers to relieve shoulder dystocia. **A.** McRoberts maneuver. The pregnant person's thighs are flexed and abducted as much as possible to straighten the pelvic curve. **B.** Suprapubic pressure. Light pressure is applied just above the pubic bone, pushing the fetal anterior shoulder downward to displace it from above the symphysis pubis. The newborn's head is depressed toward the pregnant person's anus while light suprapubic pressure is applied.

TAKE NOTE!

Prompt recognition and appropriate management of shoulder dystocia can reduce the severity of injuries to the birthing person and infant. Immediately assess the infant for signs of trauma, such as a fractured clavicle, Erb palsy, or neonatal asphyxia. Assess the birthing person for excessive vaginal bleeding and blood in the urine from bladder trauma.

Multifetal pregnancy or **multiple gestation** refers to twins, triplets, or more infants within a single pregnancy. These fetuses can result from fertilization of a single ovum or multiple ova. The incidence is increasing, primarily as a result of infertility treatment (both ovarian stimulation and in vitro fertilization) and an increased number of people giving birth at older ages. Monozygotic twins occur in 30% of twin births, while dizygotic twins occur in 70% (Chasen, 2023). The prevalence of triplet and higher order multiple births is 78.9 per 100,000 births in the United States (Hayes, 2023). Compared with singletons (one fetus), the risk of perinatal morbidity and mortality is markedly increased in multiple gestations. The most common maternal complication is postpartum hemorrhage resulting from uterine atony caused by overstretching of the uterus. Based on recent evidence from a randomized controlled study, there was no difference in newborn outcomes between a planned surgical birth and a planned vaginal birth for twins between 32 and 39 weeks' gestation. As long as the presenting twin is vertex, a vaginal birth should be considered (Chen et al., 2022). See Box 21.1 for additional information about multiple gestations.

Excessive fetal size and abnormalities can also contribute to labor and birth dysfunctions. Macrosomia ("big body"), in which a newborn weighs 4,000 to 4,500 g (8.13 to 9.15 lb) or more at birth, complicates approximately 7% of all pregnancies (Abramowicz & Ahn, 2024). It is the result of a change in body composition in the neonate with an increase in both percentage of fat and fat mass. Macrosomia is associated with later-in-life obesity, diabetes, metabolic syndrome, and cardiovascular disease (Abramowicz & Ahn, 2024). Fetal abnormalities may include hydrocephalus, ascites, or a large mass on the neck or head. Complications associated with dystocia related to excessive fetal size and anomalies include an increased risk for postpartum hemorrhage, shoulder dystocia, low Apgar scores, dysfunctional labor, fetopelvic disproportion, soft-tissue laceration during vaginal birth, fetal injuries or fractures, and perinatal asphyxia. Accurate prenatal identification of a macrosomic fetus is difficult; the American College of Obstetricians and Gynecologists (ACOG) recommends elective cesarean birth be considered after consultation with the family and not before 39 weeks' gestation unless medically indicated (Akanmode & Mahdy, 2023).

BOX **21.1 Multiple Gestation**

Monozygotic (Identical) Twins

These twins develop from one single ovum that divides into equal halves during the early cleavage phase. Monozygotic twins are genetically identical, always the same sex, and look very similar in appearance. The number of amnions and chorions depends on the timing of division (cleavage). One fertilized ovum splitting into two separate individuals is termed *natural clones*.

Dizygotic (Fraternal) Twins

Twin pregnancies that are multiple-ova conceptions result from two ova fertilized by two sperms. They are referred to as fraternal twins. Genetically, dizygotic twins are as alike (or unlike) as any other pair or siblings. There are separate amnions and chorions although the chorions and placentas may be fused. Fraternal twins account for two thirds of all twins, and there is a tendency to repeat within families. The incidence of fraternal twins is increasing secondary to advancing maternal age when pregnancy occurs and an increase in the use of fertility drugs and procedures being done.

Triplets or Higher Order

Multiple births other than twins can be of the identical type, the fraternal type, or combination of the two. Triplets can occur from the division of one zygote into two, with one dividing again, producing identical triplets, or they can come from two zygotes, one dividing into a set of identical twins, and the second zygote developing as a single fraternal sibling, or from three separate zygotes. In recent years, fertility drugs used to induce ovulation have resulted in a greater frequency of quadruplets, quintuplets, sextuplets, and even octuplets.

Problems With the Maternal Pelvis and Birth Canal

Problems with the maternal pelvis and birth canal are related to a contraction of one or more of the three planes of the maternal pelvis: inlet, midpelvis, and outlet. The female pelvis can be classified into four types based on the shape of the pelvic inlet, which is bounded anteriorly by the posterior border of the symphysis pubis, posteriorly by the sacral promontory, and laterally by the linea terminalis. The four basic types are gynecoid, anthropoid, android, and platypelloid (see Chapter 12 for additional information). Contraction of the midpelvis is more common than inlet contraction and typically causes an arrest of fetal descent. Obstructions in the maternal birth canal, such as swelling of the soft maternal tissue and cervix, termed *soft-tissue dystocia*, can also hamper fetal descent, and impede labor progression outside the maternal bony pelvis.

Problems With the Maternal Psychological Stress

Many people experience an array of emotions during labor, which may include fear, anxiety, helplessness, isolation, and weariness. These emotions can lead to psychological stress, which can indirectly cause dystocia. Hormones released in response to anxiety can cause dystocia. Intense anxiety stimulates the sympathetic nervous system, which releases catecholamines that can lead to myometrial dysfunction. Norepinephrine and epinephrine then lead to uncoordinated or increased uterine activity. Anxiety can also increase fear and tension, and reduce pain tolerance, decreasing uterine contractility and increasing surgical birth rates (Sanni et al., 2022).

Nursing Assessment

Begin the assessment by reviewing the patient's history to look for risk factors for dystocia, which may include maternal short stature, obesity, hydramnios, uterine abnormalities, fetal malpresentation, cephalopelvic disproportion, overstimulation with oxytocin, maternal exhaustion, ineffective pushing, excessive size fetus, poor maternal positioning in labor, and maternal anxiety and fear. Counsel the person early in the admission process about the risk factors that may lead to an abnormal labor pattern (Olsen & Karjane, 2022). Assess the birthing person's frame of mind to identify fear, anxiety, stress, lack of support, and pain, which can interfere with uterine contractions and impede labor progress. Helping the patient relax will promote normal labor progress.

Assess the patient's vital signs. Note any elevation in temperature (suggesting a potential infection) or changes in heart rate or blood pressure (potential hypovolemia). Evaluate the uterine contractions for frequency and intensity. Ask about any changes in the contraction pattern, such as a decrease or increase in frequency or intensity, and report them. Assess the fetal heart rate (FHR) and pattern, reporting any abnormal patterns immediately.

Assess fetal position via Leopold maneuvers (see Chapter 14 for more information) to identify any deviations in presentation or position and report any deviations. Assist with or perform a vaginal examination to determine cervical dilation, effacement, and engagement of the fetal presenting part. Evaluate for evidence of membrane rupture. Report any malodorous fluid.

Nursing Management

Nursing management of the patient with dystocia, regardless of the etiology, requires patience. The nurse should provide physical and emotional support to the patient and family. The final outcome of any labor depends on the size and shape of the maternal pelvis; the quality of the uterine contractions; and the size, presentation, and position of the fetus. Thus, dystocia is diagnosed after labor has progressed for a time, not at the beginning of labor.

Promoting the Progress of Labor

The nurse plays a major role in determining the progress of labor. Continue to assess the patient, frequently monitoring cervical dilation and effacement, uterine contractions, and fetal descent, and document that all assessed parameters are progressing. Evaluate progress in active labor by using the simple rule of 1 cm per hour for cervical dilation. When the patient's membranes rupture, if they have not already ruptured, observe for visible cord prolapse.

> ***TAKE NOTE!***
>
> If dysfunctional labor occurs, contractions will slow or fail to advance in frequency, duration, or intensity; the cervix will fail to respond to uterine contractions by dilating and effacing; and the fetus will fail to descend.

Throughout labor, assess the birthing person's fluid balance status. Check skin turgor and mucous membranes. Monitor intake and output. Also monitor the patient's bladder for distention at least every 2 hours and encourage them to empty their bladder often. In addition, monitor bowel status. A full bladder or rectum can impede descent.

Continue to monitor fetal well-being. If the fetus is in the breech position, be especially observant for visible cord prolapse and note any variable decelerations in heart rate. If either occurs, report it immediately.

Be prepared to administer a labor stimulant such as oxytocin (Pitocin) if ordered to treat hypotonic labor contractions. Anticipate the need to assist with manipulations if shoulder dystocia is diagnosed. Prepare the patient and family for the possibility of a cesarean birth if labor does not progress.

Providing Physical and Emotional Comfort

Employ physical comfort measures to promote relaxation and reduce stress. Offer blankets for warmth and a backrub if the patient wishes to reduce muscle tension. Provide an environment conducive to rest so the patient can conserve their energy. Lower the lights and reduce external noise by closing the hallway door. Offer a warm shower to promote relaxation (if not contraindicated). Use pillows to support the patient in a comfortable position, changing their position every 30 minutes to reduce tension and to enhance uterine activity and efficiency. Offer fluids and/or food as appropriate to moisten the mouth and replenish energy (Fig. 21.2).

Assist with providing counterpressure along with backrubs if the fetus is in the occiput posterior position. Encourage the patient to assume different positions to promote fetal rotation. Upright positions are helpful in facilitating fetal rotation and descent. Also encourage the patient to visualize the descent and birth of the fetus.

Assess the patient's level of pain and degree of distress. Administer analgesics as ordered or according to the facility's protocol. Evaluate the patient's level of

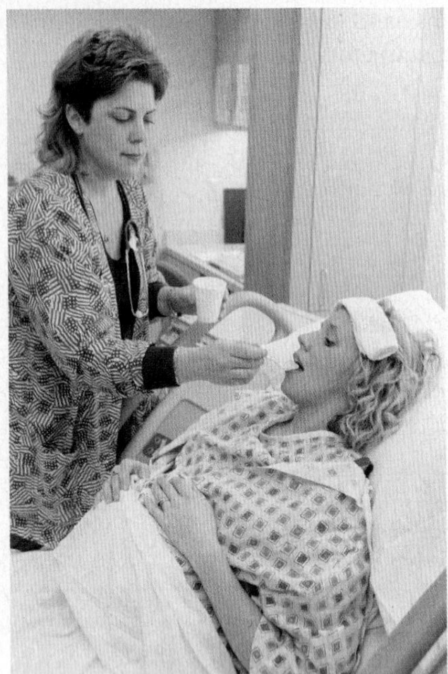

FIGURE 21.2 The nurse applies a cool, moist washcloth to the patient's forehead and offers ice chips to combat thirst and provide comfort while experiencing dystocia.

fatigue throughout labor, such as verbal expressions of feeling exhausted, inability to cope in early labor, or inability to rest or calm down between contractions. Praise the patient and any birthing partner who may be present for their efforts. Provide empathetic listening to increase the patient's coping ability and remain with the patient to demonstrate caring.

Promoting Empowerment

Educate the patient and family about dysfunctional labor and its causes and therapies. Explain therapeutic interventions that may be needed to assist with the labor process. Encourage the patient and family to participate in decision making about interventions.

Assist the patient and family in expressing their fears and anxieties. Provide encouragement to help them to maintain control. Support the patient and family in their coping efforts. Keep the patient and family informed of progress and advocate for them.

PRETERM LABOR

Preterm labor is defined as the occurrence of regular uterine contractions accompanied by cervical effacement and dilation before the end of the 37th week of gestation. If not halted, it leads to preterm birth. Preterm births remain one of the biggest contributors to perinatal morbidity and mortality in the world. Worldwide, preterm births occur in 10% of all births (Mandy, 2022). In the United States, 10% of all live births occur before the completion of 27 weeks, and 3% occur before completion of 34 weeks (Mandy, 2022). Racial disparities also occur: About 9.5% of non-Hispanic White infants are born preterm, 9.7% of Hispanic infants are born preterm, and 14.5% of non-Hispanic Black infants are born preterm (Mandy, 2022; Osterman et al., 2024). Extremely preterm infants have a mortality rate of 25% to 50%, and mortality rates decrease with increasing birth weight and gestational age (Mandy, 2022). Those who survive face an increased risk of developmental delay and disability (Mandy, 2023). Preterm births also increase the risk of neurodevelopmental disorders and other serious morbidities, as well as behavioral and social problems. Neurodevelopmental impairments include cognitive, sensory, motor, behavioral, and psychological impairments such as cerebral palsy, hearing loss, visual impairment, and significant cognitive impairment. The severity of these issues and the incidence in which they occur are inversely related to gestational age, meaning the very preterm infant is more likely to encounter these problems than the moderate or late preterm infant (Mandy, 2023). Infants born prematurely are also at risk for serious sequelae such as respiratory distress syndrome, infections, congenital heart defects, thermoregulation problems that can lead to acidosis and weight loss, intraventricular hemorrhage, jaundice, hypoglycemia, feeding difficulties resulting from diminished stomach capacity and an underdeveloped sucking reflex, and neurologic disorders related to hypoxia and trauma at birth. A single course of corticosteroids prior to birth before 34 weeks' gestation improves neurodevelopmental outcomes (Duncan et al., 2022). While the precise cause of preterm labor is not known, prevention is the goal (see Evidence-Based Practice 21.1).

Therapeutic Management

Many factors must be considered before selecting an intervention to manage preterm labor. Factors to be considered include the probability of progressive labor, gestational age, and the risks of treatment.

- There are no clear first-line **tocolytics** (drugs that promote uterine relaxation by interfering with uterine contractions) to manage preterm labor, and the results of research on their efficacy are mixed. Clinical circumstances and the health care provider's preference should dictate treatment.
- Deferring birth to the 39th week is not recommended if there is a medical or obstetric indication for an earlier delivery.
- Patients at high risk should be offered progesterone supplementation starting at 16 weeks' gestation.
- Activity restriction is not recommended to reduce the risk of preterm birth.
- Antibiotics do not appear to prolong gestation and should be reserved for group B streptococcal prophylaxis when birth is imminent.

EVIDENCE-BASED PRACTICE 21.1

Interventions to Prevent Spontaneous Preterm Birth in People With Singleton Pregnancy Who Are at High Risk: Systematic Review and Network Meta-Analysis

BACKGROUND

Preterm birth is defined as any birth before 37 weeks' gestation. Complications of preterm birth are the leading cause of neonatal mortality and responsible for approximately a third of the 2.5 million deaths annually in children and young adolescents worldwide. Many of the survivors experience long-term disability, which may include cerebral palsy, visual or hearing impairment, delayed social development, numerous behavioral problems, and increased chronic diseases in adulthood. Currently, the best predictors of spontaneous preterm birth are short cervical length and a previous history of spontaneous preterm birth. The purpose of this study was to compare the efficacy of bed rest, cervical cerclage, cervical pessary, fish oils or omega fatty acids, nutritional supplementation of zinc, progesterone, prophylactic antibiotics, prophylactic tocolytics, combination of interventions, placebo, or no treatment (control) to prevent spontaneous preterm birth.

STUDY

A total of 395 studies were screened, with 61 trials (17,273 pregnant people) selected to contribute data for this analysis. Spontaneous preterm birth is a heterogeneous disease, and it is unwise to assume that a single treatment could reduce the risk of preterm birth for every person presenting with risk factors.

Findings

Compared to the other interventions applied, vaginal progesterone is currently the best preterm birth prevention treatment for people with a singleton pregnancy who are without symptoms, but at high risk of giving preterm birth.

Nursing Implications

The findings can serve as a guide for discussions with patients who have risk factors for preterm labor. The intervention found in this study to be beneficial in preterm labor prevention can be discussed with pregnant patients prenatally to make them aware of possible interventions available to assist them. Nurses can integrate information from this study into their teaching about the risks associated with preterm labor and births. They can also use this information to help answer questions about interventions currently used and their effectiveness as well as provide anticipatory guidance about the procedure. Doing so fosters empowerment of the patient and family, promoting optimal informed decision making.

Adapted from Care, A., Nevitt, S. J., Medley, N., Donegan, S., Good, L., Hampson, L., Smith, C. T., & Alfirevic, Z. (2022). Interventions to prevent spontaneous preterm birth in women with singleton pregnancy who are at high risk: Systematic review and network meta-analysis. *British Medical Journal, 376*, e064547. https://doi.org/10.1136/bmj-2021-064547

- Tocolytics may prolong pregnancy for 2 to 7 days; during this time, steroids can be given to improve fetal lung maturity and the patient can be transported to a tertiary care center.
- A single course of corticosteroids is recommended for all pregnant people between 24 and 34 weeks' gestation who are at risk of preterm birth within 7 days (Lockwood, 2024).

With these recommendations, health care providers continue to prescribe pharmacologic treatment for preterm labor at home and in the hospital setting. This treatment often includes oral or intravenous tocolytics and varying degrees of activity restriction (Fig. 21.3). Antibiotics may also be prescribed to treat confirmed infections.

Tocolytic Therapy

The decision to stop preterm labor is based on the extent of cervical dilation, cervical length, membrane status, fetal gestational age, and presence or absence of infection. Tocolytic therapy is most likely ordered if preterm labor occurs before completion of the 34th week of gestation in an attempt to delay birth and thereby reduce the severity of respiratory distress syndrome and other complications associated with prematurity. Tocolytic therapy does not typically prevent preterm birth, but it may delay it for 2 to 7 days and works by creating a quiescent environment within the uterus. It is contraindicated for placental abruption, acute fetal distress or death, oligohydramnios, eclampsia or severe preeclampsia, active vaginal bleeding, dilation of more than 6 cm, chorioamnionitis, and maternal hemodynamic instability (Mayer & Apodaca-Ramos, 2023).

Medications commonly used for tocolysis include magnesium sulfate (which reduces the muscle's ability to contract), indomethacin (Indocin, a prostaglandin synthetase inhibitor), and nifedipine (Procardia, a calcium channel blocker). These drugs are used "off label," which means that they are effective for this purpose but have not been officially tested and developed for this purpose by the U.S. Food and Drug Administration (FDA) (UpToDate, Inc., 2024). All of these medications have serious side effects, and the patient needs close supervision when they are being administered (Drug Guide 21.1).

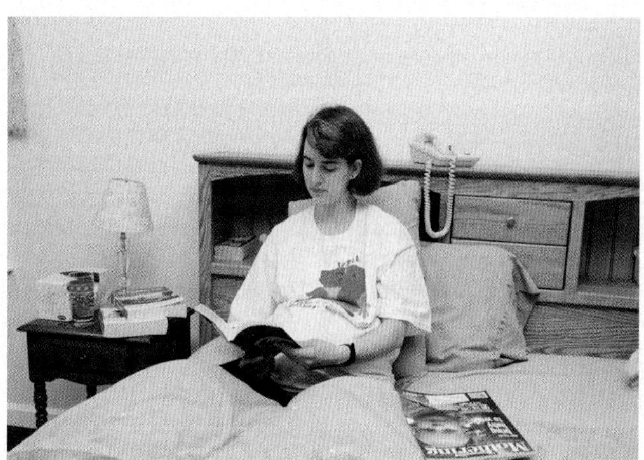

FIGURE 21.3 The pregnant person with preterm labor resting in bed at home.

DRUG GUIDE 21.1

MEDICATIONS USED WITH PRETERM LABOR

Drug	Action/Indication	Nursing Implications
Magnesium sulfate	Relaxes uterine muscles to stop irritability and contractions (off-label use) Has been used in seizure prophylaxis and treatment of seizures in preeclamptic and eclamptic patients for almost 100 years Is neuroprotective for the fetus	Administer IV with a loading dose of 4–6 g over 15–30 minutes initially and then maintain infusion at 1–4 g/h. Assess vital signs and deep tendon reflexes (DTRs) hourly; report any hypotension, depressed, or absent DTRs. Monitor level of consciousness; report any headache, blurred vision, dizziness, or altered level of consciousness. Perform continuous electronic fetal monitoring; report any decreased FHR variability, hypotonia, or respiratory depression. Monitor intake and output hourly; report any decrease in output (<30 mL/h). Assess respiratory rate; report respiratory rate <12 breaths/min; auscultate lung sounds for evidence of pulmonary edema. Monitor for common maternal side effects, including flushing, nausea and vomiting, dry mouth, lethargy, blurred vision, and headache. Assess for nausea, vomiting, transient hypotension, and lethargy. Assess for signs and symptoms of magnesium toxicity, such as decreased level of consciousness, depressed respirations and DTRs, slurred speech, weakness, and respiratory and/or cardiac arrest. Have calcium gluconate readily available at the bedside to reverse magnesium toxicity.
Indomethacin (Indocin)	Inhibits prostaglandins, which stimulate contractions; inhibits uterine activity to arrest preterm labor	Continuously assess vital signs, uterine activity, and FHR. Administer oral form with food to reduce gastrointestinal irritation. Do not give to people with peptic ulcer disease. Schedule ultrasound to assess amniotic fluid volume and function of ductus arteriosus before initiating therapy; monitor for signs of maternal hemorrhage. Be alert for maternal adverse effects such as nausea and vomiting, heartburn, rash, prolonged bleeding time, oligohydramnios, and hypertension. Monitor for neonatal adverse effects, including constriction of ductus arteriosus, premature ductus closure, necrotizing enterocolitis, oligohydramnios, and pulmonary hypertension. Contraindicated in >32 weeks' gestations, fetal growth restriction, history of asthma, urticaria, or allergic-type reactions to aspirin or nonsteroidal anti-inflammatory drugs. Use for no more than 48 hours.
Nifedipine (Procardia)	Blocks calcium movement into muscle cells and inhibits uterine activity to arrest preterm labor	Use caution if giving this drug with magnesium sulfate because of the increased risk of hypotension. Monitor blood pressure hourly if given with magnesium sulfate; report a pulse rate >110 bpm. Monitor for fetal effects such as decreased uteroplacental blood flow manifested by fetal bradycardia, which can lead to fetal hypoxia. Monitor for adverse effects, such as flushing of the skin, headache, transient tachycardia, palpitations, postural hypertension, peripheral edema, and transient fetal tachycardia. Contraindicated in people with cardiovascular disease or hemodynamic instability
Betamethasone (Celestone)	Promotes fetal lung maturity by stimulating surfactant production; prevents or reduces the risk of respiratory distress syndrome and intraventricular hemorrhage in the preterm neonate less than 34 weeks' gestation	Administer two doses intramuscularly 24 hours apart. Monitor for maternal infection or pulmonary edema. Educate parents about the potential benefits of drug to preterm infant. Assess maternal lung sounds and monitor for signs of infection.

FHR, fetal heart rate; IV, intravenous.

UpToDate, Inc. (2024). *UpToDate® Lexidrug™* (Version 8.2.0) [Mobile app]. Wolters Kluwer. https://apps.apple.com/us/app/lexicomp/id313401238

Nursing Assessment

The preterm birth rate cannot be reduced until there are ways to predict the risk for preterm birth. Because the etiology is often multifactorial, an individualized approach is needed.

Health History and Physical Examination

The signs of preterm labor are subtle and may be overlooked by the patient as well as the health care provider. Obtain a thorough health history and be alert for risk factors associated with preterm labor and birth (Box 21.2).

Frequently, patients are unaware that uterine contractions, effacement, and dilation are occurring, thus making early intervention ineffective in arresting preterm labor and preventing the birth of a premature newborn.

BOX 21.2 Risk Factors Associated With Preterm Labor and Birth

- Black race (doubles the risk)
- Maternal age extremes (<16 years and >40 years old)
- Low socioeconomic status
- Alcohol or other drug use, especially cocaine
- Poor maternal nutrition
- Maternal periodontal disease
- Cigarette smoking
- Low level of education
- History of prior preterm birth (triples the risk)
- Uterine abnormalities, such as fibroids
- Low pregnancy weight for height
- Preexisting diabetes or hypertension
- Multiple pregnancy
- Premature rupture of membranes
- Late or no prenatal care
- Short cervical length
- Sexually transmitted infections: gonorrhea, *chlamydia*, trichomoniasis
- Bacterial vaginosis (50% increased risk)
- Chorioamnionitis
- Hydramnios
- Gestational hypertension
- Cervical insufficiency
- Short interpregnancy interval (<1 year between births)
- Placental problems, such as placenta previa and abruption placenta
- Maternal anemia
- Urinary tract infection
- Domestic violence
- Stress, acute and chronic

American College of Obstetricians and Gynecologists. (2021). Prediction and prevention of spontaneous preterm birth: ACOG practice bulletin, number 234. *Obstetrics & Gynecology, 138*, e65–e90. https://doi.org/10.1097/AOG.0000000000004479; Arnold, M. J. (2022). Predicting and preventing preterm birth: Recommendations from ACOG. *American Family Physician, 106*(3), 337–339. https://www.aafp.org/pubs/afp/issues/2022/0900/practice-guidelines-preventing-preterm-birth.html; and Lockwood, C. J. (2024). Preterm labor: Clinical findings, diagnostic evaluation, and initial treatment. *UpToDate*. Retrieved May 8, 2024, from https://www.uptodate.com/contents/preterm-labor-clinical-findings-diagnostic-evaluation-and-initial-treatment

Ask the patient about any complaints, being alert for subtle symptoms of preterm labor, which may include:

- Change or increase in vaginal discharge with mucus, water, or blood in it
- Pelvic pressure (pushing-down sensation)
- Low, dull backache
- Menstrual-like cramps
- Urinary tract infection symptoms
- Feeling of pelvic pressure or fullness
- Vaginal spotting or light bleeding
- Ruptured membranes
- Gastrointestinal upset like nausea, vomiting, and diarrhea
- General sense of discomfort or unease
- Heaviness or aching in the thighs
- Uterine contractions with or without pain
- More than six contractions per hour
- Intestinal cramping with or without diarrhea (Lockwood, 2024)

Assess the pattern of the contractions; the contractions must be persistent, such that four contractions occur every 20 minutes or eight contractions occur in 1 hour. Evaluate cervical dilation and effacement; cervical effacement is 80% or greater and cervical dilation is greater than 1 cm (Baker & Hurst, 2024). Upon examination, engagement of the fetal presenting part will be noted.

Laboratory and Diagnostic Testing

Cervical length is evaluated by transvaginal ultrasound. The length of the cervix in mid-pregnancy relates to the chance of an early birth; in general, the shorter the cervix, the greater the risk of preterm birth. A cervical length measurement to identify a short cervix is obtained between 16 and 24 weeks' gestation (Berghella, 2024b). Cervical length varies during pregnancy and can be measured fairly reliably after 16 weeks' gestation using an ultrasound probe inserted in the vagina. A cervical length of 30 mm or more has a high negative predictive value for preterm birth, while a short cervical length of less than 30 mm indicates an increased risk for preterm birth in all pregnant people (Lockwood, 2024).

TAKE NOTE!

Cervical length measurement is contraindicated in the presence of placenta previa, cervical cerclage, and preterm prelabor rupture of membranes.

Fetal fibronectin (fFN), a glycoprotein produced by the chorion, is found at the junction of the chorion and decidua. It acts as biologic glue attaching the fetal sac to the uterine lining and cannot usually be detected between 24 and 34 weeks of pregnancy unless there has been a disruption between the chorion and decidua. It is present in cervicovaginal fluid prior to delivery, regardless of gestational age. A sterile applicator is used to collect a cervicovaginal sample during an examination by speculum. A positive quantitative fFN test of more than 50 ng/mL (0.05 mcg/mL) is predictive of preterm birth within 14 days, whereas a negative test suggests preterm birth is not likely (Lockwood, 2024). Interpretation of fFN results must always be viewed in conjunction with the clinical findings, particularly cervical length.

TAKE NOTE!

The accuracy of fFN is decreased in the presence of gross blood, ejaculate from coitus within the previous 24 hours, recent intercourse, or digital cervical examination.

Other tests that may be performed if indicated include:

- Complete blood count—if infection is suspected
- Urinalysis—to detect bacteria and nitrites if urinary tract infection is suspected
- Amniotic fluid analysis—to determine fetal lung maturity or chorioamnionitis

See the Healthy People 2030 box to learn more about nursing actions to reduce preterm births.

Nursing Management

Nurses play a key role in reducing preterm labor and births to improve pregnancy outcomes for both birthing parents and their infants. Early detection of preterm labor is currently the best strategy to improve outcomes. Preterm birth prevention programs for patients at high risk have used self-monitoring of symptoms and patterns, weekly cervical examinations, clinical markers, telephone monitoring, and home visiting, alone or in combination, with disappointing results.

HEALTHY PEOPLE 2030

Objective	Nursing Significance
Reduce preterm births.	• Screen pregnant people for risk factors for preterm birth. • Educate pregnant people about the symptoms of preterm labor. • Carefully provide highly skilled nursing management to the patient experiencing preterm labor.

Healthy People Objectives retrieved from http://www.healthypeople.gov

Supportive nursing care is needed for the patient in preterm labor whether the contractions are stopped with tocolytic therapy or not. Bed rest and hydration are commonly recommended but without proven efficacy. Nursing tasks include monitoring vital signs, measuring intake and output, encouraging bed rest on the left side to enhance placental perfusion, monitoring the FHR via an external monitor continuously, limiting vaginal examinations to prevent an ascending infection, and monitoring the pregnant person and fetus closely for any adverse effects from the tocolytic agents. Offering the patient ongoing explanations will help prepare them for the birth.

Administering Medications

The primary goals of tocolytics are to arrest labor and delay birth for up to 48 hours allowing time for corticosteroid therapy when indicated for stimulation of fetal lung maturity and to arrange for maternal–fetal transport to a perinatal tertiary care hospital. Refer to Drug Guide 21.1 for additional information regarding tocolytics. Absolute contraindications to administering tocolytic agents to stop labor include intrauterine infection, active hemorrhage, fetal distress, fetus before viability, fetal abnormality incompatible with life, fetal growth restriction (FGR), severe preeclampsia, heart disease, chorioamnionitis, prolonged premature rupture of the membranes (PPROM), and intrauterine demise (Mayer & Apodaca-Ramos, 2023). Administer magnesium sulfate if ordered (refer to Chapter 20 for additional information).

Educating the Patient

Ensure every pregnant person receives basic education about preterm labor, including information about harmful lifestyles, signs of genitourinary infections and preterm labor, and appropriate responses to these symptoms. Teach the patient how to palpate for and time uterine contractions. Provide written materials to support this education at a level and in a language appropriate for the patient. Also educate patients about the importance of prenatal care, risk reduction, and recognizing the signs and symptoms of preterm labor. Teaching Guidelines 21.1 highlights important instructions related to preventing preterm labor.

TEACHING GUIDELINES 21.1 Teaching to Prevent Preterm Labor

- Avoid traveling for long distances in cars, trains, planes, or buses.
- Avoid lifting heavy objects, such as laundry, groceries, or a young child.
- Avoid performing hard, physical work, such as yard work, moving furniture, or construction.

- Mild to moderate levels of exercise are permitted, such as walking daily.
- Achieve an appropriate prepregnancy weight.
- Achieve adequate iron stores through balanced nutrition.
- Wait at least 18 months between pregnancies.
- Visit a dentist in early pregnancy to evaluate and treat any periodontal disease.
- Enroll in a smoking cessation program if you are unable to quit on your own.
- Curtail sexual activity until after 37 weeks if experiencing preterm labor symptoms.
- Consume a well-balanced nutritional diet to gain appropriate weight.
- Avoid the use of substances such as cannabis, cocaine, and heroin.
- Identify factors and areas of stress in your life and use stress management techniques to reduce them.
- If you are experiencing intimate partner violence, seek resources to modify the situation.

Recognize the signs and symptoms of preterm labor and notify your birth attendant if any occur:

- Uterine contractions, cramping, or low back pain
- Feeling of pelvic pressure or fullness
- Increase in vaginal discharge
- Constant low, dull backache
- Nausea, vomiting, and diarrhea
- Leaking of fluid from the vagina

If you are experiencing any of these signs or symptoms, do the following:

- Stop what you are doing and rest for 1 hour.
- Empty your bladder.
- Lie down on your side.
- Drink two to three glasses of water.
- Feel your abdomen and make note of the hardness of the contraction. Call your health care provider and describe the contraction as:
  - Mild if it feels like the tip of the nose
  - Moderate if it feels like the tip of the chin
  - Strong if it feels like your forehead

Funai, E. F. (2022). Patient education: Preterm labor (beyond the basics). *UpToDate*. Retrieved May 8, 2024, from https://www.uptodate.com/contents/preterm-labor-beyond-the-basics; and Lockwood, C. J. (2024). Preterm labor: Clinical findings, diagnostic evaluation, and initial treatment. *UpToDate*. Retrieved May 8, 2024, from https://www.uptodate.com/contents/preterm-labor-clinical-findings-diagnostic-evaluation-and-initial-treatment

Providing Education and Psychological Support

Explain to the patient and family what is happening in terms of labor progress, the treatment regimen, and the status of the fetus to reduce the anxiety associated with the risk of giving birth to a preterm infant. Educate patients about the importance of promoting fetal lung maturity with corticosteroids. Include supportive family members in all education and allow time for the patient and family to express their concerns about possible outcomes for the infant and the possible side effects of tocolytic therapy. Encourage them to vent any feelings, fears, and anger they may experience. Provide the patient and family with an honest appraisal of the situation and plan of treatment throughout their care.

Preterm labor and birth present multifactorial changes for everyone involved. If the patient's activities are restricted, additional stress may be placed on the family, contributing to the crisis. Assess the stress levels of the patient and family and make appropriate referrals. Emphasize the need for more frequent supervision and office visits and encourage patients to talk to the health care provider for reassurance.

Every case of spontaneous preterm labor is unique. Half of all people who ultimately give birth prematurely have no identifiable risk factors, so with few exceptions, risk factors do not reliably predict preterm labor (ACOG, 2021). Nurses should be sensitive to any complaint and should provide appropriate assessment, information, and follow-up. Sensitivity to the subtle differences between normal pregnancy sensations and the prodromal symptoms of preterm labor is a key factor in ensuring timely care. Offer validation and clarification of the patient's symptoms.

If tocolytic therapy is not successful in stopping uterine contractions, support the patient and family through this stressful period to prepare for the birth. Keep them informed of all progress and changes; for example, continuously monitor maternal vital signs and FHR, especially the maternal temperature to detect signs of early infection. Offer one-on-one contact and be available throughout this difficult and anxiety-producing period.

POSTTERM PREGNANCY

A full-term pregnancy is designated as 39 weeks through 40 weeks and 6 days. A prolonged or **postterm pregnancy** is one that continues past the end of the 42nd week of gestation. Within the United States, up to 0.3% of singleton pregnancies extend beyond 42 weeks (Norwitz, 2024). Incorrect dates may account for the majority of these cases: Many people have irregular menses and thus cannot identify the date of the last menstrual period accurately. An ultrasound early in gestation provides the most accurate gestational age.

Recall Jennifer, described at the beginning of the chapter, who was at 41 weeks' gestation. What information would be most important to assess upon admission to the facility? What interventions might the nurse anticipate when she arrives?

The exact etiology of a postterm pregnancy is unknown. A person who has one prolonged pregnancy is at greater risk for another in subsequent pregnancies. Modest risk factors include nulliparity, male fetus, obesity, older maternal age, and maternal personal history of postterm birth.

Non-Hispanic White people are at higher risk of delivering postterm than other people (Norwitz, 2024). Maternal risks associated with postterm pregnancies are related to the large size of the fetus at birth (macrosomia) and include shoulder dystocia, cephalopelvic disproportion, prolonged labor, maternal trauma, and postpartum hemorrhage. These problems increase the chance of cesarean birth or forceps- or vacuum-assisted birth. In addition, maternal exhaustion and feelings of despair over prolonged gestation can add to the patient's anxiety level and reduce their coping ability. Patients often blame themselves for prolonging the pregnancy, and a person's negative feelings about themselves can bring about strained relationships with the people closest to them.

Dysmaturity, related to placental insufficiency, may occur in the fetus, resulting in FGR. Newborn complications include clavicular or brachial plexus injury, perinatal asphyxia, low Apgar scores, and neonatal encephalopathy. The postterm newborn with FGR is at increased risk for hypoglycemia and polycythemia. Postterm newborns also display an increased incidence of congenital malformations, meconium aspiration, and persistent pulmonary hypertension of the newborn as compared to term infants (Ringer, 2023).

Nursing Assessment

Obtain a thorough history to determine the estimated date of birth. Many people are unsure of the date of the last menstrual period, so the date given may be unreliable. Despite numerous methods used to date pregnancies, many are still misdated. Accurate gestational dating via ultrasound is essential.

When expectant management is chosen versus labor induction for the postterm pregnancy, the nurse should anticipate that assessments for a postterm pregnancy will typically include daily fetal movement counts done by the patient, nonstress tests with amniotic fluid assessments as part of the biophysical profile done twice weekly, and weekly cervical examinations to evaluate for ripening. Induction can be deferred until 42 weeks if the fetal surveillance is reassuring. In addition, assess the following:

- The patient's understanding of the various fetal well-being tests
- The patient's stress and anxiety concerning the prolonged pregnancy
- The patient's coping ability and support network

Nursing Management

When determining the plan of care for a person with a prolonged pregnancy, the first decision is whether to deliver the baby or wait. If the decision is to wait, fetal surveillance becomes key. If the decision is to have the patient give birth, labor induction is initiated. Both decisions remain controversial, and there is no clear answer about which option is more appropriate. Therefore, the plan must be individualized.

Think back to Jennifer, who is scheduled for labor induction. What ongoing nursing assessments would be important when providing care for her?

Providing Support

The intense surveillance is time-consuming and intrusive, adding to the anxiety and worry already being experienced by the patient about the pregnancy's status. Be alert to the patient's anxiety and allow them to discuss their feelings. Provide reassurance about the expected time range for birth and the well-being of the fetus based on the assessment tests. Validating the person's stress state due to the postterm pregnancy provides an opportunity for them to openly verbalize their feelings.

Educating the Patient and Family

Teach the patient and family about the testing required and the reasons for each test. Also describe the methods that may be used for cervical ripening if indicated. Explain the possibility of induction if labor is not spontaneous or if a dysfunctional labor pattern occurs. Also prepare them for the possibility of a surgical delivery if fetal distress occurs.

Providing Care During the Intrapartum Period

During the intrapartum period, continuously assess and monitor FHR to identify potential fetal distress early (e.g., late or variable decelerations) so that interventions can be initiated. Also monitor the patient's hydration status to ensure maximal placental perfusion. When the membranes rupture, assess amniotic fluid characteristics (color, amount, and odor) to identify previous fetal hypoxia and prepare for the prevention of meconium aspiration. Report meconium-stained amniotic fluid immediately when the patient's membranes rupture. Encourage the patient to verbalize their feelings and concerns and answer all their questions. Provide support, presence, information, and encouragement throughout this time.

PEOPLE REQUIRING LABOR INDUCTION AND AUGMENTATION

Ideally, all pregnancies go to term with labor beginning spontaneously. However, many pregnancies require help with initiating or sustaining the labor process. **Labor induction** involves the stimulation of uterine contractions by medical or surgical means before the onset of spontaneous labor. The labor induction rate is at an all-time high in the United States; 25% of all pregnant people undergo labor induction (Vrees & Kelly, 2023). Potential complications associated with labor induction include tachysystole and fetal decelerations/bradycardia (with oxytocin and prostaglandins), intrapartum vaginal bleeding, umbilical cord prolapse, pain unrelieved with regional anesthesia, perineal lacerations, postpartum hemorrhage, chorioamnionitis, postpartum endometritis, and meconium-stained amniotic fluid (Gill et al., 2023).

Labor induction is not an isolated event; it brings about a cascade of other interventions that may or may not produce favorable outcomes. It also involves intravenous therapy, bed rest, continuous electronic fetal monitoring, significant discomfort from stimulating uterine contractions, epidural analgesia and/or anesthesia, and a prolonged stay in the labor and birth unit (Gill et al., 2023). Labor augmentation (stimulating the uterus, typically with oxytocin) enhances ineffective contractions after labor has begun. Continuous electronic FHR monitoring is necessary.

The World Health Organization (WHO, 2022) has put forth recommendations regarding labor induction, including:

- Labor induction should be performed only for a clear medical indication.
- Routine induction of labor is not recommended for improving birth outcomes.
- Patients being induced should not be left unattended.
- Oxytocin use to delay labor in people with an epidural is not recommended.
- Labor induction should only be performed after cephalopelvic disproportion has been ruled out.
- Labor induction should not be applied to people with abnormal fetal presentations.
- Close monitoring is needed of the FHR and uterine contraction patterns.

There are multiple medical and obstetric reasons for inducing labor, the most common being prolonged gestation. Other indications for inductions include PPROM, gestational hypertension, chorioamnionitis, oligohydramnios, placental abruption, FGR, fetal demise, isoimmunization, intrahepatic cholestasis of pregnancy, and diabetes (Grobman, 2024a). Contraindications to labor induction include complete placenta previa, transverse fetal lie, a prolapsed umbilical cord, prior classic uterine incision that entered the uterine cavity, previous myomectomy, and active genital herpes infection (Vrees & Kelly, 2023). In general, labor induction is indicated when the benefits of birth outweigh the risks to the pregnant person or fetus for continuing the pregnancy. However, the balance between risk and benefit remains controversial.

TAKE NOTE!

Before labor induction is started, fetal maturity (dating, ultrasound, amniotic fluid studies) and cervical readiness (vaginal examination, Bishop scoring) must be assessed. Both need to be favorable for a successful induction.

Therapeutic Management

The decision to induce labor should be based on a thorough evaluation of maternal and fetal status. Typically, this includes an ultrasound to evaluate fetal size, position, and gestational age and to locate the placenta; engaged presenting fetal part; pelvimetry to rule out fetopelvic disproportion; a nonstress test to evaluate fetal well-being; a phosphatidylglycerol (PG) level to assess fetal lung maturity; confirmation of category I FHR pattern; complete blood count and urinalysis to rule out infection; and a vaginal examination to evaluate the cervix for inducibility (Grobman, 2024b). Accurate dating of the pregnancy is also essential before cervical ripening and induction are initiated to prevent a preterm birth.

Cervical Ripening

In the United States, about 25% of people who give birth undergo induction of labor, which frequently involves cervical ripening with a variety of methods (Wheeler et al., 2022). Cervical ripening is a process by which the cervix softens via the breakdown of collagen, leading to its elasticity and distensibility preceding cervical dilation. It is the first step in the process of cervical effacement and dilation so that on average, the cervix is approximately 50% effaced and 2 cm dilated at the onset of labor, though wide differences do exist. There has been increasing awareness that if the cervix is unfavorable or unripe, a successful vaginal birth is unlikely. Cervical ripeness is an important variable when labor induction is being considered. A ripe cervix is shortened, centered (anterior), softened, and partially dilated. An unripe cervix is long, closed, posterior, and firm. Cervical ripening usually begins prior to the onset of labor contractions and is necessary for cervical dilation and the passage of the fetus.

Various scoring systems to assess cervical ripeness have been introduced, but the Bishop score is most commonly used today. The Bishop score helps identify people who would be most likely to achieve a successful induction (Table 21.2). The duration of labor is inversely correlated with the Bishop score, which has a maximum score of 13; a score over 8 indicates a successful vaginal

TABLE 21.2 • Bishop Scoring System

Score	Dilation (cm)	Effacement (%)	Station	Cervical Consistency	Position of Cervix
0	Closed	0–30	−3	Firm	Posterior
1	1–2	40–50	−2	Medium	Mid position
2	3–4	60–70	−1 or 0	Soft	Anterior
3	5–6	80	+1 or +2	Very soft	Anterior

Modified from Wormer, K. C., Bauer, A., & Williford, A. E. (2023). Bishop score. *StatPearls.* https://www.ncbi.nlm.nih.gov/books/NBK470368/

birth. Bishop scores of less than 5 usually indicate that a cervical ripening method should be used prior to induction (Wheeler et al., 2022). Medical induction of labor has two components: cervical ripening and induction of contractions. When induction of labor is indicated, cervical readiness for labor is evaluated by pelvic examination and determination of a Bishop score is documented. Cervical ripening can be achieved by either mechanical or pharmacologic methods.

COMPLEMENTARY AND ALTERNATIVE MEDICINE METHODS

Nonpharmacologic methods for cervical ripening are less frequently used today, but nurses need to be aware of them and question patients about their use. Methods may include herbal agents such as evening primrose oil, black haw, black and blue cohosh, and red raspberry leaves. In addition, castor oil, hot baths, and enemas may be used for cervical ripening and labor induction. The risks and benefits of these agents are unknown. None have been evaluated scientifically, and thus, none can be recommended regarding efficacy or safety.

Another nonpharmacologic method suggested for labor induction is sexual intercourse along with breast stimulation. This promotes the release of oxytocin, which stimulates uterine contractions. In addition, human semen is a biologic source of prostaglandins used for cervical ripening. With penetration, the lower uterine segment is stimulated to release prostaglandins as well (Evbuomwan & Chowdhury, 2023). However, nipple stimulation and sexual intercourse as a method for labor induction has not been validated by research.

MECHANICAL METHODS

Mechanical methods are used to open the cervix and stimulate the progression of labor. All share a similar mechanism of action; application of local pressure stimulates the release of prostaglandins to ripen the cervix. For example, an indwelling (Foley) catheter (e.g., 26 Fr) can be inserted into the endocervical canal to ripen and dilate the cervix. The catheter is placed in the uterus, and the balloon is filled. Direct pressure is then applied to the lower segment of the uterus and the cervix. This direct pressure causes stress in the lower uterine segment and probably the local production of prostaglandins. Balloon induction reduces the risk of uterine hyperstimulation with FHR changes by 65%, and neonatal morbidity and perinatal death are reduced by half (Weeks et al., 2022).

Hygroscopic dilators absorb endocervical and local tissue fluids; as they enlarge, they expand the endocervix and provide controlled mechanical pressure. The products available include natural osmotic dilators (Laminaria, a type of dried seaweed) and synthetic dilators containing magnesium sulfate (Lamicel, Dilapan). Hygroscopic dilators are advantageous because they can be inserted on an outpatient basis and no fetal monitoring is needed. As many dilators as will fit are inserted in the cervix, they expand over 12 to 24 hours as they absorb water. Absorption of water leads to expansion of the dilators and opening of the cervix. They are a reliable alternative when prostaglandins are contraindicated or unavailable (Vrees & Kelly, 2023).

SURGICAL METHODS

Surgical methods used to ripen the cervix and induce labor include stripping the membranes and performing an amniotomy. Stripping of the membranes is accomplished by inserting a finger through the internal cervical os and moving it in a circular direction. This motion causes the membranes to detach. Manual separation of the amniotic membranes from the cervix is thought to release prostaglandins which induce cervical ripening and the onset of labor. However, there is no strong evidence at this time that membrane stripping significantly shortens the duration of pregnancy.

An amniotomy, also known as artificial rupture of membranes, involves inserting a cervical hook (Amniohook) through the cervical os to deliberately rupture the membranes. This promotes pressure of the presenting part on the cervix and stimulates an increase in the activity of prostaglandins locally. Risks associated with these procedures include umbilical cord prolapse or compression, maternal or neonatal infection, FHR deceleration, and patient discomfort (Mahdy et al., 2023).

When either of these techniques is used, amniotic fluid characteristics (such as whether it is clear or bloody, or meconium is present) and the FHR pattern must be monitored closely.

PHARMACOLOGIC METHODS

The use of pharmacologic agents has revolutionized cervical ripening. The use of prostaglandins to attain cervical ripening has been found to be highly effective in producing cervical changes independent of uterine contractions (Grobman, 2024b). In some instances, people will go into labor and require no additional stimulants for induction. Induction of labor with prostaglandins offers the advantage of promoting both cervical ripening and uterine contractility. A drawback of prostaglandins is their ability to induce excessive uterine contractions, which can increase maternal and perinatal morbidity (Grobman, 2024a). Prostaglandin analogs commonly used for cervical ripening include dinoprostone gel (Prepidil), dinoprostone inserts (Cervidil), and misoprostol (Cytotec). It is important to note that only dinoprostone is approved by the FDA for use as a cervical ripening agent (Goldberg, 2023). Misoprostol, a synthetic prostaglandin E1 (PGE1) analog, is a gastric cytoprotective agent used in the treatment and prevention of peptic ulcers. It can be administered intravaginally or orally to ripen the cervix or induce labor. It is available in 100- or 200-mcg tablets, but doses of 25 mcg are typically used, and may be reported every 4 hours. Hyperstimulation of the uterus can occur with misoprostol, progressing to uterine rupture (Drug Guide 21.2) (UpToDate, Inc., 2024). ACOG does not recommend using misoprostol for cervical ripening after prior cesarean birth or major uterine surgery because of the risk of uterine rupture (Goldberg, 2023).

Oxytocin

Oxytocin is a hormone secreted by the posterior pituitary that stimulates uterine contractions and is the most common agent used for labor induction. It is used as a potent endogenous uterotonic agent for both artificial induction and augmentation of labor, administered by intravenous infusion based on uterine contraction frequency. For people with low Bishop scores, cervical ripening is typically initiated before oxytocin is used. Once

DRUG GUIDE 21.2

DRUGS USED FOR CERVICAL RIPENING AND LABOR INDUCTION

Drug	Action/Indication	Nursing Implications
Dinoprostone (Cervidil insert; Prepidil gel)	Directly softens and dilates the cervix to ripen the cervix and induce labor FDA-approved for cervical ripening	Provide emotional support. Administer pain medications as needed. Frequently assess the degree of effacement and dilation. Monitor uterine contractions for frequency, duration, and strength. Assess maternal vital signs and FHR pattern frequently. Monitor for possible adverse effects such as headache, nausea and vomiting, and diarrhea.
Misoprostol (Cytotec)	Ripens cervix to induce labor	Instruct patient about the purpose and possible adverse effects of medication. Ensure informed consent is signed per hospital policy. Assess vital signs and FHR patterns frequently. Monitor the patient's reaction to the drug. Initiate oxytocin for labor induction at least 4 hours after the last dose was administered. Monitor for possible adverse effects such as nausea and vomiting, diarrhea, uterine hyperstimulation, and category II FHR patterns.
Oxytocin (Pitocin)	Acts on uterine myofibrils to contract to initiate or reinforce labor	Administer as an IV infusion via pump, increasing dose based on protocol until adequate labor progress is achieved. Assess baseline vital signs and FHR and then frequently after initiating oxytocin infusion. Determine frequency, duration, and strength of contractions frequently. Notify the health care provider of any uterine hypertonicity or abnormal FHR patterns. Maintain careful intake and output, being alert for water intoxication. Keep patient informed of labor progress. Monitor for possible adverse effects such as hyperstimulation of the uterus, impaired uterine blood flow leading to fetal hypoxia, rapid labor leading to cervical lacerations or uterine rupture, water intoxication (if oxytocin is given in electrolyte-free solution or at a rate exceeding 20 mU/min), and hypotension.

FDA, U.S. Food and Drug Administration; FHR, fetal heart rate; IV, intravenous.

Grobman, W. (2024a). Induction of labor: Techniques for preinduction cervical ripening. *UpToDate*. Retrieved May 9, 2024, from https://www.uptodate.com/contents/induction-of-labor-techniques-for-preinduction-cervical-ripening; and Vrees, R. A., & Kelly, B. (2023). Induction of labor. *Medscape*. https://emedicine.medscape.com/article/2500091-overview

the cervix is ripe, oxytocin is the most popular pharmacologic agent used for inducing or augmenting labor.

Frequently, a person with an unfavorable cervix is admitted the evening before induction to ripen the cervix with one of the prostaglandin agents. Then induction begins with oxytocin the next morning if they have not already gone into labor. Doing so markedly enhances the success of induction.

Response to oxytocin varies widely; some people are sensitive to even small amounts. The most common adverse effect of oxytocin is uterine hyperstimulation, leading to fetal compromise and impaired oxygenation (Grobman, 2024b). The uterus's response to the drug is closely monitored throughout labor so that the oxytocin infusion can be titrated appropriately. In addition, oxytocin has an antidiuretic effect, decreasing urine flow that may lead to water intoxication. Symptoms to watch for include headache and vomiting.

Oxytocin is administered via an intravenous infusion pump piggybacked into the main intravenous line at the port most proximal to the insertion site. Typically, 10 units of oxytocin are added to 1 L of isotonic solution. The dose is titrated according to protocol to achieve stable contractions every 2 to 3 minutes lasting 40 to 60 seconds. Recent studies suggest that a more conservative oxytocin protocol with lower doses reduces the number of neonatal intensive care unit (NICU) admissions and lower cesarean deliveries, but either regimen is acceptable for use in labor induction (Kruit et al., 2022; Olsen & Karjane, 2022).

The uterus should relax between contractions. If the resting uterine tone remains above 20 mm Hg, uteroplacental insufficiency and fetal hypoxia can result. This underscores the importance of continuous FHR monitoring. Unfortunately, neither the optimal oxytocin administration regimen nor the maximum oxytocin dose has been established or agreed upon through research or expert opinion. Nurses assisting with labor inductions need to become familiar with their hospital protocols concerning dosage, infusion rates, and frequency of change (Fig. 21.4).

Oxytocin has many advantages: It is potent and easy to titrate, it has a short half-life (1 to 5 minutes), and it is generally well tolerated. Induction using oxytocin has side effects (water intoxication, hypotension, and uterine hypertonicity), but because the drug does not cross the placental barrier, no direct fetal problems have been observed.

Remember Jennifer, the young woman described at the beginning of the chapter? After her cervix is ripened, an oxytocin infusion is started, and her progress is slow. What encouragement can the nurse offer? After a few hours, her contractions begin to increase in intensity and frequency. What typical pain management measures can the nurse implement, and how would the nurse evaluate the effectiveness of these measures?

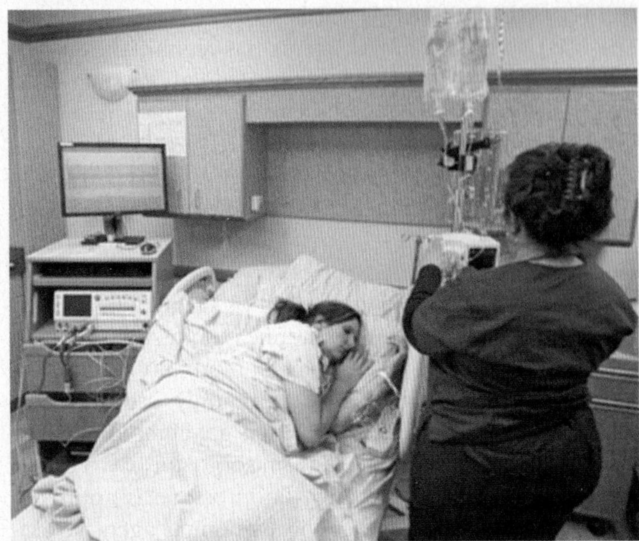

FIGURE 21.4 The nurse monitors an intravenous infusion of oxytocin being administered to a person in labor who is being induced.

Nursing Assessment

Nursing assessment of the patient who is undergoing labor induction or augmentation involves a thorough history and physical examination. Review the patient's history for relative indications for induction or augmentation, such as diabetes, hypertension, postterm status, dysfunctional labor pattern, prolonged ruptured membranes, and maternal or fetal infection, and for contraindications such as placenta previa, overdistended uterus, active genital herpes, fetopelvic disproportion, fetal malposition, or severe fetal distress.

Assist with determining the fetus's gestational age to prevent a preterm birth. Assess fetal well-being to validate the patient's and fetus's ability to withstand labor contractions. Evaluate the patient's cervical status, including cervical dilation and effacement, and station via vaginal examination as appropriate before cervical ripening or induction is started. Determine the Bishop score to determine the probable success of induction.

TAKE NOTE!

Nurses working with people in labor play an important role in acting as the eyes and ears for the birth attendant because they remain at the patient's bedside throughout the entire experience. Close, frequent assessment and follow-up interventions are essential to ensure the safety of the birthing person and unborn child during cervical ripening and labor induction or augmentation.

Nursing Management

Explain the induction or augmentation procedure clearly, using simple terms (Teaching Guidelines 21.2). Ensure an informed consent has been signed after the patient

TEACHING GUIDELINES 21.2 Teaching in Preparation for Labor Induction

- Your health care provider may recommend you have your labor induced. This may be necessary for a variety of reasons, such as elevated blood pressure, a medical condition, prolonged pregnancy over 41 weeks, or problems with fetal heart rate (FHR) patterns or fetal growth.
- Your health care provider may use one or more methods to induce labor, such as stripping the membranes, breaking the amniotic sac to release the fluid, administering medication close to or in the cervix to soften it, or administering a medication called oxytocin (Pitocin) to stimulate contractions.
- Labor induction is associated with some risks and disadvantages, such as overactivity of the uterus; nausea, vomiting, or diarrhea; and changes in FHR.
- Prior to inducing your labor, your health care provider may perform a procedure to ripen your cervix to help ensure a successful induction.
- Medication may be placed around your cervix the day before you are scheduled to be induced.
- During the induction, your contractions may feel stronger than normal. However, the length of your labor may be reduced with induction.
- Medications for pain relief and comfort measures will be readily available.
- Health care staff will be present throughout labor.

and family have received complete information about the procedure, including its advantages, disadvantages, and potential risks. Ensure that the Bishop score has been determined before proceeding. Clinical Judgment & Nursing Process 21.1 presents an overview of the nursing care for a person undergoing labor induction.

Administering Oxytocin

If not already done, prepare the oxytocin infusion by diluting 10 units of oxytocin in 1,000 mL of lactated Ringer's solution or ordered isotonic solution. Use an infusion pump on a secondary line connected to the primary infusion. Start the oxytocin infusion in mU/min or mL/h as ordered. Each hospital has its own standards and protocols for oxytocin infusion and dilution. The nurse must follow that procedure when administering this medication. Maintain the rate once the desired contraction frequency has been reached. To ensure adequate maternal and fetal surveillance during induction or augmentation, the nurse-to-patient ratio should not exceed 1:1 (Lothian, 2024).

During induction or augmentation, monitoring of the maternal and fetal status is essential. Apply an external electronic fetal monitor or assist with the placement of an internal device. Obtain the patient's vital signs and the FHR every 15 minutes during the first stage. Evaluate the contractions (frequency, duration, and intensity) and resting tone, and adjust the oxytocin infusion rate accordingly. Monitor the FHR, including baseline rate, baseline variability, and decelerations to determine whether the oxytocin rate needs adjustment. Discontinue the oxytocin and notify the health care provider

CLINICAL JUDGMENT & NURSING PROCESS 21.1 Overview of the Person Undergoing Labor Induction

Rose, a 29-year-old primipara, is admitted to the labor and birth suite at 40 weeks' gestation for induction of labor. Assessment reveals that her cervix is ripe, 80% effaced, and dilated to 2 cm. Rose says, "I'm a bit nervous about being induced. I've never been through labor before and I'm afraid that I'll have a lot of pain from the medicine used to start the contractions." She consents to being induced but wants reassurance that this procedure won't harm the baby. Upon examination, the fetus is engaged and in a cephalic presentation, with the vertex as the presenting part. Her partner is at her side. Induction is initiated with oxytocin. Rose reports that contractions have started and are beginning to get stronger.

NURSING ANALYSIS: Anxiety related to induction of labor and associated medical interventions needed as evidenced by statements about being nervous, not having gone through labor before, fear of pain, and potential harm to fetus

OUTCOME IDENTIFICATION AND EVALUATION

The patient will experience a decrease in anxiety as evidenced by the ability to verbalize understanding of the procedures involved and the use of positive coping skills to reduce the anxious state.

INTERVENTIONS: *Minimizing Anxiety*

- Provide a clear explanation of the labor induction process *to provide patient and their family with a knowledge base.*
- Maintain continuous physical presence *to provide physical and emotional support and demonstrate concern for maternal and fetal well-being.*

(*continued*)

CLINICAL JUDGMENT & NURSING PROCESS 21.1 Overview of the Person Undergoing Labor Induction (*continued*)

- Explain each procedure before carrying it out and answer questions *to promote understanding of the procedure and rationale for use and decrease fear of the unknown.*
- Review with patient measures used in the past to deal with stressful situations *to determine effectiveness;* encourage the use of past effective coping strategies *to aid in controlling anxiety.*
- Instruct patient's partner or support person in helpful measures to assist the patient in coping and encourage their use *to foster joint participation in the process and feelings of being in control and to provide support to the patient.*
- Offer frequent reassurance of fetal status and labor progress *to help alleviate patient's concerns and foster continued participation in the labor process.*

NURSING ANALYSIS: Injury risk (maternal or fetal) related to induction procedure risk factors: hypertonic uterine contractions, potential preterm birth as evidenced by patient's concerns about fetal well-being and possible adverse effects of oxytocin administration

OUTCOME IDENTIFICATION AND EVALUATION

The patient will remain free of complications associated with induction as evidenced by the progression of labor as expected, delivery of the healthy newborn, and absence of signs and symptoms of maternal and fetal adverse effects.

INTERVENTIONS: *Promoting Maternal and Fetal Safety*

- Follow agency's protocol for medication use and infusion rate *to ensure accurate, safe drug administration.*
- Set up oxytocin intravenous (IV) infusion to piggyback into the primary IV infusion line *to allow for prompt discontinuation should adverse effects occur.*
- Use an infusion pump *to deliver accurate dose as ordered.*
- Gradually increase oxytocin dose in increments based on assessment findings and protocol *to promote effective uterine contractions.*
- Maintain oxytocin rate once the desired frequency of contractions has been reached *to ensure continued progress in labor.*
- Accurately monitor contractions for frequency, duration, intensity, and resting tone *to prevent the development of hypertonic contractions.*
- Maintain a nurse-to-patient ratio of 1:2 *to ensure maternal and fetal safety.*
- Monitor fetal heart rate (FHR) via electronic fetal monitoring during induction and continuously observe the FHR response to titrated medication rate *to ensure fetal well-being and identify adverse effects immediately.*
- Obtain maternal vital signs every 1 to 2 hours or as indicated by the agency's protocol, reporting any deviations *to promote maternal well-being and allow for prompt detection of problems.*
- Communicate with birth attendant frequently concerning progress *to ensure continuity of care.*
- Discontinue oxytocin infusion if tetanic contractions (>90 seconds), uterine hyperstimulation (<2 minutes apart), elevated uterine resting tone, or a distressed FHR pattern occurs *to minimize the risk of the drug's adverse effects.*
- Provide patient with frequent reassurance of maternal and fetal status *to minimize anxiety.*

NURSING ANALYSIS: Acute pain related to uterine contractions as evidenced by patient's statements about contractions increasing in intensity and expected effect of oxytocin administration

OUTCOME IDENTIFICATION AND EVALUATION

The patient will report a decrease in pain as evidenced by statements of increased comfort and pain rating of 3 or less on the numeric pain rating scale.

INTERVENTIONS: *Promoting Maternal and Fetal Safety*

- Explain to the patient that they will experience discomfort sooner than with naturally occurring labor *to promote patient's awareness of events and prepare patient for the experience.*
- Frequently assess patient's pain using a pain rating scale *to quantify patient's level of pain and evaluate the effectiveness of pain relief measures.*
- Provide comfort measures, such as hygiene, backrubs, music, and distraction, and encourage the use of breathing and relaxation techniques *to help promote relaxation.*
- Provide support for patient's partner *to aid in alleviating stress and concerns.*
- Employ nonpharmacologic methods, such as position changes, birthing ball, hydrotherapy, visual imagery, and effleurage, *to help in managing pain and foster feelings of control over the situation.*
- Administer pharmacologic agents such as analgesia or anesthesia as appropriate and as ordered *to control pain.*
- Continuously reassess patient's pain level *to evaluate the effectiveness of the pain management techniques used.*

if uterine hyperstimulation or a category II or III FHR pattern occurs. Perform or assist with periodic vaginal examinations to determine cervical dilation and fetal descent; cervical dilation of 1 cm per hour typically indicates satisfactory progress. Continue to monitor the FHR continuously and document it every 15 minutes during the active phase of labor and every 5 minutes during the second stage. Assist with pushing efforts during the second stage. Measure and record the intake and output to prevent excess fluid volume. Encourage the patient to empty their bladder every 2 hours to prevent soft tissue obstruction.

Providing Pain Relief and Support

A person in labor experiences two types of pain—visceral and somatic. Their perception of pain is influenced by physiologic, psychological, and cultural factors (Grant & Reale, 2024). Assess the level of pain. Ask the patient frequently to rate their pain and provide pain management as needed. Offer position changes and other nonpharmacologic measures. Note their reaction to any medication given and document its effect. Monitor their need for comfort measures as contractions increase.

Throughout induction and augmentation, frequently reassure the patient and family about the fetal status and labor progress. Provide them with frequent updates on the condition of the patient and the fetus. Assess the patient's ability to cope with stronger contractions and perform pain assessments (using a validated assessment tool) for each phase and stage of labor at the frequency determined by hospital protocols (Rantala et al., 2022). Provide support and encouragement as indicated.

After a long day, Jennifer gives birth to a healthy baby boy with Apgar scores of 9 at 1 minute and 10 at 5 minutes. When transferring her to the postpartum unit, what information is essential to include for the accepting nurse? What specific nursing information should be given to the nursery nurse regarding the laboring experience? With such a lengthy labor, what assessments might the postpartum nurse need to focus on for the first few hours after birth?

VAGINAL BIRTH AFTER CESAREAN

Vaginal birth after cesarean (VBAC) describes giving birth vaginally after having at least one previous cesarean birth. Despite evidence that some people who have had a cesarean birth are candidates for vaginal birth, some who have had a cesarean birth once undergo cesarean births for subsequent pregnancies. Trial of labor after cesarean birth (TOLAC) refers to a planned attempt to give birth vaginally by a person who has had a previous surgical birth, regardless of the outcome. However, although TOLAC is appropriate for some, several risk factors increase the incidence of a failed TOLAC, which may increase maternal and fetal morbidity and mortality (Habak & Kole, 2023).

A multidisciplinary guideline group representing family medicine, epidemiology, obstetrics, and midwifery developed recommendations based on high-quality systematic evidence-based, peer-reviewed research, that individual assessment of risks and benefits be discussed with the pregnant person with a history of one or more prior cesarean births who is deciding between a planned VBAC or a repeat cesarean birth. A planned VBAC is an appropriate option for many people with histories of prior cesarean birth (Metz, 2024).

Contraindications to VBAC include a prior classic uterine incision, prior transfundal uterine surgery (myomectomy), uterine scar other than a low-transverse cesarean scar, obesity, short maternal stature, macrosomia, maternal age (over 40 years), gestational diabetes, contracted pelvis, and inadequate staff or facility if an emergency cesarean birth is required in the event of uterine rupture (Habak & Kole, 2023). Most people go through a trial of labor to see how they progress, but this must be performed in an environment capable of handling the emergency of uterine rupture. The use of cervical ripening agents increases the risk of uterine rupture and thus is contraindicated in VBAC patients. The patient considering induction of labor after a previous cesarean birth needs to be informed of the risks versus benefits of induction than with spontaneous labor (Metz, 2024).

Patients are the primary decision makers about the choice of birth method, but they need education about VBAC to make the best decisions for themselves. Management is similar for any person experiencing labor, but certain areas require special focus:

- *Consent:* Fully informed consent is essential for the patient who wants to have a TOLAC. The patient must be advised about the risks as well as the benefits. They must understand the ramifications of uterine rupture, even though the risk is small.
- *Documentation:* Record keeping is an important component of safe patient care. If and when an emergency occurs, it is imperative to not only take care of the patient but also to keep track of the plan of care, interventions and their timing, and the patient's response. Events and activities can be written on the fetal monitoring tracing to correlate with the change in fetal status.
- *Surveillance:* A distressed fetal monitor tracing in a patient undergoing a TOLAC should alert the nurse to the possibility of uterine rupture. Terminal bradycardia must be considered an emergency situation, and the nurse should prepare the team for an emergency delivery.
- *Readiness for emergency:* According to ACOG (2023) criteria for a safe trial of labor for a person who has had a previous cesarean birth, the primary provider, anesthesia provider, and operating room team must be immediately available. Anything less would place the patient and fetus at risk.

Patients and their health care providers are advised to consider VBAC in the context of potential risk, available resources, and the health care system. The ACOG (2023) guidelines state that VBACs are safe and appropriate for many patients, but they emphasize the need for thorough counseling, shared decision making, and patient autonomy. Nurses must act as advocates, giving input on the appropriate selection of people who wish to undergo VBAC. Nurses also need to become experts at reading fetal monitoring tracings to identify fetal distress and set in motion an emergency birth. Including all of these nursing strategies will make VBAC safer for all.

PEOPLE EXPERIENCING AN OBSTETRIC EMERGENCY

Obstetric emergencies are challenging to all labor and birth personnel because of the increased risk of adverse outcomes for the pregnant person and fetus. Quick clinical judgment and good critical decision making will increase the odds of a positive outcome for both the pregnant person and fetus. This section discusses a few of these emergencies: umbilical cord prolapse, placenta previa, placental abruption, uterine rupture, and anaphylactoid syndrome of pregnancy (ASP).

Umbilical Cord Prolapse

Umbilical cord prolapse is a rare obstetric emergency that occurs when the cord precedes the fetus out, increasing the risk of fetal/newborn mortality (Fig. 21.5). Its incidence has decreased over time as a result of increased cesarean use for risk factors such as fetal malpresentation (Boushra et al., 2023). This condition occurs in up to six per 1,000 births and requires prompt recognition and intervention for a positive outcome (Botezatu et al., 2022). The risk is increased further when the presenting part does not fill the lower uterine segment, as is the case with incomplete breech presentations, premature infants, hydramnios, and multiparous people.

Pathophysiology

The pathogenesis of umbilical cord prolapse is not always clear. If the presenting part doesn't adequately fill the pelvis or obstetric interventions performed dislodge the presenting part, the risk of prolapse is increased. Prolapse usually leads to total or partial occlusion of the cord. Since this is the fetus's only lifeline, fetal perfusion deteriorates rapidly. Complete occlusion renders the fetus helpless and oxygen deprived. The fetus will die if the cord compression is not relieved. It is diagnosed by seeing or palpating the prolapsed cord outside or within the vagina in addition to abnormal FHR patterns. Once diagnosed, birth should be expedited.

Nursing Assessment

Prevention is the key to managing cord prolapse by identifying patients at risk for this condition. Risk factors include fetal malpresentation (noncephalic presentation), multifetal pregnancy, long cord length, polyhydramnios, preterm labor, premature rupture of membranes, FGR, amniotomy without an engaged fetal presenting part, and placement of cervical ripening balloon (Boushra et al., 2023). Carefully assess each patient to help predict risk status. When a persistent deceleration appears on the tracing in labor, after membranes rupture, consider cord prolapse and check for it immediately. Continuously assess the patient and fetus to detect changes and to evaluate the effectiveness of any interventions performed.

TAKE NOTE!

When the presenting part does not fully occupy the pelvic inlet, prolapse is more likely to occur.

Nursing Management

Prompt recognition of a prolapsed cord is essential to reduce the risk of fetal hypoxia resulting from prolonged cord compression. Often the first sign of cord prolapse is a sudden fetal bradycardia or recurrent variable

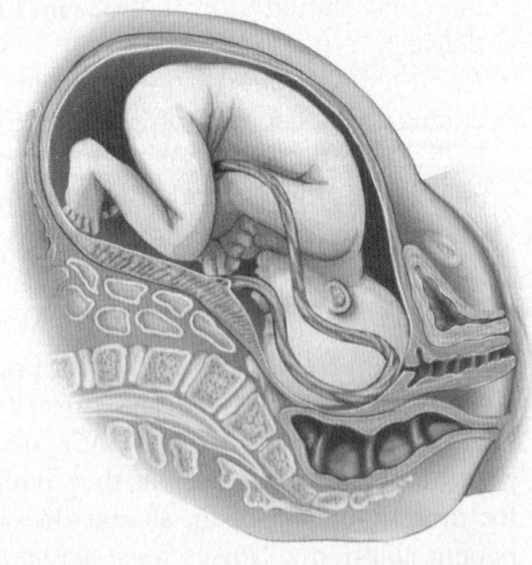

A

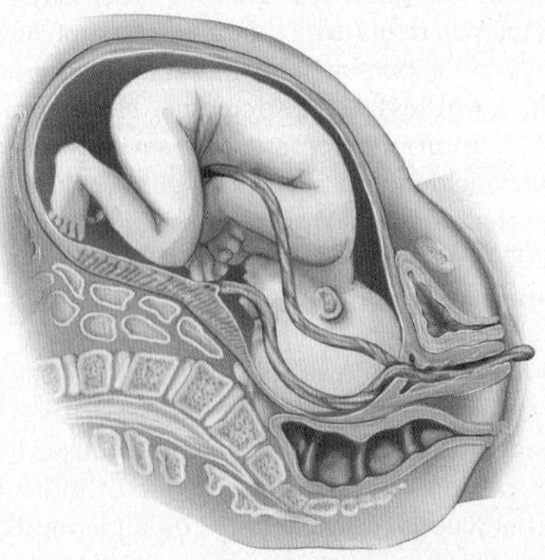

B

FIGURE 21.5 Prolapsed cord. **A.** Prolapse within the uterus. **B.** Prolapse with the cord visible at the vulva.

decelerations that become progressively more severe. Call for help immediately and do not leave the patient. Inform the patient of what is happening and what options they may discuss with the health care provider. When membranes are artificially ruptured, assist with verifying that the presenting part is well applied to the cervix and engaged into the pelvis. If pressure or compression of the cord occurs, assist with measures to relieve the compression. Typically, the examiner places a sterile gloved hand into the vagina and holds the presenting part off the umbilical cord until delivery. Changing the patient's position to a modified Sims, Trendelenburg, or knee–chest position also helps relieve cord pressure. Do not attempt to replace the cord in the uterus. Monitor FHR, maintain bed rest, and administer oxygen if ordered. Provide emotional support and explanations as to what is going on to allay the patient's fears and anxiety. If the cervix is not fully dilated, prepare the patient for an emergency cesarean birth to save the fetus's life if that is the intervention planned for by the health care provider.

Placenta Previa

Placenta previa is the complete or partial covering of the uterine internal os of the cervix with the placenta, typically identified during the second or third trimester of pregnancy. It is the most common cause of bleeding in the second half of pregnancy and should be suspected in any person beyond 24 weeks' gestation presenting with vaginal bleeding. During labor and birth, bleeding can be severe, which can place the pregnant person and fetus at risk. The reported incidence is approximately 0.5% of all U.S. pregnancies (Bakker, 2023).

All placentas covering the cervical os to any degree are termed *placenta previa*. A placenta 2 to 3.5 cm from the os is referred to as a low-lying placenta, and about 90% will ultimately resolve as the placenta grows toward the increasing blood supply of the fundus (Anderson-Bagga & Sze, 2023). The degree of occlusion of the internal cervical os may depend on the degree of cervical dilation, so what may appear to be a low-lying or marginal placenta previa prior to the onset of labor can progress to become more serious as the cervix effaces and opens up (Lockwood & Russo-Stieglitz, 2024). The incidence of maternal mortality is less than 1%, but common morbidities include septicemia, renal failure, invasive placenta, and postpartum anemia. The risk for perinatal mortality is less than 1.2%, but common neonatal morbidities include preterm birth, malpresentation, FGR, and fetal anemia (Bakker, 2023).

Management of placenta previa varies by type and gestational age. Some patients are managed with bed rest at home with frequent medical surveillance. Vaginal delivery is possible when bleeding is minimal, placenta is low lying, or labor is rapid. Pregnancy termination, early birth by cesarean delivery, or a hysterectomy may be necessary in order to control severe bleeding, especially for patients with complete placenta previa. The overall maternal prognosis is good if hemorrhage is controlled, and sepsis or other complications are prevented. Fetal prognosis is directly related to the amount of blood loss.

Nursing Assessment

Review the patient's history for placenta previa risk factors including previous cesarean delivery, infertility treatment, short interval between pregnancies, maternal age older than 34, prior placenta previa, multiparity, multiple gestation, uterine leiomyomas, prior placenta previa, cocaine use, and cigarette smoking. Determine the onset, volume, and progress of vaginal bleeding (may be episodic). The bleeding is usually sudden and painless. Assess for pallor, a rapid, weak pulse, and decreased blood pressure indicating hypovolemia. Palpate the uterus which will be soft and nontender. In some instances, placenta previa is without symptoms because there is intrauterine bleeding only without external signs. A transvaginal ultrasound will be used to diagnose placenta previa or low-lying placenta.

Nursing Management

Nursing management within the acute care setting includes monitoring maternal vital signs, intake and output, vaginal bleeding, and physiologic status for signs of hemorrhage, shock, or infection. Closely monitor FHR for distress (e.g., bradycardia, tachycardia, baseline changes). Treat fetal distress as ordered. Administer prescribed intravenous fluids, packed red blood cells, platelets, and frozen plasma for transfusion if ordered. If labor is to be induced, administer intravenous oxytocin as prescribed. When preterm labor is occurring, provide prescribed tocolytics and corticosteroids (to enhance fetal lung maturity). Administer Rho(D) immune globulin if the patient is Rh-negative. Follow facility presurgical and postsurgical protocols if the patient becomes a candidate for cesarean delivery. Reinforce presurgical and postsurgical education. Postoperatively, monitor the patient for bleeding, infection, and other complications. Assess anxiety level and coping ability, and provide emotional support and reassurance.

Placental Abruption

Placental abruption refers to premature separation of a normally implanted placenta from the maternal myometrium. Placental abruption occurs in three to 10 instances per 1,000 births in the United States, Canada, Netherlands, Spain, Finland, Sweden, Denmark, and Norway, with the United States and Canada being at the upper end (and increasing) (Ananth & Kinzler, 2023). Risk factors include preeclampsia, gestational hypertension, trauma, smoking, and cocaine use, as these conditions may force blood into the underlayer of the placenta and cause it to detach (Oyelese & Vintzileos, 2024).

Management of placental abruption depends on the gestational age, the extent of the hemorrhage, and maternal–fetal oxygenation perfusion or reserve status (see Chapter 19 for additional information on placental abruption). Treatment is based on the circumstances. Typically, once the diagnosis is established, the focus is on maintaining the cardiovascular status of the birthing person and developing a plan to deliver the fetus quickly. A cesarean birth may take place quickly if the fetus is still alive with only a partial abruption. A vaginal birth may take place if there is fetal demise secondary to a complete abruption.

Uterine Rupture

A uterine rupture is a complete division of all three layers of the uterus—endometrium, myometrium, and perimetrium. It is estimated that one rupture occurs per every 5,000 to 7,000 births, and its incidence is increasing due to the high number of surgical births worldwide (Togioka & Tonismae, 2023). Uterine rupture in pregnancy is a rare and often catastrophic complication with a high incidence of fetal and maternal morbidity. Uterine rupture is a catastrophic tearing of the uterus at the site of a previous scar into the abdominal cavity. Its onset is often marked only by sudden fetal bradycardia, and treatment requires rapid surgery for good outcomes. From the time of diagnosis to delivery, only a short amount of time is available before clinically significant fetal morbidity occurs. Fetal morbidity occurs secondary to catastrophic hemorrhage, fetal anoxia, or both.

Nursing Assessment

Review the patient's history for risk conditions such as uterine scars, prior cesarean births (fundal or longitudinal incision), prior rupture, increasing maternal age, gestation more than 40 weeks, labor induction, and birth weight greater than 4,000 g (Frey & Landon, 2024). Generally, the first and most reliable symptom of uterine rupture is sudden fetal distress. Other signs may include acute and continuous abdominal pain with or without an epidural, vaginal bleeding, hematuria, irregular abdominal wall contour, loss of station in the fetal presenting part, and hypovolemic shock in the patient, fetus, or both (Smith & Wax, 2024).

Timely management of uterine rupture depends on prompt detection. Because many people desire a TOLAC, the nurse must be familiar with the signs and symptoms of uterine rupture. It is difficult to prevent uterine rupture or to predict which people will experience rupture, so constant preparedness is necessary. Screening all patients with previous uterine surgical scars is important, and continuous electronic fetal monitoring should be used during labor because this may provide the only indication of an impending rupture.

Nursing Management

Because the presenting signs may be nonspecific, initial management will be the same as that for any other cause of acute fetal distress. Urgent delivery by cesarean birth is usually indicated. Monitor maternal vital signs and observe for hypotension and tachycardia, which might indicate hypovolemic shock. Assist in preparing for an emergency cesarean birth by alerting the operating room staff, anesthesia provider, and neonatal team. Insert an indwelling urinary catheter if one is not in place already. Inform the patient of the seriousness of this event and remind them that the health care staff will be working quickly to ensure their health and that of the fetus. Remain calm and provide reassurance that everything is being done to ensure a safe outcome for both. Maternal death is a real possibility without rapid intervention. Newborn outcome after rupture depends largely on the speed of surgical rescue. As in any case of acute obstetric emergency, preparation and timely mobilization of all necessary personnel is essential to optimizing outcomes.

> *TAKE NOTE!*
>
> When excessive bleeding occurs during the childbirth process and it persists or signs such as bruising or petechiae appear, disseminated intravascular coagulation (DIC) should be suspected.

Amniotic Fluid Embolism

Amniotic fluid embolism (AFE), also called ASP, is an unforeseeable, life-threatening complication of childbirth. AFE results in significant hypoxia rapidly. The mortality rate for AFE is 10% to 20%, and 50% of maternal survivors have significant neurologic injury (Baldisseri & Clark, 2023). When AFE occurs prior to delivery, the neonatal mortality rate is 20% to 60% and only 50% of survivors have neurologic impairment (Baldisseri & Clark, 2023).

The etiology of AFE remains an enigmatic, devastating obstetric condition associated with significant maternal and newborn morbidity and mortality. It is a rare event characterized by the sudden onset of hypotension, cardiopulmonary collapse, hypoxia, and coagulopathy. Amniotic fluid containing particles of debris (e.g., hair, skin, vernix, or meconium) enters maternal circulation and obstructs the pulmonary vessels, causing respiratory distress and circulatory collapse (Baldisseri & Clark, 2023). Prediction and diagnosis of the event are nearly impossible. However, timely recognition and response are critical in saving a person's life.

Pathophysiology

The pathophysiology of AFE continues to be researched and debated; it involves the introduction of amniotic fluid into the pregnant person's circulation and an abnormal maternal response to fetal tissue exposure associated with breaches of the maternal–fetal physiologic barrier during the postpartum period. Normally, amniotic fluid does not enter the maternal circulation because it is contained within the uterus, sealed off by the amniotic sac. An embolus occurs when the barrier between the maternal circulation and the amniotic fluid is broken and amniotic fluid enters the maternal venous system via the endocervical veins, the placental site (if the placenta is separated), or a site of uterine trauma. Within minutes after the amniotic fluid and maternal blood mix, the patient experiences dyspnea and cyanosis followed by respiratory distress and respiratory arrest. An anaphylactic-type reaction occurs when the amniotic fluid enters the circulatory system.

Although medical science has supplied many answers to questions about this condition, health care providers remain largely unable to predict or prevent AFE or to decrease its mortality rate. Recent evidence suggests at least one fifth of all cases of AFE are incorrectly diagnosed; thus, failure to rescue might contribute to the dismal outcomes of pregnancy complicated by AFE contributing to high maternal mortality (Mazza et al., 2022).

Nursing Assessment

Determine the presence of potential risk factors including preeclampsia/eclampsia, placental abnormalities (previa, abruption, accreta), instrumental vaginal delivery, and cesarean delivery (Baldisseri & Clark, 2023). However, many people who experience AFE have none of the risk factors. Carefully assess the laboring patient; the nurse's assessment skills are critical. Immediate recognition and diagnosis of this condition are essential to improving maternal and fetal outcomes. The four cardinal signs of AFE include respiratory failure, altered mental status, hypotension, and DIC. Monitor vital signs, pulse oximetry, skin color, and temperature, and observe for clinical signs of coagulopathy (vaginal bleeding, bleeding from intravenous site, bleeding from gums). There is no laboratory test that can confirm the diagnosis.

TAKE NOTE!

AFE should be suspected in any pregnant person with an acute onset of dyspnea, hypotension, and DIC. By knowing how to intervene, the nurse can promote a better chance of survival for both the birthing person and the newborn. Most patients are transferred to the intensive care unit.

Nursing Management

Early recognition and the use of immediate resuscitative measures improve the chances of survival. A team response is essential because every person will be needed. Upon recognizing the signs and symptoms of this life-threatening diagnosis, institute supportive measures: oxygenation (resuscitation and 100% oxygen), circulation (intravenous fluids, inotropic agents to maintain cardiac output and blood pressure), control of hemorrhage and coagulopathy (oxytocic agents to control uterine atony and bleeding), seizure precautions, and administration of steroids to control the inflammatory response.

Care is largely supportive and aimed at maintaining oxygenation and hemodynamic function and correcting coagulopathy. Adequate oxygenation is necessary with endotracheal intubation and mechanical ventilation for most people. Vasopressors are used to maintain hemodynamic stability. Management of DIC may involve replacement with packed red blood cells or fresh-frozen plasma as necessary. Oxytocin infusions and prostaglandin analogs can be used to address uterine atony.

Explain to the patient and family what is happening and what therapies are being instituted. The patient is usually transferred to a critical care unit for intensive observation and care. Assist the family with expressing their feelings and provide support as needed. Inform and reassure the patient and family as much as possible during this crisis. Early recognition and goal-directed treatment are critical to successful management and reduction of mortality for AFE (Arnolds, 2023).

PEOPLE REQUIRING BIRTH-RELATED PROCEDURES

Many people can give birth without the need for any operative obstetric interventions. Most do not anticipate the need for any medical intervention. However, in some situations, interventions are necessary to safeguard the health of the birthing person and fetus. The most common birth-related procedures are forceps-assisted or vacuum-assisted birth, cesarean birth, episiotomy, and VBAC (see "Vaginal Birth After Cesarean" section earlier in this chapter). Nurses play a major role in helping patients and families cope with any unanticipated procedures by offering thorough explanations of the procedure, its anticipated benefits and risks, and any other options available.

Forceps- or Vacuum-Assisted Birth

Instrument-assisted vaginal birth may be accomplished by the use of a vacuum extractor or forceps to apply traction to the fetal head or to provide a method of rotating the fetal head during birth. Overall, the rates of instrument-assisted births are decreasing in the United States,

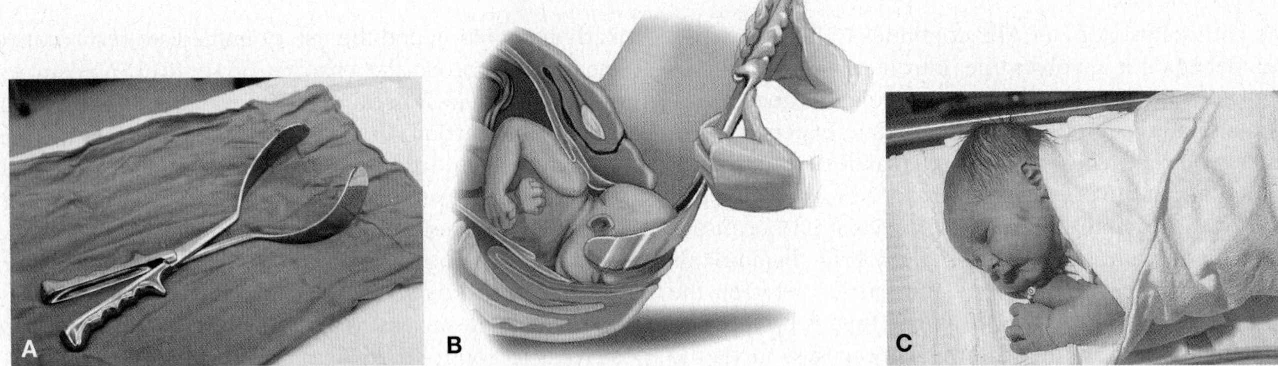

FIGURE 21.6 Forceps delivery (uncommon). **A.** Example of forceps. **B.** Forceps being applied to the fetus. **C.** Forceps marks are commonly found in newborns delivered by forceps. Such marks are transient and disappear in a day or two.

and currently occur in just over 3% of births (Bernstein & Coggin-Carr, 2024).

Forceps are stainless steel instruments, similar to tongs, with rounded edges that fit around the fetus's head. Some forceps have open blades, and some have solid blades. Outlet forceps are used when the fetal head is crowning, and low forceps are used when the fetal head is at a +2 station or lower but not yet crowning (Fig. 21.6). The forceps are applied to the sides of the fetal head. The type of forceps used is determined by the birth attendant. All forceps have a locking mechanism that prevents the blades from compressing the fetal skull. Use of forceps has declined in popularity over recent years because many obstetricians are not trained to use them in residency since they are rarely used in obstetric practice today.

A **vacuum extractor** is a cup-shaped instrument attached to a suction pump used for the extraction of the fetal head (Fig. 21.7). The suction cup is placed against the occiput of the fetal head. The pump is used to create negative pressure (suction) of approximately 50 to 60 mm Hg. The birth attendant then applies traction until the fetal head emerges from the vagina.

The indications for the use of either method are similar and include a prolonged second stage of labor, a distressed FHR pattern, failure of the presenting part to fully rotate and descend in the pelvis, limited sensation, and inability to push effectively due to the effects of regional anesthesia, presumed fetal jeopardy or fetal distress, maternal heart disease, acute pulmonary edema, intrapartum infection, maternal fatigue, or infection. There is a clear trend to choose vacuum extraction over forceps to assist delivery, but the evidence supporting that trend is unconvincing. Recent literature confirms some advantages for forceps (e.g., a lower failure rate but higher maternal pelvic floor injuries) and some disadvantages for vacuum extraction (e.g., increased neonatal injury) depending on the clinical circumstances. Collective evidence between the two operative instruments has led some authorities to recommend the vacuum extractor as the instrument of first choice for operative vaginal births, but the choice of instrument is determined by the health care provider's expertise in using them. The percentage of births delivered by forceps or vacuum extraction in the United States is 0.5% (forceps) and 2.5% (vacuum extraction) (Bernstein & Coggin-Carr, 2024).

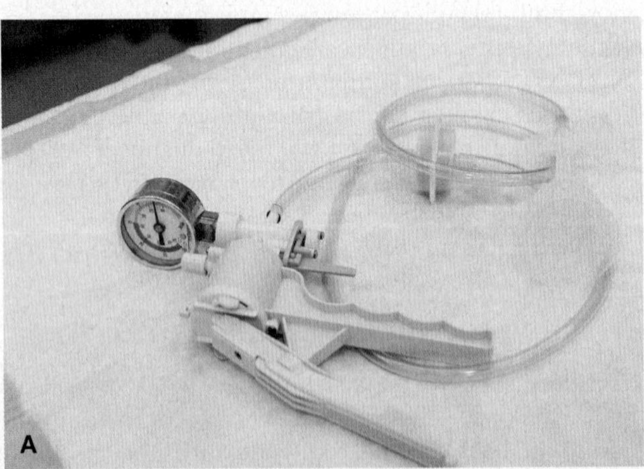

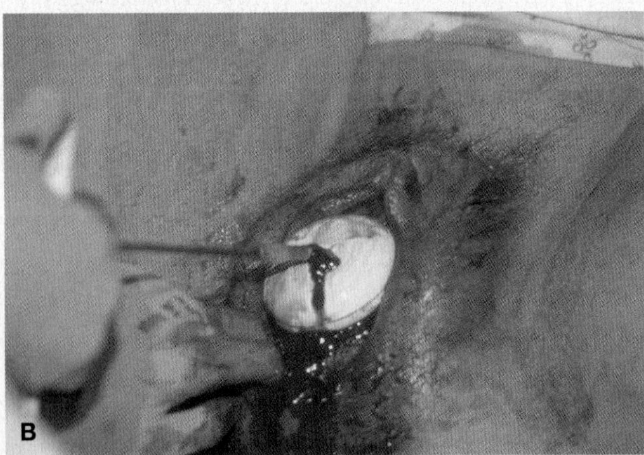

FIGURE 21.7 Vacuum extractor for delivery. **A.** Example of a vacuum extractor. **B.** Vacuum extractor applied to the fetal head to assist in delivery.

The use of forceps or a vacuum extractor poses the risk of tissue trauma to the birthing person and the newborn. Maternal lower genital tract laceration, anal sphincter injury, vulvar and vaginal hematoma, and urinary tract injury may occur. Potential trauma to the newborn includes intracranial or intraventricular hemorrhage ecchymoses, serious facial and scalp lacerations or abrasions, facial nerve injury, cephalohematoma, retinal hemorrhage, facial nerve or brachial plexus injury, and skull fracture (Bernstein & Coggin-Carr, 2024). For forceps or a vacuum extractor to be applied, the following criteria need to be met: membranes ruptured, cervix completely dilated, fetus vertex and engaged, and an adequate maternal pelvis size.

Prevention is the key to reducing the use of these techniques. Preventive measures include frequently changing the patient's position, encouraging ambulation if permitted, frequently reminding the patient to empty their bladder to allow maximum space for birth, and providing adequate hydration throughout labor. Additional measures include assessing maternal vital signs, the contraction pattern, the fetal status, and the maternal response to the procedure. Provide a thorough explanation of the procedure and the rationale for its use. Reassure the birthing person that any marks or swelling on the newborn's head or face will disappear without treatment within 2 to 3 days. Alert the postpartum nursing staff about the use of the technique so that they can observe for any bleeding or infection related to genital lacerations.

Cesarean Birth

A **cesarean birth** is the surgical birth of the fetus through an incision in the abdomen and uterine wall (Fig. 21.8). It is the most commonly performed surgery in the United States, with 30% of infants being born via cesarean birth (Patient Safety Network, 2022). The cesarean birth rate continues to rise despite several medical organizations, including the WHO and ACOG, urging medical care providers to work on lowering the cesarean birth rate (Osterman, 2022).

Cesarean births may result from maternal, fetal, or placental factors that interfere with a vaginal birth. Several factors may explain the increased incidence of cesarean deliveries: the use of electronic fetal monitoring, which identifies fetal distress early; the reduced number of forceps-assisted births; older maternal age and reduced parity; increasing maternal obesity; convenience to the patient and doctor; and an increase in malpractice suits. The leading indications for cesarean births are previous cesarean birth, breech presentation, dystocia, and fetal distress. Once a person has experienced a primary cesarean birth, they have an 85% chance of having another one in a subsequent pregnancy (Stephenson, 2022).

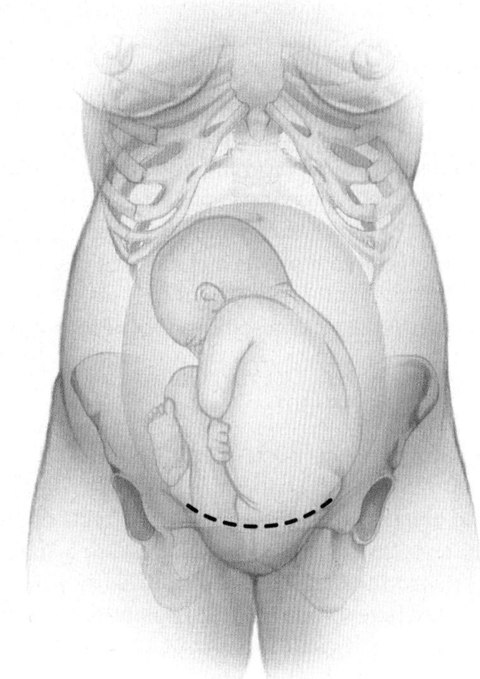

FIGURE 21.8 Low-transverse incision for cesarean birth.

Cesarean birth is a major surgical procedure with increased risks in comparison to a vaginal birth. The patient is at risk for complications such as infection, endometritis, hemorrhage, wound complications, surgical injury, and venous thromboembolism. Fetal injury and transient tachypnea of the newborn may also occur (Berghella, 2024a).

Spinal, epidural, or general anesthesia is used for cesarean births. Epidural anesthesia is most commonly used because it is associated with less risk and most people wish to be awake and aware of the birth experience.

Nursing Assessment

Review the patient's history for indications associated with cesarean birth and complete a physical examination. Any condition that prevents the safe passage of the fetus through the birth canal or that seriously compromises maternal or fetal well-being may be an indication for a cesarean birth. Controversy exists for the option of elective cesarean birth on maternal request. The Agency for Healthcare Research and Quality (AHRQ) has published a report on personal maternal request for a surgical birth, and although there is no high-quality medical evidence to support this, it is recognized that patients have the right to be actively involved in choosing the route of childbirth (Norwitz, 2023). The pregnant person who requests a surgical birth must be made aware of the associated risks and benefits for the current and any subsequent pregnancies. The clinician's role should be to provide the best evidence-based counseling possible to the patient and to respect their autonomy and decision-making capabilities when considering the route of birth.

Examples of specific indications include labor dystocia, active genital herpes, fetopelvic disproportion, prolapsed umbilical cord, placental abnormality (placenta previa or placental abruption), previous classic uterine incision or scar, and untreated human immunodeficiency virus infection. Fetal indications include fetal distress, malpresentation (nonvertex presentation), suspected fetal macrosomia, and multiple gestation (ObG Project, n.d.).

Nursing Management

Once the decision has been made to proceed with a cesarean birth, assess the patient's knowledge of the procedure and necessary preparation. Assist with obtaining diagnostic tests as ordered. These tests are usually ordered to ensure the well-being of both parties and may include a complete blood count; urinalysis to rule out infection; blood type and cross-match so that blood is available for transfusion if needed; an ultrasound to determine fetal position and placental location; and an amniocentesis to determine fetal lung maturity if needed.

Although the nurse's role in a cesarean birth can be technical and skill-oriented at times, the focus must remain on the patient, not the equipment surrounding the bed. Care should be centered on the family, not the surgery. Provide education and minimize separation of the patient, partner, and newborn. Remember that the patient is anxious and concerned about their own welfare as well as that of the child. Use touch, eye contact, therapeutic communication, and genuine caring to provide patients and families with a positive birth experience, regardless of the type of delivery.

PROVIDING PREOPERATIVE CARE

Patient preparation varies depending on whether the cesarean birth is planned or unplanned. The major difference is the time allotted for preparation and teaching. In an unplanned cesarean birth, institute measures quickly to ensure the best outcomes for the pregnant person and fetus. Ensure that the patient has signed an informed consent and allow for discussion of fears and expectations. Provide essential teaching and explanations to reduce the patient's fears and anxieties.

Ascertain the patient's and family's understanding of the surgical procedure. Reinforce the reasons for surgery provided by the surgeon. Outline the procedure and expectations of the surgical experience. Ensure that all diagnostic tests ordered have been completed and evaluate the results. Explain to the patient and family about what to expect postoperatively. Reassure the patient that pain management will be provided throughout the procedure and afterward. Encourage the patient to report any pain. Ask the patient about the time they last had anything to eat or drink. Document the time and what was consumed. Throughout the preparations, assess maternal and fetal status frequently.

Provide preoperative teaching to reduce the risk of postoperative complications. Demonstrate the use of the incentive spirometer and deep breathing and leg exercises. Instruct the patient on how to splint the incision.

Complete preoperative procedures which may include:

- Preparing the surgical site as ordered
- Starting an intravenous infusion for fluid replacement therapy as ordered
- Inserting an indwelling catheter and informing the patient about how long it will remain in place (usually 24 hours)
- Administering any preoperative medications as ordered; documenting the time administered and the patient's reaction

Maintain a calm, confident manner in all interactions with the patient and family. Help transport the patient and partner to the operative area.

PROVIDING POSTOPERATIVE CARE

Postoperative care for the person who has had a cesarean delivery is similar to that for one who has had a vaginal birth with a few additional measures. Assess vital signs and lochia flow every 15 minutes for the first hour, then every 30 minutes for the next hour, and then every 4 hours if stable. Assist with perineal care and instruct the patient in the same. Inspect the abdominal dressing and document description, including any evidence of drainage. Assess uterine tone to determine fundal firmness. Check the patency of the intravenous line and ensure the infusion is flowing at the correct rate. Inspect the infusion site frequently for redness.

Assess the level of consciousness if sedative drugs were administered. Institute safety precautions until the patient is fully alert and responsive. If a regional anesthetic was used, monitor for the return of sensation to the legs.

Assess for evidence of abdominal distention and auscultate bowel sounds. Assist with early ambulation to prevent respiratory and cardiovascular problems and to promote peristalsis. Monitor intake and output at least every 4 hours initially and then every 8 hours as indicated.

Encourage the patient to cough, perform deep breathing exercises, and use the incentive spirometer every 2 hours. Enhance comfort and general well-being. Administer analgesics as ordered and provide comfort measures, such as splinting the incision and pillows for positioning. Assist the patient with moving in bed and turning side to side to improve circulation. Also encourage the patient to ambulate to promote venous return from the extremities.

Assessment of maternal and family adjustment is crucial. The general areas to address during the early postpartum period should include homeostasis, involution, vital signs, bladder function, maternal comfort, initiation of lactation if breastfeeding, review of the birth experience to help the patient process it, and infant care. Encourage early touching and holding of the newborn to promote bonding. Promote family unity and bonding. Assist with breastfeeding initiation and offer continued support. Suggest alternate positioning techniques to reduce incisional discomfort while breastfeeding (see Chapter 18 for breastfeeding positions).

Review with the family their perception of the surgical birth experience. Allow them to verbalize their feelings and assist them in positive coping measures. Promote a positive emotional response to the birth experience and parenting role. Prior to discharge, teach the patient about the need for adequate rest, activity restrictions such as lifting, and signs and symptoms of infection. Provide information about postpartum care at home upon discharge.

PERINATAL LOSS

Pregnancy and childbirth are often associated with hope, expectations, joy, and happiness for the future. **Perinatal loss**, defined as any pregnancy loss and/or neonatal death up to 1 month of age, can be one of the most devastating events a family can experience. In the United States, the perinatal mortality rate is about 5.54 in 1,000 births (Valenzuela et al., 2023). Social determinants associated with perinatal loss include lack of education, poverty, racism, maternity care deserts, overcrowded living conditions, poor sanitation, poor air quality, poor public transportation, lack of employment, malnourishment, and war zones (Girardi, et al., 2023). It continues to be a common occurrence though major advances have taken place in perinatal health care. The prevalence of perinatal death reflects a real possibility that all nurses will meet and care for a family that has experienced the death of a baby.

Perinatal loss encompasses miscarriage, stillbirth, and neonatal deaths. *Miscarriage* is fetal death that occurs before 20 weeks' gestation. It occurs in about 10% of clinically recognized pregnancies (Prager et al., 2024). *Stillbirth* occurs when the fetus dies after 20 weeks' gestation. The cause of stillbirth is often unknown, and it occurs in one of 168 deliveries in the United States (Maslovich & Burke, 2023). *Neonatal death* is the death of the neonate within the first 28 days of life. It occurs in about 5.4 per 1,000 births annually in the United States (Hopkins et al., 2023). Fetal death can occur at any gestational age, and typically there is little or no warning other than reduced fetal movement. Early pregnancy loss may be through a spontaneous abortion (miscarriage), an induced abortion (therapeutic abortion), or a ruptured ectopic pregnancy. Fetal demise can be due to an extensive range of risk factors and possible causes, such as placental abnormalities, diabetes, postterm pregnancy, substance misuse, infection, hypertension, advanced maternal age, multiple gestation, uterine rupture, diabetes, congenital anomalies, obesity, smoking, or it may go unexplained (Maslovich & Burke, 2023). Trauma in pregnancy remains one of the major contributors to maternal and fetal morbidity and mortality. Potential complications include maternal injury or death, shock, internal hemorrhage, direct fetal injury, placental abruption, and uterine rupture. The leading causes of obstetric trauma are motor vehicle crashes, intimate partner violence, falls, assault, and gunshots, and ensuing injuries are classified as blunt abdominal trauma, pelvic fractures, or penetrating trauma. Approximately 7% of all pregnancies in the United States are affected by trauma. In view of the significant impact of trauma on the pregnant person and fetus, preventive strategies are paramount.

The moment fetal death is diagnosed can frequently be described clearly and in detail by most patients. In many instances, the death was sudden, and patients have no chance to prepare for the impending grief. Once fetal demise is confirmed, most people choose to immediately undergo induction of labor. The majority of people will go into spontaneous labor within 1 to 2 weeks of fetal death (Grunebaum & Chervenak, 2023). With the death of a fetus or neonate, a pregnant person's dreams and hopes for the expected child suddenly dissolve. Particularly, experiencing fetal death in the last trimester of pregnancy, when a pregnant person feels very close to the fetus due to its frequent movement in the uterus, can feel similar to losing a part of their own body. For people who have experienced a sudden fetal death, the following processes may take place: experiencing a quiet birth without the infant, eclipsed by emptiness, anger, anxiety, loneliness, and sorrow; living without the infant, making it difficult to see others with young infants; and experiencing differences with their partner over the loss (Weir, 2022). Grief, the typical response to the loss of a valued person or object, is not an intellectual response. Rather, it is personally experienced as a deep emotion of sadness and sorrow. Feelings such as helplessness, disbelief, unreality, and powerlessness are common. Societal expectations may limit the timeline of grief, implying the bereaved should be able to "move on" from grief, but the duration and nature of grief are unique to each person. The process of grieving a death is not completed within a specific time frame, and for some, it is never complete. Perinatal loss is a transformative experience, and the emotions accompanying it can be intense and complex with parents moving through these emotions differently, eventually accepting the reality of the loss while maintaining a healthy connection to the fetus/infant. The grief process may be ongoing for quite some time, and depression or anxiety may occur in the parent (Donegan et al., 2023).

The period following a fetal death is extremely difficult for the family. For many, emotional healing takes much longer than physical healing. The feelings of loss can be intense. The grief response in some people may be so great that their relationships become strained, and healing can become hampered unless appropriate interventions and support are provided.

Fetal death also affects the health care staff. Despite the trauma that the loss of a fetus causes, some staff members avoid dealing with the bereaved family, never talking about or acknowledging their grief. This seems to imply that not discussing the problem will allow the grief to dissolve and vanish. As a result, the family's needs go unrecognized. Failing to keep the lines of communication open with a bereaved patient and family closes off some of the channels to recovery and healing that may be desperately needed. Subsequently, the bereaved family members may feel isolated. It is important to remember that nurses have the responsibility of facilitating a healthy transition from a healthy pregnancy to nonviable pregnancy or fetal demise. Nurses who have the honor of walking alongside families experiencing perinatal loss must remember that each moment in the journey matters and sensitive communication is needed (Berry & Capuano, 2024).

Nursing Assessment

A person experiencing fetal demise is likely to seek care when they notice that the fetus is not moving or when they experience contractions, loss of fluid, or vaginal bleeding. History and physical examination frequently are of limited value in the diagnosis of fetal death since many times the only history tends to be recent absence of fetal movement and no fetal heartbeat heard. An inability to obtain fetal heart sounds on examination suggests fetal demise, but an ultrasound is necessary to confirm the absence of fetal cardiac activity. Once fetal demise is confirmed, induction of labor or expectant management is offered.

Fetal loss impacts family dynamics and the social environment of the parents. It can cause serious health problems due to the significant presence of anxiety and depression that follows, even leading to posttraumatic stress disorder (PTSD) (Fernández-Ordoñez et al., 2021). Nurses need to understand the psychological evolution of couples experiencing perinatal loss without falling into preconceived ideas about the influence of gender, cultures, and settings. For example, after pregnancy loss, men can also experience high levels of grief that require acknowledgment and validation from nurses. In short, meet the family where they are in the grieving process and support them from there.

Nursing Management

Up to 60% of bereaved parents exhibit symptoms of depression, anxiety, and PTSD (Berry, 2022). Perinatal loss is associated with PTSD, anxiety, and depression in a subsequent pregnancy (Berry, 2022). The nurse can play a major role in assisting the grieving family. Those who can deal honestly with their own feelings regarding loss will be better able to help others cope with theirs. Nurses who are aware of their personal feelings about loss and how these feelings are part of their lives and personal belief systems are best able to help grieving families. By working with couples who have suffered a significant loss, the nurse can grow personally and professionally and gain a deeper perspective on life. With skillful intervention, the bereaved family may be better prepared to resolve their grief and move forward. The nurse's continued presence and availability can provide emotional support and comfort for the patient and family. The patient and family can be encouraged to view, touch, and hold the deceased newborn and allow as much time as needed for this. Parent–newborn interaction is vital to the normal processes of attachment and bonding. The detachment process involved in a newborn's death is equally important for parents. Nurses can aid in this process by helping parents see their newborn through the maze of equipment, explaining the various procedures and equipment, encouraging them to express their feelings about the newborn's status, and providing time for them to be with their dying newborn.

Openness to talking with families about their loss and grief is the basis for support provided by nurses, which can have a positive influence on the long-term adjustment of couples and families coping with perinatal loss. Families need to talk about their loss, its meaning, and the emotions that accompany it while the nurse listens. A nurse's willingness to sit quietly and observe, to remain open and nonjudgmental, and to explore what might be helpful is a useful strategy to bridge cultural differences. Statements such as "Help me understand how your family cares for someone who is dying" or "What would be important for me to know about how best to care for your baby's body?" convey a nurse's willingness to learn what is most important to each family. Parents' answers may help guide nurses in providing culturally appropriate care for diverse populations (Hopkins et al., 2023).

TAKE NOTE!

Include the partner in planning and decision making after experiencing perinatal loss to acknowledge the partner has also lost a newborn and will need time to express feelings of loss and receive the nurse's support. Remembering that grieving is individual helps the nurse support each person at their own pace.

In a time of crisis or loss, people are often more sensitive to other people's reactions. For example, the parents may be extremely aware of the nurse's facial expressions, choice of words, and tone of voice. Talking quickly in a businesslike fashion or ignoring the loss may inhibit parents from discussing their pain or how they are coping with it. Parents may need to vent their frustrations and anger, and the nurse may become the target. Validate their feelings and attempt to reframe or refocus the anger toward the real issue of loss. An example would be to say, "I understand your frustration and anger about this situation. You have experienced a tremendous loss and it must be difficult not to have an explanation for it at this time." Doing so helps to defuse the anger while allowing them to express their feelings.

When assisting bereaved parents, start where the parents are in the grief process to avoid imposing your own agenda on them. You may feel uncomfortable at not being able to change the situation or take the pain away. However, giving families some sense of control in an otherwise hopeless situation can provide some comfort. Some ideas to provide them with a sense of control include:

- Ask the family who they wish to have present as the infant dies.
- Give the family a choice of rooms in which they can say goodbye to their infant.
- Provide privacy for the family during this time period by placing a sign on the door.
- Unless requested, the family should never be left to handle their emotions alone.
- Respect a family's wishes if they refuse to be with their infant during the dying process or afterward. Everyone grieves differently (Qian et al., 2022).

Comforting the family after the infant's death is vital to giving them a sense of closure and starting the healing process. Table 21.3 highlights other appropriate interventions for a family experiencing a perinatal loss before and after a newborn dies.

TABLE 21.3 • Assisting Parents With Coping With Perinatal Loss

Before the newborn's death	Respect variations in the family's spiritual needs and readiness. Assess cultural beliefs and practices that may bring comfort; respect culturally appropriate requests for truth telling and informed refusal. Initiate spiritual comfort by calling the hospital clergy if appropriate; offer to pray with the family if appropriate. Encourage the parents to take photographs, make memory boxes, and record their thoughts in a journal. Explore with family members how they dealt with previous losses. Discuss techniques for reducing stress, such as meditation and relaxation. Recommend that family members maintain a healthy diet and get adequate rest and exercise to preserve their health. Participate in early and repeated care conferencing to reduce family stress. Allow family to be present at both medical rounds and resuscitation; provide explanations of all procedures, treatments, and findings; answer questions honestly and as completely as possible. Provide opportunities for the family to hold the newborn if they choose to. Assess the family's support network. Provide suggestions as to how friends can be helpful to the family.
After the newborn's death	Help the family accept the reality of death by using the word "died." Acknowledge their grief and the fact that their newborn has died. Help the family work through their grief by validating and listening. Provide the family with realistic information about the causes of death. Offer condolences to the family in a sincere manner. Encourage the family to cry and grieve with the birthing parent. Provide opportunities for the family to hold the newborn if they desire.
At the time of the release of the newborn's body	Reassure the family that their feelings and grieving responses are normal. Encourage the parents to have a funeral or memorial service to bring closure. Assist the parents with the funeral arrangements or disposition of the body. Suggest the parents plant a tree or flowers to remember the infant. Address attachment issues concerning subsequent pregnancies. Provide information about local support groups, such as SHARE Pregnancy and Infant Loss Support, Inc., which is designed for those who have lost an infant through abortion, miscarriage, fetal death, stillbirth, or any tragic circumstances. Provide anticipatory guidance regarding the grieving process. Present information about any impact on future childbearing and refer the parents to appropriate specialists or genetic resources. Provide the parents with brochures offering advice about how to talk to any siblings about the loss. Make community referrals to a bereavement counselor, peer support group, or mental health professional to promote a continuum of care after discharge.
After the family is discharged	Send the family a card from the nursing staff signed by all who worked with the infant within a week of leaving the hospital. Attend the funeral to allow for a public goodbye and to support others in their time of loss. Provide the family with a memory box, which might contain an outfit worn by their infant, a blanket used to cover their infant, a lock of hair, a card with hand and footprints, a photo with someone holding the infant, etc. Remember their infant at various anniversaries by sending a card or calling the family to see how they are doing. Donate to a charity such as March of Dimes in memory of the infant.

Berry, S. N. (2022). The trauma of perinatal loss: A scoping review. *Trauma Care, 2*(3), 392–407. https://doi.org/10.3390/traumacare2030032; Hopkins, M., Davies, H., Hennessy, K., & Barry, M. (2023). Perinatal bereavement. *American Nurse Journal, 18*(2), 13–16. https://www.myamericannurse.com/perinatal-bereavement/; and Roberts, L. R., Sarpy, N. L., Peters, J., Nick, J. M., & Tamares, S. (2021). Bereavement care immediately after perinatal loss in health care facilities: A scoping review protocol. *JBI Evidence Synthesis, 20*(3), 860–866. https://doi.org/10.11124/jbies-21-00053

Nurses are a vital part of the interdisciplinary health care team caring for families who have experienced perinatal loss and continue to require timely and sensitive care throughout the grieving process. Being present during this traumatic event for families is challenging. Serving infants and their families by bearing witness to their pain and grief is a special privilege. Being present for the family with compassion, comfort, support, and resources during their time of loss is truly an honorable gesture. Nurses can help parents navigate the feelings and numerous grief-related issues that occur as a consequence of the loss, with the nurse serving as the expert guide (Berry & Capuano, 2024). Nurses are remembered years later for their kindness and guidance of the family members through this adverse event with dignity.

NONTRADITIONAL FAMILIES

Increasing acceptance of a broad definition of the term family highlights the need for nurses to provide holistic care. There are a growing number of nontraditional families in the world. If one considers family forms cross-nationally, a variety of configurations exist. Awareness requires nurses to shift away from heteronormative thinking when caring for the childbearing family. Nurses must be adequately educated about lesbian, gay, bisexual, transgender, queer, intersex, and asexual (LGBTQIA+) health issues to be empathetic and conscious of the needs of this population. With increasing numbers of LGBTQIA+ couples wanting children and the availability of alternative methods of conception, nurses are helping these families navigate the birthing process. LGBTQIA+ families may face making complex childbearing decisions, navigating a health care system designed for heterosexual couples, and confronting barriers such as insurance issues, negative attitudes from health care workers, and uncertain legal rights. It is essential for nurses to create a culture of inclusion through appropriate communication and respect as well as a nonjudgmental approach. They need to endorse quality care to all people regardless of sexual orientation or gender identity. It is paramount that nurses promote equitable care to pregnant people of any background (Croll et al., 2022).

Like any other population, the LGBTQIA+ population is not a homogeneous group, and people are shaped by a range of factors including race, sexual orientation, ethnicity, socioeconomic status, and age. This community has traditionally been marginalized in American society. Nurses caring for LGBTQIA+ patients need to facilitate them in expressing their own identities, values, and beliefs. Every patient should be treated with kindness and an individualized approach, and the nurse must be an advocate for every patient's needs. Nurses need to consider using appropriate language, identification, and cultural representation by asking patients how they wish to be identified and by personalizing care that includes all intersecting aspects of identity. Cultivating an environment of inclusion and acceptance makes patients more comfortable and more likely to seek health care (Ferreira et al., 2022).

KEY CONCEPTS

- Risk factors for dystocia include epidural analgesia, occiput posterior position, longer first stage of labor, nulliparity, short maternal stature, high birth weight, maternal age older than 35 years, gestational age more than 41 weeks, chorioamnionitis, pelvic contractions, macrosomia, and high station at complete cervical dilation.
- Dystocia may result from problems in the expulsive forces; fetal presentation, position, and development; the maternal bony pelvis or birth canal; or psychological maternal stress.
- Problems involving the powers that lead to dystocia include hypertonic uterine dysfunction, hypotonic uterine dysfunction, and precipitous labor.
- Management of hypertonic labor pattern involves therapeutic rest with the use of sedatives to promote relaxation and stop the abnormal activity of the uterus.
- Any presentation other than occiput or a slight variation of the fetal position or size increases the probability of dystocia.
- A multifetal pregnancy may result in dysfunctional labor due to uterine overdistention, which may lead to hypotonic dystocia and abnormal presentations of the fetuses.
- During labor, evaluation of fetal descent, cervical effacement and dilation, and characteristics of uterine contractions are paramount to determine progress or lack thereof.
- Antepartum assessment for a postterm pregnancy typically includes daily fetal movement counts done by the patient, nonstress tests done twice weekly, amniotic fluid assessments as part of the biophysical profile, and weekly cervical examinations to check for ripening for induction.
- Once the cervix is ripe, oxytocin is the most popular pharmacologic agent used for inducing or augmenting labor.
- Generally, the first and most reliable symptom of uterine rupture is fetal distress.
- AFE is a rare but often fatal event characterized by the sudden onset of hypotension, hypoxia, and coagulopathy.
- Cesarean births have steadily risen in the United States; today, approximately one in three births occurs this way. It is a major surgical procedure and has increased risks when compared to vaginal birth.
- Nurses working with parents experiencing a perinatal loss can help by actively listening, understanding the parents' experiences, and communicating empathy.

REFERENCES AND RECOMMENDED READINGS

Abramowicz, J. S., & Ahn, J. T. (2024). Fetal macrosomia. *UpToDate*. Retrieved May 10, 2024, from https://www.uptodate.com/contents/fetal-macrosomia

Akanmode, A. M., & Mahdy, H. (2023). Macrosomia. *StatPearls*. https://www.ncbi.nlm.nih.gov/books/NBK557577/

Allen, R. H., & Allen, E. D. G. (2023). Shoulder dystocia. *Medscape*. https://emedicine.medscape.com/article/1602970-overview#a2

American College of Obstetricians and Gynecologists. (2021). Prediction and prevention of spontaneous preterm birth: ACOG practice bulletin, number 234. *Obstetrics & Gynecology, 138*, e65–e90. https://doi.org/10.1097/AOG.0000000000004479

American College of Obstetricians and Gynecologists. (2023). *Counseling regarding approach to delivery after cesarean and the use of a vaginal birth after cesarean calculator (reaffirmed 2023)*. https://www.acog.org/clinical/clinical-guidance/practice-advisory/articles/2021/12/counseling-regarding-approach-to-delivery-after-cesarean-and-the-use-of-a-vaginal-birth-after-cesarean-calculator

Ananth, C. V., & Kinzler, W. L. (2023). Acute placental abruption: Pathophysiology, clinical features, diagnosis, and consequences. *UpToDate*. Retrieved May 10, 2024, from https://www.uptodate.com/contents/acute-placental-abruption-pathophysiology-clinical-features-diagnosis-and-consequences

Anderson-Bagga, F. M., & Sze, A. (2023). Placenta previa. *StatPearls*. https://www.ncbi.nlm.nih.gov/books/NBK539818/

Argani, C. H., & Satin, A. J. (2023). Occiput posterior position. *UpToDate*. Retrieved May 10, 2024, from https://www.uptodate.com/contents/occiput-posterior-position

Arnold, M. J. (2022). Predicting and preventing preterm birth: Recommendations from ACOG. *American Family Physician, 106*(3), 337–339. https://www.aafp.org/pubs/afp/issues/2022/0900/practice-guidelines-preventing-preterm-birth.html

Arnolds, D. E. (2023). Recognition and management of amniotic fluid embolism: A critical role for anesthesia professionals on labor and delivery. *Anesthesia Patient Safety Foundation, 37*(3). https://www.apsf.org/article/recognition-and-management-of-amniotic-fluid-embolism-a-critical-role-for-anesthesia-professionals-on-labor-and-delivery/

Baker, B., & Hurst, H. E. (2024). Labor and delivery at risk. In B. J. Baker, J. Janke, & Association of Women's Health, Obstetric and Neonatal Nurses, *Core curriculum for maternal-newborn nursing* (6th ed.). Elsevier.

Bakker, R. (2023). Placenta previa. *Medscape*. https://emedicine.medscape.com/article/262063-overview#a5

Baldisseri, M. R., & Clark, S. L. (2023). Amniotic fluid embolism. *UpToDate*. Retrieved May 8, 2024, from https://www.uptodate.com/contents/amniotic-fluid-embolism

Basit, H., Ali, C. D. M., & Madhani, N. B. (2023). Erb palsy. *StatPearls*. https://www.ncbi.nlm.nih.gov/books/NBK513260/

Berghella, V. (2024a). Cesarean birth: Postoperative care, complications, and long-term sequelae. *UpToDate*. Retrieved May 9, 2024, from https://www.uptodate.com/contents/cesarean-birth-postoperative-care-complications-and-long-term-sequelae

Berghella, V. (2024b). Short cervix before 24 weeks: Screening and management in singleton pregnancies. *UpToDate*. Retrieved May 9, 2024, from https://www.uptodate.com/contents/short-cervix-before-24-weeks-screening-and-management-in-singleton-pregnancies

Bernstein, I. M., & Coggin-Carr, D. (2024). Assisted (operative) vaginal birth: Overview. *UpToDate*. Retrieved May 9, 2024, from https://www.uptodate.com/contents/operative-vaginal-birth

Berry, S. N. (2022). The trauma of perinatal loss: A scoping review. *Trauma Care, 2*(3), 392–407. https://doi.org/10.3390/traumacare2030032

Berry, S. N., & Capuano, R. (2024). *Foundational course: Healthcare professionals*. Institute of Reproductive Grief Care. https://education.reproductivegrief.org/home.aspx?pagename=ext_product_lp&PID=96538

Botezatu, R., Gica, N., Peltecu, G., & Panaitescu, A. M. (2022). Umbilical cord prolapse—Interesting CTG traces. *Diagnostics, 12*(11). https://doi.org/10.3390/diagnostics12112845

Boushra, M., Stone, A., & Rathbun, K. M. (2023). Umbilical cord prolapse. *StatPearls*. https://www.ncbi.nlm.nih.gov/books/NBK542241/

Care, A., Nevitt, S. J., Medley, N., Donegan, S., Good, L., Hampson, L., Smith, C. T., & Alfirevic, Z. (2022). Interventions to prevent spontaneous preterm birth in women with singleton pregnancy who are at high risk: Systematic review and network meta-analysis. *British Medical Journal, 376*, e064547. https://doi.org/10.1136/bmj-2021-064547

Chasen, S. T. (2023). Twin pregnancy: Overview. *UpToDate*. Retrieved May 8, 2024, from https://www.uptodate.com/contents/twin-pregnancy-overview

Chen, J., Shen, H., Chen, Y. T., Chen, C.-H., Lee, K.-H., & Torng, P.-L. (2022). Experience in different modes of delivery in twin pregnancy. *PLoS One, 17*(3), e0265180. https://doi.org/10.1371/journal.pone.0265180

Chung, S., Alshowaikh., K., Yacoel, T., Chadha, K., & Francis, A. P. (2022). Precipitous delivery complicated by uterine artery laceration and uterine rupture in an unscarred uterus: A case report. *Case Reports in Women's Health, 36*, e00433. https://doi.org/10.1016/j.crwh.2022.e00433

Croll, J., Sanapo, L., & Bourjeily, G. (2022). LGBTQ+ individuals and pregnancy outcomes: A commentary. *BJOG: An International Journal of Obstetrics & Gynaecology, 129*(10), 1625–1629. https://doi.org/10.1111/1471-0528.17131

Cunningham, F. G., Leveno, K. J., Dashe, J. S., Hoffman, B. L., Spong, C. Y., & Casey, B. M. (2022). Abnormal labor. In F. G. Cunningham, K. J. Leveno, J. S. Dashe, B. L. Hoffman, C. Y. Spong, & B. M. Casey, *William's obstetrics* (26th ed.). McGraw Hill.

Dike, N. O., & Ibine, R. (2023). Hypotonic labor. *StatPearls*. https://www.ncbi.nlm.nih.gov/books/NBK564403/

Donegan, G., Noonan, M., & Bradshaw, C. (2023). Parents experiences of pregnancy following perinatal loss: An integrative review. *Midwifery, 121*, 103673. https://doi.org/10.1016/j.midw.2023.103673

Duncan, A. F., Malleske, D. T., & Maitre, N. L. (2022). Use of antenatal corticosteroids for risk of preterm birth—Is timing everything? *JAMA Pediatrics, 176*(6), e220480. https://doi.org/10.1001/jamapediatrics.2022.0480

Ehsanipoor, R. M., & Satin, A. J. (2023). Labor: Overview of normal and abnormal progression. *UpToDate*. Retrieved May 10, 2024, from https://www.uptodate.com/contents/labor-overview-of-normal-and-abnormal-progression

Evbuomwan, O., & Chowdhury, Y. S. (2023). Physiology, cervical dilation. *StatPearls*. https://www.ncbi.nlm.nih.gov/books/NBK557582/

Fernández-Ordoñez, E., González-Cano-Caballero, M., Guerra-Marmolejo, C., Fernández-Fernández, E., & García-Gámez, M. (2021). Perinatal grief and post-traumatic stress disorder in pregnancy after perinatal loss: A longitudinal study protocol. *International Journal of Environmental Research and Public Health, 18*(6), 2874. https://doi.org/10.3390/ijerph18062874

Ferreira, E. P. P., Fernandes, M. F. S. F., Braganca, R. A. P., & Maceiras, M. (2022). Midwife's interventions to promote positive experiences for female homosexual couples during pregnancy: A scoping review. *Journal of Nursing Education and Practice, 12*(9), 54–62. https://doi.org/10.5430/jnep.v12n9p54

Fischer, R., & Modena, A. B. (2022). Breech presentation. *Medscape*. https://emedicine.medscape.com/article/262159-overview

Frey, H., & Landon, M. B. (2024). Uterine rupture: After previous cesarean birth. *UpToDate*. Retrieved May 10, 2024, from https://www.uptodate.com/contents/uterine-rupture-after-previous-cesarean-birth

Funai, E. F. (2022). Patient education: Preterm labor (beyond the basics). *UpToDate*. Retrieved May 8, 2024, from https://www.uptodate.com/contents/preterm-labor-beyond-the-basics

Galerneau, F. (2023). Face and brow presentations in labor. *UpToDate*. Retrieved May 10, 2024, from https://www.uptodate.com/contents/face-and-brow-presentations-in-labor

Gill, P., Lende, M. N., & Van Hook, J. W. (2023). Induction of labor. *StatPearls*. https://www.ncbi.nlm.nih.gov/books/NBK459264/

Girardi, G., Longo, M., & Bremer, A. A. (2023). Social determinants of health in pregnant individuals from underrepresented, understudied, and underreported populations in the United States. *International Journal of Equity in Health, 22*(1), 186. https://doi.org/10.1186/s12939-023-01963-x

Goldberg, A. E. (2023). Cervical ripening. *Medscape*. https://emedicine.medscape.com/article/263311-overview

Grant, G. J., & Reale, S. (2024). Pharmacologic management of pain during labor and delivery. *UpToDate*. Retrieved May 10, 2024, from https://www.uptodate.com/contents/pharmacologic-management-of-pain-during-labor-and-delivery

Grobman, W. (2024a). Induction of labor: Techniques for preinduction cervical ripening. *UpToDate*. Retrieved May 9, 2024, from https://www.uptodate.com/contents/induction-of-labor-techniques-for-preinduction-cervical-ripening

Grobman, W. (2024b). Induction of labor with oxytocin. *UpToDate*. Retrieved May 9, 2024, from https://www.uptodate.com/contents/induction-of-labor-with-oxytocin

Grunebaum, A., & Chervenak, F. A. (2023). Stillbirth: Maternal care and prognosis. *UpToDate*. Retrieved May 10, 2024, from https://www.uptodate.com/contents/stillbirth-maternal-care-and-prognosis

Habak, P. J., & Kole, M. (2023). Vaginal birth after cesarean delivery. *StatPearls*. https://www.ncbi.nlm.nih.gov/books/NBK507844/

Hayes, E. J. (2023). Triplet pregnancy. *UpToDate*. Retrieved May 8, 2024, from https://www.uptodate.com/contents/triplet-pregnancy

Hill, D. A., Lense, J., & Roepcke, F. (2020). Shoulder dystocia: Managing an obstetric emergency. *American Family Physician, 102*(2), 84–90. https://www.aafp.org/dam/brand/aafp/pubs/afp/issues/2020/0715/p84.pdf

Hofmeyr, G. J. (2023). Overview of breech presentation. *UpToDate*. Retrieved May 10, 2024, from https://www.uptodate.com/contents/overview-of-breech-presentation

Hopkins, M., Davies, H., Hennessy, K., & Barry, M. (2023). Perinatal bereavement. *American Nurse Journal, 18*(2), 13–16. https://www.myamericannurse.com/perinatal-bereavement/

Hoyert, D. L. (2022). *Maternal mortality rates in the United States, 2020*. https://www.cdc.gov/nchs/data/hestat/maternal-mortality/2020/maternal-mortality-rates-2020.htm

Kissler, K., & Hurt, K. J. (2022). The pathophysiology of labor dystocia: Theme with variations. *Reproductive Sciences, 30*(3), 729–742. https://doi.org/10.1007/s43032-022-01018-6

Kruit, H., Nupponen, I., Heinonen, S., & Rahkonen, L. (2022). Comparison of delivery outcomes in low-dose and high-dose oxytocin regimens for induction of labor following cervical ripening with a balloon catheter: A retrospective observational cohort study. *PLoS One, 17*(4), e0267400. https://doi.org/10.1371/journal.pone.0267400

Lockwood, C. J. (2024). Preterm labor: Clinical findings, diagnostic evaluation, and initial treatment. *UpToDate*. Retrieved May 8, 2024, from https://www.uptodate.com/contents/preterm-labor-clinical-findings-diagnostic-evaluation-and-initial-treatment

Lockwood, C. J., & Russo-Stieglitz, K. (2024). Placenta previa: Management. *UpToDate*. Retrieved May 10, 2024, from https://www.uptodate.com/contents/placenta-previa-management

Lothian, J. (2024). Normal childbirth. In B. J. Baker, J. Janke, & Association of Women's Health, Obstetric and Neonatal Nurses, *Core curriculum for maternal-newborn nursing* (6th ed.). Elsevier.

Mahdy, H., Glowacki, C., & Eruo, F. U. (2023). Amniotomy. *StatPearls*. https://www.ncbi.nlm.nih.gov/books/NBK470167/

Mandy, G. T. (2022). Preterm birth: Definitions of prematurity, epidemiology, and risk factors for infant mortality. *UpToDate*. Retrieved May 9, 2024, from https://www.uptodate.com/contents/preterm-birth-definitions-of-prematurity-epidemiology-and-risk-factors-for-infant-mortality

Mandy, G. T. (2023). Overview of the long-term complications of preterm birth. *UpToDate*. Retrieved May 9, 2024, from https://www.uptodate.com/contents/overview-of-the-long-term-complications-of-preterm-birth

Maslovich, M. M., & Burke, L. M. (2023). Intrauterine fetal demise. *StatPearls*. https://www.ncbi.nlm.nih.gov/books/NBK557533/

Mayer, C., & Apodaca-Ramos, I. (2023). Tocolysis. *StatPearls*. https://www.ncbi.nlm.nih.gov/books/NBK562212/

Mazza, G. R., Youssefzadeh, A. C., Klar, M., Kunze, M., Matsuzaki, S., Mandelbaum, R. S., Ouzounian, J. G., & Matsuo, K. (2022). Association of pregnancy characteristics and maternal mortality with amniotic fluid embolism. *JAMA Network Open, 5*(11), e2242842. https://doi.org/10.1001/jamanetworkopen.2022.42842

Metz, T. D. (2024). Choosing the route of delivery after cesarean birth. *UpToDate*. Retrieved May 9, 2024, from https://www.uptodate.com/contents/choosing-the-route-of-delivery-after-cesarean-birth

Norwitz, E. R. (2023). Cesarean birth on patient request. *UpToDate*. Retrieved May 9, 2024, from https://www.uptodate.com/contents/cesarean-birth-on-patient-request

Norwitz, E. R. (2024). Postterm pregnancy. *UpToDate*. Retrieved May 9, 2024, from https://www.uptodate.com/contents/postterm-pregnancy

ObG Project. (n.d.). *Safe prevention of the primary cesarean delivery*. https://www.obgproject.com/2022/12/13/safe-prevention-of-the-primary-cesarean-delivery/

Olsen, N. S., & Karjane, N. W. (2022). Abnormal labor. *Medscape*. https://emedicine.medscape.com/article/273053-overview

Osterman, M. J. K. (2022). Changes in primary and repeat cesarean delivery: United States, 2016–2021. *Vital Statistics Rapid Release, 21*. https://www.cdc.gov/nchs/data/vsrr/vsrr021.pdf

Osterman, M. J. K., Hamilton, B. E., Martin, J. A., Driscoll, A. K., & Valenzuela, C. P. (2024). Births: Final data for 2022. *National Vital Statistics Reports, 73*(2). https://doi.org/10.15620/cdc:145588

Oyelese, Y., & Vintzileos, A. M. (2024). Placental abruption. *BMJ Best Practice*. https://bestpractice.bmj.com/topics/en-us/1117

Patient Safety Network. (2022). *A statewide collaborative to support vaginal birth and reduce unnecessary cesarean deliveries*. https://psnet.ahrq.gov/innovation/statewide-collaborative-support-vaginal-birth-and-reduce-unnecessary-cesarean-deliveries

Prager, S., Micks, E., & Dalton, V. K. (2024). Pregnancy loss (miscarriage): Terminology, risk factors, and etiology. *UpToDate*. Retrieved May 10, 2024, from https://www.uptodate.com/contents/pregnancy-loss-miscarriage-terminology-risk-factors-and-etiology

Qian, J., Chen, S., Jevitt, C., Sun, S., Wang, M., & Yu, X. (2023). Experiences of obstetric nurses and midwives receiving a perinatal bereavement care training programme: A qualitative study. *Frontiers in Medicine, 15*(10), 1122472. https://doi.org/10.3389/fmed.2023.1122472

Rantala, A., Hakala, M., & Polkki, T. (2022). Women's perceptions of pain assessment and non-pharmacological pain relief methods using during labor: A cross-sectional survey. *European Journal of Midwifery, 6*, 21. https://doi.org/10.18332/ejm/146136

Ringer, S. (2023). Postterm infant. *UpToDate*. Retrieved May 9, 2024, from https://www.uptodate.com/contents/postterm-infant

Roberts, L. R., Sarpy, N. L., Peters, J., Nick, J. M., & Tamares, S. (2021). Bereavement care immediately after perinatal loss in health care facilities: A scoping review protocol. *JBI Evidence Synthesis, 20*(3), 860–866. https://doi.org/10.11124/jbies-21-00053

Sanni, K.-R., Eeva, E., Noora, S. M., Laura, K. S., Linnea, K., & Hasse, K. (2022). The influence of maternal psychological distress on the mode of birth and duration of labor: Findings from the FinnBrain Birth Cohort Study. *Archives of Women's Mental Health, 25*, 463–472. https://doi.org/10.1007/s00737-022-01212-0

Simpson, K. R., & O'Brien-Abel, N. (2021). Labor and birth. In K. R. Simpson, P. A. Creehan, N. O'Brien-Abel, C. K. Roth, & A. J. Rohan (Eds.), *AWHONN's perinatal nursing* (5th ed.). Lippincott Williams & Wilkins.

Smith, J. F., & Wax, J. R. (2024). Uterine rupture: Unscarred uterus. *UpToDate*. Retrieved May 9, 2024, from https://www.uptodate.com/contents/uterine-rupture-unscarred-uterus

Stephenson, J. (2022). Rate of first-time cesarean deliveries on the rise in the US. *JAMA Health Forum, 3*(7), e222824. https://doi.org/10.1001/jamahealthforum.2022.2824

Togioka, B. M., & Tonismae, T. (2023). Uterine rupture. *StatPearls*. https://www.ncbi.nlm.nih.gov/books/NBK559209/

UpToDate, Inc. (2024). *UpToDate® Lexidrug™* (Version 8.2.0) [Mobile app]. Wolters Kluwer. https://apps.apple.com/us/app/lexicomp/id313401238

U.S. Department of Health and Human Services. (2020). *Healthy People 2030: Objectives and data: Browse objectives by topic: Infants*. https://health.gov/healthypeople/objectives-and-data/browse-objectives/infants

Valenzuela, C. P., Gregory, E. C. W., & Martin, J. A. (2023). Perinatal mortality in the United States, 2020–2021. *National Center for Health Statistics Data Brief, 489*. https://www.cdc.gov/nchs/products/databriefs/db489.htm

Vrees, R. A., & Kelly, B. (2023). Induction of labor. *Medscape*. https://emedicine.medscape.com/article/2500091-overview

Weeks, A. D., Lightly, K., Mol, B. W., Frohlich, J., Pontefract, S., & Williams, M. J. (2022). Evaluating misoprostol and mechanical methods for induction of labor. *BJOG: An International Journal of Obstetrics & Gynaecology, 129*(8), e61–e65. https://doi.org/10.1111/1471-0528.17136

Weir, L. F. (2022). *Perinatal loss: Policy updates and best practices*. https://www.dhaj7-cepo.com/sites/default/files/course/2022-02/S04_Presentation.pdf

Wheeler, V., Hoffman, A., & Bybel, M. (2022). Cervical ripening and induction of labor. *American Family Physician, 105*(2), 177–186. https://www.aafp.org/pubs/afp/issues/2022/0200/p177.html

World Health Organization. (2022). *WHO recommendations on induction of labour, at or beyond term*. https://www.who.int/publications/i/item/9789240052796

Wormer, K. C., Bauer, A., & Williford, A. E. (2023). Bishop score. *StatPearls*. https://www.ncbi.nlm.nih.gov/books/NBK470368/

DEVELOPING CLINICAL JUDGMENT

PRACTICING FOR NCLEX

1. When reviewing the medical record of a patient, the nurse notes that the patient has a condition in which the fetus cannot physically pass through the maternal pelvis. How does the nurse interpret this?
   a. Cervical insufficiency
   b. Contracted pelvis
   c. Maternal disproportion
   d. Fetopelvic disproportion

2. Active infection during pregnancy places the patient and fetus at risk. For which active infection would the nurse anticipate a cesarean birth?
   a. Hepatitis
   b. Herpes simplex virus
   c. Toxoplasmosis
   d. Human papillomavirus

3. After a vaginal examination, the nurse determines that the patient's fetus is in an occiput posterior position. Based on this assessment, what does the nurse anticipate the patient will have?
   a. Intense back pain
   b. Frequent leg cramps
   c. Nausea and vomiting
   d. A precipitous birth

4. The nurse is caring for four patients. Which patient would the nurse identify as being at the greatest risk for preterm labor?
   a. Person who had twins in a previous pregnancy
   b. Patient living in a large city close to the subway
   c. Person working full-time as a computer programmer
   d. Patient with a history of a previous preterm birth

5. The nurse has administered prostaglandin gel for a patient prior to the induction of labor. What does the nurse teach the patient the gel is for?
   a. Stimulation of uterine contractions
   b. Numbing cervical pain receptors
   c. Preventing cervical lacerations
   d. Softening and effacing the cervix

6. A patient who is in active labor and whose cervix had dilated to 6 cm experiences a weakening in the intensity and frequency of contractions and exhibits no further progress in labor. How does the nurse interpret this assessment?
   a. Hypertonic labor
   b. Precipitous labor
   c. Hypotonic labor
   d. Dysfunctional labor

7. The nurse is developing a plan of care for a patient experiencing dystocia. Which nursing intervention would be the highest priority?
   a. Changing the patient's position frequently
   b. Providing comfort measures to the patient
   c. Monitoring the FHR patterns
   d. Keeping the patient and family informed of the labor progress

8. The nurse is caring for a patient experiencing hypertonic uterine dystocia. The contractions are erratic in their frequency, duration, and of high intensity. What is the priority nursing intervention?
   a. Encourage ambulation every 30 minutes.
   b. Provide pain relief measures.
   c. Monitor the oxytocin infusion rate closely.
   d. Prepare the patient for an amniotomy.

9. The nurse is caring for a patient at 25 weeks' gestation with contractions. The Bishop score is completed. What is the Bishop score used to assess?
   a. Presence of bacterial vaginosis
   b. Amount of amniotic fluid present
   c. Overall fetal well-being in labor
   d. Cervical readiness for induction

CRITICAL THINKING EXERCISES

1. A 26-year-old multipara is admitted to the labor and birth suite in active labor. After a few hours, the nurse notices a change in their contraction pattern—poor contraction intensity and no progression of cervical dilatation beyond 7 cm. The patient keeps asking about labor progress and appears anxious about "how long this labor is taking."
   a. Based on the nurse's findings, what might be happening?
   b. How can the nurse address the patient's anxiety?
   c. What are the appropriate interventions to change this labor pattern?

2. The patient activates the call light and states, "I feel increased wetness down below."
   a. What might be occurring?
   b. How will the nurse confirm the suspicions?
   c. What interventions are appropriate for this finding?

STUDY ACTIVITIES

1. Visit the SHARE Pregnancy and Infant Loss Support, Inc., website and assess its helpfulness to parents.

2. Outline the fetal and maternal risks associated with a prolonged pregnancy.

3. An abnormal or difficult labor describes ____________.

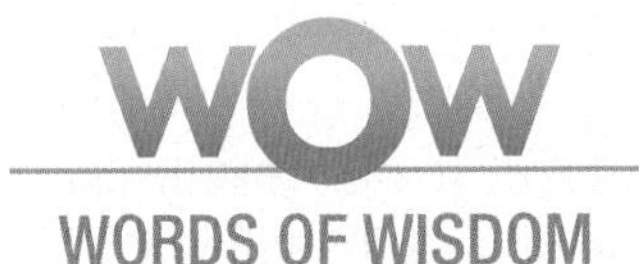

WORDS OF WISDOM

Nurses should remain vigilant and observant throughout the childbirth experience all the way through the discharge of the childbearing family.

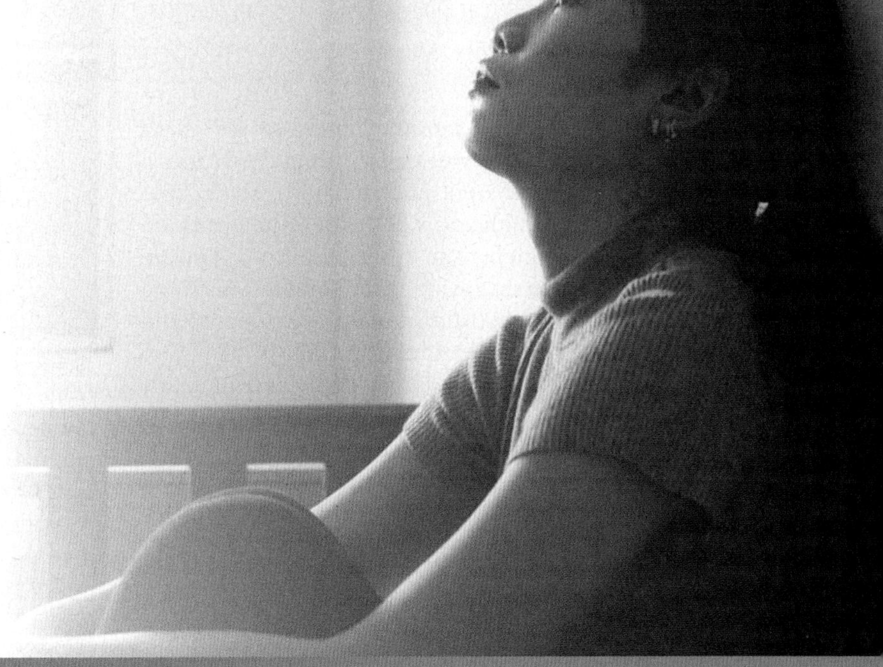

22

Nursing Management of the Postpartum Patient at Risk

LEARNING OBJECTIVES

Upon completion of the chapter, you will be able to:

1. Examine the major conditions that place the postpartum patient at risk.
2. Analyze the risk factors, assessment, preventive measures, and nursing management of common postpartum complications.
3. Differentiate the causes of postpartum hemorrhage (PPH) based on the underlying pathophysiologic mechanisms.
4. Outline the nurse's role in assessing and managing the care of a patient with a thromboembolic condition.
5. Characterize the nursing management of a patient who develops a postpartum infection.
6. Compare and contrast affective disorders that can occur in patients after birth, describing specific therapeutic management for each.

Joan gave birth about an hour ago to her fifth baby boy, who weighed 10 lb, and she is resting in bed when the nurse comes in to assess her. She tells the nurse that she feels like there is "something really wet" between her legs. She also feels a bit lightheaded. What would the nurse suspect is happening? What findings would support the nurse's suspicion? What should the nurse do first?

KEY TERMS

endometritis (en'dō-mē-trī'tis)
mastitis (mas-tī'tis)
postpartum depression (PPD)
postpartum hemorrhage (PPH)
uterine atony (yū'tĕr-in at'ŏ-nē)

INTRODUCTION

The postpartum period is the culmination of the childbearing experience. The weeks following birth are a critical period for the parent and newborn, setting the stage for long-term health and well-being. Numerous adaptations and adjustments must be made to assimilate the newborn into the established family unit. It is a time designed for patient recovery, family attachment, and new role development. The American College of Obstetricians and Gynecologists (ACOG, 2021) recommends that health care providers have contact with new parents within the first 3 weeks postpartum, previously 6 weeks, and provide ongoing care with a comprehensive visit no later than 12 weeks after birth. Typically, recovery from childbirth progresses without complications, both physiologically and psychologically. The postpartum body faces significant changes in the weeks and months following childbirth. It is a time filled with many transformations and wide-ranging emotions, and the new parent commonly experiences a great sense of accomplishment. However, they can also experience deviations from health, developing postpartum conditions that can place them at risk. These high-risk conditions or complications can become life-threatening (see the Healthy People 2030 Box). About 52% of maternal deaths occur in the postpartum period (within 1 year following childbirth) and up to 70,000 females experience severe postpartum morbidities including cardiovascular events, kidney failure, postpartum depression (PPD), anxiety, and posttraumatic stress disorder (Agency for Healthcare Research and Quality [AHRQ], 2022). This chapter addresses the nursing management of the most common conditions that place the postpartum patient at risk: hemorrhage, thromboembolic disease, infections, and postpartum affective disorders.

HEALTHY PEOPLE 2030

Objective	Nursing Significance
Reduce maternal deaths.	• Focus on thorough risk assessments for potential infections and postpartum hemorrhage in the postpartum period.

Healthy People Objectives retrieved from http://www.healthypeople.gov

POSTPARTUM HEMORRHAGE

Postpartum hemorrhage (PPH) is a potentially life-threatening complication that can occur after both vaginal and cesarean births. The incidence of PPH in the United States has been increasing (Escobar et al., 2022). It is the leading cause of maternal death worldwide, with PPH resulting in 70,000 annual maternal deaths globally (World Health Organization, 2022). In the United States, about 11.4% of maternal deaths are attributed to PPH annually (Smith, 2022). Blood loss that occurs within 24 hours of birth is termed primary (immediate or early) PPH; blood loss that occurs 24 hours to 12 weeks after birth is termed secondary (delayed or late) PPH (Belfort, 2024).

PPH is defined by ACOG as a cumulative blood loss greater than 1,000 mL with signs and symptoms of hypovolemia within 24 hours of the birth process, regardless of the route of delivery (Escobar et al., 2022). Morbidity from PPH can be severe, with sequelae including organ failure, shock, thrombosis, acute respiratory distress, and anemia. Some patients undergo hysterectomy or experience abdominal compartment syndromes (Belfort, 2024). As with many other sources of perinatal harm, a delay in recognition and diagnosis may lead to delayed treatment and a poorer patient outcome (Smith, 2022).

Pathophysiology

Excessive bleeding can occur at any time between the separation of the placenta and its expulsion or removal. The most common cause of PPH is **uterine atony**, failure of the uterus to contract and retract after birth; it causes 80% of PPH cases (Belfort, 2024). The uterus must remain contracted after birth to control bleeding from the placental site. Risk factors for uterine atony include:

- Prior PPH
- Chorioamnionitis
- Fibroids
- Labor induction or augmentation
- Therapeutic use of magnesium sulfate
- Uterine overdistention (macrosomia, multiple gestation, polyhydramnios)
- Uterine inversion
- Previous blood transfusion for PPH (Belfort, 2024)

In addition to problems with uterine tone, other causes of PPH may be related to trauma (laceration, episiotomy, surgical birth, genital or rectal hematoma), tissue problems (retained placental fragments, placenta previa, placenta accreta, uterine inversion), and thrombin issues (history of coagulopathy such as von Willebrand disease, thrombotic thrombocytopenic purpura, and disseminated intravascular coagulation [DIC]) (Belfort, 2024). Additionally, strong traction placed on the umbilical cord to expel the placenta can result in cord detachment from the placenta or uterine inversion, resulting in a massive hemorrhage.

Therapeutic Management

Uterine atony may be managed with fundal massage and uterotonic medications. Bimanual uterine compression may also be needed. For patients who are hemodynamically unstable, fluid resuscitation and blood transfusion are necessary. In some instances, uterine or hypogastric artery embolization or other surgical interventions are needed (Belfort, 2023).

Nursing Assessment

The period after birth and the first hours postpartum are crucial times for the prevention, assessment, and management of bleeding. Compared with other maternal risks such as infection, bleeding can rapidly become life-threatening, and nurses, along with other health care providers, need to identify this condition quickly and intervene appropriately.

Begin by reviewing the patient's history, including labor and birth history, for risk factors associated with PPH. Assess the patient's vital signs, noting trends over time. During pregnancy, maternal blood volume increases as much as 50%. The majority of birthing parents are generally healthy, allowing for initial blood loss without alteration in vital signs. Dizziness, palpitations, and tachycardia may occur with compensated shock (Smith, 2022).

Since the most common cause of immediate severe PPH is uterine atony, assess uterine tone after birth by palpating the fundus for firmness and location. The uterus is expected to be firm, with bright red bleeding. A soft, boggy fundus indicates uterine atony. Assess the current amount of bleeding. Keep in mind that accurate determination of blood loss is difficult because of blood pooling inside the uterus and on peripads, mattresses, and the floor. Continue to note the estimated blood loss occurring throughout the delivery.

TAKE NOTE!

A soft, boggy uterus that deviates from the midline suggests that a full bladder is interfering with uterine involution. If the uterus is not in the correct position (midline), it will not be able to contract to control bleeding.

Assess the perineal area and any surgical site for hematomas, which may require surgical treatment. Most hematomas arise from bleeding lacerations related to operative deliveries. Observe for a localized bluish bulging area just under the skin surface in the perineal area (Fig. 22.1). Often the patient will report severe perineal or pelvic pain and will have difficulty voiding.

Inspect the skin and mucous membranes for gingival bleeding or petechiae and ecchymoses. Check venipuncture sites for oozing or prolonged bleeding. These findings might suggest coagulopathy as a cause of PPH. Also assess the amount of lochia, which would be much greater than usual. Signs of shock do not appear until hemorrhage is far advanced due to the increased fluid and blood volume of pregnancy. Clinical manifestations of shock resulting from blood loss are outlined in Table 22.1.

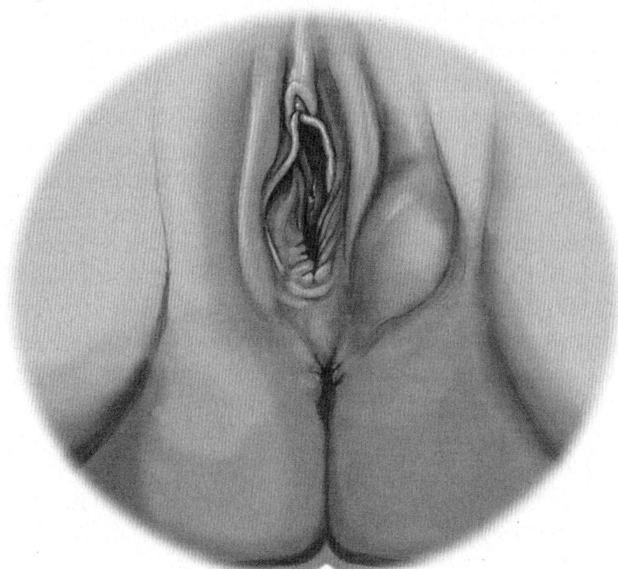

FIGURE 22.1 Perineal hematoma. Note the bulging swollen mass.

Nursing Management

PPH is a serious complication of pregnancy that is often unanticipated. Even with prompt aggressive management, postpartum bleeding can quickly evolve into a life-threatening event. Perinatal nurses are often the first to observe significant postpartum bleeding, and their prompt initial response and continued assessments are pivotal in the anticipation and coordination of necessary interventions. Multidisciplinary team support is critical because obstetric caregivers need a full array of medical and surgical strategies to manage intractable bleeding. Because all postpartum patients are at risk for hemorrhage, nurses need to possess the knowledge and skills to practice active management of the third stage of labor to prevent hemorrhage and to recognize, assess, and respond rapidly to excessive blood loss in their patients.

TABLE 22.1 • Clinical Manifestations of Shock Due to Blood Loss

Degree of Shock	Blood Volume Loss	Signs and Symptoms
Mild	15%–25%	Diaphoresis, weakness, tachycardia, slight fall in blood pressure
Moderate	25%–35%	Pallor, restlessness, oliguria, moderate fall in blood pressure
Severe	35%–50%	Hypotension (marked fall in blood pressure), agitation/confusion, hemodynamic instability, anuria

Smith, J. R. (2022). Postpartum hemorrhage. *Medscape*. https://emedicine.medscape.com/article/275038-overview#

When excessive bleeding is encountered, initial management steps are aimed at improving uterine tone: immediate fundal massage, administration of uterotonic medications, and intravenous (IV) fluid resuscitation. If these methods fail to control bleeding, additional resources are mobilized and more aggressive interventions such as bimanual compression, internal uterine packing, and/or balloon tamponade techniques are employed by the health care provider. Other potential causes of bleeding should be thoroughly explored, and laboratory tests such as a complete blood count, type and cross-match, and coagulation studies should be obtained immediately. Transfusion of blood products should be instituted without hesitation for ongoing blood loss or estimated loss in excess of 2,000 mL (Smith, 2022). Hysterectomy is a last-resort lifesaving measure for uterine bleeding that does not stop.

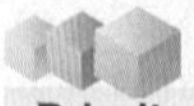

Concept Mastery Alert

Priority Intervention for Uterine Atony

Before initiating fundal massage, the nurse must first place a hand over the symphysis pubis to anchor the uterus and prevent possible uterine inversion.

Massaging the Uterus

Massage the uterus if uterine atony is noted. The uterine muscles are sensitive to touch; massage stimulates the muscle fibers to contract. Massage the boggy uterus to stimulate contractions and expression of any accumulated blood clots while supporting the lower uterine segment. As blood pools in the vagina, stasis of blood causes clots to form. These clots need to be expelled as pressure is placed on the fundus. Note, however, that overly forceful massage can tire the uterine muscles, resulting in further uterine atony and increased pain. See Nursing Procedure 22.1 for steps in massaging the fundus.

Administering a Uterotonic Drug

Administer a prescribed uterotonic drug if repeated fundal massage and expression of clots fail. Such medication is probably needed to contract the uterus in order to control bleeding from the placental site. The injection of a uterotonic drug immediately after birth is a first-line therapy and an important intervention used to prevent PPH. Oxytocin (Pitocin), misoprostol (Cytotec), dinoprostone (Prostin E2), methylergonovine maleate (Methergine), a derivative of prostaglandin (PGF2α), and carboprost (Hemabate) are drugs used to manage PPH (see Drug Guide 22.1). However, misoprostol is not approved by the U.S. Food and Drug Administration (FDA) for this purpose. The choice of which uterotonic drug to use for the management of bleeding depends on the judgment of the health care provider, the availability of drugs, and the risks and benefits of the drug.

Maintaining the Primary Intravenous Infusion

Maintain the primary IV infusion and be prepared to start a second infusion at another site if blood transfusions

NURSING PROCEDURE 22.1 Massaging the Fundus

Purpose: To Promote Uterine Contraction

1. After explaining the procedure to the patient, place one gloved hand on the area above the symphysis pubis (this helps support the lower uterine segment).
2. Place the other gloved hand (usually the dominant hand) on the fundus.
3. With the hand on the fundus, gently massage the fundus in a circular manner. Be careful not to overmassage the fundus, which could lead to muscle fatigue and uterine relaxation.
4. Assess for uterine firmness (uterine tissue responds quickly to touch).
5. If firm, apply gentle yet firm pressure in a downward motion toward the vagina to express any clots that may have accumulated.
6. Do not attempt to express clots until the fundus is firm because the application of firm pressure on an uncontracted uterus could cause uterine inversion, leading to massive hemorrhage.
7. Assist the patient with perineal care and applying a new perineal pad.
8. Remove gloves and wash hands.

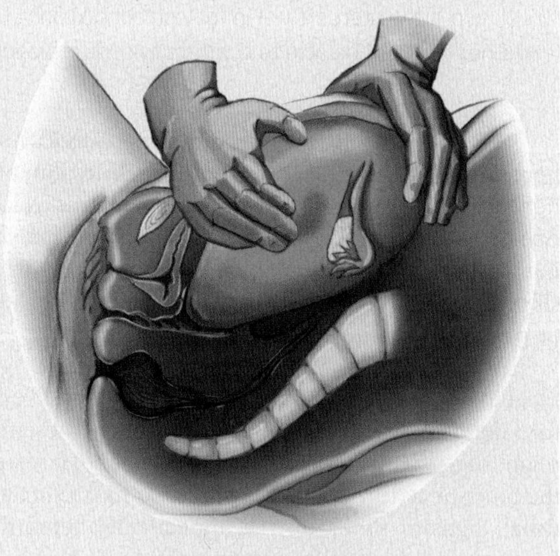

DRUG GUIDE 22.1

DRUGS USED TO CONTROL POSTPARTUM HEMORRHAGE

Drug	Action/Indication	Nursing Implications
Oxytocin (Pitocin) first-line therapy	Stimulates the uterus to contract/to contract the uterus to control bleeding from the placental site 10–40 units in a liter IV or 10 units IM	Assess the fundus for evidence of contraction and compare the amount of bleeding every 15 minutes or according to orders. Monitor vital signs every 15 minutes. Monitor uterine tone to prevent hyperstimulation. Reassure the patient about the need for uterine contraction and administer analgesics for comfort. Offer explanation to the patient and family about what is happening and the purpose of the medication. Provide nonpharmacologic comfort measures to assist with pain management. Set up the IV infusion to be piggybacked into a primary IV line. This ensures that the medication can be discontinued readily if hyperstimulation or adverse effects occur while maintaining the IV site and primary infusion. Contraindications: Never give undiluted as a bolus injection IV.
Misoprostol (Cytotec)	Stimulates the uterus to contract/to reduce bleeding; a prostaglandin analogue 600–1,000 mcg PR, PO, or SL	As above. Not FDA approved for this indication, but an effective drug therapy for acute postpartum hemorrhage Contraindications: allergy, active cardiovascular disease, pulmonary or hepatic disease; use with caution in patients with asthma.
Dinoprostone (Prostin E2)	20-mg vaginal or rectal suppository May be repeated every 2 hours	Monitor blood pressure frequently since hypotension is a frequent side effect along with vomiting and diarrhea, nausea, and temperature elevation.
Methylergonovine maleate (Methergine)	Stimulates the uterus to prevent and treat postpartum hemorrhage due to atony or subinvolution 0.2-mg IM injection May be repeated in 5 minutes Thereafter, every 2–4 hours	Assess baseline bleeding, uterine tone, and vital signs every 15 minutes or according to protocol. Offer explanation to the patient and family about what is happening and the purpose of the medication. Monitor for possible adverse effects, such as hypertension, seizures, uterine cramping, nausea, vomiting, and palpitations. Report any complaints of chest pain promptly. Contraindication: hypertension
Prostaglandin (PGF2α), Carboprost (Hemabate)	Stimulates uterine contractions/to treat postpartum hemorrhage due to uterine atony when not controlled by other methods 250-mcg IM injection May be repeated every 15–90 minutes up to eight doses	Assess vital signs, uterine contractions, patient's comfort level, and bleeding status as per protocol. Offer explanation to the patient and family about what is happening and the purpose of the medication. Monitor for possible adverse effects, such as fever, chills, headache, nausea, vomiting, diarrhea, flushing, and bronchospasm. Contraindications: asthma or active cardiovascular disease
Tranexamic acid (TXA)	Stimulates uterine contractions to reduce bleeding when not controlled by the first-line therapy of oxytocin Antifibrinolytic drug that prevents bleeding by inhibiting the enzymatic breakdown of fibrin blood clots 1 g in 10 mL (100 mg/mL) to infuse at a rate of 1 mL/min over 10 minutes If bleeding continues after 30 minutes, a second dose of 1 g can be given	Same as above Contraindications: active cardiac, pulmonary, renal, or hepatic disease TXA complements uterotonics, but it is not a substitute. It is a coagulant and antifibrinolytic agent. TXA should not be mixed with blood for transfusion or solutions containing mannitol or penicillin. Monitor for possible adverse effects, such as nasal stuffiness, abdominal discomfort, nausea, vomiting, diarrhea, hypersensitivity or anaphylactic reactions, pulmonary embolism, deep vein thrombosis, cerebral vascular accident, myocardial infarction, or seizures. TXA, administered within 3 hours of birth in addition to standard care, has been shown to significantly reduce maternal death due to PPH by about 30%. The WHO recommends TXA be used as a first-line treatment for PPH as soon as possible after childbirth and no more than 3 hours after childbirth.

FDA, U.S. Food and Drug Administration; IM, intramuscular; IV, intravenous; PO, by mouth; PR, by rectum; SL, sublingually; WHO, World Health Organization.

Belfort, M. A. (2024). Overview of postpartum hemorrhage. *UpToDate*. Retrieved April 27, 2024, from https://www.uptodate.com/contents/overview-of-postpartum-hemorrhage; ObG Project. (2022). *Postpartum hemorrhage—Medications to treat uterine atony.* https://www.obgproject.com/2022/11/01/postpartum-hemorrhage-medications-treat-uterine-atony/; UpToDate, Inc. (2024). *UpToDate Lexidrug* (Version 8.2.0) [Mobile app]. Wolters Kluwer. https://apps.apple.com/us/app/lexicomp/id313401238

are necessary. Draw blood for type and cross-match and send it to the laboratory. Administer oxytocics as ordered, correlating and titrating the infusion rate to assessment findings of uterine firmness and lochia. Assess for visible vaginal bleeding, and count or weigh perineal pads.

Remember Joan, the patient described at the beginning of the chapter? The nurse assesses her and finds that her uterus is boggy. What would the nurse do next? What additional nursing measures might be used if Joan's fundus remains boggy? When should the health care provider be notified?

Checking Vital Signs

Check vital signs every 15 to 30 minutes, depending on the acuity of the patient's health status. Monitor complete blood count to identify any deficit or assess the adequacy of replacement. Assess the patient's level of consciousness to determine changes that may result from inadequate cerebral perfusion.

An indwelling catheter is typically in place to keep the bladder empty to avoid displacement of the uterus. A fundus above the umbilicus and deviated laterally indicates a full bladder and interferes with uterine contractions to slow the bleeding.

Preparing for Removal of Retained Placental Fragments

Prepare the patient for the removal of retained placental fragments. These fragments are usually manually separated and removed by the health care provider. Be sure that the health care provider remains long enough after birth to assess the bleeding status of the patient and determine the etiology. Assist the health care provider with suturing any lacerations immediately to control hemorrhage and repair the tissue.

Nurses should anticipate and prepare the patient for transfer to the operating room for surgical intervention if tamponade techniques fail to achieve hemostasis. The blood bank should be notified that additional transfusions may be required, and the patient's condition should be closely monitored for signs of hypovolemic shock.

Assessing for Signs and Symptoms of Hemorrhagic Shock

Continually assess the patient for signs and symptoms of hemorrhagic shock, the most common form of shock encountered in obstetric practice. Assess the anxiety level of the patient; the patient going into hypovolemic shock is highly anxious and may lose consciousness. The patient's significant others experience a high level of anxiety as well and need a great deal of support.

Monitor the patient's blood pressure, pulse, capillary refill, mental status, and urinary output. These assessments allow estimation of the severity of blood loss and help direct treatment. If the patient develops hemorrhagic shock, interventions focus on controlling the source of blood loss; restoring adequate oxygen-carrying capacity; and maintaining adequate tissue perfusion. Successful treatment depends on efficient collaboration among all health care team members to meet the patient's specific needs.

Be alert for patients with abnormal bleeding tendencies, ensuring that they receive proper diagnosis and treatment. Teach them how to prevent severe hemorrhage by learning how to feel for and massage their fundus when boggy; assisting the nurse in keeping track of the number of and amount of bleeding on perineal pads; and avoiding any medications with antiplatelet activity such as aspirin, antihistamines, or nonsteroidal anti-inflammatory drugs (NSAIDs). Institute measures to avoid tissue trauma or injury, such as giving injections and drawing blood. Also provide emotional support to the patient and their family throughout this critical time by being readily available and providing explanations and reassurance. For the patient with a bleeding disorder or coagulopathy, expect to administer prescribed medications related to the particular disorder. If the patient develops DIC, institute emergency measures to control bleeding and impending shock, and prepare to transfer the patient to the intensive care unit.

TAKE NOTE!

Always remember the five causes of postpartum hemorrhage and the appropriate intervention for each: (1) uterine atony–massage and oxytocics, (2) retained placental tissue–evacuation and oxytocics, (3) lacerations or hematoma–surgical repair, (4) thrombin (bleeding disorders)–blood products, and (5) uterine inversion caused by too much cord traction–gentle replacement of the uterus and oxytocics.

Preventing Postpartum Hemorrhage

Avoid an episiotomy unless an emergency birth is necessary and the perineum is a limiting factor. It is important to have the continuous intrapartum presence of an experienced labor and birth nurse.

Frequent staff education and PPH drills will help keep skills up to date. Nurses must identify anemia and screen for coagulopathies before labor and birth. After birth, it is important to inspect the placenta (once it is delivered) for completeness. Assess the patient for lower genital tract lacerations immediately after birth and re-evaluate the patient's vital signs and vaginal flow after childbirth. Finally, it is important to be aware of the patient's beliefs about blood transfusions. Having a PPH cart and medication kit readily available decreases the time to intervention for patients with PPH, optimizing the team's ability to provide efficient treatment (Kogutt et al., 2022).

An IV oxytocin infusion is started for Joan. What assessments will need to be done frequently to make sure Joan is not losing too much blood? What discharge instructions need to be reinforced with Joan?

VENOUS THROMBOEMBOLIC CONDITIONS

Venous thromboembolism is a potentially serious complication of the postpartum period. It is one of the leading causes of maternal mortality and morbidity, with an annual incidence of 1 per 1,000 pregnancies (Blondon & Skeith, 2022). Activation of the coagulation system, endothelial trauma, and venous stasis all contribute to the high risk during pregnancy. A thrombosis (blood clot within a blood vessel) can cause inflammation of the blood vessel lining (thrombophlebitis), which in turn can lead to thromboembolism (obstruction of a blood vessel by a blood clot carried by the circulation from the site of origin). Thrombi can involve the superficial or deep veins in the legs or pelvis. Superficial vein thrombosis usually involves the saphenous venous system and is confined to the lower leg. Superficial thrombophlebitis may be caused by the use of the lithotomy position during birth. Deep vein thrombosis (DVT) can involve deep veins from the foot to the calf, thighs, or pelvis. Thrombi can dislodge and migrate to the lungs, causing a pulmonary embolism (PE).

DVT is a common condition that can have serious complications. Deep venous thrombi have a high probability of propagating and leading to pulmonary emboli, which may cause chest pain, breathlessness, and sudden death. Thus, an accurate and timely diagnosis of DVT is imperative. Although DVT is often clinically silent, it may present with a number of signs, including calf pain, edema, and venous distention.

The three most common venous thromboembolic conditions occurring during the postpartum period are superficial vein thrombosis, DVT, and PE. Although venous thromboembolic disorders occur in less than 1% of all postpartum patients, pulmonary embolus can be fatal if a clot obstructs the lung circulation; thus, early identification and treatment are paramount. Risk for postpartum venous thromboembolism is highest during the first few weeks after childbirth with risk declining by 12 weeks postpartum. Patients who have a cesarean birth or experience postpartum hemorrhage are at highest risk (Berens, 2024).

Pathophysiology

Thrombus formation typically results from venous stasis, injury to the innermost layer of the blood vessel, and hypercoagulation related to pregnancy. Both venous stasis and hypercoagulation are common in the postpartum period.

If a clot dislodges and travels to the pulmonary circulation, PE can occur. When the clot is large enough to block one or more of the pulmonary vessels that supply the lungs, it can result in sudden death. Approximately 900,000 DVTs and PEs occur yearly in the United States, resulting in 60,000 to 100,000 deaths (Centers for Disease Control and Prevention [CDC], 2023). Sudden death may be the first symptom in 25% of people who have PE (CDC, 2023). Many deaths due to PE are unrecognized, and the diagnosis is often made during autopsy. The diagnosis of PE should always be considered in any postpartum patient who presents with dyspnea or chest pain (Thompson et al., 2024). A national review of severe obstetric complications found a significant increase in the rate of PE associated with the increasing rate of cesarean births and obesity. Adequate treatment of thrombotic events in pregnancy with heparin (unfractionated or low molecular weight) is important to prevent the progression of thrombosis to the development of PE (Springel & Mahotra, 2022) (see Evidence-Based Practice 22.1).

Nursing Assessment

Assess the patient closely for risk factors and signs and symptoms of thrombophlebitis. Look for risk factors in the patient's history such as use of oral contraceptives before the pregnancy; smoking; employment that necessitates prolonged standing; history of thrombosis; thrombophlebitis or endometritis; or evidence of current varicosities. Also look for other factors that can increase a patient's risk, such as prolonged bed rest, PPH, diabetes, obesity, cesarean birth, progesterone-induced distensibility of the veins of the lower legs during pregnancy, severe anemia, varicose veins, a history of any prior VTE, age older than 34 years, and multiparity. The likelihood of thrombophlebitis is increased through most of pregnancy and for approximately 12 weeks after childbirth. This is partly due to increased platelet stickiness and partly due to reduced fibrinolytic activity.

Ask the patient if they have pain or tenderness in the lower extremities. Suspect superficial vein thrombosis in a patient with varicose veins who reports tenderness and discomfort over the site of the thrombosis, most commonly in the calf area. The area appears reddened along the vein and is warm to the touch. The patient will report increased pain in the affected leg when ambulating and bearing weight.

Manifestations of DVT are often absent and diffuse. If present, they are caused by an inflammatory process and obstruction of venous return. DVT is more common in the left lower extremity, presumably due to compression of the left iliac artery. Calf swelling and tenderness, difference in leg circumference, erythema, warmth,

EVIDENCE-BASED PRACTICE **22.1**

Venous Thromboembolism Prophylaxis in Pregnancy: Are We Adequately Identifying and Managing Risks?

BACKGROUND

Pregnancy is a risk factor for venous thromboembolism (VTE). Deep vein thrombosis (DVT) is a blood clot that forms in a vein deep in the body, usually in the leg. People who have one or more of the following risk factors are at a particularly high risk of developing DVT and pulmonary embolisms (PEs): reduced mobility, obesity, history of surgery (cesarean section), history of previous DVT, and the hypercoagulable state of pregnancy. The symptoms of DVT are pain and swelling in the leg, though it can be without symptoms as well. A blood clot caused by DVT can move from the legs to the lungs, putting the patient in danger of developing PE or even dying. In the postpartum period, the risk for developing VTE is 15 times greater when compared to the risk during the prenatal period. VTE is preventable, and it is paramount that risk assessments be done to identify those at great risk and apply appropriate preventive measures.

STUDY

The purpose of this study was to assess adherence to the guidelines for the identification of risk factors of VTE and their management. This was a retrospective review of medical notes for a cohort of 82 female patients.

Nursing Implications

Prevention of VTE can be achieved through thoroughly documented and continuing risk factor assessments. The proper documentation of all risk factors will allow for the optimal early identification and management of potential DVT risks. The nurse should complete risk assessments for DVT at the patient's first prenatal visit and then continuously throughout the pregnancy and postpartum periods. Compression stockings should be recommended to all patients at high risk of developing DVT to reduce exacerbation of varicose veins. Nurses should make this recommendation to all high-risk patients and explain the reasoning behind the recommendation. This intervention works and should be carried out to reduce the incidence of this medical condition in patients who are in high-risk categories.

Adapted from Choy, K. R., Emmett, S., & Wong, A. (2022). Venous thromboembolism prophylaxis in pregnancy: Are we adequately identifying and managing risks? *Australian and New Zealand Journal of Obstetrics and Gynecology, 62*(6), 915–920. https://doi.org/10.1111/ajo.13579

tenderness, pain with calf pressure, and pedal edema may be noted. Be alert for signs and symptoms of PE, including unexplained sudden onset of shortness of breath and severe chest pain. The patient may be apprehensive and diaphoretic. Additional manifestations may include calf or thigh pain and/or edema, cough, hemoptysis, orthopnea, or wheezing (Thompson et al., 2024).

TAKE NOTE!

PE in the postpartum period is a rare event, yet it is potentially catastrophic. Cardiac arrest occurs in up to 23% of high-risk PE pregnant and postpartum patients (Krawczyk et al., 2023).

Nursing Management

Nursing management focuses on preventing thrombotic conditions; promoting adequate circulation if thrombosis occurs; and educating the patient about preventive measures, anticoagulant therapy, and danger signs. If the patient demonstrates signs and symptoms of PE, prepare the patient for a lung scan to confirm the diagnosis.

Preventing Thrombotic Conditions

Prevention of thrombotic conditions is an essential aspect of nursing management and can be achieved with the routine use of simple measures:

- Prevent venous stasis by encouraging activity that causes leg muscles to contract and promotes venous return (leg exercises and walking).
- Facilitate dorsi/plantar flexion of feet with prolonged sitting to promote venous return.
- Use intermittent sequential compression devices to produce passive leg muscle contractions until the patient is ambulatory.
- Elevate the patient's legs above their heart level to promote venous return.
- Apply compression stockings and remove them daily for inspection of legs.
- Use postoperative deep-breathing exercises to improve venous return by relieving the negative thoracic pressure on leg veins.
- Reduce hypercoagulability with prescribed aspirin or anticoagulation therapy.
- Prevent venous pooling by avoiding pillows under the knees and not crossing the legs for long periods.
- Have the patient avoid sitting or standing in one position for prolonged periods.
- Increase the patient's fluid intake to prevent dehydration (American Heart Association, 2023).

In patients at risk, early ambulation is the easiest and most cost-effective method. Use of compression stockings decreases distal calf vein thrombosis by decreasing venous stasis and augmenting venous return. Patients who are at high risk for thromboembolic disease based on risk factors or a previous history of DVT or PE may be placed on prophylactic anticoagulation therapy during pregnancy. A low-molecular-weight heparin such as enoxaparin (Lovenox) can be given as can rivaroxaban (Xarelto), apixaban (Eliquis), or dabigatran etexilate (Pradaxa) (Blondon & Skeith, 2022). It is typically discontinued during labor and birth and then restarted during the postpartum period.

Promoting Adequate Circulation

The mainstay of venous thromboembolic conditions is anticoagulation, while interventions such as thrombolysis and inferior vena cava filters are reserved for limited circumstances. For the patient with superficial venous thrombosis, administer NSAIDs for analgesia, facilitate rest and elevation of the affected leg, apply warm compresses to the affected area to promote healing, and use antiembolism stockings to promote circulation to the extremities.

Implement bed rest or limited ambulation if ordered and elevation of the affected extremity for the patient with DVT. These actions help reduce interstitial swelling and promote venous return from that leg. Apply antiembolism stockings to both extremities as ordered. Fit the stockings correctly to avoid excess pressure and constriction and urge the patient to wear them at all times. Sequential compression devices can also be used for patients with varicose veins, a history of thrombophlebitis, or a surgical birth.

Anticoagulant therapy using a continuous IV infusion of low-molecular-weight heparin along with vitamin K antagonists is usually initiated to prolong the clotting time and prevent the extension of the thrombosis. Monitor the patient's coagulation studies closely; these might include activated partial thromboplastin time (aPTT), whole-blood partial thromboplastin time, and platelet levels. A therapeutic aPTT value typically ranges from 30 to 40 seconds, depending on which standard values are used (Pagana et al., 2023). Also apply warm, moist compresses to the affected leg and administer analgesics as ordered to decrease the discomfort.

After several days of IV low-molecular-weight heparin therapy, expect to begin oral anticoagulant therapy as ordered. In most instances, the patient will continue to take this medication for several months after discharge.

For the patient who develops a PE, institute emergency measures immediately. The objectives of treatment are to prevent the growth or multiplication of thrombi in the lower extremities, prevent more thrombi from traveling to the pulmonary vascular system, and provide cardiopulmonary support if needed. Administer oxygen via mask or cannula as ordered and initiate IV low-molecular-weight heparin therapy titrated according to the results of the coagulation studies. Maintain the patient on bed rest, and administer analgesics as ordered for pain relief. Be prepared to assist with administering thrombolytic agents, such as alteplase (tPA), which might be used to dissolve pulmonary emboli and the source of the thrombus in the pelvis or deep leg veins, thus reducing the potential for a recurrence.

Educating the Patient

Provide teaching about the use of anticoagulant therapy and danger signs that should be reported (Teaching Guidelines 22.1). Provide anticipatory guidance, support, and education about associated signs of complications and risks.

TEACHING GUIDELINES 22.1 Teaching to Prevent Bleeding Related to Anticoagulant Therapy

- Watch for possible signs of bleeding and notify your health care provider if any occur:
  - Nosebleeds
  - Bleeding from the gums or mouth
  - Black tarry stools
  - Brown "coffee grounds" vomitus
  - Red to brown speckled mucus from a cough
  - Oozing at the incision, episiotomy site, cut, or scrape
  - Pink, red, or brown-tinged urine
  - Bruises, "black and blue marks"
  - Increased lochia discharge (from present level)
- Practice measures to reduce your risk of bleeding:
  - Brush your teeth gently using a soft toothbrush.
  - Use an electric razor for shaving.
  - Avoid activities that could lead to injury, scrapes, bruising, or cuts.
  - Do not use any over-the-counter products containing aspirin or aspirinlike derivatives.
  - Avoid consuming alcohol.
  - Inform other health care providers about the use of anticoagulants, especially dentists.
- Be sure to adhere to follow-up laboratory testing as scheduled.
- If you inadvertently cut or scrape yourself, apply firm direct pressure to the site for 5–10 minutes. Do the same after receiving any injections or having blood specimens drawn.
- Wear an identification bracelet or band that indicates that you are taking an anticoagulant.
- Eliminate modifiable risk factors for DVT (smoking, use of oral contraceptives, a sedentary lifestyle, and obesity).
- Understand the importance of using compression stockings.
- Avoid constrictive clothing and prolonged standing or sitting in a motionless, leg-dependent position.
- Know the danger signs and symptoms (sudden onset of chest pain, dyspnea, and tachypnea) to report to the health care provider.

American College of Obstetricians and Gynecologists. (2022). *Preventing deep vein thrombosis.* https://www.acog.org/womens-health/faqs/preventing-deep-vein-thrombosis; Blondon, M., & Skeith, L. (2022). Preventing postpartum venous thromboembolism in 2022: A narrative review. *Frontiers in Cardiovascular Medicine*, 9. https://doi.org/10.3389/fcvm.2022.886416; and Mithoowani, S. (2022). Patient education: Deep vein thrombosis (DVT) (beyond the basics). *UpToDate*. Retrieved January 17, 2024, from https://www.uptodate.com/contents/deep-vein-thrombosis-dvt-beyond-the-basics

POSTPARTUM GENITOURINARY INFECTIONS

Infection during the postpartum period is a common cause of maternal morbidity and mortality. Overall, postpartum infection is estimated to occur in 5% to 7% of all births and accounts for 10% to 15% of global maternal mortality (Boushra & Rahman, 2023). There is a higher occurrence in cesarean births than in vaginal births. Postpartum fever is defined as a temperature of 100.4°F (38°C) or higher; in the first 24 hours after childbirth, 20% of patients with postpartum fever have a pelvic infection (Cunningham et al., 2022).

Risk factors include surgical birth, prolonged rupture of membranes, prolonged labor, multiple cervical evaluations, presence of intrapartal chorioamnionitis, lower socioeconomic status, bacterial colonization of the lower genital tract with particular organisms, general anesthesia, younger maternal age, nulliparity, obesity, meconium-stained amniotic fluid, and significant hysterotomy extension (Cunningham et al., 2022).

Infections can easily enter the female genital tract externally and ascend through the internal genital structures. Postpartum patients possess an increased risk for infection due to tissue trauma during birth, vulnerability from the placenta separation site, and the incision from cesarean section. In addition, the normal physiologic changes of childbirth increase the risk of infection by decreasing vaginal acidity due to the presence of amniotic fluid, blood, and lochia, all of which are alkaline. An alkaline environment encourages the growth of bacteria. Signs and symptoms of postpartum infection include elevated temperature, general malaise, pain, chills, increased pulse rate, abdominal pain, and malodorous lochia.

Postpartum infections usually arise from organisms that constitute the normal vaginal flora, typically a mix of aerobic and anaerobic species. Generally, they are polymicrobial and involve the following microorganisms: *Staphylococcus aureus, Escherichia coli, Klebsiella, Gardnerella vaginalis,* gonococci, coliform bacteria, group A or B hemolytic streptococci, *Chlamydia trachomatis,* and the anaerobes that are common to bacterial vaginosis. Common postpartum infections include endometritis, surgical site infections, and urinary tract infections (UTIs).

Endometritis

Endometritis is a uterine infection that typically develops within 2 to 4 days postpartum to as late as 6 weeks. It is an infectious condition that involves the endometrium, decidua, and adjacent myometrium of the uterus. Extension of endometritis into the ovaries, fallopian tubes, or pelvic peritoneum is termed pelvic inflammatory disease (Taylor et al., 2023).

The uterine cavity is sterile until the rupture of the amniotic sac. As a consequence of labor, birth, and associated manipulations, anaerobic and aerobic bacteria can contaminate the uterus. In most instances, the bacteria responsible for pelvic infections are those that normally reside in the bowel, vagina, perineum, and cervix, such as *E. coli, Klebsiella pneumoniae,* or *G. vaginalis.*

The risk of endometritis increases dramatically after a cesarean birth; puerperal endometritis is up to 20 times more common in females who underwent cesarean births versus a vaginal birth (Taylor et al., 2023). Standard practice involves one dose of prophylactic antibiotic therapy administered 1 hour before cesarean delivery (Chen, 2024). Once rupture of the amniotic membranes occurs during labor and birth, the uterus becomes more susceptible to colonization and infection, especially if it is a prolonged labor. Any area traumatized during childbirth is susceptible to infection.

When endometritis occurs, broad-spectrum antibiotics are used to treat the infection. Care also includes measures to restore and promote fluid and electrolyte balance, provide analgesia, and provide emotional support. After treatment, the patient's fever usually drops, and their symptoms cease within 48 to 72 hours after the start of antibiotic therapy.

Surgical Site Infections

Any break in the skin or mucous membranes provides a portal for bacteria. Surgical site infections are relatively common following childbirth, complicating up to 7% of cesarean deliveries. They present with erythema, purulent drainage, warmth, and pain at the surgical site (Boushra & Rahman, 2023). In the postpartum patient, sites of wound infection include cesarean surgical incisions, the episiotomy site in the perineum, and genital tract lacerations (Fig. 22.2). Wound infections are usually not identified until the patient has been discharged from the hospital because symptoms may not show up until 24 to 48 hours after birth. Treatment consists of broad-spectrum antibiotics given as soon as the diagnosis is made. The wound may also be opened to allow drainage.

Urinary Tract Infections

UTIs are most commonly caused by bacteria often found in bowel flora, including *E. coli*, *Klebsiella*, *Proteus*, and *Enterobacter* species (Wong & Rosh, 2024). Invasive manipulation of the urethra (e.g., urinary catheterization), frequent vaginal examinations, and genital trauma increase the likelihood of a UTI. Definitive diagnosis is made by a clean-catch urinalysis with culture and sensitivity, revealing the presence of a significant number of bacteria. It is treated with antibiotics.

Nursing Assessment

Perinatal nurses are the primary caregivers for postpartum patients and have a unique opportunity to identify

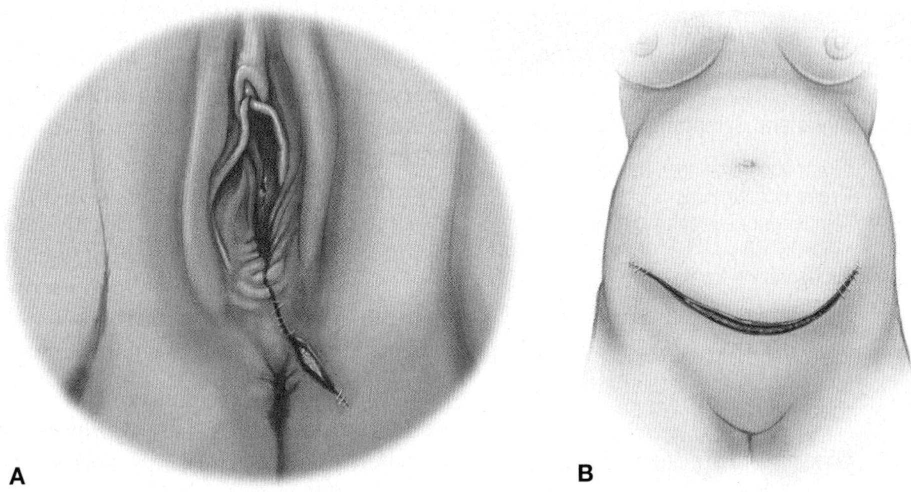

FIGURE 22.2 Postpartum wound infections. **A.** Infected episiotomy site. **B.** Infected cesarean birth incision.

subtle changes that place them at risk for infection. Nurses play a key role in identifying signs and symptoms that suggest a postpartum infection. Today, patients are commonly discharged 24 to 48 hours after giving birth. Therefore, nurses must assess patients for risk factors and identify early, subtle signs and symptoms of an infectious process. Factors that place a patient at risk for a postpartum infection are highlighted in Box 22.1.

Review the patient's history, physical examination, and labor and birth record for factors that might increase their risk for developing an infection. Then complete the assessment (using the "BUBBLE-EE" parameters discussed in Chapter 16), paying particular attention to areas such as the abdomen and fundus, breasts, urinary tract, episiotomy, lacerations, or incisions and being alert for signs and symptoms of infection (Table 22.2).

TAKE NOTE!

A postpartum infection is commonly associated with an elevated temperature. Other generalized signs and symptoms may include chills, foul-smelling vaginal discharge, headache, malaise, restlessness, anxiety, and tachycardia. In addition, the patient may have specific signs and symptoms based on the type and location of the infection.

BOX 22.1 Factors Placing a Patient at Risk for Postpartum Infection

- Prolonged (>18–24 hours) premature rupture of membranes (removes the barrier of amniotic fluid so bacteria can ascend)
- Cesarean birth (allows bacterial entry due to break in protective skin barrier)
- Urinary catheterization (could allow entry of bacteria into the bladder due to break in aseptic technique)
- Regional anesthesia that decreases the perception of the need to void (causes urinary stasis and increases the risk of urinary tract infection)
- Staff attending to patient are ill (promotes droplet infection from personnel)
- Compromised health status, such as anemia, obesity, smoking, and substance use disorder (reduces the body's immune system and decreases the ability to fight infection)
- Preexisting colonization of the lower genital tract with bacterial vaginosis, *Chlamydia trachomatis*, group B streptococci, *Staphylococcus aureus*, and *Escherichia coli* (allows microbes to ascend)
- Retained placental fragments (provides a medium for bacterial growth)
- Manual removal of a retained placenta (causes trauma to the lining of the uterus and thus opens up sites for bacterial invasion)
- Insertion of fetal scalp electrode or intrauterine pressure catheters for internal fetal monitoring during labor (provides entry into the uterine cavity)
- Instrument-assisted childbirth, such as forceps or vacuum extraction (increases risk of trauma to the genital tract, which provides bacteria access to grow)
- Trauma to the genital tract, such as episiotomy or lacerations (provides a portal of entry for bacteria)
- Prolonged labor with frequent vaginal examinations to check progress (allows time for bacteria to multiply and increases potential exposure to microorganisms or trauma)
- Poor nutritional status (reduces body's ability to repair tissue)
- Gestational diabetes (decreases the body's healing ability and provides higher glucose levels on the skin and in urine, which encourages bacterial growth)
- Break in aseptic technique during surgery or birthing process (allows entry of bacteria)

Boushra, M., & Rahman, O. (2023). Postpartum infection. *StatPearls*. https://www.ncbi.nlm.nih.gov/books/NBK560804/; and Taylor, M., Jenkins, S. M., & Pillarisetty, L. S. (2023). Endometritis. *StatPearls*. https://www.ncbi.nlm.nih.gov/books/NBK553124/

TABLE 22.2 • Signs and Symptoms of Postpartum Infections

Postpartum Infection	Signs and Symptoms
Endometritis	Lower abdominal tenderness or pain on one or both sides Temperature elevation (>100.4°F [>38°C]) Foul-smelling lochia Anorexia Nausea Fatigue and lethargy Leukocytosis and elevated sedimentation rate
Wound infection	Weeping serosanguineous or purulent drainage Separation of or unapproximated wound edges Edema Erythema Tenderness Discomfort at the site Fever Elevated white blood cell count
Urinary tract infection	Urgency Frequency Dysuria Flank pain Low-grade fever Urinary retention Hematuria Urine positive for nitrates Cloudy urine with a strong odor

Boushra, M., & Rahman, O. (2023). Postpartum infection. *StatPearls*. https://www.ncbi.nlm.nih.gov/books/NBK560804/; and Chen, K. T. (2024). Postpartum endometritis. *UpToDate*. Retrieved April 28, 2024, from https://www.uptodate.com/contents/postpartum-endometritis

The acronym REEDA is frequently used for assessing the status of the patient's perineum. It is derived from five components that have been identified to be associated with the healing process of the perineum. These include:

1. Redness—area may also feel warm to touch
2. Edema—may indicate infection or a hematoma
3. Ecchymosis—may indicate vaginal trauma
4. Discharge—should follow the expected lochia pattern
5. Approximation of skin edges—should be well aligned without gaps

Each category is assessed and a number is assigned (0 to 3 points) for a total REEDA score ranging from 0 to 15. The higher scores indicate increased tissue trauma. See Figure 22.3 for the REEDA method for assessing perineum healing.

Monitor the patient's vital signs, especially their temperature. Changes may also signal an infection.

Nursing Management

Measures to prevent a UTI include timely removal of urinary catheters used during labor or surgical births, fully emptying the bladder at each voiding, wearing loose clothing that allows airflow to the genital area, avoiding douching, wiping from front to back only, staying hydrated, and using the peribottle after each trip to the bathroom to cleanse the genital area.

Nursing management focuses on preventing postpartum infections. Use the following guidelines to reduce the incidence of postpartum infections:

- Maintain aseptic technique when performing invasive procedures such as urinary catheterization, when changing dressings, and during all surgical procedures.
- Use good hand hygiene before and after each patient care activity.
- Practice standard precautions whenever in contact with blood, body fluids, and excretions.
- Use extreme caution when handling sharp instruments, specimens, and waste disposal.
- Review the patient's history for preexisting infections or chronic conditions.
- Assess frequently for early signs of infection, especially fever and the appearance of lochia.
- Use adequate lighting and turn the patient to the side to assess the episiotomy site and perineum.
- Inspect wounds frequently for inflammation and drainage.
- Encourage rest, adequate hydration, and healthy eating habits.
- Reinforce measures for maintaining good perineal hygiene.
- Screen all visitors for any signs of active infections to reduce the patient's risk of exposure.
- Monitor laboratory results for any abnormal values.
- Reinforce preventive measures during any interaction with the patient.

If the patient develops an infection, administer prescribed antibiotics and provide analgesics for pain management. Review any special care measures, such as dressing changes, that might be needed (Clinical Judgment & Nursing Process 22.1).

Offer postpartum patients anticipatory guidance on the signs and symptoms of life-threatening conditions, including sepsis. Information should include the importance of good hand and perineal hygiene and of the need to seek immediate medical care if feeling unwell. Patient education is a priority due to today's short lengths of stay after childbirth. Some infections may not manifest until after discharge. Review the signs and symptoms of infection, emphasizing the danger signs that need to be reported to the health care provider. Most importantly, stress proper hand hygiene, especially after perineal care

REEDA Method for Assessing Perineum Healing

- **R**edness
  - None = 0 points
  - Redness within .25 cm of incision bilaterally = 1
  - Redness within .5 cm of incision bilaterally = 2
  - Redness reaching beyond .5 cm of incision bilaterally = 3
- **E**dema – the more swelling present, the high the score
  - None = 0 points
  - < 1 cm from incision = 1 point
  - 1-2 cm from incision = 2 points
  - > 2 cm from incision = 3 points
- **E**cchymosis – the more bruising observed, the higher the score
  - None = 0 points
  - 1-2 cm from incision = 1 point
  - .25 cm-1 cm bilaterally or .5-2 cm unilaterally = 2 points
  - > 1 cm bilaterally or 2 cm unilaterally = 3 points
- **D**ischarge – range would be from none present to profuse
  - None = 0 points
  - Serum discharge present = 1 point
  - Serosanguineous discharge present = 2 points
  - Bloody, purulent discharge present = 3 points
- **A**pproximation of skin edges
  - Closed, skin edges approximated well = 0 points
  - Skin separated 3 cm or less = 1 point
  - Skin and subcutaneous fat separated = 2 points
  - Skin, subcutaneous fat and facial separation = 3 points

FIGURE 22.3 REEDA method for assessing perineum healing. (Adapted from Hrelic, D. A., & Griggs, K. M. [2018]. Critically ill obstetric patients. *American Nurse Today*, *13*[11], 20–24.)

CLINICAL JUDGMENT & NURSING PROCESS 22.1 Overview of the Patient With a Postpartum Complication

Jennifer, a 16-year-old G1P1, gave birth to a boy 3 days ago. It was a cesarean birth due to cephalopelvic disproportion following 25 hours of labor with ruptured membranes. Her temperature is 102.6°F (39.2°C). She is complaining of chills and malaise and says, "My incision really hurts." Jennifer rates her pain as 7–8 out of 10. The incision site is red, swollen, and warm to the touch. A 5-cm area of purulent drainage is noted on the dressing; a 3-cm area of the incision is slightly opened, with the wound edges separated. Jennifer's lochia is scant and dark red, with a strong odor. She asks the nurse to take her baby back to the nursery because she doesn't feel well enough to care for him.

NURSING ANALYSIS: Altered thermoregulation related to bacterial invasion as evidenced by fever, complaints of chills and malaise, and statement of not feeling well

OUTCOME IDENTIFICATION AND EVALUATION

The patient will exhibit a return to normothermia as evidenced by a body temperature being maintained below 99°F (37.2°C), reports of a decrease in chills and malaise, and statements of feeling better.

INTERVENTIONS: *Promoting Fever Reduction*

- Assess vital signs every 2–4 hours and record results *to monitor the progress of infection.*
- Administer antipyretics as ordered *to reduce temperature and help combat infection.*
- Encourage fluid intake *to promote fluid balance.*
- Document intake and output *to assess hydration status.*
- Offer a cool bed bath or shower *to reduce temperature.*
- Place a cool cloth on the forehead and/or back of the neck *to provide comfort.*
- Change bed linen and gown when damp from diaphoresis *to provide comfort and hygiene.*

NURSING ANALYSIS: Altered tissue integrity related to wound infection as evidenced by purulent drainage, redness, swelling, and separation of wound edges

OUTCOME IDENTIFICATION AND EVALUATION

The patient will experience a resolution of wound infection as evidenced by a reduction in redness, swelling, and drainage from the wound; absence of purulent drainage; and beginning signs and symptoms of wound healing.

INTERVENTIONS: *Promoting Wound Healing*

- Administer antibiotic therapy as ordered *to treat infection.*
- Perform frequent dressing changes and wound care as ordered *to promote wound healing*; monitor dressing for drainage, including amount, color, and characteristics, *to evaluate for resolution of infection.*
- Use an aseptic technique *to prevent the spread of infection.*
- Encourage fluid intake *to maintain fluid balance;* encourage adequate dietary intake, including protein, *to promote healing.*

NURSING ANALYSIS: Acute pain related to infectious process

OUTCOME IDENTIFICATION AND EVALUATION

The patient will report a decrease in pain as evidenced by a pain rating of 0 or 1 on a pain scale, verbalization of relief with pain management, and statements of feeling better and ability to rest comfortably.

INTERVENTIONS: *Relieving Pain*

- Place patient in semi-Fowler position *to facilitate drainage and relieve pressure.*
- Assess pain level on a pain scale of 0–10 to quantify pain level; reassess pain level after intervening *to determine the effectiveness of intervention.*
- Assess fundus gently *to ensure appropriate involution.*
- Administer analgesics as needed and on time as ordered *to maintain pain relief.*
- Provide for rest periods *to allow for healing.*
- Assist with positioning in bed with pillows *to promote comfort.*
- Offer nonpharmacologic pain measures such as a backrub *to ease aches and discomfort if desired and enhance the effectiveness of analgesics.*

CLINICAL JUDGMENT & NURSING PROCESS 22.1 Overview of the Patient With a Postpartum Complication

NURSING ANALYSIS: Altered parent–infant attachment risk related to effects of postpartum infection as evidenced by birthing parent's request to take the baby back to the nursery

OUTCOME IDENTIFICATION AND EVALUATION

The patient will begin to bond with the newborn appropriately with each exposure as evidenced by a desire to spend time with the newborn, expression of positive feelings toward the newborn when holding him, increasing participation in care of the newborn as the patient's condition improves, and statements about help and support at home to care for self and newborn.

INTERVENTIONS: *Promoting Parent–Newborn Interaction*

- Promote adequate rest and sleep *to ensure adequate energy for interaction and wound healing.*
- Bring the newborn to the birthing parent after they are rested and have had an analgesic *to allow the birthing parent to focus their energies on the child.*
- Progressively allow the patient to care for or comfort the infant as the patient's energy level and pain level improve *to promote self-confidence in caring for the newborn.*
- Offer praise and positive reinforcement for caregiving tasks; stress positive attributes of the newborn to the birthing parent while caring for the infant *to facilitate bonding and attachment.*
- Contact family members to participate in care of the newborn *to allow the birthing parent to rest and recover from infection.*
- Encourage the birthing parent to care for themselves first and then the newborn *to ensure adequate energy for newborn's care.*
- Arrange for assistance and support after discharge from the hospital *to provide necessary backup.*
- Refer to community health nurse for follow-up care of birthing parent and newborn at home *to foster continued development of maternal–infant relationship.*

and before and after breastfeeding. Also reinforce measures to promote breastfeeding, including proper breast care (see Chapter 16). Teaching Guidelines 22.2 highlights the major teaching points for a patient with a postpartum infection.

Mastitis

Mastitis is defined as inflammation of the mammary glands associated with breastfeeding. It may occur any time during lactation but occurs most frequently in the first 4 to 6 weeks of breastfeeding and affects 2% to 20% of lactating people (Dixon & Louis-Jacques, 2023). Risk factors associated with mastitis include breastfeeding difficulties; stasis of milk due to infrequent, inconsistent breastfeeding; previous episodes of mastitis; nipple trauma; hyperlactation; and breast pump use. In addition to causing significant discomfort, it is a frequent reason for people to stop breastfeeding. It can result from any event that creates milk stasis, including insufficient drainage of the breast; rapid weaning; oversupply of milk; pressure on the breast from a poorly fitting bra;

TEACHING GUIDELINES 22.2 Teaching for the Patient With a Postpartum Infection

- Continue your antibiotic therapy as prescribed.
- Take the medication exactly as ordered and continue with the medication until it is finished.
- Do not stop taking the medication even when you are feeling better.
- Check your temperature every day and call your health care provider if it is >100.4°F (38°C).
- Watch for other signs and symptoms of infection, such as chills; increased abdominal pain; change in the color or odor of your lochia; or increased redness, warmth, swelling, or drainage from a wound site such as your cesarean incision or episiotomy. Report any of these to your health care provider immediately.
- Practice good infection prevention:
  - Always wash your hands thoroughly before and after eating, using the bathroom, touching your perineal area, or providing care for your newborn.
  - Wipe from front to back after using the bathroom.
  - Remove your perineal pad using a front-to-back motion. Fold the pad in half so that the inner sides of the pad that were touching your body are against each other. Wrap in toilet tissue or place in a plastic bag and discard.
  - Wash your hands before applying a new pad.
  - Apply a new perineal pad using a front-to-back motion. Handle the pad by the edges (top and bottom or sides) and avoid touching the inner aspect of the pad that will be against your body.
  - When performing perineal care with a peribottle, angle the spray of water so that it flows from front to back.
- Drink plenty of fluids each day and eat a variety of foods that are high in vitamins, iron, and protein.
- Be sure to get adequate rest at night and periodically throughout the day.

a blocked duct; missed feedings; and breakdown of the nipple via fissures, cracks, or blisters (La Leche League International, 2024). The most common infecting organism is *S. aureus,* which comes from the breastfeeding infant's mouth or throat. *Staphylococcus albus*, *E. coli*, and streptococci are also causative agents but are found less frequently. Ductal narrowing is the likely initiator of milk stasis, eventually resulting in infection (Dixon & Louis-Jacques, 2023). The upper outer quadrant of the breast is the most common site for mastitis to occur because most of the breast tissue is located there; the right and left breasts are equally affected (Fig. 22.4). A breast abscess may develop if mastitis is not treated adequately. Effective milk removal, pain medication, and antibiotic therapy are the mainstays of treatment.

Nursing Assessment

Note flulike symptoms such as malaise, fever, and chills; these are often the first symptoms experienced by the patient. Inspect the breasts, noting the presence of:

- Tender, firm area in one breast
- Nipple or areola cracking
- Breast distended with milk

Nursing Management

Treatment of mastitis focuses on two areas: emptying the breasts and controlling the infection. Frequent breast emptying helps both infectious and noninfectious mastitis. The breast can be emptied either by the infant sucking or by manual expression. Increasing the frequency of breastfeeding is advised. Control of infection is achieved with antibiotics. Ice or warm packs and analgesics may be needed for pain. In addition to antibiotics, management of lactational mastitis includes symptomatic treatment; assessment of the infant's attachment to the breast; and reassurance, emotional support, education, and support for ongoing breastfeeding.

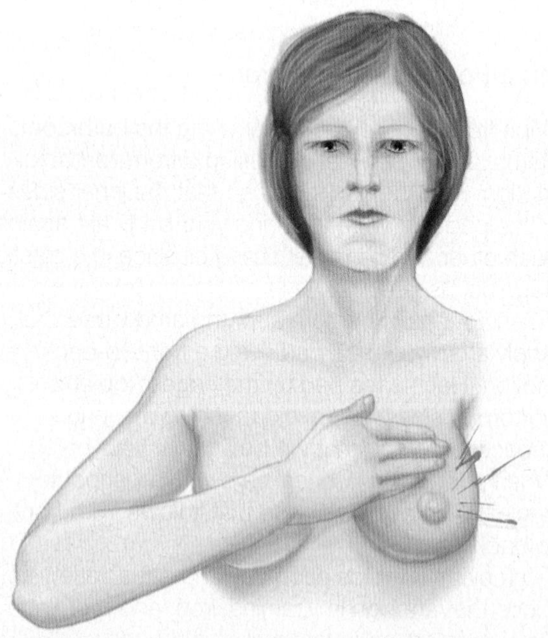

FIGURE 22.4 With mastitis, an area on one breast is tender, hot, red, and painful.

> **TAKE NOTE!**
>
> Regardless of the etiology of mastitis, the focus is on reversing milk stasis, maintaining milk supply, continuing breastfeeding, providing patient comfort, and preventing recurrence.

POSTPARTUM AFFECTIVE DISORDERS

Pregnancy and childbirth are an exciting and celebratory time for many families. However, the postpartum period involves extraordinary physiologic, psychological, and sociocultural changes in the life of the birthing parent and their family. People have varied reactions to their childbearing experiences, exhibiting a wide range of emotions. Often, the birth of a newborn is associated with positive feelings such as happiness, joy, and gratitude for the birth of a healthy infant. However, postpartum people may also feel weepy, overwhelmed, or unsure of what is happening to them. They may experience fear about loss of control and may feel scared, alone, guilty, or as if they have somehow failed. During the postpartum period, 50% to 80% of birthing parents experience some type of mood disorder (Sriraman, 2022).

Postpartum affective disorders have been documented for years, but only relatively recently have they begun to receive serious medical attention. Plummeting levels of estrogen and progesterone immediately after birth can contribute to postpartum mood disorders. Reproductive hormones influence every biologic system, and moods are sensitive to the effects of perinatal changes in hormone levels after childbirth. It is believed that the greater the change in these hormone levels between pregnancy and postpartum, the greater the chance of developing a mood disorder. Postpartum mood and anxiety disorders are huge public health issues in the United States, affecting up to a million people annually. Mood and anxiety disorders are influenced by genetics, as well as environment. They impact the entire family by disturbing the postpartum person's ability to bond with their infant and connect with their partner; they also negatively impact the child's long-term health and development (Association of Women's Health, Obstetric and Neonatal Nurses, 2022).

Many types of affective disorders occur in the postpartum period. Although their descriptions and classifications may be controversial, the disorders form a spectrum on the basis of their severity, such as postpartum or baby blues, PPD, and postpartum psychosis.

Postpartum Blues

Many postpartum people (approximately 40%) experience the postpartum blues within the first week after childbirth (Viguera, 2023). Emotional lability is the most prominent symptom of postpartum blues. The blues typically develop on postpartum Day 2 or 3 and usually resolve by 2 weeks postpartum. Although the symptoms may be distressing, they do not reflect psychopathology and usually do not affect the postpartum parent's ability to function and care for the infant. Postpartum blues are usually self-limiting and require no formal treatment other than reassurance and validation of the postpartum person's experience, as well as assistance in caring for themselves and the newborn.

Postpartum Depression

Postpartum depression (PPD) is a form of clinical depression that can affect birthing parents, and sometimes their partners, after childbirth. Unlike the postpartum blues, people with PPD feel worse over time, and changes in mood and behavior do not go away on their own. PPD may persist for a minimum of 6 months if untreated. Approximately one in seven people develop PPD (Mughal et al., 2022). The symptoms of PPD are more severe than those of the blues and require treatment.

The cause of PPD is not known, but research suggests it is multifactorial. According to ACOG (2024), PPD is caused by a combination of factors: sharp decrease in estrogen and progesterone, history of depression, volatile emotions, fatigue, and stressful life events. The levels of estrogen, progesterone, serotonin, and thyroid hormone decrease sharply and return to normal during the immediate postpartum period, which can trigger depression and change a patient's mood and behavior. Other aspects that can lead to PPD include:

- Unresolved feelings about the pregnancy
- Fatigue after delivery from lack of sleep or broken sleep
- Feelings of being less attractive
- Inadequate assistance from a partner
- Lack of social support network
- History of sexual or physical abuse
- Having a challenging infant who cries often
- Unemployment or financial insecurity
- Doubts about the ability to be a good parent
- Stressful life events
- Relationship issues
- Stress from changes in work and home routines
- Loss of freedom and former identity (American Psychological Association, 2022)

PPD may lend itself to prophylactic intervention because its onset is predictable, the risk period for illness is well defined, and patients at high risk potentially could be identified using a screening tool. This is not the case for all people, however. Prophylaxis starts with a prenatal risk assessment and education. Based on the patient's history of prior depression, prophylactic antidepressant therapy may be needed during the third trimester or immediately after giving birth. Management mirrors that of any major depression: a combination of antidepressant medication, antianxiety medication, adequate sleep and rest, and psychotherapy in an outpatient or inpatient setting (Mughal et al., 2022). PPD affects not only the patient but also the entire family. Identifying depression early can substantially improve patient and family outcomes. Marriage or couples counseling may be necessary if relationship problems are contributing to the patient's depressive symptoms (see the Healthy People 2030 box).

HEALTHY PEOPLE 2030

Objective	Nursing Significance
Increase the proportion of adults with depression who receive treatment.	• Screen postpartum patients for risk factors and symptoms indicative of postpartum depression. • Support and educate patients as they undergo treatment for depression. • Assist the postpartum parent with strategies for caring for their newborn.

Healthy People Objectives retrieved from http://www.healthypeople.gov

Depression in Partners

If the postpartum patient has a significant other or partner, the partner's emotional health should not be overlooked during the pregnancy and throughout the first postpartum year. PPD, once expected only in postpartum birthing parents, occurs in their partners as well. Up to 25% of partners also suffer from PPD (Wedajo et al., 2023). Depressive symptoms are likely to decrease their ability to provide support to the birthing parent. A partner's PPD can be difficult to identify. Partners may seem angrier and more anxious than sad, yet depression is present. When left untreated, a partner's PPD limits their capacity to provide emotional support to the postpartum parent and children. The highest rates of depression among nonbirthing parents have been reported between 3 and 6 months postpartum. Factors that increase the risk of paternal PPD include a personal history of depression and/or anxiety, marital discord, maternal depression, sleep deprivation, poverty, and unintended pregnancy (Scarff, 2019).

Assessing a partner's PPD is not easy. Nevertheless, it is important for all nurses who have contact with partners to remain open to the notion that they can be predisposed to PPD, particularly if the birthing parent is afflicted. Delving deeper into understanding behaviors of withdrawing, indecisiveness, cynicism, avoiding, drinking, using drugs, fighting, partner violence, extramarital affairs, and feelings of heightened irritation will reveal important insights. Asking birthing parents' partners candidly if they are feeling depressed, anxious, or angry can open the door to further exploration of these emotions.

Although partner depression is only now beginning to be defined and measured, sufficient evidence exists to warrant nurses' attention and concern. Nurses may be most able to help a birthing parent's partner devastated by PPD when they plant seeds of awareness that the disorder exists, they are not alone, and help is available.

CONSIDER THIS!

Even though I was an assertive practicing attorney in my 30s, my first pregnancy was filled with nagging feelings of doubt about this upcoming event in my life. Throughout my pregnancy, I was so busy with trial work that I never had time to really evaluate my feelings. I was always reading about the bodily changes that were taking place, and on one level, I was feeling excited, but on another level, I was emotionally drained. Shortly after the birth of my daughter, those suppressed nagging feelings of doubt surfaced and practically immobilized me. I felt exhausted all the time and was so glad to have someone else care for my daughter. I didn't breastfeed because I thought it would tie me down too much. Although at the time I thought this "low mood" was normal for all new birthing parents, I have since found out it was PPD. But how could anybody be depressed about the birth of a new child?

Thoughts: Now that PPD has been recognized as a real emotional disorder, it can be treated. This patient showed tendencies during their pregnancy but suppressed the feelings. Their description of depression is typical of many people who suffer in silence, hoping to get over these feelings in time. What can nurses do to promote awareness of this disorder? Can it be prevented?

Postpartum Psychosis

At the severe end of the continuum of postpartum emotional disorders is postpartum psychosis, which occurs in one to two patients per 1,000 live births (Shepherd & Davies, 2022). The onset can be abrupt and unexpected, though a previous history of mental illness is common. Symptoms of postpartum psychosis usually begin shortly after childbirth (days to weeks) and can be frightening for the people who are affected and for their families. Postpartum psychosis is considered an emergency psychiatric condition, as it can result in a significantly increased risk for suicide and infanticide. The postpartum patient frequently loses touch with reality and experiences a severe regressive breakdown associated with a high risk of suicide or infanticide (Shepherd & Davies, 2022). Anyone with postpartum psychosis should not be left alone with their infant. Most people with postpartum psychosis are hospitalized and treated with psychotropic drugs along with individual psychotherapy and support group therapy.

TAKE NOTE!

The greatest hazard of postpartum psychosis is suicide. Infanticide and child abuse are also risks if the postpartum parent is left alone with their infant. Early recognition and prompt treatment of this disorder are imperative.

Nursing Assessment

Postpartum affective disorders are often overlooked and go unrecognized despite the large percentage of people who experience them. The postpartum period is a time of increased vulnerability, but few people receive education about the possibility of depression after birth. In addition, many people may feel ashamed of having negative emotions at a time when they "should" be happy; thus, they do not seek professional help. Nurses can play a major role in providing guidance about postpartum affective disorders, detecting manifestations, and assisting patients with obtaining appropriate care.

Begin the assessment by reviewing the history to identify general risk factors that could predispose a patient to depression:

- Poor coping skills
- First pregnancy
- Low self-esteem
- History of bipolar disorder
- Sleep deprivation
- Numerous life stressors
- History of abuse
- Mood swings and emotional stress
- Previous psychological problems or a family history of psychiatric disorders
- Substance use disorder
- Limited or lack of social support network

Risk factors specific to postpartum psychosis include prior history of postpartum psychosis, personal history of schizoaffective disorder or schizophrenia, sleep deprivation, discontinuation of psychiatric medications during pregnancy, and family history of psychosis or bipolar disorder (Raza & Raza, 2023).

Also review the history for specific pregnancy and birth factors that may increase the patient's risk for depression. These may include a history of PPD, evidence of depression during the pregnancy, prenatal anxiety, a difficult or complicated pregnancy, traumatic birth experience, or birth of a high-risk infant or infant with a disability. Fifty percent or more of females with postpartum psychosis have no prior psychiatric history (Payne, 2023).

Screening for symptoms of PPD in all new parents is an important preliminary step to diagnosis and treatment. The Edinburgh Postnatal Depression Scale (EPDS) is a widely used, quick, and easy self-report screening tool for PPD that consists of 10 questions, each with four possible responses. Birthing parents and partners fill out the tool according to their symptoms during the previous 7 days. Each response is given a score of 0 to 3 points, creating a maximum score of 30. A score of 10 or higher indicates possible depression (American Academy of Pediatrics, 2022).

Early identification, screening, prevention, and treatment of PPD are crucial for improving overall outcomes for the postpartum parent and infant, as well as for decreasing mortality and morbidity. This is why it is crucial for nurses to understand and know about the risk factors, signs and symptoms, prevention, and use and interpretation of screening tools and to make appropriate referrals for treatment. Mass screening for PPD using a validated screening tool improves the rates of detection and treatment of PPD and should be implemented in obstetricians' and pediatricians' offices and in primary care settings. The Edinburgh Scale is shown in Figure 22.5.

Assess the patient's activity level, including their level of fatigue. Ask about their sleeping habits, noting any problems with insomnia. When interacting with the patient, observe for verbal and nonverbal indicators of anxiety as well as the patient's ability to concentrate during the interaction. Difficulty concentrating and anxious behaviors suggest a problem. Also assess the patient's nutritional intake; weight loss due to poor food intake may be present. The patient with postpartum blues may exhibit mild depressive symptoms (sadness, tearfulness, anxiety, irritability, mood swings), exhaustion, insomnia, and appetite changes (Balaram & Marwaha, 2023; Viguera, 2023).

Assessment can identify patients with high-risk profiles for depression, and the nurse can educate them and make referrals for individual or family counseling if needed. Some common assessment findings associated with PPD are listed in Box 22.2.

People with postpartum psychosis also experience depressive symptoms, mood lability, fatigue, and sleep disturbances. In addition, delusional beliefs, hallucinations, disorganized thinking, and hypomania can occur. The patient may be tearful, confused, and preoccupied with feelings of guilt and worthlessness. Symptoms escalate to delirium, hallucinations, extreme disorganization of thought, anger toward themselves and their infant, bizarre behavior, delusions, disorientation, depersonalization, manifestations of mania, and thoughts of hurting themselves and the infant (Raza & Raza, 2023; Shepherd & Davies, 2022).

Nursing Management

Nurses need to educate themselves about postpartum affective disorders to facilitate early recognition of signs and symptoms, which in turn would make early treatment possible, thus supporting recovery. Furthermore, greater knowledge could contribute to providing more effective and compassionate care to these patients. Nursing care focuses on assisting any postpartum patient in coping with the changes of this period. Encourage the patient to verbalize what they are going through and emphasize the importance of keeping expectations realistic. Assist them in structuring their day to regain a sense of control over the situation. Encourage them to seek professional help if necessary, using available support systems. Also reinforce the need for good nutrition and adequate exercise and sleep. Ensuring the parent's and infant's safety is paramount (Payne, 2023).

The nurse can play an important role in assisting patients and their partners with postpartum adjustment. Providing facts about the enormous changes that occur during the postpartum period is critical. This information includes expected changes in the patient's body. Review the signs and symptoms of all three affective disorders. This information is typically included as part of prenatal visits and childbirth education classes. Know the risk factors associated with these disorders and review the history of patients and their families. Use specific, nonthreatening questions to aid in early detection, such as "Have you felt down, depressed, or hopeless lately?" and "Have you felt little interest or pleasure in doing things recently?"

Discuss factors that may increase a patient's vulnerability to stress during the postpartum period, such as sleep deprivation and unrealistic expectations, so birthing parents and partners can understand and respond to those problems if they occur. Stress that many people need help after childbirth and that help is available from many sources, including people they already know. Assisting patients in learning how to ask for help is important so they can gain the support they need. Also provide educational materials about postpartum emotional disorders. Have available referral sources for psychotherapy and support groups appropriate for patients experiencing postpartum adjustment difficulties. Administer antidepressant medication (PPD) or antipsychotics (postpartum psychosis) as prescribed (see Evidence-Based Practice 22.2).

Edinburgh Postnatal Depression Scale

Name: ______________________ Address: ______________________

Your Date of Birth: ______________________ ______________________

Baby's Date of Birth: ______________________ Phone: ______________________

As you are pregnant or have recently had a baby, we would like to know how you are feeling. Please check the answer that comes closest to how you have felt **IN THE PAST 7 DAYS**, not just how you feel today.

Here is an example, already completed.

I have felt happy:
- ☐ Yes, all the time
- ☒ Yes, most of the time
- ☐ No, not very often
- ☐ No, not at all

This would mean: "I have felt happy most of the time" during the past week. Please complete the other questions in the same way.

In the past 7 days:

1. I have been able to laugh and see the funny side of things
   - ☐ As much as I always could
   - ☐ Not quite so much now
   - ☐ Definitely not so much now
   - ☐ Not at all

2. I have looked forward with enjoyment to things
   - ☐ As much as I ever did
   - ☐ Rather less than I used to
   - ☐ Definitely less than I used to
   - ☐ Hardly at all

*3. I have blamed myself unnecessarily when things went wrong
   - ☐ Yes, most of the time
   - ☐ Yes, some of the time
   - ☐ Not very often
   - ☐ No, never

4. I have been anxious or worried for no good reason
   - ☐ No, not at all
   - ☐ Hardly ever
   - ☐ Yes, sometimes
   - ☐ Yes, very often

*5. I have felt scared or panicky for no very good reason
   - ☐ Yes, quite a lot
   - ☐ Yes, sometimes
   - ☐ No, not much
   - ☐ No, not at all

*6. Things have been getting on top of me
   - ☐ Yes, most of the time I haven't been able to cope at all
   - ☐ Yes, sometimes I haven't been coping as well as usual
   - ☐ No, most of the time I have coped quite well
   - ☐ No, I have been coping as well as ever

*7. I have been so unhappy that I have had difficulty sleeping
   - ☐ Yes, most of the time
   - ☐ Yes, sometimes
   - ☐ Not very often
   - ☐ No, not at all

*8. I have felt sad or miserable
   - ☐ Yes, most of the time
   - ☐ Yes, quite often
   - ☐ Not very often
   - ☐ No, not at all

*9. I have been so unhappy that I have been crying
   - ☐ Yes, most of the time
   - ☐ Yes, quite often
   - ☐ Only occasionally
   - ☐ No, never

*10. The thought of harming myself has occurred to me
   - ☐ Yes, quite often
   - ☐ Sometimes
   - ☐ Hardly ever
   - ☐ Never

Administered/Reviewed by ______________________ Date ______________________

SCORING

QUESTIONS 1, 2, & 4 (without an *)
Are scored 0, 1, 2 or 3 with top box scored as 0 and the bottom box scored as 3.

QUESTIONS 3, 5-10 (marked with an *)
Are reverse scored, with the top box scored as a 3 and the bottom box scored as 0.

Maximum score: 30
Possible Depression: 10 or greater
Always look at item 10 (suicidal thoughts)

FIGURE 22.5 The Edinburgh Postnatal Depression Scale aims to detect postpartum depression. A score of 12 or more identifies most people with postpartum depression. (Reprinted from Cox, J. L., Holden, J. M., & Sagovsky, R. [1987]. Detection of postnatal depression: Development of the 10-item Edinburgh Postnatal Depression Scale. *British Journal of Psychiatry*, *150*[6], 782–786. https://doi.org/10.1192/bjp.150.6.782)

BOX 22.2 Common Assessment Findings Associated With Postpartum Depression

- Loss of pleasure or interest in life
- Low mood, especially in the morning, sadness, tearfulness
- Exhaustion that is not relieved by sleep
- Feelings of guilt
- Weight loss
- Low energy
- Irritability
- Poor personal hygiene
- Constipated
- Preoccupied and unfocused
- Indecisiveness
- Diminished concentration
- Anxiety
- Despair
- Compulsive thoughts
- Loss of libido
- Loss of confidence
- Sleep difficulties (insomnia)
- Loss of appetite
- Bleak and pessimistic view of the future
- Not responding to infant's cries or cues for attention
- Social isolation, won't answer the door or the phone
- Feelings of failure as a parent

Association of Women's Health, Obstetric and Neonatal Nurses. (2022). AWHONN position statement: Perinatal mood and anxiety disorders. *Journal of Obstetric, Gynecologic, & Neonatal Nursing, 51*(4), E1–E4. https://doi.org/10.1016/j.jogn.2022.03.007; American College of Obstetricians and Gynecologists. (2024). *Postpartum depression.* https://www.acog.org/womens-health/faqs/postpartum-depression; and American Psychological Association. (2022). *Postpartum depression: Causes, symptoms, risk factors, and treatment options.* https://www.apa.org/topics/women-girls/postpartum-depression

EVIDENCE-BASED PRACTICE 22.2

Screening for Partner Postpartum Depression: A Systematic Review

BACKGROUND

Partner postpartum depression (PPD) is a significant mental health condition, but most research has focused on postpartum birthing parents with little attention paid toward their partners. Research suggests that up to 20% of partners experience PPD. As partner depression is directly linked with maternal depression, any deviation in the partner's mental health could directly impact the mental and physical health of the birthing parent. The purpose of this review was to examine the current tools available to evaluate PPD in partners.

STUDY

This review provided a synthesis of the most common assessment methods for PPD, with a perspective on how nurses can leverage screening to identify partners at risk for depression. Of the 1,701 peer-reviewed studies researched, only 17 met the inclusion criteria. Seven different measures were used to evaluate PPD. The Edinburgh Postnatal Depression Scale (EPDS) was used in 16 out of the 17 studies included. The EPDS assesses important markers of depression—such as mood, self-image, enjoyment, and stress—within the last week. The tool takes less than 5 minutes to complete; it has a sensitivity of 59% to 100% and a specificity of 49% to 100% for detecting PPD.

Findings

Across the included studies, the average prevalence of partner PPD was about 15%. All except one of the included studies used the EPDS as the primary screening tool. Partners tended to exhibit higher levels of self-reported severe depression and suicidal thoughts compared to their postpartum partners. This can be attributed to traditional societal values in the United States, which especially discourage men to be open about their feelings.

Nursing Implications

Based on this study's conclusions, routine PPD screening of partners should be recommended as part of standard care. Early identification of depressive symptoms and subsequent interventions are essential measures of safe care for partners and families. Screening in the prenatal time period could help nurses identify risk factors for PPD and provide partners with more guidance throughout the gestation and postpartum periods. Nurses are critical liaisons for linking family members with appropriate referrals and available community resources.

Adapted from Le, J., Alhusen, J., & Dreisbach, C. (2023). Screening for partner postpartum depression: A systematic review. *MCN: The American Journal of Maternal/Child Nursing, 43*(3), 142–150. https://doi.org/10.1097/NMC.0000000000000907

KEY CONCEPTS

- PPH is a potentially life-threatening complication of both vaginal and cesarean births. It is the leading cause of maternal mortality in the United States.
- A good way to remember the causes of PPH is the "5 Ts:" tone, tissue, trauma, thrombin, and traction.
- Uterine atony is the most common cause of early PPH, which can lead to hypovolemic shock.
- Oxytocin (Pitocin), misoprostol (Cytotec), dinoprostone (Prostin E2), methylergonovine maleate (Methergine), prostaglandin PGF2α (carboprost [Hemabate]), and tranexamic acid are commonly used drugs used to manage PPH.
- Failure of the placenta to separate completely and be expelled interferes with the ability of the uterus to contract fully, thereby leading to hemorrhage
- Lacerations should always be suspected when the uterus is contracted and bright red blood continues to trickle out of the vagina.
- Conditions that cause coagulopathies may include thrombolytic thrombocytopenic purpura, von Willebrand disease, and DIC.

- PE is a potentially fatal condition that occurs when the pulmonary artery is obstructed by a blood clot that has traveled from another vein into the lungs, causing obstruction and infarction.
- The major causes of a thrombus formation (blood clot) are venous stasis and hypercoagulation, both of which are common in the postpartum period.
- Postpartum infection is defined as a fever of 100.4°F (38°C) or higher after the first 24 hours after childbirth, occurring on at least 2 of the first 10 days exclusive of the first 24 hours.
- Common postpartum infections include endometritis, wound infections, UTIs, and mastitis.
- Postpartum emotional disorders are commonly classified on the basis of their severity: "baby blues," PPD, and postpartum psychosis.
- Management of PPD mirrors the treatment of any major depression: a combination of antidepressant medication, antianxiety medication, and psychotherapy in an outpatient or inpatient setting.

REFERENCES AND RECOMMENDED READINGS

Agency for Healthcare Research and Quality. (2022). *Postpartum care for women up to one year after pregnancy.* https://effectivehealthcare.ahrq.gov/products/postpartum-care-one-year/protocol

American Academy of Pediatrics. (2022). *Integrating postpartum depression screening in your practice in 4 steps.* https://www.aap.org/en/patient-care/perinatal-mental-health-and-social-support/integrating-postpartum-depression-screening-in-your-practice-in-4-steps/

American College of Obstetricians and Gynecologists. (2021). *Reaffirmed ACOG committee opinion no. 736: Optimizing postpartum care.* https://www.acog.org/clinical/clinical-guidance/committee-opinion/articles/2018/05/optimizing-postpartum-care

American College of Obstetricians and Gynecologists. (2022). *Preventing deep vein thrombosis.* https://www.acog.org/womens-health/faqs/preventing-deep-vein-thrombosis

American College of Obstetricians and Gynecologists. (2024). *Postpartum depression.* https://www.acog.org/womens-health/faqs/postpartum-depression

American Heart Association. (2023). *Prevention and treatment of venous thromboembolism.* https://www.heart.org/en/health-topics/venous-thromboembolism/prevention-and-treatment-of-venous-thromboembolism-vte

American Psychological Association. (2022). *Postpartum depression: Causes, symptoms, risk factors, and treatment options.* https://www.apa.org/topics/women-girls/postpartum-depression

Association of Women's Health, Obstetric and Neonatal Nurses. (2022). AWHONN position statement: Perinatal mood and anxiety disorders. *Journal of Obstetric, Gynecologic, & Neonatal Nursing, 51*(4), E1–E4. https://doi.org/10.1016/j.jogn.2022.03.007

Balaram, K., & Marwaha, R. (2023). Postpartum blues. *StatPearls.* https://www.ncbi.nlm.nih.gov/books/NBK554546/

Belfort, M. A. (2023). Postpartum hemorrhage: Medical and minimally invasive management. *UpToDate.* Retrieved April 27, 2024, from https://www.uptodate.com/contents/postpartum-hemorrhage-medical-and-minimally-invasive-management

Belfort, M. A. (2024). Overview of postpartum hemorrhage. *UpToDate.* Retrieved April 27, 2024, from https://www.uptodate.com/contents/overview-of-postpartum-hemorrhage

Berens, P. (2024). Overview of the postpartum period: Normal physiology and routine maternal care. *UpToDate.* Retrieved July 16, 2024, from https://www.uptodate.com/contents/overview-of-the-postpartum-period-normal-physiology-and-routine-maternal-care

Blondon, M., & Skeith, L. (2022). Preventing postpartum venous thromboembolism in 2022: A narrative review. *Frontiers in Cardiovascular Medicine, 9.* https://doi.org/10.3389/fcvm.2022.886416

Boushra, M., & Rahman, O. (2023). Postpartum infection. *StatPearls.* https://www.ncbi.nlm.nih.gov/books/NBK560804/

Centers for Disease Control and Prevention. (2023). *Data and statistics on venous thromboembolism.* https://www.cdc.gov/blood-clots/data-research/facts-stats/

Chen, K. T. (2024). Postpartum endometritis. *UpToDate.* Retrieved April 28, 2024, from https://www.uptodate.com/contents/postpartum-endometritis

Choy, K. R., Emmett, S., & Wong, A. (2022). Venous thromboembolism prophylaxis in pregnancy: Are we adequately identifying and managing risks? *Australian and New Zealand Journal of Obstetrics and Gynecology, 62*(6), 915–920. https://doi.org/10.1111/ajo.13579

Cunningham, F. G., Leveno, K. J., Dashe, J. S., Hoffman, B. L., Spong, C. Y., & Casey, B. M. (2022). Puerperal infection. In F. G. Cunningham, K. J. Leveno, J. S. Dashe, B. L. Hoffman, C. Y. Spong, & B, M. Casey (Eds.), *William's obstetrics* (26th ed.). McGraw Hill.

Dixon, J. M., & Louis-Jacques, A. (2023). Lactational mastitis. *UpToDate.* Retrieved April 28, 2024, from https://www.uptodate.com/contents/lactational-mastitis

Escobar, M. F., Nassar, A. H., Theron, G., Barnea, E. R., Nicholson, W., Ramasauskaite, D., Lloyd, I., Chandraharan, E., Miller, S., Burke, T., Ossanan, G., Andres Carvajal, J., Ramos, I., Hincapie, M. A., Loaiza, S., Nasner, D., & FIGO Safe Motherhood and Newborn Health Committee. (2022). FIGO recommendations on the management of postpartum hemorrhage 2022. *International Journal of Gynecology & Obstetrics, 157*(Suppl. 1), 3–50. https://doi.org/10.1002/ijgo.14116

Kogutt, B. K., Kim, J. M., Will, S. E., & Sheffield, J. S. (2022). Development of an obstetric hemorrhage response intervention: The postpartum hemorrhage cart and medication kit. *The Joint Commission Journal on Quality and Patient Safety, 48*(2), 120–128. https://doi.org/10.1016/j.jcjq.2021.09.007.

Krawczyk, P., Huras, H., Jaworowski, A., Tyszecki, P., & Kołak, M. (2023). Cesarean section complicated with presumed massive pulmonary embolism and cardiac arrest treated with rescue thrombolytic therapy—Two case reports. *Annals of Palliative Medicine, 12*(1), 219–226. https://doi.org/10.21037/apm-22-435

La Leche League International. (2024). *Mastitis and sore breasts.* https://www.llli.org/breastfeeding-info/mastitis/

Le, J., Alhusen, J., & Dreisbach, C. (2023). Screening for partner postpartum depression: A systematic review. *MCN: The American Journal of Maternal/Child Nursing, 43*(3), 142–150. https://doi.org/10.1097/NMC.0000000000000907

Mithoowani, S. (2022). Patient education: Deep vein thrombosis (DVT) (beyond the basics). *UpToDate.* Retrieved January

17, 2024, from https://www.uptodate.com/contents/deep-vein-thrombosis-dvt-beyond-the-basics

Mughal, S., Azhar, Y., & Siddiqui, W. (2022). Postpartum depression. *StatPearls*. https://www.ncbi.nlm.nih.gov/books/NBK519070/

ObG Project. (2022). *Postpartum hemorrhage—Medications to treat uterine atony*. https://www.obgproject.com/2022/11/01/postpartum-hemorrhage-medications-treat-uterine-atony/

Pagana, K. D., Pagana, T. J., & Pagana, T. N. (2023). *Mosby's diagnostic and laboratory test reference* (16th ed.). Elsevier.

Payne, J. (2023). Treatment of postpartum psychosis. *UpToDate*. Retrieved April 28, 2024, from https://www.uptodate.com/contents/treatment-of-postpartum-psychosis

Raza, S. K., & Raza, S. (2023). Postpartum psychosis. *StatPearls*. https://www.ncbi.nlm.nih.gov/books/NBK544304/

Scarff, J. R. (2019). Postpartum depression in men. *Innovations in Clinical Neuroscience*, *16*(5–6), 11–14. https://www.ncbi.nlm.nih.gov/pmc/articles/PMC6659987/pdf/icns_16_5-6_11.pdf

Shepherd, F., & Davies, W. (2022). *An update on the presentation, nosology, and causes of postpartum psychosis*. https://www.psychiatrictimes.com/view/an-update-on-the-presentation-nosology-and-causes-of-postpartum-psychosis

Smith, J. R. (2022). Postpartum hemorrhage. *Medscape*. https://emedicine.medscape.com/article/275038-overview#

Springel, E. H., & Mahotra, T. (2022). Thromboembolism in pregnancy. *Medscape*. https://emedicine.medscape.com/article/2056380-overview?form=fpf

Sriraman, N. K. (2022). *Depression during & after pregnancy: You are not alone*. https://healthychildren.org/English/ages-stages/prenatal/delivery-beyond/Pages/understanding-motherhood-and-mood-baby-blues-and-beyond.aspx

Taylor, M., Jenkins, S. M., & Pillarisetty, L. S. (2023). Endometritis. *StatPearls*. https://www.ncbi.nlm.nih.gov/books/NBK553124/

Thompson, B. T., Kabrhel, C., & Pena, C. (2024). Clinical presentation, evaluation, and diagnosis of the nonpregnant adult with suspected acute pulmonary embolism. *UpToDate*. Retrieved July 16, 2024, from https://www.uptodate.com/contents/clinical-presentation-evaluation-and-diagnosis-of-the-nonpregnant-adult-with-suspected-acute-pulmonary-embolism

UpToDate, Inc. (2024). *UpToDate® Lexidrug™* (Version 8.2.0) [Mobile app]. Wolters Kluwer. https://apps.apple.com/us/app/lexicomp/id313401238

U.S. Department of Health and Human Services. (n.d.). *Healthy People 2030*. https://health.gov/healthypeople

Viguera, A. (2023). Postpartum blues. *UpToDate*. Retrieved April 28, 2024, from https://www.uptodate.com/contents/postpartum-blues

Wedajo, L. F., Alemu, S. S., Tola, M. A., & Teferi, S. M. (2023). Paternal postnatal depression and associated factors: Community-based cross-sectional study. *SAGE Open Medicine*, *11*, 20503121231208265. https://doi.org/10.1177/20503121231208265

Wong, A. W., & Rosh, A. J. (2024). Postpartum infections. *Medscape*. https://emedicine.medscape.com/article/796892-overview

World Health Organization. (2022). *WHO postpartum haemorrhage (PPH) summit*. https://www.who.int/publications/m/item/who-postpartum-haemorrhage-(pph)-summit#

DEVELOPING CLINICAL JUDGMENT

PRACTICING FOR NCLEX

1. A postpartum patient appears very pale and states they are bleeding heavily. What should the nurse do first?
   a. Call the patient's health care provider immediately.
   b. Begin an IV infusion of magnesium sulfate.
   c. Assess the fundus and ask about their voiding status.
   d. Reassure the patient that this is a normal finding after birth.

2. A postpartum patient reports hearing voices and says, "The voices are telling me to do bad things to my baby." The nurse should interpret these findings as being suggestive of what?
   a. Postpartum psychosis
   b. Anxiety disorder
   c. Postnatal depression
   d. Postpartum blues

3. The nurse is caring for a multigravid postpartum patient who gave birth just a few hours ago. For what will the nurse vigilantly monitor?
   a. Deep venous thrombosis
   b. Postpartum psychosis
   c. Uterine infection
   d. Postpartum hemorrhage

4. A patient with mastitis is receiving antibiotic therapy. What will the nurse include in the plan of care for this patient?
   a. Stop breastfeeding and apply lanolin.
   b. Administer analgesics and bind both breasts.
   c. Apply warm or cold compresses and administer analgesics.
   d. Remove the nursing bra and expose the breast to fresh air.

5. While assessing a postpartum multiparous patient, the nurse detects a boggy uterus midline 2 cm above the umbilicus. Which intervention would be the priority?
   a. Assessing the patient's vital signs immediately
   b. Measuring the patient's next urinary output
   c. Massaging the patient's fundus
   d. Notifying the patient's obstetrician

6. Methergine has been ordered for a postpartum patient because of excessive bleeding. The nurse should question this order if which is present?
   a. Mild abdominal cramping
   b. Tender inflamed breasts
   c. Pulse rate of 68 beats/min
   d. Blood pressure of 158/96 mm Hg

7. The nurse is caring for several patients on the postpartum unit. Which finding would lead the nurse to suspect that a patient is developing a complication?
   a. Moderate lochia rubra for the first 24 hours
   b. Clear lung sounds upon auscultation
   c. Temperature of 100°F (37.7°C)
   d. Chest pain experienced when ambulating

8. The nurse is caring for a postpartum patient. Which factor in the patient's history would lead the nurse to monitor them closely for an infection?
   a. Hemoglobin of 12 mg/dL
   b. Manually extracted placenta
   c. Labor of 10 hours length
   d. Multiparity of five pregnancies

CRITICAL THINKING EXERCISES

1. A patient had a 22-hour labor before a cesarean birth. The patient's membranes ruptured 20 hours before they came to the hospital. Their fetus showed signs of fetal distress, so internal electronic fetal monitoring was used. Their most recent test results indicate the patient is anemic.
   a. For which postpartum complication is this new parent at highest risk? Why?
   b. What assessments need to be done to detect this complication?
   c. What nursing measures will the nurse use to prevent this complication?

2. A 32-year-old G9P9 had a spontaneous vaginal birth 2 hours ago. They have been having a baby each year for the past 9 years. The patient's lochia has been heavy with some clots. The patient hasn't been up to void since they had epidural anesthesia and have decreased sensation in their legs.
   a. What factors place the patient at risk for postpartum hemorrhage?
   b. What assessments are needed before planning interventions?
   c. What nursing actions are needed to prevent a postpartum hemorrhage?

3. A 25-year-old G2P2 gave birth 2 days ago and is expected to be discharged today. The patient had severe postpartum depression 2 years ago with their first child. They have not been out of bed for the past 24 hours, are not eating, and provide no care for themselves or their newborn. The patient states they already have a boy at home and not having a girl this time is disappointing.
   a. What factors or behaviors place the patient at risk for an affective disorder?
   b. Which interventions might be appropriate at this time?
   c. What education does the family need prior to discharge?

STUDY ACTIVITIES

1. Compare and contrast postpartum blues, postpartum depression, and postpartum psychosis in terms of their characteristics and medical management.
2. Interview a person who has given birth and ask if they had any complications and what was most helpful to them during the experience.
3. The number one cause of postpartum hemorrhage is ________________.
4. When giving a report to the nurse who will be caring for a patient and their newborn in the postpartum period, what information should the labor nurse convey?

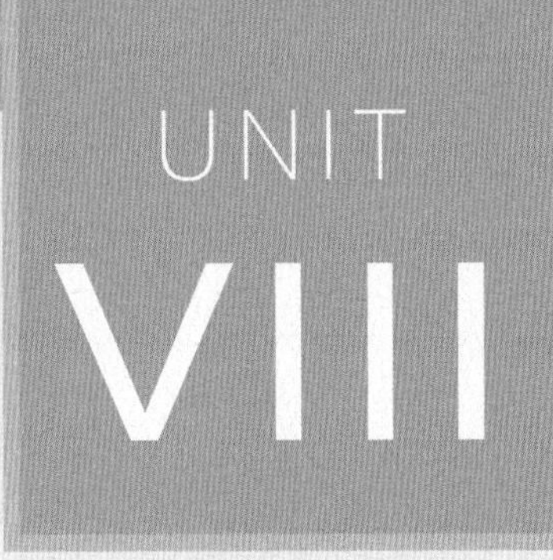

The Newborn at Risk

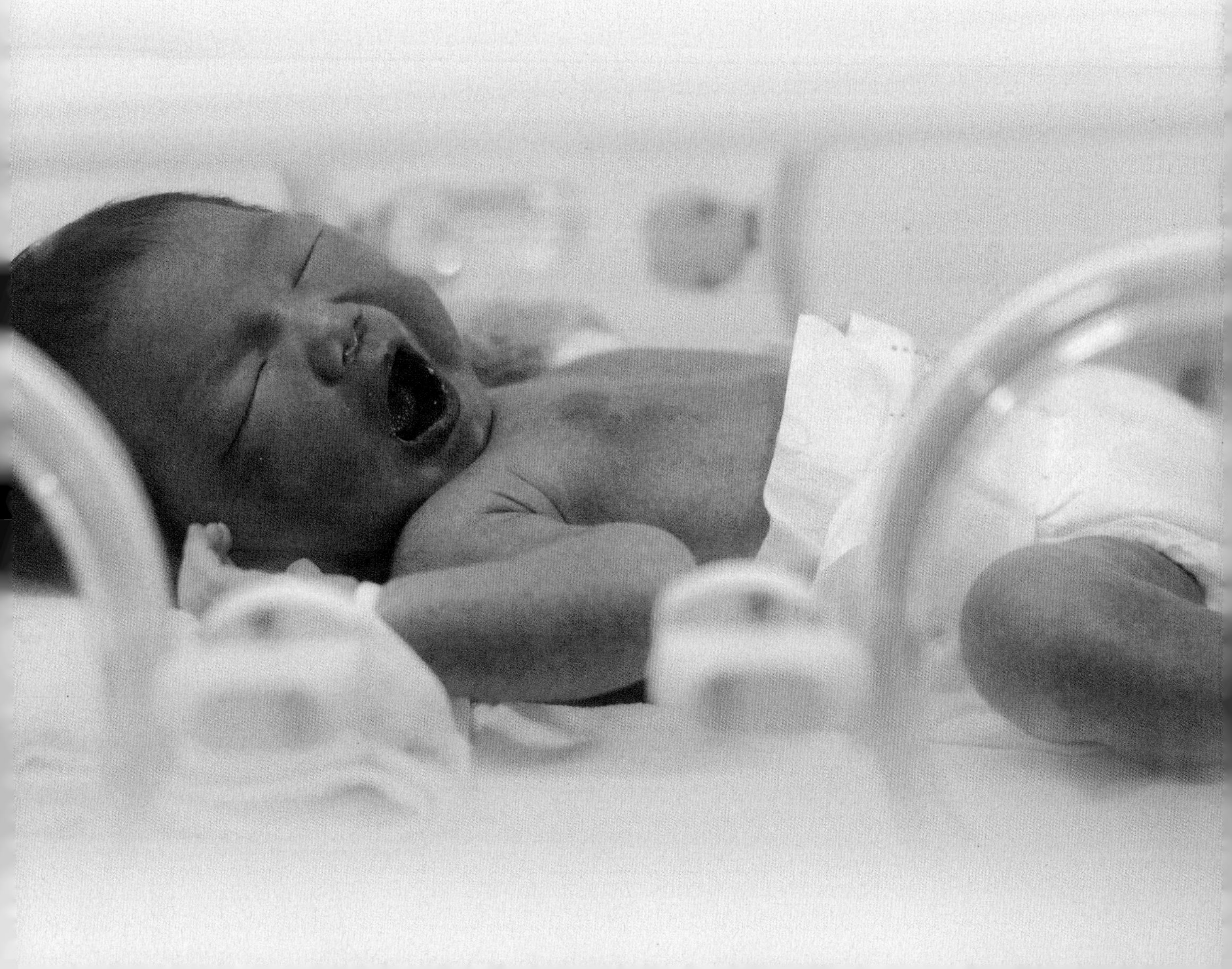

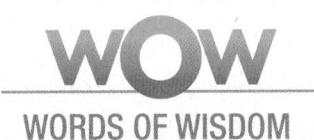

WORDS OF WISDOM

Guiding a parent's hand to touch a frail or ill newborn demonstrates courage and compassion under very difficult circumstances and is a powerful tool in helping them to deal with the newborn's special needs.

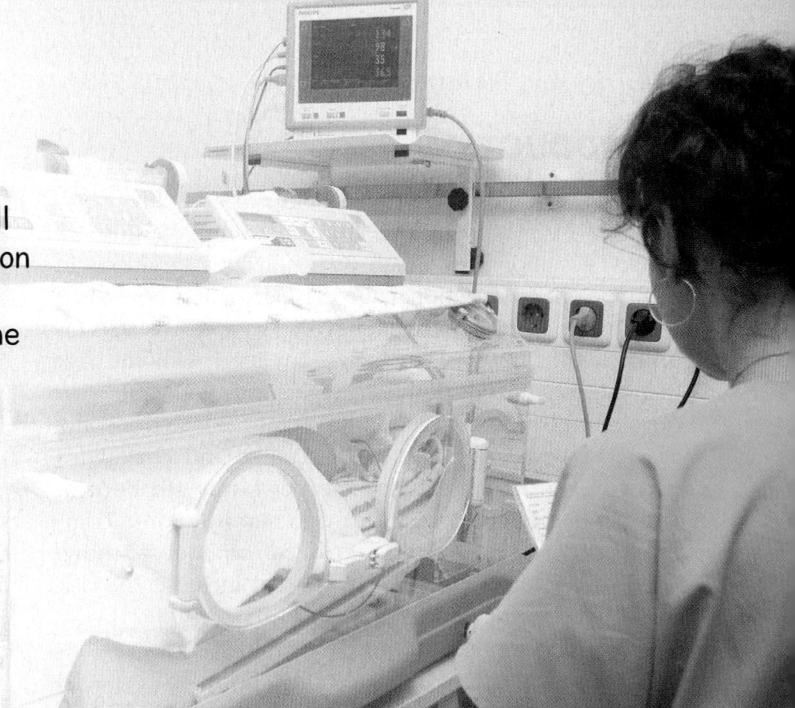

23

Nursing Care of the Newborn With Special Needs

KEY TERMS

appropriate for gestational age (AGA)
extremely low birth weight
full-term newborn
large for gestational age (LGA)
late preterm newborn
low birth weight (LBW)
postterm newborn
preterm newborn
small for gestational age (SGA)
very low birth weight

LEARNING OBJECTIVES

Upon completion of the chapter, you will be able to:

1. Examine factors that assist in identifying a newborn at risk due to variations in birth weight and gestational age.
2. Detect contributing factors and common complications associated with dysmature infants and their management.
3. Differentiate associated conditions that affect the newborn with variations in birth weight and gestational age, including appropriate management.
4. Compare and contrast a small-for-gestational-age newborn and a large-for-gestational-age newborn as well as a postterm and a preterm newborn.
5. Integrate knowledge of the risks associated with late preterm births into nursing interventions, discharge planning, and parent education.
6. Outline the nurse's role in helping parents experiencing perinatal grief or loss.

Anna and her husband were stunned when she went into labor at 7 months' gestation. They couldn't understand what would cause her to give birth early, but it happened. When they approached the neonatal intensive care unit (NICU), Anna took a deep breath and looked down at her tiny baby hooked up to tubes everywhere. What feelings might they be experiencing at this moment?

INTRODUCTION

Expecting families hope for the birth of a healthy newborn. Most newborns are born between 38 and 42 weeks' gestation and weigh 6 to 8 lb, but variations in birth weight or gestational age can occur, and newborns with these variations often have special needs. Gestational age at birth is inversely correlated with the risk that the infant will experience physical, neurologic, or developmental sequelae (Davis et al., 2023). In some cases, however, unexpected difficulties and challenges occur along the way, and some newborns are born ill and need special advanced care to survive. Some complications are unexpected and occur without warning. Other times, there are risk factors that increase the risk of problems in newborns.

The development of new technologies and regionalized care centers for the care of newborns with special needs has resulted in significant improvements. Nurses need to have a sound knowledge base to identify the newborn with special needs and to provide coordinated care.

The key to identify a newborn with special needs related to birth weight or gestational age variation is an awareness of the factors that could place a newborn at risk. These factors are similar to those that would suggest a high-risk pregnancy. Being able to anticipate the birth of a newborn at risk allows the birth to take place at a health care facility equipped with the resources to meet the needs of the birthing parent and the newborn. This is vital to reducing mortality and morbidity.

This chapter discusses the nursing management of newborns with special needs related to variations in birth weight and gestational age. It also describes select associated conditions affecting these newborns. Due to the frailty of these newborns, the care of the family experiencing perinatal loss and the role of the nurse in helping the family cope are also addressed.

BIRTH-WEIGHT VARIATIONS

Fetal growth is influenced by maternal nutrition, genetics, placental function, environment, and a multitude of other factors. Assigning size to a newborn is a way to measure and monitor the growth and development of the newborn at birth. Newborns can be classified according to their weight and weeks of gestation. At any gestational age, birth weights vary with altitude, race, country of origin, and socioeconomic class. Knowing the birth-weight group into which a newborn fits is important.

Birth weight is plotting on the growth chart based on the newborn's gestational age (most accurately determined by early ultrasound). The classifications are:

- **Appropriate for gestational age (AGA):** birth weight between the 10th and 90th percentile for gestational age on the growth chart (Trotter, 2025)

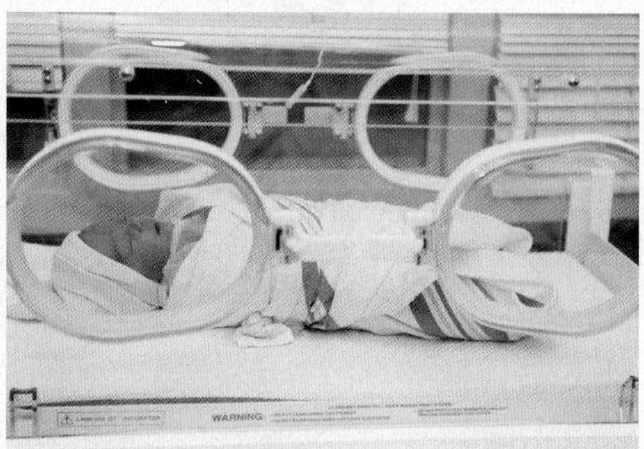

FIGURE 23.1 A low-birth-weight newborn in an isolette.

- **Small for gestational age (SGA):** birth weight below the 10th percentile for gestational age on the growth chart (Mandy, 2024a)
- **Large for gestational age (LGA):** birth weight above the 90th percentile (Mandy, 2024b)

Newborns who are AGA have the lowest risk for neonatal and childhood problems, having lower morbidity and mortality rates than other groups.

Newborns with lower birth weights can be further classified according to their weight:

- **Low birth weight (LBW):** less than 2,500 g (5.5 lb) (Fig. 23.1)
- **Very low birth weight:** less than 1,500 g (3 lb, 5 oz)
- **Extremely low birth weight:** less than 1,000 g (2 lb, 3 oz)

Small-for-Gestational-Age Newborns

The fetus is thought to have an inherent growth potential that, under normal circumstances, yields a healthy newborn of appropriate size. Fetal growth is dependent on genetic, placental, and maternal factors. The maternal–placental–fetal units act in harmony to meet the needs of the fetus during gestation. However, growth potential in the fetus can be limited. Newborns who are SGA can be preterm, term, or postterm, and they account for 8% to 10% of newborns (Mandy, 2024a). Many infants who are SGA are simply constitutionally small and experience better long-term outcomes and decreased mortality rates. Infants may be considered constitutionally small when one or both parents are small and there is an absence of or poor intrauterine growth. Most infants who are SGA demonstrate adequate catch-up growth.

Fetal Growth Restriction

Some infants who are SGA are not simply constitutionally small; they have experienced fetal growth restriction (FGR). FGR is defined as a birth weight below the 3rd percentile (severe FGR) or three or more of the following: birth weight below the 10th percentile, length below the 10th percentile, head circumference below the 10th percentile, prenatal history of a condition strongly associated with FGR (Box. 23.1), or a prenatal diagnosis of FGR (Mandy, 2024a). About 30% of newborns who are SGA have FGR (Cunningham et al., 2022). These infants are at increased risk of morbidity and mortality as compared with newborns whose birth weight is AGA.

BOX 23.1 Potential Factors Contributing to the Birth of Newborns With Fetal Growth Restriction

Maternal Causes

- Chronic hypertension
- Diabetes mellitus with vascular disease
- Autoimmune diseases
- Living at a high altitude (hypoxia)
- Smoking or exposure to passive smoke
- Periodontal disease of the mouth
- Nulliparity
- Low gestational weight gain
- Indoor or outdoor air pollution
- Heavy physical workload during pregnancy
- Birth interval of <18 months
- Vitamin D deficiency
- Maternal age of younger than 20 or older than 34 years
- Failure to seek any prenatal care
- Substandard living conditions
- Low socioeconomic status
- Abuse and violence
- Substance use disorder (heroin, cocaine, methamphetamines)
- Hemoglobinopathies (sickle cell anemia)
- Preeclampsia
- Exposure to occupational hazards
- Chronic kidney disease
- Maternal nutrition (malnutrition or higher weight)
- Extreme maternal stress
- Maternal infections—malaria, HIV, chlamydia, and trichomonas

Placental Factors

- Abnormal cord insertion
- Chronic abruption
- Decreased surface area, infarction
- Decreased placental weight
- Placenta previa
- Placental insufficiency

Fetal Factors

- Trisomies 13, 18, and 21
- Turner syndrome
- Chronic fetal infection (cytomegalovirus, rubella, syphilis, toxoplasmosis)
- Congenital anomalies (heart, diaphragmatic hernia, tracheoesophageal fistula)
- Radiation exposure
- Multiple fetal gestation

Mandy, G. T. (2024a). Fetal growth restriction (FGR) and small for gestational age (SGA) newborns. *UpToDate.* Retrieved March 16, 2024, from https://www.uptodate.com/contents/fetal-growth-restriction-fgr-and-small-for-gestational-age-sga-newborns; Simmons, R. A. (2024). Abnormalities of fetal growth. In C. A. Gleason & T. Sawyer (Eds.), *Avery's diseases of the newborn* (11th ed., pp. 33–41). Elsevier.

FGR can be further categorized as symmetric or asymmetric. Symmetric fetal growth restriction refers to fetuses whose head, body, and length are equally affected. Symmetric FGR occurs in 20% to 30% of cases (Mandy, 2024a). Asymmetric FGR refers to fetuses whose weight is negatively impacted significantly, whose length may be somewhat impacted, and whose head circumference is spared. Asymmetric FGR occurs in 70% to 80% of cases (Mandy, 2024a). These infants usually have a better prognosis than infants with symmetric FGR. Once the infant is born, optimal nutrition usually restores normal growth potential. Factors that can contribute to the newborn experiencing FGR are highlighted in Box 23.1.

Nursing Assessment

Assessment of the infant who is SGA includes reviewing the maternal history to identify risk factors such as smoking, maternal malnutrition, drug use, alcohol consumption, preeclampsia, anemia, uteroplacental insufficiency, intrauterine viral infection, cord prolapse, chronic maternal illness, hypertension, kidney disease, multiple gestation, or genetic disorders. This information allows the nurse to anticipate a possible problem and to be prepared to intervene quickly should one occur. At birth, perform a thorough physical examination, closely observing the newborn for typical characteristics, including:

- Head disproportionately large compared with rest of body (asymmetric FGR)
- Wasted appearance of extremities
- Reduced subcutaneous fat stores
- Decreased muscle mass
- Face is shrunken and wrinkled
- Widened cranial sutures with a large anterior fontanel
- Loose and dry skin that appears oversized
- Thin umbilical cord (Mandy, 2024a)

Also assess the newborn who is SGA for any congenital malformations or signs of infection. These newborns commonly face problems after birth. Table 23.1 highlights some of the common problems associated with newborns experiencing a variation in birth weight or gestational age.

Nursing Management

Anticipate the need for and provide resuscitation as indicated by the newborn's condition.

Interventions for the newborn who is SGA may include obtaining weight, length, and head circumference, comparing them with standards, and documenting the findings. Perform frequent serial blood glucose measurements as ordered and monitor vital signs, being particularly alert for changes in respiratory status that might indicate respiratory distress. Institute measures to maintain a neutral thermal environment to prevent cold stress and acidosis.

TABLE 23.1 • Common Problems Associated With Newborns Experiencing a Variation in Birth Weight or Gestational Age

Problem	Occurrence	Etiology/Pathophysiology	Nursing Implications
Perinatal asphyxia	Severe FGR	Living in hypoxic environment prior to birth due to placental insufficiency, leaving little to no oxygen reserves available to withstand stress of labor. Poor tolerance to stress of labor, frequently leading to acidosis and hypoxia	Anticipate possible problem; assess for maternal risk factors. Initiate resuscitation measures immediately at birth.
	Postterm newborn	Placental deprivation or oligohydramnios, leading to cord compression and subsequent reduction in perfusion to fetus	
	Preterm newborn	Surfactant deficiency Unstable chest wall Immaturity of respiratory control centers in the CNS Small respiratory passages, increasing risk for obstruction Inability to clear mucus from airways	
Difficulty with thermoregulation	FGR	Less muscle mass, less brown fat, less heat-preserving subcutaneous fat, and limited ability to control skin capillaries	Maintain a neutral thermal environment to promote stabilization of newborn's temperature. Assess skin temperature and respiration characteristics. Monitor ABGs and blood glucose levels. Eliminate sources of heat loss: • Dry newborn thoroughly. • Wrap in warmed blanket with stockinette cap on head. • Use radiant heat source.
	Postterm newborn	Associated with depleted glycogen stores, poor subcutaneous fat stores, and disturbances in CNS thermoregulation due to hypoxia Increased risk for acidosis and hypoglycemia secondary to metabolic stress Loss of subcutaneous fat secondary to placental insufficiency Use of stored nutrients for nutrition due to lost ability of placenta to nourish fetus Subsequent wasting of subcutaneous fat, muscle, or both Loss of natural insulation (subcutaneous fat) important in temperature regulation	
	Preterm newborn	Immaturity of CNS (temperature-regulating center) interferes with ability to regulate body temperature Inadequate amounts of subcutaneous fat Lack of muscle tone and flexion to conserve heat	
	Late preterm infant	Inadequate brown fat to generate heat Limited muscle mass activity, reducing ability to produce own heat Inability to shiver to generate heat	
Hypoglycemia	SGA, FGR	Lack of adequate glycogen stores to meet newborn's metabolic needs	Monitor blood glucose levels, initially on arrival to nursery and hourly thereafter. Maintain fluid and electrolyte balance. Watch for subtle changes. Initiate early oral feedings if possible; if not, administer IV infusion with 10% dextrose in water.
	LGA	Commonly associated with infants of birthing parent with diabetes Abrupt cessation of high-glucose maternal blood supply with birth and continued insulin production by the newborn Limited ability to release glucagon and catecholamines, which normally stimulate glucagon breakdown and glucose release	
	Postterm newborn	Hypoxia secondary to depleted glycogen reserves Placental insufficiency secondary to placental aging contributing to chronic fetal nutritional deficiency, further depleting glycogen stores	
	Preterm newborn	Immature sucking and swallowing, leading to insufficient intake Perinatal hypoxia	
	Late preterm infant	Increased energy expenditure Decreased subcutaneous and brown fat with little to no glycogen stores	

TABLE 23.1 • Common Problems Associated With Newborns Experiencing a Variation in Birth Weight or Gestational Age

Problem	Occurrence	Etiology/Pathophysiology	Nursing Implications
Polycythemia	FGR	Chronic mild hypoxia secondary to placental insufficiency Stimulation of erythropoietin release, leading to increased RBC production	Ensure adequate hydration (orally or IV). Monitor hematocrit levels (goal is ~60%). Administer partial exchange transfusion, albumin, or normal saline IV to reduce RBC volume and increase fluid volume (controversial).
	LGA	Secondary to fetal hypoxia, trauma with bleeding, increased erythropoietin production, or delayed cord clamping	
	Postterm newborn	Intrauterine hypoxia triggers increased RBC production to compensate for lower oxygen levels.	
Meconium aspiration	FGR	Release of meconium into amniotic fluid prior to birth Inhalation of meconium-containing amniotic fluid by the newborn, leading to aspiration	Initiate resuscitation measures as necessary. Suction airways and support ventilation (see Chapter 24 for more information).
	Postterm newborn	Commonly associated with chronic intrauterine hypoxia Struggling by fetus making respiratory efforts and bearing down with abdominal muscles, leading to expulsion of meconium into amniotic fluid Normal sucking and swallowing by fetus leads to meconium filling airways.	
Hyperbilirubinemia	LGA	Associated with polycythemia and RBC breakdown Inability to tolerate feedings in the first few days of life, leading to increased enterohepatic circulation of bilirubin	Ensure adequate hydration. Institute early feedings if possible. Administer phototherapy (see Chapter 24 for more information).
	Preterm newborn	Excessive bruising secondary to birth trauma, leading to higher-than-normal bilirubin levels	
	Late preterm infant	Increased breakdown of RBCs and immature liver function to handle excess load	
Birth trauma	LGA	Large size requiring use of operative birth procedure	Perform complete physical and neurologic assessment of the newborn. Note symmetry of structure and function. Assist parents in understanding situation (see Chapter 24).

ABG, arterial blood gas; CNS, central nervous system; FGR, fetal growth restriction; IV, intravenous; LGA, large for gestational age; RBC, red blood cell; SGA, small for gestational age.

Mandy, G. T. (2024a). Fetal growth restriction (FGR) and small for gestational age (SGA) newborns. *UpToDate*. https://www.uptodate.com/contents/fetal-growth-restriction-fgr-and-small-for-gestational-age-sga-newborns; Mandy, G. T. (2024b). Large-for-gestational-age (LGA) newborn. *UpToDate*. Retrieved March 16, 2024, from https://www.uptodate.com/contents/large-for-gestational-age-lga-newborn; and Mandy, G. T. (2023b). Overview of the short-term complications in preterm infants. *UpToDate*. Retrieved March 18, 2024, from https://www.uptodate.com/contents/overview-of-short-term-complications-in-preterm-infants

Metabolic needs are increased for catch-up growth. Initiate early and frequent oral feedings unless contraindicated. Monitor for hypoglycemia. With the loss of the placenta at birth, the newborn now must assume control of glucose homeostasis through intermittent oral feedings. Initiate breastfeeding as soon as possible or otherwise formula feed the infant on demand. If oral feedings are not accepted, a buccal dextrose gel or an intravenous (IV) infusion with 10% dextrose in water may be needed to maintain the glucose level above 40 mg/dL. Application of 40% dextrose gel to the buccal mucosa has emerged as an alternative to intravenous dextrose infusion (Rao, 2022). Weigh the newborn daily and ensure that they have adequate rest periods to decrease metabolic requirements. Monitor feeding tolerance, sucking, and swallowing ability.

Concept Mastery Alert

Planning Priority Care for the Small-for-Gestational-Age Infant

Infants who have SGA are different from preterm infants who often have underdeveloped respiratory systems. Infants who have SGA often have developed respiratory systems but have to be observed frequently for hypoglycemia because of their inadequate glycogen stores. This leads to the need for frequent and early feedings. Other complications include perinatal asphyxia, meconium aspiration, hypothermia, and polycythemia.

POLYCYTHEMIA

Polycythemia, also called erythrocytosis, is not uncommon and is a potentially serious disorder of newborns, though most newborns are asymptomatic. It is defined as a venous hematocrit above 65% and hemoglobin of more than 20 g/dL. Polycythemia occurs in up to 5% of neonates (Garcia-Prats, 2024). In infants with FGR, increased erythropoiesis occurs in utero in response to placental insufficiency. Most symptoms displayed in polycythemic infants are attributed to hyperviscosity or other metabolic differences.

Hyperviscosity results from the increased number of red blood cells and increases exponentially when the venous hematocrit is over 65%. Poor perfusion to organs occurs with hyperviscosity and is associated with long-term motor and cognitive neurodevelopmental disorders (Garcia-Prats, 2024). In addition to infants with FGR, infants of birthing parents with diabetes, newborns who are large for gestational age, and postterm newborns are at increased risk for hyperviscosity related to polycythemia. About one third of infants with polycythemia will also develop hyperbilirubinemia (Garcia-Prats, 2024).

Observe for clinical signs of polycythemia:

- Ruddy skin
- Abdominal distention, vomiting, poor feeding
- Cyanosis, tachycardia (less common)

Monitor hematocrit as ordered. Asymptomatic newborns with a hematocrit less than or equal to 70% may simply be supported with adequate fluid intake, close observation, and a repeat hematocrit level in 12 hours (Garcia-Prats, 2024). If the newborn is symptomatic, a partial plasma exchange transfusion may be needed to decrease the viscosity of blood and relieve symptoms (see Chapter 24 for additional information). Provide education to parents about any treatments and procedures that are being done.

Large-for-Gestational-Age Newborns

A newborn whose weight is above the 90th percentile on a growth chart based on gestational age is defined as large for gestational age (LGA) and occurs in up to 10% of births (Mandy, 2024b). Macrosomia refers to infants weighing over 4,000 g regardless of gestational age; this occurs in about 7% of births, with 1% being over 4,500 g (Mandy, 2024b). Having an infant who is LGA or macrosomic increases the risk for maternal morbidity including difficult labor, perineal lacerations, caesarean delivery, and postpartum hemorrhage. The infant is at increased risk for birth injury, asphyxia, respiratory distress, hypoglycemia, and polycythemia.

TAKE NOTE!

Maternal diabetes is commonly associated with newborns who are LGA. However, with chronic insulin-dependent diabetes, poor placental perfusion may occur leading the newborn to be SGA.

Nursing Assessment

Assessment of the newborn who is LGA begins with a review of the maternal history, which can provide clues as to whether the pregnant person has an increased risk of giving birth to a larger infant. Maternal factors that increase the chance of bearing a newborn who is LGA or macrosomic include the birthing parent having been LGA as an infant or having diabetes mellitus, higher weight, or excessive gestational weight gain. Infant factors include having a sibling who was LGA and has certain genetic syndromes (Mandy, 2024b).

Assess the newborn for characteristics of the macrosomic infant: full rosy cheeks with a ruddy skin color, round puffy face, massive shoulders, and excessive subcutaneous fat tissue (Sheanon & Muglia, 2020).

Thoroughly assess the newborn at birth to identify traumatic birth injuries such as fractured clavicles, skull fractures, or hematomas. Perform a neurologic examination to identify any nerve palsies, looking for abnormalities such as immobility of the upper arm and asymmetric extremity movement. Document any injuries discovered to allow for early intervention and improved outcomes.

Due to early depletion of glycogen stores in the liver, newborns who are LGA or macrosomic are at increased risk for hypoglycemia. Obtain frequent blood glucose levels as ordered to evaluate for hypoglycemia. Observe for clinical signs of hypoglycemia including listlessness, hypotonia, apathy, poor feeding, apneic episodes with a drop in oxygen saturation, weak or high-pitched cry, cyanosis, temperature instability, pallor and sweating, tremors, irritability, and seizures (Abramowski et al., 2023). In addition, be alert for signs of other common problems, such as polycythemia and hyperbilirubinemia (see Table 23.1).

Nursing Management

Assist in stabilizing the newborn. Screening for hypoglycemia in high-risk infants who are LGA is essential. Monitor blood glucose levels within 30 minutes of birth and repeat the screening every hour. Recheck levels before feedings and also immediately in any infant suspected of having or showing clinical signs of hypoglycemia, regardless of age. Early on-demand breastfeeding or formula feeding may help prevent hypoglycemia (Abramowski et al., 2023). Monitor and record intake and output, and obtain daily weights to aid in evaluating nutritional intake.

Observe for signs of polycythemia and hyperbilirubinemia and report immediately to the health care provider so early interventions can be taken to prevent poor long-term neurologic development outcomes. Polycythemia and hyperviscosity are associated with fine and gross motor delays, speech delays, and neurologic sequelae (Garcia-Prats, 2024). Increasing fluid volume aids in decreasing blood viscosity. Hydration, early feedings, and phototherapy are used to treat hyperbilirubinemia (see Chapter 24 for more information about hyperbilirubinemia). Provide parental guidance about the treatments and procedures being done and about the need for follow-up care for any abnormalities identified.

GESTATIONAL AGE VARIATIONS

The mean duration of pregnancy, calculated from the first day of the last normal menstrual period, is approximately 280 days, or 40 weeks. Gestational age is typically measured in weeks. An infant born with a gestational age of 39 weeks through 40 weeks and 6 days is classified as a **full-term newborn**. A newborn born before completion of 37 weeks is classified as a **preterm newborn** and one born after completion of 42 weeks is classified as a **postterm newborn**.

- Term newborn subgroups:
  - Early term: 37 to 38 6/7 weeks
  - Full term: 39 to 40 6/7 weeks
  - Late term: 41 to 41 6/7 weeks (American College of Obstetricians and Gynecologists [ACOG], 2022)
- Preterm newborn subgroups:
  - Extremely preterm: less than 28 weeks
  - Very preterm: 28 to 32 weeks
  - Moderate preterm: 32 to 33 6/7 weeks
  - **Late preterm newborn** (near term): 34 to 36 6/7 weeks (Mandy, 2022)
- Postterm newborn: more than 42 0/7 completed weeks' gestation and beyond (ACOG, 2022)

Precise knowledge of a newborn's gestational age is imperative for effective postnatal management. Determination of gestational age by the nurse assists in planning appropriate care for the newborn and provides important information regarding potential problems that need interventions. See Chapter 18 for more information on assessing gestational age.

TAKE NOTE!

Although pre- and postterm newborns may appear to be at opposite ends of the gestational age spectrum and are different in size and appearance, both are at high risk and need special care.

Preterm Newborn

Despite improved survival of preterm infants due to advancing technology and improved evidence-based perinatal care, respiratory failure, infection, congenital anomalies, intraventricular hemorrhage, and necrotizing enterocolitis continue to be the most common causes of mortality in this population (Mandy, 2022). Excellent nursing care can positively impact these causes (except congenital anomalies), thereby decreasing the mortality rate for preterm infants.

Risk factors for preterm birth include:

- Previous preterm birth or maternal history of being born preterm
- Painless cervical dilatation
- Short cervix
- Use of reproductive technologies
- Multiple gestation
- Obstetric complications
- Past history of procedural abortion
- Cervical issues
- Uterine issues
- Non-Hispanic Black or American Indian/Alaskan native race
- Infection (including periodontal disease)
- Maternal chronic disease
- Extremes of maternal age
- Maternal undernutrition
- Extremes of prepregnancy weight or gestational weight gain
- Male sex
- Lack of prenatal care
- Cigarette smoking or substance use (Robinson & Norwitz, 2024).

Tertiary centers caring for a high volume of preterm infants and who provide a high level of neonatal intensive care demonstrate a reduction in preterm newborn morbidity and mortality. Therefore, transporting high-risk pregnant person to a tertiary center for birth rather than transferring the neonate after birth is preferred (Mandy, 2022). Despite increasing survival rates, preterm infants continue to be at high risk for neurodevelopmental disorders such as cerebral palsy, cognitive delay, motor deficits, hearing or vision issues, behavioral problems and attention deficit-hyperactivity disorder, impaired social interactive skills, growth impairment, and chronic lung disease (Mandy, 2023a). Preterm birth survivors often need ongoing medical attention and education intervention. See Healthy People 2030.

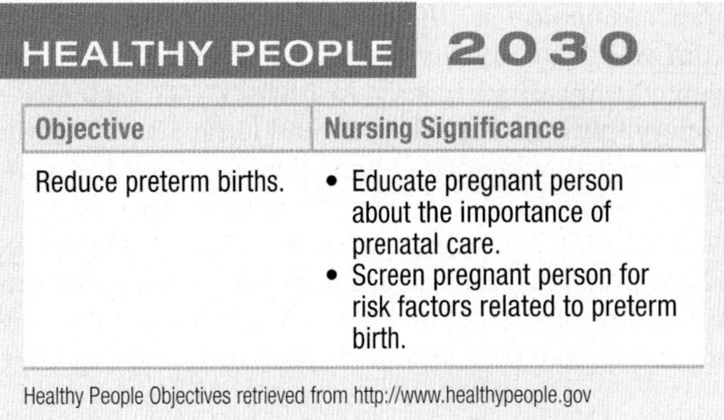

HEALTHY PEOPLE 2030

Objective	Nursing Significance
Reduce preterm births.	• Educate pregnant person about the importance of prenatal care. • Screen pregnant person for risk factors related to preterm birth.

Healthy People Objectives retrieved from http://www.healthypeople.gov

Effects of Prematurity on Body Systems

Since the preterm newborn did not remain in utero long enough, every body system may be immature, affecting the newborn's transition from intra- to extrauterine life and placing them at risk for complications. Risk is increased with decreasing gestational age. Short-term complications include:

- Hypothermia due to a relatively larger body surface area and heat production inability
- Infection
- Anemia as preterm infants have lower levels of circulating hemoglobin at birth as compared with term infants
- Glucose abnormalities
- Intraventricular hemorrhage related to the preterm infants' fragile germinal matrix
- Retinopathy of prematurity related to immature retinal vascularization
- Respiratory issues due to surfactant deficiency
- Apnea as a consequence of immature respiratory control
- Patent ductus arteriosus
- Hypotension
- Necrotizing enterocolitis
- Feeding difficulties
- Slow growth (Mandy, 2023b)

Recall Anna, who gave birth to a newborn at 7 months' gestation. What problems would you anticipate her newborn might have?

Nursing Assessment

Preterm newborns are at high risk for numerous problems and require special care. When preterm labor develops and cannot be stopped by medical interventions, plans are necessary for appropriate management of the birthing parent and the preterm newborn, such as transporting them to a regional center with facilities to care for preterm newborns or notifying the facility's neonatal intensive care unit (NICU). Depending on the degree of prematurity and health of the infant, the preterm newborn may be kept in the NICU for months.

A thorough assessment of the preterm newborn upon admission to the nursery provides a baseline from which to identify changes in clinical status. Review the maternal history to identify risk factors for preterm birth and check ante- and intrapartum records for maternal infections to anticipate the need for treatment. Maternal risk factors associated with preterm birth include a previous preterm delivery, low socioeconomic status, preeclampsia, hypertension, poor maternal nutrition, smoking, multiple gestation, infection, advanced maternal age, and substance use disorder. Be aware of the common physical characteristics and be able to identify any deviation from the expected (Fig. 23.2). Common physical characteristics of preterm infants may include:

- Birth weight of less than 5.5 lb
- Scrawny appearance
- Head disproportionately larger than chest circumference
- Poor muscle tone
- Minimal subcutaneous fat
- Undescended testes and minimal scrotal rugae in males
- Prominent clitoris and labia minora in females
- Plentiful lanugo (soft, downy hair), especially over the face and back
- Poorly formed ear pinna, with soft, pliable cartilage
- Fused eyelids (in the periviable infant, less than or equal to 25 weeks' gestation)
- Soft and spongy skull bones, especially along suture lines
- Matted scalp hair, woolly in appearance
- No or few creases in the soles and palms
- Thin, transparent skin with visible veins
- Breast and nipples not clearly delineated
- Abundant vernix caseosa (Reyna, 2024)

Be alert for evidence that might suggest that the preterm newborn is developing a complication (see Table 23.1). Note the newborn's gestational age and assess for FGR. Inspect the newborn's skin closely, especially skin color. Assess vital signs, including temperature via skin probe to identify hypothermia or fever and heart rate for tachycardia or bradycardia. Evaluate the newborn's respiratory effort and respiratory rate. Observe for periods of apnea lasting longer than 20 seconds. Monitor oxygen saturation levels by pulse oximetry to validate perfusion status. Note and report any signs of respiratory distress. Auscultate lung and heart sounds, being especially alert for possible murmur, which would indicate the presence of patent ductus arteriosus. Assess neurologic status by observing the newborn's behavior. Note any restlessness, hypotonia, or weak cry or sucking effort, and report unusual findings.

Screen for hypoglycemia upon admission and then hourly, always observing for nonspecific signs of hypoglycemia such as lethargy, poor feeding, and seizures. Evaluate serum bilirubin concentrations. Finally, assess the birthing parent and family members. Identify family strengths and coping mechanisms to establish a basis for intervention.

TAKE NOTE!

Glucose is needed by the brain and CNS to maintain and support numerous body system functions.

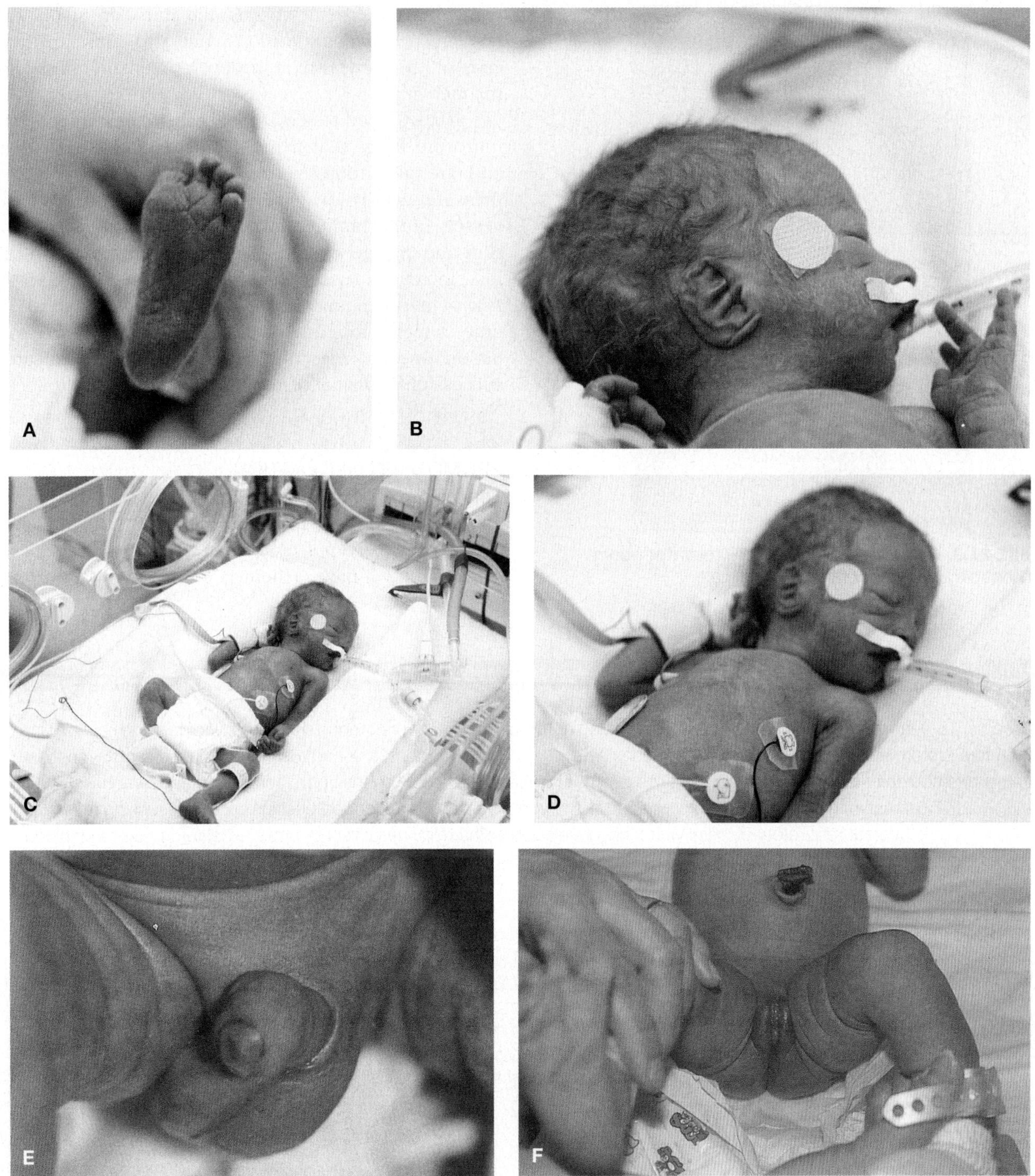

FIGURE 23.2 Characteristics of a preterm newborn. **A.** Few plantar creases. **B.** Soft, pliable ear cartilage, matted hair, and fused eyelids. **C.** Lax posture with poor muscle tone. **D.** Breast and nipple area barely visible. **E.** Male genitalia with minimal rugae on scrotum. **F.** Female genitalia with prominent labia and clitoris.

Nursing Management

Preterm newborns present with immaturity of all organ systems, abundant physiologic challenges, and significant morbidity and mortality globally (Karlsson et al., 2022). This places them at risk for complications as well as ongoing developmental concerns. The NICU environment is overstimulating, often painfully so. Preterm infants are at lifelong risk for learning problems, visual-motor-perceptual skill limitations, and emotional dysregulation. Additionally, they are at risk for attention problems and moderate to severe deficits in academic achievement, internalization, and executive function (especially in infants with very low birth weights) (Als, 2023). When

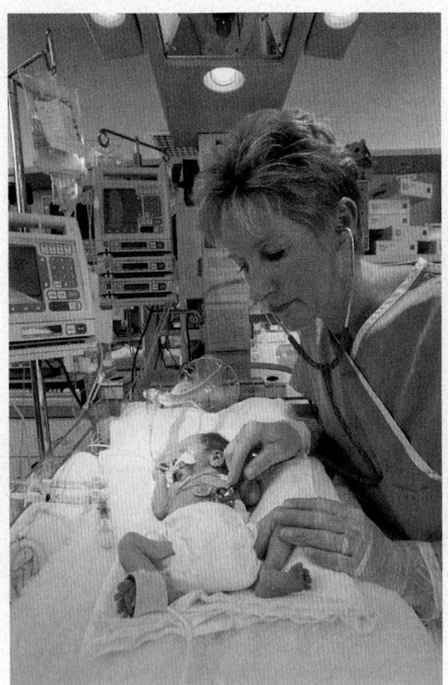

FIGURE 23.3 The physical condition of a preterm newborn demands skilled assessment and nursing care.

managing preterm newborns, the nurse must not only be vigilant for complications, but also must approach care of the newborn in a developmentally supportive manner (Fig. 23.3).

Nurses need to remember that preterm infants have immature lungs that may be more difficult to ventilate and are also more vulnerable to injury by positive-pressure ventilation. They also have immature blood vessels in the brain that are prone to hemorrhage, thin skin and a large surface area contributing to rapid heat loss, increased susceptibility to infection, and increased risk of hypovolemic shock related to small blood volume. Anticipation, adequate preparation, accurate evaluation, and prompt initiation of support are critical for successful neonatal resuscitation (Clinical Judgment & Nursing Process 23.1).

PROMOTING OXYGENATION

The preterm infant lacks surfactant, which lowers surface tension in the alveoli and stabilizes them to prevent their collapse. Even if preterm newborns can initiate respirations, they have a limited ability to retain air due

CLINICAL JUDGMENT & NURSING PROCESS 23.1 Overview of the Care of a Preterm Newborn

Alice, an 18-year-old, believed she had done everything right during her first pregnancy and certainly didn't anticipate giving birth to a preterm newborn at 32 weeks' gestation. When Mary Ellen was born, she had respiratory distress and hypoglycemia and couldn't stabilize her temperature. Assessment revealed the following: newborn scrawny in appearance; skin thin and transparent with prominent veins over abdomen; hypotonia with lax, extended positioning; weak sucking reflex when nipple is offered; respiratory distress with tachypnea (70 breaths/min), nasal flaring, and sternal retractions; low blood glucose level suggested by lethargy, tachycardia, jitteriness; axillary temperature of 96.8°F (36°C) despite warmed blanket; weight 2,146 g (4.73 lb); length 45 cm (17.72 in).

NURSING ANALYSIS: Altered breathing pattern related to immature respiratory system and respiratory distress as evidenced by tachypnea, nasal flaring, and sternal retractions.

OUTCOME IDENTIFICATION AND EVALUATION

The newborn's respiratory status will return to an adequate level of functioning as evidenced by rate remaining within 30 to 60 breaths/min, maintenance of acceptable oxygen saturation levels, and minimal to absent signs of respiratory distress.

INTERVENTIONS: *Promoting Optimal Breathing Pattern*

- Assess gestational age and risk factors for respiratory distress *to allow early detection.*
- Anticipate need for bag and mask setup and wall suction *to allow for prompt intervention should respiratory status continue to worsen.*
- Assess respiratory effort (rate, character, effort) *to identify changes.*
- Assess heart rate for tachycardia and auscultate heart sounds *to determine worsening of condition.*
- Observe for cues (grunting, shallow respirations, tachypnea, apnea, tachycardia, central cyanosis, hypotonia, increased effort) *to identify need for additional oxygen.*
- Maintain slight head elevation *to prevent upper airway obstruction.*
- Assess skin color *to evaluate tissue perfusion.*
- Monitor oxygen saturation level via pulse oximetry *to provide objective indication of perfusion status.*
- Provide supplemental oxygen as indicated and ordered *to ensure adequate tissue oxygenation.*
- Assist with any ordered diagnostic tests, such as chest x-ray and arterial blood gases (ABGs), *to determine effectiveness of treatments.*
- Cluster nursing activities *to reduce oxygen consumption.*
- Maintain a neutral thermal environment *to reduce oxygen consumption.*
- Monitor hydration status *to prevent fluid volume deficit or overload.*
- Explain all events and procedures to the parents *to help alleviate anxiety and promote understanding of the newborn's condition.*

NURSING ANALYSIS: Altered thermoregulation related to lack of fat stores and hypotonia as evidenced by extended positioning, low axillary temperature despite warmed blanket, respiratory distress, and lethargy.

CLINICAL JUDGMENT & NURSING PROCESS 23.1 Overview of the Care of a Preterm Newborn

OUTCOME IDENTIFICATION AND EVALUATION

The newborn will demonstrate ability to regulate temperature as evidenced by temperature remaining in normal range of 97.7°F to 99.5°F (36.5°C to 37.5°C) and absent signs of cold stress.

INTERVENTIONS: *Promoting Thermoregulation*

- Assess the axillary temperature every hour or use a thermistor probe *to monitor for changes.*
- Review maternal history *to identify risk factors contributing to the problem.*
- Monitor vital signs, including heart rate and respiratory rate, every hour, *to identify deviations.*
- Check radiant heat source or isolette *to ensure maintenance of appropriate temperature of the environment.*
- Assess environment for sources of heat loss or gain through evaporation, conduction, convection, or radiation *to minimize risk of heat loss.*
- Avoid bathing and exposing newborn *to prevent cold stress.*
- Warm all blankets and equipment that come in contact with newborn; place warmed cap on the newborn's head and keep it on *to minimize heat loss.*
- Encourage kangaroo care (birthing parent or partner holds preterm infant underneath clothing skin-to-skin and upright between breasts) *to provide warmth.*
- Educate parents on how to maintain a neutral thermal environment, including importance of keeping the newborn warm with a cap and double-wrapping with blankets and changing them frequently to keep dry *to promote newborn's adjustment.*
- Demonstrate ways to safeguard warmth *to prevent heat loss.*

NURSING ANALYSIS: Malnutrition risk related to poor sucking and lack of glycogen stores necessary to meet the newborn's increased metabolic demands as evidenced by weak sucking reflex, low birth weight, and signs and symptoms of hypoglycemia, including lethargy, tachycardia, and jitteriness.

OUTCOME IDENTIFICATION AND EVALUATION

The newborn will demonstrate adequate nutritional intake, remaining free of signs of hypoglycemia as evidenced by blood glucose levels being maintained above 45 mg/dL, enhanced sucking ability, and appropriate weight gain.

INTERVENTIONS: *Promoting Optimal Nutrition*

- Identify newborn at risk based on behavioral characteristics, body measurements, and gestational age *to establish a baseline and allow for early detection.*
- Assess blood glucose levels as ordered *to determine status and establish a baseline for interventions.*
- Obtain blood glucose measurements upon admission to nursery and every 1 to 2 hours as indicated *to evaluate for changes.*
- Observe behavior for signs of low blood glucose *to allow early identification.*
- Initiate early oral feedings or gavage feedings *to maintain blood glucose levels.*
- If oral or gavage feedings aren't tolerated, initiate an IV glucose infusion *to aid in stabilizing blood glucose levels.*
- Assess skin for pallor and sweating *to identify signs of hypoglycemia.*
- Assess neurologic status for tremors, seizures, jitteriness, and lethargy *to identify further drops in blood glucose levels.*
- Monitor weight daily for changes *to determine effectiveness of feedings.*
- Maintain temperature using warmed blankets, radiant warmer, or warmed isolette *to prevent heat loss and possible cold stress and reduce energy demands.*
- Monitor temperature *to prevent cold stress resulting in decreased blood glucose levels.*
- Offer opportunities for nonnutritive sucking on premature-size pacifier *to satisfy sucking needs.*
- Monitor for tolerance of oral feedings, including intake and output, *to determine effectiveness.*
- Administer IV dextrose if newborn is symptomatic *to raise blood glucose levels quickly.*
- Decrease energy requirements, including clustering care activities and providing rest periods, *to conserve glucose and glycogen stores.*
- Inform parents about procedures and treatments, including rationale for frequent blood glucose levels, *to help reduce their anxiety.*

to insufficient surfactant. Therefore, preterm newborns develop atelectasis quickly without alveoli stabilization. The inability to initiate and establish respirations leads to hypoxemia, acidosis, and hypercarbia. This change in the newborn's biochemical environment may inhibit the transition to extrauterine circulation, thus allowing fetal circulation patterns to persist.

Failure to initiate extrauterine breathing or failure to breathe well after birth leads to hypoxia. As a result, the heart rate falls, cyanosis develops, temperature decreases, blood pressure decreases, and respirations are altered (apnea, tachypnea, retractions, grunting, and nasal flaring), with the newborn eventually becoming hypotonic and unresponsive. Although this can happen with any newborn, the risk is higher in preterm newborns.

Note the newborn's Apgar score at 1 and 5 minutes. When performing newborn resuscitation, use the mnemonic "ABC" (airway, breathing, circulation) to remember the sequence of steps.

If the newborn does not respond to tactile stimulation with effective respirations and/or vigorous crying, position and clear the airway then immediately provide positive pressure ventilation (Weiner & Zaichkin, 2021). Refer to Chapter 18 for a full description of the neonatal resuscitation process. Throughout the resuscitation period, keep the parents informed of what is happening to their newborn and what is being done and why. Provide support through this initial crisis. Once the newborn has been stabilized, encourage bonding by having them stroke, touch, and, when appropriate, hold the newborn.

Administering Oxygen. Oxygen administration is a common therapy in neonatal intensive care units. When used, the target oxygen saturation level is 80% to 95%, depending on the newborn's gestational age and other factors. When saturations are above 95%, oxygen should be weaned (Vaughan et al., 2022).

Respiratory distress in preterm infants is commonly caused by a deficiency of surfactant, retained fluid in the lungs (wet lung syndrome), meconium aspiration, pneumonia, hypothermia, and/or anemia. Neonatal respiratory distress syndrome is the leading cause of death in preterm infants. Providing exogenous surfactant via nebulizer (aerosol delivery), instead of an endotracheal tube, is being advocated for to reduce the risk of bronchopulmonary dysplasia (Walther & Waring, 2022). The principles of care are the same regardless of the cause of respiratory distress:

- First, keep the newborn warm, preferably in a warmed isolette or with an overhead radiant warmer, to conserve the baby's energy and prevent cold stress.
- Handle the newborn as little as possible because stimulation often increases the oxygen requirement.
- Suction as needed to remove secretions, maintain a patent airway, and enhance oxygenation.
- Treat cyanosis with an oxygen hood or blow-by oxygen placed near the newborn's face if respiratory distress is mild and short-term therapy is needed.
- Record the following important observations every hour or more frequently if indicated, and document any deterioration or changes in respiratory status:
  - Respiratory rate, quality of respirations, and respiratory effort
  - Airway patency, including removal of secretions per facility policy
  - Skin color, including any changes to duskiness, blueness, or pallor
  - Lung sounds on auscultation to differentiate breath sounds in upper and lower fields
- Method of oxygen delivery, such as:
  - Blow-by oxygen delivered via mask or tube for short-term therapy
  - Oxygen hood (oxygen is delivered via a plastic hood placed over the newborn's head)
  - Nasal cannula (oxygen is delivered directly through the nares) (Fig. 23.4A)
  - Continuous positive airway pressure (CPAP), which prevents collapse of unstable alveoli and delivers high levels of inspired oxygen into the lungs
  - Mechanical ventilation, which delivers consistent assisted ventilation and oxygen therapy, reducing the work of breathing for the fatigued infant (but with risks) (Fig. 23.4B)
- Correct placement of endotracheal tube (if present)
- Heart rate
- The infant's respiratory status and oxygen saturation via pulse oximetry, clinically as well as by oxygen saturation, ABG, and chest x-ray (Lubbers & Eklund, 2022)

MAINTAINING THERMAL REGULATION

An optimal thermal environment is desirable for preterm infants. Worldwide, hypothermia is a major contributor to infant morbidity and mortality. Normothermia is defined as a body temperature measurement between 97.7°F and 99.5°F (36.5°C and 37.5°C) (Singh et al., 2022). When an infant becomes chilled, they attempt to conserve body heat by vasoconstriction and thermogenesis by metabolizing brown adipose tissue and increasing oxygen consumption. This increase in energy expenditure reduces the newborn's ability to gain weight. Immediately after birth, dry the newborn with a warmed towel and then place them in a second warm, dry towel before performing the assessment. Preterm newborns who are not considered stable may be placed under a radiant warmer or in a warmed isolette after they have been dried with a warmed towel.

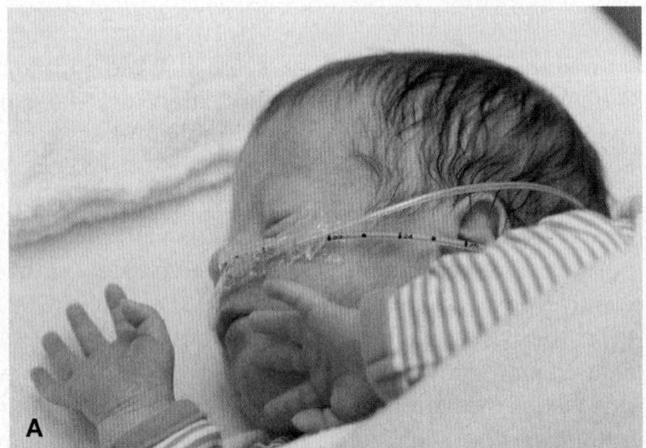

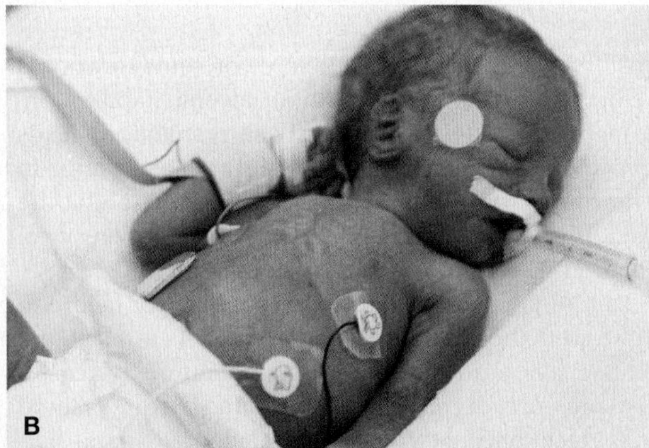

FIGURE 23.4 A. A preterm newborn receiving oxygen therapy via a nasal cannula. The newborn also has an enteral feeding tube inserted for nutrition. **B.** A preterm newborn receiving mechanical ventilation.

Typically, newborns use nonshivering thermogenesis for heat production by metabolizing their own brown adipose tissue. However, the preterm newborn has an inadequate supply of brown fat because they left the uterus early, before the supply was adequate. The preterm newborn also has decreased muscle tone and thus cannot assume the flexed fetal position, which reduces the amount of skin exposed to a cooler environment. In addition, preterm newborns have large body surface areas compared with weight. This allows an increased transfer of heat from their bodies to the environment.

When promoting thermal regulation for the preterm newborn, remember the four mechanisms for heat transfer and ways to prevent heat loss:

- *Convection*: heat loss through air currents (avoid drafts near the newborn)
- *Conduction*: heat loss through direct contact (warm everything the newborn comes into contact with, such as blankets, mattress, stethoscope)
- *Radiation*: heat loss without direct contact (keep isolettes away from cold sources and provide insulation to prevent heat transfer)
- *Evaporation*: heat loss by conversion of liquid into vapor (keep the newborn dry, and delay the first bath until the baby's temperature is stable)
- Frequently assess the temperature of the isolette or radiant warmer, adjusting the temperature as necessary to prevent hypothermia or hyperthermia.
- Encourage immediate skin-to-skin contact after birth to ensure stable thermoregulation.
- Utilize plastic wraps and bags, skin-to-skin contact, or transwarmer mattresses if available to keep infants warmer and decrease the incidence of hypothermia.
- Assess the newborn's temperature every hour until stable.
- Facilitate breastfeeding frequently.
- Cover the infant's head with a cap.
- Observe for clinical signs of cold stress, such as respiratory distress, central cyanosis, hypoglycemia, lethargy, weak cry, abdominal distention, apnea, bradycardia, and acidosis.
- Monitor the newborn for signs of hyperthermia such as tachycardia, tachypnea, apnea, warm to touch, flushed skin, lethargy, weak or absent cry, and central nervous system (CNS) depression; adjust the environmental temperature appropriately.
- Explain to the parents the need to maintain the newborn's temperature, including the measures used; demonstrate ways to safeguard warmth and prevent heat loss (Bedwell & Holtzclaw, 2022; Yadav, 2022).

PROMOTING NUTRITION

Providing nutrition is challenging for preterm newborns because their needs are great, but their ability to take in optimal amounts of energy/calories is reduced due to their small stomach capacity and compromised health status. In addition, preterm newborns have weak abdominal muscles, compromised metabolic function, limited ability to digest proteins and absorb nutrients, and weak or absent suck and gag reflexes. They often experience feeding intolerance and are at high risk of aspiration. All of these limitations place the preterm newborn at risk for nutritional deficiency and subsequent growth and development delays (Indrio et al., 2022). The preterm infant's ability to coordinate sucking, swallowing, and breathing is also challenged. Additionally, preterm infants who are ill or experiencing stressful situations have higher energy requirements. The exact nutritional needs of preterm infants depend on their gestational age, postnatal age, weight, route of nutritional intake, growth rate, activity, and thermal environment.

Depending on gestational age, preterm newborns receive nutrition orally, enterally, or parenterally via infusion. Total parenteral nutrition can be administered through a percutaneous central venous catheter for long-term venous access. Enteral feedings of breast milk (preferred) or formula may be oral, or via continuous nasogastric tube feedings or intermittent nasogastric or orogastric gavage tube feedings (Fig. 23.5). Gavage feedings are commonly used for compromised newborns to allow them to rest during the feeding process. Many have a weak suck and become fatigued and cannot consume enough calories orally to meet their needs.

Most newborns born after 34 weeks' gestation without significant complications can feed orally. Those born before 34 weeks' gestation typically start with parenteral nutrition within the first 24 hours of life. Enteral nutrition is then introduced and advanced based on the degree of maturity and clinical condition. Ultimately, enteral nutrition methods replace parenteral nutrition.

Trophic enteral feeding is used to prepare the preterm newborn's gut to overcome the many feeding

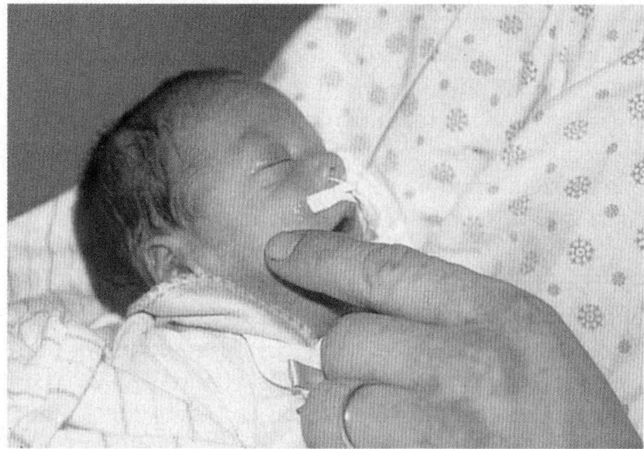

FIGURE 23.5 Infants who are ill at birth often need supplemental feedings by nasogastric or gastrostomy tubes. (Copyright Caroline Brown, RNC, MS, DEd.)

difficulties associated with gastrointestinal immaturity. It involves the introduction of very small amounts of enteral feeding (within 6 hours of birth if the newborn is stable) to induce surges in gut hormones that enhance maturation of the intestine. This minute amount of breast milk or formula given via gavage feeding prepares the gut to absorb future introduction of nutrients. It builds mucosal bulk, stimulates development of enzymes, enhances pancreatic function, stimulates maturation of gastrointestinal hormones, reduces gastrointestinal distention and malabsorption, and enhances transition to oral feedings (Hair, 2024).

To promote nutrition in the preterm newborn:

- Measure daily weight and plot it for gestational age on the preterm infant growth chart.
- Monitor intake; calculate fluid and caloric intake daily.
- Be alert for signs of dehydration, such as a decrease in urinary output, sunken fontanelles, temperature elevation, lethargy, and tachypnea.
- Continually assess for enteral feeding intolerance (measure abdominal girth, auscultate bowel sounds, and measure gastric residuals before the next tube feeding).
- Encourage and support breastfeeding by facilitating maternal breast pumping.
- Encourage nuzzling at the breast in conjunction with kangaroo care if the newborn is stable.

TAKE NOTE!

When assessing the fluid status of a preterm newborn, palpate the fontanelles. Sunken fontanelles suggest dehydration; bulging fontanelles suggest overhydration.

PREVENTING INFECTION

Preterm infants are vulnerable to bacterial infections due to prolonged hospitalization, invasive monitoring, and testing and treatments. Early birth deprives them of maternal antibodies needed for passive protection. They are also susceptible to infection because of their limited ability to produce their own antibodies, heightened risk for asphyxia at birth, and thin, friable skin that is easily traumatized, providing a portal of entry for microorganisms. Late-onset sepsis (occurring after 7 days of age) is a most common cause of morbidity and mortality in the NICU population (Flannery et al., 2022). The incidence of preterm bacterial sepsis increases with decreasing gestational age, ranging from 2% to 11% in the infant born between 25 and 34 weeks' gestation (Pammi, 2024). Prevention of infection is critical when caring for preterm newborns. Nursing assessment and early identification of problems are imperative to improve outcomes.

Clinical manifestations can be nonspecific and subtle and may include increase in apnea, respiratory distress, increased need for respiratory support, hypotonia, lethargy, poor feeding, temperature instability, hypotension, and tachycardia (Pammi, 2024). Report any of these to the primary care provider immediately so that treatment can be instituted.

Include the following interventions to prevent infection:

- Monitor for changes in vital signs such as temperature instability, tachycardia, or tachypnea, decreased oxygen saturation.
- Assess for feeding intolerance, which can be an early sign of infection.
- Encourage skin-to-skin contact to stabilize temperature.
- Avoid using tape on the newborn's skin to prevent tearing.
- Use equipment that can be discarded after use.
- Adhere to standard precautions; use clean gloves to handle dirty diapers and dispose of them properly.
- Attempt to minimize the use of invasive procedures; use sterile gloves when assisting with any invasive procedure.
- Remove all jewelry on your hands prior to washing hands; wash hands upon entering the nursery and in between caring for newborns.
- Avoid coming to work when ill, and screen all visitors for contagious infections.

Remember Anna, who entered the NICU to see her preterm baby after birth for the first time? How could the nurse have prepared her for this event? What information needs to be given at the isolette to reduce her anxiety and fear?

MANAGING PAIN

Pain is an unpleasant sensory and emotional experience felt by all humans. Unlike adults, infants are incapable of rating their pain verbally, and yet from the moment they take their first breath, newborns are exposed to heel sticks, circumcisions, injections, and immunizations, all of which cause pain. Newborns feel pain and require the same level of pain assessment and management as adults. As part of lifesaving treatments, preterm infants are typically exposed to about 300 invasive procedures during their stay in the NICU (Zhao et al., 2022). Awareness of the importance of pain in newborns has increased in recent years, but it remains a challenging area of clinical practice. Preterm infants express pain through specific signs and behaviors. Providing effective pain management for routine procedures for preterm infants in the NICU is a high priority in neonatal care. Apart from acute discomfort, there is now growing evidence that painful procedures may have adverse consequences on long-term neurologic development (Giordano et al., 2023). Pain control and prevention is imperative for ethical and clinical reasons and is required by the American Academy of Pediatrics (AAP) and The Joint Commission as a standard of excellence. Untreated pain in newborns may result in increased morbidity and length of stay in the NICU, exaggerated responses to pain in later life, decreased ability to respond to stress, and altered psychosocial development (Giordano et al., 2023). Parents commonly expect that health care providers will use appropriate measures to prevent pain in their newborns, but there are gaps in knowledge about the most effective way to accomplish this.

Assessing Pain in Newborns

Preterm infants show cortical, biochemical, physiologic, and behavioral responses to painful procedures. Common indicators of pain in the newborn who is unable to vocalize include facial expressions, body movements, and physiologic changes such as oxygen saturation (Clifton-Koeppel, 2023). Assessment of pain in the newborn remains a contentious and vexing problem as pain is difficult to validate with consistent behaviors. An international consortium established principles of newborn pain prevention and management that all nurses must be familiar with and apply (Box 23.2).

Nurses play a key role in assessing a newborn's pain level. Assess the newborn frequently. Differentiate pain from agitation by observing for changes in vital signs, behavior, facial expression, and body movement. Suspect pain if the newborn exhibits the following:

- Sudden high-pitched cry
- Facial grimace with furrowing of brow and quivering chin
- Increased muscle tone
- Oxygen desaturation
- Increase in heart rate
- Body posturing, such as squirming, kicking, and arching
- Limb withdrawal and thrashing movements
- Increase in heart rate, blood pressure, pulse, and respirations
- Fussiness and irritability (Clifton-Koeppel, 2023)

Several psychometric tools are available to assess pain in the newborn. Most are based on facial expressions, crying patterns, changes in vital signs, and body movements. Examples include:

- Pain Assessment Tool (PAT)—evaluates respirations, heart rate, oxygen saturation, and blood pressure
- Premature Infant Pain Profile Revised—assesses heart rate and oxygen saturation
- CRIES tool—evaluates cry, requires oxygen, increased vital signs, expression and sleeplessness
- Neonatal Infant Acute Pain Assessment Tool—assesses five behavioral and three physiologic indicators for pain
- Neonatal Infant Pain Scale (NIPS)—evaluates respiratory patterns

A more comprehensive neonatal pain assessment tool may be needed to address the complexity of neonatal pain (Llerena et al., 2023).

BOX 23.2 Newborn Pain Prevention and Management Guidelines

- Newborn pain frequently goes unrecognized and undertreated.
- Pain assessment is an essential activity prior to pain management.
- Newborns experience pain, and analgesics should be given.
- A procedure considered painful for an adult should also be considered painful for a newborn.
- Developmental maturity and health status must be considered when assessing for pain in newborns.
- Newborns may be more sensitive to pain than are adults.
- Pain behavior is frequently mistaken for irritability and agitation.
- Newborns are more susceptible to the long-term effects of pain.
- Adequate pain management may reduce complications and mortality.
- Nonpharmacologic measures can prevent, reduce, or eliminate newborn pain.
- Sedation does not provide pain relief and may mask pain responses.
- A newborn's response to both pharmacologic and nonpharmacologic pain therapy should be assessed within 30 minutes of administration or intervention.
- Health care professionals are responsible for pain assessment and treatment.
- Written guidelines are needed on each newborn unit.

Campbell-Yeo, M., Eriksson, M., & Benoit, B. (2022). Assessment and management of pain in preterm infants: A practice update. *Children, 9*(2), 244. https://doi.org/10.3390/children9020244; and Llerena, A., Tran, K., Choudhary, D., Hausmann, J., Goldgof, D., Sun, Y., & Prescott, S. (2023). Neonatal pain assessment: Do we have the right tools? *Frontiers in Pediatrics, 10*. https://doi.org/10.3389/fped.2022.1022751

Pain Management Strategies

Proper pain assessment, documentation, and management are needed to prevent adverse outcomes due to pain in infants. The goals of pain management are to minimize the amount, duration, and severity of pain and to assist the newborn in coping. It is essential that pain-related stress in preterm infants is accurately identified and appropriately managed and that pain management strategies are evaluated for protective or adverse effects in the long term. Effective pain management strategies for newborns include preventing, limiting, or avoiding noxious stimuli, using nonpharmacologic techniques to reduce pain, and administering pharmacologic agents when appropriate. Box 23.3 lists some of the more commonly used nonpharmacologic pain management techniques for the preterm newborn.

Nonpharmacologic pain management strategies include nonnutritive sucking, breastfeeding, skin-to-skin contact, radiant heat source, swaddling, therapeutic touch or massage, rocking, comfort positioning, and oral sucrose/glucose solutions. Administration of oral sucrose

BOX 23.3 Nonpharmacologic Techniques to Reduce Pain in the Preterm Newborn

- Gentle handling, rocking, caressing, cuddling, and massaging
- Rest periods before and after painful procedures
- Kangaroo care (skin-to-skin contact) during procedure
- Breastfeeding, if feasible, to reduce pain from minor procedures
- Use of a facilitated tuck (holding arms and legs in a flexed position)
- Application of topical anesthetics prior to venipuncture or lumbar puncture
- Swaddling and positioning to establish physical boundaries
- Nonnutritive sucking (pacifier dipped in sucrose) prior to procedure
- Minimal use of tape, with gentle removal to avoid skin tears
- Warm blankets for wrapping to facilitate relaxation
- Reduction of environmental stimuli by removing or turning down noxious stimuli such as noise from alarms, beepers, loud conversations, and bright lights
- Distraction, such as with colored objects or mobiles

Campbell-Yeo, M., Eriksson, M., & Benoit, B. (2022). Assessment and management of pain in preterm infants: A practice update. *Children, 9*(2), 244. https://doi.org/10.3390/children9020244; and Roue, J.-M. (2024). Management and prevention of pain in neonates. *UpToDate.* Retrieved March 19, 2024, from https://www.uptodate.com/contents/management-and-prevention-of-pain-in-neonates

with or without nonnutritive sucking is frequently used as a nonpharmacologic intervention for procedural pain relief in neonates. The recommended sucrose concentration is a 24% solution which is even more effective when combined with a skin-to-skin experience or nonnutritive sucking (Yamada et al., 2023).

The number of analgesics available for use with preterm newborns is limited. Morphine, ketamine, and fentanyl are the most commonly used medications for moderate to severe pain. Acetaminophen and nonsteroidal antiinflammatory drugs (NSAIDs) are effective for mild pain. Benzodiazepines are used as sedatives during painful procedures and can be combined with opioids for more effectiveness. Local or topical anesthetics may also be used before procedures such as venipuncture, lumbar puncture, and IV catheter insertion (Roue, 2023).

Be vigilant in assessing for adverse effects (respiratory depression or hypotension) when administering pharmacologic agents for pain management, especially in preterm newborns with neurologic impairment. These negative effects are usually dose and route related, so be knowledgeable about the pharmacokinetics and therapeutic dosing of any drug administered.

PROMOTING DEVELOPMENT

Preterm infants are at high risk for delayed neurodevelopment. Preterm infants admitted to the NICU are more vulnerable to stressors than their mature counterparts. Stressors that may contribute to growth development delays include exposure to light and noises, high risk of infections due to invasive procedures and fragile states of body systems, pain due to invasive procedures, and fewer parent–infant interactions. The NICU environment lends itself to persistent and unpredictable sounds that are in stark contrast to the protective sounds inside the birthing parent.

There is evidence to support the use of positive sensory exposures (music, touch, skin-to-skin) with preterm infants in the NICU on their neuromotor development. The beneficial effects of sensory stimulation while in NICU include improved feeding, visual function, and psychomotor development (Embarek-Hernández et al., 2022). Developmentally supportive care involves a framework for the delivery care process and care environment to be altered to support individualized developmental needs of the infant and family. Developmental care focuses on what newborns or infants can do at their stage of development, uses therapeutic interventions only to the point that they are beneficial, and provides for the development of the newborn–family unit (Kenner & McGrath, 2023).

Developmental care can be fostered by clustering the lights in one area so that no lights are shining directly on newborns, installing visual alarm systems and limiting overhead pages to minimize noise, and monitoring continuous and peak noise levels. In a recent study, developmental care improved outcomes and was associated with fewer cases of late-onset sepsis, retinopathy of prematurity (ROP), feeding intolerance, fewer days of ventilation support, antibiotic therapy, parenteral feeding, better weight gain, and growth parameters at discharge (Pavlyshyn et al., 2023). Nurses can play an active role by serving on committees that address these issues. In addition, nurses can provide direct developmentally supportive care. Doing so involves careful planning of nursing activities to provide the ideal environment for the newborn's development. For example:

- Dim the lights and cover isolettes at night to simulate nighttime.
- Turn down volume of noises from machines.
- Engage parents as their infant's primary caregivers.
- Support early extubation from mechanical ventilation if used.
- Encourage early and consistent feedings with breast milk.
- Administer prescribed antibiotics judiciously.
- Offer single-family rooms for privacy if available.
- Position the newborn as if they were still in utero (a nesting fetal position).
- Promote kangaroo care by encouraging parents to hold the newborn against the chest for extended periods each day.
- Coordinate care to respect sleep and awake states (Als, 2022).

Newborn stimulation involves a series of activities to encourage normal development (examples mentioned earlier). In the hospital, multisensory stimulation has shown to have a positive effect on feeding behavior, psychomotor development, and visual function (Embarek-Hernández et al., 2022). Conversely, overstimulation may have negative effects by reducing oxygenation and causing stress. A newborn reacts to stress by flaying the hands or bringing an arm up to cover the face. When overstimulated (e.g., by noise, lights, excessive handling, alarms, and procedures) and stressed, heart and respiratory rates decrease and periods of apnea or bradycardia may follow (LaRossa, 2023).

The NICU environment can be altered to provide periods of calm and rest for the newborn by dimming the lights, lowering the volume and tone of conversations, closing doors gently, setting the telephone ringer to the lowest volume possible, clustering nursing activities, and covering the isolette with a blanket to act as a light shield to promote rest at night. Nurses play a vital role in implementing a calming environment by controlling environmental stimuli, applying relaxation techniques, and therapeutic positioning when caring for preterm infants. For stable premature infants, encourage parents to hold and interact with the newborn. Demonstrate skin-to-skin care to parents to reduce stress in the infant. Doing so helps acquaint the parents with the newborn, promotes self-confidence, and fosters parent–newborn attachment (Fig. 23.6).

Think back to Anna, the woman who gave birth to a preterm newborn at 7 months' gestation. Anna will be discharged, but her newborn will be staying in the NICU for a while. What interventions would be appropriate to facilitate bonding despite their separation? What support can be provided specifically to this family?

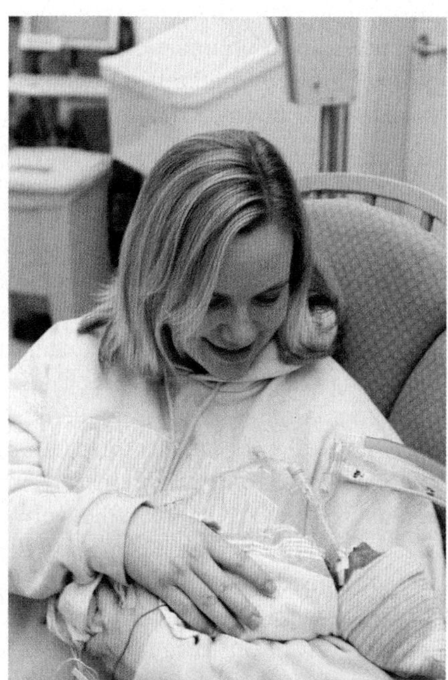

FIGURE 23.6 A parent bonding with their preterm newborn.

Family-centered care is also important. The overall principles of family-centered care involve dignity, respect, sharing of information, participation in care, and autonomy in decision making. Family presence and participation in the care in the NICU is fundamental to the recovery and well-being of the sick neonate and family. Promoting kangaroo care in the NICU for preterm infants is an example of development care and holds many benefits for the birthing parent–infant dyad (Evidence-Based Practice 23.1). Developmental care and family-centered care notably not only improve parental satisfaction but also influence the infant's health and well-being long after the NICU stay (Als, 2023).

Parents of NICU infants experience stress related to feelings of helplessness, exclusion, and isolation and lack sufficient knowledge regarding parenting and interacting with their newborn. There are several developmental interventions that nurses can do to help parents and newborns while in the NICU. Developmental care includes:

- Clustering care to promote rest and conserve the infant's energy
- Flexed positioning to simulate in utero positioning
- Active involvement of parents during painful procedures
- Environmental management to reduce noise and visual stimulation
- Kangaroo care to promote skin-to-skin sensation
- Placement of twins in the same isolette or open crib to reduce stress
- Activities to promote self-regulation and state regulation:
  - Surrounding the newborn with nesting rolls or devices
  - Swaddling with a blanket to maintain the flexed position
  - Providing sheepskin or a waterbed to simulate the uterine environment
  - Providing nonnutritive sucking (calms the infant) (Fig. 23.7)
  - Providing objects to grasp (comforts the newborn)
- Promotion of parent–infant bonding by making parents feel welcome in the NICU
- Education for parents about infant behavioral cues for feeding and fatigue
- Use of nonpharmacologic methods to reduce pain and stress
- Open, honest communication with parents and staff
- Collaboration with the parents in planning the infant's care (Altmier & White, 2023)

Throughout the newborn's stay, work with the parents to develop a collaborative partnership so they feel comfortable caring for the newborn. A successful transition from the NICU to home is imperative for the long-term health of preterm infants. Be prepared to make referrals to medical offices, clinics, and community support groups to enhance coping (Griffith et al., 2022).

EVIDENCE-BASED PRACTICE 23.1

Skin-to-Skin Contact to Support Preterm Infants and Reduce NICU-Related Stress

BACKGROUND

Recent advances in neonatal care have increased survival rates of preterm infants and those with complex medical needs, but mortality and morbidity rates continue to rise. Being hospitalized in an overstimulating environment, undergoing several painful medical interventions, and being separated from their parents leads to high stress levels for preterm infants in the NICU. The long-term consequences of high stress levels include postnatal growth restriction, cortisol activation, and disturbed brain development. Oxytocin is called the relaxation and calm hormone because it controls stress, anxiety, and autonomic functions. In addition, it helps build trust and connection with others. During times of stress cortisol is released, which stimulates the release of "fight or flight" hormones, such as adrenaline, to help people stay on high alert. In addition, cortisol raises blood sugar by releasing stored glucose, thus regulating it.

STUDY

The objective of the study was to investigate how skin-to-skin contact can influence the biologic stress levels in preterm infants in the NICU by evaluating cortisol and oxytocin levels. The study included 71 preterm infants with gestational ages <34 weeks. Saliva and urine samples were taken 1 hour before, immediately after, and 2 hours after skin-to-skin contact.

Findings

Preterm infants in NICU experience significant stress, characterized by a hormonal imbalance: an increased level of the stress hormone cortisol and a decreased level of the antistress hormone oxytocin. When the infant experiences heightened stress levels, apnea, increased arousal, anxiety, and tachycardia may result. Thus, the infant's body diverts resources away from growth and toward meeting the immediate demands of the stressed body. In addition, elevated levels of corticosteroid hormones result in poor brain growth, inhibition of bone formation, increased gastric acid secretion, and suppression of the immune system. Skin-to-skin care, or kangaroo care, has been well documented as promoting stress reduction by reducing cortisol levels and activating the release of oxytocin, otherwise known as the attachment hormone. Preterm infants receiving skin-to-skin care were found to have decreased respiratory rates, decreased heart rates, increased oxygen saturations, and better temperature regulation.

Nursing Implications

There is substantial evidence to support the use of skin-to-skin care for preterm infants receiving intensive care and undergoing painful procedures. Skin-to-skin care reduces stress by stimulating oxytocin release and blocking activation of the stress hormone cortisol. Nurses are instrumental in shaping the NICU environment and facilitating the relationship between infants and their parents. Encouraging early, frequent skin-to-skin care of sufficient duration (60 minutes or more) is important to improve the overall outcomes of vulnerable infants by reducing their stress levels.

Adapted from Pavlyshyn, H., Sarapuk, I., Horishna, I., Slyva, V., & Skubenko, N. (2022). Skin-to-skin contact to support preterm infants and reduce NICU-related stress. *International Journal of Developmental Neuroscience, 82*(7), 639–645. https://doi.org/10.1002/jdn.10216

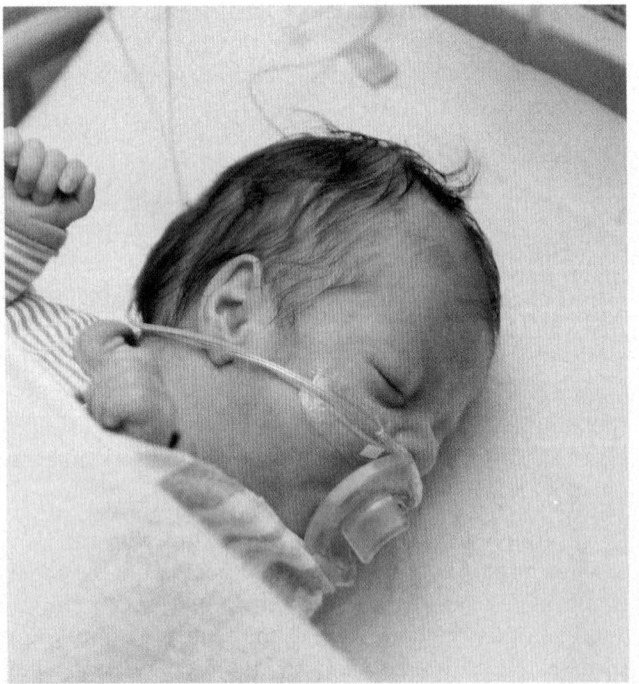

FIGURE 23.7 A preterm newborn receiving nonnutritive sucking with pacifier.

PROMOTING PARENTAL COPING

Generally, pregnancy and the birth of a newborn are exciting times, but when the newborn has serious, perhaps life-threatening, problems, the exciting experience suddenly changes to one of anxiety, fear, guilt, loss, and grief. The birth of a preterm infant is an acutely stressful event for the birthing parent, their partners, and families. Preterm birth creates a crisis for the birthing parent and family. Multiple studies have found that hospitalization for preterm newborns is often followed by negative mental health and behavioral outcomes, anxiety and depressive disorders, and long-term neurologic sequelae.

Parents are typically unprepared for the birth of a preterm newborn and commonly experience an array of emotions, including disappointment, fear for the survival of the newborn, and anxiety due to the separation from their newborn immediately after birth. Gaining insight into the experience of parents of premature infants can help nurses ensure services more effectively meet the needs of these families. Research suggests that nurses should address the needs of all family members, be more attentive to parents whose babies are experiencing long NICU stays, provide support to siblings, and address parental needs for continuity of care, follow-up, and information (Nurlaila et al., 2022).

Provide nursing interventions aimed at reducing parental anxiety:

- Review the events that have occurred since birth with the parents.
- Provide simple relaxation and calming techniques (visual imagery, breathing).
- Explore their perception of the newborn's condition, offering explanations.
- Validate their anxiety and behaviors as normal reactions to stress and trauma.
- Provide a physical presence and support during emotional outbursts.
- Explore the coping strategies they used successfully in the past and encourage their use now.
- Help parents clarify their individual needs and values in caring for a preterm infant.
- Encourage frequent visits to the NICU.
- Increase parents' self-efficacy in caring for infant.
- Encourage physical closeness of caregiver with infant.
- Involve parents in decision making.
- Provide empathetic listening and collaborative problem-solving.
- Provide individualized support to parents while the newborn is in NICU.
- Encourage parental involvement with the newborn in the NICU.
- Address their reactions to the NICU environment and explain all equipment used.
- Identify family and community resources available to them (Klawetter et al., 2022).

PREPARING FOR DISCHARGE

Discharge readiness is a key determinant of outcomes for families in the NICU. Discharge planning typically begins with evidence that recovery of the newborn is certain. However, the exact date of discharge may not be predictable. The goal of the discharge plan is to make a successful transition to home care. Essential elements for discharge are a physiologically stable infant, a family who can provide the necessary care with appropriate support services in place in the community, and a pediatrician or family practice primary provider or nurse practitioner available for ongoing care.

The care of each high-risk newborn after discharge requires careful coordination to provide ongoing multidisciplinary support for the family. The discharge planning team typically includes the parents or caregiver, primary care provider, neonatologists, neonatal nurses, and the discharge planner, case manager, or social worker. Other health care providers, such as occupational therapists, physical therapists, speech therapists, nutritionists, and home health care nurses may be included as needed. Critical components of discharge planning are summarized in Box 23.4.

BOX 23.4 Critical Components of Discharge Planning

- Parental education—involvement and support in newborn care during NICU stay will ensure their readiness to care for the infant at home.
- Evaluation of unresolved medical problems—review of the active problem list and determination of what home care and follow-up is needed.
- Implementation of primary care—completion of newborn screening tests, immunizations, examinations such as funduscopic examination for ROP, and hematologic status evaluation
- Development of home care plan, including assessment of:
  - Equipment and supplies needed for care
  - In-home caregiver's preparation and ability to care for infant
  - Adequacy of the physical facilities in the home
  - An emergency care and transport plan if needed
  - Financial resources for home care costs
  - Family needs and coping skills
  - Community resources, including how they can be accessed

NICU, neonatal intensive care unit; ROP, retinopathy of prematurity.

Boykova, M. V., Kenner, C., & Discenza, D. (2022). Transition to home and primary care. In C. Kenner & M. V. Boykova (Eds.), *Neonatal nursing care handbook: An evidence-based approach to conditions and procedures* (3rd ed.). Springer Publishing Company; and Smith, V. C., Love, K., & Goyer, E. (2022). Consensus statement: NICU discharge preparation and transition planning: Guidelines and recommendations. *Journal of Perinatology, 42*, 7–21. https://doi.org/10.1038/s41372-022-01313-9

Nurses involved in the discharge process are instrumental in bridging the gap between the hospital and home. When planning for discharge from the NICU:

- Assess the physical status of the birthing parent and the newborn.
- Start the discharge process at the time of admission to the NICU.
- Assess the physiologic markers of thermoregulation, respiratory stability, adequate weight gain, and feeding skill.
- Assess the emotional readiness of parents for the newborn's discharge.
- Discuss the early signs of complications and what to do if they occur.
- Reinforce instructions for infant care and safety.
- Stress the importance of proper car seat use.
- Assess readiness of specific technical skills needed to care for the infant.
- Provide instructions for medication administration.
- Reinforce instructions for equipment operation, maintenance, and troubleshooting.
- Teach infant cardiopulmonary resuscitation and emergency care.
- Demonstrate techniques for special care procedures such as dressings, ostomy care, artificial airway maintenance, chest physiotherapy, suctioning, and infant stimulation.
- Provide breastfeeding support or instruction on gavage feedings.
- Assist with defining roles in the adjustment period at home.

- Assess the parents' emotional stability and coping status.
- Provide support and reassurance to the family.
- Report abnormal findings to the health care team for intervention.
- Ensure parents know who to contact for any unanticipated event (Smith et al., 2022).

Late Preterm Newborn

A late preterm newborn is an infant born between 34 0/7 and 36 6/7 weeks' gestation. They may not necessarily appear premature, but they are. They have higher mortality and morbidity rates when compared with term infants due to their physiologic and metabolic immaturity, even though they are often the same size and weight of term infants. In recent years, the subject of late preterm birth has received much attention as this population of preterm newborns represents 75% of all preterm births in the United States and 7.5% of all live births (Barfield & Lee, 2023). The underlying causes are poorly understood, though genetic, social, and environmental factors all likely play a role. Reasons for this might include an increased demand for assisted reproductive technology, older women having babies, diabetes, hypertension, higher weight, preeclampsia, and higher rates of surgical births and inductions of labor (Barfield & Lee, 2023).

With birth weights typically ranging from 2,000 to 2,500 g, late preterm infants may appear physically well developed when compared with their more premature counterparts. Consequently, it may be easy for nurses to overlook the fact that biologically and developmentally these infants may be 4 to 6 weeks less mature than their full-term counterparts. Recent research has indicated that these infants are at heightened risk for a number of complications that are not normally seen in the healthy newborn population, such as respiratory distress, hypothermia, feeding difficulties, future cardiometabolic disease, and hypoglycemia (Barfield & Lee, 2023; Iacono & Regelmann, 2022).

Late preterm babies are more likely than term babies to suffer complications at birth such as respiratory distress, hypoglycemia, hypothermia, apnea, and seizures; require intensive and prolonged hospitalization; incur higher medical costs; die within the first year of life; and suffer brain injury that can result in long-term neurodevelopmental problems (Barfield & Lee, 2023).

Some additional challenges also facing the late preterm newborn include respiratory distress (secondary to cesarean births, maternal gestational diabetes, pulmonary hypertension, sepsis, chorioamnionitis, premature rupture of membranes, and fetal distress), thermoregulation issues related to limited ability to flex the trunk and extremities to decrease exposed surface area; hypoglycemia related to the first two challenges (respiratory distress and cold stress), jaundice and hyperbilirubinemia related to a gestational age of 36 weeks or less; sepsis; and feeding difficulties related to immature sucking and swallowing reflexes (Golden & Watchko, 2024).

Recent research suggests that after the neonatal period, risks of behavioral problems, particularly attention-deficit/hyperactivity disorder (ADHD), and emotional lability increase (Navalón et al., 2022). These challenges are similar to those facing the preterm newborn and require similar management. Parents should be taught about these risks so that they will be aware of the unique risks and the need to remain vigilant. Health risks for the late preterm infant include:

- Hypothermia
- Respiratory distress
- Apnea
- Hypoglycemia
- Seizure
- Perinatal asphyxia
- Hyperbilirubinemia
- Feeding difficulties
- Apgar score less than 4 (Barfield & Lee, 2023)

Nurses and parents must be aware of the risks associated with late preterm births to optimize care and outcomes for this group of newborns. Late preterm infants should not be discharged home before at least 48 hours of age. They should also have demonstrated thermal stability when clothed in an open crib, normal vital signs, the ability to take feeds orally, a weight loss of less than 7% of birth weight, and the ability to pass stools spontaneously. Other assessments before discharge include metabolic and genetic screening together with hearing screening and a successful car seat challenge (Barfield & Lee, 2023).

Encourage and empower parents of a late preterm infant with appropriate teaching and ongoing support. Stress that although the infant may seem equivalent to the term infant in many ways, there are specific risks that should be addressed not only in the first year of life but also beyond. Close surveillance, follow-up, and referral to appropriate support services can optimize outcomes.

Postterm Newborn

A pregnancy that extends beyond 42 weeks' gestation (294 days) produces a postterm newborn. About 5.5% of infants are born postterm (Ringer, 2023). Another term used to describe this late birth is *postmature infant*. Postterm newborns may be AGA, LGA, SGA, or dysmature. When the placenta continues to function well, the infant is often LGA. Placental insufficiency leads to the infant being SGA or dysmature. Without sufficient nutrition, the fetus relies on nutritional stores and FGR occurs. The dysmature infant appears long and thin, with wasted extremities (Reyna, 2024).

After 42 weeks, the placenta may begin to age. Deposits of fibrin and calcium along with hemorrhagic infarcts occur, and the placental blood vessels begin to degenerate. All of these changes affect diffusion of oxygen to the fetus. As the placenta loses its ability to nourish the fetus, the fetus uses stored nutrients to stay alive, and wasting occurs. This wasted appearance at birth is secondary to the loss of muscle mass and subcutaneous fat.

Nursing Assessment

A thorough assessment of the postterm newborn upon admission to the nursery provides a baseline from which to identify changes in clinical status. Review the maternal history for any risk factors associated with postterm birth. Also be aware of the common physical characteristics and be able to identify any deviation from the expected. Postterm newborns typically exhibit the following characteristics:

- LGA characteristics
- Evidence of placental aging:
  - Dry, cracked, peeling, and/or wrinkled skin
  - Absence of vernix caseosa and lanugo
  - Long, thin extremities
  - Creases that cover the entire soles of the feet
  - Wide-eyed, alert expression
  - Little body fat
  - Thin umbilical cord
- Abundant hair on scalp
- Long fingernails and toenails
- Limited vernix and lanugo (Reyna, 2024)

Assess the newborn's gestational age, and complete a physical examination to identify any abnormalities. Review the medical record to determine the color of the amniotic fluid when membranes ruptured and observe for a meconium-stained umbilical cord and fingernails if amniotic fluid is meconium stained. Also be alert to signs of potential complications often associated with a postterm newborn, such as perinatal asphyxia (caused by placental aging or oligohydramnios), hypoglycemia (caused by acute episodes of hypoxia related to cord compression, which exhausts carbohydrate reserves), hypothermia (caused by loss of subcutaneous fat), and polycythemia (caused by an increased production of red blood cells (RBCs) to compensate for a reduced oxygen environment). Be prepared to initiate early interventions (see Table 23.1).

Nursing Management

The birth of a postterm newborn may create stress for the birthing parent and their family. In most situations, birth of a newborn requiring special care was not anticipated. When a laboring patient is postterm, the newborn resuscitation team needs to be available in the birthing suite for immediate backup. The newborn may require transport to the NICU for continuous assessment, monitoring, and treatment, depending on their status after resuscitation.

Monitor and maintain the postterm newborn's blood glucose levels once stabilized. IV dextrose 10% and/or early initiation of feedings will help stabilize the blood glucose levels to prevent CNS sequelae. Also monitor the postterm newborn's skin temperature, respiratory characteristics, neurologic status, and results of blood studies, such as ABGs and serum bilirubin levels. Institute measures to prevent or reduce the risk of hypothermia by eliminating sources of heat loss: thoroughly dry the newborn at birth, wrap them in a warmed blanket, and place a stockinette cap on the newborn's head. Providing environmental warmth via a radiant heat source will help stabilize the newborn's temperature.

Closely assess all postterm newborns for polycythemia, which contributes to hyperbilirubinemia due to RBC destruction. Providing adequate hydration helps reduce the viscosity of the newborn's blood to prevent thrombosis. Be alert to the early, often subtle signs to promote early identification and prompt treatment to prevent any neurodevelopmental delays.

CONSIDER THIS!

I had been waiting for this baby since I can remember, and now I was told to wait even longer. I was into my 3rd week past my due date and was just told that if I didn't go into labor on my own, the doctor would induce me on Monday. As I walked out of his office into the hot summer sun, I thought about all the comments that would await me at the office: "You're not still pregnant, are you?" "Weren't you due last month?" "You look as big as a house." "Are you sure you aren't expecting triplets?" I started to get into my car when I felt warm fluid slide down my legs. Although I was embarrassed at my wetness, I was thrilled I wouldn't have to go back to the office and drove myself to the hospital. Within hours, my wait was finally over with the birth of my son, a postterm infant with a thick head of hair. He was certainly worth the wait!

Thoughts: Although most due dates are within plus or minus 2 weeks, we can't rely on that because so many factors influence the start of labor. This woman was anxious about her overdue status, but nature prevailed. The old adage "when the fruit is ripe, it will fall" doesn't always bring a good outcome though; many women need a little push to go into labor. What happens when the fetus stays inside the uterus too long? What features are typical of postterm infants?

KEY CONCEPTS

- Variations in birth weight and gestational age can place a newborn at risk for problems that require special care.
- Variations in birth weight include the following categories: SGA, AGA, and LGA. Newborns who are small or large for gestational age have special needs.
- The newborn who is SGA faces problems related to a decrease in placental function in utero; these problems may include perinatal asphyxia, hypothermia, hypoglycemia, polycythemia, and meconium aspiration.
- Risk factors for the birth of an infant who is LGA include their birthing parent having been LGA, having a sibling who was LGA, maternal diabetes mellitus,

higher weight, or excessive gestational weight gain, and certain genetic syndromes.

- Newborns who are LGA face problems such as birth trauma due to cephalopelvic disproportion, hypoglycemia, and hyperbilirubinemia.
- Variations in gestational age include extremely preterm, very preterm, moderate preterm, late preterm, early term, full term, late term, and postterm.
- The postterm newborn may develop complications after birth including perinatal asphyxia, hypoglycemia, hypothermia, polycythemia, and meconium aspiration.
- The preterm newborn is at risk for complications because their organ systems are immature, thereby impeding the transition from intrauterine life to extrauterine life.
- Newborns can experience pain, but their pain is difficult to validate with consistent behaviors.
- Newborns with gestational age variations, primarily preterm newborns, benefit from developmental care, which includes a variety of activities designed to manage the environment and individualize the care based on behavioral observations.
- Nurses play a key role in assisting the parents and family of a newborn with special needs to cope with this crisis situation, including dealing with the possibility that the newborn may not survive.
- The goal of discharge planning is to make a successful transition to home care.

REFERENCES AND RECOMMENDED READINGS

Abramowski, A., Ward, R., & Hamdan, A. H. (2023). *Neonatal hypoglycemia*. In *StatPearls*. StatPearls Publishing. https://www.ncbi.nlm.nih.gov/books/NBK537105/

Als, H. (2023). Theoretical perspective for developmentally supportive care. In C. Kenner & J. M. McGrath (Eds.), *Developmental care of newborns and infants: A guide for health professionals* (3rd ed.). National Association of Neonatal Nurses.

Altmier, L. B., & White, R. D. (2023). Single-family room design in the neonatal intensive care unit. In C. Kenner & J. M. McGrath (Eds.), *Developmental care of newborns and infants: A guide for health professionals* (3rd ed.). National Association of Neonatal Nurses.

American College of Obstetricians and Gynecologists. (2022). *Definition of term pregnancy, committee opinion 579 (reaffirmed 2022)*. https://www.acog.org/clinical/clinical-guidance/committee-opinion/articles/2013/11/definition-of-term-pregnancy

Barfield, W. D., & Lee, K. G. (2023). Late preterm infants. *UpToDate*. Retrieved March 18, 2024, from https://www.uptodate.com/contents/late-preterm-infants

Bedwell, S., & Holtzclaw, B. J. (2022). Early interventions to achieve thermal balance in term neonates. *Nursing for Women's Health, 26*(5), 389–396. https://doi.org/10.1016/j.nwh.2022.07.006

Boykova, M. V., Kenner, C., & Discenza, D. (2022). Transition to home and primary care. In C. Kenner & M. V. Boykova (Eds.), *Neonatal nursing care handbook: An evidence-based approach to conditions and procedures* (3rd ed.). Springer Publishing Company.

Campbell-Yeo, M., Eriksson, M., & Benoit, B. (2022). Assessment and management of pain in preterm infants: A practice update. *Children, 9*(2), 244. https://doi.org/10.3390/children9020244

Clifton-Koeppel, R. (2023). Pain assessment and nonpharmacologic management. In C. Kenner & J. M. McGrath (Eds.), *Developmental care of newborns and infants: A guide for health professionals* (3rd ed.). National Association of Neonatal Nurses.

Cunningham, F. G., Leveno, K. J., Dashe, J. S., Hoffman, B. L., Spong, C. Y., & Casey, B. M. (2022). Fetal growth disorders. In F. G. Cunningham, K. J. Leveno, J. S. Dashe, B. L. Hoffman, C. Y. Spong, & B. M. Casey (Eds.), *William's obstetrics* (26th ed.). McGraw-Hill.

Davis, B. E., Leppert, M. O., German, K., Lehmann, C. U., Adams-Chapman, I., Council On Children With Disabilities, and Committee on Fetus and Newborn. (2023). Primary care framework to monitor preterm infants for neurodevelopmental outcomes in early childhood. *Pediatrics, 152*(1), e2023062511. https://doi.org/10.1542/peds.2023-062511

Embarek-Hernández, M., Güeita-Rodríguez, J., & Molina-Rueda, F. (2022). Multisensory stimulation to promote feeding and psychomotor development in preterm infants: A systematic review. *Pediatrics and Neonatology, 63*(5), 452–461. https://doi.org/10.1016/j.pedneo.2022.07.001

Flannery, D. D., Edwards, E. M., Coggins, S. A., Horbar, J. D., & Puopolo, K. M. (2022). Late-onset sepsis among very preterm infants. *Pediatrics, 150*(6), e2022058813. https://doi.org/10.1542/peds.2022-058813

Garcia-Prats, J. A. (2024). Neonatal polycythemia. *UpToDate*. Retrieved March 17, 2024, from https://www.uptodate.com/contents/neonatal-polycythemia

Giordano, V., Deindl, P., Gal, E., Unterasinger, L., Fuiko, R., Steinbauer, P., Weninger, M., Berger, A., & Olischar, M. (2023). Pain and neurodevelopmental outcomes of infants born very preterm. *Developmental Medicine & Child Neurology, 65*(8), 1043–1052. https://doi.org/10.1111/dmcn.15505

Golden, W. C., & Watchko, J. F. (2024). Neonatal hyperbilirubinemia and kernicterus. In C. A. Gleason & T. Sawyer (Eds.), *Avery's diseases of the newborn* (11th ed., pp. 1044–1066). Elsevier.

Griffith, T., Singh, A., Naber, M., Hummel, P., Bartholomew, C., Amin, S., White-Traut, R., & Garfield, L. (2022). Scoping review of interventions to support families with preterm infants post-NICU discharge. *Journal of Pediatric Nursing, 67*, e135–e149. https://doi.org/10.1016/j.pedn.2022.08.014

Hair, A. B. (2024). Approach to enteral nutrition in the premature infant. *UpToDate*. Retrieved May 20, 2024, from https://www.uptodate.com/contents/approach-to-enteral-nutrition-in-the-premature-infant

Iacono, L., & Regelmann, M. O. (2022). Late preterm birth and the risk of cardiometabolic disease. *JAMA Network Open, 5*(5), e2214385. https://doi.org/10.1001/jamanetworkopen.2022.14385

Indrio, F., Neu, J., Pettoello-Mantovani, M., Marchese, F., Martini, S., Salatto, A., & Aceti, A. (2022). Development of the gastrointestinal tract in newborns as a challenge for an appropriate nutrition: A narrative review. *Nutrients, 14*(7), 1405. https://doi.org/10.3390/nu14071405

Karlsson, V., Blomqvist, Y. T., & Ågren, J. (2022). Nursing care of infants born extremely preterm. *Seminars in Fetal and Neonatal Medicine, 27*(3), 101369. https://doi.org/10.1016/j.siny.2022.101369

Kenner, C., & McGrath, J. M. (2023). *Developmental care for newborns and infants: A guide for health professionals* (3rd ed.). National Association of Neonatal Nurses.

Klawetter, S., Cetin, N., Ilea, P., McEvoy, C., Dukhovny, D., Saxton, S. N., Rincon, M., Rodriguez-JenKins, J., & Nicolaidis, C. (2022). "All these people saved her life, but she needs me too": Understanding and responding to parental mental health in the NICU. *Journal of Perinatology, 42,* 1496–1503. https://doi.org/10.1038/s41372-022-01426-1

LaRossa, M. M. (2023). *Understanding preterm infant behavior in the NICU.* https://med.emory.edu/departments/pediatrics/divisions/neonatology/dpc/nicubeh.html

Llerena, A., Tran, K., Choudhary, D., Hausmann, J., Goldgof, D., Sun, Y., & Prescott, S. M. (2023). Neonatal pain assessment: Do we have the right tools? *Frontiers in Pediatrics, 10.* https://doi.org/10.3389/fped.2022.1022751

Lubbers, L. A., & Eklund, W. M. (2022). Respiratory system. In C. Kenner & M. V. Boykova (Eds.), *Neonatal nursing care handbook: An evidence-based approach to conditions and procedures* (3rd ed.). Springer Publishing Company.

Mandy, G. T. (2022). Preterm birth: Definitions of prematurity, epidemiology, and risk factors for infant mortality. *UpToDate.* Retrieved March 18, 2024, from https://www.uptodate.com/contents/preterm-birth-definitions-of-prematurity-epidemiology-and-risk-factors-for-infant-mortality

Mandy, G. T. (2023a). Overview of the long-term complications of preterm birth. *UpToDate.* Retrieved March 18, 2024, from https://www.uptodate.com/contents/overview-of-the-long-term-complications-of-preterm-birth

Mandy, G. T. (2023b). Overview of the short-term complications in preterm infants. *UpToDate.* Retrieved March 18, 2024, from https://www.uptodate.com/contents/overview-of-short-term-complications-in-preterm-infants

Mandy, G. T. (2024a). Fetal growth restriction (FGR) and small for gestational age (SGA) newborns. *UpToDate.* Retrieved March 16, 2024, from https://www.uptodate.com/contents/fetal-growth-restriction-fgr-and-small-for-gestational-age-sga-newborns

Mandy, G. T. (2024b). Large for gestational age (LGA) newborn. *UpToDate.* Retrieved March 16, 2024, from https://www.uptodate.com/contents/large-for-gestational-age-lga-newborn

Navalón, P., Ghosn, F., Ferrín, M., Almansa, B., Moreno-Giménez, A., Campos-Berga, L., Sahuquillo-Leal, R., Diago, V., Vento, M., & García-Blanco, A. (2022). Are infants born after an episode of suspected preterm labor at risk of attention deficit hyperactivity disorder? A 30-month follow-up study. *American Journal of Obstetrics and Gynecology, 227*(757), e1–e11. https://doi.org/10.1016/j.ajog.2022.05.065

Nurlaila, Herini, E. S., Hartini, S., & Kusuma, M. T. P. L. (2022). Interventions to reduce parental stress and increase readiness of parents with preterm infants in the neonatal intensive care unit: A scoping review. *Journal of Neonatal Nursing, 29*(4), 595–601. https://doi.org/10.1016/j.jnn.2022.12.002

Pammi, M. (2024). Clinical features and diagnosis of bacterial sepsis in preterm infants <34 weeks gestation. *UpToDate.* Retrieved March 18, 2024, from https://www.uptodate.com/contents/clinical-features-and-diagnosis-of-bacterial-sepsis-in-preterm-infants-less-than34-weeks-gestation

Pavlyshyn, H., Sarapuk, I., Horishna, I., Slyva, V., & Skubenko, N. (2022). Skin-to-skin contact to support preterm infants and reduce NICU-related stress. *International Journal of Developmental Neuroscience, 82*(7), 639–645. https://doi.org/10.1002/jdn.10216

Pavlyshyn, H., Sarapuk, I., Tscherning, C., & Slyva, V. (2023). Developmental care advantages in preterm infants management. *Journal of Neonatal Nursing, 29*(1), 117–122. https://doi.org/10.1016/j.jnn.2022.03.008

Rao, R. B. (2022). Neonatal hypoglycemia. *Newborn, 1*(1), 151–157. https://www.newbornjournal.org/abstractArticleContentBrowse/JNB/27407/JPJ/fullText

Reyna, B. A. (2024). The Infant at risk. In B. J. Baker, J. Janke, & AWHONN (Eds.), *Core curriculum for maternal-newborn nursing* (6th ed.). Elsevier.

Ringer, S. (2023). Postterm infant. *UpToDate.* Retrieved March 20, 2024, from https://www.uptodate.com/contents/postterm-infant

Robinson, J. N., & Norwitz, E. R. (2024). Spontaneous preterm birth: Overview of risk factors and prognosis. *UpToDate.* Retrieved March 18, 2024, from https://www.uptodate.com/contents/spontaneous-preterm-birth-overview-of-risk-actors-and-prognosis

Roue, J.-M. (2023). Management and prevention of pain in neonates. *UpToDate.* Retrieved March 19, 2023, from https://www.uptodate.com/contents/management-and-prevention-of-pain-in-neonates

Sheanon, N. M., & Muglia, L. J. (2020). The endocrine system. In R. M. Kliegman, J. W. St. Geme, N. J. Blum, S. S. Shah, R. C. Tasker, & K. M. Wilson (Eds.), *Nelson textbook of pediatrics* (21st ed.). Elsevier Health Sciences.

Simmons, R. A. (2024). Abnormalities of fetal growth. In C. A. Gleason & T. Sawyer (Eds.), *Avery's diseases of the newborn* (11th ed., pp. 33–41). Elsevier.

Singh, T. S., Skelton, H., Baird, J., Padernia, A., Maheshwari, R., Shah, D. M., D'Cruz, D., Luig, M., & Jani, P. (2022). Improvement in thermoregulation outcomes following the implementation of a thermoregulation bundle for preterm infants. *Journal of Pediatrics and Child Health, 58*(7), 1201–1208. https://doi.org/10.1111/jpc.15949

Smith, V. C., Love, K., & Goyer, E. (2022). Consensus statement: NICU discharge preparation and transition planning: Guidelines and recommendations. *Journal of Perinatology, 42,* 7–21. https://doi.org/10.1038/s41372-022-01313-9

Trotter, C. W. (2025). Gestational age assessment. In C. L. Witt & C. M. Wallman (Eds.), *Tappero & Honeyfield's physical assessment of the newborn* (7th ed.). Springer Publishing Company.

U.S. Department of Health and Human Services. (n.d.). *Healthy People 2030.* https://health.gov/healthypeople

Vaughan, R., Greenaway, S., & Lee, G. (2022). Resuscitation of the newborn. *Anesthesia & Intensive Care Medicine, 24*(1), 45–53. https://doi.org/10.1016/j.mpaic.2022.10.018

Walther, F. J., & Waring, A. J. (2022). Aerosol delivery of lung surfactant and nasal CPAP in the treatment of neonatal respiratory distress syndrome. *Frontiers in Pediatrics, 10,* 923010. https://www.ncbi.nlm.nih.gov/pmc/articles/PMC9240419/

Weiner, G. M., & Zaichkin, J. (2021). *Textbook of neonatal resuscitation* (8th ed.). American Academy of Pediatrics.

Yadav, S. (2022). Plastic wrap to prevent hypothermia in neonates: An overall review article. *International Journal of Science and Research, 11*(7). https://doi.org/10.21275/SR22719075010

Yamada, J., Bueno, M., Santos, L., Haliburton, S., Campbell-Yeo, M., & Stevens, B. (2023). Sucrose analgesia for heel-lance procedures in neonates. *Cochrane Database of Systematic Reviews.* https://doi.org/10.1002/14651858.CD014806

Zhao, T., Starkweather, A. R., Matson, A., Lainwala, S., Xu, W., & Cong, X. (2022). Nurses' experiences of caring for preterm infants in pain: A meta-ethnography. *International Journal of Nursing Sciences, 9*(4), 533–541. https://doi.org/10.1016/j.ijnss.2022.09.003

DEVELOPING CLINICAL JUDGMENT

PRACTICING FOR NCLEX

1. The nurse documents that a newborn is postterm. How many weeks' gestation was the newborn?
   a. 38
   b. 40
   c. 42
   d. 39
2. The nurse cares for several newborns who are either SGA or LGA. What condition predisposes these newborns to develop polycythemia?
   a. Hypoxia
   b. Hypoglycemia
   c. Hypocalcemia
   d. Hypothermia
3. A newborn is SGA. Which condition in this infant does the nurse understand was caused by the use of subcutaneous and brown fat stores for survival in utero?
   a. Hyperbilirubinemia
   b. Hypothermia
   c. Polycythemia
   d. Hypoglycemia
4. A nurse is examining a preterm newborn. Which nursing assessment finding would be of greatest concern?
   a. Milia over the bridge of the nose
   b. Thin transparent skin
   c. Poor muscle tone
   d. Heart murmur
5. The nurse is providing care to several newborns with variations in gestational age and birth weight. When developing the plan of care for these newborns, the nurse focuses on energy conservation to promote growth and development. Which measures would the nurse include in the nursing plans of care? Select all that apply.
   a. Keeping the handling of the newborn to a minimum
   b. Maintaining a neutral thermal environment
   c. Decreasing environmental stimuli
   d. Initiating early oral feedings
   e. Using thermal warmers in all cribs
   f. Promoting kangaroo care by caregivers
6. The nurse is assessing pain in a newborn with special needs. Which concept would the nurse incorporate into the plan of care?
   a. Newborns experience pain primarily with surgical procedures.
   b. Preterm newborns in the NICU are at the least risk for pain.
   c. Pain assessment needs to be comprehensive and frequent.
   d. A newborn's facial expression is the primary indicator of pain.
7. A preterm infant at 6 hours old has a respiratory rate of 65, mild nasal flaring, and an expiratory grunt. The birthing parent experienced ruptured membranes 36 hours prior to giving birth. Which measure should the nurse include in the plan of care?
   a. Have a respiratory therapist set up a ventilator and obtain blood gases every hour.
   b. Monitor vital signs every 8 hours to allow for adequate rest for the infant.
   c. Place infant in radiant warmer and restrict visitation of parents and family.
   d. Observe for signs of sepsis, obtain cultures as ordered, and monitor vital signs frequently.
8. A preterm infant is placed under the radiant heat warmer after birth. The nurse evaluates the temperature frequently to prevent which condition?
   a. Cold stress
   b. Respiratory depression
   c. Tachycardia
   d. Thermogenesis
9. The nurse is caring for an infant who is LGA. Which lab value should the nurse monitor?
   a. White blood cell count
   b. Direct Coombs test
   c. Blood glucose
   d. Potassium level

CRITICAL THINKING EXERCISE

1. After fetal distress was noted on the monitor, a postterm newborn was delivered via a difficult vacuum extraction. The newborn had low Apgar scores and had to be resuscitated before being transferred to the nursery. Once admitted, the nurse observed jitteriness, tremors, hypotonia, lethargy, and rapid respirations.
   a. What might these findings indicate?
   b. For what other conditions might this newborn be at high risk?
   c. What intervention is needed to address this newborn's condition?
2. A preterm newborn was born at 35 weeks following a placental abruption due to a car crash. The newborn was transported to the NICU at a nearby regional medical center. After being stabilized, the newborn was placed in an isolette close to the door and placed on a cardiac monitor. A short time later, the nurse notices that the newborn is cool to the touch and lethargic, has a weak cry, and has an axillary temperature of 36°C.
   a. What might have contributed to this newborn's hypothermic condition?
   b. What transfer mechanism may have been a factor?
   c. What intervention would be appropriate for the nurse to initiate?

3. A term newborn weighing 4 lb was brought to the nursery for admission a short time after birth. The labor and birth nurse reports the birthing parent is a heavy smoker, addicted to cocaine, and experienced physical abuse throughout their pregnancy. After stabilizing the newborn and correcting the hypoglycemia with oral feedings, the nurse observes acrocyanosis, ruddy color, poor circulation to the extremities, tachypnea, and irritability.
   a. What complication might this newborn be manifesting?
   b. What factors may have contributed to this complication?
   c. What would be an appropriate intervention for managing this condition?

STUDY ACTIVITIES

1. At a community health department maternity clinic, secure permission to interview the parents of a child with special needs. Ask about their feelings throughout the experience. How are they managing and coping now?
2. Visit the March of Dimes website and review this group's national campaign to reduce the incidence of prematurity. Are their strategies workable or not? Explain your reasoning.
3. A common metabolic disorder present in both newborns who are SGA and those who are LGA after birth is ________________.
4. A 10-lb newborn is brought to the nursery after a difficult vaginal birth. The nursery nurse should focus on detecting birth injuries such as ________________.

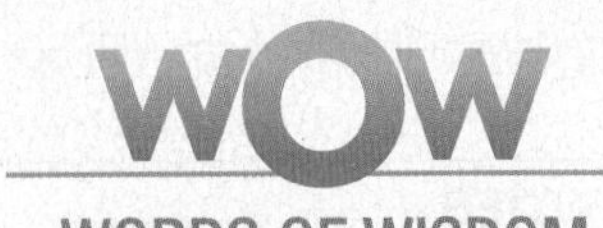

WORDS OF WISDOM

Courage and faith in oneself project onto others, giving them the strength to persevere.

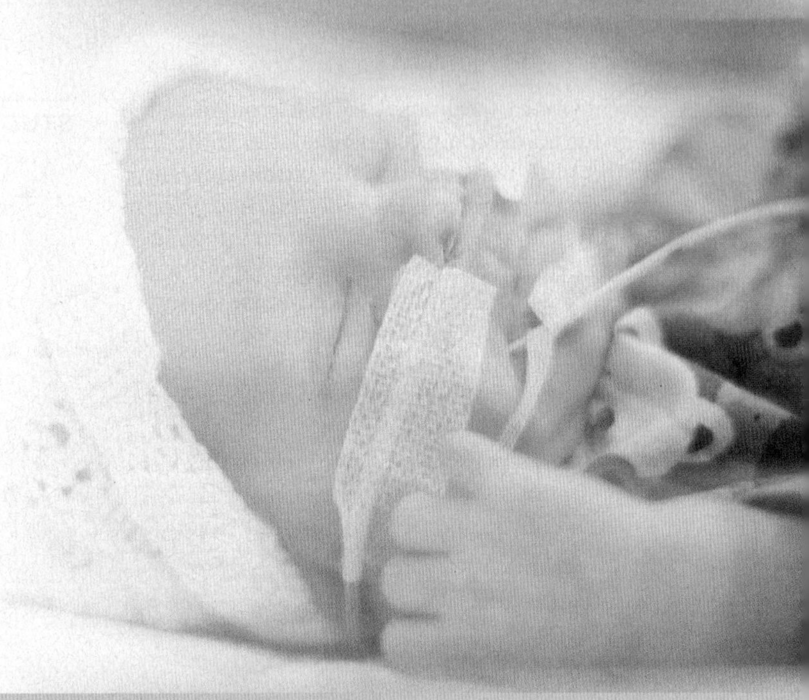

24

Nursing Management of the Newborn at Risk: Congenital and Acquired Newborn Conditions

KEY TERMS

anencephaly (an'en-sef'ă-lē)
asphyxia
birth injury
caput succedaneum (kap'ŭt sŭk-sĕ-dā'nē-ŭm)
cephalohematoma (sef'ă-lō-hē-mă-tō'mă)
gastroschisis (gas-tros'ki-sis)
hyperbilirubinemia (hī'pĕr-bil'i-rū-bi-nē'mē-ă)
infant of a mother with diabetes (IMD)
meconium aspiration syndrome (MAS)
meningocele (mĕ-ning'gō-sēl)
microcephaly (mī'krō-sef'ă-lē)
myelomeningocele (mī'ĕ-lō-mĕ-ning'gō-sēl)
neonatal opioid withdrawal syndrome (NOWS)
neonatal sepsis
neural tube defect (NTD)
omphalocele (om'fal-ō-sēl)

LEARNING OBJECTIVES

Upon completion of the chapter, you will be able to:

1. Describe the most common congenital conditions affecting the newborn.
2. Compare and contrast the four classifications of congenital heart disease.
3. Distinguish four inborn errors of metabolism.
4. Describe the most common acquired conditions affecting the newborn.
5. Outline the assessment and nursing management needed for newborns sustaining birth injury.
6. Plan the assessment, interventions, prevention, and management of hyperbilirubinemia in newborns.
7. Examine the impact of maternal diabetes on the newborn and the care needed.
8. Research the assessment and interventions for a newborn experiencing substance withdrawal after birth.
9. Summarize the interventions appropriate for a newborn with neonatal sepsis.
10. Plan the nursing management of a newborn experiencing respiratory distress syndrome (RDS).
11. Outline the birthing room preparation and procedures necessary to prevent meconium aspiration syndrome (MAS) in the newborn at birth.

12. Devise parent education for the follow-up care needed by newborns with retinopathy of prematurity (ROP).
13. Identify risk factors for the development of necrotizing enterocolitis (NEC).
14. Evaluate the major congenital and acquired anomalies affecting the central nervous system, respiratory system, gastrointestinal system, genitourinary system, and musculoskeletal system that can occur in a newborn.
15. Characterize the importance of parental participation in care of the newborn with an acquired or congenital condition, including the nurse's role in facilitating parental involvement.

Kelly, a 27-year-old G2P1, comes to the labor and birth area in active labor. She tells you she is overdue and relieved to finally be giving birth. Her membranes rupture upon admission, revealing meconium-stained fluid. What additional nursing assessments need to be performed? What risk factors need to be considered when developing Kelly's plan of care as well as her newborn's?

INTRODUCTION

Advances in prenatal and neonatal medical and nursing care throughout the world have led to a marked increase in the number of newborns who have survived high-risk pregnancies and have congenital or acquired conditions. These newborns are considered one of the most vulnerable at-risk populations; that is, they are susceptible to morbidity and mortality because of the acquired or congenital disorder. Several national health goals address the issues of acquired and congenital conditions in newborns (U.S. Department of Health and Human Services [USDHHS], 2020).

During the past several decades, technologic, genomic, and pharmacologic advances in conjunction with standardized policies and procedures have significantly improved survival rates for at-risk newborns. However, the risk of morbidity remains. For example, some of these newborns are at risk for continuing health problems that require long-term technologic support. Other newborns remain at risk for physical and developmental problems into the school years and beyond. Although challenges remain in application of these advances to improve the newborn's health, the high-risk newborn will increasingly benefit from them in the future. Providing the complex care needed to maintain the child's health and well-being will have a tremendous emotional and economic impact on the family. Nurses are challenged to provide support to families when neonatal well-being is threatened.

Congenital disorders can be defined as structural, functional, or metabolic abnormalities that are present at birth. They can be caused by single-gene defects, chromosomal disorders, multifactorial inheritance, environmental teratogens, or micronutrient deficiencies. Most congenital disorders have a complex etiology, involving many interacting genes, gene products, and social and environmental factors during organogenesis (the origin and development of organs). The most common serious congenital disorders are congenital heart defects (CHDs), neural tube defects (NTDs), and Down syndrome (World Health Organization [WHO], 2024). Some alterations can be prevented or compensated for with pharmacologic, nutritional, or other types of interventions, while others cannot be changed.

Acquired disorders typically occur at or soon after birth. They may result from problems or conditions experienced by the pregnant person during pregnancy or at birth, such as diabetes, maternal infection, or substance misuse or conditions associated with labor and birth, such as prolonged rupture of membranes or fetal distress. However, there may be no identifiable cause for the disorder.

This chapter addresses select congenital and acquired newborn conditions. In addition, it describes the nurse's role in assessment and management, emphasizing parental education and support. Nurses play a key role in helping parents cope with the stress of having an ill newborn.

CONGENITAL CONDITIONS

According to the WHO, an estimated 6% of infants are born each year globally with a congenital disorder (2024). In the United States, congenital disorders occur in 2% to 4% of live births (Bacino, 2023). Congenital conditions can arise from single-gene disorders, chromosomal aberrations, and teratogen exposure; or, they may occur sporadically. They may be isolated or occur in conjunction with other disorders, apparent or hidden, gross, or microscopic. Congenital conditions are the primary cause of death in infancy (Centers for Disease Control and Prevention [CDC], 2024a). When a serious anomaly is identified prenatally, the parents can decide whether to continue the pregnancy. When an anomaly is identified at or after birth, parents need to be informed promptly and given a realistic appraisal of the severity of the condition, the prognosis, and treatment options so they can participate in all decisions pertaining to the child.

Congenital conditions can affect virtually any body system. This section describes common congenital conditions identified at or after birth. Some of these conditions warrant immediate treatment soon after birth. Other conditions, though identified in the newborn period, are long term with ongoing effects into childhood.

Congenital Heart Defect

A *congenital heart defect* (CHD) is defined as a structural defect involving the heart, the great vessels, or both and is present at birth (American Heart Association [AHA], 2023). About 1% of newborns (about 40,000) born each year in the United States have heart defects (CDC, 2024a). The defect may be mild, with the newborn appearing healthy at birth, or it may be so severe that the newborn's life is in immediate jeopardy. Annually, about 7,200 infants with a CHD have a critical defect that needs surgery within the first year of life (CDC, 2024b). Critical congenital heart defects (CCHDs) usually present in the first few days or weeks of life while the newborn's circulation is continuing to adapt to the demands of extrauterine life. Advances in diagnosis as well as medical and surgical interventions have led to dramatic increases in survival rates for newborns with CCHDs (Jone et al., 2022; Schneider, 2023).

Pathophysiology

In most cases, the exact cause of CHD is unknown. Most CHDs develop during the first 8 weeks' of gestation and are usually the result of genetic and environmental forces (Bernstein, 2025). CCHD is a group of the eight most severe CHDs: critical coarctation of the aorta, transposition of the great arteries, hypoplastic left heart syndrome, total anomalous pulmonary venous return, pulmonary atresia with intact ventricular septum, tetralogy of Fallot, tricuspid atresia, and truncus arteriosus (Altman, 2024). Pulse oximetry screening in the neonatal period increases early identification of CCHDs. Treatment is needed soon after birth, or CCHD can be deadly (Altman, 2024).

Therapeutic Management

Though some defects can be medically managed for a period of time, most infants with CHDs need corrective surgery. CCHDs in particular require surgical correction early if the infant is to survive.

Nursing Assessment

Although most CHDs cannot be prevented, several key areas need to be addressed to ensure the optimal health status for the pregnant person and the fetus. A thorough health history and physical examination of the birthing person and newborn provide valuable information. Laboratory and diagnostic tests provide additional information about the defect and its severity.

Ideally, the nursing assessment begins prenatally by reviewing the maternal history for risk factors that might predispose the newborn to a CHD. Risk factors include family history of CHD, maternal diabetes, phenylketonuria, rubella infection during pregnancy, maternal use of angiotensin-converting enzymes or retinoic acids in the first trimester, and maternal smoking or exposure to secondhand smoke (National Heart, Lung, and Blood Institute, 2022). See the Healthy People 2030 box.

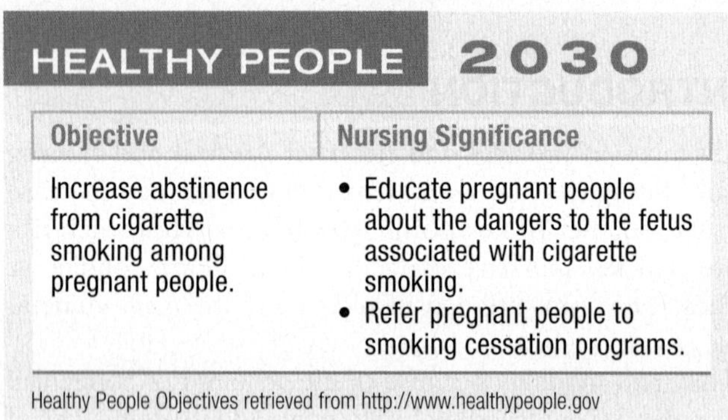
HEALTHY PEOPLE 2030

Objective	Nursing Significance
Increase abstinence from cigarette smoking among pregnant people.	• Educate pregnant people about the dangers to the fetus associated with cigarette smoking. • Refer pregnant people to smoking cessation programs.

Healthy People Objectives retrieved from http://www.healthypeople.gov

After birth, carefully assess the newborn's cardiovascular and respiratory systems. Look for respiratory distress, cyanosis, or abnormal heart rate, rhythm, or sounds. Note signs of heart failure including edema, diminished peripheral pulses, poor feeding, poor growth, cyanosis, hepatomegaly, tachycardia, diaphoresis, respiratory distress with tachypnea, peripheral pallor, and irritability. Perform pulse oximetry screening as recommended by the American Academy of Pediatrics (AAP) when the infant is at least 24 hours old (AAP, 2023). Failed oximetry screening includes any of the following:

- Any oxygen saturation below 90%
- Three separate measures (separated by 1 hour each) of oxygen saturation below 95% in the right hand and foot
- Three separate measures (separated by 1 hour each) of oxygen saturation above 3% of the absolute difference between the right hand and the foot (AAP, 2023)

Nursing Management

Infants failing CCHD screening should be immediately referred to pediatric cardiology for additional workup.

Continuously monitor the newborn's cardiac and respiratory status. Administer medications as ordered. Provide comfort measures to the newborn, who may be subjected to a variety of painful procedures. Include the parents in the plan of care. Assess their ability to cope with the diagnosis, encouraging them to verbalize their feelings about the newborn's condition and treatment. Educate them about the specific cardiac defect. Assist parents with making decisions about treatment and support their decisions for the newborn's care. If surgical correction is planned, provide the parents with preoperative teaching, and orient them to the neonatal intensive care unit (NICU) prior to surgery. Provide emotional support and guidance throughout the newborn's care. Refer parents to local support groups, national organizations, and websites. Emphasize the importance of close supervision and follow-up care.

Neural Tube Defects

Neural tube defect (NTD) is the common name used to describe congenital central nervous system structural defects. NTDs are serious malformations involving the spine (spina bifida) and brain (anencephaly). About 11.5 of 10,000 live births in the United States each year result in newborns with NTDs, with the defects occurring more often in females (Dukhovny & Wilkins-Haug, 2024).

An NTD occurs when the neural tube that develops into the brain and spinal cord fails to close properly by the fifth to sixth week of gestation (Dukhovny & Wilkins-Haug, 2024). In pregnancies in which the fetus has an NTD, the level of alpha-fetoprotein in the amniotic fluid and maternal serum is elevated. The most severe NTDs are anencephaly and myelomeningocele. It is thought that adequate maternal folic acid intake decreases the risk for the development of NTDs—see the Healthy People 2030 box.

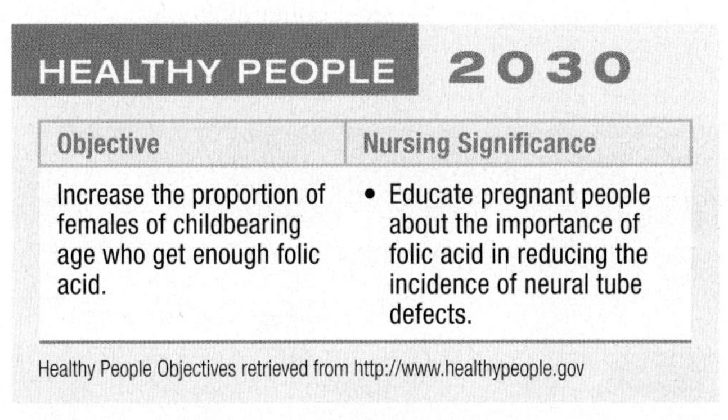

HEALTHY PEOPLE 2030

Objective	Nursing Significance
Increase the proportion of females of childbearing age who get enough folic acid.	• Educate pregnant people about the importance of folic acid in reducing the incidence of neural tube defects.

Healthy People Objectives retrieved from http://www.healthypeople.gov

Anencephaly

Anencephaly, considered the most severe fatal NTD, results from failure of the neural tube to fuse in the cranial area, with the cerebral hemispheres completely missing or reduced to small masses. The brain is replaced by an undifferentiated mass of connective tissue and vessels. Anencephaly most commonly involves the forebrain and variable amounts of the upper brain stem, where there is no brain tissue above the brain stem. Infants with this disorder are born without a brain front and a cerebrum, with the rest of the brain tissue exposed without bone or skin covering. The incidence is approximately 9.4 in 100,000 live births annually in the United States (Tomita & Ogiwara, 2022). Prenatally, alpha-fetoprotein levels are elevated late in the first trimester. Anencephaly is apparent on visual inspection after birth with exposed neural tissue without a cranium surrounding it. Because anencephaly is fatal, provide support to the parents of newborns with anencephaly and allow them to grieve the loss of their child (see Chapter 21 for suggestions related to supporting the surviving family after a perinatal loss).

Spina Bifida

Spina bifida is a general term used to refer to a spinal dysraphism. *Spinal dysraphism* refers to a caudal defect (below the level of T12) involving spinal cord tissue. The defect involves incomplete development of the spinal cord and/or its protective coverings caused by the failure of the spine to close properly during embryogenesis (around the 25th day of pregnancy) (Bowman, 2024). The spinal dysraphism may be open or closed.

Closed spinal dysraphism is termed *spina bifida occulta* and involves a defect in the vertebrae without any protrusion or herniation of the spinal cord or meninges. Spina bifida occulta is a closed defect and is not visible externally; it rarely causes disability or symptoms, and no immediate treatment is needed.

The open form of the defect may be either spina bifida cystica or spina bifida aperta (Fig. 24.1). **Meningocele** is the less severe form of spina bifida cystica and is an opening in the spine through a bony defect where the meninges and cerebrospinal fluid (CSF) have protruded. The spinal cord and nerve roots do not herniate into this dorsal dural sac. Most infants with meningocele have little or no neurologic involvement (Nehri & Ayra, 2023).

The most severe form is **myelomeningocele**. The prevalence of myelomeningocele is about 3.1 per 10,000 people up to 19 years old (Bowman, 2024). With this defect, the spinal cord and nerve roots herniate into the sac through an opening in the spine, compromising the meninges. *Cystica* refers to a thin membrane over the defect and protrusion, whereas with spina bifida aperta, there is no covering present. Leakage of CSF may occur, and infection risk exists. Hydrocephalus (abnormal accumulation of CSF within the ventricles and subarachnoid spaces) frequently accompanies myelomeningocele. Although the spinal opening can be surgically repaired shortly after birth, the nerve damage is permanent, resulting in varying degrees of paralysis of the lower limbs, as well as issues with bowel and bladder elimination.

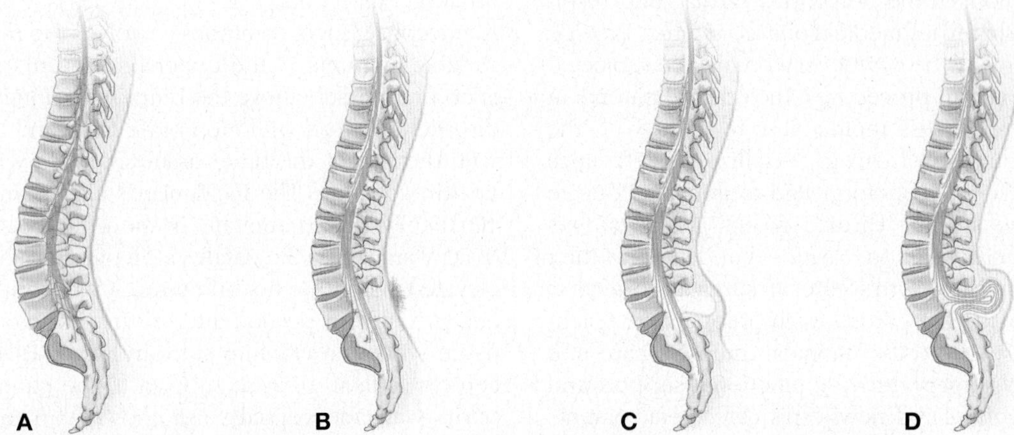

FIGURE 24.1 Neural tube defects. **A.** Normal spine. **B.** Spina bifida occulta. **C.** Meningocele. **D.** Myelomeningocele.

Fetal surgery is also an option, though not widely available (Bowman, 2024).

> **TAKE NOTE!**
>
> Myelomeningoceles can arise at any point along the vertebral column, but they most commonly occur in the lower lumbar or sacral regions, causing neurologic deficits below the level of the defect. Paralysis, bladder and bowel incontinence, and hydrocephalus are the most common complications.

NURSING ASSESSMENT

Determine the presence of any risk factors such as birth of a previous newborn with an NTD, folate deficiency or female sex in the newborn, and first-trimester fever, pregestational diabetes, or obesity in the birthing parent (Bowman, 2024). Inspect the newborn's spine for abnormalities. Spina bifida occulta may present with dimpling, a hair tuft or hairy patch, dermal sinus tract, hemangioma, or lipoma in the thoracic, lumbar, or sacral areas. Observe for a protrusion along the back that may be partially or completely covered with skin or a membrane (a sign of meningocele or myelomeningocele). Assess movement and sensation below the defect and observe for issues with urinary and bowel elimination, which may be affected based on the level of the lesion. Measure head circumference daily to observe for hydrocephalus (Fig. 24.2).

> **TAKE NOTE!**
>
> Newborns with meningocele usually have normal examination findings and a covered (closed) dural sac. They typically do not have associated neurologic complications.

NURSING MANAGEMENT

Nursing management of the newborn with spina bifida occulta is primarily supportive. Be sure that the parents understand the term used and that they do not confuse their newborn's condition with a more serious form of NTD. Teach them about the possibility of surgery in the future should complications develop. For the infant with meningocele, prepare the newborn and parents for surgery and closely monitor the skin covering the area for evidence of CSF leakage.

Nursing management for a newborn with myelomeningocele focuses on reducing the risk of infection and injury to the defect site.

- Use strict aseptic technique when caring for the defect to prevent infection.
- Avoid trauma to the sac (to prevent leakage of CSF or damage to the nerve tissue) through prone or side-lying positioning.
- Avoid placing a diaper over the sac to prevent rupture or infection by fecal contamination.

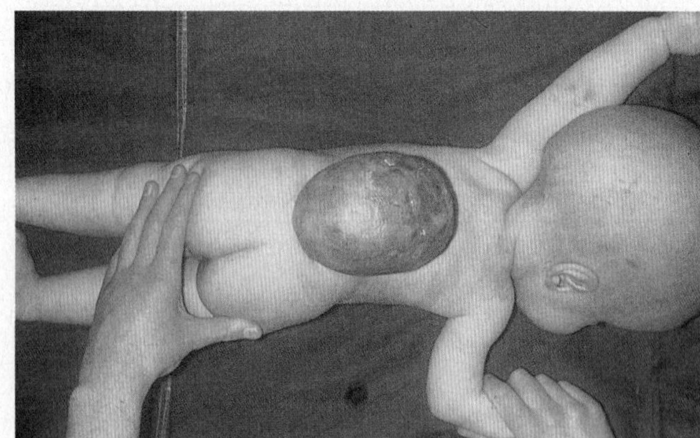

FIGURE 24.2 A newborn with myelomeningocele and hydrocephalus.

- Apply a sterile dressing or protective covering over the sac to prevent rupture and drying with frequent changes to prevent the dressing from adhering to the defect.
- Frequently monitor the sac for signs of oozing fluid or drainage.
- Preserve skin integrity on and around the spinal defect.
- Meticulously clean the genital area to avoid contamination of the sac.
- Ensure a neutral thermal environment and avoid hypothermia. Heat can be lost through the defect opening, placing the newborn at increased risk for cold stress.

Administer prescribed antibiotics to prevent infection both preoperatively and postoperatively. Prepare the infant and parents for surgery. Educate the parents about the necessity of closing the spinal defect as soon after birth as possible to preserve the neurologic function present. Provide support and information to help the parents cope. Allow them to verbalize their feelings and ask questions, encouraging open discussions regarding the baby's prognosis and long-term care. Encourage the parents to participate in their newborn's care as much as possible. Refer the parents to a support group if they desire.

TAKE NOTE!

Infants with myelomeningocele are at increased risk for developing a latex allergy due to their repeated and numerous exposures to products containing latex during surgery and other necessary treatments.

Microcephaly

Microcephaly, meaning "small head," is a rare condition affecting about one in every 1,150 infants born in the United States annually (CDC, 2024c). It is generally defined as a head circumference that is more than two standard deviations below the mean for age and sex. It can be present at birth (primary) or may develop later (secondary). Risk factors for microcephaly include genetic syndromes, intrauterine infection (cytomegalovirus, herpes simplex virus, human immunodeficiency virus [HIV], rubella, syphilis, toxoplasmosis, Zika virus), hypoxia, radiation to the maternal pelvis in the first or second trimester, and maternal phenylketonuria, hypothyroidism, and alcohol or cocaine use (Messer et al., 2022). As the brain is smaller than usual, the infant will experience neurologic issues and developmental delay. There is no treatment for microcephaly that can return an infant's brain to a normal size. Treatment focuses on ways to decrease the impact of the associated deformities and neurologic disabilities. Provide supportive care.

Educate parents about the potential cognitive impairment of the newborn. Ensure that appropriate community referrals are made to assist the parents and the child.

Hydrocephalus

The term *hydrocephalus* comes from the Greek words *hydro* (water) and *kephale* (head). Hydrocephalus is an increase in CSF in the ventricles of the brain due to overproduction or impaired circulation and absorption; it may be congenital or acquired. In the United States and Europe, congenital hydrocephalus occurs in 0.5 to 0.8 per 1,000 live births and stillbirths (Haridas & Tomita, 2022). When CSF movement is prevented at any point within the brain or around the spinal cord, fluid accumulates in the ventricles, causing them to swell. This results in compression of the surrounding tissue and increased intracranial pressure (Fig. 24.3).

The management of congenital hydrocephalus consists primarily of early shunting as soon as possible after birth. A ventriculoperitoneal (VP) shunt is inserted from the ventricle in the brain and threaded down into the peritoneal cavity to allow drainage of excess CSF. Complications include shunt malfunction and shunt infection. External ventriculostomy (endoscopic third ventriculostomy or ETV) is an alternative to VP shunting and creates an opening in the floor of the third ventricle using an endoscope placed within the ventricular system through a burr hole. This allows the movement of CSF out of the blocked ventricular system and into the interpeduncular cistern (a normal CSF space), thereby shortcutting any obstruction (Haridas & Tomita, 2024).

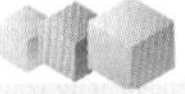
Concept Mastery Alert

Treatment of Hydrocephalus

Hydrocephalus stops CSF from moving out of the cranium. The increased fluid causes pressure on the brain and, ultimately, brain damage. The goal of treatment is to release pressure on the brain and drain the CSF. Treatment consists of surgical insertion of a shunt to halt any further damage to the brain, or an ETV procedure for infants with obstructive hydrocephalus. The success of the ETV depends on the child's age, cause of the hydrocephalus, and history of previous complications (Haridas & Tomita, 2024).

Nursing Assessment

Nursing assessment focuses on obtaining a health history and performing a physical examination. Be alert for risk factors in the maternal history, such as intrauterine infection or preterm birth. Assess the infant's head circumference and note any increases. Also note any visible scalp veins (see Fig. 24.3). Palpate the infant's head, noting any widened sutures and wide, opened fontanelles. Typically, the fontanelles will feel tense and bulging. Also

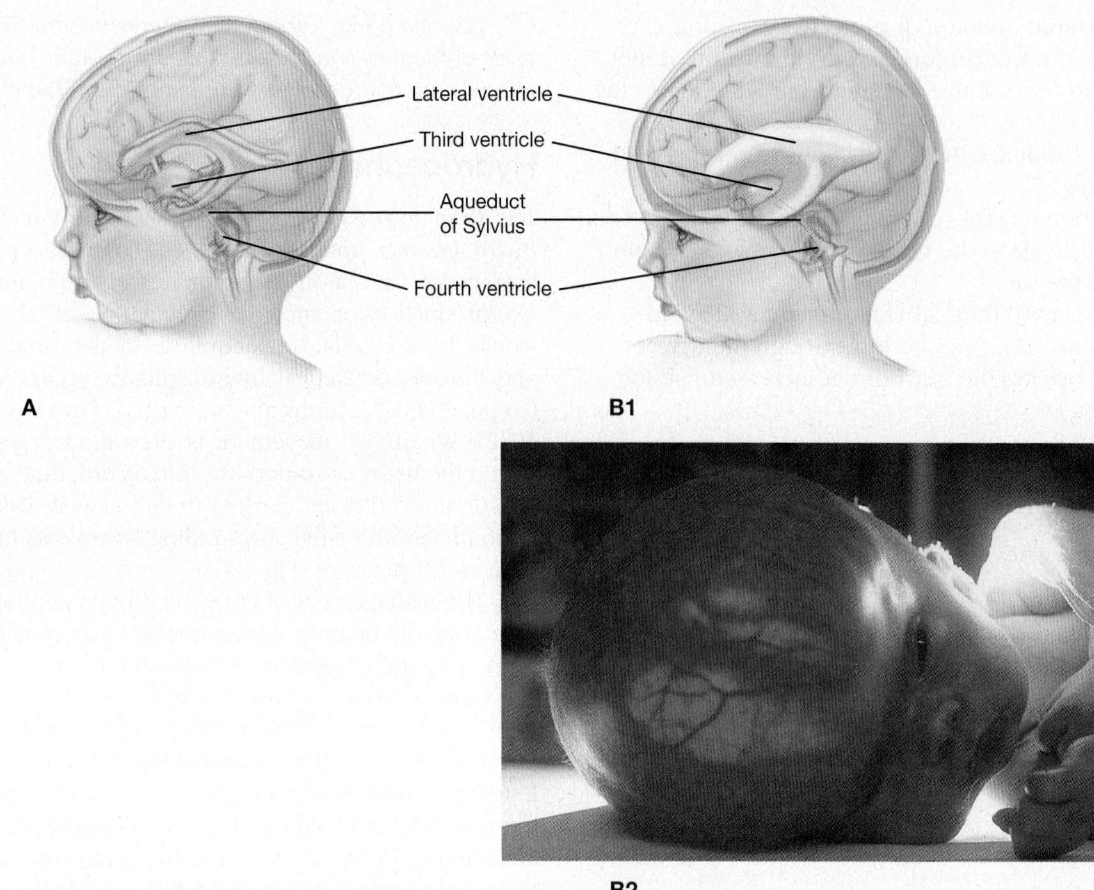

FIGURE 24.3 **A.** Infant without hydrocephalus. Note the ventricles of the brain and channels for the normal flow of cerebrospinal fluid. **B1, B2.** Infant with hydrocephalus. Note broadening of the forehead and large head size.

observe for other signs of increased intracranial pressure, including poor feeding, "setting sun" eyes, vomiting, lethargy, and irritability. A computed tomography (CT) scan or magnetic resonance imaging (MRI) confirms the diagnosis.

Nursing Management

Prior to shunt insertion or ETV, nursing management focuses on daily documentation of the newborn's head circumference and monitoring for increases in intracranial pressure noted by irritability, high-pitched cry, poor feeding and sucking, lethargy or sleepiness, vomiting, bulging anterior fontanelle when newborn is quiet, seizures or posturing, or a decrease in consciousness. Palpate the fontanelles for bulging and tenseness, and the suture lines for increasing separation. Protect the enlarged head to prevent skin breakdown. Handle the head gently and use a sheepskin, waterbed, or egg crate mattress. Change the newborn's position frequently to minimize pressure.

After surgery, continue to provide protective and comfort measures for the enlarged head. Position the newborn's head so that they do not lie on the shunt area. Strictly monitor for indications of increased intracranial pressure secondary to a blockage in the shunt, including noting pupillary dilation (increased intracranial pressure places pressure on the oculomotor nerve, producing dilation). Assess the abdomen for distention because drainage of CSF into the abdomen can cause peritonitis. Educate the parents about caring for the shunt and signs of infection or blockage. A referral for follow-up home care is appropriate. Stress the importance of close medical follow-up and prompt treatment of any health problems to prevent the spread of infections to the shunt.

Choanal Atresia

Choanal atresia is an uncommon congenital malformation that involves a narrowing of the nasal airway due to membranous or bony tissue. There is an absence of communication between the posterior nasal cavity and the nasopharynx. It can be unilateral (which occurs more often) or bilateral (Andalaro & La Mantia, 2023). If bilateral, the newborn is unable to breathe. Since newborns are obligatory nasal breathers, establishing an airway becomes an emergency. Choanal atresia typically presents with other anomalies involving the heart and central nervous system. It occurs in approximately one in 5,000 to 8,000 live births, with females affected more often (Andaloro & La Mantia, 2023).

During attempted inspiration, the tongue is pulled to the palate, and obstruction of the oral airway results. If the newborn cries and takes a breath through the mouth, the airway obstruction is momentarily relieved. When the crying stops, however, the mouth closes and the cycle of obstruction is repeated (Andaloro & La Mantia, 2023). If the nasal airway is completely obstructed, death from asphyxia may occur at birth. Surgery to remove the obstruction to establish a patent airway is needed, and full recovery is the usual outcome.

Congenital Diaphragmatic Hernia

Congenital diaphragmatic hernia (CDH) is a severe anomaly resulting in failed full development of the diaphragm. Some or all of the abdominal organs and contents protrude into the thoracic cavity, impeding fetal lung development. CDH is characterized by pulmonary hypoplasia and decreased pulmonary vasculature. Newborns with CDH often require prompt treatment of severe respiratory distress and pulmonary hypertension to prevent death. The incidence of CDH in the United States is one to four cases per 10,000 live births (Dumpa & Chandrasekharan, 2023). It is often associated with anomalies in other organ systems and single-gene disorders or other chromosomal abnormalities (Dumpa & Chandrasekharan, 2023).

Pathophysiology

The pathogenesis of CDH is complex and remains poorly understood. It is thought that the diaphragm fails to close properly during early embryonic development. The abdominal contents then herniate into the thoracic cavity through a defect in the diaphragm (Fig. 24.4). The timing of the herniation and the amount of abdominal contents in the thoracic cavity greatly influence the clinical picture at birth and the survival rate. The presence of the abdominal contents in the chest compresses the lung(s), leads to pulmonary hypoplasia, and promotes persistent pulmonary hypertension in the newborn (PPHN). Signs and symptoms of CDH include acute respiratory distress, cyanosis, sterna retractions, grunting, nasal flaring, tachycardia, rapid breathing, barrel-shaped chest, and a concave abdomen. The majority of CDHs are detected in the prenatal period using ultrasound imaging (Dumpa & Chandrasekharan, 2023).

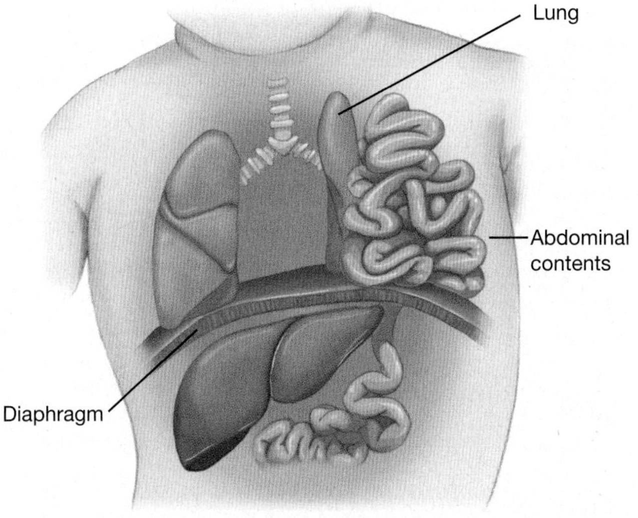

FIGURE 24.4 Congenital diaphragmatic hernia. Note how some of the abdominal contents have entered the thoracic cavity, compressing the lung.

Nursing Assessment

Assess the newborn closely for evidence of respiratory distress, including cyanosis. Affected newborns present with profound respiratory distress because at least one of the lungs cannot expand or may not have fully developed, resulting in persistent pulmonary hypertension shortly after birth. If present, institute resuscitation measures immediately.

Inspect the chest and abdomen, noting a barrel-shaped chest and scaphoid-shaped abdomen. During auscultation, note absent breath sounds on the affected side of the chest and heart sounds displaced to the right. Also listen for bowel sounds, which would be heard in the chest. Prepare the newborn for a chest x-ray or ultrasound, which will reveal evidence of air-filled bowel in the chest.

> **TAKE NOTE!**
> Prenatal diagnosis of CDH is possible through ultrasound. This diagnosis should be considered when polyhydramnios is present.

Nursing Management

Initial treatment involves respiratory support with the goal of maintaining oxygenation and cardiovascular stability. Surgery to correct the anatomic malformation is usually delayed until after the newborn's condition stabilizes. The surgical repair can also be delayed for months and done by minimally invasive surgery with the use of prosthetic material for closure of large defects. Extracorporeal membrane oxygenation (ECMO), a process that mimics the gas exchange process of the lungs, may be ordered when the surgery is undertaken.

Nursing management focuses on maintaining optimal respiratory function until surgery is performed to correct the defect. Assist with endotracheal intubation and positive-pressure ventilation to aid in lung expansion and improvement of ventilation. Position the newborn on the affected side with the head and chest elevated to promote normal lung expansion. Monitor ventilatory pressures to prevent pneumothorax. If a pneumothorax occurs, assist with insertion of a chest tube, and monitor chest tube drainage. Monitor oxygen saturation levels to evaluate systemic perfusion status. If the infant's condition does not stabilize, anticipate the use of ECMO or high-frequency oscillatory ventilation. Be cognizant of potential complications postoperatively, which might include persistent pulmonary hypertension, gastric reflux, chronic lung disease, and failure to thrive (Dumpa & Chandrasekharan, 2023).

Administer prescribed medications as ordered. For example, give inotropics (drugs that affect the force of muscle contractions) to support systemic blood pressure. Administer surfactant, steroids, and inhaled nitric oxide as ordered to correct hypoxia and acid–base imbalance. Monitor vital signs, weight, urinary output, and serum electrolytes to identify changes early. Maintain nothing by mouth (NPO) status to prevent aspiration and ensure a neutral thermal environment to prevent cold stress and reduce oxygen demands. Minimize environmental stimuli to reduce agitation and oxygen demand. Assist with placement of an orogastric tube for gastric decompression.

Counseling is an essential component in the management of CDH. Parents should be informed about the severity of this condition, the treatment plan, the risk of poor outcomes, and the potential for several long-term morbidities. Assess the parental anxiety level and coping ability; provide emotional support and educate about CDH pathophysiology, potential complications, treatment risks and benefits, long-term medical surveillance to reduce the risk of complications, and individualized prognosis. Refer for counseling on coping strategies as appropriate; provide written information on CDH to reinforce verbal education. Provide the parents with continuing updates about the newborn's condition. Encourage the parents to see and touch the infant frequently to promote bonding. Assist parents with identifying newborn cues and responding to them.

Cleft Lip and Palate

Cleft lip (CL) and cleft palate (CP) are the most common congenital malformations of the head and neck, with a prevalence of one in 690 births in the United States (Wilkins-Haug, 2024). A CL involves a congenital fissure or longitudinal opening in the lip. It may be unilateral or bilateral. A CP involves a congenital fissure or longitudinal opening in the roof of the mouth. The defects may occur either in isolation or together. About 30% of cases of CL/CP are associated with a genetic or other syndrome (Wilkins-Haug, 2024). In addition to immediate feeding difficulties, infants with CL and CP may have problems with dentition, nutrition, mental and social developmental disorders, language acquisition, and hearing (Salari et al., 2022) (Fig. 24.5).

Therapeutic Management

Repairing the facial anomaly as soon as possible is important to facilitate bonding between the newborn and the parents and to improve nutritional status. Treatment of CL is surgical repair usually by 3 months of age. Successful surgery often leaves only a thin scar on the upper lip. The outcome of surgery depends on the severity of the defect; children with more severe cases will need additional surgery in stages (Tolarova et al., 2022).

The timing of the palate repair is more controversial, and there is no universally agreed-upon recommendation.

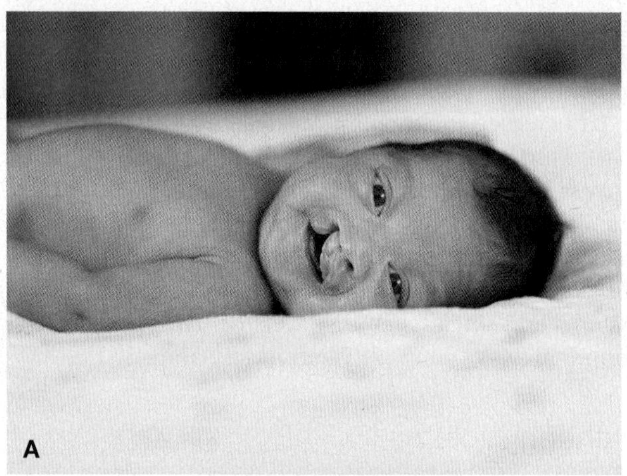

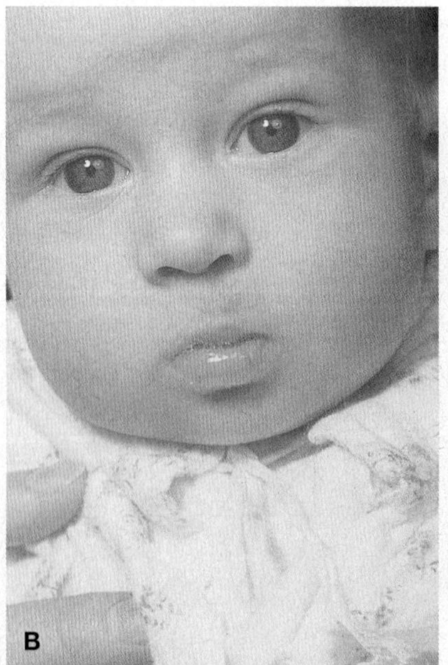

FIGURE 24.5 **A.** A newborn with a cleft lip. The defect may extend up through the roof of the palate. **B.** Infant with a surgical repair of a cleft lip. (Image **A**, PeopleImages.com—Yuri A/Shutterstock.)

Surgical correction for CP is typically done by 12 months of age to allow for developmental growth to occur. A plastic palate guard to form a synthetic palate may need to be used to allow for introduction of solid foods and to prevent aspiration in the interim.

Nursing Assessment

Obtain a thorough maternal history, noting the presence of any risk factors, such as family history, consanguinity, treatment with antibiotics during early pregnancy, advanced maternal age, and low folic acid intake (Darjazini Nahas et al., 2023). Inspect the lip for a visible deformity. Inspect and palpate the mouth for an opening, which may be small or involve the entire palate. Also observe for any feeding difficulties, which are common in newborns with CL and CP.

TAKE NOTE!

Milk flow during feeding requires negative pressure and sucking pressure. Newborns with CL and CP have feeding difficulties because they cannot generate a negative pressure in the mouth to facilitate sucking (American Cleft Palate Craniofacial Association, 2024). Use special nipples, squeezable bottles, and feeders to help meet the nutritional needs of infants with this anomaly.

Nursing Management

Nursing management focuses on providing adequate nutrition, promoting parental bonding, and providing parental education. Prevention should be considered the ultimate objective through preconception education.

PROVIDING ADEQUATE NUTRITION

Many infants born with CL and CP cannot be breastfed. Those with CP cannot produce the negative pressure necessary for suction. Infants with a unilateral CL may succeed with breastfeeding when they are positioned so that the cleft in the lip is obstructed by the breast. No single method of feeding has been identified as ideal. Parents working together with the health care provider and nursing staff should choose the method that is best for their infant.

Nurses need to instruct parents and caregivers to feed the infant in an upright position to prevent aspiration and assess for achievement of adequate suction during feeding. Use high-calorie formula to improve caloric intake. Burp the infant frequently to reduce the risk for vomiting and aspiration; burp them in the sitting position on your lap to prevent trauma to the mouth on your shoulder. Limit feeding sessions to avoid poor weight gain due to fatigue. After feeding, position the newborn on their side in an infant seat.

PROMOTING PARENTAL BONDING

Prenatal diagnosis of CL and CP may be made via ultrasound after 13 to 14 weeks' gestation (Wilkins-Haug, 2024). Prenatal diagnosis is increasing with the use of three-dimensional (3D) ultrasound, often performed around the 20th week of gestation. A 3D ultrasound may provide a better understanding and acceptance of the malformation by parents, providing them time to prepare for the birth. Nurses need to develop interventions to help parents deal with the impact of potential social stigmatization and physical concerns of the CL and CP condition.

Parents may be upset with the appearance of their newborn. Encourage the parents to express their feelings about this highly visible anomaly. Emphasize the newborn's positive features and role model nurturing behaviors when interacting with the infant. Encourage parents to interact with the newborn. Provide support to the parents, especially related to feeding difficulties. Allow them to vent their frustrations. Offer practical suggestions and continued encouragement for their efforts.

PROVIDING PARENTAL EDUCATION

The impact on the quality of life for the infant and the family can be severe, particularly for unprepared families. Emotional and psychological needs must be recognized and addressed, in addition to surgical care, by all those caring for the infant. Outline treatment modalities and explain the staging of surgical interventions. Show the family photos taken before and after surgical repair in other babies. These photos can alleviate some anxiety. Start planning for discharge as soon as the parents feel comfortable with infant care. Provide anticipatory guidance and instructions for potential challenges they may face at home and into the future, which include feeding difficulties, frequent ear infections, speech difficulties, and dental problems. As part of the discharge plan, initiate appropriate referrals for community support and counseling as needed. Nurses can help parents to trust in themselves and feel confident in their ability to nurture their newborns by listening, informing, and encouraging them.

Esophageal Atresia and Tracheoesophageal Fistula

Esophageal atresia (EA) and tracheoesophageal fistula (TEF) are common anomalies that develop before birth. The incidence of TEF and EA is one in 3,500 to 4,500 live births (Oermann, 2023). EA is a congenitally interrupted esophagus in which the proximal and distal ends do not communicate; the upper esophageal segment ends in a blind pouch, and the lower segment ends a variable distance above the diaphragm (Fig. 24.6). TEF is an abnormal communication between the trachea and the esophagus. When associated with EA, the fistula most

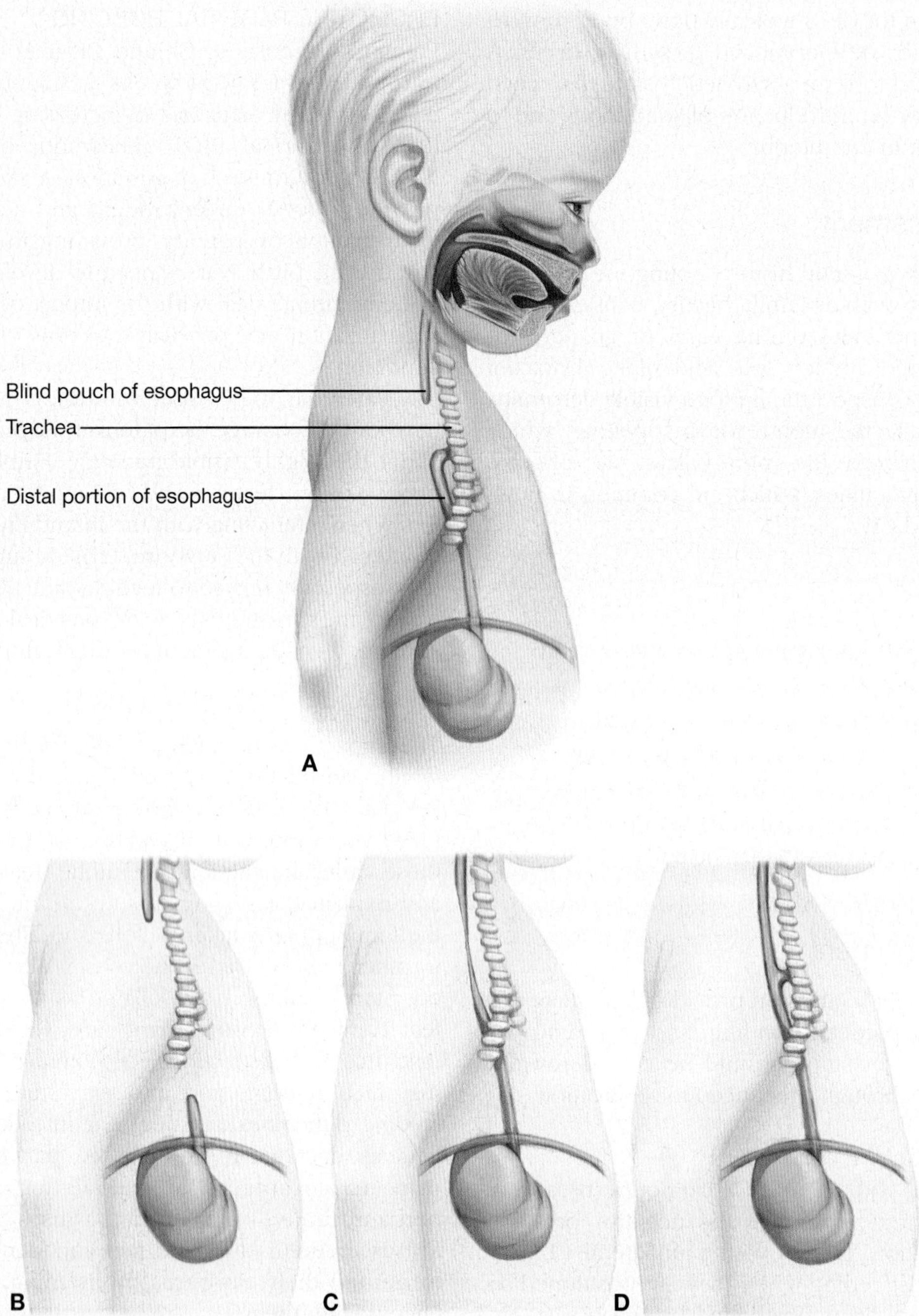

FIGURE 24.6 Esophageal atresia and tracheoesophageal fistula. **A.** The most common type of esophageal atresia, in which the esophagus ends in a blind pouch and a fistula connects the trachea with the distal portion of the esophagus. **B.** The upper and distal portions of the esophagus end in a blind pouch. **C.** The esophagus is one segment, but a portion of it is narrowed. **D.** The upper portion of the esophagus connects to the trachea via a fistula.

commonly occurs between the distal esophageal segment and the trachea. The lack of esophageal patency prevents swallowing. In addition to preventing normal feeding, this problem may cause infants to aspirate and literally drown in their own saliva, which quickly overflows the upper pouch of the obstructed esophagus. If a TEF is present, fluid (either saliva from above or gastric secretions from below) may flow directly into the lungs.

Concept Mastery Alert

Priority Concern in EA

The priority concern for the infant with EA is the risk for respiratory distress. Many infants with EA also have a TEF, which is a connection between the esophagus and the trachea. This connection can put the infant at high risk for respiratory distress, especially if the child is fed any food by mouth.

Pathophysiology

EA and TEF are multifactorial conditions due to multiple gene variations and environmental factors that contribute to their occurrences. They are thought to result from incomplete separation of the lung bed from the foregut during early fetal development. A large percentage (50% to 70%) of these newborns have other congenital anomalies involving the vertebrae, kidneys, heart, and musculoskeletal and gastrointestinal systems (Baldwin & Yadav, 2023).

Nursing Assessment

Review the maternal history for hydramnios during pregnancy. Often, this is the first sign of EA because the fetus cannot swallow and absorb amniotic fluid in utero, leading to accumulation. Soon after birth, the newborn may exhibit copious, frothy bubbles of mucus in the mouth and nose, accompanied by drooling. Abdominal distention develops as air builds up in the stomach. In EA, an orogastric tube cannot be inserted beyond a certain point because the esophagus ends in a blind pouch. The newborn may have rattling respirations, excessive salivation, drooling, and "the three Cs" (coughing, choking, and cyanosis) if feeding is attempted. The presence of a fistula increases the risk of respiratory complications such as pneumonitis and atelectasis due to aspiration of food and secretions (Oermann, 2023). Clinical manifestations of EA and TEF include:

- Excessive secretions
- Feeding intolerance
- Inability to pass orogastric tube
- Abdominal distention
- Failure to gain weight
- Coughing or choking during feeding
- Vomiting
- Respiratory distress

TAKE NOTE!

The "three Cs" of choking, coughing, and cyanosis when feeding are considered the classic signs of TEF and EA.

Prepare the newborn and parents for x-ray evaluation. Diagnosis is made by x-ray, ultrasound, or MRI of the chest and abdomen; if the gastric tube appears coiled in the upper esophageal pouch with air in the gastrointestinal tract, this indicates the presence of a fistula (Baldwin & Yadav, 2023). Once a diagnosis of EA is established, begin preparations for surgery if the newborn is stable.

Nursing Management

Once the diagnosis is established, an orogastric tube is placed in the upper esophageal pouch and set to low continuous suction to prevent aspiration of oral secretions. Nursing management focuses on preparing the newborn and parents for surgery and providing meticulous postoperative care. The type of esophageal defect dictates the surgical approach needed.

PROVIDING PREOPERATIVE CARE

Preoperative nursing interventions include the following measures:

- Initiate NPO status.
- Elevate the head of the bed 30 to 45 degrees to prevent reflux and aspiration.
- Monitor hydration status and fluid and electrolyte balance; administer and monitor parenteral intravenous (IV) fluid infusions.
- Assess and maintain the patency of the orogastric tube. Monitor the functioning of the tube, which is attached to low continuous suction. Avoid irrigation of the tube to prevent aspiration.
- Have oxygen and suctioning equipment readily available should the newborn experience respiratory distress.
- Assist with diagnostic studies to rule out other anomalies.
- Use comfort measures to minimize crying and prevent respiratory distress; provide nonnutritive sucking.
- Inform the parents about the rationales for the aspiration prevention measures.
- Document frequent observations of the newborn's condition (Savin & Phalen, 2022).

PROVIDING POSTOPERATIVE CARE

Surgery consists of closing the fistula and joining the two esophageal segments. Postoperative care involves closely observing all of the newborn's body systems to identify any complications. Expect to administer total parenteral nutrition (TPN) and antibiotics until the esophageal anastomosis is proven intact and patent. Before initiating oral feedings, an esophagram is usually ordered to verify complete anastomotic healing and the absence of any leaks. If that validates healing, then oral feedings are started, usually within a week after surgery. Feeding and swallowing difficulties are common postoperatively (Maybee et al., 2023). Keep the parents informed of the newborn's condition and progress. Closely assess the newborn during feeding and report any difficulty with swallowing. Provide parent teaching. Demonstrate and reinforce all teaching prior to discharge.

Omphalocele and Gastroschisis

Omphalocele and gastroschisis are congenital anomalies of the anterior abdominal wall at or near the umbilicus. Gastroschisis and omphalocele occur at a rate of three to four per 10,000 pregnancies (Stephenson et al., 2023).

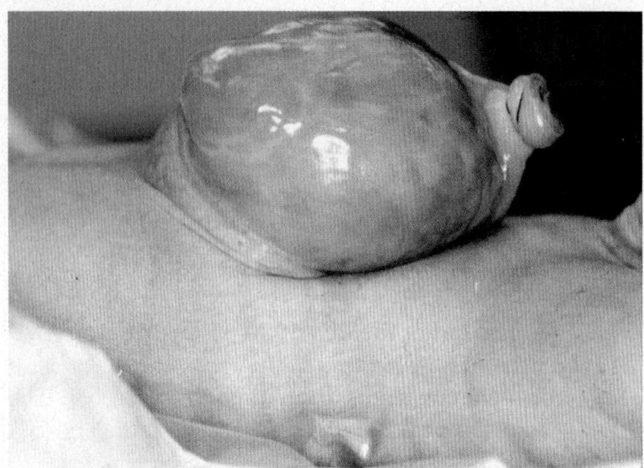

FIGURE 24.7 Omphalocele in a newborn. Note the large, protruding sac.

An **omphalocele** is a defect of the umbilical ring that allows evisceration of the abdominal contents into an external peritoneal sac. Defects vary in size; they may be limited to bowel loops or may include the entire gastrointestinal tract and liver (Fig. 24.7). Bowel malrotation is common, but the displaced organs are usually normal.

Gastroschisis is a full-thickness defect of the abdominal wall that occurs most commonly on the right side of the umbilicus exposing the extruded bowel to the amniotic fluid. It differs from omphalocele in that there is no peritoneal sac protecting the herniated organs, and thus exposure to amniotic fluid makes intestines thickened, edematous, and inflamed. Gastroschisis is associated with fetal demise and preterm birth, and, when repaired, growth restriction (Stephenson et al., 2023). Both omphalocele and gastroschisis are most often diagnosed by prenatal ultrasound and require that a pediatric surgeon be available at birth to determine the extent of the defect and complications.

Nursing Assessment

Omphalocele and gastroschisis are readily observed, noted as eviscerated bowel; gastroschisis does not have a peritoneal covering, whereas omphalocele does. Note the appearance of the protrusion on the abdomen and evidence of a sac. Inspect the sac closely for the presence of organs, most commonly the intestines but sometimes the liver. Also inspect the contents for any twisting of the intestines. Note the color of the organs within the sac and measure the size of the omphalocele.

Nursing Management

Nursing management of newborns with omphalocele or gastroschisis focuses on stabilizing the airway, preventing hypothermia, minimizing fluid loss, maintaining perfusion to the eviscerated abdominal contents, and protecting the exposed abdominal contents from trauma and infection. Keep the infant under the radiant warmer. Maintain IV access for hydration. For omphalocele with an intact sac, use a sterile warm saline-soaked gauze to loosely cover the defect, with dry gauze on top. For gastroschisis or omphalocele with ruptured sac, place the lower two thirds of the infant in a clear, polyurethane, drawstring bowel bag to provide a barrier and decrease fluid and heat loss. Carefully handle the infant to avoid injury to the intestinal wall or other exposed organs. Position the infant on the side to further prevent injury to the bowel. Maintain an orogastric tube for gastric decompression. Administer IV antibiotics as prescribed (Degrazia, 2022).

PROVIDING POSTOPERATIVE CARE

Surgical repair of both defects occurs after initial stabilization. It may have to occur in stages, depending on the defect (Box 24.1). Postoperatively, the nurse will:

- provide pain management.
- monitor respiratory and cardiac status, and intake and output.
- note color and degree of hydration.
- assess for vascular compromise noted by decreased perfusion to the legs and decreased urine output; report immediately.
- maintain an orogastric tube to low suction, noting the quantity and color of stomach contents (Degrazia, 2022).

PROMOTING PARENT–NEWBORN INTERACTION

The parents need continued support and progress reports on their newborn. They may be distraught at the sight of the anomaly, and they may be frightened to

BOX 24.1 Surgery to Repair Omphalocele and Gastroschisis

Surgical repair of gastroschisis is an emergency due to the high risk of intestinal atresia, resulting in obstruction. Primary repair of gastroschisis is usually performed without incident unless the contents are unable to fit into the abdominal cavity. If the defect is quite large, staged closure may be necessary (similar to omphalocele) (Stephenson et al. 2023). For omphalocele, closure generally occurs within 24–72 hours. Initially, a preformed silastic silo is placed by the surgeon to cover the defect and allow some portion of the herniated material to reenter the abdominal cavity. After enough of the defect is in the abdominal cavity, a surgical repair is then performed (Stephenson et al., 2022). If portions of the bowel are necrosed, they are removed during the repair. When a significant amount of small intestine is lost, then the complication of short bowel syndrome may occur.

Stephenson, C. D., Lockwood, C. J., & MacKenzie, A. P. (2023). Gastroschisis. *UpToDate.* Retrieved March 12, 2024, from https://www.uptodate.com/contents/gastroschisis; and Stephenson, C. D., Lockwood, C. J., & MacKenzie, A. P. (2022). Omphalocele: Prenatal diagnosis and pregnancy management. *UpToDate.* Retrieved June 4, 2024, from https://www.uptodate.com/contents/omphalocele-prenatal-diagnosis-and-pregnancy-management

touch their newborn. Encourage the parents to touch the newborn and participate in care as much as possible. Because of the nature of this defect, bonding opportunities will be limited initially. However, strongly encourage frequent visits. In addition, provide information to the parents about the defect, treatment modalities, and prognosis. After surgery, instruct the parents in care measures. Anticipate the need for a referral to a home health care agency and community resources for support.

Imperforate Anus

An imperforate anus is a gastrointestinal system malformation of the anorectal area that may occur in several forms. The rectum may end in a blind pouch that does not connect to the colon, or it may have fistulas (openings) between the rectum and the perineum, the vagina in females, or the urethra in males (Fig. 24.8). The malformations occur during early fetal development and may be associated with a variety of birth defects. When a malformation of the anus is present, the muscles and nerves associated with the anus are frequently malformed as well.

Imperforate anus occurs in about one of every 5,000 live births, and males are slightly more often affected than females (Singh & Mehra, 2023). The location of the fistula connection significantly influences fecal continence and management (Wood & Levitt, 2022). Surgical intervention is needed for all types. A colostomy may be placed in the newborn period, with corrective surgery performed in stages to allow for growth. Surgery involves closure of the fistula, creation of an anal opening, and repositioning of the rectal pouch into the anal opening (anoplasty). A major challenge for either type of surgical repair is finding, using, or creating adequate nerve and muscle structures around the rectum to provide for normal evacuation.

Nursing Assessment

In the newborn, observe for an appropriate anal opening. If the anal opening exists, observe for passage of meconium stool within the first 24 hours of life. Assess urine output to identify genitourinary problems. For the newborn with an imperforate anus, inspection of the perineal area would reveal the absence of the usual opening, and meconium is generally not passed or present within 24 hours of birth. Assess for common signs of intestinal obstruction, such as abdominal distention and bilious vomiting.

Nursing Management

Nursing management focuses on preparing the newborn and parents for diagnostic evaluation and surgery, as well as providing postoperative care. Preoperatively, maintain the newborn's NPO status and provide gastric decompression. Administer IV therapy and antibiotic therapy as ordered and monitor the newborn's hydration status. Provide a full explanation of the defect, surgical options, potential complications, typical postoperative course, and long-term care needed to the parents. Prepare them for the possibility that the newborn may require a colostomy. Provide support to the parents and family.

Postoperative care includes ensuring adequate pain relief, maintaining NPO status and gastric decompression until normal bowel function is restored, and providing colostomy care if applicable (Degrazia, 2022). Stoma care and parental teaching are paramount for home care of the infant.

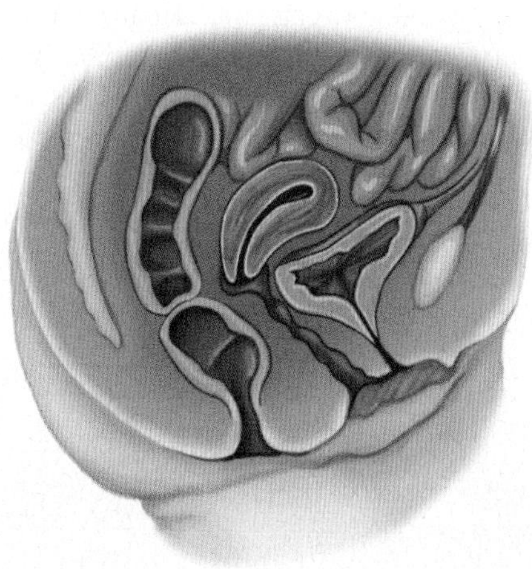

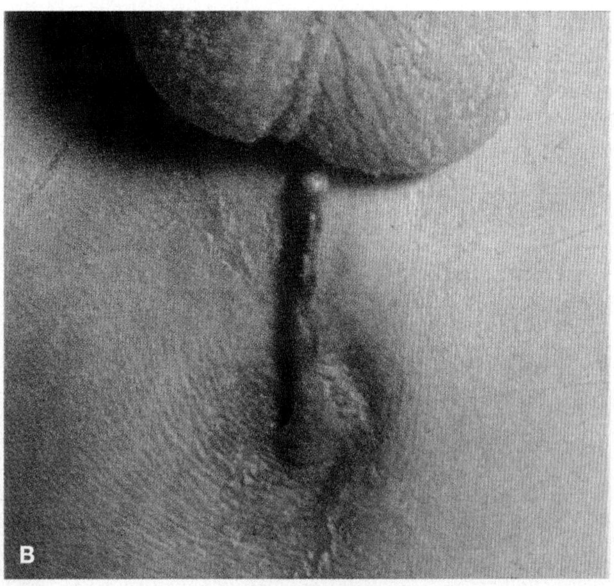

FIGURE 24.8 A. Imperforate anus, in which the rectum ends in a blind pouch. **B.** Imperforate anus without fistula. The visible meconium streak along the raphe is consistent with a low imperforate anus. (Courtesy of Kevin P. Lally, MD.)

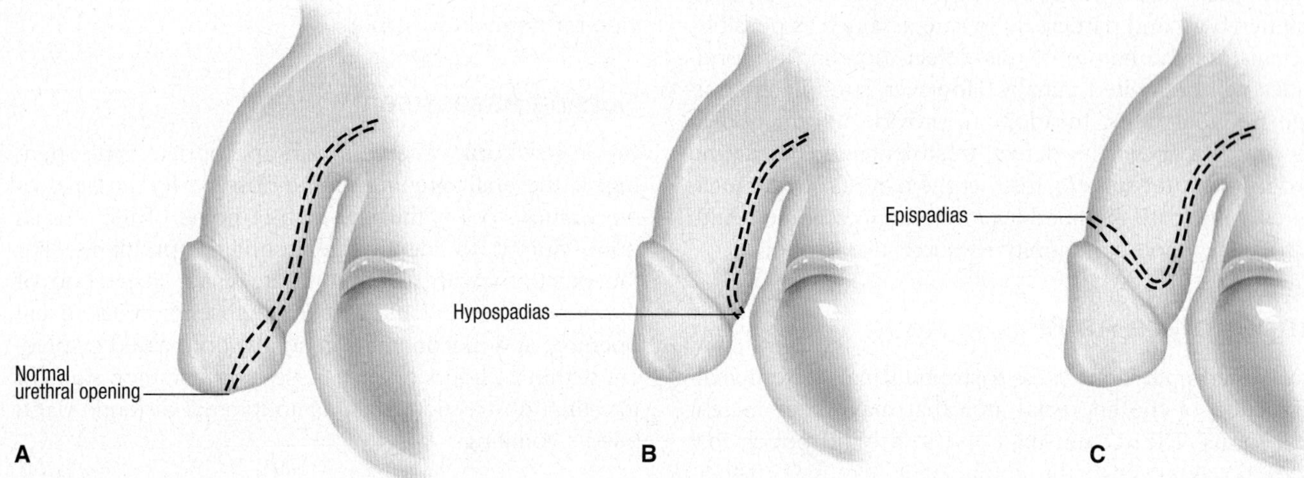

FIGURE 24.9 Genitourinary tract structural anomalies.

Hypospadias

Hypospadias is a relatively common malformation of the penis, with an incidence of one in 250 male births (Donaire & Mendez, 2023). It may be an isolated abnormality or associated with a disorder of sex development. It is an abnormal positioning of the urinary meatus on the underside (ventral) of the penis or glans (Fig. 24.9). Scrotal and testicular anomalies may also be associated. Hypospadias occurs as a result of the urethral folds failing to partially or completely close with the lack of fusion of the foreskin (Baskin, 2023). The cause is unknown, but it is thought to be influenced by genetic and environmental factors. Reported risk factors include maternal diabetes, placental insufficiency, prematurity, fetal growth restriction, advanced maternal age, and in vitro fertilization (Baskin, 2023). Epispadias is a rare defect and refers to the urinary meatal opening being located on the dorsal surface of the penile shaft or glans; it may be associated with bladder exstrophy (Suneja et al., 2020).

The degree of hypospadias/epispadias depends on the location of the opening. It is often accompanied by a downward bowing of the penis (chordee), which can lead to urination and erection problems and infertility in adulthood. When either condition is noted in the newborn, circumcision should be delayed. The defects can be surgically corrected, and any excess foreskin may be needed for the reconstruction. To limit psychological stress, surgical intervention should be completed between 6 and 18 months of age (Donaire & Mendez, 2023).

Bladder Exstrophy

In classic bladder exstrophy, a midline closure defect occurs during the embryonic period of gestation, leaving the bladder open and exposed outside the abdomen (Fig. 24.10). The bony pelvis is also malformed, resulting in an opening in the pelvic arch. Virtually all affected male infants have associated epispadias. It occurs in 2.2 of 100,000 live births (Anand & Lotfollahzadeh, 2023). Bladder exstrophy may be diagnosed by prenatal ultrasound. Complications include urinary tract infection (UTI) from ascending organisms. Treatment of bladder exstrophy involves staged surgical repair, with initial bladder closure completed within 48 hours after birth. Epispadias repair occurs at this time if possible. Further

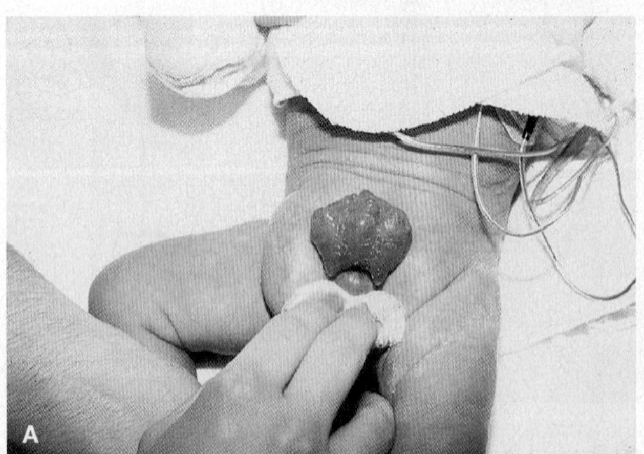

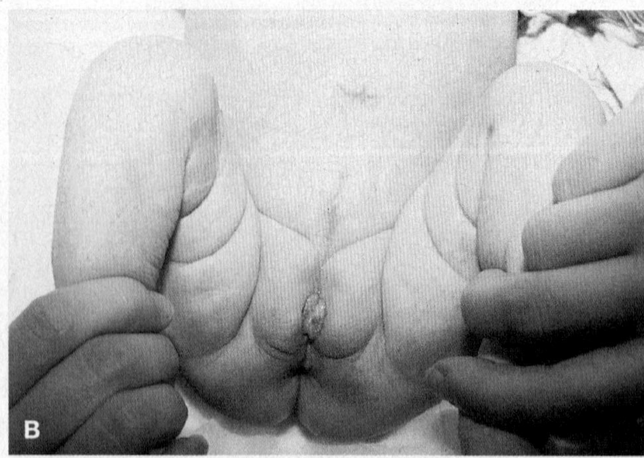

FIGURE 24.10 Bladder exstrophy. **A.** Before surgical repair. **B.** After surgery.

surgical reconstruction is performed in several stages at about 2 to 3 years of age (see Fig. 24.10). Because of the potential long-term implications of exstrophy, family education is critical. Exstrophy support groups are established at several major medical centers.

Nursing assessment of the newborn with bladder exstrophy reveals a red appearance to the bladder seen on the abdominal wall, visible draining urine, possible abdominal skin excoriation in males, and a misplaced urethra in females (Anand & Lotfollahzadeh, 2023). Preoperative nursing management focuses on preventing infection and skin breakdown by covering the bladder with a nonadherent film. After surgery, provide routine postoperative care as well as educate the parents about the care of the urinary catheter at home if applicable. Refer the parents to a support group to enhance their coping ability.

Congenital Clubfoot

Clubfoot, or talipes equinovarus, is a common congenital developmental deformity affecting approximately 0.5 to 2 cases per 1,000 live births, occurring twice as often in males (Barrie & Varacallo, 2023). The foot is excessively turned in and nonflexible (Fig. 24.11). Clubfoot has four components:

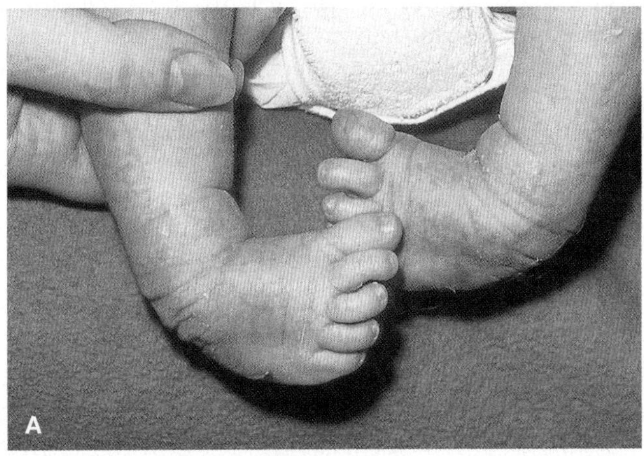

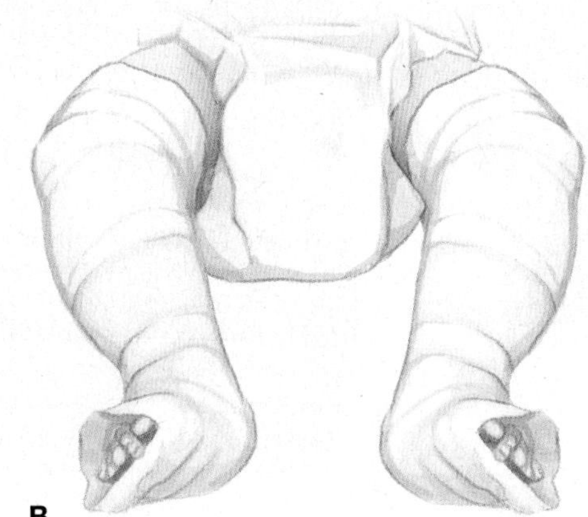

FIGURE 24.11 Clubfoot deformity. **A.** Initial appearance. **B.** Application of cast to correct clubfoot.

- Inversion of the heel (talipes varus)
- Plantarflexion of the foot; the heel is raised and would not strike the ground in a standing position (talipes equinus)
- Plantarflexion of the forefoot on the hindfoot (cavus)
- Forefoot inversion with slightly upward turning (forefoot adduction with supination) (Barrie & Varacallo, 2023).

Therapeutic Management

The management of clubfoot must begin shortly after birth, beginning with serial casting. Casts are initially changed every 5 to 7 days and are applied until the deformity responds and is fully corrected. If full correction does not occur with casting, surgery and bracing may become necessary. If serial casting is not successful in correcting the deformity, surgical intervention is necessary between 4 and 9 months of age (Zhang et al., 2022).

Nursing Assessment

On examination, the foot appears "down and in." It is smaller than a normal foot, with a flexible, softer heel because of the hypoplastic (underdeveloped) calcaneus. The heel is internally rotated, making the soles of the feet face each other when the deformity occurs bilaterally.

Nursing Management

Nursing management focuses on cast care, skin integrity maintenance, and education of the parents. Educate the parents about the newborn's condition and the treatment protocol to reduce anxiety and provide reassurance that the clubfoot is not painful and will not hinder the child's development. Discuss challenges associated with sleep, play, and dressing. Inform them that slight modifications will be necessary to accommodate the plaster casts. Review positioning, bathing, and skin care along with pain management when new casts are applied. Stress the need to provide a calm, quiet environment to promote relaxation and sleep for the newborn.

Developmental Dysplasia of the Hip

Developmental dysplasia of the hip (DDH) involves abnormal growth or development of the hip that results in instability. This includes hips that are unstable, subluxated, or dislocated (luxated) or have a malformed acetabulum. The instability allows the femoral head to become easily displaced from the acetabulum. Early diagnosis and treatment will prevent long-term complications, such as persistent dislocation and early hip osteoarthritis (Nandhagopal & De Cicco, 2023). The incidence of hip instability is about 10 per 1,000 live births and is more common in females and breech presentations (Dwan et al., 2022). The etiology of DDH is unclear.

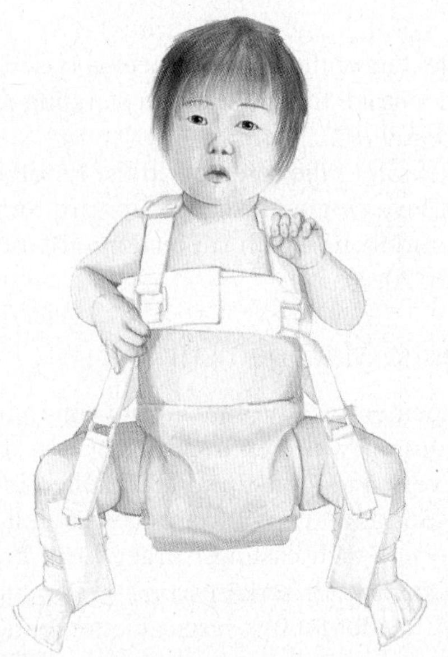

FIGURE 24.12 The Pavlik harness is used to treat developmental dysplasia of the hip.

Treatment is started as soon as DDH is identified. If the newborn examination reveals DDH, the newborn is referred to an orthopedist. The goal of treatment is to relocate the femoral head in the acetabulum to facilitate normal growth and development. The Pavlik harness is the most widely used device; it prevents adduction while allowing flexion and abduction to accomplish the treatment goal (Fig. 24.12). The harness is worn continuously until the hip is stable, which may take several months. If harnessing is not successful, surgery is necessary.

Nursing Assessment

Assess the history for risk factors, including racial background (Native Americans), genetic transmission (runs in families), intrauterine positioning (breech), sex (female), oligohydramnios, birth order (firstborn), and postnatal infant-carrying positions (swaddling, which forces the hips to be adducted). Upon physical examination, pay particular attention to assessing hip instability. Perform Ortolani and Barlow maneuvers (see Chapter 18 for more information on these maneuvers). The Ortolani maneuver elicits the sensation of the dislocated hip reducing. The Barlow maneuver detects the unstable hip dislocating from the acetabulum; "clunk" is felt in the hip when the infant's legs are abducted into a frog position. Observe for other physical signs of DDH, including an asymmetric thigh or buttock skinfolds, an apparent or true short leg, and limited hip abduction (Rosenfeld, 2022) (Fig. 24.13).

Nursing Management

Teach the parents how to care for the newborn while in the harness during treatment. Proper fit and adjustments for growth are essential for successful treatment. Teach parents to assess for skin breakdown. Inform parents that clinical assessment on an outpatient basis is needed to monitor progress.

Inborn Errors of Metabolism

Inborn errors of metabolism are biochemical genetic disorders that disrupt normal carbohydrate metabolism, protein metabolism, fatty acid oxidation, and glucose storage. Most are due to a defect in an enzyme or transport protein, resulting in a blocked metabolic pathway. Clinical symptoms are manifested secondary to toxic accumulations of substances before the block. The management of inborn errors of metabolism has traditionally consisted of diet or supportive therapy, but newer treatments include enzyme and coenzyme replacement, removal of harmful substances, cell and organ transplant, and gene therapy (Weiner, 2024). When viewed individually, inborn errors of metabolism are rare, but

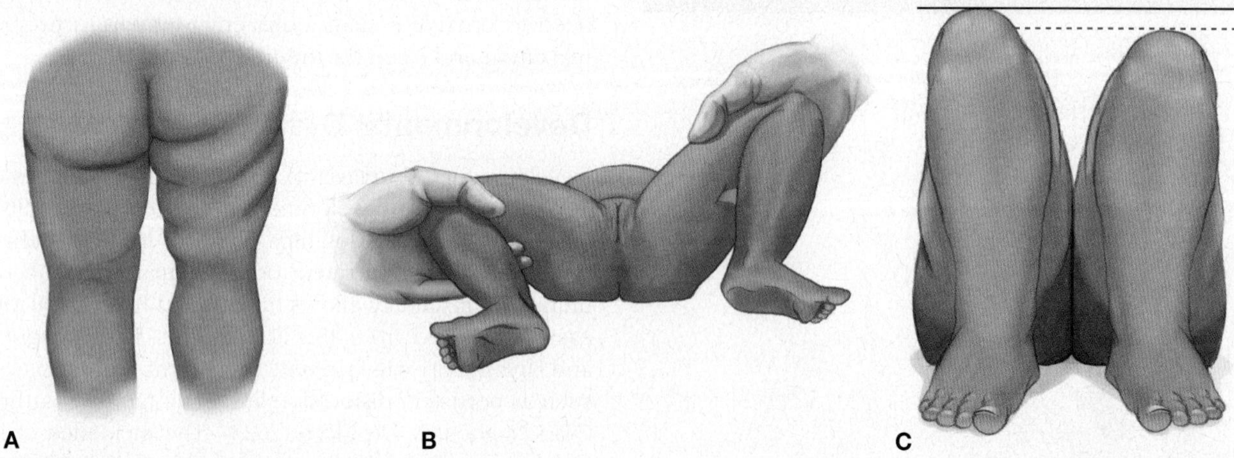

FIGURE 24.13 Characteristics of developmental dysplasia of the hip. **A.** Asymmetric number of skin folds on the thigh or buttock. **B.** Limited hip abduction. **C.** Unequal knee height.

collectively, they are responsible for significant levels of infant mortality and morbidity. The collective incidence ranges from one in 800 live births to one in 2,500 live births (Matern, 2023). Outcomes can often be good if recognized early, but diet and medication therapy are needed for life (Weiner, 2024). Table 24.1 summarizes four common inborn errors.

A successful outcome depends on early diagnosis and prompt intervention. Most inborn errors present in the newborn period with nonspecific and subtle manifestations—lethargy, hypotonia, respiratory distress, developmental delay, loss of milestones, poor feeding and weight gain, vomiting, and seizures. Identification of an inborn error of metabolism in a newborn depends largely on the awareness of the nurse and clues from the maternal history, laboratory work, and clinical examination.

ACQUIRED DISORDERS

Congenital disorders are disorders the infant is born with and may be passed genetically from a parent to the offspring or occur spontaneously due to a variety of factors. Acquired disorders are not passed genetically or caused by hereditary or developmental factors; they are obtained after birth by a reaction to in utero exposures or environmental influences outside the body. Examples include birth trauma, hyperbilirubinemia, newborn infections, respiratory distress syndrome (RDS), and retinopathy of prematurity (ROP).

Birth Injury

Birth injury is defined as an impairment of the newborn's body function or structure due to an adverse event

TABLE **24.1** • Inborn Errors of Metabolism

Condition	Etiology	Clinical Picture	Management
Phenylketonuria (PKU)	Autosomal recessive genetic disorder caused by a deficiency of the hepatic enzyme phenylalanine hydroxylase Enzyme deficiency with subsequent accumulation of amino acid phenylalanine	Newborns appear normal at birth, but by 6 months of age, signs of slow mental development are evident. Vomiting, poor feedings, failure to thrive, overactivity, irritability, musty-smelling urine If not treated, possible intellectual disability	Screening of all newborns at about 48 hours after birth to ensure adequate intake of protein Dietary restriction of phenylalanine with regular monitoring of serum phenylalanine levels (effective when started before the first month of age) Lifelong dietary restriction of phenylalanine
Maple syrup urine disease (MSUD)	Most prevalent among the Mennonite population in Lancaster, PA Autosomal recessive inherited disorder Enzyme metabolism of certain amino acids is affected with the buildup of acids causing ketoacidosis.	Lethargy, poor feeding, vomiting, weight loss, seizures, shrill cry, shallow respirations, loss of reflexes, coma, sweet maple syrup odor to urine	Dialysis to remove accumulated acids Lifelong low-protein diet to prevent neurologic deficits of disease
Galactosemia	Autosomal recessive inherited disorder in which an enzyme needed to convert galactose to glucose is missing and newborn cannot metabolize lactose	Vomiting, hypoglycemia, liver damage, hyperbilirubinemia, poor weight gain, cataracts, frequent infections	Routine newborn screening for galactosemia is performed in the majority of states. Lifelong lactose-restricted diet is needed to prevent intellectual disability, liver disease, and cataracts.
Congenital hypothyroidism	Multiple causes—absent or underdeveloped thyroid gland or biochemical defects in thyroid hormone	Large protruding tongue, slow reflexes, distended abdomen, large, open posterior fontanelle, constipation, hypothermia, poor feeding, hoarse cry, dry skin, coarse hair, goiter, and jaundice If untreated, irreversible cognitive and motor impairment occurs. Decreased levels of thyroid hormone (T_4) and elevated levels of thyroid-stimulating hormone	Newborn screening program in all states Lifelong thyroid replacement hormone therapy and continued monitoring of thyroid levels and clinical response to therapy

Sutton, V. R. (2023). Inborn errors of metabolism: Epidemiology, pathogenesis, and clinical features. *UpToDate*. Retrieved March 12, 2024, from https://www.uptodate.com/contents/inborn-errors-of-metabolism-epidemiology-pathogenesis-and-clinical-features; Matern, D. (2023). Newborn screening for inborn errors of metabolism. *UpToDate*. Retrieved June 4, 2024, from https://www.uptodate.com/contents/newborn-screening-for-inborn-errors-of-metabolism; and Weiner, D. L. (2024). Inborn errors of metabolism treatment and management. *Medscape*. https://emedicine.medscape.com/article/804757-overview

during childbirth (McKee-Garrett, 2023). Injury to a fetus or neonate during childbirth can be due to several factors, involving the fetus, placenta, birthing parent, and/or instrumentation. In the past, numerous injuries were associated with difficult births requiring external or internal version or mid or high forceps deliveries (Dump & Kamity, 2023). Today, however, cesarean births have contributed to the decline in birth injuries. Some of these injuries resolve spontaneously with little or no consequence, while others result in permanent damage and severe morbidity or mortality. Damage occurs to the tissues and organs of the newborn caused by mechanical forces during childbirth, often accompanied by impaired blood circulation and organ functioning. In the United States, birth injury occurs in about 2% to 3% of births, with the most frequent (80%) being to the scalp (McKee-Garrett, 2023).

Pathophysiology

The process of birth is a blend of compression, contractions, torque, and traction. When fetal size, presentation, or neurologic immunity complicates this process, the forces of labor and birth may lead to tissue damage, edema, hemorrhages, or fractures in the newborn. For example, birth injury may result from the pressure of birth (especially in prolonged or abrupt labor), abnormal or difficult presentation, cephalopelvic disproportion, or mechanical forces, such as forceps or vacuum used during delivery. Table 24.2 summarizes the most common types of birth injury.

TABLE 24.2 • Common Types of Birth Injury

Type	Description	Findings	Treatment
Fractures	Most often occur during breech births or shoulder dystocia in newborns with macrosomia Midclavicular fractures are the most common type of fracture, secondary to shoulder dystocia. Long bone fractures of the humerus or femur, usually midshaft, also can occur.	Midclavicular fractures: the newborn is irritable and does not move the arm on the affected side either spontaneously or when the Moro reflex is elicited. Femoral or humeral long bone fractures: the newborn shows loss of spontaneous leg or arm motion, respectively; usually swelling and pain accompany the limited movement. X-rays confirm the fracture.	Midclavicular fractures typically heal rapidly and uneventfully; arm motion may be limited by pinning the newborn's sleeve to the shirt. Femoral and humeral shaft fractures are treated with splinting. Healing and complete recovery are expected within 2–4 weeks without incident. Explanation to the parents and reassurance are needed.
Brachial plexus injury	Primarily in large babies, babies with shoulder dystocia, or breech delivery Results from stretching, hemorrhage within a nerve, or tearing of the nerve or the roots associated with cervical cord injury Associated traumatic injuries include fracture of the clavicle or humerus or subluxations of the shoulder or cervical spine. Erb palsy is an upper brachial plexus injury. Klumpke palsy is an injury to the lower brachial plexus (lower brachial injuries are less common).	In Erb palsy, the involved extremity usually presents adducted, prone, and internally rotated; shoulder movement is absent; and Moro, bicep, and radial reflexes are absent, but the grasp reflex is usually present. Klumpke palsy is manifested by weakness in the hand and wrist; grasp reflex is absent.	Erb palsy usually involves immobilization of the upper arm across the upper abdomen/chest to protect the shoulder from excessive motion for the first week; then gentle passive range of motion (ROM) exercises are performed daily to prevent contractures. There is usually no associated sensory loss, and this condition usually improves rapidly. Treatment for Klumpke palsy involves placing the hand in a neutral position and using passive ROM exercises. In some cases, deficits may persist, requiring continuing observation.
Cranial nerve trauma	Most common is facial nerve palsy Frequently attributed to pressure resulting from forceps May also result from pressure on the nerve in utero, related to fetal positioning such as the head lying against the shoulder	Physical findings include asymmetry of the face when crying; mouth may be drawn toward the unaffected side; wrinkles are deeper on the unaffected side. The paralyzed side may be smooth with a swollen appearance. The eye is persistently open on the affected side.	Most infants begin to recover in the first week, but full resolution may take up to several months; parents need reassurance about this. In most cases, treatment is not necessary, only observation. If the eye is affected and unable to close, protection with patches and synthetic tears may be necessary. Parents need instruction about how to feed the newborn since they cannot close the lips around the nipple without having milk seep out.

TABLE **24.2** • Common Types of Birth Injury

Type	Description	Findings	Treatment
Head trauma	Mild trauma can cause soft tissue injuries such as cephalohematoma and caput succedaneum; greater trauma can cause depressed skull fractures. **Cephalohematoma** (subperiosteal collection of blood secondary to the rupture of blood vessels between the skull and periosteum) occurs in 2.5% of all births and typically appears within hours after birth. **Caput succedaneum** (soft tissue swelling) is caused by edema of the head against the dilating cervix during the birth process.	In cephalohematoma, suture lines delineate its extent; usually located on one side over the parietal bone. In caput succedaneum, swelling is not limited by suture lines; it extends across the midline and is associated with head molding. It does not usually cause complications other than a misshapen head. Swelling is maximal at birth and then rapidly decreases in size.	Cephalohematoma resolves gradually over 2–3 weeks without treatment. Caput succedaneum usually resolves over the first few days without treatment. Subarachnoid hemorrhage requires minimal handling to reduce stress. Subdural hematoma requires aspiration; it can be life-threatening if it is in an inaccessible location and cannot be aspirated.
	Subarachnoid hemorrhage (one of the most common types of intracranial trauma) may be due to hypoxia/ischemia, variations in blood pressure, and the pressure exerted on the head during labor. Bleeding is of venous origin, and underlying contusions also may occur. Subdural hemorrhage (hematomas) occurs less often today because of improved obstetric techniques. Typically, tears of the major veins or venous sinuses overlying the cerebral hemispheres or cerebellum (most common in newborns of primigravida and large newborns, or after an instrumented birth) are the cause. Increased pressure on the blood vessels inside the skull leads to tears. Depressed skull fractures (rare) may result from the pressure of a forceps delivery; can also occur during spontaneous or cesarean births and may be associated with other head trauma causing subdural bleeding, subarachnoid hemorrhage, or brain trauma.	In subarachnoid hemorrhage, some red blood cells may appear in the cerebrospinal fluid (CSF) of full-term newborns. Newborns may present with apnea, seizures, lethargy, or abnormal findings on a neurologic examination. Subdural hemorrhage can be asymptomatic, or the neonate can exhibit seizures, enlarging head size, decreased level of consciousness, or abnormal findings on a neurologic examination with hypotonia, a poor Moro reflex, or extensive retinal hemorrhages. Depressed skull fractures can be observed and palpated as depressions. Confirmation by x-ray is necessary.	Depressed skull fractures typically require a neurosurgical consultation.

Dumpa, V., & Kamity, R. (2023). Birth trauma. *StatPearls*. https://www.ncbi.nlm.nih.gov/books/NBK539831/; and McKee-Garrett, T. M. (2023). Neonatal birth injuries. *UpToDate*. Retrieved March 13, 2024, from https://www.uptodate.com/contents/neonatal-birth-injuries

Nursing Assessment

Recognition of birth injuries is imperative so that early treatment can be initiated. Review the labor and birth history for risk factors, such as prolonged or abrupt labor, abnormal or difficult presentation, cephalopelvic disproportion, forceps or vacuum delivery, multiple fetus deliveries, large for gestational age (LGA) status, extreme prematurity, large fetal head, or congenital anomalies.

Complete a careful physical and neurologic assessment of every newborn admitted to the nursery to establish whether injuries exist. Inspect the head for lumps, bumps, or bruises. Note if swelling or bruising crosses the suture line. Assess the eyes and face for facial paralysis, observing for asymmetry of the face with crying or appearance of the mouth being drawn to the unaffected side. Ensure that the newborn spontaneously moves all extremities. Note any absence of or decrease in deep tendon reflexes or abnormal positioning of extremities.

Assess and document symmetry of structure and function. Be prepared to assist with scheduling diagnostic studies to confirm trauma or injuries, which will be important in determining treatment modalities.

Nursing Management

Nursing management is primarily supportive and focuses on assessing for resolution of the injury or any associated complications along with providing support and education to the parents. Provide the parents with explanations and reassurance that these injuries usually resolve with minimal or no treatment. Parents are alarmed when their newborn is unable to move an extremity or demonstrates asymmetric facial movements. Provide parents with realistic information about the situation to gain their understanding and trust. Be readily available to answer questions and teach them how to care for the newborn, including any modifications that might be necessary. Allow parents adequate time to understand the implications of the birth trauma or injury and what treatment modalities are needed, if any. Provide them with information about the length of time until the injury will resolve and when and if they need to seek further medical attention for the condition. Spending time with the parents and providing them with support, information, and teaching are important to allow them to make decisions and care for their newborn. Anticipate the need for community referral for ongoing follow-up and care if necessary.

Hyperbilirubinemia

In the newborn, **hyperbilirubinemia** is a total serum bilirubin (TSB) level above 5 mg/dL, resulting in jaundice (Kenner, 2022). The term *jaundice* is from the French word *jaune*, meaning yellow. Jaundice is a yellow discoloration of the skin and sclera of the eyes caused by the deposition of bilirubin in those areas when increased levels of unconjugated bilirubin exist in the newborn's circulation. Newborns produce large quantities of bilirubin, which is a byproduct of the breakdown of red blood cells. It is processed in the liver and normally excreted out of the body in the urine and stools. About 80% of newborns appear clinically jaundiced in the first few weeks of life (Ansong-Assoku et al., 2023). Some infants are at higher risk for developing elevated bilirubin levels. Risk factors include:

- Bruising at birth
- Prematurity
- History of a sibling with jaundice
- Inadequate breastfeeding
- Hemolytic disease
- Birth injury such as cephalohematoma
- Polycythemia
- Down syndrome
- Family history of hemolytic disorder
- Maternal diabetes (infant LGA)
- Male sex (Wong & Bhutani, 2023a)

Pathophysiology

Bilirubin is a byproduct of heme, which is produced from the breakdown of hemoglobin. Newborns are relatively polycythemic at birth with large percentages of fetal hemoglobin (HgbF). The lifespan of red blood cells containing HgbF is shorter than cells containing adult hemoglobin (HgbA). Therefore, the amount of bilirubin the newborn must process is large compared to that of an adult. Bilirubin has two forms—unconjugated or indirect, which is fat soluble and toxic to body tissues, and conjugated or direct, which is water soluble and nontoxic. Fetal unconjugated bilirubin is normally cleared by the placenta and the pregnant person's liver in utero, so total bilirubin at birth is low. After the umbilical cord is cut, the newborn must conjugate bilirubin (convert a lipid-soluble pigment into a water-soluble pigment) in the liver on their own (Wong & Bhutani, 2022).

BENIGN NEONATAL HYPERBILIRUBINEMIA

Benign neonatal hyperbilirubinemia was formerly referred to as *physiologic jaundice*. Bilirubin levels reach a high enough level after 24 hours of age to manifest as jaundice, peaking on the third to fourth day of life (Ansong-Akkoku et al., 2023). TSB levels usually peak at 8 to 14 mg/dL with resolution by 7 to 10 days of age (Wong & Bhutani, 2022). Early frequent feedings can provide the newborn with adequate calories and fluid volume (via colostrum) to stimulate peristalsis and passage of meconium to eliminate bilirubin.

A particular type of benign neonatal hyperbilirubinemia is referred to as *breast milk jaundice*. In newborns who are breastfeeding well and gaining weight, hyperbilirubinemia persists up to 3 months of age. In the breastfed newborn, the rate of bilirubin decline is less rapid compared with the bottle-fed newborn. About 34% of breastfed infants continue to have a TSB level of 5 mg/dL or higher (Kemper et al., 2022). This is a benign condition, and the recommended maternity care practice is to promote family-centered breastfeeding support within the first hour after birth with frequent feeding on demand. The AAP recommends early and exclusive breastfeeding and advises not to provide newborns with supplemental water or dextrose water because those supplements do not prevent hyperbilirubinemia and may lead to hyponatremia (Kemper et al., 2022).

SIGNIFICANT HYPERBILIRUBINEMIA

Significant hyperbilirubinemia (formerly pathologic jaundice) refers to the development of jaundice within the first 24 hours of life, regardless of gestational age (Wong & Bhutani, 2023a). In newborns, significant hyperbilirubinemia in neonates is related to increased bilirubin production, deficient bilirubin conjugation, diminished hepatic uptake, and/or heightened enterohepatic circulation of bilirubin. In addition to jaundice before 24 hours of age, significant hyperbilirubinemia occurs when the TSB level is greater than the 95th percentile for age, or if the TSB level increases by more than 5 mg/dL/day or more than 0.2 mg/dL/hour (Ansong-Akkoku et al., 2023). A TSB 25 mg/dL or higher indicates severe hyperbilirubinemia, placing the infant at risk for bilirubin-induced neurotoxicity (Wong & Bhutani, 2022). A TSB 30 mg/dL or higher places the infant at risk for bilirubin-induced neurologic disorders (BINDs) (Wong & Bhutani, 2022).

Conditions that alter the production, transport, uptake, metabolism, excretion, or reabsorption of bilirubin can cause significant hyperbilirubinemia in the newborn. Examples of these conditions include polycythemia, hemolysis due to Rh isoimmunization or ABO incompatibility, metabolic or respiratory acidosis, and congenital inherited defects of enzymes involved in bilirubin metabolism (Wong & Bhutani, 2023a). BIND (formerly termed *kernicterus*) results when free bilirubin crosses the blood–brain barrier and binds to brain tissue, resulting in selective brain damage (Wong & Bhutani, 2022). The brain damage may result in subtle dysfunction or acute or chronic bilirubin encephalopathy. Infants at increased risk for BIND include gestational age 38 weeks or less with an increasing risk associated with the degree of prematurity, albumin less than 3.0 g/dL, alloimmune hemolytic disease of the newborn, G6PD deficiency, sepsis, and significant clinical instability (Wong & Bhutani, 2023a). BIND is a preventable disorder, so immediate recognition of significantly increasing bilirubin is needed.

TAKE NOTE!

Significant jaundice in a newborn younger than 24 hours should be immediately reported to the primary care provider, because it may indicate a pathologic process.

Nursing Assessment

Neonatal jaundice first becomes visible in the face and forehead, identified by gentle pressure on the skin, since blanching reveals the underlying color. Jaundice spreads in a cephalocaudal manner (down the trunk and extremities). Jaundice resolves or disappears in the opposite direction. Nurses play an important role in early detection and identification of jaundice in the newborn. Keen observation skills are essential.

HEALTH HISTORY AND PHYSICAL EXAMINATION

Review the history for factors that might predispose the newborn to hyperbilirubinemia. Perform a complete physical examination. Assess the skin, mucous membranes, sclera, and body fluids (tears, urine) for a yellow color. Detect jaundice by observing the infant in a well-lit room and blanching the skin with digital pressure over a bony prominence. Visual inspection for jaundice should be conducted at least every 12 hours (Wong & Bhutani, 2023c). Also inspect for pallor (anemia), excessive bruising (bleeding), and dehydration (sluggish circulation), which may contribute to the development of jaundice and the risk for BIND.

Visual assessment of the extent of jaundice is not as accurate as obtaining a transcutaneous bilirubin (TCB) reading or a TSB reading via blood specimen. If an infant appears jaundiced, obtain a TCB. According to the AAP, all infants should be assessed visually or using a transcutaneous bilirubinometer at least every 12 hours following their birth until discharge (Kemper et al., 2022).

LABORATORY AND DIAGNOSTIC TESTING

Determine maternal and fetal blood types, checking for incompatibilities (Comparison Chart 24.1). Assess laboratory values for bilirubin (both unconjugated and conjugated). Bilirubin levels establish the diagnosis of hyperbilirubinemia. Additional laboratory tests to use for assessment when the TSB is rising include:

- *Direct Coombs test*—to identify hemolytic disease of the newborn; positive results indicate that the newborn's red blood cells have been coated with antibodies and thus are sensitized
- *Hemoglobin concentration*—for evidence of anemia
- *Total serum protein*—to detect reduced binding capacity of albumin
- *Reticulocyte count*—to identify an elevated level indicating increased hemolysis
- *Alkaline phosphatase, liver enzymes, prothrombin time, and partial thromboplastin time*—may also be evaluated in the newborn with significant hyperbilirubinemia to determine the cause

Assist with obtaining blood specimens. Use cord blood for hemoglobin concentration measurements; use a heel stick for direct Coombs testing and bilirubin levels. Prepare the parents and newborn for radiologic evaluation, if necessary, to determine abnormalities that may be causing the jaundice.

COMPARISON CHART 24.1 Rh Versus ABO Incompatibility

Clinical Picture	Rh Incompatibility	ABO Incompatibility
Firstborn	Rare	Common
Later pregnancies	More severe	No increase in severity
Jaundice	Moderate to severe	Mild
Hydrops fetalis	Frequent	Rare
Anemia	Frequently severe	Rare
Ascites	Frequent	Rare
Hepatosplenomegaly	Frequent	Common

Nursing Management

Nursing management of a newborn with hyperbilirubinemia requires a comprehensive approach. As members of the health care team, nurses share in the responsibility for early detection and identification, management, family education, and follow-up of the birthing parent and newborn. Documentation of the timing of onset of jaundice is essential to differentiate between benign (later than 24 hours) and significant (earlier than 24 hours) hyperbilirubinemia. Nurses can improve care by offering their presence and support and by following the AAP guidelines for preventing hyperbilirubinemia:

- Promote and support successful breastfeeding.
- Establish nursery protocols for identifying jaundice, including when a serum bilirubin can be ordered by a nurse.
- Measure TSB on infants who display jaundice in the first 24 hours.
- Assess for risk factors that may increase bilirubin levels.
- Interpret all bilirubin levels according to the infant's age in hours.
- Do not use a visual estimation of jaundice, which may be inaccurate; instead, use transcutaneous tools or lab values.
- Treat jaundiced newborns with phototherapy if prescribed.
- Provide parents with written and oral information about jaundice at discharge.
- Provide follow-up care and referrals based on the time of discharge and risk.
- Empower parents to make appropriate decisions at home (Kemper et al., 2022; Kenner, 2022).

REDUCING BILIRUBIN LEVELS

Encourage early initiation of feedings to prevent hypoglycemia and provide protein to maintain albumin levels to transport bilirubin to the liver. Ensure newborn feedings (breast milk or formula) occur every 2 to 3 hours to promote prompt emptying of bilirubin from the bowel. Encourage breastfeeding (at least eight feedings per day) to prevent inadequate intake and thus dehydration. Supplement breast milk with formula to supply protein if bilirubin levels continue to increase with breastfeeding only. Monitor serum bilirubin levels frequently to reduce the risk of severe hyperbilirubinemia. Check for at least six wet diapers daily and a transition to at least four yellow, seedy stools by Day 4 of life.

Phototherapy

Phototherapy is the use of blue LED light to provide high-intensity narrow band light for the treatment of hyperbilirubinemia in the newborn. Photons emitted by the light source convert bilirubin into water-soluble isomers that can be eliminated via bile and urine without conjugation in the liver. Phototherapy may be provided from above via the bili-light source and below via a bili-light mat. Another option is a fiberoptic blanket wrapped around the newborn, which may be left of on the infant during feedings (extending light exposure time) (Wong & Bhutani, 2023b).

For the newborn receiving phototherapy, place the newborn under the lights or on the fiberoptic blanket, exposing as much skin as possible. Cover the newborn's genitals and shield the eyes to protect them from becoming irritated or burned when using direct lights. Assess the intensity of the light source to prevent burns and excoriation (Fig. 24.14). Turn the newborn every 2 hours to maximize the area of exposure, removing the newborn from the lights only for feedings. Maintain a neutral thermal environment to decrease energy expenditure and assess the newborn's neurologic status frequently.

Assess the newborn's temperature every 4 hours. Monitor fluid intake and output closely and assess daily weights for gains or losses. Encourage breastfeeding or bottle-feeding every 2 to 3 hours. Check skin turgor for evidence of dehydration. Turn the infant every 2 hours. With feedings, remove the newborn from the lights. Remove the eye shields when not under the lights to allow interaction with the newborn and assess the eyes for discharge or corneal irritation secondary to eye shield pressure. Monitor stool for consistency and frequency. Unconjugated bilirubin excreted in the feces will produce a greenish appearance, and typically, stools are loose. Lack of frequent green stools is a cause for concern. Provide meticulous skin care. Assess skin surfaces frequently for dryness and irritation secondary to the dehydrating effects of phototherapy and irritation from highly acidic stool to prevent excoriation and skin breakdown (Kemper et al., 2022; Kenner, 2022; Wong & Bhutani, 2023b).

Exchange Transfusion

If the TSB level remains elevated or continues to rise after intensive phototherapy, or hemolytic disease or

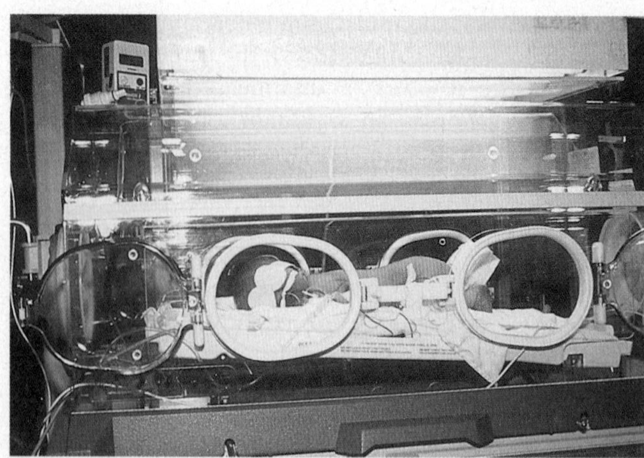

FIGURE 24.14 A newborn receiving phototherapy.

severe anemia is present, an exchange transfusion may be necessary. The exchange transfusion removes bilirubin and hemolysis-causing antibodies directly, by withdrawing the infant's blood and replacing it with nonhemolyzed red blood cells from a donor (Ansong-Assoku et al., 2023). Exchange transfusion is used only as a second-line therapy after phototherapy has failed to yield results. Intensive nursing care is needed. During the transfusion, monitor the newborn's cardiovascular status continuously because serious complications can arise, such as acid–base imbalances, infection, hypovolemia, and fluid and electrolyte imbalances.

PROVIDING PARENT TEACHING AND SUPPORT

Providing education on newborn jaundice is essential. Nurses can help parents understand the diagnostic tests and treatment modalities by offering individualized teaching. Provide culturally sensitive and developmentally appropriate education in a language that is easy to understand. Teach the parents about jaundice and its potential risks using written and verbal material. Also show the parents how to identify newborn behaviors that might indicate rising bilirubin levels. Emphasize the need to seek treatment from the pediatrician should any of the following occur:

- Lethargy, sleepiness, poor muscle tone, floppiness
- Poor sucking, lack of interest in feeding
- High-pitched cry

Teach the parents how to assess the newborn for signs of jaundice because physiologic jaundice may not occur until after the newborn is discharged. Reinforce the need for appropriate follow-up with the primary care provider within 48 hours after discharge to assess jaundice status (Kemper et al., 2022).

Some infants will need home phototherapy, which can be anxiety producing for parents. Explain the rationale for the procedure and demonstrate techniques that the parents can use to interact with the newborn. See Teaching Guidelines 24.1.

Infant of a Mother With Diabetes

Diabetes during pregnancy (whether type 1, type 2, or gestational) can negatively affect the health of the neonate. An **infant of a mother with diabetes (IMD)** is a diagnosis describing newborns born to a person with pregestational or gestational diabetes (see Chapter 20 for additional information). The IMD is at high risk for numerous health-related complications, especially hypoglycemia and congenital anomalies. In the United States, up to 8% of pregnant people have type 2 diabetes, and up to 90% of pregnant people with diabetes have gestational diabetes (Moore, 2022). In light of the increasing incidence of type 2 diabetes among people of childbearing age, as well as incidence of gestational diabetes, it is important to educate patients about the potential impact of poor glycemic control on their offspring.

TEACHING GUIDELINES 24.1 Caring for Your Newborn Receiving Home Phototherapy

- Inspect your newborn's skin, eyes, and mucous membranes for a yellow color.
- Remember that a home health nurse will come to visit and help you set up the light system.
- Keep the lights about 12–30 in above your newborn.
- Cover your newborn's eyes with patches or cotton balls and gauze to protect them.
- Keep the newborn undressed, except for the diaper area; fold the diaper down below the newborn's navel in the front and as far as possible in the back to expose as much skin as possible.
- Turn your newborn every 2 hours so that all areas of the body are exposed.
- Remove the newborn from the lights only for feeding.
- Remove the eye patches during feedings so that you can interact with your newborn.
- Record your newborn's temperature, weight, and fluid intake daily.
- Document the frequency, color, and consistency of all stools; the stools should be loose and green as the bilirubin is broken down.
- Keep the skin clean and dry to prevent irritation.

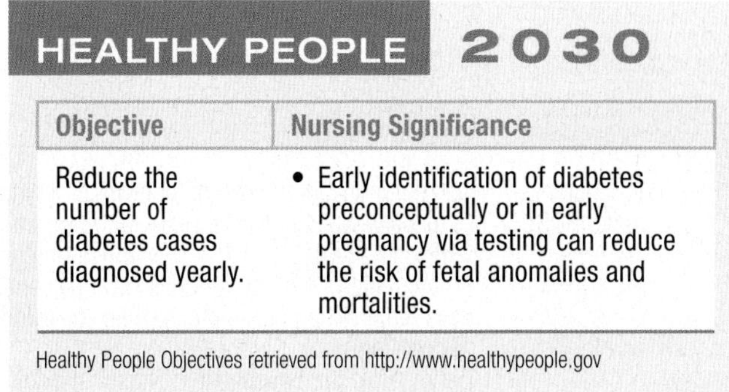
HEALTHY PEOPLE 2030

Objective	Nursing Significance
Reduce the number of diabetes cases diagnosed yearly.	• Early identification of diabetes preconceptually or in early pregnancy via testing can reduce the risk of fetal anomalies and mortalities.

Healthy People Objectives retrieved from http://www.healthypeople.gov

Impact of Diabetes on the Newborn

For decades, it has been cleared that diabetes during pregnancy can have severe adverse effects on fetal and newborn outcomes. IMDs have increased morbidity and mortality in the perinatal period. The incidence of major congenital anomalies is much greater for these newborns than for other newborns, particularly when the birthing parent requires insulin during pregnancy. About 66% of

IMDs born with a congenital anomaly have an abnormality of the cardiovascular or central nervous system, though anomalies in other systems also occur (Riskin & Garcia-Prats, 2023).

IMDs can be LGA or small for gestational age (SGA), depending on the vascular impact of glycemic control in the pregnant person prior to and during the pregnancy. Fetal macrosomia occurs in 29% to 38% of diabetic pregnancies (Akanmode & Mahdy, 2023). LGA infants (>90th percentile on the growth chart) are longer and weigh more than 4,000 g. Infants of mothers with pregestational diabetes may be SGA (<10th percentile on the growth chart) owing to long-standing insulin use and vascular compromise (Mishra et al., 2024). Despite their increased or decreased size and weight, they may be remarkably frail, showing behaviors like those of a preterm newborn. Thus, birth weight may not be a reliable criterion of maturity. They are frequently hypoglycemic in the first few hours after birth. The IMD who is LGA has increased organ weights (organomegaly) and excessive fat deposits on their shoulders and trunk, predisposing them to shoulder dystocia, perinatal asphyxia, stillbirth, brachial plexus injury, fracture, low Apgar scores, and respiratory depression (Riskin & Garcia-Prats, 2023). These newborns frequently require instrumental or cesarean births for cephalopelvic disproportion and dysfunctional labor patterns.

Pathophysiology

The large size of the IMD arises secondary to exposure to high levels of maternal glucose crossing the placenta into the fetal circulation. Maternal hyperglycemia acts as a fuel to stimulate increased production of fetal insulin, which, in turn, promotes somatic growth within the fetus. The fetus responds to these high levels by producing more insulin, which acts as a growth factor in the fetus. IMDs experience fetal hyperinsulinism and increased peripheral glucose utilization, placing them at risk for hypoglycemia in the immediate postnatal period (Abramowski et al., 2023). How the fetus will be affected and the problems that the newborn will experience depend on the severity, duration, and control of the diabetes in the pregnant person. Table 24.3 summarizes the common problems that may occur in IMDs.

TABLE 24.3 • Common Problems of Infants of Mothers With Diabetes

Condition	Description	Effects
Macrosomia	Newborn with an excessive birth weight; defined as a birth weight >4,000 g (8 lb 13 oz) to 4,500 g (9 lb 15 oz) or >90th percentile for gestational age	Increased risk for shoulder dystocia, traumatic birth injury, birth asphyxia Risks for newborn hypoglycemia and hypomagnesemia, polycythemia, and electrolyte disturbances Increased maternal risk for surgical birth, postpartum hemorrhage and infection, and birth canal lacerations Increased risk of developing type 2 diabetes later in life for both Higher weight and accumulation of fat in childhood and a higher rate of obesity in adults
Respiratory distress syndrome (RDS)	Cortisol-induced stimulation of lecithin/sphingomyelin (phospholipids) necessary for lung maturation is antagonized due to the high-insulin environment within the fetus due to birthing parent's hyperglycemia. Less mature lung development than expected for gestational age Decrease in the phospholipid phosphatidylglycerol (PG), which stabilizes surfactant, compounding risk	Most commonly, baby is breathing normally at birth but develops labored, grunting respiration with cough and a hoarse complaining cry within a few hours with chest retractions and varying degrees of cyanosis. IMDs who also have vascular disease seldom develop RDS because the chronic stress of poor intrauterine perfusion leads to increased production of steroids, which accelerates lung maturation.
Hypoglycemia	Glucose is the major source of energy for organ function. Typical characteristics: • Poor feedings • Jitteriness • Lethargy • High-pitched or weak cry • Apnea • Cyanosis and seizures Some newborns are asymptomatic.	Low blood glucose levels are problematic during the early postnatal period due to abrupt cessation of high-glucose maternal blood supply and the continuation of insulin production by the newborn. Limited ability to release glucagon and catecholamines, which normally stimulate glucagon breakdown and glucose release Prolonged and untreated hypoglycemia leads to serious, long-term adverse neurologic sequelae such as learning disabilities and intellectual disability.

TABLE 24.3 • Common Problems of Infants of Mothers With Diabetes

Condition	Description	Effects
Hypocalcemia and hypomagnesemia	Hypocalcemia (drop in calcium levels) is manifested by tremors, hypotonia, apnea, high-pitched cry, and seizures due to abrupt cessation of maternal transfer of calcium to the fetus, which occurs primarily in the third trimester and if the infant experiences birth asphyxia. Associated hypomagnesemia is directly related to the maternal level before birth. About half of infants of birthing parents with diabetes are affected.	Newborn is at risk for a prolonged delay in parathyroid hormone production and cardiac dysrhythmias.
Polycythemia	Venous hematocrit of >65% in the newborn Increased oxygen consumption by neonate secondary to fetal hyperglycemia and hyperinsulinemia Increased fetal erythropoiesis secondary to intrauterine hypoxia due to placental insufficiency from maternal diabetes Hypoxic stimulation of increased red blood cell (RBC) production as a compensatory mechanism	Increased viscosity, resulting in poor blood flow that predisposes newborn to decreased tissue oxygenation and development of microthrombi
Hyperbilirubinemia	Usually seen within the first few days after birth; manifested by a yellow appearance of the sclera and skin Excessive red cell hemolysis necessary to break down increased RBCs in circulation due to polycythemia Resultant elevated bilirubin levels Excessive bruising secondary to birth trauma of macrosomic infants, further adding to high bilirubin levels	If untreated, high levels of unconjugated bilirubin may lead to kernicterus (neurologic syndrome that results in irreversible damage) with long-term sequelae that include cerebral palsy, sensorineural hearing loss, and intellectual disability.

Riskin, A., & Garcia-Prats, J. A. (2023). Infants of mothers with diabetes (IMD). *UpToDate.* Retrieved March 14, 2024, from https://www.uptodate.com/contents/infants-of-mothers-with-diabetes; and Mishra, V., Lui, K., Schelonka, R. L., Maheshwari, A., & Jain, R. (2024). Infants of diabetic mothers. In A. Maheshwari (Ed.), *Principles of neonatology.* Elsevier.

Nursing Assessment

Assessment begins in the prenatal period by identifying pregnant people with diabetes and taking measures to control maternal glucose levels. (See Chapter 20 for information on management of the pregnant person with diabetes.)

PHYSICAL EXAMINATION

Note birth weight in comparison to gestational age. At birth, inspect the LGA newborn for full rosy cheeks with a ruddy skin color, round puffy face, massive shoulders, and excessive subcutaneous fat tissue (Yang, 2025) (Fig. 24.15).

Be alert for hypoglycemia, which may occur immediately or within an hour after birth. The AAP defines a neonatal blood glucose level below 40 mg/dL as hypoglycemic (AAP, 2022). Closely assess the newborn for signs of hypoglycemia, including listlessness, hypotonia, apathy, poor feeding, apneic episodes with a drop in oxygen saturation, weak or high-pitched cry, cyanosis,

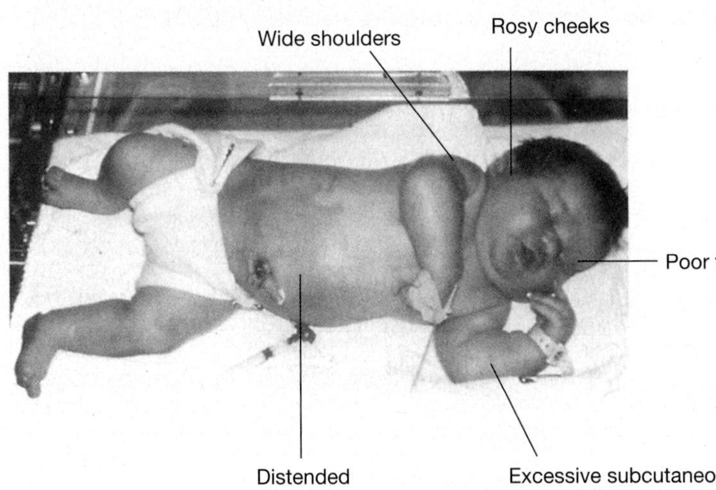

FIGURE 24.15 Characteristics of an infant of a mother with diabetes (IMD). A macrosomic IMD has head circumference and length that are at the 90th percentile; the IMD's body weight greatly exceeds the 90th percentile. The IMD has considerable fat deposition in the shoulder and intrascapular area. (Modified with permission from Boardman, J., Groves, A., & Ramasethu, J. [2021]. *Avery & MacDonald's neonatology: Pathophysiology and management of the newborn* [8th ed.] Wolters Kluwer.)

temperature instability, pallor and sweating, tremors, irritability, and seizures (Abramowski et al., 2023).

Note a ruddy appearance as the infant may be polycythemic. Assess respiratory rate and work of breathing as IMDs are at risk for the development of transient tachypnea of the newborn (TTN) and RDS. Perform a thorough cardiovascular assessment, as cardiac congenital anomalies occur at increased rate in IMDs (Riskin & Garcia-Prats, 2023). Assess the newborn for signs of birth trauma involving the head (tense or bulging fontanels, cephalohematoma, skull fractures, and facial nerve paralysis), shoulders and extremities (posturing, paralysis), and skin (bruising). Take the newborn's temperature frequently.

LABORATORY AND DIAGNOSTIC TESTING

Determine baseline serum calcium, magnesium, and bilirubin levels, and monitor them frequently for changes (Table 24.4).

TABLE 24.4 • Critical Laboratory Values for Infants of Mothers With Diabetes

Hypoglycemia	<50 mg/dL
Hypocalcemia	<7 mcg/dL
Hypomagnesemia	<1.5 mg/dL
Hyperbilirubinemia	>12 mg/dL (term infant)
Polycythemia	>65% (venous hematocrit)

O'Brien, K. (2023). Neonatal effects of maternal diabetes. In E. C. Eichenwald, A. R. Hansen, C. R. Martin, & A. R. Stark (Eds.), *Cloherty and Stark's manual of neonatal care* (9th ed.). Wolters Kluwer.

Nursing Management

Nursing management of the IMD focuses on correcting hypoglycemia and hypocalcemia, providing phototherapy for jaundice, administering fluid therapy, and maintaining oxygen and ventilation if required. It is also important to provide a neutral thermal environment to prevent cold stress, which would increase the glucose utilization and contribute to the hypoglycemic state. Refer to Clinical Judgment & Nursing Process 24.1 for additional information.

PREVENTING HYPOGLYCEMIA

Prevent and manage hypoglycemia by providing early oral feedings with breast milk (preferred) or formula at

CLINICAL JUDGMENT & NURSING PROCESS 24.1 Overview of the Infant of a Mother With Diabetes

Jamie, a 38-year-old Hispanic woman, gave birth to a term large for gestational age (LGA) newborn weighing 10 lb. She had a history of gestational diabetes but had not received any prenatal care. She arrived at the hospital in active labor. Despite macrosomia, the newborn's Apgar scores were 8 and 9 at 1 and 5 minutes, respectively. No resuscitative measures were needed.

One hour after birth, assessment revealed a pale, irritable newborn with sweating and several episodes of apnea. A glucose level obtained at this time via a heel stick was 30 mg/dL. Two hours later, the newborn begins exhibiting signs of respiratory distress—grunting, nasal flaring, retractions, tachypnea (respiratory rate 72 breaths/min), and tachycardia (heart rate 176 bpm).

NURSING ANALYSIS: Unstable glucose level risk related to hypoglycemia secondary to intrauterine hyperinsulinemic state resulting from maternal gestational diabetes as evidenced by low blood glucose level, irritability, pallor, sweating, and apnea

OUTCOME IDENTIFICATION AND EVALUATION

The newborn will exhibit adequate glucose control as evidenced by maintaining blood glucose levels >40 mg/dL and an absence of clinical signs of hypoglycemia.

INTERVENTIONS: *Promoting Glucose Control*

- Monitor blood glucose levels hourly for the first 4 hours and then every 3–4 hours or as necessary *to detect hypoglycemia, which would be <40 mg/dL.*
- Continue to observe for manifestations of hypoglycemia, such as pallor, tremors, jitteriness, lethargy, and poor feeding, *to allow for early detection and prompt intervention, thereby minimizing the risk of complications associated with hypoglycemia.*
- Monitor temperature frequently and institute measures to maintain a neutral thermal environment *to prevent cold stress, which would increase metabolic demands and further deplete glycogen stores.*
- Initiate early feedings every 2–3 hours or as appropriate or administer glucose supplements as ordered *to prevent hypoglycemia caused by the newborn's hyperinsulinemic state.*
- Administer intravenous (IV) glucose infusions as ordered *to correct hypoglycemia if glucose levels do not stabilize with feeding.*
- Cluster infant care activities and provide for rest periods *to conserve the newborn's energy and reduce use of glucose and glycogen stores.*
- Reduce environmental stimuli by dimming lights and speaking softly *to reduce energy demands and further utilization of glucose.*
- Explain all events and procedures to the parent *to help alleviate anxiety and promote understanding of the newborn's condition.*

CLINICAL JUDGMENT & NURSING PROCESS 24.1 Overview of the Infant of a Mother With Diabetes

NURSING ANALYSIS: Altered gas exchange related to respiratory distress secondary to delayed lung maturity resulting from inhibition of pulmonary surfactant production due to fetal hyperinsulinemia as evidenced by grunting, nasal flaring, retractions, tachypnea, and tachycardia

OUTCOME IDENTIFICATION AND EVALUATION

The newborn will demonstrate signs of adequate oxygenation without respiratory distress as evidenced by respiratory and heart rates within the usual newborn range; absence of nasal flaring, retractions, and grunting; and oxygen saturation and arterial blood gas (ABG) levels within acceptable parameters.

INTERVENTIONS: *Promoting Oxygenation*

- Monitor newborn's vital signs *to establish a baseline and evaluate for changes.*
- Assess airway patency and perform gentle suctioning as ordered *to ensure patency and allow for adequate oxygen intake.*
- Position the newborn prone *to optimize respiratory status and reduce stress.*
- Continuously monitor oxygen saturation levels via pulse oximetry *to determine the adequacy of tissue perfusion.* Assess lung sounds for changes *to allow early detection of change in status.*
- Administer oxygen as ordered *to promote adequate tissue perfusion.*
- Assess newborn's skin to identify cyanosis, pallor, and mottling *to detect changes indicating compromised oxygenation.*
- Assess ABG results *to detect changes indicating acidosis, hypoxemia, or hypercarbia, which would suggest hypoxia.*
- Administer medications as ordered *to correct acidosis.*
- Administer surfactant replacement therapy as ordered *to aid in stabilizing the newborn's lungs until postnatal surfactant synthesis improves.*
- Institute measures to maintain normal blood glucose levels and a neutral thermal environment, cluster care activities, and reduce excessive stimuli *to reduce oxygen demand and consumption.*

frequent intervals (every 2 to 3 hours). Feedings help control glucose levels, reduce hematocrit, and promote bilirubin excretion. Maintain a neutral thermal environment to avoid cold stress, which may stimulate the metabolic rate, thereby increasing the demand for glucose. Provide rest periods to decrease energy demand and expenditure.

Monitor blood glucose levels via heel stick every hour for the first 4 hours of life and then every 3 to 4 hours until stable. Document the results. Report unstable glucose values. If glucose levels are not stabilized, initiate oral dextrose gel or IV glucose infusions as ordered and ensure that the infusions are flowing at the prescribed rate.

MAINTAINING FLUID AND ELECTROLYTE BALANCE

Monitor serum calcium levels for changes indicating the need for supplementation, such as with oral or IV calcium gluconate. Assess the newborn for signs of hypocalcemia, such as tremors, jitteriness, twitching, seizures, and high-pitched cry. Also administer fluid therapy as ordered to maintain adequate hydration.

PROVIDING PARENTAL SUPPORT

Good communication between the nurse and the family is essential. It should be supported by evidence-based, written information tailored to meet the family's individual needs. Assist the parents and family in understanding the newborn's condition and need for frequent monitoring. Offer support and information to the parents and family about the benefits of breastfeeding for the lactating person and the infant. They may erroneously interpret the newborn's large size as an indication that the newborn is free of problems. Encourage open communication and listen with empathy to the family's fears and concerns. Provide frequent opportunities for the parents to interact with their newborn.

Newborns of Birthing Parents With Substance Use Disorder

Drug misuse and addiction have significantly increased over the past few decades to epidemic proportions. Annually, among people aged 12 years and older, about 14.5% have a diagnosable substance use disorder, with 10.2% misusing alcohol and 6.6% misusing illicit drugs (Dugosh & Cacciola, 2022). People who use tobacco, alcohol, or illicit substances during pregnancy place themselves and their newborns at risk for numerous complications before and after birth. A recent survey revealed that 15.9% of pregnant people reported smoking cigarettes, 8.5% drank alcohol, and almost 6% used illicit drugs during pregnancy (Prince et al., 2023). The type of substance used, the timing of use during embryogenesis and fetal development, and the duration and amount used all contribute to the impact on a pregnancy and to the fetal and newborn effects.

Pregnant people most frequently report using tobacco, alcohol, and cannabis, followed by opioids and cocaine (Prince et al., 2023). In utero exposure of the fetus to maternal tobacco smoking or secondhand smoke increases the risk of birth defects, stillbirths, preterm births, and sudden unexplained infant death (WHO, 2021). Infants exposed to cannabis during gestation are at increased risk for neonatal death and, possibly, poorer cognitive outcomes (Chang, 2024). Cocaine and methamphetamine use during pregnancy contributes to the development of maternal hypertension and placental abruption, as well as preterm birth, low birth weight, and miscarriage (Chang, 2024). Among the general population, opioid use has increased dramatically over the past two decades, with a resultant similar increase among pregnant people (Patrick et al., 2020). Nurses should educate all pregnant patients to avoid using these potentially harmful substances when pregnant and refer them to treatment centers.

TAKE NOTE!

Cocaine-exposed newborns are typically fussy, irritable, and inconsolable at times. They demonstrate poor coordination of sucking and swallowing, making feeding time frustrating for the newborn and caregiver alike.

Fetal Alcohol Spectrum Disorders

Alcohol misuse during pregnancy is currently among the fastest growing health care challenges in the United States. Fetal alcohol exposure remains the leading preventable cause of developmental disability and congenital birth defects. With exposure to alcohol during pregnancy, the newborn is at risk for the development of a fetal alcohol spectrum disorder (FASD). FASD is not a medical diagnosis, rather an umbrella term used to describe the effects of alcohol on the newborn and child, ranging from mild involvement to severe (fetal alcohol syndrome [FAS]), and the prevalence of FASD in the United States is 1.5% to 5% (Weitzman & Rojmahamongkol, 2024). Children with FASDs may show issues in three categories: facial dysmorphology, prenatal and postnatal growth deficiencies, and central nervous system dysfunction. Children with FAS demonstrate the highest levels of central nervous system dysfunction.

Decreasing or eliminating alcohol consumption during pregnancy is the only way to prevent FASD. No level of alcohol has been proven to be safe for the fetus, so alcohol should be completely avoided when planning for conception and during pregnancy; it is also not recommended during breastfeeding. See the Healthy People 2030 box. Newborns rarely exhibit symptoms related to alcohol withdrawal; however, when they do, symptoms may include agitation, hyperactivity, and marked tremors for the first 72 hours of life (Vaux & Chambers, 2023). Box 24.2 summarizes the clinically visible manifestations of FAS.

BOX 24.2 Clinically Visible Manifestations of Fetal Alcohol Syndrome

- Microcephaly (head circumference <10th percentile)
- Hypoplastic midface
  - Epicanthal folds (folds of skin of the upper eyelid over the eye)
  - Narrow-set eyes
  - Maxillary hypoplasia (flattened or absent)
  - Smooth and/or long philtrum
  - Thin, smooth vermilion border of the upper lip
- Short upturned nose
- Joint and limb defects
- Altered palmar crease pattern (looks like a hockey stick)
- Prenatal or postnatal growth ≤10th percentile

Weitzman, C., & Rojmahamongkol, P. (2024). Fetal alcohol spectrum disorder: Clinical features and diagnosis. *UpToDate*. Retrieved June 4, 2024, from https://www.uptodate.com/contents/fetal-alcohol-spectrum-disorder-clinical-features-and-diagnosis; and Vaux, K. K., & Chambers, C. (2023). Fetal alcohol syndrome. *Medscape*. https://emedicine.medscape.com/article/974016-overview

HEALTHY PEOPLE 2030

Objective	Nursing Significance
Increase abstinence from alcohol among pregnant people.	• Educate pregnant people about the dangers to the fetus associated with alcohol. • Encourage pregnant people to stop drinking alcohol. • Refer pregnant people to alcohol treatment programs as needed.

Healthy People Objectives retrieved from http://www.healthypeople.gov

Neonatal Opioid Withdrawal Syndrome

Prescription opioid use during pregnancy is a concern, with 7% of pregnant people reporting use and 20% of those people reporting opioid misuse during pregnancy (Ndanga et al., 2022). Opioids used may include hydrocodone, oxycodone, fentanyl, morphine, meperidine, codeine, heroin, methadone, and others. **Neonatal opioid withdrawal syndrome (NOWS)** refers to a constellation of opioid withdrawal signs and symptoms. Neonatal abstinence syndrome (NAS) may result in a similar collection of symptoms resulting from withdrawal from barbiturates, selective serotonin reuptake inhibitors (SSRI), or benzodiazepine exposure. These substances cross the placenta and may cause the fetus to develop a dependency; when fetal exposure to the substances terminates at birth, the newborn is at risk for a spectrum of withdrawal symptoms that may necessitate prolonged treatment, intensive monitoring, and extended hospitalization. NOWS is a generalized multisystem disorder of the drug-exposed newborn, which may progress to seizures. It manifests as disturbances in the central nervous system as well as disruptions in the autonomic, respiratory, and gastrointestinal systems (Anbalagan et al., 2023). See the Healthy People 2030 box.

HEALTHY PEOPLE 2030

Objective	Nursing Significance
Increase abstinence from illicit drugs among pregnant people.	• Educate pregnant people about the dangers to the fetus associated with illicit drug exposure. • Refer pregnant people to drug treatment programs. • Support people in their efforts to be successful in drug treatment.

Healthy People Objectives retrieved from http://www.healthypeople.gov

Nursing Assessment

A comprehensive prenatal medical and drug history, especially with respect to polydrug use, is vital. Fear of referral to child welfare agencies or the legal system has prompted people to conceal their drug use history. Frequently, the first inkling of drug use appears in the newborn when symptoms of withdrawal begin within 72 hours after birth. Several screening tools have been developed, and the Finnegan Neonatal Abstinence Scoring system is the widely used. It assesses 21 of the most common clinical symptoms of drug withdrawal, and the total score can range from 0 to 62. Another such tool is Eat, Sleep, Console; it is simpler and assesses the three areas in its title. Figure 24.16 shows a generic example of a screening tool for neonatal drug exposure.

The newborn's behavior often prompts the health care provider or nurse to suspect intrauterine drug exposure. Refer to Box 24.3 for clinical manifestations the drug-exposed newborn is likely to display.

Assist with obtaining diagnostic studies. Toxicology screening of the newborn's meconium (most common and considered the gold standard), urine, or umbilical cord blood identifies the substances to which the newborn has been exposed (Bagwell, 2022). The newborn physical examination may also reveal low birth weight for gestational age.

Nursing Management

Nonpharmacologic management of NOWS includes environmental control, feeding methods, social integration, and soothing techniques. Interventions include breastfeeding, swaddling, rooming-in, skin-to-skin contact, and providing quiet, nonstimulating environments. These interventions should begin at birth using a family-centered approach (Patrick et al., 2022). The objectives of nonpharmacologic treatment are to assist the neonate in self-organization, support the infant's neuromaturation, and promote newborn–parent connection (Anbalagan et al., 2023; Jansson, 2024). Nonpharmacologic treatment is recommended by the AAP as the first-line treatment for NOWS (Anbalagan et al., 2023). Implement these nonpharmacologic treatments:

- At the first sign of infant distress, limit stimulation
- Feed on demand, frequently (preferably breastfeeding)
- Provide nonnutritive sucking
- Encourage skin-to-skin contact with the parent/caregiver
- Hold the infant often
- Safely swaddle in a flexed position
- Ensure the environment is quiet and not stimulating
- Cluster nursing care
- Apply a topical skin barrier cream to prevent/treat diaper dermatitis (Bagwell, 2022)

Swaying or vertical rocking can be helpful to reduce irritability. These nonpharmacologic interventions can be effective as standalone therapy for milder cases of NOWS (Anbalagan et al., 2023; Jansson, 2024; Patrick et al., 2022).

With severe NOWS, pharmacologic treatment may be needed while the nonpharmacologic interventions above are continued. When the modified Finnegan score is greater than 8 on two occasions or greater than 12 on one occasion, or if on two consecutive assessments with the Eat, Sleep, Console tool the answer is "yes" to any question, pharmacologic intervention is warranted. Administer morphine, methadone, or buprenorphine as prescribed. Most nonopioid fetal drug exposures result in limited clinical manifestations, respond well to supportive care measures, and rarely require pharmacologic intervention. However, chronic opioid exposure does require pharmacotherapy to mitigate withdrawal signs in the newborn, especially when there has been maternal polysubstance consumption (Anbalagan et al., 2023).

MEETING NUTRITIONAL NEEDS

Newborns experiencing NOWS may have impaired feeding behaviors, such as excessive sucking, poor feeding, and regurgitation. Along with anticipated diarrhea, weight loss or failure to gain weight may occur. To improve weight gain, offer frequent feedings on demand and use high-calorie supplements as prescribed. Breastfeeding is encouraged for birthing parents who stopped nonprescribed substance use by the time of delivery unless a true contraindication exists (Harris et al., 2023). Contraindications include maternal HIV infection and maternal hepatitis C infection with cracked nipples. Birthing parents treated with methadone or buprenorphine may breastfeed. These drugs are excreted in minute quantities in breast milk and may assist with withdrawal symptoms (Patrick et al., 2022).

When bottle-feeding the newborn, use small amounts and position the newborn upright to prevent aspiration and to facilitate rhythmic sucking and swallowing. Burp

CENTRAL NERVOUS SYSTEM DISTURBANCES

SIGNS AND SYMPTOMS	SCORE	AM							PM				
Excessive high-pitched cry	2												
Continuous high-pitched cry	3												
Sleeps <1 hour after feeding	3												
Sleeps <2 hours after feeding	2												
Sleeps <3 hours after feeding	1												
Hyperactive Moro reflex	2												
Markedly hyperactive Moro reflex	3												
Mild tremors disturbed	1												
Moderate–severe tremors disturbed	2												
Mild tremors undisturbed	1												
Moderate–severe tremors undisturbed	4												
Increased muscle tone	2												
Excoloration (specify area)	1												
Myoclonic jerks	3												
Generalized convulsions	5												
METABOLIC VASOMOTOR/RESPIRATORY DISTURBANCES													
Sweating													
Fever <101 (99–100.8°F/37.2–38.2°C)	1												
Fever >101 (38.2°C and higher)	2												
Frequent yawning (>3–4 times/interval)	1												
Mottling	1												
Nasal stuffiness	1												
Sneezing (>3–4 times/interval)	1												
Nasal flaring	2												
Respiratory rate >60 min	1												
Respiratory rate >60 min, with retractions	2												
GASTROINTESTINAL DISTURBANCES													
Excessive sucking	1												
Poor feeding	2												
Regurgitation	2												
Projectile vomiting	3												
Loose stools	2												
Watery stools	3												
TOTAL SCORE													

FIGURE 24.16 Neonatal abstinence scoring system.

BOX 24.3 Manifestations of Neonatal Abstinence Syndrome

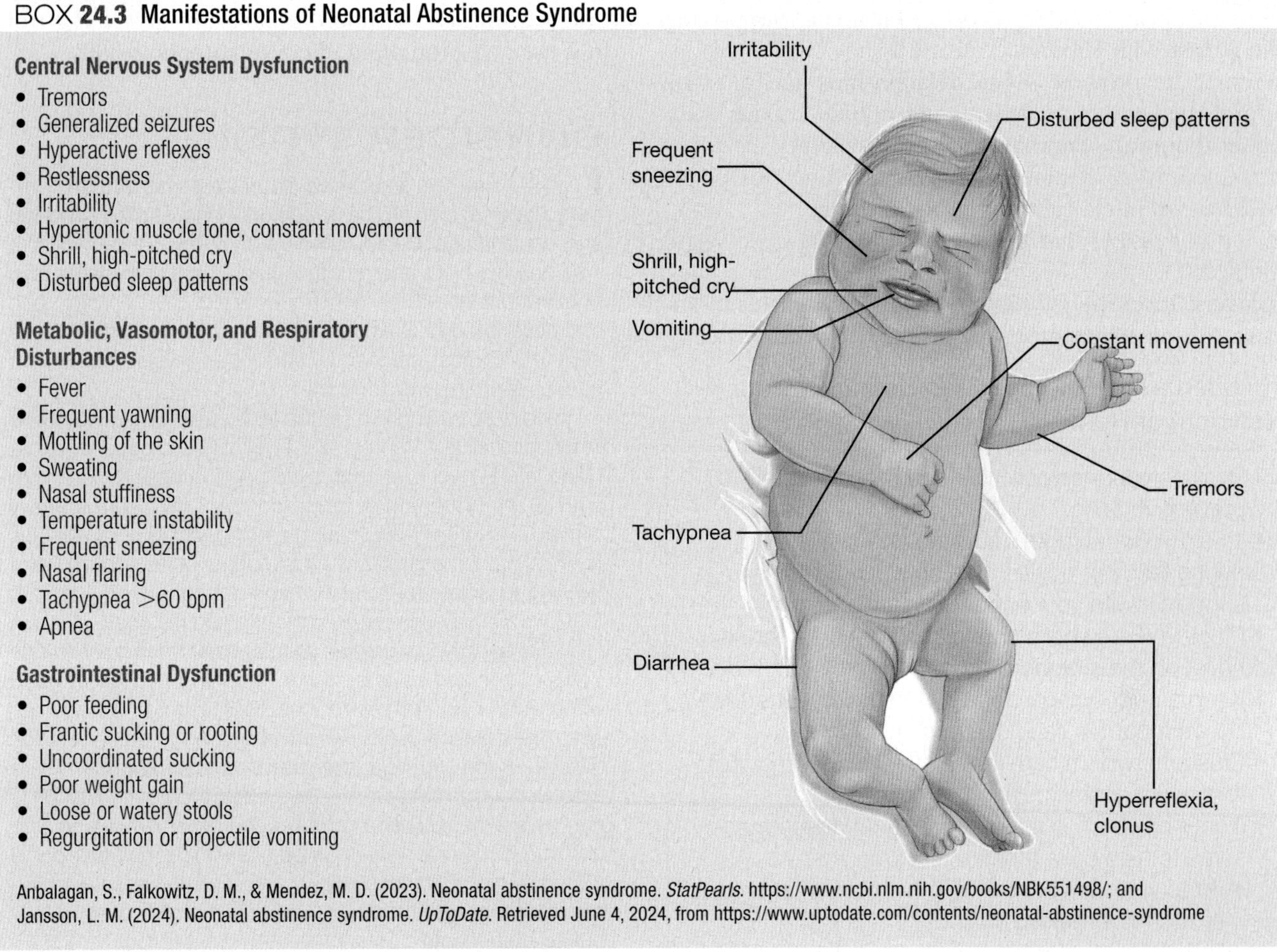

Central Nervous System Dysfunction

- Tremors
- Generalized seizures
- Hyperactive reflexes
- Restlessness
- Irritability
- Hypertonic muscle tone, constant movement
- Shrill, high-pitched cry
- Disturbed sleep patterns

Metabolic, Vasomotor, and Respiratory Disturbances

- Fever
- Frequent yawning
- Mottling of the skin
- Sweating
- Nasal stuffiness
- Temperature instability
- Frequent sneezing
- Nasal flaring
- Tachypnea >60 bpm
- Apnea

Gastrointestinal Dysfunction

- Poor feeding
- Frantic sucking or rooting
- Uncoordinated sucking
- Poor weight gain
- Loose or watery stools
- Regurgitation or projectile vomiting

Anbalagan, S., Falkowitz, D. M., & Mendez, M. D. (2023). Neonatal abstinence syndrome. *StatPearls.* https://www.ncbi.nlm.nih.gov/books/NBK551498/; and Jansson, L. M. (2024). Neonatal abstinence syndrome. *UpToDate.* Retrieved June 4, 2024, from https://www.uptodate.com/contents/neonatal-abstinence-syndrome

the infant frequently to minimize vomiting, regurgitation, and the potential for aspiration. Frequent, small feedings are preferable. Monitor the newborn's weight daily to evaluate the success of food intake. Assess hydration by evaluating perfusion and checking the fontanel remains soft and flat (sunken fontanel occurs with dehydration). Assess the frequency and characteristics of bowel movements and monitor the newborn's fluid and electrolyte and acid–base status (Bagwell, 2022).

PREVENTING COMPLICATIONS

The newborn is at risk for skin breakdown. Weight loss, diarrhea, dehydration, and irritability can contribute to this risk. Provide meticulous skin care and protect the newborn's elbows and knees against friction and abrasions. Apply barrier ointments to avoid skin breakdown and diaper rash. If breakdown becomes severe, clear transparent dressings over reddened or excoriated areas may help avoid further progression of the skin breakdown.

PROMOTING PARENT–NEWBORN INTERACTION

For a parent who misuses substances, the birth of a drug-exposed newborn is both a crisis and an opportunity. The parent may feel guilty about the newborn's condition. Many of these newborns are less responsive and have disorganized sleeping and feeding patterns. When awake, they can be easily overstimulated and irritated. Such characteristics make parent–newborn interactions difficult and frustrating, leading to possible detachment and avoidance. Some symptoms of withdrawal may last for up to 6 months (Patrick et al., 2022).

In addition, the parent may be a victim of physical or sexual abuse and may have a limited support system. Many of these parents may have had poor parenting themselves, lack information about characteristic infant behaviors, and have unrealistic expectations about the newborn's abilities. Drug-exposed infants and their parents experience a difficult early period together. Parents need assistance in recognizing early cues from the infant signaling a need for caregiving. Communicate and provide referral to social services or other community agencies for follow-up postdischarge. Nursing support is essential if maternal–infant attachment is to occur (Bagwell, 2022). Encourage the maternal–infant relationship through support for breastfeeding and rooming-in if there are no contraindications. Instruct the parent or caregiver on how to care for the newborn, including what to do after the newborn goes home. Supporting the parent with substance misuse issues creates an opportunity to promote secure relationships and must be approached with a nonjudgmental attitude. Infants without withdrawal symptoms may be discharged 24 to 48 hours following treatment. Refer to Teaching Guidelines 24.2 for parent education prior to discharge.

It is possible that the newborn may be a powerful motivator for the parent to undergo treatment and seek recovery. Refer the parent to community agencies to address the substance misuse and refer the infant for early intervention (Patrick et al., 2022). The nurse can play a pivotal role in assisting the parent in abstaining from drug use and promoting effective parenting skills.

TEACHING GUIDELINES 24.2 Caring for Your Newborn at Home

- Position your newborn with the head elevated to prevent choking.
- To aid your newborn's sucking and swallowing during feeding, position the chin downward and support it with your hand. Do not overfeed.
- Place your newborn on their back to sleep or nap, never on the stomach.
- Keep a bulb syringe close by to suction your newborn's mouth in case of choking.
- Cluster newborn care (bathing, feeding, dressing) to prevent overstimulation.
- If your newborn is fussy or crying, try these measures to help calm them:
  - Wrap your newborn snugly in a blanket and gently rock in a rocking chair.
  - Take the baby for a ride in the car (using a newborn car seat).
  - Play soothing music and "dance" with the newborn.
  - Use a wind-up swing with calming music.
- To help your newborn get to sleep, try these measures:
  - Schedule a bath with a gentle massage prior to bedtime.
  - Change diaper and clothes to make the baby comfortable.
  - Feed the baby just prior to bedtime.
  - If the newborn cries when put in the crib and all needs are met, allow them to cry.
  - Use a rocking chair to feed and sing a soft lullaby.
- Call your primary care provider if you observe heightened withdrawal behaviors such as:
  - Slight tremors (shaking) of hands and legs
  - Stiff posture when held in your arms
  - Irritability and frequent fussiness
  - High-pitched cry, excessive sucking motions
  - Erratic sleep pattern
  - Frequent yawning, nasal stuffiness, sweating
  - Prolonged time needed to feed
  - Frequent vomiting after feeding

CONSIDER THIS!

I admit I had led a reckless life since I was a teen. I rebelled against my mother's authority and started smoking and doing drugs just to "check out" of my painful world. It was one big blast after another with a high and then a low. I never considered the consequences of my behavior then and never thought it would hurt anyone until I learned I was about 4 months' pregnant. I convinced myself that if I cut back, everything would be fine.

Now, as I stand here in the NICU watching my tiny son struggle for air and tremble all over, I am not so convinced that I didn't hurt anyone, except myself. As I witness my son fight against *my* nicotine and drug addiction, my heart is heavy with guilt. I wonder how I could have thought that my troubles wouldn't become another's plight sooner or later. What was I thinking to isolate my addiction and not consider the impact that it would have on me as a mother and my son?

Thoughts: This woman regrets what her addiction has done to her son as she stands watching him go through withdrawal. Her lifestyle choices have affected others, despite her previous denial. One problem with addiction is the difficulty in getting help after deciding to finally quit. There aren't enough rehabilitation centers to deal with the large numbers of people needing their services, and it can be difficult to get into one. What can be offered to pregnant people who misuse substances? How can nurses increase community awareness about the impact of this problem, especially during pregnancy?

Neonatal Sepsis

Neonatal sepsis is defined as an infection of the bloodstream occurring within the first 28 days of life (Singh et al., 2023). In the United States, neonatal sepsis occurs in 0.5 of 1,000 live births and has a mortality rate of about 3% (Briggs-Steinberg & Roth, 2023). Newborns are susceptible to infections because of their immature immune systems. The antibodies newborns receive from the birthing parent during pregnancy and from breast milk help protect them; however, they do not provide full protection against all microorganisms.

When a pathologic organism overcomes the newborn's defenses, infection, and sepsis result. Neonatal sepsis results from the presence of bacterial, viral, or fungal microorganisms or their toxins in blood or other tissues. Newborn infections are usually grouped into three classes according to their time of onset: congenital infection acquired in utero (intrauterine infections); early-onset infections acquired by vertical transmission in the perinatal period, either shortly before or during birth; and late-onset infections acquired by horizontal transmission in the nursery. This discussion focuses on early-onset sepsis.

Early-onset neonatal sepsis is most often associated with acquisition of microorganisms from the birthing parent. Transplacental infection, an ascending infection from the cervix, or transmission via birth may be caused by organisms that colonize in the birthing parent's genitourinary tract or colonized birth canal. Group B beta-hemolytic *Streptococcus* and *Escherichia coli* are the most frequent causes of bacterial sepsis in newborns, though *Listeria monocytogenes* and *Staphylococcus aureus* infections may also occur (Cantey, 2023). Common nonbacterial causes of neonatal infection include herpes simplex virus, *Candida*, enterovirus, and parechovirus (Cantey, 2023). Preterm infants are at greater risk of sepsis than term infants, as they tend to undergo more invasive procedures than full-term infants.

TAKE NOTE!

The SARS-CoV-2 (COVID-19) virus could potentially cause acute and chronic adverse neurodevelopment in neonates exposed to the COVID-19 virus during gestation. Vertical transmission of COVID-19 from the birthing parent via the placenta is rare, but gestational COVID-19 infection has been linked to a high risk of developing placental infarcts; this may be due to the inflammatory response to COVID-19 in the birthing parent. This type of injury typically occurs in the first and second trimesters. Placental infarcts can result in decreased oxygen and nutrient delivery, fetal growth restriction, impaired fetal brain development, preterm birth, and even death (Holland et al., 2023).

Nursing Assessment

Nursing assessment focuses on early identification of a newborn at risk for infection to allow for prompt treatment, thus reducing mortality and morbidity. The most common risk factors contributing to neonatal sepsis are maternal birth canal colonization with group B streptococcal (GBS), rupture of membranes longer than 18 hours, intrapartum fever, chorioamnionitis, prematurity, and low birth weight (Mukhopadhyay & Puopolo, 2023). Few newborn infections are easy to recognize because manifestations are usually nonspecific. Often, the observation is that the newborn does not "look right." Assess the newborn for common nonspecific signs of infection, including:

- Irritability
- Temperature instability
- Poor feeding
- Lethargy
- Poor muscle tone
- Decreased movement
- Seizure
- Respiratory distress, cyanosis
- Tachycardia/bradycardia
- Poor perfusion, hypotension (late signs)
- Vomiting, diarrhea, abdominal distention
- Jaundice, rash, petechiae (Cantey, 2023; Kenner, 2022)

Since infection can be confused with other newborn conditions, laboratory and radiographic tests are needed to confirm the presence of infection. Be prepared to coordinate the timing of the various tests and assist as necessary. Evaluate the complete blood count with a differential to identify anemia, leukocytosis, or leukopenia. Elevated CRP levels may indicate inflammation. As ordered, obtain x-rays of the chest and abdomen, which may reveal infectious processes located there. Blood, CSF, and urine cultures are indicated to identify the location and type of infection present. Positive cultures confirm that the newborn has an infection.

Nursing Management

To enhance the newborn's chance of survival, early recognition and diagnosis are key. Often, the diagnosis of sepsis is based on a suspicious clinical picture. Antibiotic therapy is usually started before the laboratory results identify the infecting pathogen. Administer antibiotics as ordered, expecting a possible change when culture results are received (the most narrow-spectrum antibiotic will be ordered based on organism sensitivity). Along with antibiotic therapy, circulatory, respiratory, nutritional, and developmental support is important. Provide a neutral thermal environment. Ensure adequate fluid intake via breast milk, formula, or IV fluid as prescribed. Maintain medical asepsis for all encountering the infant. Continue to observe for subtle signs of infection. Educate the family about the treatment plan and continue support their bonding with the infant.

Perinatal infections continue to be a public health problem with severe consequences for those affected. By promoting a better understanding of newborn infections and appropriate use of therapies, nurses can lower the mortality rates associated with severe sepsis, especially with appropriate timing of interventions. The potential for nursing interventions to identify, prevent, and minimize the risk for sepsis is significant. Primary disease prevention must be a major focus for nurses. Family education plays a key role in the prevention of perinatal infections, in addition to following accepted practices in immunization.

Perinatal Asphyxia

Asphyxia is characterized by the development of fetal hypoxemia and hypercapnia, with resultant fetal acidemia (Mota-Rojas et al., 2022). Perinatal asphyxia is one of the most prevalent causes of morbidity and mortality in neonates. It occurs in association with maternal, fetal, and maternofetal factors that might include maternal chronic illness, preterm delivery, meconium aspiration syndrome (MAS), and prolonged maternal labor (Mota-Rojas et al., 2022). At birth, the lungs of newborns are filled with fluid. This fluid must be cleared and replaced with air after birth. As the newborn makes the transition to life outside the fluid-filled intrauterine environment, dramatic changes must occur to facilitate newborn respiration.

Perinatal asphyxia occurs when pulmonary oxygenation is delayed or interrupted before, during, or after the birth process. This insult can lead to death if not adequate ventilation is not reestablished. Perinatal asphyxia can result in profound systemic and neurologic sequelae that interfere with newborn development, resulting in long-term deficits associated with mental and neurologic conditions with delayed onset (Mota-Rojas et al., 2022).

Asphyxia is the most common clinical insult in the perinatal period. As many as 10% of newborns require some degree of active resuscitation to stimulate breathing at birth (Cunningham et al., 2022a). In developed countries, perinatal asphyxia occurs in about two per 100 births, with about 15% to 20% dying within the newborn period (Gillam-Krakauer & Gowen, 2023). About 25% of newborns who survive asphyxia at birth develop long-term neurologic problems, such as cerebral palsy, intellectual disability, and speaking, hearing, visual, and learning disabilities (Gillam-Krakauer & Gowen, 2023).

Think back to Kelly, described at the beginning of the chapter. She gives birth to a son weighing approximately 2,500 g; he appears postterm and SGA. His skin is stained yellow green, and he is limp, cyanotic, and apneic at birth. The initial assessment once he is under the radiant warmer indicates resuscitation and tracheal suctioning are needed. What is the nurse's role during resuscitation? What assessments will be needed during this procedure?

Pathophysiology

Physiologically, *asphyxia* can be defined as impaired gas exchange resulting in a decrease in blood oxygen levels (hypoxemia) and an excess of carbon dioxide (hypercarbia) or hypercapnia that leads to metabolic acidosis. Any condition that reduces oxygen delivery to the fetus can result in asphyxia. These conditions may include fetal heart rate (FHR) tracings categories II and III, intrauterine growth restriction, nulliparity, meconium-stained or bloody amniotic fluid, placental abruption, and prolonged second stage of labor (Tunç et al., 2022).

Initially, the newborn uses compensatory mechanisms including tachycardia and vasoconstriction to help bring oxygen to the vital organs for a time. However, without intervention, these mechanisms fail, leading to hypotension, bradycardia, and, eventually, cardiopulmonary arrest. With failure to breathe well after birth, the newborn will develop hypoxia (too little oxygen in the cells of the body). As a result, the heart rate falls, cyanosis develops, and the newborn becomes hypotonic and unresponsive. Newborn resuscitation is needed to help initiate breathing in newborns who fail to breathe spontaneously at birth.

Nursing Assessment

The key to successful treatment of newborn asphyxia is early identification and recognition of newborns who may be at risk. Review the perinatal history for risk factors, including maternal diseases (such as collagen–vascular disease, diabetes, pregnancy-induced hypertension, and heart or kidney diseases), fetal conditions (fetal anomalies, growth restriction, multiple births, prematurity), and conditions occurring during the labor and birth process (fetal distress, administration of anesthetics or opioid analgesics) (Smith, 2022).

At birth, immediately and rapidly assess the newborn. Observe the infant's color, noting any pallor or cyanosis. Assess work of breathing. Be alert for apnea, poor muscle tone, tachypnea, gasping respirations, grunting, nasal flaring, or retractions. Evaluate heart rate and note bradycardia. Assess the newborn's temperature, noting hypothermia. Based on the initial assessment if poor, begin resuscitation measures until the Apgar score is above 7.

Nursing Management

Management of the newborn experiencing asphyxia includes immediate resuscitation. Ensure the equipment needed for resuscitation is readily available and in working order. Essential equipment includes:

- Wall suction apparatus
- Stethoscope
- Oxygen source
- Newborn ventilation bag
- Infant warmer
- Pulse oximeter leads
- Surgical blue towels
- Endotracheal tubes (2 to 3 mm)
- Laryngoscope
- Ampules of naloxone (Narcan) and epinephrine with syringes and needles for administration

Effective ventilation is the key to successful newborn resuscitation. Ventilation is frequently initiated with a manual resuscitation bag and face mask followed by endotracheal intubation if respiratory depression continues. (See Chapter 23 for a more detailed discussion of resuscitation.)

Dry the newborn quickly with a prewarmed towel and then place them under a radiant heater to prevent rapid heat loss through evaporation. Handling and rubbing the newborn with a dry towel may be all that is needed to stimulate breathing. If the newborn fails to respond to stimulation, active resuscitation is needed.

The procedure for newborn resuscitation is easily remembered by the mnemonic ABC—*a*irway, *b*reathing, *c*irculation. Refer to Chapter 18 for a full description of the neonatal resuscitation process. Continue resuscitation until the newborn has a pulse above 100 bpm, a healthy cry, or good breathing efforts and a pink tongue. This last sign indicates a good oxygen supply to the brain (Weiner & Zaichkin, 2022).

TAKE NOTE!

The goals of resuscitation are to assist with the initiation and maintenance of adequate ventilation and oxygenation, adequate cardiac output and tissue perfusion, and normal core temperature and serum glucose. Resuscitation prevents neonatal morbidity and mortality and reestablishes spontaneous respiration and cardiac output (Weiner & Zaichkin, 2022).

Provide continued observation and assessment of the newborn who has been successfully resuscitated. Monitor the newborn's vital signs and oxygen saturation levels closely for changes. Maintain a neutral thermal environment to prevent hypothermia, which would increase the newborn's metabolic and oxygen demands. Check the blood glucose level and observe for signs of hypoglycemia; if this develops, it can further stress the newborn.

The need for resuscitative measures can be extremely upsetting for the parents. Explain to them the initial resuscitation activities being performed and offer ongoing explanations about any procedures being done, equipment being used, or medications given. Provide physical and emotional support to the parents through the initial crisis and throughout the newborn's stay. When the newborn is stable, allow the family to spend time with the newborn to promote bonding (Fig. 24.17). Point out the newborn's positive attributes (color, activity level, healthy cry) and give frequent updates on their status. Role model techniques for holding, interacting with, and caring for the newborn to decrease the parents' anxiety postresuscitation.

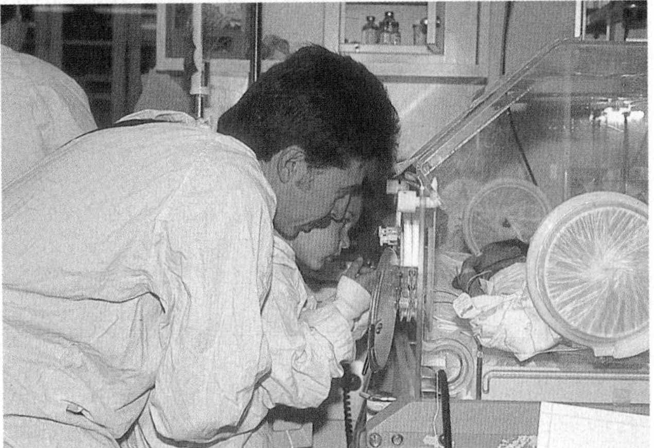

FIGURE 24.17 A parent and sibling interacting with the newborn once the newborn's condition has stabilized.

Remember Kelly, the patient described at the beginning of the chapter? Her newborn son is intubated, and tracheal suctioning is performed. Positive-pressure ventilation is also started with a self-inflating bag and 50% oxygen. Ventilation is continued for 1 minute and then gradually discontinued. His heart rate is now 120 bpm, and spontaneous respirations are noted. When free-flow oxygen is administered, the newborn begins to cry and turn pink. What continued care is needed in the special care nursery? What explanation should be offered to Kelly regarding her son's treatment?

Transient Tachypnea of the Newborn

TTN is a self-limiting condition involving a mild degree of respiratory distress with rapid breathing (≥60 breaths per minute). TTN is the result of a delay in clearance of fetal lung liquid leading to ineffective gas exchange, respiratory distress, and transient pulmonary edema. In the past, respiratory distress was thought to be a problem of relative surfactant deficiency, but it is now characterized by an airspace–fluid burden secondary to the inability to absorb fetal lung liquid. It usually occurs within a few hours of birth and resolves over 1 to 2 days, though more severe cases may need 72 hours to resolve (Johnson, 2023). It occurs in approximately 1% of live term births, and risk factors include male sex, infants who are SGA or LGA, and perinatal asphyxia (Jha et al., 2023).

Pathophysiology

Most newborns make the transition from fetal to newborn life without incident. During fetal life, the lungs are filled with a serous fluid because the placenta, not the lungs, is used for nutrient and gas exchange. During and after birth, this fluid must be removed and replaced with air. Passage through the birth canal during a vaginal birth compresses the thorax, which helps remove the majority of this fluid. An infant born by cesarean birth is at risk of having excessive pulmonary fluid as a result of not having experienced all of the stages of labor (McGillick et al., 2022). Pulmonary circulation and lymphatic drainage remove the remaining fluid shortly after birth. TTN occurs when the liquid in the lung is removed slowly or incompletely. The excess lung fluid results in decreased pulmonary compliance and tachypnea with increased work of breathing develops to compensate (Johnson, 2023).

Nursing Assessment

Astutely observe the newborn with respiratory distress because TTN is a diagnosis of exclusion. Initially, it might be difficult to distinguish this condition from RDS or GBS pneumonia, because the clinical picture is similar. Review the perinatal history for contributing factors. Closely assess the newborn for signs of TTN. Within the first few hours of birth, observe for tachypnea, retractions, expiratory grunting, nasal flaring, cyanosis, need for supplemental oxygen to maintain PaO_2 at 50 to 70 mm Hg, and paradoxical or seesaw respirations. Arterial blood gases (ABGs) may reveal hypoxemia with hypercapnia; a chest ultrasound may be used to accurately diagnose TTN (Johnson, 2023).

Nursing Management

As the retained lung fluid is absorbed by the infant's lymphatic system, the pulmonary status improves. Nursing management is supportive and focuses on providing adequate oxygenation while determining whether the newborn's respiratory manifestations are improving or persisting. Maintain a neutral thermal environment with minimal stimulation to minimize oxygen demand. Provide supplemental oxygen via a nasal cannula or oxygen hood to maintain adequate oxygen saturation. Administer IV fluids and/or gavage feedings until the respiratory rate decreases enough to allow safe oral feeding. Provide reassurance and progress reports to the parents to help them cope with this crisis. As TTN resolves, the respiratory rate declines to 60 breaths per minute or less; cyanosis, nasal flaring, and grunting resolve; and the oxygen requirement decreases.

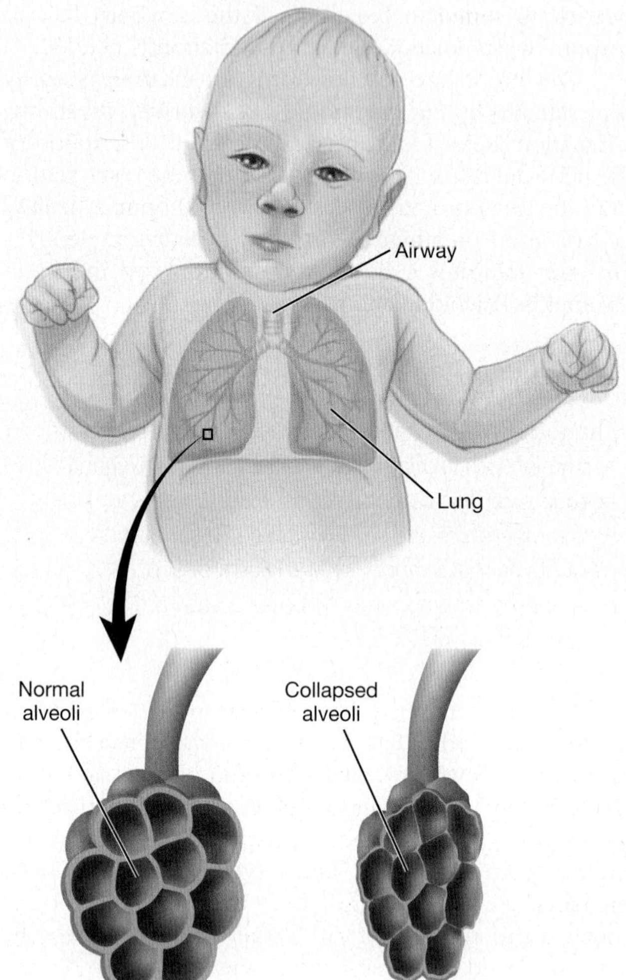

FIGURE 24.18 Pathophysiology of neonatal respiratory distress syndrome. Comparison of normal and collapsed alveoli.

Respiratory Distress Syndrome

RDS is a respiratory disorder that is specific to neonates. It results from lung immaturity and a deficiency in surfactant, so it is seen most often in premature infants. Other infants who might experience RDS include infants of birthing parents with diabetes, those delivered via cesarean birth without preceding labor, and those experiencing perinatal asphyxia (Pramanik, 2020). It is believed that each of these conditions has an impact on surfactant production, thus resulting in RDS in the term infant.

The lack of surfactant in the affected newborn's lungs results in stiff, poorly compliant lungs with poor gas exchange. Right-to-left shunting and hypoxemia result. As the disease progresses, fluid and fibrin leak from the pulmonary capillaries, causing a hyaline membrane to form in the bronchioles, alveolar ducts, and alveoli (Fig. 24.18). The presence of the membrane further decreases gas exchange. If untreated, RDS progresses to seesaw respirations, respiratory failure, and shock.

Complications of RDS include air leak syndrome, bronchopulmonary dysplasia (BPD) (also called *chronic lung disease of prematurity*), patent ductus arteriosus and congestive heart failure, intraventricular hemorrhage (IVH), ROP, necrotizing enterocolitis (NEC), complications resulting from IV catheter use (infection, thrombus formation), and developmental delay or disability. The administration of exogenous surfactant helps to decrease the incidence and severity of RDS. Intensive respiratory care is needed (often with continuous positive airway pressure [CPAP] or mechanical ventilation).

Nursing Assessment

Nursing assessment focuses on keen observation to identify the signs and symptoms of respiratory distress. Review the history for risk factors associated with RDS. These include preterm birth (including late preterm delivery), perinatal asphyxia regardless of gestational age, cesarean birth in the absence of preceding labor (due to the lack of thoracic squeezing), White race, male sex, perinatal asphyxia, and maternal diabetes (produces high levels of insulin that inhibit surfactant production).

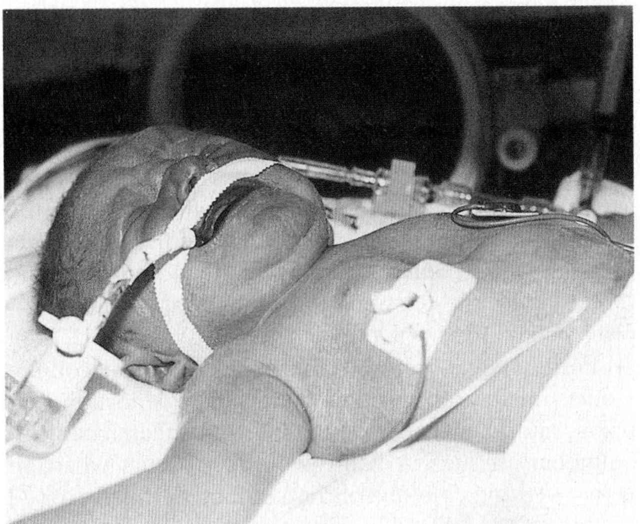

FIGURE 24.19 Sternal retractions are a sign of respiratory distress requiring immediate intervention, such as mechanical ventilation and other monitoring devices. (Copyright Caroline Brown, RNC, MS, DEd.)

It is believed that each of these conditions has an impact on surfactant production, thus resulting in RDS in the full-term infant (Yadav & Lee, 2023).

Assess the infant for the onset of RDS, which usually occurs within several hours of birth. Note signs of respiratory distress, including tachypnea (rate > 60 breaths per minute), retractions (Fig. 24.19), nasal flaring, grunting, seesaw respirations, and varying degrees of cyanosis. Auscultation reveals fine rales and diminished breath sounds. Use the Silverman–Anderson index assessment tool to determine the degree of respiratory distress and the need for respiratory support in the weaning process. The index involves observation of five features, each of which is scored as 0, 1, or 2 (Fig. 24.20). The higher the score, the greater the respiratory distress. A score over 7 suggests severe respiratory distress (Nussbaum et al., 2022).

The chest x-ray reveals hypoaeration, diffuse atelectasis, underexpansion, and a "ground-glass" pattern (Do et al., 2022).

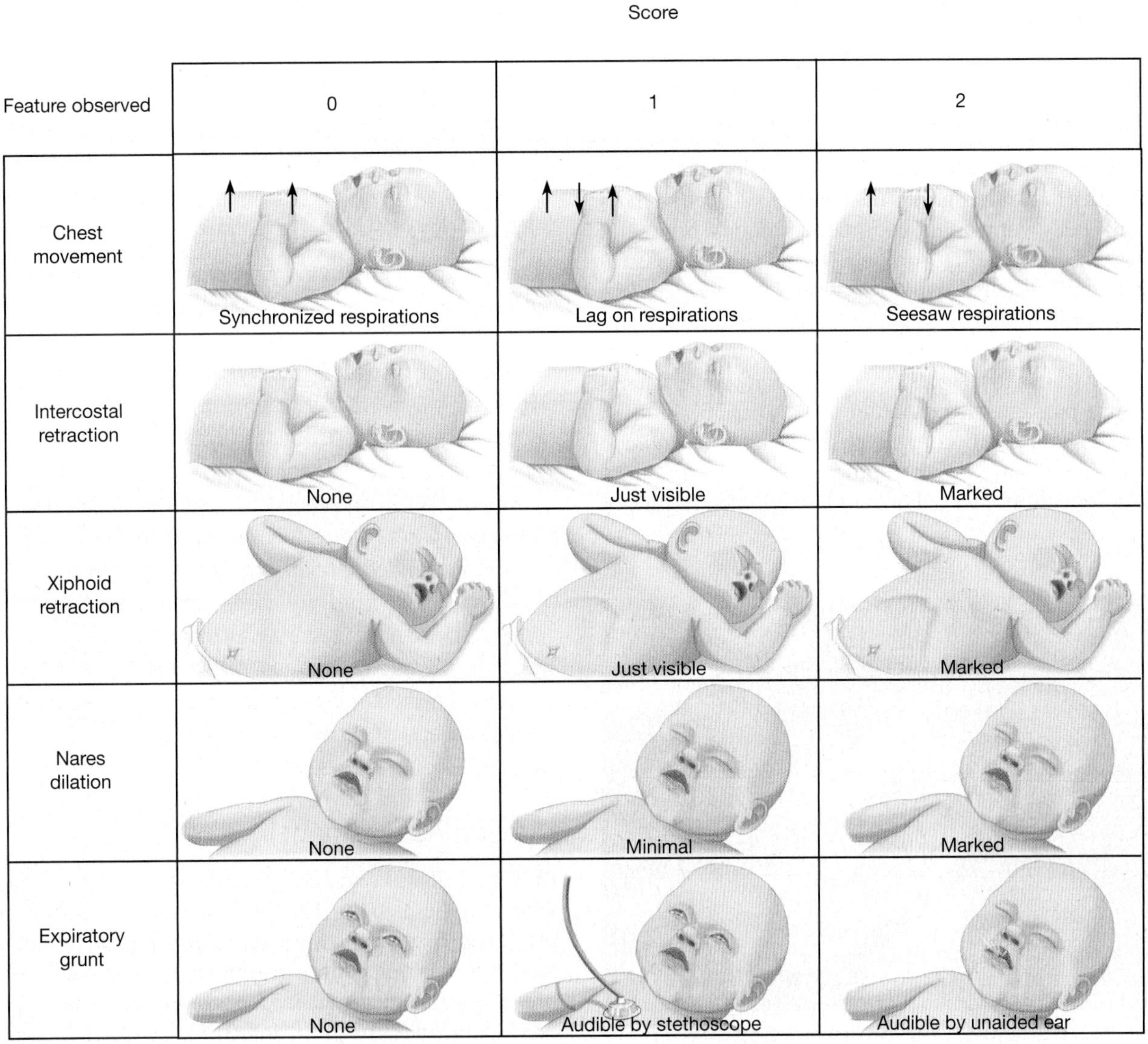

	Score		
Feature observed	0	1	2
Chest movement	Synchronized respirations	Lag on respirations	Seesaw respirations
Intercostal retraction	None	Just visible	Marked
Xiphoid retraction	None	Just visible	Marked
Nares dilation	None	Minimal	Marked
Expiratory grunt	None	Audible by stethoscope	Audible by unaided ear

FIGURE 24.20 Assessing the degree of respiratory distress.

Nursing Management

If untreated, RDS will worsen. However, it can be a self-limiting disease, with respiratory symptoms declining after 72 hours. This decline parallels the production of surfactant in the alveoli (Martin, 2022). The newborn needs supportive care until surfactant is produced. Administration of exogenous surfactant has dramatically improved morbidity and mortality in preterm infants, whether administered via endotracheal tube or via aerosol delivery (Martin, 2024). Early positive airway pressure is another important intervention. CPAP or positive end-expiratory pressure (PEEP) prevents volume loss during expiration. Some newborns will require mechanical ventilation. Closely observe the neonate placed on the ventilator after surfactant administration; though rare, mucous plugging can occur. Watch for adequate lung expansion. In addition to expert respiratory intervention, other crucial nursing goals include maintenance of normothermia, prevention of infection, maintenance of fluid and electrolyte balance, and promotion of adequate nutrition (parenterally or via gavage feeding) (Martin, 2024). Nursing care of the infant with RDS generally occurs in the intensive care unit (Fig. 24.21).

Meconium Aspiration Syndrome

Meconium is a viscous green substance composed primarily of water and other gastrointestinal secretions, such as epithelial cells, vernix, lanugo, mucus, amniotic fluid, and intestinal secretions, that can be noted in the fetal gastrointestinal tract as early as 10 to 16 weeks' gestation. Meconium is sterile and does not contain bacteria, the primary factor that differentiates it from stool. It is usually expelled as the newborn's first stool after birth. Intrauterine distress can cause passage of meconium into the amniotic fluid. Factors promoting meconium passage in utero include hypoxia or increased vagal outflow occurring umbilical cord compression. Meconium can be aspirated before or during labor and after birth. Meconium is rarely found in the amniotic fluid prior to 34 weeks' gestation, so meconium aspiration mainly affects infants born at full term and post term (Garcia-Prats, 2023b).

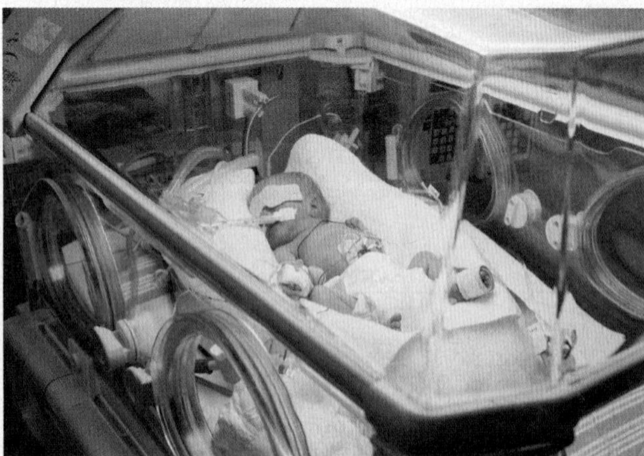

FIGURE 24.21 A newborn with respiratory distress syndrome receiving mechanical ventilation.

Meconium aspiration syndrome (MAS) is a serious condition that occurs when the newborn inhales particulate meconium mixed with amniotic fluid into the lungs while still in utero or when taking the first breath after birth. Meconium staining of the amniotic fluid (MSAF), with the possibility of aspiration, occurs in approximately 16.5% of pregnancies at term and 27% at postterm (Garcia-Prats, 2023b). Aspiration of meconium induces airway obstruction, surfactant dysfunction, hypoxia, and chemical pneumonitis with inflammation of pulmonary tissues. A ball-valve effect occurs when air is inspired into the alveoli but cannot be fully expired secondary to reduced airway diameter. In severe cases, it progresses to persistent pulmonary hypertension and death (Garcia-Prats, 2023b). Of the infants born through meconium-stained amniotic fluid, about 2% to 10% develop MAS (Garcia-Prats, 2023b). Numerous changes in therapeutic management of MSAF have occurred over the decades, and routine endotracheal suctioning is no longer recommended. Therapeutic management is primarily supportive (Garcia-Prats, 2023a). Conventional mechanical or high-frequency oscillatory ventilation, nitric oxide administration, or ECMO may be necessary.

> ***TAKE NOTE!***
>
> Standard prevention and treatment for MAS previously included suctioning the mouth and nares upon head delivery before body delivery. However, recent evidence suggests that aspiration may occur in utero, not necessarily at delivery; therefore, the infant's birth should not be impeded for suctioning. After full delivery, the infant should be handed to a neonatal team for evaluation and treatment. Although infants have previously been given intubation and airway suctioning, routine tracheal suction is not recommended. Use of orogastric suctioning to prevent MAS is not supported by evidence from current studies. Infants should no longer routinely receive intrapartum suctioning. Guidelines suggest not stimulating infants born with meconium staining at birth with vigorous sucking to avoid aspiration (Garcia-Prats, 2023a).

Nursing Assessment

Review prenatal and birth records to identify newborns who may be at high risk for meconium aspiration. Predisposing factors for MAS include postterm pregnancy, fetal hypoxia, placental insufficiency, oligohydramnios, preeclampsia, maternal hypertension, maternal tobacco or cocaine use, maternal infection, or chorioamnionitis (Geis & Clark, 2023).

Assess the amniotic fluid for meconium staining when the maternal membranes rupture. Green-stained amniotic fluid suggests the presence of meconium in the amniotic fluid and should be reported immediately. After birth, note any yellowish green staining of the umbilical cord, nails, and skin. This staining indicates meconium has been present for some time.

Consider Kelly, the 27-year-old woman who gave birth to a son who required resuscitation. What findings would lead the nurse to suspect that the newborn had aspirated meconium? What risk factors in Kelly's history would support the diagnosis of MAS?

Observe the newborn for a barrel-shaped chest; progressive respiratory distress including cyanosis; marked tachypnea, which progresses to significant respiratory distress; intercostal and subxiphoid retractions; and end-expiratory grunting. Auscultate the lungs, noting coarse crackles and rhonchi (Garcia-Prats, 2023b).

Chest x-ray initially shows streaky linear densities progressing to patchy infiltrates with a flattened diaphragm and marked hyperaeration (Garcia-Prats, 2023b). ABG analysis will indicate the presence of metabolic and respiratory acidosis (Geis & Clark, 2023). Provide supplemental oxygen as ordered to maintain oxygen saturation between 95% and 98% (Garcia-Prats, 2023a). Hypoxemia and acidosis must be avoided to prevent increasing pulmonary vascular resistance leading to PPHN. Often, this may be provided via oxygen hood or nasal cannula. Some infants will require conventional or high-frequency oscillatory ventilation (Garcia-Prats, 2023a). In addition, administer vasopressors and pulmonary vasodilators as prescribed and administer surfactant as ordered to counteract inactivation by meconium. In addition, as with any other newborn, maintain a neutral thermal environment, ensure adequate nutrition and fluid balance, and provide continuous reassurance and support to the parents throughout the experience.

Persistent Pulmonary Hypertension of the Newborn

PPHN is a cardiopulmonary disorder characterized by marked pulmonary hypertension that causes right-to-left extrapulmonary shunting of blood and severe hypoxemia and acidemia. It occurs when the newborn's circulatory system does not have a normal transition after birth. PPHN is most common in full-term infants and rare in preterm infants. It occurs in about two per 1,000 live births of term, near-term, or postterm infants (Stark & Eichenwald, 2022). PPHN can occur idiopathically or as a complication of perinatal asphyxia, MAS, pneumonia, CDH, sepsis, or RDS (Stark & Eichenwald, 2022). Current research findings also link a doubled increased risk of developing PPHN to exposure to SSRIs, a class of antidepressants, in late pregnancy (Buffoni et al., 2022). Treatment of depression with antidepressants is complicated by the pregnant person's needs. Careful consideration must be given to the risks, benefits, and alternatives of in utero medication exposure, and these must be discussed with the patient.

Normally, pulmonary artery pressure decreases when the newborn takes the first breath. However, interference with this ability to breathe allows pulmonary pressures to remain increased. Hypoxemia and acidosis also occur, leading to vasoconstriction of the pulmonary artery and increased pulmonary vascular resistance. With PPHN, elevated pulmonary vascular resistance causes venous blood to be diverted to some degree through the ductus arteriosus and foramen ovale (which remain open), resulting in systemic arterial hypoxemia.

Nursing Assessment

Assess the newborn's status closely. A newborn with persistent pulmonary hypertension demonstrates tachypnea within 12 hours after birth. Observe for marked cyanosis, grunting, respiratory distress with tachypnea, retractions, and prominent precordial impulse. Auscultate the heart, noting a harsh systolic murmur associated with tricuspid insufficiency (Stark & Eichenwald, 2022). Measure oxygen saturation via pulse oximetry and report low values. Prepare the newborn for an echocardiogram, which will reveal right-to-left shunting of blood that confirms the diagnosis.

Nursing Management

Nursing management focuses on ensuring adequate tissue perfusion and minimizing oxygen demand and energy expenditure. Caring for the newborn with PPHN includes identifying signs and symptoms associated with the disorder. Usually, the newborn is transferred to the NICU for close monitoring.

TAKE NOTE!

Almost any procedure, such as suctioning, weighing, changing diapers, or positioning, can precipitate severe hypoxemia due to the instability of the pulmonary vasculature. Therefore, minimize the newborn's exposure to stimulation as much as possible.

Bronchopulmonary Dysplasia/ Chronic Lung Disease

BPD, a serious chronic lung disease, commonly occurs in preterm infants who have experienced a lung injury, resulting in the need for continued use of oxygen after the initial neonatal period (28 days of life). BPD results from inflammation and damage to the premature infant's vulnerable lungs, resulting in disruption of lung development and leading to lung injury. BPD occurs in as many as 85% of infants born at 22 weeks' gestation, decreasing with advanced gestation to about 23% in those born at 28 weeks' gestation (Eichenwald & Stark, 2023). Newborns with BPD need intensive hospital care and home oxygen therapy after being discharged.

BPD results from injury to the highly vulnerable premature lung. The etiology of the lung injury is multifactorial, complex, and incompletely understood. The injury results in larger alveoli, which are fewer in number, thereby reducing the surface area available for gas exchange. Pulmonary vascular resistance is increased, and interstitial elastic tissue is increased and thickened (Eichenwald & Stark, 2023).

BPD remains the most common severe adverse pulmonary outcome of preterm birth. It contributes significantly to morbidity and mortality in the premature infant population (Eichenwald & Stark, 2023). Therapeutic management of the newborn with BPD includes respiratory support with the lowest levels of supplemental oxygen and least invasive method of delivery tolerated (such as CPAP), though mechanical ventilation is needed in some infants. Diuretics, bronchodilators, and/or corticosteroids are used in some infants (Stark & Eichenwald, 2023a). Frequently, BPD can be prevented by administering steroids to the pregnant person in the prenatal period and administering exogenous surfactant within 30 to 60 minutes of birth to help reduce the risk for RDS and its severity (Stark & Eichenwald, 2023b). In addition, the following practices may help reduce the incidence of BPD:

- Use a target oxygen saturation level of 90% to 95% for infants born at less than 34 weeks' gestation.
- Use lower tidal volumes on ventilators.
- Administer caffeine within the first 24 hours of life.
- Use breast milk as the preferred form of nutrition to formula (Stark & Eichenwald, 2023b).

Nursing Assessment

Although BPD is most common in preterm newborns, it can also occur in full-term newborns who had respiratory problems during their first days of life. Assess the newborn's history for risk factors related to BPD. Assess the infant for the clinical manifestations of BPD: tachypnea, tachycardia, sternal retractions (see Fig. 24.19), episodes of cyanosis, nasal flaring, bronchospasm, adventitious breath sounds (crackles, rhonchi, and wheezes), and poor weight gain related to the increased metabolic workload. ABG may demonstrate hypoxemia, hypercapnia, and acidosis. Chest x-ray shows hyperinflation, infiltrates, and cardiomegaly.

Nursing Management

The focus of management is to provide supportive care and minimize additional lung injury. Deliver continuous ventilatory and oxygen support, provide optimal nutrition to support growth, and administer bronchodilators, anti-inflammatory agents, and diuretics as ordered. Continuously monitor the newborn's respiratory status to determine the need for ongoing ventilatory assistance. When the newborn is clinically stable and ready, expect to wean them slowly so that they can compensate for the changes. Supplemental oxygen may be needed after discharge from the hospital. Some infants may require high-calorie formulas to foster adequate growth and compensate for the calories expended due to the increased work of breathing.

Newborns with BPD may require continued care at home. When planning for discharge, educate the family caregiver about how to manage a chronically ill child who may be oxygen dependent for an extended time. Successful discharge is greatly influenced by how prepared the family is to take an infant home on oxygen. Provide ongoing support to parents as they learn to meet their infant's needs. Also instruct the family about the safe use of oxygen in the home, including the need to notify emergency medical services and utility companies that a technology-dependent child is living in their district. In addition, initiate a social service referral to help the family access community resources and obtain necessary support (Blanco et al., 2021).

Retinopathy of Prematurity

ROP is a developmental proliferative vascular disorder that occurs in the retina of preterm infants born before 31 weeks with undeveloped retinal vascularization (Bhatt, 2023). In the fetus, retinal vascularization begins at 15 to 18 weeks' gestation and progresses until completion at 40 weeks. In ROP, new vessels continue to grow between the vascularized and nonvascularized retina. Growth of abnormal blood vessels occurs in an attempt to nourish the retina following an insult, such as hypoxia, hypotension, and hyperoxia. The vessels are highly fragile and bleed easily, leading to the formation of scar tissue. They can also enlarge and twist, pulling the retina away from the wall of the eye and resulting in retinal detachment.

Risk factors include prematurity, low birth weight, sepsis, hyperoxemia, mechanical ventilation for greater than 1 week, surfactant therapy, and BPD. The incidence of ROP in preterm newborns is inversely proportional to their birth weight. Among newborns born between 22 and 25 weeks' gestation, approximately 43% develop ROP, compared with 3% of infants born at 27 to 30 weeks' gestation (Bhatt, 2023). ROP is classified according to the stage, ranging from mild (stage I) to severe (stage V), and is further defined based on retinal zone affected and the extent of retina involved. Complications of ROP include myopia, glaucoma, and blindness. Premature infants should have serial examinations by an ophthalmologist until the ROP has regressed and normal vascularization is seen. If ROP continues to progress, laser photocoagulation or injection of anti-vascular endothelial growth factor (anti-VEGF) into the vitreous may be necessary to prevent blindness (Bhatt, 2024).

TAKE NOTE!

Although the precise levels of hyperoxemia that can be sustained without causing retinopathy are not known, very immature newborns who develop respiratory distress may need to be given high oxygen concentrations to maintain life (Cunningham et al., 2022c).

Nursing Assessment

The newborn who develops ROP exhibits no signs or symptoms, so assessment involves identifying the newborn at risk. Review the maternal prenatal history for risk factors. Be especially alert for newborns weighing 1,500 g or less or those born at 28 weeks' gestation or less. Evaluate the newborn's history for the duration of intubation and the use of oxygen therapy, IVH, and sepsis (Bhatt, 2023). Prepare the infant for an ophthalmologic examination.

Nursing Management

Administer supplemental oxygen as prescribed; studies have not clearly defined the role of oxygen supplementation in the development of ROP but have demonstrated decreased mortality when appropriately used (Bhatt, 2024). Assist with scheduling an ophthalmic examination for the newborn. Expect to administer a mydriatic eye agent to dilate the newborn's pupils approximately 1 hour prior to the examination as ordered. During this time, take extra care to protect the newborn's eyes from bright light. Cycloplegic eye drops are used to prevent movement of the eye during the examination. Cycloplegic eye drops and manipulation of the eye may result in adverse cardiorespiratory and gastrointestinal effects, so monitor for apnea, oxygen desaturation, bradycardia, dysrhythmia, and emesis. If necessary, aid with the examination by holding the newborn's head. Assist with scheduling follow-up eye examinations, usually every 1 to 3 weeks until ROP is resolved (Bhatt, 2023). Provide individualized support to the parents, educating them about the follow-up ophthalmologic examinations needed.

TAKE NOTE!

Any newborn with a birth weight of less than 1,500 g or born at less than 28 weeks' gestation should be examined by a pediatric ophthalmologist within 4 to 6 weeks after birth.

Periventricular–Intraventricular Hemorrhage

Periventricular–intraventricular hemorrhage (PIVH) in preterm infants continues to be a major clinical challenge associated with neurodevelopmental abnormalities manifested by cognitive, behavioral, attention, social, and motor deficits. PIVH is defined as bleeding that usually originates in the subependymal germinal matrix region of the brain with extension into the ventricular system. The germinal matrix is the embryonic structure that is unique to preterm infants, which provides vascular supply for 24 to 32 weeks' gestation. It is primitive and made of smooth endothelial cells that are highly vascular and prone to bleeding.

Very-low-birth-weight infants have the earliest onset of hemorrhage and the highest mortality rate. PIVH severity occurs at increasing rates with decreasing birth weight (correlating with gestational age), occurring in 25% to 30% of infants weighing under 1,500 g at birth and in 45% of newborns with birth weight of 1,000 g or less (Starr et al., 2023). Further risk factors for PIVH include hypocapnia, blood pressure fluctuations, IV fluid bolus receipt, and use of sodium bicarbonate (Tatawy et al., 2022). Sequelae of PIVH include posthemorrhagic hydrocephalus and lifelong neurologic deficits, such as cerebral palsy, periventricular leukomalacia (an ischemic injury resulting from inadequate perfusion of the white matter adjacent to the ventricles), attention deficit-hyperactivity disorder (ADHD), emotional and personality disorders visual and hearing impairment, cognitive disorders, developmental delay or intellectual disability, and seizures (Ditzenberger & Blackburn, 2022; Rees et al., 2022).

Nursing Assessment

The signs of PIVH vary significantly; no clinical signs may be evident. Closely monitor newborns who are at an increased risk, such as those who are preterm or of low birth weight. Evaluate the newborn for an unexplained drop in hematocrit, pallor, and poor perfusion as evidenced by respiratory distress and oxygen desaturation. Note lethargy or other changes in level of consciousness, weak sucking, high-pitched cry, hypotonia/flaccidity, seizures, or metabolic acidosis. Observe for bulging of the anterior fontanelle and palpate for tenseness. Assess vital signs, noting bradycardia and hypotension. Prepare the newborn for cranial ultrasonography, the diagnostic tool of choice to detect hemorrhage and determine severity (Ditzenberger & Blackburn, 2023).

Nursing Management

Ninety percent of cases of PIVH occur within the first 72 hours of life; thus, nursing management during this period is extremely important (Ditzenberger & Blackburn,

2022). Care for the preterm newborn at high risk of developing PIVH consists of the following measures:

- A course of prenatal corticosteroids given 24 hours apart to the birthing parent
- Delayed cord clamping for 30 to 60 seconds
- Adequate oxygenation to avoid hypocarbia, hypercarbia, and acidosis
- Maintenance of a neutral thermal environment
- Head of the newborn elevated 15 to 30 degrees and kept in midline position, with the infant flexed
- Slow administration of fluids to prevent fluctuations in blood pressure
- Minimal handling to avoid pain and stress; cover isolettes to reduce light and noise
- Serial monitoring of cranial ultrasound and increasing head circumference measurements (Ditzenberger & Blackburn, 2022; Tatawy et al., 2022)

Care of the newborn with PIVH is primarily supportive. Cluster nursing care, minimize handling of the newborn, limit environmental stimulation, and reduce noxious stimuli to avoid a fluctuation in blood pressure and energy expenditure. Provide adequate oxygenation to promote tissue perfusion. Correct anemia, acidosis, and hypotension with fluids and medications. Avoid rapid volume expansion to minimize changes in cerebral blood flow. Keep the newborn in a flexed, contained position with the head elevated to prevent or minimize fluctuations in intracranial pressure. Continuously monitor the newborn for signs of hemorrhage, such as changes in the level of consciousness, bulging fontanelle, seizures, apnea, and reduced activity level. Measure head circumference daily.

Support for the parents to cope with the diagnosis and potential long-term sequelae is essential. Provide education and emotional support for the parents throughout the newborn's stay. Discuss expectations for short- and long-term care needs with the parents and assist them in obtaining the necessary support from appropriate community resources. The long-term neurodevelopmental outcome is determined by the severity of the bleed. As the cerebral cortex is immature in the preterm infant, it may take months or years before the impact on the child's development is fully realized, necessitating long-term developmental follow-up.

Necrotizing Enterocolitis

NEC is a life-threatening illness caused by a bacterial invasion into the intestinal wall that leads to inflammation and cellular destruction of the intestinal wall. This invasion can cause ischemic and necrotic injury in the gastrointestinal tract. It is the most common and most serious acquired gastrointestinal disorder among hospitalized preterm neonates and is associated with significant acute and chronic morbidity and mortality. NEC is a significant clinical problem and affects close to 10% of infants who weigh less than 1,500 g, with mortality rates of 50% or more depending on severity (Ginglen & Butki, 2023).

The pathophysiology of NEC is poorly understood and is thought to be multifactorial in nature. Infection and infarction occur with abnormal bacterial colonization in the premature infant's gut (Kim, 2023b). The intestine of a premature infant is characterized by underdeveloped immune defenses and compromised mucosal barrier function. As a result, the immature intestine is susceptible to bacterial colonization by opportunistic pathogens when enterally fed, which, in turn, incites an inflammatory response culminating in the development of NEC (Ginglen & Butki, 2023).

During perinatal or postnatal stress, oxygen is shunted away from the gut to more important organs, such as the heart and brain. Ischemia and intestinal wall damage occur, allowing bacteria to invade. Although any region of the bowel can be affected, the distal ileum and proximal colon are the regions most commonly involved. NEC is characterized by patchy necrosis in the intestines, resulting in mild to full-thickness perforation of the intestines, which may lead to systemic sepsis (Kim, 2023b). NEC can present slowly or as a sudden, catastrophic event. The onset of NEC is heralded by the development of feeding intolerance, abdominal distention, and bloody stools in a preterm infant receiving enteral feedings. Progression may be rapid, resulting in bowel perforation with evidence of free air on the x-ray. As the disease worsens, the infant develops signs and symptoms of septic shock (respiratory distress, temperature instability, lethargy, hypotension, and oliguria).

Ways to improve gastrointestinal function and reduce the risk of NEC include enteral antibiotics, judicious administration of parenteral fluids, human breast milk feedings, antenatal corticosteroids, and slow continuous-drip feedings. See Evidence-Based Practice 24.1.

Nursing Assessment

NEC can be devastating, and astute assessment is crucial. Nurses need to be suspicious of this condition in caring for the preterm infant. Determine the risk factors for the development of NEC, including prematurity, low birth weight, and formula feeding (Ginglen & Butki, 2023). Observe the newborn for common signs and symptoms, which may include:

- Cardiorespiratory baseline changes
- Feeding intolerance
- Abdominal distention, tenderness, visible bowel loops
- Bloody or hemoccult-positive stools
- Diarrhea
- Respiratory distress or cyanosis
- Metabolic acidosis

EVIDENCE-BASED PRACTICE 24.1

Evaluation of Risk and Preventive Factors for Necrotizing Enterocolitis in Premature Newborns: A Systematic Review of the Literature

BACKGROUND

Necrotizing enterocolitis (NEC) is a leading cause of mortality affecting preterm infants when enteral feeding is initiated. The identified risk factors for NEC include prematurity, feeding with formula, and the existence of intestinal microflora imbalances. The preventive factors found were breast milk, probiotics, and administering prenatal corticosteroids to the birthing parent.

STUDY

NEC is one of the most common and devastating diseases encountered in preterm infants, but it remains poorly understood despite decades of research. Several clinical practices designed to reduce the risk of NEC have been proposed and/or implemented. This review summarizes the results of several clinical trials and meta-analyses that provide evidence aimed at identifying risk factors and prevention strategies. The search obtained 113 research articles, of which 19 were selected for final analysis. For this purpose, PubMed, MEDLINE, and Cochrane Library databases were searched.

Findings

Three prevention interventions were supported. First, it is evident that human breast milk can reduce the incidence of NEC, and all neonatal intensive care units (NICUs) should support lactation and establish more human milk banks in NICUs. Second, probiotic supplementation may also reduce the incidence of NEC in preterm infants, but optimal dosage and treatment duration have not been established. Lastly, standardized feeding protocols should be instituted in all NICUs to prevent NEC and improve postnatal growth in preterm infants.

Nursing Implications

The findings in this review were significant and should be applied in the nursing care of preterm infants to prevent NEC from occurring in the NICU. All three interventions can be employed by nurses within the units. Nurses can encourage breastfeeding or pumping to provide an adequate supply for feedings. Administering probiotics may also help in the prevention of NEC. Nurses can take the lead role in establishing standardized feeding protocols in the NICU for all at-risk preterm infants to assist in the prevention of this serious condition. In addition, being cognizant of the risk factors that contribute to NEC will be helpful in preparing for admission of a high-risk preterm.

Adapted from Campos-Martinez, A. M., Expósito-Herrera, J., Gonzalez-Bolívar, M., Fernández-Marin, E., & Uberos, J. (2022). Evaluation of risk and preventive factors for necrotizing enterocolitis in premature newborns. A systematic review of the literature. *Frontiers in Pediatrics, 10*, 874976. https://doi.org/10.3389/fped.2022.874976

- Temperature instability
- Decreased or absent bowel sounds
- Signs of sepsis
- Bile-stained emesis
- Lethargy or decreased activity level
- Apnea
- Shock (Kim, 2023a)

An abdominal x-ray may demonstrate dilated bowel loops, abnormal gas patterns, intramural air bubbles that occur from bacteria, and thickened bowel walls (Briere & Labrecque, 2022).

Nursing Management

Nursing management of the newborn with NEC focuses on maintaining fluid and nutritional status, providing supportive care, and teaching the family about the condition and prognosis. Determine residual gastric volume prior to feeding; when it is elevated, be suspicious for NEC. When NEC is diagnosed, the infant will likely be initially managed with bowel rest. The newborn will not be allowed to take anything by mouth (NPO), nor enteral tube feeding. Institute gastric decompression as ordered with an orogastric tube attached to low intermittent suction. NEC is usually limited to a short period and resolves within 48 hours of stopping oral feedings.

Administer IV fluids initially to restore proper fluid balance. Administer breast milk if possible and permitted. Administer prescribed IV antibiotics to prevent sepsis from the necrotic bowel. Carefully monitor intake and output. Restart enteral feedings once the disease has resolved (normal abdominal examination and kidney, urinary, and bladder x-rays negative for pneumatosis).

If medical treatment fails to stabilize the newborn or if free air is present on an x-ray, surgical intervention will be necessary to resect the portion of necrotic bowel while preserving as much of the intestinal length as possible. Surgery for NEC usually requires the placement of a proximal enterostomy until the anastomosis site is ready for reconnection. After surgery, postoperative supportive care includes fluids, TPN, antibiotics, and bowel rest for 10 to 14 days. Administer prescribed analgesics to manage pain. The amount of bowel that has necrosed, as determined during the bowel resection, significantly increases the likelihood of long-term medical problems. Short bowel syndrome may result from a large resection of the bowel. Provide education about ostomy care if surgery is required.

Promote parental interaction with the newborn. Nursing actions of active engagement with parents and the sick infant (providing NICU orientation and physical care), providing cautious guidance (offering information and instruction on infant care), and maintaining subtle presence (overseeing parents' interaction with their infant) all contribute to fostering a positive, trusting relationship with parents (Ginglen & Butki, 2023).

The diagnosis of NEC may cause significant family anxiety. Listen to the family's worries and fears. Answer their questions honestly.

KEY CONCEPTS

- Congenital conditions can arise from many etiologies, including single-gene disorders, chromosomal aberrations, exposure to teratogens, and many sporadic conditions of unknown cause. Congenital structural anomalies may be inherited or sporadic, isolated or multiple, apparent or hidden, and gross or microscopic.
- Congenital heart disease is commonly physiologically classified as defects that result in increased pulmonary blood flow, defects that result in decreased pulmonary blood flow, defects that cause obstruction to blood flow out of the heart, and defects that are mixed.
- A worldwide decline in NTDs has occurred during recent decades due to improved prevention secondary to preconception folic acid supplementation, maternal serum alpha-fetoprotein monitoring, and use of ultrasonography and amniocentesis.
- Congenital respiratory tract structural disorders include choanal atresia and CDH. Evidence of bowel sounds in the chest suggests CDH.
- CL with CP is the most common craniofacial birth defect. The newborn has immediate feeding difficulties and may have problems with dentition, language acquisition, and hearing.
- EA refers to a congenitally interrupted esophagus in which the proximal and distal ends do not communicate; the upper esophageal segment ends in a blind pouch, and the lower segment ends a variable distance above the diaphragm. TEF is an abnormal communication between the trachea and the esophagus.
- Omphalocele and gastroschisis are congenital anomalies of the anterior abdominal wall. An omphalocele is a defect of the umbilical ring that allows evisceration of abdominal contents into an external peritoneal sac. Gastroschisis is a herniation of abdominal contents through an abdominal wall defect, usually to the left or right of the umbilicus.
- Hypospadias and epispadias are genitourinary system structural anomalies. Epispadias often occurs in conjunction with bladder exstrophy, in which the bladder protrudes onto the abdominal wall.
- Congenital clubfoot usually involves inversion and adduction of the forefoot, inversion of the heel and hindfoot, limitation of extension of the ankle and subtalar joint, and internal rotation of the leg.
- DDH includes dislocation, subluxation, or malformation of the acetabulum. Early recognition and prompt treatment are crucial.
- Inborn errors of metabolism are genetic disorders that disrupt normal metabolic function. Most are due to a defect in an enzyme or transport protein, resulting in a blocked metabolic pathway.
- Factors that place the newborn at risk for birth injury include cephalopelvic disproportion, maternal pelvic anomalies, oligohydramnios, prolonged or rapid labor, abnormal presentation, fetal prematurity, fetal macrosomia, and fetal abnormalities.
- Physiologic jaundice is a common, normal newborn phenomenon that appears during the second or third day of life and then declines over the first week after birth. Pathologic jaundice is manifested within the first 24 hours of life when total bilirubin levels increase by more than 5 mg/dL/day and the TSB level is higher than 17 mg/dL in a full-term infant.
- IMDs are at risk for malformations most frequently involving the cardiovascular, skeletal, central nervous, gastrointestinal, and genitourinary systems; cardiac anomalies are the most common.
- People who misuse drugs during pregnancy expose their unborn children to the possibility of intrauterine growth restriction, prematurity, neurobehavioral and neurophysiologic dysfunction, birth defects, infections, and long-term developmental sequelae.
- Newborns of birthing parents who use tobacco, illicit substances, and alcohol can exhibit withdrawal behavior.
- Newborn infections are usually classified according to the time of onset and grouped into three categories: congenital infection acquired in utero by vertical transmission with onset before birth; early-onset neonatal infections acquired by vertical transmission in the perinatal period, either shortly before or during birth; and late-onset neonatal infections acquired by horizontal transmission in the nursery.
- Asphyxia, the most common clinical insult in the perinatal period, results in brain injury and may lead to intellectual disability, cerebral palsy, or seizures.
- TTN occurs when the liquid in the lung is removed slowly or incompletely.
- Common risk factors for RDS include young gestational age, perinatal asphyxia regardless of gestational age, cesarean birth in the absence of labor (related to the lack of thoracic squeeze), male sex, and maternal diabetes.
- Meconium aspiration has three major pulmonary effects: airway obstruction, surfactant dysfunction, and chemical pneumonitis.
- The management of PPHN requires meticulous attention to detail with continuous monitoring of oxygenation, blood pressure, and perfusion.
- ROP is a developmental abnormality that affects the immature vasculature of the retina; abnormal growth of blood vessels (neovascularization) takes place within the retina and vitreous.

- PIVH is bleeding that usually originates in the subependymal germinal matrix region of the brain with extension into the ventricular system.
- NEC is a serious gastrointestinal disease of unknown etiology in newborns that can result in necrosis of a segment of the bowel.

REFERENCES AND RECOMMENDED READINGS

Abramowski, A., Ward, R., & Hamdan, A. H. (2023). Neonatal hypoglycemia. *StatPearls.* https://www.ncbi.nlm.nih.gov/books/NBK537105/

Akanmode, A. M., & Mahdy, H. (2023). Macrosomia. *StatPearls.* https://www.ncbi.nlm.nih.gov/books/NBK557577/

Altman, C. A. (2024). Identifying newborns with critical congenital heart disease. *UpToDate.* Retrieved March 1, 2024, from https://www.uptodate.com/contents/identifying-newborns-with-critical-congenital-heart-disease

American Academy of Pediatrics. (2022). Standard-dose oral dextrose gel for neonatal hypoglycemia. *AAP Grand Rounds, 47*(5), 51. https://doi.org/10.1542/gr.47-5-51

American Academy of Pediatrics. (2023). *Newborn screening for critical congenital heart defect (CCHD).* https://www.aap.org/en/patient-care/congenital-heart-defects/newborn-screening-for-critical-congenital-heart-defect-cchd/

American Cleft Palate Craniofacial Association. (2024). *Your baby's first year.* https://acpacares.org/resource/your-babys-first-year/

American Heart Association. (2023). *As people born with congenital heart defects now live longer, challenges evolve over time.* https://newsroom.heart.org/news/as-people-born-with-congenital-heart-defects-now-live-longer-challenges-evolve-over-time

Anand, S., & Lotfollahzadeh, S. (2023). Bladder exstrophy. *StatPearls.* https://www.ncbi.nlm.nih.gov/books/NBK563156/

Anbalagan, S., Falkowitz, D. M., & Mendez, M. D. (2023). Neonatal abstinence syndrome. *StatPearls.* https://www.ncbi.nlm.nih.gov/books/NBK551498/

Andaloro, C., & La Mantia, I. (2023). Choanal atresia. *StatPearls.* https://www.ncbi.nlm.nih.gov/books/NBK507724/

Ansong-Assoku, B., Shah, S. D., Adnan, M., & Ankola, P. A. (2023). Neonatal jaundice. *StatPearls.* https://www.ncbi.nlm.nih.gov/books/NBK532930/

Bagwell, G. A. (2022). Neonatal abstinence syndrome/neonatal opioid withdrawal. In C. Kenner & M. V. Boykova (Eds.), *Neonatal nursing care handbook: An evidence-based approach to conditions and procedures* (3rd ed.). Springer Publishing Company.

Bacino, C. A. (2023). Congenital anomalies: Epidemiology, types, and patterns. *UpToDate.* Retrieved February 28, 2024, from https://www.uptodate.com/contents/congenital-anomalies-epidemiology-types-and-patterns

Baldwin, D., & Yadav, D. (2023). Esophageal atresia. *StatPearls.* https://www.statpearls.com/ArticleLibrary/viewarticle/21326

Barrie, A., & Varacallo, M. (2023). Clubfoot. *StatPearls.* https://www.ncbi.nlm.nih.gov/books/NBK551574/

Baskin, L. S. (2023). Hypospadias: Pathogenesis, diagnosis, and evaluation. *UpToDate.* Retrieved March 13, 2024, from https://www.uptodate.com/contents/hypospadias-pathogenesis-diagnosis-and-evaluation

Bernstein, D. (2025). Epidemiology and genetic basis of congenital heart disease. In R. M. Kliegman, J. W. St Geme III, N. J. Blum, R. C. Tasker, K. M. Wilson, A. M. Schuh, C. L. Mack, & M. A. Deardorff (Eds.), *Nelson textbook of pediatrics* (22nd ed.). Elsevier Health Sciences.

Bhatt, A. (2023). Retinopathy of prematurity (ROP): Risk factors, classification, and screening. *UpToDate.* Retrieved March 1, 2024, from https://www.uptodate.com/contents/retinopathy-of-prematurity-rop-risk-factors-classification-and-screening

Bhatt, A. (2024). Retinopathy of prematurity (ROP): Treatment and prognosis. *UpToDate.* Retrieved June 4, 2024, from https://www.uptodate.com/contents/retinopathy-of-prematurity-rop-treatment-and-prognosis

Blanco, M. A., Lilly, C. M., Bavinger, B. C., Garcia, S., & Hojnicki, M. P. (2021). Caring for medically complex children in the outpatient setting. *Advances in Pediatrics, 68,* 89–102. https://doi.org/10.1016/j.yapd.2021.05.012

Bowman, R. M. (2024). Myelomeningocele (spina bifida): Anatomy, clinical manifestations, and complications. *UpToDate.* Retrieved June 4, 2024, from https://www.uptodate.com/contents/myelomeningocele-spina-bifida-anatomy-clinical-manifestations-and-complications

Briere, J., & Labrecque, M. (2022). Gastrointestinal surgical conditions in the neonate. In C. Kenner & M. V. Boykova (Eds.), *Neonatal nursing care handbook: An evidence-based approach to conditions and procedures* (3rd ed.). Springer Publishing Company.

Briggs-Steinberg, C. & Roth, P. (2023). Early onset sepsis in newborns. *Pediatrics in Review, 44*(1), 14–22. https://doi.org/10.1542/pir.2020-001164

Buffoni, I., Buratti, S., Mallamaci, M. F., Pezzato, S., Lampugnani, E., Buffelli, F., Fulcheri, E., Fulcheri, E., & Moscatelli, A. (2022). Sudden onset of severe pulmonary hypertension in a preterm infant: A case report on the role of maternal use of serotonin re-uptake inhibitors during pregnancy and concurrent risk factors. *Frontiers in Pediatrics, 10,* 855419. https://doi.org/10.3389/fped.2022.855419

Campos-Martinez, A. M., Expósito-Herrera, J., Gonzalez-Bolívar, M., Fernández-Marin, E., & Uberos, J. (2022). Evaluation of risk and preventive factors for necrotizing enterocolitis in premature newborns. A systematic review of the literature. *Frontiers in Pediatrics, 10,* 874976. https://doi.org/10.3389/fped.2022.874976

Cantey, J. B. (2023). Clinical features, evaluation, and diagnosis of sepsis in term and late preterm neonates. *UpToDate.* Retrieved March 15, 2014, from https://www.uptodate.com/contents/clinical-features-evaluation-and-diagnosis-of-sepsis-in-term-and-late-preterm-neonates

Centers for Disease Control and Prevention. (2024a). *Birth defects or congenital anomalies.* https://www.cdc.gov/nchs/fastats/birth-defects.htm

Centers for Disease Control and Prevention. (2024b). *Congenital heart defects (CHDs): Data and statistics.* https://www.cdc.gov/heart-defects/data/?CDC_AAref_Val=https://www.cdc.gov/ncbddd/heartdefects/data.html

Centers for Disease Control and Prevention. (2024c). *Microcephaly.* https://www.cdc.gov/birth-defects/about/microcephaly.html

Chang, G. (2024). Substance use during pregnancy: Overview of selected drugs. *UpToDate.* Retrieved March 14, 2024, from https://www.uptodate.com/contents/substance-use-during-pregnancy-overview-of-selected-drugs

Cunningham, F. G., Leveno, K. J., Dashe, J. S., Hoffman, B. L., Spong, C. Y., & Casey, B. M. (2022a). The newborn. In F. G. Cunningham, K. J. Leveno, J. S. Dashe, B. L. Hoffman, C. Y., Spong, & B. M. Casey (Eds.), *William's obstetrics* (26th ed.). McGraw-Hill.

Cunningham, F. G., Leveno, K. J., Dashe, J. S., Hoffman, B. L., Spong, C. Y., & Casey, B. M. (2022b). Complications of the newborn. In F. G. Cunningham, K. J. Leveno, J. S. Dashe, B. L. Hoffman, C. Y., Spong, & B. M. Casey (Eds.), *William's obstetrics* (26th ed.). McGraw-Hill.

Cunningham, F. G., Leveno, K. J., Dashe, J. S., Hoffman, B. L., Spong, C. Y., & Casey, B. M. (2022c). The preterm newborn. In F. G. Cunningham, K. J. Leveno, J. S. Dashe, B. L. Hoffman, C. Y., Spong, & B. M. Casey (Eds.), *William's obstetrics* (26th ed.). McGraw-Hill.

Darjazini Nahas, L., Hmadieh, M., Audeh, M., Yousfan, A., Almasri, I. A., & Martini, N. (2023). Cleft lip and palate risk factors among otorhinolaryngology: Head and neck surgery patients in two hospitals. *Medicine, 102*(42), e34419. https://doi.org/10.1097/MD.0000000000034419

Degrazia, M. (2022). Surgical care of the neonate. In C. Kenner & M. V. Boykova (Eds.), *Neonatal nursing care handbook: An evidence-based approach to conditions and procedures* (3rd ed.). Springer Publishing Company.

Do, P., Ha, B. Y., & Patel, M. R. (2022). Neonatal respiratory distress syndrome (RDS) imaging. *Medscape*. https://emedicine.medscape.com/article/409409-overview#a2

Donaire, A. E., & Mendez, M. D. (2023). Hypospadias. *StatPearls*. https://www.ncbi.nlm.nih.gov/books/NBK482122/

Dugosh, K. L., & Cacciola, J. S. (2022). Substance use disorders: Clinical assessment. *UpToDate*. Retrieved March 14, 2024, from https://www.uptodate.com/contents/substance-use-disorders-clinical-assessment

Dukhovny, S., & Wilkins-Haug, L. (2024). Neural tube defects: Overview of prenatal screening, evaluation, and pregnancy management. *UpToDate*. Retrieved June 4, 2024, from https://www.uptodate.com/contents/neural-tube-defects-overview-of-prenatal-screening-evaluation-and-pregnancy-management

Dumpa, V., & Chandrasekharan, P. (2023). Congenital diaphragmatic hernia. *StatPearls*. https://www.ncbi.nlm.nih.gov/books/NBK556076/

Dumpa, V., & Kamity, R. (2023). Birth trauma. *StatPearls*. https://www.ncbi.nlm.nih.gov/books/NBK539831/

Dwan, K., Kirkham, J., Paton, R. W., Morley, E., Newton, A. W., & Perry, D. C. (2022). Splinting for the non-operative management of developmental dysplasia of the hip (DDH) in children under six months of age. *The Cochrane Database of Systematic Reviews, 10*(10), CD012717. https://doi.org/10.1002/14651858.CD012717.pub2

Eichenwald, E. C., & Stark, A. R. (2023). Bronchopulmonary dysplasia (BPD): Clinical features and diagnosis. *UpToDate*. Retrieved February 28, 2024, from https://www.uptodate.com/contents/bronchopulmonary-dysplasia-bpd-clinical-features-and-diagnosis

Garcia-Prats, J. A. (2023a). Meconium aspiration syndrome: Prevention and management. *UpToDate*. Retrieved February 28, 2024, from https://www.uptodate.com/contents/meconium-aspiration-syndrome-prevention-and-management

Garcia-Prats, J. A. (2023b). Meconium aspiration syndrome: Management and outcome. *UpToDate*. Retrieved February 28, 2024, from https://www.uptodate.com/contents/meconium-aspiration-syndrome-management-and-outcome

Geis, G. M., & Clark, D. A. (2023). Meconium aspiration syndrome. *Medscape*. https://emedicine.medscape.com/article/974110-overview

Gillam-Krakauer, M., & Gowen, C. W. (2023). Birth asphyxia. *StatPearls*. https://www.ncbi.nlm.nih.gov/books/NBK430782/

Ginglen, J. G., & Butki, N. (2023). Necrotizing enterocolitis. *StatPearls*. https://www.ncbi.nlm.nih.gov/books/NBK513357/

Haridas, A., & Tomita, T. (2022). Hydrocephalus in children: Physiology, pathogenesis, and etiology. *UpToDate*. Retrieved March 2, 2024, from https://www.uptodate.com/contents/hydrocephalus-in-children-physiology-pathogenesis-and-etiology

Haridas, A., & Tomita, T. (2024). Hydrocephalus in children: Management and prognosis. *UpToDate*. Retrieved June 4, 2024, from https://www.uptodate.com/contents/hydrocephalus-in-children-management-and-prognosis

Harris, M., Schiff, D. M., Saia, K., Muftu, S., Standish, K. R., & Wachman, E. M. (2023). Academy of Breastfeeding Medicine clinical protocol #21: Breastfeeding in the setting of substance use and substance use disorder (revised 2023). *Breastfeeding medicine, 18*(10), 715–733. https://doi.org/10.1089/bfm.2023.29256.abm

Holland, C., Hammond, C., & Richmond, M. M. (2023). COVID-19 and pregnancy: Risk and outcomes. *Nursing for Women's Health, 27*(1), 31–41. https://doi.org/10.1016/j.nwh.2022.11.004

Ito, M., Kato, S., Saito, M., Miyahara, N., Arai, H., Namba, F., Ota, E., & Nakanishi, H. (2023). Bronchopulmonary dysplasia in extremely premature infants: A scoping review for identifying risk factors. *Biomedicines, 11*(2), 553. https://doi.org/10.3390/biomedicines11020553

Jansson, L. M. (2024). Neonatal abstinence syndrome (NAS): Management and outcome. *UpToDate*. Retrieved June 4, 2024, from https://www.uptodate.com/contents/neonatal-abstinence-syndrome-nas-management-and-outcome

Jha, K., Nassar, G. N., & Makker, K. (2023). Transient tachypnea of the newborn. *StatPearls*. https://www.ncbi.nlm.nih.gov/books/NBK537354/

Johnson, K. E. (2023). Transient tachypnea of the newborn. *UpToDate*. Retrieved February 29, 2024, from https://www.uptodate.com/contents/transient-tachypnea-of-the-newborn

Jone, P.-N., Kim, J. S., Burkett, D., Jacobsen, R., & Von Alvensleben, J. (2022). Cardiovascular diseases. In M. Bunik, W. W. Hay, M. J. Levin, & M. J. Abzug. (Eds.), *Current diagnosis and treatment: Pediatrics* (26th ed.). McGraw-Hill Education.

Kemper, A. R., Newman, T. B., Slaughter, J. L., Maisels, M. J., Watchko, J. F., Downs, S. M., Grout, R. W., Bundy, D. G., Stark, A. R., Bogen, D. L., Holmes, A. V., Feldman-Winter, L. B., Bhutani, V. K., Brown, S. R., Maradiaga Panayotti, G. M., Okechukwu, K., Rappo, P. D., & Russell, T. L. (2022). Clinical practice guideline revision: Management of hyperbilirubinemia in the newborn infant 35 or more weeks of gestation. *Pediatrics, 150*(3), e2022058859. https://doi.org/10.1542/peds.2022-058859

Kenner, C. (2022). Hematologic and immune system. In C. Kenner & M. V. Boykova (Eds.), *Neonatal nursing care handbook: An evidence-based approach to conditions and procedures* (3rd ed.). Springer Publishing Company.

Kim, J. H. (2023a). Neonatal necrotizing enterocolitis: Clinical features and diagnosis. *UpToDate*. Retrieved February

29, 2024, from https://www.uptodate.com/contents/neonatal-necrotizing-enterocolitis-clinical-features-and-diagnosis

Kim, J. H. (2023b). Neonatal necrotizing enterocolitis: Pathology and pathogenesis. *UpToDate*. Retrieved February 29, 2024, from https://www.uptodate.com/contents/neonatal-necrotizing-enterocolitis-pathology-and-pathogenesis

Martin, R. (2022). Overview of neonatal respiratory distress and disorders of transition. *UpToDate*. Retrieved February 28, 2024, from https://www.uptodate.com/contents/overview-of-neonatal-respiratory-distress-and-disorders-of-transition

Martin, R. (2024). Respiratory distress syndrome (RDS) in preterm infants: Management. *UpToDate*. Retrieved February 28, 2024, from https://www.uptodate.com/contents/respiratory-distress-syndrome-rds-in-preterm-infants-management

Matern, D. (2023). Newborn screening for inborn errors of metabolism. *UpToDate*. Retrieved June 4, 2024, from https://www.uptodate.com/contents/newborn-screening-for-inborn-errors-of-metabolism

Maybee, J., Deck, J., Jensen, E., Ruiz, A., Kinder, S., & DeBoer, E. (2023). Feeding and swallowing characteristics of children with esophageal atresia and tracheoesophageal fistula. *Journal of Pediatric Gastroenterology and Nutrition, 76*(3), 288–294. https://doi.org/10.1097/MPG.0000000000003697

McGillick, E. V., Te Pas, A. B., van den Akker, T., Keus, J. M. H., Thio, M., & Hooper, S. B. (2022). Evaluating clinical outcomes and physiological perspectives in studies investigating respiratory support for babies born at term with or at risk of transient tachypnea: A narrative review. *Frontiers in Pediatrics, 10*, 878536. https://doi.org/10.3389/fped.2022.878536

McKee-Garrett, T. M. (2023). Neonatal birth injuries. *UpToDate*. Retrieved March 13, 2024, from https://www.uptodate.com/contents/neonatal-birth-injuries

Messer, R., Schreiner, T. L., Troy, E., Walleigh, D., Wright, M., & Yang, M. L. (2022). Neurologic & muscular disorders. In M. Bunik, W. W. Hay, M. J. Levin, & M. J. Abzug (Eds.), *Current diagnosis and treatment: Pediatrics* (26th ed.). McGraw-Hill Education.

Mishra, V., Lui, K., Schelonka, R. L., Maheshwari, A., & Jain, R. (2024). Infants of diabetic mothers. In A. Maheshwari (Ed.), *Principles of neonatology*. Elsevier.

Moore, T. R. (2022). Diabetes mellitus and pregnancy. *Medscape*. https://emedicine.medscape.com/article/127547-overview

Mota-Rojas, D., Villanueva-García, D., Solimano, A., Muns, R., Ibarra-Ríos, D., & Mota-Reyes, A. (2022). Pathophysiology of perinatal asphyxia in humans and animal models. *Biomedicines, 10*(2), 347. https://doi.org/10.3390/biomedicines10020347

Mukhopadhyay, S., & Puopolo, K. M. (2023). Bacterial and fungal infections. In E. C. Eichenwald, A. R. Hansen, C. R. Martin, & A. R. Stark (Eds.), *Cloherty and Stark's manual of neonatal care* (9th ed.). Wolters Kluwer.

Nandhagopal, T., & De Cicco, F. L. (2023). Developmental dysplasia of the hip. *StatPearls*. https://www.ncbi.nlm.nih.gov/books/NBK563157/

National Heart, Lung, and Blood Institute. (2022). *Congenital heart defects: Causes and risk factors*. https://www.nhlbi.nih.gov/health/congenital-heart-defects/causes

Ndanga, M., Sulley, S., & Saka, A. K. (2022). Trend analysis of substance use disorder during pregnancy. *Cureus, 14*(3), e23548. https://doi.org/10.7759/cureus.23548

Nethi, S., & Arya, K. (2023). Meningocele. *StatPearls*. https://www.ncbi.nlm.nih.gov/books/NBK562174/

Nussbaum, C., Lengauer, M., Puchwein-Schwepcke, A. F., Weiss, V. B. N., Spielberger, B., & Genzel-Boroviczény, O. (2022). Noninvasive ventilation in preterm infants: Factors influencing weaning decisions and the role of the Silverman-Andersen score. *Children, 9*(9), 1292. https://doi.org/10.3390/children9091292

O'Brien, K. (2023). Neonatal effects of maternal diabetes. In E. C. Eichenwald, A. R. Hansen, C. R. Martin, & A. R. Stark (Eds.), *Cloherty and Stark's manual of neonatal care* (9th ed.). Wolters Kluwer.

Oermann, C. M. (2023). Congenital anomalies of the intrathoracic airways and tracheoesophageal fistula. *UpToDate*. https://www.uptodate.com/contents/congenital-anomalies-of-the-intrathoracic-airways-and-tracheoesophageal-fistula

Patrick, S. W., Barfield, W. D., Poindexter, B. B., Committee on Fetus and Newborn, Committee on Substance Use and Prevention, Cummings, J., Hand, I., Adams-Chapman, I., Aucott, S. W., Puopolo, K. M., Goldsmith, J. P., Kaufman, D., Martin, C., Mowitz, M., Gonzalez, L., Camenga, D. R., Quigley, J., Ryan, S. A., & Walker-Harding, L. W. (2020). Neonatal opioid withdrawal syndrome. *Pediatrics, 146*(5), e2020029074. https://doi.org/10.1542/peds.2020-029074

Prince, M. K., Daley, S. F., & Ayers, D. (2023). Substance use in pregnancy. *StatPearls*. https://www.ncbi.nlm.nih.gov/books/NBK542330/

Rees, P., Callan, C., Chadda, K. R., Vaal, M., Diviney, J., Sabti, S., Harnden, F., Gardiner, J., Battersby, C., Gale, C., & Sutcliffe, A. (2022). Preterm brain injury and neurodevelopmental outcomes: A meta-analysis. *Pediatrics, 150*(6), e2022057442. https://doi.org/10.1542/peds.2022-057442

Riskin, A., & Garcia-Prats, J. A. (2023). Infants of mothers with diabetes (IMD). *UpToDate*. Retrieved March 14, 2024, from https://www.uptodate.com/contents/infants-of-mothers-with-diabetes-imd

Rosenfeld, S. B. (2022). Developmental dysplasia of the hip: Clinical features and diagnosis. *UpToDate*. Retrieved March 12, 2024, from https://www.uptodate.com/contents/developmental-dysplasia-of-the-hip-clinical-features-and-diagnosis

Salari, N., Darvishi, N., Heydari, M., Bokaee, S., Darvishi, F., & Mohammadi, M. (2022). Global prevalence of cleft palate, cleft lip and cleft palate and lip: A comprehensive systematic review and meta-analysis. *Journal of Stomatology, Oral and Maxillofacial Surgery, 123*(2), 110–120. https://doi.org/10.1016/j.jormas.2021.05.008

Savin, M. K., & Phalen, A. G. (2022). Gastrointestinal conditions. In C. Kenner & M. V. Boykova (Eds.), *Neonatal nursing care handbook: An evidence-based approach to conditions and procedures* (3rd ed.). Springer Publishing Company.

Schneider, D. S. (2023). The cardiovascular system. In K. J. Marcdante, & R. M. Kliegman (Eds.). *Nelson's essentials of pediatrics* (9th ed.). Elsevier.

Singh, M., Alsaleem, M., & Gray, C. P. (2023). Neonatal sepsis. *StatPearls*. https://www.ncbi.nlm.nih.gov/books/NBK531478/

Singh, M., & Mehra, K. (2023). Imperforate anus. *StatPearls*. https://www.ncbi.nlm.nih.gov/books/NBK549784/#article-17726.s3

Smith, D. (2022). The newborn infant. In M. Bunik, W. W. Hay, M. J. Levin, & M. J. Abzug (Eds.), *Current diagnosis and treatment: Pediatrics* (26th ed.). McGraw-Hill Education.

Stark, A. R., & Eichenwald, E. C. (2022). Persistent pulmonary hypertension of the newborn (PPHN): Clinical features and diagnosis. *UpToDate*. Retrieved February 28, 2024, from https://www.uptodate.com/contents/persistent-pulmonary-hypertension-of-the-newborn-pphn-clinical-features-and-diagnosis

Stark, A. R., & Eichenwald, E. C. (2023a). Bronchopulmonary dysplasia (BPD): Management and outcome. *UpToDate*. Retrieved February 28, 2024, from https://www.uptodate.com/contents/bronchopulmonary-dysplasia-bpd-management-and-outcome

Stark, A. R., & Eichenwald, E. C. (2023b). Bronchopulmonary dysplasia (BPD): Prevention. *UpToDate*. Retrieved February 28, 2024, from https://www.uptodate.com/contents/bronchopulmonary-dysplasia-bpd-prevention

Starr, R., De Jesus, O., Shah, S. D., & Borger, J. (2023). Periventricular and intraventricular hemorrhage. *StatPearls*. https://www.ncbi.nlm.nih.gov/books/NBK538310/

Stephenson, C. D., Lockwood, C. J., & MacKenzie, A. P. (2022). Omphalocele: Prenatal diagnosis and pregnancy management. *UpToDate*. Retrieved June 4, 2024, from https://www.uptodate.com/contents/omphalocele-prenatal-diagnosis-and-pregnancy-management

Stephenson, C. D., Lockwood, C. J., & MacKenzie, A. P. (2023). Gastroschisis. *UpToDate*. Retrieved March 12, 2024, from https://www.uptodate.com/contents/gastroschisis

Suneja, M., Szot, J. F., LeBlond, R. F., & Brown, D. D. (2020). The male genitalia and reproductive system. In M. Suneja, J. F. Szot, R. F. LeBlond, & D. D. Brown (Eds.), *DeGowin's diagnostic examination* (11th ed.). McGraw-Hill.

Sutton, V. R. (2023). Inborn errors of metabolism: Epidemiology, pathogenesis, and clinical features. *UpToDate*. Retrieved March 12, 2024, from https://www.uptodate.com/contents/inborn-errors-of-metabolism-epidemiology-pathogenesis-and-clinical-features

Tatawy, S. S. E., Gad, A. M., Eissa, T. S., Houchi, S. Z. E., & Sabry, A. M. (2022). Care bundle application decreases the frequency and severity of intraventricular hemorrhage in preterm neonates: Single center study. *Pediatrics Sciences Journal*, *2*(2), 112–119. https://doi.org/10.21608/cupsj.2022.142531.1061

Tolarova, M. M., Al-Kharafi, L., Tolar, M., & Boyd, C. (2022). Pediatric cleft lip & palate. *Medscape*. https://emedicine.medscape.com/article/995535-overview

Tomita, T., & Ogiwara, H. (2022). Anencephaly. *UpToDate*. Retrieved March 12, 2024, from https://www.uptodate.com/contents/anencephaly

Tunç, Ş., Oğlak, S. C., Özköse, Z. G., & Ölmez, F. (2022). The evaluation of the antepartum and intrapartum risk factors in predicting the risk of birth asphyxia. *The Journal of Obstetrics and Gynecology Research*, *48*(6), 1370–1378. https://doi.org/10.1111/jog.15214

U.S. Department of Health and Human Services. (n.d.). *Healthy People 2030*. https://health.gov/healthypeople

Vaux, K. K., & Chambers, C. (2023). Fetal alcohol syndrome. *Medscape*. https://emedicine.medscape.com/article/974016-overview

Weiner, D. L. (2024). Inborn errors of metabolism. *Medscape*. https://emedicine.medscape.com/article/804757-overview

Weiner, G. M., & Zaichkin, J. (2022). Updates for the neonatal resuscitation program and resuscitation guidelines. *NeoReviews*, *23*(4), e238–e249. https://doi.org/10.1542/neo.23-4-e238

Weitzman, C., & Rojmahamongkol, P. (2024). Fetal alcohol spectrum disorder: Clinical features and diagnosis. *UpToDate*. Retrieved June 4, 2024, from https://www.uptodate.com/contents/fetal-alcohol-spectrum-disorder-clinical-features-and-diagnosis

Wilkins-Haug, L. (2024). Etiology, prenatal diagnosis, obstetric management, and recurrence of cleft lip and/or palate. *UpToDate*. Retrieved June 4, 2024, from https://www.uptodate.com/contents/etiology-prenatal-diagnosis-obstetric-management-and-recurrence-of-cleft-lip-and-or-palate

Wong, R. J., & Bhutani, V. K. (2022). Unconjugated hyperbilirubinemia in neonates: Etiology and pathogenesis. *UpToDate*. Retrieved March 13, 2024, from https://www.uptodate.com/contents/unconjugated-hyperbilirubinemia-in-neonates-etiology-and-pathogenesis

Wong, R. J., & Bhutani, V. K. (2023a). Unconjugated hyperbilirubinemia in neonates: Risk factors, clinical manifestations, and neurologic complications. *UpToDate*. Retrieved March 13, 2024, from https://www.uptodate.com/contents/unconjugated-hyperbilirubinemia-in-neonates-risk-factors-clinical-manifestations-and-neurologic-complications

Wong, R. J., & Bhutani, V. K. (2023b). Unconjugated hyperbilirubinemia in term and late preterm newborns: Initial management. *UpToDate*. Retrieved March 13, 2024, from https://www.uptodate.com/contents/unconjugated-hyperbilirubinemia-in-term-and-late-preterm-newborns-initial-management

Wong, R. J., & Bhutani, V. K. (2023c). Unconjugated hyperbilirubinemia in term and late preterm newborns: Screening. *UpToDate*. Retrieved March 13, 2024, from https://www.uptodate.com/contents/unconjugated-hyperbilirubinemia-in-term-and-late-preterm-newborns-screening

Wood, R. J., & Levitt, M. A. (2022). Surgery for pediatric anorectal malformation (imperforate anus). *Medscape*. https://emedicine.medscape.com/article/933524

World Health Organization. (2021). *New brief outlines devastating harms from tobacco use and exposure to second-hand tobacco smoke during pregnancy and throughout childhood—Report calls for protective policies*. https://www.who.int/news/item/16-03-2021-new-brief-outlines-devastating-harms-from-tobacco-use-and-exposure-to-second-hand-tobacco-smoke-during-pregnancy-and-throughout-childhood

World Health Organization. (2024). *Congenital disorders*. https://www.who.int/health-topics/congenital-anomalies#tab=tab_1

Xiao, H., Tang, Y., & Su, Y. (2022). Risk factors of developmental dysplasia of the hip in a single clinical center. *Scientific Reports*, *12*(1), 19461. https://doi.org/10.1038/s41598-022-24025-8

Yadav, S., & Lee, B. (2023). Neonatal respiratory distress syndrome. *StatPearls*. https://www.statpearls.com/ArticleLibrary/viewarticle/37547

Yang, K. C. (2025). Infants of diabetic mothers. In R. M. Kliegman, J. W. St Geme III, N. J. Blum, R. C. Tasker, K. M. Wilson, A. M. Schuh, C. L. Mack, & M. A Deardorff (Eds.), *Nelson textbook of pediatrics* (22nd ed.). Elsevier Health Sciences.

Zhang, J., Wang, N., Lv, H., & Liu, Z. (2022). Magnetic resonance imaging of clubfoot treated with the Ponseti method: A short-term outcome study. *Frontiers in Pediatrics, 10*, 924028. https://doi.org/10.3389/fped.2022.924028

DEVELOPING CLINICAL JUDGMENT

PRACTICING FOR NCLEX

1. The nurse is caring for a premature infant in the nursery. Which finding would lead the nurse to suspect the newborn is experiencing RDS?
- **a.** Abdominal distention
- **b.** Acrocyanosis
- **c.** Depressed fontanelles
- **d.** Nasal flaring

2. A newly delivered birthing parent reports misusing opioids during the pregnancy. Which nursing assessment finding would the nurse expect in this newborn?
- **a.** Calm facial appearance
- **b.** Daily weight gain
- **c.** Increasing irritability
- **d.** Feeding and sleeping well

3. The nurse is caring for a newborn with a congenital anomaly. Which assessment finding will the nurse note with tracheoesophageal fistula?
- **a.** Subnormal temperature
- **b.** Absent Moro reflex
- **c.** Inability to swallow
- **d.** Drooling from mouth

4. In the nursery, a nurse is caring for several newborns. Which newborn would the nurse be most alert for the development of transient tachypnea?
- **a.** Infant born by cesarean birth 1 hour ago
- **b.** Newborn whose birthing parent received no sedation
- **c.** History of birthing parent with heart disease
- **d.** Neonate who is SGA

5. The nurse is teaching the parents of a newborn with CL and CP about caring for their infant. Which instruction would the nurse include in the teaching plan?
- **a.** Feed the infant in a semi-lying position.
- **b.** Continue feeding the infant for as long as it takes.
- **c.** Burp the infant frequently during feedings.
- **d.** Avoid the use of high-calorie formulas.

6. The nurse has performed a comprehensive physical examination on a newly born infant. Which finding would lead the nurse to suspect developmental dysplasia of the hip?
- **a.** Symmetrical thigh folds
- **b.** Even knee height
- **c.** Full abduction of the hip
- **d.** Audible clunk on hip abduction

7. A 30-week preterm newborn is found to have tachypnea during the first few hours of life, and oxygen administered via face mask at 100% doesn't improve the oxygen saturation level. Which substance, if administered to the pregnant person prenatally, could have prevented RDS?
- **a.** Insulin
- **b.** Lecithin
- **c.** Folic acid
- **d.** Dexamethasone

8. A preterm newborn with RDS is receiving supplemental oxygen. Which referral for consultation will the infant need?
- **a.** Pediatric cardiology
- **b.** Pediatric ophthalmology
- **c.** Pediatric otolaryngology
- **d.** Infectious disease specialist

CRITICAL THINKING EXERCISES

1. As the nursery nurse, you receive a newborn from the labor and birth suite and place them under the radiant warmer. The nurse who reports states that the birthing parent couldn't remember when their membranes broke before labor and that they ran a fever during labor for the past few hours. The Apgar scores were good, but the newborn seemed lethargic. As you begin your assessment, you note that they are pale and floppy and have a subnormal temperature; heart rate is 180 bpm, and respiratory rate is 70 breaths per minute.
- **a.** What in the birthing parent's history should raise a red flag to the nurse?
- **b.** For what condition is this newborn at high risk?
- **c.** What interventions are appropriate for this condition?

2. Terry, a day-old baby, is fretful, and calming measures do not seem to work. As the nursery nurse, you notice that they are losing weight and their formula intake is poor, even though they are manifesting hungry behaviors. The birthing parent received no prenatal care and denied drug use, but their drug screen was positive for heroin.
- **a.** What additional information do you need to obtain from the birthing parent?
- **b.** What additional laboratory work might be needed for the infant?
- **c.** What specific measures need to be made for the infant's ongoing care?

3. A term newborn is brought to the nursery. Their birthing parent received no prenatal care, but the newborn's Apgar scores were adequate. As you carry out your newborn assessment, you note an imperforate anus, and you palpate no testicles in the scrotal sac.
   a. What additional assessments should you complete?
   b. How common are anorectal agenesis and genitourinary tract anomalies?
   c. What diagnostic tests might be ordered? What might be included in the treatment plan for this newborn?

STUDY ACTIVITIES

1. Arrange for a tour of a regional NICU to see the nurse's role in caring for sick neonates. Ask the nurse to give a quick history of each newborn's condition. Was the nurse's role like what you imagined? What was your impression of the NICU, and how would you describe it to expectant parents?
2. Select and visit a website that pertains to either an acquired or a congenital newborn condition. What kind of information is given? How helpful would it be for parents with an infant diagnosed with a specific condition?
3. A herniation of a newborn's abdominal contents present at birth describes ________________.

UNIT

IX

Health Promotion of the Growing Child and Family

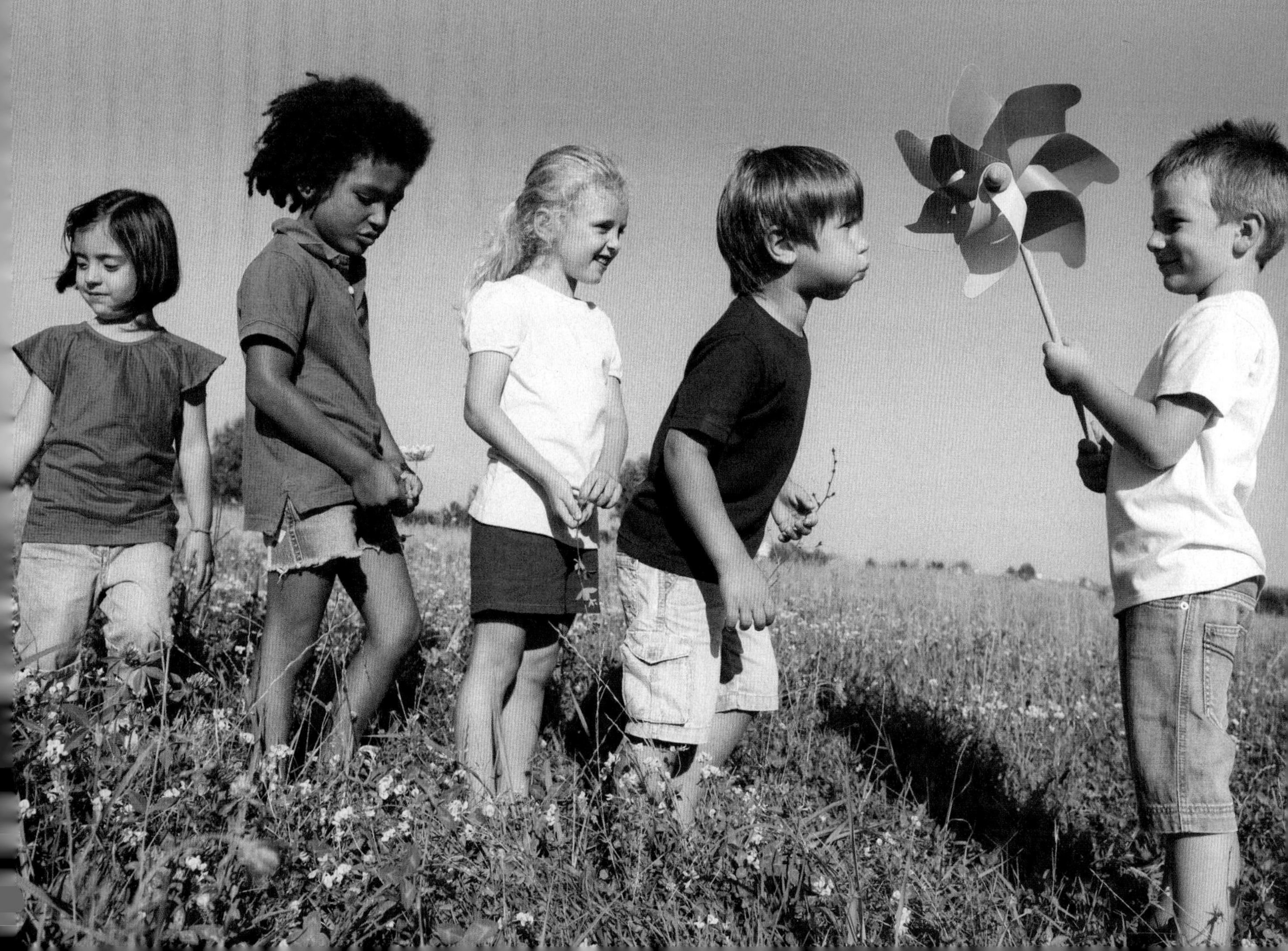

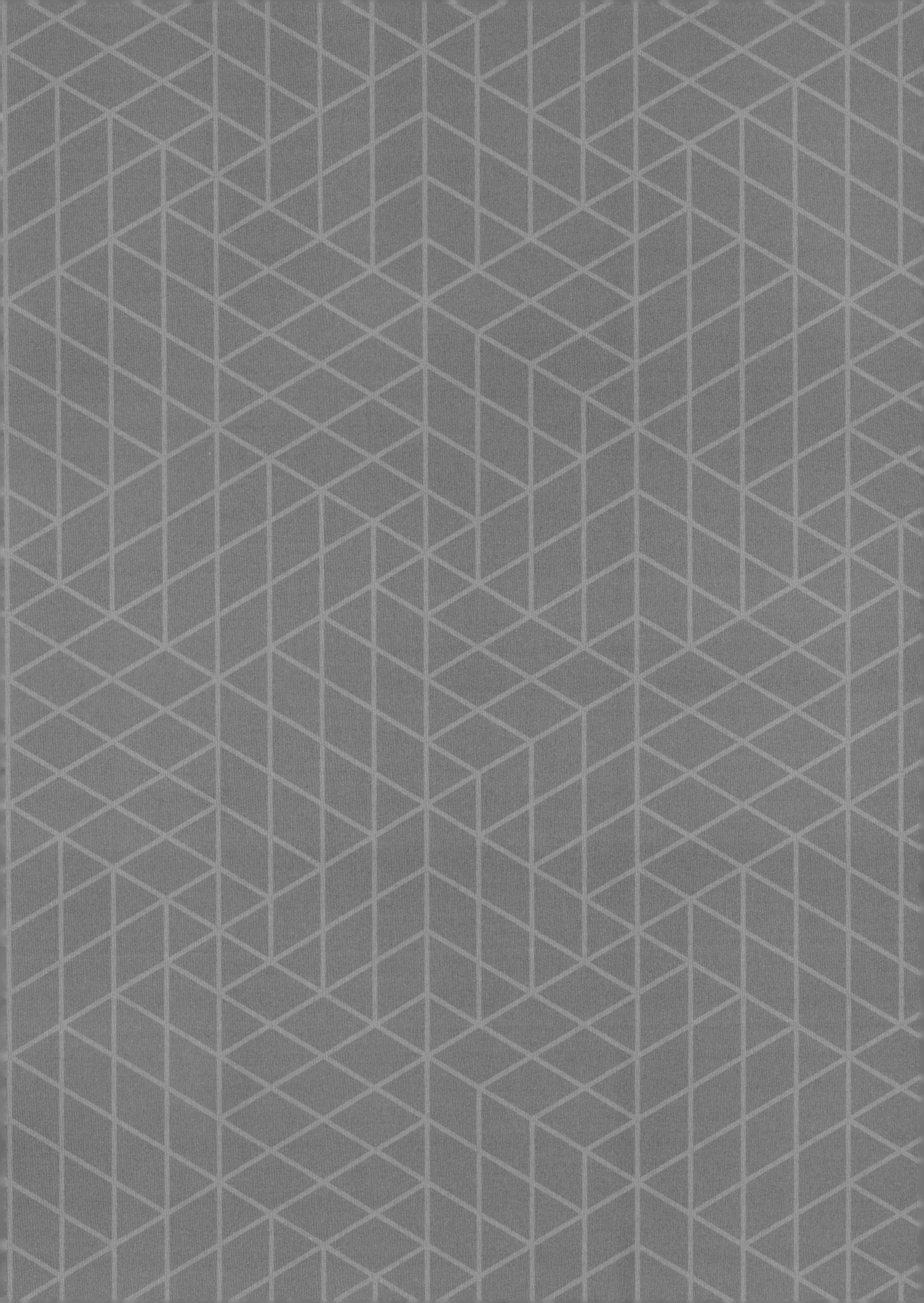

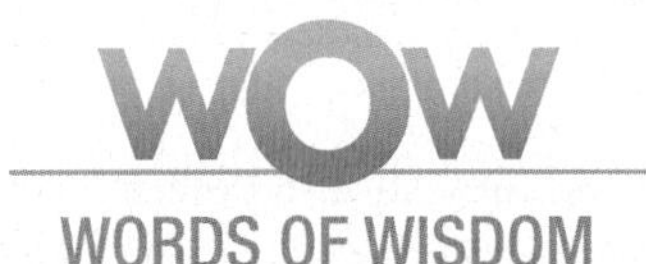

WORDS OF WISDOM

The miracle of a newborn infant... the commitment of raising a child... the nurse's presence helps guide this journey.

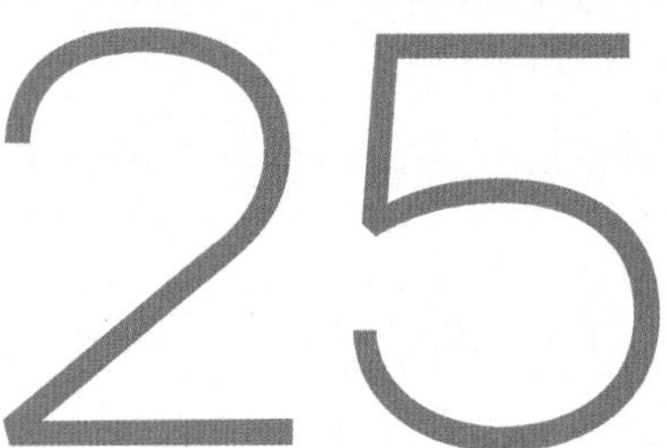

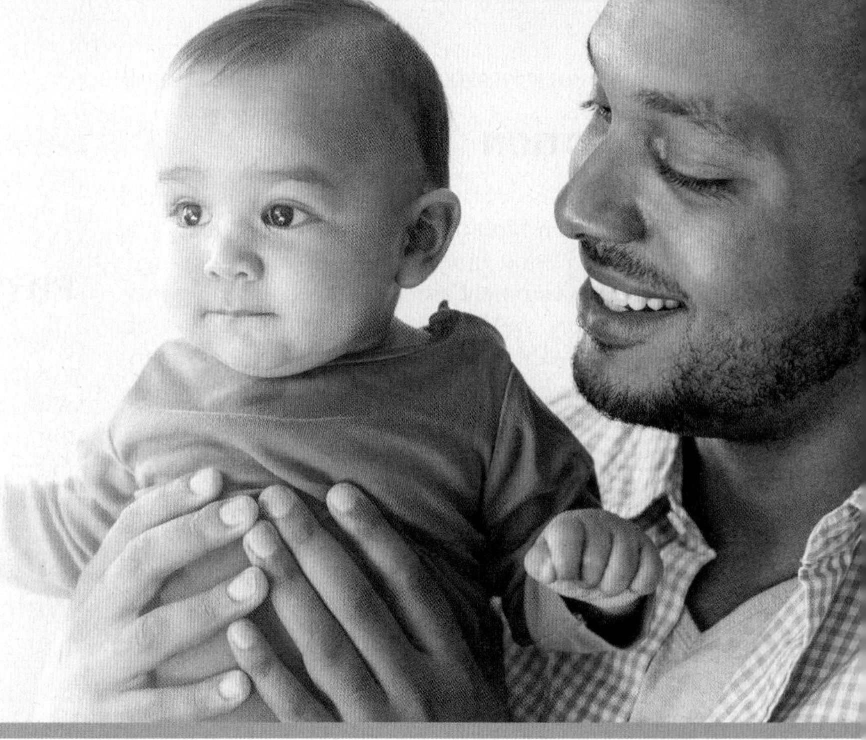

Growth and Development of the Newborn and Infant

KEY TERMS

anticipatory guidance
binocularity
cephalocaudal (sef′ă-lō-kaw′dăl)
colic
colostrum (kŏ-los′trŭm)
development
foremilk
growth
hindmilk
let-down reflex
maturation
object permanence
proximodistal (prok′si-mō-dis′tăl)
solitary play
stranger anxiety
temperament

LEARNING OBJECTIVES

Upon completion of the chapter, you will be able to:

1. Describe typical physical growth, physiologic changes, and sensory development in the newborn and infant.
2. Identify the gross and fine motor milestones of the newborn and infant.
3. Examine expected language development in the first year of life.
4. Implement a nursing care plan to address common issues related to growth and development in infancy.
5. Describe nutritional requirements of the newborn and infant.
6. Develop a nutritional plan for the first year of life.
7. Examine common issues related to growth and development in infancy.
8. Demonstrate knowledge of appropriate anticipatory guidance for common developmental issues.

Allison Johnson is a 6-month-old brought to the clinic by her parents for her 6-mo check-up. As new parents, they have a list of questions and concerns. As the n caring for Allison, assess growth and development, and then teach the parents what changes to expect in Allison over the next few months.

INTRODUCTION

The newborn or neonatal period of infancy is defined as the period from birth until 28 days of age. Infancy is defined as the period from birth to 12 months of age. Growth and development are interrelated, ongoing processes in infancy and childhood. **Growth** refers to an increase in physical size. **Development** is the sequential process by which infants and children gain various skills and functions. Heredity influences growth and development by determining the child's potential, while environment contributes to the degree of achievement. **Maturation** refers to an increase in functionality of various body systems or developmental skills.

GROWTH AND DEVELOPMENT OVERVIEW

Growth and developmental changes in the first year of life are numerous and dramatic. Physical growth, maturation of body systems, and gross and fine motor skills progress in an orderly and sequential fashion. Although timing may vary from infant to infant, the order in which developmental skills are acquired is consistent. Infants also exhibit vast amounts of learning in the psychosocial and cognitive, language and communication, and social/emotional domains. Adequate growth and development are indicative of health in the infant or young child. Nurses must be familiar with normal developmental milestones so that they can accurately assess the infant's development as well as provide age-appropriate anticipatory guidance to the parents.

Achievement of developmental milestones may be assessed in a variety of ways. While obtaining the health history, the nurse may ask the parent or caregiver if the skill is present and when it was attained. The infant may also demonstrate the skill during the interview or examination, or the nurse may elicit the skill from the infant. A number of screening tools are also used to assess development, such as the Ages and Stages Questionnaire (ASQ), Infant–Toddler Checklist (ITC), Infant Development Inventory (IDI), and Parents' Evaluation of Developmental Status-Developmental Milestones (PEDS-DM).

Ill or premature infants may exhibit delayed acquisition of physical growth and developmental skills. When assessing the growth and development of a premature infant, use the infant's adjusted age to determine expected outcomes. To determine adjusted age, subtract [illegible]e number of weeks that the infant was premature from [illegible] infant's chronologic age. Plot growth parameters and [illegible]s developmental milestones based on adjusted age. [illegible]ample, a 6-month-old who was born at 28 weeks' [illegible]n was born 12 weeks early (3 months), so sub[illegible]onths from their chronologic age of 6 months [illegible]an adjusted age of 3 months. This infant would [illegible]ate healthy growth if they were the size of a 3-month-old, and they should be expected to achieve the developmental milestones of a 3-month-old rather than a 6-month-old.

PHYSICAL GROWTH

Ongoing assessments of growth are important so that too-rapid or inadequate growth can be identified early. With early identification, the cause can be diagnosed and the potential for further appropriate growth maximized. Infants grow rapidly over the first 12 months of life. Weight, length, and head and chest circumference are all indicators of physical growth in the newborn and infant.

Weight

The average newborn weighs 3.400 kg (7.5 lb) at birth, with males being slightly heavier than females. Newborns may lose 5% to 10% of their body weight over the first week of life. The average newborn then gains about 20 to 30 g per day and regains their birth weight by 7 to 10 days of age. Most infants double their birth weight by 4 to 5 months of age and triple their birth weight by the time they are 1 year old (Branchford & Levine, 2023).

Length

The average newborn is 50 cm (20 in) long at birth. The infant grows more quickly in length over the first 6 months than during the second 6 months. By 12 months of age, the infant's length has increased by 50% (Branchford & Levine, 2023).

Head Circumference

The average head circumference of the full-term newborn is 35 cm (13.5 in). Similarly to the weight and length, the head circumference increases rapidly during the first 6 months. Head circumference increases about 10 cm from birth to 1 year of age (Branchford & Levine, 2023).

Remember Allison Johnson, the 6-month-old introduced at the beginning of the chapter? Allison's weight is 7.26 kg (16 lb), her length is 65.41 cm (25.75 in), and her head circumference is 43.18 cm (17 in).

PHYSIOLOGIC CHANGES

The newborn's and infant's organ systems undergo significant changes as the infant grows. Systems that undergo significant change include the neurologic system, the cardiovascular system, the respiratory system, the gastrointestinal (digestive) system, the renal system, the hematopoietic system, the immunologic system, and the integumentary system.

Neurologic System

The infant experiences tremendous changes in the neurologic system over the first year of life. Critical brain growth and continued myelination of the spinal cord occur. Involuntary movement progresses to voluntary control, and immature vocalizations and crying progress to the ability to speak as a result of maturational changes of the neurologic system.

States of Consciousness

The typical newborn's ability to move sequentially through states of consciousness reassures parents and health care providers that the neurologic system, though immature, is intact. An average newborn will ordinarily move through six states of consciousness:

1. Deep sleep: Sleeping with eyes closed and no movement.
2. Light sleep: Sleeping with eyes closed; rapid eye movements and irregular movements may be noticed.
3. Drowsiness: Eyes may close or be half-lidded; the infant may be dozing.
4. Quiet alert state: The infant's eyes are wide open, and the body is calm.
5. Active alert state: The infant's eyes are open; body movements occur.
6. Crying: The infant cries or screams, and it is difficult to gain the infant's attention (Olsson, 2020).

Newborns usually progress through these states slowly, rather than going from deep sleep immediately into outright crying.

Brain Growth

The nervous system continues to mature throughout infancy, and the increase in head circumference is indicative of brain growth. The brain undergoes tremendous growth during the first 2 years of life. By 6 months of age, the infant's brain weighs half that of the adult brain. At age 12 months, the brain has grown considerably, weighing 2.5 times what it did at birth. Usually, the anterior fontanel remains open until 12 to 18 months of age to accommodate this rapid brain growth. However, the fontanel may close as early as 9 months of age, and this is not of concern in the infant with age-appropriate growth and development.

In general, the neurologic system matures a significant amount over the first year of life. Myelination of the spinal cord and nerves continues over the first 2 years. Maturation of the nervous system and continued myelination are necessary for the tremendous developmental skills that are achieved in the first 12 months. During the first few months of life, reflexive behavior is replaced with purposeful action.

Reflexes

Primitive reflexes are subcortical and involve a whole-body response. Selected primitive reflexes present at birth include Moro, root, suck, asymmetric tonic neck, plantar and palmar grasp, step, and Babinski. Except for the Babinski, which disappears around 1 year of age, these primitive reflexes diminish over the first few months of life, giving way to protective reflexes. Protective reflexes (also termed postural responses or reflexes) are gross motor responses related to maintenance of equilibrium. These responses are prerequisites for appropriate motor development and remain throughout life once they are established. The protective reflexes include the righting and parachute reactions. Appropriate presence and disappearance of primitive reflexes, as well as development of protective reflexes, are indicative of a healthy neurologic system. Persistence of primitive reflexes beyond the usual age of disappearance may indicate an abnormality of the neurologic system and should be investigated.

Table 25.1 gives descriptions and illustrations of several primitive and protective reflexes, as well as the timing of appearance and disappearance of these reflexes.

Respiratory System

The respiratory system continues to mature over the first year of life. The respiratory rate slows from an average of 30 to 60 breaths in the newborn to about 20 to 30 in the 12-month-old. The newborn breathes irregularly, with periodic pauses. As the infant matures, the respiratory pattern becomes more regular and rhythmic.

In comparison with the adult, in the infant:

- The nasal passages are narrower.
- The trachea and chest wall are more compliant.
- The bronchi and bronchioles are shorter and narrower.
- The larynx is more funnel shaped.
- The tongue is larger.
- There are significantly fewer alveoli.

These anatomic differences place the infant at higher risk for respiratory compromise. The respiratory system does not reach adult levels of maturity until about 7 years of age. The lack of immunoglobulin A (IgA) in the mucosal lining of the upper respiratory tract also contributes to the frequent infections that occur in infancy.

Cardiovascular System

The heart doubles in size over the first year of life. As the cardiovascular system matures, the average pulse rate decreases from 120 to 140 in the newborn to about 100 in the 1-year-old. Blood pressure steadily increases over the first 12 months of life, from an average of 60/40 in the newborn to 100/50 in the 12-month-old. The peripheral

TABLE 25.1 • Select Primitive and Protective Reflexes in Infancy

	Description	Age Reflex Appears	Age Reflex Disappears
Primitive Reflexes			
Root 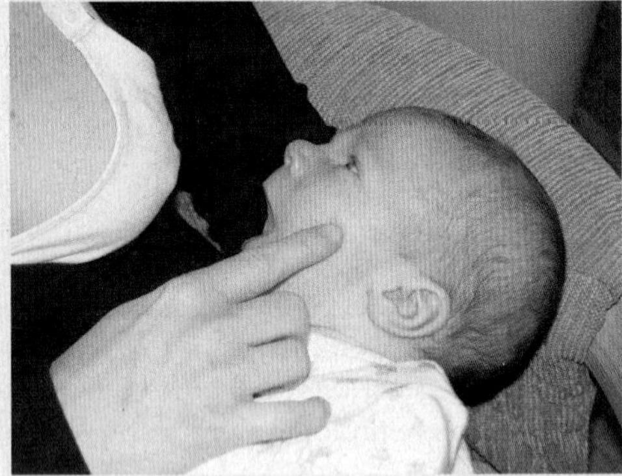	When infant's cheek is stroked, the infant turns to that side, searching with the mouth.	Birth	3 months
Suck 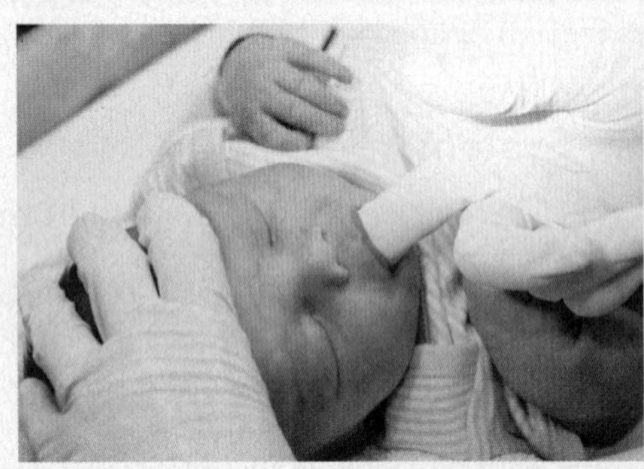	Reflexive sucking when the nipple or finger is placed in the infant's mouth	Birth	2–5 months
Moro 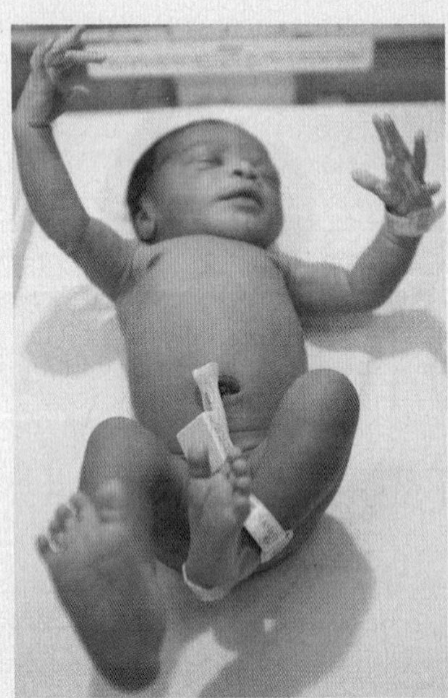	With sudden extension of the head, the arms abduct and move upward, and the hands form a "C."	Birth	4 months

TABLE 25.1 • Select Primitive and Protective Reflexes in Infancy

	Description	Age Reflex Appears	Age Reflex Disappears
Asymmetric tonic neck 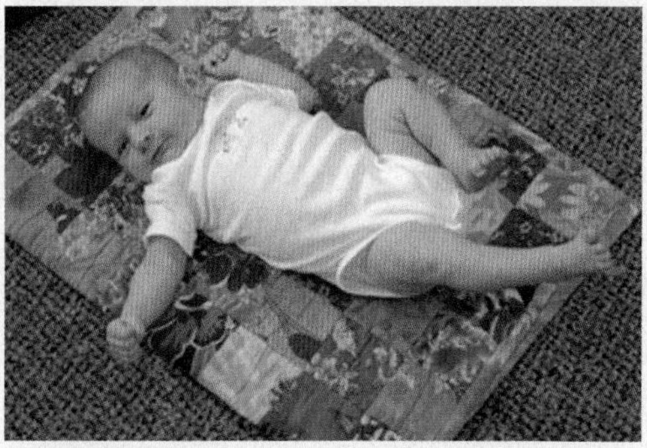	While lying supine, extremities are extended on the side of the body to which the head is turned, and opposite extremities are flexed (also called the "fencing" position).	Birth	4 months
Palmar grasp 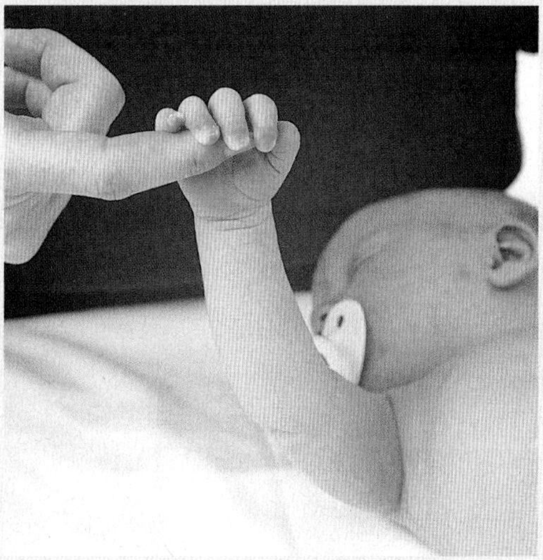	Infant reflexively grasps when the palm is touched.	Birth	4–6 months
Plantar grasp 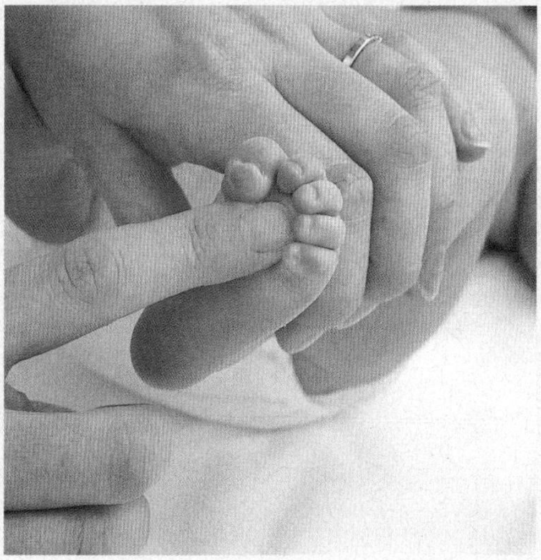	Infant reflexively grasps with the bottom of the foot when pressure is applied to the plantar surface.	Birth	9 months

(*continued*)

TABLE 25.1 • SelectPrimitive and Protective Reflexes in Infancy (*continued*)

	Description	Age Reflex Appears	Age Reflex Disappears
Babinski 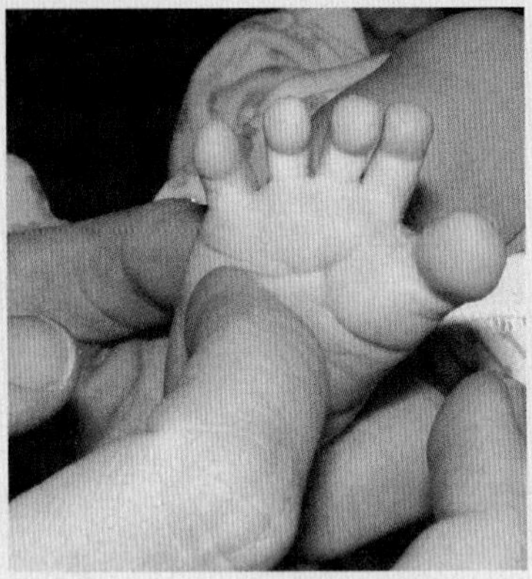	Stroking along the lateral aspect of the sole and across the plantar surface results in fanning and hyperextension of the toes.	Birth	12 months
Step 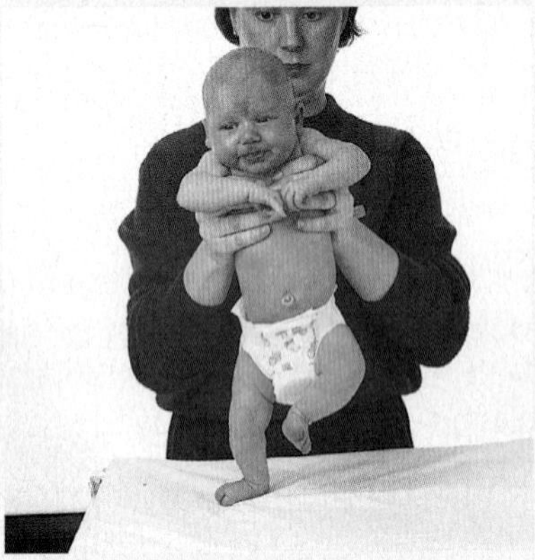	With one foot on a flat surface, the infant puts the other foot down as if to "step."	Birth	4–8 weeks
Protective Reflexes			
Neck righting	Neck keeps the head in an upright position when the body is tilted.	4–6 months	Persists
Parachute (sideways)	Protective extension with the arms when tilted to the side in a supported sitting position	6 months	Persists
Parachute (forward) 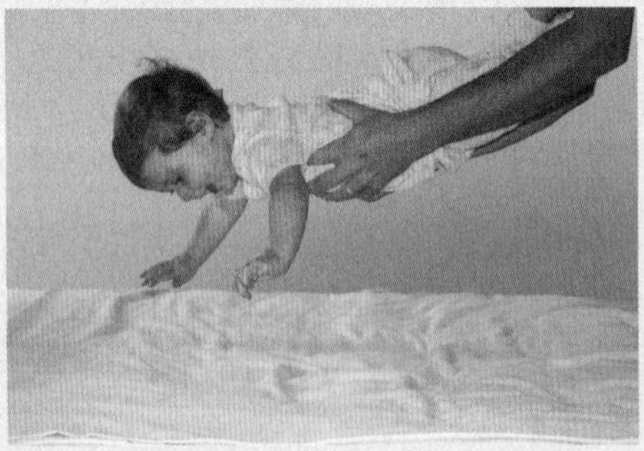	Protective extension with the arms when held up in the air and moved forward; the infant reflexively reaches forward to catch themselves.	6–7 months	Persists
Parachute (backward)	Protective extension with the arms when tilted backward	9–10 months	Persists

capillaries are closer to the surface of the skin, thus making the newborn and young infant more susceptible to heat loss. Over the first year of life, thermoregulation (the body's ability to stabilize body temperature) becomes more effective: The peripheral capillaries constrict in response to a cold environment and dilate in response to heat.

Gastrointestinal System

Teeth

The vast majority of newborns do not have teeth at birth, nor do they develop them in the first month of life. Occasionally, an infant is born with one or more teeth (termed natal teeth) or develops teeth in the first 28 days of life (termed neonatal teeth). The presence of natal or neonatal teeth may be associated with other birth anomalies. On average, the first primary teeth begin to erupt between the ages of 6 and 8 months. The primary teeth (also termed deciduous teeth) are lost later in childhood and will be replaced by the permanent teeth. The gums around the emerging tooth often swell. The lower central incisors are usually the first to appear, followed by the upper central incisors (Fig. 25.1). The average 12-month-old has four to eight teeth.

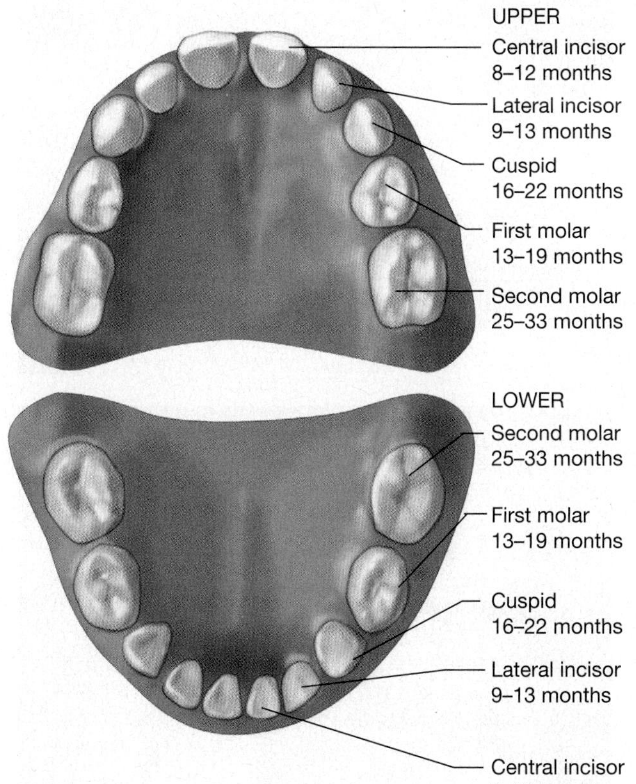

FIGURE 25.1 Sequence and average age of tooth eruption.

Digestion

The newborn's digestive system is not fully developed. Small amounts of saliva are present for the first 3 months of life, and ptyalin is present only in small amounts in the saliva. Gastric digestion occurs as a result of the presence of hydrochloric acid and rennin. The small intestine is about 270 cm (106.29 in) long and grows to the adult length by about 4 years of age (Maqbool & Liacouras, 2020). The stomach capacity is relatively small at birth, holding about 0.5 to 1 oz. However, by 1 year of age the stomach can accommodate three full meals and several snacks per day. In the duodenum, three enzymes, in particular, are important for digestion. Trypsin is available in sufficient quantities for protein digestion after birth. Amylase (needed for complex carbohydrate digestion) and lipase (essential for appropriate fat digestion) are both deficient in the infant and do not reach adult levels until about 5 months of age.

The liver is also immature at birth. The ability to conjugate bilirubin and secrete bile is present after about 2 weeks of age. Conjugation of medications may remain immature over the first year of life. Other functions of the liver, including gluconeogenesis, vitamin storage, and protein metabolism, remain immature during the first year of life.

Stools

The consistency and frequency of stools change over the first year of life. The newborn's first stools (meconium) are the result of digestion of amniotic fluid swallowed in utero. They are dark green to black and sticky (Fig. 25.2). In the first few days of life, the stools become yellowish or tan. Generally, the formula-fed infant has stools the consistency of peanut butter. Breastfed infants' stools are usually looser in texture and appear seedy. Newborns may have as many as eight to 10 stools per day or as few as one stool every day or two. After the newborn period, the number of stools may decrease, and some infants do not have a bowel movement for several days. Infrequent stooling is considered normal if the bowel movement remains soft. Due to the immaturity of the gastrointestinal system, newborns and young infants often grunt, strain, or cry while attempting to have a bowel movement. This is not of concern unless the stool is hard and dry. Stool color and texture may change depending on the foods that the infant is ingesting (Kaiser Permanente, n.d.).

> ***TAKE NOTE!***
>
> Parents should call the primary care provider if the infant's stools are red, white, or black; mucus-like; frequent and watery; frothy or foul-smelling; or hard, dry, formed, or pellet-like; or if the baby is vomiting.

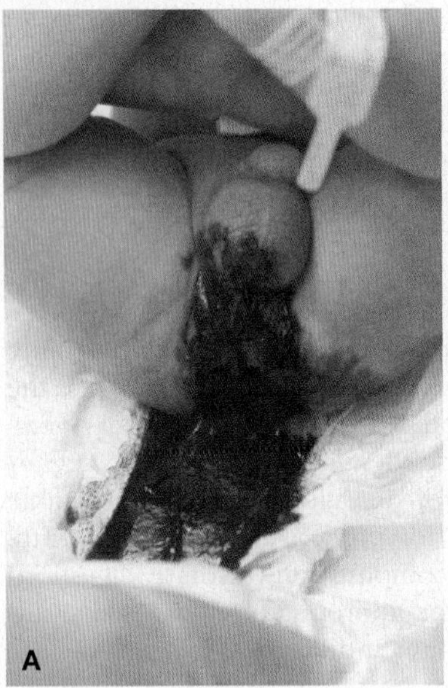

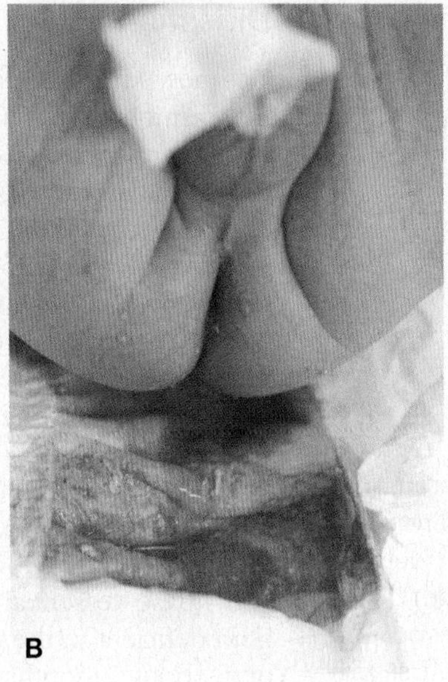

FIGURE 25.2 A. Meconium stool. **B.** Typical stool after the first few days. Note the yellowish, seedy stool of a breastfed infant.

Genitourinary System

In the infant, total body water is a greater percentage of weight than it is in the adult. Thus, the infant is more susceptible to dehydration. Over the first 12 months of life, extracellular fluid (lymph, interstitial fluid, and blood plasma) decreases, while the intracellular fluid volume increases, reaching the adult levels of 20% to 25% and 30% to 40%, respectively (Greenbaum & Londeree, 2023). Infants urinate frequently, and the urine has a relatively low specific gravity. The renal structures are immature and the glomerular filtration rate, tubular secretion, and reabsorption as well as renal perfusion are all reduced compared with those in the adult. The glomeruli reach full maturity by 2 years of age.

Integumentary System

In utero, the infant is covered with vernix caseosa, which protects the developing infant's skin. At birth, the infant may be covered with vernix (earlier gestational age), or vernix may be found in the folds of the skin, axilla, and groin areas (later gestational age). Production of vernix ceases at birth. Fine downy hair (lanugo) covers the body of many newborns. Often, this hair is lost over time and is not replaced. Darker-skinned neonates tend to have more lanugo present at birth than those with light skin.

Acrocyanosis (blueness of the hands and feet in light-skinned infants, noted on the soles and palms in darker-skinned infants) is normal in the newborn; it decreases over the first few days of life (Fig. 25.3). Newborns often experience mottling of the skin (a pink-and-white marbled appearance easily noted in light-skinned infants, more difficult to distinguish in darker-skinned infants) because of their immature circulatory system. Mottling decreases over the first few months of life (see Fig. 25.3). The newborn and young infant's skin is relatively thinner than that of the adult, with the peripheral capillaries being closer to the surface. This may cause increased absorption of topical medications.

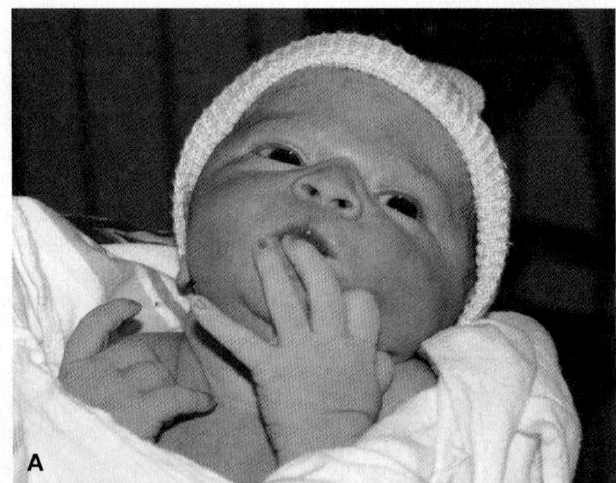

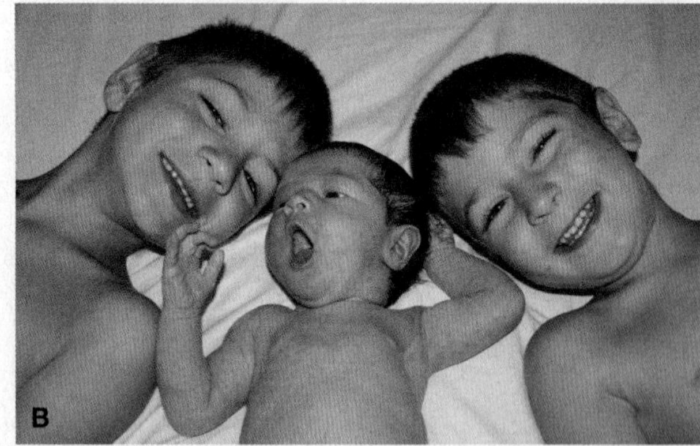

FIGURE 25.3 A. Acrocyanosis. Note blueness of the hands. **B.** Mottling of the skin in a young infant.

Hematopoietic System

Significant changes in the hematopoietic system occur over the first year of life. After birth, erythrocyte production decreases significantly, resulting in a relatively low hemoglobin and hematocrit around 2 to 3 months of age (physiologic anemia of infancy) (Nuss et al., 2022). During the last 3 months of gestation, maternal iron stores are transferred to the fetus. Healthy newborns typically have sufficient iron stores at birth. As the high hemoglobin concentration of the newborn decreases over the first 2 to 3 months, iron is reclaimed and stored. These stores may be sufficient for the first 6 to 9 months of life but will become depleted if iron intake is not sufficient (Powers, 2021).

TAKE NOTE!

Maternal iron stores are transferred to the fetus throughout the last trimester of pregnancy. Infants born prematurely miss all or at least a portion of this iron store transfer, placing them at increased risk for iron-deficiency anemia compared with term infants.

Immunologic System

Newborns receive large amounts of IgG through the placenta. This confers immunity during the first 3 to 6 months of life for antigens to which the birthing parent was previously exposed. Infants then synthesize their own IgG, reaching approximately 60% of adult levels at age 12 months (Cherry et al., 2019). IgM is produced in significant amounts after birth, reaching adult levels by 9 months of age. IgA, IgD, and IgE production increase very gradually, maturing in early childhood (Cherry et al., 2019).

PSYCHOSOCIAL DEVELOPMENT

Erik Erikson (1963) identifies the psychosocial crisis of infancy as trust versus mistrust. Development of a sense of trust is crucial in the first year, as it serves as the foundation for later psychosocial tasks. The parent or primary caregiver can have a significant impact on the infant's development of a sense of trust. When the infant's needs are consistently met, the infant develops this sense of trust. But if the parent or caregiver is inconsistent in meeting the infant's needs in a timely manner, then the infant develops a sense of mistrust. Table 25.2 lists activities that promote a sense of trust in infancy.

COGNITIVE DEVELOPMENT

The first stage of Jean Piaget's theory of cognitive development is referred to as the sensorimotor stage (birth to 2 years) (Piaget, 1969). Infants learn about themselves and the world through their developing sensory and motor capacities. Infants' development from birth to 1 year of age can be divided into four substages within the sensorimotor stage: reflexes, primary circular reactions, secondary circular reactions, and coordination of secondary schemes. Cause and effect guides most of the cognitive development seen in infancy (Table 25.2).

TABLE 25.2 • Developmental Theories

Theorist	Stage	Activities
Erikson	Trust vs. mistrust (birth to 1 year)	Caregivers respond to the infant's basic needs by feeding, changing diapers, cleaning, touching, holding, and talking to the infant. This creates a sense of trust in the infant. As the nervous system matures, infants realize they are separate beings from their caregivers. Over time, the infant learns to tolerate small amounts of frustration and trusts that although gratification may be delayed, it will eventually be provided.
Piaget	Sensorimotor (birth to 2 years)	Infant uses senses and motor skills to learn about the world.
	Substage 1: use of reflexes (birth to 1 month)	Reflexive sucking brings the pleasure of ingesting nutrition. Infant begins to gain control over reflexes and recognizes familiar objects, odors, and sounds.
	Substage 2: primary circular reactions (1–4 months)	Thumb sucking may occur by chance; then the infant repeats it on purpose to bring pleasure. Imitation begins. Object permanence begins. Infant shows affect.
	Substage 3: secondary circular reactions (4–8 months)	Infant repeats actions to achieve wanted results (e.g., shakes rattle to hear the noise it makes). The infant's actions are purposeful, but the infant does not always have an end goal in mind.
	Substage 4: coordination of secondary schemes (8–12 months)	Infants coordinate previously learned schemes with previously learned behaviors. They may grasp and shake a rattle intentionally or crawl across the room to reach a desired toy. Infant can anticipate events. Object permanence is fully present at about 8 months of age. The infant begins to associate symbols with events (e.g., waving goodbye means someone is leaving).
Freud	Oral stage (birth to 1 year)	Pleasure is focused on oral activities: feeding and sucking.

Adapted from Erikson, E. H. (1963). *Childhood and society* (2nd ed.). W. W. Norton and Company; Piaget, J. (1969). *The theory of stages in cognitive development.* McGraw-Hill; Reynolds, A., Angulo, A., Breheney, M., Green, J., & Goldson, E. (2022). Child development and behavior. In M. Bunik, W. W. Hay, M. J. Levin, & M. J. Abzug (Eds.), *Current diagnosis & treatment: Pediatrics* (26th ed.). McGraw-Hill Education.

The concept of **object permanence** begins to develop between 4 and 7 months of age and is solidified by about 8 months of age (Piaget, 1969). If an object is hidden from the infant's sight, the infant will search for it in the last place it was seen, knowing it still exists. This development of object permanence is essential for the development of self-image. By age 12 months, the infant knows they are separate from the parent or caregiver. Self-image is also promoted through the use of mirrors. By 12 months of age, infants can recognize themselves in the mirror. The 12-month-old will explore objects in different ways, such as throwing, banging, dropping, and shaking. The infant may imitate gestures and knows how to use certain objects correctly (e.g., puts phone to ear, turns up cup to drink, attempts to comb hair) (Piaget, 1969).

MOTOR SKILL DEVELOPMENT

Infants exhibit phenomenal increases in their gross and fine motor skills over the first 12 months of life.

Gross Motor Skills

The term "gross motor skills" refers to those that use the large muscles (e.g., head control, rolling, sitting, and walking). Gross motor skills develop in a **cephalocaudal** fashion (from the head to the tail) (Fig. 25.4). In other words, the baby learns to lift the head before learning to roll over and sit (Reynolds et al., 2022). At birth, babies have poor head control and need to have their necks supported when being held. They can lift their heads only slightly while in a prone position. Over the next several months, the infant's motor skills progress at a dramatic rate. First, the infant achieves head control, then the ability to roll over, sit, crawl, pull to stand, and, usually around 1 year of age, walk independently. Table 25.3 gives details on when the infant develops each specific gross motor skill. Progression of gross motor skills is illustrated in Figures 25.5 through 25.7.

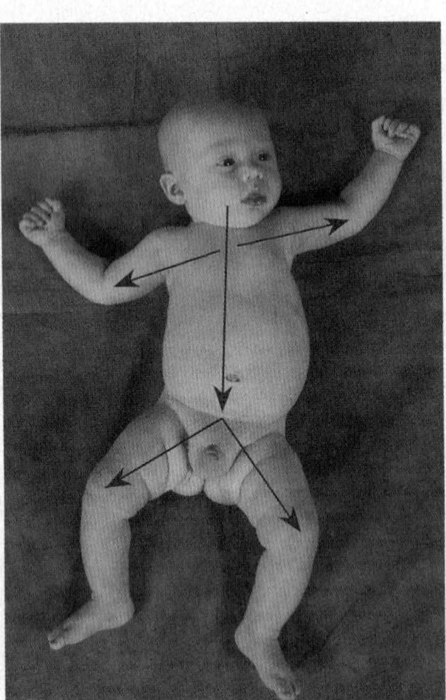

FIGURE 25.4 Gross motor skills develop in a cephalocaudal direction, fine motor skills in a proximodistal fashion.

TAKE NOTE!

Warning signs that may indicate problems with motor development include the following: arms and legs are stiff or floppy; child cannot support head at 3 to 4 months of age; child reaches with one hand only; child cannot sit with assistance at 6 months of age; child does not crawl by 12 months of age; child cannot stand supported by 12 months of age.

Fine Motor Skills

Fine motor development includes the maturation of hand and finger use. Fine motor skills develop in a **proximodistal** fashion (from the center to the periphery) (see Fig. 25.4). In other words, the infant first bats with the whole hand, eventually progressing to gross grasping, before being capable of fine fingertip grasping (Reynolds et al., 2022) (Fig. 25.8). The newborn's hand movements

TABLE 25.3 • Key Gross Motor Skills in Infancy

Age (months)	Gross Motor Skills
2	Holds head up when prone Moves all four extremities
4	Holds head steady without support When prone, pushes up on forearms/elbows
6	Rolls from prone to supine Tripod sits When prone, uses arms to push up straight
9	Sits unsupported Gets to sitting on own
12	Pulls to stand Cruises (walks holding onto furniture)

Adapted from Centers for Disease Control and Prevention. (2022b). *CDC's developmental milestones.* http://www.cdc.gov/ncbddd/actearly/milestones/index.html; Zubler, J. M., Wiggins, L. D., Macias, M. M., Whitaker, T. M., Shaw, J. S., Squires, J. K., Pajke, J. A., Wolf, R. B., Slaughter, K. S., Broughton, A. S., Gerndt, K. L., Mlodoch, B. J., & Lipkin, P. H. (2022). Evidence-informed milestones for developmental surveillance tools. *Pediatrics, 149*(3), e2021052138. https://doi.org/10.1542/peds.2021-052138

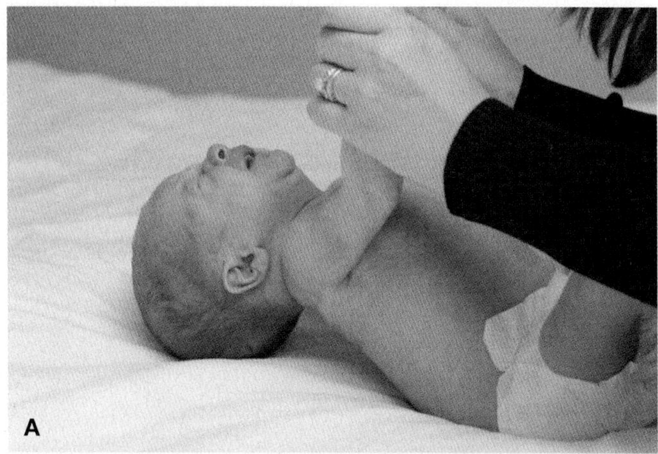

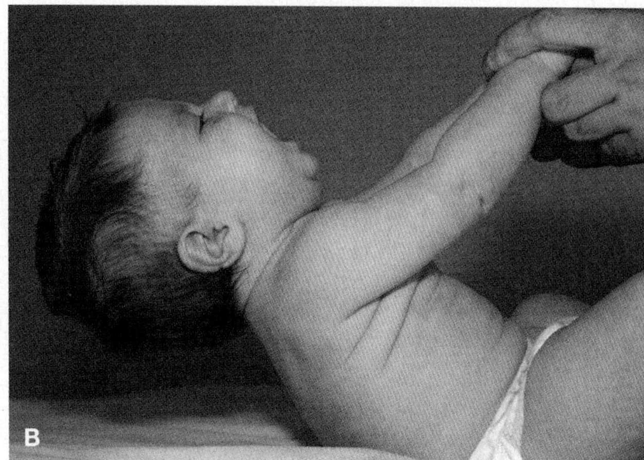

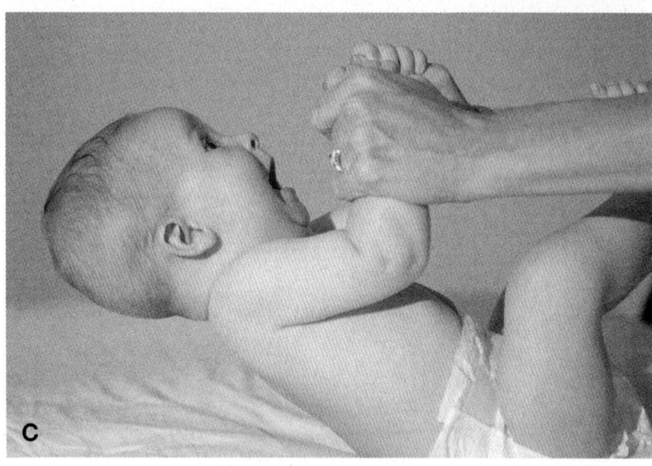

FIGURE 25.5 When pulled to sit, an infant shows significant head lag (newborn; 2 or 3 weeks old) (**A**), improving head control (2 months old) (**B**), and no head lag (4 months old) (**C**).

are involuntary in nature, whereas the 12-month-old is capable of feeding themselves with a cup and spoon. By 12 months of age, the infant should be able to eat with their fingers and assist with dressing (e.g., pushing an arm through the sleeve). Table 25.4 provides details on when the infant develops each specific fine motor skill.

SENSORY DEVELOPMENT

Although hearing should be fully developed at birth, the other senses continue to develop as the infant matures. Although they mature at different rates, sight, smell, taste, and touch all continue to develop after birth.

Sight

The newborn is nearsighted, preferring to view objects at a distance of 20 to 38 cm (8 to 15 in). Newborns prefer the human face to other objects and may even imitate the facial expressions made by those caring for them. In addition to human faces, newborns show a preference for certain objects, particularly those with contrasts such as black-and-white stripes. The newborn's eyes wander and occasionally cross. At 1 month of age, the infant can recognize by sight the people the infant knows best. The infant will study objects within their visual range closely. The ability to fuse two ocular images into one cerebral picture (**binocularity**) begins to develop at 6 weeks of age and is well established by 4 months of age. Full color vision develops by 7 months of age, as do distance vision and the ability to track objects.

Hearing

The newborn's hearing is intact at birth and as acute as that of an adult. Newborns prefer the sound of human voices to nonhuman sounds. By 1 month of age, the infant can recognize the sounds of people the infant knows best.

Smell and Taste

The sense of smell develops rapidly: The 7-day-old infant can differentiate the smell of their lactating parent's breast milk from that of another and will preferentially turn toward their parent's smell. Newborns prefer sweet tastes to all others. This persists for several months, and, eventually, the infant will accept nonsweet flavors.

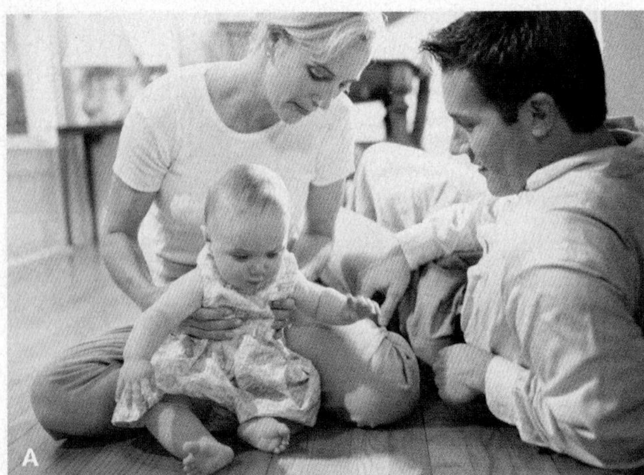

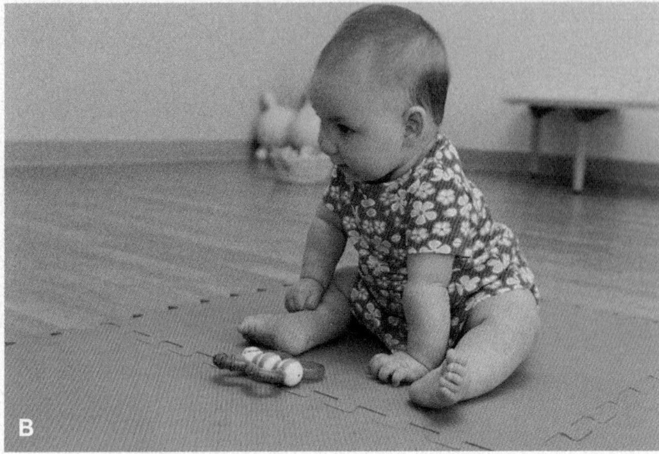

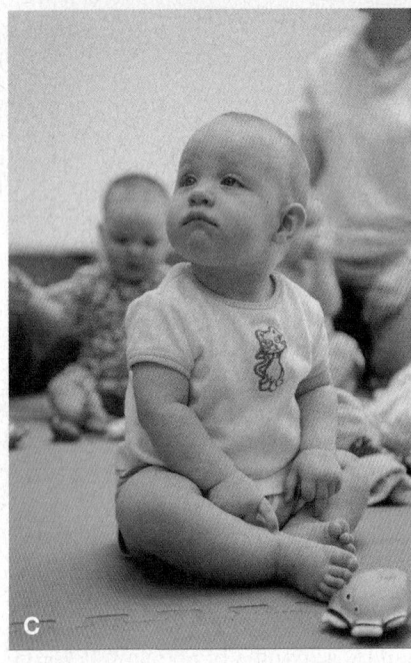

FIGURE 25.6 Development of sitting. **A.** At 4 months, the infant requires significant support. **B.** The 6-month-old infant sits in tripod fashion. **C.** The 8-month-old sits alone.

Touch

The sense of touch is perhaps the most important of all the senses for newborn communication. Even the most immature infant responds to soothing stroking. The infant prefers soft sensations to coarse sensations. The infant dislikes rough handling and may cry. Holding, stroking, rocking, or cuddling calms infants when they are upset and makes them more alert when they are drowsy. Infants learn to understand their caregiver's moods by the way they touch them.

TAKE NOTE!

Warning signs that may indicate problems with sensory development include the following: young infant does not respond to loud noises; child does not focus on a near object; infant does not start to make sounds or babble by 4 months of age; infant does not turn to locate sound at age 4 months; infant crosses eyes most of the time at age 6 months.

COMMUNICATION AND LANGUAGE DEVELOPMENT

For several months, crying is the only means of communication for the newborn and infant. The basic reason for crying is unmet needs. The 2-month-old baby reacts to loud sounds, coos, makes other vocalizations, and demonstrates differentiated crying. At 4 to 5 months of age, the infant makes simple vowel sounds, vocalizes in response to voices, and laughs aloud. The 6-month-old performs "raspberries," and squeals (in joy or displeasure). At age 9 months, babbling occurs in strings (e.g., mamama, dadada) without meaning, and the infant lifts their arms to be picked up. At 9 to 12 months of age, the infant begins to attach meaning to "mama" and "dada" and starts to imitate other speech sounds. The 12-month-old also babbles with inflection (this babbling has the rhythm and timing of spoken language, but few of the "words" make sense) (Reynolds et al., 2022; Zubler et al., 2022).

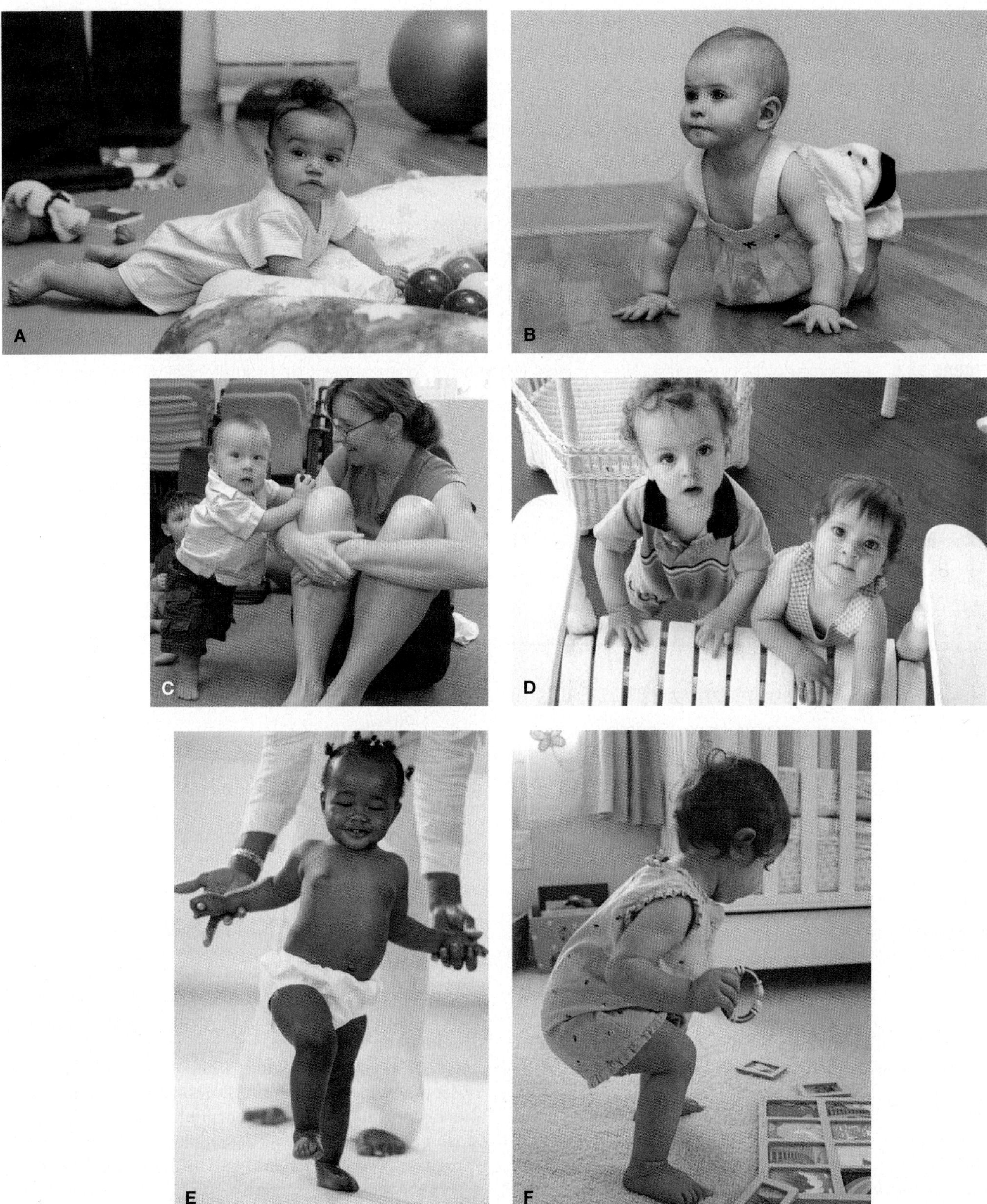

FIGURE 25.7 Development of locomotion. **A.** At 4 months, the infant pushes up from a prone position. **B.** At 8 months of age, the infant crawls with the abdomen off the floor. **C.** The infant pulls to stand by 10 months of age. **D.** The infant cruises along furniture or **(E)** takes steps with assistance at 10 to 11 months of age. **F.** The infant independently stands from a crouched position and walks around 12 months of age (+/− 3 months).

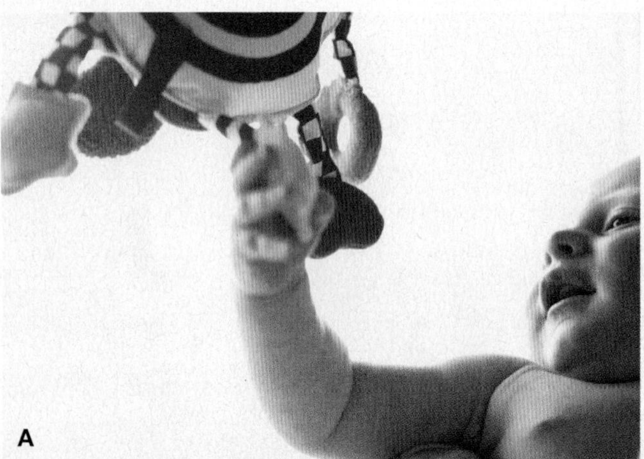

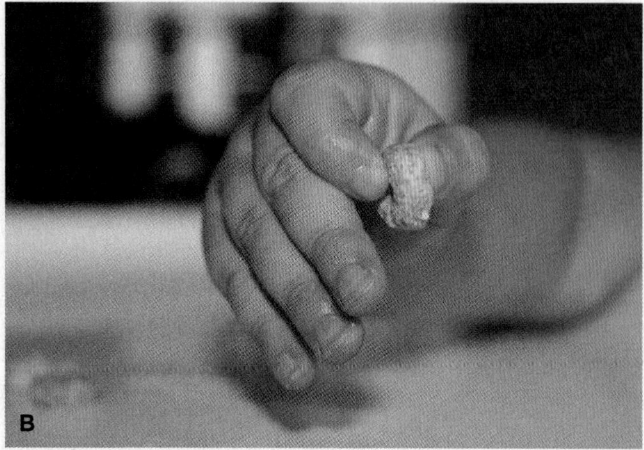

FIGURE 25.8 Development of the pincer grasp. Note the gross (whole-hand) approach to grasping a small object (**A**), compared with the fine (thumb-to-finger) ability (**B**).

TABLE 25.4 • Key Fine Motor Skills in Infancy

Age (months)	Fine Motor Skills
2	Briefly opens hands
4	Bats at objects Holds toy when put in hand Brings hands to mouth
6	Reaches for desired item
9	Gross pincer grasp (rakes) Transfers objects from one hand to the other
12	Fine pincer grasp

Adapted from Centers for Disease Control and Prevention. (2022b). *CDC's developmental milestones.* http://www.cdc.gov/ncbddd/actearly/milestones/index.html; Zubler, J. M., Wiggins, L. D., Macias, M. M., Whitaker, T. M., Shaw, J. S., Squires, J. K., Pajke, J. A., Wolf, R. B., Slaughter, K. S., Broughton, A. S., Gerndt, K. L., Mlodoch, B. J., & Lipkin, P. H. (2022). Evidence-informed milestones for developmental surveillance tools. *Pediatrics, 149*(3), e2021052138. https://doi.org/10.1542/peds.2021-052138

It is very important for the parent or caregiver to talk to the infant in order for the infant to learn communication skills. Sometimes, regression in language development occurs briefly when the child is focusing energy on other skills, such as crawling or walking. As long as the infant's hearing is normal, language acquisition should continue to progress. Infants in bilingual families may "language mix" (uses some words from each language). This is considered to be a normal progression in language development for these children (Linguistic Society of America, 2023), but it makes it more difficult for the health care provider or nurse practitioner to determine delays in communication skills.

TAKE NOTE!

Warning signs that may indicate problems in language development are as follows: infant does not make sounds at 4 months of age; infant does not laugh or squeal by 6 months of age; infant does not babble by 8 months of age; infant does not use single words with meaning at 12 months of age ("mama," "dada").

As you assess Allison (the 6-month-old introduced at the beginning of the chapter), what would you expect her gross motor, fine motor, and language skills to be at this age? How would this be different if Allison had been born 8 weeks premature?

SOCIAL AND EMOTIONAL DEVELOPMENT

The newborn spends much of the time sleeping, but by 2 months of age, the infant is ready to start socializing. The infant exhibits a first real smile at age 2 months and spends a great deal of time while awake watching and observing what is going on. By about 4 months of age, the infant will start an interaction with a caregiver by smiling widely and possibly gurgling. This prompts the caregiver to smile back and talk to the infant. The infant responds with more smiling, cooing, and gurgles as well as moving the arms and legs. The 4-month-old will also smile, chuckle, and move or vocalize to get the caregiver's attention. The baby may hesitate at first, but once the other person responds pleasantly to the infant, the infant engages and gets into the interaction. The infant may cry when the pleasant interaction stops. At 6 months of age, the infant knows familiar people, likes to look at themselves in the mirror, and laughs aloud (Zubler et al., 2022).

Stranger Anxiety

Around the age of 9 months, the infant may develop **stranger anxiety**. The previously happy and very friendly infant may become clingy and whiny when approached by strangers or people not well known. Stranger anxiety is an indicator that the infant is recognizing themselves as separate from others. As the infant becomes more aware of new people and new places, they may view an interaction with a stranger as threatening and may start crying, even if the parent is right there. Family members whom the child sees infrequently, as well as others the child does not spend a lot of time with, should approach the infant calmly and slowly, with the parent in sight. Sometimes, this will prevent a sudden crying spell (Branchford & Levine, 2023; Zubler et al., 2022).

Separation Anxiety

Separation anxiety may also start in the last few months of infancy. The infant becomes quite distressed when the parent leaves. The infant will eventually calm down and become engaged with the current caregiver. It is not until the infant is older that cognition and memory are sufficient for them to understand that the parent will come back (Reynolds et al., 2022).

TAKE NOTE!

Warning signs of possible problems with social/emotional development include: child does not smile at people at 3 months of age; child refuses to cuddle; child does not seem to enjoy people; child shows no interest in peek-a-boo at 8 months of age.

Temperament

Temperament is an individual's nature; it is the child's inborn traits that determine how they interact with the world (Child Development Institute [CDI], 2019). Temperament ranges from low or moderately active, regular, and predictable to highly active, more intense, and less adaptable. These are all considered normal along a continuum. An infant's innate temperament affects the way they respond to the environment. As parents take note of their infant's usual activity level, how intensely they react with others and the environment, and how stimulated they become with interactions, parents start to learn about their infant's temperament. The parent should note how adaptable and flexible the infant is as well as how predictable and persistent the baby is.

When parents are familiar with how the baby approaches life on a routine basis, they will be better able to recognize when the baby is not acting like themselves. Nurses can help parents interpret observations about their infant's temperament and recommend ways to support the infant's individual behavior. Some infants are slower to warm up than others; those infants should be approached slowly and calmly. Some infants exhibit increased levels of activity compared with quieter, more passive babies; those infants generally require more direct play with the parent or caregiver and will be the type of older infant who is in constant motion. Some infants are loud and some are not. The quiet infant may become overwhelmed with excessive stimulation, whereas the very active baby may need additional stimulation to be satisfied. Becoming familiar with the infant's temperament also helps the parents describe the best approach to the infant by others (e.g., child care workers or health care professionals) (CDI, 2019).

CULTURAL INFLUENCES ON GROWTH AND DEVELOPMENT

Many cultural differences have an impact on growth and development. For instance, certain groups tend to be shorter than others because of their genetic makeup (Sinha, 2021). These children will not grow to be as tall as those of another background that doesn't share the same genetic makeup. Cultural feeding practices in some cultures may lead to excess weight in some children. Some cultures and certain religions advocate for vegetarianism; those children need nutritional assessment to ensure they are getting enough protein intake for adequate growth.

Parenting styles and health promotion behaviors can also be significantly influenced by culture. Parents and extended family are the most significant influences in an infant's life in most cultures. Certain cultures place a high value on independence and may encourage their infants to develop quickly, while other cultures "baby" their infants for longer periods. Different cultures assign responsibility to major health-related decisions to different family members.

Health beliefs are often strongly influenced by an individual's religious or spiritual background. Sometimes, this creates conflict in the health care setting when the health providers have a different value system than that of the infant's family.

In some cultures, infants and children share a bed with their parents. When an infant or child is hospitalized and is accustomed to sleeping with the parents, it may be difficult and distressing for them to try to sleep alone.

The nurse should explore the family's cultural practices related to growth and development. Usually, these practices are not harmful and can be supported by the health care team, but safety must always be considered. The nurse should not make assumptions about a family's cultural practices based on their appearance or background; rather, the nurse should perform an adequate assessment for each individual and family (Centers for Disease Control and Prevention [CDC], 2021).

TAKE NOTE!

Many communities include people from a variety of cultures, so it is important for nurses to practice transcultural nursing (nursing care that is directed by cultural aspects and that respects the individual's differences). Many nurse researchers are exploring the cultural aspects of health care and the impact that cultural diversity has on health.

THE NURSE'S ROLE IN NEWBORN AND INFANT GROWTH AND DEVELOPMENT

Growth and development affect every aspect of the infant's life. As infants progress through various stages of development, they do so in a predictable fashion. Growth and development are sequential and orderly, although some children develop at faster rates than others. It is important for the nurse to understand growth and development. Health care visits through infancy often focus primarily on **anticipatory guidance** (educating parents and caregivers about what to expect in the next phase of development). The purpose of anticipatory guidance is to give parents the tools they need to support their infant's development in a safe fashion.

Clinical Judgment and the Nursing Process

After the infant's current growth and development status has been assessed, problems related to growth and development may be identified. The nurse may then identify one or more nursing diagnoses. The following nursing diagnoses with identified outcomes and interventions provide suggestions for nursing care planning or concept mapping. Care planning should be individualized based on the infant's and family's needs.

Nursing Analysis

Breastfeeding difficulty related to insufficient parental knowledge regarding breastfeeding techniques or the importance of breastfeeding, inadequate infant opportunity for breast suckling, inadequate milk supply, or parental ambivalence or anxiety as evidenced by insufficient infant weight gain or sustained weight loss, infant resistance to latching onto breast, or infant inability to correctly latch onto breast

Goal/Outcome

Lactating parent/infant dyad will experience successful breastfeeding: Infant will latch on, suck, and swallow at the breast; lactating parent will not experience sore nipples.

Promoting Effective Breastfeeding (interventions with *rationale*)

- Educate lactating parent on recognition of and response to infant hunger cues *to promote on-cue breastfeeding, which will establish milk supply.*
- Educate lactating parent on appropriate diet and fluid intake *to ensure ability to manufacture adequate supply of breast milk.*
- Demonstrate breastfeeding positions with infant at the breast (*appropriate positioning increases probability of successful latch*).
- Assess infant's latch technique, sucking motion, and audible swallowing (*an appropriately latched infant will take most of the areola in the mouth, suck in spurts, and demonstrate audible swallowing*).
- Assess infant voiding/stool patterns: *at least six voids per day and passage of stool ranging from one or more per day to one every several days is a normal pattern for breastfed infants.*
- Assess infant weight gain; *gain of 15 to 30 g per day after the second week of life indicates infant is receiving appropriate nutrition.*
- Assess lactating parent's nipples for redness or soreness; *if infant appropriately latches on, nipples will not become sore.*

Nursing Analysis

Desire for improved nutrition as evidenced by caregiver expression of readiness to enhance infant's nutrition.

Goal/Outcome

Infant will demonstrate adequate growth and appropriate feeding behaviors: steady increases in weight, length, and head circumference; infant feeds appropriately for age.

Promoting Enhanced Nutrition (interventions with *rationale*)

- Observe lactating parent/infant dyad breastfeeding or bottle-feeding *to determine need for further education or identify infant difficulties with feeding.*
- Educate parent about appropriate breastfeeding or bottle-feeding *so that they are aware of what to expect in normal feeding pattern.*

- When infant is old enough, provide education about addition of solid foods, spoon, and cup feeding: *after 6 months of age, breast milk or formula needs to be supplemented with a variety of foods.*
- Determine need for additional caloric intake if necessary (*premature infants and infants with chronic illnesses or metabolic disorders often need adjustments in caloric intake to demonstrate adequate or catch-up growth*).
- Obtain daily weights if hospitalized (weekly if outpatient) and weekly length and head circumference *to determine whether nutritional intake is sufficient to promote adequate growth.*

Nursing Analysis

Alteration in nutritional status related to insufficient dietary intake, as evidenced by failure to gain weight or by inadequate increases in weight, length, and head circumference over time.

Goal/Outcome

Infant will take in adequate nutrients using effective feeding pattern: Infant will demonstrate adequate weight gain (15 to 30 g/day) and steady increases in length and head circumference.

Promoting Adequate Nutritional Intake (interventions with *rationale*)

- Assess current feeding pattern and daily intake *to determine areas of concern.*
- Increase frequency of breastfeeding or volume of bottle-feeding *if needed to meet caloric needs.*
- Introduce solid foods on age-appropriate schedule: *introducing solids at the right time improves the chances that the child will learn to take solid foods.*
- Limit juice intake or discontinue altogether (*juice has little nutritive value and displaces nutrients from breast milk or formula*).
- Use human milk fortifier (if ordered) *to increase caloric density of breast milk.*
- Increase caloric density of formula (if ordered) by mixing to a more concentrated level or with additives (fats or carbohydrates) *to provide increased calories needed to support adequate growth.*
- If infant is taking solids already, choose higher-calorie foods *to maximize nutrient intake.*

Nursing Analysis

Altered attachment risk; risk factors include premature infant, disordered infant behavior and/or resulting parental conflict, or parental substance misuse.

Goal/Outcome

Parent and infant will demonstrate appropriate attachment via eye contact, parental response to infant cues, parental verbalization of caring for infant, and infant response to parent's caregiving behaviors.

Encouraging Appropriate Parent–Infant Attachment (interventions with *rationale*)

- Assess parent's response to infant cues *to determine degree of attachment and level of parent's knowledge about infant care.*
- Assess infant's response to parent's caregiving behaviors *to determine degree of attachment.*
- Determine infant's temperament *to counsel parent effectively about responses appropriate for that type of temperament.*
- Encourage en face positioning for holding or feeding the young infant *to encourage give-and-take response between infant and parent.*
- Encourage parent to meet infant's needs promptly and with affection *to promote sense of trust in the infant.*
- Reinforce parent's attempts at improving attachment with infant (*positive reinforcement naturally encourages appropriate behaviors*).

Nursing Analysis

Delayed growth and development risk; risk factors include prematurity, chronic illness, impaired attachment, or failure to thrive.

Goal/Outcome

Development will be maximized: Infant will make continued progress toward attainment of developmental milestones.

Maximizing Development (interventions with *rationale*)

- Perform developmental evaluation of the infant *to determine infant's current level of functioning.*
- Offer age-appropriate play, activities, and toys *to encourage further development.*
- Carry out interventions as prescribed by developmental specialist, physical therapist, occupational therapist, or speech therapist (*repeated exposure to the activities or exercises is needed to make developmental progress*).
- Provide support to parents of infants with developmental concerns, *as developmental progress can be slow and it is difficult for families to stay motivated and maintain hope.*

Nursing Analysis

Caregiver fatigue risk; risk factors include inexperience with caregiving, insufficient assistance, and not being developmentally ready for caregiving role.

Goal/Outcome

Parent will experience competence in role: will demonstrate appropriate caregiving behaviors and verbalize comfort in new role.

Preventing Caregiver Fatigue (interventions with *rationale*)

- Assess parent's knowledge of newborn/infant care and the issues that arise as a part of normal development *to determine parent's needs.*

- Provide education on normal newborn/infant care *so that parents have the knowledge they need to appropriately care for their new baby.*
- Provide anticipatory guidance related to normal infant development *to prepare parents for what to expect next and how to intervene.*
- Encourage respite for parents (*even a few hours away from the demands of an infant's care can rejuvenate the parents*).

Nursing Analysis

Injury risk; risk factors include extremes of age, infant curiosity, rapidly progressing motor abilities, or unsafe mode of transport.

Goal/Outcome

Infant safety will be maintained: Infant will remain free from injury.

Preventing Injury (interventions with *rationale*)

- Encourage car seat safety *to decrease risk of injury related to motor vehicles.*
- Childproof home; *as infant becomes more mobile, they will want to explore everything, increasing risk of injury.*
- Parents should have the Poison Control Center phone number available; *should an inadvertent ingestion occur, Poison Control can give parents the best advice for appropriate intervention.*
- Never leave an infant unattended in the sink, bathtub, or swimming pool *to prevent drowning.*
- Teach parents first aid measures and infant cardiopulmonary resuscitation (CPR) *to minimize consequences of injury should it occur.*
- Parents should watch the infant at all times (*no amount of childproofing can replace the watchful eye of a caring parent*).

PROMOTING HEALTHY GROWTH AND DEVELOPMENT

Adding a new person to the family produces both excitement and anxiety. Newborns are completely reliant on their parents or caregivers to fill every need. It is quite a burden and precious responsibility that new parents are taking on. Many parents read the latest books about caring for newborns, while others rely on information received from family and friends. Newborns and their parents spend only a short time in the hospital after delivery, so it is important that parents can care for their newborn and know when to call the primary care provider with concerns.

Periodic screening for adequate growth and development is recommended by the American Academy of Pediatrics (AAP) for all infants and children. The prevention of devastating disease is another priority for infants and children. The AAP and the Advisory Committee on Immunization Practices (ACIP) have made recommendations for immunization schedules. Immunizations are a very important part of the newborn's and infant's health visits. Nurses caring for newborns and infants should be familiar with the recommended infant/child periodic screenings (check-ups) as well as the current immunization schedule (see Chapter 31 for further information on immunizations).

Promoting Growth and Development Through Play

Experts in child development and behavior have said repeatedly that play is the work of children. Infants practice their gross and fine motor skills and language through play (Reynolds et al., 2022). Play is a natural way for infants and children to learn. Play is critical to infant development, as it gives infants the opportunity to explore their environment, practice new skills, and solve problems. The newborn prefers interacting with the parent to toys. Parents can talk to and sing to their newborns while participating in the daily activities that infants need, such as feeding, bathing, and changing diapers. Newborns and young infants love to watch people's faces and often appear to mimic the expressions they see.

As infants become older, toys may be geared toward the motor skills or language skills that the child is developing. Parents can promote fine motor development in infants by providing age-appropriate toys. For example, a rattle that a young infant can hold promotes reaching and attaining. The older infant builds fine motor skills by stacking cups or placing smaller toys inside of larger ones. Gross motor skills are reinforced and practiced over and over again when the infant wants to reach something they are interested in.

When playing with toys, the infant usually engages in **solitary play**; they do not share with other infants or directly play with other infants (Reynolds et al., 2022). A wide variety of toys are available for infants, but infants often enjoy the most basic ones, such as plastic containers of various shapes and sizes, soft balls, and wooden or plastic spoons. Books are also very important toys for infants. Reading to all ages of infants is appropriate, and the older infant develops fine motor skills by learning to turn book pages. Table 25.5 lists age-appropriate toys.

Promoting Early Learning

Research has shown that reading aloud and sharing books during early infancy are critical to the development of neural networks that are important in the later tasks of reading and word recognition. Reading books increases listening comprehension. Infants

TABLE 25.5 • Appropriate Toys for Newborns and Infants

Age	Appropriate Toys
Newborn to 1 month	Mobile with contrasting colors or patterns Unbreakable mirror Soft music Soft, brightly colored toys
1–4 months	Bright mobile Unbreakable mirror Rattles Singing by parent or caregiver, varied music High-contrast patterns in books or images
4–7 months	Fabric or board books Different types of music Easy-to-hold toys that do things or make noise (fancy rattles) Floating, squirting bath toys Soft dolls or animals
8–12 months	Plastic cups, bowls, buckets Unbreakable mirror Large building blocks Stacking toys Busy boxes (with buttons or knobs that make things happen) Balls Dolls Board books with large pictures Toy telephone Push–pull toys (older infants)

Adapted from National Association for the Education of Young Children. (n.d.). *Good toys for young children by age and stage.* http://www.naeyc.org/toys

demonstrate their excitement about picture books by kicking and waving their arms and babbling when looking at them. At 6 to 12 months, the infant reaches for books and brings them to the mouth. Over time, reading leads to acquisition of language skills. Reading picture books and simple stories to infants starts a good habit that should be continued throughout childhood (Lewis, 2019).

Promoting Safety

Hundreds of children younger than 1 year of age die each year as a result of injury (AAP, 2018a). As infants become more mobile, they risk injury from falls down stairs and off chairs, tables, and other structures. Curiosity leads the infant to explore potentially dangerous items, such as electrical outlets, hot stove or furnace vents, mop buckets, and toilets. Since infants explore so much with their mouths, small objects or hard foods pose a choking hazard. The infant will invariably pick up any accessible object and bring it to the mouth. With increasing dexterity, poisoning from medications, household cleaning products, or other substances also becomes a problem.

Safety in the Car

Motor vehicle crashes are one source of injury, particularly if the infant is improperly restrained. Infants should never be transported in a motor vehicle without proper restraint. Infant car seats should face the rear of the car throughout infancy (Smola et al., 2020). The car seat should be secured tightly in the center of the back seat. The infant should never be placed in a front seat that is equipped with an airbag.

Infants should never be left unattended in a motor vehicle. The temperature rises very quickly inside a closed vehicle, and an infant can suffocate from heat in a closed vehicle in the summer. Even during cooler weather, the heat generated within a closed vehicle can reach three to five times the exterior temperature. Kidnapping is also a concern if the baby is left unattended in a vehicle.

Safety in the Home

The baby's crib should have a firm mattress that fits snugly in the crib on a secure support. The distance between crib slats should be no wider than a soda can (6 cm [2.36 in] or less) to prevent injury (Safe Kids Worldwide, 2023). All crib edges should be smooth. Only well-fitting crib sheets should be used, not sheets intended for large beds. Crib side rails should always be raised when the parent is not right next to the crib.

Even before the infant can roll over, the baby wiggles and pushes with the feet. The infant can easily fall from a changing table, sofa, or crib with the side rails down, so the infant should never be left unattended on any surface. If infant seats, bouncy seats, or swings are used, the infant should always be restrained in the seat with the appropriate straps.

The AAP (2022) does not recommend the use of infant walkers, because the walker may tip over, and the baby may fall out of it or the infant may fall down the stairs in it. Walkers allow infants access to things they may not otherwise be capable of reaching until they are able to walk alone, such as hot stoves and items on the edge of the countertop.

As the infant becomes more mobile, learning to crawl and walk, new safety issues arise. Safety gates should be used at the tops and bottoms of stairways. Gates may also be used to block curious infants from rooms that may pose physical danger to them because of sharp-edged furniture or decorative objects. Electrical outlets should be covered with approved safety covers. Cabinets and drawers should be secured with child safety latches. Medications, household cleaning supplies, and other potentially hazardous substances should be stored completely out of reach of infants (AAP, 2018a).

Choking is a risk because infants immediately bring small items to the mouth for exploration. To avoid choking, recommend the following to parents:

- Use only toys recommended for children of 0 to 12 months of age.
- Avoid stuffed animals with eyes or buttons that can be dislodged by the persistent infant.
- Keep the floor free of small items (unintentionally dropped coins, paper clips, straight pins).
- Avoid feeding popcorn, nuts, carrot slices, grapes, and hot dog pieces to infants.

Suffocation is also a risk for infants. Cribs should not have pillows, comforters, stuffed animals, or other soft items in them. Keep plastic bags of any size away from infants. Avoid the risk of strangulation by keeping window blind and drapery cords out of the infant's reach (AAP, 2017, 2018a).

Although no safety measure is as effective as close supervision by a watchful parent or caregiver, the aforementioned safety measures can be critical to the infant's well-being.

Safety in the Water

Infants can drown in a small amount of water. Never leave an infant unattended in the sink, a baby bathtub or standard bathtub, a swimming or wading pool, or any other body of water, even if it is quite shallow. The bathroom door should be kept closed and the toilet lid down. Water should be emptied from tubs, pails, or buckets immediately after use. If the family has a swimming pool, a locked fence or locked screen enclosure should surround it. Exterior doors should be kept locked to prevent the older infant from wandering out to the pool (AAP, 2018a). The AAP recommends that parents use caution when enrolling their infant in an aquatic or swim program. Research has not sufficiently demonstrated that water survival skills taught to infants are effective (AAP, 2019). Completing an aquatic program does not decrease the risk of drowning; vigilant supervision is still always required.

> Remember Allison Johnson, the infant described at the beginning of the chapter? What anticipatory guidance related to safety would you provide to Allison's parents?

Promoting Nutrition

Adequate nutrition is essential for growth and development. Breastfeeding and bottle-feeding of infant formula are both acceptable means of nutrition in the newborn and infant. Breast milk or formula supplies all of the infant's daily nutritional requirements until 6 months of age, at which time solid foods may be introduced (Buchanan & Marquez, 2023).

Cultural Factors

Many dietary practices are affected by culture, both in the types of food eaten and in the approach to progression of infant feeding. Some groups tend to be lactose intolerant (particularly Black, Native American, and Asian individuals); therefore, alternative sources of calcium must be offered. Explore the cultural practices of the family related to infant feeding so that you can support the family's cultural values.

Nutritional Needs

Newborns and infants are experiencing tremendous growth and need diets that support these rapid changes. Table 25.6 compares fluid and caloric needs in the newborn and infant.

Breastfeeding

The National Association of Pediatric Nurse Practitioners (NAPNAP), the AAP, the American College of Obstetrics and Gynecology, the American Dietetic Association, and the U.S. Breastfeeding Committee of the Department of Health and Human Services all recommend breastfeeding as the natural and preferred method of newborn and infant feeding (Busch et al., 2019). In their position statement on breastfeeding, NAPNAP recommends exclusive breastfeeding for the first 6 months as optimal since breast milk provides complete infant nutrition (Busch et al., 2019).

Breastfeeding or feeding of expressed human milk is recommended for all infants, including sick or premature newborns (with rare exceptions). The exceptions include infants with galactosemia, maternal use of illicit drugs and a few prescription medications, maternal untreated active tuberculosis, and maternal HIV infection

TABLE 25.6 • Nutritional Requirements

Nutritional Requirements	Newborn	Infant
Fluid	140–160 mL/kg/day	100 mL/kg/day for first 10 kg 50 mL/kg/day for next 10 kg
Calories	105–108 kcal/kg/day	1–6 months: 108 kcal/kg 6–12 months: 98 kcal/kg

Adapted from Kleinman, K., McDaniel, L., & Molloy, M. (Eds.). (2021). *The Harriet Lane handbook* (22nd ed.). Elsevier.

HEALTHY PEOPLE 2030

Objective	Nursing Significance
Increase the proportion of infants who are breastfed exclusively through 6 months. Increase the proportion of infants who are breastfed at 1 year.	• Encourage breastfeeding in all birthing parents beginning with the prenatal visit if applicable. • Provide accurate education related to breastfeeding. • Be available for questions or problems related to initiation and continuation of breastfeeding. Consult a lactation consultant as needed or available. • Encourage pumping of breast milk when birthing parent returns to work in order to continue breastfeeding. • Refer to local breastfeeding support groups such as La Leche League.

Healthy People Objectives retrieved from http://www.healthypeople.gov

in developed countries. Data from the CDC's *Breastfeeding Report Card* indicate that 83.2% of U.S. infants were ever breastfed, 55.6% of infants were breastfeeding at 6 months of age, and only 35.9% were receiving some breast milk at 1 year of age (2022a). Even partial breastfeeding is helpful and offers some of the health benefits of breastfeeding. Pediatric nurses in the community and the hospital are in an excellent position to promote and support breastfeeding, thereby contributing to the Healthy People 2030 goal of increasing the proportion of birthing parents who exclusively breastfeed their babies for the first 6 months (see Evidence-Based Practice 25.1).

BOX 25.1 Benefits of Breastfeeding

Infant

- Increased bonding with parent
- Immunologic protection
- Breast milk has anti-infective properties.
- Decreased incidence and severity of diarrhea
- Decreased incidence of asthma, otitis media, bacterial meningitis, botulism, urinary tract infection
- Possible enhancement of cognitive development
- Decreased incidence of higher weight in later childhood

Parental

- Increased bonding with infant
- Lessens birthing parent blood loss in the postpartum period
- Decreased risk of ovarian and premenopausal breast cancer
- Reduced incidence of pregnancy-induced, long-term higher weight
- Possible delay of return of ovulation in some
- Always ready; no mixing
- Economic advantage

Adapted from La Leche League International. (2023). *Breastfeeding info A to Z.* https://www.llli.org/breastfeeding-info/

BREAST MILK COMPOSITION

Breast milk includes lactose, lipids, polyunsaturated fatty acids, and amino acids. The ratio of whey to casein protein in breast milk makes it readily digestible. The high concentration of fats and the balance of amino acids are believed to contribute to proper myelination of the nervous system. The concentration of iron in breast milk is less than that of formula, but the iron has increased bioavailability and is sufficient to meet the infant's requirements for the first 4 to 6 months of life. In addition to complete nutrition, immunologic protection is transferred from lactating parent to infant via breast milk, and parental–infant bonding is promoted. The benefits of breastfeeding are listed in Box 25.1.

EVIDENCE-BASED PRACTICE 25.1

Milk Boosters for Breastfeeding Term Infants

STUDY

Earlier weaning from the breast and earlier formula supplementation often occur as a result of poor milk supply (as identified by the lactating parent). The authors performed a comprehensive review of research studies related to the use of galactagogues (milk boosters) by parents breastfeeding their term infants. The authors evaluated 41 eligible studies involving 3,005 parents and 3,006 infants from at least 17 countries. The studies evaluated increased milk production in relation to the use of medications, herbal supplements, and foods.

Findings

Upon analysis of the various research studies, the authors reached the conclusion that since the studies were so varied in their approach and report, it is difficult to conclude which (if any) galactagogue increases milk supply most effectively. Minor adverse effects may occur with medication as well as natural milk boosters. The authors were unable to make a recommendation as to the most effective milk booster to use, as well as if any galactagogue was effective.

Nursing Implications

Given the importance of breastfeeding and the Healthy People goal of increasing the proportion of infants exclusively breastfeeding for the first 6 months, it is important for parents to experience adequate milk production. According to current published research studies, neither medications, herbal, nor food galactagogues reigned superior at increasing milk production. Nurses should continue to provide appropriate education and support to breastfeeding parents and ensure they consult with their health care provider or advanced practice nurse if they decide to use galactagogues. Additional research is needed in this area, which nurses could initiate.

Adapted from Foong, S. C., Tan, M. L., Foong, W. C., Marasco, L. A., Ho, J. J., & Ong, J. H. (2020). Oral galactagogues (natural therapies or drugs) for increasing breast milk production in mothers of non-hospitalised term infants. *Cochrane Database of Systematic Reviews.* https://doi.org/10.1002/14651858.CD011505.pub2

BREAST MILK SUPPLY AND DEMAND

Frequent, on-demand breastfeeding of the newborn is necessary to establish an adequate milk supply. After delivery of the placenta, levels of progesterone drop dramatically, which stimulates the anterior pituitary to produce prolactin. Prolactin stimulates the production of milk in the acinar or alveolar cells of the breast. When the infant sucks at the breast, nervous impulses stimulate further production of breast milk.

The first "milk" to be produced by the breasts is termed **colostrum**. It is produced for the first 2 to 4 days after birth. Colostrum is a thin, watery, yellowish fluid that is easy to digest, as it is high in protein and low in sugar and fat. Colostrum is complete nutrition and all that is needed by the newborn for the first 2 to 4 days of life (La Leche League International [LLLI], 2023). Transitional breast milk replaces colostrum on days 2 to 4 after birth. By day 10 after birth, mature breast milk is produced. Mature breast milk has a slightly bluish color and appears thin.

The breastfeeding parent produces milk continually. Called **foremilk**, it collects in the lactiferous sinuses, which are small tubules serving as reservoirs for milk located behind the nipples. The **let-down reflex** is responsible for the release of milk from these reservoirs. When the baby sucks at the breast, oxytocin is released from the posterior pituitary, causing the lactiferous sinuses to contract. This allows milk to "let down" into the nipples, and the infant then sucks the milk. The let-down reflex is triggered not only by suckling at the breast but also by thinking of the baby or by the sound of a baby crying. After the foremilk is let down, new, fattier milk is formed. This **hindmilk** helps the breastfed infant to grow quickly (LLLI, 2023). Parents should be informed that the production of oxytocin during suckling may also cause uterine contractions and may cause afterpains during breastfeeding.

BREASTFEEDING TECHNIQUE

Breastfeeding parents may not have established adequate breastfeeding prior to leaving the hospital after birth of the newborn. The pediatric nurse may encounter an infant–parent dyad experiencing difficulty with breastfeeding for a variety of reasons. Thus, the pediatric nurse must be competent in counseling the breastfeeding parent.

Before each breastfeeding session, the breastfeeding parent should wash their hands. It is not necessary to wash the breast in most cases. The parent should be positioned comfortably. A number of positions are possible, and they should be varied throughout the day. The parent may hold the breast in a "C" position if that is helpful (Fig. 25.9). Stroke the nipple against the baby's cheek (Fig. 25.10). This should stimulate the infant to open the mouth widely. Bring the baby's wide-open mouth to the breast

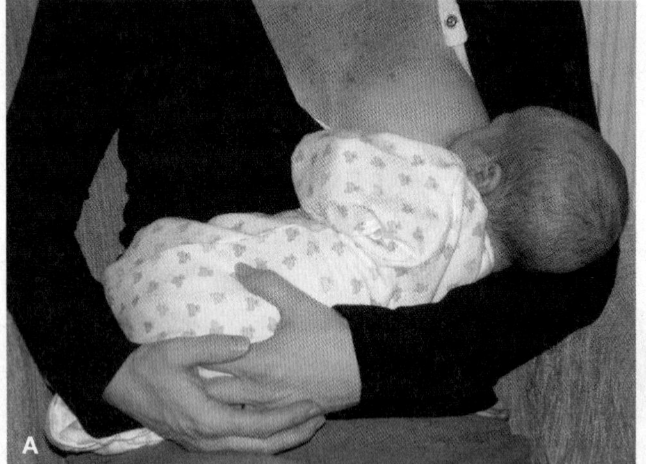

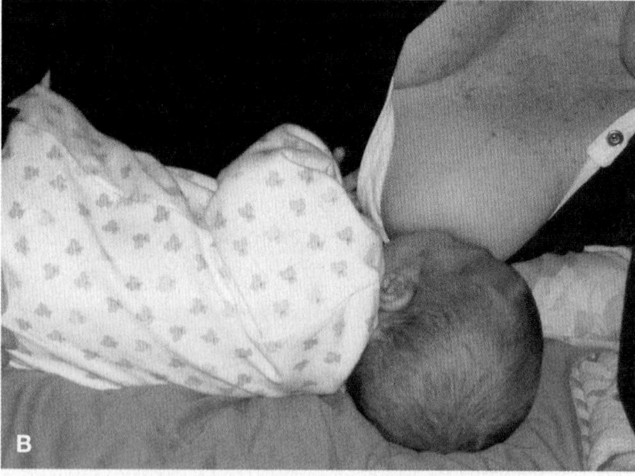

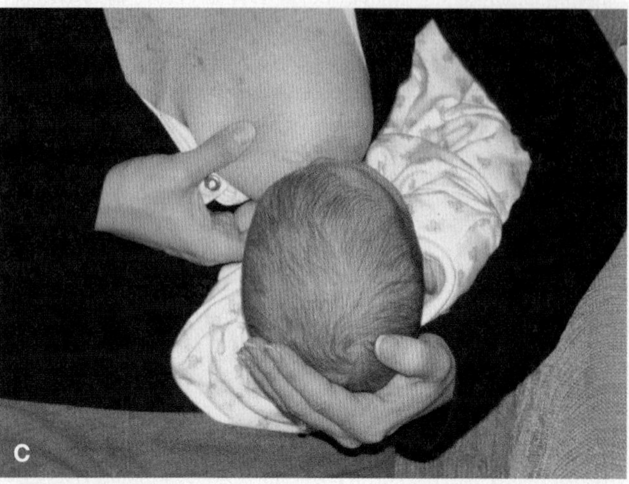

FIGURE 25.9 Various positions may be used during breastfeeding: cradle hold (**A**), side-lying (**B**), football hold (**C**). (Note the "C" position for holding the breast during latching on.)

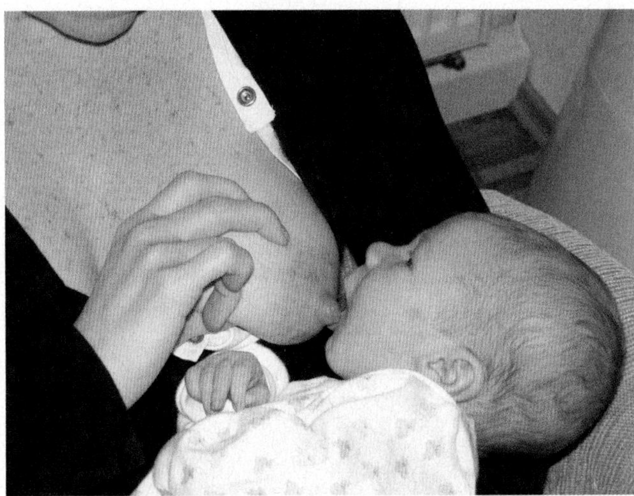

FIGURE 25.10 Stroking the infant's cheek with the nipple will elicit the rooting reflex.

to form a seal around all of the nipple and areola. When the infant is finished feeding, the parent can break the suction by inserting their finger into the baby's mouth, thus releasing the mouth from the nipple (Fig. 25.11). This technique may prevent the infant from pulling on the nipple, which can lead to soreness and cracking.

Watching and listening to the infant feed may help assess the adequacy of the baby's latch technique. The infant who is properly latched onto the breast will suck rhythmically, taking most or all of the areola into the mouth. Audible swallowing should be heard as milk is delivered into the infant's mouth. Assess the lactating parent for pain related to breastfeeding. They should not be in pain if the baby is latched on properly.

Establishment of breastfeeding is best achieved if the infant is allowed to feed on demand, whenever they are hungry. This may be as often as every 1.5 to 3 hours in the neonate. Infants may feed for 10 to 20 minutes on each breast at each feeding, or longer on just one breast, alternating the breast at each feeding. Both methods are acceptable.

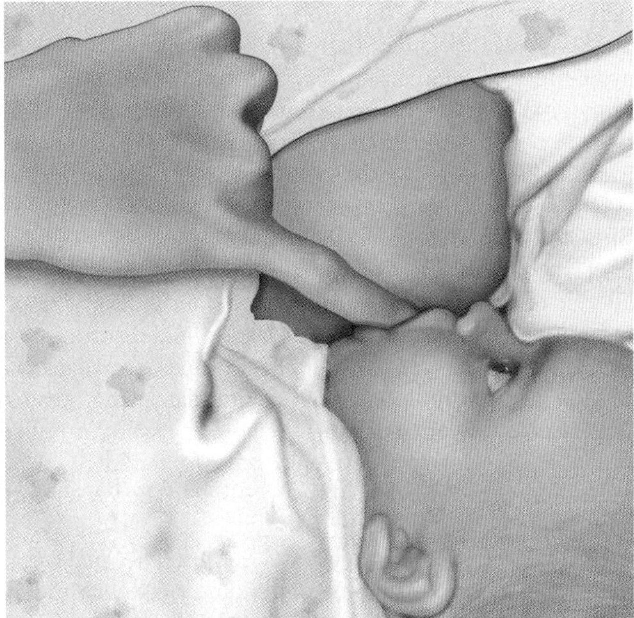

FIGURE 25.11 Inserting the little finger between the areola and the infant's mouth helps to break the suction.

The breastfeeding infant does not need supplementation with water or formula even in the first few days of life as long as the newborn continues to wet six to eight diapers per day. After several days of age, the lactating parent's milk supply should be well established. Adequate urine output and bowel movements, as well as continued weight gain in the infant, indicate the adequacy of breastfeeding. Working parents, in particular, may need additional support from the nurse in order to continue breastfeeding if they desire to do so. Common problems occurring with breastfeeding are addressed in Teaching Guidelines 25.1.

TEACHING GUIDELINES 25.1 Promoting Breastfeeding

Problem	Solutions
Sore nipples	Prevention: encourage appropriate latch-on from the beginning. Expose nipples to air between feedings. Allow breast milk to dry on nipples. Use aloe vera or vitamin E to help heal sore nipples. May use medical-grade lanolin or preservative-free lanolin
Engorgement	Apply warm compresses or encourage the lactating parent to take a warm shower prior to having the baby latch on (warmth encourages some of the milk to be released, allowing the breast to soften and making it easier for the infant to latch on).
Poor sucking	Feed on cue, not on a schedule. Encourage the sleepy infant by stroking the feet, undressing, and rubbing the head.
Inadequate milk supply	Decrease parental stress. Encourage adequate parental diet and fluid intake. Instruct working parents to pump in order to keep up milk supply when away from infant.
Other parent feels left out.	Encourage nonlactating parent to participate in other aspects of care.
Parent worries about adequacy of breast milk.	If infant is voiding six times per day and gaining weight, then the infant is receiving enough milk and appropriate nutrition.

BOTTLE-FEEDING

For the parent who does not desire to or cannot breastfeed, commercially prepared formulas are available for bottle-feeding. These formulas are designed to imitate human milk. Standard infant formulas based on cow's milk provide 20 kcal/oz and use lactose as a source for carbohydrates (Buchanan & Marquez, 2023). Vegetable oil is used as the source of fat; whey or casein provides protein. Newer cow's milk–based formulas contain long-chain polyunsaturated fatty acids that are thought to improve brain development. Ordinary cow's milk is not recommended for the first year of life.

> **TAKE NOTE!**
>
> Cow's milk does not provide an adequate balance of nutrients for the growing infant, especially iron. It may also overload the infant's renal system with inappropriate amounts of protein, sodium, and minerals.

Only formulas that are fortified with iron should be used. Iron stores that the infant received prenatally are depleted by 4 to 6 months of age. To prevent iron-deficiency anemia, poor growth patterns, and impaired development, iron-fortified formulas must be used. The AAP recommends that commercial formulas provide 10 to 12 mg of iron per liter (Buchanan & Marquez, 2023). Commercial formulas also provide an adequate blend of essential vitamins and minerals.

FEEDING PATTERNS

Infant feeding is an opportune time to establish good eating behaviors. The infant should always be held while being bottle-fed. Cradling in a semiupright position allows for additional bonding time, as the infant can see the caregiver's face while feeding (Fig. 25.12). Talking or singing during feeding time also increases bonding. As with breastfed infants, the bottle-fed infant should be fed on cue. Overfeeding with the bottle increases the incidence of spitting up and higher weight, so families need to learn their baby's cues to hunger and satiety (AAP, 2023).

It is important to feed the baby when the infant displays signs of hunger. Crying is a late sign of hunger; earlier signs include making sucking motions, sucking on hands, or putting the fist to the chin. The infant should be burped two or three times per feeding, when the infant slows feeding or stops sucking. Newborns may only take a half to 1 oz per feeding initially, working up to 2 to 3 oz in the first few days. They need to feed about six to 10 times per day. The infant will gradually be able to ingest more formula per feeding. By 6 months of age, babies feed four or five times per day and take 6 to 8 oz per feeding. Most infants will not require specific amounts per feeding; the infant should be fed until full. To prevent overfeeding, healthy bottle-fed infants should be allowed to self-regulate the amount of formula ingested per feeding. When the baby is satiated, they might fall asleep, spit out the nipple or formula, play with the nipple, or lie quietly, only sucking once in a while (AAP, 2023).

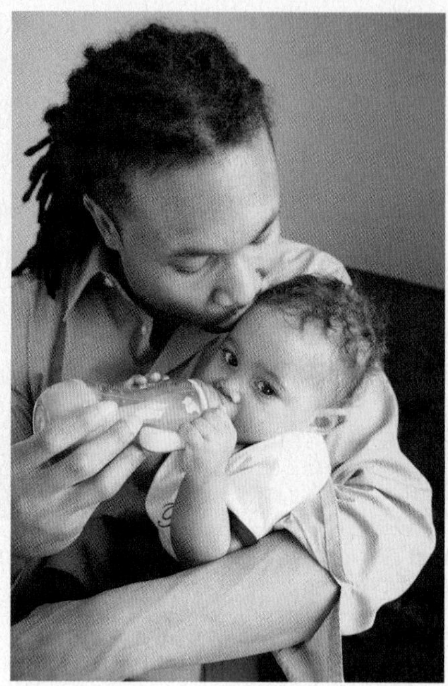

FIGURE 25.12 Technique for bottle-feeding the infant.

TYPES OF FORMULAS AND BOTTLES

Parents may choose to use commercial formulas that are ready to feed or available as a concentrate or as a powder. Parents should follow the instructions for mixing the concentrate or powder to avoid dehydration or fluid and electrolyte imbalances. Ready-to-feed formula should be used as is and never diluted (Buchanan & Marquez, 2023). A wide variety of baby bottle and nipple types are available for formula feeding, and the choice is purely individual. Few infants require special nipples or bottles. Box 25.2 gives guidelines on preparation and storage of formula and care of bottles.

SPECIAL FORMULAS

Special formulas may be needed for the infant who is allergic to a particular component of standard formula or has a renal, hepatic, metabolic, or intestinal disorder. For example, lactose-free cow's milk formulas are available for the lactose-intolerant child. Formulas using soy as the base ingredient instead of whey or casein are also available. Soy formulas are necessary for infants with a milk allergy, and they may be appealing to the vegetarian family.

These special formulas are designed to meet the nutritional needs of infants, depending on the disorder.

BOX **25.2** **Preparation and Storage of Bottles and Formula**

- Wash nipples and bottles in hot soapy water and rinse well OR run nipples and bottles through the dishwasher.
- Store the tightly covered ready-to-feed formula can after opening in refrigerator for up to 48 hours.
- After mixing concentrate or powdered formula, store tightly covered in refrigerator for up to 48 hours.
- Do not reheat and reuse partially used bottles. Throw away the unused portion after each feeding.
- Do not add cereal to the formula in the bottle.
- Do not sweeten formula with honey.
- Warm formula by placing bottle in a container of hot water.
- Do not microwave formula.

Adapted from American Academy of Pediatrics. (2023). *Formula feeding.* https://www.healthychildren.org/English/ages-stages/baby/formula-feeding/Pages/default.aspx

Infants who fail to gain weight may be placed on standard infant formula prepared to deliver a higher caloric density per ounce. Preterm infants (those born earlier than 36 weeks' gestation) need adequate nutrition to exhibit catch-up growth. Good catch-up growth (quadrupling or even quintupling the birth weight) in the first year or so of life is critical for adequate head growth and avoidance of neurodevelopmental consequences. Premature infant follow-up formulas are designed to provide additional calories, protein, and a particular calcium-to-phosphorus ratio as well as the vitamins and minerals needed for adequate catch-up growth.

Progressing to Solid Foods

After 6 months of age, infants usually require the nutrients available in solid foods in addition to their breast milk or formula. Progressing to feeding solid foods can be exciting and trying. Before solid foods are attempted, the infant should be assessed for readiness to progress. Parents need instruction in choosing appropriate solid foods and support in the progression process.

ASSESSING INFANT READINESS

Several factors contribute to the appropriate timing of solid food introduction. The tongue extrusion reflex is necessary for sucking to be an automatic reaction—that is, when a nipple or other item is placed in the mouth, the tongue extrudes and sucking begins. This reflex disappears at about 4 to 6 months of age (Duryea & Fleisher, 2022). Introducing solid food with a spoon prior to 4 to 6 months of age will result in extrusion of the tongue. The parent may think that the infant does not want the food and is spitting it out intentionally, but this is not the case; the infant simply must be mature enough to eat with a spoon (absence of extrusion reflex).

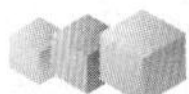

Concept Mastery Alert

Cow's milk should never be given to an infant because of its potential to cause an allergic reaction. Parents should avoid adding fruit juice to the infant's diet because the infant needs the protein and fat in breast milk or formula. Fruit juice would displace these important nutrients.

The ability to swallow solid food does not become completely functional until 4 to 6 months of age. Enzymes to appropriately digest food other than breast milk and formula are also not present in sufficient quantities until the age of 4 to 6 months.

Before the introduction of solid foods and the cup, the infant should be able to sit supported in a highchair. Solids should be fed with a spoon, with the infant in an upright position.

CHOOSING APPROPRIATE SOLID FOODS

Iron-fortified rice cereal mixed with a small amount of breast milk or formula is a good choice for the first solid food. The cereal is easily digested, and its taste is generally well accepted. The cereal should be quite thin at first; it can be mixed to a thicker consistency as the infant gets older. Once the feeding of cereal with a spoon is successful, other single foods may be introduced. The foods should be puréed to a smooth consistency, whether prepackaged "baby food" or puréed at home.

The introduction of one new food every 3 to 5 days is recommended (Buchanan & Marquez, 2023). This allows for identification of food allergies (Box 25.3). No salt, sugar, or other seasoning should be added to these first foods. Previously, avoidance of peanut-containing food until at least 12 months of age was recommended. Recent research recommends early introduction (around 6 months of age) of developmentally appropriate peanut food in skin prick-negative infants to decrease the incidence of developing peanut allergy (McCarthy, 2020).

Generally, by 8 months of age, the infant is ready for more texture in foods. Soft, smashed table food without large chunks is appropriate. Finger foods such as Cheerios, soft green bean pieces, or soft peas may also be offered. Avoid hard foods that the infant may choke on.

BOX **25.3** **Foods to Avoid in Infancy**

- Cow's milk
- Honey
- Excessive amounts of fruit juice
- Foods likely to cause choking
  - Popcorn
  - Other small hard foods (e.g., raw carrot chunks)
  - Grapes and hot dog slices (must be cut in smaller pieces)

Adapted from Schmitt, B. (2022a). *Solid foods (baby foods).* Schmitt Pediatric Guidelines LLC. https://doi.org/10.1542/ppe_schmitt_222

Strained, puréed, or mashed meats may be introduced at 10 to 12 months of age.

The cup should be introduced at 6 to 8 months of age. One ounce of breast milk or formula should be placed in the cup while the infant is learning. This will decrease the amount of mess should the cup be spilled. Old-fashioned sippy cups are generally acceptable for use, although older infants quickly learn to drink from an ordinary cup with assistance when they are thirsty. Older infants are also able to drink from a straw. Newer no-spill sippy cups are not recommended for general home use. They require sucking much like a bottle and do not really encourage the child to learn cup drinking. In addition, the no-spill sippy cup allows for juice or milk to be in constant contact with the baby's teeth, increasing the risk of dental caries (Hagan et al., 2017). Fruit juice is unnecessary and should not be introduced until 6 months of age. If juice is given, it should be limited to 2 to 4 oz per day. Fruit itself is much more nutritious than fruit juice. If infants are allowed to consume larger quantities of juice, it can displace important nutrients from breast milk or formula (Buchanan & Marquez, 2023).

PROMOTING HEALTHY EATING HABITS

Infants and children learn about food within a social context, so the family plays an important role in creating healthy eating habits. Families "model" eating behaviors; infants and children learn about eating through watching others. Lifelong eating patterns are often established in childhood, so it is important to emphasize healthy eating practices beginning in infancy. Parents should not let infants eat whatever they want (permissive feeding style); this will lead to fights over eating in the future. Infants may require as many as 20 exposures to a new food before it is accepted. On the other hand, infants should not be coerced into eating all that is provided (authoritarian feeding style). Forcing an infant to eat when they are full sets the child up for overeating in the future and may lead to more power struggles (Duryea & Fleisher, 2022). Parents need to find a balance between the permissive and authoritarian feeding styles to establish lifelong healthy eating patterns in their children. By providing education about appropriate diet and feeding behaviors, the nurse can help the family accomplish this goal.

Think back to Allison Johnson. What questions should you ask Allison's parents related to her nutritional intake? What anticipatory guidance related to nutrition would be appropriate?

Promoting Healthy Sleep and Rest

Newborns sleep about 10 to 19 hours a day, waking frequently to feed and quickly returning to sleep. By 3 months of age, most infants sleep 7 to 8 hours per night without waking. They will continue to take about three naps a day. By 6 months of age, the infant is more active and alert and may have more trouble going to sleep in the evening. Night waking may occur, but the infant should be capable of sleeping through the night and does not require a night feeding. By 12 months of age, infants sleep 9 to 12 hours per night and take one to two naps per day (Reynolds et al., 2022).

Discuss safe sleeping practices with parents of newborns and infants; the baby should sleep on a firm mattress without pillows or comforters. The baby's bed should be placed away from air conditioner vents, open windows, and open heaters. Sudden infant death syndrome (SIDS) has been associated with prone and side-lying positioning of newborns and infants, so the infant should be placed to sleep alone (no pillows, stuffed animals, fluffy blankets), on their back, and in their own crib (Moon et al., 2022). See the Healthy People 2030 box.

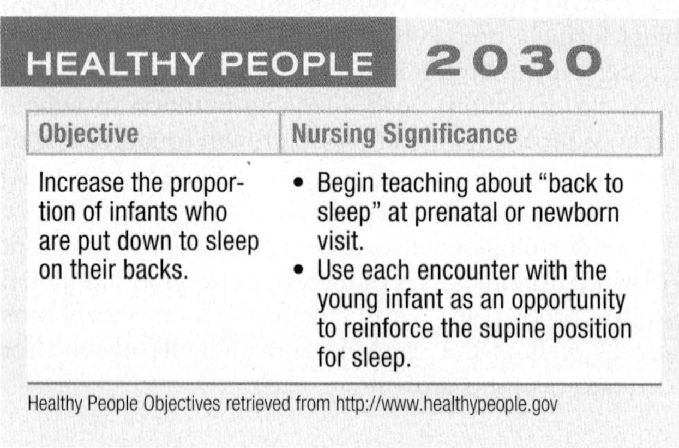
HEALTHY PEOPLE 2030

Objective	Nursing Significance
Increase the proportion of infants who are put down to sleep on their backs.	• Begin teaching about "back to sleep" at prenatal or newborn visit. • Use each encounter with the young infant as an opportunity to reinforce the supine position for sleep.

Healthy People Objectives retrieved from http://www.healthypeople.gov

TAKE NOTE!

The AAP has determined that side sleeping is not as safe as supine sleeping.

In the newborn period, the primary caregiver should try to sleep when the baby is sleeping. Since newborns need to be fed every 1.5 to 3 hours around the clock, parents may become exhausted quickly and are often eager for the infant to sleep through the night. Adding rice cereal to the evening bottle has not been proven to discourage night waking and is not recommended (CDC, 2022c). Provide support to parents of newborns and educate them on infant sleeping patterns.

It is important to establish a bedtime routine around 4 months of age due to the infant's increased alertness and activity level. The baby who is 4 months or older needs a time of calming and relaxation before going to sleep. A consistent bedtime routine should be established, perhaps a bath followed by rocking, singing, or reading. The infant should fall asleep in their own crib rather than being rocked to sleep or held until sleeping and then put in the crib. After 4 months of age, infants must learn to soothe themselves back to sleep following night waking. Older infants may exhibit head banging as a form of self-soothing and use it to fall asleep at night. Parents should minimize attention and stimulation provided during a night waking. Briefly checking on the infant to ascertain their safety, followed by placing the infant back in a lying position and telling them good night, is all that is needed. This may have to be repeated several times before the infant falls back to sleep. It is important to keep interactions brief during the night waking so that the infant learns to fall back to sleep on their own. Continued issues with night waking should be discussed with the infant's primary care provider.

Promoting Healthy Teeth and Gums

Healthy teeth and gums require proper oral hygiene and appropriate fluoride supplementation. Early childhood dental caries can result from pooling of milk or juice around teeth and gums. Before tooth eruption, parents should clean the child's gums after feeding with a damp washcloth. After teeth have erupted, parents can continue to use a soft cloth for tooth cleaning and then eventually use a small soft-bristled toothbrush. Toothpaste is unnecessary in infancy.

Infants should not be allowed to take milk or juice bottles to bed, as the high sugar content of the fluid in contact with the teeth all night leads to dental caries. Weaning from the bottle at age 12 to 15 months may help prevent dental caries. No-spill sippy cups have also been implicated in the development of dental caries and should be avoided. The American Academy of Pediatric Dentistry (AAPD) recommends that infants receive their first dental visit by the age of 1 year (2021). Children older than 6 months of age who are at risk for developing dental caries and whose drinking water source is not optimally fluoridated may require fluoride supplementation (AAPD, 2021). Excess fluoride ingestion may result in discoloration of the teeth (fluorosis), so ensure parents understand the dosage.

Promoting Appropriate Discipline

Parenting requires everchanging adaptations to the developing infant's needs. Unconditional love, patience, and compassion must be balanced with the parents' needs. Discipline refers to the molding of a child's behavior through instruction, practice, and consistency. Discipline helps build self-esteem in children as well as sets standards for social interactions. The primary goal of discipline is to teach an infant limits. Discipline should be used to help the infant solve problems. The infant's activities are based on the basic needs of food, security, warmth, love, and comfort. Misbehavior is the result of an unmet need, and the parents should respond accordingly.

As the infant is undergoing rapid changes in motor skills, safety needs increase. Nurses should encourage the parents to "childproof" their home so that the infant can develop physical skills without being at risk. In a childproof home, fewer restrictions need to be placed on the infant's behavior, and the infant can more readily explore.

Physical punishment or spanking should never be used in infancy. Infants are at increased risk for physical injury from spanking and cannot make the connection between the spanking and the undesirable behavior. Providing a safe environment, redirection away from undesirable behaviors, and saying "no" in appropriate instances are far more effective. For example, when the infant is in potential danger (e.g., inserting a key into an electrical outlet, attempting to ingest a poisonous substance, or reaching into the toilet), the parent must use a firm but calm and brisk approach. If the infant knows the parent is serious, adherence will usually come more quickly (AAP, 2018b).

Remaining calm, firm, and consistent is necessary. Immediacy is also an important component of appropriate discipline. The infant cannot make the connection between a subsequent punishment and discussion of behavior with the earlier event itself. Positive reinforcement should be used to support good behavior (AAP, 2018b).

Addressing Child Care Needs

Many parents work outside the home, there are many single-parent families, and many families live a distance away from relatives. In all of these circumstances, infants may need to be cared for outside the home, often in child care settings or home day care centers.

Parents contemplating child care must consider a number of factors. Do they want a sitter to come to their home? Will they use a traditional day care center or a home care situation with fewer children? How much can they afford? If families choose to use a freestanding day care center or a home-based day care center, they should make sure that the provider is appropriately licensed. Parents should feel comfortable with the caregiver-to-child ratio. Are the caregivers trained in infant CPR and first aid? Families may need to visit or interview several facilities before finding one that meets their requirements.

When an older infant is attending a child care situation for the first time, it may be helpful to visit the center once or twice beforehand so that the infant can get used to the caregivers from the comfort and security of the parent's lap. Warn parents that separation anxiety in late infancy can cause a disturbing crying episode when the parent leaves. Reassure parents that the infant will not suffer harm due to the separation.

ADDRESSING COMMON DEVELOPMENTAL CONCERNS

Parents commonly have multiple concerns during normal infant growth and development. Although most of these issues are not actual disease states or behavior problems, nurses must be aware of these issues to recognize them and to intervene appropriately.

Colic

Colic is defined as inconsolable crying that lasts 3 hours or longer per day and for which there is no physical cause. It may begin as early as 2 weeks of age, and healthy infants cry for a total of about 3 hours daily, 3 to 7 days per week. Crying and fussing are more prevalent in the evenings. Typically, colic resolves by 3 months of age, coinciding with the age at which infants are better able to soothe themselves (e.g., by finger sucking). The cause of colic is thought to be problems in the gastrointestinal or neurologic system (probably system immaturity), temperament, or parenting style. Some parents are overly anxious or overly attentive or, at the other extreme, may not give the infant the attention needed. Any of these may contribute to a baby's fussing and crying.

Prolonged crying leads to increased stress among caregivers. Failure to stop the crying leads to frustration, and crying that prevents the parents from sleeping contributes to the exhaustion they are already experiencing. Educate parents that normal crying increases by the time the infant is 6 weeks old and diminishes by about 12 weeks. When faced with a colicky baby, parents should develop a stepwise approach to checking that all of the infant's basic needs are met. When these needs are met, attempts at soothing the infant may be used. Reducing stimulation may decrease the length of crying. Carrying the infant more may also be helpful. Some infants respond to the motion of an infant swing or a car ride. Vibration, white noise, or swaddling may also help to decrease fussing in some infants. Pacifiers can be soothing to babies who need additional nonnutritive sucking. Parents should try one intervention at a time, taking care not to stimulate the infant excessively in the process of searching for solutions. Nurses should provide ongoing support to the parents of a colicky infant and reassure them that this is a temporary condition that will resolve in time (Reynolds et al., 2022).

Spitting Up

Spitting up (regurgitating small amounts of stomach contents) occurs in all infants, and a significant number of infants spit up excessively. Although spitting up after feeding is normal, it can be a cause of great concern to parents. Overfed babies who feed based on a parent-designed schedule and those who burp poorly are more likely to spit up. For some infants, the amount and frequency of spitting up are significant, and those babies should be evaluated by the health care provider or nurse practitioner (AAP, 2019).

Teach parents that feeding smaller amounts on a more frequent basis may help to decrease spitting-up episodes. Always burp the baby at least two or three times per feeding. Keep the baby upright for 30 minutes after feeding, and do not lay the infant prone after feeding. Avoid bouncing or excess activity immediately after feeding. Avoid compressing the stomach after meals with tummy time or positioning in an infant seat (AAP, 2019).

Reassure parents that if the infant is wetting at least six diapers per 24 hours and gaining weight, the spitting up is normal. If the infant vomits one third or more of most feedings, chokes when vomiting, or experiences forceful emesis, the primary care provider should be notified.

Thumb Sucking, Pacifiers, and Security Items

Infants demonstrate a clear need for nonnutritive sucking; even fetuses can be observed sucking their thumbs or fingers in utero. Thumb sucking is a healthy self-comforting activity. Infants who suck their thumbs or pacifiers often are better able to soothe themselves than those who do not. Studies have not shown that sucking either thumbs or pacifiers leads to the need for orthodontic braces unless the sucking continues well beyond the early school-age period. However, pacifier use has been associated with the increased incidence of otitis media (Reynolds et al., 2022). Hygiene is always a concern as pacifiers often fall on the floor. Infants may also become attached to a doll, stuffed animal, or blanket. Just like thumb sucking, the attachment item gives the infant the security to self-soothe when uncomfortable.

Families need to explore their feelings and cultural preferences about sucking habits and security items. Parents should not try to break the habit during a stressful time for the infant. When the infant is intensely trying to master a new skill such as sitting or walking, the infant may need the sucking or security item to self-soothe. Pacifiers and security items can be physically taken away at some point, but the thumb is attached. The infant who has become attached to thumb sucking should not have additional attention drawn to the issue, as that may prolong thumb sucking.

Families of infants who use pacifiers may want to wean the infant from the pacifier when the child approaches 1 year of age, as this is the time when the need for additional sucking naturally decreases. Otherwise, weaning from the pacifier should occur by 18 months of age in order to limit adverse effects upon dentition (AAPD, 2022). Attempts to wean the child from a security blanket or toy should probably be reserved for after infancy.

Teething

Discomfort is common as the tooth breaks through the periodontal membrane. Infants may drool, bite on hard objects, or increase finger sucking. Some infants may become very irritable, refuse to eat, and not sleep well. Fever, vomiting, and diarrhea are generally not considered a sign of teething but rather of illness.

Teething pain results from inflammation. Teach parents that gum massage or application of cold may be soothing to the gums. The parent should rub the inflamed gum with a clean finger for 2 minutes. The infant may chew on a chilled (not frozen) teething ring, or parents can rub an ice cube wrapped in a washcloth on the gums. Occasionally, oral acetaminophen or ibuprofen may be given to relieve pain (Schmitt, 2022b).

TAKE NOTE!

Advise against the use of over-the-counter topical anesthetics containing benzocaine (such as baby Orajel), as they can cause serious side effects, do not work very well, and are not approved for use by the Food and Drug Administration (Schmitt, 2022b).

Refer back to 6-month-old Allison Johnson. List some common developmental concerns of 6-month-old infants. What anticipatory guidance related to these concerns would you provide to her parents?

KEY CONCEPTS

- Infancy encompasses the period from birth to age 12 months.
- The infant exhibits tremendous growth, doubling the birth weight by 6 months of age and tripling it by 12 months of age.
- Most organ systems are immature at birth and develop and mature over the first year of life.
- Child development is orderly, sequential, and predictable, progressing in a cephalocaudal and proximodistal fashion.
- The infant is mastering the psychosocial task of trust versus mistrust.
- Cognitive development in infancy is sensorimotor; infants use their senses and progressing motor skills to master their environments.
- The 12-month-old babbles expressively and uses two or three words with meaning.
- Promotion of safety is of key importance throughout infancy.
- Breastfeeding is the natural and preferred method for infant feeding.
- Breastfed and bottle-fed infants should both be fed on cue rather than on a parent-designed schedule.
- Solid foods should be introduced at age 4 to 6 months. New foods should be introduced no more frequently than every 3 to 5 days.
- The cup may be introduced at 6 months of age. No-spill sippy cups are generally not recommended.
- Spitting up and colic are parts of normal development in the otherwise thriving infant and do not require medical intervention.

REFERENCES AND RECOMMENDED READINGS

American Academy of Pediatrics. (2017). *Safety for your child: Birth to 6 months.* http://www.healthychildren.org/English/tips-tools/Pages/Safety-for-Your-Child-Birth-to-6-Months.aspx

American Academy of Pediatrics. (2018a). *Safety for your child: 6 to 12 months.* http://www.healthychildren.org/English/tips-tools/Pages/Safety-for-Your-Child-6-to-12-Months.aspx

American Academy of Pediatrics. (2018b). *What's the best way to discipline my child?* http://www.healthychildren.org/English/family-life/family-dynamics/communication-discipline/Pages/Disciplining-Your-Child.aspx

American Academy of Pediatrics. (2019). *Swim lessons: When to start & what parents should know.* https://www.healthychildren.org/English/safety-prevention/at-play/Pages/swim-lessons.aspx

American Academy of Pediatrics. (2022). *Baby walkers: A dangerous choice.* https://www.healthychildren.org/English/safety-prevention/at-home/Pages/Baby-Walkers-A-Dangerous-Choice.aspx

American Academy of Pediatrics. (2023). *Formula feeding.* https://www.healthychildren.org/English/ages-stages/baby/formula-feeding/Pages/default.aspx

American Academy of Pediatric Dentistry. (2021). *Perinatal and infant oral health care: Latest revision.* https://www.aapd.org/media/Policies_Guidelines/BP_PerinatalOralHealthCare.pdf

American Academy of Pediatric Dentistry. (2022). *Policy on pacifiers.* https://www.aapd.org/globalassets/media/policies_guidelines/p_pacifiers.pdf

Branchford, B. R., & Levine, D. A. (2023). Section 2: Growth and development. In K. J. Marcdante, R. M. Kliegman, & A. M. Schuh (Eds.), *Nelson's essentials of pediatrics* (9th ed.). Elsevier.

Buchanan, A. O., & Marquez, M. L. (2023). Section 6: Pediatric nutrition and nutritional disorders. In K. J. Marcdante, R. M. Kliegman, & A. M. Schuh (Eds.), *Nelson's essentials of pediatrics* (9th ed.). Elsevier.

Busch, D. W., Silbert-Flagg, J., Ryngaert, M., & Scott, A. (2019). NAPNAP position statement on breastfeeding: National Association of Pediatric Nurse Practitioners, Breastfeeding Education Special Interest Group. *Journal of Pediatric Health Care, 33*(1), A11–A15. https://doi.org/10.1016/j.pedhc.2018.08.011

Centers for Disease Control and Prevention. (2021, September 10). *Cultural competence in health and human services.* https://npin.cdc.gov/pages/cultural-competence#what

Centers for Disease Control and Prevention. (2022a, August 31). *Breastfeeding report card.* https://www.cdc.gov/breastfeeding/data/reportcard.htm

Centers for Disease Control and Prevention. (2022b, December 29). *CDC's developmental milestones*. http://www.cdc.gov/ncbddd/actearly/milestones/index.html

Centers for Disease Control and Prevention. (2022c, May 17). *Infant and toddler nutrition, FAQs*. https://www.cdc.gov/nutrition/InfantandToddlerNutrition/faqs.html

Cherry, J., Harrison, G. J., Kaplan, S. L., Steinbach, W. J., & Hotez, P. (2019). *Feigin and Cherry's textbook of pediatric infectious diseases* (8th ed.). Elsevier.

Child Development Institute. (2019). *Temperament and your child's personality*. https://childdevelopmentinfo.com/uncategorized/temperament_and_your_child/

Duryea, T. K., & Fleisher, D. M. (2022). Patient education: Starting solid foods during infancy (beyond the basics). *UpToDate*. Retrieved September 22, 2022, from https://www.uptodate.com/contents/starting-solid-foods-during-infancy-beyond-the-basics

Erikson, E. H. (1963). *Childhood and society* (2nd ed.). W. W. Norton and Company.

Foong, S. C., Tan, M. L., Foong, W. C., Marasco, L. A., Ho, J. J., & Ong, J. H. (2020). Oral galactagogues (natural therapies or drugs) for increasing breast milk production in mothers of non-hospitalised term infants. *Cochrane Database of Systematic Reviews*. https://doi.org/10.1002/14651858.CD011505.pub2

Greenbaum, L. A., & Londeree, J. T. (2023). Maintenance fluid therapy. In K. J. Marcdante, R. M. Kliegman, & A. M. Schuh (Eds.), *Nelson's essentials of pediatrics* (9th ed.). Elsevier.

Hagan, J. F., Shaw, J. S., & Duncan, P. M. (2017). *Bright futures: Guidelines for health supervision of infants, children, and adolescents* (4th ed.). American Academy of Pediatrics.

Kaiser Permanente. (n.d.). *Bowel movements in babies*. https://healthy.kaiserpermanente.org/health-wellness/health-encyclopedia/he.bowel-movements-in-babies.abo3062

Kleinman, K., McDaniel, L., & Molloy, M. (Eds.). (2021). *The Harriet Lane handbook* (22nd ed.). Elsevier.

La Leche League International. (2023). *Breastfeeding info A to Z*. https://www.llli.org/breastfeeding-info/

Lewis, K. N. (2019). *Reading books to babies*. https://kidshealth.org/en/parents/reading-babies.html

Linguistic Society of America. (2023). *FAQ: Raising bilingual children*. https://www.linguisticsociety.org/resource/faq-raising-bilingual-children

Maqbool, A., & Liacouras, C. A. (2020). Normal development, structure, and function of the stomach and intestines. In R. M. Kliegman, J. W. St Geme, N. J. Blum, S. S. Shah, R. C. Tasker, & K. M. Wilson, *Nelson textbook of pediatrics* (21st ed.). Elsevier.

McCarthy, C. (2020). *Peanut allergies: What you should know about the latest research & guidelines*. https://www.healthychildren.org/English/health-issues/conditions/allergies-asthma/Pages/Peanut-Allergies-What-You-Should-Know-About-the-Latest-Research.aspx

Moon, R. Y., Carlin, R. F., Hand, I., & the Task Force on Sudden Infant Death Syndrome and the Committee on Fetus and Newborn. (2022). Sleep-related infant deaths: Updated 2022 recommendations for reducing infant deaths in the sleep environment. *Pediatrics, 150*(1), e2022057990. https://doi.org/10.1542/peds.2022-057990

National Association for the Education of Young Children. (n.d.). *Good toys for young children by age and stage*. http://www.naeyc.org/toys

Nuss, R., McKinney, C., & Wang, M. (2022). Hematologic disorders. In M. Bunik, W. W. Hay, M. J. Levin, & M. J. Abzug (Eds.), *Current diagnosis & treatment: Pediatrics* (26th ed.). McGraw-Hill.

Olsson, J. (2020). The newborn. In R. M. Kliegman, J. W. St Geme, N. J. Blum, S. S. Shah, R. C. Tasker, & K. M. Wilson (Eds.), *Nelson textbook of pediatrics* (21st ed.). Elsevier.

Piaget, J. (1969). *The theory of stages in cognitive development*. McGraw-Hill.

Powers, J. M. (2021). Iron deficiency in infants and children <12 years: Screening, prevention, clinical manifestations, and diagnosis. *UpToDate*. Retrieved September 21, 2022, from https://www.uptodate.com/contents/iron-deficiency-in-infants-and-children-less-than12-years-screening-prevention-clinical-manifestations-and-diagnosis

Reynolds, A., Angulo, A., Breheney, M., Green, J., & Goldson, E. (2022). Child development and behavior. In M. Bunik, W. W. Hay, M. J. Levin, & M. J. Abzug (Eds.), *Current diagnosis & treatment: Pediatrics* (26th ed.). McGraw-Hill Education.

Safe Kids Worldwide. (2023). *Baby sleep safety and suffocation prevention*. https://www.safekids.org/safetytips/field_age/babies-0–12-months/field_risks/sleep-safety

Schmitt, B. (2022a). Solid foods (baby foods). Schmitt Pediatric Guidelines LLC. https://doi.org/10.1542/ppe_schmitt_222

Schmitt, B. (2022b). Teething. Schmitt Pediatric Guidelines LLC. https://doi.org/10.1542/ppe_schmitt_235

Sinha, S. K. (2021). *Short stature*. http://emedicine.medscape.com/article/924411-overview

Smola, C., Sorrentino, A., Shah, N., Nichols, M., & Monroe, K. (2020). Child passenger safety education in the emergency department: Teen driving, car seats, booster seats, and more. *Injury Epidemiology*, *7*(Suppl. 1), 26. https://doi.org/10.1186/s40621-020-00250-5

U.S. Department of Health and Human Services. (n.d.). *Healthy People 2030*. https://health.gov/healthypeople

Zubler, J. M., Wiggins, L. D., Macias, M. M., Whitaker, T. M., Shaw, J. S., Squires, J. K., Pajke, J. A., Wolf, R. B., Slaughter, K. S., Broughton, A. S., Gerndt, K. L., Mlodoch, B. J., & Lipkin, P. H. (2022). Evidence-informed milestones for developmental surveillance tools. *Pediatrics, 149*(3), e2021052138. https://doi.org/10.1542/peds.2021-052138

DEVELOPING CLINICAL JUDGMENT

PRACTICING FOR NCLEX

1. The parent of a 3-month-old infant asks the nurse about starting solid foods. What is the most appropriate response by the nurse?
   a. "It's okay to start puréed solids at this age if fed via the bottle."
   b. "Infants don't require solid food until 12 months of age."
   c. "Solid foods should be delayed until age 6 months, when the infant can handle a spoon on their own."
   d. "The tongue extrusion reflex disappears at age 4 to 6 months, making it a good time to start solid foods."
2. The parent of a 2-month-old infant is expressing concern that the infant may be getting spoiled. What is the nurse's best response?
   a. "The baby just needs love and attention. Don't worry; the baby's too young to spoil."
   b. "Consistently meeting the infant's needs helps promote a sense of trust."
   c. "Infants need to be fed and cleaned; if you are sure those needs are met, just let your baby cry."
   d. "Consistency in meeting needs is important, but you are right, holding the infant too much will spoil the baby."
3. Parents of an 8-month-old infant express concern that the infant cries when left with the babysitter. How does the nurse best explain this behavior?
   a. "Crying when left with the sitter may indicate difficulty with building trust."
   b. "Stranger anxiety should not occur until toddlerhood; this concern should be investigated."
   c. "Separation anxiety is normal at this age; the infant recognizes parents as separate beings."
   d. "Perhaps the sitter doesn't meet the infant's needs; choose a different sitter."
4. The nurse is providing anticipatory guidance to the parent of a 6-month-old infant. What is the best instruction by the nurse in relation to the infant's oral health?
   a. "Start brushing the teeth after all the baby teeth come in."
   b. "Use a washcloth with toothpaste to clean the mouth."
   c. "Clean your baby's gums, then new teeth, with a washcloth."
   d. "Rinse your baby's mouth with water after every feeding."
5. A 9-month-old infant's parent is questioning why cow's milk is not recommended in the first year of life as it is much cheaper than formula. What rationale does the nurse include in the response?
   a. It is permissible to substitute cow's milk for formula at this age as the infant is so close to 1 year old.
   b. Cow's milk is poor in iron and does not provide the proper balance of nutrients for the infant.
   c. As long as the parent provides whole milk, rather than skim, they can start cow's milk in infancy.
   d. If the parent cannot afford the infant formula, they should dilute it to make it last longer.
6. Parents report to the nurse that their young infant breastfeeds and sleeps well on their abdomen on a soft mattress, with a light blanket covering them. The nurse determines the infant is at risk for ____ related to _____ and ______.
   Blank 1:
   a. Shaken baby syndrome (SBS)
   b. Sudden infant death syndrome (SIDS)
   c. Gastroesophageal reflux disease (GERD)
   Blanks 2 and 3:
   a. Prone sleeping
   b. Supine sleeping
   c. Soft crib mattress
   d. Breastfeeding
7. A 12-month-old infant was born full-term without any difficulties. The infant weighed 8 lb at birth. Which assessment findings would the nurse expect for this infant? (Select four items.)
   a. Current weight is 24 lb.
   b. Anterior fontanel is closed.
   c. Posterior fontanel is slightly open.
   d. The infant is now walking.
   e. The infant tries to build a two-block tower.
   f. The infant says 10 words with meaning.

CRITICAL THINKING EXERCISES

1. The parent of an 11-month-old infant who was born at 24 weeks' gestation is concerned about the infant's size and motor skills. What information should the nurse provide?
2. An infant's parent thinks there may be something wrong because "he spits up so much." What further information should the nurse obtain?

3. If you determine that the infant in the preceding question is experiencing normal spitting up associated with his developmental age, develop a brief teaching plan to review with the parent.

STUDY ACTIVITIES

1. Parents bring their 9-month-old infant to the clinic for a well-child check-up. They have questions about feeding, speech, and walking. Develop a teaching plan of anticipatory guidance for the 9-month-old infant.
2. Develop a home and car safety plan for the 12-month-old infant.
3. In the clinical setting, observe two infants of the same age, one who is developing appropriately for their age and one who is experiencing delays. Note the similarities and differences between the two infants.

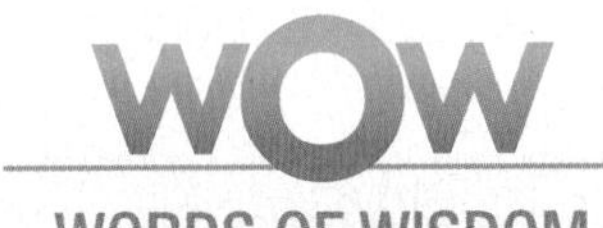

WORDS OF WISDOM

Toddlers will take risks and make many mistakes; nurses can help parents remember that both are an essential part of their growth.

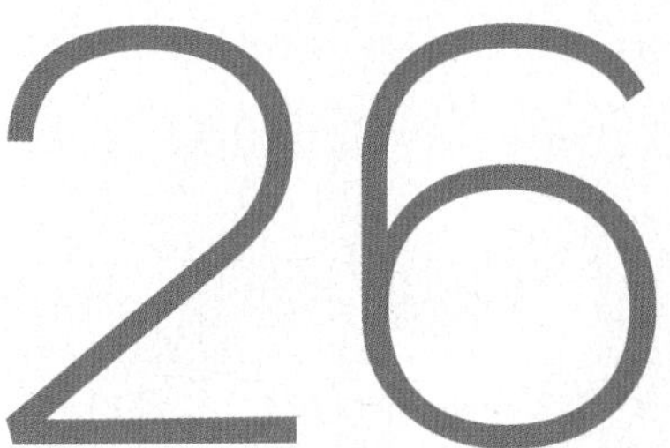

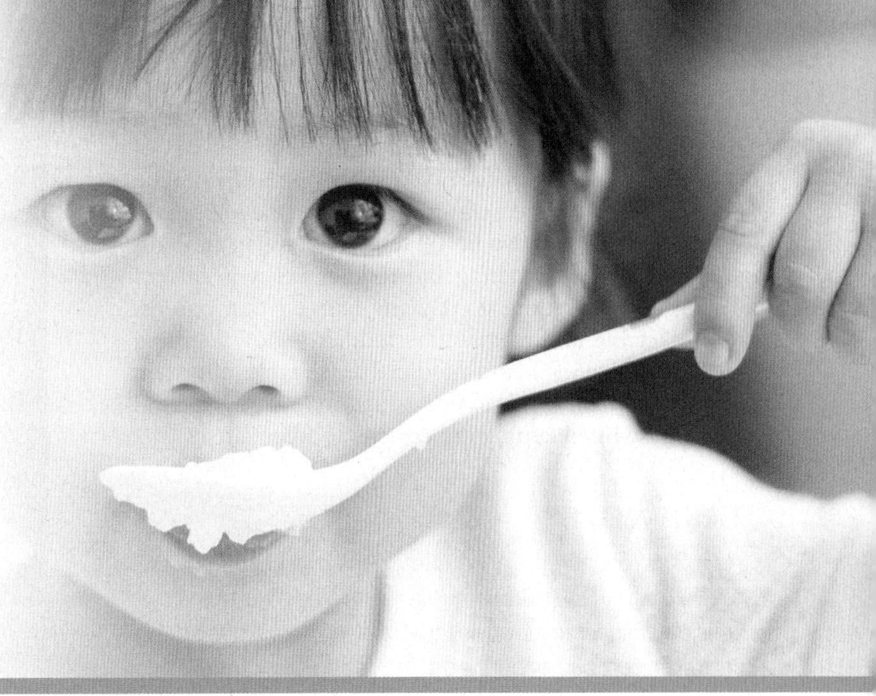

Growth and Development of the Toddler

KEY TERMS

animism (an′i-mizm)
echolalia (ek′ō-lā′lē-ă)
egocentrism (ē′gō-sen′trizm)
expressive language
food jag
individuation (in′di-vij′yū-ā′shŭn)
negativism
parallel play
physiologic anorexia (fiz′ē-ō-loj′ik an′ō-rek′sē-ă)
receptive language
regression
separation
separation anxiety
sibling rivalry
telegraphic speech

LEARNING OBJECTIVES

Upon completion of the chapter, you will be able to:

1. Describe normal physical growth, physiologic changes, and sensory development in the toddler.
2. Examine psychosocial, cognitive, social/emotional, and moral/spiritual development in the toddler.
3. Identify the gross and fine motor milestones of the toddler.
4. Explain normal language development in toddlerhood.
5. Implement a nursing care plan to address common issues or delays related to growth and development in toddlerhood.
6. Develop a teaching plan for safety promotion in the toddler period.
7. Examine common issues related to growth and development in toddlerhood.
8. Develop a nutritional plan for the toddler based on average nutritional requirements.
9. Consider appropriate methods of discipline for use during the toddler years.
10. Provide appropriate anticipatory guidance for common developmental issues that arise in the toddler period.

Jose Gonzales is a 2-year-old brought to the clinic by his parents for his 2-year-old check-up. As the nurse caring for him, assess Jose's growth and development, and then teach the parents what changes to expect in Jose over the next few months.

INTRODUCTION

The toddler period encompasses the second 2 years of life, from age 1 year to age 3 years. This period is a time of significant advancement in growth and development for the child. It can also be quite a challenging time for parents. The theme during the toddler years is one of holding on and letting go. Having learned that parents are predictable and reliable, the toddler is now learning that their behavior has a predictable, reliable effect on others. The challenge is to encourage independence and autonomy while keeping the curious toddler safe.

TAKE NOTE!

As more grandparents are assuming the primary caregiver role for their grandchildren, nurses should be alert to the possibility of increased stress that is placed upon the older caregiver, particularly during the active and sometimes trying years of toddlerhood (Smith & Segal, 2023).

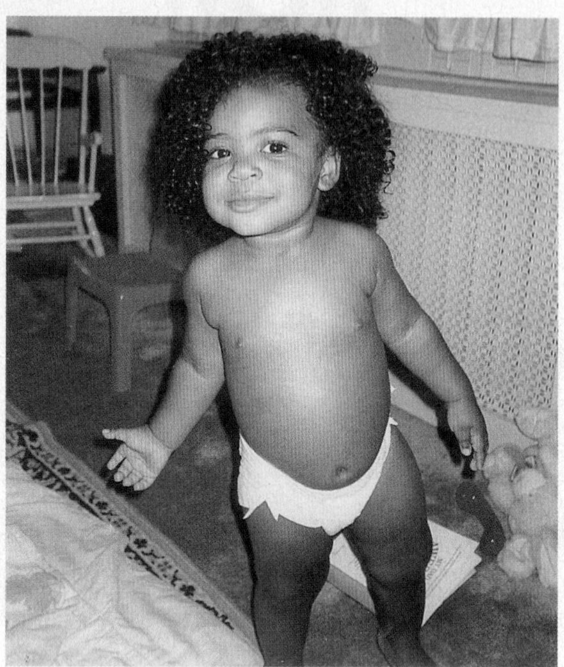

FIGURE 26.1 The typical toddler appearance is that of a rounded abdomen, a slight swayback, and a wide-based stance.

GROWTH AND DEVELOPMENT OVERVIEW

Infancy is a time of intense growth and development. Both physical growth and acquisition of new motor skills slow somewhat during the toddler years. Refinement of motor skills, continued cognitive growth, and acquisition of appropriate language skills are of prime importance during toddlerhood. The nurse uses the knowledge of normal toddler development as a roadmap for assessment of the 1- to 3-year-old child.

PHYSICAL GROWTH

The toddler's height and weight continue to increase steadily, although the increase occurs at a slower velocity compared to infancy. Toddler gains in height and weight tend to occur in spurts, rather than in a linear fashion (Fig. 26.1). The average toddler weight gain is 1.36 to 2.27 kg (3 to 5 lb) per year. Length/height increases by an average of 7.62 cm (3 in) per year. Toddlers generally reach about half of their adult height by 2 years of age. Head circumference increases about 2.54 cm (1 in) from age 1 to 2 years, then increases an average of 1.27 cm (0.5 in) per year until age 5. The anterior fontanel should be closed by the time the child is 18 months old. Head size becomes more proportional to the rest of the body near the age of 3 years (Carter & Feigelman, 2020a, 2020b; Reynolds et al., 2022).

Remember Jose Gonzales, introduced at the beginning of the chapter? During your assessment, you find that his weight is 13.6 kg (30 lb), height 83.82 cm (33 in), and head circumference 49.53 cm (19.5 in).

PHYSIOLOGIC CHANGES

Although not as pronounced as the changes occurring during infancy, the toddler's organ systems continue to grow and mature in their functioning. Significant functional changes occur within the neurologic, gastrointestinal, and genitourinary systems. The respiratory and cardiovascular systems undergo changes as well.

Neurologic System

Brain growth continues through toddlerhood, and head circumference (reflective of brain growth) reaches about 90% of its adult size by 2 years of age (Carter & Feigelman, 2020b). Myelination of the brain and spinal cord continues to progress and is complete around 24 months of age. Myelination results in improved coordination and equilibrium as well as the ability to exercise sphincter control, which is important for bowel and bladder mastery. Integration of the primitive reflexes occurs in infancy, allowing for the emergence of the protective reflexes near the end of infancy or early in toddlerhood. The forward or downward parachute reflex is particularly helpful when the child starts to toddle. Rapid increase in language skills is evidence of continued progression of cognitive development.

Respiratory System

The respiratory structures continue to grow and mature throughout toddlerhood. The alveoli continue to increase in number, not reaching the adult number until about

7 years of age. The trachea and lower airways continue to grow but remain small compared with the adult. The tongue is relatively large in comparison to the size of the mouth. Tonsils and adenoids are large, and the eustachian tubes are relatively short and straight.

Cardiovascular System

The heart rate decreases, and blood pressure increases in toddlerhood. Blood vessels are close to the skin surface and so are compressed easily when palpated.

Gastrointestinal System

The stomach continues to increase in size, allowing the toddler to consume three regular meals per day. Pepsin production matures by 2 years of age. The small intestine continues to grow in length, although it does not reach the maximum length of 2 to 3 m until adulthood. Stool passage decreases in frequency to one or more per day. The color of the stool may change (yellow, orange, brown, or green) depending on the toddler's diet. Since the toddler's intestines remain somewhat immature, the toddler often passes whole pieces of difficult-to-digest food such as corn kernels. Bowel control is generally achieved by the end of the toddler period.

Genitourinary System

Bladder and kidney function reach adult levels by 16 to 24 months of age. The bladder capacity increases, allowing the toddler to retain urine for longer periods. Urine output should be about 1 mL/kg/hour. The urethra remains short in both the male and the female toddler, making them more susceptible to urinary tract infections compared to adults.

Musculoskeletal System

During toddlerhood, the bones increase in length, and the muscles mature and become stronger. The abdominal musculature is weak in early toddlerhood, resulting in a pot-bellied appearance. The toddler appears to have a swayback along with the potbelly. Around 3 years of age, the musculature strengthens, and the abdomen is flatter in appearance.

PSYCHOSOCIAL DEVELOPMENT

Erikson defines the toddlerhood period as a time of autonomy versus shame and doubt. It is a time of asserting independence. Since the toddler developed a sense of trust in infancy, they are ready to give up dependence and to assert their sense of control and autonomy (Erikson, 1963). The toddler is struggling for self-mastery, to learn to do for themselves what others have been doing for them. Toddlers often experience ambivalence about the move from dependence to autonomy, resulting in emotional lability. The toddler may quickly change from happy and pleasant to crying and screaming. Assertion of independence also results in the toddler's favorite response, "no." The toddler will often answer "no" even when they really mean "yes." This **negativism**—always saying "no"—is a normal part of healthy development and is occurring as a result of the toddler's attempt to assert their independence. Table 26.1 gives further information related to developing a sense of autonomy.

COGNITIVE DEVELOPMENT

According to Jean Piaget (1969), toddlers move through the last two substages of the first stage of cognitive development, the sensorimotor stage, between 12 and 24 months of age. Young toddlers engage in tertiary circular reactions and progress to mental combinations. Rather than just repeating a behavior, the toddler is able to experiment with a behavior to see what happens. By 2 years of age, toddlers are capable of using symbols to allow for imitation. With increasing cognitive abilities, toddlers may now engage in delayed imitation. For example, they may imitate a household task that they observed a parent doing several days ago.

Piaget identified the second stage of cognitive development as the preoperational stage. It occurs in children between ages 2 and 7 years. During this stage, toddlers begin to become more sophisticated with symbolic thought. The thinking of the older toddler is far more advanced than that of the infant or young toddler, who views the world as a series of objects. During the preoperational stage, objects begin to have characteristics that make them unique from one another. Objects are considered large or small, having a particular color or shape, or having a unique texture. This moves beyond the connection of sensory information and physical action. Words and images allow the toddler to begin this process of developing symbolic thought by providing a label for the objects' characteristics (Piaget, 1969).

Toddlers also use symbols in dramatic play. First, they imitate life with appropriate toy objects, and then they are able to substitute objects in their play. A bowl may be used to pretend to eat from, but then later it can be used upside down on the head as a hat (Fig. 26.2). Human feelings and characteristics may also be attributed to objects (**animism**) (Martorell, 2022). See Table 26.1 for further explanation of cognitive development in toddlerhood.

TAKE NOTE!

Birthing parents who are depressed may not be as sensitive to their children as those who are not depressed. For this reason, maternal depression is a risk factor for poor cognitive development. Be alert to the mental status of a toddler's birthing parent so that appropriate referrals can be made if needed (Viguera, 2023).

TABLE 26.1 • Developmental Theories

Theorist	Stage	Activities
Erikson	Autonomy vs. shame and doubt Age: 1–3 years	Achieves autonomy and self-control Separates from parent/caregiver Withstands delayed gratification Negativism abounds. Imitates adults and playmates Spontaneously shows affection Is increasingly enthusiastic about playmates Cannot take turns in games until age 3 years
Piaget	Sensorimotor Substage 5: tertiary circular reactions Age: 12–18 months Substage 6: Mental combinations Age: 18–24 months Preoperational Age: 2–7 years	Differentiates self from objects Increased object permanence (knows that objects that are out of sight still exist [e.g., cookies in the cabinet]) Uses ALL senses to explore environment Places items in and out of containers Imitates domestic chores (domestic mimicry) Imitation is more symbolic. Starting to think before acting Understands requests and is capable of following simple directions Has a sense of ownership (my, mine) Time, space, and causality understanding is increasing. Uses mental trial and error rather than physical Makes mechanical toys work Plays make-believe with dolls, animals, and people Increased use of language for mental representation Understands concept of "two" Starting to make connections between an experience in the past and a new one that is currently occurring Sorts objects by shape and color Completes puzzles with four pieces Play becomes more complex.
Freud	Anal stage Age: 1–3 years	Focus is on achieving anal sphincter control. Satisfaction and/or frustration may occur as the toddler learns to withhold and expel stool.

Data from Erikson, E. H. (1963). *Childhood and society* (2nd ed.). W.W. Norton and Company; Reynolds, A., Angulo, A., Breheney, M., Green, J., & Goldson, E. (2022). Child development and behavior. In M. Bunik, W. W. Hay, M. J. Levin, & M. J. Abzug (Eds.), *Current diagnosis & treatment: Pediatrics* (26th ed.). McGraw-Hill Education; Piaget, J. (1969). *The theory of stages in cognitive development.* McGraw-Hill.

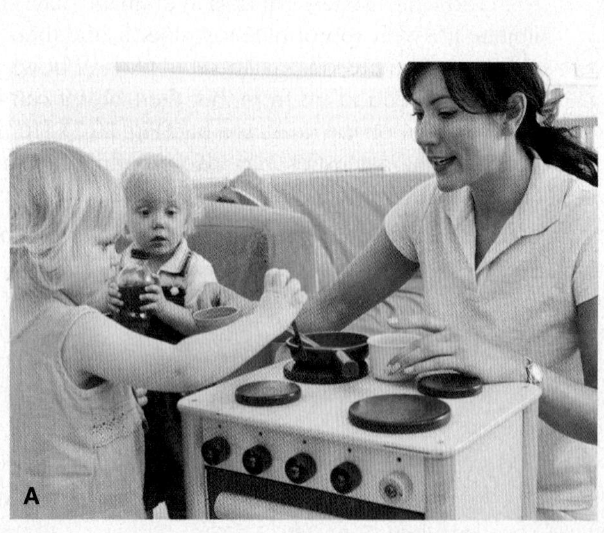

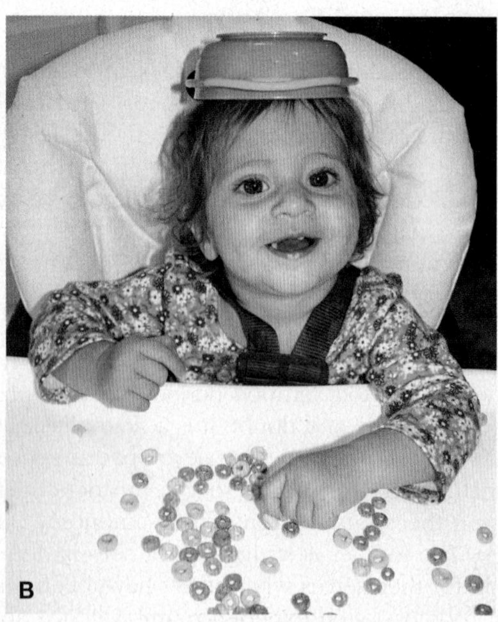

FIGURE 26.2 The toddler will pretend with items in the way they are intended to be used (**A**) as well as find other creative uses for them (**B**).

MOTOR SKILL DEVELOPMENT

Toddlers continue to gain new motor skills as well as refine others. Walking progresses to running, climbing, and jumping. Pushing or pulling a toy, throwing a ball, and pedaling a tricycle are accomplished in toddlerhood. Fine motor skills progress from holding and pinching to the ability to manage utensils, hold a crayon, string a bead, and use a computer. Development of eye–hand coordination is necessary for the refinement of fine motor skills. These increased abilities of mobility and manipulation help the curious toddler explore and learn more about their environment (Fig. 26.3). As the toddler masters a new task, they have confidence to conquer the next challenge. Thus, mastery in motor skill development contributes to the toddler's growing sense of self-esteem. The toddler who is eager to face challenges will likely develop more quickly than one who is reluctant. The senses of sight, hearing, and touch are useful in helping to coordinate gross and fine motor movement.

Gross Motor Skills

As gross motor skills are mastered and then used repeatedly, the large muscle groups in the toddler are strengthened. The "toddler gait" is characteristic of new walkers. The toddler does not walk smoothly and maturely. Instead, the legs are planted widely apart, toes are pointed forward, and the toddler seems to sway from side to side while moving forward (Fig. 26.4). Often, the toddler seems to speed along, be pitching forward, and may appear ready to topple over at any moment. The toddler may fall often but will use outstretched arms to catch themselves (parachute reflex). After about 6 months of practice walking, the toddler's gait is smoother, and the feet are closer together. By 3 years of age, the toddler walks in a heel-to-toe fashion similar to that of adults. Toddlers often use physical actions such as running, jumping, and hitting to express their emotions because they are only just learning to express their thoughts and feelings verbally. Table 26.2 lists motor skill expectations in relation to age.

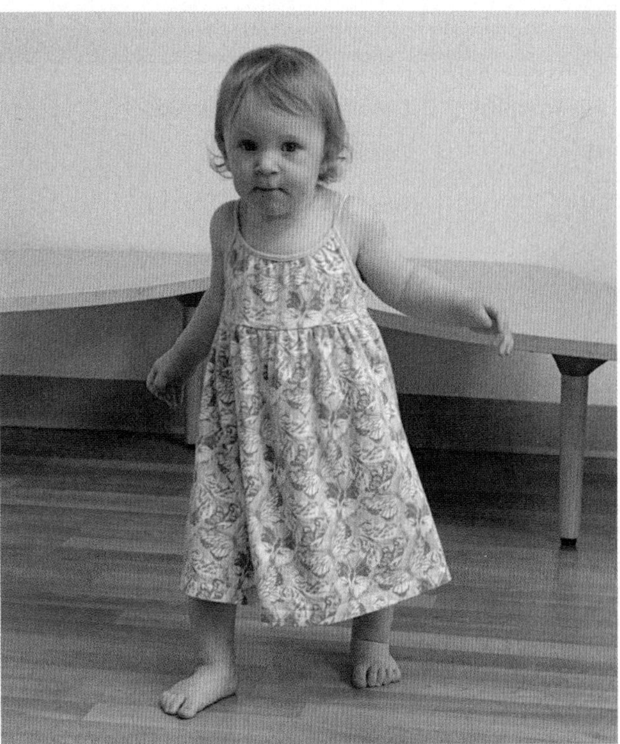

FIGURE 26.4 The young toddler (early walker) walks with a wide-based stance, feet pointing forward, and arms akimbo.

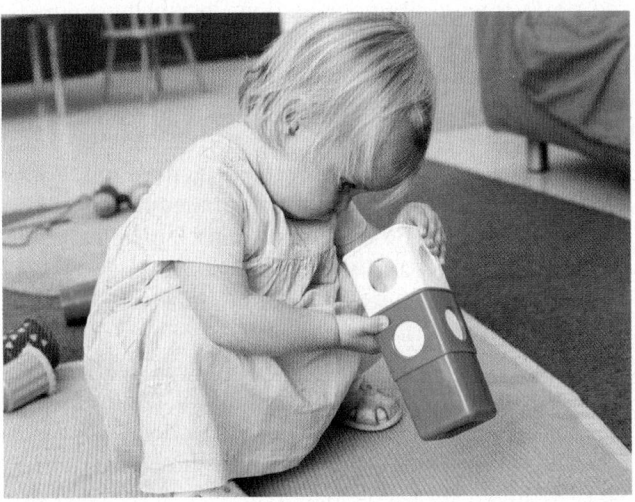

FIGURE 26.3 The toddler's curiosity about the world increases, as does their ability to explore it.

Fine Motor Skills

Fine motor skills in the toddler period are improved and perfected. Holding utensils requires some control and agility, but even more is needed for buttoning and zipping. Adequate vision is necessary for the refinement of fine motor skills because eye–hand coordination is crucial for directing the fingers, hand, and wrist to accomplish small muscle tasks such as fitting a puzzle piece or stringing a bead. See Table 26.2 for age expectations for various motor skills.

SENSORY DEVELOPMENT

Toddlers use all of their senses to explore the world around them. Toddlers examine new items by feeling them, looking at them, shaking them to hear what sound they make, smelling them, and placing them in their mouths. Toddler vision continues to progress and should be 20/50 to 20/40 in both eyes. Depth perception

TABLE 26.2 • Motor Skill Development

Age (months)	Expected Gross Motor Skill	Expected Fine Motor Skills
15	Takes few steps on own	Feeds self finger foods
18	Walks independently Climbs on/off furniture Climbs stairs with assistance Seats self in chair	Scribbles Tries to use a spoon Throws a ball Stacks three to four cubes
24	Runs Kicks ball Walks upstairs with assistance (not climbing) Kicks a ball	Eats with a spoon Stacks six to seven cubes Points to named pictures and objects Starting to turn knobs
30	Jumps with both feet	Turns knobs Turns book page one at a time Takes off some clothing items
36	Puts on some clothes by self	Strings items together Uses a fork Puts on some clothes by self Copies circle

Data from Carter, R. G., & Feigelman, S. (2020a). The preschool years. In R. M. Kliegman, J. W. St. Geme III, N. J. Blum, S. S. Shah, R. C. Tasker, K. M. Wilson, & R. E. Behrman (Eds.), *Nelson's textbook of pediatrics* (21st ed.). Elsevier; Carter, R. G., & Feigelman, S. (2020b). The second year. In R. M. Kliegman, J. W. St. Geme III, N. J. Blum, S. S. Shah, R. C. Tasker, K. M. Wilson, & R. E. Behrman (Eds.), *Nelson's textbook of pediatrics* (21st ed.). Elsevier; Reynolds, A., Angulo, A., Breheney, M., Green, J., & Goldson, E. (2022). Child development and behavior. In M. Bunik, W. W. Hay, M. J. Levin, & M. J. Abzug (Eds.), *Current diagnosis & treatment: Pediatrics* (26th ed.). McGraw-Hill Education; Zubler, J. M., Wiggins, L. D., Macias, M. M., Whitaker, T. M., Shaw, J. S., Squires, J. K., Pajke, J. A., Wolf, R. B., Slaughter, K. S., Broughton, A. S., Gerndt, K. L., Mlodoch, B. J., & Lipkin, P. H. (2022). Evidence-informed milestones for developmental surveillance tools. *Pediatrics, 149*(3), e2021052138. https://doi.org/10.1542/peds.2021-052138

also continues to mature. Hearing should be at the adult level, as infants are ordinarily born with hearing intact. The sense of smell continues to mature, and toddlers may comment if they do not care for the scent of something. Although taste discrimination is not completely developed, toddlers may exhibit preferences for certain flavors of foods. The toddler is more likely to try a new food if its appearance or smell is familiar. Lack of complete taste discrimination places the toddler at risk for inadvertent ingestion.

COMMUNICATION AND LANGUAGE DEVELOPMENT

Language development occurs rapidly during the toddler years. The acquisition of language is a dynamic and complex process. The child's age and social interactions and the types of language to which they have been exposed influence language development. **Receptive language** development (the ability to understand what is being said or asked) is typically far more advanced than **expressive language** development (the ability to communicate one's desires and feelings) (Carter & Feigelman, 2020b; Reynolds et al., 2022). In other words, the toddler understands language and is able to follow commands far sooner than they can actually use the words themselves. Language is a very important part of the toddler's ability to organize their world and actually make sense of it. Thoughtfully planned use of language can provide behavior guidance and contribute to the avoidance of power struggles. In regard to expressive language development, the young toddler begins to use short sentences and will progress to a vocabulary of 50 words by 2 years of age (Carter & Feigelman, 2020b; Reynolds et al., 2022). **Echolalia** (repetition of words and phrases without understanding) normally occurs in toddlers younger than 30 months of age. "Why" and "what" questions dominate the older toddler's language. Telegraphic speech is common in the 3-year-old. **Telegraphic speech** refers to speech that contains only the essential words to get the point across, much like a telegram. Rather than "I want a cookie and milk," the toddler might say, "Want cookie milk." In telegraphic speech, the nouns and verbs are present and are verbalized in the appropriate order (Carter & Feigelman, 2020b). Table 26.3 gives an overview of receptive and expressive language development in the toddler.

Early identification and referral of children with potential speech delays is critical. If a delay is identified, early intervention may increase the child's potential to acquire age-appropriate receptive and expressive language skills. Children with preexisting conditions

TABLE 26.3 • Language Development in Toddlers

Age (months)	Receptive Language	Expressive Language
12	Understands the word "no"	Imitates or uses gestures such as waving goodbye
15	Follows a command accompanied by a gesture	Uses a finger to point to things Looks for a familiar object when named Tries to say one to two words other than "dada" and "mama"
18	Follows a one-step command without gesture	Tries to say three or more words other than "dada" and "mama"
24	Points to named body parts Points to pictures in books	Sentences of two words ("me up," "want cookie") Uses gestures like blowing a kiss or nodding yes
30	Follows a series of two independent commands Names items when pointed to and asks, "what's this?"	Vocabulary of approximately 50 words Sentences of two words with an action word ("cat run")
36	Uses at least two back-and-forth exchanges when conversing Understands physical relationships (on, in, under)	Most outside the family understand speech. Asks "why," "where," and "what?" Verbalizes actions happening in a picture Says first name when asked

Data from Carter, R. G., & Feigelman, S. (2020a). The preschool years. In R. M. Kliegman, J. W. St. Geme III, N. J. Blum, S. S. Shah, R. C. Tasker, K. M. Wilson, & R. E. Behrman (Eds.), *Nelson's textbook of pediatrics* (21st ed.). Elsevier; Carter, R. G., & Feigelman, S. (2020b). The second year. In R. M. Kliegman, J. W. St. Geme III, N. J. Blum, S. S. Shah, R. C. Tasker, K. M. Wilson, & R. E. Behrman (Eds.), *Nelson's textbook of pediatrics* (21st ed.). Elsevier; Reynolds, A., Angulo, A., Breheney, M., Green, J., & Goldson, E. (2022). Child development and behavior. In M. Bunik, W. W. Hay, M. J. Levin, & M. J. Abzug (Eds.), *Current diagnosis & treatment: Pediatrics* (26th ed.). McGraw-Hill Education; Zubler, J. M., Wiggins, L. D., Macias, M. M., Whitaker, T. M., Shaw, J. S., Squires, J. K., Pajke, J. A., Wolf, R. B., Slaughter, K. S., Broughton, A. S., Gerndt, K. L., Mlodoch, B. J., & Lipkin, P. H. (2022). Evidence-informed milestones for developmental surveillance tools. *Pediatrics, 149*(3), e2021052138. https://doi.org/10.1542/peds.2021-052138.

such as genetic syndromes that are known to have an effect on language development should be referred to a speech–language pathologist as soon as the condition is recognized rather than waiting until the child exhibits a delay.

Of special concern in the toddler years is the development of speech and language in potentially bilingual children. At the age of 1 to 2 years, the potentially bilingual child may blend two languages—that is, parts of the word in both languages are blended into one word. At age 2 to 3 years, the potentially bilingual toddler may mix languages within a sentence. Thus, the assessment of adequate language development is more complicated in bilingual children. There are websites that may be helpful to parents of potentially bilingual children, where they can find support and resources.

TAKE NOTE!

Young children exposed to more than one language may experience simultaneous acquisition of both languages. The first word may be slightly delayed as compared with single language speakers, but still occurs within the normal range (Linguistic Society of America, 2023).

As you assess Jose (the 2-year-old introduced at the beginning of the chapter), what would you expect his gross motor, fine motor, and language skills to be at this age? How would this be different if Jose had been born 12 weeks premature?

EMOTIONAL AND SOCIAL DEVELOPMENT

Emotional development in the toddler years is focused on separation and individuation (Martorell, 2022). Seeing oneself as separate from the parent or primary caregiver (**separation**) is accompanied by forming a sense of self and learning to exert control over one's environment (**individuation**). As this need to feel in control of their world emerges, the toddler displays **egocentrism** (focus on self). This need for control results in emotional lability: happy and pleasant one moment, then overreacting to limit setting with a temper tantrum in the next moment (Lieberman, 2018). As toddlers identify the boundaries between themselves and the parent or primary caregiver, they learn to negotiate a balance between attachment and independence. Toddlers initially rely on the parents' communication and signals in order to initiate appropriate behavior or inhibit undesirable behavior. They have a difficult time choosing between sets of behaviors as

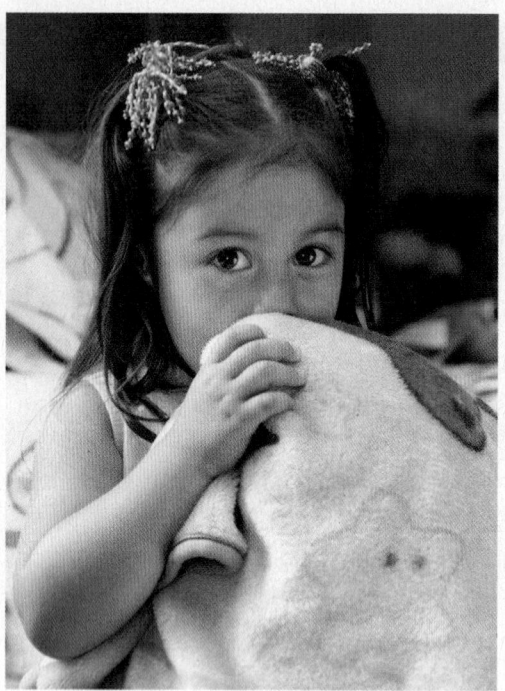

FIGURE 26.5 The toddler may be able to self-soothe and produce a sense of comfort during this stage of establishing autonomy by relying on a security item, such as a doll, bear, or blanket.

they occur in different situations. Power struggles often occur in this age group, and it is important for parents and caregivers to thoughtfully and intentionally develop the rituals and routines that will provide stability and security for the toddler (Carter & Feigelman, 2020b). Many toddlers rely on a security item (blanket, doll, or bear) to comfort themselves in stressful situations (Fig. 26.5). This ability to self-soothe is a function of autonomy and is viewed as a sign of a nurturing environment, rather than, as one might suspect, one of neglect.

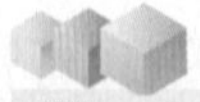 *Concept Mastery Alert*

When teaching parents interventions appropriate to the emotional development of their toddler, nurses can teach parents that they may offer a toddler limited choices (usually two are sufficient) to assist with control over their environment. Nurses should advise parents that aggressive behavior is normal in the toddler period, so parents should not blame toddlers for the behavior but should help toddlers understand the results of their behavior.

Children also begin to learn about sex and gender differences in the toddler years. They observe the differences between male and female body parts if they are exposed to them. Toddlers may question parents about these differences and may begin to explore their own genitals. Toddlers also begin to understand and mimic social gender differences. They make observations about gender-specific behavior dependent on what they are exposed to.

Aggressive behaviors are typically displayed during the toddler years. Toddlers may hit, bite, or push other children and grab toys. Adults can assist the toddler in building empathy by pointing out when someone is hurt and explaining what happened. Toddlers should not be blamed for their impulsive behavior; rather, they should be guided toward socially acceptable actions in order to foster development of appropriate social judgment. It is particularly important for the parent or caregiver to serve as a role model for appropriate behavior, rather than losing their own temper, in order for the toddler to be able to learn how to acceptably handle frustrations. Offering limited choices is one way of allowing toddlers some control over their environment and helping them to establish a sense of mastery. Since toddlers naturally have a short attention span, they tend to dawdle. As the toddlers become more self-aware, they start to develop emotions of self-consciousness such as embarrassment and shame.

Although toddlers are becoming more self-aware, they still do not have clear body boundaries. They do not clearly understand the body's functions, although they are beginning to make appropriate connections. Feces may be viewed as a part of the child, and the toddler may become upset at seeing it disappear in the toilet. The toddler will protect their body by resisting intrusive procedures such as temperature or blood pressure measurement.

Separation Anxiety

As toddlers become increasingly skilled at mobility, they realize that if they have the capability to leave, then so does the parent. As self-awareness develops and conflicts over closeness versus exploration occur, **separation anxiety** may reemerge in the 18- to 24-month period (Lieberman, 2018). Power struggles may escalate, and distress at separating from the parent may increase. Again, a predictable routine with appropriate limit setting may help toddlers to feel safer and more secure during this period. From the age of 24 to 36 months, separation anxiety again eases. The older toddler begins to have a concept of object constancy: they have an internal representation of the parent or caregiver and are better able to tolerate separation, knowing that a reunion will occur.

Temperament

Temperament is the biologic basis for personality. It is our emotional and motivational core, around which the personality develops over time (Child Development Institute, 2022). Temperament affects how the toddler interacts with the environment. The easygoing toddler may adapt more easily and not mind changes in routine as much as other toddlers. The easygoing toddler usually sleeps and eats well and has more predictable and regular behaviors. However, the toddler may still express frustration by having a temper tantrum. The challenging toddler is more likely to have intense reactions, negative or positive, with temper tantrums being more likely, more frequent, and more intense than in other toddlers. The structure and routine that toddlers need to feel secure are essential for this toddler; otherwise, the child feels insecure and, as a result, is more likely to behave inappropriately. The challenging toddler is also the most active of the three temperament types. The slow-to-warm-up toddler is more of a loner and may be very shy. They may experience more difficulty with separation anxiety. The behavior of the slow-to-warm-up toddler is more passive; the toddler may be watchful and withdrawn and may take longer to mature. Changes in routine usually do not result in as much upset, since the toddler's natural reaction is one of passivity (Lieberman, 2018).

Based on the toddler's temperament, make suggestions to the parents for interacting with the toddler in various situations. For example, to avoid temper tantrums in the challenging toddler, suggest that the parent should be especially diligent about maintaining structure and routine as well as avoiding tantrum triggers such as fatigue and hunger. Explain to parents that they may need to exercise additional patience with new activities to which the slow-to-warm-up toddler may need extra time becoming accustomed.

Fears

Common fears of toddlers include loss of parents (which contributes to separation anxiety) and fear of strangers. Some toddlers may be slow to warm up to people they do not know. The nurse caring for a toddler in the outpatient or hospital setting should take the time to establish a relationship with the toddler in order to allay the toddler's fears. Toddlers may be afraid of loud noises and large or unfamiliar animals. Going to sleep may be a scary time for toddlers as they may be afraid of the dark. A nightlight in the toddler's room may be helpful.

MORAL AND SPIRITUAL DEVELOPMENT

During the toddler years, children may feel comfort from the routine of praying, but they do not understand religious beliefs because of their limited cognitive abilities. Reading simple religious or moral allegories can lay a foundation for later related teachings. Kohlberg's (1984) description of moral development places the older toddler at the preconventional level. The toddler is only just beginning to learn right from wrong and does not understand the larger concept of morality. The toddler will base their actions on the avoidance of punishment and the attainment of pleasure. Older toddlers begin to feel empathy for others.

SOCIOCULTURAL INFLUENCES ON GROWTH AND DEVELOPMENT

Homelessness or poverty may directly influence the toddler's ability to grow adequately, as resources for the purchase and preparation of appropriate food may be lacking. Safe, appropriate toys may also not be available in those situations. Food customs continue to have an impact on the child's diet and ability to ingest appropriate nutrients. Individual families' value systems have an impact on the toddler's development as well. Some parents desire to keep their child a "baby" for a longer period, thus delaying weaning or continuing to feed the child baby food or puréed food for a longer period. Other families may highly value independence and encourage the toddler to walk everywhere on their own rather than carrying the child.

Culture may also affect emotional development. Some families start to discourage crying in male children. Ridicule for crying at this age may hurt the toddler's self-concept. Educating families about normal growth and development while continuing to value and support cultural practices is important (Martorell, 2022).

> Remember Jose Gonzales, whom you met at the beginning of the chapter? What developmental milestones would you expect him to have reached at his age?

THE NURSE'S ROLE IN TODDLER GROWTH AND DEVELOPMENT

The toddler's growth and development affect their everyday life as well as the family's. Although some toddlers may grow more quickly or reach developmental milestones sooner than others, growth and development remains orderly and sequential. Health care visits throughout toddlerhood continue to focus on growth and development. The nurse must have a good understanding of the changes that occur during the toddler years in order to provide appropriate anticipatory guidance and support to the family.

When the toddler is hospitalized, growth and development may be altered. The toddler's primary task is establishing autonomy, and the toddler's focus is mobility and language development. Hospitalization removes most opportunities for the toddler to learn through exploration of the environment. Isolation for contagious illness further constrains the toddler's ability to find some control over the environment. The nurse caring for the hospitalized toddler must use knowledge of normal growth and development to be successful in interactions with the toddler, promote continued development, and recognize delays (see Chapter 33) (Fig. 26.6).

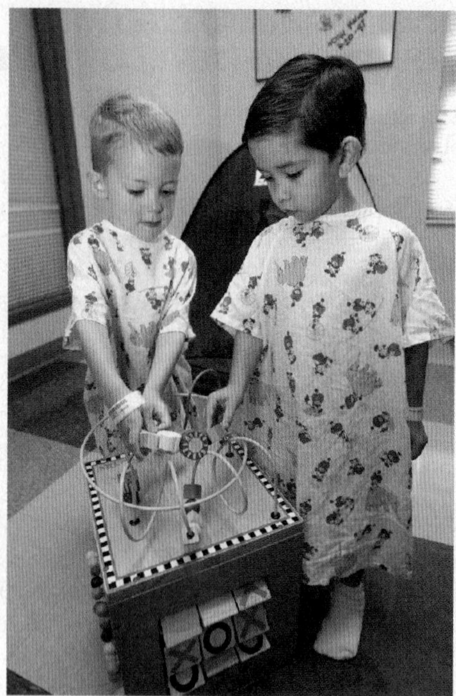

FIGURE 26.6 The hospitalized toddler continues to enjoy developmental tasks appropriate for their age, such as playing with manipulative toys.

Clinical Judgment and the Nursing Process

On completion of assessment of the toddler's current growth and development status, problems or issues related to growth and development may be identified. The nurse may then identify one or more nursing diagnoses. The following nursing diagnoses with identified outcomes and interventions provide suggestions for nursing care planning or concept mapping. Care planning should be individualized, based on the toddler's and family's needs.

Nursing Analysis

Injury risk due to extremes of age (e.g., curiosity, increased mobility, developmental immaturity) or unsafe mode of transport (e.g., lack of car seat and helmet use)

Goal/Outcome

Toddler safety will be maintained: Toddler will remain free from injury.

Preventing Injury (interventions with *rationale*)

- Teach and encourage appropriate use of rear-facing car seat until 2 years of age and forward-facing car seat after 2 years of age *to decrease risk of toddler injury related to motor vehicles.*
- Teach toddlers to stay away from the street and provide constant supervision *to prevent pedestrian injury.*
- Require bicycle helmet use while riding any wheeled toy *to prevent head injury and form habit of helmet use.*
- Childproof the home *to provide a developmentally safe environment for the curious and increasingly mobile toddler.*
- Post Poison Control Center phone number *in case of inadvertent ingestion.*
- Never leave a toddler unattended in a tub or pool or near any body of water *to prevent drowning.*
- Teach parents first-aid measures and child cardiopulmonary resuscitation (CPR) *to minimize consequences of injury should it occur.*
- Provide close observation and keep side rails up on crib/bed in hospital *because toddlers are at particularly high risk for falling or becoming entangled in tubing as they attempt mobility.*

Nursing Analysis

Alteration in nutritional status related to inappropriate nutritional intake to sustain growth needs (e.g., excess juice or milk intake, inadequate food variety intake), as evidenced by failure to attain adequate increases in length/height and weight over time.

Goal/Outcome

Toddler will consume adequate nutrients while using an appropriate feeding pattern: Toddler will demonstrate weight gain and increases in length/height.

Promoting Appropriate Nutrition (interventions with *rationale*)

- Assess current feeding schedule and usual intake, as well as methods used to feed, *to determine areas of adequacy versus inadequacy.*
- Determine toddler's ability to drink from cup, finger feed, swallow, and consume textures *to determine if additional exposure is needed or if further interventions such as speech or occupational therapy are required.*
- Weigh toddler daily on same scale if hospitalized, weekly on same scale if at home, and plot growth patterns weekly or monthly as appropriate on standardized growth charts *to determine if growth is improving.*
- Wean from bottle by 15 months of age *to discourage excess milk or juice intake in toddler who can carry bottle around.*
- Limit juice to 4 to 6 oz per day and milk to 16 to 24 oz per day *to discourage sense of fullness achieved with excess milk or juice intake, thereby increasing appetite for solid foods.*
- Provide three nutrient-dense meals and at least two healthy snacks per day *to encourage adequate nutrient consumption.*

- Feed toddler on a similar schedule daily without distractions and with the family; *toddlers respond well to routine and structure and may eat better in the social context of meals, and they become distracted easily (television should be off).*

Nursing Analysis

Delayed development risk; risk factors include inadequate nutrition, abuse, chronic illness, prematurity, technology dependence, behavioral disorder, or involvement with the foster care system.

Goal/Outcome

Development will be enhanced: Toddler will make continued progress toward realization of expected developmental milestones.

Enhancing Development (interventions with *rationale*)

- Screen for developmental capabilities *to determine toddler's current level of functioning.*
- Offer age-appropriate toys, play, and activities (including gross motor) *to encourage further development.*
- Perform interventions as prescribed by physical, occupational, or speech therapist; *participation in those activities helps to promote function and accomplish acquisition of developmental skills.*
- Provide support to families of toddlers at risk for developmental delay *(progress in achieving developmental milestones can be slow and ongoing motivation is needed).*
- Reinforce positive attributes in the toddler *to maintain motivation.*
- Model age-appropriate communication skills *to illustrate suitable means for parenting the toddler.*

Nursing Analysis

Risk for body mass index (BMI) over 85th percentile for age 2+, or weight for length approaching 95th percentile for age (1 to 2 years of age); risk factors include portion sizes larger than recommended, excess milk or juice intake, late bottle weaning, and frequent snacking.

Goal/Outcome

Toddler will grow appropriately and not become overweight or obese: Toddler will achieve weight for length less than 85th percentile for age (less than 2 years old) or BMI less than 85th percentile (greater than 2 years old).

Promoting Proportionate Growth (interventions with rationale)

- Wean from bottle and discourage use of no-spill sippy cups by 15 months of age *(will keep mobile toddler from carrying around and continually drinking from cup or bottle).*
- Provide juice (4 to 6 oz per day) and milk (16 to 24 oz per day) from a cup at meal and snack time *to encourage appropriate cup drinking and limit intake of nutrient-poor, high-calorie fluids.*
- Provide only nutrient-rich foods without high sugar content for meals and snacks; *even if the toddler will not eat, it is inappropriate to provide high-calorie junk food just so the toddler eats something.*
- Ensure adequate physical activity *to stimulate development of motor skills and provide appropriate caloric expenditure. This also sets the stage for forming lifelong habit of appropriate physical activity.*

Nursing Analysis

Altered family functioning related to shift in family roles (toddler illness or hospitalization) as evidenced by change in family satisfaction/assigned tasks/communication pattern or decrease in available emotional support.

Goal/Outcome

Family will demonstrate adequate functioning: Family will display coping and psychosocial adjustment.

Enhancing Family Functioning (interventions with *rationale*)

- Assess the family's level of stress and ability to cope *to determine family's ability to cope with multiple stressors.*
- Engage in family-centered care *to provide a holistic approach to care of the toddler and family.*
- Encourage the family to verbalize feelings (*verbalization is one method of decreasing anxiety levels*) and acknowledge feelings and emotions.
- Encourage family visitation and provide for sleeping arrangements for a parent or caregiver to stay in the hospital with the toddler (*contributes to family's sense of control of situation*).
- Involve family members in toddler's care, *giving them a feeling of control and connectedness.*

Nursing Analysis

Desire for strengthened parenting related to parental expression of desire for enhanced skills.

Goal/Outcome

Parent will provide safe and nurturing environment for the toddler.

Increasing Parenting Skill Set (interventions with *rationale*)

- Use family-centered care *to provide holistic approach.*
- Educate parent about normal toddler development *to provide basis for understanding the parenting skills needed in this time period.*

- Acknowledge and encourage parent's verbalization of feelings related to chronic illness of child or difficulty with normal toddler behavior *to validate the normalcy of the parent's feelings.*
- Encourage positive parenting with respect to toddlers and their normal development *to help parents develop approaches to toddlers that can be used in place of anger and frustration.*
- Acknowledge and admire positive parenting skills already present *to contribute to parents' confidence in their abilities to parent.*
- Role model appropriate parenting behaviors related to communicating with and disciplining the toddler *to actually show rather than just tell the parent what to do.*

PROMOTING HEALTHY GROWTH AND DEVELOPMENT

Parents who give their toddler love and respect regardless of the child's sex, behavior, or capabilities are helping to lay the foundation for self-esteem. Self-esteem is also built through familiarity with the daily routine. Routine and ritual help toddlers develop a conscience. Making expectations known through everyday routines helps to avoid confrontations. If the toddler knows the routine, they know what to expect and how they are expected to act. When routine and limits are absent, the toddler develops feelings of uncertainty and anxiety. Limit setting (and remaining consistent with those limits) helps toddlers master their behavior, develop self-esteem, and become successful participants in the family. Children are then able to learn about cooperation throughout the predictable flow of daily life. Nurses need to be aware of normal developmental expectations in order to determine whether the toddler is progressing appropriately. Table 26.4 lists potential signs of developmental delay. Any toddler with one or more of these concerns should be referred for further developmental evaluation.

TABLE 26.4 • Signs of Developmental Delay

Age or Time Frame	Concern
After independent walking for several months	• Persistent tiptoe walking • Failure to develop a mature walking pattern
By 18 months	• Not walking • Not speaking 15 words • Does not understand function of common household items
By 2 years	• Does not use two-word sentences • Does not imitate actions • Does not follow basic instructions • Cannot push a toy with wheels
By 3 years	• Difficulty with stairs • Frequent falling • Cannot build tower of more than four blocks • Difficulty manipulating small objects • Extreme difficulty in separation from parent or caregiver • Cannot copy a circle • Does not engage in make-believe play • Cannot communicate in short phrases • Does not understand simple instructions • Little interest in other children • Unclear speech, persistent drooling

Promoting Growth and Development Through Play

Play is the major socializing medium for toddlers. Parents should limit television viewing and encourage creative and physical play instead. Toddlers typically play alongside another child (**parallel play**) rather than cooperatively (Fig. 26.7). The short attention span of the toddler will make them often change toys and types of play. It is important to provide a variety of safe toys to allow the toddler many different opportunities for exploring the environment. Toddlers do not need expensive toys; in fact, regular household items sometimes make the most enjoyable toys. Toddlers are egocentric, a normal part of their development (Piaget, 1969). This makes it difficult for them to share. As they are developing a sense of self (who they are as a person), they may see their toys as an extension of themselves. Learning to share occurs in later toddlerhood. Toddlers also like dramatic play and play that recreates familiar activities in the home. Toddlers like to listen to music of all kinds and will often dance to whatever they hear on the radio. Toddlers enjoy

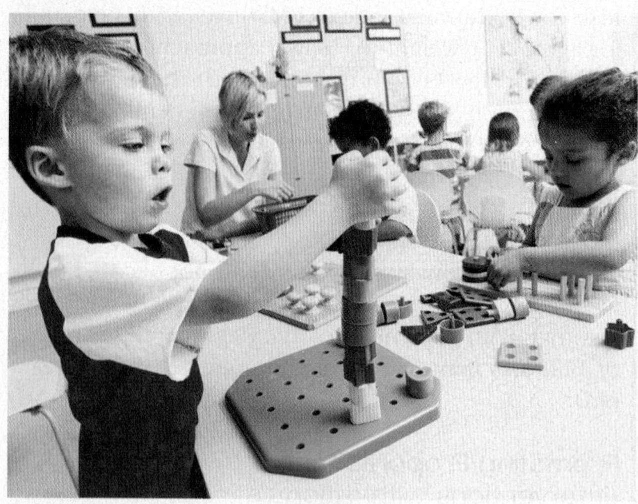

FIGURE 26.7 Parallel play. The toddler usually plays alongside another child rather than cooperatively.

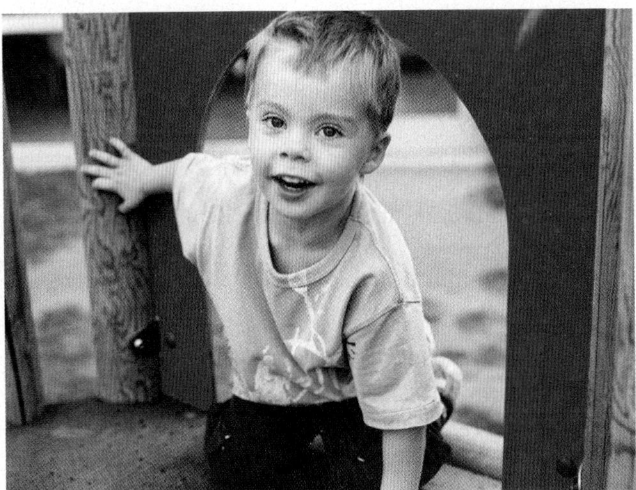

FIGURE 26.8 Toddlers love outdoor physical play, such as climbing on playground equipment. An adult should always supervise toddlers when they are playing outdoors.

BOX 26.1 Appropriate Toys for Toddlers

- Familiar household items such as plastic bowls and cups of various sizes, large plastic serving utensils, pots and pans, wooden spoons, cardboard boxes and tubes (from paper towel rolls), old magazines, baskets, purses, hats
- Child-size household item toys (kitchen, broom, vacuum cleaner, lawnmower, telephone, and so on)
- Blocks, cars and trucks, plastic animals, trains, plastic figures (family, community helpers), simple dolls, stuffed animals, balls, doll beds, and carriages
- Manipulative toys with knobs, wind-ups, and buttons that make things happen; putting large pegs or shapes into matching holes; stringing large beads on shoelaces; blocks and containers that stack; jigsaw puzzles with large pieces; toys that can be taken apart and put back together again
- Gross motor toys: play gym, push and pull toys, wagons, tricycle or other ride-on toys, tunnels
- Devices for playing music, various musical instruments
- Chalk, large crayons, finger paint, Play-Doh, washable markers
- Bucket, plastic shovel, and other containers for sand and water play
- Squeaking, floating, and squirting toys for the bath

Data from National Association for the Education of Young Children. (n.d.). *Good toys for young children by age and stage.* http://www.naeyc.org/toys

drums, xylophones, cymbals, and toy pianos. Musical instruments made at home are also enjoyed. A few pebbles or coins inside an empty water bottle with the top tightly secured is a great music maker; an empty butter tub with a lid and a pair of wooden spoons makes a nice drum.

Adequate physical activity is necessary for the development and refinement of movement skills. Toddlers need at least 60 minutes of structured physical activity and anywhere from 1 to several hours of unstructured physical activity per day (Hagan et al., 2017). Indoor and outdoor play areas should encourage play activities that use the large muscle groups. The activity must occur within a safe environment. Outdoor play structures should be positioned over surfaces that are soft enough to absorb a fall, such as sand, wood chips, or sawdust (Fig. 26.8). Box 26.1 lists recommended age-appropriate toys.

Promoting Early Learning

The parent–child relationship and the interactions between parent and child form the context for the toddler's early learning.

Promoting Language Development

Talking and singing to the toddler during routine activities such as feeding and dressing provide an environment that encourages conversation. Frequent, repetitive naming helps the toddler learn appropriate words for objects. The parent or caregiver should be attentive to what the toddler is saying as well as to their moods. Using clarification validates the toddler's emotions and ideas. Parents should listen to and answer the toddler's questions. They should sit down quietly with the toddler and gently repeat what the toddler is saying. Encouragement and elaboration convey confidence and interest to the toddler. The toddler needs time to complete their thoughts without being interrupted or rushed, because they are just starting to be able to make the connections necessary to transfer thoughts and feelings into language.

Parents should not overreact to the child's use of the word "no." They can give the toddler opportunities to use the word "no" appropriately by asking silly questions such as "Can a cat drive a car?" or "Is a banana purple?" When promoting language development, the parent or primary caregiver should teach the toddler appropriate words for body parts and objects and should help the toddler choose appropriate words to label feelings and emotions. Toddlers' receptive language and interpretation of body language and subtle signs far surpass their expressive language, especially at a younger age (Carter & Feigelman, 2020b; Reynolds et al., 2022).

Parents should avoid discussing scary or serious topics in the presence of the toddler, since the toddler is very adept at reading emotions. If the parents speak a foreign language in addition to English, both languages should be used in the home.

Encouraging Reading

Reading to the toddler every day is one of the best ways to promote language and cognitive development (Fig. 26.9). Toddlers particularly enjoy homemade or purchased books about feelings, family, friends, everyday life, animals and nature, and fun and fantasy. Board books have thick pages

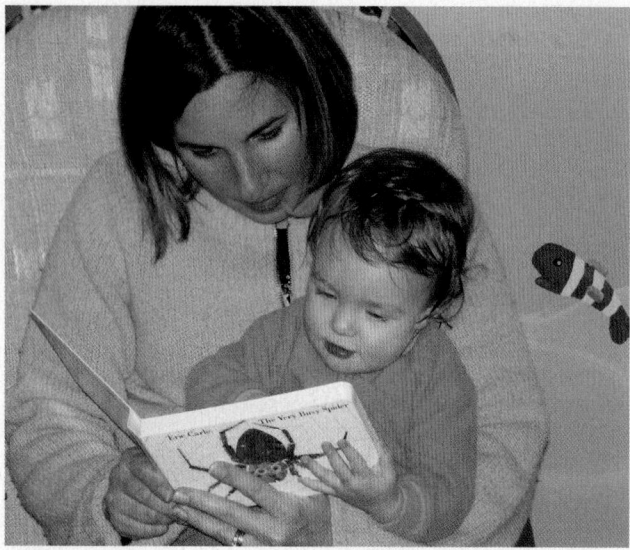

FIGURE 26.9 Reading to a toddler daily is one of the best ways to promote language development and school readiness.

that are easier for young toddlers to turn; older toddlers can turn paper pages one at a time. The toddler may also enjoy "reading" the story to the parent. Reach Out and Read, a program designed to promote early literacy, offers tips for reading with young children (see Teaching Guidelines 26.1).

Choosing a Preschool

The older toddler may benefit from the structure and socialization provided by attending preschool. Attending preschool will help the toddler become more mature and independent and give the toddler a different source for a sense of accomplishment. At this age, toddlers need supervised play with some direction that fosters their cognitive development. A strict curriculum is not necessary in this age group. When choosing a preschool, the parent or caregiver should look for an environment that has the following qualities:

- Goals and an overall philosophy with which the parents agree (promotion of independence and self-confidence through structured and free play)

TEACHING GUIDELINES 26.1 Tips for Reading With Young Children

- Read often for a short time.
- Keep reading fun, short, and simple.
- Reading stories over and over, rhyming, and singing songs help the toddler learn.
- Be engaging: use voices for the story characters.
- Use body motions during the story (toddlers will too).
- Ask questions about the story and about the pictures.

Data from Reading Rockets. (2023). *Tips for parents of toddlers*. https://www.readingrockets.org/topics/activities/articles/reading-tips-parents-toddlers

- Teachers and assistants trained in early childhood development as well as child CPR
- Small class sizes and an adult-to-child ratio with which the parent feels comfortable
- Disciplinary procedures consistent with the parents' values
- Parents can visit at any time
- School is childproofed inside and out
- Appropriate hygiene procedures, including prohibiting sick children from attending

Teach the parents how to ease the toddler's transition to attending preschool. Encourage parents to talk about going to preschool, and visit the school a couple of times. On the first day, parents should calmly and in a matter-of-fact tone tell the toddler that they will return to pick the child up. If the toddler expresses separation anxiety, the parent should remain calm and follow through with the plan for school attendance. After a few days of attendance, the toddler will be accustomed to the new routine, and crying when parting from the parent should be minimal.

Promoting Safety

Safety is of prime concern throughout the toddler period. Curiosity, mobility, and lack of impulse control all contribute to the incidence of unintentional injury in toddlerhood. Even the most watchful and caring parents have toddlers who run into the street, otherwise disappear from parents, and fall down the stairs. Toddlers require direct observation and cannot be trusted to be left alone. A childproof environment provides a safe place for the toddler to explore and learn. Motor vehicle crashes, drowning, choking, burns, falls, and poisoning are the most common injuries suffered by toddlers. Safety and injury prevention focus on these categories.

Safety in the Car

The safest place for the toddler to ride is in the back seat of the car. Parents should use the appropriate size and style of car seat for the child's weight and age as required by state law. At a minimum, toddlers should be in a rear-facing car seat with harness straps and a clip until 2 years of age (American Academy of Pediatrics [AAP], 2023b). After age 2 years, a forward-facing seat may be used if the toddler has reached the height and weight requirements. A toddler riding in a pickup truck should never ride in the cargo area or truck bed. A full rear seat in the truck is the preferred placement for the toddler car seat. If an appropriate rear seat is unavailable, the airbag should be disarmed, and the forward-facing car seat should be secured appropriately in the truck seat. The lower anchor and top tether are additionally required for all forward-facing car seats manufactured since 2002 and are accommodated by motor vehicles manufactured since that time (Fig. 26.10). In older vehicles or car seats,

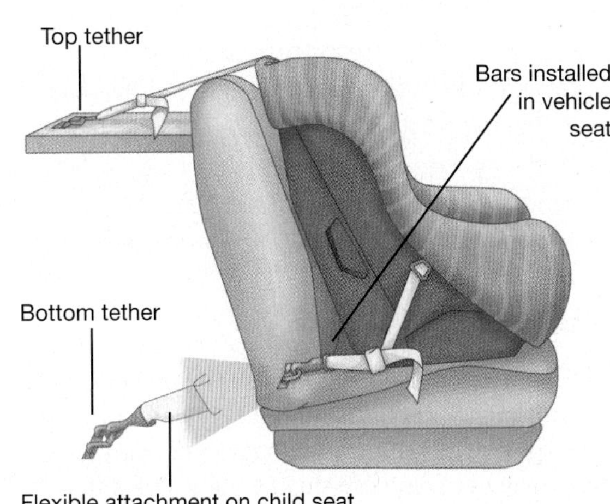

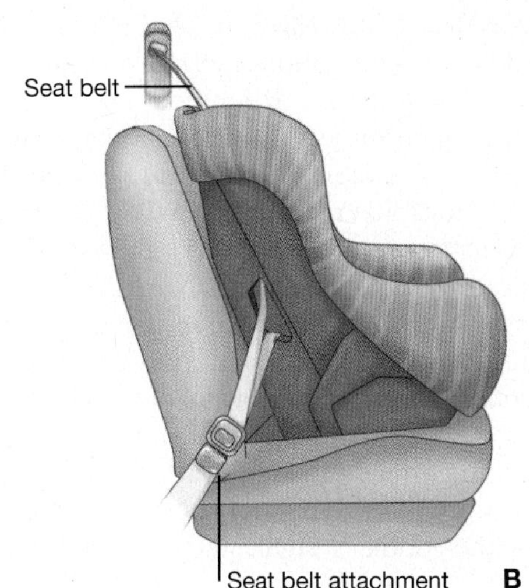

FIGURE 26.10 **A.** A lower anchor and top tether secure the forward-facing car seat. **B.** The shoulder safety strap may also be used to secure the toddler seat. (Adapted from American Academy of Pediatrics. [2021]. *Car seats: Information for families*. https://www.healthychildren.org/English/safety-prevention/on-the-go/Pages/Car-Safety-Seats-Information-for-Families.aspx)

seat belts are utilized for installation. Drivers should avoid using the cell phone or attempting to intervene with the children while they are driving.

Safety in the Home

Key areas of concern for keeping toddlers safe in the home include avoiding exposure to tobacco smoke, preventing injury, and preventing poisoning.

AVOIDING EXPOSURE TO TOBACCO SMOKE

Environmental exposure to tobacco smoke has been associated with increased risk of respiratory disease and infection, decreased lung function, and increased incidence of middle ear effusion and recurrent otitis media (Samet & Sockrider, 2023). Parents should avoid cigarette smoking entirely to best protect their children. Even smoking outside of the home is suboptimal because smoke lingers on parents' clothing, and children who are often carried (such as younger toddlers) face more exposure. Counsel parents to stop smoking (optimal), but if they continue smoking never to smoke inside the home or car with children present.

PREVENTING INJURY

The toddler is able to open drawers and doors, unlock dead bolts, and climb anywhere they want to go. Toddlers have a limited concept of body boundaries and essentially no fear of danger. Toddlers may fall from any height to which they can climb (e.g., play structures, tables, counters). They may also fall from wheeled toys such as tricycles. As toddlers gain additional height and hand dexterity, they are able to reach potentially dangerous items on the counter or stove, leading to an inadvertent ingestion, burn, or cut.

The AAP advises against having guns in homes with children. If a gun is kept in the home, it should be stored unloaded and locked away (Schaechter, 2023).

To prevent injury in the home, stress the following to parents:

- Never leave a toddler unsupervised outdoors.
- Lock doors to dangerous rooms.
- Install safety gates at the top and bottom of staircases.
- Ensure that window locks are operable; if windows are left opened, then secure all window screens.
- Keep pot handles on the stove turned inward, out of an inquisitive toddler's reach.
- Teach the toddler to avoid the oven, stove, and iron.
- Keep electrical equipment, cords, and matches out of reach.
- Remove firearms from the home or keep them in a locked cabinet out of the toddler's reach.
- Always require the child to wear a helmet approved by the Consumer Products Safety Commission (CPSC) when riding a wheeled toy. This starts the habit of helmet wearing early, so it can be more easily carried over to the bicycle-riding years of the future.
- Begin teaching the toddler about watching for cars when crossing the street, but always carry or hold the hand of the toddler when crossing the street.
- Teach the toddler to avoid unknown animals (AAP, 2021b, 2022).

TAKE NOTE!

Bernie Burn, by Sarah Cruz, RN, is a book designed to educate parents and their toddlers about burn prevention while entertaining them. It is endorsed by the *American Journal of Nursing*.

PREVENTING POISONING

As toddlers become more mobile, they are increasingly able to explore their environment and more easily and efficiently gain access to materials that may be unsafe for them to handle. Their natural curiosity leads them into situations that may place them in danger. Poor taste discrimination in this age group allows for ingestion of chemicals or other materials that older children would find too unpleasant to swallow. Box 26.2 lists most potentially dangerous ingested poisons. Discuss poison prevention in the home at each well-child visit. The AAP (2021a) recommends that potentially poisonous substances (e.g., medications, cleaners, hair care products, car care products) be stored out of the toddler's reach, out of the toddler's sight, and in a childproof, locked cabinet.

Encourage all families to take the following safety measures:

- Store all substances in original containers only.
- Never store any liquid other than water or soda in beverage containers.
- Do not allow toddlers access to baby powder, lotion, cream, or other toddler hygiene products.
- Ensure all medications have child-safety caps.
- Do not leave within the toddler's reach medications such as lozenges or samples that are not packaged in safety bottles.
- Be very careful with medications that are provided in transdermal patch form.
- Do not refer to medicines as candy, as the toddler may mistake pills for candy and ingest them.
- Do not expose toddlers to hazardous vapors such as paints, cleaners, tobacco or cannabis smoke, and especially illicit drugs.
- Keep "button" batteries secured and away from a toddler's reach.
- Keep house plants off the floor, remove them from the home, or hang them or place them on a high shelf (AAP, 2021a; American Association of Poison Control Centers, n.d.).

BOX **26.2** **Most Dangerous Potential Poisons**

- Medicines (especially iron)
- Cleaning products
- Antifreeze, windshield washer solution
- Alcohol
- Pesticides
- Gasoline, kerosene, lamp oil, furniture polish
- Wild mushrooms

Data from American Association of Poison Control Centers. (n.d.). *In the home safety tips.* https://aapcc.org/prevention/in-the-home

TAKE NOTE!

The AAP (2021a) recommends that all families post the Poison Control Center number in a readily accessible place in the home: (800) 222-1222. Since 2003, the AAP has discouraged the use of syrup of ipecac in the home to induce vomiting after an unintentional ingestion. Instead, families should call the Poison Control Center right away.

Safety in the Water

Drowning is the leading cause of unintentional injury and death in U.S. children, with nearly half of drowning victims being 4 years old and younger (Safe Kids, 2023a). Drowning may occur in very small volumes of water such as a toilet, bucket, or bathtub, as well as the obvious sites such as swimming pools and other bodies of water. Toddlers' large heads in relation to their body size place them at risk for toppling over into a body of water that they are inquisitive about. Toddlers should be supervised at all times when in or around the water. In general, most children do not have the physical and cognitive capabilities necessary to truly learn how to swim until 4 years of age. Parents who want to enroll a toddler in a swimming class should be aware that a water safety skills class would be most appropriate. However, even toddlers who have completed a swimming program still need *constant* supervision in the water (Safe Kids, 2023a). Box 26.3 gives recommendations for the prevention of drowning.

Remember Jose Gonzales, the 2-year-old described at the beginning of the chapter? What anticipatory guidance related to safety should you provide to Jose's parents?

Promoting Nutrition

The toddler's ability to chew and swallow is improving, and they learn to use utensils effectively to feed themselves. The early years lay a foundation for the future, and

BOX **26.3** **Preventing Drowning**

- Pools should be fenced with locked gates or screened with locked doors.
- Interior doors should be kept locked.
- Young children should never be left unattended in or near water.
- Water wings or "floaties" are not a substitute for adult supervision or for personal flotation devices.
- U.S. Coast Guard–approved life preservers or personal flotation devices should be available when a young child is in or near a body of water.
- Parents and caregivers should be trained in child CPR.

Data from Safe Kids. (2023b). *Water safety tips at home.* https://www.safekids.org/tip/water-safety-home-tips

a great deal of parental and societal interest is focused on nutrition and eating. Forming healthy eating habits has its foundation early in life, and diet has a significant influence on the child's future health status. By establishing healthier food choice patterns early in life, the child is better able to continue these healthy choices later in life. The child younger than 2 years should not have their fat intake restricted, but unhealthy foods and sweets should not be eaten liberally. A diet high in nutrient-rich foods and low in nutrient-poor high-calorie foods such as sweets is appropriate for children of all ages. See the Healthy People 2030 box.

HEALTHY PEOPLE 2030

Objective	Nursing Significance
Reduce household food insecurity and in doing so reduce hunger.	• Counsel families about the appropriate toddler diet. • Refer eligible families to the special supplemental nutrition program for women, infants, and children (WIC).

Healthy People Objectives retrieved from http://www.healthypeople.gov

Weaning

The timing of weaning from breastfeeding or chestfeeding is influenced by a number of factors such as cultural beliefs, local and regional ethnic beliefs, the lactating parent's work schedule, desired child spacing, or societal feelings about the nature of the lactating parent–infant relationship. The AAP recommends breastfeeding for at least 6 months, then for as long as is mutually agreeable to the breastfeeding parent and child (AAP, 2023a). Extending breastfeeding or chestfeeding into toddlerhood is believed to be beneficial to the child. It provides nutritional, immunologic, and emotional benefits to the child. Contrary to popular belief, it is biologically possible to become pregnant while breastfeeding. Breastfeeding a newborn appropriately can occur while continuing to nurse the older sibling.

Weaning from breastfeeding or chestfeeding tends to occur earlier in the United States than in countries around the world, despite recommendations on length of breastfeeding by a number of organizations. Most professional organizations recommend breastfeeding for at least 1 year (National Association of Pediatric Nurse Practitioners [NAPNAP] et al., 2019). Weaning is a highly individualized decision. Educate parents about the benefits of extended breastfeeding, and support the decision to wean at a given time.

Weaning from the bottle should occur by 12 to 15 months of age. Prolonged bottle-feeding is associated with the development of dental caries. No-spill "sippy cups" contain a valve that requires sucking by the toddler in order to obtain fluid, thus functioning similarly to a baby bottle. Hence, no-spill sippy cups can also be associated with dental caries and are not recommended (Hagan et al., 2017). Cups with spouts that do not contain valves are acceptable. The 12- to 15-month-old is developmentally capable of consuming adequate fluid amounts using a cup.

Teaching About Nutritional Needs

Adequate calcium intake and appropriate exercise lay the foundation for proper bone mineralization. The toddler requires an average intake of 700 mg of calcium per day (Ben-Joseph, 2018). Dairy products are considered the primary sources of dietary calcium. One cup of low-fat or whole milk, 8 oz of low-fat yogurt, and 1½ oz of cheddar cheese each provide 300 mg of calcium. Broccoli, oranges, sweet potatoes, tofu, and dried beans or legumes are also good sources of calcium (35- to 120-mg calcium per serving).

Iron-deficiency anemia in the first 2 years of life may be associated with developmental and psychomotor delays (Powers, 2023). Although it is important for toddlers to consume adequate amounts of iron, they tend to have the lowest daily iron intake of any age group. When breastfeeding or formula-feeding ends (most often at 1 year of age), it is often replaced with iron-poor cow's milk. Limiting milk intake to 16 oz per day, as well as limiting juice intake, can be helpful. Encourage the parents to provide iron-fortified cereals and other foods rich in iron and vitamin C.

TAKE NOTE!

Toddlers who consume a strictly vegan diet (no food from animal sources) are at risk for deficiencies in vitamin D, vitamin B_{12}, and iron. Supplementation with these nutrients should occur to promote adequate nutrition and growth (Parks et al., 2020).

Fat or cholesterol intake should not be restricted in children younger than age 2 years. The first 2 years of life require high energy intake because they are a time of very rapid growth and development. Due to daily variations and the pickiness of the toddler, fat intake should be evaluated over a period of several days. Encourage parents to feed toddlers foods containing adequate amounts of fiber and limit processed foods. Generally, toddler serving sizes should be about two thirds of that of an older child. Box 26.4 lists common sources of several nutrients.

BOX 26.4 Key Nutrients Provided by Fruits and Vegetables

Dietary fiber: Apples, artichokes, berries, oranges, green peas, pears, prunes
Folate: Asparagus, Brussels sprouts, fruits, spinach, and dark greens
Vitamin A: Fruits, leafy green vegetables, orange and yellow vegetables, tomatoes
Vitamin C: Berries, broccoli, Brussels sprouts, cauliflower, cantaloupe, citrus fruits, kiwi, mango, papaya, green peas, pineapple, sweet and white potatoes, tomatoes, watermelon, winter squash

Data from Division of Agriculture. (2023). Fruits and vegetables: Important sources of nutrients and vitamins. *University of Arkansas*. https://www.uaex.uada.edu/counties/miller/news/fcs/fruits-veggies/fruits-and-vegetables-important-sources-of-nutrients-and-vitamins.aspx

Parents should encourage toddlers to drink water. Juice intake should be limited to 4 to 6 oz per day. Milk intake should be limited to no more than 24 oz per day. Juice and milk should be served along with meals or snacks. Water should be offered for between-meal drinking. Toddlers should drink from a cup.

Advancing Solid Foods

Parents should offer three full meals and two snacks daily. Portion sizes for toddlers are about one quarter of the size of adult portions. Large portions of a new or different food on the toddler's plate may intimidate the toddler. Normal toddler behaviors of mouthing, handling, tasting, extruding the food from the mouth, and then resampling the food often occur. These behaviors are distasteful to some parents but are a normal part of toddler development. Parents need to understand and tolerate these behaviors rather than scolding the toddler for them (Lieberman, 2018).

Toddlers are often afraid to try new things anyway, so the parent or caregiver should be flexible with the toddler's acceptance or rejection of new foods. If the toddler refuses healthy food choices at meal or snack time, parents should not substitute high-fat, high-sugar, processed food just to make sure that the child eats something (Parks et al., 2020). This sets the stage for future power struggles. The parent decides which foods will be served or offered. The toddler decides how much will be eaten. The toddler self-regulates the amount of food needed to sustain and allow further growth and development. The toddler may not eat well every day but, generally, over the course of several days, will consume the foods they need (Satter, 2023).

Foods should be served near room temperature. Some of the food on the plate should be soft and moist. Food should always be cut into bite-size pieces. Teaching Guidelines 26.2 gives recommendations on ways to prevent choking.

TEACHING GUIDELINES 26.2 Avoiding Choking

- Slowly add foods that are more difficult to chew as the toddler becomes more adept at chewing.
- Cut all foods into bite-sized pieces.
- Avoid foods that are hard to chew and that may become lodged in the airway, such as:
  - Nuts
  - Gumdrops or other chewy candies, hard candy
  - Raw carrots
  - Peanut butter (by itself)
  - Popcorn
- Cut hotdogs and grapes into quarters. Cook carrots until soft; if serving raw, then grate them.
- Always supervise the toddler while they are eating.

Adapted from Durani, Y. (2023). *Preventing choking*. https://kidshealth.org/en/parents/safety-choking.html

Promoting Self-Feeding

Toddlers most often eat with their fingers, but they do need to learn to use utensils properly. The following are suggestions for parents:

- Use a child-sized spoon and fork with dull tines.
- Seat the toddler in a highchair or at a comfortable height in a secure chair. The toddler should have their feet supported rather than dangling (Fig. 26.11).
- Never leave the toddler unattended while eating.
- Minimize distractions during mealtime. Serve food to the toddler along with the other members of the family (Satter, 2023).

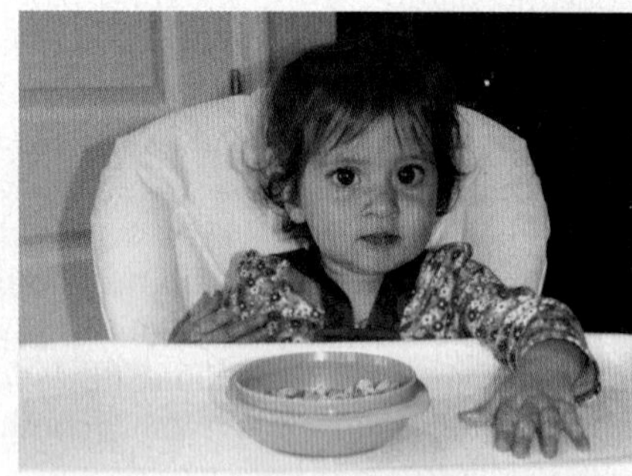

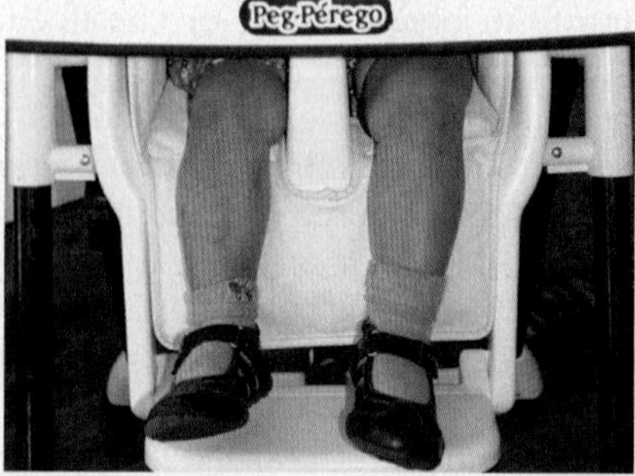

FIGURE 26.11 The toddler should be appropriately and safely seated in the highchair. The safety strap is secure, the toddler's feet are supported, and the tray table is locked in place.

Promoting Healthy Eating Habits

Since the toddler's rate of growth has slowed somewhat compared to that in infancy, the toddler requires less caloric intake for their size compared to the infant. This results in **physiologic anorexia**: toddlers simply do not require as much food intake for their size as they did in infancy. The toddler will also exhibit **food jags**. During a food jag, the toddler may prefer only one particular food for several days, then not want it for weeks. Again, it is important for the parent to continue to offer healthy food choices during a food jag and not give in by allowing the toddler to eat junk food (Satter, 2023).

The normal developmental issue of testing limits will also occur for the toddler at mealtime. Since toddlers still have limited ability to express their emotions with words, they use nonverbal behaviors to do so. While eating, the toddler may dislike the taste of a particular food or experience a feeling of fullness but will communicate that feeling by screaming or throwing food. When the child exhibits these behaviors, the parent must remain calm and remove the toddler from the situation. Meals should be eaten in a calm and pleasant environment. Parents should serve as role models for appropriate eating habits, but toddlers may also be willing to try more foods if they are exposed to other children who eat those foods. Praise the child for trying a new food, and never punish the toddler for refusing to try something new. A new food may need to be offered many times in a row before the toddler chooses to try it. Parents should be sure to include foods the child is familiar with and likes to eat at the same meal that the new food is being introduced (Satter, 2023). Teaching Guidelines 26.3 lists alternative foods that meet nutritional needs and a list of books for picky eating.

Preventing Overweight and Higher Weight

In children, the greatest risk factor for the development of overweight and higher weight is having a parent with a high BMI (Skelton & Klish, 2023). The nurse can screen for overweight and higher weight in the child older than 2 years of age by calculating the BMI and plotting the BMI on the standardized age- and sex-appropriate growth charts (see Appendix D for growth charts, and refer to Chapter 32 for BMI calculation instructions). Trends over time may be predictive of the development of overweight and higher weight. See the Healthy People 2030 box.

Another factor in the development of excess weight in young children is juice intake (Parks et al., 2020). Since most young children like the sweet taste of juice, they may drink excessive amounts of it. Toddlers who drink excess fruit juice and eat well may gain excess weight because of the high sugar content in the juice. On the other end of the spectrum, some children may feel

TEACHING GUIDELINES 26.3 Meeting Nutritional Needs for Picky Eating

Alternative Food Choices for Picky Eating

- Won't drink milk? Obtain calcium through yogurt (frozen or regular), cheese, pudding, and hot cocoa.
- Poor meat intake? Obtain iron through unsweetened iron-fortified cereals or breakfast bars, or raisins; cook with an iron skillet.
- Loves processed white bread? Encourage fiber intake with fresh fruits and vegetables, bran muffins, beans, or peas (can be in soup).
- Refuses vegetables? Encourage vitamin A intake with apricots, sweet potatoes, and vegetable juices.

Books for Picky Eating

- *Feeding with Love and Good Sense* by E. Satter. Kelcy Press, 2022.
- *First Foods* by M. Stoppard. Dorling-Kindersley Publishing, Inc., 2002.
- *Food Chaining: The Proven 6-Step Plan to Stop Picky Eating, Solve Feeding Problems, and Expand Your Child's Diet* by C. Fraker, M. Fishbein, S. Cox, & L. Walbert. Da Capo Lifelong Books, 2007.
- *Helping Your Child with Extreme Picky Eating: A Step-By-Step Guide for Overcoming Selective Eating, Food Aversion, and Feeding Disorders* by K. Rowell & J. McGlothlin. New Harbinger Publications, 2015.
- *Raising a Healthy, Happy Eater: A Parent's Handbook* by N. Fernando & M. Potock. The Experiment. 2022.
- *The No-Cry Picky Eater Solution: Gentle Ways to Encourage Your Child to Eat - and Eat Healthy* by E. Pantley. McGraw-Hill, 2011.
- *The Healthy Baby Meal Planner: Mom-Tested, Child-Approved Recipes for your Baby and Toddler* by A. Karmel. Fireside, 2005.

HEALTHY PEOPLE 2030

Objective	Nursing Significance
Reduce the proportion of children and adolescents aged 2–19 years who have higher weight.	• Counsel families about the appropriate toddler diet. • Educate families to decrease excess toddler intake of milk or juice and offer only nutrient-rich foods.

Healthy People Objectives retrieved from http://www.healthypeople.gov

full from juice consumption and decrease their intake of solid foods. These children are at risk for malnutrition. Fruit juice intake should be limited to 4 to 6 oz per day. See Evidence-Based Practice 26.1.

TAKE NOTE!

Young children should consume only pasteurized juice, as unpasteurized juice consumption places the toddler at increased risk of *Escherichia coli, Salmonella,* and *Cryptosporidium* infection.

Think back to Jose Gonzales. What questions should you ask Jose's parents related to his nutritional intake? What anticipatory guidance related to nutrition would be appropriate?

Promoting Healthy Sleep and Rest

The 18-month-old requires 13.5 hours of sleep per day, the 24-month-old 13 hours, and the 3-year-old 12 hours (Carter & Feigelman, 2020a, 2020b). A typical toddler should sleep through the night and take one daytime nap. Most children discontinue daytime napping at around 3 years of age. The toddler who slept in a crib as an infant will need to move to a youth or toddler bed or even a full-size bed usually sometime in the toddler period. When the crib becomes unsafe (i.e., when the toddler becomes physically capable of climbing over the rails), then they must make the transition to a bed.

Consistent bedtime rituals help the toddler prepare for sleep. Choose a bedtime and stick to it as much as possible. The nightly routine might include a bath followed by reading a story. The routine should be a calm period with minimal outside distractions. Toddlers often require a security item to help them get to sleep. Older toddlers may be afraid of the dark, so a nightlight is often helpful.

Night waking is a problem for some toddlers. This may occur as a result of change in routine or as a desire for nighttime attention. Attention during night waking should be minimized so that the toddler receives no reward for being awake at night. The book *No-Cry Sleep Solution,* by Elizabeth Pantley (2020) is an excellent resource for the family with a toddler who resists bedtime or is a persistent night waker. For some toddlers, night waking is caused by nightmares. As the imagination and capacity for make-believe grow, the toddler may not be able to distinguish between reality and pretend. The parent should hold and comfort the toddler after a nightmare. Limiting television viewing (especially shortly before bedtime) may be helpful in limiting nightmares.

Some families practice "co-sleeping" (when children sleep in the parents' bed). Although some professionals believe that co-sleeping may interfere with the toddler's struggle for independence, this theory has not been proven. The nurse should support the family's choice for sleep arrangements unless the co-sleeping is unsafe either physically or psychologically (SafeBedSharing.org, 2023). Refer to http://www.safebedsharing.org for bed-sharing safety guidelines.

What anticipatory guidance should you provide to Jose's parents in relation to sleep?

EVIDENCE-BASED PRACTICE **26.1**

Higher Weight in Childhood Research Demonstration Projects

STUDY

Excess weight is a reliable predictor of poor health across the lifespan. While the four protective factors of healthy eating habits, self-regulation, parental responsive feeding practices, and parental sensitive scaffolding are known to be protective against higher weight development, they are less prevalent among families living in poverty (Nix et al., 2021). Few home-based interventions have been demonstrated to decrease the development of excess weight in toddlers living in poverty.

The researchers enrolled and retained 66 families of toddlers in Early Head Start, who were aged 18 to 36 months. Families were randomly assigned to an intervention or control group. Those in the intervention group received the Recipe 4 Success curriculum during a series of home visits.

Findings

A variety of measures were used to determine toddler healthy eating habits, toddler self-regulation, parental responsive feeding practices, and parental sensitive scaffolding. The study results revealed toddlers in the intervention (Recipe 4 Success) group were more likely to eat balanced meals and snacks rather than sweets and junk food. Additionally, these toddlers showed improved self-regulation (gratification delay in the presence of highly desired food). Parents in the intervention group were more likely to engage in responsive feeding practices and to demonstrate sensitive scaffolding (structuring task for engagement without overwhelming the toddler).

Nursing Implications

Overweight and higher weight in childhood places children at risk for negative cardiovascular events and excess weight continuing into adulthood. Nurses are in an ideal position to educate and support families in their decisions related to providing nutrition to their young children. Assisting parents in making healthy food decisions and appropriately involving their toddlers in the eating process may lead to decreased incidence of excess weight in toddlerhood.

Data from Nix, R. L., Francis, L. A., Feinberg, M. E., Gill, S., Jones, D. E., Hostetler, M. L., & Stifter, C. A. (2021). Improving toddlers' healthy eating habits and self-regulation: A randomized controlled trial. *Pediatrics, 147*(1), e20193326. https://doi.org/10.1542/peds.2019-3326

Promoting Healthy Teeth and Gums

By 30 months of age, the toddler should have a full set of primary ("baby") teeth. Parents may not be aware of the importance of preventing cavities in primary teeth since they will eventually be replaced by the permanent teeth. Poor oral hygiene, prolonged use of a bottle or no-spill sippy cup, lack of fluoride intake, and delayed or absent professional dental care may all contribute to the development of dental caries (Nowak & Warren, 2023). Cleaning of the toddler's teeth should progress from brushing with water alone to using a very small amount (pea-sized) of fluoridated toothpaste, with brushing beginning at 2 years of age (Fig. 26.12). Weaning from the bottle no later than 15 months of age and severely restricting use of a no-spill sippy cup (the kind that requires sucking for fluid delivery) is recommended.

By the age of 1 year, the toddler should have their first dentist visit to establish current health of the teeth and gums. Eating should be limited to meal and snack times, as "grazing" throughout the day exposes the teeth to food throughout the day. Carbohydrate-containing foods combined with oral bacteria create a decreased oral pH level that is optimal for the development of dental caries (cavities).

Public water fluoridation is a public health initiative that ensures that most children receive adequate fluoride intake to prevent dental caries. If the water supply contains adequate fluoride, no other supplementation is necessary other than brushing with a small amount of fluoride-containing toothpaste after age 2 years. Excess fluoride ingestion should be avoided, as it contributes to the development of fluorosis (mottling of the enamel). Risk factors for fluorosis development include:

- High fluoride levels in the local water supply
- Use of fluoride-containing toothpaste prior to age 2 years
- Excessive ingestion of fluoride either in toothpaste or foods
- Fluoride-containing foods: tea, ready-to-eat infant foods containing chicken, white or purple grape juice, and beverages, processed foods, and cereals that were manufactured with fluoride-containing water

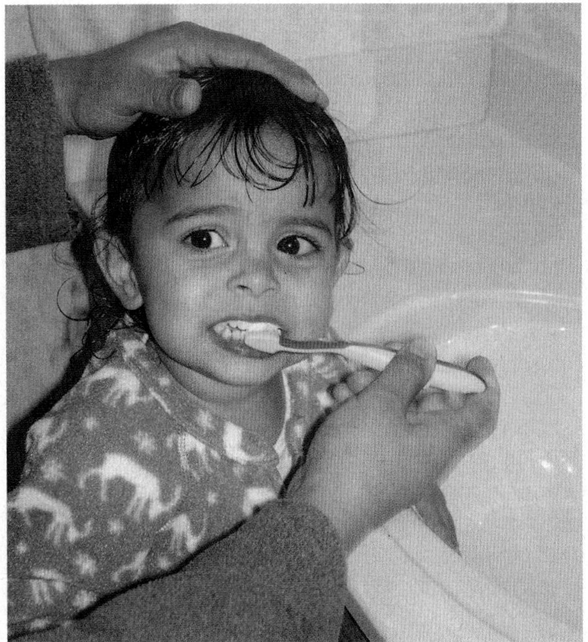

FIGURE 26.12 The parent should brush the toddler's teeth to ensure proper cleaning of the teeth, gums, and tongue. Use only water for brushing before 2 years of age and a pea-sized amount of fluoride-containing toothpaste after age 2 years.

Promoting Appropriate Discipline

Discipline is a common concern during toddlerhood. The toddler's intense personality and extreme emotional reactions can be difficult for parents to cope with and understand. The toddler needs firm, gentle guidance to learn what the expectations are and how to meet them. The parent's love and respect for the toddler teach the toddler to care about themselves and others. Affection is as important as the guidance aspect of discipline. Having realistic expectations of what the toddler is capable of learning and understanding can help the parent in the disciplinary process. The toddler's intense push for autonomy can often test a parent's limits. The easygoing infant usually becomes more challenging in toddlerhood. The toddler's continual quest for new experiences often places the toddler at risk, and their negativism often taxes the parent's patience.

In an effort to prevent the toddler from experiencing harm and in response to their continual testing of limits, parents often resort to spanking. Although commonly accepted, the AAP and the NAPNAP recommend against corporal or physical punishment (American Academy of Child and Adolescent Psychiatry, 2018; NAPNAP et al., 2022). Recent research points out the dangers inherent in the use of corporal punishment as well as the possibilities for negative effects on the child's future behavior (Box 26.5). Spanking or other forms of corporal punishment lead to a pro-violence attitude, create resentment and anger in some children, and contribute to the cycle of violence (NAPNAP et al., 2022).

TAKE NOTE!

Toddlers younger than 18 months should *never* be spanked, as there is an increased possibility of physical injury in this age group. Also, the infant/young toddler is not capable of linking the spanking with the undesired behavior (AAP, 2018).

BOX 26.5 Negative Impact of Physical Punishment

- Spanking is less effective than time-out or other disciplinary measures to reduce undesired behavior in children.
- The toddler younger than 18 months of age:
  - Is not capable of making the appropriate connections between spanking and the undesired behavior
  - Is at increased risk for physical injury from spanking than older children
- Physical punishment:
  - May lead to a pro-violence attitude
  - May create resentment in the toddler
  - Is a poor model for learning effective problem-solving
  - May be correlated with antisocial and criminal behavior later in life
  - Leads to increased aggression in preschoolers, school-age children, and adults
  - When used frequently, may weaken the parent–child relationship
- Childhood corporal punishment increases the probability of depression and substance use disorder in adulthood.
- Spanking may lead to more severe forms of punishment and to actual child abuse and maltreatment.
- The more frequently children are hit or spanked, the more likely they are to hit their own children and to be involved in spouse abuse as adults.

Data from Global Initiative to End All Corporal Punishment of Children. (2018). *Global initiative to end corporal punishment.* http://www.endcorporalpunishment.org/; National Association of Pediatric Nurse Practitioners, Child Maltreatment and Neglect Special Interest Group, VanGraafeiland, B., Hornor, G. A., Herendeen, P. A., Chiocca, E. M., Loyke, J. A., Dietzman, H., Boucher, N. L., Nielsen, A., & Record, S. C. (2022). NAPNAP position statement on using positive parenting to eliminate corporal punishment. *Journal of Pediatric Health Care, 36*, 202–204. https://doi.org/10.1016/j.pedhc.2021.09.001

Normal toddler development includes natural curiosity, which often results in dangerous or problematic activities for the toddler (Buckloh, 2023). Toddlers have a difficult time learning the rules and, in general, do not behave badly intentionally. Providing a childproof environment will allow the toddler to participate in safe exploration, which will meet their developmental needs and decrease the frequency of intervention needed on the part of the parents.

Discipline should focus on limit setting, negotiation, and techniques to assist the toddler to learn problem-solving. Parents should provide consistency and commit to the limits that are set. Offering realistic choices helps give the toddler a sense of mastery. Rules should be simple and limited in number. Maintaining the toddler's schedule of meals and rest/sleep will help to prevent conflicts that occur as a result of hunger or fatigue. Toddlers should not be made to share, as this is a concept they do not understand. Parents should encourage simple activities enjoyed by the children involved and avoid confrontation over toys. Parents should offer toddlers appropriate choices to help them develop autonomy but should not offer a choice when none exists.

Positive reinforcement should be used as much as possible. "Catching" a child being good helps to reinforce appropriate or desirable behaviors. When the toddler is displaying appropriate behavior, the parent should reward the child consistently with praise and physical affection.

"Time-out" can be used effectively at around 2.5 to 3 years of age (refer to Chapter 27 for details). "Extinction" is a particularly useful technique with 2- and 3-year-olds. Extinction involves systematically ignoring the undesired behavior. Parents sometimes unknowingly contribute to the occurrence of an unwanted behavior simply by the attention they give the toddler (even if it is negative in nature, it is still attention). Parents who want to extinguish an annoying (non-dangerous) behavior should resolve to ignore it every time it occurs. When the child withholds the behavior or performs the opposite (appropriate) behavior, parents should use compliments and praise. It may be difficult to ignore a difficult behavior, but the results are well worth the effort. Teaching Guidelines 26.4 provides tips on avoiding power struggles and offers appropriate guidance to toddlers.

TEACHING GUIDELINES 26.4 Providing Toddlers With Guidance

- When giving the toddler instructions, tell the child what to do, NOT what not to do. This allows for a positive focus. If you must say "no," "don't," or "stop," then follow with a direction of what to do instead.
- Offer limited choices, when a choice is truly available. Say, "Do you want to wear your blue hat or your red hat?" *not* "Do you want to put on your hat?" This gives the toddler some, but not all, control.
- Role model appropriate communication, but don't feel like you have to speak nicely all the time. If the situation warrants, use a firm and even tone to get the point across. Avoid yelling.
- Pay attention to the inflection in your voice. A statement or direction should not end in a questioning tone or with "Okay?" Be clear. Statements should sound like statements, and only questions should end in a questioning tone.
- When a toddler behaves aggressively, label the child's feelings calmly, but be firm and consistent with the expectation. For example, "I know you're mad at your friend, but it is not okay to hit."

Adapted from Buckloh, L. M. (2023). *Disciplining your toddler*. https://kidshealth.org/en/parents/toddler-tantrums.html#; Sears, W., & Sears, M. (2020b). *8 tools for toddler discipline*. http://www.askdrsears.com/topics/parenting/discipline-behavior/8-tools-toddler-discipline

ADDRESSING COMMON DEVELOPMENTAL CONCERNS

Common developmental concerns of the toddler period are toilet teaching, temper tantrums, thumb sucking or pacifier use, sibling rivalry, and regression. An understanding of the normalcy of negativism, temper tantrums, and sibling rivalry will help the family cope with these issues. Prepare parents for these developmental events by giving appropriate anticipatory guidance.

Toilet Teaching

When myelination of the spinal cord is achieved around age 2 years, the toddler is capable of exercising voluntary control over the sphincters. Female children may be ready for toilet teaching earlier than male children (Gavin, 2019). Toddlers are ready for toilet teaching when:

- Bowel movements occur on a fairly regular schedule.
- The toddler expresses knowledge of the need to defecate or urinate. This may be through verbalization, change in activity, or gestures such as:
  - Looks into or grabs diaper
  - Squats
  - Crosses legs
  - Grimaces and grunts
  - Hides behind a door or the couch when defecating
- The diaper is not always wet (this indicates the ability to hold the urine for a period of time).
- The toddler is willing to follow instructions.
- The toddler walks well alone and is able to pull down their pants.
- The toddler follows caregivers to the bathroom.
- The toddler climbs onto the potty chair or toilet (AAP, 2023c).

Parents should approach toilet teaching with a calm, positive, and nonthreatening manner. Initially it may be helpful to allow the toddler to observe a same-sex family member using the toilet. Start with the toddler fully clothed on the potty chair or toilet while the parent or caregiver talks about what the toilet is used for and when. The toddler will feel most comfortable with a toddler potty chair that sits on the floor (Fig. 26.13). If a potty chair is unavailable, facing toward the toilet tank may make the toddler feel more secure, as the buttocks remain on the front of the seat rather than sinking through the toilet seat opening. After a week or longer, remove a dirty diaper and place the contents in the toilet. Next, try having the toddler sit on the potty chair or toilet without pants or diaper on. The toddler may benefit from watching a caregiver or friend use the toilet. It may also be beneficial to demonstrate using the potty chair with a baby doll that wets.

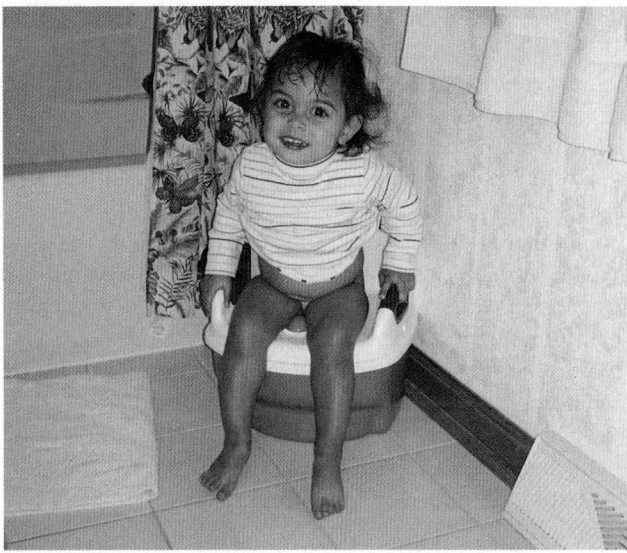

FIGURE 26.13 The toddler will feel most comfortable with a potty chair that sits on the floor.

Parents should always use gentle praise and no reproaches. Usually, the best time to achieve success with defecation on the toilet is following a meal. When the toddler has achieved success with bowel control, bladder control will come next. It may be many months before nighttime bladder control is achieved, and the toddler may still require a diaper at night. Parents should use appropriate words for body parts, urination, and defecation, then use those words consistently so the toddler understands what to say and do (AAP, 2023c).

After a couple of weeks of successful toileting, the toddler may start wearing training pants. When toddlers have an accident and do not make it to the toilet, gently remind them about toileting and let them help clean up. Toddlers should never be punished for bowel or bladder "accidents."

With so much attention focused on the genitalia during toilet teaching and the frequency of being without a diaper, it is natural for toddlers to become more focused on their own genitalia. Boys and girls both will explore their genitalia and discover the resulting pleasurable sensation. Masturbation in the toddler often causes a great deal of discomfort in the parent. The parent should not draw attention to the activity, as that may increase its frequency. The parent should calmly explain to the toddler that this is an activity that may only be done in private (Carter & Feigelman, 2020b). If the toddler is masturbating excessively or refuses to stop when in public, then there may be additional stressors in the toddler's life that should be explored.

Negativism

Negativism is common in the toddler period (Lieberman, 2018). As the toddler separates from the parent, recognizes their own individuality, and exerts autonomy, negativism abounds. Parents should understand that this negativism is a normal developmental occurrence and not necessarily deliberate defiance (although that also occurs). Avoid asking yes-or-no questions, as the toddler's usual response will be "no," whether they mean it or not. Offering the child simple choices will give the toddler a sense of control. The parent should not ask the toddler if they "want" to do something if there is actually no choice. "Do you want to use the red cup or the blue cup?" is more appropriate than "Do you want your milk now?" When it is time to go outside, don't ask, "Do you want to put your shoes on?" Instead, state in a matter-of-fact tone that shoes must be worn outside and give the toddler a choice of type of shoe or color of socks. If the child continues with negative answers, then the parent should remain calm and make the decision for the child.

Temper Tantrums

Even children who displayed an easygoing personality as infants may lose their temper frequently during the toddler years (Fig. 26.14). A toddler who was more intense as an infant may have more temper tantrums. Temper tantrums are a natural result of the frustration that toddlers experience. Toddlers are eager to explore new things, but their efforts are often thwarted (usually for safety reasons). Toddlers do not behave badly on purpose. They need time and maturity to learn the rules and regulations. Some of their frustration may come from lack of language skills to express themselves. Toddlers are just starting to learn how to verbalize feelings and to use alternative actions rather than just "pitching a fit."

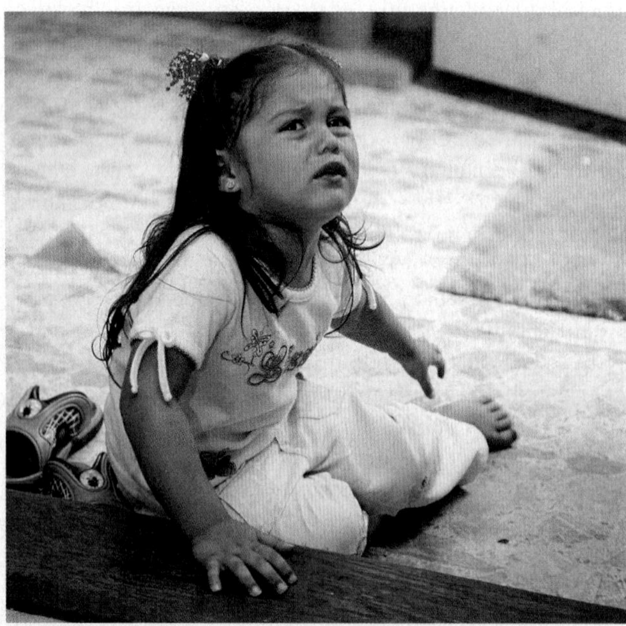

FIGURE 26.14 Tantrums are a normal component of toddler development.

The temper tantrum may be manifested as a screaming and crying fit or a full-blown episode in which the toddler throws themselves on the floor kicking, screaming, and pounding, perhaps even holding the breath. Fatigue or hunger may limit the toddler's coping abilities and promote negative behavior and temper tantrums (Buckloh, 2023).

Although tantrums are annoying to parents and caregivers, they are a normal part of the toddler's quest for independence. As toddlers mature, they become better able to express themselves and to understand their environment. Parents need to learn their toddler's behavioral cues in order to limit activity that is frustrating. When the parent notes the beginnings of frustration, a friendly warning might be given. Intervening early with an activity change might prevent a tantrum. Use distraction, refocusing, or removal from the situation.

When a temper tantrum does occur, the best course of action is to ignore the behavior and ensure that the child is safe during the tantrum. Physical punishment will probably just prolong the tantrum and, in fact, produce more intense negative behavior. If the tantrum occurs in public, it may be necessary for the parent to immobilize the child with a big bear hug and use a calm voice to soothe the toddler. It is important for parents to model self-control. Since toddlers' tantrums most often result from frustration, the role-modeled behavior of self-control helps to teach toddlers to control their temper when they can't get what they want (Buckloh, 2023).

Thumb Sucking and Pacifiers

Infants bring their hands to their mouths and begin thumb sucking as a form of self-soothing (Sears & Sears, 2020c). This habit may continue into the toddler years and beyond. The pacifier is used for the same reason. Toddlers may calm themselves in a stressful situation by thumb sucking or sucking on a pacifier. Opinions about thumb and finger sucking and pacifier use are significantly affected by family history and culture. For most children, there is no need to worry about a sucking habit until it is time for the permanent teeth to erupt. Prolonged and frequent sucking in the withdrawn child is more likely to yield changes to the tooth and jaw structure than sucking that is primarily used for self-soothing. Parents must sort through their own feelings about thumb sucking and pacifier use and then decide how they want to handle the habit.

To ensure safety with pacifier use:

- Use only one-piece pacifiers.
- Replace worn pacifiers with new ones.
- Never tie a pacifier around a toddler's neck.

Parents may want to limit thumb sucking and pacifier use to bedtime, in the car, and in stressful situations. The parent should calmly discuss these limits with the toddler and then remain consistent about enforcing them (Sears & Sears, 2020a, 2020c).

Sibling Rivalry

Many families have subsequent children when their first child is a toddler. The toddler has been accustomed to being the baby and receiving a great deal of attention, both at home and with the extended family. Since toddlers are normally egocentric, bringing a new baby into the home may be quite disruptive. To minimize issues with **sibling rivalry** (competition or jealousy between siblings), parents should attempt to keep the toddler's routine as close to normal as possible. Spend individual time with the toddler on a daily basis. Involve the toddler in the care of the baby. The toddler is capable of fetching a diaper or T-shirt, entertaining the baby with a toy, or helping sing a song to calm the baby (Schmitt, 2023). "Helping" the parent care for the baby gives the toddler a sense of importance (Fig. 26.15). The toddler will need significant support while holding the baby.

Regression

Some toddlers experience regression during a stressful event (e.g., the birth of a sibling, hospitalization). Stress in a toddler's life affects their ability to master new developmental tasks. During **regression**, the toddler may want to go back to an earlier stage. They may desire a bottle or pacifier forgotten long ago. The toddler may stop displaying previously achieved language or motor skills. A significant stress in the toddler's life may also disrupt the toilet teaching process (toilet teaching may not be achieved near the time a sibling is born). When regression occurs, parents should ignore the regressive behavior and offer praise for age-appropriate behavior or attainment of skills (AAP, 2021c).

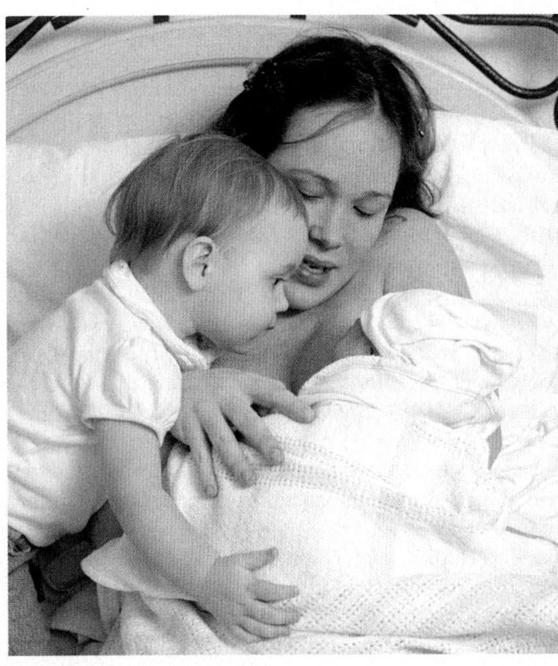

FIGURE 26.15 The toddler may be more likely to accept the new baby in a positive manner if they feel that this is "our baby," not just "Mommy's baby." This toddler is meeting their new sibling for the first time.

Refer to Jose Gonzales, the 2-year-old. List common developmental concerns of the toddler. What anticipatory guidance related to these concerns would you provide to Jose's parents?

Unfolding Patient Stories: Jackson Webber • Part 1

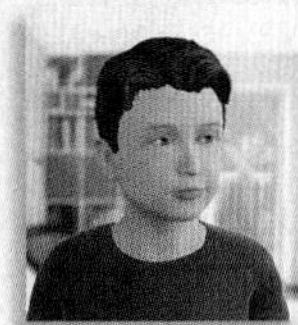

Jackson Webber, age 3, is diagnosed with generalized seizures and started on phenobarbital. His parent is single and employed full time. She is concerned about his recent developmental regression and how it will affect his return to child care. What education can the nurse provide on normal growth and development for a 3-year-old and the relationship between developmental milestones and the new onset of an illness? What questions can the nurse ask to evaluate the adequacy and safety of the child care center that Jackson attends when considering his new diagnosis of seizures? (Jackson Webber's story continues in Chapter 38.)

Care for Jackson and other patients in a realistic virtual environment: ***vSim** for Nursing* (thepoint.lww.com/vSimPediatric). Practice documenting these patients' care in DocuCare (thepoint.lww.com/DocuCareEHR).

KEY CONCEPTS

- The toddler's organ systems are continuing to mature, and growth slows during this period as compared with infancy.
- The psychosocial task of the toddler years is to attain a sense of autonomy and to experience separation and individuation.
- Cognitive development in toddlerhood progresses from sensorimotor in nature to preoperational.
- The toddler refines gross motor skills after learning to walk and builds fine motor skills through the use of utensils and various manipulative toys.
- The toddler progresses from limited expressive language capabilities to a vocabulary of 900 words by age 3 years.
- Toddlers use all of their senses to explore and learn about their environment.
- Visual acuity progresses to at least 20/50 in the toddler period.
- Negativism abounds in toddlers as they attempt to assert their independence.

- Very ritualistic, toddlers feel safer and more secure when clear limits are enforced and a structured routine is followed.
- The toddler is starting to learn right from wrong and bases actions on punishment avoidance.
- Toddler development may be promoted through active gross motor play, books, music, and block building.
- Safety is a primary concern in the toddler years as the child is more mobile, very curious, and experimenting with autonomy.
- Poisoning in the toddler period may be prevented through proper storage of medications and other potentially poisonous substances and appropriate supervision.
- Consistent bedtime rituals help ease the toddler's transition to sleep.
- All primary teeth are erupted by 30 months of age and may be kept healthy with appropriate tooth brushing and fluoride supplementation.
- The toddler may experience a decrease in appetite as growth slows, yet they still need appropriate nutritional intake for continued development.
- Toilet teaching can be achieved after myelination of the spinal cord is complete, usually around 2 years of age.
- Thumb sucking, pacifier use, security items, and temper tantrums are expected issues in the toddler years.
- Toddler discipline should focus on clear limits and consistency. It should not involve spanking. It should be balanced with a caring and nurturing environment along with frequent praise for appropriate behavior.
- Parental role modeling of appropriate behavior, especially related to dealing with frustration, is beneficial to toddlers.
- Parents play an important role in toddler development, not only by providing a loving environment but also by role modeling appropriate behavior in most areas of daily life.

REFERENCES AND RECOMMENDED READINGS

American Academy of Child and Adolescent Psychiatry. (2018). *Physical punishment*. https://www.aacap.org/aacap/families_and_youth/facts_for_families/fff-guide/Physical-Punishment-105.aspx

American Academy of Pediatrics. (2018). *Where we stand: Spanking*. https://www.healthychildren.org/English/family-life/family-dynamics/communication-discipline/Pages/Where-We-Stand-Spanking.aspx

American Academy of Pediatrics. (2021a). *Poison prevention & treatment tips for parents*. https://www.healthychildren.org/English/safety-prevention/all-around/Pages/Poison-Prevention.aspx

American Academy of Pediatrics. (2021b). *TIPP—2 to 4 years: Safety for your child*. https://doi.org/10.1542/peo_document303

American Academy of Pediatrics. (2021c). *Welcoming a new sibling: How to help your child adjust*. https://doi.org/10.1542/peo_document133

American Academy of Pediatrics. (2022). *Safety for your child: 1 to 2 years*. https://www.healthychildren.org/English/ages-stages/toddler/Pages/Safety-for-Your-Child-1-to-2-Years.aspx

American Academy of Pediatrics. (2023a). *Breastfeeding*. https://www.healthychildren.org/English/ages-stages/baby/breastfeeding/Pages/default.aspx

American Academy of Pediatrics. (2023b). *Car seats: Information for families*. https://www.healthychildren.org/English/safety-prevention/on-the-go/Pages/Car-Safety-Seats-Information-for-Families.aspx

American Academy of Pediatrics. (2023c). *Potty training*. https://www.healthychildren.org/English/ages-stages/toddler/toilet-training/Pages/default.aspx

American Association of Poison Control Centers. (n.d.). *In the home safety tips*. https://aapcc.org/prevention/in-the-home

Ben-Joseph, E. P. (2018). *Nutrition guide for toddlers*. https://kidshealth.org/en/parents/toddler-food.html

Buckloh, L. M. (2023). *Disciplining your toddler*. https://kidshealth.org/en/parents/toddler-tantrums.html#

Carter, R. G., & Feigelman, S. (2020a). The preschool years. In R. M. Kliegman, J. W. St. Geme III, N. J. Blum, S. S. Shah, R. C. Tasker, K. M. Wilson, & R. E. Behrman (Eds.), *Nelson's textbook of pediatrics* (21st ed.). Elsevier.

Carter, R. G., & Feigelman, S. (2020b). The second year. In R. M. Kliegman, J. W. St. Geme III, N. J. Blum, S. S. Shah, R. C. Tasker, K. M. Wilson, & R. E. Behrman (Eds.), *Nelson's textbook of pediatrics* (21st ed.). Elsevier.

Child Development Institute. (2022). *Temperament and your child's personality*. https://childdevelopmentinfo.com/uncategorized/temperament_and_your_child/

Division of Agriculture. (2023). Fruits and vegetables—Important sources of nutrients and vitamins. *University of Arkansas*. https://www.uaex.uada.edu/counties/miller/news/fcs/fruits-veggies/fruits-and-vegetables-important-sources-of-nutrients-and-vitamins.aspx

Durani, Y. (2023). *Preventing choking*. https://kidshealth.org/en/parents/safety-choking.html

Erikson, E. H. (1963). *Childhood and society* (2nd ed.). W. W. Norton and Company.

Gavin, M. L. (2019). *Toilet training*. https://kidshealth.org/en/parents/toilet-teaching.html

Global Initiative to End All Corporal Punishment of Children. (2018). *Global initiative to end corporal punishment*. https://endcorporalpunishment.org

Hagan, J. F., Shaw, J. S., & Duncan, P. M. (2017). *Bright futures: Guidelines for health supervision of infants, children, and adolescents* (4th ed.). American Academy of Pediatrics.

Kohlberg, L. (1984). *Moral development*. Harper & Row.

Lieberman, A. (2018). *The emotional life of a toddler*. Simon & Schuster.

Linguistic Society of America. (2023). *FAQ: Raising bilingual children*. https://www.linguisticsociety.org/resource/faq-raising-bilingual-children

Martorell, G. (2022). *Life: The essentials of human development* (2nd ed.). McGraw-Hill Publishing.

National Association for the Education of Young Children. (n.d.). *Good toys for young children by age and stage*. http://www.naeyc.org/toys

National Association of Pediatric Nurse Practitioners, Breastfeeding Education Special Interest Group, Busch, D. W., Silbert-Flagg, J., Ryngaert, M., & Scott, A. (2019). NAPNAP position statement on breastfeeding. *Journal of Pediatric Health Care, 33*(1), A11–A15. https://doi.org/10.1016/j.pedhc.2018.08.011

National Association of Pediatric Nurse Practitioners, Child Maltreatment and Neglect Special Interest Group, VanGraafeiland, B., Hornor, G. A., Herendeen, P. A., Chiocca, E. M., Loyke, J. A., Dietzman, H., Boucher, N. L., Nielsen, A., & Record, S. C. (2022). NAPNAP position statement on using positive parenting to eliminate corporal punishment. *Journal of Pediatric Health Care, 36*, 202–204. https://doi.org/10.1016/j.pedhc.2021.09.001

Nix, R. L., Francis, L. A., Feinberg, M. E., Gill, S., Jones, D. E., Hostetler, M. L., & Stifter, C. A. (2021). Improving toddlers' healthy eating habits and self-regulation: A randomized controlled trial. *Pediatrics, 147*(1), e20193326. https://doi.org/10.1542/peds.2019-3326

Nowak, A. J., & Warren, J. J. (2023). Preventive dental care and counseling for infants and young children. *UpToDate*. Retrieved September 23, 2023, from https://www.uptodate.com/contents/preventive-dental-care-and-counseling-for-infants-and-young-children

Pantley, E. (2020). The *no-cry sleep solution* (2nd ed.). McGraw Hill.

Parks, E. P., Shaikhkhalil, A., Sainath, N. N., Mitchell, J. A., Brownell, J. N., & Stallings, V. A. (2020). Feeding healthy infants, children, and adolescents. In R. M. Kliegman, J. W. St. Geme III, N. J. Blum, S. S. Shah, R. C. Tasker, K. M. Wilson, & R. E. Behrman (Eds.), *Nelson's textbook of pediatrics* (21st ed.). Elsevier.

Piaget, J. (1969). *The theory of stages in cognitive development*. McGraw-Hill.

Powers, J. M. (2023). Iron deficiency in infants and children <12 years: Screening, prevention, clinical manifestations, and diagnosis. *UpToDate*. Retrieved September 23, 2023, from https://www.uptodate.com/contents/iron-deficiency-in-infants-and-children-less-than12-years-screening-prevention-clinical-manifestations-and-diagnosis

Reading Rockets. (2023). *Reading tips for parents of toddlers*. https://www.readingrockets.org/topics/activities/articles/reading-tips-parents-toddlers

Reynolds, A., Angulo, A., Breheney, M., Green, J., & Goldson, E. (2022). Child development and behavior. In M. Bunik, W. W. Hay, M. J. Levin, & M. J. Abzug (Eds.), *Current diagnosis & treatment: Pediatrics* (26th ed.). McGraw-Hill Education.

SafeBedSharing.org. (2023). *Bed sharing or co-sleeping*. http://www.safebedsharing.org/safetyguidelines.html

Safe Kids. (2023a). *Swimming*. https://www.safekids.org/poolsafety

Safe Kids. (2023b). *Water safety tips at home*. https://www.safekids.org/tip/water-safety-home-tips

Samet, J. M., & Sockrider, M. (2023). Secondhand smoke exposure: Effects in children. *UpToDate*. Retrieved September 23, 2023, from https://www.uptodate.com/contents/secondhand-smoke-exposure-effects-in-children

Satter, E. (2023). *Child feeding ages and stages*. https://www.ellynsatterinstitute.org/how-to-feed/child-feeding-ages-and-stages/

Schaechter, J. (2023). *Guns in the home: How to keep kids safe*. https://www.healthychildren.org/English/safety-prevention/at-home/Pages/Handguns-in-the-Home.aspx

Schmitt, B. (2023). *Sibling rivalry toward a newborn*. https://doi.org/10.1542/ppe_schmitt_205

Sears, W., & Sears, M. (2020a). *Choosing & using a safe pacifier*. http://www.askdrsears.com/topics/parenting/child-rearing-and-development/bringing-baby-home/pacifiers-in-or-out/choosing-using

Sears, W., & Sears, M. (2020b). *8 tools for toddler discipline*. http://www.askdrsears.com/topics/parenting/discipline-behavior/8-tools-toddler-discipline

Sears, W., & Sears, M. (2020c). *Thumbsucking: Harmful or helpful?* http://www.askdrsears.com/topics/parenting/discipline-behavior/bothersome-behaviors/thumbsucking

Skelton, J. A., & Klish, W. J. (2023). Definition, epidemiology, and etiology of obesity in children and adolescents. *UpToDate*. Retrieved September 23, 2023, from https://www.uptodate.com/contents/definition-epidemiology-and-etiology-of-obesity-in-children-and-adolescents

Smith, M. A., & Segal, J. (2023). *Grandparents raising grandchildren: The rewards & challenges of parenting the second time around*. https://www.helpguide.org/articles/parenting-family/grandparents-raising-grandchildren.htm?pdf=13581

U.S. Department of Health and Human Services. (n.d.). *Healthy People 2030*. https://health.gov/healthypeople

Viguera, A. (2023). Postpartum depression: Adverse consequences in mothers and their children. *UpToDate*. Retrieved September 23, 2023, from https://www.uptodate.com/contents/postpartum-depression-adverse-consequences-in-mothers-and-their-children

Zubler, J. M., Wiggins, L. D., Macias, M. M., Whitaker, T. M., Shaw, J. S., Squires, J. K., Pajke, J. A., Wolf, R. B., Slaughter, K. S., Broughton, A. S., Gerndt, K. L., Mlodoch, B. J., & Lipkin, P. H. (2022). Evidence-informed milestones for developmental surveillance tools. *Pediatrics, 149*(3), e2021052138. https://doi.org/10.1542/peds.2021-052138

DEVELOPING CLINICAL JUDGMENT

PRACTICING FOR NCLEX

1. The nurse is caring for a hospitalized 30-month-old who is resistant to care, is angry, and yells "no" all the time. The nurse identifies this toddler's behavior as
   a. problematic, as it interferes with needed nursing care.
   b. normal for this stage of growth and development.
   c. normal because the child is hospitalized and out of his routine.

2. The parent of a 15-month-old is concerned about a speech delay. They describe the toddler as being able to understand what is said, sometimes following commands, but using only one or two words with any consistency. What is the nurse's best response to this information?
   a. The toddler should have a developmental evaluation as soon as possible.
   b. If the parent would read to the child, then speech would develop faster.
   c. Receptive language normally develops earlier than expressive language.
   d. The parent should ask the child's health care provider for a speech therapy evaluation.

3. A 2-year-old is having a temper tantrum. What advice should the nurse give the parent?
   a. For safety reasons, the toddler should be restrained during the tantrum.
   b. Punishment should be initiated, as tantrums should be controlled.
   c. The parent should promise the toddler a reward if the tantrum stops.
   d. The tantrum should be ignored as long as the toddler is safe.

4. What is the best advice about nutrition for the toddler?
   a. Encourage cup drinking and give water between meals and snacks.
   b. Encourage unlimited milk intake, because toddlers need the protein for growth.
   c. Avoid sugar-sweetened fruit drinks and allow as much natural fruit juice as desired.
   d. Allow the toddler unlimited access to the sippy cup to ensure adequate hydration.

5. To gain cooperation from a toddler, what is the best approach by the nurse?
   a. Immediately pick the toddler up from the parent's lap.
   b. Kneel in front of the toddler while they are on the parent's lap.
   c. Do the nursing tasks quickly so the toddler can play.
   d. Ask the toddler if it is okay if you begin the needed task.

6. The nurse is teaching the parents of a 2-year-old about toilet training. Which statements by the nurse are correct? Select all that apply.
   a. "Bowel training is usually accomplished before bladder training."
   b. "Wanting to please the parents helps motivate the child to use the toilet."
   c. "Watching older siblings use the toilet can provide role modeling for the child."
   d. "Children must be forced to sit on the toilet when first learning."
   e. "Children should never be scolded if they have an accident during toilet training."
   f. "Once toilet training is established, children never regress."

7. The nursing instructor has taught a group of nursing students about toddler physical growth and development. The nursing students verbalize the toddler is at increased risk for ___ related to ___ and ___.

   Blank 1:
   a. respiratory distress
   b. diarrhea
   c. infection

   Blanks 2 and 3:
   a. slower pulse and respiratory rate than in infancy
   b. less efficient defense mechanisms than in infancy
   c. abdominal respirations
   d. large lymphatic tissues
   e. immature intestinal functions
   f. short, straight eustachian tube

CRITICAL THINKING EXERCISES

1. Develop a teaching plan about safety to present to a toddler-age preschool class.
2. Construct a 3-day menu that is realistic and that will provide the nutrients needed for a 2-year-old.
3. Develop a plan for educating the parent of a 34-month-old who has been resistant to toilet teaching. Include assessments the nurse will make as well as the plan for teaching.

STUDY ACTIVITIES

1. Visit a preschool that provides care for toddlers with special needs as well as typical toddlers. Perform a developmental assessment on a typical toddler and one with special needs (both the same age). Compare and contrast your findings.
2. Care for two average 2-year-olds in the clinical setting. Describe each toddler's behavior, response to the parent, and response to the nurse, and list strategies used to gain adherence and minimize stress to the toddler.
3. Observe in the toddler classroom of a typical preschool. Choose two toddlers the same age with different temperaments. Record the toddlers' differences and similarities in response to structure and authority, interactions with classmates, attention levels, and language and activity levels.

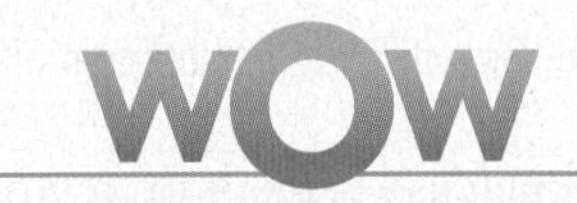

WORDS OF WISDOM

Preschoolers have been called the "little scientists" for their bold and inquisitive natures.

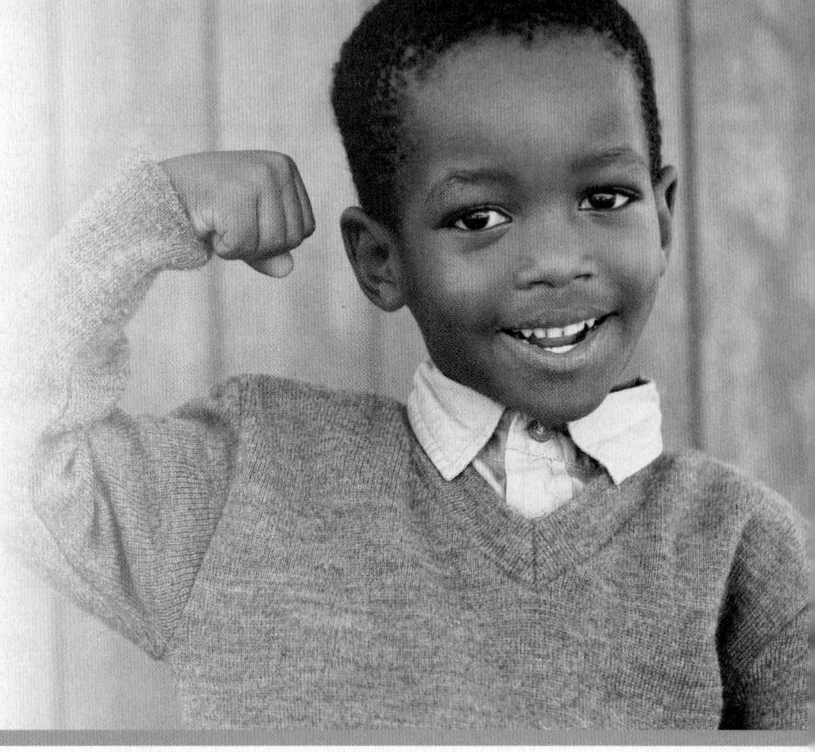

27

Growth and Development of the Preschooler

LEARNING OBJECTIVES

Upon completion of the chapter, you will be able to:

1. Describe expected physical growth, physiologic changes, and sensory development in the preschooler.
2. Examine psychosocial, cognitive, and moral/spiritual development in the preschooler.
3. Identify the gross and fine motor skills milestones of the preschooler.
4. Explain expected language and social/emotional development, and cultural influences on development in the preschool years.
5. Implement a nursing care plan that addresses common concerns or delays in the preschooler's development.
6. Develop a nutrition plan for the preschool-age child.
7. Provide appropriate anticipatory guidance for common developmental issues that arise in the preschool period.

KEY TERMS

animism (an´i-mizm)
empathy
imaginary friend
magical thinking
preoperational thought
school readiness
transduction

Nila Patel is a 4-year-old brought to the clinic by her parents for her school check-up. As the nurse caring for her, assess Nila's growth and development and then teach the parents what changes to expect in Nila over the next few months.

INTRODUCTION

The preschool period is the period between 3 and 6 years of age. This is a time of continued growth and development. Physical growth continues more slowly than in earlier years. Gains in cognitive, language, and psychosocial development are substantial throughout the preschool period. Many tasks that began during the toddler years are mastered and perfected during the preschool years. The child has learned to tolerate separation from parents, has a longer attention span, and continues to learn skills that will lead to later success in the school-age period. Preparation for success in school continues during the preschool period because most children enter elementary school by the end of the preschool period.

GROWTH AND DEVELOPMENT OVERVIEW

The healthy preschooler is slender and agile with an upright posture. The formerly clumsy toddler becomes more graceful, demonstrating the ability to run more smoothly. Athletic abilities may begin to develop. Major development occurs in the area of fine motor coordination. Psychosocial development is focused on the accomplishment of initiative. Preconceptual thought and intuitiveness dominate cognitive development. The preschooler is an inquisitive learner and absorbs new concepts like a sponge absorbs water.

PHYSICAL GROWTH

The average preschool-age child will grow 6.35 to 7.62 cm (2.5 to 3 in) per year. The average 3-year-old is 94 cm (37 in) tall, the average 4-year-old is 102.9 cm (40.5 in) tall, and the average 5-year-old is 109.2 cm (43 in) tall. Average weight gain during this time period is about 1.8 to 2.3 kg (4 to 5 lb) per year (Carter & Feigelman, 2020). The average weight of a 3-year-old is 14.5 kg (32 lb), increasing to an average weight of 18.6 kg (41 lb) by age 5. The loss of baby fat and the growth of muscle during the preschool years give the child a stronger, more mature appearance (Fig. 27.1). The length of the skull also increases slightly, with the lower jaw becoming more pronounced. The upper jaw widens through the preschool years in preparation for the emergence of permanent teeth, usually starting around age 6.

During your assessment of Nila (the 4-year-old introduced at the beginning of the chapter), you measure her weight to be 20 kg (44 lb) and her height to be 101.6 cm (40 in).

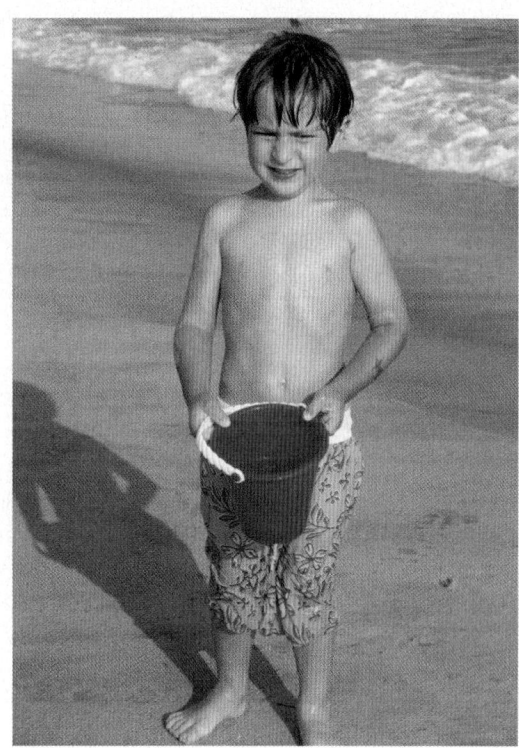

FIGURE 27.1 The preschool child has a slenderer appearance and erect posture than the toddler.

PHYSIOLOGIC CHANGES

Most of the body systems have matured by the preschool years. Myelination of the spinal cord allows for bowel and bladder control to be complete in most children by age 3 years. The respiratory structures are continuing to grow in size, and the number of alveoli continues to increase, reaching the adult number at about 7 years of age. The eustachian tubes remain relatively short and straight. Heart rate decreases and blood pressure increases slightly during the preschool years. An innocent heart murmur may be heard upon auscultation, and splitting of the second heart sound may become evident. The preschooler should have 20 deciduous teeth present.

The small intestine is continuing to grow in length. Stool passage usually occurs once or twice per day in the average preschooler. The 4-year-old generally has adequate bowel control. The urethra remains short, making preschoolers more susceptible to urinary tract infections than adults. Bladder control is usually present in 4- and 5-year-old children, but an occasional injury may occur, particularly in stressful situations or when the child is absorbed in an interesting activity.

The bones continue to increase in length, and the muscles continue to strengthen and mature. However, the musculoskeletal system is still not fully mature, making the preschooler susceptible to injury, particularly with overexertion or excess activity.

SENSORY DEVELOPMENT

Hearing is intact at birth and should remain so throughout the preschool years. The senses of smell and touch continue to develop throughout the preschool years. The young preschooler may have a less discriminating sense of taste than the older child, putting them at increased risk for inadvertent ingestion. Visual acuity continues to progress and should be equal bilaterally. The typical 5-year-old has visual acuity of 20/40 or 20/30. Color vision is intact at this age.

PSYCHOSOCIAL DEVELOPMENT

According to Erik Erikson (1963), the psychosocial task of the preschool years is establishing a sense of initiative versus guilt. The preschooler is an inquisitive learner, enthusiastic about learning new things. Preschoolers feel a sense of accomplishment when succeeding in activities (Fig. 27.2), and feeling pride in one's accomplishment helps the child to use initiative. However, when the child extends themselves further than current capabilities allow, they may feel a sense of guilt. The superego or conscience development is completed during the preschool period, and this is the basis for moral development (understanding right and wrong). Table 27.1 gives examples illustrating the stage of initiative versus guilt.

COGNITIVE DEVELOPMENT

According to Jean Piaget's theory (1969), the preschool-age child continues in the preoperational stage. **Preoperational thought** dominates during this stage and is based on a self-centered understanding of the world. In the preconceptual phase of preoperational thought, the child remains egocentric and is able to approach a problem from a single point of view only. The young preschooler may understand the concept of counting and begins to engage in fantasy play.

Magical thinking is a normal part of preschool development. In magical thinking, the preschooler believes that their thoughts are all-powerful. The fantasy experienced through magical thinking allows the preschooler to make room in their world for the actual or the real. Through make-believe and magical thinking, preschool-age children satisfy their curiosity about differences in the world around them.

The preschooler often has an **imaginary friend** as well (Reynolds et al., 2022). The imaginary friend is not real and exists only in the child's imagination. This friend serves as a creative way for the preschooler to sample different activities and behaviors and practice conversational skills. Despite this imaginative practice, the preschooler is able to switch easily between fantasy and reality throughout the day.

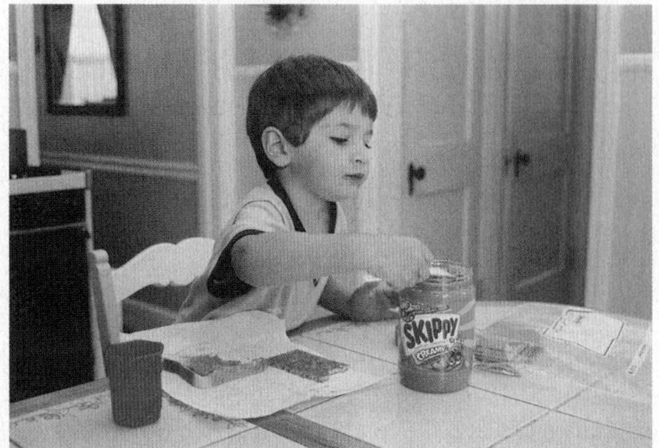

FIGURE 27.2 Allowing the preschooler to assist with simple household tasks, such as preparing a sandwich, encourages the development of initiative.

The child in the intuitive phase can count 10 or more objects, correctly name at least four colors, and better understand the concept of time. They know about things that are used in everyday life, such as appliances, money, and food. The preschooler uses **transduction** when reasoning; they extrapolate from a particular situation to another, even though the events may be unrelated. The preschooler also attributes life-like qualities to inanimate objects (**animism**). Table 27.1 gives further examples illustrating this developmental stage.

The acquisition of language skills in the toddler period is enhanced in the preschool period. The expansion of vocabulary enables the preschooler to progress further with symbolic thought. At this age, children do not completely understand the concept of death or its permanence: They may ask when their grandparent or pet who died is returning.

MORAL AND SPIRITUAL DEVELOPMENT

The preschool-age child can understand the concepts of right and wrong and is developing a conscience. That inner voice that warns or threatens is developing in the preschool years. Kohlberg (1984) identified this stage (between 2 and 7 years) as the preconventional stage, which is characterized by a punishment-and-obedience orientation. Preschool children see morality as external to themselves; they defer to power (that of the adult). The child's moral standards are those of their parents or other adults who influence them, not necessarily their own. Preschoolers adhere to those standards to gain rewards or avoid punishment. Since the preschool-age child is facing the psychosocial task of initiative versus guilt, it is natural for the child to experience guilt when something goes wrong.

TABLE 27.1 • Developmental Theories

Theorist	Stage	Activities
Erikson	Initiative vs. guilt Age: 3–6 years	Likes to please parents Begins to plan activities, make up games Initiates activities with others Acts out the roles of other people (real and imaginary) Develops sexual identity Develops conscience May take frustrations out on siblings Likes exploring new things Enjoys sports, shopping, cooking, working Feels remorse when making the wrong choice or behaving badly Cooperates with other children Negotiates solutions to conflicts
Piaget	Preoperational substage: preconceptual phase Age: 2–4 years	Exhibits egocentric thinking, which lessens as the child approaches age 4 Has a short attention span Learns through observing and imitating Displays animism Forms concepts that are not as complete or as logical as the adult's Is able to make simple classifications By age 4 understands the concept of opposites (hot/cold, soft/hard) Reasoning is that of specific to specific. Has an active imagination
	Preoperational substage: intuitive phase Age: 4–7 years	Is able to classify and relate objects Has intuitive thought processes; knows if something is right or wrong, though cannot state why Tolerates others' differences but does not understand them Is curious about facts Knows acceptable cultural rules Uses words appropriately but often without true understanding of their meaning Has a more realistic sense of causality May begin to question parents' values
Kohlberg	Punishment–obedience orientation Age: 2–7 years (preconventional morality)	Determines good vs. bad depending on associated punishment Children may learn inappropriate behavior at this stage if parental intervention does not occur (if the child hits, bites, or is verbally disrespectful but is not punished for these activities, the child will view those behaviors as good and continue to participate in them).

Data from Erikson, E. H. (1963). *Childhood and society* (2nd ed.). W. W. Norton and Company; Carter, R. G., & Feigelman, S. (2020). The preschool years. In R. M. Kliegman, J. W. St. Geme III, N. J. Blum, S. S. Shah, R. C. Tasker, K. M. Wilson, & R. E. Behrman (Eds.), *Nelson's textbook of pediatrics* (21st ed.). Elsevier; Kohlberg, L. (1984). *Moral development.* Harper & Row; Piaget, J. (1969). *The theory of stages in cognitive development.* McGraw-Hill.

As the child's moral development progresses, they learn how to deal with angry feelings. Sometimes the way the child chooses to deal with those feelings may be inappropriate, such as fighting and biting. Lying begins to occur in the preschool period. Younger preschoolers have difficulty differentiating between reality and their imagination and fantasies, whereas older preschoolers are more aware of right and wrong. Preschoolers also use their limited life experiences to make sense of and help them cope with crises. They need to learn the socially acceptable limits of behavior and are also learning the rewards of manners. The preschool-age child begins to help out in the family and begins to understand the concept of give-and-take in relationships.

During the preoperational phase of cognitive development, the preschooler's concept of faith is intuitive and projective in nature (Chromey, 2021). The preschool-age child's imagination allows for anything to be possible, so they do not have a logical view of the world as adults do. Preschool-age children have limited life experiences, so they may project a feeling onto a new person or situation. They may use this projection to help them understand what is going on around them. Preschoolers may project their parents' or caregivers' feelings or characteristics onto "God;" if Mommy gets angry, then God is probably also angry.

The family's religious beliefs may affect the child's diet, the mode of discipline that parents use, and even how the parents view their children. Knowing about a family's practices of prayer or meditation is helpful to the pediatric nurse, who can help continue the ritual when the child is ill or hospitalized (Fig. 27.3).

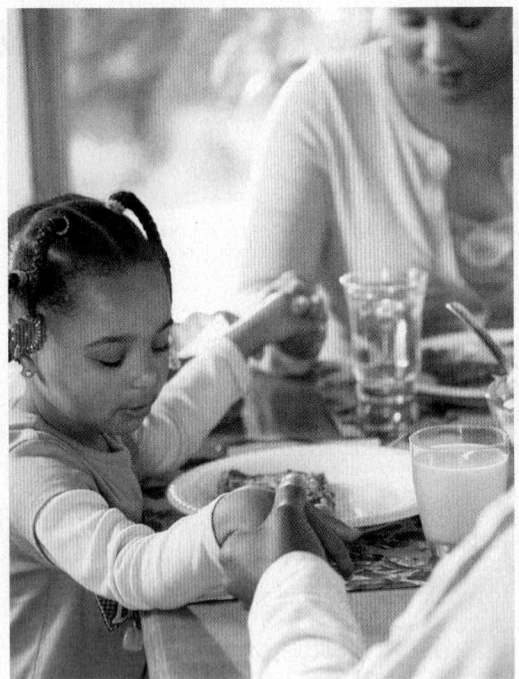

FIGURE 27.3 The preschool child may participate in religious rituals without having full understanding of their meaning.

MOTOR SKILL DEVELOPMENT

As the preschooler's musculoskeletal system continues to mature, existing motor skills become refined and new ones develop. The preschooler has more voluntary control over their movements and is less clumsy than the toddler. Significant refinement in fine motor skills occurs during the preschool period (Table 27.2).

Gross Motor Skills

The preschooler is agile while standing, walking, running, and jumping (Fig. 27.4). They can go up and down stairs and walk forward and backward easily. Standing on tiptoes or on one foot still requires extra concentration. The preschooler seems to be in constant motion. They also use the body to understand new concepts (such as using the arms in a "chug-chug" motion when describing how the train wheels work).

Fine Motor Skills

The 3-year-old can move each finger independently and is capable of grasping utensils and crayons in adult fashion, with the thumb on one side and the fingers on the other. They can also scribble freely, copy a circle, trace a square, and feed themselves without spilling much. These skills become refined over the next 2 years, and by 5 years of age, the child can write letters, cut with scissors more accurately, and tie shoelaces (Fig. 27.5).

COMMUNICATION AND LANGUAGE DEVELOPMENT

The acquisition of language allows the preschool-age child to express thoughts and creativity. The preschool years are a time of refinement of language skills. The

TABLE **27.2** • Motor Skill Development

Age	Expected Gross Motor Skills	Expected Fine Motor Skills
3 years	• Climbs well • Pedals tricycle • Runs easily • Walks up and down stairs with alternate feet • Bends over easily without falling	• Undresses self, puts on loose clothing items independently • Uses a fork • Builds a tower of 9 or 10 cubes • Strings beads or macaroni • Screws/unscrews lids, nuts, bolts • Copies circle
4 years	• Throws ball overhand • Kicks ball forward • Catches bounced ball • Stands on one foot for up to 5 seconds • Alternates feet going up and down steps • Moves backward and forward with agility	• Uses scissors successfully • Copies capital letters • Draws circles and squares • Traces a cross or diamond • Draws a person with two to four body parts • Laces shoes
5 years	• Hops on one foot • Stands on one foot for 10 seconds or longer • Swings and climbs well • May skip • Somersaults • May learn to skate and swim	• Prints some letters • Draws a person with a body and at least six parts • Fastens some buttons • Dresses/undresses without assistance • Can learn to tie laces • Uses fork, spoon, and knife (supervised) well • Copies triangle and other geometric patterns • Mostly cares for own toileting needs

Data from Carter, R. G., & Feigelman, S. (2020). The preschool years. In R. M. Kliegman, J. W. St. Geme III, N. J. Blum, S. S. Shah, R. C. Tasker, K. M. Wilson, & R. E. Behrman (Eds.), *Nelson's textbook of pediatrics* (21st ed.). Elsevier; Reynolds, A., Angulo, A., Breheney, M., Green, J., & Goldson, E. (2022). Child development and behavior. In M. Bunik, W. W. Hay, M. J. Levin, & M. J. Abzug (Eds.), *Current diagnosis & treatment: Pediatrics* (26th ed.). McGraw-Hill Education; Zubler, J. M., Wiggins, L. D., Macias, M. M., Whitaker, T. M., Shaw, J. S., Squires, J. K., Pajke, J. A., Wolf, R. B., Slaughter, K. S., Broughton, A. S., Gerndt, K. L., Mlodoch, B. J., & Lipkin, P. H. (2022). Evidence-informed milestones for developmental surveillance tools. *Pediatrics, 149*(3), e2021052138. https://doi.org/10.1542/peds.2021-052138

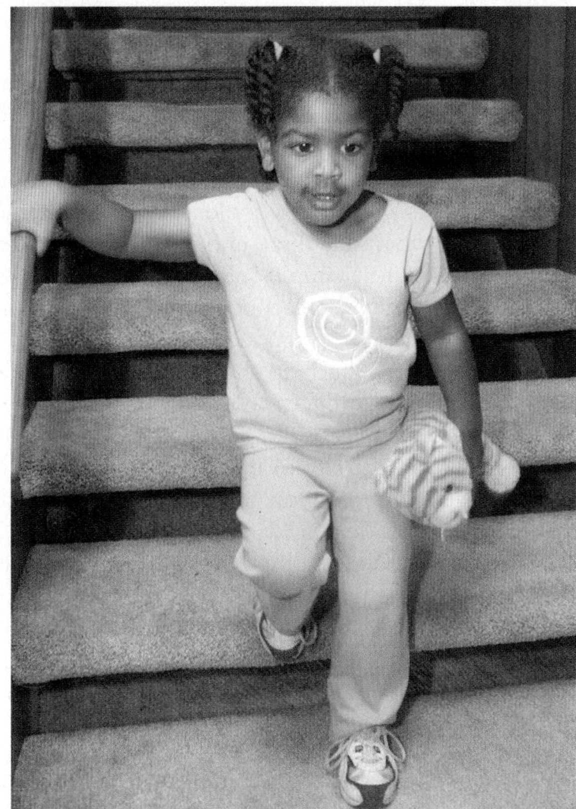

FIGURE 27.4 The preschooler runs well, navigates stairs, and can balance on one foot.

3-year-old exhibits telegraphic speech, using short sentences that contain only the essential information. Language development in the preschool years is extensive. At 2 years of age, a child uses 50 to 100 words and by 5 years of age uses about 2,000 words (Carter & Feigelman, 2020). By the end of the preschool period, the child is using sentences that are adult-like in structure (Table 27.3).

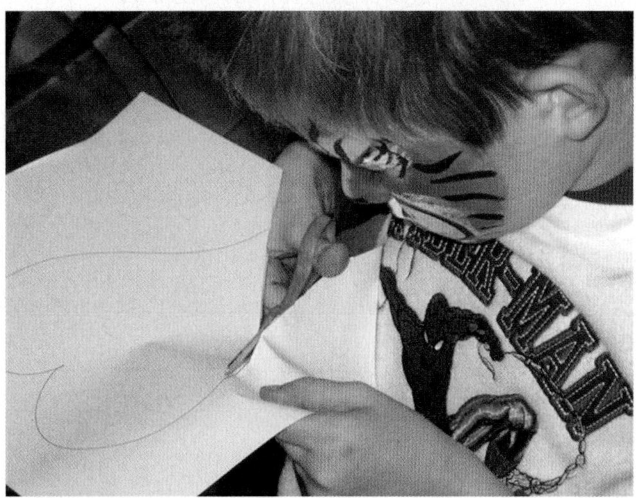

FIGURE 27.5 The 5-year-old has the fine motor dexterity to cut well with scissors.

TABLE 27.3 • Communication Skills in the Preschool Child

Age	Communication Abilities
4 years	• Speaks in complete sentences (four or more words) using adult-like grammar • Tells a story that is easy to follow • 75% of speech understood by others outside of family • Asks questions with "who," "how," and "how many" • Stays on topic in a conversation • Understands the concepts of "same" and "different" • Asks many questions • Knows names of familiar animals • Names common objects in books and magazines • Knows at least one color • Uses language to engage in make-believe • Follows a three-part command • Can count a few numbers • Vocabulary of 1,500 words
5 years	• People outside of the family can understand most of the child's speech. • Explains how an item is used • Participates in long, detailed conversations • Tells stories • Talks about past, future, and imaginary events • Answers questions that use "why" and "when" • Uses and recognizes simple rhymes • Can count to 10 • Recalls part of a story • Speech should be completely intelligible, even if the child has articulation difficulties. • Speech is generally grammatically correct. • Vocabulary of 2,100 words • Says name and address

Data from Centers for Disease Control and Prevention. (2023). *CDC's developmental milestones.* http://www.cdc.gov/ncbddd/actearly/milestones/index.html; Carter, R. G., & Feigelman, S. (2020). The preschool years. In R. M. Kliegman, J. W. St. Geme III, N. J. Blum, S. S. Shah, R. C. Tasker, K. M. Wilson, & R. E. Behrman (Eds.), *Nelson's textbook of pediatrics* (21st ed.). Elsevier; Zubler, J. M., Wiggins, L. D., Macias, M. M., Whitaker, T. M., Shaw, J. S., Squires, J. K., Pajke, J. A., Wolf, R. B., Slaughter, K. S., Broughton, A. S., Gerndt, K. L., Mlodoch, B. J., & Lipkin, P. H. (2022). Evidence-informed milestones for developmental surveillance tools. *Pediatrics, 149*(3), e2021052138. https://doi.org/10.1542/peds.2021-052138

The 3- to 6-year-old is starting to develop fluency (the ability to smoothly link sounds, syllables, and words when speaking). Initially, the child may exhibit disfluency or stuttering. Speech may sound choppy, or the child may say repeated consonants or "um." Stuttering usually has its onset in the preschool years and will resolve in 80% of children by age 8 years (Carter & Feigelman, 2020). Parents should slow down their speech and should give the child time to speak without rushing or interrupting. Some sounds remain difficult for the preschooler to enunciate properly: "f," "v," "s," and "z" sounds are usually mastered by age 5 years, but some children do not master the sounds of "sh," "l," "th," and "r" until age 6 or later. The potentially bilingual child may lag slightly behind the single-language speaker but will be able to differentiate and use both languages by the end of the preschool period (Linguistic Society of America, 2023).

Communication in preschool children is concrete in nature, as they are not yet capable of abstract thought. Despite its concrete nature, the preschooler's communication can be quite elaborate and involved; they may talk about dreams and fantasies. In addition to acquiring vocabulary and learning the correct use of grammar, the preschool child's receptive language skills are also becoming refined.

The preschooler is in tune with the parents' moods and easily picks up on negative emotions in conversations. If the preschooler hears parents discussing things that are frightening to the child, the preschooler's imagination may fuel the development of fears and lead to misinterpretation of what the child has heard.

As you assess Nila, the 4-year-old introduced at the beginning of the chapter, what would you expect her gross motor, fine motor, and language skills to be at this age?

EMOTIONAL AND SOCIAL DEVELOPMENT

By the time a child enters kindergarten, they should have developed a useful set of social skills that will help them have successful experiences in the school setting as well as in life in general. These skills include cooperation, sharing (of things and feelings), kindness, generosity, affection display, conversation, expression of feelings, helping others, and making friends.

Preschoolers tend to have strong emotions. They can be excited, happy, and giddy in one moment, then extremely disappointed in the next. The preschool-age child has a vivid imagination, and fears are very real to preschoolers. Most children this age have learned to control their behaviors. They should be able to name the feelings they are having rather than acting on them. Strong feelings may be expressed through outlets such as clay or Play-Doh, water play, drawing or painting, or dramatic play such as with puppets.

Preschoolers are developing a sense of identity. They may identify as boys or girls. They know that they belong to a particular family, community, or culture. They take pride in using self-control rather than giving in to their impulses. The preschool-age child is capable of helping others and being involved in routines and transitions.

Parents can encourage and assist preschool-age children with developing the social and emotional skills that will be needed when the child enters school. Preschool-age children thrive on one-to-one communication with a parent. During interactive communication, children learn to express their feelings and ideas. Interactive communication fosters not only emotional and moral development but also self-esteem and cognitive development. Asking the preschool child questions requires the child to think through their own intention or motivation and encourages vocabulary development. Parents may use individual communication as a time to explore right and wrong, thus further contributing to moral development. Being listened to while answering parents' questions gives preschoolers a sense that they are valued, that what they think and have to say matters.

Establishing a few simple rules and then enforcing them consistently gives preschoolers the structure and security they need while promoting moral development. Parents or caregivers can help the child give a name to the emotion that is being experienced. Fears are very real to preschoolers because of their active imaginations and may result in a variety of emotions. Parents should validate the feeling or emotion and then discuss with the child alternatives for dealing with the emotion.

Preschoolers are developing their senses of identity, and parents should encourage preschoolers to do simple things for themselves, like dressing and washing their hands and faces (Fig. 27.6). Parents should give the child the time needed to complete the task. This helps to establish a sense of accomplishment.

At this age, the child may begin to show an interest in basic sexuality. The preschooler may want to know why male and female bodies are different, how the reproductive organs function, and where babies come from. The parent should answer the child honestly and directly, using the correct anatomic terms. Long explanations are not necessary, just simple answers. This curiosity is a normal function of the preschool years, and the curiosity may also involve playing with the genitals (see the "Masturbation" section later in this chapter).

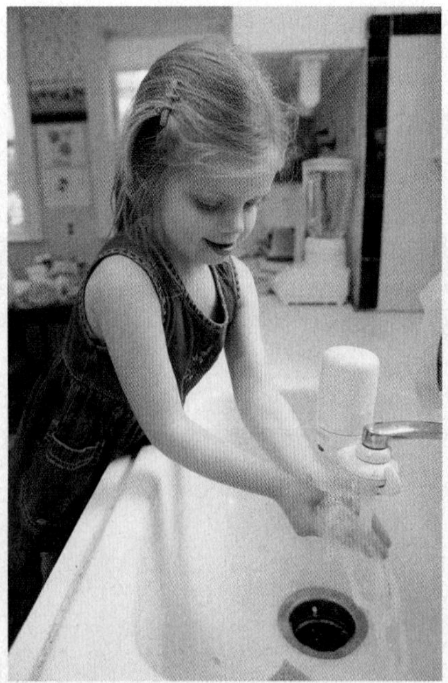

FIGURE 27.6 Encouraging the preschooler to complete simple tasks by themselves helps build self-esteem.

Friendships

Preschoolers need interactions with friends as well. Learning how to make and keep a friend is an important part of social development. Friends may be other children in the neighborhood or those at preschool or day care. A special friend is someone the preschooler can care about, talk to, and play with (Fig. 27.7). The preschooler is more likely to agree to rules and wants to please friends and be like them. The preschooler loves to sing, dance, and act and will enjoy these activities with friends. Disagreements may occur, but the parent can encourage the children to express their views, discuss and resolve conflicts, and continue being friends.

Temperament

By the time children are 3 years old, they recognize that what they do matters. It is helpful for the parent to view the child as an active participant in the parent–child relationship. The child's temperament has become a reliable indicator of how a parent might expect the child to react in a certain situation. When the parent is in tune with the preschooler's temperament, it is easier to find ways to ease transitions and changes for that child. In the area of task orientation, temperament may range from the highly attentive and persistent to the more distractible and active (Child Development Institute, 2022).

A child's social flexibility is also evident by this age. A child who is adaptable will handle stimuli from the outside world in an approaching rather than a withdrawing manner. Temperament also determines the extent of reactivity (the child's sensory threshold of responsiveness). This determines the quality of the child's mood and the intensity of reactions to stimuli, change, or situations. When the parents are familiar with the child's task orientation, social flexibility, and reactivity, they can better structure activities and situations for the child.

The 4-year-old is better at learning self-control and can use setbacks in appropriate behavior as opportunities for growth. Temper tantrums should ease by this age, as the child's language skills are more capable of keeping up with complex ideas. The 4-year-old is able to see the rewards of growing up. However, this awareness of self-power may lead to additional fears. The 5-year-old, who has a more vulnerable as opposed to a confident temperament, may be more apt to experience fears.

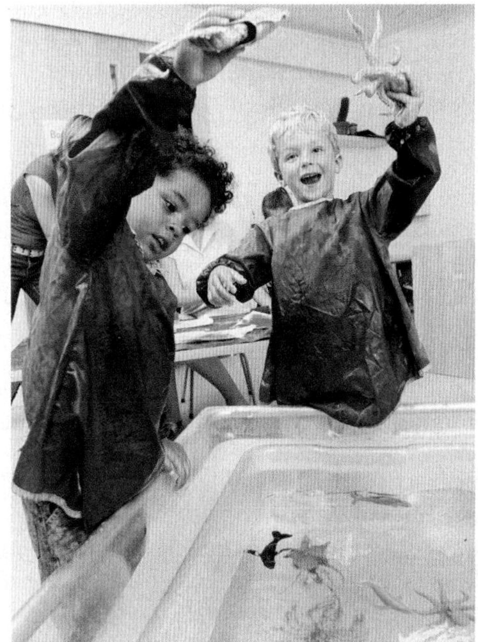

FIGURE 27.7 The preschool child begins to develop friendships.

Fears

With their vivid imaginations, preschoolers experience a variety of fears. Preschoolers may be scared of loud noises such as fire engine sirens or barking dogs. Imaginary monsters may scare the child. Preschoolers are often afraid of people they do not know and of strange people (Santa Claus or people who look or dress differently from what they are accustomed to). Many preschoolers are afraid of the dark. Preschoolers may also fear insects as well as animals they are not familiar with. The preschooler's memory is long enough that they may fear returning to the doctor's office when a painful procedure occurred during the prior visit.

Parents should acknowledge fears rather than minimizing them. They can then collaborate with the child on strategies for dealing with the fear.

CULTURAL INFLUENCES ON GROWTH AND DEVELOPMENT

Children may learn prejudice or bias at home before entering school or day care. The ways families view people of other races or cultures may be subtly or overtly demonstrated in routine daily activities. The preschool-age child is developing a conscience, so attitudes of tolerance or bias may influence the child's values. As in the toddler period, the value that the family places on independence will affect the child's development of a healthy self-concept.

Some families value reading and education more than others. If reading is not valued in the home, the preschool-age child's first experience with books may not occur until they are in school. Food served in the home is often specific to the family's cultural background. As the preschool-age child is exposed to people of other cultures in school, they may or may not like the food that is served. Exploring customs or cultural practices that the family participates in is important so that these practices may be safely incorporated into the child's plan of care.

THE NURSE'S ROLE IN THE GROWTH AND DEVELOPMENT OF PRESCHOOL-AGE CHILDREN

Growth and development in the preschool-age child remains orderly and sequential. Some preschoolers grow faster than others or reach various developmental milestones sooner than others. Nurses must be aware of the usual growth and development patterns for this age group so that they can assess preschool-age children appropriately and provide guidance to their families. The changes that the preschool-age child is experiencing affect not only the child but also the family. Health care visits throughout the preschool period continue to focus on expected growth and development and anticipatory guidance. An additional concern is the preparation for school entry (**school readiness**).

If the preschooler is hospitalized, growth and development may be altered. Hospitalization hinders the preschool-age child's ability to explore the environment and engage in make-believe play, thus presenting a challenge for the curious and inquisitive child. If the child must be isolated for a contagious illness, the opportunities for exploration and experimentation are further restricted. In addition, a sick preschooler may feel a sense of guilt, worrying that they may have caused the illness with negative thoughts or behaviors.

When caring for the hospitalized preschooler, the nurse must use knowledge of expected growth and development to recognize potential delays, promote continued appropriate growth and development, and interact successfully with the preschooler.

Clinical Judgment and the Nursing Process

After recognizing and analyzing cues from a thorough assessment of the preschool-age child's growth and development status, the nurse might identify several hypotheses, including:

- Injury risk
- Alteration in nutritional status
- Delayed growth and development risk
- Risk for body mass index (BMI) beyond 85th percentile for age
- Altered family functioning
- Desire for improved parenting skills

The above hypotheses provide suggestions for nursing care planning or concept mapping. The nurse will then generate solutions by planning interventions (suggested with rationales). Care planning should be individualized based on the preschooler's and family's needs.

Nursing Analysis

Injury risk; risk factors include extremes of age (e.g., curiosity, increased mobility, developmental immaturity) and unsafe mode of transport (e.g., lack of car seat and helmet use).

Goal/Outcome

Preschooler safety will be maintained: Preschooler will remain free from injury.

Preventing Injury (interventions with *rationale*)

- Teach and encourage appropriate use of forward-facing car seat or booster seat *to decrease risk of injury related to motor vehicles.*
- Teach preschoolers to stay away from the street and to cross the street only when holding the hand of an adult *to prevent pedestrian injury.*
- Require bicycle helmet use while riding any wheeled toy *to prevent head injury and form a habit of helmet use.*
- Teach the preschooler appropriate safety rules in the home (e.g., avoiding electric outlets); *the preschooler is able to follow simple directions and carry out directives. Limits help them organize the environment.*
- Post Poison Control Center phone number *in case of accidental ingestion; the preschool child is curious.*
- Never leave a preschool child unattended in a tub or pool or near any body of water *to prevent drowning.*
- Provide swimming lessons for children of ages 4 or 5 *to encourage water safety but not as a replacement for adult supervision.*
- Teach parents first aid measures and child cardiopulmonary resuscitation (CPR) *to minimize consequences of injury should it occur.*
- Provide close observation and keep side rails up on the bed in the hospital *because the preschool child continues to be at risk for falling or injuring themselves on equipment or tubing due to curiosity.*

Nursing Analysis

Alteration in nutritional status related to insufficient dietary intake (excess juice or milk intake, inadequate variety of food intake) as evidenced by failure to attain adequate increases in height and weight over time.

Goal/Outcome

Child will consume adequate nutrients: Child will demonstrate weight gain and increases in height.

Promoting Appropriate Nutrition (interventions with *rationale*)

- Assess current feeding schedule and usual intake as well as methods used to feed *to determine areas of adequacy versus inadequacy.*
- Determine if the preschooler is unable to drink from a cup or does not finger feed or use utensils properly or if

the child has difficulty swallowing or tolerating certain textures of foods *to determine if further interventions such as speech or occupational therapy are required.*
- Weigh child daily on the same scale if hospitalized, weekly on the same scale if at home, and plot growth patterns weekly or monthly as appropriate on standardized growth charts *to determine if growth is improving.*
- Limit juice to 4 to 6 oz per day and milk to 16 to 24 oz per day *to discourage the sense of fullness achieved with excess milk or juice intake, thereby increasing appetite for appropriate solid foods.*
- Provide three nutrient-dense meals and at least two healthy snacks per day *to encourage adequate nutrient consumption.*
- Feed the child on a similar schedule daily without distractions and with the family; *preschool children continue to respond well to routine and structure. They are more interested in the social context of meals and are still apt to become distracted easily, so the television should be off at mealtimes.*

Nursing Analysis
Delayed growth and development risk; risk factors include inadequate nutrition, abuse, chronic illness, prematurity, technology dependence, behavioral disorders, or involvement with the foster care system.

Goal/Outcome
Development will be enhanced: The child will make continued progress toward realization of expected developmental milestones.

Enhancing Development (interventions with *rationale*)
- Screen for developmental capabilities *to determine the child's current level of functioning.*
- Offer age-appropriate toys, play, and activities (including those using gross motor skills) *to encourage further development.*
- Perform interventions as prescribed by a physical, occupational, or speech therapist; *participation in those activities helps promote function and accomplish acquisition of developmental skills.*
- Provide support to families of preschoolers with developmental delay (*progress in achieving developmental milestones can be slow, and ongoing motivation is needed*).
- Reinforce positive attributes in the child *to maintain motivation.*
- Model age-appropriate communication skills *to illustrate suitable means for parenting the preschooler.*

Nursing Analysis
Risk for BMI beyond 85th percentile for age; risk factors include portion sizes larger than recommended, excess milk or juice intake, and excess snacking.

Goal/Outcome
Child will grow appropriately and achieve BMI within the fifth to 85th percentiles for age on standardized growth charts.

Promoting Appropriate Growth (interventions with *rationale*)
- Discourage use of no-spill sippy cups *which contribute to dental caries and allow unlimited access to fluids, possibly decreasing appetite for appropriate solid foods.*
- Provide juice (4 to 6 oz per day) and milk (16 to 24 oz per day) from a cup at meal and snack time and water in between *to avoid the child drinking excessive juice or milk.*
- Provide only nutrient-rich foods without high sugar content for meals and snacks; *even if the preschooler is a picky eater, it is inappropriate to provide high-calorie junk food just to get the child to eat something.*
- Teach parents to role model appropriate eating (nutrient-rich, varied diet) *to encourage the child to try and accept new foods as well as to become familiar with a variety of foods.*
- Severely limit the intake of fast foods and foods with high sugar and fat content *to decrease intake of nutrient-poor, high-calorie foods.*
- Ensure adequate physical activity *to stimulate development of motor skills and provide appropriate caloric expenditure. This also sets the stage for forming a lifelong habit of appropriate physical activity.*
- Teach parents to limit entertainment screen time to 1 hour per day *to encourage participation in physical activities.*

Nursing Analysis
Altered family functioning related to a shift in family roles (preschooler illness or hospitalization) as evidenced by a change in family satisfaction/assigned tasks/communication pattern or decrease in available emotional support.

Goal/Outcome
Family will demonstrate adequate functioning: Family will display coping and psychosocial adjustment.

Enhancing Family Functioning (interventions with *rationale*)
- Assess the family's level of stress and ability to cope *to determine family's ability to cope with multiple stressors.*
- Engage in family-centered care *to provide a holistic approach to care of the preschooler and family.*
- Encourage the family to verbalize feelings (*verbalization is one method of decreasing anxiety levels*) and acknowledge feelings and emotions.
- Use puppets or dramatic play with the child *to elicit the preschooler's feelings about the current situation.*

- Encourage family visitation and provide for sleeping arrangements for a parent or caregiver to stay in the hospital with the preschooler; *this contributes to the family's sense of control in a situation.*
- Involve family members in the preschooler's care, *giving them a feeling of control and connectedness.*

Nursing Analysis

Desire for improved parenting skills related to parental expression of readiness for enhanced skills.

Goal/Outcome

Parents will provide a safe and nurturing environment for the preschool child: Parents will verbalize new skills they will employ in the family.

Increasing Parenting Skill Set (interventions with *rationale*)

- Use family-centered care *to provide a holistic approach.*
- Educate the parent about normal preschool development *to provide a basis of understanding for parenting skills needed in this time period.*
- Acknowledge and encourage parents' verbalization of feelings related to chronic illness of the child or difficulty with normal preschool behavior; *this validates the normalcy of parents' feelings.*
- Encourage positive parenting and respect for the preschooler and their normal development *to help parents develop approaches to preschoolers that can be used in place of anger and frustration.*
- Role model appropriate parenting behaviors related to communicating with and disciplining the child; *role modeling demonstrates rather than just verbalizes what the parent should strive for.*

PROMOTING HEALTHY GROWTH AND DEVELOPMENT

The building of self-esteem continues throughout the preschool period. It is of particular importance during these years, as the preschooler's developmental task is focused on the development of initiative rather than guilt. A sense of guilt will contribute to low self-esteem, while a child who is rewarded for their initiative will have increased self-confidence. The parent who provides a loving and nurturing environment for the preschooler builds upon the earlier foundation.

Routine and ritual continue to be important throughout the preschool years, as they help the child develop a sense of time as well as provide the structure for the child to feel safe and secure. Daily routine continues to assist with the development of conscience in the preschooler. As in toddlerhood, making expectations known through everyday routines helps avoid confrontations. The preschooler is developing the maturity to know how to behave in various situations and is capable of learning manners.

Setting limits (and remaining consistent with those limits) continues to be important in the preschool period. Consistent limits provide the preschooler with expectation and guidance. As the preschooler increasingly participates in fantasy and imagination, the limits of routine and structure help guide their behavior and ability to distinguish reality.

Nurses caring for preschoolers should have knowledge of typical developmental expectations, so they can determine whether the preschool child is progressing appropriately. Table 27.4 lists potential signs of developmental delay. A preschool child with one or more of these concerns should be referred for further developmental evaluation.

Promoting Growth and Development Through Play

Providing sincere encouragement for the preschool child's efforts and accomplishments helps them develop a sense of initiative. Giving children opportunities to

TABLE 27.4 • Signs of Developmental Delay

Age	Concern
4 years	• Cannot jump in place or ride a tricycle • Cannot stack four blocks • Cannot throw ball overhand • Does not grasp crayon with thumb and fingers • Has difficulty with scribbling • Cannot copy a circle • Does not use sentences with three or more words • Cannot use the words "me" and "you" appropriately • Ignores other children or does not show interest in interactive games • Will not respond to people outside the family; still clings or cries if parents leave • Resists using the toilet, dressing, sleeping • Does not engage in fantasy play
5 years	• Is often unhappy or sad • Has little interest in playing with other children • Is unable to separate from parent without major protest • Is extremely aggressive • Is extremely fearful or timid, or unusually passive • Cannot build a tower of six to eight blocks • Is easily distracted; cannot concentrate on a single activity for 5 minutes • Rarely engages in fantasy play • Has trouble with eating, sleeping, or using the toilet • Cannot use plurals or past tense • Cannot brush teeth, wash and dry hands, or undress efficiently

decide how and with whom they want to play also helps them develop initiative. Preschool children like to write, color, draw, paint with a brush or their fingers, and trace or copy patterns (Fig. 27.8). They may start small collections that may be sorted. They like using toys for their intended purposes as well as for whatever invented purpose they can imagine.

Preschoolers begin to play cooperatively with one another. Play may be focused on a distinct theme. They define roles, make up rules, and assign jobs. They are able to work together toward a common goal such as building a house or fort with discarded boxes. Cooperative play encourages the preschool child to learn to share, take turns and compromise, listen to others' opinions, consider the feelings of others, use self-control, and overcome fears.

Preschoolers have incredible imaginations and love to play "make-believe" (Fig. 27.9). Encouraging pretend play and providing props for dress-up stimulate curiosity and creativity. Fantasy play is usually cooperative in nature. It encourages the preschooler to develop social skills such as taking turns, communication, paying attention, and responding to one another's words and actions. Fantasy play also allows preschoolers to explore complex social ideas such as power, compassion, and cruelty. Through role-play, children begin to develop their sexual identity as well.

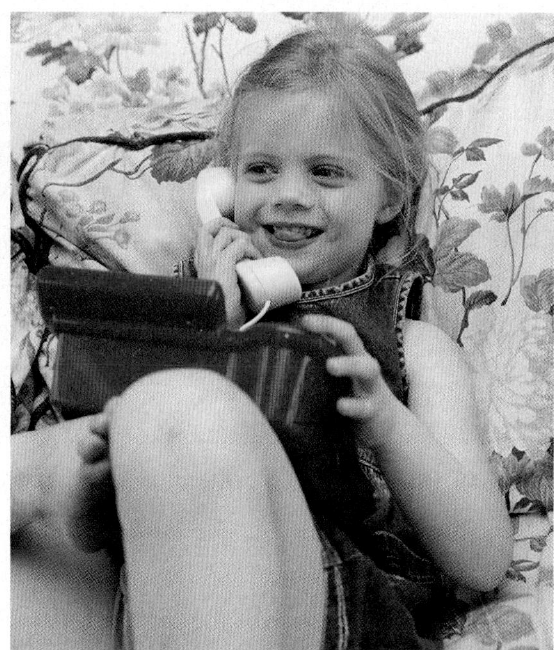

FIGURE 27.9 Preschool children enjoy imitative play.

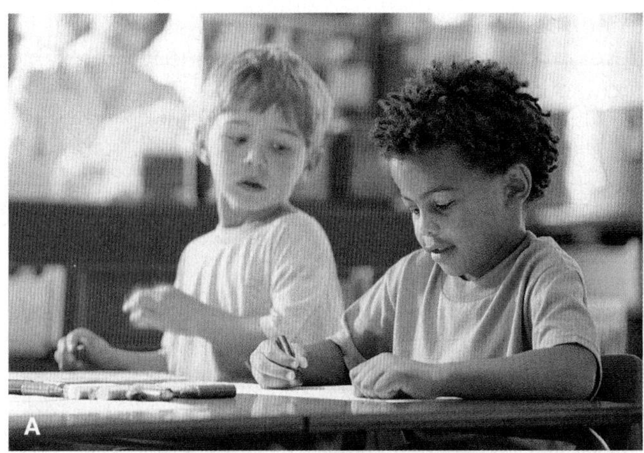

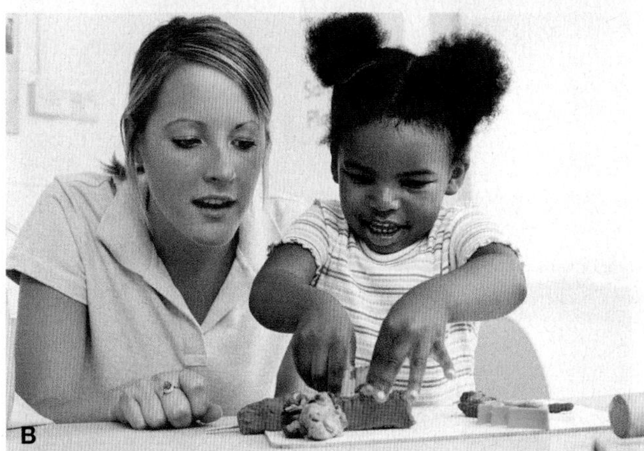

FIGURE 27.8 The preschool child loves to create things, so coloring (**A**) and molding clay (**B**) are ideal activities for children at this age.

Since preschool children have vivid imaginations, it is important to be careful about what television they watch. The preschooler should be limited to no more than 1 hour per day of quality television or other digital media programming (American Academy of Child and Adolescent Psychiatry [AACAP], 2020). The violence in some television programs may scare the preschool child or inspire them to act out the violent behavior.

Most preschoolers also engage in dramatic play, fueled by their innate curiosity and vivid imaginations. Three-year-olds may not realize that they are pretending. They run from scary creatures, make plans, and pack their backpacks (never intending to actually leave). Four-year-olds are more sophisticated with dramatic or pretend play; they know they are pretending, and they use dress-up clothes and props to act out more complex roles and scenarios (Fig. 27.10). Five-year-olds are capable of quite complex scenarios. They pretend they are real or fantasy characters. They often use dramatic play to express anxiety, try out negative feelings, or conquer their fears. For example, a child who is afraid of getting a shot at the doctor's office may work through that feeling with pretend play.

Parents should encourage physical activity in the preschool child. Regular physical activity improves gross motor skills, may enhance the child's self-confidence, and allows the child to expend excess energy. Establishing the habit of daily physical activity in the early years is important in the long-term goal of avoiding excess weight. The main goal of organized sports at this age should be

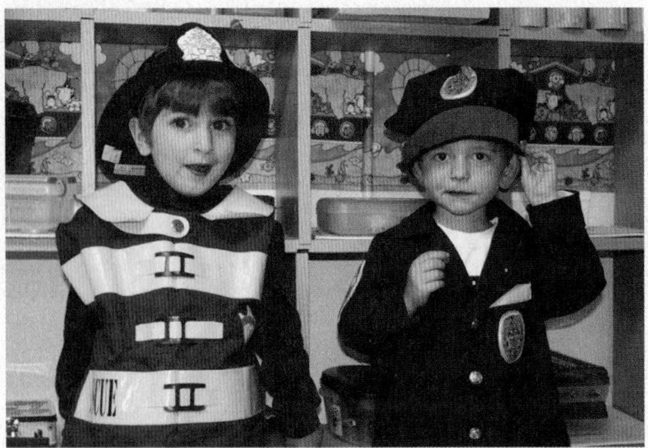

FIGURE 27.10 Preschool children love to dress up and pretend.

fun and enjoyment, though safety must remain a priority. Expensive toys that claim to teach the young child are not necessary. Toys that require interactive rather than passive play and that may include the involvement of the parent are recommended (National Association for the Education of Young Children, n.d.). Box 27.1 lists appropriate playthings for the preschool child.

Promoting Early Learning

The family is the foundation for the child's early growth and development. Parents serve as role models for behavior related to education and learning, as well as instilling values in their children. School readiness is a topic that has received a significant amount of national attention in recent years. To succeed in school, children need safe, responsive home environments that allow them to learn and explore as well as structure and limits that allow them to learn the socially acceptable behaviors that they will need in school. Language development is critical to the ability to succeed in school and can be encouraged through books and reading. Each of these components is important in readying the child for education in a more formal setting (Williams et al., 2019). Promoting language development, choosing a preschool, and making the transition to kindergarten are discussed in more detail in the sections that follow.

Promoting Language Development

The parent serves as the child's first teacher. The interactions between parent and child in relation to books and other play activities model the types of interactions that the child will later have in school. Asking open-ended questions stimulates the development of thinking as well as language in the preschool child. The preschooler is a great imitator, so the parent should serve as a role model for appropriate language. Parents should avoid swearing, as the child is sure to repeat "bad words" even if they do not understand what they mean. Allowing children to pursue interests at their own pace will help them to develop the literacy and numeric skills that will enable them to later focus on academic skills.

Preschoolers enjoy books with pictures that tell stories (Fig. 27.11). Stories with repeated phrases help keep the child's attention. Children like stories that describe experiences similar to their own. The preschool child

BOX 27.1 Appropriate Toys for Preschoolers

- Blocks, simple jigsaw puzzles (four to six large pieces), pegboards, wooden bead with string
- Supplies for creativity: chalk, large crayons, finger paint, Play-Doh or clay, washable markers, paper, paint and paintbrush, scissors, paste, or glue
- Puppets, dress-up clothes, and props for dramatic play
- Bucket, plastic shovel, and other containers for sand and water play
- Play kitchen with accessories and pretend food (Empty food boxes can be recycled for kitchen play.)
- Squeaking, floating, and squirting toys for the bath
- Sandbox with a shovel and various toys for building
- Dolls that can be dressed and undressed (large buttons, zippers, and snaps), doll care accessories (diapers, bottles, carriage, crib)
- Gross motor toys: tricycle or big wheel (with helmet), jungle gym or swing set (with supervision), Hula-Hoop, tunnel, wagon
- Blocks, Legos, cars and trucks, plastic animals, trains, plastic figures (family, community helpers), stuffed animals, balls, sewing cards
- Tape/CD/record players or streaming devices for music, various musical instruments
- Simple card and board games (older preschoolers)
- Dollhouse with furniture and accessories, people, and animals

Data from National Association for the Education of Young Children. (n.d.). *Good toys for young children by age and stage.* http://www.naeyc.org/toys

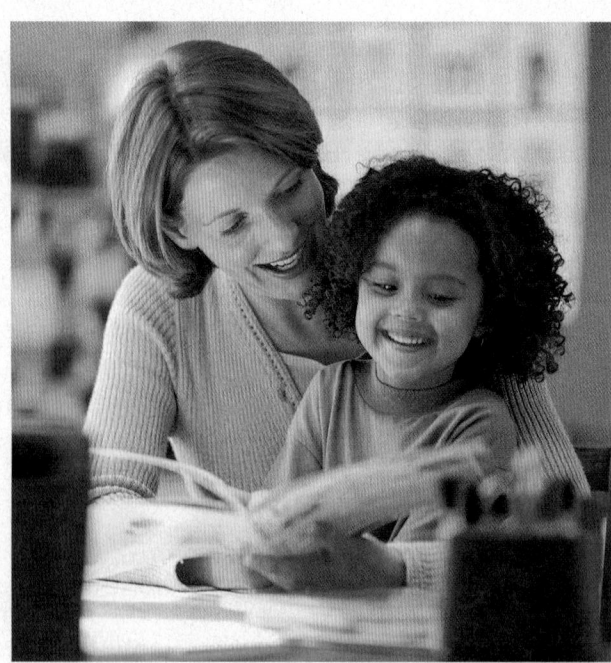

FIGURE 27.11 Preschool children enjoy being read to and looking at the pictures that go along with the story.

demonstrates early literacy skills by reciting stories or portions of books. They may also retell the story from the book, pretend to read books, and ask questions about the story. The preschool child has enough focus and expanded attention to notice when a page is skipped during reading and will call it to the parent's attention.

Choosing a Preschool and Starting Kindergarten

Many parents choose to enroll their child in preschool. Preschool should be used primarily as an opportunity to foster the child's social skills and accustom them to the group environment. When selecting a preschool, the parent may want to consider the accreditation of the school, the teachers' qualifications, and recommendations of other parents. The focus of the school environment is also important: What is the daily schedule of activities? Is the school very structured, or does it have a looser environment? The parents must decide how focused on curriculum they want the school to be. The parent should observe the classroom, evaluating the environment, noise level, and sanitary practices as well as how the children interact with each other and how the teachers interact with the children.

The type of discipline used in the school is also an important factor. Parents should not choose a preschool that uses corporal punishment. The American Academy of Pediatrics (AAP) discourages the use of corporal punishment in the school setting (Sege, 2018). Recent research demonstrates that corporal punishment may hurt a child's self-esteem, result in adverse behavioral outcomes, and result in harmful brain changes leading to cognitive differences affecting the child's ability to succeed in school (Cuartas et al., 2021). It may also lead to disruptive and violent behavior in the classroom (Sege, 2018). As preschool is the foundation for later education, the child should have the opportunity to build self-esteem and the skills needed for the more formal setting of elementary school.

Kindergarten will be the next big step. Kindergarten hours may be longer than preschool hours, and kindergarten is usually held 5 days per week. This may be a significant change for some children. For most children, the setting and personnel in kindergarten will be new. Rules and expectations are often different as well. When discussing starting kindergarten with the preschool child, parents should do so in an enthusiastic fashion, keeping the conversation light and positive. Parents should meet with the child's teacher prior to the start of school, if possible, to discuss any particular needs or concerns. Parents may want to schedule a tour of the school for the preschooler or attend the school's open house with the child to ease the transition. Practicing the new daily routine prior to the start of school will also be helpful.

Most states require up-to-date immunizations and a health screening of the child before they enter kindergarten, so advise parents to plan ahead and schedule these in a timely fashion so that school entrance is not delayed (Public Health Law Program, 2022).

TAKE NOTE!

Risk factors for lack of social and emotional readiness for school include insecure attachment in the early years, parental depression, parental substance use disorder, and low socioeconomic status. Nurses should screen for these factors and make referrals if appropriate.

Promoting Safety

In the United States, unintentional injury remains the leading cause of death for children between the ages of 1 and 14 years (National Center for Injury Prevention and Control, 2020). Preschoolers are at an ideal age to be taught about safety and safe behaviors. They are cognitively able to absorb concrete information and they desire to master the situations they are in, but they continue to display poor judgment related to safety issues. Their engagement in fantasy is so strong that it makes it difficult for them to master complicated cause-and-effect relationships. The preschool child is capable of learning safe behaviors but may not always be able to transfer those behaviors to a different situation. Parents must continue to closely supervise preschool children to avoid accidental injury during this period.

Safety in the Car

The preschooler up until 4 years of age, whose height meets the car seat size requirement, should use a forward-facing car seat with harness and top tether. All preschoolers after reaching the car seat height restriction should ride in a booster seat that uses both the lap and shoulder belts (Fig. 27.12). It is recommended that

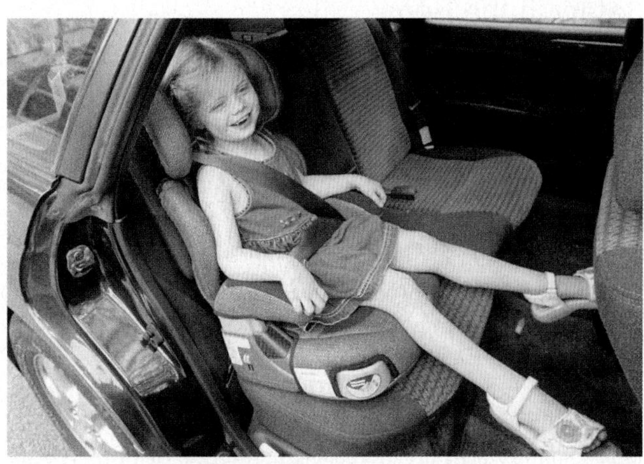

FIGURE 27.12 The older preschool child should be appropriately secured in an approved booster seat.

the booster seat continue to be used until a height of 145 cm (4 ft 9 in) and age of 8 to 12 years are reached (AAP, 2023a). The back seat of the car is always the safest place for a child to ride. If a child younger than 12 years must sit in the front seat because there are not enough rear seats available, then the front passenger seat air bag should be deactivated. Young children should never ride in the cargo area of a pickup truck as their risk for dying in the event of a crash is increased 10-fold as compared with riding appropriately restrained inside a motor vehicle (Stanford Medicine, 2023). See the Healthy People 2030 box.

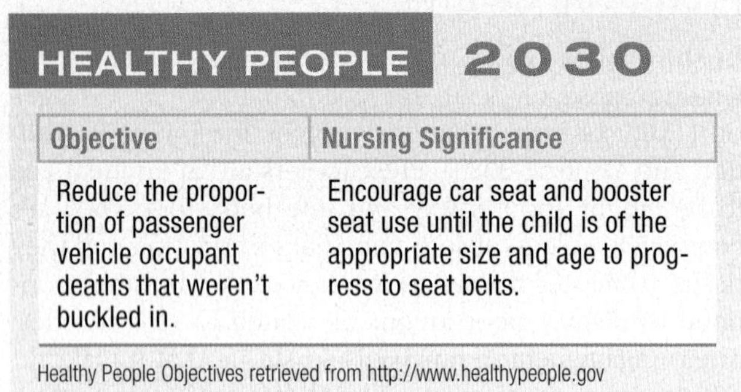

HEALTHY PEOPLE 2030

Objective	Nursing Significance
Reduce the proportion of passenger vehicle occupant deaths that weren't buckled in.	Encourage car seat and booster seat use until the child is of the appropriate size and age to progress to seat belts.

Healthy People Objectives retrieved from http://www.healthypeople.gov

TAKE NOTE!

Although motor vehicle crashes remain a major cause of injury and death in the preschool-age group, many families do not use appropriate car seat/seat belt safety with their children. Child passenger safety technicians are available to provide proper installation of car seats. To find one in your area, visit http://cert.safekids.org/ or http://www.seatcheck.org. The National Highway Traffic Safety Administration (NHTSA) Auto Safety Hotline may be reached at (888) 327-4236.

Safety in the Home

Handguns, matches, bodies of water, bicycle riding, and poisons continue to be sources of potential injury during the preschool years. Falls account for the highest percentage of nonfatal injuries among preschoolers. In this age group, drowning is responsible for the most fatal injuries followed by motor vehicle crashes. A significant number of injuries also occur in or around the home, including burns and poisoning (National Safety Council, 2023).

PREVENTING EXPOSURE TO TOBACCO SMOKE

Parents should protect their preschoolers from second-hand tobacco smoke. Exposure to tobacco smoke is associated with an increased incidence of otitis media and respiratory infections, as well as increased symptoms and medication use in children with asthma. Other effects include decreased lung function and behavioral difficulties (World Health Organization, n.d.). The preschool child should never be in an enclosed space, such as a car, where tobacco smoke is present.

PREVENTING INJURY

The preschool child who runs out into the street is at risk for being struck by a car. Teach preschoolers to stop at the curb and never go into the street without a grown-up. The preschooler may learn to ride a bicycle (with or without training wheels). The child must wear an approved bicycle helmet any time they ride the bicycle, even if it is just in the driveway. Requiring helmet use in the early years may lead to the habit of helmet use as the child gets older. Allowing the preschooler to choose their own helmet may encourage the child to use the helmet.

Bicycles should be safe for this age group. The size must be correct; the balls of the feet should reach both pedals while the child is sitting on the seat and has both hands on the handlebars. Children younger than 5 years have difficulty learning to use hand-operated brakes, so traditional pedal-back brakes are recommended in this age group. Preschoolers are not mature enough to ride a bicycle in the street even if they are riding with adults, so they should always ride on the sidewalk (AAP, 2022c).

It is important to make the inside of the home safe for the preschool child. Parents should install and maintain smoke alarms as well as carbon monoxide detectors in the home. Increased physical dexterity and refinement of motor skills enable the preschooler to strike matches or use a lighter and start a fire. The preschool child is capable of washing their hands independently, so the water heater should be set at 49°C (120°F) or below to prevent scalding (AAP, 2022b).

The preschooler's active imagination and desire to play make-believe may result in a firearm injury. The average preschooler is physically capable of handling and firing a gun, particularly a handgun, which is smaller and lighter. If present in the home, firearms should be kept in a locked cabinet with the ammunition stored elsewhere (AAP, 2022a).

PREVENTING POISONING

Though it is continuing to develop, preschoolers still have unrefined taste discrimination, placing them at risk for accidental ingestion. Parents should never try to coax a child to take a vitamin supplement, tablet, or pill by calling it "candy." Dangerous fluids should be stored in their original containers and should be kept out of reach of preschoolers; they should not be poured into containers that look like ordinary drinking glasses or cups. Potentially dangerous cleaning or personal health and beauty products, gardening and pool chemicals, and automotive materials should be kept out of reach of preschoolers and in a locked cabinet if possible.

Medications should have childproof caps and should be kept in a locked cabinet. The Poison Control Center telephone number should be posted on or near the home phone (1-800-222-1222) (American Association of Poison Control Centers, n.d.).

Safety in the Water

Children 4 years of age are able to voluntarily hold their breath, making this age an appropriate time for a child to learn to swim (AAP, 2023b). Children at this age are physically capable of this activity and have the cognitive maturity to accomplish the task of swimming and basic water safety. If developmentally appropriate, water survival skills may be started at age 1 year and can help decrease the risk of drowning (AAP, 2023b). Swimming programs should focus on appropriate swim techniques as well as safety measures. Parents and caregivers should be trained in infant/child CPR. Homes with swimming pools should have lifesaving devices readily accessible. Preschoolers should be taught never to dive into water until an adult has verified its depth. Preschoolers are still too young to be left unattended around any body of water, even if they know how to swim. Preschoolers should never be allowed to swim in a canal or any fast-moving water. Preschoolers who are riding in boats or fishing off riverbanks should wear a personal flotation device. Parents should also be cautioned about close supervision of young children walking, skating, or riding near thin or weak ice.

TAKE NOTE!

All swimming pools should be secured by a fence that is at least 5 ft in height with a self-latching gate to protect young children from entering a pool area unattended (SafeKids, 2023).

Recall Nila Patel, the 4-year-old presented at the beginning of the chapter. What anticipatory guidance related to safety should you provide to her parents?

Promoting Nutrition

The preschool child has a full set of primary teeth, is able to chew and swallow competently, and has learned to use utensils fairly effectively to feed themselves (Fig. 27.13). As in the toddler years, it is important for the preschool child to continue to learn and build upon healthy eating habits. These habits will last throughout the child's life. A diet high in nutrient-rich foods such as whole grains, vegetables, fruits, appropriate dairy foods, and lean meats is appropriate for the preschooler. Nutrient-poor, high-calorie foods such as sweets and typical fast foods should be offered only in limited amounts.

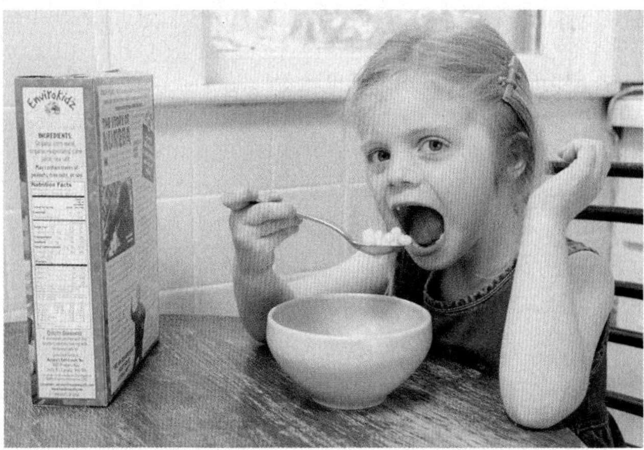

FIGURE 27.13 The preschool child has the manual dexterity to handle utensils appropriately and feed themselves independently.

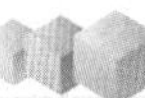

Concept Mastery Alert

Preschoolers are erratic eaters and may eat well one day and then eat little the next day. Food jags are not common in preschoolers but are common in toddlers.

Nutritional Needs

The 3- to 5-year-old requires 700 to 1,000 mg of calcium (Gavin, 2021) and 7 to 10 mg of iron daily (Powers, 2023). Box 27.2 lists calcium and iron sources. For dietary fiber, 3-year-olds should consume 8 g daily, 4-year-olds should eat 9 g, and 5-year-olds should eat 10 g (Diab et al., 2022).

BOX 27.2 Daily Calcium and Iron Recommendations for Preschool Children

Calcium: 700 mg (3-year-old), 1,000 mg (4- to 8-year-old)

Calcium in Foods

- 8 oz low-fat or whole milk: 275–300 mg
- 8 oz low-fat yogurt: 313–415 mg
- 1½ oz cheddar cheese: 307 mg
- 1 oz dried white beans (cooked): 75 mg
- ¼ c tofu: 138–253 mg
- ½ c raw broccoli: 21 mg

Iron: 7 mg (3-year-old), 10 mg (4- to 8-year-old)

Iron in Foods

- ¾ c 100% fortified prepared cereal: 18 mg
- 3 oz beef: 3 mg
- 3 oz chicken (dark meat): 1.1 mg
- ½ c cooked lentils: 3 mg
- 3 oz chicken (white meat): 0.9 mg
- 15.2-cm (6-in) slice watermelon: 0.7 mg
- ¼ c fresh cooked spinach: 1.6 mg
- ¼ c tofu: 1.7 mg
- ¼ c raisins: 1 mg
- 1 slice enriched bread: 0.8–0.9 mg
- ¼ c frozen spinach, cooked: 0.85 mg

Data from National Institutes of Health. (2023). *Iron dietary supplement fact sheet.* http://ods.od.nih.gov/factsheets/Iron-HealthProfessional/#h4; National Institutes of Health. (2022). *Calcium dietary supplement fact sheet.* http://ods.od.nih.gov/factsheets/Calcium-HealthProfessional/#h3

The typical preschooler requires about 85 kcal/kg of body weight. Saturated fats should account for less than 10% of total calories. Preschool children's diets should include a daily total fat intake of not less than 10% and not more than 35% of total calories to promote and maintain healthy cholesterol levels (Diab et al., 2022).

TAKE NOTE!

Drinking excess amounts of milk may lead to iron deficiency, as the calcium in milk blocks iron absorption.

Promoting Healthy Eating Habits

Preschool children may be selective eaters. They may eat a limited variety of foods or foods prepared in certain ways and may not be willing to try new things. The 3- or 4-year-old may exhibit "food fads," eating only certain foods over a several-day period. As the child gets older, pickiness lessens. By 5 years of age, the child is more focused on the social context of eating—table conversation and manners. The 5-year-old is generally more willing to at least try new foods and may like to help with meal preparation and clean-up as appropriate.

If the preschooler is growing well, then the pickiness is not a cause for concern. A larger concern may be the negative relationship that can develop between the parent and child relating to mealtime. The more the parent coaxes, cajoles, bribes, and threatens, the less likely the child is to try new foods or even eat the ones they like. The parent must maintain a positive and patient demeanor at mealtime.

The child should be offered a healthy diet with foods from all groups over the course of the day as recommended by the U.S. Department of Agriculture (USDA, n.d.). Parents may visit the USDA's website at https://www.myplate.gov/myplate-plan to develop a personalized daily food plan for their child based on age and activity level.

The parent should maintain a matter-of-fact approach, offer the meal or snack, and then allow the child to decide how much of the food, if any, they are going to eat. High-fat, nutrient-poor snacks should not be substituted for healthy foods just to coax the child to "eat something." See the Healthy People 2030 box.

HEALTHY PEOPLE 2030

Objective	Nursing Significance
Increase consumption of calcium in the population aged 2 years and older.	• Screen preschoolers for appropriate dietary intake of calcium. • Educate families about calcium content in foods. • Assist families with choosing a diet that meets calcium needs and is appealing to the young child.

Healthy People Objectives retrieved from http://www.healthypeople.gov

Maintaining Healthy Body Weight

Worldwide, over 22 million children younger than 5 years have BMIs classified as obese. In the past 30 years, the number of U.S. children and adolescents with overweight BMIs has doubled. According to the National Health and Nutrition Examination Survey, 13.9% of 2- to 5-year-olds have BMIs classified as obese (Centers for Disease Control and Prevention, 2022). Children are now developing traditionally adult onset-associated diseases related to higher weight such as type 2 diabetes mellitus, dyslipidemia, and nonalcoholic fatty liver disease (Cunningham et al., 2022). This risk is increased if one or both parents have overweight BMIs (Fan & Zhang, 2022).

Parents are in an opportune position to exert a positive influence on their preschooler's nutritional intake and activity level. The habits learned in early childhood will likely carry over into the school-age, adolescent, and adult years. Children whose parents take an authoritarian approach to mealtime may learn to overeat, as they are encouraged to finish the entire meal ("Clean your plate!"). If they are offered appropriate, healthy food choices and access to high-calorie, nutrient-poor food is limited, preschoolers will learn to self-regulate (eat only until full). Food should not be used as either reward or punishment.

Parents should remain positive and patient at mealtime. Mealtimes should continue to be structured. Unstructured meals lead to an increase in fat and calorie consumption. Nutrient-dense (increasingly plant-based) foods and beverages with lower fat and sugar content are recommended to decrease the incidence of developing excess weight (Fisher et al., 2022). To limit the chance that overeating will occur, preschoolers should be offered a variety of healthy foods at each meal. This may include one each of a protein source, grain, vegetable, and fruit. The preschool child's serving size is usually one third to one half of the recommended size of an adult serving. The preschool child may imitate the other eaters at the table. Parents have a prime chance to be good role models, setting an example by eating vegetables and fruits.

As with toddlers, fruit juice should be limited to 4 to 6 oz per day, as excess consumption can lead to excess weight gain. Preschoolers should be encouraged to drink water.

Limiting television viewing time and encouraging physical activity are also important strategies for maintaining a healthy weight. See Evidence-Based Practice 27.1.

Refer back to Nila Patel, the 4-year-old introduced at the beginning of the chapter. What questions should you ask Nila's parents related to nutritional intake? What anticipatory guidance related to nutrition would be appropriate? Nila's parent expresses concern regarding higher weight. How would you address these?

EVIDENCE-BASED PRACTICE **27.1**

Preventing Higher Weight in Preschoolers

STUDY

One of the most pressing public health issues is the continued rise in excess weight gain during childhood. Early childhood higher weight is associated with immediate health consequences as well as long-term issues such as adult higher weight and early-onset metabolic syndrome. Early childhood is a prime time for establishing healthy eating and activity habits that may persist into adulthood.

The authors of this study conducted a meta-analysis of existing literature on interventions for the prevention of higher weight in children.

Findings

The authors noted that during early childhood, providing a healthy diet and ensuring physical activity for children until age 5 years helps reduce BMI. Neither diet nor activity alone affects BMI as significantly as the two interventions together. The authors therefore recommend utilizing both interventions.

Nursing Implications

Nurses are in a unique position to provide ongoing, repeated education about the importance of maintaining healthy weight in preschoolers to families wherever they encounter them. Nurses should encourage families to:

- Provide meals seated with the family and in a positive atmosphere.
- Ensure the preschooler receives a varied diet with plenty of plant-based foods.
- Encourage water as the beverage of choice.
- Instruct families to avoid high-sugar foods and beverages.
- Encourage daily physical activity: structured, at least 60 minutes daily; and unstructured, 60 minutes to several hours daily.
- Teach families to limit media consumption to 30 minutes daily and to not put a television in the child's bedroom.

Data from Brown, T., Moore, T. H. M., Hooper, L., Gao, Y., Zayegh, A., Ijaz, S., Elwenspoek, M., Foxen, S. C., Magee, L., O'Malley, C., Waters, E., & Summerbell, C. D. (2019). Interventions for preventing obesity in children. *Cochrane Database of Systematic Reviews*. https://doi.org/10.1002/14651858.CD001871.pub4

Promoting Healthy Sleep and Rest

The preschool child needs about 10 to 13 hours of sleep each day, including naps if taken (AAP, 2020). Unless very tired, many preschool children will resist going to bed from time to time. Bedtime rituals continue to be reassuring to children, and it is important to continue them in the preschool years. Having a time of relaxation with a decrease in stimulation will allow the child to fall asleep more easily. Some children continue to need a security item at bedtime or naptime. A nightlight in the bedroom may be necessary, as many children this age are afraid of the dark. Teaching Guidelines 27.1 gives information about assisting parents to establish a bedtime routine.

Nightmares often occur in preschool children as a result of the child's struggle to distinguish what is real from what is not. When a child awakens from a nightmare, they are often crying and may be able to recount what the dream was about. Parents should validate the child's fear rather than discount it (Reynolds et al., 2022). Saying, "Yes, I agree, monsters are scary; it's a good thing they aren't real" is more appropriate than, "Don't be silly; monsters aren't real." Sometimes children benefit from reading stories about dreams. Recommended books include:

- *Bedtime for Frances* by Russell Hoban
- *Ben's Dream* by Chris Van Allsburg
- *In the Night Kitchen* by Maurice Sendak
- *There's a Nightmare in My Closet* by Mercer Mayer

Nightmares should not be confused with night terrors. After a nightmare, the child is aroused and interactive, but night terrors are different: A short time after falling asleep, the child partially awakens and is screaming. The child usually does not respond much to the parent's soothing, but they eventually stop screaming and go back to sleep. Night terrors are often frightening for parents because the child does not seem to be responding to them. One technique that may help to decrease the incidence of night terrors is to wake the child about 30 to 45 minutes into the sleep cycle. If continued nightly for about a week, the cycle of night terrors may be broken (Morse & Kotagal, 2021). See Comparison Chart 27.1.

TEACHING GUIDELINES **27.1** Bedtime Routines

- Establish a bedtime as well as morning wake-up time.
- Avoid sugar or caffeine consumption in the evening.
- Avoid stimulating activities such as roughhousing before bedtime.
- Do not allow television watching in bed.
- Make the child's bedroom an inviting and comfortable area of the home.
- Provide a nightlight in the child's bedroom if they are afraid of the dark.
- Conform to a nightly routine:
  - Television off at a certain time
  - Bath
  - Quiet game or story reading/telling
  - Bedtime prayer or song
- Maintain quiet in the bedroom and nearby to increase the child's ability to fall asleep.

Data from American Academy of Pediatrics. (2020). *Healthy sleep habits: How many hours does your child need?* https://www.healthychildren.org/English/healthy-living/sleep/Pages/Healthy-Sleep-Habits-How-Many-Hours-Does-Your-Child-Need.aspx; Reynolds, A., Angulo, A., Breheney, M., Green, J., & Goldson, E. (2022). Child development and behavior. In M. Bunik, W. W. Hay, M. J. Levin, & M. J. Abzug (Eds.), *Current diagnosis & treatment: Pediatrics* (26th ed.). McGraw-Hill Education.

COMPARISON CHART 27.1 Nightmares Versus Night Terrors

	Nightmare	Night Terror
Definition	Scary or bad dream followed by awakening	Partial arousal from deep sleep
When parents become aware	The child awakens the parent after episode is over.	Screaming and thrashing during the episode awakens the parent.
Timing	Usually in the second half of the night	Usually about an hour after falling asleep
Behavior	Crying, may be scared after awakening	Sits up, thrashes, cries, screams, talks, looks wild-eyed. Sweats, may have racing heartbeat
Responsiveness	Responsive to parents' soothing and reassurances	Child unaware of parents' presence, may scream and thrash more if restrained
Return to sleep	Difficulty going back to sleep if afraid	Rapidly returns to sleep without full awakening
Memory of occurrence	May remember the dream and talk about it later	No memory of the event

Data from Morse, A. M., & Kotagal, S. (2021). Sleepwalking and other parasomnias in children. *UpToDate*. Retrieved October 13, 2022, from https://www.uptodate.com/contents/sleepwalking-and-other-parasomnias-in-children#H27172832

Think back to Nila Patel. What anticipatory guidance would you provide to her parents in relation to sleep during the preschool years?

Promoting Healthy Teeth and Gums

Prevention of dental caries continues to be important for the preschool child and can be achieved through daily brushing and flossing. Parents should use only a pea-sized amount of toothpaste to prevent excess fluoride consumption, which can contribute to fluorosis (Nowak & Warren, 2023). The preschooler may brush their own teeth, but the parent must continue to supervise to ensure adequate brushing. Parents must perform flossing because the preschool child cannot perform this task adequately. Cariogenic foods should be avoided. If sugary foods are consumed, the mouth should be rinsed with water if it is not possible to brush the teeth immediately (Nowak & Warren, 2023). The preschool child should visit the dentist every 6 months.

TAKE NOTE!

Prevention of dental caries is important in the primary teeth, because loss of these teeth to caries may affect the proper formation of permanent teeth as well as the width of the dental arch.

Promoting Appropriate Discipline

Successful discipline results from a loving and nurturing environment in which the preschooler's self-esteem is fostered and limits are well chosen and enforced consistently. Spanking (striking with the open hand) is the least effective discipline practice and is discouraged by the AACAP (2018) and the National Association of Pediatric Nurse Practitioners (2022). Belts, switches, paddles, or other items should never be used to strike a child. The use of physical punishment has been associated with a number of additional problems in adulthood, such as antisocial and criminal behaviors (AACAP, 2018; see Chapter 26).

If parents are consistent with discipline while encouraging the preschooler's normal growth and development of imagination and make-believe, the child will learn to accept that certain things are not allowed. The sense of initiative can be preserved and guilt avoided if the rules are clear and enforced consistently (Sears & Sears, 2020a).

TAKE NOTE!

Corporal punishment not only causes physical and emotional pain, it also decreases learning capacity (AACAP, 2018).

Minimize the occurrence of misbehavior by anticipating conditions likely to lead to the undesired or risky action. When the situation becomes difficult, parents should use distraction to change the preschooler's focus. When discussing the misbehavior, be certain to label the behavior and not the child. This helps preserve the preschooler's self-esteem. When teaching preschoolers about undesired behavior, be sure they also understand the reason why it is wrong or unacceptable to do it. This helps encourage the child to use internal controls over behavior. Parents should serve as role models for self-control, including choice of words, the tone they are delivered in, and the actions that accompany them.

Children work harder to obtain praise than to receive punishment, so always reward positive behaviors. Preschool children are becoming capable of understanding the concept of right and wrong. They start to understand each other's feelings (**empathy**) and are cognitively capable of remembering basic rules.

Time-out or time away from the situation can be effective in this age group. This punishment should be used only for intentional misbehavior (knowing something is forbidden but doing it anyway). It is particularly helpful with dangerous or destructive behavior. The preschooler is given a warning that time-out will occur if the behavior does not stop. The preschooler is removed from the situation and must stay in time-out for a specified period of time. A particular time-out area is helpful; a boring corner of the room without distractions available is a good location. The generally recommended period of time is to require 1 minute of time-out per year of age; thus, a 4-year-old would be in time-out for 4 minutes (Sears & Sears, 2020b). Set the timer so the child will know when the time-out is over. If the child gets up before the prescribed time, replace the child in time-out and restart the timer. Time-out works best if used each and every time the undesirable behavior occurs. It is also important to praise the child when they follow the rules and behave appropriately.

A simple and clear explanation of the misbehavior should be given to the child; parents should also talk about acceptable alternative strategies that the child can use in the future instead of the undesired behavior. Removal of a privilege such as playing with a favorite toy can be as effective as time-out. Books and other media that are available to help educate parents about appropriate discipline and to help the child learn self-control are listed in Box 27.3.

BOX 27.3 Selected Resources for Parents and Preschoolers

Books for Parents (About Discipline)

- *How to Talk so Kids Will Listen and Listen so Kids Will Talk* by A. Faber & E. Mazlish (Harper Resource)
- *Kids Are Worth It: Giving Your Children the Gift of Inner Discipline* by B. Colorosos (Harper Collins Publishers)
- *Positive Discipline A to Z: 1001 Solutions to Everyday Parenting Problems* by J. Nelson, L. Lott, & S. G. Glenn (Three Rivers Press)
- *Setting Limits With Your Strong-Willed Child: Eliminating Conflict by Establishing Clear, Firm and Respectful Boundaries* by R. MacKenzie (Three Rivers Press)
- *The Case Against Spanking: How to Discipline Children Without Hitting* by I. A. Hyman (Jossey-Bass)
- *The Nurturing Parent: How to Raise Creative, Loving, Responsible Children* by J. S. Dacey & A. J. Packer (Fireside)
- *Without Spanking or Spoiling: A Practical Approach to Toddler and Preschool Guidance* by E. Crary (Parenting Press)

Books for Preschoolers (About Dealing With Feelings and Learning How to Behave)

- *Hands Are Not for Hitting* by M. Agassi (Free Spirit Publishing)
- *I Can't Wait* by E. Crary (Parenting Press)
- *I Want It* by E. Crary (Parenting Press)
- *I Want to Play* by E. Crary (Parenting Press)
- *I Was so Mad* by M. Mayer (Golden Books)
- *I Was so Mad* by N. Simon & D. Leder (Albert Whitman & Company)
- *I'm Excited* by E. Crary (Parenting Press)
- *I'm Frustrated* by E. Crary (Parenting Press)
- *I'm Mad* by E. Crary (Parenting Press)
- *I'm Scared* by E. Crary (Parenting Press)
- *Feet Are Not for Kicking* by E. Verdick (Free Spirit Publishing)
- *Teeth Are Not for Biting* by E. Verdick (Free Spirit Publishing)
- *When Sophie Gets Angry . . . Really, Really Angry* by M. Bang (Blue Sky Press)
- *Words Are Not for Hurting* by E. Verdick (Free Spirit Publishing)

ADDRESSING COMMON DEVELOPMENTAL CONCERNS

Common developmental concerns of the preschool period include lying, how to address sex education, and masturbation. Parents often express difficulty in dealing with these issues with their preschool children. Offering appropriate anticipatory guidance may give the parents the support and confidence they need to deal with these issues.

Lying

Lying is common in preschool children. It may occur because the child fears punishment, has gotten carried away with imagination, or is imitating what they see the parent do. The parent should ascertain the reason for the lie before punishing the child. If the child has broken a rule and fears punishment, then the parent must determine the truth. The child needs to learn that lying is usually worse than the misbehavior itself. The punishment for the misbehavior should be lessened if the child admits the truth. The parent should remain calm and serve as a role model of an even temper. The next time the misbehavior occurs, the child will be more apt to simply tell the truth.

If the child's lying is their imagination getting carried away, then the parent should guide the child in distinguishing between myth and reality (Sears & Sears, 2020c). The preschooler's imagination is vivid, and the child needs direction in the use of that faculty. Parents should serve as role models of appropriate behavior for their children to learn it. Children who lie because they hear their parents lying must not see or hear their parents do it.

Sex Education

Preschoolers are keen observers but are still not able to interpret all that they see correctly. The child may recognize but not understand sexual activity. Preschoolers are inquisitive and want to learn about everything around them; therefore, they are likely to ask questions about sex and where babies come from. Before attempting to answer questions, parents should try to find out first exactly what the child is asking and what the child already thinks about that subject. Then they should provide a simple, direct, and honest answer. The child needs only the information that they are requesting. Additional questions will occur in the future and should be addressed as they arise.

Masturbation

The normal curiosity of the preschool years often leads children to explore their own genitals (Carter & Feigelman, 2020). This behavior may be upsetting to some parents, but masturbation is a healthy and natural part of normal preschool development if it occurs in moderation. If the parent overreacts to this behavior, then it may occur more frequently. Masturbation should be treated in a matter-of-fact way by the parent. The child needs to learn certain rules about this activity; nudity and masturbation are not acceptable in public. The child should also be taught safety; no other person can touch the child's private parts unless it is the parent, doctor, or nurse checking to see when something is wrong.

Think back to Nila Patel. What are some developmental concerns that are common during the preschool years? What anticipatory guidance related to these concerns would you provide to Nila's parents?

Unfolding Patient Stories: Sabina Vasquez • Part 1

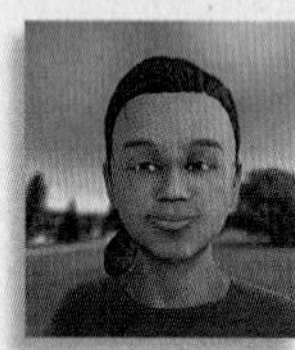

Sabina Vasquez, age 8, was diagnosed with asthma at age 4. At her first visit to the primary care provider's office with asthma symptoms as a 4-year-old, what appropriate age-related strategies would have been used in planning asthma education for this patient and her family? How would patient education strategies differ when explaining asthma to an 8-year-old compared with a 4-year-old? (Sabina Vasquez's story continues in Chapter 40.)

Care for Sabina and other patients in a realistic virtual environment: ***vSim** for Nursing* (thepoint.lww.com/vSimPediatric). Practice documenting these patients' care in DocuCare (thePoint.lww.com/DocuCareEHR).

KEY CONCEPTS

- The preschool child grows at a slower rate and takes on a more slender and upright appearance than the toddler.
- The primary psychosocial task of the preschool period is developing a sense of initiative.
- Cognitive development moves from an egocentric approach to the world toward a more empathetic understanding of what happens outside of the self.
- The preschooler gains additional motor skills and displays significant refinement of fine motor abilities.
- Cognitive and language skills that develop in the preschool years help prepare the child for success in school.
- Disfluency or hesitancy in speech is a normal finding in the preschool period and occurs as a result of the fast pace with which the preschooler is gaining language skills and vocabulary.
- The vocabulary of a preschooler increases to about 2,100 words, and the child speaks in full sentences with appropriate use of tense and prepositions.
- Appropriate growth and development should be maintained in the child who is ill or hospitalized.
- Recognizing concerns or delays in growth and development is essential so that the appropriate referrals may be made and intervention can begin.
- The preschool child requires a well-balanced diet with fat content between 20% and 30% of calories consumed.
- Adequate physical activity and provision of a nutrient-dense diet (rather than foods high in fat and sugar) are the foundation for maintaining healthy weight in the preschool child.
- Adequate dental care is important for the health of the primary teeth.
- Preschoolers need about 12 hours of sleep per day and benefit from a structured bedtime routine.
- Due to the active imagination of the preschooler, nightmares and night terrors may begin during this period.
- Safety and injury prevention remain a focus in the preschool years.
- Structure, appropriate limit setting, and consistency are the keys for effective discipline in the preschool period.
- Time-out is an effective disciplinary measure for preschoolers.
- Masturbation may occur as the preschooler discovers their body. If not excessive, it is considered a normal part of growth and development.

REFERENCES AND RECOMMENDED READINGS

American Academy of Child and Adolescent Psychiatry. (2018). *Physical punishment*. https://www.aacap.org/aacap/families_and_youth/facts_for_families/fff-guide/Physical-Punishment-105.aspx

American Academy of Child and Adolescent Psychiatry. (2020). *Screen time and children*. https://www.aacap.org/AACAP/Families_and_Youth/Facts_for_Families/FFF-Guide/Children-And-Watching-TV-054.aspx

American Academy of Pediatrics. (2020). *Healthy sleep habits: How many hours does your child need?* https://www.healthychildren.org/English/healthy-living/sleep/Pages/Healthy-Sleep-Habits-How-Many-Hours-Does-Your-Child-Need.aspx

American Academy of Pediatrics. (2022a). *Gun safety: Where we stand*. https://www.healthychildren.org/English/safety-prevention/all-around/Pages/where-we-stand-gun-safety.aspx

American Academy of Pediatrics. (2022b). *Safety for your child: 2 to 4 years.* https://www.healthychildren.org/English/ages-stages/toddler/Pages/Safety-for-Your-Child-2-to-4-Years.aspx

American Academy of Pediatrics. (2022c). *Your child's first tricycle or bike: Important safety rules.* https://www.healthychildren.org/English/safety-prevention/at-play/Pages/your-childs-first-tricycle-or-bike-teaching-them-to-ride-safely.aspx

American Academy of Pediatrics. (2023a). *Car seats: Information for families.* https://www.healthychildren.org/English/safety-prevention/on-the-go/Pages/Car-Safety-Seats-Information-for-Families.aspx

American Academy of Pediatrics. (2023b). *Swim lessons: When to start & what parents should know.* https://www.healthychildren.org/English/safety-prevention/at-play/Pages/Swim-Lessons.aspx

American Association of Poison Control Centers. (n.d.). *Prevention.* https://poisoncenters.org/prevention

Brown, T., Moore, T. H. M., Hooper, L., Gao, Y., Zayegh, A., Ijaz, S., Elwenspoek, M., Foxen, S. C., Magee, L., O'Malley, C., Waters, E., & Summerbell, C. D. (2019). Interventions for preventing obesity in children. *Cochrane Database of Systematic Reviews.* https://doi.org/10.1002/14651858.CD001871.pub4

Carter, R. G., & Feigelman, S. (2020). The preschool years. In R. M. Kliegman, J. W. St. Geme III, N. J. Blum, S. S. Shah, R. C. Tasker, K. M. Wilson, & R. E. Behrman (Eds.), *Nelson's textbook of pediatrics* (21st ed.). Elsevier.

Centers for Disease Control and Prevention. (2022, May 17). *Childhood obesity facts.* https://www.cdc.gov/obesity/data/childhood.html

Centers for Disease Control and Prevention. (2023, June 6). *CDC's developmental milestones.* http://www.cdc.gov/ncbddd/actearly/milestones/index.html

Child Development Institute. (2022). *Temperament and your child's personality.* https://childdevelopmentinfo.com/uncategorized/temperament_and_your_child/

Chromey, R. (2021). *Do you know the ABCs of spiritual growth in children?* https://childrensministry.com/abcs-spiritual-growth/

Cuartas, J., Weissman, D. G., Sheridan, M. A., Lengua, L., & McLaughlin, K. A. (2021). Corporal punishment and elevated neural response to threat in children. *Child Development, 92*(3), 831–832. https://doi.org/10.1111/cdev.13565

Cunningham, S. A., Hardy, S. T., Jones, R., Ng, C., Kramer, M. R., & Narayan, K. M. V. (2022). Changes in the incidence of childhood obesity. *Pediatrics, 150*(2), e2021053708. https://doi.org/10.1542/peds.2021-053708

Diab, L. K., Haemer, M., Primark, L. E., & Krebs, N. R. (2022). Normal childhood nutrition and its disorders. In M. Bunik, W. W. Hay, M. J. Levin, & M. J. Abzug (Eds.), *Current diagnosis & treatment: Pediatrics* (26th ed.). McGraw-Hill Education.

Erikson, E. H. (1963). *Childhood and society* (2nd ed.). W. W. Norton and Company.

Fan, H., & Zhang, X. (2022). Influence of parental weight change on the incidence of overweight and obesity in offspring. *BMC Pediatrics, 22*, 330. https://doi.org/10.1186/s12887-022-03399-8

Fisher, E. F., Lemus, T. P., Reichert, A., Alsopp, M., & Harvey, T. S. (2022). *Reframing childhood obesity: Cultural insights on nutrition, weight, and food systems.* Vanderbilt Cultural Contexts of Health Initiative. https://www.vanderbilt.edu/cultural-contexts-health/wp-content/uploads/sites/350/2022/06/Reframing-Childhood-Obesity-CCH-Report.pdf

Gavin, M. L. (2021). *Calcium.* https://kidshealth.org/en/parents/calcium.html?WT.ac=p-ra

Kohlberg, L. (1984). *Moral development.* Harper & Row.

Linguistic Society of America. (2023). *FAQ: Raising bilingual children.* https://www.linguisticsociety.org/resource/faq-raising-bilingual-children

Morse, A. M., & Kotagal, S. (2021). Sleepwalking and other parasomnias in children. *UpToDate.* Retrieved September 29, 2023, from https://www.uptodate.com/contents/sleepwalking-and-other-parasomnias-in-children#H27172832

National Association for the Education of Young Children. (n.d.). *Good toys for young children by age and stage.* https://www.naeyc.org/resources/topics/play/toys

National Association of Pediatric Nurse Practitioners, Child Maltreatment and Neglect Special Interest Group, VanGraafeiland, B., Hornor, G. A., Herendeen, P. A., Chiocca, E. M., Loyke, J. A., Dietzman, H., Boucher, N. L., Nielsen, A., & Record, S. C. (2022). NAPNAP position statement on using positive parenting to eliminate corporal punishment. *Journal of Pediatric Health Care, 36*, 202–204. https://doi.org/10.1016/j.pedhc.2021.09.001

National Center for Injury Prevention and Control. (2020). *10 leading causes of death by age group, United States 2020, all races, both sexes.* https://www.cdc.gov/injury/wisqars/pdf/leading_causes_of_death_by_age_group_2020-508.pdf

National Institutes of Health. (2022). *Calcium dietary supplement fact sheet.* https://ods.od.nih.gov/factsheets/Calcium-HealthProfessional/#h3

National Institutes of Health. (2023). *Iron dietary supplement fact sheet.* https://ods.od.nih.gov/factsheets/Iron-HealthProfessional/#h4

National Safety Council. (2023). *Top 10 preventable injuries.* https://injuryfacts.nsc.org/all-injuries/deaths-by-demographics/top-10-preventable-injuries/data-details/

Nowak, A. J., & Warren, J. J. (2023). Preventive dental care and counseling for infants and young children. *UpToDate.* Retrieved September 29, 2023, from https://www.uptodate.com/contents/preventive-dental-care-and-counseling-for-infants-and-young-children

Piaget, J. (1969). *The theory of stages in cognitive development.* McGraw-Hill.

Powers, J. M. (2023). Iron deficiency in infants and children <12 years: Screening, prevention, clinical manifestations, and diagnosis. *UpToDate.* Retrieved September 29, 2023, from https://www.uptodate.com/contents/iron-deficiency-in-infants-and-children-less-than12-years-screening-prevention-clinical-manifestations-and-diagnosis

Public Health Law Program. (2022). *State school immunization requirements and vaccine exemption laws.* Centers for Disease Control and Prevention. https://www.cdc.gov/phlp/docs/school-vaccinations.pdf

Reynolds, A., Angulo, A., Breheney, M., Green, J., & Goldson, E. (2022). Child development and behavior. In M. Bunik, W. W. Hay, M. J. Levin, & M. J. Abzug (Eds.), *Current diagnosis & treatment: Pediatrics* (26th ed.). McGraw-Hill Education.

SafeKids. (2023). *Swimming.* https://www.safekids.org/poolsafety

Sears, W., & Sears, M. (2020a). *Shape children's behavior.* https://www.askdrsears.com/topics/parenting/discipline-behavior/shape-childrens-behavior

Sears, W., & Sears, M. (2020b). *10 time-out for children techniques.* https://www.askdrsears.com/topics/parenting/discipline-behavior/10-time-out-techniques

Sears, W., & Sears, M. (2020c). *Why do kids lie?* https://www.askdrsears.com/topics/parenting/discipline-behavior/morals-manners/why-do-kids-lie

Sege, R. D. (2018). *AAP policy opposes corporal punishment, draws on recent evidence.* https://www.aappublications.org/news/2018/11/05/discipline110518

Stanford Medicine. (2023). *Motor vehicle safety for children.* https://www.stanfordchildrens.org/en/topic/default?id=motor-vehicle-safety-for-children-85-P01038

U.S. Department of Agriculture. (n.d.). *MyPlate plan.* https://www.myplate.gov/myplate-plan

Williams, P. G., Lerner, M. A., Council on Early Childhood; Council on School Health, Sells, J., Alderman, S. L., Hashikawa, A., Mendelsohn, A., McFadden, T., Navsaria, D., Peacock, G., Scholer, S., Takagishi, J., Vanderbilt, D., De Pinto, C. L., Attisha, E., Beers, N., Gibson, E., Gorski, P., … Weiss-Harrison, A. (2019). School readiness. *Pediatrics, 144*(2), e20191766. https://doi.org/10.1542/peds.2019-1766

World Health Organization. (n.d.). *Passive smoking.* http://www.who.int/tobacco/en/atlas10.pdf

Zubler, J. M., Wiggins, L. D., Macias, M. M., Whitaker, T. M., Shaw, J. S., Squires, J. K., Pajke, J. A., Wolf, R. B., Slaughter, K. S., Broughton, A. S., Gerndt, K. L., Mlodoch, B. J., & Lipkin, P. H. (2022). Evidence-informed milestones for developmental surveillance tools. *Pediatrics, 149*(3), e2021052138. https://doi.org/10.1542/peds.2021-052138

DEVELOPING CLINICAL JUDGMENT

PRACTICING FOR NCLEX

1. The nurse is caring for a 4-year-old who is hospitalized and insists on having the nurse perform every assessment and intervention on their imaginary friend first. The child then agrees to have the assessment or intervention done to themselves. The nurse identifies this preschooler's behavior as:
   a. problematic; the child is old enough to begin to have a basis in reality.
   b. normal, because the child is hospitalized and out of their routine.
   c. normal for this stage of growth and development.
   d. problematic, as it interferes with needed nursing care.
2. The parent of a 3-year-old is concerned about their child's speech. They describe the preschooler as hesitating at the beginning of sentences and repeating consonant sounds. What is the nurse's best response?
   a. "Hesitancy and disfluency are normal during this period of development."
   b. "Reading to the child will help model appropriate speech."
   c. "Expressive language concerns warrant a developmental evaluation."
   d. "You should ask your child's health care provider for a speech therapy evaluation."
3. The parent of a 4-year-old asks for advice on using time-out for discipline with their child. What advice should the nurse give the parent?
   a. If spanking is not working, then time-out is not likely to be helpful either.
   b. Place the child in time-out for 4 minutes.
   c. Use time-out only if removing privileges is unsuccessful.
   d. The child should stay in time-out until crying ceases.
4. A 5-year-old child is not gaining weight appropriately. Organic problems have been ruled out. What is the priority action by the nurse?
   a. Allow the child unlimited access to the sippy cup to ensure adequate hydration.
   b. Encourage sweets for the extra caloric content.
   c. Teach the parent about nutritional needs of the preschooler.
   d. Assess the child's usual intake pattern at home.
5. The nurse is providing teaching about accidental poisoning to the family of a 3-year-old. The nurse understands that a child of this age is at increased risk of accidental ingestion due to which sensory alteration?
   a. A lack of fully developed hearing
   b. A less discriminating sense of touch
   c. Visual acuity that has not fully developed
   d. A less discriminating sense of taste
6. The nurse is caring for a 4-year-old. Which behaviors does the nurse expect to observe in this child, indicating Piaget's stage of preoperational thought? Select all that apply.
   a. Egocentrism
   b. Temper tantrums
   c. Magical thinking
   d. Trust issues
   e. Having an imaginary friend
   f. Initiative
7. The nursing instructor has taught a group of nursing students about preschooler physical growth and development. The nursing students state that the 3-year-old should have been able to achieve control over ___ and ___ as a result of ____.
   Blanks 1 and 2:
   a. bowel elimination
   b. emotions
   c. urinary elimination
   d. utensil use
   e. social skills
   f. writing skills
   Blank 3:
   a. increased psychosocial maturity
   b. complete myelination of the spinal cord
   c. improved fine motor control
   d. skillful toilet teaching

DOSAGE CALCULATION QUESTIONS

1. A child who weighs 33 lb has an order for acetaminophen 10 mg/kg/dose, every 4 hours as needed for pain or fever.
   a. How many milligrams will the child receive per dose?
   b. Acetaminophen elixir is provided as 160 mg/5 mL. How many milliliters will the nurse administer per dose?

CRITICAL THINKING EXERCISES

1. Teach a preschool class about bicycle and street safety. Be certain to design the content at an appropriate developmental level.
2. Construct a 3-day menu for a 4-year-old who is selective about eating. Include three daily meals and two snacks. Follow the nutritional guidelines recommended by the USDA.
3. Color or draw with a preschool child. Analyze the drawings and interactions or discussions you have with the child, relating them to psychosocial and cognitive development expected at this age.

STUDY ACTIVITIES

1. Care for two average 3-, 4-, or 5-year-old children in the clinical setting (make sure both are of the same age). Describe each child's development level, response to hospitalization, and family dynamics.

2. Visit a preschool that provides care for children with developmental delays as well as children exhibiting expected development. Perform a developmental assessment on a child with expected development and one with developmental delays (both of the same age). Compare and contrast your findings.

3. Observe a 3-, 4-, or 5-year-old's classroom of a typical preschool. Choose two children who are of the same age with different temperaments. Record the differences and similarities in their response to structure and authority, interactions with classmates, attention levels, and language and activity levels.

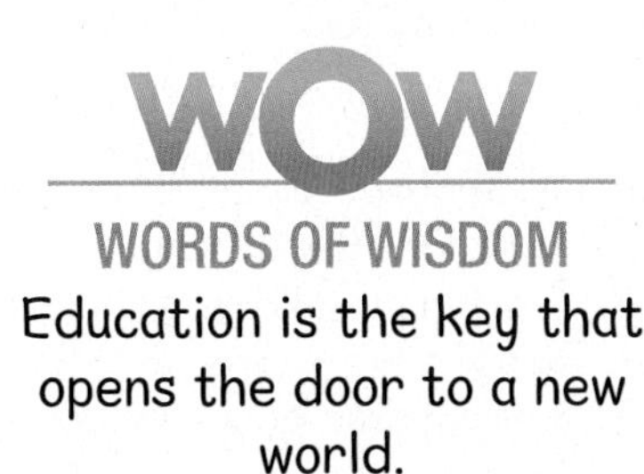

Education is the key that opens the door to a new world.

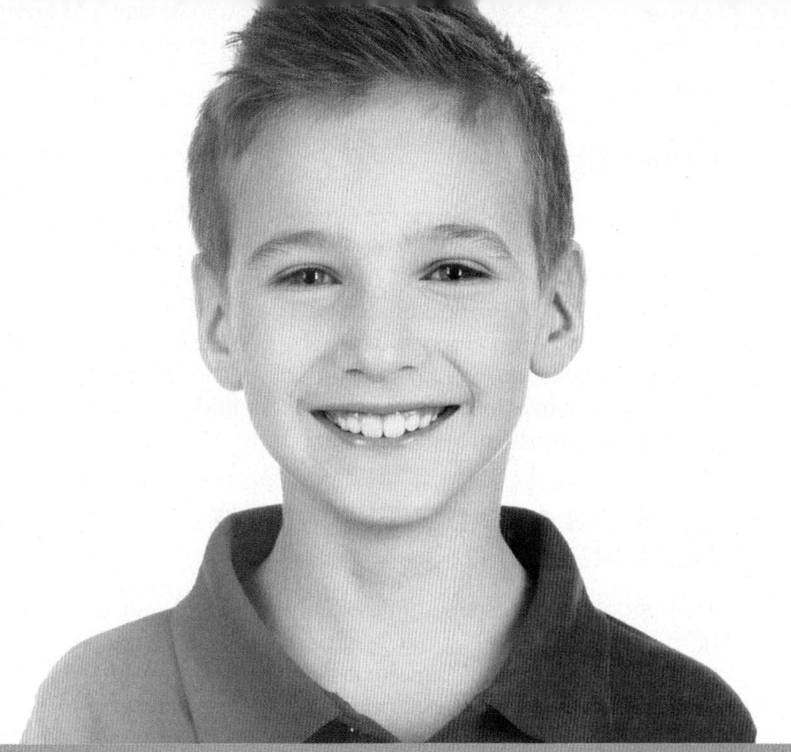

28

Growth and Development of the School-Age Child

LEARNING OBJECTIVES

Upon completion of the chapter, you will be able to:

1. Identify normal physiologic, cognitive, and moral changes occurring in the school-age child.
2. Describe the role of peers and schools in the development and socialization of the school-age child.
3. Identify the developmental milestones of the school-age child.
4. Describe the role of the nurse in promoting safety for the school-age child.
5. Demonstrate knowledge of the nutritional requirements of the school-age child.
6. Identify common developmental concerns in the school-age child.
7. Demonstrate knowledge of the appropriate nursing guidance for common developmental concerns.

KEY TERMS

bruxism (brŭk′sizm)
caries
industry
inferiority
malocclusion (mal′ō-klū′zhŭn)
prepubescence (prē′pyū-bes′ĕnt)
principle of conservation
school-age child
school refusal
self-esteem

Lawrence Jones is a 10-year-old brought to the clinic by his parent for his annual school check-up. As the nurse caring for him, assess Lawrence's growth and development, and then provide appropriate anticipatory guidance to his parent.

INTRODUCTION

School-age children, between the ages of 6 and 12 years, are experiencing a time of slow progressive physical growth, while their social and developmental growth accelerate and increase in complexity. The focus of their world expands from family to teachers, peers, and other outside influences (e.g., coaches, media). The child at this stage becomes increasingly more independent while participating in activities outside the home.

GROWTH AND DEVELOPMENT OVERVIEW

The school-age years are a time of continued maturation of the child's physical, social, and psychological characteristics. It is during this time that children move toward abstract thinking and seek approval of peers, teachers, and parents. Their eye–hand–muscle coordination allows them to participate in organized sports in school or the community. The **school-age child** typically values school attendance and school activities. The nurse uses knowledge of normal growth and development of the school-age child to assist the child in coping with disruptions and changes during this period.

PHYSICAL GROWTH

From 6 to 12 years of age, children grow an average of 6 to 7 cm (2 to 2.5 in) per year, increasing their height by at least 1 ft (CHOC, 2021). An increase of 2 to 3 kg (4 to 7 lb) per year in weight is expected (CHOC, 2021). In the early school-age years, female and male children are similar in height and weight and appear thinner and more graceful than in previous years (Cincinnati Children's, 2023). In later school-age years, most female children begin to surpass males in both height and weight (Biro & Chan, 2023; Cincinnati Children's, 2023; see Appendix D for growth charts).

Preadolescent children generally do not want to be different from peers, although there are biologic sex-based differences in physical and physiologic growth during the school-age years. These differences, especially secondary sexual characteristics, may be concerning to children and are often a source of embarrassment.

Sex-based differences are more apparent at the end of the middle school years and may become extreme and a source of emotional problems. These differences in height and weight relationships, and changes in growth patterns, should be explained to parents and children (Fig. 28.1). Physical maturity is not necessarily associated with emotional and social maturity. An 8-year-old who is the size of an 11-year-old will think and act like an 8-year-old. Many times, the expectations placed on these children are unrealistic and can impact their self-esteem and competence. This can work in reverse, to similar effect, for an 11-year-old who is the size of an 8-year-old and is therefore treated as such.

Remember Lawrence Jones, the 10-year-old introduced at the beginning of the chapter? Lawrence's weight is 28.1 kg (62 lb) and his height is 137.2 cm (54 in). Plot Lawrence's measurements on the appropriate growth chart.

PHYSIOLOGIC CHANGES

Maturation of organs may differ with age or sex. Maturation of organs remains fairly consistent until late school age. In the late school-age years (10- to 12-year-olds),

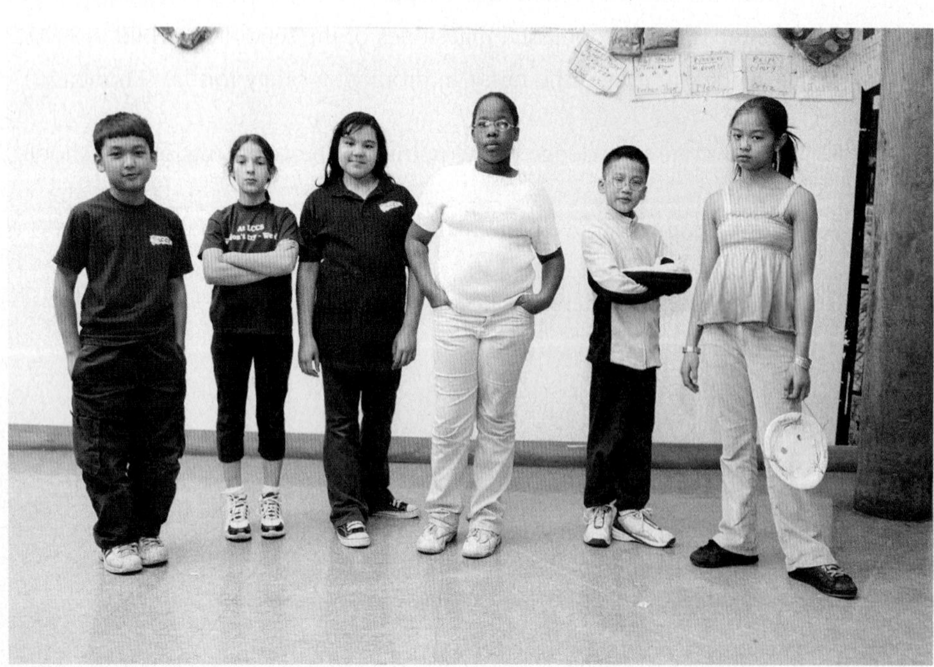

FIGURE 28.1 The different growth rates of school-age children are depicted by these same-age school-age children.

male children experience a slowed growth in height and increased weight gain, which may lead to excess weight. During this time, female children may begin to have changes in the body that soften body lines. Preadolescence is a period of rapid growth, especially for female children.

Neurologic System

The brain and skull grow slowly during the school-age years. Brain growth is complete by the time the child is 10 years of age. The shape of the head is longer, and the growth of the facial bones changes facial proportions.

Respiratory System

The respiratory system continues to mature with the development of the lungs and alveoli, resulting in fewer respiratory infections. Respiratory rates decrease, abdominal breathing disappears, and respirations become diaphragmatic in nature. The frontal sinuses are developed by 7 years of age. Tonsils decrease in size from the preschool years, but they remain larger than those of adolescents. The adenoids and tonsils may appear large normally, even in the absence of infection.

Cardiovascular System

The school-age child's blood pressure increases, and the pulse rate decreases. The heart grows more slowly during the middle years and is smaller in size in relation to the rest of the body than at any other development stage.

Gastrointestinal System

During the school-age years, all 20 primary deciduous teeth are lost and replaced by 28 of 32 permanent teeth, with the exception of the third molars (commonly known as wisdom teeth). The school-age child experiences fewer gastrointestinal upsets compared with earlier years. Stomach capacity increases, which permits retention of food for longer periods. In addition, the caloric needs of the school-age child are lower than in the earlier years.

Genitourinary System

Bladder capacity increases, but this varies among individual children. Female children generally have a greater bladder capacity than male children. Urination patterns vary with the amount of fluids ingested, the time they were ingested, and the stress level of the child. The formula for bladder capacity is age in years plus 2 oz. Therefore, the bladder capacity of the 7-year-old would be 9 oz. The larger capacity of the bladder allows for the child to experience longer periods between voiding.

Prepubescence

The late school-age years are also referred to as *preadolescence* (the time between middle childhood and the 13th birthday). During preadolescence, **prepubescence** occurs. Prepubescence typically occurs in the 2 years before the beginning of puberty and is characterized by the development of secondary sexual characteristics, a period of rapid growth for female children, and a period of continued growth for male children. There is approximately 2 years' difference in the onset of prepubescence between males and females. Sexual development, especially if there is a mismatch between timing of puberty and chronologic age, can have an effect on psychosocial functioning (Biro & Chan, 2023). Early development in female children can lead to concern over physical appearance and lower self-esteem (Biro & Chan, 2023). Delayed development in male children can lead to psychological and social issues such as depression and anxiety (Biro & Chan, 2023). It is important for the nurse and parents to educate the late school-age child about body changes to help minimize psychosocial issues such as anxiety, depression, and low self-esteem and promote comfort with these body changes.

Musculoskeletal System

Musculoskeletal growth leads to greater coordination and strength, yet the muscles are still immature and can be injured easily. Bones continue to ossify throughout childhood, but mineralization is not complete until maturity.

Immune System

Lymphatic tissues continue to grow until the child is 9 years old; immunoglobulins A and G (IgA and IgG) reach adult levels at around 10 years of age. Due to the lymphatic system becoming more competent in localizing infections and producing antibody–antigen responses, school-age children may have fewer infections. They may experience more infections during the first 1 to 2 years of school due to exposure to other children who may have infections.

PSYCHOSOCIAL DEVELOPMENT

Erikson (1963) describes the task of the school-age years to be a sense of **industry** versus **inferiority**. During this time, the child is developing their sense of self-worth by becoming involved in multiple activities at home, at school, and in the community, which develops their cognitive and social skills. The child is interested in learning how things are made and work. The school-age child's satisfaction from achieving success in developing new skills leads them to an increased sense of self-worth and level of competence. It is the role of the parents, teachers, coaches, and nurses of the school-age child to identify areas of competency and to build on the child's successful experiences to promote mastery, success, and self-esteem. If the expectations of adults are set too high, the child will develop a sense of inferiority and incompetence that can affect all aspects of their life. See Table 28.1 for a further explanation of psychosocial development in school-age children.

COGNITIVE DEVELOPMENT

Piaget's stage of cognitive development for the 7- to 11-year-old is the period of concrete operational thoughts (Piaget, 1969). In developing concrete operations, the child is able to assimilate and coordinate information about their world from different dimensions. The child is able to see things from another person's point of view and think through an action, anticipating its consequences and the possibility of having to rethink the action. They are able to use stored memories of past experiences to evaluate and interpret present situations. The school-age child also develops the ability to classify or divide things into different sets and to identify their relationships to each other. The school-age child is able to classify members of four generations on a family tree vertically and horizontally and at the same time see that one person can be a father, son, uncle, and grandson. It is at this time that the school-age child develops an interest in collecting objects. The child starts out collecting multiple objects and becomes more selective as they get older. Also, during concrete operational thinking, the school-age child develops an understanding of the **principle of conservation**—that matter does not change when its form changes. For example, if the child pours a half cup of water into a short, wide glass and into a tall, thin glass, they still only have a half cup of water even though it looks like the tall, thin glass has more (Fig. 28.2). The child learns about conserving matter in a sequence ranging from the simplest to the more complex. See Table 28.1 for further information about cognitive development of school-age children.

TABLE 28.1 • Developmental Theories

Theorist	Stage	Activities
Erikson	Industry vs. inferiority	Interested in how things are made and run Success in personal and social tasks Increased activities outside home—clubs, sports Increased interactions with peers Increased interest in knowledge Needs support and encouragement from important people in child's life Needs support when child is not successful Inferiority occurs with repeated failures with little support or trust from those who are important to the child.
Piaget	Concrete operational	Learns by manipulating concrete objects Lacks ability to think abstractly Learns that certain characteristics of objects remain constant Understands concepts of time Engages in serial ordering, addition, subtraction Classifies or groups objects by their common elements Understands relationships among objects Starts collections of items Can reverse thought process
Kohlberg	Conventional Stage 3: interpersonal conforming, "good child, bad child," age 7–10 years Stage 4: "law and order," age 10–12 years	An act is wrong because it brings punishment. Behavior is completely wrong or right. Does not understand the reason behind rules If child and adult differ in opinions, the adult is right. Can put self in another person's position Begins to exercise the "golden rule" Acts are judged in terms of intention, not just punishment.
Freud	Latency	A time of tranquility between the Oedipal phase of early childhood and adolescence—focuses on activities that develop social and cognitive skills Develops social skills in relating to same-sex friends through joining clubs like Brownies, Girl Scouts, Boy Scouts

Data from Erikson, E. (1963). *Childhood and society* (2nd ed.). Norton; Kohlberg, L. (1984). *Moral development.* Harper & Row; Piaget, J. (1969). *The theory of stages in cognitive development.* McGraw-Hill; Feigelman, S. (2020). Developmental & behavioral theories. In R. M. Kleigman, J. W. St. Geme III, N. J. Blum, S. S. Shah, R. C. Tasker, K. M. Wislon, & R. E. Behrman (Eds.), *Nelson textbook of pediatrics* (21st ed., pp. 1233–1257). Elsevier.

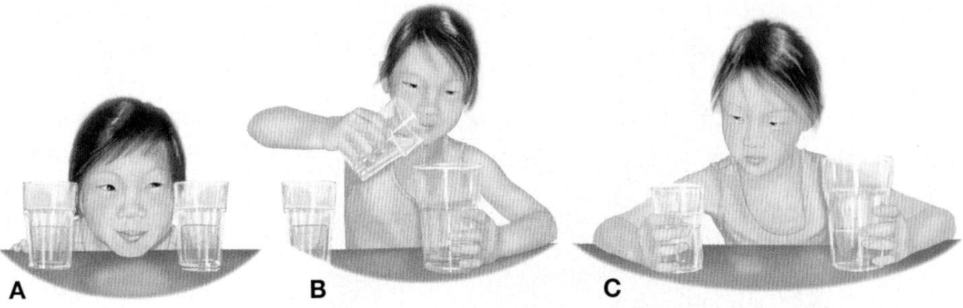

FIGURE 28.2 School-age children understand the theory of conservation (**A**). If you pour an equal amount of liquid into two glasses of unequal shape (**B**), the amount of water you have remains the same despite the unequal appearance in the two glasses (**C**).

MORAL AND SPIRITUAL DEVELOPMENT

During the school-age years, the child's sense of morality is constantly being developed. According to Kohlberg (1984), the school-age child is at the conventional stage of moral development. The 7- to 10-year-old usually follows rules out of a sense of being a "good" person. They want to be a good person to parents, friends, and teachers and to themselves. The adult is viewed as being right. This is stage 3: interpersonal conformity (good child, bad child), according to Kohlberg. The 10- to 12-year-olds progress to stage 4: the "law and order" stage. At this stage, the child can determine if an action is good or bad based on the reason for the action, not just on the possible consequences of the action. The older school-age child's behavior is guided by their desire to cooperate and by their respect for others. This leads to the school-age child's ability to understand and incorporate into their behavior the concept of the "golden rule," to treat others how you would like to be treated (Finkelstein & Feigelman, 2020). See Table 28.1 for additional information about the moral development of school-age children.

During school age, children are still concrete thinkers and are guided by their family's religious and cultural beliefs. They may be comforted by the rituals of their religion, but they are just beginning to understand the differences between natural and supernatural. Incorporating spiritual or religious practices in their lives can assist school-age children in coping with different stressors.

MOTOR SKILL DEVELOPMENT

Gross and fine motor skills continue to mature throughout the school-age years. Refinement of motor skills occurs, and speed and accuracy increase. To assess the motor skills of school-age children, ask questions about participation in sports and afterschool activities, band membership, constructing models, and writing skills.

Gross Motor Skills

During the school-age years, coordination, balance, and rhythm improve, facilitating the opportunity to ride a two-wheel bike, jump rope, dance, and participate in a variety of other sports (Fig. 28.3). Older school-age children may become awkward because their bodies grow faster than their ability to compensate.

School-age children between the ages of 6 and 8 enjoy gross motor activities such as bicycling, skating, and swimming. They are enthralled with the world and are in constant motion. Sometimes, fear is limited due to the strong impulses of exploration. Children between 8 and 10 years of age are less restless, but their energy level continues to be high, with activities more subdued and directed. These children exhibit greater rhythm and gracefulness of muscular movements, allowing them to participate in physical activities that require longer and more concentrated attention and effort, such as baseball or soccer.

Between the ages of 10 and 12 years (the pubescent years for female children), energy levels remain high but are more controlled and focused. Physical skills in this

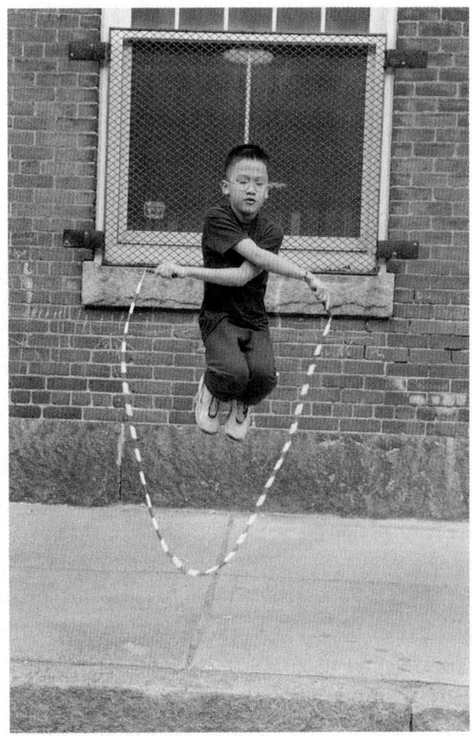

FIGURE 28.3 Jumping rope is an example of the increased development of gross motor skills of the school-age child.

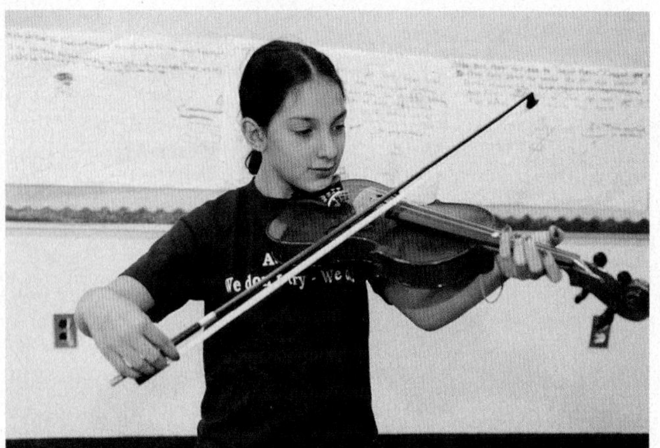

FIGURE 28.4 School-age children improve their fine motor skills so they can play musical instruments well.

age group are similar to those of adults, with strength and endurance increasing during adolescence.

All school-age children should be encouraged to engage in physical activities and learn physical skills that contribute to their health for the rest of their lives. Cardiovascular fitness, weight control, emotional tension release, and development of leadership and following skills are enhanced through physical activity and team sports.

Fine Motor Skills

Myelinization of the central nervous system is reflected by refinement of fine motor skills. Eye–hand coordination and balance improve with maturity and practice. Hand usage improves, becoming steadier and independent and granting an ease and precision that allows these children to write, print words, sew, or build models or other crafts. The child between 10 and 12 years of age begins to exhibit manipulative skills comparable to adults. School-age children take pride in activities that require dexterity and fine motor skills such as playing musical instruments (Fig. 28.4). Talent and practice become the keys to proficiency.

SENSORY DEVELOPMENT

All senses are mature early in the school-age years. Good vision is essential to the physical development and educational progression of school-age children. Vision screening programs conducted by school nurses identify problems with vision and result in appropriate referrals when warranted. Some problems frequently identified include amblyopia (lazy eye), uncorrected refractive errors or other eye defects, and malalignment of the eyes (called *strabismus*). Amblyopia is reduced vision in an eye that has not been adequately used during early development. Inadequate use can result from conditions such as strabismus, one eye being more nearsighted, farsighted, or astigmatic than the other eye. If untreated in childhood, it can persist into adulthood and cause permanent visual impairments (American Association for Pediatric Ophthalmology and Strabismus [AAPOS], 2021). This condition is correctable with glasses or patching, which forces the child to use the weaker eye. A recent study by the National Institutes for Health confirmed that older children (up to 14 years of age) can achieve some improvement in vision, but success remains higher when started at a younger age (AAPOS, 2021). Proper screening and referral, as well as notification to parents of the existing condition, are essential to the education and socialization of the school-age child.

Hearing deficits that are severe are usually diagnosed in infancy, but the less severe may not be diagnosed until the child enters school and has difficulty learning or with speech. It is important to screen children for hearing deficits to ensure proper educational and social progression.

The sense of smell is mature and can be tested in the school-age child by using scents that children are familiar with, such as chocolate or other familiar odors. In addition, the school-age child may be tested for the sense of touch with objects to discriminate cold from hot, soft from hard, and blunt from sharp.

COMMUNICATION AND LANGUAGE DEVELOPMENT

Language skills continue to accelerate during the school-age years and vocabulary expands. Culturally specific words are used, with bilingual children speaking English in school and a second language at home. The school-age child learns to read, and reading efficiency improves language skills. Reading skills are improved with increased reading exposure. School-age children begin to use more complex grammatical forms such as plurals and pronouns. Also, they develop metalinguistic awareness—an ability to think about language and comment on its properties. This enables them to enjoy jokes and riddles due to their understanding of double meanings and play on words and sounds. They are also beginning to understand metaphors such as "a stitch in time saves nine." School-age children may experiment with profanity and dirty jokes if exposed. This age group tends to imitate parents, family members, or others. Therefore, role modeling is important.

Refer back to Lawrence Jones, who was introduced at the beginning of this chapter. What developmental milestones would you expect him to have reached by this age? What would you expect his gross motor, fine motor, and language skills to be at this age?

EMOTIONAL AND SOCIAL DEVELOPMENT

Patterns of temperamental traits identified in infancy may continue to influence behavior in the school-age child. Analyzing past situations may provide clues to the way a child may react to new or different situations. Children may react differently over time due to their experiences and abilities. **Self-esteem** is the child's view of their individual worth. This view is impacted by feedback from family, teachers, and other authority figures.

Temperament

Temperament has been described as the way individuals behave. Three commonly grouped temperaments in children are *even-tempered and adaptable, slow to warm up, and challenging and easily frustrated* (Bogues & Levine, 2023). Variations and combinations of these categories are seen. Not every child can be placed into one of these groups. Understanding a child's temperament can help care providers and parents to understand the child's behavior, actions, and how they relate to the world.

The child who is even-tempered may adapt to school entry and other experiences smoothly and with little or no stress. The slow-to-warm child may be slow to adapt to changes. The slow-to-warm school-age child may exhibit discomfort when placed in different or new situations such as school. This child may need time to adjust to the new place or situation and may demonstrate frustration with tears or somatic complaints. The slow-to-warm child should be allowed time to adjust to new situations and people (such as teachers) within their own time frame. All of these factors may impact the younger school-age child upon entering the school environment, with changes in authority and the introduction of many peers. The challenging or easily distracted child may benefit from an introduction to the new experience and people by role-playing, by visiting the site and being introduced to the teachers, and by hearing stories or participating in conversations about the upcoming school experience. These children require patience, firmness, and understanding to make the transition into a new situation or experience such as school.

Assessment of temperament by a professional would include a combination of interview, observation, and a standardized questionnaire. Better understanding a child's temperament can assist parents with adjusting their parenting style to better fit their child and may help limit emotional and behavioral problems that occur when these areas are in conflict.

Self-Esteem Development

Self-esteem mirrors the child's individual self-worth and consists of both positive and negative qualities. Children strive to achieve internalized goals of attainment, although they continually receive feedback from individuals they perceive as authorities (parent or teacher). By the school-age years, children have received feedback related to their performance or tasks. The direction of this feedback influences the child's opinion of self-worth, which influences self-esteem and self-evaluation.

Children face the process of self-evaluation from a framework of either self-confidence or self-doubt. Children who have mastered the earlier developmental task of autonomy and initiative face the world with feelings of pride rather than shame (Erikson, 1963).

If school-age children regard themselves as worthwhile, they have a positive self-concept and high self-esteem. Significant adults in school-age children's lives can manipulate the environment to facilitate success. This success impacts the self-esteem of the child.

Body Image

Body image is how the school-ager perceives their body. School-age children are knowledgeable about the human body but may have different perceptions about body parts. School-age children are very interested in peers' views and acceptance of their body, body changes, and clothing. This age group may model themselves after parents, peers, and people in movies or on television. It is important for late school-agers to feel accepted by peers. If they feel different and are teased, there may be lifelong effects.

School-Age Fears

The school-age child's fears shift away from pretend things, like monsters, to things that could happen to them in real life, such as natural disasters, others hurting them, and the death of a loved one (Radcliff, 2023). School-age children are less fearful of harm to their body than in their preschool years but fear being kidnapped or undergoing surgery. They may continue to fear the dark but are less fearful of animals, such as dogs and noises. The school-age child needs reassurance that their fears are normal for this developmental age. Parents, teachers, and other caregivers should listen to the child's fears with sympathy and support. Recognize the child's fears, but do not cater to them. Help the child face their fears, and teach the child coping strategies, for instance, using positive self-statements such as "I can do this" and relaxation techniques such as deep breathing and visualization (Radcliff, 2023).

Peer Relationships

The school-age child's concept of self is shaped not only by their parents but also by relationships with others. Peer relationships influence children's independence from parents. Peers play an important role in the approval and critiquing of skills of school-age children. Previously, only adults such as parents and teachers have been authorities; now, peers influence school-age children's perceptions of themselves. Peer relationships help to support the school-age child by providing enough security to risk the parental conflict brought about when establishing independence. School-age children associate with peers of the same sex or same gender most of the time. Although games and other activities are shared by all children, the child's concept of the appropriate gender role is influenced by their relationship with peers.

Continuous peer relationships provide the most important social interaction for school-age children. Valuable lessons are learned from interactions with children of their own age. Children learn to respect differing points of view that are represented in their groups. Peer groups establish norms and standards that signify acceptance or rejection. Children may modify behavior to gain acceptance. A characteristic of school-age children is their formation of groups with rules and values.

Teacher and School Influences

School serves as a means to transmit values of society and to establish peer relationships. Secondary only to the family, school exerts a profound influence on the social development of the child. Often, school requires changes for the child and parent. The child enters an environment that requires conforming to group activities that are structured and directed by an adult other than the parent. The parent's attitude and support influence the child's transition into the school setting. Parents who are positive and supportive promote a smooth entry into school. Parents who encourage clinging behaviors may delay a successful transition into school.

To facilitate the transition from home to school, the teacher must have the personality and knowledge of development that will allow them to meet the needs of young children. Even though the teacher's responsibilities are primarily to stimulate and guide intellectual development, they must share in shaping the child's attitudes and values. The system of awards and punishment administered by teachers affects the self-concept of children and influences their response to school. Teachers and school are important in shaping the socialization, self-concept, and intellectual development of children.

Family Influences

The school-age years are a time for peer relationships, questioning of parents, and the potential for parental conflict but continued respect for family values. School-age years are the beginning of the time of peer-group influence, with testing of parental and family values. Although the peer group is influential, the family's values usually predominate when parental and peer-group values come into conflict. Even though the school-age child may question the parents' values, the child will usually incorporate the values from parents into their values.

Often, in the late school age and preadolescent period, the child may prefer to be in the company of peers and show a decreased interest in family functions. This may require an adjustment for parents. Parents' awareness of this developmental trend and their continuing support for the child are important while they continue to enforce restrictions and control of behaviors. The school-ager is beginning to strive for independence, but parental authority and controls continue to impact choices and values.

TAKE NOTE!

School-age children continue to need parenting. They do not need parents as friends.

CULTURAL INFLUENCES ON GROWTH AND DEVELOPMENT

Culture influences habits, beliefs, language, and values. School-age children thrive on learning the music, language, traditions, holidays, games, values, gender roles, and other aspects of culture. Nurses must be aware of the effects on children of various groups' family structures and traditional values. The school-age child's cultural and ethnic backgrounds must be considered when assessing growth and development. Cultural implications must be considered for all children and families in order to provide appropriate care.

THE NURSE'S ROLE IN SCHOOL-AGE GROWTH AND DEVELOPMENT

Growth and development in the school-age child occurs in irregular spurts, with a wide variation of sizes, shapes, and abilities seen. Nurses must be aware of the usual growth and development patterns for this age group so that they can assess school-age children appropriately and provide guidance to the child and their family. This is a time when children compare themselves to peers, and self-esteem is a central issue. The school-age child is separating from their parents and seeks acceptance from peers and adults outside of their family. Health care visits throughout the school-age period continue to focus on expected growth and development and anticipatory guidance. Visits are more infrequent during the school-age years; therefore, the nurse needs to assess the child's functioning not only at home but also at school and within the community.

If the school-age child is hospitalized, growth and development may be altered. The school-age child is able to understand the reason for hospitalization and what will happen. They are often worried about pain or changes that may occur to their body. It is important for health care providers and family members to be honest and open with the school-age child. The school-age child may miss school and the interactions with their peers. The school-age child may regress and exhibit behaviors of a younger child, such as needing special comfort toys or demanding attention from their parents. Hospitalization for the school-age child can bring with it a loss of control. The school-age child is used to controlling their self-care and making choices about their meals and activities.

When caring for the hospitalized school-age child, the nurse must use knowledge of normal growth and development to recognize potential delays, promote continued appropriate growth and development, and interact successfully with the school-age child. Provide opportunities for the school-age child to maintain independence, gain control, and increase self-esteem.

Clinical Judgment and the Nursing Process

On completion of assessment of the school-age child's current growth and development status, problems or issues related to growth and development may be identified. The nurse may then identify one or more nursing diagnoses. The following nursing diagnoses with identified outcomes and interventions provide suggestions for nursing care planning or concept mapping. Care planning should be individualized.

Nursing Analysis

Risk for excess weight; risk factors include average daily physical activity being less than recommended for sex and age, consumption of sugar-sweetened beverages, frequent snacking, high frequency of restaurant or fried food, insufficient knowledge of modifiable factors, sedentary behavior occurring for more than 2 hours a day, portion sizes larger than recommended, body mass index (BMI) approaching 85th percentile, and parental excess weight.

Goal/Outcome

The school-age child will maintain a healthy weight for age, BMI of less than the 85th percentile; lose weight at an appropriate rate: Increase the amount of exercise; make appropriate eating choices; and decrease caloric intake to an appropriate amount for age and sex.

Promoting Healthy Weight (interventions with *rationale*)

- Assess knowledge of parents and child about nutritional needs of school-age children *to determine deficits in knowledge.*
- Plot out height, weight, and BMI *to detect weight loss or weight gain.*
- Have child keep food and exercise diary for 1 week *to determine current patterns of eating and exercise.*
- Interview parents in relation to their eating habits and exercise habits *to determine where adjustments might need to be made.*
- Analyze preceding data, and base recommendations for changes on these data, *to best develop a further plan.*
- Educate primary caregiver about appropriate serving sizes and foods *so that primary caregiver is aware of what to expect for school-age children.*
- Discuss ways to decrease temptation to overeat and to make good meal choices *to assist the child with developing healthy eating habits* (see Teaching Guidelines 28.2).
- Have child assist in meal planning and grocery shopping *to allow them some sense of control in process.*
- Incorporate increase in daily exercise, which will stress sense of self-improvement, *to increase caloric expenditure and self-esteem.*
- Decrease television/computer/device time *to increase caloric expenditure.*
- Develop reward system *to increase self-esteem.*
- Investigate joining weight-loss program for school-age children *to increase self-esteem and to increase awareness that other children have the same problem.*

Nursing Analysis

Delayed growth and development risk; risk factors include inadequate nutrition, presence of abuse, substance misuse, technology dependence, behavioral disorder, low socioeconomic status involvement with the foster care system, prematurity, chronic illness, genetic disorder.

Goal/Outcome

Growth and development will be maximized: School-age child will make continued progress toward attainment of expected standards of school performance.

Promoting Development (interventions with *rationale*)

- Perform developmental evaluation of the school-age child *to determine current functioning.*
- Develop realistic multidisciplinary plan *to ensure maximizing resources.*
- Carry out interventions as prescribed by developmental specialist, physical therapist, occupational

therapist, or speech therapist at home and at school *to maximize benefit of interventions.*
- Have scheduled evaluation meetings *to be able to adapt interventions as soon as possible.*

Nursing Analysis

Injury risk due to exposure to toxic chemicals, insufficient knowledge of modifiable factors, unsafe mode of transport, extremes of age (e.g., developmental stage including high level of curiosity and increasing cognitive skills and motor abilities).

Goal/Outcome

School-age child's safety will be maintained: They will remain free from injury.

Preventing Injury (interventions with *rationale*)

- Discuss safety measures needed for the following: bikes, scooters, guns, skateboards, cars, water, and playground *to decrease risk of injury related to those areas.*
- Discuss and develop a fire safety plan *to decrease risk of injury related to fire.*
- Discuss appropriate safety equipment needed for each sport *to decrease risk of injury.*
- Discuss appropriate sports to participate in depending on age and maturity of child *to prevent possible injury* and *to promote child's self-esteem.*
- Instruct parents to post the Poison Control Center phone number (*in the event of accidental ingestion, Poison Control can give parents the best advice for appropriate intervention*).
- Teach parents and child first-aid measures and child cardiopulmonary resuscitation (CPR) *to minimize consequences of injury should it occur.*
- Discuss influence of peers on actions of school-age children *to prevent possible injury due to mimicking behavior.*

Nursing Analysis

Caregiver role strain risk; risk factors include dependency, discharged home with significant needs, problematic behavior, caregiver substance misuse, unstable health condition, insufficient knowledge about community resources, social isolation.

Goal/Outcome

Parent will experience competence in role: They will demonstrate appropriate caregiving behaviors and verbalize comfort in caring for a school-age child.

Preventing Caregiver Role Strain (interventions with *rationale*)

- Assess parents' knowledge of school-age children and the issues that arise as a part of normal development *to determine parents' needs.*
- Provide education on normal issues of school-age children *so that parents have the knowledge they need to appropriately care for their school-age child.*
- Provide anticipatory guidance related to upcoming expected issues related to school-age development *to prepare parents for what to expect next and how to intervene.*

PROMOTING HEALTHY GROWTH AND DEVELOPMENT

The family plays a critical role in promoting healthy growth and development of the school-age child. Respectful interchange of communication between the parent and child will foster self-esteem and self-confidence. This respect will give the child confidence in achieving personal, educational, and social goals appropriate for their age. The nurse should study interactions between parents and school-age children to observe for this respect or lack of respect ("putting the child down"). The nurse can model appropriate behaviors by listening to the child and making appropriate responses. The nurse can be a resource for parents and an advocate for the child in promoting healthy growth and development.

Promoting Growth and Development Through Play

Cooperative play is exhibited by the school-age child. Play for the school-age child includes both organized cooperative activities (such as team sports) and solitary activities. School-age children have the coordination and intellect to participate with other children of their age in sports such as soccer, baseball, football, and tennis. The school-age child comprehends that their cooperation with others will lead to a unified whole for the team. In addition, the child learns rules and the value of playing by the rules.

School-age children also enjoy solitary activities, including board, card, video, and computer games, and dollhouse and other small-figure play (Fig. 28.5). Many school-agers start collections of stamps, cars, or other valuable or not-so-valuable items. During the school-age years, children may also begin a scrapbook or keep a diary. They may participate in activities, such as dance or karate, and join clubs or special interest groups (Fig. 28.6).

Active play has decreased in recent years as television viewing, multimedia device use, and video games have increased (Oh et al., 2022). This trend has resulted in health risks such as excess weight, type 2 diabetes, and cardiovascular problems (CDC, 2022b).

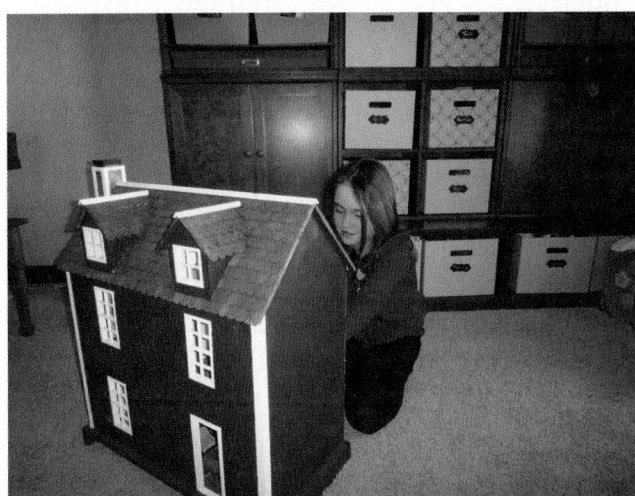

FIGURE 28.5 This school-age child enjoys solitary play with their dollhouse and dolls.

Promoting Learning

School attendance and learning are important to the school-age child. Parent–child, child–teacher, and child–peer relationships and activities influence the school-age child's learning.

Formal Education

Most children are excited about starting school and making new friends. They like the notion of getting books, having book bags, and having homework assignments. The reality of the work involved with school and homework may decrease the enthusiasm about school.

Peers are important within this age group. Both peers and teachers influence children. Attending school may be their first experience interacting with a large number of children of their own age. Through this interaction, children learn cooperation, competition, and the importance of following the rules. Peer approval and influences grow as the child matures. Teachers have significant influences on children. They help to guide the child's intellectual development by rewarding successes and helping the child deal with failures. The student–teacher relationship is a key to success. Teachers play a role in fostering feelings of industry and preventing feelings of inferiority (Fig. 28.7). School-age children also learn skills, rules, values, and other ways to work with peers and other authority figures.

Parental support is important for school adjustment and achievement. Parents must collaborate with teachers and school personnel to ensure that the child is fulfilling the expectations and requirements for this age group in school. Parents must monitor the child's homework assignments and friends and observe for any changes in behavior that would indicate school or behavioral problems.

Reading

Encouraging reading is an excellent way to promote learning in the school-age child. Trips to the library and purchasing books help to promote a love of reading. School-age children enjoy being read to as well as reading on their own. Younger school-age children (6 to 8 years) enjoy books that are simple to read, with few words on a page, such as the Dr. Seuss books. They enjoy books about animals and trains and simple mysteries. Children 8 to 10 years of age have more advanced reading skills and enjoy those books from early childhood, as well as more classic novels and adventures such as the *Harry Potter* series. Older children enjoy horror stories, mysteries, romances, and adventure stories as well as classic novels. School-age children of all ages benefit from books on topics related to things they may be experiencing, such as a visit to the hospital for a surgical procedure. See Box 28.1 for ideas for parents to promote reading in the school-age child.

FIGURE 28.6 School-age children like to join clubs. These children, in the acting club at school, are rehearsing for a play.

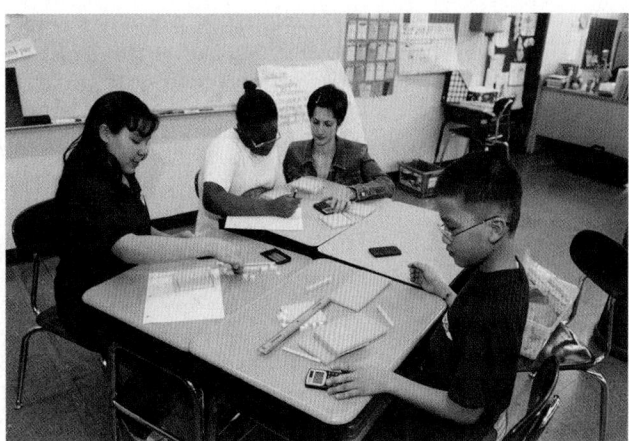

FIGURE 28.7 School is important to the school-age child.

BOX 28.1 Promotion of Reading in School-Age Children

- Parents, read to and with your children.
- Ask teachers and librarians for advice on books appropriate for your child.
- Choose stories that the child can relate to if the child has difficulty reading.
- Choose books with movement if the child has a short attention span.
- Take advantage of all reading opportunities (cereal boxes, road signs).
- Provide choices for the child to select a book of interest.
- Talk about the text and ask questions to improve understanding.
- Keep a record of what the child is reading.
- Visit a library, get a library card, and check out books.
- Parents, demonstrate role modeling through reading books.

Promoting Safety

School-age children become more independent with age. This independence leads to an increased self-confidence and decreased fears, which may contribute to accidents and injuries. School age is a time that the child may walk to school with peers who may influence their behavior. Increased independence may also increase exposure to dangerous situations such as the approach of strangers or unsafe streets. Promotion of safe habits during the school-age years is important for parents and nurses. See Teaching Guidelines 28.1 for additional information on safety education for nurses and parents.

TEACHING GUIDELINES 28.1 Safety Issues and Interventions of the School-Age Child

Safety Issue	Interventions
Car safety	• A seat belt or age- and weight-appropriate booster seat should be used at all times. The lap belt should lie low and flat on the hips, and the shoulder belt should lie on the shoulder, not the neck or face (proper fitting of adult shoulder and lap belts without a booster seat usually occurs when the child is about 144.8 cm [57 in] tall). • Seat belts should be fastened before car is started. • Children under 13 years must sit in the back seat. • Childproof locks should be used in the back seat. • Rules of conduct for car rides must be established.
Pedestrian safety	• The child should be instructed to stop at the curb and look right, left, then right again before crossing the street and to cross only at safe crossings. • Older children and adults should provide supervision of younger children. • Walking should only be done on sidewalks. • Phones, headphones, and devices should be put away when crossing the street. • In parking lots, children should know to watch for cars backing up and not dart out between parked cars. • If children are playing outside, drivers should be aware of their presence before backing up.
Bike safety: general	• The child should know to wear a properly fitted, Consumer Product Safety Commission (CPSC) or Snell-approved helmet every time they ride a bike. • A properly fitting helmet should sit level, not tilted, and firmly and comfortably on the head; have strong wide Y-shaped straps and when you open your mouth should pull down a bit; not move with sudden pulling or twisting; never be worn over anything else (hat, scarf, etc.). • Bikes should be well maintained and appropriately sized. • The child should be oriented to the bike and demonstrate ability to ride the bike safely before being allowed to ride on street. • Safe areas for bike riding should be established, as should routes to and from the area of activities. • Riding a bike barefoot, with someone else on the bike, or with clothing that might get entangled in the bike should be prohibited. • The child should know to wear sturdy, well-fitting shoes. • The bike should be inspected often to ensure it is in proper working order. • A basket should be used to carry heavy objects.
Bike safety in traffic	• All traffic signs and signals must be observed. • Avoid riding at night; if riding at night occurs, the bike should have lights and reflectors, and the rider should wear light-colored clothes. • The child should know to ride on the side of the road traveling with traffic and keep close to the side of the road in single file.

TEACHING GUIDELINES 28.1 Safety Issues and Interventions of the School-Age Child

Safety Issue	Interventions
	• The child should learn to watch and listen for cars and to stop and check for traffic in both directions when leaving driveways, alleys, or curbs. • Headphones should not be used while riding a bike. • Never hitch a ride on any vehicle.
Sports safety	• Sports should be matched to child's ability and desire. • The sports program should have a warm-up procedure. • Coaches should be trained in CPR and first aid. • Appropriate protection devices should be used for individual sports.
Skateboarding and inline skating safety	• The child should wear a helmet and protective padding on knees, elbows, and wrists. • The child should know not to skate in traffic or on streets or highways. • Homemade ramps should be assessed for hazards before skating.
All-terrain vehicle safety	• The child should be at least 16 years of age to operate vehicle. • Take a hands-on safety course before riding. • Helmets designed for motorcycles must be worn in addition to protective coverings. • No nighttime riding • No double riding • Use should be avoided on public roads. • Never stand up in the vehicle or ride in a person's lap.
Fire safety	• All homes should have working smoke detectors and fire extinguishers. Change the batteries at least twice a year. • Have a fire-escape plan. • Practice the fire-escape plan routinely. • Nobody should smoke in the home, especially in bed. • Teach what to do in case of a fire: use a fire extinguisher, call 911, and know how to put out clothing fire. • Use the stove and other cooking facilities under adult supervision. • All flammable materials and liquids should be stored safely. • Fireplaces should have protective gratings. • Teach children to avoid touching wires they might encounter while playing.
Water safety	• Teach children how to swim and to never play around or in water without adult supervision. • If swimming skill is limited, the child must wear a life preserver at all times. • The child should know never to swim alone—if at all possible, they should swim only where there is a life guard. • Understand basic CPR. • Teach the child to never run or fool around at the edge of the pool. • Drains in pool should be covered with appropriate cover. • Life jackets should be worn when on a boat. • Make sure the water is deep enough to support diving.
Firearm safety	• Teach the child never to touch guns and to tell an adult when they encounter a gun. • If there are guns in household, secure them in a safe place, use gun safety locks, and store bullets in a separate place. • Never point a gun at a person.
Toxin safety	• Teach the child the hazards of accepting recreational drugs, alcohol, or dangerous drugs. • Store potentially dangerous material in a safe place.

Data from American Academy of Pediatrics, HealthyChildren. (2021). *Booster seats for school-age children*. https://www.healthychildren.org/English/safety-prevention/on-the-go/Pages/Booster-Seats-for-School-Age-Children.aspx; Jennissen, C. (2022). *ATVs are not safe for children: AAP policy explained*. https://www.healthychildren.org/English/safety-prevention/at-play/Pages/ATV-Safety-Rules.aspx; Gill, A. C. (2022). Bicycle injuries in children: Prevention. *UpToDate*. Retrieved October 17, 2022, from https://www.uptodate.com/contents/bicycle-injuries-in-children-prevention

Unintentional injuries are the leading cause of death in children older than 1 year of age (Gill & Kelly, 2022). In 2020, more than 6 million children sought medical attention at a hospital emergency room for nonfatal unintentional injuries (Gill & Kelly, 2022). School-age children are very active at home, in the community, and at school. This increased mobility, activity, and time away from parents increase the risk of unintentional injuries. School-age children continue to need supervision and guidance. They need information and rules about car safety, pedestrian safety, bicycle and other sport safety, fire safety, and water safety.

Car Safety

Motor vehicle crashes are a common cause of injury in the school-age child. While traveling in the car, school-age children should always sit in the rear seat. The front seat is dangerous because of passenger-side airbags in most new-model cars. A school-age child over 18.1 kg (40 lb; generally 4 to 8 years of age) should use a belt-positioning, forward-facing booster seat using both lap and shoulder belts (American Academy of Pediatrics [AAP], HealthyChildren, 2021). School-age children who outgrow the convertible restraint can sit in a booster seat until the vehicle seat belt restraint fits properly over the hips and shoulder, typically when they are 144.8 cm (4 ft 9 in) or taller, usually between 8 and 12 years of age (AAP, HealthyChildren, 2021). The seat belt needs to lie low and flat over the hip bones and across the shoulder, not the neck or face. Children younger than 13 years of age should not ride in the front seat of a vehicle with an airbag (AAP, HealthyChildren, 2021).

Pedestrian Safety

In 2021, about 9,250 children were injured as pedestrians, with 385 suffering fatal injuries (Safe Kids Worldwide, 2023). The highest risk age group is 12 to 19 years (Safe Kids Worldwide, 2023). Children younger than 10 years should not be unsupervised pedestrians. Young school-age children, therefore, should walk to school or the bus with an older friend, sibling, or parent. Darting out into the street without looking both ways or from between cars is a common occurrence in the school-age years. Teach children safe street and pedestrian practices.

Bicycle and Sport Safety

Bicycling, riding scooters, skateboarding, and inline skating or roller skating are common activities of school-age children. Laws in some states require helmets for riding bicycles and scooters. In addition, when skating or skateboarding, school-age children should wear a helmet, kneepads, and elbow pads.

Research has shown that brain injuries due to bicycle crashes have been reduced by wearing a well-fitting helmet (Gill, 2022; see Healthy People 2030). It is important for children to wear helmets that fit and that do not obstruct their vision or hearing. Because school-age children have completed most of their skull growth, a helmet can be worn into adolescence. It is important for the child to have a bicycle that is appropriate for their size and age. The child should be able to plant both feet on the ground when sitting on the seat of the bike (Fig. 28.8). It is important to stress to parents the importance of appropriate size and not to get a bike for the child to “grow into.” If older school-agers are using the bike for transportation on busy streets, they should be taught to use bike lanes and to give appropriate hand signals for turning. Nonmotorized and motorized scooters also place children at risk for injury, so counsel families about the use of protective gear, including helmets, elbow pads, and kneepads.

Fire Safety

School-age children are eager to help parents with cooking and ironing. They are curious about fire and are drawn to play with fire, matches, and fireworks. Serious burns can occur from any exposure to fire. Educate children about the hazards of fire. In addition, teach children proper behavior around fires at home and outdoors.

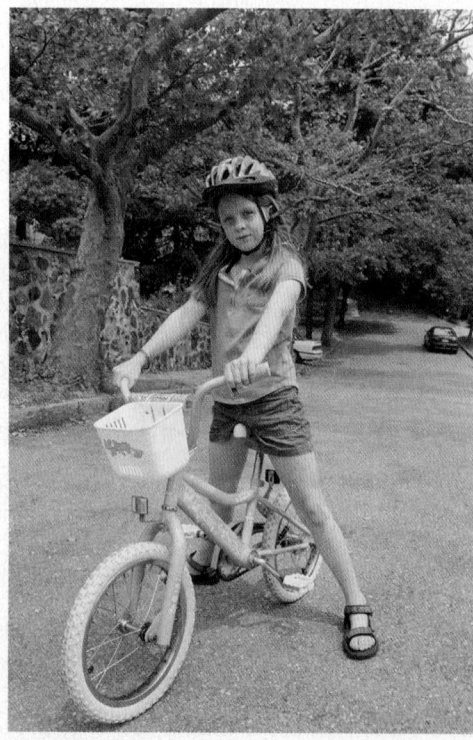

FIGURE 28.8 Wearing the appropriate safety equipment and having an appropriately sized bicycle are important to prevent injuries in school-age children.

HEALTHY PEOPLE 2030

Objective	Nursing Significance
Reduce fatal traumatic brain injuries.	• Provide education to children and their parents about avoiding head injury through helmet use. • Encourage child to choose a helmet that appeals to them (one that looks "cool").

Healthy People Objectives retrieved from http://www.healthypeople.gov

Always supervise children in the use of matches. In the home setting, parents should develop a fire safety plan with their children, teach children what to do if their clothes catch fire, and practice evacuating the house in the event of a fire. In the school setting, children should be aware of the appropriate response to fire drills, and fire drills should be conducted on a regular basis.

Water Safety

Teach school-age children swimming and water safety. An adult should always supervise children when they are swimming to prevent water-related accidents.

Remember Lawrence Jones, the 10-year-old presented in the case study? What anticipatory guidance related to safety should you provide to his parent?

Child Abuse

Child abuse, including physical abuse and sexual abuse, is a common crime of violence against children. An estimated 2.1 million reports of child abuse are made annually to child protective services in the United States (U.S. Department of Health and Human Services, Administration for Children and Families, Administration on Children, Youth and Families, Children's Bureau, 2022). Nationally, 618,000 cases were substantiated in 2020; in 76.1% the children were victims of neglect in, 16.5% they were victims of physical abuse, in 9.4% they were victims of sexual abuse, and in 6% they were victims of other abuse, such as drug or alcohol use disorder, emotional or psychological abuse (U.S. Department of Health and Human Services, Administration for Children and Families, Administration on Children, Youth and Families, Children's Bureau, 2022). The perpetrators may be family, friends, and strangers. It is important for parents to teach children the concept of "good touch" versus "bad touch" prior to school-age years. Whenever the school-age child's behavior yields suspicion of physical or sexual abuse, the nurse should report to the appropriate authorities in their state. These topics will be discussed in more depth in Chapter 50.

Promoting Nutrition

Growth, body composition, and body shape remain constant during late school-age years. Needed calories decrease while the appetite increases. In preparation for adolescence, the body fat composition of school-age children increases. This tendency toward increased body fat occurs earlier in female children than in male children, with the amount of increase greater in females. Males tend to have more lean body mass per inch of height than females.

Diet preferences established in the preschool years continue during the school-age period. As the child grows older, influences of family, media, and peers can impact the eating habits of this age group. Some of these influences are parents' work schedule, outside activities, and exercise level of the child. Decreased exercise levels and poor nutritional choices lead to the higher weight more frequently seen in this age group. See Box 28.2 for appropriate questions to ask the child and parent regarding nutritional status. Healthy People 2030 provides objectives and actions to improve the nutritional health of children.

Nutritional Needs

The school-age child's calorie needs vary based on age, sex, and activity level. Children 4 to 8 years old who are moderately active will need about 1,400 to 1,600 calories a day (U.S. Department of Agriculture [USDA] & U.S. Department of Health and Human Services [HHS],

BOX 28.2 Dietary Questions

Questions for the Child

- How often do you eat together as a family?
- What are the usual mealtimes?
- How often does the family eat out?
- Do you eat breakfast regularly?
- Where do you eat lunch?
- What do you drink/how much?
- What foods do you eat most often?
- What is your favorite food?
- How often do you eat fast foods?
- What type of exercise do you do?

Questions for the Parents

- How would you describe your child's usual appetite?
- Do you have any special cultural/religious practices regarding food?
- Has your child gained or lost weight recently?
- Do you have any concerns about their eating behaviors?
- How does your child exercise? Your family?
- Is there a family history of cancer, hypertension, diabetes, higher weight, or heart disease?

HEALTHY PEOPLE 2030

Objective	Nursing Significance
Increase fruit consumption by people aged 2 years and older. Increase vegetable consumption by people aged 2 years and older. Increase consumption of dark green vegetables, red and orange vegetables, and beans and peas by people aged 2 years and older. Increase whole grain consumption by people aged 2 years and older. Reduce consumption of added sugars by people aged 2 years and older. Reduce consumption of saturated fat by people aged 2 years and older. Reduce consumption of sodium by people aged 2 years and older. Increase calcium consumption by people aged 2 years and older. Increase potassium consumption by people aged 2 years and older.	• Educate families about the importance of whole grains, fruits, and vegetables in the diet. • Encourage the child to choose fruits and vegetables that appeal to them. • Provide creative suggestions for vegetable preparation to make them more appealing to children. • Educate families about saturated fat–containing foods. • Offer suggestions for alternative sources of proteins and fats (chicken or fish, olive oil).

Healthy People Objectives retrieved from http://www.healthypeople.gov

2020). Males 9 to 13 years old who are moderately active need about 1,800 to 2,200 calories a day, while females of this age who are moderately active need about 1,600 to 2,000 calories a day (USDA & HHS, 2020). Of these calories, 45% to 65% should come from carbohydrates, 10% to 30% from protein, and 25% to 35% from fat (USDA & HHS, 2020). The 4- to 8-year-old child needs 1,000 mg of calcium, while the 9- to 13-year-old needs 1,300 mg of calcium for maintenance of growth and good nutrition (USDA & HHS, 2020). Calcium is needed for the development of strong bones and teeth. Milk, yogurt, and cheese provide protein, vitamins, and minerals and are an excellent source of calcium. Meats, poultry, fish, and eggs provide protein, vitamins, and minerals.

Promoting Healthy Eating Habits

School-age children should choose culturally appropriate foods and snacks from the USDA's MyPlate. MyPlate illustrates the five food groups and encourages children to make half of their plate fruits and vegetables, to make half of their grains whole grains, and to choose lean proteins and calcium-rich foods. The website https://www.choosemyplate.gov/kids offers many tools for the child to use, including development of personalized goals and menus, online diet and physical activity assessment tools, games, activities, and tips for parents. School-age children need to limit intake of fat and processed sugars. A prudent diet limits the use of fatty meats, high-fat dairy products, and hydrogenated shortenings and promotes the consumption of fish and the substitution of polyunsaturated vegetable oils and margarines.

Maintaining a Healthy Body Weight

Maintenance of a healthy body weight weight remains a serious health concern for children in the United States, with 20.7% of school-age children having a BMI greater than 95% (CDC, 2022a). According to the CDC (2022a), overweight is classified as a BMI greater than 85%, and obese is classified as a BMI greater than 95% (see Healthy People 2030 objectives).

Some factors linked to higher weight include family role modeling, lack of exercise, unstructured meals, consumption of sugar-sweetened beverages, large portion sizes, lack of sleep, recreational media use such as television viewing and video gaming as well as genetic, environmental, and socioeconomic factors (Skelton & Klish, 2023). Some factors that influence lack of exercise include the decreased number of days that school systems offer physical education programs and recess. Some children live in neighborhoods or communities that lack sidewalks or parks and have no safe place to play outside; therefore, they spend time doing sedentary activities such as watching TV or playing video or computer games. Children with higher weight are at higher risk for cardiovascular diseases such as high cholesterol and hypertension; type 2 (non–insulin-dependent) diabetes; respiratory complications such as obstructive sleep apnea; mental health issues such as depression, anxiety

HEALTHY PEOPLE 2030

Objective	Nursing Significance
Reduce the proportion of children and adolescents with higher weight	• Screen all children for the development of overweight, as indicated by an increasing BMI for their age. • Provide accurate diet counseling. • Encourage daily physical activity. • Counsel parents to limit television/computer time daily.

Healthy People Objectives retrieved from http://www.healthypeople.gov

and eating disorders; and orthopedic problems (USDA & HHS, 2020). When parents do not have knowledge of nutrition, do not monitor snacks or meals, and have unstructured meals, habits are established that contribute to higher weight.

Maintaining healthy body weight in childhood is important because childhood higher weight often carries over into adolescence and adulthood and contributes to disease (Skelton & Klish, 2023). Due to the risk of higher weight, encourage parents to never use food as a reward. To achieve a healthy weight, caregivers should establish regular mealtimes and offer healthy foods and snacks. Encourage parents to praise their child's good food choices and to role model appropriate eating and exercise.

> Think back to Lawrence Jones; what questions should you ask Lawrence's parent related to nutritional intake? What anticipatory guidance related to nutrition would be appropriate?

Promoting Healthy Sleep and Rest

The number of hours of sleep required for growth and development decreases with age. Children between the ages of 6 and 8 years require about 12 hours of sleep per night, children between 8 and 10 years of age require 10 to 12 hours of sleep per night, and children between 10 and 12 years of age need 9 to 10 hours of sleep per night. Young school-age children may need an occasional brief nap for an energy boost after being in school for most of the day. Bedtime rituals and consistent schedules continue to be important throughout the school-age years. Parents must facilitate a bedtime schedule and quiet time before bed. Bedtime is a special time for parents and children. They can spend time together reading, listening to soothing music, and discussing the day's events. This time continues to be important during the school-age years as the child gains independence from their parents. Children should have bedtime expectations as well as wake-up times and methods for waking up (alarm, calling by parent, and so forth). Night terrors or sleepwalking may occur in young children but typically resolve as the child gets older (Morse & Kotagal, 2021).

> What anticipatory guidance should you provide to Lawrence Jones's parent in relation to proper sleep for their 10-year-old?

Promoting Healthy Teeth and Gums

Dental **caries** remain a leading chronic disease in children even though the incidence has declined since the 1970s, mostly due to the introduction of fluoride (Nowak & Warren, 2022). Recent statistics show that 45.8% of children have treated or untreated dental caries (Nowak & Warren, 2022). Dental caries disproportionately affect children living below 100% of the poverty level and non-Hispanic Black and Hispanic children. (Clark et al., 2020).

Dental care with emphasis on prevention of caries is important in this age group. School-age children need to brush their teeth two to three times per day for 2 to 3 minutes each time with fluorinated toothpaste (Fig. 28.9). Parents should replace the toothbrush (soft) every 3 to 4 months. Flossing the teeth at least once daily is recommended along with limiting the intake of sugar to aid in the prevention of cavities and improved oral health. Parents must monitor toothbrushing, observe for abnormal alignment of their child's teeth, and schedule regular dental examinations every 6 months to ensure good dental health and prevent dental problems. Children will need help with brushing teeth until they are between 7 and 10 years of age.

Dental sealants are an easy way to protect a child's primary or permanent teeth. The sealant is a plastic coating applied to biting surfaces to seal out tooth decay on back teeth and sometimes to cover deep pits or grooves. In addition, parents should give a fluoride supplement (as directed by the dentist) to their children if fluoride is not in the town's water supply (Clark et al., 2020). The school-age child should have an established dental home; if not, provide appropriate resources to establish one. See Healthy People 2030.

Proper alignment of teeth is important to tooth formation, speech development, and physical appearance. Many school-age children need braces or other orthodontic devices to correct **malocclusion**, a condition in which the teeth are crowded, crooked, or misaligned. **Bruxism** or teeth grinding while asleep may continue in the school-age years. Bruxism may result in grinding away of tooth enamel. Teeth grinding may be due to malalignment. A dental evaluation should be scheduled if consistent teeth grinding occurs.

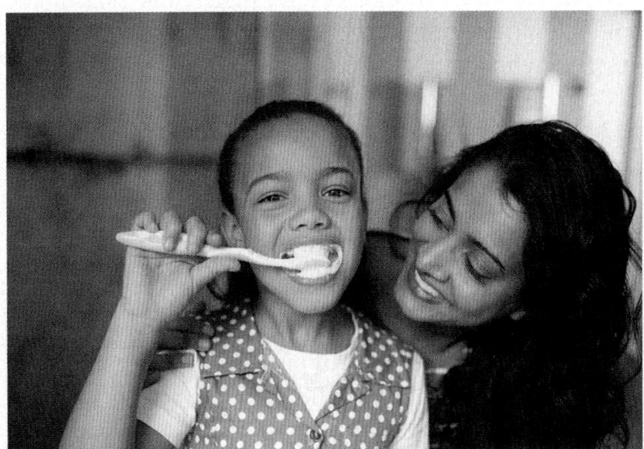

FIGURE 28.9 Using correct technique to brush the teeth is important in the prevention of cavities.

HEALTHY PEOPLE 2030

Objective	Nursing Significance
Reduce the proportion of children and adolescents with lifetime tooth decay. Reduce the proportion of children and adolescents with active and untreated tooth decay. Increase the proportion of children and adolescents who have dental sealants on one or more molars. Increase the proportion of children from families with low income who have a preventive dental visit.	• Encourage appropriate toothbrushing and flossing. • Educate child and family about fluoride use. • Refer school-age children to dentist for regular check-ups and interventions such as molar sealants. • Assist families lacking dental insurance to find resources for the provision of dental care.

Healthy People Objectives retrieved from http://www.healthypeople.gov

Children wearing braces are more prone to cavities; encourage them to brush their teeth after meals and snacks. School nurses can assist these children with brushing after lunch. In addition, the school nurse should promote dental health through education on dental care and gum problems that result from lack of proper dental care. Diet can play a part in dental health. Limiting sticky, high-sugar, and high-carbohydrate foods will decrease the possibility of cavities.

Promoting Appropriate Discipline

Because of the increasing ability of the school-age child to view situations from different angles, the school-age child should be able to see how their actions affect others. The school-age child is aware of the cause and effect of their behaviors and realizes that their behaviors have consequences. School-age children should be able to express emotions without using violence. Discipline techniques with consequences have both *natural* and *logical* consequences. Natural consequences allow the child to learn the results of their actions. For example, if the child throws a toy out of the window, they cannot play with the toy anymore. In logical consequences, if the child does not put away their bike, they do not get to ride the bike for the rest of the day.

In disciplining children, parents should teach children the rules established by the family, values, and social rules of conduct. Rules should provide the school-age child with guidelines about behavior that is acceptable and unacceptable. School-age children look to their parents for guidance and as role models. Parents should role model appropriate expressions of feelings and emotions and allow the child to express emotions and feelings. Discuss the effects of the child's temperament on their behavior, as well as what constitutes age-appropriate behavior. Include how the parents' temperament can influence the child's temperament.

Effective guidance and discipline focus on the development of the child. They can preserve the child's self-esteem and dignity. Discuss with parents guidelines regarding discipline. Explain to parents that they should never belittle the child. Children may view parents and caregivers negatively if they are consistently belittled or insulted. These negative actions can inhibit learning and teach the child to react unkindly to others. Instead, parents should discipline with praise. Positive acknowledgments of appropriate behavior and setting consistent appropriate limits are likely to encourage healthy development and appropriate behavior (Sege et al., 2018). Discuss with parents how to be realistic when planning activities so as not to overwhelm the child, resulting in misbehavior. Encourage parents to say "no" only when they mean it, to avoid a negative atmosphere in the home, and to avoid inconsistency.

When misbehaviors occur, the type and amount of discipline are based on different factors:

- Developmental level of both the child and the parents
- Severity of the misbehavior
- Established rules of the family
- Temperament of the child
- Response of the child to rewards

Keep in mind that school-age children should participate in developing a plan of action for their misbehavior. Whatever methods of discipline are chosen, it is important that parents are consistent in providing discipline in a nurturing environment.

ADDRESSING COMMON DEVELOPMENTAL CONCERNS

According to Erikson (1963), the developmental task of the school-age child is industry. The school-age child is busy learning, achieving, and exploring. As the school-age child becomes more independent, forces other than the family such as television, video games, and peers influence them. Some of these influences are positive and others are negative. Some of the common developmental concerns for the school-age child are discussed in the following sections. Guidelines to assist the parents and nurses when encountering these concerns are included in Teaching Guidelines 28.2.

TEACHING GUIDELINES 28.2 Addressing Common Developmental Concerns

Television, Video Games, and the Internet

- Establish a consistent time limit for any media use and develop a family media plan.
- Establish media-free times, such as mealtimes and car rides.
- Monitor television programs and internet activity.
- Prohibit television or video games with violence.
- Do not put television, video games, or internet-connected devices in children's bedrooms.
- Place computers in an open area that allows easy monitoring by an adult.
- Co-view television, video games, and internet content with the child.
- Encourage sports, interactive play, and reading.
- Teach your child internet safety, such as never to share personal information or meet a friend they have only met online without parental permission, never to share passwords, never to respond to a message that hurts their feelings or makes them uncomfortable, and never to send mean messages over the internet.
- Teach proper social media use.
- Be a good role model.

Maintaining Healthy Weight

- Provide healthy meals and snacks.
- Schedule and encourage daily exercise.
- Encourage involvement in sports and activities.
- Restrict TV, digital media, and video game use.
- Limit the amount of fast food intake.
- Provide education about healthy nutrition.
- Never use food as a reward.
- Be a good role model.

School Refusal

- Return the child to school.
- Investigate the cause of the fear.
- Support the child.
- Collaborate with teachers.
- Praise success in school attendance.

Children Who Are Home Alone

- Provide rules to follow and expectations, such as:
  - Not answering the door or phone
  - No friends in the house when parents are not home
  - No playing with fire
- Teach the child to call a trusted neighbor when help is needed and 911 in the event of emergency.
- Post all resource numbers (even numbers you think your child may have memorized), including afterschool help lines, if available, in a clearly viewable spot. Include the pediatrician's number and preferred hospital.
- Enroll the child in an afterschool program, if available.
- Discuss limitations of outside play.
- Discuss limitations of television viewing and video game use.
- Make sure the child knows how to contact the parent.
- Set clear homework expectations.
- *Do not* keep guns in the home.
- Teach the child where first-aid supplies are located.
- Teach the child household emergency procedures including for circuit breakers and water shut-off valves.
- Practice with your child. Have a trial run by leaving for a short time but staying close and role-playing situations that may occur.
- Always check in with your child while you are away.

Stealing

- Educate parents about the possibility of stealing.
- Discuss ways to teach the concepts of ownership and property rights.
- Handle the situation openly.
- Assist the child in developing and enacting a plan to return what was stolen.
- Make sure the punishment is appropriate for the action.

Lying

- Help parents in understanding why the child is lying.
- When the child lies, calmly confront the child and explain why the behavior is not acceptable.
- Educate parents that their behavior should reflect what they teach and expect from their child.
- Educate parents that too rigid or severe punishments can decrease the child's sense of worth.
- Seek professional help if lying persists in the older school-age child, to rule out underlying problems.

Cheating

- Educate parents that the child must be mature enough to understand the concept of rules.
- Handle cheating situations openly.
- Help parents to understand why their child is cheating and to modify the trigger.
- Develop an appropriate punishment; inappropriate punishment could undermine the child.
- Educate parents that their behavior should reflect what they expect from their child.
- Seek professional help if cheating persists in the older school-age child, to rule out underlying problems.

(*continued*)

TEACHING GUIDELINES **28.2** Addressing Common Developmental Concerns (*continued*)

Bullying

The Bullied Child

- Educate parents whose children are at risk for being bullied, such as:
  - Children who appear different from the majority
  - Children who act different from the majority
  - Children who have low self-esteem
  - Children with a mental or psychological problem
- Teach parents to role play different scenarios the child may face at school; show the child different ways to react to being bullied.
- Impress upon the child that they did not cause the bullying.
- Develop ways to increase the child's self-esteem at home.
- Discuss the situation with the teacher and develop a plan of care.

The Bullying Child

- Educate parents on reasons why it is important to correct the behavior.
- Discuss ways the child can appropriately show their anger and feelings.
- Have parents help the child to see how it feels to be bullied.
- Do not allow fighting at home.
- Reward settling of conflicts without violence.

Tobacco and Alcohol Education

- Inquire about tobacco and alcohol use.
- Discuss the physical and social dangers of tobacco and alcohol use.
- Urge parents to be good role models.
- Limit reading and media materials about alcohol and tobacco use.
- Discuss the influences of tobacco and alcohol use by peers.
- Educate the child on chewing tobacco. Let them know it is just as dangerous as smoking tobacco.
- Educate the child on e-cigarettes and the dangers associated with them.
- Advocate for a smoke-free environment in the home and other places frequented.
- Avoid having tobacco and alcohol products readily available in the home.

Television, Video Games, and the Internet

The influence of television, video games, digital media, and the internet on the school-age child is a growing concern for parents and child specialists. In today's world, the child is surrounded by digital media. School-age children use digital media for education, communication, and entertainment. They have access to thousands of apps, live streaming, streaming movies and TV shows, videos, games, and social media, all on multiple devices, from TVs and computers to smartphones and tablets. By the age of 18, a child will have seen 200,000 violent acts (Ben-Joseph, 2022). Although a school-age child can determine what is real from what is fantasy, research has shown that too much time in front of a screen—watching it or playing video games—can lead to aggressive behavior, less physical activity, and excess weight (Ben-Joseph, 2022; see Healthy People 2030).

Some television shows, video games, and internet activity can have positive influences on children, but parents should be taught guidelines on the use of TV, video games, digital media, and the internet. Parents should set limits on how much screen time the child can have. The AAP recommends that parents place consistent limits on media time and type and that there should be designated media-free times (American Academy of Pediatrics [AAP], Council on Communications and Media, 2016, reaffirmed 2022).

HEALTHY PEOPLE 2030

Objective	Nursing Significance
Increase the proportion of parents who follow AAP recommendations on limiting screen time for children aged 6 to 17 years.	• Encourage the family to develop a family media plan. • Assist families to identify activities other than television or video games for the child to participate in. • Praise craft, music, and sports participation.

Healthy People Objectives retrieved from http://www.healthypeople.gov

Television watching, internet activity, or video gaming should not be used as a reward. The parents should be aware of what the child is watching and doing online. This can be accomplished by parents and children watching programs together and parents using that opportunity to discuss the subject matter with the child. There should be no TV during dinner and no TV or internet-connected devices in the child's room. The parents need to set an example for the child by reading instead of using digital media or by doing a physical activity together as a family. If the TV or digital media causes fights or arguments, it should be turned off for a period of time.

TAKE NOTE!

According to the AAP age-based guidelines, school-age children need supervision and monitoring when using the internet to ensure they are not exposed to inappropriate material or content (AAP, Council on Communications and Media, 2016, reaffirmed 2022). Encourage parents of children in this age group to utilize internet safety tools that limit access to content and websites and that provide information on internet activities.

School Refusal

School refusal (also called *school phobia* or *school avoidance*) has been defined as a refusal to attend school or difficulty remaining in school for an entire day. Behaviors include frequent absences, skipping classes, being chronically late for school, severe misbehavior before school, or attending school with great fear. School phobia needs to be defined both symptomatically and operationally as the cause for the anxiety.

Some of the fears expressed by school-refusing children include separating from parents, riding the bus, tests, bullying, teacher reprimands, anxieties over toileting in a public bathroom, physical harm, or undressing in the locker room. Due to the emotional distress caused in these children when attending school, they are frequently classified as having school phobia. Young children may complain of stomachache or headache, and older children may complain of palpitations or feeling faint.

It is important to investigate specific causes of school refusal/school phobia and take appropriate actions. Often, school phobia is a symptom of deeper problems. The health care provider or nurse practitioner should conduct a physical examination of the child to rule out any physical illness. After these measures are taken, the parent, teacher, school counselor, and school administrator may devise a plan to assist the student to overcome a specific fear. In uncomplicated cases, parents must return the child to school as soon as possible. There may be altered schedules (partial days or decreased hours) to help promote a successful transition back to school. Another idea to help desensitize the child may be to have them spend part of the day in the counselor's or school nurse's office.

Children Who Are Home Alone

With the increasing incidence of both parents in the workforce and many children living with just one parent, children often return home alone without adult supervision for a number of hours. Most young children are not capable of handling stress or making decisions on their own before 11 or 12 years of age. However, some school-age children are more mature and can be left alone by 8 to 10 years of age; maturity is the key, not the age. Parents not only need to consider their child's maturity and readiness to be home alone but must also comply with legal requirements if present. Many states offer guidelines concerning when it is okay to leave a child alone at home, and a few states have laws with a minimum age, but these vary by state; therefore, the nurse needs to be familiar with the state and local laws in order to assist parents in making decisions about when it is appropriate for their child to be home alone (Child Welfare Information Gateway, 2018). However, the AAP continues to recommend that a school-age child come home to a parent or other responsible adult (AAP, 2022).

If children come home to no supervision, they should know the names, addresses, and phone numbers of parents and a neighbor, as well as emergency numbers. They should be given rules about answering the door and the phone. They should not answer the door and should tell anyone who calls that a parent is home but busy at this time. Directions as to the handling of the house key and fire safety should be taught and demonstrated (see Teaching Guidelines 28.2).

Stealing, Lying, and Cheating

Stealing, lying, and cheating are inappropriate behaviors that may occur during the school-age years. In most cases, these behaviors will result in a good lesson learned, and the child will outgrow them. In some cases, they may indicate a more severe psychological or behavioral problem. Parents are usually disturbed by these behaviors. In turn, they have difficulty in addressing these issues and need help providing appropriate interventions.

Children between 6 and 8 years old do not fully understand the concepts of ownership and property rights. These children may steal things because they like the look of the item. By the age of 9, the child should respect others' possessions and property and understand that stealing is wrong. The school-age child may steal because they desire the item, because they feel peer pressure and are trying to impress their peers, or because they have a sense of low self-esteem. Stealing becomes a concern if the child steals and does not have remorse or steals continuously or if stealing is accompanied by other behavioral problems (Johns Hopkins Medicine, n.d.).

Stealing and lying are both more common in boys and in children between 5 and 8 years old (Johns Hopkins Medicine, n.d.). It is acceptable for these children to tell tall tales, but they should know what truth is and what make-believe is. These younger children typically lie to avoid punishment. However, they do not like others to lie and will tell on them if they lie. Children between 8 and 12 years old typically lie because they are unable to meet expectations of family and peers, they are testing the rules and limits placed on them, or they are unable to explain bad behavior (Johns Hopkins Medicine, n.d.). If lying persists in older school-age children, if it is accompanied by other behavioral problems, or if the child does not show remorse with lying, parents should discuss the matter with a health care provider because the lying may be evidence of underlying problems.

The concept of cheating is not well understood until the child is about 6 to 7 years old. Before this age, the desire to "win" is most important, and rigid rules are hard to understand. In children between 8 and 12 years old, the concept of cheating is fully understood, and following of rules becomes more important (Johns Hopkins Medicine, n.d.). If cheating persists in older school-age children, parents should discuss the matter with a health care provider because the behavior may indicate underlying problems.

In dealing with children who exhibit stealing, lying, or cheating behaviors, parents must first realize the importance of their own behaviors in those areas. Parents are role models to the school-age child. Therefore, when the child sees or hears that parents lie, steal, or cheat (e.g., parents bragging about cheating on their taxes), they think it is all right to mimic those behaviors. Secondly, parents must directly confront any stealing, lying, or cheating behaviors and discuss (and follow through consistently with) the consequences of such behaviors (see Teaching Guideline 28.2).

Bullying

Bullying, which is inflicting unwanted, repeated verbal, emotional, or physical aggression on others and involves a power imbalance, is widespread and negatively impacts all parties involved (CDC, 2021). Utilizing e-mail, text messages, social media, and instant messaging, often referred to as cyberbullying, is a growing concern. Bullies often look for victims who appear shy, weak, and defenseless.

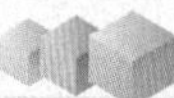

Concept Mastery Alert

Most often, children who bully have low self-esteem, poor grades, and poor interpersonal skills. Both male and female children are bullied, but male children tend to bully other male children and more often show force when bullying.

Being bullied can have negative results on children throughout life. These children often have increased episodes of headaches, stomachaches, sleep problems, anxiety, loneliness, depression, substance use, lower academic achievement, and suicidal tendencies (Moreno & Englander, 2020). After the problem of either being bullied or being the bully has been identified, parents must work with the child, the school, and the health care provider or nurse practitioner to solve the problem (see Teaching Guidelines 28.2 and Evidence-Based Practice 28.1).

Tobacco and Alcohol Education

School-age children are eager to grow up and be independent. Peers and acceptance are very important at this time. School-age children may be exposed to messages that are in conflict with their parents' values regarding smoking and alcohol. Peers often exert pressure for children to experiment with tobacco and alcohol.

School-age children are ready to absorb information that deals with drugs and alcohol. Information from parents or other adults who are major influences in the child's life is essential at this time to set clear rules and

EVIDENCE-BASED PRACTICE **28.1**

Meta-Analysis of the Effectiveness of School-Based Programs to Reduce Bullying Perpetration and Victimization

STUDY

Bullying perpetration and victimization continue to pose a problem in elementary schools. In addition to the behavioral disruption that occurs as a result of bullying perpetration and victimization, prior research has demonstrated that child bullies and victims are at increased risk for mental health problems, such as depression, anxiety, low self-esteem, suicidal ideation, and low social competence. Adverse consequences from bullying have led to prevention programs to decrease peer victimization. This systematic review and meta-analysis summarized 100 studies to evaluate the effectiveness of face-to-face school-based antibullying programs.

Findings

The results of this analysis found that school-based antibullying programs are effective in reducing bully perpetration by approximately 18% to 19% and bully victimization by approximately 15% to 16%. Variations in the effectiveness of intervention programs were found and demonstrate a need for further research to explore these variations.

Nursing Implications

Nurses should continue to educate parents and teachers about bullying. Become actively involved in the local elementary school bullying-prevention program, and encourage a whole school comprehensive approach. Further research is needed to determine which programs are most effective.

Data from Gaffney, H., Ttofi, M. M., & Farrington, D. P. (2021). Effectiveness of school-based programs to reduce bullying perpetration and victimization: An updated systematic review and meta-analysis. *Campbell Systematic Reviews, 17*(2), e1143. https://doi.org/10.1002/cl2.1143

model behaviors for children to embrace. Discussions with children need to be based on facts and focused on the present. Some topics for discussion include:

- What alcohol and drugs are like and how they harm you
- Differences in medical use versus illegal use of drugs
- How to think critically to interpret messages seen in advertising, media, and sports and from entertainment personalities

Recall Lawrence Jones, the 10-year-old presented at the beginning of the chapter. List potential developmental problems he may experience. What anticipatory guidance related to these concerns should you provide to his parent?

Unfolding Patient Stories: Charlie Snow • Part 1

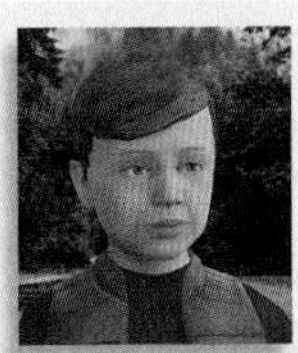

Charlie Snow, a 6-year-old with a known hypersensitivity to perfumes and dyes and an allergy to peanuts, comes for a routine clinic visit accompanied by his aunt. He is living with his aunt and uncle while his parents are serving in the military. The nurse discovers a rash in multiple areas underneath his clothing. What questions should the nurse ask to determine the cause of the rash? What education should the nurse provide for his aunt, who has limited knowledge of allergies and child care experience? (Charlie Snow's story continues in Chapter 47.)

Care for Charlie and other patients in a realistic virtual environment: ***vSim** for Nursing* (thepoint.lww.com/vSimPediatric). Practice documenting these patients' care in DocuCare (thePoint.lww.com/DocuCareEHR).

KEY CONCEPTS

- Physical growth is slow and steady, with social and cognitive development progressing rapidly, during the school-age years of 6 to 12. Height increases approximately 6 to 7 cm (2.5 in) per year, and weight gain is 3 to 3.5 kg (7 lb) per year. Males are generally taller and heavier than females during this period.
- With entrance into the school system, school-age children have the influences of peers and teachers.
- With the development of gross motor skills and involvement in sports at school and in the community, safety education and practices are required. Also, with participation in cooperative sports, injuries occur.
- Increased independence leads to increased exposure to safety hazards.
- The school-age child develops the cognitive ability to classify objects and to identify relationships among objects.
- Dental care is very important to prevent dental caries, malocclusion, and other problems. In early school age, the first primary teeth will be lost.
- The onset of puberty may occur by the later school-aged years.
- Erikson's (1963) developmental task for the age group is the development of a sense of industry.
- Peers are important, especially peers of the same gender. School-age children usually have a best friend and belong to clubs. They have collections of nonvaluable items such as rocks, clips, and so forth.
- School-age children are capable of concrete operations, solving problems, and making decisions. They continue to need guidance, rules, and direction from parents.
- The school-age child develops a conscience and knows cultural and social values. They can understand and obey rules.
- The school-age child incorporates spiritual or religious practices into their life, which may be a source of comfort during stressful times.
- The nurse's role includes educating parents and school-age children in promoting health and safety.
- Nurses should inform the school-age child about expected developmental changes in the body to promote self-esteem and self-confidence.

REFERENCES AND RECOMMENDED READINGS

American Academy of Pediatrics. (2022). *Back-to-school tips for families.* https://www.healthychildren.org/English/ages-stages/gradeschool/school/Pages/Back-to-School-Tips.aspx

American Academy of Pediatrics, Council on Communications and Media. (2016, reaffirmed 2022). Policy statement: Media use in school-aged children and adolescents. *Pediatrics, 138*(5), e20162592. https://doi.org/10.1542/peds.2016-2592

American Academy of Pediatrics, HealthyChildren. (2021). *Booster seats for school-aged children.* https://www.healthychildren.org/English/safety-prevention/on-the-go/Pages/Booster-Seats-for-School-Aged-Children.aspx

American Association for Pediatric Ophthalmology and Strabismus. (2021). *Amblyopia.* https://aapos.org/glossary/amblyopia

Ben-Joseph, E. P. (2022). *How media use can affects kids.* https://kidshealth.org/en/parents/tv-affects-child.html#catsafe-play

Biro, F. M., & Chan, Y.-M. (2023). Normal puberty. UpToDate. Retrieved October 10, 2023, from https://www.uptodate.com/contents/normal-puberty

Bogues, L., & Levine, D. A. (2023). Section 2: Growth and development. Chapter 7: Normal development. In K. J. Marcdante, R. M. Kleigman, & A. M. Schuh (Eds.), *Nelson essentials of pediatrics* (9th ed., pp. 14–16). Elsevier.

Centers for Disease Control and Prevention. (2021). *Preventing bullying.* https://www.cdc.gov/violenceprevention/pdf/yv/Bullying-factsheet_508_1.pdf

Centers for Disease Control and Prevention. (2022a). *Childhood obesity facts.* https://www.cdc.gov/obesity/data/childhood.html

Centers for Disease Control and Prevention. (2022b). *Physical activity facts.* https://www.cdc.gov/healthyschools/physicalactivity/facts.htm

Child Welfare Information Gateway. (2018). *Leaving your child home alone.* U.S. Department of Health and Human Services, Children's Bureau. https://www.childwelfare.gov/pubPDFs/homealone.pdf

CHOC. (2021). *Growth & development: 6 to 12 years (school age).* https://www.choc.org/primary-care/ages-stages/6-to-12-years/

Cincinnati Children's. (2023). *Growth, range of height and weight.* https://www.cincinnatichildrens.org/health/g/normal-growth

Clark, M. B., Keels, M. A., Slayton, R. L., & AAP Section on Oral Health. (2020). Fluoride use in caries prevention in the primary care setting. *Pediatrics, 146*(6), Article e2020034637. https://doi.org/10.1542/peds.2020-034637

Erikson, E. (1963). *Childhood and society* (2nd ed.). Norton.

Feigelman, S. (2020). Developmental & behavioral theories. In R. M. Kleigman, J. W. St. Geme, III, N. J. Blum, S. S. Shah, R. C. Tasker, K. M. Wislon, & R. E. Behrman (Eds.), *Nelson textbook of pediatrics* (21st ed., pp. 1233–1257). Elsevier.

Finkelstein, L. H., & Feigelman, S. (2020). Middle childhood. In R. M. Kleigman, J. W. St. Geme, III, N. J. Blum, S. S. Shah, R. C. Tasker, K. M. Wislon, & R. E. Behrman (Eds.), *Nelson textbook of pediatrics* (21st ed., pp. 1358–1373). Elsevier.

Gaffney, H., Ttofi, M. M., & Farrington, D. P. (2021). Effectiveness of school-based programs to reduce bullying perpetration and victimization: An updated systematic review and meta-analysis. *Campbell Systematic Reviews, 17*(2), e1143. https://doi.org/10.1002/cl2.1143

Gill, A. C. (2022). Bicycle injuries in children: Prevention. *UpToDate.* Retrieved October 17, 2022, from https://www.uptodate.com/contents/bicycle-injuries-in-children-prevention

Gill, A. C., & Kelly, N. R. (2022). Pediatric injury prevention: Epidemiology, history, and application. *UpToDate.* Retrieved October 19, 2022, from https://www.uptodate.com/contents/pediatric-injury-prevention-epidemiology-history-and-application

Jennissen, C. (2022). *ATVs are not safe for children: AAP policy explained.* https://www.healthychildren.org/English/safety-prevention/at-play/Pages/ATV-Safety-Rules.aspx

Johns Hopkins Medicine. (n.d.). *Lying and stealing. Health Library.* Retrieved October 22, 2022, from https://www.hopkinsmedicine.org/healthlibrary/conditions/pediatrics/lying_and_stealing_90,P02241

Kohlberg, L. (1984). *Moral development.* Harper & Row.

Moreno, M. A., & Englander, E. (2020). Bullying, cyberbullying, and school violence. In R. M. Kleigman, J. W. St. Geme, III, N. J. Blum, S. S. Shah, R. C. Tasker, K. M. Wislon, & R. E. Behrman (Eds.), *Nelson textbook of pediatrics* (21st ed., pp. 1083–1087). Elsevier.

Morse, A. M., & Kotagal, S. (2021). Parasomnias of childhood, including sleepwalking. *UpToDate.* Retrieved October 13, 2023, from https://www.uptodate.com/contents/parasomnias-of-childhood-including-sleepwalking

Nowak, A. J., & Warren, J. J. (2022). Preventive dental care and counseling for infants and young children. *UpToDate.* Retrieved October 17, 2022, from https://www.uptodate.com/contents/preventive-dental-care-and-counseling-for-infants-and-young-children

Oh, C., Carducci, B., Vaivada, T., & Bhutta, Z. A. (2022). Interventions to promote physical activity and healthy digital media use in children and adolescents: A systematic review. *Pediatrics, 149*(Suppl. 6), e2021053852I. https://doi.org/10.1542/peds.2021-053852I

Piaget, J. (1969). *The theory of stages in cognitive development.* McGraw-Hill.

Radcliff, Z. (2023). Childhood Fears and Worries. https://kidshealth.org/en/parents/anxiety.html

Safe Kids Worldwide. (2023). *FAST facts pedestrian injuries among children in 2021.* https://www.safekids.org/sites/default/files/documents/fast_facts_-_2021_-_pedestrian_injuries.pdf

Sege, R. D., Siegel, B. S., AAP Council on Child Abuse and Neglect, & AAP Committee on Psychosocial Aspects of Child and Family Health. (2018). Effective discipline to raise healthy children. *Pediatrics, 142*(6), Article 20183112. https://doi.org/10.1542/peds.2018-3112

Skelton, J. A., & Klish, W. J. (2023). Definition, epidemiology, and etiology of obesity in children and adolescents. *UpToDate.* Retrieved October 12, 2023, from https://www.uptodate.com/contents/definition-epidemiology-and-etiology-of-obesity-in-children-and-adolescents

U.S. Department of Agriculture, & U.S. Department of Health and Human Services. (2020). *Dietary guidelines for Americans, 2020–2025.* (9th ed.) https://www.dietaryguidelines.gov/sites/default/files/2021-03/Dietary_Guidelines_for_Americans-2020-2025.pdf

U.S. Department of Health and Human Services. (n.d.). *Healthy People 2030.* https://health.gov/healthypeople

U.S. Department of Health and Human Services, Administration for Children and Families, Administration on Children, Youth and Families, Children's Bureau. (2022). *Child maltreatment 2020.* https://www.acf.hhs.gov/cb/data-research/child-maltreatment

DEVELOPING CLINICAL JUDGMENT

PRACTICING FOR NCLEX

1. The successful resolution of developmental tasks for the school-age child, according to Erikson, would be identified by:
   a. learning from repeating tasks.
   b. developing a sense of worth and competence.
   c. using fantasy and magical thinking to cope with problems.
   d. developing a sense of trust.
2. Which of the following are reasons that school-age children steal? Select all that apply.
   a. To escape punishment
   b. High self-esteem
   c. Low expectations of family/peers
   d. Lack of sense of property
   e. Strong desire to own something
3. Which activities will promote weight loss in a school-age child with higher body weight? Select all that apply.
   a. Unlimited computer and TV time
   b. Role modeling by family
   c. Becoming active in sports
   d. Eating unstructured meals
   e. Involving the child in meal planning and grocery shopping
   f. Drinking seven to eight glasses of water per day
4. Samantha, a 10-year-old, is brought into your clinic for a well-child examination. The parent states, "Samantha's friend group seems to be so much more important to them these days." As the nurse caring for the child, how would you explain the role of peers in the school-age child?
   a. This allows them the opportunity to learn conflict management.
   b. This helps them to shape their concept of self and provides security as they gain independence from their parents.
   c. This will encourage them to remain dependent on their teachers and family.
   d. This will help them to work through their fears of body safety.
5. The parent of two children, ages 6 and 9, states the children want to play on the same baseball team. As the school nurse, what advice would you give their parent?
   a. Having the children on the same team will make it more convenient for the family.
   b. Levels of coordination and concentration differ, so the children need to be on different teams.
   c. Put the children on the same team because they are both school-age children.
   d. It is best to avoid putting the children on the same team to prevent sibling rivalry.
6. The nursing student is caring for a 9-year-old child. According to Piaget's cognitive development theory, the nurse can expect the child to understand the principle of __________ and have a concept of __________ as the school-age child is in the ______________ stage.

   Blanks 1 and 2:
   a. Spatial reasoning
   b. Space
   c. Conservation
   d. Elasticity
   e. Time
   f. Representation

   Blank 3:
   a. Preoperational
   b. Sensorimotor
   c. Formal operational
   d. Concrete operational

CRITICAL THINKING EXERCISES

1. Ms. Sams brings her 8-year-old, Frank, to the health care provider's office for his annual examination. She states that she is concerned about his recent behavior. He went to the grocery store with his friend and his friend's parent, and he came home with a Matchbox car. The friend's parent stated she had not purchased the car.
   a. What would be your response to Ms. Sams?
   b. Ms. Sams said she still has the car. What would you advise Ms. Sams to do to make Frank aware of the consequences of his actions?
2. Sally's parent is asking the nurse for advice about purchasing a two-wheeled bike for her 7-year-old. What guidance should the nurse offer this parent?
3. Ms. Shaw brings in her 11-year-old daughter for a well-child check-up. The school-ager says to the nurse, "I look different from my friends. I do not wear bras, and my friends are already wearing bras." What would be an appropriate response to this school-ager?
4. Johnny is a 9-year-old whose parents both work during the day. He returns home alone after school. How should the parents prepare Johnny for this experience? What safety rules would be included in the education for Johnny?

STUDY ACTIVITIES

1. Attend a sporting event (such as soccer or baseball) with school-age teams. Describe the coordination and gross motor functioning of this group.
2. Attend a first-grade class. Observe the behaviors exhibited by the school-age children in this class. How do these behaviors compare with expected values for this age group?

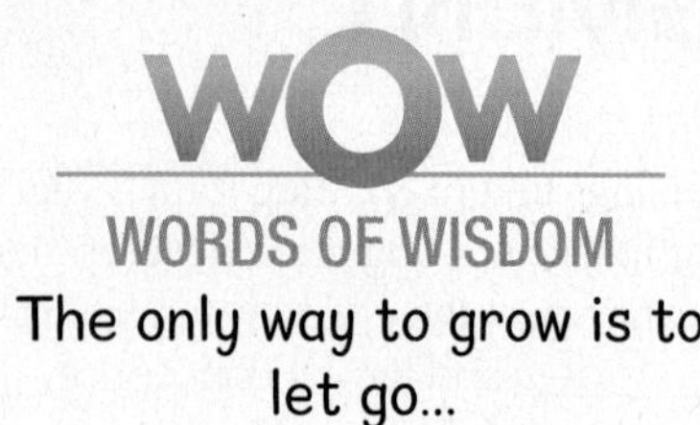

The only way to grow is to let go...

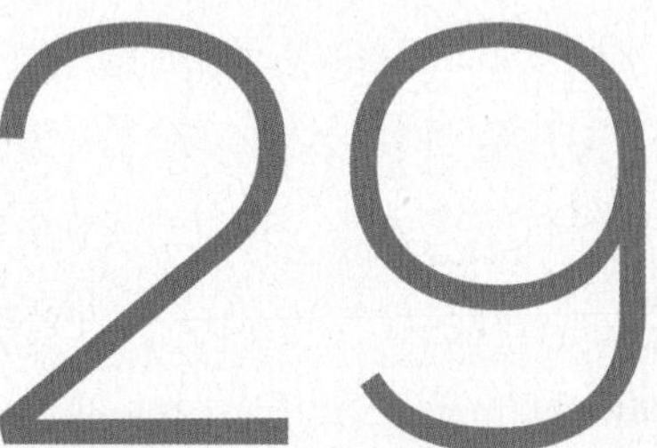

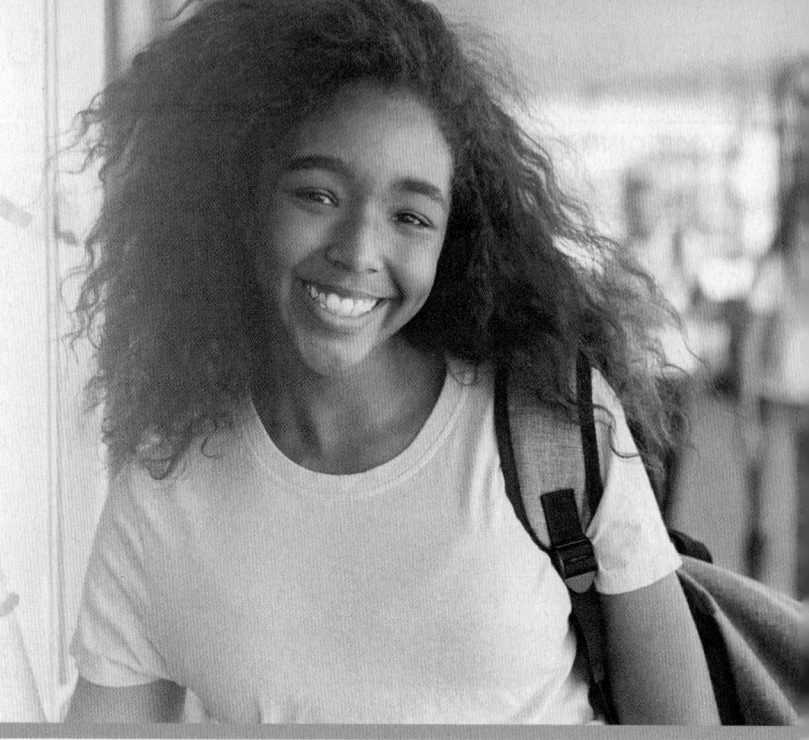

Growth and Development of the Adolescent

LEARNING OBJECTIVES

Upon completion of the chapter, you will be able to:

1. Identify normal physiologic changes, including puberty, occurring in the adolescent.
2. Discuss psychosocial, cognitive, social, and moral changes occurring in the adolescent.
3. Identify changes in relationships with peers, family, teachers, and community during adolescence.
4. Describe interventions to promote safety during adolescence.
5. Demonstrate knowledge of the nutritional requirements of the adolescent.
6. Demonstrate knowledge of the development of sexuality and its influence on dating during adolescence.
7. Identify common developmental concerns of the adolescent.
8. Demonstrate knowledge of the appropriate nursing guidance for common developmental concerns.

KEY TERMS

adolescence
menarche (men-ahr´kē)
peer groups
puberty
risk-taking behaviors
sexuality
thelarche (thē-lahr´kē)

Cho Chung is a 15-year-old brought to the clinic by her parent for her annual school check-up. As the nurse caring for her, assess Cho's growth and development, and then provide appropriate anticipatory guidance to her parent.

INTRODUCTION

Adolescence spans the years of transition from childhood to adulthood, which is usually between the ages of 11 and 20 years. There is some overlap between late school age and adolescence. The adolescent experiences drastic changes in the physical, cognitive, psychosocial, and psychosexual areas. With this rapid growth during adolescence, the development of secondary sexual characteristics, and amorous interest in peers, the adolescent needs the support and guidance of parents and nurses to facilitate a healthy lifestyle and to reduce **risk-taking behaviors** such as drinking, drug use, unsafe sexual activity, and participating in reckless behavior or dangerous activities. Not all adolescents will align with the sex they are assigned at birth; in this chapter, the term "male" will be used to refer to those born with male internal and external genitalia, and "female" will be used to refer to those born with female internal and external genitalia.

GROWTH AND DEVELOPMENT OVERVIEW

Adolescence is a time of rapid growth with dramatic changes in body size and proportions. The magnitude of these changes is second only to the growth in infancy. During this time, sexual characteristics develop, and reproductive maturity is achieved. The age of onset and the duration of the physiologic changes vary from individual to individual. Generally, females enter puberty earlier (at 9 to 10 years of age) than males (at 10 to 11 years; Table 29.1). Adolescents will represent varying levels of identity formation and will offer unique challenges to the nurse.

PHYSIOLOGIC CHANGES ASSOCIATED WITH PUBERTY

The secretion of estrogen in females and testosterone in males stimulates the development of breast tissue in females, pubic hair in both sexes, and changes in male genitalia. These biologic changes that occur during adolescence are known as **puberty**. Puberty is the result of triggers from the environment, the central nervous system, the hypothalamus, the pituitary gland, the gonads, and the adrenal glands. Gonadotropin-releasing hormone (GnRH), produced by the hypothalamus, travels to the anterior pituitary gland to stimulate the production and secretion of follicle-stimulating hormone (FSH) and luteinizing hormone (LH). The increased levels of FSH and LH stimulate the gonadal response. LH stimulates ovulation in females and acts on testicular Leydig cells in males, prompting maturation of the testicles and testosterone production. FSH with LH stimulates sperm production. Estrogen, progesterone, and testosterone and other androgens are released from the gonads and affect biologic changes and changes in various organs, including alterations in muscles, bones, skin, and hair follicles.

Females reach physical maturity before males, and **menarche**, the first menstrual period, usually begins between the ages of 9 and 15 years (average 12.8 years). Breast budding (**thelarche**) occurs at approximately age 9 to 11 years and is followed by the growth of pubic hair.

TABLE 29.1 • Physiologic Changes of Adolescence

Stage of Adolescence	Changes in Females	Changes in Males
Early adolescence (10–13 years)	Pubic hair begins to curl and spread over mons pubis; genitalia pigmentation increases. Breast bud and areola continue to enlarge; no separation of breasts. First menstrual period (average 12 years, normal range 9–16 years)	Pubic hair spreads laterally, begins to curl; pigmentation increases. Growth and enlargement of testes in scrotum (scrotum reddish in color) and continued lengthening of penis Leggy look due to extremities growing faster than the trunk
Middle adolescence (15–17 years)	Pubic hair becomes coarse in texture and continues to curl; amount of hair increases. Areola and papilla separate from the contour of the breast to form a secondary mound.	Pubic hair becomes coarser in texture and takes on adult distribution. Testes and scrotum continue to grow; scrotal skin darkens; penis grows in width, and glans penis develops. May experience breast enlargement Voice changes; more masculine due to rapid enlargement of the larynx and pharynx as well as lung changes
Late adolescence (18–21 years)	Mature pubic hair distribution and coarseness	Mature pubic hair distribution and coarseness Breast enlargement disappears Adult size and shape of testes, scrotum, and penis; scrotal skin darkening

Data from Holland-Hall, C. (2020). Adolescent physical and social development. In R. M. Kleigman, J. W. St. Geme, III, N. J. Blum, S. S. Shah, R. C. Tasker, K. M. Wilson, & R. E. Behrman (Eds.), *Nelson textbook of pediatrics* (21st ed., pp. 5550–5576). Elsevier.

TAKE NOTE!

Black females, on average, reach menarche slightly earlier than White females (Blake & Van Eyk, 2023a).

The first sign of pubertal changes in males is testicular enlargement in response to testosterone secretion, usually occurring in Tanner stage 2. As testosterone levels increase, the penis and scrotum enlarge, hair distribution increases, and scrotal skin texture changes. During late puberty, males will typically experience their first ejaculation, which may occur while they are sleeping (nocturnal emissions). Nurses should provide anticipatory guidance to adolescent males regarding involuntary nocturnal emissions (wet dreams) to assure them that this is an expected occurrence.

Tanner stages 3 to 5 usually occur during adolescence. Refer to Figures 10.28, 10.36, and 10.34 for an illustration of the increase in breast tissue and pubic hair distribution in females and scrotal and penile changes as well as hair distribution changes in males. The nurse should provide guidance to adolescents about the normalcy of the sexual feelings and evolving body changes that occur during puberty.

PHYSICAL GROWTH

Diet, exercise, and hereditary factors influence the height, weight, and body build of the adolescent. Over the past three decades, adolescents have become taller and heavier than their ancestors, and the beginning of puberty is earlier. During the early adolescent period, there is an increase in the percentage of body fat, and the head, neck, and hands reach adult proportions.

The rapid growth during adolescence is secondary only to that of the infant years and is a direct result of the hormonal changes of puberty. Adolescents experience changes in appearance and size. Height in females increases rapidly before menarche and usually ceases 2 to 2½ years after menarche. The growth spurt in males occurs later than in females and usually begins between the ages of 10½ and 16 years and ends sometime between the ages of 13½ and 17½ years. Muscle mass increases in males, and fat deposits increase in females (Fig. 29.1).

During early adolescence, growth is rapid, but it decreases in middle and late adolescence. Height for adolescent males who are between the 50th and 95th percentile ranges from 132 cm (52½ in) to 176.8 cm (69½ in). Weight of males in these percentiles ranges from 35.3 kg (77¼ lb) to 95.76 kg (211 lb). On average, males will gain 10 to 30 cm (4 to 12 in) in height and 7 to 30 kg (15 to 65 lb) in weight.

Height for females who are between the 50th and 95th percentile ranges from 144.8 cm (57 in) to 173.6 cm (68½ in), with weight ranging from 27.24 kg (60 lb) to 82.47 kg (181 lb). On average, females will gain 5 to 20 cm (2 to 8 in) in height and 7 to 25 kg (15 to 55 lb) in weight during adolescence. See Appendix D for growth charts for this age group. Refer to Chapter 32, Box 32.1, for instructions for calculating body mass index (BMI).

Remember Cho Chung, the 15-year-old introduced at the beginning of the chapter. During your assessment, you measure Cho's weight at 49.89 kg (110 lb) and her height at 152.4 cm (60 in). Plot Cho's measurements on the appropriate growth chart.

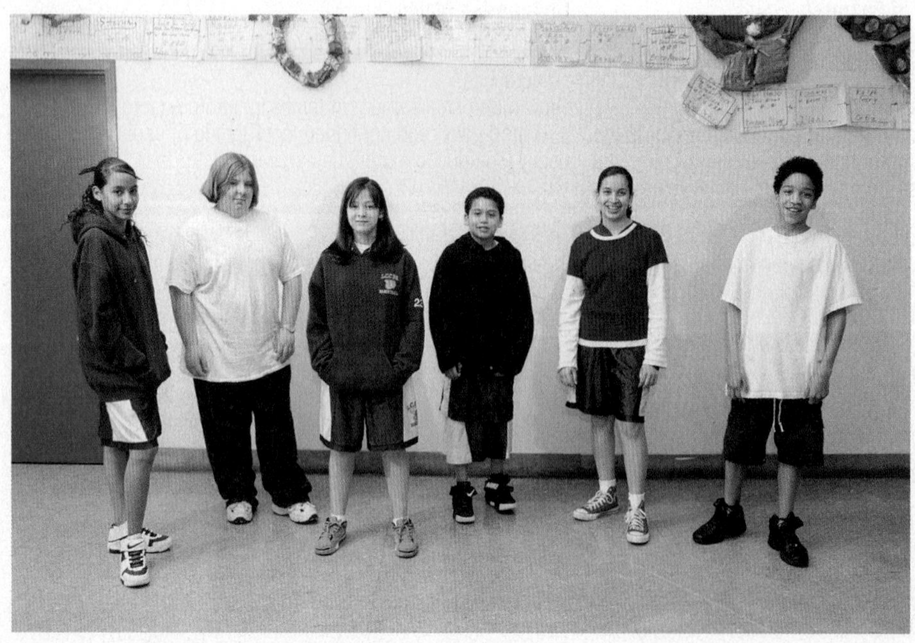

FIGURE 29.1 These adolescents reflect the differences in sizes and shapes seen in adolescents of the same age.

PHYSIOLOGIC CHANGES

Adolescence is a time of metabolic slowing and of increasing size of some organs. The basal metabolic rate (BMR) reaches the adult level during late adolescence.

Neurologic System

During adolescence, there is continued brain growth, although the size of the brain does not increase significantly. Neurons do not increase in number, but growth of the myelin sheath enables faster neural processing.

Respiratory System

The adolescent years see an increase in diameter and length of the lungs. Respiratory rate decreases and reaches the adult rate of 15 to 20 breaths/min. Respiratory volume and vital capacity increase. Volume and capacity are greater in males than females, which may be associated with increased chest and shoulder size in males. The growth of the laryngeal cartilage, larynx, pharynx, vocal cords, and lungs produces the voice changes experienced in adolescence. These changes in the quality of the child's voice are often preceded by some voice instability, where voice cracking is heard. Deepening of both male and female voices occurs but is more pronounced in males.

Cardiovascular System

There is an increase in size and strength of the heart. Systolic blood pressure increases and heart rate decreases. Blood volume reaches higher levels in males, which may be due to their greater muscle mass.

Gastrointestinal System

The adolescent has a full set of permanent teeth with the exception of the last four molars (wisdom teeth), which may erupt between the ages of 17 and 20 years. The liver, spleen, kidneys, and digestive tract enlarge during the growth spurt in early adolescence, but do not change in function. These systems are mature in early school age.

Musculoskeletal System

The ossification of the skeletal system is incomplete until late adolescence in males. Ossification is more advanced in females and occurs at an earlier age. During the growth spurt, muscle mass and strength increase. At similar stages of development, muscle development is generally greater in males. Estrogen, progesterone, and testosterone (sex steroids) and other androgens are released from the gonads and affect changes in the muscles and bones. Low estrogen levels tend to stimulate skeletal growth, while higher levels inhibit growth. During middle adolescence, shoulder, chest, and hip breadth increase.

Integumentary System

During adolescence, the skin becomes thick and tough. Under the influence of androgens, the sebaceous glands become more active, particularly on the face, back, and genitals. Due to the increased levels of testosterone during Tanner stages 4 and 5, adolescents may have increased sebum production, which may lead to the development of acne and oily hair.

The exocrine and apocrine sweat glands function at adult levels during adolescence. The exocrine glands are all over the body, and they produce sweat, which helps to eliminate body heat through evaporation. The apocrine glands are found in the axillae, genital, and anal areas and around the breasts. The apocrine sweat glands produce sweat in response to hair follicles. This sweat is produced continuously and is stored and released in response to emotional stimuli.

PSYCHOSOCIAL DEVELOPMENT

According to Erikson, it is during adolescence that individuals achieve a sense of identity (Erikson, 1963). As the adolescent is trying out many different roles in regard to their relationships with peers, family, community, and society, they are developing their own individual sense of self. If the adolescent is not successful in forming their own sense of self, they develop a sense of role confusion or diffusion. The adolescent culture becomes important to the individual. It is through their involvement with adolescent groups that the individual finds support and help with developing their own identity.

Erikson (1963) believed that during the task of developing their own sense of identity, the adolescent revisits each of the previous stages of development. The sense of trust is encountered as the adolescent strives to find out in whom and in what ideals they can have faith. In revisiting the stage of autonomy, the adolescent is seeking out ways to express their individuality in an effective manner. The adolescent would avoid behaviors that would "shame" or ridicule them in front of their peers. The sense of initiative is revisited as the adolescent develops their vision for what they might become. And the sense of industry is again encountered as the adolescent makes their choice to participate in different activities at school, in the community, at church, and in the workforce.

The ability of the adolescent to successfully form a sense of self is dependent on how well the adolescent successfully completed the former stages of development.

TABLE 29.2 • Developmental Theories

Theories	Stages	Activities
Erikson (psychosocial)	Identity vs. role confusion or diffusion Early (10–13 years)	Focuses on bodily changes Experiences frequent mood changes Importance placed on conformity to peer norms and peer acceptance Strives to master skills within peer groups Defining boundaries with parents and authority figures Early stage of emancipation—struggles to separate from parents while still desiring dependence on them Identifies with same-sex peers Takes more responsibility for own behaviors
	Middle (14–16 years)	Continues to adjust to changed body image Tries out different roles within peer groups Need for acceptance by peer group at the highest level Interested in being romantically attractive to peers Time of greatest conflict with parents/authority figures
	Late (17–20 years)	Able to understand implications of behavior and decisions Roles within peer groups established Feels secure with body image Has matured sexual identity Has idealistic career goals Importance of individual friendships emerges Process of emancipation from family almost complete
Piaget (cognitive)	Formal operations Early (10–13 years)	Limited abstract thought process Egocentrical thinking Eager to apply limited abstract process to different situations and to peer groups
	Middle (14–17 years)	Increased ability to think abstractly or in more idealistic terms Able to solve verbal and mental problems using scientific methods Thinks they are invincible—risky behaviors increase Likes making independent decisions Becomes involved/concerned with society, politics
	Late (17–20 years)	Abstract thinking establishes Develops critical thinking skills—tests different solutions to problems Less risky behaviors Develops realistic goals and career plans
Kohlberg	Postconventional level III	Morals based on peer, family, church, and societal morals
	Early (10–13 years)	Asks broad, usually unanswerable questions about life
	Middle (14–17 years)	Developing own set of morals—evaluates individual morals in relation to peer, family, and societal morals
	Late (17–20 years)	Internalizes own morals and values Continues to compare own morals and values with those of society Evaluates morals of others

Data from Erikson, E. (1963). *Childhood and society* (2nd ed.). Norton; Kohlberg, L. (1984). *Moral development.* Harper & Row; and Piaget, J. (1969). *The theory of stages in cognitive development.* McGraw-Hill.

Erikson (1963) believed that if the adolescent has been successful, they can develop resources during adolescence to overcome any gaps in previous developmental stages. If the adolescent believes that they cannot express themselves in any manner due to societal restrictions, they will develop role confusion. See Table 29.2 for additional information.

COGNITIVE DEVELOPMENT

According to Piaget, the adolescent progresses from a concrete framework of thinking to an abstract one (Piaget, 1969). During this formal operational period, the adolescent develops the ability to think outside of the present; that is, they can incorporate into thinking concepts that do exist as well as concepts that might exist. The adolescent's thinking becomes logical, organized, and consistent. They are able to think about a problem from all points of view, ranking the possible solutions while solving the problem. Not all adolescents achieve formal operational reasoning at the same time.

In the early stages of formal operational reasoning, the adolescent's thinking is egocentric, thinking they are at the center of everyone's attention. The adolescent is idealistic, constantly challenging the way things are and wondering why things cannot change. These activities lead to the adolescent's feeling of being omnipotent. The adolescent must undergo this way of thinking, even though it can frustrate adults, in their quest to reach formal operational reasoning. As the individual progresses toward middle adolescence, their thinking becomes introspective. They assume others are just as interested in what interests them, which leads them to feel unique, special, and exceptional. That feeling of "being exceptional" leads to the risk-taking behaviors for which adolescents are well known. Also, the adolescent feels very committed to their viewpoints. They try very hard to convince others of their viewpoints and strongly embrace those causes that support their opinions. This idealism can cause the adolescent to reject their family, culture, religion, and community beliefs, which can cause conflict. See Table 29.2 for additional information.

MORAL AND SPIRITUAL DEVELOPMENT

It is during the adolescent years that individuals develop their own set of values and morals. According to Kohlberg, adolescents are experiencing the postconventional stage of moral development (Kohlberg, 1984). It is only because adolescents are developing their formal operational way of thinking that they can experience the postconventional stage of moral development. At the beginning of this stage, adolescents begin to question the status quo. The majority of their choices are based on emotions while they are questioning societal standards. As they progress to developing their own set of morals, adolescents realize that moral decisions are based on rights, values, and principles that are agreeable to a given society. They also realize that those rights, values, and principles can be in conflict with the laws of the given society, but they are able to reconcile the differences. Because adolescents undergo the process of developing their own set of morals at different rates, they might find that their friends view a situation differently. This difference can lead to conflicts and the forming of different friendships. See Table 29.2 for additional information.

Adolescents may also begin to question their formal religious practices or in some cases cling to them (Ford, 2007). As they progress through adolescence, individuals may become more interested in the spiritualism of their religion than in the actual practices of their religion. Adolescents are searching for ideals and may exhibit intense emotions along with introspection (Ford, 2007). Increased spirituality and religious activities are related to increased healthy behaviors and decreased high-risk behaviors (Ford, 2007).

Referring back to Cho Chung, identify the stage of psychosocial development that she should be in according to Erikson. What approaches for assessment and teaching would be most effective based on the stage you identified?

MOTOR SKILL DEVELOPMENT

During adolescence, the individual refines and continues to develop their gross and fine motor skills. Because of this period of rapid growth spurts, adolescents may experience times of decreased coordination and have a diminished ability to perform previously learned skills, which can be worrisome for the adolescent.

Gross Motor Skills

It is usually during early adolescence that individuals begin to develop endurance. Their concentration has increased, so they can follow complicated instructions. Coordination can be a problem because of the uneven growth spurts. During middle adolescence, speed and accuracy increase while coordination also improves. Adolescents become more competitive with each other (Fig. 29.2). During late adolescence, the individual usually narrows their areas of interest and concentrates on the needed relevant skills.

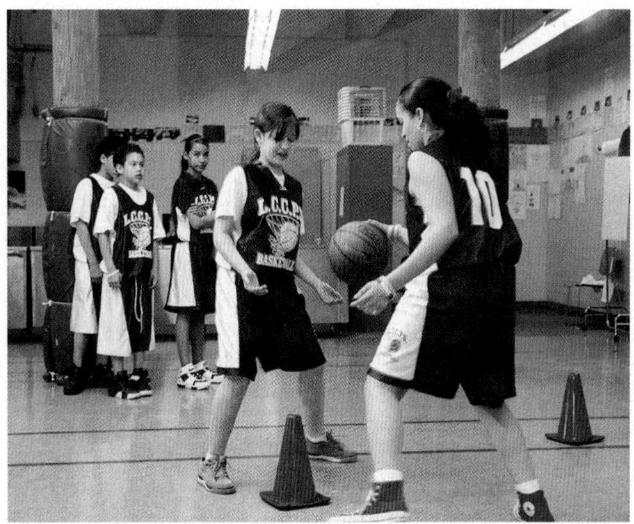

FIGURE 29.2 Adolescents become involved in competitive sports, which draw upon their gross motor skills.

Fine Motor Skills

In the early adolescent years, the individual increases their ability to manipulate objects. The adolescent's handwriting is neater, and they have increased finger dexterity. The middle adolescent years see the individual refining their dexterity skills. By late adolescence, the individual has developed precise eye–hand coordination and finger dexterity.

COMMUNICATION AND LANGUAGE DEVELOPMENT

Language skills continue to develop and be refined during adolescence. Adolescents have improved communication skills, using correct grammar and parts of speech. Vocabulary and communication skills continue to develop during middle adolescence. However, the usage of colloquial speech (slang) increases, causing communication with people other than peers to be difficult at times. By late adolescence, language skills are comparable to those of adults.

As you assess Cho (the 15-year-old introduced at the beginning of the chapter), what would you expect her gross motor, fine motor, and language skills to be at this age?

EMOTIONAL AND SOCIAL DEVELOPMENT

Adolescents undergo a great deal of change in the areas of emotional and social development as they grow and mature into adults. Areas that are affected include the adolescent's relationship with parents; self-concept and body image; importance of peers; and sexuality and dating.

Relationship With Parents

Families and parents of adolescents experience changes and conflict that require adjustments and the understanding of adolescent development. The adolescent is striving for self-identity and increased independence. They spend more time with peers and less time with family and attending family functions. Parents sense that they have less influence on the adolescent as the adolescent questions family values and becomes more mobile. This may lead to a family crisis, and the parents may respond by setting stricter limits or asking questions about the adolescent's activities and friends. Other parents may drop all rules and assume that the adolescent can manage themselves. Both of these responses increase tension in the family.

With the adolescent attempting to establish some level of independence—and the family learning to let go while focusing on aging parents, their marriage, and other children—a state of disequilibrium occurs. The family may experience more stress than at any other time.

Some families have better outcomes with their adolescents than others. Families who listen to and continue to demonstrate affection for and acceptance of their adolescent have a more positive outcome. This does not mean that the family accepts all of the adolescent's ideas or actions, but they are willing to listen and attempt to negotiate some limits. For tips to improve communication with adolescents, see Box 29.1.

Siblings experience changes in the relationship with the adolescent; the older sibling may attempt to parent, and the younger sibling may regress in an attempt to avoid the family conflict. Understanding the status of the adolescent–family relationship is essential for the nurse.

Self-Concept and Body Image

Self-concept and self-esteem are often tied to body image. Adolescents who perceive their body as being different than their peers' bodies or as less than ideal may view themselves negatively.

Sexual characteristics are important to the adolescent's self-concept and body image. Adolescents are concerned about the size of their penis or breasts, facial hair, and the onset of menstruation. Larger breasts are often considered more feminine, and menstruation is considered a rite of passage into adulthood. All of these body changes are important to the adolescent's self-concept.

Importance of Peers

Peer groups play an essential role in the identity of the adolescent (Holland-Hall, 2020). Adolescent peer relationships are important in providing opportunities to learn about negotiating differences; for recreation, companionship, and someone to share problems with; for learning peer loyalty; and for creating stability during transitions or times of stress. Learning to work out differences with peers is a skill that is important throughout life. Peers serve as someone safe to discuss family issues with, as the adolescent emotionally moves away from the

BOX 29.1 Ways to Improve Communication With Adolescents

- Set aside an appropriate amount of time to discuss subject matter without interruptions.
- Talk face-to-face. Be aware of body language.
- Ask questions to see why they feel the way they do.
- Ask them to be patient as you tell your thoughts.
- Choose words carefully so they understand you.
- Tell them exactly what you mean.
- Give praise and approval to your adolescent often.
- Speak to your adolescent as an equal—don't talk down to them.
- Be aware of your tone of voice and body language.
- Don't pretend you know all the answers.
- Admit that you do make mistakes.
- Set rules and limits fairly.

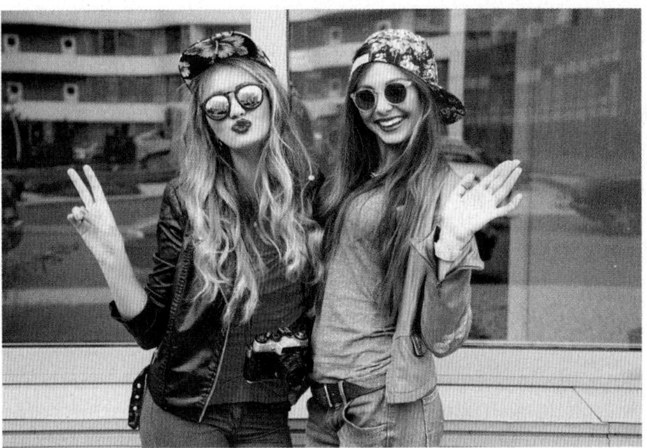

FIGURE 29.3 Peers play an important role in shaping the adolescent's identity.

family while trying to find their identity. Due to changes that have taken place within family systems in society, peer groups play a significant role in the socialization of adolescents (Fig. 29.3).

Peers serve as credible sources of information, role model social behaviors, and act as sources of social reinforcement. Friends provide an opportunity for fun and excitement. Peers impact each other's appearance, dress, social behavior, and language. Peers can also have positive influences on each other, such as promoting college attendance, or negative influences, such as involvement with alcohol, drugs, or gangs. Early and middle adolescence are periods when adolescents may consider joining gangs. Peer role modeling and peer acceptance may lead to the formation of a gang that provides a collective identity and gives a sense of belonging. Peer pressure, companionship, and protection are the most frequent reasons given for joining gangs, particularly those associated with criminal activity.

Parents must know their adolescent's friends and continue to be aware of potential problems while allowing the adolescent the independence to become their own person. Nurses must remind parents of the importance of peers and the impact they have on the adolescent's decisions and life choices. The transition to greater peer involvement requires guidance and support. Adolescents who do not have parental or adult supervision and opportunities for conversation with adults may be more susceptible to peer influences and at higher risk for poor peer selections.

Sexuality

Adolescence is a critical time in the development of sexuality. **Sexuality** includes the thoughts, feelings, and behaviors related to the adolescent's sexual identity. Adolescence is a time when individuals may begin experimentation related to their sexual identity, orientation, and behavior. This experimentation is part of the process of sorting through their sexuality and does not always define their sexual identity or orientation.

Adolescents who identify as lesbian, gay, bisexual, transgender, queer, intersex, asexual, and identities that defy discrete labels (LGBTQ+) face the same health concerns as other adolescents, but additional challenges may include questioning of their sexual identity, the complexity of coming out, and possible societal discrimination (Forcier & Olson-Kennedy, 2020). The majority of LGBTQ+ adolescents are healthy and well, but some are at an increased risk for adverse outcomes such as depression, suicide, substance use disorder, homelessness, sexually transmitted infections (STIs), unplanned pregnancy, and victimization (Forcier & Olson-Kennedy, 2020). See Evidence-Based Practice 29.1. Personal, societal, and family acceptance are crucial and lead to decreased adverse outcomes.

EVIDENCE-BASED PRACTICE 29.1

Reducing Behavioral Health Symptoms by Addressing Minority Stressors in LGBTQ+ Adolescents: A Randomized Controlled Trial of Proud & Empowered

STUDY

LGBTQ+ adolescents have an increased incidence of depression, anxiety, self-harm, suicidal attempts and ideation, and substance use. Discrimination, violence, and victimization place the LGBTQ+ adolescent at higher risk for mental health conditions. Previous studies have shown evidence that improving adolescents' ability to cope with stress improves mental health outcomes. This study was a randomized control trial (RCT) of a program called Proud & Empowered, to be delivered in school settings. It is a small group program for LGBTQ+ adolescents, consisting of 10 sessions lasting about 45 minutes each.

Nursing Implications

Nurses should support school-based programs. School staff and school officials should be educated on the increased mental health risks for LGBTQ+ youth and programs that have demonstrated effectiveness at decreasing mental health symptoms and reducing stress. Further research is needed to evaluate the effectiveness of school-based programs, utilizing larger sample sizes. Nurses should work with a multidisciplinary team that includes medical and mental health professionals, school and educational professionals, and adolescents and their families to incorporate appropriate interventions into their local schools.

Data from Goldbach, J. T., Rhoades, H., Mamey, M. R., Senese, J., Karys, P., & Marsiglia, F. F. (2021). Reducing behavioral health symptoms by addressing minority stressors in LGBTQ adolescents: A randomized controlled trial of Proud & Empowered. *BMC Public Health, 21*, 2315. https://doi.org/10.1186/s12889-021-12357-5

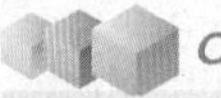
Concept Mastery Alert

When providing care to an adolescent who shares information about their sexual identity, the nurse must remember that assessment is the first step in the nursing process.

Dating

An interest in romantic partnerships occurs during adolescence (Fig. 29.4). Some of the reasons cited for this developing interest are physical development and body changes, peer-group pressure, and curiosity. During the past couple of decades, dating has become less common (Eickmeyer et al., 2020). The percentage of adolescents who date frequently increases with age. As of 2020, 51% of high school seniors reported dating, a decrease from 78% 20 years before (Eickmeyer et al., 2020). Adolescent dating can range from group dating to single dating to serious relationships.

During early adolescence, individuals tend to date for fun and recreation.

Middle and late adolescents have group and single dates. Romantic relationships become more central to the social life of this age group. Dating or spending time with a potential romantic partner is viewed as a major developmental marker for adolescents and is one of the most challenging adjustments. Both positive and negative developmental outcomes can result depending on the quality of the relationship that forms. Some adolescents who date may report slightly higher levels of self-esteem, self-worth and social support (Emerson et al., 2023; Kansky & Allen, 2018). However, other types of dating relationships may result in an adolescent having lower academic success and motivation, higher depression rates, increased anxiety, and increased risk of substance use (Emerson et al., 2023; Kansky & Allen, 2018). Trends in dating are everchanging, but dating remains a developmental milestone for the adolescent.

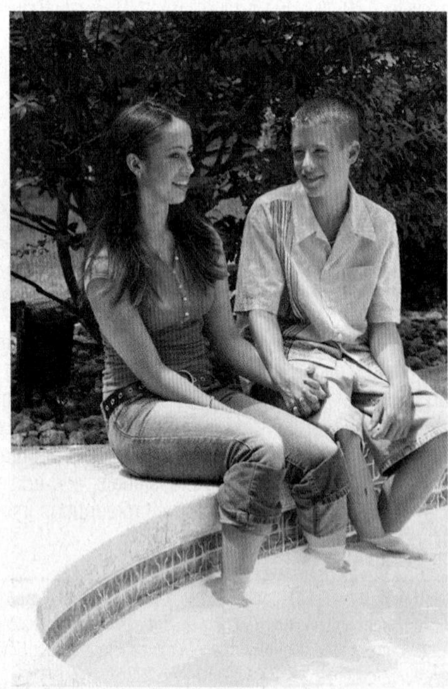

FIGURE 29.4 Dating becomes an important aspect of the adolescent's life.

Healthy romantic relationships can assist the adolescent in developing a strong sense of self-identity, self-regulation; self-expression; emotional autonomy from their family; and interpersonal skills, such as empathy; and are related to increased quality of adult relationships (Emerson et al., 2023; Kansky & Allen, 2018). The emotional ups and downs that accompany dating can help develop emotional resilience and coping skills. Romantic relationships at this stage are a great source of emotional support. Risks of being involved in unhealthy romantic relationships include dating violence and risky sexual activity such as STIs and pregnancy. Adolescents do not automatically know what makes for a healthy relationship. They need to be educated on the right and wrong behaviors of dating and what behaviors make up a healthy relationship, such as open communication, honesty, and trust. They need to know the signs of an unhealthy relationship and how to seek help if needed.

Refer back to Cho, the 15-year-old from the beginning of the chapter. Cho's parent states they are concerned about the changes that have occurred in their relationship over the past year. Cho seems much more self-centered, always wants to be with her friends, is critical of her parents, and seems to be constantly in conflict with them. Based on what you know about this stage of development, what guidance, including approaches and techniques, can you discuss with Cho's parent to address these concerns?

CULTURAL INFLUENCES ON GROWTH AND DEVELOPMENT

Although the adolescent's culture continues to influence them, the desire to be in harmony with peers becomes paramount. That desire can cause conflict with the adolescent's family and culture. Today's adolescents live in a rapidly changing, increasingly culturally diverse world. They may be exposed to people from many different cultures and ethnic groups.

Attitudes regarding adolescence vary among cultures. Certain cultures may have more permissive attitudes toward issues facing adolescents, while others are more conservative (e.g., toward sexuality). Experiencing a rite-of-passage ceremony to signal the adolescent's movement to adult status varies among cultures. American culture does not have a universal rite of passage for

support as evidenced by alteration in sleep pattern, destructive behavior toward others or self, frequent illness, inability to meet basic needs, insufficient coping strategies, risk-taking behavior, substance misuse.

Goal/Outcome

Adolescent will demonstrate adequate coping abilities as evidenced by management of stress of adolescence and no evidence of participating in risk-taking behaviors.

Ineffective Coping (interventions with *rationale*)

- Assess adolescent's knowledge of normal stress facing adolescents *to determine current knowledge.*
- Assess adolescent's present coping skills *to determine areas for improvement/support.*
- Encourage parents to accept adolescent as a unique individual *to improve self-esteem.*
- Discuss with parents and adolescent normal developmental issues facing adolescents *to give them knowledge needed to cope.*
- Provide different situations the adolescent might be faced with, and encourage adolescent to develop different solutions *to assist adolescent in developing problem-solving strategies.*
- Allow for increasing independence and opportunities to solve own problems *to improve coping skills.*
- Encourage parents to provide unconditional love *to improve self-esteem.*
- Assess for any evidence of any risk-taking behaviors (drugs, smoking, self-harm) *to identify need for early interventions.*

Nursing Analysis

Caregiver role strain risk; risk factors include dependency, discharge home with significant needs, substance misuse, unstable health condition, insufficient knowledge about community resources, and social isolation.

Goal/Outcome

Parent will experience competence in role: will demonstrate appropriate caregiving behaviors and verbalize comfort in caring for an adolescent.

Preventing Caregiver Role Strain (interventions with *rationale*)

- Assess parents' knowledge of adolescents and the issues that arise as a part of expected development *to determine parents' needs.*
- Provide education on normal issues of adolescence *so that parents are prepared with the knowledge they need to appropriately care for their adolescents.*
- Provide anticipatory guidance related to upcoming expected issues related to adolescent development *to prepare parents for what to expect next and how to intervene in an appropriate manner.*

PROMOTING HEALTHY GROWTH AND DEVELOPMENT

It takes multiple groups who address multiple issues to promote healthy growth and development in the adolescent. Some of these groups include sports teams in the school or the community, peers, teachers, band and choir members, and so forth. Also, the family's support and love will influence growth and development.

Promoting Growth and Development Through Sports and Physical Fitness

Many adolescents are involved in team sports that provide avenues for exercise. High levels of physical activity may reduce cardiovascular disease risk factors and provide disease prevention against cancer, higher weight, osteoporosis, diabetes, and depression (Centers for Disease Control and Prevention [CDC], 2022a). Adolescents probably spend more time and energy participating in sports than any other age group. Participation in sports contributes to the adolescent's development, educational process, and better health. Sports and games provide an opportunity to interact with peers while enjoying socially accepted stimulation and conflict. Competition in sports activities helps the adolescent in processing self-appraisal and in developing self-respect and concern for others.

Every sport has some potential for injury. Rapidly growing bones, muscles, joints, and tendons are more vulnerable to unusual strains and fractures. Incidence of concussions (which is considered a mild traumatic brain injury) is a growing concern in all adolescent athletes. To help prevent injury, parents and coaches need to be aware of early warning signs of fatigue, dehydration, and injury. See Chapter 44 for a discussion of sports injuries.

In relation to youth sports, the role of the nurse is to educate to prevent injuries (Fig. 29.5). This education

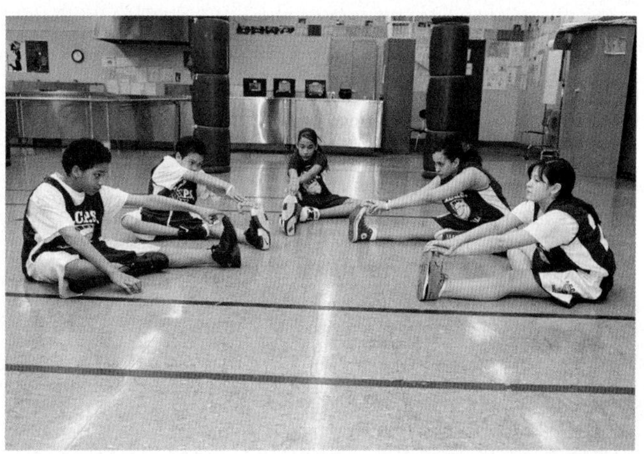

FIGURE 29.5 Stretching before exercise is an important part of exercise.

should include discouraging participation when the adolescent is tired or has an existing injury, encouraging the use of proper well-fitting protective gear, and ensuring the adolescent learns how to play a sport before participating in it.

In addition, adolescence is a good time to develop an exercise program. The U.S. Department of Health and Human Services (HHS) recommends that adolescents participate in 60 minutes of moderate to vigorous physical activity each day (CDC, 2022a). Nurses should encourage all adolescents to be physically active daily.

Promoting Learning

School, teachers, family, and peers influence education and learning for the adolescent. Also, activities such as athletics and club membership enhance learning through interactions with peers, coaches, club leaders, and others.

School

School plays an essential part in preparing adolescents for the future. Completing school prepares the adolescent for college or employment to make an adequate income. Schools in the United States may not meet the developmental needs of all adolescents. Students from historically marginalized communities may not be at the appropriate grade level, and the dropout rate may be higher than in students from communities that have not been historically marginalized. Dropout rates have declined since the 1970s but still remain a concern. Dropout rates are highest among Hispanic students (National Center for Education Statistics, 2022). Those who drop out of school may lack skills needed to function in today's society. They are more likely to be unemployed, have higher rates of incarceration, and have lower income levels and occupational status than those with a high school diploma (American Public Health Association [APHA], 2018; National Center for Education Statistics, n.d.; see Healthy People 2030).

HEALTHY PEOPLE 2030

Objective	Nursing Significance
Increase the pr[illegible]rtion of high [illegible] students who [illegible]aduate in 4 years.	• Encourage school attendance and completion when encountering adolescents for well-child or sick visits. • Refer children who have difficulty concentrating or learning for further evaluation. • Praise school accomplishments.

Healthy People Objectives retrieved from http://www.healthypeople.gov

There is evidence that the transition from elementary school to middle school, at age 12 or 13, and then the transition to high school, both of which occur at the time of physical changes, may have a negative effect on adolescents. It is important to observe for transition problems into middle or high school, which may be exhibited by failing grades or behavior problems. Also, students who experience difficulties in school, resulting in negative evaluations and failing grades, may feel alienated from school. Students with poor grades and low academic achievement exhibit more unhealthy behaviors such as physical inactivity and poor diet and are more likely to engage in risky behaviors such as early sexual initiation and substance use (CDC, 2022b). Schools that support peer-group relationships, promote health and fitness, encourage parental involvement, and strengthen community relationships have better student outcomes. Parents, teachers, and health care providers should provide guidance and support.

Other Activities

Adolescents are involved in many other activities that influence learning. Some of these activities include (1) school activities such as band, choir, or clubs; (2) athletic activities in the school and community and sometimes in the state or region; (3) art, sewing, and building classes; and (4) work activities when the late adolescent has a part-time job. These activities all contribute to the growth, development, and education of the adolescent.

Promoting Safety

Unintentional injury is the leading cause of death in adolescents (CDC, 2021a). Motor vehicle crashes are the leading cause of unintentional injury death, followed by poisoning, primarily due to drug overdose from opioids, and drowning (CDC, 2021a). Males are more likely than females to die of any type of injury (CDC, 2021a).

Influencing factors related to the prevalence of adolescent injuries include increased physical growth, insufficient psychomotor coordination for the task, abundance of energy, impulsivity, peer pressure, and inexperience. Impulsivity, inexperience, and peer pressure may place the adolescent in a vulnerable situation between knowing what is right and wanting to impress peers. On the other hand, adolescents have a feeling of invulnerability, which may contribute to negative outcomes. Alcohol and other drugs are contributing factors in automobile crashes and unintentional firearm injuries among adolescents. Most of the serious or fatal injuries in adolescents are preventable (Fig. 29.6). Nurses must educate parents and adolescents on car, gun, and water safety to prevent unintentional injuries. See Teaching Guidelines 29.1 for information on promoting safety.

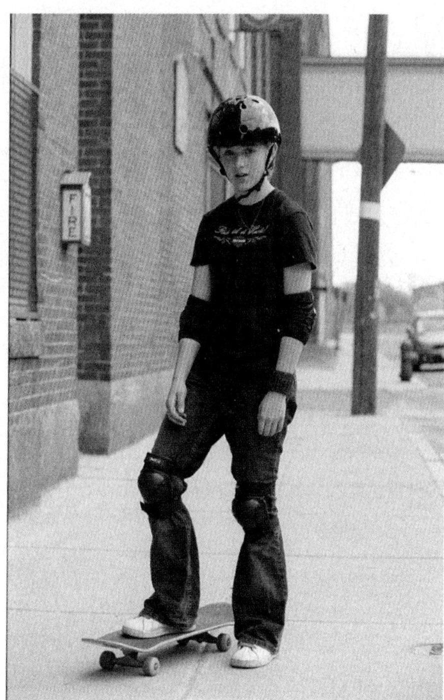

FIGURE 29.6 Wearing appropriate safety equipment can prevent injuries.

TAKE NOTE!

A sharp increase in firearm-related deaths in children 0 to 19 years of age was seen from 2019 to 2020, along with drug overdose and poisonings (CDC/National Center for Health Statistics, 2022; Goldstick et al., 2022). Nurses need to follow this trend to ensure we are providing interventions to help protect our youth from these preventable causes of death.

Motor Vehicle Safety

The largest numbers of adolescent injuries are due to motor vehicle crashes. When the adolescent passes their driving test, they are able to drive legally. However, driving is complex and requires judgments that the adolescent is often incapable of making. Also, the typical adolescent is opposed to authority and is interested in showing peers and others their independence. It is also normal for adolescents to take risks. These factors, coupled with inexperience with driving, may lead to underestimating hazardous and dangerous situations. Adolescents and young adults are the least likely age group to wear a seat belt (CDC, 2021b). Crashes involving

TEACHING GUIDELINES 29.1 Promoting Safety

Safety Issue	Activity
Motor vehicle	• Wear a seat belt at all times. • Do not drive impaired or drive with someone who is impaired. • Take a driver-education course. • Parents should drive with the adolescent for 30–50 hours prior to obtaining license, at different times of the day, in different heavy and light traffic and during different weather conditions. • Restrict nighttime driving. • Establish driving rules between parent and adolescent prior to the adolescent getting license. • Have all passengers wear seat belts. • Do not use cell phone or text while driving, drink and drive, or drive when tired. • Maintain the car's good condition. • Drive with adult supervision for a period of time after receiving a license. • Encourage a limit on the number of adolescent passengers.
Bike: General	• Have a well-maintained and appropriate-size bike for adolescent. • Adolescent should demonstrate their ability to ride the bike safely before being allowed to ride on the street. • Safe areas for bike riding should be established as well as routes to and from area of activities. • Do not ride bike barefoot, with someone else on bike, or with clothing that might get entangled in the bike. • Wear sturdy, well-fitting shoes and Consumer Product Safety Commission (CPSC) or Snell-approved helmets. • A properly fitting helmet should: sit level, not tilted, and firmly and comfortably on the head; have strong wide Y-shaped straps and when you open your mouth should pull down a bit; not move with sudden pulling or twisting; never be worn over anything else (hat, scarf, etc.). • The bike should be inspected often to ensure it is in proper working order. • A basket should be used to carry heavy objects.

(continued)

TEACHING GUIDELINES **29.1** Promoting Safety (*continued*)

Safety Issue	Activity
Bike: In traffic	• All traffic signs and signals must be observed. • If the adolescent is riding at night, the bike should have lights and reflectors, and the rider should wear light-colored clothes. • Ride on the side of the road traveling with traffic and keep close to the side of the road in single file. • Watch and listen for cars and never hitch a ride on any vehicle. • Do not wear headphones while riding a bike.
All-terrain vehicles	• The vehicle not be operated by an adolescent younger than 16 years of age. • Take a hands-on safety course before riding. • Helmet and protective coverings are required. • No nighttime or double riding • Not for use on public roads or if the adolescent has been drinking or using drugs • Do not stand up in the vehicle or ride in a person's lap.
Skateboards/skates	• Wear a helmet, and protective padding on knees, elbows, and wrists. • Do not skate in traffic or on streets or highways. • Skating on homemade ramps could be dangerous—assess ramps for any hazards before skating.
Water safety	• Learn how to swim; if swimming skill is limited, wear a life preserver at all times. • Never swim alone; if at all possible, swim only where there is a life guard. • Learn basic cardiopulmonary resuscitation (CPR). • Do not run or fool around at the edge of the pool. • Drains in the pool should be covered with appropriate cover. • Wear a life jacket when on a boat. • Make sure there is enough water to support diving. • Do not swim if drinking alcohol or using drugs.
Firearms	• If guns are in the household, take a firearm safety class, secure guns in a safe place, use gun safety locks, and store bullets in a separate place. • Never point a gun at a person.
Fire safety	• All homes should have working smoke detectors and fire extinguishers. Change the batteries at least twice a year. • Have a fire-escape plan and practice the plan routinely. • No smoking in bed • Teach what to do in case of a fire—use a fire extinguisher, call 911, and know how to put out clothing fire. • All flammable materials and liquids should be stored safely. • Fireplaces should have protective gratings. • Avoid touching any downed power lines.
Machinery	• Use safety devices. • Receive training on how to use equipment. • Do not use machinery when alone.
Sports	• Match the sport to the adolescent's ability and desire. • Sports programs should have a warm-up procedure and hydration policy. • Undergo a sports physical before start of activity. • Coaches should be trained in CPR and first aid. • Wear appropriate protection devices for the individual sport.
Sun	• Use sunscreen with both ultraviolet A (UVA) and ultraviolet B (UVB) protection. • Apply sunscreen prior to going out, and reapply sunscreen often. • Limit sun exposure, especially between 10 a.m. and 2 p.m. • Wear protective clothing and a hat and sunglasses while outside. • Do not suntan, and avoid using tanning beds.

TEACHING GUIDELINES **29.1** Promoting Safety

Safety Issue	Activity
Personal safety	• Never go with a stranger. • Do not enter a car when the driver has been drinking. • Notify an adult about where you are when out after dark. • Keep your cell phone fully charged. • Never give out personal information over the internet. • Say "no" to drugs, alcohol, smoking, and to being touched when you do not want to be touched.
Toxins	• Teach the hazards of accepting illegal drugs, alcohol, and dangerous drugs. • Store potentially dangerous material in a safe place.

Data from American Academy of Pediatrics. (2010, reaffirmed 2016). The teen driver. *Pediatrics*, *118*(6), 2570–2581. http://pediatrics.aappublications.org/content/118/6/2570.full; Centers for Disease Control and Prevention. (2021c). *Keep teen drivers safe*. https://www.cdc.gov/injury/features/teen-drivers/index.html; American Academy of Pediatrics, Council on Environmental Health and Section on Dermatology. (2011, reaffirmed 2017). Policy statement—Ultraviolet radiation: A hazard to children and adolescents. *Pediatrics*, *127*(3), 588–597. https://doi.org/10.1542/peds.2016-4205; American Academy of Pediatrics, HealthyChildren. (2022). *ATVs are not for children: AAP urges these safety rules*. https://www.healthychildren.org/English/safety-prevention/at-play/Pages/ATV-Safety-Rules.aspx; Centers for Disease Control and Prevention. (2022c). *Drowning facts*. http://www.cdc.gov/HomeandRecreationalSafety/Water-Safety/waterinjuries-factsheet.html; Gill, A. C. (2022). Bicycle injuries in children: Prevention. *UpToDate*. Retrieved October 17, 2022, from https://www.uptodate.com/contents/bicycle-injuries-in-children-prevention

adolescents are more likely to involve speeding, driving too fast for conditions, or following too close to the car in front of them (CDC, 2021b). More crashes occur when passengers, mostly other adolescents, are present in the car; during driving at night; or when driving under the influence of alcohol or drugs (American Academy of Pediatrics, 2010, reaffirmed 2016; CDC, 2021b).

It is essential to promote driver education, to teach about the importance of wearing seat belts, and to explain laws about adolescent driving and curfews (Fig. 29.7). See Teaching Guidelines 29.1 for additional information.

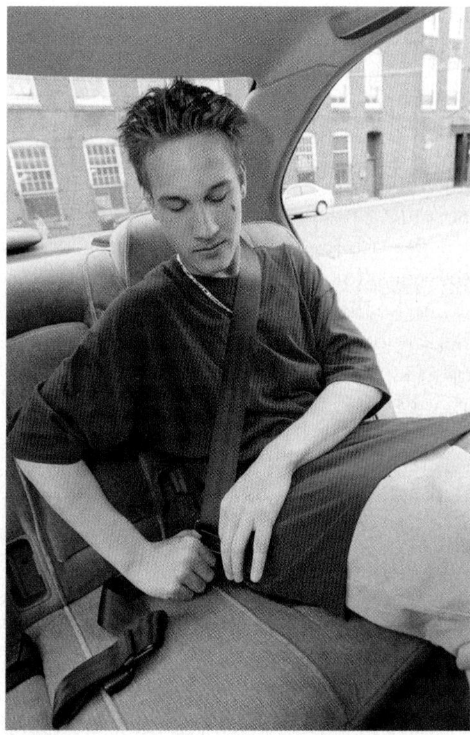

FIGURE 29.7 The use of seat belts has led to fewer fatal injuries in car crashes.

TAKE NOTE!

All states, although varied, have enacted a Graduated Driving License (GDL) program, which allows adolescents to gain driving experience and limits risky circumstances (such as nighttime driving and driving with passengers) by providing a license in three stages (learner's permit, provisional license, and full license; CDC, 2021b). Studies have shown this program to be highly effective in reducing adolescent driver crashes (CDC, 2021b).

Firearm Safety

The risk of dying from a firearm injury among 15- to 19-year-olds has been rising. In 2019, firearms became the leading cause of death in children 0 to 19 years of age, exceeding motor vehicle crashes (Naik-Mathuria & Gill, 2022). Seventy-four percent of homicides involved firearms, and 45% of suicides in children and adolescents involved firearms (Naik-Mathuria & Gill, 2022). Homicides in adolescent males account for the majority of pediatric firearm deaths (Naik-Mathuria & Gill, 2022). Provide education about gun safety. Emphasize that an absence of guns in the home is the most effective way to prevent firearm injuries. If there are guns in the home, they must be kept locked in a safe location, with ammunition kept separately. Parents must teach adolescents about the dangers of playing with firearms. See Teaching Guidelines 29.1 for additional information on gun safety.

Water Safety

Drowning is a needless cause of death in adolescents. Many drownings are a result of risk-taking behaviors. With the independence of the adolescent, adult supervision is often not prevalent, and the adolescent takes a risk that results in drowning. Provide water safety education and proper supervision to decrease the incidence of risk taking. Teach about swimming lessons for nonswimmers. See Teaching Guidelines 29.1 for additional information.

Remember Cho Chung, the 15-year-old presented at the beginning of the chapter? What anticipatory guidance related to safety should you provide to Cho and her parent?

Promoting Nutrition

Nutritional needs are increased during adolescence due to accelerated growth and sexual maturation. Adolescents may appear to be constantly hungry and need regular meals and snacks with adequate nutrients to meet the body's needs. Multiple factors influence the adolescent's diet and eating habits (Box 29.2).

According to CDC data, since the 1970s, the obesity rate in adolescents has more than tripled (CDC, 2022d). Poor diet and physical inactivity have contributed to higher weight in this age group. Excess weight in adolescence is associated with excess weight in adulthood, along with numerous adverse health conditions such as diabetes, heart disease, certain types of cancer, osteoarthritis, and overall poorer physical and mental health (CDC, 2022e).

Nutritional Needs

Adolescents have a need for increased calories, zinc, calcium, and iron for growth. However, the number of calories needed during adolescence depends on the individual's age and activity level as well as growth patterns. Female adolescents who are moderately active require about 2,000 calories per day (U.S. Department of Agriculture [USDA] & Health and Human Services [HHS], 2020). Male adolescents who are moderately active require between 2,200 and 2,800 calories per day (USDA & HHS, 2020). Of these calories, 45% to 65% should come from carbohydrates, 10% to 30% from protein, and 25% to 35% from fat (USDA & HHS, 2020). Adolescents require about 1,300 mg of calcium each day (USDA & HHS, 2020). Adolescents should be made aware of foods high in calcium, including fortified ready-to-eat cereals, cheese, yogurt, almond milk, white beans, and broccoli. Adolescent males require 11 mg of iron each day, and females require 15 mg each day (USDA & HHS, 2020). Advise adolescents about foods high in iron (Box 29.3; see Healthy People 2030). Protein requirements for adolescent females, 14 to 18 years of age, are 46 g/day, and for adolescent males, 14 to 18 years of age, 52 g/day (USDA & HHS, 2020). Some foods high in protein are meats, fish, poultry, beans, and dairy products.

BOX 29.2 Factors Influencing the Adolescent's Diet

- Peer pressure
- Busy schedules
- Concern about weight control
- Convenience of fast food

BOX 29.3 Foods High in Iron

- Beef, chicken, seafood, liver
- Tofu
- Nuts and seeds
- Lentils and legumes
- Eggs
- Dark leafy vegetables such as spinach
- Iron-fortified cereals, whole-grain breads, and pastas

HEALTHY PEOPLE 2030

Objective	Nursing Significance
Reduce iron deficiency in females aged 12–49 years. Increase calcium consumption by people aged 2 years and older. Increase vitamin D consumption by people aged 2 years and older. Increase consumption of potassium in the population aged 2 years and older. Reduce consumption of sodium in the population aged 2 years and older.	• Educate parents and adolescents about iron, calcium, vitamin D, and potassium-containing foods. • Encourage adolescent females to consume a diet high in iron-rich foods. • Educate adolescents on vitamin D–fortified foods and vitamin D supplements. • Educate the parent and adolescent about sodium reduction and high sodium-containing foods.

Healthy People Objectives retrieved from http://www.healthypeople.gov

Promoting Healthy Eating Habits

The nurse must understand expected growth and development of the adolescent in order to provide guidance that fits the quest for independence and the need for adolescents to make their own choices. Assess the eating habits and diet preferences of the adolescent. The assessment should include an evaluation of foods from the different food groups that the adolescent eats each day. Also, assess the number of times that fast foods, unhealthy snacks, and other junk food are eaten per week. This assessment will help the nurse to guide the adolescent in making better food choices at home and in fast-food establishments. Many fast-food restaurants offer baked chicken sandwiches and salads with fewer calories and less fat. Adolescents may be guided in alternating hamburgers and fries with more nutritious choices. Remember that planning should always include the adolescent.

The USDA provides a personalized food plan called MyPlatePlan based on an individual's age, sex, weight, height, and amount of physical activity. Refer to Figure 29.8

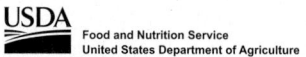

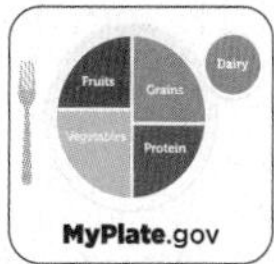

Start simple with MyPlate Plan

The benefits of healthy eating add up over time, bite by bite. Small changes matter. Start Simple with MyPlate.

A healthy eating routine is important at every stage of life and can have positive effects that add up over time. It's important to eat a variety of fruits, vegetables, grains, protein foods, and dairy or fortified soy alternatives. When deciding what to eat or drink, choose options that are full of nutrients. Make every bite count.

Food Group Amounts for 2,800 Calories a Day for Ages 14+ Years

 Fruits	 Vegetables	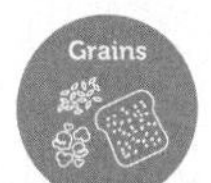 Grains	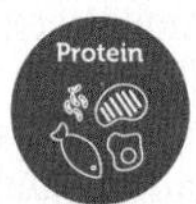 Protein	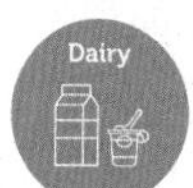 Dairy
2½ cups	**3½ cups**	**10 ounces**	**7 ounces**	**3 cups**
Focus on whole fruits	Vary your veggies	Make half your grains whole grains	Vary your protein routine	Move to low-fat or fat-free dairy milk or yogurt (or lactose-free dairy or fortified soy versions)
Focus on whole fruits that are fresh, frozen, canned, or dried.	Choose a variety of colorful fresh, frozen, and canned vegetables—make sure to include dark green, red, and orange choices.	Find whole-grain foods by reading the Nutrition Facts label and ingredients list.	Mix up your protein foods to include seafood; beans, peas, and lentils; unsalted nuts and seeds; soy products; eggs; and lean meats and poultry.	Look for ways to include dairy or fortified soy alternatives at meals and snacks throughout the day.

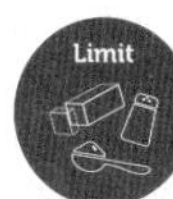

Choose foods and beverages with less added sugars, saturated fat, and sodium.
Limit:

- Added sugars to <**70 grams** a day.
- Saturated fat to <**31 grams** a day.
- Sodium to <**2,300 milligrams** a day.

Be active your way:
Children 6 to 17 years old should move **60 minutes** every day. Adults should be physically active at least **2½ hours** per week.

MyPlate Plan

Write down the foods you ate today and track your small changes, bite by bite.

Food group targets for a 2,800-calorie* pattern are:	Write down your food choices for each food group.	Did you reach your target?
Fruits: **2½ cups** 1 cup of fruits counts as • 1 cup raw or cooked fruit; or • ½ cup dried fruit; or • 1 cup 100% fruit juice.		Y N
Vegetables: **3½ cups** 1 cup of vegetables counts as • 1 cup raw or cooked vegetables; or • 2 cups leafy salad greens; or • 1 cup 100% vegetable juice.		Y N
Grains: **10-ounce equivalents** 1 ounce of grains counts as • 1 slice bread; or • 1 ounce ready-to-eat cereal; or • ½ cup cooked rice, pasta, or cereal.		Y N
Protein: **7-ounce equivalents** 1 ounce of protein foods counts as • 1 ounce seafood, lean meats, or poultry; or • 1 egg; or • 1 Tbsp peanut butter; or • ¼ cup cooked beans, peas, or lentils; or • ½ ounce unsalted nuts or seeds.		Y N
Dairy: **3 cups** 1 cup of dairy counts as • 1 cup dairy milk or yogurt; or • 1 cup lactose-free dairy milk or yogurt; or • 1 cup fortified soy milk or yogurt; or • 1½ ounces hard cheese.		Y N

Limit:

- Added sugars to <**70 grams** a day.
- Saturated fat to <**31 grams** a day.
- Sodium to <**2,300 milligrams** a day.

Y N

Activity — Be active your way:
Children 6 to 17 years old should move **60 minutes** every day. Adults should be physically active at least **2½ hours** per week.

Y N

* This 2,800-calorie pattern is only an estimate of your needs. Monitor your body weight and adjust your calories if needed.

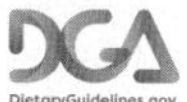

FNS-904-29
July 2021
USDA is an equal opportunity provider, employer, and lender.

FIGURE 29.8 MyPlatePlan for a 15-year-old male 63.5 kg (140 lb), 162.56 cm (5 ft 4 in), 30 to 60 minutes of exercise daily. (Retrieved November 4, 2022, from https://myplate-prod.azureedge.us/sites/default/files/2021-08/2020MyPlatePlan_2800cals_Age14%2B.pdf)

for an example. At https://www.myplate.gov/life-stages/teens, the adolescent can create their customized food plan. Nurses may use the information in MyPlatePlan to help adolescents plan a healthy diet for themselves. See Healthy People 2030.

HEALTHY PEOPLE 2030

Objective	Nursing Significance
Increase whole-grain consumption by people aged 2 years and older. Increase fruit consumption by people aged 2 years and older. Increase vegetable consumption by people aged 2 years and older. Increase consumption of dark green vegetables, red and orange vegetables, and beans and peas by people aged 2 years and older. Reduce consumption of added sugars by people aged 2 years and older. Reduce consumption of saturated fat by people aged 2 years and older.	• Educate adolescents and families about the importance of whole grains, fruits, and vegetables in the diet. • Encourage the adolescent to choose fruits and vegetables that appeal to them. • Educate adolescents and families about saturated fat–containing foods and ways to reduce them in their diet. • Educate adolescents and families about foods with added sugar and how to avoid them. • Offer suggestions for alternative sources of proteins and fats (chicken or fish, olive oil).

Healthy People Objectives retrieved from http://www.healthypeople.gov

Maintaining Healthy Body Weight

The prevalence of BMIs classified as obese in children aged 12 to 19 years old is 19.7% (CDC, 2022f). Although excess weight has increased in all segments of the U.S. population, there are differences specific to race, ethnicity, and socioeconomic status. The prevalence of BMIs classified as obese is highest in Hispanic and non-Hispanic Black children and adolescents (CDC, 2022f).

This increase in excess weight in adolescents has led to increases in hypertension, heart disease, and type 2 diabetes. Influential factors causing excess weight include poor food choices, unhealthy eating practices, and lack of exercise. Around 15% of youths reported drinking sugary beverages at least once a day, and 25.9% reported attending physical education classes in school (Merlo et al., 2020). Overall, measures of how well Americans' food choices follow the dietary guidelines have remained low (USDA & HHS, 2020). Adolescents are busy and eat on the run, with many meals from fast-food facilities. In addition, many schools have decreased or discontinued physical education, which has resulted in a more sedentary lifestyle, leading to weight gain (APHA, 2021). Interest in computer games, smartphones, and television watching at home has decreased physical activity and exercise and further contributed to weight gain and higher weight (Woessner, 2021; see Healthy People 2030).

HEALTHY PEOPLE 2030

Objective	Nursing Significance
Reduce the proportion of children and adolescents with obesity. Increase the proportion of adolescents who do enough aerobic physical activity. Increase the proportion of adolescents who do enough muscle strengthening activity. Increase the proportion of children and adolescents who play sports.	• Screen all children for the development of excess weight, as indicated by an increasing body mass index (BMI) for their age. • Provide accurate diet counseling. • Encourage daily physical activity. • Counsel adolescents and parents to limit television screen time daily. • Educate the adolescent on the health risks associated with excess weight. • For the nonexercising adolescent, advise them to start slowly by walking. • Work with the adolescent to identify physical activities that interest them. • Praise efforts to participate in a routine exercise plan. • Identify an athletic individual that the adolescent identifies with, and encourage similar activities in the adolescent. • Encourage involvement in organized sports through school or local programs.

Healthy People Objectives retrieved from http://www.healthypeople.gov

Nurses must make parents and adolescents aware of factors leading to excess weight. Nurses should recommend:

- Proper nutrition and healthy food choices
- Good eating habits, including eating a healthy breakfast daily
- Decreased fast-food intake
- Physical activity for at least 60 minutes daily
- Parents/adolescents exercising more at home
- Parents living a healthy lifestyle
- Decreasing nonactive screen viewing and use

Think back to Cho Chung. What questions should you ask Cho and her parent related to nutritional intake? What anticipatory guidance related to nutrition would be appropriate?

Promoting Healthy Sleep and Rest

The average number of hours of sleep that adolescents require per night is 9 hours (Paul & Wallace, 2023). The adolescent often experiences a change in sleep patterns that leads to feeling more awake at night and the desire to sleep later in the morning (Paul & Wallace, 2023). Also, in this independence-seeking phase of adolescence, the adolescent may stay up later to do homework, to complete projects, or to participate in activities and may have difficulty awakening in the morning. Surveys show that 72.7% of high schoolers and 57.8% of middle schoolers do not get enough sleep on school nights (CDC, 2020). Inadequate sleep leads to an increased risk of certain health and cognitive problems such as higher weight, diabetes, poor mental health, problems with attention, and negative effects on mood and motivation (CDC, 2020). Early school start times contribute to this pattern of not getting enough sleep for adolescents (see Healthy People 2030). Adolescents will often try to make up for needed sleep by sleeping longer hours on weekends. Rapid growth and increased activities may produce fatigue and the need for more rest. Parents may report that the adolescent sleeps all the time and never has the time or energy to help with household chores. Explain to parents the need to discourage late hours on school nights because they may affect school performance. Encourage the adolescent to go to bed at the same time each night and awaken at the same time in the morning, even on weekends (CDC, 2020). Provide advice to adolescents and parents about having realistic expectations; encourage them to agree on a level of normalcy and adequate rest for the adolescent so that they can still fulfill responsibilities in the home.

HEALTHY PEOPLE 2030

Objective	Nursing Significance
Increase the proportion of high school students who get enough sleep. Increase proportion of secondary schools with a start time of 8:30 a.m. or later.	• Encourage consistent bedtimes. • Encourage adolescent to make bedroom dark, relaxing, and quiet. • Encourage no electronic devices in bedroom, and limit light exposure and technology use in the evening hours. • Encourage regular exercise. • Limit caffeine and tobacco. • Educate and encourage local school officials to adopt later start schedule for adolescents.

Healthy People Objectives retrieved from http://www.healthypeople.gov

What anticipatory guidance to Cho Chung and her parent in relation to sleep during the adolescent years should you provide?

Promoting Healthy Teeth and Gums

Most permanent teeth have erupted with the possible exception of the third molars (wisdom teeth). These molars may be impacted and require surgical removal. The rate of cavities decreases, but the need for routine dental visits every 6 months and brushing two to three times per day are important. Some of the conditions that occur during adolescence include malocclusion, gingivitis, and tooth avulsion. Malocclusion (a poor bite) occurs from facial and mandibular bone growth that results in misalignment of the top teeth with the bottom teeth. It is the most common reason for referral to an orthodontist. The treatment includes braces and other dental devices. Teach the adolescent to brush the teeth more frequently if they have braces or other dental devices. Gingivitis is inflammation of the gums and breakdown of gingival epithelium due to diet and hormonal changes. The use of dental devices/braces makes cleaning more difficult and contributes to gingivitis. Tooth avulsion (knocked-out teeth) may occur during sports and other activities such as falls. The avulsed tooth should be reimplanted as soon as possible. The nurse may see the adolescent first, so it is important that nurses know the proper procedure, which is to reinsert the tooth into its socket, if possible, or to store it in cool milk or normal saline for transport to the dentist.

Promoting Personal Care

Promotion of personal care during adolescence is an important topic to cover with the adolescent and their parents. Topics to discuss include general hygiene tips, caring for body piercings and tattoos, preventing sun-tanning, and promoting a healthy sexual identity.

General Hygiene Tips

Adolescents find that frequent baths and deodorant use are important due to apocrine sweat gland secretory activity. Also, to decrease oily skin, teach the adolescent to wash their face two to three times per day with plain unscented soap. Vigorous scrubbing should be discouraged because it could irritate the skin and lead to follicular rupture. The hair should be shampooed daily or every other day to remove excess oil from the hair and scalp. Many over-the-counter medications are available for beginning acne or acne with a few lesions. These preparations may cause drying or redness. Discourage adolescents from squeezing acne lesions to prevent further irritation and permanent scarring. If the adolescent has severe acne, encourage them to ask a parent to make an appointment with a dermatologist.

Caring for Body Piercings and Tattoos

It is not uncommon for an adolescent to experiment with body piercing (Fig. 29.9). Generally, body piercing is safe, but nurses should caution adolescents about obtaining these procedures under nonsterile conditions and should educate them about potential complications. Qualified personnel using sterile needles should perform the procedure. Teach the adolescent to cleanse the pierced area twice a day and more often at some sites.

Infections from body piercing usually result from unclean tools of the trade. Some infections that may occur as a result of unclean tools include hepatitis, tetanus, tuberculosis, and human immunodeficiency virus (HIV). Also, keloid formation and allergies to metal may occur. The navel is an area prone to infection because it is a moist area that endures friction from clothing. Naval piercings, particularly after a navel infection occurs, may take up to a year to heal (Desai, 2023). Pierced ear cartilage also heals slowly and is prone to infection (Desai, 2023). Potential concerns with tongue piercing include tooth damage from biting on the jewelry or partial paralysis if the jewelry pierces a nerve.

Tattoos are continuing to grow in popularity among adolescents and are more commonplace among both adolescents and adults than in the past (Desai, 2021). Tattoos serve to define one's identity and are a form of self-expression (see Fig. 29.9). Because of the invasiveness of the tattooing procedure, it should be considered a health risk situation. Like piercings, tattoos begin as open wounds predisposing to infection.

Nurses should educate adolescents about the risk of tattooing under unsafe conditions, including bloodborne infections, such as hepatitis B and C, skin infections, scarring, bleeding, and allergic reactions to dyes used in the tattoo process (Desai, 2021). They need to encourage the adolescent to go to a licensed facility with licensed tattoo artists and to double check that all equipment used is disposable and sterilized (Desai, 2021). Teach adolescents to cleanse tattoos with an antibacterial soap and water several times a day and to keep the area moist with an ointment to prevent scab formation while it is healing. Refer to Box 29.4 for additional information about tattoos.

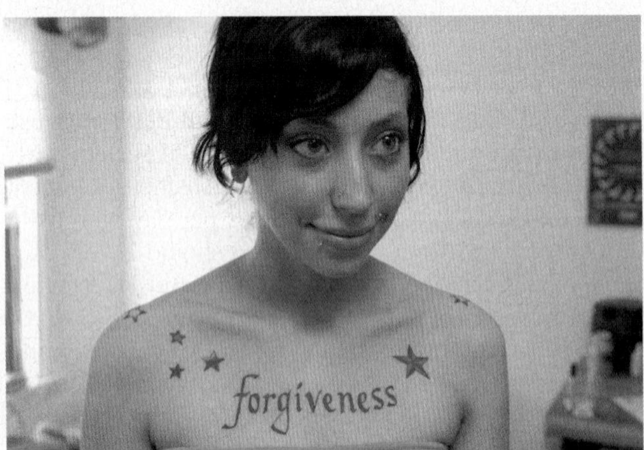

FIGURE 29.9 Having multiple piercings and tattoos can lead to certain health risks.

Preventing Sun-Tanning

Sun-tanning is popular among some adolescents and is influenced by the American media, which promotes a link between tan skin and beauty in light-skinned individuals. There is no such thing as a good tan. Most exposure to ultraviolet rays occurs during childhood and adolescence, thereby putting people at risk for the development of skin cancer. However, it can be difficult to convince adolescents that tanning is harmful to their skin and puts them at risk for skin cancer later in life (see Healthy People 2030).

HEALTHY PEOPLE 2030

Objective	Nursing Significance
Reduce the proportion of students in grades 9 through 12 who report sunburn.	• Remind adolescents to use sunscreen during outdoor organized-sports practice. • Encourage adolescents to use sunscreen-containing makeup. • Educate adolescents and families about the risks associated with sun exposure. • Educate adolescents and their families to avoid the sun between 10 a.m. and 4 p.m., wear sun-protective clothing when exposed to sunlight, use sunscreen with a sun protection factor (SPF) of 15 or higher, and avoid artificial sources of UV light.

Healthy People Objectives retrieved from http://www.healthypeople.gov

BOX 29.4 What Adolescents Need to Know About Tattooing

- Infections occur as a result of nonsterile equipment used in the procedure.
- New tattoos are open wounds predisposed to infection; sites require proper care. Keep bandaged for the first 24 hours, then wash with soap and warm water several times per day, and apply antibiotic ointment or fragrance-free lotion three times a day for the first week.
- Do not let the tattoo dry out. Do not expose it to direct sunlight until fully healed, and then keep it protected from the sun with sunscreen.
- Avoid pools, hot tubs, or long baths/showers until healed.
- For most people, a tattoo is permanent; new procedures for removal can be painful and expensive.

Educate adolescents about the benefits and effects of different sun protection products. Explain that sun damage and skin cancers can be prevented if sunscreens are used as directed on a regular basis. Encourage sunscreen or sunblock use for water sports, beach activities, and participation in outdoor sports. Also, make adolescents aware of allergies to some sunscreen products. See Teaching Guidelines 29.1 for additional information.

Promoting a Healthy Sexual Identity

Encourage parents and adolescents to have discussions about sexuality. In addition, nurses should ensure that adolescents have the knowledge, skills, and opportunities that enable them to make responsible decisions regarding sexual behaviors. Education for the adolescent should include a discussion about media influences and the use of sexuality to promote products. This discussion should make the adolescent aware of the motives of the media and the need to be an individual and not be influenced by television, magazines, and other forms of advertisement. Encourage parents to be aware of whom their adolescents are dating and where they go on their dates. Refer to Teaching Guidelines 29.2 for information on counseling related to adolescent sexuality.

Promoting Appropriate Discipline

Adolescents naturally misbehave or do not follow the rules of the house, and parents must determine how to respond. Adolescents need to know the rules and expectations. After rules are established, parents must explain to the adolescent the consequences of breaking the rules.

Offer guidance to parents related to disciplining adolescents. The parent and the adolescent should collaborate on what the consequences will be if the rules are broken. Parents must acknowledge and offer reinforcement and support when the adolescent follows the rules. Consistency and predictability are the cornerstones of discipline, and praise is the most powerful reinforcer of learning.

TEACHING GUIDELINES 29.2 Adolescent Sexuality

- It should be your choice to engage in sexual relations. Do not be influenced by peers. When you say "no," be firm and clear about your position. If someone says "no" to you, you must respect their choice.
- Pregnancy, sexually transmitted infections (STIs), and human immunodeficiency virus (HIV) infection can occur with any sexual encounter without the use of barrier methods of contraception. Use appropriate contraception if you are sexually active. Discuss abstinence as a contraceptive method.
- Sexual activity in a mature relationship should be pleasurable to both parties. If your sexual partner is not interested in your pleasure, you need to reconsider the relationship.

Promoting Proper Media Use

Television, the internet, social media, and other forms of media, are a large force in the lives of adolescents today. Adolescents are immersed daily in a variety of different media. Of adolescents, 95% report owning a smartphone, and 35% report using the top five social media platforms (i.e., YouTube, TikTok, Instagram, Snapchat, and Facebook) almost constantly (Pew Research Center, 2022). With greater technology and media access come benefits such as enhancing communication skills, increasing social connections, and improving technical skills, but risks also exist, such as cyberbullying, exposure to inappropriate content, privacy issues, internet addiction, and sleep deprivation. Health care providers need to assess media use and advise parents on ways to decrease media risks. Parents should be advised to evaluate websites their adolescent wants to participate in and verify they are age-appropriate. Parents should talk to their adolescent children daily about online use and activity and help them to balance online and offline activity. They need to discuss the dangers of sharing too much information and posting images or photographs. Parents should emphasize that once something is online, it is available for others to see and share and may be difficult to remove. Parents need to be educated on the technology their children are using and encourage the development of a family media use plan that involves establishing consistent, reasonable rules about use of cell phones, texting, the internet and social media. Such rules could include no media during meals and regular checking of privacy settings and online profiles for inappropriate content (American Academy of Pediatrics, Council on Communications and Media, 2016, reaffirmed 2022).

ADDRESSING COMMON DEVELOPMENTAL CONCERNS

Adolescence is a time of rapid growth and development with maturation of sexuality. The adolescent period begins with a child and ends with the expectation of adulthood. Many developmental concerns are present during this period, including violence, suicide, homicide, and substance misuse. The following is an overview of some of these concerns.

Violence

The CDC's Injury Center defines youth violence as occurring when young people between the ages of 10 and 24 years intentionally use physical force or power to threaten or harm others (CDC, 2022g). More than 1,000 youth are

BOX 29.5 Factors Contributing to Adolescent Violence

- Crowded conditions/housing
- Low socioeconomic status
- Limited parental supervision/involvement
- Single-parent families/both parents in workforce
- History of violent victimization
- Poor family functioning
- Access to guns or cars
- Drug or alcohol use
- Low self-esteem
- Racism
- Peer or gang pressure
- Aggression

treated in an emergency department as a result of injuries from physical violence every day (CDC, 2022g). The issue of youth violence is a growing concern in America's communities. The health and well-being of adolescents and society are threatened by this violence. See Box 29.5 for factors contributing to adolescent violence. Health care providers need to provide education on the effects and ways to prevent youth violence along with supporting programs developed to curb youth violence.

Suicide

Suicide is the third leading cause of death in people 10 to 19 years old (Kennebeck & Bonin, 2021). Certain factors can put adolescents at risk for suicide, but having these risk factors does not mean suicide will occur. Refer to Box 29.6 for risk factors for suicide in adolescents (see Healthy People 2030). Most people are not comfortable discussing the topic of suicide and therefore do not communicate openly about it. It is important that health care providers address this significant health problem and work to prevent suicide. The National Center for Injury Prevention and Control (NCIPC) is working to create awareness of suicide as a serious public health problem and is developing strategies to reduce injuries and deaths due to suicide.

BOX 29.6 Risk Factors for Suicide in Adolescents

- Depression or other mental illness
- Mental health changes
- Family history of suicide or mood disorders
- History of previous suicide attempt
- Poor school performance
- Family disorganization
- Substance misuse
- Marginalization for identifying as LGBTQ+
- Access to means to attempt suicide
- Social isolation
- History of physical or sexual abuse
- Exposure to violence or bullying
- Incarceration

Homicide

Homicide is the second leading cause of death in children between 10 and 24 years old, with the majority of victims being male and killed by firearms (CDC, 2022g; Naik-Mathuria & Gill, 2022). It is the leading cause of death for non-Hispanic Black or African American individuals 10 to 24 years old (CDC, 2022g). Refer to Box 29.5 for factors that contribute to violence among adolescents. In a nationwide survey conducted in 2019, 13% of participants reported carrying a weapon (e.g., gun, club, knife) on one or more days within the past 30 days (Sege, 2022; see Healthy People 2030).

HEALTHY PEOPLE 2030

Objective	Nursing Significance
Reduce physical fighting among adolescents. Reduce gun carrying among adolescents. Reduce suicide attempts by adolescents. Reduce suicidal thoughts in lesbian, gay, or bisexual high school students. Reduce suicidal thoughts in transgender students.	• Screen adolescents at all encounters for indications of violent behaviors. • Provide education related to decreasing school violence at middle and high schools. • Encourage alternative, appropriate methods for dispelling anger. • Screen adolescents at all encounters for indications of depression. • Assist schools to implement school-based initiatives that foster supportive, inclusive, antidiscriminatory environments.

Healthy People Objectives retrieved from http://www.healthypeople.gov

Dating Violence

Violent behavior that takes place in a context of dating is not a rare event and can have serious short-term and lifelong effects. In a recent survey, approximately 1 in 12 high school students reported physical violence, and one in 12 reported sexual violence from a dating partner in the past 12 months (CDC, 2022h). Dating violence in the adolescent years is a risk factor for continued violence exposure in adulthood. Risk factors for dating violence include inadequate parental supervision, substance misuse, history of physical or sexual abuse in childhood, early-onset puberty, early onset of sexual activity, identifying as LGBTQ+, low socioeconomic status, and risky sexual practices (Miller & Wiemann, 2020). Nurses need to assess for and provide interventions to those adolescents experiencing dating violence or those at risk for being a victim or perpetrator. Education on development of healthy relationships is important. See Healthy People 2030.

HEALTHY PEOPLE 2030

Objective	Nursing Significance
Reduce sexual or physical adolescent dating violence.	• Screen adolescents at all encounters for indications of dating violence. • Teach safe and healthy relationship skills. • Discuss with the adolescent good relationship role models in their life.

Healthy People Objectives retrieved from http://www.healthypeople.gov

Gangs

Much of youth violence is a result of the behavior of adolescent gangs. The risk factors for gang involvement are similar to those for aggressive or delinquent behavior. See Box 29.7 for risk factors for adolescent gang involvement. Gang membership occurs in cities and in suburban areas but may differ in composition. All socioeconomic groups are represented in gang membership. Gang membership may aid in the formation of identity by providing status and a sense of belonging. However, adolescents who are gang members are more likely to commit serious and violent crimes. Identifying those at risk and providing early intervention is important. Research has shown that increasing parental monitoring, increasing involvement in extracurricular activities, improving coping skills to deal with conflict, and educating about the negative consequences of gang membership may be beneficial in preventing gang membership (American Academy of Child and Adolescent Psychiatry, 2017).

Nursing Interventions to Decrease Youth Violence

Nurses working with adolescents should include violence prevention in anticipatory guidance. Violence is a learned behavior. It is often reinforced by the media, television, music, and personal example. Explain to parents, teachers, and peers the importance of being good role models. Parents should monitor video games, music, television, and other media to decrease exposure to violence. Parents need to know who their adolescent's friends are and monitor for negative behaviors and actions. Pediatric nurses play a key role in identifying at-risk youth and developing, planning, implementing, and evaluating interventions to prevent youth violence.

BOX 29.7 Risk Factors for Gang Involvement

- Delinquency involvement, especially at a young age
- History of or victim of physical violence or aggression
- Alcohol and drug use; drug dealing
- Association with violent or aggressive peers
- Low socioeconomic status
- Family with criminal history, drug or alcohol problems, violence in the home
- Poor parental supervision/involvement
- Poor academic performance
- Living in a community with a high rate of crime among adolescents and access to firearms and drugs

Substance Use

Agents commonly misused by children and adolescents include alcohol; nicotine; cannabis; prescribed medications such as Ritalin and OxyContin; hallucinogens; sedatives; analgesics; anxiolytics; steroids; inhalants (inhaling fumes of common household products); stimulants; opiates; and various club drugs such as ecstasy, gamma-hydroxybutyrate (GHB), and lysergic acid diethylamide (LSD). The substance misused is related to its availability and cost. Overall, the use of illicit drugs showed a decline in 2021 (Johnston et al., 2022). The occurrence of substance use varies by age, sex, race, ethnicity, and sociodemographic factors. Two common substances that are more accessible and have the highest incidence of use are alcohol and nicotine. Drug use often progresses from beer or wine to nicotine or hard liquor and then to cannabis, followed by illicit drugs.

Some of the long-term effects and consequences of drug and alcohol use include the possibility of overdose and death, unintentional injuries, irrational behaviors, inability to think clearly, unsafe driving and legal consequences, problems with relationships with family and friends, sexual activity and STIs, and health problems such as liver problems (hepatitis) and cardiac problems (sudden death with cocaine). Refer to Table 29.3 for commonly misused drugs and behaviors exhibited.

Tobacco/Nicotine

Smoking remains the leading preventable cause of death in the United States (CDC, 2023). Long-term consequences of adolescent smoking are reinforced by the fact that most young people who smoke regularly continue to smoke throughout adulthood. Each day in the United States, approximately 21,600 children younger than 18 years try their first cigarette, with 200 becoming regular smokers; nine out of 10 adult people who smoke started smoking before age 18 (CDC, 2022i). One in 13 Americans will die early from the effects of smoking (CDC, 2022i). The overall rate of use of any tobacco product has been declining, with the latest estimates at 4% of middle schoolers and 13.4% of high schoolers reporting use of any form of tobacco in the past 30 days (CDC, 2022i). There are many forms of tobacco use, such as e-cigarettes, flavored cigars, smokeless tobacco, hookahs, pipes, nicotine pouches, heated tobacco products,

TABLE 29.3 • Drugs Commonly Misused

Drug	Manifestations	Considerations
Cannabis	Red eyes; dry mouth; euphoria; relaxation; decreased motivation; difficulty with coordination, thinking, and problem solving; loss of inhibition; appetite stimulation	Considered a gateway drug
Synthetic cannabis	Laboratory-synthesized liquid chemicals mimic the effect of tetrahydrocannabinol (THC), the psychoactive ingredient in the naturally grown cannabis plant; relaxed feeling, mild changes in perception, extreme paranoia, anxiety, hallucinations	Unpredictable effect; not clear what chemicals are used and how they can harm the body; symptoms reported include increased heart rate, vomiting, agitation, confusion, hallucinations; has been associated with heart attacks
Cocaine and crack	Powerful stimulant; weight loss, euphoria, elation, agitation, increased motor activity, pressured speech, dilated pupils, tachycardia, hypertension, anorexia, insomnia	Psychotic behavior with large doses; if combined with other drugs can be fatal
Heroin	Elation, euphoria, detachment, drowsiness, constricted pupils, slurred speech, impaired judgment	Tolerance, dependence, and highly addictive; self-neglect with malnutrition and dehydration; criminal behaviors to get drugs; infections at injection sites; at risk for acquiring human immunodeficiency virus (HIV)/acquired immunodeficiency syndrome (AIDS) and hepatitis; highly addictive; can lead to coma or death
Prescription opiate drugs: • Oxycodone • Hydrocodone • Diphenoxylate • Morphine • Codeine • Fentanyl • Propoxyphene • Hydromorphone • Meperidine • Methadone	Feelings of relaxation and euphoria	Can lead to addiction and drug-seeking behaviors; high doses can lead to breathing complications and death
Methamphetamine	Euphoria, increased energy and alertness, agitation, weight loss, insomnia, tachycardia, hypertension	Increased risk of human immunodeficiency virus (HIV)/acquired immunodeficiency syndrome (AIDS) or hepatitis; risk for dysrhythmia and hyperthermia; repeated use can cause violent behavior and psychosis; possible paradoxical effect of depression in children
MDMA (3,4-methylenedioxymethamphetamine) and other club drugs (lysergic acid diethylamide [LSD], ketamine, phencyclidine [PCP])	Hallucinations, illusions, euphoria, hyperalertness, depersonalization, heightened sensual awareness, dilated pupils, hypertension, increased salivation, distorted perceptions. agitation, violence, antisocial behaviors, loss of sense of time, forceful clenching of the teeth	Panic flashbacks long after use of drugs; psychotic behaviors; can lead to hyperthermia as it interferes with the body's ability to regulate temperature; memory loss with long-term use; high blood levels lead to increased risk of seizures and dysrhythmia
Inhalants	Similar effects as alcohol but high only lasts a few minutes, slurred speech, lack of coordination, euphoria, dizziness	Long-term use can break down myelin and damage brain cells.
Bath salts	Similar effect as stimulants such as methamphetamines and MDMA; hallucinatory effects	Much is still unknown about how these substances affect the brain; linked to a high number of emergency room and Poison Control Center visits
Prescription stimulants such as dextroamphetamine and methylphenidate	Increased alertness, attention, and energy; feelings of exhilaration; increased heart rate and blood pressure	High doses increase risk for dysrhythmia, hyperthermia, heart failure, and seizures. If mixed with antidepressants or over-the-counter cold medicines can lead to dangerously high blood pressure and dysrhythmia.

TABLE 29.3 • Drugs Commonly Misused

Drug	Manifestations	Considerations
Prescription central nervous system depressants: • Mephobarbital; sodium pentobarbital • Diazepam • Alprazolam • Lorazepam • Estazolam • Zolpidem • Zaleplon Eszopiclone	Euphoria followed by depression or hostility, decreased anxiety, drowsiness, impaired judgment, decreased inhibitions, slurred speech, incoordination	Often used with stimulants; may have a paradoxical effect of hyperactivity in children
Dextromethorphan	Taken in very large amounts; effects similar to phencyclidine (PCP) and ketamine; feelings of being detached from oneself and the environment	Found in over-the-counter cold medicines; can lead to impaired motor function, numbness, nausea, vomiting, increased heart rate and blood pressure; risk of hypoxic brain damage

Data from Breuner, C. C. (2020). Substance abuse. In R. M. Kleigman, J. W. St. Geme, III, N. J. Blum, S. S. Shah, R. C. Tasker, K. M. Wilson, & R. E. Behrman (Eds.), *Nelson textbook of pediatrics* (21st ed., pp. 5678–5765). Elsevier; Blake, K., & Van Eyk, N. (2023b). Section 12: Adolescent medicine. Substance abuse. In K. J. Marcdante, R. M. Kleigman, & A. M. Schuh (Eds.), *Nelson essentials of pediatrics* (9th ed., pp. 297–300). Elsevier.

and bidis. Electronic nicotine delivery systems (ENDSs), such as vaporizers, vapes, and e-cigarettes, may look like conventional cigarettes or resemble things such as pens and USB flash drives. There was an upward trend in the use of ENDSs in middle and high school students from 2013 to 2019, but it has since declined (Rigotti & Reddy, 2022). Adolescents need to be aware that e-cigarettes are not a safe alternative to smoking. Nicotine, which is highly addictive, and other harmful chemicals are absorbed through the lungs and into the body with the use of e-cigarettes. Nicotine is harmful to the developing brain and can have lasting effects.

TAKE NOTE!

In 2016, the U.S. Food and Drug Administration extended their regulation on all tobacco and nicotine products and has a comprehensive plan to help better protect our youth and decrease the number of adolescents using Electronic Nicotine Delivery Systems (ENDSs). Most states have enacted minimum legal age for sales of ENDSs ranging from 18 to 21 years old.

Adolescents who smoke are more likely than those who don't to use alcohol and illegal drugs (American Cancer Society, 2020). Smoking is associated with other risky behaviors, including fighting, carrying weapons, mental health problems such as depression, attempting suicide, and engaging in unprotected sex (American Cancer Society, 2020). Studies have found that the use of e-cigarettes (or vaping) in youth is strongly linked to the use of regular cigarettes and other tobacco products in adulthood (American Cancer Society, 2022). The short-term health effects of smoking include damage to the respiratory system, addiction to nicotine, and the associated risk of other drug use. Smoking negatively impacts physical fitness and lung growth and increases the potential for addiction in adolescents. Smokeless tobacco may also cause many problems. It can lead to bleeding gums and sores in the mouth that never heal. Smokeless tobacco use leads to discoloration of the teeth and may eventually lead to cancer.

HEALTHY PEOPLE 2030

Objective	Nursing Significance
Reduce current use of tobacco products among adolescents. Reduce current use of e-cigarettes among adolescents. Reduce current use of cigarettes among adolescents. Reduce current use of cigars among adolescents. Reduce current use of flavored tobacco products among adolescent tobacco users. Reduce current use of cigarettes among adolescents. Reduce current use of smokeless tobacco products among adolescents.	• Provide education in the office, hospital, or school related to adverse effects of tobacco/nicotine. • Emphasize the dangers of tobacco/nicotine. • Praise adolescents for abstaining from the use of tobacco/nicotine products and rising above peer pressure.

Healthy People Objectives retrieved from http://www.healthypeople.gov

Alcohol

Although alcohol remains the most widely used and misused drug among youths in the United States, its use among adolescents has continued a downward trend (Johnston, 2022). A national survey on drug use found that 26% of eighth graders and 61.5% of 12th graders reported ever trying alcohol, while 7% of eighth graders, 13% of 10th graders, and 26% of 12th graders reported drinking alcohol in the past 30 days (Johnston, 2022). The incidence of alcohol use increases throughout adolescence, and adolescents who begin drinking before the age of 15 are 5.6 times more likely to develop alcohol dependence later in life (NIH/National Institute on Alcohol Abuse and Alcoholism, 2022). Alcohol use in adolescence can lead to prevailing alcohol use in adulthood; contributes to physical health problems, school problems, and legal problems; leads to increased injuries; impairs judgment; increases the risk of sexual and physical assault; and interferes with brain development (NIH/National Institute on Alcohol Abuse and Alcoholism, 2022). It may also precede other drug misuse.

HEALTHY PEOPLE 2030

Objective	Nursing Significance
Reduce the proportion of adolescents reporting use of alcohol during the past 30 days. Reduce the proportion of adolescents reporting use of any illicit drugs during the past 30 days. Reduce the proportion of adolescents reporting use of cannabis in the past 30 days. Reduce the proportion of persons under 21 engaging in binge drinking of alcoholic beverages. Reduce the proportion of motor vehicle crash deaths involving an alcohol-impaired driver with a blood alcohol concentration (BAC) of 0.08 g/dL or higher. Increase the proportion of adolescents who perceive great risk associated with substance misuse.	• Provide education in the office, hospital, or school related to adverse effects of alcohol and illicit substance use. • Emphasize the dangers of substance use and driving, and educate the adolescent to never get in a car with someone who is under the influence of alcohol or drugs. • Praise adolescents for abstaining from the above substances and rising above peer pressure.

Healthy People Objectives retrieved from http://www.healthypeople.gov

TAKE NOTE!

Research shows adolescents who have parents who are actively involved in their lives are less likely to drink alcohol (NIH/National Institute on Alcohol Abuse and Alcoholism, 2022).

Illicit Drugs

Adolescents may also experiment with or misuse illicit drugs. Substance misuse remains a widespread problem among American adolescents, even though prevalence is trending downward. Cannabis remains the most widely used illicit drug (Johnston et al., 2022). A national survey on drug use showed the annual prevalence rate for illicit drugs remaining stable at the lowest levels in over 20 years, with a significant decline seen in 2021 (Johnston et al., 2022). During this time, the COVID-19 pandemic led to changes in adolescent lives and decreased social and school activities (Johnston et al., 2022). The trends in adolescent drug use need continued monitoring to assess if the decline will persist over time.

Factors that primarily affect drug use include the psychoactive potential and benefits reported, how risky the drug is to use, how acceptable it is to peer groups, and the accessibility and availability of the drug. The riskier or less accepted a drug is by peers, the less likely the adolescent will use it.

Nursing Interventions to Decrease Substance Misuse Among Adolescents

Adolescents' brains are still developing, leaving them particularly vulnerable to the damaging effects of drugs. Substance misuse in adolescence is related to poorer health outcomes; therefore, it is important that nurses be aware of interventions to decrease these behaviors. Adolescent drug misuse is related to social factors, including times of life transitions and stress, such as changing schools, moving, or divorce, as well as peer factors such as peer pressure. Therefore, nurses need to target assessments and programs at these critical times. Based on reviews of programs and interventions, it has been found that certain methods work. Programs that reach children and adolescents through a variety of sources such as school, family, community, and media campaigns are more successful. Programs that are culturally competent and address all forms of drug use (alcohol, tobacco, and illicit drugs) tend to work well. Programs that focus on increasing awareness of the risks and health consequences of substance use are important. Certain factors have been found to help adolescents remain drug-free. These include strong connections to parents, family, school, and religion; presence of parents in the home at key times of the day; and limited access to substances such as alcohol, tobacco, and cannabis (NIH/National Institute on Alcohol Abuse and Alcoholism, 2022). Programs that focus on decreasing risk factors and increasing protective factors such as enhancing self-esteem, social and parental support, and stress-specific coping skills are beneficial. Topics that should be discussed include:

- Short- and long-term effects of alcohol, tobacco, and drugs on health
- Risk factors and implications for unintentional injuries and sexual activity

- Short- and long-term effects of alcohol, tobacco, and drugs on relationships and school performance and progression
- The how and why of chemical dependency
- Impact of substance abuse on society
- Importance of maintaining a healthy lifestyle
- Importance of resisting peer pressure to use drugs and alcohol
- Importance of having confidence in one's own judgment

Refer back to 15-year-old Cho. List some common developmental concerns of the adolescent. What anticipatory guidance related to these concerns would you provide?

KEY CONCEPTS

- Adolescence is a period of rapid and variable growth in the areas of physical, psychosocial, cognitive, and moral development.
- The adolescent is developing their own identity, becoming an abstract thinker, and developing their own set of morals and values. Inability to successfully develop an individual identity leads to poor preparation for the challenges of adulthood.
- Relationships with parents fluctuate widely during adolescence. The adolescent eventually gains independence from their parents.
- Peers become most important—guiding mainly the early and middle adolescent in their decisions—while the late adolescent can usually formulate their own decisions.
- Adolescence is a critical time in the development of sexuality. Sexuality includes the thoughts, feelings, and behaviors surrounding the adolescent's sexual identity.
- The egocentric and invincible thought processes of the adolescent can lead to injuries. Health care providers must emphasize safety regarding cars, bikes, water, firearms, and fire.
- Unintentional injury is the leading cause of death in adolescents (CDC, 2021a). Motor vehicle crashes are the leading cause of unintentional injury death followed by poisoning, primarily due to drug overdose from opioids, and drowning (CDC, 2021a).
- Nutritional habits of the adolescent lead to deficiency in vitamins and minerals needed for the rapid growth during this period.
- Excess weight in adolescents is a growing health concern. Health care providers are facing increased numbers of adolescents with hypertension, type 2 diabetes, and hyperlipidemia.
- Substance misuse and experimentation is common during adolescence; it is associated with other risk-taking behaviors such as injuries and sexual activity.
- Health care providers must work collaboratively with the adolescent in the development of interventions to promote health.

REFERENCES AND RECOMMENDED READINGS

American Academy of Child and Adolescent Psychiatry. (2017). *Gangs and children.* https://www.aacap.org/AACAP/Families_and_Youth/Facts_for_Families/FFF-Guide/Children-and-Gangs-098.aspx

American Academy of Pediatrics. (2010, reaffirmed 2016). The teen driver. *Pediatrics, 118*(6), 2570–2581. http://pediatrics.aappublications.org/content/118/6/2570.full

American Academy of Pediatrics, Council on Communications and Media. (2016, reaffirmed 2022). Policy statement: Media use in school-aged children and adolescents. *Pediatrics, 138*(5), Article e20162592. https://doi.org/10.1542/peds.2016-2592

American Academy of Pediatrics, Council on Environmental Health and Section on Dermatology. (2011, reaffirmed 2017). Policy statement—Ultraviolet radiation: A hazard to children and adolescents. *Pediatrics, 127*(3), e791–e817. https://doi.org/10.1542/peds.2010-3502

American Academy of Pediatrics, HealthyChildren. (2022). *ATVs are not safe for children: AAP policy explained.* https://www.healthychildren.org/English/safety-prevention/at-play/Pages/ATV-Safety-Rules.aspx

American Cancer Society. (2020). *Health risks of smoking tobacco.* https://www.cancer.org/content/dam/CRC/PDF/Public/8345.00.pdf

American Cancer Society. (2022). *What do we know about e-cigarettes?* https://www.cancer.org/content/dam/CRC/PDF/Public/9309.00.pdf

American Psychological Association. (2019). *Children, youth, families and socioeconomic status.* Retrieved January 21, 2019, from https://www.apa.org/pi/ses/resources/publications/children-families.aspx

American Public Health Association. (2018). *The dropout crisis: A public health problem and the role of school-based health care.* https://www.apha.org/-/media/Files/PDF/SBHC/Dropout_Crisis.ashx

American Public Health Association. (2021). *Supporting physical education in schools for all youth.* https://apha.org/Policies-and-Advocacy/Public-Health-Policy-Statements/Policy-Database/2022/01/07/Supporting-Physical-Education-in-Schools-for-All-Youth

Blake, K., & Van Eyk, N. (2023a). Adolescent medicine: Overview and assessment of adolescents. In K. J. Marcdante, R. M. Kleigman, & A. M. Schuh (Eds.), *Nelson essentials of pediatrics* (9th ed., pp. 281–287). Elsevier.

Blake, K., & Van Eyk, N. (2023b). Adolescent medicine: Substance abuse. In K. J. Marcdante, R. M. Kleigman, & A. M. Schuh (Eds.), *Nelson essentials of pediatrics* (9th ed., pp. 297–300). Elsevier.

Breuner, C. C. (2020). Substance abuse. In R. M. Kleigman, J. W. St. Geme, III, N. J. Blum, S. S. Shah, R. C. Tasker, K. M. Wilson, & R. E. Behrman (Eds.), *Nelson textbook of pediatrics* (21st ed., pp. 5678–5765). Elsevier.

Centers for Disease Control and Prevention. (2020). *Sleep in middle and high school students.* https://www.cdc.gov/healthyschools/features/students-sleep.htm

Centers for Disease Control and Prevention. (2021a). *Injuries among children and teens.* https://www.cdc.gov/injury/features/child-injury/index.html#:~:text=That%20is%20about%2020%20deaths,Child%20injury%20is%20often%20preventable

Centers for Disease Control and Prevention. (2021b). *Teen drivers: Get the facts.* https://cdctransportation.org/www.cdc.gov/transportationsafety/teen_drivers/teendrivers_factsheet.html

Centers for Disease Control and Prevention. (2021c). *Keep teen drivers safe.* https://www.cdc.gov/injury/features/teen-drivers/index.html

Centers for Disease Control and Prevention. (2022a). *CDC healthy schools: Physical activity facts.* https://www.cdc.gov/healthyschools/physicalactivity/facts.htm

Centers for Disease Control and Prevention. (2022b). *CDC healthy schools: Health & academics.* https://www.cdc.gov/healthyschools/health_and_academics/index.htm

Centers for Disease Control and Prevention. (2022c). *Drowning facts.* Replace with this link please https://www.cdc.gov/drowning/facts/index.html

Centers for Disease Control and Prevention. (2022d). *Obesity.* https://www.cdc.gov/healthyschools/obesity/facts.htm

Centers for Disease Control and Prevention. (2022e). *Consequences of obesity.* https://www.cdc.gov/obesity/basics/consequences.html

Centers for Disease Control and Prevention. (2022f). *Overweight and obesity: Childhood obesity facts.* https://www.cdc.gov/obesity/data/childhood.html#:~:text=Prevalence%20of%20Childhood%20Obesity%20in%20the%20United%20States&text=The%20prevalence%20of%20obesity%20was,to%2019%2Dyear%2Dolds

Centers for Disease Control and Prevention. (2022g). *Preventing youth violence.* https://www.cdc.gov/violenceprevention/youthviolence/fastfact.html?CDC_AA_refVal=https%3A%2F%2Fwww.cdc.gov%2Fviolenceprevention%2Fyouthviolence%2Fdefinitions.html

Centers for Disease Control and Prevention. (2022h). *Preventing teen dating violence.* https://www.cdc.gov/violenceprevention/pdf/ipv/TDV-factsheet_2022.pdf

Centers for Disease Control and Prevention. (2022i). *Smoking & tobacco use: Youth and tobacco use.* https://www.cdc.gov/tobacco/data_statistics/fact_sheets/youth_data/tobacco_use/index.htm

Centers for Disease Control and Prevention. (2023). *Smoking and tobacco use: Fast facts and fact sheets.* https://www.cdc.gov/tobacco/data_statistics/fact_sheets/fast_facts/index.htm

Centers for Disease Control and Prevention, & National Center for Health Statistics. (2022). *All injuries.* https://www.cdc.gov/nchs/fastats/injury.htm

Desai, N. (2021). Tattooing in adolescents and young adults. *UpToDate.* Retrieved November 2, 2022, from https://www.uptodate.com/contents/tattooing-in-adolescents-and-young-adults

Desai, N. (2023). *Body piercing in adolescents and young adults. UpToDate.* Retrieved October 15, 2023, from https://www.uptodate.com/contents/body-piercing-in-adolescents-and-young-adults

Eickmeyer, K., Hemez, P., Manning, W. D., Brown, S. L., & Guzzo, K. B. (2020). *Trends in relationship formation and stability in the United States dating, cohabitation, marriage, and divorce.* http://mastresearchcenter.org/wp-content/uploads/2020/05/MAST-PA1-Trends-Brief_May-2020_final.pdf

Emerson, A., Pickett, M., Moore, S., & Kelly, P. J. (2023). A scoping review of digital health interventions to promote healthy romantic relationships in adolescents. *Prevention Science, 24*(4), 625–639. https://doi.org/10.1007/s11121-022-01421-0

Erikson, E. (1963). *Childhood and society* (2nd ed.). Norton.

Forcier, M., & Olson-Kennedy, J. (2020). Lesbian, gay, bisexual, and other sexual minoritized youth: Epidemiology and health concerns. *UpToDate.* Retrieved October 23, 2022, from https://www.uptodate.com/contents/lesbian-gay-bisexual-and-other-sexual-minoritized-youth-epidemiology-and-health-concerns

Ford, G. S. (2007). Hospitalized kids: Spiritual care at their level. *Journal of Christian Nursing, 24*(3), 135–140. https://doi.org/10.1097/01.cnj.0000279357.48047.a3

Gill, A. C. (2022). Bicycle injuries in children: Prevention. *UpToDate.* Retrieved October 17, 2022, from https://www.uptodate.com/contents/bicycle-injuries-in-children-prevention

Goldbach, J. T., Rhoades, H., Mamey, M. R., Senese, J., Karys, P., & Marsiglia. F. F. (2021). Reducing behavioral health symptoms by addressing minority stressors in LGBTQ adolescents: A randomized controlled trial of proud & empowered. *BMC Public Health, 21,* 2315. https://doi.org/10.1186/s12889-021-12357-5

Goldstick, J. E., Cunningham, R. M., & Carter, P. M. (2022). Current causes of death in children and adolescents in the United States [Editorial]. *New England Journal of Medicine, 386*(20), 1955–1956. https://doi.org/10.1056/NEJMc2201761

Holland-Hall, C. (2020). Adolescent physical and social development. In R. M. Kleigman, J. W. St. Geme, III, N. J. Blum, S. S. Shah, R. C. Tasker, K. M. Wilson, & R. E. Behrman (Eds.), *Nelson textbook of pediatrics* (21st ed., pp. 5550–5576). Elsevier.

Johnston, L. D., Miech, R. A., O'Malley, P. M., Bachman, J. G., Schulenberg, J. E., & Patrick, M. E. (2022). *Monitoring the future national survey results on drug use 1975–2021: Overview, key findings on adolescent drug use.* Institute for Social Research, University of Michigan. https://monitoringthefuture.org/wp-content/uploads/2022/08/mtf-overview2021.pdf

Kansky, J., & Allen, J. P. (2018). Long-term risks and possible benefits associated with late adolescent romantic relationship quality. *Journal of Youth and Adolescents, 47*(7), 1531–1544. https://doi.org/10.1007%2Fs10964-018-0813-x

Kennebeck, S., & Bonin, L. (2021). Suicidal behavior in children and adolescents: Epidemiology and risk factors. *UpToDate.* Retrieved November 3, 2022, from https://www.uptodate.com/contents/suicidal-behavior-in-children-and-adolescents-epidemiology-and-risk-factors

Kohlberg, L. (1984). *Essays on moral development.* Harper & Row.

Mattoo, T. K. (2021). Epidemiology, risk factors, and etiology of hypertension in children and adolescents. *UpToDate.* Retrieved October 23, 2022, from https://www.uptodate.com/contents/epidemiology-risk-factors-and-etiology-of-hypertension-in-children-and-adolescents

Merlo, C. L., Jones, S. E., Michael, S. L., Chen, T. J., Sliwa, S. A., Lee, S. H, Brener, N. D., Lee, S. M., & Parket, S. (2020). Dietary and physical activity behaviors among high school students—

Youth Risk Behavior Survey, United States, 2019. *MMWR Supplements, 69*(Suppl. 1), 64–76. http://doi.org/10.15585/mmwr.su6901a8

Miller, E., & Wiemann, C. M. (2020). Adolescent relationship abuse including physical and sexual teen dating violence. *UpToDate*. Retrieved November 3, 2022, from https://www.uptodate.com/contents/adolescent-relationship-abuse-including-physical-and-sexual-teen-dating-violence

Naik-Mathuria, B., & Gill, A. C. (2022). Firearm injuries in children: Prevention. *UpToDate*. Retrieved October 31, 2022, from https://www.uptodate.com/contents/firearm-injuries-in-children-prevention

National Center for Education Statistics. (n.d.). Trends in high school dropout and completion rates in the United States. https://nces.ed.gov/programs/dropout/intro.asp

National Center for Education Statistics. (2022). *Condition of education: Status dropout rates*. U.S. Department of Education, Institute of Education Sciences. https://nces.ed.gov/programs/coe/indicator/coj

NIH/National Institute on Alcohol Abuse and Alcoholism. (2022). *Underage drinking*. https://www.niaaa.nih.gov/sites/default/files/publications/NIAAA_Underage_Drinking_1.pdf

Paul, C. R., & Wallace, C. M. (2023). Behavioral disorders: Normal sleep and pediatric sleep disorders. In K. J. Marcdante, R. M. Kleigman, & A. M. Schuh (Eds.), *Nelson essentials of pediatrics* (9th ed., pp. 54–58). Elsevier.

Pew Research Center. (2022). *Teens, social media and technology 2022*. https://www.pewresearch.org/internet/2022/08/10/teens-social-media-and-technology-2022/

Piaget, J. (1969). *The theory of stages in cognitive development*. McGraw-Hill.

Rigotti, N. A., & Reddy, K. P. (2022). Vaping and e-cigarettes. *UpToDate*. Retrieved November 3, 2022, from https://www.uptodate.com/contents/vaping-and-e-cigarettes

Sege, R. D. (2022). Peer violence and violence prevention. *UpToDate*. Retrieved November 3, 2022, from https://www.uptodate.com/contents/peer-violence-and-violence-prevention

U.S. Department of Agriculture, & U.S. Department of Health and Human Services. (2020). *Dietary guidelines for Americans, 2020–2025* (9th ed.). https://www.dietaryguidelines.gov/sites/default/files/2021-03/Dietary_Guidelines_for_Americans-2020-2025.pdf

U.S. Department of Health and Human Services. (n.d.). *Healthy people 2030*. https://health.gov/healthypeople

Woessner, M. N., Tacey, A., Levinger-Limor, A., Parker, A. G., Levinger, P., & Levinger, I. (2021). The evolution of technology and physical inactivity: The good, the bad, and the way forward. *Frontiers in Public Health, 9*, 655491. https://doi.org/10.3389/fpubh.2021.655491

DEVELOPING CLINICAL JUDGMENT

PRACTICING FOR NCLEX

1. When giving parents guidance for the adolescent years, which would the nurse advise the parents to do? Select all that apply.
a. Accept the adolescent as a unique individual.
b. Provide strict, inflexible rules.
c. Listen and try to be open to the adolescent's views.
d. Screen all of their friends.
e. Respect the adolescent's privacy.
f. Provide unconditional love.

2. In developing a weight loss plan for an adolescent, which would the nurse include? Select all that apply.
a. Have parents make all of the meal plans.
b. Eat slowly and place the fork down between each bite.
c. Have the family exercise together.
d. Refer to an adolescent weight loss program.
e. Keep a food and exercise diary.

3. Which is associated with the period of early adolescence? Select all that apply.
a. Uses scientific reasoning to solve problems
b. At times, still wants to be dependent on parents
c. Incorporates own set of morals and values
d. Is influenced by peers and values memberships in cliques

4. What has the most influence in deterring an adolescent from beginning to drink alcohol?
a. Drinking habits of parents
b. Drinking habits of peers
c. Drinking philosophy of adolescent's culture
d. Drinking philosophy of adolescent's religion

5. The nurse is teaching a parent about adolescent growth and development. After the teaching session, the parent should be able to verbalize that adolescence is a time of ___________growth and the adolescent needs ______________ and ___________.

Blank 1:
a. rapid
b. slow
c. continual
d. gradual

Blanks 2 and 3:
a. more than 8 hours of sleep
b. increased calories
c. a low-calcium diet
d. decreased calories
e. fewer than 8 hours of sleep
f. a low protein diet

6. The nurse is caring for an 11-year-old female. What changes in puberty should the nurse expect to find on assessment? Select all that apply.
a. Hip girth widening
b. Pubic hair beginning to curl
c. Breasts beginning to separate
d. Breast buds enlarging
e. Genital pigmentation increasing

CRITICAL THINKING EXERCISES

1. During a sports physical examination, Susan, a 16-year-old, tells her health care provider that she is overweight. What additional information would the nurse obtain?

2. The parents of Joe, a 14-year-old, talk to the school nurse about Joe's behavior at home. He is moody, fights with his younger siblings, only wants to be on his computer, and does not want to go on the family vacation. What advice would the nurse give the parents?

3. Jane tells the school nurse that she thinks she might be a lesbian. What additional information would the nurse obtain?

4. Alicia's parents are worried because all of Alicia's friends wear heavy makeup and have multiple piercings and hair colors. What advice would the nurse give Alicia's parents?

STUDY ACTIVITIES

1. Talk to an early, middle, and late adolescent. Compare and contrast their interactions with you. Identify what psychosocial, cognitive, and moral stage they are in, using examples from their conversations with you.

2. Have an adolescent keep a food and exercise diary for 1 week. Analyze the information. Develop with the adolescent any interventions needed to promote healthy eating and exercise habits.

3. Plan a class on the dangers of smoking and electronic nicotine delivery systems (ENDSs) for 15-year-olds.

4. Plan a class for parents on how to keep the lines of communication open for adolescents.

5. Go to https://www.myplate.gov/myplate-plan and create and compare a customized meal plan for an adolescent at a healthy weight versus an adolescent with excess weight.

UNIT

X

Foundations of Pediatric Nursing

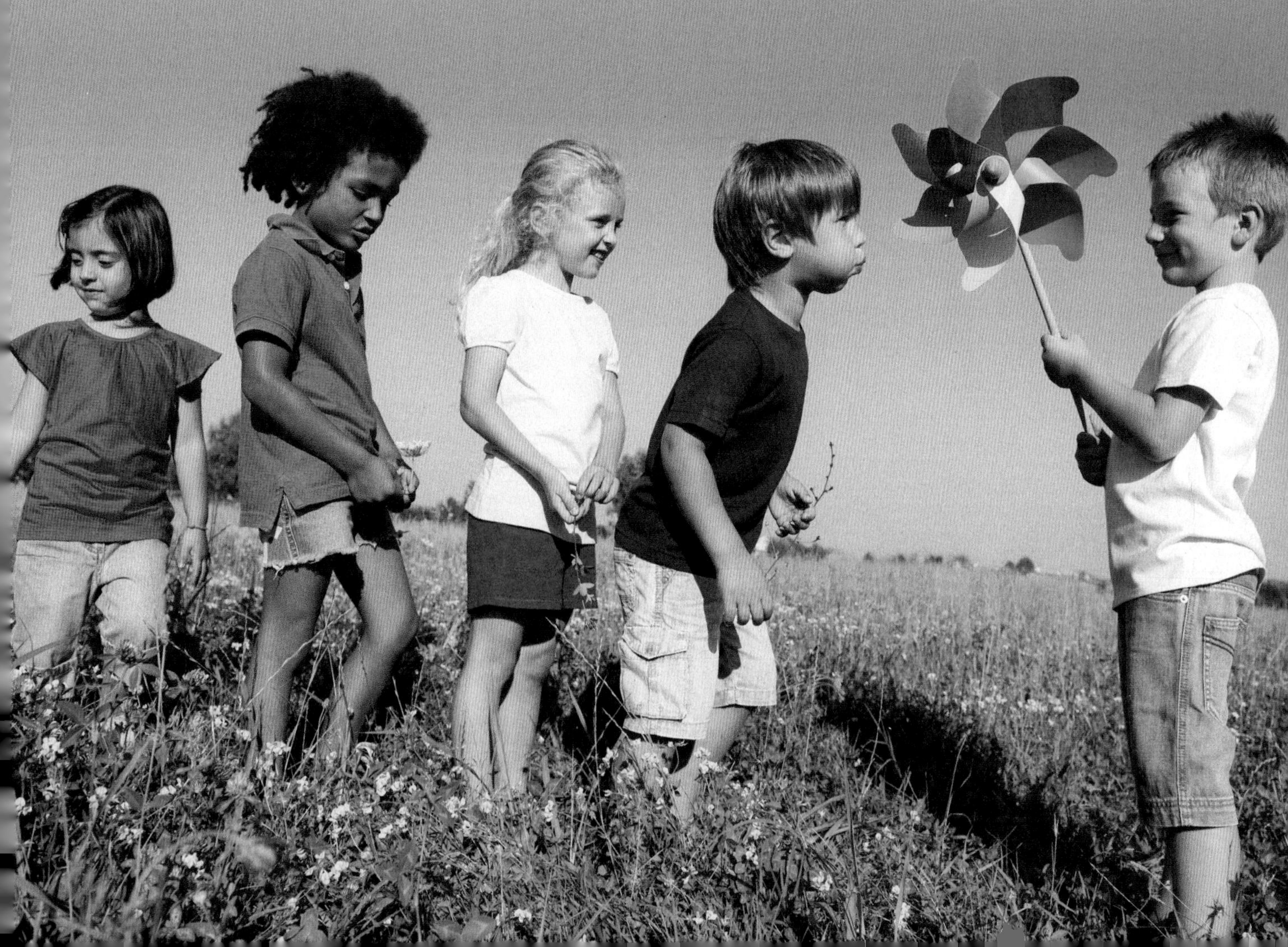

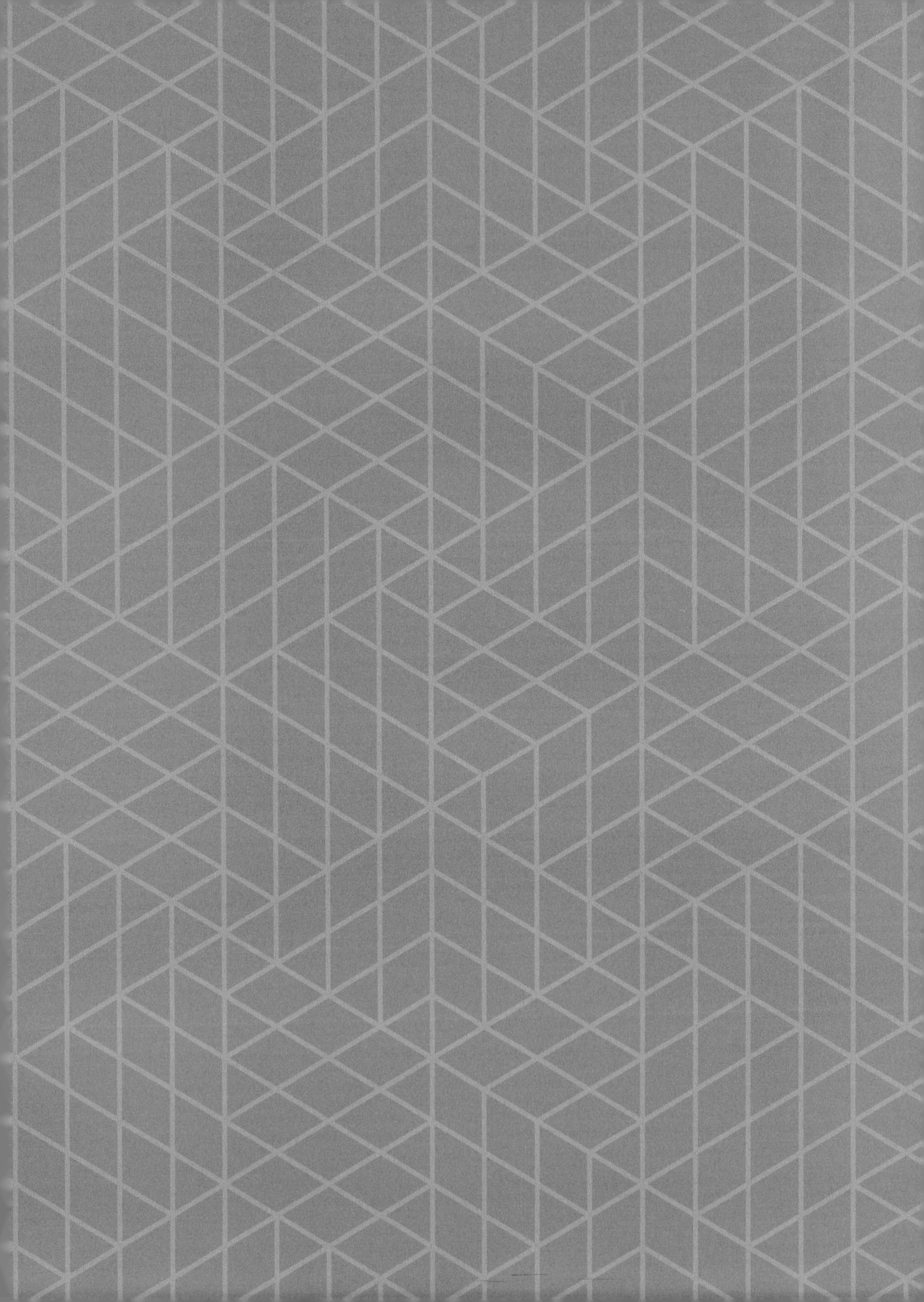

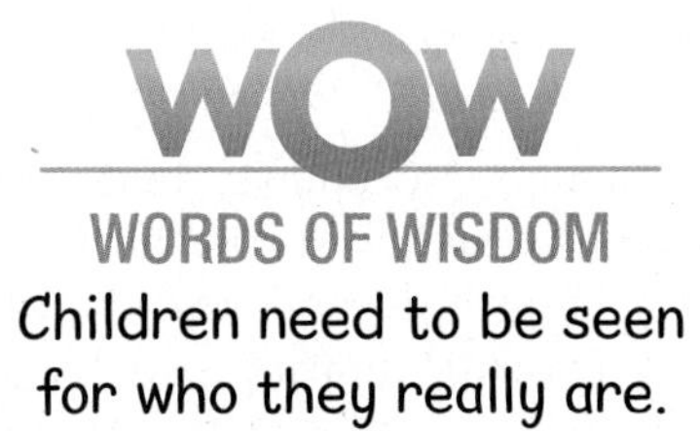

WOW
WORDS OF WISDOM
Children need to be seen
for who they really are.

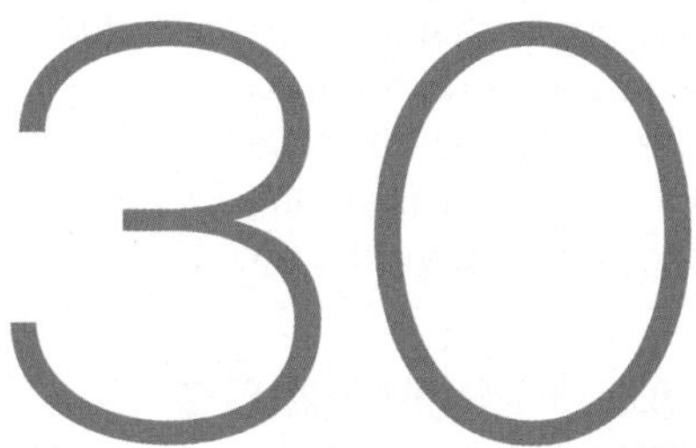

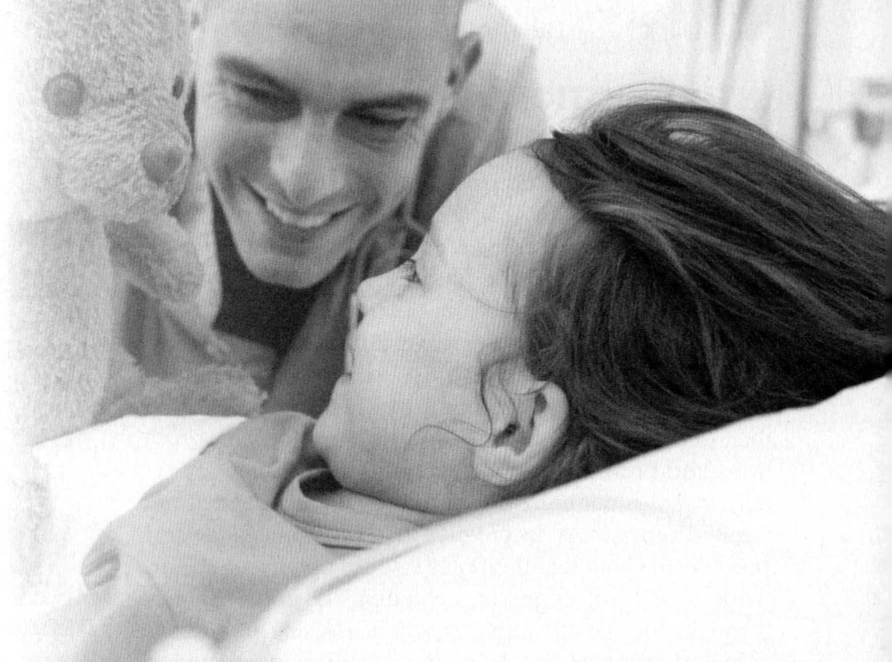

Atraumatic Care of Children and Families

LEARNING OBJECTIVES

Upon completion of the chapter, you will be able to:

1. Describe the major principles and concepts of atraumatic care.
2. Describe interventions to incorporate atraumatic care to prevent and minimize physical stress for children and families.
3. Explain the major components and concepts of family-centered care.
4. Discuss appropriate therapeutic communication skills when interacting with children and their families.
5. Describe the process of health teaching as it relates to children and their families.

Emma Moore, 4 years old, is admitted to the pediatric unit with a suspected head injury from a fall. She was playing at a playground with a babysitter and fell from the top of the slide.

KEY TERMS

atraumatic care
child life specialist
family-centered care
therapeutic hugging

INTRODUCTION

Atraumatic care is defined as therapeutic care that minimizes or eliminates the psychological and physical distress experienced by children and their families in the health care system (Wong, 1995). This concept is based on the underlying premise of "do no harm." Box 30.1 highlights the major principles of atraumatic care.

Pediatric nurses must be vigilant for any situation that may cause distress and must be able to identify potential stressors. It is important to provide nursing care that decreases the child's exposure to stressful situations and prevents or minimizes pain and bodily injury; take steps to minimize separation of the child from the family; and utilize techniques of communication and provide teaching that promotes a sense of control. Atraumatic care involves guiding children and their families through the health care experience using a family-centered approach by promoting family roles, fostering family support of the child, and providing appropriate information. Help children cope with this experience by using age-appropriate and child-specific interventions. Preparation can help children and their families adjust to illness and hospitalization. Use appropriate techniques for therapeutic communication (goal-directed, focused, purposeful communication); therapeutic play (type of play that provides an emotional outlet or improves the child's ability to cope with the stress of illness and hospitalization); and education to help the child and family understand the reason for the hospitalization and the necessary tests and procedures. In addition, help the family and other health care personnel obtain the resources and relationships they need for optimal care.

The best pediatric nursing care encompasses the concepts of atraumatic care. Minimizing physical stressors during procedures, providing family-centered care, and utilizing excellent communication skills on the part of the nurse enhance the health care experience for the child and family. Having an informed and educated family is the best way to provide optimal health care for children.

Table 30.1 gives suggestions for incorporating the principles of atraumatic care into nursing care for the child and family. Look for tips on atraumatic care as it relates to specific topics throughout the text.

BOX 30.1 Principles of Atraumatic Care

- Prevent or minimize physical stressors, including pain, discomfort, immobility, sleep deprivation, inability to eat or drink, and changes in elimination.
  - Avoid or reduce intrusive and painful procedures, such as injections, multiple punctures, and urethral catheterization.
  - Avoid or reduce other kinds of physical distress, such as noise, smells, shivering, nausea and vomiting, sleeplessness, restraints, and skin trauma.
  - Control pain via frequent assessments and use of pharmacologic and nonpharmacologic interventions.
- Prevent or minimize parent–child separation.
  - Promote family-centered care, treating the family as the patient.
  - Use core primary nursing.
  - Consider research findings related to preferences of parents and children and whether to be together.
- Promote a sense of control.
  - Elicit the family's knowledge about the child and their health condition, promoting partnerships, empowerment, and enabling.
  - Reduce fear of the unknown through education, familiar articles, and decreasing the threat of the environment.
  - Provide opportunities for control, such as participating in care, attempting to normalize a daily schedule, and providing direct suggestions.

Adapted from Wong, D. (1995). *Whaley & Wong's nursing care of infants and children* (5th ed.). Mosby.

PREVENTING AND MINIMIZING PHYSICAL STRESSORS

The health care facility or hospital is an unfamiliar environment for children and parents and may upset or intimidate them. They may feel anxiety, fear, helplessness, anger, or loss of control. Even health care procedures performed in the home or school may be perceived as threatening to children. To prevent and minimize the physical stress experienced by children and their families in relation to health care, pediatric nurses, child life specialists (CLSs), and other health care professionals recommend the use of atraumatic care.

Utilizing the Child Life Specialist

The **child life specialist** (CLS) is an individual specially trained in the developmental impact of illness, injury, and trauma who provides programs that prepare children for hospitalization, surgery, and other procedures that could be painful or distressing (Association of Child Life Professionals, 2022). The CLS is a member of the multidisciplinary team and works in conjunction with the health care provider and parents to foster an atmosphere that promotes the child's well-being. Services provided by a CLS include:

- Nonmedical preparation for hospitalization, clinic visits, tests, surgeries, and other medical procedures
- Support during medical procedures
- Therapeutic play
- Activities to support normal growth and development
- Education for the child and family about health conditions
- Teaching and support with coping and pain management strategies
- Sibling support
- Advocacy for the child and family
- Grief and bereavement support
- Emergency room interventions for children and families
- Hospital preadmission tours and information programs
- Outpatient consultation with families (Romito et al., 2021).

TABLE 30.1 • Suggestions for Atraumatic Care

Principle	Suggestions for Nursing Care
Preventing or minimizing physical stressors	• For painful injections, blood draws, or intravenous insertion, use numbing techniques (see Chapter 36). • During painful or invasive procedures, avoid traditional restraint or "holding down" of the child. Use alternative positioning such as "therapeutic hugging." • If the aforementioned positions are not an option, have the parent stand near the child's head to provide comfort. • Insert a saline lock if the child requires multiple doses of parenteral medications. • Advocate for minimal laboratory blood draws. • Minimize intramuscular or subcutaneous injections. • Provide appropriate pain management (refer to Chapter 36).
Preventing or minimizing child and family separation	• Promote family-centered care. • In the hospital, provide comfortable accommodations for the parent. • Allow the family the choice about whether to stay for an invasive procedure, and support them in their decision.
Promoting a sense of control	• Maintain the child's home routine related to activities of daily living. • In the hospital, use primary nursing. • Encourage the child to have a security item present if desired. • Involve the child and family in planning care from the moment of the first encounter. • Empower the family and child by providing knowledge. • Allow the child and family choices when they are available. • Make the environment more inviting and less intimidating.

The goal of the CLS is to decrease the child's anxiety and fear while improving and encouraging the child's understanding and cooperation. The CLS considers the needs of siblings or other children who may be affected by the child's illness or trauma. The CLS provides engaging and uplifting events by coordinating special entertainment and activities. The CLS is an excellent resource and provides education to health care providers and families. The American Academy of Pediatrics (AAP) recommends child life services because they are "a quality benchmark of an integrated patient- and family-centered health care system, a recommended component of medical education, and an indicator of excellence in pediatric care" (Romito et al., 2021, p. 5).

Minimizing Physical Stress During Procedures

Children undergo numerous diagnostic and therapeutic procedures in a wide range of settings during their development. These procedures may be performed in the community or outpatient setting or in a care facility. Regardless of the procedure and the setting, children, like adults, need thorough preparation before the procedure and support during and after the procedure to promote the best outcome and to ensure atraumatic care.

Using positions that are comforting to the child during painful procedures is an important aspect of atraumatic care (Fig. 30.1). **Therapeutic hugging** (a holding position that promotes close physical contact between the child and a parent or caregiver) may be used for certain procedures or treatments where the child must remain still. For example, the parent can hold the child in their lap snugly to prevent the child from moving during an injection or venipuncture. When using this technique, make sure the parent understands their role and knows which body parts to hold still in a safe manner. Alternatively, distraction or stimulation (such as with a toy) can help to gain the child's cooperation. Refer to Box 30.2 for distraction methods (Fig. 30.2).

Before the Procedure

Appropriate preparation for procedures helps decrease the child's and family's anxiety levels; promote the child's cooperation; support the child's and family's coping skills; improve recovery; and increase trust among the child, their family, and the health care team (Romito et al., 2021). Adequate preparation and explanation also help encourage long-term coping and build trust and rapport that will positively impact future medical situations (Romito et al., 2021).

Preparation may include preparing the child psychologically (including explanation and education) as well as physically. It is important to employ the concepts of atraumatic care when preparing children for a procedure. General guidelines for preparation include:

- Provide a description of and the reason for the procedure using age-appropriate language ("The doctor will look at your blood to see why you are sick").
- Describe where the procedure will occur ("The x-ray department has big machines that won't hurt you; it's a little cold there too").
- Introduce strange equipment the child may see ("You will lie on a special bed that moves in the big machine, but you can still see out").
- Describe how long the procedure will last ("You will be in the x-ray department until lunchtime").
- Identify unusual sensations that may occur during the procedure ("You may smell something different" or "The machine makes loud noises").

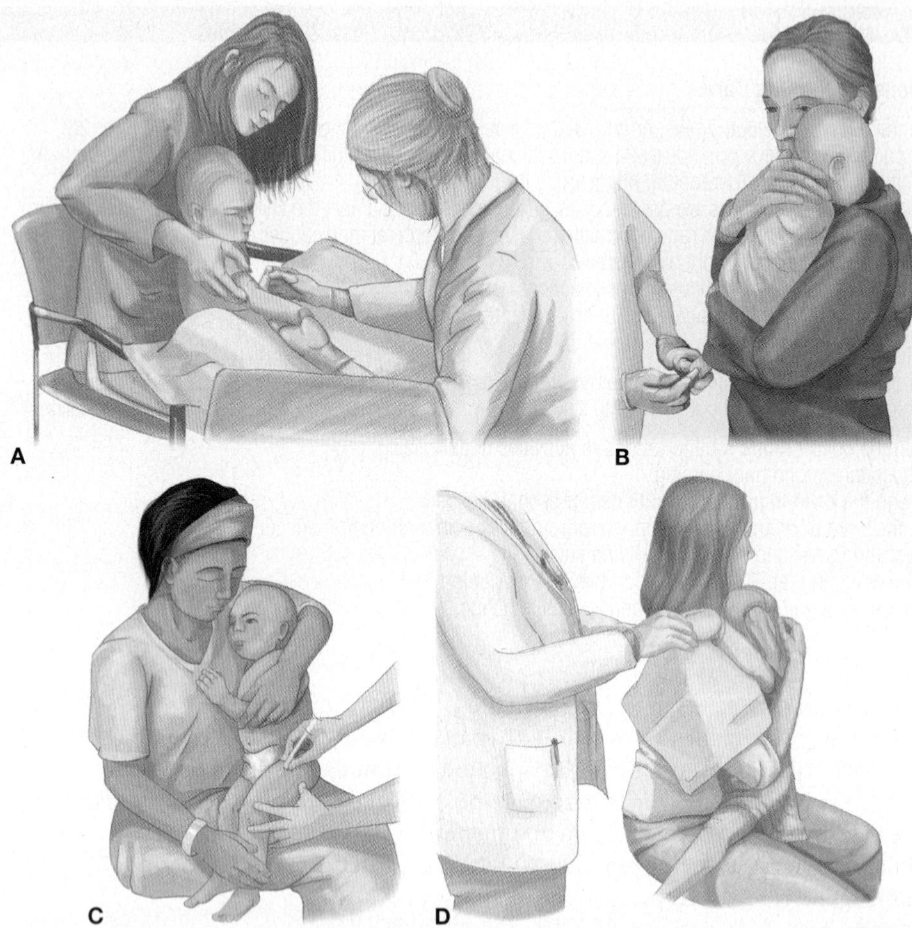

FIGURE 30.1 Positioning a child for comfort during a painful procedure. **A.** Sitting on the parent's lap while undergoing allergy testing provides this toddler with a sense of comfort. **B.** Position the infant cuddled over the parent's or the nurse's shoulder when obtaining a heel stick. The parent is preferable to the nurse. **C.** Use "therapeutic hugging" to maintain a child's position when the child is receiving an intramuscular injection. **D.** Use "therapeutic hugging" to position a child while the child is having an intravenous line inserted.

- Inform the child if any pain is involved.
- Tell the child it is okay to cry or yell.
- Identify any special care required after the procedure ("You will need to lie quietly for 15 minutes afterward").
- Discuss ways to help the child stay calm, such as using distraction methods or relaxation techniques ("During the procedure, you may want to count from 1 to 100 or sing your favorite song").

TAKE NOTE!

In the hospital, perform all invasive procedures in the treatment room or a room other than the child's room. The child's room should remain a safe and secure area (Ernst & AAP Committee on Hospital Care, 2020).

BOX 30.2 Distraction Methods

- Have the child point toes inward and wiggle them.
- Ask the child to squeeze your hand.
- Encourage the child to count aloud.
- Sing a song and have the child sing along.
- Point out the pictures on the ceiling.
- Have the child blow bubbles.
- Play music appealing to the child.

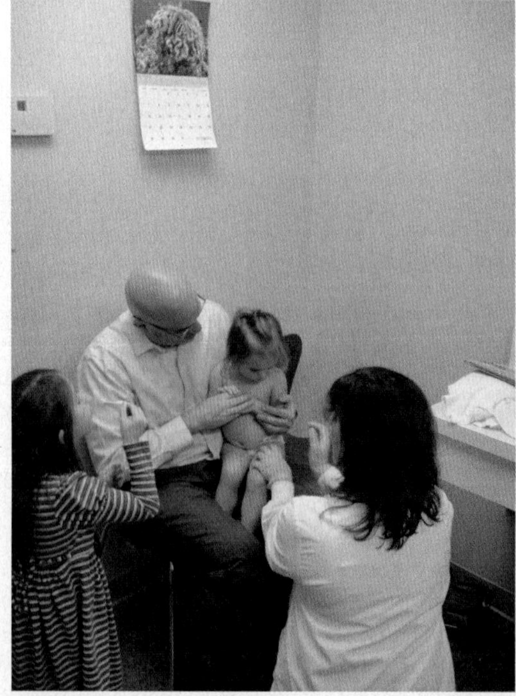

FIGURE 30.2 When possible, allow the caregiver to assist with providing positions of comfort and involve a sibling to assist with distraction techniques such as blowing bubbles, singing, or reading to the child during procedures.

A major aspect of preparation involves play. Toys and dolls provide an excellent way to demonstrate procedures that will occur. Consider the child's temperament, coping strategies, and previous experiences as well as developmental needs and cognitive abilities. First, gain trust and provide support. Include the child's parents, because parents are usually the greatest source of comfort for the child. Be short, simple, and appropriate in explaining situations at the child's level of development. Explain what is to be done and what is expected of the child. Avoid terms that have double meanings or that might be confusing. Table 30.2 lists alternative words or phrases to use for terms that may be confusing or misunderstood. Allow the child time to play with a toy or dolls and medical equipment as appropriate. Watch for signs of anxiety or fears.

During the Procedure

Use a firm, positive, confident approach that provides the child with a sense of security. Encourage cooperation by involving the child in decision making and allowing the child to select from a list or group of appropriate choices. Allow the child to express feelings of anger, anxiety, fear, frustration, or any other emotions. Often, this is how a child communicates and copes with the situation. Remind the child that it is okay to scream or cry but that it is important to hold still. Use distraction methods such as those listed in Box 30.2.

Toddlers and preschoolers often resist procedures despite preparation for them. Being held down or restrained is often more traumatizing to the young child than the procedure itself. Use alternative methods (positions that provide comfort for the child) to keep the child still during the procedure (see Fig. 30.1). The older child can be held while using a book or story for distraction.

After the Procedure

After the procedure, hold and comfort the child. Cuddle and soothe infants. Encourage children to express their feelings through play, such as dramatic play, or use of puppets. Gross motor activities such as pounding or throwing are also helpful for children to discharge pent-up feelings and energy. School-age children and adolescents may not outwardly demonstrate behavior indicating the need for comforting; however, provide them with opportunities to express their feelings and be comforted. Remember to praise children for appropriate behavior during the procedure and after all interventions are completed.

TABLE 30.2 • Alternatives for Confusing or Misunderstood Terms

Term to Avoid	How Children Might Interpret It	Use These Terms Instead
Catheter	Too technical	Tube
Deaden	Kill	Make sleepy
Dye	Die	Special medicine to help the doctor see (part of the body) better
Electrodes	Too technical	Stickers, ticklers, snaps
ICU	I see you.	Special room with your own nurse
Incision, cut open, make a hole	Too explicit	Special or small opening
Monitor	Too technical	Screen
Dressing change	To change clothes	Clean bandage/Band-Aid
Pain	May be too explicit	Child's word for hurt; "boo-boo"
Put to sleep, anesthesia	May confuse with putting a pet to sleep	Special kind of sleep
Shot	Children are scared of shots.	Medication under the skin
Stool	Like you sit on	"Poop" or child's word for it
Stretcher or gurney	"Stretch her"	Rolling bed or special bed on wheels
Take your temperature/blood pressure	Where are you going to "take" them?	See how warm you are/hug your arm.
Test	Like at school (the child will need to perform)	See how your heart is working.
Tourniquet	Too technical	Special kind of rubber band
Urine	"You're in"	"Pee" or child's word for it
X-ray	Don't understand	Picture or big camera to take pictures of the inside of your body

Based on Gaynard, L., Wolfer, J., Goldberger, J., Redbum, L., Laidley, L., & Thompson, R. (1998). *Psychosocial care of children in hospitals: Clinical practice manual from the ACCH Child Life Research Project* (1st ed.). Child Life Council.

TAKE NOTE!

Remember to utilize CLSs when available.

Remember Emma Moore, the 4-year-old introduced at the beginning of the chapter? The health care provider's orders for Emma include starting intravenous (IV) fluids and obtaining blood work upon arrival at the unit. As the admitting nurse, how will you provide atraumatic care?

PREVENTING OR MINIMIZING CHILD AND FAMILY SEPARATION: PROVIDING CHILD- AND FAMILY-CENTERED CARE

Family-centered care involves a partnership of the child, family, and health care providers in planning, providing, and evaluating care (American Academy of Pediatrics, Committee on Hospital Care, Institute for Patient and Family-Centered Care, 2012, reaffirmed 2018; Kuo & Turchi, 2023). It works well for children of any age and in all arenas of health care, from preventive care of the healthy child to long-term care of the child with a chronic or terminal illness. Family-centered care enhances parents' and caregivers' confidence in their own skills and also prepares children and young adults for assuming responsibility for their own health care needs. It is based on the concept that the family is the constant in the child's life and the primary source of strength and support for the child (American Academy of Pediatrics, Committee on Hospital Care, Institute for Patient and Family-Centered Care, 2012, reaffirmed 2018; Kuo & Turchi, 2023).

According to the American Academy of Pediatrics, Committee on Hospital Care, Institute for Patient and Family-Centered Care (2012, reaffirmed 2018), family-centered care focuses on several core principles:

- Respect for the child and family
- Recognition of the effects of cultural, racial, ethnic, and socioeconomic factors on the family's health care experience
- Identification of and expansion of the family's strengths
- Support of the family's choices related to the child's health care
- Maintenance of flexibility
- Provision of honest, unbiased information in an affirming and useful approach
- Assistance with the emotional and other support the child and family require
- Collaboration with families
- Empowerment of families

When children's health care is provided through a family-centered approach, many positive outcomes are possible, including:

- Anxiety is decreased.
- Children are calmer and pain management is enhanced.
- Recovery times are shortened.
- Families' confidence and problem-solving skills are improved.
- Communication between the health care team and the family is also improved, leading to greater satisfaction for both health care providers and health care consumers (families).
- A decrease in health care costs is seen and health care resources are used more effectively (American Academy of Pediatrics, Committee on Hospital Care, Institute for Patient and Family-Centered Care, 2012, reaffirmed 2018).

Ways to increase collaboration between the family and the health care team may include a family advisory board, a newsletter, conferences, or parent resource notebooks. Methods for increasing communication between the health care team and the family may include the use of mailboxes or dry-erase boards for updating the daily plan of care, including the parents' participation in rounds or through a daily assessment of health status by the child or family.

Vigilant parents are committed to the child's care, and most want to be present for all aspects of their child's care. They want to be part of the decision-making process regarding their child's care; they want to be heard and develop a rapport with the health care professionals caring for their child. They demonstrate resilience in their ability to make it through the emotional upheaval associated with an illness. It is important to be sensitive to the inconveniences that a child's illness may impose on the family. Address the family's emotional and spiritual needs, attend to their concerns, and provide the best accommodations possible when the child is hospitalized (Fig. 30.3). Practicing true

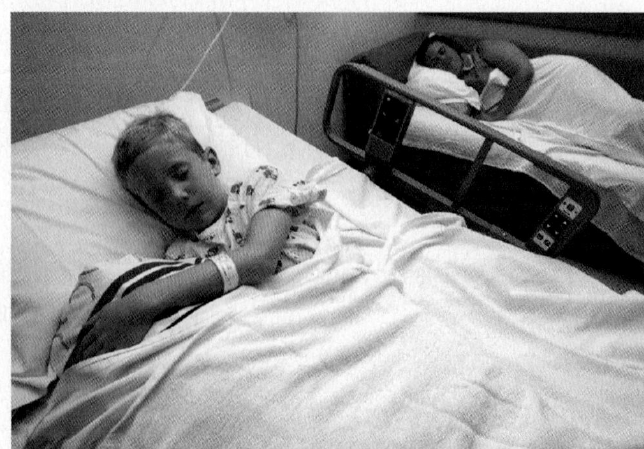

FIGURE 30.3 Providing a comfortable area for the parent to rest is an important component of family-centered care.

family-centered care may empower the family, strengthen family resources, and help the child and family feel more secure and supported throughout the process.

TAKE NOTE!

Some parents will not know how to advocate or speak up for their child; as a nurse, you must help open this door for them.

PROMOTING A SENSE OF CONTROL

During times of illness, hospitalization, or health-related interventions, the child and family can experience an extreme sense of loss of control. Providing effective communication and teaching can help foster feelings of control and improve the child's and family's ability to cope. Assisting the family with obtaining necessary information, resources, and relationships contributes to optimal health care for the child and family. Communication and teaching are skills that are used continuously in pediatric nursing, no matter what the setting or the child's state of health.

Enhancing Communication

Effective communication with children and their parents is critical to providing atraumatic quality nursing care. Child- and parent-centered communication enhances child outcomes and child and family satisfaction with nursing care. Effective communication is the foundation of the therapeutic relationship and leads to increased knowledge and health care behaviors on the part of the child and family (Betancourt et al., 2021; Levetown & American Academy of Pediatrics Committee on Bioethics, 2008, reaffirmed 2017). Nurses are in an ideal position to improve communication in the health care environment. They need to ensure inclusion of the child and family in health conversations and to clarify misconceptions following medical encounters.

Children are often socialized to be passive participants in health care, doing as they are told with or without protests. "As pediatric nurses, we have an obligation to listen, to hear, and to feel the voices of the children in our care" (McPherson & Thorne, 2000, p. 28). Children can inform nurses of their experiences in an accurate fashion, and nurses need to be able to discern this information from communication with the child. Children want to be respected, listened to, and understood.

Communication patterns can vary greatly from one child to the next. Some children are talkative, while others are quiet. Children may be more apt to communicate if they are engaged in another activity. Children often use fewer words than adults and may rely more on nonverbal communication and silence. Communicating in the pediatric setting can be complicated and more difficult than in the adult setting, but it remains crucial. The pediatric nurse needs to consider the age of the child and the child's cognitive and developmental level as well as communicating at an appropriate level with the parents. Refer to Chapter 2 for information on verbal and nonverbal communication.

Developmental Techniques for Communicating With Children

Effective communication with children involves a variety of age-appropriate methods. If the child is shy, talk to the parents first to give the child time to warm up to you. Use specific and clear phrases in an unhurried, quiet, yet confident manner. Communicate at the child's eye level (Fig. 30.4A). Spending time and incorporating play with younger children, even for just a few moments, may help them feel more at ease with you and help open the door to communication. Instead of direct questioning, use dolls, puppets, or stuffed animals with younger children (Fig. 30.4B). The use of metaphors (e.g., referring to white blood cells as "bad guy fighters") and stories can help illustrate health concepts to young and school-age children.

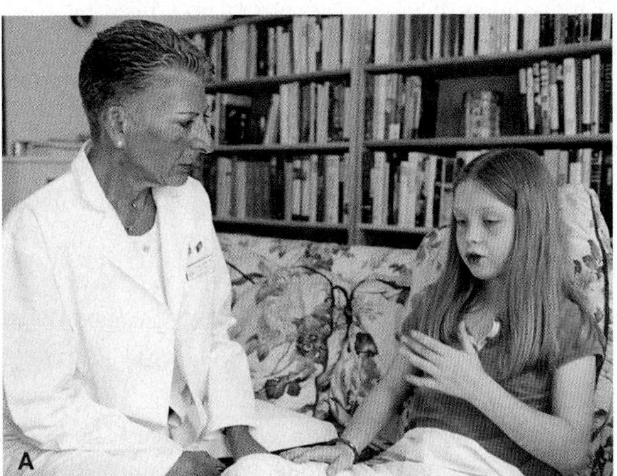

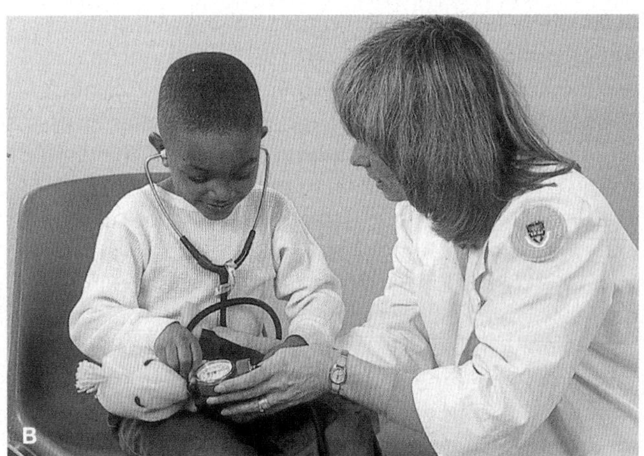

FIGURE 30.4 A. Sitting at the child's level and allowing the child time for self-expression are steps that improve therapeutic communication. **B.** Communication or teaching with dolls may be useful with younger children.

BOX 30.3 Basics for Communicating With Children

- Introduce yourself and explain your role.
- Position yourself at the child's level.
- Allow the child to remain near the parent if needed so the child can remain comfortable and relaxed.
- Smile and make eye contact with the child if culturally appropriate.
- Direct your questions and explanations to the child.
- Listen attentively and pause to allow time for the child to formulate their thoughts.
- Use the child's or family's terms for body parts and medical care when possible.
- Speak in a calm, quiet, confident, and unhurried voice.
- Use positive rather than negative statements and directions.
- Encourage the child to express their feelings and ask questions.
- Observe for nonverbal cues.
- Ask for permission if you need to approach the child to avoid appearing threatening.

Older children need privacy. Provide the child or adolescent with honest answers at a developmentally appropriate level. Allow children to express their thoughts and feelings. Offer the child choices when possible but only when they truly exist. Encourage children to write and draw about their experiences. This may increase their understanding and also draw attention to any misconceptions or fears. Box 30.3 lists requirements for communication with children and adolescents.

Children feel empowered when health care professionals communicate directly with them. Include children in discussions and avoid talking about them in their presence. Children may also desire advice about their health care and reassurance about their health status. To be effective when communicating with children of different developmental stages, the nurse must become familiar with how children of different ages communicate and then use age-appropriate techniques for effective communication.

- Infants communicate primarily through touch, sight, and hearing. Communication with the infant can occur by cuddling, holding, rocking, and singing to the infant.
- When working with toddlers and preschoolers, allow them time to complete their thoughts. Although language acquisition at this age is exponential, it often takes longer for the young child to find the right words, particularly in response to a question.
- School-age children are interested in learning and appreciate simple but honest and straightforward responses. When addressed first and allowed to respond, the school-age child may be eager to communicate. The school-age child is beginning to utilize more sophisticated language and developing problem-solving and critical thinking skills.
- Adolescents may experience strong feelings and emotions and perceive situations in extreme terms. Building a trusting, respectful rapport is essential.

For communication tips related to the child's age, see Table 30.3.

Tips for Communicating With Parents

When communicating with parents, be honest. Parents want to feel valued and should be equal partners with the health care team. Allow the parent to express concerns and ask questions. Explain equipment and procedures thoroughly. Help the parents understand the long-term as well as short-term effects of the treatment. Teach the parents what the child will feel like and how they will look during a procedure. Teach and encourage the parent to perform as much of the child's care as is reasonable and permitted. Ask the parent about their perception of the child's progress. Allowing the parents to be involved in the care of their child gives them a sense of control and lets them know they are valued by the health care team. Provide parents with positive reinforcement, reassurance, guidance, and support. Refer to Chapter 2 for more information on communication across cultures, working with interpreters, and communicating with children with hearing impairments.

At the beginning of the chapter, you were introduced to Emma Moore, a 4-year-old with a suspected head injury. Discuss ways to facilitate communication with Emma and her family.

Teaching Children and Families

Regardless of the type of practice or health care setting, nurses are in a unique position to help families manage the health care needs of their child. Indeed, the family has a right and a responsibility to participate fully in making decisions about health care processes for their child. This is true whether the child is hospitalized with a long-term, devastating illness or needs only health maintenance activities. To accomplish this, families need to be knowledgeable about their child's condition, the health care management plan, and when and how to contact health care providers. With the limited time available in all health care arenas and shortened stays in inpatient facilities, the pediatric nurse must focus on teaching goals and begin teaching at the earliest opportunity.

TAKE NOTE!

"There is no prescription more valuable than knowledge."
—C. Everett Koop, MD, former Surgeon General of the United States

Patient education occurs when nurses share information, knowledge, and skills with families, thus empowering them to take responsibility for their child's health care. Through patient education, families can

TABLE 30.3 • Communicating Effectively With Children

Age	Techniques
Infants	• Respond to crying in a timely fashion. • Allow the infant time to warm up to you. • Use a soothing and calming tone when speaking to the infant. • Talk to the infant directly. • Communication through play may be helpful with older infants. • Watch for signs of overstimulation such as closing eyes, turning away, yawning, and irritability.
Toddlers	• Approach toddlers carefully; they are often not only fearful but also can be resistant. • Use the toddler's preferred words for objects or actions so they are better able to understand. • Toddlers enjoy stories, dolls, and books. • Participate in parallel play to help start communication. • Prepare toddlers for procedures just before they are about to occur.
Preschoolers	• Use play, puppets, or storytelling via a third-party approach. • Speak honestly. • Use simple, concrete terms. • Ask specific questions. • Allow the child to have choices as appropriate. • Participate in imaginative play to help open communication. • Prepare preschoolers about 1 hour prior to a procedure.
School-age children	• Use diagrams, illustrations, books, and videos. • Allow the child to honestly express feelings. • Use third-party stories to elicit desired information (such as "some children feel anxious about…"). • Allow the child to ask questions related to care and treatment. Give the child adequate time for all of the questions to be answered. • Prepare the child a few days in advance for a procedure.
Adolescents	• Always respect the adolescent's need for privacy. • Ensure confidentiality. • Remain nonjudgmental. • Listen attentively and speak respectfully. • Use appropriate medical terminology, defining words as necessary. • Use creativity and humor. • Do not force the adolescent to talk as this may shut down communication. • Prepare the adolescent up to 1 week prior to a procedure.

overcome feelings of powerlessness and helplessness and gain the confidence and ability to step to the forefront of the health care team. Nurses spend innumerable hours teaching children and families; in fact, on some days in the hospital, more teaching than nursing care is provided. Given the importance of and the amount of time spent on child and family education, each nurse should become an expert at basic patient education principles. See the Healthy People 2030 box.

Goals of Child and Family Education

The goals of child and family education are to:

- Improve the child's and family's health literacy.
- Encourage communication with health care providers.
- Improve health outcomes and promote healthy lifestyles.
- Encourage involvement of the child and family in care and decision making about care.
- Improve adherence to the care and treatment plan.
- Promote a sense of autonomy and control.

HEALTHY PEOPLE 2030

Objective	Nursing Significance
Increase the proportion of people who report their health care provider always asked them to describe how they will follow instructions. Reduce the proportion of people who report poor patient/provider communication (e.g., listening, explanations, disrespect, time). Increase the proportion of adults with limited English proficiency who say their providers explain things clearly. Increase the health literacy of the population.	• Assess health learning needs of children and their families. • Plan health care education in collaboration with children and their families. • Provide health education at each patient encounter and evaluate for effective learning. • Practice universal literacy precautions. • Focus on providing easy-to-understand information during every patient encounter.

Healthy People Objectives retrieved from http://www.healthypeople.gov

Overall goals for the child and family include the ability of children and families to make informed decisions, perform basic health care skills, recognize when the child has a problem and know how to respond to the problem, and know how to get answers when questions arise.

TAKE NOTE!

Today, health care consumers have information available at their fingertips. It is important to steer children and their families to reliable and credible health care resources.

Refer to Chapter 2 for information on steps of patient and family education.

Teaching Children and Adolescents

Teaching children and adolescents is a vital part of pediatric nursing practice. Children and adolescents have a great need for information about their illness as they attempt to master their anxiety and restore feelings of competency, self-confidence, and hope. As with adults, they learn best when their input is valued, and they are actively involved in the learning process. The age and developmental level of the child will determine the amount, format, and timing of the information given. Before beginning to teach a child, it is important to establish rapport and lay the foundation for good communication. Refer to the "Developmental Techniques for Communicating With Children" section and Table 30.3 for additional information related to communicating well with children and adolescents.

TEACHING PRESCHOOL CHILDREN

When teaching young children, the nurse or family assumes part or all of the responsibility for what is learned, how it is learned, and when it is learned. Because they have vivid imaginations, young children often attempt to invent pieces of information, or they pick up bits and pieces of misinformation that can lead to false assumptions. Skillfully delivered and timed information can promote trust, calmness, and control in an otherwise apprehensive and uncooperative preschooler. Table 30.4 presents some general guidelines for teaching young children.

TEACHING SCHOOL-AGE CHILDREN

Unless they are quite ill, school-age children often want to participate in their care. They have a need to cooperate and achieve. When teaching, speak directly to them and include them in the education plan. Teach the school-age child and parent together, as parents can often learn by observing the care being given and taught to their child. Table 30.5 provides some general guidelines to keep in mind when teaching school-age children.

TEACHING ADOLESCENTS

Adolescents are particularly sensitive about maintaining body image and feelings of control and autonomy. This is especially important with health care processes and decisions that affect them. Table 30.6 gives some general guidelines to use when teaching adolescents.

TABLE **30.4** • General Teaching Tips for Young Children

Teaching Tips	Practical Application
Offer simple, concise, concrete explanations based on the assessed needs, questions, and developmental level of the child.	Use a child's senses and relate what a procedure will look, sound, smell, taste, or feel like ("The machine will sound very loud, like a big train").
Be honest, even when the information you need to convey is not positive. This helps the child form a bond of trust and confidence with caregivers.	Use the family's words that the child understands; use "soft words" ("This will feel warm" instead of "This will burn").
Time explanations to decrease anxiety and excess worry before the event. Avoid telling unpleasant news close to bedtime.	As a general rule, give toddlers information about procedures, medicines, and other interventions immediately beforehand; give 4- to 7-year-olds information 1 or 2 days in advance.
Parents know their child best. Eliciting information from them about their child's past behaviors and coping skills can often mean the difference between a positive and negative experience for their child.	Teach parents how to coach their child with pain management, visualization, or other methods of distraction when appropriate ("Remember when we went to the beach…").
Provide an active role for the child. This helps foster a child's sense of self-confidence and control over the situation.	Allow the child to help with simple self-care activities such as holding a dressing or piece of tape. Provide props and dolls to touch and feel as much as possible ("Your job is to keep your hands still").
Children's wishes must be respected when they verbalize or demonstrate that they do not want more information.	Keep explanations short and simple; know when to stop teaching.
Praise the child and let them know how much you appreciate their help and cooperation.	Use "please" and "thank you" often ("Thank you. I like the way you held still for me").

TABLE 30.5 • General Guidelines When Teaching School-Age Children

Teaching Tips	Practical Application
Allow the child some control and involvement in the decision-making process.	Offer choices whenever possible (taking the medicine with juice or milk), but don't offer choices when there are no alternatives (taking the medicine or not).
Children can relate present-day happenings to past experiences.	Use examples and past experiences that are familiar to the child ("Remember when you were first learning to swim...").
Achievement and accomplishment are important to children at this age, so anything they can be actively involved in will help them adjust and learn.	Provide an active role and allow the child to do as much of their care as possible. Use props, dolls, games, and computers to enhance learning.
At this age, most children are able to sequence, understand cause and effect, and make sense of time.	Teach children the steps involved and how long it will take ("Today I'm going to teach you how to change your dressing. This will help keep your cut clean. First, wash your hands...").
Gaining control over the situation and preparing mentally are important for the child's self-confidence.	Provide information 3–7 days in advance, depending on the child's age and developmental level.
Praise the child and let them know how much you appreciate their help and cooperation.	Use "please" and "thank you" often ("Thanks! You did a great job using your inhaler").

TABLE 30.6 • General Guidelines When Teaching Adolescents

Teaching Tips	Practical Application
Allow adolescents to be in control and involved in the decision-making process.	Speak directly to adolescents; consider their input in all decisions about their care and education.
Adolescents can process abstract information and understand how their actions affect long-term outcomes.	Provide reasons why something is important, and discuss how their lives will be affected by their decision to take care of their health needs ("If you take your asthma medicine, you'll be better able to play tennis").
Adolescents are concerned about how they look and how they fit in with peers.	Collaborate with the adolescent to develop acceptable solutions and strategies for dealing with health issues that affect personal appearance and peer acceptance (e.g., wigs or head scarves for hair loss from chemotherapy).
Adolescents strive for independence and have personal values and ideologies that may conflict with those of parents and the medical community.	Expect some potential lack of adherence to the care plan, despite best educational efforts. Work together to achieve win–win outcomes of educational goals.

Remember Emma Moore, the 4-year-old described at the beginning of the chapter? What teaching methods would be appropriate to facilitate learning?

Refer to Chapter 2 for information regarding evaluating learning and documenting education for the child and family.

CONSIDER THIS!

Elsa is a 5-year-old on your unit who was recently diagnosed with diabetes. She is getting ready to be discharged home at the end of the week. Her grandparents are her primary caregivers.

- What concerns regarding learning would you take into consideration during your assessment?
- Describe different teaching strategies you would utilize with Elsa and her family.
- How would you evaluate learning with Elsa and her family?

KEY CONCEPTS

- Atraumatic care focuses on minimizing stressors and separation from the family and promoting a sense of control for the child and family.
- Children and families need appropriate explanation and education before a procedure is performed. Preparation may include explaining the procedure as well as physically preparing the child. Appropriate preparation helps decrease the child's and family's anxiety, promote the child's cooperation, and support the child's and family's coping skills.
- A major aspect of preparation involves play.
- Include the child's parents in preparation because parents are usually the greatest source of comfort for the child.
- Be short, simple, and appropriate in explaining situations at the child's level of development. Explain what is to be done and what is expected of the child.

- Utilize a CLS when available.
- Family-centered care involves a beneficial partnership among the patient, family, and health care providers in planning, providing, and evaluating care.
- Family-centered care is based on the concept that the family is the primary source of strength and support for the child.
- Family-centered care includes respect for the child and family, recognition of cultural diversity, identification of the family's strengths, assistance with emotional and other support of the family, providing honest and unbiased information, and collaborating and empowering families.
- Maintain open and honest lines of communication with children and their families.
- Therapeutic communication involves the use of open-ended questions, reflection, paraphrasing, acknowledgment of emotions, and active listening.
- To communicate effectively with children, provide information and support on the child's developmental level and utilize age-appropriate methods.
- When communicating with parents, be honest. Parents want to feel valued and should be equal partners in the health care team.
- It is vital for the family to have knowledge about their child's health.
- Patient education begins with the first patient encounter and proceeds through discharge and beyond. Reassessment after each step or change in the process is critical to success.

REFERENCES AND RECOMMENDED READINGS

Agency for Healthcare Research and Quality. (2010, reviewed 2020). *AHRQ health literacy universal precautions toolkit*. https://www.ahrq.gov/health-literacy/improve/precautions/index.html

American Academy of Pediatrics. (2021). *Addressing low health literacy and limited English proficiency*. https://www.aap.org/en/practice-management/providing-patient--and-family-centered-care/addressing-low-health-literacy-and-limited-english-proficiency/

American Academy of Pediatrics, Committee on Hospital Care, Institute for Patient and Family-Centered Care. (2012, reaffirmed 2018). Policy statement: Patient and family-centered care and the pediatrician's role. *Pediatrics*, *129*(2), 394–404. https://doi.org/10.1542/peds.2011-3084

Association of Child Life Professionals. (2022). *The child life profession: What is a certified child life specialist?* https://www.childlife.org/the-child-life-profession

Betancourt, J. R., Green, A. R., & Carillo, J. E. (2021). The patient's culture and effective communication. *UpToDate*. Retrieved November 9, 2022, from https://www.uptodate.com/contents/the-patients-culture-and-effective-communication

Brega, A. G., Barnard, J., Mabachi, N. M., Weiss, B. D., DeWalt, D. A., Brach, C., Cifuentes, M., Albright, K., & West, D. R. (2015). *AHRQ health literacy universal precautions toolkit* (2nd ed.). Agency for Healthcare Research and Quality. https://www.ahrq.gov/sites/default/files/publications/files/healthlittoolkit2_4.pdf

Centers for Disease Control and Prevention. (2022a). *What is health literacy*. https://www.cdc.gov/healthliteracy/learn/index.html

Centers for Disease Control and Prevention. (2022b). *CDC's health literacy action plan*. https://www.cdc.gov/healthliteracy/planact/cdcplan.html

Ernst, K. D., & AAP Committee on Hospital Care. (2020). Recommended for the care of pediatric patients in hospitals. *Pediatrics*, *145*(4), e20200204. https://doi.org/10.1542/peds.2020-0204

Gaynard, L., Wolfer, J., Goldberger, J., Redbum, L., Laidley, L., & Thompson, R. (1998). *Psychosocial care of children in hospitals: Clinical practice manual from the ACCH Child Life Research Project* (1st ed.). Child Life Council.

Health Resources & Services Administration. (2022). *Health literacy*. https://www.hrsa.gov/about/organization/bureaus/ohe/health-literacy/index.html

Hickey, K. T., Masterson Creber, R. M., Reading, M., Sciacca, R. R., Riga, T. C., Frulla, A. P., & Casida, J. M. (2018). Low health literacy: Implications for managing cardiac patients in practice. *The Nurse Practitioner*, *43*(8), 49–55. https://doi.org/10.1097/01.NPR.0000541468.54290.49

Knowles, M. S., Holton, E. F., 3rd, & Swanson, R. A. (2015). *The adult learner: The definitive classic in adult education and human resource development* (8th ed.). Routledge.

Koh, H. K., Berwick, D. M., Clancy, C. M., Baur, C., Brach, C., Harris, L. M., & Zerhusen, E. G. (2012). New federal policy initiatives to boost health literacy can help the nation move beyond the cycle of costly "crisis care". *Health Affairs*, *31*(2), 434–443. https://doi.org/10.1377/hlthaff.2011.1169

Krontoft, A. (2021). How do patients prefer to receive patient education material about treatment, diagnosis and procedures?—A survey study of patients preferences regarding forms of patient education materials; leaflets, podcasts, and video. *Open Journal of Nursing*, *11*, 809–827. https://doi.org/10.4236/ojn.2021.1110068

Kuo, D. Z., & Turchi, R. M. (2023). Children and youth with special health care needs. *UpToDate*. Retrieved October 17, 2023, from https://www.uptodate.com/contents/children-and-youth-with-special-health-care-needs

Levetown, M., & American Academy of Pediatrics Committee on Bioethics. (2008, reaffirmed 2017). Communicating with children and families: From everyday interactions to skill in conveying distressing information. *Pediatrics*, *121*(5), e1441–e1460. https://doi.org/10.1542/peds.2008-0565

McPherson, G., & Thorne, S. (2000). Children's voices: Can we hear them? *Journal of Pediatric Nursing*, *15*(1), 22–29. https://doi.org/10.1016/S0882-5963(00)80020-2

National Association of the Deaf. (2022). *Questions and answers for healthcare providers*. http://www.nad.org/issues/health-care/providers/questions-and-answers

Romito, B., Jewell, J., Jackson, M., & AAP Committee on Hospital Care; Association of Child Life Professionals. (2021). Child life services. *Pediatrics*, *147*(1), e2020040261. https://doi.org/10.1542/peds.2020-040261

Rothwell, J. (2020). Assessing the economic gains of eradicating illiteracy nationally and regionally in the United States. *Gallup*. https://www.barbarabush.org/wp-content/uploads/2020/09/BBFoundation_GainsFromEradicatingIlliteracy_9_8.pdf

U.S. Department of Health and Human Services. (n.d.). *Healthy People 2030*. https://health.gov/healthypeople

Wong, D. (1995). *Whaley & Wong's nursing care of infants and children* (5th ed). Mosby.

DEVELOPING CLINICAL JUDGMENT

PRACTICING FOR NCLEX

1. When providing atraumatic care to a child, which action would be the most appropriate?
   a. Applying restraints for any procedure that would be uncomfortable
   b. Keeping the lights on in the child's room throughout the day and night
   c. Limiting the use of topical anesthetics for painful injections
   d. Allowing parents and children an informed choice about being together
2. When caring for children, how does the nurse best incorporate the concept of family-centered care?
   a. Encourages the family to allow the health care provider to make health care decisions for the child
   b. Uses the concepts of respect, family strengths, diversity, and collaboration with the family
   c. Advises the family to choose a pediatric provider who is on the child's insurance plan
   d. Recognizes that families undergoing stress related to the child's illness cannot make good decisions
3. When working with children and families, which are strategies for promoting therapeutic communication? Select all that apply.
   a. Detailed explanations
   b. Attentive listening
   c. Comforting touch
   d. Closed-ended questions
   e. Demonstrating empathy
   f. Acknowledging the child's emotions
4. The nurse is caring for a 2-year-old in the hospital, and the parent expresses concern that the toddler will be scared. Which response by the nurse would be most appropriate?
   a. "Don't worry; we practice family-centered and atraumatic care here."
   b. "We will do our best to minimize the stress your child experiences."
   c. "It will probably be upsetting for you as well, so you should stay home."
   d. "Our practice of atraumatic care will eliminate all pain and stress for your child."
5. A 2-year-old is scheduled to undergo an endoscopic procedure. The child's parents are asking when they should tell the child about it. Based on the nurse's understanding of the child's developmental stage, when would be the most appropriate time to prepare the child for the procedure?
   a. About 1 week before the scheduled date
   b. A few days in advance of the scheduled date
   c. About 1 hour before the procedure is to occur
   d. Just before the procedure is to be performed

CRITICAL THINKING EXERCISES

1. A 5-year-old is being admitted to your unit. The health care provider has ordered IV fluids along with laboratory work including a complete blood count, electrolytes, and a urine culture. As the nurse, how will you prepare the child and family before the procedure and support them during and after the procedure to promote the best outcomes and to ensure atraumatic care?
2. A 16-year-old is admitted to your nursing unit. Please describe some techniques and tips the nurse can use to communicate effectively with this adolescent.

STUDY ACTIVITIES

1. Develop a teaching plan for one of the families you care for in the clinical setting. Be sure to follow the appropriate steps for providing education.
2. Interview a CLS about the effects that the traditional (not atraumatic) approach to restraining a child for procedures might have on a child of various ages.
3. Research the availability of language interpreters and translators in your local community, compiling a list of the available resources.

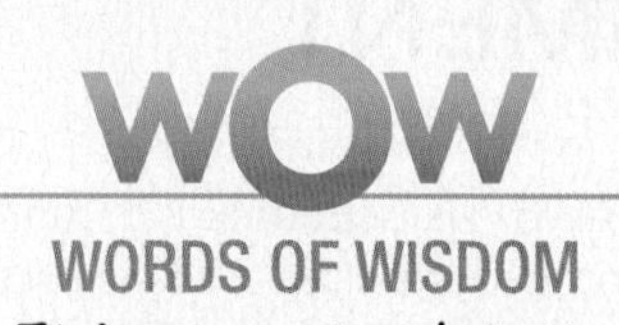

WORDS OF WISDOM

It is never too late to start prevention. It begins with a genuine desire for health improvement.

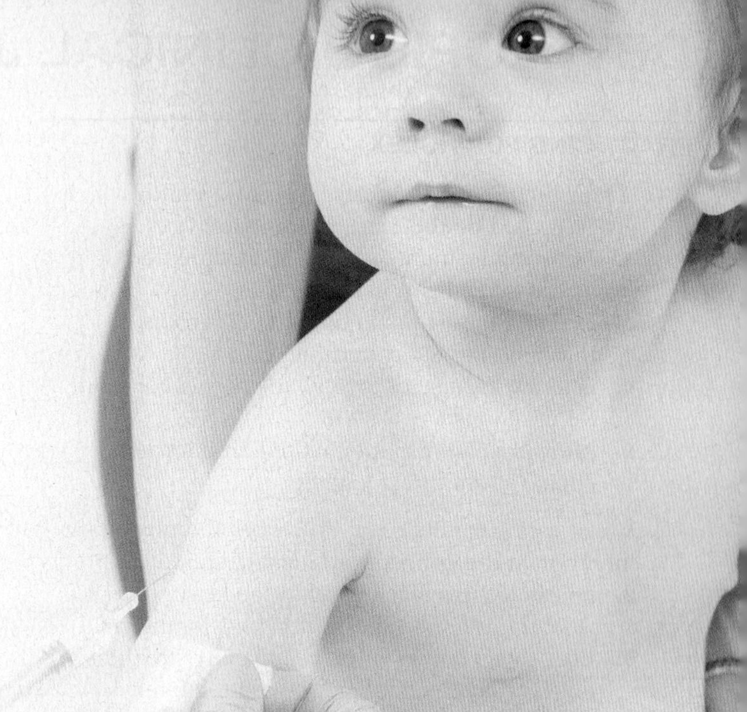

31 Health Supervision

LEARNING OBJECTIVES

Upon completion of the chapter, you will be able to:

1. Describe the principles of health supervision.
2. Identify challenges to health supervision for children with chronic illnesses.
3. List the three components of a health supervision visit.
4. Discuss developmental surveillance and developmental screening of children.
5. Demonstrate knowledge of the principles of immunization.
6. Identify barriers to immunization.
7. Explain key components of health promotion.
8. Describe the role of anticipatory guidance in health promotion.

KEY TERMS

active immunity
developmental screenings
developmental surveillance
immunity
medical home
passive immunity
risk assessment
screening tests
selective screening
universal screening

Three-year-old **Maya Randall** and 9-month-old **Evan Randall** are brought to the clinic by their parent. Maya was last seen in the clinic when she was 1 year old, and Evan has never been seen. The parent says that both children have been healthy, so they did not need to come to the clinic before this. Maya is complaining of a sore throat, which is what prompted today's visit.

PRINCIPLES OF HEALTH SUPERVISION

Health supervision involves providing services proactively with the goal of optimizing the child's level of functioning. It ensures the child is growing and developing appropriately, and it promotes the best possible health of the child by teaching parents and children about preventing injury and illness (e.g., proper immunizations and anticipatory guidance). This chapter is organized around the three components of health supervision: developmental surveillance and screening; injury and disease prevention; and health promotion. Health supervision of the child begins at birth and continues through adolescence. It is vital to every child and is most effective when the child has a centralized source of health care. Any place publicly accessible by children and families can be an appropriate setting for health supervision services—private health care providers' offices, community health departments, sliding-scale clinics, homeless shelters, day care centers, and schools. The framework for the health supervision visit is developed from national guidelines available through the U.S. Department of Health and Human Services (USDHHS), the American Medical Association (AMA), and the American Academy of Pediatrics (AAP). These organizations also provide guidelines for children with chronic illness and services and information regarding unique situations such as the internationally adopted child.

Wellness

The focus of pediatric health supervision is wellness. The health supervision visit provides an opportunity to maximize health promotion for the child, family, and community. Nurses have the ability to promote optimal health during these encounters. Health supervision visits must be viewed as part of a continuum of care, not as the accomplishment of isolated tasks.

Medical Home

A **medical home** is an approach to care that builds a long-term and comprehensive relationship with the family. This continuing relationship promotes trust between the pediatric care team and the family and leads to comprehensive, continuous, coordinated, and cost-effective care. The medical home is the setting that allows the highest level of health supervision. To be effective, the medical home must be accessible, family-centered, culturally effective, and community based. It must be integrated into the child's world, not adjacent to it. Characteristics of a medical home are displayed in Box 31.1.

BOX 31.1 Characteristics of a Medical Home

- Care accessible and in the child's community
- All insurance, including Medicaid, accepted
- Family-centered care provided
- Child or family able to speak directly to the health care provider when needed
- Partnership based on mutual trust and respect between the family and pediatric care team
- Preventive care activities provided
- Ambulatory and inpatient care are accessible.
- Continuity of care from infancy through adolescence
- Coordinated care with other care providers
- Comprehensive care where all health care needs can be met: well care, sick care, and behavioral care
- Availability of subspecialty consultation and referrals
- Work with family to meet the nonmedical and medical needs of the child and family.
- Interactive relationships with school and community agencies
- A centralized database containing all pertinent information
- Concern and compassion for the well-being of the child and family expressed
- Respect for family's cultural and religious beliefs.

Adapted from American Academy of Pediatrics, National Resource Center for Patient and Family Centered Medical Home. (2022). What is medical home. https://www.aap.org/en/practice-management/medical-home/medical-home-overview/what-is-medical-home/

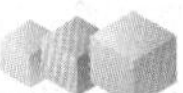
Concept Mastery Alert

Medical Home

A pediatric medical home provides continuity of care from infancy through adolescence. A medical home contains a centralized database that contains all information about a child that pertains to their health status.

Partnerships

The child is the focus of the health supervision visit. However, the child's health is linked to the needs and resources of their family and community. For instance, if the family is in turmoil because of divorce, drug misuse, or parental health problems, the child is less likely to receive the attention and energy that they need to thrive. Likewise, a community with high federal poverty levels, poor infrastructure, and lack of resources will not be able to provide the support services needed to allow children to reach their full potential. To be effective, the nurse must offer commitment and develop an ongoing partnership with the child, family, and community. These partnerships allow for mutual goal setting, marshaling of resources, and development of optimal health practices.

The partnership between the child and the health supervision team develops over time. In infancy, the family is the surrogate for the child in the partnership. The child's participation in the partnership increases at a rate that is developmentally appropriate. The child's increasing influence in the partnership allows the nurse to tailor health supervision to the child's needs. The partnership allows the child to take increasing responsibility for their personal health and optimizes health promotion.

Nurses must validate and enhance the role of family members as they influence and inform the child's concept of wellness. The health care community must involve the family to have a significant impact on a child's health. The family wants the best possible outcome for their child, and health care decisions are based on the knowledge they possess. The nurse can greatly facilitate trust by acknowledging that the family has unique insights to offer on their child's health. Nurses can also strengthen the partnership between the family and the health care community by recognizing the family's healthy practices, addressing their health issues, and strengthening their skills. By contributing to the partnership, both the nurse and the family enhance the chance of success for health care plans, but families are the ones who must implement any health care strategy and know what expected outcomes are reasonable. Their feedback is invaluable to formulating an effective long-term health supervision plan that optimizes their child's wellness.

TAKE NOTE!

Observe the parent–child interaction during the health supervision visit. The nurse can learn much about the family dynamic by observing the family for behavioral clues:

- Does the parent make eye contact with the infant?
- Does the parent anticipate and respond to the infant's needs?
- Are parents effective when dealing with a toddler's temper tantrum?
- Do the parents' comments increase the school-age child's sense of self-worth?

Behavioral observations are crucial to the proper assessment of the family's needs and issues.

Partnerships between the community and the health promotion team benefit the community as well as individual children. When nurses develop partnerships with community agencies such as schools, places of worship, and ancillary health facilities, barriers to care can be overcome. The nurse becomes aware of available resources in the community that can benefit an individual family. With input from community partners, the nurse can perform an assessment of the community's needs. The assessment then provides the foundation for the development of community-based health promotion programs. These programs expand the resources of the community, which in turn enhances the health of its members.

Special Issues in Health Supervision

Special issues in health supervision include cultural influences, community influences, health supervision and the child with a chronic illness, and health supervision and the child who was internationally adopted.

Cultural Influences on Health Supervision

A person's definition of health is influenced by their culture. Successful interactions result when the nurse is aware of the beliefs and interactive styles that are often present in members of a specific culture. If the goals of the health care plan are not consistent with the health belief system of the family, the plan has little chance of success. Optimal wellness for the child requires the nurse and the family to partner to establish a mutually acceptable plan of care. A plan must balance the cultural beliefs and practices of the family with those of the health care establishment. The nurse must possess cultural respect, humility, and sensitivity for the partnership to be successful.

Most health promotion and disease prevention strategies in the United States have a future-based orientation and view the child as an active and controlling agent in their own health. This may reflect many families in the United States, but the nurse must be prepared to develop strategies that are meaningful to children whose cultures do not align with this orientation. Significant numbers of children belong to cultures with a present-based orientation. These cultures are more concerned about what is going on now. For these children and families, health promotion activities need shorter-term goals and outcomes to be useful. Families with a fatalistic worldview will see any actions on their part as ineffective. They may feel that a higher power controls their fate and that health is a gift to be appreciated, not a goal to be pursued. Certain cultures believe health is the result of being in harmony within oneself and the larger universe. From this viewpoint, taking a medication or receiving a treatment may not be perceived as an effective way to restore health because it does not address the problem of being "out of harmony." It is important to remember that each individual does not necessarily subscribe to all of the beliefs and practices of their cultural group. The nurse should explore each child's and family's specific beliefs during the health interview.

Community Influences on Health Supervision

The child is a member of a community as well as a family and a culture. Each community has unique strengths, weaknesses, and values. A community can be a contributor to a child's health or the cause of their illnesses. The child's health cannot be totally separated from the health of the surrounding community.

Ideally, the child's medical home is within the family's community. If home and access to medical care are close, barriers such as lack of transportation, expense of travel, and time away from the parents' workplace are reduced. Having the medical home within the community facilitates bonds between the health team and schools, places of worship, and support services and agencies. Community support and resources are necessary for children with significant problems. A close working relationship between the child's health care provider and community agencies is an enormous benefit to the child (see the "Partnerships" section).

The community assessment may reveal problems that are causing or contributing to the child's health problems. A deteriorating infrastructure can contribute to decreased access to care and increased risk of injury or illness. Poverty has been linked to low birth weight and can lead to food insecurity and hunger or higher weight, among other health problems (Carlson & Neuberger, 2021). Housing is an important social determinant of health. Substandard housing can be directly related to lead poisoning and asthma, for example (Bryant-Stephens et al., 2021; National Center for Healthy Housing, 2022). A thorough knowledge of the family's community is needed before a health surveillance program can be effective.

Health Supervision and the Child With Chronic Illness

Effective health supervision must be responsive to the individual child's situation. The child with a chronic illness needs to be assessed repeatedly to determine their health maintenance needs. These assessments determine the frequency of visits and types of interventions needed. The impact of the illness on the child's functional health patterns determines whether standard health supervision visits need to be augmented.

An effective partnership among the child's medical home, family, and community is vital for a child with a chronic illness. Coordination of specialty care, community agencies, and family support networks enhances the quality of life and health of these children. Access to care and services minimizes the risk of injury from the illness. Support groups and community-based resources optimize the family's adaptation to the stressors of chronic illness.

Comprehensive health supervision includes frequent psychosocial assessments. Issues to be covered include:

- Health insurance coverage
- Transportation to health care facilities
- Financial stressors
- Family coping
- School's response to the chronic illness

These are often stressful and emotionally charged issues. The nurse with a trusting and ongoing relationship with the child and family is in the best position to help with these issues. The nurse can assist the family to find financial and medical assistance programs, take advantage of community resources, and participate in support groups. The nurse can also educate school personnel about the child's illness and assist them in maximizing the child's potential for academic success.

Health Supervision and the Child Adopted Internationally

In 2021, approximately 1,785 children were adopted from countries outside the United States, many from areas with a high prevalence of infectious diseases (Intercountry Adoption, Bureau of Consular Affairs, U.S. Department of State, 2022). International adoptions have been decreasing over the past 10 years, and many countries ceased adoptions during the COVID-19 pandemic. In 2021, Colombia supplied nearly half of all international adoptees, followed by India, Ukraine, and South Korea (Intercountry Adoption, Bureau of Consular Affairs, U.S. Department of State, 2022).

Health supervision of the child who is internationally adopted must include comprehensive screening for infectious diseases and disorders of growth and development, along with dental, vision, hearing, and any further testing based on diseases common in their country of origin (Schulte, 2020). A complete blood cell count and blood lead level screening in young infants is also recommended (Schulte, 2020). A thorough review of immunization records should be performed. Intestinal parasites are a common problem, and infected children are frequently symptom-free, so a thorough history and physical examination along with universal screening is recommended (Schulte, 2020).

Universal screening for hepatitis B, C, and A; varicella virus; HIV; syphilis; and tuberculosis infections is recommended (Schulte, 2020). Due to lack of resources in the home country, screening and treatment for these diseases are sporadic and ineffective. If testing is documented, it is likely to be unreliable. Testing supplies may have been outdated or improperly stored. Also, the test may have been performed before the child's seroconversion occurred.

Proper screening is important not only to the child's health but also to the adopting family and the larger community. Screening is recommended within the first few weeks of the child's arrival in the United States.

COMPONENTS OF HEALTH SUPERVISION

Developmental surveillance and screening, injury and disease prevention, and health promotion are the critical components of health supervision for children. Health supervision visits for children without health problems and with appropriate growth and development are recommended at birth, within the first week of life, by 1 month, then at 2 months, 4 months, 6 months, 9 months, 12 months, 15 months, 18 months, 24 months, 30 months, and then yearly until age 21 (Bright Futures/American Academy of Pediatrics [AAP], 2022). Children with disabilities or concerns will have more frequent and intensive visits. Health supervision visits include assessment of physical health along with intellectual and social development and parent–child interaction.

Each health supervision visit will include:

- A history and physical assessment, including head circumference (until 2 years of age), height, and weight
- Developmental surveillance or screening and behavioral–social–emotional screening
- Sensory screening (vision and hearing)
- Appropriate at-risk screening (such as lead screening, anemia screening, tuberculin test, hypertension screening, cholesterol screening)
- Immunizations
- Health promotion/anticipatory guidance (injury prevention, violence prevention, nutrition counseling) (Bright Futures/AAP, 2022)

Disease prevention and health promotion are concepts well established in adult health supervision. Injury prevention and developmental surveillance/screening are additional components of pediatric health supervision visits that help every child achieve their optimal state of wellness.

Developmental Surveillance and Screening

Developmental surveillance is an ongoing collection of skilled observations made over time during health care visits. Components include:

- Noting and addressing parental concerns
- Obtaining a developmental history
- Making accurate observations
- Consulting with relevant professionals

Developmental screenings are brief assessment procedures that identify children who warrant more intensive assessment and testing. Developmental screening assessments may be observational or by caregiver report (Fig. 31.1).

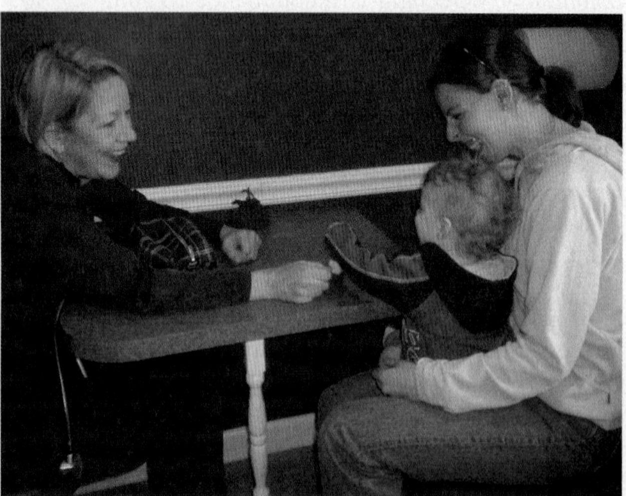

FIGURE 31.1 Developmental screening provides the opportunity for the nurse to identify problems in the child's development.

Development, or the emergence of the child's abilities, is a longitudinal process. Within the trust and security of the medical home, family and health care providers can share observations and concerns. In collaboration, the family and the health care provider observe the child's accomplishments or milestones over time. Data collection for developmental surveillance of infants and young children is performed through developmental questionnaires, health care provider observations, and a thorough physical examination. School records and test results can provide academic performance data for the older child. Input from teachers, coaches, and other adults involved with the child can give insight into the child's emotional and social development. Early identification of developmental delays leads to improved outcomes (Zubler et al., 2022).

When developmental delay is suspected, frequent developmental surveillance is warranted. Reemphasizing parental roles and responsibilities fosters cooperation and adherence. It is therefore crucial that parents understand the need for frequent assessments. A pattern of developmental delays warrants a formal evaluation.

The pediatric nurse must understand expected growth and development and become proficient at screening for problems related to development. The historical information obtained from the parent or primary caregiver about developmental milestones may identify risks for developmental delay. To access the most recent developmental milestone checklists, go to the Developmental Milestones website of the Centers for Disease Control and Prevention (CDC). Special attention to developmental surveillance is recommended at 4 to 5 years of age before a child enters school (Lipkin et al., 2020). If at any time there is a concern about development or a developmental delay is suspected, developmental screening should occur.

TAKE NOTE!

In 2022, the CDC's Learn the Signs. Act Early. program provided funding for the AAP to revise its developmental surveillance checklists. The goal was to provide milestone checklists when most children (at least 75%) would be expected to attain a milestone. In the past, the checklist incorporated milestones that 50% of children met, and this may have led to delays in diagnosis and a "wait-and-see" approach. Additional goals included aligning the developmental checklist with the recommended AAP health supervision visits by adding 15-and 30-month checklists and clarifying milestones, eliminating repetition of milestones across ages, and eliminating warning signs to minimize confusion (Zubler et al., 2022).

Factors placing the infant or toddler at risk for developmental problems include:

- Birth weight less than 1.5 kg
- Gestational age less than 33 weeks
- Central nervous system abnormality
- Hypoxic ischemic encephalopathy
- Alcohol or drug misuse by the pregnant parent
- Hypertonia
- Hypotonia
- Hyperbilirubinemia requiring exchange transfusion
- Kernicterus
- Congenital malformations
- Symmetric intrauterine growth deficiency
- Perinatal or congenital infection
- Suspected sensory impairment
- Chronic (more than 3 months) otitis media with effusion
- Inborn error of metabolism
- HIV infection
- Lead level above 5 mg/dL
- Inappropriate parental concern about developmental issues (e.g., not allowing a developmentally appropriate 3-year-old to feed themselves)
- Parent with less than high school education
- Single parent
- Sibling with developmental problems
- Parent with developmental disability or mental illness

Infants or children with any of these risk factors should be screened carefully for developmental delays. This screening should occur in a prospective manner, with screenings occurring at frequent intervals to identify concerns early.

TAKE NOTE!

Any child who "loses" a developmental milestone–for example, the child able to sit without support who now cannot–needs an immediate full evaluation, since this may indicate a significant neurologic problem.

A number of developmental screening tools are available to guide the nurse in assessing development. Screening tools can be general and covering all developmental domains or targeted and focusing on one area of development. Table 31.1 provides a few examples of

TABLE 31.1 • Common Developmental Screening Tools Used in Primary Care

Age	Screening Tool	Definition	Nursing Implications
Birth–66 months	Survey of Well-Being of Young Children	Simple questions to screen for social–emotional, developmental milestones, as well as autism and family risk (including parent mental health concerns, substance use, food insecurity, and family violence)	A parental-report tool, requires scoring manually or electronically after completion to determine risk level or presence of delays; written at sixth-grade reading level; takes about 10 minutes to complete and 5 minutes to score; available in several languages
Birth–66 months	Ages and Stages Questionnaire (ASQ), 3rd edition	Assesses communication, gross motor, fine motor, personal–social, and problem-solving skills	A parental-report screening tool, scored by the nurse after completion to determine child's progress in each of the developmental areas; written at a fourth- to sixth-grade reading level; takes 10–15 minutes to complete, 2–3 minutes to score; many languages available
Birth–7 years, 11 months	Parents' Evaluation of Developmental Status (PEDS)	Screens for a wide range of developmental, behavioral, social–emotional/mental health, self-help, early academic, and family issues	A short 10-question parental-report screening tool that can also be used in nurse interview format. Effective regardless of parents' level of education, income, race, marital status, or child's age or birth order; written at a fourth- to fifth-grade reading level; 5 minutes to complete, 2 minutes to score; available in Spanish
Birth–7 years, 11 months	Parents' Evaluation of Developmental Status -Developmental Milestones (PEDS-DM)	Screens for fine motor, gross motor, expressive and receptive language, self-help, social–emotional issues and reading and math issues for older children	A short six- to eight-question parental-report screening tool that can also be used in nurse interview format Includes an assessment level version for use in neonatal intensive care unit and early childhood intervention programs; written at a second- to fourth-grade reading level; 5 minutes to complete, 1 minute to score; available in Spanish

Adapted from Aites, J., & Schonwald, A. (2022). Developmental-behavioral surveillance and screening in primary care. *UpToDate.* Retrieved December 12, 2022, from https://www.uptodate.com/contents/developmental-behavioral-surveillance-and-screening-in-primary-care

common developmental screening tools. The AAP provides an online screening tool finder in their Screening Technical Assistance and Resource (STAR) Center, which can be found on their website. Many screening methods assist the nurse in identifying infants and children who may have developmental delays, thus allowing for prompt identification and referral for evaluation. Additional data can be used to determine a school-age child's developmental level, including handwriting samples, ability to draw, school performance, and social skills.

In addition to developmental and behavioral surveillance at every visit, the AAP recommends performing the following additional screening tests. Perform a developmental screening at 9, 18, and 30 months and a screening test for autism spectrum disorder (ASD) with a standardized developmental tool at 18 and 24 months or at any point that concerns about ASD are raised (Lipkin et al., 2020). Also, perform a risk assessment for tobacco, alcohol, and drug use at every visit from 11 to 21 years of age, as well as a depression screening at every visit from 12 to 21 years of age. For the latest recommendations for preventive pediatric health care and links to recommended screening tools, visit the AAP website for the preventive care/periodicity schedule.

Injury and Disease Prevention

Disease prevention is defined as interventions performed to protect children from a disease or to identify it at an early stage and lessen its consequences. These interventions are determined by the results of the nurse's assessment, nationally accepted practice guidelines, and the family's goals. Components of disease prevention include screening tests and immunizations.

Injury prevention is accomplished primarily through education, anticipatory guidance, and physical changes in the environment. Injuries can be unintentional (poisoning, falls, or drowning) or intentional (child abuse, homicide, or suicide). The types of injuries a child is most likely to encounter vary greatly among age groups. Although aggressive public health initiatives have decreased mortality rates of childhood unintentional injuries significantly in the past 50 years, injury is still the leading cause of death in children and adolescents, and rates remain higher in some populations. Therefore, continued vigilance and public health action remain necessary (CDC, 2021a). The nurse, in partnership with the family and the community, can have an enormous impact on child safety. Specific interventions are discussed in Chapters 25 to 29.

Screening Tests

Screening tests are procedures or laboratory analyses used to identify children with a certain condition. These tests are done to ensure that no child with the disorder is missed. They have a high sensitivity (a high false-positive rate) and a low specificity (a low false-negative rate). If a screening test is positive, follow-up tests with higher specificity are performed. A **risk assessment** is performed by the health care provider or nurse practitioner in conjunction with the child and includes objective as well as subjective data to determine the likelihood that the child will develop a condition.

In **universal screening**, an entire population is screened regardless of the child's individual risk. This type of screening is performed when a reliable risk assessment procedure is not available. In contrast, **selective screening** is done when a risk assessment indicates the child has one or more risk factors for the disorder.

> *TAKE NOTE!*
>
> To increase cooperation from young children during screenings, set up a reward system. Easy-to-do rewards include:
>
> - Stamping the back of the child's hand with a "smiley face"
> - Making an eye cover by placing two stickers back to back over a tongue blade and letting the child keep the cover after the screening
> - Copying a design onto a sheet of paper and letting the child take it home to color
> - Letting the child play with a simple device such as a penlight or stethoscope

NEWBORN SCREENING

Newborn screening is performed on every newborn at birth for health disorders that would not have been found otherwise. These disorders, if left untreated, would lead to significant morbidity or death. State law determines which metabolic screening tests are mandatory in that state. The March of Dimes would like to see all states provide newborn screening for 35 health conditions (March of Dimes, 2020). Go online to Baby's First Test to see a list of conditions tested for by state. To decrease variability across states, the United States Secretary of the USDHHS has established the Recommended Uniform Screening Panel (RUSP) (Kemper, 2021). For the latest RUSP, visit the Health Resources & Services Administration website at www.hrsa.gov. These disorders include:

- Amino acid metabolism disorders (these newborns cannot process amino acids) such as classic phenylketonuria, maple syrup urine disease, and homocystinuria
- Organic acid metabolism disorders (these newborns cannot metabolize food correctly) such as isovaleric acidemia, glutaric acidemia, and propionic acidemia
- Fatty acid oxidation disorders (these newborns cannot change fat to energy) such as medium-chain acyl-CoA

dehydrogenase deficiency, trifunctional protein deficiency, and carnitine uptake defect

- Hemoglobinopathies (these newborns have problems with their red blood cells) such as sickle cell anemia and hemoglobin S/beta-thalassemia
- Lysosomal storage disorders (these newborns cannot break down certain types of complex sugars) such as mucopolysaccharidosis type-1 (MPS 1) and Pompe disease
- Endocrine disorders (these newborns have problems with certain glands that help the body make hormones) such as congenital adrenal hyperplasia (CAH) and congenital hypothyroidism
- Others such as biotinidase deficiency, classical galactosemia, cystic fibrosis, critical congenital heart defect, severe combined immunodeficiency (SCID), spinal muscular atrophy, and hearing loss

During the initial health supervision visit, the nurse should confirm that newborn screening was performed prior to discharge from the birthing unit. If the test was not performed or was performed before 48 hours of age, the screening should be performed at that visit. The metabolic screening results need to be noted in the child's permanent record at the medical home.

HEARING SCREENING

The AAP recommends hearing screening of all infants. Hearing loss is a common condition in newborns, and even mild hearing loss can cause serious delays in social and emotional development, language acquisition, and cognitive function (Vohr, 2022). Identification of hearing loss by 6 months of age is crucial to reduce the impact on the child's development (Delaney, 2022). Refer to Healthy People 2030 box. Targeted screening based on risk factors will identify only 50% to 75% of infants with hearing loss, and with reliable screening tests available, universal screening has been implemented (Vohr, 2022). Screening should be done before discharge from the birthing unit; if not, the newborn needs to be screened before 1 month of age. Behavioral observations of the infant's response to sounds, such as a ringing bell or clapping hands, are not sensitive enough to preclude mild to moderate hearing loss (Delaney, 2022). Accepted methodologies for screening newborn hearing are displayed in Table 31.2.

TABLE 31.2 • Hearing Screening Methods

Test Name	Age Group	Characteristics	Nursing Implications
Automated auditory brain stem response (AABR)	Newborn–6 months	Measures electroencephalographic waves; electrodes placed on forehead, mastoid, and nape of neck Click stimulus delivered via earphones. Test results may be affected by ear debris.	Infant must be quiet (sedation may be needed). Can be conducted in presence of background noise
Otoacoustic emissions (OAEs)	Newborn–6 months or developmentally delayed children at the infant's level of functioning	The machine produces clicks that stimulate cilia in the cochlea and measures the response.	Infant must be quiet. Test results may be inaccurate in first 24 hours of life. Not sufficient to detect neural hearing loss
Visual reinforcement audiometry (VRA)	6 months–2 years	Visual reward is linked to a tone signal. Child looks to the visual reward in response to the tone. Reward is activated, reinforcing the response.	Child must be alert and happy for best results. Schedule for after sleep/rest period.
Tympanometry	Over 7 months	Measures tympanic membrane mobility and determines middle ear pressure	The probe must form a seal with the canal. The child must remain still to obtain a valid result.
Conditioned play audiometry (CPA)	2–4 years	Similar to VRA except uses "listening games" Child does listening game at the tone and receives social reward. May be used when developmental age is 2 years	See Nursing Implications for VRA.

(continued)

TABLE 31.2 • Hearing Screening Methods (*continued*)

Test Name	Age Group	Characteristics	Nursing Implications
Pure-tone (conventional) audiometry	4 years and older	Measures hearing acuity through a range of frequencies and intensities Child must wear earphones. Performed in a soundproof room if possible	Teach the child the desired motor response before screening. Administer conditioning trials. Offer two presentations of stimulus to ensure reliability. At a minimum, screen 1,000-, 2,000-, and 4,000-Hz levels at 20 dB
Whisper test	4 years and older	One ear is occluded. Examiner stands behind the child and whispers a word. The child must accurately repeat the whispered word.	The child must be in a quiet room and away from distractions. The child should be alert and well rested for accurate results. Consider a reward system to increase adherence.
Weber test	6 years and older	Place a vibrating tuning fork in the middle of the top of the head. Ask if the sound is in one ear or both ears. The sound should be heard in both ears.	The child must understand the instructions and be able to cooperate.
Rinne test	6 years and older	Place a vibrating tuning fork on the mastoid process to assess bone conduction. The child signals when the sound is gone. Next, place a vibrating tuning fork outside the ear to test air conduction. The child signals when the sound is gone. For a passing test, air conduction time should be twice as long as bone conduction time.	The child must understand the instructions and be able to cooperate.

HEALTHY PEOPLE 2030

Objective	Nursing Significance
Increase the proportion of newborns who are screened for hearing loss by no later than age 1 month. Increase the proportion of infants who did not pass the hearing screening test that receive diagnostic audiologic evaluation for hearing loss no later than age 3 months. Increase the proportion of infants with confirmed hearing loss who are enrolled for intervention services no later than age 6 months.	• Determine results of newborn hearing screening at first newborn check-up. • Refer any infant with possible hearing deficit for further evaluation. • Ensure infants with hearing loss receive appropriate augmentation (hearing aids). • Ensure all children and adolescents receive hearing screenings with well-child check-ups as appropriate.

Healthy People Objectives retrieved from http://www.healthypeople.gov

Screening for hearing loss in older children begins with a history from the primary caregivers. If any problems are noted, audiometry should be performed. When the child is capable of following simple commands reliably, the nurse can perform some basic procedures to screen for hearing loss. The whisper test is easy to perform but in order to be valid requires a quiet room that is away from distractions. The Weber and Rinne tests are typically performed together and can be used to screen for sensorineural or conductive hearing loss. Refer to Table 31.2, for hearing screening methods.

Universal hearing screening with objective testing is recommended at ages 4, 5, 6, 8, and 10 (Bright Futures/AAP, 2022). Screening with audiometry should occur once between the ages of 11 and 14, once between 15 and 17, and again between 18 and 21 (Bright Futures/AAP, 2022). See Box 31.2 for examples of risk assessment. More frequent screening is recommended if there is any behavior that indicates the child's hearing may be impaired. Repeated hearing screenings are recommended if a child has risk factors for acquired hearing loss such as those listed in Box 31.3.

BOX 31.2 Hearing Risk Assessment

Ages 3 Months–4 Years
- Auditory skill monitoring
- Developmental surveillance
- Assessment of parental concerns

Age 4 Years
- Difficulty hearing on the telephone
- Difficulty hearing people in a noisy background
- Frequent asking of others to repeat themselves
- Turning the television up too loudly

BOX 31.3 Risk Factors for Hearing Impairment

- Family history of hearing loss
- Prenatal or neonatal infection
- Anomalies of the head, face, or ears (craniofacial anomalies)
- Low birth weight (<1.5 kg)
- Hyperbilirubinemia requiring exchange transfusion
- Ototoxic medications
- Low Apgar scores: 4 or less at 1 minute or 6 or less at 5 minutes
- Mechanical ventilation or extracorporeal membrane oxygenation (ECMO)
- Neonatal intensive care unit admission lasting 5 days
- Syndrome associated with hearing loss
- Head trauma
- Bacterial meningitis
- Neurodegenerative disorders
- Persistent pulmonary hypertension
- Otitis media with effusion for 3 months

Adapted from Delaney, A. M. (2022). Newborn hearing screening. *eMedicine*. https://emedicine.medscape.com/article/836646-overview?form=fpf; Vohr, B. R. (2022). Screening the newborn for hearing loss. *UpToDate*. Retrieved December 13, 2022, from https://www.uptodate.com/contents/screening-the-newborn-for-hearing-loss

VISION SCREENING

Newborns with ocular structural abnormalities are at high risk for vision impairment. Vision screening with objective testing is recommended at ages 3, 4, 5, 6, 8, 10, 12, and 15 years, with risk assessment being performed at all other health supervision visits (Bright Futures/AAP, 2022). The screening procedures for children younger than 3 years of age or for nonverbal children involve evaluating the child's ability to fixate on and follow objects. The neonate should be able to fixate on an object approximately 25 to 30 cm (10 to 12 in) from the face. After fixation, the infant should be able to follow the object to the midline. By 2 months of age, the infant should be able to follow the object 180 degrees. The technique of photoscreening can help identify problems such as ocular malalignment, refractive error, and lens and retinal problems.

TAKE NOTE!

Use objects with black-and-white patterns when performing vision screening on an infant younger than 6 months. The infant's vision at this age is more attuned to high-contrast patterns than to colors. Try checkerboard patterns or concentric circles. Animal figures like pandas and Dalmatians also work well.

After the age of 3 years, a variety of standardized age-appropriate vision screening charts are available. These charts include the "tumbling E" and Allen figures (Fig. 31.2A, B). These charts allow for a more precise vision assessment and aid the nurse in identifying

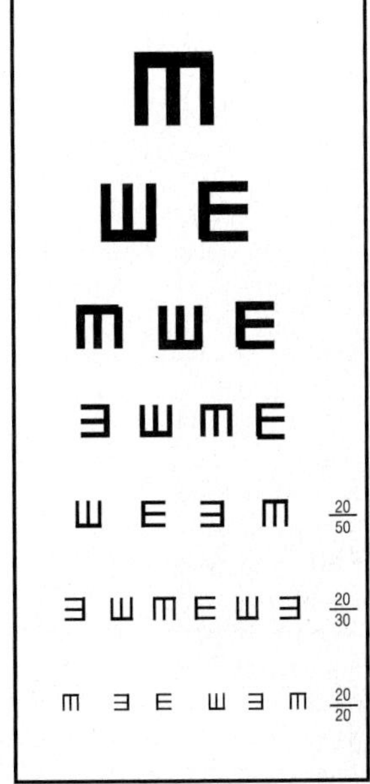

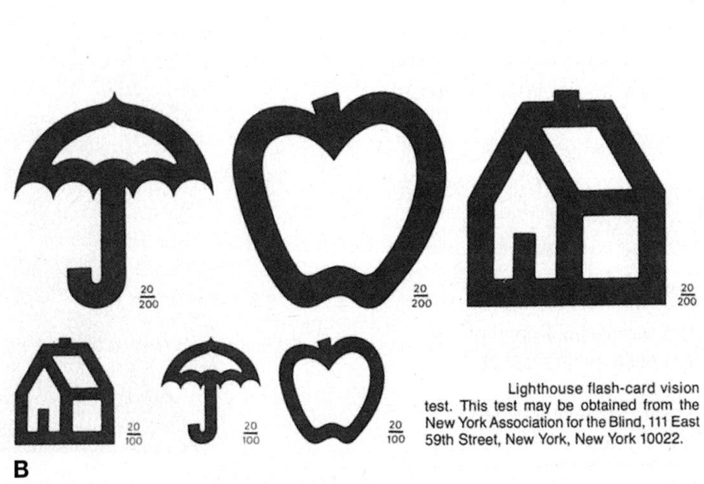

E
H N
D F N
P T X Z
U Z D T F
D T F P D H
P H U N T D Z
C

FIGURE 31.2 A. The "tumbling E" chart is appropriate for children who do not yet know the alphabet but who can follow instructions to indicate the direction in which the arms of the "E" are pointing. **B.** A picture chart similar to the Allen object recognition chart is appropriate for vision screening in the preschool-age child. **C.** The Snellen eye chart may be used for children 6 years or older who know the alphabet. The test can be obtained at www.preventblindness.org/children or by calling 1-800-331-2020.

TABLE 31.3 • Vision Screening Tools

Screening Tool	Age	Nursing Implications
Snellen letters or numbers	School-age	The child must know their letters or numbers for the test to be valid.
"Tumbling E"	Preschool	The child points in the direction that the "E" is facing.
LEA symbols or Allen figures	Preschool	The child should first identify the pictures with both eyes at a comfortable distance prior to monocular testing to ensure validity of the test.
Ishihara	School-age	Screens for color discrimination (numbers composed of dots, hidden within other dots)
Color Vision Testing Made Easy (CVTME)	Preschool	Uses dot pictures like the Ishihara, but instead of numbers has easily identified shapes embedded in the dots

preschool children with visual acuity problems. By age 5 or 6, most children know the alphabet well enough to use the traditional Snellen chart for vision screening (Fig. 31.2C). Refer to the Healthy People 2030 box. Table 31.3 gives further information about vision screening tools.

Screenings should be performed when children are alert, as fatigue and lack of interest can mimic poor vision. When using any vision screening chart, several simple steps need to be followed:

- Place the chart at the child's eye level.
- Make sure there is sufficient lighting.
- Place a mark on the floor approximately 300 to 600 cm (10 to 20 ft) from the chart (distance depends on what the tool is calibrated for).
- Align the child's heels on the mark.
- Have the child read each line, first, with one eye covered and then with the other eye covered. Explain to the child to keep the eye covered but open (Fig. 31.3).
- Have the child read each line with both eyes.

In addition to visual acuity screening, children should also be screened for color discrimination. Any child who has eye abnormalities or who has failed visual screening needs to be evaluated by a specialist appropriately trained to treat children.

HEALTHY PEOPLE 2030

Objective	Nursing Significance
Increase the proportion of preschool children aged 3–5 years who receive vision screening.	• Use a preschool-appropriate vision screening tool to assess vision. • Ensure screening begins at age 3 years.

Healthy People Objectives retrieved from http://www.healthypeople.gov

IRON-DEFICIENCY ANEMIA SCREENING

Iron deficiency is the leading nutritional deficiency in children (Powers, 2021). Iron deficiency can cause cognitive and motor deficits resulting in developmental delays and behavioral disturbances. The increased incidence of iron-deficiency anemia is directly associated with periods of diminished iron stores, rapid growth, and high metabolic demands. At 6 months of age, the in utero iron stores of a full-term infant are almost depleted (Powers, 2021). The adolescent growth spurt warrants constant iron replacement. Pregnant adolescents are at even higher risk for iron deficiency due to the demands of the adolescent's growth spurt and the needs of the developing fetus.

The AAP recommends assessing for risk factors related to iron-deficiency anemia at 4, 15, 18, 24, and 30 months and then annually and performing a hematocrit or hemoglobin at 12 months (Bright Futures/AAP, 2022). Refer to Box 31.4 for risk factors for iron-deficiency anemia.

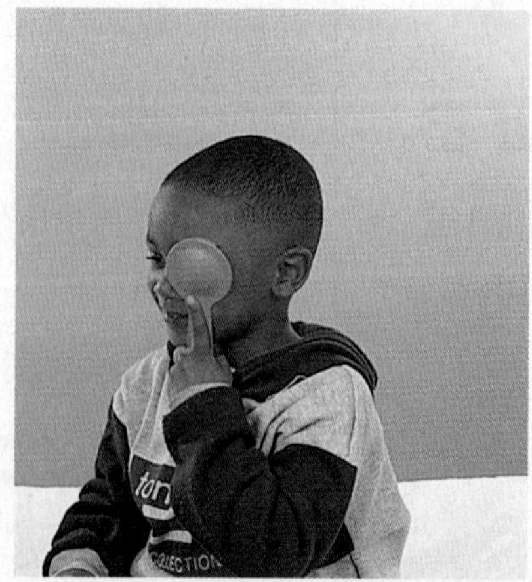

FIGURE 31.3 One eye must be covered while the other is tested in order to detect discrepancies in visual acuity between the two eyes and identify amblyopia early.

BOX 31.4 Risk Factors for Iron-Deficiency Anemia

- Periods of rapid growth
- Low-birth-weight or preterm infants
- Low dietary intake of meat, fish, poultry, and ascorbic acid
- Higher weight
- Inappropriate consumption of cow's milk
- Use of infant formula not fortified with iron
- Exclusive breastfeeding after age 4 months without iron-fortified supplemental foods
- Meal skipping, frequent dieting
- Exposure to lead
- Feeding problems
- Pregnancy or recent pregnancy
- Intensive physical training
- Recent blood loss, heavy/lengthy menstrual periods
- Chronic use of aspirin or nonsteroidal antiinflammatory drugs
- Parasitic infections

Children at High Risk for Iron-Deficiency Anemia

- Families with low income
- Those eligible for the Special Supplemental Nutrition Program for Women, Infants, and Children (WIC)
- Hispanic/Latin American and Asian American children
- Migrants or recently arrived refugees

Data from Powers, J. M. (2021). Iron deficiency in infants and children <12: Screening, prevention, clinical manifestations, and diagnosis. *UpToDate*. Retrieved December 14, 2022, from https://medilib.ir/uptodate/show/5925

LEAD SCREENING

Elevated blood lead levels (3.5 mcg/dL or higher) remain a preventable environmental health threat. Approximately half a million children have blood levels greater than 3.5 mcg/dL, which can lead to a wide variety of symptoms and problems, such as headaches, stomach pain, inattentiveness, irritability, hyperactivity, decreased bone and muscle growth, poor muscle coordination, problems with language and speech, cognitive impairments, hearing problems, and seizures (CDC, 2022a; Gavin, 2021). Although the prevalence of elevated lead levels has declined significantly over the past two decades, mainly due to the banning of lead-based paint in 1978, the elimination of lead from motor vehicle gasoline, banning the use of lead pipes for plumbing, and the removal of lead for solder in food cans, certain communities still possess a high level of lead exposure (Sample, 2022; United States Environmental Protection Agency, 2018). Lead poisoning is a problem that affects children younger than 6 years the most because children of this age are crawling on the ground and putting things in their mouths, and their developing neurologic system is more sensitive to the effects of lead. It has also been found that even low blood lead levels can harm children and result in IQ deficits, attention-related behavior problems, and poor academic achievement (Sample, 2022). Therefore, the AAP and CDC state that there is no safe blood lead level in children and that a shift to primary prevention is the key (Sample, 2022). Ensuring that no children spend time or live in homes, buildings, or environments where they are exposed to lead hazards is the key. Educate parents on lead hazards, and encourage them to avoid exposure of their children. Lead-based paint continues to be the highest hazard and most dangerous source of lead exposure in children (Gavin, 2021). Lead hazards include homes or buildings built before 1978, contaminated soil and dust, water that flows through old lead pipes or faucets, foods stored in containers that are painted with lead paint (such as lead-glazed pottery or lead crystal) or canned food that is sealed with lead (such as those imported from other countries), toys or toy jewelry that may be painted with lead paint or have lead components, and folk remedies that contain lead, such as greta and azarcon (Sample, 2022).

TAKE NOTE!

A healthy diet that includes calcium, iron, and vitamin C can also help decrease the way the body absorbs lead (Gavin, 2021).

The AAP Bright Future guidelines recommends performing a risk assessment and, if positive, screening at 6, 9, 12, 18, and 24 months and at 3, 4, 5, and 6 years (Bright Futures/AAP, 2022). At-risk children should have a blood lead level drawn at ages 12 and 24 months (Bright Futures/AAP, 2022). Refer to the Healthy People 2030 box.

HEALTHY PEOPLE 2030

Objective	Nursing Significance
Reduce blood lead level in children aged 1–5 years.	• Screen for lead exposure. • Ensure that high risk children have blood lead levels measured.

Healthy People Objectives retrieved from http://www.healthypeople.gov

TAKE NOTE!

Many cases of elevated blood lead levels have been reported in children who are recent immigrants, refugees, or international adoptees. In addition to blood lead testing for all children between ages 6 months and 6 years, it is also recommended for these children on entering the United States and again 3 to 6 months after placement in a permanent residence (Sample, 2022).

HYPERTENSION SCREENING

Higher weight and resulting hypertension have been on the rise in children and can lead to adult cardiovascular disease. Universal hypertension screening for children beginning at 3 years of age is recommended (Bright Futures/AAP, 2022). If the child has risk factors for systemic hypertension, such as preterm birth, very low birth weight, kidney disease, organ transplant, congenital heart defect, or other illnesses associated with hypertension, then screening begins when the risk factor becomes apparent (Bright Futures/AAP, 2022).

The guidelines for determining hypertension in children and adolescents utilize body size in order to be more precise. Sex and age are used to determine specific systolic and diastolic blood pressure percentiles. Refer to Appendix E for Blood Pressure Charts for Children and Adolescents. Auscultation is the preferred method of measuring blood pressure in children, and an elevated blood pressure must be confirmed on repeated visits before a diagnosis of hypertension is given. Refer to Box 31.5 for hypertension guidelines. Anticipatory guidance on activity is appropriate for any child with the inclusion of weight management for children with elevated blood pressure, stage 1 or 2 hypertension (Flynn et al., 2017). Refer to Chapter 41 for additional information on hypertension.

BOX 31.5 Childhood Hypertension Guidelines

	Children 1 to <13 Years Old	Children >13 Years Old
Optimal/normal	<90th percentile for sex, age, and height	BP <120/<80 mm Hg
Elevated blood pressure	BP 120/80 mm Hg to <95th percentile for sex, age, and height (whichever is lower) or BP ≥90th percentile to ≤95th percentile for sex, age, and height	BP 120/<80–129/<80 mm Hg
Stage 1 hypertension	≥95th percentile to <95th percentile + 12 mm Hg for sex, age, and height, or 130/80 to 139/89 mm Hg (whichever is lower) on at least three separate occasions	130/80–139/89 mm Hg
Stage 2 hypertension	≥95th percentile + 12 mm Hg for sex, age, and height or ≥140/90 mm Hg (whichever is lower) on at least three separate occasions	≥140/90 mm Hg

Data from Flynn, J. T., Kaelber, D. C., Baker-Smith, C. M., Blowey, D., Carroll, A. E., Daniels, S. R., de Ferranti, S. D., Dionne, J. M., Falkner, B., Flinn, S. K., Gidding, S. S., Goodwin, C., Leu, M. G., Powers, M. E., Rea, C., Samuels, J., Simasek, M., Thaker, V. V., Urbina, E. M., & Subcommittee on Screening and Management of High Blood Pressure in Children. (2017). Clinical practice guideline for screening and management of high blood pressure in children and adolescents. *Pediatrics, 140*(3), e20171904. https://doi.org/10.1542/peds.2017-1904

HYPERLIPIDEMIA SCREENING

Atherosclerosis has been documented in children, and a link exists between high lipid levels and the development of these lesions. Bright Futures Guidelines recommends universal screening for dyslipidemia once between 9 and 11 years of age and again between 17 and 21 years of age (Bright Futures/AAP, 2022). Performing a risk assessment screening at 24 months and 4, 6, 8, and 12 through 17 years of age is also recommended. Refer to Box 31.6 for details regarding screening for hyperlipidemia.

Remember Maya and Evan, the children introduced at the beginning of the chapter? How would you assess their growth and development? Which screening tests are warranted for them, and why? What further information would you need to determine which tests should be performed?

Immunizations

Immunization is the key disease prevention activity during childhood health supervision visits. The development of effective vaccines, beginning in the 1940s, revolutionized children's health care. Immunization allowed the focus to shift from disease treatment to disease prevention. The nurse needs to understand the principles of immunizations, the proper use of vaccines, and barriers to immunization. Armed with this knowledge, the nurse can partner with families to provide the highest level of disease protection to children (Fig. 31.4). Refer to the Healthy People 2030 box. For information on vaccine-preventable communicable diseases, refer to Chapter 37.

BOX 31.6 Hyperlipidemia Screening

Screen if parents, grandparents, aunts/uncles, siblings have/had documented:

- Coronary atherosclerosis
- Myocardial infarction
- Angina pectoris
- Peripheral vascular disease
- Cerebrovascular disease/stroke
- Coronary artery bypass graft/stent/angioplasty at <55 years in males, <65 years in females
- Sudden cardiac death

Screen if a parent's blood cholesterol level is 240 mg/dL or higher.

Screen at health care provider's discretion:

- Parental history is unobtainable.
- Child has diabetes or hypertension.
- Child has lifestyle risk factors:
  - Cigarette smoking
  - Higher weight
  - Sedentary lifestyle
  - High-fat dietary intake

Data from National Heart, Lung, and Blood Institute. (2012). *Expert panel on integrated guidelines for cardiovascular health and risk reduction in children and adolescents.* Summary Report (NIH Publication No. 12-7486). U.S. Department of Health and Human Services. http://www.nhlbi.nih.gov/guidelines/cvd_ped/peds_guidelines_sum.pdf

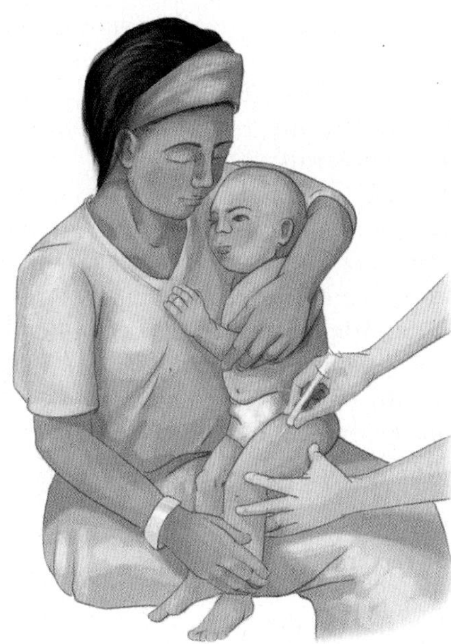

FIGURE 31.4 Nurse administering intramuscular injection into the vastus lateralis of an infant.

PRINCIPLES OF IMMUNIZATION

The immune system has the ability to recognize materials present in the body as "self" or "nonself." Foreign materials (nonself) are called antigens. When an antigen is recognized by the immune system, the immune system responds by producing antibodies (immunoglobulins) or directing special cells to destroy and remove the antigen.

HEALTHY PEOPLE 2030

Objective	Nursing Significance
Increase the vaccination coverage level of 4 doses of the diphtheria–tetanus–acellular pertussis (DTaP) vaccine among children by age 2 years. Maintain the vaccination coverage level of 2 doses of measles–mumps–rubella (MMR) vaccine for children in kindergarten. Maintain the vaccination coverage level of 1 dose of MMR among children by age 2 years. Reduce the proportion of children in the United States who receive 0 doses of recommended vaccines by age 2 years. Increase the percentage of adolescents who receive recommended doses of human papillomavirus (HPV) vaccine. Increase the proportion of people who are vaccinated annually against seasonal influenza.	• Immunize at every opportunity. If a child is due or past due for vaccinations, provide them at a sick visit if not contraindicated. • Educate families about the benefits and risks of immunization.

Healthy People Objectives retrieved from http://www.healthypeople.gov

Immunity is the ability to destroy and remove a specific antigen from the body. The acquisition of immunity can be active or passive. **Passive immunity** is produced when the immunoglobulins of one person are transferred to another. This immunity lasts only weeks or months. Passive immunity can be obtained by injection of exogenous immunoglobulins. It can also be transferred from birthing parents to infants via colostrum or the placenta. **Active immunity** is acquired when a person's own immune system generates the immune response. Active immunity lasts for many years or for a lifetime. This long-term protection is the result of immunologic memory. After the initial immune response, specialized cells for that antigen continue to exist. When an antigen returns, these memory cells rapidly produce a fresh supply of antibodies to reestablish protection. This immunity can occur after exposure to natural pathogens or after exposure to vaccines. Vaccines mimic the characteristics of the natural antigen. The immune system mounts a response and establishes an immunologic memory as it would for an infection.

The classification of vaccines is based on the characteristics of the antigen present. The antigen may be viral or bacterial. It may be live attenuated (weakened) or killed. It may be the whole antigen or a portion of it (fractional).

- Live attenuated vaccines are modified living organisms that are weakened. The organism can produce an immune response but does not produce the complications of the illness.
- Inactivated vaccines contain whole dead organisms; they are incapable of reproducing but are capable of producing an immune response.
- Toxoid vaccines contain protein products produced by bacteria called toxins. The toxin is heat-treated to weaken its effect, but it retains its ability to produce an immune response.
- Conjugate vaccines are the result of chemically linking the bacterial cell wall polysaccharide (sugar-based) portions with proteins. This dramatically increases the immune response compared to presenting the polysaccharide portion alone.
- Recombinant vaccines use genetically engineered organisms. For example, the hepatitis B vaccine (HepB) is produced by splicing a gene portion of the virus into a gene of a yeast cell. The yeast cell is then able to produce hepatitis B surface antigen to use for vaccine production.
  - Messenger RNA (mRNA) vaccines make a specific type of protein to trigger an immune response. This technology was used to make some of the COVID-19 vaccines.
  - Viral vector vaccines use a modified harmless version of a different virus as a vector to deliver protection. This type of technology was used to make some of the COVID-19 vaccines.

The safety and efficacy of existing vaccines are constantly being reviewed, and research to improve vaccines is ongoing. The goal is to refine vaccines so that a maximum immune response is produced with the least amount of risk for the child.

IMMUNIZATION MANAGEMENT

The Advisory Committee on Immunization Practices (ACIP), a branch of the CDC, reviews the recommended immunization schedules at least yearly and updates the schedule to ensure that it reflects current best practices. In addition to the recommended schedule, the ACIP publishes a "catch-up" schedule for children who have not been adequately immunized. The child's immunization record must be compared with the latest edition of these schedules when assessing the need for immunization. For the latest immunization schedule, visit the CDC immunization schedules website.

TAKE NOTE!

When obtaining an immunization history from the parent, ask, "When and where did your child receive their last immunization?" The answer will provide more information than simply asking, "Are your child's immunizations up to date?" The nurse can compare this information with that on the immunization record, discover in what settings the child is getting health care, and use the information as a starting point in a discussion of any reactions to previous immunizations.

Vaccine storage and administration affect the efficacy of a vaccine. Improperly stored or reconstituted vaccines can be ineffective (CDC, 2022b). The vaccine must be given by the correct route; not all vaccines are given intramuscularly (Fig. 31.5). The manufacturer's package insert is the best reference source for any vaccine.

TAKE NOTE!

Proper vaccine storage is critical to vaccine efficacy. If you suspect that a vaccine was not maintained at the proper storage temperature, do not use it! An ineffective vaccine is of no use in preventing disease.

Any vaccine can have side effects, and the most common ones are mild, such as redness, tenderness, and swelling at the site; low-grade fever; and fussiness. These symptoms usually resolve within a few days. The National Childhood Vaccine Injury Act (NCVIA) requires that Vaccine Information Statements (VISs) (Fig. 31.6) be provided to parents before an immunization is given (CDC, 2021b). These inform about the benefits and risks and discuss specific side effects that may be seen for each immunization. In accordance with the concept of partnership with the parents, allow ample time for them to read the VIS and to discuss their concerns. If the parents do not understand the information presented, they should feel comfortable asking questions. If the parents do not have reading literacy, present the information orally and verify that the parents understand it. If the information in the VIS is not in the parent's native language, have a translator present the information.

At this time, ask the parents about the child's reactions to previous immunizations, and screen for precautions and contraindications for each vaccine to be administered. Before the vaccine is given, the parents must sign consent forms.

Any clinically significant adverse event that occurs after an immunization should be reported to the Vaccine Adverse Event Reporting System (VAERS), which is a co-sponsored surveillance program by the CDC and the U.S. Food and Drug Administration (FDA) (VAERS, n.d.). For assistance in obtaining and completing a VAERS form, call 800-822-7967 or visit www.vaers.hhs.gov.

Documentation in the child's permanent record includes the following:

- Date the vaccine was administered
- Name of vaccine (commonly used abbreviation is acceptable)
- Lot number and expiration date of vaccine
- Manufacturer's name
- Site and route by which vaccine was administered (e.g., left deltoid, intramuscularly)
- Edition date of VIS given to the parents
- Name and address of the facility administering the vaccine (where the permanent record will be kept)
- Name of the person administering the immunization

Families should be provided with a copy of the child's immunizations. This reinforces the importance of the procedure and reminds the parents to keep the child's immunizations up to date.

Figure 31.7 shows a typical vaccine administration record.

VACCINE DESCRIPTIONS

This section reviews the most commonly used vaccines. These immunizations are recommended by the ACIP and the AAP. Each state has laws that determine which immunizations are required for school admittance. These requirements can be waived if a contraindication or precaution to the vaccine exists. *Contraindications* are conditions that justify withholding an immunization either permanently or temporarily. The majority of contraindications are temporary, and the vaccine can be administered at a later date when the contraindication has resolved. The only permanent contraindication to all vaccines is an anaphylactic or systemic allergic reaction to a vaccine component. If severe allergic reaction occurs, this is a contraindication for any subsequent doses of that specific vaccine (Kroger et al., 2022). Children who are severely immunocompromised or people who are pregnant should not receive live vaccines (such as MMR and varicella) (see further on). With pertussis immunization (DTP, DTaP, or Tdap) (see the following section), encephalopathy without an identified cause within 7 days of the immunization permanently contraindicates further immunization with pertussis-containing vaccine. Children with SCID disease or a history of intussusception are both contraindications to the immunization

Administering Vaccines: Dose, Route, Site, and Needle Size

Vaccine	Dose	Route
COVID-19 *For product and dosage information for COVID-19 vaccine primary series and booster doses for both immunocompetent and immunocompromised adults, see CDC's "COVID-19 Vaccine Interim COVID-19 Immunization Schedule for Persons 6 Months of Age and Older."**		IM
Dengue (DENV4CYD)	0.5 mL	Subcut
Diphtheria, Tetanus, Pertussis (DTaP, DT, Tdap, Td)	0.5 mL	IM
***Haemophilus influenzae* type b** (Hib)	0.5 mL	IM
Hepatitis A (HepA)	≤18 yrs: 0.5 mL ≥19 yrs: 1.0 mL	IM
Hepatitis B (HepB) *People 11–15 yrs may be given Recombivax HB(Merck) 1.0 mL adult formulation on a 2-dose schedule.*	Engerix-B; Recombivax HB ≤19 yrs: 0.5 mL ≥20 yrs: 1.0 mL Heplisav-B ≥18 yrs: 0.5 mL PreHevbrio ≥18 yrs: 1.0 mL	IM
Human papillomavirus (HPV)	0.5 mL	IM
Influenza, live attenuated (LAIV4)	0.2 mL (0.1 mL in each nostril)	Intranasal spray
Influenza, inactivated (IIV4); 6 thru 35 mos • Egg-based IIV4: Afluria, Fluzone, Fluarix, FluLaval • Cell-culture based (ccIIV4): Flucelvax	Afluria: 0.25 mL Fluzone: 0.25 or 0.5 mL Fluarix, Flucelvax, FluLaval: 0.5 mL	IM
Influenza, inactivated (IIV4) and • Cell-culture based (ccIIV4), 3+ yrs; • Recombinant (RIV4, Flublok), 18+ yrs; • Adjuvanted (aIIV4, Fluad) 65+ yrs	0.5 mL	IM
Influenza, high-dose (IIV4-HD) 65+ yrs	0.7 mL	IM
Measles, Mumps, Rubella (MMR)	0.5 mL — MMR II (Merck) 0.5 mL — Priorix (GSK)	IM or Subcut Subcut
Meningococcal serogroups A, C, W, Y (MenACWY)	0.5 mL	IM
Meningococcal serogroup B (MenB)	0.5 mL	IM
Mpox (Jynneos)	0.5 mL	Subcut†
Pneumococcal conjugate (PCV)	0.5 mL	IM
Pneumococcal polysaccharide (PPSV23)	0.5 mL	IM or Subcut
Polio, inactivated (IPV)	0.5 mL	IM or Subcut
Respiratory Syncytial Virus (RSV) vaccine	0.5 mL	IM
RSV preventive antibody (RSV-mAb)	0.5 mL, 1 mL, or 2 mL based on weight and/or age	IM
Rotavirus (RV)	Rotarix: 1.0 mL Rotateq: 2.0 mL	Oral
Varicella (VAR)	0.5 mL	IM or Subcut
Zoster (Zos)	Shingrix: 0.5‡ mL	IM
Combination Vaccines		
DTaP-HepB-IPV (Pediarix) DTaP-IPV/Hib (Pentacel) DTaP-IPV (Kinrix; Quadracel) DTaP-IPV-Hib-HepB (Vaxelis)	0.5 mL	IM
MMRV (ProQuad)	0.5 mL	IM or Subcut
HepA-HepB (Twinrix)	1.0 mL	IM

*www.cdc.gov/vaccines/covid-19/downloads/COVID-19- immunization-schedule-ages-6months-older.pdf

†Administer mpox vaccine (Jynneos) 0.5 mL Subcut or, in adults, 0.1 mL intradermally. Subcut is the route indicated on the package insert. Intradermal administration to adults is permitted under FDA emergency use authorization (see www.fda.gov/media/160774/download).

‡The Shingrix (RZV) vial may contain more than 0.5 mL. Do not administer more than 0.5 mL.

Injection Site and Needle Size

Subcutaneous (Subcut) injection

Use a 23–25 gauge needle. Choose the injection site that is appropriate to the person's age and body mass.

AGE	NEEDLE LENGTH	INJECTION SITE
Infants (1–12 mos)	⅝"	Fatty tissue over anterolateral thigh muscle
Children 12 mos or older, adolescents, and adults	⅝"	Fatty tissue over anterolateral thigh muscle or fatty tissue over triceps

Intramuscular (IM) injection

Use a 22–25 gauge needle. Choose the injection site and needle length that is appropriate to the person's age and body mass.

AGE	NEEDLE LENGTH	INJECTION SITE
Newborns (1st 28 days)	⅝[1]"	Anterolateral thigh muscle
Infants (1–12 mos)	1"	Anterolateral thigh muscle
Toddlers (1–2 yrs)	1–1¼"	Anterolateral thigh muscle[3]
	⅝[2]–1"	Deltoid muscle of arm
Children (3–10 yrs)	⅝[2]–1"	Deltoid muscle of arm[3]
	1–1¼"	Anterolateral thigh muscle
Adolescents and teens (11–18 yrs)	⅝[2]–1"	Deltoid muscle of arm[3]
	1–1½"	Anterolateral thigh muscle
Biological sex and weight of patient 19 yrs or older		
Female or male <130 lbs	⅝[2]–1"	Deltoid muscle of arm
Female or male 130–152 lbs	1"	Deltoid muscle of arm
Female 153–200 lbs Male 153–260 lbs	1–1½"	Deltoid muscle of arm
Female more than 200 lbs Male more than 260 lbs	1½"	Deltoid muscle of arm
Female or male, any weight	1[2]–1½"	Anterolateral thigh muscle

1 If skin is stretched tightly and subcutaneous tissues are not bunched.

2 Alternate needle lengths may be used if the skin is stretched tightly and subcutaneous tissues are not bunched, as follows: a) a ⅝" needle in toddlers, children, and patients weighing less than 130 lbs (less than 60 kg) for IM injection in the deltoid muscle only, or b) a 1" needle for administration in the thigh muscle for adults of any weight.

3 Preferred site

NOTE: Always refer to the package insert included with each biologic for complete vaccine administration information. CDC's Advisory Committee on Immunization Practices (ACIP) recommendations for the particular vaccine should be reviewed as well. Access the ACIP recommendations at www.immunize.org/acip.

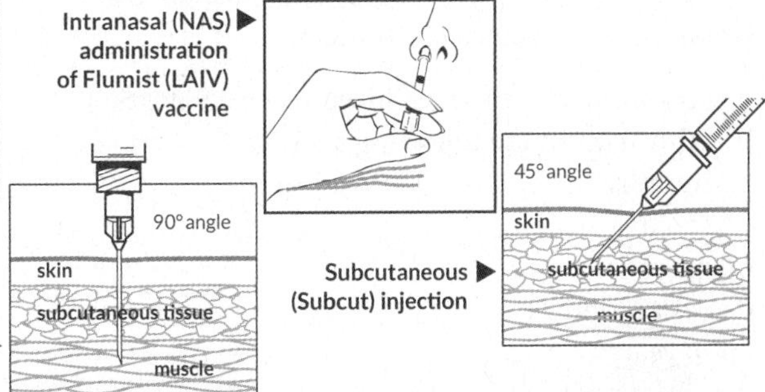

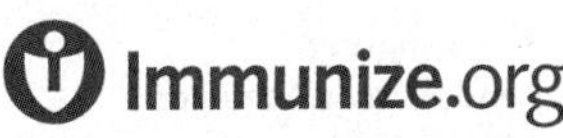

FOR PROFESSIONALS www.immunize.org / **FOR THE PUBLIC** www.vaccineinformation.org

www.immunize.org/catg.d/p3085.pdf
Item #P3085 (2/19/2024)

Scan for PDF

FIGURE 31.5 Administering vaccines: Dose, route, site, and needle size. (Reprinted from Immunize.org. (2024). *Administering vaccines: Dose, route, site, and needle size*. https://www.immunize.org/wp-content/uploads/catg.d/p3085.pdf)

VACCINE INFORMATION STATEMENT

DTaP (Diphtheria, Tetanus, Pertussis) Vaccine: *What You Need to Know*

Many vaccine information statements are available in Spanish and other languages. See www.immunize.org/vis

Hojas de información sobre vacunas están disponibles en español y en muchos otros idiomas. Visite www.immunize.org/vis

1. Why get vaccinated?

DTaP vaccine can prevent **diphtheria**, **tetanus**, and **pertussis**.

Diphtheria and pertussis spread from person to person. Tetanus enters the body through cuts or wounds.

- **DIPHTHERIA (D)** can lead to difficulty breathing, heart failure, paralysis, or death.
- **TETANUS (T)** causes painful stiffening of the muscles. Tetanus can lead to serious health problems, including being unable to open the mouth, having trouble swallowing and breathing, or death.
- **PERTUSSIS (aP)**, also known as "whooping cough," can cause uncontrollable, violent coughing that makes it hard to breathe, eat, or drink. Pertussis can be extremely serious especially in babies and young children, causing pneumonia, convulsions, traumatic brain injury, or death. In adolescents and adults, it can cause weight loss, loss of bladder control, passing out, and rib fractures from severe coughing.

2. DTaP vaccine

DTaP is only for children younger than 7 years old. Different vaccines against tetanus, diphtheria, and pertussis (Tdap and Td) are available for older children, adolescents, and adults.

It is recommended that children receive 5 doses of DTaP, usually at the following ages:

- 2 months
- 4 months
- 6 months
- 15–18 months
- 4–6 years

DTaP may be given as a stand-alone vaccine, or as part of a combination vaccine (a type of vaccine that combines more than one vaccine together into one shot).

DTaP may be given at the same time as other vaccines.

3. Talk with your health care provider

Tell your vaccination provider if the person getting the vaccine:

- Has had an **allergic reaction after a previous dose of any vaccine that protects against tetanus, diphtheria, or pertussis**, or has any **severe, life-threatening allergies**
- Has had **a coma, decreased level of consciousness, or prolonged seizures within 7 days after a previous dose of any pertussis vaccine (DTP or DTaP)**
- Has **seizures or another nervous system problem**
- Has ever had **Guillain-Barré Syndrome** (also called "GBS")
- Has had **severe pain or swelling after a previous dose of any vaccine that protects against tetanus or diphtheria**

In some cases, your child's health care provider may decide to postpone DTaP vaccination until a future visit.

Children with minor illnesses, such as a cold, may be vaccinated. Children who are moderately or severely ill should usually wait until they recover before getting DTaP vaccine.

Your child's health care provider can give you more information.

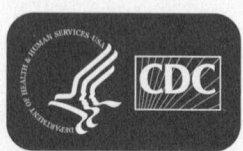

U.S. Department of Health and Human Services
Centers for Disease Control and Prevention

FIGURE 31.6 Federal law mandates the use of Vaccine Information Statements (VISs). These should be given to the parent or primary caregiver for each vaccine the child receives. (Reprinted from Centers for Disease Control and Prevention. (2021). *DTaP (Diphtheria, Tetanus, Pertussis) vaccine: What you need to know*. https://www.cdc.gov/vaccines/hcp/vis/vis-statements/dtap.pdf)

4. Risks of a vaccine reaction

- Soreness or swelling where the shot was given, fever, fussiness, feeling tired, loss of appetite, and vomiting sometimes happen after DTaP vaccination.
- More serious reactions, such as seizures, nonstop crying for 3 hours or more, or high fever (over 105°F) after DTaP vaccination happen much less often. Rarely, vaccination is followed by swelling of the entire arm or leg, especially in older children when they receive their fourth or fifth dose.

As with any medicine, there is a very remote chance of a vaccine causing a severe allergic reaction, other serious injury, or death.

5. What if there is a serious problem?

An allergic reaction could occur after the vaccinated person leaves the clinic. If you see signs of a severe allergic reaction (hives, swelling of the face and throat, difficulty breathing, a fast heartbeat, dizziness, or weakness), call **9-1-1** and get the person to the nearest hospital.

For other signs that concern you, call your health care provider.

Adverse reactions should be reported to the Vaccine Adverse Event Reporting System (VAERS). Your health care provider will usually file this report, or you can do it yourself. Visit the VAERS website at www.vaers.hhs.gov or call **1-800-822-7967**. *VAERS is only for reporting reactions, and VAERS staff members do not give medical advice.*

6. The National Vaccine Injury Compensation Program

The National Vaccine Injury Compensation Program (VICP) is a federal program that was created to compensate people who may have been injured by certain vaccines. Claims regarding alleged injury or death due to vaccination have a time limit for filing, which may be as short as two years. Visit the VICP website at www.hrsa.gov/vaccinecompensation or call **1-800-338-2382** to learn about the program and about filing a claim.

7. How can I learn more?

- Ask your health care provider.
- Call your local or state health department.
- Visit the website of the Food and Drug Administration (FDA) for vaccine package inserts and additional information at www.fda.gov/vaccines-blood-biologics/vaccines.
- Contact the Centers for Disease Control and Prevention (CDC):
  - Call **1-800-232-4636 (1-800-CDC-INFO)** or
  - Visit CDC's website at www.cdc.gov/vaccines.

Vaccine Information Statement

DTaP (Diphtheria, Tetanus, Pertussis) Vaccine

42 U.S.C. § 300aa-26

8/6/2021

OFFICE USE ONLY

FIGURE 31.6 *(continued)*

Vaccine Administration Record for Children and Teens

Patient name ____________________

Birthdate______________ Chart number ____________

PRACTICE NAME AND ADDRESS

Before administering any vaccines, give copies of all pertinent Vaccine Information Statements (VISs) to the child's parent or legal representative and make sure they understand the risks and benefits of the vaccine(s). Always provide or update the patient's personal record card.

Vaccine	Type of Vaccine[1]	Date vaccine given (mo/day/yr)	Funding Source (F,S,P)[2]	Site[3]	Vaccine		Vaccine Information Statement (VIS)		Vaccinator[6] (signature or initials and title)
					Lot #	Mfr.	Date on VIS[4]	Date given[4]	
Hepatitis B[6] (e.g., HepB, DTaP-HepB-IPV, DTaP-IPV-Hib-HepB) Give IM.[7]									
RSV-mAb[8] Give IM.[7]									
Diphtheria, Tetanus, Pertussis[6] (e.g., DTaP, DTaP-HepB-IPV, DTaP-IPV-Hib-HepB, DTaP-IPV/Hib, DTaP-IPV, Tdap, Td) Give IM.[7]									
***Haemophilus influenzae* type b**[6] (e.g., Hib, Hib-DTaP-IPV/Hib, DTaP-IPV-Hib-HepB) Give IM.[7]									
Polio[6] (e.g., IPV, DTaP-HepB-IPV, DTaP-IPV/Hib, DTaP-IPV, DTaP-IPV-Hib-HepB) Give IPV Subcut or IM.[7] Give all others IM.[7]									
Pneumococcal (e.g., PCV13, PCV15, PCV20; PPSV23) Give PCV IM.[7] Give PPSV23 Subcut or IM.[7]									
Rotavirus (RV1, RV5) Give orally (po).									

Abbreviation	Trade Name and Manufacturer
DTaP	Daptacel (Sanofi); Infanrix (GSK); Tripedia (Sanofi)
DTaP-HepB-IPV	Pediarix (GSK)
DTaP-IPV/Hib	Pentacel (Sanofi)
DTaP-IPV	Kinrix (GSK); Quadracel (Sanofi)
DTaP-IPV-Hib-HepB	Vaxelis (MCM Vaccine)
Tdap	Adacel (Sanofi); Boostrix (GSK)
Td	Tenivac (Sanofi); Tdvax (MA Biological Labs)
HepB (see note #1)	Engerix-B (GSK), Recombivax HB (Merck); Heplisav-B (Dynavax); PreHevbrio (VBI Vaccines) for 18 yrs & older
HepA-HepB	Twinrix (GSK) for teens age 18 yrs & older
Hib	ActHIB (Sanofi), Hiberix (GSK), PedvaxHIB (Merck)
IPV	IPOL (Sanofi)
RSV-mAb	Beyfortus (Sanofi & AstraZeneca)
PCV13; PCV15: PCV20	PCV13: Prevnar 13 (Pfizer); PCV15: Vaxneuvance (Merck); PCV20: Prevnar 20 (Pfizer)
PPSV23	Pneumovax 23 (Merck)
RV1; RV5	RV1: Rotarix (GSK); RV5: RotaTeq (Merck)

CONTINUED ON THE BACK ▶

How to Complete this Record

1. Record the standard abbreviation (e.g., Tdap) or the trade name for each vaccine (see table at right). Use trade name for HepB if vaccinating an older teen (schedule varies by brand).
2. Record the funding source of the vaccine given as either F (federal), S (state), or P (private).
3. Record the site where vaccine was administered as either RA (right arm), LA (left arm), RT (right thigh), LT (left thigh), or NAS (intranasal).
4. Record the publication date of each VIS as well as the date the VIS is given to the patient.
5. To meet the space constraints of this form and federal requirements for documentation, a healthcare setting should keep a reference list of vaccinators that includes their initials and titles.
6. For combination vaccines, fill in a row for each antigen in the combination.
7. IM is the abbreviation for intramuscular; Subcut is the abbreviation for subcutaneous.
8. RSV monoclonal antibody (mAb) is a passive immunization product, not a vaccine, routinely recommended for seasonal prevention of RSV disease in infants. Record administration in an equivalent manner.

www.immunize.org/catg.d/p2022.pdf
Item #P2022 (9/18/2023)

Scan for PDF

Immunize.org FOR PROFESSIONALS www.immunize.org / FOR THE PUBLIC www.vaccineinformation.org

FIGURE 31.7 Sample of a vaccine administration record. (Reprinted from Immunize.org. [2023]. *Vaccine administration record for children and teens*. http://www.immunize.org/catg.d/p2022.pdf)

Vaccine Administration Record for Children and Teens (continued)

Patient name ____________________

Birthdate ____________ Chart number ____________

PRACTICE NAME AND ADDRESS

Before administering any vaccines, give copies of all pertinent Vaccine Information Statements (VISs) to the child's parent or legal representative and make sure they understand the risks and benefits of the vaccine(s). Always provide or update the patient's personal record card.

Vaccine	Type of Vaccine[1]	Date vaccine given (mo/day/yr)	Funding Source (F,S,P)[2]	Site[3]	Vaccine		Vaccine Information Statement (VIS)		Vaccinator[5] (signature or initials and title)
					Lot #	Mfr.	Date on VIS[4]	Date given[4]	
Measles, Mumps, Rubella (e.g., MMR, MMRV) Give MMRII and MMRV Subcut or IM; give Priorix Subcut.[6]									
Varicella (e.g., VAR, MMRV) Give Subcut or IM.[6]									
Hepatitis A (HepA) Give IM.[6]									
Meningococcal ACWY (MenACWY) Give IM.[6]									
Meningococcal B (MenB-4C, MenB-FHbp) Give IM.[6]									
Human papillomavirus (HPV) Give IM.[6]									
Influenza (IIV, ccIIV, RIV, LAIV) Give IIV, ccIIV, and RIV IM.[6] Give LAIV NAS.[6]									
COVID-19 (e.g., COV-mRNA; COV-aPS) Give IM.[6]									
Other (e.g., dengue)									

Abbreviation	Trade Name and Manufacturer
MMR	MMR II (Merck); Priorix (GSK)
VAR	Varivax (Merck)
MMRV	ProQuad (Merck)
HepA	Havrix (GSK); Vaqta (Merck)
HepA-HepB	Twinrix (GSK) for teens age 18 and older
MenACWY	MenQuadfi (Sanofi); Menveo (GSK)
MenB-4C (see note #1)	Bexsero (GSK)
MenB-FHbp (see note #1)	Trumenba (Pfizer)
HPV	Gardasil 9 (Merck)
ccIIV (cell culture-based IIV)	Flucelvax (Seqirus) for teens 18 and older
IIV (inactivated influenza vaccine)	Fluarix, FluLaval (GSK); Afluria (Seqirus); Flubok (Sanofi)
LAIV (live attenuated influenza vaccine)	FluMist (AstraZeneca)
RIV (recombinant influenza vaccine)	RIV: Flublok (Sanofi) for teens 18 and older
COV-mRNA (see note #1)	Comirnaty (Pfizer-BioNTech); Spikevax (Moderna)
COV-aPS (see note #1)	Novavax (Novavax)
Other (e.g., dengue)	Dengue vaccine: Dengvaxia (Sanofi)

How to Complete this Record

1. For meningococcal B and COVID-19 vaccines, record the trade name (see table at right); for all other vaccines, record the standard abbreviation (e.g., HPV) or trade name for each vaccine (see table at right).
2. Record the funding source of the vaccine given as either F (federal), S (state), or P (private).
3. Record the site where vaccine was administered as either RA (right arm), LA (left arm), RT (right thigh), LT (left thigh), or NAS (intranasal).
4. Record the publication date of each VIS as well as the date the VIS is given to the patient.
5. To meet the space constraints of this form and federal requirements for documentation, a healthcare setting should keep a reference list of vaccinators that includes their initials and titles.
6. IM is the abbreviation for intramuscular; Subcut is the abbreviation for subcutaneous; NAS is the abbreviation for intranasal.
7. For combination vaccines, fill in a row for each antigen in the combination.

Immunize.org

www.immunize.org/catg.d/p2022.pdf / Item #P2022 (9/18/2023)

FIGURE 31.7 *(continued)*

of rotavirus vaccines (Kroger et al., 2022). Current, recent, or upcoming anesthesia, surgery, or hospitalization is not a contraindication for vaccination, and hospitalization can be used as an opportunity to provide recommended immunizations (Kroger et al., 2022).

Precautions are conditions that increase the risk of an adverse reaction, may cause diagnostic confusion, or may impair the child's ability to acquire immunity from the vaccine (Kroger et al., 2022). The presence of a moderate to severe acute illness with or without fever is a precaution for all vaccines (Kroger et al., 2022). However, with minor illness the safety and efficacy of immunizations has been documented (Kroger et al., 2022). In general, immunizations should be postponed when a precaution is present; however, on an individualized basis, providers must weigh the benefits of immunization against the likelihood of an adverse event (Kroger et al., 2022).

Diphtheria, Tetanus, and Pertussis Vaccines

Immunization against diphtheria, tetanus, and pertussis diseases is given via a combination vaccine. The vaccine currently used for children younger than 7 years is diphtheria, tetanus, acellular pertussis (DTaP). It contains diphtheria and tetanus toxoids and pertussis cell wall proteins. The older version of this vaccine—diphtheria, tetanus, pertussis (DPT)—contained killed whole cells of pertussis bacteria and caused more frequent and severe adverse reactions than DTaP. Diphtheria and tetanus (DT) vaccine is used for children younger than 7 years who have contraindications to pertussis immunization. Full-strength diphtheria toxoid causes significant adverse reactions in people older than 7 years. For this group, the Tdap adolescent preparation vaccine is used: it contains tetanus toxoid, reduced diphtheria toxoid, and acellular pertussis vaccine. The lowercase "d" is used to designate the lower dose of diphtheria toxoid. The ACIP recommends that Tdap be used for all tetanus boosters in older children (11 to 12 years) and adolescents because Tdap provides a boost to diphtheria and pertussis immunization.

Haemophilus Influenzae Type B Vaccines

Haemophilus influenzae type B is a bacterium that causes several life-threatening illnesses in children younger than 5 years. These infections include meningitis, epiglottitis, and septic arthritis. *H. influenzae* type B conjugate vaccines (Hib) have been extremely effective in cutting the rates of these diseases in children. There are several different types of Hib conjugate vaccines. Two or three doses are needed for the primary infant series depending on the vaccine product used (e.g., PedvaxHIB requires two doses, while ActHIB, Hiberix, Vaxelis, and Pentacel require three doses) (CDC, 2022c). A booster vaccine is needed at 12 to 15 months. These vaccine products are interchangeable, but if different brands are administered to a child, then a total of three doses is necessary to complete the primary series in infants. Hib vaccine is not routinely given to children aged 5 years or older and is contraindicated in children younger than 6 weeks (CDC, 2021d).

Polio Vaccine

Wild polio has been eliminated in the United States, and since 2000, inactivated polio vaccine (IPV) is the only polio vaccine currently recommended (ACIP, 2000; CDC, 2021e, 2022g). It is a killed virus vaccine that poses no risk of vaccine-acquired disease. The CDC recommends four doses of IPV. IPV is available in combination vaccines, which has several vaccines in one injection; this may result in a child getting five doses of IPV. This has been determined to be safe in children. Children who will be traveling to an area outside of the United States where polio is prevalent should complete the series before leaving, and an accelerated schedule is encouraged to accomplish this if necessary (CDC, 2022c).

Measles, Mumps, and Rubella Vaccines

MMR is a live attenuated virus combination vaccine. It is the one most commonly used in childhood immunizations. MMR can be given the same day as other live attenuated virus vaccines such as varicella vaccine (Var). However, if not given on the same day, the immunizations should be spaced at least 28 days apart (Kroger et al., 2022). Anaphylactic reactions are believed to be associated with the neomycin or gelatin components of the vaccine rather than the egg component. The vaccine is not prepared from the allergenic albumen portion of the egg, so egg allergy is no longer a contraindication for measles vaccine (Kroger et al., 2022). Pregnancy in a child's parent is not a contraindication to the vaccination of the child (Kroger et al., 2022).

> **TAKE NOTE!**
>
> During mumps outbreaks, children in the area who are identified as high risk, such as those living in close, prolonged contact at universities, schools, or close-knit communities, should receive a third dose of a mumps-containing vaccine (CDC, 2021f).

Hepatitis A Vaccine

Hepatitis A vaccine (HepA) is an inactivated whole virus vaccine. Hepatitis A is spread through close physical contact and by eating or drinking contaminated food or water. It is one of the most frequently reported vaccine-preventable diseases in the United States. Young children are particularly susceptible to hepatitis A because of their close contact with other children, inadequate hygiene practices, and tendency to place everything in their mouths. HepA is recommended to be given to all children at age 12 months, followed by a repeat dose with a minimum interval of 6 to 18 months (CDC, 2022c).

Hepatitis B Vaccine

The hepatitis B vaccine (HepB) is a recombinant vaccine. Hepatitis B virus can result in a serious infection that affects the liver. It is spread through contact with blood and body fluids and can be spread from an infected gestational parent to a newborn at birth. Hepatitis B vaccination is recommended at birth, preferably within the first 12 hours, then at 1 to 2 months and 6 to 18 months (CDC, 2022c). A total of four doses is acceptable when a combination vaccine with hepatitis B is used after birth (CDC, 2022c). Because hepatitis B is a sexually transmitted infection, it is important to verify the immunization status of all adolescents.

Varicella Vaccine

Varicella vaccine is a live attenuated virus vaccine. All children aged 12 to 15 months who have not had varicella (chickenpox) should be immunized. A second dose is recommended at age 4 to 6 years. The vaccine provides effective postexposure prophylaxis if administered within 3 to 5 days after exposure. The ACIP does recommend vaccination even if exposure is greater than 5 days in children without evidence of immunity and eligible for the vaccination (not recommended for children younger than 12 months of age) (Immunization Action Coalition, 2022b). Varicella may be given the same day as other live attenuated virus vaccines. However, if not given on the same day, the immunizations should be spaced at least 28 days apart (Kroger et al., 2022). Pregnancy in a child's parent is not a contraindication to the vaccination of the child (Kroger et al., 2022).

Pneumococcal Vaccines

Streptococcus pneumoniae (pneumococcus) is a common cause of pneumonia, sepsis, meningitis, and otitis media in young children (CDC, 2022d). In 2022, the ACIP recommended PCV15 or PCV13 for use in routine vaccination for children (Kobayashi et al., 2022). It stimulates an immune response in infants and is given at 2, 4, 6, and 12 to 15 months of age as part of the initial immunization series (CDC, 2022d). PPSV contains 23 strains of *S. pneumoniae.* It does not provoke an immune response in children under 2 years of age (Kobayashi et al., 2022). PPSV is given to children over 2 years of age who are at high risk for pneumococcal sepsis. This group includes children with anatomic/functional asplenia; sickle cell disease; chronic cardiac, pulmonary, or kidney disease; diabetes mellitus; cerebrospinal fluid leak or HIV infection; children getting or who have cochlear implants; and children with immunosuppression (Kobayashi et al., 2022).

Influenza Vaccines

Influenza immunization is recommended yearly for all people 6 months of age or older. All children 6 months to 8 years of age who have not received at least two doses of the influenza vaccine will require two doses separated by 4 weeks (CDC, 2022c). The ACIP provides yearly recommendations for the use of the influenza vaccine. Ensure you are aware of the most up-to-date recommendations available.

There are three influenza vaccines available: the inactivated influenza vaccine (IIV), recombinant influenza vaccine (RIV), and live attenuated influenza vaccine (LAIV). These vaccines are available as trivalent or quadrivalent, depending on the number of virus strains they vaccinate against. Quadrivalent seasonal influenza vaccine protects against two B virus strains and provides broader protection against influenza. LAIV is given intranasally and should not be given to anyone who is immunocompromised or who will be in close contact with an immunosuppressed person. It is also contraindicated in children 2 to 4 years old diagnosed with asthma or with a history of wheezing or medically attended wheezing in the past 12 months, children who have received influenza antiviral therapy in the past 48 hours, or children who are taking aspirin or other salicylates (Grohskopf et al., 2022). The ACIP provides no preference of which type of age-appropriate, licensed influenza vaccine is administered (Grohskopf et al., 2022).

Rotavirus Vaccine

Prior to the availability of the rotavirus vaccine, rotavirus was the most common cause of severe gastroenteritis among young children (CDC, 2021g). The virus is shed in the stool and easily spreads via the fecal–oral route. Severe, watery, crampy diarrhea quickly leads to dehydration in the infected child. The rotavirus vaccine is a live vaccine targeting five strains of rotavirus and is given via the oral route to infants. Two vaccine products are currently available. Rotarix requires two doses (at 2 and 4 months) and RotaTeq requires three doses (at 2, 4, and 6 months) (CDC, 2022c). If RotaTeq was used for any doses or the vaccine product is unknown, a total of three doses should be administered (CDC, 2022c). Administration of rotavirus vaccine is contraindicated in children with SCID or a history of intussusception (Kroger et al., 2022).

Human Papillomavirus Vaccine

Human papillomavirus (HPV) is a DNA tumor virus transmitted through direct skin-to-skin contact. HPV is contracted most often during vaginal or anal penetrative sexual acts. HPV infection is the most common sexually transmitted infection in the United States (CDC, 2022e). HPV causes genital warts and is responsible for the development of cancer. For these reasons, the ACIP and AAP have recommended that HPV vaccination occur in all preadolescent children (CDC, 2022c). Children 11 to 12 years old, and as young as 9 years old, should receive two shots 6 to 12 months apart. If the child is 15 years or older, they will need to receive the three-dose series (CDC, 2022c).

Meningococcal Vaccine

Meningococcal disease may manifest as meningitis, a deadly blood infection (meningococcemia), or bacteremic pneumonia. It is caused by the bacterium *Neisseria meningitidis*, which is spread through direct contact or by air droplets. It develops quickly, usually in healthy children and adolescents, and results in high rates of morbidity and mortality. For these reasons, the meningococcal conjugate vaccine is recommended for all previously unvaccinated children at age 11 to 12 years with a booster dose at the age of 16 years (CDC, 2022c). Routine vaccination is also recommended for children 2 months to 10 years old who are at an increased risk for the disease due to certain medical conditions such as anatomic or functional asplenia (including sickle cell disease); taking a medicine called Soliris; complement component deficiency; HIV infection; part of a community where there is an outbreak of serogroup A, C, W, or Y meningococcal disease; or traveling to a country where meningococcal disease is common (CDC, 2021h). Vaccination with serogroup B meningococcal vaccine is recommended in adolescents and preadolescents who are at an increased risk for the disease due to certain medical conditions such as anatomic or functional asplenia (including sickle cell disease), taking a medicine called a complement inhibitor such as Soliris, complement component deficiency, or part of a community where there is an outbreak of serogroup B meningococcal disease (CDC, 2021h). Specific populations such as military recruits and first-year college students living in residence halls who are unvaccinated or incompletely vaccinated need the immunization (CDC, 2023a).

TAKE NOTE!

In October 2023, the CDC recommended that if meningococcal groups A,C,Y & W-135 (MenACWY) and serogroup B meningococcal (MenB) are both indicated at the same visit, a new vaccine pentavalent meningococcal (MenABCWY) may be given (CDC, 2023b).

Respiratory Syncytial Virus Vaccine

Respiratory syncytial virus (RSV) is a common respiratory virus that causes mild, cold like symptoms in people of all ages. In some infants and young children, it can be dangerous and lead to difficulty breathing, low oxygen levels, dehydration, and severe lung complications. RSV is the most common cause of bronchiolitis and hospitalization among infants in the United States (CDC, 2023c). It is easily spread through contact with infected respiratory secretions or objects contaminated with the virus. Seasonal outbreaks occur (refer to Chapter 40 for further information regarding bronchiolitis and RSV).

The RSV preventive antibody (nirsevimab) can help prevent severe illness in infants and young children. The ACIP released new recommendations in August 2023 (CDC, 2023b). All infants younger than 8 months and born shortly before or during the RSV season should receive one dose of nirsevimab within 1 week of birth (in most infants, if the parent received the RSV vaccine during pregnancy, they do not need to receive nirsevimab). Those not born during the RSV season should receive one dose of nirsevimab shortly before the start of their first RSV season (CDC, 2023b, 2023c). Infants aged 8 to 19 months who are at increased risk for severe RSV disease should receive nirsevimab before the start of their second RSV season (CDC, 2023b).

TAKE NOTE!

The ACIP recommends COVID-19 vaccination for everyone 6 months or older. It is safe to administer the COVID-19 vaccine on the same day as other vaccines. Refer to the CDC website for updated COVID-19 vaccine information.

Recall the Randall children, introduced at the beginning of the chapter. What immunizations would be appropriate for them to receive? Explain how you would administer the injections, and discuss any contraindications or precautions.

BARRIERS TO IMMUNIZATION

A fully immunized child is protected from the discomforts and complications of many infectious diseases. Disease prevention spares the family the emotional and financial burdens that serious illnesses can cause. Immunization programs prevent devastating epidemics in a community. Health care dollars not spent treating preventable diseases can be used for other urgent issues. Immunization rates for routine, recommended pediatric vaccines remain above 90%, with the exception of the influenza and HPV vaccines (USDHHS, 2021). Despite the numerous advantages of immunization and these high immunization rates, gaps among children receiving vaccines still exist. Disparities in immunization rates by race, sex geography, ethnicity, and social determinants of health, such as employment, income, housing, education, and transportation, reflect health inequities in the United States (USDHHS, 2021).

Many factors lead to children not being fully immunized. Parental concerns about vaccine safety and side effects are a significant cause of inadequate immunization (Boom & Healy, 2020). Other parental objections include "vaccines do not work," "my child is not at risk," "the disease prevented by the vaccine is not dangerous," and "natural immunity is better" (Boom & Healy, 2020). Parents may also have a lack of trust in governmental and health organizations, as well as pharmaceutical companies (Boom & Healy, 2020). See Evidence-Based Practice 31.1. Parents may want to postpone some of the scheduled immunizations because they are concerned about the effects of multiple injections on their child. Postponing a portion of the immunizations puts the child at risk for contracting disease. Disrupting the optimal spacing of the immunizations can decrease the efficacy of vaccine, putting the child at further risk.

Misconceptions of what constitutes a contraindication to vaccination and having more than one health care provider are major contributors to inadequate immunization

EVIDENCE-BASED PRACTICE 31.1

COVID-19 Vaccine Hesitancy Among Racially Diverse Parents

STUDY

As of October 2021, 1.9 million cases of COVID-19 were diagnosed in children 5 to 11 years of age in the United States. Underrepresented groups have borne the greatest burden of COVID-19 infections and hospitalization in the United States. Non-Hispanic Black children experienced higher rates of hospitalization and higher incidence of the COVID-19–associated complication, multisystem inflammatory syndrome. The COVID-19 pandemic seems to have worsened and magnified the already existing health disparities in the United States. Early research in the general population has shown a high rate of vaccine hesitancy. This study was an online survey of 400 English-speaking racially diverse female guardians of children 5 to 10 years of age. The aim of the study was to understand how race/ethnicity influenced the decision of a parent to vaccinate their child against the COVID-19 infection.

Findings

Overall, 34.5% of parents surveyed would not vaccinate their child against COVID-19, while 40.85% would vaccinate and 24.75% were unsure. In parents who did not plan to vaccinate their child, the study found significantly higher levels of COVID-19 misconceptions, including the perception that children are less susceptible to infection, the belief that symptoms were less severe, a general mistrust of vaccines, a lower confidence in the safety and efficacy of the COVID-19 vaccine, less community support for the vaccine, and a lower likelihood of being influenced by the FDA or doctor recommendation for the vaccine. Analysis of the findings found that race/ethnicity, parental vaccine status, education, financial security, perceived childhood COVID-19 susceptibility and severity, vaccine safety and efficacy concerns, community support, and FDA and health care provider recommendations accounted for 70.3% of the differences for vaccine hesitancy. The study found 62% of non-Hispanic Asian parents, 45% of Hispanic parents, 31% of non-Hispanic Black parents, and 25% of non-Hispanic White parents planned to vaccinate their child. A higher number of non-Hispanic Asian parents were vaccinated themselves compared to other racial/ethnic groups. A significantly higher number of non-Hispanic Asian parents intended to vaccinate their child, while more non-Hispanic Black parents were unsure, and a higher proportion of non-Hispanic White parents did not plan to vaccinate their child.

Nursing Implications

Parents often have concerns regarding immunizations. The findings of this study emphasize the importance of understanding and addressing racial and ethnic differences when designing public health strategies regarding immunizations. Nurses are in a unique position to educate families and the community about current research findings. Even though the number of routine immunizations has increased dramatically over the past two decades, the total number of antigens the child is exposed to is actually less. This is due to the fact that newer vaccines are less crude and less antigenic than before.

Data from Fisher, C. B., Gray, A., & Sheck, I. (2021). COVID-19 pediatric vaccine hesitancy among racially diverse parents in the United States. *Vaccines, 10*(1), 31. https://doi.org/10.3390/vaccines10010031

status. The more children there are in a family, the less likely the children are to be fully vaccinated. The costs of vaccines or lack of access to health services can also deter families from obtaining immunizations.

OVERCOMING BARRIERS TO IMMUNIZATION

The use of a manufacturer-produced combination vaccine is encouraged when appropriate, particularly whenever it will reduce the number of injections at a visit (CDC, 2022c). These combination vaccines have been studied and approved by the FDA. The nurse should never mix separate vaccines in the same syringe unless expressly permitted in the product insert for all vaccines involved. Examples of combination vaccines are:

- ProQuad: measles, mumps, rubella, varicella
- Kinrix/Quadracel: DTaP–IPV
- Pediarix: DTaP–HepB–IPV
- Pentacel: DTaP–IPV/Hib
- Vaxelis: DTaP–IPV–Hib–HepB (CDC, 2022c)

Vaccines for Children (VFC) is a federally funded program that was implemented in 1994 in response to the 1989–1991 measles epidemic (CDC, 2016). Prior to this program, free vaccines were available only through public health agencies. The goal of this program is to improve immunization rates by providing free vaccines to families with low income and uninsured through private health care providers who are registered VFC providers. Additional information on the VFC program is available at http://www.cdc.gov/vaccines/programs/vfc/. The Affordable Care Act of 2010 requires new health plans to cover preventive services, including ACIP-approved immunizations, without charging a deductible, copayment, or coinsurance (USDHHS, 2022). The goal of these programs is to increase access to vaccines.

Establishing a medical home for every child will alleviate many of the factors associated with lack of immunization. Parents who have a long-term, trusting relationship with a health care provider are more likely to have their concerns about vaccine safety discussed and removed. Missed opportunities for immunizations can be reduced by:

- Maintaining a centralized immunization record
- Verifying immunization status at every visit, not just health supervision visits
- Verifying the status of siblings accompanying the child to the appointment
- Providing parents with up-to-date information on vaccines geared to their concerns and needs

Two excellent resources for vaccination recommendations in the United States are the CDC's Vaccines and Immunizations website (https://www.cdc.gov/vaccines/) and the CDC Hotline (800-232-4636 or 800-CDC-INFO).

What are some potential barriers to the Randall children being fully immunized? As a nurse, how can you help overcome these barriers?

Health Promotion

Health promotion focuses on maintaining or enhancing the physical and mental health of children. The principal components of health promotion are identifying risk factors for a disease, facilitating lifestyle changes to eliminate or reduce those risk factors, and empowering children at the individual and community level to develop resources to optimize their health. The nurse implements health promotion through education and anticipatory guidance.

Partnership development is the key strategy for success when implementing a health promotion activity. Identifying key stakeholders from the community allows problems to be solved and provides additional venues for disseminating information. Health promotion messages can be reinforced at schools, dayHealthy People Objectives retrieved from http://www.healthypeople.govcare centers, community agencies, and places of worship. If families have difficulty getting to health care facilities, the community arenas may be the primary source of health promotion.

Providing Anticipatory Guidance

Anticipatory guidance is primary prevention. The nurse partners with the parents to create a "road map" to optimal health for the child. The Healthy People 2030 box provides a framework for determining health promotion goals. *Bright Futures: Guidelines for Health Supervision of Infants, Children, and Adolescents* (Hagan et al., 2017) is another valuable resource.

The "skeleton" of the guidance provided involves common childhood health problems. The nurse fleshes out that information using the results of risk assessments and screening tests, health concerns unique to the child, and the interests and concerns of the parents. Age-related anticipatory guidance information is provided in Chapters 25 to 29.

Provide appropriate anticipatory guidance for 3-year-old Maya and 9-month-old Evan.

Promoting Oral Health Care

Effective oral health practices are essential to the overall health of children and adolescents. Dental caries are one of the most common chronic illnesses seen in children (Nowak & Warren, 2022). Poor oral health can have significant negative effects on systemic health. Children who suffer from untreated dental caries have an increased incidence of pain and infections and may have problems with eating and playing, difficulty at school, and sleep pattern disturbances (CDC, 2022f). Refer to the Healthy People 2030 box.

Optimal oral health is not limited to the prevention and treatment of dental caries. It includes anticipatory guidance about nonnutritive sucking habits, injury

HEALTHY PEOPLE 2030

Objective	Nursing Significance
Reduce the proportion of children and adolescents with lifetime tooth decay experience in their primary or permanent teeth. Reduce the proportion of children and adolescents with active and currently untreated tooth decay in their primary or permanent teeth. Increase the proportion of youth from families with low income who have a preventive dental visit.	• Teach children and adolescents appropriate tooth brushing and flossing techniques. • Encourage use of fluoride-containing toothpastes. • Encourage routine dental visits.

Healthy People Objectives retrieved from http://www.healthypeople.gov

prevention, oral cancer prevention, and tongue and lip piercing. Preventing and treating malocclusion can have a significant benefit for children. Comprehensive health care is not possible if oral health is not a priority in the health delivery system.

Optimizing oral health can benefit the community as well as the individual child. The cost of pediatric oral health care can be reduced by 50% with the proper use of fluoride treatments coupled with other preventive measures (AAPD, 2018a). These health care dollar savings will enhance community resources.

Having a dental home enhances the likelihood that the child will obtain appropriate preventive and routine care. The AAPD adopted the policy of the dental home in 2001 (AAPD, 2018b). It is modeled on the AAP medical home policy. The dental home provides the same benefits to the child as the medical home. Characteristics of a dental home are listed in Box 31.7. The AAPD (2018b) recommends that the dental home be established by the infant's first birthday.

Promoting Healthy Weight

Higher weight in children is an important public health issue. The number of children with higher weight has continued to rise over the past 20 years. The principal causes

BOX 31.7 Characteristics of the Dental Home

- Preventive health program based on risk assessment
- Anticipatory guidance on oral health developmental issues, including dietary counseling related to oral health
- Plans for emergency dental trauma, management of oral pain and infection
- Anticipatory guidance on oral hygiene
- Comprehensive, evidence-based dental care (acute and preventive services)
- Comprehensive assessment for oral diseases
- Referral to specialists for care not available at the dental home

Based on American Academy of Pediatric Dentistry. (2018b). *Policy on the dental home.* http://www.aapd.org/media/Policies_Guidelines/P_DentalHome.pdf

of this increase are unhealthy eating habits and decreased physical activity. Weight is best managed by balancing calories with a combination of diet and exercise. Nurses can have the maximum effect in promoting healthy weight in children by encouraging activities that address both healthy eating patterns and physical fitness. Children, parents, and communities are all targets for healthy weight promotion by nurses. Refer to the Healthy People 2030 box.

HEALTHY PEOPLE 2030

Objective	Nursing Significance
Reduce the proportion of children and adolescents with higher weight	• Screen all children for the development of overweight as indicated by an increasing body mass index (BMI) for their age. • Provide accurate diet counseling. • Encourage daily physical activity. • Counsel parents to limit television/computer time daily.

Healthy People Objectives retrieved from http://www.healthypeople.gov

The focus of healthy weight promotion should be health centered, not weight centered. Linking success to numbers on a scale increases the possibility of developing eating disorders, nutritional deficiencies, and body hatred. Instead, emphasizing the benefits of health through an active lifestyle and nutritious eating creates a nurturing environment for the child. This allows the child to maintain their self-esteem. In addition, a health-centered orientation also allows the family to develop a lifestyle that incorporates its cultural food patterns and traditions.

Parents who have a healthy eating pattern are likely to maintain and encourage those patterns in their children. The nurse provides parents with anticipatory guidance about age-related eating patterns during each health supervision visit. Parents with toddlers and preschoolers may need training in ways to cope with the child's growing autonomy while providing a variety of nutritious options.

The nurse can begin directly advising the young child on healthy foods. Information and teaching modalities need to be age appropriate. With colorful posters and games, the nurse can teach the preschool child the difference between healthy and unhealthy food choices. As children enter school, group and peer-led activities can be effective. The nurse must gear material toward the adolescent's growing autonomy in making self-care decisions.

Before providing education to school-age and adolescent children, it is important to obtain nutritional histories directly from them because increasingly they are eating meals away from the family table. As they spend more time away from their parents, they need to develop the ability to make nutritious choices. The goal is to help older children develop strategies for making healthy choices as part of their increasingly independent lifestyle. Detailed anticipatory guidance is provided in Teaching Guidelines 31.1 and in Chapters 25 to 29.

TEACHING GUIDELINES 31.1 Healthy Eating

Breakfast

1. Don't skip breakfast. You will not have enough energy to play well later in the day. Skipping breakfast can also lower your grades in school.
2. Avoid eating high-sugar foods at breakfast. They will make you sleepy during the day.
3. Start your breakfast with some fruit. A small glass of juice, berries on your cereal, or a banana is a good choice.
4. Protein is important at breakfast. Milk, either in a glass or on cereal, is a good source of protein; so is yogurt or peanut butter.

Lunch

1. Check the quality of school-provided lunches. If they are high in fat or sugar, bring your lunch. Many schools publish their daily menus in advance. Check online or ask the school for a copy.
2. Add a variety of healthy alternatives to your lunches.
   a. Try different types of breads. Pitas, wraps, bagels, and taco shells can be a good change of pace in the sandwich routine.
   b. Freeze fruits before putting them in the lunch box. This will keep the lunch items cool and the fruit fresh tasting. Canned pineapple and grapes freeze well; so do bananas.
   c. Try alternatives to high-fat chips. Dried fruits, baked pretzels, and animal crackers are a few examples of tasty, healthy treats.
   d. Low-fat chocolate milk is more nutritious than prepackaged juice boxes, which have high sugar concentrations.

Snacks

1. Limit snacks to afterschool and bedtime. Light snacks such as yogurt or fruit provide good hunger management. A very hungry child will tend to overeat at meals.
2. Children need to learn to eat only when they are hungry. Children often eat out of boredom. Discourage nonstop grazing by planning activities to occupy the child.
3. A small bedtime snack is okay if the child is hungry but should not become a habit. A light carbohydrate such as graham crackers or a piece of fruit works well.

(*continued*)

(continued)

Dinner

1. Plan your menu a week ahead. Planning ahead reduces the likelihood of eating out or getting take-out food. Restaurant foods are more likely to be high in fats and refined carbohydrates.
2. Prepare homemade healthy versions of take-out favorites. Top prepared pizza crust with cooked chicken, vegetables, mushrooms, and cheese. Serve the pizza with a salad for a complete and healthy meal. "Make your own tacos" nights, using lean hamburger and low-fat sour cream, can be a lot of fun for children.
3. Don't turn dinner into a battle zone. Forcing children to eat foods they do not like will only deepen their dislike of them. Give them the healthy foods they do enjoy, and eventually they will explore more options.
4. Lead by example. Children eventually adopt the eating patterns of their parents. If they see their parents eat vegetables, they will eventually try them.

Promoting Healthy Activity

Healthy physical activity can take many forms. During the preschool years, encourage parents to provide a wide variety of physical activities. This exposure to multiple types of exercise allows the child to find the one that is most enjoyable and increases the chances that they will maintain an active lifestyle. The focus should be on noncompetitive, fun activities. When the child enters school, the lure of television and computers can significantly diminish the amount of time spent in physical activity. Parents can encourage their children to stay physically active in several ways. They can limit the amount of time spent in sedentary activities and actively encourage the child to pursue any exercise that they enjoy. In addition to verbal encouragement, parents can promote exercise by participating in exercise with the child. A simple family walk can increase physical fitness while providing time for interaction between parent and child. Refer to the Healthy People 2030 box. Teaching Guidelines 31.2 gives additional suggestions for promoting physical activity.

TEACHING GUIDELINES 31.2 Healthy Activity

1. Plan physical activities that your family can do as a group.
2. Write exercise activities on your family's daily schedule.
3. Look for activities that appeal to your child's interest, such as dance, team sports, or swimming.
4. Place value on noncompetitive as well as competitive activities.
5. Show your child you believe exercise is important. Exercise daily yourself.
6. Encourage the community to develop safe areas for spontaneous games and activities.

TAKE NOTE!

The USDHHS recommends all children 6 to 17 years of age participate in at least 60 minutes of physical activity every day (U.S. Department of Agriculture & USDHHS, 2020).

HEALTHY PEOPLE 2030

Objective	Nursing Significance
Increase the proportion of children and adolescents who meet the current aerobic physical activity guideline. Increase the proportion of adolescents who meet the current muscle strengthening activity guideline. Increase the proportion of adolescents who walk or use a bicycle to get to and from places. Increase the proportion of children and adolescents who participate on a sports team or take sports lessons afterschool or on weekends.	• For the adolescent who does not exercise, advise them to start slowly by walking. • Work with the adolescent to identify physical activities that interest them. • Praise efforts to participate in a routine exercise plan. • Identify an athletic individual with whom the adolescent identifies, and encourage similar activities in the adolescent.

Healthy People Objectives retrieved from http://www.healthypeople.gov

Promoting Personal Hygiene

Handwashing is the first personal hygiene topic that needs to be introduced to children. Handwashing prevents disease by limiting a child's exposure to pathogens. The nurse can introduce the topic to preschool children using cartoons and games. Have the child sing "Twinkle, Twinkle Little Star" while washing their hands; this encourages adequate cleansing time. Use soap containers and towels with colorful characters to make the experience more fun. The school-age child can understand the concepts of germs and disease. Slogans such as "Let's drown a germ" can serve as a reminder of the importance of handwashing. The Glo Germ program (n.d.) is effective in this age group. A nontoxic substance that shines under a black light is placed on the children's hands. The children can follow how germs travel from object to object. After washing their hands, the children can see if they did a good job (Glo Germ, n.d.).

In response to peer pressure, adolescents are usually stringent about personal hygiene. Younger adolescents may need guidance in dealing with pubescent body changes such as body odor, fungal infections such as tinea pedis (athlete's foot), and acne.

Promoting Safe-Sun Exposure

Skin cancer is a significant health problem in the United States. Blistering sunburns in children substantially increase the risk of melanoma and other skin cancers (American Academy of Dermatology, 2022). People with fair skin are at highest risk for skin cancers, but anyone can become sunburned and develop skin cancer. When teaching children about safe-sun exposure, remind them that harmful ultraviolet (UV) rays can reflect off water, snow, sand, and concrete, so being in the shade or under an awning does not guarantee protection. Adequate sun protection requires using sunscreen, avoiding peak sun hours, and wearing proper clothing. Teaching Guidelines 31.3 gives more detailed instructions. Refer to the Healthy People 2030 box.

TEACHING GUIDELINES 31.3 Safe-Sun Exposure

Sunscreen

1. Use sunscreen lotions every day. Harmful UV rays penetrate clouds and cause damaging sunburns.
2. Use sunscreens with a sun protection factor (SPF) of 30 or higher and with UVA and UVB protection. An adequate amount for an average-sized child is half an ounce.
3. Apply sunscreens half an hour before sun exposure.
4. Reapply every hour if the child is perspiring heavily.
5. Reapply immediately after swimming.
6. Infants 6 months old or younger should not use sunscreens. Take steps to avoid sun exposure completely with this age group.

Clothing

1. Wear hats. The brim of the hat should be 10.16 cm (4 in) or more and should shade the ears. Straw hats need to have a sunproof liner to be effective. Children introduced to hats as infants usually accept hats as part of the "outfit."
2. Wear UV-blocking sunglasses. The eye is the second most common site for melanoma.
3. Wear long, loose, and lightweight clothing for maximum sun protection.

Lifestyle

1. Avoid sun exposure between 10 a.m. and 4 p.m. This is when UV rays are the strongest.
2. Ask your health care provider if your medication will increase your sensitivity to UV rays. If the answer is yes, take extra precautions to reduce sun exposure.
3. Avoid tanning beds. The devices emit UV rays just like the sun and can cause damage.
4. Check the UV index before going out. The higher the index, the more precautions you should take. UV index figures are available online and in TV and radio weather reports.
5. Advocate for safe-sun scheduling of recreational activities. Talk to others about scheduling outdoor activities before 10 a.m., after 4 p.m., or in the shade.
6. Consider UV-blocking plastic film for your house and car windows.

HEALTHY PEOPLE 2030

Objective	Nursing Significance
Reduce the proportion of students in grades 9–12 who report sunburn.	• Educate families to start skin protection from the sun in childhood to reduce the risk of skin cancer as an adult. • Teach parents to use PABA-free sunscreen (formulated specifically for children) after age 6 months with an SPF of 15 or greater and to reapply sunscreen frequently while the child is out of doors. • Advocate for schools to encourage a sun-safe environment.

Healthy People Objectives retrieved from http://www.healthypeople.gov

TAKE NOTE!

Give children the following physical reference when doing health promotion on safe-sun exposure. Tell the child, "Play outside only when your shadow is taller than you are." The child's shadow will be "taller" before 10 a.m. and after 2 p.m. The nurse can demonstrate this concept by placing a ruler on end and shining a bright light over it. As the nurse moves the light, the child will see the ruler's shadow lengthen.

KEY CONCEPTS

- Health supervision for children is a dynamic process. Optimal wellness for the child can occur only if the nurse forms meaningful partnerships with the child, the family, and the community. These partnerships allow for free exchange of information and the establishment of mutually agreed upon goals. The medical home exists when there is a single primary care provider for the child. The medical home establishes a trusting long-term relationship with the child and family. This relationship leads to comprehensive, coordinated, and cost-effective care for the child.
- Children with chronic illnesses have a critical need for comprehensive and coordinated health supervision. Children with chronic illnesses require more frequent health supervision assessments. These children must have a medical home. The location of that medical home may be with a knowledgeable primary health care provider or at a multidisciplinary specialty facility. The location is determined by the child's needs and the family's preferences.
- The nurse incorporates frequent assessments of the many psychosocial stressors faced by families of children with chronic illnesses when establishing health care plans for them.

- Health supervision has three components: developmental surveillance and screening; injury and disease prevention; and health promotion.
- Developmental surveillance is an ongoing process requiring a skilled observer and interviewer. To be effective, the nurse must understand normal growth and development expectations and be proficient at developmental screening procedures and techniques. Caregivers are most likely to reveal risk factors for developmental delay when the nurse has a long-term and trusting relationship with the family.
- Screening tests are part of injury and disease prevention. They are modalities that identify treatable disease in an early or asymptomatic state and allow for cure or lessening of the disease's injury.
- Vision and hearing screening are functional testing modalities that the nurse must be proficient in administering in order for the child's results to be valid.
- Immunizations are a cornerstone of pediatric disease prevention. The nurse increases the effectiveness of immunization by understanding the principles of immunization and applying them to the child's individual circumstances. Adhering to good immunization management practices, as outlined by the ACIP and the AAP, enhances the benefits and reduces the risks of immunization.
- Barriers to full immunization include fragmentation of health care, concerns about vaccine safety, financial constraints, and lack of knowledge. The nurse can be pivotal in ensuring that children and adolescents are fully immunized by serving as child educator and advocate.
- The principal components of health promotion are identifying risk factors for a disease, facilitating lifestyle changes to eliminate or reduce those risk factors, and empowering children at the individual and community level to develop resources to optimize their health.
- The nurse implements health promotion through education and anticipatory guidance.
- Anticipatory guidance provided involves common childhood health problems and seeks to prevent or improve the health of children.
- The nurse uses the results of risk assessments and screening tests, health concerns unique to the child, and the interests and concerns of the parents to develop appropriate anticipatory guidance for each child and family.

REFERENCES AND RECOMMENDED READINGS

Advisory Committee on Immunization Practices. (2000). Recommendations and reports: Poliomyelitis prevention in the United States: Updated recommendations of the Advisory Committee on Immunization Practices (ACIP). *Morbidity and Mortality Weekly Report (MMWR), 49*(RR05), 1–22. http://www.cdc.gov/mmwr/preview/mmwrhtml/rr4905a1.htm

Aites, J., & Schonwald, A. (2022). Developmental-behavioral surveillance and screening in primary care. *UpToDate*. Retrieved December 12, 2022, from https://www.uptodate.com/contents/developmental-behavioral-surveillance-and-screening-in-primary-care

American Academy of Dermatology. (2022). *Skin cancer*. https://www.aad.org/media/stats/conditions/skin-cancer

American Academy of Pediatric Dentistry. (2018a). *Policy on use of fluoride*. http://www.aapd.org/media/Policies_Guidelines/P_FluorideUse.pdf

American Academy of Pediatric Dentistry. (2018b). *Policy on the dental home*. http://www.aapd.org/media/Policies_Guidelines/P_DentalHome.pdf

American Academy of Pediatrics, National Resource Center for Patient and Family Centered Medical Home. (2022). *What is medical home*. https://www.aap.org/en/practice-management/medical-home/medical-home-overview/what-is-medical-home/

Boom, J. A., & Healy, C. M. (2020). Standard childhood vaccines: Caregiver hesitancy or refusal. *UpToDate*. Retrieved December 20, 2022, from https://www.uptodate.com/contents/standard-childhood-vaccines-parental-hesitancy-or-refusal

Bright Futures/American Academy of Pediatrics. (2022). *Recommendations for preventive pediatric health care*. https://downloads.aap.org/AAP/PDF/periodicity_schedule.pdf?_ga=2.17675389.55149517.1670352585-1010168752.1655126485&_gac=1.21185481.1667484109.CjwKCAjwzY2bBhB6EiwAPpUpZvGVWommkXC3nD4TQGqyFG8j5TGVRbeF_LzRU01f-VGezeqJ-uf2ExoCRJEQAvD_BwE

Bryant-Stephens, T. C., Strane, D., Robinson, E. K., Bhambhani, S., & Kenyon, C. C. (2021). Housing and asthma disparities. *The Journal of Allergy and Clinical Immunology, 148*(5), 1121–1129. https://doi.org/10.1016/j.jaci.2021.09.023

Carlson, S., & Neuberger, Z. (2021). *WIC works: Addressing the nutrition and health needs of low-income families for more than four decades*. https://www.cbpp.org/research/food-assistance/wic-works-addressing-the-nutrition-and-health-needs-of-low-income-families

Centers for Disease Control and Prevention. (2016). *Vaccines for children program (VFC)*. http://www.cdc.gov/vaccines/programs/vfc/about/index.html

Centers for Disease Control and Prevention. (2021a). *Injuries among children and teens*. https://www.cdc.gov/injury/features/child-injury/index.html

Centers for Disease Control and Prevention. (2021b). *Vaccine information statements (VIS): Facts about VISs*. http://www.cdc.gov/vaccines/hcp/vis/about/facts-vis.html

Centers for Disease Control and Prevention. (2021c). *DTaP (diphtheria, tetanus, pertussis) vaccine: What you need to know*. https://www.cdc.gov/vaccines/hcp/vis/vis-statements/dtap.pdf

Centers for Disease Control and Prevention. (2021d). *Vaccines and preventable diseases: Hib vaccination: Information for healthcare professionals*. https://www.cdc.gov/vaccines/vpd/hib/hcp/index.html

Centers for Disease Control and Prevention. (2021e). *Vaccines and preventable diseases: Polio vaccination*. https://www.cdc.gov/vaccines/vpd/polio/index.html

Centers for Disease Control and Prevention. (2021f). *Vaccines and preventable diseases: Mumps vaccination*. https://www.cdc.gov/vaccines/vpd/mumps/index.html

Centers for Disease Control and Prevention. (2021g). *Rotavirus in the U.S.* https://www.cdc.gov/rotavirus/surveillance.html

Centers for Disease Control and Prevention. (2021h). *Vaccines and preventable diseases: Meningococcal vaccination: What everyone should know.* https://www.cdc.gov/vaccines/vpd/mening/public/index.html

Centers for Disease Control and Prevention. (2022a). *Overview of childhood lead poisoning prevention.* https://www.cdc.gov/nceh/lead/overview.html

Centers for Disease Control and Prevention. (2022b). *Vaccine storage and handling tool kit.* https://www.cdc.gov/vaccines/hcp/admin/storage/toolkit/storage-handling-toolkit.pdf

Centers for Disease Control and Prevention. (2022c). *Recommended child and adolescent immunization schedule, United States.* https://www.cdc.gov/vaccines/schedules/hcp/imz/child-adolescent.html

Centers for Disease Control and Prevention. (2022d). *Pneumococcal vaccination: Information for health professional.* https://www.cdc.gov/vaccines/vpd/pneumo/hcp/index.html

Centers for Disease Control and Prevention. (2022e). *Human papillomavirus (HPV): Genital HPV infection—Basic fact sheet.* http://www.cdc.gov/std/HPV/STDFact-HPV.htm

Centers for Disease Control and Prevention. (2022f). *Oral health: Children's oral health.* https://www.cdc.gov/oralhealth/basics/childrens-oral-health/index.html

Centers for Disease Control and Prevention. (2022g). *Polio in the United States.* https://www.cdc.gov/polio/us/index.html

Centers for Disease Control and Prevention. (2023a). *Meningococcal disease: Risk factors.* https://www.cdc.gov/meningococcal/about/risk-factors.html

Centers for Disease Control and Prevention. (2023b). *Addendum—Child and adolescent recommended immunization schedule for ages 18 years or younger, United States, 2023.* https://www.cdc.gov/vaccines/schedules/hcp/imz/child-adolescent.html#addendum-child

Centers for Disease Control and Prevention. (2023c). *Respiratory syncytial virus (RSV) preventive antibody: Immunization information statement (IIS): What you need to know.* https://www.cdc.gov/vaccines/vpd/rsv/immunization-information-statement.html

Delaney, A. M. (2022). Newborn hearing screening. *eMedicine.* https://emedicine.medscape.com/article/836646-overview#a1

Fisher, C. B., Gray, A., & Sheck, I. (2021). COVID-19 pediatric vaccine hesitancy among racially diverse parents in the United States. *Vaccines, 10*(1), 31. https://doi.org/10.3390/vaccines10010031

Flynn, J. T., Kaelber, D. C., Baker-Smith, C. M., Blowey, D., Carroll, A. E., Daniels, S. R., de Ferranti, S. D., Dionne, J. M., Falkner, B., Flinn, S. K., Gidding, S. S., Goodwin, C., Leu, M. G., Powers, M. E., Rea, C., Samuels, J., Simasek, M., Thaker, V. V., Urbina, E. M., & Subcommittee on Screening and Management of High Blood Pressure in Children. (2017). Clinical practice guideline for screening and management of high blood pressure in children and adolescents. *Pediatrics, 140*(3), e20171904. https://doi.org/10.1542/peds.2017-1904

Gavin, M. L. (2021). *Lead poisoning.* http://kidshealth.org/parent/medical/brain/lead_poisoning.html#

Glo Germ. (n.d.). *Glo Germ.* http://www.glogerm.com

Grohskopf, L. A., Blanton, L. H., Ferdinands, J. M., Chung, J. R., Broder, K. R., Talbot, H. K., Morgan, R. L., & Fry, A. M. (2022). Prevention and control of seasonal influenza with vaccines: Recommendations of the advisory committee on immunization practices—United States, 2022–23 Influenza Season. *Morbidity and Mortality Weekly Report (MMWR), 71*(RR-1), 1–28. http://doi.org/10.15585/mmwr.rr7101a1

Hagan, J. F., Shaw, J. S., & Duncan, P. M. (Eds.). (2017). *Bright futures: Guidelines for health supervision of infants, children, and adolescents* (4th ed.). American Academy of Pediatrics. https://brightfutures.aap.org/materials-and-tools/guidelines-and-pocket-guide/Pages/default.aspx

Immunization Action Coalition. (2022a). *Administering vaccines: Dose, route, site, and needle size.* http://www.immunize.org/catg.d/p3085.pdf

Immunization Action Coalition. (2022b). *Ask the experts: Varicella (chickenpox).* http://www.immunize.org/askexperts/experts_var.asp

Immunization Action Coalition. (2023). *Vaccine administration record for children and teens.* http://www.immunize.org/catg.d/p2022.pdf

Intercountry Adoption, Bureau of Consular Affairs, U.S. Department of State. (2022). *Annual report on intercountry adoption—FY 2021.* https://travel.state.gov/content/dam/NEWadoptionassets/pdfs/FY21%20Annual%20Report%20on%20Intercountry%20Adoption.pdf

Kemper, A. R. (2021). Newborn screening. *UpToDate.* Retrieved December 13, 2022, from https://www.uptodate.com/contents/newborn-screening

Kobayashi, M., Farrar, J. L., Gierke, R., Leidner, A. J., Campos-Outcalt, D., Morgan, R. L., Long, S. S., Poehling, K. A., Cohen, A. L., ACIP Pneumococcal Vaccines Work Group, & CDC Contributors. (2022). Use of 15-Valent pneumococcal conjugate vaccine among U.S. children: Updated recommendations of the advisory committee on immunization practices—United States. *Morbidity and Mortality Weekly Report (MMWR), 71*(37), 1174–1181. http://doi.org/10.15585/mmwr.mm7137a3

Kroger A, Bahta L, & Hunter P. (2022). *General best practice guidelines for immunization. Best practices guidance of the Advisory Committee on Immunization Practices (ACIP).* www.cdc.gov/vaccines/hcp/acip-recs/general-recs/downloads/general-recs.pdf

Lipkin, P. H., Macias, M. M., Norwood, K. W., Brei, T. J., Davidson, L. F., Davis, B. E., Ellerbeck, K. A., Houtrow, A. J., Hyman, S. L., Kuo, D. Z., Noritz, G. H., Yin, L., Murphy, N. A., Levy, S. E., Weitzman, C. C., Bauer, N. S., Childers D. O. Jr., Levine, J. M., Peralta-Carcelen, A. M., & AAP Council on Children with Disabilities, Section on Developmental and Behavioral Pediatrics. (2020). Promoting optimal development: Identifying infants and young children with developmental disorders through developmental surveillance and screening. *Pediatrics, 145*(1), e20193449. https://doi.org/10.1542/peds.2019-3449

March of Dimes. (2020). *Newborn screening tests for your baby.* https://www.marchofdimes.org/baby/newborn-screening-tests-for-your-baby.aspx

National Center for Healthy Housing. (2022). *Lead.* https://nchh.org/information-and-evidence/learn-about-healthy-housing/health-hazards-prevention-and-solutions/lead/

National Heart, Lung, and Blood Institute. (2012). *Expert panel on integrated guidelines for cardiovascular health and risk reduction in children and adolescents.* Summary report (NIH Publication No. 12-7486). U.S. Department of Health and Human Services. http://www.nhlbi.nih.gov/guidelines/cvd_ped/peds_guidelines_sum.pdf

Nowak, A. J., & Warren, J. J. (2022). Preventive dental care and counselling for infants and young children. *UpToDate.*

Retrieved December 21, 2022, from https://www.uptodate.com/contents/preventive-dental-care-and-counseling-for-infants-and-young-children

Powers, J. M. (2021). Iron deficiency in infants and children <12: Screening, prevention, clinical manifestations, and diagnosis. *UpToDate*. Retrieved December 14, 2022, from https://www.uptodate.com/contents/iron-deficiency-in-infants-and-children-less-than12-years-screening-prevention-clinical-manifestations-and-diagnosis

Sample, J. A. (2022). Childhood lead poisoning: Clinical manifestations and diagnosis. *UpToDate*. Retrieved December 14, 2022, from https://www.uptodate.com/contents/childhood-lead-poisoning-clinical-manifestations-and-diagnosis

Schulte, E. E. (2020). Domestic and international adoption. In R. M. Kleigman, J. W. St. Geme III, N. J. Blum, S. S. Shah, R. C. Tasker, K. M. Wilson, & R. E. Behrman (Eds.), *Nelson textbook of pediatrics* (21st ed., pp. 960–976). Elsevier.

U.S. Department of Agriculture, & U.S. Department of Health and Human Services. (2020). *Dietary guidelines for Americans, 2020–2025* (9th ed.). DietaryGuidelines.gov

U.S. Department of Health and Human Services. (2021). *Vaccines National Strategic Plan 2021–2025*. https://www.hhs.gov/sites/default/files/HHS-Vaccines-Report.pdf

U.S. Department of Health and Human Services. (2022). *About ACA: Preventative care*. https://www.hhs.gov/healthcare/about-the-aca/preventive-care/index.html

U.S. Department of Health and Human Services. (n.d.). *Healthy People 2030*. https://health.gov/healthypeople

United States Environmental Protection Agency. (2018). *Protecting children from lead exposures*. https://www.epa.gov/sites/production/files/2018-10/documents/leadpreventionbooklet2018-v11_web.pdf

Vaccine Adverse Event Reporting System. (n.d.). *About the VAERS program*. https://vaers.hhs.gov/index.html

Vohr, B. R. (2022). Screening the newborn for hearing loss. *UpToDate*. Retrieved December 13, 2022, from https://www.uptodate.com/contents/screening-the-newborn-for-hearing-loss

Zubler, J. M., Wiggins, L. D., Macias, M. M., Whitaker, T. M., Shaw, J. S., Squires, J. K., Pajek, J. A., Wolf, R. B., Slaughter, K. S., Broughton, A. S., Gerndt, K. L., Mlodoch, B. J., & Lipkin, P. H. (2022). Evidence-informed milestones for developmental surveillance tools. *Pediatrics, 149*(3), e2021052138. https://doi.org/10.1542/peds.2021-052138

DEVELOPING CLINICAL JUDGMENT

PRACTICING FOR NCLEX

1. During the health interview, the parent of a 4-month-old says, "I'm not sure my baby is doing what they should be." What is the nurse's best response?
   a. "I'll be able to tell you more after I do the physical."
   b. "Fill out this developmental screening questionnaire and then I can let you know."
   c. "Tell me more about your concerns."
   d. "All parents worry about their babies. I'm sure they're doing well."
2. An infant is at your facility for their initial health supervision visit. They are 2 weeks old and respond to a bell during the examination. You review all the birth records and find no documentation that a newborn hearing screening was performed. What is the best action by the nurse?
   a. Do nothing; responding to the bell proves the infant does not have a hearing deficit.
   b. Schedule the infant immediately for newborn hearing screening.
   c. Ask the parent to observe for signs that the infant is not hearing well.
   d. Screen again with the bell at the infant's 2-month health supervision visit.
3. A 15-month-old is having their first health supervision visit at your facility. Their parent has not brought a copy of the child's immunization record but believes the child is fully immunized: "They had immunizations 3 months ago at the local health department." Which would be the best action by the nurse?
   a. Ask the parent to bring the records to the 18-month health supervision visit.
   b. Start the "catch-up" schedule because there are no immunization records.
   c. Keep the child at the facility while the parent returns home for the records.
   d. Call the local health department and verify the child's immunization status.
4. A 4-year-old child is having a vision screening performed. Which screening chart would be best for determining the child's visual acuity?
   a. Snellen
   b. Ishihara
   c. Allen figures
   d. CVTME
5. Which facility fulfills the characteristics of a medical home?
   a. Urgent care center
   b. Primary care pediatric practice
   c. Mobile outreach immunization program
   d. Dermatology practice
6. The nurse understands that a live attenuated vaccine is contraindicated in which children? Select all that apply.
   a. A child currently being treated with antibiotics due to an ear infection
   b. A child who received the rotavirus vaccine last week
   c. A pregnant adolescent
   d. A child currently receiving chemotherapy
   e. A child who is scheduled for surgery next week

CRITICAL THINKING EXERCISES

1. During a health supervision visit for a 5-year-old, the parent tells you they are worried about the child's hearing. Your facility has been his medical home since birth. The child was the product of a normal pregnancy and delivery. They have had frequent ear infections since the age of 8 months. Six months ago, the child had a ruptured appendix and was treated with an aminoglycoside. The child has been fully recovered for 4 months.
   a. During the health interview, what information should the nurse elicit from the parent?
   b. What information should the nurse verify from the permanent medical record?
   c. What risk factors for hearing loss does this child have?
   d. What is the best course of action at this time?
2. The nurse is examining a 4-year-old to determine their readiness for school. Describe the developmental, vision, and hearing screening tools that will help the nurse to identify any problems.

STUDY ACTIVITIES

1. Develop an immunization plan for the following well children: a 2-month-old, an 18-month-old who has never been immunized, and a 5-year-old who was current with all immunizations at age 2.
2. This is the first health supervision visit for a 3-year-old adoptee from Russia since arriving in this country 1 week ago. Develop a plan for this visit.
3. Develop a healthy weight program for the following: a preschool class, a family in which the parents and the two school-age children have mildly overweight BMIs, and an adolescent girl who is of healthy weight but fears "getting fat."

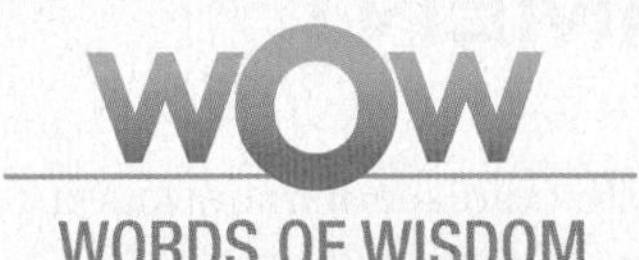

WORDS OF WISDOM

Astute nursing assessment of the child provides a snapshot of the child's overall health, growth, and development.

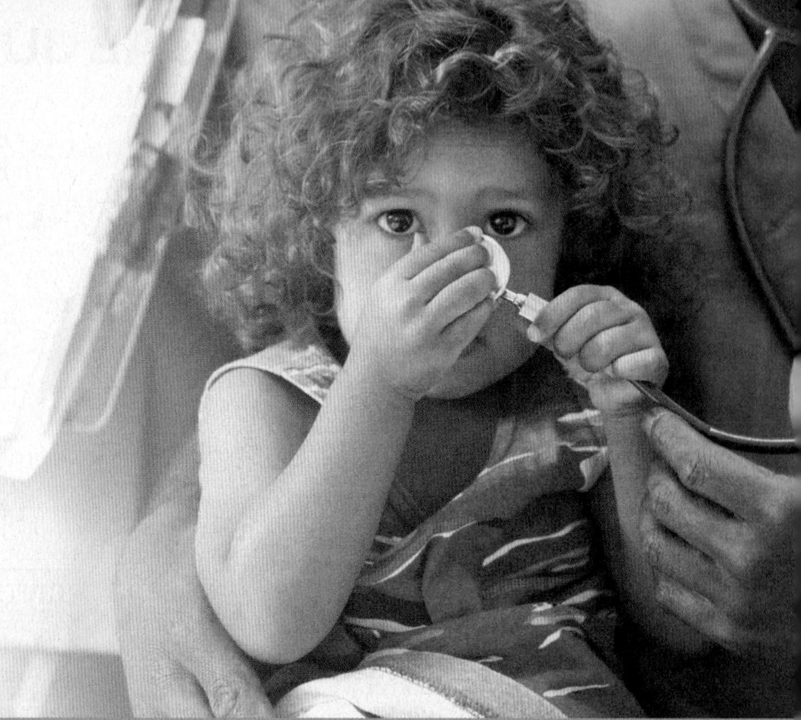

32

Health Assessment of Children

KEY TERMS

accommodation
acrocyanosis (ak′rō-sī-ă-nō′sis)
body mass index (BMI)
chief complaint
fontanels
lanugo
obligate nose breather
PERRLA
point of maximum intensity (PMI)
stadiometer
Tanner stages
tympanometer

LEARNING OBJECTIVES

Upon completion of the chapter, you will be able to:

1. Demonstrate an understanding of the appropriate health history to obtain from the child and the parent or primary caregiver.
2. Individualize elements of the health history depending on the age of the child.
3. Discuss important concepts related to health assessment in children.
4. Identify health assessment approaches that relate to the age and developmental stage of the child.
5. Describe the appropriate sequence of the physical examination in the context of the child's developmental stage.
6. Distinguish normal variations in the physical examination from differences that may indicate serious alterations in health status.
7. Determine sexual maturity based on evaluation of the secondary sex characteristics.

Elliot Simmons, 3 years old, is brought to the clinic for his annual examination. His parent states that he is very fearful and anxious about this visit.

INTRODUCTION

Assessment of the child's health status involves many components: the health interview and history; observation of the parent–child interaction; assessment of the child's emotional, physiologic, cognitive, and social development; and physical examination. The nurse's skills are vital to the success of the assessment process. The nurse must:

- Establish rapport and trust.
- Demonstrate respect for the child and the parent or caregiver.
- Communicate effectively by listening actively, demonstrating empathy, and providing feedback.
- Observe systematically (especially while the child is quiet).
- Obtain accurate data.
- Validate and interpret data accurately (Treitz et al., 2022).

The focus of the assessment process depends on the purpose of the visit and the needs of the child. Assessment is an ongoing process and is repeated to varying degrees at every encounter. The expert nurse is constantly evaluating the children in their care, whether directly or indirectly as part of conversation and play. Indeed, some of the most subtle developmental signs may express themselves only during relaxed and casual interaction with a child (Brazelton & Sparrow, n.d.). The nurse may observe gait while watching a child run down the hall, assess fine motor skills and social adaptation while the child is playing a board game, or observe balance and coordination while the child is bouncing a ball. Play activities can give the nurse feedback related to upper body strength, such as when the child pushes the nurse's arms away when tickled. The nurse must also learn to perform a comprehensive and thorough examination of a child in an efficient manner.

A thorough and thoughtful assessment of a child is the foundation on which the nurse determines the needs of the child. A comprehensive history, a thorough examination, and developmental or cognitive testing as appropriate will provide practical information about the health of a child and guide the nurse's plan of care (developmental testing is covered in Chapter 31). The history and physical examination also provide a time for health education, teaching about expected growth and development, and discussing healthy lifestyle choices. The nurse uses critical thinking skills to analyze the data and establish priorities for nursing intervention or follow-up care (Chiocca, 2020).

The health assessment may be documented using a number of formats such as a written narrative, a written flow sheet, or an electronic health record. The information should be easily retrievable and available to all members of the child's health care team.

HEALTH HISTORY

The health history provides the nurse with an overall picture of what the child has experienced, highlighting areas of concern such as recurrent upper respiratory infections or headaches. This not only helps the nurse to assess those specific areas more comprehensively but also provides the opportunity to ask focused questions and identify areas where education may be needed. The time used to obtain the health history also gives the nurse an opportunity to interact with the child in a nonthreatening manner while the child watches the interactions between the nurse and the primary caregiver (Drutz & White-Satcher, 2023; Miller, n.d.).

Preparing for the Health History

Appropriate materials and a suitable environment are needed when performing a thorough health history. Take into account family roles and values. Consider the age and developmental stage of the child in order to approach the child appropriately and possibly involve them in the health history. Observe the child–parent interaction. Determine the extent of the health history that is needed in a given situation. Being well organized and staying flexible will help ensure success (Chiocca, 2020).

Gathering Materials

Before beginning, make sure the following are available: materials to record the history data (either a computer or chart paper and a pen), a private space with adequate lighting, chairs for adults and the nurse, and a bed or examination table for the child. The space should be safe for the child's developmental stage. Sit down for as much of the history taking as possible to demonstrate a relaxed and welcoming manner.

Approaching the Parent or Caregiver

Greet the parent or caregiver by name. While interviewing the parent, provide toys or books to occupy the child, allowing the parent to concentrate on the questions. Use open-ended questions and avoid making judgmental comments. Show respect by remaining approachable. Remember that the structure of the family and its roles and dynamics will affect how the family communicates and how they make decisions about health care. Demonstrate patience and help the parent stay on track when there are several children in the family. Throughout the interview, refer to the child by name and use the preferred gender when referring to the child, demonstrating interest and competence.

> *TAKE NOTE!*
>
> Illness can cause great stress in families and individuals, so nurses must remember to protect themselves from potentially threatening behavior on the part of the family. Sit close to the door, and if uncomfortable with a family member, ask for assistance. The nurse may need to alert security personnel in certain cases (Mento et al., 2020).

Approaching the Child

Show a professional demeanor while still being warm and friendly to the caregivers and child. To have a positive impact on the interaction, wear a child-friendly lab coat, uniform, or character pins, or use a colorful stethoscope cover. These may allow the child to see the nurse as friendly or nonthreatening (Drutz & White-Satcher, 2023). Make eye contact if possible and address the child by name. Use slow deliberate gestures rather than very quick or grand ones, which may be frightening to shy children.

Some young children will warm up when given time to be invisible in the room, such as hiding behind a parent before they tentatively appear. Make physical contact with the child in a nonthreatening way at first. Briefly cuddling a newborn before returning them to the caregiver, laying a hand on the head or arm of toddlers and preschoolers, and warmly shaking the hand of older children and adolescents will convey a gentle demeanor. A joke, a puppet, a silly story, or even a simple magic trick may coax the child into warming up. Being at the same eye level as the child can also be more reassuring than standing over the child (Miller, n.d.). This may require having extra seating for the nurse at the same level as the child and parent or caregiver. Aim to be seen as a trustworthy adult who is the child's partner in feeling better and staying healthy.

Elicit the child's cooperation by allowing them control over the pace and order of the health history, or anything else that the child can control while still allowing the nurse to obtain the information needed. All of this establishes a personal relationship with the child and helps gain their cooperation (Miller, n.d.).

Communicating With the Child During the Health History

Give the child opportunities to actively participate in the health history and assessment process. For young children, such as toddlers and preschoolers, ask them to point to where it hurts and allow them to answer questions. Validation of the information by the parent or caregiver is essential because of the limited comprehension and language use of children at these ages. The school-age child can answer more accurately because of their increased language skills and maturity level.

Initially, address the child and obtain as much information from them as possible. School-age children should be able to answer questions about interactions with friends and siblings and school and activities they enjoy or in which they are involved. Ask the parent or caregiver if any additional information or observations should be included.

Adolescents may not feel comfortable addressing health issues, answering questions, or being examined in the presence of the parent or caregiver. The nurse must establish a trusting relationship with the adolescent to provide them with optimal health care. Ask adolescents whether they would be more comfortable answering questions alone in the examination area or whether they prefer their parents to be present. Either way, the parent or caregiver will have an opportunity to talk with the nurse after the health history and assessment are completed (Sass & Richards, 2022).

Demonstrate an interest in the adolescent by asking questions about school, work, hobbies or activities, and friendships. Begin with these topics to make the adolescent feel comfortable in communicating with the nurse. Communicate honestly with the adolescent and explain the rationale for various aspects of the health history. Adolescents can be sensitive to nonverbal communication, so be aware of gestures and expressions (Sass & Richards, 2022). Once a rapport has been established, move on to more emotionally charged questions that relate to sexuality, substance use, depression, and suicide.

Always assure the adolescent that complete confidentiality will be maintained to the extent possible. Current state law will determine the types of information that may be withheld from parents. If the information that the nurse receives indicates that the adolescent may be in danger, then the nurse must inform the adolescent that the information will be shared with other providers and the parents (Sass & Richards, 2022).

TAKE NOTE!

Do not try to become the adolescent's peer. Remain in the role of the nurse while demonstrating respect and acceptance toward the adolescent. Clarify the meaning of jargon or slang that the adolescent uses, but do not use these words yourself; the adolescent will simply not accept the nurse as a peer.

Observing the Parent–Child Interaction

Observation of the parent–child interaction begins during the focused conversation of the health interview and continues throughout the physical examination. Explore the family dynamics, not only through questions but also by observing the family for behavioral clues. Does the parent make eye contact with the infant? Does the parent anticipate and respond to the infant's needs? Are the parents ineffective when dealing with a toddler's temper tantrum? The plan of care may need to be adjusted to teach appropriate responses to the infant's needs or toddler's behavior. Do the parents' comments increase the school-age child's sense of self-worth? Behavioral observations are crucial to proper assessment of the family's needs (Columbia University, College of Physicians and Surgeons, n.d.; Drutz & White-Satcher, 2023).

Further observe the parent–child interaction to determine if the parent appears to be overwhelmed and if their behavior seems appropriate. Monitor the child's behavioral cues. Does the child look at the parent or caregiver before answering? Does the child seem relaxed and happy with the parent or caregiver, or is the child tense? The infant will appear calm and relaxed if their needs are generally met. Crying may occur when the baby is ill or frightened but may also indicate discomfort with the parent or caregiver. Use a calm and comforting voice with the infant. Infants respond well to higher-pitched and soothing voices.

When observing the relationship between the adolescent and the parent or caregiver, does the parent or caregiver allow the adolescent to speak, or do they frequently interrupt? Does the parent or caregiver contradict what is being said? Observe the body language of the adolescent: does the adolescent seem relaxed or tense? Since adolescents are between childhood and adulthood, they have unique needs. They are experiencing a time of multiple physical and emotional changes, many of which they cannot control. They need to know that the nurse is interested in what they have to say (Sass & Richards, 2022). The use of open-ended questions allows the adolescent to talk. "Tell me about your ..." or "What have you noticed about ...?" are comfortable phrases to use to elicit the information needed. Be aware of your own reactions to the adolescent's questions or behaviors, such as nonverbal and facial expressions. Talk with the adolescent using accurate language that is developmentally and age appropriate.

Determining the Type of History Needed

The purpose of the examination will determine how comprehensive the history must be. If the health care provider or nurse practitioner rarely sees the child or if the child is critically ill, a complete and detailed history is in order, no matter what the setting. The child who has received routine health care and presents with a mild illness may need only a problem-focused history. In critical situations, some of the history taking must be delayed until after the child's condition is stabilized. Evaluate the situation to determine the best timing and the extent of the history (Quinlin & Gawlik, 2021). Also, be sensitive to repetitive interviews in hospital situations, and collaborate with health care providers or other members of the health care team to ensure that a family already under stress does not need to undergo prolonged or repetitive questioning.

CLINICAL REASONING ALERT!

Immediately report absence of the red reflex in one or both eyes, as this may indicate the presence of cataracts (Chiocca, 2020).

Performing a Health History

The health interview is the foundation of an accurate health assessment. Careful conversation and interview with the child or the caregiver will provide important information about the child's health. Depending on the intent of the health assessment, many of the questions will be direct, and many will require the caregiver or child to answer simply "yes" or "no." In other than emergency situations, though, asking open-ended questions offers an excellent opportunity to learn more about the patient's life. For example, "Are you happy at school?" may elicit a brief nod of the head, whereas "Tell me what it's like on your school playground" may result in a story about the child's friends, the kind of activities the child enjoys, any bullying that goes on, and so forth. These stories will provide the nurse with clues to the child's stage of physical, emotional, and moral development as well as their functional status (Columbia University, College of Physicians and Surgeons, n.d.; Drutz & White-Satcher, 2023).

Establish a therapeutic relationship with the child and family. Without the trust that comes from this therapeutic relationship, the family may not reveal vital information due to fear, embarrassment, or mistrust (Treitz et al., 2022). Use therapeutic communication techniques such as active listening, open-ended questions, and eliminating barriers to communication. Establishing a "medical home" where ongoing health supervision occurs encourages trust through continuity of care and the family's continuing relationships with primary care providers (see Chapter 31).

The structure of the health interview is determined by the nature of the visit. At an initial visit, large amounts of historical data are collected. Having the family fill out a questionnaire can save time, but a questionnaire is not a substitute for the health interview. The questionnaire may serve as a springboard to begin structured conversations between the family and the nurse. At subsequent visits, the health interview can focus on the pertinent issues of that visit as well as any health issues that are being monitored.

The health history includes demographics, chief complaint and history of present illness, past health history, review of systems, family health history, developmental history, functional history, and family composition, resources, and home environment.

TAKE NOTE!

Any questionnaires used in the health care setting should be written at a fourth- to sixth-grade reading level and be in the primary language of the person completing them (National Institutes of Health, 2021).

Demographics

Initially, questions should be simple and nonintrusive; once a rapport between the nurse and the patient has started, sensitive questions can be asked. First, obtain data such as the child's name, nickname, birth date, and sex and gender. Determine the child's race or ethnicity, the language the child understands, and the language the child speaks. Record the child's address and home telephone number and the parent's or caregiver's work telephone number. Identify who the historian is (the child or the parent or caregiver) and note how reliable this source of information is considered to be. Do not assume that an adult with the child is the child's parent. Establish the relationship of the adult to the child, and ask who cares for the child if that person does not. Determine the composition of the household, including other children and other family members or other people who live there.

Chief Complaint and History of Present Illness

Next, ask about the **chief complaint** (reason for the visit). The reason may not always be apparent to you. A question such as "What can I help you with today?" or "What did you notice in your baby or child that you wanted to have checked today?" is welcoming. The response from the child or parent may be a functional problem, a developmental concern, or a disease. Record the chief complaint in the child's or parent's own words.

Next, address the history related to the present illness. For each concern, determine its onset, duration, characteristics, and course (location, signs, symptoms, exposures, and so on), previous episodes in the patient or the family, previous testing or therapies, what makes it better or worse, and what the concern means to the child and the family. Inquire about any exposure to infectious agents.

Past Health History

Ask about the prenatal history (any problems with pregnancy), perinatal history (any problems with labor and delivery), past illnesses, or any other health or developmental problems. Document the child's prior history of illnesses (recurrent, chronic, or serious) and any accidents or injuries in the past. Inquire about any operations or hospitalizations the child has had. Document the child's diet. Note the child's allergies to foods, medications, animals, environmental or contact agents, or latex products. Determine the child's reaction to the allergen as well as its severity. Determine the child's immunization status (refer to Chapter 31 for further information on immunizations). Record any medications the child is taking, the dosage and schedule, as well as when the last dose was given. Determine menstrual history as appropriate.

Family Health History

Obtaining information about the family's health is a key part of a health interview. Perform a three-generation

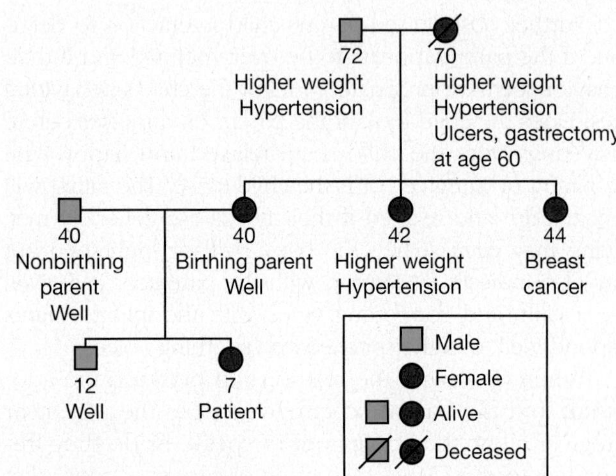

FIGURE 32.1 Genogram.

family health history. This information may be documented in a genogram (Fig. 32.1). Asking about the age and health status of parents, siblings, and other family members helps to identify trends and specific health issues (Bryant & Speck, 2022). For example, do the grandparents have early-onset coronary artery disease? If they do, the child may benefit from additional health screening. Siblings may exhibit a genetic disease or carry a trait for the disease. This family health information helps to guide future health planning.

Review of Systems

Inquire about current or past history of problems related to:

- Growth and development
- Skin
- Head and neck
- Eyes and vision
- Ears and hearing
- Mouth, teeth, and throat
- Respiratory system and breasts
- Cardiovascular system
- Gastrointestinal system
- Genitourinary system
- Musculoskeletal system
- Neurologic system
- Endocrine system
- Hematologic system

Table 32.1 provides specific questions related to each of these systems.

Developmental History

Determine the age when landmarks in gross motor control were achieved, such as sitting, standing, walking, pedaling, and so on. Ask whether the child has attained

TABLE 32.1 • Questions for the Review of Systems

Systems	Has the Child Experienced
Growth and development	Weight loss or gain; appropriate energy and activity levels; fatigue; behavioral changes such as irritability, nervousness, anger, or increased crying
Skin	Easy bruising or bleeding, rash, lesion, skin disease, pruritus, birthmarks, or change in mole, pigment, hair, or nails
Head and neck	Head injury, headache, dizziness, syncope
Eyes and vision	Pain, redness, discharge, diplopia, strabismus, cataracts, vision changes, reading difficulties, need to sit close to the board at school or close to the TV at home
Ears and hearing	Earache, recurrent ear infection, tubes in eardrums, discharge, difficulty hearing, ringing, excess cerumen
Mouth, teeth, and throat	Swollen gums, pain with teething, caries, tooth loss, toothache, sores, difficulty with chewing or swallowing, hoarseness, sore throat, mouth breathing, change in voice
Respiratory system and breasts	Nasal congestion or discharge, cough, wheeze, noisy breathing, snoring, shortness of breath or other difficulty breathing, problems with or changes in breasts
Cardiovascular system	Murmur, color change (cyanosis), exertional dyspnea, activity intolerance, palpitations, extremity coldness, high blood pressure, high cholesterol
Gastrointestinal system	Nausea, vomiting, abdominal pain, cramping, diarrhea, constipation, stool holding, anal pain or itching
Genitourinary system	Dysuria; polyuria; oliguria; narrow urine stream; dark, cloudy, or discolored urine; difficulty with toilet training; bedwetting Undescended testicles, pain in penis or scrotum, sores or lesions, discharge, scrotal swelling when crying, changes in scrotum or penis size, addition of pubic hair Vaginal discharge, itching rash, problems with menstruation or menstrual cycle, development of pubic hair
Musculoskeletal system	Joint or bone pain, stiffness, swelling, injury (e.g., broken bones or sprains), movement limitation, decreased strength, altered gait, changes in coordination, back pain, posture changes or spinal curvature
Neurologic system	Numbness, tingling, difficulty learning, altered mood or ability to stay alert, tremors, tics, seizures
Endocrine system	Increased thirst, excessive appetite, delayed or early pubertal changes, problems with growth
Hematologic system	Swelling of lymph nodes, pale color, excessive bruising

Data from Bryant, P., & Speck, P. M. (2022). Health assessment. In T. Kyle (Ed.), *Primary care pediatrics for the nurse practitioner.* Springer; Jarvis, C., & Eckhardt, A. (2020). *Physical examination and health assessment* (8th ed.). Elsevier.

fine motor skills such as grasping, releasing, pincer grasp, crayon or utensil use, and handwriting skills. Note the child's age and extent of language acquisition. Document speech problems such as a lisp or stuttering. The rate of developmental skill acquisition may vary from child to child, but the sequence of skill attainment should remain the same. Inquire about self-care ability (e.g., tying shoes, dressing, brushing teeth) and, in the younger child, how toilet training is progressing. Question the parents about the child's feeding skills, including how well the child drinks from a cup and uses utensils or whether the child has any special requirements. Inquire about social skills and comfort articles (e.g., blankets, stuffed animals). Note whether the child has a habit of thumb or finger sucking or using a pacifier. Document day care attendance and preschool or school adjustment and achievements.

Functional History

The functional history should contain information about the child's daily routine. Inquire about:

- Safety measures (e.g., car seats and their placement, use of seat belts, smoke detectors, bike helmets)
- Routine health care and dental care (including dates of dental care and what was done)
- Nutrition, including a 24-hour dietary recall or week-long food diary, use of supplements and vitamins, feeding pattern and satisfaction with diet, amount of "junk food" consumed, food likes and dislikes, and the parent's perception of the child's nutrition (refer to Chapters 25 to 29 for nutritional needs at various ages)
- Physical activity, recreation, play, and organized sports
- Television and computer habits
- Sleep behavior and bedtime

- Elimination patterns and any concerns
- Hearing or vision problems (dates of last screenings and results)
- Relationships with other family members and friends, coping and temperament, discipline strategies, attention or school behavior problems
- Religious involvement and other spiritual practices
- Use of adaptive and assistive devices such as eyeglasses or contact lenses, hearing aids, walker, braces, wheelchair
- Sexual practices (Bryant & Speck, 2022)

Family Composition, Resources, and Home Environment

Determine the marital status of the parents. Does the child live with the parents, a stepparent, or other family member? Is the child adopted or in foster care? Are the parents the primary caregivers for the child? If not, the primary caregiver should be included in the interview process if possible. Parents may not know some of the child's routines if the child spends much of the time being cared for by someone else. Working parents may learn about a health or behavior issue only after being alerted by the child's day care center or babysitter. It may be helpful to expand the family history to include the grandparents and their interaction with the child.

Determine the employment status of the parents and their occupations, as this can affect the child's overall well-being; for example, the parents' work schedule may not allow them to spend much time with the child. Assess family income and financial resources, including health insurance and Supplemental Nutrition Assistance Program (SNAP); Special Supplemental Nutrition Program for Women, Infants, and Children (WIC); or other governmental supplemental income. Major family changes can also affect how the parents and child interact, so evaluate for relationship problems or changes.

Ask about the family's home and its age and environment. Is there a safe outdoor play area? If there is a pool, are safety features in place? Determine whether the home has electricity and an indoor water supply. Also determine whether the home has heating, air conditioning, and refrigeration. What pets does the family have? How are they housed? Are there infestations of insects or rodents in the home?

TAKE NOTE!

Homes or apartments built prior to 1978 may contain lead-based paint, and children who live there are at an increased risk for the development of lead poisoning (Centers for Disease Control and Prevention [CDC], 2023).

PHYSICAL EXAMINATION

The next step after the health history is the physical examination. It should focus on the chief complaint or any of the systems that engaged the nurse's critical thinking while obtaining the history. The examination will reflect the nurse's general practice style, the developmental stage and age of the child, the temperament of the child and caregiver, and the health status of the child. For example, a very ill child will not waste energy protesting the examination, so the nurse can move quickly in that situation. A healthy child, however, will express their expected developmental stage and will show varying degrees of resistance to the examination (Columbia University, College of Physicians and Surgeons, n.d.; Miller, n.d.).

Preparing for the Physical Examination

When performing the physical examination, being prepared and organized ensures that the needed information will be obtained efficiently. The appropriate methods to use and ways to approach the child depend on the child's developmental stage.

Gathering Materials

The examination area should include an examination table or the child's hospital crib or bed. Appropriate lighting is necessary for adequate observation and inspection. Gather the equipment necessary for the examination such as clean gloves, stethoscope, thermometer, sphygmomanometer, tape measure, reflex hammer, penlight, otoscope/ophthalmoscope, tongue depressor, and cotton ball. An infant or adult scale is needed, as well as a stadiometer for children capable of standing independently. Young children may be frightened by seeing a large amount of equipment, so take out one piece of equipment at a time. Some children can be very resistant to what they see as a threat or an invasion of their privacy, so it may help to have washable toys in the examination area to use as distractions during the assessment (Drutz & White-Satcher, 2023; Miller, n.d.).

Children and their parents may be able to sense any frustration or anxiety on the part of the examiner, so display a confident and matter-of-fact approach. If the child is not cooperative, do not become discouraged; more time and explanation will usually do the trick.

Regardless of the child's age, if the examination room is cold, the child will be uncomfortable and possibly less cooperative. Provide appropriate covers to ensure the child's comfort, or have the child remain dressed until the time of the examination (Miller, n.d.).

Approaching the Child

Approach the child according to their developmental age and stage. Table 32.2 outlines a general approach to

TABLE **32.2** • Developmental Considerations for Examination

	Newborn	Infant	Toddler	Preschool	School-Age	Early Adolescent	Late Adolescent
Place to perform examination	May lie on examination table or in caregiver's lap	In caregiver's lap or on examination table with caregiver right beside infant	Allow some freedom of movement when possible; child may stand between seated caregiver's legs or sit on the lap.	Some may be willing to sit on examination table with caregiver standing close by with hand on the leg.	Sitting on examination table where they still have eye contact with caregiver	Some may be willing to have their caregiver wait outside the examination room.	Explain to the caregiver that the adolescent needs privacy and that they should wait outside the examination room.
Examination direction	Keep up a running dialogue with the caregiver, explaining each step as you do it.	Continue to explain each step to the caregiver; address child by name. Perform most invasive parts last.	Introduce yourself to caregiver and child; explain most steps to the child and all steps to caregiver; allow child to handle instruments. Perform most invasive parts last.	Allow child to decide the order of the examination; explain what the instruments do and let the child try them; speak to the caregiver before and after the examination.	Include the child in all parts of the examination; use head-to-toe approach with genital examination last. Speak to the caregiver before and after the examination.	Speak to the child using mature language; appeal to their desire for self-care. Use a head-to-toe approach, with genital examination last.	Explain confidentiality to caregiver and adolescent; allow time talking with them together and separately. Use a head-to-toe approach, with genital examination last.

Data from Chiocca, E. M. (2020). *Advanced pediatric assessment* (3rd ed.). Springer Publishing Company; Miller, S. (n.d.). *Pediatric physical exam video* [Video]. http://www.columbia.edu/itc/hs/medical/clerkships/peds/Student_Information/Reference_Materials/PE_Video.html; Columbia University, College of Physicians and Surgeons. (n.d.). *Points on the pediatric physical exam*. http://www.columbia.edu/itc/hs/medical/clerkships/peds/Student_Information/Reference_Materials/Pediatric_PE.html

the physical examination in each broad developmental category.

If several children are to be seen at the same time, begin with the child who will be most cooperative. If the other children do not see anything scary and realize that their sibling was examined without a problem, it sets the stage for better cooperation from the younger ones.

NEWBORNS AND INFANTS

If the infant is asleep, auscultate the heart, lungs, and abdomen first while the baby is quiet. Count the heart rate and respiratory rate before undressing the baby. Completely undress newborns and infants down to their diaper, removing it just at the end to examine the genitalia, anus, spine, and hips. It is best to examine the infant 1 to 2 hours before a feeding. Having the parent or caregiver hold the child during the examination can help to alleviate fears and anxieties (Fig. 32.2). Allow the parent or caregiver to be a nurturer rather than assisting with painful procedures, unless there are no other choices available (Miller, n.d.).

Perform the assessment in a head-to-toe manner, leaving the most traumatic procedures, such as examination of the ears, nose, mouth, and throat, until the end (Bryant & Speck, 2022; Miller, n.d.). Also delay eliciting the Moro reflex until the end of the examination, as the startling sensation may make the infant cry. Use firm, gentle handling while examining the infant. Make sure your hands and the stethoscope are warm. Perform the assessment as quickly and completely as possible. Use a soft and crooning voice, smile, and engage the infant in eye contact. In addition, use brightly colored objects to help distract them. If the baby is crying, a pacifier may be useful.

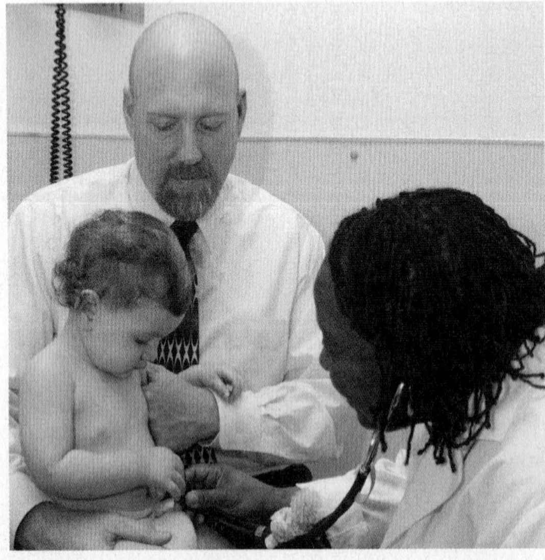

FIGURE 32.2 The infant or toddler may feel more comfortable and secure being examined while sitting in the parent or caregiver's lap.

TAKE NOTE!

Many older infants demonstrate stranger anxiety as a normal part of development. If the parent is not holding the infant, make sure the parent is within the infant's view; this will increase the baby's comfort and cooperation (Miller, n.d.).

TODDLERS

Toddlers usually prefer to remove their clothing one item at a time as needed for the examination. After one area is examined, the child may feel more comfortable replacing that item of clothing before removing another one (Treitz et al., 2022). An examination gown is usually not necessary before school age. Again, make certain the room temperature is comfortable.

When the nurse enters the room, a child of this age is often sitting or standing by the parent. Incorporate play as appropriate during the health assessment. Remember your own facial expressions and tone. Use little touch at the beginning of the encounter with the child and the caregiver.

Introduce the equipment to be used slowly, explaining briefly what is going to happen. Let the child touch and hold the equipment whenever possible, even taking a parent's temperature or putting the blood pressure cuff on a teddy bear (Fig. 32.3). The toddler will prefer to sit on the caregiver's lap. When the toddler must be supine for the abdominal examination, sit in your chair knee-to-knee with the caregiver so the toddler may lie back on the caregiver's and your laps. Praise the child for being cooperative during the examination. "You did such a good job holding still while I listened to your chest" and similar phrases give positive feedback to the child.

If the child is uncooperative, assess as thoroughly as possible and move on to the next area to be assessed. The caregiver may need to place an arm around the toddler's body to provide restraint for invasive procedures. Use

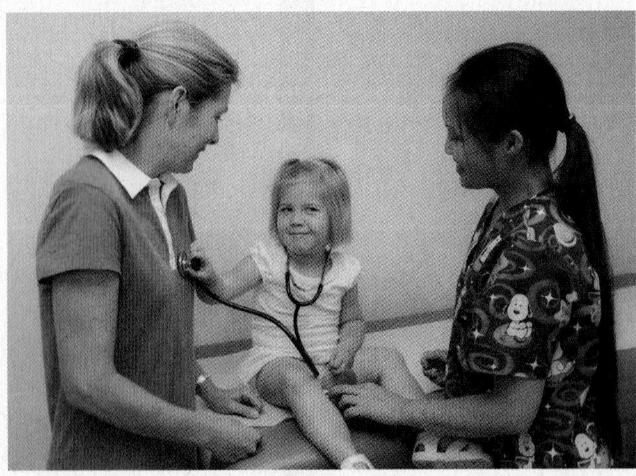

FIGURE 32.3 The preschooler enjoys listening to the parent's heart first.

short phrases to tell the toddler what you are going to do, rather than asking if it is okay (Chiocca, 2020; Miller, n.d.).

TAKE NOTE!

Toddlers are egocentric. Telling a toddler how well another child behaved probably will not be helpful in gaining the young child's cooperation.

PRESCHOOLER

The preschooler may fear body invasion and mutilation and will withdraw from any procedure or assessment that is viewed as intrusive. Otherwise, the sense of initiative often leads the preschooler to be cooperative. Use simple explanations to inform the child about each step of the examination, offering reassurance as appropriate. Allow them to "help" by holding the stethoscope or penlight. If choices are available, offer them to the child. Again, always compliment the child on their cooperation.

TAKE NOTE!

Preschoolers like to play games. To encourage deep breathing during lung auscultation, hold up a finger or a lit penlight and instruct the child to "blow it out" (Miller, n.d.).

SCHOOL-AGE CHILDREN

The school-age child's thinking is still very concrete, but they can be objective and realistic. Avoid using medical jargon and words that may have a double meaning to a young child. Instead of "take your temperature," "take your blood pressure," "hit your knee," or "test," say, "Let's see how warm you are," "I want to listen to you breathe," and other phrases that describe, in words the child can understand, what you are preparing to do. The school-age child may be interested in how things work and why certain things need to be done and will be responsive to truthful and simple explanations. Instruments that are colorful or look like toys are helpful throughout early childhood and the early school-age period (Drutz & White-Satcher, 2023; Miller, n.d.).

Always respect a child's desire to avoid pain and insult. Allow children to wear their underpants under the examination gown to provide a sense of security until the genitalia need to be examined. Allow the child to replace their clothing as soon as possible. Privacy and respect for the child's feelings are important to children of this age (Treitz et al., 2022).

TAKE NOTE!

Describing and commenting on your findings during the physical examination is interesting to the school-age child, as children of this age like to learn about how the body works (Miller, n.d.).

ADOLESCENTS

Provide privacy while the adolescent is undressing and putting on a gown. Demonstrate an attitude of respect. Perform the assessment in a head-to-toe manner, exposing only the area to be examined. Provide information about physical changes in a matter-of-fact way, such as "The hair on your legs is what is expected at this time." This provides information related to sensitive areas that the adolescent may be reluctant to ask about. It also provides the adolescent with information about the sexual development that is normal and expected. Allow opportunities for the adolescent to ask questions without the caregiver being present. Assure the adolescent that there are no "dumb questions" about the changes being experienced. The nurse should ask adolescents to remove their bras so that the nurse can perform a breast examination, teach breast self-examination, and check for scoliosis. During the breast and genital examination, it is appropriate to have a staff member present whose gender the adolescent is comfortable with, such as having a female staff member present when a male nurse examines a female patient (Sass & Richards, 2022).

Steps of the Physical Examination

The physical examination of children, just as for adults, begins with a systematic inspection: checking color, warmth, characteristics, and texture visually and smelling for any odor. Palpation follows inspection to validate your observations. Percussion is a useful tool for determining the location, size, and density of organs or masses. Tapping with the reflex hammer elicits deep tendon reflexes. The stethoscope is used to auscultate the heart, lungs, and abdomen.

Performing a Physical Examination

A complete examination includes assessment of the general appearance, vital signs, body measurements, and pain, as well as examination of the head, neck, eyes, ears, nose, mouth and throat, skin, thorax and lungs, breasts, heart and peripheral perfusion, abdomen, genitalia and rectum, musculoskeletal system, and neurologic system. The nurse in most settings will not be assessing the breasts, genitalia, eyes, or ears in detail. Be aware of the role of the nurse in different settings and how the nurse can facilitate the assessment process.

General Appearance

Never discount first impressions. Does the child give an impression of being ill or well? What is the child's expression and energy level? Note lethargy, listlessness, excessive activity, or inappropriate attention span for the child's age. Observe the child's state of alertness and whether they are responding appropriately to the stress of the situation. Note the child's posture and positioning:

- The newborn's posture is flexed, with arms and legs tucked in.
- The older infant should have improving head and then trunk control.
- The toddler demonstrates lordosis (swayback) and bowlegs, with a relatively large head and protuberant belly.
- The preschooler is slenderer and upright in appearance.
- The school-age child and adolescent should demonstrate an upright, straight, and well-balanced posture.

Note whether the child's development appears appropriate. Observing the child initially may yield a wealth of information about the child's development. Is the child active, moving about the room? Does the child's speech seem appropriate for their age? Notice whether the family interacts appropriately with one another and the child. Does the child appear clean and well cared for? Does the child appear well nourished or small for age, or is higher weight a concern? Note the scent of tobacco smoke or alcohol on family members. Notice if the baby bottle or pacifier is nearby and whether the child has a toy or transitional object. Assess whether the siblings appear equally well cared for. Observe for tension in the room between adults and children or adolescents. This initial quick assessment of general appearance will serve the nurse well if it is objective; delay interpretation of this assessment until additional data are gathered.

Measurement of Vital Signs

Measure, document, and interpret the vital signs of children using age-appropriate equipment and approaches. The child's age and size, as well as knowledge of underlying health conditions, will affect analysis of the vital signs. Vital signs are the temperature, pulse rate, respiratory rate, and blood pressure. These measurements fluctuate normally in children; assessing vital signs while the child is quiet is most appropriate. Comforting an infant or distracting a young child may be necessary while obtaining vital signs. If the child is crying or otherwise active during the assessment, document that fact. Many acute care settings require continuous measurement of vital signs using specific monitoring equipment. Also assess the child's pain level when assessing the vital signs.

TEMPERATURE

Temperature is measured as it is in adults. Thermometers are available in electronic and digital types. Use the same type of equipment consistently to allow reliable comparisons to be made and to permit tracking of temperatures during the course of illness. No matter which type of thermometer is used, ensure accuracy by carefully following the manufacturer's instructions.

The routes for taking the child's temperature are tympanic, temporal, oral, axillary, and rectal. Numerous research studies have been undertaken to determine the best method for temperature assessment in children. Take the child's temperature using the least invasive method that is best accepted by the child, parent, and health care provider or nurse practitioner.

> ***TAKE NOTE!***
>
> Although they may continue to be available in some instances, glass thermometers are not recommended for use due to the mercury they contain (Vorvick et al., 2022).

Choosing a method of measuring temperature depends on what is available at the facility and the child's age and physical condition. Tympanic temperature reflects the pulmonary artery temperature and can be measured with the tympanic thermometer within seconds. The accuracy of a tympanic temperature reading depends on the user's technique and can be safely and effectively used in children 6 months of age and older (American Academy of Pediatrics [AAP], 2021). Refer to Nursing Procedure 32.1.

Temporal scanning uses infrared scanning on the skin over the temporal artery combined with a

NURSING PROCEDURE 32.1 Measuring Tympanic Temperature

1. Note age of child. If younger than 3 years, pull the earlobe back and down.
2. Insert the tympanic thermometer gently into the ear canal with the infrared sensor beam directed toward the center of the tympanic membrane rather than the sides of the ear canal.
3. Push the button to take the temperature and hold until a reading is obtained. The length of time required for the temperature to register varies per manufacturer but is only a few seconds at most.

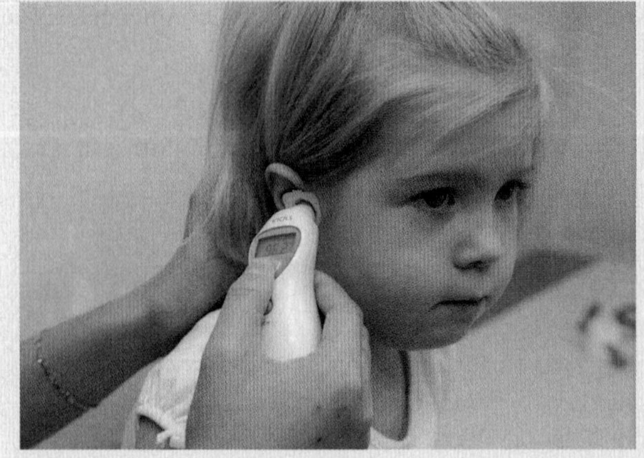

mathematical computation to determine the child's arterial temperature. Temporal artery thermometry may be used with any child over the age of 3 months (AAP, 2021). Measure temperature on the exposed side of the head (not the side that has been lying on a pillow or covered by a hat). Depress the sensor button and slide the sensor tip externally in a horizontal line across the child's forehead, midway between the eyebrows and hairline and ending at the lateral hairline (Fig. 32.4). Continuing to depress the button, lift the sensor from the forehead and then place it on the soft spot behind the ear lobe. Hold it there until the device registers the temperature reading, which usually requires 1 second. Accuracy may be affected by excessive sweating (Exergen Corporation, n.d.).

Oral temperature is highly reliable if the child can cooperate. By 5 years of age, the child can hold an electronic oral thermometer in the mouth well enough to obtain a reading. Place the probe under the tongue, and ensure the child's mouth remains closed until the device registers the temperature. Oral intake, oxygen administration, and nebulized medications or treatments may affect oral temperature.

The axillary method may be used for children who have difficulty cooperating, neurologic impairment, immunosuppression, or injuries or recent surgery to the oral cavity. Place the tip of the electronic or digital thermometer in the axilla to obtain the reading. Make sure the tip is indeed in the axilla and not just between the arm and the child's side. Hold the thermometer parallel rather than perpendicular to the child's side to obtain the most accurate reading. Keep the child's arm pressed down to the side until the thermometer registers, which will be as little as 10 seconds with certain electronic models but 2 or 3 minutes with digital models commonly used at home.

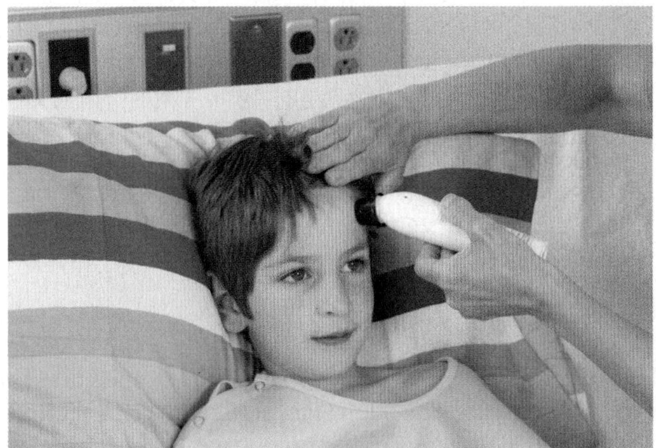

FIGURE 32.4 Temporal artery thermometers are noninvasive and well tolerated by young children. For an accurate reading, move hair to expose forehead and hairline.

Although long considered to reflect core temperature, the rectal route is invasive, not well accepted by some children, and probably unnecessary with the modern alternative methods now available (Chiocca, 2020). To take the rectal temperature, position the young infant supine with legs flexed. The older infant or child should be prone or side-lying. Small children may lie across the parent's lap for additional comfort. Apply a water-soluble jelly to the covered probe, insert the thermometer past the anal sphincter no more than 2.5 cm (1 in), and hold it there until the temperature registers (as little as 15 seconds with certain electronic models but longer with digital models).

TAKE NOTE!

Avoid the rectal route of temperature measurement in the child with immunosuppression or neutropenia, as well as the child who has diarrhea, a bleeding disorder, or a history of rectal surgery (Perry et al., 2022).

PULSE

Assess the heart rate while the child is resting or sleeping. The heart rate in infants is much faster than in adults. It also varies in infants and children who are anxious, fearful, or crying. As the child grows, the heart rate slows, and the range of normal values narrows. Table 32.3 lists heart rate ranges according to the child's age. The radial pulse is difficult to palpate accurately in children younger than 2 years of age because the blood vessels lie close to the skin surface and are easily obliterated (Bryant & Speck, 2022). For children younger than 10 years of age, auscultate the apical pulse with the stethoscope for a full minute (Jarvis & Eckhardt, 2020). In older children, palpate the radial pulse for a full minute (Fig. 32.5).

TABLE 32.3 • Heart Rate and Respiratory Rate Ranges by Age Group

	Infant	Toddler	Preschooler	School-Age	Adolescent
Heart rate	80–150	70–120	65–110	60–100	55–95
Respiratory rate	25–55	20–30	20–25	14–26	12–20

Data from Kleinman, K., McDaniel, L., & Molloy, M. (2021). *The Harriet Lane handbook: A manual for pediatric house officers* (22nd ed.). Elsevier; Chiocca, E. M. (2020). *Advanced pediatric assessment* (3rd ed.). Springer Publishing Company.

Note any irregularities in strength or rhythm. Finally, document the method used to obtain pulse measurement as well as any activity of the child during the assessment and any action taken.

TAKE NOTE!

In the infant and young child, the heart rate is often quite elevated due to fear or anxiety when the stethoscope is placed on the chest initially. For an accurate heart rate, wait several seconds until the rate slows, and then count for 1 full minute.

RESPIRATORY RATE

Assess respirations when the child is resting or sitting quietly, since respiratory rate often changes when infants or young children cry, feed, or become more active. They also tend to breathe faster when they are anxious or scared. The most accurate respiratory rate is obtained before disturbing the infant or child. This can often be done easily when the parent or caregiver is holding the child before any clothing is removed. Count the respiratory rate for a full minute to ensure accuracy. Infants' respirations are primarily diaphragmatic, so count the abdominal movements. After 1 year of age, count the thoracic movements. Table 32.3 lists ranges of respiratory rate according to the child's age. Document the rate, activity of the child, any deviations from normal, and any action taken.

TAKE NOTE!

Infants normally display an uneven or irregular breathing pattern, with short pauses between some breaths. This may be accentuated when they are ill (Kyle, 2022).

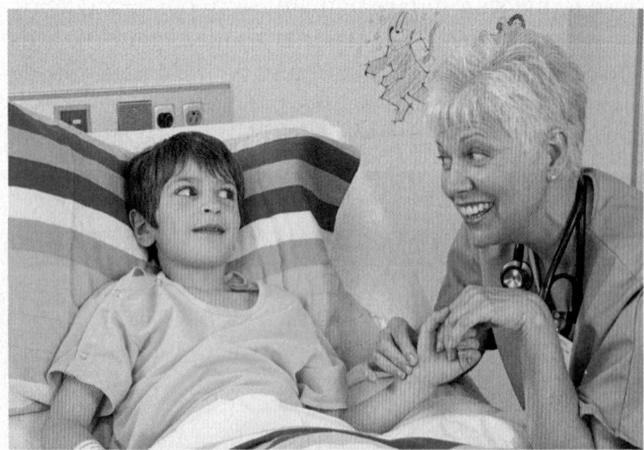

FIGURE 32.5 Assessing the radial pulse of a young child.

MEASURING OXYGEN SATURATION

Since the incidence of respiratory dysfunction is high in children during an illness, pulse oximetry is often routinely included in the vital signs assessment. This method is reliable and noninvasive. Pulse oximetry determines the oxygen saturation (SaO_2) in blood by using a sensor that measures the absorption of light waves as they pass through highly perfused areas of the body. The pulse rate on the oximeter should coincide with the apical pulse rate to ensure that the oxygen saturation reading is accurate. Nursing Procedure 32.2 details how to use the pulse oximeter. Identify whether pulse oximetry monitoring will be continuous or intermittent (as with vital signs).

A few guidelines to follow when using pulse oximetry are as follows:

- The probe may be placed on the finger, toe, ear, foot, or forehead. Avoid placing the probe on the same extremity with a blood pressure cuff or an intravenous or other type of line.
- Use the health care provider's or nurse practitioner's orders or health care agency guidelines to set parameters for high and low pulse rate as well as high and low oxygen saturation. Never turn off the alarm settings.
- Ensure that the probe is not applied too tightly, as this will prevent venous flow and cause inaccurate readings.
- It is helpful to use the provided cover over the sensor to prevent disruption from ambient light.

Potential sources of errors in pulse oximeter readings include abnormal hemoglobin value, poor perfusion, ambient light interference, motion artifact, and skin breakdown. Falsely low readings may be associated with a nonsecure connection (movement of child's foot or hand), and poor perfusion. Falsely normal readings may be associated with carbon monoxide poisoning and severe anemia (Mechem, 2022).

BLOOD PRESSURE

The AAP recommends that children older than 3 years have their blood pressure measured at least once during every health care episode (Flynn et al., 2017). Children younger than 3 years old should have blood pressure measured if they have one of the following risk factors:

- History of prematurity, very low birth weight, or other neonatal intensive care complication
- Congenital heart defect
- Recurrent urinary tract infections, hematuria, proteinuria, known kidney disease or urologic malformations, family history of congenital kidney disease
- Malignancy, bone marrow transplant, or solid organ transplant
- Treatment with medications that raise blood pressure
- Systemic illnesses associated with hypertension such as neurofibromatosis and tuberous sclerosis
- Increased intracranial pressure (Flynn et al., 2017)

NURSING PROCEDURE 32.2 Pulse Oximetry Monitoring

1. Explain the procedure to the child and family (use a penlight to show how the sensor "looks through the skin").
2. Attach the probe to the child and connect to the monitor.
3. Set the parameters for the alarm if monitoring pulse oximetry continuously.
4. Observe and record pulse rate and oxygen saturation.
5. Record the activity level of the child and the percentage of oxygen in use.
6. Check skin condition and rotate sensor position every few hours if adhesive type used.

Types of Sensors

a. Nonadhesive for infants (continuous use)

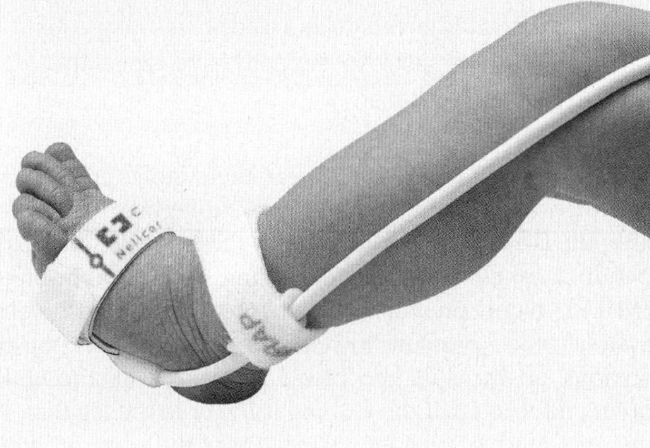

b. Finger adhesive (continuous use)

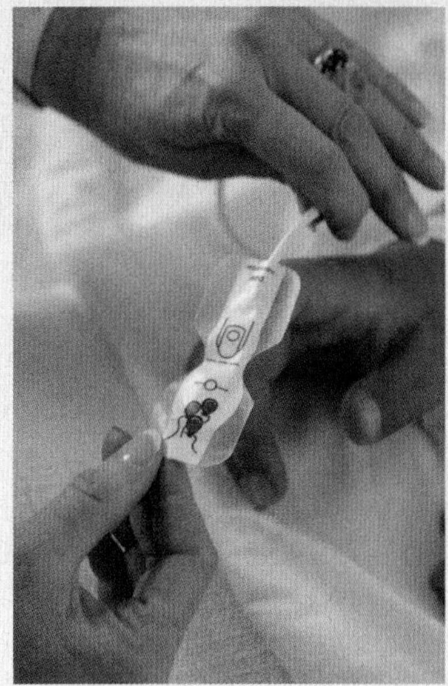

c. Finger reusable (intermittent use)

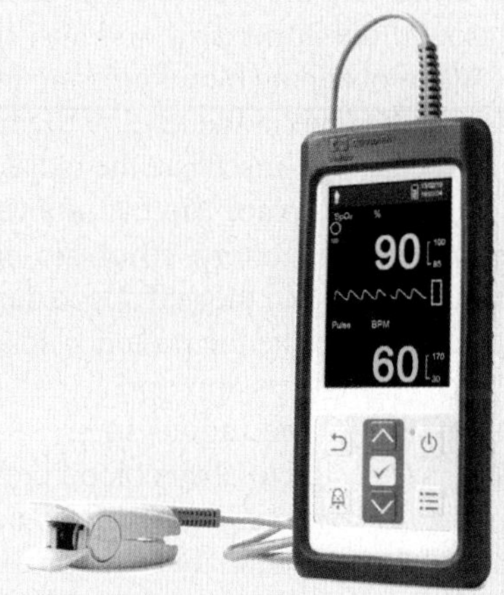

Copyright © 2024 Medtronic. All rights reserved. Used with the permission of Medtronic.

In the hospital or outpatient setting when a child is ill or undergoing surgery or a procedure, the frequency of blood pressure measurement will depend on the child's physical status. Measurement of blood pressure can be frightening to a young child, so include an age-appropriate explanation and perform the procedure after obtaining the pulse rate and respirations (Fig. 32.6). Accuracy of blood pressure measurement depends on the cuff size, as well as the operator's skill and accurate calibration of an electronic device. The cuff bladder width should be at least 40% of the circumference of the upper arm at its midpoint, and the cuff bladder length should cover 80% to 100% of the circumference of the upper arm (Flynn et al., 2017). Various pediatric and infant cuffs are available, as well as larger thigh cuffs that may be used on an arm in an adolescent with higher weight.

TAKE NOTE!

Using an accurate cuff size is important: a wider cuff yields a lower reading, and a narrower cuff yields a higher reading.

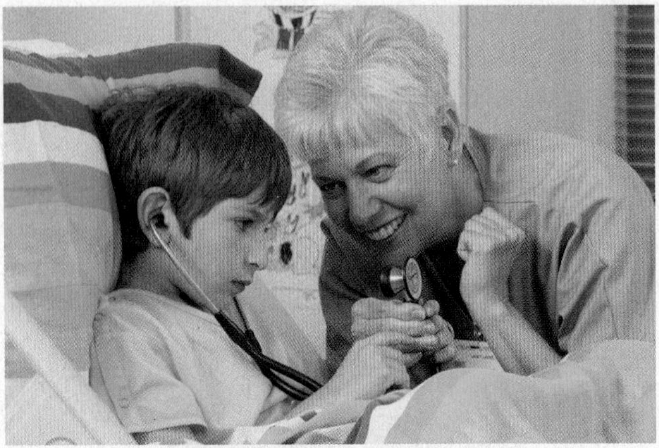

FIGURE 32.6 Allowing children to handle the equipment gives them some control over the situation.

Measure blood pressure in the upper arm, lower arm, thigh, or calf/ankle. The size of the cuff should match the extremity used. The measurement should be taken in the same limb, at the same place, and in the same position with each subsequent measurement to ensure consistency in tracking the blood pressure. To measure blood pressure using the upper arm, place the limb at the level of the heart, place the cuff around the upper arm, and auscultate at the brachial artery. When obtaining blood pressure in the lower arm, again, position the limb at the level of the heart, place the cuff above the wrist, and auscultate the radial artery. For measurement in the thigh, place the cuff above the knee and auscultate the popliteal artery. To obtain blood pressure on the calf or ankle, place the cuff above the malleolus or at the midcalf and auscultate the posterior tibial or dorsal pedal artery. Figure 32.7 shows appropriate cuff placement and auscultation points for the various sites.

When using auscultation to obtain blood pressure readings in children, note systolic pressure at the moment the first Korotkoff sound is heard as the manometer pressure is lowered (Fig. 32.8). The point at which the sound disappears is the diastolic pressure. The systolic blood pressure can sometimes be heard to a measurement of zero, so document the reading as systolic pressure over "P" for pulse.

Alternative methods for obtaining blood pressure measurements in children include the use of Doppler or oscillometric devices. The Doppler ultrasound method uses high-frequency sound waves that bounce off body parts to obtain blood pressure. Apply the gel to the Doppler end, and listen with the Doppler device where Korotkoff sounds would normally be auscultated.

With either the Doppler method or auscultation, inflate the cuff 20 mm Hg past the point where the distal pulse disappears. Oscillometric equipment measures the mean arterial pulse and then calculates the systolic and diastolic readings. The accuracy of this method depends heavily on ongoing validation and calibration. Also, the cuff inflates to a preset value often far higher than the infant or child's blood pressure, resulting in a tight, uncomfortable cuff being in place for a longer period of time.

TAKE NOTE!

If the oscillometric device yields a blood pressure greater than the 90th percentile for sex and height, repeat the reading using auscultation.

In children older than 1 year, the systolic pressure in the thigh tends to be 10 to 40 mm Hg higher than in the arm; the diastolic pressure remains the same. Refer to Appendix E for the National Heart, Lung, and Blood Institute (NHLBI) blood pressure levels based on sex and height. Systolic blood pressure increases if the child is crying or anxious, so measure the blood pressure with the child quiet and relaxed. If the reading is lower in the leg than in the arm, always consider coarctation of the aorta or interference with circulation to the lower extremities.

Pain Assessment

Pain is considered to be the fifth vital sign. Use the Face, Legs, Activity, Cry, Consolability (FLACC) pain scale to measure pain in children who are too young to verbally or conceptually quantify their pain or when there is a

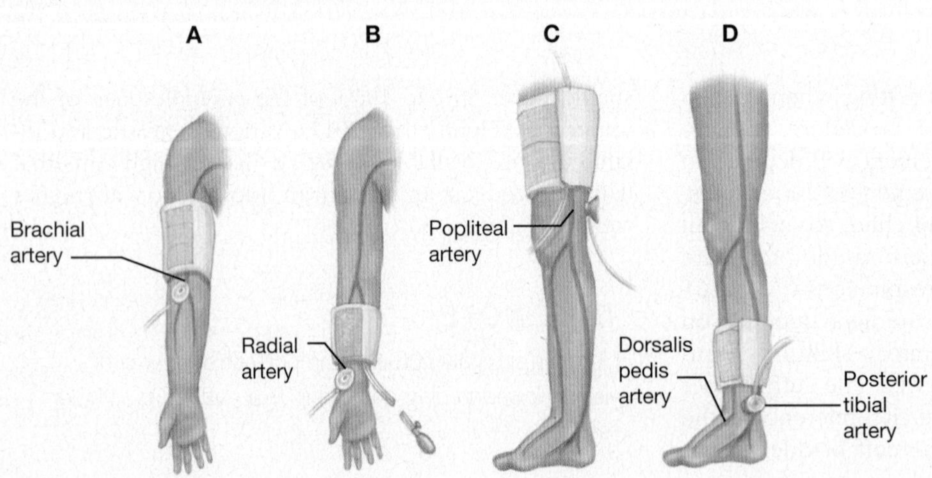

FIGURE 32.7 Various positions of cuff placement and auscultation area for obtaining blood pressure. **A.** Upper arm. **B.** Lower arm. **C.** Thigh. **D.** Calf/ankle.

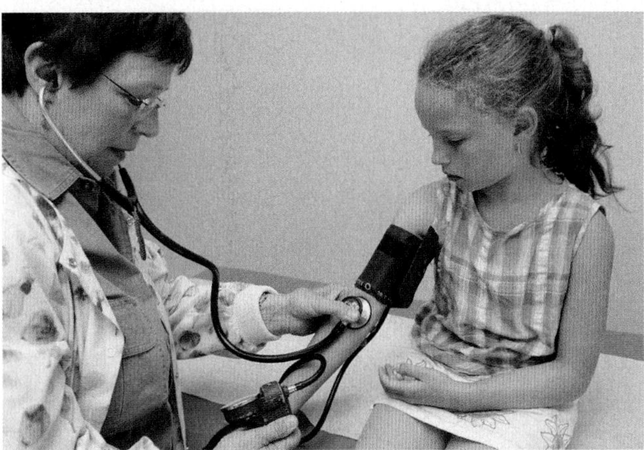

FIGURE 32.8 Auscultation is the preferred method for measuring blood pressure in children.

language barrier (Choueiry et al., 2020). The FLACC pain scale consists of a possible 10 points, with 0, 1, or 2 points given for each of five clinical signs (see Table 36.7).

Children who are older and can express that pain is worsening or improving should use the Pain Faces Scale (see Fig. 36.3). Explain that each face represents a person who is happy or sad, depending on how much or how little pain they have: 0 is for a person who is "very happy because they don't hurt at all;" 1 means "it hurts just a little bit;" 2, "it hurts a little more;" 3, "it hurts even more;" 4, "it hurts a whole lot;" and 5, "it hurts as much as you can imagine—but you don't have to be crying to feel this bad." Then ask the child to point to the face that best describes the amount of pain being felt (Wong & Baker, 1988).

For additional information related to pain assessment, refer to Chapter 36.

Body Measurements

Appropriate growth in children is usually an indicator of good health. A child who is not growing well may be in poor health, have inappropriate or inadequate dietary intake, or have a chronic disease. Accurate assessment of growth is a critical skill for the pediatric nurse.

Determine the child's height or length, weight, and weight for length or **body mass index (BMI)**. BMI is a reflection of weight in relation to height. Measure the head circumference for healthy children younger than age 2. Plot these measurements on a graph so they can be compared with earlier measurements and those of the child's peers' measurements. Additional anthropometric measurements used in children may include the chest circumference, midupper arm circumference, and skinfold measurement at the triceps, abdomen, or subscapular regions, but these are not performed routinely and are usually used only when a nutritionist consultation is necessary.

The growth chart is a screening tool for nutritional problems as well as a useful screen for chronic illness. Record each measurement in ink with a small dot at the correct location for the child's age and the date of the measurement written above it. Then use a plastic straightedge to connect the previous measurement to the most current one. Children grow at variable rates; in infancy and prepuberty, the growth velocity is normally more rapid. The growth chart allows the nurse to compare the child to other children of the same age and sex while allowing for normal genetic variation. When measurements fall close to the same percentiles over time, growth is normal for that child. Measurements falling within the following percentiles for age are generally considered the expected growth range:

- World Health Organization (WHO) growth charts (age birth to 2 years)—2nd to 98th percentile
- CDC growth charts (age 2 to 20 years)—5th to 85th percentile (CDC, 2022)

Sudden or sustained changes in percentile may indicate a chronic disorder, emotional difficulty, or nutritional intake problem. These findings require further assessment of the physical status of the child as well as other types of evaluations such as dietary intake or serum laboratory measurements. Appendix D provides growth charts for ages birth to 24 months and 2 to 20 years. The AAP and CDC recommend the use of these growth charts with all children, although special growth charts are also available for children with specific conditions (CDC, 2017). Look for a trend over time of healthy growth that is neither too fast nor too slow.

LENGTH OR HEIGHT

Calculate the length of the infant and toddler in a lying position until the age of 24 months. Use a measuring board (Fig. 32.9) or a cloth or paper measuring tape. Stretch out the legs to get a full extension of the body. Marking the examination paper at the child's head and extended foot is an option. Make sure that the growth chart where the measurement is plotted is marked for length and not height, as the two measurements differ. Document the length in centimeters and inches.

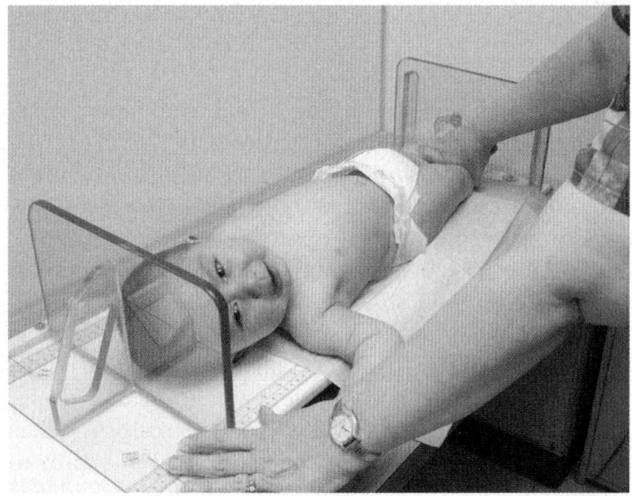

FIGURE 32.9 The recumbent measuring board is the most accurate method for obtaining a length measurement in infants and very young children.

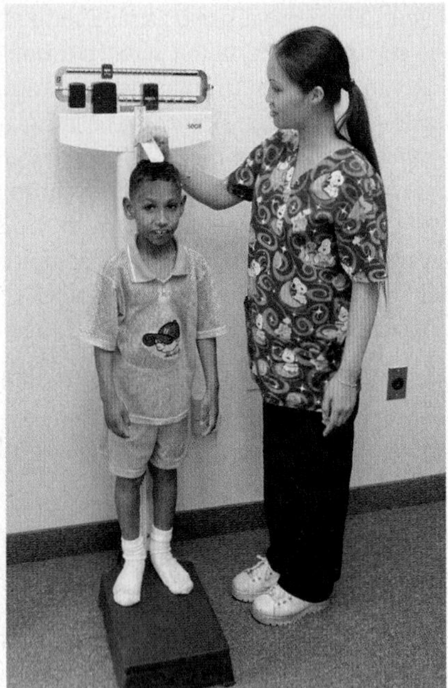

FIGURE 32.10 Standing height is most accurately measured with the stadiometer.

Once the child can cooperate and stand independently, begin measuring the standing height. Using a **stadiometer** is best (Fig. 32.10), but a cloth or paper tape can be used. Ask the child to remove their shoes and check that the back, shoulders, buttocks, and heels are against the wall, with the pelvis tucked as much as possible to correct for lordosis. The chin should be parallel to the floor. Plot this measurement on a growth chart marked for height rather than length. Record the height in centimeters as well as feet and inches.

TAKE NOTE!

Cloth and paper measuring tapes may stretch over time. Periodically replace or recalibrate all measuring tools.

WEIGHT

Measure weight on a scale that is calibrated between every measurement. Just before placing the child on the electronic scale, press the "zero" or "tare" button and make sure the reading is 0. Calibrate the balance-type scale by setting the weight at zero, observing the beam balance, and making adjustments as necessary. Infants and toddlers should be weighed on a platform-type electronic or balance scale, with an examination paper placed between the child and the scale surface. Calibrate the scale with the examination paper in place. Remove the infant's diaper immediately before placing them on the scale. Toddlers may sit on the scale with the nurse or caregiver nearby to avoid falls (Fig. 32.11). Weigh older children and adolescents on a standing scale (Fig. 32.12). They may keep their underpants on and wear a lightweight examination gown.

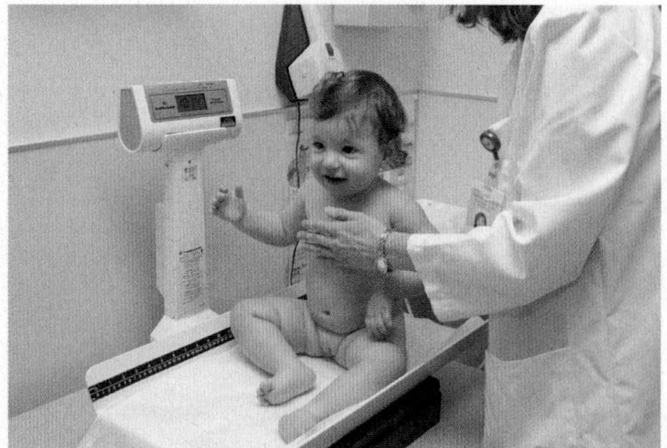

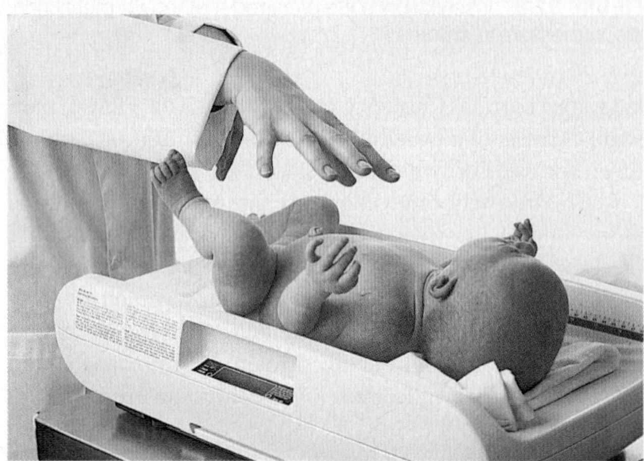

FIGURE 32.11 A nurse or caregiver should remain nearby while weighing the infant or toddler.

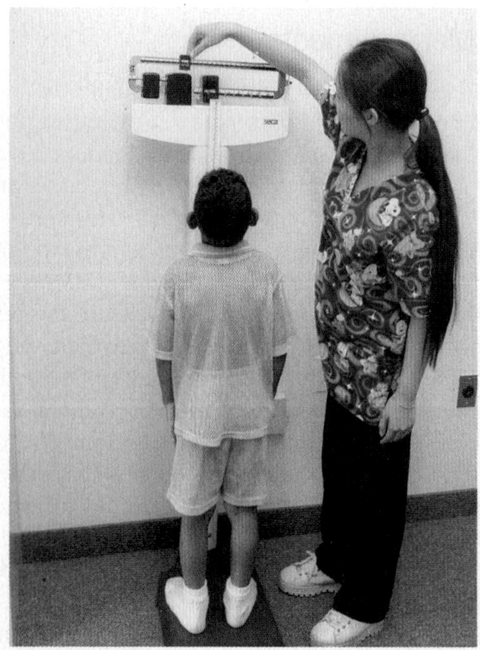

FIGURE 32.12 Children who can stand independently can be weighed on a regular standing balance scale.

An alternate method for obtaining weight, although much less accurate, is to weigh the caregiver initially and then weigh the caregiver holding the child. The difference between the two weights is the child's weight. Regardless of the method used, weigh the infant to the nearest 10 g (or half-ounce) and the toddler and older child to the nearest 100 g (or quarter pound). Record the weight in kilograms and in pounds.

WEIGHT FOR LENGTH

For children between the ages of newborn and 24 months, plot weight on the growth chart in comparison to the child's length. This allows the nurse to determine whether the child is a healthy weight for how long they are. Children placing less than the fifth percentile on the weight-for-length chart are considered lower weight. Those placing greater than the 95th percentile are considered to be overweight.

BODY MASS INDEX

BMI is determined by comparing the child's height and weight. Calculate the BMI using the child's weight and height by either the English or the metric method. Box 32.1 provides BMI calculation formulas. BMI is included on the charts for children ages 2 to 20 years. Plot the BMI on the growth chart according to the child's age. A child whose BMI for age plots at less than the fifth percentile is considered to be lower weight. BMI for age between the 85th and 95th percentiles indicates risk of overweight. BMI for age greater than the 95th percentile indicates the child is higher weight (CDC, 2022).

The growth chart can indicate when a child is not growing adequately and can also be used to predict the development of overweight and higher weight. Refer to the Healthy People 2030 box.

HEAD CIRCUMFERENCE

Measure head circumference at well-child visits and upon hospital admission until the third birthday. Then measure it at the annual well-child visit until 6 years old if there are problems such as microcephaly or macrocephaly present at age 3. Measure the largest point across the skull, not including the ears, with a nonstretching cloth or paper tape. Begin at the forehead just above the eyebrows and bring the tape around the head in a taut circle just above the occipital prominence at the back of the head (Fig. 32.13). Plot this measurement in relation to the child's age on the appropriate standardized growth chart (usual growth charts include head circumference only up to age 2 years).

BOX 32.1 Calculation of Body Mass Index (BMI)

English Formula

$$\frac{\text{weight in pounds}}{(\text{height in inches}) \times (\text{height in inches})} \times 703$$

Metric Formula

$$\frac{\text{weight in kilograms}}{(\text{height in meters}) \times (\text{height in meters})} \times 10{,}000$$

HEALTHY PEOPLE 2030

Objective	Nursing Significance
Reduce the proportion of children and adolescents with higher weight.	• Screen for overweight in all children by plotting weight for length of children younger than 24 months and body mass index for age for children aged 2–20 years. • Assess dietary intake and activity level in all children at risk for or overweight. • Provide diet and activity recommendations to attain a healthy weight or BMI. • Refer children with significant higher weight to a pediatric endocrinologist.

Healthy People Objectives retrieved from http://www.healthypeople.gov

Monitoring Equipment

Sometimes, children in acute care settings require continuous monitoring of vital signs. This monitoring could be via an apnea monitor or a cardiopulmonary monitor. The apnea monitor measures abnormal or irregular breathing in infants. The cardiopulmonary monitor generally measures heart rate and respiratory rate. Additional equipment on this monitor also allows for blood pressure and temperature monitoring. Set high and low alarm limits according to the health care facility's policies. Figure 32.14 indicates the placement of electrodes for the apnea and cardiopulmonary

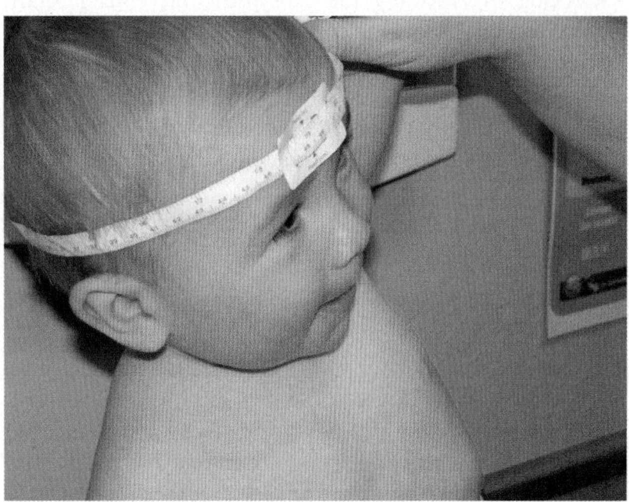

FIGURE 32.13 Measure occipitofrontal head circumference at the largest point.

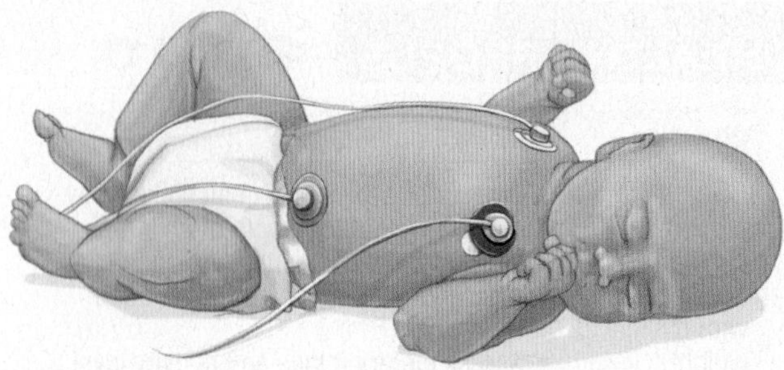

FIGURE 32.14 Placement of cardiac apnea monitor leads: white on the right upper chest, black on the left upper chest, green or red on the abdomen (not over bone).

monitors. Assess the skin where the electrodes are placed to ensure there is no skin breakdown. If the alarm sounds, immediately check the child to ensure the leads are not disconnected or the child is not in distress.

Skin

The skin is the body's largest organ and reveals information about a child's nutrition, respiratory, cardiac, endocrine, and hydration status at a glance. A careful skin examination provides an invaluable understanding of a child's health (Chiocca, 2020).

INSPECTION

Inspect the color of the skin. The color should be appropriate to the child's racial or ethnic background, with the nail beds, conjunctivae, soles of the feet, and palms of the hands appearing pink. Normal variations include the following:

- Blueness of the hands and feet, known as **acrocyanosis**, is normal in babies up to several days of age and results from an immature circulatory system completing the switch from fetal to extrauterine life (see Fig. 25.3A).
- Cooling or warming the newborn and young infant may produce a vasomotor response that causes a mottling of the skin over the trunk and extremities (see Fig. 25.3B).
- Babies of darkly pigmented parents will be paler than their parents for many months until the melanocytes in the epidermis begin production.
- Dark-skinned infants commonly have hyperpigmented areolas, genitals, and linea nigra.

Other variations related to skin color are discussed in Box 32.2.

Inspect the skin for the presence of lanugo. All infants display some degree of **lanugo** (soft, downy hair on the body, particularly the face and back). Lanugo is more abundant in infants of Hispanic descent and in premature infants and recedes over the first few weeks of life.

Inspect the entire body for nevi and vascular and other lesions. Note their location, size, distribution, characteristics, and color. Pigmented nevi (also termed "birthmarks") are indicated by a darker patch of skin and generally do not fade over time. Note the presence of hyperpigmented nevi (formerly called Mongolian spots), which appear as blue or gray, variably and irregularly shaped macules (Fig. 32.15). These are a common finding in dark-skinned infants. These nevi fade over months to years as the child's skin pigment darkens. Do not mistake hyperpigmented nevi for bruises. Inspect the skin for vascular lesions. Table 32.4 describes vascular lesions and their significance.

Rashes are common in children and are often associated with communicable diseases. Describe the rash in detail, noting types of lesions, distribution, drying, scabbing, scaling, and any drainage. The newborn and young infant may display milia (small white papules) on the forehead, chin, nose, and cheeks. These recede spontaneously. In adolescents, the skin examination may reveal open or closed comedones (pimples or blackheads) across the face, chest, and back. Adolescents may sport

BOX 32.2 Variations in Skin Color and Their Causes

- **Pallor** (defined as decreased pinkness in light-skinned patients, ashy-gray in dark-skinned) is caused by anemia, shock, fever, or syncope.
- **Central cyanosis** (blueness of the lips, tongue, oral mucosa, trunk) is caused by hypoxia or circulatory collapse.
- Overall yellow color (**jaundice**) may be physiologic in the newborn or related to liver or hematopoietic disease in any age child.
- **Yellowing** of nose, palms, and soles may result from excess intake of yellow vegetables.
- **Redness** of the skin results from blushing, exposure to cold, hyperthermia, inflammation (localized), or alcohol ingestion.
- **Lack of color** in skin, hair, and eyes is related to albinism

Data from Chiocca, E. M. (2020). *Advanced pediatric assessment* (3rd ed.). Springer Publishing Company; Jarvis, C., & Eckhardt, A. (2020). *Physical examination and health assessment* (8th ed.). Elsevier.

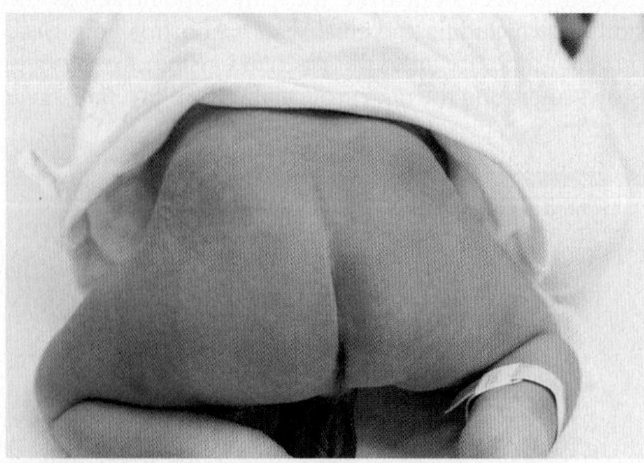

FIGURE 32.15 Transient hyperpigmentation most often occurs in darker-skinned infants.

TABLE 32.4 • Vascular Lesions and Their Significance

Description	Significance
Salmon nevi: light pink macule usually on eyelids, nasal bridge, back of neck ("stork bite")	Usually fade over time but may never go away completely. No complications
Strawberry nevus: raised reddish papule made of blood vessels (hemangiomas)	Present at or develop after birth; recede over time, usually by the age of 9 years. Usually no complications
Nevus flammeus: dark purple-red flat patch, grows with the child ("port-wine stain")	May be associated with Sturge–Weber syndrome. May be disfiguring; may be removed with laser therapy
Ecchymosis: purplish discoloration, changing to blue, brown, black (bruise)	Common on lower extremities in young children. Should correlate with the injury
Petechiae: pinpoint reddish-purple macules that do not blanch when pressed	Broken tiny blood vessels; occur with coughing, bleeding disorders, meningococcemia
Purpura: larger purple macules that do not blanch when pressed	Bleeding under the skin; occur with bleeding disorders, meningococcemia

Data from Chiocca, E. M. (2020). *Advanced pediatric assessment* (3rd ed.). Springer Publishing Company; Jarvis, C., & Eckhardt, A. (2020). *Physical examination and health assessment* (8th ed.). Elsevier.

tattoos, brandings, or various body piercings; inspect these areas for signs of infection such as erythema or drainage (Fig. 32.16).

Document the presence of any lacerations, abrasions, or burns. Note the distribution of the injury and whether it seems consistent with the mechanism described in the health history. Be alert to the possibility of child abuse if the type or number of burns, lacerations, or bruises seems unusual for the situation.

TAKE NOTE!

Petechiae or ecchymosis may be found over areas traumatized by the birth process; these may take a few weeks to resolve. Certain cultures use "cupping" or "coining" when a child is ill, and these practices may yield bruises or mild burns (Boos, 2022).

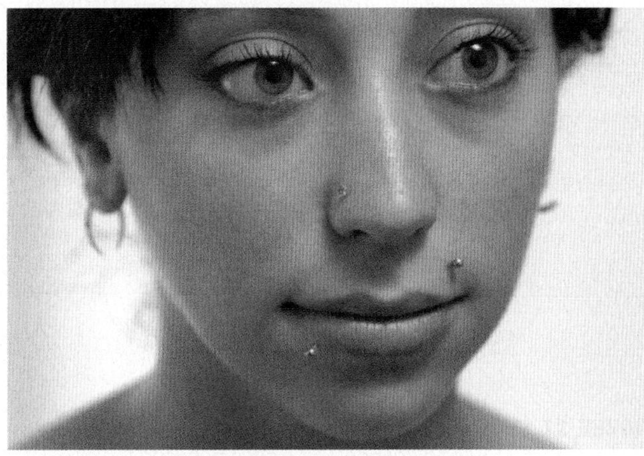

FIGURE 32.16 Adolescent with multiple piercings.

PALPATION

Palpate the skin for temperature, moisture, texture, turgor, and edema. Use the back of your hand to assess the skin's temperature, comparing the right side of the body to the left and the upper body to the lower. The skin should feel uniformly warm. Cool extremities are associated with environmentally cool temperatures as well as impending circulatory collapse and shock. Warm skin may be associated with fever or sunburn, or locally a burn or infectious process. The skin should feel fairly dry, occasionally moister in the creases. Dry, flaking skin may occur in the young infant, particularly if born postmaturely. Overall skin dryness in the well-hydrated child may occur with excess sun exposure, poor nutrition, or overbathing. Moist skin occurs with perspiration, fever resolution, and shock. The infant's and young child's skin is ordinarily soft. Older children should continue to have a smooth and even skin texture. The preadolescent and adolescent may have oily-feeling skin on the face, shoulders, or back.

Assess skin turgor by elevating the skin on the abdomen in the infant or on the back of the hand in the older child or adolescent. The "pinched-up" skin should quickly return to place. Skin that remains tented is strongly suggestive of moderate to severe dehydration. When edema is present, palpate the edematous area to determine its extent. Palpate any lumps or protrusions to determine firmness or tenderness. Palpate lesions or rashes with a gloved hand to document the size and extent of the lesions.

Hair and Nails

Inspect the hair and scalp, noting distribution of hair as well as color, texture, amount, and quality. The young infant's hair may be entirely absent or quite thick; it will be replaced by hair that is of a texture and color closer to what the child will have throughout childhood. Coarse, dry hair at any age may indicate a thyroid disorder or nutritional deficiency. Inspect the scalp thoroughly; it should be free from lesions and infestations. Note the presence of a greasy, scaly plaque on the scalp of infants; termed "seborrheic dermatitis" or "cradle cap," it is benign and easily treated.

Inspect the nails for color, shape, and condition. Full-term infants may have long, papery fingernails that can scratch their skin if not trimmed. Children should have healthy nails. Dry, brittle nails may indicate a nutritional deficiency. Inspect the skin around the nails to ensure that it is intact and without signs of infection. Many children (especially school-age children) have a nervous habit of nail biting or hangnail biting or pulling.

Inspect the school-age child's or adolescent's toenails to ensure they are trimmed in a horizontal fashion. Self-trimming of toenails either too low or in a curved fashion places the child at risk for the development of ingrown nails. Clubbing of the nails indicates chronic hypoxemia related to respiratory or cardiac disease. Nails that curve inward or outward may be hereditary or linked with injury, infection, or iron-deficiency anemia.

Head

Examining the head is critical in the newborn and infant periods but should not be overlooked in older children as an opportunity to check for diseases of the scalp and functional and developmental problems that are reflected in poor hygiene of the head and scalp. Note hair distribution and any bald or thinning areas. Use of gloves may be indicated, depending on the overall scalp cleanliness and chance of infestation by head lice (seen as small grayish specks near the base of hair shafts).

INSPECTION

Examine the head and face for shape and symmetry. In newborns, the head may be temporarily misshapen from uterine positioning or a lengthy vaginal delivery. Some infants have a slight flattening of the back of the head since the recommended sleeping position is supine. Note any irregularities or asymmetry. Observe the infant's head shape by looking down on it from above. Observe whether the head appears centered on the neck or tilts to one side. After 4 months of age, the infant should have achieved enough head control to hold the head erect and in midline when placed in a vertical position. Pull the infant from the supine position into sitting to determine the extent of head lag. To determine the extent of head control in older infants and children, ask the child to turn the head in different directions, either by simple commands or by following a colorful object.

Observe the infant's face when crying, smiling, or babbling for symmetry of muscle movement. In children who are old enough to follow directions, a game of "Simon Says" is a playful way to determine facial symmetry and strength; ask them to puff out their cheeks, make kisses, look surprised, stick out their tongue, and so on (effectively testing function of cranial nerve VII [facial]) (Chiocca, 2020).

> **TAKE NOTE!**
>
> When you note a flattened occiput in an infant, encourage the parent or caregiver to allow the infant "tummy time" while awake and observed and to change the infant's head position frequently when upright in an infant seat (Fahrenkopf et al., 2020).

PALPATION

Gently palpate the anterior and posterior fontanels (Fig. 32.17). The **fontanels** are the soft areas on the skull that remain open in infancy to allow for rapid brain growth in the first few months of life. Note the size of the fontanels. The anterior fontanel's size is 1 to 4 cm in either direction until it can no longer be felt when it is closed by the age of 9 to 18 months (Chiocca, 2020). The posterior fontanel is much smaller and may close any time between shortly after birth and approximately 2 months of age. The fontanels should not be depressed or taut and bulging, although it is not uncommon to see them pulsate or briefly bulge if the baby cries. In an acutely ill infant, assess the fontanels while obtaining the vital signs. Dehydration can cause the fontanels to be sunken; increased intracranial pressure and overhydration can cause them to bulge. Palpate the skull for asymmetry, overriding or open sutures, and lumps or other deformities. Palpate the jaw joints as the child bites down to assess cranial nerve V (trigeminal). Use the fingertips to palpate for occipital, postauricular, preauricular, submental, and submandibular lymph nodes, noting their size, mobility, and consistency (Fig. 32.18).

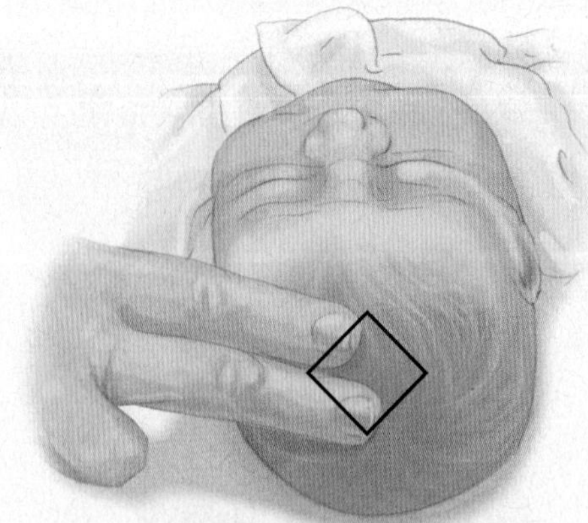

FIGURE 32.17 Note location and size of the fontanels. The anterior fontanel is diamond shaped and closes between the ages of 9 and 18 months.

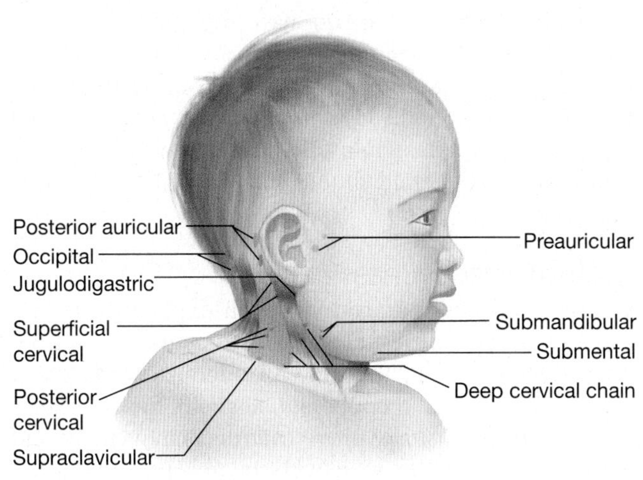

FIGURE 32.18 Location of lymph nodes.

> **TAKE NOTE!**
> A large fontanel may be associated with congenital hypothyroidism. Sagittal fontanel presence may occur with Down syndrome. A fontanel that becomes larger over time rather than smaller may indicate the development of hydrocephalus, especially if accompanied by an accelerated increase in head circumference (Chiocca, 2020).

Neck

Inspect the neck for symmetry. The infant's neck is short, but by 4 years of age the child's neck should be similar in appearance to the adult's. Webbing or excessive neck skinfolds may be associated with Turner syndrome, and lax neck skin may occur with Down syndrome. Assess the flexibility of the neck through a full range of motion. Take younger children through a passive range of motion. Older children will be able to look in all directions on command and stretch their chins to their chests themselves. Test cranial nerve XI (accessory) in the older child by having the child attempt to turn the head against resistance. Assessment of neck mobility is particularly important when infections of the central nervous system are suspected. Pain or resistance to range of motion may indicate meningeal irritation. Do not assess neck mobility in the trauma victim.

> **TAKE NOTE!**
> The infant or child who has experienced trauma should have the cervical spine maintained completely immobile until a radiologist has determined that the spinal cord is not damaged.

Palpate the neck for masses and lymph nodes. Palpate the cervical and clavicular lymph nodes with the distal part of the fingers using gentle but firm pressure in a circular motion. Tilt the child's head upward slightly to allow better access. Assess the lymph nodes for swelling, mobility, temperature, and tenderness. In healthy infants and adolescents, the cervical lymph nodes are usually not palpable; in healthy children between 1 and 11 years, the cervical nodes are often found to be small, nontender, and mobile (see Fig. 32.18 for locations of lymph nodes). Enlarged cervical lymph nodes frequently occur in association with upper respiratory infections and otitis media. Report significant enlargement to the health care provider or nurse practitioner. Palpate the trachea; the thyroid is usually palpable only in older children.

Eyes

Assessment of the eyes includes evaluation of the external and internal structures as well as screening for visual acuity. Any nurse caring for a child should be adept at examining the external structures. Assessment of the internal structures will also be covered later but is usually performed only by the advanced nurse practitioner. Refer to Chapter 31 for information on vision screening. Determination of visual acuity tests the function of cranial nerve II (optic).

EXTERNAL STRUCTURES

Observe the eyes for symmetry and spacing, even distribution of eyelashes and eyelids, and presence of epicanthal folds. Note the child's ability to blink and report an inability to do so. The eyes should look symmetric, and both should be facing forward in the midline when the child is looking directly ahead. The iris should be perfectly round, and the sclerae should be clear. The cornea should be uniformly transparent. Inspect the corners of the eye (medial and lateral canthus) and the conjunctiva (lining of the eyelids). They should be free of discharge, inflammation, or swelling. Epicanthal folds may be present in children of Asian descent, children with genetic abnormalities, or those with fetal alcohol spectrum disorder. Using a small penlight or ophthalmoscope, inspect the function and clarity of the pupil by putting your nondominant hand on the child's forehead and moving the light toward and away from each eye. This will elicit the blink reflex. Next, observe whether the pupil contracts with the light and expands when the light is removed. Make the same motion with a small toy or object, and direct the child to look at it. The eyes demonstrate **accommodation**, or focusing at different distances, if the pupil constricts as the object moves closer. If normal findings are present, report **PERRLA** (pupils are equal, round, reactive to light and accommodation) (Fig. 32.19). This is a particularly important assessment in head and eye injuries, as well as when other neurologic concerns are present.

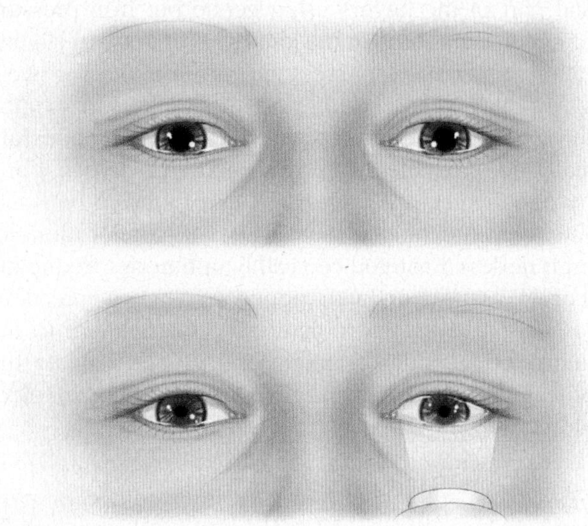

FIGURE 32.19 The pupils should be equal, round, and reactive to light and accommodation (PERRLA).

TAKE NOTE!

The infant may exhibit intermittent strabismus (crossing of the eyes) until about 4 months of age. However, persistent strabismus at any age or intermittent strabismus after 4 months of age should be evaluated by a pediatric ophthalmologist (Andre & Rockwell, 2022).

Check extraocular muscle motility and function of cranial nerves III and IV (oculomotor and abducens) by instructing the child to follow the light through the six cardinal positions of gaze. Infants and very young children will follow an interesting object. Instruct the older child to look downward and inward (testing cranial nerve IV [trochlear]). Assess eye muscle strength using two tests. Using the Hirschberg test, bring the penlight to the middle of your face and direct the child to look at it. The small dot of reflected light seen in the iris should be placed symmetrically in each eye (Fig. 32.20). The cover test also assesses eye muscle strength. Cover one of the child's eyes and instruct the child to focus on an interesting object. The eye should not waver. While the child is still focusing with the first eye, remove the cover from the second. Observe the uncovered eye for movement. Report any movement or drift.

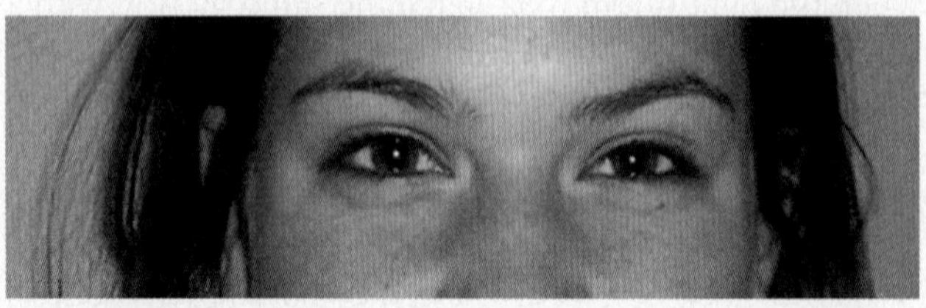

FIGURE 32.20 Note reflected light falling symmetrically on each pupil with the Hirschberg test.

To test peripheral vision, have the child focus on a specific point or object directly in front. Bring a finger or a small object from beyond the range of vision into the area of the peripheral vision. When the child sees the object from the side, while still focusing on the object or point in front, the child should say "stop." This also tests cranial nerve II (optic).

INTERNAL STRUCTURES

An advanced nurse practitioner with experience in this type of assessment best accomplishes assessment of the internal structures of the eye. An adequate assessment requires that the child cooperate. Restraint for eye examination does not usually prove fruitful, as movement and tearing of the eyes interfere with the accuracy of the examination. Use the ophthalmoscope to inspect the internal eye structures. Observe the glow of the pupil, which appears red (creamy colored in children with very dark eye color). Inspect the optic disc, macula, fovea, and blood vessels. Refer any child with blurring or bulging of the optic disc or hemorrhage of vessels to a pediatric ophthalmologist for further evaluation.

CLINICAL REASONING ALERT!

A child in an emergent situation should have a health history that is focused on the child's most immediate need. On the other hand, a comprehensive health history is appropriate for the child who is having his first visit at a pediatrician's office, for example.

Remember Elliot, the 3-year-old being seen for his annual examination? When you enter the room, he is hiding behind his parent's legs.

Ears

Assessment of the ears includes evaluation of the external and internal structures as well as screening for hearing. Any nurse caring for a child should be adept at examining the external structures. Assessment of the internal structures will also be covered further on but is usually performed only by the advanced nurse practitioner. Refer to Chapter 31 for information on hearing screening. Testing of hearing also tests the function of cranial nerve VIII (acoustic).

EXTERNAL STRUCTURES

Assess the placement of the external ears on the head. They should be symmetric and placed no lower than the eyes. The pinna should deviate no more than 10 degrees from an imaginary line that is perpendicular to a line drawn between the outer canthus of the eye and the top of the ear. Low-set ears may be associated with genetic abnormalities or syndromes (Fig. 32.21). Note protrusion or flattening of the ears, which may be normal for that child or may indicate inflammation (protrusion) or persistent side-lying

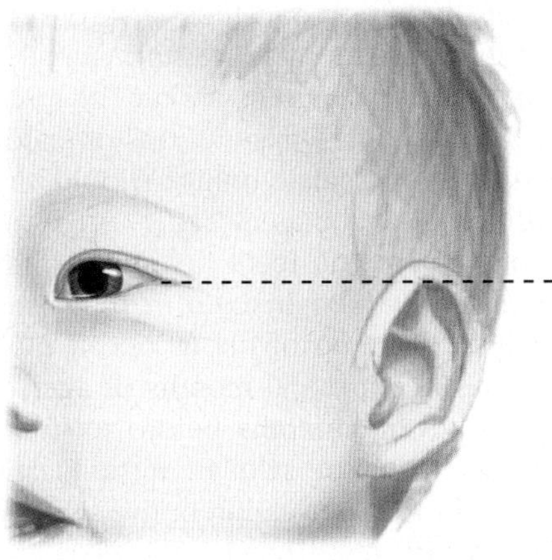

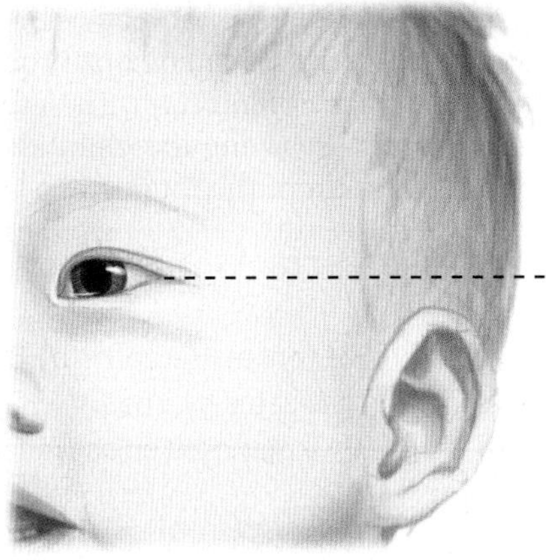

FIGURE 32.21 Low-set ears may be associated with chromosomal or other genetic anomalies.

(flattening). Note the presence of pits or skin tags in the preauricular area. Observe the exterior ear canal. A waxy cerumen that is soft and an orangish-brown color is normally found lubricating and protecting the external ear canal and should be left in place or washed gently away when bathing. Note drainage from the ear canal, which is always considered abnormal. Pull on the auricle and palpate the mastoid process, neither of which should result in pain in the healthy child.

TAKE NOTE!

Impacted and dry cerumen can be softened with a few drops of peanut, olive, or almond oil and then gently irrigated from the canal with an ear syringe and warm water (Sevy et al., 2023).

INTERNAL STRUCTURES

Use a **tympanometer** to assess the mobility of the eardrum (tympanic membrane). Gently pull down on the earlobe of infants and toddlers and up on the outer edge of the pinna in older children to straighten the ear canal, and press the tip of the tympanometer over the external canal. A reading of air pressure is recorded by the instrument, and this is useful to assess middle ear disease. Many tympanometers record a wave pattern that may be printed to include in the child's chart.

A nurse practitioner or health care provider generally performs inspection of the ear canal and tympanic membrane with an otoscope (Fig. 32.22). The otoscopic examination is usually performed near the end of the physical assessment for infants and young children, as they are often quite resistant to this intrusive procedure. The infant or toddler may require restraint in the parent's lap for the otoscopic evaluation. The preschooler may cooperate if the nurse uses a game such as looking for pretend puppies or potatoes in the child's ear. As with the tympanometer, gently pull down on the earlobe of the infant or toddler and up on the outer edge of the pinna in older children to straighten the ear canal. Use an otoscopic speculum appropriate to the size of the child's ear canal. Insert the speculum into the ear canal to visualize the canal and the tympanic membrane. The canal should be pink, should have tiny hairs, and should be free from scratches, drainage, foreign bodies, and edema. The tympanic membrane should appear pearly pink or gray and should be translucent, allowing visualization of the bony landmarks. It may be red if the child has been crying recently. Compress the pneumatic insufflator bulb to provide a puff of air; this causes motion of the tympanic membrane when the middle ear is healthy. Note abnormalities such as a fluid level; bubble or pus behind the tympanic membrane; tympanic membrane immobility; holes or perforations in the tympanic membrane; and the presence of tympanostomy tubes, scarring, or vesicles.

TAKE NOTE!

Never attempt to flush a foreign object out with water until it has been identified, because small pieces of sponge, clay, or vegetative material like peas or beans swell with water, further obstructing the ear canal (Yoon et al., 2022).

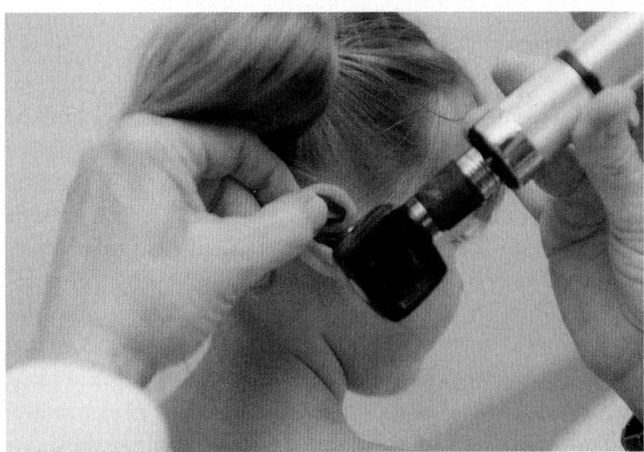

FIGURE 32.22 Otoscopic examination allows visualization of the internal structures of the ear.

Nose and Sinuses

The nose, as with all facial features in a child, should be symmetric, but it can be displaced temporarily by birth trauma in newborns. Ensure the nares provide unobstructed airflow by alternately occluding one nostril at a time and observing for air movement through the other nostril. If the child is breathing comfortably, there should be little nostril movement visible. Adolescents may have pierced their nose or nasal septum; ensure that the site is free from infection or loose jewelry that could migrate into the sinuses. Ideally, the nose should not be draining, although clear mucus may be present if the child has been crying. Assess the amount, color, thickness, and presence of any odor if drainage is present. Inspect the interior of the nose by tilting the child's head backward and pushing the tip of the nose upward. Direct the beam of a penlight in the nostril. The nasal mucosa should be uniformly firm, pink, and free from edema, excoriation, or masses. Test the older child's sense of smell by having the child close the eyes and identify a familiar scent such as peppermint or coffee (cranial nerve I [olfactory]). Palpate the sinuses for tenderness.

> ***TAKE NOTE!***
>
> Infants younger than 1 month of age are **obligate nose breathers**, which allows for swallowing without aspiration during breast or artificial nipple feeding (Smith, 2022).

Mouth and Throat

Wear a powder-free glove to examine the mouth, teeth, and throat. Inspection of the exterior of the mouth may be done at any point in the examination. Infants and young children may find assessment of the mouth and particularly the pharynx and uvula to be quite intrusive, so delay that part of the assessment until the end of the examination, after otoscopic evaluation. Assess the character and quality of the child's voice and the infant's cry. It should be neither too hoarse nor too shrill.

INSPECTION OF THE MOUTH

Observe the lips for color, symmetry, and absence of inflammation or edema. Salivation in infants begins at about 3 months of age; drooling occurs because the infant does not learn to swallow saliva until several months later. Next, inspect the interior of the mouth. The mouth is the first part of the digestive system, and a pink, moist, healthy mucosal lining is indicative of a healthy gastrointestinal tract. In infants, the tongue should lie within the mouth at rest and should be capable of extending over the lower gum line to help the baby feed. The tongue extrusion reflex is normal in infants until the age of 6 months and allows the infant to suckle easily from birth. Observe movement of the tongue when the infant or young child babbles or cries. Ask the older child to touch the tongue to the roof of the mouth and then stick out the tongue and move it from side to side (testing cranial nerve XII [hypoglossal]). Full movement should be present, and the tongue should be free from lesions or exudate. Visualize the hard and soft palate (which should be intact) or palpate with the gloved finger.

Most infants have no teeth before the fifth to sixth month. When the teeth begin to erupt, they usually erupt symmetrically at the rate of about one a month, until toddlers have 20 teeth by 30 months of age. The infant may drool for several months before teething. During teething, the gums will be swollen at the location of the impending tooth. In older children, the secondary teeth replace the primary teeth much more slowly and with little discomfort from ages 5 to 20. Figure 32.23 shows the usual permanent tooth eruption pattern.

Look for dental caries or alignment problems, and inspect the gums for signs of infection. Test cranial nerve IX (glossopharyngeal) by having the child identify taste with the posterior portion of the tongue.

> ***TAKE NOTE!***
>
> Natal (present at birth) or neonatal (erupting by 30 days of age) teeth should be evaluated by a pediatric dentist for potential extraction, as they may pose an aspiration risk (Smith, 2022).

INSPECTION OF THE THROAT

Inspect the tonsils, uvula, and oropharynx. Assess the infant's throat during a yawn or cry, as any forcible attempt to depress the tongue with a tongue depressor produces a strong reflex elevation of the base of the tongue that completely blocks the view of the pharynx. The young child will require restraint so that the nurse can depress the tongue and visualize the back of the mouth without injuring the child (Fig. 32.24). Asking the older child to open wide, stick out the tongue, and say "aaaah" simultaneously will allow for a quick look at the tonsils and pharynx without the need to use a tongue depressor, but the nurse must be quick because the tongue rises rapidly after those maneuvers are performed.

Tonsils usually cannot be seen in the infant. As the child becomes a toddler, the tonsils become dramatically larger and then begin to decrease in size again by age 9. The tonsils should be pink and often have crypts on their surfaces, which are sometimes filled with debris. Ensure that the uvula is midline and rises if the gag reflex is elicited (cranial nerve X [vagus]). Inspect the oropharynx, which should be pink and free from exudate.

Thorax and Lungs

Assessment of the thorax and lungs begins by observing the shape and contour of the thorax and determining the

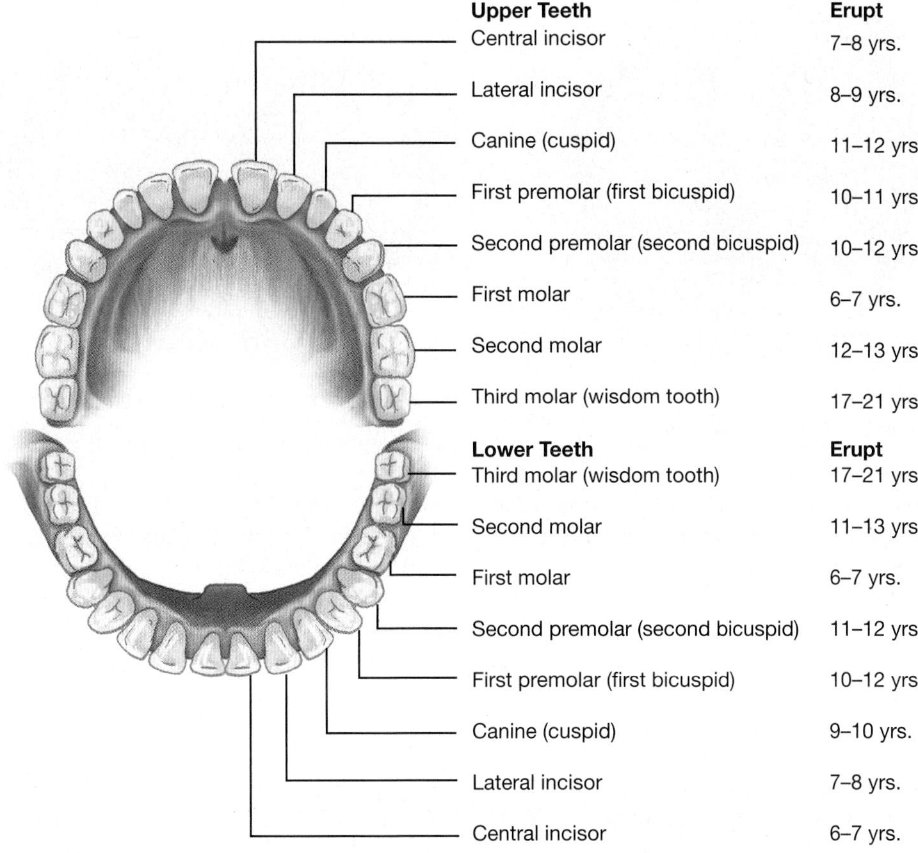

FIGURE 32.23 Usual sequence of permanent tooth eruption.

work of breathing. Accurate auscultation of the lungs is essential since children often have respiratory infections and disorders and may exhibit alterations in respiratory effort and breath sounds. Note the child's color, which should be pink; cyanosis indicates hypoxia. Listen for audible stridor (inspiratory high-pitched sound), expiratory grunting or snoring, audible wheezing (heard with the naked ear), or cough. Document type and extent of cough. Observe the nail beds for clubbing, which occurs with diseases inducing chronic hypoxic states.

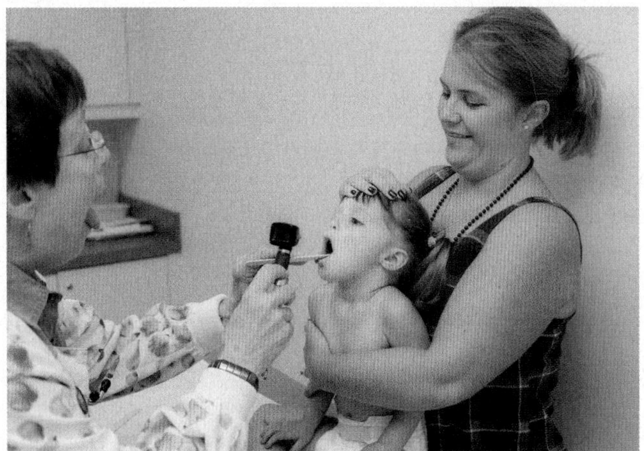

FIGURE 32.24 The young child may need to be restrained so that the throat examination can be done safely.

THORAX

Examine the chest with the head in a midline position to determine size and shape as well as symmetry, movement, and bony landmarks. The newborn's chest should be smooth and round, with the transverse diameter nearly equal to the anterior–posterior diameter. The shape of the chest progresses to that of the adult by the age of 5 to 6 years. At that time, the anterior–posterior diameter is about half the transverse diameter (Fig. 32.25). At the point where the xiphoid process and the right and left costal margins meet, the costal angle should measure 90 degrees or less. Inspect for structural deformity such as pectus excavatum (depressed sternum) or pectus carinatum (protuberant sternum) (Fig. 32.26). Note symmetric movement of the chest wall with respiration. Infants and younger children are primarily diaphragmatic breathers, so the abdomen and chest will rise and fall together. Older children, particularly adolescent females, demonstrate thoracic breathing, yet the abdomen and chest should continue to rise and fall together. Asymmetry of chest wall movement is an abnormal finding.

Observe the depth and regularity of respirations, noting the length of the inspiratory and expiratory phases

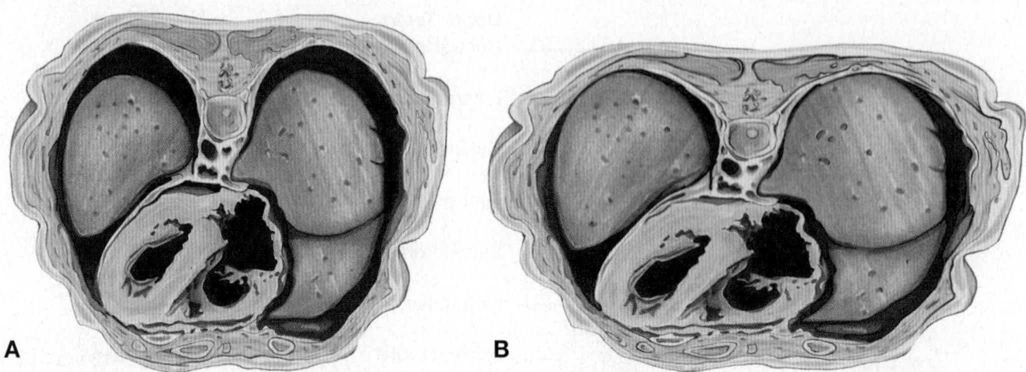

FIGURE 32.25 **A.** The newborn's chest is round. **B.** The adult chest has an anterior–posterior diameter about half the transverse diameter.

in relation to each other. The newborn and young infant demonstrate an irregular respiratory pattern. Older infants and children should have a more regular respiratory pattern.

Assess the child's respiratory effort by first observing for nasal flaring, which indicates labored breathing. Observe the chest wall and shoulders for accessory muscle use, which normally is not present. If retractions are present, note their location and severity. Typical locations for retraction include the intercostal, subcostal, substernal, suprasternal, and clavicular regions (Fig. 32.27). Pay attention to the position the child naturally assumes to breathe comfortably; children in respiratory distress often sit forward and are uncomfortable lying down or talking (Jarvis & Eckhardt, 2020).

LUNGS

Experienced examiners may palpate and percuss the lungs before using auscultation to evaluate the breath sounds.

Palpation and Percussion

Palpate for symmetric respiratory excursion by placing the thumbs and fingers together along the costal margin on the chest or back. Movement should be symmetric with each breath. Palpate for the normal presence of tactile fremitus with the palms or fingertips while the infant is crying or while the older child says "99." Indirectly percuss the lungs of older children, noting resonance over lung fields. Hyperresonance may be present in conditions resulting in hyperaeration of the lungs, such as asthma.

Auscultation

Use the bell of the stethoscope or switch to a small diaphragm to auscultate lung sounds in the infant or child. The adult-sized diaphragm may be used for the adolescent. Auscultate the lung fields with the infant or child in a sitting position, even if that requires propping the infant in a parent's lap. Infants and young children have loud breath sounds because of their thin chest walls. Breath sounds should be clear with adequate aeration throughout all lung fields. Listen to a full inspiration and expiration at the apices of the lungs as well as symmetrically across the entire lung field, systematically comparing the right to the left side. Listen on the anterior chest, on the posterior chest, and in the axillary regions.

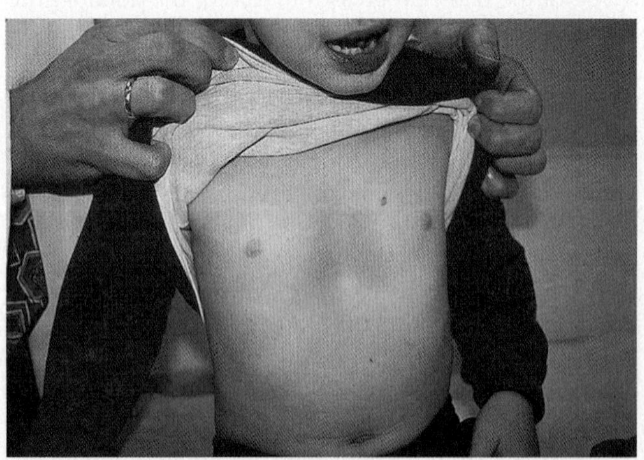

FIGURE 32.26 Pectus excavatum: note depression in xiphoid area.

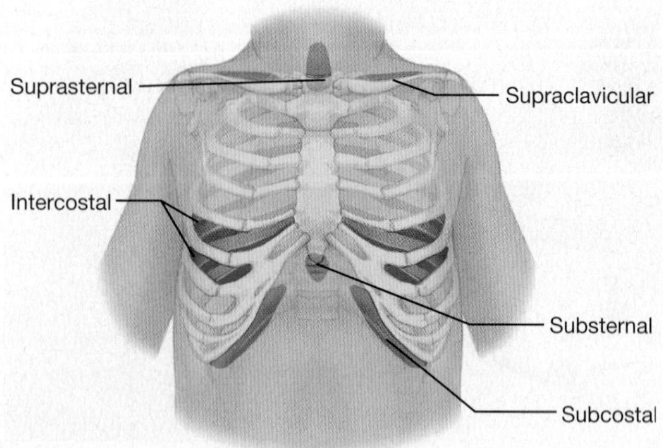

FIGURE 32.27 Location of retractions.

Playing games may encourage younger children to cooperate with deep breathing during lung assessment. The child can blow a cotton ball up in the air, blow a pinwheel, or "blow out" the light of the penlight (Miller, n.d.). Older children are capable of deep breathing when instructed to do so.

The child who has a respiratory disorder or who is experiencing respiratory distress may exhibit diminished breath sounds, most often in the lung bases. Diminished breath sounds are softer and quieter than lung sounds demonstrating adequate aeration. In the healthy infant or child, no adventitious sounds should be heard. If noisy breath sounds are heard in the infant or young child, particularly over all lung fields, compare the sound to the noises heard over the trachea or below the nares. Infants and young children with secretions in the nasopharyngeal area may have those sounds transmitted over the lung fields. These sounds usually clear with coughing or airway suctioning; they are not true adventitious sounds. Note adventitious breath sounds such as wheezes or crackles, documenting their location and whether they are present on inspiration, expiration, or both. It is most important to describe the abnormal breath sounds being heard rather than attempting to classify the sounds. Adventitious lung sounds are associated with a variety of disorders, and extensive experience is required to appropriately classify lung sounds. Adventitious breath sounds should be reported for further evaluation.

Breasts

Assess the breasts of children of all ages and sexes. Note the size of the breasts in relation to the age of the child. Palpate the axillary lymph nodes during the breast assessment.

INSPECTION

Observe the breasts for position, shape, size, symmetry, and color. Newborns of any sex may have swollen nipples from the influence of maternal estrogen, but by several weeks of age, the nipples should be flat and should continue to be so in all prepubertal children. In children, the nipples are located lateral to the midclavicular line, usually between the fourth and fifth ribs. The areola becomes darker in color as the child approaches puberty. Children with higher weight may appear to have enlarged breasts due to adipose tissue. Note the location of additional (supernumerary) nipples if present (usually located along the mammary ridge); they may appear as darkly pigmented, elevated, or nipple like spots. These are usually of no concern as they do not change over time, but they may be associated with kidney disorders.

Inspect the breasts for the current stage of development: widening of the areola, elevation of the nipple, and increase in breast size. Female breast development may begin as early as age 8 but usually starts by age 13. Breast development then continues in a characteristic, but usually asymmetric, pattern, with one breast larger than the other throughout the lifespan. The sexual maturity rating scale developed by Tanner in 1962 is used to describe breast development (**Tanner stages**) (Fig. 32.28). Adolescent males may develop gynecomastia (enlargement of the breast tissue) due to hormonal pubertal changes. When the hormone levels stabilize, male adolescents then have flat nipples. Occasionally, gynecomastia is caused by cannabis use, H_2 blockers, phenytoin, or hormonal dysfunction (Gilmore & Hay, 2021).

PALPATION

Palpate the breasts in a systematic fashion. A tender nodule palpated just under the nipple confirms pubertal changes. This change may be difficult to assess in patients with excessive adipose tissue. Normal breast tissue should feel smooth, firm, and elastic. Note masses or nodules if present. Palpate for axillary lymph nodes with the child's arms relaxed at the side but slightly abducted. Note size and texture of nodes if present.

Heart and Peripheral Perfusion

The examination of the heart in children is identical to that of adults except for the focus of the examiner's attention. Congenital heart defects are the most common cause of heart problems in children, and children with these defects present differently than adults with heart disease.

> ***TAKE NOTE!***
>
> The younger the child, the more responsive the heart rate is to activity changes. It increases with fever, fear, crying, or anxiety and decreases with sleep, sedation, or vagal stimulation (Jarvis & Eckhardt, 2020).

INSPECTION

Observe the child's posture. Note the presence of pallor, cyanosis, mottling, or edema, which may indicate a cardiovascular problem. Inspect the anterior chest from the side or at an angle, noting symmetry in shape as well as movement. Observe for the apical impulse, which is visible in about half of children. It occurs at the **point of maximum intensity (PMI)**, which is located at the third to fourth intercostal space just medial of the child's left midclavicular line until the age of 4 years, at the fourth intercostal space at the left midclavicular line in children ages 4 to 6 years, and then lateral to the left midclavicular line at the fifth intercostal space in children ages 7 years and older (Fig. 32.29). Note clubbing of the fingertips or distention of neck veins, both of which may be associated with congenital heart defect.

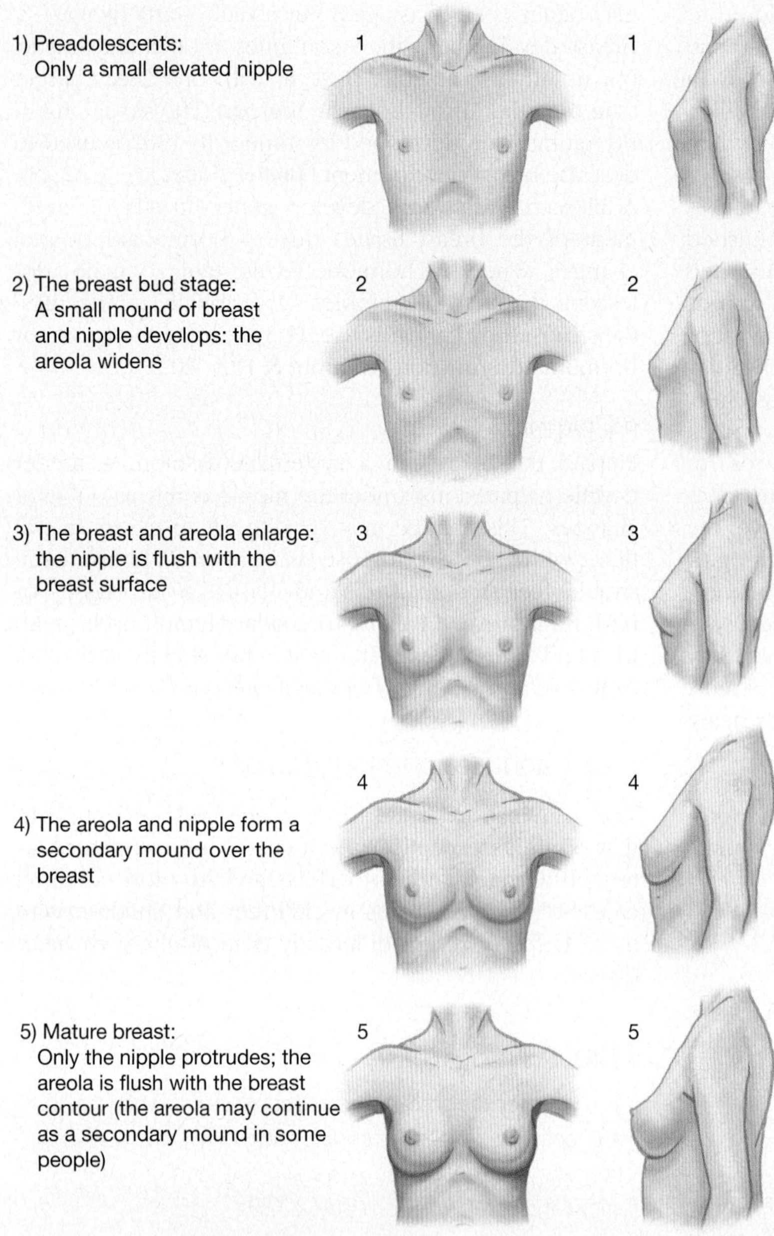

1) Preadolescents:
Only a small elevated nipple
1
1
2) The breast bud stage:
A small mound of breast and nipple develops: the areola widens
2
2
3) The breast and areola enlarge:
the nipple is flush with the breast surface
3
3
4) The areola and nipple form a secondary mound over the breast
4
4
5) Mature breast:
Only the nipple protrudes; the areola is flush with the breast contour (the areola may continue as a secondary mound in some people)
5
5

FIGURE 32.28 Tanner sexual maturity rating for breast development. (Adapted from Tanner, J. M. [1962]. *Growth at adolescence*. Blackwell Scientific Publications.)

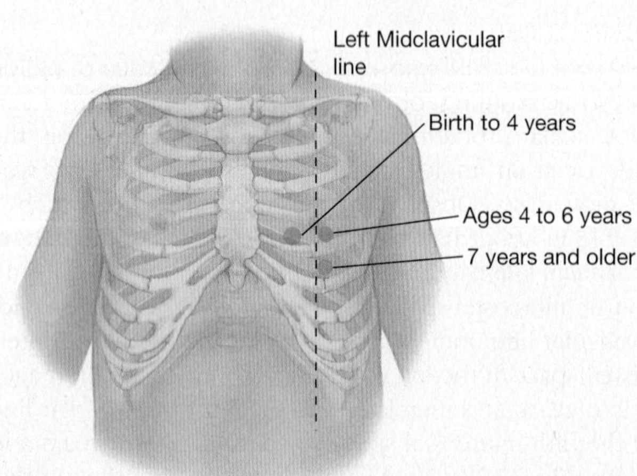

FIGURE 32.29 The point of maximum intensity (PMI) or apical impulse.

PALPATION

Using the fingertips, palpate the chest for lifts and heaves or thrills, which are not normal. Palpate the apical pulse in the area of the PMI (see Fig. 32.29). Check the pulses and compare the upper body to the lower body pulses, as well as left versus right, noting strength and quality (Fig. 32.30). The pedal, brachial, and femoral pulses are usually easily palpated. The radial pulse is very difficult to palpate in children younger than 2 years. Note the warmth of the distal extremities. To assess capillary refill time, place slight pressure on the nail beds and quickly release it. Observe the length of time required for refill and return to original color. Compare capillary refill time of the fingers to the toes. A capillary refill time of less than 3 seconds indicates adequacy of perfusion.

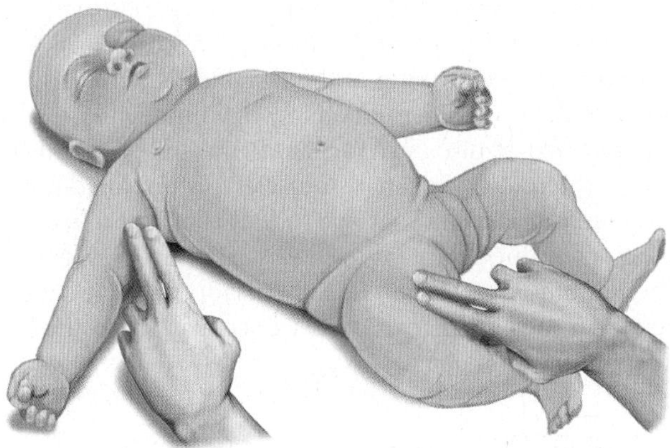

FIGURE 32.30 It is important to assess brachial and femoral pulses simultaneously to determine equality or differences in strength and intensity.

AUSCULTATION

Perform auscultation of the heart with the child in two different positions, upright and reclined (Fig. 32.31). Auscultate the heart rate in the area of the PMI as this is the point on the chest wall where the heartbeat is heard most distinctly (see Fig. 32.29). As you begin auscultation, listen first for respirations and note their timing so as not to confuse the heart sounds with the lung sounds. A crying infant may help by briefly holding their breath between cries. Once you are confident that you are listening to the heart, be sure to listen for 1 full minute because of the irregularity of rhythms in some children. Count the heart rate, which should be consistent with the palpated pulse (either radial or brachial, depending on the child's age).

Develop a systematic approach to auscultation of the heart. Listen over all four valvular areas anteriorly (Fig. 32.32). In the infant or younger child, also auscultate the heart in the axillary region and posteriorly (certain murmurs radiate to these areas). Note S_1, S_2, extra heart sounds, or murmurs. S_1 is usually loudest at the mitral and tricuspid areas and increases in intensity with fever, exercise, and anemia. S_2 is usually most intense at the aortic and pulmonic areas. A split S_2 heard at the apex occurs in many infants and young children. S_3 may be heard in many healthy children and is considered normal, although the child with a chronic cardiac condition may develop an S_3 when congestive heart failure is present. S_4 is usually considered abnormal, most often occurring with cardiac disease.

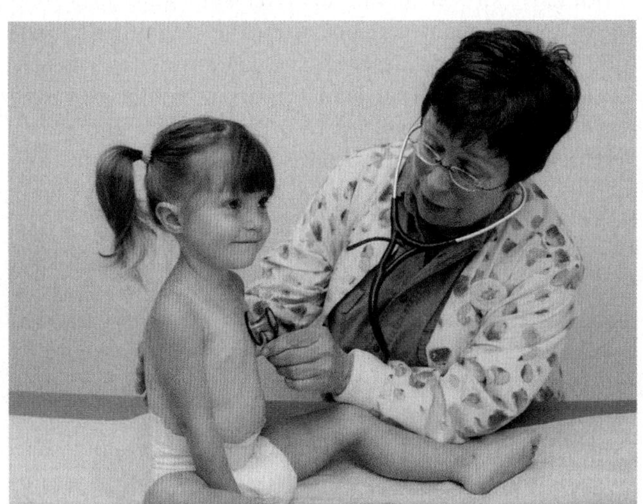

FIGURE 32.31 Auscultating the child's heart.

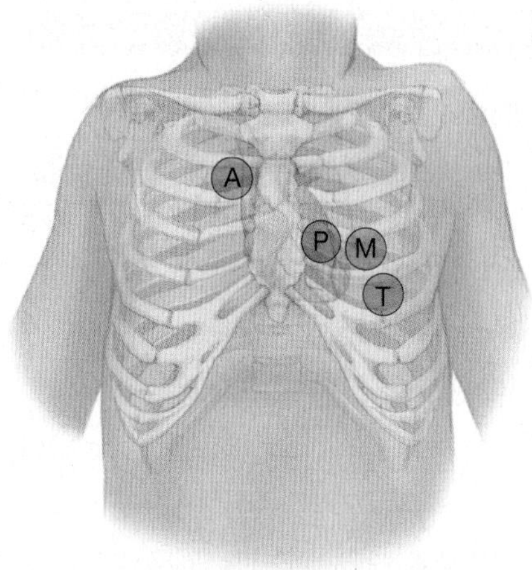

FIGURE 32.32 Areas where the sounds of heart valves radiate. A, Aortic valve—second intercostal space, just right of sternum; P, Pulmonic valve—second intercostal space, just left of sternum; T, Tricuspid valve—fourth intercostal space, just left of sternum; M, Mitral valve—fourth intercostal space at left midclavicular line.

Sinus arrhythmia is a common and normal finding in children and adolescents. It results in an irregular heart rhythm: the heart rate increases with inhalation and decreases with exhalation. If the child holds their breath, the rhythm becomes regular.

Auscultate for murmurs. Note the location (where it is heard best or loudest) and timing of the murmur. A systolic murmur occurs in association with S_1 (closure of the atrioventricular valves), a diastolic murmur in association with S_2 (closure of the semilunar valves). Also note the duration of murmur. Does it occur early or late in diastole or systole? Does it occur all the way across systole (holosystolic)? Note the intensity of the murmur. Table 32.5 discusses grading of murmur intensity.

Innocent murmurs occur in about 40% to 50% of children at some point throughout childhood. A Still murmur is most common, usually occurring between 2 and 7 years of age. It occurs in early systole, is best heard between the apex and left lower sternal border, and is usually medium pitched and musical. A venous hum that is heard in the infraclavicular area and possibly radiating down the chest is considered an innocent murmur. Often an innocent murmur disappears when the child changes position. Refer any child with a murmur to an experienced practitioner for further evaluation (Jone et al., 2022).

TABLE 32.5 • Grading Heart Murmurs in Children

Grade	Sound
1	Barely audible; sometimes heard, sometimes not. Usually heard only with intense concentration
2	Quiet, soft; heard each time the chest is auscultated
3	Audible, intermediate intensity
4	Audible, with a palpable thrill
5	Loud, audible with edge of the stethoscope lifted off the chest
6	Very loud, audible with the stethoscope placed near but not touching the chest

Data from Jone, P.-N., Kim, J. S., Burkett, D., Jacobson, R., & Von Alvensleben, J. (2022). Cardiovascular diseases. In M. Bunik, W. W. Hay, M. J. Levin, & M. J. Abzug (Eds.), *Current diagnosis & treatment: Pediatrics* (26th ed.). McGraw-Hill.

Abdomen

The abdomen contains organs related to the genitourinary and lymphatic systems, in addition to the gastrointestinal system. These structures lie within the abdomen in approximately the same location as they do in adults. Dividing the abdomen into quadrants simplifies the description of normal organ location and the reporting of abnormalities. Draw an imaginary vertical line from the xiphoid process to the symphysis pubis. Cross this with an imaginary perpendicular line through the umbilicus. The sequence of physical examination is altered for the abdominal assessment: auscultation is done before percussion and palpation because manipulation of the lower abdomen may affect the bowel sounds (Chiocca, 2020).

INSPECTION

Inspect the abdomen for size, shape, and symmetry. The abdomen in the infant and toddler is rounded and protuberant until the abdominal musculature becomes well developed. Although rounded, the abdomen should not be distended (at any age). By adolescence, the stature is more erect, and the abdomen begins to appear flat when standing and concave when supine. The thin skin of a young child may allow the visualization of superficial venous circulation across the abdomen. Inspect the abdomen for movement. At eye level with the abdomen, note abdomen and thorax movement occurring simultaneously. Visible peristaltic waves are abnormal and should be reported immediately.

Inspect the newborn's umbilicus for color, bleeding, odor, and drainage. The umbilical stump should slowly dry, become black and hard, and fall away from the cutaneous navel by the end of the second week of life. Note drainage or granulation at the umbilical site, indicating delayed drying of the umbilical stump. Inspect the umbilicus in older infants and young children for the presence of umbilical hernia. Because the umbilicus divides the rectus abdominis muscle, it is not uncommon to see an umbilical hernia protrude through and become larger when the infant or toddler strains or cries. This is a benign finding and will usually disappear as the abdomen becomes stronger. Adolescents may have jewelry piercing the umbilicus.

AUSCULTATION

Auscultate the abdomen using the diaphragm or the bell of the stethoscope pressed firmly against the abdomen. Count the bowel sounds in each of the four quadrants for a full minute. Bowel sounds should be present by a few hours after birth and should remain active throughout life. Note whether bowel sounds are normally active, hyperactive, hypoactive, or absent. Normal bowel sounds can be described as growls, gurgles, and clicking sounds. Hypoactive bowel sounds may occur postoperatively. Hyperactive bowels sounds are common with diarrhea. Classify bowel sounds as absent after listening for 5 full minutes in each area. Absent bowel sounds may indicate ileus or peritonitis.

PERCUSSION

Indirectly percuss all areas of the abdomen. Normal findings include dullness along the costal margins and tympany over the remainder of the abdomen. A full bladder may yield dullness to percussion.

PALPATION

Palpate the abdomen with the child in a supine position. If the child's legs are small enough, the knees may be brought up with the nondominant hand to flex the hips and relax the abdomen. Palpate all four quadrants of the abdomen in a systematic fashion, first lightly and then deeply. Apply light pressure with the fingertips to perform light palpation, assessing for tenderness and muscle tone (Fig. 32.33). Note skin turgor by gently elevating a piece of skin and allowing it to fall back into place. Perform deep palpation to assess the organs and any masses. Place one hand on top of the other and palpate from the lower quadrants to the upper (see Fig. 32.33). The edge of the liver may be felt at the right costal margin, and the tip of the spleen can be felt at the left costal margin. The descending colon may be felt in the left lower quadrant as a small column and the bladder as a soft balloon below the umbilicus. The kidneys are rarely palpable. The abdomen should be soft and nontender to palpation. Report firmness, tenderness, or masses. Palpate the inguinal area for the presence of hernia or enlarged lymph nodes.

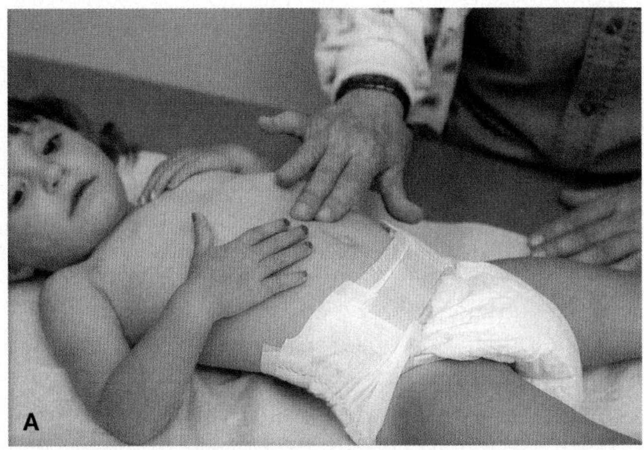

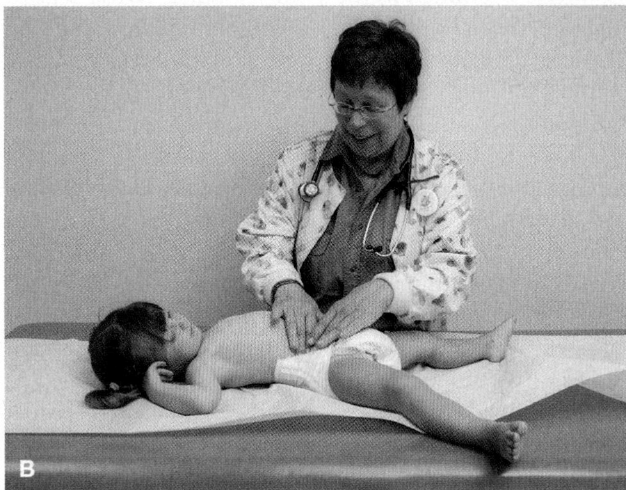

FIGURE 32.33 (**A**) Light and (**B**) deep palpation of the abdomen.

TAKE NOTE!

To decrease ticklishness with abdominal palpation, place a flat, warm, still hand on the abdomen while distracting the child before palpation begins. An alternate technique is to first palpate with the child's hand over the examiner's hand.

Genitalia and Anus

Examination of the genitals should immediately follow the abdominal assessment in the younger child and should be reserved for the end of the assessment in the adolescent. Although the anus is part of the gastrointestinal tract, it is best assessed during the genital examination. The AAP recommends that a parent chaperone the genitalia and anus examination of the infant and the child. In the case of the adolescent, a medical provider chaperone is recommended (Dev & Cruz, 2017).

Ensure privacy for the older child and adolescent. Keep the child covered as much as possible. Use a casual, matter-of-fact approach to place the child or adolescent at ease. During the genital examination, teach the child or adolescent about normal variations and changes with puberty, as well as issues related to health promotion.

MALE

Inspect the penis and scrotum for size, color, skin integrity, and obvious masses. With higher weight, the penis may appear small because of additional skinfolds. Penis size should correlate with pubertal stage (Fig. 32.34). The penis may have a foreskin that covers the glans, protecting and lubricating it. If present, do not forcibly retract the foreskin. In circumcised penises, the urinary meatus is

From top to bottom:

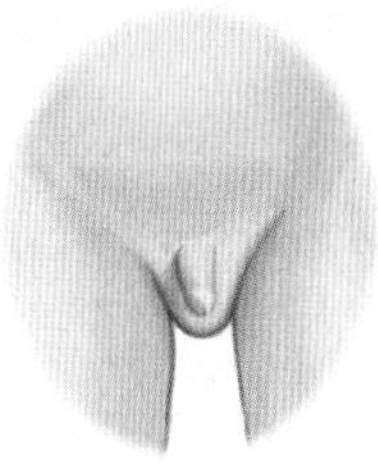

1) No pubic hair and scrotum size and proportion the same as during childhood

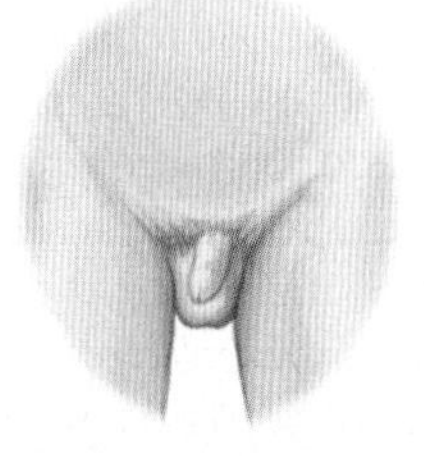

2) Few straight hairs at base of penis, little or no penis enlargement, testes/scrotum begin to enlarge

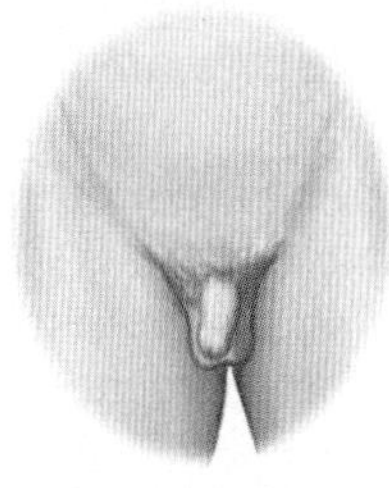

3) Sparse pubic hair growth over entire pubis, penis begins to lengthen, scrotum continues to enlarge

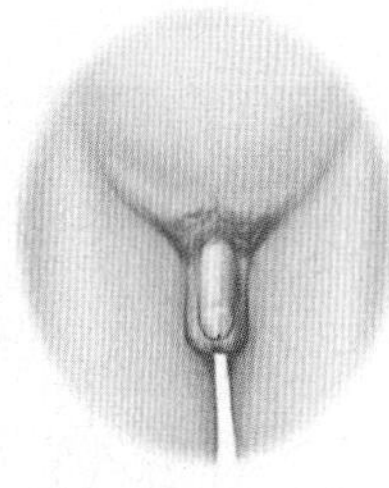

4) Thick pubic hair growth but not on thighs, penis grows in length and diameter, testes almost full grown

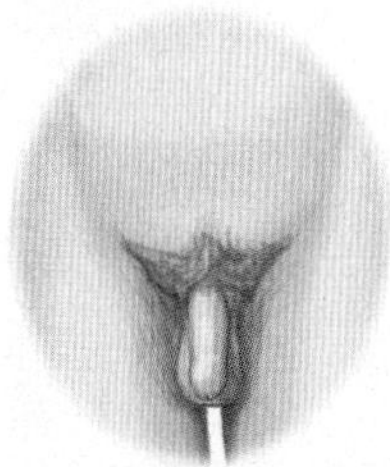

5) Pubic hair growth spread over medial thighs, penis and scrotum are adult size and shape

FIGURE 32.34 Tanner male sexual maturity rating for genitalia and pubic hair. (Adapted from Tanner, J. M. [1962]. *Growth at adolescence*. Blackwell Scientific Publications.)

exposed and should be at the tip of the glans. Assess the meatus for absence of discharge. If possible, observe the stream of urine for strength of flow and patency of the urethral orifice. Skin lesions may indicate sexually transmitted infection. A foreskin that cannot be retracted in a person older than 3 years may indicate phimosis. Report abnormal findings.

TAKE NOTE!

When you first remove a male infant's diaper, this is the ideal time to assess the force of the urine stream and the erection reflex, as the cool air may make the infant void and briefly experience an erection.

Assess the presence and distribution of pubic hair. Inspect the scrotum for size, slight asymmetry, color, and absence of edema. The scrotum may initially be swollen from birth trauma or maternal hormones, but this swelling should decrease in the first few days of life. The scrotum is ordinarily more deeply pigmented than the rest of the skin. Figure 32.34 illustrates scrotal changes that occur with puberty. Assess the testicles by placing one finger over the inguinal canal and palpating the scrotum with the other. This prevents the retractile testes in a young child from slipping back up the inguinal canal. The testicles should be smooth, of similar sizes, and freely movable. The infant's testicles may be palpated in the scrotum or in the inguinal canal, where they can be easily moved into the scrotum with gentle pressure from the examiner's nondominant hand (Fig. 32.35). Beyond infancy, allow the child to sit cross-legged to reduce the cremasteric reflex that retracts the testicles during palpation. An adolescent may need to stand for the nurse to fully palpate the scrotum. Document the presence of both testicles in the scrotal sac, if they are retractile, or if they are absent. Report undescended testicle or other abnormal findings.

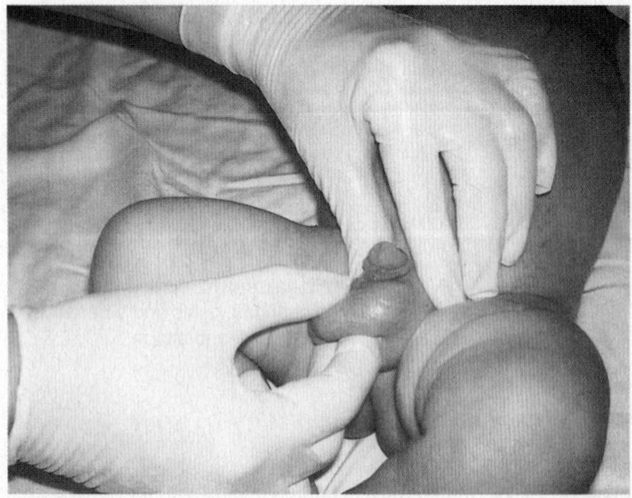

FIGURE 32.35 Placing a digit over the inguinal canal during testicular palpation prevents retraction of the testis into the canal.

FEMALE

In most cases, the female genitalia examination is limited to assessment of the external genitalia. Internal examination is not routinely performed before maturity unless the adolescent anticipates becoming or is sexually active or requests birth control, or if pathology is suspected. If an internal examination is needed, refer the child or adolescent to the appropriate advanced nurse practitioner or health care provider.

Position the infant in the parent's lap or on the examination table or crib. The toddler or preschooler should be examined in the parent's lap, in a frog-legged position. The school-age or adolescent female should lie on the examination table or bed. Provide for privacy by keeping the genital area covered until it is time for the examination.

Perform the assessment of the external genitalia in a systematic fashion. First, determine the presence and distribution of pubic hair. Infants and young females may have a small amount of downy pubic hair. Otherwise, the appearance of pubic hair indicates the onset of pubertal changes, sometimes prior to breast changes. Pubic hair generally begins to appear by age 11 years, with age 13 being the latest. Figure 32.36 illustrates the development of pubic hair on the vulva through puberty.

Inspect the labia majora and minora for size, color, and skin integrity. The newborn's labia minora are swollen from the effects of maternal estrogen but will decrease in size and be hidden by the labia majora within the first few weeks of life. Redness or swelling of the labia may occur with infection, sexual abuse, or masturbation. Lesions on the external genitalia may indicate sexually transmitted infection. Gently spread the labia to inspect the clitoris, urethral meatus, and vaginal opening. Some children may prefer to spread the labia themselves. The urinary meatus and vaginal orifice should be visible and not occluded by the hymen. It is not uncommon to see a hymenal tag. Note clitoral size. Inspect the urinary meatus and vaginal opening for edema or redness, which should not be present. Observe for any vaginal discharge. A small amount of blood-tinged or mucoid discharge may be noted in the first few weeks of life as a result of maternal hormone exposure. A small amount of clear mucous like discharge is normal in all females. If present, document labial adhesion or other abnormal findings.

ANUS

Inspect the anal area for fissures, rash, hemorrhoids, prolapse, or skin tags. Examine the infant's anal area while examining the genitalia. The younger child may lie back in the parent's lap and flex the knees to the chest. The

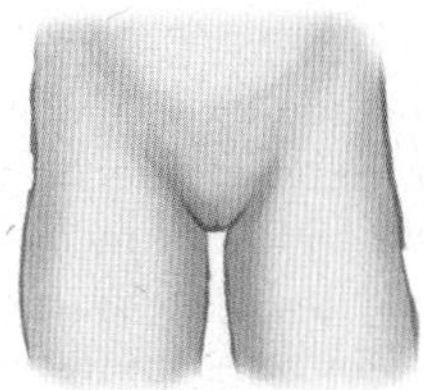

Stage 1 Preadolescents.
No pubic hair. Mons and labia covered with fine vellus hair as on abdomen.

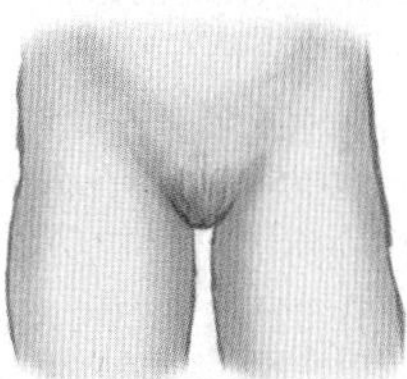

Stage 2 Growth sparse and mostly on labia. Long, downy hair, slightly pigmented, straight or only slightly curly.

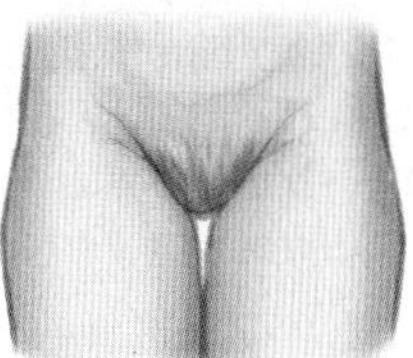

Stage 3 Growth sparse and spreading over mons pubis. Hair darker, coarser, curlier.

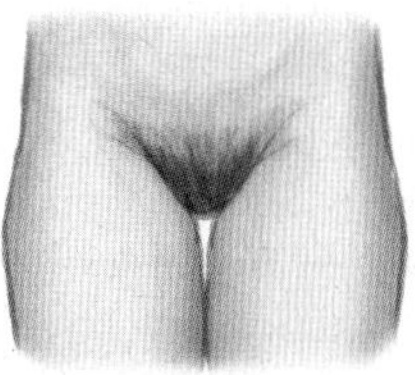

Stage 4 Hair is adult in type but over smaller area; none on medial thigh.

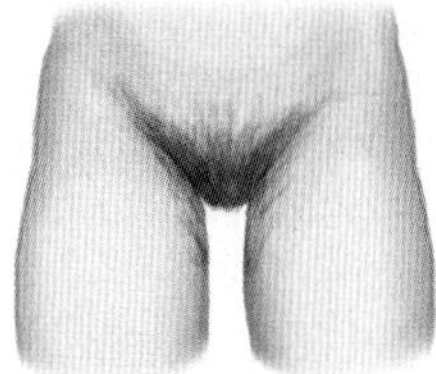

Stage 5 Adult in type and pattern; inverse triangle. Also on medial thigh surface.

FIGURE 32.36 Tanner female sexual maturity rating for pubic hair. (Adapted from Tanner, J. M. [1962]. *Growth at adolescence*. Blackwell Scientific Publications.)

older child or adolescent may be prone or in a side-lying position. If the adolescent is already standing for the scrotal assessment, have them bend forward so that you can assess the anal area. The anus should appear moist and hairless. Gently stroke the anal area to elicit the anal reflex (quick contraction). If indicated, inspect anal sphincter tone by inserting a gloved finger lubricated with water-soluble jelly just inside the anal sphincter.

Musculoskeletal

Assessment of the musculoskeletal system includes examination of the clavicles and shoulders, spine, extremities, joints, and hips. Determining the child's ability to move all extremities through the full range of motion is also important.

CLAVICLES AND SHOULDERS

Palpate the clavicles. In the newborn, tenderness or crepitus reveals a fracture sustained at birth. In the older infant or child, a bump indicates callus formation with clavicle fracture. Test shoulder strength and the function of cranial nerve XI in the older child by requesting that the child shrug the shoulders while you apply downward pressure.

SPINE

Observe the child's resting posture and alignment of the trunk. The newborn's position will look like the position the baby preferred in utero and is one of general flexion. The older infant moves more and can sit unassisted in the second half of the first year. Toddlers stand with a wide-based gait, a slightly swayed back, and the abdomen slightly protruding. The posture straightens in the preschool and school-age years. Adolescents often demonstrate kyphosis as the skeleton and muscles are both growing rapidly (Fig. 32.37).

Inspect the child's spine. The newborn's spine has a single C-shaped curve and remains rounded for the first 3 months of life. The cervical curve begins to develop around 3 to 4 months of age as the baby gains head control. By 12 to 18 months of age, the lumbar curve develops, which corresponds to the onset of walking. The S-shaped spine in older children and adolescents is similar to that of the adult. The spine should be flexible, with good muscle tone and no rigidity. Assess the back, and hip and shoulder heights for symmetry.

Examine the preadolescent and adolescent for the development of scoliosis. Refer to Chapter 44 for information about scoliosis screening. Scoliosis screening is

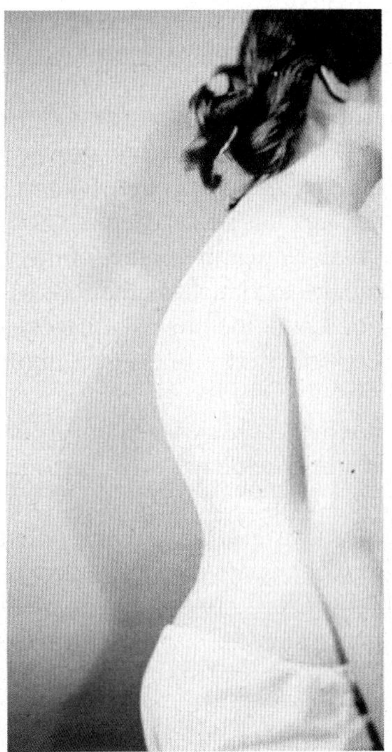

FIGURE 32.37 The adolescent's posture often demonstrates kyphosis.

generally performed during well-child examinations by the health care provider or nurse practitioner or by the middle or high school nurse on a particular day of the school year.

Note mobility of the vertebral column by having the child bend forward and side to side. Flex the neck and move it from side to side. No resistance or pain should occur. Inspect the back for discoloration, tufts of hair, or dimples. A normal pilonidal dimple is sometimes seen at the base of the spine, but there should be no tuft of hair or nevi along the spine. Document and report unexpected findings.

EXTREMITIES

All children, even newborns, should be able to move all extremities spontaneously. Screen the infant younger than 6 months for developmental dysplasia of the hip by performing the Ortolani and Barlow maneuvers (refer to Chapter 44 for additional information). These maneuvers are usually best performed by a proficient examiner. Inspect and palpate the child's upper and lower extremities. Assess for symmetry in size, contour, movement, warmth, and color of the extremities. The infant's feet and legs appear bowed secondary to in utero positioning but can be straightened through passive range of motion. Observe the child in a standing position. Bowing of the lower legs (internal tibial torsion) lessens as the toddler begins to bear weight and usually resolves in the second or third year of life as the strength of the muscles and bones increases. When it persists past that time, it is termed "genu varum" (bow legs). Genu valgum (knock knee) is usually present until the child is 7 years old. Observe the child walking, noting any difficulty with leg position or balance. If the child is reluctant to walk, use play as a way to elicit the behavior. The school-age child should have gait and leg appearance similar to that of the adult.

Note the normal flat foot in the toddler and young child. The arch develops as the child grows, and the muscles become less lax, although some children may continue with flexible flat feet; this is considered a normal variation.

Perform passive range of motion of the young infant's extremities. Inability to straighten the foot to midline may indicate clubfoot. Count the fingers and toes, noting abnormalities such as polydactyly (increased number of digits) or syndactyly (webbing of the digits). Palpate the joints for warmth or tenderness. Check the mobility of the joints of the upper and lower extremities by performing range of motion. Determine lower extremity muscle strength by having the child push against the examiner's hands with the soles of the forefoot. Assess upper extremity strength by having the child squeeze the examiner's crossed fingers or push up or down against the examiner's outstretched hands.

TAKE NOTE!

Slight tremors may be noticed in the infant's extremities in the first month of life.

Neurologic

The neurologic examination should include level of consciousness, balance and coordination, sensory function, reflexes, and a developmental screening. Motor function is assessed within the musculoskeletal section. Cranial nerve function is generally tested within other portions of the physical assessment as it applies to that section.

LEVEL OF CONSCIOUSNESS

Note the state of alertness and attentiveness to parents and the environment in the newborn and infant. Older infants become interactive with other people, as do toddlers and preschoolers. Younger children demonstrate orientation by positive interaction with family members and by crying or fussing when they feel threatened. By school age, the child should be oriented to name and place and a few years later should be able to state the date as well (even if only the day of the week).

BALANCE AND COORDINATION

The cerebellum controls balance and coordination. Observe the child's gait to assess balance and coordination. Observe toddlers and older children rising and walking from a seated and supine position. They should be able to stand and balance without straining or holding on to objects. Continue to test cerebellar function by having the younger child skip or hop and requesting that the older child or adolescent walk heel to toe. Further tests of cerebellar function responsible for balance and coordination are discussed in Box 32.3. Demonstrate each test and make sure the child understands your instructions.

BOX 32.3 Cerebellar Function Testing

- **Romberg:** Ask the school-age or older child to stand still with eyes closed and arms down by the sides. Observe the child for leaning (stand close in case this does occur). This is considered a positive Romberg test, indicating cerebellar dysfunction.
- For the following tests, the child should demonstrate accuracy and smoothness:
- **Heel-to-shin:** Have the child lie in a supine position, place one heel on the opposite knee, and run it down the shin.
- **Rapid alternating movements:** The child pats the thighs with the hands, lifts them, turns them over, pats the thighs with the back of the hands, and repeats the process multiple times. An alternate test is for the child to touch the thumb to each finger of the same hand, starting at the index finger, then reverse the direction and repeat.
- **Finger-to-finger:** The child's eyes are open. The child touches the examiner's outstretched finger with the index finger, then touches their own nose. The examiner moves the finger to a different spot, and the child repeats this process several times.
- **Finger-to-nose:** The child's eyes are closed. The child stretches the arm with the index finger extended, then touches their nose with that finger, keeping the eyes closed.

Data from Chiocca, E. M. (2020). *Advanced pediatric assessment* (3rd ed.). Springer Publishing Company; Jarvis, C., & Eckhardt, A. (2020). *Physical examination and health assessment* (8th ed.). Elsevier.

SENSORY TESTING

Portions of sensory testing related to most of the cranial nerves, vision, hearing, taste, and smell have already been incorporated into other sections as appropriate within the physical assessment. Test cranial nerve V (trigeminal) by lightly touching the child's cheek with a cotton ball. The young infant will root toward the side that is touched. With the child's eyes closed, ask the child to identify other locations where they are lightly touched (several different ones) to assess sensation. Ask the child to tell you when they are touched. Make a game of this activity to encourage cooperation in younger children. In the older child who knows the definition of sharp and dull, test for these sensations with the child's eyes closed. Use the rounded end of a tongue blade for dull and the broken edge of a tongue blade for the sharp sensation. The child should be able to discriminate the sensations of sharp and dull.

REFLEXES

Assess the infant's primitive and protective reflexes. The primitive reflexes involve a whole-body response and are subcortical in nature. Selected primitive reflexes present at birth include Moro, root, suck, asymmetric tonic neck, plantar and palmar grasp, step, and Babinski. Most of the primitive reflexes diminish over the first few months of life, giving way to protective or postural reflexes. Protective reflexes are motor responses related to maintenance of equilibrium. They are necessary for appropriate motor development and remain throughout life once they are established. The protective reflexes include the righting and parachute reactions.

Place one finger in each of the infant's hands to elicit the palmar grasp reflex (usually disappears by the age of 3 to 4 months). Touch the thumb to the ball of the infant's foot to elicit the plantar grasp reflex. The infant's toes will curl down (this reflex disappears by the age of 8 to 10 months). Refer to Table 3.1 for illustrations and additional explanation of the other reflexes. Appropriate presence and disappearance of primitive reflexes, as well as development of protective reflexes, is indicative of a healthy neurologic system. Primitive reflexes that persist beyond the usual age of disappearance may indicate an abnormality of the neurologic system and should be further investigated (Kotagal & Morse, 2022).

Assess deep tendon reflexes in all infants and children. Appropriate responses indicate that the reflex arc is intact. Use the reflex hammer in all ages or the curved tips of the two first fingers to elicit the responses in infants. The limb must be relaxed and the muscle partly stretched. Use a snapping motion of the wrist to tap with the fingertips or the reflex hammer. Test the biceps, triceps, patellar, and Achilles reflexes as you would in the adult. It may help to place a finger under the infant's knee to encourage relaxation. Young children who tense up when their reflexes are being tested may relax the area if you have them focus on another area, so have the child clasp the hands while testing the Achilles and patellar reflexes. As the child focuses on the hands, the lower extremities relax (Jarvis & Eckhardt, 2020). Distraction may also be helpful.

Grade the strength of the response using the standard scale from 0 to 4+:

- 0: no response
- 1+: diminished or sluggish
- 2+: average
- 3+: brisker than average
- 4+: very brisk, may involve clonus

The newborn's deep tendon reflexes are normally brisk (3+). They decrease to average (2+) usually by 4 months of age. Healthy children should have reflexes of 2+ if the reflex has been elicited properly. Absent, sluggish, or hyperreactive responses usually indicate disease (Bryant & Speck, 2022).

DEVELOPMENTAL SCREENING

An important component of the neurologic assessment and a comprehensive child health assessment is developmental screening. Developmental screening may be used to identify children whose developmental status may warrant additional evaluation. Become comfortable with the developmental screening tools used and what the results of the screening mean. On completion of the screening, discuss the child's abilities with the parent or caregiver. Developmental screening is often performed separately from the physical examination and is discussed in further detail in Chapter 31.

Refer back to Elliot, the 3-year-old from the beginning of the chapter. What are some important considerations when performing his physical examination?

Unfolding Patient Stories: Eva Madison • Part 1

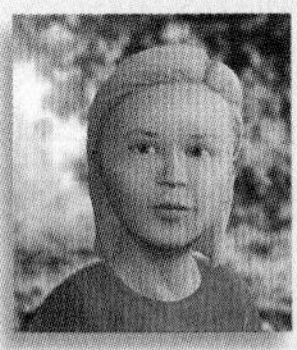

Eva Madison, a 5-year-old, is at the clinic with their parent for a routine check-up. How can the nurse create an environment that is conducive to obtaining health information? How can the nurse prepare the child and the parent for the physical examination? What key areas of the health history and physical assessment should the nurse evaluate in this 5-year-old? (Eva Madison's story continues in Chapter 42.)

Care for Eva and other patients in a realistic virtual environment: ***vSim** for Nursing* (thepoint.lww.com/vSimPediatric). Practice documenting these patients' care in DocuCare (thePoint.lww.com/DocuCareEHR).

KEY CONCEPTS

- The health history in children includes more than just the chief complaint, history of present illness, and past medical history; it is important to include the perinatal history and developmental milestones.
- Allow the chief complaint to determine which parts of the history require more in-depth investigation.
- The developmental history will warrant more attention in the younger child, while school performance and adjustment will be more important in the school-age child and adolescent.
- Although the parent will provide most of the health history for the infant and the young child, allow the young verbal child to answer questions during the health history as appropriate.
- Direct health history questions to the school-age child and adolescent, seeking clarification from the parents as needed.
- Provide confidentiality and privacy for the adolescent during the health history.
- Weight and length or height should be assessed at each well-child visit to determine adequacy of growth.
- Measure head circumference until age 3 years to monitor brain growth.
- Perform hearing and vision screenings for children of all ages.
- BMI can be used to identify children who are overweight or at risk for being overweight.
- The normal range of vital signs varies based on the child's age.
- The sequence of the physical examination in children should be based on the child's developmental age, their level of cooperation, and the severity of the illness.
- Obtain heart rate and respiratory rate, and auscultate the heart and lungs while the infant or young child is quiet.
- Perform intrusive procedures such as examination of the ears, mouth, and throat last in the infant or young child.
- Perform the health assessment in a head-to-toe fashion in the school-age child or adolescent, reserving the genitalia and anus examination for last.
- Plan the health assessment in such a way as to minimize trauma to the child or adolescent.
- Use age-appropriate measurement tools to assess pain in children.
- Allow the infant or young child to remain in the parent's lap for as much of the assessment as possible so that the child feels secure.
- Use age-appropriate games during the health assessment to gain cooperation in the younger child.
- Having the young child sit cross-legged for a testicular examination may reduce the cremasteric reflex.
- The newborn may exhibit a wide variety of normal skin variations.
- The infant's fontanels should be soft and flat; report a bulging fontanel immediately.
- Jaundice (outside of the newborn period), pallor, cyanosis, and poor skin turgor indicate illness and may need immediate intervention.
- Heart murmurs should be assessed for intensity, location, and duration. They may be innocent or may indicate a congenital heart defect.
- The infant's chest wall is relatively thin, allowing upper airway sounds to be transmitted throughout the lung fields.
- Substernal or xiphoid retractions indicate that the child is laboring to breathe, whereas a fixed, depressed sternum (pectus excavatum) is a structural abnormality.
- The Tanner stages of sexual maturity provide a basis for assessing pubertal development. Use the breast and pubic hair charts for females and the pubic hair and penis and scrotum size chart for males.

REFERENCES AND RECOMMENDED READINGS

American Academy of Pediatrics. (2021). *Fever and your child.* https://publications.aap.org/patiented/article/doi/10.1542/peo_document040/80029/Fever-and-Your-Child

Andre, J. H., & Rockwell, M. (2022). Management of eye disorders. In T. Kyle (Ed.), *Primary care pediatrics for the nurse practitioner* (pp. 269–285). Springer.

Boos, S. (2022). Differential diagnosis of suspected child physical abuse. *UpToDate.* Retrieved November 3, 2023, from https://www.uptodate.com/contents/differential-diagnosis-of-suspected-child-physical-abuse

Brazelton, T. B., & Sparrow, J. (n.d.). *The Touchpoints model of development.* https://www.brazeltontouchpoints.org/wp-content/uploads/2011/09/Touchpoints-Model-of-Development-April-2015.pdf

Bryant, P., & Speck, P. M. (2022). Health assessment. In T. Kyle (Ed.), *Primary care pediatrics for the nurse practitioner* (pp. 25–47). Springer.

Centers for Disease Control and Prevention. (2017, June 16). *Clinical growth charts.* https://www.cdc.gov/growthcharts/clinical_charts.htm

Centers for Disease Control and Prevention. (2022, September 24). *About child & teen BMI.* https://www.cdc.gov/healthyweight/assessing/bmi/childrens_bmi/about_childrens_bmi.html

Centers for Disease Control and Prevention. (2023, January 10). *Childhood lead poisoning prevention program.* http://www.cdc.gov/nceh/lead/

Chiocca, E. M. (2020). *Advanced pediatric assessment* (3rd ed.). Springer Publishing Company.

Choueiry, J., Reszel, J., Hamid, J. S., Wilding, J., Martelli, B., & Harrison, D. (2020). Development and pilot evaluation of an educational tool for the FLACC pain scale. *Pain Management Nursing, 21*(6), 523–529. https://doi.org/10.1016/j.pmn.2020.06.002

Columbia University, College of Physicians and Surgeons. (n.d.). *Points on the pediatric physical exam.* http://www.columbia.edu/itc/hs/medical/clerkships/peds/Student_Information/Reference_Materials/Pediatric_PE.html#PhysicalExam

Dev, L. S., & Cruz, M. (2017). Healthy sexual development and sexuality. In T. K. McInerny, H. M. Adam, D. E. Campbell, J. M. Foy, & D. M. Kamat (Eds.), *American Academy of Pediatrics textbook of pediatric care* (2nd ed.). American Academy of Pediatrics.

Drutz, J. E., & White-Satcher, D. (2023). The pediatric physical examination: General principles and standard measurements. *UpToDate.* Retrieved November 3, 2023, from https://www.uptodate.com/contents/the-pediatric-physical-examination-general-principles-and-standard-measurements

Exergen Corporation. (n.d.). *Nurse's center.* https://medical.exergen.com/nurses-center/

Fahrenkopf, M. P., Adams, N. S., Mann, R. J., & Girotto, J. A. (2020). Deformational plagiocephaly. In R. M. Kliegman, J. W. St Geme, N. J. Blum, S. S. Shah, R. C. Tasker, & K. M. Wilson (Eds.), *Nelson textbook of pediatrics* (21st ed.). Elsevier.

Flynn, J. T., Kaelber, D. C., Baker-Smith, C. M., Blowey, D., Carrol, A. E., Daniels, S. R., de Ferranti, S. D., Dionne, J. M., Leu, M. G., Powers, M. E., Rea, C., Samuels, J., Simasek, M., Thaker, V. V., Urbina, E. M., & The Subcommittee on Screening and Management of High Blood Pressure in Children. (2017). Clinical practice guideline for screening and management of high blood pressure in children and adolescents. *Pediatrics, 140*(3), e20171904. https://doi.org/10.1542/peds.2017-1904

Gilmore, B. M., & Hay, B. B. (2021). Evidence-based assessment of the breasts and axillae. In K. S. Gawlik, B. M. Melnyk, & A. M. Teall (Eds.), *Evidence-based physical examination: Best practices for health and well-being assessment* (pp. 483–501). Springer.

Jarvis, C., & Eckhardt, A. (2020). *Physical examination and health assessment* (8th ed.). Elsevier.

Jone, P.-N., Kim, J. S., Burkett, D., Jacobson, R., & Von Alvensleben, J. (2022). Cardiovascular diseases. In M. Bunik, W. W. Hay, M. J. Levin, & M. J. Abzug (Eds.), *Current diagnosis & treatment: Pediatrics* (26th ed.). McGraw-Hill.

Kleinman, K., McDaniel, L., & Molloy, M. (2021). *The Harriet Lane handbook: A manual for pediatric house officers* (22nd ed.). Elsevier.

Kotagal, S., & Morse, A. M. (2022). Detailed neurologic assessment of infants and children. *UpToDate.* Retrieved November 3, 2023, from https://www.uptodate.com/contents/detailed-neurologic-assessment-of-infants-and-children

Kyle, T. (2022). Well-child visits during infancy. In T. Kyle (Ed.), *Primary care pediatrics for the nurse practitioner* (pp. 161-169). Springer.

Mechem, C. C. (2022). Pulse oximetry. *UpToDate.* Retrieved November 3, 2023, from https://www.uptodate.com/contents/pulse-oximetry

Medtronic. (2023). *Pulse oximetry.* https://www.medtronic.com/covidien/en-us/products/pulse-oximetry.html

Mento, C., Silvestri, M. C., Bruno, A., Muscatello, M. R. A., Cedro, C., Pandolfo, G., & Zoccali, R. A. (2020). Workplace violence against healthcare professionals: A systematic review. *Aggression and Violent Behavior, 51*, 101381. https://doi.org/10.1016/j.avb.2020.101381

Miller, S. (n.d.). *Pediatric physical exam video* [Video]. http://www.columbia.edu/itc/hs/medical/clerkships/peds/Student_Information/Reference_Materials/PE_Video.html

National Institutes of Health. (2021). *Clear & simple.* https://www.nih.gov/institutes-nih/nih-office-director/office-communications-public-liaison/clear-communication/clear-simple

Perry, A. G., Potter, P. A., Ostendorf, W. R., & Laplante, N. (2022). Chapter 5: Vital signs. In A. G. Perry, P. A. Potter, W. R. Ostendorf, & N. Laplante (Eds.), *Clinical nursing skills and tecchniques* (10th ed., pp. 68-107). Elsevier.

Quinlin, L., & Gawlik, K. (2021). Evidence-base history-taking approach for wellness exams, episodic visits and chronic care management. In K. S. Gawlik, B. M. Melnyk, & A. M. Teall (Eds.), *Evidence-based physical examination: Best practices for health and well-being assessment* (pp. 17-42). Springer.

Sass, A. E., & Richards, M. J. (2022). Adolescence. In M. Bunik, W. W. Hay, M. J. Levin, & M. J. Abzug (Eds.), *Current diagnosis & treatment: Pediatrics* (26th ed.). McGraw-Hill.

Sevy, J. O., Hohman, M. H., & Singh, A. (2023). Cerumen impaction removal. *StatPearls.* StatPearls Publishing. Retrieved November 3, 2023, from https://www.ncbi.nlm.nih.gov/books/NBK448155/

Smith, D. (2022). The newborn infant. In M. Bunik, W. W. Hay, M. J. Levin, & M. J. Abzug (Eds.), *Current diagnosis & treatment: Pediatrics* (26th ed.). McGraw-Hill.

Tanner, J. M. (1962). *Growth at adolescence.* Blackwell Scientific Publications.

Treitz, M., Nicklas, D., & Fox, D. (2022). Ambulatory & office pediatrics. In M. Bunik, W. W. Hay, M. J. Levin, & M. J. Abzug (Eds.), *Current diagnosis & treatment: Pediatrics* (26th ed.). McGraw-Hill.

U.S. Department of Health and Human Services. (n.d.). *Healthy People 2030.* https://health.gov/healthypeople

Vorvick, L. J., Zieve, D., Conaway, B., & the A.D.A.M. Editorial Team. (2022). *Temperature measurement.* https://medlineplus.gov/ency/article/003400.htm

Wong, D. L., & Baker, C. M. (1988). Pain in children: Comparison of assessment scales. *Pediatric Nursing, 14*(1), 9–17. https://pubmed.ncbi.nlm.nih.gov/3344163/

Yoon, P. J., Scholes, M. A., & Herrmann, B. W. (2022). Chapter 18: Ear, nose, & throat. In M. Bunik, W. W. Hay, M. J. Levin, & M. J. Abzug (Eds.), *Current diagnosis & treatment: Pediatrics* (26th ed.). McGraw-Hill.

DEVELOPING CLINICAL JUDGMENT

PRACTICING FOR NCLEX

1. A 5-year-old visits the pediatric office with an upper respiratory infection. Which approach would give the nurse the most information about the child's developmental level?
   a. Playing a game with the child
   b. Talking with the child about the teddy bear next to them
   c. Using a screening tool during a follow-up office visit
   d. Asking the 10-year-old sibling about the child
2. Which statement indicates the best sequence for the nurse to conduct an assessment in a nonemergency situation?
   a. Introduce yourself, ask about any problems, take a history, and do the physical examination.
   b. Perform the physical examination and then ask the family if there are any problems in the child's life.
   c. Do the physical examination while at the same time asking about the child's previous illnesses; then talk about the family's concerns.
   d. Get a complete history of the family's health beliefs and practices, and then assess the child.
3. What approach by the nurse would most likely encourage a child to cooperate with an assessment of physical and developmental health?
   a. Explain to the child what's going to happen when the child asks questions.
   b. Explain what is going to happen in words the child can understand.
   c. Force the child to cooperate by having a parent hold them down.
   d. Give the child a sticker before beginning the examination.
4. A sleeping 5-month-old is being held by the parent when the nurse comes in to do a physical examination. What assessment should be done initially?
   a. Listening to the bowel sounds
   b. Counting the heart rate
   c. Checking the temperature
   d. Looking in the ears
5. Which assessment finding is considered normal in children?
   a. Irregular respiratory rate and rhythm
   b. Split S_2 and sinus arrhythmia
   c. Decreased heart rate with crying
   d. Genu varum past the age of 5 years
6. A child's weight is 35 lb, 7 oz. Convert the weight to kilograms.
7. A child's height is 41 in. Convert the height to centimeters.

CRITICAL THINKING EXERCISES

1. A soft and muffled heart murmur is heard in a 4-year-old patient. The parent states that they have never been told that the child has a murmur. What should the nurse do?
2. A nurse is helping a new parent breastfeed their 4-day-old baby. The parent notices that the baby has a bluish cast to the skin on their hands and that sometimes the infant has a tremor. They ask the nurse if the baby is cold, although the baby is swaddled and comfortably resting against the parent's skin. How might the nurse help teach this parent?
3. Devise a plan for encouraging cooperation of the toddler or preschooler during various parts of the physical examination.

STUDY ACTIVITIES

1. In the clinical setting, obtain a health history on an infant, child, or adolescent.
2. In the clinical setting, compare the approach you use for the physical examination of a toddler versus a school-age child or adolescent.
3. No matter how thoughtfully and appropriately you plan your assessment, odds are good that you will have difficulty assessing a 2-year-old. Discuss with your classmates the strategies that you have used for success, and brainstorm with them about their ideas for assessing a crying or resistant young child.

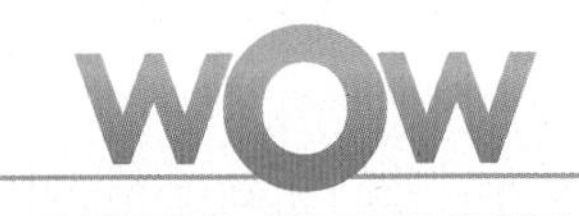

WORDS OF WISDOM

Nurses should leave their "comfort zone" of practice and reach out to children on their turf to make a difference.

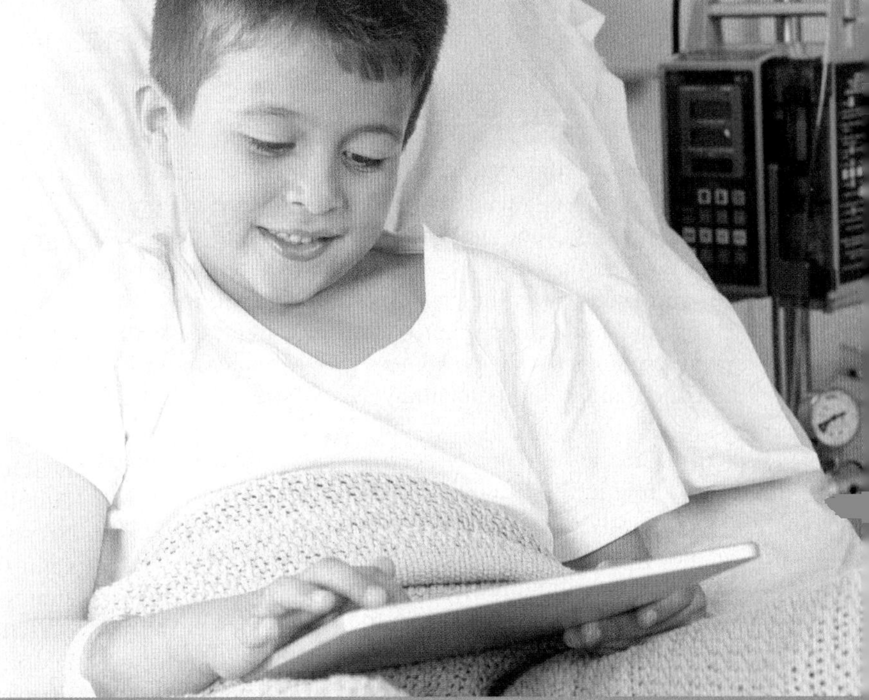

33

Caring for Children in Diverse Settings

LEARNING OBJECTIVES

Upon completion of the chapter, you will be able to:

1. Discuss the variety of settings in which nursing care occurs.
2. Describe the various roles of the nurse, including hospital and community settings and home care nurses.
3. Examine the nurse's role in home health care.
4. Explain the major stressors of illness and hospitalization for children.
5. Identify the reactions and responses of children and their families during illness and hospitalization.
6. Describe the nursing care that minimizes stressors for children who are ill or hospitalized.
7. Delineate the major components of admission for children to the hospital.
8. Discuss appropriate safety measures to use with hospitalized children.
9. Identify nursing responsibilities related to patients discharged from the hospital.

KEY TERMS

child with medical complexity
community
individualized health plan
therapeutic play

Jake Jorgenson, 8 years old, was brought to the clinic with a history of headaches, vomiting not related to feeding, and changes in his gait. Initial testing leads to a suspected brain tumor. Jake is to be admitted to the neurologic service at a pediatric hospital for further testing and treatment. Up to this point, he has been a healthy child with no previous hospitalizations. He lives at home with his parents and two siblings, Jenny, age 11, and Joshua, age 5.

INTRODUCTION

Nursing care of the child occurs in a variety of settings, from acute care in a hospital to well and ill care in community settings, such as health care providers' offices, schools, churches, health departments, community centers, and even within the child's own home. Within each setting, the nurse incorporates basic nursing care with specific strategies to help promote positive outcomes for the child, family, and community as a whole.

Children receive most of their health care, well and ill care, in the community setting. Nurses play an important role in the health and wellness of a community. They not only meet the health care needs of individuals but also go beyond to create interventions that affect the community. Community health nursing refers to nursing care that strives to improve the health of a specific community as a whole. For example, community health nurses working in the Department of Health and Human Services would strive to make sure that all children in their particular community were up-to-date on immunizations. Community-based nursing focuses more on providing care to the individual or family (which, of course, impacts the community) in settings outside of acute care. For example, a community-based nurse would work in the local public school to care for students' health needs. Nurses practicing in the community promote the health of individuals, families, groups, communities, and populations and promote an environment that supports health.

COMMUNITY HEALTH NURSING

Nursing in the community is aimed at disease prevention and improvement of the health of populations and communities. "Population" refers to all of the people occupying an area who may not necessarily interact, such as the population of the United States, or to all of those who share one or more characteristics, for example, the pediatric population (Rector, 2022). **Community** can be defined as a "collection of people who interact with one another and whose common interests or characteristics form the basis for a sense of unity or belonging" (Rector, 2022, p. 5). Community health nurses work in geographically and culturally diverse settings. They address current and potential health needs of the population or community. They promote and preserve the health of a population and are not limited to particular age groups or diagnoses. Public health nursing is a specialized area of community health nursing.

Epidemiology can help determine the health and health needs of a population and assist in planning health services. Community health nurses perform epidemiologic investigations to help analyze and develop health policy and community health initiatives. Community health initiatives can be focused on the community as a whole or a specific target population with specific needs. Healthy People 2030 is an example of national health initiatives developed using the epidemiologic process (U.S. Department of Health and Human Services, n.d.). Healthy People 2030 ensures that health care professionals look at the individual as well as the community. It addresses the link between the individual's health and the health of the community. Nurses play a key role in the health of a community and the individuals who reside in it.

Healthy People 2030 is the fifth edition of national health goals, which were launched in 1979. Healthy People 2030 is a comprehensive health initiatives plan. Nurses can help the nation meet these objectives by educating those in the community on appropriate prevention strategies, such as proper immunization and smoking cessation (see individual chapters for relevant Healthy People objectives and nursing implications). Healthy People 2030 is available online at https://www.healthypeople.gov. Refer to Chapter 23 for more information.

COMMUNITY-BASED NURSING

In the past, the major role of the nurse in the community was that of the community health nurse or public health nurse. Today, nurses practice in a variety of settings within a community, such as clinics and health care providers' offices, schools, camps, shelters, places of worship, health departments, community health centers, and homes.

Shifting Responsibilities From Hospital-Based to Community-Based Nursing Care

Over the past century, changes in health care such as strained health care funding, shorter hospital stays, and cost containment, have led to a shift in responsibilities of care for children from the hospital to homes and communities. Community care, especially home care, is a rapidly growing service in the United States. Community-based care has been shown to be a cost-effective way to provide care. It emphasizes wellness and prevention. Increases in disposable income and the longevity of children with chronic and debilitating health conditions have also contributed to the continued shift of health care to the community and home setting. Advances in technology have allowed for improved monitoring of children in community settings and at home, as well as allowing complicated procedures, such as intravenous administration of antibiotics, to be done at home.

Another major reason for the increase in community care of children, especially home care, is the understanding that an acute care setting is not an ideal environment for children's development. Caring for children at home and within their community not only improves their physical health but also allows for adequate growth and development while keeping them within their family. When they are in a familiar environment with the comfort and support of family, there is a better opportunity for improved care and quality of life.

Role of the Community-Based Nurse

With the shift in responsibilities from hospital care to community care have come changes in nursing care. More opportunities exist for nurses to provide direct care to children in the community setting, especially the home. Community-based nursing care differs from nursing care in the acute setting. In the community or home care setting, the nurse provides direct care for the child but spends more time in the role of educator, communicator, and manager than the nurse in the acute care setting. In home care, the nurse spends a significant amount of time in the supervision or management role. Community-based nursing focuses on the practice of nursing that provides personal care to individuals and families in the community. Community-based nurses focus on promoting and preserving health as well as preventing disease or injury. They are educators, managers of care, and advocates along with being direct providers of care.

Communication and Education

The community-based nurse must use the principles and techniques of interpersonal communication. The nurse must be able to assess the child's and family's learning needs and their readiness to learn. As hospital stays become shorter and admissions to the hospital become less frequent, teaching now begins wherever the child or family enters the health care system. Often, initial teaching occurs in the community setting, especially the home. In the community-based setting, teaching is often focused on assisting the child and family to achieve independence.

Discharge Planning and Care Coordination

Due to the short lengths of stay in acute settings and the shift to community settings for children with complex health needs, discharge planning and care coordination have become important nursing roles. Discharge planning involves the development and implementation of a comprehensive plan for the safe discharge of a child from a health care facility and for continuing safe and effective care in the community and at home. Successful discharge planning begins upon the child's admission to the facility.

Modern pediatric health care focuses on an interdisciplinary plan of care designed to meet the child's physical, developmental, educational, spiritual, and psychosocial needs. Nurses provide care coordination through the implementation of this interdisciplinary plan in a collaborative manner to ensure continuity of care that is cost-effective, quality oriented, and outcome focused.

Advocacy and Resource Management

Another important role of the community-based nurse is to advocate for the child and family to ensure that their needs are being met and that they have available resources and appropriate health care services. Working in a child's and family's home can lead a nurse to become overly involved or attached. To best serve the child and family, the community-based nurse must be an advocate and educator but avoid becoming a personal friend by maintaining professional boundaries and a therapeutic nurse–patient relationship (National Council of State Boards of Nursing [NCSBN], 2018).

Nurses must have a basic understanding of community, state, and federal resources to ensure they are providing families with the resources they may need. One such resource important in the community-based care of children with complex medical needs is Medicaid. Medicaid is a national program providing medical assistance for children and families with low incomes. It is jointly run by the federal and state governments but is administered at the state level; therefore, provisions vary widely. Additionally, medical model waivers are state-run programs that use federal and state funds to pay for health care for people with certain medical conditions. These waivers will refrain from enforcing one or more Medicaid rules to extend eligibility or services to children who qualify. Home- and community-based waiver programs, such as the Katie Beckett waiver (also known as the Deeming waiver), allow children and young adults with complex medical needs to be cared for at home and make them eligible for Medicaid based on their own income and assets, regardless of their parents' income (Kids' Waivers, 2022). Without medical waiver programs, many children with special needs would either go without health care or would be institutionalized in order to qualify for Medicaid.

Physical Care

The community-based nurse performs less direct physical care than the nurse in the acute care setting. Many times, the nurse observes the child or caregiver performing physical care tasks. Excellent assessment skills are especially important in the community care setting. The nurse often functions in a more autonomous role; after data collection, the community-based nurse will often decide whether to initiate, continue, alter, or end physical nursing care. Assessment will go beyond physical assessment of the child to include the environment and the community.

ILLNESS AND HOSPITALIZATION IN CHILDHOOD

In today's health care environment, children receive much of their care for illnesses in community health settings, as discussed previously. As a result of this trend, fewer children may actually be admitted to a hospital unit, and those who are hospitalized are generally acutely ill. In addition, hospital stays are often shorter due to economic trends in the health care environment, such as the delivery system of managed care and other factors that attempt to control costs. In all of the varied settings where health care is administered, nurses provide well care, episodic ill care, and chronic care. They work to promote, preserve, and improve the health of children and families in all these settings.

General Inpatient Unit

With inpatient unit stays for children that are shorter and that involve more acute conditions, there is little time for admission preparation. Often, the admission procedure and treatment actually occur simultaneously. Sometimes, the stay is in a special 23-hour observation unit, so the child is in the setting for less than 24 hours. General hospital stays may be in a pediatric hospital, a pediatric unit in a general hospital, or a general unit that occasionally admits children. General units often lack child-oriented services, such as play areas, child-size equipment, and staff familiar with caring for children.

Emergency Departments

A major cause of illness and hospitalization in children is injuries from accidents; the top seven nonfatal injuries are all unintentional (National Center for Injury Prevention and Control, Centers for Disease Control and Prevention [CDC], 2020). Many times, a family's first experience with the acute care setting is the emergency department. Due to the situation, the child and family may experience increased anxiety, and it may become overwhelming as uncertainties develop and critical decisions must be made. The family may be frightened, insecure, and in a state of shock.

Procedures and tests are performed quickly, with minimal time for preparation. The family is often ill-prepared for the visit, having little money or clothing with them. Siblings may be present if the parents did not have time to arrange other child care.

Due to the fast pace of the emergency department, the family may be hesitant to ask questions; hence, it is important for the nurse to keep the family and child well informed. Allow the family to stay with the child, provide support, and allow the family, and when appropriate the child, to participate in decisions.

Families may have a strong fear of the unknown and may be terrified that the child will die or be permanently disabled. Help the family to identify their concerns and their support systems. Prepare them for what they will experience. Provide comfort such as holding, touching, talking softly, and other appropriate interventions according to age, developmental level, and culture.

Pediatric Intensive Care Units

The pediatric intensive care unit (PICU) specializes in caring for children in crisis. The same principles and concepts of general care of children apply to this setting, but everything is intensified. Families will be faced with an unfamiliar, high-tech environment and interaction with a large team of care providers.

Families must deal with the critical situation that brought them to the PICU. The child will likely experience pain, unusual noises, and increased stimulation and will probably undergo uncomfortable procedures. Parents may face the possibility of losing their child. Sometimes, the child cannot talk, eat, or display other appropriate developmental behaviors. Sensory overload (increased stimulation) or sensory deprivation (lack of stimulation) can affect both child and family.

The nurse should welcome families (if institutional policy permits) and encourage them to stay with the child and participate in care. Explain everything to the parents and, when appropriate, to the child. Frequently touch the child and encourage the parents to comfort them. Listen for clues about what the child and family need during the PICU stay.

Rehabilitation Units/Facilities

The rehabilitation unit/facility provides care for children beyond the initial period of illness or injury. The care involves an interdisciplinary approach that assists the child to reach their potential and achieve developmental skills. For example, rehabilitation units help children regain abilities lost due to neurologic injuries or serious burns. The facilities often resemble a home environment, with special services to help children to relearn activities of daily living and to help them deal with the physical or mental challenges associated with the original illness or injury. Typically, families are encouraged to participate and are given support for their child's eventual return home. There is a balance of nurturing and firm discipline while the child reclaims independence.

Outpatient Facilities

Outpatient care is health care provided to individuals who do not require care in an acute setting. Due to advances in medical technology, more medical procedures (such as diagnostic tests, treatments, and surgeries) can be administered on an outpatient basis and do not require children to be hospitalized. Outpatient care delivers convenient and cost-effective health care to children and their families, often right within their own community. These settings allow for increased independence and permit children to return to their normal routine as quickly as possible. More and more outpatient care centers are opening, sponsored by health maintenance organizations (HMOs), health care providers' groups, community agencies and public health departments, and hospitals.

Outpatient units are used to keep hospital stays short and decrease the cost of hospitalization. Outpatient units may be a part of the hospital or a freestanding facility. The child and family arrive in the morning; the child undergoes the procedure, test, or surgery and then goes home in the evening. Examples of surgeries and procedures performed in outpatient settings include tympanostomy tube placement, hernia repair, tonsillectomy, cystoscopy, bronchoscopy, blood transfusions, dialysis, and chemotherapy. The advantages of this environment include minimal separation of the child from the family, minimal disruption of the family pattern, decreased risk of infection, and decreased cost. Disadvantages include lack of equipment for overnight stays, so if there are complications, the child will need to be transported to the hospital.

Many centers offer preoperative health assessment and teaching sessions. These allow the parent and child to ask questions and resolve them before the procedure. On the day of the procedure, parents should be allowed to be with their child until the procedure begins. Parents should also be allowed to be with their child in the postanesthesia recovery unit as quickly as possible. This provides reassurance and comfort to the child while meeting their physical and emotional needs.

The role of the nurse in the outpatient or ambulatory setting includes admission and assessment, preoperative teaching and preparation, patient assessment and support, postoperative monitoring, case management, discharge planning, and teaching. Before the procedure, the nurse reviews with the family the routine to be followed and any special instructions (such as NPO orders) and familiarizes the child with the setting to help alleviate fears. This may occur during the preoperative health assessment.

TAKE NOTE!

Encourage the parent to bring one of the child's favorite toys, blankets, or games to make the child feel more comfortable.

The nurse performs any surgical preparation and discusses intraoperative procedures as necessary. The nurse provides postoperative care and assessment of the child. Once the child's condition is stable and they meet the discharge criteria of the facility, the nurse reviews with the parent postoperative instructions, including pain management; care of the incision if appropriate; diet; activity, including return to school; necessary follow-up; and when to call the health care provider or nurse practitioner.

Health Care Provider's Office or Clinic, Health Departments, and Urgent Care Centers

Health care providers' offices, clinics, health departments, and urgent care centers are used by children and their families for well care, episodic ill care, acute care, and care of chronic conditions. For well care and illness or injury, children are often seen by their primary care health care provider. They may visit a health care provider's office or clinic or the health department. In more acute situations or for after-hours issues that cannot wait until clinic operating hours, a child may be seen in an urgent care center or may be referred to the emergency department. The American Academy of Pediatrics discourages children and families from using urgent care centers or the emergency department for routine care, since it is difficult to provide coordinated, comprehensive family-centered care consistent with a "medical home" concept (see "Medical Homes" section on Chapter 31) (Conners et al., 2017).

The nurse's role in these settings includes preparing patients, collecting pertinent health information, performing assessments, assisting the health care provider with diagnostic testing and procedures, administering injections and medications, changing wound dressings, assisting with minor surgery, helping to maintain records, and educating the child and family about home care and when to call the health care provider or nurse practitioner or return to be seen.

An essential component of primary care practice is telephone or virtual triage. Pediatric office nurses often fill this role. When parents feel comfortable with the providers in their child's medical home office, they often call or message for advice to treat their child at home. A triage nurse needs excellent assessment and critical thinking skills along with solid training and education. The triage nurse needs to assess the child's entire situation, including current signs and symptoms, history, and home treatment.

Protocols, standardized policies and procedures, and professional judgment guide the triage nurse in the decision-making process. Pediatric telephone protocols are available for purchase through the American Academy of Pediatrics (http://www.aap.org/). The triage nurse needs to determine whether the child requires emergency care, an office visit, or home management. Good listening and the ability to maintain a calm voice when talking to parents are skills necessary for successful telephone triage. The triage nurse should not discourage parents from bringing the child into the office to be seen; triage is not meant to keep children out of the office, and if a parent is concerned, that is reason enough to be seen.

TAKE NOTE!

Parents can often pick up on subtle problems in their children. They may not be able to accurately describe signs and symptoms, but they know that their child "isn't acting right." Nurses must listen to parents and act on their concerns.

Medical Care Centers

The **child with medical complexity** (CMC) is defined as a child with "substantial health care needs, one or more chronic conditions, functional limitations often associated with technology assistance, and health care use" (Elias et al., 2012, reaffirmed 2022, p. 997). The number of children with medical complexity accounts for less than 1% of the children in the United States, but they make up more than a third of the total pediatric health care costs (Murphy et al., 2020). The number of children with medical complexity is growing. Reasons include improvements in the treatment and care of complex medical conditions and increased sophistication of medical technology, which has led to infants and children surviving and thriving with previously fatal conditions (Gallo et al., 2021). For many years, these children lived in hospitals their entire lives. Due to concerns about the high cost of long-term hospitalization and the diminished quality of life for these children, alternative care settings in the community, such as medical day care centers, have been developed.

Medical day care centers are specifically designed to meet the needs of these children. Most centers accept children who have complicated medical needs or who are dependent on technology. Examples include children with multiple congenital anomalies, children who are ventilator dependent, children with respiratory conditions, children with cardiac conditions, and children with cancer. Some centers accept children with less complicated needs, such as cardiorespiratory monitoring or asthma, and some enroll children without health care needs to promote peer relationships and acceptance. Just as at a regular day care center, the parents or caregivers can drop the child off in the morning and pick the child up in the afternoon. Some centers offer afterschool, weekend, or respite services. The centers usually provide needed therapies and have indoor and outdoor play areas, educational activities, and arts and crafts.

Health professionals are present at these centers to provide for the children's medical, emotional, and developmental needs. Nurses trained in pediatric and neonatal care, physical therapists, occupational therapists, speech therapists, child-life specialists (CLSs), and social workers staff the centers; some centers have respiratory therapists on site. Children are able to receive all of their prescribed therapies while at the center. Nursing care includes direct care such as administering medication and changing dressings, assessing and evaluating the child's overall condition, identifying potential medical emergencies, determining the need for changes in care or treatment and monitoring, and providing frequent treatments or interventions to maintain life and health.

Most centers are located in the community to help ease transportation issues. Some centers provide transportation to and from home or school. Centers are licensed by the state day care licensing authorities or, in some states, prescribed pediatric extended care (PPEC) agencies. Families may be able to obtain financial assistance from their private insurance or Medicaid.

Schools

School nursing is a specialized practice of professional nursing and focuses on improving students' health, development, and safety to improve their achievement and success. School nurses work to remove or minimize health barriers to learning to provide students with the best opportunity for academic success. School nurses help bridge the gap between health care and education (National Association of School Nurses [NASN], 2023).

School nurses provide direct health care to students along with screening and referrals for health conditions. They provide leadership for health services, such as identifying health and safety concerns in the school environment and planning and training for emergencies and disasters. School nurses promote a healthy school environment by supporting healthy food services and promoting proper physical education and sports policies and practices. They promote health education through health counseling and education of students and staff. School nurses coordinate school health programs and link health service programs within the school and community. School nurses carry out a variety of roles in providing health care to children (Fig. 33.1). Box 33.1 lists some of the activities of the school nurse.

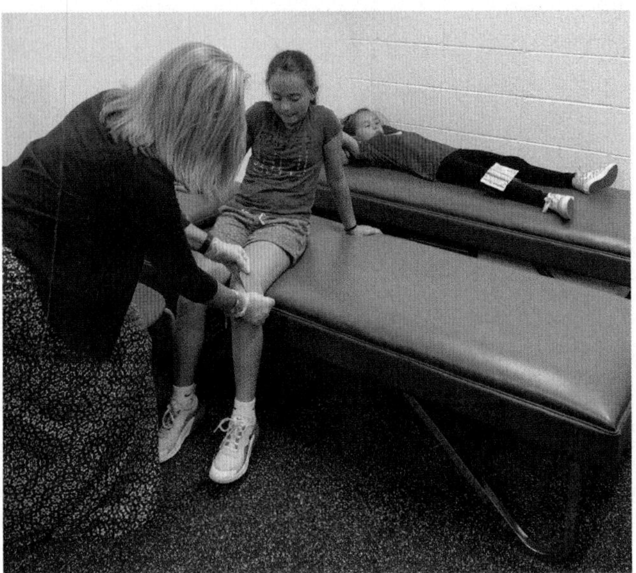

FIGURE 33.1 The school nurse provides nursing assessment as well as health education to students in the school setting.

The population of students has changed over the years. Access to public schools for children with disabilities is mandated. Due to improvements in technology, children with chronic conditions or special needs live longer and enter school. There has been an increase in the number of children with psychiatric conditions such as depression, attention-deficit/hyperactivity disorder, and more serious conditions such as bipolar disorder. All have contributed to an increase in the number of children with diverse and sometimes complex health needs in the school system. The essential role of the school nurse has not changed, but the responsibilities and expectations have. School nurses are challenged to meet the growing needs of the changing school population.

BOX **33.1 Examples of Activities of the School Nurse**

- Conduct health screenings (such as vision, hearing, and scoliosis).
- Assess growth and development.
- Provide emergency first aid, care for acute and chronic illnesses, such as medication administration and diabetes monitoring.
- Train and educate staff on cardiopulmonary resuscitation (CPR), first aid, and health issues.
- Assess, monitor, and refer students with communicable diseases.
- Educate on health promotion and disease prevention (such as immunizations; bike and car safety; decreasing high-risk behaviors, such as smoking, drinking, drug use, and sexual activity).
- Serve as a resource for health issues and education.
- Act as a liaison between health care provider and school.
- Reinforce patient and family health education (such as discharge instructions, self-care measures).
- Monitor long-term illness in students.
- Network with community agencies and make necessary referrals.

Nurses in the school setting develop **individualized health plans** (IHPs). It is the position of the National Association of School Nurses that school nurses develop an IHP to formalize the plan of support for a student with complex health care needs (NASN, 2020). It is a written agreement developed as part of an interdisciplinary collaboration of school staff along with the student, the student's family, and the student's health care provider. The plan describes the student's needs and how the school plans to meet these needs. The nurse plays a critical role in developing these plans. The nurse will use the nursing process and then, based on the nursing assessment and analysis, will develop goals and interventions to ensure that the child's needs are being met. Examples of students who may need an IHP are students with asthma, serious allergies, chronic conditions such as type 1 diabetes, physical disabilities, attention-deficit/hyperactivity disorder, and medication needs.

TAKE NOTE!

The IHP needs to include directions for care while the child is at school and must also take into account circumstances that may affect the student's health care needs, such as variations in school routine, absence of staff, special outings such as field trips and extracurricular activities, and a plan in case of emergency.

Home Health Care

Home care provides short- or long-term services for children and their families in the home. It is also used for medically needy and technology-dependent children, such as ventilator-dependent children. Among those who often benefit from home care are children with acute illness, such as a child with osteomyelitis requiring intravenous antibiotics, or chronic health care issues, such as a child with bronchopulmonary dysplasia, who may have required traditional in-hospital care.

It is important that the nurse practices family-centered home care that focuses on increasing support for the emotional and developmental needs of the child. This type of care encourages families to care for their children at home while health care professionals provide the support, empowerment, education, and expertise in caring for the child that they need. In family-centered home care, the family and health care professionals build a partnership of trust to meet the needs of the child. The nurse must value the role of the family and regard family members as the ultimate experts in caring for their child. In home care, the family is extensively involved in the child's care, and the home care nurse is there to facilitate.

Any illness, especially a chronic illness, affects the entire family and can disrupt family structure. There is a change in the role of the parent when they must care for an ill child. These role changes can result in stress for the family members and can affect their participation in the child's care. It is important for home care nurses to seek a partnership role with the family regarding care of the child. This can be difficult for both parties. Often, nurses set limits on parental involvement and do not consider the parents' perspective. Many nurses are concerned that the parents may not be able to care for the child safely. It is important for nurses to use self-awareness and reflective practice to help them understand and empower families as well as to develop a partnership for care. A communication framework, developed by Berlin and Fowkes (1983), that can assist nurses in the home care setting is the LEARN framework, which can help create cross-cultural collaboration and communication between nurses and families (Box 33.2).

Home care is geared toward the needs of the child and family. Private-duty nursing care is used when more extensive care is needed; it may be delivered hourly (several hours per day) or on a full-time, live-in basis. Periodic visiting nurse care is used when the child needs intermittent interventions such as intravenous antibiotic administration, follow-up with child and family teaching, and periodic monitoring, such as bilirubin monitoring. The goals of nursing care in the home setting include promoting, restoring, and maintaining the health of the child. Home care focuses on minimizing the effects of the illness or disability, along with providing the child or family with the means to care for the illness or disability at home. Nurses in the home care setting are direct providers of care, child and family educators, child and family advocates, and case managers.

There are some disadvantages to home care. The presence of health care professionals in the home can be an intrusion on family privacy. Also, caring for children with complex medical needs can be overwhelming for some families. Financial issues can become a large burden: families may have higher out-of-pocket costs if their insurance does not reimburse for home care. Having one parent at home full time and not earning an income can contribute to increased financial strain, not to mention social isolation of that parent. All of these factors can lead to increased stress on family members. The advantages of home care usually outweigh the disadvantages, but nurses need to be aware of these potential disadvantages and provide support and resources as necessary.

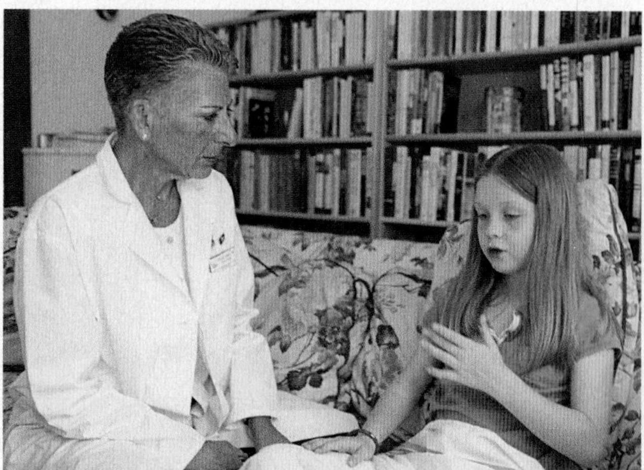

FIGURE 33.2 Listening to the child helps to develop a trusting relationship between the home care nurse and the child and her family.

The Nurse's Role in Home Care

Early discharge planning, teaching, and case management are keys to promoting a successful transition from the hospital setting to home. The environment differs greatly between the acute setting and home setting. In the acute setting, the nurse is in control of the environment; in the home setting, the nurse is a guest in the home. It is important for the nurse to establish a trusting relationship with both the child and the family (Fig. 33.2). A trusting therapeutic relationship will make all aspects of care more effective. Box 33.3 gives hints on building this relationship.

NURSING ASSESSMENT IN THE HOME SETTING

Nursing in the home care setting can be challenging. The focus is on meeting the child's physical and psychological needs while involving the family. In this role, the nurse uses the nursing process. Assessment in the home is similar to that in the acute care setting but also involves obtaining first-hand data about the family and

BOX 33.2 LEARN Framework

- L: Listen empathetically and with understanding to the family's perception of the situation.
- E: Explain your perception of the situation.
- A: Acknowledge and discuss the similarities as well as differences between the two perceptions.
- R: Recommend interventions.
- N: Negotiate and agree on the interventions.

Adapted from Berlin, E. A., & Fowkes, W. C., Jr. (1983). A teaching framework for cross-cultural health care—Application to practice. *The Western Journal of Medicine, 139*(6), 934–938.

BOX 33.3 Hints to Establishing a Trusting Relationship in Home Care

- Include the child in the conversation and make them feel a part of the interaction.
- Address caregivers formally unless otherwise instructed.
- Be friendly. Use a soft, calm voice.
- Be interested in the child's activities.
- Have the primary caregiver present at the initial visit.
- Listen to and show respect to the child and the family.

the way it functions. Assess the child's growth and development, and thoroughly assess the home environment (refer to Chapters 25 to 29 and 31 for additional information). Ensure that the home offers a safe and nurturing environment for the child. The U.S. Environmental Protection Agency (EPA) provides online training and resources for health care providers, including nurses (U.S. Environmental Protection Agency, 2022). These resources can be accessed on the EPA website under "Resources for Healthcare Providers about Children's Environmental Health."

Assess resources available to the family. This includes necessary equipment such as a hospital bed and oxygen, suitable physical and emotional surroundings (are the family members able to deal with the stress of the situation?), ability to contact emergency services, power backup if needed, and ease of evacuation of the child in case of a fire. Determine whether electricity, sanitary conditions, heat, air conditioning, and telephone access are present. If there is no phone in the home, the family needs to have plans for accessing a phone in case of emergency (perhaps a neighbor's phone). Identify areas of priority and provide appropriate referrals to resources.

During the assessment phase, the nurse identifies the person who is the primary caregiver; this may be a parent, grandparent, or older sibling. It is essential to include this person when developing the plan of care, as they are the expert on the child and family. The primary caregiver can provide insight into direct care and which strategies will be most effective with this child, taking into account the physical layout of the home, the financial ability of the family, and the way the family functions. The home care nurse must also assess the family's teaching and learning needs.

After the assessment is complete, develop appropriate nursing diagnoses, outcomes, and goals. This will include the frequency and duration of the home visits. Consider the individual needs of each patient in conjunction with state, federal, and agency policies, certification standards, and payer guidelines from private insurance and/or Medicaid regulations to assist in the development of the plan. The nurse may be the provider of direct care to the child, or the care may be indirect, in which case the nurse plans and supervises the care that is given by others, such as unlicensed personnel and parents.

NURSING MANAGEMENT IN THE HOME SETTING

Nursing care in the home requires excellent critical thinking skills. The nurse has a great deal of independence since there are no other nurses, supervisors, or health care providers on site. When complex care is provided in the home, the nurse may need to adjust procedures to fit the setting. For example, feeding schedules may be adjusted to fit a child's school schedule, or equipment may be adjusted to allow a child to receive feedings continuously while at school (Fig. 33.3).

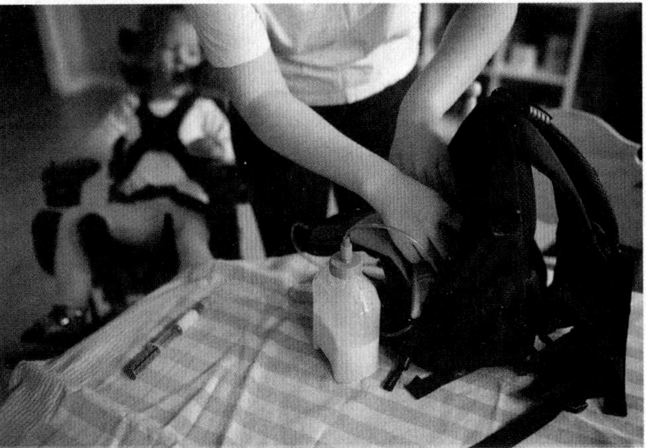

FIGURE 33.3 The home care nurse may have to adjust procedures and equipment use to fit the home setting. Placing a feeding pump in a backpack allows this child to receive feedings continuously while at school. (Shutterstock/Johner Images.)

Educating the Child and Family

An important role of the home care nurse is empowering children and their families through education (refer to Chapter 30 for further information related to teaching). Encourage the family to participate in the child's care. In many situations, parents or caregivers must learn caregiving procedures immediately so the child can be cared for at home, such as a child who needs dressing changes four times a day or a child who is ventilator dependent. A child newly diagnosed with diabetes will have some immediate teaching needs, but as the child grows and their condition changes, additional care will need to be taught.

As with any nursing care, the effectiveness of nursing interventions along with changes in the child's or family's status needs to be continuously evaluated and the plan of care altered as needed.

Other Community Settings

The primary focus of nursing in other community settings continues to be on promoting health, preventing disease and injury, and ensuring a safe environment. Nurses play important roles in child care centers, camps, health department clinics, and shelters. In child care centers, nurses help address infection control issues and assess for a safe environment. They provide education and training to staff members. A camp nurse ensures a safe environment for all campers and provides first-aid and acute illness care as needed. Camps for children with special needs exist, staffed by specially trained nurses. These camps cater to children with complex health care needs, such as diabetes, cancer, head injuries, and physical disabilities, and allow the children the opportunity to experience camp life while providing a safe environment and necessary medical care. Health department and shelter nurses focus on health supervision services and connecting patients to needed community resources.

TAKE NOTE!

Nurses have a unique opportunity to give back to their community by volunteering their services in various settings, such as shelters and clinics in medically underserved areas.

CHILDREN'S REACTIONS TO ILLNESS AND HOSPITALIZATION

In general, children are more vulnerable to the effects of illness and hospitalization because this is a change from their usual state of health and routine. They also have limited understanding and coping mechanisms to assist them in resolving the stressors that might occur during this time. Hospitalization and illness create a series of traumatic and stressful events in a climate of uncertainty for children and their families, whether it is an elective procedure that is planned in advance or an emergency situation resulting from trauma. The stressors that children experience in relation to hospitalization and illness may result in various reactions. Children react to the stresses of hospitalization before admission, during hospitalization, and after discharge.

Besides the physiologic effects of the health problem, the psychological effects of illness and hospitalization on a child include anxiety and fear related to the overall process and the potential for bodily injury, physical harm, and pain. In addition, children are separated from their homes, families, and friends and what is familiar to them, which may result in separation anxiety (distress related to removal from family and familiar surroundings). There is a general loss of control over their lives and sometimes their emotions and behaviors. The result may be feelings of anger and guilt, regression (return to a previous stage of development), acting out, and other types of defense mechanisms to cope with these effects. Children's typical coping strategies are tested during this experience.

Anxiety and Fear

For many children, entering a health care setting is like entering a foreign world. The result is anxiety and fear. Anxiety often stems from the rapid onset of the illness or injury, particularly when the child has limited experiences with disease or injury. Normal fears of childhood include the fear of separation from their parents and family or guardians, loss of control, and bodily injury, mutilation, or harm. Children's fears are similar to adult fears of the unknown, including fear of unfamiliar environments and losing control.

Therefore, when the child is in the hospital, they become distressed about the unfamiliar environment; health care procedures, especially the use of needles or associated pain that may occur; and situations such as the strange words being used, ominous-looking equipment, strangers in unusual attire (e.g., surgical caps, masks, gowns), unfamiliar and frightening noises and smells, or the sounds of other children crying. This exposure to people, situations, and procedures that may be new to them and that cause them pain leads to increased anxiety and fear (Fig. 33.4). Overall, illness and hospitalization are a difficult experience for children.

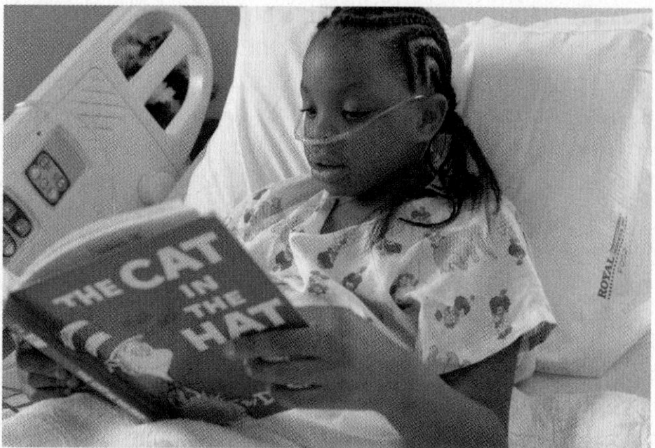

FIGURE 33.4 The presence of familiar objects and home routines normalizes the environment and helps the child cope with hospitalization. Reading a favorite bedtime story can be comforting.

Separation Anxiety

Separation anxiety is a major stressor for children of certain ages. Timing of separation anxiety varies among children. It typically begins once a child has developed object permanence (an understanding that things exist even when they are out of sight), which is usually around 4 to 8 months (Piaget, 1969).

James Robertson and John Bowlby described three stages that the infant and child goes through during separation anxiety—protest, despair, and detachment (Robertson & Bowlby, 1952). The first phase, protest, occurs when the child is separated from the parents or primary caregiver. This phase may last from a few hours to several days. The child reacts aggressively to this separation and exhibits great distress by crying, expressing agitation, and rejecting others who attempt to offer comfort. The child may also display anger and inconsolable grief.

If the parents do not return within a short time, the child exhibits the second phase, despair. The child displays hopelessness by withdrawing from others; becoming quiet without crying; and exhibiting apathy, depression, lack of interest in play and food, and overall feelings of sadness.

Detachment (also known as denial) is the third and final phase of separation anxiety. During this phase, the child forms coping mechanisms to protect against further emotional pain. This occurs more often in long-term separations. During this stage, the child shows interest in the environment, starts to play again, and forms superficial relationships with the nurses and other children. If the parents return, the child ignores them. A child in this phase of separation anxiety exhibits resignation, not contentment. It is more difficult to reverse this stage, and developmental delays may occur.

Today, health care providers primarily observe the first and second stages because of the shorter hospital stays and the more common use of a family-centered approach to care.

Loss of Control

When ill or hospitalized, children experience a significant loss of control. This loss of control increases the perception of threat and affects their coping skills. They lose control over routine self-care and their usual tasks and play as well as decisions related to the care of their own bodies. In the hospital, the child's usual routine is disrupted. They cannot choose what to do and at what time. The child can no longer accomplish simple tasks independently as they do at home or school. Confinement to the bed or crib worsens this loss of control. For example, if connected to tubes or intravenous lines, the child may not even be able to visit the bathroom alone.

Hospitalization also affects the child's control over decisions related to their own body. Many of the procedures and treatments that occur in the hospital are invasive or are at least disturbing to children, and much of the time they do not have the option to refuse to undergo them. Adults are presumed to be competent to make health care decisions, but, generally, children are not. Although the parents and nurses of hospitalized children have the children's best interest in mind, children often feel powerless when in the hospital, not having their feelings and wishes respected and having minimal control over events.

> *TAKE NOTE!*
> When advocating for a child, make sure to include the child's voice. Do not assume what their wishes may be; ask about them directly.

FACTORS AFFECTING CHILDREN'S REACTION TO ILLNESS AND HOSPITALIZATION

Various factors have a great impact on the ability of children to handle illness and hospitalization. These factors may increase or diminish the fears of the child who is ill and hospitalized. Each child responds differently and will perceive the hospital experience differently. Box 33.4 lists the various factors affecting a child's response to illness and hospitalization.

BOX 33.4 Factors Affecting a Child's Response to Illness and Hospitalization

- Amount of separation from parent/caregiver
- Age
- Developmental level
- Cognitive level
- Previous experience with illness and hospitalization
- Recent life stresses and changes
- Type and amount of preparation
- Temperament
- Innate and acquired coping skills
- Seriousness of the diagnosis/onset of illness or injury (e.g., acute or chronic)
- Support systems available, including the family and health care professionals
- Cultural background
- Parents' reaction to illness and hospitalization

Developmental Level

The child's age, cognitive level, and developmental level will affect their perceptions of actual events, and this in turn will affect their reaction to illness and hospitalization. Children's responses to the stressors of fear, separation anxiety, and loss of control vary depending on their age and developmental level. Younger children, with their limited life experience and immature intellectual capacities, have a more difficult time comprehending what is happening to them. This can be particularly true for toddlers and preschoolers, who perceive the intactness of their bodies to be exposed during physical intrusions. In addition, they frequently interpret illness as punishment for wrongdoing or hospital procedures as hostile, mutilating acts. Although children are increasingly able to adapt as they grow older, lack of understanding about the need for hospitalization and threatened sense of control can make adaptation difficult.

Infants

Newborns and infants are adapting to life outside the womb with rapid growth and development and establishment of a healthy attachment to parents or primary caregivers. They are dependent on others for nurturance and protection. They gain a sense of trust in the world through rhythmic and reciprocal patterns of contact and feeding, resulting in bonding to the primary caregiver. They need a secure pattern of restful sleep, satisfaction of oral and nutritional needs, relaxation of body systems, and spontaneous response to communication and gentle stimuli. The caregiver–infant attachment is critical for psychological health, especially during periods of illness and hospitalization.

Unfortunately, during illness and hospitalization, these critical patterns of feeding, contact, comfort, sleeping, elimination, and stimulation are disrupted, resulting in fear, separation anxiety, and loss of control. By 5 to 6 months of age, infants have developed an awareness of self as separate from the birthing parent. As a result, infants of this age are acutely aware of the absence of their primary caregiver and become fearful of unfamiliar people. Infants may be separated from their parents when hospitalized if the parents cannot room-in because of hospital policy or if they must work or care for other children. This results in separation anxiety.

The infant's oral needs, the basic source of infant satisfaction, are often not met in the hospital due to the condition of the child or the procedures that must be performed. The infant is accustomed to having their basic needs met by the parent when they cry or gesture. The constraints of hospitalization result in loss of control over the environment, leading to additional anxiety in the infant.

Toddlers

Toddlers are more aware of self and can communicate their desires. Because their autonomy is developing, toddlers need to master accomplishments to minimize the development of shame and doubt. Control becomes an issue for toddlers. Toddlers also need opportunities to explore, and they need consistent routines. In addition, toddlers are aware of the need for care and protection from others, so they need familiarity and closeness to the primary caregiver. When the toddler is ill or hospitalized, disruption occurs in this development of autonomy.

Toddlers are often fearful of strangers and can recall traumatic events. Simply walking toward the room where a traumatic procedure previously occurred may upset the toddler. Ordinarily, a resurgence in separation anxiety occurs during the toddler years. When the toddler is separated from their parents or caregivers in an unfamiliar environment, separation anxiety is compounded. In response to this anxiety, toddlers may demonstrate behaviors such as pleading for the parents to stay, physically trying to go after the parents, throwing temper tantrums, and refusing to comply with usual routines. Restrictions related to mobility and new skill acquisition result in loss of control. Disruption in usual routines also contributes to loss of control, and the toddler feels insecure. As a result, regression in toilet training and refusal to eat are common reactions in toddlers.

Preschoolers

The preschooler has better verbal and developmental skills to adapt to various situations, but illness and hospitalization can still be stressful. Preschoolers may understand that they are in the hospital because they are sick, but they may not understand the cause of their illness. Preschoolers fear mutilation and are afraid of intrusive procedures since they do not understand the body's integrity. They interpret words literally and have an active imagination. Therefore, when the nurse says, "I need to take some blood," preschoolers' fantasies may run wild. They may not understand the concept of blood and may think everything will come out of their body. They may think that blood is "taken" the same way a child picks up a toy to take it out of the room. Preschoolers' thinking is egocentric; they believe that some personal deed or thought caused their illness, which can lead to guilt and shame. These feelings may be internalized. Overall, preschoolers' concrete, egocentric, and magical thinking (type of thinking that allows for fantasies and creativity) limits their ability to understand, so communication and interventions must be on their level.

Separation anxiety may not be as much of an issue as it is for toddlers since preschoolers may already be spending time away from parents in preschool. They are, however, still acutely aware of the comfort and security that their family provides for them, so disruptions in these relationships lead to challenges. The preschooler may constantly ask for their parents or ask to call the parents. They may quietly cry, refuse to eat or take medication, or generally be uncooperative.

In addition, the ill or hospitalized preschooler loses control over the environment. The preschooler is naturally curious about their surroundings and learns best by observing and working with objects. This might be limited during illness or hospitalization. Because the preschooler cannot participate in typical activities and explore the environment as usual, the child's normal creative, curious nature may give rise to a variety of fantasies that may present challenges.

School-Age

School-age children, generally, are hospitalized because of long-term illnesses or trauma. The general task of their development stage, to develop confidence through a sense of industry, can be disrupted during illness or hospitalization. Even at this time, they generally want to continue to learn and maintain their skills and abilities. The stress of illness or anxiety related to diagnostic tests and therapeutic interventions may lead to inward or outward expressions of distress. If they have learned various coping skills, this distress may be minimized. After 11 years of age, there is an increased awareness of physiologic, psychological, and behavioral causes of illness and injury. Typically, the school-age child has a more realistic understanding of the reasons for the illness and can better comprehend explanations. School-age children are concerned about disability and death, and they fear injury and pain. They want to know why procedures and tests are being performed. They can understand cause and effect and how it relates to their illness. They are uncomfortable with any type of genital examination.

Separation anxiety is not as much of an issue for school-age children. They are accustomed to periods of separation and may already be experiencing some separation anxiety related to being in school. At the same time, they may be missing school and friends as they try to adjust to the unfamiliar environment. They may feel that friends will forget them if they remain ill or in the hospital for a long time. Some school-age children may regress and become needy, demanding their parents' attention or playing with special "comfort toys" they used at a younger age.

Since school-age children are accustomed to controlling self-care and are typically highly social, they like being involved. They are used to making choices about meals and activities. Illness or hospitalization presents loss of control by limiting their activities, making them feel helpless and dependent. This may result in feelings of loneliness, boredom, isolation, and depression. The key is to give them opportunities to maintain independence, retain a sense of control, enhance self-esteem, and continue to work toward achieving a sense of industry.

Adolescents

Adolescents fear injury and pain. Since appearance is important to them, they are concerned with how the illness or injury will affect their body image. Anything that changes their perceptions of themselves has a major impact on their response. Typically, adolescents do not like to be different; they like "being cool," which means being in control and not showing how afraid they really are. They may also feel ambivalent about wanting their parents. Adolescents typically do not experience separation anxiety from being away from their parents; instead, their anxiety comes from being separated from friends.

Loss of control is a key factor affecting the behavior of adolescents who are ill or hospitalized. Anger, withdrawal, or general lack of cooperation may occur due to the feelings of loss of control. In addition, their desire to appear confident may lead them to question everything that is being done or that they are asked to do. Their feelings of invincibility may cause them to take risks and be noncompliant with treatment. Overall, adolescents strive for independence, self-assertion, and liberation while developing their identity.

Previous Experiences

In general, children's lack of understanding and experience of illness, hospitalization, and hospital procedures contributes to their anxiety level. However, previous experience with hospitalization and other health-related experiences can either facilitate preparation or impair it if the experiences were perceived as negative. For example, the child who associates the hospital with the birth of a sibling may view this experience as positive. However, the child who associates the hospital with the serious illness or death of a relative or close friend will probably view the experience as negative.

The type of experience may contribute to increased anxiety and fear if the child must be admitted to the hospital. If children have had previous experiences, how the experience unfolded and their response to it will determine many of their reactions to illness or hospitalization. Older children may cling to their parents, kick, or create a scene because of their previous experience.

Recent Stresses and Changes and Individual Coping Skills

The effects of illness hospitalization on children are influenced by the nature and severity of the health problem, the condition of the child, and the degree to which activities and routines differ from those of everyday life. A lack of sensory stimulation in the hospital environment can lead to listlessness, indifference, unhappiness, and even appetite changes. When the child's motor activity is restricted, anger and hyperactivity may result. Play, recreation, and educational opportunities can provide an outlet to distract the child from the illness, provide pleasant experiences, and help the child understand their condition.

The child's ability to work through a situation will also affect their responses to illness and hospitalization. This ability depends on the age of the child, their perceptions of the event, previous encounters with health care personnel, and support from significant others. Box 33.5 lists various coping skills used by children and suggestions for promoting positive coping.

Parents' Response to Child's Illness and Hospitalization

Parents who do not tell children the truth or who do not answer their questions confuse and frighten them and may weaken the child's trust in the parents. Children take in their parents' anxiety and concern. Even whispers can set off children's imaginations. For example, preschoolers may invent elaborate stories to explain what is

BOX 33.5 Children and Coping

Behavior/Methods for Coping	Suggestions to Promote Coping
Ignore or negate the problem.	Breathing techniques such as blowing bubbles, pinwheels, or party noise makers
Stoicism, passive acceptance	Distraction with books or games
Acting out—yelling, kicking, screaming, crying	Imagery with tapes or scenarios
Anger, withdrawal, rejection	Music
Intellectualizing	Teaching before events or procedures

happening to them. It is important for children to believe that someone is in control and that the person can be trusted. Some parents, however, have their own fears and insecurities. Thus, a child's reaction is often related to the parents' reaction to the illness and hospitalization.

The relationship between the family and the health care staff may either add to or ease the child's stress. This relationship can contribute significantly to the quality of the environment. Health care personnel must assume responsibility for the care of ill or hospitalized children by maintaining good partnerships with families.

FAMILY'S REACTIONS TO THE CHILD'S ILLNESS AND HOSPITALIZATION

Whether planned or unplanned, hospitalization increases the family's stress and anxiety level. The illness or serious injury of one family member affects all members of the family because the process disrupts the family's usual routines and may alter family roles. Parents and siblings have their own reactions to this experience.

Reactions of Parents

Watching a child in pain is difficult, especially when the parent is assisting with the procedure by holding the child. The parent may feel guilty for not seeking care sooner. Parents may also exhibit other feelings such as denial, anger, depression, and confusion. Parents may deny that the child is ill. They may express anger, especially directed at the nursing staff, another family member, or a higher power, because of their loss of control in caring for the child. Depression may occur because of exhaustion and the psychological and physical requirements of spending long hours in a hospital caring for a child. Confusion may develop because of dealing with an unfamiliar environment or the loss of a parental role. Finally, the parents' relationship may be strained because of dual roles, long separation, and increased stress.

Reactions of Siblings

Siblings of children who are hospitalized may experience jealousy, insecurity, resentment, confusion, and anxiety. They may have difficulty understanding why their sibling is ill or getting all the attention, leaving little for them. They may wonder if their sibling is going to die or ever return home. They may worry that their sibling's illness is going to happen to them. Certain age groups, such as preschoolers, may feel that they caused the illness. Little information or understanding about what is happening, combined with their magical and egocentric thinking, contributes to their fears that they may have caused the illness or injury by their thoughts, wishes, or behaviors. If the family roles or routines change significantly, the siblings may feel insecure or anxious. They may develop changes in behavior or in school performance. See Evidence-Based Practice 33.1.

EVIDENCE-BASED PRACTICE **33.1**

What Personal Challenges Do Caregivers Face During Pediatric Hospitalization?

The stressors of an ill child in the hospital can affect all family members. Strong parent–provider partnerships can improve patient- and family-centered care and patient outcomes. Limited data are available describing challenges caregivers face in general pediatric hospitalization regardless of illness or diagnosis. Unaddressed caregiver needs may influence understanding and perceptions of the plan of care, caregiver decision-making skills, and caregiver engagement in care. Addressing caregiver needs optimizes family-centered care.

STUDY

A small qualitative study was performed. Caregivers at a children's hospital were interviewed to learn about their hospital experience and the personal challenges they faced and to obtain feedback on possible interventions to minimize their challenges.

Findings

The study found caregiver difficulties with their child's hospitalization were connected to physiologic challenges, including lack of sleep and inability to eat and tend to personal care; psychosocial challenges, including isolation, stress, and juggling multiple roles; and communication challenges between the family and medical team.

Nursing Considerations

Recognize that caregivers of a hospitalized child often experience personal challenges. Nurses are in the unique position to help caregivers overcome these challenges. Helping address caregivers' physiologic, psychosocial, and communication needs may be critical to improving the experience of hospitalization. Meeting caregiver's basic needs is crucial to assisting them to function as an advocate for their child. This study also sought out interventions that caregivers felt the hospital could implement to help address these challenges. Examples of interventions nurses could implement include clustering care and posting signs alerting staff to when the child or caregiver is sleeping. The nurse can offer personal hygiene items and improve access to food by educating the caregiver on food options available to them. Nurses can help uncover and address transportation issues and improve communication by using white boards in patient rooms to share key information, help caregivers sign up for the patient portal, thoroughly review all discharge paperwork with the caregiver, and answer all questions the caregiver or patient may have. Further research is warranted and needs to be focused on developing evidence-based interventions that address the challenges faced by caregivers of hospitalized children.

Based on Vaz, L. E., Jungbauer, R. M., Jenisch, C., Austin, J. P., Wagner, D. V., Everist, S. J., Libak, A. J., Harris, M. A., & Zuckerman; K. E. (2022). Caregiver experiences in pediatric hospitalizations: Challenges and opportunities for improvement. *Hospital Pediatrics, 12*(12), 1073–1080. https://doi.org/10.1542/hpeds.2022-006645

Factors Influencing Family Reactions

The parenting style and the family–child relationship can influence the hospital experience as well as the family members' coping skills. Cultural, ethnic, and religious variations, values, and practices related to illness; general response to stress; and attitudes about the care of a sick child have a significant influence on the family's response. For example, religious beliefs can increase problems or can be a source of strength to the family and child. Families already in crisis or without support systems have a more difficult time dealing with the added stress of hospitalization. Chapter 24 gives further explanations of some of these influences on children and their families.

> Remember Jake, the 8-year-old with a suspected brain tumor introduced at the beginning of the chapter? What reactions to illness and hospitalization might you see from him and his family?

Clinical Judgment and the Nursing Process

In most instances, the nurse is the primary person involved in the care of a hospitalized or ill child. The nurse is probably the first one to see the child and family and will spend more time with them than other health care personnel. Nurses are part of a medical community that makes decisions in the child's best interest, but the nurse needs to bear in mind the child's rights and must try to minimize the child's distress so that the hospital stay will be as pleasant an experience as possible. When establishing strategies to care for children, nurses should examine the general effects of hospitalization and illness on children in each developmental stage and should strive to understand both the reactions of the child and family to illness and hospitalization and the factors affecting these reactions.

Nursing Analysis

After recognizing and analyzing cues from a thorough assessment, the nurse may identify several hypotheses, including:

- Anxiety
- Risk for powerlessness
- Decreased diversional activity engagement
- Interrupted family processes
- Bathing/dressing/feeding self-care deficit
- Risk for delayed development
- Deficient knowledge
- Risk for caregiver role strain

These hypotheses provide suggestions for nursing care planning or concept mapping. The nurse will then generate solutions by planning interventions (suggested along with rationales further on). The plan of care should be individualized, based on the child's and family's needs.

Nursing Analysis

Anxiety related to stressors (from hospital situation or illness, fear of injury or bodily mutilation, separation from family or friends, changes in routine, painful procedures and treatments, and unfamiliar events and surroundings) as evidenced by crying, fussing, withdrawal, or resistance

Goal/Outcome

Child and family will exhibit a decrease in anxiety level as evidenced by positive coping strategies, verbalization or playing out of feelings, appropriate behaviors, positive interactions with staff, child and parent cooperation and participation, and absence of signs and symptoms of increasing anxiety and fear.

Minimizing Anxiety (interventions with *rationale*)

- Orient child and family to the unit and the child's room *to familiarize them with the facility.*
- Assess for signs and symptoms of anxiety and fear *to establish a baseline and assess effectiveness of interventions.*
- Place the child in a room with another child of a similar age, developmental level, and condition severity *to promote sharing.*
- Provide atraumatic care *to minimize exposure to distress, which would increase anxiety.*
- Explain all events, treatments, procedures, and activities to the parents and child (at a level the child can understand) in a calm, relaxed manner *to help the child prepare for what is to come and decrease fear of the unknown. A calm, relaxed manner helps to establish rapport and instill trust.*
- Enlist the aid of a CLS *to assist in age-appropriate preparation for all events, treatments, and procedures.*
- Encourage parents to room-in if possible *to provide the child with support;* if parents cannot stay, encourage them to call *to reduce the child's fear of being alone.*
- Urge parents to inform the child when they will be leaving and when they are expected to return *to help the child cope with their absence and promote trust.*
- Assess child's usual routine at home and attempt to incorporate aspects of usual routine into hospital routine *to ease the transition to the hospital and promote the child's participation in routine.*
- Offer comfort measures such as holding, stroking, and rocking *to relieve distress.*
- Encourage the child to play (unstructured and therapeutic play as necessary) *to allow for expression of feelings and fears and promote energy expenditure.*

- Suggest that parents bring in a special toy or object from home *to promote feelings of security.*
- Provide positive reinforcement for participation in care activities *to foster self-esteem.*
- Assess for regression behaviors and inform parents that such behaviors are common *to alleviate their concerns about this behavior.*
- Provide consistency with care measures *to facilitate trust and acceptance.*

Nursing Analysis

Risk for powerlessness; risk factors include insufficient knowledge to manage a situation, ineffective coping strategies, pain, anxiety (lack of control over procedures, treatments, and care, changes in usual routine, continual hospital readmissions)

Goal/Outcome

Child and family will demonstrate an increase in control over the situation as evidenced by participation in care activities, identification of needs and choices, and incorporation of appropriate aspects of child's usual routine with that of the hospital routine.

Promoting Control (interventions with *rationale*)

- Encourage child and parents to identify areas of concern *to help determine priority needs.*
- Encourage parent and child to participate in care activities *to promote feelings of control.*
- Incorporate aspects of child's routine at home and use terms similar to those used at home *to foster a sense of normalcy.*
- Offer child choices as much as possible, such as options for foods, drinks, hygiene, activities, or clothing (if appropriate) *to promote feelings of individuality and control.*
- Allow child opportunities for being out of bed or room within limitations as appropriate *to foster independence.*
- Work with child, as age and development allow, and family to set up a schedule *to promote structure and routine.*

Nursing Analysis

Decreased diversional activity engagement related to the current setting/situation not allowing engagement in activity (confinement in bed or health care facility, lack of appropriate stimulation from toys or peers), impaired mobility (activity restrictions or equipment such as IV pump), insufficient energy, insufficient motivation, or physical discomfort as evidenced by verbalization of boredom or lack of participation in play, reading, or school work.

Goal/Outcome

Child will participate in diversional activities as evidenced by engagement in unstructured and therapeutic play that is developmentally appropriate and by interaction with family, staff, and other children.

Promoting Adequate Diversional Activities (interventions with *rationale*)

- Question child and family about favorite types of activities *to establish a baseline for developing appropriate choices during hospitalization.*
- Assist with planning activities within the limits of the child's condition *to maintain muscle tone and strength without overexerting the child.*
- Spend time with the child *to provide stimulation and foster trust.*
- Enlist the aid of a CLS *to provide suggestions for appropriate activities.*
- Encourage interaction with other children *to promote sharing and avoid loneliness.*
- Provide developmentally appropriate opportunities for unstructured and therapeutic play *to facilitate expression of feelings.*
- Encourage short trips to the playroom or activity room *to provide a change of scenery and sensory stimulation.*
- Integrate play activities with nursing care *to achieve therapeutic effect.*

Nursing Analysis

Interrupted family processes related to power shift among family members and shift in family roles (separation from child due to hospitalization, increased demands of caring for an ill child, changes in role function and routine, and effect of hospitalization on other family members such as siblings), as evidenced by parental verbalization of issues, parental presence in hospital, or child's hospitalization requiring parent to miss work.

Goal/Outcome

Family will demonstrate positive coping strategies and mutual support for one another as evidenced by visiting frequently and staying with the child as necessary, sharing of family responsibilities, obtaining assistance for relief or respite, and visiting by other members of the child's family and friends.

Maximizing Family Functioning (interventions with *rationale*)

- Encourage parents and family members to verbalize concerns about child's illness, diagnosis, and prognosis *to promote family-centered care and identify areas where intervention may be needed.*
- Explain therapies, procedures, child's behaviors, and plan of care to parents *to promote understanding of the child's status and plan of care, which helps to decrease anxiety.*
- Encourage parental involvement in care *to promote feelings of the parents being needed and valued,*

providing them with a sense of control over their child's health.

- Identify support system for family and child *to identify resources available for coping.*
- Educate family and child on additional resources available *to promote a wider base of support to deal with the situation.*
- Suggest ways that parents can divide time between child and other siblings *to prevent feelings of guilt.*
- Provide support and positive reinforcement *to promote family coping and foster family strength.*
- Encourage frequent visits by family members, including siblings as appropriate, *to promote ongoing family functioning.*
- Stress the need for adequate rest, sleep, exercise, and nutrition for family members *to promote family health and minimize stress of hospitalization on family.*
- Assist with referrals for resources and help from additional family members and friends as necessary *to allow for respite or relief of care responsibilities.*
- Encourage family to maintain usual routine as much as possible *to minimize the effects of hospitalization on family functioning.*
- Enlist the aid of a CLS to work with any siblings *to provide support and education and to address the needs of a sibling of a hospitalized child.*

Nursing Analysis

Bathing/dressing/feeding self-care deficit related to anxiety, decrease in motivation (regression), discomfort, environmental barrier (such as activity restrictions, immobility or use of equipment, devices, or prescribed treatments), fatigue, pain, or weakness as evidenced by inability to feed, bathe, or dress self or accomplish other activities of daily living.

Goal/Outcome

Child will participate in self-care within limitations of condition as evidenced by assisting with bathing and hygiene, feeding, toileting, and dressing and grooming.

Promoting Self-Care (interventions with *rationale*)

- Assess child's usual routine for self-care and self-care abilities *to provide a baseline for individualizing interventions.*
- Provide child-sized equipment and devices *to promote child's ability to complete the self-care task.*
- Encourage parents and child to do as much self-care as possible, within limitations of the child's condition and developmental level, *to promote feelings of independence and foster growth and development.*
- Offer praise and encouragement for activities performed *to foster self-esteem, confidence, and competence.*
- Ensure adequate rest periods *to minimize energy expenditure associated with self-care activities.*

Nursing Analysis

Risk for delayed development; risk factors include chronic illness and treatment regimen (resultant stressors associated with hospitalization, current condition or illness, separation from family, and sensory overload or sensory deprivation).

Goal/Outcome

Child will demonstrate developmentally appropriate milestones as evidenced by age-appropriate behaviors and activities.

Promoting Growth and Development (interventions with *rationale*)

- Assess child's developmental stage *to establish a baseline and determine appropriate strategies.*
- Use unstructured and therapeutic play and adaptive toys *to promote developmental functioning.*
- Provide stimulating environment when possible *to maximize potential for growth and development.*
- Praise accomplishments and emphasize child's abilities *to foster self-esteem and encourage feelings of confidence and competence.*
- Include parents in techniques to foster growth and development *to promote feelings of control in their child's care.*

Nursing Analysis

Deficient knowledge related to insufficient knowledge (regarding hospitalization, surgery, treatments, procedures, required care, and follow-up) as evidenced by questioning and verbalization, lack of prior exposure.

Goal/Outcome

Child and family will demonstrate understanding of all aspects of child's current situation as evidenced by identification of child's and family's needs, verbal statements of understanding and/or need for additional information, return demonstration of procedures and treatments, and verbalization of instructions for follow-up and continued care.

Providing Child and Family Teaching (interventions with *rationale*)

- Assess child's and family's willingness to learn *to ensure effective teaching.*
- Provide family with time to adjust to diagnosis *to facilitate their ability to learn and participate in the child's care.*
- Repeat information *to promote multiple opportunities for child and family to learn.*
- Teach in short sessions *to prevent overloading the child and parents with information.*

- Gear teaching to appropriate level of understanding for the child and the family (depends on age of child, physical condition, memory) *to promote learning*.
- Provide reinforcement and rewards *to facilitate the teaching/learning process*.
- Use multiple modes of learning, such as written information, verbal instruction, demonstrations, and media, when possible *to facilitate learning and retention of information*.
- Provide the child and family with written step-by-step instructions for procedures or care *to provide a reference, if needed, at a later date*.
- Have child and family provide return demonstrations of care procedures *to ensure effectiveness of teaching*.
- Arrange for trial home care during hospitalization and after discharge as appropriate *to ensure understanding and provide opportunities for additional teaching and learning*.

Nursing Analysis

Risk for caregiver role strain; risk factors include child's increased care needs, unstable health condition, competing role commitments, inexperience with caregiving, stressors, change in nature or complexity of care activities.

Goal/Outcome

Caregiver will exhibit emotional health: *verbalizes concerns calmly, participates in child's care, and demonstrates knowledge of resources*.

Easing Caregiver Role Strain (interventions with *rationale*)

- Assess parental behavior *to identify role strain*.
- Provide emotional support and encourage talking about feelings, fears, and concerns *to promote trust in nurse as a source of emotional support*.
- Arrange for and/or encourage respite care for child: *provides parent with time away from continual care*.
- Consult social services *to identify community resources available for caregiver support (home health, support group, etc.)*.
- Encourage parent to meet own needs and find personal time *to increase energy level and self-esteem, ultimately enhancing the quality of care given*.

PREPARING THE CHILD AND FAMILY FOR SURGERY

If the child is to undergo a surgical procedure, whether in the hospital or an outpatient setting, special interventions are necessary. Preparation provides reassurance and comfort to the child and allows them to know what will happen and what is expected of them. The parents should be allowed to stay with the child until surgery begins. Parents should also be allowed to be with the child when they wake up in the postanesthesia recovery area.

Preoperative care for the child who is to undergo surgery is similar to that for an adult. The major difference is that the preparation and teaching must be geared to the child's age and developmental level. Many facilities offer special programs to help prepare children and families for the surgical experience. Preoperative preparation programs allow children and their families to experience a "trial run" in a supportive environment to help reduce anxiety, increase knowledge, increase comfort level, and enhance coping skills (Romito et al., 2021). The American Society of Anesthesiologists has prepared a coloring and activity book entitled *My Surgery Journey* (American Society of Anesthesiologists, n.d.). This book is designed to alleviate some of the fears that younger children may have related to the hospital experience. It describes the process from admission (whether it be to the hospital or the ambulatory surgery center) through discharge.

Many facilities have coloring or activity books specific to the facility and procedures that allow children to prepare and learn about their surgical and hospital experience through interactive activities like word searches, mazes, and matching games. These activities help the child and family prepare for what to expect and can provide a place to express thoughts, feelings, and questions through interactive and fun activities.

Providing Preoperative Teaching

Teaching the child and family is essential. Table 33.1 discusses strategies for preoperative teaching. Like any intervention, adapt the teaching to the child's developmental level. For example, when teaching a toddler or preschooler about breathing exercises, have the child blow a pinwheel or cotton balls across the table through a straw. The child will enjoy the activity while also reaping the respiratory benefits of the activity.

In preparation for surgery, use items such as stuffed animals or dolls to help children understand what is going to happen to them (Fig. 33.5). Allow

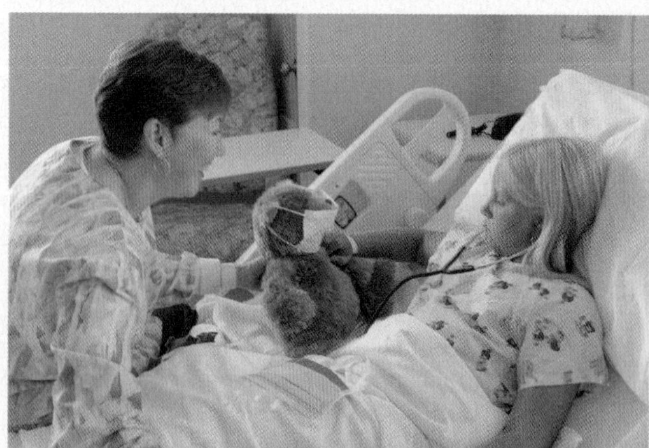

FIGURE 33.5 Using a stuffed animal to explain a surgical procedure to the child.

TABLE 33.1 • Strategies for Preoperative Teaching

Developmental Level	Implications for Teaching
Infants and toddlers	Encourage parents to use a soft tone of voice and stroking and secure, comfortable holding positions to promote calm. Remind parents to use positive facial expressions. Encourage the parent or caregiver to stay with the child as much as possible. Use terms that the child and parents can understand. For toddlers, provide information as close to the day of surgery as possible to prevent undue anxiety.
Preschoolers and school-age children	Provide factual explanations using terms the child and parents can understand. Incorporate pictures and other visual aids in explanation. Tailor the timing of education to meet the child's learning needs, allowing enough time for the child to ask questions. For preschoolers, provide information 1–2 days before surgery. For school-age children, provide information 3–5 days before surgery.
Adolescents	Provide detailed explanations of the procedure at least 7–10 days beforehand. Answer questions honestly, ensuring privacy at all times. Remain available for questions or concerns arising before or after surgery.

the child to role-play various experiences with dolls. Dolls designed to simulate surgical experiences have been developed. For example, Shadow Buddies are custom-made dolls that have the same illness or surgery as the child; the doll may have an ostomy, a scar, or a catheter (Shadow Buddies Foundation, n.d.). The dolls were developed to help children cope with their illness or disease and send the message that it is okay to be different. These dolls also provide the child with a companion to talk to.

SAFETY DURING HOSPITALIZATION OR PROCEDURES

Safety is a critical aspect of care of the child. Due to their age and developmental level, children are vulnerable to harm.

Maintaining the Child's Safety

Ensure the child has an identification band in place at all times. Sometimes, in implementing interventions, an armband is removed, so make sure it is attached to another extremity. Monitor children closely to avoid accidents such as a child pushing the wrong knob, picking up a piece of equipment or supplies left in the bed or room, or climbing out of bed (Fig. 33.6). Table 33.2 highlights nursing goals for ensuring safe, developmentally appropriate care for the hospitalized child.

Use of Restraints

When caring for children, some type of restriction may be necessary. The restriction, often referred to as a restraint, may be needed to ensure the child's safety, allow a therapeutic or diagnostic procedure to be done, immobilize a body part or limit movement, or prevent disruption of prescribed therapy. However, restraints can be overused and are not without risks to the child's safety and should be used as a last resort (Centers for Medicare & Medicaid Services [CMS], 2020). As a result, each facility will have specific procedures and policies in place related to the use of restraints based on standards developed by The Joint Commission, regulations developed by the CMS, state law, and facility requirements. These procedures and policies are designed to safeguard children's physical safety and psychological well-being.

TAKE NOTE!

Always refer to your institution's policy regarding restraint use.

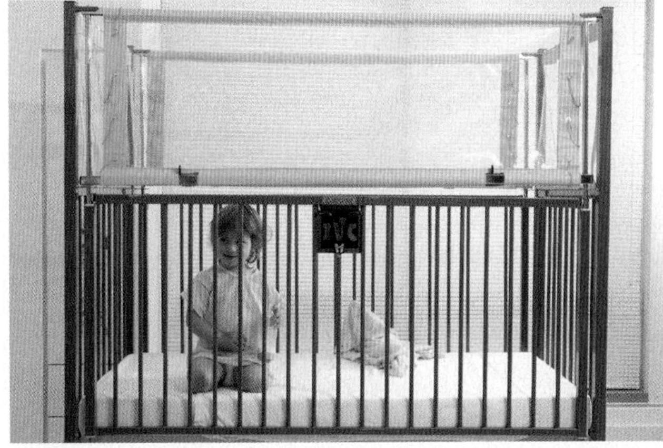

FIGURE 33.6 Safety is an essential aspect of pediatric nursing. A clear plastic cover over the crib prevents the older infant or toddler from climbing out and falling.

TABLE 33.2 • Nursing Considerations for Providing Safe, Developmentally Appropriate Care

	Ensuring Safety	Promoting Healthy Growth and Development
Infants	• Maintain close supervision of the infant. • Keep one hand on the infant when crib sides are down. • Keep crib rails up all the way when the infant is in the crib. • Avoid leaving small objects that are harmful or that can be swallowed in the crib. • Provide safe and appropriate toys for the infant. • Place infants in rooms close to the nurses' station. • Encourage a family member to stay with the infant at all times.	• Use the en face position when holding newborns. • Smile and talk to the infant during bathing, feeding, and other interactions. • Minimize the number of painful or uncomfortable procedures. • Provide comfort during and after procedures by holding or talking, using soothing tones and movements. • When handling the infant, use smooth, continuous movements. • Use gentle stroking and holding, which may reduce stress. • Serve as a role model for first-time parents. • Encourage the family to maintain home routines while in the hospital, planning nursing care around the usual feeding and sleep times. • Use the pacifier between feedings to satisfy nonnutritive sucking needs.
Toddlers	• Keep crib side rails up with overhead crib protection intact when the toddler is in the crib. • Never leave a toddler alone in the room unless secured in the crib. • Use a bed only for the older toddler who has an adult present in the room at all times. • Avoid leaving small objects that can be swallowed or are harmful in the crib or bed. • Place crib out of reach of cords, equipment, and electrical outlets. • Provide safe and appropriate toys for the toddler. • Place toddlers in rooms close to the nurses' station. • Always have someone with the toddler when ambulating.	• Encourage the parent to stay with the toddler to decrease separation anxiety. • To promote autonomy, allow the toddler to make appropriate choices, such as which juice to take the medicine with. • Encourage active play in the playroom or with push/pull toys in the hallway (accompanied by an adult). • Expect and plan for regression in areas of toilet training, eating, and other behaviors. • Expect increased temper tantrums, in general, and intense reactions to intrusive procedures. • Maintain home routine while in the hospital, planning nursing care around the usual feeding and sleep times. • Give simple directions with choices appropriate to the hospital situation. • Provide close supervision while encouraging independence.
Preschoolers	• Keep bed in low position with the side rails up when the preschooler is in the bed. • Instruct the child to call the nurse or caregiver for help getting out of bed. • Keep harmful objects out of reach of the child.	• Encourage parents to stay with the preschooler in the room as well as other areas of the hospital. • Encourage the preschooler to be involved in care by providing choices and opportunities for the child to help. • Use play as an opportunity to work through the preschooler's fears. • Explain activities in simple, concrete terms, being cautious with the words you use because of the preschooler's fantasies and magical thinking. • Expect reactions to pain and bodily injury to be verbally aggressive and specific. • Try to maintain home routines while the child is in the hospital, working them into the plan of care when possible.
School-Age Children	• Keep the bed in the low position with the side rails up while the child is in the bed, explaining that this is a hospital rule, not a punishment.	• Provide opportunities for the child to be involved in care. • Allow children to select their meals, assist with treatments, and keep their rooms neat. • Allow visits with other children if the condition allows. • Encourage parents to tell the child when they will return. • Plan care around the child's usual home routines (meals, sleep). • Encourage the child to do school work.
Adolescents	• Be aware of the adolescent's whereabouts. The adolescent may not wish to stay in the room but may become confused about where the room or unit is located in the hospital.	• Allow adolescents to interact with others. • Alter hospital routines as possible to allow the adolescent to sleep in or stay up later at night. • Provide others close to their age as roommates. • Encourage visits from friends. • Provide emotional support for feelings of being alone or away from friends; be alert for regression, which may result in the adolescent becoming emotional. • Answer questions honestly and with appropriate information. • Give the adolescent a sense of control by allowing choices. • Be sensitive to concerns about being "different."

Restraints can promote physical distress in a child and be stressful for the parents as well. Children may also view restraints as punishment. Before a restraint is used, other measures need to be considered and alternative attempts or rationales for not using alternatives need to be documented (CMS, 2020).

Restraining Children to Maintain Safety

When deciding whether it is necessary to restrain a child, consider the child's age, developmental level, mental status, and threat to others and self. If it is determined that a restraint is needed, select the most appropriate, least restrictive type of restraint (CMS, 2020). For example, if the child has an intravenous catheter in the antecubital space that stops flowing when the child bends the arm, an elbow restraint or arm board, rather than a soft wrist restraint or four-point extremity restraint, would be appropriate. Table 33.3 lists the types of restraints and the major issues associated with the use of restraints in children.

Explain why the child should not touch the intravenous site or should maintain a certain position so that they have a basic understanding of what is necessary. This may be all that is necessary for an older child. One-to-one supervision and behavior modification techniques may be other alternatives to the use of restraints.

• • • ATRAUMATIC CARE • • •

Therapeutic hugging should be used for procedures and treatments such as intravenous line insertion for which the child needs to remain still. Refer to Chapter 30 for further information.

TAKE NOTE!

When selecting a restraint, the nurse must choose the least restrictive type and apply it for the shortest time necessary (CMS, 2020).

TABLE 33.3 • Types of Restraints and Associated Safety Concerns

Type of Restraint	Purpose	Safety Concerns
Soft limb restraint 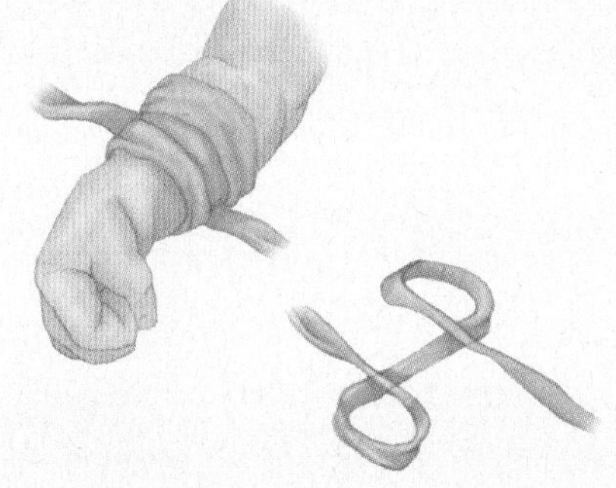	Wrist or ankle restraint to prevent range of motion of extremities	Check wrist or ankle for any sign of circulatory, integumentary, or neurologic compromise.
Elbow restraint 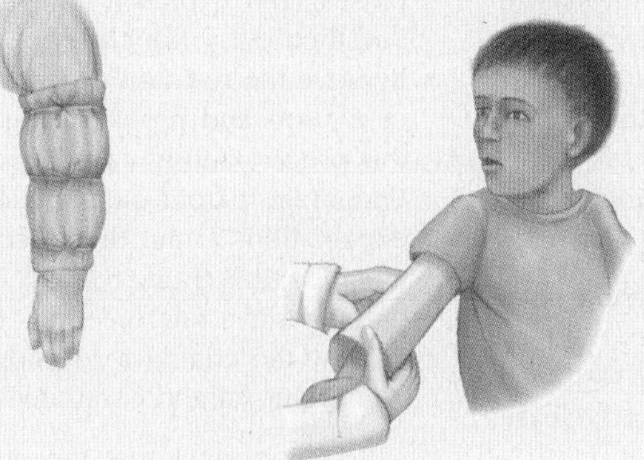	Prevents child from flexing and reaching face, head, IV, and other tubes	Position the restraint so that it does not rub against axilla. Check pulse, temperature, and capillary refill of the extremity.

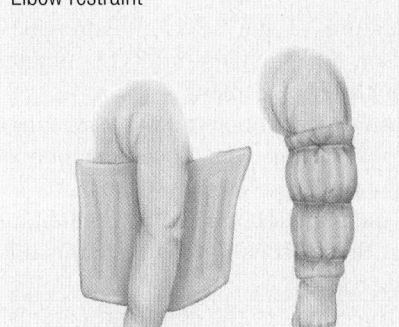

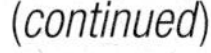
(continued)

TABLE 33.3 • Types of Restraints and Associated Safety Concerns (*continued*)

Type of Restraint	Purpose	Safety Concerns
Mummy restraint	Body restraint using a sheet/blanket folded in a square appropriate to size of infant or young child to secure the whole body of the child or every extremity except for one	Ensure that all extremities are secured within the sheet. Ensure face is not covered or airway restricted.
Jacket (vest) restraint	Jacket worn by child with ties attached to the child's back and to side of bed. Used to keep children flat in bed, such as after surgery, or safe in chair	Ensure the child can turn head to side and that the head of the bed is elevated, if possible. Place ties in back so child cannot manipulate them. Ensure attached to nonmovable part of bed frame.

Before applying a restraint, explain the reason for the restraint to the child and the parents. Emphasize that the rationale is to maintain the child's safety; the restraint is not punishment. Having the child and parents state the reason for the restraint demonstrates their understanding.

In addition, the nurse must do the following:

- Ensure that the restraint fits properly.
- Secure the restraints with ties to the bed or crib frame, not the side rails.
- Use a clove-hitch type of knot to secure the restraints with ties (this allows for quick, easy access and release of the restraint).
- Check restraints 15 minutes following initial placement and then every hour for proper placement.
- Assess the temperature of the affected extremities, pulses, and capillary refill, initially after 15 minutes and then every hour after placement.
- Remove the restraint every 2 hours to allow for range of motion and repositioning, with documentation of this process and any findings.
- Encourage parent participation, providing continuous explanations about the reasons for the restraints and tentative time frame for use.
- Offer positive reinforcement to the child and parents.
- Review the criteria for removing the restraints; document removal and continued assessment.

It is important that the nurse is familiar with federal standards and regulations and state laws, and they should always follow facility policy and procedures.

TAKE NOTE!

Appropriate safety interventions that are age and developmentally appropriate and that would be used outside of the health care setting to protect an infant, toddler, or preschool child such as stroller, swing, highchair safety belts, and crib rails, crib covers, and enclosed or domed cribs, and raised padded side rails used for seizure precautions are not considered restraints (CMS, 2020).

Transport of the Child

Children may need to be transported to other units for diagnostic tests or surgery; to different areas in the same unit, such as the playroom or treatment room; or for discharge. When the child is transported to other areas, specific guidelines need to address safety issues, the age and developmental level of the child, the child's physical condition, and the destination. These factors need to be considered before transport so that the appropriate method can be used with the least amount of risk for the child. Various methods to transport children include carrying the infant and using strollers, wagons, or rolling beds (Fig. 33.7). If possible, the parents should accompany the child to offer support and comfort.

Providing Safe Transportation Within the Hospital

When carrying an infant, good support of the back and head is vital. Rails should be up on all beds and wagons. Use safety belts with strollers and wheelchairs.

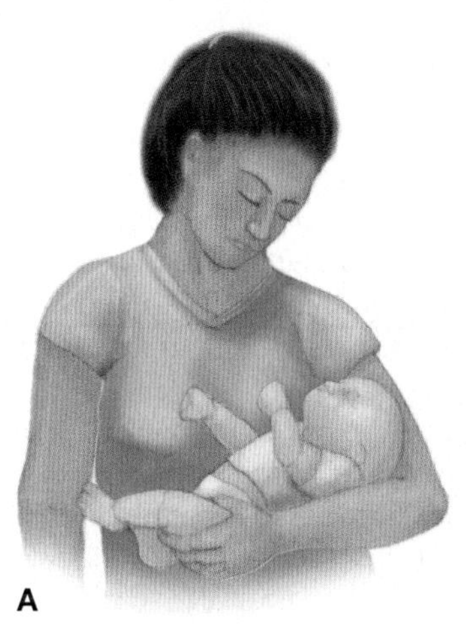

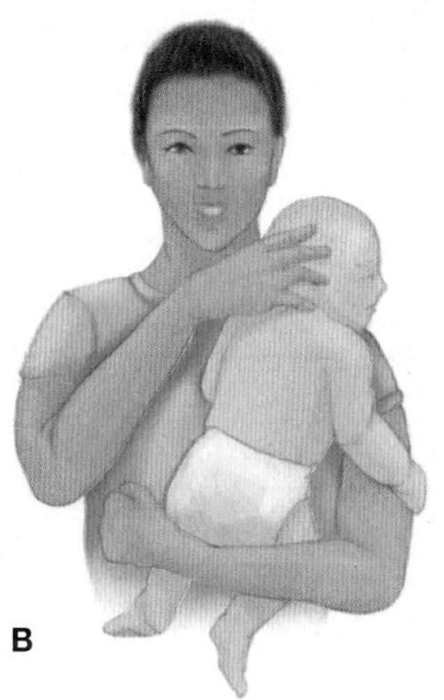

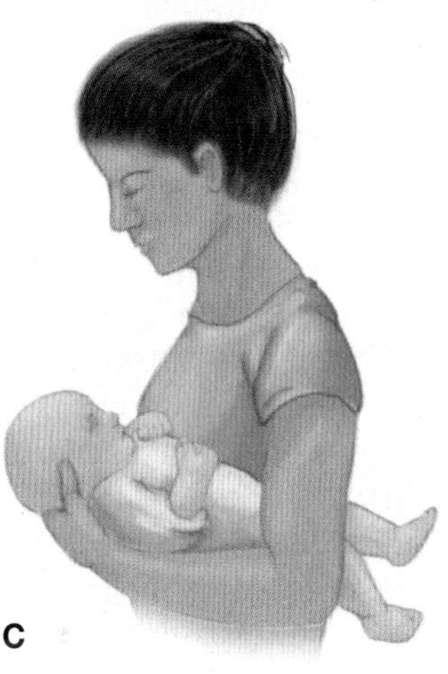

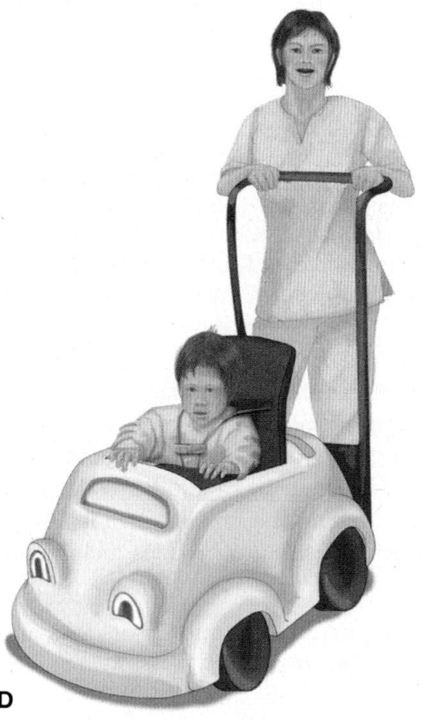

FIGURE 33.7 Methods for transporting the infant or child. **A.** Cradle method for carrying infants up to 3 months of age. One hand grasps the infant's thighs; the other arm supports the infant's head and back. **B.** The "over-the-shoulder" method for carrying infants up to 7 months of age. Support the head if the infant does not have head control. **C.** Football method for carrying infants up to 2 months of age. The forearm and hand support the body and head of the infant. **D.** A wagon with rails and padding is used to transport small children.

TAKE NOTE!

Never leave a child unattended during transport. Keep the child visible at all times during the transport.

THINKING ABOUT DEVELOPMENT

Discuss ways to maintain safety for an 8-year-old child in the hospital. How would this differ if the child was 3 years old?

HOSPITALIZATION IN CHILDHOOD

Hospitalization is often confusing, complex, and overwhelming for children and their families. Reactions and responses to illness and hospitalization depend on a number of factors, including the child's developmental stage. Nursing strategies are needed to prepare children and their families for this experience while minimizing negative effects. These strategies include identifying the needs of children and families through astute assessment of nonverbal and verbal behaviors, then validating the information with accurate interpretation and providing appropriate responses and interventions.

Although the nurse implements these strategies throughout the interaction with the child and family, a critical time to ensure the best outcome for the child and family is during the admission process. The nurse assesses the learning needs and abilities of the child and family. For the interventions to be successful, the nurse must communicate and teach in the most effective method for the individual child and family. The nurse also evaluates the child's and family's competence in performing specific activities prior to discharge.

In a study of hospitalized children, Crole and Smith (2002) found that the nursing care for a hospitalized child occurred in four phases: introduction, building a trusting relationship, decision-making phase, and providing comfort and reassurance. These phases remain relevant today. All of these phases are interconnected. For example, if trust is not established, it becomes difficult to move to the next phase.

The introduction phase involves the initial contact with children and their families, and it establishes the foundation for a trusting relationship. Use favorite toys and common television shows to establish rapport. Allow the child to participate in the conversation without the pressure of having to comply with requests or undergo any procedures. Next, a trusting relationship can be built by using appropriate language, games, and play such as singing a song during a procedure, preparing the child adequately for procedures, and providing explanations and encouragement. Get down to the child's level and play on their terms.

In the decision-making phase, the nurse gives some control over to the child by allowing them to participate in making certain decisions. This phase is critical to maintaining the trust the child has developed. For example, it is imperative to decide how much control the child will have during treatment, how much information to share with the child about upcoming events, and whether parents should participate. Reinforce the child's use of coping strategies that lead to healthy outcomes by providing options whenever it is safe to do so. Finally, the comfort and reassurance phase uses techniques such as praising the child and providing opportunities to cuddle with a favorite toy. This phase helps the nurse re-establish trust and provide comfort to the child to increase positive outcomes.

Preparing Children and Families for Hospitalization

When preparing children for hospitalization, be aware of the situations that may create distress in a child and try to minimize or eliminate them. Even the most minor situations may be frightening to young children. Remember, new experiences, unfamiliar sights and sounds, disruption of sleep patterns, and pain associated with procedures and treatments are major causes of stress for the hospitalized child and family.

Table 33.4 presents some hospital activities that may seem scary or stressful to a child and gives suggestions for preparing the child and family. Thoughtful preparation for these situations may help relieve stress. Educate children about what to expect so they can cope with their imagination and distinguish reality from fantasy. Describe the intervention and the sequence of steps that will occur, and include sensory information such as how the child will feel.

 *Concept Mastery Alert*

Preparing the Child for Hospitalization

To help ease the stress of hospitalization in a child, encourage the parents and child to work with a child-life specialist at the hospital who can give the child a comprehensive preparation for the hospitalization.

Reduce the child's fears and increase their ability to cope with the hospital experience through good preparation. Preparation should include exploring the child's perceptions, reviewing previous experiences, and identifying coping strategies. The goal should be to decrease fear and anxiety by allowing the child to better understand what is happening. Useful techniques include the following:

- Perform nursing care on stuffed animals or dolls and allow the child to do the same.
- Avoid the use of medical terms.

TABLE 33.4 • Strategies to Reduce Fear of Common Hospitalization Situations

Situation	Strategies to Reduce Fear
Procedure involving intrusion into the body or use of equipment or technology	Describe the procedure and equipment in terms the child can understand. Review the steps of the procedure or steps involved with the use of the equipment. Explain what the child's role will be and what is or isn't allowed. If appropriate, have the child rehearse with the equipment or role-play.
Darkness, such as with radiologic examinations or at night	Keep a light on in the examination area. Use a nightlight in the child's room. If possible, allow the child to hold the caregiver's or nurse's hand or a favorite toy.
Transport to other areas of the hospital	Allow caregiver to accompany child, if possible. Inform the child of where they are going, about how long they will be there, and approximately when they will return. Introduce the child to the person who will be transporting the child.
Numerous personnel in and out of child's room	Identify all staff members working with the child (each shift and each day). Place a small board in the child's room with the name of the nurse caring for the child that shift or day. Inform the child how long the nurse will be caring for the child (adapt this information according to the child's cognitive level; for example, instead of saying that you'll be there for 8 hours, say, "I'll be your nurse until just before dinnertime" or "I'll be your nurse until you go for your test"). Say goodbye to the child when leaving for the day; tell the child about their new nurse; inform the child of when you will return.

- Allow the child to handle some equipment.
- Teach the child the steps of the procedure or inform them exactly what will happen during the hospital stay.
- Show the child the room where they will be staying.
- Introduce the child to the health care personnel with whom they will come in contact.
- Explain the sounds the child may hear.
- Let the child sample the food that will be served.

All techniques used to prepare the child for hospitalization should emphasize the philosophy of atraumatic care. Adapt all information to the cognitive and developmental level of the child. Identify what role the child will play in the situation: it is always helpful for children to have something to do, since it shows them that they are included. A rehearsal of what will occur in the hospital allows the child to become comfortable with the situation. If time permits, provide pamphlets that describe the procedure, and suggest preparation activities for the child at home before admission.

The child and family may be able to take a tour of the hospital unit or the surgical facility. Videos, photographs, and books on hospitalization and surgery can serve as resources for the family and child. Many institutions offer programs to familiarize children and families with the hospital experience with a guided tour. During the tour, opportunities are provided for role-playing, and during stops along the way the child can see, touch, and feel the equipment that may be used (Fig. 33.8). If the tour guide notes a child or family member is really scared or concerned about something, the pediatric staff can be alerted and therefore address this issue, leading to improved family-centered care.

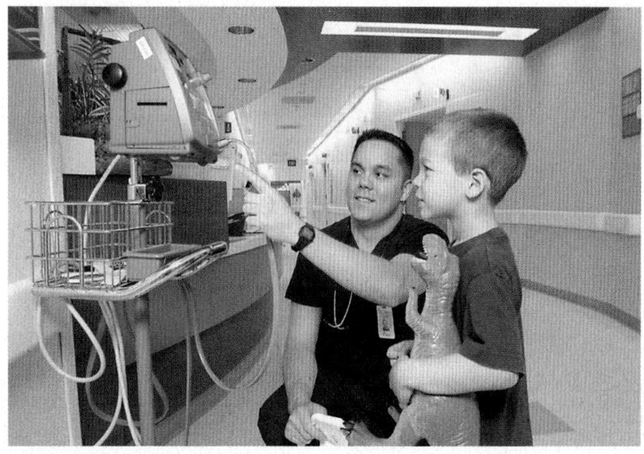

FIGURE 33.8 A child is being prepared for hospitalization by becoming familiar with some of the equipment that might be used.

Several children's books are available that focus on hospital stays and procedures, such as the coloring and activity book by Johns Hopkins Children's Center (2023), *My Trip to the Hospital* in the Little Critter Series by Mercer Mayer, and *Clifford Visits the Hospital* by Norman Bridwell. A list may be available at the hospital from the child-life department. Be familiar with these resources at your particular setting.

Parents are instrumental in preparing children by reviewing the materials that are given, answering questions,

TEACHING GUIDELINES 33.1 Preparing Your Child for Hospitalization

- Read stories about experiences with hospitals or surgery.
- Talk about going to the hospital and what it will be like coming home.
- Be honest and encourage the child to ask questions.
- Visit the hospital and go through the preadmission tour if time permits.
- Provide support to the child via your presence, phone or video calls, and special items brought from home.
- Encourage the child to draw pictures to express how they are feeling.
- Include siblings in the preparation.

and being truthful and supportive. Teaching Guidelines 33.1 provides suggestions for parents in preparing their child for hospitalization.

Remember Jake, the 8-year-old introduced at the beginning of the chapter? How can you help prepare Jake and his family for hospitalization?

Admitting the Child to the Facility

Admitting the child to the facility involves preparing them for admission and introducing the child to the unit where they will be staying. Use the appropriate hospital forms. Chapter 30 gives general information about communicating with and teaching children and families.

In today's health care environment, the admission process occurs quickly, with little time for extensive preparation; this is why preparation before admission is so important. Of course, the urgency of the child's medical condition may also limit the amount of preparation that can be done in advance.

TAKE NOTE!

When a child is admitted to a general unit, take extra time to orient and explain the routines and procedures to the child and family. Emphasize that the parents can stay with the child (if institutional policy permits). If possible, place the child in a room close to the nurses' station, and order food appropriate for the child's age and developmental level.

Types of Admissions and Nursing Care

The hospital units to which a child may be admitted include:

- General inpatient unit
- Emergency and urgent care department
- PICU
- Outpatient or special procedures unit
- Rehabilitation unit or hospital

ADMISSION ASSESSMENT

Obtain information about the child's history, routines, and reason for admission. Determine baseline vital signs and height and weight, and perform a physical assessment. Follow the facility's admission policy or procedure. Recognize the needs of the family and child during this process. If some of this information already exists, do not ask for it again, except to confirm vital information such as allergies, medications taken at home, and history of the illness. Typically, the information is collected immediately if the child's condition is urgent; otherwise, the information is collected within 8 hours, except for the information that is required for safe care.

COMMUNICATING WITH THE CHILD AND FAMILY

Regardless of the site of care, nursing care must begin by establishing a trusting, caring relationship with the child and family. Smile, introduce yourself, and give your title. Let the child and family know what will happen and what is expected of them. Ask the family and child what names they prefer to be called by. Maintain eye contact at the appropriate level. With a younger child, start with the family first so the child can see that the family trusts you. Communicate with children at age-appropriate levels. Orient the child and family to the hospital unit. Briefly explain policies and routines and the personnel who will be involved in the care of the child.

Isolation Rooms

Isolation rooms are used for situations involving the risk for infection. When a child is admitted with an infectious disease, or to rule out an infectious disease, or if the child has impaired immune function, isolation will be instituted. Children in this setting may experience sensory deprivation due to the limited contact with others and the use of personal protective equipment such as gloves, masks, and gowns.

CARING FOR THE CHILD IN ISOLATION

Encourage the family to visit often, and help them understand the reason for the isolation and any special procedures that are required. Introduce yourself before entering the room, and allow the child to view your face before applying a mask if possible. Continue to have contact with the child, and hold or touch the child often, especially if the parents are not present.

Addressing the Effects of Hospitalization Developmentally

When addressing the fears, separation anxiety, and loss of control that occur in hospitalized children, the nurse should consider the child's age and cognitive or developmental level. Interventions are then based on how the child experiences these stressors at that age or developmental level. The content, timing, setting, and method of preparation are also based on the child's age and cognitive or developmental level. General guidelines for addressing fear and anxiety, separation anxiety, and loss of control are provided in Box 33.6.

Caring for Newborns and Infants Who Are Hospitalized

Assess the developmental stage of the infant, and assess the baby's attachment to the parents or primary caregivers. Assess the infant's facial expression as it is the most consistent indicator of pain or bodily injury. Avoid separation from the primary caregiver, if possible, in order to decrease fear and minimize separation anxiety; this will also promote healthy attachment. Arrange for volunteers to provide consistent comfort to the baby if the parent or primary caregiver cannot stay with the infant. Maintain the infant's home routine related to sleep and feeding to help decrease feelings of loss of control. Weigh the infant daily, at the same time, on the same scale. Monitor intake and output closely. Be alert to signs of discomfort other than crying, such as a furrowed brow or tense body posture. Additional nursing considerations related to ensuring safety and promoting growth and development of the infant are presented in Table 33.2.

BOX 33.6 Guidelines to Address the General Effects of Hospitalization

Minimizing Fear and Anxiety

- Prepare the child and family for hospitalization and procedures.
- Explain everything to the child and their families before it occurs (see Chapter 30).
- Use age-appropriate communication techniques. Include the family in this process so they can help the child cope with fears.
- Allow time for children to play out their fears and concerns.
- Talk to the child and parents using a soft, friendly, comforting tone of voice.
- Have a calm, empathetic approach when caring for the child.

Addressing/Minimizing Separation Anxiety

- Know the stages of separation anxiety and be able to recognize them.
- Remember that behaviors demonstrated during the first stage do not indicate that the child is "bad."
- Encourage the family to stay with the child, and always use a family-centered approach to care.
- Help the child cope, and intervene before the behaviors of detachment occur.

Addressing Loss of Control

- Minimize physical restrictions, altered routines and rituals, and dependency issues, because they produce loss of control.
- Allow as much independence as possible within the constraints of the diagnosis.
- Allow the child to participate in care and decisions regarding care whenever possible.

Caring for Hospitalized Toddlers

Key nursing concerns when caring for toddlers are separation anxiety, growth and development, and autonomy. Establish a trusting relationship with the toddler through nonthreatening play to decrease the amount of fear the toddler feels. Be alert to subtle, nonverbal indicators of grief or discontent.

Encourage the parent or primary caregiver to stay with the toddler in the hospital to decrease separation anxiety. Maintain the home routine related to meals and sleep or a nap to provide structure, and help decrease the toddler's feelings of loss of control. If indicated, weigh the toddler daily. Closely monitor intake and output. Refer to Table 33.2 for additional nursing considerations related to ensuring safety and promoting growth and development in the hospitalized toddler.

Caring for Preschoolers Who Are Hospitalized

Nursing care for preschoolers who are hospitalized focuses on their special needs, fears, and fantasies. When working with preschoolers, remember that they use magical thinking and fantasy. Be honest and specific, providing information just prior to the intervention to allay the child's fears. As with toddlers, encourage parental involvement to decrease the amount of separation anxiety the preschooler experiences while in the hospital. Allow the preschooler to make simple decisions such as which color bandage to use or whether to take medicine from a cup or syringe. This will help the child to feel some sense of control. Table 33.2 gives specific nursing considerations related to ensuring safety and promoting growth and development for the preschooler in the hospital.

Caring for School-Age Children Who Are Hospitalized

Provide honest information using concrete, meaningful words to the school-age child to minimize fear of the unknown. Encourage parental involvement or rooming-in to decrease separation anxiety as school-age children are still very attached to their parents. Involve the child in making simple decisions and planning the schedule as appropriate to give them a sense of control. Table 33.2 provides additional nursing considerations when caring for hospitalized school-age children that include ensuring safety and promoting growth and development.

Caring for Adolescents Who Are Hospitalized

The adolescent may or may not express fears. Educate the adolescent honestly; younger adolescents require more concrete explanations, while older adolescents can process more abstract concepts. Respect the adolescent's need for privacy. Encourage visits from the adolescent's friends to minimize anxiety related to separation. Prepare a mutually agreeable schedule with the adolescent, as appropriate, that includes their preferences while incorporating the required nursing care. Collaborating with the adolescent will provide them with increased control. Refer to Table 33.2 for additional nursing considerations related to care of the adolescent in the hospital.

Providing Basic Care for the Child Who Is Hospitalized

Basic care involves general hygiene measures, including bathing, hair care, oral care, and nutritional care. Young children are dependent on an adult for most, if not all, of their self-care needs. If parents are present, allow them to provide care for the child to decrease the child's stress. Older children may perform hygiene measures themselves but may need some assistance from the nurse.

General Hygiene Measures

General hygiene measures help to maintain healthy skin, hair, and teeth. Skin is a complex structure; its primary function is to protect the tissues that it encloses and to protect itself. Injury to the child's skin may occur when inserting and maintaining an intravenous line, removing a dressing, positioning a child in bed, changing a diaper, using and removing electrode patches, and maintaining restraints. Risk factors for problems include impaired mobility, protein malnutrition, edema, incontinence, sensory loss, anemia, and infection. A good time to assess the skin is during bath time.

BATHING

Bathing infants and children is a common daily hygiene measure in the health care environment. Although a parent or primary caregiver often does this in today's family-centered environment, the nurse is still responsible for ensuring that bathing is done safely and hygienically. Adhere to safety principles to prevent falls, burns, and aspiration of water. Never leave a child alone in a bathtub. Use a gentle, pH-balanced soap with moisturizer if there is a need to rehydrate the skin. Note any condition that might require special considerations or further assessment, such as paralysis, loss of sensation, surgical incisions, skin traction/cast, external lines (intravenous lines, urinary catheters, or feeding tubes), or other alterations in skin integrity. Pay close attention to the ears, between skin folds, the neck, the back, and the genital area for alterations in skin integrity. Table 33.5 highlights specific developmental considerations for bathing.

Before bathing and performing other hygiene measures, assess the family's preferences and home practices for the child, such as time of day, rituals, special equipment, and allergies to products. This is a good time to assess the amount of assistance that might be required by the parents and to address learning needs related to hygiene. Follow general guidelines in bathing any patient with regard to equipment, room temperature, privacy, and use of products such as deodorant and lotion.

PROVIDING HAIR CARE

Lying in bed can make the hair matted and tangled. Avoid pulling on the child's hair when combing or brushing it. If necessary, use commercial detangling solutions to ease combing.

If the hair requires washing, this is often done during the daily bath for infants. Typically, shampooing once or twice a week is sufficient for younger children. Adolescents may need more frequent shampooing due to the increase in sebaceous gland secretion. The frequency of shampooing also varies based on the child's condition; for example, if the child has experienced diaphoresis, more frequent shampooing may be indicated.

Shampooing may be done at the bedside with specially adapted equipment, at a readily accessible sink while the child is sitting in a chair or lying on a stretcher, or in a tub or shower. Commercial no-rinse shampoos may be available for use. With these products, the shampoo is applied to the hair and then brushed or combed out.

If the child uses a tub or shower for hair care, monitor the child's safety throughout to ensure that the child does not slip and fall due to the slippery surface or is burned because of improper water temperature.

TABLE 33.5 • Developmental Considerations for Bathing

Age of Child	Special Considerations
Infants	Use a sponge bath or tub bath to bathe young infants who cannot sit unaided. Support the infant's body at all times. Ensure appropriate water temperature. Avoid use of talcum powder.
Toddlers	Bathe older infants and toddlers at the bedside or in a regular bathtub, depending on their health condition.
School-age children and adolescents	Older children may prefer a shower, if available and acceptable for their health condition. Assess whether a shower would be safe. Provide privacy.

The child's ethnicity may require special measures for hair care. For example, a child of African descent may use a broad-toothed comb for hair care. Ask the child's parents to bring one from home if one is not available. Also ask the child and parents about any products used on the hair that the child prefers; the parents can bring some from home. Encourage the parents to help with braiding or plaiting of the hair if desired.

PROVIDING ORAL HYGIENE

Oral hygiene is an important part of basic care. Wipe the infant's gums with a wet cloth after each feeding. Assist children in brushing and flossing their teeth after each feeding or meal and before bedtime. Provide special attention to oral hygiene of the immunosuppressed, such as using soft toothbrushes and moistened gauze sponges to prevent bleeding, and carefully inspect the oral cavity for areas of breakdown.

Nutrition

Adequate nutrition is necessary for growth and development and tissue repair, so it is an essential component of care for the ill or hospitalized child. Frequently, the ill or hospitalized child experiences a loss of appetite, which can affect the child's nutritional status. This may be compounded by other problems such as nausea and vomiting and nothing by mouth (NPO) restrictions for testing or surgery. The hospitalized child may adopt feeding habits that do not fit their age or stage of development, such as use of a bottle in an older infant/child or a child capable of self-feeding wanting to be fed. Readoption of these feeding habits should be accommodated when possible.

CLINICAL REASONING ALERT!

Relieve pain and nausea before meals are served.

PROVIDING NUTRITIONAL CARE

If possible, schedule procedures or treatments away from mealtimes. In younger children, refusing to eat may be related to the child's feeling of separation; in others, refusing to eat may reflect the child's attempt to control the situation. Encourage parents to use gentle persuasion instead of force to assist with intake. The use of force can lead to an aversion for food that carries beyond the hospital stay into the home environment. Give the child choices about what to eat; this reinforces the child's sense of control. Remind parents that the child's appetite will probably improve as their condition improves. Teaching Guidelines 33.2 provides tips for promoting nutrition in the hospitalized child. Although geared to parents, nurses can also incorporate these guidelines into the child's plan of care.

TEACHING GUIDELINES 33.2 Promoting Nutrition for Your Hospitalized Child

- Check with the nurse about any restrictions related to your child's diet. Find out if intake and output are being monitored.
- Encourage your child to eat their favorite foods.
- Assist your child with eating or drinking as necessary; be present at mealtimes to promote socialization.
- Frequently offer small cups of fluid and finger foods; avoid giving large quantities at one time.
- Try offering fluids at different temperatures at different times for variety.
- Remember that children can ingest greater amounts of thin liquids (e.g., gelatin or carbonated drinks) than thicker liquids (e.g., cream soups or milkshakes).
- Include ice chips as fluid intake. Ice is approximately equivalent to half the same amount of water (e.g., 1 cup of ice equals a half-cup of water).
- Use straws (unless not allowed) and brightly colored utensils, cups, or dishes to provide contrast and stimulation.
- Offer the child choices; allow the child to choose what they want from the menu.
- Talk with the dietitian to see if any special preferences can be addressed.
- Offer praise to your child for what they eat or drink.
- Never punish the child for not eating or drinking.
- Encourage the older child to help keep track of what they eat and drink.

Providing Play, Activities, and Recreation for the Child Who Is Hospitalized

Play is an important component in the child's plan of care. Today, many health care settings providing care for children have playrooms with age-appropriate toys, equipment, and other creative activities (Fig. 33.9). If the facility is large enough, there may even be a separate area for adolescents where they can listen to music, play video games, and visit with peers.

TAKE NOTE!

Avoid using the term "playroom" when caring for older school-age children and adolescents. Instead, call it the "activity room" or "social room." Doing so promotes a greater feeling of maturity and makes it more likely that they will use the area.

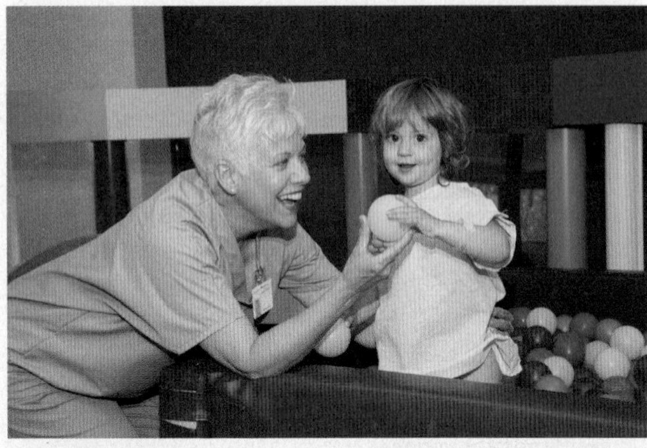

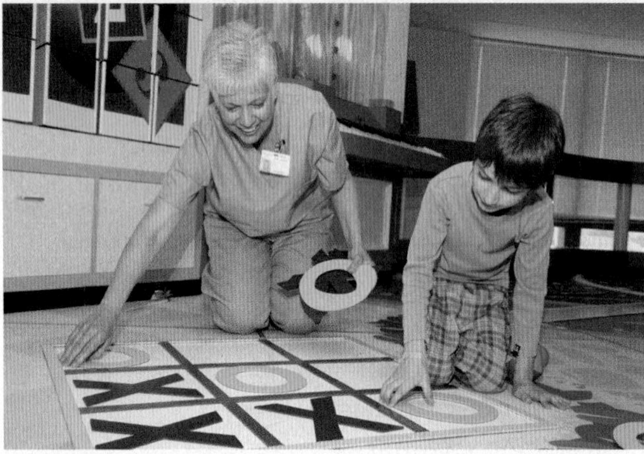

FIGURE 33.9 Children occupied in a hospital playroom. It is important to provide age-appropriate activities for younger and older children alike.

Obviously, some children will not be able to use these facilities if their activity level is restricted or if isolation is necessary. Children may also play in their rooms. Ensure that opportunities for unstructured play are provided to all children who can engage in play. Therapeutic play may be used to teach children about their health status or to allow them to work through issues in their lives.

TAKE NOTE!

Keep the bed or crib and playroom as "safe" places. Perform invasive procedures such as venipunctures in the treatment room, if possible. Never perform any nursing interventions in the playroom, no matter how nonthreatening they may appear to the nurse.

The nurse's greatest ally in the hospital in relation to atraumatic care is the CLS. They not only prepare the child for procedures but also provide activities and events to encourage play and normal growth and development.

Providing Unstructured Play

Encourage unstructured play as it allows children to control events, ideas, and relationships. Encourage parents to bring small toys and favorite stuffed animals from home to make the child feel more comfortable in the strange environment of the hospital. Children also enjoy receiving small new toys as surprises when they are hospitalized. Many children enjoy diversional activities such as playing board games or electronic games, reading books, and watching TV or videos. Quiet activities appropriate to the child's developmental level provide the opportunity for play and encourage the use and development of fine motor skills even if the child is confined to bed. Infants and toddlers enjoy manipulating blocks and playing with stacking toys. The preschooler may enjoy coloring, dollhouses, or playing with plastic building blocks such as Legos. School-age children and adolescents may enjoy playing video games, putting together a puzzle, or building a model geared toward their developmental level.

Play as Part of Nursing Care

Play is also an important part of nursing care. Use play as appropriate while providing routine nursing care to the child. An example of the use of play in nursing care involves the school-age child's love of competition and games. To increase range of motion in a school-age child who is hospitalized for traction due to a fracture, have the child throw a soft sponge ball or beanbag ball into a hoop, and compete against the child. To increase deep breathing, encourage the child to blow bubbles or blow a whistle. To increase intake of fluids, help the child create a graph to chart the number of glasses of fluids they drink over a period of time. Award the child a sticker, baseball card, special pencil, or other small item if they reach a certain level.

When using play as part of nursing care, it is important to evaluate the outcome of play. Play used in the manner described previously should enhance the child's outcome. For example, for the child blowing bubbles, determine whether this activity enhanced coughing and deep breathing.

Therapeutic Play

Another important aspect of play is **therapeutic play**. Therapeutic play is nondirected and focuses on helping the child cope with feelings and fears. Health care professionals use therapeutic play to help the child deal with the physical and psychological challenges of illness and hospitalization. Supervised play with medical equipment in the hospital environment can help children work through their feelings about what has happened to them (Fig. 33.10). In a large hospital or a children's hospital, the CLS typically coordinates these activities. Goals include maintaining normal living patterns, minimizing psychological trauma, and promoting optimal development of the child. If a CLS is not

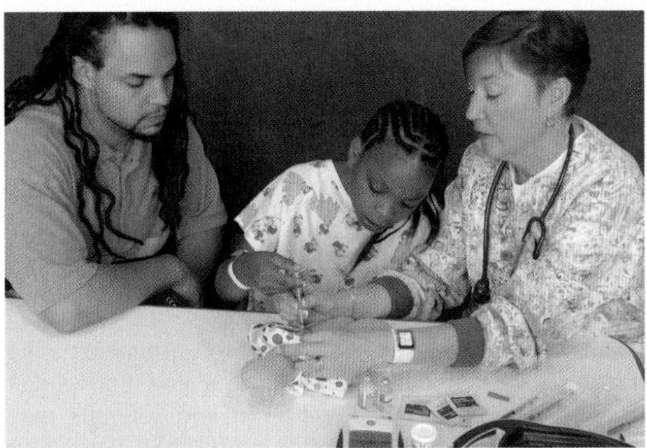

FIGURE 33.10 The nurse supervises play with medical equipment to help the child work through her feelings about being hospitalized.

available, the nurse provides this type of activity. There is a greater emphasis on the developmental and psychosocial implications of illness and hospitalization and validation of the child's voice.

In emotional outlet play or traumatic play, the child acts out or dramatizes real-life stressors. For example, using a wooden hammer and pegs, a soft sponge ball, or boxing gloves can allow the child to express anger over separation from family and friends. Commercial toys such as anatomically correct dolls and puppets have removable parts so children can see various organs of the body. Sometimes, younger children "talk" to puppets and dolls, allowing them to express their feelings to a nonthreatening "person" about a specific situation or what they want from the health care provider. For example, the Shadow Buddies dolls mentioned earlier in the chapter provide a way of coping with a specific condition. The company creates an ostomy buddy who has a stoma, a cancer buddy with thinning hair and a chest catheter for chemotherapy treatments, and a heart buddy who has a chest incision and a repaired heart (Shadow Buddies Foundation, n.d.).

Other types of therapeutic play include drawing and supervised "needle play." Drawing is a way for the child to express their thoughts and feelings. Supervised "needle play" assists children who must undergo frequent blood work, injections, or intravenous procedures. A doll can receive an injection as the child works out their anger and anxiety. Keep in mind safety and the child's growth and development level before planning this type of directed play; an adult must always be present.

Promoting School Work and Education During Hospitalization

Promote school work while the child is in the hospital. Determine the amount of school work that can be done by assessing the child's condition, the availability of teachers, and the family situation. Many children's hospitals have teachers at the hospitals; there may be classrooms too. These teachers work closely with the child's school to continue school work as the child's condition permits. Hospitals without an educational staff will rely on parents to coordinate with the child's school. Parents may bring in schoolbooks and the child's homework for completion while in the hospital. This connection to the child's school helps maintain normalcy for the child and minimizes the disruption of everyday life. Nurses and other health care providers, such as social workers, should help facilitate this process.

> Think back to Jake, the 8-year-old, from the beginning of the chapter. What nursing care could you provide that will help minimize stressors?

Family Members' Needs

Many factors may influence the family's reaction to the child's hospitalization. Parents or caregivers and siblings experience many emotions when a child is hospitalized, including disbelief, anger, guilt, fear, anxiety, frustration, and depression. Visiting restrictions, unexpected changes in the child's health status, lack of information or understanding of their child's health condition, changes in their routine and roles, financial stress, and feelings of being undervalued in the care of their child all contribute to the parents' or caregivers' feelings.

Family-centered care recognizes the need to treat the child in the context of the family, including siblings. Important questions that will affect how siblings deal with the hospitalization of the child include:

- Was the admission an emergency?
- Were there previous admissions, and how did the siblings perceive those hospitalizations?
- How serious is the illness or trauma?
- Is the prognosis known?

Addressing Parents' Needs

Assess the factors that may influence the family's reaction to the child's hospitalization and plan the care of the child to accommodate some of these issues. Encourage families to have support systems in place before, during, and after hospitalization. Help parents and caregivers to work through their feelings in order to decrease anxiety, thus decreasing the child's anxiety level. The philosophy of family-centered care places the family at the core of care; the family is the primary and continuing provider of care for the child. Practice family-centered care, which addresses the child's and family's needs and preferences and increases the child's and parents' satisfaction with the health care setting (American Academy of Pediatrics, Committee on Hospital Care, Institute for Patient and Family-Centered Care, 2012, reaffirmed 2018).

Encourage parents to room-in with the child throughout the hospital stay, if possible. Facilities can be designed to welcome family participation. For example, having charging ports, internet, and printers or scanners available and providing extra meals and beds for the parents can encourage parents to participate in care. View the parents as vital members of the health care team and partners in the care of the child who is ill.

Addressing Siblings' Needs

Address the siblings' possible feelings of guilt. Use educational materials, allow time for visits, send photographs back and forth between siblings, and allow siblings to talk on the phone.

Child and Family Teaching

Not all experiences with hospitalization are negative; in fact, the experience may enhance the child's and family's coping skills, bolster self-esteem, and provide new socialization experiences. It may allow the child to master self-care skills and provides an opportunity for the child and family to learn new information. Parents may learn more about their child's growth and development skills as well as additional parenting or caregiving skills, resulting in improved parenting abilities. In addition, the child's overall health may be improved because of the hospital stay if the child receives current immunizations and the parents learn more about health care practices.

The overall goals of child and family teaching are to minimize the child's and family's stress, educate them about treatment and nursing care in the hospital, and ensure the family can provide appropriate care at home on discharge. Providing support before, during, and after hospitalization may minimize stress. Preadmission programs can introduce the child and family to the setting. During the hospital stay, forming partnerships with the child and family, using strategies to promote coping, and providing appropriate preparation for procedures, tests, and surgery serve to decrease stress.

Educating the Child and Family

Assess the child's and family's knowledge of the illness and hospital experience. This provides a baseline for teaching. Include hospital rules in child and family teaching. Behavioral changes in hospitalized children often disturb parents or caregivers. Determine the child's usual patterns of behavior and explain to the parents about the child's reaction to hospitalization. Encourage the family to maintain consistent discipline even while in the hospital to provide structure for the child as well as to prevent discipline issues after discharge. Also discuss how siblings may react to the hospitalization, and provide appropriate teaching to the siblings. Every interaction the nurse has with the child or family provides an opportunity for teaching. Explain the purpose of even simple procedures such as vital signs assessment to the child and family. Provide ongoing information about the child's illness or trauma, treatment plan, and expected outcomes. Chapter 30 provides general principles related to teaching children and their families.

Preparing the Child and Family for Discharge

Discharge planning actually begins on admission. The nurse assesses the family's resources and knowledge level to determine what education and referrals they may need. On discharge, children and their parents or caregivers receive written instructions about home care, and a copy is retained in the medical record. These instructions are individualized for the child. Generally, discharge instructions should include:

- Follow-up appointment information
- Guidelines about when to contact the health care provider or nurse practitioner (e.g., new or worsening symptoms or indications that the child is not improving)
- Diet
- Activity level allowed
- Medications, including dose, times to be given, route, adverse effects, and special instructions; any prescriptions should be included
- Information on additional treatments the child requires at home
- Specific dates for when the child may return to school or day care
- Names and phone numbers of agencies the family has been referred to, such as durable medical equipment providers

Provide and review educational booklets that give basic health information or general care for a child with a particular disease (Fig. 33.11). Media such as videos may also be used, if available. The ability to watch a

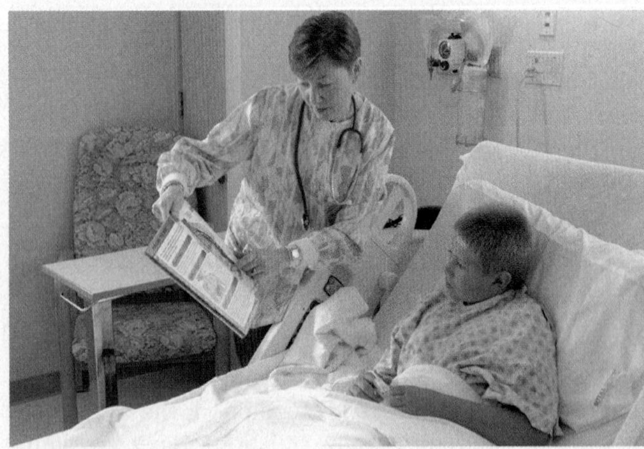

FIGURE 33.11 The nurse uses charts with pictures to perform patient teaching before the child goes home.

procedure over and over is helpful to some families. Explain, demonstrate, and request a return demonstration of any treatments or procedures to be done at home. Provide a written schedule if the child is to receive multiple medications, tube feedings, or other medical treatments. For complicated cases, a written teaching plan may be used to provide continuity of child/family education between various nurses. As the family attempts to perform each task, document whether the caregiver continues to require assistance or prompting with the task or whether they can perform the task independently.

Parents of children with multiple medical needs may benefit from a trial period of home care. This occurs while the child is still in the hospital, but the parents or caregivers provide all of the care that the child requires. Support the family and praise their accomplishments during this trial period.

KEY CONCEPTS

- Nursing care of the child occurs in a variety of settings, from acute care in a hospital to well and ill care in community settings, such as health care providers' offices, schools, places of worship, health departments, community centers, and even within the child's own home. Within each setting, the nurse incorporates basic nursing care with specific strategies to help promote positive outcomes for the child, family, and community as a whole.
- Advantages of community-based care, especially home care, include shorter hospital stays and decreased health care costs, but the major advantage of home care is the comfort and family support it provides, promoting an improved quality of life for these children. Caring for children at home not only improves their physical health but also allows for adequate growth and development while keeping them within their family.
- Community-based nurses focus on the practice of nursing that provides personal care to children and families in the community. These nurses focus on promoting and preserving health as well as preventing disease or injury. They help children and their families cope with illness and disease. They are direct providers of care as well as advocates and educators working to minimize and remove barriers to allow the child to develop to their full potential.
- Due to the short lengths of stay in acute settings and the shift to home care for children with complex health needs, discharge planning and care coordination have become important nursing roles. Discharge planning provides a comprehensive plan for the safe discharge of a child from a health care facility and for continuing safe and effective care at home. Care coordination focuses on coordinating health care services while balancing quality and cost outcomes. Both contribute to improved transitions from hospital to home for children, their families, and the health care team.
- In all of the varied settings where health care is administered, nurses provide well care, episodic ill care, and chronic care. They work to promote, preserve, and improve the health of children and families in these settings.
- Goals of the nurse in the home care setting include promoting, restoring, and maintaining the health of the child. Home care focuses on minimizing the effects of the illness or disability and providing the child or family with the means to care for the illness or disability at home. Nurses in the home care setting are direct providers of care, child and family educators, child and family advocates, and case managers.
- Disadvantages to home care include intrusion on family privacy. Caring for children with complex medical needs can be overwhelming for some families, and financial issues related to home care can become a large burden to families.
- Nursing in the home care setting can be challenging. The focus is on meeting the child's physical and psychological needs while involving the family. Health care professionals provide the support, empowerment, education, and expertise in caring for the child that families need.
- Stressors associated with hospitalization and illness include separation from family and routines; fear of an unknown environment; potential for pain, bodily injury, or mutilation; and loss of control.
- Responses of children to the general stressors of hospitalization include anxiety, fear, anger, guilt, and regression.
- The responses of children and families to illness and hospitalization can be influenced by the age and developmental level of the child, their perceptions of the situation, previous experiences, separation from family and peers, coping skills, and the preparation and support provided by the family, facility, and health care providers.
- Family-centered care and atraumatic care are philosophies that pay special attention to the concerns of the family and child during hospitalization.
- Providing support to children who are hospitalized and their families is critical for minimizing stress.
- Whatever the reason for admission, preparation for admission is vital.
- Upon admission to the hospital or outpatient unit, orient the child and family to the unit, discuss unit policies and routines and the personnel who will be involved in the care of the child, and begin child/family teaching.
- Establish a trusting, caring relationship with the child and family. Let the child and family know what will happen and what is expected of them. Obtain information about the child's history, routines, and reason for admission. Obtain baseline vital signs and height and weight, and perform a physical assessment. Each health care setting has its own policies and procedures for this.
- Due to their age and developmental level, children may be vulnerable to harm, and the nurse must use

appropriate safety measures in caring for children (e.g., identification of children, use of restraints and transportation, basic hygiene measures). These measures need to address developmental risks, such as that the infants, toddlers, and preschoolers require close supervision, and the nurse must avoid leaving small objects within reach.

- Play, including therapeutic play, is an important strategy to prepare children for hospitalization and to help them adapt to the effects of illness and hospitalization. It provides an emotional outlet, opportunities for teaching and learning, and the ability to become familiar with a situation and improve physiologic abilities. A CLS is a specially trained individual who is a member of the child's multidisciplinary team. They work in conjunction with the child's health care providers and parents to foster an atmosphere that promotes the child's well-being.
- Parents may experience anger or guilt related to the hospitalization of their child.
- Discharge planning begins on admission. Each interaction with the family is an opportunity for child and family teaching.
- Provide and review discharge instructions with the child and primary caregiver. Use educational booklets or media such as videos that give basic health information or general care for a child with a particular disease.
- Explain, demonstrate, and request a return demonstration of any treatments or procedures to be done at home. Provide a written schedule if the child is to receive multiple medications, tube feedings, or other medical treatments.

REFERENCES AND RECOMMENDED READINGS

American Academy of Pediatrics, Committee on Hospital Care, Institute for Patient and Family-Centered Care. (2012, reaffirmed 2018). Policy statement: Patient and family-centered care and the pediatrician's role. *Pediatrics, 129*(2), 394–404. https://doi.org/10.1542/peds.2011-3084

American Society of Anesthesiologists. (n.d.). My Surgery Journal. https://www.asahq.org/madeforthismoment/wp-content/uploads/2020/10/ASA-239-MFTM-Coloring-Book_BOY.pdf

Berlin, E. A., & Fowkes, W. C., Jr. (1983). A teaching framework for cross-cultural health care. Application in family practice. *The Western Journal of Medicine, 139*(6), 934–938. https://www.ncbi.nlm.nih.gov/pmc/articles/PMC1011028/pdf/westjmed00196-0164.pdf

Centers for Medicare & Medicaid Services. (2020). *State Operations Manual Appendix A—Survey protocol, regulations and interpretive guidelines for hospitals.* https://www.cms.gov/Regulations-and-Guidance/Guidance/Manuals/downloads/som107ap_a_hospitals.pdf

Conners, G. P., Kressly, S. J., Perrin, J. M., Richerson, J. E., Usha, M., Sankrithi, U. M., Committee on Practice and Ambulatory Medicine, Committee On Pediatric Emergency Medicine, Section On Telehealth Care, Section On Emergency Medicine, Subcommittee On Urgent Care, & Task Force On Pediatric Practice Change. (2017). Nonemergency acute care: When it's not the medical home. *Pediatrics, 139*(5), e20170629. https://doi.org/10.1542/peds.2017-0629

Crole, N., & Smith, L. (2002). Examining the phases of nursing care of the hospitalized child. *Australian Nursing Journal, 9*(8), 30–31.

Elias, E. R., Murphy, N. A., & the Council on Children with Disabilities. (2012, reaffirmed 2022). Clinical report: Home care of children and youth with complex health care needs and technology dependencies. *Pediatrics, 129*(5), 996–1005. https://doi.org/10.1542/peds.2012-0606

Gallo, M., Agostiniani, R., Pintus, R., & Fanos, V. (2021). The child with medical complexity. *Italian Journal of Pediatrics, 47*(1), 1. https://doi.org/10.1186/s13052-020-00935-z

John Hopkins Children Center. (2023). *Hopkins children's guide to surgery coloring book.* https://www.hopkinsmedicine.org/johns-hopkins-childrens-center/patients-and-families/your-visit/abcs-surgery/surgery-coloring-book.html

Kids' Waivers. (2022). *Full list.* http://www.kidswaivers.org/full-list/

Murphy, N. A., Alvey, J., Valentine, K. J., Mann, K., Wilkes, J., & Clark, E. B. (2020). Children with medical complexity: The 10-year experience of a single center. *Hospital Pediatrics, 10*(8), 702–708. https://doi.org/10.1542/hpeds.2020-0085

National Association of School Nurses. (2020). *Individualized healthcare plans: The role of the school nurse (Position Statement).* Author.

National Association of School Nurses. (2023). *About NASN: Definition of school nursing.* https://www.nasn.org/about-nasn/about

National Center for Injury Prevention and Control, Centers for Disease Control and Prevention. (2020). *WISQARS leading causes of nonfatal injury.* https://wisqars.cdc.gov/lcnf/

National Council of State Boards of Nursing. (2018). *A nurse's guide to professional boundaries.* https://www.ncsbn.org/public-files/ProfessionalBoundaries_Complete.pdf

Piaget, J. (1969). *The theory of stages in cognitive development.* McGraw-Hill.

Rector, C. (2022). The journey begins: Introduction. In C. Rector & M. J. Stanley (Eds.), *Community and public health nursing. Promoting the public's health* (10th ed., pp. xxiv–22). Wolters Kluwer Health.

Robertson, J., & Bowlby, J. (1952). Responses of young children to separation from their mothers II: Observations of the sequences of response of children aged 18 to 24 months during the course of separation. *Courrier du Centre International de l'Enfance, 2,* 131–142.

Romito, B., Jewell, J., Jackson, M., & AAP Committee on Hospital Care; Association of Child Life Professionals. (2021). Child life services. *Pediatrics, 147*(1), e2020040261. https://doi.org/10.1542/peds.2020-040261

Shadow Buddies Foundation. (n.d.). *Shadow buddies foundation.* http://www.shadowbuddies.org/

U.S. Department of Health and Human Services. (n.d.). *Healthy People 2030.* https://health.gov/healthypeople

United States Environmental Protection Agency. (2022). *Resources for healthcare providers about children's environmental health.* https://www.epa.gov/children/resources-healthcare-providers-about-childrens-environmental-health

Vaz, L. E., Jungbauer, R. M., Jenisch, C., Austin, J. P., Wagner, D. V., Everist, S. J., Libak, A. J., Harris, M. A., & Zuckerman, K. E. (2022). Caregiver experiences in pediatric hospitalizations: Challenges and opportunities for improvement. *Hospital Pediatrics, 12*(12), 1073–1080. https://doi.org/10.1542/hpeds.2022-006645

DEVELOPING CLINICAL JUDGMENT

PRACTICING FOR NCLEX

1. The nurse is preparing a 5-year-old for surgery on their lower leg. The parent is helping them into the hospital gown, and the child fights removal of their underwear. What is the most appropriate nursing action?
   a. Allow the parent to remove the underwear.
   b. Tell the child they are acting childishly.
   c. Notify the operating room that the underwear is on.
   d. Allow the child to keep their underwear on.

2. A 6-month-old infant requires restraint to prevent removal of a nasogastric tube. What is the priority nursing intervention?
   a. Tie the restraint loosely to prevent skin breakdown.
   b. Leave the baby unrestrained when directly observed.
   c. Position the restrained infant prone to prevent aspiration.
   d. Place the infant in a room near the nurses' station.

3. A 10-year-old child on a regular diet refuses to eat the food on the meal tray. They request chicken nuggets, French fries, and ice cream. What is the best nursing action?
   a. Ask that the child's desired foods be sent up from the kitchen.
   b. Negotiate with the child to eat at least part of the food on the tray.
   c. Remove a privilege.
   d. Offer the child cereal and milk from stock on the nursing unit.

4. The nurse providing home care to a 2-year-old listens to the child's parents talk about how the child and family are adjusting to the child's current illness. Which role is the nurse providing?
   a. Case management
   b. Child and family advocacy
   c. Direct nursing care
   d. Child and family education

5. A child is to undergo a tympanostomy tube placement in a freestanding outpatient surgery center. What are the major advantages associated with this location? Select all that apply.
   a. Decreased risk for infection
   b. Decreased health care costs
   c. Ability to be transferred if overnight stay is required
   d. Decreased disruption of family functioning
   e. Decreased risk of complications
   f. Ability to return to normal routine for the child quickly

CRITICAL THINKING EXERCISES

1. Becky, an 8-year-old, is admitted to the pediatric unit for an emergency surgery. She is in third grade and very active in afterschool programs. Her parent is with her during the admission process but will have to return to work shortly after Becky returns from surgery to the pediatric unit. Would the nurse expect Becky to show separation anxiety? What are the three top nursing concerns for Becky relating to the effects of hospitalization?

2. A 6-year-old is admitted to the general pediatric unit after spending several hours in the emergency department with an acute asthma attack. A parent and two younger siblings are present, but the parent plans to leave shortly to take the siblings home. The other parent will visit in about 2 hours, after work. What is the overall goal for this child's care? What could the nurse say to promote coping in this child? What would be the best answer if the parent asks if they should stay rather than take the siblings home?

3. A child with cerebral palsy is discharged from the hospital, where they have been receiving treatment for pneumonia. Home health care nurses, through a local agency, are to help the family administer intravenous antibiotic therapy and to monitor the child's health status.
   a. As the home health nurse assigned to this child, what should your nursing assessment include?
   b. In this situation, what are some nursing interventions that will help ensure family-centered care?
   c. When this child is stable and can go back to school, what will be the role of the school nurse in caring for this child?

STUDY ACTIVITIES

1. Follow a child and family during the admission process, from preadmission to initial time on the unit, to identify the procedures and tasks involved. Examine the response of the child and family and how the nursing staff responds to their needs.

2. Develop a teaching plan to orient a toddler or preschooler and their family to a nursing unit. Include the resources, personnel, and techniques to include in the teaching plan.

3. Shadow a nurse working in a community setting, such as a camp, school, shelter, or health department. Identify the role the nurse plays in the health of the children and families in the setting and the community.

4. Spend a day in a medical day care setting. Identify the needs of one child and their family, how they may differ from those of a child in a traditional day care setting, and the role of the nurse in meeting those needs.

5. Develop an IHP for a child with diabetes.

6. Shadow a nurse working in a home health care setting. Identify ways they help the family to promote the child's growth and development and to ensure that the child has normal a childhood as possible. Identify interventions that embody the key concepts of family-centered care.

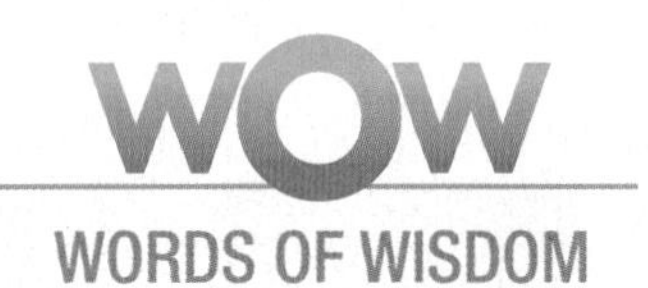

WORDS OF WISDOM

The touch of a parent's hand and the sound of their voice bring comfort to the child with special health care needs, and when the nurse brings comfort, you strengthen both of them.

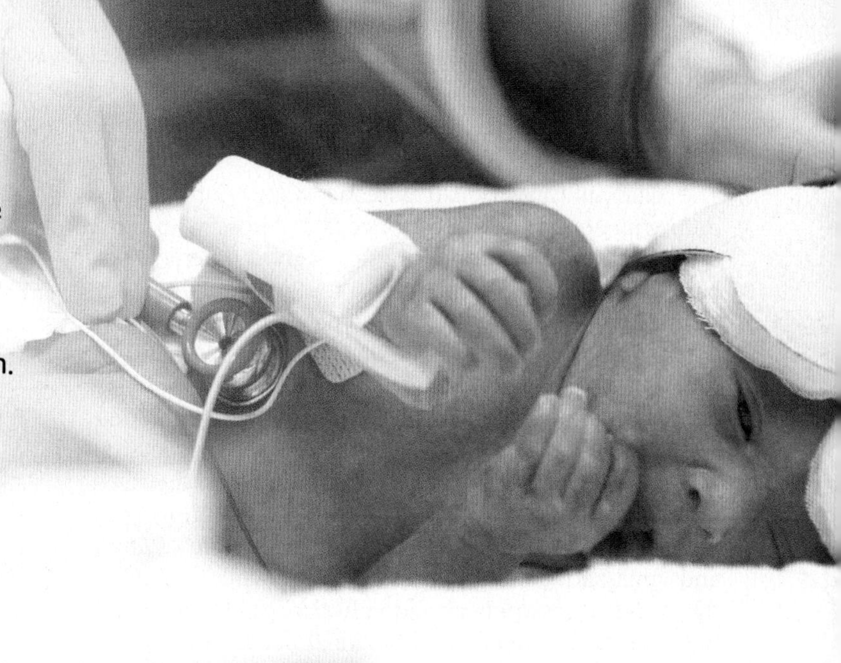

34

Caring for the Child With Special Health Care Needs

LEARNING OBJECTIVES

Upon completion of the chapter, you will be able to:

1. Analyze the impact that special health care needs has on the child and family.
2. Identify anticipated times when the child and family will require additional support.
3. Describe ways that nurses assist children with special health care needs and their families to obtain optimal functioning.
4. Discuss early intervention and public school education for the child with special health care needs.
5. Plan for transition of the child with special health care needs from the inpatient facility to the home and from pediatric to adult medical care.
6. Discuss key elements related to pediatric end-of-life care.
7. Differentiate developmental responses to death and appropriate interventions.

KEY TERMS

chronic illness
developmental delay
developmental disability
palliative care (pal´ē-ă-tiv kār)
respite care (res´pit kār)
terminal illness

Preet Singh, an 18-month-old who was born at 28 weeks' gestation, is seen in your clinic for the first time. He has a history of hydrocephalus and developmental delay. During the examination, his parent states, "I'm concerned about finding a good, affordable preschool for Preet. His older brother attends public school, but I can't imagine Preet going there."

INTRODUCTION

The Maternal Child Health Bureau (MCHB) defines children with special health care needs as "those who have or are at risk for chronic physical, developmental, behavioral, or emotional conditions" and who "also require health and related services of a type or amount beyond that required by children generally" (MCHB, 2023, para. 4). Children who have a terminal illness or are otherwise dying also require additional care. Nurses are in a unique position, in both the inpatient and the outpatient setting, to have a significant and positive influence on the lives of these children and their families. In addition to providing direct care, the nurse fills the critical role of child and family advocate and case manager. When a child is dying, nurses not only provide physical care to the child but also strive to meet the emotional needs of the child and family.

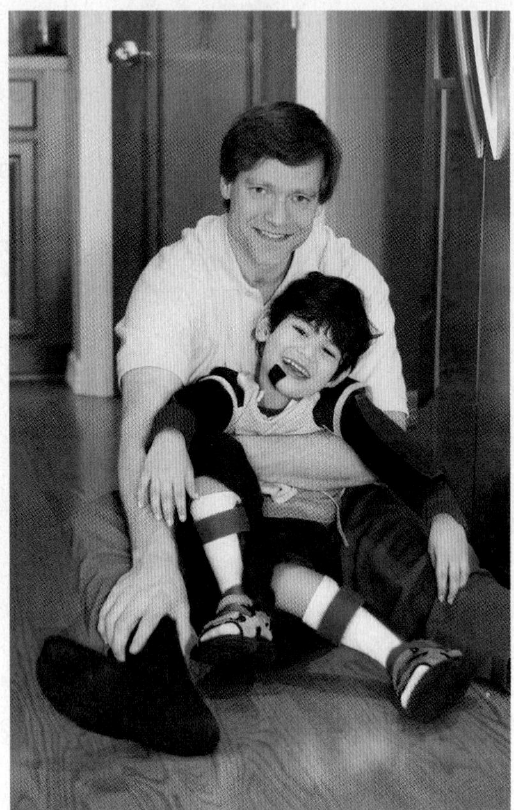

FIGURE 34.1 The child with special health care needs often requires a significant amount of care at home throughout life.

THE CHILD WITH SPECIAL HEALTH CARE NEEDS

The numbers of children with **chronic illnesses** (long-lasting or recurrent illnesses) are increasing. Children with special health care needs make up about 19% of the population of children in the United States, and nearly one in five families has a child with a special health care need (MCHB, 2023). Increasing numbers of children are being diagnosed with physical and mental disorders (Abdi et al., 2020), and larger numbers of children are living with the assistance of high-tech treatments and equipment (Brenner et al., 2021).

Impact of the Problem

Children with chronic physical, developmental, behavioral, or emotional conditions may use or need prescription medication, medical care, mental health services, or education services more than other children of the same age. They may need physical, occupational, or speech therapy (Fig. 34.1). Alternatively, they may require ongoing treatment for emotional, developmental, or behavioral problems (MCHB, 2023). These children and their families may be inadequately insured, have financial needs and unmet family support needs, or have difficulty obtaining the specialty care that the child requires (Kuo & Turchi, 2023). It can be challenging for the family of a child with these needs to navigate the system and obtain all of the services the child requires.

When an infant is born very prematurely, when a child is injured and requires long-term rehabilitation and special care, or when a child is diagnosed with a complex chronic health condition, the parents are often initially devastated. The parents may feel they must adapt to the risk and protect their child. They are interested in preserving their family while compensating for the past, and they cautiously look to the future and become hopeful again. While the infant or child is in the hospital, nurses can help families build on their strengths, empowering them to care for their medically fragile infant or special needs child. Education is paramount and should begin as early in hospitalization as possible (Cincinnati Children's Hospital Medical Center [CCHMC], 2023). In many situations, particular discharge needs are known early in the course of the hospitalization. Nurses should provide anticipatory guidance about the course of treatment and the expected outcome.

Most children with chronic illnesses or those who require technology progress through stages of growth and development just as typical children do, although sometimes at a slower pace. The exception is the child with significant psychomotor delays, although some developmental progression may occur. Children with developmental or functional needs desire to be treated as normal, and they want to experience the same events that other children do.

Remember Preet, the 18-month-old former 28-week premature neonate introduced at the beginning of the chapter? What would you expect his gross motor, fine motor, and language skills to be at this age?

Effects of Special Health Care Needs on the Child

When a child has a chronic physical, developmental, behavioral, or emotional condition, the child's coping ability is affected. In addition, the child's ability to cope is significantly affected by the family's response to stressors, which can be numerous for these families. Children experience differing effects of the chronic illness or disability based on their developmental level, which naturally changes over time for most children. These differences in their health and needs may lead to alterations in social–emotional development (Population Reference Bureau [PRB], 2023).

Infants may fail to develop a sense of trust, while the toddler may experience difficulty developing autonomy. The preschooler may experience limited opportunities for socialization. The school-age child may have limited opportunities to achieve a sense of industry because of school absence and inability to participate in activities or competitive events. Many school-age children who have medically complex conditions may often be absent from school, affecting their academic achievement (PRB, 2023).

Adolescents may feel as though they are different from their peers because of their different skills, abilities, or appearance. This may hinder the adolescent's ability to form a sense of personal identity. Since the adolescent may require significant amounts of support from the family, it may be difficult for the adolescent to achieve independence. If the earlier stages of cognitive development have been delayed, then reaching the level of abstract thinking may be blocked (American Academy of Child and Adolescent Psychiatry [AACAP], 2023).

The child with special health care needs may be able to focus on the positive experiences in their life as a method of coping, leading to as much independence as possible. Other children may always feel different from their peers in a negative sense and withdraw. Irritability and acting out may also occur. Some children may be compliant and seek support for themselves. The child's coping pattern may change over time or with certain situations, such as relapse or worsening of the condition. Children with more protective parents may display marked dependence and may be fearful (Schmitz, 2019). Children whose parents have been more indulgent may be more independent and defiant. The nurse must assess the child's individual response to the current health care status and intervene as appropriate.

Effects on the Family

Each member of the family experiences effects related to the child's situation. Family members' experiences and their responses influence each other directly (Fig. 34.2).

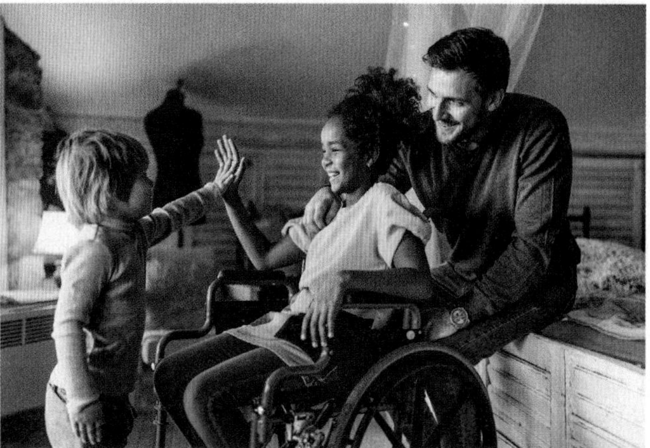

FIGURE 34.2 A child with special health care needs with their family. (Shutterstock/NDAB Creativity.)

Effects on Parents

Raising a child with special health care needs is generally not what parents expected. Some parents may adapt over time and accept the child's illness or disability. Others may adapt but do not find acceptance and experience the continual fading and reemergence of chronic sorrow. Denial of problems may prevent parents from progressing through grief, but it also gives them a sense of hope (Bally et al., 2018).

Caring for the child at home rather than in a facility may decrease the parents' feelings of anxiety and helplessness. As with healthy children, parents enjoy witnessing the emotional and social growth of the child. Parents of children with special health care needs experience a multitude of emotions and changes in their lives. They worry about the child's and family's well-being and, as experts in their child's care, often feel burdened with the demands of continual care. They may feel helpless and overwhelmed when their child is discharged from the hospital. Although willing to carry out the responsibility for care, they may experience fear, anger, sadness, guilt, frustration, or resentment. Many parents experience grief as a result of losing the child they expected (Bally et al., 2018).

STRESSORS OF DAILY LIVING

Families with children who have special health care needs experience life differently from other families. They may have to change their housing situations to accommodate the child's functional needs. Sleep may be affected. Constant supervision of a child who requests technologic assistive devices makes it difficult to carry out other basic household activities. In addition to basic child care and running of the household, medical and technical care must be incorporated into daily life. The family's identity and the parents' employment may be radically altered. Holidays and vacations may be affected, as it can be difficult to plan activities. Nursing and other health care professional visits can be disruptive to family life.

The extended caregiving responsibilities can also have adverse health effects on caregivers; often, families report emotional and physical burdens of their own (Blanco et al., 2021). In addition, these parents are at increased risk for the development of depression (Blanco et al., 2021). Parents may experience role conflicts, financial burdens, and difficulty balancing the independence of providing care with the isolation associated with it. It can be difficult to enjoy spontaneous events outside the home since extra planning is necessary.

The degree of independence can be influenced by mobility issues, education, and assistive technology. Although education for all children is federally mandated, parents have anxiety about educational decisions and may find it difficult to obtain the support and educational services the child needs.

Additional stress is associated with transition times in the care of a child with special health care needs. These transition times include:

- Initial diagnosis or change in prognosis
- Increased symptoms
- When the child moves to a new setting (hospital, school)
- During a parent's absence
- During periods of developmental change

VULNERABLE CHILD SYNDROME

Vulnerable child syndrome is a clinical state in which the parents' reactions to a serious illness or event in the child's past continue to have long-term psychologically harmful effects on the child and parents for many years (Schmitz, 2019). The parents view the child as being at higher risk for medical, developmental, or behavioral problems than the child may actually be. Parents exhibit excessive unwarranted concerns and seek health care for their child frequently. Risk factors for the development of vulnerable child syndrome include pregnancy-related problems (e.g., illness, history of miscarriage, infertility), preterm birth, low birth weight, and an illness or threat to life while the child is quite young (Verbeek et al., 2021). Parental fears result in extreme concern and overprotection, inability to trust another caregiver with their children, and lack of setting age-appropriate boundaries, thereby threatening the child's development (Verbeek et al., 2021). The child may also develop difficult behaviors such as aggression, conduct issues, or hyperactivity, or they may develop a disease role and have sleep issues, anxiety, and chronic physical complaints (Verbeek et al., 2021).

Effects on Siblings

The siblings of children with special health care needs may also be dramatically affected. Their relationship with their parents is different from what it would have been if their sibling had been healthy. Parents often need to spend more time with the child with special health care needs and have less time with the siblings (Sewell-Roberts, 2021). Children exhibit emotional and psychological responses to a sibling's long-term needs (Lummer-Aikey & Goldstein, 2021). The sibling's knowledge about the illness, their attitude toward and adjustment to it, their own self-esteem, how socially supported they are, and the parents' awareness of their feelings are all related to how well the sibling adjusts.

Nursing Management of the Child With Special Health Care Needs and Their Family

Family-centered care provides the optimal framework for caring for all children and their families. Family-centered care can also minimize the impact of chronic illness and maximize the child's developmental potential. To provide the best nursing care for children with special health care needs and their families, the nurse must first develop a trusting relationship with the family.

To ensure optimal functioning, children with special health care needs require comprehensive and coordinated services from multiple professionals. These professionals should work collaboratively to address the child's health, educational, psychological, and social service needs. In addition to case management and advocacy, nursing management focuses on screening and ongoing assessment of the child, provision of home care, care of the child with technology needs, education and support of the child and family, and referral for resources.

Developing a Therapeutic Relationship

Raising children always has the potential to be challenging, but a child's additional health care needs can completely overwhelm a parent. The parents' needs change continuously, so it is best if the family has a stable, long-term relationship with a primary health care provider. This promotes trust and a more efficient two-way flow of information.

Respect the parents' range of emotions and work with them as a team to manage the child's care. Nurses should recognize when parents are successful in adhering to the treatment plan or when other small gains are made. Empowering the family strengthens them and gives them self-confidence. Feeling supported and invigorated gives parents and caregivers strength, energy, and hope. Box 34.1 lists principles related to family involvement.

Screening and Ongoing Assessment

Nurses should perform screening to identify children with unmet health care needs. Children with special health care needs may attain developmental milestones

BOX 34.1 Principles Related to Family Involvement

Families:

- Are the constant in a child's life
- Need to have access to information and training
- Deserve to receive culturally respectful care
- Know their strengths, limitations, and fears
- Merit mutual respect and responsibility for outcomes

Adapted from de Leon Siantz, M. L., Kilanowski, J. F., & Thomas, T. L. (2018). Cultural values, beliefs, and preference are integral to family-centered care. In C. L. Betz, M. J. Krajicek, & M. Craft-Rosenberg (Eds.), *Guidelines for nursing excellence in the care of children, youth, and families* (2nd ed.). Springer Publishing Company.

more slowly than other children. If a developmental screening tool is used for ongoing developmental surveillance of the young child, then the results should be compared visit to visit to determine progress rather than using it as a screening tool. Assess these families for vulnerable child syndrome.

Promoting Home Care

Home is the most developmentally appropriate environment for all children, even those who have technology needs. The child's home can be an emotionally nurturing and socially stimulating environment. Receiving care in the home allows children with technology needs to display improved physical, emotional, psychological, and social status (Mitchell et al., 2022).

Technology needs for children may include supplemental oxygen, assisted ventilation, tracheostomy care, assisted enteral or parenteral feeding, or parenteral medication administration. With advances in technology, children with extensive medical and developmental needs may be cared for at home, and the decision for home care should be undertaken seriously by the health care team and family (Blanco et al., 2021). Early discharge planning is important, and parents will need detailed instructions and support in caring for children using these devices at home (CCHMC, 2022).

EARLY DISCHARGE PLANNING

Early discharge planning and ongoing inclusion and education of the family facilitates continuity of care. Box 34.2 provides information about preparing the child with special health care needs for discharge.

BOX 34.2 Preparing for Home Care Before Discharge

- Promote liaison with community resources. Develop communication between various services. Plan appointments. Set up home nursing care (either private duty or visits).
- Teach skills, encouraging active caregiving in the hospital setting to increase the caregivers' self-confidence.
- Discuss psychological and emotional issues with parents.
- Obtain and organize equipment and supplies (running out of supplies may cause significant stress on families).
- Refer the family for necessary financial resources.
- Ensure the family's home environment is adequate (e.g., enough room for equipment, electricity on, air conditioner for warm weather, heater for cold weather, refrigeration for food).
- For the baby being discharged from the neonatal intensive care unit (NICU):
  - Teach the parents about the infant's cues and behaviors and the different sleep–wake patterns.
  - Encourage kangaroo care and infant massage while in the NICU (as the infant's condition allows).
  - Educate the parents about possible effects on short- and long-term neurodevelopment.
  - Refer to a local early intervention program.
  - Assist the family with finding a primary care provider who is experienced in the ongoing follow-up of high-risk infants.

Adapted from Smith, V. C., & Stewart, J. (2023). Discharge planning for high-risk newborns. UpToDate. Retrieved on November 5, 2023, from https://www.uptodate.com/contents/discharge-planning-for-high-risk-newborns

CARING FOR THE CHILD WITH TECHNOLOGY NEEDS AT HOME

Home care nurses are often involved in the care of children with technology needs. Caring for a child who requires these devices at home can be a complex process, but children thrive in the home care setting with appropriate intervention and care. Improved collaboration between parents and home care nurses may decrease the parents' stress and maximize opportunities for appropriate growth and development in the child with technology needs. Thus, a strong relationship, good communication, and effective negotiation skills are assets to the family and child.

Help the family incorporate the medical regimen into daily life to minimize the child's potential perception of being different from other children. Teach families about the technical processes related to home and travel oxygen therapy, use of the ventilator, suctioning, chest percussion and postural drainage, tube feedings and care of the feeding tube, and medications. Assist parents with the planning and management of routine care, respiratory treatments, nutritional support, and developmental interventions. Reinforce exercises and techniques as prescribed by developmental therapists. Refer to Chapter 33 for additional information about home care nursing.

Providing Care Coordination

Once a child with special health care needs has been discharged to the home setting, the nurse plays a vital role in care coordination. Any child with special health care needs benefits from a medical home for their primary care, as it provides continuous, accessible, comprehensive services (National Resource Center for Patient/Family-Centered Medical Home, 2020). See the Healthy People 2030 box.

HEALTHY PEOPLE 2030

Objective	Nursing Significance
Increase the proportion of children with special health care needs who have a system of care that is family-centered, comprehensive, and coordinated.	Refer the child and family with special needs to an integrated health program that provides interdisciplinary, collaborative care for children requiring complex, coordinated care.

Healthy People Objectives retrieved from http://www.healthypeople.gov

The nurse in the medical home is a critical team member, providing ongoing care coordination and follow-up. The nurse can best benefit the family by being available to the family as needed and providing the support they need as they learn how to deal with the child's care needs at home. Refer to Box 34.3 for nursing interventions for families of children with special health care needs.

Providing Ongoing Follow-Up of the Former Premature Infant

Many former premature infants experience medical and developmental problems throughout infancy, early childhood, and beyond. Upon or following discharge, many former premature infants display one or more of the following medical or developmental problems:

- Chronic lung disease (bronchopulmonary dysplasia)
- Cardiac changes such as right ventricular hypertrophy and pulmonary artery hypertension
- Growth delays, poor feeding, anemia of prematurity, other nutrient deficiencies
- Apnea of prematurity, gastroesophageal reflux disease, bradycardia
- Sudden unexplained infant death (SUID)
- Osteopenia (rickets) of prematurity
- Hydrocephalus, ventriculomegaly, abnormal head magnetic resonance imaging results, ventriculoperitoneal shunt
- Inguinal or umbilical hernias
- Retinopathy of prematurity, strabismus, decreased visual acuity
- Hearing deficits
- Delayed dentition
- Gross motor skills, fine motor skills, and language development delay; sensory integration issues (Stewart, 2023)

Over the long term, former premature infants are at higher risk than full-term infants of developing cognitive delay, cerebral palsy, attention-deficit/hyperactivity disorder, learning disabilities, difficulties with socialization, and vulnerable child syndrome (Mandy, 2023; Stewart, 2023). In addition, many former premature infants display alterations in muscle tone at or shortly after discharge from the neonatal intensive care unit (NICU) that require physical therapy intervention.

For these reasons, former premature infants require special attention and thorough, appropriate assessment to discern subtle changes that may affect their long-term physical, cognitive, emotional, and social outcome. The pediatric nurse should have an understanding of the special concerns that former premature infants and children as well as their families may face (Fig. 34.3).

From the beginning, encourage families to keep all of the infant's pertinent check-up, insurance, and medical and developmental information; this will serve as a resource for the parents, and they will be able to supply complete information when visiting various providers.

BOX 34.3 Nursing Interventions for Families of Children With Special Health Care Needs

- Develop written health plans.
- Provide care coordination and collaboration with specialists in other disciplines, early intervention, schools, and public agencies.
- Address needs for prior authorization for treatments, medications, or specialist referrals; retain copies in the child's chart of authorization forms and approvals.
- Modify office routines to promote family and child comfort.
- Assist parents with child care decisions.
- Know community resources available to children with special health care needs.
- When the child is hospitalized, encourage high levels of parental participation.
- Provide care coordination across multiple health settings.
- Educate child care providers on child health needs.
- Help parents get involved with parent support networks.

Adapted from Cincinnati Children's Hospital Medical Center. (2023). *Ongoing support resources. https://www.cincinnatichildrens.org/patients/child/special-needs*; Kuo, D. Z., & Turchi, R. M. (2023). Children and youth with special health care needs. UpToDate. Retrieved on November 5, 2023, from https://www.uptodate.com/contents/children-and-youth-with-special-health-care-needs

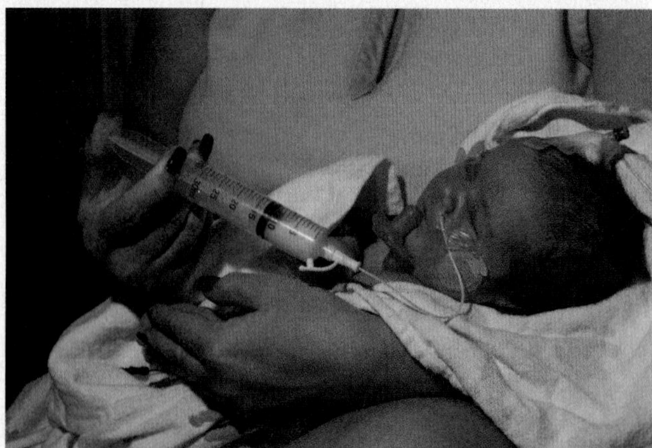

FIGURE 34.3 Parents of an infant discharged from the neonatal intensive care unit (NICU) may need to administer special care, such as feeding.

PROVIDING ROUTINE WELL-CHILD CARE TO THE FORMER PREMATURE INFANT

Former premature infants require similar well-child care as full-term infants do, with additional visits for management of any complex medical issues and developmental screenings or interventions. Teach families routine newborn care, including bathing, dressing, and avoidance of cigarette smoke. All visits for primary care follow-up will be scheduled based on the infant's chronologic age.

Prior to discharge from the NICU, the infant will be tested for oxygen desaturation while seated in the car seat (Smith & Stewart, 2023). Clearance will be obtained prior to the infant's discharge. Former premature infants require car seat use just as other infants do. Help the parents find methods of padding the car seat or adding an additional semifirm cushion inside the seat for the infant to ride in the car safely. Some infants may need to continue cardiac/apnea monitoring while in the car seat. Since the former premature infant is at increased risk for SUID compared to the general population, it is critical to teach parents to put the infant on their back to sleep (Stewart, 2023).

Give immunizations according to the current immunization schedule recommended by the Centers for Disease Control and Prevention (CDC) based on the infant's chronologic age. All former premature infants should receive the flu vaccine as recommended after 6 months' chronologic age. Respiratory syncytial virus (RSV) prophylaxis is critical for certain groups of premature infants (Stewart, 2023). Therefore, administer the palivizumab (Synagis) vaccine according to the recommended schedule (refer to Chapter 40 for additional information about RSV prophylaxis).

ASSESSING GROWTH AND DEVELOPMENT OF THE FORMER PREMATURE INFANT

When assessing growth and development of the infant or child who was born prematurely, determine the child's adjusted or corrected age so that you can perform an accurate assessment. The corrected or adjusted age should be used for evaluating progression in growth as well as development. For example, if a 6-month-old infant was born at 28 weeks' gestation (12 weeks, or 3 months early), their growth and development expectations are those of a 3-month-old (corrected age). Continue to correct age for growth and development until the child is 3 years old.

Although breast milk is the preferred form of nutrition for former premature infants, many require special diets to foster catch-up growth (Stewart, 2023). Extra calories are necessary for increased growth needs. Additional calcium and phosphorus are required for bone mineralization. For these reasons, former premature infants should be fed breast milk fortified with additional nutrients or a commercially prepared formula specifically for premature infants. When former premature infants demonstrate consistent adequate growth (usually by 6 months corrected age), they may be switched to a "term infant formula" such as Similac or Enfamil, concentrated to a higher caloric density if needed. Assess the infant's ability to suck efficiently and refer them to occupational or speech therapy if the infant is a slow feeder or has difficulty feeding.

All anticipatory guidance related to nutrition is based on the child's corrected age (The Warren Center, 2023). In other words, begin solid foods at 6 months' corrected age, not chronologic age, and delay the addition of whole milk until 12 months' corrected age, rather than chronologic age. Signs that the former premature infant may be ready to attempt spoon-feeding include interest in feeding, decrease in tongue thrust, and adequate head control.

Early screening and intervention for issues related to development are critical to the attainment of optimal development in the former premature infant. The comorbidities that they exhibit in the form of prior and current medical problems place these infants at high risk for **developmental delay** (lag in meeting developmental milestones). Even mild developmental delays warrant evaluation and intervention. Developmental screening tools may be used to screen for developmental concerns in the former premature infant, although they do not always identify children at risk. Parent-report questionnaires demonstrate fairly accurate estimations of developmental problems and are simple to use. Most importantly, assess the child's development based on corrected age until the child is 3 years old. Refer infants and children early if developmental concerns are suspected.

Identifying and Managing Undernutrition and Feeding Disorders in Children With Special Health Care Needs

Undernutrition can cause inadequate growth in infants and children. The child fails to demonstrate appropriate weight gain over a prolonged period of time. Length or height velocity and head circumference growth may also be affected. Risk factors for undernutrition include malignancy, developmental disability, and chronic illness, among others (Bamberger et al., 2022). Adequate nutrition is critical for appropriate brain growth in the first 3 years of life and for growth in general throughout childhood and adolescence (Seymour, 2021).

Undernutrition can be a multifactorial problem. **Developmental disability** (mental or physical or combination impairment resulting in lifelong disability) may contribute to undernutrition, as the child's ability to consume adequate nutrition is impaired because of sensory or motor delays, such as with cerebral palsy. Other organic causes of undernutrition include inability to suck or swallow correctly, malabsorption, diarrhea, vomiting, or alterations in metabolism and caloric/nutrient needs associated with a variety of chronic illnesses. Infants and children with cardiac or metabolic disease, chronic lung disease (bronchopulmonary dysplasia), cleft palate, or gastroesophageal reflux disease are at particular risk. Feeding disorders or food refusal may occur in infants or children who have required prolonged mechanical ventilation, long-term enteral tube feedings, or an unpleasant event such as a choking episode. Additional causes of undernutrition include family income below the poverty threshold, neglect, abuse, behavioral problems, lack of appropriate parental interaction, poor feeding techniques, lack of parental knowledge, or parental mental illness (Bamberger et al., 2022).

Screen all children for undernutrition to identify it early. In addition to poor growth, the infant or child with undernutrition may present with a history of developmental delay or loss of acquired milestones. Infants or children with feeding problems may display nipple, spoon, or food refusal; difficulty sucking; disinterest in feeding; or difficulty progressing from liquid to puréed to textured food. Perform a detailed dietary history, and instruct the parents to complete a 3-day food diary to identify what the child actually eats and drinks. Assess the parent–child interaction, with particular attention to the parent's ability to read and respond to the infant's or child's cues. Observe feeding, noting the child's oral interest or aversion, oral–motor coordination, and swallowing ability, as well as parent–child interactions before, during, and after the feeding (Bamberger et al., 2022).

Significant undernutrition may require hospitalization for evaluation and management. Sometimes, enteral tube feedings are necessary in order for children with undernutrition or feeding disorders to demonstrate adequate growth (Duryea, 2023). Box 34.4 lists nursing interventions for the hospitalized child with undernutrition.

TAKE NOTE!

Infants and children who have experienced neglect may not interact appropriately with their environment or caregiver (lack of eye contact) (Duryea, 2023).

BOX 34.4 Nursing Interventions During Hospitalization for Undernutrition

- Observe parent–child interactions, especially during feedings.
- Develop an appropriate feeding schedule.
- Provide feedings as prescribed (usually, 120 kcal/kg/day is needed to demonstrate proper weight gain).
- Weigh the child daily and maintain strict records of intake and output.
- Educate parents about proper feeding techniques and volumes.
- Provide extensive support to alleviate parental anxiety related to the child's inability to gain weight.

Adapted from Duryea, T. K. (2023). Poor weight gain in children younger than two years in resource-abundant countries: Management. *UpToDate.* Retrieved on November 5, 2023, from https://www.uptodate.com/contents/poor-weight-gain-in-children-younger-than-two-years-in-resource-abundant-countries-management

Promoting Growth and Development

When caring for the infant with special health care needs in the hospital, provide consistent caregivers to encourage the infant to develop a sense of trust. Allow and encourage the parent to stay with the infant, providing a comfortable place for the parent to sleep. To promote attachment, emphasize the baby's positive qualities. Encourage developmentally appropriate skills, and allow the infant to have pleasurable experiences through all of the senses.

For the toddler, begin developmentally appropriate limit setting and discipline. Encourage independence as the toddler is able. Modify gross motor and sensory activities to accommodate the toddler's limitations. To encourage a sense of control, offer the toddler simple choices.

As the preschooler develops, encourage mastery of self-help skills as the child is able. Encourage socialization with same-age peers to develop a sense of friendship. Reinforce to the child that an illness or disability is not a punishment for wrongdoing or the child's fault in any way.

Encourage the school-age child to attend school and make up work that must be missed for medical treatments or appointments. Provide education to the school staff and other students about the child's special needs. Promote involvement in appropriate sports activities; music, drama, or art activities; and clubs such as Boy Scouts or Girl Scouts. Educate the child about the illness or disability and the course of treatment.

Inform parents of adolescents that those with chronic illnesses often participate in the same activities as those without, such as risk taking, rebelling, and trying out different identities. Assist the adolescent with coping and interpersonal skills. Promote involvement in activities with other adolescents with special health care needs as well as those without. Ensure that the adolescent participates in rites of passage as able, such as attending the prom or obtaining a driver's license. Discuss future plans with the adolescent, such as college or vocation, as well as transition to a nonpediatric health care provider (Blanco et al., 2021).

Providing Resources to the Child and Family

Nurses should be familiar with community resources available to children with special health care needs. Educational opportunities for children with special health care needs include early intervention programs and programs offered through the public school system. Financial resources, respite care, and complementary therapies are other areas with which the nurse should become familiar.

EDUCATIONAL OPPORTUNITIES FOR THE CHILD WITH SPECIAL HEALTH CARE NEEDS

The foundation for health and development in children is laid during the first few years of life. Children with special health care needs often require multiple developmental interventions and special education in the early years in order to reach their developmental potential later in childhood. Children learn best when they are at the stage of maximal readiness, and the early years must not be missed as an opportunity for development. See the Healthy People 2030 box.

HEALTHY PEOPLE 2030

Objective	Nursing Significance
Increase the proportion of children and youth with disabilities who are usually in regular education programs.	• Ensure that children younger than 3 years who may qualify are referred to the local early intervention program. • Encourage families to advocate for their child's needs on the individualized education plan.

Healthy People Objectives retrieved from http://www.healthypeople.gov

Early intervention programs are intended to enhance the development of infants and toddlers with or at risk for disabilities, thereby minimizing educational costs and special education. Early intervention is also directed toward enhancing the capacity of families to meet their children's needs as well as to maximize the likelihood of independent living (CDC, 2022).

The Individuals with Disabilities Education Improvement Act of 2004 (formerly called Public Law 99–457) mandates government-funded care coordination and special education for children up to 3 years of age. This early intervention program is administered through each state. Federal law allows each state to define developmental disability differently, but, in general, qualified personnel perform an evaluation of the child's physical, language, emotional, and social capabilities to determine eligibility (U.S. Department of Education [USDE], n.d.). The law guarantees that eligible children will obtain access to services that will enhance their development. Children who qualify for services receive care coordination, and an individualized family service plan is developed by the service coordinator in conjunction with the family. The service coordinator manages the developmental services and special education that the child requires.

The intent of the program is that the child receives services in a nonmedical environment, so most services occur in the home or day care center. Home visits by the service coordinator and maintenance of regular contact with the family ensure the success of the program.

Refer children who may have developmental delay to the local early intervention program. For children receiving these services, collaborate with the service coordinator on an ongoing basis with particular involvement at hospital discharge and when transition of services occurs at age 3 years.

> Think back to Preet, the 2-year-old boy with a history of hydrocephalus and developmental delay, from the beginning of the chapter. After further discussion with Preet's parent, you realize he has not been involved in an early intervention program. Discuss with his parent the educational opportunities that are available for Preet and why they are important.

Schools may have a profound impact on the child's overall health and development. Some children with special needs do not require additional services to succeed in school. For these children, the nurse's role is to assess for school success or failure and determine the effect of the school environment on the child's health. The Individuals with Disabilities Education Act, reauthorized in 2004, provides for the education of children with special needs through the public school system, from ages 3 to 21 years. These services are provided within the public school system.

According to the law, each student with special health care needs is entitled to an individualized education program (IEP), which is a written plan designed to meet the preschool, primary, or secondary school student's individual needs. A committee consisting of the child's parent, a regular teacher, a special education teacher, and various other specialists develops the IEP. Nurses may be called to serve on this committee. The IEP must include measurable short- and long-term goals. Parents are informed of the student's progress routinely, and the IEP is reviewed at least annually (USDE, n.d.).

Preschool special education through the local public school system is provided from ages 3 to 5 years; access to the curriculum is ensured for all children. A child is eligible for special education preschool when a significant delay is present in the cognitive, language, adaptive, social–emotional, or motor development domains to the extent that it adversely affects the child's learning ability. In the school setting, the child receives developmental therapy as needed to augment their ability to participate in the education process. The least restrictive environment is preferred, with children with special health care needs participating in classes containing age-appropriate peers without special health care needs whenever possible (USDE, n.d.). Special education preschool services are often offered in the elementary school setting.

FINANCIAL AND INSURANCE RESOURCES

Many children with special health care needs whose families demonstrate financial need may be eligible for Supplemental Security Income (SSI). This program was created in 1972 through Public Law 92–603. SSI is a cash assistance program, and monthly benefits vary per individual. SSI qualification usually makes the child eligible for state-administered Medicaid (Social Security Administration [SSA], n.d.-a). Medicaid benefits vary slightly from state to state, but generally cover medical visits, medication, hospitalization, and limited adjuvant therapies. The Children's Health Insurance Program (CHIP) provides low-cost health insurance to eligible children. Eligibility and the extent of benefits provided by CHIP vary by state (Centers for Medicare and Medicaid Services, n.d.). Title V programs under the MCHB block grant program provide funds to the individual states for administration of services. State Title V programs provide community-based, comprehensive service coordination for children with special health care needs (SSA, n.d.-b). Online directories providing a wealth of links to resources for children with special health care needs include Children's Disabilities Information and Special Child.

RESPITE CARE

Primary caregivers of children with special health care needs must be dedicated, skillful, vigilant, and knowledgeable. Constant care can be a stress on the primary caregiver, who needs temporary relief from the daily caregiving demands. **Respite care** provides an opportunity for families to take a break from the daily intensive caregiving responsibilities. Respite care should meet the child's health care needs and offer the child developmental opportunities. Finding and using respite care that the family is comfortable with and trusts may decrease the family's stress and lead to an enhanced quality of life for these families. Nurses can facilitate access to respite care, educate respite providers, and ensure quality respite care practices through involvement in community agencies.

COMPLEMENTARY THERAPIES

Families of children with special health care needs often use adjuvant therapies. These may include homeopathic and herbal medicine, pet therapy, hippotherapy, music, and massage, among others. Many families may want to blend complementary and alternative therapies with mainstream medicine in search of palliation or a cure. When obtaining the health history, ask specifically about homeopathy or herbal medications the child may be taking.

> ***TAKE NOTE!***
>
> Become familiar with the risks and benefits of homeopathic and herbal medications as well as any contraindications, as many families use these treatments in an effort to improve their child's quality of life or outcome.

Hippotherapy is the use of equine movement for the engagement of the sensory, neuromuscular, and cognitive systems resulting in achievement of functional outcomes. Occupational and physical therapists as well as speech-language pathologists utilize evidence-based practice and clinical reasoning to provide purposeful movement of the horse with the child riding. Hippotherapy should not be confused with therapeutic horseback riding or adaptive horseback riding. In hippotherapy, the pathologist or therapist chooses specific horse movements for therapeutic exercise, neuromuscular re-education, therapeutic activities, or treatment of speech, language, voice, communication, and auditory processing disorder. Additional information may be obtained through the American Hippotherapy Association (2022) at www.americanhippotherapyassociation.org.

Pet therapy may be used to decrease stress or as a component of psychotherapy. Music may be used to induce positive behavioral changes, reduce pain or stress, or induce various other positive effects (American Music Therapy Association, 2023). Massage therapy may be beneficial to a wide variety of children. It may be used to reduce pain, promote relaxation, decrease fear, and demonstrate a specific positive effect related to the child's particular medical condition (Genik et al., 2020).

Providing Support and Education

At the time of initial diagnosis, allow and encourage the family to express their feelings. Parents of children with special health care needs require emotional, practical, economic, and social support. Encourage parents to obtain help with daily routines. Encourage stress reduction for the parents through exercise and allowing time for themselves. Be a supportive and encouraging listener, and be sure to nurture the whole child, rather than just treating their condition. Refer to Evidence-Based Practice Box 34.1.

Parents may value peer support groups, sometimes feeling that only other parents in similar situations could understand the emotions they experience (Foster et al., 2022). Pediatric nurses should be proactive in helping families find support systems.

Each parent may react differently. It is important for nurses to involve each parent in the child's care. Teach skills to each parent, and actively involve both parents by asking about their observations and opinions.

Parents become the experts on their child's needs and care, and they should be recognized as such. Parents want to be taken seriously and do not like being ignored. They should be viewed as having reliable and valuable information about their children. By being an active and reflective listener, the nurse can demonstrate to the parents that their opinion is valued, in addition to finding out what the child really needs. Some parents may hesitate to volunteer information, unsure about what information the nurse needs. Show respect for the parents' knowledge of their child's needs by seeking advice on the child's daily care, medical and physical needs, and current developmental level, no matter what the site of care is (Foster et al., 2022).

Families may need additional support from the nurse at times of transition. As the equipment or treatment needs change, adjust the teaching plan. Educate the child and family about the use of adaptive equipment.

EVIDENCE-BASED PRACTICE **34.1**

Caring for Children With Technology Needs at Home

STUDY

Caring for a child who has technology needs at home can be an overwhelming task for parents. A qualitative descriptive study examined parents' perceptions of what was most helpful versus what wasn't in providing this care. A convenience sample of 103 participants was utilized.

Findings

Items identified as helpful included emotional support from partners, other family members, and nurses; positive thoughts; hope; self-care; respite care; and work flexibility.

NURSING IMPLICATIONS

Provide emotional support to families caring for children with technology needs at home. Encourage parents to incorporate positivity and self-care into their daily routines. Assist families with obtaining resources for respite care.

Data from Toly, V. B., Blanchette, J. E., & Musil, C. M. (2019). Mothers caring for technology-dependent children at home: What is most helpful and least helpful? *Applied Nursing Research, 46*, 24–27. https://doi.org/10.1016/j.apnr.2019.02.001

Ensure families understand how specific activities must be modified to accommodate the child's needs. Provide anticipatory guidance related to expected developmental changes, including resources and laws related to education. Act as a liaison between the family and the day care center or school. As the child grows and matures, encourage parents to relinquish caregiving tasks to the child as appropriate to encourage independence and promote self-esteem.

Assisting the Adolescent With Special Health Care Needs Making the Transition to Adulthood

Adolescence is a time of physical changes, psychosocial challenges, and initiation of independence from parents. The adolescent with a chronic illness or one who has technology needs may experience this period differently from others. Puberty can be affected by chronic illness, either delaying it or expediting it. Chronic illness may lead to isolation from peers at a time when peer interaction is the core of psychosocial development. Adolescents may struggle to fit in with their peers by hiding their illness or health care needs, not adhering well to treatment regimens, or participating in risky behaviors. At a time when the child should be developing independence from the parents, they may be experiencing significant dependence related to their health condition. For these reasons, the adolescent with special health care needs may require increased amounts of support from the nurse.

Making the transition to adult care for a child with special health care needs can be difficult, and advance planning leads to a smoother transition. Transition planning involves multidisciplinary care coordination; acknowledgment of the changing roles among the adolescent, family, and health care professionals; and fostering of the adolescent's self-determination skills. A written plan for transition to adult care should be initiated in midadolescence. Have ongoing conversations with the adolescent about this transition. Issues to be resolved prior to the transition include financial resources for medical care, college or vocational school attendance, living arrangements, and caregiving arrangements (Ellison et al., 2022).

Recommendations for successful transition include:

- At age 12 to 14 years, ensure that the adolescent is aware of the facility's transition policy, and continue to reinforce at visits.
- Track the adolescent's transition progress via a registry.
- Plan for transition services with the adolescent and family, including health care goals, emergency planning, and legal changes.
- With the adolescent and family, identify an adult provider.
- Complete a full transition plan/packet (Ellison et al., 2022).

Before moving to adult care with an adult medical provider, ensure that the adolescent understands the treatment rationale, symptoms of worsening condition, and especially danger signs. Teach the adolescent about when to seek help from a health professional. Introduce the adolescent to the medical insurance process. At transition, coordinate a seamless transfer by providing a detailed written plan to the care coordinator or advanced practice nurse after verbal collaboration. After the transition, serve as a consultant to the adult office in relation to the adolescent's needs. Consult with a transition services coordinator or other service agency as available in the local community. See the Healthy People 2030 box.

HEALTHY PEOPLE **2030**

Objective	Nursing Significance
Increase the proportion of youth (ages 12–17) with or without special health care needs, who receive services to support their transition to adult health care.	• In the primary care setting, assist families with planning for transition beginning in early adolescence. • If available, refer families to multidisciplinary programs for children with medically complex needs.

Healthy People Objectives retrieved from http://www.healthypeople.gov

THE CHILD WHO IS DYING

Each year, the death rate for children 1 to 14 years of age is 17.2 per 100,000 children (Kaiser Family Foundation [KFF], 2023a). The death rate for infants is much higher, at 5.4 per 1,000 live births (KFF, 2023b). A child's chronic illness may progress to the point of becoming a **terminal illness**, one deemed to be noncurable, ultimately leading to death. Despite the increased survival rates for children with cancer as a result of improved treatment options and protocols, cancer remains the leading cause of death from disease in all children older than 1 year (CDC, n.d.). Less frequently, other diseases also lead to terminal illness in children, such as congenital defects and cardiovascular and neurologic disorders (Adistie et al., 2020). Pediatric nurses will inevitably encounter situations in which a child dies. These situations are extremely difficult for all people involved, and the nurse plays a key role in caring for the dying child and their family. Caring for the child who is dying is a family-centered, multidisciplinary process. Nurses must respond to the child's and family's physiologic, emotional, and spiritual needs during this difficult time. Children display differing responses to the dying process and impending death, depending on their developmental level. Children and their families need significant amounts of support throughout the process of dying.

End-of-Life Decision Making

Parents are obligated not only to protect their children from harm but also to do as much good for them as possible, from both an ethical and a legal standpoint. When the time comes for end-of-life decision making, parents are often torn about the "right" course of action. Parents may be asked to make decisions about stopping treatment, withdrawing treatment, providing palliative care, or consenting to "do not resuscitate" (DNR) orders. Children, parents, and health care providers are generally in agreement that continued suffering is not desired for any child with a terminal illness. When all possible curative attempts have been made, then survival is no longer possible (Shaw et al., 2021).

Nurses involved in this process must examine their own values related to dying and consider the American Nurses Association's *Code of Ethics for Nurses* (2015) as well. The family's feelings must also be acknowledged. During the process of end-of-life decision making, health care providers must assure families that the focus of care is changing and that the child is not being abandoned. Emphasize to parents that no matter what their decision is, the health care team is dedicated to the comfort and expert care of their child (Stokes, 2021).

Ensure communication is family-centered. Quality of life must be taken into consideration when making decisions to continue or withhold treatment. Provide parents facing end-of-life decisions with honest information and education from the time of the diagnosis and prognosis forward. Anticipate that parents may vacillate in the decision-making process. Clarify information for them and allow them private time to discuss the options. Do not make judgments about or question the parents' decision. Be sensitive to any ethnic, spiritual, or cultural preferences during the terminal stage of the illness. Encourage parents to interact with other parents who have a child with a terminal illness (Cacciatore et al., 2019).

Allowing Natural Death

The decision to institute a DNR order is one of the most difficult decisions a family may make. DNR refers to withholding cardiopulmonary resuscitation should the child's heart stop beating. Parents may initially feel like this means they are giving up on their child. Nurses must educate families that resuscitation may be inappropriate and lead to more suffering than if death were allowed to occur naturally. The parents need to understand that when a **palliative care** (specialized care for a serious or terminal illness) route is chosen, rather than continuing a curative or treatment route, the focus of the child's care is changing, but the child and family are not being abandoned. Families may wish to specify a certain extent of resuscitation that they feel more comfortable with (e.g., allowing supplemental oxygen but not providing chest compressions). Some institutions are now replacing the DNR terminology with "allow natural death" (AND), which may be more acceptable to families facing the decision to withhold resuscitation.

Involving the Child Who Is Dying in the Decision-Making Process

End-of-life decision making often involves ethical dilemmas for the child, family, and health care team. This is particularly true when the parents' wishes conflict with the child's or adolescent's desires. Children should be involved in decision making to the extent that they are able. Discuss intervention within the context of the child's condition and wishes. Children of sufficient maturity may assent to the continuation or withdrawal of treatment (National Association of Pediatric Nurse Practitioners et al., 2020). Be available to the older child or adolescent to provide support and information if they desire. Talk with the child or adolescent with the parents present, as well as in private. Maintain the child's comfort and dignity. Encourage the child to spend time with other children with a terminal illness. Assure the child that everything will be done to make them comfortable. Consult parents about the timing and depth of end-of-life discussions. Just as parents do, the child with a terminal illness may vacillate in the decision-making process. Remain sensitive and respect the child's decisions.

Organ or Tissue Donation

With large numbers of organ transplant candidates on waiting lists and the shortage of viable organs, pediatric organ and tissue donation is a priority (Vyas & Nakagawa, 2023). For many families, knowing that a child's organs or tissues may save another child's life provides a way to help others despite their own loss. A healthy child who dies unexpectedly is a good candidate for organ donation. Many chronic illnesses in children preclude the option of organ or tissue donation, although individual determinations of eligibility should be made.

The discussion of organ donation should be separated from the discussion of impending death or brain death notification. Written consent is necessary for organ donation, so the family must be appropriately informed and educated. Many families who never thought about it before may consider the option of donation if adequately educated about the process. All expenses for organ procurement are borne by the recipient's family, not the donor's. Ask whether the child who is dying ever expressed a wish to donate organs and whether the parents have considered it.

Families need to know that procurement of the organs does not mar the child's appearance, so an open casket at the child's funeral is still possible if the family desires. The donating child will not suffer further because of organ donation. The organs or tissues will be harvested in a timely fashion after the declaration of death, so the family need not worry about delay of end-of-life rituals. The family's cultural and religious beliefs must be considered, and the team discussing organ donation with the family must do so in a sensitive and ethical manner (Vyas & Nakagawa, 2023).

Palliative Care of the Child Who Is Dying

Appropriate palliative care is essential for any child with a life-threatening or progressive incurable condition (Hauer, 2023). Whether palliative care is provided in the home, hospital, or hospice setting, the goal is to provide the best quality of life possible at the end of life while alleviating physical, psychological, emotional, and spiritual suffering (Hauer, 2023). Palliative care of children should be based on the following principles:

- Respect for the child's goals, preferences, and choices
- Acknowledgment and addressing of caregiver's concerns
- Provision of a comprehensive, interdisciplinary continuum of care in the community
- Competent and ethical care

Hospice Care

Hospice allows for family-centered care in the child's home or a hospice facility. As with adult hospice care, the comfort of the entire family is important. The goal of pediatric hospice care is enhancement of quality of life for the child and family through an individualized plan of care. The recommended standards for pediatric hospice care allow for palliative care to be given concurrently with potentially curative treatments, and thus hope is not lessened (Hauer, 2023). Parents are educated on ways to comfort and interact with their dying child, such as massage, movement, or singing. Spiritual support is available through a chaplain, a social worker, or the family's minister. The nurse not only educates the family about the dying process but also assists them with providing basic care and pain management. The decision to withhold nutrition or hydration may be made in certain instances. Anticipating and preventing symptoms, including pain, while managing them if they do occur is of the utmost importance (Hauer, 2023). Ongoing bereavement care is also provided to the family by the hospice after the child's death.

Nursing Management of the Child Who Is Dying

Although interdisciplinary care is essential for quality care at the end of life, it is the nurse who plays the key role of child/family advocate and who is usually the constant presence throughout the dying process. Nursing management of the child who is dying focuses on managing pain and discomfort, providing nutrition, providing emotional support to the child and family, and assisting the family through the grief process. Throughout the process, it is important to focus on the family as the unit of care.

Managing Pain and Discomfort

Pain management is an essential component of care for the child with a terminal illness. Adequately managing pain may enhance the child's quality of life and minimize suffering. Assess pain using a developmentally appropriate tool (see Chapter 36 for further information). Provide pain medication around the clock rather than on an as-needed basis to prevent recurrence or escalation of pain. Determine the child's preferred comfort measures and use them to provide additional relief. Change the child's position frequently but gently to minimize discomfort. Limit nursing care to comfort measures that ease the child's discomfort. Maintain a calm environment, minimizing noise and light. Include integrative care interventions such as massage or healing touch as requested and tolerated.

Providing Nutrition

Since the body naturally requires less nutrition as the child is dying, do not excessively coax the child to eat or drink. Offer frequent small meals or snacks of the child's choosing. Soups and shakes require less energy to eat and so may be desirable. If the child desires a different food, provide that one. Keep strong odors away from the child to decrease nausea. Administer antiemetics as needed. Provide mouth care and keep the lips lubricated to keep the mouth feeling clean and prevent the discomfort associated with chapped lips. Make sure the environment is a pleasant one for eating.

Providing Emotional Support to the Child and Family

Be attuned to the entire family's needs and emotions in order to foster a holistic connection with the child and family. Nurses provide physical care through specific tasks and interventions for the child who is dying, but they also need to be fully present emotionally with the child and family. Many people are uncomfortable with the concept of a dying child. Nurses should work through their own feelings about the situation in order to stay fully present with the child and family, attending to their individualized needs. Families and children who are dying benefit from the presence of the nurse, not just the interventions they perform.

Ask yourself what you need to do in order to be fully present with the child and family. Listen to the child and family; be still and silent for a time to accomplish this. Foster respect for the whole child by attending to them as such (Broden et al., 2020).

Respect the parents by helping them honor the commitments they have made to their child. Acknowledge that parents have diverse needs for information and participation in decision making. Allow and encourage family customs or rituals in relation to death and dying. Families may want a faith leader to be present when the child's death is imminent. Certain rituals may be desired, depending on the family's religious or spiritual background. Ensure that these important events occur, and alter nursing care routines as needed to accommodate them. Respect the family's need to participate in these rituals and customs (Hauer, 2023).

Work collaboratively with the family and health care team to provide for the needs of the child and family. Resources for these families are listed in Box 34.5. The Make-a-Wish Foundation works to grant the wishes of children who are terminally ill, giving the child and family an experience of hope, strength, and love.

EASING ANXIETY OR FEARS

Parents may be afraid about the child dying alone or not know what to expect in the death process. This fear may contribute to increased anxiety, which the child may sense. Younger children may fear separation from their parents, and older children may not want to die alone or experience pain or discomfort associated with dying. Each child and family is individual; discuss their particular fears and anxieties in order to determine the child's and family's needs for education and support (Hauer, 2023).

Involve the parents and other family members in all phases of the child's care. Explain all aspects of care to the child to minimize anxiety related to nursing interventions. Answer the child's questions honestly. Involve the child in decision making whenever possible. Limit interventions to those related to palliation, rather than treatment, advocating for the child as needed. Remain with the child when a parent or family member is not in the room, so the child will not fear dying alone.

BOX 34.5 Resources for Families of a Dying Child

Websites

- Project Joy and Hope: www.joyandhope.org
- Children's Hospice International: www.chionline.org
- Compassionate Friends: www.compassionatefriends.org

Books

- *Gentle Willow: A Story for Children About Dying* by Joyce Mills
- *35 Ways to Help a Grieving Child* by the Dougy Center for Grieving Children
- *Sad Isn't Bad* by Michaeline Mundy
- *A Child Asks … What Does Dying Mean?* by Lake Pylant Monhollon
- *Talking with Children and Young People About Death and Dying: A Workbook* by Mary Turner
- *The Worst Loss: How Families Heal from the Death of a Child* by Barbara Rosof
- *I Have No Intention of Saying Goodbye: Parents Share Their Stories of Hope and Healing After a Child's Death* by Sandy Fox
- *Stars in the Deepest Night: After the Death of a Child* by Genesse Gentry
- *The Bereaved Parent* by Harriet Schiff
- *You Are Special* by Max Lucado

MEETING THE CHILD'S NEEDS ACCORDING TO DEVELOPMENTAL STAGE

It is important to provide the type of support and education that the child who is dying needs according to their developmental stage. For the infant, unconditional love and trust are of utmost importance. Ensure that the infant's family is available to the child. The toddler, 1 to 3 years old, thrives on familiarity and routine. Maximize the toddler's time with parents, be consistent, provide favorite toys, and ensure physical comfort. Spirituality in the preschool years focuses on the concept of right versus wrong. The 3- to 5-year-old may see death as punishment for wrongdoing; correct this misunderstanding. Use honest and precise language (Hauer, 2023). Help the parents teach the child that although the family will miss the child, it will continue to function without them.

The school-age child has a concrete understanding of death. Children who are 5 to 10 years old need specific, honest details as desired. Encourage the child to help make decisions and help the child establish a sense of control (Hauer, 2023). The young adolescent (10 to 14 years old) will benefit from reinforcement of self-esteem, self-respect, and a sense of worth. Respect the child's need for privacy and time alone as well as time requested with peers. Support the need for independence and encourage the child to participate in decision making. The older adolescent (14 to 18 years of age) has a more adult-like understanding of death and will need further support through honest, detailed explanations and will want to feel truly involved and listened to. They may also benefit from group activities away from family and unrelated to their medical diagnosis (Hauer, 2023).

Assisting the Family Through the Grief Process

The family may experience anticipatory grief when the diagnosis of a terminal illness is made. Family members may deny the prognosis, become angry at the health care system or a higher power, or experience depression. Acute grief is an intense process that occurs around the time of the actual death. Family members may feel short of breath or as though the throat is tight. They may verbalize that the situation is unreal to them or search for reasons why death was not prevented. Families may also display hostility or restlessness. Each individual will express grief in their own manner. Mourning the death of a loved one takes a long time, and families should be supported throughout the process (Broden et al., 2020). Local and national resources are available for grieving parents. Refer parents to bereavement resources as appropriate.

KEY CONCEPTS

- Children with special health care needs are those who have or who are at risk for a chronic physical, developmental, behavioral, or emotional condition that generally requires more intensive and diverse health services, as well as coordination of those services, than do other children.
- Most children with chronic illnesses or who are dependent on technology progress through stages of growth and development just as healthy children do, although possibly at a slower pace.
- Parents of children with special needs experience a multitude of emotions and changes in their lives, often carrying a heavy caregiving burden. They become the experts on their child's care and should be empowered and supported in their efforts.
- The child with special health care needs and their family may require additional support during times of transition, such as at initial diagnosis or change in prognosis, when symptoms increase, when the child moves to a new setting (hospital, school), during periods of developmental change, or during a parent's absence.
- Children with special health care needs and their families are at increased risk for the development of vulnerable child syndrome, which may have psychologically harmful effects on the child and family for many years.
- Home is the most developmentally appropriate environment for children with special health care needs. Children display an improved physical, emotional, psychological, and social status when they are cared for at home.
- Family-centered care provides the optimal framework for caring for children with special health care needs and their families. Empowering the family strengthens them. A medical home or a permanent relationship with the health care provider or nurse practitioner benefits the family as care coordination and advocacy are provided.
- Use adjusted or corrected age when assessing growth and development of the infant or child who was born prematurely. Provide early screening and intervention for issues related to development to maximize the former premature infant's potential for growth and development.
- Become familiar with the risks and benefits of adjuvant therapies used by some families of children with special health care needs.
- Screen children with special health care needs for undernutrition or a feeding disorder.
- Screening helps identify children with unmet health needs so that intervention may begin.
- Early intervention provides care coordination (developmental services and special education), as well as an individualized family service plan for qualifying children and their families.
- Each student with special health care needs is entitled to an IEP, which is a written plan that is designed to meet the preschool, primary, or secondary school student's needs.
- Early discharge planning and ongoing inclusion and education of the family facilitate continuity of care. During midadolescence, initiate a written plan to help the child make the transition to adult care.
- Support the child who is dying and their family throughout the end-of-life decision-making process, providing facts as desired about palliative care, hospice, and organ donation.
- Younger children who are dying generally need their families to be close and to trust their needs will be provided for. Older children require honest explanations given at a level appropriate for the child's age or developmental stage.

REFERENCES AND RECOMMENDED READINGS

Abdi, F. M., Seok, D., & Murphey, D. (2020). *Children with special health care needs face challenges accessing information, support, and services*. Child Trends. https://cms.childtrends.org/wp-content/uploads/2020/02/CYSHCN-Brief_ChildTrends_February2020.pdf

Adistie, F., Lumbantobing, V. B. M., & Maryam, N. N. A. (2020). The needs of children with terminal illness: A qualitative study. *Child Care in Practice*, *26*(3), 257–271. https://doi.org/10.1080/13575279.2018.1555136

American Academy of Child and Adolescent Psychiatry. (2023). *Chronic illness and children*. https://www.aacap.org/AACAP/Families_and_Youth/Facts_for_Families/FFF-Guide/The-Child-With-A-Long-Term-Illness-019.aspx

American Hippotherapy Association. (2022). *FAQs for families*. https://www.americanhippotherapyassociation.org/frequently-asked-questions

American Music Therapy Association. (2023). *What is music therapy?* https://www.musictherapy.org/about/musictherapy/

American Nurses Association. (2015). *Code of ethics for nurses with interpretive statements (view only for members and non-members)*. https://www.nursingworld.org/practice-policy/nursing-excellence/ethics/code-of-ethics-for-nurses/coe-view-only/

Bally, J., Smith, N., Holtslander, L., Duncan, V., Hodgson-Viden, H., Mpofu, C., & Zimmer, M. (2018). A metasynthesis: Uncovering what is known about the experiences of families with children who have life-limiting and life-threatening illnesses. *Journal of Pediatric Nursing*, *38*, 88–98. https://doi.org/10.1016/j.pedn.2017.11.004

Bamberger, J. M., Nelson, C. S., & Westry, M. F. G. (2022). Management of nutritional disorders. In T. Kyle (Ed.), *Primary care pediatrics for the nursing practitioner* (p. 419-456). Springer.

Blanco, M. A., Lilly, C. M., Bavinger, B. C., Garcia, S., & Hojnicki, M. P. (2021). Caring for medically complex children in the outpatient setting. *Advances in Pediatrics*, *68*, 89–102. https://doi.org/10.1016/j.yapd.2021.05.012

Brenner, M., Alexander, D., Quirke, M. B., Eustace-Cook, J., Leroy, P., Berry, J., Healy, M., Doyle, C., & Masterson, K. (2021). A systematic concept analysis of 'technology dependent': Challenging the terminology. *European Journal of Pediatrics*, *180*(1), 1–12. https://doi.org/10.1007/s00431-020-03737-x

Broden, E. G., Deatrick, J., Ulrich, C., & Curley, M. A. Q. (2020). Defining a "good death" in the pediatric intensive care unit. *American Journal of Critical Care*, *29*(2), 111–121. https://doi.org/10.4037/ajcc2020466

Cacciatore, J., Thieleman, K., Lieber, A. S., Blood, C., & Goldman, R. (2019). The long road to farewell: The needs of families with dying children. *Omega: Journal of Death & Dying*, *78*(4), 404–420. https://doi.org/10.1177/0030222817697418

Centers for Disease Control and Prevention. (n.d.). *WISQARS leading causes of death visualization tool*. https://wisqars.cdc.gov/data/lcd/home

Centers for Disease Control and Prevention. (2022). *What is "early intervention"?* https://www.cdc.gov/ncbddd/actearly/parents/states.html

Centers for Medicare and Medicaid Services. (n.d.). *Children's health insurance program (CHIP)*. https://www.medicaid.gov/chip/index.html

Cincinnati Children's Hospital Medical Center. (2023). *Ongoing support resources*. https://www.cincinnatichildrens.org/patients/child/special-needs

de Leon Siantz, M. L., Kilanowski, J. F., & Thomas, T. L. (2018). Cultural values, beliefs, and preference are integral to family-centered care. In C. L. Betz, M. J. Krajicek, & M. Craft-Rosenberg (Eds.), *Guidelines for nursing excellence in the care of children, youth, and families* (2nd ed., pp. 57-75). Springer Publishing Company.

Duryea, T. K. (2023). Poor weight gain in children younger than two years in resource-abundant settings: Management. *UpToDate*. Retrieved on November 5, 2023, from https://www.uptodate.com/contents/poor-weight-gain-in-children-younger-than-two-years-in-resource-abundant-countries-management

Ellison, J. L., Brown, R. E., & Ameringer, S. (2022). Parents' experiences with health care transition of their adolescents and young adults with medically complex conditions: A scoping review. *Journal of Pediatric Nursing*, *66*, 70–78. https://doi.org/10.1016/j.pedn.2022.04.018

Foster, C. C., Shaunfield, S., Black, L. E., Labellarte, P. Z., & Davis, M. M. (2022). Improving support for care at home: Parental needs and preferences when caring for children with medical complexity. *Journal of Pediatric Health Care*, *36*(2), 154–164. https://doi.org/10.1016/j.pedhc.2020.08.005

Genik, L. M., McMurty, M., Marshall, S., Rapoport, A., & Stinson, J. (2020). Massage therapy for symptom reduction and improved quality of life in children with cancer in palliative care: A pilot study. *Complementary Therapies in Medicine*, *48*, 102263. https://doi.org/10.1016/j.ctim.2019.102263

Hauer, J. (2023). Pediatric palliative care. *UpToDate*. Retrieved on November 5, 2023, from https://www.uptodate.com/contents/pediatric-palliative-care

Kaiser Family Foundation. (2023a). *Rate of child deaths (1-14) per 100,000 children*. https://www.kff.org/other/state-indicator/child-death-rate/?currentTimeframe=0&sortModel=%7B%22colId%22:%22Location%22,%22sort%22:%22asc%22%7D

Kaiser Family Foundation. (2023b). *Total infant deaths*. https://www.kff.org/other/state-indicator/infant-death-rate/?dataView=1¤tTimeframe=0&sortModel=%7B%22colId%22:%22Location%22,%22sort%22:%22asc%22%7D

Kuo, D. Z., & Turchi, R. M. (2023). Children and youth with special health care needs. *UpToDate*. Retrieved on November 5, 2023, from https://www.uptodate.com/contents/children-and-youth-with-special-health-care-needs

Lummer-Aikey, S., & Goldstein, S. (2021). Sibling adjustment to childhood chronic illness: An integrative review. *Journal of Family Nursing*, *27*(2), 136–153. https://doi.org/10.1177/1074840720977177

Mandy, G. T. (2023). Overview of the long-term complications of preterm birth. *UpToDate*. Retrieved on December 29, 2023, from https://www.uptodate.com/contents/overview-of-the-long-term-complications-of-preterm-birth

Maternal and Child Health Bureau. (2023). *Children with special health care needs*. Health Resources and Services Administration. https://mchb.hrsa.gov/maternal-child-health-topics/children-and-youth-special-health-needs

Mitchell, T. K., Bray, L., Blake, L., Dickinson, A., & Carter, B. (2022). 'I feel like my house was taken away from me': Parents' experiences of having home adaptations for their medically complex, technology-dependent child. *Health and Social Care in the Community*, *30*(6), e4639–e4651. https://doi.org/10.1111/hsc.13870

National Association of Pediatric Nurse Practitioners, Research Committee, Ordway, M. R., Bahorski, J., Spratling, R., Sonney, J. T., & Danford, C. A. (2020). NAPNAP position statement on protection of children involved in research studies. *Journal of Pediatric Health Care, 34*(5), 510–513. https://doi.org/10.1016/j.pedhc.2020.04.012

National Resource Center for Patient/Family-Centered Medical Home. (2020). *Implementing medical homes for children and youth with special health care needs (CYSHCN) within Medicaid managed care*. National Academy for State Health Policy. https://downloads.aap.org/MedHome/pdf/Medical%20Home%20CYSHCN%20Fact%20Sheet5.pdf

Population Reference Bureau. (2023). *Summary: Impacts of special health care needs on children and families*. https://www.kidsdata.org/topic/15/impacts-of-special-health-care-needs-on-children-and-families/summary

Schmitz, K. (2019). Vulnerable child syndrome. *Pediatrics in Review, 40*(6), 313–315. https://doi.org/10.1542/pir.2017-0243

Sewell-Roberts, C. (2021). *Caring for siblings of kids with disabilities*. https://kidshealth.org/en/parents/siblings-special-needs.html

Seymour, K. (2021). *Supporting healthy brain development in children through nutrition*. https://ks.childcareaware.org/supporting-healthy-brain-development-in-children-through-nutrition/

Shaw, T., Winegard, B., & Timmons, Z. (2021). Determining futility—One free-standing children's hospital's experience with a policy. *Pediatrics, 147*(3_MeetingAbstract), 525–527. https://doi.org/10.1542/peds.147.3MA5.525

Smith, V. C., & Stewart, J. (2023). Discharge planning for high-risk newborns. *UpToDate*. Retrieved on November 5, 2023, from https://www.uptodate.com/contents/discharge-planning-for-high-risk-newborns

Social Security Administration. (n.d.-a). *Supplemental security income (SSI) for children*. https://www.ssa.gov/ssi/text-child-ussi.htm

Social Security Administration. (n.d.-b). *Title V—Maternal and child health services block grant*. https://www.ssa.gov/OP_Home/ssact/title05/0500.htm

Stewart, J. (2023). Care of the neonatal intensive care unit graduate. *UpToDate*. Retrieved on November 5, 2023, from https://www.uptodate.com/contents/care-of-the-neonatal-intensive-care-unit-graduate

Stokes, L. (2021). ANA position statement: Nursing care and do-not-resuscitate (DNR) decisions. *The Online Journal of Issues in Nursing, 26*(1). https://doi.org/10.3912/OJIN.Vol26No01PoSCol02

The Warren Center. (2023). *Corrected (adjusted) age for preemies*. https://thewarrencenter.org/help-information/premature-birth/corrected-adjusted-age-for-preemies/

Toly, V. B., Blanchette, J. E., & Musil, C. M. (2019). Mothers caring for technology-dependent children at home: What is most helpful and least helpful? *Applied Nursing Research, 46*, 24–27. https://doi.org/10.1016/j.apnr.2019.02.001

U.S. Department of Education. (n.d.). *IDEA*. https://sites.ed.gov/idea/

U.S. Department of Health and Human Services. (n.d.). *Healthy people 2030*. https://health.gov/healthypeople

Verbeek, I. N. E., van Onzenoort-Bokken, L., Hermanus, S., & Zegers, J. (2021). Vulnerable child syndrome in everyday paediatric practice: A condition deserving attention and new perspective. *Acta Paediatrica, 110*(2), 397–399. https://doi.org./10.1111/apa.15505

Vyas, H., & Nakagawa, T. A. (2023). Management of the potential pediatric organ donor following neurologic death. *UpToDate*. Retrieved on November 5, 2023, from https://www.uptodate.com/contents/management-of-the-potential-pediatric-organ-donor

DEVELOPING CLINICAL JUDGMENT

PRACTICING FOR NCLEX

1. The parents of a 5-year-old with special health care needs talk to the parents of a 10-year-old with a similar condition for quite a while each day. What is the nurse's interpretation of this behavior?
   a. The nurse has not provided enough emotional support for the parents.
   b. This relationship between the two families is potentially unhealthy.
   c. Support between families of children with special health care needs is extremely valuable.
   d. Confidentiality is a pressing issue in this particular situation.
2. The nurse is caring for a child who has received all possible medical care for cancer yet continues to experience relapse and metastasis. It is time to make the transition from curative care attempts to palliative care. What is the most important nursing consideration at this time?
   a. The health care professionals should make the decision about the child's care.
   b. The family may lose a sense of hope, so cancer treatments should continue.
   c. Involve the family in the decision-making process about the shift to palliative care.
   d. Palliative care can take place only at home, so the child should be discharged.
3. The nurse is caring for a 3-year-old with a gastrostomy tube and tracheostomy who is on supplemental oxygen and multiple medications. The parent is rooming in during this hospitalization. What is the priority nursing action?
   a. Incorporate the parent's assistance in care when convenient.
   b. Recognize the parent as the expert on the child's needs and care.
   c. Recommend that the parent go home to get some rest.
   d. Provide family-centered care since the parent is there.
4. The nurse is caring for a child with a developmental disability who is starting kindergarten this year. The parent is tearful and doesn't want the child to go to school. What is the best response by the nurse?
   a. "Do you need some time alone to collect yourself?"
   b. "You've known for a while this time would come."
   c. "Can I call your partner or a friend for you?"
   d. "It is normal to feel stressed or sad at this time."
5. The parents of a child with a developmental disability ask the nurse for advice about disciplining their child. What is the best response by the nurse?
   a. "You should choose methods that are most congruent with your values about discipline."
   b. "Children like this really can't follow directions, so they may be hard to discipline."
   c. "Punish your child only for socially unacceptable or offending behaviors."
   d. "Spanking works well for this type of child, as they really don't like pain."

CRITICAL THINKING EXERCISES

1. A 15-year-old is dying of cancer after all medical care options have been exhausted. Describe the plan of care for this child and family. What strategies should the nurse use to support the child and family through this difficult process?
2. A 5-month-old infant who was born at 24 weeks' gestation is ready to be discharged from the NICU. The infant will be going home on oxygen, gastrostomy tube feedings, and eight medications. Develop a teaching plan for the family.

STUDY ACTIVITIES

1. In the clinical setting, care for a child with a terminal illness. Reflect in your clinical journal about the feelings you had during the care of the child as well as the feelings and behaviors that you noticed in the child, siblings, parents, and nursing staff.
2. Visit a preschool that provides care for both children who have developmental delays and children developing as expected. Choose two same-age children, one with a disability and the other without. Perform a developmental screening on each of the two children. Compare your findings.
3. Spend the day with a home care nurse providing care for a child with technology needs. What obstacles has the family overcome to have this child at home? What adjustments does the nurse make to provide family-centered care in the home (as compared to the hospital setting)?

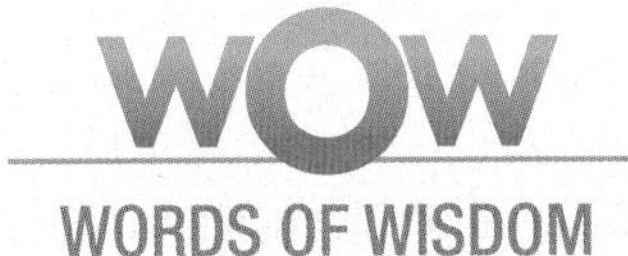

WORDS OF WISDOM

Quality technical skills delivered by a caring hand are a vital part of good nursing care.

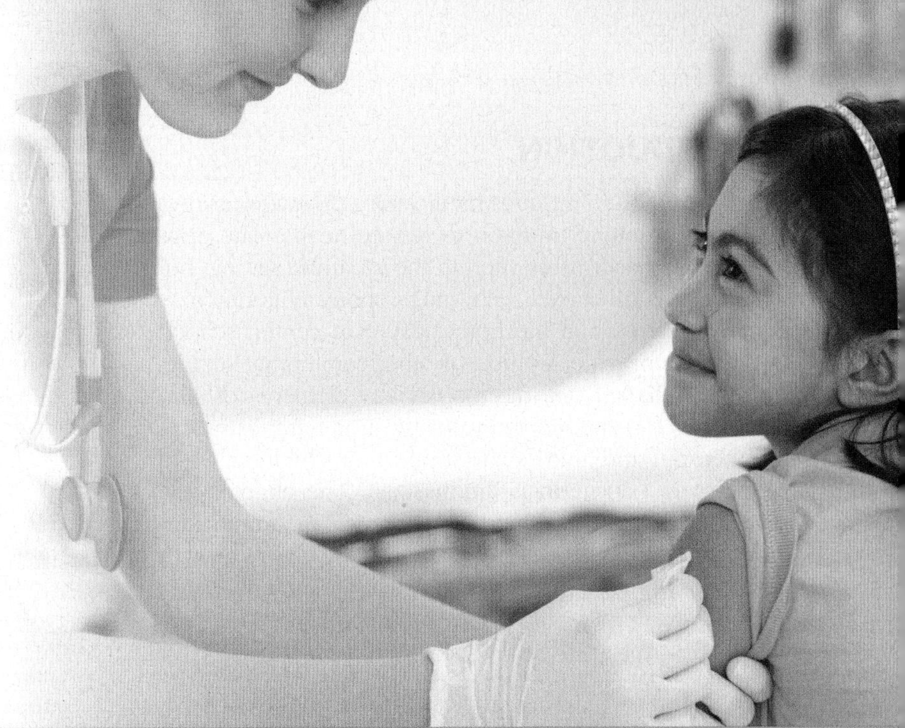

35

Key Pediatric Nursing Interventions

KEY TERMS

bolus feeding

enteral nutrition (en´tĕr-ăl nū-trish´ŭn)

gastric residual

gastrostomy (gas-tros´tŏ-mē)

gavage feedings (gă-vahzh´ fēd´ingz)

infiltration

parenteral nutrition (pă-ren´tĕr-ăl nū-trish´ŭn)

pharmacodynamics (fahr´mă-kō-dī-nam´iks)

pharmacokinetics (fahr´mă-kō-ki-net´iks)

total parenteral nutrition

LEARNING OBJECTIVES

Upon completion of the chapter, you will be able to:

1. Describe the "rights" of pediatric medication administration.
2. Explain the physiologic differences in children affecting a medication's pharmacodynamic and pharmacokinetic properties.
3. Accurately determine recommended pediatric medication doses.
4. Explain the proper technique for administering medication to children via the oral, rectal, ophthalmic, otic, intravenous, intramuscular, and subcutaneous routes.
5. Discuss atraumatic approaches to care in medication administration in children.
6. Identify the preferred sites for peripheral and central intravenous medication administration.
7. Describe nursing management related to maintenance of intravenous infusions and prevention of complications in children.
8. Explain nursing care related to enteral tube feedings.
9. Describe nursing management of the child receiving total parenteral nutrition.

Lily Kline, a 9-month-old, is admitted to your unit for malnutrition. The health care provider has ordered insertion of a nasogastric tube to begin gavage feedings. The parents are nervous and upset about this. They ask, "What will this tube do for Lily? It sounds uncomfortable. What do you have to do to insert it? Will it have to stay in all the time? Won't it move?" How would you address their concerns?

INTRODUCTION

The ill child often requires medications, intravenous (IV) therapy, or enteral nutrition to restore health. These interventions occur most often in the inpatient setting, but with today's advanced technology, many children may receive treatment in the home, day care center, school, health care provider's office, or other community setting.

This chapter will discuss the key elements of, and guidelines for, care related to medication administration, IV therapy, and nutritional support in children. Child and parent education is emphasized. The chapter will focus on adapting and modifying medication administration and nursing procedures based on the child's growth and development and providing these treatments using a family-centered, atraumatic approach. Refer back to Chapter 30 for an overview of the important aspects of caring for a child who is to undergo a procedure.

MEDICATION ADMINISTRATION

At one time or another, every child will need to receive medication. As with adults, pediatric medication administration is a critical component of safe and effective nursing care. The pediatric nurse must adapt administration principles and techniques to meet the child's needs. Medication administration, regardless of the route, requires a solid knowledge base about the drug and its action. As with medication administration to any person, the nurse must adhere to the "rights" of medication administration (Box 35.1). These rights were developed to ensure patient safety by decreasing the occurrence of medication errors. Some experts have added additional rights, such as right documentation, right to be educated, right to refuse, right approach, and right form. These additional rights are important to consider to increase patient safety and satisfaction.

BOX 35.1 Rights of Pediatric Medication Administration

Right Patient

- Confirm child identity by two ways. Children may deny their identity in an attempt to avoid an unpleasant situation, play in another child's bed, or remove ID bracelet.
- Confirm identity each time medication is given.
- Verify child's name with caregiver to provide additional verification.
- Use technology when available (i.e., bar code systems).

Right Medication

- Check order and expiration dates.
- Know action of medication and potential side effects (use pharmacy, drug formulary).
- Ensure that the medication provided is the medication that is ordered.

Right Route of Administration

- Check ordered route and ensure this is the most effective and safest route for this child; clarify any order that is confusing or unclear.
- Give the medication by the route ordered. If there is a need to change route, always check with prescriber (e.g., if a child is vomiting and has an order for an oral medication, the medication may need to be given via the IV or rectal route).

Right Time

- Give within 20 to 30 minutes of the ordered time.
- For a medication given on an as-needed (PRN) basis, know when it was last given and how much was given during the past 24 hours.

Right Dose

- Calculate the recommended dose according to child's weight, and double-check your calculations.
- Always question the pharmacist and/or prescriber if the ordered dose falls outside the recommended dose range.
- Unusually large or small volumes or dosages should always be verified.

Differences in Pharmacodynamics and Pharmacokinetics

Although a drug's mechanism of action is the same in any individual, the physiologic immaturity of some body systems in a child can affect a drug's **pharmacodynamics** (behavior of the medication at the cellular level). As a result, the body may not respond to the drug as intended. The intended effect may be enhanced or diminished, necessitating a change in the dosage to ensure optimal effectiveness without increasing the child's risk for toxicity.

The child's age, weight, body surface area (BSA), and body composition can also affect the drug's **pharmacokinetics** (movement of drugs throughout the body via absorption, distribution, metabolism, and excretion). Drugs are administered to children via many of the same routes that are used for adults. However, this similarity ends once the drug is administered. During the absorption process, drugs move from the administration site into the bloodstream. In infants and young children, the absorption of orally administered medications is affected by slower gastric emptying, increased intestinal motility, a proportionately larger small intestine surface area, higher gastric pH, and decreased lipase and amylase secretion compared with adults. Intramuscular (IM) absorption in infants and young children is affected by the amount of muscle mass, muscle tone and perfusion, and vasomotor instability. Similarly, decreased perfusion alters subcutaneous (SQ) absorption. Absorption by these routes is erratic and may be decreased. In contrast, topical absorption of medications is increased in infants and young children, which can result in adverse effects not seen in adults. Infants and young children have a greater BSA, leading to increased absorption of topical medications. Absorption in infants is also increased due to greater permeability of the infant's skin.

The distribution (movement of a drug from the blood to interstitial spaces and then into cells) of medications is also altered in infants and young children. Medication distribution in children is affected by the following:

- Higher percentage of body water than adults
- More rapid extracellular fluid exchange
- Decreased body fat
- Liver immaturity, altering first-pass elimination
- Decreased amounts of plasma proteins available for drug binding
- Immature blood–brain barrier, especially in neonates, allowing permeation by certain medications

Metabolism of medications in children is altered because of differences in hepatic enzyme production and the child's increased metabolic rate. Biotransformation (the alteration of chemical structures from their original form, which allows for the eventual excretion of the substance) is affected by the same variations affecting distribution in children. In addition, the immaturity of the kidneys until the age of 1 to 2 years affects renal blood flow, glomerular filtration, and active tubular secretion. This results in a longer half-life and increases the potential for toxicity of drugs primarily excreted by the kidneys.

Developmental Issues and Concerns

Children are constantly growing and developing. The specific psychosocial, cognitive, physical, and motor developmental levels of children are important. Nurses need a solid understanding of growth and development to ensure safe administration of medications to children. Table 35.1 details some growth and development issues related to administering medications to children. Always give developmentally appropriate, truthful explanations before administering medications to children, including:

- Why the drug is needed
- What the child will experience
- What is expected of the child
- How the parents can participate and support their child

Refer to Chapters 25 to 29 for further information about growth and developmental issues.

The child's past experiences with taking medications and the approaches that may have been used will often affect how the child reacts. Always approach children positively; let your manner convey the belief that they can accomplish this needed behavior. Never label the child as "bad" if they did not fully cooperate in taking medication. When medications must be administered with a needle (intramuscularly or subcutaneously), assure the child that this method is not a consequence of the child's behavior. Help parents to work through the feelings of frustration that may result from the child's

TABLE 35.1 • Growth and Development Issues Related to Pediatric Medication Administration

Stage of Development	Issue/Concern	Nursing Interventions
Infant	Development of trust, which is fostered by consistent care; development of stranger anxiety later in infancy	Involve parents in medication administration to reduce stress for infant. Ensure that parents hold and comfort infant during intervention.
Toddler	Development of autonomy with displays of negativism; rituals, routines, and choices necessary to maintain some sense of control	Follow routines and rituals from home in giving medications if these are safe and positive approaches. Involve parents in medication administration. Offer simple choices (e.g., "Do you want Mom or me to give you your medicine?"). Allow child to touch or handle equipment as appropriate.
Preschooler	Development of initiative, which is fostered when they sense they are helping	Provide an opportunity to play with the equipment and respond positively to explanations and comforting. Provide choices that are possible, and keep them simple (e.g., "Do you want juice or water with your medication?" or "Which medication do you want to take first?"). Do not ask, "Will you take your medicine now?" Involve parents in medication administration. Be aware that giving suppositories is particularly upsetting to this age group because of their fears of bodily intrusion and mutilation.
School-age child	Development of industry, benefiting from being a part of their care; generally cooperative	Explain to child in simple terms the purpose of the medication. Seek their assistance, such as putting pills in cup or opening the packet, and allow a broader range of choices. Establish a reward system to enhance their cooperation, if necessary.
Adolescent	Development of identity, benefiting from much more control over their care	Approach in same manner as adults, with respect and sensitivity to their needs. Maintain the adolescent's privacy as much as possible.

refusal to cooperate with medication administration. Provide parents with facts about growth and developmental issues and children's fears and anxiety related to medication administration. Model alternative ways for the parents to deal with undesirable behavior.

> *TAKE NOTE!*
>
> Always administer medications promptly, assist the child in holding still using a comforting position for the child, and reward positive behavior.

Determination of Correct Dose

Administering the correct dose is a key component of medication administration. Children are more vulnerable to medication errors due to the individual dosing necessary for proper medication administration. Improper dosing is a more common medication error reported in the pediatric population than the adult population (The Joint Commission, 2021). Many drug references list recommended pediatric dosages, and nurses are responsible for checking doses to ensure that they are appropriate for the child. Two common methods for determining pediatric doses are based on the unit of drug per kilogram of body weight or BSA.

Dose Determination by Body Weight

The most common method for calculating pediatric medication doses is based on body weight. The recommended dosage is usually expressed as the amount of drug to be given over a 24-hour period (mg/kg/day) or as a single dose (mg/kg/dose). It is important to differentiate between the 24-hour dosage and the single dose. Use these guidelines to determine the correct dose by body weight:

1. Weigh the child.
2. If the child's weight is in pounds, convert it to kilograms (divide the child's weight in pounds by 2.2).
3. Check a drug reference for the safe dose range (e.g., 10 to 20 mg/kg of body weight).
4. Calculate the low safe dose (Box 35.2).
5. Calculate the high safe dose (Box 35.2).
6. Determine if the dose ordered is within this range.

> *TAKE NOTE!*
>
> Pay close attention to ensure if the safe range dose is for 24 hours (mg/day) or a single dose period (mg/dose).

The pediatric dosage should not exceed the minimum recommended adult dosage. With many medications, once a child or adolescent weighs 40 to 50 kg or greater, the adult dose is frequently prescribed. However, it remains important to always verify that the dose does not exceed the recommended adult dose.

BOX 35.2 Dosage Calculation Using Body Weight

After converting the child's weight in pounds to kilograms and checking the safe dose range:

- Calculate the low safe dose range (e.g., 10 to 20 mg/kg, and the child weighs 30 kg):
  - Set up a proportion using the low safe dose range
    10 mg/1 kg = x mg/30 kg
    Solve for x by cross-multiplying:
    $1 \times x = 10 \times 30$
    $x = 300$ mg
- Calculate the high safe dose range:
  - Set up a proportion using the high safe dose range
    20 mg/1 kg = x mg/30 kg
    Solve for x by cross-multiplying:
    $1 \times x = 20 \times 30$
    $x = 600$ mg
- Compare the safe dose range (for this, e.g., 300 to 600 mg) with the ordered dose. If the dose falls within the range, the dose is safe. If the dose falls outside the range, notify the prescriber.

Dose Determination by BSA

Calculating the dosage based on BSA takes into account the child's metabolic rate and growth. It is commonly used for chemotherapeutic agents. Some recommended medication doses may read "mg/BSA/dose." To determine the dose using BSA, you will need to know the child's height and weight, which will be plotted on a nomogram (Fig. 35.1). A nomogram is a graph divided into three columns: height (left column), surface area (middle column), and weight (right column).

Use these guidelines to determine BSA:

1. Measure the child's height.
2. Determine the child's weight.
3. Using the nomogram, draw a line to connect the height measurement in the left column and the weight measurement in the right column.
4. Determine the point where this line intersects the line in the surface area column. This is the BSA, expressed in meters squared (m^2).

Once you have determined the BSA, use the recommended dosage range to calculate the safe dosage.

> *TAKE NOTE!*
>
> Prior to administration of any medication, wash hands and don gloves if necessary. Adhere to the rights of medication administration.

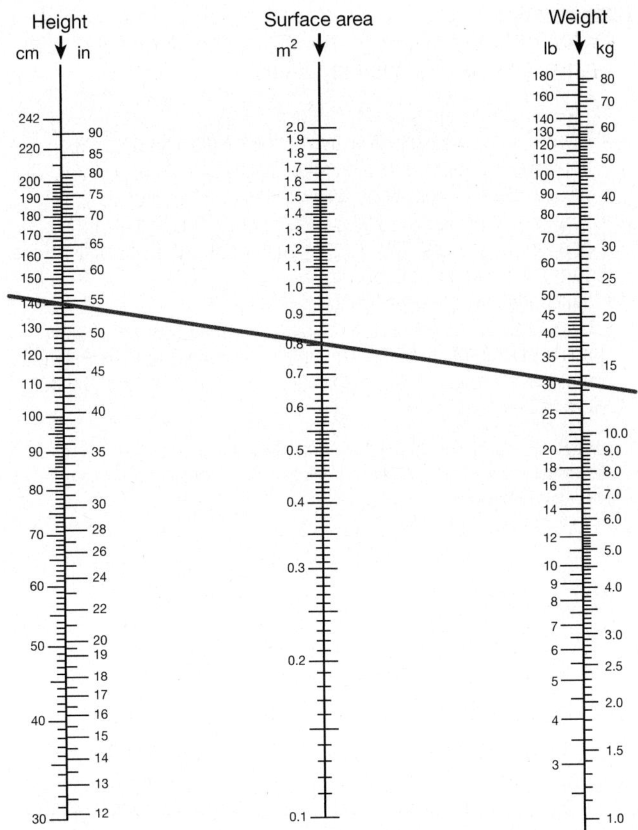

FIGURE 35.1 A nomogram to determine body surface area.

Oral Administration

Medications to be given via the oral route are supplied in many forms, including liquids (elixirs, syrups, or suspensions), powders, tablets, and capsules. Generally, children younger than 5 to 6 years are at risk for aspiration because they have difficulty swallowing tablets or capsules. Therefore, if a tablet or capsule is the only oral form available, it needs to be crushed or opened and mixed with a pleasant-tasting liquid or a small amount (generally no more than a tablespoon) of a nonessential food such as applesauce. However, never crush or open an enteric-coated or time-release tablet or capsule. The crushed tablet or inside of a capsule may taste bitter, so never mix it with formula or other essential foods. Otherwise, the child may associate the bitter taste with the food and later refuse to eat it.

CLINICAL REASONING ALERT!

Certain drug formulations should not be crushed. Before crushing a pill or opening a capsule, always check that this will not alter the intended effects of the drug. Crushing a time-release medication allows immediate absorption of the entire dose of the medication and can have lethal consequences.

Liquid medications, primarily suspensions, may be less concentrated at the top of the bottle than at the bottom of the bottle. Always shake the liquid to ensure even drug distribution. The key to administering liquid forms of oral medications is to use calibrated equipment such as a medicine cup, spoon, plastic oral syringe, or dropper (Fig. 35.2).

TAKE NOTE!

Use the medicine cup or syringe with proper calibration instead of household cups or measuring spoons, since they are not calibrated and may deliver an incorrect dose of medication.

If a dropper is packaged with a certain medication, never use it to administer another medication, since the drop size may vary from one dropper to another. If using a syringe for oral administration, only use the type intended for oral medications, not the one designed for parenteral administration. When using a dropper or oral syringe (without a needle) for infants or young children, direct the liquid toward the posterior side of the mouth. Give the drug slowly in small amounts (0.2 to 0.5 mL), and allow the child to swallow before more medication is placed in the mouth (Fig. 35.3). A nipple without the bottle attached is sometimes used to administer medication to infants. Place the medication directly in the nipple, and keep the nipple filled with medication as the infant sucks so no air is taken in while the infant takes the medication. Always place the infant or young child upright (at least a 45-degree angle) to avoid aspiration. The toddler or young preschooler may enjoy using the oral syringe to squirt the medicine into their own mouth. Older children can take oral medication from a medicine cup or measured medicine spoon.

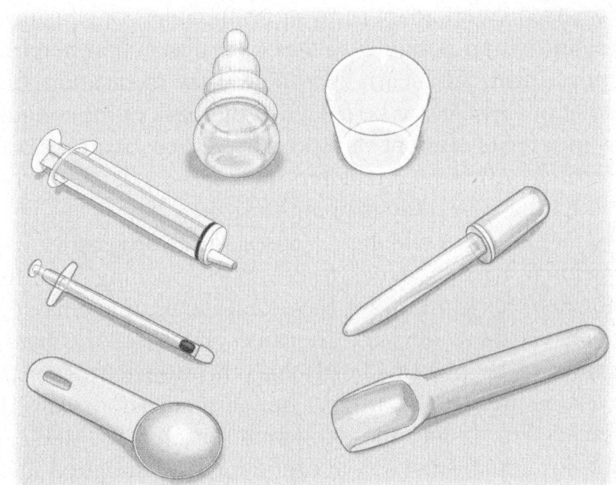

FIGURE 35.2 Devices used to administer oral medications to children.

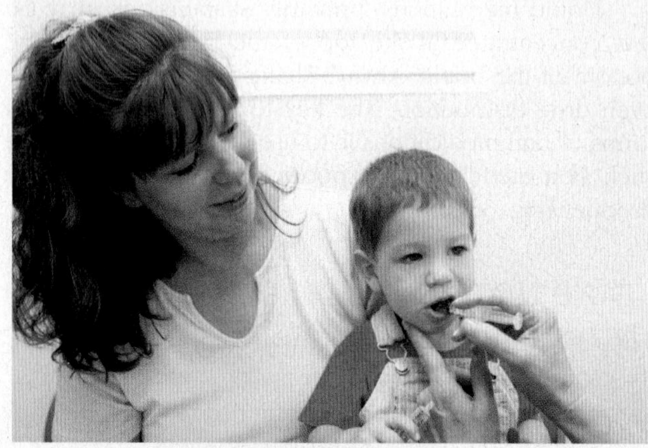

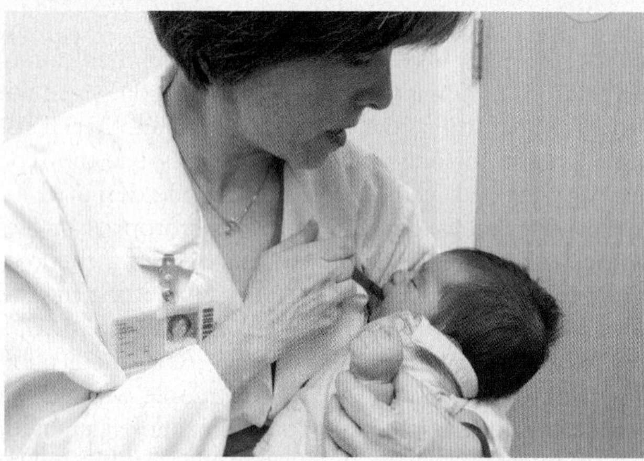

FIGURE 35.3 Position the infant or young child with head elevated for safe medication administration. Holding the child or having a parent hold the child is preferred unless contraindicated.

TAKE NOTE!

Never force an oral medication into a child's mouth or pinch the child's nose. Doing so increases the risk of aspiration and interferes with the development of a trusting relationship.

As children adapt to swallowing tablets or capsules, administration is similar to that of adults. When helping the younger child learn how to swallow medication, the tablet or capsule can be placed at the back of the tongue or in a small amount of food such as ice cream or applesauce. Always tell children if there is medicine in the food; otherwise, they may not trust you.

When the child has a nasogastric, orogastric, nasojejunal, nasoduodenal, **gastrostomy** (opening into the stomach), or jejunostomy tube, oral medications may be given via these devices. The tube allows for the medication to be placed directly into the stomach or small intestine area. Be aware that not all medications can be placed directly into the duodenum or jejunum. Medication for administration via a tube must be supplied in a liquid form, or a crushed tablet or opened capsule can be mixed with a liquid (Box 35.3). Always check tube placement before administering the medication. After administration, flush the tube to maintain patency.

BOX 35.3 Guidelines for Administering Medications via Gastrostomy or Jejunostomy Tubes

Verify correct placement (refer to Box 35.4).

- Give liquid medications directly into the medication port. Draw appropriate amount into syringe and clear air.
- Mix powdered medications well with warm water first.
- If medication is in pill or capsule form, verify it is okay to crush or open. Then, crush tablets or open capsules and mix with warm water to prevent tube occlusion.
- Label each syringe appropriately.
- Give medications one at a time. Flush the tube with water after administering each medication unless contraindicated to ensure that the entire amount of medication has been given and to prevent tube occlusion.

Adapted from Cincinnati Children's Hospital Medical Center. (2022). *Gastrostomy tube (G-tube) home care.* https://www.cincinnatichildrens.org/health/g/g-tube-care

TAKE NOTE!

Parental involvement in medication administration when possible helps decrease stress on the child and provides an opportunity for teaching and evaluating parental techniques.

Rectal Administration

Rectal medications are typically supplied in the form of suppositories. The rectal route is not a preferred route for medication administration in children because the drug's absorption may be erratic and unpredictable, and the method is invasive. The rectal route can be extremely upsetting to the toddler and preschooler because of age-related fears and may be embarrassing to the school-age child or adolescent. However, the rectal route may be used when the child is vomiting or receiving nothing by mouth (NPO). Use age-appropriate explanations and reassurance. Helping the child to maintain the correct position may be necessary to ensure proper insertion and safety of rectal suppositories.

Lubricate the suppository well with a water-soluble lubricant. With the child in the side-lying position, insert the suppository into the rectum quickly but gently. Use a gloved finger or a finger cot to insert the suppository. Insert the suppository above the anal sphincter. For an infant or child younger than 3 years, use the fifth finger for insertion. For an older child, use the index finger. To prevent expulsion of the suppository, hold the buttocks together for several minutes or until the child loses the urge to defecate. If the child has a bowel movement within 10 to 30 minutes after administration of the medication, examine the stool for the presence of the suppository. If it is observed, notify the health care provider or nurse practitioner to determine if the drug needs to be administered again.

Ophthalmic Administration

Ophthalmic medications are typically supplied in the form of drops or ointment. Many children have a fear of having anything placed in their eyes. Therefore, provide an age-appropriate explanation to gain their cooperation. Also, have the child keep their eyes closed until you are ready to administer the medication. Ensure that the medication is at room temperature, as chilled medication may be uncomfortable to the child. Proper positioning of the child is necessary to control the child's head, keep the child's hands from interfering, and prevent injury to the eye. Attempt to administer the medication when the child is not crying to ensure that the medication reaches its intended target area.

Place the child in the supine position, slightly hyperextending the neck with the head lower than the body so the medication will be dispersed over the cornea. Rest the heel of your hand on the child's forehead to stabilize it. Retract the lower eyelid, and place the medication in the conjunctival sac; maintain sterile technique by being careful not to touch the tip of the tube or dropper to the sac. For eye drops, place the prescribed number of drops into the lower conjunctival sac (Fig. 35.4). For ointment, apply the medication in a thin ribbon from the inner canthus outward without touching the eye or eyelashes. If the child is old enough to cooperate, instruct the child to gently close the eyes to allow the medication to be dispersed.

If a child is uncooperative, they may need to be immobilized in order to administer the eye drops. Alternatively, one or two drops on the inner canthus of the closed eye can be administered while the child is lying supine. Then instruct the child to open their eyes, and the drops will enter the eye. Wipe any excess medication from the skin. Punctal occlusion after application is also important to slow systemic absorption and ensure that the medicine stays in the eye.

Children often require ophthalmic medications at home. Parents or caregivers need instruction about how to administer this type of medication. Teaching Guidelines 35.1 provides information on administering eye drops and eye ointments.

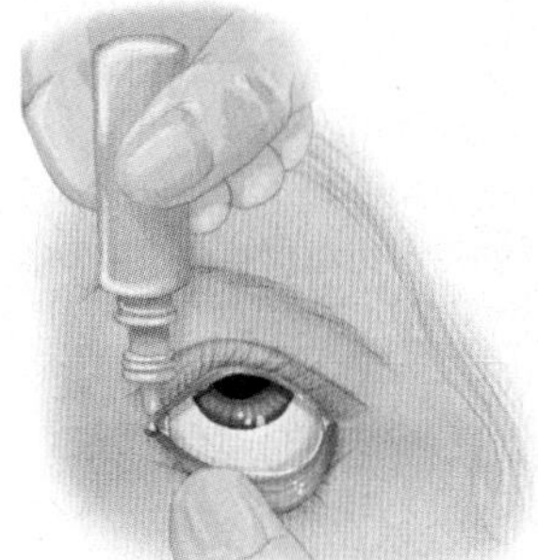

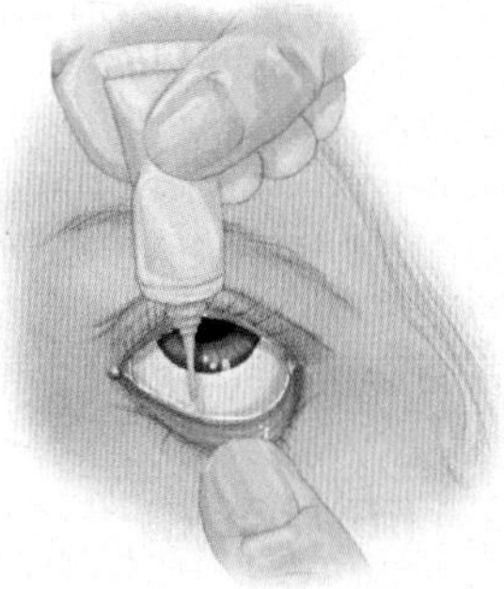

FIGURE 35.4 Administering eye medication: gently press the lower lid down, and have the child look up as the medication is instilled into the lower conjunctival sac.

TEACHING GUIDELINES 35.1 Applying Eye Medications

- Wash your hands with soap and water. Dry them thoroughly using a clean cloth.
- Cleanse the eye. Move from the nose side of the eye outward. Use a clean area of the cloth each time you wipe and a separate cloth for each eye. Use warm water to help clear crusty eye drainage. Wash your hands again.
- Allow the eye drops or ointment to come to room temperature (if the medication was stored in the refrigerator). If necessary, warm the eye drops or ointment tube in the palm of your hand. Keep the cap on to avoid any spillage. Make sure medication is well mixed if needed.
- Remove the cap, placing it on a dry, clean surface.
- For young children (3 years or younger), obtain assistance from an additional adult to keep their arms and fingers away during the procedure. If doing this procedure alone, wrap the child in a towel or blanket, keeping the arms inside.
- Have the child look up and to the other side. The eye drops should flow away from the child's nose.
- Place the wrist of the hand you will be using to give the drops against the child's forehead. With the other hand, gently pull down the lower eyelid. Have the medication about 2.54 cm (1 in) away from the eye.
- Gently squeeze the eye drop bottle, dispensing the proper number of drops away from the tear ducts that are in the inner corner of the eye, or gently squeeze the ointment tube, dispensing a small trail (about 2 cm) of ointment into the gap between the lower portion of the eye and the bottom eyelid. Twist or rotate the tube when you reach the outer eye to help disconnect the ointment from the tube.
- Make sure the tip of the bottle or tube does not make contact with the eye or any other surface.
- For eye drops, gently press your finger against the inside corner where the eye meets the nose for about 1 to 3 minutes, blocking the tears and medication from exiting through the tear duct. This will help the eye retain more of the medication. If the child is old enough, they may be able to do this unassisted.
- For ointment, have the child close their eye and not rub the area.
- Ask the child to close their eyes gently and not to blink or squeeze the eye shut more than normal, as this may wash away the medication prematurely.
- Gently dab away any tears or excess medication on the face with a clean tissue.
- Wash your hands again and dry them thoroughly.

Adapted from Lippincott Williams & Wilkins. (2023). *Lippincott nursing procedures* (9th ed.). Wolters Kluwer.

Otic Administration

Medications for otic administration are typically in the form of ear drops. This route of administration can be upsetting to the child because they cannot see what is happening. The child often receives otic drugs for an earache, and they may fear that the ear drops will increase the pain. Explain the procedure to the younger child in terms that they can understand to help allay these fears. Gain the older child's cooperation by explaining the purpose of the medication and the procedure for administration.

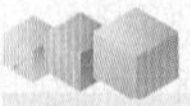

Concept Mastery Alert

Administering Pediatric Ear Drops

When administering pediatric ear drops, pulling the pinna down and back is correct if the child is under 3 years of age. To administer ear drops to a child who is 4 years old, the nurse should pull the pinna up and back.

Reinforce the need for the child to keep the head still. Younger children may require assistance to do so. Be sure that the ear drops are at room temperature. If necessary, roll the container between the palms of your hands to help warm the drops. Using cold ear drops can cause pain and possibly vertigo when they reach the eardrum (Cleveland Clinic, 2023).

Place the child in a supine or side-lying position with the affected ear exposed (Fig. 35.5). Pull the pinna downward and back in children under age 3 and upward and back in older children. Instill the prescribed amount of medication using a dropper, being careful not to contaminate the tip of the dropper. Then, have the child remain in the same position for several minutes to ensure that the medication stays in the ear canal. Soothe, comfort, and distract the child to allow the medication to instill. Massage the area anterior to the affected ear to promote passage of the medication into the ear canal. If necessary, place a piece of cotton or a cotton ball loosely in the ear canal to prevent the medication from leaking.

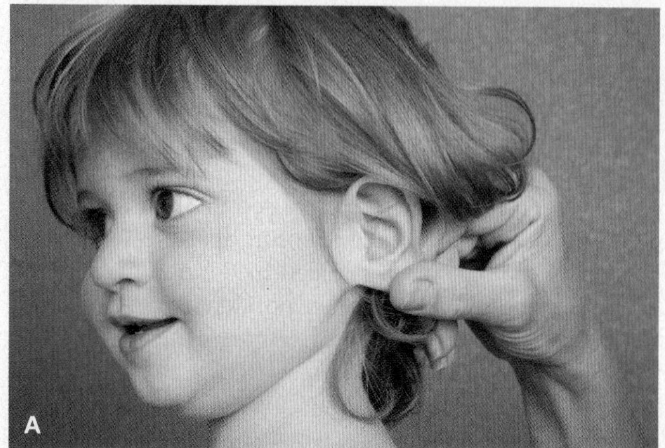

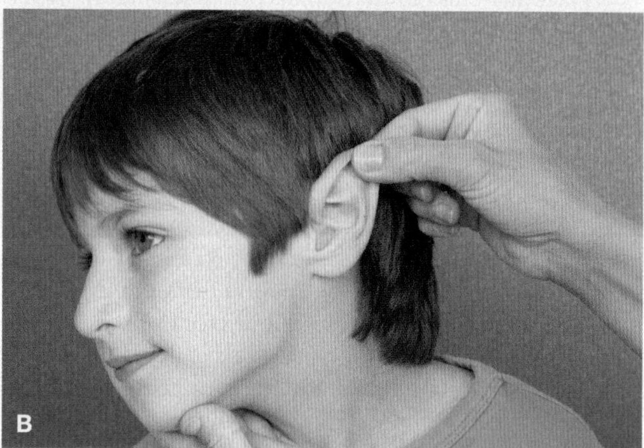

FIGURE 35.5 Administering ear drops. **A.** For the child younger than 3 years, the nurse pulls the pinna of the ear down and back. **B.** For a child older than 3 years, the nurse pulls the pinna of the affected ear up and back.

Nasal Administration

Nasally administered medications are typically drops and sprays. Administering nose drops to infants and young children may be difficult, and additional help may be needed to help maintain the child's position. Ensure medication is at room temperature. Have the child blow their nose or use a bulb syringe to clear nasal passage of secretions. For nose drops, position the child supine with the head hyperextended to ensure that the drops will flow back into the nares. A pillow or folded towel can be used to facilitate this hyperextension. Place the tip of the dropper just at or inside the nasal opening, taking care not to touch the nares with the dropper (Fig. 35.6). Doing so might stimulate the child to sneeze. Although the nasal membranes are not sterile, the drop solution is, and sneezing would contaminate the dropper, leading to contamination of the drop solution when the dropper is returned to the bottle. Once the drops are instilled, maintain the child's head in hyperextension for at least 1 minute to ensure that the drops have come in contact with the nasal membranes.

For nasal sprays, position the child upright with head tilted slightly back, and place the tip of the spray bottle just inside the nasal opening and tilted toward the back. Hold one nostril closed (or have the child do this if appropriate) and instruct the child to take a deep breath through the nostril while the medication is being administered. Squeeze the container, providing just enough force for the spray to be expelled from the container. Using too great a force can push the spray solution and secretions into the sinuses or eustachian tube.

TAKE NOTE!

In young infants, instill the medication in one naris at a time, since they are obligate nose breathers.

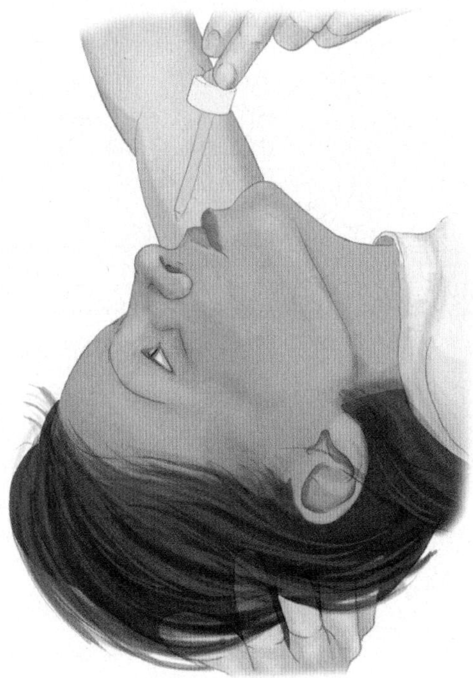

FIGURE 35.6 Administering nose drops. Tilt the head down and back to instill nose drops.

Intramuscular Administration

IM administration delivers medication to the muscle. In children, this method of medication administration is used as infrequently as possible because it is painful, and children often lack adequate muscle mass for medication absorption. However, IM administration is used to administer certain medications, such as many immunizations.

Muscle development and the amount of fluid to be injected determine IM injection sites in children. Needle size (gauge and length) is determined by the size of the muscle and the viscosity of the medication. For example, more viscous medications often require a larger-gauge needle. In addition, the needle must be long enough to ensure that the medication reaches the muscle.

The preferred injection site for infants 12 months or less is the vastus lateralis or anterolateral thigh muscle; in certain circumstances (such as physical obstruction of the anterolateral thigh), the gluteal muscle can be considered (Immunization Action Coalition, 2022; Kroger et al., 2023). In infants and children greater than 12 months, the vastus lateralis or anterolateral thigh muscle remains the preferred site, but the deltoid can be considered if sufficient mass is present (Immunization Action Coalition, 2022; Kroger et al., 2023).

TAKE NOTE!

Many experts no longer recommend use of the dorsogluteal site at any age due to the risk of damaging nerves and vasculature and the possibility of a suboptimal immune response (Drutz, 2023).

The deltoid muscle is used as an IM injection site in children older than 3 years and may be used in toddlers if the muscle mass is sufficient (Immunization Action Coalition, 2022; Kroger et al., 2023). Figure 35.7 illustrates IM injection sites.

Select the needle size and gauge based on the size of the child's muscle. The goal is to use the smallest length and gauge that will deposit the medication in the muscle. Table 35.2 provides general guidelines for solution amount, needle size, and needle gauge when administering IM medications.

Insert the needle into the skin at a 90-degree angle. Aspirating and, if no blood was present, injecting the medication was the traditional procedure. However, recent research has shown decreased discomfort and no associated complications with rapid injection of IM immunizations without aspiration (Centers for Disease Control and Prevention [CDC], 2021). In addition, there are no large blood vessels present in the currently recommended injection sites, the vastus lateralis and deltoid muscles (CDC, 2021). Therefore, the CDC and the Advisory Committee on Immunization Practices (ACIP) no longer recommend aspiration before injection of vaccines (CDC, 2021; Kroger et al., 2023).

Subcutaneous and Intradermal Administration

SQ administration distributes medication into the fatty layers of the body. It is used primarily for insulin administration, heparin, and certain immunizations, such as Measles, Mumps, Rubella (MMR). The amount of SQ tissue differs among individuals. Therefore, when selecting a site and needle size, choose the most appropriate based on adequacy and condition of the SQ tissue and the frequency and duration of the therapy. The preferred sites for SQ administration include the anterior thigh for infants younger than 12 months and the lateral upper triceps area (Kroger et al., 2023). Use a 3/8- or 5/8-in, 23- to 25-gauge needle. With the nondominant hand, pinch up the skin to isolate the tissue from the muscle or pull it taut depending on the amount of adipose tissue present and the length of needle. Insert the needle at a 45- to 90-degree angle, release the skin if pinched, and inject the medication. Remove the needle at the same angle it was inserted.

Intradermal (ID) administration deposits medication just under the epidermis. The forearm is the usual site for administration. ID administration is used primarily for tuberculosis screening and allergy testing. A 1-mL syringe with a 5/8-in, 25- or 27-gauge needle is commonly used to administer the medication. Insert the needle, with the bevel up, beneath the skin at a 5- to 15-degree angle. Keep the fingers and thumb resting on the sides of the syringe to ensure the proper angle.

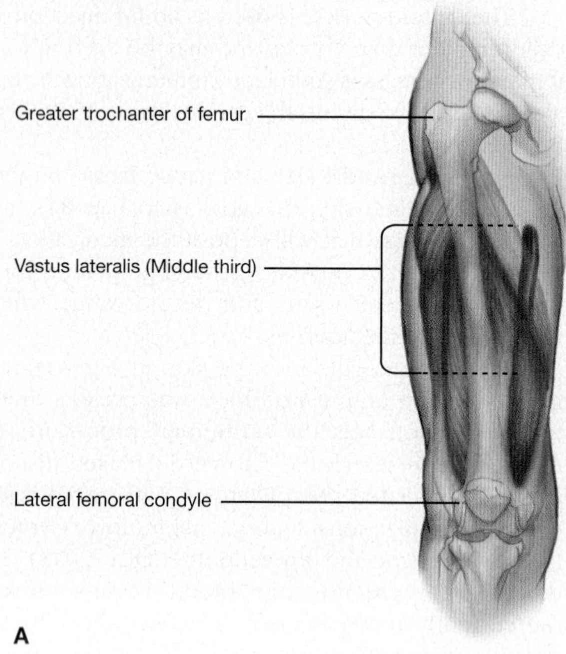

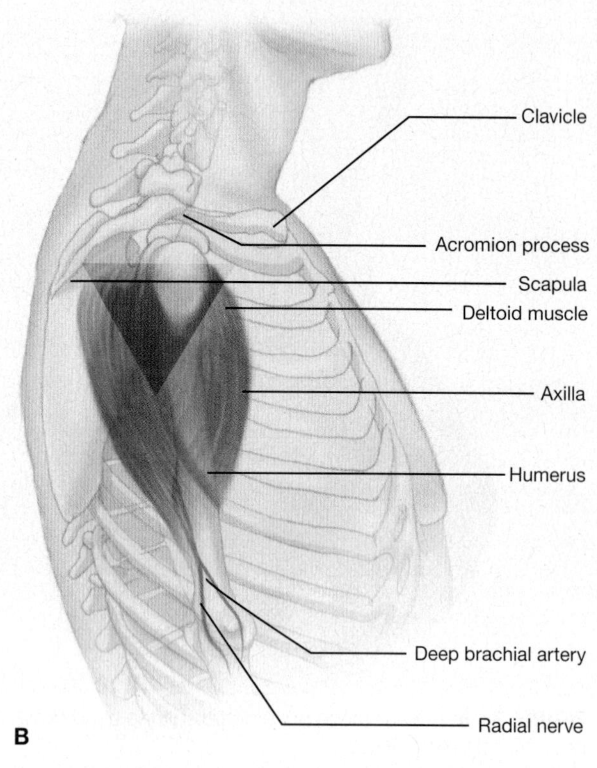

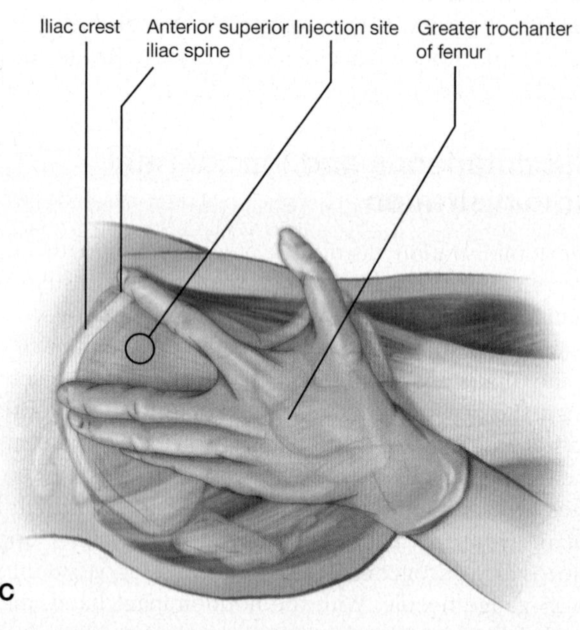

FIGURE 35.7 Locating intramuscular injection sites. **A.** Vastus lateralis: identify the greater trochanter and the lateral femoral condyle; inject in middle third and anterior lateral aspect. **B.** Deltoid: locate the lateral side of the humerus, one to two finger widths below the acromion process. Inject into upper third of muscle. **C.** Ventrogluteal: place palm of left hand on right greater trochanter so index finger points toward anterosuperior iliac spine, spread middle finger to form a V, and inject in the middle of the V.

Intravenous Administration

IV medication administration is commonly used with children, especially when a rapid response to a drug is desired or when absorption via other routes is difficult due to the child's illness or condition. In some cases, the IV route is the only effective method for administering a medication. Use of the IV route requires that the child have an IV device inserted, peripherally or centrally. Although insertion of this device is invasive and traumatic for the child, IV medication administration is considered to be less traumatic when compared to the trauma associated with multiple injections. Unfortunately, the veins of a child are small and easily irritated.

Most medications given by the IV route must be given at a specified rate and diluted properly to prevent overdose or toxicity due to the rapid onset of action that occurs with this route. Therefore, when administering medications via the IV route, knowledge of the drug, the amount of drug to be administered, the minimum dilution of the drug, the type of solution for dilution or infusion, the compatibility of various solutions and medications, the length of time for infusion, and the rate of infusion is required. Careful maintenance of the IV site is required to prevent complications.

TABLE 35.2 • Guidelines for Solution Amount, Needle Length, and Needle Gauge for Intramuscular Injections

	Solution Amount				
	Vastus Lateralis (Anterolateral)	**Deltoid**	**Ventrogluteal**	**Length**	**Gauge**
Infant <12 months old	0.5 mL	Not recommended	Not recommended until 7 months; then 0.5 mL	5/8 to 1 in	22–25
Toddler 12 months to 2 years	0.5–1 mL (preferred site)	0.5 mL	1 mL	5/8 to 1 in	22–25
Preschooler 3–5 years old	1 mL	0.5 mL (preferred site)	1.5 mL	5/8 to 1 in	22–25
School age 6–10 years old	1.5–2 mL	0.5–1 mL (preferred site)	1.5–2 mL	5/8 to 1.25 in	22–25
Late school-age/adolescent (11–18 years old)	Up to 3 mL	1–2 mL (preferred site)	1–5 mL	5/8 to 1.5 in	22–25

Needle size and site need to be individualized based on the size of the muscle, amount of adipose tissue, and amount of solution to be administered.

Data from Kroger, A., Bahta, L., Long, S., & Sanchez, P. (2023). *General best practice guidelines for immunization.* www.cdc.gov/vaccines/hcp/acip-recs/general-recs/downloads/general-recs.pdf; Schneider, M. (2022). *Clinical guidelines (Nursing): Intramuscular injections.* https://www.rch.org.au/rchcpg/hospital_clinical_guideline_index/Intramuscular_Injections/#:~:text=The%20anterolateral%20aspect%20of%20the,anaphylaxis%20management%20in%20all%20ages

The primary method for IV medication administration is a syringe pump. This method provides a highly precise rate of infusion. Nursing Procedure 35.1 outlines the steps for administering medication via a syringe pump.

If a pump is unavailable, the medication may be administered via a volume control device. The medication is added to the device with a specified amount of compatible fluid and then infused at the ordered rate.

Direct IV push medication is typically reserved for emergency situations and when therapeutic blood levels must be reached quickly to achieve the desired effect. Direct IV push administration requires that the drug be diluted appropriately and given at a specified rate, such as over 2 to 3 minutes. Care must be taken to prevent fluid overload, which may occur due to flushing needed to maintain IV patency and prevent drug incompatibilities, and from the administration of multiple drug therapies.

TAKE NOTE!

The use of clinical judgment is necessary when selecting injection or intravenous sites, needle length and gauge, and appropriate infusion devices.

NURSING PROCEDURE 35.1 Administering Medication via a Syringe Pump

Purpose: To provide accurate and safe administration of IV medication

1. Verify the medication order.
2. Gather the medication and necessary equipment and supplies.
3. Wash hands and put on gloves.
4. Attach the syringe pump tubing to the medication syringe, and purge air from the tubing by gently filling the tubing with medication from the syringe.
5. Insert the syringe into the pump according to the manufacturer's directions.
6. Clean the appropriate port on the child's IV access device or tubing, flush the device or tubing if appropriate (e.g., an intermittent infusion device [saline lock or heparin lock]), and attach the syringe tubing to the IV tubing or device.
7. Set the infusion rate on the pump as ordered.
8. When the medication infusion is completed, flush the syringe pump tubing to deliver any medication remaining in the tubing, according to institution protocol.
9. Document the procedure and the child's response to it.

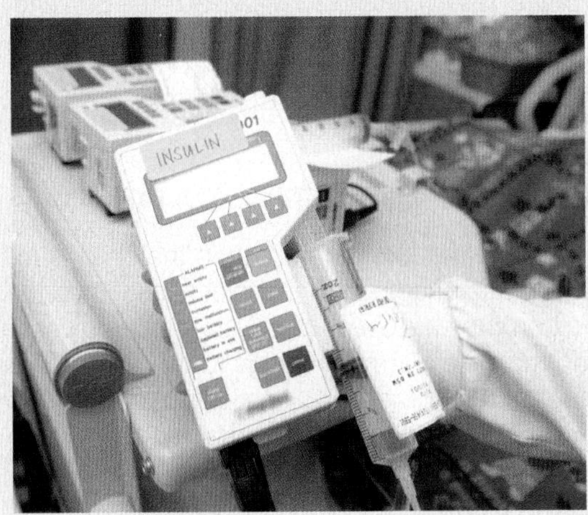

Providing Atraumatic Care

When administering any medication, including oral medications, use the principles of atraumatic care (see Chapter 30 for more information). Children can experience stress and fear or upset when they must take medications. The child may become upset or stressed when they must be secured snugly or positioned to minimize movement. The child may experience further discomfort if the medication has an unpleasant taste or results in pain, such as with an injection.

• • • ATRAUMATIC CARE • • •

Encourage the child to participate in care, and provide the child with developmentally appropriate options, such as which fluid to drink with the medication or which flavor of ice pop to suck on before or after the administration (see Table 35.1).

To decrease discomfort and pain for the child who is to receive an injection, apply a topical anesthetic such as a eutectic mixture of local anesthetic (EMLA) cream or vapocoolant spray to the site before injection when possible (Kroger et al., 2023), and inject the most painful medication last (see Chapter 36 for additional information). Also, utilize developmentally appropriate distraction techniques, such as music, books, blowing bubbles or a pinwheel, and deep breathing exercises (see Chapter 30 for additional information).

Ensuring that the child doesn't move is essential to prevent injury when administering an injection. When administering an injection to a young child, at least two adults should hold the child; this may also be necessary to help an older child to remain still.

TAKE NOTE!

According to research, children experience less pain and decreased fear if they are sitting versus lying down when receiving an injection (CDC, 2021).

• • • ATRAUMATIC CARE • • •

Use positions that are comforting to the child, such as therapeutic hugging, during injections. Have the child sit on the caregiver's lap, with the caregiver holding the child's arms and legs to their body. Refer to Chapter 30, Figure 30.1. After administration, encourage the parents or caregivers to hold and cuddle the child and offer praise.

Educating the Child and Parents

Teaching the child and parents or caregivers about medication administration is key. Many medications are given in the home, making the parents or caregivers responsible for administration. They need to know what medications they are giving and why, how to give them, and what to expect from the drug, including adverse effects. Caregivers and parents often make medication errors at home, such as incorrectly dosing over-the-counter medications and prescription medications or failing to follow or understand medication instructions given, for example, not completing the full course of the medication or missing doses (Lopez-Pineda et al., 2021). Therefore, ensure thorough instruction, including frequency of administration, when the next dose is due, and length of time the medication is to be given. Emphasize the importance of completing the prescribed dose. Demonstrate use with an actual syringe if possible, encourage return demonstration of medication administration, advise against the use of home-measuring devices (such as a spoon), and emphasize the importance of always using the calibrated dispensing device that was given with the medication. If the medication is to be given via injection, parents and caregivers need to learn how to administer the injection properly. Encourage questions or concerns from parents or caregivers.

Parents and caregivers commonly need suggestions about the best ways to administer the medication to their child. Provide them with tips for administration, such as mixing unpleasant-tasting medications with applesauce or yogurt or offering a favorite liquid as a chaser. Also teach the parents how to properly measure the amount of drug to be given. Teaching Guidelines 35.2 gives pointers about oral medication administration. Refer to Chapter 30 for further information on teaching children and families about medication administration.

Preventing Medication Errors

Experts agree that the incidence of potentially harmful medication errors is higher in the pediatric population compared to adults (The Joint Commission, 2021). This can be related to weight-based dosing calculations, fractional dosing, and the need for the use of decimal points. Children are also more susceptible because many drugs used in pediatrics are formulated and packaged for adults and lack U.S. Food and Drug Administration (FDA) approval and dosing guidelines for children. Recent legislative changes have led to a dramatic increase in pediatric drug studies and improvement in accurate pediatric dosing and labeling (FDA, 2023).

The need for safety takes on even greater importance due to the physiologic, psychological, and cognitive differences inherent in children. Children are more vulnerable to medication errors as they vary in weight,

TEACHING GUIDELINES 35.2 Administering Oral Medications

- Be firm when telling your child that it is time for their medication. State, "It's time for your medicine" instead of asking, "Will you take your medicine?" or "Can you take your medicine for me?"
- Allow your child to choose an appropriate liquid to help swallow the medication or drink after taking it. Limit the choices to two or three.
- Never bribe or threaten your child to take their medication.
- Never refer to the medication as "candy."
- Be honest about the taste of the medication. If necessary, mix it with another food such as applesauce, yogurt, or syrup to help mask the taste.
- Do not mix the medication with formula or baby food.
- Always check with your health care provider or nurse practitioner and pharmacy about opening capsules or crushing tablets and mixing them with food. Some medications should not be opened or crushed.
- If you are giving a liquid using an oral syringe or dropper, place the medication slowly along the inside of the cheek. Never squirt the medication forcibly to the back of the child's throat. It may cause the child to gag and spit out the medication or aspirate it into their lungs.
- Always praise the child after taking the medication and provide comfort and cuddling.

BSA, and organ maturity, which affect their ability to metabolize and excrete medications; they depend on others for medication administration; they are often unable to communicate if an adverse reaction is occurring; and they need special compound medication formulations (The Joint Commission, 2023). Confirming the child's identity and double-checking the dosage before administration of any medication are two critical safeguards that play a major role in preventing medication errors. Other ways to prevent medication errors include the following:

- Confirm that the children's weight is accurate.
- Always weigh children in kilograms.
- Double-check medication calculations; utilize another health care provider when possible, especially for high-risk medications.
- If a dose seems unusually small or large, verify the order.
- Utilize medication ordering and dispensing systems, if available.
- Always report medication errors or near-miss errors to help prevent future mistakes.
- Utilize The Joint Commission's official "Do Not Use" list. (The up-to-date list can be found on The Joint Commission's website.)

TAKE NOTE!

If a parent, caregiver, or child questions whether a medication should be given, listen attentively, answer their questions, and double-check the order.

INTRAVENOUS THERAPY

IV access provides a route for the administration of medications and fluids. It is commonly used for children because it is the quickest, and often the most effective, method of administration. As with adults, numerous sites and various devices and equipment may be used to provide IV therapy over a short or long period of time. When administering IV therapy, safety is crucial. The nurse must have a solid knowledge base about the fluids or medications to be given as well as a thorough understanding of the child's physical and emotional development. Venipuncture can be a terrifying and painful experience for children and their families. Nurses play a crucial role in providing support and education to the child and family before, during, and after the procedure (refer to Chapter 30 for additional information related to provision of atraumatic care with procedures).

Sites

IV therapy may be administered via a peripheral vein or a central vein. Peripheral IV therapy sites commonly include the hands, feet, and forearms (Fig. 35.8). In

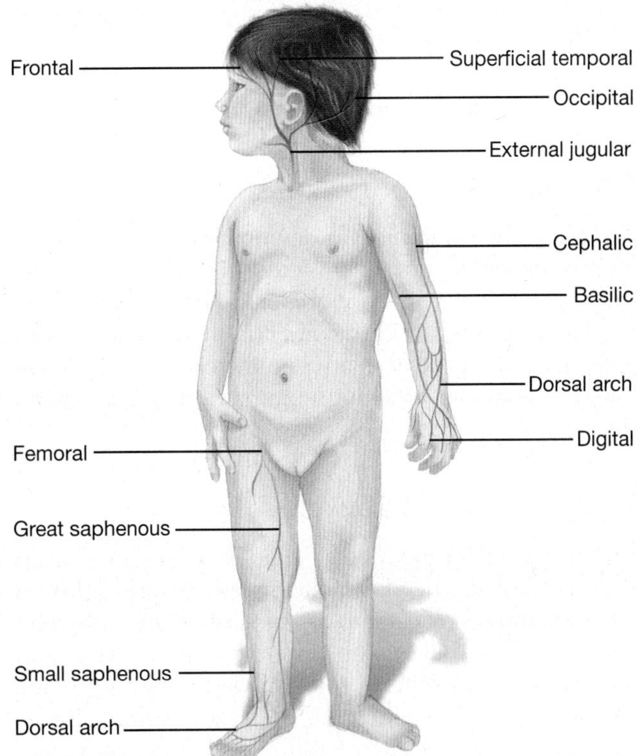

FIGURE 35.8 Preferred peripheral sites for IV insertion.

neonates and young infants, the scalp veins may be used (Doyle et al., 2022). The scalp veins are easily visualized, being covered only by a thin layer of SQ tissue. These veins do not have valves, so the device may be inserted in either direction, although the preference would be in the direction of blood flow. However, use of a scalp vein requires that that area of the infant's head be cleared of hair to enhance visualization. In addition, use of the scalp veins can be frightening to parents, who may think the fluid is infusing into the infant's brain. Thus, scalp veins are usually used only if other sites are assessed to be inferior or attempts at other sites have been unsuccessful (Doyle et al., 2022). When used, ensure appropriate education of the parents prior to insertion, and, if shaving the child's hair is needed, inquire if parents would like to keep the child's hair.

TAKE NOTE!

When selecting an IV site in an extremity, always choose the most distal site. Doing so prevents injury to the veins superior to the site and allows additional access sites should complications develop in the most distal site.

Central IV therapy is usually administered through a large vein, such as the subclavian, femoral, or jugular vein or the vena cava. The tip of the device lies in the superior vena cava just at the entrance to the right atrium. The device is inserted surgically or percutaneously and exits the body typically in the chest area, just below the clavicle. A device can be inserted via a peripheral vein, such as the median, cephalic, or basilic vein, and then threaded into the superior vena cava.

Equipment

The choice of equipment is determined by the solution or medication to be administered, the duration of the therapy, the age and developmental level of the child, the child's status, and the condition of their veins. Various types of IV devices are commercially available. In addition, different types of tubing and infusion control devices may be necessary.

Peripheral Access Devices

Devices used for peripheral venous access in a child include over-the-needle catheters or winged-infusion sets, commonly referred to as "butterflies" or scalp vein needles. These devices are inserted into the vein and then connected to the IV solution via tubing to provide a continuous infusion of fluid. These devices can also be inserted for intermittent use if the child does not require a continuous fluid infusion. Typically, the hub of the device is capped or plugged to allow intermittent access, such as for administering medications or obtaining blood specimens. When used in this manner, these devices are termed peripheral intermittent infusion devices or saline or heparin locks.

Needle size on the device also varies. Typically, the needle ranges from 21- to 25-gauge, depending on the child's size. Use the smallest-gauge catheter with the shortest length possible to prevent traumatizing the child's fragile veins. Typically, peripheral IV devices are used for short-term therapy, usually averaging 3 to 5 days. Midline catheters or peripherally inserted central catheters (PICCs) are also available and recommended for use if therapy is to exceed 7 days (Paterson et al., 2020).

Central Access Devices

Numerous devices for central venous access are available. The type chosen depends on several factors, including the duration of the therapy, the child's diagnosis, the risks to the child from insertion, and the ability of the child and family to care for the device. The device may have one or multiple lumens. Although central venous access devices can be used short term, the majority are used for moderate- to long-term therapy.

Central venous access devices are indicated when the child lacks suitable peripheral access, requires IV fluid or medication for a prolonged period of time, or is to receive specific treatments, such as the administration of highly concentrated solutions or irritating drugs like chemotherapeutic agents, parenteral nutrition, or blood and blood products. Child preference is also a consideration. Central venous access is advantageous because it provides vascular access without the need for multiple IV starts, thus decreasing discomfort and fear. However, central venous access devices are associated with complications such as infection at the site, sepsis due to the direct access to the central circulation, and thrombosis due to partial occlusion of the vessel. Typically, a chest radiograph is performed after a central venous access device is inserted to verify proper placement. No fluids are administered until correct placement is confirmed. Table 35.3 describes the major types of central venous access devices.

Infusion Control Devices

Infants and young children are at increased risk for fluid volume overload compared with adults. Also, malfunction at the IV insertion site, such as infiltration, may result in much greater injury than a similar incident would cause in an adult. Therefore, IV fluids must be carefully administered and monitored. To ensure accurate fluid administration, infusion control devices such as infusion

TABLE 35.3 • Types of Central Venous Access Devices

Device	Description
Peripherally inserted central catheter (PICC)	Short- to moderate-term therapy (few weeks to a few months) Insertion via a peripheral vein such as basilic, cephalic, or brachial vein Catheter typically threaded into superior vena cava; distal tip terminates in the superior vena cava, inferior vena cava, or proximal right atrium Insertion via saphenous vein with tip terminating in inferior vena cava above the diaphragm for infants Single or multiple lumens Can be inserted at the bedside; requires additional training and advanced skill Blood sampling is possible; child can be sent home with the line in place
Nontunneled central venous catheter (CVC)	Usually used short term (1–2 weeks) One or more lumens Percutaneous insertion most commonly via the subclavian, internal jugular, or femoral vein with the tip of the catheter at the top of the superior vena cava just above the right atrium Useful for emergency situations Catheter sutured in place at the exit site Increased rate of central line–associated bloodstream infection than tunneled CVC
Tunneled central venous catheter (e.g., Groshong, Hickman/Broviac)	Usually for long-term use (1–6 months) Catheter inserted by a health care provider via small incision in jugular or subclavian vein and tunneled in the subcutaneous tissue under the skin Initially sutured in place to stabilize position; sutures removed after approximately 1–2 weeks when cuff on catheter attaches to subcutaneous tissue Single or multiple lumens Some have valves that prevent backflow of blood and air entrance Radiologic confirmation of placement needed Blood sampling is possible; child can be sent home with the line in place Requires surgical removal
Implanted ports (e.g., Port-a-Cath, Infuse-a-Port, Mediport)	Long-term use (>3 months to years) Surgically inserted by a health care provider Stainless steel port with a polyurethane or silicone catheter attached Catheter tip lying in subclavian or jugular vein; port implanted under skin in a subcutaneous pocket, usually on the upper chest wall Port covered completely by skin and visible only as a slight bulging on the chest; possibly more appealing to the older child and adolescent because there are no visible parts or dressings Access to port via a specially angled, noncoring needle (Huber needle) Site preparation and pain relief measures necessary before accessing the port Lowest risk for central line–associated bloodstream infection Blood sampling is possible; child can be sent home with the line in place Surgical removal is required

Adapted from Naik, V. M., Mantha, S. S. P., & Rayani, B. K. (2019). Vascular access in children. *Indian Journal of Anaesthesia*, *63*(9), 737–745. https://doi.org/10.4103/ija.IJA_489_19

pumps, syringe pumps, and volume control sets may be used.

Infusion pumps used for children are similar to those used for adults. In addition, syringe pumps are often used to deliver fluid and medications to children. These pumps can be programmed to deliver minute amounts of fluid over controlled periods of time (syringe pumps are discussed further in the next section).

An IV solution bag may be attached to a calibrated volume control set that has been filled with a specified amount of IV solution (Fig. 35.9). The fluid chamber holds a maximum of 100 to 150 mL of fluid that can be infused over a specified period of time as ordered. Usually, a maximum of a 2-hour infusion amount in the chamber avoids accidental fluid overload in the pediatric population. This chamber can be filled every 1 to 2 hours so only small amounts of ordered quantities of fluid can infuse and the child is protected from receiving too much fluid volume. Due to the advances in pump technology and the introduction of "smart pumps," which include dose error reduction systems such as hospital-defined drug libraries (drug lists) with standard drug concentrations, and dose limits to potentially improve the safety of IV medication administration, the use of volume control devices has been reduced or eliminated in many facilities. Concerns include inability to identify the

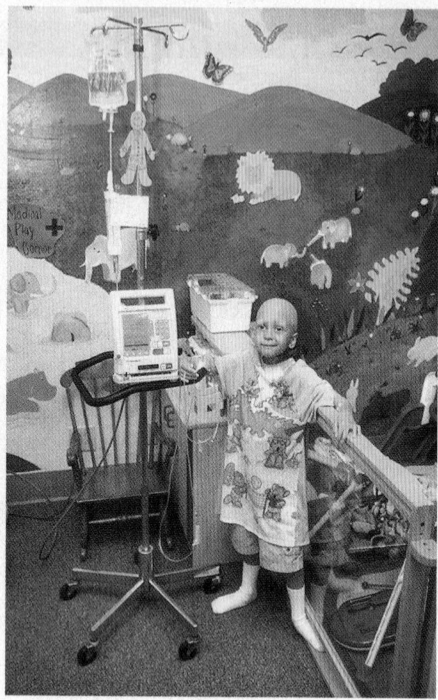

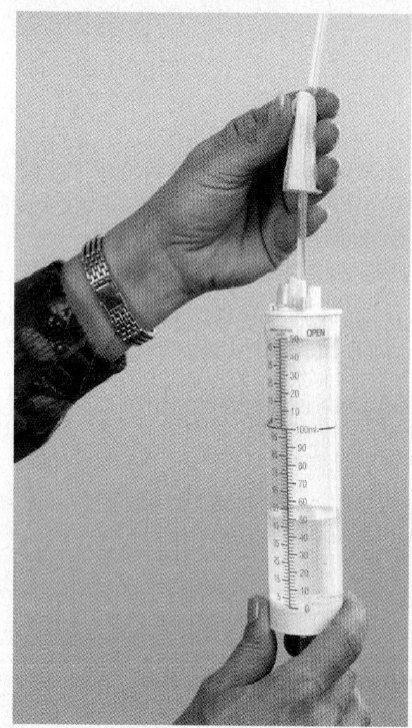

FIGURE 35.9 Volume control infusion device.

medication in the volume control device and the potential for interaction or precipitation that may occur when multiple medications are administered using the same volume control device. However, they are still available as a safety device for controlling the volume of fluid administered to children; therefore, nurses should be familiar with how to use them. Be familiar with your facility's policies and procedures. When using a volume control device, label the chamber when medications are added, and check for incompatibilities and potential interactions when multiple medications are given.

Inserting Peripheral IV Access Devices

Peripheral IV devices are used for most IV therapies. Prior to insertion, review the child's diagnosis and medical history for information that may affect therapy, such as site selection or insertion. For example, a child who has a history of chronic illness may have heightened fears and anxieties related to insertion due to previous experiences or difficulty in accessing IV sites. Typically, the nondominant extremity should be used for insertion, but this may not be possible in certain situations, such as if a right-handed child has a cast on their left arm.

Check the orders for the prescribed therapy. Determine the purpose and length of the IV therapy and the type of fluid or medication that is to be administered. This information aids in selecting the best device and insertion site. For example, the device needs to be of an adequate gauge to allow the solution or medication to infuse into the vein while at the same time allowing enough blood flow around the device to promote dilution of the infusion.

Establish rapport with the child and parents. Inform them about IV therapy and what to expect. Be honest with the child. Explain that the venipuncture will hurt but only for a short time. Provide the child with a time frame that they can understand, such as the time it takes to brush their teeth or eat a snack.

• • • ATRAUMATIC CARE • • •

Use therapeutic play to assist the child in preparing and coping for the procedure (see Chapter 33 for more information).

Insertion of an IV therapy device is traumatic. Follow the principles of atraumatic care, including the following:

- Gather all equipment needed before approaching the child.
- If possible, select a site using hand veins rather than wrist or upper arm veins to reduce the risk of phlebitis. Avoid sites where excessive movement may occur, such as the lower extremity veins and areas of joint flexion, if possible, because these are associated with an increased risk of thrombophlebitis and other complications (Lippincott Williams & Wilkins, 2023).
- Ensure adequate pain relief using pharmacologic and nonpharmacologic methods prior to insertion of the device (see Chapter 36 for more information about management of pain related to procedures).
- Allow the antiseptic used to prepare the site to dry completely before attempting insertion.
- Use a barrier such as gauze or a washcloth or the sleeve of the child's gown under the tourniquet to avoid pinching or damaging the skin.
- If the child's veins are difficult to locate, use a device to transilluminate the vein (utilizes a bright light, which illuminates the vein's size and direction of travel).

- Make only two attempts to gain access; if you are unsuccessful after two attempts, allow another individual two attempts to access a site. If still unsuccessful, evaluate the need for insertion of another device.
- Encourage parental participation as appropriate in helping to position the child or to provide comfort positioning, such as therapeutic hugging.
- Coordinate care with other departments such as the laboratory for blood specimen collection to minimize the number of venipunctures for the child.
- Secure the IV line using a minimal amount of tape or transparent dressing.
- Protect the site from bumping by using a security device such as the IV house dressing (Fig. 35.10).

TAKE NOTE!

Some facilities have policies in place allowing only one stick per nurse, with a maximum of two sticks; then the doctor needs to be notified unless the situation is an emergency.

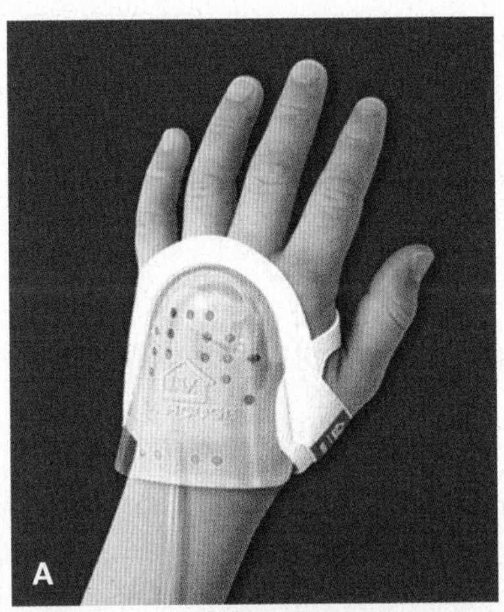

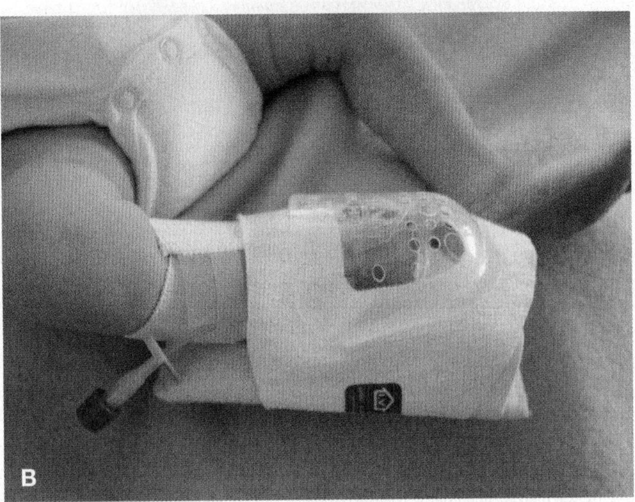

FIGURE 35.10 A. IV house over the IV site on a child's hand. **B.** IV house over the site on an infant's foot.

IV Fluid Administration

Administering IV fluids to an infant or child requires close attention to the child's fluid status. Typically, the amount of fluid to be administered in a day (24 hours) is determined by the child's weight (in kilograms) using the following approach:

- 100 mL/kg of body weight for the first 10 kg
- 50 mL/kg of body weight for the next 10 kg
- 20 mL/kg of body weight for the remainder of body weight in kilograms

Table 35.4 gives examples of calculating a child's fluid requirements using body weight. Once the 24-hour total fluid requirement is determined, this amount is divided by 24 hours to arrive at the correct hourly rate of infusion.

Maintaining IV Fluid Therapy

Throughout the course of therapy, monitor the fluid infusion rate and volume closely, as often as every hour. If a volume control set is used to administer the IV infusion, fill the device with the allotted amount of fluid that the child is to receive in 1 hour. Doing so prevents inadvertent administration of too much fluid. Never assume that just because an infusion pump is in use, the infusion is being administered without problems. Pumps can malfunction. The tubing can become blocked, or the IV device can move out of the vein lumen. Not enough fluid, fluid overload, or infiltration of the solution into the tissues can occur.

In addition to monitoring the fluid infusion, closely monitor the child's output. Expected urine output for children and adolescents is 1 to 2 mL/kg/hour.

TAKE NOTE!

When measuring the output of an infant or child who is not toilet trained or who is incontinent, weigh the diaper to determine the output. Remember that 1 g of weight is equal to 1 mL of fluid.

Flushing the IV line when the device is used intermittently may be necessary to maintain patency, such as before and/or after medication is administered and after obtaining blood specimens. However, there is much debate as to how often flushing should be done and the best flush solution to use, heparin or saline. Saline has been found to be more compatible with the numerous solutions and medications administered intravenously and is less expensive and less irritating to the vein. In addition, using saline lessens the incidence of pain and phlebitis. Heparin is expensive and incompatible with numerous medications and solutions, and it can affect clotting time, depending on the concentration of the flush solution used. However, it has also been found to increase catheter patency and decrease infusion failures. Evidence appears to support the effectiveness of both heparin and normal saline for maintaining

TABLE 35.4 • Intravenous Maintenance Fluid Calculations by Body Weight

<10 kg in weight	100 mL/kg of weight = # mL for 24 hours Example: A child weighs 7.4 kg 7.4 × 100 = 740 mL (daily requirement) 740/24 = 30.8 or 31 mL/hour
11–20 kg in weight	100 mL/kg of weight for the first 10 kg + 50 mL/kg for the next 10 kg = # mL for 24 hours Example: A child weighs 16 kg (10 × 100 = 1,000) plus (6 × 50 = 300) Total = 1,300 mL (daily requirement) 1,300/24 = 54 mL/hour
>20 kg in weight	100 mL/kg for the first 10 kg + 50 mL/kg for the next 10 kg + 20 mL/kg for each kg >20 kg = # mL for 24 hours Example: A child weighs 30 kg (10 × 100 = 1,000) plus (10 × 50 = 500) plus (10 × 20 = 200) Total = 1,700 mL (daily requirement) 1,700/24 = 70.8 or 71 mL/hour

patency of peripheral IV catheters, and which fluid is used will depend on provider and agency preference. The most effective flushing solution may depend on individual factors, such as catheter type, patient condition, and medications being infused. Additional research is needed to determine the best solution, volume and concentration of the flush solution, and interval for flushing. Flushing solutions and procedure will vary; therefore, it is important to always follow your agency's policy or provider order for flushing IV lines. See Evidence-Based Practice 35.1

If the child is receiving IV therapy via a central venous access device, provide site care using sterile technique and flush the device according to agency policy. Note the exit site for the device, and inspect it frequently for signs of infection. If the device has multiple lumens, label each lumen with its use (i.e., blood specimen, medication, or fluid). Always check the compatibilities of solutions and medications being given simultaneously.

TAKE NOTE!

When flushing or administering medications through a PICC line, follow the manufacturer's recommended syringe size, because PICC lines are fragile. Using a larger-volume syringe (i.e., 10 mL or larger) exerts less pressure on the PICC, thereby reducing the risk of rupture (Lippincott Williams & Wilkins, 2023).

Preventing Complications

IV therapy is an invasive procedure that is associated with numerous complications. Strict aseptic technique is necessary when inserting the device and caring for the site.

EVIDENCE-BASED PRACTICE 35.1

Which Is More Effective—Normal Saline or Heparin for Maintaining Patency and Avoiding Complications in Peripheral Intravenous Catheters (PIVC)?

The debate on flushing with heparin or saline has been investigated in a number of research studies for many years, with controversial results. Many differences in the maintenance of PIVCs exist even within the same facilities.

STUDY

A systematic review of research studies involving hospitalized patients with PIVC was performed to evaluate the efficacy of normal saline versus heparin in maintaining patency and preventing complications of peripheral venous catheters.

Findings

The review found that it is not fully documented if normal saline is superior to heparin in maintaining patency and preventing complications. Researchers tend to support the use of normal saline over heparin as it is safer, more compatible with other medications, more efficient, easier to use, and cost effective.

Nursing Implications

The use of normal saline (NS) seems to have more advantages over the use of heparin. These findings cannot be generalized due to the small number of studies. Therefore, further research is warranted. Nurses must be aware of and follow their agency policy and procedures. Nursing care needs to be based on current scientific evidence. Nurses need to continuously question their care practices and review current research and perform research on topics they feel need it.

Data from Sotnikova, C., Fasoi, G., Efstathiou, F., Kaba, E., Bourazani, M., & Kelesi, M. (2020). The efficacy of normal saline (N/S 0.9%) versus heparin solution in maintaining patency of peripheral venous catheter and avoiding complications: A systematic review. *Materia Socio-Medica*, *32*(1), 29–34. https://doi.org/10.5455/msm.2020.32.29-34

Adherence to standard precautions is key. Inspect the insertion site every 1 to 2 hours for inflammation or **infiltration** (inadvertent infusion of a nonirritant solution or medication into the surrounding tissue). Note signs of inflammation such as warmth, redness, induration, or tender skin. Check closely for signs of infiltration such as cool, blanched, or puffy skin. Use of a transparent dressing or IV house dressing provides easy access for assessing the IV insertion site. These types of dressings also help to prevent movement of the catheter hub, thus minimizing the risk of mechanical irritation, dislodgement, and complications such as phlebitis or infection (see Fig. 35.10).

Typically, in adults, an IV site is changed every 72 to 96 hours and at any time when the integrity of the system has been compromised or contamination is suspected (CDC, 2017). Recent clinical trials have suggested that routine replacement of a PIVC does not decrease the risk of infection (Ullman & Chopra, 2022). Current recommendations include replacement in children only when clinically indicated (CDC, 2017; Ullman & Chopra, 2022). Follow the agency's policies and procedures related to site changes. Consider an alternative route for fluid and medication administration or the insertion of an alternative IV device, such as a PICC line. Catheter-related bloodstream infections can often occur with the use of central venous lines. These infections result in increased morbidity, mortality, and health care costs (Haddadin et al., 2022). Prevention is paramount. Nurses need to practice proper hand hygiene, use maximal barrier protection during insertion, assess the site frequently, provide proper site care using strict sterile technique, and ensure that the child's central venous catheter is removed as soon as it is no longer needed. In children, it is also important to prevent the child from touching and playing with the central venous line site or dressing. The CDC and Healthcare Infection Control Practices Advisory Committee (HICPAC) currently recommends changing administration sets that are continuously used no more frequently than every 96 hours but at least every 7 days, except if fluids that increase microbial growth, such as blood, blood products, or parenteral nutrition, have been administered (CDC, 2017; Ullman & Chopra, 2022). In these cases, changing the administration sets every 24 hours is recommended (CDC, 2017; Ullman & Chopra, 2022). Replace administration sets per agency policy. Ensure proper disinfecting of all catheter hubs, needleless connectors, and injection ports before accessing them to minimize contamination.

TAKE NOTE!

Chlorhexidine-impregnated sponge (Biopatch) dressings may be used to help prevent infection in children over 2 months old (Ullman & Chopra, 2022). Always follow agency or institution policy and procedures regarding site care.

Discontinuing the IV Device

Prepare the child for removal of the IV device in much the same manner as for insertion. Many children may fear the removal of the device to the same extent that they feared its insertion. Explain what is to occur, and enlist the child's help in the removal.

• • • ATRAUMATIC CARE • • •

If appropriate, allow the child to assist in removing the tape or dressing. This gives the child a sense of control over the situation and also encourages their cooperation.

In addition, practice atraumatic care by doing the following:

- Use water or adhesive remover to help loosen the tape.
- If a transparent dressing is in place, gently lift off the dressing by pulling up opposite corners using a motion parallel to the skin surface.
- Avoid using scissors to cut the tape, but if cutting the tape is necessary, be sure that the child's fingers are clear of the tape and scissors.
- Turn off the infusion solution and pump.
- Once all tape and dressings are removed, gently slide the IV device out using a motion opposite to that used for the insertion.
- Apply pressure to the site with a dry gauze dressing, and then cover with a small adhesive bandage. If possible, allow the child to choose the bandage.

TAKE NOTE!

If the IV site was in the arm at or near the antecubital space, apply pressure until the bleeding stops. Do not have the child bend their arm after removal of the device as this is not sufficient pressure to prevent hematoma formation.

PROVIDING NUTRITIONAL SUPPORT

Adequate nutrition is important for all individuals but especially for children. During the growing years, the quality of a child's nutrition affects their overall health and development. The presence of a chronic illness, disease, or trauma can increase the child's nutritional demands; if the child cannot meet these even with oral supplementation, other measures may be necessary to provide nutritional support. Such measures may include **enteral nutrition** (delivery of nutrition into the gastrointestinal tract via a tube) and **parenteral nutrition** (IV delivery of nutritional substances). The nutritional plan is determined by the child's age, developmental level, and health status.

Enteral Nutrition

Enteral nutrition, commonly called tube feedings, involves the insertion of a tube so that feedings can be delivered directly into the child's gastrointestinal tract. The tube may be inserted via the nose or mouth or through an opening in the abdominal area, with the tube ending in the stomach or small intestine. Nasogastric or orogastric tube feedings, a tube from the nose to the stomach or from the mouth to the stomach, respectively, are commonly referred to as **gavage feedings**. Nasoduodenal or nasojejunal feedings involve a tube that is inserted through the nose and ends in either the duodenum or the jejunum. Gastrostomy feedings involve the insertion of a gastrostomy tube through an opening in the abdominal wall and into the stomach. Jejunostomy feedings are similar to gastrostomy feedings except that the tube lies in the jejunum.

Enteral nutrition is indicated for children who have a functioning gastrointestinal tract but cannot ingest enough nutrients orally. The child may be unconscious or have a severely debilitating condition that interferes with their ability to consume adequate food and fluids. Other conditions that may warrant the use of enteral nutrition include the following:

- Failure to thrive
- Inability to suck or tiring easily during sucking
- Abnormalities of the throat or esophagus
- Swallowing difficulties or risk of aspiration
- Respiratory distress
- Metabolic conditions
- Severe gastroesophageal reflux disease (GERD)
- Surgery
- Severe trauma

Enteral feedings may be given via nasogastric, orogastric, nasojejunal, nasoduodenal, gastrostomy, or jejunostomy tubes (Fig. 35.11). Table 35.5 provides additional information about these types of feeding tubes. Enteral feedings cost less, are associated with fewer complications, and are considered safer than parenteral feedings. However, tube misplacement is a serious complication.

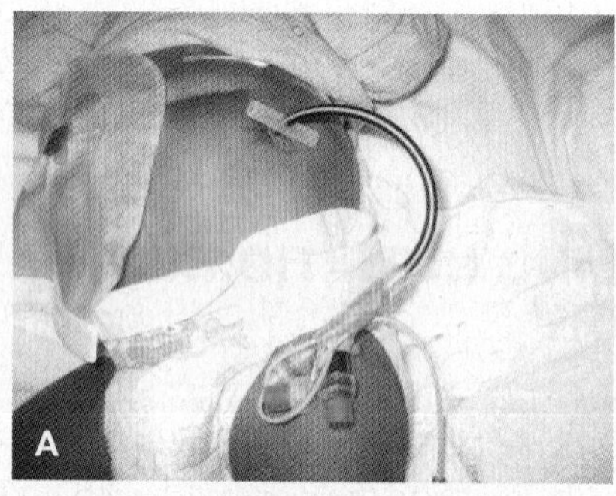

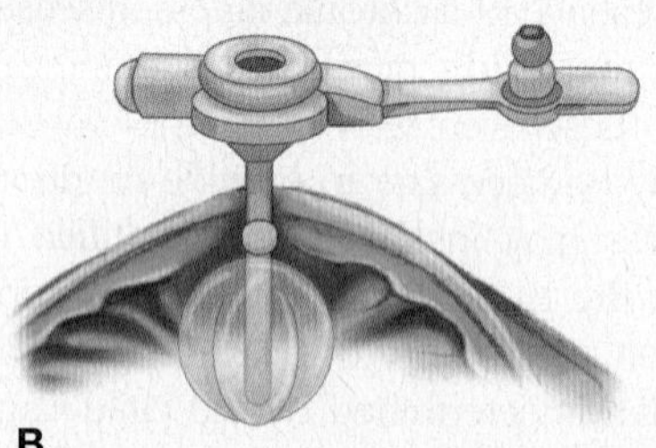

FIGURE 35.11 **A.** Gastrostomy tube. **B.** Low-profile (button) gastrostomy tube. The filled balloon keeps the tube in place inside the stomach.

Inserting a Nasogastric or Orogastric Feeding Tube

Tubes for gavage feeding can be inserted via the nose or mouth. For infants, who are obligate nose breathers, insertion via the mouth may be appropriate. Oral insertion also promotes sucking in the infant. For the older child, nasal insertion is usually the preferred method. If the tube is to remain in place, the nose is also considered to be more comfortable. Nursing Procedure 35.2 gives the steps for inserting a gavage feeding tube.

DETERMINING TUBING LENGTH FOR INSERTION

Several methods exist for determining proper tube length, and significant variation in clinical practice is common. Therefore, it is imperative to know your institution's policy and procedures and be up-to-date on current evidence-based practice guidelines. Traditionally, morphologic methods, measuring from the nose to ear to mid-xiphoid to umbilicus (NEMU) or just nose to ear to mid-xiphoid (NEX), have been used to determine tube length for insertion. Research supports the use of the NEMU method over the NEX method, as it demonstrates consistent placement into the body of the stomach (Irving et al., 2018).

Improving the accuracy of predicting tube length will lead to an increase in successful nasogastric tube placements and, therefore, improved outcomes and decreased health care costs.

Determining tubing length for insertion of a nasogastric tube has also been done by using age-related height-based (ARHB) methods. Recent research has shown this method may be more accurate for measuring tube length (Manzo et al., 2023). Refer to Table 35.7 for ARHB equations. Continued research is warranted, and nurses need to ensure they are following best evidence-based practices.

CHECKING TUBE PLACEMENT

Once the gavage feeding tube is inserted, checking for placement is essential. Tube placement must be confirmed each time the tube is inserted and before each use. Radiologic confirmation of tube placement is considered the most accurate method, but the risks associated with repeated radiation exposure, high costs, and the impractical nature of obtaining a radiograph before feeding tube use make it unrealistic (Irving et al., 2018). Several methods have been proposed as reliable for checking tube placement, but no single method has

TABLE 35.5 • Types of Enteral Feeding Tubes

Type of Tube	Indication	Nursing Implications
Nasogastric (inserted via the nose into the stomach) Orogastric (inserted via the mouth into the stomach)	Short-term enteral feeding Orogastric usually limited to young infants only	• Long-term use or repeated insertion causes irritation and discomfort. • Silicone and polyurethane tubes are very flexible and more comfortable; they require a stylet or guidewire for insertion. • Length of long-term use varies according to the type of tube used and the institution protocol. Periodically, a nasogastric tube is removed and reinserted via the opposite nostril to prevent pressure on the nasal mucosa. • Maintaining orogastric placement between feedings can be difficult due to oral secretions.
Nasoduodenal (inserted via the nose to the duodenum) or nasojejunal (inserted via the nose to the jejunum)	Short-term enteral feeding. Indicated if child has trouble digesting food, cannot use their gastrointestinal tract secondary to congenital anomalies or surgery, or is at risk for or has a history of severe reflux or aspiration	• Silicone and polyurethane tubes with weighted tip allow tube to pass from pylorus into small intestines. • Agency may require special training in order to place at bedside; may also be performed in radiology • Length of use same as nasogastric or orogastric tubes
Gastrostomy (surgically inserted through the abdominal wall into the stomach) Jejunostomy (surgically inserted through the abdominal wall into the jejunum)	Long-term enteral feeding or when esophageal atresia or stricture is present Jejunostomy tubes are indicated when gastric feeding is not tolerated.	• The inner section of the tube is below the skin surface, with the tip located in the stomach or jejunum (may be balloon, winged, or mushroom shaped). The outer section appears above the skin surface at the insertion site and has an opening or feeding port to which the feeding solution is attached. • Low-profile gastrostomy device (gastrostomy button) is flush with the abdominal surface. The flip-top opening is anchored by a dome that fits against the stomach wall. Less conspicuous, it allows the child to be more active and mobile. • After initial insertion, the tube length is measured from the insertion site to the far end of the tube and recorded. This measurement is checked at least daily to ensure that the tube has not moved. • There are many different devices available. For any gastrostomy or jejunostomy tube, the type and size of tube inserted as well as the amount required to fill the balloon, if present, should be known.

been shown to be consistently accurate for continually assessing tube placement.

Research has suggested alternative methods such as using measurements of bilirubin, trypsin, and pepsin levels, CO_2 monitoring, transillumination, and magnetic detection to enhance assessment of tube placement, but insufficient evidence is available to support these methods. Also, these methods have other limitations such as the cost, the availability of equipment, and the limited availability for bedside testing of these levels.

Refer to Box 35.4 for methods to verify feeding tube placement. However, keep in mind that even with these methods, tube malpositioning can occur. Therefore, nurses need to be vigilant in checking for tube placement using the recommended methods and be cautious and proactive if there is any suspicion that the tube may be misplaced.

TAKE NOTE!

Radiologic verification is recommended if bedside methods are conflicting, the nasogastric tube (NGT) was difficult to place, or the child is at high risk, such as children with swallowing problems, children with altered levels of consciousness, or children in the intensive care unit (Irving et al., 2018).

If the gavage feeding tube is to remain in place, secure it to the child's cheek. Do not tape the tube to the child's forehead, because this could lead to irritation and pressure on, and possible breakdown of, the nasal mucosa. Also, measure the length of the tube extending from the nose or mouth to the end, and record this information. Double-check this measurement before administering each intermittent tube feeding to verify that

NURSING PROCEDURE 35.2 Inserting a Gavage Feeding Tube

Purpose: To provide a means for delivering nutrition to the child's functioning gastrointestinal tract

1. Verify the order for gavage feeding, confirm identity, and review child's medical history for any contraindications to placing a feeding tube.
2. Explain the procedure to the child and parents using appropriate language geared to the child's development level.
3. Gather the necessary equipment; remove formula for feeding from refrigerator if appropriate, and allow it to come to room temperature.
4. Wash hands and put on gloves.
5. Inspect the child's nose and mouth for deformities that may interfere with the passage of the tube.
6. Position the infant supine with the head slightly elevated and with the neck slightly hyperextended so that the nose is pointed upward. If necessary, place a rolled towel or blanket under the neck to help in maintaining this position. Assist the older child to a sitting position, if appropriate. Alternatively, have the parent or another person hold the child to promote comfort and reassurance. Enlist the aid of additional people, such as a parent or other health care team member, to assist in maintaining the child's position.
7. Determine the proper tube circumference or French. This will depend on the indication for use of the tube (suction or nutrition), the expected duration the tube will be in place, and the size and age of the child. Use clinical judgment to determine the correct tube type and size. Refer to Table 35.6.
8. Determine the tubing length for insertion: Use morphologic measurement from the tip of the nose to the earlobe to the middle of the area between the xiphoid process and umbilicus or age-related height-based (ARHB) method, ensuring accurate height and calculations (Table 35.7). Mark this measurement on the tube with an indelible pen or with a piece of tape.
9. Lubricate the tube with a generous amount of sterile water (many small-bore feeding tubes have a water-activated lubricant) or water-soluble lubricant to promote passage of the tube and minimize trauma to the child's mucosa.
10. Insert the tube into one of the nares or the mouth. Direct a nasally inserted tube straight back toward the occiput; direct an orally inserted tube toward the back of the throat.
11. Advance the tube slowly to the designated length; encourage the child (if capable) to swallow frequently to assist with advancing the tube. If not contraindicated, the child can sip on water through a straw to help facilitate swallowing and advancement of the tube.
12. Watch for signs of distress, such as gasping, coughing, or cyanosis, indicating that the tube is in the airway. If these signs develop, withdraw the tube and allow the child to rest before attempting reinsertion.
13. Temporarily secure tube, remove stylet if applicable, and check for proper placement of the tube. Refer to Box 35.4.
14. Document the type of tube inserted; length of tubing inserted; measurement of external tubing length, from nares to end of tube, after insertion; and confirmation of placement.

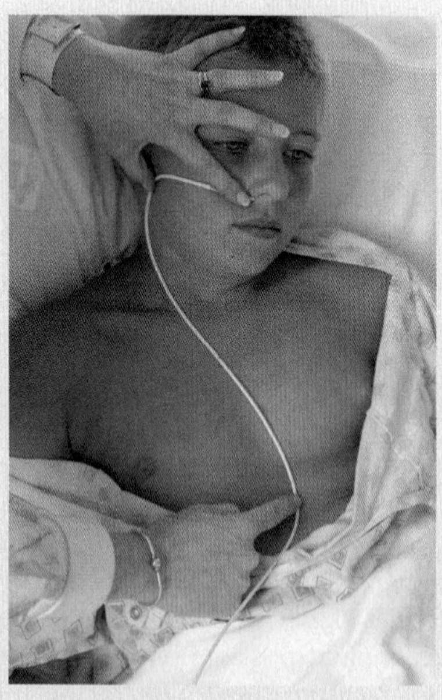

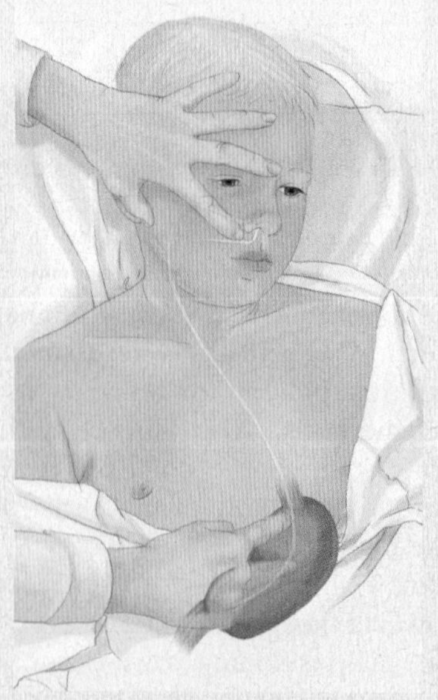

Adapted from Lippincott Williams & Wilkins. (2023). *Lippincott nursing procedures* (9th ed.). Wolters Kluwer.

TABLE 35.6 • General Gavage Feeding Tube Size Based on Age

Age	Size of Tube (Fr)
Newborn	6–8
0–5 years	6–10
6–12 years	8–12
>12 years	10–14

A larger tube will be utilized if tube is used for suction.

the feeding tube is in the proper position. Once the position of the gavage feeding tube is confirmed, the feeding solution or medication can be administered.

Remember Lily, the 9-month-old infant diagnosed with malnutrition who is to receive gavage feedings with a nasogastric tube? What equipment will be needed, and what steps will you take to complete the procedure?

Administering Enteral Feedings

Enteral feedings can be given continuously or intermittently, regardless of the type of tube used. Intermittent feedings are commonly called bolus feedings. With a **bolus feeding**, a specified amount of feeding solution is given at specific intervals, usually over a short period of time such as 15 to 30 minutes. Given via a syringe, feeding bag, or infusion pump, bolus feedings most closely resemble regular meals. Continuous feedings are given at a slower rate over a longer period of time. In some cases, the feeding may be given during the night so that the child can be free to move about and participate in activities during the day. For continuous feedings, an enteral feeding pump is used to administer the solution at a prescribed rate.

Checking for tube placement is a priority before administering any intermittent tube feeding and periodically during continuous tube feedings, regardless of the type of tube being used. (Refer to Box 35.4.) For gastrostomy and jejunostomy tubes, ensure that the calibration, if present, has not changed. Measure the length of the tube daily from the exit site on the stomach to the end of the tube. Assess the abdomen for distension and bowel sounds. Also, measure the **gastric residual** (the amount remaining in the stomach, which indicates gastric emptying time) by aspirating the gastric contents with a syringe, measuring it, and then replacing the contents. Check the residuals periodically, according to the facility's policy, such as every 4 to 6 hours, and before each intermittent feeding. If the residual volume exceeds the amount specified by the health care provider's order, hold the feeding and notify the health care provider or nurse practitioner.

Begin the feeding by placing the child in a supine position with the head and shoulders elevated approximately 30 degrees so that the feeding will remain in the stomach area. Flush the tube with a small amount of water to clear it and prevent occlusion. This is not necessary for a gavage feeding if the tube is being inserted each time a feeding is given. Ensure that the feeding solution is at room temperature. Administer the feeding per the facility's policy.

Feeding solutions may be placed into the barrel of a syringe or into a feeding bag attached to the feeding tube and allowed to flow by gravity. The rate of flow for gravity-assisted feedings can be increased or decreased by raising or lowering the feeding solution container,

TABLE 35.7 • Age-Related Height-Based Equations for Predicting Orogastric/Nasogastric Tube Insertion Lengths

Route	Age Group	Predicted Internal Distance to the Body of the Stomach Determined by:
Oral	Age ≤28 months	16.6 + 0.183 (height, cm)
	Between ages 28 months and 100 months (8 years 4 months)	20.1 + 0.183 (height, cm)
	Between ages 100 months (8 years 4 months) and 121 months (~10 years)	17 + 0.218 (height, cm)
	Greater than 121 months (~10 years)	18.5 + 0.218 (height, cm)
Nasal	Age <28 months	17.6 + 0.197 (height, cm)
	Between ages 28 months and 100 months (8 years 4 months)	21.1 + 0.197 (height, cm)
	Between ages 100 months (8 years 4 months) and 121 months (~10 years)	18.7 + 0.218 (height, cm)
	Greater than 121 months (~10 years)	21.2 + 0.218 (height, cm)

Data from Cincinnati Children's Hospital Medical Center. (2011). *Best Evidence Statement (BESt). Confirmation of nasogastric/orogastric tube (NGT/OGT) placement.* Cincinnati Children's Hospital Medical Center. https://rightbiometrics.com/wp-content/uploads/2023/02/Confirmation-of-Nasogastric-Tube-NGT-Placement.pdf

BOX 35.4 Methods for Verification of Feeding Tube Placement

- Obtain radiographic confirmation of proper tube placement in children who are considered high risk for aspiration, such as children with neurologic impairment, children obtunded, sedated, unconscious, critically ill, having reduced gag reflex or static encephalopathy, or when nonradiologic methods are not feasible or bedside results are conflicting.
- Nonradiologic verification is used in children who are not considered high risk for aspiration; document pH of aspirate; document insertion distance and external length of tube in the chart. Mark and document the tube's exit site from the nose or mouth.
- Use bedside techniques at regular intervals to determine proper tube positioning.
  - Measuring pH: Gastric secretions have a pH less than 5. Small intestine secretions will usually have a pH greater than 6, but this does not reliably predict proper tube placement. A pH greater than 6 can occur with respiratory or esophageal placement, with proper tube placement (gastric or intestinal) when feedings are given continuously, or if the child is receiving acid-inhibiting medications. Therefore, if the pH is greater than 5, additional assessment is warranted.
  - Observing appearance of fluid aspirated from tube (can be used in conjunction with pH testing but is not a reliable single verification method)
    - Gastric secretions are usually grassy green or clear and colorless and can have off-white or tan mucous shreds. It may also be brown tinged if blood is present.
    - Intestinal secretions are often bile stained, light golden yellow to brownish green. They tend to be thicker and more translucent than gastric secretions.
    - Respiratory secretions can be white, yellow, straw colored, or clear.
  - Instill air into the tube, and then auscultate for the sound (gastric auscultation) (can be used in conjunction with other assessment methods).
  - Check external markings on tube and external tube length (tube remaining from nares to end of tube) to determine if the tube seems to have migrated or been misplaced.
- Continually assess for signs indicative of feeding tube misplacement, such as unexplained gagging, vomiting, or coughing; signs and symptoms of respiratory distress; and decreased oxygen saturations.
- If bedside techniques reveal conflicting results or the child is at high risk, radiologic confirmation is recommended.
- Review routine chest and abdominal radiographs (if obtained) to double-check correct tube position. Always follow agencies' policy and procedures.

Adapted from Irving, S. Y., Rempel, G., Lyman, B., Sevilla, W. M., Northington, L., Guenter, P., & The American Society for Parenteral and Enteral Nutrition. (2018). Pediatric nasogastric tube placement and verification: Best practice recommendations from the NOVEL Project. *Nutrition in Clinical Practice, 33*(6), 921–927; Lippincott Williams & Wilkins (2023). *Lippincott nursing procedures* (9th ed.). Wolters Kluwer.

respectively. Typically, intermittent feedings last from 15 to 30 minutes. A feeding bag may also be attached to a pump to control the rate of flow. Monitor the child's tolerance to the feeding.

Once the feeding is complete, but before the formula completely empties from the container, flush the tube with water. As the water leaves the syringe or tubing, clamp the tube to prevent air from entering the stomach. Then disconnect the syringe or tube-feeding bag from the tube.

CLINICAL REASONING ALERT!

If the child vomits during the feeding, stop the feeding immediately and turn the child onto their side or sit them up.

If the child has a gastrostomy button, open the cap and connect an adaptor or insert extension tubing through the one-way valve. This allows access to the gastric conduit. The feeding solution container is connected to the extension tubing or adaptor, and the feeding is given as described previously. After the feeding is completed, the extension tubing or adaptor is flushed with water and the flip-top opening is closed.

Burp the infant during and after any type of tube feeding in the same manner as for an infant who is bottle- or breast-fed. Also, position the child on their right side with the head slightly elevated, approximately 30 degrees, for about 1 hour after the feeding to facilitate gastric emptying and reduce the risk of aspiration and regurgitation. Some children have a difficult time with gas and burping on their own after tube placement. Venting, which helps relieve gas, may be ordered by the health care provider or nurse practitioner. It removes excess air and can be helpful if the child is bloated or the abdomen is distended. Use a catheter-tip syringe with the plunger removed and attach to the end of the tube. Hold the syringe above the child's stomach for a few minutes. Once the air or gas is removed, allow any stomach contents or formula to flow back into the stomach.

Weigh the child daily throughout enteral nutrition therapy to determine the effectiveness of the therapy.

Providing Skin and Insertion Site Care

Skin around the gastrostomy or jejunostomy insertion site may become irritated from movement of the tube, moisture, leakage of stomach or intestinal contents, or the adhesive device holding the tube in place. Keeping the skin clean and dry is important and will help prevent most of these problems.

The skin around a gastrostomy or jejunostomy tube requires cleaning at least once a day. Routine site care includes, for newly placed tubes, gentle cleansing with sterile water or saline or, for established tubes, soap and water, followed by rinsing or cleaning with water alone. To clean under an external disk or bumper, a cotton-tipped applicator may be used. During insertion site care, rotate the gastrostomy tube or button a quarter-turn to prevent skin adherence and irritation. Always follow agency or institution policies and procedures.

TAKE NOTE!

Do not rotate a jejunal or gastrojejunal tube because it can cause kinking.

Assess the insertion site and condition of the surrounding skin for signs and symptoms of infection, such as erythema, induration, foul drainage, or pain. A small amount of clear or tan drainage is normal. If any drainage is present, a dressing can be placed. Use a presplit 2 × 2 gauze, and place it loosely around the site. Change this dressing when it is soiled. If no drainage is present, do not place a dressing as it can cause undue pressure and trap moisture, leading to skin irritation.

Preventing movement of the tube also helps reduce skin irritation. Check the volume of the balloon with a balloon-tipped device about once or twice a week, and reinflate the balloon to the initial volume if needed. The tube should be able to move slightly in and out of the child's stomach. The plastic disk should be snug against the skin but not tight enough to cause pressure. Tube stabilization methods help prevent the tube from moving around and sliding further into the stomach or jejunum. Stabilize the tube by pulling gently on the tubing and sliding the stabilizer bar or disk snugly against the abdomen.

TAKE NOTE!

Rotate sites where the tube is secured to the abdomen to prevent tension on the stoma or skin breakdown.

Measure and record the length of the tube from the exit site of the abdominal wall to the end of the tube. All future measurements should be the same unless the tube length is changed. For tubes without a stabilizer bar or disk or for additional stabilization needs, several other methods may be used, including cut baby bottle nipples, taping methods, and commercially available stabilizers (Fig. 35.12). It is always important to follow agency policy.

TAKE NOTE!

When using the nipple method, make sure to cut several holes in the base of the nipple to allow air circulation and site assessment.

Promoting Growth and Development

Some children receive all of their nutritional needs through tube feedings, whereas other children use tube feedings as a supplement to eating by mouth. Feeding time is a special time for infants and children. Occasionally, babies who are fed solely through an enteral feeding tube may forget or lose the desire to eat by mouth. Use a pacifier to help avoid this, allowing the infant to associate the pacifier in their mouth with a feeding. The sucking motion will also exercise the jaw and promote the flow of the feedings. The saliva produced during sucking aids in digestion. Combined with holding the infant and cuddling, rocking, and talking to them, this promotes a more normal feeding time.

Talking with children, playing music, or reading a story promotes an active feeding time. At home, encourage parents to include the feeding as a part of regular family mealtime together to provide socialization for the child. Allow the child to participate in the feedings by gathering supplies and administering the actual feeding so that the child may experience independence and adaptation. If the child also eats food by mouth, feed them by mouth first and then administer the tube feeding. Children with feeding tubes should be allowed as normal a routine as possible. For example, they can crawl, walk, and jump just like children of the same age and developmental level. However, in some cases, contact sports such as football, hockey, and wrestling should be avoided because of

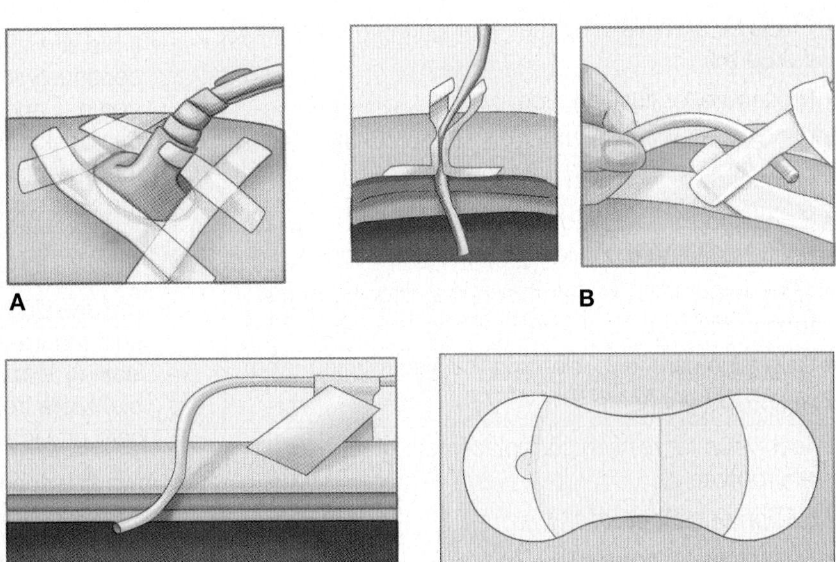

FIGURE 35.12 Methods to stabilize a gastrostomy tube include (**A**) the nipple method, (**B**) taping methods, (**C**) the tension loop method, and (**D**) commercially available stabilizing devices (GripLok; pictured here).

the higher risk of injury. Securing the tubing under the child's clothing will prevent it from becoming accidentally dislodged and prevent the child from pulling and playing with it. Using one-piece outfits, an Ace wrap, or stretchy gauze to cover the tube can help protect it.

Educating the Child and Family

Educate children receiving enteral feedings and their parents thoroughly about this method of nutritional support. Reinforce the reason for the therapy, and provide the child and parents with opportunities to verbalize their concerns and ask questions. Ensure that the parents understand the risks and benefits of the therapy and the expected duration.

Provide the child, if developmentally appropriate, and parents with opportunities to participate in the feeding sessions. This helps allay some of their fears and anxieties and promotes a sense of control over the situation. They will also gain valuable practice in learning the skill should the feedings be required at home. Teaching Guidelines 35.3 identifies important topics to include in the teaching plan for a child receiving enteral nutrition at home. Troubleshooting problems at home is an important topic to cover. Refer to Teaching Guidelines 35.4. Education also involves helping the family develop appropriate coping strategies to adapt, solve problems, and access the support and services they will need after discharge.

TEACHING GUIDELINES 35.3 Topics to be Covered for Home Enteral Nutrition

- Type and size of tube
- Type of nutritional support
- Rationale for therapy
- Expected results from therapy
- Duration of therapy
- Frequency of feedings
- Feeding solution and equipment
- Tube insertion technique (if appropriate)
- Methods to check for correct placement
- Steps for administering the feeding (and medication, if ordered)
- Procedure for flushing tube
- Procedure for venting the tube, if appropriate
- Frequency of weighing the child
- Signs and symptoms of complications and when to notify health care provider or nurse practitioner
- Troubleshooting problems, such as clogging of the tube or dislodgement (see Teaching Guidelines 35.4)
- Daily tube care (e.g., cleaning the site, rotating tube)
- Site assessment
- Technique for reinsertion/replacement of tube as appropriate
- Equipment suppliers
- Resources for support
- Follow-up visits and referrals

Remember Lily from the beginning of the chapter? She is to be discharged home after having a gastrostomy tube inserted to continue feedings at home. What teaching is needed for her family prior to discharge?

TEACHING GUIDELINES 35.4 Troubleshooting Complications at Home

- If a tube becomes clogged, instruct caregivers to slowly push warm water into the tube. Amount and size of syringe will vary based on child's size and facility policy. Repeat if necessary. Instruct caregivers to never use an object or put anything into the tube. They should call the doctor or nurse if they are unable to unclog the tube. Declogging medications may be prescribed.
- If a tube is inadvertently removed, instruct the caregiver to try to replace the tube into the opening 1 to 2 in, tape the tube to the child's abdomen, and do not use the tube. If unable to do this, cover the site with a small clean dressing tape. They should then call the health care provider or nurse immediately; the tube needs to be replaced as soon as possible (within 1 to 4 hours), or the tract will close. Some institutions may instruct the family on how to replace the tube once the tube is more than 6 weeks old and has formed an established G-tube tract.
- If the site is red or irritated, instruct caregivers to continue with routine cleaning, keep the area clean and dry, and call the health care provider. An antibiotic or skin barrier cream may be ordered. Assess for leakage and try to minimize, if possible. Check the tube's position, and ensure tube is stabilized and secure and not dangling.
- If the tube is leaking, the caregiver needs to keep the dressing clean and dry. Assess tube position and secure the tube to avoid dangling. Assess if leaking is from stoma area or tube valve, if applicable. More frequent venting may help, and the health care provider should be notified.

Always teach following the instructions per agency policy and procedure regarding home care.

Adapted from Cincinnati Children's Hospital Medical Center. (2022). *Gastrostomy tube (G-tube) home care*. https://www.cincinnatichildrens.org/health/g/g-tube-care

Parenteral Nutrition

Nutritional support can be administered IV through a peripheral or central venous catheter. The concentration and components of the solution determine the type of parenteral nutrition. Parenteral nutrition given via a central venous access device is termed **total parenteral nutrition** (TPN). Comparison Chart 35.1 gives information about peripheral and central parenteral nutrition.

Administering TPN

Typically, the health care provider or nurse practitioner determines the concentration and components of the TPN solution based on a thorough assessment of the child's status, including the results of laboratory testing. This information is used as a baseline for evaluating the effectiveness of therapy.

The solution is prepared under sterile conditions in the pharmacy. For TPN, a central venous access device is inserted and secured, if one is not already in place. Use specialized tubing with an in-line filter (to prevent small microparticles from entering the circulation).

TPN solutions may be refrigerated until they are to be used. Once started, a single solution of TPN should hang for no longer than 24 hours (Lippincott Williams & Wilkins, 2023). The infusion of the solution is initiated at a slow rate that is gradually increased as ordered based on how the child tolerates the therapy. TPN solutions are highly concentrated glucose solutions that can cause hyperglycemia if given too rapidly. Use of an infusion pump is essential to control the rate of infusion. Fat emulsions are administered periodically to meet the child's need for essential fatty acids. These solutions are given as a piggyback solution into the TPN line but below the in-line filter.

Throughout TPN therapy, be vigilant in monitoring the infusion rate, and report any changes in the infusion rate to the health care provider or nurse practitioner immediately. Gradual adjustments may be made to the rate, but only as ordered by the health care provider or nurse practitioner.

Initially, check blood glucose levels frequently, such as every 4 to 6 hours, to evaluate for hyperglycemia. These levels can be obtained with a bedside glucose meter. Minimize the trauma and discomfort associated with frequent invasive procedures by using the principles of atraumatic care. If blood glucose levels are elevated, SQ administration of insulin may be needed. Once the child's glucose levels stabilize, the frequency of blood glucose level testing decreases, such as every 8 to 12 hours, based on the facility's policy.

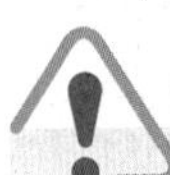

CLINICAL REASONING ALERT!

If for any reason the TPN infusion is interrupted or stops, be prepared to begin an infusion of a 5% to 10% dextrose solution at the same infusion rate as the TPN (Lippincott Williams & Wilkins, 2023). This helps to prevent rebound hypoglycemia that may occur due to the increased insulin secretion by the child's body in response to the use of the highly concentrated TPN solution.

Perform catheter site care, tubing and filter changes, and dressing changes according to the facility's policy. Inspect the insertion site closely for signs of infection.

COMPARISON CHART 35.1 Peripheral Parenteral Nutrition Versus Total Parenteral Nutrition

	Peripheral Parenteral Nutrition	Total Parenteral Nutrition
Indications/use	Primarily supplemental Short-term use to supply additional calories and nutrients (2 weeks or less)	Provides all nutrients to meet child's needs Enough calories supplied to restore nitrogen balance[a] Longer-term use (2 weeks or more)
Route	Peripheral vein	Central venous access to allow rapid dilution of hypertonic solution
Child's status	Nutritional status usually within acceptable parameters Oral intake decreased or absent	Child with a nonfunctioning gastrointestinal (GI) tract, such as a congenital or acquired GI disorder Severe failure to thrive Multisystem trauma or organ involvement Preterm newborns
Components	Less concentrated mixture of fluid, electrolytes, carbohydrates (dextrose), amino acids, vitamins, and minerals Carbohydrate concentration usually limited to 10% or less and osmolarity of <600 mOsm[a]	Highly concentrated solution of carbohydrates, electrolytes, vitamins, and minerals Lipid emulsion to supply need for essential fatty acids Total nutrient admixture (TNA) with components of TPN plus lipids and other additives in one container

[a]Lippincott Williams & Wilkins. (2023). *Lippincott nursing procedures* (9th ed.). Wolters Kluwer; Baker, R. D., Baker, S. S. & Bojczuk, G. (2022). Parenteral nutrition in infants and children. *UpToDate.* Retrieved March 1, 2023, from https://www.uptodate.com/contents/parenteral-nutrition-in-infants-and-children

Also, monitor the child's vital signs, daily weights, and intake and output closely for changes. In addition, review laboratory test results, which can aid in early detection of problems, such as infection or electrolyte excesses or deficits.

TPN can be administered continuously over a 24-hour period, or after initiation it may be given on a cyclic basis, such as over a 12-hour period during the night. When administering cycled TPN, the solution is infused at half the prescribed rate for the first and last hour to prevent hyper- and hypoglycemia.

Preventing Complications

Nurses play a key role in minimizing the risk for complications related to use of central venous access devices and TPN. Box 35.5 describes these complications. Key measures to reduce the risk of complications include the following:

- Monitor the child's vital signs closely for changes.
- Adhere to strict aseptic technique when caring for the catheter and administering TPN.
- Ensure that the system remains a closed system at all times. Secure all connections, and clamp the catheter or have the child perform the Valsalva maneuver during tubing and cap changes.
- Use occlusive dressings. Chlorhexidine-impregnated sponge (Biopatch) dressings may be used to help prevent infection. Always follow agency or institution policy and procedures.
- Adhere to agency policy for flushing of the catheter and maintaining catheter patency.
- Assess intake and output frequently.
- Monitor blood glucose levels and obtain laboratory tests as ordered to evaluate for changes in fluid and electrolytes.

BOX 35.5 Complications That Can Occur With Central Venous Access Devices and Total Parenteral Nutrition (TPN)

- Air embolism from inadvertent entry of air into the system during tubing or cap changes or accidental disconnection
- Cardiac tamponade due to catheter advancement with movement of the arm, neck, or shoulder
- Catheter occlusion from the development of a fibrin sheath or thrombus at the catheter tip, malpositioning or kinking, or the deposition of precipitates or a blood clot
- Venous thrombosis from injury to the vessel wall during insertion or movement of the catheter after insertion or from chemical irritation due to administration of concentrated solutions, vesicants, and other medications through the catheter
- Hyperglycemia, typically with too rapid an infusion of TPN
- Hypoglycemia, which may occur with rapid cessation
- Dehydration as the child's body attempts to rid itself of excess glucose through renal excretion
- Electrolyte imbalance (particularly potassium, sodium, calcium, magnesium, and phosphorus)
- Infection at the skin insertion site, along the catheter pathway, or in the bloodstream. Organisms can arise from the skin, hands of caregivers, or other areas such as wound drainage, droplets from the lungs, or urine. For example, connection sites can be contaminated during tubing or dressing changes.

Promoting Growth and Development

Meals are a time for meeting nutritional needs as well as a time for love, comfort, support, and socialization. TPN meets the child's nutritional needs, but the child's need for love and support also must be met. Implement measures similar to those for children receiving enteral nutrition (see discussion earlier in this chapter). Also provide opportunities for holding and cuddling the child. Allow the older child to participate in activities that can help to occupy the time associated with meals. When administering cyclic TPN, run the TPN over the nighttime hours, whenever possible, to allow the child to participate in developmentally appropriate activities during the day. Encourage the child and parents to participate in the care to promote a sense of independence as well as a sense of control over the situation.

Educating the Child and Family

Children who require long-term TPN therapy may receive TPN in the home. Administering TPN at home requires thorough education of the child and parents. This teaching can occur in the health care agency or in the child's home. The amount of information to be taught can be overwhelming, so ensure that ample time is available. Allow time for questions and concerns. Offer emotional support and guidance whenever necessary.

Provide written and verbal instructions about the care involved. Have the child (if appropriate) and parents demonstrate the care needed, including care of the central venous access device. Review with them the measures for obtaining, storing, and handling the solutions and supplies. Develop plans for troubleshooting problems with devices and equipment, and give instructions on how to recognize and treat complications. Also teach them about danger signs and symptoms that require immediate notification. Be sure they have the name and number of a contact person in case of emergency situations.

Initiate the appropriate referrals for support. Specialized home care infusion services are available for follow-up in the home. In addition, social services can be helpful in providing assistance with finances, health insurance reimbursement, scheduling, transportation, emotional support, and community resources.

Unfolding Patient Stories: Brittany Long • Part 1

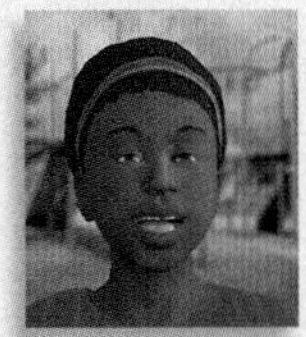

Brittany Long, a 5-year-old child diagnosed with sickle cell anemia, is having an acute pain crisis, and her parent brings her to the emergency department (ED). Her last visit to the ED was 1 year ago, when she was hospitalized for a vaso-occlusive crisis episode. How would the nurse prepare Brittany for insertion of an IV line and administration of IV fluids? How would the explanation differ for her parent? What nursing interventions safeguard the IV line and administration of fluids? (Brittany Long's story continues in Chapter 46.)

Care for Brittany and other patients in a realistic virtual environment: ***vSim** for Nursing* (thepoint.lww.com/vSimPediatric). Practice documenting these patients' care in DocuCare (thePoint.lww.com/DocuCareEHR).

KEY CONCEPTS

- The "rights" of pediatric medication administration are the right drug, right dose, right route, right time, and right patient. Some experts have added additional rights, such as right documentation, right to be educated, right to refuse, right form, and right approach. These additional rights are important to consider to increase patient safety and satisfaction.
- The physiologic immaturity of some body systems in children can affect a drug's pharmacodynamics, leading to differences in the body's response to the drug and thus enhancing or diminishing the drug's effects. The child's age, weight, BSA, and body composition can affect the drug's pharmacokinetics.
- The two most common methods for determining pediatric drug doses involve the use of the child's body weight and BSA.
- Children younger than 5 to 6 years are at risk for aspiration when receiving tablets or capsules because they have difficulty swallowing them; liquids may be more appropriate. When administering oral medications to children, always tell them whether a medication is being mixed with food.
- Medication administration via the rectal route is not preferred because the drug's absorption may be erratic and unpredictable, and children find this route extremely upsetting or embarrassing.
- When administering otic medications, pull the pinna downward and back if the child is under age 3, and up and back for older children.
- IM administration is used infrequently in children because it is painful and children often lack the adequate muscle mass. When used with infants up to 12 months old, the preferred site is the vastus lateralis muscle or anterolateral thigh muscle. In infants and children older than 12 months, the vastus lateralis or anterolateral thigh muscle remains the preferred site, but the deltoid can be considered if sufficient mass is present.
- Administration of medication via the IV route is common with children, especially when a rapid response to the drug is desired or when absorption via other routes is difficult or impossible. The primary method for IV medication administration is via a syringe pump.
- Preferred sites for peripheral IV therapy include the veins of the hands, feet, and forearms. The scalp vein may be used in infants but only if attempts at other sites have been unsuccessful. The general guideline for insertion of any peripheral devices is to use the smallest-gauge catheter for the shortest length of time possible to prevent trauma to the child's fragile veins.
- Central venous therapy is usually administered through a large vein, such as the subclavian, femoral, or jugular vein or vena cava. The tip of the device lies in the superior vena cava just at the entrance to the right atrium. Devices include single- or multiple-lumen short- and long-term catheters, PICCs, tunneled catheters, and vascular access ports.
- Monitoring intake and output is important when a child is receiving IV therapy. Site inspection, proper care of the site, and proper dressing changes are key to preventing complications.
- Nutritional support can be administered enterally via a nasogastric or orogastric tube (gavage feeding) or via a gastrostomy or jejunostomy device or administered parenterally through a peripheral or central venous access device.
- Enteral nutrition is indicated for children who have a functioning gastrointestinal tract but cannot consume adequate amounts of nutrients orally.
- Prior to any enteral feeding, placement of the feeding tube must be confirmed. The gold standard for confirming placement is with a radiograph. At the bedside, nonradiologic methods are used to confirm placement, including checking the color and pH of the aspirate, checking external markings on the tube and verifying external tube length, continually assessing for signs indicative of feeding tube misplacement, such as unexplained gagging, vomiting, or coughing; signs and symptoms of respiratory distress; and decreased oxygen saturations.
- Children receiving TPN require close monitoring of the infusion rate and volume, intake and output, vital signs, and blood glucose levels. Strict aseptic technique is necessary when caring for the central venous access site and TPN infusion.

REFERENCES AND RECOMMENDED READINGS

Baker, R. D., Baker, S. S. & Bojczuk, G. (2022). Parenteral nutrition in infants and children. *UpToDate*. Retrieved March 1, 2023, from https://www.uptodate.com/contents/parenteral-nutrition-in-infants-and-children

Centers for Disease Control and Prevention. (2017). *Guidelines for the prevention of intravascular catheter-related infections (2011)*. (Edit [February 2017]). https://www.cdc.gov/infectioncontrol/guidelines/bsi/recommendations.html#rec2

Centers for Disease Control and Prevention. (2021). *Epidemiology and prevention of vaccine-preventable diseases* (14th ed). In E. Hall, A. P. Wodi, J. Hamborsky, V. Morelli, & S. Schillies (Eds.). Public Health Foundation.

Cincinnati Children's Hospital Medical Center. (2011). *Best Evidence Statement (BESt). Confirmation of nasogastric/orogastric tube (NGT/OGT) placement*. Cincinnati Children's Hospital Medical Center. https://rightbiometrics.com/wp-content/uploads/2023/02/Confirmation-of-Nasogastric-Tube-NGT-Placement.pdf

Cincinnati Children's Hospital Medical Center. (2022). *Gastrostomy tube (G-tube) home care*. https://www.cincinnatichildrens.org/health/g/g-tube-care

Cleveland Clinic. (2023). *Ear drops*. https://my.clevelandclinic.org/health/treatments/24654-ear-drops

Doyle, T. D., Anand, S., & Edens, M. A. (2022). Scalp catheterization. *StatPearls* [Internet]. StatPearls Publishing. https://www.ncbi.nlm.nih.gov/books/NBK507856/

Drutz, J. E. (2023). Standard immunizations for children and adolescents: Overview. *UpToDate*. Retrieved February 22, 2023, from https://www.uptodate.com/contents/standard-immunizations-for-children-and-adolescents-overview

Haddadin, Y., Annamaraju, P., & Regunath, H. (2022). Central line associated blood stream infections. *StatPearls* [Internet]. StatPearls Publishing. https://www.ncbi.nlm.nih.gov/books/NBK430891/

Immunization Action Coalition. (2022). *How to administer intramuscular (IM) and how to administer subcutaneous (SC) injections*. http://www.immunize.org/catg.d/p2020.pdf

Irving, S. Y., Rempel, G., Lyman, B., Sevilla, W. M., Northington, L., Guenter, P., & The American Society for Parenteral and Enteral Nutrition. (2018). Pediatric nasogastric tube placement and verification: Best practice recommendations from the NOVEL project. *Nutrition in Clinical Practice, 33*(6), 921–927. https://doi.org/10.1002/ncp.10189

Kroger, A., Bahta, L., Long, S., & Sanchez, P. (2023). *General best practice guidelines for immunization*. https://www.cdc.gov/vaccines/hcp/acip-recs/general-recs/index.html

Lippincott Williams & Wilkins. (2023). *Lippincott nursing procedures* (9th ed.). Wolters Kluwer.

Lopez-Pineda, A., Gonzalez de Dios, J., Guilabert, M., Mira-Perceval Juan, G., & Joaquín Mira Solves, J. (2021). A systematic review on pediatric medication errors by parents or caregivers at home, *Expert Opinion on Drug Safety, 21*(1), 95–105. https://doi.org/10.1080/14740338.2021.1950138

Manzo, B. F., Marcatto, J. O., Ferreira, B., Galvão Diniz, C., & Parker, L. A. (2023). Comparison of 3 methods for measuring gastric tube length in newborns: A randomized clinical trial. *Advances in Neonatal Care, 23*(3), E79–E86. https://doi.org/10.1097/ANC.0000000000001065

Naik, V. M., Mantha, S. S. P., & Rayani, B. K. (2019). Vascular access in children. *Indian Journal of Anaesthesia, 63*(9), 737–745. https://doi.org/10.4103/ija.IJA_489_19

Paterson, R. S., Chopra, V., Brown, E., Kleidon, T. M., Cooke, M., Rickard, C. M., Bernstein, S. J., & Ullman, A. J. (2020). Selection and insertion of vascular access devices in pediatrics: A systematic review. *Pediatrics, 145*(Suppl. 3), S243–S268. https://doi.org/10.1542/peds.2019-3474H

Schneider, M. (2022). *Clinical guidelines (Nursing): Intramuscular injections*. https://www.rch.org.au/rchcpg/hospital_clinical_guideline_index/Intramuscular_Injections/#:~:text=The%20anterolateral%20aspect%20of%20the,anaphylaxis%20management%20in%20all%20ages

The Joint Commission. (2021). Preventing pediatric medication errors. *Sentinel Event Alert,* Issue 39. https://www.jointcommission.org/-/media/tjc/documents/resources/patient-safety-topics/sentinel-event/sea-39-ped-med-errors-rev-final-4-14-21.pdf

The Joint Commission. (2023). *Facts about the official "do not use" list*. https://www.jointcommission.org/resources/news-and-multimedia/fact-sheets/facts-about-do-not-use-list/

Ullman, A. J., & Chopra, V. (2022). Routine care and maintenance of intravenous devices. *UpToDate*. Retrieved February 28, 2023, from https://www.uptodate.com/contents/routine-care-and-maintenance-of-intravenous-devices

U.S. Food and Drug Administration. (2023). *Pediatric labeling changes*. https://www.fda.gov/science-research/pediatrics/pediatric-labeling-changes

DEVELOPING CLINICAL JUDGMENT

PRACTICING FOR NCLEX

1. A 3-year-old child is to receive a medication that is supplied as an enteric-coated tablet. What is the best nursing action?
   a. Crush the tablet and mix it with applesauce.
   b. Dissolve the medication in the child's milk.
   c. Place a pill in the posterior part of the pharynx, and tell the child to swallow.
   d. Check with the prescriber to see if an alternative form can be used.
2. The nurse is caring for an infant who weighs 8.2 kg and is NPO and receiving IV fluid therapy. What rate does the nurse calculate as meeting the child's daily fluid requirements?
   a. 82 mL per hour
   b. 41 mL per hour
   c. 34 mL per hour
   d. 22 mL per hour
3. When administering ear drops to a 2-year-old, which action would be most appropriate?
   a. Tell the child that the drops are to treat their infection.
   b. Pull the pinna of the child's ear down and back.
   c. Have the child turn their head to the opposite side after giving the drops.
   d. Massage the child's forehead to facilitate absorption of the medication.
4. An infant is to receive intermittent gavage feedings via a nasogastric tube every 6 hours. The feeding tube was inserted with a previous feeding and remains in place. The nurse is preparing to administer the next scheduled feeding. Place the events in the proper sequence.
   a. Check the placement of the feeding tube.
   b. Position the infant on their right side with the head of the bed slightly elevated.
   c. Allow the feeding to come to room temperature.
   d. Flush the tube with water.
   e. Clamp the tube to prevent air from entering the stomach.
   f. Pour the solution into the barrel of the syringe.
5. Which statements are appropriate when administering medication to children? Select all that apply.
   a. Prior to administering a liquid medication, always shake the bottle.
   b. If the child is upset or crying, administer oral liquid medication into the posterior side of the child's mouth, and pinch their nose to assist them to swallow.
   c. When administering a crushable medicine to an infant, place the medication in the infant's bottle before their next feeding.
   d. When administering liquid medication to a toddler, make sure the child is sitting at a 45-degree angle.
   e. When administering a medication using a dropper, ensure that the dropper is the one that was packaged with the medication.
   f. The nurse must administer all medications to ensure that the parents do not make an error.

CRITICAL THINKING EXERCISES

1. When reviewing the medical record of a child, the nurse notes that the ordered dose of medication is different from the recommended dose. How should the nurse proceed?
2. While caring for a 5-year-old child who is receiving IV fluid therapy at a rate of 100 mL per hour, the nurse notes that the infusion is running slowly. The insertion site appears slightly reddened and swollen. What should the nurse do next?
3. A school-age child is to be discharged, continuing TPN therapy at home. The child lives with their parents and two younger siblings. How would the nurse prepare this child and family for discharge? How could the nurse promote growth and development for this child during TPN therapy?

STUDY ACTIVITIES

1. Review the medical records of several children who are on a pediatric unit in your agency. Note the type of medication, route ordered, and what specific interventions are needed for each child related to the medication administration and developmental age of the child, including atraumatic care interventions. Compile a list of the most commonly used routes.
2. Interview several parents about their experiences in giving medications to their children. From these interviews, develop a teaching sheet that provides tips to facilitate oral medication administration to children.
3. Create a chart that compares the SQ, IM, and IV methods of medication administration. Include examples of medications given via these routes, onset of action, appropriate sites, and necessary safety measures for each.

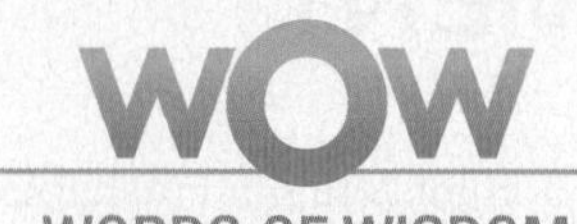

WORDS OF WISDOM

All of our children in pain deserve as much comfort as we can give.

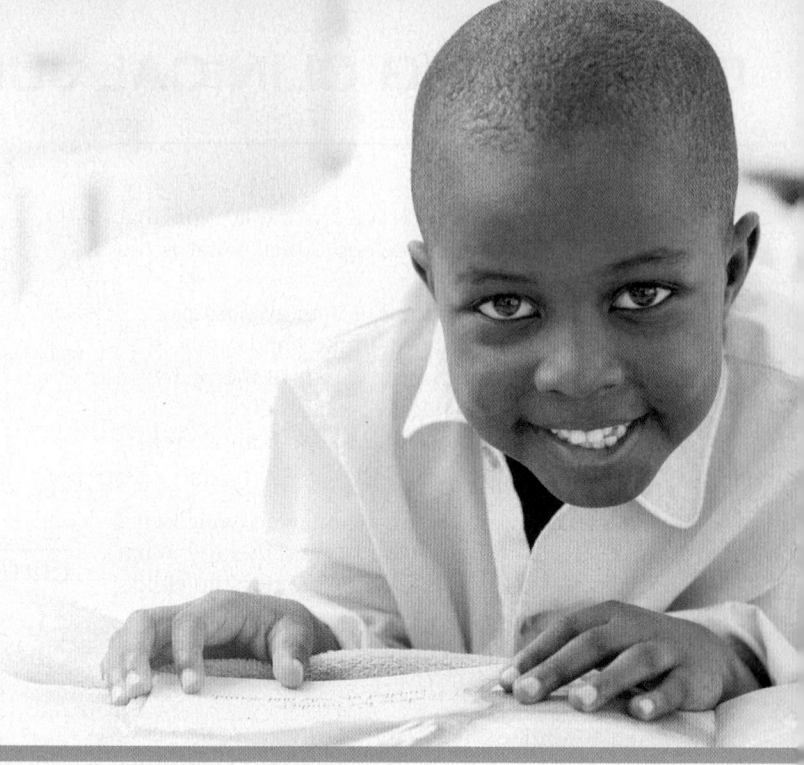

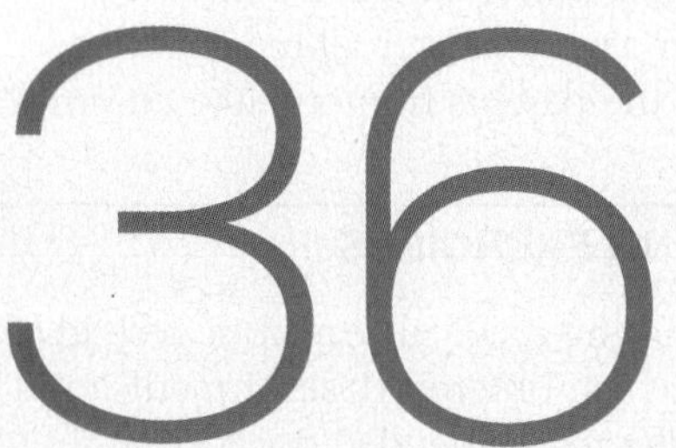

Nursing Care of the Child With an Alteration in Comfort–Pain Assessment and Management

KEY TERMS

acute pain
chronic pain
drug tolerance
epidural analgesia (ep′i-dūr′ăl an′ăl-jē′zē-ă)
moderate sedation
neuromodulators (nŭr′ō-mod′yū-lā′tōrz)
neuropathic pain (nŭr′ō-path′ik pān)
nociceptive pain (nō′si-sep′tiv pān)
nociceptors (nō′si-sep′tŏrz)
pain
pain threshold
patient-controlled analgesia (PCA)
physical dependence
somatic pain (sō-mat′ik pān)
transduction
visceral pain (vis′ĕr-ăl pān)

LEARNING OBJECTIVES

Upon completion of the chapter, you will be able to:

1. Identify the major physiologic events associated with the perception of pain.
2. Distinguish different types of pain based on duration, etiology, and source or location.
3. Discuss the factors that influence the pain response.
4. Identify the developmental considerations for the effects and management of pain.
5. Explain the principles of pain assessment as they relate to children.
6. Understand the use of the various pain rating scales and physiologic monitoring for children.
7. Establish a nursing plan of care for children related to management of pain, including pharmacologic and nonpharmacologic techniques and strategies.

Aiden Russell is a 6-year-old on the pediatric unit admitted for a wound infection. He requires twice-daily (BID) dressing changes. In report, you are told that Aiden cries and fights during the dressing change but otherwise seems to be playing and not experiencing much pain.

INTRODUCTION

A child's comfort is affected by many factors such as hunger, sleep, temperature, presence of caregivers and family, presence of strangers, and the presence of pain. Alteration in comfort in children incorporates all of these factors. A major issue affecting a child's comfort is pain, and nurses have an integral role in helping children and families deal with pain. Therefore, in this chapter, the main focus will be pain assessment and pain management in children.

Pain is a highly individualized, subjective experience that can affect any person of any age. It is a complex phenomenon that involves multiple components and is influenced by myriad factors. **Pain** is defined by the International Association for the Study of Pain (2011) as "an unpleasant sensory and emotional experience associated with, or resembling that associated with, actual or potential tissue damage" (Hauer & Jones, 2021). Another definition of pain that is commonly used is as follows: It is whatever the person experiencing it says it is, existing whenever the person says it does (McCaffery, 1968). The person experiencing the pain is the only one who can identify pain and know what the pain is like.

Pain is a universal experience. Pain affects adults and children of all ages, even preterm infants. Pain can result from numerous causes, including disease processes, injuries, procedures, and surgical interventions. In 1995, the American Pain Society (1995) labeled it "the fifth vital sign." The American Pain Society's goal was to encourage health care professionals to assess pain every time temperature, pulse, respirations, and blood pressure were assessed and to institute measures to manage it.

Unlike adults, however, children may lack the verbal capacity to describe their pain effectively. In addition, many caregivers and health care providers have misconceptions about pain in children, it is difficult to assess the complex nature of the pain experience, and limited resources and research are available related to pain relief strategies for children. Therefore, pain is a major source of distress for children and their families as well as for health care providers.

If left unmanaged, pain in children can lead to serious physical and emotional consequences, such as increased oxygen consumption and alterations in blood glucose metabolism. In addition, the experience of untreated pain early in life may lead to long-term physiologic and psychological consequences for the child (Roué, 2023). For example, inadequately controlled pain can have long-lasting negative outcomes, such as increased distress during later procedures, nonadherence to treatment regimens, inactivity, prolonged bed rest, and the development of chronic pain. Detrimental effects on the course of a disease itself may also be seen with untreated pain. Preterm infants are at a greater risk due to long hospitalizations and numerous painful and invasive procedures (Roué, 2023).

All these factors make pain management a critical element in the plan of care for children. Pain management in children has improved, but underestimation and inadequate management still remain a problem (American Academy of Pediatrics [AAP] et al., 2016, reaffirmed 2020). Various national health associations have issued position papers and guidelines related to the need to treat pain and suffering in children. Effective pain management involves initial pain assessment, therapeutic interventions, and reassessment for all children in any health care setting.

This chapter describes the pain experience in children, including the types of pain, factors influencing pain, and common fallacies and myths associated with pain in children. The nursing process is applied to provide an overview of the care for a child in pain. Various pain management strategies are described, including nonpharmacologic and pharmacologic interventions and measures to address procedure-related and chronic pain.

PHYSIOLOGY OF PAIN

The sensation of pain is a complex phenomenon that involves a sequence of physiologic events in the nervous system. These events are transduction, transmission, perception, and modulation.

Transduction

Peripheral nerve fibers extend from the spinal cord to various locations in and throughout the body's tissues, such as the skin, joints, bones, and membranes covering the internal organs. At the end of these fibers are specialized receptors, called **nociceptors**, which become activated when they are exposed to noxious stimuli. The noxious stimuli can be mechanical, chemical, or thermal. Mechanical stimuli may include intense pressure to an area, a strong muscular contraction, or extensive pressure due to muscular overstretching. Chemical stimulation may involve the release of mediators, such as histamine, prostaglandins, leukotrienes, or bradykinin, as a response to tissue trauma, ischemia, or inflammation. Thermal stimuli typically involve extremes of heat and cold. This process of nociceptor activation is called **transduction**.

Transmission

When nociceptors are activated by noxious stimuli, the stimuli are converted to electrical impulses that are relayed along the peripheral nerves to the spinal cord and brain. Specialized afferent nerve fibers are responsible for moving the electrical impulse along. Myelinated A-delta fibers are large fibers that conduct the impulse at very rapid rates. The pain transmitted by these fibers is often referred to as "fast pain," most commonly associated with mechanical or thermal stimuli (Nath, 2023). Pain is also transmitted by unmyelinated small C fibers. These fibers transmit the impulse slowly and are often activated by chemical stimuli or continued mechanical or thermal stimuli (Nath, 2023). These fibers carry the impulse to the spinal cord via the dorsal horn. Neurotransmitters are released to facilitate the transmission process to the brain.

Several theories have been proposed in an attempt to explain the process of pain transmission. The best known of these is gate control theory. According to this theory, the dorsal horn of the spinal cord contains interneuronal or interconnecting fibers. Large-diameter, faster fibers carry nonnociceptive, tactile information, while smaller nerve fibers carry nociceptive or pain signals. Large fibers, when stimulated, close the gate or pathway to the brain, thereby inhibiting or blocking the transmission of the pain impulse. Subsequently, the impulse does not reach the brain, where it would be interpreted as pain. It is now known that pain modulation is a more complex process, but this theory helps explain why some nonpharmacologic therapies, such as massage and pressure, are effective in reducing pain (Nath, 2023).

Perception

Once in the dorsal horn of the spinal cord, the nerve fibers divide and then cross to the opposite side and rise upward to the thalamus. The thalamus responds quickly and sends a message to the somatosensory cortex of the brain, where the impulse is interpreted as the physical sensation of pain. The impulses carried by the fast A-delta fibers lead to the perception of sharp, stabbing localized pain that also commonly involves a reflex response to withdraw from the stimulus. The impulses carried by the slow C fibers lead to the perception of diffuse, dull, burning, or aching pain. The point at which the person first feels the lowest intensity of the painful stimulus is termed the **pain threshold**. In addition to sending a message to the cerebral cortex, the thalamus also sends a message to the limbic system, where the sensation is interpreted emotionally, and to the brain stem centers, where autonomic nervous system responses begin.

Modulation

Research has identified substances called **neuromodulators** that appear to modify the pain sensation. These substances have been found to change a person's perception of pain. Examples of these neuromodulators include serotonin, endorphins, enkephalins, and dynorphins.

Pain perception can be modified peripherally or centrally. In the peripheral nerve fibers, chemical substances are released that either stimulate the nerve fibers or sensitize them. Peripheral sensitization allows the nerve fibers to react to a stimulus that is of lower intensity than would be needed to cause pain. As a result, the person perceives more pain. Actions that block or inhibit the release of these substances can lead to a decrease in pain perception.

Modification of pain perception can occur centrally in the spinal cord at the dorsal horn. Substances released by the excited interneurons can potentiate the pain sensation. Other neurochemicals, through their binding to specific receptors, can inhibit the perception of pain. Figure 36.1 illustrates the physiology of pain.

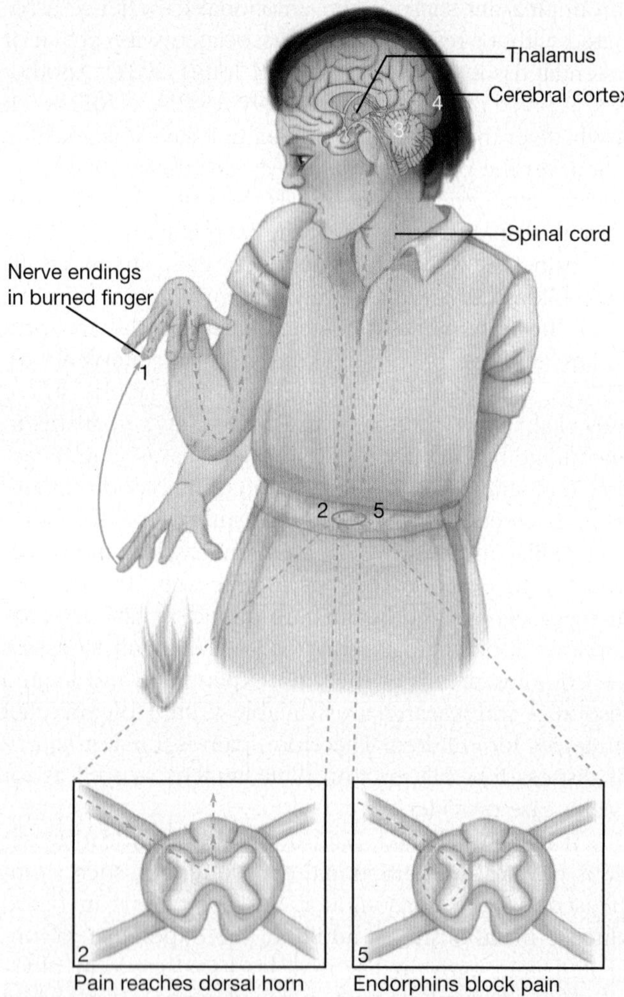

FIGURE 36.1 Physiology of pain. (*1*) Exposure to thermal noxious stimuli results in activation of nociception (transduction). (*2*) Impulses are relayed along the peripheral nerves to the spinal cord through the dorsal horn (transmission). (*3, 4*) This results in the individual feeling the sensation of pain (perception). (*5*) Neurons in the brain stem send signals back down to the dorsal horn, and these fibers release substances such as endorphins, which can inhibit painful impulses in the dorsal horn (modulation). These neurotransmitters are taken back by the body, therefore limiting the analgesic value.

TYPES OF PAIN

Many different systems can be used to classify pain. Most commonly, pain is classified based on its duration, etiology, or source or location.

Classification by Duration

Pain is classified by duration as either acute or chronic.

Acute Pain

Acute pain is defined as pain that is associated with a rapid onset of varying intensity. It usually indicates tissue damage and resolves with healing of the injury. Acute pain reflects stimulation of nociceptors and serves a protective function (i.e., alerting the person to a problem). Examples of causes of acute pain include trauma, invasive procedures, acute illnesses such as sore throat or appendicitis, and surgery. This type of pain generally lasts a few days.

TAKE NOTE!

Children often experience pain associated with various procedures done in health care settings. This type of pain is usually short in duration. Preparation of the child and family will help decrease fears or anxiety. Depending on the type of procedure and the child's age, cognitive level, and temperament, various techniques and methods can be used. Advocating for atraumatic care and adhering to its guidelines will help minimize procedure-related pain.

Chronic Pain

Chronic pain is defined as pain that continues past the expected point of healing for injured tissue. It provides no protective function. It may be continuous or intermittent, with and without periods of exacerbation or remission. It often interferes with sleep and performance of activities of daily living. It can result in loss of appetite and depression. Thus, chronic pain impairs a person's ability to function. In contrast to acute pain, environmental and psychological factors influence behaviors associated with chronic pain. In children, chronic, recurrent pain is most commonly associated with abdominal pain, nonspecific headache, limb pain, or chest pain. Some conditions, such as sickle cell disease and migraines, have characteristics of both acute and chronic pain. Children with chronic pain may not exhibit the same physical or emotional responses as seen with acute pain. As pain becomes prolonged and continuous, the autonomic nervous system response tends to diminish.

Classification by Etiology

Pain can be classified by etiology as nociceptive or neuropathic.

Nociceptive Pain

Nociceptive pain reflects pain due to noxious stimuli that damage normal tissues or have the potential to do so if the pain is prolonged. The pain perceived often correlates closely with the degree or intensity of the stimulus and the extent of real or possible tissue damage. With nociceptive pain, nervous system functioning is intact. Reports of nociceptive pain vary depending on the location of the nociceptors being stimulated. Nociceptive pain ranges from sharp or burning, to dull, aching, or cramping, and to deep aching or sharp stabbing. Examples of conditions that result in nociceptive pain include chemical burns, sunburn, cuts, appendicitis, and bladder distention.

Neuropathic Pain

Neuropathic pain is pain due to malfunctioning of the peripheral or central nervous system. It may be continuous or intermittent and is commonly described as burning, tingling, shooting, squeezing, or spasm-like pain. Examples of neuropathic pain include posttraumatic and postsurgical peripheral nerve injuries, pain after spinal cord injury, metabolic neuropathies, phantom limb pain after amputation, and poststroke pain.

Classification by Source or Location

Pain may also be classified by the source or location of the area involved. It can be somatic pain (superficial and deep) or visceral pain. These classifications typically indicate nociceptive pain.

Somatic Pain

Somatic pain refers to pain that develops in the tissues. It can be further divided into two groups—superficial and deep. Superficial somatic pain, often called cutaneous pain, involves stimulation of nociceptors in the skin, subcutaneous tissue, or mucous membranes. Typically, the pain is well localized and described as a sharp, pricking, or burning sensation. Superficial somatic pain may be due to external mechanical, chemical, or thermal injury or skin disorders. Tenderness is commonly present.

Deep somatic pain typically involves the muscles, tendons, joints, fasciae, and bones. It can be localized or diffuse and is usually described as dull, aching, or cramping. Deep somatic pain may be due to strain from overuse or direct injury, ischemia, and inflammation. Tenderness and reflex spasm may be present. In addition, the person may exhibit sympathetic nervous system activation such as tachycardia, hypertension, tachypnea, diaphoresis, pallor, and pupillary dilation.

Visceral Pain

Visceral pain is pain that develops within organs such as the heart, lungs, gastrointestinal (GI) tract, pancreas, liver, gallbladder, kidneys, or bladder. It is often produced by disease. It is usually diffuse and poorly localized and is described as a deep ache or sharp stabbing sensation that may be referred to other areas. Visceral pain may be due to distention of the organ, organ muscular spasm, contraction, pulling, ischemia, or inflammation. Tenderness, nausea, vomiting, and diaphoresis may be present.

FACTORS INFLUENCING PAIN

Children, like adults, experience neurologic events that result in the perception of pain. However, research has found that environmental and psychological factors may exert a greater influence on the child's perception of pain (McGrath, 2005). Certain factors such as age, sex, cognitive level, temperament, previous pain experiences, and family and cultural backgrounds cannot be changed. However, situational factors involving behavioral, cognitive, and emotional aspects can be modified.

Age and Sex

Research has demonstrated that the nervous system structures needed for pain impulse transmission and perception are present before birth (Roué, 2023). Therefore, children of any age, including preterm newborns, are capable of experiencing pain. Early on, children can interpret pain as an unpleasant sensation, but this interpretation is based on their comparison with other sensations. As they get older, they learn to use words to describe their pain more fully.

Gender and sex may also play a role in a child's perception of pain. It has been suggested that males and females differ in how they perceive, experience, express, and cope with pain and respond to analgesics (Osborne & Davis, 2022). This may be influenced by various factors, including genetics, hormones, family, and culture. Further research is warranted in this area to facilitate more focused care in pain management.

Cognitive Level

Cognitive level is a key factor affecting a child's pain perception and response and usually goes hand in hand with the child's age. Cognitive level typically increases with age, thereby influencing the child's understanding of the pain and its impact and their choices for coping strategies. In addition, as the child's cognitive level increases, their ability to communicate information about pain increases. However, this increased understanding and ability to communicate with advancing age may not apply to the child experiencing developmental delays. For example, a school-age child or adolescent with developmental delays may have the same cognitive level as a toddler or preschooler. Health care providers need to be cognizant of these differences when caring for the child in pain.

Temperament

Literature suggests that temperament plays a role in predicting distress and pain levels in a child during painful events (Favaretto et al., 2022; Horton et al., 2015). For example, a child with a challenging temperament is more likely to have an increased distress response to pain. Nurses can personalize interventions in the clinical environment and during the pain experience to better fit the child's temperament and other personality traits of the child and family.

Previous Pain Experiences

A child identifies pain based on their experiences with pain in the past. The number of episodes of pain, the type of pain, the severity or intensity of the previous pain experience, the effectiveness of treatment of pain, and how the child responded all affect how the child will perceive and respond to the current experience. Research suggests that severe pain experiences in the neonate or young infant can lead to increased pain sensitivity and chronic pain syndrome later in life (Roué, 2023). Previous pain experiences with inadequate pain control may lead to increased distress during future painful procedures. For example, research studies have demonstrated that neonates who had undergone painful procedures such as circumcision and heel lancing showed a stronger negative response to routine immunizations and venipuncture weeks to months later (Roué, 2023).

Family and Culture

The child's cultural and family background will influence how they will express and manage pain. Some cultures transmit the standard of accepting pain stoically; others encourage outward expression. Parents have a strong influence on the child's ability to cope. For example, if a parent reacts to the child's pain in a positive manner and offers comfort measures, the child may have an easier time coping. If the parent shows anger or disapproval, the pain experience may be intensified for the child.

Situational Factors

Situational factors involve factors or elements that interact with the child and their current situation involving the experience of pain. These factors are highly variable and dependent on the specific situation. Situational factors result from the context in which the child is experiencing pain and include cognitive factors, or what the child understands and believes about the pain experience; behavioral factors, or how the child and family react and what they do about the pain experience; and emotional factors, or how the child and family feel about the pain experience (McGrath, 2005). Due to children's limited experience with pain, situational factors may affect them more than adults (McGrath, 2005). A thorough pain assessment must include assessment for situational factors that may exacerbate pain. Examples of situational factors include:

- Child's lack of understanding of the source of pain
- Child's lack of ability to use coping mechanisms or pain-relieving strategies to decrease pain
- Stress and anxiety in anticipation of pain
- Child's lack of control of cause of pain
- Child's lack of ability to understand what to expect from potentially painful experiences
- Increased anxiety exhibited by the family
- Overly protective behaviors exhibited by the family
- Presence of emotions such as fear, anxiety, frustration, distress, underlying anxiety, and depression (McGrath, 2005).

DEVELOPMENTAL CONSIDERATIONS

Since children of various developmental ages respond differently to pain and perceive pain in different ways, it is important to review developmental considerations. Refer to Chapters 25 through 29 for a more complete understanding of childhood development. Nurses must understand how children of various ages respond to painful stimuli and what behaviors may be expected on the basis of their developmental level. By understanding these developmental considerations, the nurse can appropriately assess the child's pain and provide effective interventions.

Infants

Research has demonstrated that infants, including preterm infants, experience pain and can distinguish pain from other tactile experiences (Roué, 2023). Much of this research focuses on pain related to invasive procedures, such as heel sticks and intravenous catheter insertion. Research suggests that neonates actually have a lower pain threshold and pain tolerance and experience pain at a greater intensity than older-age children and adults (Luo et al., 2023).

Concept Mastery Alert

Levels of Pain

When obtaining a blood sample with a heel stick, the nurse should remember that neonates, and, in particular, preterm infants, feel pain and feel it with greater intensity than do older infants.

In preterm and term newborns, behavioral and physiologic indicators are used for determining pain. Behavioral indicators include facial expression, such as brow contracting and chin quivering; body movements; and crying (Roué, 2023). Physiologic signs include changes in heart rate, respiratory rate, blood pressure, oxygen saturation levels, breathing pattern, skin color, pupillary size, intracranial pressure, vagal tone, and palmar sweating (Roué, 2023).

In the younger infant, facial expression is the most common response to pain (Fig. 36.2). The brows may be lowered and drawn together, with the eyes tightly closed. The mouth is open, often forming a square. The body may be stiff, and thrashing may be seen. When the area is stimulated, the infant may demonstrate a generalized reflex withdrawal. The infant may exhibit a high-pitched, shrill cry.

The older infant often displays similar behavioral manifestations of pain. The older infant may display an angry facial expression, but the eyes are open. They often demonstrate a definite withdrawal response when

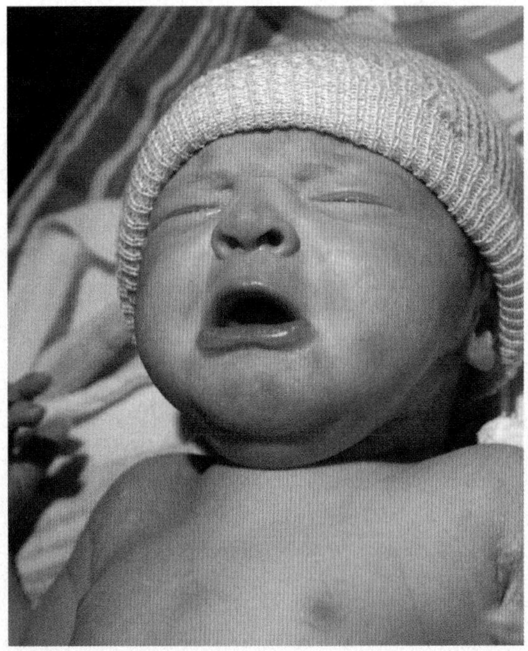

FIGURE 36.2 In the younger infant, facial expression is the most common response to pain.

the area is stimulated. The older infant cries loudly and tries to push away the stimulus that is causing the pain. Other manifestations include irritability, restless sleeping, and poor feeding.

> **TAKE NOTE!**
>
> Remember that anything that causes pain in an adult or older child will cause pain in a neonate or infant regardless of whether the neonate or infant exhibits typical behaviors indicating pain (Roué, 2023). The response to pain is highly variable.

Infants also demonstrate physiologic responses to pain. These may include:

- Increased heart rate, usually averaging approximately 10 bpm; possibly bradycardia in preterm newborns
- Decreased vagal tone
- Decreased oxygen saturation
- Palmar or plantar sweating (as measured by skin conductivity testing); not reliable in infants before 37 weeks' gestation

Toddlers

Toddlers can react to painless procedures as intensely as painful ones, with intense emotional upset and physical resistance or aggression. They may bite, hit, scream, or kick. Other behaviors may include being quiet, pointing to where it hurts, or saying such words as "ow." Facial grimacing and teeth clenching may be noted. They may also react with fear and try to hide or leave the room. They often have limited vocabularies, so it may be difficult for them to express pain. It is important to ask about and encourage the child to verbalize their pain. Ensure the use of words the toddler understands, such as "owie" or "boo-boo." Toddlers may demonstrate regressive behaviors, such as clinging to the parent or crying loudly.

> **TAKE NOTE!**
>
> Young children express pain by using simple words such as "hurt" or "ouchie" or by pointing to the area that hurts. By the age of 3 to 7 years, they can express the presence of pain, and they can usually describe it and its intensity, location, and quality (Zeltzer et al., 2020).

Preschoolers

Preschoolers may become quiet or try to withdraw and hide in response to actual or perceived pain. For example, the child may say they need to go to the bathroom or to get something from another room. Because of their magical thinking, preschoolers may believe pain is a punishment for misbehaving or having bad thoughts. Preschoolers may not verbally report their pain, thinking that pain is something to be expected or that the adults are aware of their pain. They can tell someone where it hurts and can use various tools to describe the severity of pain. However, because they may have limited experience with pain, they may have difficulty distinguishing among types of pain (e.g., sharp or dull), describing the intensity of the pain, and determining whether the pain is worse or better.

School-Age Children

School-age children can usually communicate the type, location, and severity of pain. Children older than the age of 8 can use specific words, such as "sharp as a knife," "burning," or "pulling" to describe their pain. However, they may deny pain in an attempt to appear brave or to avoid further pain related to a procedure or intervention. They may be more concerned with their fear about the illness and its effects rather than the pain. They may also fear being embarrassed by acting out behaviors in response to pain, such as screaming or thrashing. Thus, a typical response might be to withdraw by staring at the television. Other behaviors that may indicate pain in a school-age child include muscular rigidity, such as clenching the fists, stiffening the body, closing the eyes, wrinkling the forehead, or gritting the teeth.

Adolescents

Adolescents may be concerned primarily about body image and fear losing control over their behavior. This may result in denial or refusal of medications. Their mood and what they think is expected of them will also affect their response to pain. Adolescents often ask numerous questions and pay close attention to how others respond to them. Fearing that their behavior may be viewed as juvenile, they may attempt to remain stoic and not exhibit any emotion. Subtle changes such as increased muscle tension with clenched fists and teeth, rapid breathing, and guarding the affected body part may occur. They may also show lack of interest in everyday activities or a decreased ability to concentrate.

Common Fallacies and Myths About Pain in Children

In general, children respond to pain based on the type of pain, the extent of pain, and their age and developmental level. Table 36.1 highlights some common myths and misconceptions related to pain in children. Because of these myths, children have historically been medicated less than adults with similar diagnoses, leading to inadequate pain management (Gai et al., 2020; Roué, 2023).

TABLE 36.1 • Myths and Misconceptions About Children and Pain

Myth or Misconception	Fact
Newborns do not feel pain.	Newborns, including preterm newborns, do feel pain. The neurologic and hormonal systems needed for the transmission of painful stimuli are sufficiently developed.
Exposure to pain at an early age has little to no effect on the child.	Prolonged or severe pain can lead to increased newborn morbidity. Infants who have experienced pain during the neonatal period respond differently to subsequent painful events.[a]
Infants and small children have little memory of pain.	Repeated exposure to painful procedures and events can have long-term consequences. Memories of pain may be stored in the child's nervous system, influencing later reactions to painful stimuli.[a]
The intensity of a child's behavioral reaction indicates the intensity of the child's pain.	Numerous factors affect a child's response to pain. Each child is an individual with their own set of responses.
A child who is sleeping or playing is not in pain.	Sleep or play may be a coping strategy for the child in pain. Sleep may reflect exhaustion of the child who is coping with pain.
Children are truthful when they are asked if they are experiencing pain.	Often, children deny pain to avoid a painful situation or procedure, embarrassment, or loss of control. Children may assume that others know how they are feeling and will thus not verbalize their complaints.
Children learn to adapt to pain and painful procedures.	Repeated exposure to pain or painful procedures can result in an increase in behavioral manifestations.
Children experience more adverse effects of narcotic analgesics than adults do.	The risk of adverse effects of narcotic analgesics is the same for children as for adults.
Children are more prone to addiction to narcotic analgesics.	There is no increased risk of addiction to narcotics when used appropriately to treat children's pain.[b]

[a]Roué, J.-M. (2023). Assessment of neonatal pain. *UpToDate*. Retrieved March 13, 2023, from https://www.uptodate.com/contents/assessment-of-neonatal-pain

[b]Zeltzer, L. K., Krane, E. J., & Levy, R. L. (2020). Pediatric pain management. In R. M. Kleigman, J. W. St. Geme III, N. J. Blum, S. S. Shah, R. C. Tasker, K. M. Wilson, & R. E. Behrman (Eds.), *Nelson textbook of pediatrics* (21st ed., pp. 2915–3011). Elsevier.

Clinical Judgment and the Nursing Process

Nursing care of the child with pain includes nursing assessment, analysis, planning, interventions, and evaluation. Each step of this process must be individualized for each child. A general understanding of the physiology of pain, factors that influence pain, and effective pain management techniques can help to individualize the child's plan of care.

Assessment

Assessment of pain in children consists of both subjective and objective data collection. The acronym "QUESTT" is an excellent way to remember the key principles of pain assessment (Baker & Wong, 1987):

- *Q*uestion the child.
- *U*se a reliable and valid pain scale.
- *E*valuate the child's behavior and physiologic changes to establish a baseline and determine the effectiveness of the intervention. The child's behavior and motor activity may include irritability and protection as well as withdrawal of the affected painful area.
- *S*ecure the parent's involvement.
- *T*ake the cause of pain into account when intervening.
- *T*ake action.

TAKE NOTE!

Children do experience pain. Pain management techniques work just as well with children as they do with adults.

Health History

When assessing pain in children, tailor the assessment to the child's developmental level, and ask questions geared toward the child's cognitive ability. During the health history, determine the child's previous exposure to pain, if any, and how the child responded. This information will provide clues about how the child copes and their current response. Attempt to determine what word the child uses to denote pain. Some children may not understand the term "pain" but do understand terms such as "ouchie" or "boo-boo."

The health history also includes questioning the parents about their cultural beliefs related to pain and their child's usual responses. This information aids in planning developmentally and culturally appropriate family-centered care.

Questioning the Child

When questioning the child, phrase the questions in a manner that the child will be able to understand based on their developmental level. Some input from the child's family may be helpful in determining where best to focus the questions.

Ask the child what pain means to them. Use words that the child may comprehend more easily, such as "hurt," "boo-boo," or "ouch," as appropriate. Inquire about similar experiences in the past and how they responded. Determine whether the child let others know that they were hurting and how this message was conveyed (e.g., crying, acting out, or pointing to the hurting area).

Review the history of the pain and various influences such as cultural aspects, caregiver attitudes or expectations, previous experiences, and any education or teaching related to pain management. Continue to formulate questions to ascertain the following:

- Location, quality, severity, and onset of the pain, as well as the circumstances in which the child experiences the pain. Have the child point to the area where it hurts, or identify the location on a diagram or doll.
- Conditions, if any, that preceded the onset of pain and the conditions that followed the onset of pain
- Any associated symptoms, such as weight loss, fever, vomiting, or diarrhea, that may indicate a current illness.
- Any recent trauma, including any interventions that were used in an attempt to relieve the pain.

Continue the health history by inquiring about what the child wants others, including the nurse, to do when the child hurts. Conversely, ask the child what they don't want others to do. Finally, question the child about measures that seem to be most effective in relieving the pain. Ask if there is anything special the child wants to tell the nurse, such as a special pain relief technique or a specific comfort object.

If the child is experiencing chronic or recurrent pain, suggest the child and family record information in a symptom diary. Explain that this will be helpful in identifying the best ways to manage the pain.

Questioning the Parents

Parents play a key role in assessing pain in children. Often, it is the parents who provide information about the child's current and past experiences with pain. In addition, parents can provide information about how the child exhibits and responds to pain. Parents may be aware of subtle changes in the child's behavior that may precede the pain, occur with the pain, or indicate relief of pain. Including the parents in this process helps create a positive experience for all involved and promotes feelings of control over the situation.

The questions posed to the parents are similar in focus to those posed to the child. However, more detailed information may be obtained from the parents because they are usually able to describe events more fully or in greater detail owing to their higher cognitive level. Parents typically know their child best.

TAKE NOTE!

Parents may assume that nurses have greater expertise when it comes to assessing their child's pain and taking appropriate action. Thus, they may not always report when they notice changes suggesting that their child is uncomfortable. Emphasize the important role parents play in reporting any changes in their child so that pain relief measures can be instituted as soon as possible.

When questioning the parents, use the following examples as a guide for assessing the child's pain:

- Has your child ever been in pain before? If so, what was the cause of the pain? How long did they have the pain? Where was the pain located?
- How did your child react to the pain? What did you do to lessen the pain?
- Did your child let you know that they were in pain? Did they tell you or did you notice something?
- Are there any special signs that let you know that your child is hurting? If so, what are they?
- Is there anything that your child does or that you do when they are hurting that helps relieve the pain?
- Does one thing work better than another when your child is hurting?
- Is there any special information that you want to tell me about your child?

Using Pain Rating Scales

Various pain assessment, or pain rating, scales are available. These scales allow the child to report their pain, and the pain level is quantified. These standardized rating scales provide a greater alignment between the child's pain and the nurse's assessment of the severity of the pain. Self-report is the preferred source for the measurement of pain in verbal children (Gai et al., 2020). Self-report measures should be used in conjunction with observation and discussion with the child and family, especially in young children or in children with cognitive impairments (Hauer & Jones, 2021). Some children as young as 3 years of age can accurately use self-report tools to quantify their pain levels (Hauer & Jones, 2021). The reliability of these tools will increase as the child grows older and more cognitively mature. It is important to assess young children's ability to perform self-report tasks rather than rely solely on their chronologic age.

Many health care facilities have specific policies and procedures related to pain assessment, including the frequency of assessment, the rating tool to use, and nursing interventions to be instituted on the basis of the rating. For example, many facilities require assessment of the child using a specific tool with documentation at least once a shift and 30 minutes to 1 hour after a nonpharmacologic or pharmacologic pain relief intervention. This process provides a more objective method to determine whether the pain is increasing or decreasing and whether pain relief methods are effective.

TAKE NOTE!

Typically, different pain rating scales are appropriate for different developmental levels. However, children may regress when in pain, so a simpler tool may be needed to make sure that the child understands what is being asked. Regardless of the tool used, nurses need to be consistent in using the same tool so that appropriate comparisons can be made and effective interventions can be planned and implemented. Using the most appropriate tool consistently allows the most accurate assessment of the child's pain.

FACES Pain Rating Scale. The FACES pain rating scale (Fig. 36.3) is a self-report tool that is typically used in children 3 to 8 years of age (Hauer & Jones, 2021). The scale consists of six illustrations of faces arranged horizontally, with expressions ranging from smiling (indicating no hurt) to crying with frowning (indicating hurts worst). Under each face is a short description such as "hurts little bit" and a number. The number scale can be 0, 1, 2, 3, 4, and 5 or 0, 2, 4, 6, 8, and 10. The nurse explains the words associated with each face to the child. Then, the nurse asks the child to select the facial expression that best describes the level of pain they are feeling. The nurse then documents the number corresponding to the word description and face.

Oucher Pain Rating Scale. The Oucher pain rating scale is similar to the FACES scale in that it uses facial expressions to indicate increasing degrees of hurt. However, instead of illustrations, six photographs are used: "no hurt" is placed at the bottom of the arrangement and "most hurt" at the top. Alongside the photos is a scale ranging from 0 to 10 that corresponds to the facial expressions in the photographs (Fig. 36.4). After explaining the photos and numeric scale, the child is asked to point to the number that best describes their level of pain (Beyer et al., 1992).

This scale is useful for self-reporting of pain in children between 3 and 12 years of age (Beyer et al., 1992). Different versions have been developed for use with children of different racial and ethnic backgrounds (Beyer et al., 1992).

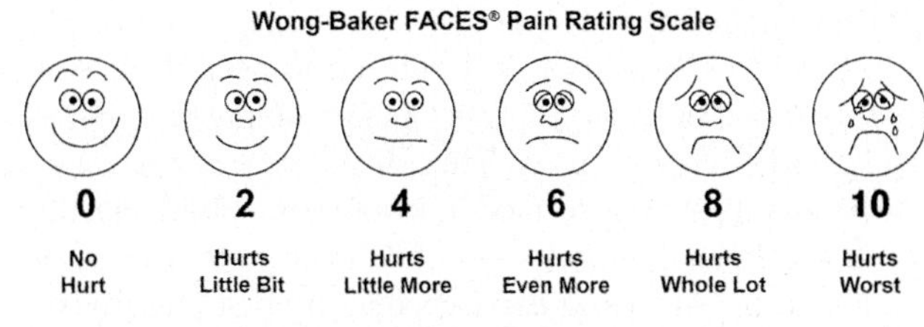

FIGURE 36.3 FACES pain rating scale. (Copyright © 1983 Wong-Baker FACES Foundation. www.WongBakerFACES.org. Used with permission. Originally published in Whaley & Wong's Nursing Care of Infants and Children. Copyright © Elsevier Inc.)

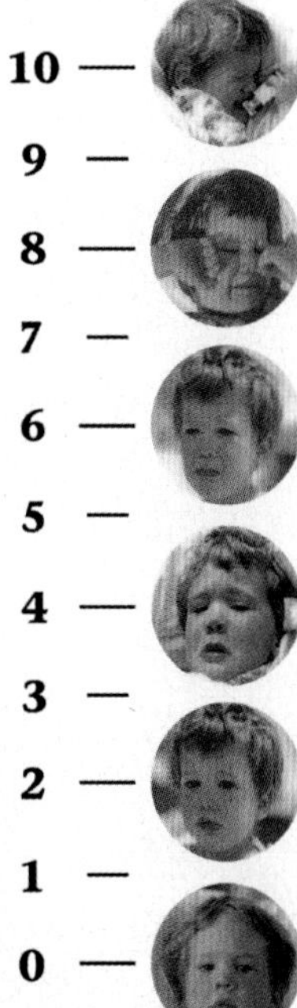

FIGURE 36.4 Oucher pain rating scale. (Reprinted with permission of Pain Associates in Nursing 2024.)

Poker Chip Tool. The poker chip tool, also known as the pieces of hurt tool, is a self-reporting pain assessment tool that uses four red poker chips to quantify the child's level of pain. The chips are arranged in a horizontal line on a surface in front of the child. Starting with the chip closest to the child's left side, the nurse points to the chip and explains that the first chip means a little hurt, the next chip means more hurt, the third chip means more hurt, and the fourth chip means the worst hurt ever. Then, the nurse asks the child how many "pieces of hurt" they are having (Fig. 36.5). If the child is not experiencing any pain, typically the child will state that they are not having any. When the child identifies the number of "pieces of hurt," the nurse follows up by asking the child to tell the nurse more about their hurt (Hester, 1979).

The poker chip tool is useful for assessing pain in preschool-age children and can be used in children 3 to 18 years of age (Thirion et al., 2015). Children may view this assessment tool as a game since it involves poker chips. However, the nurse needs to ensure that the child has the cognitive ability to distinguish the numbers.

TAKE NOTE!

Toddlers and preschoolers may not be used to being asked questions by strangers and may not understand quantitative ratings or estimation. Preschoolers will often construct an answer even if they do not understand the question. They will also often use extremes of scales, such as no pain or the worst pain (Thirion et al., 2015).

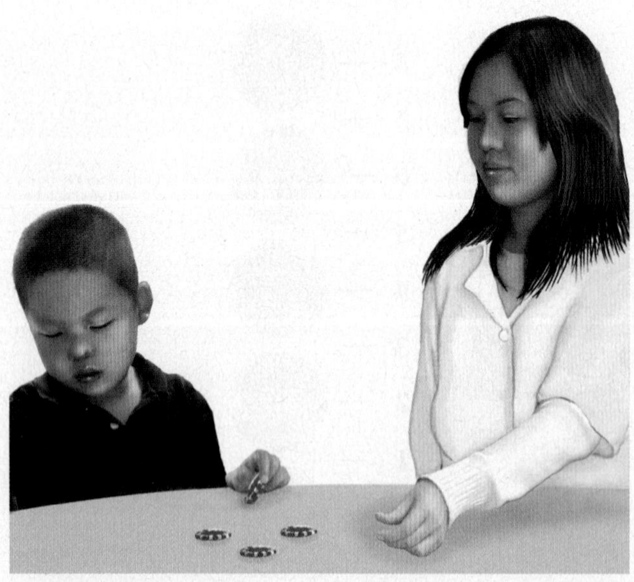

FIGURE 36.5 The poker chip tool. Here, the nurse asks the child to identify the number of chips that indicate their degree of "hurt."

Visual Analog and Numeric Scales. Visual analog and numeric scales involve a horizontal or vertical line with marked endpoints. With a visual analog scale, the endpoints are identified as no pain and worst pain. A numeric scale typically has endpoints of 0 and 10, reflecting no pain and worst pain, respectively (Fig. 36.6). The nurse explains the scale to the child. With the visual analog scale, the child makes a line that best describes the level of pain. The nurse then measures the distance from the "no pain" endpoint to the child's mark and records this as the pain score. With the numeric scale, the nurse asks the child to pick the number that best describes their level of pain.

The visual analog scale can be used in children 6 years or older (Zeltzer et al., 2020). The numeric scale can be used with children 7 years or older (Gai et al., 2020). Even though a younger child may be able to count and give numbers on the scale, they have not yet developed an understanding of the quantitative significance of the numbers.

Adolescent Pediatric Pain Tool. The Adolescent Pediatric Pain Tool is a multidimensional self-report type of tool useful for older children, usually between 8 and 17 years of age (Boitor et al., 2019). The tool involves three aspects of assessment. In the first assessment, the child identifies the location of the pain on two illustrations of the body—front and back views (Fig. 36.7).

The child is instructed to color the areas where they are hurting. The child is also instructed to color the area as big or as small as how much they are hurting. For example, if the hurt is mild or moderate, the child would color a moderate area of the location; if the pain is severe, they would color a much larger area. The second portion of the tool involves a scale that ranges from "no pain" to "worst possible pain." The nurse instructs the child to identify the severity of their pain. The third assessment is a list of words that may be used to describe pain, such as "throbbing,"

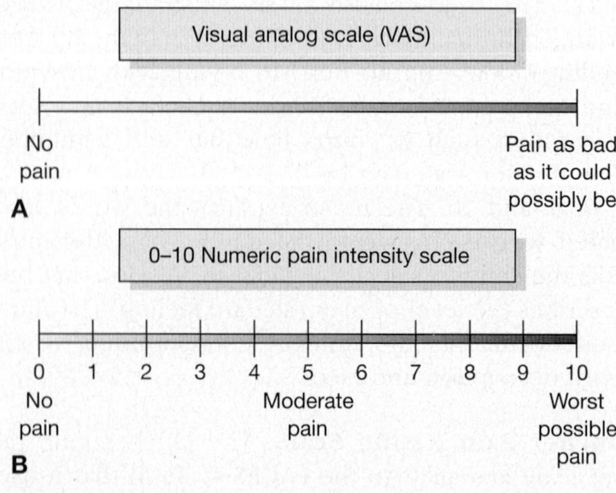

FIGURE 36.6 A. Visual analog scale. **B.** Numeric scale.

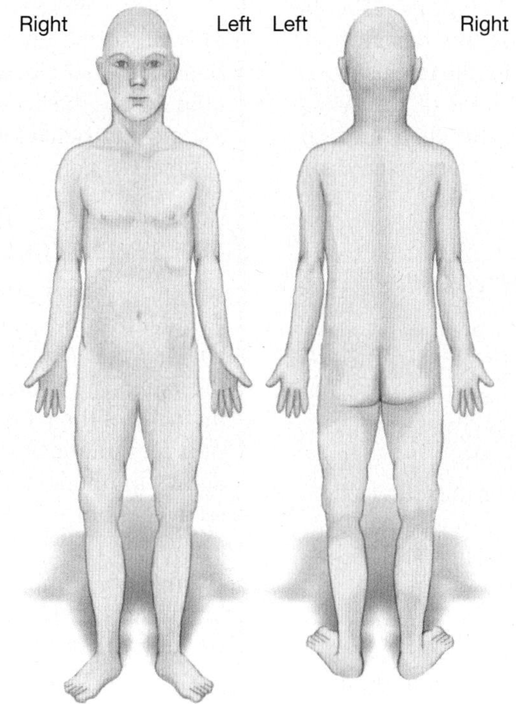

Sensory	**Affective**	**Evaluative**	**Temporal**
Aching ("pain all over")	Awful ("cannot do anything")	Annoying ("cannot sleep")	Always ("pain always there")
Hurting ("pain all over")	Crying ("hurts so bad")	Bad ("cannot stop the hurting")	Comes and goes ("always pain")
Sore ("like a cut")	Frightening ("scared it won't stop")	Miserable ("cannot sleep or do stuff")	Comes on all of a sudden ("no warning")
Beating (procedural pain "spots")	Screaming (afraid of "going to the hospital")	Terrible ("don't like it")	Constant ("never goes away")
Pounding ("gets on your nerves")	Terrifying ("cannot sleep," "really tired," "not going to live")	Uncomfortable ("can't stay in one spot")	Continuous ("pain not going away")
Cutting ("hurts more than a cut")		Uncontrollable ("cannot stop it")	Forever ("never will go away")
Like a sharp knife ("stabbing and sharp")	Dizzy ("don't know where I am")		Once in a while ("in a month sometimes pain; sometimes not")
Sharp (no meaning)			Sneaks up ("don't know when the pain will happen")
Stabbing (no meaning)			Sometimes ("goes away sometimes; sometimes not")
Cramping ("everywhere like a plane crash")			
Crushing (no meaning)			
Pressure ("pushing all over")			
Itching ("all over")			
Scratching ("helps sometimes")			
Shocking (pain "surprises" them)			
Splitting (body "splitting in half")			
Numb ("knows pain is there"/procedural pain)			
Stiff ("cannot move")			
Swollen ("meds do not help")			
Tight ("cannot move")			

FIGURE 36.7 Adolescent Pediatric Assessment Tool. (Top) Adolescent Pediatric Pain Tool (APPT): body outline. (Bottom) Pain Quality: Words chosen and meaning of words. (Used with permission from Crandall, M., & Savedra, M. [2005]. Multidimensional assessment using the adolescent pediatric pain tool: A case report. *Journal for Specialists in Pediatric Nursing*, *10*[3], 115–123. https://doi.org/10.1111/j.1744-6155.2005.00023.x)

"pounding," "stabbing," or "sharp." The nurse asks the child to point to or circle the words that describe the current pain. Children with limited reading skills or vocabulary may have difficulty with some of the words listed to describe pain. Work with the child and encourage the parents to help the child understand the various descriptive words.

THINKING ABOUT **DEVELOPMENT**

Kaylee Cooper is a 4-year-old with a fractured femur. She has been in traction since arriving in the emergency room last night. When you enter her room at the beginning of your shift, you note she is quiet and withdrawn. How will Kaylee's developmental stage affect the use of self-report? What special considerations must the nurse think about when using self-report of pain with Kaylee? What is the most appropriate pain rating scale for Kaylee?

Physical Examination

Physical examination of the child for pain primarily involves the skills of observation and inspection. These skills are used to assess for physiologic and behavioral changes that indicate pain. Auscultation may also be used to assess for changes in vital signs, specifically heart rate and blood pressure.

OBSERVE FOR MANIFESTATIONS OF PAIN

Observe for physical signs and symptoms of pain, keeping in mind the child's developmental level. Look for facial expressions of discomfort, grimacing, or crying. Be alert for movements that may suggest pain. For example, an infant or toddler may pull on the ear when experiencing ear pain. The child may move the head from side to side, suggesting head pain. Typically, children with abdominal pain will lie on one side and draw their knees up to the abdomen. Inspect the child's gait; a limp or avoidance of weight bearing may suggest leg pain. Immobility, guarding of a particular body area, or refusal to move an area may be observed. Inspect the skin for flushing or diaphoresis, possible indicators of pain. Also monitor vital signs for changes. Pulse or heart rate, respiratory rate, and blood pressure may increase. Other physiologic parameters that suggest pain may include elevated intracranial pressure and pulmonary vascular resistance and decreased oxygen saturation levels.

The child may also exhibit behavioral changes indicating pain. Be alert for irritability and restlessness. Watch for clenching of teeth or fists, body stiffening, or increased muscle tension. Note any changes in the child's behavior. For example, a child who was previously talkative and playful may become quiet and withdrawn in response to pain. Remember, a child in pain may sleep or play in order to cope with the pain. In addition, pay close attention to the child's cultural background and how these beliefs may be affecting the behavioral response to pain.

Each child is an individual with unique responses to pain, so the nurse must ensure that observations of behavior do indeed reflect the child's pain level. To help ensure the accuracy of observations, several physiologic and behavioral assessment tools have been developed to help quantify the observations.

USING PHYSIOLOGIC AND BEHAVIORAL PAIN ASSESSMENT TOOLS

Use of physiologic and behavioral pain assessment tools allows measurement of specific parameters and changes that would indicate that the child is experiencing pain. These measurements aid in determining the intensity of the pain experience. Along with the self-report pain rating scales, measurement of these changes allows the nurse to objectively assess pain and the effectiveness of pain management measures.

Premature Infant Pain Profile. The Premature Infant Pain Profile (PIPP) is an assessment tool that is useful for measuring pain in term or preterm neonates. It looks at behavioral indicators, such as facial expressions, and physiologic changes, such as changes in heart rate and oxygen saturation. It also takes into account gestational age. See Table 36.2. Each parameter is scored as 0, 1, 2, or 3. The score is then totaled, and the maximum score that can be achieved is 21. The higher the total score, the more intense the pain.

Neonatal Infant Pain Scale. The Neonatal Infant Pain Scale (NIPS) is a behavioral assessment tool that is useful for measuring pain in term and preterm neonates (Lawrence et al., 1993). Six parameters are measured: facial expression, cry, breathing patterns, arms, legs, and state of arousal (Table 36.3). Each parameter, except for cry, is scored as 0 or 1; cry is scored as 0, 1, or 2. The scores are then totaled, and the maximum score that can be achieved is 7. A higher score indicates increased pain.

Riley Infant Pain Scale. The Riley Infant Pain Scale (RIPS) is a behavioral assessment tool useful for infants who lack verbal ability (Schade et al., 1996). Like NIPS, RIPS measures six parameters: facial expression, body movement, sleep, verbal or vocal ability, consolability, and response to movements and touch (Table 36.4). Each parameter is scored as 0, 1, 2, or 3. The score is then totaled, and the maximum score that can be achieved is 18. The higher the total score, the more intense the pain.

Pain Observation Scale for Young Children. The Pain Observation Scale for Young Children (POCIS) is a behavioral assessment tool designed for use in children between 1 and 4 years of age (Boelen-van der Loo et al., 1999). This tool measures seven parameters: facial expression, cry, breathing, torso, arms and fingers, legs and toes, and state of arousal (Table 36.5).

TABLE 36.2 • Premature Infant Pain Profile (PIPP)

Parameter	Finding		Score
Gestational age	36 weeks or more		0
	32–35 weeks + 6 days		1
	28–31 weeks + 6 days		2
	<28 weeks		3
Observe infant for 15 seconds	Behavioral state	Active, awake, eyes open, facial movements	0
		Quiet, awake, eyes open, no facial movements	1
		Active, awake, eyes closed, facial movements	2
		Quiet, asleep, eyes closed, no facial movements	3
Observe baseline heart rate and O_2 saturation for 30 seconds	Maximum heart rate	0–4 bpm increase	0
		5–15 bpm increase	1
		15–24 bpm increase	2
		24 bpm increase	3
	Oxygen saturation	92%–100%	0
		89%–91%	1
		85%–88%	2
		84% or less	3
Observe infant's facial action for 30 seconds	Brow bulge	None	0
		Minimum	1
		Moderate	2
		Maximum	3
	Eye squeeze	None	0
		Minimum	1
		Moderate	2
		Maximum	3
	Nasolabial furrow	None	0
		Minimum	1
		Moderate	2
		Maximum	3

Adapted with permission from Stevens, B., Johnston, C., Petryshen, P., & Taddio, A. (1996). Premature infant pain profile: Development and initial validation. *Clinical Journal of Pain*, *12*(1), 13–22. https://doi.org/10.1097/00002508-199603000-00004

TABLE 36.3 • The Neonatal Infant Pain Scale (NIPS)

Parameter	Finding	Score
Facial expression	Relaxed (restful face; neutral expression)	0
	Grimace (tight facial muscles; furrowed brow, chin, or jaw; negative facial expression)	1
Cry	No cry (quiet; not crying)	0
	Whimper (mild intermittent moaning)	1
	Vigorous crying (loud screaming, shrill, continuous)	2
Breathing patterns	Relaxed	0
	Change in breathing (irregular; faster than usual; gagging; breath holding)	1
Arms	Relaxed (no muscular rigidity; occasional random movements of arm)	0
	Flexed/extended (tense, straight, rigid, or rapid flexion or extension)	1
Legs	Relaxed (no muscular rigidity; occasional random movements of leg)	0
	Flexed/extended (tense, straight, rigid, or rapid flexion or extension)	1
State of arousal	Sleeping/awake (quiet, peaceful; settled)	0
	Fussy (alert, restless, thrashing)	1

Copyright © 1989, Children's Hospital of Eastern Ontario. Adapted with permission.

TABLE 36.4 • The Riley Infant Pain Scale

Parameter	Score
Facial expression	
• Neutral/smiling	0
• Frowning/grimacing	1
• Clenched teeth	2
• Full cry expression	3
Body movement	
• Calm, relaxed	0
• Restless, fidgeting	1
• Moderate agitation or mobility; thrashing, flailing, incessant agitation or strong voluntary mobility	2
	3
• Voluntary immobility	
Sleep	
• Sleeping quietly with easy respirations	0
• Restless while asleep	1
• Sleeping intermittently (sleep/awake)	2
• Sleeping for prolonged periods of time interrupted by jerky movements or inability to sleep	3
Verbal/vocal	
• No cry	0
• Whimpering, complaining	1
• Pain crying	2
• Screaming, high-pitched cry	3
Consolability	
• Neutral	0
• Easy to console	1
• Not easy to console	2
• Inconsolable	3
Response to movement/touch	
• Moves easily	0
• Winces when touched or moved	1
• Cries out when moved or touched	2
• High-pitched cry or scream when touched or moved	3

Adapted with permission from Schade, J. G., Joyce, B. A., Gerkensmeyer, J., & Keck, J. F. (1996). Comparison of three preverbal scales for postoperative pain assessment in a diverse pediatric sample. *Journal of Pain and Symptom Management, 12*(6), 348–359. https://doi.org/10.1016/s0885-3924(96)00182-0

TABLE 36.5 • The Pain Observation Scale for Young Children (POCIS)

Parameter	Finding	Score
Facial expression	Neutral	0
	Grimace (negative)	1
Cry	No cry	0
	Moan, scream	1
Breathing	Relaxed and regular	0
	Irregular and indrawn	1
Torso	At rest, inactive	0
	Tense, shivering	1
Arms and fingers	At rest, inactive	0
	Tense, restless	1
Legs and toes	At rest, inactive	0
	Tense, restless	1
State of arousal	Calm, sleepy	0
	Fussy	1

Reprinted with permission from Boelen-van der Loo, W. J. C., Scheffer, E., de Haan, R. J., & de Groot, C. J. (1999). Clinimetric evaluation of the pain observation scale for young children in children aged between 1 and 4 years after ear, nose, and throat surgery. *Developmental and Behavioral Pediatrics, 20*(4):222–227. https://doi.org/10.1097/00004703-199908000-00004

Each parameter is scored as 0 or 1; the maximum score achievable is 7. The higher the score, the greater the pain being experienced by the child.

CRIES Scale for Neonatal Postoperative Pain Assessment. The CRIES scale is a behavioral assessment tool that also includes measures of physiologic parameters (Krechel & Bildner, 1995). It was developed to quantify postoperative pain in the newborn. The tool may also be used to monitor the infant's progress over time during recovery or after interventions. The tool assesses five parameters that create the "CRIES" acronym: *c*ry; oxygen *r*equired for saturation levels less than 95%; *i*ncreased vital signs; facial *e*xpression; and *s*leeplessness (Table 36.6). Each parameter is scored as 0, 1, or 2 and then totaled. As with other assessment tools, the higher the score, the greater the infant's pain.

r-FLACC Behavioral Scale for Pain in Nonverbal Young Children and Children With Cognitive Impairment. The original FLACC behavioral scale is a behavioral assessment tool that is useful in assessing a child's pain when the child cannot accurately report their level of pain (Merkel et al., 1997). It has been demonstrated to be a reliable tool for children from age 2 months to 7 years (Merkel et al., 1997). This tool measures five parameters that create the "FLACC" acronym: *f*acial expression, *l*egs, *a*ctivity, *c*ry, and *c*onsolability (Table 36.7). Observe the child with the legs and body uncovered. If the child is awake, observe them for 1 to 2 minutes; if sleeping, observe the child for 2 minutes or longer. Each parameter is scored as 0, 1, or 2. The scores are totaled, with a maximum achievable score of 10. As with other assessment tools, the higher the score, the greater the pain.

The revised FLACC (r-FLACC) is used in the same manner as the original FLACC, but it includes additional descriptors of behaviors most commonly associated with pain that have been validated in children with cognitive impairment (Hauer & Jones, 2021). Refer to Table 36.7. Pain assessment tools are a supplement to pain assessment and are not meant to replace caregiver or parent input. Review the descriptor terms with parents and caregivers, and individualize the scale by adding pain-related behaviors that are specific indicators of pain observed in the child in the appropriate categories (Hauer & Jones, 2021).

TABLE 36.6 • The Cries Scale for Neonatal Postoperative Pain Assessment

Assessment	0	1	2
Crying	No	High-pitched, but consolable	High-pitched, inconsolable
Oxygen required for saturation above 95%	No	<30%	>30%
Increased vital signs	Heart rate and blood pressure within 10% of preoperative values	Heart rate or blood pressure 11%–20% higher than preoperative values	Heart rate or blood pressure 21% or more above preoperative values
Expression	No grimace	Grimace	Grimace with grunt
Sleepless	No	Waking at frequent intervals	Constantly awake
Total infant score			

Reprinted with permission from Krechel, S. W., & Bildner, J. (1995). CRIES: A new neonatal postoperative pain measurement score. Initial testing of validity and reliability. *Paediatric Anaesthesia*, *5*, 53–61. https://doi.org/10.1111/j.1460-9592.1995.tb00242.x

Nursing Analysis

After recognizing and analyzing cues from a thorough assessment, the nurse may identify several hypotheses. The most commonly identified nursing hypotheses would be acute pain and, in some cases, chronic pain, such as in a child with prolonged illness or injury, from effects of cancer on surrounding tissues or from treatment-related effects. However, the related factors and defining characteristics can vary widely. Nursing hypotheses will focus on the effects of pain on the child; for example, the stress incurred as a result of the pain or the fear or anxiety associated with the pain or events causing the pain. Moreover, pain can affect physiologic functions, such as sleep, nutrition, mobility, and elimination. Examples of common nursing hypotheses may include:

- Acute pain
- Anxiety

TABLE 36.7 • rFLACC Behavioral Scale

		SCORE (circle most appropriate)
FACE	0=No particular expression or smile	**0**
	1=Occasional grimace/frown; withdrawn or disinterested; **appears sad or worried**	**1**
	2=Consistent grimace or frown; Frequent/constant quivering chin, clenched jaw; **Distressed-looking face; Expression of fright or panic**	**2**
	Individual behavior: ______	
LEGS	0=Normal position or relaxed; Usual tone & motion to limbs	**0**
	1=Uneasy, restless, tense; **occasional tremors**	**1**
	2=Kicking, or legs drawn up; **marked increase in spasticity, constant tremors or jerking**	**2**
	Individual behavior: ______	
ACTIVITY	0=Lying quietly, normal position, moves easily; Regular, rhythmic respirations	**0**
	1=Squirming, shifting back and forth, tense or guarded movements; **mildly agitated (eg. head back & forth, aggression); Shallow, splinting respirations, intermittent sighs.**	**1**
	2=Arched, rigid or jerking; **severe agitation; head banging; shivering (not rigors); Breath holding, gasping or sharp intake of breaths, severe splinting**	**2**
	Individual behavior: ______	
CRY	0=No cry	**0**
	1=Moans or whimpers; **occasional complaint; occasional verbal outburst or grunt**	**1**
	2=Crying steadily, screams or sobs, frequent complaints; **repeated outbursts, constant grunting**	**2**
	Individual behavior: ______	
CONSOLABILITY	0=Content and relaxed	**0**
	1=Reassured by occasional touching, hugging or being talked to. Distractable	**1**
	2=Difficult to console or comfort; **pushing away caregiver, resisting care or comfort measures**	**2**
	Individual behavior: ______	
		Total:

Copyright © 2002, The Regents of the University of Michigan. All rights reserved.

- Risk of constipation
- Deficient knowledge
- Sleep deprivation
- Risk of injury

The foregoing hypotheses provide suggestions for nursing care planning or concept mapping. The nurse will then generate solutions by planning interventions (suggested further on with rationales). The plan of care should be individualized, based on the child's and family's needs.

Goal/Outcome

When caring for a child experiencing pain, the ultimate goal is that the child will be free of pain, as evidenced by participation in age-appropriate activities of daily living and vital signs within age-appropriate parameters. However, at times, this may be unrealistic, especially if the child is experiencing chronic pain. Therefore, a more appropriate and realistic goal would be that the child reports that their pain has decreased to a tolerable level. Pain assessment tools can be used to quantify the amount by which the child's pain has decreased. For example, if the child has rated the pain as 7 out of 10, a realistic goal might be that the child reports a pain rating of no more than 4 out of 10. Additional goals would reflect improvement or resolution of the identified problem. For example, a short-term goal for a child experiencing disturbed sleep due to pain might be that the child sleeps for a minimum of 4 consecutive hours through the night. A long-term goal might be that the child sleeps for 7 to 8 hours undisturbed through the night.

Interventions

Various interventions can be used for pain management. These interventions include nonpharmacologic and pharmacologic measures. A guiding principle when caring for the child experiencing pain is the provision of atraumatic care (see Chapter 30 for more information). For example, cognitive and behavioral approaches are appropriate for pain management, including pain management related to procedures. In addition to nonpharmacologic measures, pharmacologic measures may be appropriate for pain management. For example, applying a topical anesthetic cream to a site early enough before a venipuncture can be effective. Another example is to use an intermittent infusion device to obtain multiple blood specimen samples rather than perform repeated venipunctures. In addition, it is a good idea to consider the use of sedation for more painful procedures.

Throughout the child's care, be sure to discuss specific goals and interventions with the child and family as appropriate. Include the family in developing appropriate interventions so they can continue to support the child. Education of the child and family about interventions, including various therapies, is key. Ongoing assessment is needed to determine the effectiveness of the pain relief measures in achieving the desired goals.

The previously listed hypotheses provide suggestions for nursing care planning or concept mapping. The nurse will then generate solutions by planning interventions (suggested next with rationales). The plan of care should be individualized, based on the child's and family's needs. Specific information related to pain management and the nurse's role will be discussed later in the chapter.

Nursing Analysis

Acute pain related to physical or biologic injury agents (such as invasive procedures, surgery, recent trauma, or infection) as evidenced by pain rating scale, facial grimacing, crying, irritability, withdrawal activity, or changes in vital signs.

Goal/Outcome

Child will achieve adequate comfort level, as evidenced by a decrease in rating number on a pain rating scale, quietness, calm resting behaviors, decrease in crying and irritability, and vital signs within acceptable parameters.

Promoting Pain Relief (interventions with *rationale*)

- Assess pain level using a developmentally appropriate pain rating tool *to establish a baseline.*
- Assess for verbal and nonverbal indicators of pain *to help determine child's pain level;* question parents about child's typical behaviors and previous experiences with pain *to determine factors that may be influencing child's response to pain.*
- Institute nonpharmacologic methods for pain control based on the child's age and cognitive level *to help decrease pain;* encourage parental participation in use of methods *to provide additional support and pain relief for the child.*
- Administer pharmacologic agents as ordered using the least traumatic route possible *to alter pain impulse transmission and minimize distress while promoting effective pain relief.*
- Explain the action of the drug and what the child should expect from the medication at a level that the child can understand *to promote trust and reduce fear while providing effective pain relief.*
- Give analgesics around the clock if pain is continuous and can be predicted *to maintain steady blood levels of the drug, thereby maximizing the drug's effect.*
- Perform atraumatic care at all times *to minimize the child's exposure to physical and psychological distress and pain.*
- Anticipate timing of procedures or situations that may lead to pain, and provide appropriate analgesic therapy as ordered *to ensure therapy is most effective at the time of the procedure.*
- Ensure the child's environment is quiet and conducive to rest, dim the lights, and close the door or

curtain *to reduce sensory overload that would increase the child's pain sensation.*
- Encourage the parents to stroke, touch, caress, and hold the child *to reduce discomfort and promote feelings of security.*
- Reassess the child's pain level after use of nonpharmacologic and pharmacologic methods *to determine effectiveness;* anticipate the need to modify or adapt nonpharmacologic methods or adjust analgesic dosage, route, or frequency *to promote maximum pain relief.*
- Perform nursing care activities after administering analgesics *to prevent exacerbating the child's pain.*
- Use diversional activities, distraction, and play appropriate to the child's age and cognitive level *to promote additional pain relief.*

Nursing Analysis
Anxiety related to stress and unmet needs (such as uncertainty of the situation; unknown cause of pain; lack of familiarity with procedures, testing, and health care facility; and painful procedures), as evidenced by crying, irritability, withdrawal, and/or stoic or aggressive behaviors

Goal/Outcome
Child and family will demonstrate a decrease in anxiety level, as evidenced by age-appropriate positive coping behaviors, verbalization of feelings, playing out of feelings, child and family cooperation with plan of care, and absence of signs and symptoms associated with escalating anxiety.

Minimizing Anxiety (interventions with *rationale*)
- Assess child's and parents' understanding of the situation, including their understanding of what may be causing the pain and the reasons for the procedures and testing *to provide baseline information about the child's and parents' knowledge and possible causes of anxiety.*
- Spend time with the child and parents discussing what they think might be happening, encouraging the child and parents to talk openly about their feelings to facilitate continued expressions and communication. Allow time for questions, and answer questions honestly *to establish rapport and build trust.*
- Approach the child and family in a calm, relaxed manner *to foster trust and communication and decrease anxiety.*
- Allow the child options related to interventions as much as possible, such as fluids to drink or snacks to eat, extremity to use for venipuncture (right or left), color of bandage, or holding tape or dressing, *to foster feelings of control.*
- Provide atraumatic care *to reduce exposure to distress, which would exacerbate the child's anxiety level.*
- Explain any procedures, tests, or activities at a level the child can understand *to reduce fear of the unknown.*
- Incorporate aspects of the child's routine at home as much as possible *to reduce feelings of separation and promote feelings of normalcy.*
- Ensure consistency in care *to facilitate trust and acceptance.*
- Encourage parents to use comfort measures such as stroking, cuddling, holding, and rocking *to promote feelings of security and minimize stress.*
- Provide positive reinforcement for choices, participation in activities, and use of appropriate coping methods *to foster self-esteem.*
- Encourage the child's participation in play (unstructured and therapeutic play as needed) *to promote expression of feelings and fears.*

Nursing Analysis
Risk of constipation; risk factors include decrease in GI motility (a side effect of some pain medications is decreased motility and hard, dry stools), and average daily physical activity is less than recommended for age (limited mobility due to pain).

Goal/Outcome
Child will pass soft bowel movements on a regular basis without pain or straining.

Preventing Constipation (interventions with *rationale*)
- Palpate for abdominal distention, percuss for dullness, and auscultate for bowel sounds *to assess for signs of constipation.*
- Encourage adequate fluid intake *to soften the stool.*
- Encourage adequate fiber intake: *fiber helps increase stool bulk and increase movement through the GI tract.*
- Administer medications as ordered *to keep stool moving on a regular basis.*
- Encourage activity as tolerated; *immobility contributes to constipation.*

Nursing Analysis
Deficient knowledge related to insufficient information or knowledge of resources (about current condition and appropriate methods for managing pain), as evidenced by crying, irritability, pushing away, and questions and verbalizations about pain and relief methods

Goal/Outcome
The child and parents will demonstrate adequate knowledge about the child's current condition and use of pain relief methods, as evidenced by statements about the cause of the child's pain, demonstration of chosen nonpharmacologic relief methods, use of pharmacologic agents, and statements related to signs and symptoms of increased and decreased pain.

Educating the Child and Family (interventions with *rationale*)

- Assess the child's and parents' knowledge and understanding of the child's current condition and current pain level *to establish a baseline for teaching.*
- Provide time for the child and parents to ask questions; answer questions honestly and in terms they can understand *to promote learning.*
- Explain in simplified terms how the child's condition is associated with pain or the rationale for procedures needed that may contribute to pain *to promote understanding and foster trust.*
- Teach in short sessions *to prevent overloading the child and parents with information.*
- Provide reinforcement and rewards *to help facilitate the teaching and learning process.*
- Use multiple modes of learning, such as written information, verbal instruction, demonstrations, and media when possible, *to facilitate learning and retention of information.*
- Instruct the parents and child as appropriate in nonpharmacologic methods for pain relief; encourage practice and participation by parents in methods chosen *to foster independence and use of method when necessary.*
- Teach the child as appropriate and parents about pharmacologic methods for pain relief; review specific information about the drug to be used, including action, duration, administration, possible adverse effects, and care necessary when the drug is used, *to promote learning;* have the child and parents report back information or demonstrate administration *to evaluate effectiveness of teaching.*
- Provide parents with written information about pain relief methods for use at home if indicated *to allow for reference at a later date.*

Nursing Analysis

Sleep deprivation related to prolonged discomfort (inability to manage pain effectively), as evidenced by frequent waking during the night; signs and symptoms of pain, including irritability and restlessness; statements about being tired; and pain rating scale remaining the same

Goal/Outcome

The child will exhibit increased ability to sleep during the night, as evidenced by increasing periods of calm and restfulness (initially starting at 2 hours and gradually increasing to 7 to 8 hours), decreased pain level on pain rating scale, and statements of decreased fatigue.

Promoting Sleep and Rest (interventions with *rationale*)

- Assist the child in using nonpharmacologic methods of pain relief, such as imagery, distraction, and muscle relaxation, *to promote relaxation.*
- Administer pharmacologic pain relief as ordered *to minimize pain interfering with sleep;* anticipate a change in drug therapy if pain relief is inadequate.
- Cluster nursing care activities *to minimize energy expenditure and disruptions in the child's ability to rest.*
- Help the child with a nighttime routine similar to one they use at home *to promote feelings of security.*
- Offer the child a back rub, warm bath, or warm liquids; reading a story; or listening to music *to facilitate relaxation;* provide stroking, hugging, cuddling, rocking, and light touch *to promote a sense of security and calm.*
- Dim the lights and close the curtain or door to the room *to provide a quiet, restful environment.*
- Ensure around-the-clock pain relief for the child through the night *to minimize the risk of pain.*

Nursing Analysis

Risk of injury; risk factors include unsafe mode of transport and alteration in cognitive and psychomotor functioning (possible adverse effects of analgesics).

Goal/Outcome

Child will remain free of any injury related to signs and symptoms of adverse effects of analgesic therapy, as evidenced by respiratory rate appropriate for age and no complaints of GI upset; dizziness; or sedation; or episodes of constipation, nausea, vomiting, or pruritus.

Promoting Safety (interventions with *rationale*)

- Ensure the child's call light is within reach *to allow for notification of health care personnel should the child need assistance.*
- Administer analgesic exactly as prescribed *to reduce the risk of error and development of adverse effects.*
- Assess the child's respiratory status closely for changes *to allow for early detection of respiratory depression.*
- If an opioid analgesic is being given, have naloxone readily available *to reverse the action of the narcotic if respiratory depression occurs.*
- Monitor appetite and assess bowel sounds for changes; note any abdominal distention or decreased bowel sounds, which would suggest decreased peristalsis, *to allow for early detection of constipation.*
- Ensure adequate fluid and fiber intake *to reduce risk of constipation.*
- Offer small frequent meals and give medication with food *to minimize the risk of GI upset.*
- Assess for nausea and vomiting; if necessary, withhold food and fluids *to rest the GI tract,* and administer antiemetics until nausea and vomiting resolve *to decrease nausea and vomiting.*
- Instruct the child to remain in bed after receiving analgesic, raise crib or side rails as appropriate, and instruct the child and parents to have someone

accompany the child to the bathroom, if allowed, *to reduce the risk of falls from sedation.*
- Assess for complaints of itching, and observe for rash or reddened areas; if pruritus occurs, urge the child not to scratch, and expect to administer an antihistamine as ordered *to reduce pruritus.*
- Provide the child with distraction *to assist in helping reduce the effects of pruritus.*

TAKE NOTE!

The National Database of Nursing Quality Indicators (NDNQI) was established by the American Nurses Association to evaluate nursing-sensitive care. One indicator that can help improve pain management is the pediatric pain assessment, intervention, and reassessment (AIR) cycle (NDNQI, n.d.).

Remember Aiden, the 6-year-old introduced at the beginning of the chapter? The nurse reporting off duty states, "Aiden's parents keep requesting pain medication for him. They say he's complaining of pain most of the time. I'm not sure if I believe them; when I see Aiden, he's playing video games or watching television and seems to be fine. I've tried to hold off on his pain medication as long as I can." When you enter Aiden's room, he is crying and says his leg hurts. What will be your initial action? What will be your plan of care to manage Aiden's pain (refer to the QUESTT assessment)? How would you address the statements made by the nurse in report? What approaches can you use to change staff behavior about pain management?

MANAGEMENT OF PAIN

Management of pain begins with assessment of the child's comfort level. If pain or the potential for pain, such as that caused by an invasive procedure, is identified, steps must be taken to minimize or treat the pain. Three general principles guide pain management in children:

1. Individualize interventions based on the amount of pain experienced and the child's characteristics, such as developmental level, temperament, previous pain experience, and coping strategies.
2. Use nonpharmacologic and pharmacologic approaches to ease or eliminate the pain.
3. Teach the child and family about pain relief interventions and techniques, and discuss with the child and family expectations of pain management.

Specific strategies for pain management include nonpharmacologic interventions, such as relaxation, distraction, and guided imagery, and pharmacologic interventions, such as analgesics, patient-controlled analgesia, local analgesia, epidural analgesia, and moderate sedation.

Nonpharmacologic Management

Various techniques may be available to assist in managing mild pain in children or to augment the effectiveness of medications for moderate or severe pain. Many of these nonpharmacologic techniques assist children in coping with pain and give them an opportunity to feel a sense of mastery or control over the situation. Two types of techniques are cognitive behavioral strategies and biophysical strategies. It is important to involve the parents in the process when using these techniques.

Behavioral Cognitive Strategies

Behavioral cognitive strategies for pain management involve measures that require the child to focus on a specific area rather than the pain. These strategies help change the interpretation of the painful stimuli, reducing pain perception or making pain more tolerable. In addition, these strategies help decrease negative attitudes, thoughts, and anxieties, thereby improving the child's coping mechanisms. Use of these strategies before procedures has resulted in decreased anxiety and has improved the transition to sedation and may result in a decreased amount of medication needed for sedation (Cravero & Roback, 2022). Typically, these interventions work well with older children, but younger children also benefit from these techniques if they are adapted to the child's age and developmental level. Common behavioral cognitive strategies include relaxation, distraction, imagery, biofeedback, thought stopping, and positive self-talk.

RELAXATION

Relaxation aids in reducing muscle tension and anxiety. A wide variety of techniques can be used. Relaxation can be as simple as holding an infant or young child closely while stroking the child or speaking in a soft soothing manner or having the child inhale and exhale slowly using rhythmically controlled deep breathing. It can also involve more sophisticated techniques such as progressive relaxation. With this technique, the child is asked to focus on one area of the body and let that body part go limp. Then, in an organized fashion, usually working from the toes to the head or vice versa, the child is asked to focus on another body part, making it go limp. Eventually, the exercises work through all body areas, leading to relaxation of the entire body.

DISTRACTION

Distraction involves having the child focus on another stimulus, thereby attempting to shield them from pain. Research has shown distraction to be associated with lower parental perception of pain and distress in younger children and decreased situational anxiety in older children (Cravero & Roback, 2022).

This technique does not eliminate the pain but can help to make it more tolerable. Various methods can be used for distraction, including:

- Counting
- Repeating specific phrases or words, such as "ouch"
- Listening to music or singing
- Playing games, including video games
- Blowing bubbles or blowing pinwheels or party favors
- Listening to or reading favorite stories (Fig. 36.8)
- Watching cartoons, television shows, or movies
- Playing on mobile devices
- Visiting with friends
- Humor

Humor has been demonstrated to be an effective distracting technique for pain management (Osincup, 2020; Strean, 2009). However, be sure to use an age-appropriate technique and to determine what or who will make the child laugh. If possible, allow the child and their family to choose the materials that they consider humorous.

The type of distraction used depends on the age of the child. For example, a younger child may enjoy blowing pinwheels and blowing bubbles. They also may enjoy listening to favorite stories or books. Older children may enjoy computer or video games, listening to favorite music, or visiting with friends.

• • • ATRAUMATIC CARE • • •

Play therapy may be helpful in allowing the child to express their feelings and adapt to the stressors of the current situation.

IMAGERY

Imagery involves the use of the imagination to create a mental image. This mental image is usually a positive, pleasurable image, but it doesn't need to be real. The child is encouraged to include details and sensations that are associated with the image, such as specific descriptions of the image, colors, sounds, feelings, and smells. In some instances, the child may write down or record the image on a tape or compact disc. When pain occurs, the child is encouraged to create the mental image or read or listen to the description.

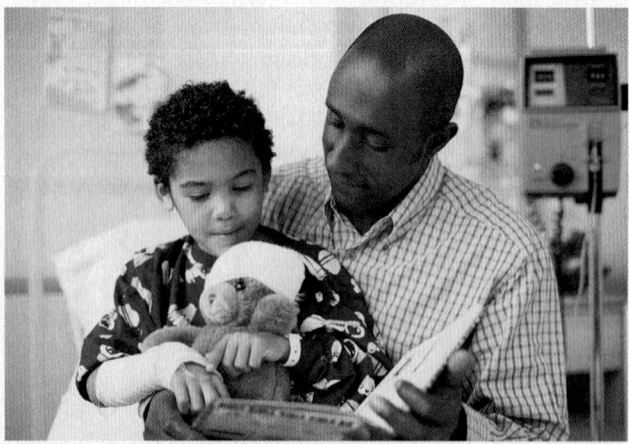

FIGURE 36.8 A child using distraction for pain management.

BIOFEEDBACK

Biofeedback involves having the child gain an awareness of their body functions and learn ways to modify them voluntarily. The child is usually taught specific skills about how to modify body functions using an apparatus that measures pain-related changes in muscle tone or physiologic data, such as blood pressure or pulse rate. This teaching is usually performed by a specialized health care provider and occurs over several sessions in advance of the pain experience. With practice, the child learns to control the changes without the apparatus. This technique can be used by older children, such as adolescents, who can concentrate for longer periods of time.

THOUGHT STOPPING

Thought stopping involves substituting a pleasurable or positive thought for the painful experience. Examples of positive thoughts might be, "It's only for a short time" or "It's important so I get better." The negative component of the pain is not ignored or suppressed; rather, it is transformed into something positive. Thought stopping can also involve the use of short, positive phrases. For example, the child may repeat "quick stick, feel better, go home soon" when they anticipate or experience pain.

Thought stopping is a useful method for reducing anxiety before and during events associated with pain. Children can be taught to use this technique anytime they experience anxiety related to a painful experience. Doing so helps promote the child's sense of control over the situation.

POSITIVE SELF-TALK

Positive self-talk is similar to thought stopping in that it involves the use of positive statements. With positive self-talk, the child is taught to say positive statements when they are experiencing pain. For example, the child may be taught to say, "I will feel better and be able to go home and play with my friends."

Biophysical Interventions

Biophysical interventions focus on interfering with the transmission of pain impulses reaching the brain. The interventions involve some type of cutaneous stimulation near the site of the pain. This stimulation decreases the ability of the A-delta and C fibers to transmit pain impulses. Examples of biophysical interventions include application of heat and cold, massage and pressure, and transcutaneous electrical nerve stimulation (TENS).

SUCKING AND SUCROSE

Sucking is a behavior from which infants derive satisfaction. Therefore, nonnutritive sucking (NNS) (e.g., sucking a pacifier) can be used to reduce pain behaviors in neonates undergoing painful procedures. In addition, infants show reduced pain behaviors after ingestion of sucrose or other sweet-tasting solutions, such as glucose, during single-event procedures, such as heel lancing (Roué, 2022). Optimal dosing for sucrose needs further research, and caution must be used in extremely low–birth-weight infants and infants with unstable blood glucose levels. Combining nonpharmacologic measures such as NNS, oral sucrose, skin-to-skin contact, and swaddling has been shown to increase the analgesic effectiveness of measures used alone (Roué, 2022). See Evidence-Based Practice 36.1.

• • • ATRAUMATIC CARE • • •

Breastfeeding is also a noninvasive, natural, and feasible way to use sucking to reduce pain in infants.

HEAT AND COLD APPLICATIONS

Heat and cold applications alter physiologic mechanisms associated with pain. Cold results in vasoconstriction and alters capillary permeability, leading to a decrease in edema at the site of the injury. Owing to vasoconstriction, blood flow is reduced, and the release of pain-producing substances such as histamine and serotonin is also decreased. Moreover, transmission of painful stimuli via peripheral nerve fibers is decreased.

Heat results in vasodilation and increases blood flow to the area. It also leads to a decrease in nociceptive stimulation and removal of chemical substances that can stimulate nociceptive fibers. The increase in blood flow alters capillary permeability, leading to a reduction in swelling and pressure on nociceptive nerve fibers. Heat may also trigger the release of endogenous opioids, which mediate the pain response.

MASSAGE AND PRESSURE

Massage and pressure, like other biophysical interventions, are believed to inhibit stimulation of the A-delta and C fibers. These methods are helpful in relaxing muscles and reducing tension. In addition, these techniques can aid in distracting the child. Massage can be as simple as rubbing a body part or pressing on an area such as an injection site for about 10 seconds. It can also be more involved, requiring the use of another person to perform the massage. Lotion or ointment can be used during the massage and may provide a comforting effect. Contralateral pressure or massage of the opposite area may be used, especially if the area of pain cannot be accessed or if the affected area is too painful to touch.

A more formal method of pressure application is acupressure. In acupressure, the fingertip, the thumb, or a blunt instrument is used to apply gentle, firm pressure to specifically designated sites to control pain. The pressure may be applied in one motion followed by releasing, in a circular motion for several minutes and then releasing, or with a vibrating motion using the fingertips. The motion of applying and then releasing pressure is thought to facilitate the release of endogenous endorphins and enkephalins.

EVIDENCE-BASED PRACTICE 36.1

What Is the Effect of the Use of Swaddling and Sucrose on the Intensity of Pain in Neonates During Venous Blood Sampling?

Neonates who are hospitalized undergo numerous painful experiences. It is well established that neonates feel pain. Pain in neonates has been found to have short- and long-term effects on the neonates' behavioral and neurologic development. Nonpharmacologic interventions used to decrease neonatal procedural pain include swaddling, NNS, sucrose, breastfeeding, and skin-to-skin contact. Some evidence has shown that combining sucrose with other nonpharmacologic interventions can be more effective than sucrose ingestion alone. This study aimed to evaluate the effectiveness of swaddling and sucrose ingestion on pain intensity during venous blood sampling.

STUDY

This study was a clinical trial. Sixty term infants were randomly divided into four groups. The first group was swaddled before blood sampling; the second group had sucrose administered; the third group was swaddled and given sucrose; and the fourth group was the control group.

Findings

The results showed that neonatal pain intensity mean scores during and after blood sampling were significantly different between the groups, with the control group having the highest scores. The results showed that pain intensity was lower in the intervention groups versus the control group and that the combined sucrose and swaddle group scores were lower than either intervention alone.

Nursing Implications

The use of swaddle and sucrose together is a safe and effective way to decrease procedural pain in neonates. Nurses should consider combining nonpharmacologic interventions with sucrose administration when performing painful procedures in neonates. More randomized controlled trials or well-designed studies are needed. Further research is warranted to determine safe and effective concentration, dosing, and dosing intervals of sucrose in the neonatal population.

Data from Talebi, M., Amiri, S. R. J., Roshan, P. A., Zabihi, A., Zahedpasha, Y., & Chehrazi, M. (2022). The effect of concurrent use of swaddle and sucrose on the intensity of pain during venous blood sampling in neonate: a clinical trial study. *BMC Pediatrics, 22*(1), 263. https://doi.org/10.1186/s12887-022-03323-0

The techniques of pressure and massage are easy to learn and use and can be taught to children and parents.

The Nurse's Role in Nonpharmacologic Pain Intervention

The nurse plays a major role in teaching the child and family about nonpharmacologic pain interventions. Help the child and family choose the most appropriate and most effective methods, and ensure that the child and parents use the methods before pain occurs as well as before the pain increases. Teaching Guidelines 36.1 lists some helpful instructions for the parents and child about nonpharmacologic pain management.

It is also important to assist the child and parents when using the technique in order to make sure that they are using the technique correctly. Offer suggestions for modifications or adaptations as necessary.

Parents are important to the pain management program. Give them the option to stay with the child, or let them know that someone else will support the child if they opt not to stay. Offer simple, concrete ways to assist and help the child manage pain. Many of the nonpharmacologic techniques can be done by parents, and children may respond better if their parents demonstrate the technique and encourage them to use it. Invite parents to participate in decisions as well as act as a coach to their child during procedures. Prepare the parents, and explain the most appropriate pain management approaches and strategies. Discuss the type and amount of pain expected as well as the potential complications associated with pain management approaches. Ask how the parent predicts the child will react to a painful situation. Finally, offer techniques and strategies to the parents as they act as the coach during these situations.

Although parents want to help their children and some are able to act as coaches, the responses of the child and parent to pain and stress and to different interventions are highly variable. Some children appear to be soothed by their parents' actions; others appear to become distressed. The nurse must be alert to these reactions and provide necessary support and education to ensure effectiveness of pain-relieving interventions.

TEACHING GUIDELINES **36.1** Teaching Nonpharmacologic Pain Management

- Review the methods available, and choose the method(s) that you and your child find best for your situation.
- Learn to identify the ways in which your child shows pain or demonstrates they are anxious about the possibility of pain. For example, do they get restless, make a face, or get flushed in the face?
- Begin using the technique chosen before your child experiences pain or when your child first indicates they are anxious about or beginning to experience pain.
- Practice the technique with your child, and encourage the child to use the technique when they feel anxious about pain or anticipate that a procedure or experience will be painful.
- Perform the technique with your child. For example, take the deep breath in and out or blow bubbles with them; listen to music or play a game with your child.
- Avoid using terms such as "hurt" or "pain" that suggest or cause your child to expect pain.
- Use descriptive terms like "pushing," "pulling," "pinching," or "heat."
- Avoid overly descriptive or biased statements such as "This will really hurt a lot" or "This will be terrible."
- Stay with your child as much as possible; speak softly and gently stroke or cuddle your child.
- Offer praise, positive reinforcement, hugs, and support for using the technique even if it was not effective.

Pharmacologic Management

Pharmacologic interventions involve the administration of drugs for pain relief. Administration may occur using a wide variety of methods. The selection of the method is determined by the drug being administered; the child's status; the type, intensity, and location of the pain; and any factors that may be influencing the child's pain. Research overwhelmingly supports the appropriate use of analgesics to reduce pain perception in children.

Medications Used for Pain Management

Analgesics (medications for pain relief) typically fall into one of two categories—nonopioid analgesics and opioid analgesics. The choice of analgesic medication is based on the child's pain intensity and the child's response to previously administered pain medications (Hauer & Jones, 2021). In general, mild pain can be treated with nonopioid medications, while moderate to severe pain may require opioid medications. Anesthetics may also be used. Drugs such as sedatives and hypnotics may be used as adjuvant medications to help minimize anxiety or provide or assist with pain relief when typical analgesics are ineffective.

NONOPIOID ANALGESICS

Nonopioid analgesics include acetaminophen and nonsteroidal antiinflammatory drugs (NSAIDs) such as ibuprofen, ketorolac, naproxen, and indomethacin (Drug Guide 36.1). These agents may be used to treat mild to moderate pain, often for conditions such as arthritis; joint, bone, and muscle pain; headache; dental pain; and menstrual pain. Acetaminophen and ibuprofen are also commonly used to treat fever in children.

DRUG GUIDE 36.1

COMMON DRUGS FOR PAIN MANAGEMENT

Drug	Actions/Indications	Nursing Implications
Acetaminophen (Tylenol)	Possible inhibition of cyclo-oxygenase in the central nervous system Direct action on hypothalamic heat-regulating center Mild to moderate pain, fever, arthritis, musculoskeletal pain, headache	• Administer orally, rectally, or intravenously. • Maximum daily dose ≤ 75 mg/kg/day in ≤ 5 divided doses (not to exceed 4,000 mg/day). • Do not exceed five intravenous doses or 60 mg/kg/day of drug in 24 hours. • Caution parents to read labels of other over-the-counter (OTC) drugs carefully; some may contain acetaminophen and, if given in conjunction, may lead to overdose and toxicity.
Ibuprofen (Motrin, Advil)	Inhibition of prostaglandin synthesis Mild to moderate pain, fever, treatment of inflammatory diseases	• Administer orally. • Give with food or after meals if GI upset occurs. • Assess for easy bruising, bleeding gums, or frank or occult blood in urine or stool. • Monitor for nausea, vomiting, GI upset, diarrhea or constipation, dizziness, or drowsiness. • Caution parents to read labels of OTC medications closely; some may contain ibuprofen or other NSAIDs and, if given in conjunction, may lead to overdose.
Other NSAIDs: ketorolac (Toradol), diclofenac (Voltaren), indomethacin (Indocin), naproxen (Naprosyn, Aleve)	Inhibition of prostaglandin synthesis Moderate to severe pain	• Administer oral form with food or after meals if GI upset occurs. • Monitor for headache, dizziness, nausea, vomiting, constipation, or diarrhea. • Assess for signs and symptoms of bleeding, such as bruising, epistaxis, gingival bleeding, or frank or occult blood in urine or stool. • Naproxen is also available in combination products (caution parents to read OTC labels carefully). • When administering indomethacin intravenously, report oliguria or anuria. • Diclofenac may also be given rectally.
Opioid agents: morphine, fentanyl (Sublimaze, Duragesic), hydromorphone (Dilaudid), oxycodone (OxyContin), methadone	Opioid agonist acting primarily at mu-receptor sites (morphine, fentanyl, hydromorphone, oxycodone, methadone) Moderate to severe acute and chronic pain Morphine: Intractable pain, preoperative sedation Fentanyl: Pain associated with short procedures such as bone marrow aspiration, fracture reductions, suturing	• Assess respiratory status frequently, noting any decrease in ventilatory rate or changes in breathing patterns; have naloxone readily available in case of respiratory depression (particularly with morphine, fentanyl, hydromorphone). • Monitor for sedation dizziness, lethargy, or confusion. • Educate parents and child that the drug may make the child sleepy, drowsy, or lightheaded. • Institute safety measures to prevent injury to the child. • Assess bowel sounds for decreased peristalsis; observe for abdominal distention. • Ensure adequate fiber intake and administer stool softeners as prescribed to minimize risk for constipation. • Monitor urine output for changes and report. • Morphine may cause itching, particularly of the face. • With fentanyl, observe for chest wall rigidity, which can occur with rapid intravenous infusion. • Oxycodone is the opioid component of brand-name products such as Tylox, Roxicet, and Percocet.

Data from Lexicomp. (2023b). Pediatric drug information. *UpToDate*. Retrieved April 5, 2023, from https://www.uptodate.com/contents/table-of-contents/drug-information/pediatric-drug-information

CLINICAL REASONING ALERT

Aspirin or products containing aspirin should not be used in infants or children for analgesic or antipyretic purposes because of the high risk of Reye syndrome.

Nonopioid agents are typically administered orally or rectally. In some cases, such as with postoperative pain, they may be administered intravenously as a continuous infusion or as bolus doses. Administration via intramuscular injection is not recommended because the injection can cause significant pain and the onset of pain relief is not increased.

Acetaminophen is a relatively safe medication, and it does not have the same GI or antiplatelet effects of NSAIDs; therefore, it is useful in children with cancer, with bleeding or clotting disorders, or children on anticoagulants. Acetaminophen toxicity and resulting hepatotoxicity can occur with misuse and overdosing. NSAIDs, owing to their antiinflammatory abilities, may be more effective in reducing pain caused by inflammatory conditions, such as musculoskeletal injuries and rheumatic diseases. Adverse effects associated with NSAIDs are uncommon but include GI irritation, blood clotting problems, and renal dysfunction. Nonopioids are relatively safe, have few incompatibilities with other medications, and do not depress the central nervous system. However, after a certain level, they do not provide increasing pain relief even when administered at increased doses. As a result, they may be combined with opioids for more effective pain relief.

OPIOID ANALGESICS

Opioid analgesics are typically used for moderate to severe pain. They are classified as either agonists (when they act as the neurotransmitter at the receptor site) or antagonists (when they block the action at the receptor site). Opioid agents that act as agonists include morphine, fentanyl, hydromorphone, oxycodone, and hydrocodone. Opioids that act as mixed agonists–antagonists include pentazocine, butorphanol, and nalbuphine. See Drug Guide 36.1. Opioids can be administered orally, rectally, intramuscularly, or intravenously. In addition, some agents such as fentanyl can be administered transdermally or transmucosally. Morphine is considered the "gold standard" and is the most commonly used of all opioid agonists; it is the drug of choice for severe pain (Hauer & Jones, 2021).

> **TAKE NOTE!**
>
> In 2017, the U.S. Food and Drug Administration (FDA) made the use of codeine or tramadol contraindicated in children younger than 12 years due to serious safety concerns related to the genetic variability in the metabolism of children (some children have slow metabolisms, while others have rapid metabolisms) (Hauer & Jones, 2021).

Opioid agonists, such as morphine, are associated with numerous adverse effects, resulting primarily from their depressant action on the central nervous system.

CLINICAL REASONING ALERT

When administering parenteral or epidural opioids, always have naloxone (Narcan) readily available to reverse the opioid's effects should respiratory depression occur.

Opioids stimulate the chemoreceptor trigger zone (CTZ), leading to nausea and vomiting. Moreover, **drug tolerance** (increased dosage required for the same pain relief previously achieved with a lower dose) and **physical dependence** (need for continued administration of the drug to prevent withdrawal symptoms) are commonly noted when opioids are given repeatedly (Yin, 2022). Drug Guide 36.1 gives additional information related to the opioid analgesics.

CLINICAL REASONING ALERT

Meperidine (Demerol), an opioid agonist, is not recommended as a first-choice agent for pain relief in children due to its toxicity on the central nervous system (Lexicomp, 2023a).

ADJUVANT DRUGS

Adjuvant drugs are drugs used to promote more effective pain relief, either alone or in combination with nonopioids or opioids. Their primary indications are for diagnoses other than pain. These agents are not classified as analgesics but may provide a coanalgesic effect or may treat side effects. Benzodiazepines, such as diazepam and midazolam, help relieve anxiety. Midazolam also produces amnesia. Anticonvulsants, such as gabapentin, and tricyclic antidepressants, such as amitriptyline and nortriptyline, may be used to treat neuropathic pain.

LOCAL ANESTHETICS

Local anesthetics are commonly used to provide analgesia for procedures. They are effective in providing successful pain relief, with only minimal risk of systemic adverse effects. However, local anesthetics such as lidocaine were not historically used in children because these drugs need to be injected. The belief was that children feared needles, and use of a local anesthetic subjected the child to two needlesticks instead of one. Advances in technology have led to the development of improved methods of delivery such as topical ointments and iontophoresis for administration of local anesthetics, thereby promoting atraumatic care. (For a more detailed discussion, see the next section on drug administration methods and later in the chapter on the nurse's role in managing procedure-related pain.)

Drug Administration Methods

With any medication administered for pain management, the timing of administration is vital. It is essential and more effective to stay ahead of pain and anticipate it, as opposed to treating it once it is present. Timing depends on the type of pain. For continuous or severe pain, administration of analgesia around the clock at scheduled intervals may be needed to achieve the necessary effect (Schechter, 2022). As-needed (PRN) dosing for continuous pain can lead to inadequate pain relief because of the delay before the drug reaches its peak effectiveness, and as a result, the child continues to experience pain, possibly necessitating a higher dose of analgesic to achieve relief. This then places the child at risk for overmedication and toxic effects.

For pain that can be predicted or considered temporary, such as with a procedure, analgesia is administered so that the peak action of the drug matches the time of the painful event.

There are various methods for administering pain medications to children. The preferred methods are the oral, rectal, intravenous, topical, or local nerve block routes. Epidural administration and moderate sedation may also be used.

ORAL METHOD

The oral method is often preferred because it is simple, easy, and convenient. The medication may be in the form of a pill, capsule, tablet, syrup, or elixir. Oral administration provides relatively steady blood levels of the drug when administered as a scheduled dose. Effectiveness typically occurs 1 to 2 hours after administration. As soon as possible, switch the child to oral dosing from parenteral dosing. However, keep in mind that higher doses of the oral medication may be needed to achieve the same effect.

RECTAL METHOD

The rectal method may be used when the child cannot take the medication orally, such as when the child has difficulty swallowing or is experiencing nausea and vomiting. It is a viable alternative for drug administration. Some analgesics are available in suppository form. For others that are not, the drug can be compounded into a suppository form. The absorption rate varies with rectal administration. Children may find insertion of a suppository uncomfortable and embarrassing.

INTRAVENOUS METHOD

Intravenous analgesia administration is the method of choice in emergency situations and when pain is severe and quick relief is needed. With intravenous administration, the drug usually takes effect within 5 minutes. Intravenous administration can be accomplished with bolus injections or continuous infusions. Continuous infusions may be preferred over bolus doses because steady blood levels are more easily maintained, thereby enhancing the drug's effect in relieving pain. Typically, opioids such as morphine, hydromorphone, and fentanyl are used due to their short half-life and decreased risk of toxicity.

PATIENT-CONTROLLED ANALGESIA

In **patient-controlled analgesia (PCA)**, a computerized pump is programmed to deliver an infusion of analgesics via a catheter inserted intravenously, epidurally, or subcutaneously. The analgesic may be given as a continuous infusion, as a continuous infusion supplemented by patient-delivered bolus doses, or as patient-delivered bolus doses only. Typically, the child presses a button to administer a bolus dose. The pump has a lockout function that is preset with the dose and time interval. If the child presses the button before the preset time, they will not receive an overdose of medication. By delivering small, frequent doses of opioids, the child can experience pain relief without the effects of oversedation. The child also experiences a sense of control over the pain experience.

The Institute for Safe Medication Practices (ISMP) has identified infants and young children as not being good candidates for PCA usage (2021). It may be appropriate for children starting around the age of 7 to 8 years (Schechter, 2022). It is essential to assess each child individually and consider the child's developmental level and psychosocial factors in determining appropriate PCA use. The child must have the necessary intellect, manual dexterity, and strength to operate the device.

PCA has been used to control postoperative pain and the pain associated with trauma, cancer, and sickle cell crisis. It can be used in acute care settings or in the home. Most commonly, morphine, hydromorphone, and fentanyl are the drugs used with PCA. The dosage is based on the child's response. Dosages for infusions depend on the child's age, the opioid used, and the type of pain.

The dangers and effectiveness of authorized agent–controlled analgesia, when family members or caregivers who are not authorized administer PCA doses "by proxy," warrant further research. In most circumstances, authorized agent–controlled analgesia by a family member should be avoided (Schechter, 2022). Health care providers who can assess pain and vital signs before and after each dose may be an alternative to activate the device. It is recommended that facilities develop specific criteria in any situation where authorized agent–activated PCA is being used (Schechter, 2022). Proper education and instruction are crucial in any situation in which someone other than the child may be administering PCA doses. Thorough assessment is necessary to ensure the child's pain is neither undertreated nor overtreated. To ensure safety with PCA use, each institution must have policies and procedures in place, appropriate education of health care staff, quality control measures, and quality machines.

LOCAL ANESTHETIC APPLICATION

A local anesthetic may sometimes be used to alleviate the pain associated with procedures such as venipuncture, injections, wound repair, lumbar puncture, or accessing of implanted ports. Local anesthesia is a type of regional analgesia that blocks or numbs specific nerves in a region of the body. Medications called local anesthetics include topical forms, such as creams, agents delivered by iontophoresis, vapocoolants, and skin refrigerants, as well as injectable forms.

Topical Forms

A common choice for effective, painless local anesthesia is a eutectic mixture of local anesthetics (EMLA). The mix is of lidocaine and prilocaine. It achieves anesthesia to a depth of 2 to 4 mm, so it reduces pain related to phlebotomy, venous cannulation, and intramuscular injections for up to 24 hours after the injection. However, it requires a 60- to 90-minute application time to intact skin using an occlusive dressing for superficial procedures and up to 2 to 3 hours for deeper, more invasive procedures (Box 36.1). EMLA is approved for use in infants born at 37 weeks' gestation or more (Lexicomp, 2023b). Maximum dosage and maximum area of application are based on the child's weight. Parents can be taught how to apply EMLA at home in preparation for a procedure (Fig. 36.9).

Sometimes, EMLA is not used due to the expense and the time needed to allow the drug to act. New approaches to EMLA delivery have been developed. Examples include other drug formulations and a patch delivery with a heat-activated system (Synera) that enhances the delivery of lidocaine and prilocaine. Synera is labeled for children older than 3 years and needs to be applied only 20 to 30 minutes before the procedure (Lexicomp, 2023b).

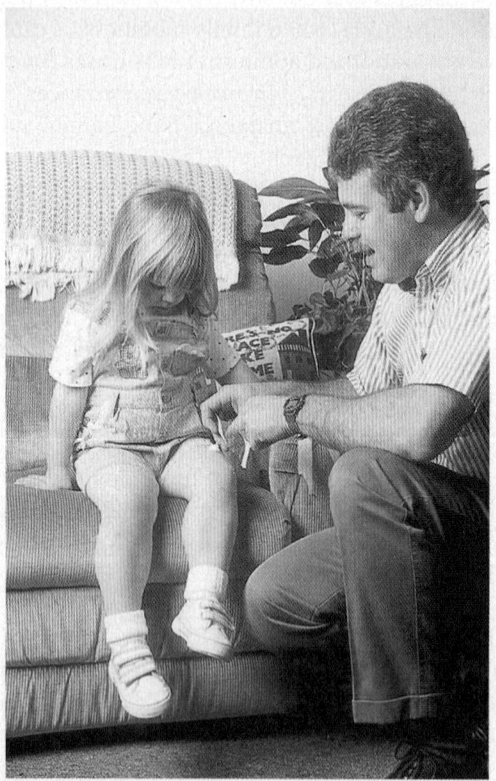

FIGURE 36.9 A parent applies EMLA cream to the child at home in preparation for a procedure. EMLA, eutectic mixture of local anesthetics.

BOX 36.1 Applying Eutectic Mixture of Local Anesthetics (EMLA)

Follow these guidelines when applying EMLA:

- Explain the purpose of the medication to the child and parents, reinforcing that it will help the pain go away.
- Check the scheduled time for the procedure; plan to apply the cream 60 minutes before a superficial procedure such as an intramuscular injection or a venipuncture or 2 to 3 hours before a deeper procedure such as a lumbar puncture or bone marrow aspiration.
- Place a thick layer of the cream on the skin at the intended site of the procedure, making sure that the area where the cream is being applied is free of any breaks. Do not rub the cream in once it is applied to the skin.
- Cover the site with a transparent dressing, and secure it so that the dressing is occlusive. Alternatively, use plastic film wrap and tape the edges to secure the dressing.
- Instruct the child not to touch the dressing once it is secured. If necessary, cover the occlusive dressing with a protection device or a loosely applied gauze or elastic bandage.
- After the allotted time, remove the occlusive dressing, and wipe the cream from the skin. Inspect the skin for a change in color (blanching or redness), which indicates the medication has penetrated the skin adequately.
- Verify that sensation is absent by lightly tapping or scratching the area. Use this technique also to demonstrate to the child that the anesthetic is effective. If sensation is present, reapply the cream.
- Prepare the child for the procedure. Assess the child's pain after the procedure to evaluate for pain and to differentiate pain from fear and anxiety.

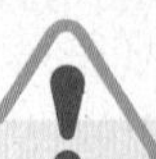

CLINICAL REASONING ALERT

EMLA is used with caution in children younger than 3 to 6 months and other susceptible patients because it may be associated with methemoglobinemia caused by prilocaine toxicity (Lexicomp, 2023b). It is contraindicated in children who have congenital or idiopathic methemoglobinemia (Lexicomp, 2023b). It must be used cautiously in children younger than 12 months who are receiving methemoglobin-inducing agents, such as sulfonamides, phenytoin, phenobarbital, and acetaminophen (Lexicomp, 2023b). Use of these agents in combination with EMLA increases the child's risk for methemoglobinemia, a condition that could lead to cyanosis and hypoxemia.

Other examples of topical anesthetics are tetracaine, epinephrine, cocaine (TAC) and lidocaine, epinephrine, tetracaine (LET). These are commonly used for lacerations that require suturing. The agent is applied directly to the wound with a cotton ball or swab for 20 to 30 minutes until the area is numb. These methods are not used in children with known sensitivity to any of these medications.

Lidocaine can also be dispersed in liposomes to allow for transcutaneous delivery (liposomal lidocaine). OTC lidocaine 4% (LMX4) or lidocaine 5% (LMX5), formerly called ELA-Max, is massaged into the skin without the use of an occlusive dressing. Anesthesia to the area is reached in 15 to 30 minutes and lasts about 60 minutes.

Needle-free powder lidocaine (Zingo or J-Tip) is another topical analgesic. It is labeled for use in children 3 to 18 years of age. It is a single-use, prefilled disposable system that provides analgesia in 1 to 3 minutes.

Another choice for local anesthesia is iontophoresis. Iontophoretic lidocaine (Numby Stuff) provides a deeper analgesia in a shorter duration (~10 to 25 minutes) and is used over intact skin. A mild electrical current from a small battery-powered generator and two iontophoretic drug-delivery electrodes push drug molecules (lidocaine hydrochloric acid 2% with epinephrine 1:100,000) into the skin. A mild tingling sensation may be felt during drug delivery, with an increase in tingling noted with higher currents. This type of local anesthesia is not recommended for use in children who have a history of allergy or sensitivity to these drugs, electrically sensitive equipment such as a pacemaker, or damaged skin or scar tissue. There is limited use of this anesthetic due to the discomfort associated with the procedure and local skin reactions, including blisters and burn-like reactions (Hsu, 2022).

Vapocoolant spray can be applied to the skin, but efficacy is highly dependent on spraying time, and it can cause discomfort (Hsu, 2022). The duration of analgesia is short, approximately 1 to 2 minutes, which may not allow enough time for a procedure to be completed.

> *TAKE NOTE!*
>
> Studies comparing lidocaine–prilocaine products to other topical anesthetics (such as liposomal lidocaine and heated lidocaine) have shown equal or better pain relief with a shorter onset of action (Hsu, 2022).

Injectable Forms

Injectable forms of lidocaine or procaine can be administered subcutaneously or intradermally around the procedural area approximately 5 to 10 minutes before the procedure. Common problems with this form of anesthetic include the pain associated with the subcutaneous injection and some burning associated with lidocaine administration, as well as blanching of the skin.

> *TAKE NOTE!*
>
> The burning that lidocaine causes on injection may be diminished by buffering lidocaine with sodium bicarbonate, using 10 parts lidocaine and one part sodium bicarbonate (1 mL of 1% to 2% lidocaine and 0.1 mL of 8.4% sodium bicarbonate). Then, inject 0.1 mL or less of the solution intradermally at the site of venipuncture. Anesthetic action is almost immediate. The solution is stable for only approximately 1 week if not refrigerated.

EPIDURAL ANALGESIA

For **epidural analgesia**, a catheter is inserted into the epidural space, usually between the lumbar (L3) and the thoracic (T3) areas. The drug, usually fentanyl or morphine, diffuses into the cerebrospinal fluid and crosses the dura mater to the spinal cord. Then, it binds with the opioid receptors located at the dorsal horn. The drugs can be administered as bolus injections (a one-time bolus or on an intermittent schedule), a continuous infusion, or PCA. Usually, an opioid such as morphine, fentanyl, or hydromorphone is given in conjunction with a long-acting local anesthetic such as bupivacaine.

Epidural analgesia is typically used postoperatively, providing analgesia to the lower body for approximately 12 to 14 hours. The small amount of medication used with this type of analgesia causes less sedation, thereby allowing the child to participate more actively in postoperative care activities. This type of analgesia is also effective for children undergoing upper or lower abdominal surgeries because it controls localized intense pain, somatic pain, and visceral pain.

When epidural analgesia is being administered, additional narcotic analgesics are not given in order to prevent complications such as respiratory depression, pruritus, nausea, vomiting, and urinary retention.

> **CLINICAL REASONING ALERT!**
>
> Respiratory depression, although rare when epidural analgesia is used, is always a possibility. When it does occur, it usually occurs gradually over a period of several hours after the medication is initiated. This allows adequate time for early detection and prompt intervention.

Constant assessment is essential because insertion of an epidural catheter and epidural analgesia can lead to infection at the site of the insertion, epidural hematoma, arachnoiditis, neuritis, spinal headache (rare) due to a cerebrospinal fluid leak, and respiratory depression. Frequent assessment, typically every 1 to 2 hours, of heart rate, respiratory rate, and depth of sedation, and every 2 to 4 hours of blood pressure, pain level, and motor function, is imperative. Assessing for adverse reactions such as nausea and vomiting and pruritus, checking the tubing and catheter site, and ensuring the occlusive dressing is intact are all important nursing interventions. The dermatome, which is the area of the body associated with supply by a particular nerve, that innervates the diaphragm can become suppressed during continuous epidural analgesia, resulting in respiratory depression. It is important to assess the child's sensory level frequently. Using cool water or an alcohol pad, bilaterally touch the child's body every 2 to 3 cm. The level at which the child states they feel the temperature change is the level of anesthesia. (Refer to Fig. 36.10 for dermatome levels.)

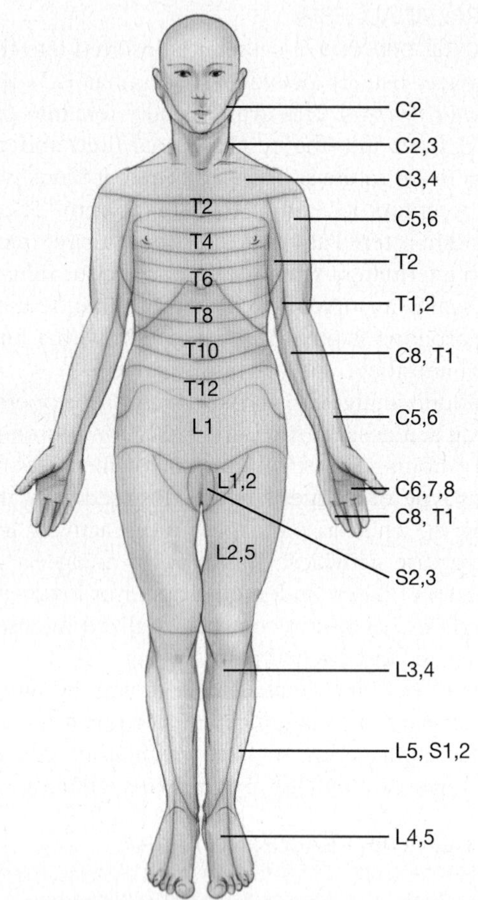

FIGURE 36.10 The level of anesthesia should not go higher than T4, the nipple line, in children.

MODERATE SEDATION

Moderate sedation used to be called conscious sedation, but the term "conscious" has been replaced since it can be misleading (Cravero & Roback, 2022). It is a medically controlled state of depressed consciousness that allows protective reflexes to be maintained so the child has the ability to maintain a patent airway and respond to physical or verbal stimulation.

Sedation in children is different than in adults as it is often administered to help control behavior in order to complete procedures or diagnostic studies. Moderate sedation requires adherence to specific protocols, and many regulatory bodies, such as The Joint Commission, and societies, including the AAP, American Academy of Pediatric Dentistry (AAPD), American Society of Anesthesiologists, and American College of Emergency Physicians, have published standards and guidelines to improve patient safety and outcomes. The depressed state is obtained by using various agents such as morphine, fentanyl, midazolam, ketamine, chloral hydrate, diazepam, pentobarbital, nitrous oxide, or propofol. The medication used will depend on the expected degree of pain and discomfort, amount of motion restriction needed, and individual factors such as age, ability to cooperate, and medical history.

Moderate sedation is used for procedures that are painful and stressful. For example, moderate sedation is suggested instead of restraints, especially for toddlers and preschool children undergoing frightening or invasive procedures who are manifesting extreme anxiety and behavioral upset. Other indications include situations involving:

- Evidence the child is experiencing a heightened stress reaction (e.g., attempting to flee, crying inconsolably, or flailing)
- Verbalization by the child that they are frightened and do not want to be touched
- Inability to remain immobilized, such as during laceration repair or computed tomography
- Any procedure that is painful and fear-provoking

The route of administering the medications for sedation should follow the guidelines of atraumatic care. Oral, topical, or an existing intravenous route should be used. The child may pass from the intended level of sedation to a deeper unintended level of sedation; therefore, personnel administering moderate sedation must be specially trained, with strong resuscitation and advanced pediatric life support skills, and emergency equipment and medications must be readily available (Cravero & Roback, 2022).

The Nurse's Role in Pharmacologic Pain Management

The nurse plays a major role in providing pharmacologic pain relief. As with any medication, the nurse is responsible for adhering to the rights of medication administration—right drug, right dose, right route, right time, right patient, and right approach. The nurse also adheres to additional rights, such as the right of the child and parents to be educated, the right of the child to refuse the medication, the right documentation, and the right form. The nurse must also have a solid knowledge base about the medications used for pain relief. This knowledge includes information about the drug's pharmacokinetics (absorption, distribution, metabolism, and excretion) and pharmacodynamics (mechanism of action, including adverse effects). Refer to Chapter 35 for further information.

Assessment is crucial when pharmacologic pain interventions are used. An initial assessment of pain provides a baseline from which options for relief can be chosen. Factors that can affect the choice of analgesic, such as the child's age, pain intensity, physiologic status, or previous experiences with pain, also need to be considered. The nurse acts as an advocate for the child and the family to ensure that the most appropriate pharmacologic agent is chosen for the situation.

Assessment is ongoing once the agent is administered. Monitor physiologic parameters such as level of consciousness, vital signs, oxygen saturation levels, and urinary output for changes that might indicate an adverse reaction to the agent. More intensive monitoring is needed when agents are administered intravenously or epidurally or by moderate sedation. For example, if the child is receiving moderate sedation, interventions include:

- Ensuring emergency equipment is readily available
- Maintaining a patent airway
- Monitoring the child's level of consciousness and responsiveness
- Assessing the child's vital signs (especially heart rate, blood pressure, and respiratory rate)
- Monitoring oxygen saturation levels

Typically, a specially trained health care provider is specifically designated to perform these activities during the administration of the sedation. Afterward, the nurse is responsible for ongoing monitoring of the child's status.

Monitor the child closely for evidence of adverse effects. Table 36.8 describes the interventions useful for responding to these adverse effects. Be alert for signs and symptoms of respiratory depression secondary to opioid administration. Have an opioid antagonist such as naloxone and the benzodiazepine antagonist flumazenil readily available should the child experience respiratory depression.

In addition to assessing physiologic parameters, assess the child's and parents' emotional status before and after the agent is administered. For example, increased anxiety and fear may necessitate a change in method of administration, such as topical application instead of an intradermal injection of a local anesthetic. Use nonpharmacologic methods to help lessen anxiety, thereby promoting more effective relief from the drug.

Nurses are also responsible for ensuring that the child and parents are adequately prepared for the use of the pharmacologic agent. Teach the child and parents about the drug, why it is being used, its intended effects, and possible adverse effects, tailoring the teaching to the child's cognitive level. Provide opportunities for the child and parents to ask questions, offering support and guidance throughout the experience. Provide a demonstration or use visual aids so that the child and parents know exactly what to expect. Encourage the use of play to help the child express fears and anxieties related to the administration.

TABLE 36.8 • Interventions for Common Opioid-Induced Adverse Effects

Adverse Effect	Nursing Interventions
Constipation	Encourage fluid intake unless contraindicated. Ensure intake of high-fiber foods, including fruits, if allowed. Encourage activity, including ambulation if possible. Obtain order for stool softener, and administer laxative as ordered.
Pruritus	Apply cool compresses and lotions. Administer antihistamine as ordered.
Nausea and vomiting	Inform child and parents that these symptoms usually subside in 1–2 days. Encourage small frequent meals with bland foods. Administer antiemetic if ordered. Notify health care provider for possible change in pain medication.

Management of Procedure-Related Pain

One of the most common causes of pain in children is procedure-related pain. The procedure may be minor, such as an intramuscular injection, heel stick, or venipuncture, or it may be more involved, such as lumbar puncture, bone marrow aspiration, or wound care. Regardless, pain is real for children, and painful procedures are often extremely distressing. Variables that affect pain include the intensity or length of the procedure and the skill of the health care provider performing it.

The Nurse's Role in Managing Procedure-Related Pain

Through the use of behavioral and pharmacologic approaches, nurses can significantly reduce the pain and distress of procedures. Use the guiding principles of atraumatic care, which include:

- Use topical EMLA or other topical analgesics such as liposomal lidocaine or tetracaine gel, iontophoretic lidocaine, vapocoolant spray, or buffered lidocaine at the intended site of a skin or vessel puncture.
- Incorporate the use of nonpharmacologic strategies for pain relief in conjunction with pharmacologic methods.
- Prepare the child and parents about the procedure, and then keep all equipment out of sight until it is ready to be used.
- Use therapeutic hugging (see Chapter 30) to secure the child.
- Use the smallest-gauge needle possible or an automated lancet device to puncture the skin.
- Use an intermittent infusion device or peripherally inserted central catheter (PICC) if multiple or repeated blood samples are necessary. Coordinate care so that several tests can be performed from one sample if possible.

- Opt for venipuncture in newborns instead of heel sticks if the amount of blood needed would require much squeezing.
- Use kangaroo care (skin-to-skin contact) for newborns before and after a heel stick.
- Provide NNS with sucrose solution, if appropriate; pacifier; or breastfeeding for newborns several minutes before the procedure.

TAKE NOTE!

Individualize interventions based on the painfulness of the procedure and the child's developmental age and personality. Use behavioral cognitive approaches and pharmacologic interventions. For example, encouraging the school-age child to assist during painful procedures in age-appropriate ways may help ease some of the pain related to a heightened state of anxiety or at least assist the child in coping with the situation. Always use appropriate pharmacologic treatment, especially for the first procedure, to provide as painless an experience as possible for the child.

Nursing care for the child with procedure-related pain includes the child as well as the parents. Be sure to prepare them for the procedure using an appropriate developmental approach. Promote environmental comfort, too. Ensure the child's privacy is maintained and the lighting is adequate for the procedure but not so bright as to cause the child discomfort.

Painful procedures performed in the child's room can lead to an association of pain or fear with the room or bed. Many hospitals have a special treatment room where procedures can be performed. These rooms are usually equipped with many activities, toys, and decorations to help distract the child. The use of a treatment room may not be feasible or desirable in all situations or for all procedures. The ultimate goal is to do what is best for the child; therefore, the nurse should consider the needs of the child, the demands of the procedures, and the conditions that would facilitate the best outcome.

Unless contraindicated, encourage the parents to be present before, during, and after the procedure to provide comforting support to the child. Also encourage the child and parents to use nonpharmacologic methods to help maximize pain relief and reduce anxiety. For example, nonpharmacologic methods that are helpful for the toddler and preschooler may include positioning the child on the lap and hugging the child, distracting the child with toys or interactive books, and blowing bubbles.

Play therapy can be useful when preparing children for painful procedures. Encourage children to make decisions about their care related to pain management if their condition or procedure allows. It is also helpful to anticipate and recognize painful situations and provide pain medication before the actual procedure to ensure comfort. Many nonpharmacologic strategies can be enhanced and better implemented with the help of the child life specialist or play therapist, who have specialized training in these techniques.

Recall Aiden from the beginning of the chapter. What are some interventions that may be helpful prior to, during, and after his dressing change?

Management of Chronic Pain

Typically, pain in children is acute, but chronic pain is a significant problem in the pediatric population as well. Chronic pain is ongoing and recurrent pain that persists beyond the expected healing time (World Health Organization [WHO], 2020). Chronic pain is the result of a complex interplay of biologic, psychological, and sociocultural factors. Children with chronic pain and their families may experience significant physical, emotional, and social consequences, including notable economic burdens from the pain and disability (WHO, 2020). Children with chronic pain have an increased risk of depression and anxiety, sleep problems, and problems with school functioning, and the experience of chronic pain in childhood may predispose the individual to chronic pain in adulthood (WHO, 2020).

The Nurse's Role in Managing Chronic Pain

The nurse's role in managing chronic pain in children is similar to that for the child experiencing acute pain or procedure-related pain. Assessment of the child's pain is key and should include a history of the present problem. Questions should focus on the onset of the pain; its intensity, duration, and location; and any factors that alleviate or exacerbate it. In addition, it is important to question the child and parents about the impact of the pain on the child's daily life, such as sleep; play; eating; school; and interactions with peers, other family members, and friends. Also address the impact of the child's chronic pain on the family's life.

Another key area of assessment is determining how the pain affects the child's and family's level of stress. Areas to address include the child's and parents' feelings of hopelessness, anxiety, and depression. Also question the child and parents about what they think has caused the pain and how they have coped with it. In addition, ascertain what methods the child and parents have used to alleviate the pain and the success of these methods. Inquire about any home remedies or alternative therapies that may have been used.

Review past physical examination findings for clues to the underlying problem. Observe the child's overall appearance, gait, and posture. Assess the child's cognitive level and emotional response, especially related to the experience of pain. Expect to complete a neurologic examination, and observe for muscle spasms, trigger points, and increased sensitivity to light touch. Abnormal body postures assumed by the child due to chronic pain may result in the development of secondary pain in the muscles and fascia. When children tense their muscles due to fear of examination, somatic pain may occur.

Various nonpharmacologic and pharmacologic strategies are used to manage chronic pain. Often, multiple strategies are combined to address pain relief as well as the pain's impact on other areas, such as sleep or school functioning. When pharmacologic agents are used, the oral form is the method of choice. As with any pain management strategy, education of the child and family is paramount. A referral to a pediatric pain specialist may be needed if the child's pain is not controlled effectively.

KEY CONCEPTS

- Pain is a highly individualized subjective experience affecting people of all ages. It is a universal experience and may be considered the fifth vital sign.
- Pain management is a critical element in a child's plan of care because children may lack the verbal capacity to describe their pain experience; caregivers and health care providers often have misconceptions about pain; assessment of the complex nature of the pain experience is difficult; if left unmanaged, pain in children can lead to serious physical and emotional consequences; and available resources and research related to pain relief strategies in children are limited.
- The sensation of pain involves a sequence of physiologic events: transduction, transmission, perception, and modulation.
- Pain can be classified by duration as acute or chronic, by etiology as nociceptive or neuropathic, or by source or location as somatic or visceral.
- Factors influencing a child's perception of pain include age and gender or sex, cognitive level, temperament, previous pain experiences, and family and cultural background, all of which cannot be changed. Situational factors involve behavioral, cognitive, and emotional aspects and can be changed.
- Infants, including preterm infants, experience pain. Behavioral and physiologic indicators are used to assess pain. Toddlers commonly react with intense emotional upset and physical resistance or aggression. Preschoolers may believe pain is a punishment for misbehaving or having bad thoughts. School-age children can communicate the type, location, and severity of pain but may deny having pain so as to appear brave or avoid further pain. Adolescents, with their focus on body image and fear of loss of control, often ask numerous questions and may attempt to remain stoic to avoid being viewed as childish.
- Assessment of pain in children includes both subjective and objective data. Nurses need to tailor the assessment to the child's developmental level and ask appropriate questions geared to the child's cognitive level. Parental questioning during the health history is also important.
- Self-report pain rating scales are valuable assessment tools that allow the child's level of pain to be quantified. Examples include the FACES pain rating scale, the Oucher pain rating scale, the poker chip tool, the visual analog and numeric scales, and the Adolescent Pediatric Pain Tool.
- Different pain rating scales are appropriate for different developmental levels. However, children may regress when in pain, so a simpler tool may be needed to make sure that the child understands what is being asked. Consistency in using the same tool is essential so that appropriate comparisons can be made and effective interventions can be planned and implemented.
- Physical examination of the child for pain primarily involves the skills of observation and inspection. These skills are used to assess for physiologic and behavioral changes that indicate pain. Auscultation may also be used to assess for changes in vital signs, specifically heart rate and blood pressure. Physiologic and behavioral pain assessment tools, such as the PIPP, NIPS, RIPS, Pain Observation Scale for Young Children, CRIES Scale for Neonatal Postoperative Pain Assessment, and r-FLACC Behavioral Scale, measure specific parameters and changes that would indicate the child is in pain.
- Nonpharmacologic pain management strategies aim to assist children in coping with pain and to give them a sense of mastery or control over the situation. These strategies may be categorized as behavioral cognitive, in which the child focuses on a specific area or aspect rather than the pain (e.g., relaxation, distraction, imagery, biofeedback, thought stopping, and positive self-talk), or biophysical, in which the focus is on interfering with the transmission of pain impulses reaching the brain (e.g., heat and cold applications, massage, and pressure).
- The nurse plays a major role in teaching the child and family about available nonpharmacologic pain interventions, helping them choose the most appropriate and most effective methods and ensuring the child and parents use the methods before the pain occurs as well as before it increases.
- Pharmacologic interventions involve the administration of drugs for pain relief, most commonly, nonopioids and opioid analgesics. The selection of the

method is determined by the drug being administered; the child's status; the type, intensity, and location of the pain; and any factors that may be influencing the child's pain. The preferred methods for administering analgesics include the oral, rectal, intravenous, or local nerve block routes; epidural administration; and moderate sedation.

- Nonopioid analgesics used to treat mild to moderate pain include acetaminophen and NSAIDs such as ibuprofen, ketorolac, naproxen, and, less commonly, indomethacin, diclofenac, and piroxicam.
- Morphine is considered the "gold standard" for all opioid agonists; it is the drug to which all other opioids are compared and is usually the drug of choice for severe pain (Hauer & Jones, 2021).
- Local anesthetics are commonly used to provide analgesia for procedures. They are effective in providing successful pain relief, with only minimal risk of systemic adverse effects. The first choice for the most effective, painless local anesthesia is EMLA. It achieves anesthesia to a depth of 2 to 4 mm, so it reduces pain associated with phlebotomy, venous cannulation, and intramuscular injections up to 24 hours after injection.
- Epidural analgesia involves the insertion of a catheter into the epidural space through which drugs can be administered as bolus injections (a one-time bolus or on an intermittent schedule), as a continuous infusion, or as PCA. Usually an opioid, such as morphine, fentanyl, or hydromorphone, is given in conjunction with a long-acting local anesthetic, such as bupivacaine.
- Moderate sedation is a medically controlled state of depressed consciousness that allows protective reflexes to be maintained so the child has the ability to maintain a patent airway and respond to physical or verbal stimulation.
- When providing pharmacologic pain relief, the nurse must adhere to the rights of medication administration and have a solid knowledge base about the medications used for pain relief and the drug's pharmacokinetics (absorption, distribution, metabolism, and excretion) and pharmacodynamics (mechanism of action, including adverse effects). Initial and ongoing assessment is crucial.
- The principles of atraumatic care guide nursing interventions for providing pain relief, especially for procedure-related pain.
- Chronic pain in children can significantly affect the child's daily life and activities as well as the family's life.

REFERENCES AND RECOMMENDED READINGS

American Academy of Pediatrics (AAP), Committee on Fetus and Newborn, & Section on Anesthesiology and Pain Medicine. (2016, reaffirmed 2020). Prevention and management of procedural pain in the neonate: An update. *Pediatrics, 137*(2). https://doi.org/ 10.1542/peds.2015-4271

American Pain Society. (1995). *Pain: The fifth vital sign.* Author.

Baker, C. M., & Wong, D. L. (1987). Q.U.E.S.T.: A process of pain assessment in children. *Orthopaedic Nursing, 6*(1), 11–21. https://doi.org/10.1097/00006416-198701000-00003

Beyer, J. E., Denyes, M. J., & Villarruel, A. M. (1992). The creation, validation, and continuing development of the Oucher: A measure of pain intensity in children. *Journal of Pediatric Nursing, 7*(5), 335–346.

Boelen-van der Loo, W. J., Scheffer, E., de Haan, R. J., & de Groot, C. J. (1999). Clinimetric evaluation of the pain observation scale for young children in children aged between 1 and 4 years after ear, nose, and throat surgery. *Journal of Developmental and Behavioral Pediatrics, 20*(4), 222–227. https://doi.org/10.1097/00004703-199908000-00004

Boitor, M., Gélinas, C., Rauch, F., Jacob, E., LeMay, S., Carrier, J. I., Bilodeau, C., & Tsimicalis, A. (2019). Validation of the adolescent pediatric pain tool for the multidimensional measurement of pain in children and adolescents diagnosed with osteogenesis imperfecta. *Canadian Journal of Pain, 3*(1), 148–156. https://doi.org/10.1080/24740527.2019.1626705

Crandall, M., & Savedra, M. (2005). Multidimensional assessment using the adolescent pediatric pain tool: A case report. *Journal for Specialists in Pediatric Nursing, 10*(3), 115–123. https://doi.org/10.1111/j.1744-6155.2005.00023.x

Cravero, J. P., & Roback, M. G. (2022). Procedural sedation in children: Approach. *UpToDate.* Retrieved March 22, 2023, from https://www.uptodate.com/contents/procedural-sedation-in-children-approach

Favaretto, E., Gögele, M., Bedani, F., Hicks, A. A., Erfurth, A., Perugi, G., Pramstaller, P. P., & Melotti, R. (2022). Pain sensitivity is modulated by affective temperament: Results from the population-based CHRIS Affective Disorder (CHRIS-AD) study. *Journal of Affective Disorders, 316*, 209–216. https://doi.org/10.1016/j.jad.2022.08.015

Gai, N., Naser, B., Hanley, J., Peliowski, A., Hayes, J., & Aoyama, K. (2020). A practical guide to acute pain management in children. *Journal of Anesthesia, 34*(3), 421–433. https://doi.org/10.1007/s00540-020-02767-x

Hauer, J., & Jones, B. L. (2021). Pain in children: Approach to pain assessment and overview of management principles. *UpToDate.* Retrieved March 13, 2023, from https://www.uptodate.com/contents/pain-in-children-approach-to-pain-assessment-and-overview-of-management-principles

Hester, N. K. (1979). The preoperational child's reaction to immunization. *Nursing Research, 28*(4), 250–255. https://doi.org/10.1097/00006199-197907000-00017

Hockenberry, M. J., & Wilson, D. (2009). *Wong's essentials of pediatric nursing* (8th ed., p. 162). Elsevier Mosby.

Horton, R. E., Pillai Riddell, R., Flora, D., Moran, G., & Pederson, D. (2015). Distress regulation in infancy: Attachment and temperament in the context of acute pain. *Journal of Developmental and Behavioral Pediatrics, 36*, 35–44. https://doi.org/10.1097/DBP.0000000000000119

Hsu, D. C. (2022). Clinical use of topical anesthetics in children. *UpToDate.* Retrieved April 8, 2023, from https://www.uptodate.com/contents/clinical-use-of-topical-anesthetics-in-children

Institute for Safe Medication Practices. (2021). *ISMP medication safety self-assessment for perioperative settings.* https://www.ismp.org/sites/default/files/attachments/2021-05/FAQs.pdf

International Association for the Study of Pain. (2011). *IASP pain terminology.* https://www.iasp-pain.org/Education/Content.aspx?ItemNumber=1698#Pain

Krechel, S. W., & Bildner, J. (1995). CRIES: A new neonatal postoperative pain measurement score. Initial testing of validity and reliability. *Paediatric Anaesthesia, 5*, 53–61. https://doi.org/10.1111/j.1460-9592.1995.tb00242.x

Lawrence, J., Alcock, D., McGrath, P., Kay, J., MacMurray, S. B., & Dulberg, C. (1993). The development of a tool to assess neonatal pain. *Neonatal Network, 12*(6), 59–66.

Lexicomp. (2023a). *Meperidine (pethidine): Pediatric drug information. UpToDate.* Retrieved April 5, 2023, from https://www.uptodate.com/contents/meperidine-pethidine-pediatric-druginformation

Lexicomp. (2023b). *Pediatric drug information. UpToDate.* Retrieved April 5, 2023, from https://www.uptodate.com/contents/table-of-contents/drug-information/pediatric-drug-information

Luo, F., Zhu, H., Mei, L., Shu, Q., Cheng, X., Chen, X., Zhao, Y., Chen, S., & Pan, Y. (2023). Evaluation of procedural pain for neonates in a neonatal intensive care unit: A single-centre study. *BMJ Paediatrics Open, 7*(1):e002107. https://doi.org/10.1136/bmjpo-2023-002107

McCaffery, M. (1968). *Nursing practice theories related to cognition, bodily pain and main environment interactions.* University of California, Los Angeles.

McGrath, P. A. (2005). Children—Not simply "little adults." In H. Merskey, J. D. Loeser, & R. Dubner (Eds.), *The paths of pain 1975–2005* (pp. 433–446). IASP Press.

Merkel, S. I., Voepel-Lewis, T., Shayevitz, J. R., & Malviya, S. (1997). The FLACC: A behavioral scale for scoring postoperative pain in young children. *Pediatric Nursing, 23*(3), 293–297.

Nath, J. (2023). *Applied pathophysiology* (4th ed.). Wolters Kluwer.

National Database of Nursing Quality Indicators. (n.d.). *NDNQI nursing-sensitive indicators.* Retrieved March 20, 2023, from https://nursingandndnqi.weebly.com/ndnqi-indicators.html

Osborne, N. R., & Davis, K. D. (2022). Chapter Eight—Sex and gender differences in pain. *International Review of Neurobiology, 164*: 277–307. https://doi.org/10.1016/bs.irn.2022.06.013

Osincup, P. (2020). How to use humor in clinical settings. *AMA Journal of Ethics, 22*(7):E588–E595. https://doi.org/10.1001/amajethics.2020.588

Roué, J.-M. (2022). Prevention and treatment of neonatal pain. *UpToDate.* Retrieved March 13, 2023, from https://www.uptodate.com/contents/prevention-and-treatment-of-neonatal-pain

Roué, J.-M. (2023). Assessment of neonatal pain. *UpToDate.* Retrieved March 13, 2023, from https://www.uptodate.com/contents/assessment-of-neonatal-pain

Schade, J. G., Joyce, B. A., Gerkensmeyer, J., & Keck, J. F. (1996). Comparison of three preverbal scales for postoperative pain assessment in a diverse pediatric sample. *Journal of Pain and Symptom Management, 12*(6), 348–359. https://doi.org/10.1016/S0885-3924(96)00182-0

Schechter, W. (2023). Pharmacologic management of acute perioperative pain in infants and children. *UpToDate.* Retrieved April 7, 2023, from https://www.uptodate.com/contents/pharmacologic-management-of-acute-perioperative-pain-in-infants-and-children

Strean, W. B. (2009). Laughter prescription. *Canadian Family Physician/Medecin de Famille Canadien, 55*(10), 965–967. https://www.cfp.ca/content/cfp/55/10/965.full.pdf

Talebi, M., Amiri, S. R. J., Roshan, P. A., Zabihi, A., Zahedpasha, Y., & Chehrazi, M. (2022). The effect of concurrent use of swaddle and sucrose on the intensity of pain during venous blood sampling in neonate: A clinical trial study. *BMC Pediatrics, 22*(1), 263. https://doi.org/10.1186/s12887-022-03323-0

Thirion, J., O'Riordan, M. A., & Stormorken, A. (2015). Commentary revisiting the pieces of hurt pain assessment tool—Do the pieces matter? *Pediatric Pain Letter, 17*(1), 1–4. http://childpain.org/ppl/issues/v17n1_2015/v17n1_thirion.pdf

World Health Organization. (2020). *Guidelines on the management of chronic pain in children.* https://www.who.int/publications/i/item/9789240017870

Yin, S. (2022). Opioid withdrawal in adolescents. *UpToDate.* Retrieved November 10, 2023, from https://www.uptodate.com/contents/opioid-withdrawal-in-adolescents

Zeltzer, L. K., Krane, E. J., & Levy, R. L. (2020). Pediatric pain management. In R. M. Kleigman, J. W. St. Geme III, N. J. Blum, S. S. Shah, R. C. Tasker, K. M. Wilson, & R. E. Behrman (Eds.), *Nelson textbook of pediatrics* (21st ed., pp. 2915–3011). Elsevier.

DEVELOPING CLINICAL JUDGMENT

PRACTICING FOR NCLEX

1. The nurse is preparing to assess the pain of a 3-year-old child who had surgery the day before. Which pain assessment methods would be most appropriate for the nurse to use? Select all that apply.
- **a.** FACES pain rating scale
- **b.** Numeric pain scale
- **c.** Asking the parents to report their child's pain scale
- **d.** Visual analog scale
- **e.** Observation of the child

2. When developing the plan of care for a child in pain, the nurse identifies appropriate strategies aimed at modifying which factors that influence pain? Select all that apply.
- **a.** Lack of control
- **b.** Cognitive level
- **c.** Previous pain experiences
- **d.** Anticipatory anxiety
- **e.** Gender
- **f.** Fear

3. An adolescent who is a competitive swimmer comes to the emergency department complaining of localized aching pain in their shoulder, stating, "I've been practicing really hard and long to get myself ready for my meet this weekend." The area is tender to the touch. The nurse determines that the adolescent is most likely experiencing which type of pain?
- **a.** Cutaneous pain
- **b.** Deep somatic pain
- **c.** Visceral pain
- **d.** Neuropathic pain

4. After teaching a child's parents about the different methods of distraction that can be used for pain management, which statement by the parents indicates a need for additional teaching?
- **a.** "We'll have her focus on her hand and count each finger slowly."
- **b.** "We'll read some of her favorite stories to her."
- **c.** "We'll have her imagine that she's at the beach this summer."
- **d.** "She likes to play video games, so we'll bring in some from home."

5. A child is scheduled for a bone marrow aspiration at 4 p.m. The nurse would plan to apply EMLA cream to the intended site at which time?
- **a.** 1:30 p.m.
- **b.** 3:00 p.m.
- **c.** 3:30 p.m.
- **d.** 4:00 p.m.

6. The patient is postoperative day 1 after cardiac surgery. The nurse understands that in a(n)____________ the most consistent indicator of pain is______________.

Blank 1:
- **a.** infant
- **b.** preschooler
- **c.** adolescent
- **d.** school-age child

Blank 2:
- **e.** increased heart rate
- **f.** high-pitched cry
- **g.** increased heart rate
- **h.** facial expression

CRITICAL THINKING EXERCISES

1. The nurse asks a 12-year-old if she is having pain. She denies pain, even though she is lying on her left side, holding her abdomen, with her knees flexed up to it. What might be some underlying factors leading the child to deny her pain? How would the nurse go about assessing this child's pain?

2. The nurse comes into the room of a 6-year-old who is sleeping. His parent states, "He's asleep, so he's not in pain." How should the nurse respond?

3. A child who is receiving ibuprofen is experiencing increased pain. The dosage of ibuprofen is increased but is no longer effective in providing adequate pain relief. What is occurring? What would be most likely to happen next?

STUDY ACTIVITIES

1. Interview nurses who work on a pediatric unit about their experiences with managing pain in children. Ask them how they assess pain in children and the major methods they use to assist the children in managing their pain.

2. Interview families of children with chronic illnesses who experience pain. Ask the parents how they assess their children's pain level and what methods they have used in assisting their children in managing pain.

3. Compare the drugs fentanyl and midazolam when used for moderate sedation in terms of onset of action, duration, primary effects, and antidotes.

4. A child is receiving epidural analgesia with morphine. The nurse would be alert for which adverse effects? Select all that apply.
   a. Respiratory depression
   b. Pruritus
   c. Constipation
   d. Vomiting
   e. Amnesia
   f. Hematoma

DOSAGE CALCULATION QUESTIONS

After you have performed your nonpharmacologic interventions, your patient, who is an infant, is exhibiting kicking, is not reaching for toys, and is occasionally crying. There is an order for morphine sulfate 1 mg IV every 3 to 4 hours. The safe dose range for morphine sulfate is 0.1 to 0.2 mg/kg/dose every 3 to 4 hours. Morphine sulfate is supplied as 1 mg/mL.

1. Is this a safe dose?

2. Describe how you will administer this medication and what you would assess for after giving it.

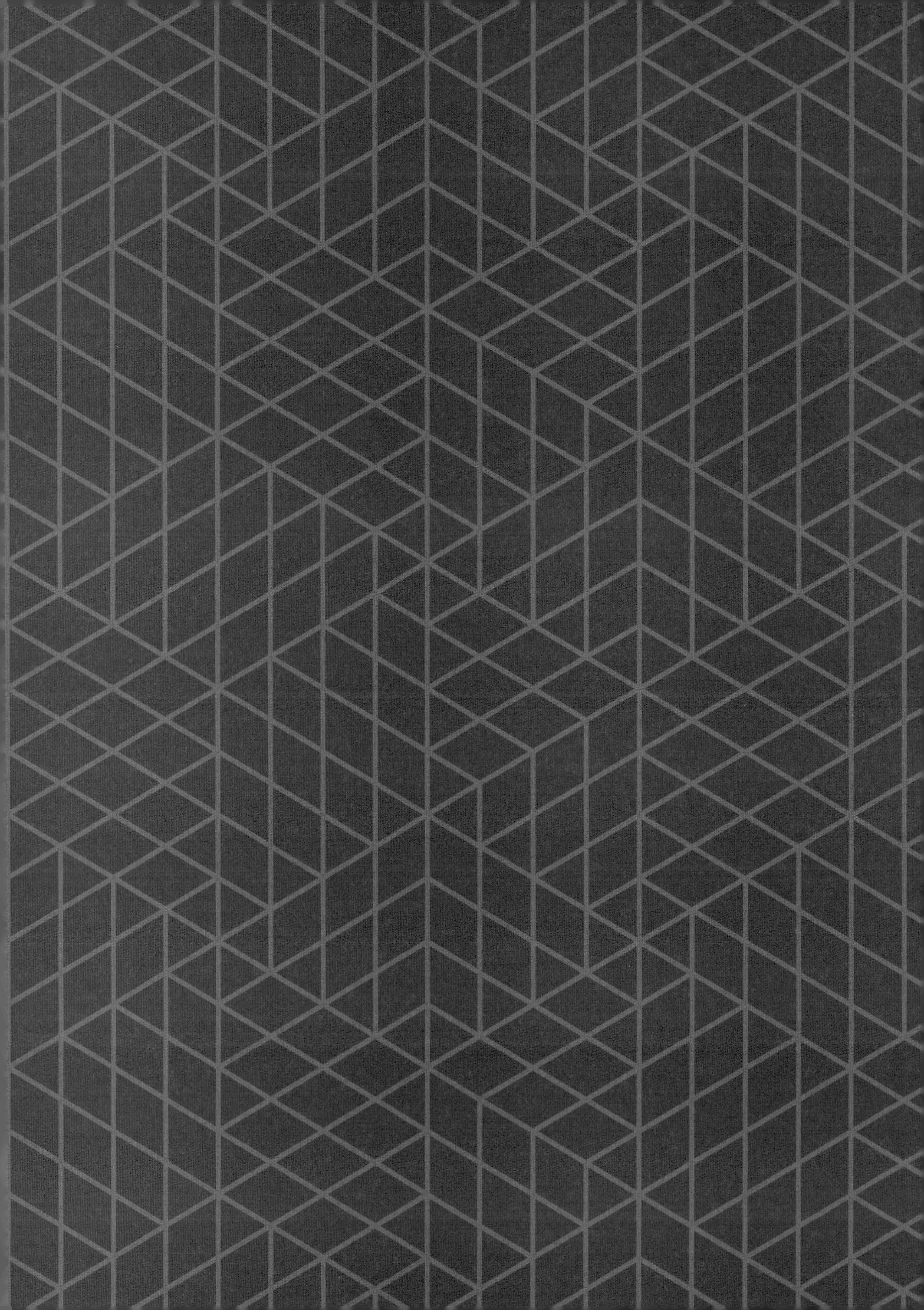

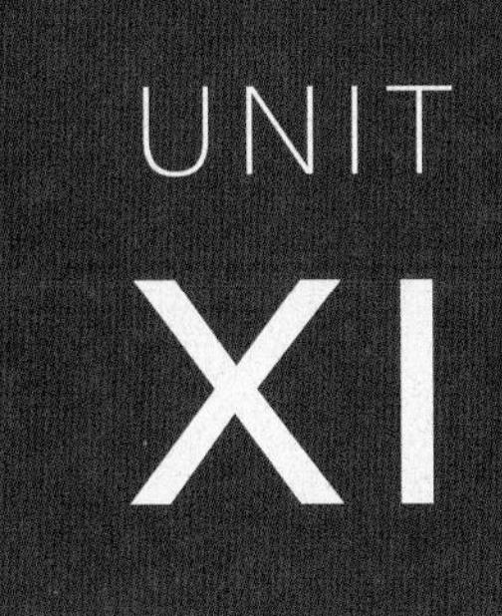

Nursing Care of the Child With a Health Disorder

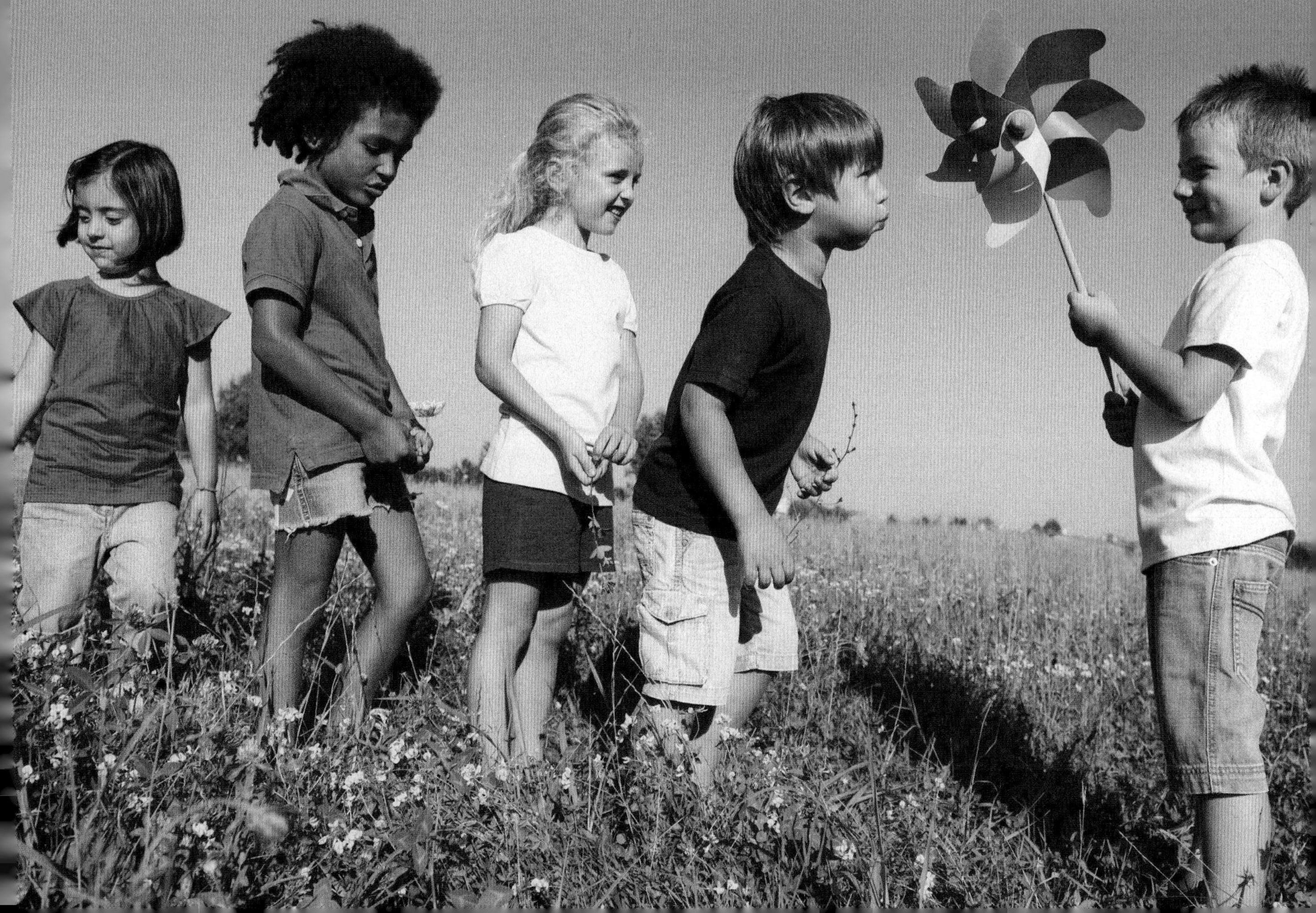

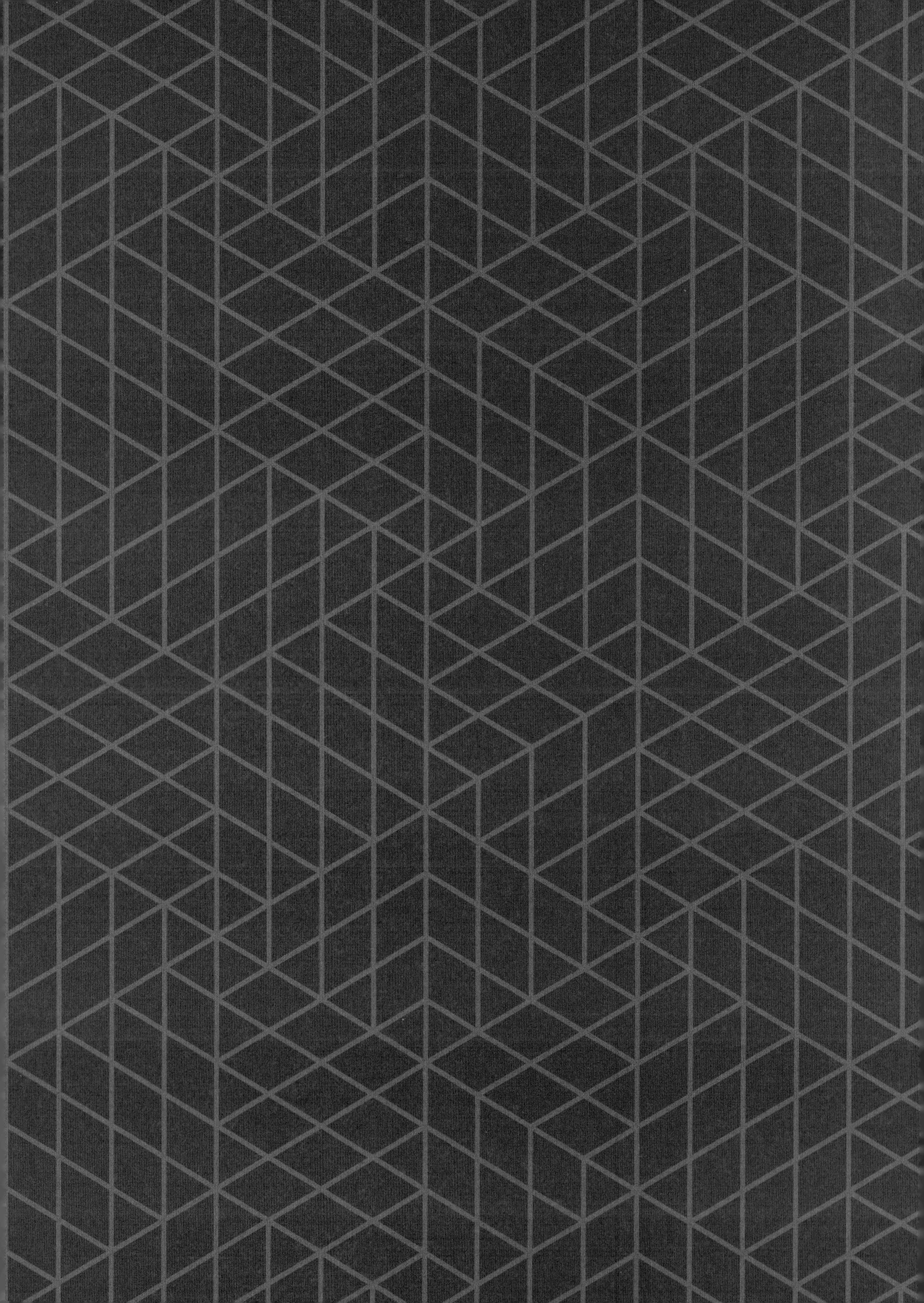

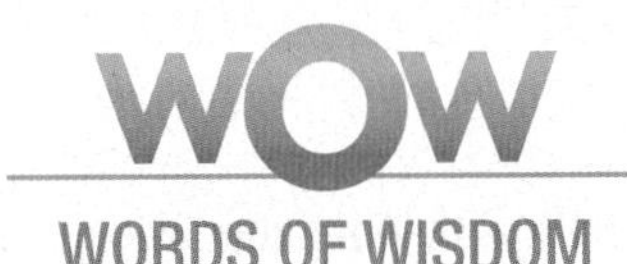

WORDS OF WISDOM

Complete and lasting freedom from infectious disease remains a dream, but one worth fighting a hard battle for.

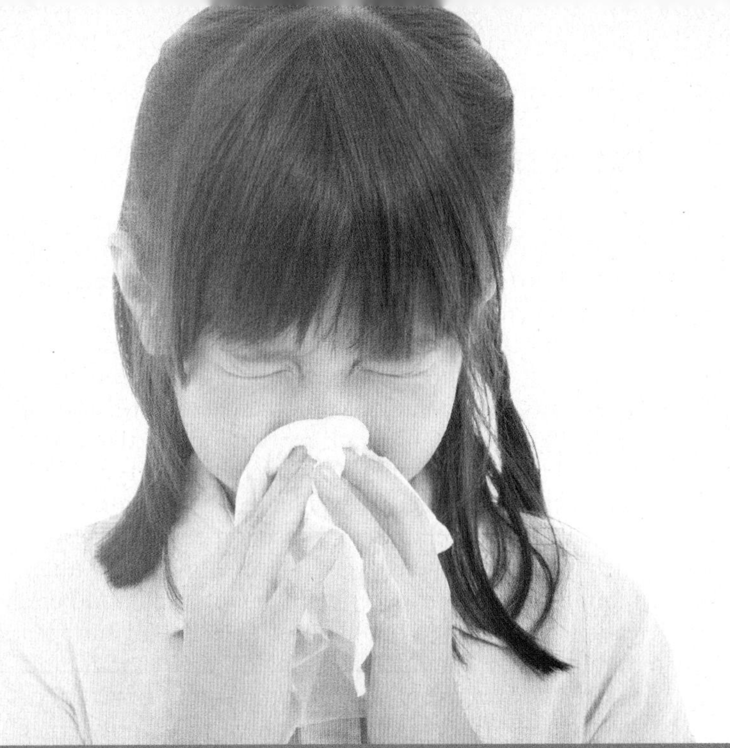

37

Nursing Care of the Child With an Infection

KEY TERMS

antibodies
antigen
chain of infection
communicability
endogenous pyrogens (en-doj′ĕ-nŭs pī′rō-jenz)
exanthem (eg-zan′thĕm)
phagocytosis (făg′ō-sī-tō′sis)
vector-borne
zoonotic (zō′ō-not′ik)

LEARNING OBJECTIVES

Upon completion of the chapter, you will be able to:

1. Discuss anatomic and physiologic differences in children versus adults in relation to the infectious process.
2. Identify nursing interventions related to common laboratory and diagnostic tests used in the diagnosis and management of infectious conditions.
3. Identify appropriate nursing assessments and interventions related to medications and treatments for childhood infectious and communicable disorders.
4. Distinguish various infectious illnesses occurring in childhood.
5. Devise an individualized plan of care for the child with an infectious or communicable disorder.
6. Develop child and family teaching plans for the child with an infectious or communicable disorder.

Samuel, 2 years old, is brought by his parent into the clinic. He presents with a history of fever and nasal congestion. His parent tells you, "He's been very irritable, crying more than usual and refusing to drink."

INTRODUCTION

Infection refers to the invasion of body cells and tissues by microorganisms with the potential to cause illness or disease (Nath, 2023). Nurses encounter potential or actual infections in all types of patients and must detect problems and intervene early to prevent life-threatening complications. Infections (infectious and communicable diseases) are one of the leading causes of death worldwide. As the world has become increasingly connected, infectious diseases have presented new challenges. Children are particularly vulnerable to these types of illnesses. Their immune systems are still developing and their natural curiosity, especially in infants and toddlers, leads to wide-range handling of objects and surfaces coupled with a tendency to place their hands and objects in their mouths without washing first. Infectious diseases in children can range in severity from mild with few or no symptoms to serious illness, such as damage to organs, and even death. Infectious and communicable diseases include bacterial infections (e.g., sepsis), viral infections (e.g., viral exanthems and rabies), zoonotic infections, vector-borne infections, parasitic and helminthic infections (e.g., roundworm and pediculosis capitis [head lice]), and sexually transmitted infections (STIs, e.g., chlamydia and gonorrhea).

There has been a dramatic decrease in the incidence and severity of infectious and communicable diseases since the advent of vaccines, antibiotics, antiviral drugs, and antitoxins. Some diseases have been effectively controlled, but the vast majority will not be eliminated. New diseases emerge and old diseases are reappearing, sometimes in a drug-resistant form. The Centers for Disease Control and Prevention (CDC) tracks certain infectious diseases. This list of nationally reportable diseases is revised periodically to add new pathogens or remove diseases as their incidence declines. Reporting by each state to the CDC is voluntary. Therefore, slight variations exist from state to state. Box 37.1 lists nationally reportable diseases.

Nurses, particularly those working in schools, child care centers, and outpatient settings, are often the first to see the signs of infectious or communicable diseases in children. These signs are often vague at first (e.g., a sore throat or rash). Therefore, nurses must have accurate assessment skills and be familiar with the signs and symptoms of common childhood infectious diseases so that they can provide prompt recognition, treatment, guidance, and support to families. Identifying the infectious agent is of primary importance to prevent further spread.

Many infectious diseases can be prevented through simple and inexpensive methods such as handwashing, adequate immunization, proper handling and preparation of food, and judicious antibiotic use. Nurses play a key role in educating parents and the community on ways to prevent infectious and communicable diseases.

BOX 37.1 Nationally Notifiable Diseases

- Botulism
- *Chlamydia trachomatis*
- COVID-19
- Diphtheria
- Ehrlichiosis
- Gonorrhea
- Hepatitis A, B, and C
- Influenza (pediatric mortality)
- Lyme disease
- Malaria
- Measles
- Meningococcal disease
- Mumps
- Pertussis
- Poliomyelitis, paralytic
- Poliovirus infection, nonparalytic
- Q fever
- Rabies
- Rocky Mountain spotted fever (spotted fever rickettsiosis)
- Rubella
- Syphilis
- Tetanus
- Tuberculosis
- Varicella (morbidity)
- Varicella (deaths only)

For a complete list of nationally notifiable diseases in the United States, go to https://ndc.services.cdc.gov/search-results-year.

HEALTHY PEOPLE 2030

Objective	Nursing Significance
Reduce the proportion of children who get no doses of recommended vaccines by age 2 years. Reduce cases of pertussis among infants. Maintain elimination of measles, rubella, congenital rubella syndrome (CRS), and acute paralytic poliomyelitis.	• Educate children and their families on the importance of proper immunizations. • Assess immunization status at every health encounter. • Provide families with a written record of immunizations given. • Promptly recognize infectious diseases, and provide child and family education regarding ways to prevent spread.

Healthy People Objectives retrieved from http://www.healthypeople.gov

INFECTIOUS PROCESS

Infection occurs when an organism enters the body and multiplies, causing damage to the tissues and cells. The body's response to this damage due to infection or injury is inflammation. The body delivers fluid, blood, and nutrients to the area of infection or injury and attempts to eliminate the pathogens and repair the tissues. The body does this through vascular and cellular reactions. The vascular response is an initial period of vasoconstriction followed by vasodilation. This vasodilation allows for the increase of fluids, blood, and nutrients to the area.

The cellular response involves the arrival of white blood cells (WBCs) to the area. WBCs are the body's defense against infection or injury. The types of WBCs are neutrophils, basophils, eosinophils, lymphocytes, and monocytes. Elevations in certain portions of the WBC count reflect different processes occurring in the body, such as infection, allergic reaction, or leukemia. Table 37.1 explains the function of each type of WBC. Each type is generally present in a balanced state; the types are reported as a percentage of the total WBC count or as the number per certain volume of blood.

TABLE **37.1** • Function of White Blood Cells by Leukocyte Type

Type of White Blood Cell	Function
Granulocytes • Neutrophils (polymorphonuclear leukocytes or PMNs, segs) • Eosinophils • Basophils	Phagocytic cells • First line of defense upon invasion of bacteria, fungus, cell debris, and other foreign substances • Respond to allergic disorders, parasitic infections, and chronic immune responses • Respond to allergic disorders and hypersensitivity reactions; used to study chronic inflammation
Lymphocytes (B lymphocytes, T lymphocytes, and natural killer cells)	Main source of producing an immune response; respond to viral infections (measles, rubella, chickenpox, infectious mononucleosis); tumors
Monocytes	Second line of defense; respond to larger and more severe infections than neutrophils by phagocytosis; leukemias and lymphomas; chronic inflammation

Data from Fischbach, F. T., Fischbach, M. A., & Stout, K. (2022). *A manual of laboratory and diagnostic tests* (11th ed.). Wolters Kluwer.

WBCs use **phagocytosis** to ingest and destroy the pathogen. If bacteria escape the action of phagocytosis, they enter the bloodstream and lymph system, and the immune system is activated. With activation of the immune system, B lymphocytes (humoral immunity) and T lymphocytes (cell-mediated immunity) are matured and activated. B and T cells recognize and attack infectious pathogens. B cells, which mature in the bone marrow, produce specific **antibodies** (specialized immune proteins) that bind to and neutralize a specific offending **antigen** (a substance that the body recognizes as foreign). T cells, which mature in the thymus, attack the antigen directly. Once B and T cells have been exposed to an antigen, some cells will remember the antigen. Therefore, if the particular antigen invades again, the body will act more quickly. A third type of lymphocyte, natural killer cells are a part of the innate immune system and function to destroy foreign material present.

Fever

Infection or inflammation caused by bacteria, viruses, or other pathogens stimulates the release of **endogenous pyrogens** (interleukins, tumor necrosis factor, and interferon). The pyrogens act on the hypothalamus, where they trigger prostaglandin production and increase the body's temperature set point. This triggers the cold response, resulting in shivering, vasoconstriction, and a decrease in peripheral perfusion to help decrease heat loss and allow the body's temperature to rise to the new set point, therefore resulting in fever. The definition of fever varies based on the age of the child, the method of temperature measurement, and the presence of any underlying conditions. There is no single value defined for fever due to individual variations, but Box 37.2 shows generally accepted guidelines based on measurement route in an otherwise healthy child. Refer to Chapter 32 for further information on measurement of temperature.

It is important to distinguish between fever and hyperthermia. Hyperthermia occurs when normal thermoregulation fails, resulting in an unregulated rise in core temperature. Hyperthermia may occur if the central nervous system of the child becomes impaired by disease, drugs, and abnormalities of heat production or thermal

BOX **37.2** **General Guideline of Fever Based on Measurement Route**

- Oral: >37.8°C (100°F)
- Rectal: >38°C (100.4°F)
- Axillary: >37.2°C (99°F)
- Tympanic: >38°C (100.4°F)
- Temporal: >38°C (100.4°F)

stressors, such as being left in a hot automobile or exertional heat stroke. In the absence of hyperthermia or neurologic impairment, the body does not allow fever to rise to lethal levels. The body actually produces a natural antipyretic, called cryogen. If there is no hyperthermic insult, it is rare to see a child's temperature rise above 41°C (105.8°F) (Ward, 2022).

Fever in their children is one of the most common reasons parents seek medical attention (Sullivan et al., 2011, reaffirmed 2023). Most infections or communicable diseases are accompanied by fever. Many parents have great concerns about fever. For example, they fear febrile seizures, neurologic complications, and a potential serious underlying disease. Many health care providers share these fears. This leads to the common recommendation to intervene and reduce fever. These fears and misconceptions about fever can lead to mismanagement of fever, such as inappropriate dosing of antipyretics, awakening the child during sleep to give antipyretics, or inappropriate use of nonpharmacologic treatments such as sponging the child with alcohol or cold water (Sullivan et al., 2011, reaffirmed 2023).

Fever is a protective mechanism the body uses to fight infection. Evidence exists that an elevated body temperature actually enhances various components of the immune response (Sullivan et al., 2011, reaffirmed 2023). Fever can slow the growth of bacteria and viruses and increase neutrophil production and T-cell proliferation (Sullivan et al., 2011, reaffirmed 2023). Another concern is that reducing fever may hide signs of serious bacterial illness (Sullivan et al., 2011, reaffirmed 2023).

TAKE NOTE!

Infants younger than 3 months with a rectal temperature greater than 38°C (100.4°F) should be seen by a health care provider or nurse practitioner.

Antipyretics are often used to lower fever and increase comfort. They decrease the temperature set point by inhibiting the production of prostaglandins. As a result, sweating and vasodilation occur, and there is heat loss and a drop in temperature. Antipyretics provide symptomatic relief but do not change the course of the infection. The major benefits of decreasing fever are increasing comfort in the child and decreasing fluid requirements, which helps to prevent dehydration. Children with certain underlying conditions, such as cardiovascular disease or pulmonary disease, also benefit from treating fever because such treatment decreases demands on the body. The use of acetaminophen or ibuprofen to reduce fever in children has been shown to be safe and effective when the appropriate dose is administered at the appropriate interval (Ward, 2022). However, some studies have shown that ibuprofen is superior

BOX 37.3 Dose Recommendations for Oral Acetaminophen and Ibuprofen

Acetaminophen, 10–15 mg/kg/dose
- No more than every 4 hours
- No more than five doses in a 24-hour period
- Not to exceed 4,000 mg/day

Ibuprofen, 4–10 mg/kg/dose
- Only children older than 6 months of age
- Given every 6–8 hours; no more than four doses in a 24-hour period
- Maximum daily dose: 2,400 mg/day

Source: Lexicomp. (2023). Pediatric drug information. *UpToDate*. Retrieved April 5, 2023, from https://www.uptodate.com/contents/table-of-contents/drug-information/pediatric-drug-information

in reducing fever and lasts longer than acetaminophen (Ward, 2022). Box 37.3 gives dosing recommendations for both medications.

CLINICAL REASONING ALERT!

Never give aspirin or aspirin-containing products to children to reduce fever, due to the risk of Reye syndrome.

Acetaminophen is widely used and accepted, with a long track record of safety and efficacy when used according to the label directions, but overdose can lead to toxic reactions (Ward, 2022). Causes of acetaminophen toxicity include overdosing or incorrect dosing due to failure to read and understand the label instructions, use of an incorrect measuring device or concentration, and coadministration with an over-the-counter, fixed-dose combination medication (the parent may not recognize that it has acetaminophen in it).

Another factor that may cause acetaminophen toxicity is the controversial, but common, practice of alternating acetaminophen and ibuprofen to help reduce fever. Although insufficient evidence exists to support or refute alternating or combining acetaminophen with ibuprofen to treat fever, safety concerns remain (Sullivan et al., 2011, reaffirmed 2023). This practice can result in overdose or improper administration. It can be hard for parents to keep track of the time each medication is due. Parents may confuse which medication is given every 4 hours and which is given every 6 hours. They may exceed the recommended daily doses or may confuse the strength or dosage of the medicines. In some cases, alternating or combining acetaminophen and ibuprofen may be needed if the child's distress or discomfort persists or recurs before the next dose is due. In these cases, careful and thorough dosing instructions and intervals are imperative. See Evidence-Based Practice 37.1.

EVIDENCE-BASED PRACTICE 37.1

Which Is More Effective in Treating Fever in Children—Ibuprofen or Acetaminophen? Combined, Alternating, or Alone?

Fever is one of the most common health concerns seen in pediatrics, and it is an important component of the body's response to infection. Although ibuprofen (IBU) and acetaminophen (APAP) are the most widely used antipyretics and are recommended by the American Academy of Pediatrics (AAP), the question of safety and efficacy of one over the other and combining or alternating for fever reduction continues.

STUDY

This study was a narrative review of randomized, blinded, controlled studies assessing the effectiveness of IBU versus APAP, combined, alternating, or alone in reducing fever in children. This review compared health care provider dosing (IBU 10/mg; APAP 15 mg/kg) to over-the-counter (OTC) dosing (IBU 5 to 10 mg/kg; APAP 10 to 15 mg/kg) for both IBU and APAP.

Findings

This study suggests a modest improvement in fever reduction with IBU over APAP at OTC dosing but similar effectiveness in health care provider dosing. Combining or alternating IBU and APAP seems to provide a better reduction in fever and to be well tolerated.

Nursing Implications

According to the AAP, improvement of the child's overall comfort, not just reducing fever, should be the goal of antipyretic therapy. Therefore, future research is warranted focusing on this outcome. Future research also needs to focus on evaluating the effectiveness of combined versus alternating antipyretic therapy and safety concerns with these approaches. Nurses need to continue to educate parents regarding why fever occurs, fever facts and myths, when treatment of fever is necessary, and best treatment options.

Data from Paul, I. M., & Walson, P. D. (2021). Acetaminophen and ibuprofen in the treatment of pediatric fever: a narrative review. *Current Medical Research and Opinion, 37*(8), 1363–1375. https://doi.org/10.1080/03007995.2021.1928617

DOSAGE CALCULATION BOX 37.1

The nurse is caring for a toddler who is 2 years old and 28 lb. The order reads ibuprofen 100 mg po every 6 hours as needed for temperature greater than 38°C (100.4°F). Is this a safe and effective dose?

Stages of Infectious Disease

Infectious diseases follow a similar pattern. They progress through certain stages (Table 37.2) in which **communicability** (ability to spread to others) can be predicted. It is important for nurses to understand these stages to help control and manage infectious diseases.

TABLE 37.2 • Stages of Infectious Disease

Stage	Explanation
Incubation	Time from entrance of pathogen into the body to appearance of first symptoms; during this time, pathogens grow and multiply.
Prodrome	Time from onset of nonspecific symptoms such as fever, malaise, and fatigue to more specific symptoms
Illness	Time during which child demonstrates signs and symptoms specific to an infection type
Convalescence	Time when acute symptoms of illness disappear

Chain of Infection

The **chain of infection** is the process by which an organism is spread. Behaviors of infants and young children, mainly pertaining to hygiene, increase their risk for infection by promoting the chain of infection. Poor hygiene habits, including lack of handwashing, placing toys and hands in the mouth, drooling, and leaking diapers, all can contribute to the spread of infection and communicable diseases. Table 37.3 reviews the chain of infection and nursing implications related to it.

Preventing the Spread of Infection

Nurses play a key role in breaking the chain of infection and preventing the spread of diseases. It is important to follow infection control and prevention practices. It is also very important to educate parents and children on the measures they can take to prevent the spread of infection.

TAKE NOTE!

Frequent handwashing is the most important way to prevent the spread of infection.

Isolation precautions help nurses break the chain of infection and provide strategies to prevent the spread of pathogens among hospitalized children. Guidelines can be found on the CDC website (http://www.cdc.gov/hicpac/2007IP/2007isolationPrecautions.html). Additional guidelines are available from various infection control societies and regulatory agencies such as the

TABLE 37.3 • Chain of Infection

Chain Link	Explanation	Nursing Implications
Infectious agent	Any agent capable of causing infection; examples: bacteria, viruses, rickettsiae, protozoa, and fungi	Control or eliminate infectious agents through: • Handwashing • Wearing gloves • Cleaning, disinfecting, or sterilizing equipment
Reservoir	A place where the pathogen can thrive and reproduce; examples: human body, animals, insects, food, water, inanimate objects (e.g., stethoscopes)	• Control or eliminate reservoirs. • Control sources of body fluids, drainage, or solutions that may harbor pathogens. • Follow institutional guidelines for disposing of infectious wastes. • Provide proper wound care; change dressings or bandages when soiled. • Assist children to carry out appropriate skin and oral care. • Keep linens clean and dry.
Portal of exit	A way for the pathogen to exit the reservoir; examples: skin and mucous membranes, respiratory tract, urinary tract, gastrointestinal tract, reproductive tract	• Control portals of exit and educate children and families. • Cover mouth and nose when sneezing or coughing. • Avoid talking, coughing, or sneezing over open wounds or sterile fields. • Use personal protective equipment.
Modes of transmission	Direct transmission: body-to-body contact Indirect transmission: transferred by fomite or vector; spread by droplet or airborne transmission	• Wash hands before and after child contact, invasive procedures, or touching open wounds. • Use personal protective equipment when necessary. • Urge children and family to wash hands frequently, especially before eating or handling food, after eliminating, and after touching infectious material.
Portal of entry	A way for the pathogen to enter the host; examples: skin and mucous membranes, respiratory tract, urinary tract, gastrointestinal tract, reproductive tract	• Use proper sterile technique during invasive procedures. • Provide appropriate wound care. • Dispose of needles and sharps in puncture-resistant containers. • Provide all children with their own personal care items.
Susceptible host	Any person who cannot resist the pathogen	• Protect susceptible host by promoting normal body defenses against infection. • Maintain integrity of the child's skin and mucous membranes. • Protect normal defenses by regular bathing and oral care, adequate fluid intake and nutrition, and proper immunization.

Occupational Safety and Health Administration (OSHA) agency. The Joint Commission has also developed infection control standards. This leads to an array of complex guidelines that all health professionals need to be familiar with.

The Hospital Infection Control Practices Advisory Committee (HICPAC) has presented guidelines for hospitalized children that include two tiers (Siegel et al., 2007, updated 2022). Tier 1 is standard precautions, which are designed for the care of all children in the hospital regardless of their diagnosis. Tier 2 is transmission-based precautions, designed for children who are known, or suspected, to be infected with epidemiologically important pathogens. These pathogens can be spread by airborne, droplet, or contact transmission. Box 37.4 gives an overview of standard and transmission-based precautions.

TAKE NOTE!

Hand hygiene includes both handwashing with soap and water and the use of alcohol-based products (gels, rinses, foams) that do not require water. If there is no visible soiling of the hands, approved alcohol-based products are preferred because of their superior microbicidal activity, reduced drying of the skin, and convenience (Anderson, 2023; CDC, 2020a).

BOX 37.4 Standard Precautions and Isolation Precautions

Standard Precautions (Tier 1)

- Apply to all children.
- Apply to all body fluids, secretions, and excretions except sweat, nonintact skin, and mucous membranes.
- Designed to reduce the risk of transmission of microorganisms from recognized and unrecognized sources
- Techniques include:
  - Proper hand hygiene
  - Use of gloves (clean or sterile) when touching blood, body fluids, secretions or excretions, and contaminated items
  - Masks, eye protection, and face shields when patient care may include splashing or sprays of blood, body fluid secretions, or excretions, and during bronchoscopy, endotracheal intubation, and open suctioning of the respiratory tract
  - Fluid-resistant nonsterile gowns, to protect skin and clothing, when patient care may include splashing or sprays of blood, body fluid secretions, or excretions
  - Patient care equipment handled in a manner that prevents skin or mucous membrane exposure and contamination of clothing
  - All used linen is considered contaminated and needs to be handled and disposed of appropriately.
  - Mouthpieces, resuscitation bags with one-way valves, and other ventilation devices should be readily available.
  - Cleaning and disinfecting noncritical surfaces in patient care areas
  - Respiratory hygiene/cough etiquette: applies to any person with signs of illness including cough, congestion, rhinorrhea, or increased respiratory secretions that is entering a health care facility. It includes education regarding covering the mouth/nose with a tissue; prompt disposal of used tissues, along with surgical masks used by a person who is coughing when appropriate; hand hygiene after contact with respiratory secretions; and separation, ideally greater than 3 ft, of people with respiratory infections in common waiting areas when possible.
  - Safe injection practices: use of sterile single-use disposable needle. When possible, use of single-dose vials; precautions used to prevent injury when using, cleaning, or disposing of needles and sharps
  - Use of masks for insertion of catheters or injection into the spinal or epidural space via lumbar puncture procedures

Transmission-Based Precautions (Tier 2)

Designed for children with known or suspected infection with pathogens for which additional precautions are warranted to interrupt transmission

Airborne

- Designed to reduce the risk of infectious agents transmitted by airborne droplet nuclei or dust particles that may contain the infectious agent
- Examples of such illnesses include measles, varicella, and tuberculosis.
- Techniques include standard precautions as well as:
  - Room with negative air pressure ventilation, with air externally exhausted or high-efficiency particulate air filtered if recirculated; if unavailable, mask the child and place in private room with the door closed.
  - Wear a mask or respirator depending on specific recommendations based on disease, such as if infectious pulmonary tuberculosis is suspected or proven, wear a respiratory protective device, such as an N95 respirator, while in the child's room.
  - Susceptible health care personnel should not enter the room of children with measles or varicella zoster infections. Those with proven immunity to these viruses need not wear a mask.

Droplet

- Intended to prevent transmission of pathogens spread through close respiratory or mucous membrane contact with respiratory secretions. Designed to reduce the risk of infectious agents transmitted by contact of the conjunctivae or the mucous membranes of the nose or mouth of a susceptible person with large-particle droplets containing pathogens generated from a person (generally through coughing, sneezing, talking, or procedures such as suctioning) who has a clinical disease or who is a carrier of the disease
- Examples of such illnesses include diphtheria, pertussis, group A streptococcal disease, influenza, mumps, rubella, and scarlet fever.
- Techniques include standard precautions as well as:
  - Private room (if unavailable, consider cohorting children with the same disease. If this is not possible, separation of at least 3 ft between other children and visitors should be maintained.)
  - Wear a mask if within 3 ft of the child.

Contact

- Most important and most common route of transmission of health care–associated infections
- Designed to reduce the risk of infectious agents transmitted by direct or indirect contact. Direct-contact transmission involves skin-to-skin contact and physical transfer of pathogens between a susceptible host and an infected or colonized person. Examples include patient care activities that involve physical contact such as turning and bathing. Direct-contact transmission also can occur between two children, where one serves as the source of infectious pathogen and the other as a susceptible host. Indirect-contact transmission involves contact of a susceptible host with a contaminated intermediate object, usually inanimate, in the child's environment.
- Examples of such illnesses include diphtheria,[a] pediculosis, scabies, and multidrug-resistant bacteria.
- Techniques include standard precautions as well as:
  - Private room (if unavailable, consultation with infection control personnel is recommended. Consider cohorting children with the same disease. If this is not possible, separation of at least 3 ft between other children and visitors should be maintained.)
  - Gloves (clean or sterile) should be used at all times.
  - Proper hand hygiene after glove removal
  - Use gloves and gowns for all interactions that involve contact with the child or potentially contaminated areas. Don before entering and remove before leaving the child's room.

Prevention standards are applied in all health care settings and are modified to meet each setting's unique needs. Health care workers must practice within the specific institution's guidelines.

[a]Certain infections require more than one precaution.

Data from Siegel, J. D., Rhinehart, E., Jackson, M., Chiarello, L., & The Healthcare Infection Control Practices Advisory Committee. (2007, updated 2022). Guideline for isolation precautions: Preventing transmission of infectious agents in healthcare settings. https://www.cdc.gov/infectioncontrol/pdf/guidelines/isolation-guidelines-H.pdf

CLINICAL REASONING ALERT!

When caring for a child with suspected or confirmed norovirus or *Clostridioides* (formerly *Clostridium*) *difficile* ensure handwashing is performed using soap and water as alcohol does not kill these microorganisms (Anderson, 2023).

When caring for children, these guidelines may need to be modified. For instance, diaper changing is routine in the pediatric setting. Since it does not usually soil hands, it is not mandatory to wear gloves (except if gloves are required due to transmission-based precautions). According to the standard precaution guidelines, single rooms are required for those who are incontinent and cannot control bodily excretions. Since the majority of young children are incontinent, obviously this guideline is inappropriate in the pediatric setting. Pediatric units often have common rooms, such as playrooms and schoolrooms. Children placed on transmission-based isolation are not allowed to leave their rooms and therefore are not allowed to use these common rooms.

VARIATIONS IN PEDIATRIC ANATOMY AND PHYSIOLOGY

Normal immune function is an amazing protective response by the body. It involves complex responses including phagocytosis, humoral immunity, cellular immunity, and activation of the complement system. Blood and lymph are responsible for transporting the agents of the immune system. Due to the immature responses of the immune system, infants and young children are more susceptible to infection. The newborn displays a decreased inflammatory response to invading organisms, contributing to an increased risk for infection. Cellular immunity is generally functional at birth, and humoral immunity occurs when the body encounters and then develops immunity to new diseases. Since the infant has had limited exposure to disease and is losing the passive immunity acquired from maternal antibodies, the risk of infection is higher. Young children continue to have an increased risk for infection and communicable disorders because disease protection from immunizations is not complete. (Refer to Chapter 31 for further details.)

COMMON MEDICAL TREATMENTS

A variety of medications and other medical treatments are used to treat infectious disorders in children. Most of these treatments will require a health care provider's or nurse practitioner's order when the child is in the hospital. The most common treatments and medications are listed in Common Medical Treatments 37.1 and Drug Guide 37.1. The nurse caring for the child with an infectious disorder should be familiar with what the procedures are, how they work, and common nursing implications related to use of these modalities.

COMMON MEDICAL TREATMENTS 37.1

Treatment	Explanation	Indications	Nursing Implications
Hydration	Promoting proper fluid balance either orally or intravenously	Child who can't replace insensible loss due to fever, child who is vomiting or has diarrhea	• Encourage oral fluids, if possible. • Offer child preferred fluid; try popsicles or games to promote fluid intake. • If administering IV fluids, ensure proper fluid and rate per order and assess IV site and fluid intake every hour. • Maintain strict record of intake and output.
Fever reduction	Reducing temperature by use of antipyretics or nonpharmacologic interventions	Febrile child who is uncomfortable or who can't keep up with the increased metabolic demands associated with fever	• Administer antipyretics, such as ibuprofen and acetaminophen. • Avoid aspirin use in children and adolescents. • Use nonpharmacologic interventions such as dressing lightly, removing blankets, use of a fan, tepid bath, and cooling blanket. Make sure that nonpharmacologic measures do not induce shivering or discomfort. If they do, they should be stopped immediately.

IV, intravenous.

DRUG GUIDE 37.1

COMMON DRUGS FOR COMMUNICABLE DISORDERS

Medication	Actions/Indications	Nursing Implications
Antibiotics	Kill and prevent the growth of bacteria. Used for the treatment of bacterial infections such as sepsis	• Check for antibiotic allergies. • Give as prescribed for the length of time prescribed.
Antivirals (e.g., acyclovir)	Kill and prevent the growth of viruses. Used for the treatment of viral infections such as herpes simplex type 2	• Observe infusion site for signs of tissue damage. • If administering topically, clean and dry area before application and wear gloves. • Give as prescribed for the length of time prescribed.
Antipyretics (acetaminophen, ibuprofen)	Decrease the temperature set point (only in a child with a raised temperature) by inhibiting the production of prostaglandins, leading to heat loss (through vasodilation and sweating) and resulting in a reduction in fever. Used to decrease temperature in the febrile child who is uncomfortable or who can't keep up with the increased metabolic demands associated with fever	• Ensure proper dosing, concentration, and dosing interval. • Avoid aspirin use in children and adolescents. • Avoid ibuprofen use in children with a bleeding disorder. • Assess fever and any related symptoms such as tachycardia, shivering, or diaphoresis. • Properly educate caregivers on appropriate dosing, concentration, dosing interval, and use of accurate measuring device.
Antipruritics (usually antihistamines)	Given orally or topically to block the histamine reaction Used to relieve discomfort associated with itching	• When applying topically, wear gloves. • Do not apply to open wounds. • Oral antihistamines may cause drowsiness.

Adapted from Lexicomp. (2023). Pediatric drug information. *UpToDate*. Retrieved April 5, 2023, from https://www.uptodate.com/contents/table-of-contents/drug-information/pediatric-drug-information

Clinical Judgment and the Nursing Process for the Child With an Infection

Care of the child with an infectious or communicable disorder includes assessment, nursing analysis, planning, interventions, and evaluation. There are a number of general concepts related to the nursing process that may be applied to the care of children with infectious disorders. From a general understanding of the care involved for a child with an infectious disorder, the nurse can then individualize the care based on the child's specifics.

Assessment

Assessment of the child with a communicable or infectious disorder includes health history, physical examination, and laboratory and diagnostic testing.

Health History

The health history consists of the past medical history, including the birthing parent's pregnancy history; family history; and history of present illness (when the symptoms started and how they have progressed), as well as treatments used at home. The past medical history might be significant for lack of recommended immunizations, prematurity, infection during birthing parent's pregnancy or labor, prolonged difficult delivery, or immunocompromise. Family history might be significant for lack of immunization or recent infectious or communicable disease. When eliciting the history of the present illness, inquire about the following:

- Any known exposure to infectious or communicable disease
- Immunization history
- History of having any common childhood communicable diseases
- Fever
- Sore throat
- Lethargy
- Malaise
- Poor feeding or decreased appetite
- Vomiting
- Diarrhea
- Cough
- Rash (in the older child ask for a description [i.e., Is it painful? Does it itch?])

TAKE NOTE!

Many childhood infections and communicable diseases involve a rash. Rashes can be difficult to identify. Therefore, it is important to obtain a thorough description and history from the caregiver.

Physical Examination

Physical examination of the child with an infectious disorder includes inspection, observation, and palpation.

INSPECTION AND OBSERVATION

Begin the physical examination with inspection and observation. Assess the child's skin, mouth, throat, and hair for lesions or wounds. Note the color, shape, and distribution of any lesions or wounds. Assess whether there is any exudate from the lesions or wounds. A thorough and accurate description is important to assist in identifying the rash and causative organism. Observe for scratching, restlessness, avoidance of the use of a body part, or guarding of a body part. Observe the child's affect, energy level, and interaction with caregivers. Lethargy can indicate serious infection or sepsis. Observe if there is any discharge from the nose, cough, or respiratory difficulty.

Assess hydration status. Inspect the oral mucosa; dry and pale mucous membranes can indicate dehydration. Observe for other signs of dehydration, such as sunken eyes and no tears with crying.

Assessment of vital signs can provide more information about the child's condition. Elevated temperature can indicate infection. Often tachypnea and tachycardia accompany fever. Hypotension may also occur, but it is usually a late sign with sepsis.

CLINICAL REASONING ALERT!

Neonates and young infants may not present with fever; some may present with normal or low temperatures and have serious infections (Cantey, 2023; Scarfone & Cho, 2022).

PALPATION

Palpate the skin to assess temperature, moisture, texture, and turgor. In a child with an infectious or communicable disease, the skin may be warm and moist due to fever. Turgor may be decreased secondary to dehydration. In infants, palpate the fontanels; if they are sunken, the infant may be dehydrated. Palpate the rash to determine if it is raised or flat. A thorough picture of the presenting rash can help identify the child's illness. Palpate the lymph nodes and note any that are swollen and tender.

Laboratory and Diagnostic Testing

Common Laboratory and Diagnostic Tests 37.1 discusses the tests used most commonly when communicable disorders are suspected. The tests can assist the health care provider or nurse practitioner in diagnosing the disorder and/or be used as guidelines in determining ongoing treatment. Laboratory or non-nursing personnel obtain some of the tests, while the nurse might obtain others. In either instance, the nurse should be familiar with how the tests are obtained, what they

COMMON LABORATORY AND DIAGNOSTIC TESTS 37.1

Test	Explanation	Indications	Nursing Implications
Complete blood count (CBC)	Evaluate white blood cell count (particularly the percentage of individual white cells).	Detect the presence of inflammation, infection.	• Normal values vary according to age and sex. • White blood cell count differential is helpful in differentiating source of infection. • May be affected by myelosuppressive drugs
Erythrocyte sedimentation rate (ESR)	Nonspecific test used in conjunction with other tests to determine presence of infection or inflammation	Detect the presence of inflammation, infection.	Send to laboratory quickly; specimens allowed to stand for longer than 24 hours may produce a falsely low result.
Standard C-reactive protein (CRP)	Nonspecific test that measures a type of protein produced in the liver that is present during episodes of acute inflammation or infection Usually used to diagnose acute infections	To detect the presence of infection, CRP is a more sensitive and rapidly responding indicator than ESR.	Do not confuse it with high-sensitivity CRP, which measures a different range and is used to evaluate cardiovascular risk.
Blood culture and sensitivity	Deliberate growing of microorganism in a solid or liquid medium. Once it has grown, it is tested against various antibiotics to determine which antibiotics will kill it.	Detect the presence of bacteria or yeast, which may have spread from a certain site in the body into the bloodstream. Determine which antibiotics the bacteria or yeast is sensitive to.	• Follow aseptic technique and hospital protocol to prevent contamination. • Two cultures obtained from two different sites are preferred. • Ideally obtain before administering antibiotics; if child is taking antibiotics, notify laboratory and draw specimen shortly before next dose. • Draw below intravenous line, if possible, to prevent dilution of sample.

COMMON LABORATORY AND DIAGNOSTIC TESTS 37.1

Test	Explanation	Indications	Nursing Implications
Stool culture (including stool for ova and parasites [O&P])	To determine if bacteria or parasite have infected the intestines	Detect pathogens, including parasites or overgrowth of normal flora in the bowel. Indicated for children with diarrhea, fever, or abdominal pain.	• Stool must be free of urine, water, and toilet paper. • Do not retrieve out of toilet water. • Obtain freshly passed stool. • Deliver to laboratory immediately. • Mineral oil, barium, and bismuth interfere with the detection of parasites; specimen collection should be delayed for 7–10 days. • Often a minimum of three specimens on 3 separate days are required for adequate examination, since many parasites and worm eggs are shed intermittently.
Urine culture	Collection of urine to detect the presence of bacteria in the urine	Detect the presence of bacteria in the urinary tract. Indicated for children with fever of unknown origin, dysuria, frequency, or urgency, or if urinalysis suggests infection.	• Should be obtained by midstream clean-catch, catheterization, or suprapubic aspiration. Avoid contamination with stool, vaginal secretions, hands, or clothing. • Placing bags on the perineum is not preferred due to high chance of contamination; if used, analyze specimen as soon as possible. • Obtain before antibiotics are administered. • Deliver to laboratory immediately (preferable) or refrigerate.
Wound culture	Allows for microbial growth and identification of specific organism	Identification of specific organism	• Do not take from exudate or eschar. • If moderate to heavy drainage is present, irrigate the wound with sterile saline. Disinfect the surface of the wound. • Specimens taken from wounds can harbor a variety of organisms. Pathogenicity depends on the quantity of organisms present. • Avoid touching intact skin at the wound edges. • Culture highly vascular granulation tissue.
Throat culture	Vigorous swabbing of the tonsillar area and posterior pharynx to detect the presence of invasive organisms	Most reliable method of detecting group A streptococcal pharyngitis Will also detect *Bordetella pertussis*, *Corynebacterium diphtheriae*; viral infections May be performed in those with fever of unknown origin	• Ensure specimen is of secretions in the pharyngeal or tonsillar area. Avoid touching tongue or lips with swab. • When performing on young children, have adult hold child in lap. • Health care worker needs to stabilize head by placing hand on the child's forehead.
Nasal swabs (nasopharyngeal)	Insertion of swabs into the nose until reaching the nasopharynx to detect the presence of invasive organisms	Optimal method for detecting *B. pertussis*. Also used to detect *Corynebacterium diphtheriae* and viral illnesses such as *respiratory syncytial virus* (RSV), *parainfluenza*	• The distance from the child's nose to ear gives an estimate of how far to insert the swab into the nostril to reach the nasopharynx. • Insert swab straight back, not up, and leave in nasopharynx for several seconds. • When performing on young children, have adult hold child in lap. • Health care worker needs to stabilize head as child will likely try to pull away.

Data from Fischbach, F. T., Fischbach, M. A., & Stout, K. (2022). *A manual of laboratory and diagnostic tests* (11th ed.). Wolters Kluwer.

are used for, and normal versus abnormal results. This knowledge will also be necessary when providing child and family education related to the testing.

OBTAINING BLOOD SPECIMENS

Giving a blood specimen may be frightening to children because of the fear of needles, pain, and blood loss. Provide atraumatic care when performing venipunctures and other needlesticks in children (refer to Chapter 30 for further information). Whether the laboratory technician or the nurse is drawing the blood, the procedure should be performed in an area other than the child's bed, such as the treatment room; the child's bed should be kept as a "safe" area. Provide teaching about the procedure based on the child's developmental level and readiness to learn. In infants and younger children, additional assistance with positioning and restraint will be needed to perform the procedure safely and to ensure proper collection. Use a topical anesthetic cream or gel (preferred), refrigerant spray, or iontophoresis before venipuncture. Refer to Chapter 36 for additional information about decreasing venipuncture-related pain in infants and children.

The usual sites for obtaining blood specimens via venipuncture are the superficial veins of the dorsal surface of the hand or the antecubital fossa, although other locations may also be used. In specific situations, the jugular or femoral vein may be used; in this case either the health care provider or the nurse practitioner will perform the venipuncture.

Capillary puncture of the child's fingertip, the great toe, or the infant's heel may also be used to obtain blood specimens. Fingertip puncture is similar to that in the adult, directed to the sides of the fingertip. Great toe puncture is performed in the same way. Capillary heel puncture must be performed in the proper location to avoid striking the medial plantar artery or periosteum (see Nursing Procedure 37.1). Automatic lancet devices can be used to deliver a more precise puncture depth.

• • • ATRAUMATIC CARE • • •

The young infant will benefit from the use of oral sucrose combined with nonnutritive sucking, skin-to-skin contact, and/or swaddling before and during the capillary puncture (Roué, 2022).

Occasionally, blood samples may be obtained from an artery rather than a vein or capillary. Blood gases in particular are usually obtained by arterial puncture. Arterial puncture requires additional training and in many institutions is performed only by the respiratory therapist, health care provider, or nurse practitioner.

Children with indwelling venous access devices may be spared the trauma of puncture for blood specimens. Follow your institution's guidelines for withdrawing blood from peripherally inserted venous

NURSING PROCEDURE 37.1 Capillary Heel Puncture

1. Choose the collection site and apply a commercial heel warmer or warm pack for several minutes prior to specimen collection.
2. Assemble equipment:
   - Gloves
   - Automatic lancet
   - Antiseptic wipe
   - Cotton ball or dry gauze
   - Capillary blood collection tube
   - Band-aid
3. Perform hand hygiene and don gloves. Remove the warm pack.
4. Cleanse the site with antiseptic prep pad and allow to dry.
5. Hold the dorsum of the foot with the nondominant hand; with the dominant hand, pierce the heel with the lancet. Place the extremity in the dependent position.
6. Wipe away the first drop of blood with the cotton ball or dry gauze.
7. Collect the blood specimen with a capillary specimen collection tube. Avoid squeezing the foot during specimen collection if possible, as it may contribute to hemolysis of the specimen.
8. Hold dry gauze over the site until bleeding stops, elevate extremity above the level of the heart, and then apply a Band-Aid.

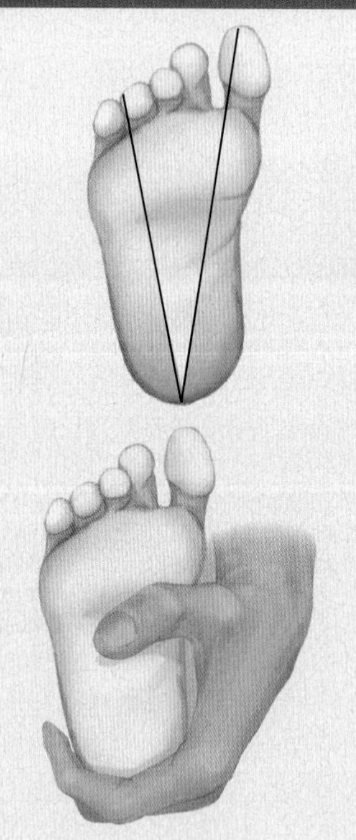

catheters or central venous catheters. The initial blood will be discarded to prevent contamination with intravenous fluids or medications such as heparin. The amount discarded depends on the size of the catheter, the weight of the child, and the institution's guidelines. After aspirating the specimen, flush the venous access device with normal saline to prevent clogging. The device may then be reconnected to the intravenous fluid or flushed according to the institution's protocol.

Remember Samuel, the child with fever, congestion, and irritability? What additional health history and physical examination assessment information should you obtain?

Nursing Analysis

After recognizing and analyzing cues from a thorough assessment, the nurse may identify several patient problems, including:

- Impaired comfort
- Infection risk
- Dehydration risk
- Social isolation
- Knowledge deficiency (specify)

After completing an assessment of Samuel, you note the following: rectal temperature of 39°C (102.2°F), poor sucking, and lethargy. Based on these assessment findings, what would your top three patient problems be for Samuel?

The patient problems provide suggestions for developing a nursing plan of care or concept mapping. The nurse will then generate solutions by planning interventions (suggested with rationales). The plan of care should be individualized, based on the child's and family's needs. Refer to Chapter 36 for the nursing process for pain management and to Chapter 33 for nursing interventions related to interrupted family processes and risk for caregiver role strain. Additional information will be included later in the chapter as it relates to specific disorders.

Nursing Analysis

Impaired comfort related to illness-related symptoms (infectious and/or inflammatory process) as evidenced by rectal temperature greater than 38°C (100.4°F), pruritus, rash or skin lesions, sore throat, or joint pain

Goal/Outcome

Pain or discomfort will be reduced to levels acceptable to the child. Child will verbalize absence or decrease of pain using a pain scale (FLACC, FACES, or linear pain scale), will verbalize or exhibit signs of comfort during febrile episode, will verbalize decrease in uncomfortable sensations such as itching and aches; infants will exhibit decreased crying and ability to rest quietly.

Improving Comfort (interventions with *rationale*)

- Assess pain and response to interventions frequently with use of pain scales or other pain measurement tools: *provides baseline of pain and allows for evaluation of effectiveness of interventions.*
- Administer analgesics and antipruritics as ordered *to relieve pain via interruption of central nervous system pathways and to decrease discomfort related to itching.*
- Administer antipyretics per health care provider order when the child is experiencing discomfort or cannot keep up with the metabolic demands of the fever. *Fever is a protective response of the body to fight infection. Antipyretics provide symptomatic relief but do not change the course of the infection. The major benefits to decreasing fever are increasing comfort in the child and decreasing fluid requirements, helping to prevent dehydration.*
- Keep linens and clothing clean and dry: *diaphoresis can leave clothing and linen soaked, increasing discomfort for the child.*
- Use of nonpharmacologic measures such as tepid bath and removal of clothing and blankets *to decrease temperature and increase comfort.* If used, discontinue if shivering begins *as this will increase temperature and increase discomfort.*
- Apply cool compresses to areas of pruritus or provide a cool bath *to decrease inflammation and soothe pruritus.*
- Keep child's fingernails short (use mitts, gloves, or socks over hands if necessary) to prevent injury *to the skin, which leads to increased pain.*
- Encourage child to press on rather than scratch the area of pruritus: *pressing on the area that itches can soothe the itching and prevent scratching, which can lead to skin injury.*
- Provide fluids frequently and offer warm fluids such as soup or cold foods such as popsicles *to ease the discomfort of a sore throat.*
- Provide cool mist humidification *to ease the discomfort of a sore throat.*
- Dress the child in light clothing: *restrictive clothing and diaphoresis can lead to increased pruritus.*
- Use diversional activities and distraction appropriate to developmental level: *distraction from pain can reduce the need for pharmacologic agents, and distraction from pruritus can minimize scratching.*

Nursing Analysis

Infection risk; risk factors include insufficient knowledge to avoid exposure to pathogens, inadequate vaccination, and exposure to disease outbreak.

Goal/Outcome

Child will exhibit no signs or symptoms of local or systemic infection. Child will not spread infection to others. Symptoms of infection will decrease over time; others will remain free of infection. Child and family will demonstrate appropriate hygiene measures using proper technique, such as handwashing, to prevent the spread of infection.

Preventing and Controlling Infection (interventions with *rationale*)

- Monitor vital signs: *elevation in temperature may indicate infection.*
- Monitor skin lesions for signs of local infection: redness, warmth, drainage, swelling, and pain at lesions: *can indicate infection.*
- Maintain aseptic technique and practice good handwashing: *to prevent introduction of further infectious agents and prevent transmission to others.*
- Administer antibiotics as prescribed: *to prevent or treat bacterial infection.*
- Encourage nutritious diet and proper hydration according to child's preferences and ability to feed orally: *to assist body's natural defenses against infection.*
- Isolate child as required based on transmission-based precautions: *to prevent nosocomial spread of infection.*
- Teach child and family preventive measures such as good handwashing, covering mouth and nose with cough or sneeze, and proper disposal of used tissues: *to prevent nosocomial or community spread of infection.*

Nursing Analysis

Dehydration risk due to insufficient fluid intake to meet fluid loss due to conditions such as increased metabolic demands and insensible loss due to fever, diaphoresis, vomiting, or poor feeding/fluid intake

Goal/Outcome

Fluid volume will be maintained and balanced. Oral mucosa is moist and pink, skin turgor is elastic, urine output is at least 1 to 2 mL/kg/hour.

Promoting Adequate Fluid Balance (interventions with *rationale*)

- Administer intravenous fluids if ordered *to maintain adequate hydration in children who are (nothing by mouth) NPO, unable to tolerate oral intake, or unable to keep up with fluid losses.*
- When oral intake is allowed and tolerated, encourage oral fluids *to promote intake and maintain hydration.*
- Assess for signs of adequate hydration such as pink and moist oral mucosa, elastic skin turgor, and adequate urine output *to detect fluid imbalance.*
- Monitor intake and output *to identify fluid imbalance.*
- Assess urine specific gravity, urine and serum electrolytes, blood urea nitrogen, creatinine, and osmolality and daily weights *to monitor fluid status.*

Nursing Analysis

Social isolation related to inability to engage in satisfying personal relationships (required isolation from peers secondary to transmission-based precautions) as evidenced by disruption in usual play secondary to inability to leave hospital room, activity intolerance, and fatigue

Goal/Outcome

Child will participate in stimulating activities. Child is able to verbalize reason for isolation and length of isolation (if developmentally appropriate); child verbalizes interest in activities.

Preventing Social Isolation (interventions with *rationale*)

- Explain reasons for transmission-based precautions and length of time: *this helps increase understanding and decrease anxiety about isolation. Children sometimes mistake isolation as punishment. Explaining length of time gives child an endpoint they can work toward.*
- Visit child frequently, at least every hour, and try to spend some uninterrupted time to play and allow child time to verbalize feelings about separation from others: *helps establish a therapeutic relationship and demonstrates caring.*
- Let child see caregiver's face before applying mask if appropriate: *to help child identify and relate to those caring for them and minimize anxiety about strangers and the unknown.*
- Consult child life specialist to arrange for stimulating activities child enjoys: *can help child to understand reasons for isolation and minimize feelings of social isolation.*
- Contact volunteers to spend time with child, if appropriate: *gives child attention and support, which will help child to cope and decrease stress.*

Nursing Analysis

Knowledge deficiency related to insufficient information (regarding medical condition, prognosis, and medical needs) as evidenced by verbalization, questions, or actions demonstrating lack of understanding regarding child's condition or care

Goal/Outcome

Child and family will verbalize accurate information and understanding about condition, prognosis, and medical needs. Child and family demonstrate knowledge of condition and prognosis and medical needs, including possible causes, contributing factors, and treatment measures.

Providing Child and Family Teaching (interventions with *rationale*)

- Assess the child's and family's willingness to learn: *child and family must be willing to learn in order for teaching to be effective.*
- Provide the family with time to adjust to diagnosis: *to facilitate adjustment and ability to learn and participate in child's care.*
- Repeat information: *to give family and child time to learn and understand.*
- Teach in short sessions: *many short sessions are more helpful and facilitate learning compared to one long session.*
- Gear teaching to level of understanding of the child and family (depends on age of child, physical condition, memory): *to ensure understanding.*
- Provide reinforcement and rewards: *to facilitate the teaching/learning process.*
- Use multiple modes of learning involving many senses (provide written, verbal, demonstration, and videos) when possible: *the child and family are more likely to retain information when it is presented in different ways using many senses.*

Managing Fever

Fever is typically managed at home, so it is important to give guidance and instruction at well-child visits and review this information at subsequent visits. Written and video materials about fever management may be effective in increasing caregivers' knowledge. Parents can refer to the written instructions when needed (see Teaching Guidelines 37.1).

Managing Skin Rashes

Skin rashes accompany many infectious or communicable diseases. These rashes can be uncomfortable and irritating for the child. Management often occurs at home, so it is important to educate parents on ways to relieve the discomfort and protect and maintain skin integrity. The health care provider may prescribe antipruritics, including oral medications or topical creams or ointments (see Drug Guide 37.1). Instruct parents on the importance of maintaining skin integrity to prevent infection or scarring. Teach parents to keep their child's fingernails short and hands clean. Explain the importance of discouraging scratching, and discuss distraction techniques they can use with the child. Cool compresses or cool baths can relieve itching. Encourage the child to press on rather than scratch the itchy area; this can relieve discomfort while maintaining skin integrity. Refer to Chapter 45 for more information on managing skin rashes.

TEACHING GUIDELINES 37.1 Fever Management

- Fever is a sign of illness, not a disease; it is the body's weapon to fight infection.
- Diurnal variation may allow temperature changes as much as 1°C (33.8°F) over a 24-hour period, peaking in the evening.
- Initially fever should be managed by trying to decrease the child's temperature by increasing fluid intake and decreasing activity.
- Antipyretics are used if the child demonstrates discomfort. Always check correct doses before administration. Never give aspirin or aspirin-containing products to a child younger than 19 years with a fever due to the risk of Reye syndrome.
- In some children fever can be associated with a seizure or dehydration, but this will not lead to brain damage or death. Discuss the facts about febrile seizures (see Chapter 38 for further information on febrile seizures).
- Watch for the signs and symptoms of dehydration; it is important to provide oral rehydration by increasing fluid intake.
- Dress the child lightly and avoid warm, binding clothing or blankets.
- The use of sponging with tepid water is controversial; if used, encourage the parent to give an antipyretic prior to sponging. Ensure the sponging does not produce shivering (which causes the body to produce heat and maintain the elevated set point), and reinforce the importance of using tepid water, not cold water or alcohol. Instruct the parent to stop if the child experiences discomfort.
- Call the provider for:
  - Any child younger than 3 months who has a rectal temperature above 38°C (100.4°F).
  - Any child who is lethargic or listless, regardless of temperature.
  - Fever lasting more than 3–5 days.
  - Fever greater than 40.6°C (105°F).
  - Any child who is immunocompromised by illness, such as cancer or human immunodeficiency virus (will need further evaluation and treatment).

> **THINKING ABOUT DEVELOPMENT**
>
> Lisa Hernandez is a 4-year-old with a history of fever and cold-like symptoms who presents currently with an itchy rash. Based on her developmental stage, how will you instruct her and her caregiver on managing her rash at home? How would your instructions change if the child was 12 years old?

> Based on your top three nursing concerns for Samuel, describe appropriate nursing interventions.

SEPSIS

Sepsis is a systemic overresponse to infection resulting from bacteria and viruses (most commonly), fungi, viruses, rickettsiae, or parasites. It can lead to septic shock, which results in hypotension, low blood flow, and multisystem organ failure. Septic shock is a medical emergency, and children are usually admitted to an intensive care unit (see Chapter 51). The cause of sepsis may not be known, but common causative organisms in infants and children include *Escherichia coli*, group B streptococcus, *Staphylococcus aureus*, and *Streptococcus pneumoniae* (Pomerantz & Weiss, 2022). Sepsis can affect any age group, but infants less than 1 month of age, immunocompromised children, children with a debilitating chronic condition, children with a serious injury or large incision site, children with urinary tract abnormalities and frequent infections, and children with an indwelling vascular catheter are at higher risk (Pomerantz & Weiss, 2022).

Neonates and young infants have a higher susceptibility due to their immature immune system, inability to localize infections, and lack of immunoglobulin M (IgM), which is necessary to protect against bacterial infections.

The prognosis for sepsis is variable and depends on the child's age and the cause of the sepsis. Neonates are at highest risk for a poor outcome. Due to this high mortality rate, when an ill-appearing febrile neonate presents, a full workup is indicated (Kronman et al., 2023a). Usually, admission to the hospital to rule out sepsis is the standard of practice.

Pathophysiology

Sepsis results in the systemic inflammatory response syndrome (SIRS) due to infection. The pathophysiology of sepsis is complex. It results from the effects of circulating bacterial products or toxins, mediated by cytokine release, occurring as a result of sustained bacteremia. The pathogens cause an overproduction of proinflammatory cytokines, previously termed endotoxins. These cytokines are responsible for the clinically observable effects of the sepsis. Impaired pulmonary, hepatic, or renal function may result from excessive cytokine release during the septic process.

Therapeutic Management

Therapeutic management of sepsis in infants, especially neonates, is more aggressive than for older children. Neonates and infants with sepsis or even suspected sepsis are treated in the hospital. The infant or child with sepsis is admitted for close monitoring along with antibiotic therapy. Intravenous antibiotics are started immediately after the blood, urine, and cerebrospinal fluid cultures have been obtained. The length of therapy and the specific antibiotic used will be determined based on the source of the positive culture and the results of the culture and sensitivity. If final culture reports are negative and symptoms have subsided, antibiotics may be discontinued (usually after 72 hours of treatment). If the child is not responding to therapy and symptoms worsen, sepsis may be progressing to shock. Management of the child with septic shock is usually done in the intensive care unit.

Nursing Assessment

For a full description of the assessment phase of the nursing process, refer to the "Clinical Judgment and the Nursing Process" box earlier in this chapter. Assessment findings pertinent to sepsis are discussed further.

Health History

Elicit a description of the present illness and chief complaint. Signs of sepsis can vary with each child. Some common signs and symptoms reported during the health history might include:

- Child just does not look or act right.
- Crying more than usual, inconsolable
- Fever
- Hypothermia (in neonates and those with severe disease)
- Lethargic and less interactive or playful
- Increased irritability
- Poor feeding or poor suck
- Rash (e.g., petechiae, ecchymosis, diffuse erythema)
- Difficulty breathing
- Nasal congestion
- Diarrhea
- Vomiting
- Decreased urine output
- Hypotonia
- Changes in mental status (confused, anxious, excited)
- Seizures
- Older child may complain of heart racing.

Explore the child's current and past medical history for risk factors such as:

- Prematurity
- Lack of immunizations
- Immunocompromise
- Exposure to communicable pathogens

In neonates and young infants, seek pregnancy and labor risk factors such as:

- Premature rupture of membranes or prolonged rupture
- Difficult delivery
- Maternal infection or fever, including STIs
- Resuscitation and other invasive procedures
- Positive maternal group beta-streptococcal vaginosis

Sepsis may occur in the hospitalized child. Assess for risk factors such as:

- Intensive care unit stay
- Presence of central line or other invasive lines or tubes
- Immunosuppression

TAKE NOTE!

Listen to the parents' descriptions of their child's behavior and appearance, as well as changes they have observed. Many times, they are the first to notice when their child is not acting right, even before clinical signs of infection are seen.

Physical Examination

Perform a thorough physical examination of the infant or child with proven or suspected sepsis. Specific findings related to inspection and observation are noted further.

Inspection and Observation

Observe the child's general appearance, color, level of arousal, and hydration status. The child with sepsis may appear lethargic and pale and show signs of dehydration. In neonates and infants, observe the quality of their cry and reaction to parental stimulation, noting weak cry, lack of smile or facial expression, or lack of responsiveness. Inspect the skin for petechiae or other skin lesions. Petechiae may indicate a serious bacterial infection (often *Neisseria meningitidis*), and other skin lesion patterns may help identify the cause of the fever. Observe respiratory effort and rate. The infant or child with sepsis may demonstrate tachypnea and increased work of breathing, such as nasal flaring, grunting, and retractions.

Assess vital signs, noting abnormalities. Note elevation in temperature or hypothermia in the young infant. Note tachypnea or tachycardia in the child or apnea or bradycardia in the infant. Document blood pressure. Hypotension, especially when accompanied by signs of poor perfusion, can be a sign of worsening sepsis with progression to shock (refer to Chapter 51).

Laboratory and Diagnostic Tests

Symptoms of sepsis can be vague in infants. Therefore, laboratory tests play a crucial role in confirming or ruling out sepsis. Common laboratory and diagnostic studies ordered for the assessment of sepsis include:

- Complete blood count: WBC levels will be elevated; in severe cases they may be decreased (this is an ominous sign).
- C-reactive protein: elevated
- Blood culture: positive in septicemia, indicating bacteria is present in the blood
- Urine culture: may be positive, indicating presence of bacteria in the urine
- Cerebrospinal fluid analysis: may reveal increased WBCs and protein and low glucose
- Stool culture: may be positive for bacteria or other infectious organisms
- Culture of tubes, catheters, or shunts suspected to be infected: the fluid inside these tubes may be tested for bacteria.
- Chest radiograph: may reveal signs of pneumonia such as hyperinflation and patchy areas of atelectasis or infiltration

Nursing Management

Monitor the infant or child closely for changes in condition, especially the development of shock. Administer antibiotics as ordered. Refer to the "Clinical Judgment and the Nursing Process" section for patient problems and related interventions. In addition to these interventions, it is important to prevent infection and provide education to the child and family.

Preventing Infection

Sepsis is a potentially life-threatening illness, and prevention is important. Handwashing is the most effective intervention against nosocomial infection. Nurses play a key role in minimizing environmental sources by cleaning equipment, disposing of soiled linens and dressings properly, and adhering to proper aseptic technique with all invasive procedures. Follow your institution's policies, and use evidence-based practice guidelines for interventions such as invasive line dressing changes and intravenous tubing changes to reduce the risk of infection. Encourage immunization as recommended. To reduce group B streptococcus infection in neonates, screen pregnant patients. If the results are positive, administer intrapartum antibiotics.

TAKE NOTE!

There has been a dramatic reduction in invasive *Haemophilus influenzae* type B diseases since the widespread use of the Hib vaccine (CDC, 2022k).

Educating the Child and Family

Early recognition of the signs of sepsis is essential in preventing morbidity and mortality. Educate parents about the significance of fever, especially in neonates and infants younger than 3 months. Instruct parents to contact their health care provider or nurse practitioner if their infant or neonate has a fever. A health care provider or nurse practitioner should see any child with a fever accompanied by lethargy, poor responsiveness, or lack of facial expressions. Signs and symptoms of sepsis can be vague and vary from child to child. Encourage parents to contact their health care provider or nurse practitioner if they feel their febrile child is "just not acting right."

BACTERIAL INFECTIONS

Bacteria are one-celled organisms that can live, grow, and reproduce. They exist everywhere. Most are completely harmless and some are useful. Others can lead to disease either because they are in the wrong place in the body or they invade and cause disease in humans and animals. Children are at a high risk of developing bacterial infections, which can result in life-threatening illness. Fortunately, many bacterial diseases, such as diphtheria, pertussis, and tetanus, can be prevented by immunization (see Chapter 31 for more information on immunizations).

Community-Acquired Methicillin-Resistant *Staphylococcus aureus*

Community-acquired methicillin-resistant *Staphylococcus aureus* (CAMRSA) is a staphylococcal infection that is resistant to certain antibiotics. Methicillin-resistant *S. aureus* (MRSA) was originally a nosocomial acquired infection (hospital-acquired [HA]-MRSA) with few cases acquired in the community. However, community-acquired infection, in seemingly healthy individuals, is increasing in occurrence throughout the United States (Kaplan, 2023). These infections range from minor skin rashes to abscesses to serious, complicated, life-threatening infections. Serious and invasive infections, such as sepsis, necrotizing pneumonia, and osteomyelitis, often are secondary to a skin or soft tissue infection.

Transmission occurs through direct person-to-person contact, respiratory droplets, blood, or sharing personal items, such as hair brushes, towels, and sports equipment, and touching surfaces or items contaminated with MRSA. Clusters of MRSA have been found in day care centers and among athletic teams. Staphylococci are resistant to heat and drying and can be found on environmental surfaces months after contamination. Intact skin and mucous membranes, along with proper hand hygiene, are the best barriers to MRSA.

Nursing Assessment

In the child, skin and tissue infections are common infections caused by CAMRSA. Symptoms include a bump or skin area that is red, swollen, painful, and warm to touch. It may also include fever, fluctuance, and purulent drainage. The lesion may have appeared suddenly and be red and raised, resembling an insect bite. Necrotic areas may develop. Abscesses, especially abscessed hair follicles, and pimples are common presentations. Assessment needs to include a thorough past medical history to determine history of recurrent skin infections with or without complete resolution along with assessment for risk factors. Risk factors include frequent skin-to-skin contact; openings in the skin/skin trauma, such as abrasions and cuts; contact with potentially contaminated personal items, equipment, and surfaces; poor hygiene; limited access to health care; frequent exposure to antimicrobial agents; and crowded living conditions (Kaplan, 2023).

Diagnosis is determined through culture. Diagnostic tests include incision and drainage (I&D), aspiration of the abscess, and culturing the fluid or tissue. Antimicrobial susceptibility along with culture is critical.

Nursing Management

Care of the child with CAMRSA will typically occur at home. Antibiotics with microbial susceptibility will often be prescribed. Comprehensive wound care, which may include I&D, may occur. Follow-up for reassessment is key. Child and family education is crucial. Include the following in the teaching plan:

- Educate the family on the importance of taking the antibiotics as directed and finishing all the medicine. Emphasize that this will help slow the creation of antimicrobial-resistant organisms.
- Teach the child and parents proper hand hygiene and handwashing.
- Discourage family members from sharing personal items.
- Explain the risk factors involved in transmission.
- Explain the importance of keeping cuts and scrapes cleaned and covered.
- Review the signs of MRSA and emphasize the importance of early recognition and treatment.

Scarlet Fever

Scarlet fever is an infection resulting from group A streptococci. It usually occurs with a group A streptococci throat infection (i.e., strep throat) or rarely streptococcal skin infection. However, in the case of scarlet fever, the bacteria produce a toxin that causes a rash. Not all children with a group A streptococci infection will develop the rash of scarlet fever. Only children who are infected with streptococci that produce pyrogenic exotoxins and do not have antitoxin antibodies, making them sensitive to the bacterial toxin, will develop scarlet fever (Shulman & Reuter, 2020). Scarlet fever is usually seen in children 5 to 15 years of age and is rare in children younger than 3 years (CDC, 2022a). Transmission is through droplets and follows contact with respiratory tract secretions. Transmission is facilitated by the type of close contact that occurs in schools and child care centers. Food-borne outbreaks have occurred due to human contamination of food. After exposure, the incubation period is 2 to 5 days (Shulman & Reuter, 2020). Communicability is highest during acute infection, and the child is no longer contagious 24 hours after the initiation of appropriate antimicrobial therapy (Shulman & Reuter, 2020).

There has been a dramatic decrease in the mortality rate from scarlet fever due to antibiotic use, and scarlet fever today is seen less frequently and typically follows a benign course (Sotoodian, 2020). Rare but serious complications such as rheumatic fever, glomerulonephritis, skin infections, abscesses of the throat, pneumonia, and arthritis can still occur; therefore, prompt recognition and proper treatment are important (CDC, 2022a).

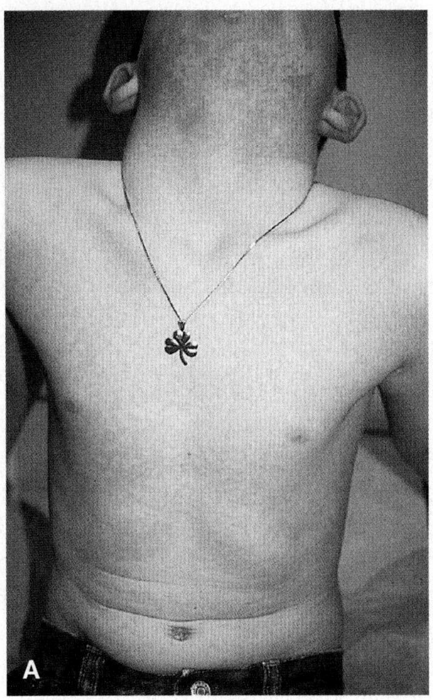

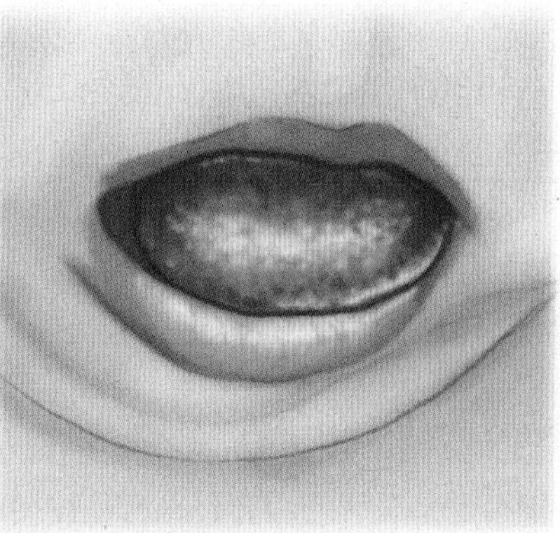

FIGURE 37.1 **A.** Rash of scarlet fever. **B.** Strawberry tongue.

Nursing Assessment

Symptoms of scarlet fever begin abruptly. The health history may reveal a fever greater than 38.3°C (101°F), chills, body aches, loss of appetite, nausea, and vomiting. Inspect the pharynx, which is usually very red and swollen. The tonsils may have yellow or white specks of pus, and cervical lymph nodes may be swollen. Inspect the skin for the most striking symptom of scarlet fever, which is an erythematous rash appearing on the face, trunk, and extremities. The rash is typically absent from the palms and soles of the feet. It looks like a sunburn but feels like sandpaper (Fig. 37.1A). The rash lasts approximately 5 days and is followed by desquamation, typically on the fingers and toes. Early in the illness the tongue develops a thick coat with a strawberry appearance. The tongue will later lose the coating and become bright red (Fig. 37.1B).

Diagnosis is made by identification of group A streptococcus on throat culture. Several rapid tests for group A streptococcal pharyngitis are available. The accuracy of these tests depends on the quality of the specimen. It is important that the secretions obtained are pharyngeal or tonsillar (see Common Medical Treatments 37.1 for more information on throat cultures).

Nursing Management

Children with scarlet fever are usually cared for at home. Penicillin and amoxicillin are the antibiotics of choice (Shulman & Reuter, 2020). In those sensitive to penicillin, erythromycin may be used. Educate the family on the importance of taking the antibiotic as directed and finishing all the medicine.

Encourage fluid intake to maintain adequate hydration due to fever. Teach parents ways to provide comfort for the child. A cool mist humidifier can soothe the child's sore throat. Soft foods, warm liquids like soup, or cold foods like popsicles may also be helpful. If the child is hospitalized, droplet precautions, along with standard precautions, are necessary.

Diphtheria

Diphtheria is caused by infection with *Corynebacterium diphtheriae* and may affect the nose, larynx, tonsils, or pharynx. Tonsillar and pharyngeal infections are the most common and will be the focus of this discussion. A pseudomembrane forms over the pharynx, uvula, tonsils, and soft palate (Fig. 37.2). The neck becomes edematous, and lymphadenopathy develops. The pseudomembrane causes airway obstruction and suffocation. Diphtheria is rare in developed countries but is reappearing in some regions and continues to be a serious disease worldwide due to lack of routine immunization (Barroso & Pegram, 2023). Risk factors include children and adults who are unimmunized or underimmunized, living in crowded or unsanitary living conditions, having a compromised immune system, and traveling to developing countries where diphtheria remains endemic (Barroso & Pegram, 2023). Routine infant immunization can prevent the disease. Therapeutic management involves administration of antibiotics and antitoxin, as well as airway management.

Nursing Assessment

Assess immunization history as children at risk for diphtheria are those who are unimmunized. Note history of sore throat and fever, usually less than 38.9°C (102°F). As the pseudomembrane forms, swallowing becomes difficult and signs of airway obstruction become apparent. A specimen of the membrane may be cultured for *C. diphtheriae*.

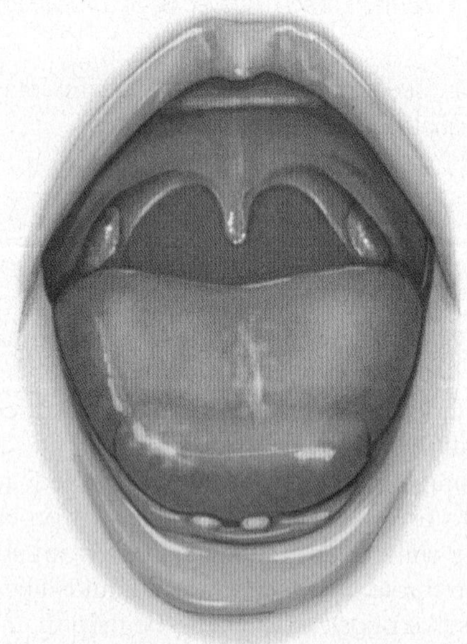

FIGURE 37.2 In diphtheria, a pseudomembrane forms over the pharynx, uvula, tonsils, and soft palate.

Nursing Management

Close observation of respiratory status is of utmost importance. Administration of antibiotics and the antitoxin is critical to encourage sloughing of the membrane. The child should remain on strict droplet precautions in addition to standard precautions and should maintain bed rest.

Pertussis

Pertussis is an acute respiratory disorder characterized by paroxysmal cough (whooping cough) and copious secretions. The highest incidence and the greatest risk for severe disease and death are seen in children younger than 1 year (Yeh & Mink, 2022). The disease is caused by *Bordetella pertussis*. The incubation period is 6 to 20 days, usually 7 to 10 days. Pertussis usually starts with 7 to 10 days of cold symptoms. The paroxysmal coughing spells then begin and can last 1 to 4 weeks. Convalescence occurs over the course of several weeks to months. Initially, immunization decreased the incidence of pertussis, but an increase has occurred since the 1990s (Yeh & Mink, 2022). Recent trends show pertussis as an increasing endemic with cycling epidemics and a shifting burden of disease to young infants, adolescents, and adults. Many factors contribute to this increase in pertussis such as changes in diagnostic testing, increase in recognition and reporting of pertussis, changes in the molecular makeup of the organism, and waning vaccine-induced immunity (CDC, 2021a). Infants and young children continue to be advised to get four doses of DTaP (diphtheria, tetanus, and pertussis) at 2, 4, 6, and 15 to 18 months; a fifth booster dose at 4 to 6 years before entering school; and an additional Tdap (tetanus, diphtheria, and acellular pertussis) booster at age 11. Complications of pertussis include hypoxia, apnea, secondary infections such as pneumonia and otitis media, seizures, encephalopathy, and death.

TAKE NOTE!

Rates of pertussis hospitalization in infants less than 2 months have decreased since the Advisory Committee on Immunization Practices (ACIP) advised pertussis immunization for pregnant people, preferably during their third trimester (Yeh & Mink, 2022).

Therapeutic Management

Therapeutic management of pertussis focuses on eradicating the bacterial infection and providing respiratory support. CDC guidelines recommend antimicrobial treatment early in the course of disease. Ideally, antibiotics are initiated during the first 1 to 2 weeks of illness prior to the occurrence of paroxysmal cough for the best treatment results (CDC, 2022b). For infants older than 1 month, macrolide drugs, including erythromycin, clarithromycin, and azithromycin, are the drugs of choice (CDC, 2022b). For younger infants, azithromycin should be used and erythromycin and clarithromycin avoided (CDC, 2022b). An alternative to macrolides in children older than 2 months is trimethoprim–sulfamethoxazole (TMP-SMZ) (CDC, 2022b). A course of macrolide antibiotics is also recommended to treat all close contacts regardless of age or immunization status (CDC, 2021a). Also, all close contacts who are younger than 7 years and who are unimmunized or underimmunized should have pertussis immunization initiated or the series completed according to the recommended dosing schedule (CDC, 2021a).

CLINICAL REASONING ALERT!

Monitor infants less than 1 month of age who receive macrolide antibiotics (particularly erythromycin) for signs of the development of infantile hypertrophic pyloric stenosis, such as projectile vomiting (Souder & Long, 2020).

Nursing Assessment

Assess for lack of immunization as this is the most important risk factor for the development of pertussis. Obtain history that may reveal cold and cough symptoms, progressing to paroxysmal coughing spells. During the paroxysms, the child might cough 10 to 30 times in a row, followed by a whooping sound. This might be accompanied by redness in the face, progressive cyanosis, and protrusion of the tongue. Saliva, mucus, and tears flow from the mouth, nose, and eyes. Between the paroxysmal episodes, the child might rest well and appear relatively unaffected. Assess oxygen levels, and auscultate the lungs to assess air exchange. The diagnosis may be confirmed by a variety of laboratory tests, such as culture, polymerase chain reaction, and serology, accompanied by clinical history.

Nursing Management

Nursing care will focus on providing a high-humidity environment and frequent suctioning to mobilize secretions. Observe for signs of airway obstruction and respiratory distress. Encourage fluids to keep secretions thin and maintain adequate hydration. Offer reassurance to the child and family; the coughing episodes can be very frightening. Droplet precautions along with standard precautions are necessary for the hospitalized child.

Tetanus

Tetanus is an acute, often fatal neurologic disease caused by the toxins produced by *Clostridium tetani*. Tetanus is rare in the United States but continues to be significant worldwide due to lack of routine immunization (Thwaites, 2022). It is characterized by increased muscle tone and spasm. *C. tetani* spores can live anywhere but are found most commonly in soil, dust, and feces from humans or animals, such as sheep, cattle, chickens, dogs, cats, and rats. The spores can enter the body through a wound that is contaminated, through a burn, or by injecting contaminated street drugs. Once it enters the body, an anaerobic environment allows it to multiply and a poisonous toxin is released.

There are four forms of tetanus. Neonatal tetanus affects newborns in the first week of life secondary to an infected umbilical stump in infants whose birthing parents were poorly immunized (CDC, 2021a). Most adults in the United States have been immunized and will pass the immunity to their fetus. Along with proper hygiene during delivery and adequate cord care, this makes this type rare in the United States, but in underdeveloped countries it remains a significant problem (CDC, 2021a). The second form is local tetanus. This rare form is characterized by local muscle spasms within the same area/extremity of the wound. The third type is cephalic tetanus, which is associated with recurrent otitis media or head trauma. It is also rare and affects the cranial nerves, especially facial nerves. Generalized tetanus is the most common and severe form, and patients will often present first with trismus (masseter muscle spasm or lockjaw) (CDC, 2021a). Symptoms then progress in a descending fashion with tonic contraction of the skeletal muscles and intermittent intense, painful muscular spasms. The most profoundly affected muscles are those of the neck and back.

The general incubation period is 1 to 21 days, with an average of 8 days (CDC, 2021a). Recovery can be long and difficult, and children with tetanus may have to spend several weeks in the hospital in an intensive care setting. It has been suggested that the shorter the incubation period, the higher the risk of more severe illness and poorer prognosis (CDC, 2021a). Complications associated with tetanus include breathing problems, fractures, elevated blood pressure, dysrhythmias, clotting in the blood vessels of the lung, pneumonia, and coma.

Therapeutic Management

Therapeutic management is directed toward supporting respiratory and cardiovascular function, stopping toxin production, neutralizing unbound toxins, and controlling muscle spasms. Tetanus immunoglobulin may be given as well as the tetanus vaccine. Removal of the offending organism, by debridement of the wound, may occur, and intravenous antibiotics such as metronidazole may be initiated. In severe cases, the child may require intensive nursing care with mechanical ventilation.

Nursing Assessment

Note history of initial signs such as headache, spasms, crankiness, and cramping of the jaw (lockjaw), which are followed by difficulty swallowing and a stiff neck. Tetanus progresses in a descending fashion to other muscle groups, causing spasms of the neck, arms, legs, and stomach; seizures may result. Document the presence of fever along with an elevated blood pressure and tachycardia. Opisthotonos (refer to Fig. 38.12 in Chapter 38) may be noted due to severe spasms of the neck and back. The spasms or muscle contractions in children may be strong enough to result in fractures. The diagnosis of tetanus is based on the clinical findings of the history and physical examination. There is no laboratory test to confirm tetanus.

Nursing Management

Nursing management focuses on observing for signs of respiratory distress. Provide a quiet environment with reduced external stimuli to decrease the incidence of spasms. Appropriately manage pain. Encourage adequate nutrition and hydration. Administer sedatives and muscle relaxants as ordered to reduce the pain associated with the muscle spasms and to prevent seizures. Encourage the parents to stay with their child. The child's mental status is unaffected by the disease, so the child is aware of what is happening. Efforts need to be made to reduce the child's anxiety and to provide reassuring, sympathetic care to the child and family. Tetanus is not contagious from person to person; therefore, standard precautions are sufficient.

Tetanus is a preventable but potentially fatal disease. Education is essential regarding the importance of receiving this routine immunization (refer to Chapter 31 for immunization schedule) as well as a booster every 10 years. Instructing parents on proper wound care can also help prevent tetanus. All wounds should be cleaned thoroughly and a proper antiseptic used. If a wound is deep and contamination is suspected, the child should be seen by a health care provider or nurse practitioner. If it has been more than 5 years since the last tetanus dose, a booster may be needed. This can help to neutralize the poison and prevent it from entering the nervous system.

Botulism

Botulism is a disease that is caused by a toxin produced in the immature intestines of young children resulting from infection with the bacterium *Clostridium botulinum*. It is rare but can cause serious paralytic illness. There are several types of botulism. Food-borne botulism results from ingestion of food contaminated with botulinum toxin. Wound botulism results from wounds infected with *C. botulinum*. Infant botulism is the most common in the United States and results from the ingestion of spores of *C. botulinum*, most often from environmental dust and soil. *C. botulinum* is common in soil and can also be found in a variety of foods, such as improperly preserved home-canned foods. Although recently thought to be a minor reservoir, *C. botulinum* spores can be found in raw honey. Botulism has been associated with feeding raw honey to infants; thus, this should be avoided in children younger than 1 year (CDC, 2022c; Pegram & Stone, 2023). The disease is not infectious; to become infected, the child must ingest the bacterial spores. These spores then multiply in the intestinal tract and produce the toxin, which is absorbed in the immature intestines of the infant. It is generally not a problem for older children because the bacteria do not grow well in mature intestines due to the presence of the normal intestinal flora. Prognosis is good, but if treatment is not initiated, paralysis of the arms, legs, trunk, and respiratory system can develop. Therapeutic management is usually supportive but may involve administration of botulinum immune globulin or botulism antitoxin.

Nursing Assessment

For a full description of the assessment phase of the nursing process, refer to the "Clinical Judgment and the Nursing Process" section earlier in this chapter. Assessment findings pertinent to botulism are discussed further.

HEALTH HISTORY

Elicit a description of the present illness and chief complaint. Signs and symptoms usually occur soon after ingestion of the bacteria. Common signs and symptoms in infants reported during the health history might include:

- Constipation
- Poor feeding
- Listlessness
- Generalized weakness
- Weak cry

Common signs and symptoms in older children reported during the health history might include:

- Double vision
- Blurred vision
- Drooping eyelids
- Difficulty swallowing
- Slurred speech
- Muscle weakness

PHYSICAL EXAMINATION AND LABORATORY AND DIAGNOSTIC TESTS

Assess for a diminished gag reflex, which is indicative of botulism. Diagnostic tests include cultures of stool and serum. Botulism is a rare disease and is difficult to diagnose since its symptoms are similar to those of other neuromuscular diseases. Therefore, assessment may include diagnostic tests to help rule out other diseases, such as Guillain–Barré syndrome, stroke, and myasthenia gravis.

Nursing Management

Treatment is mainly supportive and focuses on maintaining respiratory status and nutritional status. Administration of an antitoxin is the main therapeutic treatment and should occur as early as possible (Pegram & Stone, 2023). If ordered, administer botulinum immune globulin early in the disease to reduce its severity and progression.

Osteomyelitis

Osteomyelitis is a bacterial infection of the bone and soft tissue surrounding the bone. *S. aureus* is the most common infecting organism, with MRSA accounting for a third of these infections (Krogstad, 2022a). Additional causes in infants and children include group A and B streptococci, *E. coli*, *S. pneumoniae*, *Kingella kingae*, and *Haemophilus influenzae* (which is now rare due to improvements in immunizations) (Krogstad, 2022a). Children usually present for evaluation within a few days to a week of onset of symptoms, though some may present later.

Osteomyelitis acquired hematogenously (spread through the blood) is the most common mechanism in children (Kronman et al., 2023b). Bacteria from the bloodstream mainly invade the most rapidly growing portion of the bone. The invading bacteria trigger an inflammatory response, formation of pus and edema, and vascular congestion. Small blood vessels thrombose, and the infection extends into the metaphyseal marrow cavity. As the infection progresses, the inflammation extends throughout the bone and blood supply is disrupted, resulting in death of the bone tissues (Fig. 37.3).

Therapeutic Management

Aspiration is necessary to confirm diagnosis and identify specific microorganisms. Treatment includes a 4- to 6-week course of antibiotics. Some children may receive 1 to 2 weeks of intravenous antibiotics and then be switched to oral antibiotics for the remainder of the course. Surgical debridement is rarely necessary. Early treatment may prevent the complications of bone destruction, fracture, and growth arrest. Additional complications include recurrent infection, septic arthritis, and systemic infection.

Nursing Assessment

For a full description of the assessment phase of the nursing process, refer to the "Clinical Judgment and the Nursing Process" section earlier in this chapter. Assessment findings pertinent to osteomyelitis are discussed here.

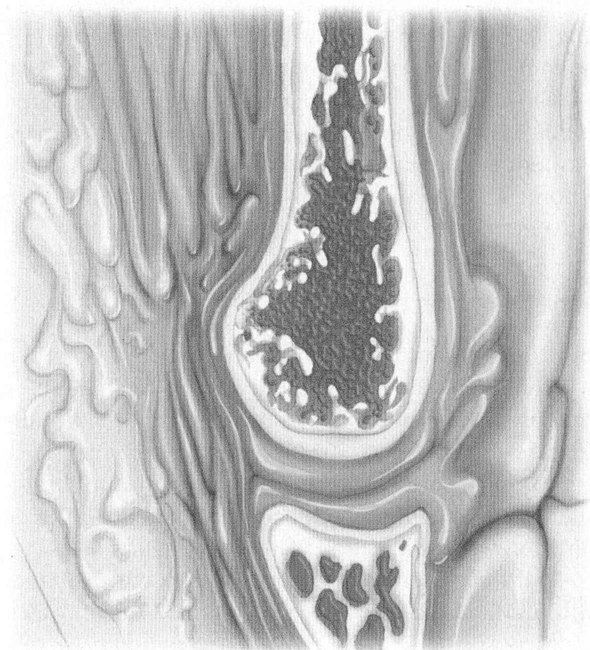

FIGURE 37.3 In osteomyelitis, bacterial invasion leads to infection within the bone.

Explore the health history for risk factors and symptoms. Risk factors include impetigo, infected varicella lesions, furunculosis, recent trauma, infected burns, prolonged intravenous line use, primary or acquired immune deficiency, and sepsis. Obtain history of current or recent antibiotic therapy and response. Note history of irritability, lethargy, possible fever, and onset of pain or change in activity level. The child usually refuses to walk and demonstrates decreased range of motion in the affected extremity. Inspect the affected extremity for swelling. Palpate for local warmth and tenderness. Note point tenderness over affected bone.

Laboratory and diagnostic testing may reveal:

- Elevated WBC count, erythrocyte sedimentation rate, and C-reactive protein level
- Positive blood cultures
- Deep soft tissue swelling on radiography
- Changes in ultrasound, computed tomography (CT) scan, or magnetic resonance imaging (MRI)

Nursing Management

Nursing management of the child with osteomyelitis focuses on assessment, pain management, and maintenance of intravenous access for administration of antibiotics. Individualize care based on the child's and family's response to the illness. Maintain bed rest initially to prevent injury and promote comfort. Administer antipyretics as ordered if the child is febrile in the initial stage of the illness. Encourage the use of unaffected extremities by providing developmentally appropriate toys and games.

Instruct the child and family on safe and proper use of crutches or walker if prescribed. Some children will be discharged home on intravenous antibiotics, while others will finish an oral antibiotic course. Teach parents proper administration of medications and maintenance of a peripherally inserted central catheter or central line at home if the child is finishing the antibiotic course intravenously.

Septic Arthritis

Acute septic arthritis is a condition in which bacteria invade the joint space, most often the hip or knee. It can occur at any age but usually occurs in children younger than 5 years (Krogstad, 2022b). Usually, bacteria gain access to the joint through the bloodstream but can also get access through direct puncture from injections, venipuncture, wound infection, surgery, or injury.

S. aureus is the most common causative organism with CAMRSA on the rise (Krogstad, 2022b). Various streptococci species, *K. kingae*, *N. meningitidis* (with or without an associated meningitis), *H. influenzae* (in unvaccinated children), and *Neisseria gonorrhoeae* are also responsible organisms (Krogstad, 2022b). Sepsis of the hip joint may cause avascular necrosis of the femoral head due to pressure on blood vessels and cartilage within the joint space. Septic arthritis is considered a medical emergency, as destruction of the joint cartilage may occur within just a few days. Additional complications of septic arthritis include permanent deformity, leg-length discrepancy, and long-term decreased range of motion and disability.

The goals of treatment of septic arthritis are to prevent destruction of the joint cartilage and maintain function, motion, and strength. Septic arthritis is treated rapidly with joint aspiration or arthrotomy, followed by intravenous antibiotic therapy while in the hospital and oral antibiotics at home.

Nursing Assessment

Note a history of predisposing factors such as respiratory infection or otitis media, skin or soft tissue infections, or, in the neonate, traumatic puncture wounds and femoral venipunctures. The history is usually significant for sudden onset of fever and moderate to severe pain.

Upon physical examination, the infant or child appears ill. Note extent of fever, reports of pain, refusal to bear weight or straighten the joint, and limited range of motion (the child usually maintains the joint in flexion and will not allow the leg to be straightened). The child will generally hold the joint in a position of comfort and the child or infant will appear without pain as long as the joint is immobile. Any attempt at passive range of motion will reveal pain. Palpate the affected joint for warmth and swelling.

Laboratory findings may include:

- WBC count normal or elevated with elevated neutrophil counts.
- Elevated erythrocyte sedimentation rate and C-reactive protein levels.
- Fluid from joint aspiration demonstrates elevated WBC count; culture determines responsible organism.
- Joint radiograph may show subtle soft tissue changes or increase in the joint space.
- Positive blood culture for the causative organism (40% of cases) (Krogstad, 2023).

Nursing Management

Assess aspiration wound for signs of infection. Monitor vital signs for resolution of fever. Pain management with ibuprofen or acetaminophen will be sufficient for some children; others may initially require an opioid, such as morphine. Assess the affected joint for a decrease in swelling, increasing range of motion, and decreasing or absent pain. The child may be discharged after 72 hours of intravenous antibiotics following joint aspiration if they are improving and can tolerate oral antibiotics. Some children may be discharged home on intravenous antibiotics. At discharge, if the child cannot ambulate, physical therapy may be consulted for short-term use of crutches or a wheelchair. Teach families how to assess for signs and symptoms of wound infection, how to administer oral antibiotics and pain medication, and how to assist their child with crutch walking.

VIRAL INFECTIONS

Viruses are very small particles that infect cells. They cannot multiply on their own and require a living host, such as humans, animals, or plants. They can reproduce only by invading and taking over the host cells. Young children are highly sensitive to viruses; their resistance is low and exposure is high. Viruses are hard to destroy without damaging or killing the living cells they infect. Therefore, drugs are not used to control them. However, many viral diseases can be prevented by immunization, such as measles, rubella, varicella, mumps, and poliomyelitis (see Chapter 31 for more information on immunizations).

Viral Exanthems

Many viral infections of the skin in childhood are called viral exanthems. **Exanthem** means rash or skin eruption. Viral exanthems of childhood often present with a distinct rash pattern that assists in the diagnosis of the virus. Table 37.4 discusses common childhood exanthems. Immunizations have led to a decrease in the incidence of certain viral exanthems, such as measles, rubella, and varicella.

TABLE 37.4 • Common Viral Exanthems of Childhood

Disease	Clinical Manifestations	Management/Complications	Nursing Implications
Rubella (German Measles)			
• Caused by rubella virus • Transmission: by direct or indirect contact with droplets, primarily by nasopharyngeal secretions, but also in blood, stool, and urine. Also transmitted from birthing parent to fetus • Peak incidence: late winter and early spring • Incubation period: 12–23 days (usually 14 days) • Communicable: 7 days before to 7 days after onset of rash 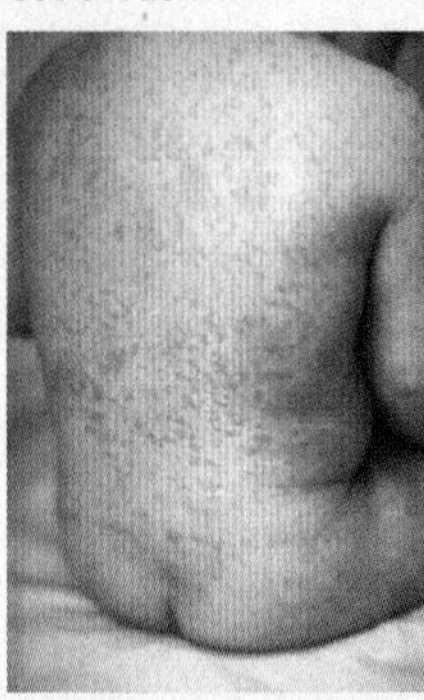 Rubella rash. (Courtesy of Centers for Disease Control and Prevention. [1978]. *Public health image library [PHIL]: Details.* https://phil.cdc.gov/Details.aspx?pid=712)	• Rash usually first sign. Maculopapular rash that begins on face and spreads head to foot; disappears in same order it spread, usually by the third day. On the second day, the rash may appear pinpoint. Desquamation is minimal. • In older children: lymphadenopathy (retroauricular, posterior cervical, postoccipital) 24 hours before the onset of the rash; lasting up to 1 week; low-grade fever, malaise, upper respiratory symptoms • Mild pruritus • Polyarthralgia and polyarthritis (rare in children but common in adolescents) • Half of cases may be subclinical or inapparent.	• Usually mild and self-limiting • Treatment is mainly supportive. • Complications: encephalitis and thrombocytopenia (rare) • Maternal rubella during pregnancy can result in miscarriage, fetal death, or congenital malformations.	• Comfort measures such as antipyretics, antipruritics, and analgesics for joint pain • Droplet precautions until 7 days after onset of rash
Rubeola (Measles)			
• Caused by measles virus • Transmission: direct or indirect contact with droplets, primarily by nasopharyngeal secretions and airborne (virus can stay in air for up to 2 hours after infected person leaves the area); highly contagious • Peak incidence: late winter and spring • Incubation period: 6–21 days, usually 13 days • Communicable 1–2 days before the onset of symptoms (4 days before onset of rash) until 4 days after rash has appeared 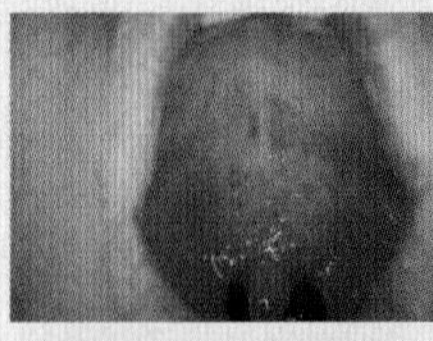 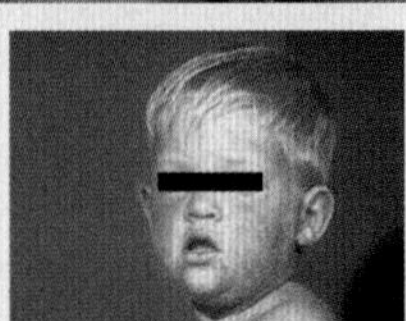 Koplik spots. (Courtesy of Centers for Disease Control and Prevention, & Eichenwald, H. F. [1958]. https://phil.cdc.gov/Details.aspx?pid=3187); (Courtesy of Centers for Disease Control and Prevention. [1963]. *Public health image library [PHIL]: Details.* https://phil.cdc.gov/Details.aspx?pid=1150)	• Prodromal phase: 2–4 days, consisting of fever, cough, coryza, conjunctivitis • Followed by Koplik spots (bright red spots with blue white centers on mucous membranes, mainly buccal mucosa; look like tiny grains of white sand surrounded by red rings) • Erythematous maculopapular, blanching rash appears 3–4 days after the onset of fever. Rash gradually proceeds from head downward and outward.	• Treatment is mainly supportive, including antipyretics, bed rest, adequate fluid intake, and antibiotics to treat secondary bacterial infections such as pneumonia and otitis media. • Postexposure vaccination of unimmunized child within 72 hours of exposure may prevent or reduce illness severity and duration. • Immune serum globulin (IG) given within 6 days of exposure may prevent or make symptoms less severe. • Possible vitamin A supplementation in children hospitalized for severe measles or its complications or those with immunodeficiency • Complications: diarrhea, otitis media, and pneumonia common in young children; acute encephalitis	• Comfort measures, such as antipyretics and antipruritics • Clean eyes with warm, moist cloth to remove secretions. • Cool mist humidification to alleviate coryza and cough • Airborne precautions until 4 days after the onset of rash

(continued)

TABLE 37.4 • Common Viral Exanthems of Childhood (*continued*)

Disease	Clinical Manifestations	Management/Complications	Nursing Implications
Varicella Zoster (Chickenpox)			
• Caused by varicella zoster virus, human herpes virus 3 • Transmission: direct contact with infected people's nasopharyngeal secretions or via airborne spread, to a lesser degree by contact with unscabbed lesions. Highly contagious. Also transmitted from birthing parent to fetus • Peak incidence: winter and early spring • Incubation period: 10–21 days, usually 14–16 days • Communicable 1–2 days before the onset of rash until all vesicles have crusted over (about 3–7 days after the onset of rash) 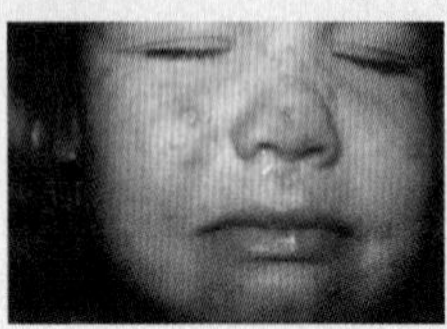 Varicella. (Courtesy of Centers for Disease Control and Prevention, & Noble, J. [1968]. *Public health image library [PHIL]: Details.* https://phil.cdc.gov/Details.aspx?pid=10486)	• Prodromal symptoms (fever, malaise, anorexia, headache, mild abdominal pain) may be present 24–48 hours before the onset of the rash. In children, rash is often the first sign of disease. • Lesions often appear first on scalp, face, trunk, then extremities; initially intensely pruritic erythematous macules that evolve to papules and then form clear, fluid-filled vesicles • Vesicles eventually erupt, and then lesions scab and crust. A variety of lesions are present at one time. • More severe in adolescents and adults than in young children	• Usually self-limiting; treatment is mainly supportive: fever reduction, antipruritics, and skin care to prevent infection of lesions • Antiviral therapy and varicella zoster IG may be used in those considered to be at high risk (immunocompromised, pregnant people, and newborns exposed to maternal varicella). Routine antiviral therapy is not recommended for the treatment of uncomplicated varicella infection in otherwise healthy children. • Complications: bacterial superinfection of skin lesions, thrombocytopenia, arthritis, hepatitis, cerebellar ataxia, encephalitis, meningitis, pneumonia, glomerulonephritis, congenital infection, and life-threatening perinatal infection • Lifelong latent infection occurs; reactivation results in herpes zoster (shingles), uncommon in childhood.	• Comfort measures, such as antipyretics and antipruritics • For those with exposure to susceptible people, airborne and contact precautions, from 8 to 21 days after exposure • Children may return to school or child care once lesions have crusted. • Airborne and contact precautions in the hospitalized child for a minimum of 5 days after the onset of rash and as long as vesicular lesions are present
Exanthem Subitum (Roseola Infantum or Sixth Disease)			
• Caused by B variant of human herpes virus 6 (HHV-6); (less frequently human herpes virus 7 [HHV-7], adenoviruses, enteroviruses, parainfluenza virus) • Transmission: little is known and depends on causative virus but HHV-6 suspected to be from saliva of infected person and enters the host through the oral, nasal, or conjunctival mucosa • Peak incidence: ages 7–13 months, spring and fall • Incubation period: 5–15 days, average of 10 days • Communicability is unknown, but most likely contagious before symptoms appear 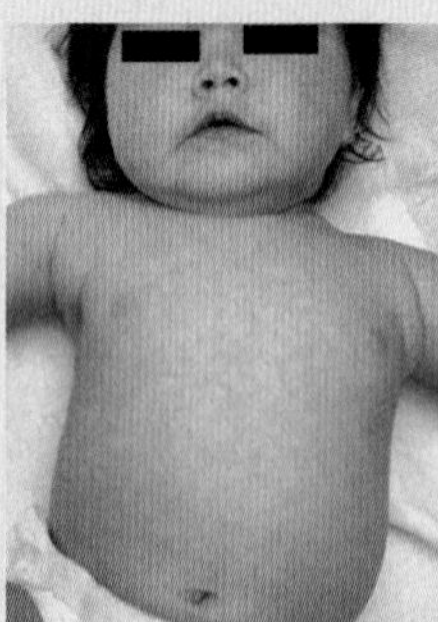 Exanthem subitum (roseola infantum).	• Prodromal phase: usually asymptomatic but may include upper respiratory signs • Clinical illness: high fever ranging from 37.9 to 40°C (101–106°F) for 3–5 days; resolves abruptly; rash appears 12–24 hours later, lasting about 1–3 days. Rash is pinkish red, flat or raised spots that blanch when touched.	• Course is generally benign. • In children who are uncomfortable or irritable or have a history of febrile seizures, antipyretics may be warranted. • Complications: HSV-6 may be responsible for some febrile seizures, encephalitis, aseptic meningitis, and thrombocytopenia purpura.	• Comfort measures, such as antipyretics, antipruritics • Standard precautions are sufficient in the hospitalized child.

TABLE 37.4 • Common Viral Exanthems of Childhood

Disease	Clinical Manifestations	Management/Complications	Nursing Implications
Erythema Infectiosum (Fifth Disease)			

• Caused by human parvovirus B19
• Transmitted by large droplet spread from nasopharyngeal viral shedding or percutaneous exposure to blood and blood products. Also transmitted from birthing parent to fetus
• Peak incidence late winter and spring
• Incubation period: 4–28 days, average 16–17 days
• Communicability is uncertain, but most children are no longer infectious by the time the rash appears and diagnosis is made, so isolation or exclusion from school, once the child is diagnosed, is unnecessary (those with aplastic crisis may be communicable up to 1 week after the onset of symptoms and those who are immunosuppressed with chronic infection and severe anemia may be communicable for months to years).
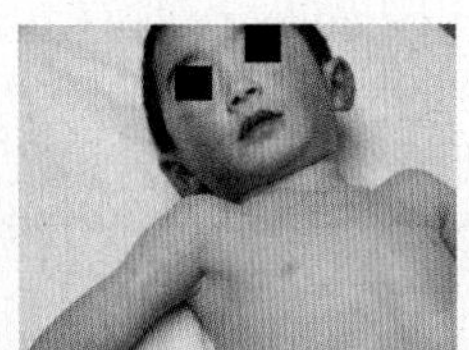
Erythema infectiosum (fifth disease).
	• Prodromal phase: mild symptoms, low-grade fever, headache, mild upper respiratory infection
	• Characteristic rash occurs in three stages:
	  • Begins with erythematous flushing often described as "slapped-cheek" appearance, often with circumoral pallor
	  • Spreads to trunk
	  • Moves peripherally, appearing as a maculopapular, lace-like appearance; often pruritic
	• Palms and soles are usually spared. Rash fluctuates in intensity and will disappear and reappear with environmental changes such as exposure to sunlight.
	• Resolves spontaneously over 1–3 weeks
	• Pain or swelling in joints may be present (more common in older adolescents).
	• Children with preexisting anemias may develop aplastic crisis (will have fever, malaise, myalgia, but usually no rash).
		• Usually benign and self-limited; supportive treatment is all that is needed.
		• Blood transfusion may be necessary in children with aplastic crisis.
		• Intravenous immunoglobulin (IVIG) many be given if child is immunocompromised.
		• Complications: arthritis and arthralgia
		• May result in fetal loss, hydrops fetalis in pregnant person
			• Comfort measures, such as antipyretics, antipruritics
			• Inform pregnant people (including health care workers) of the potential risks to the fetus and preventive measures to decrease these risks (strict infection control practices, not caring for those likely to be contagious). The CDC does not recommend routine exclusion from a workplace where an outbreak is occurring.
			• Droplet precautions are required in the hospitalized child.

Hand, Foot, and Mouth Disease, or Herpangina (if Only Mouth Involvement)			
• Caused by viruses belonging to *Enterovirus* genus. Coxsackie A viruses (especially A16) is the most common. Transmitted by direct contact with infected fecal, oral secretions; spread mostly through saliva • Peak incidence during fall and summer, particularly in children who wear diapers and children <5 years old • Incubation period: 3–6 days • Communicable from time of infection until fever resolves; virus is shed for several weeks after the infection begins.	• High fever usually occurs first. • Vesicles on tongue and oral mucosa erode to shallow ulcers; vesicles on hands and feet are football shaped, with erythematous rims. • Extensive mouth lesions may lead to anorexia, dehydration, and drooling.	• Usually mild and self-limiting, resolving within 1 week • Treatment is mainly supportive. • Complications: dehydration, meningitis, encephalitis, and possible fingernail/toenail loss	• Encourage oral fluids of preference, such as popsicles. • Provide analgesics as needed. • Mouthwash or sprays to numb the mouth may be needed. • Standard precautions and good hand hygiene are necessary. Contact precautions for diapered or incontinent children

Data from Siegel, J. D., Rhinehart, E., Jackson, M., Chiarello, L., & The Healthcare Infection Control Practices Advisory Committee. (2007, updated 2022). Guideline for isolation precautions: Preventing transmission of infectious agents in healthcare settings. https://www.cdc.gov/infectioncontrol/pdf/guidelines/isolation-guidelines-H.pdf; Centers for Disease Control and Prevention. (2021a). In E. Hall, A. P. Wodi, J. Hamborsky, V. Morelli, & S. Schillie (Eds.), *Epidemiology and prevention of vaccine-preventable diseases* (14th ed.). Public Health Foundation. https://www.cdc.gov/vaccines/pubs/pinkbook/index.html; Centers for Disease Control and Prevention. (2020b). Measles (rubeola): For healthcare professionals. Retrieved April 27, 2023, from https://www.cdc.gov/measles/hcp/index.html; Centers for Disease Control and Prevention. (2022d). Chickenpox (varicella): For healthcare professionals. Retrieved April 27, 2023, from https://www.cdc.gov/chickenpox/hcp/; Tremblay, C., & Brady, M. T. (2023). Roseola infantum (exanthem subitum). *UpToDate.* Retrieved April 27, 2023, from https://www.uptodate.com/contents/roseola-infantum-exanthem-subitum; Koch, W. C. (2020). Parvoviruses. In R. M. Kleigman, J. W. St. Geme III, N. J. Blum, S. S. Shah, R. C. Tasker, K. M. Wilson, & R. E. Behrman (Eds.), *Nelson textbook of pediatrics* (21st ed., pp. 9133–9154). Elsevier; Centers for Disease Control and Prevention (CDC). (2021b). *Hand, foot and mouth disease (HFMD).* Retrieved April 27, 2023, from https://www.cdc.gov/hand-foot-mouth/index.html#:~:text=Hand%2C%20Foot%2C%20and%20Mouth%20Disease%20(HFMD),-Espa%C3%B1ol%20(Spanish)&text=The%20illness%20is%20usually%20not,schools%20and%20day%20care%20centers.&text=Hand%2C%20foot%2C%20and%20mouth%20disease%20spreads%20easily.&text=Symptoms%20can%20include%20mouth%20sores%2C%20skin%20rash%2C%20and%20more

Typically, children with viral exanthems are cared for at home, but there are times when a child may be hospitalized or may develop the disease while being hospitalized. Appropriate transmission-based precautions must be taken. Therapeutic management of the viral exanthems focuses on fever management and relief of discomfort.

Nursing Assessment

Obtain the history of the present illness, noting the onset of rash in relation to the onset of fever. Note accompanying symptoms such as respiratory complaints. Document known exposure to childhood diseases. Note immunization status. Inspect the skin for rash, noting the distribution, type, and extent of lesions. Table 37.4 describes the rash as well as accompanying symptoms for each of the viral exanthems.

Nursing Management

Nursing management of viral exanthems focuses on fever reduction, relief of discomfort, and protection of skin integrity. Encourage hydration. Administer antipyretics and antipruritics as needed (refer to Drug Guide 37.1). Nonpharmacologic interventions to reduce fever, such as tepid sponging and cool compresses, may be used. Refer to the "Clinical Judgment and the Nursing Process" section earlier in the chapter. Care should be individualized based on the child's and family's response to the illness.

TAKE NOTE!

Trim the child's fingernails or cover hands with mitts, gloves, or socks (which work well with younger infants and children) if the rash itches to help prevent breaks in the skin, which can lead to discomfort and infection.

Mumps

Mumps, a contagious disease caused by Paramyxovirus, is characterized by fever and parotitis (inflammation and swelling of the parotid gland). Mumps is spread via airborne droplets or contact with infected droplets. The incubation period is 12 to 25 days, usually 16 to 18 days (Albrecht, 2021). Infected individuals are contagious several days prior to the onset of parotitis and for 6 to 9 days after parotid swelling begins (Albrecht, 2021). The most common complication in postpubertal boys is orchitis (inflammation of the testicle) (Albrecht, 2021). This may lead to some degree of testicular atrophy, but rarely sterility. In about 5% of females oophoritis (ovarian inflammation) occurs, with the relationship to fertility unknown (Albrecht, 2021). Complications of mumps include meningitis with or without encephalitis with seizures, pancreatitis, and auditory neuritis, which can result in hearing loss. Therapeutic management is supportive.

Since the recommendation of the two-dose MMR (measles, mumps, rubella) vaccine, the incidence of mumps has declined and made mumps a rare disease in the United States (CDC, 2021a). The AAP and the ACIP recommend immunization against mumps for all children (CDC, 2021a). Current recommendations include first mumps immunization between 12 and 15 months of age, followed by a second vaccine between 4 and 6 years of age (CDC, 2021a). According to the CDC (2021a), research shows that one dose of MMR prevents 78% of cases and two doses prevent approximately 88% of cases (see Chapter 31 for information on mumps vaccination).

Nursing Assessment

Note history of exposure to infected individuals as well as immunization status. Determine history of low-grade fever and onset and progression of parotid swelling. History may also include malaise, anorexia, headache, and abdominal pain. The parotid swelling is easily observed as swelling of the neck either bilaterally or unilaterally (Fig. 37.4). In boys, note orchitis. The diagnosis is usually based on the history and clinical presentation, but serum may be tested for the presence of mumps IgG or IgM antibody.

Nursing Management

Nursing management of mumps is primarily supportive. Acetaminophen or ibuprofen is used for fever management, and occasionally narcotic analgesics are required

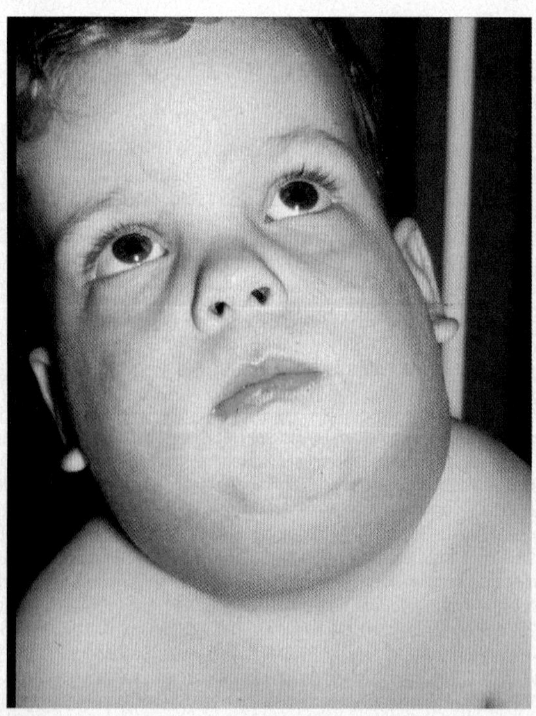

FIGURE 37.4 Parotitis associated with mumps.

for pain management. Oral fluids are encouraged to prevent dehydration. If orchitis is present, ice packs to the testicles and gentle testicular support may be helpful. Hospitalized children should be confined to respiratory isolation to prevent spread of the disease until 6 to 9 days following the onset of parotid swelling (Albrecht, 2021).

TAKE NOTE!

In recent years mumps outbreaks have occurred, mainly in settings where prolonged close contact with other people occurs, such as college campuses, camps, athletic teams, and worship groups (CDC, 2021a). The mumps vaccine is not 100% effective, and mumps infection can occur in vaccinated individuals. During an outbreak it is essential to define the population at risk and transmission setting, identify and isolate suspected cases, and identify and vaccinate susceptible individuals.

ZOONOTIC INFECTIONS

Zoonotic and **vector-borne** infections are diseases caused by infectious agents that are transmitted directly or indirectly from animals or vectors, such as ticks, mosquitoes, or other insect vectors, to humans. Zoonotic infections are responsible for about 75% of emerging infectious diseases, with approximately 60% of all human pathogens originating from animals (CDC, 2021c).

Children are at a particular risk for contracting zoonotic or vector-borne diseases. Young children are unaware of the health risks around them and cannot take protective measures. Their immature immune system leads to a decreased capacity to resist zoonotic or vector-borne diseases. These diseases can be severe and even fatal, although most are treatable if identified early. Many times, the child presents initially with nonspecific symptoms. Coupled with the fact that there are few definitive diagnostic tests available, this can lead to difficulty in promptly recognizing and treating these diseases. Tick-borne diseases are common vector-borne illnesses in the United States. Determining the incidence of zoonotic and vector-borne diseases is difficult due to the complexity of the transmission cycle and geographic climate variability. Table 37.5 discusses other zoonotic and vector-borne diseases. Nurses need to be aware of zoonotic and vector-borne diseases common in the area they are practicing as well as the impact of patient travel and the risk of these diseases. Nurses need to tap into state and local resources as well as national and international resources, such as the CDC and the World Health Organization (WHO).

TABLE **37.5** • Other Zoonotic and Vector-Borne Illnesses

Disease	Causative Organism	Geographic Distribution	Vector of Transmission	Manifestations
West Nile virus	*Flavivirus*	Throughout United States with higher rates found in Great Plains and mountain regions; seasonal epidemic from summer to fall	Mosquito bites Rare cases spread through blood transfusions, transplants, and birthing parent to baby during pregnancy and breastfeeding	No symptoms in majority of cases Symptoms include febrile illness, headache, joint pain, body aches, vomiting, diarrhea, and rash; in rare cases serious symptoms such as meningitis, encephalitis, or acute flaccid paralysis are seen.
Dengue	*Dengue viruses (flaviviruses)*	Tropics and subtropics Asia, India, Southeast Asia, Latin America, the Pacific Islands, United States (mostly Florida and Texas), US territories (mostly Puerto Rico), and Africa	Mosquito	Sudden-onset high fever, headache, severe pain behind eyes, joint, muscle and bone pain, rash, mild bleeding such as nose or gums bleeding and bruising easily, leukopenia, thrombocytopenia, and hemorrhagic manifestations Symptoms can be mild to severe and life threatening.
Zika	*Flavivirus*	Americas, Caribbean, the Pacific, Africa, and Southeast Asia	Mosquito	Acute onset of low-grade fever, maculopapular rash, arthralgia, conjunctivitis Can be passed to fetus in utero Infection during pregnancy can lead to birth defects and neurologic complications of fetus.

(continued)

TABLE 37.5 • Other Zoonotic and Vector-Borne Illnesses (*continued*)

Disease	Causative Organism	Geographic Distribution	Vector of Transmission	Manifestations
Anaplasmosis	*Anaplasma phagocytophilum*	Mostly upper Midwest and northeast United States	Black-legged tick	Headache, fever, malaise, chills, muscle aches, nausea, abdominal pain, cough, and confusion Rash is rarely seen. Symptoms appear 1–2 weeks after infected tick bite.
Ehrlichiosis	Three pathogens: *Ehrlichia chaffeensis*, *Ehrlichia ewingii*, *Ehrlichia muris*	Mostly in southeastern and south-central United States	Black-legged and lone star tick	Fever, headaches, fatigue, muscle aches, chills, nausea, vomiting, diarrhea, confusion, red eyes. Clinical signs similar to Rocky Mountain spotted fever. Rash is less commonly associated but is more common in children. May also present with leukopenia, anemia, and hepatitis
Malaria	*Plasmodium* (five species exist that infect humans: *P. falciparum*, *P. vivax*, *P. ovale*, *P. malariae*, *P. knowlesi*)	Endemic in tropical areas of the world Highest incidence in Africa, Asia, and South America. Cases in the United States are usually in travelers and immigrants returning from countries where malaria transmission occurs.	Bite of *Anopheles* species of mosquito	High fever with chills, rigors, sweats, and headache, which may be paroxysmal Nausea, vomiting, diarrhea, cough, arthralgia, and abdominal and back pain may also occur. Anemia and thrombocytopenia with pallor and jaundice may be seen. May occur in a cyclic pattern, and depending on the species fever may occur every other day or every third day.

Adapted from Centers for Disease Control and Prevention. (2023a). West Nile virus. https://www.cdc.gov/westnile/index.html; Centers for Disease Control and Prevention. (2023d). Dengue. http://www.cdc.gov/Dengue/; Centers for Disease Control and Prevention. (2022h). Zika virus. https://www.cdc.gov/zika/index.html; Centers for Disease Control and Prevention. (2022i); Anaplasmosis. http://www.cdc.gov/anaplasmosis/; Centers for Disease Control and Prevention. (2022j). Ehrlichiosis. http://www.cdc.gov/ehrlichiosis/; Centers for Disease Control and Prevention. (2023e). Malaria. https://www.cdc.gov/parasites/malaria/index.html

TAKE NOTE!

The CDC lists the current infectious disease outbreaks that are being reported at http://www.cdc.gov/outbreaks.

TAKE NOTE!

In 2016 large outbreaks of Zika occurred with increasing cases in the United States. In 2017 cases in the United States began declining, and from 2018 to 2022 there were no reports of Zika virus in the United States (CDC, 2022h).

Cat-Scratch Disease

Cat-scratch disease is a relatively common and occasionally serious disease caused by the bacteria *Bartonella henselae*. It occurs in both children and adults but is more common in children (Orscheln, 2020). Cats can carry the bacteria in their saliva. In 87% to 99% of cases, the child has had a recent interaction with cats and often kittens (Orscheln, 2020). *B. henselae* is transmitted between cats via the cat flea. The incubation period is 7 to 12 days, with lymphadenopathy appearing in 1 to 4 weeks (Orscheln, 2020). Therapeutic management is supportive and is aimed at management of symptoms. The disease itself is usually self-limited, resolving on its own in 2 to 4 months. If lymphadenopathy persists or if the child is immunocompromised, antibiotics may be needed. Painful, swollen nodes may be treated with needle aspiration to provide symptom relief.

Nursing Assessment

Note history of headaches, fever, anorexia, and fatigue. The history may also include interaction or rough play with cats or kittens, resulting in a scratch. Document temperature, noting fever. Palpate for enlarged lymph nodes, noting their location. A skin papule or pustule may be present or reported at the site of the bite or scratch. Diagnostic tests are available to detect serum antibodies to antigens of *Bartonella* species.

Nursing Management

Administer antibiotics if ordered. No transmission-based isolation is required; standard precautions are sufficient. Educate the child and family about prevention and control measures. Teach children to avoid rough play with cats and kittens. Teach parents and children to immediately wash any bites or scratches with soap and running water. Explain that cats should never lick open wounds on the child. Control of fleas in cats is important to prevent the spread of *B. henselae*.

Rabies

Rabies is a preventable viral infection of the central nervous system. It is transmitted to other animals and humans through close contact with the saliva of a rabid animal, usually by a bite. It is rare in the United States and Western Europe due to routine vaccination of domestic animals, such as dogs, and the availability of effective postexposure prophylaxis (PEP). Now most cases of rabies in these areas are due to wild animals such as raccoons, skunks, bats, and foxes (Brown & DeMaria, 2022). Rabies continues to be a major health problem in other parts of the world, especially in areas where dogs are not controlled.

Most cases of rabies occur in children younger than 15 years, and most human deaths occur in Asia and Africa (Brown & DeMaria, 2022; WHO, 2023). Children have an increased susceptibility to rabies due to their fearlessness around animals, eagerness to play with animals, shorter stature, and inability to protect themselves. The incubation period for rabies is extremely variable. Typically, it is 1 to 3 months but can range from days to years (Brown & DeMaria, 2022). The incubation period tends to be shorter in children. Once symptoms of rabies have developed, the prognosis is poor. Death usually occurs within days of the onset of symptoms. Prevention is of paramount importance, and eliminating infection in animal vectors is essential. Successful animal vaccination and animal control campaigns in the United States have led to a very low rate of human rabies cases. Recently, rabies transmitted from other animals, especially bats, has become a cause for concern (WHO, 2023).

It is important to contact the local health department whenever there is an exposure, or suspected exposure, to rabies. Several factors need to be considered when deciding to provide PEP, such as local epidemiology, type of animal involved, availability of the responsible animal for testing or quarantine, and the circumstances of the exposure, such as a provoked versus an unprovoked attack. Algorithms are available to help health care providers decide if PEP is warranted (Brown & DeMaria, 2023). In a previously unvaccinated child, PEP should begin with a thorough cleansing of all wounds with soap and water followed by a virucidal agent, such as povidone–iodine solution, if available. Animal studies have shown a 90% reduction in the likelihood of developing rabies with proper wound cleaning (Brown & DeMaria, 2023). In the United States, concurrent use of passive (rabies immune globulin) and active (rabies vaccine) immunoprophylaxis is then recommended. It consists of a regimen of one dose of immune globulin and four doses of human rabies vaccine. Rabies immune globulin and the first dose of rabies vaccine should be given as soon as possible after exposure, ideally within 24 hours. Additional doses of rabies vaccine should be given on days 3, 7, and 14 after the first vaccination. Rabies immune globulin is infiltrated into and around the wound, with any remaining volume administered intramuscularly at a site distant from the vaccine inoculation. Human rabies vaccine is administered intramuscularly into the anterolateral thigh or deltoid, depending on the age and size of the child. Administration into the gluteus muscle should be avoided, since this site has been associated with vaccine failure (Brown & DeMaria, 2023). Preexposure vaccination can be given to prevent rabies in people at high risk, such as veterinarians, laboratory technicians working with the virus, and people exposed to wild animals (Brown & DeMaria, 2023).

Nursing Assessment

Note the history of an animal bite, especially if it was unprovoked, and exposure to bats. Document history of early symptoms of rabies infection, which are nonspecific and flu-like, such as fever, headache, and general malaise. The child may complain of pain, pruritus, and paresthesia at the bite site. As the virus spreads to the central nervous system, encephalitis develops. The disease will have progressive neurologic manifestations, which may include insomnia, confusion, anxiety, changes in behavior, agitation or excitation, hallucinations, hypersalivation, dysphagia, and hydrophobia, which results from aspiration when swallowing liquid or saliva. In some cases, progressive paralysis may be present. The child may have periods of lucidity alternating with these neurologic changes.

Laboratory testing may include hair and saliva specimens from which the virus may be isolated. Serum and cerebrospinal fluid can be tested for antibodies to the rabies virus. Direct fluorescent antibody testing can be done to diagnose rabies in a suspected animal. The test can only be done postmortem and requires brain tissue from the potentially rabid animal.

Nursing Management

Few people survive once symptomatic rabies infection develops. Intensive supportive care is required, but recovery is extremely rare. Therefore, it is vital to educate children and families about the importance of seeking medical care after any animal bite to prevent death from rabies infection. Also, teach children to avoid wild animals, stray animals, and any animal with unusual behavior. Teach children not to provoke or attempt to capture wild or stray animals.

TAKE NOTE!

There have been 17 survivors of rabies once symptoms developed using a treatment protocol developed by Dr. Rodney Willoughby, Jr. called the Milwaukee Protocol at the Children's Hospital of Wisconsin. In half of the survivors, neurologic outcomes were poor (Willoughby, 2020).

Regardless of whether immunoprophylaxis is initiated, appropriate wound management is necessary in all victims of a bite from a potentially rabid animal. This includes a thorough cleansing of all wounds with soap and water. Irrigation of wounds with large volumes of a virucidal agent, such as povidone–iodine solution, along with avoiding closure of the wound is recommended (Willoughby, 2020).

When caring for a child requiring PEP, provide support and education to the child and family. Due to the seriousness and urgency surrounding this disease and treatment, the child and family are often very frightened. Consider comfort measures, such as EMLA (eutectic mixture of local anesthetic) cream and positioning, when giving immunizations.

Lyme Disease

Lyme disease, the most commonly reported vector-borne disease in the United States, is caused primarily by the spirochete *Borrelia burgdorferi* (Mead, 2021). It is transmitted to humans via the bite of an infected black-legged (deer) tick. Ninety-three percent of reported Lyme disease cases occurred in 14 states, mainly in the northeast (Pennsylvania, New Jersey, New York, Massachusetts, Connecticut, Maryland, New Hampshire, Delaware, Maine, Rhode Island, Vermont, and Virginia) and the upper Midwest (Minnesota and Wisconsin) (Mead, 2021).

Lyme disease can affect any age group, but the incidence is highest among children between 5 and 14 years of age and adults 45 to 55 years old (Mead, 2021). The prognosis for recovery in children who are treated is excellent.

Therapeutic Management

In most cases Lyme disease can be cured by antibiotics, especially if they are started early in the illness. Doxycycline is the drug of choice for children followed by amoxicillin and cefuroxime (Hu & Shapiro, 2023). In the past doxycycline was not recommended in children less than 8 years of age due to the risk that it could cause permanent discoloration of the teeth. The AAP and CDC now support the use of doxycycline in young children if treatment duration is less than 21 days as studies have shown that short courses of doxycycline do not lead to tooth staining or weakening of tooth enamel (CDC, 2019). Duration of treatment is usually 10 to 28 days, depending on the stage of disease.

Nursing Assessment

The clinical signs of Lyme disease are divided into three stages—early localized, early disseminated, and late disease. Untreated children may progress through the three stages or may present with early disseminated or late disease without having any symptoms of the earlier stages. If children are treated in the early stage, it is uncommon to see them with late disease. Nursing assessment for Lyme disease includes an accurate health history as well as physical examination.

HEALTH HISTORY

Explore the health history for a tick bite. Document onset of rash. In early localized disease, the rash usually occurs 7 to 14 days after the tick bite (though it can appear 3 to 32 days after the bite). In early disseminated disease, the rash usually begins 3 to 5 weeks after the tick bite. Note complaints of fever, malaise, mild neck stiffness, headache, fatigue, myalgia, and arthralgia or pain in the joints. In late disease, note recurrent arthritis of the large joints, such as the knees, beginning weeks to months after the tick bite. The child with late disease may or may not have a history of earlier stages of the disease, including erythema migrans.

PHYSICAL EXAMINATION

Observe for a rash. A ring-like rash at the site of the tick bite (erythema migrans) characterizes early local disease (Fig. 37.5). If untreated, the rash gradually expands and will remain for 1 to 2 weeks. Suspect early disseminated disease if multiple areas of erythema migrans are found. The multiple lesions are usually smaller than the primary lesions. Note cranial nerve palsies (especially cranial nerve VII), conjunctivitis, or signs of meningeal irritation, which occur in early disseminated disease.

LABORATORY AND DIAGNOSTIC TESTING

When diagnosing Lyme disease health care providers need to consider presence of signs and symptoms of Lyme disease, likelihood of exposure, and other illnesses that may cause similar symptoms along with results of laboratory tests. Immunoglobulin-specific antibody tests may not be positive in the early stage of the disease but may be useful in the later stages. The CDC recommends

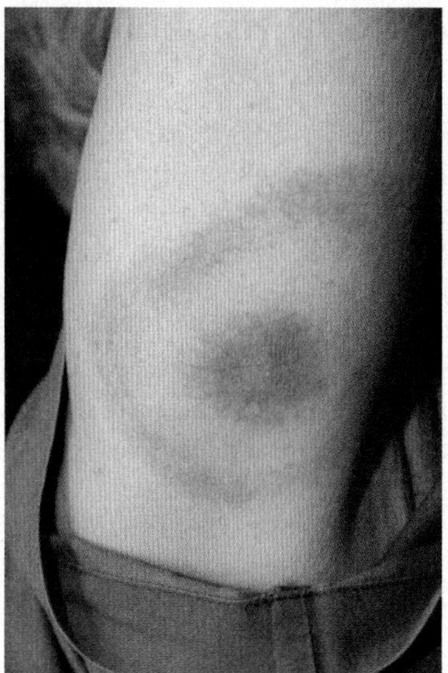

FIGURE 37.5 Erythema migrans, a ring-like rash at the site of the tick bite, occurs in Lyme disease. (Courtesy of Centers for Disease Control and Prevention, & Gathany, J. [2007]. *Public health image library [PHIL]: Details*. https://phil.cdc.gov/Details.aspx?pid=9875)

a two-step test, where both steps are required and use the same blood sample (CDC, 2021d). If these are negative, no further testing is indicated.

Nursing Management

Administer antibiotics as ordered. In the hospitalized child, no transmission-based precautions are necessary. Educate the child and family on the importance of taking the antibiotic as directed and finishing all the medicine. Another important nursing function is educating the child, family, and community on prevention measures (Box 37.5). For infection to occur, typically the tick must be attached for 36 to 48 hours (CDC, 2023b). Therefore, prompt removal (within 24 hours) of ticks is essential to the prevention of Lyme disease. Teaching Guidelines 37.2 gives information on tick removal.

Rocky Mountain Spotted Fever

Rocky Mountain spotted fever (RMSF) is the most severe and frequently reported rickettsial illness in the United States and is the second most common vector-borne disease after Lyme disease (Reller & Dumler, 2020). RMSF is caused by the bacteria *Rickettsia rickettsii*. The American dog tick and Rocky Mountain wood tick are the primary vectors, although others have been implicated. RMSF can be fatal without prompt and appropriate treatment (Reller & Dumler, 2020). Most cases occur between April and September (Reller & Dumler, 2020).

RMSF occurs throughout the United States. Its name is derived from the fact that it was discovered in the Rocky Mountain region, though few cases are found there today. It occurs in all age groups but most frequently in children, with the peak incidence in children older than 10 years (Reller & Dumler, 2020).

Complications of RMSF include noncardiogenic pulmonary edema, cerebral edema, and multiorgan damage. Long-term neurologic involvement, such as partial paralysis of the lower extremities, hearing loss, loss of bladder and bowel control, movement disorders, and language disorders, may be seen, especially in children with severe illness who require long hospital stays.

Therapeutic Management

The fatality rate from RMSF has decreased with the widespread use of antimicrobial therapy (Reller & Dumler, 2020). However, delays in diagnosis and therapy are significant factors associated with severity of disease and death. In most cases RMSF resolves rapidly with appropriate antibiotic therapy, especially if it is started early. Treatment of choice for children of all ages is doxycycline (Sexton & McClain, 2021). Length of treatment is typically 5 to 7 days (Sexton & McClain, 2021).

Nursing Assessment

Note history of early signs of RMSF, such as sudden onset of fever, headache, malaise, nausea and vomiting, muscle pain, and anorexia. The incubation period varies from 2

TEACHING GUIDELINES 37.2 Tick Removal

- Use clean, fine-tipped tweezers.
- Protect fingers with a tissue, paper towel, or latex gloves.
- Grasp tick as close to the skin as possible and pull upward with steady, even pressure.
- Do not twist or jerk the tick.
- Once the tick is removed, clean site with soap and water, rubbing alcohol, or iodine scrub and wash your hands.
- Save the tick for identification in case the child becomes sick. Place in a sealable plastic bag and put it in your freezer. Write date of bite on the bag.

BOX 37.5 Prevention of Tick-Borne Illnesses

- Wear appropriate protective clothing when entering tick-infested areas. Clothing should fit tightly around wrists, waists, and ankles. Tuck pants into socks if possible.
- After leaving the area, do a full body check for ticks and remove them promptly.
- Examine gear, clothes, and pets for ticks. Tumble dry clothes and appropriate gear on high heat for an hour.
- Insect repellent may provide temporary relief but may produce toxicity, especially in children, if used frequently or in large doses.

to 14 days, with the average being around 7 days after the tick bite (Reller & Dumler, 2020). Other signs include a rash, usually seen 1 to 3 days after the onset of the fever, abdominal pain, joint pain, and diarrhea. Inspect the skin for a rash, which starts as small, pink, macular, nonitchy, blanchable spots on the wrists, forearms, and ankles. The rash then spreads rapidly over the entire body, including the soles and palms. After several days the rash will appear red, spotted, and petechial or hemorrhagic (Fig. 37.6). Approximately 3% to 5% of children with RMSF do not have a rash (Reller & Dumler, 20120). Laboratory findings may include a low leukocyte count, low or decreasing platelet count, and hyponatremia. Biopsy of the rash with immunofluorescent assay and serologic tests may also be used.

Nursing Management

Nursing management is similar to that for Lyme disease. Educate the family about completing the antibiotic course, preventing tick bites, and appropriate tick removal (refer to Box 37.5 and Teaching Guidelines 37.2).

TAKE NOTE!

Many folklore remedies exist for tick removal such as use of petroleum jelly, nail polish, or hot matches. These often do little to get the tick to detach and may actually irritate the tick and stimulate it to release more saliva or gut contents, therefore increasing the chance of disease. The goal of tick removal is to detach it as quickly as possible (CDC, 2022e).

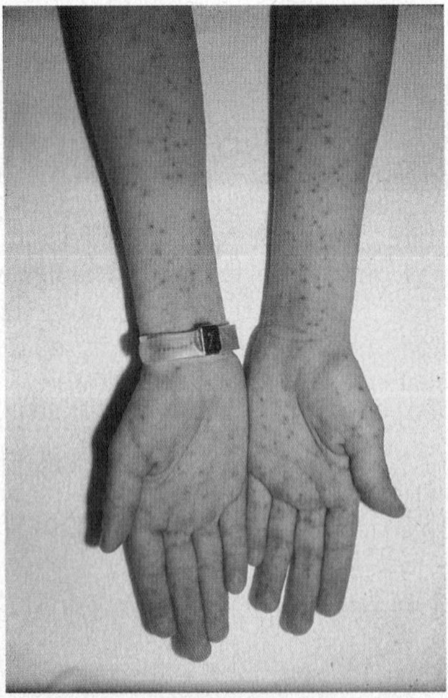

FIGURE 37.6 Rash associated with Rocky Mountain spotted fever.

PARASITIC AND HELMINTHIC INFECTION

Parasites are organisms larger than yeast or bacteria that can cause infection. They live in or on a host. Parasites receive nourishment from the host without benefiting or killing the host. Parasites frequently seen in children are scabies and head lice. A helminth is a parasitic intestinal worm. Helminthic infections seen in children include pinworms, roundworms, and hookworms. Children are at an increased risk for parasitic or helminthic infections due to poor hygiene practices. For example, children typically are more careless about handwashing and they tend to put things in their mouths and share toys and objects with other children.

Nursing Assessment and Management

Parents are often embarrassed when they find out that their child has a parasitic or helminthic infection. Reassure them that these infections can occur in any child. Tables 37.6 and 37.7 give nursing assessment and management information related to specific common parasitic and helminthic infections in children.

TAKE NOTE!

The head louse becoming resistant to pediculicides is a growing concern (Goldstein & Goldstein, 2022a).

CONSIDER THIS!

After cheerleading practice, I noticed my head was itchy. When I got home, I told my mom. She looked at my head and said she found lice. What am I going to do? Am I going to have to cut off all my hair? I love my hair! What are my friends on my team going to say if they find out? How could this happen to me?

Thoughts: Why is this adolescent so upset? How does her developmental age affect her reaction to this discovery? How would you respond to her concerns?

TAKE NOTE!

Prescription-only treatments have been approved by the Food and Drug Administration (FDA) for the treatment of head lice, including spinosad, malathion, and ivermectin tablets. Over-the-counter permethrin or pyrethrins remain the first line of treatment, but the new medications may be helpful with difficult-to-get-rid-of cases or cases of resistant lice (Nolt et al., 2022).

TABLE 37.6 • Common Parasitic Infections in Children

Infection/Causative Organism	Transmission	Clinical Manifestations	Diagnosis/Treatment	Isolation/Control Measures/Concerns
Pediculosis capitis (head lice) Caused by *Pediculus humanus capitis* (head louse)	Direct contact with hair of infested people, less commonly with personal belongings, such as combs and hats, of those infested Incubation period from laying of eggs to hatching of nymph is 6–10 days; adult lice will appear 2–3 weeks later.	Extreme pruritus is the most common symptom. Adult eggs (nits) or lice may be seen, especially behind the ears and at the nape of the neck.	Diagnosis by identification of eggs, nymph, and lice with the naked eye is possible; adult lice are rarely seen. Treatment: washing hair with a pediculicide such as pyrethroids (permethrin and pyrethrins) is preferred, or malathion, spinosad, and ivermectin. Wet combing (manual removal of lice) primarily used for young infants and patients who prefer to avoid pediculicides Careful instructions on proper use of any product should be given and strict adherence to application instructions encouraged. Retreatment is usually recommended 9 days after first treatment, depending on treatment used. Detection of living lice 24 hours after treatment suggests incorrect use, a very heavy infestation, reinfestation, or resistance to treatment.	Contact precautions After treatment check hair and comb nits and lice from hair shafts every 2–3 days to prevent reinfestation. Control measures: Household and other close contacts should be examined and if infested treated. Bedmates should be treated prophylactically. Head lice do not survive long once they have fallen off. Most children can be treated effectively without treating their clothing and bedding. But to help avoid reinfestation, disinfection of clothing, headgear, pillowcases, towels, and other items used by the individual within the past 2 days by washing in hot water and drying on the hot cycle may be helpful. Dry-cleaning nonwashable items or simply sealing them in a plastic bag for 10 days is effective. Soak combs and hairbrushes in pediculicide, shampoo, or hot water. Lice infestation is not a sign of poor hygiene; all socioeconomic groups are affected.
Pediculosis pubis (pubic lice) Caused by *Pthirus pubis*	Transmission usually occurs through sexual contact; also can be through contaminated items such as towels Adolescents and young adults most commonly affected	Pruritus of anogenital area; other hairy areas of the body, including eyelashes, eyebrows, axilla, legs, and beard, can be affected.	Diagnosis by identification of eggs, nymph, and lice with the naked eye is possible; adult lice are rarely seen. Same as treatment with pediculicides to treat head lice Retreat 9–10 days later. To treat eyelashes and eyebrows: if only a few nits are present, remove these with fingernails or a nit comb; if additional treatment is needed, apply ophthalmic-grade petrolatum ointment (prescription).	Standard precautions Control measures similar to head lice All sexual contacts should be treated simultaneously. Avoid sexual contact with partners until both they and their partners have been successfully treated and reevaluated. Evaluation for the presence of other sexually transmitted infections Bedding and clothing should be machine washed and dried at a high temperature or bagged for 2 weeks. If found on children, may be a sign of sexual exposure or abuse

(continued)

TABLE 37.6 • Common Parasitic Infections in Children (*continued*)

Infection/Causative Organism	Transmission	Clinical Manifestations	Diagnosis/Treatment	Isolation/Control Measures/Concerns
Scabies Caused by *Sarcoptes scabiei*	Incubation period from laying of eggs to hatching of nymph is 3–4 days; adult lice will appear 2–4 weeks later. Incubation period in those without previous exposure is 4–6 weeks. Usually no symptoms are present during this time but transmission to others can occur. People who were previously infested can develop symptoms in 1–4 days. Transmission usually occurs through prolonged, close personal contact.	Intense pruritus (especially at night) with the presence of erythematous, papular rash with excoriations. The lesions are generally distributed but often are concentrated on the hands and feet and in body folds. May be found on head and neck In infants and young children the rash is often heavy on palms, soles, and fingers, and it may include vesicles, pustules, or bullous lesions.	Diagnosis can be made by a history of itching (especially at night), classic rash, and reports of itching in household or sexual contacts. Mites can be seen on microscopic examination of skin scrapings to confirm diagnosis. Treatment: A scabicide, such as permethrin or lindane, should be applied to the entire body below the head. Treatment of infants and young children should include the head, neck, and body. In infants younger than 2 months, permethrin is not approved; therefore, a topical sulfur treatment cream is used and left on for a specified time (usually 8–14 hours) depending on the type of scabicide. Retreatment 1–2 weeks later may be needed. Oral ivermectin (cannot be used in children <15 kg) Careful instructions on proper use of any product should be given and strict adherence to application instructions should be urged. Itching may not subside for several weeks, even after successful treatment.	Contact precautions Prophylactic therapy for household members and sexual contacts Bedding and clothing used by infested person or household, sexual, or close contacts within 3–4 days before treatment should be laundered in hot water and dried on the hot cycle (mites do not survive more than 3–4 days without skin contact). Avoid direct skin-to-skin contact with person or items used by those infested. Room used by an infected person, especially if they have crusted scabies, should be thoroughly cleaned and vacuumed.

Data from Goldstein, A. O., & Goldstein, B. O. (2022a). Pediculosis capitis. *UpToDate.* Retrieved May 1, 2023, from https://www.uptodate.com/contents/pediculosis-capitis Nolt, D., Moore, S., Yan, A. C., Melnick, L., & Committee on Infectious Diseases, Committee on Practice and Ambulatory Medicine, Section on Dermatology (2022). Head lice. *Pediatrics, 150*(4), e2022059282. https://doi.org/10.1542/peds.2022-059282; Goldstein, A. O., & Goldstein, B. G. (2023). Pediculosis pubis and pediculosis ciliaris. *UpToDate.* Retrieved May 1, 20123, from https://www.uptodate.com/contents/pediculosis-pubis-and-pediculosis-ciliaris; Goldstein, B. G., & Goldstein, A. O. (2022b). Scabies: Epidemiology, clinical features, and diagnosis. *UpToDate.* Retrieved May 1, 2023, from https://www.uptodate.com/contents/scabies-epidemiology-clinical-features-and-diagnosis; Goldstein, B. G., & Goldstein, A. O. (2022c). Scabies: Management. *UpToDate.* Retrieved May 1, 2023, from https://www.uptodate.com/contents/scabies-management; Siegel, J. D., Rhinehart, E., Jackson, M., Chiarello, L., & The Healthcare Infection Control Practices Advisory Committee. (2007, updated 2022). Guideline for isolation precautions: Preventing transmission of infectious agents in healthcare settings. Retrieved March 19, 2019, from https://www.cdc.gov/infectioncontrol/pdf/guidelines/isolation-guidelines-H.pdf

SEXUALLY TRANSMITTED INFECTIONS

STIs, commonly called sexually transmitted diseases, are infectious diseases transmitted through sexual contact, including oral, vaginal, or anal intercourse. Certain infections can be transmitted in utero to the fetus or during childbirth to the newborn leading to miscarriage, stillbirth, ectopic pregnancy, preterm delivery, low birth weight, birth defects, and congenital infection (Rietmeijer, 2023).

STIs are a major health concern for adolescents. The rates of many STIs are highest in adolescents (Fortenberry, 2022). Adolescents are at a greater risk for developing STIs for a variety of reasons, including frequency of unprotected intercourse, being biologically more susceptible to infection, and engaging in partnerships of limited duration (Fortenberry, 2022). Table 37.8 discusses common clinical manifestations of specific STIs in adolescents.

Detection of STIs in infants and children is an important warning sign of potential sexual abuse. Due to the serious implications that a diagnosis of an STI can have in children, only tests that have high specificities and that can isolate an organism should be used. Also, treatment for the child with a suspected STI may be delayed until a definitive diagnosis can be made. Refer to Chapter 5 for further information on STIs and adolescents. Chapter 47 provides information related to HIV.

TABLE **37.7** • Common Helminthic Infections in Children

Infection/Causative Organism	Clinical Manifestations	Transmission	Diagnosis/Treatment	Isolation/Control Measures
Ascariasis Most commonly caused by *Ascaris lumbricoides*, common in temperate and tropical areas, especially in areas with unsanitary conditions	Most people are asymptomatic, may demonstrate slower growth and weight gain In more severe infections, loss of appetite, nausea, vomiting, and abdominal pain may be seen. Cough and difficulty breathing may be present as immature worms migrate through the lungs. In significant infestation, partial or complete intestinal obstruction may occur. The more worms, the worse the symptoms.	Human feces are the major source of infected eggs. Hand to mouth is the usual route of transmission. The eggs are swallowed due to unclean hands or contaminated food or water. They pass into the intestine; larvae then hatch, penetrate the intestinal wall, enter the circulatory system, and migrate to other body tissues, primarily the lungs first.	Diagnosis: once female worms are in the intestine, eggs can be visualized by microscopic evaluation of the stool. Occasionally a worm may be coughed up and visualized or seen in vomit, stool, or urine. Imaging can also be used. Mainstay of treatment is with mebendazole, albendazole, or pyrantel pamoate.	Standard precautions are sufficient. Sanitary disposal of feces Proper hand hygiene
Hookworm Caused by *Ancylostoma duodenale* (roundworm) and *Necator americanus* (roundworm); *Ancylostoma ceylanicum* (a hookworm found in cats and dogs that can cause human infections) common in tropics and subtropics especially in areas with unsanitary conditions; rare in areas with <40 in of annual rainfall	Most often people are asymptomatic until significant worms are established. May see pruritic erythematous papular rash at entry site (referred to as ground itch) or pulmonary symptoms as the larvae migrate One of the greatest concerns in chronic infection is anemia (microcytic hypochromic anemia) secondary to blood loss as the worms suck blood and juices from the intestines. This can lead to hypoproteinemia, edema, pica, and wasting. The infection may result in physical or intellectual disability in children.	Hookworms are found in soil and enter the host through pores, hair follicles, and even intact skin (hands and feet are major sites of entry). The maturing larvae travel through the circulatory system into the lungs and then up the bronchial tree and are swallowed with secretions. They then migrate into the intestinal tract and attach to the wall of the small intestines, where they feed and reproduce.	Diagnosis: through microscopic examination of feces that reveals hookworm eggs Treatment: albendazole (preferred), mebendazole, and pyrantel pamoate Iron supplementation and possible blood transfusion in severe cases	Standard precautions are sufficient. Proper sanitation and disposal of feces Treatment of all known infested people Screening of high-risk individuals Encourage the wearing of shoes and avoiding going barefoot.

(*continued*)

TABLE 37.7 • Common Helminthic Infections in Children (*continued*)

Infection/Causative Organism	Clinical Manifestations	Transmission	Diagnosis/Treatment	Isolation/Control Measures
Pinworm Caused by *Enterobius vermicularis* (roundworm); found in tropical and temperate climates; most common helminthic infection found in the United States	Most people are asymptomatic. May cause anal itching (pruritus ani), especially at night Other clinical findings may include restlessness and teeth grinding at night, weight loss, enuresis, abdominal pain, nausea and vomiting. Most frequently seen in children 5–10 years of age	Fecal–oral route directly, indirectly, or inadvertently by contaminated hands or shared toys, bedding, clothing, toilet seats Incubation period is 1–2 months or longer.	Diagnosis: when adult worms are visualized in the perianal region; they are best viewed when the child is sleeping. Very few ova are present in stool, so examination of stool is not recommended. Transparent tape pressed to perianal area and then viewed under a microscope may reveal eggs. Three consecutive specimens should be obtained when the child first awakens in the morning. Treatment of choice is mebendazole, pyrantel pamoate, and albendazole, usually single doses and repeated in 2 weeks.	Standard precautions are sufficient. Reinfection occurs easily. Infected people should bathe, preferably in a shower, in the morning, which will remove a large portion of the eggs. Frequent changing of underclothes and bedding Personal hygiene measures such as keeping fingernails short, avoiding scratching of perianal area, and nail biting Good hand hygiene is the most effective preventive measure, especially after using the bathroom and before eating. All family members should be treated since transmission from person to person is very easy.

Data from Leder, K., & Weller, P. F. (2022a). Ascariasis. *UpToDate*. Retrieved May 1, 2023, from https://www.uptodate.com/contents/ascariasis; Weller, P. F., & Leder, K. (2021). Hookworm. *UpToDate*. Retrieved May 1, 2023, from https://www.uptodate.com/contents/hookworm-infection

Leder, K., & Weller, P. F. (2022b). Enterobiasis (pinworm) and trichuriasis (whipworm). In E. L. Baron (Ed.), *UpToDate*. Retrieved May 1, 2023, from https://www.uptodate.com/contents/enterobiasis-pinworm-and-trichuriasis-whipworm; Siegel, J. D., Rhinehart, E., Jackson, M., Chiarello, L. & The Healthcare Infection Control Practices Advisory Committee. (2007, updated 2022). Guideline for isolation precautions: Preventing transmission of infectious agents in healthcare settings. https://www.cdc.gov/infectioncontrol/pdf/guidelines/isolation-guidelines-H.pdf

KEY CONCEPTS

- Infants and young children are more susceptible to infection due to their immature immune system. Young children continue to have an increased risk for infections and communicable disorders because disease protection from immunizations is not complete.
- Health care providers need to remember to educate parents that fever is a protective mechanism the body uses to fight infection.
- When obtaining blood cultures, follow aseptic technique and hospital protocol to prevent contamination. Obtain the specimen before administering antibiotics.
- When administering antipyretics, proper education must be given to caregivers on appropriate dosing, concentration, dosing interval, and use of proper measuring device.
- Promoting proper fluid balance and reducing temperature in a febrile child are important nursing interventions when caring for a child with an infection or communicable illness.
- Many childhood infectious and communicable diseases involve a rash. Rashes can be difficult to identify, so a thorough description and history from the caregiver is important.
- Sepsis, a systemic overresponse to infection resulting from bacteria, fungi, viruses, or parasites, can lead to septic shock. Any infant younger than 3 months with a fever or any child with a fever accompanied by extreme lethargy, unresponsiveness, or lack of facial expressions should be seen by a health care provider or nurse practitioner.
- Many bacterial and viral infections, such as diphtheria, tetanus, pertussis, mumps, measles, rubella, varicella, and poliomyelitis, can be prevented by vaccination.
- Viral exanthems of childhood often present with a distinct rash pattern that assists in the diagnosis of the virus. Common childhood exanthems include exanthem subitum (roseola infantum), rubella (German measles), rubeola (measles), varicella (chickenpox), and erythema infectiosum (fifth disease).
- Nurses play a key role in educating the public on the importance of immunizations.

TABLE 37.8 • Sexually Transmitted Infections (STIs) Common in Adolescents

Disease	Causative Organism	Transmission Mode	Diagnostic Testing and Recommended Screening for Sexually Active Adolescents	Female Symptoms	Male Symptoms	Recommended Treatment
Chlamydia Curable STI Seen frequently among sexually active adolescents and young adults	*Chlamydia trachomatis* (bacteria)	Vaginal, anal, and oral sex and by childbirth	Preferred method: Noninvasive, non–culture-based testing is available using nucleic acid amplification and testing (NAAT) from urine—single test can test for chlamydia and gonorrhea. Culture fluid from urethral swabs in males or endocervical swabs for females. Conjunctival secretions in neonates Females (sexually active, <25 years old): screen annually. Males: screen high-risk adolescents.	May be asymptomatic Dysuria, urinary frequency, dyspareunia Cervical discharge (mucus or pus) Endocervicitis May lead to pelvic inflammatory disease, ectopic pregnancy, infertility Can cause inflammation of the rectum and conjunctiva Can infect the throat from oral sexual contact with an infected partner	May be asymptomatic Dysuria, urethral itching Penile discharge (mucus or pus) Urethral tingling May lead to epididymitis and sterility Can cause inflammation of the rectum and conjunctiva Can infect the throat from oral sexual contact with an infected partner	Preferred: Doxycycline (Vibramycin) Main Alternative: Azithromycin (Zithromax) Alternatives: Erythromycin (EES) Levofloxacin, Ofloxacin (Floxin) Sexual partners also need evaluation, testing, and treatment. Abstinence from sexual activity until therapy complete and symptoms no longer present Retesting in 3 months to rule out recurrence
Gonorrhea Curable STI Adolescent often coinfected with *Chlamydia trachomatis*	*Neisseria gonorrhoeae* (bacteria)	Vaginal, anal, and oral sex and by childbirth	Same noninvasive, non–culture-based test using NAAT from urine as chlamydia Gram stain or culture directly for the bacterium Females (sexually active, <25 years old): screen annually. Males: screen high-risk adolescents.	May be asymptomatic or no recognizable symptoms until serious complications such as pelvic inflammatory disease Dysuria Urinary frequency Vaginal discharge (yellow and foul) Dyspareunia Endocervicitis Arthritis May lead to pelvic inflammatory disease, ectopic pregnancy, infertility Symptoms of rectal infection include discharge, anal itching, and occasional painful bowel movements with fresh blood.	Most produce symptoms, but can be asymptomatic Dysuria Penile discharge (pus) Arthritis May lead to epididymitis and sterility Symptoms of rectal infection include discharge, anal itching, and occasional painful bowel movements with fresh blood.	Intramuscular ceftriaxone Alternatives: Other cephalosporins and Azithromycin Sexual partners also need evaluation, testing, and treatment. Abstinence from sexual activity until therapy complete and symptoms no longer present Retesting in 3 months to rule out recurrence

(*continued*)

TABLE 37.8 • Sexually Transmitted Infections (STIs) Common in Adolescents (*continued*)

Disease	Causative Organism	Transmission Mode	Diagnostic Testing and Recommended Screening for Sexually Active Adolescents	Female Symptoms	Male Symptoms	Recommended Treatment
Herpes type 2 (genital herpes) Lifelong recurrent viral disease Most people have not been diagnosed. There is no cure.	Herpes simplex virus 1 and 2 (HSV-1 and HSV-2)	HSV-1 is spread through oral secretions; can be spread to genitals through poor hand-washing of infected person or oral–genital contact HSV-2 is spread by having sexual contact (vaginal, oral, or anal) with someone who is shedding the herpes virus either during an outbreak or during a period with no symptoms; can be spread to an infant through childbirth.	Visual inspection and symptoms or culture from swabs taken from lesions (success depends on stage of lesion—optimum is during vesicular stage) Polymerase chain reaction is more sensitive than culture. Serologic tests, such as antibody-based testing (herpes Western blot assay is the most sensitive) Type-specific laboratory testing important Routine screening not recommended	Initial symptoms include itching, tingling, and pain in genital area followed by small pustules and blister-like genital lesions that then crust over and gradually heal. Recurrence episodes are usually milder than the initial episode. Dysuria, dyspareunia, and urinary retention Fever, headache, malaise, muscle aches	Same as for females	Antivirals used to treat first episode, recurrence, and suppression Acyclovir, valacyclovir, and famciclovir mainstay in treatment Does not cure; just controls symptoms Counseling important to help adolescents cope and to prevent transmission Sexual partners benefit from evaluation and counseling. If symptomatic, need treatment If asymptomatic, offer testing and education.
Syphilis	*Treponema pallidum* (spirochete bacteria)	Sexual contact with an infected person	Serologic testing mainstay for diagnosis Venereal Disease Research Laboratory (VDRL), rapid plasma reagin (RPR), and treponemal tests (e.g., fluorescent treponemal antibody absorbed [FTA-ABS]) can lead to a presumptive diagnosis and are useful for screening. Use of two tests required Darkfield examination and direct fluorescent antibody tests of lesion exudate or tissue provide definitive diagnosis of early syphilis. New tests such as enzyme immunoassay are in development. Screen based on epidemiology and personal risk factors.	Course of disease divided into stages: **Primary infection:** • Chancre on place of entrance of bacteria (usually vulva or vagina but can develop in other parts of the body) **Secondary infection:** • Maculopapular rash (hands and feet) • Sore throat • Lymphadenopathy • Flu-like symptoms **Latent infection:** • No symptoms • Can be infective during first 1–2 years of latency • Many people if not treated will suffer no further signs and symptoms. • Some people will go on to develop tertiary or late syphilis. **Tertiary infections:** • Tumors of skin, bones, and liver • Central nervous system symptoms • Cardiovascular symptoms • Usually not reversible at this stage	Course of disease divided into stages: **Primary infection:** • Chancre on place of entrance of bacteria (usually on penis but can develop in other parts of the body) **Secondary, latent, and tertiary infections:** All similar to those of female symptoms	Benzathine penicillin G injection (if penicillin allergy, doxycycline, tetracycline, or azithromycin) Sexual partners need evaluation and testing.

Trichomoniasis	*Trichomonas vaginalis* (protozoa)	Vaginal intercourse with an infected partner May be picked up from direct genital contact with damp or moist objects, such as towels or wet clothing	Highly sensitive and specific testing, such as NAAT, available and recommended, Microscopic evaluation of vaginal secretions or culture still common but less sensitive	Many females have symptoms but some may be asymptomatic. Dysuria Frequency Vaginal discharge (yellow, green, or gray and foul odor) Dyspareunia Irritation or itching of genital area	Most males infected are asymptomatic. Dysuria Penile discharge (watery white)	Metronidazole (Flagyl) or tinidazole Sexual partners also need evaluation, testing, and treatment. Abstinence recommended until therapy complete
Venereal warts (condylomata acuminata) One of the most common STIs in the United States Could lead to cancers of the cervix, vulva, vagina, anus, or penis No cure; warts can be removed but virus remains	Human papillomavirus	Vaginal, anal, or oral sex with an infected partner	Visual inspection Abnormal Pap smear may indicate cervical infection of human papillomavirus (HPV)	Wart-like lesions that are soft, moist, or flesh colored and appear on the vulva and cervix, and inside and surrounding the vagina and anus Sometimes appear in clusters that resemble cauliflower-like bumps, and are either raised or flat, small or large	Wart-like lesions that are soft, moist, or flesh colored and appear on the scrotum or penis. They sometimes appear in clusters that resemble cauliflower-like bumps, and are either raised or flat, small or large.	May disappear without treatment Treatment is aimed at removing the lesions rather than HPV itself. No optimal treatment has been identified, but there are several ways to treat depending on size and location. Most methods rely on chemical or physical destruction of the lesion: Imiquimod cream 20% Podophyllin antimitotic solution 0.5% Podofilox solution 5% 5-fluorouracil cream Trichloroacetic acid (TCA) Small warts can be removed by: • Freezing (cryosurgery) • Burning (electrocautery) • Laser treatment • Surgical excision Large warts that have not responded to treatment may be removed surgically. Vaccination recommended starting around age 12 and may lead to decrease in cancer associated with HPV Abstinence from sexual activity during treatment to promote healing

Data from Burnstein, G. R. (2020). Sexually transmitted infections. In R. M. Kleigman, J. W. St. Geme III, N. J. Blum, S. S. Shah, R. C. Tasker, K. M. Wilson, & R. E. Behrman (Eds.), *Nelson textbook of pediatrics* (21st ed., pp. 6011-6057); Elsevier; Shafii, T., & Levine, D. (2020). Office-based screening for sexually transmitted infections in adolescents. *Pediatrics*, *145* (Suppl_2), S219–S224. https://doi.org/10.1542/peds.2019-2056K

- Zoonotic infections are diseases caused by infectious agents that are transmitted directly or indirectly from animals to humans. Cat-scratch disease and rabies are types of zoonotic infections.
- Children are at a particular risk for contracting vector-borne diseases, which are diseases transmitted by ticks, mosquitoes, or other insect vectors. Two of the most commonly seen are Lyme disease and RMSF.
- Parasites frequently seen in children are scabies and head lice. Helminthic infections seen in children include pinworms, roundworms, and hookworms.
- STIs are infectious diseases transmitted through sexual contact, including oral, vaginal, or anal intercourse. Certain infections can be transmitted in utero to the fetus or during childbirth to the newborn.
- STIs are a major health concern for adolescents. Adolescents are at a greater risk for developing STIs for a variety of reasons, including frequency of unprotected intercourse, being biologically more susceptible to infection, and engaging in partnerships of limited duration (Fortenberry, 2022).

REFERENCES AND RECOMMENDED READINGS

Albrecht, M. A. (2021). Mumps. *UpToDate*. Retrieved April 25, 2023, from https://www.uptodate.com/contents/mumps

Anderson, D. J. (2023). Infection prevention: Precautions for preventing transmission of infection. *UpToDate*. Retrieved April 13, 2023, from https://www.uptodate.com/contents/infection-prevention-precautions-for-preventing-transmission-of-infection

Barroso, L. F., & Pegram, P. S. (2023). Epidemiology and pathophysiology of diphtheria. *UpToDate*. Retrieved April 17, 2023, from https://www.uptodate.com/contents/epidemiology-and-pathophysiology-of-diphtheria

Brown, C. M., & DeMaria, A., Jr. (2022). Clinical manifestations and diagnosis of rabies. *UpToDate*. Retrieved April 28, 2023, from https://www.uptodate.com/contents/clinical-manifestations-and-diagnosis-of-rabies

Brown, C. M., & DeMaria, A., Jr. (2023). Rabies immune globulin and vaccine. *UpToDate*. Retrieved April 28, 2023, from https://www.uptodate.com/contents/rabies-immune-globulin-and-vaccine

Burnstein, G. R. (2020). Sexually transmitted infections. In R. M. Kleigman, J. W. St. Geme III, N. J. Blum, S. S. Shah, R. C. Tasker, K. M. Wilson, & R. E. Behrman (Eds.), *Nelson textbook of pediatrics* (21st ed., pp. 6011–6057). Elsevier.

Cantey, J. B. (2023). Clinical features, evaluation, and diagnosis of sepsis in term and late preterm neonates. *UpToDate*. Retrieved April 13, 2023, from https://www.uptodate.com/contents/clinical-features-evaluation-and-diagnosis-of-sepsis-in-term-and-late-preterm-neonates

Centers for Disease Control and Prevention. (2019). *Research on doxycycline and tooth staining*. https://www.cdc.gov/rmsf/doxycycline/index.html

Centers for Disease Control and Prevention. (2020a). *Hand hygiene in healthcare settings: Hand hygiene guidance*. https://www.cdc.gov/handhygiene/providers/guideline.html

Centers for Disease Control and Prevention. (2020b). *Measles (rubeola): For healthcare providers*. https://www.cdc.gov/measles/hcp/index.html

Centers for Disease Control and Prevention. (2021a). In E. Hall, A. P. Wodi, J. Hamborsky, V. Morelli, & S. Schillie (Eds.), *Epidemiology and prevention of vaccine-preventable diseases* (14th ed.). Public Health Foundation. https://www.cdc.gov/vaccines/pubs/pinkbook/index.html

Centers for Disease Control and Prevention. (2021b). *Hand, foot and mouth disease (HFMD)*. https://www.cdc.gov/hand-foot-mouth/index.html#:~:text=Hand%2C%20Foot%2C%20and%20Mouth%20Disease%20(HFMD),-Espa%C3%B1ol%20(Spanish)&text=The%20illness%20is%20usually%20not,schools%20and%20day%20care%20centers.&text=Hand%2C%20foot%2C%20and%20mouth%20disease%20spreads%20easily.&text=Symptoms%20can%20include%20mouth%20sores%2C%20skin%20rash%2C%20and%20more

Centers for Disease Control and Prevention. (2021c). *Zoonotic diseases*. https://www.cdc.gov/onehealth/basics/zoonotic-diseases.html

Centers for Disease Control and Prevention. (2021d). *Lyme disease: Diagnosis and testing*. http://www.cdc.gov/lyme/diagnosistesting/LabTest/TwoStep/index.html

Centers for Disease Control and Prevention. (2022a). *Group A streptococcal (GAS) disease: Scarlet fever: All you need to know*. https://www.cdc.gov/groupastrep/diseases-public/scarlet-fever.html?CDC_AA_refVal=https%3A%2F%2Fwww.cdc.gov%2Ffeatures%2Fscarletfever%2Findex.html

Centers for Disease Control and Prevention. (2022b). *Pertussis (whooping cough)*. https://www.cdc.gov/pertussis/clinical/treatment.html

Centers for Disease Control and Prevention. (2022c). *Botulism*. Retrieved April 19, 2023, from https://www.cdc.gov/botulism/index.html

Centers for Disease Control and Prevention. (2022d). *Chickenpox (varicella): For healthcare professionals*. https://www.cdc.gov/chickenpox/hcp/

Centers for Disease Control and Prevention. (2022e). *Ticks: Tick removal*. http://www.cdc.gov/ticks/removing_a_tick.html

Centers for Disease Control and Prevention. (2022f). *Condom effectiveness: Male (external) condom use*. https://www.cdc.gov/condomeffectiveness/external-condom-use.html?CDC_AA_refVal=https%3A%2F%2Fwww.cdc.gov%2Fcondomeffectiveness%2Fmale-condom-use.html

Centers for Disease Control and Prevention. (2022g). *Condom effectiveness: Female (internal) condom use*. https://www.cdc.gov/condomeffectiveness/internal-condom-use.html?CDC_AA_refVal=https%3A%2F%2Fwww.cdc.gov%2Fcondomeffectiveness%2FFemale-condom-use.html

Centers for Disease Control and Prevention. (2022h). *Zika virus*. https://www.cdc.gov/zika/index.html

Centers for Disease Control and Prevention. (2022i); *Anaplasmosis*. http://www.cdc.gov/anaplasmosis/

Centers for Disease Control and Prevention. (2022j). *Ehrlichiosis*. http://www.cdc.gov/ehrlichiosis/

Centers for Disease Control and Prevention. (2022k). *Haemophilus influenzae disease (including Hib): For clinicians*. https://www.cdc.gov/hi-disease/clinicians.html

Centers for Disease Control and Prevention. (2023a). *West Nile virus* https://www.cdc.gov/westnile/index.html

Centers for Disease Control and Prevention. (2023b). *Lyme disease: Transmission*. Retrieved April 29, 2023, from http://www.cdc.gov/lyme/transmission/index.html

Centers for Disease Control and Prevention. (2023c). *Sexually transmitted diseases (STDs): STDs during pregnancy—CDC detailed fact sheet*. https://www.cdc.gov/std/pregnancy/stdfact-pregnancy-detailed.htm

Centers for Disease Control and Prevention. (2023d). *Dengue*. http://www.cdc.gov/Dengue/

Centers for Disease Control and Prevention. (2023e). *Malaria*. https://www.cdc.gov/parasites/malaria/index.html

Expert Working Group on the Canadian Guidelines for Sexually Transmitted Infections. (2008). *Canadian guidelines on sexually transmitted infections*. Public Health Agency of Canada.

Fischbach, F. T., Fischbach, M. A., & Stout, K. (2022). *A manual of laboratory and diagnostic tests* (11th ed.). Wolters Kluwer.

Fortenberry, J. D. (2022). Sexually transmitted infections: Issues specific to adolescents. *UpToDate*. Retrieved May 1, 2023, from https://www.uptodate.com/contents/sexually-transmitted-infections-issues-specific-to-adolescents

Goldstein, A. O., & Goldstein, B. G. (2022a). Pediculosis capitis. *UpToDate*. Retrieved May 1, 2023, from https://www.uptodate.com/contents/pediculosis-capitis

Goldstein, B. G., & Goldstein, A. O. (2022b). Scabies: Epidemiology, clinical features, and diagnosis. *UpToDate*. Retrieved May 1, 2023, from https://www.uptodate.com/contents/scabies-epidemiology-clinical-features-and-diagnosis

Goldstein, B. G., & Goldstein, A. O. (2022c). Scabies: Management. *UpToDate*. Retrieved May 1, 2023 from https://www.uptodate.com/contents/scabies-management

Goldstein, A. O., & Goldstein, B. G. (2023). Pediculosis pubis and pediculosis ciliaris. *UpToDate*. Retrieved May 1, 20123, from https://www.uptodate.com/contents/pediculosis-pubis-and-pediculosis-ciliaris

Hu, L., & Shapiro, E. D. (2023). Treatment of Lyme disease. *UpToDate*. Retrieved April 29, 2023, from https://www.uptodate.com/contents/treatment-of-lyme-disease

Kaplan, S. L. (2023). Methicillin-resistant *Staphylococcus aureus* infections in children: Epidemiology and clinical spectrum. *UpToDate*. Retrieved April 16, 2023, from https://www.uptodate.com/contents/methicillin-resistant-staphylococcus-aureus-infections-in-children-epidemiology-and-clinical-spectrum?

Koch, W. C. (2020). Parvoviruses. In R. M. Kleigman, J. W. St. Geme III, N. J. Blum, S. S. Shah, R. C. Tasker, K. M. Wilson, & R. E. Behrman (Eds.), *Nelson textbook of pediatrics* (21st ed., pp. 9133–9154). Elsevier.

Krogstad, P. (2022a). Hematogenous osteomyelitis in children: Epidemiology, pathogenesis, and microbiology. *UpToDate*. Retrieved April 18, 2023, from https://www.uptodate.com/contents/hematogenous-osteomyelitis-in-children-epidemiology-pathogenesis-and-microbiology

Krogstad, P. (2022b). Bacterial arthritis: Epidemiology, pathogenesis, and microbiology in infants and children. *UpToDate*. Retrieved April 18, 2023, from https://www.uptodate.com/contents/bacterial-arthritis-epidemiology-pathogenesis-and-microbiology-in-infants-and-children

Krogstad, P. (2023). Bacterial arthritis: Clinical features and diagnosis in infants and children. *UpToDate*. Retrieved April 18, 2023, from https://www.uptodate.com/contents/bacterial-arthritis-clinical-features-and-diagnosis-in-infants-and-children

Kronman, M. P., Crowell, C. S., & Vora, S. B. (2023a). Section 16: Infectious diseases. Chapter 96: Fever without a focus. In K. J. Marcdante, R. M. Kleigman, & A. M. Schuh (Eds.), *Nelson essentials of pediatrics* (9th ed., pp. 386–390). Elsevier.

Kronman, M. P., Crowell, C. S., & Vora, S. B. (2023b). Section 16: Infectious diseases. Chapter 117: Osteomyelitis. In K. J. Marcdante, R. M. Kleigman, & A. M. Schuh (Eds.), *Nelson essentials of pediatrics* (9th ed., pp. 443–445). Elsevier.

Leder, K., & Weller, P. F. (2022a). Ascariasis. *UpToDate*. Retrieved May 1, 2023, from https://www.uptodate.com/contents/ascariasis

Leder, K., & Weller, P. F. (2022b). Enterobiasis (pinworm) and trichuriasis (whipworm). In E. L. Baron (Ed.), *UpToDate*. Retrieved May 1, 2023, from https://www.uptodate.com/contents/enterobiasis-pinworm-and-trichuriasis-whipworm

Lexicomp. (2023). Pediatric drug information. *UpToDate*. Retrieved April 5, 2023, from https://www.uptodate.com/contents/table-of-contents/drug-information/pediatric-drug-information

Mead, P. (2021). Epidemiology of Lyme disease. *UpToDate*. Retrieved April 29, 2023, from https://www.uptodate.com/contents/epidemiology-of-lyme-disease

Nath, J. (2023). *Applied pathophysiology* (4th ed.). Wolters Kluwer.

Nolt, D., Moore, S., Yan, A. C., Melnick, L., & Committee on Infectious Diseases, Committee on Practice and Ambulatory Medicine, Section on Dermatology. (2022). Head lice. *Pediatrics, 150*(4), e2022059282. https://doi.org/10.1542/peds.2022–059282

Orscheln, R. C. (2020). Cat-scratch disease (Bartonella henselae). In R. M. Kleigman, J. W. St. Geme III, N. J. Blum, S. S. Shah, R. C. Tasker, K. M. Wilson, & R. E. Behrman (Eds.), *Nelson textbook of pediatrics* (21st ed., pp. 8275–8288). Elsevier.

Paul, I. M., & Walson, P. D. (2021). Acetaminophen and ibuprofen in the treatment of pediatric fever: A narrative review. *Current Medical Research and Opinion, 37*(8), 1363–1375. https://doi.org/10.1080/03007995.2021.1928617

Pegram, P. S., & Stone, S. M. (2023). Botulism. *UpToDate*. Retrieved April 18, 2023, from https://www.uptodate.com/contents/botulism

Pomerantz, W. J., & Weiss, S. L. (2022). Systemic inflammatory response syndrome (SIRS) and sepsis in children: Definitions, epidemiology, clinical manifestations, and diagnosis. *UpToDate*. Retrieved April 16, 2023, from https://www.uptodate.com/contents/systemic-inflammatory-response-syndrome-sirs-and-sepsis-in-children-definitions-epidemiology-clinical-manifestations-and-diagnosis

Reller, M. E., & Dumler, J. S. (2020). Rocky Mountain spotted fever (Rickettsia rickettsii). In R. M. Kleigman, J. W. St. Geme III, N. J. Blum, S. S. Shah, R. C. Tasker, K. M. Wilson, & R. E. Behrman (Eds.), *Nelson textbook of pediatrics* (21st ed., pp. 8693–8714). Elsevier.

Rietmeijer, K. (2023). Prevention of sexually transmitted infections. *UpToDate*. Retrieved March 13, 2023, from https://www.uptodate.com/contents/prevention-of-sexually-transmitted-infections

Roué, J.-M. (2022). Prevention and treatment of neonatal pain. *UpToDate*. Retrieved March 13, 2023, from https://www.uptodate.com/contents/prevention-and-treatment-of-neonatal-pain

Scarfone, R. J., & Cho, C. (2022). Approach to the ill-appearing infant (younger than 90 days of age). *UpToDate*. Retrieved April 13, 2023, from https://www.uptodate.com/contents/approach-to-the-ill-appearing-infant-younger-than-90-days-of-age

Sexton, D. J., & McClain, M. T. (2021). Treatment of Rocky Mountain spotted fever. *UpToDate*. Retrieved April 29, 2023, from https://www.uptodate.com/contents/treatment-of-rocky-mountain-spotted-fever

Shafii, T., & Levine, D. (2020). Office-based screening for sexually transmitted infections in adolescents. *Pediatrics*, *145*(Suppl_2), S219–S224. https://doi.org/10.1542/peds.2019-2056K

Shulman, S. T., & Reuter, C. H. (2020). Group A streptococcus. In R. M. Kleigman, J. W. St. Geme III, N. J. Blum, S. S. Shah, R. C. Tasker, K. M. Wilson, & R. E. Behrman (Eds.), *Nelson textbook of pediatrics* (21st ed., pp. 7617–7670). Elsevier.

Siegel, J. D., Rhinehart, E., Jackson, M., Chiarello, L., & The Healthcare Infection Control Practices Advisory Committee. (2007, updated 2022). *Guideline for isolation precautions: Preventing transmission of infectious agents in healthcare settings*. https://www.cdc.gov/infectioncontrol/pdf/guidelines/isolation-guidelines-H.pdf

Souder, E., & Long, S. S. (2020). Pertussis (*Bordetella pertussis* and *Bordetella parapertussis*). In R. M. Kleigman, J. W. St. Geme III, N. J. Blum, S. S. Shah, R. C. Tasker, K. M. Wilson, & R. E. Behrman (Eds.), *Nelson textbook of pediatrics* (21st ed., pp. 8020–8041). Elsevier.

Sotoodian, B. (2020). *Scarlet fever*. https://emedicine.medscape.com/article/1053253-overview#a6

Sullivan, J. E., Farrar, H. C., & The AAP's Section on Clinical Pharmacology and Therapeutics, and Committee on Drugs. (2011, reaffirmed 2023). Clinical report: Fever and antipyretic use in children. *Pediatrics*, *127*(3), 580–587. https://doi.org/10.1542/peds.2010-3852

Thwaites, L. (2022). Tetanus. *UpToDate*. Retrieved April 18, 2023, from https://www.uptodate.com/contents/tetanus

Tremblay, C., & Brady, M. T. (2023). Roseola infantum (exanthem subitum). *UpToDate*. Retrieved April 27, 2023, from https://www.uptodate.com/contents/roseola-infantum-exanthem-subitum

U.S. Department of Health and Human Services. (n.d.). *Healthy People 2030*. https://health.gov/healthypeople

Ward, M. A. (2022). Fever in infants and children: Pathophysiology and management. *UpToDate*. Retrieved April 11, 2023, from https://www.uptodate.com/contents/fever-in-infants-and-children-pathophysiology-and-management

Weller, P. F., & Leder, K. (2021). Hookworm infection. *UpToDate*. Retrieved May 1, 2023, from https://www.uptodate.com/contents/hookworm-infection

Willoughby, R. E., Jr. (2020). Rabies. In R. M. Kleigman, J. W. St. Geme III, N. J. Blum, S. S. Shah, R. C. Tasker, K. M. Wilson, & R. E. Behrman (Eds.), *Nelson textbook of pediatrics* (21st ed., pp. 9562–9576). Elsevier.

World Health Organization. (2023). *Rabies: Fact sheet*. http://www.who.int/mediacentre/factsheets/fs099/en/

Yeh, S., & Mink, C. M. (2022). Pertussis infection in infants and children: Clinical features and diagnosis. *UpToDate*. Retrieved April 17, 2023, from https://www.uptodate.com/contents/pertussis-infection-in-infants-and-children-clinical-features-and-diagnosis

DEVELOPING CLINICAL JUDGMENT

PRACTICING FOR NCLEX

1. Compared with adults, why are infants and children at an increased risk for infectious and communicable diseases?
   a. The infant has had limited exposure to disease and is losing the passive immunity acquired from maternal antibodies.
   b. The infant demonstrates an increased inflammatory response.
   c. Cellular immunity is not functional at birth.
   d. Infants have an increased risk for infection until they receive their first set of immunizations.
2. A parent calls the clinic because their 2-year-old child has a rectal temperature of 37.8°C (100°F). The parent wonders how high a fever should be before they should give medications to reduce it. What is the best response by the nurse?
   a. "All fevers should be treated to prevent seizures."
   b. "Antipyretics should be used with any rise in temperature. They can help change the course of the infection."
   c. "Give your child aspirin when their fever is above 38°C (100.4°F)."
   d. "In a normal healthy child, if your child is not uncomfortable, fevers less than 39°C (102.2°F) do not require medication."
3. A neonate should be evaluated by a health care provider if which sign or symptom is present?
   a. Acting fussier than normal
   b. Refusing the pacifier
   c. Rectal temperature above 38°C (100.4°F)
   d. Mottling that is present during bathing
4. The public health nurse has been asked to provide information to local child care centers on controlling the spread of infectious diseases. What is the best information the nurse can provide?
   a. The etiology of common infectious diseases
   b. Proper handwashing techniques
   c. The physiology of the immune system
   d. Why children are at a higher risk of infection than adults
5. When teaching a group of adolescents about STIs, which of the following points are important to include? Select all that apply.
   a. Many people infected with chlamydia are unaware and have no symptoms.
   b. Gonorrhea is the least common of all STIs.
   c. Adolescent females who are sexually active should be screened annually for chlamydia.
   d. Genital herpes is a lifelong viral illness.
   e. Practicing good handwashing is the best way to prevent STIs.
   f. STIs are a major health concern for adolescents.
6. Parents of a 4-month-old infant tell the health care provider their child has had a mild fever, cough, and runny nose for the past 2 weeks and now the cough is worse. Upon assessment the nurse finds the infant's heart rate to be 152 bpm, respiratory rate 64, coughing spells with a whooping sound, and axillary temperature 38.3°C (101°F). Which two nursing actions are the priority?
   a. Promote mobility.
   b. Assess oxygen level.
   c. Assess pain level.
   d. Monitor elimination.
   e. Encourage rest.

DOSAGE CALCULATION QUESTIONS

1. The nurse is caring for a child who has a rash and is complaining of feeling itchy and is continually scratching. The child weighs 32 lb. The medication order reads: Diphenhydramine 6.25 mg po every 4 to 6 hours as needed for itching. Diphenhydramine is supplied as 12.5 mg/5 mL. How many milliliters will the nurse administer? Round to the nearest tenth.

CRITICAL THINKING EXERCISES

1. A 12-year-old child presents with a very sore throat and fever. On assessment you find an erythematous rash on the child's face that feels like sandpaper. You obtain a throat culture, which is positive for group A streptococcus. What instructions would you give the parents regarding the child's care at home?
2. A 1-month-old infant is admitted to the hospital to rule out sepsis. What would be your priority nursing interventions?

3. A 4-year-old child presents with a fever and rash. What three of the following items should the nurse obtain during the health history?
   a. Immunization history
   b. Any exposure to communicable or infectious diseases
   c. Whether the child takes a daily vitamin
   d. Thorough description and history of the rash
   e. Birthing parent's immunization history

STUDY ACTIVITIES

1. The 4-year-old presented in Question 3 of the Critical Thinking Exercises was diagnosed with varicella zoster virus. Write a nursing plan of care or concept map for a child with varicella.
2. You are asked to give a presentation to a group of adolescents on STIs, including transmission, symptoms, treatment, and prevention. What information would you include?
3. A child is brought to the school nurse with intense itching. Upon assessment the nurse finds an erythematous, papular rash with excoriations on the child's hands and feet. As suspected, the diagnosis of scabies is confirmed. What teaching is necessary for the parents, family, and classmates of the child?

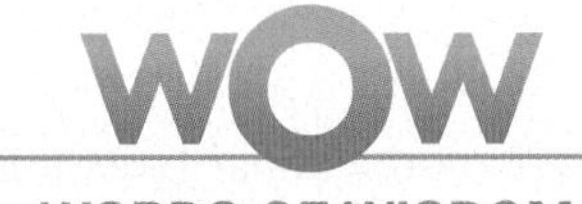

WORDS OF WISDOM

Listen to the parents of the children you care for; their insight and knowledge about their child is invaluable.

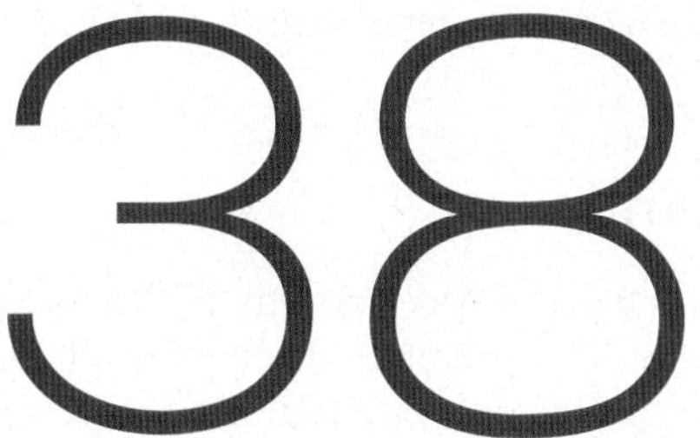

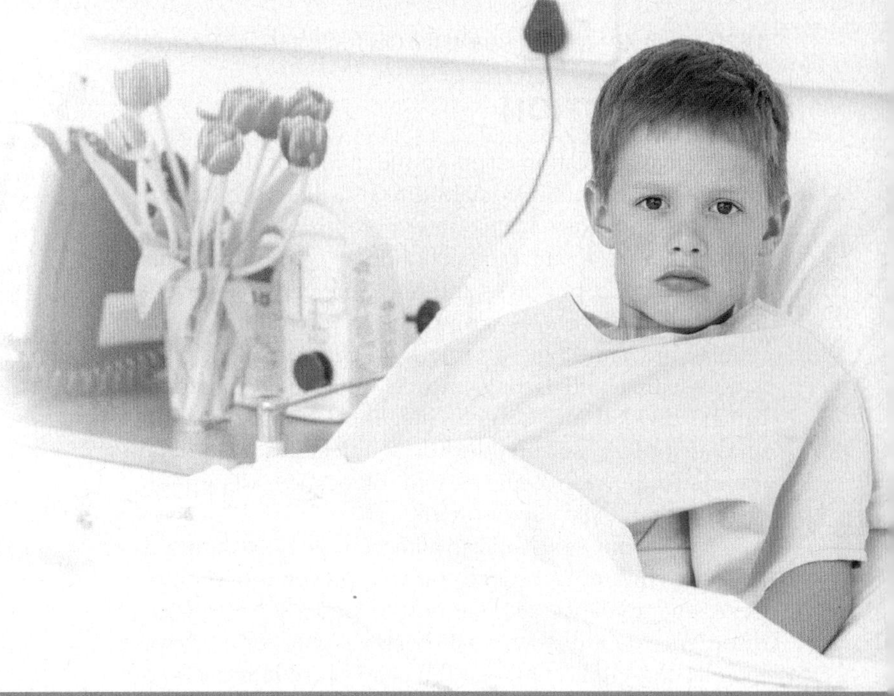

38 Nursing Care of the Child With an Alteration in Intracranial Regulation or Neurologic Disorder

KEY TERMS

- central nervous system (CNS)
- decerebrate posturing (dē-ser′ĕ-brāt pos′chŭr-ing)
- decorticate posturing (dē-kōr′ti-kāt pos′chŭr-ing)
- head circumference
- intracranial pressure (ICP)
- lumbar puncture (LP)
- myelinization (mī′ĕ-li-nī-zā′shun)
- neural tube
- opisthotonic (ō′pis-thot′ŏ-nik)
- postictal (post-ik′tăl)
- teratogen (ter′ă-tō-jen)

LEARNING OBJECTIVES

Upon completion of the chapter, you will be able to:

1. Compare how the anatomy and physiology of the neurologic system in children differ from those of adults.
2. Identify various factors associated with neurologic disease in infants and children.
3. Discuss common laboratory and other diagnostic tests useful in the diagnosis of neurologic conditions.
4. Discuss common medications and other treatments used for treatment and palliation of neurologic conditions.
5. Recognize risk factors associated with various neurologic disorders.
6. Distinguish among different neurologic illnesses based on the signs and symptoms associated with them.
7. Discuss nursing interventions commonly used for neurologic illnesses.
8. Devise an individualized plan of care or concept map for the child with a neurologic disorder.
9. Develop child and family teaching plans for the child with a neurologic disorder.
10. Describe the psychosocial impact of chronic neurologic disorders on children.

Antonio Chapman, 3 months old, has had increased irritability, poor sucking and feeding, and a fever for the past 24 hours. Today, he is lethargic with a weak cry and is vomiting his feeds.

INTRODUCTION

Intracranial regulation refers to the ability of the cranial contents to maintain equilibrium and therefore neurologic function. Nurses encounter potential and actual alterations in intracranial regulation in all types of patients and must detect problems and intervene early to prevent life-threatening complications. Alterations in intracranial regulation (neurologic disorders) in children often have a devastating and lasting impact. Neurologic disorders can be divided into several categories, including structural disorders, seizure disorders, infectious disorders, trauma to the neurologic system, blood flow disruption disorders, and chronic disorders.

Nurses must be familiar with neurologic conditions affecting children in order to provide prevention, prompt treatment, guidance, and support to families. Neurologic disorders require acute interventions, but often have long-lasting implications for the child's health and development. Due to the potentially devastating effects that neurologic disorders can have on children and their families, nurses need to be skilled in assessment and interventions in this area and must be able to provide support throughout the course of the illness and beyond.

VARIATIONS IN PEDIATRIC ANATOMY AND PHYSIOLOGY

Neurologic disorders can result from congenital problems as well as from infections or traumas. Certain neurologic conditions occur in children more often than in adults, and these conditions will affect their growth and development. In addition, children are at an increased risk for different neurologic problems compared to adults due to anatomic and physiologic differences.

Brain and Spinal Cord Development

The brain and spinal cord make up the **central nervous system (CNS)**. Development of these structures occurs in the first 3 to 4 weeks of gestation from the **neural tube**. Infection, trauma, **teratogens** (any environmental substance that can cause physical defects in the developing embryo and fetus), and malnutrition during this period can result in malformations in brain and spinal cord development and may affect normal CNS development.

At birth, the cranial bones are not well developed and are not fused. Therefore, there is an increased risk for fracture. The brain is highly vascular, leading to an increased risk of hemorrhage. Premature infants are at greater risk for brain damage; the more premature the infant, the greater the risk. The premature infant has more capillaries in the periventricular area, which is the brain tissue that lines the outside of the lateral ventricles. These capillaries are fragile and at greater risk for rupture, leading to intracranial bleeding. Also, because the cranium is very soft in the preterm infant, external pressure can change its shape and cause increased pressure in areas of the brain and possible hemorrhage.

The sutures and fontanels present in the newborn help make the skull more flexible and help to accommodate for brain growth that continues after birth. Closure of the fontanels too early or too late can be indicative of problems with brain growth. The child's spine is very mobile, especially the cervical spine region, resulting in a high risk of cervical spine injury.

Nervous System

The development of the nervous system is complete but immature at birth. The infant is born with all the nerve cells that they will have throughout life. However, **myelinization**, the formation of myelin, which covers and protects the nerves, is incomplete. The speed and accuracy of nerve impulses increases as myelinization increases. This process accounts for the acquisition of fine and gross motor movements and coordination in early childhood. Myelinization proceeds in the cephalocaudal direction. For example, infants are able to control the head and neck before the trunk and extremities.

The immaturity of the CNS in preterm infants can result in delayed development of motor skills. Premature newborns may have difficulty coordinating sucking and swallowing, leading to feeding and growth issues. Also, episodes of apnea can be problematic in the preterm newborn due to the underdevelopment of the nervous system.

Head Size

The head of the infant and young child is large in proportion to the body. The head of an infant accounts for a quarter of the body height; in adults, it accounts for one eighth of the body height (Fig. 38.1). In addition, the infant's and child's neck muscles are not well developed. Both of these differences lead to an increased incidence of head injury from falls. The head is the fastest growing body part during infancy and continues to grow until the child is 5 years old.

COMMON MEDICAL TREATMENTS

A variety of interventions, including medical treatments and medications, are used to treat neurologic illness in children. Most of these treatments will require a health care provider's or nurse practitioner's order when the child is hospitalized. The most common treatments and medications used for neurologic disorders are listed in Common Medical Treatments 38.1 and Drug Guide 38.1.

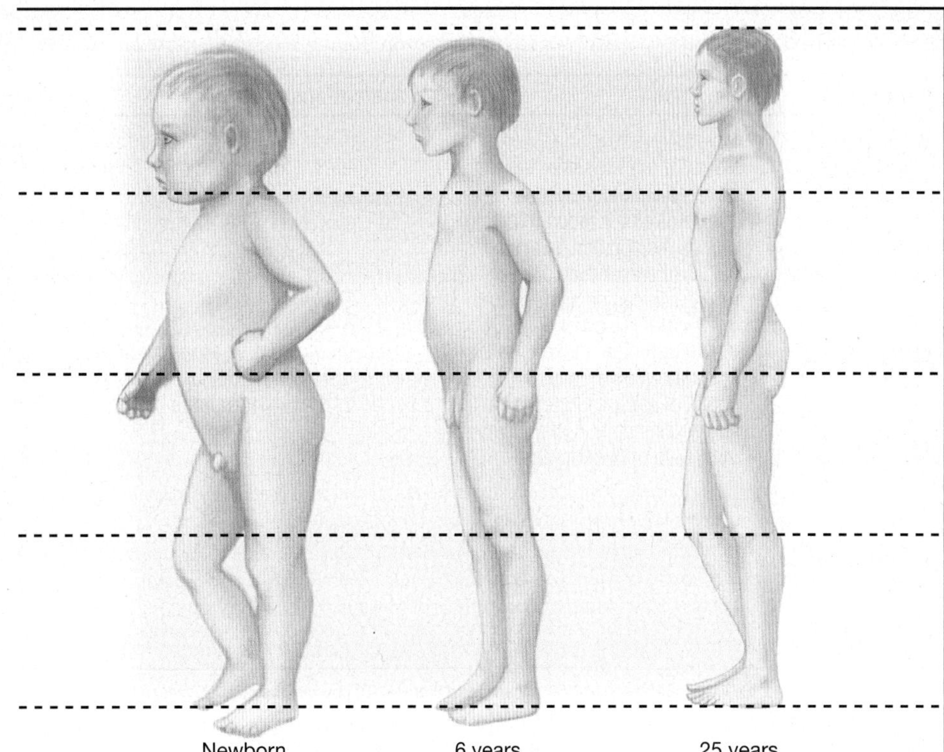

FIGURE 38.1 Proportion of head to body height in the newborn, child, and adult.

COMMON MEDICAL TREATMENTS 38.1

Treatment	Explanation	Indications	Nursing Implications
Shunt placement	A catheter is placed in the ventricle to pass the CSF to the peritoneal cavity, atrium of the heart, or pleural spaces. (Ventriculoperitoneal shunts are commonly used.)	Hydrocephalus, increased ICP	Monitor: • For signs and symptoms of increased ICP • Neurologic status closely • Level of consciousness and vital signs • For signs and symptoms of infection
Ventilation	Hyperventilation to decrease $PaCO_2$, which will result in vasoconstriction and therefore decrease in ICP Adequate oxygenation to prevent hypoxia and further damage to the brain	Increased ICP	Monitor: • Arterial blood gases • For signs and symptoms of increased ICP • Pulse oximetry
PT/OT/ST	Therapies are used to improve motor function and ability of children with neurologic disorders.	Head injury, intellectual disability	Ensure adequate communication exists within the interdisciplinary team.
External ventricular drainage (EVD)	A catheter is temporarily placed in the ventricle, and CSF is drained in a closed system to an external reservoir.	Most commonly used with shunt infections until CSF is sterile and shunt can be replaced; treats acute-onset hydrocephalus, meningitis, encephalitis, tumors that cause blockage of CSF, closed head injury, subarachnoid hemorrhage, increased ICP; also can be used to monitor ICP	Monitor: • For signs and symptoms of increased ICP • Neurologic status closely • Level of consciousness and vital signs • For signs and symptoms of infection • Level of collection container when drain is unclamped
Ventricular tap	To reduce accumulation of CSF and decrease ICP	Increased ICP	Monitor: • Level of consciousness • Neurologic status

(continued)

COMMON MEDICAL TREATMENTS 38.1 (*continued*)

Treatment	Explanation	Indications	Nursing Implications
Vagal nerve stimulator	A nerve stimulator is implanted, and a lead wire running under the skin is wrapped around the vagus nerve. The stimulator is programmed to provide the appropriate dose of stimulation at preset intervals; additional stimulation can be administered.	Short- and long-term seizure management in children over 12 years of age	Monitor: • For signs and symptoms of infection • For seizure activity
Ketogenic diet	Diet involving high intake of fats, adequate protein, and a very low intake of carbohydrates, resulting in a ketosis state. Child is kept in a mild state of dehydration.	Prevention, control, and reduction of seizures, in particular for children with difficult-to-control seizures	Monitor: • Input and output closely • For seizure activity • Growth and nutritional status • The diet is time-consuming, and many children find it unpalatable; therefore, all families and children do not accept it. • Recommended for a minimum of 3 months, reevaluate every 1–2 years • Alternative diets include: the medium chain triglyceride diet, modified Atkins diet, and a low glycemic index diet

CSF, cerebrospinal fluid; ICP, intracranial pressure; OT, occupational therapy; PT, physical therapy; ST, speech therapy.

Data from Kossoff, E. H. W. (2022). The ketogenic diet and other diet therapies for the treatment of epilepsy. *UpToDate*. Retrieved May 9, 2023, from https://www.uptodate.com/contents/ketogenic-dietary-therapies-for-the-treatment-of-epilepsy

DRUG GUIDE 38.1

Medication	Actions/Indications	Nursing Implications
Antibiotics (oral, parenteral, intrathecal)	Treatment of bacterial meningitis and shunt infections; kill and prevent the growth of bacteria.	Check for antibiotic allergies. Monitor serum levels to ensure therapeutic dosing, if indicated. Give as prescribed for the length of time prescribed.
Anticonvulsants (oral, parenteral)	Decrease hyperexcitability of nerves. Treatment and prevention of seizures	Maintain seizure precautions. Monitor for drug interactions and long-term adverse effects. Monitor and document all seizure activity. Many are used in combination, but patient and family need to be aware of interactions and long-term adverse effects. Stopping drug abruptly may precipitate seizures or even status epilepticus.
Benzodiazepines Diazepam (oral, rectal, IV, or IO) Lorazepam (oral, IV, or IO) Midazolam (IM, intranasal or buccal)	Minor sedative that prevents or stops seizures by slowing down the CNS, making abnormal electrical activity unlikely Treatment for status epilepticus	Diazepam is available in rectal form to stop prolonged seizures in children. Useful for home management; nurses must educate family members on administration and when to call health care provider or nurse practitioner. Monitor sedation level and for cessation of seizure activity.
Analgesics (acetaminophen, ibuprofen, ketorolac, morphine)	Block pain impulse in response to inhibition of prostaglandin synthesis Narcotic analgesics (i.e., morphine) act on receptors in the brain to alter perception of pain. Used to treat pain. Used to help avoid increase in ICP	Monitor for improvements in pain. Monitor sedation and respiratory status with narcotics. Monitor neurologic status closely. Used cautiously because loss of accurate neurologic evaluation can occur
Osmotic diuretics (i.e., mannitol)	Increase plasma osmolality, therefore inducing diffusion back into plasma and extravascular space/reduces ICP.	Monitor electrolytes. Monitor I/O closely. Monitor vital signs. Monitor for signs and symptoms of increased ICP.
Corticosteroids (i.e., dexamethasone)	Suppress inflammation and normal immune response/reduce cerebral edema.	Give oral doses with food. Dosage must be tapered before discontinuing.

I/O, intake/output; IO, intraosseous; IM, intramuscular; IV, intravenous

Data from Lexicomp. (2023). Pediatric drug information. *UpToDate*. Retrieved April 5, 2023, from https://www.uptodate.com/contents/table-of-contents/drug-information/pediatric-drug-information

Clinical Judgment and the Nursing Process for the Child With a Neurologic Disorder

Care of the child with a neurologic disorder includes assessment, nursing analysis, planning, intervention, and evaluation. There are a number of general concepts related to the nursing process that can be applied to the management of neurologic disorders. From an overall understanding of the care involved for a child with an alteration in intracranial regulation, the nurse can then individualize the care based on specifics for the particular child.

Assessment

Assessment of neurologic dysfunction in children includes health history, physical examination, and laboratory and diagnostic testing.

TAKE NOTE!

Neurologic assessment should proceed from least invasive to most invasive. The use of toys and familiar objects, as well as incorporating play, will help promote cooperation from the child.

Health History

The health history consists of past medical history, including the birthing parent's pregnancy history, family history, and history of present illness (when the symptoms started and how they have progressed), as well as treatments used at home. The past medical history might be significant for prematurity, difficult birth, infection during pregnancy, nausea, vomiting, headaches, changes in gait, falls, visual disturbances, or recent trauma. Family history might be significant for genetic disorders with neurologic manifestations, seizure disorders, or headaches. When eliciting the history of the present illness, inquire about the following:

- Nausea
- Vomiting
- Changes in gait
- Visual disturbances
- Complaints of headaches
- Recent trauma
- Changes in cognition
- Change in consciousness, including any loss of consciousness
- Poor feeding
- Lethargy
- Increased irritability
- Fever
- Pain
- Altered muscle tonicity
- Delays in growth and development
- Ingestion or inhalation of neurotoxic substances or chemicals

Physical Examination

Physical examination of the nervous system consists of inspection and observation, palpation, and auscultation.

Inspection and Observation

Specific areas to inspect and observe include:

- Level of consciousness (LOC)
- Vital signs
- Head, face, and neck
- Cranial nerve function
- Motor function
- Reflexes
- Sensory function
- Increased **intracranial pressure (ICP)** (a rise in the normal pressure within the skull)

Level of Consciousness. Begin the physical examination with inspection and observation. Observe the child's LOC, noting a decrease or significant changes. LOC is the earliest indicator of improvement or deterioration of neurologic status. Extreme irritability or lethargy is considered an abnormal finding. Consciousness consists of alertness, which is a wakeful state and includes the ability to respond to stimuli, and cognition, which includes the ability to process stimuli and demonstrate a verbal or motor response. Five different states constitute the levels of consciousness:

1. *Full consciousness* is defined as a state in which the child is awake and alert; is oriented to time, place, and person; and exhibits age-appropriate behaviors.
2. *Confusion* is defined as a state in which disorientation exists. The child may be alert but responds inappropriately to questions.
3. *Obtunded* is defined as a state in which the child has limited responses to the environment and falls asleep unless stimulation is provided.
4. *Stupor* exists when the child responds only to vigorous stimulation.
5. *Coma* defines a state in which the child cannot be aroused, even with painful stimuli.

CLINICAL REASONING ALERT!

Lack of response to painful stimuli is abnormal and can indicate a life-threatening condition. Report this finding immediately.

The Pediatric Glasgow Coma Scale is a popular scale used to standardize degree of consciousness. It consists of three parts: eye opening, verbal response, and motor response (Fig. 38.2). When assessing LOC in children, consider that the infant or child may not respond to unfamiliar voices in an unfamiliar environment. Therefore, it may be helpful to have a parent present to elicit the response.

TAKE NOTE!

Parents will often be the first to notice changes in their child's LOC. Listen to parents and respond to their concerns.

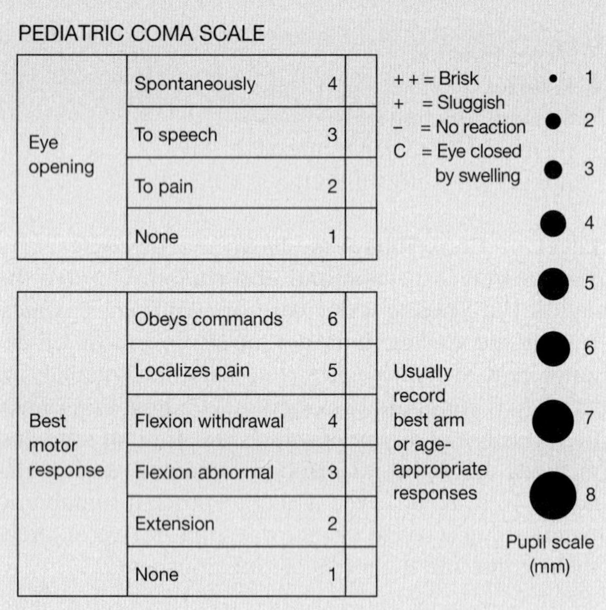

PEDIATRIC COMA SCALE

Eye opening	Spontaneously	4	
	To speech	3	
	To pain	2	
	None	1	

++ = Brisk
+ = Sluggish
− = No reaction
C = Eye closed by swelling

Best motor response	Obeys commands	6	
	Localizes pain	5	
	Flexion withdrawal	4	
	Flexion abnormal	3	
	Extension	2	
	None	1	

Usually record best arm or age-appropriate responses

	>2 years			<2 years
Best response to auditory and/or verbal stimulus	Oriented	5		5 Smiles, listens, follows
	Confused	4		4 Cries, consolable
	Inappropriate words	3		3 Inappropriate, persistent cry
	Incomprehensible words	2		2 Agitated, restless
	None	1		1 None
	Tracheal tube	T		T Tracheal tube

Pediatric coma scale total	

FIGURE 38.2 Pediatric Glasgow Coma Scale (GCS). The Pediatric GCS provides for developmentally appropriate cues to assess level of consciousness (LOC) in infants and children. Numeric values are assigned to the levels of response, and the sum provides an overall picture, as well as an objective measure, of the child's LOC. The lower the score, the less responsive the child.

Vital Signs. Assessment of vital signs can provide probable underlying causes for altered LOC as well as reveal the adequacy of oxygenation and circulation. Certain neurologic conditions like cerebral infections, increased ICP, coma, brain stem injury, or head injuries can cause alterations in the child's vital signs.

Head, Face, and Neck. Inspect and observe the head for size and shape. Abnormal skull shape can result from premature closure or widening of sutures. Inspect and observe the face for symmetry. Asymmetry may occur due to paralysis of certain cranial nerves, position in utero, or swelling caused by trauma. Assess range of motion (ROM) of the neck. Alterations in ROM can indicate CNS infections such as meningitis.

The most dramatic increase in brain volume occurs during the last 3 months of fetal development and the first 2 years of life. The relationship between head and brain growth explains why **head circumference** (measurement of the child's head around the largest area) is a standard assessment made in children younger than 3 years of age. All children younger than 3 years old, and any child whose head size is questionable, should have their head circumference measured and plotted on a growth chart (see Appendix D for growth charts).

Assessment of the growth trend of the head is important in detecting potential neurologic conditions. Report and investigate any variation in head circumference percentiles over time because variations may indicate abnormal brain or skull growth. A smaller than normal head circumference, which measures around the child's head at the largest area, may indicate microcephaly, and a larger than normal head circumference may indicate hydrocephalus.

CLINICAL REASONING ALERT!

Do not attempt any assessment that involves movement of the head and neck in cases of trauma or suspected trauma until cervical injury is ruled out. Maintain complete immobilization of the cervical spine until that time.

Cranial Nerve Function. Techniques of assessment of cranial nerve function are similar to techniques for adult assessment. The method of obtaining responses may vary based on age and developmental level of the child. Certain elements of the adult assessment may be omitted. Alterations in cranial nerve function can be the result of compression of a specific nerve, infection, or trauma leading to brain injury. Refer to Table 38.1 for an explanation of cranial nerve assessment in children.

Use the doll's eyes maneuver to evaluate cranial nerves III, IV, and VI. This maneuver can be helpful when assessing an infant, uncooperative child, or comatose child. It examines horizontal and vertical eye movements by turning the head in one direction and

TABLE 38.1 • Assessment of Cranial Nerves in Infants and Children

Cranial Nerve	Function	Assessment Procedure
I (olfactory)	Sense of smell	Not evaluated in infants and young children. In children, assess child's ability to recognize common smells (i.e., an orange) while eyes are closed.
II (optic), III (oculomotor), IV (trochlear), VI (abducens)	Vision, motor control and sensation of eye muscles, movement of major eye muscles	Assess oculomotor ability by having child follow object (toy or brightly colored object). Assess vision fields and visual acuity in older child. Assess pupil reaction same as adult. May need to talk to child or have parent in visual field while applying light stimulus
V (trigeminal)	Mastication muscles and facial sensation	Note strength of infant's suck on pacifier, examiner's thumb, or bottle. In children, assess strength of bite and ability to discern light touch on face.
VII (facial)	Facial muscles, salivation, and taste	Note symmetry of facial expressions; in infant, monitor during spontaneous cries or smiles. In older child, test as in adults. Assess taste by asking to discern certain common tastes (salt, sugar).
VIII (acoustic)	Hearing	In infant, note response to voice. In children, use whisper test or Weber or Rinne test.
IX (glossopharyngeal), X (vagus)	Motor impulses to heart and other organs, swallowing, and gag reflex	Gag reflex and swallowing tested as in adults. Check time of last feeding, especially in the infant, to avoid vomiting when gag reflex is tested.
XI (accessory)	Impulses to muscles of shoulders and pharynx	In infants, note symmetry of head position when placed in the sitting position. In children, same as adults
XII (hypoglossal)	Motor impulses to tongue and skeletal muscles	In infants, note spontaneous tongue movements. In children, same as adults

assessing if the eyes move symmetrically in the other direction. For example, if you suddenly turn the child's head to the right, the child's eyes should look to the left symmetrically. Assess vertical eye movements in a similar manner by flexing or extending the neck. Absence of expected eye movements may indicate increased ICP.

When assessing oculomotor function, be sure to note nystagmus or sunset appearance of the eyes. Observe for nystagmus by looking for involuntary, rapid, rhythmic eye movements that may be present at rest or with eye movement. Horizontal nystagmus may occur with lesions in the brain stem and can be the result of certain medications (phenytoin in particular). Vertical nystagmus indicates brain stem dysfunction. *Sunsetting* is when the sclera of the eyes is showing over the top of the iris (Fig. 38.3). Sunset eyes may indicate increased ICP as seen in hydrocephalus. Pupillary response is often abnormal when a neurologic disorder is present. Refer to Figure 38.4 for illustrations of varied pupillary responses.

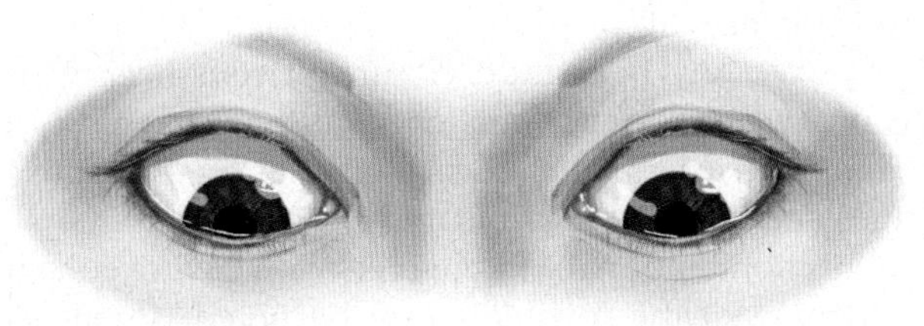

FIGURE 38.3 Sunsetting of the eyes is a sign of increased intracranial pressure.

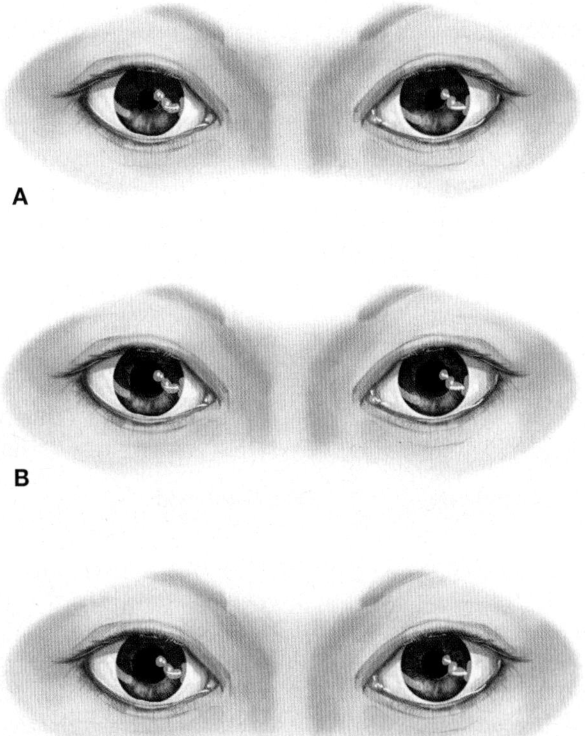

FIGURE 38.4 Assessing pupil size and reaction. **A.** *Pinpoint* is commonly observed in poisonings, brain stem dysfunction, and opiate use. **B.** *Dilated but reactive* is seen after seizures. *Fixed and dilated* is associated with brain stem herniation secondary to increased intracranial pressure. **C.** *One dilated (left eye) but reactive* is associated with intracranial mass.

CLINICAL REASONING ALERT!

Immediately report the sudden presence of fixed and dilated pupils.

Motor Function. Observe muscle strength, size, and tone in the infant or child. Assess bilaterally and compare. Observe spontaneous activity, posture, and balance, and assess for asymmetric movements. In the infant, observe resting posture, which will normally be a slightly flexed posture. The infant should be able to extend extremities to a normal stretch. Alterations in motor function, like changes in gait, muscle tone, or strength, may indicate certain neurologic problems such as increased ICP, head injury, and cerebral infections. Because cortical control of motor function is lost in certain neurologic disorders, postural reflexes reemerge and are directly related to the area of the brain that is damaged. Therefore, it is important to assess for two distinct types of posturing that may occur. **Decorticate posturing** occurs with damage of the cerebral cortex (Fig. 38.5A). **Decerebrate posturing** occurs with damage at the level of the brain stem (Fig. 38.5B). Both types of posturing are characterized by extremely rigid muscle tone.

Reflexes. Testing of deep tendon reflexes is part of the neurologic assessment, just as it is in adults. Testing of primitive and protective reflexes in the infant is important because infants cannot perform tasks on command. The Moro, tonic neck, and withdrawal reflexes are important in assessing neurologic health in infants. Refer to Chapter 25 for a further explanation of primitive and protective reflexes in infants (see Chapter 25, Table 25.1). Absence of certain reflexes, persistence of primitive reflexes after age of normal disappearance, or increases in reflexes may be present in specific neurologic conditions.

Decorticate Extremities flexed

A

Decerebrate Extremities extended and pronated

B

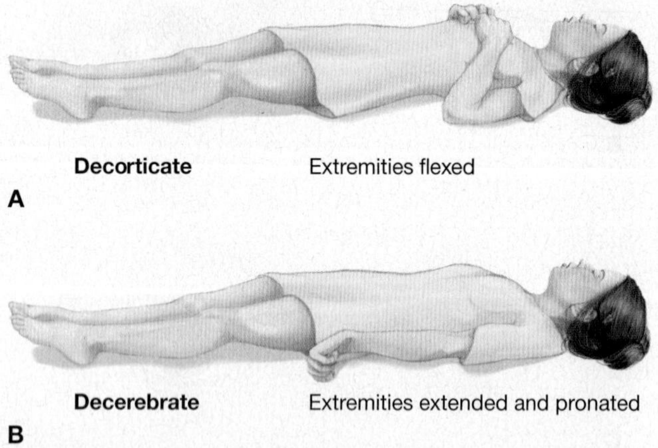

FIGURE 38.5 A. Decorticate posturing occurs with damage of the cerebral cortex and includes adduction of the arms, flexion at the elbows with arms held over chest, and flexion of the wrists with hands fisted. Lower extremities are adducted and extended. **B.** Decerebrate posturing occurs with damage to the midbrain and includes extension and pronation of the arms and legs.

Sensory Function. When assessing the child, use techniques similar to those used in the adult assessment. Be sure to explain what you are doing to the child, especially before the pinprick test, to gain continued cooperation. When assessing sensory function, the child should be able to distinguish between light touch, pain, vibration, heat, and cold. When assessing an infant, limit the examination to responses to touch or pain. The normal response in a 4-month-old infant will be movement away from the stimulus. Alterations in sensory function can result from brain or spinal cord lesions.

Increased Intracranial Pressure. Observe for signs and symptoms associated with increased ICP while caring for a child with a potential or suspected neurologic disorder. Refer to Comparison Chart 38.1 for early versus late signs and symptoms of increased ICP. Increased ICP is a sign that may occur with many neurologic disorders. It may result from head trauma, birth trauma, hydrocephalus, infection, and brain tumors. As ICP increases, LOC decreases, and the signs and symptoms will become more pronounced. It is essential to recognize early signs and symptoms of increased ICP and intervene immediately to prevent long-term damage and possible death.

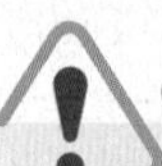

CLINICAL REASONING ALERT!

Presence of hypertension with a widening pulse pressure, bradycardia, and irregular respirations (referred to as Cushing triad) is a sign of impending herniation and a medical emergency.

Palpation

Palpation of the newborn and infant skull and fontanels is an important function of the neurologic examination. Changes in size or fullness of the fontanels may exist in certain neurologic conditions and must be noted. A bulging fontanel can be a sign of increased ICP and is seen in such neurologic disorders as hydrocephalus and head traumas. It is normal for the fontanels to be full or bulging during crying; take this into consideration during assessment.

Note any premature closure of fontanels, which can indicate skull deformities such as craniosynostosis. The posterior fontanel normally closes by 2 months of age, and the anterior fontanel normally closes by 12 to 18 months of age. In children with hydrocephalus, widening of the fontanels may be noted, along with a tense appearance and a resulting increase in head circumference.

Auscultation

Health care providers or nurse practitioners may perform auscultation of the skull. Soft, symmetric bruits may be found in children under 4 years of age or in children with acute febrile illness. A finding of a loud or localized bruit is usually significant and requires immediate further investigation. Increased ICP, resulting from conditions such as hydrocephalus, tumor, or meningitis, frequently produces intracranial bruits. Arterial venous malformations may also produce large bruits.

Laboratory and Diagnostic Testing

Common Laboratory and Diagnostic Tests 38.1 offers an explanation of the most commonly used laboratory and diagnostic tests utilized when considering neurologic disorders. The tests can assist the health care provider or nurse practitioner in diagnosing the disorder and/or serve as guidelines in determining ongoing treatment. Laboratory or nonnursing personnel obtain some of the tests, while the nurse might obtain others. In either instance, it is important to be familiar with how the tests are obtained, what they are used for, and normal versus abnormal results. This knowledge will also be necessary when providing child and family education related to the testing. Many of these tests, such as **lumbar puncture (LP)** (Fig. 38.6), can be frightening to parents and the child. Prepare the family and the child and provide support and reassurance during and after the test or procedure.

• • • ATRAUMATIC CARE • • •

During an LP, use distraction technique such as storytelling or music that will allow the child to remain in the proper position. Encourage parental involvement and enlist the help of a child life specialist, if possible.

COMMON LABORATORY AND DIAGNOSTIC TESTS 38.1

Test	Explanation	Indications	Nursing Implications
Lumbar puncture (LP)	Withdrawal of cerebrospinal fluid (CSF) from the subarachnoid space for analysis	To diagnose hemorrhage, infection, obstruction, tumor or malignancy, autoimmune disease, or multiple sclerosis Can obtain measurement of spinal fluid pressure	Assist with proper positioning (see Fig. 38.6). Help child maintain position and remain still. Maintain strict asepsis. Assist with collection and transport of specimen. Monitor respiratory status, changes in consciousness, heart rate, pain level. Encourage fluids after procedure, if not contraindicated. Keep child flat for 1 hour if ordered. Apply EMLA cream to puncture site 30–60 minutes before procedure to reduce pain, if ordered.
Head and neck x-ray	Radiographic image of the head and neck will show skull and spine structures	Detects skull and spinal fractures; shows location and course of ventricular catheters; reveals information about increased ICP and skull defects	Children may be afraid. Allow a parent or family member to accompany the child. If the child is unable or unwilling to stay still for the radiograph, restraint may be necessary. The time of restraint should be limited to the amount of time needed for the radiograph.
Fluoroscopy	Radiographic examination that uses continuous x-rays to show live up-to-date images	Can assess cervical spine for instability during movement	Same as head and neck radiographs. Child will need to cooperate with flexion and extension of neck.
Cerebral angiography	X-ray study of cerebral blood vessels. Involves injection of a contrast medium and use of fluoroscopy	Can assess for vessel defects or space-occupying lesions	Same as head and neck radiographs. Assess for allergy to contrast medium and possible NPO status. Push fluids following procedure, if not contraindicated, to help flush out contrast medium.

(*continued*)

COMMON LABORATORY AND DIAGNOSTIC TESTS 38.1 (*continued*)

Test	Explanation	Indications	Nursing Implications
Ultrasound	Use of sound waves to locate the depth and structure within soft tissues and fluid	Used to assess intracranial hemorrhage in newborns and ventricular size	Better tolerated by children who are not sedated than CT or MRI Can be performed portably at bedside
Computed tomography (CT)	Noninvasive x-ray study that looks at tissue density and structures. Images a "slice" of child's tissue	To diagnose congenital abnormalities, such as neural tube defects, hemorrhage, tumors, fractures	Machine is large and can be frightening to children. Procedure can be lengthy, and child must remain still. If unable to do so, sedation may be necessary. Can be performed with or without use of contrast medium; if used, assess for allergy and possible NPO status. Encourage fluids postprocedure, if not contraindicated.
Electroencephalogram (EEG)	Measures electrical activity of the brain	To diagnose seizures and brain death; to evaluate brain tumors, subdural hematomas, intracranial hemorrhages	Must remain still. If unable to do so, sedation may be necessary, but should be avoided, if possible, because sedatives can alter the EEG reading. Inform technician of what anticonvulsants the child is taking. Morning anticonvulsants may need to be held.
Magnetic resonance imaging (MRI)	Use of magnetic field to show different tissue compositions	Used to assess tumors and inflammation; used to diagnose congenital abnormalities, such as neural tube defects; shows normal versus abnormal brain tissue	Child may not have any metal devices, internal or external, while undergoing MRI (ensure hospital gown does not have metal snaps). Most new surgical implants are now MRI compatible; consult imaging center. Procedure can be lengthy, and child must remain still. Child is placed in long narrow tube, and the machine makes a booming noise when it is turned on and off during the procedure; therefore, can be difficult to gain cooperation. If the child is unable to remain still, sedation may be necessary. Can be performed with or without use of a contrast medium. If contrast medium is used, assess for allergy and possible NPO status. Encourage fluids postprocedure, if not contraindicated.
Positron emission tomography (PET)	Similar to CT or MRI, but radioisotope is added. Measures physiologic function	Provides information on brain functional development. Can assist in identifying seizure foci. Can assess tumors and brain metabolism	Procedure can be lengthy, and child must remain still. If unable to do so, sedation may be necessary. Intravenous access will be needed for the procedure. Encourage fluids postprocedure, if not contraindicated, to help body eliminate radioisotopes.
Single-photon emission computed tomography (SPECT)	Use of radiopharmaceuticals to provide three-dimensional splices; less expensive and more available than PET	Used to detect brain death, presence of encephalitis, hydrocephalus, to localize epileptic foci, assess metabolic activity, evaluate brain tumors, assessment of childhood development disorders	Similar to PET In children who are not cooperating, do not use sedation until after injection because it may affect brain activity Secure child's head. Sudden distractions or loud noises can alter the distribution of radionuclide.

COMMON LABORATORY AND DIAGNOSTIC TESTS 38.1

Test	Explanation	Indications	Nursing Implications
Cisternography	Radiopharmaceuticals injected intrathecally during a lumbar puncture to assess flow and reabsorption of CSF	Can assist in selection of type of shunt and pathway to use in treating hydrocephalus	Sterile LP performed and radionuclide injected into cerebrospinal circulation Imaging performed at specified times Child must lie flat after puncture.
Intracranial pressure (ICP) monitoring (intraventricular catheter, subarachnoid screw or bolt, epidural sensor, anterior fontanel pressure monitor)	A sensing device is placed in the head that monitors the pressure intracranially.	Used to monitor ICP resulting from hydrocephalus, acute head trauma, and brain tumors. Ventricular catheter also allows for draining of CSF to help reduce ICP.	Usually monitored in critical care setting Monitor for signs and symptoms of increased ICP. Monitor for infection. Keep head of bed elevated 15–30 degrees. Alarms for monitoring device should remain on at all times. Reduce stimulation and avoid interventions that may cause pain or stress and result in an increased ICP.
Video EEG	Measures electrical activity of the brain continuously along with recorded video of actions and behaviors	Can help determine precise localization of seizure area before surgery. Assists in diagnosis and management of seizures by correlating behaviors with abnormal EEG activity	Ensure that seizure precautions are in place. Parent or caregiver must be with child at all times. The child's movements are limited and usually confined to the room. When the child changes position, ensure they are still seen by video camera. Boredom can be a problem. Must notify nurse if seizure activity occurs; push the alert button to highlight attack on EEG recoding. Nurse must immediately go to the room, expose as much of the child as possible (remove covers; if at night, turn on light), and avoid blocking the camera. Ask questions (i.e., what is your name, can you raise your left arm, remember the word banana) to help assess responsiveness more accurately. Stay with the child until a full recovery has occurred. Ask the child what word you asked them to remember, and document all findings and time of the event.

Adapted from Fischbach, F. T., Fischbach, M. A., & Stout, K. (2022). *A manual of laboratory and diagnostic tests* (11th ed.). Wolters Kluwer.

Remember Antonio, the 3-month-old with lethargy, a weak cry, and vomiting? What additional health history and physical examination assessment information should the nurse obtain?

Nursing Analysis

After recognizing and analyzing cues from a thorough assessment, the nurse may identify several patient problems, including:

- Decreased intracranial adaptive capacity
- Altered tissue perfusion: cerebral
- Injury risk
- Infection risk
- Pain
- Activities of daily living (ADL) deficit (specify)
- Impaired physical mobility
- Delayed development risk
- Malnutrition
- Dehydration risk
- Knowledge deficiency
- Interrupted family processes

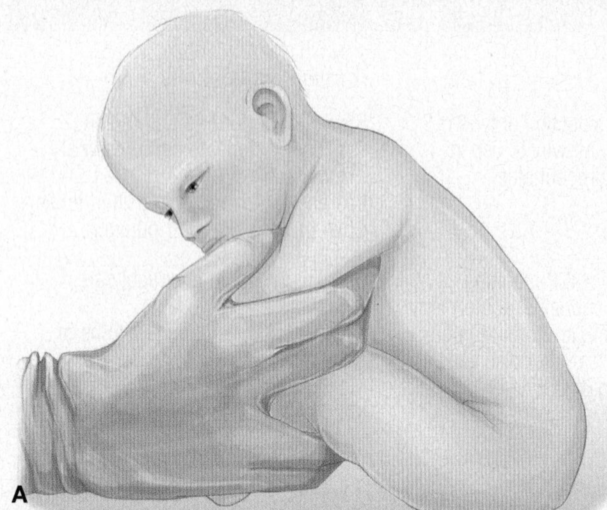

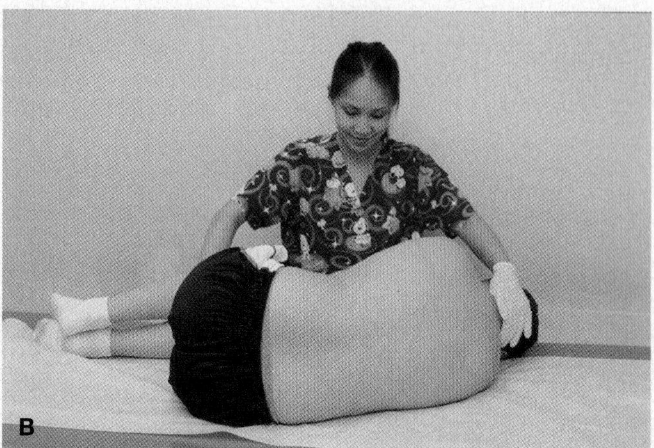

FIGURE 38.6 Proper positioning for a lumbar puncture. **A.** The newborn is positioned upright with head flexed forward. **B.** Child or older infant is positioned on the side with head flexed forward and knees flexed to abdomen.

After completing an assessment of Antonio, the nurse noted the following: a full anterior fontanel; when being held, Antonio was inconsolable; when lying still, he was calmer and in the opisthotonic position. Based on the assessment findings, what would be your top three prioritized patient problems for Antonio?

The previous patient problems or concerns provide suggestions for developing a nursing plan of care or concept mapping. The nurse will then generate solutions by planning interventions (suggested further on with rationales). The plan of care should be individualized, based on the child's and family's needs. Refer to Chapter 36 for the nursing process for pain management and to Chapter 33 for nursing interventions related to interrupted family processes and risk of caregiver role strain. Additional information will be included later in the chapter as it relates to specific disorders.

Nursing Analysis

Decreased intracranial adaptive capacity related to brain injury, sustained increase in ICP of 10 to 15 mm Hg (compression of brain tissue due to increased CSF or cerebral edema secondary to increased ICP resulting from brain injury, congenital structural defects, brain tumor, decreased reabsorption of CSF, or shunt malfunction) as evidenced by vomiting, headache, complaints of visual disturbances, elevated blood pressure, changes in LOC, increased head circumference, or bulging fontanel.

Goal/Outcome

Child will remain free of signs and symptoms of increased ICP, as evidenced by remaining free of headache, vomiting, vision disturbances, vital signs within parameters for age, no signs of altered levels of consciousness, able to maintain effective breathing pattern, free of excessive irritability or lethargy, head circumference within parameters for age.

Promoting Adequate Intracranial Adaptive Capacity (interventions with *rationale*)

- Assess neurologic status closely, and monitor for signs and symptoms of increased ICP; *changes in LOC, signs of irritability or lethargy, and changes in pupillary reaction can indicate changes in ICP.*
- Monitor vital signs; *decreased pulse and irregular respiratory rate and increased blood pressure or widening pulse pressure (Cushing triad) can indicate increased ICP and medical emergency.*
- Measure head circumference in children younger than 3 years of age; *increases in head circumference outside parameters for age can indicate increased ICP.*
- Elevate head of bed 15 to 30 degrees *to facilitate venous return and help to reduce ICP.*
- Minimize environmental stimuli and noise, and avoid pain-producing procedures, if possible; *these factors can increase ICP.*
- Have emergency equipment ready and available; *increased ICP can result in respiratory or cardiac failure.*
- Notify health care provider or nurse practitioner immediately if changes in assessment are noted; *early intervention is critical to prevent neurologic damage and death.*

Nursing Analysis

Altered (cerebral) tissue perfusion risk due to brain injury caused by increased ICP, alteration in blood flow secondary to hemorrhage, vessel malformation, or cerebral edema

Goal/Outcome

Child will exhibit adequate cerebral tissue perfusion through course of illness and childhood: child will remain alert and oriented with no signs of altered LOC; vital signs will be within parameters for age; motor, sensory, and cognitive function will be within parameters for age; head circumference will remain within parameters for age.

Promoting Adequate Tissue Perfusion (interventions with *rationale*)

- Assess neurologic status closely, and monitor for signs and symptoms of increased ICP. *Changes in LOC, signs of irritability or lethargy, and changes in pupillary reaction can indicate decreased cerebral tissue perfusion.*
- Monitor vital signs; *decreased pulse and irregular respiratory rate and increased blood pressure or widening pulse pressure (Cushing triad) can indicate increased ICP and a medical emergency, which can lead to decreased cerebral perfusion.*
- Have emergency equipment ready and available; *decreased cerebral perfusion can result in respiratory or cardiac failure.*
- Notify health care provider or nurse practitioner immediately if changes in assessment are noted; *early intervention is critical to prevent neurologic damage and death.*

Nursing Analysis

Injury risk; risk factors include alteration in cognitive functioning, alteration in psychomotor functioning (altered LOC, weakness, dizziness, ataxia, loss of muscle coordination secondary to seizure activity).

Goal/Outcome

Child will remain free of injury, as evidenced by no signs of aspiration or traumatic injury.

Preventing Injury (interventions with *rationale*)

- Ensure child has patent airway and adequate oxygenation (have suction, oxygen available at bedside) and place child in sidelying position, if possible. *A child with altered LOC may not be able to manage their secretions and is at risk for aspiration and ineffective airway clearance; providing suction and oxygenation can help ensure an open airway, and the sidelying position can help secretions drain and prevent obstruction of airway or aspiration.*
- Protect child from hurting self during seizures or changes in LOC by removing environmental obstacles, easing child to lying position, and padding side rails *to help keep the environment safe.*
- Institute seizure precautions for any child at risk for seizure activity (Box 38.1) *to help prevent injury that can result from acute seizure activity.*
- With seizure activity, do not insert a tongue blade or restrain child; *this can lead to injury to caregiver and child.*
- Administer anticonvulsant medications as ordered *to promote cessation and prevention of seizure activity.*
- Assist the child with ambulation *to help prevent injury in child with weakness, dizziness, or ataxia.*
- Allow for periods of rest *to prevent fatigue and decrease risk of injury.*

Nursing Analysis

Infection risk; risk factors include alteration in skin integrity, invasive procedure, malnutrition, stasis of body fluid (caused by surgical interventions, presence of foreign body like a shunt, trauma to the skull, nutritional deficiencies, stasis of pulmonary secretions and urine, and/or presence of infectious organisms).

Goal/Outcome

Child will exhibit no signs or symptoms of local or systemic infection and will not spread infection to others. Symptoms of infection will decrease over time; others will remain free of infection.

Preventing Infection (interventions with *rationale*)

- Monitor vital signs; *elevation in temperature can indicate presence of infection.*
- Monitor incision sites for signs of local infection; *redness, warmth, drainage, swelling, and pain at incision site can indicate presence of infection.*
- Maintain aseptic technique—practice good handwashing and use proper technique when managing postoperative incisions and external shunts *to prevent introduction of further infectious agents.*
- Administer antibiotics as prescribed *to prevent or treat bacterial infection.*

BOX 38.1 Seizure Precautions

- Padding of side rails and other hard objects
- Side rails raised on bed at all times when child is in bed
- Oxygen and suction at bedside
- Supervision, especially during bathing, ambulation, or other potentially hazardous activities
- Use of a protective helmet during activity may be appropriate.
- Child should wear a medical alert bracelet.

- Encourage nutritious diet and proper hydration according to child's preferences and ability to feed orally *to assist body's natural defenses against infection.*
- Isolate the child as required *to prevent nosocomial spread of infection.*
- Teach the child and family preventive measures such as good handwashing, covering the mouth and nose upon cough or sneeze, and adequate disposal of used tissues *to prevent nosocomial or community spread of infection.*

Nursing Analysis

Bathing, dressing, feeding ADL deficit related to pain, alteration in cognitive functioning, neuromuscular impairments, as evidenced by an inability to perform hygiene care and transfer self independently.

Goal/Outcome

Child will demonstrate ability to care for themselves within age parameters and limits of disease: Child is able to feed, dress, and manage elimination within limits of disease and age.

Maximizing Self-Care (interventions with *rationale*)

- Introduce child and family to self-help methods as soon as possible *to promote independence from the beginning.*
- Encourage family and staff to allow child to do as much as possible *to allow child to gain confidence and independence.*
- Teach specific measures for bowel and urinary elimination as needed *to promote independence and increase self-care abilities and self-esteem.*
- Collaborate with physical therapy, occupational therapy, and speech therapy departments to provide child and family with appropriate tools to modify environment and methods to promote transferring and self-care *to allow for maximum functioning.*
- Praise accomplishments and emphasize child's abilities *to help improve self-esteem and encourage feeling of confidence and competence.*
- Balance activity with periods to rest so as *to reduce fatigue and increase energy for self-care.*

Nursing Analysis

Impaired physical mobility related to decrease in muscle control, mass and strength; contractures (hypertonicity), neuromuscular, musculoskeletal impairment (impaired coordination), as evidenced by an inability to move extremities, to ambulate without assistance, to move without limitations.

Goal/Outcome

Child will be able to engage in activities within age parameters and limits of disease: Child is able to move extremities, move about environment, and participate in exercise programs within limits of age and disease.

Maximizing Physical Mobility (interventions with *rationale*)

- Encourage gross and fine motor skill activities *to facilitate motor development.*
- Collaborate with physical therapy, occupational therapy, and speech therapy departments to strengthen muscles and promote optimal mobility *to facilitate motor development.*
- Utilize passive and active ROM, and teach child and family how to perform them so as *to prevent contractures and facilitate joint mobility and muscle development (active ROM) to help increase mobility.*
- Praise accomplishments and emphasize child's abilities *to help improve self-esteem and encourage feeling of confidence and competence.*

Nursing Analysis

Delayed development risk; risk factors include brain injury, chronic illness, and seizure disorder (physical disability, cognitive deficits, activity restrictions).

Goal/Outcome

Child will demonstrate developmental milestones within age parameters and limits of disease: child expresses interest in the environment and people around them and interacts with environment age appropriately.

Maximizing Development (interventions with *rationale*)

- Use therapeutic play and adaptive toys *to help facilitate developmental functioning.*
- Provide stimulating environment when possible *to maximize potential for growth and development.*
- Praise accomplishments and emphasize child's abilities *to help improve self-esteem and encourage feeling of confidence and competence.*

Nursing Analysis

Malnutrition risk related to insufficient dietary intake (vomiting and difficulty feeding secondary to increased ICP; difficulty sucking, swallowing, or chewing; surgical incision pain or difficulty assuming normal feeding position; inability to feed themselves), as evidenced by decreased oral intake, impaired swallowing, weight loss

Goal/Outcome

Child will exhibit signs of adequate nutrition: Weight will remain within parameters for age, skin turgor will be good, intake/output (I/O) will be within normal limits, adequate calories will be ingested, and vomiting will cease or decrease.

Promoting Adequate Nutrition (interventions with *rationale*)

- Monitor height and weight; *insufficient intake will lead to impaired growth and weight gain.*
- Monitor hydration status (moist mucous membranes, elastic skin turgor, adequate urine output); *insufficient intake can lead to dehydration.*
- Use techniques to promote caloric and nutritional intake and teach family (i.e., positioning, modified utensils, soft or blended foods, allow extra time) *to facilitate intake.*
- Assess respiratory system frequently *to assess for aspiration.*
- Monitor for nausea and vomiting, and medicate if ordered *to help reduce vomiting and increase intake.*
- Monitor for pain, and medicate if ordered *to help reduce pain related to surgical incisions and trauma, and increase intake.*
- Assist family to assume as normal a feeding position as possible *to help increase oral intake.*

Nursing Analysis

Dehydration risk; risk factors include insufficient fluid intake, active fluid volume loss, deviations affecting fluid intake from vomiting, altered LOC, poor feeding or intake, insensible loss due to fever, and/or failure of regulatory mechanisms (as in diabetes insipidus [DI]).

Goal/Outcome

Fluid volume will be maintained and balanced: oral mucosa moist and pink, skin turgor elastic, urine output at least 1 to 2 mL/kg/h.

Promoting Adequate Fluid Balance (interventions with *rationale*)

- Administer intravenous (IV) fluids, if ordered *to maintain adequate hydration in children who are nothing by mouth (NPO) or unable to tolerate oral intake.*
- When oral intake is allowed and tolerated, encourage oral (PO) fluids *to promote intake and maintain hydration.*
- Strict intake and output monitoring *can help identify fluid imbalance and also detect signs of abnormal pituitary secretions, resulting in conditions like syndrome of inappropriate antidiuretic hormone secretion (SIADH) and diabetes insipidus (DI)* (see Chapter 48 for further information).
- Maintain minimum hydration and avoid overhydration in children for whom cerebral edema is a concern; *fluid overload can contribute to cerebral edema.*
- Monitor urine specific gravity, urine and serum electrolytes (especially serum sodium), blood urea nitrogen, creatinine and osmolality, and daily weights as ordered; *these are reliable indicators of fluid status and can also detect signs of abnormal pituitary secretions, resulting in conditions such as SIADH and DI.*

Nursing Analysis

Knowledge deficiency related to insufficient information (regarding complex medical condition, prognosis, and medical needs), as evidenced by verbalization, questions, or actions demonstrating lack of understanding regarding child's condition or care

Goal/Outcome

Child and family will verbalize accurate information and understanding about condition, prognosis, and medical needs: child and family demonstrate knowledge of condition and prognosis and medical needs, including possible causes, contributing factors, and treatment measures.

Providing Child and Family Teaching (interventions with *rationale*)

- Assess child's and family's willingness to learn; *child and family must be willing to learn for teaching to be effective.*
- Provide family with time to adjust to diagnosis *to help facilitate adjustment and ability to learn and participate in child's care.*
- Repeat information *to allow family and child time to learn and understand.*
- Teach in short sessions; *many short sessions are found to be more helpful than one long session.*
- Gear teaching to a level of understanding of the child and also the family (depends on age of child, physical condition, memory) *to ensure understanding.*
- Provide reinforcement and rewards *to help facilitate the teaching–learning process.*
- Use multiple modes of learning involving many senses (provide written, verbal, demonstration, and videos) when possible; *the child and family are more likely to retain information when presented in different ways using many senses.*

Based on your top three patient problems for Antonio, describe appropriate nursing interventions.

SEIZURE DISORDERS

Approximately 4% to 10% of children experience one seizure, with a lifetime incidence of epilepsy being 3%, with half of these starting in childhood (Mikati & Tchapyjnikov, 2020). Most seizures are caused by disorders that originate outside of the brain such as a high fever, infection, head trauma, hypoxia, toxins, or cardiac dysrhythmias. Seizure disorders discussed further on include epilepsy, febrile seizures, and neonatal seizures.

Epilepsy

Epilepsy is a condition in which seizures are triggered recurrently from within the brain. Epilepsy is a common neurologic disorder discovered in childhood, although brain injury or infection can cause epilepsy at any age. The International League Against Epilepsy (ILAE) defines epilepsy by the presence of any of the following conditions:

- Two or more unprovoked (or reflex) seizures, which occur more than 24 hours apart
- One unprovoked (or reflex) seizure and a chance of further seizures the same as the general recurrence risk (at least 60%) after two unprovoked seizures, happening over the next 10 years
- Diagnosis of an epilepsy syndrome (Wilfong, 2022)

The prognosis for most children with seizures associated with epilepsy is good. Many children will outgrow epilepsy, but some children will have persistent seizures that are difficult to manage and may be unresponsive to pharmacologic interventions. Living with a seizure disorder may have a devastating impact on the quality of life of the child and family.

Pathophysiology

Epilepsy is a complex disorder of the CNS in which brain function is affected. Recurrent or unprovoked seizures are the clinical manifestation of epilepsy and result from a disruption of electrical communication among the neurons of the brain. This disruption results from an imbalance between the excitatory and inhibitory mechanisms in the brain, causing the neurons to either fire when they are not supposed to or not fire when they should. Epilepsy has numerous causes. It may be acquired and related to brain injury, or it may be a familial tendency, but in some cases the cause is unknown (Mikati & Tchapyjnikov, 2020).

The ILAE revised their system of classification in 2017 in the hopes of providing greater flexibility and transparency when classifying seizure types (Fisher et al., 2017; Wilfong, 2022). The ILAE classification is used by most neurologists to classify seizure types. There are three categories of seizures—focal (previously known as partial), generalized, and unknown seizures (i.e., epileptic spasms). In focal seizures, only one hemisphere of the brain is involved, while general seizures involve the entire brain. "Unknown" is used for epileptic spasms, tonic–clonic, and behavior arrest, where it is unclear whether the mode of onset is generalized or focal (Fisher et al., 2017; Wilfong, 2022). "Focal to bilateral tonic–clonic seizures" replaces the term "secondarily generalized seizures" to describe seizures that start on one side of the brain and spread to both sides (Fisher et al., 2017; Wilfong, 2022). There are many different types of seizures, and the classification of the type of seizure is crucial in assisting with the management and control of seizures. Not all cases are easily classified.

The new classification system is based on three key elements: where the seizure began within the brain (one side [focal], both sides [generalized], or unknown); LOC/awareness during the seizure (only for focal seizure classification as generalized seizures are assumed to affect consciousness in some way); and describing features of the seizure, including movement such as stiffening, jerking or automatisms (motor) or no movement (nonmotor) characteristics. The most common seizure types are discussed in Table 38.2.

TABLE 38.2 • Common Types of Seizures

Onset	Type	Description	Characteristics
Unknown	Motor: Tonic–clonic; Epileptic spasm Nonmotor: Behavior arrest	Mode of seizure onset unknown, whether focal or generalized Mode of seizure onset unknown, whether focal or generalized Type of epileptic spasm seen in infancy Usually seen between 3 and 12 months of age, peak incidence 3–7 months and rarely seen after the age of 18 months	Occurs in series or clusters Presents as symmetrical flexing or extending, in variant clinical patterns, of the neck, arms, legs, and trunk May see: • Extension of neck, trunk, arms, and legs • Flexion of neck, trunk, and extremities with contracting of abdominal muscles (may cause body to bend forward, often referred to as "jackknife seizures") • Cry may precede or follow. Majority of infants have some brain disorder before seizures begin. The infant seems to stop developing and may lose skills that they have already attained after the onset of infantile spasms. Hormonal therapy (mainly corticotropin) and anticonvulsants (most commonly, vigabatrin) are common forms of treatment. A decrease or ceasing of an ongoing motor activity during a seizure

TABLE 38.2 • Common Types of Seizures

Onset	Type	Description	Characteristics
Generalized onset Nonmotor	Absence (formerly *petit mal*) • Typical • Atypical • Myoclonic • Eyelid myoclonic	Type of generalized seizure where motor activity is not prominent; presents with autonomic, behavior arrest, cognitive, emotional or sensory dysfunction	Abrupt onset and offset Sudden cessation of motor activity or speech with a blank facial expression or rhythmic twitching of the mouth, eyebrows, chin, eyelids, or other parts of the face Child may experience countless seizures in a day. Not associated with a postictal (after seizure) state May go unrecognized or mistaken for inattentiveness because of subtle change in child's behavior Myoclonic absence seizure consists of jerks of the shoulder and arms may result in lifting of the arms. Eyelid myoclonia brief (6 seconds) jerking of the eyelids with eyeballs rolling back; multiple seizures occur daily
Generalized onset Motor	Clonic	Type of generalized seizure that presents with repeated jerking movements	Muscles will spasm, jerk, then relax. Spasm/jerking cannot be stopped by restraining or repositioning. Clonic seizures alone are rare; may precede a tonic–clonic seizure
Generalized onset Motor	Tonic	Type of generalized seizures that present with stiffening of the muscles, typically the back, legs, arms	Consciousness usually preserved Tightening of chest muscles may lead to cyanosis; seen in children with Lennox–Gastaut syndrome
Generalized onset Motor	Tonic–clonic (formerly *grand mal*)	Extremely common generalized seizures; most dramatic seizure type	Associated with an aura Loss of consciousness occurs and may be preceded by a piercing cry. Presents with entire body experiencing tonic contractions followed by rhythmic clonic contractions alternating with relaxation of all muscle groups Cyanosis may be noted due to apnea. Saliva may collect in the mouth due to inability to swallow. Child may bite tongue. Loss of sphincter control, especially the bladder, is common. Postictal phase: child will be semicomatose or in a deep sleep for approximately 30 minutes–2 hours; usually responds only to painful stimuli Child will have no memory of the seizure; may complain of headache and feeling of fatigue Safety of the child is a primary concern. See Teaching Guidelines 38.1.
Generalized onset Motor	Myoclonic Myoclonic–tonic–clonic Myoclonic–atonic Epileptic spasm	Type of generalized seizure that involves the motor cortex of the brain. May occur along with other seizure forms	Sudden, brief, massive muscle jerks that may involve the whole body or one body part Child may or may not lose consciousness.
Generalized onset Motor	Atonic	Type of generalized seizure often referred to as "drop attacks" Seen in children with Lennox–Gastaut syndrome	Sudden loss of muscle tone. In children, may only be a sudden drop of the head. Child will regain consciousness within a few seconds to a minute. Can result in injury related to violent fall

(*continued*)

TABLE 38.2 • Common Types of Seizures (*continued*)

Onset	Type	Description	Characteristics
Focal onset with retained consciousness/awareness (previously referred to as simple partial seizure)	Motor: Automatisms, atonic, clonic, hyperkinetic, myoclonic, tonic, epileptic spasm Nonmotor: autonomic, behavior arrest, cognitive, emotional, sensory	Seizure that occurs in one part of the brain. The symptoms seen will depend on which area of the brain is affected.	Motor activity characterized by clonic or tonic movements involving the face, neck, and extremities Can include sensory signs such as numbness, tingling, paresthesia, changes in vision and hearing, possible hallucinations, or pain Can include autonomic symptoms such as changes in blood pressure, heart rhythm, bowel function Can include psychic symptoms such as triggering emotions of fear, anxiety, joy, sadness Child remains conscious and may verbalize during the seizure. No postictal state
Focal seizure with impaired consciousness/awareness (previously known as complex partial seizure) Focal seizure may also be classified with unknown awareness (often seen with epileptic spasm)	Motor: Automatisms, atonic, clonic, hyperkinetic, myoclonic, tonic, epileptic spasm Nonmotor: autonomic, behavior arrest, cognitive, emotional, sensory	May begin with a focal seizure without impaired consciousness, then progress	May or may not have a preceding aura Consciousness will be impaired. Automatisms and complex purposeful movements are common features in infants and children. Infants will present with behaviors such as lip smacking, chewing, swallowing, and excessive salivation; can be difficult to distinguish from normal infant behavior In older children, will see picking or pulling at bed sheets or clothing, rubbing objects, or running or walking in a nondirective and repetitive fashion These seizures can be difficult to control.
Onset may be generalized, focal or absence	Status epilepticus	Common neurologic emergency in children. Can occur with any seizure activity. Febrile seizures are the most common type in young children. In children with epilepsy, it commonly occurs early in the course of epilepsy. Can be life threatening	Prolonged or clustered seizures where consciousness does not return between seizures The age of the child, cause of the seizures, and duration of status epilepticus influence prognosis. Prompt medical intervention is essential to reduce morbidity and mortality. Treatment: • Basic life support—ABCs (airway, breathing, circulation) • Administration of anticonvulsants to cease seizures is crucial. Common medications include benzodiazepines such as lorazepam and diazepam, and fosphenytoin (see Drug Guide 38.1 and Table 38.3). • Blood glucose levels and electrolytes along with evaluation of the underlying cause should be initiated.

Adapted from Fisher, R. S., Cross, J. H., French, J. A., Higurashi, N., Hirsch, E., Jansen, F. E., Lagae, L., Moshé, S. L., Peltola, J., Roulet Perez, E., Scheffer, I. E., & Zuberi, S. M. (2017). Operational classification of seizure types by the International League Against Epilepsy: Position paper of the ILAE Commission for Classification and Terminology. *Epilepsia*, *58*, 522–530. https://doi.org/10.1111/epi.13670; Wilfong, A. (2022). Seizures and epilepsy in children: Classification, etiology, and clinical features. *UpToDate*. Retrieved May 4, 2023, from https://www.uptodate.com/contents/seizures-and-epilepsy-in-children-classification-etiology-and-clinical-features

Therapeutic Management

Management of epilepsy focuses on controlling seizures or reducing their frequency. Another focus of epilepsy management involves helping the child who has recurrent seizures and their family to learn to live with the seizures. The primary mode of treatment is the use of anticonvulsants. The goal for every child should be the use of the fewest drugs with the fewest possible side effects for the control of seizures. There have been significant advances in the treatment of epilepsy due to the many new anticonvulsant medications that have become available in recent years (see Table 38.3). Most anticonvulsants are taken orally and are often used in combination,

TABLE 38.3 • Common Anticonvulsant Medications

Medication	Nursing Implications
Phenytoin (IV and PO; IM administration is contraindicated)	Monitor serum levels to ensure therapeutic dosing. Be aware that gingival hyperplasia appears most commonly in children and adolescents. If on prolonged therapy, ensure adequate intake of vitamin D–containing foods. Monitor serum calcium, magnesium, folate, and vitamin B levels. IV form given in normal saline to prevent precipitation
Fosphenytoin (IM or IV only)	Adverse effects are said to be less common than with phenytoin. It does not cause local irritation, but it is typically a more expensive drug than phenytoin. It is water-soluble, therefore allowing faster and easier administration than phenytoin. All dosing is in phenytoin sodium equivalents. It does not precipitate in commonly used IV diluents.
Phenobarbital	Assess for excessive sedation. Monitor serum levels to ensure therapeutic dosing. Monitor for drug interactions. Monitor folate, vitamin B, vitamin D, and calcium levels. Increase vitamin D–fortified foods or administer supplement, if prescribed. Withdrawal symptoms will occur if drug is stopped abruptly. Valproic acid interferes with this drug, causing increased phenobarbital levels.
Felbamate	Monitor for drug interactions, especially if child is taking barbiturates, phenytoin, or carbamazepine.
Valproic acid (divalproex sodium, sodium valproate, Depakote)	Monitor serum levels to ensure therapeutic dosing. Depakote sprinkles are available and useful for children who are unable to tolerate valproate suspension, tablets, or capsules. The contents can be sprinkled on food that does not require chewing.
Carbamazepine	Monitor serum levels to ensure therapeutic dosing; toxicity can occur even with levels slightly above therapeutic range. Monitor folate and vitamin B levels. Serum levels may be increased if taken with food and grapefruit juice Plasma concentration decreased by phenytoin and may be increased by valproic acid
Gabapentin	Do not administer within 2 hours of antacids. Rapidly absorbed in the gastrointestinal tract
Topiramate	Phenytoin, carbamazepine, and valproate products may decrease concentration of topiramate Decreased bone mineral density may occur.
Oxcarbazepine	Monitor phenytoin levels, if administering concurrently. Monitor serum sodium.
Zonisamide	Phenobarbital may increase the metabolism of this drug and decrease serum concentration.
Lamotrigine	Severe and serious skin reactions have been noted. Valproate inhibits metabolism and enhances adverse effects; therefore, monitor serum blood values and decrease the dose, if necessary.
Levetiracetam	Increased incidence of psychiatric symptoms seen in children. Monitor for difficulty with gait or coordination. Plasma concentration decreased by phenytoin, phenobarbital, and carbamazepine
Ethosuximide	Give with food if GI upset occurs. Monitor closely during periods of dosage adjustment or addition of new medications. Plasma concentration decreased by phenytoin and may be increased by valproate products.
Rufinamide	Give with food, helps increase absorption. Valproic acid may increase serum levels of rufinamide; phenytoin, carbamazepine, and phenobarbital may decrease serum levels of rufinamide.

GI, gastrointestinal; IM, intramuscular; IV, intravenous; PO, by mouth.

Data from Mikati, M. A., & Tchapyjnikov, D. (2020). Chapter 611. Seizures in childhood. In R. M. Kliegman, J. W. St. Geme III, N. J. Blum, S.S. Shah, R.C. Tasker, K.M. Wilson, & R. E. Behrman (Eds.), *Nelson textbook of pediatrics* (21st ed., pp. 16312–16492). Elsevier.

Lexicomp. (2023). Pediatric drug information. *UpToDate.* Retrieved April 5, 2023, from https://www.uptodate.com/contents/table-of-contents/drug-information/pediatric-drug-information

but the goal is single-drug therapy if possible. Different medications control different types of seizures, which may be due to individual variation. It can take time to find the right medication to best control an individual's seizures.

If seizures remain uncontrolled, another option for managing them is surgery. Depending on the area of the brain that is affected, it may be possible to remove the area that is responsible for the seizure activity or to interrupt the impulses from spreading and therefore stop or reduce the seizures. The adverse effects of surgery range from mild to severe, depending on the area of the brain that is affected. Other nonpharmacologic treatments that may be considered in children with intractable seizures include a ketogenic diet or placement of a vagal nerve stimulator. Refer to Common Medical Treatments 38.1.

Nursing Assessment

For a full description of the assessment phase of the nursing process, refer to the "Clinical Judgment and the Nursing Process" section earlier in the chapter. Assessment findings pertinent to epilepsy are discussed further on.

HEALTH HISTORY

Elicit a description of the present illness and chief complaint, which will usually involve a seizure episode. Gain information to help characterize the episode as a seizure or as a nonepileptic event (see Box 38.2 for a list of nonepileptic events). It is rare to actually observe the child having a seizure; therefore, a complete, accurate, and detailed history from a reliable source is essential. Questions should include:

- Where did the event occur—while sleeping, eating, playing, or just after waking?
- Description of child's behavior during the event—what types of movements, progression, length, respiratory status, apnea?
- How did the child act after the event?
- Have the episodes been recurrent? If so, how frequent?
- Any precipitating factors such as a fever, fall, activity, anxiety, infection, or exposure to strong stimuli such as flashing lights or loud noises?

BOX 38.2 Nonepileptic Events

- Syncope
- Breath holding
- Jitteriness
- Apnea
- Gastroesophageal reflux
- Cardiac conduction abnormalities
- Migraines
- Tics
- Night terrors
- Benign sleep movements

Explore the child's current and past medical history for risk factors such as:

- Family history of seizures or epilepsy
- Any complications during the prenatal, perinatal, or postnatal periods
- Changes in developmental status or delays in developmental milestones
- Any recent illness, fever, trauma, or toxin exposure

Children known to have epilepsy are often admitted to the hospital for other health-related issues or complications and treatment of their seizure disorder. The health history should include questions related to:

- Age of onset of seizures
- Seizure control—what medications is the child taking, and have they been able to take them; when was their last seizure?
- Description and classification of seizures—does the child lose consciousness; does the child become apneic?
- Precipitating factors that may contribute to onset of seizures
- Adverse effects related to anticonvulsant medications
- Compliance with medication regimen

PHYSICAL EXAMINATION

Perform a complete neurologic examination. Careful assessment of the child's mental status, language, learning, behavior, and motor abilities can help provide information about any neurologic deficits. If you observe seizure activity directly, provide a thorough and accurate description of the event. This description needs to include:

- Time of onset and length of seizure activity
- Alterations in behavior such as a cry or changes in facial expression, motor abilities, or sensory alterations before the seizure that may indicate an aura
- Precipitating factors such as fever, anxiety, just waking, or eating
- Description of movements and any progression
- Description of respiratory effort and any apnea noted
- Changes in color (pallor or cyanosis) noted
- Position of mouth, any injury to mouth or tongue, inability to swallow, or excessive salivation
- Loss of bladder or bowel control
- State of consciousness during seizure and **postictal** (after seizure) state—during the seizure, the nurse may ask the child to remember a word; after the seizure, assess if child is able to recall it, to help accurately establish current mental state
- Assess orientation to person, place, and time; motor abilities; speech; behavior; alterations in sensation postictally
- Duration of postictal state

LABORATORY AND DIAGNOSTIC TESTS

Laboratory and diagnostic tests are used to evaluate the cause of, and aid in identifying the type of, seizure activity (refer to Common Laboratory and Diagnostic Tests 38.1). Common laboratory and diagnostic studies ordered for the diagnosis and assessment of epilepsy include:

- Serum glucose, electrolytes, and calcium—to rule out metabolic causes such as hypoglycemia and hypocalcemia
- LP—to analyze cerebrospinal fluid (CSF) to rule out meningitis or encephalitis
- Skull x-ray examinations—to evaluate for the presence of fracture or trauma
- Computed tomography (CT) and magnetic resonance imaging (MRI) studies—to identify abnormalities and intracranial bleeds and rule out tumors
- Electroencephalographs (EEGs)—EEG findings may be noted with certain seizure types, but a normal EEG does not rule out epilepsy because seizure activity rarely occurs during the actual testing time. EEGs are useful in evaluating seizure type and assisting in medication selection. They can be useful in differentiating seizures from nonepileptic activity.
- Video EEGs—provide the opportunity to see the child's actual behavior on video, accompanied with EEG changes; can improve the chance of catching a seizure because the monitoring is done over a period of time.

Nursing Management

Nursing management focuses on preventing injury during seizures, administering appropriate medication and treatments to prevent or reduce seizures, and providing education and support to the child and family to help them cope with the challenges of living with a chronic seizure disorder. See Box 38.1 for a list of basic seizure precautions. In most cases, antiseizure medication should not be discontinued abruptly due to the possibility of increased seizure activity and the risk of status epilepticus. In addition to the patient problems and related interventions discussed in the "Clinical Judgment and the Nursing Process" section, earlier in the chapter, interventions common to epilepsy follow.

DOSAGE CALCULATION 38.1

Child's weight: 9.98 kg (22 lb)

Medication order: Phenobarbital 50 mg PO twice a day

As per the Pediatric Dosage Handbook, the recommended dose is 6 to 8 mg/kg/day in one to two divided doses. Is the ordered dose safe?

RELIEVING ANXIETY

Seizures produce fear and anxiety due to their unpredictable nature along with their uncontrolled, forceful, and, at times, violent appearance. Instruct parents and family members, along with those in the community who may care for the child, on how to respond in case of a seizure (see Teaching Guidelines 38.1). This will help to empower the parents, family, and other caregivers, and, in turn, alleviate some of the anxiety that they may feel.

MANAGING TREATMENT

Provide child and family teaching and instruction regarding the administration of anticonvulsant therapy and its importance. Included in this discussion should be common adverse effects, the need to continue the medication unless instructed otherwise by the health care provider or nurse practitioner, and the need to call the health care provider or nurse practitioner if the child is ill and vomiting and unable to take their medication. Encourage parents to discuss unwanted adverse effects with the health care provider or nurse practitioner so that they can be addressed and noncompliance with the medication regimen can be reduced. A common cause of breakthrough seizures is medication noncompliance.

TEACHING GUIDELINES 38.1 How to Respond When Your Child Has a Seizure

Instruct parents and caregivers:

- Remain calm.
- If child is standing or sitting, ease child to the ground, if possible.
- Time seizure episode.
- Tight clothing and jewelry around the neck should be loosened, if possible.
- Place child on one side and open airway, if possible.
- Do not restrain the child.
- Remove hazards in the area.
- Do not forcibly open jaw with a tongue blade or fingers.
- Document length of seizure, awareness level, and movements, also cyanosis or loss of bladder or bowel control and any other characteristics.
- Remain with child until fully conscious.
- Call emergency medical services (EMS) if:
  - The child stops breathing.
  - Any injury has occurred.
  - Seizure lasts for more than 5 minutes.
  - This is the child's first seizure.
  - Child is unresponsive to painful stimuli after seizure.

PROVIDING FAMILY SUPPORT AND EDUCATION

Having a child with a chronic seizure disorder can place stress and anxiety on the family. This stress and anxiety are often due to fears and misconceptions they may have. An important nursing function is to educate not only the child and family but also the community, including the child's teachers and caregivers, on the reality and facts of the disorder. Encourage parents to be involved in the management of their child's seizures, but encourage allowing the child to learn about the disorder and its management as soon as they are old enough. Encourage parents to treat the child with epilepsy just as they would treat a child without this disorder. Children who are brought up no differently than children without epilepsy will be more likely to develop a positive self-image and have increased self-esteem. Any activity restrictions, such as limiting swimming or participation in sports, will be based on the type, frequency, and severity of the seizures the child has. Educate parents and children on any restrictions, and encourage parents to place only the necessary restrictions on the child.

The needs of the child and family will change as the child grows and develops. The nurse needs to recognize these changes and provide appropriate education and support. Referral to support groups is appropriate.

CONSIDER THIS!

I am so worried about having a seizure at school. I think the other kids will tease me and not play with me if they see me having a seizure. I just don't want to go to school.

Thoughts: How would you respond to this child's concerns?

How can you work with the school, family, and child to help ease these concerns?

Febrile Seizures

Febrile seizures are the most common type of seizure seen in children under 5 years of age (Millichap, 2022a). They usually affect children who are under 5 years of age, with the peak incidence occurring in children between 12 and 18 months old (Millichap, 2022a). Febrile seizures are slightly more commonly seen in male children, and children who have a family history of febrile seizures are at an increased risk (Millichap, 2022a). Febrile seizures are associated with a fever that is not the result of an intracranial infection or metabolic imbalance and is usually related to a viral illness. These seizures are usually benign but can be frightening for both the child and the family. In most cases, the prognosis is excellent. However, febrile seizures may be a sign of a dangerous underlying infection, such as meningitis or sepsis. Although rare, complications associated with febrile seizures include status epilepticus, motor coordination deficits, intellectual disability, and behavioral problems.

Therapeutic Management

Therapeutic management includes determination and treatment of the cause of the fever and interventions to control the fever. The American Academy of Pediatrics (AAP) does not recommend long-term or intermittent anticonvulsant therapy for the child who has suffered one or more simple febrile seizures (American Academy of Pediatrics [AAP] et al., 2008; Millichap, 2022b). Due to the benign nature of febrile seizures, the risks of side effects from the antiepileptic agents outweigh the benefits (Millichap, 2022b). Rectal diazepam has been shown to be safe and effective in terminating febrile seizures and may be used in children at high risk for febrile seizures or in children whose parents are extremely anxious. Buccal and intranasal midazolam, if available, have also been found to be effective, and intranasal lorazepam is an additional option (Millichap, 2022b).

Nursing Assessment

A febrile seizure is usually associated with a rapid rise in core temperature to 39°C (102.2°F) or higher. The degree of fever seems to be the causing stimulus, as opposed to the rapid rate of the fever rising (Millichap, 2022a). A simple febrile seizure is the most common type and will be discussed here. It is defined as a generalized seizure lasting less than 15 minutes (usually a few seconds to 10 minutes) that occurs once in a 24-hour period and is accompanied by a fever without any CNS infection present (Millichap, 2022a). A brief postictal period is often seen when the child appears drowsy. The seizure is likely to have stopped by the time a child receives medical attention. Diagnosis is made based on a thorough history and physical examination, accompanied by a determination of the source of the fever. In some cases, an LP and/or neuroimaging may be performed to rule out meningitis or encephalitis. This will be based on the age and the clinical presentation of the child.

Risk factors for recurrence of a febrile seizure include young age at first febrile seizure and family history of febrile seizures and high fever. Children who experience one or more simple febrile seizures have a slightly greater risk of developing epilepsy than the general population (AAP et al., 2008; Millichap, 2022a). No evidence exists that febrile seizures cause structural damage or cognitive declines (AAP et al., 2008; Millichap, 2022b).

Nursing Management

Provide parental support and education regarding febrile seizures. Reassure parents of the benign nature of febrile seizures. Counsel parents on controlling fever, discuss how to keep a child safe during a seizure, and provide instruction and demonstration in the administration of rectal diazepam at the onset of a seizure (if applicable).

Instruct parents when to call their health care provider or nurse practitioner and when to take their child to the emergency room. Reinforce that any recurrent seizure activity will require prompt medical attention.

Neonatal Seizures

There is a high incidence of seizures during the neonatal period. The immature brain is more prone to seizure activity, and metabolic, infectious, structural, and toxic diseases are more likely to be seen in this age group (Mikati & Tchapyjnikov, 2020). Neonatal seizures are seizures that occur within the first 4 weeks of life and are most commonly seen within the first 10 days. Most seizures in newborns are associated with a specific underlying cause such as hypoxic ischemic encephalopathy (most common), metabolic disorders (hypoglycemia and hypocalcemia), neonatal infection (meningitis and encephalitis), cerebral infarction, and intracranial hemorrhage. The prognosis depends mainly on the underlying cause of the seizures and the severity of the insult. There is evidence that neonatal seizures have an adverse effect on neurodevelopment and may predispose the infant to cognitive, behavioral, or epileptic complications later in life (Shellhaas, 2022b). About 13% to 27% of neonates with seizures will go on to develop postnatal epilepsy (Shellhaas, 2022b). Neonatal epileptic syndromes are rare but are a well-recognized cause of neonatal seizures (Shellhaas, 2022b). Our discussion will focus on the more common symptomatic neonatal seizure related to a specific underlying cause.

Therapeutic Management

Acute neonatal seizures should be treated aggressively because repeated seizure activity may result in injury to the brain. Treatment focuses on addressing the underlying cause, such as correcting metabolic disturbances, treating CNS infections, ensuring adequate ventilation and cardiovascular support, and possibly administering anticonvulsant therapy. Phenobarbital is often used in the initial management of neonatal seizures, but efficacy remains uncertain. Antiepileptic medications may not be effective if the underlying cause is not treated (Shellhaas, 2022a). The dosage of anticonvulsants may be higher in the neonate because neonates metabolize drugs more rapidly than older infants.

Nursing Assessment

Neonatal seizures may be hard to recognize clinically and may be accompanied by a normal EEG, while in some cases, there may be no clinical signs but only EEG changes (Mikati & Tchapyjnikov, 2020). Neonatal seizures have to be distinguished from nonseizure behaviors seen in newborns, such as stretching, sudden random movements, and random sucking movements, coughing, or gagging (Shellhaas, 2023). Therefore, clinical recognition of newborn seizures is critical, and the use of EEG confirmation is now widely recognized. Assessment of neonatal seizures will include a detailed clinical characterization of the seizure activity, including appearance of the neonate; location and involvement of arms, legs, trunk, and face; sequence of clinical changes; and duration and frequency of seizure activity. If seizure activity is not witnessed by a health care provider a detailed history is essential. Assessment of the cause of the seizure is a priority.

Laboratory and diagnostic tests, including serum testing (e.g., serum glucose, electrolytes, calcium), LP (to analyze CSF), cranial ultrasound, CT, and MRI, may be performed to help determine the cause of the seizures. EEGs and video EEGs may assist in the characterization of neonatal seizures and their medical management.

Nursing Management

Nursing management will focus on carrying out interventions to cease seizure activity, monitoring neurologic status closely, recognizing the seizures, preventing injury during seizure activity, and providing support and education to the parents and family.

STRUCTURAL DEFECTS

Due to the sensitivity of the development of the neurologic system in the first few weeks of embryonic life, there exists a potential for defects to occur. These structural defects include neural tube defects (NTDs), microcephaly, Chiari malformation, hydrocephalus, intracranial arteriovenous malformation (AVM), and craniosynostosis.

Neural Tube Defects

NTDs account for the majority of congenital anomalies of the CNS (Kinsman & Johnston, 2020). NTDs are serious birth defects of the spine and the brain and include disorders such as spina bifida occulta, myelomeningocele, meningocele, anencephaly, and encephalocele. The neural tube closes between the third and fourth weeks in utero. The cause of NTDs is not known, but many factors such as drugs, malnutrition, chemicals, and genetics can adversely affect normal CNS development. It is well established that maternal preconception supplementation of folic acid can decrease the incidence of NTDs in pregnancies at risk by 50% (AAP & Committee on Genetics, 1999, reaffirmed 2017; Kinsman & Johnston, 2020). In 1992, the U.S. Public Health Service recommended that all people of childbearing age who are capable of becoming pregnant take 0.4 mg (400 mcg) of folic acid daily (Centers for Disease Control and Prevention [CDC], 2022a). Pregnant people with a history of pregnancies affected by NTDs are recommended to take a higher dosage. Prenatal screening of maternal serum for alpha-fetoprotein (AFP) and ultrasound examination can help identify fetuses at risk. Encephalocele is discussed next. Refer to Chapter 44 for information on spina bifida occulta, anencephaly, meningocele, and myelomeningocele.

Encephalocele

Encephalocele is a protrusion of the brain and meninges through a skull defect. It results from failure of the anterior portion of the neural tube to close. The prognosis, including the extent of complications and cognitive deficits, will depend on the size and location of the encephalocele and involvement of other brain structures. Encephaloceles are often accompanied by craniofacial and other abnormalities such as hydrocephalus, microcephaly, spastic quadriplegia, ataxia, visual problems, developmental delay, mental and growth retardation, and seizures. Some children who are affected may display normal intelligence.

Therapeutic management consists of surgical repair, including placement of tissues back into the skull and removal of the sac; possible shunt placement to correct associated hydrocephalus; and corrective repair of any craniofacial abnormalities.

NURSING ASSESSMENT

Initial assessment after delivery will reveal a visible external sac protruding from the skull area. It occurs most commonly in the occipital region, but can occur elsewhere, such as frontally or nasofrontally. Generally, the lesion is covered by skin, but it may also be open. Therefore, assessment to ensure that the sac covering is intact remains important. Assess neurologic status carefully. Before surgical correction, the infant will be examined thoroughly to determine brain tissue involvement or associated anomalies. Diagnostic procedures such as CT, MRI, and ultrasound may be performed.

NURSING MANAGEMENT

Nursing management will consist of preoperative and postoperative care, along with symptomatic and supportive care. Preoperative and postoperative care will be similar to that for the child with myelomeningocele (refer to Chapter 44), with a focus on preventing rupture of the sac, preventing infection, and providing adequate nutrition and hydration. Infants with an encephalocele are at an increased risk for developing hydrocephalus. Therefore, monitor for signs and symptoms of increased ICP and head circumference.

Microcephaly

Microcephaly is defined as a head circumference that is more than three standard deviations below the mean for the age and sex of the infant (Kinsman & Johnston, 2020). It may be congenital, or it may be acquired and develop in the first few years of life. It generally results in intellectual disability due to the lack of functioning brain tissue. There are many causes. Microcephaly can be caused by abnormal development during gestation or follow intrauterine infections such as rubella, toxoplasmosis, and cytomegalovirus. It can also be caused by chromosomal abnormalities or be associated with other syndromes. Acquired microcephaly may occur due to severe malnutrition, perinatal infections, or anoxia in early infancy.

Nursing Assessment

Microcephalic infants will present at birth with a normal or reduced head size. As the child ages, head growth will fail, while the face will continue to grow at a normal rate. This results in a small head, a large face, and a loose, often wrinkled, scalp. As the child grows older, this smallness of the skull becomes more pronounced. Development of motor functions and speech may be delayed. The degree of intellectual disability varies, but it is a common occurrence. Convulsions may be present, and motor deficit ranges from clumsiness to spastic quadriplegia.

Nursing Management

There is no treatment. Nursing care will be supportive and focus on determining the extent of neurologic and cognitive deficits, as well as teaching parents how to care for a child with such impairments.

Chiari Malformation

Chiari malformations are classified into different groups and subgroups based on anatomic anomalies of the cerebellum, brain stem, and craniocervical junction along with downward displacement of the cerebellar structures (Khoury, 2023). The most common, type I and type II, are discussed here. Type I is usually not associated with hydrocephalus and is the more benign form. The deformity is a result of the cerebellar tonsils displacing into the upper cervical canal (Kinsman & Johnston, 2020). Type II (also referred to as Arnold–Chiari) is the most common and is usually associated with hydrocephalus and myelomeningocele. The deformity results from the cerebellum, the medulla oblongata, and the fourth ventricle displacing into the cervical canal, resulting in an obstruction of the CSF and causing hydrocephalus. The prognosis depends on the extent of the defect. Therapeutic management of the type II Chiari malformation includes surgical decompression.

Nursing Assessment

In type I, symptoms are typically seen in adolescence and adulthood. The patient will usually complain of neck pain; recurrent headaches that increase with physical activity or with Valsalva maneuvers such as coughing, laughing, or sneezing; and lower extremity spasticity (Khoury, 2023). Type II is almost always associated with myelomeningocele; therefore, it is typically detected prenatally or at birth. Symptoms seen in infancy include a weak cry, stridor, and apnea (Kinsman & Johnston, 2020). These symptoms require prompt medical treatment to reduce mortality. Gastrointestinal disturbances along with a history of chronic aspiration, choking, gagging, prolonged feeding times, and weight loss may also be present. In later infancy and childhood, progressive hydrocephalus is a common problem (Khoury, 2023). Assessment of shunt function is extremely important in the infant and older child presenting with type II Chiari malformation and associated hydrocephalus (refer to Hydrocephalus section). An MRI may be performed to help evaluate and diagnose Chiari malformations.

Nursing Management

Nursing management will focus on preoperative and postoperative care, prevention of infection, monitoring of blood loss, improvement of preoperative symptoms in the postoperative period, identification of any signs and symptoms of increased ICP, and identification of any resultant CNS injury.

Hydrocephalus

Hydrocephalus is not a specific illness but instead results from underlying brain disorders. It is a frequently seen disorder of the nervous system occurring in 0.5 to 0.8 per 1,000 live births (Haridas & Tomita, 2022a). It results from an imbalance in the production and absorption of CSF. In hydrocephalus, CSF accumulates within the ventricular system and causes the ventricles to enlarge and increases in ICP to occur.

Hydrocephalus may be congenital or acquired. Congenital hydrocephalus is present at birth and is often due to a genetic predisposition or environmental influences during fetal development. Causes of congenital hydrocephalus include abnormal intrauterine development, as is the case with myelomeningocele or other NTDs, or intrauterine infections. Acquired hydrocephalus develops at the time of birth or at some point after. It can occur at any age and can result from injury or disease. Acquired hydrocephalus can result from intentional or nonintentional trauma, intraventricular hemorrhage (IVH) in premature infants, neoplasms (e.g., posterior fossa brain tumor), infections (e.g., meningitis), or malformations (e.g., Chiari malformations).

Prognosis for the child with hydrocephalus depends mainly on the cause and whether or not brain damage has occurred prior to recognition and treatment. Children with hydrocephalus are at increased risk for developmental disabilities, visual problems, abnormalities in memory, and reduced intelligence. Long-term follow-up and multidisciplinary care are necessary.

Pathophysiology

CSF is formed primarily in the ventricular system by the choroid plexus. It flows because of the pressure gradient that exists between the ventricular system and the venous channels. CSF is absorbed primarily by the arachnoid villi. Hydrocephalus results when there is an obstruction in the ventricular system or obliteration or malfunction of the arachnoid villi. This results in impaired absorption or circulation of the CSF.

Hydrocephalus is classified as obstructive or noncommunicating versus nonobstructive or communicating. Obstructive or noncommunicating hydrocephalus occurs when the flow of CSF is blocked within the ventricular system. This is the most common type in children and is often associated with an increased ICP (Haridas & Tomita, 2022a). NTDs, neonatal meningitis, trauma, tumors, or Chiari malformations usually result in this type of hydrocephalus. One of the most common causes of obstructive or noncommunicating hydrocephalus in children is aqueductal stenosis, which results from the narrowing of the aqueduct of Sylvius (a passageway between the third and fourth ventricles in the middle brain) (Haridas & Tomita, 2022a). Nonobstructive or communicating hydrocephalus occurs when the flow of CSF is blocked after it exits from the ventricles. This form of hydrocephalus, in which the CSF can still flow between the ventricles, is most often caused by defective absorption of CSF. Examples include hydrocephalus that results from subarachnoid hemorrhage (most common), certain types of meningitis, and leukemia infiltrates (Kinsman & Johnston, 2020).

Therapeutic Management

Hydrocephalus must be identified early. Treatment needs to be initiated to prevent brain tissue damage that can result from the increased ICP that hydrocephalus creates. Specific treatment will depend on the underlying etiology. The goals of treatment include relieving hydrocephalus and managing complications associated with the disorder, such as growth and developmental delay. Most cases of hydrocephalus are treated with the surgical placement of an extracranial shunt. Most often, a ventriculoperitoneal (VP) shunt is placed. See Figure 38.7 for an illustration of a shunt. The shunt will need to be replaced as the child grows. Therefore, the child will undergo shunt revision surgery at various times during their life. It is important for health care professionals and parents to be able to recognize when a shunt needs replacing or when complications are occurring to decrease the possibility of death or disability that may occur due to increased ICP.

Although shunts have been the mainstay of treatment for hydrocephalus, they are not without complications such as infection, obstruction, and need for revision as the child grows. Endoscopic third ventriculostomy (EVT) is an alternative to shunt placement to treat hydrocephalus in select children. It has several advantages over VP shunts, such as fewer complications (infection and malfunction) and lower cost (Haridas & Tomita, 2022b). A small perforation is made in the thinned floor of the third ventricle, which allows for egress of CSF from the ventricle to the subarachnoid space. No permanently implanted hardware is needed. Success of the EVT depends on the child's age, cause of hydrocephalus, and history of previous complications.

Nursing Assessment

For a full description of the assessment phase of the nursing process, refer to the "Clinical Judgment and the Nursing Process" section. Assessment findings pertinent to hydrocephalus are discussed further on.

Health History

Explore the pregnancy history and past medical history for:

- Intrauterine infections
- Prematurity with intracranial hemorrhage
- Meningitis
- Mumps encephalitis

Elicit a description of the present illness and chief complaint. Common signs and symptoms reported during the health history of the undiagnosed child might include:

- Irritability
- Lethargy
- Poor feeding
- Vomiting
- Complaints of headache in older children
- Altered, diminished, or changes in LOC

Children known to have hydrocephalus are often admitted to the hospital for shunt malfunctions or other complications of the disease. The health history should include questions related to:

- Neurologic status—have there been changes or decreases in LOC, changes in personality, or deterioration in school performance?
- Complaints of headache
- Vomiting
- Visual disturbances
- Any other changes in physical or cognitive state

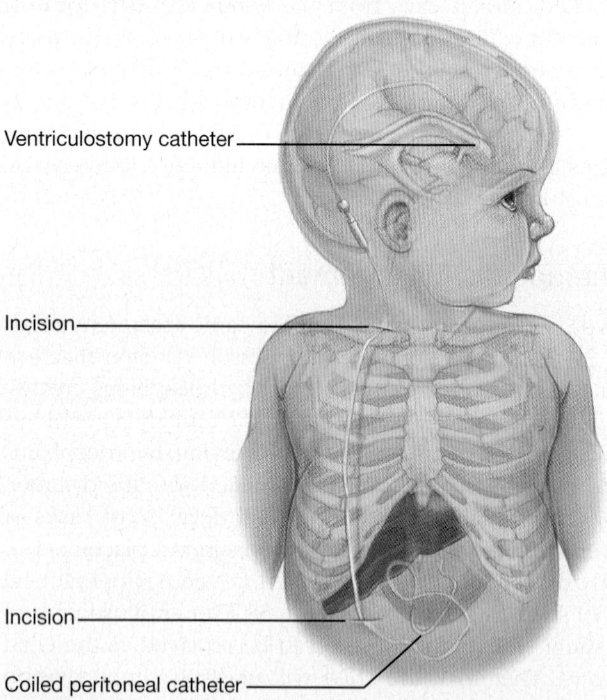

FIGURE 38.7 To treat hydrocephalus, a ventriculoperitoneal (VP) shunt catheter is placed in an enlarged ventricle. The shunt diverts the flow of cerebrospinal fluid (CSF) within the central nervous system to the peritoneum, where CSF is now absorbed across the peritoneal membrane into the body's circulation.

Physical Examination

Physical examination of the infant or child with hydrocephalus will include inspection and observation, palpation, and percussion.

INSPECTION AND OBSERVATION

Observe general appearance and affect. Pay particular attention to the size of the skull, and note any asymmetry. Note LOC and motor function. Changes or decreases in LOC may be noted along with brisk reflexes and spasticity of the lower extremities. Symptoms seen vary by age, primarily because the infant's skull is able to accommodate the buildup of CSF because the sutures have not closed. In the infant, the most obvious indication is often a rapid increase in head circumference (Fig. 38.8). In the older child, loss of development and changes in personality may be seen. Signs and symptoms associated with increased ICP may be seen (refer to Comparison Chart 38.1).

PALPATION

In the infant, palpation of the fontanels may reveal wide-open, bulging fontanels. They will be nonpulsatile and feel tense and very full.

PERCUSSION

Upon percussion of the skull, by health care providers or nurse practitioners, a positive Macewen sign may be noted. This is when a "cracked pot" sound is heard during percussion and can indicate separation of the sutures.

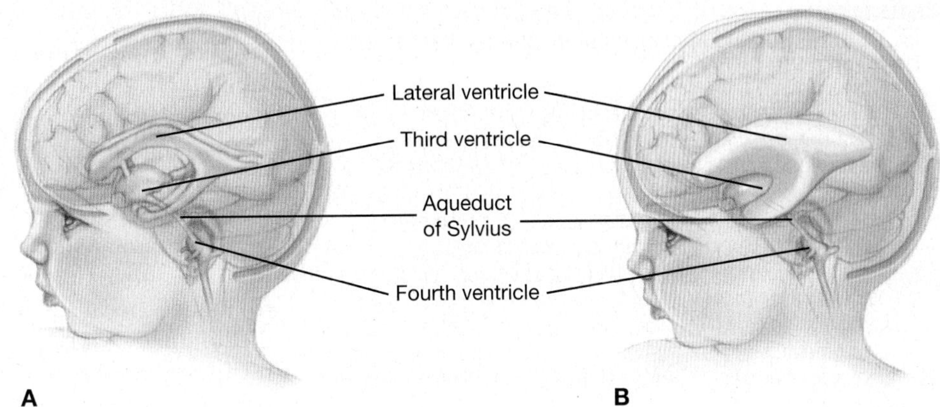

FIGURE 38.8 **A.** Infant without hydrocephalus. **B.** Infant with hydrocephalus. Note broadening of the forehead, bulging fontanel, and large head size.

Laboratory and Diagnostic Tests

Common laboratory and diagnostic tests ordered for the diagnosis and assessment of hydrocephalus include:

- Skull x-ray studies (may reveal separation of sutures)
- CT
- MRI

CT and MRI are used to evaluate for the presence of hydrocephalus and can also aid in identifying the cause of hydrocephalus. Refer to Common Laboratory and Diagnostic Tests 38.1.

Nursing Management

Nursing management of the child with hydrocephalus will focus on maintaining cerebral perfusion, minimizing neurologic complications, maintaining adequate nutrition, promoting growth and development, and supporting and educating the child and family. In addition to the patient problems and related interventions discussed in the "Clinical Judgment and the Nursing Process" section earlier in the chapter, interventions common to hydrocephalus are discussed later.

PREVENTING AND RECOGNIZING SHUNT INFECTION AND MALFUNCTION

The major complications associated with shunts are infection and malfunction. Due to the serious nature and potentially devastating effects of shunt infection or malfunction, parents and health professionals need to be aware of the signs and symptoms to provide early recognition and prompt treatment. Signs and symptoms of a shunt infection include elevated vital signs, poor feeding, vomiting, decreased responsiveness, seizure activity, and signs of local inflammation along the shunt tract. Signs and symptoms of shunt malfunction include vomiting, drowsiness, and headache. Signs and symptoms of increased ICP, as listed in Comparison Chart 38.1, can also be indicative of shunt complications.

Infection can occur at any time but is more common 1 to 2 months after placement. Infection is treated with IV antibiotics, and, if the infection is persistent, the shunt will be removed and an external ventricular drainage

COMPARISON CHART 38.1 Early Versus Late Signs of Increased Intracranial Pressure

Early Signs	Late Signs

• Headache
• Vomiting, possibly projectile
• Blurred vision, double vision (diplopia)
• Dizziness
• Increased blood pressure
• Pupil reaction time decreased and unequal
• Sunset eyes
• Changes in level of consciousness, irritability
• Seizure activity
• In infant, will also see:
  • Bulging, tense fontanel
  • Wide sutures and increased head circumference
  • Dilated scalp veins
  • High-pitched cry
	• Lowered level of consciousness
	• Decreased motor and sensory responses
	• Bradycardia
	• Irregular respirations
	• Hypertension and widening pulse pressure
	• Cheyne–Stokes respirations
	• Decerebrate or decorticate posturing
	• Fixed and dilated pupils

BOX 38.3 Nursing Management of External Ventricular Drainage (EVD) Device

- Ensure all connections are secure and label line as EVD.
- Regularly check that drip chamber of manometer is set at the height prescribed in relation to the child (i.e., zero at clavicle).
- Clamp the drain in the event of child movement or movement anticipated with care. Rezero and open clamps when done.
- Accurately document volume and color of cerebrospinal fluid (CSF) every hour (CSF is normally clear and colorless; cloudiness indicates infection). Notify health care provider, nurse practitioner, or charge nurse of any significant increase in amount of drainage (if exceeds 10 mL more than previous volumes).
- If minimal or no drainage, check tubing for kinks, blockage, or closed clamps. Check to see if CSF is oscillating in tubing. If blockage is suspected, notify neurosurgery department immediately.
- Dress the entry site into the skull with a sterile occlusive dressing; change the dressing if it is soiled or nonocclusive.
- Routine CSF samples may be sent for culture and analysis.
- Child may be taking prophylactic antibiotics due to increased risk of infection from the drain.

(EVD) system put into place until the CSF is sterile (refer to Common Medical Treatments 38.1 and Box 38.3).

TAKE NOTE!

Rapid drainage of CSF, which may occur if the child sits up without the EVD system being clamped, will decrease ICP and can lead to extreme headache, collapse of the ventricles, formation of subdural hematomas, and neurologic deterioration.

A new shunt will be placed after the infection has cleared. Intrathecal administration of antibiotics may be performed by the health care provider or nurse practitioner. Keeping the peritoneal surgical incision free of feces and urine can help prevent infection. In addition, inspect surgical incisions after shunt placement for signs and symptoms of infection and any signs of leaking CSF.

Malfunction of the shunt can occur due to kinking, clogging, or separation of the tubing. Blockage is the most common reported complication. A shunt that has been placed within the past year is at higher risk of malfunction. Early recognition and operative intervention are essential to prevent neurologic deficits or possible death from occurring.

SUPPORTING AND EDUCATING THE CHILD AND FAMILY

Hydrocephalus is a serious and chronic illness. It will require lifelong follow-up and regular evaluations. It requires early recognition of complications to prevent neurologic damage. Children will require future surgeries and hospitalizations, which can place a strain on the family and its finances. Potential growth and developmental disabilities are an additional strain. The support of the family in establishing realistic goals and helping the child to achieve their developmental and educational potential is important.

The family should be involved in the child's care from the time of diagnosis. Initially, parents may be frightened because shunt placement involves entering the brain. Provide parents with accurate information regarding the procedure and be available to listen to parents' concerns and to answer questions that arise. Ongoing education about the illness and its treatment is important, including signs and symptoms of shunt complications. As the family becomes more comfortable with the diagnosis, treatment, and signs and symptoms of complications, they will become experts on the child's care and will often recognize subtle changes that may be indicative of shunt complications. Referral to support groups can be helpful for both the family and the child.

Intracranial AVM

Intracranial AVM is a rare congenital disorder. It is caused by an abnormal development of blood vessels and can occur in the brain, brain stem, or spinal cord. AVMs that hemorrhage can lead to serious neurologic deficits and even death. However, some cases of AVMs never cause problems.

Therapeutic Management

More aggressive treatment strategies are used in children. Treatment options include surgical excision; endovascular embolization, which involves closing off the vessels of the AVM by injecting glue into them; and radiosurgery, which involves focusing radiation on the AVM. The therapeutic management approach will be based on the age of the child and size and location of the malformation in the brain. The child will usually require at least 24 hours of intensive care monitoring following surgery.

Nursing Assessment

The most common symptoms include intracranial hemorrhage (children are more likely to present with hemorrhage than adults), seizures, headaches, and progressive neurologic deficits such as vision problems, loss of speech, problems with memory, and paralysis (Singer et al., 2022). In children under 2 years of age, presentation may include cardiac failure due to arteriovenous shunting in neonates and infants; a large head secondary to hydrocephalus; and seizure activity. Diagnosis is made using diagnostic imaging procedures such as MRI, CT, and arteriography.

Nursing Management

Nursing management for these children is aimed at supportive care. Monitor for changes in neurologic status, noting any seizure activity, signs or symptoms of increased ICP, or signs and symptoms of intracranial hemorrhage. Hydrocephalus may occur as a result of intracranial hemorrhage secondary to the AVM. An EVD and eventual shunt placement may be necessary (refer to the "Hydrocephalus" section).

Craniosynostosis

Craniosynostosis is premature closure of the cranial sutures (Fig. 38.9). Complete closure of all sutures does not normally occur until late in childhood. Premature closure can inhibit brain growth, and a distorted skull appearance will be evident. In cases where only one suture is fused, neurologic impairments are rarely seen. When two or more sutures are fused, neurologic complications such as hydrocephalus with increased ICP are more likely to occur. The incidence of craniosynostosis is approximately one in 2,000 births (Kinsman & Johnston, 2020). The cause is unknown, but in 10% to 20% of cases a genetic disorder such as Carpenter syndrome or Apert, Crouzon, or Pfeiffer disease is present (Kinsman & Johnston, 2020). There are numerous types of craniosynostosis; they are listed and illustrated in Table 38.4.

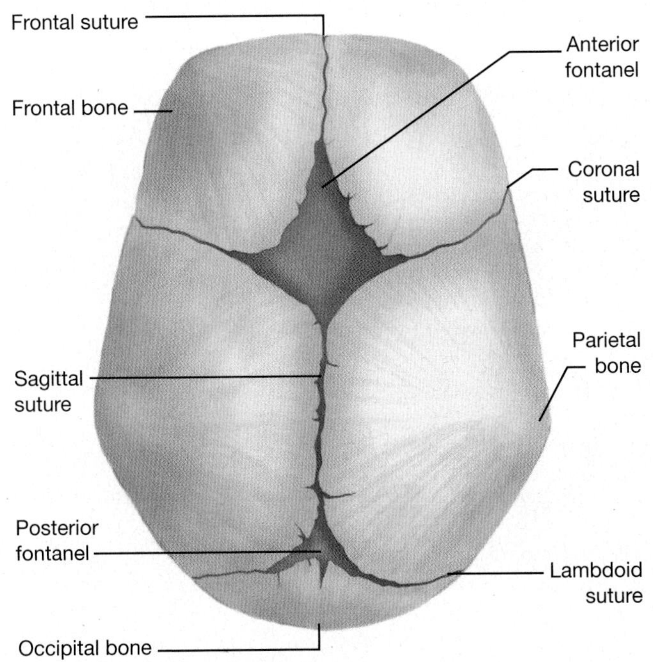

FIGURE 38.9 Skull sutures in the infant.

The prognosis is good for the majority of infants presenting with craniosynostosis, and normal brain development will occur. Exceptions to this are the infant or child who has associated genetic disorders that involve brain function and development.

Surgical correction may be done and allows for normal expansion of the brain and acceptable appearance of the head and skull. If one suture is fused, the surgical intervention is done mainly for cosmetic reasons. If more than one suture is fused, operative intervention is essential to prevent neurologic complications.

Nursing Assessment

Most cases of craniosynostosis are present at birth. Skull deformity is evident, and a prominent bony ridge can be palpated. X-ray studies can confirm fusion of the sutures. It is important that craniosynostosis be detected early if it is not evident at birth because premature closure of the suture lines will inhibit brain development. Therefore, measure head circumference in all children under 3 years old, and compare findings with normal head circumference parameters as well as past measurements of the infant or child.

Nursing Management

Nursing management focuses on postoperative care. This includes observing hemoglobin and hematocrit levels due to large volumes of blood loss that can occur and observing for pain, hemorrhage, fever, infection, and swelling. Due to the location of the surgery and incision line, large amounts of facial swelling may be present. This can result in an inability of the child to open their eyes for a few days postoperatively. Make sure that parents are aware of this. Encourage the parents to talk to, hold, and comfort their child during this time. Provide support and education to the parents before, during, and after the procedure.

Positional Plagiocephaly

Since the inception of the "back to sleep" program, which recommends placing all infants supine to sleep to decrease the risk of sudden unexplained infant death (SUID), there has been an increase in the incidence of positional plagiocephaly (Buchanan, 2021). Positional plagiocephaly refers to asymmetry in head shape without fused sutures. It results from gravitational force exertion on the developing cranium. Torticollis, which is when the neck muscles are too tight, have inadequate tone, or are shorter on one side, can contribute to plagiocephaly. Each condition, plagiocephaly and torticollis, exacerbates the other. Refer to Chapter 44 for further information on torticollis.

TABLE 38.4 • Types of Craniosynostosis

Types	Description	Illustration
Sagittal synostosis (scaphocephaly)	Sagittal suture is closed. Head grows long and narrow in anterior–posterior direction. Broad forehead and a prominent occiput are present. Most common form	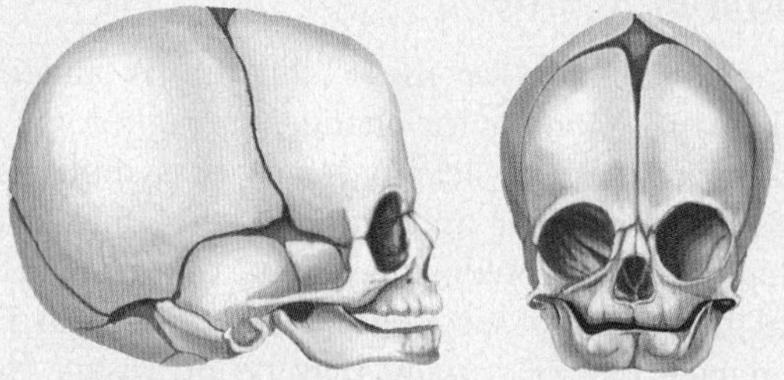
Metopic synostosis (trigonocephaly)	Metopic suture is closed. Usually a ridge down the forehead can be seen or felt. Triangular-shaped forehead Eyebrows may appear "pinched" on either side. Eyes may also appear close together.	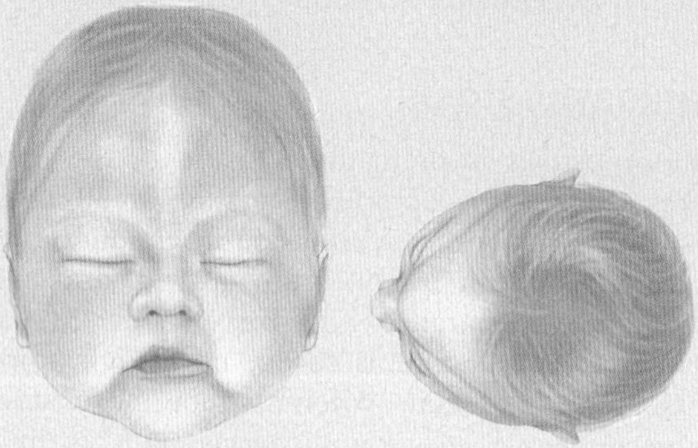
Unilateral coronal synostosis (anterior plagiocephaly)	Early closure of one side of the coronal suture Forehead and orbital rim (eyebrow) have a flattened appearance on that side. Eye on affected side has a different shape.	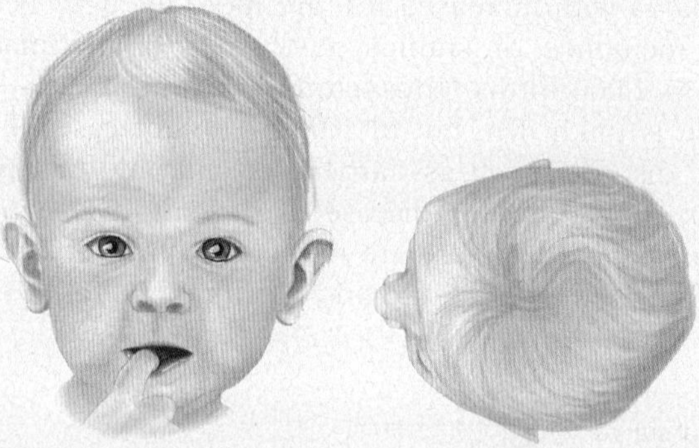
Bicoronal synostosis (brachycephaly)	Very flat, tall, recessed forehead Skull is shortened in the anterior–posterior direction. Wide-shaped head Commonly seen in Apert and Crouzon disease	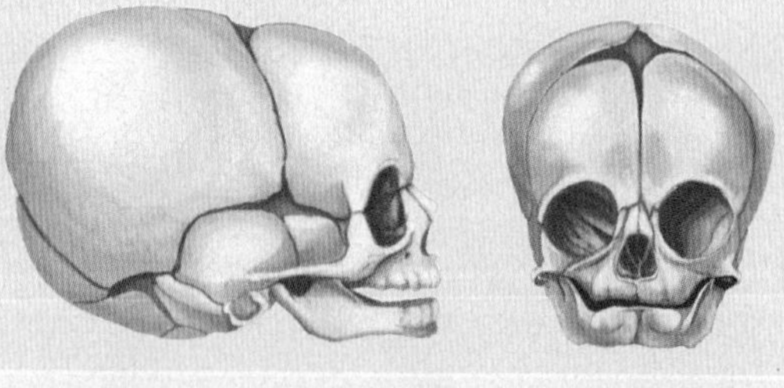
Lambdoid (posterior plagiocephaly)	Early closure of one lambdoid suture Flattening of back of head. Similar to shape found in positional molding or positional plagiocephaly	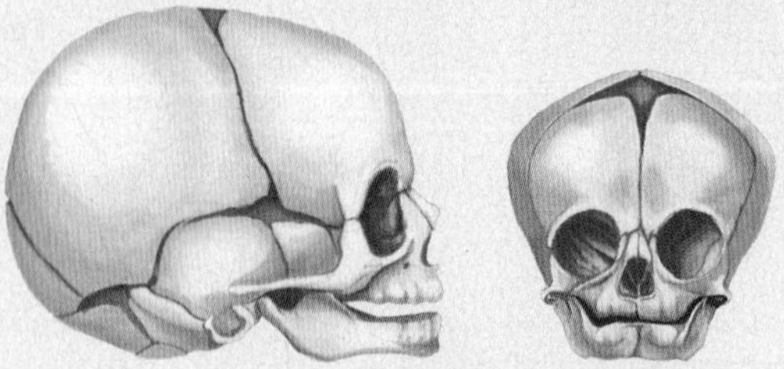

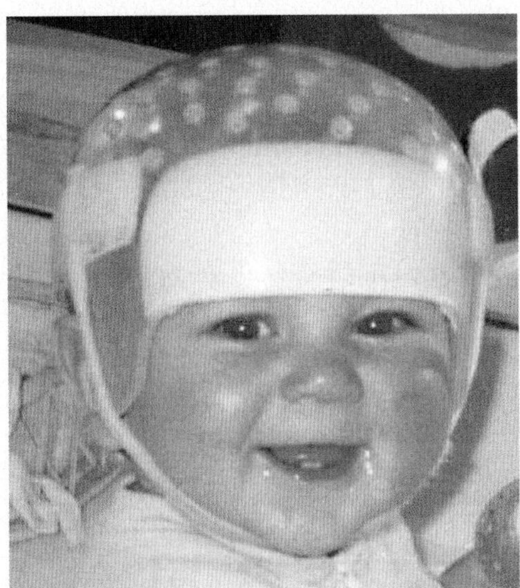

FIGURE 38.10 Molding helmet for positional plagiocephaly.

Therapeutic management for positional plagiocephaly is generally conservative, such as changing the infant's position, encouraging "tummy time," and avoiding excessive use of the car seat for infant seating outside of the automobile. Some infants may benefit from the use of a molding helmet (Fig. 38.10).

Nursing Assessment

View the infant's head from the top, noting asymmetry ranging from flattening on one side posteriorly to posterior flattening associated with anterior bulging (Fig. 38.11). Assess neck ROM to determine if torticollis is also present. Palpate the cranial sutures, which will not feel overlapped as they do when they are fused. Skull x-ray examination or head CT scan will rule out craniosynostosis by demonstrating evidence of open sutures.

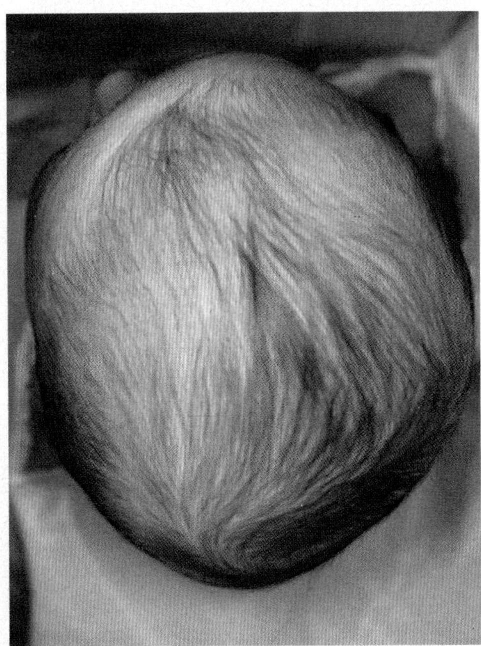

FIGURE 38.11 Note flattening of the right posterior parietal and occipital regions of the skull in this infant with positional plagiocephaly.

Nursing Management

Nursing management is directed toward repositioning the infant to decrease time spent with the flattened area in the dependent position. Position the infant so that turning away from the affected side is necessary for them to view objects of interest. Place the infant on the abdomen when awake and supervised. Discourage use of the car seat outside of the automobile. Place a rolled washcloth along the affected side of the head to discourage turning the head in that direction. Hold the child upright over the shoulder at times throughout the day, rotate feeding positions, and change the direction in which the infant lies in the crib. Following these recommendations may prevent positional plagiocephaly in the infant without congenital torticollis.

INFECTIOUS DISORDERS

Infectious disorders of the neurologic system include bacterial meningitis, aseptic meningitis, encephalitis, and Reye syndrome.

Bacterial Meningitis

Bacterial meningitis is an infection of the meninges, the lining that surrounds the brain and spinal cord. It is a serious illness in children and can lead to brain damage, nerve damage, deafness, stroke, and even death. It requires rapid assessment and treatment. See Table 38.5 for the most common types of meningitis seen in different age groups. In developed countries, disease resulting from *Haemophilus influenzae* type B, once the most common cause of meningitis in children, has decreased

TABLE 38.5 • Common Causes of Meningitis in Different Age Groups

Age Affected	Causative Organism
Newborns and infants (birth–3 months)	*Escherichia coli; Streptococcus* group B; *Listeria monocytogenes; Streptococcus pneumonia*
Infants and children (3 months–6 years)	*S. pneumonia; Neisseria meningitides (meningococcal meningitis); Haemophilus influenzae* type B; *Streptococcus* group B; *Mycobacterium tuberculosis*
Older children and adolescents (6–16 years)	*S. pneumonia; N. meningitides (meningococcal meningitis)*

Data from Centers for Disease Control and Prevention. (2021a). *Meningitis: Bacterial meningitis.* http://www.cdc.gov/meningitis/bacterial.html

dramatically since the introduction of the Hib vaccine. In less developed countries, infection with *H. influenzae* type B remains a concern.

Pathophysiology

Bacterial meningitis causes inflammation, swelling, purulent exudates, and tissue damage to the brain. It can occur as a secondary infection to upper respiratory infections, sinus infections, or ear infections and can also be the result of direct introduction through LP; skull fracture or severe head injury; neurosurgical intervention; congenital structural abnormalities, such as spina bifida; or the presence of foreign bodies, such as a ventricular shunt or cochlear implants.

Therapeutic Management

Bacterial meningitis is a medical emergency and requires prompt hospitalization and treatment. Deterioration may be rapid and occur in less than 24 hours, leading to long-term neurologic damage and even death. IV antibiotics will be started immediately after the LP and blood cultures have been obtained if bacterial meningitis is suspected. The length of therapy and specific antibiotic will be determined based on the analysis and the culture and sensitivity of the CSF. Corticosteroids may be ordered to help reduce the inflammatory process. Specific medical treatment varies based on the suspected causative organism and will be determined by the health care provider or nurse practitioner.

Nursing Assessment

For a full description of the assessment phase of the nursing process, refer to the "Clinical Judgment and the the Nursing Process" section. Assessment findings pertinent to bacterial meningitis are discussed further on.

Health History

Elicit a description of the present illness and chief complaint. Common signs and symptoms reported during the health history might include:

- Sudden onset of symptoms
- Preceding respiratory illness or sore throat
- Presence of fever, chills
- Headache
- Vomiting
- Photophobia
- Stiff neck
- Rash
- Irritability
- Drowsiness
- Lethargy
- Muscle rigidity
- Seizures

Symptoms in infants can be more subtle and atypical, but the history may reveal:

- Poor sucking and feeding
- Weak cry
- Lethargy
- Vomiting

Explore the child's current and past medical history for risk factors such as:

- Young age: 1 month to 5 years, with most cases in children younger than 1 year of age and young adults 15 to 24 years of age
- Any fever or illness during pregnancy or around delivery (for infants younger than 3 months of age)
- Exposure to ill people
- Exposure to tuberculosis
- Travel history
- History of maternal illness
- Recent neurosurgical procedure or head trauma
- Presence of a foreign body, such as a shunt or a cochlear implant
- Immunocompromised status
- Close-contact living spaces such as dormitories or military bases
- Day care attendance

Physical Examination

Observe the general appearance of the child. The infant with bacterial meningitis may rest in the **opisthotonic** position (Fig. 38.12), and the older child may complain of neck pain. In the infant, a bulging fontanel may be present, which is often a late sign, and the infant may be consolable when lying still as opposed to being held. Presence of positive Kernig and Brudzinski signs can indicate irritation of the meninges (Fig. 38.13). Inspect the child for presence of a rash; a petechial, vesicular, or macular rash may be seen.

CLINICAL REASONING ALERT!

Abrupt eruption of a petechial or purplish rash can be indicative of meningococcemia (infection with *N. meningitidis*). Immediate medical attention is warranted.

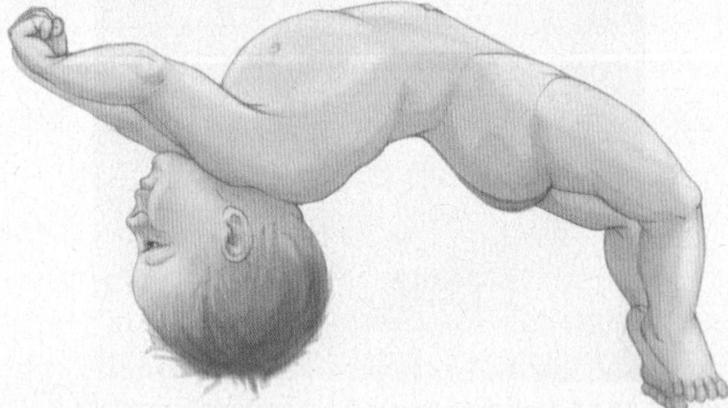

FIGURE 38.12 Infant in opisthotonic position: head and neck are hyperextended to relieve discomfort.

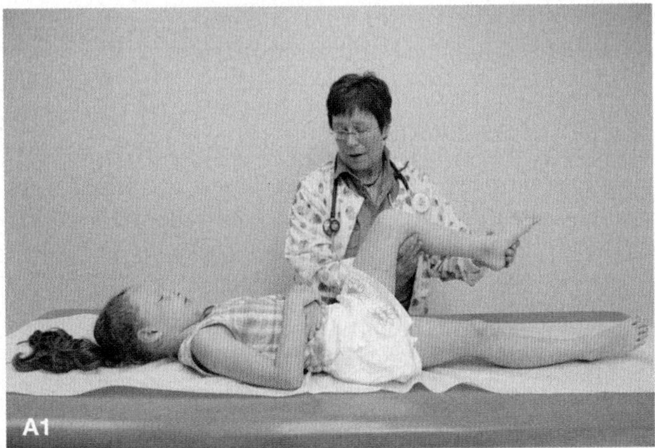

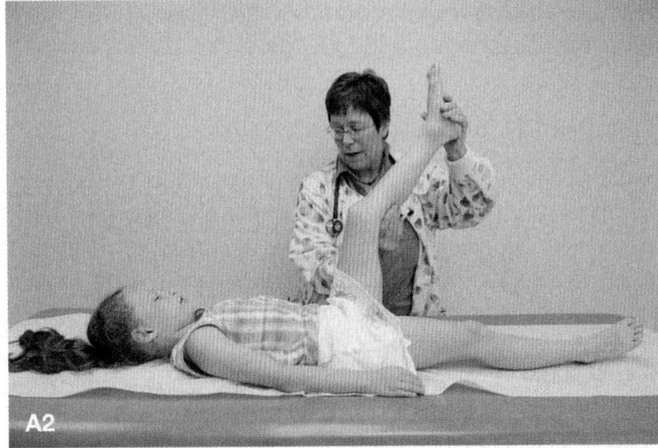

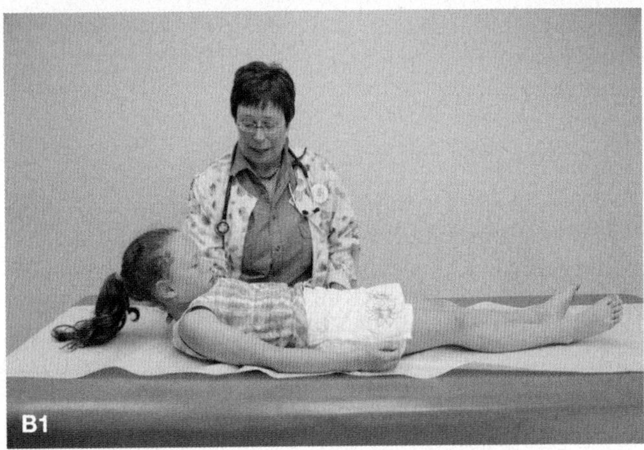

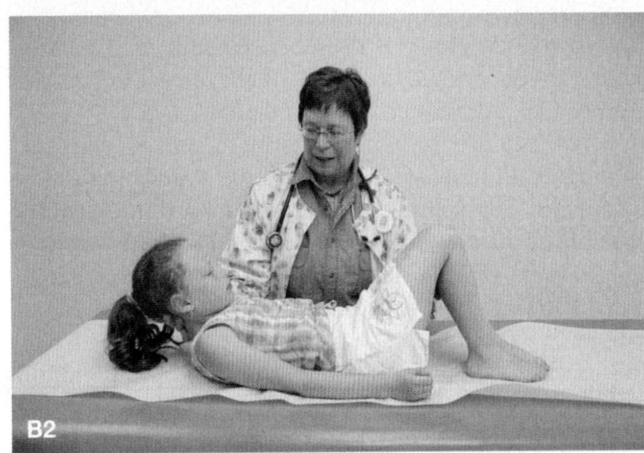

FIGURE 38.13 **A.** Kernig sign is tested by flexing legs at the hip and knee (**A1**), then extending the knee (**A2**). A positive report of pain along the vertebral column and/or inability to extend knee is a positive sign and indicates irritation of meninges. **B.** Brudzinski sign is tested by the child lying supine with the neck flexed (**B1**). A positive sign occurs if resistance or pain is met. The child may also passively flex hip and knees in reaction, indicating meningeal irritation (**B2**).

Laboratory and Diagnostic Tests

Common laboratory and diagnostic studies ordered for the assessment of bacterial meningitis include:

- LP—Fluid pressure will be measured, and a sample is obtained for analysis and culture. CSF pressure will usually be elevated, and CSF will reveal increased white blood cells (WBCs) and protein and low glucose (the bacteria present feed on the glucose).
- Complete blood count (CBC)—WBCs will be elevated.
- Blood, urine, and nasopharyngeal culture—Performed to look for source of infection and to rule out sepsis. Blood culture will be positive in cases of septicemia.

Nursing Management

Administer prescribed antibiotics as soon as possible after obtaining cultures. Quickly initiate supportive measures to ensure proper ventilation, reduce the inflammatory response, and help prevent injury to the brain. Interventions are aimed at reducing ICP and maintaining cerebral perfusion along with treating fluid volume deficit, controlling seizures, and preventing injury that may result from altered LOC or seizure activity. Initiate appropriate isolation precautions. In addition to standard precautions, infants and children diagnosed with bacterial meningitis will be placed on droplet isolation until 24 hours of antibiotics have been received to help prevent transmission to others. Refer to the "Clinical Judgment and the Nursing Process" section earlier in the chapter for patient problems and related interventions. In addition to those problems and interventions, note any measures taken to reduce fever and prevent bacterial meningitis.

Reducing Fever

Increased body temperature; warm, flushed skin; and tachycardia may be present. Reducing fever is important to help maintain optimal cerebral perfusion by reducing the metabolic needs of the brain. Administer antipyretics such as acetaminophen and nonsteroidal antiinflammatory drugs (NSAIDs) such as ibuprofen, per order. Institute nonpharmacologic measures, if needed. Reduce environmental temperature and use cooling blankets, fans, cold compresses, and tepid baths to help reduce fever. Avoid measures that cause shivering because it increases heat production and is therefore counterproductive and uncomfortable for the child.

Preventing Bacterial Meningitis

Bacterial meningitis is a serious illness, and prevention is important. It is transmitted by direct close contact with respiratory droplets from the nose or throat. Most at risk are those living with the child or anyone with whom the child played or was in close contact. Postexposure prophylaxis and postexposure immunization may be effective. Control measures should be initiated in environments where risk exists. Disinfect toys and other shared objects to decrease transmission of the microorganisms to others.

To reduce group B streptococcus infection in neonates, screen pregnant people. If the screening results are positive, administer intrapartal antibiotics.

Vaccines are an important way to prevent bacterial meningitis and are available for some specific causative organisms, but complete vaccination prevention is not possible at this time. The Hib vaccine is routine, starting at 2 months of age, and all children should be immunized to continue the reduction of bacterial meningitis caused by *H. influenzae* type B. The pneumococcal vaccine is also routine for all children, starting at 2 months of age.

Meningococcal vaccination is routine for all children 11 to 12 years of age, with a booster at age 16. Adolescents aged 16 to 18 may be vaccinated with serogroup B meningococcal vaccines if they are part of certain at-risk groups. Refer back to Chapter 31 for further information regarding immunizations.

Aseptic Meningitis

Aseptic meningitis is the most common type of meningitis, and the majority of children affected are under 5 years of age (CDC, 2021b). If the causative organism can be identified, it is usually a virus. Enteroviruses, such as echovirus and coxsackievirus, account for the majority of cases of aseptic meningitis (CDC, 2021b). Less common causes include mumps; herpesviruses; measles; influenza; vector-borne viruses, such as West Nile virus; and lymphocytic choriomeningitis virus (CDC, 2021b).

Therapeutic Management

Prompt diagnosis and treatment are essential to improve outcomes. The child is treated aggressively as if they have bacterial meningitis until the diagnosis is confirmed. Antibiotics are administered and continued until the causative organism is recognized. If the cause is viral, antibiotics may be discontinued, and antiviral agents may be started at this time. After diagnosis is confirmed, treatment is mainly supportive in nature, and the illness is usually self-limiting, lasting 3 to 10 days.

Nursing Assessment

Elicit a description of the present illness and chief complaint. Common signs and symptoms reported during the health history might include:

- Fever
- General malaise
- Headache
- Photophobia
- Poor feeding
- Nausea
- Vomiting
- Irritability
- Lethargy
- Neck pain
- Positive Kernig and Brudzinski signs

The onset of symptoms may be abrupt or gradual. Assessment is similar to that of the child with bacterial meningitis. Signs and symptoms are similar to those seen in bacterial meningitis, but the child is usually less ill.

Nursing Management

Nursing management is similar to the nursing care of the child with bacterial meningitis and will focus on comfort measures to reduce pain and fever. Aseptic meningitis can be managed successfully at home if the child's neurologic status is stable and they are tolerating oral intake.

Encephalitis

Encephalitis is an inflammation of the brain that may also include an inflammation of the meninges. It is a rare complication and can be caused by protozoan, bacterial, fungal, or viral invasion. Viral illness and autoimmune disorders are the most commonly diagnosed cause in children, although in the majority of cases the cause remains unknown (Hardarson & Messacar, 2022). In the United States, common causative organisms include enteroviruses, such as poliovirus and coxsackievirus; herpes simplex virus 1 and 2; and vector-borne viruses. Recovery from encephalitis can occur in a few days or may be complicated and involve severe neurologic damage with residual effects. Prognosis depends on the age of the child and the causative organism. Prompt diagnosis and treatment are essential. The child suspected of having encephalitis should be hospitalized. Therapeutic management is mainly supportive in nature and focuses on maintaining optimal cerebral perfusion; hydration and nutrition; and injury prevention.

Nursing Assessment

Elicit a description of the present illness and chief complaint. Common signs and symptoms reported during the health history might include:

- Fever
- Flu-like symptoms
- Altered LOC
- Headache
- Lethargy
- Drowsiness
- Generalized weakness
- Seizure activity

Explore the child's current history for risk factors such as:

- Recent travel
- Recreational activities, such as hiking and camping
- Animal contacts

Physical Examination

Perform a neurologic examination to distinguish between encephalitis and viral meningitis. In encephalitis, a neurologic examination will reveal changes in sensorium and focal neurologic changes. Neurologic findings vary and reflect the areas of the brain that are involved.

Laboratory and Diagnostic Tests

An LP may be done, and the CSF may show an elevated leukocyte count and elevated protein and glucose levels. However, in some cases, levels may be normal. MRI, CT, and EEG procedures may be performed to help identify early changes and provide useful clues in developing a diagnosis.

Nursing Management

Nursing management is similar to nursing care for the child with meningitis. Specific antiviral therapy may be used for diseases caused by the herpes simplex virus. Teach children and their families how to prevent encephalitis. Encephalitis can result from complications of childhood illnesses such as measles, mumps, or chickenpox. Explain the importance of keeping children up-to-date in their immunizations. Effective vaccines are available for a few viral pathogens that cause encephalitis (such as rabies virus and Japanese encephalitis virus), but these vaccines are not routine; they are recommended for those at high risk. For example, postexposure rabies vaccines can be administered to a child who was bitten by a suspected rabid animal. Also, those traveling to areas where Japanese encephalitis is endemic, such as India and China, and planning a prolonged stay or extreme outdoor activity should receive the appropriate vaccine.

Vector control and avoiding mosquito and tick bites are the best prevention of vector-borne infection. Preventive measures include:

- Using insect repellent (repellents containing DEET [*N,N*-diethyl-meta-toluamide] should be used cautiously in children under 12 years of age and not at all in children under 1 year of age)
- Wearing clothing that covers the arms and legs
- Controlling mosquito populations by eliminating areas of standing water where mosquitoes can breed
- Using insect traps and public measures such as sprayed insecticides to reduce the mosquito population

Reye Syndrome

Reye syndrome is an extremely rare disease that primarily affects children under 15 years of age who are recovering from a viral illness. The exact cause of Reye syndrome is unknown. It has been found that Reye syndrome is a reaction that is triggered by the use of salicylates or salicylate-containing products to treat a viral infection. This reaction causes brain swelling, liver failure, and death in hours, if treatment in not initiated. In the 1980s, the adverse effects of salicylates used to treat viral illnesses began to be publicized, and the U.S. Food and Drug Administration (FDA) required warning labels to be placed on all salicylate-containing products, such as aspirin. Since then, there has been a dramatic decrease in the occurrence of Reye syndrome.

Nursing Assessment

Elicit a description of the present illness and chief complaint. Common signs and symptoms reported during the health history might include:

- Severe and continual vomiting
- Changes in mental status
- Lethargy
- Irritability
- Confusion
- Hyperreflexia

Explore the child's current and past medical history for risk factors such as:

- A prodromal viral illness, like chickenpox, croup, flu, or an upper respiratory infection
- Ingestion of salicylate-containing products within 3 weeks of the start of the viral illness

Elevated liver function tests and elevated serum ammonia levels can confirm diagnosis.

Nursing Management

Early recognition and treatment are the most important aspects of managing this illness. Nursing management is aimed at maintaining cerebral perfusion, managing and preventing increased ICP, providing safety measures due to changes in LOC and risk for seizures, and monitoring fluid status to prevent dehydration and overhydration.

Education is an important aspect of preventing this disease. Salicylates are found in many products, including many over-the-counter products, such as Alka-Seltzer and Pepto-Bismol. Recovery from Reye syndrome is dependent on the severity of swelling of the brain. Some children will make a full recovery, while others may suffer long-term neurologic damage.

TRAUMA

Trauma or injury is a leading cause of childhood morbidity and mortality in the United States (Gill & Kelly, 2022). The child faces significant risk of trauma to their developing neurologic system, often leading to neurologic disorders with life-threatening and lasting effects. Neurologic trauma may include head trauma, nonaccidental head trauma, birth injuries, and near-drowning.

Head Trauma

In the United States, injury causes more death in children than disease (CDC, 2021c). Of these injuries, head injury is a frequent cause of death and disability in childhood. Common causes of head trauma in children include falls, motor vehicle accidents, pedestrian and bicycle accidents, and child abuse (see next section, Nonaccidental Head Trauma). Many factors make children more susceptible to head trauma than adults. Larger head size in relation to the body, coupled with a higher center of gravity, causes the child to hit their head more readily when involved in motor vehicle accidents, bicycle accidents, and falls. Children are also at risk for injury related to psychosocial factors such as their high activity level, curiosity, incomplete motor development, and lack of knowledge and judgment skills.

Head trauma is a broad term that can include specific patterns of injury. Traumatic brain injury (TBI) occurs when a head trauma results in a disruption of the normal function of the brain. Not all head traumas result in a TBI. See Table 38.6 for descriptions of common head injuries seen in children. Head trauma in children is serious because it can cause an immediate threat to the child's life and many complications that can lead to lifelong impairment of an individual's physical, cognitive, and psychosocial functioning. Prognosis for the child who has suffered a head trauma depends on the extent and severity of the injury and any complications (see the Healthy People 2030 box).

HEALTHY PEOPLE 2030

Objective	Nursing Significance
Reduce fatal traumatic brain injuries.	• Educate children and families about safety such as helmet use when inline skating, skateboarding, bicycling, and playing football or other sports that may result in head injury. • Encourage appropriate child car seat and seat belt use. • Use every encounter with a child and family as an opportunity to provide education related to injury prevention.

Healthy People Objectives retrieved from http://www.healthypeople.gov

Nursing Assessment

For a full description of the assessment phase of the nursing process, refer to the "Clinical Judgment and the Nursing Process" section earlier in the chapter. Assessment findings pertinent to head trauma are discussed here.

HEALTH HISTORY

Take a detailed history, including past medical history along with details of the events surrounding the injury such as mental status at the time of the injury, any loss of consciousness, irritability, lethargy, abnormal behavior, vomiting (if so, how many times), any seizure activity, and any complaints of headache, visual changes, or neck pain.

PHYSICAL EXAMINATION

Perform a thorough physical examination. Initial physical assessment will focus on the ABCs (airway, breathing, and circulation) (refer to Chapter 40 for further information on emergency management). All children who experience head trauma need an assessment of their neurologic function as soon as they are seen. This includes LOC, pupillary response, and any seizure activity. Fixed and dilated pupils, fixed and constricted pupils, or sluggish pupillary reaction to light will warrant prompt intervention.

CLINICAL REASONING ALERT!

A child's spine must remain stabilized after a head injury until spinal cord injury is ruled out.

LABORATORY AND DIAGNOSTIC TESTS

Diagnostic tests that may be utilized include x-ray examinations of the head and neck and CT and MRI scans. These procedures can assist in providing a more definitive diagnosis of the severity and type of trauma.

TABLE 38.6 • Common Head Injuries Seen in Children

Types	Description	Characteristics
Skull fractures	A break in the bone surrounding the brain	In infants and children under 2 years old, a great deal of force is needed to produce a skull fracture. Due to the flexibility of the immature skull, it is able to withstand a great degree of deformation before a fracture will occur. Can result in little or no brain damage but may have serious consequences if the underlying brain tissue is injured
Linear skull fracture	A simple break in the skull that follows a relatively straight line	Most common skull fracture. Can result from minor head injuries such as being struck by a rock, stick, or other object; falls; or motor vehicle accidents. Not usually serious unless there is additional injury to the brain
Depressed skull fractures	The bone is locally broken and pushed inward, causing pressure on the brain.	Can result from forceful impact from a blunt object, such as a hammer or another heavy but fairly small object Surgery is often required to elevate the bony pieces and inspect the brain for evidence of injury.
Diastatic skull fracture	A fracture through the skull sutures	Most commonly occurs in the lambdoid sutures (refer to Fig. 38.9 for location of sutures) Usually, treatment is not required but observation will be necessary.
Compound skull fracture	A laceration of the skin and splintering of the bone	The fracture can be linear or depressed. Generally is the result of blunt force. Usually requires medical intervention, and surgery may be necessary
Basilar skull fracture	A fracture of the bones that form the base of the skull	Can result from severe blunt head trauma with significant force. Due to the proximity to the brain stem, this is a serious head injury. Findings include CSF rhinorrhea and otorrhea, bleeding from the ear, and orbital or postauricular ecchymosis (bruising behind ear is referred to as Battle sign), and these children are at increased risk for infection because the fracture may allow a portal of entry into the central nervous system.
Concussion	A type of traumatic brain injury that is caused by a bump, blow, jolt, jarring, or shaking and results in disruption or malfunction of the electrical activities of the brain	Most common head injury. Results from a blow or jolt to the head caused by sports injuries, motor vehicle accidents, and falls. Confusion and amnesia after the head injury are seen. Loss of consciousness may or may not occur. Noted symptoms may include increased distractibility and difficulty with concentration. Treatment includes rest and monitoring for neurologic changes that could indicate a more severe injury, such as increased sleepiness, worsening headache, increased vomiting, worsening confusion, difficulty walking or talking, changes in LOC, and seizures.
Contusion	Bruising of cerebral tissue	Results from a blow to the head from incidents such as a motor vehicle accident, falls, or abuse such as shaken baby syndrome. May cause focal disturbances in vision, strength, and sensation. The signs and symptoms will vary based on the extent of vascular injury and can range from mild weakness to prolonged unconsciousness and paralysis. Treatment includes close monitoring for neurologic changes. Surgery is usually not necessary.
Subdural hematoma	Collection of blood between the dura and cerebrum	Low incidence of fracture. Most common in children younger than 2 years old, especially infants. Results from birth trauma, falls, bicycle injuries, and abuse such as shaken baby syndrome. Usually consists of venous bleeding. Symptoms may occur within 3 days of trauma or as late as 20 days. Symptoms include vomiting, undernutrition, changes in LOC, seizures, and retinal hemorrhage. Treatment depends on clinical symptoms, size of clot, and area of the brain involved. In some cases, the bleed may be closely monitored for resolution. In other cases, treatment may include subdural taps in infants and surgical evacuation in older children. Close monitoring of neurologic status and for signs of increased ICP is indicated.
Epidural hematoma	Collection of blood located outside the dura but within the skull	Relatively uncommon. Often results from skull fracture. Seen when head trauma is severe. Usually arterial bleeding; therefore, brain compression occurs rapidly and can result in impairment of the brain stem and respiratory or cardiovascular function. Symptoms include vomiting, headache, and lethargy. Treatment depends on clinical symptoms, the size of the clot, and the area of the brain involved. Treatment includes prompt surgical evacuation and cauterization of the artery. The earlier the bleed is recognized and treated, the more favorable the outcome. Close monitoring of neurologic status is indicated.

CLINICAL REASONING ALERT!

If clear liquid fluid is noted draining from the ears or nose, notify the health care provider or nurse practitioner. If the fluid tests positive for glucose, this is indicative of leaking CSF.

Nursing Management

Nursing management of the child with head trauma depends on the seriousness of the injury. For all head trauma, however, the nurse provides support and education to the family and provides teaching on ways to prevent future head injuries.

CARING FOR THE CHILD WITH MILD TO MODERATE HEAD INJURY

Mild to moderate closed head injury is defined as brain injury without any penetrating injury to the brain, no loss of consciousness, no other injury to the head or body, normal behavior after the injury, and healthy status before the injury. Most children with this type of injury can be cared for and observed at home. Provide parents and caregivers with clear instructions regarding the care of their child at home. Explain that they must seek medical attention if the child's condition worsens at any time during the first several days after injury. See Teaching Guidelines 38.2.

Children with mild closed head injury may exhibit some cognitive and behavioral symptoms, such as difficulty paying attention, problems making sense of what has been seen or heard, and forgetting things, in the early days after the injury. The majority make a full recovery. However, some may experience ongoing cognitive and behavioral difficulties, including slow information processing and attention difficulties.

TEACHING GUIDELINES 38.2 Monitoring the Child With Closed Head Injury at Home

Instruct parents and caregivers:

- Stay with the child for the first 24 hours, and be ready to take the child to the hospital, if necessary.
- Instructions for waking the child, if necessary, and at what frequency will be given based on child's symptoms and exam. If instructed, wake the child every 2–4 hours to ensure that they move normally, wake enough to recognize the caregiver, and respond to the caregiver appropriately.
- Closely observe the child for a few days.
- Call the medical provider or bring the child to the emergency room if the child exhibits any of the following:
  - Constant headache that gets worse
  - Slurred speech
  - Dizziness that does not go away or happens repeatedly
  - Extreme irritability or other abnormal behavior
  - Vomiting more than two times
  - Clumsiness or difficulty walking
  - Oozing blood or watery fluid from ears or nose
  - Difficulty waking up
  - Unequal-sized pupils
  - Unusual paleness that lasts longer than 1 hour
  - Seizures
  - Review signs and symptoms of increased intracranial pressure and provide parents with a number they can call if they have questions or concerns.

Adapted from Schutzman, S. (2021). Minor head trauma in infants and children: Management. *UpToDate*. Retrieved May 5, 2023, from https://www.uptodate.com/contents/minor-head-trauma-in-infants-and-children-management

THINKING ABOUT DEVELOPMENT

Antonio Blackman is an 11-year-old who suffered a concussion during his soccer game. Based on his developmental stage, how will you instruct him and his caregivers on managing his head injury at home? How would your instructions change if the child were 5 years old?

CARING FOR THE CHILD WITH SEVERE HEAD INJURY

Severe head injuries can range from a temporary unconsciousness that resolves quickly to children who may remain in a comatose state for a prolonged time. Nursing management of the comatose child is similar to nursing care of the comatose adult.

Children with more severe head injury may require intensive care initially until stabilized. Focus will be on maintaining the child's airway; monitoring breathing, circulation, and neurologic status closely; preventing and ceasing any seizure activity; and treating any other injuries that may have occurred because of the trauma. Nursing management will continue to focus on evaluation of neurologic status and assessing for changes in LOC and signs and symptoms of increased ICP. Initiate seizure precautions as ordered.

Individualize care to the specific needs of the child. Maintain a quiet environment to help reduce restlessness and irritability. Manage pain and administer sedation as ordered. Observe the level of sedation closely to ensure that LOC will not become altered, which would hinder the ability to assess adequately for neurologic changes. Monitor for the development of complications, which include hemorrhage, infection, cerebral edema, and herniation.

TAKE NOTE!

Parents are extremely helpful resources in evaluating a child's behavior for changes or abnormalities. They can provide insight into whether a behavior seen is normal or abnormal for this child. Examples include the ease at which a child is normally aroused, how much the child normally sleeps during the day, and what is the child's normal visual and hearing acuity.

PROVIDING SUPPORT AND EDUCATION

Provide support and education for the family of a child who has suffered a head trauma. Encourage involvement in the child's care. The extent of residual neurologic damage and recovery may be unclear for the child with a head injury. This can be frustrating and stressful for parents and family. Encourage verbalization of their feelings and concerns. Rehabilitation of the child with permanent brain damage is an essential component of their care. It should begin as soon as possible in the hospital setting and may continue for months to years. This can place a strain on the family and its finances. Families need to be involved in the rehabilitation process. The nurse will be a key member in ensuring the parents and family are involved with the interdisciplinary team.

PREVENTING HEAD INJURIES

Prevention of head injuries provides the greatest benefit to children and the community. Nurses play a key role in educating the public on topics such as helmet use with certain sports; bicycle and motorcycle safety; car seat and seat belt use; and providing adequate supervision of children to help prevent injuries and accidents—and resultant head trauma—from occurring.

TAKE NOTE!

Sports-related traumatic brain injuries, including concussions, in children and adolescents are a growing concern, particularly related to the long-term effects of these injuries. Increasing education, awareness, and research about concussions will help to improve prevention, recognition, and treatment of this injury among school professionals, parents, coaches, and children and adolescents. See Evidence-Based Practice 38.1.

Nonaccidental Head Trauma

In the United States, inflicted or nonaccidental head trauma is the leading cause of traumatic death and morbidity resulting from physical abuse in childhood (Christian, 2023). Children's dependence on others to care for them places them at a high risk for injuries caused by child abuse.

The infant's large head size and weak neck muscles place them at an increased risk for head trauma due to violent shaking or cranial impacts compared with adults. In addition, children under 3 years of age have a very mobile spine, especially in the cervical region, along with immature neck muscles. This places them at

EVIDENCE-BASED PRACTICE 38.1
How Does Screen Time Affect Recovery From Concussion?

The high incidence of concussion and the potential for short- and long-term complications make concussions in student athletes an important topic. General treatment protocol post sport-related concussion includes a period of cognitive and physical rest for the first 24 to 48 hours until symptom free and then a gradual, graded return to activity. Children and adolescents often spend several hours a day using screens, such as computers, tablets, and televisions. Parents and children frequently ask if screen time is permitted during the acute rest period post-concussion, and recommendations are often inconsistent. This study looks at what the evidence tells us about the effects of screen time on the duration of time until symptom recovery.

STUDY

This study was a randomized clinical trial involving 125 patients 12 to 25 years of age seen in an emergency department in a tertiary medical center.

Findings

This study found that avoiding screen time during the acute recovery phase may shorten the duration of concussion symptoms and lead to a faster recovery.

Nursing Implications

Nurses can educate children and their families on the benefits of cognitive and physical rest, which should include abstinence from screen time in the acute period, 48 hours post-concussion. Nurses can educate the child and families about signs and symptoms that would warrant further evaluation, treatment, and rehabilitation. Future clinical trials are needed on a larger scale. Further research is also needed on rest and active treatment and rehabilitation post sport-related concussion, preferably randomized controlled studies. The exact amount and duration of rest and the optimal timing, mode, duration, intensity, and frequency of active treatment warrant further studies.

Data from Macnow, T., Curran, T., Tolliday, C., Martin, K., McCarthy, M., Ayturk, D., Babu, K.M., & Mannix, R. (2021). Effect of screen time on recovery from concussion: A randomized clinical trial. *JAMA Pediatrics, 175*(11), 1124–1131. https://doi.org/10.1001/jamapediatrics.2021.2782

a higher risk for injury from acceleration/deceleration injuries, which occur when the head receives a blow or is shaken. The sudden acceleration causes deformation of the skull and movement of the brain, allowing brain contents to strike parts of the skull. Bruising of the brain can occur at the point of impact or at that point distant from the impact where the brain collides with the skull. Another result of brain movement is hemorrhages in the brain, which are caused by the shearing forces that may tear small arteries. The child's thin skull places them at increased risk for skull fractures and penetrating injuries resulting from head trauma.

Causes of nonaccidental head trauma include violent shaking, referred to as shaken baby syndrome (SBS); blows to the head; and intentional cranial impacts against the wall, furniture, or the floor. SBS is a form of child abuse, and a significant number of head traumas result from it. However, it differs from many other forms of child abuse in that frequently, there was no intent to harm the child. Shaking happens when the parent or caregiver becomes frustrated or angry because they cannot get the baby to stop crying.

The full appearance of neurologic deficits resulting from nonaccidental head trauma may take several years to identify, and recovery can be slow. Long-term outcomes are not known, but many of these infants and children have poor outcomes and may suffer neurologic defects such as profound intellectual disability, spastic quadriplegia, severe motor dysfunction, and blindness. The majority of children with inflicted head injuries have some impairment of motor and cognitive abilities, language, vision, and behavior. These injuries may also contribute to later problems with education and social attainment.

Nursing Assessment

The infant who has been a victim of nonaccidental trauma can present in many ways. Symptoms and physical findings may be similar to those seen in children with accidental head trauma or increased ICP related to infection. Therefore, many nonaccidental traumas remain unidentified. Nurses are mandatory reporters of abuse (for further information on this, see Chapter 50). Early recognition of suspected child abuse is essential to prevent death and disability from repetitive inflicted head trauma.

HEALTH HISTORY

It is important to review the child's history closely and pay particular attention to the caregivers' explanation of the child's injury. Be alert to any discrepancies between the physical injuries and the history of injury given by the parent, especially if the stories are conflicting, or if the caregivers are unable to give an explanation for the injury. Also, note any previous intracranial or skeletal injuries that cannot be explained.

In less severe cases, common signs and symptoms may include:

- Poor feeding or sucking
- Vomiting
- Lethargy or irritability
- Undernutrition/malnutrition
- Increased sleeping
- Difficulty arousing

In more severe cases, the symptoms will be more acute and may consist of:

- Seizure activity
- Apnea
- Bradycardia
- Decreased LOC
- Bulging fontanel

PHYSICAL EXAMINATION

External bruising of the head and face may be evident in some inflicted head traumas. However, no evidence of external trauma, but the presence of intracranial or intraocular hemorrhages, is the classic presentation of SBS. Retinal hemorrhages are seen in most cases, which is a rare finding in accidental or nontraumatic events.

LABORATORY AND DIAGNOSTIC TESTS

Diagnostic tests, including CT, MRI, ophthalmologic examination to rule out retinal hemorrhages, and skeletal survey x-rays to rule out or confirm other injuries may be performed to help determine the extent and type of injury.

Nursing Management

Treatment and nursing management will be similar to that for the child with accidental head trauma (see earlier section, Head Trauma). Prevention of nonaccidental head trauma, including SBS, is a major concern for all health care professionals. Be aware of risk factors related to the potential for SBS to occur. Recognizing these risk factors will allow appropriate intervention and protection of the child to take place. See Box 38.4 for risk factors related to SBS.

Educating parents and caregivers on appropriate ways to handle stress and ways to cope with a crying

BOX 38.4 Risk Factors Associated With Abusive Head Trauma (Shaken Baby Syndrome)

- Single parent
- Young parent
- Substance misuse by a parent
- Any external factors present such as financial, social, or physical burdens that place stress on the parent
- Premature or sick infant
- Infant with colic

infant can help to prevent nonaccidental head trauma (Teaching Guidelines 38.3). Many parents and caregivers may perceive shaking a child as a less violent way to react than other means of enforcing discipline. They need to be aware that shaking a baby, even for only a few seconds, can cause serious brain damage and death. Decreasing mortality and morbidity associated with SBS and nonaccidental injury through early preventive education is an essential nursing concern. Information about the dangers of shaking a baby should be a part of prenatal care and standard discharge teaching on postpartum units. In addition, this information should be provided to the community and in health education classes to reach young potential child care providers.

Nonfatal Drowning (Near-Drowning)

Drowning is a preventable problem that is far too common, especially in children. Drowning is the second leading cause of unintentional injury-related death in children between the ages of 1 and 14 years (CDC, 2022b). Those at greatest risk of drowning are children 1 to 4 years of age and adolescent males (CDC, 2022b).

TEACHING GUIDELINES 38.3 Tips to Calm a Crying Baby

Instruct parents and caregivers:

- Try to figure out what is upsetting the baby.
  - Is the baby hungry?
  - Is the baby's diaper dry?
  - Is the baby cold or hot?
  - Is the baby overtired or overstimulated?
  - Is the baby in pain?
  - Is the baby sick or running a fever?
- Try to help the baby relax.
  - Turn down the lights.
  - Swaddle the baby.
  - Walk the baby.
  - Rock the baby.
  - Give the baby a breast, bottle, or pacifier.
  - Hush, talk to, or sing to the baby.
  - Take the baby for a stroller or car ride.
- Sometimes, the baby may continue to cry after all your efforts. If you feel overwhelmed, frustrated, or angry, focus on keeping the baby safe.
  - Stop what you are doing, take a deep breath, and count to 10.
  - Place the baby in a safe place, such as the crib or playpen.
  - Leave the room and shut the door, and find a quiet place for yourself.
  - Check on the baby every 5–15 minutes.
  - Do not be afraid to call for help; call a friend, relative, or neighbor.

Nonfatal or near-drowning is described as an incident in which a child has suffered a submersion injury and has survived for at least 24 hours. Nonfatal drowning events result in a significant number of injured children and can result in long-term neurologic deficits. Children under 1 year old most often drown in bathtubs, buckets, or toilets. Children between the ages of 1 and 4 years are more likely to drown or have a nonfatal drowning incident in residential swimming pools (CDC, 2022b). In children older than 15 years, most drownings occur in natural water settings, such as oceans or lakes (CDC, 2022b). Most incidents are accidental and result from inadequately supervising children who are in or near water, lack of use of personal flotation devices while on recreational water apparatus such as boats, and diving accidents.

Nursing Assessment

Hypoxia is the primary problem resulting from nonfatal drowning. Nursing assessment needs to begin with resuscitative measures. The child may be comatose, be hypothermic, lack spontaneous respirations, and present with hypoxia and hypercapnia. Gain information about the site of submersion (was it fresh or salt water?), the water temperature, the time of submersion, and how long it was until the child received interventions such as cardiopulmonary resuscitation (CPR) and EMS.

Nursing Management

Resuscitative measures should be started as soon as the child is pulled from the water, and the child should be transported to a hospital immediately. Management will be based on the degree of cerebral insult that has occurred. The child who has been successfully resuscitated will usually require intensive nursing care and monitoring. Promotion of oxygenation and monitoring for infection related to aspiration of water are primary nursing concerns. Chronic neurologic damage occurs in many nonfatal drownings secondary to hypoxia. The child may need rehabilitation and long-term follow-up. Provide parents with support and education relating to their child's condition. Educating children, families, and the community is an important nursing intervention to help prevent drowning (see Teaching Guidelines 38.4).

BLOOD FLOW DISRUPTION

Pediatric cerebral vascular disorders occur less often than in adults, but they are still an important cause of mortality and chronic morbidity in children (Fox & Smith, 2023). Many children will develop lifelong cognitive and motor impairments. Childhood cerebral vascular disorders (stroke) are usually seen after the first month of life. Periventricular/intraventricular hemorrhage is seen in preterm infants and in infants up to 1 month of age.

TEACHING GUIDELINES 38.4 Teaching to Prevent Drowning

Instruct parents and caregivers:
- Install proper pool fencing.
- Start water safety training at a young age.
- Have your child learn swimming skills.
- Never leave an infant or child without close adult supervision in or near water (this includes bathtubs).
- Empty water from all containers, such as 5-gallon buckets, immediately after use.
- Use proper-fitting, Coast Guard–approved personal flotation devices at all times when near water.
- Never allow children to walk, skate, or ride on thinning or thawing ice.
- Learn CPR and keep emergency numbers handy (make sure babysitters are CPR qualified).
- Know the depth of water before permitting a child to jump or dive.

Cerebral Vascular Disorders (Stroke)

A cerebral vascular disorder is a sudden disruption of the blood supply to the brain. It affects neurologic functioning, such as movement and speech. Two major types of adult cerebral vascular disorders are seen in children—ischemic stroke and hemorrhagic stroke. Ischemic stroke is more common than hemorrhagic stroke in children. In children, there are a wide array of risk factors and causes as compared with adults (see Comparison Chart 38.2), but in many cases the cause remains unidentified. The outcomes reported for cerebral vascular disorders in children vary, but many children will develop some neurologic or cognitive deficit.

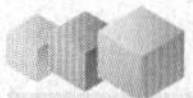

Concept Mastery Alert

Children are more likely to experience an ischemic stroke than a hemorrhagic stroke. If a child experiences a stroke, the symptoms are similar to those that an adult would experience.

Historically, children have been excluded from adult stroke studies. Therefore, many treatments used in children have had to be adapted from adult studies. Acute treatment is supportive and requires intensive care. The exact treatment will depend on the underlying cause.

Nursing Assessment

The clinical presentation will vary according to age, the underlying cause, and the location of the stroke. Signs and symptoms of acute stroke are similar to those seen in the adult and depend on the area of the brain that has been affected. Common signs include:

- Weakness on one side or hemiplegia
- Facial droop
- Slurred speech
- Speech deficits
- Seizures
- Headaches
- Lethargy

COMPARISON CHART 38.2 Risk Factors and Causes of Stroke in Children and Adults

	Risk Factors and Causes in Children	Risk Factors and Causes in Adults
Ischemic stroke	Cardiac disorders and intracardiac defects (congenital such as ventricular septal defect, atrial septal defect, and aortic stenosis, or acquired such as rheumatic heart disease) Coagulation abnormalities that lead to thrombosis Sickle cell disease Infection, such as meningitis Arterial dissection Genetic disorders	Cardiac disease, including atherosclerosis Diabetes mellitus Hyperlipidemia Hypercoagulability states Polycythemia Sickle cell disease Smoking Increased age Male sex Obesity Excessive alcohol consumption
Hemorrhagic stroke	Vascular malformations such as intracranial arteriovenous malformation (AVM) Aneurysms Warfarin therapy Cavernous malformations Malignancy Trauma Coagulation disorders such as hemophilia Thrombocytopenia Liver failure Leukemia Intracranial tumors such as medulloblastomas	Hypertension Aneurysms Use of anticoagulant medications Smoking Increased age Male sex Obesity Excessive alcohol consumption

Strokes in children are diagnosed in the same manner as strokes in adults. However, further tests may need to be run in the child, such as metabolic studies, coagulation tests, echocardiogram, and LP to help identify the cause of the stroke.

Nursing Management

Nursing management will be similar to that for the adult patient who has suffered a stroke. Care will focus on assessing neurologic status, increasing mobility, providing adequate nutrition and hydration, and encouraging self-care. Rehabilitative care may be initiated, depending on the long-term deficits, to help the child attain optimal function. Parental support and education will be essential in helping them care for a child who has new disabilities.

CHRONIC DISORDERS

Chronic disorders in children necessitate multidisciplinary care. Parents and children are in need of a large amount of education and support from the health care team. Chronic neurologic disorders commonly seen in children include headaches and breath holding.

Headaches

Acute and chronic headaches, including migraines, are common reasons why children miss school, visit their health care provider or nurse practitioner, and receive subsequent referrals to neurologists. Children with reports or symptoms of headaches need to be examined thoroughly. Headaches may result from sinusitis or eyestrain or can be indicative of more serious conditions such as brain tumors, acute meningitis, or increased ICP. Migraines are a specific type of headache. They are benign, recurrent, throbbing headaches often accompanied by nausea, vomiting, and photophobia. Acute migraines can occur in children as young as 3 to 4 years. The cause of migraine headaches is not well understood.

After other acute or chronic conditions are ruled out, management will focus on treating the child's pain. Pharmacologic measures may be utilized in the treatment of chronic headaches and migraines. Medications used in children to treat and prevent headaches are similar to the medications used to treat adults. Recent attention has been paid to headaches caused by medication overuse. The child may have a primary headache disorder that is exacerbated by the frequent use of medications. Although medication overuse headaches are common in children, they are frequently underrecognized and underdiagnosed.

Nursing Assessment

Elicit a description of the present illness and chief complaint. Important health history information to obtain is onset of the pain, aggravating and alleviating factors, frequency and duration of the pain, time of day the pain usually occurs, location of the pain, and quality and intensity of the pain.

In young children, symptoms of headache may be hard to recognize. However, common signs and symptoms may include:

- Irritability
- Lethargy
- Head holding
- Head banging
- Sensitivity to sound or light

Assessment also includes a thorough physical examination to rule out any life-threatening illness, such as a brain tumor or increased ICP. A detailed neurologic examination is warranted. Neuroimaging may be performed based on the child's history and physical examination, if needed, to rule out a brain tumor or mass as the cause of the headaches.

Nursing Management

Nursing measures will focus on support and education. After serious illness has been ruled out, reassure the child and family that no serious medical or neurologic disease is present. Because headaches are recurring and the cause may be unknown, pain management can be difficult. Provide education to help the child and parents gain control over the headaches. Teach the child and family to keep accurate records of headaches and activities surrounding the headaches to help establish a pattern of occurrence and identify triggering factors. Encourage parents and the child to recognize the triggering factors and to avoid them (Box 38.5). Teach the child and family about pain medications and how to use them. Teach other management techniques, which may include exercise, sleep regulation, proper diet with regularly spaced meals, avoiding caffeine, avoiding inadequate hydration, regular attendance at school, use of biofeedback, stress reduction techniques, and possible psychiatric assessment.

BOX 38.5 Potential Headache Triggers

- Foods, such as chocolate, caffeine, or monosodium glutamate (MSG)–containing foods
- Changes in hormone levels, around menses and ovulation
- Changes in:
  - Weather
  - Season
  - Sleep patterns
  - Meal schedule
- Stress
- Intense activity
- Bright or flickering lights
- Odors, such as strong perfumes

Breath Holding

Breath holding is a benign behavior of childhood, although it is extremely frightening for parents. It is normally seen in children 6 months to 6 years of age and is typically outgrown by 4 to 8 years of age (Nguyen et al., 2021). Breath holding is usually triggered by the child becoming angry or stressed after not getting their way and can also occur as a reflexive response to fear, pain, or being startled. The child stops inhaling and exhaling or hyperventilates, the brain becomes anoxic, and the child becomes cyanotic and may pass out. In some cases, a change in muscle tone, seizure-like activity, or hypoxic convulsions may be observed. This does not mean the child has a seizure disorder, but it must be ruled out. The spell usually resolves spontaneously. With the loss of consciousness, the child will begin breathing on their own and will often begin crying, screaming, and trying to catch their breath. The spells usually last only 30 to 60 seconds and, as long as the child does not sustain an injury while falling, have no consequences.

If no underlying condition is found, the child needs no therapy. The condition is self-limiting, and the child will outgrow it. Iron deficiency may play a role; therefore, iron supplementation may be prescribed (Nguyen et al., 2021).

Nursing Assessment

The first time a spell occurs, a primary care provider should evaluate the child because the event could indicate a seizure. Breath holding has also been shown to be aggravated by iron-deficiency anemia, and, in rare cases, it could indicate a more serious neurologic condition and therefore warrants a full evaluation. Elicit a full description of the episode and events leading up to it. Also, collect a thorough past medical history and perform a complete physical examination.

Nursing Management

Nursing management should focus on educating and supporting the parents. Breath holding is a scary event, and parents will want information on the effects of the behavior and how to prevent the behavior from recurring. Reinforce that the spells are involuntary and that they should not intervene to stop them. Encourage parents to maintain a safe environment when an episode is occurring, such as holding the child or placing them in the sidelying position. Reassure parents that the child will suffer no ill effects from breath holding and that they should not reinforce the breath-holding behavior or give in to the child. Children with breath-holding spells may benefit from structure and consistency to avoid unnecessary frustration and overtiredness.

Unfolding Patient Stories: Jackson Weber • Part 2

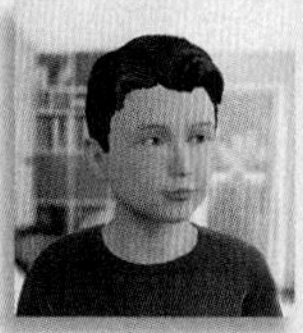

Think back to Chapter 26 where you met Jackson Weber. Jackson was diagnosed with generalized seizures 2 years ago at age 3. He had another seizure, and his parent brought him to the hospital. How would the nurse differentiate tonic–clonic seizures from other types of seizures? Compare and contrast the characteristics of each type of seizure.

Care for Jackson and other patients in a realistic virtual environment: ***vSim** for Nursing* (thepoint.lww.com/vSimPediatric). Practice documenting these patients' care in DocuCare (thePoint.lww.com/DocuCareEHR).

KEY CONCEPTS

- Development of the brain and spinal cord occurs early in gestation, in the first 3 to 4 weeks. Infection, trauma, teratogens, and malnutrition during this period can result in malformations and may affect normal CNS development.
- The brain of the newborn is highly vascular, leading to an increased risk of hemorrhage.
- The head of the infant and young child is large in proportion to the body, and the neck muscles are not well developed, placing the infant at an increased risk of head injury from falls and accidents.
- Neurologic disorders in children can result from congenital problems as well as infections or trauma.
- LP and CSF analysis can be useful in the diagnosis of hemorrhage, infection, or obstruction.
- CT and MRI studies can be useful in diagnosing congenital abnormalities such as NTDs, hemorrhage, tumors, fractures, demyelination, or inflammation.
- EEGs measure the electrical activity of the brain and can be used in diagnosing seizures or brain death.
- Antibiotics are utilized in the treatment of bacterial meningitis and shunt infections.
- Anticonvulsants are used in the treatment and prevention of seizures and are often used in combination.
- Corticosteroids are used to reduce cerebral edema and must be tapered before discontinuing.
- Risk factors associated with neurologic disorders include prematurity, difficult birth, infection during pregnancy, family history of genetic disorders with a neurologic manifestation, seizure disorders, and headaches.
- Alterations in motor function, such as changes in gait or muscle tone or strength, may indicate certain neurologic problems such as increased ICP, head injury, and cerebral infections.
- Increased ICP is a sign that may occur with many neurologic disorders. It may result from head trauma, birth trauma, hydrocephalus, infection, and brain

tumors. It is essential that the nurse observes for signs and symptoms associated with increased ICP while caring for a child with a potential or suspected neurologic disorder.

- Sunset eyes may indicate increased ICP, as seen in hydrocephalus.
- A bulging fontanel can be a sign of increased ICP and is seen in such neurologic disorders as hydrocephalus and head traumas.
- Cortical control of motor function is lost in certain neurologic disorders; postural reflexes reemerge and are directly related to the area of the brain that is damaged. Decorticate posturing occurs with damage of the cerebral cortex. Decerebrate posturing occurs with damage at the level of the brain stem.
- Nursing management of seizures focuses on preventing injury during seizures, instituting seizure precautions, maintaining a patent airway, administering appropriate medication and treatments to prevent or reduce seizures, and providing education and support to the child and family to help them cope with the challenges of living with a chronic seizure disorder.
- Hydrocephalus results from an imbalance in the production and absorption of CSF. Key assessment findings include a rapid increase in head circumference seen in the infant or loss of development and changes in personality in the older child. Signs and symptoms associated with increased ICP may be seen.
- Nursing management of the child with hydrocephalus will focus on maintaining cerebral perfusion, minimizing neurologic complications, recognizing and preventing shunt infection and malfunction, maintaining adequate nutrition, promoting growth and development, and supporting and educating the child and family.
- Bacterial meningitis requires rapid assessment and treatment. On assessment, the nurse may find the infant with bacterial meningitis resting in the opisthotonic position, and the older child may complain of neck pain.
- Nursing management of the child with bacterial meningitis will include administration of IV antibiotics, reducing ICP, and maintaining cerebral perfusion along with treating fluid volume deficit, controlling seizures, and preventing injury that may result from altered LOC or seizure activity.
- Nurses play a key role in educating the public on topics such as helmet use with certain sports, bicycle and motorcycle safety, car seat and seat belt use, and provision of adequate supervision of children to help prevent injuries and accidents and resultant head trauma from occurring.
- Many neurologic disorders affect multiple body systems with lifelong deficits that require long-term rehabilitation. Adjusting to the demands this condition places on the child and family is difficult. Parents may need time to accept their child's condition, but as soon as possible they should be involved in the child's care.
- Children with neurologic disorders and their families often need large amounts of education and support throughout the child's lifetime. As the child grows, the needs of the family and child will change. The nurse needs to provide ongoing education and support.
- Some neurologic disorders require complete intensive daily care. Adjusting to these demands can be difficult for the family. Encourage respite care and provide meaningful education programs that emphasize independence for the child in the least restrictive educational environment. Refer caregivers to local resources, including education services and support groups.

REFERENCES AND RECOMMENDED READINGS

American Academy of Pediatrics & Committee on Genetics. (1999, reaffirmed 2017). Policy statement. Folic acid for the prevention of neural tube defects. *Pediatrics*. http://pediatrics.aappublications.org/content/104/2/325.full

American Academy of Pediatrics, Steering Committee on Quality Improvement and Management, & Subcommittee on Febrile Seizures. (2008). Febrile seizures: Clinical practice guideline for the long-term management of the child with simple febrile seizures. *Pediatrics, 121*(6), 1281–1286. https://doi.org/10.1542/peds.2008-0939

Buchanan, E. P. (2021). Overview of craniosynostosis. *UpToDate*. Retrieved May 6, 2023, from https://www.uptodate.com/contents/overview-of-craniosynostosis

Centers for Disease Control and Prevention. (2021a). *Meningitis: Bacterial meningitis*. http://www.cdc.gov/meningitis/bacterial.html

Centers for Disease Control and Prevention. (2021b). *Meningitis: Viral meningitis*. Retrieved May 8, 2023, from http://www.cdc.gov/meningitis/viral.html

Centers for Disease Control and Prevention. (2021c). *Injury prevention and control: Injuries among children and teens*. https://www.cdc.gov/injury/features/child-injury/index.html

Centers for Disease Control and Prevention. (2022a). *Folic acid recommendations*. http://www.cdc.gov/ncbddd/folicacid/recommendations.html

Centers for Disease Control and Prevention. (2022b). *Drowning facts*. https://www.cdc.gov/drowning/facts/index.html

Christian, C. (2023). Child abuse: Evaluation and diagnosis of abusive head trauma in infants and children. *UpToDate*. Retrieved May 8, 2023, from https://www.uptodate.com/contents/child-abuse-evaluation-and-diagnosis-of-abusive-head-trauma-in-infants-and-children

Fischbach, F. T., Fischbach, M. A., & Stout, K. (2022). *A manual of laboratory and diagnostic tests* (11th ed.). Wolters Kluwer.

Fisher, R. S., Cross, J. H., French, J. A., Higurashi, N., Hirsch, E., Jansen, F. E., Lagae, L., Moshé, S. L., Peltola, J., Roulet Perez, E., Scheffer, I. E., & Zuberi, S. M. (2017). Operational classification of seizure types by the International League Against Epilepsy: Position paper of the ILAE Commission for Classification and Terminology. *Epilepsia, 58*, 522–530. https://doi.org/10.1111/epi.13670

Fox, C., & Smith, S. E. (2023). Ischemic stroke in children and young adults: Epidemiology, etiology, and risk factors. *UpToDate*. Retrieved May 8, 2023, from https://www.uptodate.com/contents/ischemic-stroke-in-children-and-young-adults-epidemiology-etiology-and-risk-factors

Gill, A. C., & Kelly, N. R. (2022). Pediatric injury prevention: Epidemiology, history, and application. *UpToDate*. Retrieved May 8, 2023, from https://www.uptodate.com/contents/pediatric-injury-prevention-epidemiology-history-and-application

Hardarson, H. S., & Messacar, K. (2022). Acute viral encephalitis in children: Pathogenesis, incidence, and etiology. *UpToDate*. Retrieved May 8, 2023, from https://www.uptodate.com/contents/acute-viral-encephalitis-in-children-pathogenesis-epidemiology-and-etiology

Haridas, A., & Tomita, T. (2022a). Hydrocephalus in children: Physiology, pathogenesis, and etiology. *UpToDate*. Retrieved May 6, 2023, from https://www.uptodate.com/contents/hydrocephalus-in-children-physiology-pathogenesis-and-etiology

Haridas, A., & Tomita, T. (2022b). Hydrocephalus in children: Management & prognosis. *UpToDate*. Retrieved May 6, 2023, from https://www.uptodate.com/contents/hydrocephalus-in-children-management-and-prognosis

Khoury, C. (2023). *Chiari malformations*. *UpToDate*. Retrieved May 6, 2023, from https://www.uptodate.com/contents/chiari-malformations

Kinsman, S. L., & Johnston, M. V. (2020). Chapter 609: Congenital anomalies of the central nervous system. In R. M. Kliegman, J. W. St. Geme III, N. J. Blum, S. S. Shah, R. C. Tasker, K. M. Wilson, & R. E. Behrman (Eds.), *Nelson textbook of pediatrics* (21st ed., pp. 16200–16290). Elsevier.

Kossoff, E. H. W. (2022). The ketogenic diet and other diet therapies for the treatment of epilepsy. *UpToDate*. Retrieved May 9, 2023, from https://www.uptodate.com/contents/ketogenic-dietary-therapies-for-the-treatment-of-epilepsy

Lexicomp. (2023). Pediatric drug information. *UpToDate*. Retrieved April 5, 2023, from https://www.uptodate.com/contents/table-of-contents/drug-information/pediatric-drug-information

Macnow, T., Curran, T., Tolliday, C., Martin, K., McCarthy, M., Ayturk, D., Babu, K. M., & Mannix, R. (2021). Effect of screen time on recovery from concussion: A randomized clinical trial. *JAMA Pediatrics*, *175*(11), 1124–1131. https://doi.org/10.1001/jamapediatrics.2021.2782

Mikati, M. A., & Tchapyjnikov, D. (2020). Chapter 611. Seizures in childhood. In R. M. Kliegman, J. W. St. Geme III, N. J. Blum, S. S. Shah, R. C. Tasker, K. M. Wilson, & R. E. Behrman (Eds.), *Nelson textbook of pediatrics* (21st ed., pp. 16312–16492). Elsevier.

Millichap, J. J. (2022a). Clinical features and evaluation of febrile seizures. *UpToDate*. Retrieved May 5, 2023, from https://www.uptodate.com/contents/clinical-features-and-evaluation-of-febrile-seizures

Millichap, J. J. (2022b). Treatment and prognosis of febrile seizures. *UpToDate*. Retrieved May 5, 2023, from https://www.uptodate.com/contents/treatment-and-prognosis-of-febrile-seizures

Nguyen, T. T., Kaplan, P. W., & Wilfong, A. (2021). Nonepileptic paroxysmal disorders in infancy. *UpToDate*. Retrieved on May 8, 2023, from https://www.uptodate.com/contents/nonepileptic-paroxysmal-disorders-in-infancy

Schutzman, S. (2021). Minor head trauma in infants and children: Management. *UpToDate*. Retrieved May 5, 2023, from https://www.uptodate.com/contents/minor-head-trauma-in-infants-and-children-management

Shellhaas, R. (2022a). Treatment of neonatal seizures. *UpToDate*. Retrieved May 5, 2023, from https://www.uptodate.com/contents/treatment-of-neonatal-seizures

Shellhaas, R. (2022b). Etiology and prognosis of neonatal seizures. *UpToDate*. Retrieved May 5, 2023, from https://www.uptodate.com/contents/etiology-and-prognosis-of-neonatal-seizures

Shellhaas, R. (2023). Clinical features, evaluation and diagnosis of neonatal seizures. *UpToDate*. Retrieved on May 5, 2023, from https://www.uptodate.com/contents/clinical-features-evaluation-and-diagnosis-of-neonatal-seizures

Singer, R. J., Ogilvy, C. S., & Rordorf, G. (2022). Brain arteriovenous malformations. *UpToDate*. Retrieved May 5, 2023, from https://www.uptodate.com/contents/brain-arteriovenous-malformations

U.S. Department of Health and Human Services. (n.d.). *Healthy People 2030*. https://health.gov/healthypeople

Wilfong, A. (2022). Seizures and epilepsy in children: Classification, etiology, and clinical features. *UpToDate*. Retrieved May 4, 2023, from https://www.uptodate.com/contents/seizures-and-epilepsy-in-children-classification-etiology-and-clinical-features

DEVELOPING CLINICAL JUDGMENT

PRACTICING FOR NCLEX

1. When compared with adults, why are infants and children at an increased risk of head trauma? Select all that apply.
- **a.** The head of the infant and young child is large in proportion to the body.
- **b.** The development of the nervous system is complete at birth but remains immature.
- **c.** The spine is very immobile in infants and young children.
- **d.** The skull is more flexible due to the presence of sutures and fontanels.
- **e.** The neck muscles are not well developed.
- **f.** Infants and children have a high activity level.

2. At a well-child visit, hydrocephalus may be suspected in an infant if upon assessment the nurse finds:
- **a.** Narrow sutures
- **b.** Sunken fontanels
- **c.** A rapid increase in head circumference
- **d.** Increase in weight since last visit

3. A 10-year-old child is admitted to the hospital due to history of seizure activity. As the child's nurse, you are called into the room by their parent, who states the child is having a seizure. What would be the priority nursing intervention?
- **a.** Prevention of injury by removing the child from their bed
- **b.** Prevention of injury by placing a tongue blade in the child's mouth
- **c.** Prevention of injury by restraining the child
- **d.** Prevention of injury by placing the child on their side and opening their airway

4. A 6-month-old infant is admitted to the hospital with suspected bacterial meningitis. The child is crying, irritable, and lying in the opisthotonic position. The priority nursing intervention would be:
- **a.** Educate the family on ways to prevent bacterial meningitis.
- **b.** Initiate appropriate isolation precautions and begin intravenous antibiotics.
- **c.** Assess the infant's fontanels.
- **d.** Encourage the parent to hold the infant and feed the child.

5. The nurse is caring for an 8-year-old child involved in a bicycle accident. The child was not wearing a helmet, and a head injury has been diagnosed.

Nurse's Notes

Time	Notes
1200	Spontaneously opens eyes, vomited x1, c/o headache and dizziness
1300	Sleeping, respiratory rate irregular

Vital signs

Time	Temperature	Pulse	Respiratory Rate	Blood Pressure
1200	37.1°C (98.8°F)	76 beats per minute	16 breaths per minute	129/85
1300	36.9°C (98.4°F)	52 beats per minute	12 breaths per minute	148/92

Which assessment findings indicate the child's condition is worsening? Select all that apply.
- **a.** Pulse of 52 bpm
- **b.** Dizziness
- **c.** Headache
- **d.** Irregular respiratory rate
- **e.** Vomited × 1
- **f.** BP 148/92 mm Hg
- **g.** Sleeping
- **h.** Spontaneously opens eyes
- **i.** 12 breaths per minute

6. The nurse is caring for a child in the emergency department. The parent reports the child had a seizure at home about an hour ago. Which assessment findings support a diagnosis of a simple febrile seizure? Select all that apply.
- **a.** A history of a respiratory illness for the past 24 hours
- **b.** No family history of seizures
- **c.** A fever of 39.5°C (103.1°F)
- **d.** Child is currently lethargic.
- **e.** The seizure lasted less than 2 minutes
- **f.** Child is 18 months old.

DOSAGE CALCULATION QUESTION

The nurse is caring for a child who is in status epilepticus. The child weighs 14.97 kg (33 lb). The medication order reads: Diazepam 3 mg IV push now. Per the Pediatric Dosage Handbook, the recommended dose is 0.1 to 0.3 mg/kg/dose. Diazepam is supplied as 5 mg/mL.

How many milliliters will the nurse administer? Round to the nearest tenth.

CRITICAL THINKING EXERCISES

1. A child is seen in the doctor's office after hitting their head while skateboarding. The child suffered no loss of consciousness and has no external injuries and no significant past medical history. The child is acting appropriately at this time. Their only complaint is a dull headache. What instructions would you give the parents regarding the child's care at home? Include when they should seek further medical care.

2. A 10-year-old child is admitted to the pediatric unit after experiencing a seizure. A complete, accurate, and detailed history from a reliable source is essential. What information would you ask for while obtaining the history?
3. A 6-year-old child is admitted to the hospital because of a possible seizure. The child's parent calls the nurse to the room because the child is "jerking all over" and won't respond when they call the child's name. List appropriate nursing interventions for this child. Prioritize the list of interventions.
4. Describe the impact of a cerebral vascular accident in the child as compared with the adult. How does it affect the child's future? How will the nurse provide care differently for the child stroke victim as compared with the adult?

STUDY ACTIVITIES

1. A 4-month-old child with a history of hydrocephalus has undergone surgery for placement of a VP shunt. What information would you include in the teaching plan?
2. Develop an example of a "headache log" that could be used by the family for chronicling the child's headaches, including triggers, relieving factors, and precipitating events. Ensure that the log is developed at a 6th-grade reading level to make it practical for parents with low literacy levels.
3. In the clinical setting, interview the parent of a child who has suffered significant brain trauma or injury (such as head trauma, IVH, or stroke). Talk with the family about the types of care the child requires. Reflect on this interview in your clinical journal, and compare how the ongoing care for this child compares with that for a typical child.

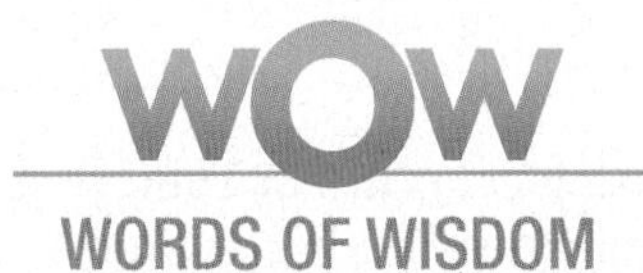

WORDS OF WISDOM

The child's senses provide an opportunity to explore the world.

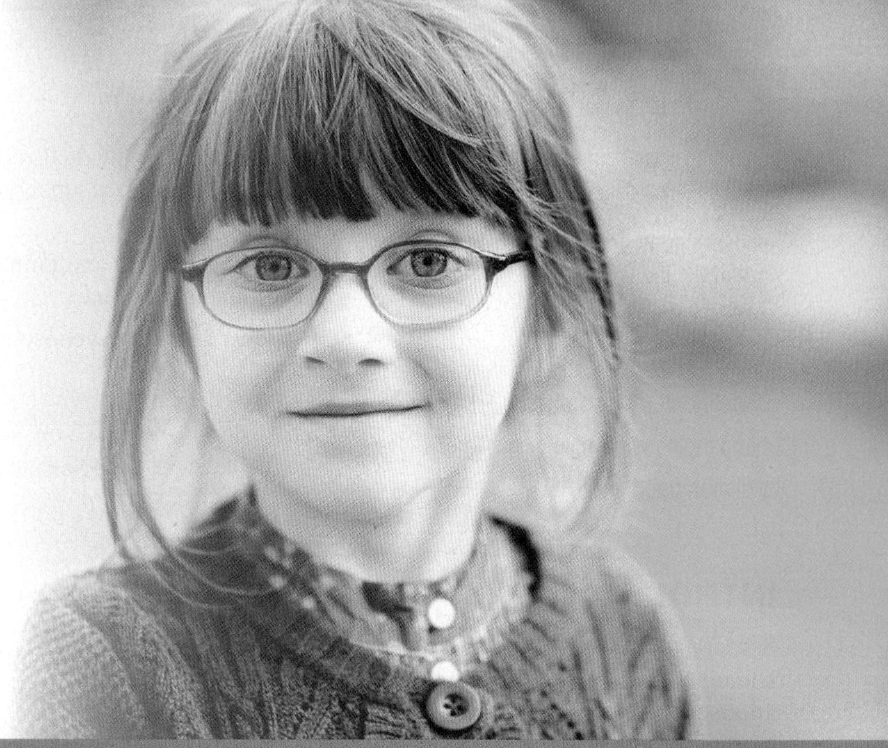

39

Nursing Care of the Child With an Alteration in Sensory Perception/ Disorder of the Eyes or Ears

LEARNING OBJECTIVES

Upon completion of the chapter, you will be able to:

1. Differentiate between the anatomic and physiologic differences of the eyes and ears in children as compared to adults.
2. Identify various factors associated with disorders of the eyes and ears in infants and children.
3. Discuss common laboratory and other diagnostic tests useful in the diagnosis of disorders of the eyes and ears.
4. Discuss common medications and other treatments used for treatment and palliation of conditions affecting the eyes and ears.
5. Recognize risk factors associated with various disorders of the eyes and ears.
6. Distinguish between different disorders of the eyes and ears based on the signs and symptoms associated with them.
7. Discuss nursing interventions commonly used in regard to disorders of the eyes and ears.

KEY TERMS

acuity
amblyopia (am′blē-ō′pē-ă)
blindness
conductive hearing loss
deafness
decibel (des′i-bĕl)
hearing impairment
nystagmus (nis-tag′mŭs)

pressure-equalizing (PE) tubes
ptosis (tō´sis)
sensorineural hearing loss (sen´sŏr-ē-nŭr´ăl hēr´ing laws)
sensory perception
strabismus (stră-biz´mŭs)
tympanometry (tim´pă-nom´ĕ-trē)
tympanostomy (tim´pă-nos´tŏ-mē)
vision impairment

8. Devise an individualized nursing care plan or concept map for the child with a sensory impairment or other disorders of the eyes or ears.
9. Develop child and family teaching plans for the child with a disorder of the eyes or ears.
10. Describe the psychosocial impact of sensory impairments on children.

Enrique Baxter, a 9-month-old, is brought to the clinic by his parent. His parent tells you, "Enrique has been fussy and not eating or sleeping well for the past 2 days."

INTRODUCTION

Sensory perception refers to receiving and interpreting stimuli. Disorders of the eyes or ears may lead to alterations in sensory perception. It is important for nurses to understand how to appropriately intervene for sensory perception alterations as well as other eye and ear disorders.

Children commonly suffer from disorders related to the eyes and ears. Conjunctivitis and otitis media are two common infectious and inflammatory disorders that affect the child's eyes or ears. Various alterations such as refractive error, strabismus, and amblyopia affect the development of visual acuity in children. Any alteration in the ear that contributes to the sensory perception alteration of hearing loss may have a significant impact on the child's language acquisition. It is important for the nurse to understand the impact of eye and ear disorders on the child's development.

Some children may be born with anomalies of the eyes or ears that will have a significant impact on vision and hearing, as well as psychomotor development. Disorders affecting the eyes or ears, particularly if chronic or recurrent, can have a significant impact on the development of visual acuity or may cause **hearing impairment** (varying degrees of hearing loss). In addition, the nurse may be caring for a child with another problem who is also either visually or hearing impaired. The nurse must take these developmental differences into account when planning care for these children.

VARIATIONS IN PEDIATRIC ANATOMY AND PHYSIOLOGY

The anatomy of children's eyes and ears differs somewhat from that of adults. In addition, visual **acuity** (sharpness of vision) develops from birth throughout early childhood. Hearing is intact at birth, but recurrent ear disorders may adversely affect the child's hearing.

Eyes

Light-skinned children are often born with blue eyes. The iris becomes pigmented over time, and eye color is determined by 6 to 12 months of age. The newborn's sclera may be slightly bluish tinged but becomes white within weeks. The eyeball of the infant and young child occupies a relatively larger space within the orbit than the adult's does, making it more susceptible to injury (Fig. 39.1).

Newborns have immature vision. The optic nerve is not fully myelinated until age 3 months, and the spherical shape of the newborn's lens negatively affects distance

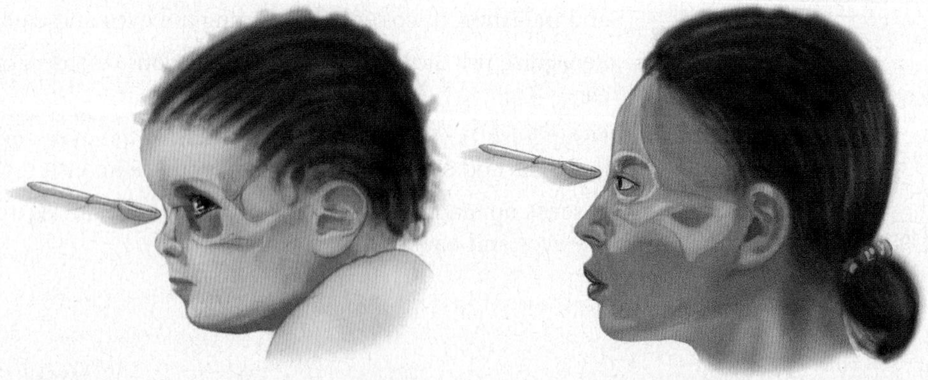

FIGURE 39.1 The relatively larger space that the infant's and young child's eyeball occupies within the orbit makes it more susceptible to injury as compared with the adult's eye.

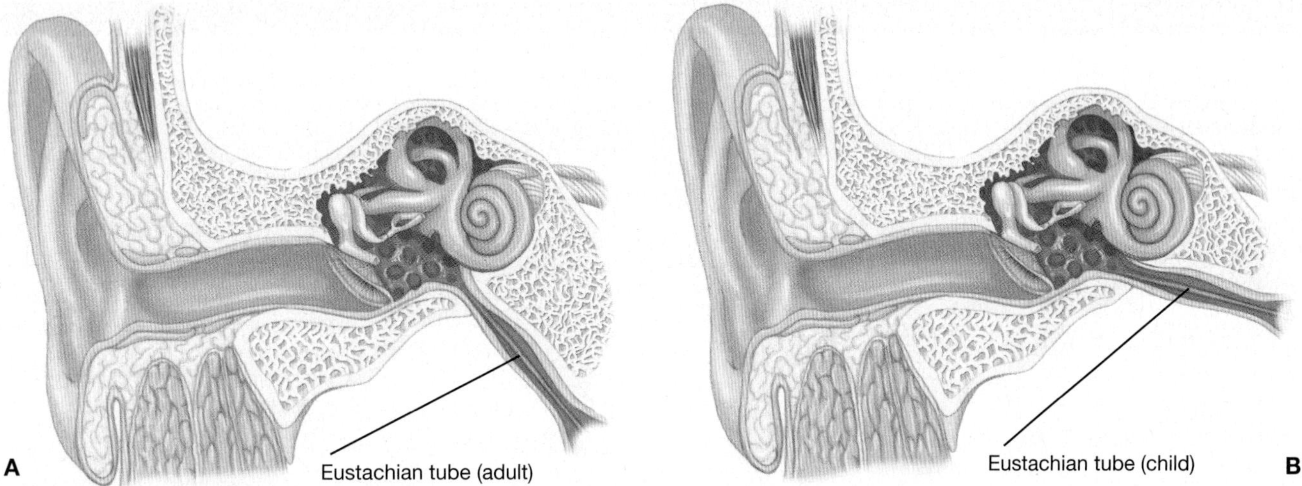

FIGURE 39.2 Note the child's relatively shorter, wider eustachian tubes and their horizontal positioning (**B**) as compared with the adult's (**A**).

accommodation (Olitsky & Marsh, 2020). At birth, visual acuity range is around 20/400. Visual acuity improves over the first few years of the child's life, with 20/20 usually achieved by age 5 years (Coats, 2023). The rectus muscles are uncoordinated at birth and mature over time so that binocular vision (the ability to focus with both eyes simultaneously) may be achieved between 3 and 7 months of age (Coats, 2023). In the preterm infant, retinal vascularization is incomplete, so visual acuity may be affected (Bhatt, 2023).

Ears

Congenital deformities of the ear are often associated with other body system anomalies and genetic syndromes. The presence of ear anomalies may lead to the search for, and subsequent diagnosis of, the other anomalies or syndromes. The infant's relatively short, wide, and horizontally placed eustachian tubes allow bacteria and viruses to gain access to the middle ear easily, resulting in increased numbers of ear infections as compared to the adult (Yoon et al., 2022). As the child matures, the tubes assume a more slanted position. Therefore, older children and adults generally have fewer cases of middle ear effusion and infection (Fig. 39.2). Sometimes enlargement of the adenoids contributes to obstruction of the eustachian tubes, leading to infection.

COMMON MEDICAL TREATMENTS

A variety of interventions are used to treat disorders of the eyes and ears in children. The treatments listed in Common Medical Treatments 39.1 and Drug Guide 39.1 usually require a health care provider's order when a child is hospitalized.

COMMON MEDICAL TREATMENTS 39.1

Treatment	Explanation	Indications	Nursing Implications
Warm compress	Warm, moist washcloth	Conjunctivitis	• Use very warm water from the tap (to avoid risk of burning, do not microwave).
Corrective lenses	In eyeglass form or as contact lenses	Correction of astigmatism, refractive error, strabismus	• Use a safety strap to help young children wear their eyeglasses.
Patching	An adhesive patch is applied to the healthier eye for several hours each day.	Strabismus, amblyopia, any other eye condition that results in one eye being weaker than the other	• Inform parents that though difficult to obtain, compliance with patching is critical. • A "pirate patch" may coax preschoolers into compliance.
Eye muscle surgery	Surgical alignment of the eyes	Strabismus	• Protect the operative site with patching. • Use elbow restraints if necessary.

(*continued*)

COMMON MEDICAL TREATMENTS 39.1 (*continued*)

Treatment	Explanation	Indications	Nursing Implications
Pressure-equalizing tubes (tympanostomy tubes)	Tiny plastic tubes inserted in the tympanic membrane	Chronic otitis media with effusion	• Teach parents dry ears precautions if prescribed or preferred by the surgeon. • Dry ears can be achieved by placing a cotton ball coated in petroleum jelly over the ear canal, in order to create a watertight seal.
Hearing aids	Amplification device worn in the ear	Hearing impairment	• Ensure appropriate fit and adequate amplification. • Direct families to outfitters that provide loaner aids of various brands and styles to determine best fit and amplification for the child.
Cochlear implants	Surgically inserted electronic prosthetic device	Sensorineural hearing loss	• Inform families that the usual minimum age for this procedure is 12 months.

Data from National Institute on Deafness and Other Communication Disorders. (2021). *Cochlear implants.* https://www.nidcd.nih.gov/health/cochlear-implants; Yoon, P. J., Scholes, M. A., & Herrmann, B. W. (2022). Ear, nose, & throat. In M. Bunik, W. W. Hay, M. J. Levin, & M. J. Abzug (Eds.), *Current diagnosis & treatment: Pediatrics* (26th ed.). McGraw-Hill Education.

DRUG GUIDE 39.1

COMMON DRUGS FOR EAR AND EYE DISORDERS

Medication	Actions	Indications	Nursing Implications
Antibiotics (oral, otic, ophthalmic)	Treatment of bacterial infections of the eyes and ears	Acute otitis media, otitis externa, conjunctivitis	Teach families to complete the entire course as prescribed. Check for drug allergies prior to administration.
Antihistamines	Block histamine reaction	Allergic conjunctivitis	Topical drops used. Oral agents usually prescribed if allergic rhinitis accompanies the conjunctivitis.
Analgesics	Pain relief	Otitis media, otitis externa, after eye or ear surgery	Narcotic analgesics may be necessary in some instances.

Data from UpToDate, Inc. (2024). *Lexicomp®* (Version 7.7.0) [Mobile app]. Wolters Kluwer. https://apps.apple.com/us/app/lexicomp/id313401238

COMMON LABORATORY AND DIAGNOSTIC TESTS 39.1

Test	Explanation	Indications	Nursing Implications
Culture of eye or ear discharge	Fluid draining from the eye or ear is cultured.	To determine specific bacteria present and appropriate antibiotic coverage	Easy to collect, relatively pain free. If drainage must be removed from within the ear canal, more likely to be painful
Tympanic fluid culture	Culture of fluid aspirated from the middle ear	To determine specific bacteria present and appropriate antibiotic coverage	Painful; usually performed only by specially trained health care providers
Tympanometry	Probe in ear canal measures movement of the eardrum.	Determines extent of effusion of the middle ear	Quick and easy to perform (seconds). Requires accurate-sized probe for adequate seal of the ear canal

Data from Yoon, P. J., Scholes, M. A., & Herrmann, B. W. (2022). Ear, nose, & throat. In M. Bunik, W. W. Hay, M. J. Levin, & M. J. Abzug (Eds.), *Current diagnosis & treatment: Pediatrics* (26th ed.). McGraw-Hill Education.

Clinical Judgment and the Nursing Process

Nursing care of the child with a disorder of the eyes or ears includes assessment, nursing analysis, planning, interventions, and evaluation. There are a number of general concepts related to the nursing process that can be applied to disorders of the eyes and ears. From an overall understanding of the care involved for a child with alterations in the eyes or ears, the nurse can then individualize care based on child and family specifics.

Assessment

Assessment of disorders of the eyes and ears in children includes health history, physical assessment, and laboratory or diagnostic testing.

Health History

The health history consists of past medical history, family history, history of present illness, and treatments used at home. The past medical history may be significant for prematurity, genetic defect, eye or ear deformities, visual acuity deficit or blindness, hearing impairment or **deafness** (the complete inability to hear sound), recurrent ear infections, or ear surgeries. Family history might be significant for eye or ear deformities or vision or hearing impairment or may reveal contacts for infectious exposure.

When eliciting the history of the present illness, inquire about its onset and progression and the presence of fever, nasal congestion, eye or ear pain, eye rubbing, ear pulling, headache, lethargy, or behavioral changes. Document if the child has corrective lenses or hearing aids prescribed and to what extent these devices are actually used.

Physical Examination

When assessing the eyes and ears, begin with inspection and observation. In addition, testing of visual activity and hearing may be performed.

INSPECTION AND OBSERVATION

Begin the physical examination with inspection and observation. Note whether the child uses eyeglasses, corrective lenses, or a hearing aid. Observe the eyes: note their positioning and symmetry and the presence of strabismus, nystagmus, and squinting. The eyelids should open equally (failure to open fully is termed **ptosis**). Note variations in eye slant and the presence of epicanthal folds. Assess the eyes for the presence of eyelid edema, sclera color, discharge, tearing, and pupillary equality, as well as the size and shape of the pupils.

Evert the eyelid to inspect the palpebral conjunctivae for redness. Test for extraocular movements and pupillary light response and accommodation. Note the symmetry of the corneal light reflex. Note the presence of the red reflex with an ophthalmoscope. Perform an age-appropriate visual acuity test. Refer to Chapter 31 for more detailed information related to visual acuity testing.

TAKE NOTE!

Attempts to inspect the palpebral conjunctivae may be frightening to children. Ask the older, cooperative child to evert the eyelid themselves while the nurse inspects the conjunctivae.

Inspect the ears: note their size and shape, position, and the presence of skin tags, dimples, or other anomalies (Fig. 39.3). Note that otoscopic examination is usually only performed by the advanced practice nurse. Upon otoscopic examination, note the presence of cerumen, discharge, inflammation, or a foreign body in the ear canal. Visualize the tympanic membrane and observe its color, landmarks, and light reflex, as well as the presence of perforation, scars, bulging, or retraction. Tympanic membrane mobility may be tested with

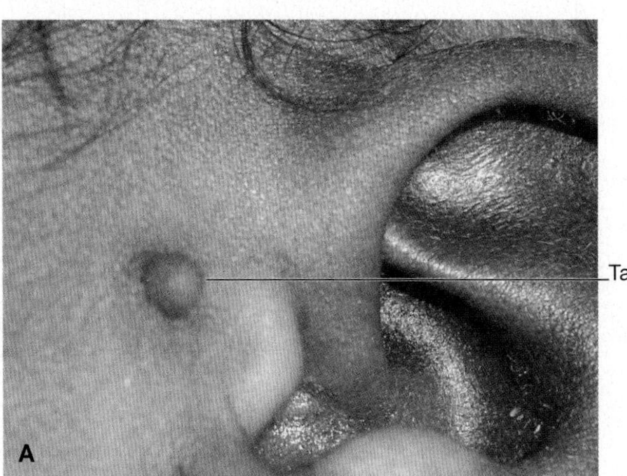

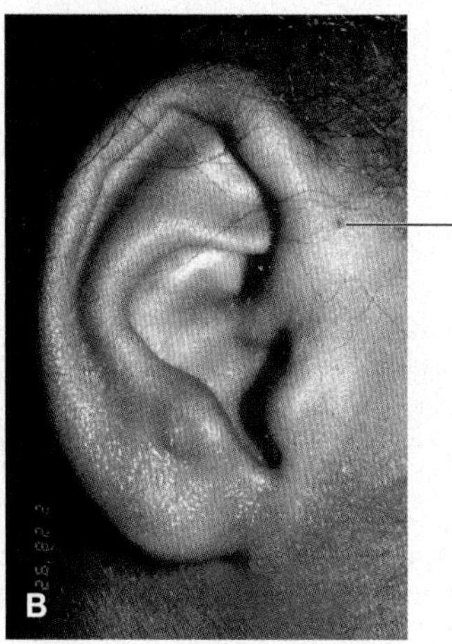

FIGURE 39.3 Note the skin tag (**A**) and preauricular pit (**B**) (in front of the ear).

pneumatic otoscopy. Auditory acuity is tested via the whisper test, audiometry, or other age-appropriate tests (refer to Chapter 31 for a more detailed explanation of hearing testing).

PALPATION

Usually, the eyes are not palpated. In the case of injury, the upper eyelid may be everted for examination purposes. Palpate the ear for tenderness over the tragus or pinna. Note the presence of tenderness over the mastoid area (tenderness may be present when otitis media progresses to mastoiditis). Palpate for enlarged cervical lymph nodes (this occurs when the eyes or ears are infected).

Laboratory and Diagnostic Testing

Common Laboratory and Diagnostic Tests 39.1 offers an explanation of the laboratory and diagnostic tests most commonly used for disorders of the eyes and ears. These tests can assist the health care provider or nurse practitioner in diagnosing the disorder and can be used as guidelines in determining ongoing treatment. Laboratory or nonnursing personnel obtain some of the tests, while the nurse may obtain others. In either instance, be familiar with how the tests are obtained, what they are used for, and normal versus abnormal results. This knowledge will also be necessary when providing child and family education related to the testing.

> Remember Enrique, the 9-month-old with fussiness and poor feeding who was not sleeping well? What additional health history and physical examination assessment information should you obtain?

Nursing Analysis

After recognizing and analyzing cues from a thorough assessment, the nurse might identify several patient problems, including the following:

- Physical trauma risk
- Fear
- Delayed development risk
- Impaired verbal communication
- Deficient knowledge
- Pain
- Interrupted family processes

> After completing an assessment of Enrique, the nurse noted the following: fever, tugging at his ears, and increased crying when lying down. Based on the assessment findings, what would your top three problems be for Enrique?

The preceding nursing analyses provide suggestions for nursing care planning or concept mapping. Suggested interventions with rationales are provided further. Care planning or concept mapping should be individualized, based on the child's and family's needs. Refer to Chapter 36 for the nursing care plan for pain management and to Chapter 33 for nursing interventions related to interrupted family processes. Additional information will be included later in the chapter as it relates to nursing management of children with specific disorders, as well as specific nursing interventions for deficient knowledge depending upon the disorder.

Nursing Analysis

Physical trauma risk related to insufficient vision

Goal/Outcome

The infant or child will remain free from physical trauma.

Preventing Physical Trauma (interventions with *rationale*)

- Orient the child to hospital surroundings *because awareness is the first step to preventing injury.*
- Encourage parent to be at bedside *so that the child feels more comfortable.*
- Encourage use of assistive devise *to promote safety.*

Nursing Analysis

Fear related to sensory deficit (severe visual impairment or blindness) and unfamiliar setting as evidenced by apprehensiveness or verbalization of feeling of alarm

Goal/Outcome

Child will experience decreased fear: child will verbalize comfort with environment or react calmly to interventions.

Decreasing Fear (interventions with *rationale*)

- Allow the verbal child to share their feelings *to promote coping in the child.*
- For the child who is severely impaired or the child who is blind, identify yourself via voice, and name items in the environment for the child *so that the child is aware of their surroundings.*
- Engage the parents in bedside caregiving *because the parents' voice and presence are reassuring to the child.*
- Encourage nutritious diet according to child's preferences *to assist body's natural infection-fighting mechanisms.*
- Isolate the child as required *to prevent nosocomial spread of infection.*
- Teach child and family preventive measures such as good handwashing, covering mouth and nose when coughing or sneezing, and adequate disposal of used tissues *to prevent nosocomial or community spread of infection.*

Nursing Analysis

Delayed development risk related to impaired vision or hearing impairment

Goal/Outcome

Child will achieve optimum independence for age: child participates in age-appropriate developmental activities.

Encouraging Development (interventions with *rationale*)

- Encourage attainment of developmental milestones with use of assistive devices as needed *for timely developmental achievements.*
- Foster independence in activities of daily living (ADLs) *to promote sense of accomplishment.*
- Encourage participation in play with another child or within a group *to promote socialization.*
- Assist family to set limits and apply discipline *because structure and routine provide a secure environment in which the developing child can grow.*
- Encourage friendships with other children with a sensory impairment *to promote socialization and let the child know that they are not the only one with these challenges.*

Nursing Analysis

Impaired verbal communication related to physiologic condition (hearing loss) as evidenced by difficulty verbalizing or inappropriate verbalization

Goal/Outcome

The child will communicate effectively with the method chosen by the family (this may be sign language, oral/deaf speech, cued speech, or augmentative alternative communication device).

Improving Communication (interventions with *rationale*)

- Encourage choice of and attendance at communication habilitation program *to promote continued learning.*
- Provide consistency between home and hospital in regard to communication style/devices *to optimize communication.*
- Support the child's efforts at correct speech *to promote speech development through reinforcement and praise.*
- Encourage family to use spoken language and read books at home *to continue to promote appropriate language development.*

Nursing Analysis

Deficient knowledge related to insufficient information or knowledge of resources (about sensory impairment)

Goal/Outcome

Parents express understanding of medical diagnosis and care of child: parents verbalize understanding, demonstrate use of assistive devices, or independently perform medical treatments.

Educating the Family (interventions with *rationale*)

- Review medical diagnosis and plan of care with the parents *to promote understanding of the disease process.*
- Refer family to resources available for children with sensory impairment *to provide further education and support to the parents.*
- Demonstrate medical treatments prescribed or use of assistive devices, requiring a return demonstration, *which shows the parents' ability to provide the prescribed care for the child.*
- Encourage exploration of different communication and learning modes available for the child with sensory impairment *to allow the child and family to find the right educational and communication style fit.*

Based on your top three problems for Enrique, describe appropriate nursing interventions.

INFECTIOUS AND INFLAMMATORY DISORDERS OF THE EYES

Infectious and inflammatory disorders of the eyes include conjunctivitis, nasolacrimal duct obstruction, eyelid lesions, and periorbital cellulitis.

Conjunctivitis

Inflammation of the bulbar or palpebral conjunctiva is referred to as conjunctivitis. It can be infectious, allergic, or chemical in nature. Viruses or bacteria may cause infectious conjunctivitis. Adenoviruses and influenza account for the bulk of cases of viral conjunctivitis. The most common bacterial causes are *Staphylococcus aureus*, *Streptococcus pneumoniae*, and *Haemophilus influenzae* (Howard & de St. Maurice, 2021). In the newborn, *Chlamydia trachomatis* and *Neisseria gonorrhoeae* are more common causes. Infectious conjunctivitis is very contagious, so epidemics are common, particularly in young children. Risk factors for acute infectious conjunctivitis include age younger than 2 weeks; day care, preschool, or school attendance; concomitant viral upper respiratory infection; pharyngitis; or otitis media. Concurrent acute otitis media (AOM) may occur depending on the bacterial cause. Complications from simple infectious conjunctivitis are uncommon. Neonates with chlamydial conjunctivitis may be at risk for the development of chlamydial pneumonia.

Allergic conjunctivitis results from exposure to particular allergens. Allergic conjunctivitis may be a seasonal or year-round complaint. A genetic predisposition to allergic conjunctivitis exists, just as it does for asthma, allergic rhinitis, and atopic dermatitis. Allergic conjunctivitis occurs more frequently in school-age children and adolescents than it does in infants and young children because of repeat exposure to allergens over time. In the case of seasonal allergic conjunctivitis, the severity of symptoms and the number of children affected are directly related to the pollen count in the area.

Pathophysiology

When bacteria or viruses come in contact with the bulbar or palpebral conjunctiva, they are recognized as foreign antigens and an antigen–antibody immune reaction occurs, resulting in inflammation. Allergic conjunctivitis occurs through a different mechanism. Contact with the allergen results in an allergic response (overreaction of the immune response). The mast cell and histamine mediators are then activated, resulting in inflammation.

Therapeutic Management

Therapeutic management of conjunctivitis is prescribed depending on the cause. Bacterial conjunctivitis is generally treated with an ophthalmic antibiotic preparation (drops or ointment). Viral conjunctivitis is a self-limiting disease and does not require topical medication. Eye drops with an antihistamine or mast cell stabilization effect may be helpful in alleviating symptoms of allergic conjunctivitis. If other allergy signs and symptoms are also present, an oral antihistamine may also be prescribed. Table 39.1 compares bacterial, viral, and allergic conjunctivitis.

Nursing Assessment

Nursing assessment of the child with conjunctivitis, regardless of the cause, is similar. It includes health history, physical examination, and, in rare instances, laboratory testing.

Health History

Elicit a description of the present illness and chief complaint. Common signs and symptoms reported during the health history might include the following:

- Redness
- Edema
- Tearing
- Discharge
- Eye pain
- Itching of the eyes (usually with allergic conjunctivitis)

Determine the onset of symptoms and their progression as well as response to treatments used at home. Assess for risk factors for infectious conjunctivitis, such as day care or school attendance. Note any history of an upper respiratory infection, sore throat, or earache. Question parents about possible infectious exposure. Review the health history for risk factors for allergic conjunctivitis, such as a family history and a history of asthma, allergic rhinitis, or atopic dermatitis. Determine seasonality related to the symptoms and whether the symptoms occur after exposure to particular allergens, such as pollen, hay, or animals.

Physical Examination

Observe for eyelid swelling or redness. Inspect the conjunctivae for redness (Fig. 39.4). Note quantity, color, and consistency of discharge. Bacterial infections generally result in a thick, colored discharge, whereas a clear or white discharge is generally seen with viral conjunctivitis. Allergic conjunctivitis often results in a watery discharge, sometimes profuse, which is usually present bilaterally. Contact with an allergen rubbed into one of the eyes may result in unilateral symptoms. Observe the child for other signs of allergic or atopic disease and document the presence of a runny nose or cough as well.

Laboratory and Diagnostic Tests

Cases of bacterial, viral, and allergic conjunctivitis are generally diagnosed based on history and clinical presentation. Cases of viral and allergic conjunctivitis do not warrant laboratory testing. If bacterial conjunctivitis is suspected, then a bacterial culture of the eye drainage may be performed to determine the exact causative organism, thus allowing the most appropriate antibiotic to be prescribed.

Nursing Management

Nursing management of the various types of conjunctivitis focuses on alleviating symptoms and, for infectious causes, preventing spread.

TABLE 39.1 • Types of Conjunctivitis

Type of Conjunctivitis	Conjunctivae	Discharge	Additional Findings	Eyelid Edema	Treatment
Bacterial	Inflamed	Purulent, mucoid	Mild pain	Occasional	Antibiotic drops or ointment
Viral	Inflamed	Watery, mucoid	Lymphadenopathy, photophobia, tearing	Usually present	Symptom relief; antiherpetic agent if cause is herpes
Allergic	Inflamed	Watery or stringy	Itching	Usually present	Antihistamine and/or mast cell stabilizer drops

Data from Mehner, L., & Jung, J. L. (2022). Eye. In M. Bunik, W. W. Hay, M. J. Levin, & M. J. Abzug (Eds.), *Current diagnosis & treatment: Pediatrics* (26th ed.). McGraw-Hill Education.

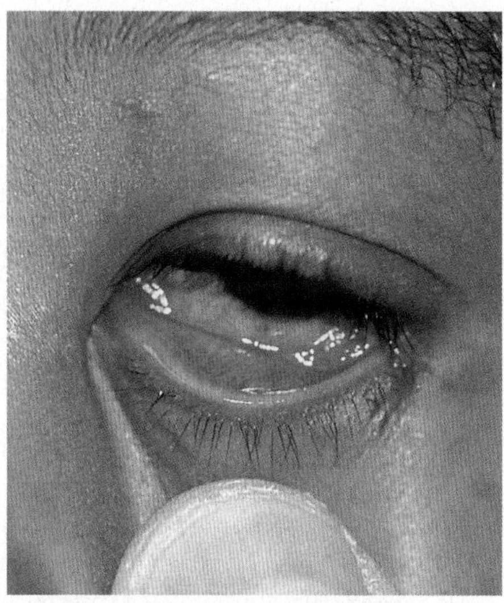

FIGURE 39.4 Note redness of conjunctiva.

Alleviating Symptoms

Teach parents how to apply eye drops or ointment (antibiotic for bacterial causes and antihistamine or mast cell stabilizer for allergic causes). Warm compresses may be used to help loosen the crust that accumulates on the eyelids overnight when drainage is copious, particularly with bacterial conjunctivitis.

• • • ATRAUMATIC CARE • • •

When instilling ear drops in the young child, use distraction (a song, a favorite toy) to decrease perceived trauma to the child.

The child with allergic conjunctivitis may experience perennial or seasonal allergies (or both). Encourage the child to avoid perennial allergens once the offending allergen is determined (refer to Chapter 40 for additional information related to education about perennial allergen avoidance). Seasonal allergies may include tree pollen in the winter or spring, grass pollen in the summer, and ragweed or flower pollen in the fall.

It is impossible to completely eliminate seasonal allergic responses, partly because it is important for children to participate in physical activity outdoors. Teach families to minimize seasonal allergens on the child's skin and hair. Educate families to:

- Encourage the child not to rub or touch the eyes.
- Rinse the child's eyelids periodically with a clean washcloth and cool water.
- Wash the child's face and hands when the child comes in from outdoors.
- Ensure that the child showers and shampoos before bedtime.

TAKE NOTE!

The itching of allergic conjunctivitis may be relieved with cool compresses. An easy way to accomplish this is to have the child hold a tube of yogurt over the affected eye.

Preventing Infectious Spread

Because infectious conjunctivitis is extremely contagious, the parent must wash hands diligently after caring for the child. Teach parents and children about appropriate handwashing and discourage them from sharing towels and washcloths. Children with viral conjunctivitis may return to school or day care when symptoms lessen. When mucopurulent drainage is no longer present (usually after 24 to 48 hours of treatment with a topical antibiotic), the child with bacterial conjunctivitis may safely return to day care or school (Jacobs, 2023a).

TAKE NOTE!

Avoid the use of vasoconstricting eye drops such as Visine to rid the eyes of redness. Rebound vasodilation may occur, and with it the redness returns. This leads to repeated frequent use of the drops to keep the eyes from being red but does not treat the actual cause of the redness (Lexicomp, 2024).

THINKING ABOUT **DEVELOPMENT**

Raisa Jordan is a 3-year-old who has been diagnosed with bacterial conjunctivitis and prescribed antibiotic eye drops. Based on her developmental stage, how will you assist her caregivers to administer the eye drops? How would this assistance change if the child was 12 years old?

Nasolacrimal Duct Obstruction

Stenosis or simple obstruction of the nasolacrimal duct is a common disorder of infancy, occurring in about 6% of newborns and infants (Paysse & Coats, 2023). Chronic tearing occurs, and buildup in the lacrimal sac causes a mucoid or mucopurulent drainage. About 66% of all cases resolve spontaneously by 6 months of age (Paysse & Coats, 2023). No apparent risk factors exist for the development of nasolacrimal duct obstruction or stenosis. Therapeutic management involves a watchful waiting approach. Massage may be prescribed, and if secondary bacterial infection is suspected or confirmed, antibiotic ointment or drops may be ordered. If the obstruction does not resolve spontaneously, then the pediatric ophthalmologist may probe the duct to relieve the obstruction (a brief outpatient procedure) (Paysse & Coats, 2023).

Nursing Assessment

Tearing or discharge from one or both eyes is often first noted at the 2-week check-up. Obtain a thorough history about the eye drainage to distinguish it from neonatal conjunctivitis. Determine the onset and progression of symptoms, as well as the newborn's response to any interventions attempted so far. Upon physical examination, note redness of the lower lid of the affected eye. If drainage is present, note its consistency, color, and quantity. Nasolacrimal duct obstruction is usually a diagnosis based on clinical presentation, but culture of the eye drainage may be used to rule out conjunctivitis or secondary bacterial infection (Fig. 39.5).

Nursing Management

Teach parents to clean the eye area frequently with a moist cloth. In addition, teach parents to massage the nasolacrimal duct, which may change the pressure and cause it to open, allowing drainage to occur. Refer to Teaching Guidelines 39.1 for appropriate nasolacrimal duct massage technique. Ensure that parents are educated about when and how to administer antibiotic eye drops if ordered.

Eyelid Disorders

Disorders of the eyelid include hordeolum (stye), chalazion, and blepharitis. Hordeolum is a localized infection of the sebaceous gland of the eyelid follicle, usually caused by bacterial invasion. Chalazion is a chronic painless infection of the meibomian gland. Blepharitis refers to chronic scaling and discharges along the eyelid

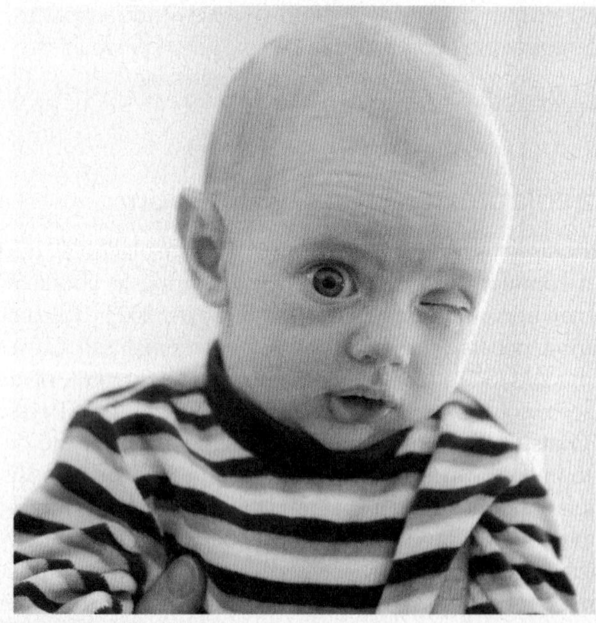

FIGURE 39.5 Mild eyelid redness and crusting are present in the infant with nasolacrimal duct stenosis.

TEACHING GUIDELINES 39.1 Nasolacrimal Duct Massage

- Using the forefinger or little finger, push on top of the bone (the puncta must be blocked).

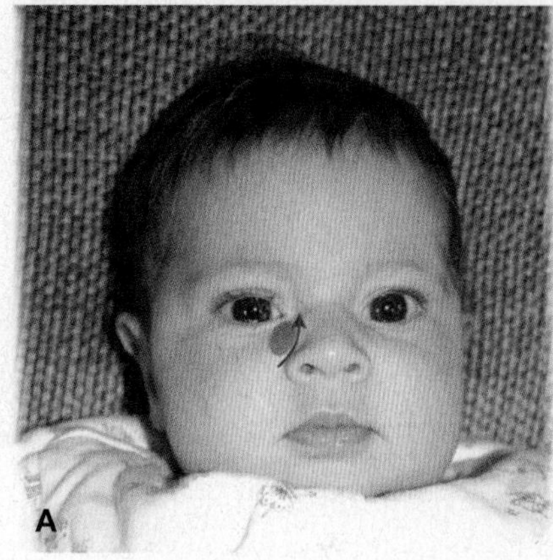

- Gently push in and up.

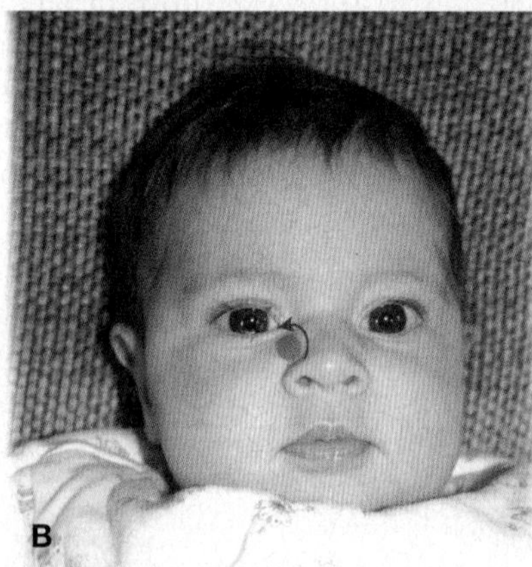

- Then gently push downward along the side of the nose.

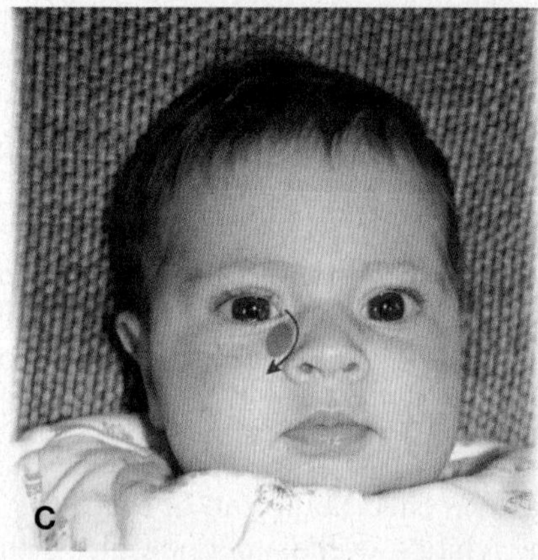

Adapted from Paysse, E. A., & Coats, D. K. (2023). Nasolacrimal duct obstruction (dacryostenosis) and dacryocystocele. *UpToDate*. Retrieved January 23, 2024, from https://www.uptodate.com/contents/congenital-nasolacrimal-duct-obstruction-dacryostenosis-and-dacryocystocele

margin. Chalazion may resolve spontaneously. Therapeutic management of hordeolum and blepharitis usually involves the use of antibiotic ointment.

Nursing Assessment

Determine the child's health history, noting onset of symptoms, extent and character of eye discharge, and presence of pain (hordeolum is usually painful). Inspect the eyelids, noting redness along the eyelid margin and presence of eyelid edema (hordeolum, blepharitis). Hordeolum may also be quite visible as an enlarged lesion along the lid margin, with purulent drainage present (Fig. 39.6). Chalazion may be visible as a small nodule on the lid margin. The conjunctivae remain clear with all three of these disorders.

Nursing Management

For hordeolum and blepharitis, instruct parents on how to administer antibiotic ointment. Encourage the use of hot, moist compresses. Inform parents that the stye may require several weeks to resolve completely. Also inform parents that chalazion will usually resolve spontaneously; if it does not, it may require minor surgical drainage.

EYE INJURIES

As mentioned earlier, infants and young children are more susceptible to eye injuries than adults since the eyeball is relatively larger in relation to the space within the orbit. Developmental maturity may also play a part in eye injuries. For example, as infants and toddlers learn to walk and run, they do not have the awareness and maturity to avert disaster. Older children involved in sports and school science experiments are also at risk for eye injuries. A few of the more common eye injuries are eyelid injuries, contusion, scleral hemorrhage, corneal abrasion, a foreign body in the eye, and chemical injury (Mehner & Jung, 2022).

Therapeutic management depends on the type of injury. Eyelid lacerations may require suturing. Deep lacerations may result in ptosis at a later date, so these children should be referred to an ophthalmologist. Simple contusions (black eye) usually need only observation, ice, and analgesics. Scleral hemorrhages resolve gradually without intervention over a few weeks. Corneal abrasions may be allowed to self-heal, or antibiotic ointment may be prescribed. Foreign bodies in the eye require removal to prevent further irritation or abrasion. Chemical injuries require irrigation and vision evaluation.

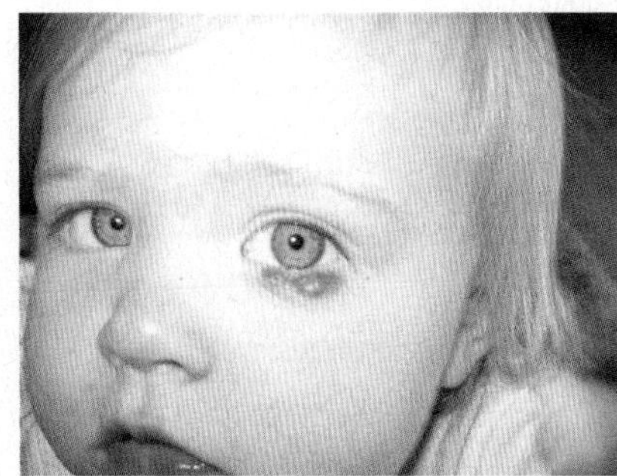

FIGURE 39.6 Hordeolum.

Nursing Assessment

When a child presents with an eye injury, it is important to obtain an accurate history related to the injury. Follow the history by performing a focused physical examination, which consists mostly of inspection and observation. It is important to determine whether an eye injury is nonemergent or emergent in order to provide rapid and appropriate treatment in the case of an emergency so that vision may be preserved.

Health History

Obtain an accurate history. Determine the mechanism of injury, and obtain as much detail about the injury as possible. Questions to ask during the health history include the following:

- When did the injury occur?
- What exactly happened?
- Was an object involved? If so, what type of object, and how fast was it going?
- Was it a splash injury?
- Was the child wearing eye protective gear or eyeglasses when the injury occurred?

Determine the extent of pain if present. Document photosensitivity, sensation of a foreign body in the eye, and blurry or lost vision. Inquire about past medical history, including previous eye injury or surgery or vision problems. Determine the child's immunization status.

Physical Examination

Regardless of the type of eye injury, the examination of the child's eye can be difficult. The nurse plays an important role in assisting the child and family to cope with the examination. Children with an eye injury often are in acute pain. The area surrounding the eye swells quickly after blunt trauma. Edema and tearing make the eye examination more difficult. Children are very frightened because of the pain and difficulty seeing. Approach the child in a calm and gentle manner. Soothe and coax the child as the eye is examined. Younger children may need to be restrained briefly in order for the examination to proceed safely.

Note the eyelid placement and look for signs of trauma such as bleeding, edema, and eyelid malformation. Evaluate the child's ability to open the eyes. Use a penlight to evaluate the pupils' response to light and

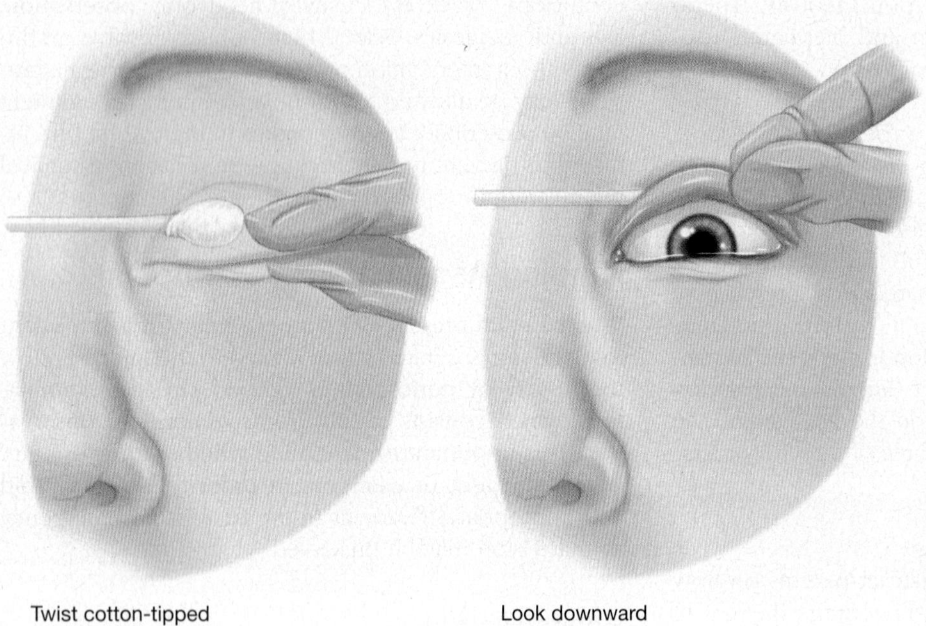

FIGURE 39.7 Eversion of the eyelid for examination. Place a cotton-tipped applicator over the eyelid. Pull the eyelid outward and up over the applicator.

accommodation (in the case of nonemergent eye trauma, the pupils should remain equally round and reactive to light and accommodation [PERRLA]). Note redness or irritation of the sclerae and/or conjunctivae. Observe for excessive tearing. Figure 39.7 shows the appropriate technique for eversion and examination of the interior of the eyelid.

In a nonemergent situation, evaluate visual acuity via the use of an age-appropriate vision screening tool (refer to Chapter 31 for additional information related to visual acuity screening). Table 39.2 provides assessment information specific to eyelid laceration, simple contusion, scleral hemorrhage, corneal abrasion, and foreign body in the eye.

TABLE 39.2 • Assessment of Eye Injuries

Description of Injury	Nursing Assessment
Eyelid injuries: May occur as laceration to the eyelid	• Laceration is noted at any point along the lid. • Vision is unaffected.
Simple contusion (black eye): Occurs as a result of blunt trauma to the eye area	• Bruising and edema of lids or area surrounding eye • PERRLA • Extraocular movements intact • Visual acuity intact • No diplopia or blurred vision • Pain surrounding eye but not within the eye
Scleral hemorrhage: Caused by blunt trauma or increased pressure such as with coughing	• Painless • Appears as erythema in the sclera; can be quite large initially • Vision unaffected
Corneal abrasion: Results from foreign body such as sand, grit, or other small object scratching the cornea	• May have tearing • Eye pain • PERRLA • Vision may be blurry. • Photophobia may be present.
Foreign body: May be dirt, glass, or other small particle	• Tearing • Complaint of "something in the eye" • PERRLA • Vision may be blurry.

PERRLA, pupils equally round and reactive to light and accommodation.

Data from Howard, L. M., & Annabelle de St. Maurice, A. (2021). Unraveling the impact of pneumococcal conjugate vaccines on bacterial conjunctivitis in children. *Clinical Infectious Diseases, 72*(7), 1208–1210. https://doi.org/10.1093/cid/ciaa202; Mehner, L., & Jung, J. L. (2022). Eye. In M. Bunik, W. W. Hay, M. J. Levin, & M. J. Abzug (Eds.), *Current diagnosis & treatment: Pediatrics* (26th ed.). McGraw-Hill Education.

TAKE NOTE!

If pupillary reaction is abnormal, vision is affected (decreased acuity from the child's norm, diplopia, or blurriness), or extraocular movements are affected, the child should be immediately referred to an ophthalmologist for further evaluation (Mehner & Jung, 2022).

Nursing Management

Refer children with urgent or emergent conditions to an ophthalmologist immediately to preserve vision. Non-emergent eye injuries usually need only simple management. Assist the health care provider or nurse practitioner with positioning and distraction of the child for eyelid laceration suturing. The child may require sedation or pain medication for this procedure.

To decrease edema in the child with a black eye (simple contusion), instruct the parent to apply an ice pack to the area for 20 minutes, then remove it for 20 minutes, and continue to repeat the cycle as often as possible during the first 24 hours. Tell the parents and child that bruising of the surrounding eye area may take up to 3 weeks to resolve.

Instruct the parents and child about the benign nature of the scleral hemorrhage (the appearance may be frightening). Educate parents about the natural history of resolution of the scleral hemorrhage without intervention over a period of a few weeks.

If the child with a corneal abrasion has pain, administer analgesics as needed. Tell parents that most corneal abrasions heal on their own. If an antibiotic ointment is prescribed, instruct the parents on how to administer the ointment appropriately.

TAKE NOTE!

Patching of the eye with a small, uncomplicated corneal abrasion or abrasion from a contact lens is not recommended. Patching does not result in decreased pain nor promote faster healing. In addition, it may place the child at risk for injury due to visual field loss while patched (Jacobs, 2023b).

Foreign bodies may be removed from the eye by gently everting the eyelid and wiping the foreign body away with a sterile cotton-tipped applicator. Irrigation with normal saline may also wash the foreign body away.

For chemical injury, irrigate the eye with copious amounts of water. Consult ophthalmology for further evaluation and management.

CLINICAL REASONING ALERT!

Refer the child with a large foreign body in the eye or one that is embedded in the globe of the eye to the ophthalmologist for appropriate, safe removal.

Eye injuries can be prevented, and nurses play a vital role in educating the public about prevention of eye injuries and use of appropriate safety equipment. See Evidence-Based Practice 39.1.

VISUAL DISORDERS

Adequate visual development requires appropriate sensory stimulation to both eyes over the first few years of life (Coats, 2023). When one or both eyes are deprived of this stimulation, visual development does not progress appropriately, and visual impairment or blindness may result. This may occur when the eyes are not aligned properly, visual acuity between the eyes is disparate, or other problems with the eyes exist (Coats, 2023). If vision disorders are diagnosed at an early age and treatment is begun, then vision may progress normally. However, when these disorders go untreated, the young child's developing vision may be reduced significantly. Therefore, it is important to appropriately screen children for these disorders. Common visual disorders in childhood include refractive errors, strabismus, amblyopia, nystagmus, glaucoma, and cataracts.

Refractive Errors

The most common cause of visual difficulties in children is refractive errors. When the light that enters the lens does not bend appropriately to allow it to fall directly

EVIDENCE-BASED PRACTICE 39.1
Antibiotic Ointment for Corneal Abrasions

STUDY

Simple corneal abrasions are a common eye complaint. Antibiotic ointment is often used for treatment. The authors reviewed randomized controlled trials comparing antibiotic use to other antibiotics and to placebo. Two trials with a total of 527 participants were included in the review.

Findings

The authors found the evidence lacking. The review did not demonstrate prevention of ocular infection nor acceleration of corneal abrasion healing with ophthalmic antibiotic use. It also did not find ill effects from antibiotic use.

Nursing Implications

Parents worry significantly when their child experiences even a very mild eye injury. Teach parents about the ability of the cornea to heal quickly from a minor abrasion.

Data from Algarni, A., Guyatt, G. H., Turner, A., & Alamri, S. (2022). Antibiotic patching for corneal abrasion. *Cochrane Database of Systematic Reviews, 5*, CD014617. https://doi.org/10.1002/14651858.CD014617.pub2

on the retina, a refractive error occurs. Infants and young children naturally have mild hyperopia (farsightedness) because the depth of the eye globe is not fully developed until about 5 years of age (Coats & Paysse, 2023c). These children may have blurriness at close range, but by school age this blurriness usually resolves. When the light entering the eye focuses in front of the retina, it results in myopia (nearsightedness). Children who are nearsighted may see well at close range but have difficulty focusing on the blackboard or other objects at a distance.

Therapeutic management for both hyperopia and myopia is prescription eyeglasses or contact lenses. Generally, a child 12 years of age can demonstrate the responsibility necessary to wear and care for contact lenses. Contact lenses may be used in younger children but are lost or damaged more readily. Because of the continuing refractive development in the child's vision through adolescence, laser surgery for vision correction is not recommended for most children (Mehner & Jung, 2022).

Nursing Assessment

Elicit the health history, noting blurred vision, complaints of eye fatigue with reading, or complaints of eye strain (headache, pulling sensation, or eye burning). Note complaints of difficulty concentrating on or maintaining a clear focus on objects up close, avoidance of up close work, or poor work performance (hyperopia). Note the risk factor of family history of myopia. Observe for squinting when the child looks at objects at a distance. Observe the hyperopic child for the presence of esotropia. Readily observable physical findings are not noted in the myopic child. Test visual acuity using an age-appropriate screening tool (for more information related to visual acuity screening, refer to Chapter 31). Hyperopia is usually not identified with visual acuity screening alone; it usually requires a retinal examination by an ophthalmologist.

Nursing Management

Nursing management of the child with a refractive error focuses on providing education about corrective lens use and monitoring for the need for new eyeglasses or contact lenses.

EDUCATING ABOUT EYEGLASS USE

Encourage the child with newly prescribed eyeglasses to wear them by having the parent spend "special time" with the child doing an activity that requires the glasses (such as reading or drawing). Provide positive reinforcement for wearing the glasses. Teach the parent and child to remove eyeglasses with both hands and to lay them on their side (not directly on the lens on any surface). Instruct the child and family about cleaning the glasses daily with mild soap and water or a commercial cleansing agent provided by the optometrist. Use a soft cloth to clean the glasses, not paper towels, tissues, or toilet paper.

CONSIDER THIS!

I can't believe I have to start wearing glasses! I have heard the other kids mock my classmates and call them "four-eyes." I'm old enough now to start wearing makeup and how will that look with glasses? I'll look like a nerd....

Thoughts: How will you respond to her worries? With this early adolescent, what will your approach be to ensure she wears her glasses as prescribed?

EDUCATING ABOUT CONTACT LENS USE

Teach the older child or adolescent how to care for the contact lenses properly, including lens hygiene and lens insertion and removal. Inform the child and parents that protective eyewear should be worn when the child is participating in contact sports. If the eye becomes inflamed, remove the contact lens and wear eyeglasses until the eye is improved. Consult with the child's eye care provider to determine if medications prescribed for an eye problem can be used while the contact lens is in.

MONITORING FOR FIT AND VISUAL CORRECTION

Encourage the family to complete visual assessments as scheduled. Since the child's vision is continuing to develop and refraction is not stable, the corrective lens prescription may change more frequently than it does in an adult. As the young child in particular is continuing to grow at a rapid rate, the head size is also changing (American Association for Pediatric Ophthalmology and Strabismus [AAPOS], 2023). Eyeglass frames may hurt or pinch the child as the child's head becomes larger. Teach families to check the fit of the glasses monthly. Monitor for signs of ill fit, such as constant removal of the glasses in an older child or rubbing at the glasses or eyes in the very young child. Monitor for squinting, eye fatigue or strain, and complaints of headache or dizziness, which may indicate the need for a change in the lens prescription. See the Healthy People 2030 box.

HEALTHY PEOPLE 2030

Objective	Nursing Significance
Increase the proportion of children aged 3–5 years who receive vision screening. Reduce visual loss from refractive errors. Reduce vision loss in children and adolescents.	• Ensure that visual acuity testing begins with an age-appropriate screening tool by 3 years of age and continues yearly throughout childhood and adolescence. • Refer for an eye evaluation any children with complaints of difficulty seeing the front of the classroom or complaints of eye strain or difficulty with close work. • Screen infants and children for asymmetric corneal light reflex for early detection of amblyopia.

Healthy People Objectives retrieved from http://www.healthypeople.gov

Strabismus

Strabismus refers to misalignment of the eyes. It is common and occurs in up to 4% of the population (Coats & Paysse, 2023b). The most common types of strabismus are exotropia and esotropia. In exotropia, the eyes turn outward; in esotropia, they turn inward. Because of this unequal alignment, visual development in each eye may proceed at different rates. Diplopia (double vision) may result, so vision in one eye may be "turned off" by the brain to avoid diplopia. Many infants have strabismus intermittently, but this usually resolves by 3 to 6 months of age. Persistent esotropia that persists past 4 months of age or constant strabismus at any age warrants referral to an ophthalmologist for further evaluation (Coats & Paysse, 2023b).

It is extremely important to treat strabismus appropriately in the developing years so that equal visual acuity may be achieved in both eyes. Therapeutic management of strabismus may include patching of the stronger eye or eye muscle surgery. Corrective lenses are also used for strabismus. Complications of strabismus include amblyopia and visual deficits.

Nursing Assessment

Parents may be the first people to notice that the child's eyes do not face in the same direction. Question parents about the onset of the problem and whether it is continuous or intermittent. If intermittent, does it occur more often when the child is tired? Elicit the health history, noting complaints of blurred vision, tired eyes, squinting or closing one eye in bright sunlight, tilting the head to focus on an object, or a history of bumping into objects (depth perception may be limited).

Observe the child's eyes for obvious exotropia or esotropia. In the absence of an obvious finding, assessment of the symmetry of the corneal light reflex is extremely helpful (Fig. 39.8). The "cover test" is also a useful tool for the identification of strabismus.

True strabismus should not be confused with pseudostrabismus. In pseudostrabismus, the eyes may appear slightly crossed (as in the child with a wide nasal bridge and epicanthal folds), but the corneal light reflex remains symmetric (Coats & Paysse, 2023b).

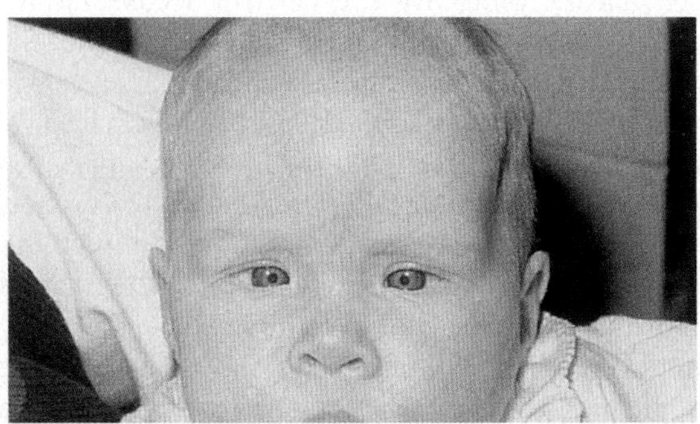

FIGURE 39.8 Esotropia. Test for strabismus by observing symmetry of the corneal light reflex. The reflex falls to the left of one pupil and to the right of the other.

Nursing Management

When patching is prescribed, encourage the family to comply with this modality. Encourage eyeglass wearing if prescribed. Provide appropriate postoperative care by protecting the operative site with eye patching.

Amblyopia

Amblyopia refers to poor visual development in the otherwise structurally normal eye. It develops within the first decade of life and, if left untreated, is the most common cause of vision loss in children and young adults, occurring in about 1% to 4% of children (Coats & Paysse, 2022). The vision in one eye is reduced because the eye and the brain are not working together properly. While the eyes are fighting to focus differently because of their differences in visual acuity, one eye is stronger than the other. This is why amblyopia is often referred to as "lazy eye."

Amblyopia may be caused by any disorder that affects normal visual development, including strabismus, differences in visual acuity between the two eyes, or astigmatism (cornea or lens is not perfectly spherical). It may also result from eye trauma, ptosis, or cataract. If untreated, children with amblyopia will have worsening acuity of the poorer eye and strain in the better eye, which may also lead to worsening of acuity in that eye. Eventually, blindness will result in one or both eyes.

It is important for children with amblyopia to receive appropriate treatment during the early years of visual development. Therapeutic management of amblyopia focuses on strengthening the weaker eye. This may be achieved through patching for several hours per day, using atropine drops in the better eye (once daily), vision therapy, or eye muscle surgery if the cause is strabismus. Patching the better eye for several hours each day encourages the eye with poorer vision to be used appropriately and promotes visual development in that eye. The once-daily use of atropine drops in the better eye results in blurring in that eye, similarly encouraging use and development of the weaker eye (Coats & Paysse, 2023a).

Nursing Assessment

One of the most important functions of the nurse is to identify the preschool child with amblyopia on screening. Begin visual acuity testing using an age-appropriate tool by 3 years of age. Observe for asymmetry of the corneal light reflex in the child of any age. This may be the only sign in the preverbal child.

Nursing Management

Support and encourage children and parents to comply with the patching protocol or atropine drop use. Promoting eye safety is extremely important for the child with amblyopia; if the better eye suffers a serious injury, both eyes may become blind.

Nystagmus

Nystagmus refers to a rapid, irregular eye movement. It is described by some as "bouncing" of the eyes. It may occur in children with congenital cataracts, but the most common cause is a neurologic problem. It is difficult for the brain and eyes to communicate when the eyes are in continuous motion; thus, visual development may be affected. Children with nystagmus must receive further evaluation by an ophthalmologist and possibly a neurologist.

Infantile Glaucoma

Infantile glaucoma is an autosomal recessive disorder that is more common in interrelated parents. It is often associated with other genetic disorders. It occurs in about one of 10,000 live births (Reynolds & Reynolds, 2023). Infantile glaucoma is characterized by obstruction of aqueous humor flow and increased intraocular pressure that results in large, prominent eyes. Vision loss may occur as a result of corneal scarring, optic nerve damage, or, most commonly, amblyopia.

Unlike adult glaucoma, in which medical management is the first step, therapeutic management of infantile glaucoma is focused on surgical intervention. Infantile glaucoma is treated surgically via goniotomy (removal of obstruction of the aqueous humor). Laser surgery is being used as well. Sometimes several surgeries may be necessary to correct the problem. Ongoing medication therapy may also be required.

Nursing Assessment

Note any family history of infantile glaucoma or other genetic disorders. Elicit the health history, noting history of the infant keeping the eyes closed most of the time or rubbing the eyes. Observe the eye for corneal enlargement and clouding; the eye may appear enlarged. Photophobia may occur, so bright light may bother the infant. Tearing or conjunctivitis and eyelid squeezing or spasm may also occur. The pediatric ophthalmologist may use a tonometer to measure the intraocular pressure during the diagnostic phase.

Nursing Management

The main goals of nursing care for the infant with glaucoma are providing postoperative care and educating the family. Postoperatively, focus on protection of the surgical site. Maintain eye patching and ensure the child remains on bedrest. If necessary, for infants and toddlers, use elbow restraints to prevent them from rubbing the affected eye. Use a calm and soothing approach, as well as distraction and developmentally appropriate play activities to calm the anxiety associated with being unable to see while patched.

Before the first surgery occurs, prepare parents for the possibility that three or four operations may be necessary. Postoperatively, teach families how to administer medications. Instruct parents and children to make sure the child avoids roughhousing and contact sports for at least 2 weeks after surgery. Encourage parents to comply with ongoing recommended visual assessments.

Congenital Cataract

A congenital cataract is an opacity of the lens of the eye that is present at birth. Sensory amblyopia will result if the infant goes untreated. Complications include visual developmental delay related to amblyopia. The disruption in visual development makes cataracts one of the leading causes of visual impairment in children (McCreery, 2023). Bilateral cataracts may be associated with metabolic or genetic syndromes. Surgery to remove the opaque lens can be done as early as 2 weeks of age. An intraocular lens implant is used, or the infant is fitted with a contact lens (McCreery, 2023). The best visual outcomes occur when cataracts are removed prior to 3 months of age. Glaucoma may occur as a complication after cataract surgery.

Nursing Assessment

Note history of lack of visual awareness. Observe the eyes for apparent cloudiness of the cornea (not always visible). Upon ophthalmoscopic examination, the red reflex will not be observed in the affected eye.

Nursing Management

Postoperative care focuses on protecting the operative site and providing developmentally appropriate activities. Ensure that the protective eye patch is secure. Elbow restraints may be necessary in the older infant to prevent accidental injury to the operative site. Teach families how to administer antibiotic or corticosteroid ophthalmic drops if prescribed for postoperative use. Once the surgical site is healed, the healthy eye may be patched for several hours a day to promote visual development in the eye with the intraocular lens or contact. Remind parents that regular visual assessments are critical for determining the adequacy of visual development after cataract removal. Instruct parents about the importance of using sunglasses that block ultraviolet rays in the child who has had a lens removed. See the Healthy People 2030 box.

HEALTHY PEOPLE 2030

Objective	Nursing Significance
Reduce visual impairment due to glaucoma.	• Appropriately screen infants and children for glaucoma or cataract.
Reduce visual impairment due to cataract.	• Refer suspected cases to a pediatric ophthalmologist for further evaluation.

Healthy People Objectives retrieved from http://www.healthypeople.gov

Retinopathy of Prematurity

Retinopathy of prematurity (ROP) is a disorder characterized by rapid growth of retinal blood vessels in the premature infant. In the fetus, retinal vascularization begins at 4 months and progresses until completion at 9 months or shortly after birth. The premature infant is born with incomplete retinal vascularization, yet new vessels continue to grow between the vascularized and nonvascularized retina. Risk factors include low birthweight, early gestational age, sepsis, high light intensity, and hypothermia. Changes in oxygen tension resulting from hypoxia, oxyhemoglobin dissociation curve changes that occur when adult blood is transfused to the premature infant, and the duration/concentration of supplemental oxygen are thought to play an important role in the development of ROP.

Premature infants should have serial examinations by an ophthalmologist until the ROP has regressed and normal vascularization is seen. If ROP continues to progress, laser surgery may be necessary to prevent blindness. Complications of ROP include myopia, glaucoma, and blindness. Strabismus may occur even in cases of regressed (resolved) ROP. Refractive errors and amblyopia may occur as early as 3 months corrected age. In the first year of life, ophthalmologic examinations should occur frequently so that if corrective lenses are needed, they may be prescribed at the earliest possible time. After 1 year corrected age, former premature infants should continue to have yearly ophthalmologic examinations to detect and treat visual deficits early.

Nursing Assessment

Ensure that all former premature infants are routinely screened for visual deficits. Discuss developmental progress with the parents. Observe for the development of strabismus, manifested by an asymmetric corneal light reflex.

Nursing Management

Nursing management of infants with ROP mainly focuses on ensuring that the family is compliant with the ophthalmologist's follow-up recommendations. Recurrent illness or rehospitalization of premature infants may interfere with scheduled eye follow-up appointments. Ensure that these appointments are rescheduled and that the family understands the importance of them. Many children who have regressed ROP or who require cryotherapy have refractive errors, so even when the ROP is considered resolved, these children should still maintain appropriate ophthalmology follow-up.

Visual Impairment

Vision impairment in children refers to acuity between 20/60 and 20/200 in the better eye on examination. "Legal **blindness**" is a term used to refer to vision of less than 20/200 or peripheral vision less than 20 degrees. In most cases, vision may be augmented with corrective lenses. Some children with blindness can differentiate light versus dark, while others live in total darkness.

Visual impairment in children may result from a number of different causes. In the United States, visual impairment and blindness may be caused by a number of disorders including but not limited to refractive error, astigmatism, strabismus, amblyopia, nystagmus, infantile glaucoma, congenital cataract, and ROP (Bregman et al., 2023). Factors that increase the risk for developing visual impairment include prematurity, developmental delay, genetic syndrome, family history of eye disease, African American heritage, previous serious eye injury, diabetes, human immunodeficiency virus (HIV), and chronic corticosteroid use. Trauma is also an important cause of blindness in children. Visual impairments are associated with many other syndromes. For example, many children with genetic syndromes have visual impairments, and albinism is associated with blindness (Bregman et al., 2023).

Children with visual impairments often exhibit motor and cognitive delays as well (World Health Organization [WHO], 2023b). With one less sense with which to experience their environment, these children may lag behind in developmental milestones. Children with blindness, since they lack the visual stimulation that children usually receive, may develop self-stimulatory actions in compensation, often called blindisms. Examples of blindisms are eye pressing, rocking, spinning, bouncing, and head banging. These repetitive behaviors may indicate an effort to communicate, and they may interfere with the child's ability to socialize (Hammer, n.d.).

TAKE NOTE!

Laser pointers pose a risk of retinal damage in infants and young children. Damage occurs if the child stares at the red light for longer than 10 seconds. They should not be used as toys (U.S. Food and Drug Administration, 2023).

Nursing Assessment

Nursing assessment for visual impairment includes a careful health history, physical examination, and visual acuity testing.

HEALTH HISTORY

Parents and nurses alike should be alert to signs of potential visual impairment. One of the most important functions of the nurse is to recognize signs of visual impairment as early as possible. These signs may include:

- At any age, a dull, vacant stare
- Infants:
  - Do not "fix and follow"
  - Do not make eye contact
  - Are unaffected by bright light
  - Do not imitate facial expression
- Toddlers and older children:
  - Rub, shut, and cover eyes
  - Squinting
  - Frequent blinking
  - Hold objects close or sit close to television
  - Bumping into objects
  - Head tilt or forward thrust

PHYSICAL EXAMINATION

Assess for symmetry or asymmetry of the corneal light reflex. Perform the "cover test." Use an age-appropriate visual acuity screening tool (refer to Chapter 31 for additional information on visual acuity screening).

Nursing Management

For the child with visual impairment, encourage the use of corrective lenses for enhancement of vision (if applicable). Encourage parents to comply with vision screening appointments in order to determine visual acuity progression or problems. Support the family's efforts at vision therapy and other habilitation programs to promote vision enhancement. Important nursing functions in relation to visual impairment and blindness are supporting the child and family and promoting socialization, development, and education. In addition, when the child with a visual impairment is hospitalized for any reason, the nurse must plan appropriate care for that child, taking into consideration the child's level of disability. Box 39.1 provides tips on working with the visually impaired child. It is important to teach these tips to families.

BOX 39.1 Tips for Interacting With the Child With Visual Impairment

- Use the child's name to gain attention.
- Identify yourself and let the child know you are there before you touch the child.
- Encourage the child to be independent while maintaining safety.
- Name and describe people/objects to make the child more aware of what is happening.
- Discuss upcoming activities with the child.
- Explain what other children or individuals are doing.
- Make directions simple and specific.
- Allow the child additional time to think about the response to a question or statement.
- Use touch and tone of voice appropriate to the situation.
- Use parts of the child's body as reference points for the location of items.
- Encourage exploration of objects through touch.
- Describe unfamiliar environments and provide reference points.
- Use the sighted-guide technique when walking with a visually impaired child.

Data from VisionServe Alliance. (2023). *Interacting with children who are visually impaired.* https://visionservealliance.org/interacting-with-children-who-are-visually-impaired/

Supporting the Child and Family

Provide emotional support to the family with a visually impaired child. Ensure that the child's environment provides familiarity and security. Encourage activities that stimulate development; these activities will vary from child to child depending on whether the child also demonstrates impairment in other areas, such as hearing or motor skills. The infant with blindness will not provide the eye contact that parents are looking for, so educate the parents about other indicators that the infant is acknowledging the parents' presence, such as:

- Increased motor activity
- Eyelid movement
- Changes in breathing pattern
- Making sounds

Encourage the family of a child with visual impairment to display affection through touch and tone of voice. Refer families to support networks and other resources for people with blindness and visual impairment.

Promoting Socialization, Development, and Education

Work with the parents to determine whether a strategy for the development of alternative behaviors specific to the individual child would be helpful. Refer the child with blindness or visual impairment who is younger than 3 years to the local district of Early Intervention to establish case management services for the child's developmental needs. After age 3, state laws provide for public education and related services for children with disabilities. An individualized education plan (IEP) should be developed to maximize the child's learning ability. Nurses may be one of the professionals involved in the development of the IEP. Refer the child with severe visual impairment or blindness for Braille training and for education on navigation of the environment with the use of a cane or other method.

INFECTIOUS AND INFLAMMATORY DISORDERS OF THE EARS

Infectious and inflammatory disorders of the ears include otitis externa and types of otitis media. Otitis media is defined as inflammation of the middle ear with the presence of fluid. It can be subdivided into two categories: AOM and otitis media with effusion (OME). AOM refers to an acute infectious process of the middle ear that may produce a rapid onset of ear pain and possibly fever. OME refers to a collection of fluid in the middle ear space without signs and symptoms of infection. Chronic OME is defined as OME lasting longer than 3 months. Otitis externa refers to inflammation of the external ear canal.

Acute Otitis Media

AOM is a common illness in children, resulting from infection (bacterial or viral) of fluid in the middle ear. Increased susceptibility in infants and young children may be partly explained by the short length and horizontal positioning of the eustachian tube, limited response to antigens, and lack of previous exposure to common pathogens (Yoon et al., 2022). AOM occurs mostly in the fall through spring, with the highest incidence in the winter. AOM often recurs in infants and young children when the fluid in the middle ear becomes reinfected. The most significant risk factors for otitis media are eustachian tube dysfunction and susceptibility to recurrent upper respiratory infections.

Pathophysiology

An upper respiratory infection frequently precedes AOM. Fluid and pathogens travel upward from the nasopharyngeal area, invading the middle ear space. Fluid behind the eardrum has difficulty draining back out toward the nasopharyngeal area because of the horizontal positioning of the eustachian tube. A viral upper respiratory infection may cause AOM or may place the child at risk for bacterial invasion. Pathogens gain access to the eustachian tube, where they proliferate and invade the mucosa. Fever and pain occur acutely. Increased pressure behind the tympanic membrane may result in perforation. This may result in decreased pain and drainage in the ear canal. Most perforations heal spontaneously and are completely benign.

AOM is most commonly caused by viral pathogens, *Streptococcus pneumoniae*, *Haemophilus influenzae*, and *Moraxella catarrhalis*. Viral causes of AOM resolve spontaneously.

After clearance of the infection, fluid remains in the middle ear space behind the tympanic membrane, sometimes for several months (OME). This may occur because of the positioning of the eustachian tubes, resulting in difficulty in draining fluid back to the nasopharyngeal area. OME may also occur because of the high frequency of upper respiratory infections in infants and young children, which again result in backup of fluid from the nasopharyngeal area.

The most common complications of AOM include:

- Hearing loss
- Expressive speech delay
- Tympanosclerosis (scarring of the tympanic membrane; usually has no effect on hearing)
- Tympanic membrane perforation (acute with resolution or chronic)
- Chronic suppurative otitis media (chronic drainage via perforation or tympanostomy tubes)
- Acute mastoiditis (infection of the mastoid process)
- Intracranial infections, including bacterial meningitis and abscesses

Therapeutic Management

Viral causes of AOM usually resolve spontaneously, but bacterial causes may require treatment with an antibiotic. It is unreasonable to obtain a culture of middle ear fluid with every episode of AOM to determine the specific cause. Scientific studies of fluid obtained via **tympanostomy** (creation of a hole in the tympanic membrane) in children with AOM have been performed, and clinical decision making is based on this research. Antibiotic resistance develops due to the overuse of antibiotics (WHO, 2023a). For this reason, clinical practice guidelines have been developed for a number of disorders based on large quantities of research.

Certain diagnosis of AOM is based on:

- Signs of fluid in the middle ear: moderate to severe bulging of the tympanic membrane, or mild bulging of the tympanic membrane with recent (within 48 hours) complaint of ear pain, and presence of middle ear infusion noted on pneumatic otoscopy or tympanometry

and

- Signs or symptoms of inflammation in the middle ear: complaint of ear pain or intense erythema of the tympanic membrane

or

- New-onset otorrhea in the absence of otitis externa (Yoon et al., 2022)

The choice of antibiotic will depend on the timing, the child's age, and whether the episode is a first or subsequent infection. The current recommendations by the American Academy of Pediatrics (AAP) allow for a period of observation or watchful waiting in certain children. This allows for natural resolution of AOM related to viral causes and decreases the overuse of antibiotics in the pediatric population (Yoon et al., 2022) (see Dosage Calculation Box 39.1).

DOSAGE CALCULATION 39.1

Child's weight: 12 lb, 4 oz

Medication order: cefuroxime 100 mg PO twice a day

Per the Pediatric Dosage Handbook, the recommended dose is 20–30 mg/kg/day in two divided doses.

Is the ordered dose safe?

Recommendations for AOM treatment in previously healthy children are found in Table 39.3. Pain management is also an important component of AOM treatment, as is appropriate follow-up to ensure disease resolution.

Nursing Assessment

Nursing assessment of the child with AOM consists of health history and physical examination.

HEALTH HISTORY

Elicit a description of the present illness and chief complaint. Note acute, abrupt onset of signs and symptoms. Common signs and symptoms reported during the health history might include:

- Fever (may be low grade or higher)
- Complaints of otalgia (ear pain)
- Fussiness or irritability
- Crying inconsolably, particularly when lying down
- Batting or tugging at the ears (may also occur with teething or OME, or may be a habit)
- Rolling the head from side to side
- Poor feeding or loss of appetite
- Lethargy
- Difficulty sleeping or awakening crying in the night
- Fluid draining from the ear

Determine the child's response to any treatments used thus far. Explore the child's current and past medical history for risk factors such as:

- Young age
- Day care attendance
- Previous history of AOM or OME
- Antecedent or concurrent upper respiratory infection
- Other risk factors (Box 39.2)

BOX 39.2 Risk Factors for AOM

- Eustachian tube dysfunction
- Recurrent upper respiratory infection
- First episode of AOM before 3 months of age
- Day care attendance (increases exposure to viruses causing upper respiratory infections)
- Previous episodes of AOM
- Family history
- Passive smoking
- Crowding in the home or large family size
- Native American, Inuit, or Aboriginal Australian ethnicity
- Absence of infant breastfeeding
- Immunocompromise
- Poor nutrition
- Craniofacial anomalies
- Presence of allergies (possibly)

AOM, acute otitis media.

Data from Yoon, P. J., Scholes, M. A., & Herrmann, B. W. (2022). Ear, nose, & throat. In M. Bunik, W. W. Hay, M. J. Levin, & M. J. Abzug (Eds.), *Current diagnosis & treatment: Pediatrics* (26th ed.). McGraw-Hill Education.

PHYSICAL EXAMINATION

The child may complain of pain when the ear is examined. On otoscopic examination, the tympanic membrane will have a dull or opaque appearance and is bulging and/or red (Fig. 39.9). Sometimes pus (greenish or yellowish) may be visible behind the eardrum. Upon

TABLE 39.3 • Treatment Recommendations for AOM

Age	Unilateral or Bilateral AOM?	Severe Signs and Symptoms?[a]	Otorrhea Present?	Treatment
6 months–2 years	Either		Yes	Antibiotics
6 months–2 years	Either	Yes		Antibiotics
6 months–2 years	Bilateral	No	No	Antibiotics
6 months–2 years	Unilateral	No	No	Antibiotics or observation[b]
>2 years	Either		Yes	Antibiotics
>2 years	Either	Yes		Antibiotics
>2 years	Bilateral	No	No	Antibiotics or observation[b]
>2 years	Unilateral	No	No	Antibiotics or observation[b]

AOM, acute otitis media.

[a]Severe illness is defined as temperature 39°C (102.2°F) or higher or moderate to severe otalgia or otalgia for at least 48 hours. Nonsevere illness is defined as mild otalgia for less than 48 hours and fever less than 39°C (102.2°F).

[b]Observation is appropriate when follow-up can be ensured in order that antibiotic therapy may begin if the child fails to improve or worsens within 48 to 72 hours.

Data from Yoon, P. J., Scholes, M. A., & Herrmann, B. W. (2022). Ear, nose, & throat. In M. Bunik, W. W. Hay, M. J. Levin, & M. J. Abzug (Eds.), *Current diagnosis & treatment: Pediatrics* (26th ed.). McGraw-Hill Education.

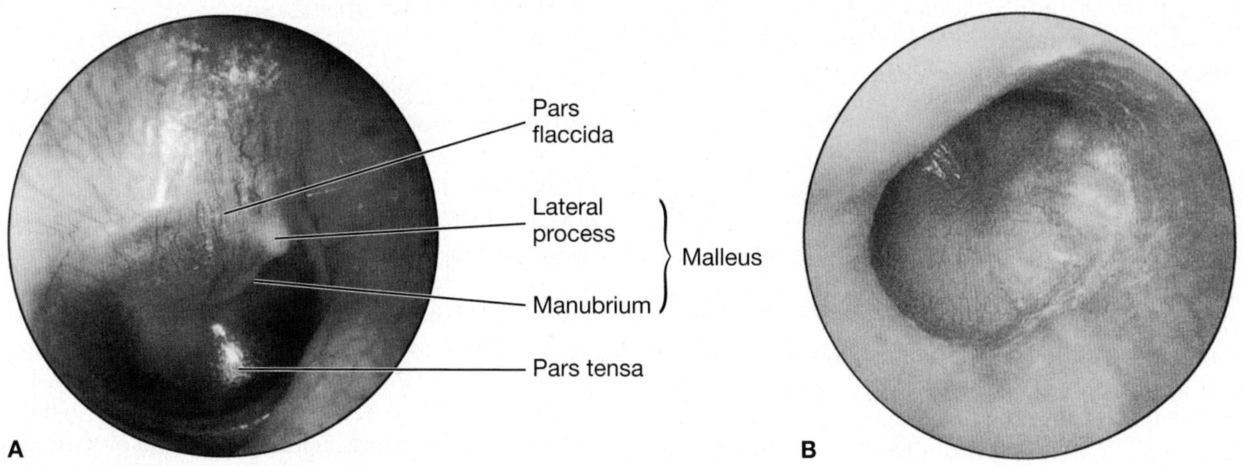

FIGURE 39.9 **A.** Normal tympanic membrane. **B.** Acute otitis media: note opacity of the tympanic membrane.

pneumatic otoscopy, the eardrum will be immobile. (A health care provider or nurse practitioner usually performs the otoscopic examination.) If the tympanic membrane has become perforated, drainage may be present in the ear canal, but the canal will otherwise appear normal. Palpate for possible cervical lymphadenopathy. Tympanometry is used to determine the presence of middle ear effusion (Yoon et al., 2022).

Nursing Management

Nursing management of the child with AOM is mainly supportive in nature. It focuses on pain management, family education, and prevention of AOM.

MANAGING PAIN ASSOCIATED WITH AOM

Administer analgesics such as acetaminophen and ibuprofen as they have been shown to be effective at managing mild to moderate pain associated with AOM and have the added benefit of reducing fever. Occasionally, narcotic analgesics may be prescribed for severe pain. Apply a warm or cool compress if helpful to the child. Instruct the family to have the child lie on the affected side with the heating pad or a covered ice pack in place against that ear.

EDUCATING THE FAMILY

If the treatment selected for AOM is observation or watchful waiting, explain the rationale for this to the family. Ensure that the family understands the importance of returning for reevaluation if the child is not improving within 48 to 72 hours or if the AOM progresses to severe illness. When antibiotics are prescribed, ensure the family understands the importance of completing the entire course of antibiotics. Families are tempted to stop giving the antibiotic because the child is usually vastly improved after taking the medication for 24 to 48 hours. Follow-up for resolution of AOM is necessary for all children and the health care provider or nurse practitioner will determine the timing of that follow-up. Emphasize the importance of follow-up to the parents, educating them about OME and its potential impact on hearing and speech. See the Healthy People 2030 box.

HEALTHY PEOPLE 2030

Objective	Nursing Significance
Reduce ear infections (otitis media) in children.	• Teach children and families the importance of handwashing to avoid the common cold (often a precursor to otitis media). • Teach families the importance of appropriate follow-up for eradication of otitis media. • Educate families about the importance of using antibiotics only for true bacterial infections (in order to decrease the development of resistant organisms, many of which cause otitis media).

Healthy People Objectives retrieved from http://www.healthypeople.gov

PREVENTING AOM

Encourage breastfeeding for at least 6 to 12 months, as breastfed infants have a lower incidence of AOM than formula-fed infants, and breast milk's immunologic benefits are well known (Yoon et al., 2022). Instruct families to avoid excess exposure to individuals with upper respiratory infections to decrease the incidence of these infections in their child. Educate families that infants and children should not be exposed to second-hand smoke. Encourage parents to stop smoking. If quitting smoking is not possible, then instruct parents not to smoke inside the house or automobile. Encourage the parents to have the child immunized with Prevnar and the influenza vaccine. When families question the protective benefits of xylitol, educate them that studies thus far have been inconclusive, and with excessive dosing, xylitol can cause diarrhea (Pelton & Marchisio, 2023).

Otitis Media With Effusion

OME refers to the presence of fluid within the middle ear space, without signs or symptoms of infection. It may occur independent of AOM or may persist after the infectious process of AOM has resolved. Risk factors for OME include passive smoking, absence of breastfeeding, frequent viral upper respiratory infections, allergy, young age, male sex, adenoid hypertrophy, eustachian tube dysfunction, and certain congenital disorders (Yoon et al., 2022). Complications of OME include AOM, hearing loss, and deafness.

Nursing Assessment

Nursing assessment of the child with OME includes health history, physical examination, and diagnostic testing.

HEALTH HISTORY

Determine the extent of symptoms. Children may be asymptomatic or may experience a popping sensation or fullness behind the eardrum. Explore the health history for risk factors such as passive smoking, absence of breastfeeding, frequent viral upper respiratory infections, allergy, or recent history of AOM.

PHYSICAL EXAMINATION AND DIAGNOSTIC TESTING

Otoscopic examination may reveal a dull, opaque tympanic membrane that may be white, gray, or bluish (Fig. 39.10). If the tympanic membrane is not opaque, a fluid level or air bubble may be visualized. Mobility may be absent or diminished upon pneumatic otoscopy. Tympanometry may be used to confirm the diagnosis of OME.

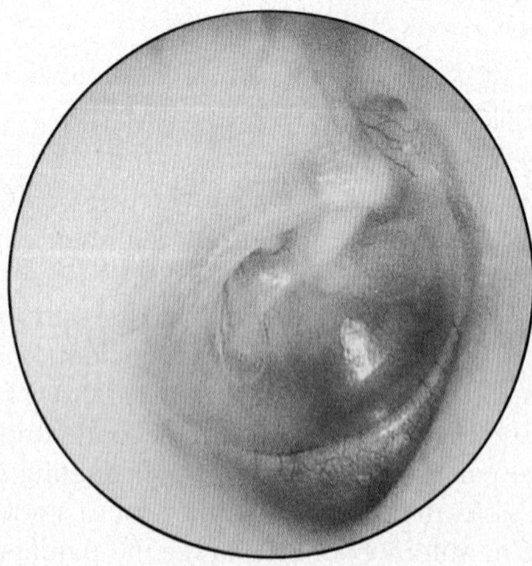

FIGURE 39.10 Otitis media with effusion; note dull white tympanic membrane.

Nursing Management

OME may take several months to resolve. Nursing management during the resolution phase focuses on education and monitoring for hearing loss.

EDUCATING THE FAMILY

Educate the family about the natural history of OME and the anatomic differences in young children that contribute to OME. Inform parents that antihistamines, decongestants, antibiotics, and corticosteroids have not been proven to hasten the resolution of OME and thus are not recommended. OME usually resolves spontaneously, but children should be rechecked every 4 weeks while this resolution is occurring. Teach parents not to feed infants in a supine position and to avoid bottle propping.

MONITORING FOR HEARING LOSS

When OME persists, the primary concern is its effect on hearing. In the infant or toddler who should be experiencing rapid language development, impaired hearing can depress language acquisition significantly (Yoon et al., 2022). Children with OME who are at risk for speech, language, or learning problems may be referred for evaluation of hearing earlier than a child with OME who is not at risk (Box 39.3). Children with chronic OME (persistent OME of 3 months' duration or longer) should be referred to a specialist for hearing evaluation (Pelton & Marom, 2022). Children who are not already at risk for speech concerns and are not experiencing difficulty with language acquisition may be reassessed every 3 to 6 months as long as hearing loss is not identified. At-risk children may require treatment earlier.

To communicate more effectively with children with OME who have hearing loss:

- Turn off music or television.
- Position yourself within 3 ft of the child before speaking.
- Face the child while speaking.
- Use visual cues.

BOX 39.3 Children at Risk for Speech, Language, or Learning Difficulties

- Permanent hearing loss (without otitis media with effusion)
- Speech/language delay (suspected or diagnosed)
- Craniofacial disorder that may interfere with speech
- Any pervasive developmental disorder
- Genetic disorders or syndromes associated with speech or learning problems
- Cleft palate
- Blindness or significant visual impairment

Data from Pelton, S., & Marom, T. (2022). Otitis media with effusion (serous otitis media) in children: Management. *UpToDate.* Retrieved January 23, 2024, from https://www.uptodate.com/contents/otitis-media-with-effusion-serous-otitis-media-in-children-management

- Increase the volume of your speech only slightly.
- Speak clearly.
- Request preferential classroom seating.

TAKE NOTE!

Evaluation of hearing is recommended when OME lasts 3 months or more if language delay, hearing loss, or a learning problem is suspected (Pelton & Marom, 2022).

PROVIDING POSTOPERATIVE CARE FOR THE CHILD WITH PRESSURE-EQUALIZING TUBES

Educate parents about the surgical insertion of **pressure-equalizing (PE) tubes** into the tympanic membrane (via myringotomy). Cover the following:

- PE tubes equalize the pressure behind the eardrum, allowing for tympanic membrane movement. This allows for adequate hearing, which in turn encourages speech development.
- The procedure is usually done as an outpatient surgery and the child returns home in the evening.
- The tubes stay in place for at least several months and generally fall out on their own (Fig. 39.11).
- Teach the parents to administer ear drops postoperatively if prescribed.
- Advise parents to have the child wear earplugs when swimming in potentially contaminated water such as lakes or rivers.
- Teach parents if the middle ear becomes infected with PE tubes in place, the tubes allow infected fluid to drain from the ear (if this occurs, they should contact their health care provider or nurse practitioner).

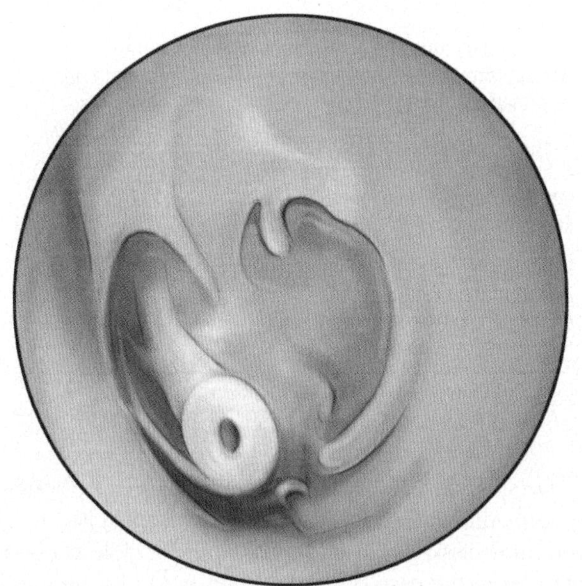

FIGURE 39.11 Pressure-equalizing tube in place in the tympanic membrane.

Otitis Externa

Otitis externa is defined as an infection and inflammation of the skin of the external ear canal. *Pseudomonas aeruginosa* and *Staphylococcus aureus* are typical causative agents, though fungi such as *Aspergillus* and other bacteria also may be implicated. Moisture in the canal contributes to pathogen growth (Yoon et al., 2022). Otitis externa is commonly known as "swimmer's ear" since it occurs more frequently in those who swim often (and thus have wet ear canals). Changing the pH in the ear canal contributes to the inflammatory process.

Nursing Assessment

Nursing assessment of the child with otitis externa focuses on the health history and physical examination.

HEALTH HISTORY

Elicit a description of the present illness and chief complaint. Note history of ear itching or pain, ear drainage, or a feeling of fullness in the ear canal, with possible difficulty hearing. Note onset and progression of symptoms, as well as the child's response to treatments. Explore the child's current and past medical history for risk factors such as previous episodes of otitis externa or history of recent swimming in a pool, lake, or ocean.

TAKE NOTE!

The child with otitis externa usually has significant ear pain. Pressure on the tragus should be avoided, as it can worsen the pain.

PHYSICAL EXAMINATION

Typically, a white or colored discharge can be seen in the ear canal or running from the ear. On otoscopy, the canal is red and edematous, often too swollen for insertion of the speculum and viewing of the tympanic membrane (Fig. 39.12). Diagnosis is based on clinical findings. Occasionally the ear drainage is cultured for bacteria or fungus, particularly if otitis externa is not improving with treatment.

Nursing Management

The primary goals of nursing management for otitis externa are pain relief, treatment of the infection, and prevention of recurrence.

MANAGING PAIN

Administer analgesics (possibly narcotics) to manage the pain. Apply a warm compress or heating pad to the affected ear as it is helpful in some children.

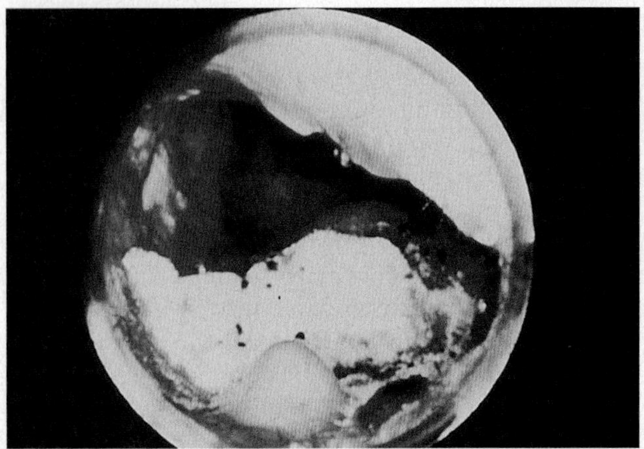

FIGURE 39.12 Note edema and erythema of the ear canal as well as purulent discharge in the child with otitis externa.

TREATING THE INFECTION

Administer antibiotic or antifungal eardrops as prescribed. If a wick is placed in the ear canal, teach the parents that it keeps the antibiotic drops in contact with the skin of the ear canal and promotes healing. Assist with wick insertion as it can be extremely painful, and younger children will need to be restrained during insertion for their safety.

PREVENTING REINFECTION

Teach children and their parents about prevention of further episodes once the infection has resolved. Since moisture contributes to otitis externa, explain the importance of keeping the ear canals dry. Encourage the child and parents to use one of the methods described in Teaching Guidelines 39.2 after swimming or showering.

TEACHING GUIDELINES 39.2 Preventing Otitis Externa

- Avoid the use of cotton swabs, headphones, and earphones.
- Wear earplugs when swimming.
- Promote ear canal dryness and alternate pH. Use one or more of the following methods:
  - Dry the ear canals using a hair dryer set on a lower setting.
  - Administer solutions that have a drying effect on the auditory canal skin and change the pH of the canal to discourage organism growth in susceptible children. The following solutions can be used:
    - A few drops of Domeboro solution can be placed in the canal and then allowed to run out.
    - A mixture of half rubbing alcohol and half vinegar (squirted into the canal and then allowed to run out). The alcohol solution should be used only when the ear canals are healthy. Using it while the canals are inflamed will cause stinging and increased pain.

Adapted from Johns Hopkins Medicine. (2023). *Swimmer's ear*. https://www.hopkinsmedicine.org/health/conditions-and-diseases/swimmers-ear

HEARING LOSS AND DEAFNESS

Infants are ordinarily born with the sense of hearing fully developed. Language development in infancy and early childhood is dependent upon adequate hearing, and even the fluctuating hearing loss associated with intermittent bouts of AOM can hinder language development (Pelton & Marom, 2022). Hearing loss may be unilateral (involving one ear) or bilateral (involving both ears). The extent of hearing loss is defined based on the softest intensity of sound that is perceived, described in **decibels** (dB). Levels of hearing loss are:

- 0 to 20 dB: normal
- 20 to 40 dB: mild loss
- 40 to 60 dB: moderate loss
- 60 to 80 dB: severe loss
- Greater than 80 dB: profound loss (American Speech-Language-Hearing Association [ASHA], 2024b)

Hearing loss may be congenital or acquired. Most congenital hearing loss is inherited through a single gene, or associated with a syndrome, though it also occurs as a result of prenatal infection (ASHA, 2024c). Premature infants and those with persistent pulmonary hypertension of the newborn are at increased risk for hearing loss compared with other infants. A variety of newborn universal hearing screening mandates have been passed by legislation in 43 states, thus allowing for earlier identification of infants with congenital hearing loss (National Center for Hearing Assessment and Management, 2024). See the Healthy People 2030 box.

HEALTHY PEOPLE 2030

Objective	Nursing Significance
Increase the proportion of newborns who are screened for hearing loss no later than age 1 month. Increase the proportion of infants who did not pass the hearing screening test who get evaluated for hearing loss no later than age 3 months. Increase the proportion of infants with confirmed hearing loss who are enrolled for intervention services no later than age 6 months.	• Encourage appropriate hearing assessments. • Refer children who are diagnosed with a hearing deficit to appropriate local services.

Healthy People Objectives retrieved from http://www.healthypeople.gov

Delayed-onset (acquired) hearing loss may be conductive, sensorineural, or mixed. **Conductive hearing loss** results when transmission of sound through the middle ear is disrupted, as in the case of OME. When fluid fills the middle ear, the tympanic membrane is unable to move properly, and partial or complete hearing loss occurs. **Sensorineural hearing loss** is caused by damage to the hair cells in the cochlea or along the auditory pathway. This may result from kernicterus, use of ototoxic medication, intrauterine infection with cytomegalovirus or rubella, neonatal or postnatal infection such as meningitis, severe neonatal respiratory depression, or exposure to excess noise. Mixed hearing loss occurs when the cause may be attributed to both conductive and sensorineural problems. Regardless of the cause of hearing loss, early intervention can make a difference in the child's ability to communicate. Once the hearing loss has been determined, intervention can begin. Hearing aids, cochlear implants, communication devices, and speech education may enable these children to communicate verbally. Improved communication beginning in infancy and early childhood may also improve the child's school achievement.

Nursing Assessment

Nursing assessment of the child with hearing loss or impairment focuses on the health history, physical examination, and diagnostic hearing testing.

Health History

Common symptoms reported during the health history might include:

- Infant:
  - Wakes only to touch, not environmental noises
  - Does not startle to loud noises
  - Does not turn to sound by 4 months of age
  - Does not babble at 6 months of age
  - Does not progress with speech development
- Young child:
  - Does not speak by 2 years of age
  - Communicates needs through gestures
  - Does not speak distinctly, as appropriate for their age
  - Displays developmental (cognitive) delays
  - Prefers solitary play
  - Displays immature emotional behavior
  - Does not respond to ringing of the telephone or doorbell
  - Focuses on facial expressions when communicating
- Older child:
  - Often asks for statements to be repeated
  - Is inattentive or daydreams
  - Performs poorly at school
  - Displays monotone or other abnormal speech
  - Gives inappropriate answers to questions except when able to view face of speaker
- At any age:
  - Speaks loudly
  - Sits close to the TV or radio or turns volume up too loud
  - Responds only to moderate or loud voices

Investigate signs of hearing loss as early as possible in order for appropriate intervention to begin. Explore the child's current and past medical history for risk factors such as congenital anomalies, genetic syndrome, infection, family history, kernicterus, neonatal ventilator use, ototoxic medication, or exposure to excess noise. Note whether newborn hearing screening was done and, if so, what the results were.

Physical Examination and Diagnostic Testing

Determine the child's level of interaction with the environment. For preschoolers and older children, administer the whisper test, keeping in mind that this is a gross screening test only. Perform the Weber and Rinne tests (refer to Chapter 31 for further explanation). If further evaluation is needed, the nurse may be responsible for administering an otoacoustic emissions test or auditory brain stem evoked response test, either in the hospital or in the outpatient office.

Nursing Management

The primary goal of nursing care for the child with a hearing impairment is to provide education and support to the family and child. Individualize care for the child with a hearing impairment and the family based on their specific responses to the hearing impairment.

Augmenting Hearing

Educate the family that compliance with hearing aids and communication curricula is critical so that the child can develop hearing and speech. Teach the child and family that hearing aids should be cleaned daily with a damp cloth and to change batteries weekly. For safety purposes, ensure parents understand that hearing aid batteries are a serious aspiration risk and should always be kept out of reach of young children. Teach parents when inserting the aid, the volume should be turned down, then adjusted to the appropriate level after insertion. Also teach families that as the infant or child grows, the hearing aid will need to be reassessed for proper fit. Many deaf schools and other organizations provide loaner hearing aids so that the best fit and amplification may be determined prior to purchase. Assist the family to explore this type of option in the local community. When cochlear implants are used, the nurse focuses on postoperative care of the incision site and pain management.

Promoting Communication and Education

Talk with families about how they need to learn how to communicate effectively with their child. If the child learns American Sign Language, for instance, the parents and siblings should as well. Table 39.4 provides information on communication options for hearing-impaired children and their families. Teach families that communication may also be enhanced by the use of text telephone service in the home, closed-caption television, and lights rather than bells or alarms to alert the child. Provide a sign language interpreter for the child at health care visits if the parent is not present for interpretation.

TABLE 39.4 • Comparing Communication Options for the Hearing Impaired

Spoken Language	
Oral deaf education (auditory-verbal therapy)	Uses technology to boost auditory potential; teaches children to notice sound and give it meaning. Develops oral speech
Cued speech	A system using hand signs to clarify lip-reading; gives the person clues about the sounds the speaker is making
Signed Language	
American Sign Language (ASL)	Entirely communicated through hand signs, gestures, and facial expressions. Has its own grammar and syntax
Combination: total communication	Combines auditory training and teaching of spoken language with "signing exact English" (corresponds to the words and syntax of English)
Augmentative and Alternative Communication (AAC)	
May use gestural communication	Can also include physical devices such as notebooks, communication boards, charts, or computers. Ranges from very low-tech to technologically complex

Data from American Speech-Language-Hearing Association. (2024a). *Augmentative and alternative communication.* http://www.asha.org/public/speech/disorders/AAC.htm

Encouraging Education

Refer the child younger than 3 years to the local district of Early Intervention for case management of developmental needs. Educate families that at 3 years of age and beyond, state laws provide for public education and related services for children with disabilities. Communicate to families that an IEP should be developed to maximize the child's learning ability. Contribute to the development of the IEP as appropriate.

Refer families to schools specifically geared toward deaf students depending upon the family's preferences and resources.

Providing Support

Encourage families to express their feelings as the diagnosis of a significant disability can be extremely stressful. Provide emotional support. Ensure that the needs of any siblings are also attended to. When the family is ready, encourage them to network with other families who have children with similar needs. Educate the family about the child's prescribed plan of care. Refer families to resources and support groups.

KEY CONCEPTS

- Though hearing is fully developed at birth, visual development continues to progress until about age 7 years.
- Binocular vision develops by age 4 months; visual acuity progresses to 20/50 by age 3 years and usually reaches 20/20 by about age 5 years.
- The relatively short and horizontally positioned eustachian tubes of infants and young children make them more susceptible to otitis media than adults.
- To maximize speech and language development, hearing loss should be identified early, and intervention begun immediately.
- Children with genetic syndromes or family history are at increased risk of visual and hearing impairments.
- The corneal light reflex test and cover test are useful tools for identifying strabismus and amblyopia.
- Tympanometry is used to determine the presence of fluid behind the eardrum (such as with OME).
- Topical ophthalmic medications are used to treat certain infectious eye disorders.
- Appropriate handwashing is the single most important factor to reduce the spread of acute viral or bacterial conjunctivitis.
- Systemic antibiotics are used for the treatment of periorbital cellulitis.
- Strabismus, glaucoma, and cataracts may all lead to visual impairment if left untreated.
- Asymmetry of the corneal light reflex occurs with true strabismus.
- Amblyopia must be identified early and treated with patching, corrective lenses, or surgery to prevent visual deterioration and promote appropriate vision development.
- A cloudy cornea indicates the presence of cataract.
- Very premature infants are at high risk of developing visual deficits related to ROP and are also at increased risk of hearing impairment compared to other infants.
- Eye strain, eye rubbing, and headaches may indicate a visual deficit.
- Children with visual disorders should be encouraged to use prescribed corrective lenses.
- Recurrent episodes of AOM may negatively affect the child's hearing.
- Recurrent or constant nasal congestion contributes to OME.
- Otitis externa can be prevented by keeping the ear canal dry and altering canal pH.
- The fluctuating hearing loss associated with recurrent otitis media and the hearing loss associated with

chronic OME can both significantly hinder language development in the infant and toddler.

- The child with hearing loss should receive early intervention with hearing aids or other augmentative devices.

REFERENCES AND RECOMMENDED READINGS

Algarni, A., Guyatt, G. H., Turner, A., & Alamri, S. (2022). Antibiotic patching for corneal abrasion. *Cochrane Database of Systematic Reviews, 5*, CD014617. https://doi.org/10.1002/14651858.CD014617.pub2

American Association for Pediatric Ophthalmology and Strabismus. (2023). *Glasses fitting for children*. https://aapos.org/viewdocument/glasses-fitting-for-children

American Speech-Language-Hearing Association. (2024a). *Augmentative and alternative communication*. https://www.asha.org/practice-portal/professional-issues/augmentative-and-alternative-communication/

American Speech-Language-Hearing Association. (2024b). *Degree of hearing loss*. https://www.asha.org/public/hearing/degree-of-hearing-loss/

American Speech-Language-Hearing Association. (2024c). *Hearing loss at birth (congenital hearing loss)*. https://www.asha.org/public/hearing/congenital-hearing-loss/

Bhatt, A. (2023). Retinopathy of prematurity: Risk factors, classification, and screening. *UpToDate*. Retrieved January 23, 2024, from https://www.uptodate.com/contents/retinopathy-of-prematurity-rop-risk-factors-classification-and-screening

Bregman, J., Sohal, P., Mishra, S., deBeaufort, H., Prakalapakorn, G., Bregman, J., Kumar, P., & Rodriguez, S. (2023). *Pediatric low vision*. https://eyewiki.aao.org/Pediatric_Low_Vision#Causes_of_Pediatric_Low_Vision

Coats, D. K. (2023). Vision screening and assessment in infants and children. *UpToDate*. Retrieved January 23, 2024, from https://www.uptodate.com/contents/vision-screening-and-assessment-in-infants-and-children

Coats, D. K., & Paysse, E. A. (2022). Amblyopia in children: Classification, screening, and evaluation. *UpToDate*. Retrieved January 23, 2024, from https://www.uptodate.com/contents/amblyopia-in-children-classification-screening-and-evaluation

Coats, D. K., & Paysse, E. A. (2023a). Amblyopia in children: Management and outcome. *UpToDate*. Retrieved January 23, 2024, from https://www.uptodate.com/contents/amblyopia-in-children-management-and-outcome

Coats, D. K., & Paysse, E. A. (2023b). Evaluation and management of strabismus in children. *UpToDate*. Retrieved January 23, 2024, from https://www.uptodate.com/contents/evaluation-and-management-of-strabismus-in-children

Coats, D. K., & Paysse, E. A. (2023c). Refractive errors in children. *UpToDate*. Retrieved January 23, 2024, from https://www.uptodate.com/contents/refractive-errors-in-children

Hammer, E. (n.d.). *Self-stimulation: Dr. Hammer responds*. http://www.nfb.org/images/nfb/Publications/fr/fr17/Issue3/F170308.htm

Howard, L. M., & Annabelle de St. Maurice, A. (2021). Unraveling the impact of pneumococcal conjugate vaccines on bacterial conjunctivitis in children. *Clinical Infectious Diseases, 72*(7), 1208–1210. https://doi.org/10.1093/cid/ciaa202

Jacobs, D. S. (2023a). Conjunctivitis. *UpToDate*. Retrieved January 23, 2024, from https://www.uptodate.com/contents/conjunctivitis

Jacobs, D. S. (2023b). Corneal abrasions and corneal foreign bodies: Management. *UpToDate*. Retrieved January 23, 2024, from http://www.uptodate.com/contents/corneal-abrasions-and-corneal-foreign-bodies-management

Johns Hopkins Medicine. (2023). *Swimmer's ear*. https://www.hopkinsmedicine.org/health/conditions-and-diseases/swimmers-ear

Lexicomp®. (2024). *Lexi-Drugs/tetrahydrozoline (ophthalmic)*. (Version 7.7.0) [Mobile app]. Wolters Kluwer. https://apps.apple.com/us/app/lexicomp/id313401238

McCreery, K. M. (2023). Cataract in children. *UpToDate*. Retrieved January 23, 2024, from https://www.uptodate.com/contents/cataract-in-children

Mehner, L., & Jung, J. L. (2022). Eye. In M. Bunik, W. W. Hay, M. J. Levin, & M. J. Abzug (Eds.), *Current diagnosis & treatment: Pediatrics* (26th ed.). McGraw-Hill Education.

National Center for Hearing Assessment and Management. (2024). *EDHI legislation: Overview*. http://www.infanthearing.org/legislation/

National Institute on Deafness and Other Communication Disorders. (2021). *Cochlear implants*. https://www.nidcd.nih.gov/health/cochlear-implants

Olitsky, S. E., & Marsh, J. D. (2020). Growth and development of the eye. In R. M. Kliegman, J. W. St. Geme, N. J. Blum, S. S. Shah, R. C. Tasker, & K. M. Wilson (Eds.), *Nelson textbook of pediatrics* (21st ed.). Elsevier Health Sciences.

Paysse, E. A., & Coats, D. K. (2023). Nasolacrimal duct obstruction (dacryostenosis) and dacryocystocele. *UpToDate*. Retrieved January 23, 2024, from https://www.uptodate.com/contents/congenital-nasolacrimal-duct-obstruction-dacryostenosis-and-dacryocystocele

Pelton, S., & Marchisio, P. (2023). Acute otitis media: Prevention of recurrence. *UpToDate*. Retrieved January 23, 2024, from https://www.uptodate.com/contents/acute-otitis-media-in-children-prevention-of-recurrence

Pelton, S., & Marom, T. (2022). Otitis media with effusion (serous otitis media) in children: Management. *UpToDate*. Retrieved January 23, 2024, from https://www.uptodate.com/contents/otitis-media-with-effusion-serous-otitis-media-in-children-management

Reynolds, J. D., & Reynolds, A. L. (2023). Primary infantile glaucoma. *UpToDate*. Retrieved November 17, 2023, from https://www.uptodate.com/contents/primary-infantile-glaucoma

UpToDate, Inc. (2024). *Lexicomp®* (Version 7.7.0) [Mobile app]. Wolters Kluwer. https://apps.apple.com/us/app/lexicomp/id313401238

U.S. Department of Health and Human Services. (n.d.). *Healthy People 2030*. https://health.gov/healthypeople

U.S. Food and Drug Administration. (2023). *Laser toys: How to keep kids safe*. https://www.fda.gov/consumers/consumer-updates/laser-toys-how-keep-kids-safe

VisionServe Alliance. (2023). *Interacting with children who are visually impaired*. https://visionservealliance.org/interacting-with-children-who-are-visually-impaired/

World Health Organization. (2023a). *Antibiotic resistance*. https://www.who.int/news-room/fact-sheets/detail/antimicrobial-resistance

World Health Organization. (2023b). *Blindness and vision impairment*. https://www.who.int/news-room/fact-sheets/detail/blindness-and-visual-impairment

Yoon, P. J., Scholes, M. A., & Herrmann, B. W. (2022). Ear, nose, & throat. In M. Bunik, W. W. Hay, M. J. Levin, & M. J. Abzug (Eds.), *Current diagnosis & treatment: Pediatrics* (26th ed.). McGraw-Hill Education.

DEVELOPING CLINICAL JUDGMENT

PRACTICING FOR NCLEX

1. Which situation would cause the nurse to become concerned about possible hearing loss?
   - **a.** A 12-month-old who babbles incessantly, making no sense
   - **b.** An 8-month-old who says only "da"
   - **c.** A 3-month-old who startles easily to sound
   - **d.** A 3-year-old who drops the letter "s"
2. A 4-year-old complains of extreme pain when the tragus is touched. Though not diagnostic, this sign is most indicative of which disorder?
   - **a.** AOM
   - **b.** Acute tympanic effusion
   - **c.** Otitis interna
   - **d.** Otitis externa
3. The nurse is caring for an infant who has undergone surgery for infantile glaucoma. What is the priority nursing intervention?
   - **a.** Place the child prone postoperatively for comfort.
   - **b.** Teach the family use of the contact lens.
   - **c.** Place elbow restraints on the infant.
   - **d.** Provide a mobile for optical stimulation.
4. A 2-year-old has been prescribed eye patching for strabismus 6 hours per day. What teaching does the nurse provide for the parent?
   - **a.** Try to patch 6 hours per day, but if you miss some it is okay.
   - **b.** Patching is necessary to strengthen vision in the weaker eye.
   - **c.** Patching will keep the eye from turning in.
   - **d.** Since the child is so young, patching can be delayed until school age.
5. The nurse is caring for a toddler with recurrent AOM. Which are risk factors for AOM? Select all that apply.
   - **a.** Recurrent upper respiratory infection
   - **b.** African American ethnicity
   - **c.** Passive smoking
   - **d.** Day care avoidance
   - **e.** Absence of infant breastfeeding
   - **f.** First episode of AOM after 12 months of age
6. A 16-month-old toddler was treated with amoxicillin for otitis media at 14 months of age. After non-resolution of the infection, the toddler was then prescribed amoxicillin-clavulanate. Two weeks later the toddler had OME. One month following that, OME persisted. Today, the toddler has a cold, is irritable and febrile, and is diagnosed with AOM. The toddler is at risk for ___ and ___ as a result of ___.

   Blanks 1 and 2:
   - **a.** tympanic membrane perforation
   - **b.** hearing impairment
   - **c.** antibiotic resistance
   - **d.** speech delay

   Blank 3:
   - **a.** otitis externa
   - **b.** upper respiratory infection
   - **c.** persistent middle ear effusion
   - **d.** lack of antibiotic adherence

DOSAGE CALCULATION QUESTION

The nurse is caring for a child with AOM. The child weighs 22 lb. The medication order reads: amoxicillin 160 mg PO every 8 hours. Amoxicillin is supplied as 200 mg/5 mL. How many milliliters will the nurse administer? Round to the nearest whole number.

CRITICAL THINKING EXERCISES

1. A 16-month-old toddler is being seen for his sixth ear infection. What particular information about his growth and development must the nurse ask about? Be specific about the questions you would ask.
2. How would you distinguish allergic conjunctivitis from acute bacterial conjunctivitis?
3. A 13-month-old has been diagnosed with severe visual impairment. Develop a list of sample nursing problems or concerns for this situation.

STUDY ACTIVITIES

1. Develop a sample plan for teaching a low-literacy parent about the etiology, treatment, and complications of recurrent AOM.
2. While in the pediatric clinical setting, compare the play styles of a sighted child with those of a visually impaired child.
3. Research hearing and vision resources in your local community.

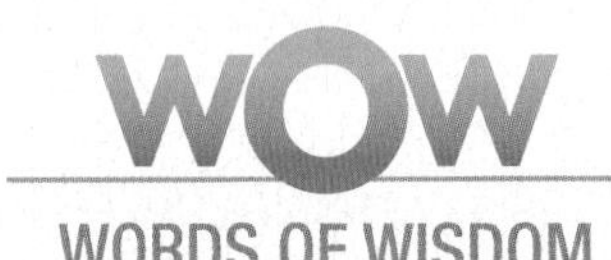

WORDS OF WISDOM

Similar to adults, children may take breathing easily for granted.

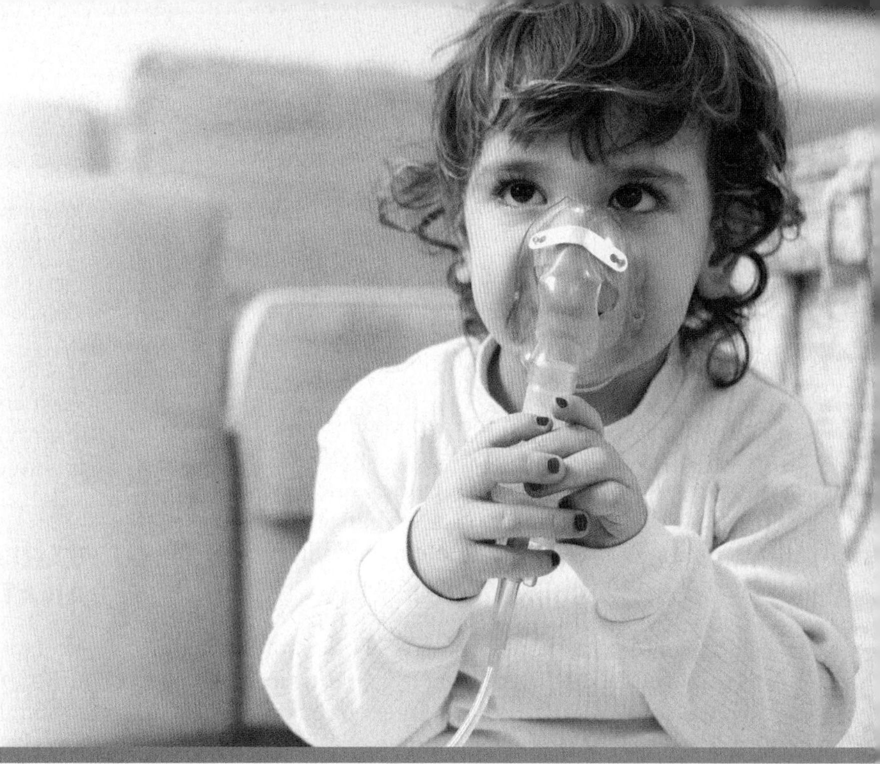

40

Nursing Care of the Child With an Alteration in Gas Exchange/Respiratory Disorder

KEY TERMS

atelectasis (at′ĕ-lek′tă-sis)
atopy
clubbing
coryza (kō-rī′ză)
cyanosis
hypoxemia
hypoxia
infiltrates
oxygenation
pulse oximetry
rales (rahls)
retractions
rhinorrhea (rī′nōr-ē′ă)
stridor
suctioning
tachypnea (tak′ip-nē′ă)
tracheostomy
ventilation
wheezing
work of breathing

LEARNING OBJECTIVES

Upon completion of the chapter, you will be able to:

1. Distinguish between the anatomy and the physiology of the respiratory system in children versus adults.
2. Identify various factors associated with respiratory illness in infants and children.
3. Discuss common laboratory and other diagnostic tests useful in the diagnosis of respiratory conditions.
4. Describe nursing care related to common medications and other treatments used for management and palliation of respiratory conditions.
5. Recognize risk factors associated with various respiratory disorders.
6. Distinguish various respiratory disorders based on their signs and symptoms.
7. Discuss nursing interventions commonly used for respiratory illnesses.
8. Devise an individualized nursing care plan or concept map for the child with a respiratory disorder.
9. Develop child/family teaching plans for the child with a respiratory disorder.
10. Describe the psychosocial impact of chronic respiratory disorders on children.

Alexander Roberts, a 4-month-old, is brought to the clinic by his parent. He has a cold and has been coughing a great deal for 2 days. Today, the infant has had difficulty taking a bottle and is breathing very quickly. The parent says Alexander seems tired.

INTRODUCTION

Gas exchange refers to the process by which oxygen is transported to cells and carbon dioxide is transported from cells (Giddens, 2021). Nurses encounter potential and actual alterations in gas exchange in all types of patients and must detect problems and intervene early to prevent life-threatening complications.

Alterations in gas exchange (respiratory disorders) are the most common causes of illness and hospitalization in children. These illnesses range from mild, nonacute disorders (such as the common cold or sore throat) to serious life-threatening conditions (such as epiglottitis). Chronic disorders, such as allergic rhinitis or asthma, can affect the quality of life, but frequent acute or recurrent infections can also interfere significantly with the well-being of some children.

Children experience numerous respiratory infections. The child's age, socioeconomic status, and general health status can influence both the development of respiratory disorders and the course of the illness. Infants and younger children are more likely to deteriorate quickly from a respiratory illness, and children with chronic disorders such as diabetes, congenital heart disease, sickle cell anemia, cystic fibrosis, and cerebral palsy tend to be more severely affected with respiratory disorders.

In addition, the season of the year can influence the development of respiratory disorders and the course of the illness. For example, certain viruses are more prevalent in the winter, whereas allergen-related respiratory diseases are more prevalent in the spring and fall.

Parents may have difficulty determining the severity of their child's condition and might either seek care very early in the course of the illness (when it is still very mild) or wait, presenting to the health care setting when the child is very ill. Nurses must be familiar with respiratory conditions affecting children so that they can provide guidance and support to families. Difficulty with breathing can be very frightening for both the child and the parents. Nurses must be able to ask questions that can help establish the severity of the child's illness and determine whether the family should seek care at a health care facility.

Since respiratory illnesses account for most pediatric admissions to general hospitals, nurses caring for children need to have expert assessment and intervention skills in this area. Detection of worsening respiratory status early during deterioration allows for timely treatment and the chance to prevent a minor problem from becoming a critical illness. Nurses are also in a unique position to provide education about respiratory illnesses and to promote efforts to prevent these illnesses.

VARIATIONS IN PEDIATRIC ANATOMY AND PHYSIOLOGY

Alterations in gas exchange/respiratory conditions often affect both the upper and the lower respiratory tract, although some affect primarily one or the other. Respiratory dysfunction in children tends to be more severe than in adults, and several differences in the infant's or child's respiratory system account for this increased severity.

Nose

Newborns are preferential nose breathers until at least 4 weeks of age (Smith, D. 2022). The young infant cannot automatically open their mouth to breathe if the nose is obstructed. The nares must be patent for breathing to be successful while feeding. Newborns breathe through their mouths only while crying.

The upper respiratory mucus serves as a cleansing agent, yet newborns produce very little mucus, making them more susceptible to infection. However, the newborn and young infant have very small nasal passages, so when excess mucus is present, airway obstruction is more likely.

Infants are born with maxillary and ethmoid sinuses present. The frontal sinuses (most often associated with sinus infection) and the sphenoid sinuses develop by age 6 to 8 years. Therefore, younger children are less apt to acquire sinus infections compared to adults.

Throat

The tongue of the infant relative to the oropharynx is larger than in adults. Posterior displacement of the tongue can quickly lead to severe airway obstruction. Through early school age, children tend to have enlarged tonsillar and adenoidal tissue even in the absence of illness. This can contribute to an increased incidence of airway obstruction.

Trachea

The airway lumen is smaller in infants and children than in adults. The infant's trachea is approximately 4 mm wide compared with the width of 20 mm in adults. When edema, mucus, or bronchospasm is present, the capacity for air passage is greatly diminished. A small reduction in the diameter of a child's airway (resulting from the presence of edema or mucus) will result in an exponential increase in resistance to airflow (Fig. 40.1). Increased **work of breathing** (effort or labor associated with respiration) then occurs.

In teenagers and adults, the larynx is cylindrical and fairly uniform in width. In infants and children younger than 10 years old, the cricoid cartilage is underdeveloped, resulting in laryngeal narrowing (Nagler, 2022). Thus, in infants and children, the larynx is funnel shaped. In addition, the larynx and glottis are located higher in the neck, increasing the chance of aspiration of foreign material into the lower airways. Congenital laryngomalacia occurs in some infants and results in the laryngeal structure being weaker than normal, yielding greater collapse on inspiration. Box 40.1 discusses congenital laryngomalacia.

The child's airway is highly compliant, making it quite susceptible to dynamic collapse in the presence of airway obstruction (Nagler, 2022). The muscles supporting the airway are less functional than those in the adult. Children have a large amount of soft tissue surrounding the trachea, and the mucous membranes lining the airway are less securely attached as compared with adults. This increases the risk for airway edema and obstruction. Upper airway obstruction resulting from a foreign body, croup, or epiglottitis can result in tracheal collapse during inspiration.

A B

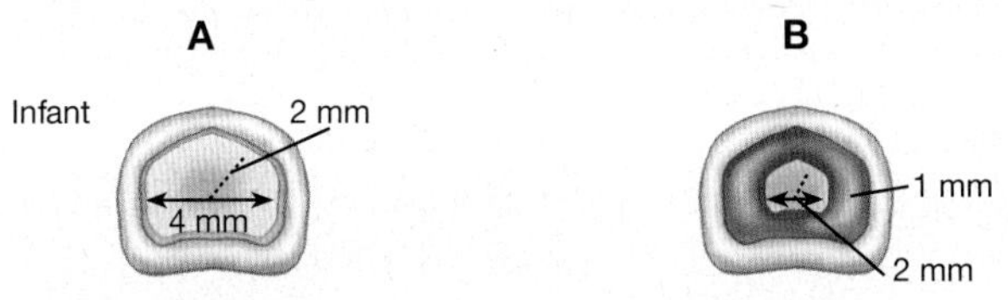

1-mm circumferential edema causes 50% reduction of diameter and radius, increasing pulmonary resistance by a factor of 16.

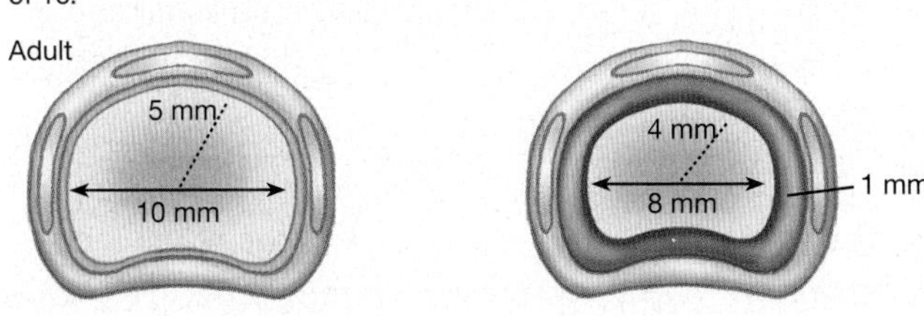

1-mm circumferential edema causes 20% reduction of diameter and radius, increasing pulmonary resistance by a factor of 2.4.

FIGURE 40.1 **A.** Note the smaller diameter of the child's airway under normal circumstances. **B.** With 1 mm of edema present, note the exponential decrease in airway lumen diameter as compared with the adult.

BOX **40.1** **Congenital Laryngomalacia**

- Inspiratory stridor is present and is intensified with certain positions.
- Suprasternal retractions may be present, but the infant exhibits no other signs of respiratory distress.
- Congenital laryngomalacia is generally a benign condition that improves as the cartilage in the larynx matures. It usually disappears by age 1 year.
- The crowing noise heard with breathing can make parents very anxious. Reassure parents that the condition will improve with time.
- Parents become very familiar with the "normal" sound their infant makes and are often able to identify intensification or change in the stridor. Airway obstruction may occur earlier in infants with this condition, so intensification of stridor or symptoms of respiratory illness should be evaluated early by the primary provider or nurse practitioner.

Lower Respiratory Structures

The bifurcation of the trachea occurs at the level of the third thoracic vertebra in children, compared to the level of the sixth thoracic vertebra in adults (Nagler, 2022). This anatomic difference is important when suctioning children and when endotracheal intubation is required (see Chapter 51 for further discussion). This difference in placement also contributes to risk of foreign material aspiration. The bronchi and bronchioles of infants and children are narrower in diameter than the adult's, placing them at increased risk for lower airway obstruction (see Fig. 40.1). Lower airway obstruction during exhalation often results from bronchiolitis or asthma or is caused by foreign body aspiration into the lower airway.

Alveoli are developed at approximately 24 weeks' gestation. Term infants are born with about 150 million alveoli. At some point between the age of 3 and 8 years, the child has developed the adult number of alveoli of around 300 million (Moore et al., 2020). Alveoli make up most of the lung tissue and are the major sites for gas exchange. Oxygen moves from the alveolar air to the blood, while carbon dioxide moves from the blood into the alveolar air. Smaller numbers of alveoli, particularly in the premature and/or young infant, place the child at a higher risk of hypoxemia (deficiency in the concentration of oxygen in arterial blood) and carbon dioxide retention.

Chest Wall

In older children and adults, the ribs and sternum support the lungs and help keep them well expanded. The movement of the diaphragm and intercostal muscles alters volume and pressure within the chest cavity, resulting in air movement into the lungs. Infants' chest walls are highly compliant (pliable) and fail to support the lungs adequately. Functional residual capacity can be greatly reduced if respiratory effort is diminished. This lack of lung support also makes the tidal volume of infants and toddlers almost completely dependent on movement of the diaphragm. If diaphragm movement is impaired (as in states of hyperinflation, such as asthma), the intercostal muscles cannot lift the chest wall, and respiration is further compromised.

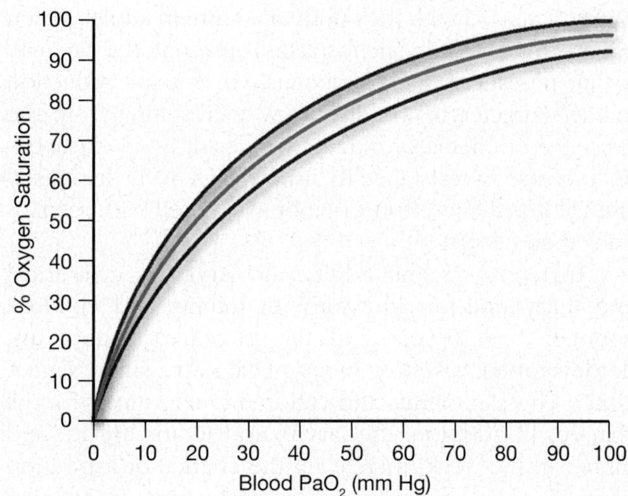

FIGURE 40.2 Normal hemoglobin dissociation curve (green), shift to the right (red), and shift to the left (blue).

Metabolic Rate and Oxygen Need

Children have a significantly higher metabolic rate than adults. Their resting respiratory rates are faster and their demand for oxygen is higher. Adult oxygen consumption is 3 to 4 L/min, while infants consume 6 to 8 L/min. In any situation of respiratory distress, infants and children will develop hypoxemia more rapidly than adults (Weiner, 2022). This may be attributed not only to the child's increased oxygen requirement but also to the effect that certain conditions have on the oxyhemoglobin dissociation curve.

Normal oxygen transport relies on binding of oxygen to hemoglobin in areas of high partial pressure of oxygen (PaO_2) (pulmonary arterial beds) and release of oxygen from hemoglobin when the PaO_2 is low (peripheral tissues). Normally, a PaO_2 of 95 mm Hg results in an oxygen saturation of 97%. A decrease in oxygen saturation results in a disproportionate (much larger) decrease in PaO_2 (Fig. 40.2). Thus, a small decrease in oxygen saturation reflects a larger decrease in PaO_2. Conditions such as alkalosis, hypothermia, hypocarbia, anemia, and fetal hemoglobin cause oxygen to become more tightly bound to hemoglobin, resulting in the curve shifting to the left. Common pediatric conditions such as acidosis, hyperthermia, and hypercarbia cause hemoglobin to decrease its affinity for oxygen, further shifting the curve to the right.

COMMON MEDICAL TREATMENTS

A variety of interventions are used to treat respiratory illness in children. The treatments listed in Common Medical Treatments 40.1 and Drug Guide 40.1 usually require a primary provider's or nurse practitioner's order when a child is hospitalized.

COMMON MEDICAL TREATMENTS 40.1 Respiratory Disorders

Treatment	Explanation	Indications	Nursing Implications
Oxygen	Supplemented via mask, nasal cannula, hood, or tent or via endotracheal or nasotracheal tube	Hypoxemia, respiratory distress	Monitor response via work of breathing and pulse oximetry.
High humidity	Addition of moisture to inspired air	Common cold, croup, tonsillectomy	Infant may require extra blankets with cool mist and frequent changes of bedclothes under oxygen hood or tent as they become damp.
Suctioning	Removal of secretions via bulb syringe or suction catheter	Excessive airway secretions (common cold, flu, bronchiolitis, pertussis)	Should be done carefully and only as far as recommended for age or tracheostomy tube size, or until cough or gag occurs
Chest physiotherapy (CPT) and postural drainage	Promotes mucus clearance by mobilizing secretions with the assistance of percussion or vibration accompanied by postural drainage	Bronchiolitis, pneumonia, cystic fibrosis, or other conditions resulting in increased mucus production. Not effective in inflammatory conditions without increased mucus	May be performed by respiratory therapist in some institutions, by nurses in others; in either case, nurses must be familiar with the technique and able to educate families on its use.

COMMON MEDICAL TREATMENTS 40.1 Respiratory Disorders

Treatment	Explanation	Indications	Nursing Implications
Saline gargles	Relieves throat pain via saltwater gargle	Pharyngitis, tonsillitis	Recommended for children old enough to understand the concept of gargling (to avoid choking)
Saline lavage	Normal saline introduced into the airway, followed by suctioning	Common cold, flu, bronchiolitis, any condition resulting in increased mucus production in the upper airway	Very helpful for loosening thick mucus; child may need to be in semi-upright position to avoid aspiration.
Chest tube	Insertion of a drainage tube into the pleural cavity to facilitate removal of air or fluid and allow full lung expansion	Pneumothorax, empyema	Should tube become dislodged from container, the chest tube must be clamped immediately or the open end placed into a container of sterile water to avoid further air entry into the chest cavity.
Bronchoscopy	Introduction of a bronchoscope into the bronchial tree for diagnostic purposes; also allows for bronchiolar lavage	Removal of foreign body, cleansing of bronchial tree	Watch for postprocedure airway swelling, complaints of sore throat.

DRUG GUIDE 40.1

COMMON DRUGS FOR RESPIRATORY DISORDERS

Medication	Actions/Indications	Nursing Implications
Expectorant (guaifenesin)	Reduces viscosity of thickened secretions by increasing respiratory tract fluid Used for the common cold, pneumonia, and other conditions requiring mobilization and subsequent expectoration of mucus	Encourage deep breathing before coughing to mobilize secretions. Maintain adequate fluid intake. Assess breath sounds frequently.
Cough suppressants (dextromethorphan, codeine, hydrocodone)	Relieve irritating, nonproductive cough by direct effect on the cough center in the medulla, which suppresses the cough reflex Used for the common cold, sinusitis, pneumonia, bronchitis	Should be used only with nonproductive coughs in the absence of wheezing
Antihistamines	Treatment of allergic conditions such as allergic rhinitis, asthma	May cause drowsiness or dry mouth
Antibiotics (oral, parenteral)	Treatment of bacterial infections of the respiratory tract such as pharyngitis, tonsillitis, sinusitis, bacterial pneumonia, cystic fibrosis, empyema, abscess, tuberculosis	Check for antibiotic allergies. Should be given as prescribed for the length of time prescribed
Antibiotics (inhaled)	Treatment of bacterial infections of the respiratory tract in children with cystic fibrosis	Can be given via nebulizer
Beta$_2$-Adrenergic agonists (short acting) (i.e., albuterol, levalbuterol, pirbuterol)	Relax airway smooth muscle, resulting in bronchodilation Used for acute and chronic treatment of wheezing and bronchospasm in asthma, bronchiolitis, cystic fibrosis, chronic lung disease; also used to prevent wheezing in exercise-induced asthma	Administered via inhalation Can be used for acute relief of bronchospasm May cause nervousness, tachycardia, and jitteriness Inhaled agents result in fewer systemic side effects.
Beta$_2$-Adrenergic agonists (long acting) (i.e., formoterol, salmeterol)	Long-acting bronchodilator used in chronic asthma management and for prevention of exercise-induced asthma Long-term control in chronic asthma Prevention of exercise-induced asthma	Administered via inhalation Used only for long-term control or for exercise-induced asthma, not for relief of bronchospasm in an acute wheezing episode

(continued)

DRUG GUIDE 40.1 (*continued*)

COMMON DRUGS FOR GI DISORDERS

Medication	Actions/Indications	Nursing Implications
Racemic epinephrine	Produces bronchodilation Indicated for croup	Assess lung sounds and work of breathing. Observe for rebound bronchospasm.
Anticholinergic (ipratropium)	Produces bronchodilation in asthma or chronic lung disease	In children, generally used as an adjunct to beta$_2$-adrenergic agonists for treatment of bronchospasm
Antiviral agents (oral: amantadine, rimantadine, oseltamivir: inhaled zanamivir)	Treatment and prevention of influenza A	Amantadine, rimantadine: monitor for confusion, nervousness, and jitteriness Oseltamivir, zanamivir: well tolerated but expensive
Corticosteroids (inhaled) (beclomethasone, budesonide, fluticasone, mometasone)	Exert a potent, locally acting antiinflammatory effect to decrease the frequency and severity of asthma attacks; may also delay pulmonary damage that occurs with chronic asthma; also used for chronic lung disease and croup syndromes	Not for treatment of acute wheezing Rinse mouth after inhalation to decrease incidence of fungal infections, dry mouth, and hoarseness. Minimal systemic absorption makes inhaled steroids the treatment of choice for asthma maintenance program.
Corticosteroids (oral, parenteral) (prednisolone, prednisone)	Suppress inflammation and normal immune response Used for acute asthma exacerbations, wheezing with chronic lung disease, and severe croup	May cause hyperglycemia May suppress reaction to allergy tests Consult primary provider or nurse practitioner if vaccinations are ordered during course of systemic corticosteroid therapy. Short courses of therapy are generally safe. Very effective, but long-term or chronic use can result in peptic ulceration, altered growth, and numerous other side effects. Children on long-term dosing should have growth assessed.
Decongestants (e.g., pseudoephedrine)	Treatment of runny or stuffy nose associated with the common cold, sinusitis, or allergic rhinitis in children older than age 6	Assess child periodically for nasal congestion. Some children react to decongestants with excessive sleepiness or increased activity.
Leukotriene receptor antagonists (montelukast, zafirlukast)	Decrease inflammatory response by antagonizing the effects of leukotrienes to control asthma in children age 1 year and older Montelukast: for allergic rhinitis in children 6 months and older	Given once daily, in the evening Not for relief of bronchospasm during an acute wheezing episode, but may be continued during the episode
Mast cell stabilizers (cromolyn, nedocromil)	Prevent release of histamine from sensitized mast cells, resulting in decreased frequency and intensity of allergic reactions in children with asthma or chronic lung disease; also used as pre-exposure treatment for allergens	Administered via inhalation For prophylactic use, not to relieve bronchospasm during an acute wheezing episode Can be used 10–15 minutes prior to exposure to allergen, to decrease reaction to allergen
Respiratory stimulants (methylxanthines: theophylline, aminophylline, caffeine)	To provide for continuous airway relaxation in moderate or severe asthma to achieve long-term control (methylxanthines)	Administered orally or intravenously; sustained-release oral preparation can be used to prevent nocturnal symptoms. Monitor drug levels routinely. Report signs of toxicity immediately: tachycardia, nausea, vomiting, diarrhea, stomach cramps, anorexia, confusion, headache, restlessness, flushing, increased urination, seizures, arrhythmias, insomnia.
Inhaled pulmonary enzyme (dornase alfa)	Enzyme that hydrolyzes the DNA in sputum, reducing sputum viscosity in children with cystic fibrosis	Administered via nebulizer Monitor for dysphonia and pharyngitis.

Data from UpToDate, Inc. (2024). *Lexi-comp®* (Version 8.1.2) [Mobile app]. Wolters Kluwer Health. https://apps.apple.com/us/app/lexicomp/id313401238.

Clinical Judgment and the Nursing Process

Care of the child with a respiratory disorder includes assessment, nursing analysis, planning, interventions, and evaluation. There are several general concepts related to the nursing process that can be applied to respiratory disorders. From an overall understanding of the care involved for a child with an alteration in gas exchange, the nurse can then individualize the care based on specifics for the particular child.

Assessment

Assessment of respiratory dysfunction in children includes health history, physical examination, and laboratory or diagnostic testing.

Health History

The health history consists of the past medical history, family history, and history of present illness (when the symptoms started and how they have progressed), as well as treatments used at home. Ascertain immunization history. The past medical history might be significant for recurrent colds or sore throats, **atopy** (genetic tendency toward asthma, allergic rhinitis, or atopic dermatitis), prematurity, respiratory dysfunction at birth, poor weight gain, or history of recurrent respiratory illnesses or chronic lung disease. Family history might be significant for chronic respiratory disorders such as asthma or might reveal contacts for infectious exposure. When eliciting the history of the present illness, inquire about onset and progression; fever; nasal congestion; noisy breathing; presence and description of cough; rapid respirations; increased work of breathing; ear, nose, sinus, or throat pain; ear pulling; headache; vomiting with coughing; poor feeding; and lethargy. Also inquire about exposure to secondhand smoke. Children exposed to environmental smoke have an increased incidence of respiratory infections, acute otitis media, and asthma exacerbations (Centers for Disease Control and Prevention [CDC], 2022). See Healthy People 2030 box.

HEALTHY PEOPLE 2030

Objective	Nursing Significance
Reduce the proportion of people exposed to secondhand smoke.	• Educate the family about the effects that passive smoking has on children. • Encourage families to join smoking cessation programs.

Healthy People Objectives retrieved from http://www.healthypeople.gov

Physical Examination

Physical examination of the respiratory system includes inspection and observation, auscultation, percussion, and palpation.

Inspection and Observation

Inspection and observation of the respiratory system includes assessing color, overall appearance, respiratory rate, and hydration status, inspecting the nose and oral cavity as well as the nail beds for clubbing, observing work of breathing, and audibly listening for cough and other airway noises.

Color. Observe the child's skin color, noting pallor or cyanosis (circumoral or central). Pallor (pale appearance) occurs as a result of peripheral vasoconstriction in an effort to conserve oxygen for vital functions. **Cyanosis** (a bluish tinge to the skin and mucous membranes) occurs because of hypoxia (oxygen deficiency). It might first present circumorally (just around the mouth) and progress to central cyanosis. Newborns might have blue hands and feet (acrocyanosis), a normal finding. The infant might have pale hands and feet when cold or when ill, as peripheral circulation is not well developed in early infancy. It is important, then, to note if the cyanosis is central (involving the midline), as this is a true sign of hypoxia. Children with low red blood cell counts might not demonstrate cyanosis as early in the course of hypoxemia as children with normal hemoglobin levels. Therefore, absence of cyanosis or the degree of cyanosis present is not always an accurate indication of the severity of respiratory involvement.

Note the rate and depth of respiration as well as work of breathing. Often, the first sign of respiratory illness in infants and children is **tachypnea** (increased respiratory rate for age).

TAKE NOTE!

A slow or irregular respiratory rate in an acutely ill infant or child is an ominous sign (Weiner, 2022). See Chapter 51.

Nose and Oral Cavity. Inspect the nose and oral cavity. Note nasal drainage and redness or swelling in the nose. Note the color of the pharynx, presence of exudate, tonsil size, and status and presence of lesions anywhere in the oral cavity.

Cough and Other Airway Noises. Note the sound of the cough (Is it wet or productive, dry and hacking, tight? When does the cough occur? Is it only or mainly at night?). Also note if noises associated with breathing are present (e.g., grunting, stridor, or audible wheeze). Grunting occurs on expiration and is produced by premature glottic closure. It is an attempt to preserve or increase functional residual capacity. Grunting might occur with alveolar collapse or loss of lung volume, such as in **atelectasis** (a collapsed or airless portion of the lung), pneumonia, and pulmonary edema. **Stridor**, a high-pitched, readily audible inspiratory noise, is a sign of upper airway obstruction. Sometimes, wheezes can be heard with the naked ear; these are referred to as audible wheezes.

Respiratory Effort. Assess respiratory effort for depth and quality. Is breathing labored? Infants and children with significant nasal congestion may have tachypnea, which usually resolves when the nose is cleared of mucus. Mouth breathing may occur when a large amount of nasal congestion is present. Increased work of breathing, particularly if associated with restlessness and anxiety, usually indicates lower respiratory involvement. Assess for the presence of nasal flaring, retractions, or bobbing of the head with each breath. Nasal flaring can occur early in the course of respiratory illness and is an effort to inhale greater amounts of oxygen.

Retractions. Retractions (the inward pulling of soft tissues with respiration) can occur in the intercostal, subcostal, substernal, supraclavicular, or suprasternal regions (Fig. 40.3). Document the severity of the retractions: mild, moderate, or severe. Also note the use of accessory neck muscles. Note the presence of paradoxical breathing (lack of simultaneous chest and abdominal rise with the inspiratory phase).

TAKE NOTE!

Seesaw (or paradoxical) respirations are very ineffective for **ventilation** (gas exchange) and **oxygenation** (binding of oxygen). The chest falls on inspiration and rises on expiration.

Anxiety and Restlessness. Is the child anxious or restless? Restlessness, irritability, and anxiety result from difficulty in securing adequate oxygen. These might be very early signs of respiratory distress, especially if accompanied by tachypnea. Restlessness might progress to listlessness and lethargy if the respiratory dysfunction is not corrected.

Clubbing. Inspect the fingertips for the presence of **clubbing**, an enlargement of the terminal phalanx of the finger, resulting in a change in the angle of the nail to the fingertip (Fig. 40.4). Clubbing might occur in children with a chronic respiratory illness. It is the result of increased capillary growth as the body attempts to supply more oxygen to distal body cells.

Hydration Status. Note the child's hydration status. Palpate the infant's fontanels to determine if sunken. Assess the oral mucosa for color and moisture. Note skin turgor, presence of tears, and adequacy of urine output. The child with a respiratory illness is at risk for dehydration. Pain related to sore throat or mouth lesions may prevent the child from drinking properly. Nasal congestion interferes with the infant's ability to suck effectively at the breast or bottle. Tachypnea and increased work of breathing interfere with the ability to safely ingest fluids.

Palpation

Palpate the sinuses for tenderness in the older child. Assess for enlargement or tenderness of the lymph nodes of the head and neck. Document alterations in tactile fremitus detected on palpation. Increased tactile fremitus might occur in the case of pneumonia or

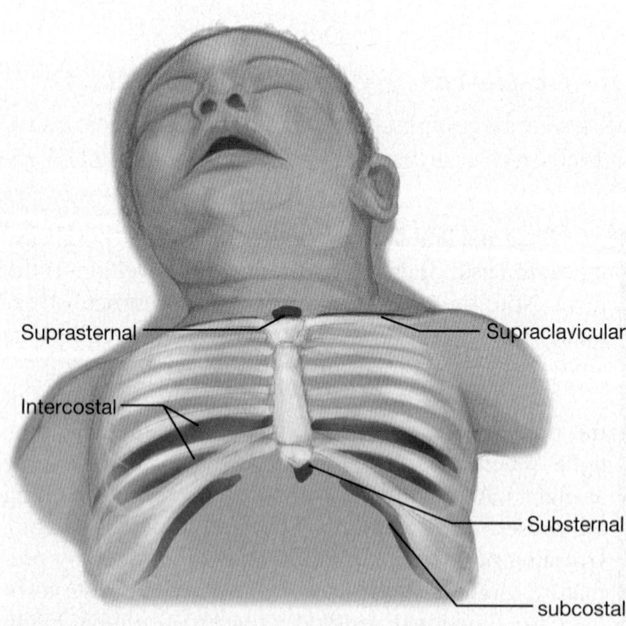

FIGURE 40.3 Location of retractions.

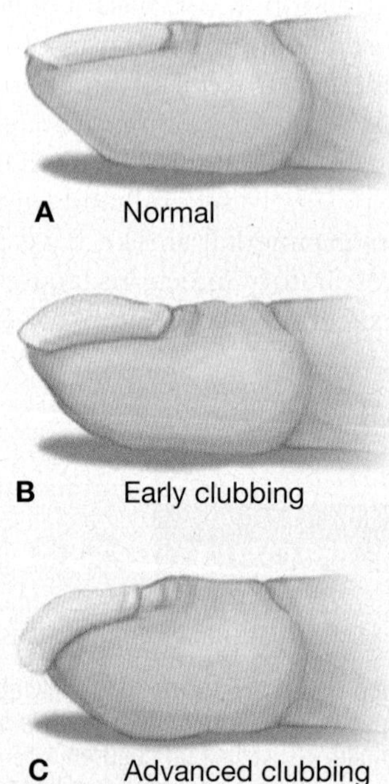

FIGURE 40.4 Normal fingertip **(A)**. Early clubbing **(B)** may progress eventually to advanced clubbing **(C)** because of chronic hypoxemia.

pleural effusion. Fremitus might be decreased in the case of barrel chest, as with cystic fibrosis. Absent fremitus might be noted with pneumothorax or atelectasis.

Compare central and peripheral pulses. Note the quality of the pulse as well as the rate. With significant respiratory distress, perfusion often becomes compromised. Poor perfusion might be reflected in weaker peripheral pulses (radial, pedal) when compared to central pulses.

Percussion

When percussing, note sounds that are not resonant in nature. Flat or dull sounds might be percussed over partially consolidated lung tissue, as in pneumonia. Tympany might be percussed with a pneumothorax. Note the presence of hyperresonance (as might be apparent with asthma).

Auscultation

Assess lung sounds via auscultation. Evaluate breath sounds over the anterior and posterior chest, as well as in the axillary areas. Note the adequacy of aeration. Breath sounds should be equal bilaterally. The intensity and pitch should be equal throughout the lungs; document diminished breath sounds. In the absence of concurrent lower respiratory illness, the breath sounds should be clear throughout all lung fields. During normal respiration, the inspiratory phase is usually softer and longer than the expiratory phase. Prolonged expiration is a sign of bronchial or bronchiolar obstruction. Bronchiolitis, asthma, pulmonary edema, and an intrathoracic foreign body can cause prolonged expiratory phases.

Infants and young children have thin chest walls. When the upper airway is congested (as in a severe cold), the noise produced in the upper airway might be transmitted throughout the lung fields. When upper airway congestion is transmitted to the lung fields, the congested sounding noise heard over the trachea is the same type of noise heard over the lungs but is much louder and more intense. To ascertain if these sounds are truly adventitious lung sounds or if they are transmitted from the upper airway, auscultate again after the child coughs or their nose has been suctioned. Another way to discern the difference is to compare auscultatory findings over the trachea to the lung fields to determine if the abnormal sound is truly from within the lung or is actually a sound transmitted from the upper airway.

Note adventitious sounds heard on auscultation. **Wheezing**, a high-pitched sound that usually occurs on expiration, results from obstruction in the lower trachea or bronchioles. Wheezing that clears with coughing is most likely a result of secretions in the lower trachea. Wheezing resulting from obstruction of the bronchioles, as in bronchiolitis, asthma, chronic lung disease, or cystic fibrosis, does not clear with coughing. **Rales** (crackling sounds) result when the alveoli become fluid filled, such as in pneumonia. Note the location of the adventitious sounds as well as the timing (on inspiration, expiration, or both). Tachycardia might also be present. An increase in heart rate often initially accompanies hypoxemia.

Laboratory and Diagnostic Testing

Common Laboratory and Diagnostic Tests 40.1 explains the laboratory and diagnostic tests most commonly used for a child with a respiratory disorder. The tests can assist the primary provider or nurse practitioner in diagnosing the disorder and/or be used as guidelines in

COMMON LABORATORY AND DIAGNOSTIC TESTS 40.1 Alterations in Oxygenation/Respiratory Disorders

Test	Explanation	Indications	Nursing Implications
Allergy skin testing	Suggested allergen is applied to skin via scratch, pin, or prick. A wheal response indicates allergy to the substance.	Allergic rhinitis, asthma	Antihistamines must be discontinued before testing, as they inhibit the test. Close observation for anaphylaxis is necessary. Epinephrine and emergency equipment should be readily available. Some children react to the skin test almost immediately; others take several minutes.
Arterial blood gases	Invasive method (requires blood sampling) of measuring arterial pH, partial pressure of oxygen and carbon dioxide, and base excess in blood	Usually reserved for severe illness, the intubated child, or suspected carbon dioxide retention	Hold pressure for several minutes after a peripheral arterial stick to avoid bleeding. Radial arterial sticks are common and can be very painful. Note if the child is crying excessively during the blood draw, as this affects the carbon dioxide level.

(continued)

COMMON LABORATORY AND DIAGNOSTIC TESTS 40.1 Alterations in Oxygenation/Respiratory Disorders (*continued*)

Test	Explanation	Indications	Nursing Implications
Chest x-ray	X-ray image of the expanded lungs: can show hyperinflation, atelectasis, pneumonia, foreign body, pleural effusion, abnormal heart or lung size	Bronchiolitis, pneumonia, tuberculosis, asthma, cystic fibrosis, bronchopulmonary dysplasia	Children may be afraid of the x-ray equipment. If a parent or familiar adult can accompany the child, often the child is less afraid. If the child is unable or unwilling to hold still for the x-ray, restraint may be necessary. Restraint should be limited to the amount of time needed for the x-ray.
Fluorescent antibody testing	Determines presence of respiratory syncytial virus (RSV), adenovirus, influenza, parainfluenza, or *Chlamydia* in nasopharyngeal secretions	Bronchiolitis, pneumonia	To obtain a nasopharyngeal specimen, instill 1–3 mL of sterile normal saline into one nostril, aspirate the contents using a small sterile bulb syringe, place the contents in sterile container, and immediately send them to the lab.
Fluoroscopy	X-ray examination that uses a fluorescent screen—"real-time" imaging	Identification of masses, abscesses	Requires the child to lie still. Equipment can be frightening. Children may respond to presence of parent or familiar adult.
Gastric washings for AFB (acid-fast bacilli)	Determines presence of AFB in stomach (children often swallow sputum)	Tuberculosis	Nasogastric tube is inserted, and saline is instilled and suctioned out of the stomach to obtain the specimen.
Peak expiratory flow	Measures the maximum flow of air (in L/s) that can be forcefully exhaled in 1 second	Daily use can indicate adequacy of asthma control.	It is important to establish the child's "personal best" by taking twice-daily readings over a 2-week period while well. The average of these is termed "personal best." Charts based on height and age are also available to determine expected peak expiratory flow.
Pulmonary function tests	Measure respiratory flow and lung volumes	Asthma, cystic fibrosis, chronic lung disease	Usually performed by a respiratory therapist trained to do the full spectrum of tests. Spirometry can be obtained by the trained nurse in the outpatient setting.
Pulse oximetry	Noninvasive method of continuously (or intermittently) measuring oxygen saturation	Can be useful in any situation in which a child is experiencing respiratory distress	Probe must be applied correctly to finger, toe, foot, hand, forehead, or ear for the machine to appropriately pick up the pulse and oxygen saturation.
Rapid flu test	Rapid test for detection of influenza A or B	Influenza	Should be done in first 24 hours of illness so that medication administration can begin Have the child gargle with sterile normal saline and then spit into a sterile container. Send immediately to the lab.
Rapid strep test	Instant test for presence of streptococcus A antibody in pharyngeal secretions	Pharyngitis, tonsillitis	Results in 5–10 minutes. Negative tests should be backed up with throat culture.
RAST (radioallergosorbent test)	Measures minute quantities of immunoglobulin E in the blood Carries no risk of anaphylaxis but is not as sensitive as skin testing	Asthma (food allergies)	Blood test that is usually sent out to a reference laboratory
Sinus x-rays, computed tomography (CT), or magnetic resonance imaging (MRI)	Radiologic tests that may show sinus involvement	Sinusitis, recurrent colds	X-ray results are usually received more quickly than CT or MRI results.

COMMON LABORATORY AND DIAGNOSTIC TESTS 40.1 Alterations in Oxygenation/Respiratory Disorders

Test	Explanation	Indications	Nursing Implications
Sputum culture	Bacterial culture of invasive organisms in the sputum	Pneumonia, cystic fibrosis, tuberculosis	Must be true sputum, not mucus from the mouth or nose; child can deep breathe, cough, and spit, or specimen may be obtained via suctioning of the artificial airway.
Sweat chloride test	Collection of sweat on filter paper after stimulation of skin with pilocarpine Measures concentration of chloride in the sweat	Cystic fibrosis	May be difficult to obtain sweat in a young infant.
Throat culture	Bacterial culture (minimum of 24–48 hours required) to determine presence of streptococcus A or other bacteria	Pharyngitis, tonsillitis	Can be obtained on separate swab at same time as rapid strep test to decrease trauma to the child (swab both applicators at once) Do not perform immediately after the child has had medication or something to eat or drink
Tuberculin skin test	Mantoux test (intradermal injection of purified protein derivative)	Tuberculosis, chronic cough	Must be given intradermally; not a valid test if injected incorrectly

Data from Corbett, J. A., & Banks, A. D. (2019). *Laboratory tests and diagnostic procedures with nursing diagnoses* (9th ed.). Pearson Education Inc.; Medtronic. (2024). *Pulse oximetry.* https://www.medtronic.com/covidien/en-us/products/pulse-oximetry.html

determining ongoing treatment. Laboratory or nonnursing personnel obtain some of the tests, while the nurse might obtain others. In either instance, it is important for the nurse to be familiar with how the tests are obtained, what they are used for, and normal versus abnormal results. This knowledge will also be necessary when providing child and family education related to the testing.

Remember Alexander, the 4-month-old with the cold, cough, fatigue, feeding difficulty, and fast breathing? What additional health history and physical examination assessment information should the nurse obtain?

Nursing Analysis

After recognizing and analyzing cues from a thorough assessment, the nurse may identify several patient problems, including:

- Ineffective airway clearance
- Altered breathing pattern
- Altered gas exchange
- Dehydration risk
- Malnutrition risk
- Activity intolerance
- Fear
- Pain
- Altered family functioning
- Caregiver role strain risk
- Knowledge deficiency

After completing an assessment of Alexander, what would your top three patient problems be?

The preceding patient problems provide suggestions for nursing care planning or concept mapping. Suggested interventions with rationales are provided further on. Care planning should be individualized, based on the child's and family's needs. Refer to Chapter 36 for the nursing process for pain management and to Chapter 33 for nursing interventions related to altered family functioning and caregiver role strain risk. Additional information will be included later in the chapter as it relates to nursing management of children with specific disorders, as well as particular nursing interventions for knowledge deficiency.

Nursing Analysis

Ineffective airway clearance related to excessive mucous, exudate in the alveoli, foreign body in airway, or presence of artificial airway as evidenced by adventitious breath sounds, alteration in respiratory pattern or rate, dyspnea, or excessive sputum.

Goal/Outcome

Child will maintain patent airway, free from secretions or obstruction, with easy work of breathing, and respiratory rate within parameters for age.

Maintaining a Patent Airway (interventions with *rationale*)

- Position with airway open (sniffing position if supine) and/or elevate head of bed *to allow for adequate ventilation.*
- Humidify oxygen or room air, and ensure adequate fluid intake (intravenous or oral) *to liquefy secretions for ease in clearance.*

- Suction with bulb syringe or via nasopharyngeal catheter as needed, particularly prior to bottle-feeding, *to promote clearance of secretions.*
- If tachypneic, maintain nothing by mouth (NPO) status *to avoid aspiration.*
- In older child, encourage expectoration of sputum with coughing *to promote airway clearance.*
- Perform chest physiotherapy (CPT) if ordered *to mobilize secretions.*
- Ensure emergency equipment is readily available *to avoid delay should airway become unmaintainable.*

Nursing Analysis

Altered breathing pattern related to respiratory muscle fatigue as evidenced by abnormal breathing pattern, bradypnea, nasal flaring, tachypnea, use of accessory muscles to breathe, dyspnea, or prolonged expiratory phase.

Goal/Outcome

Child will demonstrate effective breathing pattern: respiratory rate within parameters for age, easy work of breathing (absence of retractions, accessory muscle use, grunting, and nasal flaring), or appropriate expiratory phase.

Promoting an Effective Breathing Pattern (interventions with *rationale*)

- Assess respiratory rate, breath sounds, and work of breathing frequently *to ensure progress with treatment and so that deterioration can be noted early.*
- Position for comfort with open airway and room for lung expansion (usually with head of bed elevated). Use pillows or padding if necessary to maintain position *to ensure optimal ventilation via maximum lung expansion.*
- Allow for adequate sleep and rest periods *to conserve energy.*
- Administer antibiotics as ordered: *may be indicated in the case of bacterial respiratory infection.*
- Encourage incentive spirometry and coughing with deep breathing (can be accomplished through play) *to maximize ventilation (play enhances the child's participation).*

Nursing Analysis

Altered gas exchange related to airway plugging, hyperinflation, or atelectasis, as evidenced by abnormal skin color (duskiness or cyanosis), hypoxia, irritability, restlessness, or alterations in arterial blood gases.

Goal/Outcome

Gas exchange will be adequate: pulse oximetry reading on room air is within normal parameters for age, blood gases within normal limits, absence of cyanosis, irritability, restlessness.

Promoting Adequate Gas Exchange (interventions with *rationale*)

- Monitor oxygen saturation via pulse oximetry *to detect alterations in oxygenation.*
- Administer oxygen as ordered *to improve oxygenation.*
- Encourage clearance of secretions via coughing, expectoration, CPT, and suctioning *to improve gas exchange.*
- Administer bronchodilators if ordered (albuterol, levalbuterol, or racemic epinephrine) *to treat bronchospasm and improve gas exchange.*
- Provide frequent contact and support for the child and family *to decrease anxiety, which increases the child's oxygen demands.*
- Assess and monitor mental status (confusion, lethargy, restlessness, combativeness): *hypoxemia can lead to changes in mental status.*

Nursing Analysis

Dehydration risk related to insufficient fluid intake and/or insensible losses via fever, tachypnea, or diaphoresis.

Goal/Outcome

Fluid volume will be maintained: oral mucosa moist and pink, skin turgor elastic, urine output at least 1 to 2 mL/kg/h.

Maintaining Adequate Fluid Volume (interventions with *rationale*)

- Administer intravenous fluids if ordered *to maintain adequate hydration in NPO state.*
- When allowed oral intake, encourage oral fluids. Popsicles, favorite fluids, and games can be used *to promote intake.*
- Assess for signs of *adequate hydration* (flat fontanels, elastic skin turgor, moist mucosa, adequate urine output).
- Monitor intake and output *to identify fluid imbalance.*
- Monitor urine specific gravity, urine and serum electrolytes, blood urea nitrogen, creatinine, and osmolality *to determine fluid status.*

Nursing Analysis

Malnutrition risk factors include insufficient dietary intake.

Goal/Outcome

Child will maintain adequate nutritional intake: weight is gained or maintained. Child consumes adequate diet for age.

Promoting Adequate Nutritional Intake (interventions with *rationale*)

- Weigh on same scale at same time daily *so that measurements are consistent.*
- Perform calorie counts over a 3-day period *to determine whether caloric intake is sufficient.*
- Encourage child to choose higher-calorie, protein-rich foods *to optimize growth potential.*
- Coax young children to eat better by playing games and offering favorite foods *to improve intake.*

Nursing Analysis

Activity intolerance related to imbalance between oxygen supply and demand as evidenced by exertional dyspnea (need for frequent rest while playing), fatigue, or generalized weakness.

Goal/Outcome

Child will resume normal activity level: activity is tolerated without difficulty breathing. Pulse oximetry readings and vital signs are within parameters for age and activity level.

Increasing Activity Tolerance (interventions with *rationale*)

- Provide rest periods balanced with periods of activity, and group nursing activities and visits *to allow for sufficient rest.*
- Provide small, frequent meals *to prevent overtiring (energy is expended while eating).*
- Encourage quiet activities that do not require exertion *to prevent boredom.*
- Allow gradual increase in activity as tolerated, keeping pulse oximetry reading within normal parameters, *to minimize risk of further respiratory compromise.*

Nursing Analysis

Fear related to unfamiliar setting or learned response to difficulty breathing as evidenced by apprehensiveness (clinging, crying, fussing, lack of cooperation) or verbalization.

Goal/Outcome

Fear will be reduced: decreased episodes of crying or fussing, happy and playful at times.

Relieving Fear (interventions with *rationale*)

- Establish trusting relationship with child and family *to decrease anxiety and fear.*
- Utilize play *to gain child's cooperation and trust.*
- Explain procedures to child at developmentally appropriate level *to decrease fear of unknown.*
- Provide favorite blanket or bear as well as comfort measures preferred by child such as rocking or music *for added security.*
- Involve parents in care *to give child reassurance and decrease fear.*

Based on the top three patient problems for Alexander, describe appropriate nursing interventions.

Providing Oxygen Supplementation

Oxygen may be delivered to the child by a variety of methods (Fig. 40.5). Since oxygen administration is considered a drug, it requires a primary provider's or nurse practitioner's order, except when following emergency protocols outlined in a health care facility's policies and procedures. Many health care settings

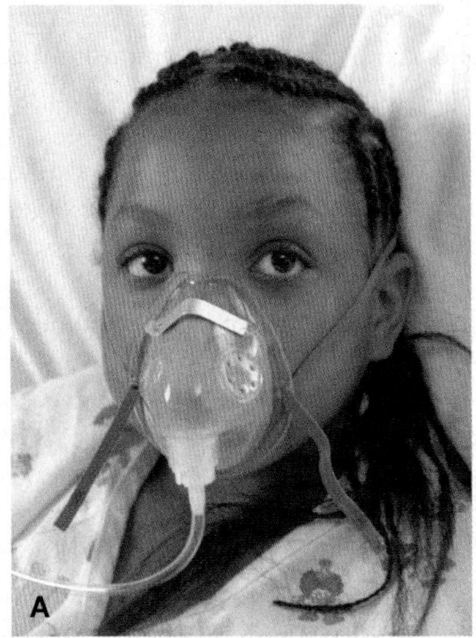

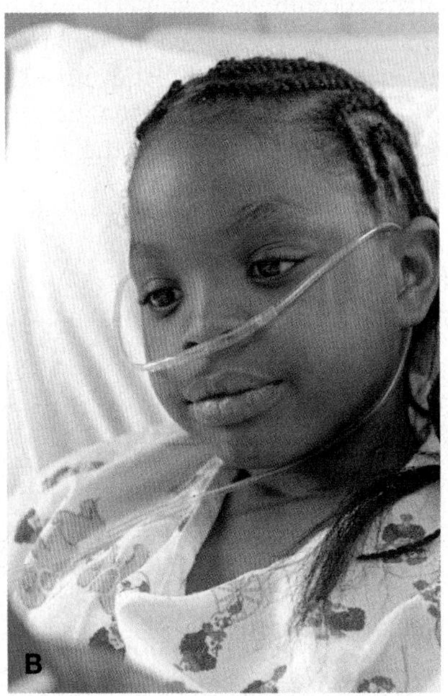

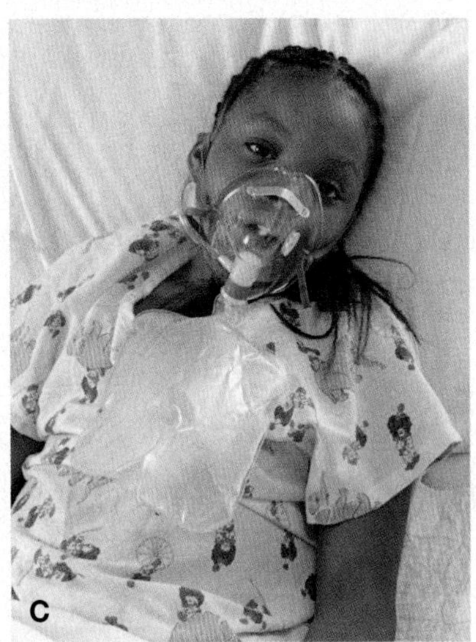

FIGURE 40.5 A. Simple oxygen mask provides about 40% oxygen. **B.** The nasal cannula provides an additional 4% oxygen per 1 L of oxygen flow (i.e., 1 L will deliver 25% oxygen). **C.** The nonrebreather mask provides 80% to 100% oxygen.

develop specific guidelines for oxygen administration that are often coordinated by respiratory therapists, yet the nurse remains responsible for ensuring that oxygen is administered properly.

Oxygen sources include wall-mounted systems as well as cylinders. The supply of oxygen available from a wall-mounted source is limitless, but use of a wall-mounted source restricts the child to the hospital room. Cylinders are portable oxygen tanks; the D-cylinder holds a little less than 400 L of oxygen, and the E-cylinder holds about 650 L of oxygen. Cylinders turn on with a gauge attached to the top of the tank. The cylinder is useful for the child on low-flow oxygen because it allows for mobility.

The tank empties relatively quickly if the child requires a high flow of oxygen, so this is not the best oxygen source in an emergency. Respiratory therapists usually maintain the respiratory equipment that is found in the emergency room or hospital. However, in an outpatient setting, the nurse may be responsible for maintaining respiratory equipment and checking the level of oxygen in the office's oxygen tanks each day.

TAKE NOTE!

Oxygen is highly flammable, so use safety precautions. Post signs ("Oxygen in Use"); inform the family to avoid matches, lighters, and flammable or volatile materials; and use only facility-approved equipment.

The efficiency of oxygen delivery systems is affected by several variables, including the child's respiratory effort, the liter flow of oxygen delivered, and whether the equipment is being used appropriately. In general, oxygen facemasks come in infant, child, and adult sizes. Select the mask that best fits the child. In addition, ensure that the mask is sealed properly to decrease the amount of oxygen that escapes from the mask. Ensure that the liter flow is set according to the manufacturer's recommendations for use with that particular delivery method. The oxygen flow rate or concentration is usually determined by the primary provider's or nurse practitioner's order. Whichever method of delivery is used, provide humidification during oxygen delivery to prevent drying of nasal passages and to assist with liquefying secretions. Table 40.1 provides details on oxygen delivery methods.

CLINICAL REASONING ALERT!

Monitor vital signs, color, respiratory effort, pulse oximetry, and level of consciousness before, during, and after oxygen therapy to evaluate its effectiveness.

ACUTE INFECTIOUS DISORDERS

Acute infectious disorders include the common cold, sinusitis, influenza, pharyngitis, tonsillitis, laryngitis, croup syndromes, respiratory syncytial virus (RSV), pneumonia, and bronchitis.

TABLE 40.1 • Oxygen Delivery Methods

Delivery Method	Description	Nursing Implications
Simple mask	Provides 35%–60% oxygen with a flow rate of 6–10 L/min; oxygen delivery percentage is affected by respiratory rate, inspiratory flow, and adequacy of mask fit.	• Must maintain oxygen flow rate of at least 6 L/min to maintain inspired oxygen concentration and prevent rebreathing of carbon dioxide • Mask must fit snugly to be effective but should not be so tight as to irritate the face.
Venturi mask	Provides 24%–50% oxygen by using a special gauge at the base of the mask that allows mixing of room air with oxygen flow.	• Set oxygen flow rate according to percentage of oxygen desired as indicated on the gauge/dial. • As with simple mask, must fit snugly
Nasal cannula	Provides low oxygen concentration (22%–44%)	• Must be used with humidification to prevent drying and irritation of airways • Can provide very small amounts of oxygen (as low as 25 mL/min) • Maximum recommended liter flow in children is 4 L/min. • Children can eat or talk while on oxygen. • Inspired oxygen concentration affected by mouth breathing • Requires patent nasal passages
Oxygen tent	Provides high-humidity environment with up to 50% oxygen concentration	• Oxygen level drops when tent is opened. • Must change linen frequently as it becomes damp from the humidity. • Secure edges of tent with blankets or by tucking edges under mattress. • Young children may be fearful and resistant. • Mist may interfere with visualization of child inside tent.
Oxygen hood	Provides high concentration (up to 80%–90%) for infants only; allows easy access to chest and lower body	• Liter flow must be set at 10–15 L/min. • Good method for infant but need to remove for feeding • Can and should be humidified

TABLE **40.1** • Oxygen Delivery Methods

Delivery Method	Description	Nursing Implications
Partial rebreathing mask	Simple facemask with an oxygen reservoir bag. Provides 50%–60% oxygen concentration	• Must set liter flow rate at 10–12 L/min to prevent rebreathing of carbon dioxide • The reservoir bag does not completely empty when child inspires if flow rate is set properly.
Nonrebreathing mask	Simple facemask with valves at the exhalation ports and an oxygen reservoir bag with a valve to prevent exhaled air from entering the reservoir; provides 95% oxygen concentration	• Must set liter flow rate at 10–12 L/min to prevent rebreathing of carbon dioxide • The reservoir bag does not completely empty when child inspires if flow rate is set properly.

Data from American Heart Association, & American Academy of Pediatrics. (2020). *Pediatric advanced life support: Provider manual.* American Heart Association; Wolters Kluwer Health. (2023). *Lippincott nursing procedures* (9th ed.). Author.

Common Cold

The common cold is also referred to as a viral upper respiratory infection (URI) or nasopharyngitis. Colds can be caused by rhinoviruses, parainfluenza, RSV, enteroviruses, adenoviruses, and human metapneumovirus. Viral particles spread through the air or from person-to-person contact. Colds occur more frequently in the winter. They affect children of all ages and have a higher incidence among children who attend day care and school-age children (Yoon et al., 2022). It is not unusual for a child to have six to nine colds per year. Spontaneous resolution of the common cold occurs after about 7 to 10 days. Potential complications include secondary bacterial infections of the ears, throat, sinuses, or lungs.

Therapeutic management of the common cold is directed toward symptom relief. Nasal congestion may be relieved via humidity and use of normal saline nasal wash or spray followed by suctioning. Antihistamines are not indicated, as they dry secretions further. Over-the-counter cold preparations are available singly and in combinations. These preparations have not been proven to reduce the length or severity of the cold but may offer symptomatic relief in some children older than 6 years of age (they are not recommended in children younger than the age of 4 due to side effects) (Yoon et al., 2022). See Healthy People 2030 box.

HEALTHY PEOPLE **2030**

Objective	Nursing Significance
Reduce inappropriate antibiotic use in outpatient settings.	• Appropriately educate families that the cause of the common cold is several viruses and that antibiotics are inappropriate for the treatment of viral infections. • Encourage families to use measures such as normal saline nasal washes to decrease symptoms associated with the common cold more quickly.

Healthy People Objectives retrieved from http://www.healthypeople.gov

TAKE NOTE!

Over-the-counter cold preparations containing decongestants intended for use in infants and toddlers are no longer on the market. The products are labeled "not for use in children under 4 years of age" (U.S. Food and Drug Administration, 2023).

Nursing Assessment

The child may have either a stuffy or runny nose. Nasal discharge is usually thin and watery at first but may become thicker and discolored. The color of nasal discharge is not an accurate indicator of viral versus bacterial infection. The child may be hoarse and complain of a sore throat. Cough usually produces very little sputum. Fever, fatigue, watery eyes, and appetite loss may also occur. Symptoms are generally at their worst over the first few days and then decrease over the course of the illness.

Assess for risk factors such as day care or school attendance. Inspect for edema and vasodilation of the mucosa. Diagnosis is based on clinical presentation rather than laboratory or x-ray studies. Comparison Chart 40.1 differentiates causes of nasal congestion.

Nursing Management

Nursing management of the child with a common cold consists of promoting comfort, providing family education, and preventing spread of the cold.

Promoting Comfort

Provide supportive measures such as normal saline nose drops and bulb syringe suctioning for the relief of nasal congestion in infants and toddlers. Teach older children to use a normal saline nose spray to mobilize secretions. A cool mist humidifier also helps with nasal congestion. If over-the-counter nose sprays are used in children,

COMPARISON CHART 40.1 Causes of Nasal Congestion

Sign or Symptom	Allergic Rhinitis	Common Cold	Sinusitis
Length of illness	Varies; may have year-round symptoms	10 days or less	Longer than 10–14 days
Nasal discharge	Thin, watery, clear	Thick, white, yellow, or green; can be thin	Thick, yellow or green
Nasal congestion	Varies	Present	Present
Sneezing	Varies	Present	Absent
Cough	Varies	Present	Varies
Headache	Varies	Varies	Varies
Fever	Absent	Varies	Varies
Bad breath	Absent	Absent	Varies

remind parents they are only for very short-term use. Promote adequate oral fluid intake to liquefy secretions.

Educate parents about the use of cold and cough medications. Although they may offer some symptomatic relief, they have not been proven to shorten the length of cold symptoms. Counsel parents to use the appropriate product depending on the symptom relief desired, rather than a combination product. Products containing acetaminophen combined with other "cold symptom" medications may mask a fever in the child who is developing a secondary bacterial infection. As with all viral infections in children, teach parents that aspirin use should be avoided because of its association with Reye syndrome (Stanford Children's Health, 2024).

Providing Family Education

Currently, there are no medications available to treat the viruses that cause the common cold, so symptomatic treatment is all that is necessary. Antibiotics are not indicated unless the child also has a bacterial infection. Explain to parents the importance of reserving antibiotic use for appropriate illnesses. Provide education about the use of normal saline nose drops and bulb suctioning to clear the infant's nose of secretions. Normal saline nasal wash using a bulb syringe to instill the solution is also helpful for children of all ages with nasal congestion. Although normal saline for nasal administration is available commercially, parents can also make it at home (Box 40.2). Teaching Guidelines 40.1 gives instructions on use of the bulb syringe.

BOX 40.2 Homemade Saltwater Nose Drops

Mix 8 oz distilled water, a half teaspoon of sea salt, and a quarter teaspoon of baking soda. Keep for 24 hours in the refrigerator but allow to come to room temperature prior to use.

Counsel parents about how to recognize complications of the common cold, which include:

- Prolonged fever
- Increased throat pain or enlarged, painful lymph nodes
- Increased or worsening cough, cough lasting longer than 10 days, chest pain, difficulty breathing
- Earache, headache, toothache, or sinus pain
- Unusual irritability or lethargy
- Skin rash

If complications do occur, tell parents to notify the primary provider or nurse practitioner for further instructions or reassessment.

Preventing the Common Cold

Teaching about ways to prevent the common cold is a vital nursing intervention. Explain that frequent handwashing helps to decrease the spread of viruses that cause the common cold. Teach parents and family to avoid secondhand smoke as well as crowded places, especially during the winter. Avoid close contact with individuals known to have a cold. Encourage parents and families to consume a healthy diet and get enough rest.

CONSIDER THIS!

Corey Davis, a 3-year-old, is brought to the clinic by their parent. They present with a runny nose, congestion, and a nonproductive cough. The parent says, "My child's miserable." "I just don't know what to do." "Ever since I put them in day care, they get sick every few weeks." "This is all my fault."

How should the nurse respond? How would you feel if your child was healthy until entering day care? What type of support can the nurse provide to Corey's parent?

TEACHING GUIDELINES 40.1 Using the Bulb Syringe to Suction Nasal Secretions

1. Hold the infant on your lap or on the bed with the head tilted slightly back.

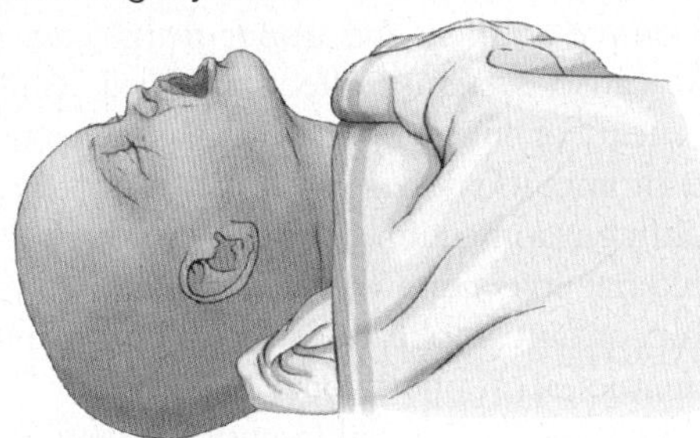

2. If using saline, instill several drops of saline solution in one of the infant's nostrils.

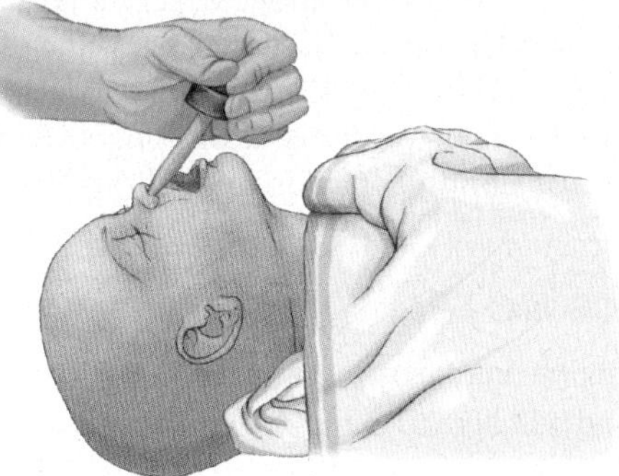

3. Compress the sides of the bulb syringe completely. Use only a rubber-tipped bulb syringe. Place the rubber tip in the infant's nose.

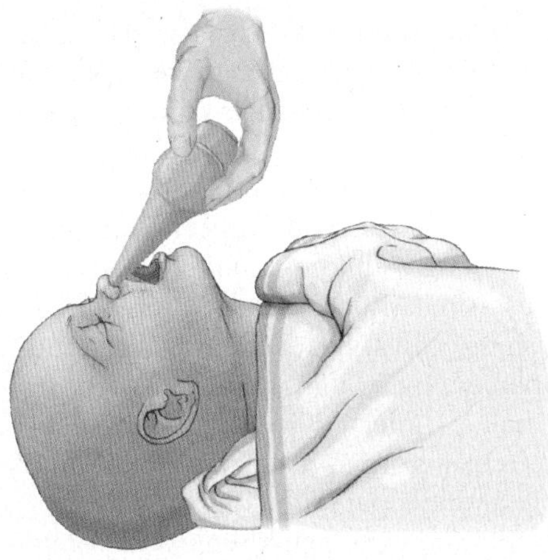

4. Release pressure on the bulb.

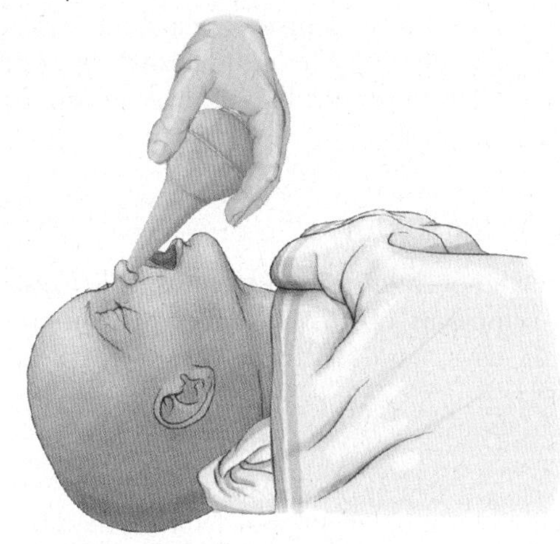

5. Remove the syringe, and squeeze bulb over tissue or the sink to empty it of secretions.

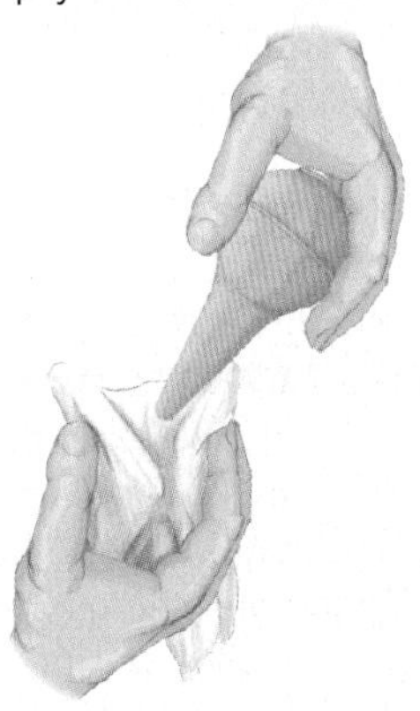

6. Repeat on other nostril if necessary. Using a bulb syringe prior to bottle-feeding or breastfeeding may relieve congestion enough to allow the infant to suck more efficiently.
7. Clean the bulb syringe thoroughly with warm water after each use and allow to air dry.

Sinusitis

Sinusitis (also called rhinosinusitis) generally refers to a bacterial infection of the paranasal sinuses. The disease may be either acute or chronic in nature. In young children, the maxillary and ethmoid sinuses are the main sites of infection. After age 10 years, the frontal sinuses may be more commonly involved (Yoon et al., 2022). Mucosal swelling, decreased ciliary movement, and thickened nasal discharge all contribute to bacterial invasion of the nose. Nasal polyps also place the child at risk for bacterial sinusitis. Complications include orbital cellulitis and intracranial infections, such as subdural empyemas.

Symptoms lasting less than 30 days generally indicate acute sinusitis, whereas symptoms persisting longer than 4 to 6 weeks usually indicate chronic sinusitis.

Sinusitis is managed with antibiotic treatment. The therapeutic management approach varies with chronicity. The course of treatment is usually 14 days. Naturally, chronic sinusitis requires a longer course of treatment than acute sinusitis. Surgical therapy may be indicated for children with chronic sinusitis, particularly if it is recurrent or if nasal polyps are present.

Nursing Assessment

The most common presentation of sinusitis is persistent signs and symptoms of a cold. Rather than improving after 7 to 10 days, nasal discharge persists. Explore the history for:

- Cough
- Fever
- In preschoolers or older children, halitosis (bad breath)
- Facial pain may or may not be present so is not a reliable indicator of disease
- Eyelid edema (in the case of ethmoid sinus involvement)
- Irritability
- Poor appetite

Assess for risk factors such as a history of recurrent cold symptoms or a history of nasal polyps.

On physical examination, note eyelid swelling, extent of nasal drainage, and halitosis. Inspect the throat for postnasal drainage. Inspect the nasal mucosa for erythema. Palpate the sinuses, noting pain with mild pressure. The diagnosis may be made based on the history and clinical presentation. The use of x-ray, CT scan, or MRI is not necessary as they are not specific and do not distinguish viral from bacterial infection (Yoon et al., 2022). (Refer to Comparison Chart 40.1, which differentiates the causes of nasal congestion.)

Nursing Management

Normal saline nose drops or spray, cool mist humidifiers, and adequate oral fluid intake are recommended for children with sinusitis. Teach families the importance of continuing the full course of antibiotics to eradicate the cause of infection. Also educate the family that the use of decongestants and antihistamines as adjuncts in the treatment of sinusitis has not been shown to be beneficial, although intranasal steroids may benefit those with allergic rhinitis (Yoon et al., 2022). Advise parents that normal saline nose spray or nasal washes may promote drainage.

Influenza

Influenza viral infection (known commonly as the "flu") occurs primarily during the winter. It is spread through inhalation of droplets or contact with fine-particle aerosols. Infected children shed the virus for 1 to 2 days before symptoms begin and may continue shedding the virus in increased amounts (as compared to adults) for as long as 2 weeks. Average annual infection rates in children range from 10% to 40% (Munoz & Edwards, 2023). Influenza viruses primarily affect the upper respiratory epithelium but can cause systemic effects as well. Children with chronic heart or lung conditions, diabetes, chronic renal disease, or immune deficiency are at higher risk for more severe influenza infection compared to other children.

Bacterial infections of the respiratory system commonly occur as complications of influenza infection, severe pneumococcal pneumonia in particular. Otitis media occurs in 10% to 50% of children with influenza (Munoz & Edwards, 2023). Rarely, Reye syndrome occurs in children with influenza who have taken aspirin. Acute myositis is a rare and severe complication, which is particular to children. A sudden onset of severe pain and tenderness in both calves causes the child to refuse to walk. Due to the potential for complications, a prolonged fever or a fever that returns during convalescence should be investigated.

TAKE NOTE!

Current recommendations are for all children older than 6 months of age to be immunized yearly against influenza (CDC, 2023c).

Nursing Assessment

Children who attend day care or school are at higher risk for influenza infection than those who are routinely at home. Note the presence of risk factors for severe disease, such as chronic heart or lung disease (such as asthma), diabetes, chronic renal disease, or immune deficiency or children with cancer receiving chemotherapy. School-age children and adolescents experience the illness similarly to adults. Abrupt onset of fever, facial flushing, chills, headache, myalgia, and malaise are accompanied by cough and **coryza** (nasal discharge). About half of infected individuals have a dry or sore throat. Ocular symptoms such as photophobia, tearing, burning, and eye pain are common.

Infants and young children exhibit symptoms similar to other respiratory illnesses. Fever greater than 39.5°C is common. Infants may be mildly toxic in appearance and irritable and have a cough, coryza, and pharyngitis. Wheezing may occur, as influenza can also cause bronchiolitis. An erythematous rash may be present, and diarrhea may also occur. The diagnosis may be confirmed by a rapid assay test.

Nursing Management

Nursing management of influenza is mainly supportive. Provide symptomatic treatment of cough and fever. Instruct parents on the maintenance of hydration. Administer antiviral drugs as prescribed as they can reduce the symptoms associated with influenza if they are started within the first 48 hours of the illness (UpToDate, Inc., 2024).

Pharyngitis

Inflammation of the throat mucosa (pharynx) is referred to as pharyngitis. A sore throat may accompany nasal congestion and is often viral in nature. A bacterial sore throat most often occurs without nasal symptoms. Group A streptococci account for 20% to 30% of cases, with the remainder being caused by other viruses or bacteria (Yoon et al., 2022).

Suppurative complications of group A streptococcal infection include peritonsillar or retropharyngeal abscess. Peritonsillar abscess may be noted by asymmetric swelling of the tonsils, shifting of the uvula to one side, and palatal edema. Retropharyngeal abscess may progress to the point of airway obstruction, hence requiring careful evaluation and appropriate treatment. Additional complications include acute rheumatic fever (see Chapter 41) and acute glomerulonephritis (see Chapter 43).

Viral pharyngitis is usually self-limited and does not require therapy beyond symptomatic relief. Group A streptococcal pharyngitis requires antibiotic therapy. If either the rapid diagnostic test or throat culture (described below) is positive for group A streptococci, penicillin is generally prescribed. Appropriate alternative antibiotics include amoxicillin and, for those allergic to penicillin, macrolides and cephalosporins.

TAKE NOTE!

A "strep carrier" is a child who has a positive throat culture for streptococci when asymptomatic. Strep carriers are not at risk for complications from streptococci, as are those who are acutely infected with streptococci and are symptomatic (Yoon et al., 2022).

Nursing Assessment

Inquire about sudden onset of pharyngitis. The history may include a fever, sore throat and difficulty swallowing, headache, and abdominal pain. Ask about recent incidence of viral or strep throat in the family, day care center, or school.

Inspect the pharynx and tonsils, which may demonstrate varying degrees of inflammation (Fig. 40.6). Exudate may be present but is not diagnostic of bacterial infection. Note the presence of petechiae on the palate. Inspect the tongue for a strawberry appearance. Palpate for enlargement and tenderness of the anterior cervical nodes. Inspect the skin for a fine, red, sandpaper-like rash (called scarlatiniform), particularly on the trunk or abdomen, a common finding with streptococcus A infection.

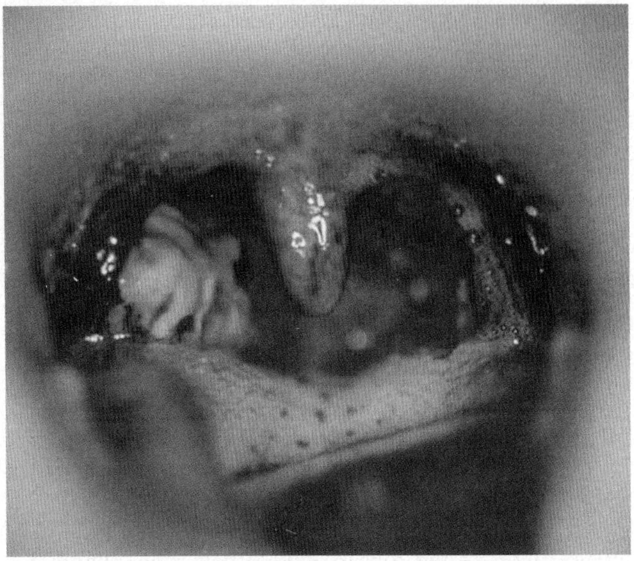

FIGURE 40.6 Note the redness of the pharynx, tonsillar exudate, and white strawberry tongue coating.

The nurse may obtain a throat swab for rapid diagnostic testing and throat culture. The rapid strep test is a sensitive and reliable measure, rarely resulting in false-positive readings (Yoon et al., 2022). If the rapid strep test is negative, the second swab may be sent for a throat culture.

• • • ATRAUMATIC CARE • • •

When obtaining two swabs for rapid strep testing and throat culture, swab the applicators simultaneously to decrease perceived trauma to the child.

Nursing Management

Nursing management of the child with pharyngitis focuses on promoting comfort and providing family education.

Promoting Comfort

Teach families that saline gargles (made with 8 oz of warm water and a half teaspoon of table salt) are soothing for children old enough to cooperate. Administering analgesics such as acetaminophen and ibuprofen may ease fever and pain. Educate families that sucking on throat lozenges or hard candy may also ease pain. Providing cool mist humidity helps to keep the mucosa moist in the event of mouth breathing. Encourage the child to ingest popsicles, cool liquids, and ice chips to maintain hydration.

Providing Family Education

Parents may often need additional education about treatments as they may be accustomed to "sore throats" being treated with antibiotics. However, teach parents that in the case of a viral cause, antibiotics will not be necessary and the pharyngitis will resolve in a few days. For the child with streptococcal pharyngitis, urge parents to have the child complete the entire prescribed course of antibiotics. After 24 hours of antibiotic therapy, instruct the parents to discard the child's toothbrush to avoid reinfection. Educate parents that children may return to day care or school after they have been receiving antibiotics for 24 hours; they are considered noncontagious at that point.

Tonsillitis

Inflammation of the tonsils often occurs with pharyngitis and, thus, may also be viral or bacterial in nature. Viral infections require only symptomatic treatment. Treatment for bacterial tonsillitis is the same as for bacterial pharyngitis. Occasionally, surgical intervention is warranted. Tonsillectomy (surgical removal of the palatine tonsils) may be indicated for the child with recurrent streptococcal tonsillitis or massive tonsillar hypertrophy or for other reasons. When hypertrophied adenoids obstruct breathing, then adenoidectomy (surgical removal of the adenoids) may be indicated.

Nursing Assessment

Note whether fever is present currently or by history. Inquire about the history of recurrent pharyngitis or tonsillitis. Note if the child's voice sounds muffled or hoarse. Inspect the pharynx for redness and enlargement of the tonsils. As the tonsils enlarge, the child may experience difficulty breathing and swallowing. When tonsils touch at the midline ("kissing tonsils" or 4+ in size), the airway may become obstructed. Also, if the adenoids are enlarged, the posterior nares become obstructed. The child may breathe through the mouth and may snore. Palpate the anterior cervical nodes for enlargement and tenderness. Rapid test or culture may be positive for streptococcus A.

Nursing Management

Tonsillitis that is medically treated requires the same nursing management as pharyngitis. Nursing care for the child after tonsillectomy is described further on.

Promoting Airway Clearance

Until fully awake, place the child in a side-lying or prone position to facilitate safe drainage of secretions. Once alert, the child may prefer to sit up or have the head of the bed elevated. Suctioning, if necessary, should be done carefully to avoid trauma to the surgical site. Note that dried blood may be present on the teeth and the nares, with old blood present in emesis. Since the presence of blood can be very frightening to parents, alert them to this possibility.

Maintaining Fluid Volume

Although unusual postoperatively, monitor for hemorrhage as it may occur any time from the immediate postoperative period to as late as 10 days after surgery. Inspect the throat for bleeding. Mucus tinged with blood may be expected, but fresh blood in the secretions indicates bleeding. Watch for continuous swallowing of small amounts of blood while awake or sleeping as this may indicate early bleeding. Monitor for other signs of hemorrhage, including tachycardia, pallor, restlessness, frequent throat clearing, and emesis of bright red blood.

To avoid trauma to the surgical site, discourage the child from coughing, clearing the throat, blowing the nose, and using straws. Upon discharge, instruct the parents to immediately report any sign of bleeding to the primary provider or nurse practitioner. To maintain fluid volume postoperatively, encourage children to take any fluids they desire; popsicles and ice chips are particularly soothing. Citrus juice and brown or red fluids should be avoided: the acid in citrus juice may irritate the throat, and red or brown fluids may be confused with blood if vomiting occurs.

Relieving Pain

Educate families that for the first 24 hours after surgery, the throat is very sore. Provide adequate pain relief (may be with or without narcotics) to establish adequate oral fluid intake. Apply an ice collar if prescribed. Counsel parents to maintain pain control upon discharge from the facility, not only for the child's sake but also to enable the child to continue to drink fluids.

Infectious Mononucleosis

Infectious mononucleosis is a self-limited illness caused by the Epstein–Barr virus. It is characterized by fever, malaise, sore throat, and lymphadenopathy. Mononucleosis is commonly called the "kissing disease" since it is transmitted by oropharyngeal secretions. It can occur at any age but is most often diagnosed in adolescents and young adults (Aronson & Auwaerter, 2023). Some infected individuals may have concomitant streptococcal pharyngitis. Complications include splenic rupture, Guillain–Barré syndrome, and aseptic meningitis.

Nursing Assessment

Note any history of exposure to infected individuals. Determine history of fever and onset and progression of sore throat, malaise, and other complaints. Observe for periorbital edema. Inspect the pharynx and tonsils for inflammation and patches of gray exudate. Petechiae may be present on the palate. Palpate for bilateral nontender enlargement of the posterior cervical lymph nodes. After 3 to 5 days of illness, the pharynx may become edematous and the tonsillar exudate more extensive. Lymphadenopathy may progress to include the anterior cervical nodes, which may become tender. Palpate the abdomen for splenomegaly or hepatomegaly. An erythematous maculopapular rash may appear as the illness progresses. Definitive diagnosis may be made by Monospot or Epstein–Barr virus titers.

TAKE NOTE!

The Monospot may be negative if obtained within the first 7 days of illness with infectious mononucleosis. Epstein–Barr virus titer is reliable at any point in the illness (Aronson & Auwaerter, 2023).

Nursing Management

Nursing management of mononucleosis is primarily symptomatic. The throat may be very sore, so encourage families to administer analgesics and provide the child with saltwater gargles. Encourage bed rest while the child is febrile. Instruct the child and family that frequent rest periods may be necessary for several weeks after the onset of illness, as fatigue may persist as long as 6 weeks. During the acute phase, if tonsillar or pharyngeal edema threatens to obstruct the airway, administer corticosteroids as prescribed to decrease the inflammation. When children or teens have splenomegaly or hepatomegaly, educate the child and family that strenuous activity and contact sports should be avoided. Ensure parents understand that the appearance of a rash or jaundice should be reported to the primary provider or nurse practitioner.

Laryngitis

Inflammation of the larynx is termed laryngitis. It may occur alone or in conjunction with other respiratory symptoms. It is characterized by a hoarse voice or loss of the voice (so soft as to make it difficult to hear). Oral fluids might offer relief, but resting the voice for 24 hours will allow the inflammation to subside. Laryngitis alone requires no further intervention.

Croup

Children between 3 months and 3 years of age are the most frequently affected with croup, rarely affecting children over age 6 (Woods, 2023). Croup is also referred to as laryngotracheobronchitis because inflammation and edema of the larynx, trachea, and bronchi occur as a result of viral infection. Parainfluenza is responsible for most cases of croup, although other viruses may also be implicated (Woods, 2023). The inflammation and edema obstruct the airway, resulting in symptoms. Mucus production also occurs, further contributing to obstruction of the airway. Narrowing of the subglottic area of the trachea results in audible inspiratory stridor. Edema of the larynx causes hoarseness. Inflammation in the larynx and trachea causes the characteristic barking cough of croup.

Symptoms occur most often at night, presenting suddenly, with resolution of symptoms in the morning. Croup is usually self-limited, lasting only about 3 to 5 days. Complications of croup are rare but may include worsening respiratory distress, hypoxia, or bacterial superinfection (as in the case of bacterial tracheitis).

Croup is usually managed on an outpatient basis, with affected children rarely requiring hospitalization. Corticosteroids (usually a single dose) are used to decrease inflammation, and racemic epinephrine aerosols demonstrate the alpha-adrenergic effect of mucosal vasoconstriction, helping to decrease edema. Children with croup may be hospitalized if they have significant stridor at rest or severe retractions after a several-hour period of observation. Comparison Chart 40.2 compares croup to epiglottitis.

COMPARISON CHART 40.2 Croup Versus Epiglottitis

	Spasmodic Croup	Epiglottitis
Preceding illness	None or minimal coryza	None or mild upper respiratory infection
Age group usually affected	3 months to 3 years	1–8 years
Onset	Usually sudden, often at night	Rapid (within hours)
Fever	Variable	High
Barking cough, hoarseness	Yes	No
Dysphagia	No	Yes
Toxic appearance	No	Yes
Cause	Viral	*Haemophilus influenzae type B*

Nursing Assessment

Note the age of the child; children between 3 months and 3 years of age are most likely to present with viral croup (laryngotracheobronchitis). History may reveal a cough that developed during the night (most common presentation) and that sounds like barking (or a seal). Inspect for the presence of mild URI symptoms. Temperature may be normal or elevated mildly. Listen for inspiratory stridor, and observe for suprasternal retractions. Auscultate the lungs for adequacy of breath sounds. Croup is usually diagnosed based on history and clinical presentation, but a lateral neck radiograph may be obtained to rule out epiglottitis.

CLINICAL REASONING ALERT!

The child with fever, a toxic appearance, and increasing respiratory distress despite appropriate croup treatment may have bacterial tracheitis (Woods, 2023). Notify the primary provider or nurse practitioner of these findings in a child with croup.

Nursing Management

If the child's care is being managed at home, advise parents about the symptoms of respiratory distress, and instruct them to seek treatment if the child's respiratory condition worsens. Teach parents to expose their child to humidified air (via a cool mist humidifier or steamy bathroom). Although never clinically proven, use of humidified air has long been recommended for alleviating coughing jags and has anecdotally been reported as helpful (particularly exposure to cooler air). Administer dexamethasone if ordered or teach parents about home administration. Explain to parents that the effects of racemic epinephrine last about 2 hours and that the child must be observed closely as occasionally a child will worsen again, requiring another aerosol. Teaching Guidelines 40.2 provides information about home care of croup.

Epiglottitis

Epiglottitis (inflammation and swelling of the epiglottis) is most often caused by *Haemophilus influenzae* type b and has become a rare occurrence with the extensive use of the Hib vaccine since the 1980s (Houin et al., 2022). Respiratory arrest and death may occur if the airway becomes completely occluded. Additional complications include pneumothorax and pulmonary edema. Therapeutic management focuses on airway maintenance and support. Intravenous antibiotic therapy is necessary. The child will be managed in the intensive care unit. See Comparison Chart 40.2 for information comparing croup to epiglottitis.

TEACHING GUIDELINES 40.2 Home Care of Croup

- Keep the child quiet and discourage crying.
- Allow the child to sit up (in your arms).
- Encourage rest and fluid intake.
- If stridor occurs, take the child into a steamy bathroom for 10 minutes.
- Administer medication (corticosteroid) as directed.
- Watch the child closely. Call the primary provider or nurse practitioner if:
  - the child breathes faster, has retractions, or has any other difficulty breathing.
  - the nostrils flare or the lips or nails have a bluish tint.
  - the cough or stridor does not improve with exposure to moist air.
  - restlessness increases or the child is confused.
  - the child begins to drool or cannot swallow.

Adapted from Schare, R. S. (2021). *Croup.* https://kidshealth.org/en/parents/croup.html

Nursing Assessment

Carefully assess the child with suspected epiglottitis. Note sudden onset of symptoms and high fever. The child has an overall toxic appearance. They may refuse to speak or may speak only with a very soft voice. The child may refuse to lie down and may assume the characteristic position: sitting forward with the neck extended. Drooling may be present. Note anxiety or a frightened appearance. Note the child's color. Cough is usually absent. A lateral neck radiograph may be performed to determine whether epiglottitis is present. This is done cautiously, so as not to induce airway obstruction with changes in position of the child's neck.

CLINICAL REASONING ALERT!

Do not under any circumstance attempt to visualize the throat: reflex laryngospasm may occur, precipitating immediate airway occlusion.

Nursing Management

Do not leave the child unattended. Keep the child and parents as calm as possible. Allow the child to assume a position of comfort. Do not place the child in a supine position, as airway occlusion may occur. Provide 100% oxygen in the least invasive manner that is acceptable to the child. If the child with epiglottitis experiences complete airway occlusion, an emergency **tracheostomy** (incision in trachea to permit breathing) may be necessary. Ensure that emergency equipment is available and that personnel trained in intubation of the pediatric occluded airway and percutaneous tracheostomy are notified of the child's presence in the facility.

CLINICAL REASONING ALERT!

Epiglottitis is characterized by dysphagia, drooling, anxiety, irritability, and significant respiratory distress. Prepare for the event of sudden airway occlusion.

Bronchiolitis

Bronchiolitis is an acute inflammatory process of the bronchioles and small bronchi. Nearly always caused by a viral pathogen, RSV accounts for the majority of cases of bronchiolitis, with adenovirus, parainfluenza, and human meta-pneumovirus also being important causative agents. This discussion will focus on RSV bronchiolitis.

The peak incidence of bronchiolitis is in the fall and winter, coinciding with RSV season, which in the United States and Canada generally begins in September or October and continues through early spring. Virtually all children will contract RSV infection within the first few years of life. RSV bronchiolitis occurs most often in infants and toddlers (Piedra, 2023). The severity of disease is related inversely to the age of the child. The frequency and severity of RSV infection decrease with age. Repeated RSV infections occur throughout life but are usually localized to the upper respiratory tract after toddlerhood.

Pathophysiology

RSV is a highly contagious virus and may be contracted through direct contact with respiratory secretions or from particles on objects contaminated with the virus. RSV invades the nasopharynx, where it replicates and then spreads down to the lower airway via aspiration of upper airway secretions. RSV infection causes necrosis of the respiratory epithelium of the small airways, peribronchiolar mononuclear infiltration, and plugging of the lumens with mucus and exudate. The small airways become variably obstructed; this allows adequate inspiratory volume but prevents full expiration. This leads to hyperinflation and atelectasis. Serious alterations in gas exchange occur, with arterial hypoxemia and carbon dioxide retention resulting from mismatching of pulmonary ventilation and perfusion. Hypoventilation occurs secondary to markedly increased work of breathing.

Therapeutic Management

Management of RSV focuses on supportive treatment. Supplemental oxygen, nasal and/or nasopharyngeal suctioning, and oral or intravenous hydration are used. Many infants are managed at home with close observation and adequate hydration. Hospitalization is required for children with more severe disease. The infant with tachypnea, significant retractions, poor oral intake, or lethargy can deteriorate quickly, to the point of requiring ventilatory support, and thus warrants hospital admission.

Nursing Assessment

For a full description of the assessment phase of the nursing process, refer to the "Clinical Judgment and the Nursing Process" section earlier in the chapter. Assessment findings pertinent to RSV bronchiolitis are discussed further on.

Health History

Elicit a description of the present illness and chief complaint. Common signs and symptoms reported during the health history might include:

- Onset of illness with a clear runny nose (sometimes profuse)
- Pharyngitis
- Low-grade fever
- Development of cough 1 to 3 days into the illness, followed by a wheeze shortly thereafter
- Poor feeding

Explore the child's current and past medical history for risk factors such as:

- Young age (younger than 2 years old), more severe disease in a child younger than 6 months old
- Prematurity
- Multiple birth
- Birth during April to September
- History of chronic lung disease (bronchopulmonary disease)
- Cyanotic or complicated congenital heart disease
- Immunocompromise
- Male sex
- Exposure to passive tobacco smoke
- Crowded living conditions
- Day care attendance
- School-age siblings
- Low socioeconomic status
- Lack of breastfeeding

Physical Examination

Examination of the child with RSV involves inspection, observation, and auscultation.

INSPECTION AND OBSERVATION

Observe the child's general appearance and color (centrally and peripherally). The infant with RSV bronchiolitis might appear air-hungry, exhibiting various degrees of cyanosis and respiratory distress, including tachypnea, retractions, accessory muscle use, grunting, and periods of apnea. Cough and audible wheeze might be heard. The infant might appear listless and uninterested in feeding, surroundings, or parents.

AUSCULTATION

Auscultate the lungs, noting adventitious sounds and determining the quality of aeration of the lung fields.

Earlier in the illness, wheezes might be heard scattered throughout the lung fields. In more serious cases, the chest might sound quiet and without wheeze. This is due to significant hyperexpansion with very poor air exchange.

Laboratory and Diagnostic Tests

Common laboratory and diagnostic studies ordered for the assessment of RSV bronchiolitis include:

- Pulse oximetry: oxygen saturation might be decreased significantly.
- Chest radiograph: might reveal hyperinflation and patchy areas of atelectasis or infiltration.
- Blood gases: might show carbon dioxide retention and **hypoxemia** (low oxygen concentration in blood).
- Nasal-pharyngeal washings: positive identification of RSV can be made via enzyme-linked immunosorbent assay (ELISA) or immunofluorescent antibody (IFA) testing.

Nursing Management

RSV infection is usually self-limited, and patient problems, goals, and interventions for the child with bronchiolitis are aimed at supportive care. Children with less severe disease might require only antipyretics, adequate hydration, and close observation. They can often be successfully managed at home, provided the primary caregiver is reliable and comfortable with close observation. Teach parents or caregivers to watch for signs of worsening and to seek care quickly should the child's condition deteriorate.

Hospitalization is required for children with more severe disease, and children admitted with RSV bronchiolitis warrant close observation. In addition to the patient problems and related interventions discussed in the "Clinical Judgment and the Nursing Process" section earlier in this chapter, interventions common to bronchiolitis follow.

Maintaining Patent Airway

Position the child with the head of the bed elevated to facilitate an open airway. Frequently assess airway patency and suction as needed. Use a Yankauer or tonsil-tip suction catheter to suction the mouth or pharynx of older infants or children, rinsing the catheter after each suctioning. Nasal bulb suctioning may be sufficient to clear the airway in some infants, while others will require nasopharyngeal suctioning with a suction catheter. Nursing Procedure 40.1 gives further information. Adjust the pressure ranges for suctioning infants and children between 60 and 100 mm Hg (40 to 60 mm Hg for premature infants).

NURSING PROCEDURE 40.1 Nasopharyngeal or Artificial Airway Suction Technique

1. Make sure the suction equipment works properly before starting.
2. After washing your hands, assemble the equipment needed:
   - Appropriate-size sterile suction catheter
   - Sterile gloves
   - Supplemental oxygen
   - Sterile water–based lubricant
   - Sterile normal saline if indicated
3. Don sterile gloves, keeping dominant hand sterile and nondominant hand clean.
4. Preoxygenate the infant or child if indicated.
5. Apply lubricant to the end of the suction catheter.
6. If indicated for loosening of secretions, instill sterile saline.
7. Maintaining sterile technique, insert the suction catheter into the child's nostril or airway.
   - Insert only to the point of gagging if inserting via the nostril.
   - Insert only 0.5 cm farther than the length of the artificial airway.
8. Intermittently apply suction for no longer than 10 seconds while twisting and removing the catheter.
9. Supplement with oxygen after suctioning.

Promoting Adequate Gas Exchange

Assess work of breathing, respiratory rate, and oxygen saturation as infants and children with RSV bronchiolitis might deteriorate quickly as the disease progresses. Adjust the percentage of inspired oxygen (FiO_2) as needed to maintain oxygen saturation within the prescribed range. Position the infant with the head of the bed elevated to improve gas exchange. Frequent assessment is necessary for the hospitalized child with bronchiolitis.

CLINICAL REASONING ALERT!

In the tachypneic infant, slowing of the respiratory rate does not necessarily indicate improvement: often, a slower respiratory rate is an indication of tiring, and carbon dioxide retention may soon be followed by apnea (Weiner, 2022).

Reducing Infection Risk

Since RSV is easily spread through contact with droplets, isolate inpatients according to hospital policy to decrease the risk of nosocomial spread to other children. Safely cohort children with RSV. Maintain attention to handwashing, as droplets might enter the eyes, nose, or mouth via the hands.

Providing Family Education

Educate parents so they can recognize signs of worsening distress. Tell parents to call the primary provider or nurse practitioner if the child's breathing becomes rapid or more difficult or if the child cannot eat secondary to tachypnea. Inform families that children who are younger than 1 year of age or who are at higher risk (those who were born prematurely or who have chronic heart or lung conditions) might have a longer course of illness. Instruct parents that cough can persist for several days to weeks after resolution of the disease but that infants usually act well otherwise.

Preventing RSV Disease

Teach strict adherence to handwashing policies in day care centers and when exposed to individuals with cold symptoms for all age groups. It is recommended that all pregnant people receive the RSV vaccine between 32 and 36 weeks' gestation for protection of newborns and infants through 6 months of age (CDC, 2023b). The vaccine provides 5 months of protection against serious RSV disease. If the birth parent did not receive the RSV vaccine during pregnancy, the infant should receive one dose of nirsevimab (Barr & Graham, 2024). During their second RSV season, infants at increased risk for severe RSV infection who are 8 to 19 months of age should receive a second dose of nirsevimab. Those at high risk include infants and toddlers who have chronic lung disease of prematurity, are immunocompromised, have cystic fibrosis, or are of Native Alaskan or Native American descent (Barr & Graham, 2024). Healthy children over 8 months of age do not require a second dose.

Pneumonia

Pneumonia is an inflammation of the lung parenchyma. It can be caused by a virus, bacteria, *Mycoplasma,* or a fungus. Respiratory viruses are the most common cause of pneumonia in younger children and the least common cause in older children. Viral pneumonia is usually better tolerated in children of all ages. Children with bacterial pneumonia are more apt to present with a toxic appearance, but they generally recover rapidly if appropriate antibiotic treatment is instituted early. *Streptococcus pneumoniae* is a common cause of bacterial pneumonia in all ages of children, and *M. pneumoniae* is a common causative agent in the school-age child and adolescent. Fungal infection may also result in pneumonia. Aspiration pneumonia may result from aspiration of foreign material into the lower respiratory tract. Pneumonia occurs more often in winter and early spring. It is common in children but is seen most frequently in infants and young toddlers.

TAKE NOTE!

Community-acquired pneumonia (CAP) refers to pneumonia in a previously healthy person that is contracted outside of the hospital setting (Barson, 2022).

Pneumonia is usually a self-limited disease. A child who presents with recurrent pneumonia should be evaluated for chronic lung disease such as asthma or cystic fibrosis. Potential complications of pneumonia include bacteremia, pleural effusion, empyema, lung abscess, and pneumothorax. Excluding bacteremia, these complications are often treated with thoracentesis and/or chest tubes as well as antibiotics if appropriate. Pneumatoceles (thin-walled cavities developing in the lung) might occur with certain bacterial pneumonias and usually resolve spontaneously over time.

Therapeutic management of children with less severe disease includes antipyretics, adequate hydration, and close observation. Even bacterial pneumonia can be successfully managed at home if the work of breathing is not severe and oxygen saturation is within normal limits. However, hospitalization is required for children with more severe disease. The child with tachypnea, significant retractions, poor oral intake, or lethargy might require hospital admission for the administration of supplemental oxygen, intravenous hydration, and antibiotics.

Nursing Assessment

For a full description of the assessment phase of the nursing process, refer to the "Clinical Judgment and the Nursing Process" section earlier in the chapter. Assessment findings pertinent to pneumonia are discussed further on.

Health History

Elicit a description of the present illness and chief complaint. Note onset and progression of symptoms. Common signs and symptoms reported during the health history include:

- Antecedent viral URI
- Fever
- Cough (note type and whether productive or not)
- Increased respiratory rate

- History of lethargy, poor feeding, vomiting, or diarrhea in infants
- Chills, headache, dyspnea, chest pain, abdominal pain, and nausea or vomiting in older children

Explore the child's past and current medical history for risk factors known to be associated with an increase in the severity of pneumonia, such as:

- Prematurity
- Malnutrition
- Passive smoke exposure
- Low socioeconomic status
- Day care attendance
- Underlying cardiopulmonary, immune, or nervous system disease (Houin et al., 2022)

Physical Examination

Observe the child's general appearance and color (centrally and peripherally), as the child with bacterial pneumonia may appear ill, and cyanosis might accompany coughing spells. Assess work of breathing, noting substernal, subcostal, or intercostal retractions. Tachypnea and nasal flaring may be present. Describe cough and quality of sputum if produced.

Auscultate the lungs for wheezes or rales in the younger child or local or diffuse rales in the older child. Document diminished breath sounds. Percuss for local dullness over a consolidated area in the older child (percussion is much less valuable in the infant or younger child). Palpate for tactile fremitus, which may be increased with pneumonia.

Laboratory and Diagnostic Tests

Common laboratory and diagnostic studies ordered for the assessment of pneumonia include:

- Pulse oximetry: oxygen saturation might be decreased significantly or within normal range.
- Chest radiograph: varies according to child age and causative agent. In infants and young children, bilateral air trapping and perihilar **infiltrates** (collection of inflammatory cells, cellular debris, and foreign organisms) are the most common findings. Patchy areas of consolidation might also be present. In older children, lobar consolidation is seen more frequently.
- Sputum culture: may be useful in determining causative bacteria in older children and adolescents.
- White blood cell count: might be elevated in the case of bacterial pneumonia.

Nursing Management

Patient problems, goals, and interventions for the child with pneumonia are aimed primarily at providing supportive care and education about the illness and its treatment. Prevention of pneumococcal infection is also important. Children with more severe disease will require hospitalization. Refer to the "Clinical Judgment and the Nursing Process" section earlier in the chapter for patient problems and related interventions. In addition to the interventions listed there, the following should be noted.

Providing Supportive Care

Ensure adequate hydration, and assist in thinning of secretions by encouraging oral fluid intake in the child whose respiratory status is stable. Provide intravenous fluids as ordered to children with increased work of breathing to maintain hydration. Allow and encourage the child to assume a position of comfort, usually with the head of the bed elevated to promote aeration of the lungs. If pain due to coughing or pneumonia itself is severe, administer analgesics as prescribed. Provide supplemental oxygen to the child with respiratory distress or **hypoxia** (low oxygen concentration in the tissues) as needed.

Providing Family Education

Educate the family about the importance of adhering to the prescribed antibiotic regimen. Antibiotics may be given intravenously if the child is hospitalized. Oral antibiotics are used on discharge or if the child is managed on an outpatient basis.

Teach the parents of a child with bacterial pneumonia to expect that for 1 to 2 weeks following resolution of the acute illness, the child might continue to tire easily and that the infant might continue to need small, frequent feedings. Cough may also persist after the acute recovery period but should lessen over time.

If the child is diagnosed with viral pneumonia, provide parents with an explanation that antibiotics are not utilized in viral infections (pneumonia is often perceived by the public as a bacterial infection). As with bacterial pneumonia, the child may experience a week or two of weakness or fatigue following resolution of the acute illness.

Teach parents of young children about the risk of the development of aspiration pneumonia. Parents need to understand that the child might be at risk for injury related to their age and developmental stage. To prevent recurrent or further aspiration, teach the parents the safety measures in Teaching Guidelines 40.3.

Preventing Pneumococcal Infection

Provide immunization to children at high risk for severe pneumococcal infection. This includes all children between 0 and 23 months of age, as well as children between 24 and 59 months of age who either never received the vaccine before age 2 or did not receive a booster dose between 12 and 23 months of age.

TEACHING GUIDELINES 40.3 Preventing Aspiration

- Keep toxic substances such as lighter fluid, solvents, and hydrocarbons out of reach of young children. Toddlers and preschoolers cannot distinguish safe from unsafe fluids due to their developmental stage.
- Avoid oily nose drops and oil-based vitamins or home remedies to avoid lipid aspiration into the lungs.
- Avoid oral feedings if the infant's respiratory rate is 60 or greater to minimize the risk of aspiration of the feeding.
- Discourage parents from "force-feeding" in the event of poor oral intake or severe illness to minimize the risk of aspiration of the feeding.
- Position infants and ill children on their right side after feeding to minimize the risk of aspirating emesis or regurgitated feeding.

In addition, children between 24 and 59 months of age with certain conditions such as immune deficiency, sickle cell disease, asplenia, chronic cardiac conditions, chronic lung problems, cerebrospinal fluid leaks, chronic renal insufficiency, diabetes mellitus, and organ transplants should receive the vaccine (CDC, 2023a). For additional information on immunization, refer to Chapter 31.

Bronchitis

Bronchitis is an inflammation of the trachea and major bronchi. It is often associated with a URI. Bronchitis is usually viral in nature, although *M. pneumoniae* and other bacterial organisms are causative in about 10% of cases (Carolan, 2023). Recovery usually occurs within 5 to 10 days. Therapeutic management involves mainly supportive care. Expectorant administration and adequate hydration are important. If bacterial infection is the cause, antibiotics are indicated.

Nursing Assessment

Ascertain the history, which usually begins with a mild URI. Note development of fever, followed by a dry, hacking cough that might become productive in older children. Determine if the cough wakes the child at night. Auscultate the lungs to determine if coarse rales are present. Note that respirations remain unlabored. The chest radiograph might show diffuse alveolar hyperinflation and perihilar markings.

Nursing Management

Nursing management is aimed at providing supportive care. Teach parents that expectorants will help loosen secretions and that antipyretics will help reduce the fever, making the child more comfortable. Encourage adequate hydration. Inform parents that antibiotics are prescribed only in cases believed to be bacterial in nature (infrequent). Discourage the use of cough suppressants: it is important for accumulated sputum to be raised.

Tuberculosis

Tuberculosis (TB) is a highly contagious disease caused by inhalation of droplets of *Mycobacterium tuberculosis* or *Mycobacterium bovis*. Children usually contract the disease from an immediate household member. Children who are unhoused or living in poverty are at higher risk, as are those exposed to an adult with TB infection (Batra & Ang, 2022). After exposure to an infected individual, the incubation period is 2 to 10 weeks. The inhaled tubercle bacilli multiply in the alveoli and alveolar ducts, forming an inflammatory exudate. The bacilli are spread by the bloodstream and lymphatic system to various parts of the body. Although pulmonary TB is the most common, children may also have infection in other parts of the body, such as the gastrointestinal tract or central nervous system. Children who test positive for TB but who do not have symptoms or radiographic/laboratory evidence of disease are considered to have latent infection.

In the case of drug-sensitive TB, the American Academy of Pediatrics (AAP) recommends a 4-month course of oral therapy. In the first 2 months isoniazid, rifampin, pyrazinamide, and ethambutol are given daily. This is followed by twice-weekly isoniazid and rifampin; administration must be observed directly (usually by a public health nurse). In the case of multidrug-resistant TB, a TB specialist is consulted, and intramuscular injection may be given (Kimberlin et al., 2021). Children with latent TB are treated with isoniazid or other drugs for 9 months to prevent progression to active disease. See Healthy People 2030 box.

Nursing Assessment

Children considered to be at high risk for contracting TB should be screened using the Mantoux test. High-risk children are those who:

- are infected with human immunodeficiency virus (HIV)
- are incarcerated or institutionalized
- have a positive recent history of latent TB infection
- are immigrants from or have a history of travel to endemic countries
- are exposed at home to people living with HIV, unhoused individuals, people who use illicit drugs, people who were recently incarcerated, migrant farm workers, or nursing home residents

HEALTHY PEOPLE 2030

Objective	Nursing Significance
Reduce tuberculosis.	• Assess the health history of all infants, children, and adolescents for risk factors for tuberculosis infection. • Provide tuberculosis screening as recommended. • Refer all tuberculosis infections to the local public health department. • Educate families about the importance of completing medication therapy as prescribed for active and latent tuberculosis and the need for appropriate follow-up and retesting for tuberculosis infection.

Healthy People Objectives retrieved from http://www.healthypeople.gov

Evaluate the health history for symptoms such as fever, malaise, weight loss, anorexia, pain and tightness in the chest, and rarely hemoptysis. Note whether cough is present or not, and if present, whether it has progressed slowly over several weeks to months. As TB progresses, note an increase in respiratory rate, diminished breath sounds and crackles with poor aeration in the affected lung. Percussion may reveal dullness. Keep in mind that some children are asymptomatic. Diagnosis is confirmed with a positive Mantoux test, positive gastric washings for acid-fast bacillus, interferon-gamma release assay (IGRA), and/or a chest radiograph consistent with TB.

Nursing Management

Hospitalization of children with TB is necessary only for the most serious cases. Nursing management is aimed at providing supportive care and encouraging adherence to the treatment regimen. Most nursing care for childhood TB is provided in outpatient clinics, schools, or a public health setting. Supportive care includes ensuring adequate nutrition and adequate rest, providing comfort measures such as fever reduction, preventing exposure to other infectious diseases, and preventing reinfection. Isolate hospitalized children with TB according to hospital policy to prevent nosocomial spread of TB infection.

TAKE NOTE!

Administration of Bacille Calmette–Guérin (BCG) vaccine can provide incomplete protection against TB, and it is not widely used in the United States (Kimberlin et al., 2021).

COVID-19

URI have long been known to be caused by the *Coronaviridae* family of viruses, among many others. In 2020, COVID-19 quickly spread worldwide, causing significant morbidity and mortality, particularly in certain populations (S. Smith, 2022). COVID-19 infection may be mild, lead to respiratory failure, or result in multisystem inflammatory syndrome (MIS-C) 4 to 6 weeks after an initial mild or unidentified infection (Zachariah, 2022). During the COVID-19 pandemic, a vaccine was made available, first to older adults or those vulnerable to severe infection, later to all adults, then, finally, to children as young as 6 months of age. The CDC recommends that every person 6 months of age and older receive the updated COVID-19 vaccine (2024).

Quarantines were implemented nationwide (and across most parts of the world) in early 2020 as a result of the quickly increasing morbidity and mortality rates. Quarantines resulted in job and income losses for some adults and lack of socialization for children who were unable to attend day care or school. As the COVID-19 pandemic has eased, morbidity and mortality rates have decreased significantly. Thus, quarantines and social distancing requirements have been lifted, and people have returned to work and school as they did prior to the pandemic. In 2023, some states still required certain populations (e.g., those who work in health care and/or certain state agencies) to either be vaccinated against COVID-19 or to submit to regular testing for the virus (Markowitz & Rough, 2024).

Nursing Assessment

About 50% of children infected with the COVID-19 virus are asymptomatic. Evaluate the health history for symptoms such as fever (may or may not be present), cough, runny nose, sore throat, nausea, vomiting, or diarrhea. The infected infant may be apneic, and the older child or adolescent may experience loss of smell and taste. Headache may be present in the older child. Determine the child's immunization status.

Nursing Management

Provide supportive care to the child with mild COVID-19 infection. Antipyretics and symptomatic relief of other clinical manifestations will make the child more comfortable. Educate families about proper hand hygiene, as well as social distancing (6 ft apart) and the proper use of masks if the child is 2 years of age or older (Rabinowicz et al., 2020). Refer families to the World Health Organization's (2021) website of updated COVID-19 information for the public at this link: https://www.who.int/emergencies/diseases/novel-coronavirus-2019/advice-for-public/myth-busters.

ACUTE NONINFECTIOUS DISORDERS

Acute noninfectious disorders include epistaxis, foreign body aspiration, acute respiratory distress syndrome (ARDS), and pneumothorax.

Epistaxis

Epistaxis (a nosebleed) occurs most frequently in children before adolescence. Bleeding of the nasal mucosa occurs most often from the anterior portion of the septum. Epistaxis may be recurrent and idiopathic (meaning there is no cause). Most cases are benign, but in children with bleeding disorders or other hematologic concerns, epistaxis should be further investigated and treated.

Nursing Assessment

Explore the child's history for initiating factors such as local inflammation, mucosal drying, or local trauma (usually nose picking). Inspect the nasal cavity for blood.

Nursing Management

Remain calm and encourage the parents to do so as well since the presence of blood often frightens children and their parents. Have the child sit up and lean forward (lying down may allow aspiration of the blood). Apply continuous pressure to the anterior portion of the nose by pinching it closed. Encourage the child to breathe through the mouth during this portion of the treatment. Ice or a cold cloth applied to the bridge of the nose may also be helpful. The bleeding usually stops within 10 to 15 minutes. Apply water-soluble gel to the nasal mucosa with a cotton-tipped applicator to moisten the mucosa and prevent recurrence.

CLINICAL REASONING ALERT!

The child with recurrent epistaxis or epistaxis that is difficult to control should be further evaluated for underlying bleeding or platelet concerns.

Foreign Body Aspiration

Foreign body aspiration occurs when any solid or liquid substance is inhaled into the respiratory tract. It is common in infants and young children and can present in a life-threatening manner. The object may lodge in the upper or lower airway, causing varying degrees of respiratory difficulty. Small, smooth objects such as peanuts are the most frequently aspirated, but any small toy, article, or piece of food smaller than the diameter of the young child's airway can be aspirated.

TAKE NOTE!

Items smaller than 1.25 in (3.2 cm) can be aspirated easily. A simple way for parents to estimate the safe size of a small item or toy piece is to gauge its size against a standard toilet paper roll (not double roll), which is generally about 1.5 in in diameter.

Foreign body aspiration occurs most frequently in children between 6 months and 3 years of age (Houin et al., 2022). Children this age are growing and developing rapidly. They tend to explore things with their mouths and can easily aspirate small items.

The child often coughs out foreign bodies from the upper airway. If the foreign body reaches the bronchus, then it may need to be surgically removed via bronchoscopy. Postoperative antibiotics are used if an infection is also present. Complications of foreign body aspiration include pneumonia or abscess formation, hypoxia, respiratory failure, and death.

Nursing Assessment

Evaluate the history of the infant or young child for usually sudden onset of cough, wheeze, or stridor, although the onset of respiratory symptoms can be more gradual. Stridor suggests that the foreign body is lodged in the upper airway. Auscultate the lungs for wheezing, rhonchi, and decreased aeration (can be heard on the affected side). A chest radiograph will demonstrate the foreign body only if it is radiopaque (Fig. 40.7).

Nursing Management

The most important nursing intervention related to foreign body aspiration is prevention. Anticipatory guidance for families with 6-month-olds should include a discussion of aspiration avoidance. Repeat this information at each subsequent well-child visit through age 5. Tell parents to avoid letting their child play with toys with small parts and to keep coins and other small objects

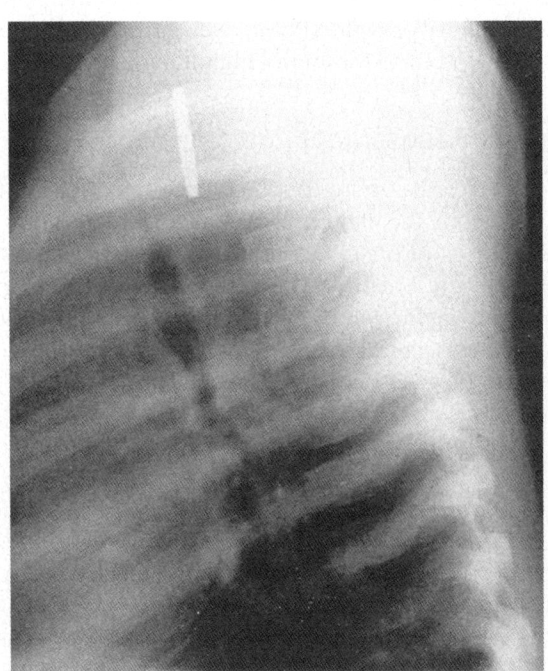

FIGURE 40.7 Foreign body is noted in the bronchus on a chest radiograph.

out of the reach of children. Teach parents not to feed peanuts and popcorn to their child until they are at least 4 years old (Durani, 2023). When children progress to table food, teach parents to chop all foods so that they are small enough to pass down the trachea should the child neglect to chew them up thoroughly. Carrots, grapes, and hot dogs should be cut into small pieces. Harmful liquids should be kept out of the reach of children.

TAKE NOTE!

Prevent young children from playing with latex balloons. When popped, small pieces pose an aspiration danger (Durani, 2023).

Acute Respiratory Distress Syndrome

ARDS occurs following a primary insult such as sepsis, infectious or aspiration pneumonia, or COVID-19 in infants and children with previously healthy lungs (Purohit et al., 2023; Zachariah, 2022). The alveolar–capillary membrane becomes more permeable, and pulmonary edema develops. Hyaline membrane formation over the alveolar surfaces and decreased surfactant production cause lung stiffness. Mucosal swelling and cellular debris lead to atelectasis. Gas diffusion is impaired significantly. Some children have residual lung disease, and some recover completely. However, ARDS can progress to respiratory failure and death.

Therapeutic management is aimed at improving oxygenation and ventilation. Mechanical ventilation is used, with special attention to lung volumes and positive end-expiratory pressure (PEEP). Newer treatment modalities show promise for improving outcomes of ARDS.

Nursing Assessment

Note tachycardia and tachypnea occurring over the first few hours of the illness. Observe for significantly increased work of breathing, nasal flaring, and retractions. Auscultate the breath sounds, which might range from normal to high-pitched crackles throughout the lung fields. Note decreased oxygen saturation. Bilateral infiltrates can be seen on a chest radiograph.

Nursing Management

Nursing care of the child with ARDS is mainly supportive and occurs in the intensive care unit. Closely monitor respiratory and cardiovascular status. Comfort measures such as hygiene and positioning as well as pain and anxiety management, maintenance of nutrition, and prevention of infection are also key nursing interventions. Soothe the child's fears as the acute phase of worsening respiratory distress can be frightening for a child of any age. As the disease worsens and progresses, especially when ventilatory support is required, it is especially important to provide psychological support of the family as well as education about the intensive care unit procedures.

Pneumothorax

A collection of air in the pleural space is called a pneumothorax. It can occur spontaneously in an otherwise healthy child or as a result of chronic lung disease, cardiopulmonary resuscitation (CPR), surgery, or trauma. Trapped air consumes space within the pleural cavity, and the affected lung suffers at least partial collapse. Needle aspiration and/or placement of a chest tube are used to evacuate the air from the chest. Some small pneumothoraces resolve independently, without intervention.

Nursing Assessment

The infant or child with a pneumothorax might have a sudden or gradual onset of symptoms. Determine risk factors for acquiring a pneumothorax, including chest trauma or surgery, intubation and mechanical ventilation, or a history of chronic lung disease such as cystic fibrosis. Note the presence of chest pain, tachypnea, retractions, nasal flaring, grunting, pallor, or cyanosis. Auscultate for tachycardia and absent or diminished breath sounds on the affected side. The radiograph reveals air within the thoracic cavity (Fig. 40.8).

Nursing Management

Frequently assess the child's respiratory status. Administer 100% oxygen as ordered as it hastens the reabsorption of air (generally used only for a few hours) (Janahi, 2024). Assist with needle aspiration and/or chest tube insertion. If a chest tube is connected to a dry suction or water seal apparatus, provide care of the drainage apparatus as appropriate (Fig. 40.9). Keep a pair of hemostats at the bedside to clamp the tube should it become dislodged from the drainage container, or the open end may be placed in a container of sterile water. The dressing around the chest tube is occlusive and is not routinely changed. If the tube becomes dislodged from the child's chest, apply Vaseline gauze and an occlusive dressing, immediately perform appropriate respiratory assessment, and notify the primary provider or nurse practitioner.

CHRONIC RESPIRATORY DISORDERS

Chronic respiratory disorders include allergic rhinitis, asthma, chronic lung disease (bronchopulmonary dysplasia), cystic fibrosis, and apnea.

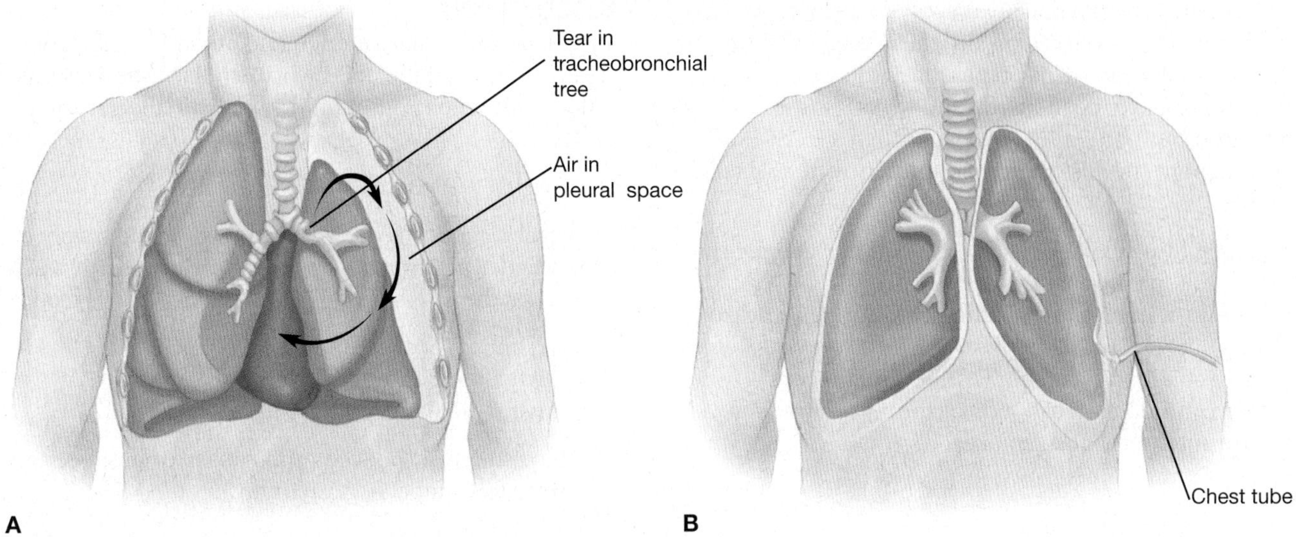

FIGURE 40.8 **A.** Pneumothorax. **B.** Note reinflation of the lung when the chest tube is present.

Allergic Rhinitis

Allergic rhinitis is a common chronic condition in childhood, affecting a significant number of children. Allergic rhinitis is associated with atopic dermatitis and asthma. Perennial allergic rhinitis occurs year-round and is associated with indoor environments. Allergens commonly implicated in perennial allergic rhinitis include dust mites, pet dander, cockroach antigens, and molds. Seasonal allergic rhinitis is caused by elevations in outdoor levels of allergens. It is typically caused by certain pollens, trees, weeds, fungi, and molds. Complications from allergic rhinitis include exacerbation of asthma symptoms, recurrent sinusitis and otitis media, and dental malocclusion.

Pathophysiology

Allergic rhinitis is an intermittent or persistent inflammatory state that is mediated by immunoglobulin E (IgE). In response to contact with an airborne allergen protein, the nasal mucosa mounts an immune response. The antigen (from the allergen) binds to a specific IgE on the surface of mast cells, releasing the chemical mediators of histamine and leukotrienes. Shortly thereafter, various white blood cells release chemical mediators, and inflammation results. IgE binds to receptors on the surfaces of mast cells and basophils, creating the sensitization memory that causes the reaction with subsequent allergen exposures. Allergen exposure then results in the inflammatory response. Histamine and other factors cause nasal vasodilation, watery **rhinorrhea** (runny nose), nasal congestion, pruritus, and sneezing. Treatment of allergic rhinitis is aimed at decreasing response to these allergic mediators as well as treating inflammation.

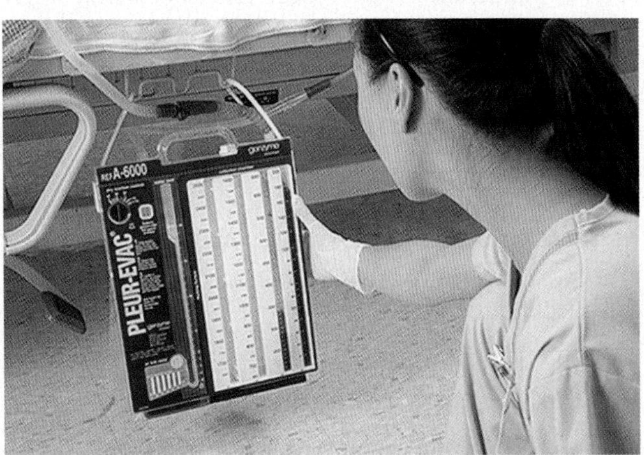

FIGURE 40.9 The chest tube is connected to a suction or water seal via a drainage container.

Nursing Assessment

For a full description of the assessment phase of the nursing process, refer to the "Clinical Judgment and the Nursing Process" section earlier in the chapter. Assessment findings pertinent to allergic rhinitis are discussed further on.

Health History

Elicit a description of the present illness and chief complaint. Common signs and symptoms reported during the health history might include:

- Mild, intermittent, to chronic nasal stuffiness
- Thin, runny nasal discharge
- Sneezing
- Itching of nose, eyes, palate
- Mouth breathing and snoring

Determine the seasonality of symptoms. Are they perennial (year-round) or do they occur during certain seasons only? What types of medications or other treatments have been used, and what was the child's response?

Explore the history for the presence of risk factors such as:

- Family history of atopic disease (asthma, allergic rhinitis, or atopic dermatitis)
- Known allergy to dust mites, pet dander, cockroach antigens, pollens, or molds
- Early childhood exposure to indoor allergens
- Early introduction to foods or formula in infancy
- Exposure to tobacco smoke

Physical Examination

Physical examination of the child with allergic rhinitis includes inspection, observation, and auscultation.

INSPECTION AND OBSERVATION

Observe the child's facies for red-rimmed eyes or tearing, mild eyelid edema, "allergic shiners" (bluish or grayish cast beneath the eyes), and "allergic salute" (a transverse nasal crease between the lower and middle thirds of the nose that results from repeated nose rubbing) (Fig. 40.10). Inspect the nasal cavity. The turbinates may be swollen and gray/blue. Clear mucoid nasal drainage may be observed. Inspect the skin for rash. Listen for nasal phonation with speech.

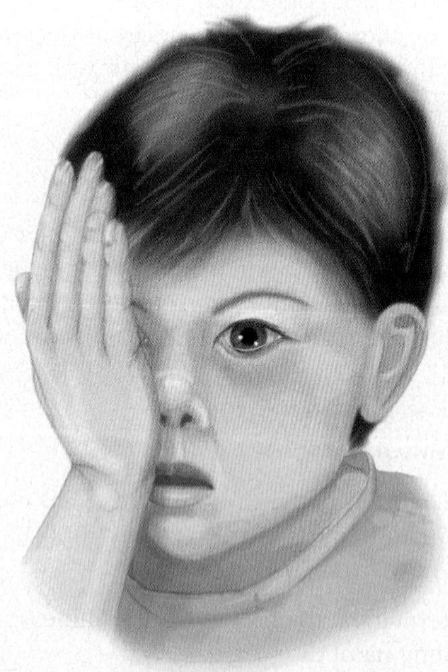

FIGURE 40.10 Allergic shiners beneath the eyes and allergic salute across the nose.

AUSCULTATION

Auscultate the lungs for adequate aeration and clarity of breath sounds. In the child who also has asthma, exacerbation with wheezing often occurs with allergic rhinitis.

Laboratory and Diagnostic Tests

The initial diagnosis is often made based on the history and clinical findings. Common laboratory and diagnostic studies ordered for the assessment of allergic rhinitis may include:

- Nasal smear (positive for eosinophilia)
- Positive allergy skin test
- Positive radioallergosorbent test (RAST)

To distinguish between the causes of nasal congestion, refer to Comparison Chart 40.1.

Nursing Management

In addition to the patient problems and related interventions discussed in the "Clinical Judgment and the Nursing Process" section earlier in the chapter, interventions common to allergic rhinitis follow.

Maintaining Patent Airway

Perform nasal washes with normal saline to keep the nasal mucus from becoming thickened and to lessen nasal obstruction. Thickened, immobile secretions often lead to a secondary bacterial infection. The nasal wash also decongests the nose, allowing for improved nasal airflow. Administer antiinflammatory (corticosteroid) nasal sprays as prescribed to decrease the inflammatory response to allergens and/or mast cell stabilizing nasal spray such as cromolyn sodium to decrease the intensity and frequency of allergic responses. Teach families about nasal medications as well as other recommended drugs such as once-daily oral antihistamines, combined antihistamine/nasal decongestants, or leukotriene modifiers such as montelukast. See Dosage Calculation Box 40.1.

DOSAGE CALCULATION BOX 40.1

Child's weight: 30 lb

Medication order: cetirizine 2.5 mg PO every morning.

Cetirizine is supplied as 5 mg/5 mL.

How many milliliters will the nurse administer? Round to the nearest tenth.

Providing Family Education

One of the most important tools in the treatment of allergic rhinitis is learning to avoid known allergens. Teaching Guidelines 40.4 gives information on educating families

TEACHING GUIDELINES 40.4 Controlling Exposure to Allergens

Tobacco
- Avoid all exposure to tobacco smoke.
- No parental smoking inside the home or car.

Dust Mites
- Use pillow and mattress covers.
- Wash bed linens once a week in 130°F water.
- Use blinds rather than curtains in bedroom.
- Remove stuffed animals from bedroom, or minimize number and wash weekly.
- Reduce indoor humidity to <50%.
- Remove carpet from bedroom.
- Clean solid-surface floors with wet mop each week.

Pet Dander
- Remove pets from home permanently.
- If unable to remove them, keep them out of bedroom and off carpet and upholstered furniture.

Cockroaches
- Keep kitchen very clean.
- Avoiding leaving food or drinks out.
- Use pesticides if necessary, but ensure that the asthmatic child is not inside the home when the pesticide is sprayed.

Indoor Molds
- Repair water leaks.
- Use dehumidifier to keep basement dry.
- Reduce indoor humidity to <50%.

Outdoor Molds, Pollen, and Air Pollution
- Avoid going outdoors when mold and pollen counts are high.
- Avoid outdoor activity when pollution levels are high.

Adapted from Houin, P., Stillwell, P., Deboer, E. M., & Hoppe, J. (2022). Respiratory tract & mediastinum. In M. Bunik, W. W. Hay, M. J. Levin, & M. J. Abzug (Eds.), *Current diagnosis and treatment: Pediatrics* (26th ed.). McGraw-Hill Education; Volkman, K. K., & Chiu, A. M. (2023). Allergy. In K. J. Marcdante, & R. M. Kliegman (Eds.), *Nelson's essentials of pediatrics* (9th ed.). Elsevier.

about avoidance of allergens. Children may be referred to a specialist for allergen desensitization (allergy shots). Products helpful with control of allergies are available from a number of vendors.

Asthma

Asthma is a chronic inflammatory airway disorder characterized by airway hyperresponsiveness, airway edema, and mucus production. Airway obstruction resulting from asthma might be partially or completely reversed. Severity ranges from long periods of control with infrequent acute exacerbations in some children to the presence of persistent daily symptoms in others. It is the most common chronic illness of childhood, with 7 million American children diagnosed before age 18 years (Volkman & Chiu, 2023). The incidence and severity of asthma are increasing; this might be attributed to increased urbanization, increased air pollution, and more accurate diagnosis. See Healthy People 2030.

HEALTHY PEOPLE 2030

Objective	Nursing Significance
Reduce asthma deaths, hospitalizations for asthma, hospital emergency department visits for asthma.	• Appropriately educate children with asthma and their families about the ongoing management of asthma. • Provide appropriate education and triage to families of children with asthma, particularly when the child is experiencing symptoms or a decreased peak flow rate.

Healthy People Objectives retrieved from http://www.healthypeople.gov

Severity ranges from symptoms associated only with vigorous activity (exercise-induced bronchospasm) to daily symptoms that interfere with quality of life (such as severe persistent asthma resulting in nighttime symptoms occurring every day). Although uncommon, childhood death related to asthma is also on the rise worldwide. Many children with asthma also have gastroesophageal disease, although the relationship between the two diseases is not clearly understood. Children with asthma are more susceptible to serious bacterial and viral respiratory infections. Acute complications include status asthmaticus and respiratory failure.

PATHOPHYSIOLOGY

In asthma, the inflammatory process contributes to increased airway activity. Thus, control or prevention of inflammation is the core of asthma management. Asthma results from a complex variety of responses in relation to a trigger. When the process begins, mast cells, T lymphocytes, macrophages, and epithelial cells are involved in the release of inflammatory mediators. Eosinophils and neutrophils migrate to the airway, causing injury. Chemical mediators such as leukotrienes, bradykinin, histamine, and platelet-activating factor also contribute to the inflammatory response. The presence of leukotrienes contributes to prolonged airway constriction. Autonomic neural control of airway tone is affected, airway mucus secretion is increased, mucociliary function changes, and airway smooth muscle responsiveness increases. As a result, acute bronchoconstriction, airway edema, and mucus plugging occur (Fig. 40.11).

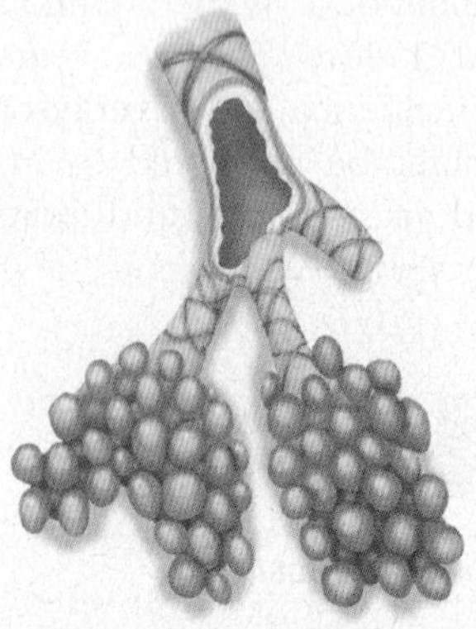

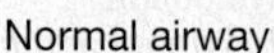

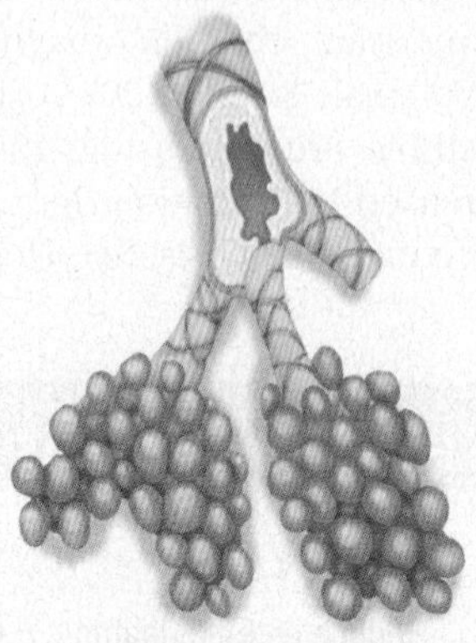

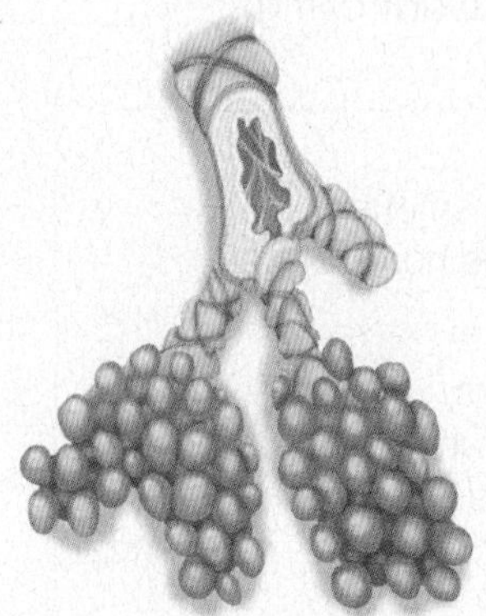

FIGURE 40.11 Note airway edema, mucus production, and bronchospasm occurring with asthma.

In most children, this process is considered reversible, and until recently it was not considered to have long-standing effects on lung function. Current research and scientific thought, however, recognize the concept of airway remodeling as a significant long-term complication. Over time, with repeat asthma exacerbations, irreversible structural airway changes occur, and pulmonary function decreases with this remodeling (Volkman & Chiu, 2023). In some individuals with poorly controlled asthma, these changes may be permanent, resulting in decreased responsiveness to therapy.

Therapeutic Management

Current goals of medical therapy are avoidance of asthma triggers and reduction or control of inflammatory episodes. The most recent recommendations by the National Asthma Education and Prevention Program (NAEPP) and the Global Initiative for Asthma (GINA) suggest a stepwise approach to medication management as well as control of environmental factors (allergens) and comorbid conditions that affect asthma. The NAEPP and GINA guidelines stress periodic assessment of asthma control. Treatment decisions may then be made based on the individual's level of asthma control, rather than on the severity at diagnosis.

The stepwise approach to asthma treatment involves increasing medications as the child's condition worsens, then backing off treatment as they improve (Box 40.3).

Short-acting bronchodilators may be used in the acute treatment of bronchoconstriction, and long-acting forms may be used to prevent bronchospasm. Exercise-induced bronchospasm may occur in any child with asthma or as the only symptom in the child with mild intermittent asthma. Most children may avoid exercise-induced bronchospasm by using a longer warm-up period prior to vigorous exercise and, if necessary, inhaling a short-acting bronchodilator just prior to exercise. Long-term prevention usually involves inhaled steroids. Leukotriene modifiers may be used as an alternative but are not preferred for mild persistent asthma (Covar et al., 2022).

Nursing Assessment

For a full description of the assessment phase of the nursing process, refer to the "Clinical Judgment and the Nursing Process" section earlier in the chapter. Assessment findings pertinent to asthma are discussed further on.

BOX 40.3 Stepwise Approach to Asthma Management

All children: child education, environmental control, and management of comorbidities at each step. Consider referral to asthma specialist at step 3. (Step 2 and above are persistent asthma.)

Step 1 (intermittent asthma)
- Preferred: short-acting beta-2 agonist PRN

Step 2
- Preferred: low-dose inhaled corticosteroid
- Alternative: cromolyn or leukotriene modifier

Step 3
- Preferred: medium-dose inhaled corticosteroid (all ages) OR low-dose inhaled corticosteroid and leukotriene modifier or long-acting beta-2 agonist (children older than 4 years)

Step 4
- Preferred: medium-dose inhaled corticosteroids and long-acting beta-2 agonist (can use leukotriene modifier in children younger than 4 years)

Step 5
- Preferred: high-dose inhaled corticosteroids and long-acting beta-2 agonist (or leukotriene modifier or theophylline)

Step 6
- Preferred: high-dose inhaled corticosteroids, long-acting beta-2 agonist, and oral systemic corticosteroids

Adapted from Houin, P., Stillwell, P., Deboer, E. M., & Hoppe, J. (2022). Respiratory tract & mediastinum. In M. Bunik, W. W. Hay, M. J. Levin, & M. J. Abzug (Eds.), *Current diagnosis and treatment: Pediatrics* (26th ed.). McGraw-Hill Education; Volkman, K. K., & Chiu, A. M. (2023). Allergy. In K. J. Marcdante, & R. M. Kliegman (Eds.), *Nelson's essentials of pediatrics* (9th ed.). Elsevier.

Health History

Elicit a description of the present illness and chief complaint. Common signs and symptoms reported during the health history might include:

- Cough, particularly at night: hacking cough that is initially nonproductive, becoming productive of frothy sputum
- Difficulty breathing: shortness of breath, chest tightness or pain, dyspnea with exercise
- Wheezing

Explore the child's current and past medical history for risk factors such as:

- History of allergic rhinitis or atopic dermatitis
- Family history of atopy (asthma, allergic rhinitis, atopic dermatitis)
- Recurrent episodes diagnosed as wheezing, bronchiolitis, or bronchitis
- Known allergies
- Seasonal response to environmental pollen
- Tobacco smoke exposure
- Poverty

Physical Examination

Physical examination of the child with asthma includes inspection, auscultation, and percussion.

INSPECTION

Observe the child's general appearance and color. During mild exacerbations, the child's color might remain pink, but as the child worsens, cyanosis might result. Assess work of breathing, which is variable, ranging from mild retractions to significant accessory muscle use and eventually head bobbing if not treated effectively. Note lethargy, irritability, or the appearance of anxiety or fearfulness. An audible wheeze might be present. Children with persistent severe asthma may have a barrel chest and routinely demonstrate mildly increased work of breathing.

AUSCULTATION AND PERCUSSION

A thorough assessment of lung fields is necessary. Wheezing is the hallmark of airway obstruction and might vary throughout the lung fields. Coarseness might also be present. Assess the adequacy of aeration. Breath sounds might be diminished in the bases or throughout. A quiet chest in an asthmatic child can be an ominous sign. With severe airway obstruction, air movement can be so poor that wheezes might not be heard on auscultation. Percussion may yield hyperresonance.

Laboratory and Diagnostic Tests

Laboratory and diagnostic studies commonly ordered for the assessment of asthma include:

- Pulse oximetry: oxygen saturation may be decreased significantly or normal during a mild exacerbation.
- Chest radiograph: usually reveals hyperinflation.
- Blood gases: might show carbon dioxide retention and hypoxemia.
- Pulmonary function tests (PFTs): can be very useful in determining the degree of disease but are not useful during an acute attack. Children as young as 5 to 6 years might be able to comply with spirometry.
- Peak expiratory flow rate (PEFR): is decreased during an exacerbation.
- Allergy testing: skin test or RAST can determine allergic triggers for the asthmatic child.

Nursing Management

Initial nursing management of the child with an acute exacerbation of asthma is aimed at restoring a clear airway and effective breathing pattern as well as promoting adequate oxygenation and ventilation (gas exchange). Ongoing management focuses on adherence to the maintenance treatment plan and supporting the child and family. Refer to the "Clinical Judgment and the Nursing Process" section earlier in the chapter for suggested nursing patient problems and interventions. Additional specific considerations are reviewed further on.

• • • ATRAUMATIC CARE • • •

When caring for a young child who must receive a nebulizer treatment by mask, play make-believe about the mask, and utilize other distraction techniques such as reading a book. Making activities into games and utilizing distraction both help to minimize trauma when providing necessary care to young children.

Educating the Child and Family

Teach families of children with asthma, and the children themselves, how to care for the disease; they need to understand the chronicity of asthma. Help families to understand that symptom-free periods (often very long) are interspersed with episodes of exacerbation. Educate parents and children about the importance of maintenance medications for long-term control. Teach them that the episodes of exacerbation (sometimes requiring hospitalization or emergency room visits) should not be viewed as an acute illness. While parents may be relieved when an episode resolves, they should not view the child as disease-free during the periods between acute episodes. Educate families that the long-term maintenance schedules must be maintained during those periods as well. Inform families that the prolonged inflammatory process occurring in the absence of symptoms, primarily in children with moderate to severe asthma, can lead to airway remodeling and eventual irreversible disease.

Educate the child and family about the management plan in place to determine when to step up or step down treatment. Figure 40.12 provides an example of an action plan that may be helpful to families in the management of asthma. Instruct parents to ensure the action plan is kept on file at the child's school and that relief medication is always available to the child. Children who experience exercise-induced bronchospasm may still participate in physical education or athletics but may need to be allowed to use their medicine before the activity. Provide appropriate education to the child and family based on the child's individualized stepwise treatment plan. Stress the concept of maintenance medications for the prevention of future serious disease in addition to controlling or preventing current symptoms.

Educate families and children on the appropriate use of nebulizers, metered-dose inhalers, spacers, dry-powder inhalers, and Diskus, as well as the purposes, functions, and side effects of the medications they deliver. Require return demonstrations of equipment use to ensure that children and families can use the equipment properly (Teaching Guidelines 40.5).

TAKE NOTE!

It is recommended to use an age-appropriate spacer or holding chamber with metered-dose inhalers to increase the bioavailability of medication in the lungs (Volkman & Chiu, 2023).

In children who have more severe asthma, the use of the PEFR helps to determine daily control. PEFR measurements obtained via a home peak flow meter can be very helpful if the meter is used appropriately (Volkman & Chiu, 2023). Teaching Guidelines 40.6 gives instructions on peak flow meter use. The child's "personal best" is determined collaboratively with the primary provider or nurse practitioner during a symptom-free period. PEFR is measured daily at home using the peak flow meter. The

AAAAI
AMERICAN ACADEMY OF ALLERGY ASTHMA & IMMUNOLOGY
www.aaaai.org

ASTHMA ACTION PLAN

Name: ____________ Date: ____________
Emergency Contact: ____________ Relationship: ____________
Cell phone: ____________ Work phone: ____________
Health Care Provider: ____________ Phone number: ____________
Personal Best Peak Flow: ____________

GREEN ZONE:
Doing Well
- ✓ No coughing, wheezing, chest tightness, or difficulty breathing
- ✓ Can work, play, exercise, perform usual activities without symptoms

OR
- ✓ Peak flow ____ to ____ *(80% to 100% of personal best)*

Take these medicines every day for control and maintenance:

Medicine	How much to take	When and how often

YELLOW ZONE:
Caution/Getting Worse
- ✓ Coughing, wheezing, chest tightness, or difficulty breathing
- ✓ Symptoms with daily activities, work, play, and exercise
- ✓ Nighttime awakenings with symptoms

OR
- ✓ Peak flow ____ to ____ *(50% to 80% of personal best)*

CONTINUE your Green Zone medicines PLUS take these quick-relief medicines:

Medicine	How much to take	When and how often

Call your doctor if you have been in the Yellow Zone for more than 24 hours.

Also call your doctor if: ____________

RED ZONE:
Alert!
- ✓ Difficulty breathing, coughing, wheezing not helped with medications
- ✓ Trouble walking or talking due to asthma symptoms
- ✓ Not responding to quick relief medication

OR
- ✓ Peak flow is less than ____ *(50% of personal best)*

FOR EXTREME TROUBLE BREATHING/SHORTNESS OF BREATH GET IMMEDIATE HELP!

Take these quick-relief medicines:

Medicine	How much to take	When and how often

CALL your doctor NOW.
GO to the hospital/emergency department or CALL for an ambulance NOW!

This information is for general purposes and is not intended to replace the advice of a qualified health professional. For more information on asthma, visit www.aaaai.org. © 2009 American Academy of Allergy, Asthma & Immunology

FIGURE 40.12 Asthma action plan. (Used with permission from the American Academy of Allergy, Asthma & Immunology. [2011]. *Asthma action plan*. http://www.aaaai.org/professionals/asthma-action-plan.pdf. Visit AAAAI.org for additional information and updates.)

TEACHING GUIDELINES 40.5 Using Asthma Medication Delivery Devices

Nebulizer

1. Plug in the nebulizer and connect the air compressor tubing.

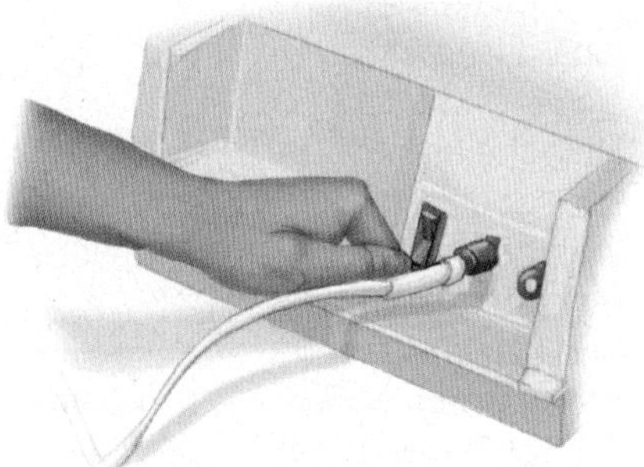

2. Add the medication to the medicine cup.

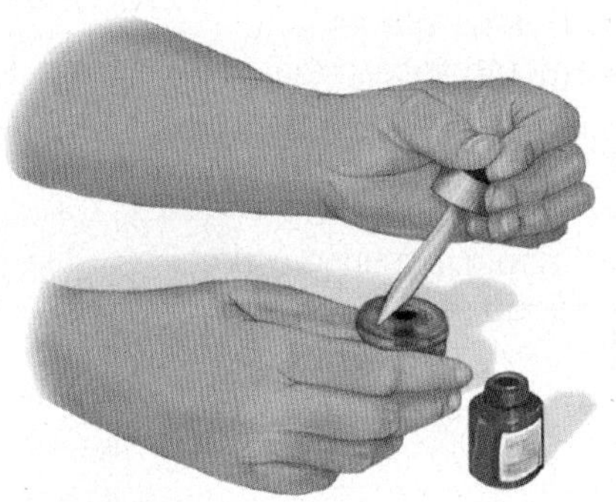

3. Attach the mask or the mouthpiece and hose to the medicine cup.

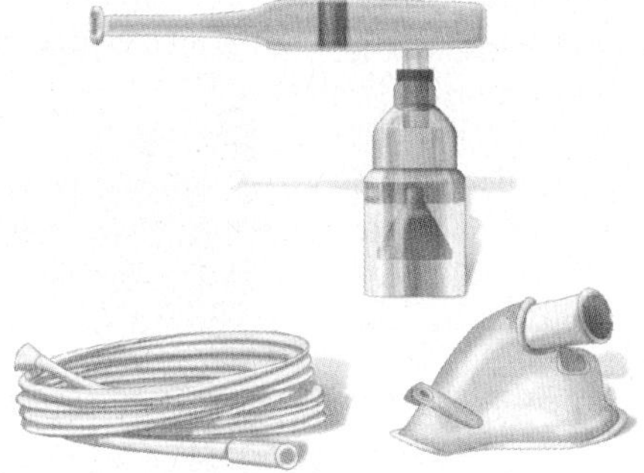

4. Place the mask on the child or (see step 5).

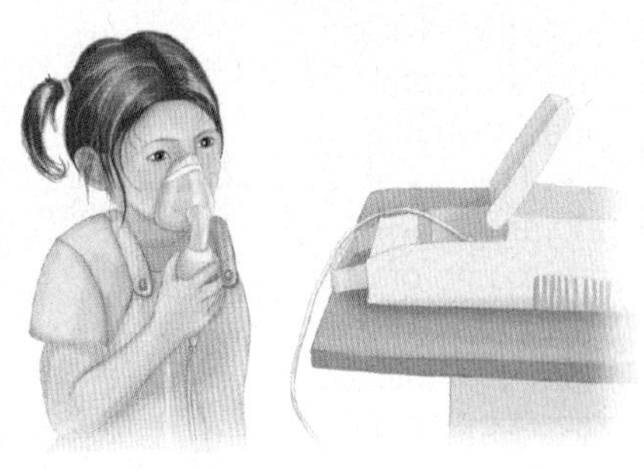

5. Instruct the child to close the lips around the mouthpiece and breathe through the mouth.

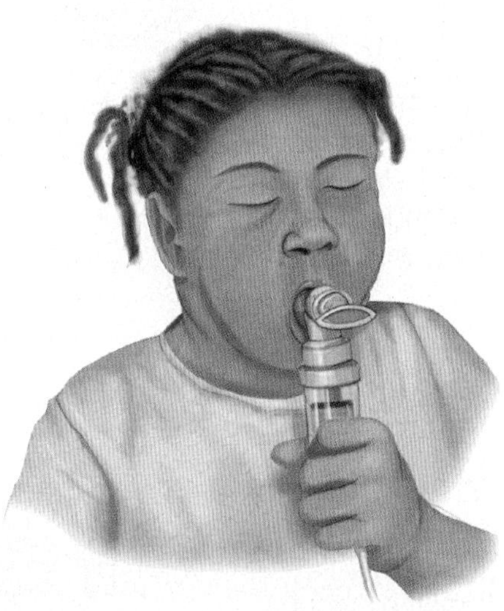

6. After use, wash the mouthpiece and medicine cup with water and allow to air dry.

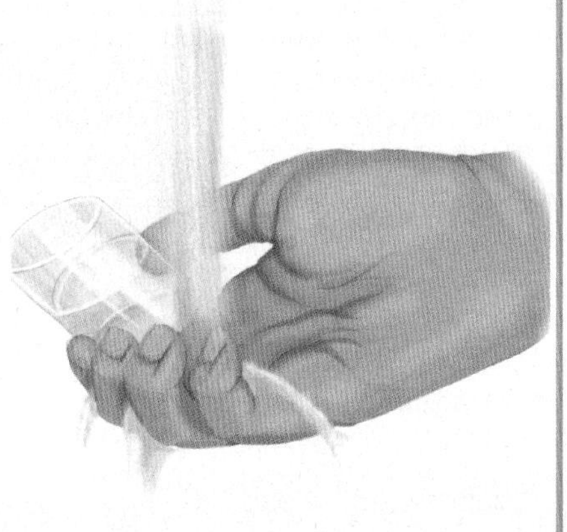

Metered-Dose Inhaler

1. Shake the inhaler and take off the cap.

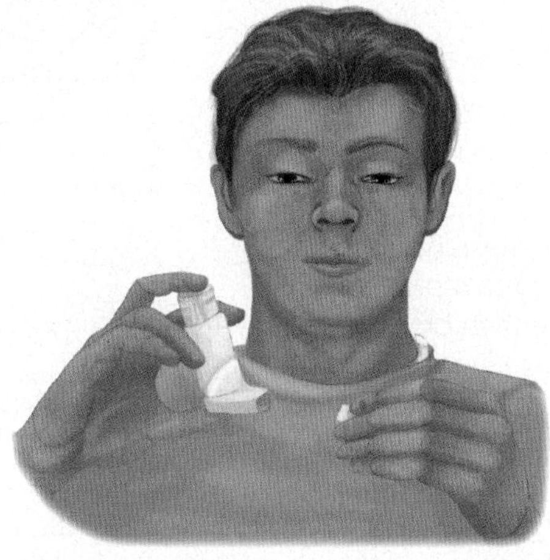

2. Attach the inhaler to the spacer or holding chamber.
3. Breathe out completely.

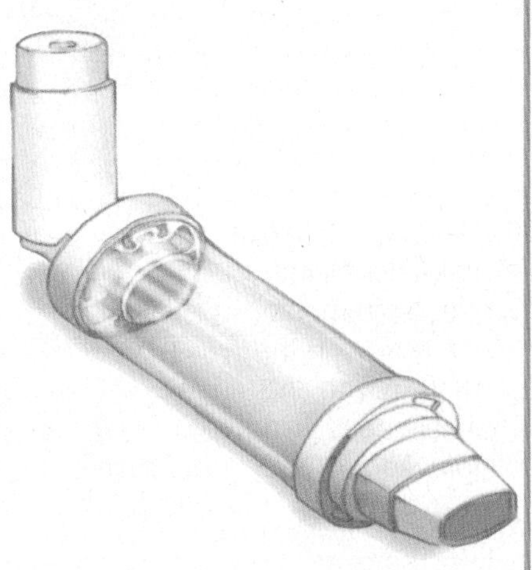

(*continued*)

TEACHING GUIDELINES 40.5 Using Asthma Medication Delivery Devices (*continued*)

4. Put the spacer mouthpiece in the mouth (or place the mask over the child's nose and mouth, ensuring a good seal).

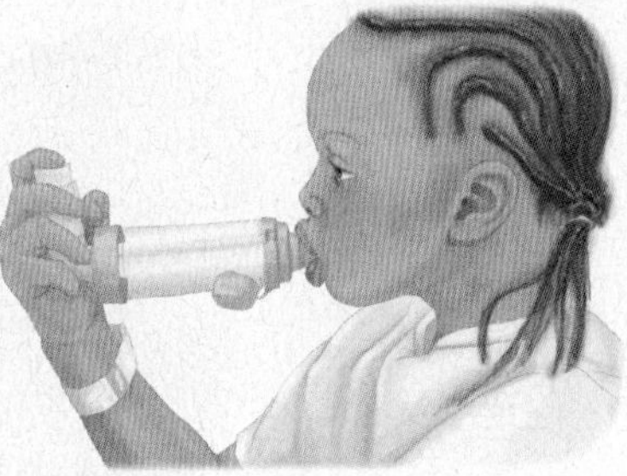

5. Compress the inhaler and inhale slowly and deeply. Hold the breath for a count of 10.
6. Wait one full minute before second inhalation, if prescribed.

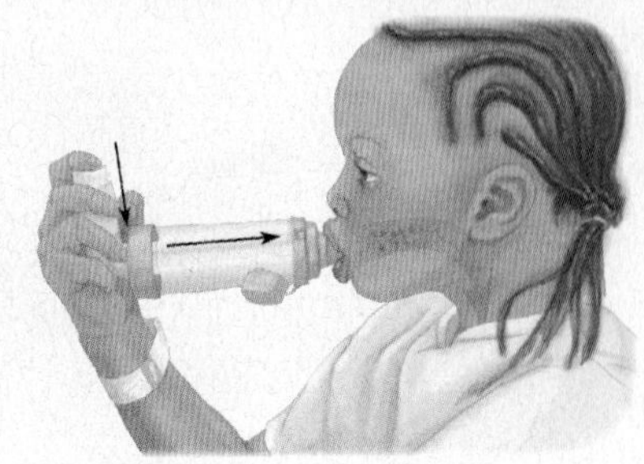

Diskus

1. Hold the Diskus in a horizontal position in one hand and push the thumb grip with the thumb of your other hand away from you until the mouthpiece is exposed.

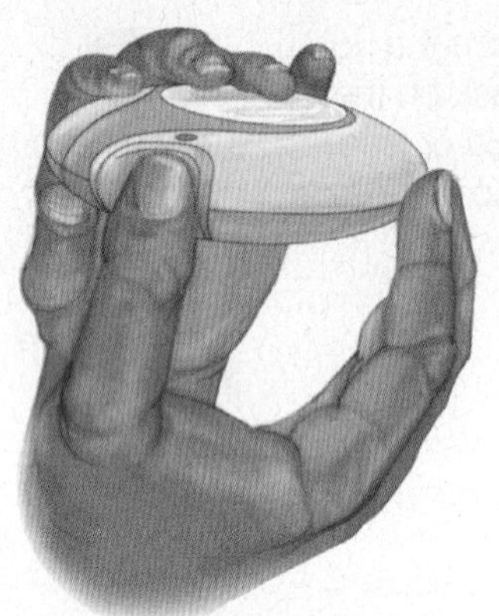

2. Push the lever until it clicks (the dose is now loaded).
3. Breathe out fully.

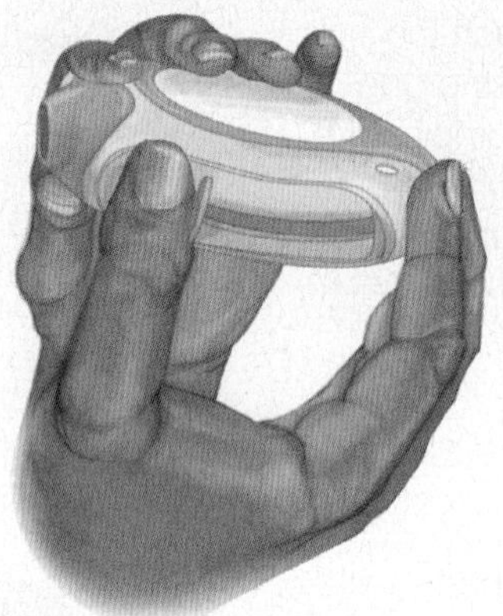

4. Place your mouth securely around the mouthpiece and then inhale.

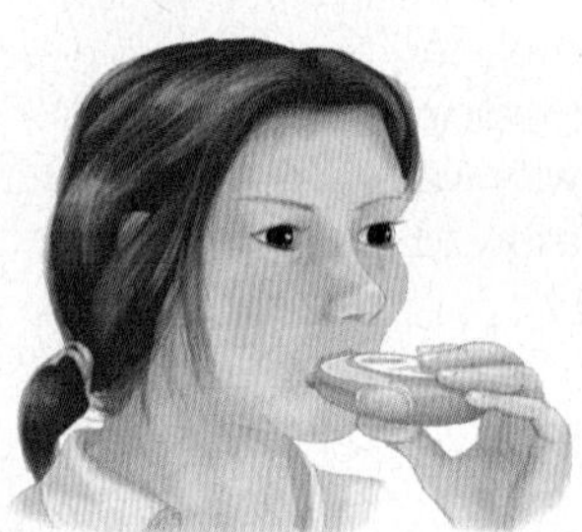

5. Remove the Diskus, hold the breath for 10 seconds, and then breathe out.

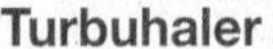

Turbuhaler

1. Hold the Turbuhaler upright. Load the dose by twisting the brown grip fully to the right.

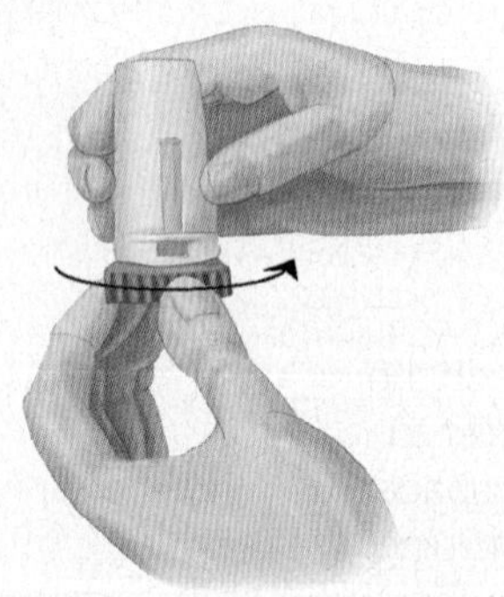

2. Then twist it to the left until you hear it click.
3. Breathe out fully.

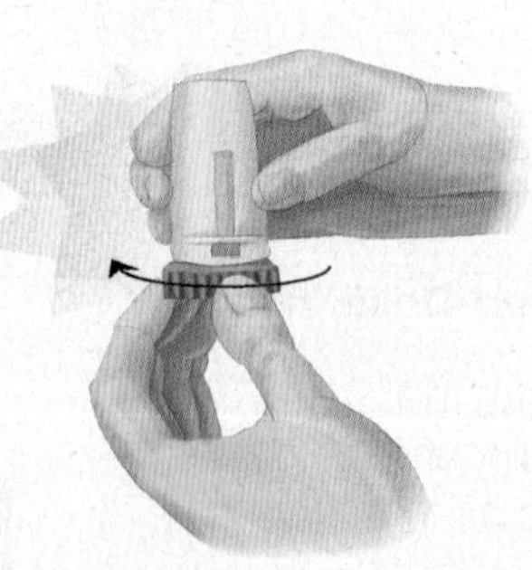

4. Holding the Turbuhaler horizontally, place the mouth firmly around the mouthpiece and inhale deeply and forcefully.

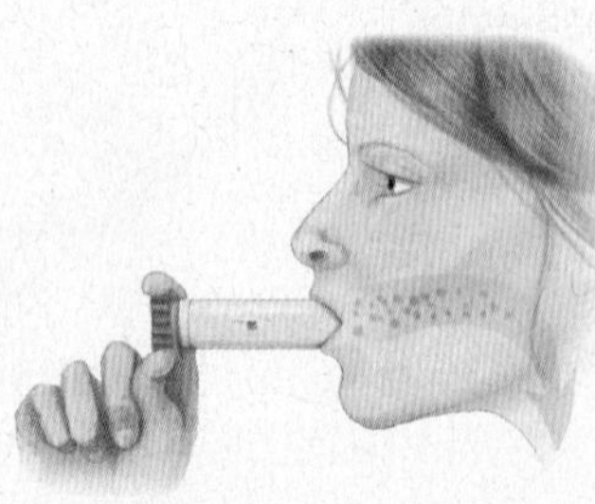

5. Remove the Turbuhaler from the mouth and then breathe out.

TEACHING GUIDELINES 40.6 Using a Peak Flow Meter

- Slide the arrow down to "zero."
- Stand up straight.
- Take a deep breath and close the lips tightly around the mouthpiece.
- Blow out hard and fast.
- Note the number the arrow moves to.
- Repeat three times and record the highest reading.
- Keep a record of daily readings, being sure to measure peak flow at the same time each day.

Adapted from Gerald, L. B., & Carr, T. (2022). Patient education: How to use a peak flow meter (beyond the basics). *UpToDate*. Retrieved March 11, 2024, from https://www.uptodate.com/contents/how-to-use-a-peak-flow-meter-beyond-the-basics

asthma management plan then gives specific instructions based on the PEFR measurement (Table 40.2).

TAKE NOTE!

Young children with asthma receiving inhaled medications via a nebulizer should use a snugly fitting mask to ensure accurate deposition of medication to the lungs and reduce loss of medication to the ambient air (Volkman & Chiu, 2023).

Avoidance of allergens is another key component of asthma management. Avoiding known triggers helps to prevent exacerbations as well as long-term inflammatory changes. This can be a difficult task for most families, particularly if the affected child suffers from several allergies. Refer to Teaching Guidelines 40.4 for strategies of allergen avoidance.

TAKE NOTE!

Teach the child and family that exposure to cigarette smoke increases the need for medications in children with asthma as well as the frequency of asthma exacerbations. Both indoor air quality and environmental pollution contribute to asthma in children.

Asthma education is a critical component in ensuring optimal health in children with asthma. This education is not limited to the hospital or clinic setting. Nurses can become involved in community asthma education: community-centered education in schools, churches, and day care centers or through peer educators has been shown to be effective. Education should include pathophysiology, asthma triggers, and prevention and treatment strategies. With so many children affected with this chronic disease, community education has the potential to make a broad impact.

School nurses must also become experts in asthma management as well as being committed to ongoing education of the child and family. See Evidence-Based Practice 40.1. Resources for schools include:

- Open airways for schools: an educational program presented by the American Lung Association or its local chapter, focusing on increasing asthma awareness and compliance with asthma action plans and decreasing asthma emergencies. Contact the local lung association or call 1-800-LUNG-USA.
- Indoor air repair at school: a kit available from Allergy and Asthma Network Mothers of Asthmatics (AANMA); and Healthy School Environments Assessment Tool.

Promoting the Child's Self-Esteem

The importance of education in the use of controller medications is well known, as increased use leads to decreased emergency room visits (Carey et al., 2019). In addition to quality asthma education, offer emotional support to children with asthma and their families. As children transition to assuming more control over their asthma, provide additional support for the child in their efforts and for the parent while helping them to let go a little more. Shared management of asthma care changes over time in a developmental fashion, as the child becomes more capable of taking responsibility for their own health. The school-age years are known to be a particular transition time (Sonney et al., 2019). An agreement related to asthma management being shared between the child and the parent my result in higher quality asthma control (Sonney et al., 2019). In

TABLE 40.2 • Assessment of Peak Expiratory Flow Rate (PEFR)

Zone[a]	PEFR	Symptoms	Action
Green: Good control	>80% personal best	None	Take usual medications.
Yellow: Caution	50%–80% personal best	Possibly present	Take short-acting inhaled beta$_2$-agonist right away. Talk to your primary provider or nurse practitioner.
Red: Medical alert	<50% personal best	Usually present	Take short-acting inhaled beta$_2$-agonist right away. Go to office or emergency department.

[a]The National Asthma Education and Prevention Program recommended the "traffic light" approach for educating individuals on PEFRs and management plans.

Data from Houin, P., Stillwell, P., Deboer, E. M., & Hoppe, J. (2022). Respiratory tract & mediastinum. In M. Bunik, W. W. Hay, M. J. Levin, & M. J. Abzug (Eds.), *Current diagnosis and treatment: Pediatrics* (26th ed.). McGraw-Hill Education; Volkman, K. K., & Chiu, A. M. (2023). Allergy. In K. J. Marcdante, & R. M. Kliegman (Eds.), *Nelson's essentials of pediatrics* (9th ed.). Elsevier.

EVIDENCE-BASED PRACTICE 40.1

School-Based Interventions for Asthma

STUDY

Asthma is a common respiratory condition in children and adolescents. Theoretically, acquisition of skills for self-management of asthma could occur with the school (a place where children already participate in learning). The review included 55 studies, with over 20,000 child and adolescent participants. The objectives of the review were to identify intervention features aligned with successful intervention and to determine effectiveness in school-based interventions in relation to child/adolescent asthma self-management.

Findings

Compared with no school intervention, school-based interventions mildly decreased the numbers of hospitalizations and emergency department visits for participants. In addition, the intervention may be responsible for slightly increasing the participants' quality of life.

Nursing Implications

Nurses should consider the results of this review. School nurses could implement interventions for self-management. Nurses outside of the school system have the opportunity to reinforce the self-management interventions as structured by the school.

Data from Harris, K., Kneale, D., Lasserson, T., McDonald, V. M., Grigg, J., & Thomas, J. (2019). School-based self-management interventions for asthma in children and adolescents: A mixed methods systematic review. ***Cochrane Database of Systematic Reviews.*** https://doi.org//10.1002/14651858.CD011651.pub2

addition to coping with a chronic illness, the child with asthma must often also cope with school-related issues. As compared to children without asthma, children with asthma often experience impaired sleep and participate less often in physical activity. They also experience increased stress and anxiety (Lack et al., 2020). Performing yoga increases physical activity in children with asthma and has been shown to improve lung function over time. Mindfulness training may also be beneficial, as increased mindfulness in children with asthma leads to improved quality of life as a result of increased asthma control (Lack et al., 2020).

Through education and support, the child can gain a sense of control. Children need to learn to master their disease. Accurate evaluation of asthma symptoms and improvement of self-esteem may help the child to experience less panic with an acute episode. Improved self-esteem might also help the child cope with the disease, in general, and with being different from their peers. The school-age child has the cognitive ability to begin taking responsibility for asthma management, with continued involvement on the part of the parents. Transferring control of asthma care to the child is an important developmental process that will increase the child's feeling of control over the illness.

Promoting Family Coping

Parent denial is an issue in many families. The family, through education and encouragement, can become the experts on the child's illness as well as advocates for the child's well-being. The resilient child is better able to cope with the challenges facing them, including asthma. Cohesiveness and warmth in the family environment can improve a child's resiliency as well as contribute to family hardiness. Parents need to be allowed to ask questions and voice their concerns. A nurse who understands the family's issues and concerns is better able to plan for support and education. Provide culturally sensitive education and interventions that focus on increasing the family's commitment to, and control of, asthma management. As the child and parents become confident in their ability to recognize asthma symptoms and cope with asthma and its periodic episodes, the family's ability to cope will improve.

THINKING ABOUT **DEVELOPMENT**

Ryan Jennings is a 13-year-old with a history of moderate asthma. They have been prescribed a long-term control medication to be taken routinely and a rescue medicine to be used as needed and before exercise. The adolescent is a talented pitcher and would like to participate with the school's baseball team.

How will Ryan's developmental stage affect self-care related to their asthma? What is the most appropriate approach for the nurse to take to educate Ryan about the medications and disease process?

How will the nurse foster compliance in Ryan?

Cystic Fibrosis

Cystic fibrosis is an autosomal recessive disorder that affects 40,000 children and adults in the United States (Cystic Fibrosis Foundation [CFF], n.d.). A deletion occurring on the long arm of chromosome 7 at the cystic fibrosis transmembrane conductance regulator (CFTR) is the responsible gene mutation. DNA testing can be used prenatally and in newborns to identify the presence of the mutation. The American College of Obstetricians and Gynecologists (2021) currently recommends screening for cystic fibrosis to any person seeking preconception or prenatal care. At present, all states include testing for cystic fibrosis as part of newborn screening.

Cystic fibrosis is the most common debilitating disease of childhood among those of European descent. Medical advances in recent years have greatly increased the length and quality of life for affected children, with median age for survival being 39.3 years (Katkin, 2023). Complications include hemoptysis, pneumothorax, bacterial colonization, cor pulmonale, volvulus, intussusception, intestinal obstruction, rectal prolapse, gastroesophageal reflux disease, diabetes, portal hypertension, liver failure, gallstones, and decreased fertility.

Pathophysiology

In cystic fibrosis, the CFTR mutation causes alterations in epithelial ion transport on mucosal surfaces, resulting in generalized dysfunction of the exocrine glands. The epithelial cells fail to conduct chloride, and water transport abnormalities occur. This results in thickened, tenacious secretions in the sweat glands, gastrointestinal tract, pancreas, respiratory tract, and other exocrine tissues. The increased viscosity of these secretions makes them difficult to clear. The sweat glands produce a larger amount of chloride, leading to a salty taste of the skin and alterations in electrolyte balance and dehydration. The pancreas, intrahepatic bile ducts, intestinal glands, gallbladder, and submaxillary glands become obstructed by viscous mucus and eosinophilic material. Pancreatic enzyme activity is lost, and malabsorption of fats, proteins, and carbohydrates occurs, resulting in poor growth and large, malodorous stools. Excess mucus is produced by the tracheobronchial glands. Abnormally thick mucus plugs the small airways, and then bronchiolitis and further plugging of the airways occur. Secondary bacterial infection with *Staphylococcus aureus*, *Pseudomonas aeruginosa*, and *Burkholderia cepacia* often occurs. This contributes to obstruction and inflammation, leading to chronic infection, tissue damage, and respiratory failure. Nasal polyps and recurrent sinusitis are common. Tenacious seminal fluid and blocking of the vas deferens often make males with cystic fibrosis infertile. In females, thick cervical secretions might limit penetration of sperm (Katkin, 2023). Table 40.3 gives further details of the pathophysiology and resulting respiratory and gastrointestinal clinical manifestations of cystic fibrosis.

Therapeutic Management

Therapeutic management of cystic fibrosis is aimed toward minimizing pulmonary complications, maximizing lung function, preventing infection, and facilitating growth. All children with cystic fibrosis who

TABLE **40.3** • Pathophysiology of Cystic Fibrosis and Resultant Respiratory and Gastrointestinal Clinical Manifestations

Defect in the CFTR Gene Effects	Pathophysiology	Clinical Manifestations
Respiratory tract	• Infection leads to neutrophilic inflammation. • Cleavage of complement receptors and immunoglobulin G leads to opsonophagocytosis failure. • Chemoattractant interleukin-8 and elastin degradase contribute to inflammatory response. • Thick, tenacious sputum that is chronically colonized with bacteria results. • Air trapping related to airway obstruction occurs. • Pulmonary parenchyma is eventually destroyed.	• Airway obstruction • Difficulty clearing secretions • Respiratory distress and impaired gas exchange • Chronic cough • Barrel-shaped chest • Decreased pulmonary function • Clubbing • Recurrent pneumonia • Hemoptysis • Pneumothorax • Chronic sinusitis • Nasal polyps • Cor pulmonale (right-sided heart failure)
Gastrointestinal tract	• Decreased chloride and water secretion into the intestine (causing dehydration of the intestinal material) and into the bile ducts (causing increased bile viscosity) • Reduced pancreatic bicarbonate secretion • Hypersecretion of gastric acid • Insufficiency of pancreatic enzymes (amylase, lipase, pancrease) necessary for digestion and absorption • Pancreas secretes thick mucus.	• Meconium ileus • Retention of fecal matter in distal intestine, resulting in vomiting, abdominal distention and cramping, anorexia, right lower quadrant pain • Sludging of intestinal contents may lead to fecal impaction, rectal prolapse, bowel obstruction, and intussusception. • Obstructive cirrhosis with esophageal varices, and splenomegaly • Gallstones • Gastroesophageal reflux disease (compounded by postural drainage with chest physiotherapy) • Inadequate protein absorption • Altered absorption of iron and vitamins A, D, E, and K • Failure to thrive • Hyperglycemia and development of diabetes later in life

Data from Houin, P., Stillwell, P., Deboer, E. M., & Hoppe, J. (2022). Respiratory tract & mediastinum. In M. Bunik, W. W. Hay, M. J. Levin, & M. J. Abzug (Eds.), *Current diagnosis and treatment: Pediatrics* (26th ed.). McGraw-Hill Education; Katkin, J. P. (2023). Cystic fibrosis: Clinical manifestations and diagnosis. *UpToDate.* Retrieved March 11, 2024, from https://www.uptodate.com/contents/cystic-fibrosis-clinical-manifestations-and-diagnosis

have pulmonary involvement require CPT with postural drainage (or an alternate method) several times daily to mobilize secretions from the lungs. Physical exercise is encouraged. Recombinant human DNase (Pulmozyme) is given daily using a nebulizer to decrease sputum viscosity and help clear secretions. Inhaled bronchodilators and antiinflammatory agents are prescribed for some children. Aerosolized antibiotics are often prescribed and may be given at home as well as in the hospital. Choice of antibiotic is determined by sputum culture and sensitivity results. Pancreatic enzymes and supplemental fat-soluble vitamins are prescribed to promote adequate digestion and absorption of nutrients and optimize nutritional status. Increased-calorie, high-protein diets are recommended, and sometimes supplemental high-calorie formula, either orally or via feeding tube, is needed. Some children require total parenteral nutrition to maintain or gain weight. Lung transplantation has been successful in some children with cystic fibrosis.

TAKE NOTE!

Children 6 years and older who have particular mutations of the cystic fibrosis gene may be prescribed a CFTR modulator such as ivacaftor or lumacaftor. Use of the CFTR modulator results in thinning of lung mucus, resulting in easier airway clearance via coughing (Simon, 2023).

Nursing Assessment

For a full description of the assessment phase of the nursing process, refer to the "Clinical Judgment and the Nursing Process" section earlier in the chapter. Assessment findings pertinent to cystic fibrosis are discussed further on.

Health History

Elicit a description of the present illness and chief complaint. Common signs and symptoms reported during the health history in the undiagnosed child might include:

- A salty taste to the child's skin (resulting from excess chloride loss via perspiration)
- Meconium ileus or late, difficult passage of meconium stool in the newborn period
- Abdominal pain or difficulty passing stool (infants or toddlers might present with intestinal obstruction or intussusception at the time of diagnosis)
- Bulky, greasy stools
- Poor weight gain and growth despite good appetite
- Chronic or recurrent cough and/or upper or lower respiratory infections

Children known to have cystic fibrosis are often admitted to the hospital for pulmonary exacerbations or other complications of the disease. The health history should include questions related to:

- respiratory status: has cough, sputum production, or work of breathing increased?
- appetite and weight gain.
- activity tolerance.
- increased need for pulmonary or pancreatic medications.
- presence of fever.
- presence of bone pain.
- any other changes in physical state or medication regimen.

Physical Examination

The physical examination includes inspection, percussion, palpation, and auscultation.

INSPECTION

Observe the child's general appearance and color. Check the nasal passages for polyps. Note respiratory rate, work of breathing, use of accessory muscles, position of comfort, frequency and severity of cough, and quality and quantity of sputum produced. The child with cystic fibrosis often has a barrel chest (anterior–posterior diameter approximates transverse diameter) (Fig. 40.13). Clubbing of the nail beds might also be present. Note whether rectal prolapse is present. Does the child appear small or thin for their age? The child might have a protuberant abdomen and thin extremities, with decreased amounts of subcutaneous fat. Observe for the

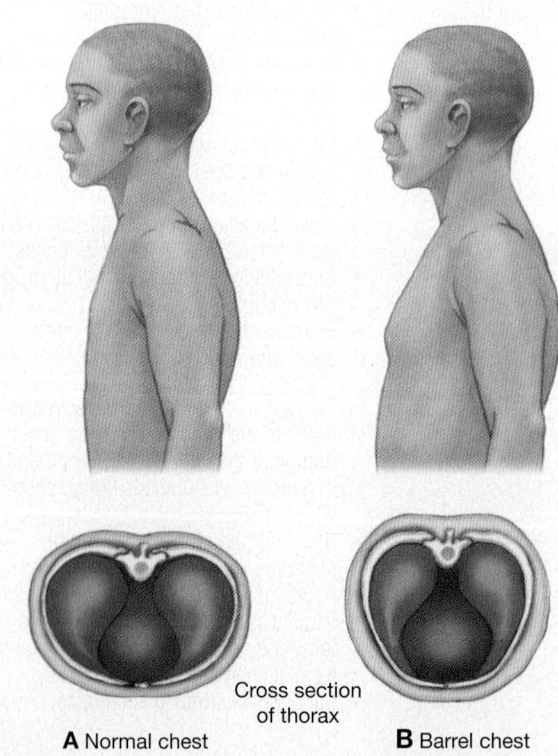

FIGURE 40.13 **A.** Normal chest shape—transverse diameter is greater than anterior–posterior diameter. **B.** Barrel chest—transverse diameter equals anterior–posterior diameter.

presence of edema (sign of cardiac or liver failure). Note distended neck veins or the presence of a heave (signs of cor pulmonale).

PERCUSSION AND PALPATION

Percussion over the lung fields usually yields hyperresonance due to air trapping. Diaphragmatic excursion might be decreased. Percussion of the abdomen might reveal dullness over an enlarged liver or mass related to intestinal obstruction. Palpation might yield a finding of asymmetric chest excursion if atelectasis is present. Tactile fremitus may be decreased over areas of atelectasis. Note if tenderness is present over the liver (might be an early sign of cor pulmonale).

AUSCULTATION

Auscultation may reveal a variety of adventitious breath sounds. Fine or coarse crackles and scattered or localized wheezing might be present. With progressive obstructive pulmonary involvement, breath sounds might be diminished. Tachycardia might be present. Note the presence of a gallop (might occur with cor pulmonale). Note the adequacy of bowel sounds.

Laboratory and Diagnostic Tests

Common laboratory and diagnostic studies ordered for the diagnosis and assessment of cystic fibrosis include:

- Sweat chloride test: considered suspicious if the level of chloride in collected sweat is above 50 mEq/L and diagnostic if the level is above 60 mEq/L.
- Pulse oximetry: oxygen saturation might be decreased, particularly during a pulmonary exacerbation.
- Chest radiograph: may reveal hyperinflation, bronchial wall thickening, atelectasis, or infiltration.
- PFTs: might reveal a decrease in forced vital capacity and forced expiratory volume, with increases in residual volume.

Nursing Management

Management of cystic fibrosis focuses on minimizing pulmonary complications, promoting growth and development, and facilitating coping and adjustment by the child and family. In addition to the patient problems and related interventions discussed in the "Clinical Judgment and the Nursing Process" section earlier in the chapter, interventions common to cystic fibrosis follow.

Maintaining Patent Airway

Provide CPT, use of the vest airway clearance system, use of the flutter-valve device, and/or positive expiratory pressure therapy to clear secretions and maintain airway patency. For children with cystic fibrosis, CPT is a critical intervention. CPT involves percussion, vibration, and postural drainage, and either it or another bronchial hygiene therapy must be performed several times a day to assist with mobilization of secretions. Nursing Procedure 40.2 gives instructions on the CPT technique. The vest airway clearance system provides high-frequency chest wall oscillation to increase airflow velocity to create repetitive cough-like shear forces and to decrease the viscosity of secretions (Hill-Rom, 2021).

For older children and adolescents, the flutter-valve device provides high-frequency oscillation to the airway as the child exhales into a mouthpiece that contains a steel ball. Positive expiratory pressure therapy involves exhaling through a flow resistor, which creates positive

NURSING PROCEDURE 40.2 Performing Chest Physiotherapy

May be preceded by an inhalation treatment; should not be performed after eating.

1. Provide percussion via a cupped hand or an infant percussion device. Appropriate percussion yields a hollow sound, not a slapping sound.

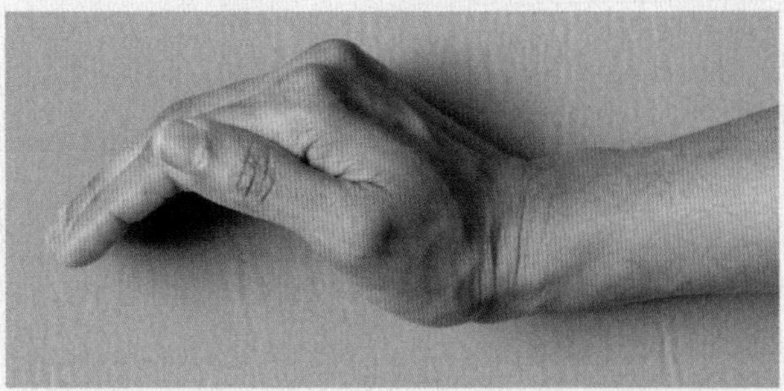

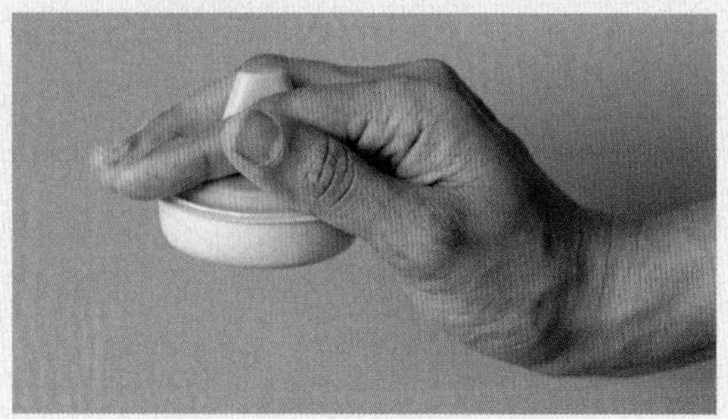

(continued)

NURSING PROCEDURE 40.2 Performing Chest Physiotherapy (*continued*)

2. Percuss each segment of the lung for 1 to 2 minutes.

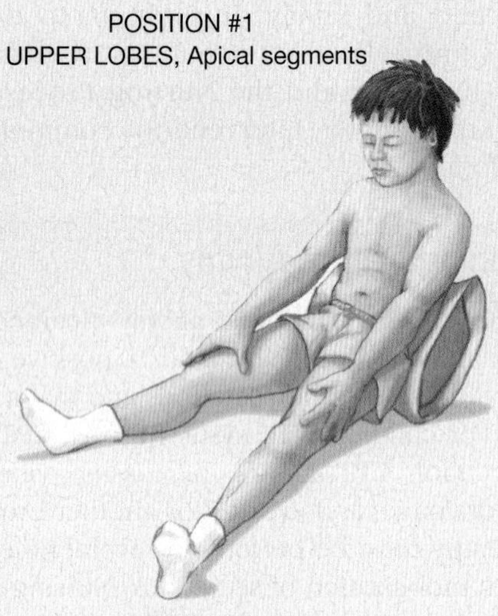

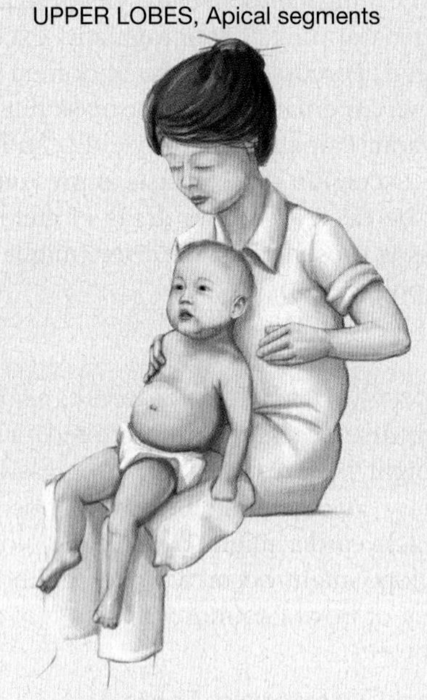

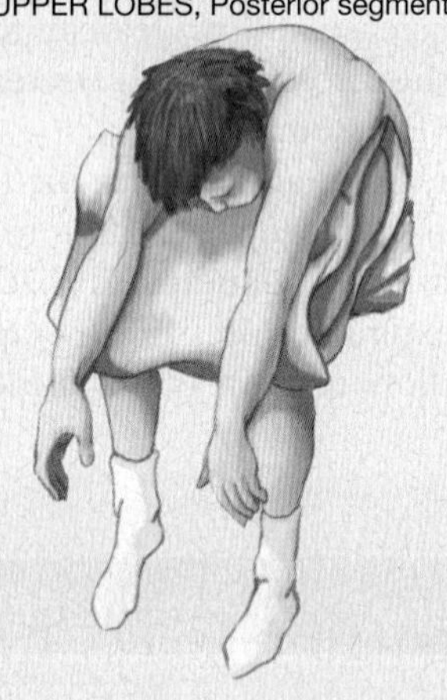

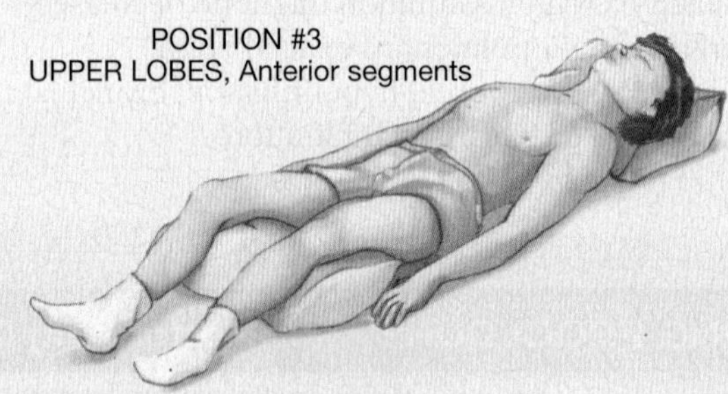

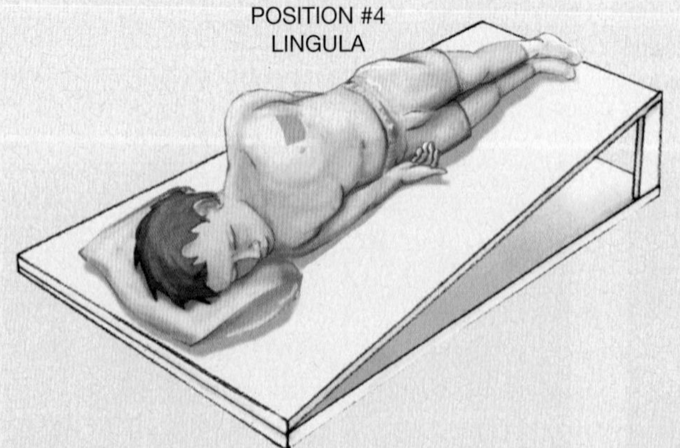

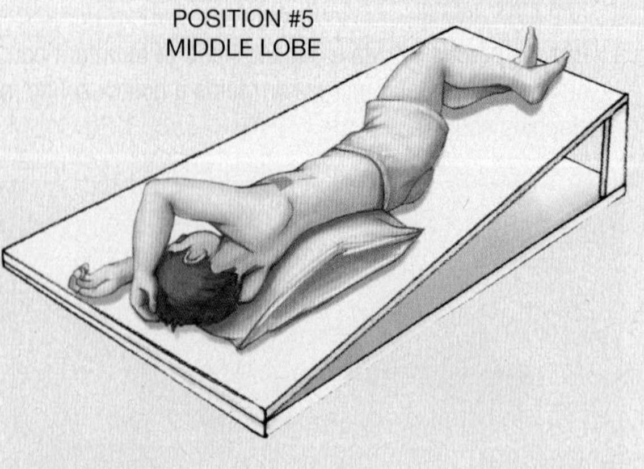

NURSING PROCEDURE 40.2 Performing Chest Physiotherapy

POSITION #6
LOWER LOBES, Anterior basal segments

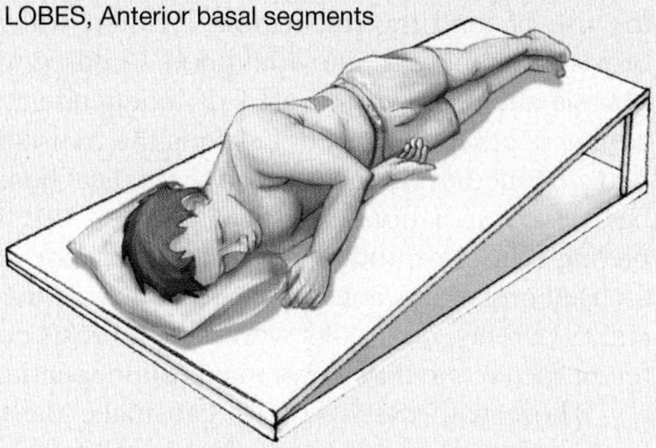

POSITION #7
LOWER LOBES, Posterior basal segments

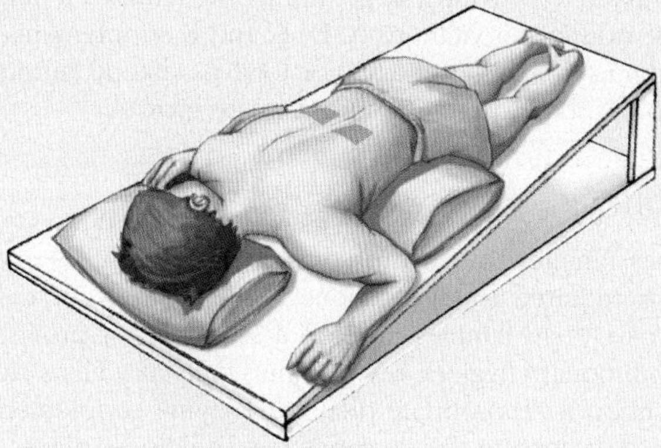

POSITION #8 & 9
LOWER LOBES, Lateral basal segments

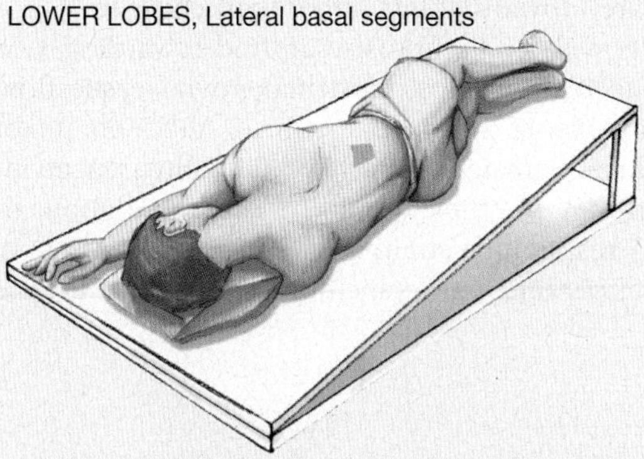

POSITION #10
LOWER LOBES, Superior segments

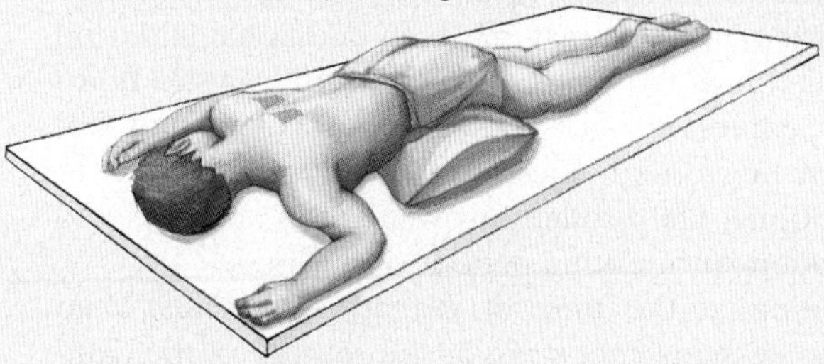

3. Place the ball of the hand on the lung segment, keeping the arm and shoulder straight. Vibrate by tensing and relaxing your arms during the child's exhalation. Vibrate each lung segment for at least five exhalations.
4. Encourage the child to deep breathe and cough.
5. Change drainage positions, and repeat percussion and vibration.

expiratory pressure. The cycles of exhalation are repeated until coughing yields expectoration of secretions. Breathing exercises are also helpful in promoting mucus clearance. Encourage physical exercise, as it helps to promote mucus secretion as well as providing cardiopulmonary conditioning. Ensure that Pulmozyme is administered, as well as inhaled bronchodilators and antiinflammatory agents, if prescribed.

Preventing Infection

Ensure parents and older children understand that vigorous pulmonary hygiene to mobilize secretions is critical to preventing infection. Administer aerosolized antibiotics as prescribed either in the hospital or teach parents to provide them at home. Children with frequent or severe respiratory exacerbations might require lengthy courses of intravenous antibiotics.

Maintaining Growth

Administer pancreatic enzyme supplements (pancrelipase [Creon, Pancreaze, Zenpep]) with all meals and snacks to promote adequate digestion and absorption of nutrients. The number of capsules required depends on the extent of pancreatic insufficiency and the amount of food being ingested. The dosage can be adjusted until an adequate growth pattern is established and the number of stools is consistent at one or two per day. Children will need additional enzyme capsules when high-fat foods are being eaten. In the infant or young child, the enzyme capsule can be opened and sprinkled on cereal or applesauce. Provide a well-balanced, high-calorie, high-protein diet to ensure adequate growth. Some children require up to one and a half times the recommended daily allowance of calories for children their age. A number of commercially available nutritional formulas and shakes are available for diet supplementation.

In infants, breastfeeding should be continued with enzyme administration. Some infants will require fortification of breast milk or supplementation with high-calorie formulas. Commercially available infant formulas can continue to be used for the formula-fed infant and can be mixed to provide a larger number of calories if necessary. Administer vitamins A, D, E, and K supplementally. Administer gavage feedings or total parenteral nutrition as prescribed to provide for adequate growth.

Promoting Family Coping

Assist families to learn to cope with the daily interventions required for the serious chronic illness of cystic fibrosis. Help families develop a schedule for provision of pulmonary hygiene several times daily as well as close attention to appropriate diet and enzyme supplementation. Adjusting to the demands that the illness places on the child and family is difficult. Continual adjustments within the family must occur. Children are frequently hospitalized, and this may place an additional strain on the family and its finances. Children with cystic fibrosis may express fear or feelings of isolation, and siblings may be worried or jealous. Encourage the family to lead a normal life through involvement in activities and school attendance during periods of wellness.

Starting at the time of diagnosis, families often demonstrate significant stress as the severity of the diagnosis and the significance of disease chronicity become real for them. Involve the family in the child's care from the time of diagnosis, whether in the outpatient setting or in the hospital. Ongoing education about the illness and its treatments is necessary. Once the initial shock of diagnosis has passed and the family has adjusted to initial care, the family usually learns how to manage the requirements of care. Powerlessness gives way to adaptation. As family members become more comfortable with their understanding of the illness and the required treatments, they will eventually become the experts on the child's care. It is important for the nurse to recognize and respect the family's changing needs over time.

Providing daily intense care can be tiring, and noncompliance on the part of the family or child might occur because of this fatigue. Hypervigilance may also occur as parents attempt to control the difficult situation and protect the child. Families welcome support and encouragement. Most families eventually progress past the stages of fear, guilt, and powerlessness to a way of living that is different than what they anticipated but is something that they can manage.

Refer parents to a local support group for families of children with cystic fibrosis. The CFF has chapters throughout the United States. Parents of children with a terminal illness might face the death of their child at an earlier age than expected. Assisting with anticipatory grieving and making decisions related to end-of-life care are other important nursing interventions.

Preparing the Child and Family for Adulthood with Cystic Fibrosis

With current technologic and medication advances and the use of lung transplantation, children with cystic fibrosis are living well into adulthood. Children with cystic fibrosis should have the goal of independent living as adults, as other children do. Making the transition from a pediatric medical home to an adult medical home should be viewed as a normal part of growing up, like completing school or finding a first job. Pediatric clinics are focused on family-centered care that heavily involves the child's parents, but adults with cystic fibrosis need a different focus, one that views them as independent adults.

Those with cystic fibrosis can make the transition from pediatric to adult care with thoughtful preparation and coordination. They desire and deserve a smooth transition in care that will result in appropriate ongoing medical management of cystic fibrosis in an environment that is geared toward adults rather than children.

Adults with cystic fibrosis can find rewarding work and pursue relationships. Most males with cystic fibrosis are capable of sexual intercourse, although unable to reproduce. Females might have difficulty conceiving, and when they do, they should be cautioned about the additional respiratory strain that pregnancy causes. All children of parents with cystic fibrosis will be carriers of the gene.

Apnea

Apnea is defined as absence of breathing for longer than 20 seconds; it might be accompanied by bradycardia. Sometimes, apnea presents in the form of a brief, resolved, unexplained event (BRUE) in which the infant or child exhibits some combination of apnea, color change, muscle tone alteration, coughing, or gagging. Apnea may also occur acutely at any age because of respiratory distress. This discussion will focus on apnea that is chronic or recurrent in nature or that occurs as part of a BRUE.

Apnea in infants may be central (unrelated to any other cause) or may occur with other illnesses such as sepsis and respiratory infection. Apnea in newborns might be associated with hypothermia, hypoglycemia, infection, or hyperbilirubinemia. Apnea of prematurity occurs secondary to an immature respiratory system. Apnea should not be considered a predecessor to sudden unexplained infant death (SUID). Current research has not proven this theory, and SUID generally occurs in otherwise healthy young infants (Moon et al., 2022). Box 40.4 gives more information about SUID and its prevention.

Therapeutic management of apnea varies depending on the cause. When apnea occurs as a result of another disorder or infection, treatment is directed toward that cause. In the event of apnea, stimulation may trigger

BOX **40.4 Sudden Unexplained Infant Death (SUID)**

Definition

Sudden death of a previously healthy infant younger than 1 year of age

Prevention

- Place all infants in the supine position to sleep.
- Provide a firm sleep surface and avoid soft bedding, bumper pads, excess covers, pillows, and stuffed animals in the crib.
- Avoid maternal prenatal smoking and exposure of the infant to secondhand smoke.
- Avoid maternal prenatal alcohol and illicit drug exposure.
- Ensure the infant sleeps in a separate bed from the parents, in the parents' room, for the first 6 months of life.
- Avoid overdressing the infant and using head coverings.
- Encourage pacifier use during naps and at bedtime if the infant is receptive to it (AAP, 2024).

Support and Information

- American SIDS Institute: www.sids.org
- National SUID/SIDS Resource Center: www.sidscenter.org
- SIDS Network, Inc.: http://sids-network.org/

the infant to take a breath. If breathing does not resume, rescue breathing, or bag-valve-mask ventilation is necessary. Infants and children who have experienced a BRUE or who have chronic apnea may require ongoing cardiac/apnea monitoring. Caffeine citrate is sometimes administered, primarily in premature infants, to stimulate respirations (S. Smith, 2022).

Nursing Assessment

Question the parents about the infant's position and activities preceding the apneic episode. Did the infant experience a color change? Did the infant self-stimulate (breathe again on their own), or did they require stimulation from the caregiver? Assess risk factors for apnea, which may include prematurity, anemia, and history of metabolic disorders. Apnea may occur in association with cardiac or neurologic disturbances, respiratory infection, sepsis, child abuse, or poisoning.

In the hospitalized infant, note absence of respiration, position, color, and other associated findings, such as emesis on the bedclothes. If an infant who is apneic fails to be stimulated and does not breathe again, pulselessness will result.

Nursing Management

When an infant is noted to be apneic, gently stimulate them to take a breath again. If gentle stimulation is unsuccessful, then rescue breathing or bag-valve-mask ventilation must be started. To avoid apnea in the newborn, maintain a neutral thermal environment. Administer caffeine or theophylline if prescribed, and teach families about the use of these medications.

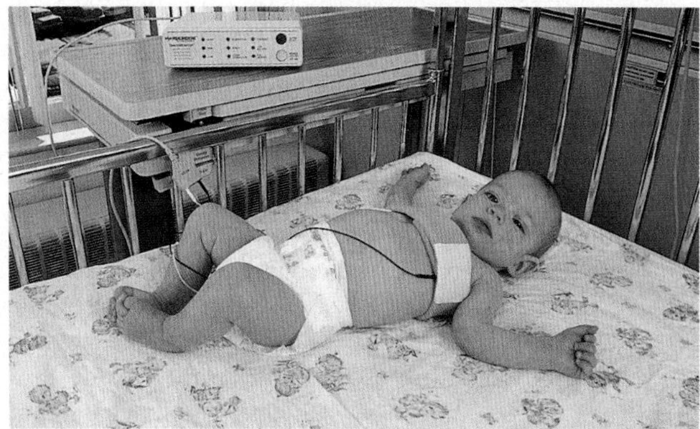

FIGURE 40.14 The home apnea monitor uses a soft belt with a Velcro attachment to hold two leads in the appropriate position on the chest.

Infants with recurrent apnea or BRUE may be discharged on a home apnea monitor (Fig. 40.14). Provide education on use of the monitor, guidance about when to notify the primary provider or nurse practitioner or monitor service about alarms, and training in infant CPR. The monitor is usually discontinued after 3 months without a significant event of apnea or bradycardia. In some ways, the monitor gives parents peace of mind, but in others it can make them more nervous about the well-being of their child. When apnea monitors are used in the home, parental sleep may be disrupted by machine alarms. Parents often express increased fear, anxiety, and depressive symptoms associated with home monitoring (Corwin, 2023). Providing appropriate education to the parents about the nature of the child's disorder as well as action to take in the event of apnea may give the family a sense of mastery over the situation, thus decreasing their anxiety. Refer families to local support groups such as those offered by Parent to Parent and Parents Helping Parents.

TRACHEOSTOMY

A tracheostomy is an artificial opening in the airway; usually, a plastic tracheostomy tube is in place to form a patent airway. Tracheostomies are performed to relieve airway obstruction, such as with subglottic stenosis (narrowing of the airway sometimes resulting from long-term intubation). They are also used for pulmonary hygiene and in the child who requires chronic mechanical ventilation. The tracheostomy facilitates secretion removal, reduces work of breathing, and increases the child's comfort. In some cases, the tracheostomy facilitates mechanical ventilation weaning. It may be permanent or temporary, depending on the indication. The tracheostomy tube varies in size and type depending on the child's airway size and health and the length of time the child will require the tracheostomy. Silastic tracheostomy tubes are soft and flexible; they are available with a single lumen or may have an outer and inner lumen. Both types have an obturator (the guide used during tube changes). Uncuffed tubes are used more often in the pediatric population. Figure 40.15 shows various types of tracheostomy tubes.

Complications immediately after surgery include hemorrhage, air entry, pulmonary edema, anatomic damage, and respiratory arrest. At any point in time, the tracheostomy tube may become occluded, which compromises ventilation. Complications of chronic tracheostomy include infection, cellulitis, and formation of granulation tissue around the insertion site.

Nursing Assessment

When obtaining the history for a child with a tracheostomy, note the reason for the tracheostomy, as well as the size and type of tracheostomy tube. Inspect the site. The stoma should appear pink and without bleeding or drainage. The tube itself should be clean and free from secretions. The tracheostomy ties should fit securely, allowing one finger to slide beneath the ties. Inspect the skin under the ties for rash or redness. Observe work of breathing.

When caring for the infant or child with a tracheostomy, whether in the hospital, home, or community setting, a thorough respiratory assessment is necessary. Note the presence of secretions and their color, thickness, and amount. Auscultate for breath sounds, which should be clear and equal throughout all lung fields. Measure pulse oximetry. When infection is suspected or secretions are discolored or have a foul odor, a sputum culture may be obtained.

TAKE NOTE!

Keep small toys (risk of aspiration), plastic bibs or bedding (risk of airway occlusion), and talcum powder (risk of inhalation injury) out of reach of the child with a tracheostomy.

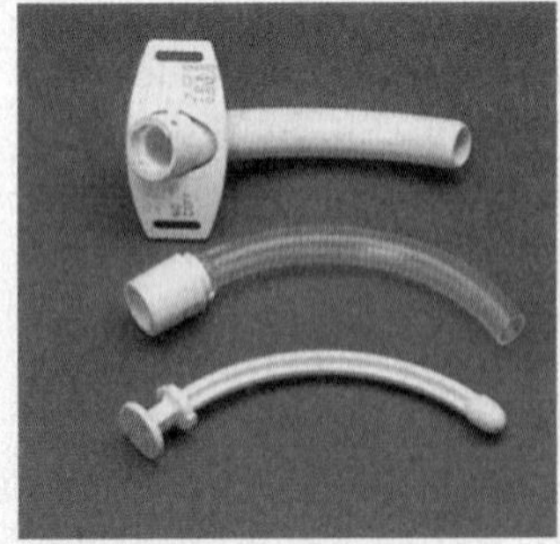

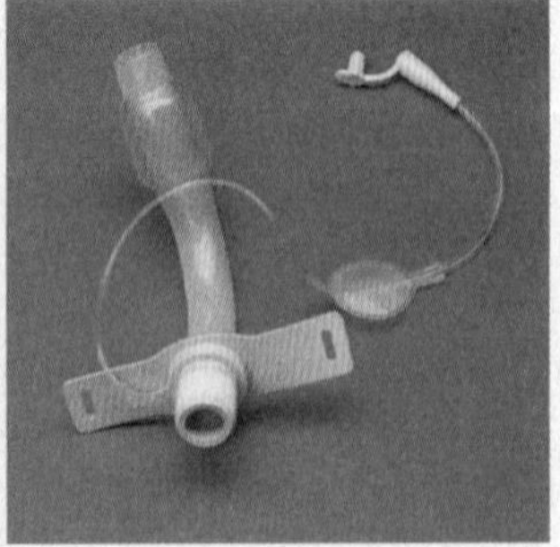

FIGURE 40.15 Note smaller size and absence of inner cannula on particular brands of pediatric tracheostomy tubes.

Nursing Management

In the immediate postoperative period, the infant or child may require restraints to avoid accidental dislodgment of the tracheostomy tube. Infants and children who have had a tracheostomy for a period of time become accustomed to it and usually do not attempt to remove the tube. Since air inspired via the tracheostomy tube bypasses the upper airway, it lacks humidification, and this lack of humidity can lead to a mucous plug in the tracheostomy and resultant hypoxia. Provide humidity to either room air or oxygen via a tracheostomy collar or ventilator, depending on the child's need (Fig. 40.16). Box 40.5 lists the equipment that should be available at the bedside of any child who has a tracheostomy.

Tracheostomies require frequent suctioning to maintain patency. The appropriate length for insertion of the suction catheter depends on the size of the tracheostomy and the child's needs. Place a sign at the head of the child's bed indicating the suction catheter size and the length (in centimeters) that it should be inserted for suctioning. Keep an extra tracheostomy tube of the same size and one size smaller at the bedside in the event of an emergency.

Many pediatric tracheostomy tubes do not have an inner cannula that requires periodic removal and cleaning, so periodic removal and replacement of the chronic tracheostomy tube is required. Clean the removed tracheostomy tube with half-strength hydrogen peroxide and pipe cleaners. Rinse with distilled water and allow it to dry. The tracheostomy tube can be reused many times if adequately cleaned between uses.

Perform tracheostomy care every 8 hours or per institution protocol. Change the tracheostomy tube only as needed or per institution protocol. Nursing Procedure 40.3 gives information about tracheostomy care. Always change tracheostomy ties with an assistant to avoid accidental dislodgement of the tube.

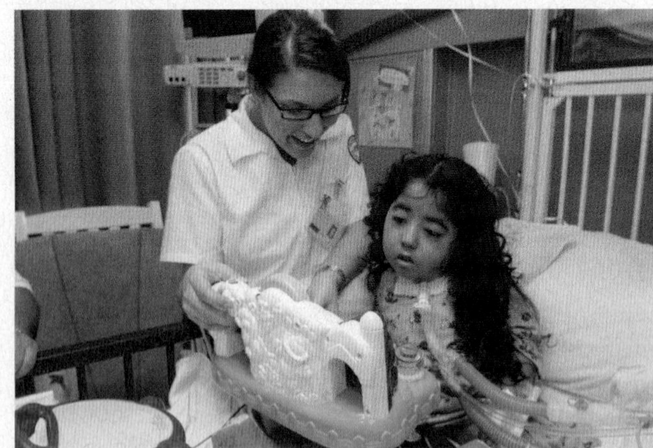

FIGURE 40.16 The trach collar allows for humidification of inspired air or supplemental oxygen.

BOX **40.5** **Emergency Equipment (Available at Bedside)**

- Two spare tracheostomy tubes (one the same size and one a size smaller)
- Suction equipment
- Stitch cutter (new tracheostomy)
- Spare tracheostomy ties
- Lubricating jelly
- Bag-valve-mask device
- Call bell within child's/parent's reach

If the older child or teen has a tracheostomy tube with an inner cannula, care of the inner cannula is similar to that of an adult. Involve parents in care of the tracheostomy and begin education about caring for the tracheostomy tube at home as soon as the child is stable. The child with a tracheostomy often qualifies for a Medicaid waiver that will provide a certain amount of home nursing care. Refer the family to local support groups.

NURSING PROCEDURE 40.1 Tracheostomy Care

1. Gather the necessary equipment:
   - Cleaning solution
   - Gloves
   - Precut gauze pad
   - Cotton-tipped applicators
   - Clean tracheostomy ties
   - Extra tracheostomy tube in case of accidental dislodgement
2. Position the infant/child supine with a blanket or towel roll to extend the neck.
3. Open all packaging and cut tracheostomy ties to appropriate length if necessary.
4. Cleanse around the tracheostomy site with prescribed solution (half-strength hydrogen peroxide or acetic acid, normal saline or soap and water if at home) and cotton-tipped applicators, working from just around the tracheostomy tube outward.
5. Rinse with sterile water and cotton-tipped applicator in similar fashion.
6. Place the precut sterile gauze under the tracheostomy tube.
7. With the assistant holding the tube in place, cut the ties and remove from the tube.
8. Attach the clean ties to the tube, and tie or secure in place with Velcro (Fig. 40.17).

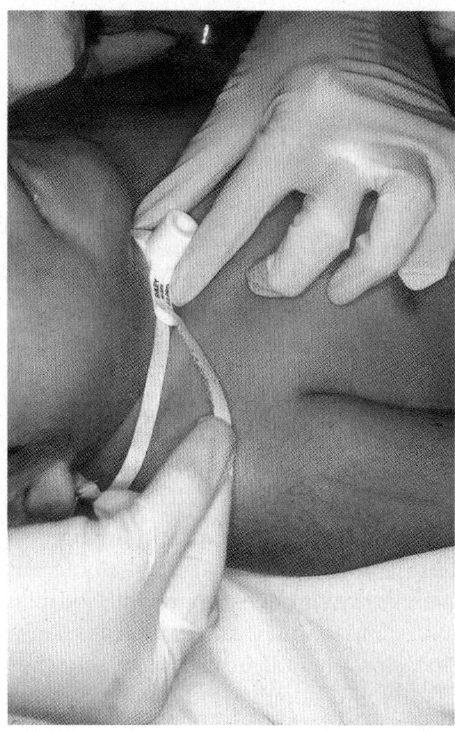

FIGURE 40.17 Trach ties are attached to the tube and secured in place with Velcro.

Unfolding Patient Stories: Sabina Vasquez • Part 2

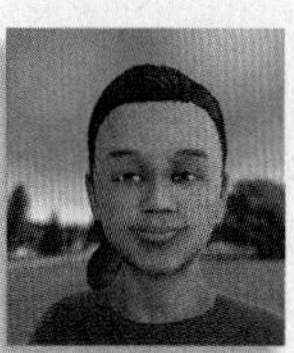

Recall Sabina Vasquez from Chapter 27, a 5-year-old diagnosed with asthma who uses an albuterol inhaler. What questions and assessments help the nurse evaluate her current respiratory status during a routine clinic visit? What methods can the nurse use to guide asthma management and determine how well Sabina's asthma is managed at home?

Care for Sabina and other patients in a realistic virtual environment: ***vSim** for Nursing* (thepoint.lww.com/vSimPediatric). Practice documenting these patients' care in DocuCare (thePoint.lww.com/DocuCareEHR).

KEY CONCEPTS

- Respiratory infections account for the majority of acute illnesses in children.
- The upper and lower airways are smaller in children than in adults, making them more susceptible to obstruction in the presence of mucus, debris, or edema.
- Newborns are preferential nose breathers.
- The child's highly compliant airway is quite susceptible to dynamic collapse in the presence of airway obstruction.
- Because they have fewer alveoli, children have a higher risk of hypoxemia than adults.
- Generally, disorders of the nose and throat do not result in increased work of breathing or affect the

lungs. Thus, if the lungs are involved, lower respiratory disease must be considered.

- Wheezing may be associated with a variety of lower respiratory disorders, such as asthma, bronchiolitis, and cystic fibrosis.
- Pulse oximetry is a useful tool for determining the extent of hypoxia. Findings should be correlated with the child's clinical presentation.
- Rapid streptococcus and rapid influenza tests are very useful for the quick diagnosis of strep throat or influenza so that appropriate treatment may be instituted early in the illness.
- Supplemental oxygen is often necessary in the child who is hospitalized (particularly with lower respiratory disease). Oxygen should be humidified to prevent drying of secretions.
- Suctioning, whether with a bulb syringe or suction catheter, is very effective at maintaining airway patency, especially in the younger child or infant.
- Normal saline nasal wash is an inexpensive, simple, and safe method for decongesting the nose in the case of the common cold, allergic rhinitis, and sinusitis.
- Infants who were born prematurely; children with a chronic illness such as diabetes, congenital heart disease, sickle cell anemia, or cystic fibrosis; and children with developmental disorders such as cerebral palsy tend to be more severely affected with respiratory disorders.
- Passive cigarette smoke exposure increases the infant's and child's risk of respiratory disease.
- Continual swallowing while awake or asleep is an indication of bleeding in the postoperative tonsillectomy child.
- Positioning to ease work of breathing and maintaining a patent airway are priorities for the child with a respiratory disorder.
- To avoid Reye syndrome, aspirin should not be given to treat fever or pain in the infant or child with a viral infection.
- Infants younger than 8 months of age whose birth parent did not receive the RSV vaccine during pregnancy should receive one dose of nirsevimab just prior to or at the onset of the RSV season.
- Children older than 6 months of age should be immunized against influenza yearly.
- Children at high risk for exposure to TB should be screened for infection.
- Promoting airway clearance and maintenance, effective breathing patterns, and adequate gas exchange is the priority focus of nursing intervention in pediatric respiratory disease.
- Children with any degree of respiratory distress require frequent assessment and early intervention to prevent progression to respiratory failure.
- Avoidance of allergens is critical in the treatment plan for the child with allergic rhinitis.
- Avoidance of allergic triggers, control of the inflammatory process, and education of the child and family are the focus of asthma management.
- CPT is extremely useful for mobilizing secretions in any condition resulting in an increase in mucus production and is required in children with cystic fibrosis.
- Children with chronic respiratory disorders and their families often need large amounts of education and psychosocial support: children often experience fear and isolation, while families must learn to balance care of the chronically ill child with other family life.

REFERENCES AND RECOMMENDED READINGS

American Academy of Allergy, & Asthma and Immunology. (2011). *Asthma action plan.* http://www.aaaai.org/professionals/asthma-action-plan.pdf

American Academy of Pediatrics. (2024). *Safe sleep.* https://www.aap.org/en/patient-care/safe-sleep/

American College of Obstetricians and Gynecologists. (2021). *Cystic fibrosis: Prenatal screening and diagnosis.* https://www.acog.org/patient-resources/faqs/pregnancy/cystic-fibrosis-prenatal-screening-and-diagnosis

American Heart Association, & American Academy of Pediatrics. (2020). *Pediatric advanced life support: Provider manual.* American Heart Association.

Aronson, M. D., & Auwaerter, P. G. (2023). Infectious mononucleosis. *UpToDate.* Retrieved November 4, 2023, from https://www.uptodate.com/contents/infectious-mononucleosis

Barr, F. E., & Graham, B. S. (2024). Respiratory syncytial virus infection: Prevention in infants and children. *UpToDate.* Retrieved March 11, 2024, from https://www.uptodate.com/contents/respiratory-syncytial-virus-infection-prevention-in-infants-and-children

Barson, W. J. (2022). Community-acquired pneumonia in children: Outpatient treatment. *UpToDate.* Retrieved March 11, 2024, from https://www.uptodate.com/contents/community-acquired-pneumonia-in-children-outpatient-treatment

Batra, V., & Ang, J. Y. (2022). Pediatric tuberculosis. *eMedicine.* Retrieved March 11, 2024, from https://emedicine.medscape.com/article/969401-overview

Carey, S. K., Edds-McAfee, C., Martinez, V., Gutierrez de Blume, A. P., & Thornton, K. M. (2019). An examination of factors affecting quality of life for children with asthma and their caregivers in southeastern Georgia. *Journal of Pediatric Health Care, 33*(5), 529–536. https://doi.org/10.1016/j.pedhc.2019.01.008

Carolan, P. L. (2023). Pediatric bronchitis. *eMedicine.* Retrieved March 11, 2024, from https://emedicine.medscape.com/article/1001332-overview

Centers for Disease Control and Prevention. (2022). *Health problems caused by secondhand smoke.* https://www.cdc.gov/tobacco/secondhand-smoke/health.html

Centers for Disease Control and Prevention. (2023a). *Pneumococcal vaccination.* Retrieved November 4, 2023, from https://www.cdc.gov/vaccines/vpd/pneumo/index.html

Centers for Disease Control and Prevention. (2023b). *Respiratory syncytial virus (RSV) vaccine VIS.* Retrieved November 6, 2023, from https://www.cdc.gov/vaccines/hcp/vis/vis-statements/rsv.html

Centers for Disease Control and Prevention. (2023c). *Seasonal influenza vaccination resources for health professionals*. Retrieved November 4, 2023, from https://www.cdc.gov/flu/professionals/vaccination/index.htm

Centers for Disease Control and Prevention. (2024). *Interim clinical considerations for use of covid-19 vaccines in the United States*. Retrieved November 4, 2023, from https://www.cdc.gov/vaccines/covid-19/clinical-considerations/interim-considerations-us.html#table-01

Corbett, J. A., & Banks, A. D. (2019). *Laboratory tests and diagnostic procedures with nursing diagnoses* (9th ed.). Pearson Education Inc.

Corwin, M. J. (2023). Use of home cardiorespiratory monitors in infants. *UpToDate*. Retrieved March 11, 2024, from https://www.uptodate.com/contents/use-of-home-cardiorespiratory-monitors-in-infants

Covar, R. A., Fleisher, M., Cho, C., & Boguniewicz, M. (2022). Allergic disorders. In M. Bunik, W. W. Hay, M. J. Levin, & M. J. Abzug (Eds.), *Current diagnosis and treatment: Pediatrics* (26th ed.). McGraw-Hill Education.

Cystic Fibrosis Foundation. (n.d.). *Intro to CF*. https://www.cff.org/What-is-CF/

Durani, Y. (2023). *Preventing choking*. https://kidshealth.org/en/parents/safety-choking.html

Gerald, L. B., & Carr, T. (2022). Patient education: How to use a peak flow meter (beyond the basics). *UpToDate*. Retrieved March 11, 2024, from https://www.uptodate.com/contents/how-to-use-a-peak-flow-meter-beyond-the-basics

Giddens, J. F. (2021). *Concepts for nursing practice* (3rd ed.). Elsevier.

Harris, K., Kneale, D., Lasserson, T., McDonald, V. M., Grigg, J., & Thomas, J. (2019). School-based self-management interventions for asthma in children and adolescents: A mixed methods systematic review. *Cochrane Database of Systematic Reviews*. https://doi.org//10.1002/14651858.CD011651.pub2

Hill-Rom, Inc. (2021). *Comparison guide*. https://respiratorycare.hill-rom.com/en/patients/comparison/

Houin, P., Stillwell, P., Deboer, E. M., & Hoppe, J. (2022). Respiratory tract & mediastinum. In M. Bunik, W. W. Hay, M. J. Levin, & M. J. Abzug (Eds.), *Current diagnosis and treatment: Pediatrics* (26th ed.). McGraw-Hill Education.

Janahi, I. A. (2024). Spontaneous pneumothorax in children. *UpToDate*. Retrieved March 11, 2024, from https://www.uptodate.com/contents/spontaneous-pneumothorax-in-children

Katkin, J. P. (2023). Cystic fibrosis: Clinical manifestations and diagnosis. *UpToDate*. Retrieved March 11, 2024, from https://www.uptodate.com/contents/cystic-fibrosis-clinical-manifestations-and-diagnosis

Kimberlin, D. W., Barnett, E. D., Lynfield, R., & Sawyer, M. H. (Eds.). (2021). *Red book 2021-2024: Report of the committee on infectious diseases* (32nd ed.). American Academy of Pediatrics.

Lack, S. Brown, R., & Kinser, P. A. (2020). An integrative review of yoga and mindfulness-based approaches for children and adolescents with asthma. *Journal of Pediatric Nursing, 52*, 76–91. https://doi.org/10.106/j.pedn.2020.03.006

Markowitz, A., & Rough, J. (2024). *List of coronavirus-related restrictions in every state*. https://www.aarp.org/politics-society/government-elections/info-2020/coronavirus-state-restrictions.html#Florida

Medtronic. (2024). *Pulse oximetry*. https://www.medtronic.com/covidien/en-us/products/pulse-oximetry.html

Moon, R. Y., Carlin, R. F., Hand, I., Task Force on Sudden Infant Death Syndrome, & The Committee on Fetus and Newborn. (2022). Sleep-related infant deaths: Updated 2022 recommendations for reducing infant deaths in the sleep environment. *Pediatrics, 150*(1), e2022057990. https://doi.org/10.1542/peds.2022-057990

Moore, K. L., Persaud, T. V. N., & Torchia, M. G. (2020). *The developing human: Clinically oriented embryology* (11th ed.). Elsevier.

Munoz, F. M., & Edwards, M. S. (2023). Seasonal influenza in children: Clinical features and diagnosis. *UpToDate*. Retrieved March 11, 2024, from https://www.uptodate.com/contents/seasonal-influenza-in-children-clinical-features-and-diagnosis

Nagler, J. (2022). Emergency airway management in children: Unique pediatric considerations. *UpToDate*. Retrieved March 11, 2024, from https://www.uptodate.com/contents/emergency-airway-management-in-children-unique-pediatric-considerations

Piedra, P. A. (2023). Bronchiolitis in infants and children: Clinical features and diagnosis. *UpToDate*. Retrieved March 11, 2024, from https://www.uptodate.com/contents/bronchiolitis-in-infants-and-children-clinical-features-and-diagnosis

Purohit, P., Steele, D. W., Cantwell, G. P., & Huang, L. H. (2023). Pediatric acute respiratory distress syndrome. *Medscape*. Retrieved March 11, 2024, from https://emedicine.medscape.com/article/803573-overview#a7

Rabinowicz, S., Leshem, E., & Pessach, I. M. (2020). COVID-19 in the pediatric population – review and current evidence. *Current Infectious Disease Reports, 22*, article number: 29. https://doi.org/10.1007/s11908-020-00739-6

Schare, R. S. (2021). *Croup*. https://kidshealth.org/en/parents/croup.html

Simon, R. H. (2023). Cystic fibrosis: Treatment with CFTR modulators. *UpToDate*. Retrieved March 11, 2024, from https://www.uptodate.com/contents/cystic-fibrosis-treatment-with-cftr-modulators

Smith, D. (2022). The newborn infant. In M. Bunik, W. W. Hay, M. J. Levin, & M. J. Abzug (Eds.), *Current diagnosis and treatment: Pediatrics* (26th ed.). McGraw-Hill Education.

Smith, S. (2022). Management of lower respiratory disorders. In T. Kyle (Ed.), *Primary care pediatrics for the nurse practitioner: A practical approach*. Springer.

Sonney, J., Segrin, C., & Kolstad, T. (2019). Parent- and child-reported asthma responsibility in school-age children: Examining agreement, disagreement, and family functioning. *Journal of Pediatric Health Care, 33*, 386–393. https://doi.org/10.1016/jpedhc.2018.11.005

Stanford Children's Health. (2024). *Reye syndrome in children*. https://www.stanfordchildrens.org/en/topic/default?id=reye-syndrome-in-children-90-P02620

UpToDate, Inc. (2024). *Lexi-comp®* (Version 8.1.2) [Mobile app]. Wolters Kluwer Health. https://apps.apple.com/us/app/lexicomp/id313401238

U.S. Food and Drug Administration. (2023). *Should you give kids medicine for coughs and colds?* https://www.fda.gov/consumers/consumer-updates/should-you-give-kids-medicine-coughs-and-colds

Volkman, K. K., & Chiu, A. M. (2023). Allergy. In K. J. Marcdante, & R. M. Kliegman (Eds.), *Nelson's essentials of pediatrics* (9th ed.). Elsevier.

Weiner, D. L. (2022). Acute respiratory distress in children: Emergency evaluation and initial stabilization. *UpToDate*. Retrieved November 4, 2023, from https://www.uptodate.com/contents/acute-respiratory-distress-in-children-emergency-evaluation-and-initial-stabilization

Wolters Kluwer Health. (2023). *Lippincott nursing procedures* (9th ed.). Author.

Woods, C. R. (2023). Croup: Clinical features, evaluation, and diagnosis. *UpToDate*. Retrieved March 11, 2024, from https://www.uptodate.com/contents/croup-clinical-features-evaluation-and-diagnosis

World Health Organization. (2021). *New brief outlines devastating harms from tobacco use and exposure to second-hand tobacco smoke during pregnancy and throughout childhood—Report calls for protective policies.* https://www.who.int/news/item/16-03-2021-new-brief-outlines-devastating-harms-from-tobacco-use-and-exposure-to-second-hand-tobacco-smoke-during-pregnancy-and-throughout-childhood

Yoon, P. J., Scholes, M. A., & Herrmann, B. W. (2022). Ear, nose, & throat. In M. Bunik, W. W. Hay, M. J. Levin, & Abzug, M. J. (Eds.), *Current diagnosis & treatment: Pediatrics* (26th ed.). McGraw-Hill Education.

Zachariah, P. (2022). COVID-19 in children. *Infectious Disease Clinics of North America, 36*(1), 1–14. https://doi.org/10.1016/j.idc.2021.11.002

DEVELOPING CLINICAL JUDGMENT

PRACTICING FOR NCLEX

1. A 5-month-old infant with RSV bronchiolitis is in respiratory distress. The infant has copious secretions, increased work of breathing, cyanosis, and a respiratory rate of 78. What is the most appropriate initial nursing intervention?
   a. Attempt to calm the infant by placing them in the parent's lap and offering them a bottle.
   b. Alert the primary provider or nurse practitioner to the situation, and ask for an order for a stat chest radiograph.
   c. Suction secretions, provide 100% oxygen via mask, and anticipate respiratory failure.
   d. Bring the emergency equipment to the room and begin bag-valve-mask ventilation.

2. A toddler has moderate respiratory distress, is mildly cyanotic, and has increased work of breathing, with a respiratory rate of 40. What is the priority nursing intervention?
   a. Airway maintenance and 100% oxygen by mask
   b. 100% oxygen and pulse oximetry monitoring
   c. Airway maintenance and continued reassessment
   d. 100% oxygen and provision of comfort

3. The nurse is caring for a child with cystic fibrosis who receives pancreatic enzymes. Which statement by the child's parent indicates an understanding of how to administer the supplemental enzymes?
   a. "I will stop the enzymes if my child is receiving antibiotics."
   b. "I will decrease the dose by half if my child is having frequent, bulky stools."
   c. "Between meals is the best time for me to give the enzymes."
   d. "The enzymes should be given at the beginning of each meal and snack."

4. Which of these factors contributes to infants' and children's increased risk for upper airway obstruction as compared with adults?
   a. Underdeveloped cricoid cartilage and narrow nasal passages
   b. Small tonsils and narrow nasal passages
   c. Cylinder-shaped larynx and underdeveloped sinuses
   d. Underdeveloped cricoid cartilage and smaller tongue

5. The school nurse is presented with a child whose nose began bleeding a few moments ago. Which is the appropriate nursing intervention?
   a. Have the child lie down and breathe through the mouth; then apply pressure to the bridge of the nose.
   b. Have the child lie down and breathe through the mouth; then pinch the lower third of the nose closed.
   c. Instruct the child to sit up and lean forward; then apply pressure to the bridge of the nose.
   d. Instruct the child to sit up and lean forward; then pinch the lower third of the nose closed.

6. The nurse is caring for a toddler who was admitted for observation because of respiratory changes. The parent states the child doesn't want to eat and seems tired.

NURSE'S NOTES

Time	Notes
1200	Alert, fearful of RN, resists examination. Color pink. Skin warm, dry, intact. Heart rate regular without murmur. Minimal intercostal retractions. Harsh cough.
1400	Parent called RN to room as toddler is restless. Does not resist examination. Color pink. Skin warm, diaphoretic. Heart rate regular with murmur. Moderate intercostal retractions, with mild nasal flaring. Harsh cough.

VITAL SIGNS

Time	Temperature	Pulse	Respiratory Rate	Blood Pressure
1200	37.4°C (99.4°F)	100 (beats per minute)	28 (breaths per minute)	118/70
1400	37.2°C (99.0°F)	110 (beats per minute)	34 (breaths per minute)	Not taken

Which assessment findings indicate the toddler is progressing to respiratory distress? Select all that apply.
   a. Cough
   b. Diaphoresis
   c. Heart rate
   d. Malaise
   e. Nasal flaring
   f. Respiratory rate
   g. Restlessness
   h. Retractions

1. A young infant has been diagnosed with bronchiolitis in the clinic. The infant will be cared for at home. What should the nurse include when teaching the parent about home care? Select all that apply.
   a. Offer small amounts of fluids frequently.
   b. Use the nebulizer machine as instructed.
   c. Allow the infant to sleep prone for comfort.
   d. Call the clinic if the infant vomits.
   e. Perform chest physiotherapy every 4 hours.
   f. Watch for difficulty breathing.

DOSAGE CALCULATION QUESTION

1. The nurse is caring for a child with acute asthma. The child weighs 37½ lb. The medication order reads: methylprednisolone 20 mg IV twice a day. The Pediatric Dosage Handbook provides a recommended dose for acute asthma of 1 to 2 mg/kg/day in two divided doses. Is the ordered dose safe?

CRITICAL THINKING EXERCISES

1. A 10-month-old infant is admitted to the pediatric unit with a history of recurrent pneumonia and failure to thrive. The sweat chloride test confirms the diagnosis of cystic fibrosis. The infant is frail in appearance with thin extremities and a slightly protuberant abdomen. The infant is tachypneic, has retractions, and coughs frequently. Based on the limited information given here and your knowledge of cystic fibrosis, choose three of the following categories as priorities to focus on when planning the infant's care:
   a. Prevention of bronchospasm
   b. Promotion of adequate nutrition
   c. Education of the child and family
   d. Prevention of pulmonary infection
   e. Balancing fluid and electrolytes
   f. Management of excess weight gain
   g. Prevention of spread of infection
   h. Promoting adequate sleep and rest
2. A child with asthma is admitted to the pediatric unit for the fourth time this year. The parent expresses frustration that the child is getting sick so often. Besides information about onset of symptoms and events leading up to this present episode, what other types of information would you ask for while obtaining the history?
3. The parent of the child in the previous question tells you that they smoke (but never around the child), the family has a cat that comes inside sometimes, and they always give the child the medication prescribed. The parent gives salmeterol and budesonide as soon as they start to cough. When the child is not having an episode, the parent gives them albuterol before baseball games. Diphenhydramine helps the runny nose in the springtime. Based on this new information, what advice/instructions would you give the parent?
4. A 7-year-old presents with a history of recurrent nasal discharge. The child sneezes every time they visit their cousins, who have pets. The child lives in an older home that is carpeted. Tobacco smokers live in the home. The parent reports that the child snores and is a mouth breather. They say the child has symptoms nearly year-round but that they are worse in the fall and the spring. The parent reports that diphenhydramine is somewhat helpful with the symptoms, but they do not like to give it to them on school days because it makes them drowsy. Based on the foregoing history, develop a teaching plan for this child.
5. The nurse is caring for a 4-year-old child who returned from the recovery room after a tonsillectomy 3 hours ago. The child has cried off and on over the past 2 hours and is now sleeping. What areas should the nurse assess and focus on for this child?

STUDY ACTIVITIES

1. While caring for children in the pediatric setting, compare the signs and symptoms of a child with asthma to those of an infant with bronchiolitis. What are the most notable differences? How does the history of the two children differ?
2. A child with asthma has been prescribed Advair (fluticasone and salmeterol), albuterol, and prednisone. Develop a sample teaching plan for the child and family. Include appropriate use of the devices used to deliver the medications, as well as important information about the medications (uses and adverse effects).
3. While caring for children in the pediatric setting, compare the signs and symptoms and presentation of a child with the common cold to those of a child with either sinusitis or allergic rhinitis.
4. While caring for children in the pediatric setting, review the census of children and identify those at risk for severe influenza and thus those who would benefit from annual influenza vaccination.
5. Compare the differences in oxygen administration between a young infant and an older child.

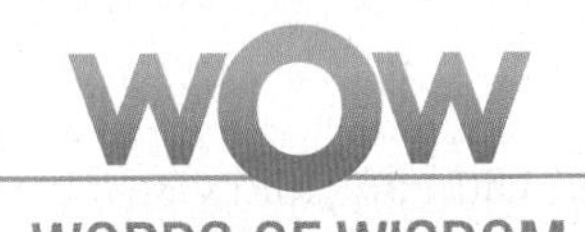

WORDS OF WISDOM

The heart of the matter is healing the child's heart so they can embrace life to its fullest.

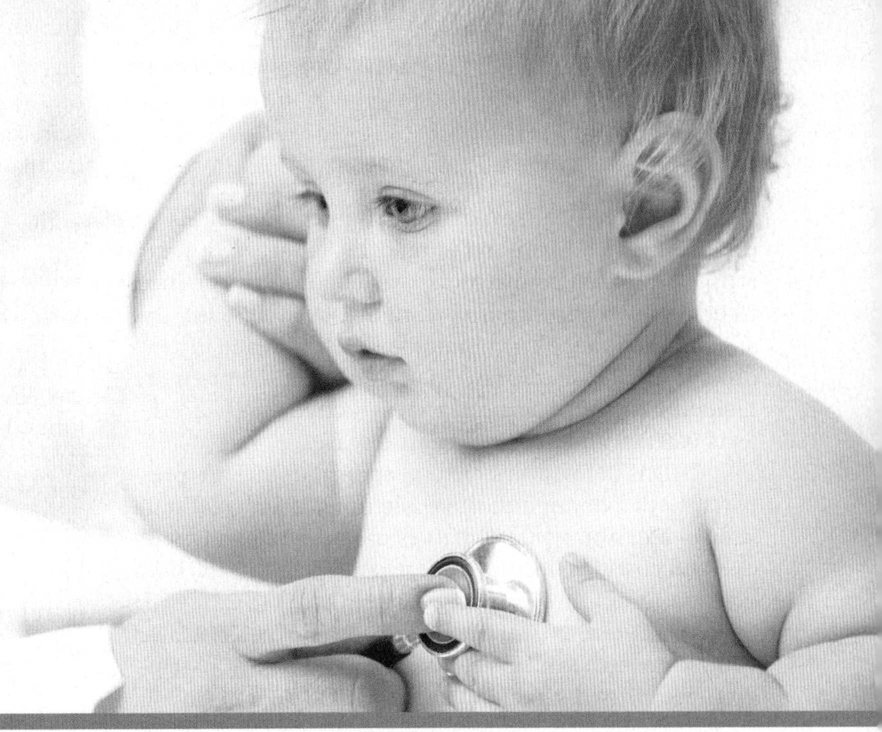

41

Nursing Care of the Child With an Alteration in Perfusion/Cardiovascular Disorder

LEARNING OBJECTIVES

Upon completion of the chapter, you will be able to:

1. Compare anatomy and physiology of the cardiovascular system in infants and children with that of adults.
2. Describe nursing care related to common laboratory and diagnostic tests used in the medical diagnosis of pediatric cardiovascular conditions.
3. Distinguish cardiovascular disorders common in infants, children, and adolescents.
4. Identify appropriate nursing assessments and interventions related to medications and treatments for pediatric cardiovascular disorders.
5. Develop an individualized nursing care plan or concept map for the child with a cardiovascular disorder.
6. Describe the psychosocial impact of chronic cardiovascular disorders on children.
7. Devise a nutrition plan for the child with cardiovascular disease.
8. Develop child and family teaching plans for the child with a cardiovascular disorder.

KEY TERMS

arrhythmia
cardiomegaly (kahr′dē-ō-meg′ă-lē)
clubbing
echocardiography
electrocardiogram
heart failure
orthotopic (ōr′thō-tō′pik)
polycythemia (pol′ē-sī-thē′mē-ă)

Logan Bernstein, 6 weeks old, is brought to the clinic by his parent. He presents with poor feeding. His parent states, "Logan falls asleep while feeding, and he's always sweaty during feedings."

INTRODUCTION

Perfusion refers to the mechanisms that facilitate blood through tissue. Nurses may encounter alterations in perfusion in children and should be familiar with various cardiovascular disorders that children experience. Alterations in perfusion, or cardiovascular disease, are a significant cause of chronic illness and death in children. Typically, cardiovascular disorders in children are divided into two major categories—congenital heart defects (CHDs) and acquired heart disease.

CHD is defined as structural anomalies that are present at birth, although they are often not diagnosed until later in life. About 40,000 babies are born annually with CHD, accounting for the largest percentage of all birth defects (American Heart Association [AHA], 2022). CHD may result from a genetic abnormality or be associated with a genetic syndrome. About 40% to 50% of children with Down syndrome have a CHD (Nees & Chung, 2020). Many CHDs result in **heart failure** (inability of the heart to pump blood sufficiently) and chronic cyanosis, leading to failure to thrive.

Acquired heart disease includes disorders that occur after birth. These disorders develop from a wide range of causes, or they can occur as a complication or long-term effect of CHD.

The diagnosis of a cardiovascular disorder in any person can be extremely frightening and overwhelming. Early on, children learn that the heart is necessary for life, so knowing that there is a heart problem can promote feelings of dread. These feelings are compounded by the child's age, the view of the child as being vulnerable and defenseless, and the stressors associated with the disorder itself. The child and parents need much support and reassurance (Gaskin & Kennedy, 2019).

Nurses need to have a sound knowledge base about cardiovascular conditions affecting children so that they can provide appropriate assessment, intervention, guidance, and support to the child and family. Cardiovascular disorders require acute interventions that often have long-term implications for the child's health and growth and development. Due to the potentially overwhelming and devastating effects that cardiovascular disorders can have on children and their families, nurses need to be skilled in assessment and interventions in this area and able to provide support throughout the course of the illness and beyond.

VARIATIONS IN PEDIATRIC ANATOMY AND PHYSIOLOGY

The cardiovascular system undergoes numerous changes at birth. Structures that were vital to the fetus are no longer needed. Circulation via the umbilical arteries and vein is replaced with the child's own closed independent circulation. Changes in the size of the heart, pulse rate, and blood pressure (BP) also occur.

Circulatory Changes From Gestation to Birth

The fetal heart rate is present on about postconceptual day 17. The four chambers of the heart and arteries are formed during gestational weeks 2 through 8, with maturation of the structures occurring throughout the remainder of gestation. During fetal development, oxygenation of the fetus occurs via the placenta; the lungs, although perfused, do not perform oxygenation and ventilation. The foramen ovale, an opening between the atria, allows blood flow from the right to the left atrium. The ductus arteriosus allows blood flow between the pulmonary artery and the aorta, shunting blood away from the pulmonary circulation (Cunningham et al., 2022). Figure 41.1 illustrates fetal circulation.

With the newborn's first breath, several changes occur in the cardiopulmonary system that enable the newborn to make the transition from fetal circulation to normal circulation. As the newborn breathes for the first time, the lungs inflate, reducing pulmonary vascular resistance to blood flow. As a result, pulmonary artery pressure drops. Subsequently, pressure in the right atrium decreases. Blood flow to the left side of the heart increases the pressure in the left atrium. This change in pressure leads to closure of the foramen ovale. The drop in pressure of the pulmonary artery promotes closure of the ductus arteriosus, which is located between the aorta and the pulmonary artery. The ductus venosus, located between the left umbilical vein and the inferior vena cava, closes because of a lack of blood flow and vasoconstriction. The closed ductus arteriosus and ductus venosus eventually become ligaments. With the lack of blood flow to the umbilical arteries and vein, these structures atrophy (Cunningham et al., 2022).

Structural and Functional Differences

The structure and function of the infant's and child's cardiovascular system differ from those of adults, depending on age. In infants and children younger than 7 years, the heart lies more horizontally, resulting in the apex lying higher in the chest, below the fourth intercostal space. As the lungs grow over time, the heart is displaced downward. Between ages 1 and 6 years, the heart is four times the birth size. Between 6 and 12 years of age, the child's heart is 10 times the size it was at birth. However, the heart is smaller proportionally at this time than at any other stage in life. During the school-age years, the heart

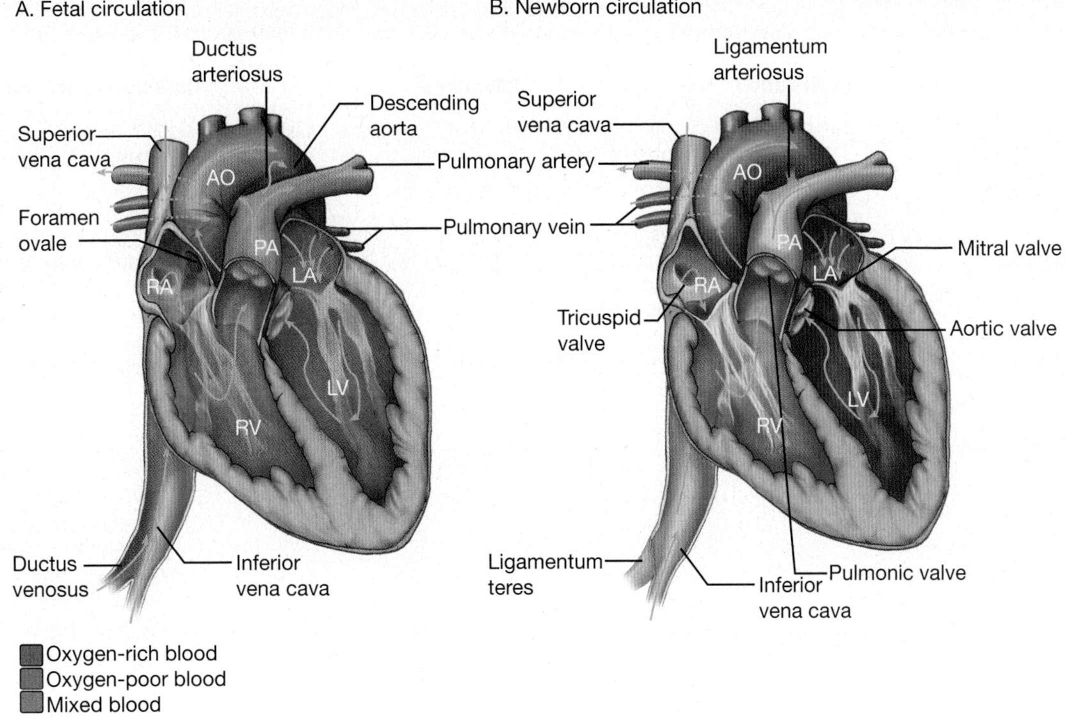

FIGURE 41.1 Fetal and newborn circulation.

grows more vertically within the thoracic cavity. During adolescence, the heart continues to grow in relation to the adolescent's rapid growth.

At birth, the ventricle walls are similar in thickness, but with time the left ventricular wall thickens. The immature myocytes of the infant's heart are thinner and less compliant than those of the adult. Right ventricular function dominates at birth, and over the first few months of life, left ventricular function becomes dominant. The infant's heart at rest exhibits a greater resting tension than the adult's, so volume loading or increased stretch may actually lead to decreased cardiac output. The infant's sarcoplasmic reticulum is less well organized than the adult's, making the infant dependent on serum calcium for contraction. Inotropic response to calcium in the actin and myosin (contractile proteins) increases with age.

The normal heart rate is higher in infancy than in adulthood, limiting the infant's ability to increase cardiac output by increasing the heart rate. The heart's efficiency increases as the child ages and the heart rate drops over time. The normal infant heart rate ranges from 90 to 160 beats per minute (bpm), the toddler's or preschooler's is 80 to 115 bpm, and the school-age child's and the adolescent's ranges from 60 to 100 bpm. Innocent murmurs and physiologic splitting of heart sounds may be noted in infancy or childhood. These findings are related to the change in the size of the heart in relation to the thoracic cavity. The infant's and child's blood vessels widen and increase in length over time. The average infant's BP is about 80/55 mm Hg; BP is usually lower in the younger infant and can be slightly higher in the older infant. The BP increases over time to the adult level. The toddler or preschooler's BP averages 90 to 110/55 to 75 mm Hg, the school-age child's 100 to 120/60 to 75 mm Hg, and the adolescent's 100 to 120/70 to 80 mm Hg (Kleinman et al., 2021).

COMMON MEDICAL TREATMENTS

A variety of medications as well as other medical treatments and surgical procedures are used to treat cardiovascular problems in children. Most of these treatments will require a health care provider's order when the child is in the hospital. The most common treatments and medications are listed in Common Medical Treatments 41.1 and Drug Guide 41.1. The nurse caring for the child with a cardiovascular disorder should be familiar with what the procedures and medications are and how they work as well as common nursing implications related to use of these modalities.

TAKE NOTE!

Give digoxin at regular intervals, every 12 hours, such as at 8 a.m. and 8 p.m., 1 hour before or 2 hours after a feeding. If a digoxin dose is missed, give the dose as soon as it is realized the dose was missed. If it is close to the next dose's time, hold the missed dose. Monitor potassium levels, as a decrease enhances the effects of digitalis, causing toxicity (UpToDate, Inc., 2024).

COMMON MEDICAL TREATMENTS 41.1

Treatment	Explanation	Indications	Nursing Implications
Oxygen	Supplemented via mask, nasal cannula, hood, tent, or endotracheal/nasotracheal tube	Hypoxemia, respiratory distress, heart failure	Monitor response via work of breathing and pulse oximetry.
Chest physiotherapy (CPT) and postural drainage	Promotes mucus clearance by mobilizing secretions with the assistance of percussion or vibration accompanied by postural drainage (refer to Chapter 40 for additional information related to CPT and postural drainage)	Mobilization of secretions, particularly in postoperative period or with heart failure	May be performed by respiratory therapist in some institutions, by nurses in others; in either case, nurses must be familiar with the technique and able to educate families on its use.
Chest tube	Drainage tube is inserted into the pleural cavity to facilitate removal of air or fluid and allow full lung expansion.	After open heart surgery, pneumothorax	If tube becomes dislodged from container, the chest tube must be clamped immediately to avoid further air entry into the chest cavity. Alternatively, the end may be immediately placed into a container of sterile water or saline to create a water seal.
Pacing	External wiring connected to a small generator used to electrophysiologically correct cardiac arrhythmias or heart block (temporary).Permanent pacing achieved with an implantable internal pacemaker.	Bradyarrhythmias, heart block, cardiomyopathy, sinoatrial or atrioventricular node malfunction	Provide close observation of the child, pacing unit, and ECG. Maintain asepsis at pacing lead insertion site. Explain to the child and family that the permanent pacemaker may be felt under the skin. Advise against participation in contact sports.[a]

ECG, electrocardiogram

[a]Children's Hospital of Wisconsin. (2024). *Living with a pediatric pacemaker.* https://childrenswi.org/medical-care/herma-heart/conditions/living-with-a-pacemaker

DRUG GUIDE 41.1

Medication	Actions/Indications	Nursing Implications
Alprostadil (prostaglandin)	Direct vasodilation of the ductus arteriosus smooth muscle Indicated for temporary maintenance of ductus arteriosus patency in infants with ductal-dependent congenital heart defects	• Apnea occurs in 10%–20% of neonates within first hour of infusion. • Monitor arterial BP, respiratory rate, heart rate, ECG, temperature, and pO2; watch for abdominal distention. • Fresh IV solution required every 24 hours. • Reposition catheter if facial or arm flushing occurs. • Use with caution in neonate with bleeding tendency. • Contraindicated in respiratory distress syndrome or persistent fetal circulation
Digoxin (cardiac glycoside, antiarrhythmic agent)	Increases contractility of the heart muscle by decreasing conduction and increasing force Used for heart failure, atrial fibrillation, atrial flutter, supraventricular tachycardia	• Prior to administering each dose, count apical pulse for one full minute, noting rate, rhythm, and quality. Withhold if apical pulse is <60 in an adolescent, <90 in an infant. • Avoid giving oral form with meals, as altered absorption may occur. • Monitor serum digoxin levels (therapeutic range: 0.8–2 ng/mL). • Note signs of toxicity: nausea, vomiting, diarrhea, lethargy, and bradycardia. • Ginseng, hawthorn, and licorice intake increase risk of drug toxicity. • Note contraindications (ventricular fibrillation and hypersensitivity to digitalis). • Avoid rapid IV administration, as this may lead to systemic and coronary artery vasoconstriction.

DRUG GUIDE 41.1

Medication	Actions/Indications	Nursing Implications
Furosemide (loop diuretic)	Inhibits resorption of sodium and chloride Used to manage edema associated with heart failure, and hypertension in combination with antihypertensives	• Administer with food or milk to decrease GI upset. • Monitor BP, kidney function, electrolytes (particularly potassium), and hearing. • May cause photosensitivity
Heparin (anticoagulant)	Interferes with conversion of prothrombin to thrombin, preventing clot formation Indicated for the prophylaxis and treatment of thromboembolic disorders, especially after cardiac surgery	• Administer SQ, not IM. • Dose is adjusted according to coagulation test results. • Monitor for signs of bleeding, platelet counts. • Ensure that the antidote, protamine sulfate, is available. • Do not administer with uncontrolled bleeding or if subacute bacterial endocarditis is suspected.
Indomethacin (nonsteroidal antiinflammatory agent)	Inhibits prostaglandin synthesis in order to close patent ductus arteriosus	• Monitor heart rate, BP, ECG, and urine output; monitor for murmur. • Monitor serum sodium, glucose, platelet count, BUN, creatinine, potassium, and liver enzymes. • May mask signs of infection • Note development of edema.
Spironolactone (potassium-sparing diuretic)	Competes with aldosterone to result in increased water and sodium excretion (spares potassium) Used to manage edema due to heart failure and for treatment of hypertension	• Administer with food. • Monitor serum potassium, sodium, and kidney function. • May cause drowsiness, headache, and arrhythmia • May cause false elevations in digitalis level • Teach children to avoid high-potassium diets, salt substitutes, and natural licorice. • Contraindicated in hyperkalemia, kidney failure, and anuria
Antibiotics		
Penicillin G benzathine Penicillin V potassium	Inhibits bacterial wall synthesis in susceptible organisms. Indicated in mild to moderate infections, for prophylaxis of endocarditis and rheumatic fever	• Contraindications include hypersensitivity to penicillins. • Report hypersensitivity reactions (chills, fever, wheezing, pruritus, anaphylaxis) immediately. • PCN-G: administer IM. • Pen-VK: administer orally on empty stomach 1 hour before or 2 hours after a meal.
Erythromycin (macrolide)	Inhibits ribonucleic acid transcription in susceptible organisms. Used in children with penicillin allergy, mild to moderate infections, or endocarditis, and for rheumatic fever prophylaxis	• Contraindicated in preexisting liver disease • IV administration may result in CV abnormalities. • Abdominal distress common with oral use. • Fever, dizziness, and rash may occur.
Antihypertensive Drugs		
Angiotensin-converting enzyme (ACE) inhibitors (captopril, enalapril)	Competitive inhibition of ACE for management of hypertension Heart failure management in conjunction with digitalis and diuretics	• Monitor BP, kidney function, WBC count, and serum potassium. • Discontinue if angioedema occurs. • Captopril: administer orally on empty stomach 1 hour before or 2 hours after meals. • Enalapril: may administer orally without regard to food
Beta-adrenergic blockers (propranolol, atenolol, sotalol)	Competitively block response to beta-adrenergic stimulation, decreasing heart rate, and force of contraction. Used for management of hypertension, arrhythmias, and prevention of myocardial infarction	• Monitor ECG and BP. • Propranolol: administer with food. • Atenolol, sotalol: administer without regard to food. Do not stop drug abruptly. • May result in bradycardia, dizziness, nausea and vomiting, dyspnea, and hypoglycemia (propranolol) • Contraindications: heart block, uncompensated heart failure, cardiogenic shock, asthma, or hypersensitivity
Hydralazine (vasodilator)	Direct vasodilation of arterioles to manage moderate to severe hypertension, heart failure	• Monitor heart rate and BP. • Closely monitor BP with IV use. • Administer oral dose with food. • May cause palpitations, flushing, tachycardia, dizziness, nausea, and vomiting • Notify health care provider or nurse practitioner if flu-like symptoms occur. • Contraindicated in rheumatic valvular disease

BP, blood pressure; BUN, blood urea nitrogen; CV, cardiovascular; ECG, electrocardiogram; GI, gastrointestinal; IM, intramuscularly; IV, intravenous; pO2, partial pressure of oxygen; SQ, subcutaneously; WBC, white blood cell.

Source: UpToDate, Inc. (2024). *UpToDate® Lexidrug™* (Version 8.2.0) [Mobile app]. Wolters Kluwer. https://apps.apple.com/us/app/lexicomp/id313401238

COMMON LABORATORY AND DIAGNOSTIC TESTS 41.1

Test	Explanation	Indications	Nursing Implications
Arteriogram (angiogram: visualization of arteries or veins)	Radiopaque contrast solution is injected through a catheter and into the circulation. Radiographs are then taken to visualize the structure of the heart and blood vessels.	To observe blood flow to parts of body and detect lesions; to confirm a diagnosis Catheters can be used to remove plaques.	• Make sure the parent signs a consent form. • Administer premedication as ordered. • Obtain child's weight to determine amount of dye needed. • Keep the child NPO before the procedure according to institutional protocol. • After the procedure, maintain the child on bed rest. • Observe the puncture site for bleeding. • Monitor vital signs frequently and check the pulse distal to the site.
Ambulatory electrocardiographic monitoring (Holter)	Monitoring of the heart's electrical patterns for 24 hours using a portable compact unit	To identify and quantify arrhythmias in a 24-hour period during normal daily activities	• Instruct the child and parent to push the "event button" whenever chest pain, syncope, or palpitations occur. • Normal daily activities should be carried out during the testing period. • Having the child wear a snug undershirt over the leads helps to keep them in place.
Chest radiograph	A radiographic film of the chest area; will determine size of the heart and its chambers and pulmonary blood flow	Serves as a baseline for comparison with films taken after surgery; used to identify abnormalities of the lungs, heart, and other structures in the chest	• Instruct child not to wear jewelry or any metal around neck or on the hospital gown. • Explain to the child and family that no pain or discomfort should result. • If a portable radiograph at bedside is done, remove electrodes temporarily.
Echocardiogram	Noninvasive ultrasound procedure used to assess heart wall thickness, size of heart chambers, motion of valves and septa, and relationship of great vessels to other cardiac structures	Specific diagnosis of structural defects; determines hemodynamics and detects valvular defects	• Assure the child that the echo does not hurt. • Instruct the child about ECG lead placement and use of gel on the scope's wand during the procedure. • Encourage the child to lie still throughout the test.
Electrocardiogram (ECG)	A graphic record produced by an electrocardiograph (device used to record the electrical activity of the myocardium to detect transmission of the cardiac impulse through the conductive tissues of the muscle) Facilitates evaluation of the heart rate, rhythm, conduction, and musculature.	To detect heart rhythm and chamber overload; also serves as a baseline for measuring postoperative complications.	• Assure the child that monitoring is a painless procedure. • Place electrodes in the appropriate location. • The child must lie still during the ECG recording period (usually about 5 minutes). • Wipe electrode paste or jelly off after procedure.
Exercise stress test	Monitoring of heart rate, blood pressure, ECG, and oxygen consumption at rest and during exercise	Quantifies exercise tolerance; can be used to provoke symptoms or arrhythmias	• Child should be NPO for 4 hours prior to test. • Obtain baseline ECG and vital signs. • Instruct child to verbalize symptoms during testing. • Usually takes about 45 minutes.
Hemoglobin (Hgb) and hematocrit (Hct)	Measures the total amount of hemoglobin in the blood and indirectly measures the red blood cell number and volume.	To detect anemia or polycythemia (may occur with CHD resulting in cyanosis)	• False elevations occur with dehydration. • May be obtained quickly via capillary puncture • Normal values vary with age.
Partial pressure of oxygen (pO2)	Measures the amount of oxygen in the blood.	To determine the presence and degree of hypoxia	• Most accurate result is with arterial specimen (venous and capillary specimens demonstrate lower levels). • Observe child for cyanosis. • Supplement with oxygen per protocol.
Pulse oximetry screening	Noninvasive method of measuring oxygen saturation in the blood	To detect critical congenital heart disease in the newborn	• Take measurements in the right hand and in either foot. Apply the probe correctly and securely, being sure to minimize movement and ambient light interference.

CHD, congenital heart defect; NPO, nothing by mouth

Data from Children's Heart Institute. (2023). *Heart tests? When do* you *need them?* https://www.childrensheartinstitute.org/health-library/health-wise/?DOCHWID=aba5713; Corbett, J. A., & Banks, A. D. (2019). *Laboratory tests and diagnostic procedures with nursing diagnoses* (9th ed.). Pearson Education Inc; Oster, M. (2023). Newborn screening for critical congenital heart disease using pulse oximetry. *UpToDate*. Retrieved March 31, 2023, from https://www.uptodate.com/contents/newborn-screening-for-critical-congenital-heart-disease-using-pulse-oximetry

CARDIAC CATHETERIZATION

Cardiac catheterization is the definitive study for infants and children with cardiac disease. It has become almost a routine diagnostic procedure and may be performed on an outpatient basis. However, it is highly invasive and not without risks, especially in sick infants and children. Indications for cardiac catheterization include:

- Cardiovascular disease, causing cyanosis in infants; these infants need to be catheterized as soon as they are in a reasonably stable condition.
- Severe heart failure or progressive problems such as pulmonary edema
- Questionable anatomic or physiologic abnormalities
- Planned cardiac surgery
- Progressive monitoring related to pulmonary hypertension
- Periodic assessment after repair of a cardiac defect
- Therapeutic interventions such as septostomy or balloon valvotomy

Cardiac catheterization may be categorized as diagnostic or interventional. The type of catheterization performed varies based on the individual needs of the child. The procedure lasts from 2 to 5 hours (UPMC, 2024).

In cardiac catheterization, a radiopaque catheter is inserted into a blood vessel and is then guided through the vessel to the heart with the aid of fluoroscopy. For a right-sided catheterization, the catheter is threaded to the right atrium via a major vein such as the femoral vein. With a left-sided catheterization, the catheter is threaded to the aorta and heart via an artery. Once the tip of the catheter is in the heart, contrast material is injected via the catheter, and radiographic images are taken.

While the catheter is in the heart, several procedures can be performed. The BP, changes in cardiac output or stroke volume, and oxygen saturation in each heart chamber and major blood vessels are recorded. With the injection of contrast material, information is revealed about the heart anatomy, ventricular wall motion and ejection fraction, intracardiac pressures and hemodynamic parameters, cardiac valve function, and structural abnormalities. The movement of the contrast material is filmed so that the details of the cardiac procedure are recorded. Samples of heart tissue to evaluate for infection, muscular dysfunction, or rejection after a transplant may also be obtained (UPMC, 2024).

Clinical Judgment and the Nursing Process

Care of the child with a cardiovascular disorder includes all steps of the nursing process: assessment, nursing analysis, planning, interventions, and evaluation. There are a number of general concepts related to the nursing process that may be applied to any child with a cardiovascular disorder. The nurse should be knowledgeable about the procedures, treatments, and medications as well as familiar with the nursing implications related to these interventions. With an understanding of these concepts, the nurse can individualize the care based on the child's and family's needs.

Assessment

When assessing a child with a cardiovascular disorder, expect to obtain a health history, perform a physical examination, and prepare the child for laboratory and diagnostic testing.

Health History

The health history consists of a history of the present illness, past medical history, and family history. Depending on their age, the child should be included in the health history interview; the child's age will determine the degree of involvement and the terminology used. Table 41.1 gives examples of typical questions that can be used when obtaining the child's health history.

HISTORY OF PRESENT ILLNESS

Elicit the history of the present illness, which addresses when the symptoms started and how they have progressed. Inquire about any treatments and medications used at home. Ask parents about history of orthopnea, dyspnea, easy fatigability, growth delays, squatting, edema, dizziness, and/or frequent occurrences of pneumonia, which can be significant signs of pediatric heart disease. The history of present illness may reveal a history of poor feeding, including fatigue, lethargy, and/or vomiting, or failure to thrive, even with adequate caloric intake. The parents may report diaphoresis, which is often seen in early heart failure. The parent or caregiver may also report delays in gross motor development, cyanosis (possibly reported by the parents as more of a gray color than blue), and tachypnea (indicative of heart failure).

PAST MEDICAL HISTORY

The past medical history includes information about the child and the birthing parent's pregnancy history. Assess the child's past medical history for:

- Problems occurring after birth (history of the child's condition after birth may reveal evidence of an associated congenital malformation or other disorder.)
- Frequent infections
- Chromosomal abnormalities
- Prematurity
- Autoimmune disorders
- Use of medications, such as corticosteroids

Assess the birthing parent's pregnancy, labor, and delivery history. Be sure to include information about the status of the neonate at birth. Also inquire about the birthing parent's use of medications, including illicit

TABLE 41.1 • Examples of Questions for Obtaining a Child's Health History

Questions	Provides Information About
• What types and amounts (dosages) of medications has the child received? What were they used for? • Who prescribed them?	• Possible underlying conditions that may be related to the child's current status • Other healthcare personnel involved in the child's care as well as the parents' health care beliefs and patterns
• Were they effective? Did the child experience any adverse effects?	• How the medications may be affecting the child's health
• To whom does the child go for medical evaluation? How often? Were the visits for regular health check-ups or for situational problems? Were there previous hospitalizations? What for?	• The child's health status and the parents' healthcare knowledge, practices, and beliefs
• Has the child experienced any growth delay? Does the child have any problems with activity and coordination?	• Problems that may result from impaired cardiac output, adequacy of tissue oxygenation, and concomitant disorders associated with heart disease
• Does the child's skin color change when crying? If so, what color do you see?	• Effectiveness of tissue oxygenation. A blue or gray skin color may be due to cyanosis.
• Does the child stop frequently during play to sit or squat?	• The child's exercise tolerance and tissue oxygenation
• Does the child have feeding difficulty? Does the child tire easily or sleep excessively?	• The child's energy expenditure, ability to tolerate activity, and tissue oxygenation
• Does the child frequently develop strep throat?	• The child's risk for developing rheumatic fever and heart disease

Data from Hueckel, R. M. (2019). Pediatric patient with congenital heart disease. *Journal for Nurse Practitioners*, *15*(1), 118–124. https://doi.org/10.1016/j.nurpra.2018.10.017

or over-the-counter drugs and alcohol; exposure to radiation; presence of hypertension; and viral illnesses such as coxsackievirus, cytomegalovirus, influenza, mumps, or rubella. A history of significant problems related to labor and delivery is also important: stress or asphyxia at birth may be related to cardiac dysfunction and pulmonary hypertension in the newborn.

Assess for additional risk factors such as:

- Family history of heart disease or CHD (investigate the history further if heart disease occurred in a first-degree relative)
- Hyperlipidemia
- Diabetes mellitus
- Obesity
- Inactivity
- Stress
- High-cholesterol diet

PHYSICAL EXAMINATION

Physical examination of the child with a cardiovascular condition consists of inspection, palpation, and auscultation. In addition, obtain the child's vital signs and measure the child's height and weight. Plot this information on a standard growth chart to evaluate nutritional status and growth. If the child is younger than 3 years, measure and plot the head circumference also.

INSPECTION

Assess the child's overall appearance. Inspect the color of the skin, noting cyanosis. Inspect the skin for edema. In infants, peripheral edema occurs first in the face, then the presacral region, and then the extremities. Edema of the lower extremities is characteristic of right ventricular heart failure in older children.

CLINICAL REASONING ALERT!

Suspect CHD in the cyanotic newborn who does not improve with oxygen administration (Weiner et al., 2021).

Inspect the fingers and toes for clubbing. Clubbing (which usually does not appear until after 1 year of age) implies chronic hypoxia due to severe CHD. The first sign of **clubbing** is softening of the nail beds, followed by rounding of the fingernails, followed by shininess and thickening of the nail ends (see Fig. 41.5 in Chapter 40). Obtain the child's temperature; fever would suggest infection. Assess respirations, including rate, rhythm, and effort. Note location and severity of retractions if present. Inspect the chest configuration, noting any prominence of the precordial chest wall, which is often seen in infants and children with **cardiomegaly** (abnormal heart enlargement). Note visible pulsations, which may indicate increased heart activity. Also inspect the neck veins for engorgement or abnormal pulsations. Note abdominal distention.

CLINICAL REASONING ALERT!

Children with cardiac conditions resulting in cyanosis will often have baseline oxygen saturations that are relatively low because of the mixing of oxygenated with deoxygenated blood.

PALPATION

Palpate the right and left radial or brachial pulse to assess cardiac rate and rhythm. Throughout infancy and childhood, the rate may vary. Palpate the femoral pulse; it should be readily palpable and equal in amplitude and strength to the brachial or radial pulse. A femoral pulse that is weak or absent in comparison to the brachial pulse is associated with coarctation of the aorta. Significant variations in pulse occur with activity, so the most accurate heart rate may be determined during sleep. In older children, exercise and emotional factors may influence the heart rate. A bounding pulse is characteristic of patent ductus arteriosus (PDA) or aortic regurgitation. Narrow or thready pulses may occur in children with heart failure or severe aortic stenosis (Driscoll, 2022). Note tachycardia, bradycardia, rhythm irregularities, diminished peripheral pulses, or thready pulse. Palpate the child's abdomen for hepatomegaly, a sign of right-sided heart failure in the infant and child.

AUSCULTATION

Auscultate the apical pulse for a full minute to determine heart rate and rhythm. Note irregularities in rhythm, tachycardia, or bradycardia. Auscultate the heart for murmurs. Many children have functional or innocent murmurs, but all murmurs must be evaluated on the basis of the following characteristics:

- Location
- Relation to the heart cycle and duration
- Intensity: grade I, soft and hard to hear; grade II, soft and easily heard; grade III, loud without thrill; grade IV, loud with a precordial thrill; grade V, loud with a precordial thrill, audible with a stethoscope partially off chest; grade VI, very loud, audible with a stethoscope or with the naked ear
- Quality: harsh, musical, or rough; high, medium, or low pitch
- Variation with position (sitting, lying, standing) (Driscoll, 2022)

Auscultate for the character of heart sounds. Note distinct, muffled, or distant heart sounds. Abnormal splitting or intensifying of S_2 sounds occurs in children with major heart problems. Ejection clicks, which are high pitched, are related to problems with dilated vessels and/or valve abnormalities. Heard throughout systole, they can be early, moderate, or late. Clicks on the upper left sternal border are related to the pulmonary area. Aortic clicks are best heard at the apex and can be mitral or aortic in origin. A mild to late ejection click at the apex is typical of a mitral valve prolapse. The S_3 heart sound may be heard in children, diminishing when moving from supine to upright, and a pathologic S_3 may occur with poor cardiac function. The S_4 heart sound is not normally audible and is associated with cardiomyopathy or diastolic dysfunction (Jone et al., 2022).

Auscultate the BP in the upper extremities and lower extremities, and compare the findings; there should be no major differences between the upper and lower extremities. Determine the pulse pressure by subtracting the diastolic pressure from the systolic pressure. The pulse pressure is less than 50 mm Hg, or less than half the systolic pressure. A widened pulse pressure, which is usually accompanied by a bounding pulse, is associated with PDA, aortic insufficiency, fever, anemia, or complete heart block. A narrowed pulse pressure is associated with aortic stenosis. Note hypotension or hypertension.

TAKE NOTE!

Alert children and parents if a heart murmur is detected, even if it is benign.

Laboratory and Diagnostic Testing

Common Laboratory and Diagnostic Tests 41.1 explains the laboratory and diagnostic tests most commonly used when considering cardiovascular disorders in children. The tests can assist the health care provider in diagnosing the disorder or can be used as guidelines in determining ongoing treatment. Laboratory or nonnursing personnel obtain some of the tests, while the nurse might obtain others. In either instance, the nurse should be familiar with how the tests are obtained, what they are used for, and normal versus abnormal results. This knowledge will also be necessary when providing child and family education related to the testing.

Remember Logan, the 6-week-old with poor feeding? What additional health history and physical examination assessment information should the nurse obtain?

Nursing Analysis

After recognizing and analyzing cues from a thorough assessment, the nurse might identify several patient problems, including:

- Decreased cardiac output
- Excess fluid volume
- Activity intolerance
- Imbalanced nutrition, less than body requirements
- Risk of delayed development
- Pain
- Interrupted family processes
- Deficient knowledge

After completing Logan's assessment, the nurse noted the following: poor weight gain, tachypnea with occasional nasal flaring, crackles heard on auscultation, and edema noted in the face, presacral area, and extremities. Based on these assessment findings, what would your top three concerns be for Logan?

The foregoing patient issues provide suggestions for nursing care planning or concept mapping. Suggested interventions with rationales are provided later. Care planning should be individualized, based on the child's and family's needs. Refer to Chapter 36 for the nursing process for pain management and to Chapter 33 for nursing interventions related to interrupted family processes. Additional information will be included later in the chapter as it relates to nursing management of children with specific disorders, as well as particular nursing interventions for deficient knowledge.

• • • ATRAUMATIC CARE • • •

When a child is diagnosed with congenital heart disease, involve the child life specialist early in the course of treatment. The child will likely have been undergoing diagnostic procedures such as electrocardiograms and echocardiograms, as well as open heart surgery. The child life specialist can be very helpful with providing atraumatic care.

Nursing Analysis

Decreased cardiac output related to structural defect, congenital anomaly, or ineffective heart pumping as evidenced by arrhythmias, edema, murmur, abnormal heart rate, or abnormal heart sounds

Goal/Outcome

Child or infant will demonstrate adequate cardiac output as evidenced by elastic skin turgor, brisk capillary refill, demonstrate pink color, pulse, and BP within normal limits for age, regular heart rhythm, adequate urinary output.

Increasing Cardiac Output (interventions with *rationale*)

- Monitor vital signs closely, especially BP and heart rate, *to detect increases or decreases.*
- Monitor cardiac rhythm via cardiac monitor *to detect arrhythmias quickly.*
- Observe for signs of hypoxia such as tachypnea, cyanosis, tachycardia, bradycardia, dizziness, and/or restlessness *to identify this change early.*
- Administer oxygen as needed *to correct hypoxia.*
- Place child in knee-to-chest or squatting position as needed *to increase systemic vascular resistance.*
- Administer antiarrhythmics, vasopressors, angiotensin-converting enzyme (ACE) inhibitors, beta-blockers, corticosteroids, or diuretics as prescribed *to improve cardiac output.*
- Monitor for signs of thrombosis such as restlessness, seizure, coma, oliguria, anuria, edema, hematuria, or paralysis *to identify this condition early.*
- Administer adequate hydration *to decrease possibility of thrombosis formation.*
- Cluster nursing care and other activities *to allow adequate periods of rest.*
- Anticipate child's needs *to decrease the child's stress, thereby decreasing oxygen consumption requirement.*

Nursing Analysis

Excess fluid volume related to compromised regulatory mechanism (ineffective cardiac muscle function) as evidenced by weight gain, edema, jugular vein distention, dyspnea, or adventitious breath sounds

Goal/Outcome

Child will attain appropriate fluid balance, will lose weight (fluid), edema or bloating will decrease, lung sounds will be clear, and heart sounds will be normal.

Encouraging Fluid Loss (interventions with *rationale*)

- Weigh daily on the same scale in a similar amount of clothing; *in children, weight is the best indicator of changes in fluid status.*
- Monitor location and extent of edema (measure abdominal girth daily if ascites is present); *a decrease in edema indicates positive increase in oncotic pressure.*
- Protect edematous areas from skin breakdown; *edema leads to increased risk for alterations in skin integrity.*
- Auscultate lungs carefully *to identify crackles, indicating pulmonary edema.*
- Assess work of breathing and respiratory rate; increased *work of breathing is associated with pulmonary edema.*
- Assess heart sounds for gallop; *the presence of S_3 may indicate fluid overload.*
- Maintain fluid restriction as ordered *to decrease intravascular volume and workload on the heart.*
- Strictly monitor intake and output *to quickly note discrepancies and provide intervention.*
- Provide sodium-restricted diet as ordered; *restricting sodium intake allows better kidney excretion of extra fluid.*
- Administer diuretics as ordered, and monitor for adverse effects *to encourage excretion of fluid and elimination of edema, reduce cardiac filling pressures, and increase kidney blood flow. Adverse effects include electrolyte imbalance as well as orthostatic hypotension.*

Nursing Analysis

Activity intolerance related to imbalanced oxygen supply and demand (ineffective cardiac muscle function, increased energy expenditure) as evidenced by exertional discomfort (squatting position), exertional dyspnea, weakness, or fatigue

Goal/Outcome

Child will increase activity level as tolerated: Child participates in play and activities (specify particular activities and level as individualized for each child).

Promoting Activity (interventions with *rationale*)

- Assess level of fatigue and activity tolerance *to determine baseline for comparison.*

- Note extent of dyspnea, oxygen requirement, or color change with exertion *to provide baseline for comparison.*
- Cluster care activities, allowing rest periods in between, *to conserve child's energy.*
- Work with the parent and child to determine a mutually satisfactory daily schedule *to allow adequate rest and energy conservation.*
- Instruct family and child in prescribed activity restrictions *to prevent fatigue while allowing some activity.*
- In the infant, avoid long periods of crying or prolonged nipple feeding; *these expend excessive calories.*
- Provide neutral thermal environment *to avoid increased oxygen and energy needs associated with excessive heat or cold.*

Nursing Analysis

Imbalanced nutrition (less than body requirements) related to the inability to increase adequate calories (due to increased energy expenditure and fatigue) as evidenced by food intake less than recommended daily allowance, weight loss or length/height and weight below accepted standards

Goal/Outcome

Child will improve nutritional intake, resulting in steady increase in weight and length/height and will feed without tiring easily.

Promoting Adequate Nutrition (interventions with *rationale*)

- Determine body weight and length/height norm for age *to determine a goal to work toward.*
- Assess child for food preferences that fall within dietary restrictions; *the child will be more likely to consume adequate amounts of foods that they like.*
- Weigh the child daily or weekly (according to health care provider order or institutional standard), and measure length/height weekly *to monitor for increased growth.*
- Offer highest-calorie meals at the time of day when the child's appetite is the greatest *to increase likelihood of increased caloric intake.*
- Provide increased-calorie shakes or puddings within diet restriction; *high-calorie foods increase weight gain.*
- Consult with the pediatric dietician *to provide optimal caloric intake within dietary restrictions.*
- Provide small, frequent feedings *to discourage tiring with feeding.*
- Feed infants with special nipple as needed *to decrease amount of energy expended for sucking.*
- Administer vitamin and mineral supplements as prescribed *to attain/maintain vitamin and mineral balance in the body.*

Nursing Analysis

Delayed development risk related to congenital disorder or chronic illness (effects of cardiac disease and necessary treatments, inadequate nutrition, or frequent separation from caregivers secondary to illness)

Goal/Outcome

Child will display development appropriate for age with evidence of cognitive and motor function within normal limits (individualized for each child)

Promoting Appropriate Development (interventions with *rationale*)

- Promote adequate caloric intake *to stimulate growth and provide adequate energy.*
- Provide age-appropriate developmental activities *to stimulate development.*
- Consult with the physical or occupational therapist or child life specialist *to determine activities most appropriate for the child within the constraints of the child's illness.*
- Schedule daily activities to allow for essential rest periods *for energy conservation.*
- Encourage parents, teachers, and playmates to be sensitive to child's self-image, using positive comments *to improve the child's self-concept.*
- As energy allows, encourage participation in all activities as feasible *to allow the child to feel normal.*

Based on your top three issues for Logan, describe appropriate nursing interventions.

Cardiac Catheterization

Nursing management of the child undergoing cardiac catheterization includes preprocedure nursing assessment and preparation of the child and family, postprocedural nursing care, and discharge teaching.

Assessment Before the Procedure

Obtain a thorough history and physical examination to establish a baseline. Measure vital signs. Note fever or other signs and symptoms of infection, which may necessitate rescheduling the procedure. Obtain the child's height and weight to aid in determining medication dosages. Assess the child for any allergies, especially to iodine and shellfish, because some contrast materials contain iodine as a base. Review the child's medications; medications such as anticoagulants are typically withheld for several days or longer prior to the procedure to reduce the child's risk for bleeding. Check the results of any laboratory tests, such as hemoglobin and hematocrit levels.

Perform a complete physical examination. Pay particular attention to assessing the child's peripheral pulses, including pedal pulses. Use an indelible pen to mark the location of the child's pedal pulses so they can be easily assessed after the procedure. Document the location and quality in the child's medical record.

Educating the Child and Family Before the Procedure

Teach the parents and, if age-appropriate, the child, about all aspects of the procedure in order to decrease their anxiety. Let them know the procedure is commonly performed on an outpatient basis but that some health care providers or nurse practitioners require the child to be admitted for an overnight stay for observation. Include information about what the procedure involves, how long it will take, and any special instructions from the health care provider or nurse practitioner. Use a variety of teaching methods as appropriate, such as videos, books, and pamphlets.

Adapt these teaching methods to the child's developmental stage. For example, introduce the younger child to equipment through play therapy. For school-age and older children and their parents, offer a tour of the cardiac catheterization laboratory. Mention sounds and sights they may experience during the procedure. Explain the use of intravenous (IV) fluid therapy, sedation, and, if ordered, anesthesia to the child and parents. Tell the child that they may feel a sensation of the heart racing when the catheter is inserted. Also warn the older child that they may experience a feeling of warmth or stinging when the contrast material is injected. Encourage the child to use familiar ways to relax. If necessary, teach the child simple relaxation measures.

Tell families to withhold food and fluid for 4 to 6 hours before the procedure (as ordered). The parent should administer prescribed medications with a sip of water. On the day of the procedure, check to ensure that a signed informed consent form is on the child's medical record and that all necessary assessment data have been included. Just before the procedure, ask the child to void, and administer a sedative, as ordered. If appropriate and permitted, allow the parents to accompany the child to the catheterization area.

Teach the child and family what to expect after the procedure is completed. Inform the parents of the possible complications that might occur, such as bleeding, low-grade fever, loss of pulse in the extremity used for the catheterization, and development of **arrhythmia** (abnormal heart rhythm). Explain to the child that they will have a dressing over the catheter site and that they will need to keep the leg straight for several hours after the procedure. Teach the child and parent that frequent monitoring will be required after the procedure.

Assessment After the Procedure

Throughout the postprocedure period, closely monitor the child for complications of bleeding, arrhythmia, hematoma, and thrombus formation and infection. Evaluate the child's vital signs, the neurovascular status of the lower extremities, and the pressure dressing over the catheterization site every 15 minutes for the first hour and then every 30 minutes for 1 hour. Vital signs should remain within acceptable parameters. Hypotension may signify hemorrhage due to perforation of the heart muscle or bleeding from the insertion site. Expect to monitor cardiac rhythm and oxygen saturation levels via pulse oximetry for the first few hours after the procedure to help identify possible complications.

Assess the child's distal pulses bilaterally for presence and quality. The pulse of the affected extremity may be slightly less than that of the other extremity in the initial postprocedure period, but it should gradually return to baseline. Also assess the color and temperature of the extremity; pallor or blanching would indicate an obstruction in blood flow. Check capillary refill and sensation to evaluate blood flow to the area.

Nursing Interventions Following Cardiac Catheterization

Maintain bed rest in the immediate postprocedure period. Ensure that the child maintains the extremity in a straight position for approximately 4 to 8 hours, depending on the approach used and the facility's policy. Inspect the pressure dressing frequently. Check to make sure that it is dry and intact, without evidence of bleeding. Reinforce the dressing as necessary and report any evidence of drainage on the dressing. If there is a risk of the dressing becoming soiled or wet, cover it with plastic.

TAKE NOTE!

If bleeding occurs after a cardiac catheterization, apply pressure 1 in above the site to create pressure over the vessel, thereby reducing the blood flow to the area.

Monitor the child's intake and output closely to ensure adequate hydration. The contrast material has a diuretic effect, so assess the child for signs and symptoms of dehydration and hypovolemia. Typically, the child resumes oral intake as tolerated, beginning with sips of clear liquids and progressing to their preprocedure diet. Continue IV fluids as ordered, and encourage oral fluid intake as allowed and ordered to promote elimination of the contrast material. Allow the child to talk about the experience and how and what they felt. Provide positive reinforcement for the child's actions.

Educating About Home Care Following Cardiac Catheterization

Provide child and family education before the child is discharged home (see Teaching Guidelines 41.1). Areas

TEACHING GUIDELINES 41.1 Providing Care After a Cardiac Catheterization

- Change the pressure dressing on the day after the procedure. Apply a dry sterile dressing or adhesive bandage for the next several days. Keep the dressing dry; cover it with plastic if there is a chance that the dressing could become wet or soiled.
- When changing the dressing, inspect the insertion site for redness, irritation, swelling, drainage, and bleeding. Report any of these to the health care provider or nurse practitioner.
- Check the temperature, color, sensation, and pulses on the child's extremities and compare. Report any changes to the health care provider or nurse practitioner.
- Resume the child's usual diet after the procedure; report any nausea or vomiting.
- Check the child's temperature at least once a day for approximately 3 days after the procedure. Report any temperature elevation of 100.4°F or greater.
- Avoid giving the child a tub bath for approximately 3 days after the procedure; use sponge baths or showers instead.
- Discourage strenuous exercise or activity for approximately 3 days after the procedure.
- Watch for changes in the child's appearance, such as changes in skin color, reports of the heart "fluttering" or "skipping a beat," fever, or difficulty breathing.
- Give acetaminophen (Tylenol) or ibuprofen (Motrin) for complaints of pain.
- Schedule a follow-up appointment with the health care provider or nurse practitioner in the time specified.

Based on KidsHealth Medical Experts. (2023). *Cardiac catheterization*. https://kidshealth.org/en/parents/cardiac-catheter.html; UCSF Benioff Children's Hospital. (2024). *Cardiac catheterization*. https://www.ucsfbenioff-childrens.org/education/cardiac_catheterization/

to address include site care, signs and symptoms of complications (especially within 24 hours after the catheterization, such as fever; bleeding or bruising at the catheterization site; or changes in color, temperature, or sensation in the extremity used), diet, and activity level.

THINKING ABOUT DEVELOPMENT

Jeremy Titus is a 2-year-old with congenital heart disease. He is having a cardiac catheterization today. How will the nurse encourage Jeremy to stay in bed and keep his leg straight for several hours following the catheterization? What types of activities would be appropriate for occupying Jeremy while he is confined to bed? How would the nurse's approach differ if Jeremy were an older child?

CONGENITAL HEART DEFECTS

In North America, more than 1% of newborn infants have CHD resulting from numerous causes. The prevalence of CHD ranges from six to 13 per 1,000 live births; premature infants have a higher rate (Altman, 2022). About one third of infants with CHD will have disease serious enough to result in death or will require cardiac catheterization or cardiac surgery within the first year of life. Complications of CHD include heart failure, hypoxemia, growth delay, developmental delay, and pulmonary vascular disease. Children with severe anomalies frequently experience failure to thrive.

With advances in palliative and corrective surgery over the past 60 years, many more children are now able to survive into adulthood. About 90% of children with CHD grow to be adults (Jone et al., 2022). As compared to healthy children, children with CHD tend to have poorer health overall and more frequently have additional morbidities either physical or neurodevelopmental in nature (Centers for Disease Control and Prevention [CDC], 2022). Due to the potential long-term effects that CHD may have on these children, nurses must be expertly equipped to care for them.

Pathophysiology

The exact cause of CHD is unknown. However, the belief is that it results from the interplay of several factors, including genetics (e.g., chromosomal alterations) and exposure during pregnancy to environmental factors (e.g., toxins, infections, chronic illnesses, and alcohol).

CHDs result from some interference in the development of the heart structure during fetal life. Subsequently, the septal walls or valves may fail to develop completely, or vessels or valves may be stenotic, narrowed, or transposed. Structures that formed to allow fetal circulation may fail to close after birth, altering the pressures necessary to maintain adequate blood flow.

After birth, with the change from fetal to newborn circulation, pressures within the chambers of the right side of the heart are less than those of the left side, and pulmonary vascular resistance is less than that for the systemic circulation. These normal pressure gradients are necessary for adequate circulation to the lungs and the rest of the body. However, these pressure gradients become disrupted if a structure has failed to develop, a fetal structure has failed to close, or a narrowing, stenosis, or transposition of a vessel has occurred. For example, blood typically flows from an area of higher pressure to one of lower pressure. If the ductus arteriosus fails to close, blood will move from the aorta to the pulmonary artery, ultimately increasing right atrial pressure. With this shunting of blood, highly oxygenated blood can mix with less oxygenated blood, interfering with the amount available to the tissues via the systemic circulation. Some of the defects may result in significant hypoxemia, the sequelae of which include clubbing, **polycythemia** (excess amount of red blood cells [RBCs]), exercise intolerance, hypercyanotic spells, brain abscess, and cerebrovascular accident (CVA) (Jone et al., 2022; Schneider, 2023).

CHDs are categorized based on hemodynamic characteristics (blood flow patterns in the heart):

- Disorders with decreased pulmonary blood flow: tetralogy of Fallot and tricuspid atresia
- Disorders with increased pulmonary blood flow: PDA, atrial septal defect (ASD), and ventricular septal defect (VSD)
- Obstructive disorders: coarctation of the aorta, aortic stenosis, and pulmonic stenosis
- Mixed disorders: transposition of the great arteries (TGA), total anomalous pulmonary venous return (TAPVR), truncus arteriosus, and hypoplastic left heart syndrome (HLHS)

Therapeutic Management

Prenatal education about avoiding certain substances or preventing infection is essential to promote optimal outcomes for the fetus. Encourage parents of children with CHD to receive genetic counseling because of the probability of having subsequent children with a CHD. Children with small septal defects are urged to lead normal lives and often require no medical intervention. Therapeutic management of other forms of CHDs focuses on palliative care or a surgical corrective approach necessary for most of the defects. In newborns and very young infants with severe cyanosis (tricuspid atresia, TGA), a prostaglandin infusion will maintain patency of the ductus arteriosus, improving pulmonary blood flow. Definitive correction of structural disorders requires surgical intervention. Table 41.2 describes the surgical procedures used for the various CHDs and the relevant nursing measures. Nursing management for the child with CHD will be provided following the disorders section.

Disorders With Decreased Pulmonary Blood Flow

Defects involving decreased pulmonary blood flow occur when there is some obstruction of blood flow to the lungs. As a result of the obstruction, pressure in the right side of the heart increases and becomes greater than that in the left side of the heart. Blood from the higher-pressure right side of the heart then shunts to the lower-pressure left side through a structural defect. Subsequently, deoxygenated blood mixes with oxygenated blood on the left side of the heart. This mixed blood, which is low in oxygen, is pumped via the systemic circulation to the body tissues.

Defects with decreased pulmonary blood flow are characterized by mild to severe oxygen desaturation. Typically, the child exhibits oxygen saturation levels ranging from 50% to 90%, which can produce severe cyanosis. To compensate for low blood oxygen levels, the kidneys produce the hormone erythropoietin to stimulate the bone marrow to produce more RBCs. This increase in RBCs is called polycythemia. Polycythemia can lead to an increase

TABLE 41.2 • Common Surgical Procedures and Nursing Measures for Congenital Heart Defects

Disorder	Surgical Procedure	Nursing Measures
Tetralogy of Fallot	Palliation with systemic-to-pulmonary anastomoses: • Blalock–Taussig shunt: an end-to-side anastomosis (or connection with a small Gore-Tex tube) of the subclavian artery and the pulmonary artery • Waterston shunt: anastomosis of the ascending aorta and the pulmonary artery • Definitive correction involves patch closure of the VSD and repair of the pulmonary valve and right ventricular outflow tract	• Avoid BP measurements and venipunctures in the affected arm after a Blalock–Taussig shunt. Pulse will not be palpable in that arm because of use of the subclavian artery for the shunt. • Monitor for ventricular arrhythmias after corrective repair.
Tricuspid atresia	• Palliation with Blalock–Taussig shunt or pulmonary artery banding may be performed. • At 3–6 months of age, the superior vena cava is detached from the heart and connected to the pulmonary artery (Glenn procedure). • By age 2–5 years, a modified Fontan procedure may be performed. Systemic venous return is redirected to the pulmonary artery directly.	• Monitor for atrial arrhythmias, left ventricular dysfunction, and protein-losing enteropathy. • Some children may eventually require a pacemaker.
Atrial septal defect (ASD)	• If small, the defect may be sutured closed. Larger defects may require a patch of pericardium or synthetic material. • Ostium secundum ASD may be repaired percutaneously via cardiac catheterization with a septal occluder.	• Monitor for atrial arrhythmias (lifelong) after surgical closure. • With the septal occluders, strenuous activity should be avoided for 2 weeks after the procedure.[a]

TABLE 41.2 • Common Surgical Procedures and Nursing Measures for Congenital Heart Defects

Disorder	Surgical Procedure	Nursing Measures
Ventricular septal defect (VSD)	• If surgical closure is required, it should be performed before permanent pulmonary vascular changes develop. • Surgical closure may be in the form of suture closure of the VSD, transcatheter placement of a device in the defect, or Dacron patch closure.	• Monitor for ventricular dysrhythmias or atrioventricular block. • With the clamshell occluding or Amplatzer device, strenuous activity should be avoided for 1 month after the procedure.[b]
Atrioventricular canal defect	• Pulmonary artery banding as palliation in very young infants • Surgical correction by 3–18 months of age • Patch closure of the septal defects and suturing of the valve leaflets or valve reconstruction are performed.	• Monitor for complete heart block postoperatively. • Teach parents that mitral regurgitation is a long-term complication and may require valve replacement.
Patent ductus arteriosus (PDA)	• PDA is closed by coil embolization or device via cardiac catheterization. • May also be surgically ligated	• Monitor for bleeding and laryngeal nerve damage.
Coarctation of the aorta	• Balloon angioplasty via cardiac catheterization is possible in some children. • Most common surgical repair is resection of the narrowed portion of the aorta, followed by end-to-end reanastomosis.	• Preoperatively, administer prostaglandin medications as ordered to relax the ductal tissue. • Postoperatively, measure and compare BP in all four extremities and quality of upper vs. lower pulses.
Aortic stenosis	• Balloon dilation is accomplished via the umbilical artery in the newborn or the femoral artery via cardiac catheterization in the older child.	• Provide routine postcatheterization care. • Teach parents that long-term aortic regurgitation requiring valve replacement may occur.
Pulmonic stenosis	• Balloon dilation valvuloplasty is performed via cardiac catheterization to dilate the valve. This is effective in all but the most severe of cases, which will require surgical valvotomy.	• Provide routine postcatheterization care for balloon dilation. • Explain to parents that prognosis is excellent.
Transposition of the great vessels (arteries)	• Balloon atrial septotomy is usually done as soon as the diagnosis is made. A balloon-tipped catheter is passed through the atrial septum to enlarge the atrial septum. • Surgical correction involves switching the arteries into their normal anatomic positions.	• Administer prostaglandin to maintain the open state of the ductus arteriosus, which will allow the mixing of poorly oxygenated blood with well-oxygenated blood. • Monitor for rapid respirations and cyanosis. • Administer oxygen as needed preoperatively.
Total anomalous pulmonary venous return	• The pulmonary vein is repositioned to the back of the left atrium, and the ASD is closed.	• Monitor for dysrhythmias, heart block, and persistent heart failure.
Truncus arteriosus	• VSD repair, separation of the pulmonary arteries from the aorta, with subsequent connection to the right ventricle with a valve conduit	• Preoperatively, administer prostaglandin infusion to prevent closing of the ductus arteriosus.
Hypoplastic left heart syndrome	• Heart transplantation is the treatment of choice. • Palliative staged treatment. First, Norwood procedure, reconstruction of the aorta and pulmonary arteries, includes a cardiac transplant. Second, bidirectional Glenn procedure, connection of the superior vena cava to the right pulmonary artery to increase the blood flow to the lungs. Third, modified Fontan procedure	• Preoperatively, administer prostaglandin infusion to prevent closing of the ductus arteriosus. • After palliative repairs, monitor for dysrhythmias or worsening ventricular function.
Valve disorders	• The incompetent valve is replaced with valve prosthesis.	• Lifelong anticoagulation therapy is necessary with prosthetic valves. • Monitor prothrombin times. • Monitor heart sounds for alterations.

[a]Cleveland Clinic. (2023). *Cardiac closure devices.* https://my.clevelandclinic.org/health/treatments/16838-cardiac-implant-closure-devices-in-adults
[b]Abbott. (2023). *Amplatzer septal occluder.* https://www.myamplatzer.com/hcp/congenital-heart-defect-solutions/ventricular-septal-defects-vsd/
Based on Jone, P.-N., Kim, J. S., Burkett, D., Jacobsen, R., & VonAlvensleben, J., (2022). Cardiovascular disease. In M. Bunik, W. W. Hay, M. J. Levin, & M. J. Abzug (Eds.), *Current diagnosis and treatment: Pediatrics* (26th ed.). McGraw-Hill Education; Schneider, D. S. (2023). The cardiovascular system. In K. J. Marcdante & R. M. Kliegman (Eds.), *Nelson's essentials of pediatrics* (8th ed.). Elsevier.

in blood volume and possibly blood viscosity, further taxing the workload of the heart. Although the number of RBCs increases, there is no change in the amount of blood that reaches the lungs for oxygenation. Disorders within this classification include tetralogy of Fallot and tricuspid atresia.

Tetralogy of Fallot

Tetralogy of Fallot is a CHD composed of four heart defects: pulmonic stenosis (a narrowing of the pulmonary valve and outflow tract, creating an obstruction of blood flow from the right ventricle to the pulmonary artery); VSD; overriding aorta (enlargement of the aortic valve to the extent that it appears to arise from the right and left ventricles rather than the anatomically correct left ventricle); and right ventricular hypertrophy (the muscle walls of the right ventricle increase in size due to continued overuse as the right ventricle attempts to overcome a high-pressure gradient). Surgical intervention is usually required during the first year of life (Jone et al., 2022; Schneider, 2023).

Pathophysiology

With pulmonic stenosis, the blood flow from the right ventricle is obstructed and slowed, resulting in a decrease in blood flow to the lungs for oxygenation and a decrease in the amount of oxygenated blood returning to the left atrium from the lungs. The obstructed flow also increases the pressure in the right ventricle. This blood, which is poorly oxygenated, is then shunted across the VSD into the left atrium. Poorly oxygenated blood also travels through the overriding aorta (if it extends to both ventricles). In some cases when the VSD is large, the pressure in the right ventricle may be equal to that of the left ventricle. In this case, the path of blood shunting depends on which circulation is exerting the higher pressure, pulmonary or systemic.

Regardless of which way shunting occurs, a mixing of oxygenated and poorly oxygenated blood occurs, with this blood ultimately being pumped into the systemic circulation. The oxygen saturation of the blood in the systemic circulation is reduced, leading to cyanosis. The degree of cyanosis depends on the extent of the pulmonic stenosis, the size of the VSD, and the vascular resistance of the pulmonary and systemic circulations.

Tetralogy of Fallot is usually diagnosed during the first few weeks of life due to the presence of a murmur and/or cyanosis. Some newborns may be acutely cyanotic, while others may exhibit only mild cyanosis that gradually becomes more severe, particularly during times of stress as the child grows older. Most often, infants with tetralogy of Fallot have a PDA at birth, providing additional pulmonary blood flow and thereby decreasing the severity of the initial cyanosis. Later, as the ductus arteriosus closes, such as within the first few days of life, more severe cyanosis can occur (Fig. 41.2) (Jone et al., 2022; Schneider, 2023).

Nursing Assessment

Nursing assessment consists of the health history, physical examination, and laboratory and diagnostic tests.

HEALTH HISTORY AND PHYSICAL EXAMINATION

Obtain the health history, noting a history of color changes associated with feeding, activity, or crying. Determine if the infant or child is demonstrating hypercyanotic spells. Hypercyanosis develops suddenly and is manifested as increased cyanosis, hypoxemia, dyspnea, and agitation. If the infant's oxygen demand is greater than the supply, such as with crying or during feeding, then the spell progresses to anoxia. When the degree of cyanosis is severe and persistent, the infant may become unresponsive. As the infant gets older, they may use specific postures, such as bending at the knees or assuming the fetal position, to relieve a hypercyanotic spell. The walking infant or toddler may squat periodically. These positions improve pulmonary blood flow by increasing systemic vascular resistance. Ask the parents if they have noticed any of these unusual positions. Note history of irritability, sleepiness, or difficulty breathing.

During the physical examination, observe the skin color and note any evidence of cyanosis. Also observe for changes in skin color with positional changes, and inspect the fingers for clubbing. Note if the child has a hypercyanotic spell during the assessment. Count the child's respiratory rate and observe work of breathing, noting retractions, shortness of breath, or noisy breathing. Document oxygen saturation via pulse oximetry; it will likely be decreased. Auscultate the chest for adventitious breath sounds, which may suggest the development of heart failure. Auscultate the heart, noting a loud, harsh murmur characteristic of this disorder.

LABORATORY AND DIAGNOSTIC TESTS

Note increased hematocrit, hemoglobin, and RBC count associated with polycythemia. Additional testing may include:

- **Echocardiography** (ultrasound study of structure and motion of heart), possibly revealing right ventricular hypertrophy, decreased pulmonary blood flow, and reduced size of the pulmonary artery
- Electrocardiogram (ECG), indicating right ventricular hypertrophy
- Cardiac catheterization and angiography, which reveal the extent of the structural defects

Tricuspid Atresia

Tricuspid atresia is a CHD in which the valve between the right atrium and right ventricle fails to develop. As a result, there is no opening to allow blood to flow from the right atrium to the right ventricle and subsequently through the pulmonary artery into the lungs (Jone et al., 2022; Schneider, 2023).

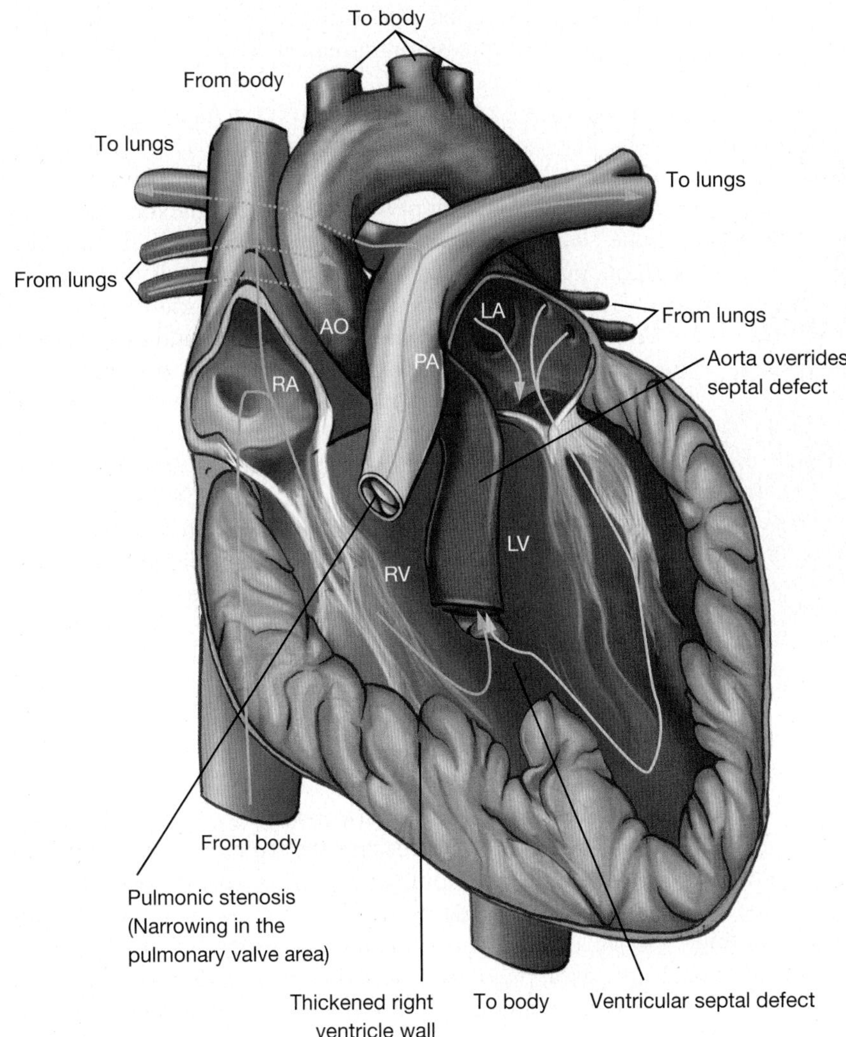

FIGURE 41.2 Tetralogy of Fallot.

> **CONSIDER THIS!**
>
> Ava Gardener, 2 weeks old, is brought to the clinic by her parent. She presents with trouble feeding. Her parent states, "When Ava eats, she seems to have trouble breathing, and a couple of times she has looked a little bluish." As the nurse takes Ava into her arms, Ava has a hypercyanotic spell.
>
> Ava is to be admitted to the hospital secondary to suspected tetralogy of Fallot. Ava's parent is very upset about the diagnosis. They say, "My poor baby, she'll never ever be able to run and play like a normal child."
>
> How should the nurse respond? How would you feel if your young baby was diagnosed with a serious disorder? What type of support can the nurse provide to Ava's parent?

Pathophysiology

In tricuspid atresia, blood returning from the systemic circulation to the right atrium cannot directly enter the right ventricle due to agenesis of the tricuspid valve. Subsequently, deoxygenated blood may pass through an opening in the atrial septum (patent foramen ovale) into the left atrium, never entering the pulmonary vasculature. Thus, deoxygenated blood mixes with oxygenated blood in the left atrium. The blood then travels to the lungs through a PDA. Most cases of tricuspid atresia are associated with a VSD, and the newborn receives inadequately oxygenated blood (Fig. 41.3) (Jone et al., 2022; Schneider, 2023).

Nursing Assessment

Nursing assessment consists of the health history, physical examination, and laboratory and diagnostic tests.

HEALTH HISTORY AND PHYSICAL EXAMINATION

Note the infant's history since birth. Document history of cyanosis either at birth or a few days later when the ductus arteriosus closed. Note history of rapid respirations and difficulty with feeding. Inspect the skin for cyanosis or a pale gray color. Observe the apical impulse, noting overactivity. Evaluate the baby's sucking strength (will usually have a weak or poor suck). Count the respiratory rate, noting tachypnea. Note increased work

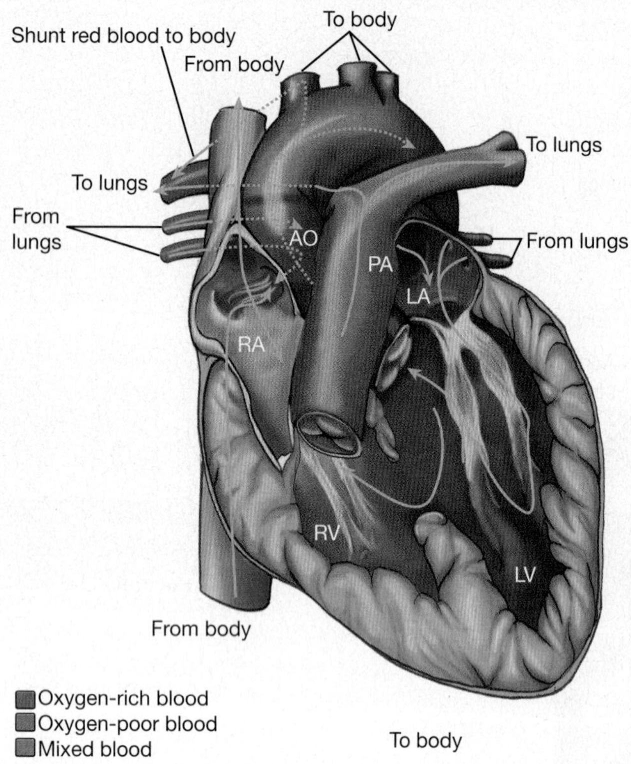

FIGURE 41.3 Tricuspid atresia.

of breathing. Auscultate the lungs, noting crackles or wheezes if heart failure is beginning to develop. Auscultate the heart, noting a murmur. Palpate the skin, noting coolness and clamminess of the extremities. Document the presence of clubbing in the older infant or child.

LABORATORY AND DIAGNOSTIC TESTING

Laboratory and diagnostic testing is similar to that for tetralogy of Fallot. A complete blood cell (CBC) count is needed to assess compensatory increases in hematocrit, hemoglobin, and erythrocyte (RBC) count, indicating the development of polycythemia. Pulse oximetry or arterial blood gas tests may be used to determine oxygen saturation levels (typically reduced). Additional testing may include:

- Echocardiography, revealing absence of tricuspid valve or underdeveloped right ventricle
- ECG, indicating possible heart failure
- Cardiac catheterization and angiography, which reveal the extent of the structural defects

Disorders With Increased Pulmonary Flow

Most CHDs involve increased pulmonary blood flow. Normally, the left side of the heart has a higher pressure than the right side. Defects with connections involving the left and right sides will shunt blood from the higher-pressure left side to the lower-pressure right side. Even a small pressure gradient such as a 1- to 3-mm difference between the left and the right sides will produce a movement of blood from the left to the right. In turn, the increase in blood on the right side of the heart will cause a greater amount of blood to move through the heart. If the amount of blood flowing to the lungs is large, the child may develop heart failure early in life. In addition, right ventricular hypertrophy may result. Sometimes, with ventricular hypertrophy, the right side of the heart pumps so forcefully that left-to-right shunting is reversed to right-to-left shunting. If this occurs, deoxygenated blood mixes with oxygenated blood, thereby lowering the overall blood oxygen saturation level.

Excessive blood flow to the lungs can produce a compensatory response such as tachypnea or tachycardia. Tachypnea increases caloric expenditure; poor cellular nutrition from decreased peripheral blood flow leads to feeding problems. Subsequently, the infant experiences poor weight gain, which delays overall growth and development. Increased pulmonary blood flow results in decreased systemic blood flow, so sodium and fluid retention may occur. Increased pulmonary blood flow also places the child at higher risk for pulmonary infections. As the child grows, the continuous increased pulmonary blood flow will cause vasoconstriction of the pulmonary vessels, actually decreasing the pulmonary blood flow. This may lead to pulmonary hypertension. For children with congenital defects with increased pulmonary blood flow, oxygen supplementation is not helpful. Oxygen acts as a pulmonary vasodilator. If pulmonary dilation occurs, pulmonary blood flow is even greater, causing tachypnea, increasing lung fluid retention, and eventually causing a much greater problem with oxygenation. Over time, continuous increased pulmonary blood flow may cause pulmonary vasoconstriction and pulmonary hypertension. Therefore, preventing the development of pulmonary disease via early surgical correction is essential.

Examples of defects with increased pulmonary blood flow are ASD, VSD, atrioventricular canal defect, and PDA.

Atrial Septal Defect

An ASD is a passageway or hole in the wall (septum) that divides the right atrium from the left atrium (Fig. 41.4). Three types of ASDs are identified based on the location of the opening:

- Ostium primum (ASD1): The opening is at the lower portion of the septum.
- Ostium secundum (ASD2): The opening is near the center of the septum.
- Sinus venosus defect: The opening is near the junction of the superior vena cava and the right atrium.

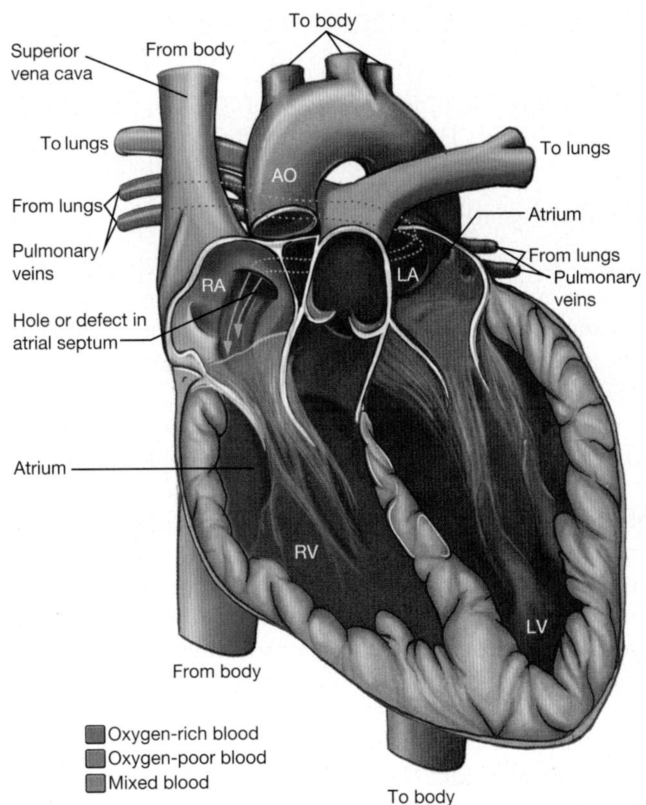

FIGURE 41.4 Atrial septal defect; note the opening between the two atria.

When the ASD is small, most infants may have a spontaneous closure within the first 18 months of life. If it does not spontaneously close by age 3, the child will most likely need corrective surgery (Jone et al., 2022; Schneider, 2023).

Pathophysiology

With ASD, blood flows through the opening from the left atrium to the right atrium due to pressure differences. The shunting increases the blood volume entering the right atrium. This, in turn, leads to increased blood flow into the lungs. If untreated, the defect can cause problems such as pulmonary hypertension, heart failure, atrial arrhythmias, or stroke (Jone et al., 2022; Schneider, 2023).

Nursing Assessment

Most children with ASDs are asymptomatic. However, a very large defect can cause increased blood flow, leading to heart failure, which results in shortness of breath, easy fatigability, or poor growth.

HEALTH HISTORY AND PHYSICAL EXAMINATION

Obtain the health history, noting poor feeding as an infant, decreased ability to keep up with peers, or history of difficulty growing. Observe the child's chest, noting a hyperdynamic precordium. Auscultate the heart, noting a fixed split-second heart sound and a systolic ejection murmur, best heard in the pulmonic valve area. Palpate along the left sternal border for a right ventricular heave.

LABORATORY AND DIAGNOSTIC TESTS

Echocardiography is done to confirm the diagnosis. An **electrocardiogram** (graphic recording of the heart's electrical activity) may show normal sinus rhythm or prolonged PR intervals. The chest radiograph may show enlargement of the heart and increased vascularity of the lungs.

Ventricular Septal Defect

A VSD is an opening between the right and left ventricular chambers of the heart (Fig. 41.5). It is one of the most common CHDs and accounts for about 30% of all CHDs. Spontaneous closure of small VSDs occurs in about half of children by age 2 years. Long-term outcomes for surgically repaired VSDs are good. Repair of larger defects by 2 years of age is recommended to prevent the development of pulmonary vascular disease (Jone et al., 2022; Schneider, 2023).

Pathophysiology

In VSD, there is an abnormal opening between the right and the left ventricles. The opening varies in size, from

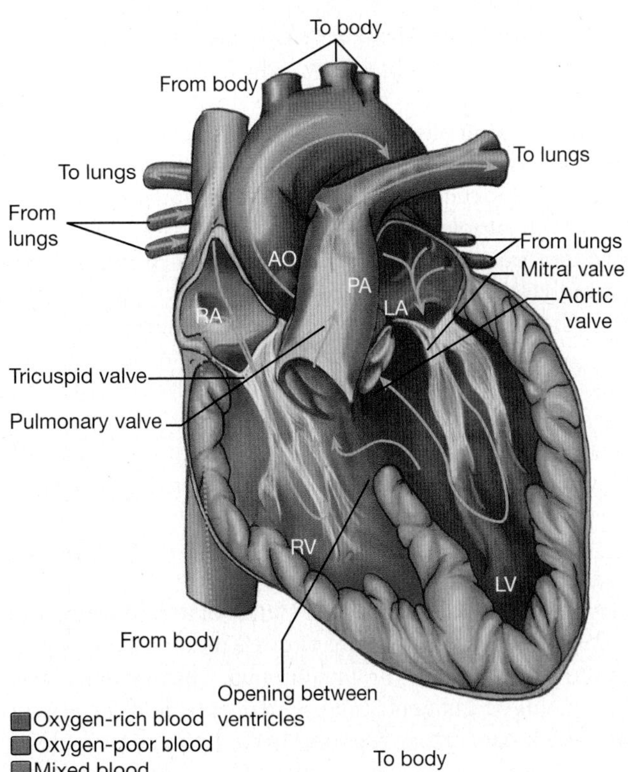

FIGURE 41.5 Ventricular septal defect; note the opening between the ventricles.

as small as a pinhole to a complete opening between the ventricles so that the right and the left sides are as one. Children with small VSDs may remain asymptomatic. In other children, blood shunts across the opening in the septum. Pulmonary vascular resistance and systemic vascular resistance determine the direction of blood flow. A left-to-right shunt results when pulmonary vascular resistance is low. Increased amounts of blood flowing into the right ventricle are then pumped to the pulmonary circulation, eventually causing an increase in pulmonary vascular resistance. Increased pulmonary vascular resistance leads to increased pulmonary artery pressure (pulmonary hypertension) and right ventricular hypertrophy. When the pulmonary vascular resistance exceeds the systemic vascular resistance, right-to-left shunting of blood across the VSD occurs, resulting in Eisenmenger syndrome (pulmonary hypertension and cyanosis). Heart failure commonly occurs in children with moderate to severe unrepaired VSDs. Children with VSDs are also at risk for the development of aortic valve regurgitation as well as infective endocarditis (Jone et al., 2022; Schneider, 2023).

Nursing Assessment

Initially, the newborn may not exhibit any signs and symptoms at birth because left-to-right shunting is most likely minimal due to the high pulmonary resistance common after birth.

HEALTH HISTORY AND PHYSICAL EXAMINATION

Determine the health history, which commonly reveals signs of heart failure around 4 to 8 weeks of age. Note history of tiring easily, particularly with exertion or feeding. Document the child's growth history, noting difficulty thriving. Ask the parent about color change or diaphoresis with nipple feeding in the infant. Note history of frequent pulmonary infections, shortness of breath, and possibly edema. Inspect the extremities for edema, noting whether pitting is present. Note mild tachypnea.

Auscultate the heart, noting a characteristic holosystolic harsh murmur along the left sternal border. In some instances, a murmur may be noted only with excessive blood flow across the opening. Adventitious lung sounds may be auscultated if the child is experiencing heart failure. Palpate the chest for a thrill.

LABORATORY AND DIAGNOSTIC TESTS

Magnetic resonance imaging (MRI) or echocardiogram with color flow Doppler may reveal the opening as well as the extent of left-to-right shunting. These studies may also identify right ventricular hypertrophy and dilation of the pulmonary artery resulting from the increased blood flow. Cardiac catheterization may be used to evaluate the extent of blood flow being pumped to the pulmonary circulation and to evaluate hemodynamic pressures.

Atrioventricular Septal Defect

Atrioventricular septal defect (AVSD) accounts for 4% of CHD. Thirty-five to forty percent of children with Down syndrome and CHD have this defect (Jone et al., 2022).

Pathophysiology

AVSD occurs because of failure of the endocardial cushions to fuse (Fig. 41.6). These cushions are needed to separate the central parts of the heart near the tricuspid and mitral (AV) valves. The complete AVSD involves ASDs and VSDs as well as a common AV orifice and a common AV valve. Partial and transitional forms of AVSD also occur, involving variations of the complete form.

The complete AVSD permits oxygenated blood from the lungs to enter the left atrium and ventricle, crossing over the atrial or ventricular septum and returning to the lungs via the pulmonary artery. This recirculation problem, which typically involves a left-to-right shunt, is inefficient because the left ventricle must pump blood back to the lungs and also meet the body's peripheral demand for oxygenated blood. Subsequently, the left ventricle must pump two to three times more blood than in a normal heart. Therefore, this specific type of cardiac defect causes a large left-to-right shunt; an increased workload of the left ventricle; and high pulmonary arterial pressure, resulting in an increased amount of blood in the lungs and causing pulmonary edema (Jone et al., 2022; Schneider, 2023).

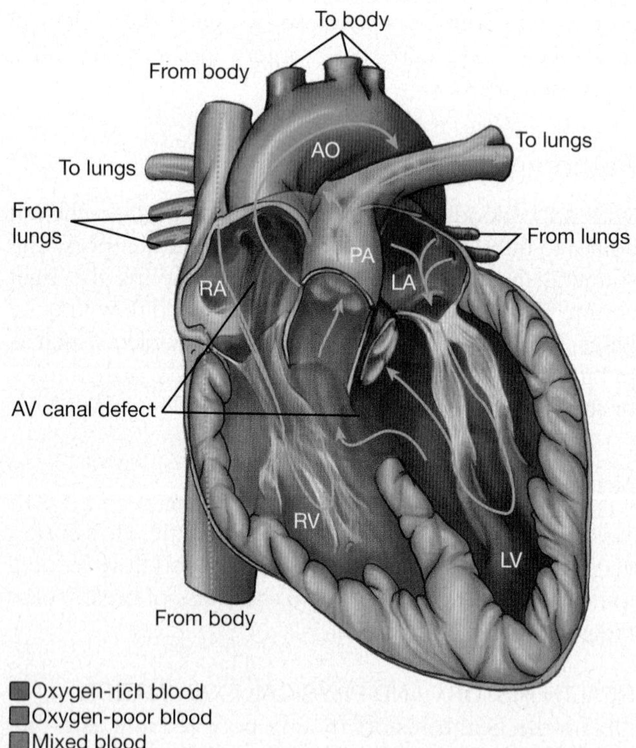

FIGURE 41.6 Atrioventricular canal defect.

Nursing Assessment

The infant with a complete AVSD commonly exhibits moderate to severe signs and symptoms of heart failure. However, for infants with a partial or transitional AVSD, the signs and symptoms will be subtler.

HEALTH HISTORY AND PHYSICAL EXAMINATION

Obtain the health history, noting frequent respiratory infections and difficulty gaining weight. Ask the parent if the infant has been experiencing difficulty feeding or increased work of breathing.

Inspect the skin, fingernails, and lips for cyanosis. Observe for retractions, tachypnea, and nasal flaring. Auscultate the lungs and heart, noting rales and a loud murmur. The murmur is commonly noted within the first 2 weeks of life. Infants with a partial or transitional AVSD defect may display more subtle signs.

LABORATORY AND DIAGNOSTIC TESTS

Echocardiography will reveal the extent of the defect and shunting as well as right ventricular hypertrophy. ECG may indicate right ventricular hypertrophy and possible first-degree heart block due to impulse blocking before reaching the AV node.

Patent Ductus Arteriosus

PDA is failure of the ductus arteriosus, a fetal circulatory structure, to close within the first few weeks of life (Fig. 41.7).

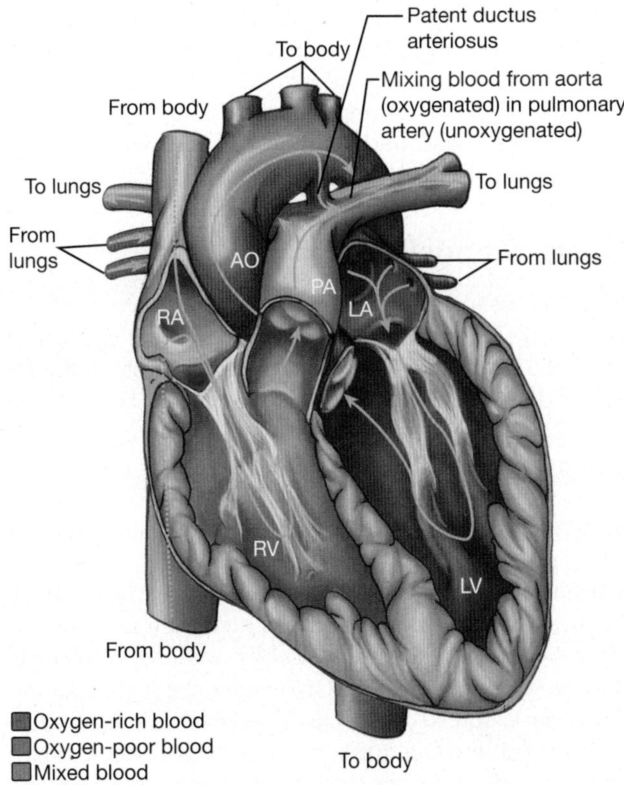

FIGURE 41.7 Patent ductus arteriosus.

As a result, there is a connection between the aorta and pulmonary artery. PDA is the second most common CHD and accounts for 10% of CHD cases (Jone et al., 2022). PDA occurs much more frequently in premature than in term infants and in infants born at high altitudes compared with those born at sea level. Infants with other CHDs that result in right-to-left shunting of blood and cyanosis may additionally display a PDA. In these infants, the PDA allows for some level of oxygenated blood to reach the systemic circulation (Jone et al., 2022; Schneider, 2023).

Pathophysiology

Failure of the ductus arteriosus to close leads to continued blood flow from the aorta to the pulmonary artery. Blood returning to the left atrium passes to the left ventricle, enters the aorta, and then travels to the pulmonary artery via the PDA instead of entering the systemic circulation. This altered blood flow pattern increases the workload of the left side of the heart. Pulmonary vascular congestion occurs, causing an increase in pressure. Right ventricular pressure increases in an attempt to overcome this increase in pulmonary pressure. Eventually, right ventricular hypertrophy occurs (Jone et al., 2022; Schneider, 2023).

Nursing Assessment

The symptoms of PDA depend on the size of the ductus arteriosus and the amount of blood flow it carries. If it is small, the infant may be asymptomatic. Some infants demonstrate signs and symptoms of heart failure.

HEALTH HISTORY AND PHYSICAL EXAMINATION

Determine the health history, which may reveal frequent respiratory infections, fatigue, and poor growth and development. On physical examination, note tachycardia, tachypnea, bounding peripheral pulses, and a widened pulse pressure. The diastolic BP typically is low due to the shunting. Auscultate the lungs and heart, noting rales if heart failure is present. Note a harsh, continuous, machine-like murmur, usually loudest under the left clavicle at the first and second intercostal spaces.

LABORATORY AND DIAGNOSTIC TESTS

Echocardiogram reveals the extent of the defective opening and confirms the diagnosis. ECG may be normal, or it may indicate ventricular hypertrophy, especially if the defect is large. Chest radiography demonstrates cardiomegaly.

Obstructive Disorders

Another group of CHDs is classified as obstructive disorders. These disorders involve some type of narrowing of a major vessel, interfering with the ability of the blood to flow freely through the vessel. As a result, peripheral circulation or blood flow to the lungs is affected. Increased pressure backing up toward the heart causes an increased workload on the heart. Examples of defects in this group include coarctation of the aorta, aortic stenosis, and pulmonic stenosis (PS).

Coarctation of the Aorta

Coarctation of the aorta is narrowing of the aorta, the major blood vessel carrying highly oxygenated blood from the left ventricle of the heart to the rest of the body (Fig. 41.8). It accounts for about 10% of CHDs (Schneider, 2023).

Pathophysiology

Coarctation of the aorta occurs most often in the area near the ductus arteriosus. The narrowing can be preductal (between the subclavian artery and the ductus arteriosus) or postductal (after the ductus arteriosus). As a result of the narrowing, blood flow is impeded, causing pressure to increase in the area proximal to the defect and to decrease in the area distal to it. Thus, BP is increased in the heart and the upper portions of the body and decreased in the lower portions of the body. Left ventricular afterload is increased, and in some children, this may lead to heart failure. Collateral circulation may also develop as the body attempts to ensure adequate blood flow to the descending aorta. Due to the elevation in BP, the child is also at risk for aortic rupture, aortic aneurysm, and CVA (Jone et al., 2022; Schneider, 2023).

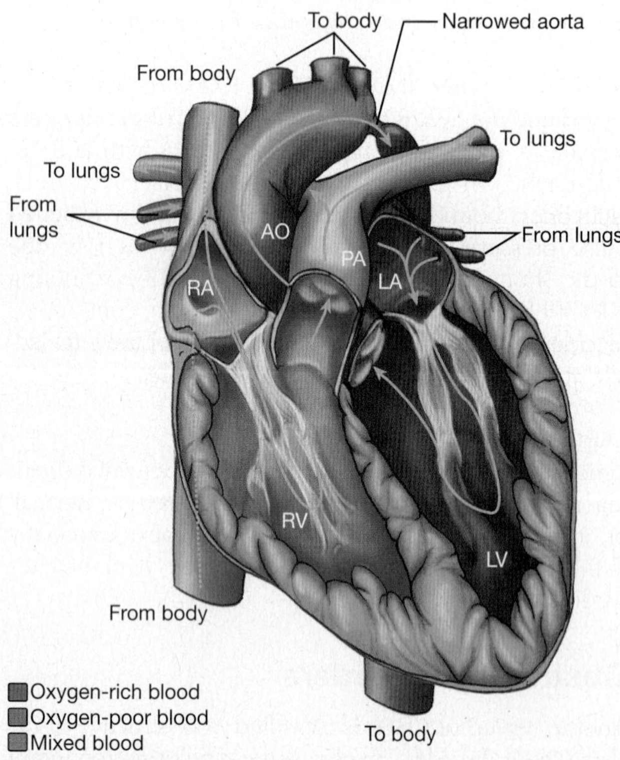

FIGURE 41.8 Coarctation of the aorta.

Nursing Assessment

The extent of the symptoms depends on the severity of the coarctation. Some children with coarctation of the aorta grow well into the school-age years before the defect is discovered.

HEALTH HISTORY AND PHYSICAL EXAMINATION

Determine the health history, noting problems with irritability and frequent epistaxis. In older children, there may also be reports of leg pain with activity, dizziness, fainting, and headaches. Assess pulses throughout, noting full, bounding pulses in the upper extremities with weak or absent pulses in the lower extremities. Determine BP in all four extremities. BP in the upper extremities may be 20 mm Hg or higher than that in the lower extremities. Inspect the school-age child's chest, noting notching of the ribs. Auscultate the heart for a soft or moderately loud systolic murmur, most often heard at the base of the heart (on the back or in the left axilla) (Jone et al., 2022).

LABORATORY AND DIAGNOSTIC TESTS

Diagnosis of coarctation of the aorta is based primarily on the history and physical examination. In addition, an echocardiogram may disclose the extent of narrowing and evidence of collateral circulation. Chest radiography may reveal left-sided cardiac enlargement and rib notching, indicative of collateral arterial enlargement. Other tests, such as ECG, computed tomography, or MRI, may be done to provide additional evidence about the extent of the coarctation and subsequent effects.

Aortic Stenosis

Aortic stenosis is a condition causing obstruction of the blood flow between the left ventricle and the aorta. The incidence of aortic stenosis is about 5% of all CHDs (Schneider, 2023).

Pathophysiology

Aortic stenosis can be caused by a muscle obstruction below the aortic valve, an obstruction at the valve itself, or an aortic narrowing just above the valve (Fig. 41.9). The most common type is an obstruction of the valve itself, called aortic valve stenosis. The aortic valve consists of three very pliable leaflets. Normally, the leaflets of the aortic valve spread open easily when the left ventricle ejects blood into the aorta. Aortic stenosis occurs when the aortic valve narrows, causing an obstruction between the left ventricle and the aorta. As a result, cardiac output

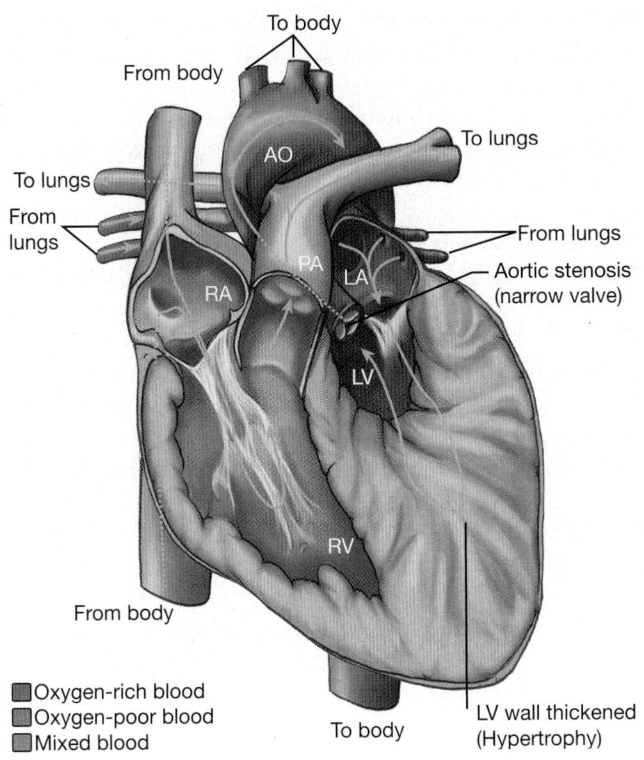

FIGURE 41.9 Aortic stenosis.

decreases. When the aortic valve does not function properly, the left ventricle must work harder to pump blood into the aorta. Because of the increased workload, the left ventricular muscle hypertrophies. If this continues, left ventricular failure can occur, leading to a backup of pressure in the pulmonary circulation and pulmonary edema. Heart failure may occur, but this is more commonly seen in the infant (Jone et al., 2022; Schneider, 2023).

Nursing Assessment

Typically, the child with aortic stenosis is asymptomatic. However, it is important to obtain an accurate health history and perform a physical examination.

HEALTH HISTORY AND PHYSICAL EXAMINATION

Obtain the child's health history, noting easy fatigability or complaints of chest pain similar to anginal pain when active. Dizziness with prolonged standing may also be reported. In the infant, note difficulty with feeding. Palpate the child's pulse; if aortic stenosis is severe, the pulses may be faint. Palpate the child's chest, noting a thrill at the base of the heart. Auscultate the heart, noting a systolic murmur best heard along the left sternal border with radiation to the right upper sternal border.

LABORATORY AND DIAGNOSTIC TESTS

The echocardiogram is the most important noninvasive test to identify aortic stenosis. An ECG may be normal in children with mild to moderate forms of aortic stenosis. For children with severe aortic stenosis, left ventricular hypertrophy may be determined from the ECG. For children experiencing easy fatigability and chest pain, an exercise stress test may be done to evaluate the degree of cardiac compromise.

Pulmonic Stenosis

PS is a condition that causes an obstruction in blood flow between the right ventricle and the pulmonary arteries. Pulmonic stenosis occurs in 0.6 to 0.8 per 1,000 live births (Peng, 2022). It is often associated with other heart anomalies and with genetic syndromes. Children may be asymptomatic, although some children with severe pulmonic stenosis may demonstrate cyanosis (Peng, 2022).

Pathophysiology

Pulmonic stenosis may occur as a muscular obstruction below the pulmonary valve, an obstruction at the valve, or a narrowing of the pulmonary artery above the valve (Fig. 41.10). Valve obstruction is the most common form of PS. Normally, the pulmonary valve is constructed with three thin and pliable valve leaflets; they spread apart easily, allowing the right ventricle to eject blood freely into the pulmonary artery. The most common problem

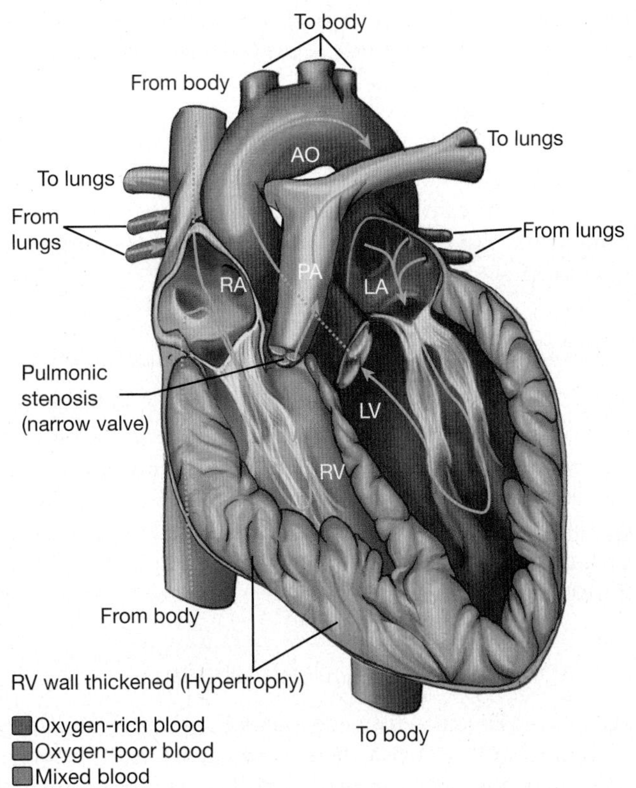

FIGURE 41.10 Pulmonic stenosis.

causing pulmonic stenosis is that the pulmonary valve leaflets are thickened and fused together along their separation lines, causing the obstruction to blood flow. The right ventricle has an additional workload, causing the muscle to thicken, resulting in right ventricular hypertrophy and decreased pulmonary blood flow. When the pulmonary valve is severely obstructed, the right ventricle cannot eject sufficient blood into the pulmonary artery. As a result, pressure in the right atrium increases, which could lead to a reopening of the foramen ovale. If this occurs, deoxygenated blood would pass through the foramen ovale into the left side of the heart and would then be pumped to the systemic circulation. In some cases, a PDA may be present, thus allowing for some compensation by shunting blood from the aorta to the pulmonary circulation for oxygenation (Peng, 2022).

Nursing Assessment

The child with pulmonic stenosis may be asymptomatic or may exhibit signs and symptoms of mild heart failure. If the stenosis is severe, the child may demonstrate cyanosis. Therefore, it is important for the nurse to obtain an accurate health history and physical examination.

HEALTH HISTORY AND PHYSICAL EXAMINATION

Elicit the health history, noting mild dyspnea or cyanosis with exertion. Document the child's growth history, which is typically normal. Carefully palpate the sternal border for a thrill (not always present). Auscultate the heart, noting a high-pitched click following the second heart sound and a systolic ejection murmur loudest at the upper left sternal border.

LABORATORY AND DIAGNOSTIC TESTS

An echocardiogram reveals the extent of obstruction present at the valve, as well as right ventricular hypertrophy. An ECG also helps to detect right ventricular hypertrophy.

Mixed Defects

Mixed defects are CHDs that involve a mixing of well-oxygenated blood with poorly oxygenated blood. As a result, systemic blood flow contains a lower oxygen content. Cardiac output is decreased, and heart failure occurs. Examples of mixed defects include TGA, total anomalous pulmonary venous connection (TAPVC), truncus arteriosus, and HLHS.

Transposition of the Great Arteries

TGA is a CHD in which the pulmonary artery and the aorta are transposed from their normal positions. The aorta arises from the right ventricle instead of the left ventricle, and the pulmonary artery arises from the left ventricle instead of the right ventricle. TGA accounts about 5% of all CHD cases (Schneider, 2023). It is most often diagnosed in the first few days of life when the infant manifests cyanosis, which indicates decreased oxygenation. As the ductus arteriosus closes, the symptoms will worsen. Corrective surgery is usually performed by age 4 to 7 days.

PATHOPHYSIOLOGY

TGV creates a situation in which poorly oxygenated blood returning to the right atrium and ventricle is then pumped out to the aorta and back to the body (Fig. 41.11). Oxygenated blood returning from the lungs to the left atrium and ventricle is then sent back to the lungs through the pulmonary artery. Unless there is a connection somewhere in the circulation where the oxygen-rich and oxygen-poor blood can mix, all the organs of the body will be poorly oxygenated. Often, the ductus arteriosus remains patent, allowing for some mixing of blood. Similarly, if a VSD is also present, mixing of blood may occur, and cyanosis will be delayed. However, these associated defects can lead to increased pulmonary blood flow that increases pressure in the pulmonary circulation. This predisposes the child to heart failure (Jone et al., 2022; Schneider, 2023).

NURSING ASSESSMENT

Significant cyanosis without a murmur in the newborn period is highly indicative of TGA. In some infants, cyanosis will not develop until several days of age as the PDA closes. In infants with septal defects, cyanosis may be further delayed.

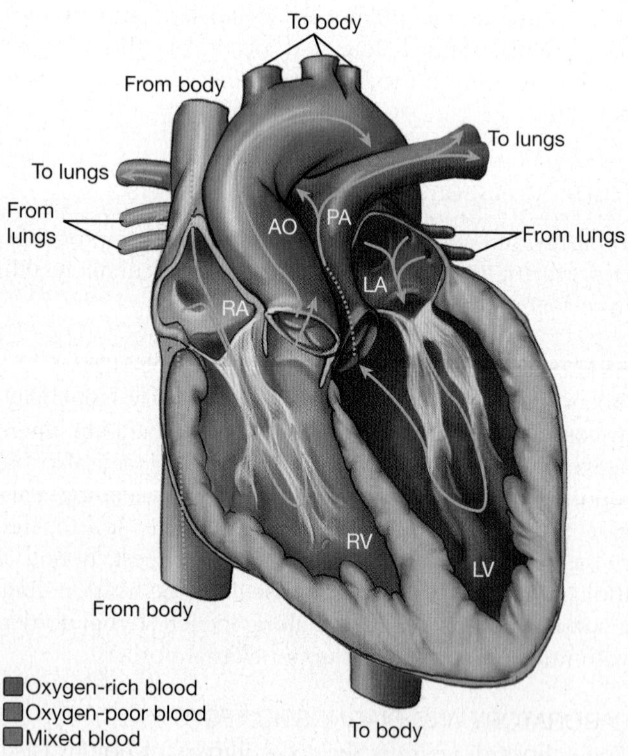

FIGURE 41.11 Transposition of the great vessels.

Health History and Physical Examination

Elicit the health history, noting onset of cyanosis with feeding or crying. Observe the infant for cyanosis while active and at rest. Observe the chest, noting a prominent ventricular impulse. Auscultate the heart, noting a loud second heart sound. A murmur may be heard if the ductus remains open or a septal defect is present. If heart failure is present, note edema, tachypnea, and adventitious lung sounds.

Laboratory and Diagnostic Tests

Echocardiography clearly reveals evidence of the transposition. Cardiac catheterization may be performed to determine whether oxygen saturation levels are low due to the mixing of the blood.

Total Anomalous Pulmonary Venous Connection

TAPVC is a CHD in which the pulmonary veins do not connect normally to the left atrium. Instead, they connect to the right atrium, often by way of the superior vena cava. Relatively rare, it accounts for up to 1.5% of all CHD (Soriano & Fulton, 2022). TAPVC may also be referred to as TAPVR.

PATHOPHYSIOLOGY

Oxygenated blood that would normally enter the left atrium now enters the right atrium and passes to the right ventricle. As a result, the pressure on the right side of the heart increases, leading to hypertrophy. TAPVC is incompatible with life unless there is an associated defect present that allows for shunting of blood from the highly pressured right side of the heart. A patent foramen ovale or an ASD is usually present. Since none of the pulmonary veins connect normally to the left atrium, the only source of blood to the left atrium is blood that is shunted from the right atrium across the defect to the left side of the heart (Fig. 41.12). The highly oxygenated blood from the lungs completely mixes with the poorly oxygenated blood returning from the systemic circulation. This causes an overload of the right atrium and right ventricle. The increased blood volume going into the lungs can lead to pulmonary hypertension and pulmonary edema (Soriano & Fulton, 2022).

NURSING ASSESSMENT

The degree of cyanosis present with TAPVC depends on the extent of the associated defects. For example, if the foramen ovale closes or the ASD is small, significant cyanosis will be present. The physical examination findings will vary depending on the type of TAPVC the infant has, whether obstruction is present, and whether other associated cardiac anomalies are present.

Health History and Physical Examination

Note history of cyanosis, tiring easily, and difficulty feeding. Observe the chest for prominence of the right ventricular impulse and retractions with tachypnea. Auscultate the heart, noting fixed splitting of the second heart sound and a murmur. Palpate the abdomen for hepatomegaly.

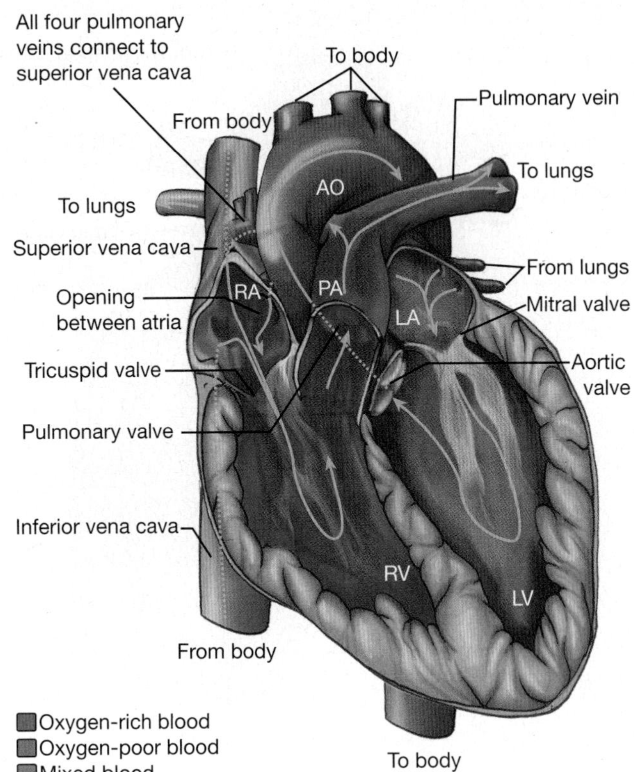

FIGURE 41.12 Total anomalous pulmonary venous connection.

Laboratory and Diagnostic Tests

An echocardiogram will reveal the abnormal connection of the pulmonary veins, enlargement of the right atrium and right ventricle, and an ASD if present. The chest radiograph will demonstrate an enlarged heart and pulmonary edema. Cardiac catheterization can also be useful to visualize the abnormal connection of the pulmonary veins, particularly if an obstruction is present.

Truncus Arteriosus

Truncus arteriosus is a CHD in which only one major artery leaves the heart and supplies blood to the pulmonary and systemic circulations. It accounts for less than 1% of all CHD cases (Jone et al., 2022; Schneider, 2023). A VSD is almost always present as well.

PATHOPHYSIOLOGY

The one great vessel contains one valve. This valve consists of two to five leaflets and is positioned over both the left and the right ventricles (Fig. 41.13). Due to the location of the valve, blood from the left ventricle mixes with blood from the right ventricle. Pressure

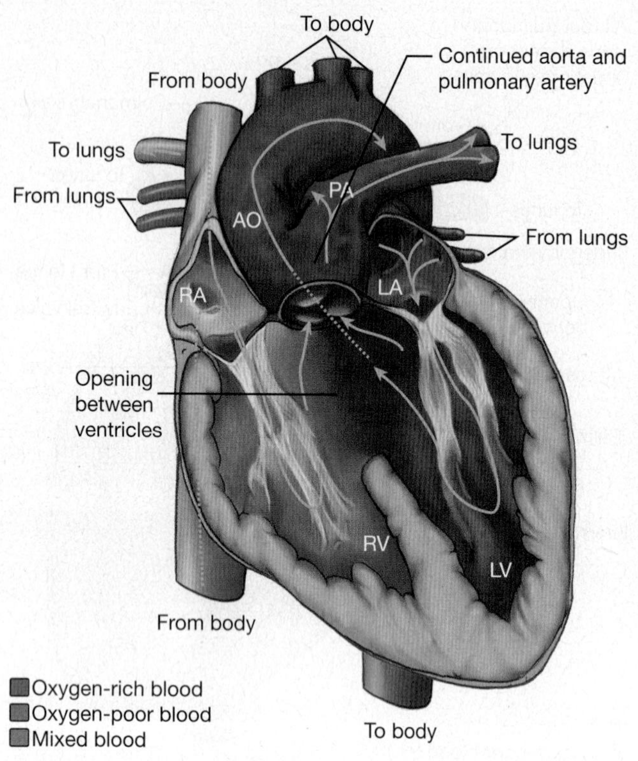

FIGURE 41.13 Truncus arteriosus.

in the pulmonary circulation is typically less than that of the systemic circulation, leading to increased blood flow to the lungs. As a result, systemic blood flow is decreased. Over time, the increased pulmonary blood flow can lead to pulmonary vascular disease (Jone et al., 2022; Schneider, 2023).

NURSING ASSESSMENT

Typically, the infant demonstrates cyanosis in varying degrees, depending on the extent of compromise in the systemic circulation. Obtain an accurate health history and perform a physical examination.

Health History and Physical Examination

Elicit the health history, noting history of cyanosis that increases with periods of activity such as feeding. Also note history of tiring easily, difficulty in feeding, and poor growth. Count the respiratory rate, which may be elevated. Observe for nasal flaring, grunting or noisy breathing, retractions, and restlessness. Auscultate the lungs, noting adventitious breath sounds, and the heart, noting a murmur associated with a VSD.

Laboratory and Diagnostic Tests

An echocardiogram will confirm the presence of truncus arteriosus as the anatomy of the great vessels, the single truncal valve, and the VSD will be seen. On rare occasions, a cardiac catheterization may be done to determine pressures in the pulmonary arteries.

Hypoplastic Left Heart Syndrome

HLHS is a CHD in which all structures on the left side of the heart are severely underdeveloped (Fig. 41.14). The mitral and aortic valves are completely closed or very small. The left ventricle is nonfunctional. Thus, the left side of the heart is completely unable to supply blood to the systemic circulation. HLHS is the fourth most common CHD. It appears to have a multifactorial and autosomal recessive inheritance pattern and occurs in 1.4% to 3.8% of cases of CHD (Jone et al., 2022). The options for treatment include palliative care, cardiac transplantation within the first few weeks of life, or palliative reconstructive surgery consisting of three stages, beginning within days to weeks of birth.

PATHOPHYSIOLOGY

With HLHS, the right side of the heart is the main working part of the heart. Blood returning from the lungs into the left atrium must pass through an ASD to the right side of the heart. The right ventricle must then pump blood to the lungs and to the systemic circulation through the PDA. A few days after birth, when the ductus arteriosus closes, the heart cannot pump blood into the systemic circulation, causing poor perfusion of the vital organs and shock. Death will occur rapidly without intervention (Jone et al., 2022; Schneider, 2023).

NURSING ASSESSMENT

Initially after birth, the newborn may be asymptomatic because the ductus arteriosus is still patent. However, as

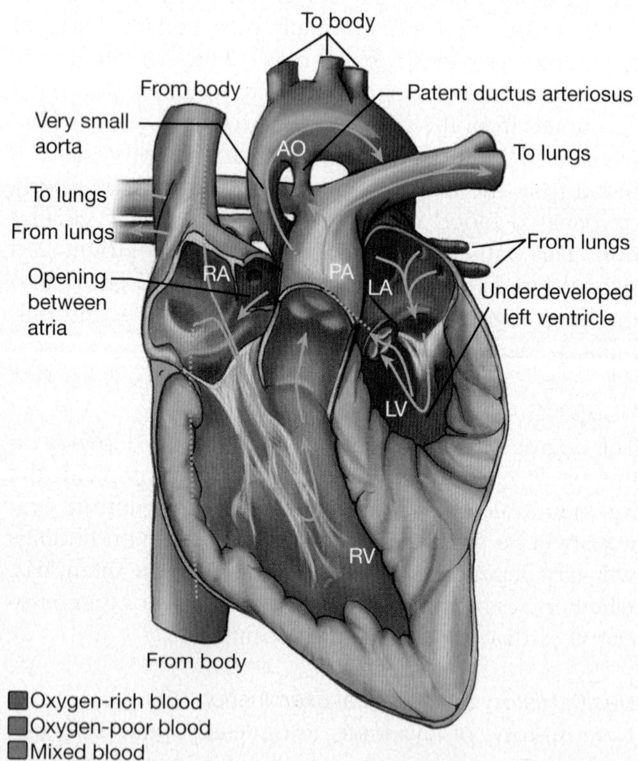

FIGURE 41.14 Hypoplastic left heart syndrome.

the ductus begins to close at a few days of age, the newborn will begin to exhibit cyanosis. Some infants may present with circulatory collapse (shock) and must be resuscitated emergently.

Health History and Physical Examination

Obtain the health history, noting onset of cyanosis. Note poor feeding and history of tiring easily. Evaluate the vital signs, noting tachycardia, tachypnea, and hypothermia. Observe for increased work of breathing and gradually increasing cyanosis. Note pallor of the extremities and decreased oxygen saturation via pulse oximetry. Auscultate the heart and lungs. Note adventitious breath sounds, a gallop rhythm, a single second heart sound, and a soft systolic ejection or holosystolic murmur.

Laboratory and Diagnostic Tests

Prenatally, a fetal echocardiogram can diagnose this syndrome, as can an ultrasound of the pregnant person. After birth, the echocardiogram illustrates the defect.

Nursing Management of the Child With a Congenital Heart Defect

The child with a CHD has multiple needs and requires comprehensive, multidisciplinary care. Nurses play a key role in helping the child and family during this intensely stressful time. Nursing care focuses on improving oxygenation, promoting adequate nutrition, assisting the child and family with coping, providing postoperative nursing care, preventing infection, and providing child and family education. An important component of education involves preparing the child and parents for discharge. In addition to the nursing management presented further on, refer to the "Clinical Judgment and the Nursing Process" section for additional interventions appropriate for the child with CHD. Individualize nursing care specific to the child's needs.

Improving Oxygenation

Provide frequent ongoing assessment of the child's cardiopulmonary status as oxygenation status varies due to the hemodynamic changes accompanying the underlying structural defect. Assess airway patency and suction as needed. Position the child in the Fowler or semi-Fowler position to facilitate lung expansion. Monitor vital signs, especially heart and respiratory rates. Monitor the child's color and oxygen saturation levels closely, using these to guide oxygen administration. Observe for tachypnea and other signs of respiratory distress, such as nasal flaring, grunting, and retractions. Auscultate the lungs for adventitious sounds. Provide humidified supplemental oxygen as ordered, warming it to prevent wide temperature fluctuations. Anticipate the need for assisted ventilation if the child has difficulty maintaining the airway or experiences deterioration in oxygenation capacity. Box 41.1 lists interventions related to relief of hypercyanotic spells.

BOX 41.1 Relieving Hypercyanotic Spells

- Use a calm, comforting approach.
- Place the infant or child in a knee-to-chest position.
- Provide supplemental oxygen.
- Administer morphine sulfate (0.1 mg/kg IV, IM, or SQ).
- Supply IV fluids.
- Administer propranolol (0.1 mg/kg IV).

IM, intramuscularly; IV, intravenously; SQ, subcutaneously.

Data from Doyle, T., & Kavanaugh-McHugh, A. (2023). Management and outcome of tetralogy of Fallot. *UptoDate*. Retrieved January 12, 2024, from http://www.uptodate.com/contents/management-and-outcome-of-tetralogy-of-fallot

DOSAGE CALCULATION BOX 41.1

Child's weight: 12 lb 12 oz

Medication order: digoxin 60 mcg by mouth every 12 hours.

Per the Pediatric Dosage Handbook, the recommended dose is 10–15 mcg/kg/day in two divided doses.

Is the ordered dose safe?

Promoting Adequate Nutrition

Provide nutrition orally, enterally, or parenterally in order to foster growth and development as well as to reduce the risk of infection. The nutritional method will vary depending on the individual child's energy expenditure associated with increased cardiac and respiratory workloads. In addition, for example, for the newborn or infant, nutrition via breast milk or formula may be provided orally or via gavage feedings. Breastfeeding is usually associated with decreased energy expenditure during the act of feeding, yet some infants in intensive care are not stable enough to breastfeed. Gavage with breast milk is possible, and the use of human milk fortifier (either with breastfeeding or added to the gavage feed) adds additional calories that the infant requires. Formula-fed infants may also require increased-calorie formula, which may be achieved by more concentrated mixing of the formula or through the use of additives such as Polycose or vegetable oil. Consult the nutritionist to determine the individual infant's caloric needs and prescription of appropriate feeding.

Cutting a larger hole in the nipple or cross-cutting the nipple decreases the work of feeding for some infants. Generally, nipple feedings should be limited to a 20-minute duration, as feeding for longer periods results in excess caloric expenditure. Many infants may feed orally for 20 minutes, receiving the remainder of that feeding via orogastric or nasogastric tube. Offer older children small, frequent feedings to reduce the amount of energy required to feed or eat and to prevent overtiring the child. When needed, administer and monitor total parenteral nutrition as prescribed.

TAKE NOTE!

Breastfeeding a child before and after cardiac surgery may boost the infant's immune system, which can help fight postoperative infection. If breastfeeding is not possible, pumped breast milk may be given via bottle, dropper, or gavage feeding.

Assisting the Child and Family With Coping

Support the family's efforts to cope with the diagnosis of CHD as it can be overwhelming for the child and the parents. The numerous examinations, diagnostic tests, and procedures are sources of stress for the infant or child regardless of age and for the parents. The parents may fear long-term disability or death or may worry that allowing the child to engage in any activity will worsen their status. Thus, the parents may tend to overprotect the child. It is important for the parents to continue parenting the child, even when the child requires extended hospitalizations or intensive care. Explain all that is happening with the child, using language the parents and child can understand. Allow the parents and child to voice their feelings, concerns, or questions. Provide ample time to address these questions and concerns. Encourage the parents and the child, as developmentally appropriate, to participate in the child's care.

If the child is a newborn or infant, encourage attachment and bonding. Emphasize the child's positive attributes, including the normal aspects of the infant. Help the parents to experience the joy of a new infant and see the beauty of the child, no matter how ill the infant is. Urge the parents to touch, stroke, pat, and talk to the infant. Encourage them to hold the infant close, using kangaroo care as appropriate. If the child is older, offer suggestions as to how the parents can meet the child's emotional needs. For example, encourage them to bring a favorite toy or object from home while the child is hospitalized.

Provide developmentally appropriate explanations to the child. Encourage play therapy to help the child understand what is happening.

Preventing Infection

Teach parents proper hand hygiene. Provide appropriate dental care. Make sure the child receives prophylaxis for infective endocarditis as needed. Ensure that children 24 months or younger who are undergoing heart transplantation during respiratory syncytial virus (RSV) season receive appropriate prophylaxis via vaccination with palivizumab (Kimberlin et al., 2021).

Providing Care for the Child Undergoing Cardiac Surgery

Cardiac surgery may be necessary to correct a congenital defect or to provide symptomatic relief. The surgery may be planned as an elective procedure or done as an emergency. Open heart surgery involves an incision of the heart muscle to repair the internal structures. This may require cardiopulmonary bypass. Closed heart surgery involves structures related to the heart but not the heart muscle itself and may be performed with or without cardiopulmonary bypass.

PROVIDING PREOPERATIVE CARE

Complete the preoperative assessment to provide important baseline information for comparison during the postoperative period. Establish a relationship with the child and parents. Identify problems that may require particular nursing interventions during the postoperative period. Before cardiac surgery, interview the parents and, if age appropriate, the child. Focus the interview on the history of the present illness, cardiac risk factors, the child's present physical and functional status, additional medical problems, current medications and drug allergies, the child's and family's understanding of the illness and planned procedure, and the family support system.

The preoperative physical assessment includes:

- Temperature and weight measurements
- Examination of extremities for peripheral edema, clubbing, and evaluation of peripheral pulses
- Auscultation of the heart (rate, rhythm, heart sounds, murmurs, clicks, and rubs)
- Respiratory assessment, including respiratory rate, work of breathing, and auscultation of the lungs for breath sounds

Obtain any necessary laboratory and diagnostic tests to establish a baseline. In addition, review the results of any tests done previously. Testing may include CBC count, electrolyte levels, clotting studies, urinalysis, cultures of blood and other body secretions, kidney and hepatic function tests, chest radiography, ECG, echocardiogram, and cardiac catheterization.

In most nonemergent cases, preoperative assessment is performed in an outpatient setting, and the child is admitted to the hospital on the day of surgery. Nursing care during this phase focuses on thorough child and parent education. If the surgery is an emergency, teaching must be done quickly, emphasizing the most important elements of the child's care (Beke et al., 2021).

Child and parent education typically includes the following topics:

- Heart anatomy and its function, including what area is involved with the defect that is to be corrected
- Events before surgery, including any testing or preparation such as a skin scrub
- Location of the child after surgery, such as a pediatric intensive care unit, which may include a visit to the unit, if appropriate, and explanation of the sights and sounds that may be present
- Appearance of the child after surgery (equipment or devices used for monitoring, such as oxygen

administration, ECG leads, pulse oximeter, chest tubes, mechanical ventilation, or IV lines)
- Approximate location of the incision and coverage with dressings
- Postoperative activity level, including measures to reduce the risk of complications, such as coughing and deep-breathing exercises, incentive spirometry, early ambulation, and leg exercises
- Nutritional restrictions, such as nothing by mouth for a specified time before surgery and use of IV fluids
- Medications, such as anesthesia, sedation, and analgesics as well as medications the child is taking now that need to be continued or withheld (Beke et al., 2021)

Prepare and educate the child at an age- and developmentally appropriate level. Advise parents to read books with their child about CHD and hospitalization such as:

- *Clifford Visits the Hospital* by N. Bridwell, 2000 (Scholastic Inc.)
- *Franklin Goes to the Hospital* by P. Bourgeois, 2000 (Scholastic Paperbacks)
- *Pump the Bear* by G. O. Whittington, 2000 (Brown Books)
- *Blue Lewis and Sasha the Great* by C. D. Newell, 2005 (Cally Press)
- *Cardiac Kids: A Book for Families Who Have a Child with Heart Disease* by V. Elder, 1994 (Dayton Area Heart and Cancer Association)
- *When Molly Was in the Hospital: A Book for Brothers and Sisters of Hospitalized Children* by D. Duncan, 1994 (Rayve Productions) (siblings)
- *A Night Without Stars* by J. Howe, 1993 (Camelot) (older children)

In addition, parents may order *It's My Heart,* a parent resource book, free of charge from the Children's Heart Foundation via this link: https://www.childrensheartfoundation.org/about-chds/resources.html.

Parents may also help their child by buying a small thrift store suitcase, spray painting it, and allowing the child to decorate it with their name, pictures of family, stickers, or favorite story characters. This will be the child's "hospital suitcase" that the child may pack with toys and videos to bring to the hospital. Hospital tours are appropriate for school-age children, and older children and adolescents may benefit from an intensive care unit tour before surgery.

Instruct parents to stop food and liquids at the designated time, depending on the child's age, and to give all medications as directed. Some medications may be withheld before surgery. If the child's nutritional status is poor or questionable, nutritional supplementation may be ordered for a period preoperatively to ensure that the child has the best possible nutritional status before surgery. When it is time for the child to be transported to the surgical area, allow the parents to accompany the child as far as possible, depending on the institution's policy. Also reinforce with the child that their parents will be present at the bedside when they awaken from surgery (Beke et al., 2021).

PROVIDING POSTOPERATIVE CARE

Postoperative nursing care for the child after cardiac surgery includes the following measures:

- Assess vital signs frequently, as often as every 1 hour, until stable.
- Assess the color of the skin and mucous membranes, check capillary refill, and palpate peripheral pulses.
- Observe cardiac rate and rhythm via electronic monitoring, and auscultate heart rate and rhythm and heart sounds frequently.
- Monitor hemodynamic status via arterial and/or central venous lines (left and right atrial and pulmonary artery pressures, pulmonary artery oxygen saturation).
- Provide site care and tubing changes according to the institution's policy.
- Auscultate lungs for adventitious, diminished, or absent breath sounds.
- Assess oxygen saturation levels via pulse oximetry and arterial blood gases as well as work of breathing and level of consciousness frequently.
- Administer supplemental oxygen as needed.
- Monitor mechanical ventilation and suction as ordered.
- Inspect chest tube functioning, noting amount, color, and character of drainage.
- Inspect the dressing (incision and chest tube) for drainage and intactness. Reinforce or change the dressing as ordered.
- Assess the incision for redness, irritation, drainage, or separation.
- Monitor intake and output hourly.
- Maintain accurate IV infusion rate; restrict fluids as ordered to prevent hypervolemia.
- Assess for changes in level of consciousness. Report restlessness, irritability, or seizures.
- Obtain ordered laboratory tests, such as CBC, coagulation studies, cardiac enzyme levels, and electrolyte levels. Report abnormal results.
- Administer medications, such as digoxin or inotropic or vasopressor agents, as ordered, watching the child closely for possible adverse effects.
- Encourage the child to turn, cough, deep breathe, use the incentive spirometer, and splint the incisional area with pillows.
- Assess the child's pain level and administer analgesics as ordered. Allow time for the child to rest and sleep.
- Assist the child to get out of bed as soon as possible and as ordered.
- Assess daily weights.
- Administer small, frequent feedings or meals when oral intake is allowed.

BOX 41.2 Possible Complications After Cardiac Surgery

- Atelectasis
- Bacterial endocarditis
- Cardiac arrhythmias
- Cardiac tamponade
- Cerebrovascular accident
- Heart failure
- Hemorrhage
- Pleural effusion
- Pneumonia
- Pneumothorax
- Postperfusion syndrome
- Postcardiac surgery syndrome
- Pulmonary edema
- Seizures
- Wound infection

Data from Fleitman, J. (2023). Postoperative complications among patients undergoing cardiac surgery. *UpToDate*. Retrieved January 12, 2024, from https://www.uptodate.com/contents/postoperative-complications-among-patients-undergoing-cardiac-surgery

- Position the child in a comfortable position, one that maximizes chest expansion. Change position frequently.
- Assess the child for complications (Box 41.2).
- Provide emotional and physical support to the child and family, making appropriate referrals, such as to social services for assistance.
- Prepare the child and family for discharge (Beke et al., 2021).

TAKE NOTE!

Abrupt cessation of chest tube output accompanied by an increase in heart rate and increased filling pressure (right atrial) may indicate cardiac tamponade (Beke et al., 2021).

Providing Child and Family Education

Provide child and family education throughout the child's stay. Initially, teaching focuses on the underlying defect and measures to treat or control the problem. If the child requires surgery, teaching shifts to preoperative and postoperative events. Emphasize discharge teaching for each admission. Teaching Guidelines 41.2 highlights the major areas to be addressed in child and family education.

TEACHING GUIDELINES 41.2 Caring for the Child With a Congenital Heart Disease

- Give medications, if ordered, exactly as prescribed.
- Weigh the child at least once a week or as ordered at approximately the same time of the day with the same scale and wearing the same amount of clothing.
- Allow the child to engage in activity as directed. Provide time for the child to rest frequently throughout the day to prevent overexertion.
- Provide a nutritious diet, taking into account any restrictions for fluids or foods.
- Use measures to prevent infection, such as frequent handwashing, prophylactic antibiotics, and skin care.
- Adhere to schedule for follow-up diagnostic tests and procedures.
- Support the child's growth and development needs.
- Use available community support services.
- Notify the health care provider or nurse practitioner if the child has increasing episodes of respiratory distress, cyanosis, or difficulty breathing; fever; increased edema of the hands, feet, or face; decreased urinary output; weight loss or difficulty eating or drinking; increased fatigue or irritability; decreased level of alertness; or vomiting or diarrhea (Gaskin & Kennedy, 2019; Hueckel, 2019).

ACQUIRED CARDIOVASCULAR DISORDERS

Acquired cardiovascular disorders occur in children because of an underlying cardiovascular problem or may refer to other cardiac disorders that are not congenital. The most common type of acquired cardiovascular disorder in children is heart failure. Other acquired disorders include rheumatic fever, cardiomyopathy, infective endocarditis, hyperlipidemia, hypertension, and Kawasaki disease.

Heart Failure

Heart failure refers to a set of clinical signs and symptoms that reflect the heart's inability to pump effectively to provide adequate blood, oxygen, and nutrients to the body organs and tissues (Kusumoto, 2019). Heart failure occurs most often in children with CHD and is the most common reason for admission to the hospital for children with CHD. The estimated number of children experiencing heart failure annually is 12,000 to 25,000 (Singh & Singh, 2022). Heart failure also occurs secondary to other conditions such as myocardial dysfunction following surgical intervention for CHD, cardiomyopathy, myocarditis, fluid volume overload, hypertension, anemia, or sepsis or as a toxic effect of certain chemotherapeutic agents used in the treatment of cancer.

The child experiencing heart failure requires a multidisciplinary approach to care. Collaboration is necessary to achieve improved cardiac function, restored fluid balance, decreased cardiac workload, and improved oxygen delivery to the tissues.

Pathophysiology

Cardiac output is controlled by preload (diastolic volume), afterload (ventricular wall tension), myocardial contractility (inotropic state), and heart rate. Protracted alterations in any of these factors may lead to heart failure. In the event of reduced cardiac output, multiple compensatory mechanisms are activated. When the ventricular contraction is impaired (systolic dysfunction), reduced ejection of blood occurs, and therefore cardiac output is reduced. Diminished ability to receive venous return (diastolic dysfunction) occurs when high venous pressures are required to support ventricular function. As a result of decreased cardiac output, the renin–angiotensin–aldosterone system is activated as a compensatory mechanism. Fluid and sodium retention as well as improved contractility and vasoconstriction then occur. Initially, BP is supported, and organ perfusion is maintained, but increased afterload worsens systolic dysfunction. As the heart chambers dilate, myocardial oxygen consumption increases, and cardiac output is limited by excessive wall stretch. Over time, the capacity of the heart to respond to these compensatory mechanisms fails, and cardiac output is further decreased (Kusumoto, 2019). Figure 41.15 shows the clinical manifestations that occur related to the mechanisms of heart failure.

Therapeutic Management

Management of heart failure is supportive. Promotion of oxygenation and ventilation is of utmost importance. Digitalis, diuretics, inotropic agents, vasodilators, antiarrhythmics, and antithrombotics have been widely used in children for palliation of symptoms. Many children with heart failure require management in the intensive care unit until they are stabilized. Augmenting nutrition and ensuring adequate rest are also key components of management.

Nursing Assessment

For a full description of the assessment phase of the nursing process, refer to the "Clinical Judgment and the

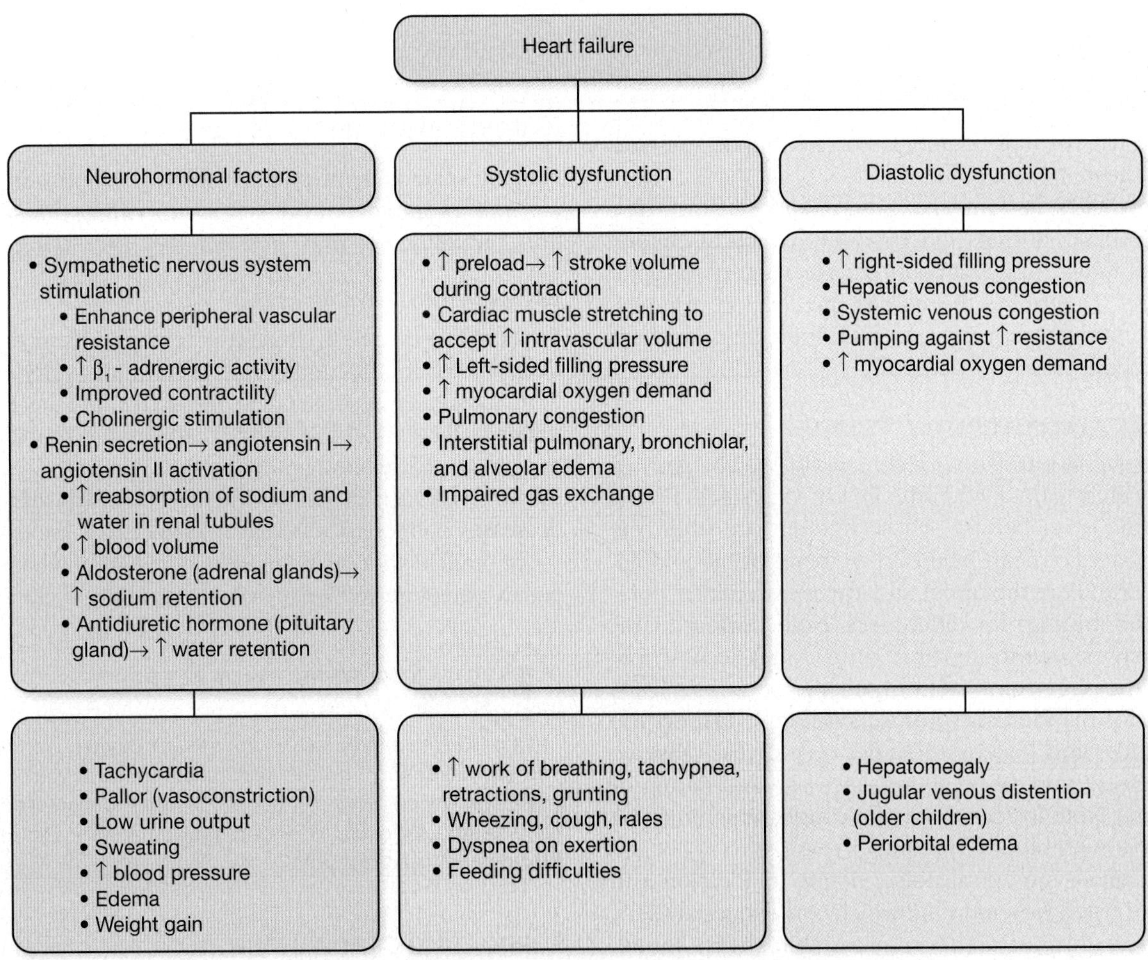

FIGURE 41.15 Pathophysiology of heart failure. (Data from Kusumoto, F. M. [2019]. Cardiovascular disorders: Heart disease. In G. D. Hammer & S. J. McPhee [Eds.], *Pathophysiology of disease: An introduction to clinical medicine* [8th ed.]. McGraw-Hill Education.)

Nursing Process" section earlier in the chapter. Specific assessment findings related to heart failure are discussed further on.

HEALTH HISTORY

When obtaining the health history, elicit a description of the present illness and chief complaint. Common complaints reported during the health history might include:

- Failure to gain weight or rapid weight gain
- Failure to thrive
- Difficulty feeding
- Fatigue
- Dizziness, irritability
- Exercise intolerance
- Shortness of breath
- Sucking and then tiring quickly
- Syncope
- Decreased number of wet diapers

Infants with heart failure often display subtle signs such as difficulty feeding and tiring easily. Pay close attention to reports of these problems from the parents. Also be alert for statements such as "The baby drinks a small amount of breast milk (or formula) and stops but then wants to eat again very soon afterwards;" "The baby seems to perspire a lot during feedings;" or "The baby seems to be more comfortable when he's sitting up or on my shoulder than when he's lying flat." In addition, the parents may report episodes of rapid breathing and grunting.

The child's current and past medical history also provide additional clues. Question the parents about any history of CHDs and treatments such as surgery to repair the defect. Determine the current medication regimen. Also ask about any recent or past infections, such as streptococcal infections or fever.

PHYSICAL EXAMINATION

Weigh the child and note recent rapid weight gain or lack of weight gain. Obtain the child's vital signs, noting tachycardia or tachypnea. These findings are often the first indicators of heart failure in an infant or older child. Measure the BP in the upper and lower extremities, comparing the findings for differences. Note decreased BP, which may be due to impaired cardiac muscle function. Inspect the skin color, noting pallor or cyanosis. Also observe for diaphoresis (profuse sweating). Inspect the face, hands, and lower extremities for edema. Observe for increased work of breathing, such as nasal flaring or retractions. Note the presence of a cough, which may be productive with bloody sputum.

Auscultate the apical pulse, noting its location and character. Listen for a murmur, which may suggest a CHD, a gallop rhythm, or an accentuated third heart sound, suggesting sudden ventricular distention. Auscultate the lungs, noting crackles or wheezes suggestive of pulmonary congestion. Palpate the peripheral pulses, noting weak or thready pulses. Note the temperature and color of the extremities; they may be cool, clammy, and pale. Assess the child's abdomen, looking for distention indicative of ascites. Gently palpate the abdomen to identify hepatomegaly or splenomegaly.

LABORATORY AND DIAGNOSTIC TESTS

The diagnosis of heart failure is based on the child's signs and symptoms and is confirmed with several laboratory and diagnostic tests. These include:

- Chest radiograph, revealing an enlarged heart and/or pulmonary edema
- ECG, indicating ventricular hypertrophy
- Echocardiogram, revealing the underlying cause of heart failure, such as a CHD

Other tests may be done to support the diagnosis. For example, the CBC count may show evidence of anemia or infection. Electrolyte levels may reveal hyponatremia secondary to fluid retention and hyperkalemia secondary to tissue destruction or impaired kidney function. Arterial blood gas results may demonstrate respiratory alkalosis in mild heart failure or metabolic acidosis. Tissue hypoxia may be evidenced by increased lactic acid and decreased bicarbonate levels.

Nursing Management

Nursing management of the child with heart failure focuses on promoting oxygenation, supporting cardiac function, providing adequate nutrition, and promoting rest.

PROMOTING OXYGENATION

Position the infant or child in a semi-upright position to decrease work of breathing and lessen pulmonary congestion. Suction as needed. Chest physiotherapy and postural drainage may also be beneficial. Administer supplemental oxygen as ordered and monitor oxygen saturation via pulse oximetry. Oxygen also serves the function of vasodilator and decreases pulmonary vascular resistance. Occasionally, the infant or child with heart failure may require intubation and positive-pressure ventilation to normalize blood gas tension.

CLINICAL REASONING ALERT!

In a child with a large left-to-right shunt, oxygen will decrease pulmonary vascular resistance while increasing the systemic vascular resistance, which leads to increased left-to-right shunting. Monitor the child carefully and use oxygen only as prescribed.

SUPPORTING CARDIAC FUNCTION

Administer digitalis, ACE inhibitors, and diuretics as prescribed. Digoxin therapy begins with a digitalizing dose divided into several doses (oral or IV) over a

24-hour period to reach maximum cardiac effect. During digitalization, monitor the ECG for a prolonged PR interval and decreased ventricular rate. Doses are then administered every 12 hours. Monitor the child for signs of digoxin toxicity. Measure BP before and after administration of ACE inhibitors, holding the dose and notifying the health care provider if the BP falls more than 15 mm Hg. Observe for signs of hypotension such as lightheadedness, dizziness, or fainting. Weigh the child daily to determine fluid loss. Maintain accurate records of intake and output, restricting fluid intake if ordered. Carefully monitor potassium levels, administering potassium supplements if prescribed. Sodium intake is not usually restricted in the child with heart failure.

PROVIDING ADEQUATE NUTRITION

Due to the increased metabolic rate associated with heart failure, the infant may require as much as 150 calories/kg/day. Older children will also require higher caloric intake than typical children. Offer small, frequent feedings if the child can tolerate them. During the acute phase of heart failure, many infants in particular will require continuous or intermittent gavage feeding to maintain or gain weight. Concentrate infant formula to 24 to 28 calories/oz as instructed by the nutritionist.

PROMOTING REST

Minimize metabolic needs to decrease cardiac demand. The infant or older child with heart failure will usually limit activities based on energy level. Ensure adequate time for sleep, and attempt to limit disturbing interventions. Provide age-appropriate activities that can be performed quietly or in bed, such as books, coloring or drawing, and video or board games. The older child or adolescent with significant heart failure may require home schooling. As the child improves, a rehabilitation program may be helpful for maximizing activity within the child's cardiovascular status limits.

Infective Endocarditis

Infective endocarditis is a microbial infection of the endothelial surfaces of the heart's chambers, septum, or valves (most common). Children with CHDs (septum or valve defects) or prosthetic valves are at increased risk for acquiring bacterial endocarditis, which is potentially fatal in these children. Other risk factors for endocarditis include central venous catheters and IV drug use. Infective endocarditis occurs when bacteria or fungi gain access to a damaged epithelium. Turbulence in blood flow associated with narrowed or incompetent valves or with a communication between the systemic and pulmonary circulation leads to damage of the endothelium. Thrombi and platelets then adhere to the endothelium, forming vegetations. When a microbe gains access to the bloodstream, it colonizes the vegetation, using the thrombi as a breeding ground. Clumps may separate from the vegetative patch and travel to other organs of the body, causing significant damage (septic emboli). Bacteria (particularly alpha-hemolytic streptococcus or *Staphylococcus aureus*) are the most common pathogens responsible for infective endocarditis, and, although rare, *Candida* species may also be found (O'Brien, 2023).

Complete antibiotic or antifungal treatment of the causative organism is necessary, and treatment generally lasts 4 to 6 weeks. Prevention of infective endocarditis in the susceptible child with CHD or a valvular disorder undergoing an invasive procedure is of the utmost importance (O'Brien, 2023).

Nursing Assessment

For a full description of the assessment phase of the nursing process, refer to "Clinical Judgment and the Nursing Process" section. Assessment findings related to endocarditis are discussed further on.

HEALTH HISTORY

Obtain the health history, noting intermittent, unexplained low-grade fever. Document history of fatigue, anorexia, weight loss, or flu-like symptoms (e.g., arthralgia, myalgia, chills, night sweats). Note history of CHD, valve disorder, or heart failure.

PHYSICAL EXAMINATION

Measure the child's temperature, noting low-grade fever. Observe for edema if heart failure is also present. Note petechiae on the palpebral conjunctiva, the oral mucosa, or the extremities. Inspect for signs of extracardiac emboli:

- Roth spots: splinter hemorrhages with pale centers on sclerae, palate, buccal mucosa, chest, fingers, or toes
- Janeway lesions: painless, flat, red or blue hemorrhagic lesions on the palms or the soles
- Osler nodes: small, tender nodules on the pads of the toes or fingers
- Black lines (splinter hemorrhages) under the nails (O'Brien, 2023)

Evaluate the ECG for a prolonged PR interval or dysrhythmias. Auscultate the heart for a new or changing murmur. Auscultate the lungs for adventitious breath sounds. Palpate the abdomen for splenomegaly.

LABORATORY AND DIAGNOSTIC TESTS

Diagnosis is usually based on the clinical presentation. Laboratory tests may reveal the following:

- Blood culture: bacteria or fungus
- CBC: anemia, leukocytosis
- Urinalysis: microscopic hematuria
- Echocardiogram: cardiomegaly, abnormal valve function, area of vegetation

Nursing Management

Nursing management focuses on maintaining IV access for at least 4 weeks to appropriately administer the antibiotic or antifungal course of therapy. Monitor the child's temperature and subsequent blood culture results.

Ideally, infective endocarditis in children should be prevented. Children at increased risk for the development of infective endocarditis include those with:

- Prosthetic cardiac valve or prosthetic material used for cardiac valve repair
- Previous endocarditis
- Unrepaired cyanotic CHD
- Completely repaired CHD with prosthetic material or device within the first 6 months after the procedure
- Repaired CHD with residual defects at the site or adjacent to the site of a prosthetic patch or prosthetic device
- Cardiac transplantation recipients who develop cardiac valve abnormalities (AHA, 2021)

Children at high risk should practice good oral hygiene, including regular toothbrushing and flossing. Instruct parents or the older child to carry emergency medical identification at all times (wallet card is available from the AHA). The card may be presented to any health care provider or nurse practitioner and includes the recommended antibiotic prophylactic regimen (AHA, 2024a). Instruct the parents to notify the primary care provider or cardiologist if the child develops flu-like symptoms or a fever.

High-risk children (as noted previously) who are undergoing dental procedures should receive prophylaxis as recommended by the AHA. Antibiotics typically used for prophylaxis may include ampicillin, amoxicillin, gentamicin, or vancomycin.

Acute Rheumatic Fever

Acute rheumatic fever (ARF) is a delayed sequela of group A streptococcal pharyngeal infection. In the United States, this disease occurs more often in school-age children between 5 and 15 years of age in areas where streptococcal pharyngitis is more prevalent, especially during the colder months. It usually develops 2 to 4 weeks after the initial streptococcal infection. Current understanding of the disease process of ARF is that the child develops an antibody response to surface proteins of the bacteria. The antibodies then cross-react with antigens in cardiac muscle and neuronal and synovial tissues, causing carditis, arthritis, and chorea (involuntary random, jerking movements). ARF affects the joints, central nervous system, skin, and subcutaneous tissue and causes chronic, progressive damage to the heart and valves. Most episodes of ARF resolve, but rheumatic fever may recur with subsequent streptococcal infections (Jone et al., 2022).

Diagnosis of ARF is based on the modified Jones criteria (Box 41.3). Therapeutic management is directed toward managing inflammation and fever, eradicating the bacteria, preventing permanent heart damage, and preventing recurrences. A full 10-day course of penicillin therapy (or equivalent) is used along with corticosteroids and nonsteroidal antiinflammatory drugs. Children without valvular disease will receive continued prophylaxis with monthly intramuscular injections of penicillin G benzathine or daily oral doses of penicillin or erythromycin following the initial illness to prevent a new streptococcal infection and recurrent ARF. Prophylaxis is usually continued until age 21 years (Jone et al., 2022).

Nursing Assessment

Elicit a description of the present illness and chief complaint, noting fever and joint pain. Explore the child's recent medical history for risk factors, such as documented streptococcal infection or sore throat within the past 2 to 3 weeks, or for history of ARF. Observe the child for Sydenham chorea, a movement disorder of the face and upper extremities. Inspect the skin for evidence of the classic rash, erythema marginatum, a maculopapular red rash with central clearing and elevated edges. Auscultate the heart, noting a murmur. Palpate the surfaces of the wrist, elbows, and knees for firm, painless, subcutaneous nodules. Note prolonged PR interval on the ECG. Throat culture will provide definitive diagnosis of current streptococcal infection, while streptococcal antibody tests may yield evidence of recent infection. Echocardiogram is required to determine if carditis is present.

Nursing Management

Nursing management of the child with ARF focuses on ensuring compliance with the acute course of antibiotics

BOX 41.3 Modified Jones Criteria

Diagnosis of ARF requires the presence of either two major criteria or one major plus two minor criteria.

Major Criteria

- Carditis
- Migratory polyarthritis
- Subcutaneous nodules
- Erythema marginatum
- Sydenham chorea

Minor Criteria

- Polyarthralgia
- Elevated ESR or CRP
- Prolonged PR interval (unless carditis is a major criterion)

ARF, acute rheumatic fever; CRP, C-reactive protein; ESR, erythrocyte sedimentation

Data from Jone, P.-N., Kim, J. S., Burkett, D., Jacobsen, R., & VonAlvensleben, J. (2022). Cardiovascular diseases. In M. Bunik, W. W. Hay, M. J. Levin, & M. J. Abzug (Eds.), *Current diagnosis and treatment: Pediatrics* (26th ed.). McGraw-Hill Education.

as well as prophylaxis following initial recovery from ARF. Allow the child to verbalize the frustration they may be feeling in relation to chorea symptoms. Offer support for dealing with the abnormal movements. Educate the child and others that the sudden jerky movements of chorea will eventually disappear, although they may last as long as several months. Some children may require a neuroleptic agent such as haloperidol (Haldol) for management of chorea. Administer corticosteroids or nonsteroidal antiinflammatory agents for control of joint pain and swelling.

Cardiomyopathy

Cardiomyopathy is a condition in which the myocardium cannot contract properly. The incidence of cardiomyopathy among children is increasing; it occurs at a rate of one per 100,000 (AHA, 2024b). Cardiomyopathy may occur in children with genetic disorders or CHDs, as a result of an inflammatory or infectious process or hypertension, or after cardiac transplantation or surgery, but most commonly, it is idiopathic. Cardiomyopathy occurs predominantly in clusters in infancy and adolescence. Three types of cardiomyopathy exist—restrictive, dilated, and hypertrophic. Restrictive cardiomyopathy is rare in children and results in atrial relaxation. Dilated cardiomyopathy is the most common type in childhood and may result in heart failure (it may be their presentation) because of ventricular dilation with decreased contractility (Jone et al., 2022). There is also some familial tendency toward dilated cardiomyopathy (Cooper, 2022). Hypertrophic cardiomyopathy is more common in adolescence and results in hypertrophy of the heart muscle, particularly the left ventricle, affecting the heart's ability to fill. About two-thirds of all cases of hypertrophic cardiomyopathy are familial, with some inherited in an autosomal dominant fashion (Cooper, 2022).

There is no cure for cardiomyopathy, meaning that currently, heart muscle function cannot be restored. Therapeutic management is directed toward improving heart function and BP. Mechanical ventilation and vasoactive medications are needed in many children. ACE inhibitors, beta-blockers, or calcium channel blockers may be used. Pacemakers or surgery may be helpful in some children. For children in whom medical management is unsuccessful, heart transplantation is the only viable long-term treatment option (Jone et al., 2022).

Nursing Assessment

Explore the health history for risk factors such as:

- CHD, cardiac transplantation, or surgery
- Duchenne or Becker muscular dystrophy
- History of myocarditis, HIV infection, or Kawasaki disease
- Hypertension
- Drugs, alcohol, or radiation exposure
- Connective tissue, autoimmune, or endocrine disease
- Maternal diabetes
- Familial history of sudden death

Inquire about a history of respiratory distress, fatigue, poor growth (dilated), chest pain, dizziness, or syncope (hypertrophic). Observe the child for extremity edema and abdominal distention. Note increased work of breathing. Auscultate the heart, noting tachycardia and irregular rhythm. Evaluate heart rhythm via ECG, noting dysrhythmias or indications of left ventricular hypertrophy.

Chest radiography may reveal cardiomegaly or congested lungs. Echocardiogram demonstrates increased heart size, poor contractility, decreased ejection fraction, or asymmetric septal hypertrophy. Cardiac catheterization is usually performed to aid in the diagnosis.

Nursing Management

Many children with cardiomyopathy require intensive care initially. Monitor for complications such as blood clots or arrhythmias, which could lead to cardiac arrest. Refer to the previous section on heart failure for nursing interventions related to heart failure, which may be present with dilated cardiomyopathy. Administer vasoactive and other medications as prescribed, monitoring the child closely for response to these therapies as well as for complications. Support the child in choosing activities that fit within the prescribed restrictions. Provide extensive emotional support to the child and family, who may experience significant stress as they realize the severity of this illness.

Hypertension

Hypertension has seen a rise in prevalence among children and adolescents. It has been found to be independently associated with body mass index and waist circumference. Childhood or adolescent hypertension often leads to long-term health consequences such as cardiovascular disease and left ventricular hypertrophy (Mattoo, 2023). In children, acceptable BP values are based on sex, age, and height. For children age 1 to 13 years, stage 1 hypertension is defined as BP persistently greater than or equal to the 95th percentile for sex, age, and height or less than the 95th percentile plus 12 mm Hg (whichever is lower). Stage 2 hypertension in children is identified as BP greater than or equal to the 95th percentile plus 12 mm Hg or 140/90, whichever is lower. For adolescents 13 years and older, stage 1 hypertension is defined as BP 130/80 to 139/89, while stage 2 hypertension is identified as BP greater than or equal to 140/90. The term "elevated blood pressure" refers to BP that is persistently between the 90th and 95th percentiles or 130/80 (whichever is lower) in children up to age 13 years. In adolescents 13 years of age or older, elevated BP refers to systolic blood pressure of 120 to 129, with diastolic BP less than 80. BP is considered normal when the systolic and diastolic values are less than the 90th percentile for sex, age, and height in the child 1 to 13 years of age or less than 120/80 in the adolescent 13 years and older (Flynn et al., 2017).

Childhood hypertension may be further defined as primary or secondary. Primary hypertension in children is found more commonly in non-Hispanic African Americans and children with overweight or obesity (Mattoo, 2023). Secondary hypertension in children most frequently occurs with an underlying medical problem such as kidney or cardiac disease (Mattoo, 2023). Mild to moderate hypertension in childhood is usually asymptomatic and is usually determined only upon BP screening during a well-child visit or during follow-up for known risk factors. Refer to Box 31.5 in Chapter 31 for a synopsis of childhood hypertension guidelines.

It is important to screen for and treat prehypertension and hypertension in children and adolescents, as they are more likely to experience hypertension as adults progressing to further cardiovascular disease (Mattoo, 2021). Therapeutic management depends on the extent of the hypertension and the length of time it has existed. Weight reduction, appropriate diet (including sodium restriction in some children), and increased physical activity are important components of management of prehypertensive and asymptomatic hypertensive children. Some children are candidates for and require antihypertensive medications or diuretics (Mattoo, 2021).

Pathophysiology

The balance between cardiac output and vascular resistance determines the BP. An increase in either of these variables, in the absence of a compensatory decrease in the other, increases the mean BP. Factors regulating cardiac output and vascular resistance include changes in electrolyte balance, particularly sodium, calcium, and potassium.

Nursing Assessment

Nursing assessment consists of the health history, physical examination, and laboratory and diagnostic tests.

HEALTH HISTORY

Elicit the health history, determining the presence of risk factors for hypertension such as:

- Family history
- Obesity
- Hyperlipidemia
- Kidney disease (including frequent urinary tract infections)
- Systemic lupus erythematosus
- CHD
- Neurofibromatosis, Turner syndrome, and other genetic disorders
- Prematurity
- Prolonged neonatal ventilation
- Umbilical artery catheterization
- Diabetes mellitus
- Increased intracranial pressure
- Malignancy
- Solid organ transplant
- Medications known to raise BP

Signs and symptoms reported during the health history might include:

- Growth delays (with certain chronic medical conditions)
- Obesity
- Signs and symptoms seen particularly in older children
- Headache
- Subtle behavioral or school performance changes
- Fatigue
- Blurred vision
- Nosebleed
- Bell palsy

PHYSICAL EXAMINATION

Determine the child's weight and height/length. Plot these growth parameters on the sex-appropriate chart for the child's age. Note the percentile for height/length, as it will be used to determine the BP percentile (see Appendix E, "Blood Pressure Charts for Children and Adolescents"). Measure the BP in all four extremities (to rule out coarctation of the aorta). Ensure that the child is relaxed and sitting or reclined. Refer to Chapter 32 for specific information related to accurate BP measurement in children.

Inspect the skin for:

- Acne, hirsutism, or striae (associated with anabolic steroid use)
- Café-au-lait spots (associated with neurofibromatosis)
- Malar rash (associated with lupus)
- Pallor, diaphoresis, or flushing (associated with pheochromocytoma)

Observe the extremities for edema (kidney disease) or joint swelling (lupus). Inspect the chest for apical heave (ventricular hypertrophy) or wide-spaced nipples (Turner syndrome). Auscultate heart sounds, noting tachycardia (associated with primary hypertension) or murmur (associated with coarctation of the aorta). Palpate the abdomen for a mass or enlarged kidney.

LABORATORY AND DIAGNOSTIC TESTING

Although diagnosis of hypertension is based on BP measurements, additional laboratory or diagnostic tests may be used to evaluate the underlying cause of secondary hypertension, including:

- Urinalysis, blood urea nitrogen, and serum creatinine: may determine the presence of kidney disease
- Renal ultrasound or angiography: may reveal kidney or genitourinary tract abnormalities
- Echocardiogram: may show left ventricular hypertrophy
- Lipid profile: determines the presence of hyperlipidemia

Nursing Management

Salt restriction and potassium or calcium supplements have not been scientifically shown to decrease BP in children. However, children with obesity may benefit from salt restriction, as those children seem to be sensitive to salt intake. Assist the child and family to develop a plan for weight reduction if the child has overweight or obesity. Encourage the child and family to control portion sizes, decrease the intake of sugary beverages and snacks, eat more fresh fruits and vegetables, and eat a healthy breakfast. Consult the nutritionist for additional assistance with meal planning. To increase physical activity, encourage the child to find a sport or type of exercise in which they are interested. Aerobic activities involving running, walking, or cycling are particularly helpful. When a child requires antihypertensive therapy, teach the child and family how to administer the medication. Caution the parents about side effects related to antihypertensives. Teach the parent to measure the child's BP as determined by the health care provider or nurse practitioner, as well as to keep appointments for BP follow-up.

Kawasaki Disease

Kawasaki disease is an acute systemic vasculitis occurring mostly in children 6 months to 5 years of age. It is the leading cause of acquired heart disease among children and in the United States, occurs more than 19 times per year per 100,000 children (Lo et al., 2025). Although Kawasaki disease affects all ethnic groups, it occurs more frequently in those of Asian or Pacific descent. It is a self-limited syndrome but can cause cardiovascular complications, such as coronary artery aneurysm and cardiomyopathy (Lo et al., 2025).

Therapeutic management of acute Kawasaki disease focuses on reducing inflammation in the walls of the coronary arteries and preventing coronary thrombosis. Chronic management of children developing aneurysms during the initial phase is directed toward preventing myocardial ischemia. In the acute phase, high-dose aspirin in four divided doses daily and a single infusion of intravenous immunoglobulin (IVIG) are used (Lo et al., 2025). See Evidence-Based Practice 41.1.

Pathophysiology

Although the etiology is still unknown, current thought is that some infectious organism (as yet unidentified) causes disease in genetically susceptible people. Kawasaki disease appears to be an autoimmune response mediated by cytokine-induced endothelial cell surface antigens that leads to vasculitis in the medium-size arteries, including the coronary arteries. Neutrophils, mononuclear cells, T lymphocytes, and immunoglobulin A–producing plasma cells infiltrate the vessels. Then, elastin and collagen fibers fragment, and the structural integrity of the vessel wall are impaired. Generalized systemic vasculitis occurs in the blood vessels throughout the body due to the inflammation and edema and can lead to coronary dilation or aneurysm. Some children never develop coronary artery changes, while others develop an aneurysm in either the acute phase or as a long-term sequela (Lo et al., 2025).

EVIDENCE-BASED PRACTICE 41.1

Treating Kawasaki Disease With Intravenous Immunoglobulin (IVIG)

STUDY

Coronary artery abnormalities remain the most serious complication of the acute vasculitis occurring in Kawasaki disease. Historically, IVIG of varying doses and other medications such as aspirin and corticosteroids have been used to reduce the risk of coronary artery anomaly (CAA) development. The study explored the use of IVIG in the acute phase. In their review, the authors included 31 studies with 4,609 participants.

Findings

It was determined that high-dose IVIG provided during the acute phase probably reduced the risk of development of CAA as compared to the use of moderate- or low-dose IVIG, aspirin, or corticosteroids. The occurrence of adverse effects was low for all treatment regimens.

Nursing Implications

The study results are consistent with the current recommendations for treatment of Kawasaki disease. Teach families that administration of IVIG is safe and that it is used to reduce the risk of CAA development. Refer to Chapter 47 for additional information related to IVIG administration.

Based on Broderick, C., Kobayashi, S., Suto, M., Ito, S., & Kobayashi, T. (2023). Intravenous immunoglobulin for the treatment of Kawasaki disease. *Cochrane Database of Systematic Reviews, 1*, CD014884. https://doi.org/10.1002/14651858.CD014884.pub2

Nursing Assessment

Nursing assessment consists of determining the health history, physical examination, and laboratory and diagnostic testing.

HEALTH HISTORY

Elicit the health history, noting any:

- Fever
- Chills
- Headache
- Malaise
- Extreme irritability
- Vomiting
- Diarrhea
- Abdominal pain
- Joint pain

Of note is a history of high fever (39.9°C [103.8°F]) of at least 5 days' duration that is unresponsive to antibiotics.

PHYSICAL EXAMINATION

Observe for significant bilateral conjunctivitis without exudate. Inspect the mouth and throat for dry, fissured lips; strawberry (cracked and reddened) tongue; and pharyngeal and oral mucosa erythema. Note hyperdynamic precordium. Evaluate the skin for:

- Diffuse, erythematous, polymorphous rash
- Edema of the hands and feet
- Erythema and painful induration of the palms and soles
- Desquamation (peeling) of the perineal region, fingers, and toes, extending to the palms and soles
- Possible jaundice

Palpate the neck for cervical lymphadenopathy (usually unilateral) and the joints for tenderness. Palpate the abdomen for liver enlargement. Auscultate the heart, noting tachycardia, gallop, or murmur.

LABORATORY AND DIAGNOSTIC TESTING

The CBC may reveal mild to moderate anemia, an elevated white blood cell count during the acute phase, and significant thrombocytosis (elevated platelet count [500,000 to 1 million]) in the later phase. The erythrocyte sedimentation rate (ESR) and the C-reactive protein (CRP) level are elevated. Echocardiogram is performed as soon as possible after the diagnosis is confirmed to provide a baseline of a healthy heart or to evaluate for coronary artery involvement. Echocardiograms may be repeated during the illness and as part of long-term follow-up. Occasionally, cardiac involvement warrants cardiac catheterization.

Nursing Management

In addition to the administration of aspirin and immunoglobulin, nursing management of the child with Kawasaki disease focuses on monitoring cardiac status, promoting comfort, and providing family education.

MONITORING CARDIAC STATUS

Administer IV and oral fluids as ordered, evaluating intake and output carefully. Prepare the child for the echocardiogram. Assess frequently for signs of developing heart failure such as tachycardia, gallop, decreased urine output, or respiratory distress. Evaluate quality and strength of pulses. Provide cardiac monitoring as ordered, reporting arrhythmias.

PROMOTING COMFORT

Provide acetaminophen for fever management, and apply cool cloths as tolerated. Keep the environment quiet, and cluster nursing care activities to decrease stimulation and hence irritability. Teach parents that irritability is a prominent feature of Kawasaki disease, and support their efforts to console the child. Apply petrolatum jelly or another lubricating ointment to the lips. Encourage the older child to suck on ice chips; the younger child may suck on a cool, moist washcloth. Popsicles are also soothing. Provide comfortable positioning, particularly if the child has joint pain or arthritis.

PROVIDING CHILD AND FAMILY EDUCATION

Teach parents to continue to monitor the child's temperature after discharge until the child has been afebrile for several days. Children with prolonged or recurrent fever may require a second dose of IVIG. Inform parents that irritability may last for up to 2 months after initial diagnosis with Kawasaki disease. Report any toxic effects of aspirin therapy, such as headache, confusion, dizziness, or tinnitus to the health care provider or nurse practitioner. It is important to avoid nonsteroidal antiinflammatory agents while aspirin therapy is ongoing. For children with continued arthritis (which resolves in several weeks), range-of-motion exercises with a morning bath may help to decrease stiffness. Instruct parents to avoid measles and varicella vaccination for 11 months after high-dose IVIG administration. It is critical that the family comply with regularly scheduled cardiology follow-up appointments to determine development or progression of coronary artery ectasia or aneurysm. If the child has severe cardiac involvement, teach the parents about infant and/or child cardiopulmonary resuscitation before discharge from the hospital.

Dyslipidemia

Dyslipidemia refers to high levels of lipids (fats/cholesterol) in the blood. High lipid levels are a risk factor for the development of atherosclerosis, which can result in coronary artery disease, a serious cardiovascular disorder occurring in adults. Children with high lipid levels, although remaining asymptomatic, are likely to have high levels as adults, which increases their risk for coronary artery disease. Therefore, detection, screening, and early intervention are important, especially if there is a family tendency toward heart disease (de Ferranti & Newburger, 2023b).

Pathophysiology

Cholesterol is a building block for hormones and cell membranes. It occurs naturally in foods derived from animals such as eggs, dairy products, meat, poultry, and seafood. Cholesterol is also manufactured in the body. Together, cholesterol and triglycerides are known as lipids. Very low–density lipoprotein (VLDL) is a lipoprotein composed mainly of triglycerides with only small amounts of cholesterol, phospholipid, and protein. VLDLs are easily converted to low-density lipoproteins (LDLs). Cholesterol is expressed in terms of LDL cholesterol or high-density lipoprotein (HDL) cholesterol. LDLs contain relatively more cholesterol and triglycerides than they do protein. HDLs contain about 50% protein, with the rest being cholesterol, triglyceride, and phospholipid. High levels of cholesterol and triglycerides place a person at risk for atherosclerosis. Elevated VLDL and LDL levels and decreased HDL levels produce a particular increase in the risk for atherosclerosis (de Ferranti & Newburger, 2023b).

Therapeutic Management

Screening children for hyperlipidemia is of prime importance for early detection, intervention, and subsequent prevention of adult atherosclerosis. The American Academy of Pediatrics recommends universal screening for dyslipidemia between 9 and 11 years of age and again between 18 and 21 years of age (Hagan et al., 2017). Performing a risk assessment screening at 24 months and at 4, 6, 8, and 12 through 17 years of age is also recommended. Selectively screening children at high risk for hyperlipidemia can reduce their lifelong risk of coronary artery disease. The risk assessment focuses on the child's family history. Screen if parents, grandparents, aunts and uncles, or siblings, have or have had documented:

- Coronary atherosclerosis
- Myocardial infarction
- Angina pectoris
- Peripheral vascular disease
- Cerebrovascular disease/stroke
- Coronary artery bypass graft/stent/angioplasty at less than 55 years of age in males and less than 65 years in females
- Sudden cardiac death
- Blood cholesterol level of 240 mg/dL or higher

The child should be screened at the health care provider's discretion if the parental history is unobtainable, the child has diabetes or hypertension, or the child has any lifestyle risk factors (cigarette smoking, obesity, sedentary lifestyle, or high-fat dietary intake) (de Ferranti & Newburger, 2023b).

All children should eat a diet with the appropriate amount of fats (see the section on nursing management further on) and should participate in physical activity. When diet and exercise are not enough to lower cholesterol to appropriate levels, medications such as statins may be used (Jone et al., 2022).

Nursing Assessment

Elicit the health history, noting risk factors such as family history of hyperlipidemia, early heart disease, hypertension, diabetes or other endocrine abnormality, cerebral vascular accident, or sudden death. Note prior lipid levels if available. Measure the child's height and weight, plotting them on standardized growth charts. Note if the child has overweight or obesity, as these are risk factors associated with hyperlipidemia. Typically, there are no other particular physical findings associated with hyperlipidemia. Table 41.3 gives details about the interpretation of cholesterol levels.

Nursing Management

Instruct families that the child must fast for 12 hours before lipid screening (initially and on follow-up samples). Dietary management is the first step in the prevention and management of hyperlipidemia in children older than 2 years. The diet should consist primarily of fruits, vegetables, low-fat dairy products, whole grains, beans, lean meat, poultry, and fish. As in adults, fat should account for no more than 30% of daily caloric intake. Fat intake may vary over a period of days, as many young children are picky eaters. Limit saturated fats by choosing lean meats; removing skin from poultry before cooking; and avoiding palm, palm kernel, and coconut oils as well as hydrogenated fats. Teach families to read nutrition labels to determine the content of the food. Limit intake of processed or refined foods as well as high-sugar drinks; these products provide minimal nutrition and significant

TABLE 41.3 • Interpretation of Cholesterol Levels for Children and Adolescents

Total Cholesterol (mg/dL)	Interpretation	LDL (mg/dL)	Interpretation	HDL (mg/dL)	Interpretation
<170	Desirable	<110	Optimal	35	Desirable
170–199	Borderline			110–129	Borderline
≥200	High			>130	High

HDL, high-density lipoprotein; LDL, low-density lipoprotein

Data from de Ferranti, S. D., & Newburger, J. W. (2023b). Dyslipidemia in children and adolescents: Definition, screening, and diagnosis. *UpToDate.* Retrieved January 12, 2024, from https://www.uptodate.com/contents/dyslipidemia-in-children-and-adolescents-definition-screening-and-diagnosis

calories. Children 5 to 10 years of age need vigorous play or physical activity for 1 hour per day, three times per week, while children older than 10 years of age should participate in vigorous activity 60 minutes daily (de Ferranti & Newburger, 2023a). Refer parents to "Healthy Habits for Healthy Kids—A Nutrition and Activity Guide for Parents" published by the American Dietetic Association and available at http://www.clocc.net/wp-content/uploads/Healthy_Habits_Healthy_Kids.pdf.

If medications are required, teach the child and family about the dose, administration, and possible adverse effects. Assist the family to develop a medication-dosing plan that is compatible with school and work schedules to increase compliance.

HEART TRANSPLANTATION

Heart transplantation is indicated in children with inoperable CHD or with end-stage heart disease related to cardiomyopathy or palliated CHD. Worldwide, 600 to 700 children receive a heart transplant each year (Bock & Chinnock, 2022). The 5-year survival rate is greater than 70%, and 20-year survival has been achieved in some instances (Bock & Chinnock, 2022).

A comprehensive evaluation is performed to determine whether the child is a candidate for heart transplant. The evaluation includes:

- Chest radiograph, ECG, echocardiogram, exercise stress test, cardiac catheterization, and pulmonary function tests
- CBC with differential, prothrombin and partial thromboplastin time, serum chemistries and electrolytes, blood urea nitrogen, and creatinine
- Urinalysis and urine creatinine clearance
- Blood, throat, urine, stool, and sputum cultures for bacteria, viruses, fungi, and parasites
- Epstein–Barr virus, cytomegalovirus, varicella, herpes, hepatitis, and HIV titers
- Human leukocyte antigen (HLA) typing and panel reactive antibody typing and titer
- Computed tomography or MRI scan and electroencephalogram
- Consults with neurology, psychology, genetics, social work, nutritionist, physical and occupational therapy, and financial coordinator or case manager (Bock & Chinnock, 2022)

Children with irreversible lung, liver, kidney, or central nervous system disease; recent malignancy (past 5 years); or chronic viral infection may be excluded as candidates.

Once candidacy is determined, the transplant center registers the child as a potential recipient with the United Network for Organ Sharing (UNOS). Blood type, body size, length of time on the waiting list, and medical urgency are used to evaluate compatibility. Children awaiting transplantation may need continuous or intermittent hospitalization. Coordination of organ procurement and the transplantation procedure is essential.

Surgical Procedure and Postoperative Therapeutic Management

Most transplantation procedures are **orthotopic**, which means that the recipient's heart is removed and the donor heart is implanted in its place in the normal anatomic position. Cardiopulmonary bypass and hypothermia are used to maintain circulation, protect the brain, and oxygenate the recipient during the procedure. Postoperatively, the child may have near-normal heart function and capacity for exercise and may be able to return to school.

Immunosuppressive therapy is necessary for the rest of the child's life to avoid rejection of the transplanted heart. Usually, a three-drug regimen is used that includes calcineurin inhibitors (cyclosporine, tacrolimus), cell toxins (mycophenolate mofetil, azathioprine), and corticosteroids. The cardiologist and transplant surgeon provide ongoing follow-up. Complications of heart transplantation include infection, pulmonary hypertension, arrhythmia, heart failure, hypertension, kidney dysfunction, and organ rejection. Neoplasm may occur as a result of chronic immunosuppression.

Nursing Management

Preoperative nursing care for the child undergoing a heart transplant is similar for children undergoing other types of heart surgery. In addition, the nurse should assist with the comprehensive pretransplant evaluation. Care for the child in the posttransplant period is intense and complex. Evaluate the family's ability to perform the tasks that will be necessary. Teach families about the evaluation and transplantation process, as well as the waiting period. In the immediate preoperative period, perform a thorough history and physical examination, and obtain last-minute blood work. Provide preoperative teaching similar to other cardiac surgeries. Older children, adolescents, and parents may enjoy the book *Future Conditional* by J. Hatton (1996, Yorkshire Art Circus), which was written by one of the first heart transplant survivors.

Postoperatively, provide frequent assessments and routine care for children who have had cardiac surgery. In addition, monitor the child closely for infection or signs of rejection. Acute rejection may be indicated by low-grade fever, fatigue, tachycardia, nausea, vomiting, abdominal pain, and decreased activity tolerance, although some children will be asymptomatic. Maintain strict handwashing techniques and isolate the child from other children with infections. Although live vaccines are contraindicated in children with immunosuppression, inactivated vaccines should be given as recommended (CDC, 2020). Teach children and families that the child may return to school and usual activities about 3 months after the transplant. Provide emotional support to the child related to body image changes such as hair growth, gum hyperplasia, weight gain, moon facies, acne, and rashes that occur due to long-term immunosuppressive therapy.

KEY CONCEPTS

- At birth, when the umbilical cord is cut and the neonate's first breath occurs, the ductus venosus closes with the foramen ovale, and the ductus arteriosus closes shortly thereafter. Pulmonary vascular resistance decreases, and systemic vascular resistance increases.
- The infant's heart rate averages 120 to 130 bpm and decreases throughout childhood, reaching the adult rate in adolescence. Conversely, the infant's and child's BP is significantly lower than the adult's, increasing as the child ages.
- Check the infant's apical pulse prior to digoxin administration, and hold the dose if the heart rate is less than 90.
- Poor weight gain, failure to thrive, and increased fatigability commonly occur with congestive heart failure.
- Clubbing of the fingernails occurs because of chronic hypoxia in the child with severe CHD.
- Children with cardiac conditions resulting in cyanosis often have baseline oxygen saturations that are relatively low, because of the mixing of oxygenated with deoxygenated blood.
- Document the presence of a murmur by grading its intensity (I through IV), describing where it occurs within the cardiac cycle, and noting the location where the murmur is best heard.
- CHD should be suspected in the cyanotic newborn who does not improve with oxygen administration.
- Cardiac catheterization postprocedure care focuses on evaluation of the child's vital signs and condition of the pressure dressing, as well as assessment of the distal pulses bilaterally for presence and quality.
- Congenital heart disorders resulting in decreased pulmonary blood flow (tetralogy of Fallot, tricuspid atresia) result in cyanosis.
- Disorders with increased pulmonary blood flow (PDA, ASD, and VSD) may result in pulmonary edema if the defect is severe.
- A decrease in the lower extremity pulses or BP as compared with the upper extremities may be indicative of coarctation of the aorta.
- It is important to remain calm when an infant or child demonstrates a hypercyanotic spell. Place the child in a knee-chest position, administer oxygen and/or morphine or propranolol, and supply IV fluids.
- Children with certain CHDs and/or heart failure require additional calories to display adequate growth.
- Children with hypertrophic cardiomyopathy, certain CHDs, valve dysfunction, or prosthetic valves require prophylaxis for infective endocarditis when undergoing procedures or invasive dental work.
- Hypertension in the child or adolescent often leads to long-term health consequences such as cardiovascular disease and left ventricular hypertrophy.
- Kawasaki disease may result in severe cardiac sequelae, so these children need ongoing cardiac follow-up to screen for development of problems.
- It is important to screen for hyperlipidemia in high-risk children.
- Abrupt cessation of chest tube output, accompanied by an increase in the heart rate and increased filling pressure, may indicate cardiac tamponade.

REFERENCES AND RECOMMENDED READINGS

Abbott. (2023). *Amplatzer septal occluder.* https://www.myamplatzer.com/hcp/congenital-heart-defect-solutions/ventricular-septal-defects-vsd/

Altman, C. A. (2022). Identifying newborns with critical congenital heart disease. *UpToDate.* Retrieved January 12, 2024, from http://www.uptodate.com/contents/identifying-newborns-with-critical-congenital-heart-disease

American Heart Association. (2021). *Infective endocarditis.* https://www.heart.org/en/health-topics/infective-endocarditis

American Heart Association. (2022). *Understand your risk for congenital heart defects.* https://www.heart.org/en/health-topics/congenital-heart-defects/understand-your-risk-for-congenital-heart-defects

American Heart Association. (2024a). *Infective endocarditis wallet card.* https://www.heart.org/en/health-topics/consumer-healthcare/order-american-heart-association-educational-brochures/infective-bacterial-endocarditis-wallet-card

American Heart Association. (2024b). *Pediatric cardiomyopathies.* https://www.heart.org/en/health-topics/cardiomyopathy/pediatric-cardiomyopathies

Beke, D., Jowa, M., & Rummell, M. (2021). *Nurse curriculum.* The Pediatric Cardiac Intensive Care Society.

Bock, M., & Chinnock, R. E. (2022). Pediatric heart transplantation. *Medscape.* Retrieved March 31, 2023, from http://emedicine.medscape.com/article/1011927-overview

Broderick, C., Kobayashi, S., Suto, M., Ito, S., & Kobayashi, T. (2023). Intravenous immunoglobulin for the treatment of Kawasaki disease. *Cochrane Database of Systematic Reviews, 1,* CD014884. https://doi.org/10.1002/14651858.CD014884.pub2

Centers for Disease Control and Prevention. (2020). *Who should not get vaccinated with these vaccines?* https://www.cdc.gov/vaccines/vpd/should-not-vacc.html

Centers for Disease Control and Prevention. (2022). *Long term outcomes in children with congenital heart disease.* https://www.cdc.gov/ncbddd/heartdefects/features/keyfinding-chd-longterm-outcomes.html

Children's Hospital of Wisconsin. (2024). *Living with a pediatric pacemaker.* https://childrenswi.org/medical-care/herma-heart/conditions/living-with-a-pacemaker

Cleveland Clinic. (2023). *Cardiac closure devices.* https://my.clevelandclinic.org/health/treatments/16838-cardiac-implant-closure-devices-in-adults

Cooper, L. T. (2022). Definition and classification of the cardiomyopathies. *UpToDate.* Retrieved January 12, 2024, from https://www.uptodate.com/contents/definition-and-classification-of-the-cardiomyopathies

Corbett, J. A., & Banks, A. D. (2019). *Laboratory tests and diagnostic procedures with nursing diagnoses* (9th ed.). Pearson Education Inc.

Cunningham, F. G., Leveno, S. L., Dashe, J. S., Hoffman, B. L., Spong, C. Y., & Casey, B. M. (2022). *Williams obstetrics* (26th ed.). McGraw-Hill Education.

de Ferranti, S. D., & Newburger, J. W. (2023a). Dyslipidemia in children and adolescents: Management. *UpToDate*. Retrieved January 12, 2024, from https://www.uptodate.com/contents/dyslipidemia-in-children-and-adolescents-management

de Ferranti, S. D., & Newburger, J. W. (2023b). Dyslipidemia in children and adolescents: Definition, screening, and diagnosis. *UpToDate*. Retrieved January 12, 2024, from https://www.uptodate.com/contents/dyslipidemia-in-children-and-adolescents-definition-screening-and-diagnosis

Doyle, T., & Kavanaugh-McHugh, A. (2023). Management and outcome of tetralogy of Fallot. *UpToDate*. Retrieved January 12, 2024, from http://www.uptodate.com/contents/management-and-outcome-of-tetralogy-of-fallot

Driscoll, D. (2022). History and physical examination. In R. E. Shaddy, D. J. Penny, T. F. Feltes, F. Cetta, & S. Mital (Eds.), *Moss and Adams' heart disease in infants, children, and adolescents: Including the fetus and young adult* (10th ed., pp. 243-250). Wolters Kluwer Health.

Fleitman, J. (2023). Postoperative complications among patients undergoing cardiac surgery. *UpToDate*. Retrieved January 12, 2024, from https://www.uptodate.com/contents/postoperative-complications-among-patients-undergoing-cardiac-surgery

Flynn, J. T., Kaelber, D. C., Baker-Smith, C. M., Blowey, D., Carroll, A. E., Daniels, S. R., de Ferranti, S. D., Dionne, J. M., Falkner, B., Flinn, S. K., Gidding, S. S., Goodwin, C., Leu, M. G., Powers, M. E., Rea, C., Samuels, J., Simasek, M., Thaker, V. V., Urbina E. M., & the Subcommittee on Screening and Management of High Blood Pressure in Children. (2017). Clinical practice guideline for screening and management of high blood pressure in children and adolescents. *Pediatrics, 140*(3), e20171904. https://doi.org/10.1542/peds.2017-1904

Gaskin, K., & Kennedy, F. (2019). Care of infants, children and adults with congenital heart disease. *Nursing Standard, 34*(8), 37–42. https://doi.org/10.7748/ns.2019.e11405

Hagan, J. F., Shaw, J. S., & Duncan, P. M. (Eds.). (2017). *Bright futures: Guidelines for health supervision of infants, children, and adolescents* (4th ed.). American Academy of Pediatrics.

Hueckel, R. M. (2019). Pediatric patient with congenital heart disease. *Journal for Nurse Practitioners, 15*(1), 118–124. https://doi.org/10.1016/j.nurpra.2018.10.017

Jone, P.-N., Kim, J. S., Burkett, D., Jacobsen, R., & VonAlvensleben, J. (2022). Cardiovascular diseases. In M. Bunik, W. W. Hay, M. J. Levin, & M. J. Abzug (Eds.), *Current diagnosis and treatment: Pediatrics* (26th ed., pp. 541-604). McGraw-Hill Education.

KidsHealth Medical Experts. (2023). *Cardiac catheterization*. https://kidshealth.org/en/parents/cardiac-catheter.html

Kimberlin, D. W., Barnett, E. D., Lynfield, R., & Sawyer, M. H. (Eds.). (2021). *Red book 2021-2024: Report of the committee on infectious diseases* (32nd ed.). American Academy of Pediatrics.

Kleinman, K., McDaniel, L., & Malloy, M. (2021). *The Harriet Lane handbook* (22nd ed.). Elsevier.

Kusumoto, F. M. (2019). Cardiovascular disorders: Heart disease. In G. D. Hammer & S. J. McPhee (Eds.), *Pathophysiology of disease: An introduction to clinical medicine* (8th ed.). McGraw-Hill Education.

Lo, M. S., Son, M. B. F., & Newburger, J. W. (2025). Chapter 208: Kawasaki disease. In R. M. Kliegman, J. W. St Geme, N. J. Blum, R. C. Tasker, K. M. Wilson, A. M. Schuh, & C. L. Mack, *Nelson textbook of pediatrics* (22nd ed., pp. 1540-1548). Elsevier.

Mattoo, T. K. (2021). Nonemergent treatment of hypertension in children and adolescents. *UpToDate*. Retrieved January 12, 2024, from https://www.uptodate.com/contents/nonemergent-treatment-of-hypertension-in-children-and-adolescents

Mattoo, T. K. (2023). Epidemiology, risk factors, and etiology of hypertension in children and adolescents. *UpToDate*. Retrieved January 12, 2024, from http://www.uptodate.com/contents/epidemiology-risk-factors-and-etiology-of-hypertension-in-children-and-adolescents

Nees, S. N., & Chung, W. K. (2020). Genetic basis of human congenital heart disease. *Cold Spring Harbor Perspectives in Biology, 12*(9), a036749. https://doi.org/10.1101/cshperspect.a036749

O'Brien, S. E. (2023). Infective endocarditis in children. *UpToDate*. Retrieved January 12, 2024, from https://www.uptodate.com/contents/infective-endocarditis-in-children

Oster, M. (2023). Newborn screening for critical congenital heart disease using pulse oximetry. *UpToDate*. Retrieved January 12, 2024, from https://www.uptodate.com/contents/newborn-screening-for-critical-congenital-heart-disease-using-pulse-oximetry

Peng, L. F. (2022). Pulmonic stenosis in infants and children: Clinical manifestations and diagnosis. *UpToDate*. Retrieved January 12, 2024, from https://www.uptodate.com/contents/pulmonic-stenosis-in-infants-and-children-clinical-manifestations-and-diagnosis

Schneider, D. S. (2023). The cardiovascular system. In K. J. Marcdante & R. M. Kliegman (Eds.), *Nelson's essentials of pediatrics* (9th ed.). Elsevier.

Singh, R. K., & Singh, T. P. (2022). Heart failure in children: Etiology, clinical manifestations, and diagnosis. *UpToDate*. Retrieved January 12, 2024, from https://www.uptodate.com/contents/heart-failure-in-children-etiology-clinical-manifestations-and-diagnosis

Soriano, B. D., & Fulton, D. R. (2022). Total anomalous pulmonary venous connection. *UpToDate*. Retrieved January 12, 2024, from https://www.uptodate.com/contents/total-anomalous-pulmonary-venous-connection

UCSF Benioff Children's Hospital. (2024). *Cardiac catheterization*. https://www.ucsfbenioffchildrens.org/education/cardiac_catheterization/

University of Pittsburgh Medical Center. (2024). *Heart catheterization*. https://www.chp.edu/our-services/heart/patient-procedures/catheterization

UpToDate, Inc. (2024). *UpToDate® Lexidrug™* (Version 8.2.0) [Mobile app]. Wolters Kluwer. https://apps.apple.com/us/app/lexicomp/id313401238

Weiner, G. M., Zaichkin, J., Kattwinkel, J., Byrne, B., Escobedo, M., Finan, E., Foglia, E., Goldsmith, J., Gupta, A., Halamek, L. P., Illuzi, J., Kapadia, V., Lakshminrusimha, S., Lee, H. C., Leone, T., Perlman, J. M., Rhein, M. D., Sawyer, T., Strand, M. L., … Olech Smith, M. J. (2021). *Textbook of neonatal resuscitation* (8th ed.). American Academy of Pediatrics.

DEVELOPING CLINICAL JUDGMENT

PRACTICING FOR NCLEX

1. The nurse is caring for a 5-year-old child with a congenital heart anomaly causing chronic cyanosis. When performing the history and physical examination, what is the nurse least likely to assess?
   a. Obesity from overeating
   b. Clubbing of the nail beds
   c. Squatting during play activities
   d. Exercise intolerance
2. A 2-day-old infant was just diagnosed with aortic stenosis. What is the most likely nursing assessment finding?
   a. Gallop and rales
   b. Blood pressure discrepancies in the extremities
   c. Right ventricular hypertrophy on ECG
   d. Heart murmur
3. Sam, age 11, has a diagnosis of rheumatic fever and has missed school for a week. What is the most likely cause of this problem?
   a. Previous streptococcal throat infection
   b. History of open heart surgery at 5 years of age
   c. Playing too much soccer and not getting enough rest
   d. Exposure to a sibling with pneumonia
4. The nurse is caring for a child after a cardiac catheterization. What is the nursing priority?
   a. Allow early ambulation to encourage activity participation.
   b. Check pulses above the catheter insertion site for strength and quality.
   c. Assess extremity distal to the insertion site for temperature and color.
   d. Change the dressing to evaluate the site for infection.
5. While assessing a 4-month-old infant, the nurse notes that the baby experiences a hypercyanotic spell. What is the priority nursing action?
   a. Provide supplemental oxygen by face mask.
   b. Administer a dose of IV morphine sulfate.
   c. Begin cardiopulmonary resuscitation.
   d. Place the infant in a knee-to-chest position.
6. The nurse is providing discharge instructions to the parent of a 2-month-old infant who has been prescribed digoxin to be administered every 12 hours orally. Which instructions should the nurse include in the discharge instructions? Select three items.
   a. Notify the health care provider or nurse practitioner if more than two consecutive doses are missed.
   b. Mix the medication with a small amount of formula or breast milk.
   c. If the infant demonstrates poor feeding or vomiting, notify the health care provider or nurse practitioner.
   d. If the child vomits immediately after administration, repeat the dose.
   e. As soon as it is noted that a dose has been missed, give the medication.
   f. Always give the medication at regular intervals.
7. An adolescent patient was admitted with a sore throat, a red rash on the trunk, swollen and painful joints, and aimless movements of the extremities. The diagnosis of ARF is made.

Vital Signs

Time	Temperature	Apical Heart Rate	Respiratory Rate	Blood Pressure
0800	38.0°C	94	22	110/80
1200	37.1°C	142	24	120/84

What should the nurse do first?
   a. Administer prescribed acetaminophen.
   b. Apply moisturizer to the adolescent's rash.
   c. Notify the health care provider or nurse practitioner of the vital signs change.
   d. Splint the affected joints to relieve pain.

DOSAGE CALCULATION QUESTION

The nurse is caring for an infant with a VSD who has heart failure. The infant weighs 11 lb. The medication order reads: spironolactone 5 mg PO every 12 hours. Spironolactone is provided by the pharmacy in a solution of 2.5 mg/1 mL. How many milliliters will the nurse administer? Round to the nearest whole number.

CRITICAL THINKING EXERCISES

1. A baby was born at 26 weeks' gestation to 15-year-old parents with substance use disorder. The infant weighed 1.5 kg at birth and was diagnosed with AV canal defect and Down syndrome. Discuss some of the major issues in planning for care. Include a care plan and a list of teaching needs for the family.
2. A 4-year-old has parents with less than a high school education, and the child has Medicaid coverage. Another child is 7 years old and has parents with advanced degrees and private insurance coverage. Both children need a heart transplant, and a heart is available that is a good match for both children. Discuss some of the issues involved in deciding which child should receive the heart.
3. A 13-year-old was diagnosed with hypertension more than 2 years ago. He is nonadherent to his antihypertensive medication regimen.

He is 5 ft tall and weighs 170 lb. His favorite activity is video games. Develop a teaching plan for this adolescent, providing creative approaches at the appropriate developmental level.

STUDY ACTIVITIES

1. Teach a class of sixth graders about healthy activities to prevent high cholesterol levels, hypertension, and heart disease. Use visual materials.
2. Spend the day with a nurse practitioner in the pediatric cardiology clinic. Report to the clinical group your observations about the children's quality of life, growth, and development.
3. Observe in the pediatric cardiothoracic intensive care unit or telemetry unit. Note the different cardiac rhythms displayed by children with a variety of cardiovascular disorders.

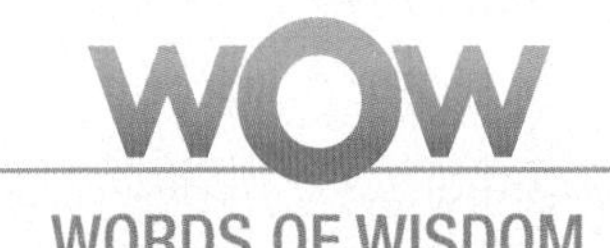

WORDS OF WISDOM

Children instinctively eat to live, and the nurse can help them devour the joys that life brings.

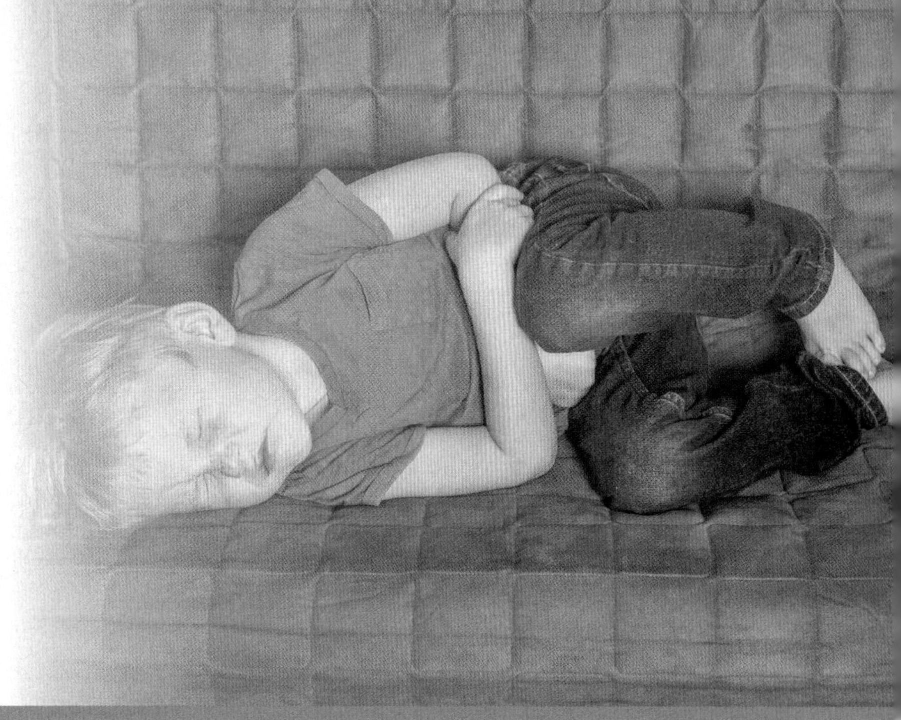

42

Nursing Care of the Child With an Alteration in Bowel Elimination/ Gastrointestinal Disorder

LEARNING OBJECTIVES

Upon completion of the chapter, you will be able to:

1. Compare the differences in the anatomy and physiology of the gastrointestinal system between children and adults.
2. Discuss common medical treatments for infants and children with alterations in bowel elimination (gastrointestinal disorders).
3. Distinguish common laboratory and diagnostic tests used to identify disorders of the gastrointestinal tract.
4. Discuss medication therapy used in infants and children with alterations in bowel elimination (gastrointestinal disorders).
5. Recognize risk factors associated with various gastrointestinal illnesses.
6. Differentiate between acute and chronic gastrointestinal disorders.
7. Distinguish common gastrointestinal illnesses of childhood.
8. Discuss nursing interventions commonly used for gastrointestinal illnesses.
9. Devise an individualized nursing care plan or concept map for infants/children with an alteration in bowel elimination/gastrointestinal disorder.
10. Develop teaching plans for family/child education for children with gastrointestinal illnesses.
11. Describe the psychosocial impact that chronic gastrointestinal illnesses have on children.

KEY TERMS

cholestasis (kō′lĕ-stā′sis)
dysphagia (dis-fā′jē-ă)
fecal impaction
guarding
icteric (ik-ter′ik)
lethargy
protuberant (prō-tū′bĕr-ănt)
rebound tenderness
regurgitation
steatorrhea (stē′ă-tŏr-ē′ă)

Ethan Richardson, 2 months old, is brought to the clinic by his birthing parent. He has been vomiting for the past 3 days. His birthing parent states that she switched the formula to see if that would help, but the vomiting worsened. Since last night she has attempted to feed him only Pedialyte. Mrs. Richardson says, "They can't keep anything down and they're very irritable." The weight at birth was 8 lb 9 oz, length 21 in, and head circumference 37 cm. At the 2-month checkup last week, the infant weighed 13 lb.

INTRODUCTION

Bowel elimination refers to the secretion and excretion of body waste through the intestinal system. Nurses may encounter children with alterations in bowel elimination and should be familiar with various gastrointestinal (GI) disorders that children experience. Alterations in bowel elimination or GI disorders affect children of all ages. GI illnesses range from acute to chronic and from non-life-threatening to life-threatening problems. However, even acute, non-life-threatening illnesses (e.g., diarrhea or vomiting) can become life threatening without proper nursing assessment and interventions. The most common result of a GI illness is dehydration, requiring fluid therapy at home, or in more extreme cases, in a hospital setting. It is important to take all GI disorders seriously until symptoms are well controlled.

Child and family education related to the treatment of GI disorders is often the key to preventing the illness from progressing to an emergency. Therefore, the nurse's knowledge of the disorders that affect the GI system is crucial. Most often, the parents or child, if the child is older, will contact the primary provider or nurse practitioner in an outpatient setting to seek help. The nurse is usually the person to triage the phone call to determine the next step in the situation, which may be determining whether the child should be managed at home, brought to the office for assessment, or sent directly to an emergency room for evaluation. Most GI disorders can be handled in an outpatient setting to avoid unnecessary hospitalizations. However, some life-threatening problems (e.g., bowel obstruction) require emergency care in the hospital. The knowledge base of the nurse is instrumental in obtaining the proper information by taking a thorough and accurate health history from the parents or child (if the child is older).

VARIATIONS IN PEDIATRIC ANATOMY AND PHYSIOLOGY

The GI tract includes all structures from the mouth to the anus. The primary functions of the GI system are the digestion and absorption of nutrients and water, elimination of waste products, and secretion of various substances required for digestion. Babies are born with immature GI tracts that are not fully mature until age 2. Due to this immaturity, there are many differences between the digestive tract of the young child and that of the older child or adult.

Mouth

The mouth is highly vascular, making it a common entry point for infectious invaders. In addition, infants and young children repeatedly bring objects to their mouths and explore them in that fashion. This behavior increases the infant's and young child's risk for contracting infectious agents via the mouth.

Esophagus

The esophagus provides a passageway from the mouth to the stomach for food. The lower esophageal sphincter (LES) prevents **regurgitation** (backflow) of stomach contents up into the esophagus and oral cavity. The muscle tone of the LES is not fully developed until age 1 month, so infants younger than 1 month frequently regurgitate after feedings. Many children younger than 1 year continue to regurgitate for several months, but this usually disappears with age. If edema or narrowing of the esophagus occurs in a child with undeveloped esophageal muscle tone, **dysphagia** (difficult or painful swallowing) may occur.

Stomach

Newborns have a stomach capacity of only 10 to 20 mL. At 2 months of age, an infant has the capacity to hold up to 200 mL, though most young infants cannot tolerate 200 mL feedings. By age 16, the stomach capacity is 1,500 mL; by adulthood, it is 2,000 to 3,000 mL. Hydrochloric acid, which is found in gastric contents to aid in digestion, reaches the adult level by the time the child is 6 months old.

Intestines

The small intestine is not functionally mature at birth. A full-term infant has approximately 250 cm of small intestine; an adult has up to 600 cm. Infants who have small bowel loss during early infancy have more problems with absorption and diarrhea than adults who have the same amount of small bowel loss.

Biliary System

The liver is relatively large at birth, allowing for the smooth edge of the liver to be easily palpated in infancy, as much as 2 cm below the costal margin. The pancreatic enzymes continue to develop postnatally, reaching adult levels around 2 years of age.

Fluid Balance and Losses

Compared with adults, children exhibit differences in how fluid volume is maintained. These differences are evident in body fluid balance and insensible fluid losses.

Body Fluid Balance

Infants and children have a proportionately greater amount of body water than do adults. Infants and young children require a larger relative fluid intake than adults and excrete a relatively greater amount of fluid. This places them at increased risk for fluid loss with illness compared to adults. Until age 2 years, the extracellular fluid, with its larger proportion of sodium and chloride, makes up about half of the child's total body water. Therefore, when potential fluid-loss states occur, water loss occurs more rapidly and in larger amounts than in adults.

Insensible Fluid Losses

Fever increases fluid loss at a rate of about 7 mL/kg/24-hour period for every sustained 1°C rise in temperature. Since children become febrile with illness more readily and their fevers are higher than those of adults, infants and young children are more apt than adults to experience insensible fluid loss with fever when ill.

Fluid loss via the skin accounts for about two thirds of insensible fluid loss. Infants have a larger body surface area (BSA) relative to their body mass as compared to older children and adults. The newborn's BSA ratio to body mass is about two or three times greater than the adult's, and the preterm infant's is about five times greater than the adult's. This places infants, especially young infants, at increased risk of insensible fluid loss as compared to older children and adults.

The basal metabolic rate in infants and children is higher than that of adults to support growth. This higher metabolic rate, even in states of wellness, accounts for increased insensible fluid losses and increased need for water for excretory functions. The young infant's renal immaturity does not allow the kidneys to concentrate urine as well as in older children and adults. This puts infants at risk for dehydration or overhydration, depending on the circumstances.

COMMON MEDICAL TREATMENTS

There are many different forms of medical treatment for GI disorders. In the hospital setting, most medical treatments will require a primary provider's order. The most common treatments and medications used for GI disorders are listed in Common Medical Treatments 42.1 and Drug Guide 42.1. Both boxes provide essential information about medical treatments and medications used in pediatric GI disorders. Refer to these boxes as needed while completing the remainder of the chapter.

COMMON MEDICAL TREATMENTS 42.1 GI Disorders

Treatment	Explanation	Indications	Nursing Implications
Cleansing enema	Insertion of fluid into the rectum to soften the stool and stimulate bowel activity	Fecal impaction, severe constipation	Explain the procedure to the child before enema. With multiple enemas, observe for electrolyte imbalances.
Bowel preparation	Use of highly osmotic fluids to induce severe diarrhea to cleanse the entire bowel	Preparation for colonoscopy or bowel surgery	Some children may need to have a nasogastric tube placed so they can consume the needed amounts of fluids. Observe for signs and symptoms of dehydration/electrolyte imbalance.
Feeding tubes	Flexible tubes used for enteral feeding when the infant or child is incapable of swallowing safely or for augmenting nutrition. May be orogastric, nasogastric, gastrostomy, or jejunostomy	Feeding difficulties, failure to thrive, gastroesophageal reflux disease (GERD), chronic illness	Orogastric and nasogastric tubes must be checked for placement before each use. If required long term, use a softer, flexible tube intended for long-term use. Stomahesive® or DuoDERM® applied to the cheek may decrease the risk of skin breakdown from tape. Gastrostomy tubes vary in type. Keep the insertion site clean and dry.
IV therapy	Administration of fluids via a catheter that delivers electrolytes and fluids into the venous system	Dehydration, bowel rest, NPO status	Monitor the IV site for redness, swelling, and pain. Assess urine output to evaluate hydration status.

(continued)

COMMON MEDICAL TREATMENTS 42.1 GI Disorders (*continued*)

Treatment	Explanation	Indications	Nursing Implications
Ostomy	A portion of the intestine is brought to the level of the skin to allow passage of stool.	Imperforate anus, gastroschisis, omphalocele, Hirschsprung disease, necrotizing enterocolitis, Crohn disease, ulcerative colitis	Ostomy contents may be acidic and irritate the skin. Use Stomahesive® or DuoDERM® under the pouch to avoid tape irritation to the skin. Pouch should fit the stoma correctly. Assess stoma for pinkness and moist appearance.
Oral rehydration therapy	Administration by mouth of fluids that contain certain amounts of electrolytes and glucose to prevent dehydration and promote rehydration	Diarrhea, acute gastroenteritis, vomiting	Fluid administration should begin before the onset of dehydration. Urine output should be monitored to evaluate hydration status.
Probiotics (lactobacillus, acidophilus)	Food supplements containing dormant bacteria that when activated may alter the intestinal microflora.	Treatment/prevention of diarrhea	Particularly helpful in the prevention of or decreasing the incidence of antibiotic-induced diarrhea
Total parenteral nutrition (TPN)	IV complete nutrition. Provides glucose, protein, lipids, vitamins, and minerals	Long-term NPO status, swallowing difficulties, difficulties tolerating enteral feeding (short bowel syndrome, necrotizing enterocolitis)	Higher glucose and protein concentrations and solutions containing calcium require central venous access. Monitor blood glucose levels with initiation, rate changes, and discontinuation. Blood chemistries should be monitored on a regular basis.

GI, gastrointestinal; IV, intravenous; NPO, nothing by mouth

DRUG GUIDE 42.1

COMMON DRUGS FOR GI DISORDERS

Classification	Actions/Indications	Nursing Implications
Histamine-2 blockers (ranitidine, famotidine, cimetidine, nizatidine)	Decrease histamine production, thereby reducing gastric acid secretion Used for heartburn, esophagitis, GERD, benign duodenal or gastric ulcers	May cause drowsiness or dizziness
Proton-pump inhibitors (omeprazole, lansoprazole, esomeprazole, pantoprazole, rabeprazole)	Block the pump that produces gastric acids. Indicated for erosive esophagitis, symptomatic GERD, *Helicobacter pylori* eradication	Adverse effects include headache, nausea, abdominal pain, or diarrhea.
Prokinetics (metoclopramide, cisapride)	Stimulate GI motility to help empty the stomach faster and promote intestinal motility.	Metoclopramide may have central nervous system adverse effects. Cisapride is available only in limited-access protocol studies.
Antibacterials/antibiotics (metronidazole, vancomycin)	Treatment of bacterial infections of the GI tract Used for suspected or proven bacterial infections of the GI tract, such as *Clostridium difficile* or parasitic infections	May cause GI upset, diarrhea. Very important to finish the entire course of treatment
Immunosuppressants (6-mercaptopurine [6-MP], azathioprine)	Suppress the immune system to keep autoimmune disorders in remission such as Crohn disease, ulcerative colitis, autoimmune hepatitis.	Drug levels should be checked to determine drug metabolite levels and potential for hepatotoxicity or bone marrow suppression.
Stimulants (senna, docusate sodium)	Stimulate peristalsis in the large intestine to produce a bowel movement. Used to relieve constipation	May cause cramping or diarrhea. Stool patterns should be constantly assessed.
Laxatives (polyethylene glycol, milk of magnesia, lactulose)	Soften the stool to allow for easier passage through the colon. Used to relieve constipation	Stool patterns should be monitored. Doses may need to be readjusted frequently to find the correct dose for the child.

DRUG GUIDE 42.1

COMMON DRUGS FOR GI DISORDERS

Classification	Actions/Indications	Nursing Implications
Antidiarrheals (loperamide, diphenoxylate/atropine)	Decrease peristalsis, thus prolonging the transit time of stool through the intestines. Indicated to treat diarrhea related to short bowel syndrome, chronic nonspecific diarrhea, IBS	May cause drowsiness or constipation
Corticosteroids (prednisone)	Act systemically to reduce inflammation and suppress the normal immune response. Used in IBD, autoimmune disorders	Systemic adverse effects include hirsutism, osteoporosis, GI upset, cushingoid appearance, increased intraocular pressure, irritability, and personality changes. Should be taken as directed. Stopping the medication suddenly may cause adrenal insufficiency.
Antiemetics (promethazine, metoclopramide)	Act on the central nervous system transmitters to prevent nausea and vomiting.	May have central nervous system adverse effects, such as drowsiness or irritability
Anticholinergic/antispasmodics (hyoscyamine, dicyclomine, glycopyrrolate)	Used to control abdominal spasms and cramping associated with IBS, functional bowel disorders	May cause excessive thirst or dizziness. Encourage plenty of fluids while taking these medications.
Antiinflammatories (mesalamine, balsalazide, hydrocortisone enemas/suppositories, olsalazine, sulfasalazine)	Reduce inflammation in the colon associated with ulcerative colitis, proctitis.	Stool output should be monitored to assess for the presence of oral medications (indicating poor absorption).

"GERD, gastroesophageal reflux disease; GI, gastrointestinal; IBD, inflammatory bowel disease; IBS, irritable bowel syndrome

Source: UpToDate, Inc. (2024). *Lexi-comp*® (Version 8.1.2) [Mobile app]. Wolters Kluwer. https://apps.apple.com/us/app/lexicomp/id313401238

Clinical Judgment and the Nursing Process

Nursing care of the child with a GI disorder or alteration in bowel elimination includes nursing assessment, nursing analysis, planning, interventions, and evaluation. It is important to individualize each step of this process for each child.

Assessment

The assessment of the child with a GI disorder includes a health history, physical examination, and laboratory and diagnostic testing.

Health History

A thorough health history is very important in the assessment of a child with a GI disorder. In the health history, include past history (previous illnesses/surgeries), past family history, present illness (when the symptoms began and how this differs from the child's normal status), and how the child's symptoms have been managed up to this point (relevant medical records/home treatments). Determine the child's historical growth patterns. Assess the family history to identify common genetic or familial GI symptoms or disorders such as irritable bowel syndrome (IBS), inflammatory bowel disease (IBD), or food allergies. Details within the history of the present illness can often distinguish chronic problems from acute disorders. Ask descriptive questions of the child and family.

Physical Examination

Perform the physical examination of the child from the least invasive part of the examination to the most invasive. It is important for the child to remain as relaxed as possible during this part of the assessment.

Inspection and Observation

Inspect and observe the child's color, hydration status, abdominal size and shape, and mental status.

Color. First observe the child's skin, eye, and lip color, as pallor may be a sign of anemia or dehydration. Note the presence of jaundiced skin or **icteric** (yellowed in color) sclerae which indicate elevated bilirubin levels related to liver dysfunction. Inspect the abdomen for distended veins, indicating abdominal or vascular obstruction or distention. As in any part of a physical assessment, watch for areas of ecchymosis (bruising), which may be a sign of abuse.

Hydration Status. Carefully assess the child's hydration status as it may indicate how severe the current GI illness is. Decreased turgor and skin turgor tenting indicate dehydration. During crying, especially in infants, the absence of tears may indicate dehydration. Assess the amount of urine output the child has had in the past 24 hours.

Abdominal Size and Shape. Inspect the size and shape of the abdomen while the child is standing and while the child is lying supine. The abdomen should be flat when the child is supine. An especially **protuberant** (bulging outward) abdomen suggests the presence of ascites, fluid retention, gaseous distention, or even a tumor. A depressed or concave abdomen could indicate a high abdominal obstruction or dehydration. Inspect the umbilicus for color, odor, discharge, inflammation, and herniation.

Mental Status. Perform a brief mental status examination as mental status changes can occur with severe dehydration, anaphylactic reactions to foods or medicines, and elevated ammonia levels. Irritability and restlessness are usually the early signs of mental status changes. **Lethargy** (sluggishness or abnormal drowsiness) and listlessness can occur much more rapidly in children than in adults. It is important to identify this promptly and treat it emergently.

Auscultation

Auscultate bowel sounds in all four quadrants. Hyperactive bowel sounds may be noted in children with diarrhea or gastroenteritis. Hypoactive or absent bowel sounds may signify an obstructive process. The nurse can determine the absence of bowel sounds after a 5-minute period of auscultation. This can be extremely difficult to perform with children and infants, who may be uncooperative during the examination.

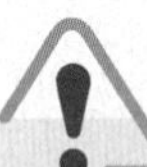

CLINICAL REASONING ALERT!

Immediately report hypoactive or absent bowel sound findings to the primary provider or nurse practitioner.

Percussion

Percuss the abdomen to reveal the normal finding of dullness or flatness along the right costal margin and 1 to 3 cm below the costal margin of the liver. The area above the symphysis pubis may be dull in young children with full bladders, which is a normal finding. Percussion of the remainder of the abdomen should reveal tympany. Note any abnormal findings.

Palpation

Reserve palpation for last in the sequence of abdominal examination. First, lightly palpate the abdomen to assess for areas of tenderness, lesions, muscle tone, turgor, and cutaneous hyperesthesia (a finding in acute peritonitis). Then perform deep palpation from the lower quadrants upward to best feel the liver edge, which should be firm and smooth. In infants and children, palpate the liver during inspiration below the right costal margin. The tip of the spleen may be palpated also during inspiration; it should be 1 to 2 cm below the left costal margin. Palpable kidneys, except in neonates, may indicate tumor or hydronephrosis. The sigmoid colon can be palpated in the left lower quadrant. The cecum may be felt in the right lower quadrant as a soft mass. Areas of firmness or masses may indicate tumors or stool in the abdomen.

Tenderness in the abdomen is not a normal physical finding. Right upper quadrant tenderness could indicate liver enlargement. Right lower quadrant pain, including **rebound tenderness** (pain upon release of pressure during palpation), can be a warning sign of appendicitis; immediately report any positive findings to a primary provider. Palpate the external inguinal canals for the presence of inguinal hernias, often elicited by having the child turn the head and cough or blow up a balloon.

Laboratory and Diagnostic Testing

Common Laboratory and Diagnostic Tests 42.1 gives information about the tests most often ordered by primary providers for children with GI illnesses. Some of these tests are ordered in the hospital setting; others are done on an outpatient basis. Typically, the nurse may be directly involved in specimen collection while a specifically trained person performs the diagnostic tests. Regardless of who performs the test, nurses must be familiar with preparation guidelines for the child, how each test is performed, and normal and abnormal findings and their significance to provide appropriate child and family education. Box 42.1 gives tips on collecting stool specimens.

Remember Ethan, the 2-month-old with vomiting and irritability? What additional health history and physical examination assessment information should you obtain?

Nursing Analysis, Goals, Interventions, and Evaluation

After recognizing and analyzing cues from a thorough assessment, the nurse may identify patient problems, including:

- Dehydration risk
- Diarrhea
- Constipation
- Malnutrition risk

BOX 42.1 Stool Specimen Collection Variations

- If the child is in diapers, use a tongue blade to scrape a specimen into the collection container.
- If the child has a runny stool, a piece of plastic wrap in the diaper may catch the stool specimen. Very liquid stool may require the application of a urine bag to the anal area to collect the stool.
- The older ambulatory child may first urinate in the toilet, and then the stool specimen may be retrieved from the new or clean collection container that fits under the seat at the back of the toilet.
- For the bedridden child, collect the stool specimen from a clean bedpan (do not allow urine to contaminate the stool specimen).
- Send the specimen to the laboratory immediately for accuracy of results.

COMMON LABORATORY AND DIAGNOSTIC TESTS 42.1

Test	Explanation	Indications	Nursing Implications
Abdominal ultrasonography	Visualizes abdominal organs and related vessels	Abdominal pain, vomiting, pregnancy, abnormal liver tests, abdominal mass, enlarged organs on palpation	Barium decreases the visualization of organs on ultrasound.
Abdominal radiograph (KUB [kidneys, ureters, and bladder])	Plain radiograph of the abdomen without contrast media	Constipation, abdominal pain, abdominal distention, ascites, foreign body, palpable mass	Usually ordered as flat and upright to allow for free air and fluid levels in the bowel to be detected
Amylase (serum)	An enzyme that changes starch to sugar, which enters the blood with inflammation of the pancreas	Acute pancreatitis, pancreatic trauma, acute cholecystitis	Increased levels are seen after 3–6 hours of the onset of abdominal pain.
Barium enema	After the instillation of barium, it fluoroscopically allows visualization of the colon.	Constipation, rectal prolapse, bleeding, suspected intussusception	Bowel preparation before the examination may be ordered. Stool will be light colored due to barium for a few days.
Electrolytes (serum)	Sodium, potassium, CO_2, chloride, blood urea nitrogen (BUN), creatinine	To determine the extent of dehydration	BUN and creatinine may be elevated with dehydration. Sodium, potassium, chloride, and CO_2 levels can be greatly affected with dehydration.
Barium swallow/upper gastrointestinal (GI) series	Visualizes the form, position, mucosal folds, peristaltic activity, and motility of the esophagus, stomach, and upper GI tract	Foreign body ingestion, abdominal pain, vomiting, dysphagia, malrotation	Females of reproductive age must be screened for pregnancy. Infants may need to be given barium via a syringe.
Small bowel series	Done in conjunction with upper GI series to visualize the small intestine contour, position, and motility.	Suspected inflammatory bowel disease (IBD) (bowel wall thickening), intussusception	Very important to encourage large amounts of water/fluids after the test to avoid barium-induced constipation.
Endoscopic retrograde cholangiopancreatography (ERCP)	A fiberoptic endoscope is used to view the hepatobiliary system by instilling contrast to outline the pancreatic and common bile ducts.	Pancreatitis, jaundice, pancreatic tumors, common duct stones, biliary tract disease	Monitor for infection, urinary retention, cholangitis, or pancreatitis after the procedure. Done only occasionally in children.
Esophageal manometry	Tests the esophagus for normal contractile activity and effectiveness of swallowing by measurement of intraluminal pressures and acid sensors	Abnormal esophageal muscle function, dysphagia, chest pain of unknown cause, esophagitis, vomiting	Often done in conjunction with a pH probe. The manometric catheter is placed through the nose into the esophagus. May cause nasal irritation/sore throat
Esophageal pH probe	A single- or double-channeled probe placed into the esophagus to monitor the pH of the contents that are regurgitated into the esophagus from the stomach	Vomiting, gastroesophageal reflux (GER), correlation of symptoms to GER events, and high risk for problems, as in asthma, apparent life-threatening event, sinusitis, or choking/gagging episodes	24-hour study is the most accurate. Special diet during study is often used. Accurate diary of symptoms and feedings during the study is essential. May cause nasal irritation/sore throat
Gastric emptying scan	Assesses the rate at which the stomach empties food into the small intestine by adding isotopes to food and visualizing with scans	Unexplained nausea, vomiting, diarrhea, abdominal cramping	Medications may alter gastric emptying times. Crying or stress during the examination may cause a delay in emptying and should be documented.
Hemoccult	Checks for occult blood in the stool	Crohn disease, ulcerative colitis, malabsorption syndromes, diarrhea, abdominal pain	Indicates bleeding in the GI tract
Hepatobiliary scan (HIDA [hepatobiliary iminodiacetic acid] scan)	Visualizes the gallbladder and determines patency of the biliary system by use of a radionuclide. The amount of radionuclide ejected from the gallbladder (ejection fraction) is calculated.	Differentiate between biliary atresia and neonatal hepatitis; assess liver trauma, right upper quadrant pain, and congenital malformations.	Intravenous (IV) line will be established to give radionuclides. Pain during injection should be assessed and documented.

(continued)

COMMON LABORATORY AND DIAGNOSTIC TESTS 42.1 (*continued*)

Test	Explanation	Indications	Nursing Implications
Lactose tolerance test	After ingesting lactose, this tests the hydrogen levels in the breath, which will increase with lactose buildup in the intestines.	Postprandial diarrhea, gassiness, bloating, abdominal pain	May produce similar symptoms during the test itself. A positive test will require diet modification and education regarding lactose intolerance.
Lipase (serum)	An enzyme that changes fat to fatty acids and glycerol appearing in the blood with pancreatic change	Pancreatitis, pancreatic carcinoma, cholecystitis, peritonitis	Lipase levels stay elevated longer with acute pancreatitis.
Liver biopsy	A test done to evaluate the microscopic hepatic structures	Hyperbilirubinemia, jaundice, chronic liver disease, hepatitis	Monitor after procedure for bleeding complications; must maintain strict bed rest for up to 8 hours
Liver function tests (LFTs) (AST [aspartate aminotransferase]/ALT [alanine aminotransferase]/GGT [gamma-glutamyl transferase])	Enzymes that have high concentrations in the liver	Elevations may indicate the severity of liver disease.	May be affected by drugs or viral illnesses
Lower endoscopy (colonoscopy)	Allows visualization and biopsies of the lower GI tract from the anus to the terminal ileum with a fiberoptic instrument	Rectal bleeding, lower abdominal pain, suspected tumors or strictures, foreign body removal	The child must undergo a bowel cleansing before the examination. Encourage fluids to prevent dehydration. Conscious sedation or anesthesia care; monitor for possible complications of perforation, bleeding, and increased abdominal pain.
Meckel scan	A gamma camera is used to identify gastric mucosa seen in the distal portion of the ileum after injection of radiopharmaceuticals.	Rectal bleeding, anemia, used only to identify a Meckel diverticulum	Gloves are worn by nurses during and after scans when radiopharmaceuticals are given.
Oropharyngeal motility study (OPMS)	A study done with different textures to evaluate the dynamics of swallowing and reveal transient abnormalities	Dysphagia, recurrent aspiration	Usually done in combination with therapists and nutritionists
Rectal suction biopsy	Biopsy is taken of the rectum at different levels to assess for the presence of ganglion cells.	Absence of ganglion cells indicates Hirschsprung disease.	Infants/children should be assessed for rectal bleeding after examination.
Stool culture	Stool is smeared on a culture medium and assessed for the growth of bacteria over a period of days.	To determine the bacterial cause of diarrhea	Requires a minimum of 48 hours for growth, several days to weeks in some cases. Can be done with a small amount of stool
Stool for ova and parasites (O&P)	Checks for the presence of parasites or their eggs in the stool	To determine the cause of diarrhea or abdominal pain	Requires about two tablespoons of stool
Upper endoscopy (EGD [esophagogastroduodenoscopy])	Allows visualization and biopsies of the upper GI tract (mouth to upper jejunum) with a fiberoptic instrument	Dysphagia, foreign body removal, epigastric/abdominal pain, suspected celiac disease	Conscious sedation or anesthesia care; monitor for complications of perforation/bleeding.
Urea breath test	Used to detect the presence of *Helicobacter pylori* in the exhaled breath	*H. pylori* infection	Child must not take proton-pump inhibitors for 5 days, all antibiotic therapy and Pepto-Bismol for 14 days.

Data from Corbett, J. A., & Banks, A. D. (2019). *Laboratory tests and diagnostic procedures with nursing diagnoses* (9th ed.). Pearson Education Inc.; CHOC Children's. (2024). *Stool tests.* https://www.choc.org/programs-services/gastroenterology/digestive-disorder-diagnostics/stool-tests/

- Altered skin integrity risk
- Altered breathing pattern
- Altered body image perception
- Pain
- Interrupted family processes
- Caregiver role strain risk
- Knowledge deficiency

After completing an assessment on Ethan, you note the following: weight 10 lb, length 23.5 in, head circumference 40.75 cm. Head is round with sunken anterior fontanel, eyes appear sunken, mucous membranes are dry, heart rate 158, breath sounds clear with a respiratory rate of 42, positive bowel sounds in all four quadrants, difficulty palpating abdomen due to crying. Based on these assessment findings, what would your top three issues or concerns be for Ethan?

The above patient problems provide suggestions for nursing care planning or concept mapping. Suggested interventions with rationales are provided later. Care planning should be individualized, based on the child's and family's needs. Refer to Chapter 36 for the nursing process for pain management and to Chapter 33 for nursing interventions related to interrupted family processes and caregiver role strain risk. Additional information will be included later in the chapter as it relates to nursing management of children with specific disorders, as well as particular nursing interventions for lack of knowledge.

Nursing Analysis

Dehydration risk; risk factors include vomiting, diarrhea, insufficient fluid intake, possible NPO [Nil Per Os/nothing by mouth] status.

Goal/Outcome

The child will maintain adequate hydration status as evidenced by elastic skin turgor; moist, pink oral mucosa; presence of tears; urine output of 1 mL/kg/h or more.

Maintaining Fluid Balance (interventions with *rationale*)

- Weigh child daily: *Accurate weight is one of the best indicators of fluid volume status in children.*
- Maintain intravenous (IV) line and administer IV fluid as ordered *to maintain fluid volume.*
- Offer small amounts of oral rehydration solution (ORS) frequently *to maintain fluid volume. Small amounts are usually well tolerated by children with diarrhea and vomiting.*
- When symptoms have lessened or resolved, reintroduce a regular diet *to reduce the number of stools, provide adequate nutrition, and shorten the duration of effects of illness.*
- Avoid high-carbohydrate fluids such as Kool-Aid and fruit juice, *as they are low in electrolytes, and increased simple carbohydrate consumption can decrease stool transit time.*
- Assess hydration status (skin turgor, oral mucosa, presence of tears) every 4 to 8 hours *to evaluate maintenance of adequate fluid volume.*
- Assess the adequacy of urine output *to assess end-organ perfusion.*
- Maintain strict intake and output records and weigh the child daily *to evaluate the effectiveness of rehydration.*
- Discourage milk products and fluids that contain high levels of sugar during the acute phase of illness, *as these products may worsen diarrhea.*

Nursing Analysis

Diarrhea related to GI inflammation, infection, or exposure to toxin, as evidenced by loose liquid stools, hyperactive bowel sounds, or abdominal cramping.

Goal/Outcome

The child will experience a decrease in diarrhea: will have bulkier stool as per normal routine.

Relieving Diarrhea (interventions with *rationale*)

- Maintain a clear liquid diet no longer than 24 hours, *as prolonged clear liquids will result in continued liquid ("starvation") stools.*
- Avoid milk products until diarrhea improves: *Temporary poor absorption from villus injury follows viral diarrhea.*
- Encourage complex carbohydrate foods *to bulk up the stools.*
- Add fat to carbohydrates to increase intestinal transit time *to encourage water absorption (bulks up stool).*

Nursing Analysis

Constipation related to irregular defecation, decrease in GI motility (obstructive lesion), or insufficient fluid or fiber intake as evidenced by abdominal pain, decrease in stool frequency or volume, distended abdomen, liquid stool, pain with defecation, hard, formed stool, or palpable abdominal mass.

Goal/Outcome

The child will experience improvement in constipation by passing daily soft bowel movements without pain or straining.

Relieving Constipation (interventions with *rationale*)

- Palpate for abdominal distention, percuss for dullness, and auscultate for bowel sounds *to assess for signs of constipation.*
- Encourage adequate fluid intake *to soften the stool.*
- Administer medications as ordered *to keep stool moving on a daily basis.*

- Encourage activity as tolerated: *Immobility contributes to constipation.*
- The child with stool withholding should sit on the toilet twice daily, preferably after breakfast and dinner, *to maximize chances for successful stool passage by taking advantage of the gastrocolic reflex.*
- For behavioral stool holding, use rewards or stickers *to encourage appropriate toileting.*

Nursing Analysis

Malnutrition risk; risk factors include insufficient dietary intake, inability to ingest or digest food, inability to absorb nutrients, and psychological disorders.

Goal/Outcome

Nutritional status will be maximized: Child will maintain or gain weight appropriately.

Maintaining Appropriate Nutrition (interventions with *rationale*)

- Encourage favorite foods (within prescribed diet restrictions if present) *to maximize oral intake.*
- Administer enteral tube feedings as ordered *to maximize caloric intake.*
- Add butter, gravy, or cheese as appropriate to foods (if allowed within diet restrictions) *to increase caloric intake.*
- Encourage high-quality, high-calorie snacks between meals, *so as not to interfere with meal intake.*
- Document response to feeding *to determine feeding tolerance.*
- Limit intake of calorie-free beverages: *Beverages should contain nutrients and calories.*
- Consult a nutritionist *for appropriate diet supplementation recommendations.*

Nursing Analysis

Altered skin integrity risk; risk factors include the presence of moisture on the skin, frequent loose stools, presence of stoma, or gastrostomy tube.

Goal/Outcome

Child's skin will remain intact: Buttocks skin will be free from rash, excoriation. In the child with an ostomy/gastrostomy: Skin surrounding stoma or tube will remain intact and free from redness, rash, excoriation.

Maintaining Skin Integrity (interventions with *rationale*)

- Change diapers frequently *to limit acidic stool content contact with skin.*
- Use barrier diaper cream *to protect skin.*
- Assess skin integrity at every diaper change to recognize skin changes early *so that corrective measures can begin.*
- Leave the diaper area open to air several times a day if redness is present *so that air can circulate, and skin healing can be facilitated.*
- Use plain water or only mild soap to cleanse the skin with diaper changes *to avoid pH changes that contribute to diaper area skin breakdown.*
- Avoid diaper wipes that contain fragrance or alcohol if the skin is red or has a rash, *as both alcohol and perfume cause stinging if used on nonintact skin and can worsen skin breakdown.*

For the child with an ostomy:

- Ensure proper fit of the ostomy appliance/pouch *to avoid acidic stool contact with skin.*
- Use a barrier wafer (e.g., Stomahesive or DuoDERM®) to attach the appliance: *Avoid repeated pulling of adhesive tape from the skin.*
- If redness occurs, use barrier/healing cream or paste on the skin around the stoma *to promote healing and prevent further skin breakdown.*
- Consult enterostomal therapy nurse as needed *to provide additional support.*

Nursing Analysis

Altered breathing pattern related to pain, or postoperative immobility as evidenced by bradypnea, dyspnea, tachypnea, nasal flaring, or use of accessory muscles to breathe.

Goal/Outcome

The child will demonstrate an effective breathing pattern: respiratory rate normal for age, absence of accessory muscle use, adequate aeration with clear breath sounds throughout all lung fields.

Promoting an Effective Breathing Pattern (interventions with *rationale*)

- Turn, cough, and deep breathe every 2 hours *to encourage adequate aeration and discourage fluid pooling in the lungs.* In the infant or toddler, turn every 2 hours and use percussor or chest physiotherapy *to prevent the pooling of secretions.*
- Play games to encourage deep breathing (blow out penlight, blow cotton ball across bedside table with straw, etc.): *Children are more likely to cooperate with interventions if play is involved.*
- In the developmentally able child, encourage incentive spirometer use every 2 hours *to improve lung aeration.*
- Demonstrate/encourage the use of pillow splinting with coughing *to decrease the abdominal pain and stress on incision.*

Nursing Analysis

Altered body image perception related to surgical procedure (presence of stoma, scars), alteration in body function (loss of control of bowel elimination), or treatment regimen as evidenced by verbalization of negative feelings about body or refusal to look at stoma.

Goal/Outcome

The child or teen will demonstrate acceptance of change in body image by verbalization of adjustment;

looking at, touching, and caring for body; and returning to previous social involvement.

Promoting Appropriate Body Image (interventions with *rationale*)

- Observe child's coping mechanisms *to reinforce their use in times of stress.*
- Acknowledge denial, anger, and other feelings as normal *to support child/teen through difficult transition.*
- Allow child gradual introduction to stoma *to ease transition.*
- Encourage child/teen to participate in care, *as this sense of control will contribute to positive self-esteem.*

Based on your top three patient problems for Ethan, describe appropriate nursing interventions.

Stool Diversions

Children may undergo stool diversions for a variety of GI disorders. Surgical procedures involve the creation of an ostomy, primarily an *ileostomy* or a *colostomy*, by bringing a portion of the small or large intestine to the surface of the abdomen (Fig. 42.1). Ostomy pouches are worn over the ostomy site to collect stool. The pouch must be of an appropriate size, and it should fit around the stoma properly (Fig. 42.2). The pouch may be tucked inside the diaper or underwear or angled to fit outside of the diaper/underwear. Contemporary pouches cannot be seen under most clothing because they are designed to lie flat against the body.

Providing Ostomy Care

Empty the ostomy pouch and measure for stool output several times per day. The stool may be semisolid to very liquid in consistency depending on the location of the stoma. Liquid stool output can be acidic, causing irritation and severe burnlike areas on the surrounding skin, so special attention to skin care around the ostomy site is essential. Products such as powders and pastes are available to help protect the skin. The stoma should be moist and pink or red, demonstrating proper circulation to the intestine (Fig. 42.3). Notify the provider if the volume of stool output is greatly increased, or if the stoma is prolapsed or retracted.

Perform ostomy care as needed; pouches usually need to be changed every 1 to 4 days. Refer to Nursing Procedure 42.1 for an explanation of the steps for changing an ostomy pouch.

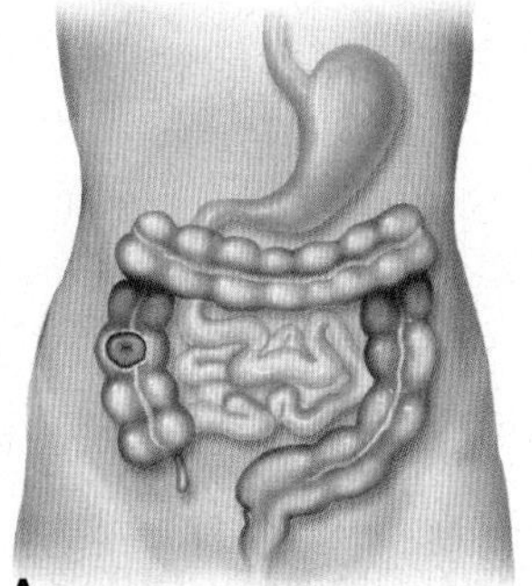

A

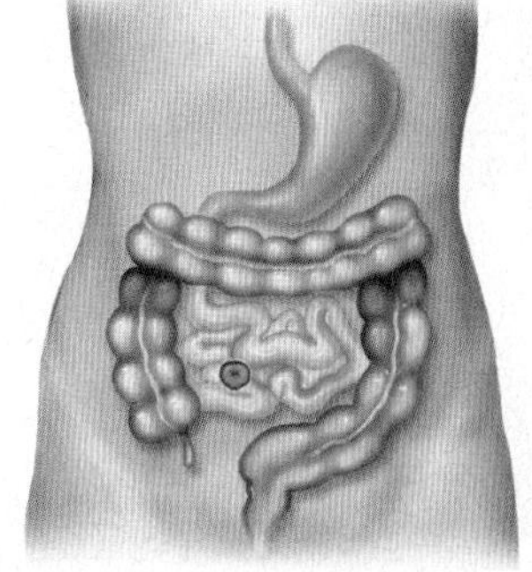

B

FIGURE 42.1 A colostomy is a stoma from the colon **(A)**; an ileostomy is a stoma from the ileum **(B)**.

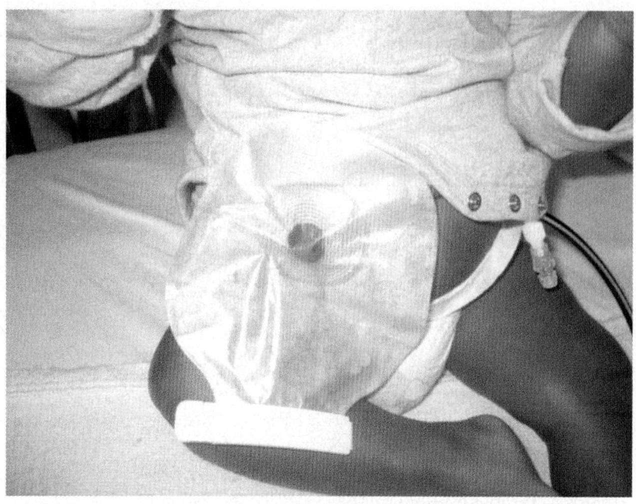

FIGURE 42.2 Ensure that the ostomy pouch fits closely around the stoma to prevent irritation of the surrounding skin.

CLINICAL REASONING ALERT!

Immediately notify the provider if the stoma is not moist and pink or red.

Educating the Child and Family About Ostomy Care

Educate the child and parent to avoid tight or constricting clothing around the stoma site. Teach families to store

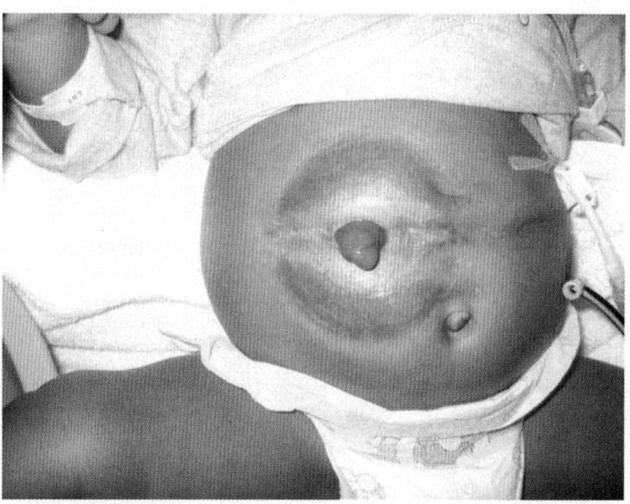

FIGURE 42.3 The healthy stoma is pink and moist.

NURSING PROCEDURE 42.1
Performing Ostomy Care

1. Set up the equipment:
   - Warm, wet washcloths or paper towels
   - Clean pouch and clamp
   - Skin barrier powder, paste, and sealant
   - Pencil or pen
   - Scissors
   - Pattern to measure stoma size
2. Take off the pouch (may need to use adhesive remover or wet washcloth to ease pouch removal).
3. Observe the stoma and surrounding skin. Clean the stoma and skin as needed, allowing it to dry thoroughly.
4. Measure the stoma, mark the new pouch backing, and cut the new backing to size.
5. Apply the new pouch.

Based on University of California, San Francisco. (2024). *Colostomy.* https://surgery.ucsf.edu/conditions--procedures/colostomy-(pediatric).aspx

ostomy supplies in a cool, dry place. Educate parents to inform school staff that the child should be allowed to use the water fountain and the bathroom without restriction, and the school nurse should have extra ostomy supplies available.

STRUCTURAL ANOMALIES OF THE GI TRACT

Structural anomalies of the GI tract include cleft lip and palate and hernias (discussed here), as well as omphalocele gastroschisis, esophageal atresia, tracheoesophageal fistula, and anorectal malformations (covered in Chapter 24).

Cleft Lip and Palate

Cleft lip and palate (Fig. 42.4) is the most common congenital craniofacial anomaly, occurring once in every 700 births worldwide. It occurs frequently in association with other anomalies, and 30% of children with cleft lip or palate have a genetic syndrome (Bishop & Ebach, 2023). Cleft lip and cleft palate, and cleft palate only, occur in association with other anomalies and appear in about 200 syndromes (Phalke & Goldman, 2022).

Complications of cleft lip and palate include feeding difficulties, altered dentition, delayed or altered speech development, and otitis media. The infant with cleft lip may have difficulty forming an adequate seal around a nipple to create the necessary suction for feeding and may also experience excessive air intake. Gagging, choking, and nasal regurgitation of milk may occur in babies with cleft palate. Excessive feeding time, inadequate intake, and fatigue contribute to insufficient growth. Primary or permanent teeth may be missing, malformed, or unusually positioned. Children with cleft palate may have a nasal quality to the speech as well as delays in speech development. Optimally, speech articulation should be clear by 4 years of age, or additional surgical intervention may be necessary. The opening in the cleft palate contributes to build up of fluid in the middle ear (otitis media with effusion), which can lead to an acute infection (acute otitis media). Otitis media with effusion leads to intermittent hearing and language delays (Meeks et al., 2022).

Pathophysiology

Development of the cleft occurs early in pregnancy. Cleft lip results from failure of the mesenchymal tissue to properly fuse during the embryonic stage, usually by week 5, and cleft palate results when there is an absence of midline fusion by week 7 (Meeks et al., 2022). Cleft lip or cleft palate may occur in isolation from one another or may occur together. The cleft may be unilateral or bilateral.

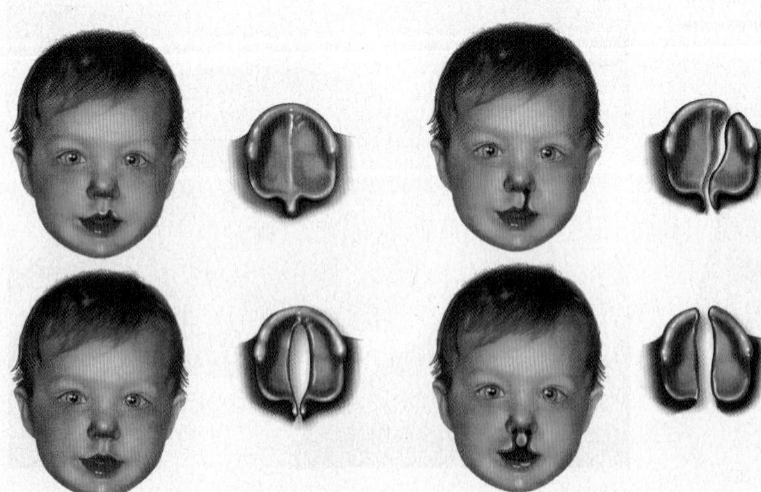

FIGURE 42.4 The cleft lip may extend all the way through the vermilion border and up into the nostril, or it may be significantly smaller. The cleft palate may be a small opening or may involve the entire palate.

Therapeutic Management

Babies with cleft lip and cleft palate are usually managed by a specialized team that may include a plastic surgeon or craniofacial specialist, oral surgeon, dentist or orthodontist, prosthodontist, psychologist, otolaryngologist, nurse, social worker, audiologist, and speech-language pathologist. Many children's hospitals offer these services in one location, such as a craniofacial specialty center. Cleft lip is usually surgically repaired by the age of 3 months and cleft palate around 12 months (Bishop & Ebach, 2023). Early repair of the cleft lip restores a normal appearance to the child's face and may improve parent–infant bonding. Regardless of the timing of the surgical repair, however, surgical revision of the palate may be required as the child grows.

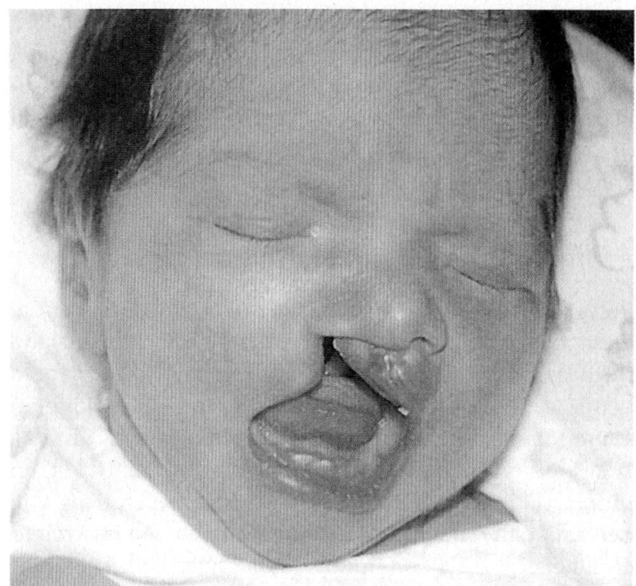

FIGURE 42.5 Cleft lip.

Nursing Assessment

For a full description of the assessment phase of the nursing process, refer to the "Clinical Judgment and the Nursing Process" section earlier in the chapter. Assessment findings pertinent to cleft lip and palate are discussed later.

Health History

For the newborn, explore pregnancy history for risk factors for the development of cleft lip and cleft palate, which include:

- Maternal smoking
- Prenatal infection
- Advanced maternal age
- Use of anticonvulsants, steroids, and other medications during early pregnancy

When an infant or child with cleft lip or palate returns for a clinic visit or hospitalization, inquire about feeding difficulties, respiratory difficulties, speech development, and otitis media.

Physical Examination

Observe the infant for the presence of the characteristic physical appearance of cleft lip. The cleft may involve the lip only or extend up into the nostril (Fig. 42.5). Cleft palate may be visualized on examination of the mouth. Palpate with a gloved finger to discover mild clefts.

Nursing Management

Refer to the "Clinical Judgment and the Nursing Process" section earlier in the chapter for patient problems and interventions related to hydration promotion, and to Chapter 36 for pain management. These should be individualized for the particular child. In addition to the patient problems and related interventions discussed in "Clinical Judgment and the Nursing Process" section, interventions common to cleft lip and cleft palate follow.

CONSIDER THIS!

The nurse is caring for a 2-week-old infant with a cleft lip who presents for a well-child check. The parent states, "I can't believe she looks like this; I always wanted a perfect baby girl! I feel like I can't go anywhere with her, other people will look at her like she's a monster. And after the surgery, there will be an ugly scar over her lip." The parent then begins crying.

How will you respond as the nurse? Are you concerned about anything other than the parent's feelings in the situation? What would it feel like if you had a baby with this facial difference? Think about the best ways to respond to this parent in a therapeutic manner.

Preventing Injury to the Suture Line

It is critical to prevent injury to the facial suture line or to the palatal operative sites. Do not allow the infant to rub the facial suture line. To prevent this, position the infant in a supine or side-lying position. It may be necessary to use arm restraints to stop the hands from touching the face or entering the mouth. Clean the suture line as ordered by the surgeon. Possible care options include using petroleum jelly on the facial suture line or a lip-protective device such as a Logan bow (thin curved metal apparatus) or a butterfly adhesive, both of which protect and maintain the suture line. Protect the palate operative site. Avoid putting items in the mouth that might disrupt the sutures (e.g., suction catheter, spoon, straw, pacifier, or plastic syringe).

Prevent vigorous or sustained crying in the infant because this may cause tension on either suture line. Ways to prevent crying include administering medications as needed for pain and providing other comfort or distraction measures, such as cuddling, rocking, and anticipation of needs.

Promoting Adequate Nutrition

Preoperatively, the baby with a cleft lip may demonstrate enhanced growth patterns if breastfed. The contour and softness of the breast against the lip may allow for a better seal to be maintained for adequate sucking in some infants (Cleft Lip and Palate Association [CLAPA], 2024). Some infants will be fed with a special cleft lip nipple (Fig. 42.6). Parent and surgeon preferences will determine the method of feeding. Burp the infant well to expel excess air taken in during difficulty with sucking.

The infant with unrepaired cleft palate is at risk for aspiration with oral feeding. In some instances, a prosthodontic device may be created to form a false palate covering. This device may prevent breast milk or formula from being aspirated. Breastfeeding may be effective in the infant with a small cleft palate due to the pliability of the breast and the fact that soft breast tissue may cover the opening in the palate (CLAPA, 2024). In the bottle-fed infant, special nipples or feeders may have to be used. When the suture line is healed, ordinary feeding may resume.

Encouraging Infant–Parent Bonding

For some parents, the appearance of a cleft lip is appalling. Encourage parents to hold the medically stable infant immediately after delivery to encourage bonding. Acknowledge normal feelings of guilt, anger, and sadness. Support the parents in providing care for the infant, particularly feeding, which is viewed as a significant nurturing function. Provide education about the anticipated surgical procedure and eventual normal appearance of the infant's lip.

Providing Emotional Support

Many families will benefit from support in addition to that received from the craniofacial team. Refer parents to the Cleft Palate Foundation or a parent-to-parent support network.

Meckel Diverticulum

Meckel diverticulum is the result of an incomplete fusion of the omphalomesenteric duct during embryonic development. This causes a fibrous band to connect the small intestine to the umbilicus, known as a Meckel diverticulum. It is the most common congenital anomaly of the GI tract, occurring in 1.5% of the population (Brumbaugh et al., 2022). Complications associated with Meckel diverticulum include bleeding, anemia, and intestinal obstruction such as volvulus and intussusception, half of which occur within the first 2 years of life (Brumbaugh et al., 2022). Surgical correction of the Meckel diverticulum is necessary in children who have complications. The surgery is usually done to remove the diverticulum itself. At times, ileal resection is necessary.

Nursing Assessment

Elicit a description of the present illness and chief complaint. Common signs and symptoms reported during the health history might include bleeding, anemia, or severe colicky abdominal pain (in children with associated intestinal obstruction). Assess the child for an acute abdomen. Observe for abdominal distention, auscultate

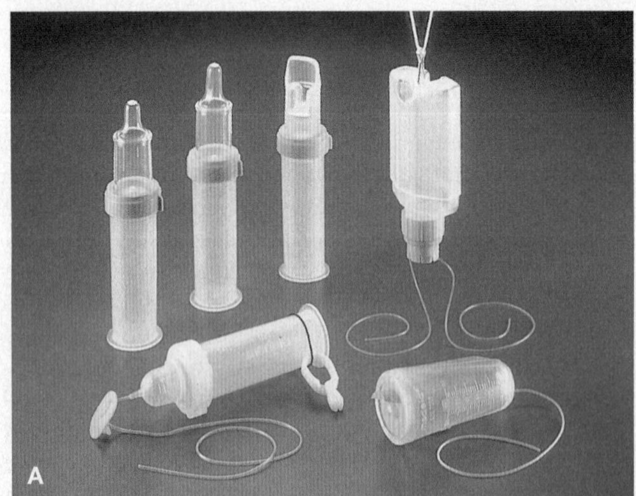

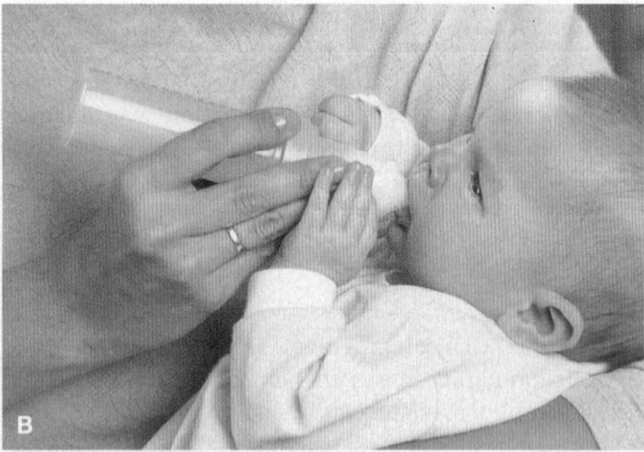

FIGURE 42.6 **A.** Specialty feeding devices used for infants with cleft lip and cleft palate. **B.** An infant uses a Haberman feeder.

for hypoactive bowel sounds, and then palpate for an abdominal mass, **guarding** (tensing of the abdominal wall muscles), and rebound tenderness. Stool for occult blood is usually positive and a complete blood count (CBC) may reveal anemia. A positive Meckel scan is conclusive.

Nursing Management

If anemia is significant, administer ordered blood products (packed red blood cells) to stabilize the child before surgery. Administer IV fluids and maintain NPO status for symptomatic children while further evaluation is being performed. Immediately report an acute abdomen to a primary provider or nurse practitioner. Postoperative care will vary depending on the surgery that was performed. Provide child and family education as necessary to relieve anxiety related to the diagnosis and surgical intervention. Refer to the "Clinical Judgment and the Nursing Process" section earlier in this chapter for additional information.

Inguinal and Umbilical Hernias

Inguinal and umbilical hernias are defects that occur during fetal development. Either may be visible at birth, and inguinal hernias may be noted later in life (Brumbaugh et al., 2022).

Inguinal Hernia

When the processus vaginalis fails to close completely during embryonal development, an inguinal hernia may occur. This allows the abdominal or pelvic viscera to travel through the internal inguinal ring into the inguinal canal. The hernia sacs that develop most often contain bowel in males and fallopian tubes or ovaries in females. Males are more likely than females to develop an inguinal hernia, and premature infants demonstrate an increased incidence overall (Brumbaugh et al., 2022). Surgical correction of the inguinal hernia is usually performed when the infant is several weeks old and has been thriving.

Nursing Assessment

Assess infants and children with an inguinal hernia for the presence of a bulging mass in the lower abdomen or groin area (Fig. 42.7). It may be possible to visualize the mass, but often the mass is seen only during crying or straining, making it difficult to actually identify in the clinic setting.

Nursing Management

If a mass is felt upon palpation, the primary provider or nurse practitioner may attempt to reduce the hernia by pushing it back through the external inguinal ring. The primary provider or nurse practitioner may ask the nurse to assist in a reduction, most likely helping to hold the child in a position that will allow the primary provider or nurse practitioner to reduce the hernia. Reduction is only a temporary method of managing inguinal hernias; they must be corrected surgically. If reduction is not possible even with sedation, the hernia could be incarcerated (Brumbaugh et al., 2022). An incarcerated hernia could eventually lead to bowel strangulation.

The hernia should be manually reduced as needed until the time of the surgery, so teach the family how to reduce the hernia. Instruct the family to contact the surgeon immediately if the hernia becomes irreducible. Provide routine pre- and postoperative care during inguinal hernia surgical repair, including child and family education to relieve anxiety.

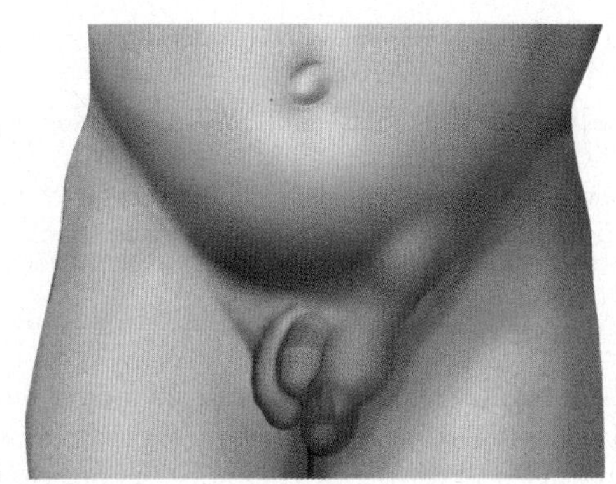

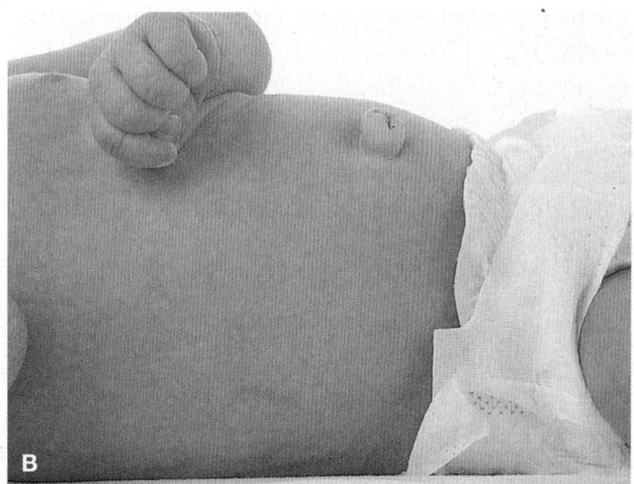

FIGURE 42.7 **A.** Inguinal hernia: note the bulge in the inguinal (groin) area. **B.** Umbilical hernia: note the protrusion in the umbilical area.

CLINICAL REASONING ALERT!

Tell the parents that if the child's inguinal hernia becomes hard, discolored, or painful (evidenced by inconsolable crying), they should immediately call the primary provider or nurse practitioner to determine the next course of action (office visit or emergency room visit).

Umbilical Hernia

Umbilical hernia occurs commonly in full-term infants and much more frequently in African Americans compared to White people (Brumbaugh et al., 2022). An umbilical hernia is caused by an incomplete closure of the umbilical ring, allowing intestinal contents to herniate through the opening. Most children will have spontaneous closure of the umbilical hernia by 4 to 5 years of age, and those not spontaneously closed may have surgical correction at that time (Brumbaugh et al., 2022). Surgical correction is necessary only for the largest umbilical hernias that have failed to close by the time the child is 4 years old.

Nursing Assessment

Assess whether the hernia can be reduced. Notify the surgeon if the hernia will not reduce. Incarceration is extremely rare, but when it does occur, the child will report abdominal pain, tenderness, or redness at the umbilicus (see Fig. 42.7).

Nursing Management

Since operative repair is not as likely with umbilical hernias as with inguinal hernias, the aim of nursing management is education. Teach the child and family how to reduce the hernia. The child may have some self-esteem issues related to the large protrusion of the unrepaired umbilical hernia. Teach the child coping skills to help relieve anxiety.

TAKE NOTE!

The use of home remedies to reduce an umbilical hernia should be discouraged because of the risk of skin maceration. This includes taping a quarter over a reduced umbilical hernia and the use of "belly bands" (Palazzi & Brandt, 2023).

ACUTE GI DISORDERS

Acute GI disorders include dehydration, vomiting, diarrhea, oral candidiasis, oral lesions, hypertrophic pyloric stenosis, necrotizing enterocolitis, intussusception, malrotation and volvulus, and appendicitis.

Dehydration

Dehydration occurs more readily in infants and young children than it does in adults. The risk is increased in infants and young children because they have an increased extracellular fluid percentage and a relative increase in body water compared to adults. Increased basal metabolic rate, increased ratio of BSA to body mass, immature renal function, and increased insensible fluid loss through temperature elevation also contribute to the increased risk for dehydration in infants and young children as compared to adults. Dehydration left unchecked leads to shock, so early recognition and treatment of dehydration is critical to prevent progression to hypovolemic shock. The goals of therapeutic management of dehydration are to restore appropriate fluid balance and to prevent complications.

Nursing Assessment

For a full description of the assessment phase of the nursing process, refer to the "Clinical Judgment and the Nursing Process" section earlier in the chapter. Assessment findings pertinent to dehydration are discussed later.

Health History

Elicit a description of the present illness and chief complaint. Common signs and symptoms reported during the health history are included in Comparison Chart 42.1, which compares the clinical manifestations of mild, moderate, and severe dehydration.

Explore the child's current and past medical history for risk factors for dehydration such as:

- Diarrhea
- Vomiting
- Decreased oral intake
- Sustained high fever
- Diabetic ketoacidosis
- Extensive burns

CLINICAL REASONING ALERT!

Nurses must be able to assess a child's hydration status accurately and intervene quickly. Children are at higher risk than adults for hypovolemic shock. Dehydrated children may deteriorate very quickly and experience shock.

Physical Examination

Assess the child's hydration status, including heart rate, blood pressure, skin turgor, fontanels, oral mucosa, eyes, temperature and color of extremities, mental status, and urine output. Children usually compensate well initially; their heart rate increases in moderate dehydration, but

COMPARISON CHART 42.1 Dehydration

	Mild	Moderate	Severe
Mental status	Alert	Alert to listless	Alert to comatose
Fontanels	Soft and flat	Sunken	Sunken
Eyes	Normal	Mildly sunken orbits	Deeply sunken orbits
Oral mucosa	Pink and moist	Pale and slightly dry	Dry
Skin turgor	Elastic	Decreased	Tenting
Heart rate	Normal	May be increased	Increased, progressing to bradycardia
Blood pressure	Normal	Normal	Normal, progressing to hypotension
Extremities	Warm, pink, brisk capillary refill	Delayed capillary refill	Cool, mottled, or dusky, significantly delayed capillary refill
Urine output	May be slightly decreased	<1 mL/kg/h	Significantly <1 mL/kg/h

Data from Anderson, C. C., Kapoor, S., & Mark, T. E. (2024). *The Harriet Lane handbook* (23rd ed.). Elsevier; Hanna, M. G., & Bock, M. (2022). Fluid, electrolyte, and acid-base disorders and therapy. In M. Bunik, W. W. Hay, M. J. Levin, & M. J. Abzug (Eds.), *Current pediatric diagnosis and treatment* (26th ed.). McGraw-Hill Education.

blood pressure remains normal until it decreases in severe dehydration.

Nursing Management

Nursing goals for the infant or child with dehydration are aimed at restoring fluid volume and preventing progression to hypovolemia. Provide oral rehydration to children for mild to moderate states of dehydration (see Teaching Guidelines 42.1). Children with severe dehydration should receive IV fluids. Initially, administer 20 mL/kg of normal saline or lactated Ringer's, and then reassess the hydration status (refer to Chapter 51 for further specifics regarding hypovolemic shock).

TEACHING GUIDELINES 42.1 Oral Rehydration Therapy

- Oral rehydration solution (ORS) should contain 75 mmol/L sodium chloride and 13.5 g/L glucose (standard ORS solutions include Pedialyte, Infalyte, and Ricelyte).
- Tap water, milk, undiluted fruit juice, soup, and broth are NOT appropriate for oral rehydration.
- Children with mild to moderate dehydration require 50 to 100 mL/kg of ORS over 4 hours.
- After reevaluation, oral rehydration may need to be continued if the child is still dehydrated.
- When rehydrated, the child can resume a regular diet.

Data from Freedman, S. (2023). Oral rehydration therapy. *UpToDate*. Retrieved November 5, 2023, from https://www.uptodate.com/contents/oral-rehydration-therapy

Once the initial fluid balance is restored, the primary provider or nurse practitioner may order IV fluids at the maintenance rate or as much as 1.5 times the maintenance. Maintenance fluid requirements refer to the amount needed under conditions of normal hydration. Maintenance fluid requirements may be determined with the use of the formula found in Box 42.2. In the example provided in Box 42.2, a 23-kg child will need maintenance fluid equivalent to 65 mL/h.

The same anatomic and physiologic differences that make infants and young children susceptible to dehydration also make them susceptible to overhydration. Thus, continuously evaluate hydration status and be aware of the appropriateness of IV fluid orders.

BOX 42.2 Formula for Fluid Maintenance

- 100 mL/kg for first 10 kg
- 50 mL/kg for next 10 kg
- 20 mL/kg for remaining kg
- Add together for total milliliters needed per 24-hour period.
- Divide by 24 for mL/h fluid requirement.

Thus, for a 23-kg child:

- 100 × 10 = 1,000
- 50 × 10 = 500
- 20 × 3 = 60
- 1,000 + 500 + 60 = 1,560
  1,560/24 = 65 mL/h

Data from Anderson, C. C., Kapoor, S., & Mark, T. E. (2024). *The Harriet Lane handbook* (23rd ed.). Elsevier.

Vomiting

Vomiting is the forceful expulsion of gastric contents through the mouth. It occurs as a reflex with three different phases:

- Prodromal period: nausea and signs of autonomic nervous system stimulation
- Retching
- Vomiting

Vomiting in infants and children has many different causes and is considered to be a symptom of some other conditions. Table 42.1 lists common causes of vomiting.

Therapeutic management of vomiting most often involves slow oral rehydration and at times may require administration of antiemetics.

Nursing Assessment

For a full description of the assessment phase of the nursing process, refer to the "Clinical Judgment and the Nursing Process" section earlier in the chapter. Assessment findings pertinent to vomiting are discussed later.

Health History

Elicit a description of the present illness and chief complaint. Note the onset and progression of symptoms. Determine the timing of the vomiting episodes as vomiting several hours after a meal could signify delayed gastric emptying and vomiting in the middle of the night or upon awakening may be associated with an intracranial lesion. Ask whether the vomiting seems effortless (as seen with gastroesophageal reflux [GER]) or if it is projectile (such as with pyloric stenosis). Inquire about the contents and character of the emesis. Bilious vomiting is never considered normal and suggests an obstruction, whereas bloody emesis can signify esophageal or GI bleeding (Brumbaugh et al., 2022). Note any events associated with the vomiting, such as diarrhea or pain.

Assess the child's past medical history to identify preexisting illnesses, drug misuse, trauma, prescribed medications, and previous abdominal surgery. Risk factors for vomiting include exposure to viruses, certain medication use, and overfeeding in an infant.

Physical Examination

Perform a physical examination, noting the child's general appearance. Note hydration status, as well as mental status changes. Note the quality of bowel sounds upon auscultation. Palpate the abdomen for the presence of abdominal masses, tenderness, or signs of trauma.

Nursing Management

Nursing management focuses on promoting fluid and electrolyte balance. Oral rehydration is accomplished successfully in most outpatient cases of simple vomiting. Teach the primary caregiver about oral rehydration (refer to Teaching Guidelines 42.1). In the child with mild to moderate dehydration resulting from vomiting, withhold oral feeding for 1 to 2 hours after emesis, after which time oral rehydration can begin. Give the infant or child 0.5 to 2 oz of ORS every 15 minutes, depending on the child's age and size. Most infants and children can retain

TABLE 42.1 • Causes of Vomiting by Temporal Pattern

Category	Acute	Chronic	Cyclic
Infectious	Gastroenteritis, otitis media, pharyngitis, sinusitis (acute), hepatitis, pyelonephritis, meningitis	*Helicobacter pylori*, *Giardia*, sinusitis (chronic)	Chronic sinusitis
GI	Intussusception, malrotation with volvulus, appendicitis, cholecystitis, pancreatitis	GERD, gastritis, peptic ulcer disease	GERD, malrotation with volvulus
Genitourinary	Ureteropelvic junction obstruction, pyelonephritis	Pregnancy, pyelonephritis	Hydronephrosis
Endocrine/metabolic	Diabetic ketoacidosis	Adrenal hyperplasia	Diabetic ketoacidosis, Addison disease, acute intermittent porphyria
Neurologic	Concussion, subdural hematoma, brain tumor	Brain tumor, Arnold–Chiari malformation	Migraines, Arnold–Chiari malformation, brain tumor
Other	Food poisoning, toxic ingestion	Bulimia, rumination	Cyclic vomiting syndrome

GERD, gastroesophageal reflux disease; GI, gastrointestinal.

this small amount of fluid if fed the restricted amount every 15 minutes. As the child improves, larger amounts will be tolerated.

TAKE NOTE!

Homemade ORS can be made by combining 1 quart of water (can be water poured from cooking rice if desired), eight teaspoons sugar, and one teaspoon salt.

If oral rehydration is not possible due to continued nausea and vomiting, IV fluids will likely be ordered. In some cases, antiemetics may be used to help control the vomiting, and ondansetron is preferred over promethazine due to lesser side effects. Educate the family regarding the prevention of vomiting and use of antiemetic therapy.

TAKE NOTE!

Ginger capsules (10 mg), ginger tea, and candied ginger are generally useful in reducing nausea, are safe for use in children over the age of 2 years, and usually produce no side effects (Canani, 2018).

Diarrhea

Diarrhea is either an increase in the frequency or a decrease in the consistency of stool. Diarrhea in children can either be acute or chronic. In the developed world, viruses cause most cases of diarrhea (Bishop & Ebach, 2023).

Pathophysiology

Acute diarrhea in children is most commonly caused by viruses, but it may also be related to bacterial or parasitic enteropathogens. Viruses injure the absorptive surface of mature villous cells, resulting in decreased fluid absorption and disaccharidase deficiency. Bacteria produce intestinal injury by directly invading the mucosa, damaging the villous surface, or releasing toxins. Acute diarrhea may be bloody or nonbloody. The viral, bacterial, and parasitic causes of acute infectious diarrhea are discussed in Box 42.3. Diarrhea may also occur in relation to antibiotic use. Risk factors for acute diarrhea include recent ingestion of undercooked meats, foreign travel, day care attendance, and well water use.

Since most cases of diarrhea are acute and viral in nature, therapeutic management of diarrhea is usually supportive (maintaining fluid balance and nutrition). Probiotic supplementation may be useful in the prevention of diarrhea but has not been shown to be effective in its treatment (Levy, 2022).

Though most cases of diarrhea in children are of acute origin, diarrhea may also occur chronically. Chronic diarrhea is diarrhea that lasts for more than 2 weeks. This type of diarrhea is not usually caused by serious illnesses. The causes of chronic diarrhea are listed according to age groups in Box 42.4.

Nursing Assessment

For a full description of the assessment phase of the nursing process, refer to the "Clinical Judgment and the Nursing Process" section earlier in the chapter. Assessment findings pertinent to diarrhea are discussed later.

BOX **42.3** **Acute Infectious Diarrhea**

Causes	Manifestations	Distinguishing Features	Treatment
Viruses: Rotavirus, adenovirus, norovirus, parvovirus, pestivirus, calicivirus, astrovirus, cytomegalovirus	Loose, watery stools, fever, vomiting	Rotavirus most common, especially in young children; norovirus more common in older children	Supportive care: oral rehydration, electrolyte replacement in some cases, early refeeding of diet. Antidiarrheals are not effective.
Bacteria: *Salmonella, Shigella, Escherichia coli* 0157:H7, *Campylobacter, Clostridium difficile, Yersinia enterocolitica*	Stools may be bloody or mucousy.	*Salmonella* may be shed for a year. *E. coli* 0157:H7 causes hemolytic anemia. *C. difficile* results from antibiotic use.	Rehydration, early refeeding of diet. Some but not all cases require antibiotic therapy.
Parasites: *Giardia lamblia, Entamoeba histolytica, Cryptosporidium*	Fever, watery stools	Oral–fecal transmission, *Cryptosporidium* spread by farm animals.	Some cases require antiparasitic therapy.

Data from Brumbaugh, D., Furuta, G. T., Hoffenberg, E., Kobak, G., Kramer, R., Walker, T., Septer, S., Shull, M., Soden, J., & Walker, T. (2022). Gastrointestinal tract. In M. Bunik, W. W. Hay, M. J. Levin, & M. J. Abzug (Eds.), *Current diagnosis and treatment: Pediatrics* (26th ed.). McGraw-Hill Education; and Thiagarajah, J. R., & Martin, M. G. (2023). Pathogenesis of acute diarrhea in children. *UpToDate.* Retrieved November 5, 2023, from http://www.uptodate.com/contents/pathogenesis-of-acute-diarrhea-in-children

BOX **42.4** **Causes of Chronic Diarrhea by Age**

Infants	Toddlers	School-Age Children
Intractable diarrhea in infancy Milk and soy protein intolerance Infectious enteritis Hirschsprung disease Nutrient malabsorption	Chronic nonspecific diarrhea Viral enteritis *Giardia* Tumors (secretory diarrhea) Ulcerative colitis Celiac disease	Inflammatory bowel disease Appendiceal abscess Lactase deficiency Constipation with encopresis

Health History

Elicit a description of the present illness and chief complaint. Important information related to the course of the diarrhea includes:

- Number and frequency of stools
- Duration of symptoms
- Stool volume
- Associated symptoms (abdominal pain, cramping, nausea, vomiting, fever)
- Presence of blood or mucus in the stool

Ask about the child's urine output (decreased with dehydration). Explore the child's current and past medical history for risk factors such as:

- Likelihood of exposure to infectious agents (well water, farm animals, day care attendance)
- Dietary history
- Family history of similar symptoms
- Recent travel
- Child's age (to identify common etiology for that age group)

Physical Examination

Note the child's general appearance and color. Note decreased tear production, sunken orbits, or dry mucous membranes with moderate to severe dehydration. Determine mental status; listlessness or lethargy may occur with moderate to severe dehydration. Evaluate skin turgor, noting that nonelasticity or tenting may occur with moderate to severe dehydration. Note abdominal distention or concavity. Stool output may be available to assess for color and consistency. Inspect the anal area for the presence of redness or rash related to increased stool volumes and increased frequency.

Auscultate bowel sounds to assess for the presence of hypoactive (obstruction or peritonitis) or hyperactive bowel sounds (diarrhea or gastroenteritis). Percuss the abdomen, noting any abnormality as it could indicate a pathologic process. Note tenderness to palpation in the lower quadrants, though rebound tenderness should not be present.

Laboratory and Diagnostic Tests

Common laboratory and diagnostic studies ordered for the assessment of diarrhea include:

- Stool culture: may indicate the presence of bacteria
- Stool for ova and parasites (O&P): may indicate the presence of parasites
- Stool viral panel or culture: to determine the presence of rotavirus or other viruses
- Stool for occult blood: may be positive if inflammation or ulceration is present in the GI tract
- Stool for leukocytes: may be positive in cases of inflammation or infection
- Stool pH/reducing substances: to see if the diarrhea is caused by carbohydrate intolerance
- Electrolyte panel: may indicate dehydration
- Abdominal radiographs (kidneys, ureters, and bladder [KUB]): Presence of stool in the colon may indicate constipation or **fecal impaction** (hardened immobile bulk of stool); air–fluid levels may indicate intestinal obstruction.

Nursing Management

Nursing management of the child with diarrhea focuses on restoring fluid and electrolyte balance and providing family education.

Restoring Fluid and Electrolyte Balance

Continue the child's regular diet if the child is not dehydrated. Initial nursing management of the dehydrated child with diarrhea is focused on fluid and electrolyte balance restoration. After rehydration is achieved, it is important to encourage the child to consume a regular diet to maintain energy and growth.

TAKE NOTE!

Avoid fluids high in glucose, such as fruit juice, gelatin, and soda, which may worsen diarrhea.

Providing Family Education

Teach the parents the importance of oral rehydration therapy (see Teaching Guidelines 42.1). The primary provider may order medication therapy. In such instances, teach the importance of finishing all prescribed antibiotic therapy. After the cause of the diarrhea is known, teach the child and family how to prevent further occurrences. As most cases of acute diarrhea are infectious, provide education about proper handwashing techniques and transmission routes. Chronic diarrhea is often a result of excessive intake of formula, water, or fruit juice, so teach the parents about appropriate fluid intake.

Oral Candidiasis (Thrush)

Oral candidiasis (thrush) is a fungal infection of the oral mucosa. It is most common in newborns and infants. Children at risk for thrush include those with immune disorders, those using corticosteroid inhalers, and those receiving therapy that suppresses the immune system (e.g., chemotherapy for cancer). Antibiotic use may also contribute to thrush. In addition, fungal infection may be transmitted between the infant and the breastfeeding parent (Campbell & Palazzi, 2023).

Therapeutic management includes treatment with oral antifungal agents such as nystatin or fluconazole.

Nursing Assessment

Assess for risk factors for oral candidiasis such as young age, immune suppression, antibiotic use, use of corticosteroid inhalers, or presence of fungal infection in the birthing or breastfeeding parent. Inspect the oral mucosa. Thrush appears as thick white patches on the tongue, mucosa, or palate, resembling curdled milk (Fig. 42.8). Unlike milk retained in the mouth, the patches do not easily wipe off with a swab or washcloth. Also, assess for the presence of candidal diaper rash (beefy-red rash with satellite lesions). Determine the extent to which the presence of the lesions is interfering with the infant's ability to feed. The lesions may cause significant discomfort.

Diagnosis is usually based on clinical presentation. However, a careful scraping of the lesions can be sent out for fungal culture.

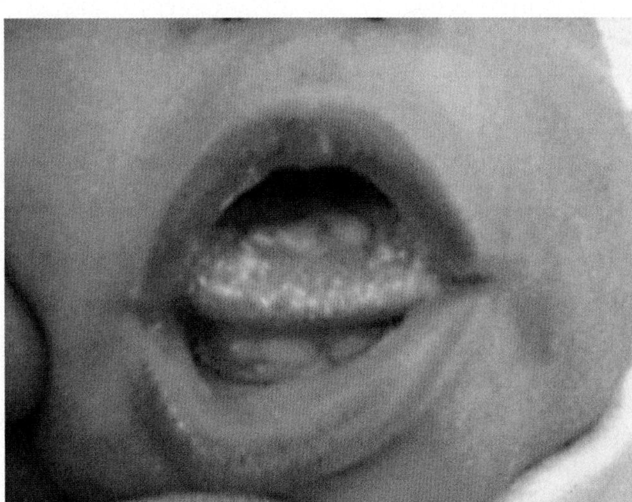

FIGURE 42.8 Thick white patches in the infant with oral candidiasis (thrush).

Nursing Management

Nursing management of the child with thrush includes administering medications and providing family education.

Administering Medications

Ensure appropriate administration of oral antifungal agents. Administer nystatin suspension four times per day following feeding to allow the medication to remain in contact with the lesions. In the younger infant, apply nystatin to the lesions with a cotton-tipped applicator. The older infant or child can easily swallow the pleasantly flavored suspension. An advantage of fluconazole is its once-daily dosing, but monitor infants and children receiving it for hepatotoxicity. Unlike nystatin, it is important to administer fluconazole with food to decrease the side effects of nausea and vomiting.

Educating the Family

If the breastfeeding parent is also infected, they must receive antifungal treatment as well. Fungal infection of the breast can cause the parent a great deal of pain with nursing, but if appropriately treated breastfeeding can continue without interruption. Stress appropriate handwashing. It is important to keep bottle nipples and pacifiers clean. Infants and young children often mouth their toys, so it is important to clean them appropriately. Explain to parents of infants with thrush the importance of reporting diaper rash because fungal infections in the diaper area often occur concomitantly with thrush and also need to be treated.

TAKE NOTE!

Geographic tongue is a benign, noncontagious condition. A reduction in the filiform papillae (bumps on the tongue) occurs in patches that migrate periodically, thus giving a maplike appearance to the tongue, with darker and lighter, higher and lower patches. Do not confuse the lighter patches of geographic tongue with the thick white plaques that form on the tongue with thrush.

Oral Lesions

A number of oral lesions may affect infants and children. A few of the most common are aphthous ulcers, gingivostomatitis (from herpes simplex virus [HSV]), and herpangina. Table 42.2 lists the causes of common oral lesions. Regardless of type, oral lesions are often painful and can interfere with the child's ability to eat. Therapeutic management of oral lesions varies depending on the cause.

TABLE **42.2** • Oral Lesions

	Aphthous Ulcers	Gingivostomatitis	Herpangina
Cause	Trauma, vitamin deficiency, celiac disease, Crohn disease	Herpes simplex virus	Enterovirus (Coxsackie)
Appearance	Erythematous border, often yellow appearance to the ulcer, anywhere on the oral mucosa or lips	Vesicular lesions on erythematous base, anywhere in the oral cavity, including lips	Bright-red ulcers, generally in the posterior oral cavity
Fever	Generally absent	May have high fever with initial outbreak	Abrupt onset of high fever (up to 39.4–40.6°C), lasting 1–4 days
Length of illness	Generally, heal within 7–14 days; may recur	10–12 days initially; may recur with stress, febrile illness, or intense sunlight exposure (as virus lies dormant in system)	Generally resolves within 5–7 days
Therapeutic management	Topical corticosteroid in dental paste may help.	Acyclovir	Supportive treatment only

Data from Kyle, T. (2022). Management of mouth disorders. In T. Kyle (Ed.), *Primary care pediatrics for the nurse practitioner: A practical approach.* Springer; Schare, R. S. (2021). *Canker sores.* http://kidshealth.org/parent/general/aches/canker.html#; Keels, M. A., & Clements, D. A. (2022). Herpetic gingivostomatitis in young children. *UpToDate.* Retrieved March 12, 2024, from https://www.uptodate.com/contents/herpetic-gingivostomatitis-in-young-children; and Romero, J. R. (2022). Hand, foot, and mouth disease and herpangina. *UpToDate.* Retrieved March 12, 2024, from https://www.uptodate.com/contents/hand-foot-and-mouth-disease-and-herpangina

Nursing Assessment

Explore the health history for the presence of risk factors such as immune deficiency, cancer chemotherapy treatment, exposure to infectious agents, trauma, stress, or celiac or Crohn disease. Note the onset of the lesion(s) and progression over time. Question the parent or child about the presence of sore throat or dysphagia (occurs with herpangina). Inspect the oral cavity, including the tongue, buccal mucosa, palate, and hypoglossal area. Note the presence of lesions and their distribution. Refer to Table 42.2 for descriptions and illustrations of various oral lesions. Inspect the pharynx, which may be red with herpangina. Generally, the diagnosis is based on the history and clinical presentation, but occasionally oral lesions are cultured for HSV.

Nursing Management

The primary concerns with oral lesions are pain management and maintenance of hydration. A corticosteroid-containing dental paste used for aphthous ulcers is formulated to "stick" to mucous membranes, so the lesion area should be as dry as possible before application of the paste. Children do not care for having the paste applied and will often resist. Older children with herpangina or stomatitis can "swish and spit" various formulations of "magic mouthwash" (typically a combination of liquid diphenhydramine, liquid acetaminophen, and milk of magnesia); they may offer some pain relief. Common over-the-counter medications such as Anbesol, Orajel, and Kank-A may be helpful for topical pain relief, though oral analgesics are often necessary.

The child with herpangina is typically an infant or young child (Kyle, 2022). It may be very difficult to coach a young child to drink fluids when their mouth is hurting. Playing games and offering favorite fluids and popsicles may encourage adequate oral intake. It is important to avoid carbonated beverages and citrus juices when oral lesions are present as they can cause further stinging and burning.

> **TAKE NOTE!**
>
> Viscous lidocaine should be used with caution in younger children as a topical treatment for numbing the lesions or as a swish-and-spit treatment because they may swallow the lidocaine (Lexicomp, 2024).

Hypertrophic Pyloric Stenosis

In hypertrophic pyloric stenosis, the circular muscle of the pylorus becomes hypertrophied, causing thickness in the luminal side of the pyloric canal (Fig. 42.9). This thickness creates a gastric outlet obstruction, causing nonbilious vomiting that presents between weeks 3 and 6 of life. The vomiting becomes more frequent and

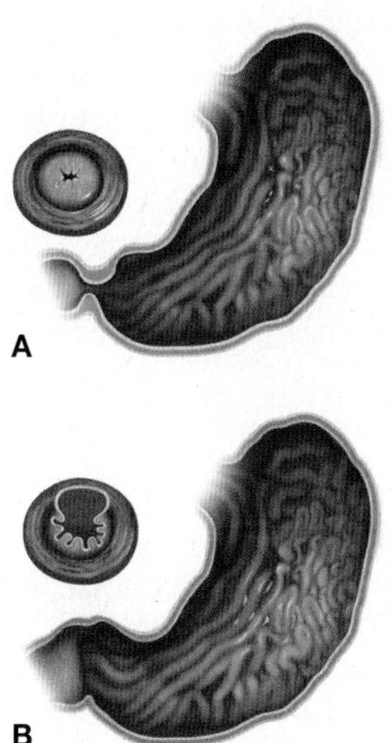

FIGURE 42.9 A. Hypertrophied pylorus muscle and narrowed stomach outlet. **B.** In pyloromyotomy, the pylorus is incised, thus increasing the diameter of the pyloric outlet.

forceful as time goes on and is often projectile. The incidence is 1 to 3.5 per 1,000 live births, and it occurs more in males than females (5:1), with first-born infants being affected up to 1.5 times more often (Endom et al., 2023). The cause of pyloric stenosis is probably multifactorial.

Pyloric stenosis requires surgical intervention. A pyloromyotomy is performed to cut the muscle of the pylorus and relieve the gastric outlet obstruction (see Fig. 42.9). Postoperative complications are rare.

Nursing Assessment

For a full description of the assessment phase of the nursing process, refer to the "Clinical Judgment and the Nursing Process" section earlier in the chapter.

Elicit a description of the present illness and chief complaint. Common symptoms reported during the health history might include:

- Forceful, nonbilious vomiting, unrelated to the feeding position
- Hunger soon after the vomiting episode
- Weight loss due to vomiting
- Progressive dehydration with subsequent lethargy
- Possible positive family history

Palpate for a hard, movable "olive" in the right upper quadrant (hypertrophied pylorus). If an easily palpable mass is felt, no further testing is necessary, and a surgical consult is called. If no mass is identified, a pyloric ultrasound may be ordered to identify a thickened hypoechoic ring in the region of the pylorus. Assess laboratory values to determine if the infant has metabolic alkalosis resulting from dehydration.

TAKE NOTE!

It may be difficult to examine the infant's abdomen when pyloric stenosis is suspected because of the infant's extreme irritability. A pacifier or nipple dipped in glucose water may soothe the infant long enough to perform the abdominal examination.

Nursing Management

Preoperative management of infants with pyloric stenosis is aimed at fluid management and correcting abnormal electrolyte values. Family anxiety is high during this time because of the impending surgery for an otherwise healthy infant. Provide emotional support to the family. Teach them about the surgical procedure and what to expect postoperatively. After surgery, infants usually resume oral feedings after 1 to 2 days.

Intussusception

Intussusception is a process that occurs when a proximal segment of bowel "telescopes" into a more distal segment, causing edema, vascular compromise, and, ultimately, partial or total bowel obstruction (Fig. 42.10). Most cases occur in toddlers 1 to 2 years of age (Bishop & Ebach, 2023). A lead point (i.e., pathologic point) may cause the telescoping. Examples of lead points are Meckel diverticulum, duplication cysts, polyps, hemangiomas, tumors, or the appendix. Typically, symptoms flare and then regress. Between episodes, children may have no symptoms of intussusception. This return to a normal state is due to the intussusception reducing on its own. The child may be without symptoms and may appear well when presenting to the primary provider, nurse practitioner, or emergency room. Again, this may be a sign that the bowel has reduced spontaneously. A pneumatic (air) enema is successful at reducing up to 90% of intussusception cases; other cases are reduced

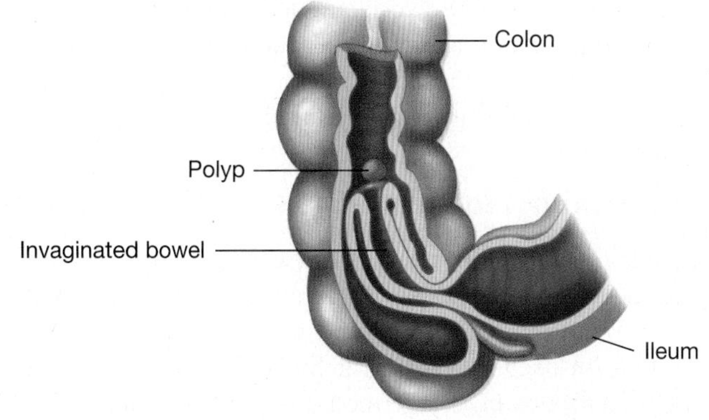

FIGURE 42.10 In intussusception, the intestine telescopes upon itself.

surgically (Bishop & Ebach, 2023). If surgical reduction is unsuccessful or bowel necrosis has occurred, a portion of the bowel must be resected.

Nursing Assessment

Elicit a description of the present illness and chief complaint. Common symptoms reported during the health history might include:

- Sudden onset of intermittent, crampy abdominal pain
- Severe pain (children usually draw up their knees and scream)
- Vomiting
- Diarrhea
- Currant-jelly stools, gross blood, or hemoccult-positive stools
- Lethargy

Determine risk factors such as cystic fibrosis or celiac disease. Determine the severity of pain, length of time the symptoms have been present, presence of vomiting, and stool patterns and color.

Palpate the abdomen for the presence of a sausage-shaped mass in the upper midabdomen (a hallmark sign of intussusception). Note any mental status changes. Intussusception is usually diagnosed with a pneumatic (air) enema. White blood cell elevation may occur, and electrolytes may show signs of dehydration.

CLINICAL REASONING ALERT!

Immediately report the presence of bilious vomiting, which occurs only in an obstructive situation.

Nursing Management

Administer IV fluids and antibiotics before the diagnostic laboratory and radiograph studies are performed. Refer to the "Clinical Judgment and the Nursing Process" section earlier in the chapter for nursing management of the postoperative child. Offer emotional support to the parents as they may be very fatigued after dealing with a crying child and quite anxious about surgery in an otherwise healthy child. Provide appropriate preoperative and postoperative education to the family.

Malrotation and Volvulus

Intestinal malrotation results from a disruption in embryonic development. When malrotation occurs, the intestine is abnormally attached and the mesentery narrows, twisting on itself (volvulus). If the volvulus involves the entire small bowel, it is termed a midgut volvulus.

The main symptom of malrotation is bilious vomiting. Many children also have abdominal pain, shock symptoms, abdominal distention, tachycardia, and bloody stools. Most cases of malrotation will present in the first few weeks of life, but symptoms may occur in older infants, children, or adults (Bishop & Ebach, 2023).

Therapeutic management of malrotation and volvulus is accomplished surgically. A Ladd procedure is performed, during which the intestine is straightened out and bands contributing to the misalignment are divided. If bowel necrosis has occurred (rare), then an ostomy may be necessary.

Nursing Assessment

Elicit a description of the present illness and chief complaint. Common symptoms reported during the health history might include vomiting and abdominal pain. Note the severity of pain, auscultate for hypoactive bowel sounds, and palpate for abdominal guarding or rebound tenderness. A KUB may reveal obstruction. An upper GI series can identify the location of the duodenojejunal junction and the corkscrew appearance of the twisted bowel.

Nursing Management

When diagnostic testing reveals malrotation/volvulus, administer ordered IV fluids and IV antibiotics. Place a nasogastric tube to decompress the stomach if ordered. Prepare the child and parents for surgery as it is performed as soon as possible. After surgery, provide postoperative care for the child. Provide continuous emotional support and family education.

Appendicitis

Appendicitis is an acute inflammation of the appendix. It is the most common cause of emergent abdominal surgery in children and peaks in prevalence at 15 to 30 years of age (Brumbaugh et al., 2022). If left untreated the appendix may rupture.

Pathophysiology

Appendicitis is due to a closed-loop obstruction of the appendix (Fig. 42.11). It is thought that the obstruction is due to fecal material impacted into the relatively narrow appendix, though other causes such as ingested foreign bodies may exist. This causes a subsequent increase in the intraluminal pressure of the appendix, resulting in mucosal edema, bacterial overgrowth, and eventual perforation. Due to the fecal material in the appendix, perforation causes inflammatory fluid and bacterial contents to leak into the abdominal cavity, resulting in peritonitis. Diffuse peritonitis is more likely in younger children. Older children and adolescents have a more developed omentum, which walls off the inflamed or perforated appendix, often causing a focal abscess.

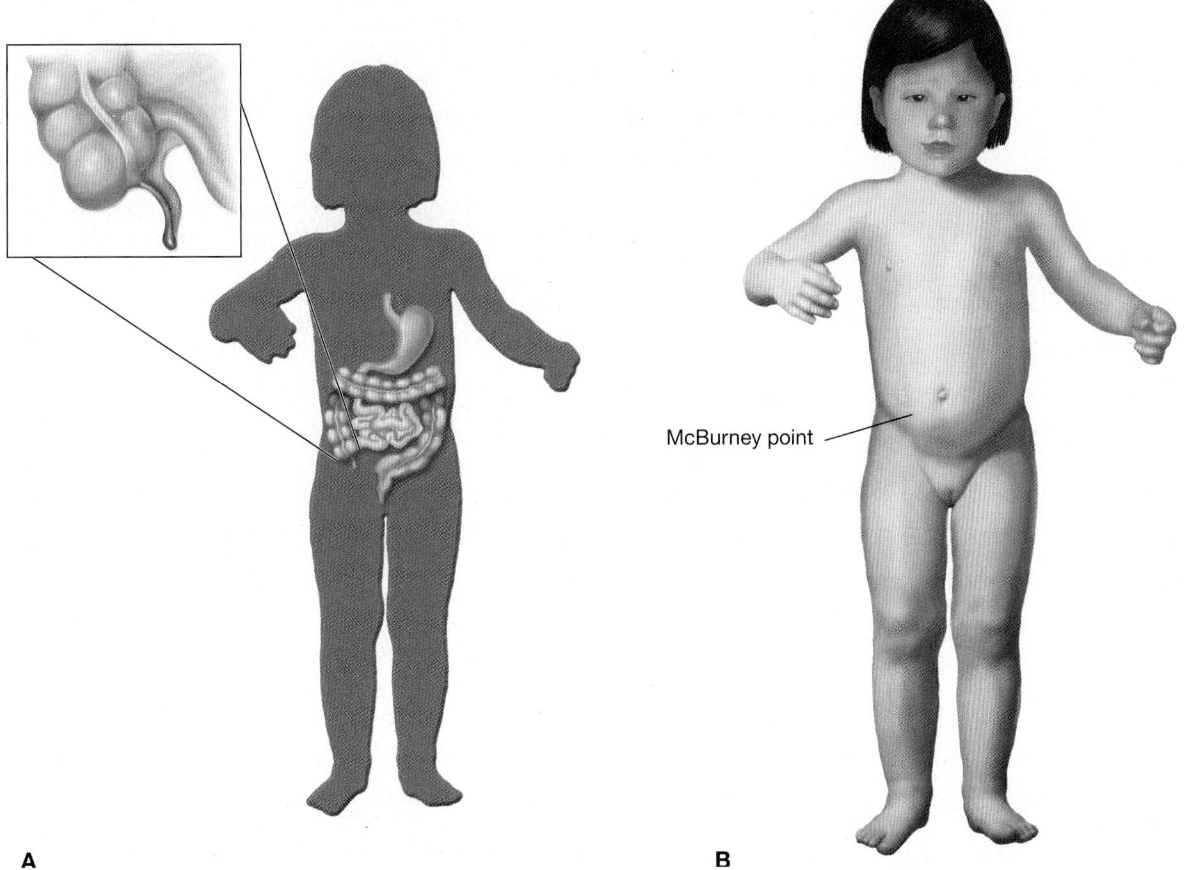

FIGURE 42.11 **A.** In appendicitis, the lumen of the appendix is obstructed, resulting in edema and compressed blood vessels. **B.** As appendicitis progresses, pain may become localized at McBurney point (a point midway between the anterior superior iliac crest and the umbilicus).

Therapeutic Management

Appendicitis is considered a surgical emergency due to the likelihood of perforation if left uncorrected. Surgical removal of the appendix is necessary and is often accomplished via a minimally invasive laparoscopic technique. In the case of perforation, an open surgical procedure is usually required, and lavage of the abdominal cavity may be performed to cleanse it of the infected fluid released from the appendix.

Nursing Assessment

Early diagnosis and intervention are the key elements to avoid perforation. For a full description of the assessment phase of the nursing process, refer to the "Clinical Judgment and the Nursing Process" section earlier in the chapter.

Assessment findings pertinent to appendicitis are discussed later.

Health History

Elicit a description of the present illness and chief complaint. Appendicitis may be gradual, but symptoms usually do not come and go; they remain persistent and intensify. Common symptoms reported during the health history might include:

- Vague abdominal pain in the initial stages, localizing to the right lower quadrant over a few hours
- Nausea and vomiting (which usually develop after the onset of pain)
- Small-volume, frequent, soft stools, often confused with diarrhea
- Fever (usually low grade unless perforation occurs, which results in high fever)

THINKING ABOUT **DEVELOPMENT**

Children with appendicitis often experience referred pain. How will you accurately assess pain location in a school-age child, as compared with a toddler?

Physical Examination

Note an ill appearance to the child. The child often cannot walk or climb up onto the examination table without assistance. Upon palpation, maximal tenderness occurs over McBurney point in the right lower quadrant (see Fig. 42.11). Diffuse abdominal tenderness or distention may indicate peritonitis.

CLINICAL REASONING ALERT!

If the child's abdominal pain is suddenly relieved without intervention, suspect perforation and notify the primary provider immediately.

Laboratory and Diagnostic Tests

Common laboratory and diagnostic studies ordered for the assessment of appendicitis include:

- Abdominal computed tomography (CT) scan: performed to visualize the appendix for further evaluation
- Laboratory testing: may reveal an elevated white blood cell count
- C-reactive protein: may be elevated

Nursing Management

Provide pre- and postoperative care and child and family education (see the "Clinical Judgment and the Nursing Process" section earlier in the chapter).

A nonruptured, nongangrenous appendix usually requires no antibiotic therapy, so provide routine postsurgical care. In addition to routine postoperative care, administer 48 to 72 hours of ordered antibiotics to the child with a suppurative or gangrenous (nonperforated) appendix to decrease the risk of postoperative infection. The child with a perforated appendix may require 7 to 14 days of IV antibiotic therapy in addition to normal postoperative care. Provide family teaching because the child is often discharged home while still receiving IV antibiotic therapy.

• • • ATRAUMATIC CARE • • •

For the child requiring a postsurgical dressing change, make sure to premedicate the child with prescribed pain medication. Employ distraction techniques appropriate for age and personal preference. For a complex dressing change, it may be necessary to additionally consult the child life specialist to determine how best to proceed with the dressing change in the most atraumatic fashion possible.

CHRONIC GI DISORDERS

Chronic GI disorders include gastroesophageal reflux disease (GERD), peptic ulcer disease (PUD), constipation/encopresis, Hirschsprung disease, short bowel syndrome, IBD, celiac disease, functional abdominal pain, failure to thrive, and chronic feeding problems.

Gastroesophageal Reflux Disease

GER is the passage of gastric contents into the esophagus. It is considered a normal physiologic process that occurs in healthy infants and children. However, when complications develop from the reflux of gastric contents back into the esophagus or oropharynx, it becomes more of a pathologic process known as GERD. GER occurs frequently during the first year of life, is considered benign, and usually resolves by 12 to 18 months of age (Brumbaugh et al., 2022). GER is particularly common in premature infants.

Pathophysiology

The process of GER occurs during episodes of transient relaxation of the LES, which can occur during swallowing, crying, or other Valsalva maneuvers that increase intra-abdominal pressure. Delayed esophageal clearance and gastric emptying, highly acidic gastric contents, hiatal hernia (protrusion of the stomach upward into the mediastinal cavity through the esophageal hiatus of the diaphragm), or neurologic disease may also be contributing factors associated with reflux.

The signs and symptoms of GERD are often seen as a result of the damaging components of the refluxate (the pH of the gastric contents, bile acids, and pepsin). GERD may cause esophagitis, esophageal stricture, Barrett esophagus (a precancerous condition), or anemia from chronic esophageal erosion. In addition, complications such as laryngitis, recurrent pneumonia, or asthma may occur.

Therapeutic Management

Conservative medical management begins with appropriate positioning, such as elevating the head of the bed and keeping the infant or child upright for 30 minutes after feeding. Smaller, more frequent feedings may be helpful. If reflux does not improve with these measures, medications such as histamine blockers or proton-pump inhibitors are prescribed to decrease acid production and stabilize the pH of the gastric contents (Brumbaugh et al., 2022) (Dosage Calculation Box 42.1).

If the GERD cannot be medically managed effectively or requires long-term medication therapy, surgical intervention may be necessary. A Nissen fundoplication is the most common surgical procedure performed for antireflux

DOSAGE CALCULATION BOX 42.1

Infant's weight: 11 lb, 8 oz

Medication order: omeprazole 4 mg PO once a day

Per the *Pediatric and Neonatal Dosage Handbook*, the recommended dose is 0.7 mg/kg/dose.

Is the ordered dose safe?

therapy. The gastric fundus is wrapped around the lower 2 to 3 cm of the esophagus (Fig. 42.12). Laparoscopic fundoplications are being performed as a way to minimize the recovery period and reduce potential complications.

Nursing Assessment

A full description of the assessment phase is provided in the "Clinical Judgment and the Nursing Process" section earlier in the chapter. Assessment findings pertinent to GER and GERD are discussed later.

Health History

Elicit a description of the present illness and chief complaint. Note the onset and progression of symptoms. Common symptoms reported during the health history include:

- Recurrent vomiting or regurgitation
- Weight loss or poor weight gain
- Irritability in infants
- Respiratory symptoms (chronic cough, wheezing, stridor, asthma, apnea)
- Hoarseness/sore throat
- Halitosis (mostly in older children)
- Heartburn or chest pain
- Abdominal pain
- Abnormal neck posturing (Sandifer syndrome)
- Hematemesis
- Dysphagia or feeding refusal
- Chronic sinusitis, otitis media
- Poor dentition (caused by acid erosion)

Explore the child's current and past medical history for risk factors such as:

- Prematurity, noting prolonged ventilator use or chronic lung disease
- Dietary habits (e.g., chocolate, coffee, spicy or fatty foods, caffeine, formula-fed or breastfed, overeating or overfeeding)
- Current medications
- Smoking/alcohol use (older children)
- Food allergies
- Other GI disorders (gastric outlet dysfunction/hiatal hernia) or congenital abnormalities
- Feeding positions and patterns (especially important in infants)
- Sleeping positions/patterns
- Other medical history, such as asthma or recurrent infections/pneumonia

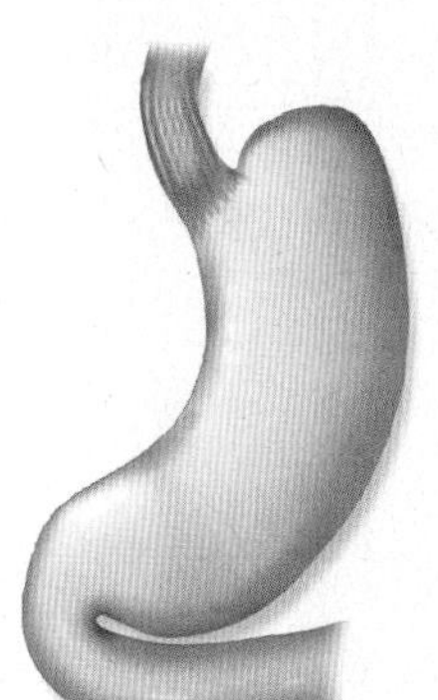
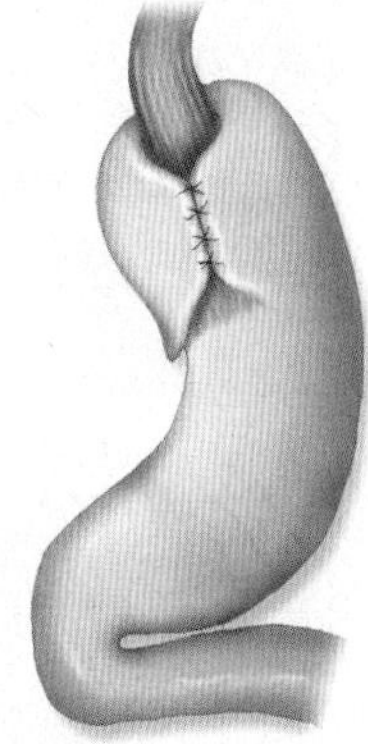

FIGURE 42.12 In the Nissen fundoplication, the fundus (upper portion of the stomach) is wrapped around the lower segment of the esophagus.

Physical Examination

Note an underweight or malnourished appearance in infants and children with uncontrolled GER for a period of time. Determine if the infant is irritable due to painful regurgitation/reflux events. Note the breathing pattern, because reflux-induced asthma may have developed. Observe the child for cyanosis, altered mental status, and alterations in tone. Inspect emesis for blood or bile. Auscultate the lung fields for the presence of adventitious breath sounds related to GERD complications. Use caution when palpating the abdomen, especially in infants with GERD, because it may induce vomiting. No abnormalities should be identified on palpation.

CLINICAL REASONING ALERT!

Not all children with GERD actually vomit. Some may only demonstrate irritability associated with feeding or posturing (arching back during or after feeding [termed Sandifer syndrome]) and grimacing. Episodes of GERD often cause bradycardia, so if the signs mentioned earlier occur, they should be reported to the primary provider or nurse practitioner, even if the baby is not vomiting (Winter, 2023a).

Laboratory and Diagnostic Tests

Common laboratory and diagnostic studies ordered for the assessment of GER include:

- Upper GI series: though not sensitive or specific to GER, may show some reflux; studies are used to narrow down the differential diagnosis.
- Esophageal pH probe study: quantifies GER episodes as they correlate to symptoms
- EGD: shows esophageal and gastric tissue damage from GERD
- CBC: may demonstrate anemia if chronic esophagitis or hematemesis is present
- Hemoccult: may be positive if chronic esophagitis is present

Nursing Management

As with most GI disorders, initial nursing management is aimed at restoring proper fluid balance and nutrition.

Refer to the "Clinical Judgment and the Nursing Process" section earlier in the chapter for information regarding individualized care. Additional considerations are reviewed later.

Promoting Safe Feeding Techniques and Positioning

Feeding adjustments are an essential part of reflux management. Give infants smaller, more frequent feedings using a nipple that controls flow well. Frequently burp the infant during feeds to control reflux. Thickening of the formula with products such as rice or oatmeal cereal can significantly help keep the formula and gastric contents down. Positioning after feedings is important. Keep infants upright for 30 to 45 minutes after feeding by holding them and elevating the head of the crib 30 degrees. Placing in infant seats or swings is not recommended as this increases intra-abdominal pressure (Winter, 2023b). For older children, elevate the head of the bed as much as possible and restrict meals for several hours before bedtime.

Maintaining a Patent Airway

GERD symptoms often involve the airway. Maximize reflux precautions to keep the risk of airway involvement to a minimum. If GERD causes apnea or there is a history of brief resolved unexplained events (BRUEs), use an apnea or bradycardia monitor to monitor for such episodes. The monitor requires a primary provider's order and can be ordered through a home health company. Teach parents how to deal with these episodes, as their anxiety is very high. Provide cardiopulmonary resuscitation (CPR) instruction to all parents whose children have had a BRUE previously.

Educating the Family and Child

The goals for the infant and child with GERD are a decrease in symptoms, a decrease in the frequency and duration of reflux episodes, healing of the injured mucosa, and prevention of further complications of GERD. Teach the parents the signs and symptoms of complications. Explain that reflux is usually limited to the first year of life, though in some cases it persists. If medications are prescribed, thoroughly explain their use and their side effects (see Drug Guide 42.1).

Providing Postoperative Care

If the child requires fundoplication, a gastrostomy tube is often placed for use in the immediate postoperative period or for long-term feeding. In the immediate postoperative period, assess for pain, abdominal distention, and return of bowel sounds. If a gastrostomy tube is placed, it is often open to straight drain for a period of time postoperatively to keep the stomach empty and allow for the internal incision to heal. When bowel sounds have returned and the infant or child is stable, introduce feedings slowly (typically via the gastrostomy tube). Assess for tolerance of feedings (absence of abdominal distention or pain, minimal residual, and passage of stool). If the abdomen does become distended or the child has discomfort, open the gastrostomy tube to air to decompress the stomach. Assess the insertion site of the gastrostomy tube for redness, edema, or drainage. Keep the site clean and dry per surgeon or hospital protocol. Teach the parents how to care for the gastrostomy tube and insertion site and how to use the tube for feeding.

Promoting Family and Child Coping

Parents may experience a great deal of anxiety. Teach the family about all aspects of GERD to help promote coping. School-age children often have reflux episodes exhibited by postprandial vomiting, which can be very embarrassing for the children. Notify the school about the medical issues related to GER to minimize the situation for the child.

Peptic Ulcer Disease

PUD is a term used to describe a variety of disorders of the upper GI tract that result from the action of gastric secretions (Fig. 42.13). Mucosal inflammation and subsequent ulceration occur as a result of either a primary or a secondary factor. Primary ulcers are usually associated

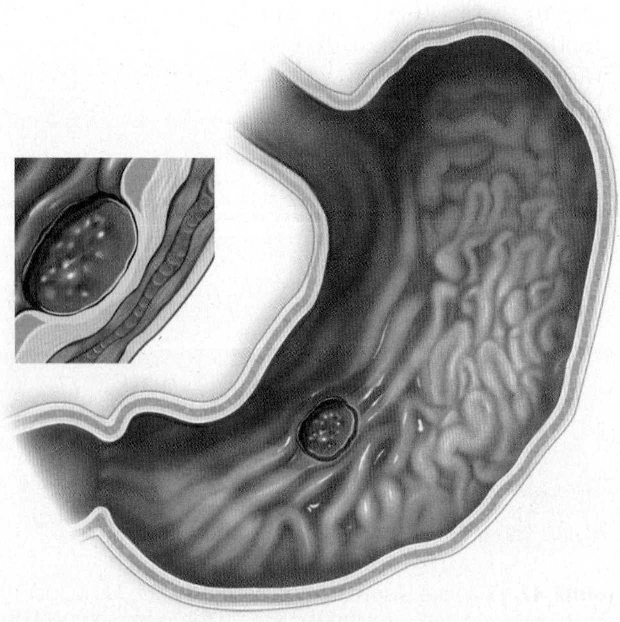

FIGURE 42.13 Peptic ulcer disease.

with *Helicobacter pylori*, a Gram-negative organism that causes mucosal inflammation and in some cases more severe disease (Bishop & Ebach, 2023). *H. pylori* is found mostly in the duodenum. Secondary peptic ulcers may occur as a result of an identifiable factor, such as excess acid production, stress, medications, or the presence of other underlying conditions. Secondary ulcers tend to be gastric in location as opposed to duodenal.

TAKE NOTE!

Severe stress, such as burns or another illness necessitating critical care, can contribute to the development of a peptic ulcer in children (Brumbaugh et al., 2022).

Therapeutic Management

PUD may be treated with antibiotics (if *H. pylori* is verified), histamine agonists, and proton-pump inhibitors. If the child presents with a severe esophageal or gastric hemorrhage, a nasogastric tube may be placed to decompress the stomach. The child may require IV infusion of a histamine-2 receptor antagonist or a proton-pump inhibitor initially until the bleeding has stopped and the disease is stabilized.

Nursing Assessment

Elicit a description of the present illness and chief complaint. Common symptoms reported during the health history might include abdominal pain (most common), vomiting, or GI bleeding. The pain of PUD tends to be dull and vague, mostly epigastric, or periumbilical, worsening after meals, and wakes the child at night. Explore the child's current and past medical history for risk factors such as a family history of PUD or other GI diseases, or chronic salicylate or prednisone use.

Palpate the abdomen for the location of the pain, which is usually epigastric or periumbilical. Note the presence of blood in emesis or stools, as GI bleeding may occur. Diagnostic studies used to identify *H. pylori* include antibody testing, urea breath test, or biopsy. An upper GI series or upper endoscopy may detect the presence of ulcerations.

Nursing Management

Hemodynamic stabilization should be the focus of nursing management if significant GI bleeding occurs. Once children are stabilized and tolerating oral feeds, they may be discharged to home. Provide discharge instructions on the following topics:

- Medications
- Dietary management (especially when allergic gastroenteropathy is found)
- Safety precautions (in cases of ingested substances)
- Stressors
- Prevention of disease recurrence

Constipation and Encopresis

Constipation is a very common problem among children, affecting up to 30% of the pediatric population, and accounting for 3% to 5% of all pediatric outpatient visits (Sood, 2023b). It may be defined as failure to achieve complete evacuation of the lower colon. Breastfed infants may produce a stool with each feeding, though some will skip a few days between stools. Most bottle-fed babies will produce a stool one or two times per day, but they may go 2 to 3 days without producing a stool. The bowel habits of both infants and children vary widely, so assess and treat each child on a case-by-case basis.

Functional constipation may be defined by the presence of at least two of the following over the course of 1 month:

- Less than three bowel movements weekly
- At least one episode of fecal incontinence weekly (after toilet training)
- Excessive stool retention history
- Hard or painful bowel movements
- Large fecal rectal mass
- Stool passage of a volume to clog the toilet
- Stool withholding behavior (retentive posturing) (children aged 4 years or older)

Encopresis is a term used to describe soiling of fecal contents into the underwear beyond the age of expected toilet training (4 to 5 years of age). Encopresis is often seen as a result of chronic constipation and withholding of stool. As stool is withheld in the rectum, the rectal muscle can stretch over time, and this stretching of the rectum causes fecal impactions. Children who have a stretched rectal vault may experience liquid stool leakage around a fecal mass. This is often an embarrassing issue that occurs with school-age children, and the child may hide their underwear to avoid punishment.

Pathophysiology

As stool passes through the colon, water is reabsorbed into the colon, resulting in a formed stool by the time it reaches the rectum. At this point, the anal sphincter relaxes to allow the passage of stool from the anus. In constipation, however, this relaxation does not occur.

Most causes of constipation are functional in nature (inorganic) (Sood, 2023b). Children with functional constipation usually present with this problem during the toilet-training years. Children have a painful experience during defecation, which in turn creates a fear of defecation, resulting in further withholding of stool. Organic causes of constipation rarely occur in children. When they do occur, they may be a sign of a disease such as spina bifida or sacral agenesis. The causes of pediatric constipation are discussed in Table 42.3.

Therapeutic Management

Once any organic process is ruled out as a cause, constipation may initially be managed with dietary manipulation such as increasing fiber and fluids. However, behavior modification is necessary for most children. Children need to relearn to allow bowel evacuation when stool is present. Children with severe constipation and withholding behaviors may not benefit from dietary management and may require laxative therapy. Sometimes mechanical disimpaction is required initially, followed by the above measures.

Nursing Assessment

For a full description of the assessment phase of the nursing process, refer to the "Clinical Judgment and the Nursing Process" section earlier in the chapter. Assessment findings pertinent to constipation/encopresis are discussed later.

Health History

Elicit a description of the present illness and chief complaint. Note the onset of symptoms as described by the parent/child. Common symptoms reported during the health history may include:

- Altered stooling patterns (size, frequency, amount, and color)
- Pain with defecation
- Withholding behaviors (postures to try to withhold the stool, such as crossing the legs, squatting or hiding in a corner, or "dancing")
- Complaints of abdominal pain and cramping and poor appetite
- Diarrhea leakage
- Soiling of undergarments

It is important to note the duration of the symptoms to determine an acute onset versus a chronic disorder. Explore the child's past and current medical history for risk factors such as:

- Family history of GI disorders
- History of rectal bleeding or anal fissures
- Report of first meconium stool after 24 hours of age
- History of sexual abuse

Determine the child's dietary habits, history of fluid intake, and current medication or laxative use.

Physical Examination

Note whether the abdomen appears distended or rounded. Observe the lower back for a deep pilonidal dimple with hair tuft, which is suggestive of spina bifida occulta, or for flat buttocks suggestive of sacral agenesis. Inspect the anus for signs of fissures or soiling. Inspect the child's underwear for stains or smears, which are indicative of soiling. Auscultate bowel sounds to determine the possibility of an obstruction (hypoactive or absent bowel sounds) in the child with an acute case of constipation. Percuss the abdomen to reveal dullness, indicating a fecal mass. Palpate the abdomen for any tenderness or masses. The nurse may assist the primary provider or nurse practitioner with the performance of a rectal examination to assess for rectal tone and rectal vault size.

TABLE 42.3 • Causes of Pediatric Constipation by Age

Newborn/Infant	Toddler and Ages 2–4 Years	School Age	Adolescent	Any Age
• Meconium plug • Hirschsprung disease • Cystic fibrosis • Congenital anorectal malformations • Pseudo-obstruction • Endocrine: hypothyroidism • Metabolic: diabetes insipidus, renal tubular acidosis • Withholding • Dietary changes	• Anal fissures • Withholding • Toilet refusal • Short-segment Hirschsprung disease • Neurologic disorders • Spinal cord: meningomyelocele, tumors, tethered cord	• Toilet or bathroom access limited or unavailable • Limited ability to recognize physiologic cues, preoccupation with other activities • Tethered cord • Withholding	• Spinal cord injury (accidents, trauma) • Dieting • Anorexia • Pregnancy • Idiopathic slow transit constipation, particularly in females • Laxative use • Irritable bowel syndrome, constipation variant	• Medication side effects, dietary, postoperative state • Previous anorectal surgery • Withholding and overflow from chronic rectal distention • Relatively rapid change to sedentary state, dehydration • Hypothyroidism

Data from Bishop, W. P., & Ebach, D. R. (2023). Digestive system. In K. J. Marcdante, R. M. Kliegman, & A. M Schuh (Eds.), *Nelson's essentials of pediatrics* (9th ed.). Elsevier; Brumbaugh, D., Furuta, G. T., Hoffenberg, E., Kobak, G., Kramer, R., Walker, T., Septer, S., Shull, M., Soden, J., & Walker, T. (2022). Gastrointestinal tract. In M. Bunik, W. W. Hay, M. J. Levin, & M. J. Abzug (Eds.), *Current diagnosis and treatment: Pediatrics* (26th ed.). McGraw-Hill Education; and Philichi, L. (2018). Management of childhood functional constipation. *Journal of Pediatric Health Care, 32*(1), 103–113. https://doi.org/10.1016/j.pedhc.2017.08.008

Laboratory and Diagnostic Tests

Laboratory and diagnostic tests are not routine with the diagnosis of functional constipation, but if an organic cause is suspected, the following laboratory and diagnostic tests may be ordered:

- Stool for occult blood: The presence of blood could indicate some other disease process.
- Abdominal radiograph: Large quantities of stool may be seen in the colon.
- Sitz marker study: to detect colonic dysmotility
- Barium enema: to rule out a stricture or Hirschsprung disease
- Rectal manometry: to evaluate rectal musculature dysfunction
- Rectal suction biopsy: to rule out Hirschsprung disease

Nursing Management

Nursing management for the infant or child with constipation is aimed at educating the child and family and promoting child and family coping. Individualize care based on the patient problems and interventions presented earlier in the chapter in the "Clinical Judgment and the Nursing Process" section earlier in the chapter. Additional considerations are reviewed later.

Educating the Family and Child

Teach parents how to assess for signs of constipation and withholding behaviors. Also, provide guidelines on scheduling and supervising bowel habits in reconditioning the child to use the toilet regularly. Teach parents to use positive reinforcement techniques. For example, when the child produces an adequate-volume bowel movement, reward them with stickers, extra playtime, or television time, and so on.

Educate parents that dietary changes may help some children as high-fiber diets help to regulate bowel activity. Encourage the parent to increase the child's fluid intake to aid in bringing extra water into the bowel, thereby softening the stool. If a formula or milk change is recommended for the infant or toddler, educate the family that the change may result in better bowel habits. Teach families about the importance of adherence with medication use if medication is ordered. Parents often are very anxious about the use of these medications, but stress to them that adherence is essential.

Many children present to their primary provider or nurse practitioner with fecal impaction or partial impaction. Teach parents how to disimpact their children at home; this often requires an enema or stimulation therapy. Nursing Procedure 42.2 gives instructions on enema administration in children. Explain the procedure to the child in developmentally appropriate terms. Enema administration can be uncomfortable, but calming measures, such as distraction and praise, provide a comforting environment. After the impaction is removed, promote regular bowel habits to keep the impaction from recurring.

NURSING PROCEDURE 42.2 Administering an Enema

1. Gather supplies (enema bag, lubricant, enema solution).
2. Wash hands and apply gloves.
3. Position the child:
   - Infant or toddler on abdomen with knees bent
   - Child or adolescent on the left side with right leg flexed toward the chest
4. Clamp the enema tubing, remove the cap, and apply lubricant to the tip.
5. Insert the tube into the rectum:
   - 2.5 to 4 cm (1 to 1.5 in) in the infant
   - 5 to 7.5 cm (2 to 3 in) in the child
6. Unclamp the tubing and administer the prescribed volume of enema solution at a rate of about 100 mL/min. Recommended volumes:
   - 250 mL or less for the infant
   - 250 to 500 mL for the toddler or preschooler
   - 500 to 1,000 mL for the school-age child
7. Hold the child's buttocks together if needed to encourage retention of the enema for 5 to 10 minutes.

Data from Cincinnati Children's. (2024). *Enema administration.* http://www.cincinnatichildrens.org/health/e/enema/

Promoting Child and Family Coping

Childhood constipation can be a very stressful process for both the child and family. Behavior modification is necessary for many children. To facilitate daily bowel evacuation, the child should sit on the toilet twice a day (after breakfast and dinner) for 5 to 15 minutes with their feet on a stool as necessary. Instruct the family to keep a "star" or reward chart to encourage adherence. Parents should award the star for adherence with time sitting on the toilet and should not reserve rewards for successful bowel movements only. Weeks to months may be required to change the stooling pattern (Sood, 2023a).

Many parents seek counselors to help the entire family deal with the issues. Counseling is geared toward allaying the fears of a child who is afraid to defecate due to pain. Also, children who are older may have behavioral issues that need to be addressed. Psychological evaluation and possible behavioral therapy may need to be implemented if constipation becomes a power struggle.

Hirschsprung Disease (Congenital Aganglionic Megacolon)

Hirschsprung disease is a disorder of motility of the intestinal tract resulting in obstruction (Bishop & Ebach, 2023). See Figure 42.14. The disease is most commonly characterized by failure to pass a stool (meconium) within the first 24 hours of life. This is due to a lack of ganglion cells in the intestine, which causes inadequate motility in part of the intestine. These ganglion cells can be absent from the rectosigmoid colon all the way into the small intestine. Hirschsprung disease occurs in one of every 5,000 live births, being about four times more common in males than in females (Brumbaugh et al., 2022).

Therapeutic Management

Surgical resection of the aganglionic bowel and reanastomosis of the remaining intestine are necessary to promote proper bowel function. There are several types of surgical procedures to correct this, usually performed in stages. The surgical resection requires the child to have an ostomy to divert the stool through a stoma on the abdomen. This allows the area of the resected bowel and anastomosis to heal before it is used. The ostomy is closed at a later date.

Nursing Assessment

When eliciting the history of the present illness, keep in mind that newborn stool patterns are a key element related to this diagnosis. Assess whether the newborn passed a meconium stool within the first 24 to 48 hours of life. Determine if the newborn required rectal stimulation to pass their first meconium stool or pass a meconium plug. Explore the child's current and past medical history for risk factors such as Down syndrome or other chromosomal abnormality, or a family history of Hirschsprung disease or Down syndrome (Brumbaugh et al., 2022).

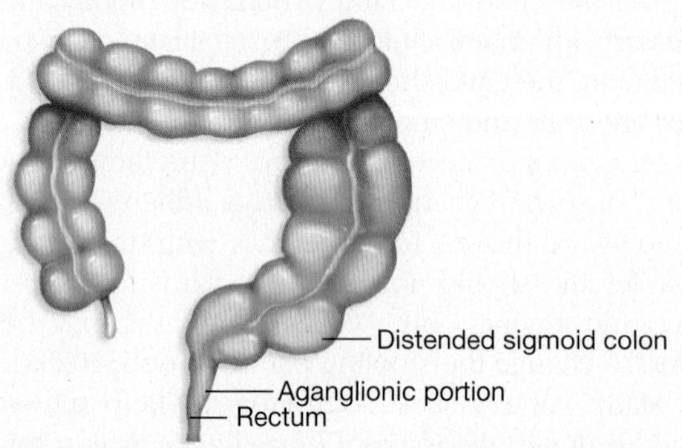

FIGURE 42.14 Enlarged megacolon of Hirschsprung disease.

Inspect the abdomen for distention. Palpate the abdomen for the presence of stool masses. Perform a rectal examination to assess for rectal tone and the presence of stool in the rectum. Often with Hirschsprung disease, no stool is present in the rectum. However, at the end of the rectal examination, when the finger is being withdrawn, a child with Hirschsprung disease may have a forceful expulsion of fecal material. Barium enema may reveal intestinal narrowing.

Rectal suction biopsy will demonstrate an absence of ganglion cells and provides the definitive diagnosis.

Nursing Management

Nursing management includes providing postoperative care, performing ostomy care, and providing child and family education.

Providing Postoperative and Ostomy Care

Provide routine postoperative care and observe for the possible complications of enterocolitis. The child with Hirschsprung disease may have either a colostomy or an ileostomy, depending on the extent of disease in the intestine. In either case, perform proper ostomy care to avoid skin breakdown. Accurately measure stool output to assess the child's fluid volume status.

Observe for the following signs and symptoms of enterocolitis: fever, abdominal distention, chronic diarrhea or explosive stools, rectal bleeding, or straining. If any of the above symptoms are noted, immediately notify the primary physician or nurse practitioner, maintain bowel rest, and administer IV fluids and antibiotics to prevent the development of shock and possibly death.

Providing Child and Family Education

The family may be anxious and fearful about upcoming surgeries and possible complications. Help to relieve their anxiety by providing information about the diagnosis and the stages of surgical procedures the child will undergo. Provide postoperative teaching to educate parents on proper stoma care as well as medication management (to avoid dehydration, most children with Hirschsprung disease will be prescribed medications to slow stool output). Arrange for the family to consult with a wound care nurse to help them deal with the anxieties and care of newly placed stomas. Provide education about possible postsurgical problems, emphasizing the importance of prompt medical treatment for signs of enterocolitis.

Short Bowel Syndrome

Short bowel syndrome is a clinical syndrome of nutrient malabsorption and excessive intestinal fluid and electrolyte losses that occur following massive small intestinal loss or surgical resection. The degree of malabsorption is usually related to the extent of resection of small bowel, absence of ileocecal valve or colon, and small bowel bacterial overgrowth (Brumbaugh et al., 2022). If the terminal ileum is lost, vitamin B_{12} deficiency and bile salt malabsorption may occur. The most common causes of short bowel syndrome are necrotizing enterocolitis, small intestinal atresia, gastroschisis, malrotation with volvulus, and trauma to the small intestine.

Therapeutic Management

The child with short bowel syndrome is at risk for chronic complications. The goals of therapeutic management are to minimize bacterial overgrowth and to maximize the child's nutritional status. Antibiotics may be used to control bacterial overgrowth. Vitamin and mineral supplementation is necessary because the small intestine is usually where fat-soluble vitamins, calcium, magnesium, and zinc are absorbed. Antidiarrheal agents such as loperamide and gastric acid–suppressive medications may be used to decrease stool output. Many children with short bowel syndrome require TPN for extended periods to achieve adequate growth. Progression to enteral feeding may occur extremely slowly, depending on the intestine's response. Despite a markedly improved prognosis for these children, some will not do as well and may ultimately require intestinal and liver transplantation due to irreversible liver damage from long-term use of total parenteral nutrition (TPN).

Nursing Assessment

Elicit the health history, noting diarrhea, which is the primary symptom of short bowel syndrome. Note past history of bowel loss or resection as noted earlier. Assess the child's hydration state. Inspect the stool for consistency, color, odor, and volume. Review laboratory results, particularly chemistries, to evaluate hydration status, and liver function tests (LFTs), which may reveal evolving **cholestasis** (impairment of bile flow) secondary to long-term TPN use.

Nursing Management

Nursing management focuses on encouraging adequate nutrition and promoting effective family coping.

Encouraging Adequate Nutrition

Treatment for short bowel syndrome can be a slow and tedious process. Most children will require TPN until they can tolerate enteral feeds without significant malabsorption. TPN is usually required for a lengthy time, so most children will require long-term IV access. Long-term IV access places the child at high risk for infection and resulting sepsis. Therefore, closely monitor for signs and symptoms of infection. Immediately report to the primary provider or nurse practitioner any fevers or redness or drainage at the IV site.

When started, enteral feeding must be administered very slowly to avoid further malabsorption. Usually, the feeding is started continuously, 24 hours/day, via a feeding pump. Most children have long-term feeding tubes, usually gastrostomy tubes. Most of these children will require special formulas to promote absorption. Assess for feeding tube residuals and abdominal distention or discomfort. Strictly monitor intake and output to avoid dehydration. Assess the stool for signs of carbohydrate malabsorption. Administer vitamin and mineral supplementation, antidiarrheals, and antibiotics as ordered. Teach the family about the use of enteral feeding tubes, feeding pumps, and medication administration.

Promoting Effective Family Coping

Children with a short bowel syndrome are considered to be medically fragile for a lengthy period. There is much anxiety related to the initial bowel resection that resulted in short bowel. Long-term hospitalization is almost always required, causing parents to miss work and cut down on the time they have to spend with other children. This can lead to even more anxiety about finances and relationships. Encourage families to become the experts on their child's needs and condition via education and participation in care. Provide teaching so that the family is better able to care for the child in an outpatient setting. Education focuses on information about TPN and central line care, enteral feedings, assessing for hydration status, and managing medications.

TAKE NOTE!

Maintaining long-term central venous access for TPN in infants can present a challenge. One-piece clothing with the central venous line (CVL) tubing exiting and secured on the back of the outfit can help discourage the infant from pulling on (and subsequently dislodging) the line.

Inflammatory Bowel Disease

Crohn disease and ulcerative colitis are the two major idiopathic IBDs in children. The causes are unknown. However, they may be due to an abnormal or uncontrolled genetically determined immunologic or inflammatory response to an environmental antigenic trigger, possibly a virus or bacterium (Bishop & Ebach, 2023). The features of Crohn disease and ulcerative colitis are listed in Comparison Chart 42.2.

COMPARISON CHART 42.2 Features of Crohn Disease and Ulcerative Colitis

Feature	Crohn Disease	Ulcerative Colitis
Age at onset	10–20 years	10–20 years
Incidence	4–6 per 100,000	3–15 per 100,000
Area of bowel affected	Oropharynx, esophagus, and stomach, rare: small bowel only, 25%–30%; colon and anus only, 25%; ileocolitis, 40%; diffuse disease, 5%	Total colon, 90%; proctitis, 10%
Distribution	Segmental; disease-free skip areas common	Continuous; distal to proximal
Pathology	Full-thickness, acute, and chronic inflammation; noncaseating granulomas (50%), extraintestinal fistulas, abscesses, stricture, and fibrosis may be present.	Superficial, acute inflammation of mucosa with microscopic crypt abscess
Radiography findings	Segmental lesions; thickened, circular folds; cobblestone appearance of bowel wall secondary to longitudinal ulcers and transverse fissures; fixation and separation of loops; narrowed lumen; "sting sign"; fistulas	Superficial colitis; loss of haustra; shortened colon and pseudopolyps (islands of normal tissue surrounded by denuded mucosa) are late findings.
Intestinal symptoms	Abdominal pain, diarrhea (usually loose with blood if colon involved), perianal disease, enteroenteric or enterocutaneous fistula, abscess, anorexia	Abdominal pain, bloody diarrhea, urgency, tenesmus
Extraintestinal symptoms:		
Arthritis/arthralgia	15%	9%
Fever	40%–50%	40%–50%
Stomatitis	9%	2%
Weight loss	90% (mean 5.7 kg)	68% (mean 4.1 kg)
Delayed growth and sexual development	30%	5%–10%
Uveitis, conjunctivitis	15% (in Crohn colitis)	4%
Sclerosing cholangitis	—	4%
Renal stones	6% (oxalate)	6% (urate)
Pyoderma gangrenosum	1%–3%	5%
Erythema nodosum	8%–15%	4%
Laboratory findings	High erythrocyte sedimentation rate; microcytic anemia; low serum iron and total iron-binding capacity; increased fecal protein loss; low serum albumin; antineutrophil cytoplasmic antibodies present in 10%–20%; *Saccharomyces cerevisiae* antibodies positive in 60%.	High erythrocyte sedimentation rate; microcytic anemia; high white blood cell count with left shift; antineutrophil cytoplasmic antibodies present in 80%.

Data from Bishop, W. P., & Ebach, D. R. (2023). Digestive system. In K. J. Marcdante, R. M. Kliegman, & A. M. Schuh (Eds.), *Nelson's essentials of pediatrics* (9th ed.). Elsevier; and Brumbaugh, D., Furuta, G. T., Hoffenberg, E., Kobak, G., Kramer, R., Walker, T., Septer, S., Shull, M., Soden, J., & Walker, T. (2022). Gastrointestinal tract. In M. Bunik, W. W. Hay, M. J. Levin, & M. J. Abzug (Eds.), *Current diagnosis and treatment: Pediatrics* (26th ed.). McGraw-Hill Education.

Therapeutic Management

Medication is used to control inflammation and symptoms. Medications commonly used include 5-aminosalicylates (5-ASA), antibiotics, immunomodulators, immunosuppressives, and anti–tumor necrosis antibody therapy. Dietary manipulation is also very important.

Failure to respond to medical therapy may result in surgical intervention. Many children with ulcerative colitis eventually undergo a total proctocolectomy, with resulting ostomy, as a curative measure. Children or adolescents with Crohn disease may require surgery to relieve obstruction, drain an abscess, or relieve intractable symptoms.

Nursing Assessment

For a full description of the assessment phase of the nursing process, refer to the "Clinical Judgment and the Nursing Process" section earlier in the chapter. Assessment findings pertinent to Crohn disease and ulcerative colitis are discussed later.

Health History

Elicit a description of the present illness and chief complaint. Common symptoms reported during the health history include:

- Abdominal cramping
- Nighttime symptoms, including waking due to abdominal pain or urge to defecate
- Fever
- Weight loss
- Poor growth
- Delayed sexual development

Children may be reluctant or unwilling to talk about their bowel movements, so explain the importance of doing so. Assess stool pattern history, including frequency, presence of blood or mucus, and duration of symptoms. Explore the child's family history for risk factors such as IBD, colon cancer, or immunologic disorders.

Physical Examination

Assess the child's growth using growth charts to identify any poor growth patterns. Perform a full abdominal examination, noting tenderness, masses, or fullness. Inspect the perianal area to look for skin tags or fissures, which would be highly suspicious for Crohn disease. Assist the primary provider in performing a rectal examination to further assess the rectal area for blood or other lesions. Laboratory test results may be normal. Results for children with Crohn disease and ulcerative colitis are found in Comparison Chart 42.2. An upper GI series with small bowel series may identify evidence of intestinal inflammation, estimate the distribution and extent of disease, and help distinguish between Crohn disease and ulcerative colitis. An upper endoscopy or colonoscopy may rule out affected mucosal tissue and diagnose IBD. A CT scan may be used to rule out suspected abscesses.

Nursing Management

Nursing management focuses on teaching about disease management, teaching about nutritional management, teaching about medication therapy, and promoting family and child coping.

Teaching About Disease Management

The diagnosis of Crohn disease or ulcerative colitis can be very difficult for the child and family to comprehend. Provide teaching about the disease process and medication therapy to help the child and family understand the seriousness of the disease. The primary provider may discuss surgical options during uncontrolled flare-ups, but the nurse may be the person to whom the family members or child address their questions regarding surgery. Provide the family with information to help answer some of their questions and allay fears.

Teaching About Nutritional Management

Teach the child and family about nutritional management of the disease. For example, adequate nutrition with a high-protein and high-carbohydrate diet may be recommended. When the disease is active, lactose may be tolerated poorly, and vitamin and iron supplements will most likely be recommended. Explain that in severe cases enteral feeding tubes or TPN may be needed; this is rare but often induces remission.

Teaching About Medication Therapy

Medications are extremely important in controlling IBD. Provide information about the following common medications used to control the disease:

- 5-ASA: used to prevent relapse (usually used in ulcerative colitis)
- Antibiotics (usually metronidazole and ciprofloxacin): typically used in children who have perianal Crohn disease
- Immunomodulators (usually 6-mercaptopurine [6-MP] or azathioprine): used to help maintain remission. Monitor children for neutropenia and hepatotoxicity.
- Cyclosporine or tacrolimus: used occasionally in conjunction with 6-MP or azathioprine to maintain remission in fulminant ulcerative colitis
- Methotrexate: sometimes used to manage severe Crohn disease
- Anti–tumor necrosis antibody therapy: widely used for children with Crohn disease; occasionally used for children with ulcerative colitis

Promoting Family and Child Coping

IBD is a chronic and often debilitating illness. Many children with this diagnosis can lead normal lives, but frequent illnesses can cause school absences, which in turn add stress to the situation. Because schools have become much less tolerant of absences and tardiness, it may be necessary to write letters to the school explaining the frequent absences or in-school needs. Bathroom privileges should be very flexible for children during flare-ups. Affected children and adolescents may experience stunted growth and delayed puberty so will need additional emotional support. Children with ostomies as a result of surgical resection may have self-esteem issues related to the presence and care of the ostomy. Arrange for counseling for both the child and family to discuss fears and anxiety related to a chronic disease.

Celiac Disease

Celiac disease, also known as celiac sprue, is an immunologic disorder in which gluten, a component of some grains, causes damage to the small intestine. The villi of the small intestine are damaged due to the body's immunologic response to the digestion of gluten. The function of the villi is to absorb nutrients into the bloodstream. When the villi are blunted or damaged, malnutrition occurs.

Celiac disease is one of the most common chronic disorders in Europe and the United States, with a prevalence of over 0.3% to 0.9% with increasing incidence (Bamberger et al., 2022). Increased incidence occurs in those with a family history of celiac disease and in people with autoimmune or genetic disorders.

The only current treatment for celiac disease is a strict gluten-free diet. Eliminating gluten will cause the villi of the intestines to heal and function normally, with subsequent improvement of symptoms. Even very small amounts of gluten introduced back into the diet can cause damage to the villi, so the child must adhere to the diet throughout life (Bamberger et al., 2022).

Nursing Assessment

The child with symptoms of celiac disease often presents for evaluation by age 2, though diagnosis in older children is increasingly occurring.

Elicit a description of the present illness noting the classic symptoms of celiac disease:

- Diarrhea
- **Steatorrhea** (fatty stools)
- Constipation
- Failure to thrive or weight loss
- Abdominal distention or bloating
- Poor muscle tone
- Irritability and listlessness
- Dental disorders
- Anemia
- Delayed onset of puberty or amenorrhea
- Nutritional deficiencies

Explore the child's current and past medical history for risk factors such as genetic predisposition (presence of HLS-DQ2 or DQ8 gene) and first-degree relative with celiac disease. Assess for the typical appearance of children with celiac disease: distended abdomen, wasted buttocks, and very thin extremities (Fig. 42.15). Tissue transglutaminase IgA is a sensitive screening test, yet if the result is negative, the endomysial antibodies test is specific for celiac disease. Small bowel biopsy may reveal partial or subtotal villous atrophy or blunting of the villi of the small intestine. Genetic testing for celiac disease includes DQ2 and DQ8 human leukocyte antigen (HLA) haplotypes (Bamberger et al., 2022).

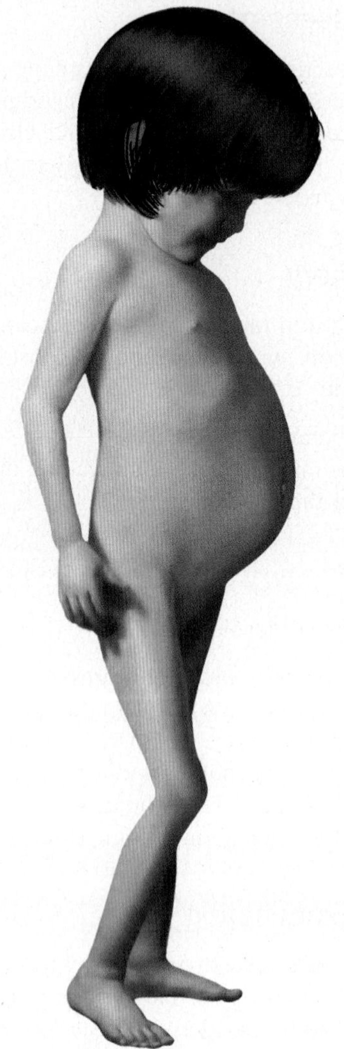

FIGURE 42.15 The child with celiac disease typically displays a distended abdomen and wasted extremities.

Nursing Management

Providing child and family education is the key nursing role in managing children with celiac disease. The child must adhere to a strict gluten-free diet for their entire life. This is often very challenging because gluten is found in most wheat products, rye, barley, and possibly oats. Encourage the parents and child to maintain this gluten-free diet. Often, families consult a dietitian to learn about the gluten-free diet (Teaching Guidelines 42.2).

Provide educational materials and resources to the parents. Many resources are available today about celiac disease because it is becoming more commonly diagnosed. Links to several resources are located on. These resources can offer information on all aspects of celiac disease, including dietary guidelines and resources

TEACHING GUIDELINES **42.2** Dietary Considerations in a Gluten-Free Diet

Foods Allowed	Foods to Avoid
Potato, soy, rice, or bean flour; rice bran, cornmeal, arrowroot, corn or potato starch, sago, tapioca, buckwheat, millet, flax, teff, sorghum, amaranth, quinoa	All wheat products; rye, triticale, barley, oats, or oat bran; graham, gluten, spelt, or durum flour; bulgur, farina, or kamut; malt extract; hydrolyzed vegetable protein
Plain, fresh, frozen, or canned vegetables made with allowed ingredients	Any creamed or breaded vegetables, canned baked beans, some French fries
All fruits and fruit juices	Some commercial fruit pie fillings and dried fruit
All milk and milk products except those made with gluten additives, aged cheese	Malted milk, flavored or frozen yogurt
All meat, poultry, fish, and shellfish; dried peas and beans, nuts; peanut butter; soybean; cold cuts, frankfurters, or sausage without fillers	Any meats or poultry prepared with wheat, rye, oats, barley, gluten stabilizers, or fillers for meats; canned meats; self-basting turkey; some egg substitutes
Butter, margarine, salad dressings, sauces, soups, and desserts with allowable ingredients; sugar, honey, jelly, jam, hard candy, plain chocolate, coconut, molasses, marshmallows, meringues, pure instant or ground coffee, tea, carbonated drinks, wine (from the United States)	Commercial salad dressings, prepared soups, condiments, sauces, and seasonings made with avoided products; nondairy cream substitutes, flavored instant coffee, alcohol distilled from cereals, licorice

Source: Celiac Disease Foundation. (2024). *Gluten-free foods.* http://celiac.org/live-gluten-free/glutenfreediet/

for food shopping and eating in restaurants. A reading source appropriate for school-age children is *Gluten-free Friends: An Activity Book for Kids* by Nancy Patin Falini.

Functional Abdominal Pain Disorders

Functional abdominal pain is a common GI complaint in children and adolescents. It affects children of all ages, and about 2% to 4% of all pediatric outpatient visits are related to recurrent abdominal pain (Brumbaugh et al., 2022). The etiology remains unclear. Functional abdominal pain in children should not be confused with IBS. Box 42.5 outlines the Rome Committee's criteria for IBS and information on the treatment of IBS.

Pathophysiology

The etiology of functional abdominal pain is likely multifactorial regulatory factors in both the enteric and central nervous systems. Functional abdominal pain may occur as referred pain following rectal distention, impaired gastric relaxation response to pain, or heightened sensitivity to visceral pain. Psychological symptoms may occur as a result of persistent or recurrent pain experiences. Therapeutic management focuses on avoidance of triggers and increasing the child's coping skills (see Evidence-Based Practice 42.1). Returning to normal activity is an important component of management (Chacko & Chiou, 2023).

Nursing Assessment

Determine the details of the pain which is usually periumbilical and described as attacks of pain. The pain does not cause night awakening. Obtain a dietary history and a detailed medication history. Identifying social and school stressors is essential. Note the child's body positioning

BOX **42.5** Rome Committee Criteria for IBS

All of the following occur at least once per week minimum for at least 2 months before diagnosis:

- Abdominal pain relieved 25% of the time by defecation.
- Onset of discomfort associated with a change in frequency of stool
- Onset of discomfort associated with a change in appearance of the stool
- No structural, neoplastic, inflammatory, or metabolic explanation for this abdominal pain

Treatment of IBS

For some children, dietary manipulation or medications may help to control diarrhea.

IBS, irritable bowel syndrome.

Data from Bishop, W. P., & Ebach, D. R. (2023). Digestive system. In K. J. Marcdante, R. M. Kliegman, & A. M. Schuh (Eds.), *Nelson's essentials of pediatrics* (9th ed.). Elsevier; Brumbaugh, D., Furuta, G. T., Hoffenberg, E., Kobak, G., Kramer, R., Walker, T., Septer, S., Shull, M., Soden, J., & Walker, T. (2022). Gastrointestinal tract. In M. Bunik, W. W. Hay, M. J. Levin, & M. J. Abzug (Eds.), *Current diagnosis and treatment: Pediatrics* (26th ed.). McGraw-Hill Education.

EVIDENCE-BASED PRACTICE **42.1**

STUDY

Acute diarrhea in children is a worldwide problem. The authors reviewed the published literature to determine how supplementation with probiotics affects the length of the diarrheal episode. They reviewed 82 studies involving over 12,000 participants who were mostly children.

Findings

The authors were unable to find a difference in the length of diarrhea when comparing probiotics to placebo to no treatment. In addition, for those hospitalized with diarrhea, the use of probiotics did not shorten the length of stay. No serious side effects from probiotics were noted.

Nursing Implications

While probiotics are likely not harmful to infants, children, and adolescents with diarrhea, the evidence does not warrant their use in functional abdominal pain. Educate families to follow the primary provider's or nurse practitioner's recommendations for the treatment of diarrhea, in particular focusing on maintaining hydration, rather than attempting to shorten the course of diarrhea with probiotics.

Data from Collinson, S., Deans, A., Padua-Zamora, A., Gregorio, G. V., Li, C., Dans L. F., & Allen, S. J. (2020). Probiotics for treating acute infectious diarrhoea (Review). *Cochrane Database of Systematic Reviews*, (12), CD003048. https://doi.org/10.1002/14651858.CD003048.pub4

and facial expressions. Interactions with family members during the interview may provide more details regarding social stressors. Palpate the abdomen for tenderness. Laboratory and diagnostic testing may be performed to rule out organic causes of abdominal pain.

Nursing Management

Once the diagnosis of functional abdominal pain with no organic cause is made, the majority of the nursing management is focused on promoting coping skills. Often the primary provider or nurse practitioner performs a battery of tests to rule out organic causes, especially when the child's and family's anxiety is high. After these tests are complete, teach the family about the factors that exacerbate the pain and how to deal with these factors. If a specific dietary trigger is identified, teach the child and family to avoid the trigger, offering suggestions for an alternative food.

Arrange for behavioral therapies as ordered and support the child's and family's efforts to follow through with those. Help families determine a plan for school management if pain occurs, to normalize the child's life and ensure they are returned to school in a timely fashion (Chacko & Chiou, 2023).

HEPATOBILIARY DISORDERS

Hepatobiliary disorders include pancreatitis, gallbladder disease, jaundice, biliary atresia, hepatitis, cirrhosis and portal hypertension, and liver transplantation.

Pancreatitis

Pancreatitis is increasingly being recognized as a childhood problem (Sokol et al., 2022). It is classified into two categories—acute and chronic. Acute pancreatitis is an acute inflammatory process that occurs within the pancreas, with variable involvement of localized tissues and remote organ systems. Most common causes of acute pancreatitis include abdominal trauma, drugs and alcohol (though probably rare in children), multisystem disease (such as IBD or systemic lupus erythematosus), infections (usually viruses such as cytomegalovirus [CMV] or hepatitis), congenital anomalies (ductal or pancreatic malformations), obstruction (most likely gallstones or tumors in children), or metabolic disorders. Chronic pancreatitis is defined based on the structural and functional permanent changes that occur in the pancreas.

When pancreatitis is suspected, the child is placed on immediate bowel rest (NPO). Often, a nasogastric tube placed for suction will be needed to keep the stomach decompressed. Serial monitoring of serum amylase levels will determine when oral feeding may be restarted.

Nursing Assessment

For a full description of the assessment phase of the nursing process, refer to the "Clinical Judgment and the Nursing Process" section earlier in the chapter. Assessment findings pertinent to pancreatitis are discussed later.

Health History

Elicit a description of the present illness and chief complaint. Common symptoms reported during the health history include:

- Acute onset of persistent midepigastric and periumbilical abdominal pain, often with radiation to the back or chest
- Vomiting, especially after meals
- Fever

Explore the child's current and past medical history for risk factors such as cystic fibrosis, history of gallstones, traumatic injury, or family history of hereditary pancreatitis.

Physical Examination

Upon auscultation, the bowel sounds may be diminished, suggesting peritonitis. The abdomen may be tender, and distention may occur in younger children and infants.

In severe cases, jaundice, ascites, or pleural effusions may occur. Bluish discoloration around the umbilicus or flanks is seen in the most severe cases of pancreatitis when hemorrhage is present.

Laboratory and Diagnostic Tests

Common laboratory and diagnostic studies ordered for the assessment and monitoring of pancreatitis include:

- Serum amylase and lipase: Levels three times the normal values are extremely indicative of pancreatitis.
- Liver profile: often done to check for increased liver functions and bilirubin levels.
- Blood work: Leukocytosis is common with acute pancreatitis. Hyperglycemia and hypocalcemia may also be noted.
- C-reactive protein: Levels may be elevated.

Diagnostic imaging studies performed to identify malformations or cysts on the pancreas include:

- Plain abdominal radiograph: may show a localized ileus
- Ultrasound: allows direct visualization of the pancreas and the surrounding structures
- Endoscopic retrograde cholangiopancreatography (ERCP): used in some children who may have ductal anomalies, usually with chronic pancreatitis

Nursing Management

Maintain NPO status and nasogastric tube suction and patency. Administer IV fluids to keep the child hydrated and correct any alterations in fluid and electrolyte balance. Pain management is crucial in children with pancreatitis. If hemorrhagic pancreatitis has occurred, blood products and IV antibiotics may be needed. Oral feedings are restarted only after the serum amylase level has returned to normal (usually in 2 to 4 days). Often, pancreatic enzymes are given with oral feedings if pain occurs after oral feeds are restarted.

Surgery is rarely needed in children with pancreatitis, except in those with severe abdominal trauma or major ductal abnormalities. Though chronic pancreatitis is rare in children, provide child and family education regarding the signs and symptoms of recurrence and complications.

Gallbladder Disease

Cholelithiasis is the presence of stones in the gallbladder. Cholesterol stones are usually associated with hyperlipidemia, higher weight, pregnancy, birth control pill use, or cystic fibrosis (Schwarz & Hebra, 2022). They are seen more often in females than males, and increased risk occurs with age and onset of puberty (Schwarz & Hebra, 2022). These stones occur in the gallbladder and may be found in the common bile duct. Pigment stones are found in prepubertal children and occur about equally in males and females. They are usually found in the common bile duct (associated with bacterial or parasitic infections) or the gallbladder itself (associated with hemolytic anemia or liver cirrhosis).

Cholecystitis is an inflammation of the gallbladder that is caused by the chemical irritation due to the obstruction of bile flow from the gallbladder into the cystic ducts. This inflammation is typically associated with gallstones in children. The most common complication in children with gallstone disease is pancreatitis. If cholelithiasis results in symptomatic cholecystitis, then surgical removal of the gallbladder (cholecystectomy) will be necessary. This is often accomplished laparoscopically.

Nursing Assessment

Common symptoms reported during the health history include right upper quadrant pain, often radiating substernally or to the right shoulder, nausea and vomiting, and jaundice and fever (with cholecystitis). Pain episodes usually occur postprandially, especially after the ingestion of fatty or greasy foods. Younger children may present with more nonspecific symptoms, most often due to their lack of ability to communicate their symptoms to others. Explore the child's current and past medical history for risk factors such as chronic TPN use or sickle cell disease.

Palpate the abdomen for tenderness localized in the area of the gallbladder. Assess skin and sclerae color for jaundice. Determine the presence of fever. Note elevated LFTs, serum bilirubin, and C-reactive protein. Ultrasound, ERCP, or hepatobiliary iminodiacetic acid (HIDA) scan may be performed to evaluate the function of the gallbladder and determine the presence of stones.

Nursing Management

The child with symptomatic cholecystitis will usually be hospitalized. Administer IV fluids, maintain NPO status and gastric decompression, and administer pain medications. If ordered, administer IV antibiotics to treat clinically worsening symptoms of cholecystitis, such as persistent fever. Provide routine postoperative care after cholecystectomy is performed. Provide pre- and postoperative teaching for families of children undergoing gallbladder removal.

Biliary Atresia

Biliary atresia is an absence of some or all of the major biliary ducts, resulting in obstruction of bile flow. The ensuing obstruction to bile flow causes cholestasis resulting in jaundice and eventual progressive fibrosis with end-stage cirrhosis of the liver. Biliary atresia affects one in 12,000 infants (Sokol et al., 2022). The etiology of biliary atresia is unknown, but there are several theories, including infectious, autoimmune, or ischemic causes.

Therapeutic Management

If there is a high suspicion of biliary atresia, the infant will undergo exploratory laparotomy. If biliary atresia is found, a Kasai procedure (hepatoportoenterostomy) is performed to connect the bowel lumen to the bile duct remnants found at the porta hepatis. This procedure is most successful for infants 30 to 45 days of age, as bile flow restoration after this age is minimal (Sokol et al., 2022). Infants who are not identified early enough or those who have failed to respond to the Kasai procedure will need to undergo liver transplantation (Sokol et al., 2022).

Nursing Assessment

Determine the history of persistent or recurring jaundice in the young infant. Note jaundice of the skin and sclerae (yellow discoloration caused by bile pigment deposition). Palpate the abdomen for a hardened and enlarged liver and possibly splenomegaly. Note stools are acholic (chalky and white due to the lack of bile pigment). Serum bilirubin, alkaline phosphatase, liver enzymes, and gamma-glutamyl transferase (GGT) will be elevated. Ultrasound, biliary scan, and liver biopsy may be performed.

Nursing Management

Nursing management of infants who have biliary atresia will focus on vitamin and caloric support. Administer fat-soluble vitamins A, D, E, and K. Special formulas containing medium-chain triglycerides are used because significant fat malabsorption occurs when cholestasis is present. Administer feedings via nasogastric tube as needed to ensure increased caloric intake. Identify infections as quickly as possible and administer IV antibiotics as ordered. Manage ascites with diuretics and dietary restrictions. Preoperative management before a Kasai procedure is focused on preparation for surgery; infants who have suspected biliary atresia require immediate surgery to optimize outcomes. Provide extensive emotional support if the family is likely to have extreme anxiety due to the implications of the diagnosis and outcomes.

Hepatitis

Hepatitis is an inflammation of the liver that is caused by a variety of agents, including viral infections, bacterial invasion, metabolic disorders, chemical toxicity, and trauma. The most common viral causes of hepatitis are listed in Table 42.4. Other viruses that may cause hepatitis are CMV, Epstein–Barr virus (EBV), and adenovirus. Fulminant hepatitis is thought to be caused by a non-A, non-B, or non-C virus. Children who present with fulminant hepatitis have

TABLE 42.4 • Hepatitis Viruses A–E

	Hepatitis A (HAV)	Hepatitis B (HBV)	Hepatitis C (HCV)	Hepatitis D (HDV)	Hepatitis E (HEV)
Transmission route	Oral–fecal route, poor sanitation, waterborne	Sexual, intravenous drug use, blood transfusion, perinatally transmitted from parent to infant	Blood product transfusion, intravenous drug use	Same as HBV; HBV markers in serum must be present.	Oral–fecal
Incubation period (days)	15–30	50–150	30–160	50–150	15–65
Signs and symptoms	Flulike symptoms Pre-icteric phase: headache, fatigue, fever, anorexia Icteric phase: jaundice, dark urine, tender liver (right upper quadrant pain)	Some cases are without symptoms; others present with anorexia, abdominal pain, and fatigue, rash, slight fever, visible jaundice, enlarged liver.	Chronic cases usually present without symptoms; others with flulike symptoms, jaundice, hepatosplenomegaly	Same as HBV	Same as HAV, more severe in pregnant people
Prognosis	Rarely develops into fulminant liver failure; 95% of children recover without sequelae.	Chronic disease state likely; increased risk of hepatic cancer	Many will develop chronic hepatitis and cirrhosis.	Same as HBV, but increased likelihood of chronic active hepatitis and cirrhosis	Same as HAV; high mortality in pregnant people

Data from Sokol, R. J., Mark, J. A., Mack, C. L., Felman, A. G., & Sundaram, S. S. (2022). Liver and pancreas. In M. Bunik, W. W. Hay, M. J. Levin, & M. J. Abzug (Eds.), *Current pediatric diagnosis and treatment* (26th ed.). McGraw-Hill Education.

acute massive hepatic necrosis. The disease progresses rapidly to severe jaundice, coagulopathy, elevated ammonia levels, significantly elevated liver enzyme levels (aspartate aminotransferase [AST] and alanine aminotransferase [ALT]), and progressive coma, resulting in death without liver transplantation. Autoimmune hepatitis is a chronic disorder, affecting mostly adolescent females. The clinical presentation of a child with autoimmune hepatitis includes hepatosplenomegaly, jaundice, fever, fatigue, and right upper quadrant pain.

Therapeutic Management

Acute hepatitis is treated with rest, hydration, and nutrition. Control of bleeding may also be necessary. Chronic hepatitis often eventually requires liver transplantation. Corticosteroids and immunosuppressants may be used for autoimmune hepatitis. The child with fulminant hepatitis usually requires intensive care with cardiorespiratory support. See Healthy People 2030.

HEALTHY PEOPLE 2030

Objective	Nursing Significance
Reduce hepatitis A and hepatitis B infection.	• Educate families about hepatitis B and its transmission. • Encourage routine infant and childhood vaccination against hepatitis A and hepatitis B as recommended. • For hepatitis A prevention, educate families about appropriate hygiene and handwashing.

Healthy People Objectives retrieved from http://www.healthypeople.gov

Nursing Assessment

Elicit the health history, noting likely symptoms of fever, fatigue, abdominal pain, and jaundice.

Explore the child's current and past medical history for risk factors such as:

- Recent foreign travel
- Sick contacts
- Medication use
- Abdominal trauma
- Sexual activity
- IV drug use
- Blood product transfusion

Observe the skin for jaundice and the sclerae for icterus. Palpate the abdomen to reveal abnormal liver and spleen size or tenderness. Laboratory studies may reveal elevated liver enzymes, GGT, and ammonia levels (in the presence of encephalopathy). Prothrombin time (PT)/partial thromboplastin time (PTT) will be prolonged. Viral and autoimmune studies may be used to identify the cause of the hepatitis. An ultrasound or liver biopsy may also be performed.

Nursing Management

Acute hepatitis requires rest, hydration, and nutrition. If the child develops vomiting, dehydration, elevated-bleeding times (PT/PTT), or mental status changes (encephalopathy), hospitalization may be required. When caring for children with infectious hepatitis, provide education about transmission and prevention, including proper hygiene, safe sexual activity, careful handwashing techniques, and blood/bodily fluid precautions.

Fulminant hepatitis treatment is aggressive and will require NPO status, nasogastric tube administration of lactulose to decrease ammonia levels that lead to encephalopathic conditions, TPN administration, vitamin K injections to help with coagulopathies, and, ultimately, liver transplantation. Fear and anxiety of the child and parents will likely be very high. Teach the child and family about the diagnosis and what to expect during treatment. Provide immunoglobulin therapy and vaccinations to close contacts of children with infectious hepatitis.

Cirrhosis and Portal Hypertension

Cirrhosis of the liver occurs as a result of the destructive processes that occur during liver damage, leading to the formation of nodules. These nodules can be small (micronodular [less than 3 mm]) or large (macronodular [greater than 3 mm]) and distort the vasculature of the liver, leading to further complications. Causes of cirrhosis in children include biliary malformations, α_1-antitrypsin deficiency, Wilson disease, galactosemia, tyrosinemia, and chronic active hepatitis (Sokol et al., 2022).

Major complications may exist due to cirrhosis of the liver, including portal hypertension. In portal hypertension, the blood flow to, through, or from the liver meets resistance, causing portal blood flow pressures to rise. As these pressures rise, collateral veins form between the portal and systemic venous circulations. The most significant complication of portal hypertension is GI bleeding, from shunting to submucosal veins (varices) in the stomach and esophagus. Esophageal varices may be treated with sclerotherapy during endoscopy to stop acute bleeding. Often blood product administration and vasopressive drugs are needed. In the long term, the only cure for cirrhosis is liver transplantation.

Nursing Assessment

During the health history, note the common symptoms of nausea and vomiting, weakness, jaundice, swelling, and weight loss. Explore the child's current and past medical history for risk factors such as hepatitis, cystic fibrosis, Wilson disease, hemochromatosis, and biliary atresia.

Inspect for jaundice, ascites, spider angiomas, and palmar erythema. Note gynecomastia in males. Palpate the liver; typically, it is enlarged and hard, but occasionally it is small and shrunken. Evaluate mental status to determine the presence of hepatic encephalopathy. Laboratory and diagnostic testing will be similar to that of a child with hepatitis.

Nursing Management

Nursing management is very similar to the care of the child with hepatitis. In cases of cirrhosis causing portal hypertension and bleeding varices, GI bleeding must be controlled. This is usually done by replacing blood loss and providing vasopressive therapy to constrict the shunted blood flow. As with all liver disorders and GI bleeding, address and manage family and child anxiety. Be honest about the child's treatment plan and prognosis. Involve the family in the care of the child and educate them as needed.

Liver Transplantation

Hepatobiliary disorders that result in failure of the liver to function result in the need for liver transplantation. Liver transplantation in children has become increasingly successful in the past several years due to advances in immunosuppression, better selection of transplant candidates, and improvements in surgical techniques and postoperative care (Sokol et al., 2022). Transplant centers now offer both cadaveric and living-related liver transplants for children. Rejection of the transplanted liver is the most significant complication. Most children will require immunosuppressive therapy for a lifetime, putting them at risk for infections.

Nursing Assessment

Many children will be admitted to a transplant center for a preoperative workup to determine the best possible tissue and blood match for the child. There is much anxiety among family members when a cadaveric transplant is the only possibility for survival. This puts a child on a waiting list that is prioritized based on several criteria. Because there are a limited number of pediatric liver transplant centers throughout the country, there may be many issues regarding transportation, finances, job loss, and lodging. Assess the need for social work intervention; a social worker is almost always involved with these children. A liver transplant coordinator will assist with coordinating the care for pre- and posttransplant children.

Nursing Management

Preoperatively, assist with the transplant workup and teach the child and family what to expect during and after the liver transplantation. Postoperatively, the child will be in the intensive care unit for several days until they are stabilized from the actual surgery. After the child is sent to a regular unit in the hospital, monitor the child for several days to weeks for signs and symptoms of rejection and infection, including fever, increasing LFT results and GGT, and increasing pain, redness, and swelling at the incision site. Child and family education is an important element of nursing management in the posttransplant child. Assess and reassess medication knowledge throughout the entire hospitalization, as these children usually require medications for a lifetime.

Unfolding Patient Stories: Eva Madison • Part 2

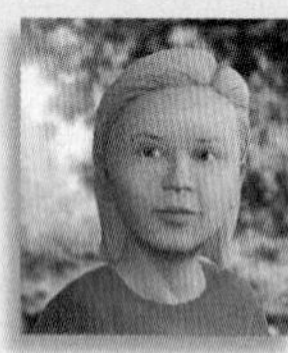

Recall Eva Madison, the 5-year-old child you met in Chapter 32. She is diagnosed with bacterial gastroenteritis. How would the nurse prepare Eva and her parents for hospitalization? What nursing actions can promote a more favorable hospital experience in this age group?

Care for Eva and other patients in a realistic virtual environment: ***vSim** for Nursing*(thepoint.lww.com/vSimPediatric). Practice documenting these patients' care in DocuCare (thePoint.lww.com/DocuCareEHR).

KEY CONCEPTS

- The esophagus of the young child exhibits underdeveloped muscle tone compared with the adult.
- A major difference between children and adults is the reduced stomach capacity in the child and the significantly shorter length of the small intestine (250 cm in the child versus 600 cm in the adult).
- Infants and children have a proportionately greater amount of body water than adults, resulting in a relatively greater fluid intake requirement than adults and placing infants and children at higher risk for fluid loss as compared with adults.
- The most common result of GI illnesses in infants and children is dehydration.
- The mildly or moderately dehydrated child must be identified and receive rehydration therapy to prevent progression to hypovolemic shock.
- Rehydration is a key medical treatment for dehydration as a result of many different GI disorders. Oral rehydration is most common, but in cases requiring hospitalization, IV fluid therapy is key.
- Promotion of adequate nutrition is another significant treatment component. The child with a chronic GI disorder may require IV TPN or enteral tube feedings to exhibit appropriate growth.

- Surgical intervention is necessary for many acute or congenital GI disorders, such as pyloric stenosis, omphalocele, gastroschisis, cleft lip and palate, appendicitis, Hirschsprung disease, and intestinal malrotation.
- Monitoring the blood count, electrolyte levels, and LFTs is necessary in many pediatric GI disorders.
- Histamine-2 blockers, proton-pump inhibitors, and prokinetic agents are used to treat disorders in which gastric acid is a problem, such as esophagitis, GERD, and ulcers.
- Close monitoring for infection is important in children with IBD, autoimmune hepatitis, or liver transplant who are being treated with immunosuppressants and corticosteroids.
- GI stimulants and laxatives may be necessary for treating constipation and encopresis.
- Diarrhea, vomiting, decreased oral intake, sustained high fever, diabetic ketoacidosis, and extensive burns place the infant or child at risk for the development of dehydration.
- Risk factors for vomiting include exposure to viruses, use of certain medications, and overfeeding in the infant.
- Risk factors for acute diarrhea include recent ingestion of undercooked meats, foreign travel, day care attendance, and well water ingestion.
- Vomiting is a symptom and should be characterized in terms of volume, color, relation to meals, duration, and associated symptoms.
- Bleeding may occur as a result of a GI disorder, particularly from the intestine with Meckel diverticulum and from esophageal varices with portal hypertension.
- Acute GI disorders are those that usually have a rapid onset and a short course, which at times may be severe. Examples include dehydration, vomiting, diarrhea, hypertrophic pyloric stenosis, and appendicitis.
- Chronic GI disorders are those that are long lasting or recur over time. Examples include constipation, GERD, IBD, functional abdominal pain, and failure to thrive.
- Right lower quadrant pain and rebound tenderness of the abdomen found on physical examination are telltale signs of appendicitis, which is considered a surgical emergency.
- Bilious vomiting is the main symptom of conditions resulting in bowel obstruction, such as malrotation with volvulus.
- The focus of nursing management of the child with diarrhea or vomiting is restoring proper fluid and electrolyte balance through oral rehydration therapy or IV fluids if necessary.
- Reduction of inguinal and umbilical hernias should be attempted; if reduction of the hernia is impossible, immediately notify the primary provider.
- Small, frequent, and thickened feedings and proper positioning after feedings are key elements in the treatment of GER.
- A crucial nursing intervention related to cleft lip and palate repair is protection of the surgical site while it is healing.
- Palpation of the abdomen should be the last part of the physical examination of an infant or child.
- A key element of nursing care for the child with a GI disorder is the promotion of appropriate bowel elimination.
- Maximizing nutritional status is a critical nursing function for the child with a GI disorder.
- For the child who has undergone surgical repair for correction of a GI disorder, promoting effective breathing patterns and managing pain are important nursing goals.
- Counseling families about how to manage the child with vomiting or diarrhea at home, including oral rehydration therapy, is a key component of child/family education.
- Education of the child and family regarding the importance of medication adherence for the management of IBD is critical.
- Behavioral therapy and counseling may be necessary for children who have functional constipation and stool withholding.
- The child or adolescent with ineffective bowel control, poor growth, or an ostomy may have poor self-esteem and body image.

REFERENCES AND RECOMMENDED READINGS

Anderson, C. C., Kapoor, S., & Mark, T. E. (2024). *The Harriet Lane handbook* (23rd ed.). Elsevier.

Bamberger, J. M., Nelson, S. S., & Westry, M. F. G. (2022). Management of nutritional disorders. In T. Kyle (Ed.), *Primary care pediatrics for the nurse practitioner: A practical approach*. Springer.

Bishop, W. P., & Ebach, D. R. (2023). Digestive system. In K. J. Marcdante, R. M. Kliegman, & A. M. Schuh (Eds.), *Nelson's essentials of pediatrics* (9th ed.). Elsevier.

Brumbaugh, D., Furuta, G. T., Hoffenberg, E., Kobak, G., Kramer, R., Walker, T., Septer, S., Shull, M., Soden, J., & Walker, T. (2022). Gastrointestinal tract. In M. Bunik, W. W. Hay, M. J. Levin, & M. J. Abzug (Eds.), *Current diagnosis and treatment: Pediatrics* (26th ed.). McGraw-Hill Education.

Campbell, J. R., & Palazzi, D. L. (2023). Candida infections in children. *UpToDate*. Retrieved March 12, 2024, from https://www.uptodate.com/contents/candida-infections-in-children

Canani, R. B. (2018). *Abstract G-O-053*. Presented at ESPGHAN 51st Annual Meeting, Geneva, Switzerland. https://www.healio.com/gastroenterology/therapeutics-diagnostics/news/online/%7B2723f19c-6f91-4656-a80b-d6d6125f7e37%7D/ginger-effective-for-treating-vomiting-in-children-with-acute-gastroenteritis

Celiac Disease Foundation. (2024). *Gluten-free foods*. https://celiac.org/gluten-free-living/gluten-free-foods/

Chacko, M. R., & Chiou, E. (2023). Functional abdominal pain in children and adolescents: Management in primary care. *UpToDate*. Retrieved March 12, 2024, from https://www.uptodate.com/contents/functional-abdominal-pain-in-children-and-adolescents-management-in-primary-care

CHOC Children's. (2024). *Stool tests*. https://www.choc.org/programs-services/gastroenterology/digestive-disorder-diagnostics/stool-tests/

Cincinnati Children's. (2024). *Enema administration*. https://www.cincinnatichildrens.org/health/e/enema

Cleft Lip and Palate Association. (2024). *Breastfeeding*. https://www.clapa.com/treatment/feeding/breastfeeding/

Collinson, S., Deans, A., Padua-Zamora, A., Gregorio, G. V., Li, C., Dans L. F., & Allen, S. J. (2020). Probiotics for treating acute infectious diarrhoea (Review). *Cochrane Database of Systematic Reviews*, (12), CD003048. https://doi.org/10.1002/14651858.CD003048.pub4

Corbett, J. A., & Banks, A. D. (2019). *Laboratory tests and diagnostic procedures with nursing diagnoses* (9th ed.). Pearson Education Inc.

Endom, E. E., Dorfma, S. R., & Olivé, A. P. (2023). Infantile hypertrophic pyloric stenosis. *UpToDate*. Retrieved March 12, 2024, from https://www.uptodate.com/contents/infantile-hypertrophic-pyloric-stenosis

Freedman, S. (2023). Oral rehydration therapy. *UpToDate*. Retrieved March 12, 2024, from https://www.uptodate.com/contents/oral-rehydration-therapy

Hanna, M. G., & Bock, M. (2022). Fluid, electrolyte, and acid-base disorders and therapy. In M Bunik, W. W. Hay, M. J. Levin, & M. J. Abzug (Eds.), *Current diagnosis and treatment: Pediatrics* (26th ed.). McGraw-Hill Education.

Keels, M. A., & Clements, D. A. (2022). Herpetic gingivostomatitis in young children. *UpToDate*. Retrieved March 12, 2024, from https://www.uptodate.com/contents/herpetic-gingivostomatitis-in-young-children

Levy, J. (2022). Diagnostic approach to diarrhea in children in resource-rich countries. *UpToDate*. Retrieved March 12, 2024, from https://www.uptodate.com/contents/diagnostic-approach-to-diarrhea-in-children-in-resource-rich-countries

Lexicomp®. (2024). *Lexi-Drugs/viscous lidocaine* (Version 8.1.2) [Mobile app]. Wolters Kluwer. https://apps.apple.com/us/app/lexicomp/id313401238

Meeks, N. J. L., Kochlar, A., Duis, J., & Saenz, M. (2022). Genetics and dysmorphology. In M. Bunik, W. W. Hay, M. J. Levin, & M. J. Abzug (Eds.), *Current diagnosis and treatment: Pediatrics* (26th ed.). McGraw-Hill Education.

Palazzi, D. L., & Brandt, M. L. (2023). Care of the umbilicus and management of umbilical disorders. *UpToDate*. Retrieved March 12, 2024, from https://www.uptodate.com/contents/care-of-the-umbilicus-and-management-of-umbilical-disorders

Phalke, N., & Goldman, J. J. (2023). *Cleft palate*. StatPearls. https://www.ncbi.nlm.nih.gov/books/NBK563128/

Philichi, L. (2018). Management of childhood functional constipation. *Journal of Pediatric Health Care*, *32*(1), 103–113. https://doi.org/10.1016/j.pedhc.2017.08.008

Romero, J. R. (2022). Hand, foot, and mouth disease and herpangina. *UpToDate*. Retrieved March 12, 2024, from https://www.uptodate.com/contents/hand-foot-and-mouth-disease-and-herpangina

Schare, R. S. (2021). *Canker sores*. https://kidshealth.org/en/parents/canker.html

Schwarz, S. M., & Hebra, A. (2022). Pediatric cholecystitis. *eMedicine*. https://emedicine.medscape.com/article/927340-overview

Sokol, R. J., Mark, J. A., Mack, C. L., Felman, A. G., & Sundaram, S. S. (2022). Liver and pancreas. In M. Bunik, W. W. Hay, M. J. Levin, & M. J. Abzug (Eds.), *Current diagnosis and treatment: Pediatrics* (26th ed.). McGraw-Hill Education.

Sood, M. R. (2023a). Chronic functional constipation and fecal incontinence in infants, children, and adolescents: Treatment. *UpToDate*. Retrieved March 12, 2024, from https://www.uptodate.com/contents/chronic-functional-constipation-and-fecal-incontinence-in-infants-children-and-adolescents-treatment

Sood, M. R. (2023b). Functional constipation in infants, children, and adolescents: Clinical features and diagnosis. *UpToDate*. Retrieved March 12, 2024, from https://www.uptodate.com/contents/functional-constipation-in-infants-children-and-adolescents-clinical-features-and-diagnosis

Thiagarajah, J. R., & Martin, M. G. (2023). Pathogenesis of acute diarrhea in children. *UpToDate*. Retrieved March 12, 2024, from http://www.uptodate.com/contents/pathogenesis-of-acute-diarrhea-in-children

University of California, San Francisco. (2024). *Colostomy*. https://surgery.ucsf.edu/conditions--procedures/colostomy-(pediatric).aspx

U.S. Department of Health and Human Services. (n.d.). *Healthy People 2030*. https://health.gov/healthypeople

Winter, H. S. (2023a). *Clinical manifestations and diagnosis of gastroesophageal reflux disease in children and adolescents*. *UpToDate*. Retrieved March 12, 2024, from https://www.uptodate.com/contents/clinical-manifestations-and-diagnosis-of-gastroesophageal-reflux-disease-in-children-and-adolescents

Winter, H. S. (2023b). *Gastroesophageal reflux in infants*. *UpToDate*. Retrieved March 12, 2024, from https://www.uptodate.com/contents/gastroesophageal-reflux-in-infants

DEVELOPING CLINICAL JUDGMENT

PRACTICING FOR NCLEX

1. A parent brings their 6-month-old infant to the clinic. The child has been vomiting since early morning and has had diarrhea since the day before. The temperature is 38°C, pulse 140, and respiratory rate 38. The infant has lost 6 oz since their well-child visit 4 days ago, cries before passing a bowel movement, and refuses to breastfeed today. What is the priority patient problem?
   a. Altered thermoregulation
   b. Pain (abdominal) related to diarrhea
   c. Dehydration risk (excessive losses and inadequate intake)
   d. Malnutrition risk (decreased oral intake)
2. A child presents with a 2-day history of fever, abdominal pain, occasional vomiting, and decreased oral intake. Which finding would the nurse prioritize for immediate reporting to the health care provider?
   a. Temperature 101.9°F
   b. Rebound tenderness and abdominal guarding
   c. Parents will be leaving the child alone in the hospital.
   d. Child can tolerate only sips of fluid without nausea.
3. A 3-day-old infant presenting with physiologic jaundice is hospitalized and placed under phototherapy. Which response indicates to the nurse that the parent needs more teaching?
   a. "These lights place my infant at risk for dehydration."
   b. "My infant needs to stay under the lights, except during feeding time."
   c. "I will be able to continue to breastfeed during this time."
   d. "I am so upset my infant has a serious liver disease."
4. A 3-month-old infant presents with a history of vomiting after feeding. The plan for the infant is to rule out GERD. What information from the history would lead the nurse to believe that this infant may need further intervention?
   a. Poor weight gain
   b. Small "spits" after feeding
   c. Sleeps through the night
   d. Difficult to burp
5. The nurse is caring for a child who has had diarrhea and vomiting for the past several days. What is the priority nursing assessment?
   a. Determine the child's weight.
   b. Ask if the family has traveled outside of the country.
   c. Assess circulation and perfusion.
   d. Send a stool specimen to the laboratory.
6. The nurse is caring for a 2-year-old with dehydration secondary to rotavirus infection who was admitted at 2:00 p.m. the day prior. The child is not toilet trained. Their weight is 15 kg. The child's IV line fell out during the night. After reviewing the intake and output chart, the nurse uses the situation background assessment recommendation (SBAR) communication technique to call the health care provider with the recommendation for which prescription?
   Intake and Output Record

Date	Time	Oral	Type	IV	Type	Urine	Stool	Emesis
Total 6/12		120	Pedialyte	500	D5 ¼ NS with 20 meq KCl/L	440	X2	0
6/13	0100	15	Pedialyte	50				
6/13	0200			50		30		Mod.
6/13	0300			0				Mod.
6/13	0400			0			Large	
6/13	0500			0				Mod.
6/13	0600			0		Diaper dry		

   a. An indwelling urinary catheter
   b. IV antibiotic
   c. Normal saline IV fluid bolus
   d. One-time dose of loperamide
7. An infant has vomited six times in the past 24 hours. The parent attempted to feed the infant Pedialyte without success. The infant's stools are watery and coat the entire diaper, sometimes with leakage. The infant is at risk for ______ related to ______.
   First blank:
   a. impaired urinary elimination
   b. deficient fluid volume
   c. impaired parenting
   d. pain
   Second blank:
   a. excessive losses from severe diarrhea
   b. infant refusing feeding
   c. vomiting and diarrhea

DOSAGE CALCULATION QUESTION

A child is NPO during the preoperative period and requires IV fluid maintenance. The child weighs 31 lb 4 oz. What is the child's recommended hourly IV fluid rate?

CRITICAL THINKING EXERCISES

1. A 6-month-old is brought to the primary provider's office with a history of diarrhea. The infant has had six watery stools in the past 18 hours and is vomiting the formula. The parent states the infant has had no fever.

a. Upon completion of the history and physical examination, what signs and symptoms would you expect to find that would indicate that the baby is experiencing mild dehydration?
b. What is the priority patient problem for this infant?
c. Identify a plan for this patient problem; include a teaching plan for the parent.

2. A 14-kg child with moderate dehydration has received two boluses of normal saline in the emergency room before being admitted to the pediatric nursing unit. The primary provider orders D5 ½ NS @ 1½ maintenance.
   a. What would the IV fluid rate be?
   b. What will the nurse assess for to determine whether the child is becoming overhydrated?
3. An infant requires a temporary colostomy. What discharge instructions would you provide to the parents about how to take care of the colostomy and when to call their child's primary provider or nurse practitioner?

STUDY ACTIVITIES

1. In the clinical setting, compare the growth records of a child with celiac disease to those of a similar-aged child without disease.
2. While caring for children in the clinical setting, compare and contrast the medical history, signs and symptoms of illness, and prescribed treatment for a child with Crohn disease and one with ulcerative colitis.
3. In the clinical setting, observe the behavioral responses of an infant or young child with inorganic failure to thrive.
4. enzymes continue to develop postnatally, reaching adult levels around 2 years of age.

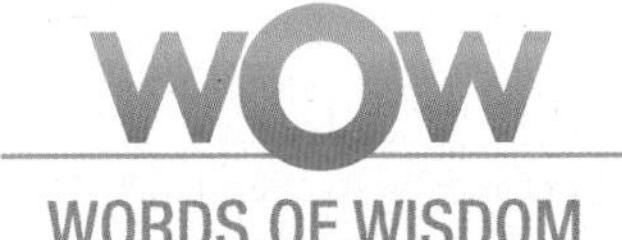

WORDS OF WISDOM

A child's essential bodily processes of elimination can be a major event of wonder and creative accomplishment.

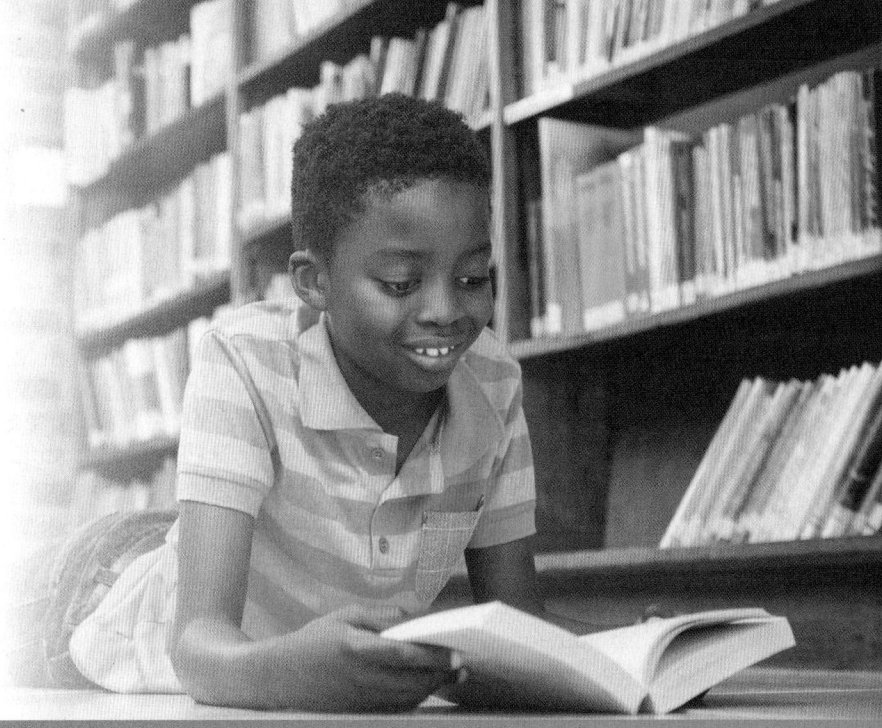

43

Nursing Care of the Child With an Alteration in Urinary Elimination/ Genitourinary Disorder

LEARNING OBJECTIVES

Upon completion of the chapter, you will be able to:

1. Compare anatomic and physiologic differences of the genitourinary system in infants and children versus adults.
2. Describe nursing care related to common laboratory and diagnostic testing used in the medical diagnosis of pediatric genitourinary and reproductive system conditions.
3. Distinguish alterations in urinary elimination and genitourinary disorders common in infants, children, and adolescents.
4. Identify appropriate nursing assessments and interventions related to medications and treatments for alterations in urinary elimination, genitourinary, and reproductive system disorders in children.
5. Develop an individualized nursing care plan or concept map for the child with an alteration in urinary elimination or genitourinary disorder.
6. Describe the psychosocial impact of chronic genitourinary disorders on children.
7. Devise a nutrition plan for the child with abnormal kidney function.
8. Develop child/family teaching plans for the child with an alteration in urinary elimination or genitourinary disorder.

KEY TERMS

anasarca (an′ah-sahr′kă)
anuria
bacteriuria
dysuria
hematuria
oliguria (ol′i-gyūr′ē-ă)
proteinuria
urgency
urinary frequency

Corey Bond, 5 years old, is brought to the clinic by her parent. She presents with fever and lethargy for the past 24 hours. Her parent states, "Corey has had a few accidents in her pants over the past few days, which is unusual for her. She also has been getting up at night more often to use the bathroom."

INTRODUCTION

Urinary elimination refers to the secretion and excretion of body waste through the urinary/renal system. Nurses may encounter children with alterations in urinary elimination and should be familiar with various genitourinary (GU) disorders that children experience. Alterations in urinary elimination or GU disorders in children and adolescents may occur because of abnormalities in fetal development, infectious processes, trauma, neurologic deficit, genetic influences, or other causes.

Congenital disorders account for a large proportion of GU disorders in infants. External GU malformations are easily identified at birth, but internal structural defects may not be identified until later in infancy or childhood when symptoms or complications arise. Enuresis and urinary tract infection (UTI) also occur in a significant number of children.

Some alterations in urinary elimination directly involve the kidney from the outset, while others involve other parts of the urinary tract and may have a long-term effect on kidney function, particularly if left untreated or treated inadequately. Disorders affecting the reproductive organs often require early diagnosis and management to preserve future reproductive capabilities.

Nurses must be knowledgeable about pediatric GU conditions to provide prompt recognition, nursing care, education, and support to children and their families. Though some disorders are acute and resolve quickly, many have a long-term effect on quality of life and will require more intense, extended support. Management of acute or common pediatric GU disorders may be provided in the pediatric or family practice outpatient setting, while specialists such as pediatric nephrologists or urologists usually manage chronic or complex GU disorders.

VARIATIONS IN PEDIATRIC ANATOMY AND PHYSIOLOGY

Although the urinary tract and reproductive organs are present at birth, their initial functioning is immature. The infant or child is at increased risk for the development of certain urinary elimination alterations because of the anatomic and physiologic differences between children and adults.

Structural Differences

The kidney is large in relation to the size of the abdomen until the child reaches adolescence. Due to this increased size, the kidneys of the child are less protected from injury by the ribs and fat padding than they are in the adult. The urethra is naturally shorter in all ages of females compared with males, placing them at increased risk for the entry of bacteria into the bladder via the urethra. In the female infant or young child, this risk is compounded by the physical proximity of the urethral opening to the rectum. The male infant or young child's urethra is much shorter than an adult male's, placing the male infant or young child at increased risk of UTI compared with the adult male.

Urinary Concentration

Blood flow through the kidneys (glomerular filtration rate [GFR]) is slower in the infant and young toddler compared with the adult. The kidney is less able to concentrate urine and reabsorb amino acids, placing the infant and young toddler at increased risk for dehydration during times when fluid loss or decreased fluid intake occurs. The normal range for serum blood urea nitrogen (BUN) and creatinine of the healthy infant or young toddler is usually less than the older child's or adult's. The renal system usually reaches functional maturity at around 2 years of age.

Urine Output

Bladder capacity is about 30 mL in the newborn; it increases to the usual adult capacity of about 270 mL by 1 year of age. The expected urine output in the infant and child is 0.5 to 2 mL/kg/h, with the average 1-year-old voiding about 400 to 500 mL/day. The average urine output for an adolescent is about 800 to 1,400 mL/day. The infant and toddler may void as often as nine or 10 times per day. By age 3, the average number of voids per day is the same as an adult (3 to 8).

Reproductive Organ Maturity

The reproductive organs are also immature at birth. The gonads are not mature until adolescence in most children. The hormonal changes that occur with puberty account for some of the reproductive concerns, particularly for female adolescents.

COMMON MEDICAL TREATMENTS

A variety of medications as well as other medical treatments and surgical procedures are used to treat urinary elimination alterations and GU problems in children. Most of these treatments will require a primary provider's or nurse practitioner's order when the child is in the hospital. The most common treatments and medications are listed in Common Medical Treatments 43.1 and Drug Guide 43.1. The nurse caring for the child with a GU disorder should be familiar with what the procedures are, how the treatments and medications work, and common nursing implications related to use of these modalities.

COMMON MEDICAL TREATMENTS 43.1 Genitourinary Disorders

Treatment	Explanation	Indications	Nursing Implications
Urinary diversion	Surgical diversion of ureters to the abdominal wall. Continent diversion uses a piece of intestine to create a bladder that can be catheterized. Noncontinent diversion involves a stoma on the abdominal wall that requires use of an ostomy pouch.	Any situation in which the bladder needs to be removed or does not function correctly (bladder exstrophy or prune belly).	Meticulous skin care is necessary to prevent breakdown around stoma. Teach families how to care for ostomy pouch or how to catheterize continent stoma. Expect mucus in urine if intestine is used for urinary reservoir. Monitor for signs of urinary tract infection.
Foley catheter	An indwelling urinary catheter stays in place by means of an inflated balloon.	Usually used only during the postoperative period	Monitor for urethral drainage or irritation. Keep area clean and dry. Monitor color, consistency, clarity, and amount of urine in drainage bag. Monitor for infection, checking results of urinalysis and urine cultures.
Ureteral stent	A thin catheter temporarily placed in the ureter to drain urine. It is removed via cystoscopy when it is time for discontinuation.	Urinary tract anomalies	Monitor urine output carefully. Check for bleeding postoperatively.
Nephrostomy tube	Tube is placed directly into the kidney to drain urine externally to a bag.	Urinary tract anomalies	Monitor urine output carefully.
Suprapubic tube	Catheter is placed in the bladder via the abdominal wall above the symphysis pubis.	Postoperative urine drainage with reconstructive surgeries	Monitor for blood in urine, adequate urine output. Minimize manipulation of suprapubic tube to avoid triggering bladder spasms.
Vesicostomy	Stoma in the abdominal wall to the bladder	Urinary tract anomalies, neurogenic bladder	Constant urine drainage requires diaper use. Monitor urine output. Assess skin around stoma for breakdown.
Appendicovesicostomy (Mitrofanoff procedure)	Uses appendix to create a stoma on the abdominal wall that allows for catheterization of the bladder	Urinary tract anomalies, neurogenic bladder	Allows for urinary continence, which improves the child's self-esteem. Teach family and child how to catheterize stoma.
Bladder augmentation	Uses a piece of stomach or intestine to enlarge bladder capacity	Decreased bladder capacity	Since a portion of the gastrointestinal tract is used, urine is often mucuslike.

DRUG GUIDE 43.1

COMMON DRUGS FOR GENITOURINARY DISORDERS

Medication	Actions/Indications	Nursing Implications
Anticholinergic agents (oxybutynin, propantheline bromide, belladonna, and opium suppository)	Cause smooth muscle relaxation of the bladder, used for urinary tract spasms or contractions related to surgical procedure or use of catheters. Control of nocturnal enuresis	Increase fluid intake (limit to during the day in the child with nocturnal enuresis). Avoid use in febrile child.
Antibiotics (oral, parenteral)	Kill bacteria or arrest their growth. Used for urinary tract infection	Check for antibiotic allergies. Should be given as prescribed for the length of time indicated
Desmopressin	Antidiuretic hormone effects by causing kidney tubule to absorb more water, decreasing volume of urine in children with nocturnal enuresis	Nasal spray may cause nasal irritation, nausea, flushing, or headache. Administer at bedtime; alternate nares. Associated with a high relapse rate

(continued)

DRUG GUIDE 43.1 (continued)

COMMON DRUGS FOR GENITOURINARY DISORDERS

Medication	Actions/Indications	Nursing Implications
Human chorionic gonadotropin (hCG)	Stimulates production of gonadal steroids to precipitate testicular descent	Monitor for signs of precocious puberty if used long term.
Corticosteroids	Antiinflammatory and immunosuppressive action to induce remission and promote diuresis in nephrotic syndrome. High-dose intravenous therapy used when nephrotic syndrome is resistant to conventional doses	Administer with food to decrease gastrointestinal (GI) upset. May mask signs of infection Do not stop treatment abruptly, or acute adrenal insufficiency may occur. Monitor for Cushing syndrome.
Cytotoxic drugs (cyclophosphamide and chlorambucil)	Interfere with normal function of DNA by alkylation. Used to induce prolonged remission in nephrotic syndrome	Doses may be tapered over time. Monitor for hypertension during infusion. Causes bone marrow suppression. Monitor for signs of infection. Cyclophosphamide: administer in the morning; provide adequate hydration; have child void frequently during and after infusion to decrease risk of hemorrhagic cystitis. Chlorambucil: administer with nonspicy, nonacidic foods; rarely seizures occur.
Immunosuppressant drugs (cyclosporine A [CyA], azathioprine, tacrolimus, mycophenolate)	Cause immune suppression to prevent rejection of kidney transplants. CyA and tacrolimus may be used for steroid-dependent nephrotic syndrome.	Monitor complete blood count, serum creatinine, potassium, and magnesium. Monitor blood pressure and observe for signs of infection. Blood levels should be drawn prior to morning dose. CyA: do not give with grapefruit juice. Azathioprine and mycophenolate: give on empty stomach; do not open capsule or crush tablet. Tacrolimus: give on empty stomach; assess for development of hyperglycemia. Relapse of nephrotic syndrome may occur after withdrawal of CyA or tacrolimus therapy.
Muromonab-CD3	Removal of all CD3 molecules from T lymphocyte surface so it has inability to act. Used for the treatment of acute kidney transplant rejection	Monitor for the development of pulmonary edema. First-dose effect may cause fever, chills, chest tightness, wheezing, nausea, and vomiting.
Angiotensin-converting enzyme (ACE) inhibitors (captopril, enalapril)	Potent vasoconstrictor, prevent conversion of angiotensin I to angiotensin II. Used to treat renal causes of hypertension	Monitor blood pressure frequently. May cause cough, hyperkalemia Captopril: administer on empty stomach. Enalapril: administer without regard to food.
Imipramine (tricyclic antidepressant)	Increases the synaptic concentration of serotonin and norepinephrine. Treatment of enuresis	Monitor for urinary retention. May cause decreased appetite
Diuretics: furosemide, hydrochlorothiazide	Inhibit resorption of sodium and chloride leading to increased excretion of water and electrolytes. Used in nephrotic syndrome, acute glomerulonephritis, hemolytic uremic syndrome, or other instances of fluid overload with normal kidney function	Administer with food or milk to decrease GI upset. Monitor blood pressure, kidney function, and electrolytes (particularly potassium). May cause photosensitivity
Vasodilators: hydralazine, minoxidil	Direct vasodilation of arterioles, resulting in decreased systemic resistance. Used to treat renal causes of hypertension	May cause fluid retention Hydralazine: administer with food. Monitor heart rate and blood pressure (closely with intravenous use). Minoxidil: may be administered without regard to food. May cause dizziness
Calcium channel blocker: nifedipine	Prevents calcium from entering voltage-sensitive channels, resulting in coronary vasodilation. Used to treat renal causes of hypertension	Administer with food; avoid grapefruit juice. Insoluble shell of extended-release tablet may pass in stool. Use caution when administering liquid-filled capsule sublingually or by bite-and-swallow method, as significant hypotension may occur.
Albumin (intravenous)	Increases intravascular oncotic pressure, resulting in movement of fluid from interstitial to intravascular space. Indicated for fluid volume excess associated with nephrotic syndrome	May require a filter depending on brand used Rapid infusion can result in vascular overload. Monitor vital signs; observe for pulmonary edema and cardiac failure.

Source: UpToDate, Inc. (2024). *Lexi-comp®* (Version 8.1.2) [Mobile app]. Wolters Kluwer. https://apps.apple.com/us/app/lexicomp/id313401238

Clinical Judgment and the Nursing Process

Care of the child with an alteration in urinary elimination or GU disorder includes assessment, nursing analysis, planning, interventions, and evaluation. It is important to individualize each step of this process for each child.

Assessment

Assessment of the urinary tract, kidney, or reproductive dysfunction includes health history, physical examination, and laboratory and diagnostic testing.

Health History

The health history consists of the birthing parent's pregnancy history; family history; and history of present illness (when the symptoms started and how they have progressed), as well as medications and treatments used at home. The medical history may be significant for polyhydramnios, oligohydramnios, diabetes, hypertension, or alcohol or cocaine ingestion. Neonatal history may include the presence of a single umbilical artery or an abdominal mass, chromosome abnormality, or congenital malformation. Document medical history of UTI or other problems with the GU tract.

Family history may be significant for kidney disease or uropathology, chronic UTIs, kidney calculi, or a history of parental enuresis. Determine age of successful toilet training, pattern of incontinent episodes (having "accidents"), and toileting hygiene self-care routines. Note myelomeningocele or other spinal disturbance that may affect the child's ability to urinate. Note previous urologic surgeries or ongoing renal interventions (e.g., dialysis). For the adolescent female, obtain a thorough menstrual history, including sexual behavior and pregnancy history.

When determining the history of the present illness, inquire about the following:

- Burning during urination
- Changes in voiding patterns
- Foul-smelling urine
- Vaginal or urethral discharge
- Genital pain, irritation, or discomfort
- Blood in the urine
- Edema
- Masses in the groin, scrotum, or abdomen
- Flank or abdominal pain
- Cramps
- Nausea and vomiting
- Poor growth
- Weight gain
- Fever
- Infectious exposure (particularly *Streptococcus* A or *Escherichia coli*)
- Trauma

Record medications used for acute or chronic conditions, or for contraception.

Physical Examination

Physical examination of the GU system includes inspection and observation, auscultation, percussion, and palpation.

Inspection and Observation

Observe the child's general appearance, noting growth retardation or unusual weight gain. Inspect the skin for the presence of pruritus, edema (generalized or periorbital), or bruising. Note pallor of the skin or dysmorphic features (associated with genetic conditions). Document the presence of lethargy, fatigue, rapid respirations, confusion, or developmental delay. Observe the external genital area for infant diaper rash, constant urine dribble, displaced or reddened urethral opening, or discharge. In females, note vaginal irritation or labial fusion. In males, observe the scrotal sac for enlargement or discoloration. Note the condition of a urinary stoma or diversion if present. With the child lying flat, observe the abdomen for distention, ascites, or slack abdominal musculature.

Auscultation

Listen carefully to heart sounds, as a flow murmur may be present in the anemic child with a kidney disorder (Klabunde, 2024). Note elevated heart rate. Auscultate blood pressure with the appropriate-size cuff, noting elevation or depression. In the edematous child, carefully auscultate the lungs, noting the presence of adventitious sounds. Note the absence of bowel sounds, as this may indicate peritonitis. In the child who receives chronic hemodialysis, auscultate the fistula for the presence of a bruit (desired normal finding).

TAKE NOTE!

Use the bell of the stethoscope when auscultating the infant's or child's blood pressure so that you can hear the softer Korotkoff sounds more accurately.

Percussion

Percuss the abdomen. Note unusual dullness or flatness (dullness is usually heard over the spleen in the left costal margin, over the kidneys, and 1 to 3 cm below the ribs on the right). A full bladder may yield dullness above the symphysis pubis.

Palpation

Palpate the abdomen. Note the presence of palpable kidneys (indicating enlargement or mass, as they are usually difficult to palpate in the older infant or child).

Note the presence of abdominal masses or a distended bladder. Document tenderness to palpation or along the costovertebral angle. Palpate the scrotum for the presence of descended testicles, masses, or other abnormalities. Note whether the foreskin, if present, can be retracted. In the child who receives chronic hemodialysis, palpate the fistula or graft for the presence of a thrill (desired normal finding).

Laboratory and Diagnostic Testing

Common Laboratory and Diagnostic Tests 43.1 explains the most commonly used laboratory and diagnostic tests for a child suspected of having a GU disorder. The test results can help the primary provider or nurse practitioner to diagnose the disorder or to determine treatment. Laboratory or nonnursing personnel obtain some of the tests, while the nurse might obtain others. In either instance, the nurse should be familiar with how the tests are obtained, what they are used for, and normal versus abnormal results. This knowledge will also be necessary when providing child and family education related to the tests and results.

Remember Corey, the 5-year-old with fever and lethargy? What additional health history and physical examination assessment information should you obtain?

COMMON LABORATORY AND DIAGNOSTIC TESTS 43.1

Test	Explanation	Indications	Nursing Implications
Complete blood count	Evaluate hemoglobin and hematocrit, white blood cell count, and platelet count.	Any condition in which anemia, infection, or thrombocytopenia is suspected	Normal values vary according to age and sex. White blood cell count differential is helpful in evaluating source of infection.
Blood urea nitrogen (BUN) (serum)	Indirect measurement of kidney function and glomerular filtration in the presence of adequate liver function	Nephrotic syndrome, hemolytic uremic syndrome, kidney failure, acute glomerulonephritis, or other kidney diseases	BUN may be elevated with high-protein diet or dehydration, may be decreased with overhydration or malnutrition.
Creatinine (serum)	A more direct measurement of kidney function, only minimally affected by liver function. Generally, doubling of the creatinine level is suggestive of a 50% reduction in glomerular filtration rate.	Used to diagnose impaired kidney function	A diet high in meat may cause a transient though not pronounced increase in creatinine. There are also slight diurnal variations in levels. Draw at same time each day if serial evaluations are ordered.
Creatinine clearance (urine and serum)	A 24-hour urine collection is evaluated for the presence of creatinine, then compared with the serum creatinine level to determine creatinine clearance.	Used to diagnose impaired kidney function	Discard the first void and then begin the 24-hour urine collection. Keep the specimen on ice during the collection period. Collect all urine passed in the 24-hour period. Ensure that a venous blood sample is drawn during the 24-hour period. The urine specimen should be sent promptly to the laboratory at the end of the 24-hour period.
Potassium (serum)	Measures the concentration of potassium in the blood	Any suspected kidney disease; followed routinely in kidney failure	Avoid hemolysis and allow child to open and close the hand with a tourniquet in place, as these can cause elevation in potassium levels. Evaluate the child with increased or decreased potassium levels for cardiac arrhythmias. Immediately notify primary provider or nurse practitioner of critically high potassium levels.
Total protein, globulin, albumin (serum)	Protein electrophoresis separates the various components into zones according to their electrical charge.	Used to diagnose, evaluate, and monitor chronic kidney disease	Significantly low levels of albumin contribute to extent of edema, as albumin is necessary in the blood to maintain colloidal osmotic pressure.
Calcium (serum)	Measurement of calcium level in the blood; half of all calcium is protein bound, so the level will decrease with hypoalbuminemia.	Kidney diseases associated with hypoalbuminemia and edema	Avoid prolonged tourniquet use during blood draw, as this may falsely increase the calcium level.

COMMON LABORATORY AND DIAGNOSTIC TESTS 43.1

Test	Explanation	Indications	Nursing Implications
Phosphorus (serum)	Measurement of phosphate level in the blood. Phosphorus levels are inversely related to calcium levels (they increase when calcium levels decrease).	Kidney disease, ongoing monitoring, particularly in the child with hypocalcemia	Child should be nothing by mouth (NPO) past midnight prior to the morning of the blood draw. Avoid hemolysis, as it can falsely elevate the phosphate level.
Urinalysis (urine)	Evaluates color, pH, specific gravity, and odor of urine. Also assess for the presence of protein, glucose, ketones, blood, leukocyte esterase, red and white blood cells, bacteria, crystals, and casts.	Reveals preliminary information about the urinary tract. Useful in children with fever, dysuria, flank pain, urgency, or hematuria. Proteinuria may be noted in kidney disorders.	Be aware of the many drugs affecting urine color and notify laboratory if child is taking one. Notify laboratory if female is menstruating. Refrigerate specimen if not processed promptly. While proteinuria may occur with various kidney disorders, it may also occur as either transient or orthostatic proteinuria, both of which are benign events.
Cystoscopy	Endoscopic visualization of the urethra and bladder	Evaluate hematuria, recurrent urinary tract infection; determine ureteral reflux; measure bladder capacity.	Encourage fluids. Monitor vital signs. Child may feel burning with voiding after procedure. Pink tinge to urine is common after procedure.
Urine culture and sensitivity	Urine is plated in the laboratory and evaluated every day for the presence of bacteria. A final report is usually issued after 48–72 hours. Sensitivity testing is performed to determine the best choice of antibiotic.	Used to diagnose urinary tract infection	Obtain culture specimen prior to starting antibiotics if possible. Avoid contamination of the specimen with stool. May be obtained by catheterization, clean-catch specimen, or sterile U-bag. In some institutions, suprapubic tap is performed in neonates and young infants by the primary provider or nurse practitioner.
Urodynamic studies	Measure the urine flow during micturition via a urine flow meter.	Dysfunctional voiding	The child must have a full bladder. The child then urinates into the urine flow meter. There is no discomfort associated with the test.
Voiding cystourethrogram (VCUG)	The bladder is filled with contrast material via catheterization. Fluoroscopy is performed to demonstrate filling of the bladder and collapsing after emptying.	Hematuria, urinary tract infections, vesicoureteral reflux, suspected structural anomalies	Just prior to the test, insert the Foley catheter. Ensure that the adolescent female is not pregnant. After the test, encourage the child to drink fluids to prevent bacterial accumulation and aid in dye elimination.
Intravenous pyelogram (IVP)	Radiopaque contrast material is injected intravenously and filtered by the kidneys. X-ray films are obtained at set intervals to show passage of the dye through the kidneys, ureters, and bladder.	Urinary outlet obstruction, hematuria, trauma to the kidney system, suspected kidney tumor	Contraindicated in children allergic to shellfish or iodine. If the dye infiltrates at the intravenous site, hyaluronidase may be used to speed absorption of the iodine. Ensure adequate hydration before and after the test. Some institutions require enema or laxative evacuation of the bowel prior to the study to ensure adequate visualization of the urinary tract.
Kidney biopsy	Usually a percutaneous specimen is obtained by inserting a needle through the skin and into the kidney. The sample of kidney tissue obtained is then microscopically examined.	Diagnosis of kidney disease or assessment of kidney transplant rejection	After the biopsy, carefully assess for signs or symptoms of bleeding: increased heart rate, pale color, flank pain or backache, shoulder pain, lightheadedness. Inspect urine for gross hematuria. Child will be on bed rest, preferably supine for 24 hours.
Kidney ultrasound	Reflected sound waves allow visualization of the kidneys, ureters, and bladder.	Useful in determining kidney size (as with hydronephrosis and polycystic kidney), presence of cysts or tumors, or rejection of kidney transplant	No fasting is required prior to the procedure. Does not require contrast material. The child should feel no discomfort during the ultrasound.

Data from Corbett, J. A., & Banks, A. D. (2019). *Laboratory tests and diagnostic procedures with nursing diagnoses* (9th ed.). Pearson Education Inc.

Nursing Analysis and Related Interventions

After recognizing and analyzing cues from a thorough assessment, the nurse may identify patient problems, such as:

- Fluid overload
- Malnutrition risk
- Altered urinary elimination
- Activity intolerance
- Altered body image perception
- Pain
- Interrupted family processes
- Knowledge deficiency

After completing an assessment of Corey, you note the following: foul-smelling urine, abdominal tenderness, redness in her perineal area, and slightly blood-tinged, cloudy urine. Based on these assessment findings, what would your top three issues or concerns be for Corey?

The above patient problems provide suggestions for nursing care planning or concept mapping. Suggested interventions with rationales are provided next. Care planning should be individualized, based on the child's and family's needs. Refer to Chapter 36 for the nursing process for pain management and to Chapter 33 for nursing interventions related to interrupted family processes. Additional information will be included later in the chapter as it relates to nursing management of children with specific disorders, as well as particular nursing interventions for knowledge deficiency.

Nursing Analysis

Fluid overload related to decreased protein in the bloodstream, decreased urine output, sodium retention, or possible inappropriate fluid intake, as evidenced by edema, anasarca, weight gain, oliguria, azotemia, pulmonary congestion, or presence of S_3 heart sound

Goal/Outcome

Child will attain appropriate fluid balance, will lose weight (fluid), edema or anasarca will decrease, lung sounds will be clear, and heart sounds will be normal.

Encouraging Fluid Loss (interventions with *rationale*)

- Weigh child daily on same scale in similar amount of clothing: *in children, weight is the best indicator of changes in fluid status.*
- Monitor location and extent of edema (measure abdominal girth daily if ascites is present): *decrease in edema indicates positive increase in oncotic pressure.*
- Auscultate lungs carefully to determine presence of crackles *(indicating pulmonary edema).*
- Assess work of breathing and respiratory rate: *increased work of breathing is associated with pulmonary edema.*
- Assess heart sounds for presence or absence of gallop: *presence of S_3 may indicate fluid overload.*
- Maintain fluid restriction as ordered *to decrease intravascular volume and workload on the heart.*
- Strictly monitor intake and output *to quickly note discrepancies and provide intervention.*
- Provide sodium-restricted diet as ordered: *restricting sodium in the diet allows for better renal excretion of extra fluid.*
- Administer diuretics as ordered and monitor for side effects of those medications. *Diuretics encourage excretion of fluid and elimination of edema, reduce cardiac filling pressures, and increase renal blood flow. Side effects include electrolyte imbalance and orthostatic hypotension.*

Nursing Analysis

Malnutrition risk; risk factors include protein loss or insufficient dietary intake (anorexia).

Goal/Outcome

Child will improve nutritional intake, resulting in steady increase in weight and length/height.

Promoting Adequate Nutrition (interventions with *rationale*)

- Determine body weight and length/height norm for age *to determine goal to work toward.*
- Assess child for food preferences that fall within dietary restrictions, *as the child will be more likely to consume adequate amounts of foods that they like.*
- Weigh daily or weekly (according to primary provider or nurse practitioner's order or institutional standard) and measure length/height weekly *to monitor for increased growth.*
- Offer highest calorie meals at the time of day when the child's appetite is the greatest *to increase likelihood of increased caloric intake.*
- Provide increased-calorie shakes or puddings within diet restriction: *high-calorie foods increase weight gain.*
- Administer vitamin and mineral supplements as prescribed *to attain/maintain vitamin and mineral balance in the body.*

Nursing Analysis

Altered urinary elimination related to pathologic process, anatomic obstruction, sensory motor impairment, or dysfunctional voiding as evidenced by dysuria, or urinary retention or incontinence or urgency

Goal/Outcome

Child's bladder will empty adequately, according to preestablished quantities and frequencies individualized for the child (usual urine output is 0.5 to 2 mL/kg/h).

Promoting Adequate Urinary Elimination and Successful Bladder Emptying (interventions with *rationale*)

- Assess the child's usual voiding pattern and success within that pattern *to determine baseline.*
- Assess child's ability to adequately empty bladder via history focused on character and duration of lower urinary symptoms *to determine baseline.*
- Develop a schedule for bladder emptying *to decrease bladder overdistention and to encourage voiding in the toilet.*
- Maintain adequate hydration, *to avoid irritating effects of dehydration on the bladder.*
- Avoid constipation, encopresis, or fecal impaction *as alterations in bowel elimination may have a negative impact on urinary elimination.*
- Assess for bladder distention by palpation or urinary retention by postvoid residual obtained via catheterization or bladder ultrasound *to determine extent of retention.*
- Teach parents to restrict child's fluid intake after dinner *to avoid bedwetting.*
- Ensure child voids prior to going to bed *to avoid bedwetting.*
- Teach bladder-stretching exercises as prescribed per primary provider or nurse practitioner *to increase bladder capacity.*
- In the child with significant urinary retention, teach parents/child the technique of clean intermittent catheterization, *which allows for regular complete bladder emptying.*

Nursing Analysis

Activity intolerance related to generalized edema, weakness, or anemia as evidenced by abnormal heart rate response with activity, exertional discomfort, or dyspnea (elevated respiratory rate, complaint of shortness of breath with play or activity), fatigue, or generalized weakness

Goal/Outcome

Child will display increased activity tolerance, desire to play without developing symptoms of exertion.

Promoting Activity (interventions with *rationale*)

- Encourage activity or ambulation per primary provider's or nurse practitioner's orders: *early mobilization results in better outcomes.*
- Observe child for symptoms of activity intolerance such as pallor, nausea, lightheadedness, or dizziness or changes in vital signs *to determine level of tolerance.*
- If child is on bed rest, perform range-of-motion exercises and frequent position changes, *as negative changes to the musculoskeletal system occur quickly with inactivity and immobility.*
- Cluster nursing care activities and plan for periods of rest before and after exertional activities *to decrease oxygen need and consumption.*
- Refer the child to physical therapy *for exercise prescription to increase skeletal muscle strength.*

Nursing Analysis

Altered body image perception related to short stature, or effects of long-term corticosteroid use as evidenced by negative feeling about body

Goal/Outcome

Child or adolescent will display appropriate body image, will look at self in mirror, and participate in social activities.

Promoting Body Image (interventions with *rationale*)

- Acknowledge feelings of anger over body changes and illness: *venting feelings is associated with less body image disturbance.*
- Support the child's or adolescent's choices of comfortable, fashionable clothing *that may disguise anatomic abnormalities and dialysis tubing.*
- Involve the child and especially the adolescent in the decision-making process, *as a sense of control of their own body will improve body image.*
- Encourage children or adolescents to spend time with others of their own age who have short stature or other effects of renal disorders: *a peer's opinions are often better accepted than those of people in authority, such as parents or health care professionals.*

Based on your top three patient problems for Corey, describe appropriate nursing interventions.

Collecting Urine Specimens in Children

Urine specimens may be collected using a variety of different methods in infants and children. Suprapubic aspiration is a useful method for obtaining a sterile urine specimen from the neonate or young infant. A sterile needle is inserted into the bladder through the anterior wall of the abdomen and the urine is then aspirated. The primary provider or nurse practitioner generally performs this method. Infants and toddlers who are not toilet trained may require a urine bag for urine collection. A sterile urine bag is required for a urine culture, a clean bag for routine urinalysis. A 24-hour urine collection bag is also available. Nursing Procedure 43.1 gives details on the use of the urine bag.

NURSING PROCEDURE 43.1 Applying the Urine Bag

1. Cleanse the perineal area well and pat dry (Fig. A). If a culture is to be obtained, cleanse the genital area with povidone-iodine (Betadine) or per institutional protocol.

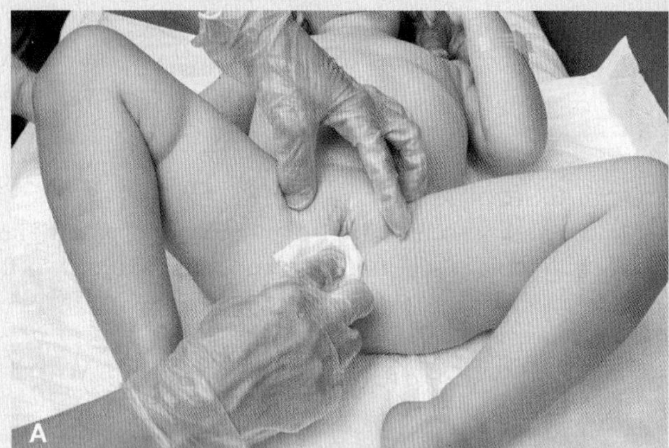

2. Apply benzoin around the scrotum or the vulvar area to aid with urine bag adhesion.
3. Allow the benzoin to dry.
4. Apply the urine bag.
   - For males: Ensure that the penis is fully inside the bag; a portion of the scrotum may or may not be inside the bag, depending on scrotal size.
   - For females: Apply the narrow portion of the bag on the perineal space between the anal and vulvar areas first for best adhesion, and then spread the remaining adhesive section (Fig. B).

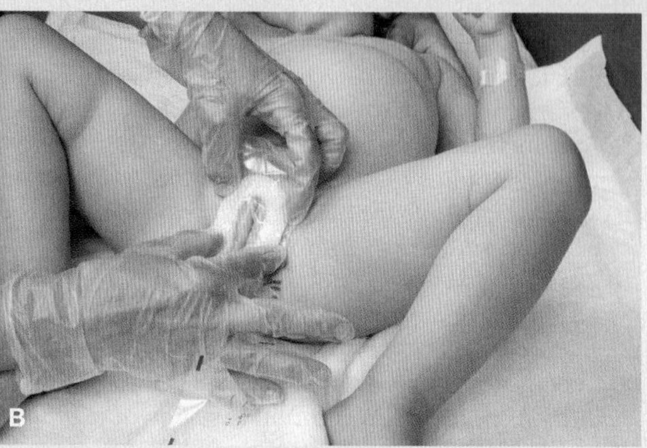

5. Tuck the bag downward inside the diaper to discourage leaking.
6. Check the bag frequently for urine (Fig. C).

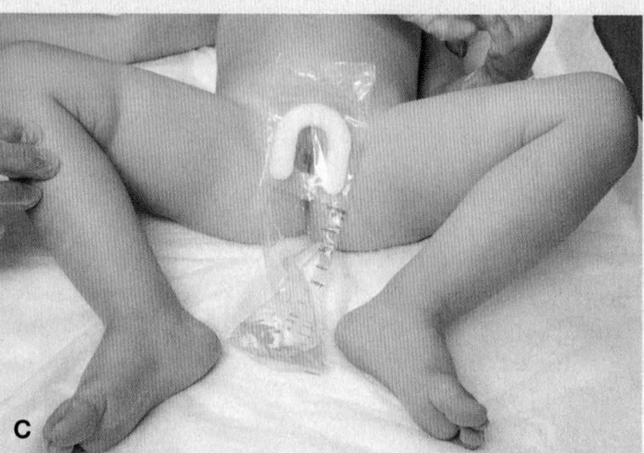

Adapted from Nationwide Children's Hospital. (2024). *U-bag urine collection guidelines for males and females.* https://www.nationwidechildrens.org/family-resources-education/health-wellness-and-safety-resources/helping-hands/ubag-urine-collection-guidelines-for-males-and-females

Sterile urinary catheterization is performed similar to that in adults. The size of the catheter varies depending on the size of the child. General size recommendations are:

- 6 to 8 Fr: Birth to 1 year old
- 8 to 10 Fr: 1 to 8 years old
- 10 to 12 Fr: 8 to 12 years old
- 12 to 14 Fr: 12 years and older (Hucker & Lawson-Wood, 2023)

• • • ATRAUMATIC CARE • • •

When examining the genital area or performing urinary catheterization of the young female, allow the child to sit with the parent on the examination table to decrease anxiety. Have the child lie back on the parent's chest, seated on the table between the parent's legs. Encourage the parent to console and hug the child while the invasive examination or procedure is being performed.

TAKE NOTE!

Use familiar terms such as "pee-pee," "tinkle," or "potty" to explain to the child what is needed and to gain their cooperation.

URINARY TRACT AND KIDNEY DISORDERS

The urinary tract and kidney disorders discussed here include structural disorders, UTI, enuresis, and acquired disorders that result in altered kidney function.

Structural Disorders

Numerous urologic conditions are congenital (present at birth) and occur because of altered fetal development. Many of these defects are apparent at birth, yet some are not recognized until later in infancy or childhood when symptoms or complications arise.

These disorders include bladder exstrophy (covered in Chapter 24), hypospadias/epispadias, obstructive uropathy, hydronephrosis, and vesicoureteral reflux (VUR).

TAKE NOTE!

Children with congenital urologic malformations are at high risk for the development of latex allergy (Hamilton, 2023). Latex allergy can result in anaphylaxis. Primary prevention of latex allergy is warranted in all children with urologic malformations, so use latex-free gloves, tubes, and catheters in these children.

Hypospadias/Epispadias

Hypospadias is a urethral defect in which the opening is on the ventral surface of the penis rather than at the end of the penis (Fig. 43.1). Epispadias is a urethral defect in which the opening is on the dorsal surface of the penis. In either case, the opening may be near the glans of the penis, midway along the penis, or near the base. If left uncorrected, the male may not be capable of appropriately aiming a urinary stream from a standing position. In addition, the abnormal placement of the urethral opening may result in erectile dysfunction or interfere with the deposition of sperm during intercourse, leaving the male infertile. For these reasons, the defect is usually repaired at 6 months and 1 year of age (Baskin, 2023a). The goal of surgical correction for either condition is to provide for an appropriately placed meatus that allows for normal voiding and ejaculation. The meatus is moved to the glans penis and the urethra is reconstructed as needed. Most repairs are accomplished in one surgery. More extensive reconstructions may require two stages.

Nursing Assessment

Note history of an unusual urine stream. Inspect the penis for placement of the urethral meatus: it may be slightly off center of the glans or may be present somewhere along the shaft of the penis. Inspect for chordee, a fibrous band causing the penis to curve downward. Palpate for the presence or absence of testicles in the scrotal sac because cryptorchidism (undescended testicles) often occurs with hypospadias, as do hydrocele and inguinal hernia.

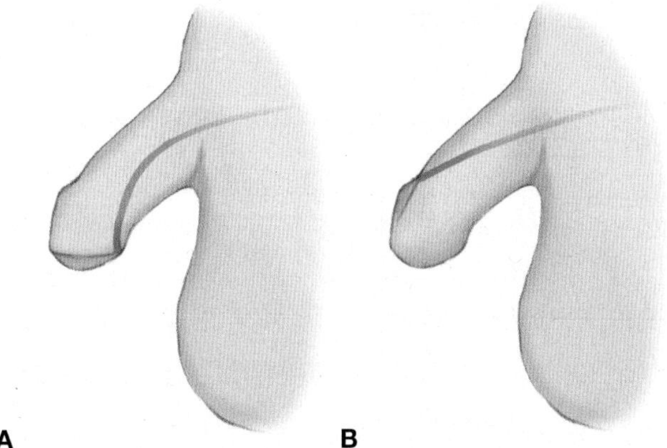

FIGURE 43.1 A. Hypospadias: The urethral opening is located on the ventral side of the penis. **B.** Epispadias: The urethral opening is located on the dorsal side of the penis.

Nursing Management

The newborn with hypospadias or epispadias should not undergo circumcision until after surgical repair of the urethral meatus. In more extreme cases, the surgeon may need to use some of the excess foreskin while reconstructing the meatus. Nursing management of the infant who has undergone a hypospadias or epispadias repair focuses on providing routine postoperative care and parent education.

PROVIDING POSTOPERATIVE CARE

Postoperatively, assess urinary drainage from the urethral stent or drainage tube, which allows for discharge of urine without stress along the surgical site. Ensure that the urinary drainage tube remains carefully taped with the penis in an upright position to prevent stress on the urethral incision. The penile dressing is usually a compression type, used to decrease edema and bruising. Administer antibiotics if prescribed. Assess for pain, which is usually not extensive, and administer analgesics or antispasmodics (oral oxybutynin or belladonna and opium [B&O] suppository) as needed for bladder spasms. See Dosage Calculation Box 43.1. Bladder spasms may also be managed effectively through the use of epidural analgesia.

DOSAGE CALCULATION BOX 43.1

Child's weight: 17 lb, 12 oz

Medication order: oxybutynin 1.6 mg PO three times a day.

Per the *Pediatric and Neonatal Dosage Handbook*, the recommended dose is 0.2 mg/kg/dose two to three times daily.

Is the ordered dose safe?

Double diapering is a method used to protect the urethra and stent or catheter after surgery; it also helps keep the area clean and free from infection. The inner diaper contains stool, and the outer diaper contains urine, allowing separation between the bowel and bladder output. Nursing Procedure 43.2 details the double-diapering technique. Change the outside (larger) diaper when the child is wet; change both diapers when the child has a bowel movement.

NURSING PROCEDURE 43.2 Double Diapering

1. Cut a hole or a cross-shaped slit in the front of the smaller diaper.
2. Unfold both diapers and place the smaller diaper (with the hole) inside the larger one.
3. Place both diapers under the child.
4. Carefully bring the penis (if applicable) and catheter/stent through the hole in the smaller diaper and close the diaper.
5. Close the larger diaper, making sure the tip of the catheter/stent is inside the larger diaper.

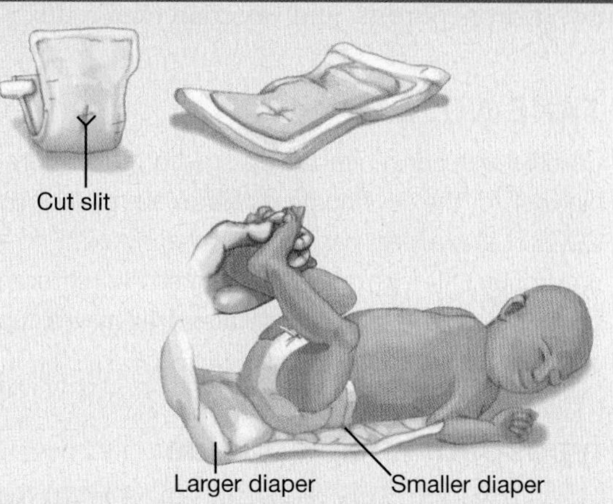

Pictures and text adapted from St. Lukes. (n.d.). *When your child needs surgery for hypospadias.* https://www.saintlukeskc.org/health-library/when-your-child-needs-surgery-hypospadias

EDUCATING THE FAMILY

If the child is to be discharged with the urinary catheter in place (which is common), teach the parents how to care for the catheter and drainage system. Have parents demonstrate their ability to irrigate the catheter should a mucus plug occur. Tub baths are generally prohibited until it is time to remove the penile dressing. Roughhousing, ride-on toys, or any activity involving straddling is not allowed for 4 weeks (Baskin, 2023a).

Obstructive Uropathy

Obstructive uropathy is an obstruction at any level along the upper or lower urinary tract. This discussion will focus on congenital structural defects, though obstruction can also occur as a result of other disease processes (acquired obstructive uropathy). The most common sites of obstruction are listed in Table 43.1. The defect may be unilateral or bilateral and can cause partial or complete

TABLE 43.1 • Common Sites of Obstructive Uropathy

Disorder	Site	Illustration
Ureteropelvic junction (UPJ) obstruction	Junction of the upper ureter with the pelvis of the kidney	Urinary tract with unilateral hydronephrosis and narrowing of the UPJ on that side Renal pelvis; Site of obstruction; Kidney; Ureter; Bladder
Ureterovesical junction (UVJ) obstruction	Junction of the lower ureter and the bladder	Urinary tract with unilateral hydronephrosis and dilated ureters with narrowing of the UVJ on that side Kidney; Bladder; Ureter; Obstruction

TABLE 43.1 • Common Sites of Obstructive Uropathy

Ureterocele	Ureter swells into the bladder	Bladder with cystic pouch where ureters insert (unilateral) 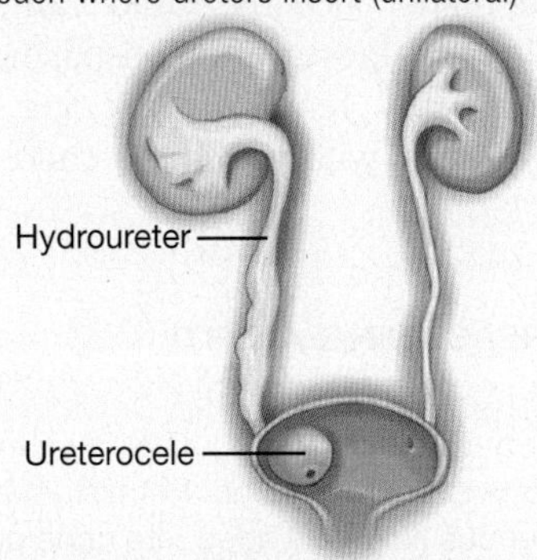
Posterior urethral valves (males only)	Flaps of tissue in the proximal urethra	Distended proximal urethra, bladder, ureters, and hydronephrosis 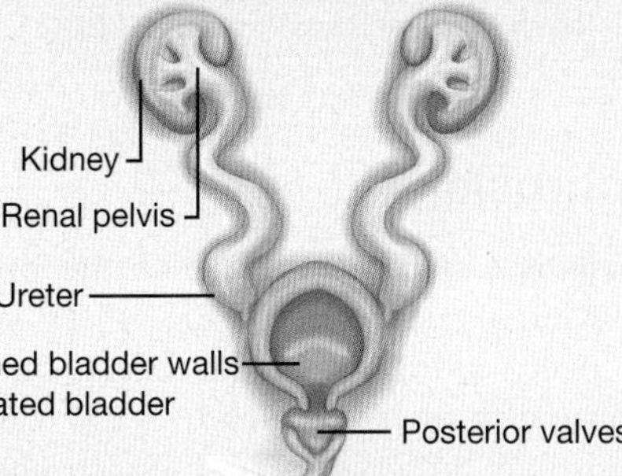

Data from Elder, J. R. (2020). Obstruction of the urinary tract. In R. M. Kliegman, J. W. St Geme, N. J. Blum, S. S. Shah, R. C. Tasker, & K. M. Wilson (Eds.), *Nelson textbook of pediatrics* (21st ed.). Elsevier.

obstruction of urine flow, resulting in dilation of the affected kidney (hydronephrosis). Complications include recurrent UTI, abnormal kidney function, and progressive damage to the kidney resulting in kidney failure.

Nursing Assessment

For a full description of the assessment phase of the nursing process, refer to the "Clinical Judgment and the Nursing Process" section earlier in the chapter. Assessment findings pertinent to obstructive uropathy are discussed next.

Health History

Elicit a description of the present illness and chief complaint. Common symptoms reported during the health history might include:

- Recurrent UTI
- Incontinence
- Fever
- Foul-smelling urine
- Flank pain
- Abdominal pain
- **Urinary frequency** (needing to void often)
- Urinary **urgency** (urge to void immediately)
- **Dysuria** (difficulty or pain with voiding)
- **Hematuria** (blood in the urine)

Explore the child's current and past medical history for risk factors such as:

- "Prune belly" syndrome
- Chromosome abnormalities
- Anorectal malformations
- Ear defects

Physical Examination and Laboratory and Diagnostic Tests

Palpate the abdomen for the presence of an abdominal mass (hydronephrotic kidney). Assess the blood pressure; elevation may occur if abnormal kidney function is present. Many cases of obstructive uropathy may be diagnosed with prenatal ultrasound if the obstruction has been significant enough to cause hydronephrosis or dilation elsewhere along the urinary tract.

Nursing Management

Surgical correction is specific to the type of obstruction and generally consists of removal of the obstruction, reimplantation of the ureters as necessary, and, occasionally, creation of a urinary diversion. Postoperatively, assess urine output via vesicostomy, nephrostomy, suprapubic tube, or urethral catheter for color, clots, clarity, and amount. Encourage fluids once the child can tolerate them orally. Administer analgesics and antispasmodics as needed for bladder spasms. Teach parents care of vesicostomy or drainage tubes, with which the child may be discharged.

CLINICAL REASONING ALERT!

Upon return from surgery, most children have intravenous fluids without added potassium infusion. Potassium is withheld from the intravenous fluid until adequate urine output is established postoperatively to avoid the development of hyperkalemia should the kidneys fail to function properly (University of Texas Medical Branch Health, 2024).

Hydronephrosis

Hydronephrosis is a condition in which the pelvis and calyces of the kidney are dilated (Fig. 43.2). Hydronephrosis may occur as a congenital defect, because of obstructive uropathy or secondary to VUR. Congenital hydronephrosis may be revealed on prenatal ultrasound. Complications of hydronephrosis include abnormal kidney function, hypertension, and eventually kidney failure.

Nursing Assessment

The infant may be asymptomatic, but symptoms reported during the health history might include failure to thrive, intermittent hematuria, presence of an abdominal mass, or symptoms associated with a UTI such as fever, vomiting, poor feeding, and irritability.

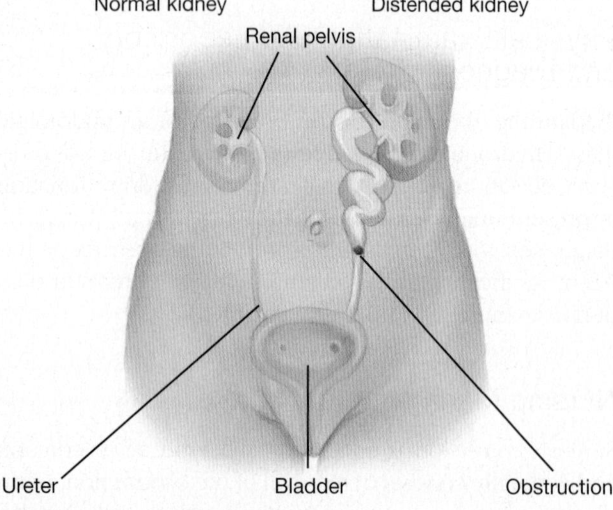

FIGURE 43.2 Hydronephrosis.

Explore the child's current and past medical history for risk factors for congenital hydronephrosis such as maternal oligohydramnios or polyhydramnios or elevated levels of serum alpha-fetoprotein.

Monitor the blood pressure of infants and children suspected of having hydronephrosis. Palpation of the abdomen may reveal enlarged kidney(s) or a distended bladder. A voiding cystourethrogram (VCUG) will be performed to determine the presence of a structural defect that may be causing the hydronephrosis. Other diagnostic tests, such as a renal ultrasound or an intravenous pyelogram, may also be performed to clarify the diagnosis.

Nursing Management

Teach the parents signs and symptoms of UTI and sepsis, as these complications may occur. Explain to the parents that they should observe the child for adequacy of urine output and hydration status. Teach the parents to perform appropriate perineal hygiene and to avoid using irritants in the genital area. The infant or child with hydronephrosis will need follow-up with a pediatric nephrologist or urologist.

Vesicoureteral Reflux

VUR is a condition in which urine from the bladder flows back up the ureters. This reflux of urine occurs during bladder contraction with voiding (Fig. 43.3). Reflux may occur in one or both ureters. If reflux occurs when the urine is infected, the kidney is exposed to bacteria and pyelonephritis may result. The increased pressure placed upon the kidney with reflux can cause renal scarring and lead to hypertension later in life and, if severe, abnormal kidney function or failure.

Primary VUR results from a congenital abnormality at the vesicoureteral junction that results in incompetence of the valve. Secondary VUR is related to other structural or functional problems such as neurogenic bladder, bladder dysfunction, or bladder outlet obstruction.

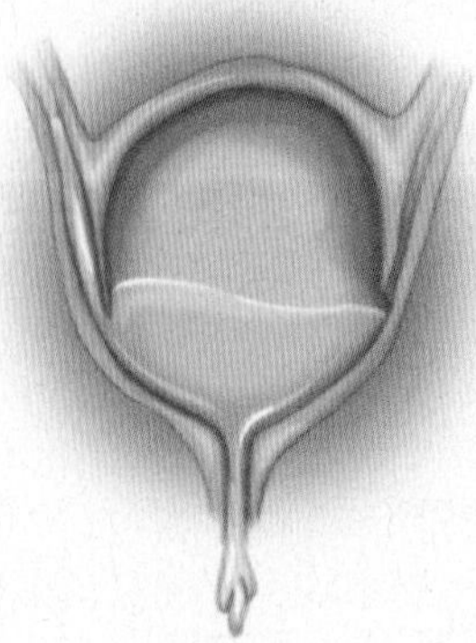

FIGURE 43.3 Note retrograde flow of urine up the ureter upon bladder contraction.

About 30% to 40% of all children diagnosed with a febrile UTI have VUR (Estrada & Cendron, 2021). VUR is graded according to its severity, from grade I, which is characterized by minor dilation of the proximal ureter, to grade V, which is characterized by severe dilation of the ureter and pelvis of the kidney. Grade I to III VUR cases usually resolve spontaneously by age 5, but grade IV through V VUR cases may be associated with recurrent UTIs, hydronephrosis, and renal issues necessitating surgical repair (Estrada & Cendron, 2021).

The goal of therapeutic management of VUR is prevention of pyelonephritis and subsequent renal scarring, which may contribute to the development of hypertension later in life. Management includes antibiotic prophylaxis to prevent breakthrough UTIs (Estrada & Cendron, 2021). Additionally, hygiene and voiding practices are used to assist with prevention of UTI. Serial urine cultures are used to determine recurrence of UTI. Biannual, annual, or biennial radionuclide VCUGs are performed to determine the status of VUR. Grade III, IV, and V cases usually warrant surgical intervention. The ureters are resected from the bladder and reimplanted elsewhere in the bladder wall to regain functionality.

TAKE NOTE!

The keys to prevention of long-term sequelae such as hypertension in children with urologic conditions are early diagnosis and intervention, prevention of infection, and close clinical follow-up. Nurses play a key role in monitoring and education.

Nursing Assessment

Common symptoms reported during the health history might include:

- fever
- dysuria
- frequency or urgency
- nocturia
- hematuria
- back, abdomen, or flank pain

Explore the child's current and past medical history for risk factors such as history of UTI, congenital defect, or family history of VUR. For the child who is receiving ongoing follow-up for VUR, determine whether UTIs have occurred since the last visit, as well as the name and dose of prophylactic antibiotic.

Monitor the blood pressure for elevation. Palpate the abdomen for presence of a mass (if hydronephrosis is present). VCUG may be used to diagnose VUR.

Nursing Management

Nursing management for the child with VUR includes preventing infection and providing postoperative care.

PREVENTING INFECTION

When VUR is present, the goal is to avoid urine infection so that infected urine cannot gain access to the kidneys. Initially, most cases of VUR are managed medically. Teach the child to empty the bladder completely. Teach the child and parents appropriate perineal hygiene as well as toileting hygiene to prevent recurrence of UTI. Teach parents about the antibiotic therapy prescribed; the child will be maintained on a low daily dose to prevent UTI. The drug is most effective when given at bedtime because of urinary stasis overnight. Inform parents of the schedule for serial urine cultures and follow-up VCUG.

PROVIDING POSTOPERATIVE CARE

If VUR is severe or if UTI is recurrent, surgical correction will be necessary. In the first 24 to 48 hours after surgery, maintain the intravenous fluid rate at 1.5 times maintenance to encourage a high urinary output. Monitor urine output via the Foley catheter; urine should be bloody initially, clearing within 2 to 3 days. If ureteral stents are present, monitor urine output from those as well. Administer analgesics for incisional pain relief and antispasmodics or B&O suppositories as needed for bladder spasms. Encourage ambulation and advancement of diet as ordered to promote return of appropriate bowel function. Teach parents that prophylactic antibiotics will be given until 1 to 2 months after surgery, when the VCUG demonstrates absence of reflux.

TAKE NOTE!

When caring for the child who has undergone urologic surgery, avoid manipulating the Foley or suprapubic catheter: catheter manipulation contributes to bladder spasms.

URINARY DISORDERS

Urinary Tract Infection

UTI is an infection of the urinary tract, most commonly affecting the bladder. UTI occurs most often because of bacteria ascending to the bladder via the urethra. About 8% of females and 2% of males will experience at least one UTI during childhood (Bock et al., 2022). One explanation for the more common occurrence in females is that the female's shorter urethra allows bacteria to have easier access to the bladder. The urethra is also located quite close to the vagina and anus in females, allowing spread of bacteria from those areas. The sexually active female adolescent is at risk for the development of UTI, as bacteria may be forced into the urethra by pressure from intercourse. The adolescent male may be somewhat protected from UTI by the antibacterial properties of prostate secretions.

UTI presents differently in infants than it does in children. Infants may exhibit fever, irritability, vomiting, failure to thrive, or jaundice. Children may experience fever and vomiting but also may have dysuria, frequency, hesitancy, urgency, and pain.

Pathophysiology

E. coli most commonly causes UTI, as it is usually found in the perineal and anal regions, close to the urethral opening. Other organisms include *Klebsiella*, *Staphylococcus aureus*, *Proteus*, *Pseudomonas*, and *Haemophilus*. Numerous factors may contribute to bacterial proliferation. Urinary stasis contributes to the development of a UTI once the bacteria have gained entry. Urine that remains in the bladder after voiding allows bacteria to grow rapidly. A decreased fluid intake also contributes to bacterial growth, as the bacteria become more concentrated. If the urine is alkaline, bacteria are better able to flourish. Untreated bladder infection may allow reflux of infected urine up the ureters to the kidneys and result in pyelonephritis, a more serious infection.

Therapeutic Management

UTIs are treated with either oral or intravenous antibiotics, depending on the severity of the infection. Urine culture and sensitivity determine the appropriate antibiotic. A 7- to 14-day course of antibiotics is often prescribed, though 2- to 5-day courses may be as effective. Adequate fluid intake is necessary to flush the bacteria from the bladder. Fever management may also be needed.

Nursing Assessment

For a full description of the assessment phase of the nursing process, refer to the "Clinical Judgment and the Nursing Process" section earlier in the chapter. Assessment findings pertinent to UTI are discussed next.

Health History

Elicit a description of the present illness and chief complaint. Common symptoms reported during the health history might include:

- Fever
- Nausea or vomiting
- Chills
- Abdomen, back, or flank pain
- Lethargy
- Jaundice (in the neonate)
- Poor feeding or "just not acting right" (in the infant)
- Urinary urgency or frequency
- Burning or stinging with urination (the infant may cry with urination; the toddler may grab the diaper)
- Foul-smelling urine
- Poor appetite (child)
- Enuresis or incontinence in a previously toilet-trained child
- Blood in the urine

Explore the child's current and past medical history for risk factors such as:

- Previous UTI
- Obstructive uropathy
- Inadequate toileting hygiene (often occurs with preschool females)
- VUR
- Constipation
- Urine holding or dysfunctional voiding
- Neurogenic bladder
- Uncircumcised male
- Sexual intercourse
- Pregnancy
- Chronic illness

Physical Examination

In the neonate or young infant, observe for jaundice or increased respiratory rate. In infants and children, inspect the perineal area for redness or irritation. Observe the urine for visible blood, cloudiness, dark color, sediment, mucus, or foul odor. Note pallor, edema, or elevated blood pressure. Palpate the abdomen. Note distended bladder, abdominal mass, or tenderness, particularly in the flank area.

Laboratory and Diagnostic Tests

Common laboratory and diagnostic studies ordered for the assessment of UTI include:

- Urinalysis (clean-catch, suprapubic, or catheterized): may be positive for blood, nitrites, leukocyte esterase, white blood cells, or bacteria (**bacteriuria**)
- Urine culture: will be positive for infecting organism
- Renal ultrasound: may show hydronephrosis if child also has a structural defect
- VCUG: not usually performed until the child has been treated with antibiotics for at least 48 hours, as infected urine tends to reflux up the ureters anyway. VCUG performed once the urine has regained sterility may be positive for VUR.

Renal ultrasound or VCUG may be indicated in certain populations. The primary provider or nurse practitioner will determine the need for radiologic testing.

Nursing Management

Goals for nursing management include eradicating infection, promoting comfort, and preventing recurrence of infection.

ERADICATING INFECTION

The child who can tolerate oral intake will be prescribed an oral antibiotic. The child who has protracted vomiting related to the UTI or who has suspected pyelonephritis will require hospitalization and intravenous antibiotics. Children younger than 3 months, and those with dehydration, a toxic appearance, or sepsis should also be hospitalized for administration of intravenous antibiotics (Bock et al., 2022). Administer oral or intravenous antibiotics as prescribed. Urge the parent to complete the entire course of oral antibiotic at home, even though the child is feeling better. Administer intravenous fluids as ordered or encourage generous oral fluid intake to help flush the bacteria from the bladder.

PROMOTING COMFORT

Administer antipyretics such as acetaminophen or ibuprofen to reduce fever. A heating pad or warm compress may help relieve abdomen or flank pain. If the child is afraid to urinate due to burning or stinging, encourage voiding in a warm sitz or tub bath.

PREVENTING RECURRENCE OF INFECTION

Encourage the parents to return as ordered for a repeat urine culture after completion of the antibiotic course to ensure eradication of bacteria. Teaching Guidelines 43.1 gives further information on preventing UTI.

TEACHING GUIDELINES 43.1 Preventing Urinary Tract Infection in Females

- Drink enough fluid (to keep urine flushed through bladder).
- Drink cranberry juice to acidify the urine.
- Avoid colas and caffeine, which irritate the bladder.
- Urinate frequently and do not "hold" urine (to discourage urinary stasis).
- Avoid bubble baths (they contribute to vulvar and perineal irritation).
- Wipe from front to back after voiding (to avoid contaminating the urethra with rectal material).
- Wear cotton underwear (to decrease the incidence of perineal irritation).
- Avoid wearing tight jeans or pants.
- Wash the perineal area daily with soap and water.
- While menstruating, change sanitary pads frequently to discourage bacterial growth.
- Void immediately after sexual intercourse.

Enuresis

Enuresis is continued incontinence of urine past the age of toilet training. Nocturnal enuresis refers to bedwetting and occurs in about 15% of children at age 5 years, decreasing to 5% of children by 10 years of age (Paul & Wallace, 2023). Nocturnal enuresis may persist in some children into late childhood and adolescence, causing significant distress for the affected child and family. Occasional daytime wetting or dribbling of urine is usually not a cause for concern, but frequent daytime wetting concerns both the child and the parents.

In some children, enuresis may occur secondary to a physical disorder such as diabetes mellitus or diabetes insipidus, sickle cell anemia, ectopic ureter, or urethral obstruction. Other causes common to both diurnal and nocturnal enuresis include a urine-concentrating defect, UTI, constipation, and emotional distress (sometimes serious). The most frequent cause of daytime enuresis is dysfunctional voiding or holding of urine, although giggle incontinence and stress incontinence also occur. Nocturnal enuresis may be related to a high fluid intake in the evening, obstructive sleep apnea, sexual abuse, a family history of enuresis, or inappropriate family expectations. Physical causes of enuresis must be treated; further management of the disorder focuses on behavioral training, which may be augmented with the use of enuresis alarms or medications.

Nursing Assessment

Elicit a description of the present illness and chief complaint. Determine the age of toilet training and when or if the child achieved successful daytime and nighttime dryness. Inquire about urine-holding behaviors such as squatting, dancing, or staring as well as rushing to the bathroom (diurnal enuresis). Inquire about the amount and types of fluid the child typically consumes before bedtime (nocturnal enuresis). Assess for risk factors such as:

- Family disruption or other stressors
- Chronic constipation (carefully assess bowel movement patterns)
- Excessive family demands related to toileting patterns
- History of being difficult to arouse from sleep
- Family history of enuresis

Assess the child's cognitive status: developmentally delayed children may take significantly longer to achieve urine continence than their typical same-age peers. Assess for short stature or elevated blood pressure, as these may occur when renal abnormalities are present.

Nursing Management

For the child with diurnal enuresis, encourage them to increase the amount of fluid consumed during the day to increase the frequency of the urge to void. Set a fixed schedule for the child to attempt to void throughout the day. These practices will usually be sufficient to retrain the child's voiding patterns.

See Evidence-Based Practice 43.1.

EVIDENCE-BASED PRACTICE 43.1

Interventions for Enuresis

STUDY

Nocturnal enuresis (bedwetting) may affect the child's psychosocial well-being and relationship with the parents. Parents and children seek resolution of this annoying problem, though most cases of nocturnal enuresis spontaneously resolve by 15 years of age. In their critical review, the authors included four studies with a total of 269 child participants (aged 5 to 15 years). The studies compared monotherapy (bedwetting alarms) with combined therapy (bedwetting alarms and medication).

Findings

Use of a bedwetting alarm is as effective as the use of an alarm with a medication. The only difference noted was with combined therapy, in which there was slightly quicker resolution of enuresis though the result was not statistically significant.

Nursing Implications

Educate parents and the child about appropriate use of the bedwetting alarm as this treatment results in the best long-term resolution. Even when medications are prescribed, the alarm should still be used. Families may see a quicker response with combination therapy, so it may be the choice of some families.

Data from Aksakall, T., Cinislioğlu, A. E., & Aksoy, Y. (2022). The efficacy of combined alarm therapy versus alarm monotherapy in the treatment of monosymptomatic nocturnal enuresis: a review of current literature. *Eurasian Journal of Medicine, 54*(Suppl. 1), S164–S167. https://doi.org/10.5152/eurasianjmed.2022.22311

EDUCATING THE CHILD AND FAMILY ABOUT NOCTURNAL ENURESIS

Teach the family that the child is not lazy, nor do they wet the bed intentionally. Encourage the child and family to read books such as *Dry All Night: The Picture Book Technique That Stops Bedwetting* by Alison Mack or *Waking Up Dry: A Guide to Help Children Overcome Bedwetting* by Dr. Howard Bennett. Encourage the parents to limit intake of bladder irritants such as chocolate and caffeine. Teach parents to limit fluid intake after dinner and ensure that the child voids just before going to bed. Waking the child to void at 11 p.m. may also be helpful. Teach the parents to use bed pads and to make the bed with two sets of sheets and pads to decrease the workload in the middle of the night. When sleeping at home, the child should wear their usual underwear or pajamas. If away on a family vacation, pull-ups may decrease the stress on both the child and the parents.

PROVIDING SUPPORT AND ENCOURAGEMENT

Enuresis may be source of shame for children and adolescents. It is important for the child to understand that they are not alone. Depending on the child's developmental level, explain that as many as 5 million people have enuresis (this can be done in terms the child can relate to, such as a proportion within a school or 100 times the number of children in one school, etc.). It is not only "little kids" who wet the bed, and all kids who wet the bed need help overcoming this problem. Parents should include the child in plans for nighttime urinary control; this helps to increase the child's motivation to become dry. Parents should set up a reward system for dry nights. Parents should include the child in bed linen changes when they wet the bed but should do so in a matter-of-fact manner rather than in a punitive way; in fact, it is important to always avoid punishment for bedwetting. Though enuresis may cause family disruption, with patience, consistency, and time, dryness will be achieved. Provide ongoing emotional support and positive reinforcement to the child and family.

DECREASING NIGHTTIME VOIDING

Teach the family using an enuresis alarm system how to use the alarm as well as the previously mentioned techniques (Fig. 43.4). Most of these devices work by sounding an alarm when the first few drops of urine appear; the child then awakens and stops the urine flow. Over time, the child becomes conditioned to either awaken when the bladder is full or stop the urine flow when sleeping.

When behavioral and motivational therapies are unsuccessful, particularly in the older child, medications may be prescribed. Teach the child and parents about the use of medications such as oxybutynin, imipramine, and desmopressin if these are prescribed (refer to Drug Guide 43.1).

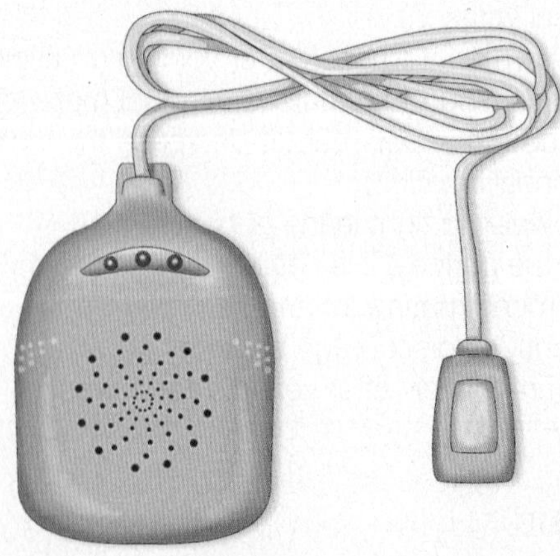

FIGURE 43.4 Some children and families find great success with the use of an enuresis alarm. The alarm wakes the child at the first sign of wetness. Over time, the child learns to awaken at night in response to the sensation of a full bladder.

ACQUIRED DISORDERS RESULTING IN ALTERED KIDNEY FUNCTION

A number of acquired disorders are responsible for alterations in kidney function. They may occur as an autoimmune response or in relation to a bacterial infection. Kidney dysfunction may also occur because of obstructive disorders or repeated VUR, as discussed earlier. Left untreated, these disorders may lead to kidney failure. Even when treated appropriately, sometimes the appropriate response is not achieved, and acute or chronic kidney disease (CKD) develops. Renal disorders are the most frequent cause of hypertension in children.

CLINICAL REASONING ALERT!

Severe ambulatory hypertension (blood pressure higher than the 95th percentile for age and sex) places the child at risk for damage to the eyes or vital organs (kidney, brain, or heart), or even death (Flynn, 2023). Nurses must be adept at accurately measuring blood pressure in children.

Nephrotic Syndrome

Nephrotic syndrome occurs as a result of increased glomerular basement membrane permeability, which allows abnormal loss of protein in the urine. Nephrotic syndrome generally occurs in three forms—congenital, idiopathic, and secondary.

Congenital nephrotic syndrome is an inherited disorder; it is rare and occurs primarily in families of Finnish descent. The prognosis is poor, though some success has occurred with early, aggressive treatment and with the advances in kidney transplantation in infants (Bock et al., 2022). Nephrotic syndrome may also occur secondary to another condition such as systemic lupus erythematosus, Henoch–Schönlein purpura, or diabetes.

Idiopathic nephrotic syndrome is the most commonly occurring type in children and is also called minimal change nephrotic disease (MCD). Idiopathic nephrotic syndrome most often has its onset in children by age 10 years (Bock et al., 2022). This discussion will focus primarily on MCD. Complications of nephrotic syndrome include anemia, infection, poor growth, peritonitis, thrombosis, and kidney failure.

Pathophysiology

Increased glomerular permeability results in the passage of larger plasma proteins through the glomerular basement membrane. This results in excess loss of protein (albumin) in the urine (**proteinuria**) and decreased protein and albumin (hypoalbuminemia) in the bloodstream. Protein loss in nephrotic syndrome tends to be almost exclusively albumin. Hypoalbuminemia results in a change in osmotic pressure, and fluid shifts from the bloodstream into the interstitial tissue (causing edema). This decrease in blood volume triggers the kidneys to respond by conserving sodium and water, leading to further edema. The liver senses the protein loss and increases production of lipoproteins. Hyperlipidemia then develops as the excess lipids cannot be excreted in the urine. Hyperlipidemia associated with nephrotic syndrome may be quite severe, yet cholesterol levels may decrease when the nephrotic syndrome is in remission, only to rise significantly again with a relapse.

Children with nephrotic syndrome are at increased risk for clotting (thromboembolism) because of the decreased intravascular volume. They are also at increased risk for the development of serious infection, most commonly pneumococcal pneumonia, sepsis, or spontaneous peritonitis. Steroid-resistant nephrotic syndrome may result in acute kidney failure.

Therapeutic Management

Medical management of MCD usually involves the use of corticosteroids. Intravenous albumin may be used in the severely edematous child. Diuretics are also required in the edematous phase. Long-term therapy is usually required to induce remission. The nephrologist will determine the length of therapy based on the child's response. Children who have steroid-responsive MCD generally have a favorable prognosis. Some children with MCD exhibit a minimal response to steroid therapy or experience remissions and the MCD is steroid resistant (Bock et al., 2022). Immunosuppressive therapy such as cyclophosphamide, cyclosporine A, or mycophenolate mofetil may be necessary.

Nursing Assessment

For a full description of the assessment phase of the nursing process, refer to the "Clinical Judgment and the Nursing Process" section earlier in the chapter. Assessment findings pertinent to MCD are discussed next.

Health History

Elicit a description of the present illness and chief complaint. Common symptoms reported during the health history might include:

- Nausea or vomiting (may be related to ascites)
- Recent weight gain
- History of periorbital edema upon waking, progressing to generalized edema throughout the day
- Weakness or fatigue
- Irritability or fussiness

Physical Examination

Observe the child for edema (periorbital, generalized [**anasarca**], or abdominal ascites). As the disease progresses, the edema also progresses to become more generalized, eventually becoming severe. Inspect the skin for a stretched, tight appearance; pallor; or skin breakdown related to significant edema (Fig. 43.5). Document height (or length) and weight. Note increased respiratory rate or increased work of breathing related to ascites and edema.

Note the blood pressure; it may be elevated in the child with nephrotic syndrome, though it is most often either normal or decreased unless the child is progressing to kidney failure. Auscultate heart and lung sounds, noting abnormalities related to fluid overload. Palpate the skin, noting tautness. Palpate the abdomen and document the presence of ascites.

Laboratory and Diagnostic Tests

Urine dipstick will reveal marked proteinuria. Infrequently, mild hematuria is also present. Serum protein and albumin levels will be low (often markedly so). Serum cholesterol and triglyceride levels are elevated. With continued nephrotic syndrome, creatinine and BUN may become elevated.

Nursing Management

Goals for nursing management include promoting diuresis, preventing infection, promoting adequate nutrition, and educating the parents about ongoing care at home. As with other chronic disorders, provide ongoing emotional support to the child and family.

PROMOTING DIURESIS

Administer corticosteroids as ordered. Tapering or weaning doses are required when the time comes to stop corticosteroid therapy. Administer diuretics if ordered, usually furosemide. Children may develop hypokalemia because of potassium loss as an adverse effect of furosemide. Those children may require potassium supplementation or a diet higher in potassium-containing foods. Monitor urine output and the amount of protein in the urine (by dipstick). Weigh the child daily on the same scale either naked or wearing the same amount of clothing. Assess for resolution of edema. Measure pulse rate and blood pressure every 4 hours to detect hypovolemia resulting from excessive fluid shifts. Enforce oral fluid restrictions if ordered.

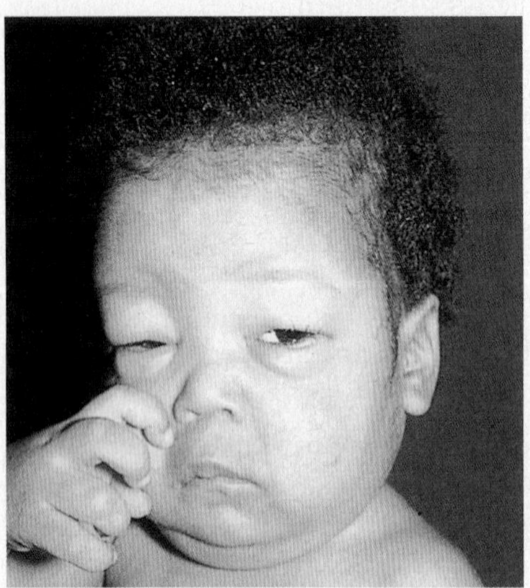

FIGURE 43.5 Note marked edema associated with nephrotic syndrome.

In cases of severe hypoalbuminemia, intravenous albumin may be administered. Increases in the serum albumin level cause fluid to shift from the subcutaneous spaces back into the bloodstream. A diuretic such as furosemide administered immediately after the albumin infusion allows for optimal diuresis and prevents fluid overload. Refer to Drug Guide 43.1 for the nursing implications related to use of these medications.

CONSIDER THIS!

Thirteen-year-old Jimmy Sanderson has a history of steroid-responsive nephrotic syndrome. In the clinic today he tells you, "I am not going to take those steroids anymore!" "I am shorter than everyone in my class, my 11-year-old brother is taller than me." "It's just not fair. I'll never get a girlfriend if I'm a shorty."

Think back to when you were an adolescent. How would you have felt if you had a chronic illness, and your necessary medications stunted your growth? As the nurse, how can you help Jimmy in this situation?

PREVENTING INFECTION

Monitor the child's temperature. Administer pneumococcal vaccine as prescribed (see Chapter 31 for information on immunizations). Administer prophylactic antibiotics, if prescribed. Delay administering live vaccines until at least 2 weeks after corticosteroid or other immunosuppressive medication therapy ceases. Teach parents that if the child is unimmunized and is exposed to chickenpox, the parents should notify the child's pediatrician, nurse practitioner, or nephrologist immediately so that the child may receive varicella zoster immunoglobulin.

ENCOURAGING ADEQUATE NUTRITION AND GROWTH

Encourage a nutrient-rich diet within prescribed restrictions. Fluid restriction is reserved for children with massive edema. Sodium intake may be restricted in the edematous child to prevent further fluid retention. Consultation with the dietitian is often helpful in meal planning because many of the foods that children like are high in sodium. Encourage protein-rich snacks. Consult with the child and family in planning meals and snacks that the child likes and will be likely to consume. Use of nutritional supplement shakes may be helpful for some children.

EDUCATING THE FAMILY

Teach parents how to give medications and monitor for adverse effects. Demonstrate the urine dipstick technique for detecting protein and encourage the family to keep a chart of dipstick results. The child may return to school but should avoid contact with sick playmates. If the child is exposed to another child with an infectious illness, explain to the parents that they should monitor temperature and urine dipstick results more frequently to identify a relapse in nephrotic syndrome early so that treatment can begin.

PROVIDING EMOTIONAL SUPPORT

Nephrotic syndrome is often a chronic condition, and children who are responsive to steroid treatment may enter remission only to experience relapse. This cycle of relapse and remission takes an emotional toll on the child and family. Frequent hospitalizations require the child to miss school and the parents to miss work; this creates further stress for the family. The child may experience social isolation because they must avoid exposure to infections or because of self-esteem problems. The child may be dissatisfied with their appearance because of edema and weight gain, short stature, and the classic "moon face" associated with chronic steroid use.

Provide emotional support to the child and family. Encourage them in their efforts to maintain the treatment plan. Introduce the child to other youngsters with chronic renal conditions. Refer families to the National Kidney Foundation for information about local support groups and resources.

Acute Poststreptococcal Glomerulonephritis

Acute poststreptococcal glomerulonephritis (APSGN) is a condition in which immune processes injure the glomeruli. Immune mechanisms cause inflammation, which results in altered glomerular structure and function in both kidneys. It often occurs following an infection, usually an upper respiratory or skin infection. APSGN is caused by an antibody–antigen reaction secondary to an infection with a nephritogenic strain of group A beta-hemolytic streptococcus (Flores, 2020). The most serious complication is progression to uremia and kidney failure (either acute or chronic).

There is no specific medical treatment for APSGN. Treatment is aimed at maintaining fluid volume and managing hypertension. If there is evidence of a current streptococcal infection, antibiotic therapy will be necessary.

Nursing Assessment

Refer to the "Clinical Judgment and the Nursing Process" section earlier in the chapter for a full description of the assessment phase of the nursing process. Assessment findings pertinent to acute glomerulonephritis are discussed next.

Health History

Elicit a description of the present illness and chief complaint. Common symptoms reported during the health history might include:

- Fever
- Lethargy
- Headache
- Decreased urine output
- Abdominal pain
- Vomiting
- Anorexia

Assess the child's current and past medical history for risk factors such as a recent episode of pharyngitis or other streptococcal infection, age older than 3 years, or male sex.

Physical Examination and Laboratory and Diagnostic Tests

Assess the child's blood pressure for elevation, which is common. Note the presence of mild edema. Observe for signs of cardiopulmonary congestion such as increased work of breathing or cough. Auscultate the lungs for crackles and the heart for gallop. The urine dipstick test will reveal proteinuria as well as hematuria. Inspect the urine for gross hematuria, which will cause the urine to appear tea colored, cola colored, or even a dirty green color. Serum creatinine and BUN may be normal or elevated, the serum complement level is depressed, and the erythrocyte sedimentation rate is elevated. Laboratory findings specific to streptococcus include an elevated antistreptolysin O (ASO) titer and an elevated DNase B antigen titer.

Nursing Management

Administer antihypertensives such as labetalol or nifedipine and diuretics as ordered. Monitor blood pressure frequently. Maintain sodium and fluid restrictions as prescribed during the initial edematous phase. Weigh the child daily on the same scale wearing the same amount of clothing. Monitor increasing urine output and note improvement in the urine color. Document resolution of edema. Provide a careful neurologic evaluation, as hypertension may cause encephalopathy and seizures. Children with APSGN generally are fatigued and choose bed rest during the acute phase. Provide the child with age-appropriate activities and cluster care to allow rest periods.

Some children may be managed at home if edema is mild and they are not hypertensive. Teach the family to monitor urine output and color, take blood pressure measurements, and restrict the diet as prescribed. The child cared for at home should not participate in strenuous activity until proteinuria and hematuria are resolved. If renal involvement progresses, dialysis may become necessary.

> **TAKE NOTE!**
>
> Avoid use of nonsteroidal antiinflammatory drugs (NSAIDs) in children with questionable kidney function, as they worsen kidney disease (Solomon, 2022).

Hemolytic Uremic Syndrome

Hemolytic uremic syndrome (HUS) is defined by three features—hemolytic anemia, thrombocytopenia, and acute kidney failure. Typical HUS features an antecedent diarrheal illness. Other causes of HUS include idiopathic, inherited, drug-related, association with malignancies, transplantation, and malignant hypertension. This discussion will focus on typical HUS, the type preceded by a diarrheal illness. Watery diarrhea progresses to hemorrhagic colitis, then to the triad of HUS. The features of HUS, as well as effects on other organs, are caused primarily by microthrombi and ischemic changes within the organs. The thrombotic events in the small blood vessels of the glomerulus lead to occlusion of the glomerular capillary loops and glomerulosclerosis, resulting in kidney failure.

A verotoxin-producing strain of *E. coli*, O157:H7, causes the majority of cases, although *Streptococcus pneumoniae*, *Shigella dysenteriae*, and other bacteria may also be the cause (Tan & Silverberg, 2021). It is thought that antibiotic treatment for the bacteria may contribute to release of the verotoxin. Undercooked ground beef accounts for most cases of *E. coli* O157:H7 infection, but it is also transmitted via the feces of numerous animals as well as unpasteurized dairy and fruit products. Transmission also occurs via human feces, and cases have been linked to public swimming pools. HUS occurs most often in children up to age 5 years (Tan & Silverberg, 2021). Complications include CKD, seizures and coma, pancreatitis, intussusception, rectal prolapse, cardiomyopathy, congestive heart failure, and acute respiratory distress syndrome.

Therapeutic management of HUS is directed toward maintaining fluid balance; correcting hypertension, acidosis, and electrolyte abnormalities; replenishing circulating red blood cells; and providing dialysis if needed. Recently, the monoclonal antibody eculizumab has been successful in terminating the microangiopathic process associated with HUS (Tan & Silverberg, 2021). Children receiving this medication are at high risk for meningococcal infection so should receive the meningococcal vaccine.

Nursing Assessment

Elicit a description of the present illness and chief complaint. Common symptoms reported during the health history might include watery diarrhea accompanied by cramping and sometimes vomiting. After several days, the diarrhea becomes bloody and eventually improves.

Explore the child's current and past medical history for risk factors such as ingestion of ground beef, visits to a water park or to a petting zoo before the onset of the diarrheal illness, or use of antidiarrheal medications or antibiotics.

Observe the child for pallor, toxic appearance, edema, **oliguria** (decreased urine output), or **anuria** (absent urine output). Assess for elevated blood pressure and tenderness in the abdomen. Assess the child for neurologic involvement, which may include irritability, altered level of consciousness, seizures, posturing, or coma.

Laboratory and Diagnostic Tests

Urinalysis may reveal the presence of blood, protein, pus, and casts. Serum laboratory abnormalities are numerous and may include:

- Elevated BUN and creatinine
- Moderate to severe anemia (with the presence of Burr cells, schistocytes, spherocytes, or helmet cells), mild to severe thrombocytopenia
- Increased reticulocyte count
- Increased bilirubin and lactic dehydrogenase (LDH) levels
- Negative Coombs test (except in cases of *S. pneumoniae* infection)
- Leukocytosis with left shift
- Hyponatremia
- Hyperkalemia
- Hyperphosphatemia
- Metabolic acidosis

Nursing Management

Nursing management of the child with HUS focuses on close observation and monitoring of the child's status. Institute and maintain contact precautions to prevent spread of *E. coli* O157:H7 to other children (bacteria are shed for up to 17 days after resolution of the diarrhea). Close attention must be paid to fluid volume status. Prevention of HUS is also an important nursing function.

MAINTAINING APPROPRIATE FLUID VOLUME BALANCE

Maintain strict intake and output monitoring and recording to evaluate the progression toward kidney failure. Carefully monitor intravenous infusions and blood chemistries. Administer diuretics as ordered. Assess blood pressure frequently and report elevations to the primary provider or nurse practitioner. Administer antihypertensives as ordered and monitor their effectiveness. Encourage adequate nutritional intake within the constraints of prescribed dietary restrictions. Monitor for bleeding as well as for fatigue and pallor. Follow institutional protocol for transfusion of packed red blood cells and platelets (platelets are usually transfused only if active bleeding or severe thrombocytopenia occurs). Report progressive deterioration in laboratory findings to the primary provider or nurse practitioner. Some children with HUS will require dialysis for at least several days.

PREVENTING HUS

Proper handwashing is necessary. Teach children to wash their hands after using the bathroom, before eating, and after petting farm animals. Encourage the use of "swim diapers," which contain feces, for children who are not toilet trained. Teach parents to thoroughly cook all meats to a core temperature of 155°F, or until the meat is gray or brown throughout and the juices from the meat are clear rather than pink. Wash all fruits and vegetables thoroughly. Ensure that drinking water and water used for recreation are treated appropriately. Avoid unpasteurized dairy products and fruit juices (including cider).

KIDNEY FAILURE

Kidney failure is a condition in which the kidneys cannot concentrate urine, conserve electrolytes, or excrete waste products. As in adults, kidney failure in children may occur as an acute or chronic condition. Some cases of acute kidney failure resolve without further complications, while dialysis is necessary in other children. When acute kidney failure continues to progress, it becomes chronic (also known as kidney failure with replacement therapy [KFRT]). Dialysis and kidney transplantation are treatment modalities used for KFRT.

Acute Kidney Failure

Acute kidney failure is defined as a sudden, often reversible, decline in kidney function that results in the accumulation of metabolic toxins (particularly nitrogenous wastes) as well as fluid and electrolyte imbalance. Fluid overload may lead to hypertension, pulmonary edema, and congestive heart failure. Additional complications include hyperkalemia, metabolic acidosis, hyperphosphatemia, and uremia. In children, acute kidney failure most commonly occurs because of decreased renal perfusion, as occurs in hypovolemic or septic shock. It may also occur in children with hemolytic anemia or as a result of nephrotoxicity from medications. Complications include anemia, hyperkalemia, hypertension, pulmonary edema, cardiac failure, and altered level of consciousness or seizures. In addition, acute kidney failure may also progress to a chronic state.

Therapeutic management is aimed at treating the underlying cause, managing the fluid and electrolyte disturbances, and decreasing blood pressure.

TAKE NOTE!

Medications commonly used in children can reduce kidney function. Cephalosporins may cause a transient increase in BUN and creatinine. Truly nephrotoxic drugs often used in children include aminoglycosides, sulfonamides, vancomycin, and NSAIDs. Make sure that potentially nephrotoxic drugs are administered according to published safe guidelines (dosage, frequency, and rate of administration).

UpToDate, Inc. (2024). *Lexi-comp®* (Version 8.1.2) [Mobile app]. Wolters Kluwer. https://apps.apple.com/us/app/lexicomp/id313401238

Nursing Assessment

The health history may reveal the following common symptoms: nausea, vomiting, diarrhea, lethargy, fever, and decreased urine output. Assess the child's current and past medical history for risk factors such as history of shock, trauma, burns, urologic abnormalities, kidney disease, use of nephrotoxic medications, or severe blood transfusion reaction.

Note decreased skin elasticity, dry mucous membranes, or edema. Auscultate the lungs for crackles, which may occur with pulmonary edema. Document tachypnea. Note cardiac rhythm disturbances. Evaluate the child's level of consciousness. Laboratory tests will reveal increased serum creatinine levels and possible electrolyte disturbances, such as hyperkalemia or hypocalcemia. Urinalysis may reveal proteinuria or hematuria.

CLINICAL REASONING ALERT!

Monitor the infant or child with kidney failure carefully for signs of congestive heart failure, such as edema accompanied by bounding pulse, presence of an S_3 heart sound, adventitious lung sounds, and shortness of breath.

Nursing Management

Nursing care focuses on managing hypertension, restoring fluid and electrolyte balance, and educating the family.

MANAGING HYPERTENSION

Carefully monitor the child's blood pressure. Administer antihypertensives as prescribed. When a fast-acting drug such as nifedipine (Procardia) sublingually or labetalol intravenously is used, stay with the child, and frequently monitor blood pressure. Immediately notify the primary provider or nurse practitioner if high blood pressure is resistant to medication and the blood pressure remains elevated.

RESTORING FLUID AND ELECTROLYTE BALANCE

Monitor vital signs frequently and assess urine specific gravity. Maintain strict records of intake and output. Administer diuretics as ordered. When urine output is restored, diuresis may be significant. Monitor for signs of hyperkalemia (weak, irregular pulse; muscle weakness; abdominal cramping) and hypocalcemia (muscle twitching or tetany). Administer polystyrene sulfonate as ordered orally, rectally, or through a nasogastric tube to decrease potassium levels. Polystyrene sulfonate removes potassium primarily by exchanging sodium for it, which is then eliminated in the feces. Administer packed red blood cell transfusions as ordered (may need to be followed by a dose of diuretic). Dialysis may become necessary if oliguria is sustained and leads to significant fluid overload, the electrolyte imbalance reaches dangerous levels, or uremia results in depression of the central nervous system.

PROVIDING FAMILY EDUCATION

Educate the family about the plan of care and the need for fluid restriction, if ordered. Instruct the family to save all voids for observation and measurement by the nurse. Provide education about the use of dialysis if relevant.

Kidney Failure With Replacement Therapy

KFRT is a CKD requiring long-term dialysis or renal transplantation. CKD in children most often results from congenital structural defects such as obstructive uropathy. It may also be caused by an inherited condition such as familial nephritis or may result from an acquired problem such as glomerulonephritis or HUS (Patel & Vogt, 2023). This contrasts with CKD in adults, which primarily results from diabetes or hypertension.

Uremia, hypocalcemia, hyperkalemia, and metabolic acidosis occur. Complications of KFRT are many. Uremic toxins deplete erythrocytes, and the failing kidneys cannot produce erythropoietin, so severe anemia results. Hypertension is common and heart failure may occur. Hypocalcemia results in renal rickets (brittle bones). Growth is retarded and sexual maturation may be delayed or absent. Children with KFRT may experience increased rates of depression, as compared to healthy children (Stahl et al., 2022). See Healthy People 2030.

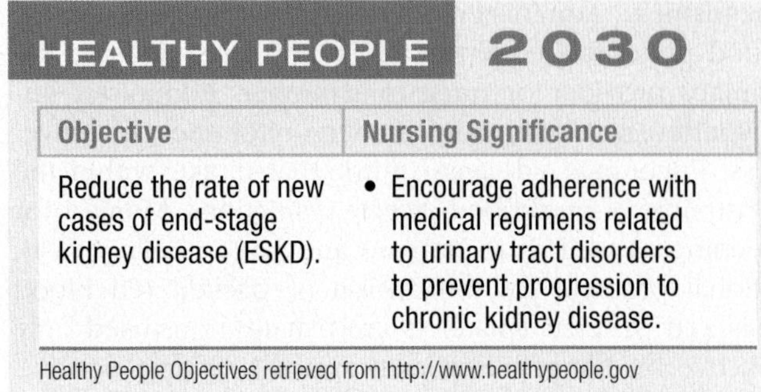

HEALTHY PEOPLE 2030

Objective	Nursing Significance
Reduce the rate of new cases of end-stage kidney disease (ESKD).	• Encourage adherence with medical regimens related to urinary tract disorders to prevent progression to chronic kidney disease.

Healthy People Objectives retrieved from http://www.healthypeople.gov

Nursing Assessment

Explore the health history for low birth weight (associated with kidney dysfunction and anatomic alterations), poor growth (weight, length/height, and head circumference), and regimen of dialysis. Note decreased appetite or energy level, dry or itchy skin, or bone or joint pain.

Perform a thorough physical assessment, noting any abnormalities (may vary from child to child). If present, assess the peritoneal catheter site for absence of drainage, bleeding, or redness. If the child undergoes hemodialysis, assess the fistula or graft site for the presence of a bruit and a thrill. Laboratory tests may reveal low hemoglobin and hematocrit, increased serum phosphorus and potassium levels, and decreased sodium, calcium, and bicarbonate levels. BUN, uric acid, and creatinine levels will be elevated. A 24-hour urine creatinine clearance test will show increased amounts of creatinine in the urine, reflecting decreasing kidney function.

CLINICAL REASONING ALERT!

Carefully assess children with KFRT for worsening uremia or metabolic acidosis. Uremia may result in central nervous system symptoms such as headache or coma, or gastrointestinal or neuromuscular disturbances. Metabolic acidosis causes lethargy, dull headache, and confusion.

Nursing Management

Nursing goals for the child with KFRT include promoting growth, removing waste products, maintaining fluid balance via dialysis, encouraging psychosocial well-being, and supporting and educating the family.

PROMOTING GROWTH

Encourage the child to choose foods they like that are within the imposed dietary restrictions. Daily protein requirements for adequate growth range from 0.9 to 1.5 g of protein per kilogram of weight. Sodium and potassium restrictions may also be necessary. Enforce fluid restrictions if prescribed. Administer medications such as erythropoietin, growth hormone, and vitamin and mineral supplements to augment nutritional status and

TABLE 43.2 • Medications and Supplements Commonly Used to Treat Kidney Failure With Replacement Therapy Complications

Medication or Supplement	Purpose
Vitamin D and calcium	Correction of hypocalcemia and hyperphosphatemia
Ferrous sulfate	Treatment of anemia
Bicitra or sodium bicarbonate tablets	Correction of acidosis
Multivitamin	Augment nutritional status
Erythropoietin injections	Stimulate red blood cell growth
Growth hormone injections	Stimulate growth in stature

Data from UpToDate, Inc. (2024). *Lexi-comp®* (Version 8.1.2) [Mobile app]. Wolters Kluwer. https://apps.apple.com/us/app/lexicomp/id313401238

promote growth. Table 43.2 lists medications and supplements used to support growth.

ENCOURAGING PSYCHOSOCIAL WELL-BEING

Refer children and their families to the hospital social worker or counselor as needed for depression or anxiety issues. The chronic need for dialysis (daily with peritoneal dialysis or three or four times per week with hemodialysis) confers long-term stress on the child and family. The child usually demonstrates poor growth and often experiences body image disturbance. Frequent medical appointments and hospitalizations interfere with the child's scholastic achievements. Introduce the child to other children with KFRT (this often happens anyway at the hemodialysis center).

Ensure that the family is aware of financial and support resources within the community and refer them to the National Kidney Foundation. Also suggest the American Kidney Fund, which provides financial aid and access to summer camps for children with renal problems. Camp is an excellent way for children to demonstrate that they have mastered some of the loss-of-control issues related to their disease.

There are also several websites that provide forums for children and adolescents with kidney failure or transplantation so they can learn about their disease, access resources, and communicate with other children.

DIALYSIS AND TRANSPLANTATION

Peritoneal dialysis or hemodialysis is required on a long-term basis for children with CKD or KFRT. Once the child has progressed to KFRT, kidney transplantation is needed for the child to progress with normal growth and development.

Peritoneal Dialysis

Peritoneal dialysis uses the child's abdominal cavity as a semipermeable membrane to help remove excess fluid and waste products (Figs. 43.6 and 43.7). The parent or caregiver performs peritoneal dialysis at home after completing a training course. The process is either completed overnight with the use of a machine (continuous cyclic peritoneal dialysis) or in increments throughout the day for a total of 4 to 8 hours (continuous ambulatory peritoneal dialysis). Comparison Chart 43.1 compares these two methods of peritoneal dialysis.

The advantages of peritoneal dialysis over hemodialysis include improved growth because of more dietary freedom, increased independence in daily activities, and a steadier state of electrolyte balance. However, the risk for infection (peritonitis and sepsis) is a continual concern with peritoneal dialysis (Chua & Warady, 2024).

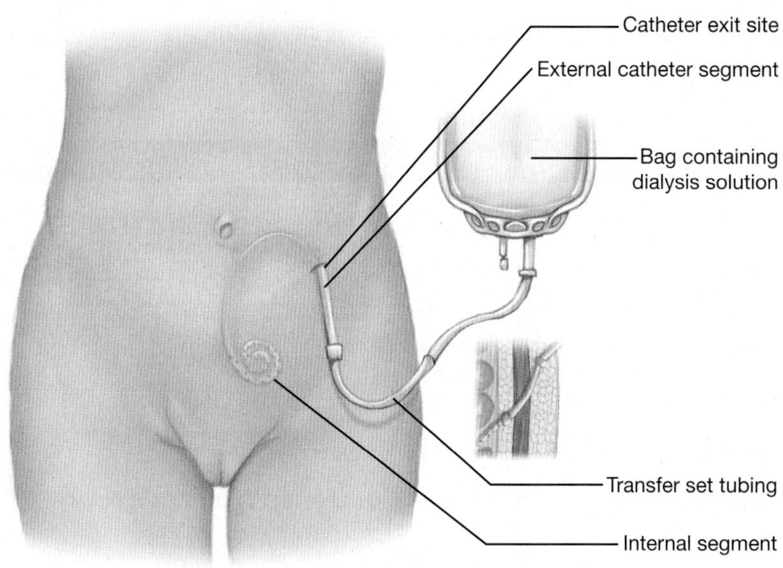

FIGURE 43.6 The peritoneal dialysis catheter is tunneled under the skin into the peritoneal cavity.

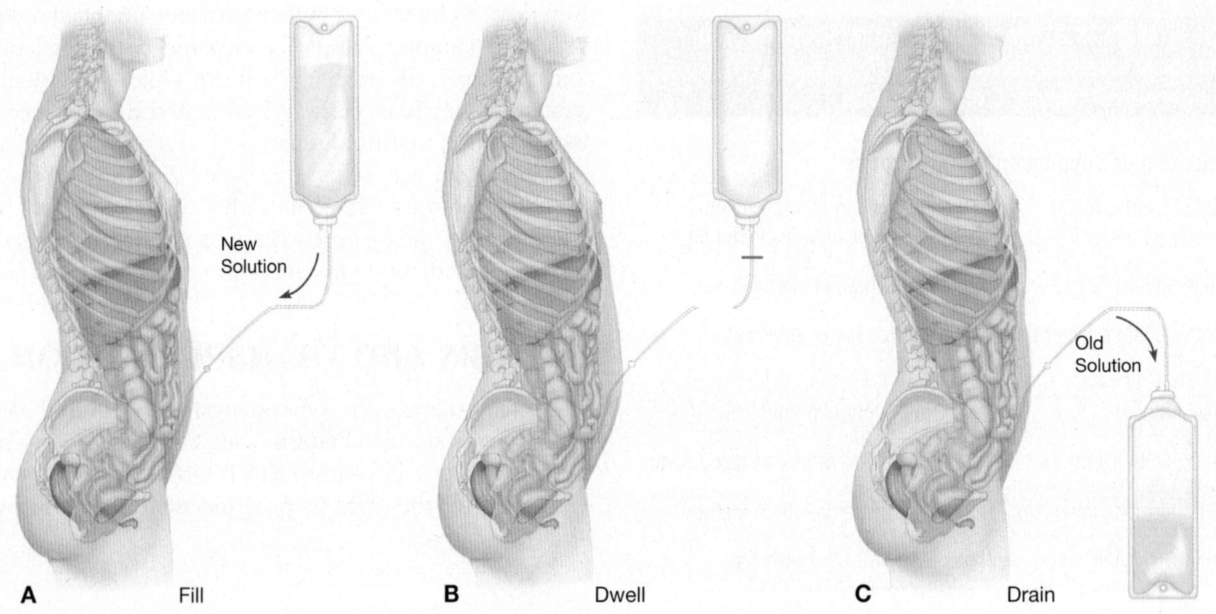

FIGURE 43.7 **A.** During the "fill" phase of peritoneal dialysis, dialysate fluid is instilled into the peritoneal cavity. **B.** During the "dwell" phase, the child may be up out of bed with the empty dialysate bag folded up with the tubing under their clothing. **C.** During the "drain" phase, the old dialysate is drained from the peritoneum by gravity, bringing with it waste products and excess fluid. The dialysate bags are weighed prior to filling and after draining to determine the amount of fluid removed from the child.

Dialysate exchange protocols, care of the catheter in the abdomen, and dressing changes must all be performed using sterile technique to avoid introducing microorganisms into the peritoneal cavity. Box 43.1 lists additional risks associated with peritoneal dialysis.

Hemodialysis

Hemodialysis removes toxins and excess fluid from the blood by pumping the child's blood through a hemodialysis machine and then reinfusing the blood into the child. Needles to remove and reinfuse the blood are inserted into an arteriovenous fistula or graft, usually located in the child's arm (Figs. 43.8 and 43.9).

Hemodialysis frees the parent from the need to perform daily dialysis, but the procedure, which takes 3 to 6 hours, must be done two to four times per week

BOX 43.1 Risks Associated With Peritoneal Dialysis

- Hypertension and other cardiac complications
- Seizures
- Obstructed catheter
- Dialysate leakage
- Hyperglycemia
- Increased triglyceride levels
- Increased protein loss
- Parental stress and burnout related to repetitive nature of daily intervention

COMPARISON CHART 43.1 Methods of Peritoneal Dialysis

	Continuous Ambulatory Peritoneal Dialysis (CAPD)	Continuous Cyclic Peritoneal Dialysis (CCPD)
When performed	Throughout the day, with exchanges every 3–6 hours. Fluid is usually allowed to dwell overnight to allow child to sleep.	Usually overnight while child is sleeping
Method	Manual instillation and draining and changing of dialysate bags with each exchange	Automated via CCPD machine; bags and tubing are attached when started, then disconnected in the morning.
Dwell time	3–6 hours	Usually 30 minutes to 1 hour
Mobility	Allows for mobility and permits child to participate in activities between exchanges	Child is confined to bed during the night while CCPD is ongoing but completely mobile while off CCPD during the day.

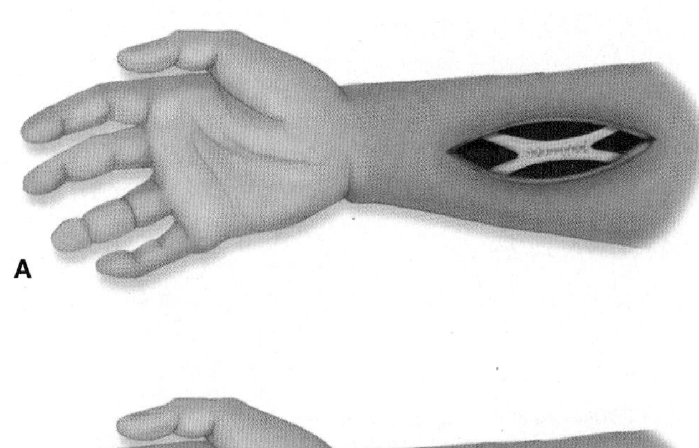

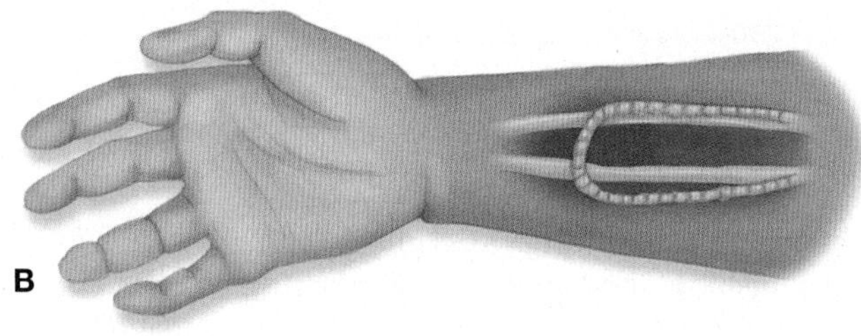

FIGURE 43.8 **A.** Arteriovenous fistula. **B.** Arteriovenous graft.

(usually three) at a pediatric hemodialysis center. This requires time away from school and other activities for the child and from work and other family responsibilities for the parent. Since hemodialysis is usually performed only every other day, larger amounts of waste products build up in the child's blood (uremia), placing the child at higher risk for seizures. The access site may become infected, and occlusion is also possible. The child must follow a stricter diet between hemodialysis treatments, although dietary restrictions are usually lifted while the child is undergoing the treatment.

Nursing Assessment

Refer to the "Nursing Assessment" under "Kidney Failure" section, as it is similar to assessment of the child undergoing dialysis. Assess for alterations in blood pressure and laboratory values following dialysis. Monitor for signs and symptoms of infection.

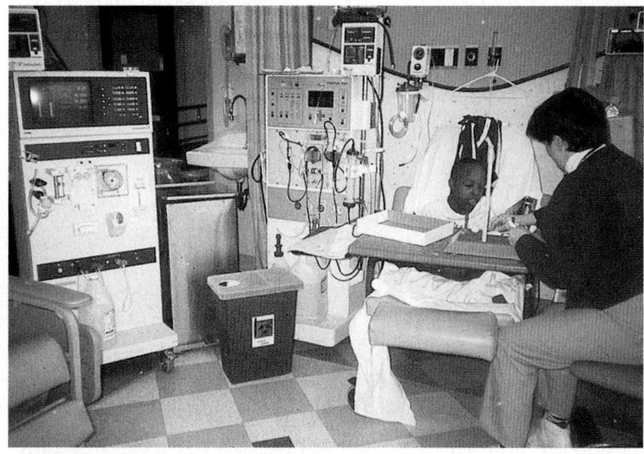

FIGURE 43.9 Pediatric hemodialysis.

Assess the child receiving peritoneal dialysis for toleration of the fluid volume instilled within the peritoneum. The abdomen will remain distended while the fluid is indwelling and will be significantly flatter when the fluid is drained. Assess the Tenckhoff catheter site for signs of infection. Monitor the child's temperature. Inspect the dialysate effluent for fibrin or cloudiness, which may indicate infection. Weigh the child daily (in the drain phase if on peritoneal dialysis).

For the child who receives hemodialysis, assess the arteriovenous fistula or graft site with each set of vital signs. Auscultate the site for the presence of a bruit and palpate for the presence of a thrill. Notify the primary provider or nurse practitioner immediately if either is absent.

TAKE NOTE!

Avoid taking blood pressure, performing venipuncture, or using a tourniquet in the extremity with the arteriovenous fistula or graft; these procedures may cause occlusion and subsequent malfunction of the fistula or graft. Teach parents and children to inform all health care providers they come in contact with about the presence of the fistula or graft.

Nursing Management

Specially trained and certified nurses perform both peritoneal dialysis and hemodialysis. The general pediatric nurse's role is related to the ongoing care of the child. The child undergoing peritoneal dialysis usually is allowed a more liberal diet and intake of fluid than the child undergoing hemodialysis. Peritoneal dialysis removes waste and excess fluids on a daily basis, whereas hemodialysis occurs about every other day. Most routine medications are withheld on the morning that hemodialysis is scheduled, since they would be filtered out through the dialysis process anyway. Administer these medications as soon as the child returns from the dialysis unit.

THINKING ABOUT **DEVELOPMENT**

Trevon Smith is a 17-year-old male football player who was on track for a college scholarship. Following an episode of acute glomerulonephritis, Trevon has progressed to CKD and is dependent upon hemodialysis. He is listed for a kidney transplant.

How will Trevon's developmental stage affect his desire to comply with the medical regimen? What types of psychosocial issues might Trevon be experiencing and how can the nurse best support Trevon at this time?

How will the nurse educate Trevon about self-care?

Kidney Transplantation

Kidney transplantation is the optimal treatment for KFRT and offers the best opportunity for the child to live a normal life. Vigilant medication administration is necessary after the transplant to prevent organ rejection. The child achieves improved kidney function with the transplant and may demonstrate improved growth, enhanced cognitive development, and improved psychosocial development and quality of life.

Kidneys are obtained from a cadaver (a patient declared brain-dead who had previously given consent to organ donation) or from a blood relative (living-related). The transplanted kidney must match the child's blood type and the child's human leukocyte antigens (HLAs). The cadaver kidney or living-related kidney is implanted surgically in the abdomen and the blood vessels are anastomosed to the aorta and superior vena cava.

Generally, living-related transplants have a decreased rejection rate compared to cadaver transplants (McDonald, 2023). Living-related kidney donation and subsequent transplantation can be planned ahead and scheduled in advance. In contrast, cadaver kidneys become available suddenly, leaving less time for preoperative preparation. For either type, last-minute blood tissue typing is required before the final decision is made to move forward with transplantation. Often the child's native kidneys are removed before or at the time of the renal transplant because of their association with hypertension in the child (McDonald, 2023).

> *TAKE NOTE!*
>
> Cadaver kidneys are allocated to potential recipients based on the age of the child with kidney failure, the time that they have been awaiting a transplant, blood type, HLA antibody matching, panel reactive antibodies, and region of the country (so that the donated kidney can be received expeditiously).

Nursing Assessment

A thorough physical assessment is warranted for any child undergoing renal transplant, whether in the initial postoperative period, at a clinic visit, or when admitted to the hospital, to rule out transplant rejection. Note recent health history, medications and their doses, and any symptoms the child has been having. In the initial postoperative period, assess the incision for redness, edema, or drainage. If any of these signs of infection or rejection occur, notify the transplant surgeon and nephrologist immediately. Monitor blood pressure and other vital signs closely. Document resolution of edema. Record intake and output accurately. Assess for signs and symptoms of transplant rejection such as malaise, fever, unexplained weight gain, or pain over the transplant area.

Nursing Management

Postoperative care focuses on preventing rejection, monitoring kidney function, maintaining fluid and electrolyte balance, and educating the child and family.

> *TAKE NOTE!*
>
> Encourage the child with a renal transplant to wear a medical alert necklace or bracelet and urge the parents to inform community emergency services of the child's transplant status.

PREVENTING REJECTION AND PROMOTING KIDNEY FUNCTION

Administer immunosuppressants accurately and in a timely fashion. Obtain and monitor serum levels of these medications per protocol. Immediately report significant alterations in vital signs or edema at the surgical site, as they may indicate transplant rejection. Maintain strict documentation of intake and output. Once adequate urine output is established, intake is usually liberalized.

EDUCATING THE CHILD AND FAMILY

Develop a schedule to cluster care so that the child may receive the rest needed for recovery despite the many and frequent assessments and interventions. With the family, develop a medication schedule that will be compatible with the family's life at home as well as the restrictions related to some medications. Begin teaching with the family as soon as the child's condition is stable. Accurate medication administration and home monitoring are necessary to prevent rejection. The child may return to school when discharged from the hospital, but the family will need to communicate closely with the school nurse about the child's immunosuppressed status. The American Nephrology Nurses Association has developed a renal transplant fact sheet that can be shared with the school nurse (link: https://www.annanurse.org/download/reference/practice/pedTransplantFactSheet.pdf).

> *TAKE NOTE!*
>
> Tell the parents to inform their child's primary provider or nurse practitioner about the child's long-term corticosteroid use and immunosuppressed status, as the child should not receive any live vaccines.

REPRODUCTIVE ORGAN DISORDERS

A number of disorders may occur within the female or male genitalia and internal reproductive organs in children. These problems may be structural or infectious.

FEMALE DISORDERS

Disorders of the female reproductive organs that occur in children and adolescents include structural disorders, infectious disorders, and menstrual disorders (covered in Chapter 4).

Labial Adhesions

Labial adhesion or labial fusion is partial or complete adherence of the labia minora (Fig. 43.10). UTI may result from urinary stasis behind the labia; if the adhesions are left untreated, the vaginal orifice may become inaccessible, presenting difficulty with sexual intercourse in the future.

Nursing Assessment

The peak incidence of labial adhesions occurs in the second year of life (Laufer & Emans, 2022). Assess the history for dysuria or urinary frequency. Inspect the genitalia for fusion or adherence of the labia minora.

Nursing Management

Administer topical estrogen cream as prescribed, usually once or twice daily. Teach the parents to continue cream application until the labia separate. Encourage use of petroleum jelly daily for 1 month following labial separation to prevent recurrence of adhesion.

Vulvovaginitis

Vulvovaginitis is inflammation of the vulva and vagina. Inflammation may occur as a result of bacterial or yeast overgrowth or from chemical factors such as bubble bath, soaps, or perfumes found in personal care products. Poor hygiene may also cause vulvovaginitis. Tight clothing may cause a heat rash in the perineal area. Persistent scratching of the irritated area may result in the complication of superficial skin infection.

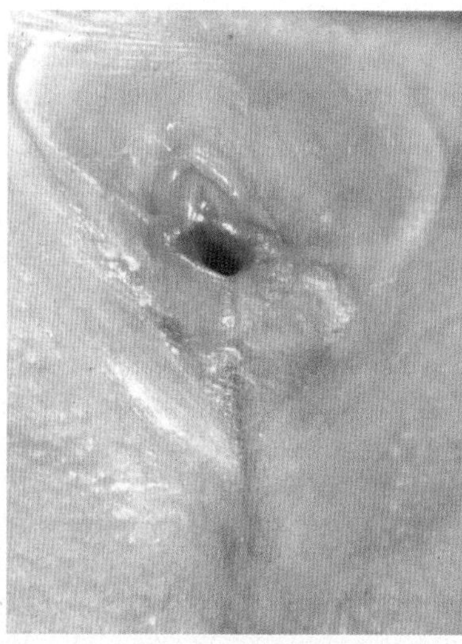

FIGURE 43.10 Labial adhesions: Note fusion of the labia minora. (Reprinted with permission from Emans, S. J., Laufer, M. R., & DiVasta, A. [2019]. *Emans, Laufer, Goldstein's pediatric and adolescent gynecology* [7th ed.]. Wolters Kluwer.)

Nursing Assessment

Eliciting the health history may reveal the common symptoms of itching or burning in the perineal area. Explore the child's current and past medical history for risk factors, which may include young age (toilet-trained preschooler), poor hygiene, sexual activity, immune disorders, or diabetes mellitus. Inspect the perineum for redness, edema, irritation, rash, or vaginal discharge (note color, consistency, and odor).

Nursing Management

Teach appropriate hygiene (daily and toileting). Females (or their parents) should thoroughly wash the genital area daily with mild soap and water. Rinse the area well. Encourage females to wipe after urinating and after bowel movements to wipe in a front-to-back motion. The female should wear cotton underwear and should change it at least once a day. Administer topical or oral medications as ordered. Table 43.3 lists treatments related to specific types of vulvovaginitis.

MALE DISORDERS

Male reproductive disorders include structural disorders and disorders caused by infection or inflammation. Circumcision will also be discussed.

Phimosis and Paraphimosis

In phimosis, the foreskin of the penis cannot be retracted. Although this is normal in the newborn, it can be pathologic later. Over time, the prepuce (foreskin) naturally becomes retractable. Local irritation, balanitis, or UTI may occur if urine is retained within the foreskin after voiding. Paraphimosis (Fig. 43.11) is a more serious disorder characterized by retraction of the phimotic prepuce, which causes a constricting band behind the glans of the penis and results in incarceration if left untreated.

Topical steroid cream applied twice a day for 1 month may be prescribed for phimosis. Paraphimosis requires reduction of the prepuce or a small dorsal incision to release the foreskin. Circumcision may be used to treat either condition (Tews, 2022).

Nursing Assessment

Common symptoms reported when eliciting the health history might include irritation or bleeding from the opening of the prepuce or dysuria (with phimosis), or

TABLE 43.3 • Vulvovaginitis: Types and Treatments

Cause	Assessment Findings	Treatment
Unhygienic practices	Irritation of labia and vaginal opening May have foul brownish-green discharge if infected with bacteria from rectum	Good hygiene Sometimes a mild antiinflammatory cream is prescribed. Assess for signs and symptoms of urinary tract infection, which may occur as a complication.
Candida albicans	Red bumpy perineal rash in infants White cottage cheeselike discharge Intense itching	Antifungal cream or vaginal suppository Prevent by ingesting probiotics (found in yogurt and kefir) daily and supplementing with a probiotic such as Lactinex when taking antibiotics.
Bordetella, Gardnerella	Thin gray vaginal discharge with fishy odor	Metronidazole orally
Trichomonas vaginalis	Foul yellow-gray or green vaginal discharge	Metronidazole orally. Sexually transmitted, so can be prevented with the use of condoms

Data from Bauman, D. (2019). Pediatric & adolescent gynecology. In A. H. DeCherney, L. Nathan, N. Laufer, & A. S. Roman (Eds.), *Current diagnosis & treatment: Obstetrics & gynecology* (12th ed., pp. 589–620). McGraw-Hill Education; Bernstein, J. (2019). Benign disorders of the vulva and vagina. In A. H. DeCherney, L. Nathan, N. Laufer, & A. S. Roman (Eds.), *Current diagnosis & treatment: Obstetrics & gynecology* (12th ed., pp. 631–657). McGraw-Hill Education.

pain and swollen penis (with paraphimosis). Determine the onset of symptoms and inspect the penis for irritation, erythema, edema, or discharge.

CLINICAL REASONING ALERT!

A swollen, reddened penis (paraphimosis) is a medical emergency and can quickly result in necrosis of the tip of the penis if left untreated.

Nursing Management

Apply topical steroid medication as prescribed for phimosis, following gentle retraction to stretch the foreskin back. Topical vitamin E cream may also help to soften

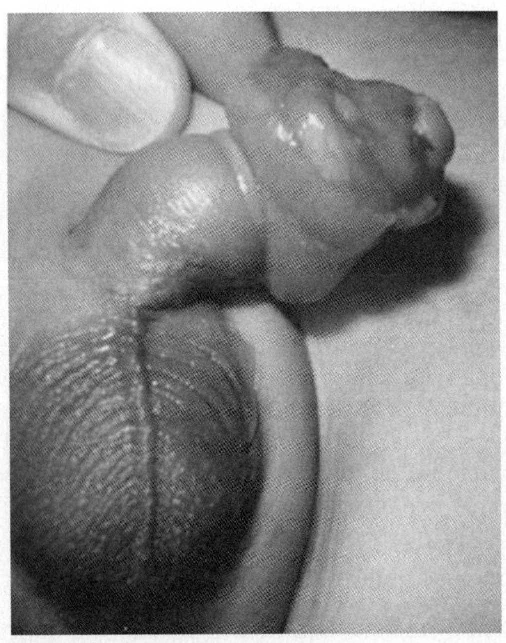

FIGURE 43.11 Paraphimosis: Note the swollen prepuce. (Reprinted with permission from Shaw, K. N., & Bachur, R. G. [2020]. *Fleisher & Ludwig's textbook of pediatric emergency medicine* [8th ed.]. Wolters Kluwer.)

the phimotic ring. When surgical intervention is necessary, provide routine postprocedural care and pain management (refer to the "Circumcision" section). Teach the parents and uncircumcised male proper hygiene, which will help to prevent phimosis and paraphimosis (Teaching Guidelines 43.2).

TEACHING GUIDELINES **43.2** Hygiene in the Uncircumcised Male

- The foreskin does not normally retract in the newborn male, so do not force it to do so.
- Change the diaper frequently and wash the penis daily with water and mild soap.
- When the infant is older and the foreskin easily retracts, gently retract the foreskin and clean around the glans with water and mild soap once a week.
- Dry the area prior to replacing the foreskin.
- Always replace the foreskin after retraction.
- Teach the preschool-age male to retract the foreskin and clean the penis during each bath or shower.

Circumcision

Circumcision is the removal of the excess foreskin of the penis. Some newborn males are circumcised shortly after birth before going home from the hospital. Some parents elect not to have their newborn male circumcised at that time but may desire it later. Neonatal circumcision may be performed in the newborn nursery, hospital unit treatment room, or outpatient office. Circumcision is indicated later for the conditions of phimosis and paraphimosis. Circumcision done after the newborn period usually requires general anesthesia.

The benefits of circumcision include a decreased incidence of UTI, sexually transmitted diseases, AIDS, and penile cancer, and in female partners a decreased occurrence of cervical cancer. Complications of circumcision are rare and include bleeding, penile adhesions, imperfect amount of foreskin removal, and meatal stenosis (Baskin, 2023b). Whether to circumcise or not is a personal decision and often based on religious beliefs or social or cultural customs. Nurses should support and educate the parents in either case.

Nursing Assessment

Prior to the procedure, assess for normal placement of the urinary meatus on the glans penis (in males with hypospadias, circumcision should be delayed until evaluation by the pediatric urologist). After the circumcision, assess for redness, edema, or active bleeding. Note signs of infection, such as purulent drainage. Assess pain level.

Nursing Management

Nursing care of the male undergoing circumcision focuses on managing pain, providing postprocedural care, and educating the parents.

MANAGING PAIN

Whether circumcision is performed in the obstetric area of the hospital before newborn discharge or in the outpatient setting at a few days of age, pain management during the procedure must not be neglected. Advocate for appropriate pain management for the infant undergoing circumcision. Pain management techniques during the procedure may include a subcutaneous ring block with lidocaine, local anesthetic with lidocaine/prilocaine, or a dorsal nerve block to the penis. Playing calming music during the procedure may also help to soothe the infant, providing distraction. A sucrose-dipped pacifier may also be used as adjuvant therapy for pain management.

• • • ATRAUMATIC CARE • • •

Restrain the infant in a padded circumcision chair with blankets covering the legs and upper body to provide a sense of comfort. If a padded restraint chair is not available, provide atraumatic care by padding the circumcision board and covering the infant as previously described.

PROVIDING POSTPROCEDURAL CARE

Usual care after circumcision depends on the type of appliance used (Gomco or Mogen clamp or Plastibell apparatus). Cleanse the penis with clear water for the first few days and avoid using alcohol-containing wipes. To avoid irritation to the penis, fasten diapers loosely. Notify the primary provider or nurse practitioner if excessive redness, active bleeding, or purulent discharge occurs. Assess for the first void following the procedure, or if performed in the outpatient setting instruct parents to call the primary provider or nurse practitioner if the infant has not voided within 6 to 8 hours after the circumcision. Apply antibiotic ointment or petroleum jelly to the penile head with each diaper change as prescribed, based on the circumcision method used and the preference of the primary provider or nurse practitioner.

CLINICAL REASONING ALERT!

If excess bleeding occurs after the circumcision, apply direct pressure, and notify the primary provider or nurse practitioner immediately.

EDUCATING THE PARENTS

Instruct parents to give sponge baths until the circumcision is healed. Describe the normal granulation tissue that will be present during the healing process. Teach parents to apply ointment or petroleum jelly if indicated. Instruct the parents to call the primary provider or nurse practitioner if any of the following occur:

- The infant does not urinate within 6 to 8 hours after the procedure.
- Heavy bleeding occurs (more than small spots on the diaper or bleeding that requires direct pressure to stop it).
- There is purulent or serous drainage from the circumcised area.
- There is redness or swelling of the penile shaft.

TAKE NOTE!

If the Plastibell is used, teach parents NOT to use petroleum jelly, as it may cause the ring to be dislodged. A yellowish crust may form that should be allowed to fall off on its own after several days.

Cryptorchidism

Cryptorchidism (also known as undescended testicles) occurs when one or both testicles do not descend into the scrotal sac. Ordinarily the testes, which in the fetus develop in the abdomen, make their descent into the scrotal sac during the seventh month of gestation. The cause for this failure to descend may be mechanical, hormonal, chromosomal, or enzymatic. The disorder may occur unilaterally or bilaterally. Up to 3.4% of term male infants exhibit cryptorchidism (Patel & Vogt, 2023).

Complications associated with cryptorchidism that is allowed to progress into the school-age years include sterility and an increased risk for testicular cancer in adolescence or the young adult years. Therapeutic management is surgical. An orchiopexy is performed to release the spermatic cord, and the testes are then pulled into the scrotum and tacked into place.

Nursing Assessment

Explore the health history for risk factors such as prematurity, first-born child, cesarean birth, low birth weight, or hypospadias. Palpate for the presence (or absence) of both testes in the scrotal sac.

> **TAKE NOTE!**
> A retractile testis is one that may be brought into the scrotum, remains for a time, and then retracts back up the inguinal canal. This should not be confused with true cryptorchidism.

Nursing Management

If the testes are not descended by 12 months of age, the infant should be referred for surgical repair. Postoperatively, observe the incision for signs of bleeding or infection.

Hydrocele and Varicocele

Hydrocele (fluid in the scrotal sac) is usually a benign and self-limiting disorder. It is usually noted early in infancy and often resolves spontaneously by 1 year of age. Varicocele (a venous varicosity along the spermatic cord) is often noted as a swelling of the scrotal sac. Complications of varicocele include low sperm count or reduced sperm motility, which can result in infertility.

Nursing Assessment

Elicit a description of the present illness and chief complaint. The male with hydrocele will have an enlarged scrotum that may decrease in size when he is lying down. Inspect the scrotum for a fluid-filled appearance.

The male with varicocele will have a mass on one or both sides of the scrotum and bluish discoloration. Inspect the scrotum for masses; the spermatic vein feels wormlike on palpation. The male with varicocele may have pain.

Nursing Management

Both hydrocele and painless varicocele require watchful waiting, as these conditions will usually resolve spontaneously. If they do not resolve, or if the difference in testicular volume is marked in the male with varicocele, refer the child to a urologist, as surgery may be indicated. Reassure parents that hydrocele is not associated with the development of infertility. Varicocele may lead to infertility if left untreated, so instruct parents to seek care if pain occurs or if there is a large difference in testicular size. Either condition may be surgically corrected on an outpatient basis. Provide routine postoperative care following either surgery.

Testicular Torsion

In testicular torsion, a testicle is abnormally attached to the scrotum and twisted. It requires immediate attention because ischemia can result if the torsion is left untreated, leading to infertility. Testicular torsion may occur at any age but most commonly occurs in males aged 12 to 18 years (Brenner & Ojo, 2023).

Nursing Assessment

Symptoms of testicular torsion include sudden, severe scrotal pain. Inspect the affected side for significant swelling, which may appear hemorrhagic or blue-black.

Nursing Management

Surgical correction is necessary immediately. Administer pain medication prior to surgery. Reassure the child and family that surgery will alleviate the problem and is performed to restore adequate blood flow to the testicle. After surgical repair, provide routine postoperative care.

> **TAKE NOTE!**
> Testicular torsion is considered a surgical emergency, as necrosis of the testis may occur, and gangrene may set in.

Epididymitis

Epididymitis (inflammation of the epididymis) is caused by infection with bacteria. It is the most common cause of pain in the scrotum. It rarely occurs before puberty, but if it does it may occur because of a urethral or bladder infection related to a urogenital anomaly. Therapeutic management is directed toward eradicating the bacteria. If left untreated, a scrotal abscess, testicular infarction, or infertility may occur.

Nursing Assessment

Note history of painful swelling of the scrotum, which may be gradual or acute. If the male is sexually active, explore history of sexual encounters prior to the onset of symptoms. Document history of dysuria or urethral discharge. Note fever, which may last from days to weeks. On inspection, note edema and erythema of the scrotum. Gently palpate the scrotum for a hardened and tender epididymis. Note urethral discharge if present. Palpate the inguinal lymph nodes for enlargement. Urinalysis may be positive for bacteria and white blood cells. The culture of urethral discharge may be positive for a sexually transmitted infection such as gonorrhea or *Chlamydia*. The complete blood count may reveal an elevated white blood cell count.

Nursing Management

Encourage the male to rest in bed with the scrotum elevated. Ice packs to the scrotum may help with pain relief. Administer pain medications such as NSAIDs or other analgesics as needed. Administer antibiotics as prescribed. Educate the male and his family to complete the entire course of antibiotics as prescribed to eradicate the infection. Advise the child and family to notify the primary provider or nurse practitioner if the condition is not improving or if the pain and swelling worsen.

KEY CONCEPTS

- Though present at birth, the reproductive organs do not reach functional maturity until puberty.
- The short length of the urethra in females and its proximity to the vagina and anus place the young female at higher risk for the development of UTIs compared with the adult.
- The urinary tract is immature in infants and young children, with a slower GFR and a decreased ability to concentrate urine and reabsorb amino acids compared with the adult.
- The expected urine output in the infant and child is 0.5 to 2 mL/kg/h.
- Obtaining a clean or sterile urine specimen is necessary for accurate urine culture results.
- A urinary catheter must be inserted just prior to the VCUG.
- Close monitoring of serum blood counts and electrolytes is a critical component of nursing care related to renal disorders.
- The treatment for nocturnal enuresis may include the use of desmopressin nasal spray or an enuresis alarm to train the child to awaken to the sensation of a filling bladder.
- Nephrotic syndrome results in significant proteinuria and edema.
- Acute glomerulonephritis most often follows a group A streptococcal infection and commonly results in hematuria, proteinuria, and hypertension.
- The most common cause of HUS is infection with *E. coli* O157:H7. It can be prevented by adequately cooking ground meat, washing hands and produce well, and making sure that an appropriate chemical balance is maintained in public recreational water sources such as swimming pools and water parks.
- Corticosteroids can cause gastrointestinal upset. If used on a long-term basis, they should be tapered rather than discontinued abruptly to avoid adrenal crisis.
- In children, CKD is most often the result of congenital structural defects, or infectious, inflammatory, or immune processes that damage the kidney, whereas in adults it usually results from hypertension or diabetes.
- Children taking immunosuppressants for nephrotic syndrome or for renal transplant are at increased risk for the development of overwhelming infection.
- Peritoneal dialysis may be accomplished at home by the parent. Close attention to sterile technique is needed.
- Hemodialysis requires an arteriovenous fistula or graft that is accessed with needles three or four times per week at a hemodialysis center. This is disruptive to the child's academic, social, and family lives.
- Renal transplantation is the best option for the treatment of end-stage kidney disease in children, but vigilant medication administration is needed to prevent organ rejection.
- Children with kidney failure experience anemia, poor growth, depression, anxiety, and low self-esteem.
- The diet for a child with a renal disorder must be individualized according to prescribed sodium, fluid, and protein restrictions.
- Postoperative care for the child undergoing urologic surgery includes pain management, avoidance or treatment of bladder spasms, and monitoring of urine output.

REFERENCES AND RECOMMENDED READINGS

Aksakall, T., Cinislioğlu, A. E., & Aksoy, Y. (2022). The efficacy of combined alarm therapy versus alarm monotherapy in the treatment of monosymptomatic nocturnal enuresis: A review of current literature. *Eurasian Journal of Medicine, 54*(Suppl. 1), S164–S167. https://doi.org/10.5152/eurasianjmed.2022.22311

American Nephrology Nurses' Association. (2021). *Pediatric ESRD renal transplantation fact sheet.* https://www.annanurse.org/download/reference/practice/pedTransplantFactSheet.pdf

Baskin, L. S. (2023a). Hypospadias: Management and outcome. *UpToDate.* Retrieved March 13, 2024, from https://www.uptodate.com/contents/hypospadias-management-and-outcome

Baskin, L. S. (2023b). Patient education: Circumcision in baby boys (beyond the basics). *UpToDate.* Retrieved March 13, 2024, from https://www.uptodate.com/contents/circumcision-in-baby-boys-beyond-the-basics

Bauman, D. (2019). Pediatric & adolescent gynecology. In A. H. DeCherney, L. Nathan, N. Laufer, & A. S. Roman (Eds.), *Current diagnosis & treatment: Obstetrics & gynecology* (12th ed., pp. 589–620). McGraw-Hill Education.

Bernstein, J. (2019). Benign disorders of the vulva and vagina. In A. H. DeCherney, L. Nathan, N. Laufer, & A. S. Roman (Eds.), *Current diagnosis & treatment: Obstetrics & gynecology* (12th ed., pp. 631–657). McGraw-Hill Education.

Bock, M. E., Blanchette, E., & Hanna, M. G. (2022). Kidney & urinary tract. In M. Bunik, W. W. Hay, M. J. Levin, & M. J. Abzug (Eds.), *Current diagnosis & treatment: Pediatrics* (26th ed.). McGraw-Hill Education.

Brenner, J. S., & Ojo, A. (2023). Causes of scrotal pain in children and adolescents. *UpToDate.* Retrieved March 13, 2024, from https://www.uptodate.com/contents/causes-of-scrotal-pain-in-children-and-adolescents

Chua, A., & Warady, B. A. (2024). Chronic peritoneal dialysis in children. *UpToDate*. Retrieved March 13, 2024, from https://www.uptodate.com/contents/chronic-peritoneal-dialysis-in-children

Corbett, J. A., & Banks, A. D. (2019). *Laboratory tests and diagnostic procedures with nursing diagnoses* (9th ed.). Pearson Education Inc.

Elder, J. R. (2020). Obstruction of the urinary tract. In R. M. Kliegman, J. W. St Geme, N. J. Blum, S. S. Shah, R. C. Tasker, & K. M. Wilson (Eds.), *Nelson textbook of pediatrics* (21st ed.). Elsevier.

Estrada, C. R., & Cendron, M. (2021). *Vesicoureteral reflux*. Medscape. https://emedicine.medscape.com/article/439403-overview

Flores, F. X. (2020). Isolated glomerular diseases associated with recurrent gross hematuria. In R. M. Kliegman, J. W. St Geme, N. J. Blum, S. S. Shah, R. C. Tasker, & K. M. Wilson (Eds.), *Nelson textbook of pediatrics* (21st ed.). Elsevier.

Flynn, J. T. (2023). Ambulatory blood pressure monitoring in children. *UpToDate*. Retrieved March 13, 2024, from https://www.uptodate.com/contents/ambulatory-blood-pressure-monitoring-in-children

Hamilton, R. G. (2023). Latex allergy: Epidemiology, clinical manifestations, and diagnosis. *UpToDate*. Retrieved March 13, 2024, from http://www.uptodate.com/contents/latex-allergy-epidemiology-clinical-manifestations-and-diagnosis

Hucker, J., & Lawson-Wood, H. (2023). *Indwelling urinary catheter insertion 1: Children and young people*. Nursing Times. https://www.nursingtimes.net/roles/childrens-nurses/indwelling-urinary-catheter-insertion-1-children-and-young-people-20-02-2023/

Klabunde, P. (2024). *Functional cardiac murmurs*. https://cvphysiology.com/heart-disease/hd006

Laufer, M. R., & Emans, S. J. (2022). Overview of vulvovaginal conditions in the prepubertal child. *UpToDate*. Retrieved March 13, 2024, from https://www.uptodate.com/contents/overview-of-vulvovaginal-conditions-in-the-prepubertal-child

McDonald, R. A. (2023). Kidney transplantation in children: General principles. *UpToDate*. Retrieved March 13, 2024, from https://www.uptodate.com/contents/kidney-transplantation-in-children-general-principles

Nationwide Children's Hospital. (2024). *U-bag urine collection guidelines for males and females*. https://www.nationwidechildrens.org/family-resources-education/health-wellness-and-safety-resources/helping-hands/ubag-urine-collection-guidelines-for-males-and-females

Patel, H. P., & Vogt, B. A. (2023). Nephrology and urology. In K. J. Marcdante, R. M. Kliegman, & A. M. Schuh (Eds.), *Nelson's essentials of pediatrics* (9th ed.). Elsevier.

Paul, C. R., & Wallace, C. M. (2023). Control of elimination. In K. J. Marcdante, R. M. Kliegman, & A. M. Schuh (Eds.), *Nelson's essentials of pediatrics* (9th ed.). Elsevier.

Solomon, D. H. (2022). Patient education: Nonsteroidal anti-inflammatory drugs (NSAIDs) (beyond the basics). *UpToDate*. Retrieved March 13, 2024, from https://www.uptodate.com/contents/nonsteroidal-antiinflammatory-drugs-nsaids-beyond-the-basics

St. Lukes. (n.d.). *When your child needs surgery for hypospadias*. https://www.saintlukeskc.org/health-library/when-your-child-needs-surgery-hypospadias

Stahl, J. L., Wightman, A. G., Flythe, J. E., Weiss, N. S., Hingorani, S. R., & Vander Stoep, A. (2022). Psychiatric diagnoses in children with CKD compared to the general population. *Kidney Medicine*, *4*(6). https://doi.org/10.1016/j.xkme.2022.100451

Tan, A. J., & Silverberg, M. A. (2021). *Hemolytic uremic syndrome in emergency medicine*. eMedicine. Retrieved March 13, 2024, from https://emedicine.medscape.com/article/779218-overview

Tews, M. (2022). Paraphimosis: Clinical manifestations, diagnosis, and treatment. *UpToDate*. Retrieved March 13, 2024, from https://www.uptodate.com/contents/paraphimosis-clinical-manifestations-diagnosis-and-treatment

U.S. Department of Health and Human Services. (n.d.). *Healthy People 2030*. https://health.gov/healthypeople

University of Texas Medical Branch Health. (2024). *Replacement fluid therapy*. https://www.utmb.edu/Pedi_Ed/CoreV2/Fluids/Fluids10.html

UpToDate, Inc. (2024). *Lexi-comp®* (Version 8.1.2) [Mobile app]. Wolters Kluwer. https://apps.apple.com/us/app/lexicomp/id313401238

DEVELOPING CLINICAL JUDGMENT

PRACTICING FOR NCLEX

1. A 4-year-old female presents with recurrent UTIs. A prior workup did not reveal any urinary tract abnormalities. What is the priority nursing action?
   a. Obtain a sterile urine sample after completion of antibiotics.
   b. Teach appropriate toileting hygiene.
   c. Prepare the child for surgery to reimplant the ureters.
   d. Administer antibiotics intramuscularly.

2. A 5-year-old who had a renal transplant 9 months ago and has no history of chickenpox presents to the pediatric clinic for their vaccinations. Which is the most appropriate set to give?
   a. DTaP, IPV
   b. DTaP, IPV, MMR, varicella
   c. DTaP, IPV, varicella
   d. IPV only

3. When the nurse is caring for a child with HUS or acute glomerulonephritis and the child is not yet toilet trained, which action by the nurse would best determine fluid retention?
   a. Test urine for specific gravity.
   b. Weigh child daily.
   c. Weigh the wet diapers.
   d. Measure abdominal girth daily.

4. An 8-year-old had a cold and sore throat that resolved about a week and a half ago. The parent is concerned as the child does not seem to be urinating as frequently as usual, has been tired, and looks pale. The child ordinarily does well in school and is very active. Upon physical examination, the nurse notes periorbital edema, blood pressure of 134/88, decreased urine output, pallor, and fatigue. Based on these findings, the child is admitted to the pediatric unit. Choose the correct options for each of the blanks in the statements below. Patients presenting with acute __________1__________ glomerulonephritis may have a history of a __________2__________ infection. Urine laboratory testing will reveal __________3__________.

   First blank
   a. post-pneumococcal
   b. post-staphylococcal
   c. poststreptococcal
   d. lupus erythematosus

   Second blank
   a. group A beta-hemolytic streptococcus
   b. group B beta-hemolytic streptococcus
   c. acute lung
   d. respiratory syncytial viral

   Third blank
   a. increased glucose
   b. increased white blood cells
   c. high leukocyte esterase
   d. increased red blood cells

5. A 4-year-old says it hurts "when I tinkle." The child has been toilet trained since age 28 months. The parent reports the child felt warm today and the urine is strong-smelling, with increased frequency and pain on urination. A urinalysis and culture is ordered. Which of the following does the nurse consider as true regarding obtaining the specimen? Select two items.
   a. Obtaining a clean voided urine sample is appropriate in children who are toilet trained.
   b. To maintain sterility, the urine specimen should be obtained through suprapubic aspiration.
   c. Since the child has a fever, an antibiotic should be started prior to obtaining the specimen.
   d. Painful urination can be resolved if the child drinks a large amount of fluid.
   e. Have the child begin urinating in the toilet, then collect the urine midway in a sterile container.

6. The nurse is caring for a 9-month-old who has had surgical correction for hypospadias. The infant will have a stent in place to drain urine for the next 5 to 10 days. Which of the following should the nurse include in the discharge teaching? Select all that apply.
   a. "The catheter will allow urine to drain into the diaper."
   b. "Administer pain medication around the clock for 10 days."
   c. "Use the double-diapering method while the stent is in place."
   d. "To prevent infection, be sure to give the antibiotic as prescribed."
   e. "Allowing tub baths may help with the child's pain control."
   f. "Avoid ride-on toys and roughhousing until cleared by the surgeon."

DOSAGE CALCULATION QUESTION

1. The nurse is caring for a child who has had a kidney transplant. The child weighs 47 lb. The medication order reads: cyclosporine 96 mg PO every 12 hours. Cyclosporine is supplied as 100 mg/mL. How many milliliters will the nurse administer? Round to the nearest whole number.

CRITICAL THINKING EXERCISES

1. Devise a meal plan for a 5-year-old child with a kidney disorder that requires a 2-g sodium restriction per day. Keep in mind the child's developmental level and feeding idiosyncrasies at this age.
2. Develop a discharge teaching plan for a 3-year-old with nephrotic syndrome who will be taking corticosteroids long term.
3. Devise a developmental stimulation plan for an 11-month-old who has had significant urinary tract reconstruction surgery and is facing a prolonged period of confinement to the crib.

STUDY ACTIVITIES

1. In the clinical setting, compare the growth and development of two children of the same age, one with CKD and one who has been healthy.
2. While caring for children in the clinical setting, compare and contrast the medical history, signs and symptoms of illness, and prescribed treatments for a child with nephrotic syndrome and one with acute glomerulonephritis.
3. Observe peritoneal dialysis in the hospital or hemodialysis in a hospital or outpatient center. Record observations about the children's psychosocial and developmental status.

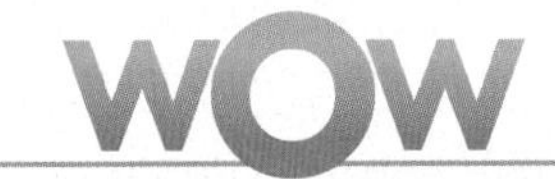

WORDS OF WISDOM

Enhancing a child's abilities may enhance their strength to overcome anything.

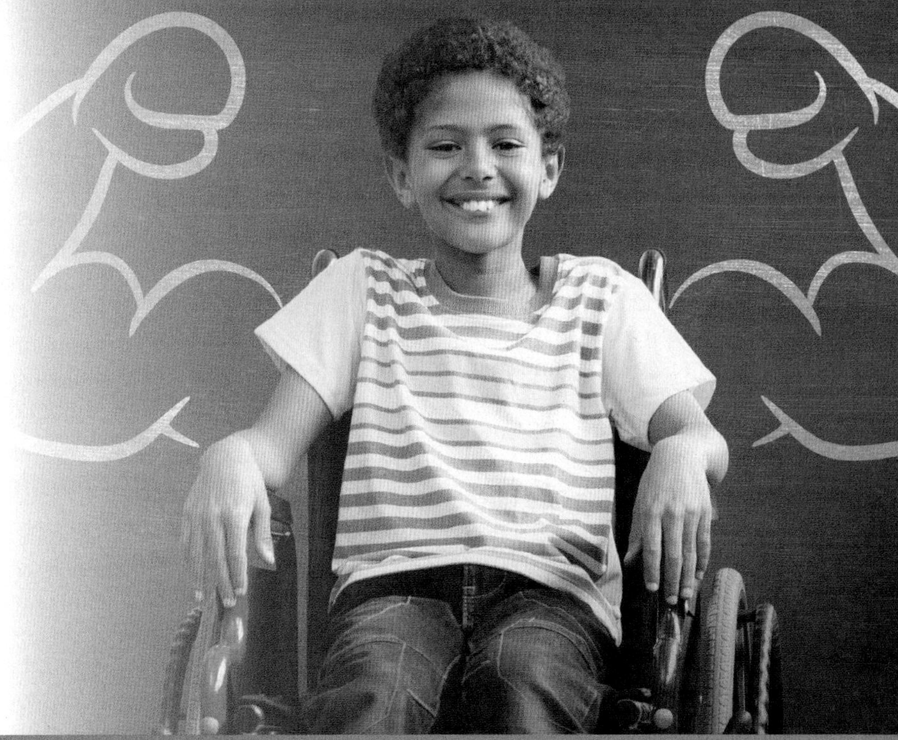

44

Nursing Care of the Child With an Alteration in Mobility/Neuromuscular or Musculoskeletal Disorder

KEY TERMS

ataxia (ă-tak´sē-ă)

clonus (klō´nŭs)

contracture (kŏn-trak´shŭr)

epiphysis (e-pif´i-sis)

external fixation

hypertonia

hypotonia

kyphosis (kī-fō´sis)

lordosis (lōr-dō´sis)

ossification (os´i-fi-kā´shŭn)

spasticity

traction

Trendelenburg gait

LEARNING OBJECTIVES

Upon completion of the chapter, you will be able to:

1. Compare the anatomy and physiology of the neuromuscular and musculoskeletal systems in children with that of adults.
2. Identify nursing interventions related to common laboratory and diagnostic tests used in the diagnosis and management of neuromuscular and musculoskeletal conditions.
3. Identify appropriate nursing assessments and interventions related to medications and treatments used for childhood neuromuscular and musculoskeletal conditions.
4. Distinguish various neuromuscular and musculoskeletal disorders occurring in childhood.
5. Devise an individualized plan of care or concept map for the child with a neuromuscular and musculoskeletal disorder.
6. Develop child and family teaching plans for the child with a neuromuscular and musculoskeletal disorder.
7. Describe the psychosocial impact of chronic neuromuscular and musculoskeletal disorders on the growth and development of children.

Frederick Stevens, 4 years old, seems to be falling often and has started to have difficulty climbing the stairs on his own. His parent states, "Recently, he hasn't been able to keep up with his 6-year-old sister when we're playing at the park. He usually ends up sitting on the bench with me." The parent is concerned about the changes they have seen in their child.

INTRODUCTION

Mobility refers to mechanisms that facilitate or impair a person's ability to move. Nurses encounter potential or actual alterations in mobility in all types of patients and must detect problems and intervene early to prevent complications. A variety of alterations in mobility (neuromuscular or musculoskeletal disorders) may affect children, but the result of each is muscular and/or skeletal dysfunction. Some of the disorders result from a neurologic insult such as trauma or hypoxia to the brain or spinal cord. Others occur as a result of genetic dysfunction or structural abnormality that is present from birth but may not be identified until later in childhood or adolescence. Infants and young children have resilient soft tissue, so sprains and strains are less common in this age group. Older school-age children and adolescents often participate in sports, resulting in an increased risk of injuries such as sprains, fractures, and torn ligaments.

The immobility associated with most neuromuscular and musculoskeletal disorders may affect the child's development and acquisition of motor skills, leading to motor dysfunction. Many neuromuscular and musculoskeletal disorders are chronic, lasting the child's entire life and resulting in disability.

The nurse caring for a child with altered mobility plays an important role in the management of these disorders. Not only must the nurse provide direct intervention in response to health alterations that result, but also the nurse is often part of the larger multidisciplinary team and may serve as the coordinator of many specialists or interventions. Understanding the most common responses to these disorders gives the nurse the foundation required to plan care for any child with any neuromuscular or musculoskeletal disorder.

VARIATIONS IN PEDIATRIC ANATOMY AND PHYSIOLOGY

The neuromuscular system is the combination of the nervous system and the muscles working together to create movement. The musculoskeletal system provides the body with form, support, stability, protection, and the ability to move. It is made up of bones, muscles, cartilage, tendons, ligaments, joints, and connective tissue. Anatomic and physiologic differences in infants and children, such as the immaturity of the neurologic and musculoskeletal systems, place them at increased risk for the development of a neuromuscular and musculoskeletal disorder and may hinder the child's growth and movement.

Brain and Spinal Cord Development

Early in gestation, around 3 to 4 weeks, the neural tube of the embryo begins to differentiate into the brain and spinal cord. If the fetus suffers infection, trauma, malnutrition, or teratogen exposure during this critical period of growth and differentiation, brain or spinal cord development may be altered. The premature infant's central nervous system is less mature than the term newborn's. Such immaturity in the preterm infant places them at a higher risk of central nervous insult within the neonatal period, which may result in delayed motor skill attainment or cerebral palsy. Compared with the adult, the child's spine is very mobile, especially the cervical spine region, resulting in a higher risk for cervical spine injury.

Myelinization

Though development of the structures of the nervous system is complete at birth, myelinization is incomplete. Myelinization continues to progress and is complete by about 2 years of age. Myelinization proceeds in a cephalocaudal and proximodistal fashion, allowing the infant to gain head and neck control before becoming able to control the trunk and the extremities. As myelinization proceeds, the speed and accuracy of nerve impulses increase. Primitive reflexes are replaced with voluntary movement.

Muscular Development

The muscular system, including tendons, ligaments, and cartilage, arises from the mesoderm in early embryonic development. At birth (term or preterm), the muscles, tendons, ligaments, and cartilage are all present and functional. The newborn infant is capable of spontaneous movement but lacks purposeful control. Full range of motion (ROM) is present at birth. Healthy infants and children demonstrate normal muscle tone; **hypertonia** (increased muscle tone) or **hypotonia** (low muscle tone) is an abnormal finding. Deep tendon reflexes are present at birth and are initially brisk in the newborn and progress to average over the first few months. Sluggish deep tendon reflexes indicate an abnormality. As the infant matures and becomes mobile, the muscles develop further and become stronger. The infant's muscles account for approximately 25% of total body weight, as compared with the adult's muscle mass, which accounts for about 40% of total body weight (Neudauer, 2019). Muscles grow rapidly in adolescence; this contributes to clumsiness, which places the adolescent at increased risk for injury. In response to testosterone release, the adolescent male experiences a growth spurt, particularly in the trunk and legs, and develops bulkier muscles. Female infants tend to have laxer ligaments than male infants, possibly due to the presence of female hormones, placing them at increased risk for developmental dysplasia of the hip (DDH) (Sankar et al., 2020).

Skeletal Development

The infant's skeleton is not fully ossified at birth. The infant's and young child's bones are more flexible and more porous and have a lower mineral content than the adult's. These structural differences in a young child's bones allow for greater shock absorption, so the bones will often bend rather than break when an injury occurs. The thick, strong periosteum of the child's bones allows for a greater absorption of force than is seen in adults. As a result, the cortex of the bone does not always break, sometimes buckling or bending only. The skeleton contains increased amounts of cartilage compared with adolescents and adults. **Ossification**, the conversion of cartilage to bone, continues throughout childhood and is complete in adolescence.

During fetal development, the spine displays **kyphosis**, an outward curvature. Cervical **lordosis**, inward curvature, develops as the infant starts to hold the head up. When the infant or toddler assumes an upright position, the primary and secondary curves of the spine begin to develop. The balance of the curves allows the head to be centered over the pelvis. During the toddler years, the period of early walking, lumbar lordosis may be significant (also termed toddler lordosis), and the toddler appears quite swaybacked and potbellied. As the child develops, the spine takes on more adult-like curves. During adolescence, thoracic kyphosis may become evident. This is most often a postural effect, and as the adolescent matures, the posture appears similar to that of an adult.

Growth Plate

The ends of the bones in young children are composed of the **epiphysis**, the end of a long bone, and the physis, in combination termed the growth plate. In infants, the epiphyses are cartilaginous and ossify over time. In children, the epiphysis is the secondary ossification center at the end of the bone. The physis is a cartilaginous area between the epiphysis and the metaphysis. Growth of the bones occurs primarily in the epiphyseal region. This area is vulnerable and structurally weak. Traumatic force applied to the epiphysis during injury may result in a fracture in that area of the bone. Epiphyseal injury may result in early, incomplete, or partial closure of the growth plate, leading to deformity or shortening of the bone. Epiphyseal growth continues until skeletal maturity is reached during adolescence. Production of androgens in adolescence gradually causes the growth plates to fuse, and thus long bone growth is complete (Fig. 44.1).

Bone Healing

The child's bones have a thick, strong periosteum with an abundant blood supply. Bone healing occurs in the same fashion as in the adult, but because of the rich nutrient supply to the periosteum, it occurs more quickly in children. Children's bones produce callus more rapidly and in larger quantities than do adults. As new bone cells quickly form, a bulge of new bone growth occurs at the site of the fracture. The younger the child, the more quickly the bone heals. Also, the closer the fracture is to the growth plate (epiphysis), the more quickly the fracture heals. The capacity for remodeling (the process of breaking down and forming new bone) is increased in children as compared with adults. This means that straightening of the bone over time occurs more easily in children.

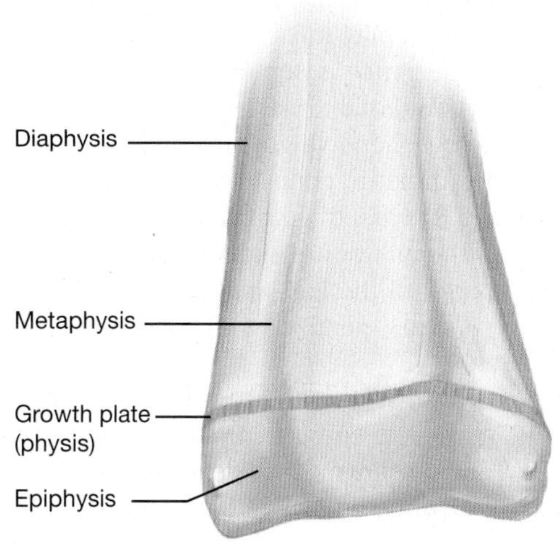

FIGURE 44.1 Anatomic areas of growing bone.

Positional Alterations

The lower extremities of the infant tend to have a bowed appearance, attributed to in-utero positioning. In utero, the fetus's hips are usually flexed, abducted, and externally rotated, with the knees also flexed and the lower limbs inwardly rotated. This normal developmental variation is termed internal tibial torsion. The legs straighten with passive motion, and internal tibial torsion should not be confused with "bowlegs" (Fig. 44.2). Internal tibial torsion usually resolves independently within the

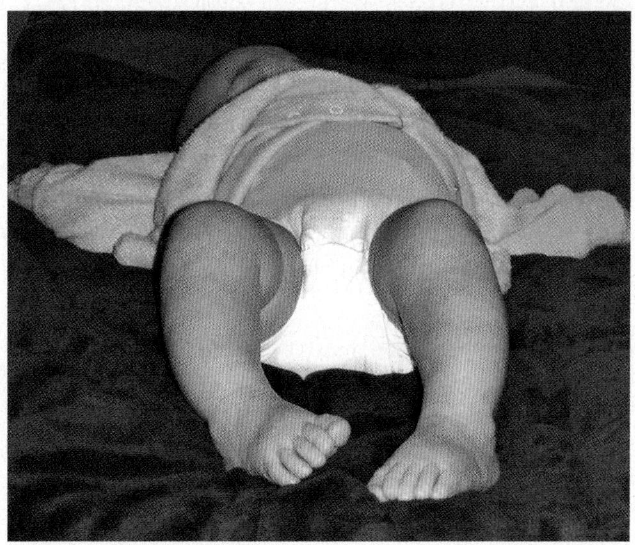

FIGURE 44.2 Internal tibial torsion with metatarsus adductus—normal findings in the infant.

second or third year of life as the toddler bears weight and the lower extremity muscles and bones mature. The bowlegged appearance is sometimes also referred to as genu varum. As internal tibial torsion or genu varum resolves, physiologic genu valgum occurs. Children usually demonstrate symmetric genu valgum (knock-knees) by the age of 2 to 3 years. In genu valgum, when the knees are touching, the ankles are significantly separated, with the lower portion of the legs angled outward (Fig. 44.3). By age 7 or 8 years, genu valgum gradually resolves in most children.

The newborn's feet also display in-toeing (metatarsus adductus) as a result of in-utero positioning (see Fig. 44.2). The feet remain flexible and may be passively moved to the midline and in a straight position. This also resolves as the infant's musculoskeletal system matures. Pes planus (flat feet) is noted in infants when they begin to walk. The long arch of the foot is not yet developed and makes contact with the floor, resulting in a medial bulge. As the child grows and the muscles become less lax, the arch generally develops. Some children may continue with flexible flat feet, and this is considered a normal variation.

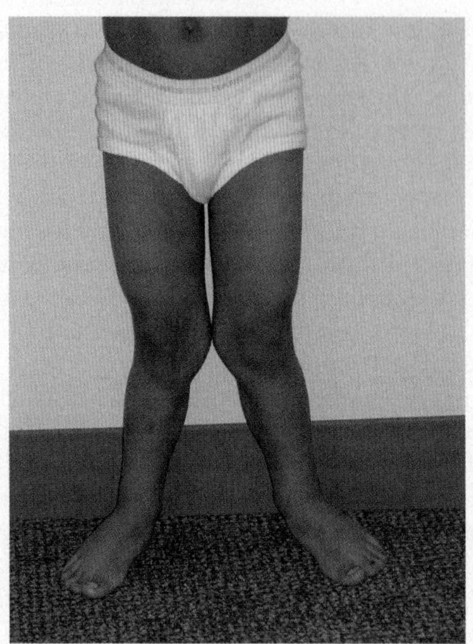

FIGURE 44.3 Genu valgum (knock-knees): Note knees touching at midline and outward angle of the lower half of the legs.

COMMON MEDICAL TREATMENTS

A variety of medications as well as other medical treatments are used to treat neuromuscular and musculoskeletal disorders in children. Most of these treatments will require a primary provider's or nurse practitioner's order when the child is in the hospital. The most common treatments and medications are listed in Common Medical Treatments 44.1 and Drug Guide 44.1. The nurse caring for the child with a neuromuscular or musculoskeletal disorder should become familiar with what these procedures are and how they work as well as common nursing implications related to the use of these modalities. The treatment of musculoskeletal disorders often involves immobilization via casting, bracing, splinting, or traction to allow healing with the bones in appropriate alignment. The length of treatment with these immobilization methods varies from weeks to months depending on the type of disorder being treated and its severity. Complications related to casting and traction include neurovascular compromise, skin integrity impairment, soft tissue injury, compartment syndrome, and, with skeletal traction, pin site infection or osteomyelitis.

COMMON MEDICAL TREATMENTS 44.1

Treatment	Explanation	Indications	Nursing Implications
Casting	Application of plaster or fiberglass material to form a rigid apparatus to immobilize a body part	Fracture reduction, dislocations, correction of deformities	Assess frequently for neurovascular compromise and skin impairment at cast edges. Protect cast from moisture. Teach family how to care for cast at home.
Splinting	Temporary stiff support of the injured area	Temporary fracture reduction, immobilization, and support of sprains	Similar to cast care. Some splints are removable and are replaced when the child is up and out of bed. Teach family the appropriate use of splints.
Fixation	Surgical reduction of a fracture or skeletal deformity with an internal or external pin or fixation device	Fractures, skeletal deformities	No additional care for internal fixation External fixation: Perform pin care as prescribed by the surgeon. Assess for excess drainage or pin slippage, and notify primary provider or nurse practitioner if this occurs. Velcro or snaps on sleeves and pant legs help with dressing.

COMMON MEDICAL TREATMENTS 44.1

Treatment	Explanation	Indications	Nursing Implications
Cold therapy	Application of ice bags, commercial cold packs, or cold compresses	Most often used in acute injuries to cause vasoconstriction, thereby decreasing pain and swelling	Apply for 20–30 minutes, remove for 1 hour, and then reapply for 20–30 minutes. Discontinue when numbness occurs. Place a towel between the cold pack and the skin to prevent thermal injury.
Crutches	Ambulatory devices that transfer body weight from lower to upper extremities	Used whenever weight bearing is contraindicated	Top of crutch should reach 2–3 fingerbreadths below the axillae to prevent nerve palsy. Teach child appropriate ambulation with crutches or reinforce teaching if performed by a physical therapist.
Skeletal or cervical traction	Traction is an application of a pulling force on an extremity or body part.	To minimize or prevent trauma to the spinal cord; fracture reduction, dislocations, correction of deformities	To maintain even, constant traction: • Ensure weights hang free at all times and ropes remain in the pulley grooves. • Keep weights out of the child's reach. • Maintain prescribed weight. • Elevate the head or foot of bed only with primary provider's order. Monitor for complications: • Perform neurovascular checks at least every 4 hours. • Monitor neurologic status closely. • Assess for signs and symptoms of infection or impaired skin integrity. • Provide appropriate pin site care.
Physical therapy, occupational therapy, or speech therapy	Physical therapy focuses on the attainment or improvement of gross motor skills. Occupational therapy focuses on the refinement of fine motor skills, feeding, and activities of daily living. Speech therapy is warranted for a child with a speech impairment or feeding difficulty related to oral muscular issues.	Cerebral palsy, spina bifida, spinal cord injury, muscular dystrophy, spinal muscular atrophy; restore function after injury or surgery; promote developmental activities when limb use is compromised, as in limb deficiency.	Provide follow-through with prescribed exercises or supportive equipment. Success of therapy is dependent on continued adherence to the prescribed regimen. Ensure that adequate communication exists within the interdisciplinary team.
Orthotics, braces	Adaptive positioning devices are specially fitted for each child by the physical or occupational therapist or orthotist. Used to maintain proper body or extremity alignment, improve mobility, and prevent contractures	Cerebral palsy, spinal cord injury, spina bifida, muscular dystrophy, spinal muscular atrophy; used to immobilize a body part or prevent deformity through positioning. Used to treat developmental dysplasia of the hip and scoliosis; may also be used for a period of time after cast removal	Provide frequent assessments of skin covered by the device to avoid skin breakdown. Cotton undergarment worn under the brace helps to maintain skin integrity. Follow the therapist's schedule of recommended "on" and "off" times. Encourage families to comply with use.

DRUG GUIDE 44.1

COMMON DRUGS FOR NEUROMUSCULAR DISORDERS

Medication	Actions/Indications	Nursing Implications
Benzodiazepines (diazepam, lorazepam)	Anticonvulsant; enhance the inhibition of GABA Used adjunctively for relief of skeletal muscle spasm associated with cerebral palsy, paralysis resulting from spinal cord injury, traction, and casting	Monitor sedation level. May cause dizziness Paradoxical excitement may occur. Assess for improvements in spasticity.

(continued)

DRUG GUIDE 44.1

COMMON DRUGS FOR NEUROMUSCULAR DISORDERS (*continued*)

Medication	Actions/Indications	Nursing Implications
Baclofen (oral or intrathecal)	Central-acting skeletal muscle relaxant; precise mechanism unknown Used to treat painful spasms and decrease spasticity in children with motor neuron lesions, such as cerebral palsy and spinal cord injury	Assess motor function. Monitor for a decrease in spasticity. Observe for mental confusion, depression, or hallucinations. Dosage must be tapered before discontinuing because withdrawal symptoms may occur.
Corticosteroids	Antiinflammatory and immunosuppressive action Duchenne muscular dystrophy, myasthenia gravis, dermatomyositis	Administer with food to decrease GI upset. May mask signs of infection Do not stop treatment abruptly or acute adrenal insufficiency may occur. Monitor for Cushing syndrome. Dosage may be tapered over time.
Botulin toxin	Neurotoxin produced by *Clostridium botulinum* that blocks neuromuscular conduction Relief of spasticity in cerebral palsy, occasionally for torticollis	Injected into the muscle by an advanced provider May cause dry mouth
Acetaminophen	Blocks pain impulses in response to inhibition of prostaglandin synthesis. Relief of mild pain if used alone, moderate or severe pain if used with a narcotic analgesic	Often combined with a narcotic such as codeine or oxycodone for increased analgesic effect Monitor pain levels and response to medication.
Narcotic analgesics	Act on receptors in the brain to alter the perception of pain. Relief of moderate to severe pain associated with injuries, orthopedic procedures	Assess pain location, quality, intensity, and duration. Assess respiratory rate prior to and periodically after administration. Monitor sedation level. May cause nausea, vomiting, constipation, pupil constriction
Nonsteroidal antiinflammatory drugs (NSAIDs: ibuprofen, ketorolac)	Inhibit prostaglandin synthesis, having a direct inhibitory effect on pain perception. Relief of mild to moderate pain, treatment of Legg–Calvé–Perthes disease	Monitor for nausea, vomiting, diarrhea, and constipation. Administer with water or food to decrease GI upset.
Bisphosphonate: IV—pamidronate, zoledronic acid; oral—alendronate, risedronate	Increase bone mineral density, decrease incidence of fractures in moderate to severe osteogenesis imperfecta	IV: given at 4-month intervals, causes a decrease in serum calcium level, influenzalike reaction with first IV dose. Oral: Side effects include heartburn, regurgitation, and upper abdominal discomfort.

GABA, gamma-aminobutyric acid; GI, gastrointestinal; IV, intravenously.

Source: Lexicomp. (2023). Pediatric drug information. *UpToDate.* Retrieved May 10, 2023, from https://www.uptodate.com/contents/table-of-contents/drug-information/pediatric-drug-information

Casts

Casts are used to immobilize a bone that has been injured or a diseased joint. When a fracture has occurred, a cast serves to hold the bone in reduction, thus preventing deformity as the fracture heals. Casts are constructed of a hard material, traditionally plaster but now more commonly fiberglass. The hard nature of the cast keeps the bone aligned so that healing may occur more quickly. In a fracture that would heal on its own without specific immobilization, a cast may be used to reduce pain and to allow the child increased mobility. The choice of cast material and type of cast will be determined by the primary provider, nurse practitioner, or orthopedic surgeon. Figure 44.4 shows selected casts used in children.

TAKE NOTE!

Gore-Tex is a special material that can be used to line casts and make them waterproof. These casts can get completely wet in the bath, shower, or during swimming. These casts cannot be used for all types of fractures, and they have an increased cost that may not be covered by insurance.

Traction

Traction, another common method of immobilization, may be used to reduce and/or immobilize a fracture, to align an injured extremity, and to allow the extremity to be restored to its normal length. Traction may

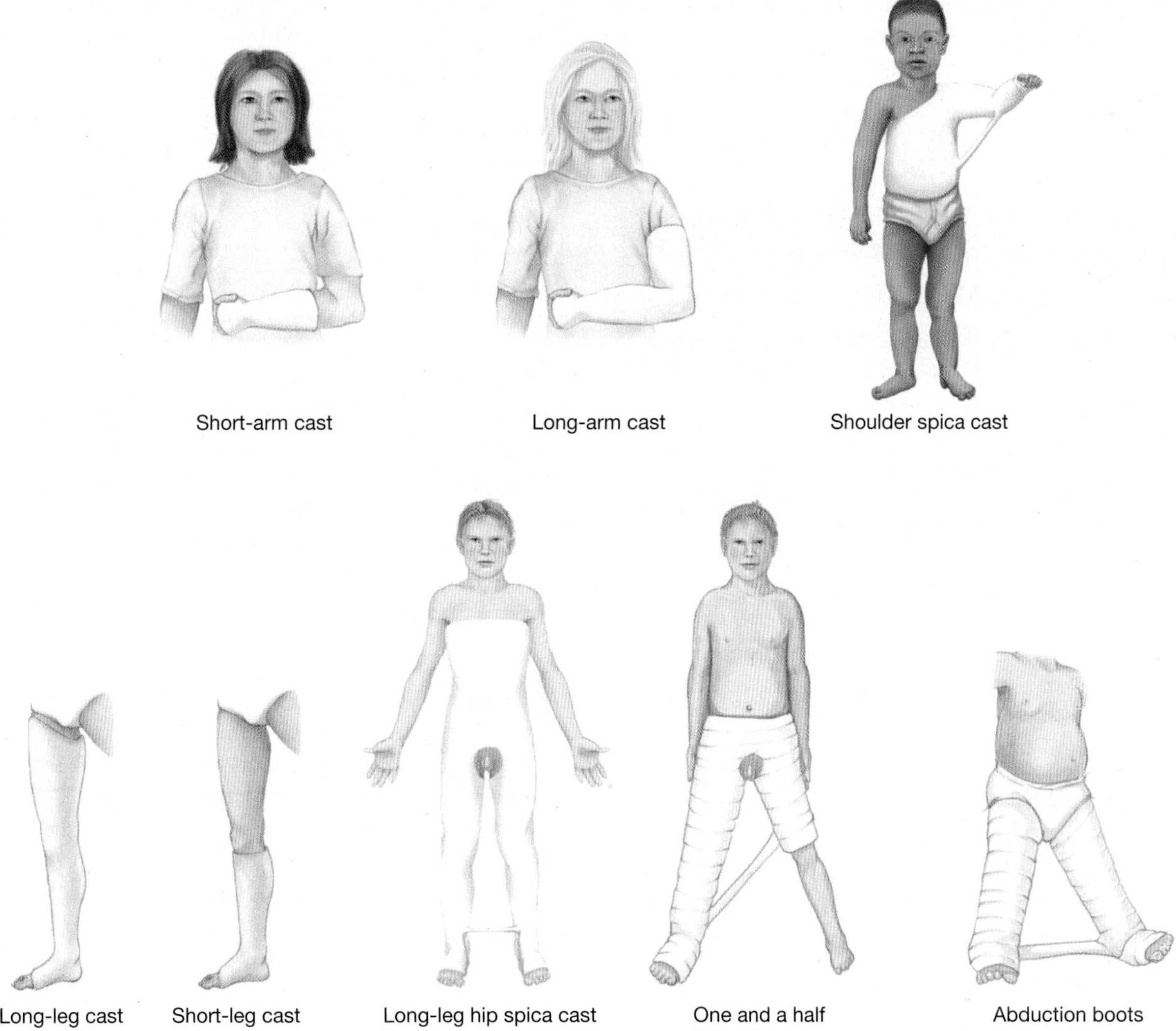

FIGURE 44.4 Selected casts used in children.

also reduce pain by decreasing the incidence of muscle spasm. In running traction, the weight pulls directly on the extremity in only one plane. This may be achieved with either skin or skeletal traction. In balanced suspension traction, additional weights are used to provide a counterbalance to the force of traction. This allows for constant pull on the extremity even if the child changes position somewhat. Comparison Chart 44.1 discusses skin versus skeletal traction.

External Fixation

External fixation may be used for complicated fractures, especially open fractures with soft tissue damage. A series of pins or wires are inserted into the bone and then attached to an external frame. The fixator apparatus may be adjusted as needed by the primary provider or nurse practitioner. Once the desired level of correction is achieved, no further adjustment occurs, and the bone is

COMPARISON CHART 44.1 Skin Versus Skeletal Traction

	Skin Traction	**Skeletal Traction**
Application of force	To the skin via strips or tapes secured with Ace bandages or traction boots	To the body part directly by fixation into or through the bone
Length of treatment	Usually limited	Allows for longer periods of traction
Amount of force	Less	More

allowed to heal. Advantages of external fixation include increased comfort for the injured child and improved function of muscles and joints when a complicated fracture occurs.

Clinical Judgment and the Nursing Process for the Child With a Neuromuscular or Musculoskeletal Disorder

Care of the child with a neuromuscular or musculoskeletal disorder includes assessment, nursing analysis, planning, interventions, and evaluation. There are many general concepts related to the nursing process that may be applied to neuromuscular and musculoskeletal dysfunction in children. From an overall understanding of the care involved for a child with an alteration in mobility, the nurse can then individualize the care based on specifics particular for that child. The nursing care of immobilized children is similar to that of adults, yet developmental and age-appropriate effects must be taken into account. Prevention of complications is a key nursing function.

Assessment

Assessment of neuromuscular and musculoskeletal dysfunction in children includes health history, physical examination, and laboratory and diagnostic testing.

Health History

The health history consists of the past medical history, including the birthing parent's pregnancy history, family history, and history of present illness (when the symptoms started and how they have progressed), as well as treatments used at home. The past medical history might be significant for prematurity, difficult birth, infection during pregnancy, changes in gait, falls, delayed development, poor growth, musculoskeletal congenital anomaly, or orthopedic injury during the birthing process. Breech delivery may be associated with DDH. Inquire about the child's usual level of physical activity, participation in sports, and use of protective equipment. Family history might be significant for neuromuscular disorders that are genetic or orthopedic problems. Determine the child's history of attainment of developmental milestones. Note the age at which milestones such as sitting, crawling, and walking were attained, and determine whether the pace of attainment of milestones has decreased. Some children may progress normally at first and then demonstrate decreased velocity of development of achievements or even loss of abilities. Obtain a clear description of weakness; is it fatigue, or is the child truly not as strong as they were in the past?

When eliciting the history of the present illness, inquire about the following:

- Changes in gait or limp
- Recent trauma (determine the mechanism of injury)
- Recent strenuous exercise
- Poor feeding
- Lethargy
- Fever
- Weakness
- Alteration in muscle tone
- Areas of redness or swelling

Physical Examination

Physical examination of the nervous and musculoskeletal systems consists of inspection, observation, and palpation. It should also include auscultation of the heart and lungs, as the function of these organs may be affected by certain neuromuscular conditions.

INSPECTION AND OBSERVATION

Observe the infant or child playing with toys, crawling, or walking to obtain significant information about cranial nerve, cerebellar, and motor function. Observe the child's general appearance, noting any asymmetry in muscle development. Observe the child's posture and alignment of the trunk. Inspect the extremities for symmetry and positioning and for absence, duplication, or webbing of any digits. Note any obvious extremity deformity or limb-length discrepancy. When extremities are not used, muscular atrophy develops, so a shortened limb may indicate chronic hemiparesis. Observe gait in the child who has achieved the developmental skill of walking. Note refusal to walk, limping, in-toeing, out-toeing, or foot slap. Inspect injured joints for ecchymosis or swelling. In the injured extremity, note the color of the fingertips or toes. Observe spontaneous ROM. Perform scoliosis screening to determine spinal alignment. Note the symmetry of thigh folds. Note the symmetry of spontaneous movement of extremities as well as facial muscles. Determine cranial nerve function (refer to Chapter 38 for a complete description of assessment of cranial nerves). Inspect the skin for redness, warmth, bruises, and puncture sites. Inspect the spine for cutaneous abnormalities such as dimples or hair tufts, which may be associated with spinal cord abnormalities. Observe the child's level of consciousness (LOC), noting a decrease or significant changes. Note the presence of lethargy. Refer to Chapter 38 for a complete description of the evaluation of LOC.

Motor Function. Observe spontaneous activity, posture, and balance, and assess for asymmetric movements. In the infant, observe resting posture, which will normally be a slightly flexed posture. The infant should be able to extend extremities to a normal stretch. Note the position of comfort of the infant's or child's neck.

Reflexes. Note sluggish or brisk deep tendon reflexes. Note the persistence of primitive reflexes in the older infant or child, such as Moro or tonic neck. Assess for the development of protective reflexes, which is often delayed in infants with motor disorders.

Sensory Function. Alterations in sensory function accompany many neuromuscular disorders. Assess sensory function in a similar fashion to that used in the adult. The sensory functions of light touch, pain, vibration, heat, and cold are distinguishable by a child. In the infant, assess for response to light touch or pain. The usual response to pain will be withdrawal from the stimulus. Always prepare the child for the sensory examination in order to gain cooperation. The pinprick test may be particularly frightening, but most children will cooperate if educated appropriately.

PALPATION

Assess muscle strength and tone in the infant or child. Compare strength and tone bilaterally. Evaluate neck tone by pulling the infant from a supine position to a sitting position (Fig. 44.5). By 4 to 5 months, the infant should be able to maintain the head in a neutral position. Perform passive ROM of the neck. Alterations in ROM may indicate a neuromuscular disorder or torticollis. Note trunk tone in the infant by holding the infant under the axillae and palpating for trunk tone. The hypotonic infant will feel as though they are slipping through the examiner's hands. Generalized hypotonia is a common sign of neuromuscular disease in the infant and young child (Sarant, 2020). The hypertonic infant will feel rigid, extending the trunk and legs. Assess leg tone in the infant by placing the infant in the vertical position with the feet on a flat surface; the 4-month-old infant should be able to momentarily support their weight (Fig. 44.6). Assess the strength of the infant or young child by noting the ability to move the muscles against gravity. In older children, have the child push against the examiner's hand with the sole of the foot to determine muscle strength (Fig. 44.7). Note any hypertonia or **spasticity**, which is involuntary muscle contractions that are not coordinated with other muscles (e.g., when you stretch out your forearm the triceps contract and the biceps stretch; in spasticity, they both contract at the same time). These may be an early indication of cerebral palsy or another neuromuscular disorder.

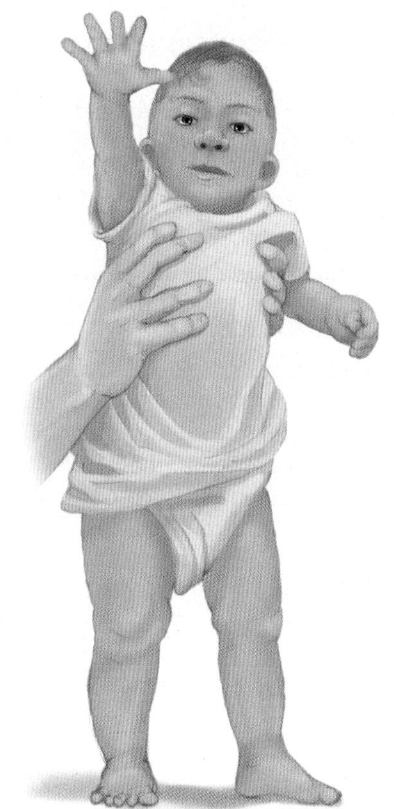

FIGURE 44.6 Assessing leg tone in an infant.

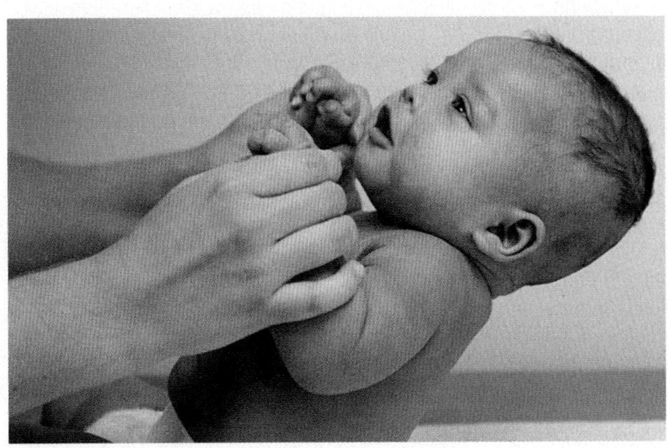

FIGURE 44.5 Assessing neck tone in an infant.

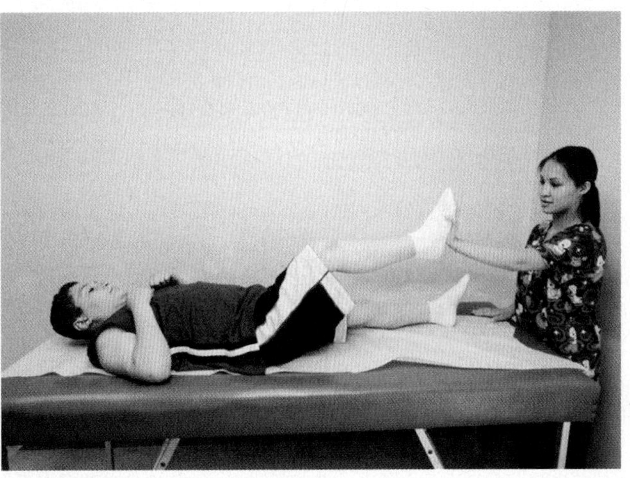

FIGURE 44.7 Assessing leg strength of the child.

CLINICAL REASONING ALERT!

In cases of trauma or suspected trauma, do not perform any assessment that involves movement of the head and neck until cervical injury is ruled out. Maintain complete immobilization of the cervical spine until that time.

Palpate the clavicles in the newborn or young infant for tenderness or a bump that indicates callus formation with clavicle fracture. Perform active ROM to determine if a joint position is fixed (e.g., clubfoot). Palpate the affected joint or extremity to detect warmth or tenderness. In the injured child or the child with a cast or splint, thoroughly assess the neurovascular status of the affected extremities. Palpate the fingers or toes for warmth. Determine the capillary refill time. Note the presence of sensation or motion. Evaluate muscle strength. Palpate pulses distal to the injury, noting their strength and quality. Perform the Ortolani and Barlow maneuvers (see the section on "Developmental Dysplasia of the Hip" later in this chapter) to assess for DDH.

TAKE NOTE!

Assess the injured site last and do so gently.

AUSCULTATION

Auscultate the child's lungs; adventitious sounds are often present when respiratory muscle function is impaired.

Laboratory and Diagnostic Testing

Common Laboratory and Diagnostic Tests 44.1 offers an explanation of the laboratory and diagnostic tests most commonly used in neuromuscular and musculoskeletal disorders. The tests can assist the primary provider or nurse practitioner in diagnosing the disorder and/or be used as guidelines in determining ongoing treatment. Laboratory or nonnursing personnel perform some of the tests, while the nurse might perform others. In either instance, the nurse should be familiar with how the tests are performed, what they are used for, and normal versus abnormal results. This knowledge will also be necessary when providing child and family education related to the testing.

Remember Frederick, the 4-year-old who has been falling and having difficulty climbing stairs and who seems to tire easily when playing with his sibling? What additional health history and physical examination assessment information should the nurse obtain?

COMMON LABORATORY AND DIAGNOSTIC TESTS 44.1

Test	Explanation	Indications	Nursing Implications
Radiographs (x-rays)	Radiographic image; usually, two views are obtained of the affected extremity (lateral and anteroposterior)	To detect fractures and other anomalies	Child must hold still. Enlist the family's help in calming the child. In the patient who has experienced trauma, the cervical spine should remain immobilized until cleared after cervical spine radiographs.
Fluoroscopy	Radiographic examination that uses continuous x-rays to show live, real-time images	Assessment of cervical spine instability during movement	Children may be afraid of the x-ray machine but will need to cooperate with flexion and extension of the neck. Allow a parent or family member to accompany the child.
Myelography	X-ray study of the spinal cord allowing visualization of the cord, nerve roots, and surrounding meninges	Detection of space-occupying lesions of the spinal cord; visualization of neural tube defects; evaluation of traumatic injury	Involves injection of contrast medium into the cerebrospinal fluid (CSF) via lumbar puncture. Postprocedure interventions vary based on the type of contrast medium; therefore, determine which one was used. After the procedure, bed rest is necessary for 4–24 hours; keep the head of the bed elevated for several hours. Encourage hydration. Observe for signs of meningeal irritation.
Ultrasound	Use of sound waves to locate the depth and structure within soft tissues and fluid	Assessment of spinal abnormalities; to diagnose Legg–Calvé–Perthes disease, slipped capital femoral epiphysis, fractures, ligament or soft tissue injuries Monitoring and follow-up of fractures and remodeling	Better tolerated than computed tomography (CT) or magnetic resonance imaging (MRI) by children who are not sedated Can be performed with a portable unit at the bedside

COMMON LABORATORY AND DIAGNOSTIC TESTS 44.1

Test	Explanation	Indications	Nursing Implications
CT	Noninvasive x-ray study that looks at tissue density and structures. Images a "slice" of tissue	Evaluation of congenital abnormalities such as neural tube defects, fractures, demyelinization, or inflammation; to evaluate the extent of Legg–Calvé–Perthes disease, or slipped capital femoral epiphysis, or to rule out other problems	Machine is large and can be frightening to children. Procedure can be lengthy, and the child must remain still. If unable to do so, sedation may be necessary. If performed with contrast medium, assess for allergy. Encourage fluids after the procedure if not contraindicated.
MRI	Based on how hydrogen atoms behave in a magnetic field when disturbed by radiofrequency signals. Does not require ionizing radiation. Provides a 3D view of the body part being scanned	Assessment of inflammation, congenital abnormalities such as neural tube defects; to assess hard and soft tissue, as well as bone marrow; to evaluate extent of Legg–Calvé–Perthes disease, or slipped capital femoral epiphysis; or to rule out other problems	Remove all metal objects from the child. Child must remain motionless for the entire scan; parent can stay in the room with the child. Younger children will require sedation in order to be still. A loud thumping sound occurs inside the machine during the procedure, which can be frightening to children. Most new surgical implants are now MRI compatible; consult the imaging center.
Creatine kinase	Reflects muscle damage: It leaks from muscle into plasma as muscles deteriorate.	Diagnosis of muscular dystrophy, spinal muscular atrophy	Draw a sample before an electromyogram or muscle biopsy, as those tests may lead to the release of creatine kinase.
Electromyography (EMG)	A recording electrode is placed in the skeletal muscle, and electrical activity is recorded.	Differentiates muscular disorders from those that are neurologic in origin	Requires insertion of short needles into the muscles. Sedation or analgesia may be ordered.
Nerve conduction velocity	Measures the speed of nerve conduction. Patchlike electrodes are attached to the skin at various nerve locations.	Differentiation of muscular disorders	Feels like mild electric shocks EMG often performed at the same time
Muscle biopsy	Removal of a piece of muscular tissue either by needle or by open biopsy	Determination of the type of muscular dystrophy or spinal muscular atrophy	Postbiopsy care is similar to that for other types of biopsies. Involves a small incision with one or two sutures
Complete blood count	Evaluates hemoglobin and hematocrit, white blood cell count, platelet count	To evaluate hemoglobin and hematocrit with a fracture with potential bleeding. To determine toxic synovitis	Normal values vary according to age and sex. White blood cell count differential is helpful in evaluating for infection. May be affected by myelosuppressive drugs
Arthrography	Multiple radiographic images of a joint after direct injection with a radiopaque substance	To assess ligaments, muscles, tendons, and cartilage, particularly after injury	Should not be performed if joint infection is present. The joint should be rested for 12 hours. Apply cold therapy afterward and assess for swelling and pain. Crepitus may be present in the joint for 1–2 days after the procedure.
Genetic testing	Tests for the presence of the gene for the disease or for carrier status	Determination of disease or carrier status of inherited muscular disorder	Entire family should be tested, even those unaffected, because carrier status should be determined, and genetic counseling related to reproduction provided.

Data from Fischbach, F. T., Fischbach, M. A., & Stout, K. (2022). *A manual of laboratory and diagnostic tests* (11th ed.). Wolters Kluwer.

Nursing Analysis

After recognizing and analyzing cues from a thorough assessment, the nurse might identify several patient problems, including:

- Pain
- Impaired physical mobility
- Malnutrition risk
- Urinary retention
- Constipation risk
- Activities of daily living (ADLs) deficit (specify)
- Altered skin integrity risk
- Chronic sorrow
- Injury risk
- Knowledge deficiency (specify)
- Delayed development risk
- Family processes, interrupted

After completing an assessment of Frederick, the nurse noted the following: He started walking at 2 years of age, he has difficulty jumping, his gait has a waddling appearance, and he does not rise from the floor in the usual fashion. Based on these assessment findings, what would your top three patient problems be for Frederick?

These patient problems or concerns provide suggestions for developing a nursing plan of care or concept map. The nurse will then generate solutions by planning interventions (suggested below with rationales). The plan of care should be individualized, based on the child's and family's needs. Refer to Chapter 36 for the nursing process for pain management and to Chapter 33 for nursing interventions related to interrupted family processes and risk for caregiver role strain. Additional information will be included later in the chapter as it relates to specific disorders.

Nursing Analysis

Impaired physical mobility related to a decrease in muscle control, mass, and/or strength; pain; joint stiffness; contractures; musculoskeletal or neuromuscular impairment as evidenced by an inability to move extremities, to ambulate without assistance, to move without limitations

Goal/Outcome

Child will be able to engage in activities within age parameters and limits of injury or disease: The child is able to move extremities, move about the environment, assist with transfers and positioning in bed, and/or participate in exercise programs within limits of age and disease.

Maximizing Physical Mobility (interventions with *rationale*)

- Assess the child's ability to move based on injury or disease and within limits of prescribed treatment *to determine baseline.*
- Prior to prescribed exercise or major position changes, ensure that pain medication is given; *relief of pain increases the child's ability to tolerate and participate in activity.*
- Encourage gross and fine motor activities *to facilitate motor development.*
- Collaborate with physical therapy, occupational therapy, and speech therapy to strengthen muscles and promote optimal mobility. Support therapy activities by using the same equipment and technique *to help rehabilitate musculoskeletal deficits, improve mobility, facilitate motor development, and allow for maximum functioning.*
- Use passive and active ROM exercises and teach the child and family how to perform them *to prevent contractures, facilitate joint mobility and muscle development (active ROM), and help increase mobility.*
- Praise accomplishments and emphasize the child's abilities *to improve self-esteem and encourage feelings of confidence and competence.*
- Teach child and family necessary care related to mobility issues *so the family can continue with these measures at home.*

Nursing Analysis

Malnutrition risk related to insufficient dietary intake (difficulty feeding secondary to deficient sucking, swallowing, or chewing; difficulty assuming normal feeding position; inability to feed self) as evidenced by decreased oral intake, impaired swallowing, weight loss, or plateau

Goal/Outcome

Child will exhibit signs of adequate nutrition as evidenced by appropriate weight gain, intake and output within normal limits, and adequate ingestion of calories.

Promoting Adequate Nutrition (interventions with *rationale*)

- Monitor height and weight: *insufficient intake will lead to impaired growth and weight gain.*
- Monitor hydration status (moist mucous membranes, elastic skin turgor, adequate urine output): *insufficient intake can lead to dehydration.*
- Use techniques to promote caloric and nutritional intake and teach family about these techniques (e.g., positioning, modified utensils, soft or blended foods, allowing extra time) *to facilitate intake.*
- Assess the respiratory system frequently *to assess for aspiration.*
- Assist family to help child assume as normal a feeding position as possible *to help increase oral intake.*

Nursing Analysis

Urinary retention related to sensory motor impairment as evidenced by dribbling, inadequate bladder emptying

Goal/Outcome

Child's bladder will empty adequately, according to preestablished quantities and frequencies individualized for the child (usual urine output is 0.5 to 2 mL/kg/h).

Promoting Successful Bladder Emptying (interventions with *rationale*)

- Assess the child's ability to empty the bladder via history focused on character and duration of lower urinary symptoms *to establish a baseline.*
- Assess for history of fecal impaction or constipation, *as alterations in bowel elimination may hinder urinary elimination.*
- Assess for bladder distention by palpation or urinary retention by postvoid residual obtained via catheterization or bladder ultrasound *to determine the extent of retention.*
- Maintain adequate hydration *to avoid irritating effects that dehydration has on the bladder.*
- Schedule voiding *to decrease bladder overdistention.*
- Teach the family (and the child if old enough) with significant urinary retention the technique of clean intermittent catheterization *to allow regular, complete bladder emptying.*

Nursing Analysis

Constipation risk (risk factors: average daily physical activity is less than recommended for sex and age, decreased gastrointestinal motility [immobility, loss of sensation, and/or use of narcotic analgesics].)

Goal/Outcome

Child will demonstrate adequate stool passage: will pass soft, formed stool every 1 to 3 days without straining or other adverse effects.

Promoting Appropriate Bowel Elimination (interventions with *rationale*)

- Assess the usual pattern of stooling *to determine baseline and identify potential problems with elimination.*
- Palpate for abdominal fullness and auscultate for bowel sounds *to assess for bowel function and presence of constipation.*
- Encourage fiber intake *to increase the frequency of stools.*
- Ensure adequate fluid intake *to prevent the formation of hard, dry stools.*
- Encourage activity within child's limits or restrictions: *even minimal activity increases peristalsis.*
- Administer medications or enemas as ordered *to promote bowel training/evacuation (especially in the child with myelomeningocele or spinal cord injury).*

Nursing Analysis

ADLs; bathing; dressing; feeding; deficit related to muscular, skeletal, and/or neuromuscular impairments; alteration in cognitive functioning; weakness; pain; and fatigue, as evidenced by an inability to perform hygiene care and transfer oneself independently.

Goal/Outcome

Child will demonstrate the ability to care for self within age parameters and limits of injury or disease: The child is able to feed, dress, and manage elimination within limits of injury, disease, and age.

Maximizing Self-Care (interventions with *rationale*)

- Introduce child and family to self-help methods as soon as possible *to promote independence from the beginning.*
- Encourage family and staff to allow the child to do as much as possible *to allow the child to gain confidence and independence.*
- Teach specific measures for bowel and urinary elimination as needed *to promote independence and increase self-care abilities and self-esteem.*
- Collaborate with physical therapy, occupational therapy, and speech therapy to provide the child and family with appropriate tools to modify the environment and methods to promote transferring and self-care *to allow for maximum functioning.*
- Praise accomplishments and emphasize the child's abilities *to improve self-esteem and encourage feelings of confidence and competence.*
- Balance activity with periods of rest *to reduce fatigue and increase energy for self-care.*

Nursing Analysis

Altered skin integrity risk (risk factors: pressure over bony prominences, alteration in sensation, impaired circulation [immobility, casting, traction, and use of braces or adaptive devices])

Goal/Outcome

Child's skin will remain intact, without evidence of redness or breakdown.

Promoting Skin Integrity (interventions with *rationale*)

- Monitor the condition of entire skin surface at least daily *to provide a baseline and allow for early identification of areas at risk.*
- Avoid excessive friction or harsh cleaning products *that may increase the risk of breakdown in child with susceptible skin.*
- Keep child's skin free from stool and urine *to decrease the risk of breakdown.*
- Keep linen clean, dry, and free from food crumbs and wrinkles *to prevent pressure areas from forming.*
- Change child's position frequently *to decrease pressure to susceptible areas.*

- Monitor skin condition affected by braces or adaptive equipment frequently *to prevent skin breakdown related to poor fit.*

For the child in traction:

- Pad bony prominences with cotton padding before applying traction *to protect skin from injury.*
- Gently massage child's back and sacrum with lotion *to stimulate circulation.*

For the child in a spica cast:

- Apply plastic wrap to the perineal edges of the cast *to prevent soiling of cast edges, which can contribute to cast breakdown.*
- Use a fracture bedpan *to facilitate toileting without a soiling cast.*
- For the child still in diapers, tuck a smaller diaper under the perineal edges of cast and cover with a larger diaper *to prevent cast soiling.*

Nursing Analysis

Chronic sorrow related to the presence of chronic disability, missed milestones, and missed opportunities as evidenced by child's or family's expression of sadness, anger, disappointment, or feeling overwhelmed

Goal/Outcome

Child and/or family will accept the situation: The child and/or family will appropriately identify feelings, function at a normal developmental level, and plan for the future.

Easing Sorrow (interventions with *rationale*)

- Assess the degree of sorrow *to provide a baseline for intervention.*
- Identify problems with eating or sleeping, *often affected when grief or sorrow is present.*
- Spend time with the child and family: *an empathetic presence is valued by suffering families.*
- Encourage the use of positive coping techniques: *taking action, expressing feelings, and intentional attempts at coping are helpful techniques.*
- Refer to appropriate support groups: *can be helpful to talk to others in similar situations.*
- Refer for spiritual counseling as desired: *many families experience grief resolution in a timelier fashion if spiritual needs are addressed.*

Nursing Analysis

Injury risk (risk factors: unsafe mode of transport [muscle weakness])

Goal/Outcome

Child will remain free from injury: The child will not fall or experience other injuries.

Preventing Injury (interventions with *rationale*)

- Ensure that the side rails of the bed are elevated when the caregiver is not directly at bedside *to prevent fall from the bed.*
- Use appropriate safety restraints with adaptive equipment and wheelchairs *to prevent fall or slipping from equipment.*
- Do not leave the child unattended in a tub *as weakness may cause the child to slip under the water.*
- Avoid restraint use if at all possible. Close observation is more appropriate. *It is in the best interest of the child to use the least restrictive measure while maintaining the child's safety.*

Nursing Analysis

Knowledge deficiency related to insufficient information (regarding cast care, activity restrictions, complex medical condition, prognosis, and medical needs) as evidenced by verbalization, questions, or actions demonstrating a lack of understanding regarding child's condition or care

Goal/Outcome

Child and family will verbalize accurate information and understanding about the condition, prognosis, and medical needs: The child and family demonstrate knowledge of the condition, prognosis, and medical needs, including possible causes, contributing factors, and treatment measures through verbalization and return demonstration.

Providing Child and Family Teaching (interventions with *rationale*)

- Assess child's and family's willingness to learn: *child and family must be willing to learn for teaching to be effective.*
- Provide family with time to adjust to diagnosis *to facilitate adjustment and ability to learn and participate in child's care.*
- Repeat information *to allow family and child time to learn and understand.*
- Teach in short sessions: *many short sessions are more helpful than one long session.*
- Gear teaching to the level of understanding of the child and family (depends on the age of the child, physical condition, and memory) *to ensure understanding.*
- Provide reinforcement and rewards *to facilitate the teaching and learning process.*
- Use multiple modes of learning involving many senses (provide written, verbal, demonstration, and videos) when possible: *child and family are more likely to retain information when it is presented in different ways using many senses.*

Nursing Analysis

Delayed development risk (risk factors: treatment regimen, chronic illness [immobility, alterations in extremities])

Goal/Outcome

Development will be enhanced: The child will make continued progress toward developmental milestones and will not show regression in abilities.

Promoting Development (interventions with *rationale*)

- Screen for developmental capabilities *to determine the child's current level of functioning.*
- Offer age-appropriate toys, play, and activities (including gross motor) *to encourage further development.*
- Perform exercises or interventions as prescribed by physical or occupational therapist: *repeat participation in those activities helps to promote function and acquisition of developmental skills.*
- Provide support to child and families: *immobility and extremity deficits may lead to slow progress in achieving developmental milestones, so ongoing motivation is needed.*

Assisting With Cast Application

Before cast or splint application, perform baseline neurovascular assessment for comparison after immobilization. Include:

- Color (note cyanosis or other discoloration)
- Movement (note inability to move fingers or toes)
- Sensation (note whether loss of sensation is present)
- Edema
- Quality of pulses

Enlist the cooperation of the child and reduce their fear by showing the child the cast materials and using an age-appropriate approach to describe the cast application. Premedicate as ordered to reduce pain when manual traction is applied to align the bone. Use distraction throughout the cast application and assist with the application of the cast or splint (Fig. 44.8).

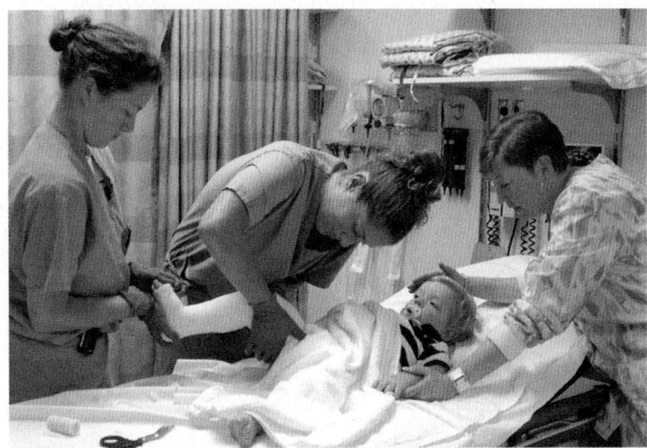

FIGURE 44.8 Assist with cast application by distracting or comforting the child.

TAKE NOTE!

Modern fiberglass cast materials are available in a variety of colors, as well as a few patterns. Allowing the child to choose the color will increase the child's cooperation with the procedure.

After the cast or splint is applied, drying time will vary based on the type of material used. Splints and fiberglass casts usually take only a few minutes to dry and will cause a very warm feeling inside the cast, so warn the child that it will begin to feel warm. Plaster requires 24 to 48 hours to dry. Take care not to cause depressions in the plaster cast while drying, as those may cause skin pressure and breakdown. Instruct the child and family to keep the cast still, positioning it with pillows as needed.

Caring for the Child With a Cast

Perform frequent neurovascular checks of the casted extremity to identify signs of compromise early. These signs include:

- Increased pain
- Increased edema
- Pale or blue color
- Skin coolness
- Numbness or tingling
- Prolonged capillary refill
- Decreased pulse strength (or absence of pulse)

Notify the primary provider or nurse practitioner of changes in neurovascular status or odor or drainage from the cast.

Fiberglass casts usually have a soft fabric edge, so they usually do not cause skin rubbing at the edges of the cast. On the other hand, plaster casts require special treatment of the cast edge to prevent skin rubbing. This may be accomplished through a technique called petaling: Cut rounded-edge strips of moleskin or another soft material with an adhesive backing and apply them to the edge of cast, as shown in Figure 44.9.

TAKE NOTE!

If a cast is lined with Gore-Tex, do not petal it.

Position the child with the casted extremity elevated on pillows. Ice may be applied during the first 24 to 48 hours after casting if needed. Teaching the child to use crutches is an important nursing intervention for

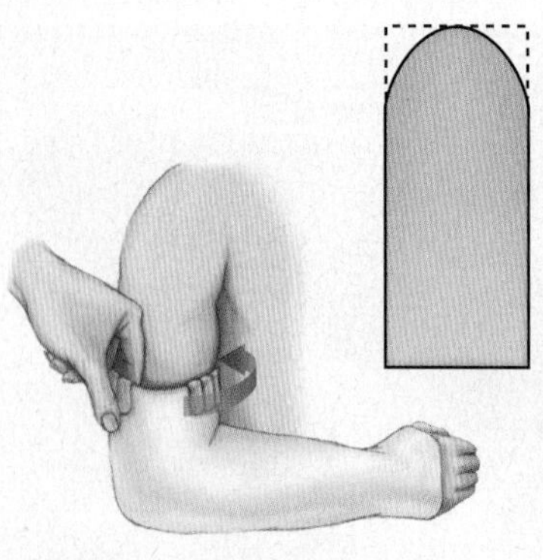

To petal a cast:

1. Cut several strips of adhesive tape or Moleskin 3 to 4 in in length. Use 1-in tape for smaller areas (e.g., infant's foot) and 2-in tape for larger areas (e.g., adolescent's waist).
2. Round one end of each strip to keep the corners from rolling.
3. Apply the first strip by tucking the straight end inside the cast and by bringing the rounded end over the cast edge to the outside.
4. Repeat the procedure, overlapping each additional strip, until all rough edges are completely covered.

FIGURE 44.9 Petaling the cast.

any child with lower extremity immobilization so that the child can maintain mobility (Fig. 44.10). Provide home care instructions to the family about cast care (see Teaching Guidelines 44.1).

CLINICAL REASONING ALERT!

Persistent complaints of pain may indicate compromised skin integrity under the cast.

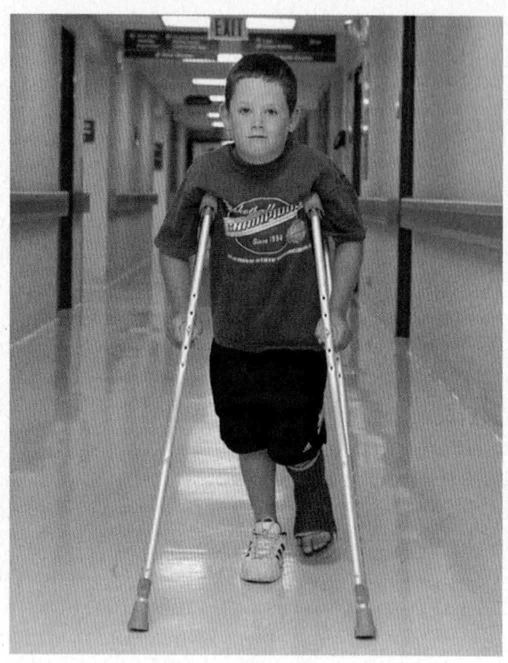

FIGURE 44.10 Reinforce appropriate crutch walking for children with lower extremity immobilization.

TEACHING GUIDELINES 44.1 Home Cast Care

- For the first 48 hours, elevate the extremity above the level of the heart and apply cold therapy for 20 minutes, then off for 2 hours, and repeat while awake.
- Take your prescribed pain medication for at least the first 48 hours.
- Assess for swelling, and have the child wiggle the fingers or toes frequently (hourly while awake).
- For itching inside the cast:
  - Never insert anything into the cast for the purposes of scratching.
  - Blow cool air in from a hair dryer set on the lowest setting or tap lightly on the cast.
  - Do not use lotions or powders.
- Do not pull padding out from the inside of the cast.
- Protect the cast from wetness.
  - Apply two plastic bags around the cast and tape each bag separately and securely for bathing or showering. Continue to avoid placing the cast directly in water (unless it is Gore-Tex lined).
  - Waterproof cast covers are available through medical supply stores (still remain cautious about submerging cast in water).
  - Cover it when your child eats or drinks.
  - If a cast becomes soiled, it can be wiped clean with a slightly damp clean cloth.
  - If the cast gets wet, dry it with a blow dryer on the cold setting (if a warm setting is used, the child could get burned). Use of a vacuum cleaner with a hose attachment to pull air through may speed drying; be careful to avoid the skin.
- If the child has a large cast, change position every 2 hours during the day, and while sleeping change position as often as possible.
- Check the skin for irritation.
  - Press the skin back around the edges of the cast.
  - Use a flashlight to look for reddened or irritated areas.
  - Feel for blisters or sores.
- Call the primary provider or nurse practitioner if:
  - The casted extremity is cool to the touch, pale, blue, or very swollen.
  - The child cannot move the fingers or toes.
  - Severe pain occurs when the child attempts to move the fingers or toes.
  - Persistent numbness or tingling occurs.
  - Drainage or a foul smell comes from under the cast.
  - Severe itching occurs inside the cast.
  - The child runs a fever greater than 101.5°F for longer than 24 hours.
  - Skin edges are red and swollen or exhibit breakdown.
  - Child complains of rubbing or burning under cast.
  - The cast gets wet and does not dry or is cracked, split, or softened.

Data from Schweich, P. (2021). Patient education: Cast and splint care (Beyond the Basics). *UpToDate*. Retrieved May 11, 2023, from https://www.uptodate.com/contents/cast-and-splint-care-beyond-the-basics

Assisting With Cast Removal

Children may be frightened by cast removal. Prepare the child using age-appropriate terminology:

- The cast cutter will make a loud noise (Fig. 44.11).
- The skin or extremity will not be injured (demonstrate by touching the cast cutter lightly to your palm).
- The child will feel warmth or vibration during cast removal.

Teaching Guidelines 44.2 gives instructions related to skin care after cast removal.

Caring for the Child in Traction

Nursing care of the child in any type of traction focuses not only on appropriate application and maintenance of traction but also on promoting normal growth and development and preventing complications (Table 44.1). Apply skin traction over intact skin only so that the pull of the traction is effective. Prepare the skin with

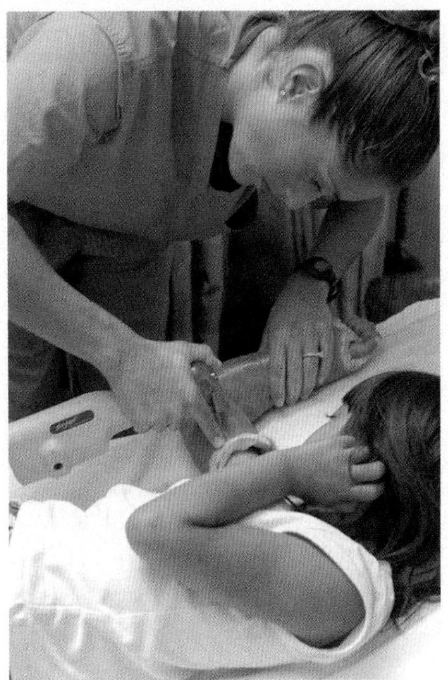

FIGURE 44.11 The loud noise of the cast saw may frighten the child.

TEACHING GUIDELINES 44.2 Skin Care After Cast Removal

- Brown, flaky skin is normal and occurs as dead skin and secretions accumulate under the cast.
- New skin may be tender.
- Soak with warm water daily.
- Wash with warm soapy water, avoiding excessive rubbing, which may traumatize the skin.
- Discourage the child from scratching the dry skin.
- Apply moisturizing lotion to relieve dry skin.
- Encourage activity to regain strength and motion of the extremity.

TABLE 44.1 • Types of Traction and Nursing Implications

Type of Traction	Description	Nursing Implications
Bryant traction 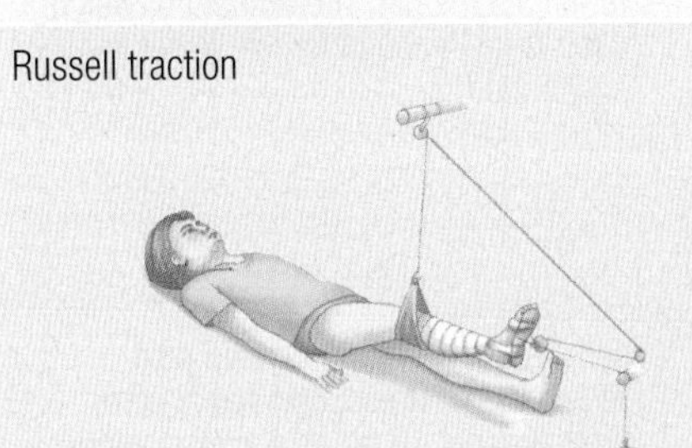	Both legs are extended vertically, with child's weight serving as countertraction. Skin traction is applied to both legs. Used to reduce femur fracture in children younger than 2 years or with developmental dysplasia of the hip.	Maintain appropriate position. Ensure heels and ankles are free from pressure. Assess condition and position of elastic bandages every shift and rewrap elastic bandages as ordered.
Russell traction	Skin traction for femur fracture, hip, and specific types of knee injuries or contractures. Uses a knee sling. In split Russell traction, a portion of the traction weight may be redistributed via a pulley from the sling to the head of the bed (used for femur fracture, Legg–Calvé–Perthes disease, slipped capital femoral epiphysis).	Wrap bandages from ankle to thigh on children younger than age 2 years, from ankle to knee on children older than 2 years. Use a foot support to prevent foot drop. Ensure heel is free from bed. Assess popliteal region for skin breakdown from the sling. Mark leg to ensure proper replacement of sling.

(*continued*)

TABLE 44.1 • Types of Traction and Nursing Implications (*continued*)

Type of Traction	Description	Nursing Implications
Buck traction	Skin traction for hip and knee contractures, Legg–Calvé–Perthes disease, slipped capital femoral epiphysis. Used to rest an injured limb or to prevent spasms of injured muscles or joints Traction force delivered in straight line	Remove traction boot every 8 hours to assess skin. Leg may be slightly abducted.
Cervical skin traction	Skin traction applied with a skin strap (head halter). Used for neck sprains/strains, torticollis, or nerve trauma	Ensure that head halter or skin strap does not place pressure on ears or throat. Limit of 5–7 lb of weight
Side-arm 90–90	Skin traction used to treat fractures of the humerus and injuries in or around the shoulder girdle	Maintain elbow flexed at 90 degrees. Fingers and hand may feel cool because of elevation. Child may turn to affected side only.
Dunlop side-arm 00–90 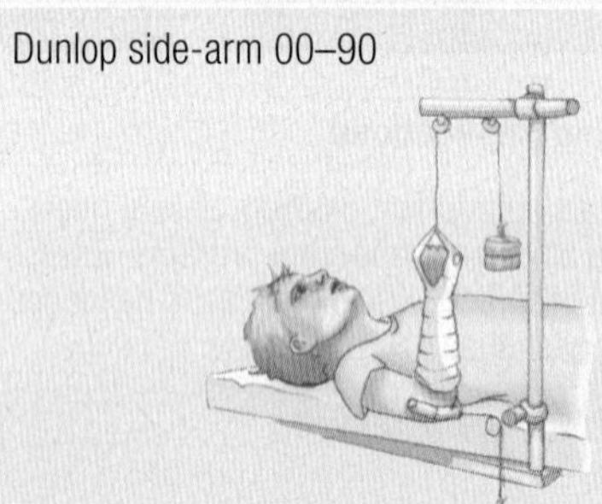	Skeletal traction through an olecranon screw or pin in distal humerus. Lower arm is held in balanced suspension.	See side-arm 90–90. In addition, provide appropriate pin site care.
Knee 90–90 traction 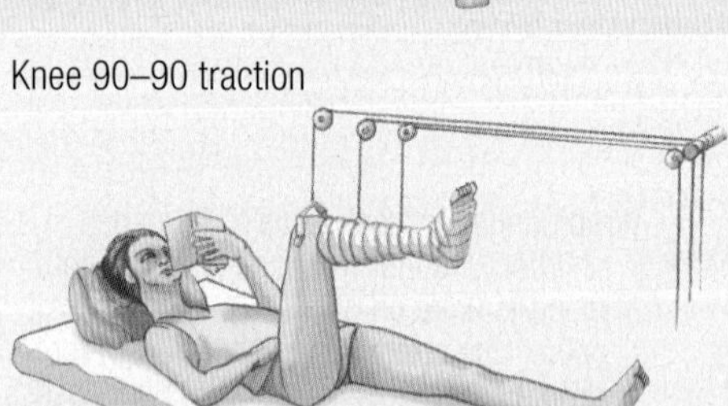 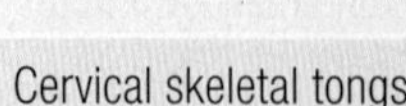	For femur fracture reduction when skin traction is inadequate. Skeletal traction with force applied through pin in distal femur	A foam boot may be used for suspension of the lower leg. Force of traction applied to femur via the pin. The amount of weight used is just enough to hold lower limb suspended.
Cervical skeletal tongs 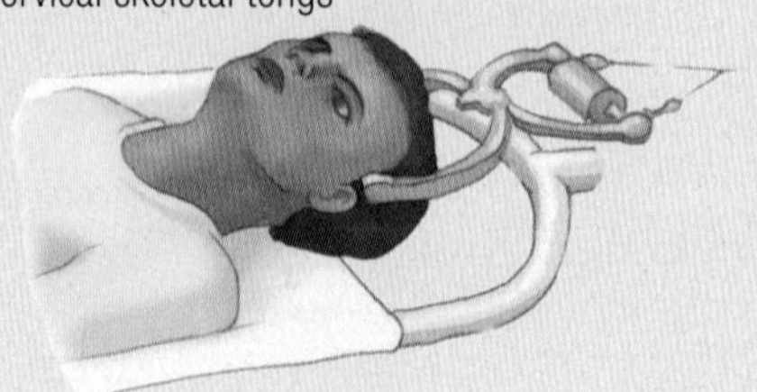	Tongs attached to skull via pins. Used with fractures or dislocations of the cervical or high thoracic vertebrae	Assess frequently for increased pain, respiratory distress, and spinal cord, cranial nerve, or brachial plexus injury. Place on Stryker frame or specially equipped bed to ease positioning without disruption of alignment.

TABLE 44.1 • Types of Traction and Nursing Implications

Type of Traction	Description	Nursing Implications
Halo traction	Metal halo attached to skull via pins. Used for cervical or high thoracic vertebrae fracture or dislocation and for postoperative immobilization following cervical fusion	Refer to nursing implications for cervical tongs. Tape small wrench to front of brace so that front panel can be quickly removed in an emergency. May become ambulatory in this type of traction; will be top-heavy so may need assistance with balance Assess pin sites and provide pin care as ordered.
Balanced suspension traction	Used for femur, hip, or tibial fracture. Thomas splint suspends the thigh while the Pearson attachment allows knee flexion and supports the leg below the knee.	Avoid pressure to popliteal area.

an appropriate adhesive before applying the traction tapes to ensure that the tapes adhere well, preventing skin friction. After application of the traction tapes, apply the elastic bandage or use the foam boot. Attach the traction spreader block and then apply the prescribed amount of weight via a rope attached to the spreader block. Ensure that the rope moves without obstruction and that the weights hang freely without touching the floor.

In skeletal traction, apply weight via ropes attached to the skeletal pins. Treat the pin sites as surgical wounds (see section on "Providing pin care"). Protect the exposed ends of the pins to avoid injury. Whether skin or skeletal traction is used, be sure that constant and even traction is maintained.

TAKE NOTE!

Avoid sudden bumping or movement of the bed. This can disturb traction alignment and cause additional pain to the child as the weights are jostled.

Preventing Complications

Refer to the "Clinical Judgment and the Nursing Process" section in Chapter 36 for interventions related to pain management, and refer to earlier discussions in this chapter for interventions related to the prevention of complications of immobility such as skin integrity impairment. To prevent **contractures** (the shortening and hardening of muscles, tendons, or tissues leading to fixated and stiff joints) and atrophy that may result from the disuse of muscles, ensure that unaffected extremities are exercised. Assist the child to exercise the unaffected joints and to use the unaffected extremity if this does not disrupt traction alignment. Promote the use of a trapeze if not contraindicated to involve the child in repositioning and assist with movement. Encourage deep-breathing exercises to prevent the pulmonary complications of long-term immobilization.

Promote normal growth and development by:

- Placing age-appropriate toys within the child's reach
- Encouraging visits from friends
- Providing diversional activities such as drawing, coloring, or video games (Fig. 44.12)

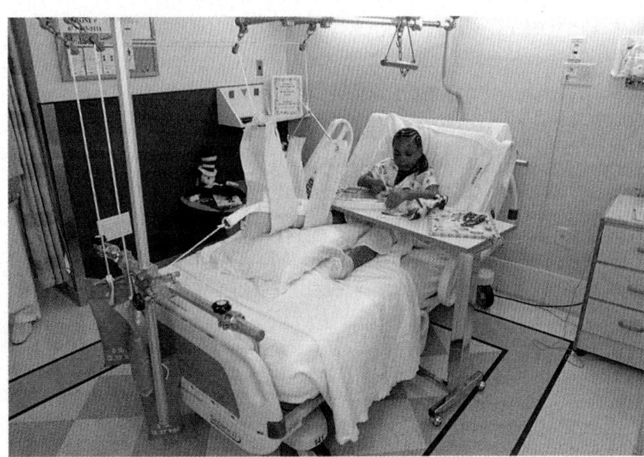

FIGURE 44.12 Provide age-appropriate diversional activities and school work for children confined to bed in traction.

CLINICAL REASONING ALERT!

Ongoing, careful neurovascular assessments are critical in the child with a cast or in skeletal traction. Notify the primary provider or nurse practitioner immediately if these signs of compartment syndrome occur: extreme pain (out of proportion to the situation), pain with passive ROM of digits, distal extremity pallor, inability to move digits, or loss of pulses.

Caring for the Child With an External Fixator

Care of an external fixator involves maintaining skin integrity, preventing infection, and preventing injury. Routine neurovascular and skin assessment is essential. Skin care is similar to a child in skeletal traction and includes pin care daily. Elevation of the extremity can help prevent swelling. The fixator may be moved by grasping the frame, as the fixator can tolerate ordinary movement. Encourage weight bearing as prescribed. Provide appropriate education to the child and family. Encourage the child to look at the apparatus. Teach the child not to pick or manipulate the pins. Baggy or loose clothing can be worn over the device. Velcro sewn into the seams can be helpful and allows clothes to slip over the device.

Providing Pin Care

Whether pins are inserted for skeletal traction or as part of an external fixator (see section titled "Fracture"), keeping the pin sites clean is important to prevent infection. Cleaning of the pin sites prevents infection by promoting comfort and preventing healing skin from adhering to the metal pin. Notify the orthopedic surgeon if signs of pin site infection are present or if pin slippage occurs.

Thus far, there is insufficient evidence to support a particular strategy of pin care, and more randomized trials are needed (Iobst, 2017; Shields et al., 2022). The National Association of Orthopaedic Nurses has published minimal guidelines, which include:

- Perform pin care weekly after the first 48 to 72 hours. Perform earlier if a large amount of drainage is present, dressing becomes wet, or infection is suspected.
- The most effective solution for pin site care may be chlorhexidine 2 mg/mL in alcohol. If the child has a sensitivity to this, use normal saline.
- Use a nonshedding material for cleaning.
- Cover pin sites with a nonshedding dressing.
- Teach children and their families pin site care along with instructions on the signs and symptoms of infection before discharge (Holmes et al., 2005; Walker, 2018).

Since the research available is minimal, these recommendations are made tentatively (Holmes et al., 2005). Therefore, interventions for pin care need to be individualized based on the child's condition and response to treatment and according to institutional policy or the primary provider's or nurse practitioner's orders. Certain primary providers or nurse practitioners prefer the site to be cleaned with normal saline; others choose a solution with antibacterial properties. Some institutions recommend the removal of all crusts formed on the skin around the pin; others do not. The rationale for crust removal is to promote free drainage and prevent the surrounding skin from adhering to the pin. A keyhole dressing may be necessary around the pin if drainage is present. No matter which procedure is ordered or preferred, perform pin care as necessary to prevent infection at the pin site. The Ilizarov fixator uses wires that are thinner than ordinary pins, so simply cleansing by showering is usually sufficient to keep the pin site clean. If drainage is present, cleanse the skin around the wires with a dry gauze pad.

TAKE NOTE!

When caring for children in the hospital, particularly those with complex medical needs, follow their home care routines as much as possible.

Based on your top three patient problems for Frederick, describe appropriate nursing interventions.

CONGENITAL AND DEVELOPMENTAL DISORDERS

Several disorders with neuromuscular and musculoskeletal effects are congenital in nature. These include neural tube defects and genetic neuromuscular disorders. The structural disorders are spina bifida occulta, meningocele, and myelomeningocele (neural tube defects). Congenital anomalies of the musculoskeletal system are usually readily identified at birth. Congenital structural anomalies involving the skeleton include pectus excavatum, pectus carinatum, limb deficiencies, polydactyly or syndactyly, metatarsus adductus, congenital clubfoot, and osteogenesis imperfecta (OI). A developmental anomaly that may be diagnosed at birth or later in life is DDH. A muscular condition, torticollis, most often presents as a congenital condition but may also develop after birth. Tibia vara is a developmental disorder affecting young children. Rarely, a developmental positional alteration such as genu varum, genu valgum, or pes planus will persist past the usual age of resolution or cause the child pain. If those situations occur, bracing, orthotics, or surgical correction may become necessary. The genetic neuromuscular disorders include various types of muscular dystrophy and spinal muscular atrophy (SMA). These disorders are not always recognized at birth because signs and symptoms are not evident until months or even years after birth. However, they are still considered to be congenital as they have a genetic basis.

NEURAL TUBE DEFECTS

Neural tube defects account for the majority of congenital anomalies of the central nervous system. The neural tube closes between the third and fourth week of gestation. The cause of neural tube defects is not known, but many factors, such as drugs, malnutrition, chemicals, and genetics, can hinder normal central nervous system development. It is well established that maternal preconception supplementation of folic acid can decrease the incidence of neural tube defects in pregnancies by 50% or more (American Academy of Pediatrics [AAP] & Committee on Genetics, 1999 [reaffirmed 2017]; Kinsman & Johnston, 2020). Beginning in 1992 and continuing until today, the U.S. Public Health Service along with the Centers for Disease Control and Prevention (CDC) recommends that anyone of childbearing age who is capable of becoming pregnant takes 0.4 mg (400 mcg) of folic acid daily (CDC, 2022a). Pregnant people who had a previous child with a neural tube defect are recommended to take a higher dosage and should consult with their primary provider or nurse practitioner (AAP & Committee on Genetics, 1999 [reaffirmed 2017]). Prenatal screening of maternal serum for alpha-fetoprotein (AFP) and ultrasound examination can help identify fetuses at risk. Neural tube defects primarily affecting spinal cord development include spina bifida occulta, meningocele, and myelomeningocele (Fig. 44.13). Neural tube defects primarily affecting brain development are discussed in Chapter 38.

Spina Bifida Occulta

Spina bifida is a term that is often used to refer to all neural tube disorders that affect the spinal cord. This can be confusing and a cause of concern for parents. There are well-defined degrees of spinal cord involvement, and it is important for health care professionals to use the correct terminology.

Spina bifida occulta is a defect of the vertebral bodies without protrusion of the spinal cord or meninges. This defect is not visible externally and, in most cases, has no adverse effects (see Fig. 44.13). Children with spina bifida occulta need no immediate medical intervention. Complications are rare but may include more significant abnormalities of the spinal cord such as tethered cord, syringomyelia, or diastematomyelia.

Nursing Assessment

In most cases, spina bifida occulta is benign and without symptoms and produces no neurologic signs. The defect, which is usually present in the lumbosacral area, often goes undetected. However, there may be noticeable dimpling, abnormal patches of hair, or discoloration of skin at the defect site. If so, further investigation, including magnetic resonance imaging (MRI), may be warranted.

Nursing Management

Nursing care will focus on educating the family. Inform parents of its presence and what the diagnosis means. Many times, parents will confuse this diagnosis with spina bifida cystica, a much more serious defect. Occasionally, children with spina bifida occulta eventually need surgical intervention due to degenerative changes or involvement of the spine and nerve roots, resulting in complications such as tethered cord, syringomyelia, or diastematomyelia. When these associated problems occur, the condition is often termed "occult spinal dysraphism" to avoid confusion.

Meningocele

Meningocele, the less serious form of spina bifida cystica, occurs when the meninges herniate through a defect in the vertebrae. The spinal cord is usually normal,

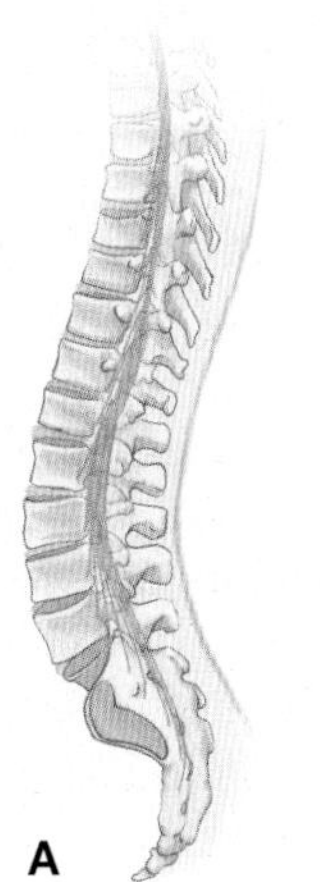

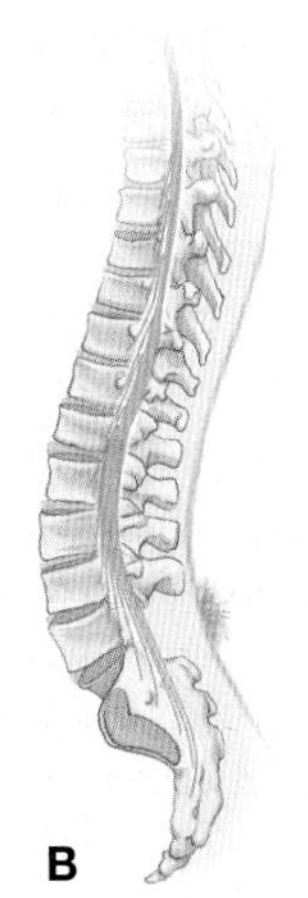

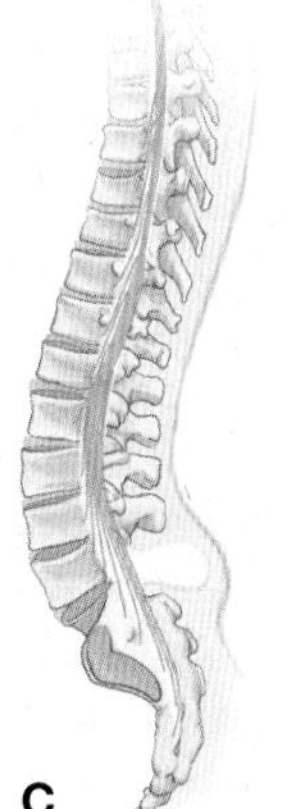

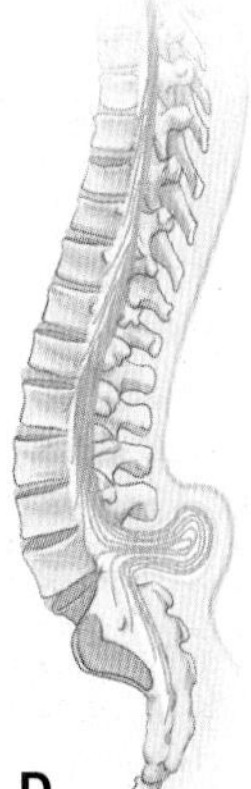

FIGURE 44.13 **A.** Normal spine. **B.** Spina bifida occulta. **C.** Meningocele. **D.** Myelomeningocele.

and there are typically minor or no associated neurologic deficits. Treatment for meningocele involves surgical correction of the lesion (see Fig. 44.13).

Nursing Assessment

Initial assessment after delivery will reveal a visible external sac protruding from the spinal area. It is most often seen in the lumbar region but can be anywhere along the spinal canal. Most are covered with skin and pose no threat to the child. However, assessment to ensure that the sac covering is intact remains important. Assess neurologic status carefully. Before surgical correction, the infant will be thoroughly examined to determine whether there is any neural involvement or associated anomalies. Diagnostic procedures such as computed tomography (CT), MRI, and ultrasound may be performed.

Nursing Management

Surgical correction may be delayed if the skin covering the sac is intact and the child has normal neurologic functioning (Kinsman & Johnston, 2020). However, as in a child with myelomeningocele, immediately report any evidence of leaking cerebrospinal fluid (CSF) to ensure prompt intervention to prevent infection. A child with leaking CSF or a thin skin covering will require immediate surgical correction (Kinsman & Johnston, 2020). Nursing management will be supportive. Provide pre- and postoperative care similar to the child with myelomeningocele to prevent rupture of the sac, to prevent infection, and to provide adequate nutrition and hydration. Monitor for symptoms of constipation or bladder dysfunction that may result due to the increasing size of the lesion. The resulting hydrocephalus has been associated with some cases of meningocele (Kinsman & Johnston, 2020). Therefore, monitor head circumference and watch for signs and symptoms of increased intracranial pressure (ICP).

Myelomeningocele

Myelomeningocele, the most severe form of neural tube defect, occurs in approximately 1 in 4,000 live births (Kinsman & Johnston, 2020). Myelomeningocele is a type of spina bifida cystica, and clinically the term "spina bifida" is often used to refer to myelomeningocele. It may be diagnosed in utero via ultrasound. Otherwise, it is visually obvious at birth. The newborn with myelomeningocele is at increased risk for meningitis, hypoxia, and hemorrhage.

In myelomeningocele, the spinal cord often ends at the point of the defect, resulting in absent motor and sensory function beyond that point (Fig. 44.14). Therefore, the long-term complications of paralysis, orthopedic deformities, and bladder and bowel incontinence are often seen in children with myelomeningocele. The presence of a neurogenic bladder and frequent catheterization put the child at an increased risk for urinary tract infections, pyelonephritis, and hydronephrosis, which may result in long-term renal damage if managed inappropriately. Accompanying hydrocephalus associated with type II Chiari defect is seen in 80% of children with myelomeningocele (Kinsman & Johnston, 2020). Due to the improper development and the downward displacement of the brain into the cervical spine, CSF flow is blocked, resulting in hydrocephalus. The lower the deformity is on the spine, the lower the risk of developing hydrocephalus (Kinsman & Johnston, 2020).

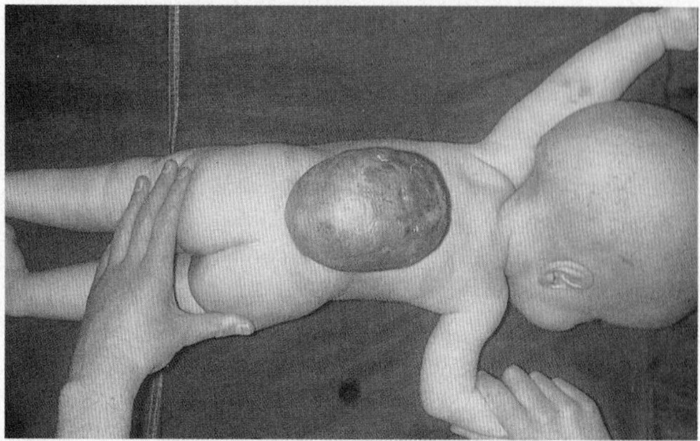

FIGURE 44.14 Usually a sac covers the deformity of myelomeningocele and is visible at birth.

Children with myelomeningocele usually require multiple surgical procedures. In addition, due to frequent catheterizations, these children are at an increased risk of developing a latex allergy (Kinsman & Johnston, 2020). Learning problems and seizures are common in these children, but the majority of those surviving with myelomeningocele have average intelligence (Kinsman & Johnston, 2020). Ambulation is possible for some children, depending on the level of the lesion.

Pathophysiology

The cause of myelomeningocele is unknown, but risk factors are consistent with other neural tube defects, such as maternal drug use, malnutrition, and a genetic predisposition (Kinsman & Johnston, 2016). In myelomeningocele, the neural tube fails to close at the end of the fourth week of gestation. As a result, an external saclike protrusion that encases the meninges, spinal fluid, and in some cases, nerves are present on the spine (see Fig. 44.13). A myelomeningocele can be located anywhere along the spinal cord, but the highest incidence occurs in the lumbosacral region (Kinsman & Johnston, 2020). The degree of neurologic deficit will depend on the location and size of the lesion (Kinsman & Johnston, 2020). An increase in neurologic deficit is seen with higher lesions as more nerves are affected.

Therapeutic Management

Surgical closure will be performed as soon as possible after birth, especially if a CSF leak is present or if there is a danger of the sac rupturing. The goal of early surgical intervention is to prevent infection and to minimize further loss of function, which can result from the stretching of nerve roots as the meningeal sac expands after birth. In-utero fetal surgery to repair the myelomeningocele has been successful, showing improved outcomes for the fetuses, such as improved psychomotor function and lower need for shunt placement, but is not without risks to the pregnant person and fetus (Bowman, 2022). Ongoing management of this disorder remains complex. A multidisciplinary approach is needed, involving specialists in neurology, neurosurgery, urology, orthopedics, therapy, and rehabilitation along with intense nursing care. The chronic nature of this disorder necessitates lifelong follow-up.

Nursing Assessment

For a full description of the assessment phase of the nursing process, refer to the "Clinical Judgment and the Nursing Process" section earlier in the chapter. Assessment findings pertinent to myelomeningocele are discussed below.

HEALTH HISTORY

High-risk deliveries should be identified. Explore the pregnancy history and past medical history for risk factors such as:

- Lack of prenatal care
- Lack of preconception and/or prenatal folic acid supplementation
- Previous child born with neural tube defect or family history of neural tube defects
- Maternal consumption of certain drugs that antagonize folic acid, such as anticonvulsants (carbamazepine and phenobarbital)

The older infant or child with a history of myelomeningocele requires numerous surgical procedures and lifelong follow-up. In an infant or child returning for a clinic visit or hospitalization, the health history should include questions related to:

- Current mobility status and any changes in motor abilities
- Genitourinary function and regimen
- Bowel function and regimen
- Signs or symptoms of urinary infections
- History of hydrocephalus with presence of shunt
- Signs or symptoms of shunt infection or malfunction (refer to the section on "Hydrocephalus" in Chapter 38)
- Latex sensitivity
- Nutritional status, including changes in weight
- Any other changes in physical or cognitive state
- Resources available and used by the family

PHYSICAL EXAMINATION

Initial assessment after delivery will reveal a visible external sac protruding from the spinal area (see Fig. 44.14). This will be repaired shortly after birth. Observe the baby's general appearance. Assess neurologic status and look for associated anomalies. Assess for movement of extremities and anal reflex, which will help determine the level of neurologic involvement. Flaccid paralysis, absence of deep tendon reflexes, lack of response to touch and pain stimuli, skeletal abnormalities such as club feet, constant dribbling of urine, and a relaxed anal sphincter may be found.

In the older infant or child, perform a thorough physical examination and focus on the functional assessment. Note the level of paralysis or paresthesia. Inspect the skin for breakdown. Determine the child's motor capabilities.

LABORATORY AND DIAGNOSTIC TESTS

A myelomeningocele may be detected prenatally around 16 to 18 weeks' gestation by ultrasound, by a blood test that detects AFP increases, or by analysis of amniotic fluid for AFP increases. Common laboratory and diagnostic studies ordered for the assessment of myelomeningocele include:

- MRI
- CT
- Ultrasound
- Myelography

These diagnostic tests are used to evaluate brain and spinal cord involvement (refer to Common Laboratory and Diagnostic Tests 44.1).

Nursing Management

Initial nursing management of the child with myelomeningocele involves preventing trauma to the meningeal sac and preventing infection before surgical repair of the defect. For initial newborn nursing management, refer to Chapter 24. Refer to the "Clinical Judgment and the Nursing Process" section earlier in this chapter. Children with myelomeningocele will have varying degrees of paralysis of the lower limbs and lifelong issues relating to the paralysis. Additional nursing considerations are reviewed below.

PROMOTING URINARY ELIMINATION

Children with myelomeningocele often have bladder incontinence, though some children may achieve normal urinary continence. The level of the lesion will influence the amount of dysfunction. Myelomeningocele remains one of the most common causes of neurogenic bladder in children. Therefore, evaluation of renal function by a pediatric urologist should be performed on each child with myelomeningocele. Refer to Chapter 43 for further information regarding neurogenic bladder and appropriate nursing interventions, including clean intermittent catheterization.

PROMOTING BOWEL ELIMINATION

Children with myelomeningocele often have bowel incontinence as well; the level of the lesion affects the amount of dysfunction. Many children with myelomeningocele can achieve some degree of bowel continence. Bowel training with the use of timed enemas or suppositories along with diet modifications can allow for defecation at predetermined times once or twice a day. Although bowel incontinence can be difficult for children as they grow older due to social concerns and self-esteem and body image disturbances, it does not pose the same health risks as urinary incontinence.

PROMOTING ADEQUATE NUTRITION

The risk for altered nutrition related to the restrictions on positioning of the infant before and after surgery is another nursing concern. Assist the family in assuming as normal a feeding position as possible. Preoperatively, the risk of rupture may be too high to warrant holding. Therefore, the infant's head can be turned to the side or the infant can be placed in the sidelying position to facilitate feeding. If the infant is held, special care needs to be taken to avoid pressure on the sac or postoperative incision. Encourage the parents to interact as much as possible with the infant by talking to and touching the infant during feeding to help promote intake. If the parent was planning on breastfeeding the infant, assist them in meeting this goal, if possible. If the infant can be held, encourage the parent to do this, or assist them in pumping and saving breast milk to be given to the infant via bottle until the infant is able to be held. Feeding an infant in an unusual position can be difficult, and it is the nurse's role to provide support, education, and modeling for the parents and family when needed.

PREVENTING LATEX ALLERGIC REACTION

Sensitivity to latex or natural rubber is common among children with myelomeningocele. They are at an increased risk of developing an allergy to latex related to multiple exposures to latex products during surgical procedures and bladder catheterizations. A latex-free environment should be created for all procedures performed on children with myelomeningocele to prevent latex allergy. Also, children with a known latex allergy must be identified and managed in a latex-free environment. The nurse must ensure that these children do not come into direct contact with latex or equipment and supplies that contain latex. Be familiar with those products and equipment at your facility that contain latex and those that are latex free. The Food and Drug Administration (FDA) requires that all medical supplies be labeled if they contain latex (FDA, 2014), but this is not the case for consumer products. Many resources exist that list products that are latex free, and each hospital should have such a list readily available to health care professionals.

Children who are at a high risk for latex sensitivity should wear medical alert identification. Education programs regarding latex sensitivity and ways to prevent it need to be directed at those who care for high-risk children, including teachers, school nurses, relatives, babysitters, and all health care professionals.

MAINTAINING SKIN INTEGRITY

Address the risk for altered skin integrity related to the infant's prone position and impaired mobility. The prone position puts constant pressure on the knees and elbows, and it may be difficult to keep the infant clean of urine and feces. Diapering may be contraindicated preoperatively to avoid pressure on the sac. Therefore, ensure that the infant is kept as clean and dry as possible. This is made more difficult by the constant dribbling of stool and urine that may be present. Placing a pad beneath the diaper area and changing it frequently is important. Perform meticulous skin care. Place the infant on a special care mattress, and place synthetic sheepskin under the infant to help reduce friction. Special attention to the infant's legs is needed when positioning them, since paralysis may be present. Using a folded diaper between the legs can help reduce pressure and friction from the legs rubbing together.

EDUCATING AND SUPPORTING THE CHILD AND FAMILY

Myelomeningocele is a serious disorder that affects multiple body systems and produces varying degrees of deficits. It is a disorder that has lifelong effects. Thanks to medical advances and technology, most children born with myelomeningocele can expect to live a normal life, but challenges remain for the family and child as they learn to cope and live with this physical condition. Adjusting to the demands this condition places on the child and family is difficult. Parents may need time to accept their infant's condition, but as soon as possible they should be involved in the infant's care.

Teaching should begin immediately in the hospital. Teaching should include positioning, preventing infection, feeding, promoting urinary elimination through clean intermittent catheterization, preventing latex allergy, and identifying the signs and symptoms of complications such as increased ICP. Due to the chronic nature of this condition, long-term planning needs to begin in the hospital. These children usually require multiple surgical procedures and hospitalizations, and this can place stress on the family and their finances. The nurse has an important role in providing ongoing education about the illness and its treatments and the plan of care. As the family becomes more comfortable with the condition, they will become the experts in the child's care. Respect and recognize the family's changing needs. Providing intense daily care can take its toll on a family, and continual support and encouragement are needed. Referral to the Spina Bifida Association and a local support group for families of children with myelomeningocele is appropriate. See the Healthy People 2030 box.

HEALTHY PEOPLE 2030

Objective	Nursing Significance
Increase the proportion of students with disabilities who spend at least 80% of their time in regular education programs.	Become familiar with local schools' offerings and capabilities so that you can refer families to an educational site appropriate for their child.

Healthy People Objectives retrieved from http://www.healthypeople.gov

CONSIDER THIS!

After learning that our new baby will be born with spina bifida I felt so alone. I feel scared and sad; I am angry too. I wish I knew how this could happen.

Thoughts: How would you respond to their concerns? What local resources could you refer them to?

Pectus Excavatum

Pectus excavatum and pectus carinatum are anterior chest wall deformities. Pectus excavatum, a funnel-shaped chest, accounts for greater than 90% of all congenital chest wall deformities (Boas, 2020). A depression that sinks inward is apparent in the xiphoid process (Fig. 44.15). Pectus carinatum, a protuberance of the chest wall, accounts for only 5% to 15% of anterior chest wall deformities (Boas, 2020). The remainder are mixed deformities. Male predominance is evident in both types (Boas, 2020).

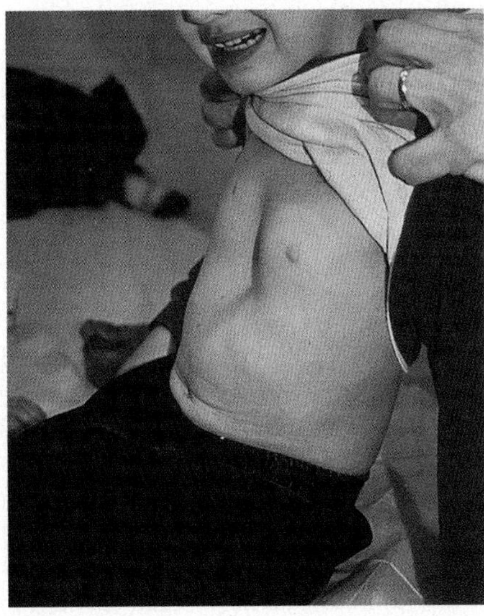

FIGURE 44.15 Pectus excavatum: Note the depression in the chest wall at the xiphoid process.

Pectus excavatum does not resolve as the child grows; rather, it progresses with growth. The chest depression may be minimal or marked. When the pectus is more pronounced, cardiac and pulmonary compression occurs. Symptoms of this compression are most often present during puberty, when the pectus quickly worsens. Children may complain of shortness of breath, withdraw from physical activities, and have a poor body image.

Therapeutic Management

Therapeutic management of pectus excavatum is based on the severity and physiologic compromise. Options include observation, use of physical therapy to work on musculoskeletal compromise, and surgical correction, preferably before puberty, when the skeleton is more pliable. Various surgical techniques may be used and generally involve either the placement of a surgical steel bar or using a piece of bone in the rib cage to lift the depression. This discussion will focus on the care of the child who undergoes surgical steel bar placement for pectus correction. This procedure, referred to as the Nuss procedure, is performed more often and is considered minimally invasive (Mayer, 2022).

Nursing Assessment

Elicit the health history, noting progression of the defect and its effects on the child's cardiopulmonary function. Note shortness of breath, exercise intolerance, or chest pain. Observe the child's chest for anterior wall deformity, noting depth and severity. Auscultate the lungs to determine the adequacy of aeration. Radiographs, CT, or MRI may be used to determine the extent of the anomaly and compression of inner structures.

Nursing Management

Prepare the child preoperatively by allowing a tour of the surgical area and the pediatric intensive care unit. Introduce the child to the pain scale that will be used in the postoperative period.

Postoperatively, nursing management focuses on assessment, protection of the surgical site, and pain management. Auscultate lung sounds frequently to determine the adequacy of aeration and to monitor for the development of the complication of pneumothorax. Assess for signs of wound infection that would necessitate removal of the curved bar. During the first few postoperative days, positioning is challenging; do not allow the child to roll in bed, lie on either side, or rotate or flex the spine (these positions may disrupt the bar's position). Administer analgesics as needed either intravenously or via the epidural catheter. Teach families that the child will not be allowed to lie on their side at home for 4 weeks after the surgery to ensure that the band does not shift. Encourage aerobic activity at home after being cleared by the surgeon (this will increase the child's vital capacity, previously hindered by the pectus). The bar will be removed 2 to 4 years after the initial placement.

Limb Deficiencies

Limb deficiencies, either complete absence of a limb or a portion of it or deformity, occur as the fetus is developing. The limb either fails to form normally or does not form at all. The cause is unknown. Certain behaviors and exposures can increase the risk of limb deficiencies such as exposure to certain chemicals, viruses, medications, and possible maternal exposure to tobacco smoke (CDC, 2022b). These defects can be attributed to an amniotic band constricting the limb, resulting in either incomplete development or amputation of the limb. Many children born with limb deformities also have congenital anomalies such as craniofacial abnormalities and cardiac and abdominal wall defects (CDC, 2022b).

Therapeutic management is aimed at improving the child's functional ability. Physical therapy and occupational therapy may be helpful. Adaptive equipment such as a prosthesis also may be prescribed.

Nursing Assessment

Note the extent of limb deformity, providing an accurate description of the presence or absence of a portion of the arm or leg, or missing fingers or toes. Assess the child's ability to use the extremity as a helper (arms) or in ambulation (legs). Determine the status of acquisition of developmental skills.

Nursing Management

Reinforce prescribed activities that are meant to improve the child's function. Provide activities in which the child is capable of participating. If the limb deficiency is significant, refer the infant to the local early intervention office as soon as possible after birth. Early intervention, available in all 50 states, is designed to promote development from birth to age 3 years. Absence of a limb or a significant portion of a limb will have a considerable impact on the child's ability to meet developmental milestones as expected.

Polydactyly and Syndactyly

Polydactyly is the presence of extra digits on the hand or foot (Fig. 44.16). One third of the time, polydactyly occurs in both the hand and foot and 50% of the time it is seen bilaterally (Winell & Davidson, 2020). It usually involves digits at the border of the hand or foot but can also occur by a central digit (Winell & Davidson, 2020). Syndactyly is webbing of the fingers and toes. Both polydactyly and syndactyly can be normal variants in the newborn and can also be inherited and associated with other genetic syndromes (Winell & Davidson, 2020).

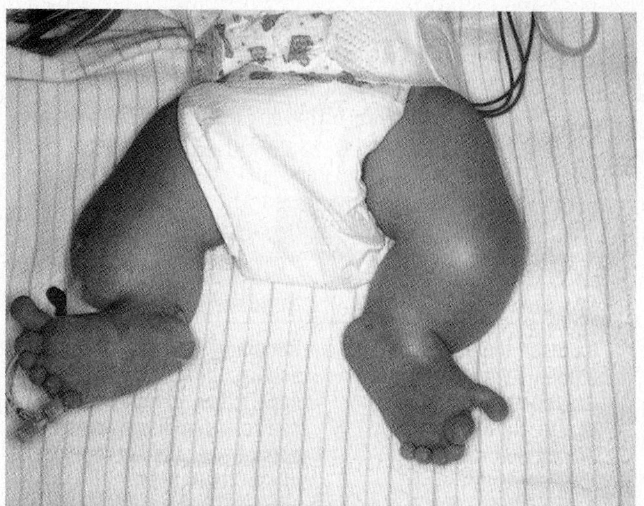

FIGURE 44.16 Note additional digits (toes) of polydactyly.

Therapeutic management includes surgical removal of the digit. No treatment is usually required for syndactyly, though surgical repair is sometimes performed for cosmetic reasons.

Nursing Assessment

Inspect the hands and feet for the presence of extra digits. Note whether the additional digits are soft (without bone) or are full or partial digits with bone present. Note the location of webbing.

Nursing Management

When surgical removal is necessary, provide routine preoperative and postoperative care as appropriate.

Metatarsus Adductus

Metatarsus adductus, a medial deviation of the forefoot, is one of the most common foot deformities of childhood (Fig. 44.17). It occurs most commonly as a result of in-utero positioning (Winell & Davidson, 2020). Half of all cases occur bilaterally (Winell & Davidson, 2020). The degree of flexibility is important and determines treatment. If the forefoot is flexible past neutral manipulation passively, observation is often sufficient. If the forefoot is flexible only to neutral manipulation, stretching exercises may be beneficial. If the forefoot is rigid and is not flexible to neutral manipulation, serial casting, preferably before the age of 8 months, may be required (Winell & Davidson, 2020). Surgical intervention is rarely needed.

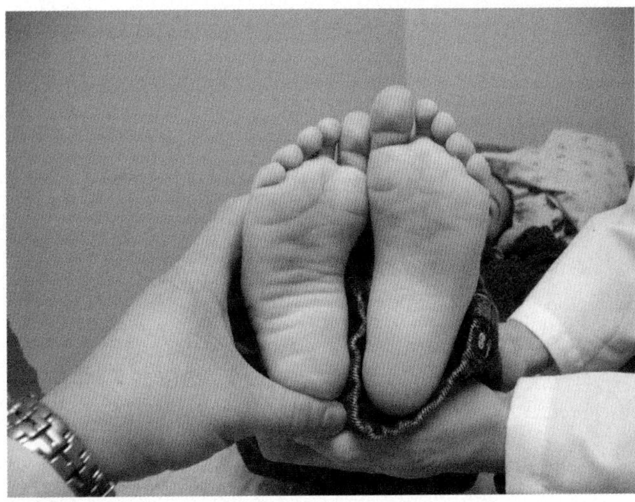

FIGURE 44.17 Metatarsus adductus: Note medial deviation of the forefoot.

Nursing Assessment

The deformity is usually noted at birth. Note inward deviation of the forefoot with the hindfoot remaining in normal position. The great and second toes might be separated. Determine forefoot flexibility. ROM of the ankle, hindfoot, and midfoot is normal.

Nursing Management

Most cases will resolve without treatment, and nursing care is aimed at education and reassurance of the parents. Nursing care for the child with severe metatarsus adductus is similar to that of the child with clubfoot (see the next section).

Congenital Clubfoot

Congenital clubfoot (also termed congenital talipes equinovarus) is a congenital anomaly that occurs in about 1 of 1,000 live births (Winell & Davidson, 2020). Clubfoot consists of:

- Talipes varus (inversion of the heel)
- Talipes equinus (plantar flexion of the foot; the heel is raised and would not strike the ground in a standing position)
- Cavus (plantar flexion of the forefoot on the hindfoot)
- Forefoot adduction with supination (the forefoot is inverted and turned slightly upward)

The foot resembles the head of a golf club (Fig. 44.18). Half of all cases occur bilaterally, and males are affected more frequently than females (Winell & Davidson, 2020). The exact etiology of clubfoot is unknown.

Clubfoot may be classified into four categories: postural, neurogenic, syndromic, and idiopathic. Postural clubfoot often resolves with a short series of manipulative casting. Neurogenic clubfoot occurs in infants with myelomeningocele. Clubfoot in association with other syndromes (syndromic) is often resistant to treatment. Idiopathic clubfoot occurs in otherwise normal healthy infants. The approach to treatment is similar regardless of the classification.

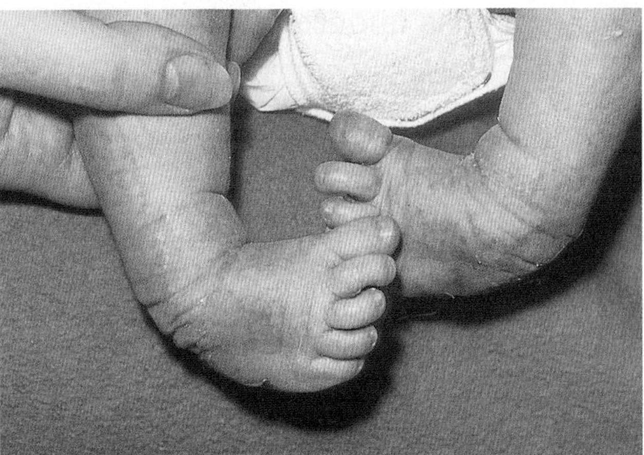

FIGURE 44.18 Note inverted heel, ankle equinus, and forefoot adduction in this infant with bilateral clubfoot.

Therapeutic Management

The goal of therapeutic management of clubfoot is the achievement of a functional foot; treatment starts as soon after birth as possible. Weekly manipulation with serial cast changes is performed; later, cast changes occur every 2 weeks. Other infants require corrective shoes or bracing. In some infants, surgical release of soft tissue may be necessary. Following surgery, the foot is immobilized with a cast for up to 12 weeks, and then ankle–foot orthoses (AFOs) or corrective shoes are used for several years.

Complications of clubfoot and its treatment include residual deformity, rocker-bottom foot, awkward gait, weight bearing on the lateral portion of the foot if uncorrected, and disturbance to the epiphysis.

Nursing Assessment

Note family history of foot deformities and obstetric history of breech position. Inspect the foot for position at rest. Perform active ROM, noting inability to move foot into normal positioning at the midline. X-rays are obtained to determine bony abnormality and note progress during treatment.

Nursing Management

Perform neurovascular assessment and cast care for infants requiring casting. Provide emotional support, as treatment often begins in the newborn period and families may have a difficult time adjusting to the diagnosis and treatment required for their new baby. Teach families cast care and about the use of orthotics or braces as prescribed.

Osteogenesis Imperfecta

OI is a genetic bone disorder that results in low bone mass, increased fragility of the bones, and other connective tissue problems such as joint hypermobility, resulting in instability of the joints. All of these contribute to fracture occurrence. Dentinogenesis imperfecta may also occur. This is characterized by the tooth enamel wearing easily and brittle and discolored teeth.

The disorder usually occurs as a result of a defect in the collagen type 1 gene, usually through an autosomal dominant inheritance pattern, but some types are inherited in a recessive manner (Balasubramanian, 2022). The types of OI range from mild to severe connective tissue and bone involvement. Originally, OI was classified into four types based on observable clinical characteristics. Since then, over 20 types have been defined (Balasubramanian, 2022). Table 44.2 discusses several types and their characteristic findings. Subtypes A and B exist depending on (A) the absence or (B) the presence of dentinogenesis imperfecta (Marini, 2020). In children with moderate to severe disease, fractures are more likely to occur, and short stature is common. In addition to multiple fractures, other complications include early hearing loss, acute and chronic pain, scoliosis, and respiratory problems.

TABLE 44.2 • Classification of Osteogenesis Imperfecta

Classification	Characteristics
I	Mild Accounts for 70%–75% of osteogenesis imperfecta (OI) cases Blue sclera Hearing loss Frequent shoulder and elbow dislocations Recurrent fractures in childhood After growth is complete, incidence of fractures diminishes dramatically. Average or slightly shorter stature compared to family members Gross motor development delays
II	Most severe form Lethal in perinatal period or die within first year of life Low birth weight, very short limbs, small chest, and soft skull Intrauterine fractures evident Very dark blue/gray sclera
III	Most severe nonlethal form Sclera ranges from white to blue. Fractures in utero and at birth with progressive deformity Bone fragility and fracture rate vary Results in significant disability Marked short stature
IV	Moderately severe Sclera may be light blue in infancy and lighten to white during childhood. Fragile bones May present at birth with in-utero fractures or bowing of lower long bones Height may be less than average for age.
V and VI	Clinically within type IV, but microscopic studies reveal distinct bone patterns; do not involve deficits of type I collagen Moderate in severity Similar to type IV in degree of fractures and skeletal deformity Type VI is extremely rare.
VII, VIII, and IX	Recessive inheritance patterns Type VII and VIII resemble type II or III, except infants have white sclera: Stature is short. IX is very rare; severity ranges from moderate to lethal.

Adapted from Marini, J. C. (2020). Osteogenesis imperfecta. In R. M. Kleigman, J. W. St. Geme III, N. J. Blum, S. S. Shah, R. C. Tasker, K. M. Wilson, & R. E. Behrman (Eds.), *Nelson textbook of pediatrics* (21st ed., pp. 19520–19539). Elsevier; Balasubramanian, M. (2022). Osteogenesis Imperfecta: An overview. *UpToDate.* Retrieved May 14, 2023, from https://www.uptodate.com/contents/osteogenesis-imperfecta-an-overview

TAKE NOTE!

Blue/gray sclera is not diagnostic of OI, but it is a common finding (Balasubramanian, 2022). However, there are some people with blue sclerae who do not have OI. Keep in mind that the sclerae of newborns tend to be bluish, progressing to white over the first few weeks of life.

Therapeutic Management

The goal of medical and surgical management is to decrease the incidence of fractures and maintain mobility. Bisphosphonate administration is used for moderate to severe disease. Fracture care is often required. Physical therapy and occupational therapy prevent contractures and maximize mobility. Standing with bracing is encouraged. Lightweight splints or braces may allow the child to bear weight earlier. Severe cases may require surgical insertion of rods into the long bones.

Nursing Assessment

Elicit a health history, which may reveal a family history of OI, a pattern of frequent fractures, or screaming associated with routine care and handling of the newborn. Inspect the eyes for sclerae that have a blue, purple, or gray tint. Note abnormalities of the primary teeth. Inspect skin for bruising and note joint hypermobility with active ROM. Laboratory tests may include a skin biopsy (which reveals abnormalities in type 1 collagen) or DNA testing (locating the genetic mutation).

Nursing Management

Handle the child carefully and teach the family to avoid trauma (Teaching Guidelines 44.3). The site includes an online store with excellent books and booklets.

Encourage safe mobility. Reinforce physical and occupational therapists' recommendations for the promotion of fine motor skills and independence in ADLs, as well as the use of adaptive equipment and appropriate promotion of mobility. Adapted physical education is important to promote mobility and maintain bone and muscle mass. If the child is ambulatory, even with adaptive equipment use, walking is a good form of exercise. Swimming and water therapy are appropriate, allowing independent movement with little fracture risk.

> *TAKE NOTE!*
>
> Use caution when inserting an intravenous line or taking a blood pressure measurement, as pressure on the arm or leg can lead to bruising and fractures.

Developmental Dysplasia of the Hip

DDH refers to abnormalities of the developing hip that include dislocation, subluxation, and dysplasia of the hip joint. In DDH, the femoral head has an abnormal relationship to the acetabulum. Frank dislocation of the hip may occur, in which there is no contact between the femoral head and acetabulum. Subluxation is a partial dislocation, meaning that the acetabulum is not fully seated within the hip joint. Dysplasia refers to an acetabulum that is shallow or sloping instead of cup shaped. DDH may affect just one or both hips. The dysplastic hip may be provoked to subluxation or dislocated and then reduced again (Fig. 44.19).

Pathophysiology

While dislocation may occur during a growth period in utero, the laxity of the newborn's hip allows dislocation

TEACHING GUIDELINES 44.3 Preventing Injury in Children With Osteogenesis Imperfecta

- Never push or pull on an arm or leg.
- Do not bend an arm or leg into an awkward position.
- Lift a baby by placing one hand under the legs and buttocks and the other hand under the shoulders, head, and neck.
- Do not lift a baby's legs by the ankles to change the diaper.
- Do not lift a baby or small child from under the armpits.
- Provide supported positioning.
- If fracture is suspected, handle the limb minimally.

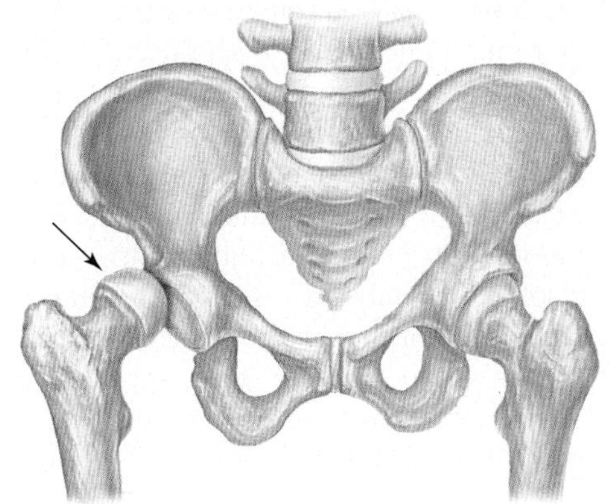

FIGURE 44.19 Developmental dysplasia of the hip.

and relocation of the hip to occur. The hip can develop normally only if the femoral head is appropriately and deeply seated within the acetabulum. If subluxation and periodic or continued dislocation occur, then structural changes in the hip's anatomy occur. Continued dysplasia of the hip leads to limited abduction of the hip and contracture of muscles. DDH is more common in females, probably due to the greater susceptibility of the female newborn to maternal hormones that contribute to laxity of the ligaments (Sankar et al., 2020). Mechanical factors such as breech positioning, the presence of oligohydramnios, or large birth weight also contribute to the development of DDH. Genetic factors also play a role. There is an increased incidence of DDH among people of Native American and Eastern Europe descent, with very low rates among people of African or Chinese heritage (Sankar et al., 2020). Complications of DDH include avascular necrosis of the femoral head, loss of ROM, recurrently unstable hip, femoral nerve palsy, leg-length discrepancy, and early osteoarthritis.

Therapeutic Management

The goal of therapeutic management is to maintain the hip joint in reduction so that the femoral head and acetabulum can develop properly.

Treatment varies based on the child's age and the severity of DDH. In newborns less than 4 weeks, the hip will often stabilize on its own in a few weeks, requiring only observation (Sankar et al., 2020). Infants younger than 6 months of age may be treated with a Pavlik harness, which reduces and stabilizes the hip by preventing hip extension and adduction and maintaining the hip in flexion and abduction (Sankar et al., 2020). The Pavlik harness is successful in the treatment of DDH in the majority of infants younger than 6 months of age if it is used on a full-time basis and applied properly (Sankar et al., 2020). Children from 6 months to 2 years of age often require closed reduction (Sankar et al., 2020). Skin or skeletal traction may be used first to gradually stretch the associated soft tissue structures. Closed reduction occurs under general anesthesia, with the hip being gently maneuvered back into the acetabulum. A spica cast worn for 12 weeks maintains reduction of the hip. After the cast is removed, the child may wear an abduction brace full-time (except for baths) (Sankar et al., 2020). Then the brace is worn at night and during naps until the development of the acetabulum is normal. Children older than 2 years of age or those who have failed to respond to prior treatment require an open surgical reduction followed by a period of casting (Sankar et al., 2020). Follow-up continues until the age of skeletal maturity.

Nursing Assessment

Nursing assessment of children with DDH includes obtaining a health history and inspecting, observing, and palpating for findings common to DDH.

HEALTH HISTORY

Assess the health history for risk factors such as:

- Family history of DDH
- Female sex
- Oligohydramnios, large birth weight, or breech birth
- Native American or Eastern European descent
- Associated lower limb deformity, metatarsus adductus, hip asymmetry, torticollis, or other congenital musculoskeletal deformity

Previously undiagnosed older children may complain of hip pain.

PHYSICAL ASSESSMENT

The physical examination for DDH includes inspection, observation, and palpation. Since DDH is a developmental process, ongoing screening assessments are required throughout at least the first several months of the infant's life.

Inspection and Observation

Ensure that the infant is on a flat surface and is relaxed. Note asymmetry of the thigh or gluteal folds with the infant in a prone position. Document shortening of the affected femur observed as a limb-length discrepancy. Older children may exhibit **Trendelenburg gait**; due to the weakness of the hip abductors, the child's trunk is shifted over the affected hip during ambulation.

Palpation

Note limited hip abduction while performing passive ROM. Abduction should ordinarily occur at 75 degrees and adduction to within 30 degrees with the infant's pelvis stabilized. Perform Barlow and Ortolani tests, feeling for, or noting, a "clunk" as the femoral head dislocates (positive Barlow) or reduces (positive Ortolani) back into the acetabulum. Force is not necessary when performing the Barlow and Ortolani maneuvers. Refer to Chapter 18 for more information on performing these maneuvers.

LABORATORY AND DIAGNOSTIC TESTING

Ultrasound of the hip allows for visualization of the femoral head and the outer edge of the acetabulum. Plain hip x-rays may be used in the infant or child older than 6 months of age.

Nursing Management

Earlier recognition of hip dysplasia with earlier harness use results in better correction of the anomaly. Excellent assessment skills and reporting of any abnormal findings are critical. Initially, the infant will need to wear the Pavlik harness continuously (Fig. 44.20). The primary provider or nurse practitioner makes all appropriate adjustments to the harness when applied so that the hips are held in the optimal position for appropriate development. Teach parents the use of the harness and assessment of the baby's skin. If started early, harness use usually continues for about 3 months (Teaching Guidelines 44.4). Breastfeeding can continue throughout the harness treatment period, but creative positioning of the infant may be needed.

For infants or children diagnosed later than 6 months of age or those who do not improve with harness use, surgical reduction may be performed (Sankar et al., 2020). Postoperative casting followed by bracing or orthotic use is common. Caring for the child in the

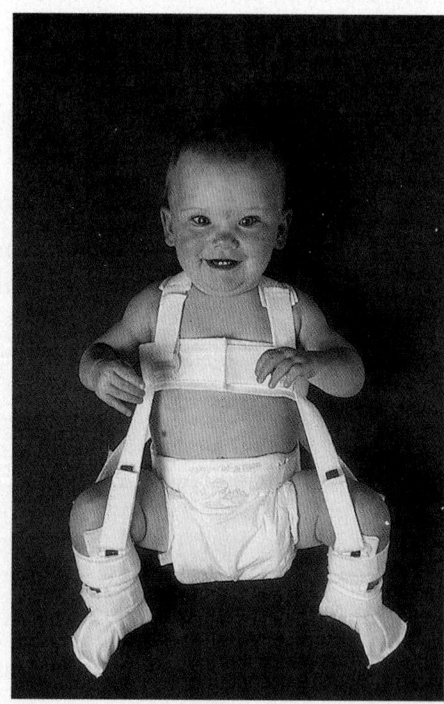

FIGURE 44.20 Pavlik harness used to keep the knees flexed and hips abducted to allow the hips to grow normally in a child with developmental dysplasia of the hip.

TEACHING GUIDELINES 44.4 Caring for a Child in a Pavlik Harness

- Do not adjust the straps without checking with the primary provider or nurse practitioner first.
- Until your primary provider or nurse practitioner instructs you to take the harness off for a period of time each day, it must be used continuously (for the first week or sometimes longer).
- Change your baby's diaper while they are in the harness.
- Place your baby to sleep on their back.
- Check skin folds, especially behind the knees and diaper area, for redness, irritation, or breakdown. Keep these areas clean and dry.
- Once the baby is permitted to be out of the harness for a short period, you may bathe your baby while the harness is off.
- Long knee socks and an undershirt are recommended to prevent rubbing of the skin against the brace.
- Note location of the markings on the straps for appropriate placement of the harness.
- Wash the harness with mild detergent by hand and air dry. If using the dryer, use *only* the air fluffing setting (no heat).
- Call the doctor if:
  - Your baby's feet are swollen or bluish.
  - The harness appears too small.
  - Skin is raw or a rash develops.
  - Your baby is unable to actively kick their legs.

postoperative period is similar to caring of any child in a cast. Pain management and monitoring for bleeding are priority activities. Teach families to care for the cast at home.

Torticollis

Torticollis is a painless muscular condition presenting in infants or in children with certain syndromes. Congenital muscular torticollis may result from in-utero positioning or difficult birth. Preferential turning of the head to one side while in the supine position after birth may also lead to torticollis. Torticollis results from tightness of the sternocleidomastoid muscle, resulting in the infant's head being tilted to one side.

Therapeutic management involves passive stretching exercises. These exercises should be effective in 90% of cases of congenital torticollis, especially if treatment is started within the first 3 months of life (Mistovich & Spiegel, 2020a). Physical therapy may be prescribed and a tubular orthosis for torticollis (TOT) collar may also be used. Surgery is not common but may be done in the preschool years if other methods have been unsuccessful. Plagiocephaly may result from the continued pressure on the side of the skull to which the neck is turned.

Nursing Assessment

Note history of head tilt and infant's lack of desire to turn the head in the opposite direction. Observe the infant for wryneck (tilting of the head to one side; Fig. 44.21). Note limited movement of the neck while performing passive ROM. Palpate the neck, noting a mass in the sternocleidomastoid muscle on the affected side. Examine the head for evidence of plagiocephaly. Accompanying hip dysplasia is seen in 8% to 20% of cases. Therefore, careful examination of the hips is warranted (Mistovich & Spiegel, 2020a).

Nursing Management

Teach parents gentle neck-stretching exercises to be performed several times a day. While immobilizing the shoulder on the affected side, gently sustain a side-to-side stretch toward the unaffected side, holding the stretch for 10 to 30 seconds. Repeat 10 to 15 times per session. Perform an ear-to-shoulder stretch in a similar fashion. To prevent the development of torticollis in the unaffected infant, prevent positional plagiocephaly. Prevent flatness of one side of the head by varying the infant's head position, and do not always turn the infant's head to one side while they are in the infant seat, in the swing, or lying supine.

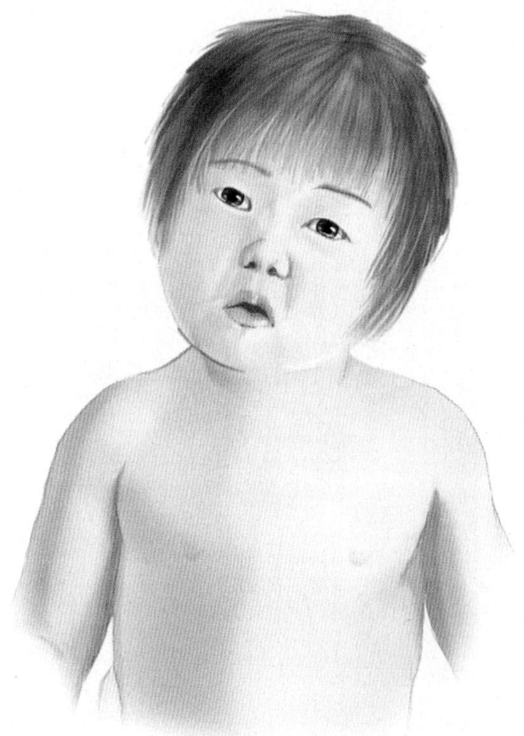

FIGURE 44.21 Note wryneck or head tilt in the infant with torticollis.

Tibia Vara (Blount Disease)

Tibia vara (Blount disease) is a developmental disorder affecting young children. There are three types: infantile (1 to 3 years), juvenile (4 to 10 years), and adolescent (11 years or older) (Winell et al., 2020). Infantile is the most common and is discussed here (Winell et al., 2020). The normal physiologic bowing or genu varum becomes more pronounced in the child with tibia vara. The cause of tibia vara is unknown, but it is considered to be a developmental disorder because it occurs most frequently in children who are early walkers. Most cases occur in Black females, and both extremities are affected (Winell et al., 2020). In addition to early walking, obesity is a risk factor. If left untreated, the growth plate of the upper tibia ceases bone production. Asymmetric growth at the knee then occurs and the bowing progresses. Severe degenerative arthritis of the knee is an additional long-term complication.

Therapeutic management is aimed at stopping the progression of the disease through bracing or surgical treatment. Medical or surgical treatment should begin early, before 4 years of age.

Nursing Assessment

Elicit a health history and determine the age at which the child started walking. Assess growth parameters to determine whether the risk factor of obesity is present. Note significant bowing of the legs while the child is standing and ambulating (Fig. 44.22).

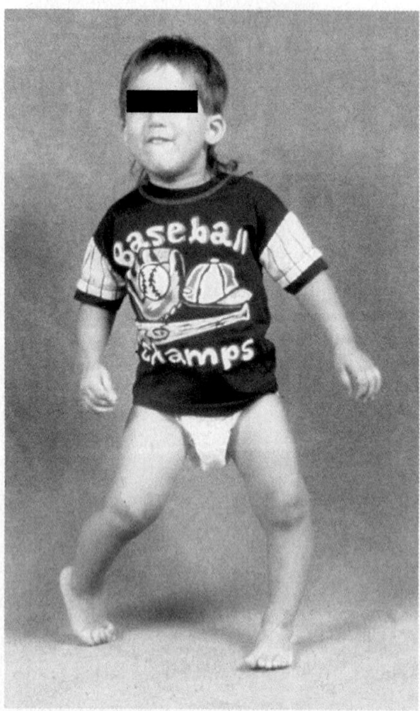

FIGURE 44.22 Note extreme bowing of the legs in tibia vara.

Nursing Management

Bracing may include a modified knee–ankle–foot orthosis that relieves the compression forces on the growth plate, allowing bone growth resumption and correction of bowlegs. To be successful, bracing must be continued for months to years and the brace must be worn 23 hours per day. Compliance is the most significant barrier to successful treatment. Parents have a difficult time forcing their toddler to stay in a brace that inhibits mobility for the bulk of the day (particularly a bilateral brace). Support parents by encouraging and praising their compliance with bracing. Teach parents to assess for potential skin impairment from brace rubbing.

When surgical treatment is required, the leg(s) will be immobilized in a long-leg bent knee or spica cast after the osteotomy is performed. Perform routine cast care. Refer to the Nursing Process section earlier in the chapter for additional interventions related to care of the immobilized child.

Muscular Dystrophy

Muscular dystrophy refers to a group of inherited conditions that result in progressive muscle weakness and wasting. The muscles affected are primarily the skeletal (voluntary) muscles. Various types of muscular dystrophy exist. All include muscle weakness over the lifetime; it is progressive in all cases but more severe in others. The various muscular dystrophies are most often diagnosed in childhood and affect a variety of muscle groups. The inheritance pattern for muscular dystrophy differs for each type but may be X-linked, autosomal dominant, or recessive. The genetic mutation in muscular dystrophy results in the absence or decrease of a specific muscle protein that prevents normal function of the muscle. The skeletal muscle fibers are affected, yet there are no structural abnormalities in the spinal cord or the peripheral nerves. Table 44.3 gives specifics related to the common types of muscular dystrophy.

Duchenne muscular dystrophy, the most common neuromuscular disorder of childhood, results in a shortened life expectancy (Darras, 2022). Due to advances in medical care, such as improvements in noninvasive mechanical ventilation, better management of cardiac dysfunction using angiotensin-converting enzyme (ACE) inhibitors, and the use of steroids, survival into their 30s, with some cases into their 40s is becoming more common (Darras, 2022). The incidence is about one in 3,600 live male births (Bharucha-Goebel, 2020). For these reasons, this discussion will focus on Duchenne muscular dystrophy.

Pathophysiology

The gene mutation in Duchenne muscular dystrophy results in the absence of dystrophin, a protein that is

TABLE 44.3 • Types of Muscular Dystrophy

Type	Onset	Inheritance	Muscle Involvement
Duchenne (pseudohypertrophic)	Early childhood (usually 3–6 years)	X-linked recessive (primarily only males; female carriers may show mild symptoms)	Generalized weakness, muscle wasting; limb and trunk first
Becker	2–16 years	X-linked recessive (primarily only males; female carriers may show mild symptoms)	Similar but less severe than Duchenne
Congenital (severe involvement at birth)	At birth to 2 years	Most forms are autosomal recessive (primarily affects males).	Generalized muscular weakness, possible joint deformities, contractures, and hypotonia noted at birth
Emery–Dreifuss	Childhood to early adolescence (usually by 10 years)	Most often X-linked recessive (primarily affects males)	Weakness, wasting of shoulder, upper arm, and shin muscles
Limb-girdle	Late adolescence to middle age	Most often autosomal recessive but may be dominant (primarily affects males)	Weakness, wasting of shoulder, and pelvic girdles first
Facioscapulohumeral	Usually late childhood to early adulthood (usually by age 20)	Autosomal dominant	Facial muscles weaken first, then shoulders and upper arms
Myotonic	Infancy to adult years	Autosomal dominant	Generalized weakness, wasting of face, feet, hands, and neck first Delayed relaxation of muscles after contraction

Data from Bharucha-Goebel, D. X. (2020). Muscular dystrophies. In R. M. Kleigman, J. W. St. Geme III, N. J. Blum, S. S. Shah, R. C. Tasker, K. M. Wilson, & R. E. Behrman (Eds.), *Nelson textbook of pediatrics* (21st ed., pp. 17216–17284). Elsevier; Darras, B. T. (2021). Patient education: Overview of muscular dystrophies (Beyond the Basics). *UpToDate.* Retrieved May 16, 2023, from https://www.uptodate.com/contents/overview-of-muscular-dystrophies-beyond-the-basics

critical for the maintenance of muscle cells. The gene is X-linked recessive, meaning that mainly males are affected, and they receive the gene from their female parent (females are carriers but have mild to no symptoms). Absence of dystrophin leads to generalized weakness of voluntary muscles, and the weakness progresses over time. The hips, thighs, pelvis, and shoulders are affected initially; as the disease progresses, all voluntary muscles as well as cardiac and respiratory muscles are affected.

Children with Duchenne muscular dystrophy are often late in learning to walk. As toddlers, they may display pseudohypertrophy (enlarged appearance) of the calves. During the preschool years, they fall often and are quite clumsy. The affected child has difficulty climbing stairs and running and cannot get up from the floor in the usual fashion. The school-age child walks on the toes or balls of the feet with a rolling or waddling gait. Balance is disturbed significantly, and the child's belly may stick out when the shoulders are pulled back to stay upright and keep from falling over. During the school-age years, it also becomes difficult for the child to raise their arms. Sometime between the ages of 7 and 12 years, nearly all children with Duchenne muscular dystrophy lose the ability to ambulate, and by adolescence, any activity of the arms, legs, or trunk requires assistance or support (Darras, 2022). Most children with Duchenne muscular dystrophy have some degree of intellectual impairment although intelligence level is often normal, but many may exhibit a specific learning disability (Bharucha-Goebel, 2020).

Therapeutic Management

There is no cure for Duchenne muscular dystrophy. However, the use of glucocorticoids may slow the progression of the disease (Darras, 2023). The side effects of glucocorticoids are many, including weight gain, short stature, osteoporosis, hirsutism, cushingoid appearance, and mood changes (Darras, 2023). Calcium supplements and vitamin D are prescribed to prevent osteoporosis, and antidepressants may be helpful when depression occurs related to the chronicity of the disease and/or as an effect of corticosteroid use (Darras, 2022). Medications to decrease the workload of the heart, such as beta blockers and ACE inhibitors may be prescribed.

TAKE NOTE!

Researchers continue to search for a way to stop or reverse this disease. Gene therapy, exon skipping or codon read through, and gene repair are some new strategies being investigated. The FDA has approved some medications, such as eteplirsen, golodirsen, viltolarsen, and ataluren, that have shown the ability to increase dystrophin. Studies are underway to establish clinical benefit (Darras, 2023).

Braces or orthoses and mobility and positioning aids are necessary. As the muscles deteriorate, joints may become fixated, resulting in contractures. Contractures restrict flexibility and mobility and cause discomfort. Sometimes contractures require surgical tendon release. Spinal curvatures result over time. The child with Duchenne muscular dystrophy who can still walk may develop lordosis. More frequently, scoliosis or kyphosis develops with this disorder. Surgical spinal fixation with rod implantation is often required by adolescence (Darras, 2022). Additional complications include pulmonary, urinary, or systemic infections; depression; learning or behavioral disorders; aspiration pneumonia (as oropharyngeal muscles become affected); cardiac dysrhythmias; and, eventually, respiratory insufficiency and failure (as weakness of the chest muscles and diaphragm progresses).

Nursing Assessment

For a full description of the assessment phase of the nursing process, refer to the "Clinical Judgment and the Nursing Process" section earlier in the chapter. Assessment findings pertinent to Duchenne muscular dystrophy are discussed below.

HEALTH HISTORY

Examine the health history for a family history of neuromuscular disorders. Note pregnancy and delivery history, as this information may be useful in ruling out a pregnancy problem or birth trauma as a cause for motor dysfunction. Determine the status of developmental milestone achievement. Children with Duchenne muscular dystrophy learn to walk but over time become unable to do so. If the child was previously diagnosed with muscular dystrophy, determine progression of the disease. Inquire about functional status and need for assistive or adaptive equipment such as braces or wheelchairs. Determine skills related to ADLs. Note history of cough or frequent respiratory infections, which occur as the respiratory muscles weaken. While talking with the child and family, determine whether psychosocial issues such as decreased self-esteem, depression, alterations in socialization, or altered family processes might be present.

PHYSICAL EXAMINATION

Perform a thorough physical examination on the child with suspected muscular dystrophy or the child with a known history of the disorder. Particular findings related to inspection, observation, auscultation, and palpation are presented below.

Inspection and Observation

Observe the child's ability to rise from the floor. A hallmark finding of Duchenne muscular dystrophy is the presence of the Gower sign: The child cannot rise from the floor in standard fashion because of increasing weakness (Fig. 44.23). Observe the child's gait. Determine effectiveness of cough.

Auscultation and Palpation

Auscultate the heart and lungs. Note tachycardia, which develops as the heart muscle weakens. Note adequacy of breath sounds, which may diminish with decreasing respiratory function. Note muscle strength with resistance testing. Palpate muscle tone.

LABORATORY AND DIAGNOSTIC TESTS

Electromyography (EMG) demonstrates that the problem lies in the muscles, not in the nerves. Serum creatine kinase (CK) levels are elevated early in the disorder when significant muscle wasting is actively occurring. Muscle biopsy provides a definitive diagnosis, demonstrating the absence of dystrophin. DNA testing reveals the presence of the gene.

Nursing Management

Nursing management is aimed at promoting mobility, maintaining cardiopulmonary function, preventing complications, and maximizing quality of life. Interventions directed at maintaining mobility and cardiopulmonary function also help to prevent complications. Refer to the "Clinical Judgment and the Nursing Process" section earlier in the chapter, and individualize nursing care based on the child's and family's response to the illness. Additional specifics related to care of the child with muscular dystrophy are discussed in the following sections.

PROMOTING MOBILITY

Administer glucocorticoids and calcium supplements as ordered. Encourage at least minimal weight bearing in a standing position to promote improved circulation, healthier bones, and a straight spine. Children with Duchenne muscular dystrophy may use a standing walker or standing frame to maintain an upright position. Perform passive stretching or strengthening exercises as recommended by the physical therapist. These exercises preserve mobility and may help to prevent muscle atrophy. Use orthotic supports such as hand braces or AFOs to prevent contractures of joints. Schedule activities

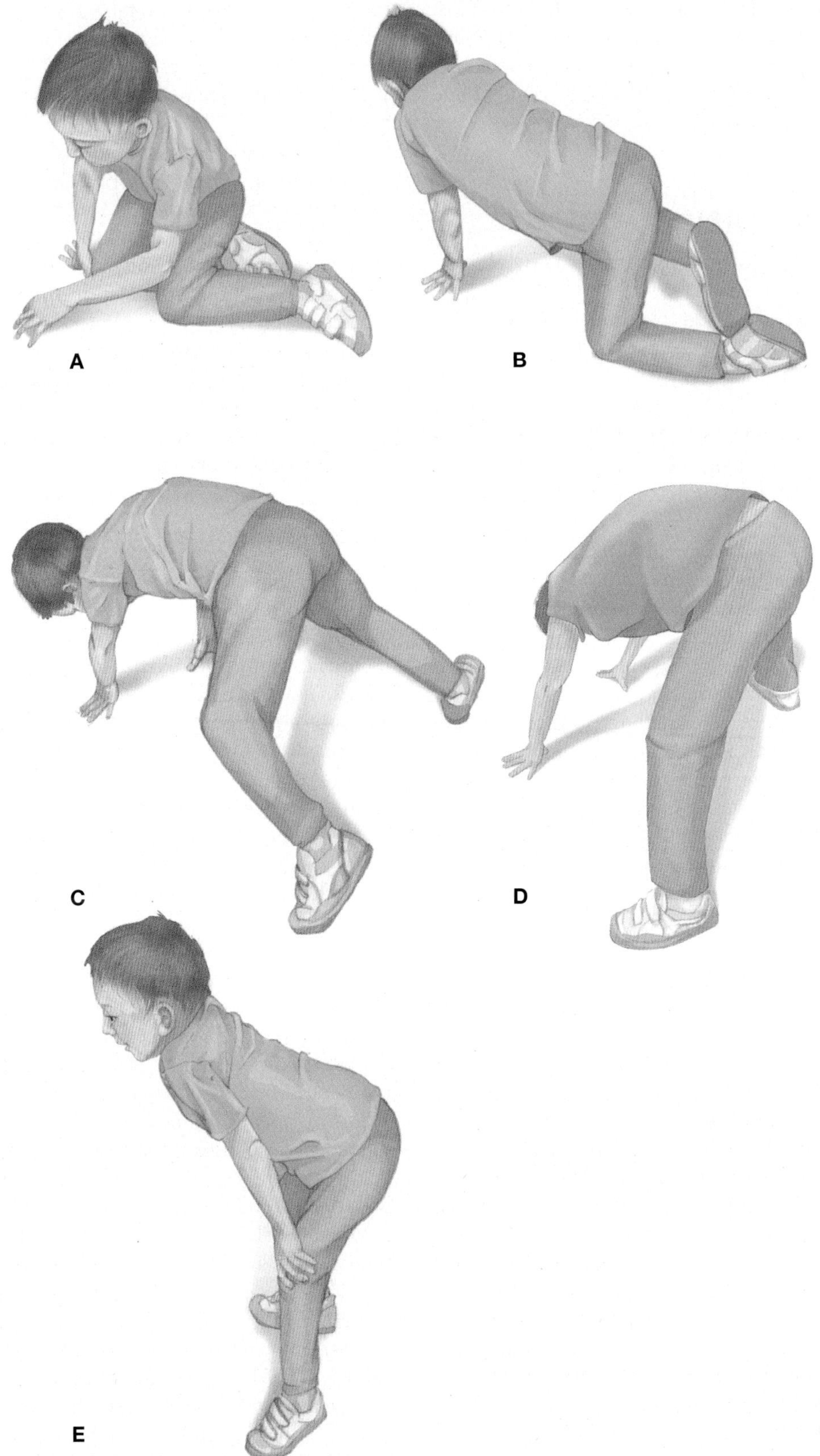

FIGURE 44.23 The Gower sign. **A.** First the child must roll onto their hands and knees. **B.** Then they must bear weight by using their hands to support some of their weight, while raising their posterior. **C–E.** The child then uses their hands to "walk" up their legs to assume an upright position.

during the part of the day when the child has the most energy. Teach parents the use of positioning, exercises, orthoses, and adaptive equipment. Use of a wheelchair full-time typically occurs between 10 and 14 years of age (Bharucha-Goebel, 2020).

> **THINKING ABOUT DEVELOPMENT**
>
> You are caring for a 6-year-old with Duchenne muscular dystrophy. How can you best help them meet developmental milestones? How would this differ if they were a 12-year-old?

MAINTAINING CARDIOPULMONARY FUNCTION

Assess respiratory rate, depth of respirations, and work of breathing. Auscultate the lungs to determine whether aeration is sufficient and to assess clarity of breath sounds. Position the child for maximum chest expansion, usually in the upright position. Teach the child and family deep-breathing exercises to strengthen or maintain respiratory muscles and encourage coughing to clear the airways. Perform chest physical therapy or assist with chest percussion. Monitor the results of pulmonary function testing. Use of intermittent positive-pressure ventilation and mechanically assisted coughing will become necessary in adolescence for some, possibly later for others. Teach parents the monitoring of respiratory status and use of these modalities in conjunction with the respiratory therapist. Monitor cardiac status closely to identify heart failure early. Assess for edema, weight gain, or crackles. Strictly monitor fluid intake and output.

MAXIMIZING QUALITY OF LIFE

Long periods of bed rest may contribute to further weakness. Work with the family and child to develop a schedule for diversional activities that provide appropriate developmental stimulation but avoid overexertion or frustration (related to inability to perform the activity). Periods of adequate rest must be balanced with activities. Walking or riding a stationary bike is appropriate for the child who has upper extremity involvement. For the child with lower extremity involvement, a wheelchair may become necessary for mobility, and the child may participate in crafts, drawing, and computer activities. Participating in the Special Olympics may be appropriate for some children. Do not place limits on the child but encourage activities they are interested in that can be modified as needed to fit their abilities.

Provide emotional support to the child and family. Long-term direct care is stressful for families and becomes more complex as the child gets older. Families often need respite from continual caregiving duties. When a child is hospitalized, the caregiver may feel comfortable allowing nurses and other health care professionals to assume more of the child's daily care; this can be an opportunity for the caregiver to obtain respite from daily care. Respite care may also be offered in the home by various community services, so explore these resources with families.

Assess the child's educational status. Some children attend school; others may opt for home schooling. Administer antidepressants as ordered; managing depression may increase the child's desire to participate in activities and self-care. Refer the child and family to the Muscular Dystrophy Association (MDA), which provides multidisciplinary care via clinics located throughout the United States. The association is also a clearinghouse for resources for people with muscular dystrophy. Ensure that families receive genetic counseling for family planning purposes as well as determining which family members may be carriers for muscular dystrophy.

Spinal Muscular Atrophy

SMA is a genetic motor neuron disease that affects the spinal nerves' ability to communicate with the muscles. It is inherited via an autosomal recessive mechanism. The motor neuron protein survival of motor neurons (SMNs) is deficient as a result of a faulty gene on chromosome 5. The motor neurons are located mostly in the spinal cord. Without adequate SMN, the signals from the neurons to the muscles instructing them to contract are ineffective, so the muscles lose function and over time atrophy. The proximal muscles, those closer to the body's center, are usually more affected than the distal muscles. Cognition is unaffected by this disease (Bodamer, 2023).

There are several types of SMA, classified as type 0 to type 4, based on age of onset, severity of weakness, and clinical course. SMA0 and SMA1 are the most common and most severe (Bodamer, 2023). Their usual progression and prognosis are compared in Table 44.4.

Respiratory muscle weakness may occur with all types of SMA and is usually the cause of death in type 1 SMA. Upper respiratory tract infections and aspiration related to dysphagia or gastroesophageal reflux often develop into pneumonia and eventual respiratory failure, as the affected child cannot effectively cough independently in order to clear the airway. Many children with severe type 1 SMA are ventilator dependent. Pectus excavatum develops in children with type 1 and type 2 SMA who exhibit paradoxical breathing (use of the diaphragm without intercostal muscle support). The chest becomes funnel shaped and the xiphoid process is retracted (pectus excavatum), further restricting respiratory development. Inability to appropriately suck and swallow leads to difficulty feeding in the child with type 1 SMA. Weak back muscles affect the developing spine, resulting in the complication of scoliosis, kyphosis, or both.

Therapeutic management of SMA is supportive and aimed at promoting mobility, maintaining adequate

TABLE 44.4 • Features of Spinal Muscular Atrophy

Features	Type 0 (Prenatal SMA)	Type 1 SMA (Werdnig–Hoffmann Disease, Infantile SMA)	Type 2 SMA (Intermediate SMA)	Type 3 SMA (Kugelberg–Welander Disease, Juvenile SMA)	Type 4 SMA (Late Onset)
Onset	Prenatal	Less than 6 months of age	6–18 months of age	After 18 months of age; child has started walking or has taken at least five independent steps.	Age not strictly defined, typically adult onset
Symptoms	• Loss of or decreased fetal movement later in pregnancy • At birth severe hypotonia • Joint contractures may be present.	• Generalized weakness; cannot sit without support • Weak cry • Difficulty sucking, swallowing, and breathing	• Proximal muscles are more affected; that is, thighs are weaker than lower legs; legs tend to be weaker than arms. • Respiratory muscles may be involved. • Scoliosis may occur.	• Weakness that is most severe in the shoulders, hips, thighs, and upper back • Respiratory muscles may be involved. • Scoliosis may occur.	• Symptoms are mild; all motor milestones achieved • Ambulation maintained
Progression	Rapidly progresses to early death by 6 months of age (typically by 1 month)	Rapidly progresses to early childhood death. Use of ventilators and gastrostomy feeding tubes may prolong life expectancy but typically death occurring by age 2	Slower progression. Life expectancy related to age of onset (the younger the onset, the more severe the disease and the shorter the life expectancy) Survival into adulthood common if respiratory status maintained appropriately	Slow progression. Lifespan usually unaffected. Walking ability maintained until at least adolescence; may need wheelchair later in life	Normal lifespan

Data from Bodamer, O. A. (2023). Spinal muscular atrophy. *UpToDate*. Retrieved May 16, 2023, from https://www.uptodate.com/contents/spinal-muscular-atrophy

nutrition and pulmonary function, and preventing complications. Spinal fusion may be performed in older children with significant scoliosis. Since the discovery of the disease-causing gene for SMA, further research and improved diagnostic techniques have occurred. Therapies, such as nusinersen (which is an intrathecally injected medication) and gene replacement, such as onasemnogene abeparvovec, have both shown promising results (Bodamer, 2023).

Nursing Assessment

Note history of attainment of developmental milestones, as well as loss of milestones. SMA should be suspected in a child showing symmetric, unexplained weakness that is more proximal than distal and greater in the legs than arms, diminished or absent tendon reflexes, history of difficulty with motor skills, or loss of motor skills (Bodamer, 2023). In the infant or child with known SMA, assess for recent hospitalizations or respiratory illness. Determine the respiratory support regimen used at home (if any). Note the level of motor ability and identify the orthoses or adaptive equipment used. Elicit history related to feeding patterns at home. Assess for floppy appearance in the infant with SMA. Note decreased ability to initiate spontaneous muscle movement. In the infant or young child with SMA, note narrow chest with decreased excursion, relatively protuberant abdomen, and paradoxical breathing pattern (Fig. 44.24). Observe the chest for the formation of pectus excavatum. Auscultate the lungs for diminished or adventitious breath sounds. Monitor laboratory testing, which may include:

- CK: elevated when muscular damage is occurring
- Genetic testing: identifies the presence of gene for SMA
- Muscle biopsy: shows the muscle abnormality
- Nerve conduction velocity test and electromyogram: to determine the extent of involvement

Nursing Management

Nursing management of type 2 and type 3 SMA focuses on promoting mobility, maintaining pulmonary function, and preventing complications. Children with type 1 SMA

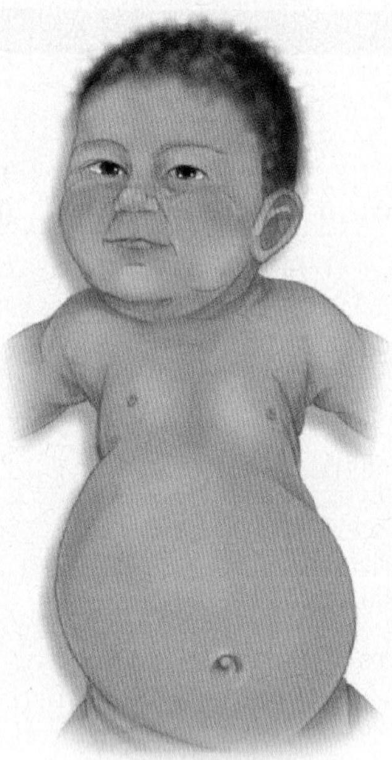

FIGURE 44.24 Note the very narrow chest, beginning xiphoid depression, and relatively enlarged appearance of the abdomen in this infant with type 1 spinal muscular atrophy (SMA).

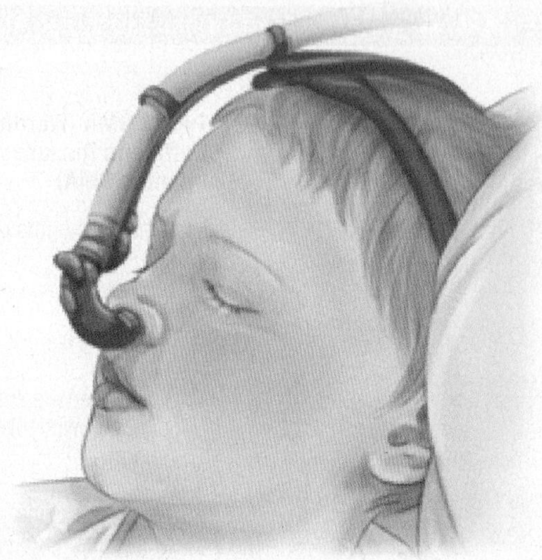

FIGURE 44.25 Use of noninvasive positive-pressure monitoring via nasal prongs can maximize respiration and may help prevent pulmonary complications.

need additional interventions related to the prevention of complications from immobility and assistance with nutrition. Refer to the "Clinical Judgment and the Nursing Process" section earlier in the chapter for interventions related to these areas. Individualize the nursing plan of care based on the individual child's responses to the disorder.

Promote mobility through the use of ROM exercises, lightweight orthotics, standing frames, and wheelchair use as appropriate. Support parents in their efforts to comply with physical and occupational therapy regimens. Older children may exercise with assistance in a warm pool. Position the child in a fashion that maintains appropriate body alignment.

Provide airway clearance techniques such as manual or mechanical cough assistance, chest percussion, and postural drainage to assist with the clearance of secretions. In collaboration with respiratory therapy, teach families the use of noninvasive ventilation support, in which positive pressure is delivered to the lungs through a mask or mouthpiece (Fig. 44.25). Provide routine tracheostomy care if the child has a tracheostomy (refer to "Tracheostomy" section of Chapter 40).

Administer gastrostomy tube feedings if ordered, and teach families gastrostomy tube care. Use bracing as prescribed to prevent spinal curvature. Make frequent inspections for skin breakdown in areas affected by bracing.

Cerebral Palsy

Cerebral palsy is a term used to describe a range of nonspecific clinical symptoms characterized by abnormal motor pattern and postures caused by nonprogressive abnormal brain function. The majority of causes occur before delivery (80%) but can also occur in the natal and postnatal periods (Box 44.1) (Johnston, 2020). Many times, no specific cause can be identified (Barkoudah & Aravamuthan, 2023). Cerebral palsy is the most common movement disorder of childhood; it is a lifelong condition and one of the most common causes of physical disability in children (Johnston, 2020). The incidence is about two in every 1,000 live births and is higher in premature and low birth weight infants (Barkoudah & Aravamuthan, 2023). See the Healthy People 2030 box.

HEALTHY PEOPLE 2030

Objective	Nursing Significance
Reduce preterm births.	• Encourage appropriate birth control use among adolescents to decrease the incidence of adolescent pregnancy (adolescents have an increased incidence of preterm delivery). • If an adolescent does become pregnant, encourage early appropriate prenatal care. • Discourage substance use among pregnant adolescents. • Teach pregnant adolescents about an appropriate diet.

Healthy People Objectives retrieved from http://www.healthypeople.gov

Most affected children will develop symptoms in infancy or early childhood. There is a large variation in symptoms and disability. For some children it may be as mild as a slight limp; for others it may result in severe motor and neurologic impairments. Primary signs include motor impairments such as spasticity, muscle weakness,

BOX 44.1 Causes of Cerebral Palsy

Prenatal

- Congenital malformation
- Hypoxia
- Fever in the pregnant parent
- Seizures in the pregnant parent
- Bleeding in the pregnant parent
- Exposure to radiation
- Environmental toxins
- Genetic abnormalities
- Metabolic disorders
- Intrauterine growth restriction
- Intrauterine infection, such as cytomegalovirus and toxoplasmosis
- Nutritional deficits
- Preeclampsia
- Multiple births
- Prematurity
- Low birth weight
- Malformation of brain structure
- Abnormalities of blood flow to the brain
- Abdominal insults
- Accidental maternal injury
- Heavy alcohol consumption by the pregnant parent
- Smoking during pregnancy

Perinatal

- Prematurity (<32 weeks)
- Asphyxia
- Hypoxia
- Abnormal fetal presentation
- Sepsis or central nervous system infection
- Placental complications
- Electrolyte disturbance
- Cerebral hemorrhage
- Chorioamnionitis (infection of the placental tissues and amniotic fluid)

Postnatal

- Kernicterus (a type of brain damage that may result from neonatal hyperbilirubinemia)
- Asphyxia
- Head trauma (e.g., motor vehicle crashes, abuse)
- Seizures
- Toxins
- Viral or bacterial infection of the central nervous system (e.g., meningitis)
- Cerebral infarcts
- Intraventricular hemorrhage

and **ataxia**, which is lack of coordination of muscle movements during voluntary movements such as walking or picking up objects. Complications include mental impairments, seizures, growth problems, impaired vision or hearing, abnormal sensation or perception, and hydrocephalus. Most children can survive into adulthood, but function and quality of life can vary from near normal to substantial impairments (Barkoudah, 2023).

Pathophysiology

Cerebral palsy is a disorder caused by abnormal development of, or damage to, the motor areas of the brain, resulting in a neurologic lesion. It is difficult to establish an exact location of the neurologic lesion, but it causes a disruption in the brain's ability to control movement and posture. The lesion itself does not change over time; thus, the disorder is considered nonprogressive since the brain injury does not progress. However, the clinical manifestations of the lesion change as the child grows. Some children may improve, but many either plateau in their attainment of motor skills or demonstrate worsening of motor abilities because it is difficult to maintain the ability to move over time.

Cerebral palsy is classified in several ways. One common way is by the type of movement disturbance (Table 44.5).

Therapeutic Management

Management of cerebral palsy involves multiple disciplines, including a primary provider, specialty primary providers such as a neurologist and an orthopedic surgeon, nurses, physical therapists, occupational therapists, speech therapists, dietitians, psychologists, counselors, teachers, and parents. There is no standard treatment for all children. The overall focus of therapeutic management will be to assist the child to gain optimal development and function within the limits of the disease. Treatment is mainly preventive, symptomatic, and supportive. Spasticity management will be a primary concern and will be determined by clinical findings.

Medical management is focused on promoting mobility through the use of therapeutic modalities and medications. Surgical management is often required and is used to correct deformities related to spasticity.

PHYSICAL, OCCUPATIONAL, AND SPEECH THERAPY

The use of therapeutic modalities such as physical therapy, occupational therapy, and speech therapy will be essential in promoting mobility and development in the child with cerebral palsy. The earlier the treatment begins, the better chance the child has of overcoming developmental disabilities (NINDS, 2023).

Physical therapists work with children to assist in the development of gross motor movements such as walking and positioning, and they help the child develop independent movement. They also assist in preventing contractures, and they instruct children and caregivers in the use of assistive devices such as walkers and wheelchairs. Occupational therapists may be responsible for fashioning orthotics and splints. AFOs are the most common orthotic used by children with cerebral palsy (Fig. 44.26) (Barkoudah & Whitaker, 2022). AFOs help prevent deformity from conditions such as contractures and help reduce the effects of existing deformities. They

TABLE 44.5 • Classification of Cerebral Palsy

Types	Description	Characteristics
Spastic	Hypertonicity and permanent contractures; different types based on which limbs are affected: • Hemiplegia: both extremities on one side • Quadriplegia: all four extremities • Diplegia or paraplegia: lower extremities	• Most common form • Poor control of posture, balance, and movement • Exaggeration of deep tendon reflexes • Hypertonicity of affected extremities • Continuation of primitive reflexes • In some children, failure to progress to protective reflexes
Dyskinetic or athetoid	Abnormal involuntary movements	• Infant is limp and flaccid. • Uncontrolled, slow, wormlike writhing or twisting movements • Affects all four extremities and possible involvement of face, neck, and tongue • Movements increase during periods of stress. • Dysarthria and drooling may be present.
Ataxic	Affects balance and depth perception	• Poor coordination • Unsteady gait • Wide-based gait • Motor milestones and language skills delayed
Mixed	Combination of the above	Most common is spastic and dyskinetic.

can help improve a child's mobility by assisting in control of alignment and helping to increase the efficiency of the child's gait. Spinal orthotics such as braces are used in young children with cerebral palsy to combat scoliosis that develops due to spasticity. These braces are used to delay surgical management of the scoliosis until the child reaches skeletal maturity. Splinting is used to maintain muscle length. Serial casting may also be used to increase muscle and tendon length.

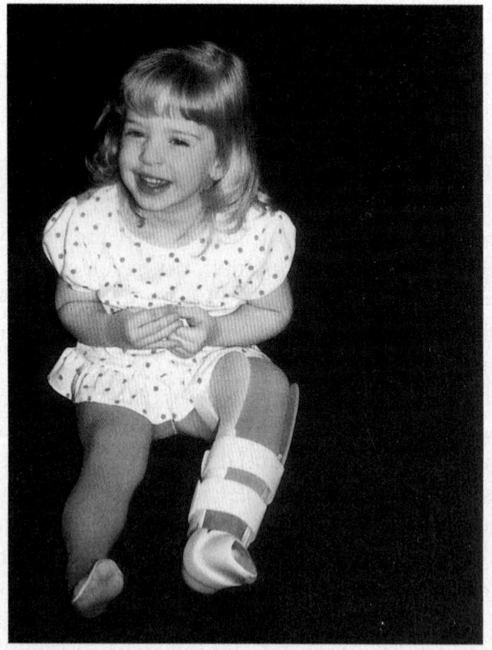

FIGURE 44.26 The child with cerebral palsy may benefit from wearing ankle–foot orthotics (AFOs) to provide support needed for independent or assisted walking.

Occupational therapy also assists in the development of fine motor skills and will help the child to perform optimal self-care by working on skills such as ADLs. Speech therapy assists in the development of receptive and expressive language and addresses the use of appropriate feeding techniques in the child who has swallowing problems. Speech therapists may teach augmented communication strategies to children who are nonverbal or who have articulation problems. Many children may not communicate verbally but can use alternative means such as communication books or boards and computers with voice synthesizers to make their desires known or to participate in conversation.

PHARMACOLOGIC MANAGEMENT

Various pharmacologic options are available to manage spasticity (see Drug Guide 44.1). Oral medications used to treat spasticity include baclofen, dantrolene sodium, and diazepam. Children with dyskinetic/athetoid cerebral palsy may be given anticholinergics to help decrease abnormal movements. Anticholinergic agents, such as scopolamine (also known as hyoscine) or glycopyrrolate, decrease saliva and are used to help control drooling.

TAKE NOTE!

Pathologic drooling is a problem for many children with cerebral palsy. It can lead to dehydration, dental enamel erosion, and maceration of the skin, and an odor can result, along with social stigmatization. Recent research has shown that intraglandular injection of botulinum toxin type A can improve drooling with few side effects in children with neurologic disorders (Barkoudah, 2023).

DOSAGE CALCULATION BOX 44.1

Child's weight: 87 lb

Medication order: Glycopyrrolate 0.8 mg per gastrostomy tube three times a day

Per the *Pediatric Dosage Handbook*, the recommended dose is 20 mcg/kg/dose three times daily and may titrate to a maximum dose of 100 mcg/kg/dose three times daily (not to exceed 1,500 to 3,000 mcg/dose).

Is this ordered dose safe?

Parenterally administered medications such as botulin toxins and baclofen are also used to manage spasticity. Botulinum toxin is injected into the spastic muscle to balance the muscle forces across joints and to decrease spasticity. It is useful in managing focal spasticity in which the spasticity is interfering with function, producing pain, or contributing to a progressive deformity. It can also help reduce drooling when injected into the salivary glands. Botulin toxin injection is performed by the primary provider or nurse practitioner and can be done in the clinic or outpatient setting. Phenol or ethanol block, a neurolytic agent that provides a temporary reduction in spasticity, may be used in conjunction with botulinum toxin or alone if botulinum toxin has been proved to be ineffective or contraindicated for the child (Barkoudah & Whitaker, 2022).

Intrathecal administration of baclofen has been shown to decrease tone, but it must be infused continuously due to its short half-life. Surgical placement of a baclofen pump will be considered in children with general spasticity that is limiting function, comfort, ADLs, and endurance. To test whether it is a suitable option, an intrathecal test dose of baclofen will be administered. If the trial is successful, a baclofen pump will be implanted. Once inserted, delivery of the drug can be individualized to meet the child's unique needs. The pump needs to be replaced every 5 to 7 years and must be refilled with medication approximately every 2 to 6 months, depending on the type of pump. Complications with baclofen pump placement include infection, rupture, dislodgment, or blockage of the catheter.

Medications are also used to treat seizure disorders in children with cerebral palsy (refer to Chapter 38 for information related to seizure management).

SURGICAL MANAGEMENT

Many children will require surgical procedures to correct deformities related to spasticity. Multiple corrective surgeries may be required; they usually are orthopedic or neurosurgical. Surgery may be used to correct contractures that are severe enough to cause movement limitations. Common orthopedic procedures include tendon lengthening procedures, correction of hip and adductor muscle spasticity, and fusion of unstable joints to help improve locomotion, correct bony deformities, decrease painful spasticity, and maintain, restore, or stabilize a spinal deformity. Neurosurgical interventions may include placement of a shunt in children who have developed hydrocephalus, or surgical interventions to decrease spasticity. Selective dorsal root rhizotomy is used to decrease spasticity in the lower extremities by reducing the amount of stimulation that reaches the muscles via the nerves.

Nursing Assessment

For a full description of the assessment phase of the nursing process, refer to the "Clinical Judgment and the Nursing Process" section earlier in the chapter. Assessment findings pertinent to cerebral palsy are discussed below.

HEALTH HISTORY

Elicit a description of the present illness and chief complaint. Obtain a detailed account of gestational and perinatal events (see Box 44.1). Common signs and symptoms reported during the health history of the undiagnosed child might include:

- Intrauterine infections
- Prematurity with intracranial hemorrhage
- Difficult, complicated, or prolonged labor and delivery
- Multiple births
- History of possible anoxia during prenatal life or birth
- History of head trauma
- Delayed attainment of developmental milestones
- Muscle weakness or rigidity
- Poor feeding
- Hips and knees feel rigid and unbending when pulled to a sitting position
- Seizure activity
- Subnormal learning
- Abnormal motor performance, scoots on back instead of crawling on the abdomen, walks or stands on toes

Children known to have cerebral palsy are often admitted to the hospital for corrective surgeries or other complications of the disease, such as aspiration pneumonia and urinary tract infections. The health history should include questions related to:

- Respiratory status: Has a cough, sputum production, or increased work of breathing developed?
- Motor function: Has there been a change in muscle tone or increase in spasticity?
- Presence of fever
- Feeding and weight loss
- Any other changes in physical state or medication regimen

PHYSICAL EXAMINATION

Observe general appearance. Pay close attention to the neurologic assessment and motor assessment. Assess for delayed development, size for age, and sensory alterations such as strabismus, vision problems, and speech disorders. Abnormal postures may be present. While lying supine, the infant may demonstrate scissor crossing of the legs with plantar flexion. In the prone position, the infant may raise their head higher than normal due to arching of the back, or the opisthotonic position may be noted. The infant may also abnormally flex the arms and legs under the trunk. Primitive reflexes may persist beyond the point at which they disappear in a healthy infant. Evolution of protective reflexes may be delayed. Watch the infant or child play, crawl, walk, or climb to determine motor function and capability. Note any movement disorder. Infants with cerebral palsy may demonstrate abnormal use of muscle groups such as scooting on their back instead of crawling or walking.

Assess active and passive ROM. Pay particular attention to muscle tone. Though an increased or decreased resistance may be noted with passive movements, hypertonicity is most often seen. Increased resistance to dorsiflexion and passive hip abduction are the most common early signs. Sustained **clonus** (muscular spasm) may be present after forced dorsiflexion. Lift the child by placing your hands in the infant's or child's axillary area to assess shoulder girdle function and tone. Infants with cerebral palsy often demonstrate prolonged standing on their toes when supported in an upright standing position in this fashion. Lift the young child off the ground while the child holds your thumbs to test hand strength. Observe for the presence of limb deformity, as decreased use of an extremity (as in the case of hemiparesis) may result in shortening of the extremity compared to the other one.

LABORATORY AND DIAGNOSTIC TESTS

A complete history, physical examination, and ancillary investigations are the primary modality for establishing a diagnosis of cerebral palsy. The following laboratory and diagnostic tests will help determine whether cerebral palsy is the likely cause or whether another condition may be the cause of the child's symptoms. These tests also will be important in evaluating the severity of the child's physical disabilities. Common supplementary laboratory and diagnostic tests ordered for the diagnosis and assessment of cerebral palsy include:

- Electroencephalogram: usually abnormal but the pattern is highly variable
- Cranial radiographs or ultrasound: may show cerebral asymmetry
- MRI or CT: may show area of damage or abnormal development but may be normal
- Screening for metabolic defects and genetic testing may be performed to help determine the cause of cerebral palsy.

Nursing Management

In addition to the patient problems and related interventions discussed in the "Clinical Judgment and the Nursing Process" section earlier in the chapter, nursing management focuses on promoting growth and development by promoting mobility and maintaining optimal nutritional intake. Providing support and education to the child and family is also an important nursing function.

PROMOTING MOBILITY

Mobility is critical to the development of the child with cerebral palsy. Treatment modalities to promote mobility include physiotherapy, pharmacologic management, and surgery. Surgical procedures are discussed previously. Physical or occupational therapy as well as medications may be used to address musculoskeletal abnormalities, to facilitate ROM, to delay or prevent deformities such as contractures, to provide joint stability, to maximize activity, and to encourage the use of adaptive devices. The nurse's role in relation to the various therapies is to provide ongoing follow-through with prescribed exercises, positioning, or bracing.

When casting, splinting, or orthotics are used, assess skin integrity frequently. Pain management may also be necessary. Nursing management of children receiving botulin toxin focuses on assisting with the procedure and providing education and support to the child and family. Nursing interventions related to baclofen include assisting with the test dose and providing preoperative and postoperative care if a pump is placed, as well as providing support and education to the child and family. Teaching Guidelines 44.5 gives information related to baclofen pump insertion.

PROMOTING NUTRITION

Children with cerebral palsy may have difficulty eating and swallowing due to poor motor control of the mouth,

TEACHING GUIDELINES 44.5 Baclofen Pump: Child/Family Education

- Check the incisions daily for redness, drainage, or swelling.
- Notify the primary provider or nurse practitioner if the child has a temperature greater than 101.5°F, or if the child has persistent incision pain.
- Avoid tub baths for 2 weeks.
- Do not allow the child to sleep on the stomach for 4 weeks after pump insertion.
- Discourage twisting at the waist, reaching high overhead, stretching, or bending forward or backward for 4 weeks.
- When the incisions have healed, normal activity may be resumed.
- Wear loose clothing to prevent irritation at the incision site.
- Carry implanted device identification and emergency information cards at all times.

tongue, and throat. This may lead to poor nutrition and problems with growth. The child may require a longer time to eat because of poor motor control. Special diets, such as soft or puréed, may make swallowing easier. Proper positioning during feeding is essential to facilitate swallowing and reduce the risk of aspiration. Speech or occupational therapists can assist in working on strengthening swallowing muscles as well as assisting in developing accommodations to facilitate nutritional intake. Consult a dietitian to ensure adequate nutrition for children with cerebral palsy. In children with severe swallowing problems or malnutrition, a feeding tube such as a gastrostomy tube may be placed.

PROVIDING SUPPORT AND EDUCATION

Cerebral palsy is a lifelong disorder that can result in severe physical and cognitive disability. In some cases, disability may require complete intensive daily care of the child. Adjusting to the demands of this multifaceted illness is difficult. Children are frequently hospitalized and need numerous corrective surgeries, which places strain on the family and its finances. From the time of diagnosis, the family should be involved in the child's care. It is important to include parents in the planning of interventions and care of this child. In most cases, they are the primary caregivers and will assist the child in the development of functioning and skills as well as providing daily care. They will provide essential information to the health care team and will be advocates for their child throughout their life. It is important that nurses provide ongoing education for the child and family.

As the child grows, the needs of the family and child will change. Recognize and respect these needs. Providing daily intense care can be demanding and tiring. When a child with cerebral palsy is admitted to the hospital, this may serve as a time of respite for family and primary caregivers. Encourage respite care and provide support and encouragement. Because cerebral palsy is a lifelong condition, children will need meaningful education programs that emphasize independence in the least restrictive educational environment. Refer caregivers to local resources, including education services and support groups.

Refer children younger than age 3 years to the local early intervention service. Early intervention provides case management of developmental services for children with special needs. Each state has a coordinator for early intervention. The office of the early intervention coordinator can then direct the health care professional to the local or district early intervention office.

ACQUIRED DISORDERS

A number of neuromuscular and musculoskeletal disorders may be acquired during childhood or adolescence. These include rickets, slipped capital femoral epiphysis (SCFE), Legg–Calvé–Perthes disease, transient synovitis of the hip, and scoliosis (spinal curvature), which may occur as a result of a neuromuscular disorder or idiopathically.

Injuries throughout childhood are inevitable. Trauma or unintentional injury is a leading cause of childhood morbidity and mortality in the United States (Gill & Kelly, 2022). The child is at increased risk for trauma based on the developmental factors of physical and emotional immaturity; additionally, adolescents often display belief of invincibility. The developing neuromuscular system, if injured, may be irreparable, so the injury may result in life-threatening or lifelong effects. Neuromuscular trauma includes spinal cord injury and birth trauma. Birth trauma is discussed in Chapter 24. Younger children tend to suffer contusions, sprains, and simple upper extremity fractures; adolescents more frequently experience lower extremity trauma. As the number of children participating in youth sports increases and the intensity of training and the level of competition also increase, the incidence of injury is also likely to increase. Many types of musculoskeletal injuries exist. This discussion will focus on fractures, sprains, overuse syndromes, and dislocated radial head.

Rickets

Rickets is a condition in which there is softening or weakening of the bones. Childhood rickets may occur as a result of nutritional deficiencies such as inadequate consumption of calcium or vitamin D or limited exposure to sunlight (required for adequate production of vitamin D). Rickets caused by vitamin D deficiency is a preventable condition, but cases continue to be reported in infants, children, and adolescents (Misra, 2022). Rickets may also occur if the body cannot regulate calcium and phosphorus in the appropriate balance, such as in chronic kidney disease. Gastrointestinal disorders in which fat absorption is altered (e.g., Crohn disease, celiac disease, and cystic fibrosis) may lead to rickets, as vitamin D is a fat-soluble vitamin.

Calcium is primarily laid down in the bones of the fetus during the third trimester. Premature infants miss this period of calcium accumulation and also suffer from inadequate calcium intake in the neonatal period. Thus, premature infants often demonstrate rickets of prematurity. Regardless of the underlying cause, rickets is most likely to occur during periods of rapid growth.

Vitamin D regulates calcium absorption from the small intestine and levels of calcium and phosphate in the bones. When calcium and phosphate levels in the blood are imbalanced, calcium is released from the bones into the blood, resulting in the loss of the supportive bony matrix.

Therapeutic Management

Treatment of rickets is aimed at correcting the calcium imbalance so that the skeleton may develop properly and without deformity. Calcium and phosphorus supplements are given, and some children also require vitamin D supplements. If rickets is not corrected while the child is still growing, permanent skeletal deformities and short stature may result.

> **TAKE NOTE!**
>
> The Academy of Pediatrics currently recommends all infants have a minimum daily intake of 400 IU of vitamin D beginning soon after birth and children 1 to 18 years of age have a minimum daily intake of 600 IU of vitamin D (Misra, 2022).

Nursing Assessment

Obtain a health history, determining risk factors such as:

- Limited exposure to sunlight
- Strict vegetarian diet or lactose intolerance (either one without milk product ingestion)
- Exclusive chest or breastfeeding by a person who has a vitamin D deficiency
- Dark-pigmented skin
- Prematurity
- Malabsorptive gastrointestinal disorder
- Chronic kidney disease

Note history of fractures or bone pain. Observe for dental deformities and bowlegs. Decreased muscle tone may also be present. Note low serum calcium and phosphate levels and high alkaline phosphatase levels. Radiographs may show changes in the shape and structure of the bone.

Nursing Management

Administer calcium and phosphorus supplements at alternate times to promote proper absorption of both of these supplements. Encourage exposure to moderate amounts of sunlight and administer vitamin D supplements as prescribed. Teach families that good dietary sources of vitamin D are fish, liver, and processed milk.

Slipped Capital Femoral Epiphysis

SCFE is a condition in which the femoral head dislocates from the neck and shaft of the femur at the level of the epiphyseal plate. The epiphysis slips downward and backward. The left hip is more often affected (Kienstra & Macias, 2022a; Sankar et al., 2020). The exact cause is unknown, but it is thought that during the adolescent growth spurt, the femoral growth plate weakens and becomes less resistant to stressors. Hormonal alterations during this period may also play a role.

SCFE is classified based on its severity and whether the slip is acute or chronic. Chronic SCFE may lead to shortening of the affected leg and thigh atrophy.

Therapeutic Management

Promptly refer the child with SCFE to an orthopedic surgeon, as early surgical intervention will decrease the risk of long-term deformity. The goals of therapeutic management are to prevent further slippage, minimize deformity, and avoid the complications of cartilage necrosis (chondrolysis) and avascular necrosis of the femoral head. Surgical intervention may include in situ pinning, in which a pin or screw is inserted percutaneously into the femoral head to hold it in place. Osteotomy may be used for more severe cases. Osteoarthritis may be a long-term complication of SCFE.

Nursing Assessment

Elicit a health history, determining the onset and extent of pain. In acute SCFE, the pain is usually sudden in onset and results in an inability to bear weight. Chronic SCFE may present with an insidious onset of pain and limp. Note risk factors for SCFE, including obesity (significant risk factor), age 9 to 16 years, African American or Polynesian heritage, sedentary lifestyle, rapid growth spurt, and male sex (slightly higher incidence seen in males) (Kienstra & Macias, 2022a; Sankar et al., 2020). Observe ambulation, noting Trendelenburg gait. Assess for pain that is in the hip or that is referred to the groin, medial thigh, or knee. Note decreased ROM in the affected hip with external rotation. Radiographs will be obtained to confirm the diagnosis (anteroposterior and lateral frog-leg views of hips). Bone scan can rule out avascular necrosis, and CT scan helps define the extent of slippage.

> **TAKE NOTE!**
>
> Do not attempt to perform passive ROM to determine the extent of limitation in the child with SCFE; this may cause worsening of the condition.

Nursing Management

Enforce bed rest and activity restriction. If traction is used for a period before surgery, perform routine traction care and neurovascular assessments. Provide routine pre- and postoperative care. Assess pain and administer analgesics as needed. After in situ pinning, assist the child with crutch walking. Teach the family that weight bearing is usually resumed about a week after the surgery and that the pin will be removed later. Prolonged immobility may isolate the adolescent from usual peer interactions, so encourage phone calls or texting, and visits with friends. Provide books, games, electronic devices, and magazines for distraction during the period of immobility. Provide education and support to the child and family.

Legg–Calvé–Perthes Disease

Legg–Calvé–Perthes disease is a self-limiting condition that involves avascular necrosis of the femoral head. It most often affects males between 4 and 8 years of age (Sankar et al., 2020). The etiology is unknown, but interruption of the blood supply to the femoral head results in bone death, and the spherical shape of the femoral head may be lost. Swelling of the soft tissues around the hip may occur. As new blood vessels develop, the area is supplied with circulation, allowing bone resorption and deposition to take place. During this period of revascularization, which takes 18 to 24 months, the bone is soft and more likely to fracture. Over time, the femoral head reforms.

Therapeutic Management

The goal of therapeutic management is to maintain normal femoral head shape and to restore appropriate motion. Treatment of Legg–Calvé–Perthes disease includes antiinflammatory medication to decrease muscle spasms around the hip joint and to relieve pain. Activity limitation may be prescribed, and sometimes bracing, casting, or traction is recommended to contain the femoral head. Serial x-ray follow-up determines the progress of the disease. If surgery becomes warranted, which is rarely done, then osteotomy may be performed. Complications include joint deformity, early degenerative joint disease, persistent pain, loss of hip motion or function, and gait disturbance.

Nursing Assessment

Explore the health history for short stature, delayed bone maturation, related trauma, or a family history of Legg–Calvé–Perthes disease. Note painless limp, which may be intermittent over a period of months. Mild hip pain may result and may be referred to the knee or the thigh. Pain may be aggravated by exercise. Observe the child walking and note Trendelenburg gait. Perform ROM, noting internal rotation of the hip and limited abduction. Muscle spasm may result with hip extension and rotation. Hip radiographs are obtained to evaluate the extent of epiphyseal involvement. MRI or bone scan may also be used to differentiate Legg–Calvé–Perthes disease from other disorders. Ultrasound and arthrograms may also be useful.

Nursing Management

Nursing care of Legg–Calvé–Perthes disease is highly variable and depends on the stage of the disease and its severity. Administer antiinflammatory medications, noting their effect on pain. If activities are restricted, exercise the unaffected body parts. Assist families with the use of the brace if prescribed. The brace may be wiped with a damp cloth if it becomes dirty. Some children will be prescribed no treatment other than avoidance of contact or high-impact sports. Swimming and bicycle riding help to maintain ROM with little risk. If mobility equipment is needed, educate the child and family on its use. If osteotomy is performed, provide routine postoperative care, including education and support of the child and family.

Transient Synovitis of the Hip

Transient synovitis of the hip (also termed toxic synovitis) is a common cause of hip pain and limping in children in the United States, typically occurring in children between 3 and 8 years of age (Sankar et al., 2020). The exact cause is unclear, but it is thought to be associated with recent or active infection, trauma, or allergic hypersensitivity (Sankar et al., 2020). It is a self-limiting disease, and most cases resolve within a week, but it may last as long as 3 to 6 weeks.

Typically, it is a clinical diagnosis with laboratory and radiographic tests used to rule out other serious conditions. Therapeutic management involves nonsteroidal antiinflammatory medications, analgesics, and bed rest to relieve weight bearing on the affected hip joint.

Nursing Assessment

Explore the health history for risk factors such as antecedent trauma, concurrent or recent upper respiratory tract infection, pharyngitis, or otitis media. Note sudden acute onset of moderate to severe pain in one hip. Sometimes pain is referred to the anterior thigh or knee. Pain is usually the worst upon arising in the morning, and the child refuses to walk; pain then decreases throughout the day. Temperature usually will be normal or low grade (less than 38°C). Observe for a limp or for refusal to bear weight. Observe position of the affected hip: It will be held in a flexed and externally rotated position. Note restricted ROM for abduction and internal rotation.

Nursing Management

Nursing care focuses on educating the family including instructions on administering nonsteroidal antiinflammatory medications, analgesics, and bed rest. Parents are very concerned when their child refuses to walk; therefore, provide significant support and reassure the child and family of the self-limiting nature of the disease.

TABLE 44.6 • Types of Scoliosis

Type	Associated Factors
Idiopathic	Unknown cause Infantile: occurs in the first 3 years of life Juvenile: diagnosed between age 4 and 10 years, or prior to adolescence Adolescent: age 11–17 years
Neuromuscular	Associated with neurologic or muscular disease such as cerebral palsy, myelomeningocele, spinal cord tumors, spinal muscular atrophy, muscular dystrophies
Congenital	Results from anomalous vertebral development

Scoliosis

Scoliosis is a lateral curvature of the spine that exceeds 10 degrees. It may be congenital, associated with other disorders, or idiopathic. Table 44.6 explains the types of scoliosis. Idiopathic scoliosis, with the majority of cases occurring during adolescence, is the most common scoliosis (Mistovich & Spiegel, 2020b). Hence, this discussion will focus on adolescent idiopathic scoliosis. The etiology of idiopathic scoliosis is not known, but genetic factors, growth abnormalities, and bone, muscle, disk, or central nervous system disorders may contribute to its development. Early screening and detection of scoliosis result in improved outcomes.

Pathophysiology

In the rapidly growing adolescent, the involved vertebrae rotate around a vertical axis, resulting in lateral curvature, and asymmetry of the shoulder and waistline is evident. The vertebrae rotate to the convex side of the curve, with the spinous processes rotating toward the concave side, resulting in displacement of the ribs and rib asymmetry (Mistovich & Spiegel, 2020b). As the curve progresses, the shape of the thoracic cage continues to change, and respiratory and cardiovascular compromise may occur (the main complications of severe scoliosis).

BOX 44.2 Types of Braces Used to Treat Scoliosis

- Underarm (thoracolumbosacral orthosis [TLSO], Boston, Wilmington): for low thoracic and thoracolumbar curves; less conspicuous, no visible neckpiece
- Milwaukee: for thoracic or major double curves; traditional, standard, has a visible neckpiece with chin rest
- Nighttime bending (Charleston): creates a curve so severe that walking is not possible, so can be worn only at night

Therapeutic Management

Treatment of scoliosis is aimed at preventing progression of the curve and decreasing the impact on pulmonary and cardiac function. Treatment is based on the age of the child, expected future growth, and severity of the curve. Observation with serial examinations and spine radiographs is used to monitor curve progression. For curves of 25 to 45 degrees, bracing may be sufficient to decrease progression of the curve (Mistovich & Spiegel, 2020b). Box 44.2 describes types of scoliosis braces, and Figure 44.27 shows examples of braces. The choice of brace will depend on the location and severity of the curve. Some curves will progress despite appropriate bracing and compliance.

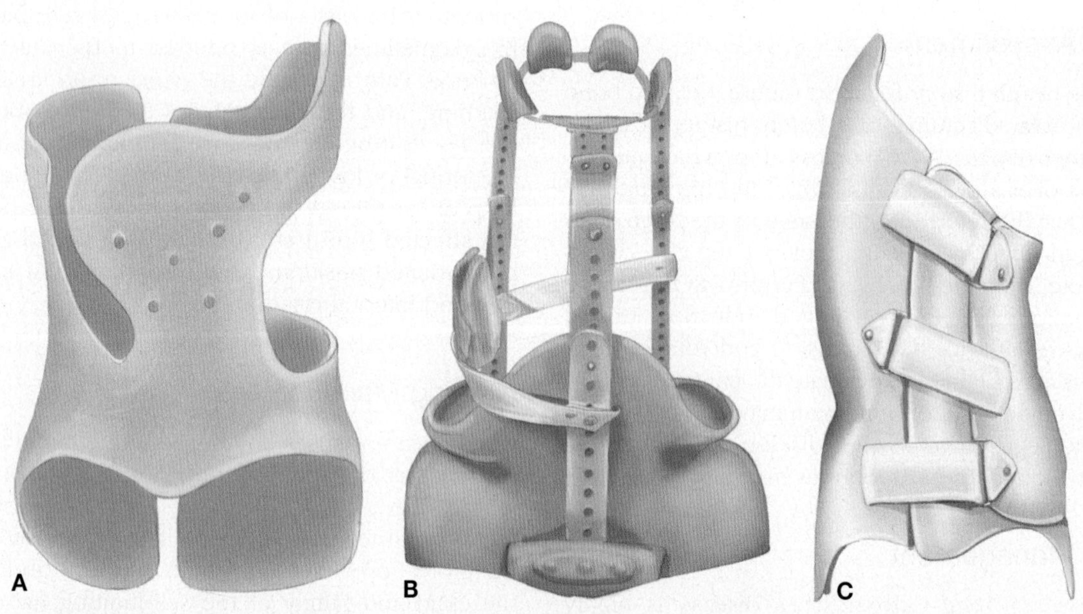

FIGURE 44.27 **A.** Boston brace. **B.** Milwaukee brace. **C.** Nighttime bending brace.

Surgical correction is often required for curves greater than 45 degrees; it is achieved with rod placement and bone grafting (Mistovich & Spiegel, 2020b). Partial spinal fusion accompanies many of the corrective surgeries. Multiple surgical approaches and techniques with various instrumentation methods exist for fusion and rod placement. The surgical approach may be anterior, posterior, or both. Traditional rod placement (Harrington rod) involves a single rod fused to the vertebrae, resulting in curve correction but also a flat-backed appearance. Newer rod instrumentations allow for scoliosis curve correction with maintenance of normal back curvature. The rods are shorter, and several are wired or grafted to the appropriate vertebrae to achieve correction. Figure 44.28 shows one example of surgical rod instrumentation. Newer minimally invasive techniques also exist, such as growth modulation techniques (Scherl & Hasley, 2023).

Nursing Assessment

For a full description of the assessment phase of the nursing process, refer to the "Clinical Judgment and the Nursing Process" section earlier in the chapter. Assessment findings pertinent to scoliosis are discussed below.

HEALTH HISTORY

Determine why the child is presenting for evaluation of scoliosis. Commonly the child or adolescent will not report back pain; only mild discomfort is associated with idiopathic scoliosis until the curve becomes severe. Often the family recognizes asymmetry in the hips or shoulders or the child is screened for scoliosis at school and determined to be at risk. Explore the child's current and past medical history for risk factors such as:

- Family history of scoliosis
- Recent growth spurt
- Physical changes related to puberty

Determine the age of development of secondary sex characteristics and the age of menarche, as these signs of pubertal development indicate the expected velocity and length of remaining growth.

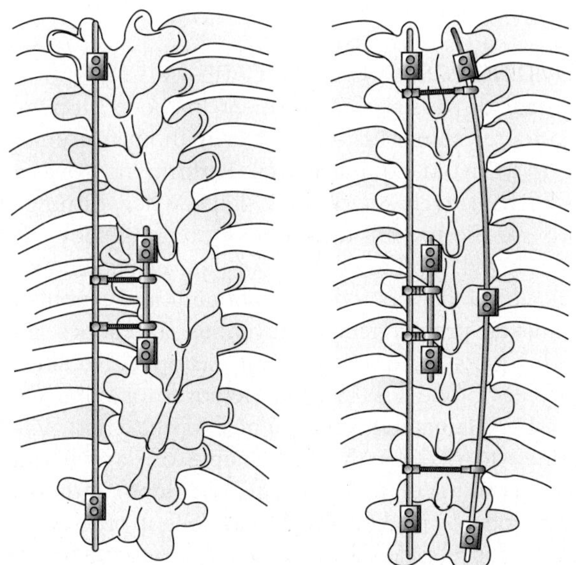

FIGURE 44.28 Rods are fused to the vertebrae and connected to a distracting rod to rotate the vertebral column (Cotrel–Dubousset method is shown).

PHYSICAL EXAMINATION

The physical assessment of a child with possible or actual scoliosis involves mainly inspection and observation. Auscultate the heart and lungs to determine compromise related to severe curvature.

Observe the child at rest, sitting, and standing for evidence of poor posture. Inspect the child's back in a standing position. Note asymmetries such as shoulder elevation, prominence of one scapula, uneven curve at the waistline, or a rib hump on one side. Measure shoulder levels from the floor to the acromioclavicular joints. Note the difference between the height of the high and low shoulder in centimeters. Measure heights of anterior and posterior iliac spines and note the difference in centimeters. View the child from the side, noting abnormalities in the spinal curve. With the child bending forward, arms hanging freely, note asymmetry of the back (pronounced hump on one side). Figure 44.29 shows scoliosis noted upon visual inspection. Note leg-length discrepancy if present. During the neurologic examination, balance, motor strength, sensation, and reflexes should all be normal.

LABORATORY AND DIAGNOSTIC TESTS

Full-spine radiographs are necessary to determine the degree of curvature. The radiologist will determine the extent of the curve based on specific formulas and techniques of measurement.

Nursing Management

The "Clinical Judgment and the Nursing Process" section earlier in the chapter lists general interventions. Tailor nursing care based on the adolescent's response to the disease and its treatment. Additional nursing interventions specific to scoliosis are discussed here.

ENCOURAGING COMPLIANCE WITH BRACING

Bracing is intended to prevent progression of the curve but does not correct the current curve. Although modern braces display an improved appearance, with no visible neckpiece, and can be worn under clothes, many adolescents are not compliant with brace wear. The brace is recommended to be worn 18 hours per day to prevent curve progression, although recent studies have found

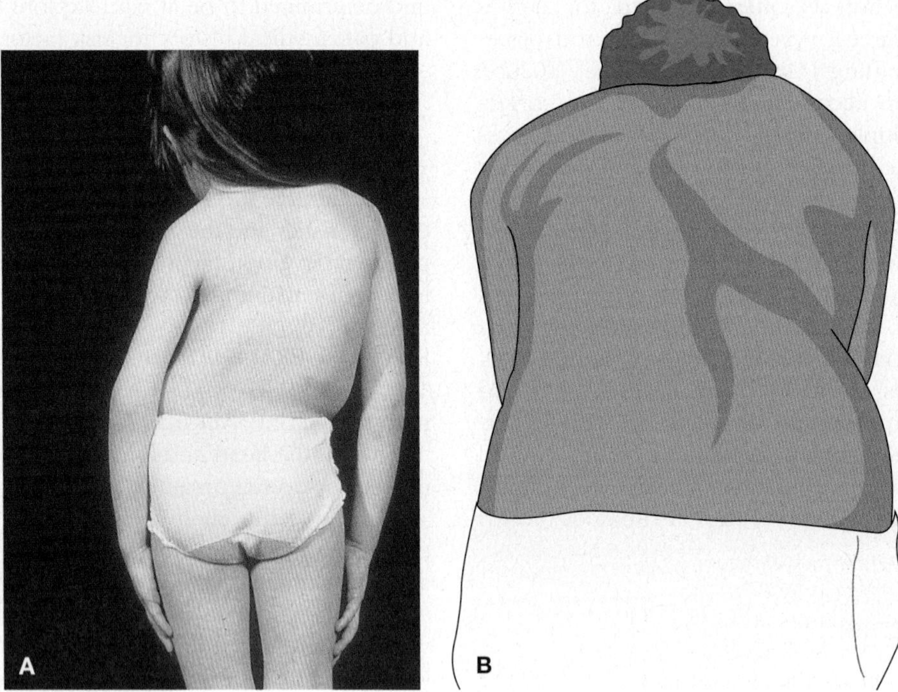

FIGURE 44.29 **A.** Note right shoulder, scapula, and hip elevation as well as discrepancy in waist curvature. **B.** Note right upper back hump.

13 hours to be sufficient in some cases (Scherl & Hasley, 2023). Many factors may contribute to noncompliance, including the discomfort associated with brace wear such as pain, heat, and poor fit. The family environment may not be conducive to compliance with brace wear, and adolescents are concerned about body image.

Inspect the skin for evidence of rubbing by the brace that may impair skin integrity. Teach families appropriate skin care and recommend they check the brace daily for fit and breakage. Encourage the adolescent to shower during the time of day that the brace is off and to ensure that the skin is clean and dry before putting the brace back on. Wearing a cotton T-shirt under the brace may decrease some of the discomfort associated with brace wear. Exercises to strengthen back muscles may prevent muscle atrophy from prolonged bracing and maintain spine flexibility.

PROMOTING POSITIVE BODY IMAGE

Encourage the adolescent to express their feelings or concerns about wearing the brace. Give the adolescent ways to explain scoliosis and its treatment to their peers. Wearing stylish baggy clothes may help the adolescent to conceal the brace if desired. Refer adolescents and their families to the National Scoliosis Foundation for additional support.

PROVIDING PREOPERATIVE CARE

If the curve progresses despite bracing or causes pulmonary or cardiac compromise, surgical intervention will be warranted. Before surgery, teach the adolescent the importance of turning, coughing, and deep breathing in the postoperative period. Explain the tubes and lines that will be present immediately after the surgery. Review positioning guidelines: Back flexion or extension will not be allowed. Introduce the child to the patient-controlled analgesia pump and explain pain scales. There is a high risk for significant blood loss with spinal fusion and instrumentation, so if possible, arrange for preoperative autologous blood donation.

PROVIDING POSTOPERATIVE CARE

The goal of nursing management in the postoperative period after spinal fusion with or without instrumentation is to avoid complications. Perform neurovascular checks with each set of vital signs. When turning the child, use the log-roll technique to avoid flexion of the back (Fig. 44.30). Provide proper pain management and medicate for pain before repositioning and ambulation. Administer prophylactic intravenous antibiotics if ordered. Assess for drainage from the operative site and for excess blood loss via the Hemovac or other drainage tube. Maintain Foley patency, as the child will be confined to bed for the first couple of days. Maintain strict recording of fluid intake and output. Administer transfusions of packed red blood cells if ordered. Ambulation, once ordered, should be done slowly to avoid orthostatic hypotension. Assist the family with arrangements to continue the adolescent's school work while hospitalized and/or arrange for home tutoring during the several-week recovery period.

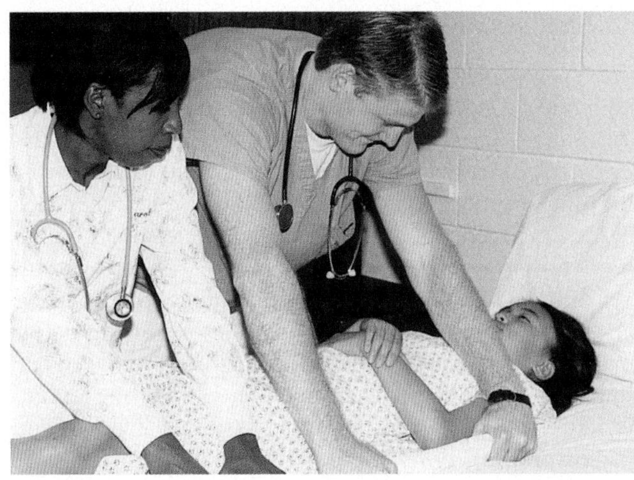

FIGURE 44.30 Log-roll the postoperative spinal fusion child to prevent spine flexion.

CONSIDER THIS!

I have been diagnosed with scoliosis and the doctor told me I have to wear a brace at night. How did this happen? I will never be able to go to another sleepover; all the other kids will laugh at me.

Thoughts: How would you respond to their concerns? What education will be necessary and how can you promote compliance?

What local resources could you refer them to?

Spinal Cord Injury

Spinal cord injury is damage to the spinal cord that results in loss of function. Frequent causes are trauma, such as car accidents, falls, diving into shallow water, gunshot or stab wounds, sports injuries, child abuse, or birth injuries. Spinal cord injuries are relatively uncommon in children, but when they do occur, they have a devastating impact on the child's physical and functional status, social and emotional development, and family functioning.

Spinal cord injury is a medical emergency, and immediate medical attention is required. Cervical traction is often used initially, and surgical intervention is sometimes necessary. Ongoing medical treatment will be based on the child's age and overall health and the extent and location of the injury. Therapeutic management focuses on rehabilitation and prevention of complications. Spinal cord injury in children is managed similarly to that in adults.

Nursing Assessment

Symptoms vary based on the location and severity of the injury. Common signs and symptoms associated with spinal cord injury include:

- Inability to move or feel extremities
- Numbness
- Tingling
- Weakness

Paralysis depends on the location of the injury to the spinal cord; the higher the injury in the spinal cord, the more extensive the damage and the greater the loss of function. High cervical injury will result in damage to the phrenic nerve, which innervates the diaphragm. Damage to this nerve will leave the child unable to breathe without assistance.

The diagnosis of spinal cord injury is made by clinical signs and diagnostic tests, which may include radiographs, CT scans, and MRI.

Nursing Management

Any child who requires hospitalization due to trauma should be considered at risk for a spinal cord injury. Immobilization of the spine is essential until full evaluation of the injury is complete and spinal cord damage is ruled out. Nursing management will be similar to the management of the adult with a spinal cord injury and will focus on optimizing mobility, promoting bladder and bowel management, promoting adequate nutritional status, preventing complications associated with extreme immobility such as contractures and muscle atrophy, managing pain, and providing support and education to the child and family. Refer to the "Myelomeningocele" section of this chapter for information related to urinary and bowel elimination.

The nurse plays an important role not only in the acute care of children with spinal cord injury but also during rehabilitation. Recovery from a spinal cord injury requires long-term hospitalization and rehabilitation. An interdisciplinary team of primary providers, nurses, therapists, social workers, and case managers will work to manage the child's complex and long-term needs. Promoting communication among the interdisciplinary team is essential and will be a key nursing function. Rehabilitation will need to focus on the everchanging developmental needs of the child as they grow.

Prevention of spinal cord injuries is an important nursing consideration. Educate the public on vehicular safety, including seat belt use and the proper use of age-appropriate safety seats. Additional education topics include bicycle, sports, and recreation safety; prevention of falls; violence prevention including gun safety; and water safety, including the risk of diving. This education can help decrease the incidence of spinal cord injury in children.

Fracture

Fractures occur frequently in children and adolescents, and common sites include fingers, the forearm, and wrist (Baldwin et al., 2020). Most pediatric fractures heal well with minimal treatment (Baldwin et al., 2020). Midclavicular, humerus, or femur fractures can occur as a result of birth trauma. They typically heal well but may require limiting mobility or splinting. Several factors contribute to differences in pediatric fractures compared to adult fractures. Different fracture patterns are seen due to the anatomic, biomechanical, and physiologic differences in the pediatric immature skeleton (see "Pathophysiology" sectiont) (Baldwin et al., 2020). When caring for children with fractures, the caregiver must consider their high activity level and their continued skeletal growth and development. Fractures in children result most frequently from accidental trauma (Baldwin et al., 2020). Nonaccidental trauma (child abuse) and other disease processes are the other causes of fractures.

CLINICAL REASONING ALERT!

Fracture in the newborn (with the exception of birth trauma) or infant should raise a high index of suspicion for abuse, as fractures are very unusual in children who cannot yet walk.

Pathophysiology

The growth plate is the most vulnerable portion of the child's bone and is frequently the site of injury. The Salter–Harris classification system is used to describe fractures involving the growth plate (Table 44.7). The thicker, more elastic periosteum in children yields to the force encountered with trauma, resulting more frequently in nondisplaced fractures in children. The increased vascularity and decreased mineral content make the child's bones more flexible. Plastic or bowing deformities and buckle and greenstick fractures are the result. Complete fractures do occur in children, but they tend to be more stable than in the adult, resulting in improved healing and function. Spiral, pelvic, and hip fractures are rare in children. Table 44.8 explains common types of fractures in children.

Fractures in children heal more rapidly and result in less disability and deformity than adults. The younger the child, the more quickly the bone heals. However,

TABLE 44.7 • The Salter–Harris Classification System

Type	Description	Illustration
I	Fracture is through the physis, widening it.	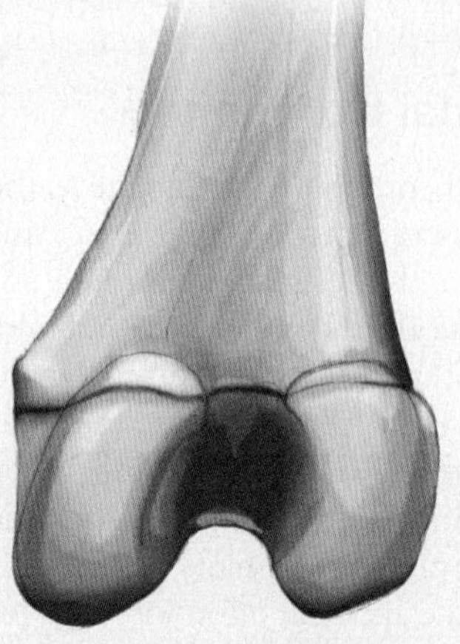
II	Fracture is partially through the physis, extending into the metaphysis.	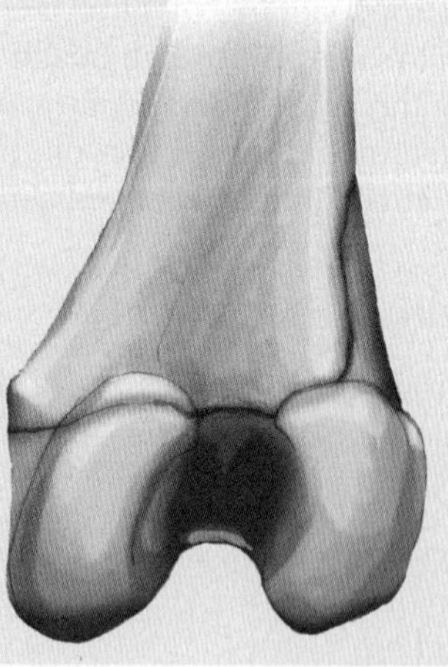

TABLE 44.7 • The Salter–Harris Classification System

Type	Description	Illustration
III	Fracture is partially through the epiphysis, extending into the epiphysis.	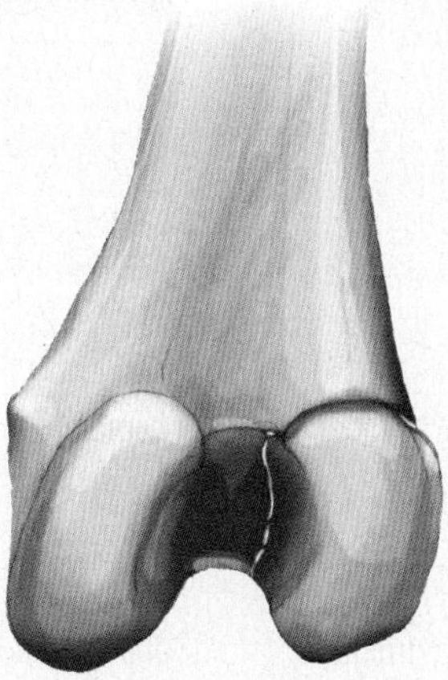
IV	Fracture is through the metaphysis, physis, and epiphysis.	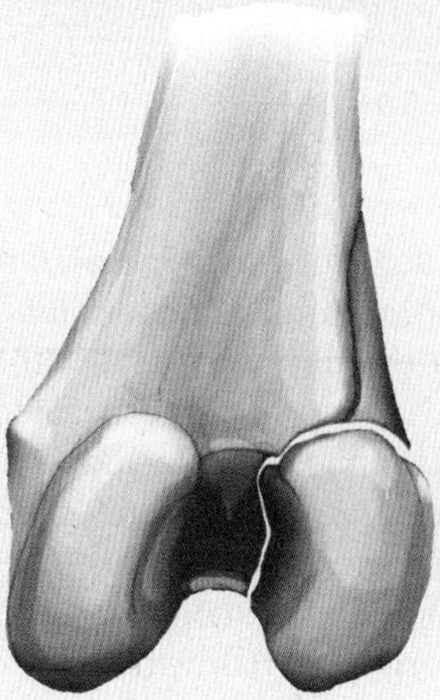
V	Crushing injury to the physis	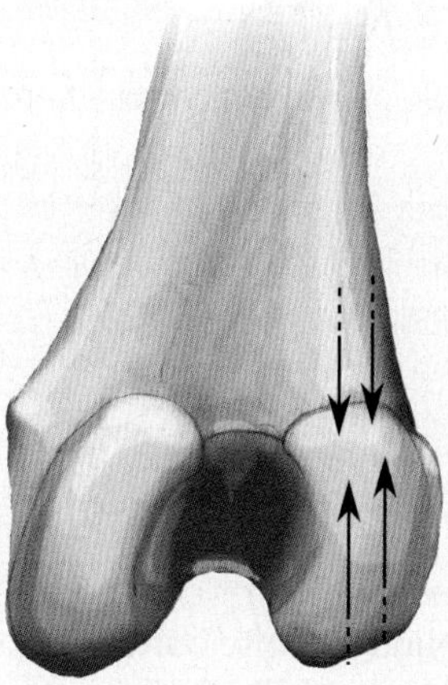

TABLE 44.8 • Types of Fractures in Children

Fracture Type	Description	Illustration
Plastic or bowing deformity	Significant bending without breaking of the bone	A
Buckle fracture	Compression injury; the bone buckles rather than breaks.	B
Greenstick fracture	Incomplete fracture of the bone	C
Complete fracture	Bone breaks into two pieces.	D

plastic deformity and Salter–Harris type IV fractures may result in an angular deformity. Though healing of fractures is usually quick and without incident in children, delayed union, nonunion, or malunion can occur. Additional complications include infection, avascular necrosis, bone shortening from epiphyseal arrest, vascular or nerve injuries, fat embolism, reflex sympathetic dystrophy, and compartment syndrome, which is an orthopedic emergency (Baldwin et al., 2020).

TAKE NOTE!

Any type of fracture can be the result of child abuse, but spiral femur fractures, rib fractures, and humerus fractures, particularly in the child younger than 2 years of age, should always be thoroughly investigated to rule out the possibility of abuse (Baldwin et al., 2020).

Therapeutic Management

The vast majority of childhood fractures would heal well with splinting only, but casting of these fractures is performed to provide further comfort to the child and to allow for increased activity while the fracture is healing. Displaced fractures require manual traction to align the bones, followed by casting. More severe fractures may require traction for a period of time, usually followed by casting. Severe or complicated fractures may alternatively require open reduction and internal fixation for healing to occur. Complex fractures are often treated with external fixation (Fig. 44.31).

TAKE NOTE!

Significant swelling may occur initially after immobilization with a splint. Delaying casting for a few days provides time for some of the swelling to subside, allowing for successful casting a few days after the injury.

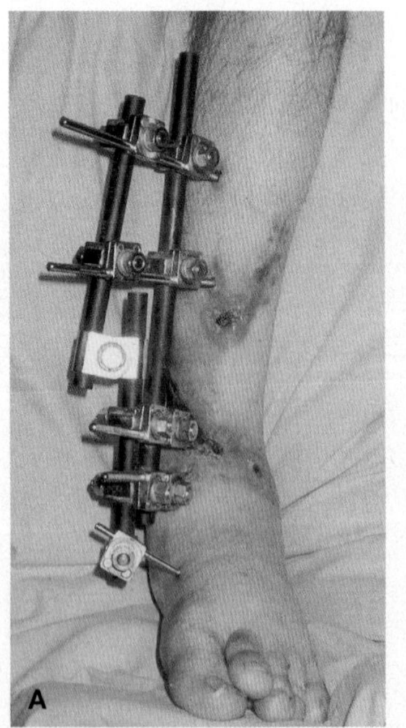

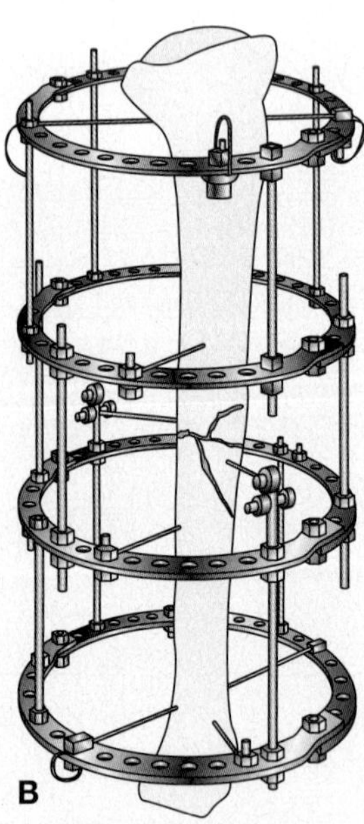

FIGURE 44.31 **A.** External fixation is required for complicated fractures. **B.** The Ilizarov fixator is a circular apparatus usually used for complicated lower extremity fractures. The pins are smaller in diameter, more like wires, than those used in other fixators.

Nursing Assessment

For a full description of the assessment phase of the nursing process, refer to the "Clinical Judgment and the Nursing Process" section earlier in the chapter. Assessment findings pertinent to fractures are discussed below.

HEALTH HISTORY

Elicit a description of the present illness and chief complaint. Common signs and symptoms reported during the health history might include recent injury, trauma, or fall; complaint of pain; difficulty bearing weight; limp; or refusal to use an extremity. Young children often demonstrate sudden onset of irritability and refusal to bear weight. Ask about the mechanism of injury and obtain a description of the traumatic event. Be alert to inconsistencies between the history and the clinical picture or mechanism of injury; inconsistency may be an indicator of child abuse. Explore the child's current and past medical history for risk factors such as:

- Rickets
- Renal osteodystrophy
- OI
- Participation in sports, particularly contact sports
- Failure to use protective equipment as recommended for various physical activities and sports (e.g., wrist guards while rollerblading)

PHYSICAL EXAMINATION

Perform the physical examination of the child with a potential fracture carefully, so as not to cause further pain or trauma. The physical examination particular to fractures includes inspection, observation, and palpation.

> **TAKE NOTE!**
>
> Do not attempt to straighten or manipulate an injured limb.

Inspection and Observation

Inspect the skin for bruising, erythema, or swelling. Observe the extremities for deformity. Note neglect of an extremity or an inability to bear weight. If ambulating, note any limp.

Palpation

Carefully palpate the joint or injured part. Distract the young child with a toy or activity while palpating. Note point tenderness, which is a reliable indicator of fracture in children. Assess neurovascular status, noting distal extremity temperature, spontaneous movement, sensation, numbness, capillary refill time, and quality of pulses. The neurovascular assessment is critical to providing a baseline so that any changes associated with compartment syndrome can be identified quickly.

LABORATORY AND DIAGNOSTIC TESTS

Usually, plain x-ray films are all that is required to identify a simple fracture. Complicated fractures that require surgical intervention may require further evaluation with CT or MRI.

Nursing Management

Immediately after the injury, immobilize the limb above and below the site of injury in the most comfortable position with a splint. Use cold therapy to reduce swelling in the first 48 hours after injury. Elevate the injured extremity above the level of the heart. Perform frequent neurovascular checks.

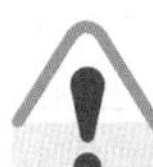

> **CLINICAL REASONING ALERT!**
>
> Assess the injured, splinted, or casted extremity frequently for the "5 Ps," which may indicate compartment syndrome: pain (increased out of proportion), pulselessness, pallor, paresthesia, and paralysis. Report these findings immediately.

Assess pain level and administer pain medications as needed. Utilize nonpharmacologic methods of pain relief as needed. Administer tetanus vaccine in the child with an open fracture if they have not received a tetanus booster within the past 5 years. Additional nursing interventions include providing family education and teaching on fracture prevention.

PROVIDING FAMILY EDUCATION

Unless bed rest is prescribed, children with upper extremity casts and "walking" leg casts can resume increased levels of activity as the pain subsides. Children who require crutches while in a cast may return to school, but those in spica casts will be at home for several weeks. Providing distraction and finding ways to keep up with school work are important. Teach families to care for the cast (see Teaching Guidelines 44.1).

PREVENTING FRACTURES

Discourage risky behavior such as climbing trees and performing tricks on bicycles. Provide appropriate supervision, particularly with outdoor activity. Encourage appropriate use of protective equipment, such as wrist guards with rollerblading and shin guards with soccer. Ensure that playground equipment is in good working order and intact; there should not be protruding screws or unbalanced portions of equipment, which may increase the risk for falling.

Sprains

Sprains result from a twisting or turning motion of the affected body part. The tendons and ligaments stretch excessively and may tear slightly. They are uncommon in young children as their growth plates are weaker than their muscles and tendons, making them more prone to fracture. They may occur at any joint, but the most common are ankle and knee sprains. Therapeutic management of sprains includes rest, ice, compression, and elevation (RICE). Other treatment options may include activity restrictions, splints or casts, crutches or wheelchair, and physical therapy. On initial evaluation, sprains need to be differentiated from torn ligaments and meniscal tears, as those conditions are more serious and may require surgical intervention.

Nursing Assessment

Elicit a health history, determining the mechanism of injury (whether it occurred during sports or simply a misstep or fall). Determine what treatment the family has used so far. Inspect the affected body part for edema, which is frequently present, and bruising, which sometimes occurs. Note limp or inability to bear weight. Do not attempt to perform passive ROM on the affected body part. Assess neurovascular status distal to the injury (usually normal).

Nursing Management

Instruct the child and family on appropriate treatment of sprains, which includes:

- Rest: Limit activity.
- Ice: Apply cold packs for 20 to 30 minutes, remove for 1 hour, and repeat (for the first 24 to 48 hours).
- Compression: Apply an Ace wrap or other elastic bandage or brace; check skin for alterations when rewrapping.
- Elevation: Elevate the injured extremity above the level of the heart to decrease swelling (Fig. 44.32).

The child may require instruction in crutch walking as well. Teach families that to prevent sprains during sports, it is important for the child to perform appropriate stretching and warm-up activities.

> **TAKE NOTE!**
>
> If the child's fingers or toes become increasingly swollen or discolored, remove the Ace wrap immediately.

Overuse Syndromes

The term "overuse syndrome" refers to a group of disorders that result from repeated force applied to normal tissue. The connective tissues fail in response to repetitive stress, leading to a small amount of tissue breakdown. They develop over the course of weeks to months. There is usually no identifiable injury associated with overuse syndromes. Pain is usually associated with the activity and worsens with continued participation in the activity. The incidence of overuse injuries in the young athlete has increased as participation of youths in organized sports has grown along with children today participating in sports year-round and sometimes in multiple sports simultaneously, the increased competitive nature of youth sports, and the early specialization in a particular sport with inadequate periods of rest (Brenner & The Council on Sports Medicine and Fitness, 2007 [reaffirmed 2021]). The young athlete is at risk for more serious overuse injuries due to the following:

- The growing bones of the young athlete cannot handle as much stress as mature bones in adults. Growth

RICE

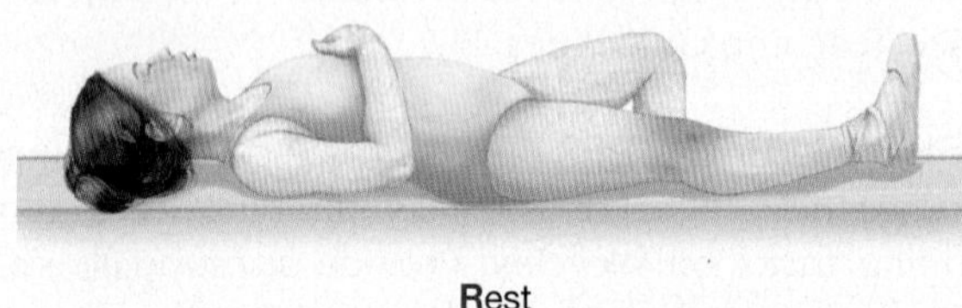

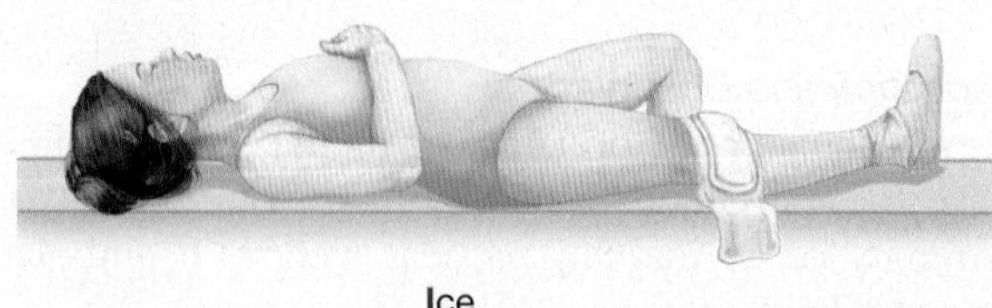

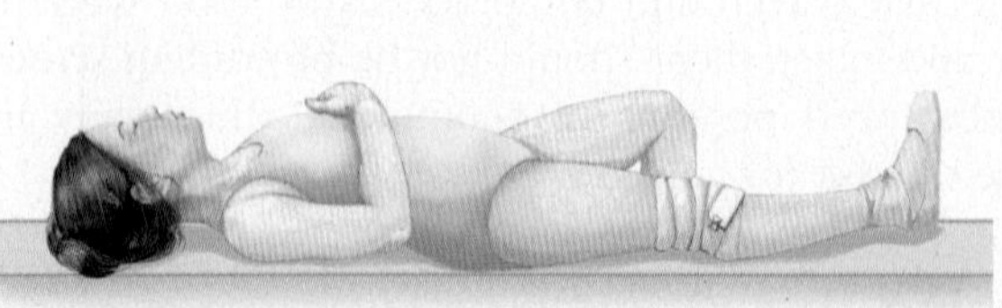
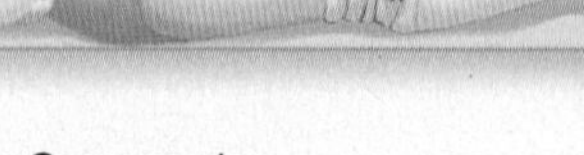

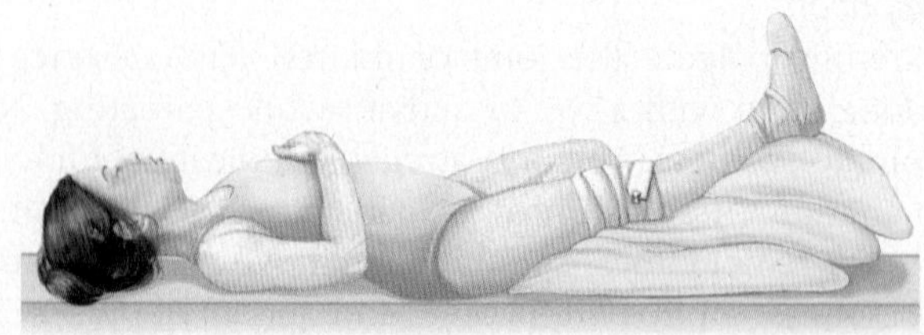

FIGURE 44.32 RICE (rest, ice, compression, elevation) is the appropriate treatment for sprains.

patterns are often uneven. Bones grow faster than muscles, leaving the child more susceptible to injury.
- The child is just learning the proper mechanisms for skills, such as throwing a baseball.
- The child is unable to recognize vague signs of injury such as fatigue and poor performance (Brenner & The Council on Sports Medicine and Fitness, 2007 [reaffirmed 2021]).

Table 44.9 gives details on several common overuse syndromes. Therapeutic management is aimed at reassurance, pain management, and limiting rather than eliminating activity.

Nursing Assessment

Elicit a health history to determine the extent of involvement in sports. Note the onset of pain, duration, intensity, aggravating factors, and treatments used at home. Examine the painful part, noting findings similar to those noted for each syndrome in Table 44.9.

Nursing Management

Initially, apply ice when the pain is severe. Antiinflammatory medications such as ibuprofen may be helpful. Encourage the child to limit exercise and participate in a different activity. After a few weeks, most overuse syndromes resolve; at that point, the athlete may resume the prior activity. Osgood–Schlatter disease is the exception and may require 6 to 18 months to resolve (Kienstra & Macias, 2022b). Using pads or braces that are appropriate to the painful body part is also helpful. Supporting the arm with a sling may relieve stress on the proximal humerus when epiphysiolysis occurs. Heel cups used in athletic shoes help relieve stress on the heels associated with Sever disease. To prevent overuse syndromes, encourage athletes to perform appropriate stretching exercises during a 20- to 30-minute warm-up period before each practice or game. Also encourage several weeks of conditioning training before the season begins.

There is currently limited research pertaining to overuse injuries in the young athlete. The AAP has developed some guidelines to help prevent these injuries such as the following: Encourage 1 to 2 days off per week of competitive athletics, sports training, and competitive practice; encourage 2 to 3 months away from a specific sport during the year; and educate to increase weekly training time, number of repetitions, or total distance by no more than 10% a week; participation in sports should be about fun, skill acquisition, sportsmanship, and safety (Brenner & The Council on Sports Medicine and Fitness, 2007 [reaffirmed 2021]). See Evidence-Based Practice 44.1.

TAKE NOTE!

"Energy healing" such as therapeutic touch and Reiki may provide a nonpharmacologic adjunct to pain management for musculoskeletal injuries.

TABLE 44.9 • Overuse Disorders

Disorder	Anatomic Area Affected	Most Commonly Occurs in	Symptoms
Osgood–Schlatter disease	Partial avulsion of the ossification center of the tibial tubercle	Active adolescents, most often males. Most frequently during periods of rapid growth	• Mild to moderate pain, activity related • Tibial tubercle is tender when palpated. • Painful swelling or prominence of the anterior portion of the tibial tubercle
Epiphysiolysis of proximal humerus	Proximal humerus (widening of growth plate)	Occurs with rigorous upper extremity activity, such as baseball pitching	• Tenderness in the shoulder or proximal humerus • Pain with active internal rotation • Full shoulder range of motion continues.
Epiphysiolysis of distal radius	Distal radius (widening of growth plate)	Occurs with overuse of the distal radius, such as in gymnasts	• Wrist pain that worsens with activity
Sever disease (calcaneal apophysitis)	Calcaneus (heel)	Usually in 9- to 14-year-olds	• Pain over the posterior aspect of the calcaneus • Limited active and passive dorsiflexion of foot
Shin splints	Refer to a variety of overuse syndromes associated with the shin (stress fracture, tibial stress, muscular issues)	Occur with activities that place repeated exertion on the lower leg, as in runners, dancers, elite soccer players	• Exercise-induced pain of the anterior aspect of the middle part of the lower leg • May be sharp pain • Worsens with exercise • With stress fracture, may have a limp that worsens with activity

EVIDENCE-BASED PRACTICE 44.1

Are Overuse Injuries Associated With Sport-Specific Specialization and Sex of the Athlete?

Youth sports provide many positive benefits to children. In recent years, there has been an increased focus on scholarships and playing time that has resulted in youth focusing more training (more hours/week and months/year) on a single sport, referred to as sport specialization. Evidence exists that sport specialization is associated with an increased risk of overuse injuries in youth athletes. This study examined if the risks of overuse are sport-specific, particularly sports that are more technical and repetitive, such as volleyball, compared with sports that have a broader movement profile, such as soccer. It also examined if the sex of an athlete influenced the risk of overuse injury associated with sport specialization.

STUDY

This was a cross-sectional study that used a self-administered, anonymous questionnaire given at club team tournaments in youth soccer, volleyball, and basketball. It included athletes aged 12 to 18 years of age, and 716 youth athletes completed the questionnaire.

Findings

The study found that the influence of sex, sport specialization, and excessive sport volume on overuse injury may be sport-specific. The results showed that high levels of specialization were only associated with overuse injury in volleyball, not basketball or soccer. Female basketball athletes were more likely than male athletes to report an overuse injury. In soccer athletes, the trend was toward more females with overuse injuries, but the association was not significant.

Nursing Implications

Nurses need to assess youth athlete's specialization level, including hours of training per week, months of training per year, and information on specific sport specialization. This study had limitations but does demonstrate the need for future research focused on sports that are more repetitive and limited in their movement profile, such as volleyball, along with examining the role of sex and the risk of overuse injuries. Nurses are in a unique position to counsel youth on the importance of diversified training and the benefits of being a well-rounded athlete. Educate youth and caregivers on the evidence that exists supporting delayed specialization until late adolescence and that the sport an athlete plays and specializes in may influence their risk for overuse injuries.

Data from Post, E. G., Biese, K. M., Schaefer, D. A., Watson, A. M., McGuine, T. A., Brooks, M. A., & Bell, D. R. (2020). Sport-specific associations of specialization and sex with overuse injury in youth athletes. *Sports Health, 12*(1), 36–42. https://doi.org/10.1177/1941738119886855

Radial Head Subluxation

Subluxation of the radial head ("nursemaid's elbow") occurs when a pulling motion on the arm causes the annular ligament surrounding the radial head to stretch or tear, therefore displacing the radial head. The ligament becomes entrapped within the joint, preventing spontaneous reduction. It usually occurs in children younger than 5 years of age (Carrigan, 2020). In most cases, a parent, sibling, or caregiver inadvertently injures the child while holding or pulling on a pronated upper extremity. Radiologic examination may be done, especially if the mechanism of injury is not clear, to rule out fracture or dislocation. To reduce the injury, the elbow is flexed to 90 degrees and then the forearm is fully and firmly supinated, causing the ligament to snap back into place. With appropriate reduction of the radial head, no complications result.

Nursing Assessment

Elicit a health history to help determine the mechanism of injury. Common precipitators of this injury include pulling on the child's arm while leading them in one direction, helping the child up the stairs, a child dropping or falling to the ground while an adult is holding the hand, or swinging or lifting the child by the hands. Assess neurovascular status and examine the extremity. The child will hold the arm slightly flexed at the side or across the abdomen and refuse to move it. When the arm is still, the child apparently has no discomfort. Neurovascular status is normally intact with no bruising or swelling present.

Nursing Management

After treatment, usually hyperpronation to reduce the dislocation, assess the child's ability to use the arm without pain. Typically, after reduction, the child will demonstrate less pain almost immediately. Educate parents that once a radial head subluxation occurs, it may recur. Teach parents to avoid excessive pulling or pulling up on the child's arm, particularly in an abrupt jerking fashion, to prevent recurrence. Encourage parents and caregivers to always lift the child under their arms.

KEY CONCEPTS

- Muscles, tendons, ligaments, and cartilage are all present and functional at birth, though intentional, purposeful movement develops only as the infant matures.
- The spine is very mobile in the newborn and infant, especially the cervical spine region, resulting in a high risk for cervical spine injury.
- Rapid muscle growth in the adolescent years places the adolescent at increased risk for injury compared with other age groups.

- The bones of the infant and young child are more flexible and have a thicker periosteum and more abundant blood supply than the adult's; as a result, bending occurs more frequently than breaking of the bone, and the fractured bone heals more quickly.
- The epiphysis of long bones is the growth center of the bones in children. Injury to this area may result in long-term extremity deformity.
- The nurse's role in laboratory and diagnostic testing for neuromuscular or musculoskeletal disorders is mainly that of educating the child and family about and preparing the child for the test or procedure.
- Plain radiographs are usually sufficient for diagnosing injuries in children. If CT or MRI scans are required, the nurse may need to help the child stay calm and still during the procedure.
- Apply a pressure dressing following joint aspiration to prevent hematoma formation or fluid recollection.
- Perform frequent assessments of pain status and the effect of pain medication in the child with a musculoskeletal disorder.
- Diazepam may be helpful in relieving muscle spasm associated with traction.
- Maintain traction and the appropriate amount of weight as ordered.
- The bulk of cast care occurs in the home. Teach the family of a child with a cast to perform neurovascular assessments, prevent the cast from getting wet, and care for the skin appropriately.
- Assessment of ROM and muscle tone is critical in the child with a neuromuscular disorder. Hypertonia or hypotonia is an abnormal finding in the infant or child.
- Assessment of neurovascular status is an essential component of care for a child with a musculoskeletal disorder.
- Determining attainment of developmental milestones and subsequent progression or loss of those milestones is useful in distinguishing various neuromuscular disorders.
- The nurse reinforces and carries out the exercise plans and adaptive equipment use as prescribed by the physical or occupational therapist in order to maintain neuromuscular and musculoskeletal function and to prevent complications.
- Nursing management of a child with myelomeningocele focuses on preventing infection, promoting bowel and urinary elimination, promoting adequate nutrition, preventing latex allergy reaction, maintaining skin integrity, providing education and support to the family, and recognizing complications, such as hydrocephalus or increased ICP, associated with the disorder.
- Cerebral palsy may result in significant motor impairment. Children with cerebral palsy require ongoing physical therapy as well as nutritional intervention.
- Children with Duchenne muscular dystrophy initially learn to walk but later lose this ability.
- Respiratory compromise occurs in muscular dystrophy and SMA and eventually leads to death.
- Children with chronic disorders such as OI may demonstrate slower or lesser growth than other children and may also be unable to participate in certain activities because of bone fragility.
- Congenital or developmental disorders such as DDH or clubfoot require bracing or casting for correction and to prevent deformity later in life.
- Torticollis may be treated by teaching the family to perform daily neck muscle–stretching exercises.
- To prevent complications after a spinal fusion for scoliosis correction, use the log-roll method for turning the child so that back flexion is avoided.
- Children with spinal cord injury require intense nursing management and lengthy rehabilitation to maintain or regain function.
- Children with neuromuscular disorders often suffer depression related to the chronic nature of the disorder.
- School attendance and participation in activities such as the Special Olympics are important for children with neuromuscular dysfunction.
- Fractures may occur as a result of unintentional or intentional injury, or because the bones are fragile, as in rickets or OI.
- Sprains, fractures, and overuse syndromes occur frequently in young athletes. Appropriate warm-up and stretching may help prevent some of these injuries.
- RICE is the appropriate treatment for sprains.

REFERENCES AND RECOMMENDED READINGS

American Academy of Pediatrics, & Committee on Genetics. (1999).Folic acid for the prevention of neural tube defects [Reaffirmed (2017). Policy statement: AAP publications reaffirmed or retired. *Pediatrics*, *139*(3): e20164205.]. *Pediatrics*, *104*(2), 325–327. http://pediatrics.aappublications.org/content/104/2/325.full

Balasubramanian, M. (2022). Osteogenesis imperfecta: An overview. *UpToDate*. Retrieved May 14, 2023, from https://www.uptodate.com/contents/osteogenesis-imperfecta-an-overview

Baldwin, K. D., Shah, U. L., & Arkader, A. (2020). Common fractures. In R. M. Kleigman, J. W. St. Geme III, N. J. Blum, S. S. Shah, R. C. Tasker, K. M. Wilson, & R. E. Behrman (Eds.), *Nelson textbook of pediatrics* (21st ed., pp. 19134–19180). Elsevier.

Barkoudah, E. (2023). Cerebral palsy: Overview of management and prognosis. *UpToDate*. Retrieved May 16, 2023, from https://www.uptodate.com/contents/cerebral-palsy-overview-of-management-and-prognosis

Barkoudah, E., & Aravamuthan, B. (2023). Cerebral palsy: Epidemiology, etiology, and prevention. *UpToDate*. Retrieved May 16, 2023, https://www.uptodate.com/contents/cerebral-palsy-epidemiology-etiology-and-prevention

Barkoudah, E., & Whitaker, A. (2022). Cerebral palsy: Treatment of spasticity, dystonia, and associated orthopedic issues. *UpToDate*. Retrieved May 16, 2023, from https://www.uptodate.com/contents/cerebral-palsy-treatment-of-spasticity-dystonia-and-associated-orthopedic-issues

Bharucha-Goebel, D. X. (2020). Muscular dystrophies. In R. M. Kleigman, J. W. St. Geme III, N. J. Blum, S. S. Shah, R. C. Tasker, K. M. Wilson, & R. E. Behrman (Eds.), *Nelson textbook of pediatrics* (21st ed., pp. 17216–17284). Elsevier.

Boas, S. R. (2020). Skeletal diseases influencing pulmonary function. In R. M. Kleigman, J. W. St. Geme III, N. J. Blum, S. S. Shah, R. C. Tasker, K. M. Wilson, & R. E. Behrman (Eds.), *Nelson textbook of pediatrics* (21st ed., pp. 12375–12398). Elsevier.

Bodamer, O. A. (2023). Spinal muscular atrophy. *UpToDate*. Retrieved May 16, 2023, from https://www.uptodate.com/contents/spinal-muscular-atrophy

Bowman, R. M. (2022). Myelomeningocele (spina bifida): Management and outcome. *UpToDate*. Retrieved May 12, 2023, from https://www.uptodate.com/contents/myelomeningocele-spina-bifida-management-and-outcome

Brenner, J. S., & The Council on Sports Medicine and Fitness. (2007). Overuse injuries, overtraining, and burnout in child and adolescent athletes [Reaffirmed (2021). Policy statement: AAP publications reaffirmed or retired. *Pediatrics, 148*(2):e2021052583.]. *Pediatrics, 119*(6), 1242–1245. https://doi.org/10.1542/peds.2007-0887

Carrigan, R. B. (2020). The upper limb. In R. M. Kleigman, J. W. St. Geme III, N. J. Blum, S. S. Shah, R. C. Tasker, K. M. Wilson, & R. E. Behrman (Eds.), *Nelson textbook of pediatrics* (21st ed., pp. 9075–19106). Elsevier.

Centers for Disease Control and Prevention. (2022a). *Folic acid recommendations*. http://www.cdc.gov/ncbddd/folicacid/recommendations.html

Centers for Disease Control and Prevention. (2022b). *Birth defects: Limb reduction defects*. http://www.cdc.gov/ncbddd/birthdefects/UL-LimbReductionDefects.html

Darras, B. T. (2021). Patient education: Overview of muscular dystrophies (Beyond the Basics). *UpToDate*. Retrieved May 16, 2023, from https://www.uptodate.com/contents/overview-of-muscular-dystrophies-beyond-the-basics

Darras, B. T. (2022). Duchenne and Becker muscular dystrophy: Management and prognosis. *UpToDate*. Retrieved May 16, 2023, from https://www.uptodate.com/contents/duchenne-and-becker-muscular-dystrophy-management-and-prognosis

Darras, B. T. (2023). Duchenne and Becker muscular dystrophy: Glucocorticoid and disease-modifying treatment. *UpToDate*. Retrieved May 16, 2023, from https://www.uptodate.com/contents/duchenne-and-becker-muscular-dystrophy-glucocorticoid-and-disease-modifying-treatment

Fischbach, F. T., Fischbach, M. A., & Stout, K. (2022). *A manual of laboratory and diagnostic tests* (11th ed.). Wolters Kluwer.

Gill, A. C., & Kelly, N. R. (2022). Pediatric injury prevention: Epidemiology, history, and application. UpToDate. Retrieved May 15, 2023, from https://www.uptodate.com/contents/pediatric-injury-prevention-epidemiology-history-and-application

Holmes, S. B., Brown, S. J., & Pin Site Care Expert Panel. (2005). Skeletal pin site care: National Association of Orthopaedic Nurses guidelines for orthopaedic nursing. *Orthopaedic Nursing, 24*(2), 99–107. https://doi.org/10.1097/00006416-200503000-00003

Iobst, C. A. (2017). Pin-track infections: Past, present, and future. *Journal of Limb Lengthening and Reconstruction, 3*, 78–84. https://journals.lww.com/jllr/Fulltext/2017/03020/Pin_Track_Infections__Past,_Present,_and_Future.4.aspx

Johnston, M. V. (2020). Cerebral palsy. In R. M. Kleigman, J. W. St. Geme III, N. J. Blum, S. S. Shah, R. C. Tasker, K. M. Wilson, & R. E. Behrman (Eds.), *Nelson textbook of pediatrics* (21st ed., pp. 16718–16741). Elsevier.

Kienstra, A. J., & Macias, C. G. (2022a). Evaluation and management of slipped capital femoral epiphysis (SCFE). *UpToDate*. Retrieved May 16, 2023, from https://www.uptodate.com/contents/evaluation-and-management-of-slipped-capital-femoral-epiphysis-scfe

Kienstra, A. J., & Macias, C. G. (2022b). Osgood-Schlatter disease (tibial tuberosity avulsion). *UpToDate*. Retrieved May 16, 2023, from https://www.uptodate.com/contents/osgood-schlatter-disease-tibial-tuberosity-avulsion

Kinsman, S. L., & Johnston, M. V. (2020). Congenital anomalies of the central nervous system. In R. M. Kleigman, J. W. St. Geme III, N. J. Blum, S. S. Shah, R. C. Tasker, K. M. Wilson, & R. E. Behrman (Eds.), *Nelson textbook of pediatrics* (21st ed., pp. 16200–16290). Elsevier.

Lexicomp. (2023). Pediatric drug information. *UpToDate*. Retrieved May 10, 2023, from https://www.uptodate.com/contents/table-of-contents/drug-information/pediatric-drug-information

Marini, J. C. (2020). Osteogenesis imperfecta. In R. M. Kleigman, J. W. St. Geme III, N. J. Blum, S. S. Shah, R. C. Tasker, K. M. Wilson, & R. E. Behrman (Eds.), *Nelson textbook of pediatrics* (21st ed., pp. 19520–19539). Elsevier.

Mayer, O. H. (2022). Pectus excavatum: Treatment. *UpToDate*. Retrieved May 14, 2023, from https://www.uptodate.com/contents/pectus-excavatum-treatment

Misra, M. (2022). Vitamin D insufficiency and deficiency in children and adolescents. *UpToDate*. Retrieved May 17, 2023, from https://www.uptodate.com/contents/vitamin-d-insufficiency-and-deficiency-in-children-and-adolescents

Mistovich, R. J., & Spiegel, D. A. (2020a). The neck. In R. M. Kleigman, J. W. St. Geme III, N. J. Blum, S. S. Shah, R. C. Tasker, K. M. Wilson, & R. E. Behrman (Eds.), *Nelson textbook of pediatrics* (21st ed., pp. 19051–19074). Elsevier.

Mistovich, R. J., & Spiegel, D. A. (2020b). The spine. In R. M. Kleigman, J. W. St. Geme III, N. J. Blum, S. S. Shah, R. C. Tasker, K. M. Wilson, & R. E. Behrman (Eds.), *Nelson textbook of pediatrics* (21st ed., pp. 18972–19049). Elsevier.

National Institute of Neurological Disorders and Stroke. (2023). *Cerebral palsy*. https://www.ninds.nih.gov/Disorders/All-Disorders/Cerebral-Palsy-Information-Page

Neudauer, C. (2019). Cell and tissue characteristics. In T. L. Norris (Ed.), *Porth's pathophysiology: Concepts of altered health states* (10th ed., pp. 13–45). Wolters Kluwer Health.

Post, E. G., Biese, K. M., Schaefer, D. A., Watson, A. M., McGuine, T. A., Brooks, M. A., & Bell, D. R. (2020). Sport-specific associations of specialization and sex with overuse injury in youth athletes. *Sports Health, 12*(1), 36–42. https://doi.org/10.1177/1941738119886855

Sankar, W. N., Horn, B. D., Winell, J. J., & Wells, L. (2020). The hip. In R. M. Kleigman, J. W. St. Geme III, N. J. Blum, S. S. Shah, R. C. Tasker, K. M. Wilson, & R. E. Behrman (Eds.), *Nelson textbook of pediatrics* (21st ed., pp. 18924–18971). Elsevier.

Sarant, H. B. (2020). Evaluation and investigation of neuromuscular disorders. In R. M. Kleigman, J. W. St. Geme III, N. J. Blum, S. S. Shah, R. C. Tasker, K. M. Wilson, & R. E. Behrman (Eds.), *Nelson textbook of pediatrics* (21st ed., pp. 17070–17111). Elsevier.

Scherl, S. A., & Hasley, B. P. (2023). Adolescent idiopathic scoliosis: Management and prognosis. *UpToDate*. Retrieved May 17, 2023, from https://www.uptodate.com/contents/adolescent-idiopathic-scoliosis-management-and-prognosis

Schweich, P. (2021). Patient education: Cast and splint care (Beyond the Basics). *UpToDate*. Retrieved May 11, 2023, from https://www.uptodate.com/contents/cast-and-splint-care-beyond-the-basics

Shields, D. W., Iliadis, A. D., Kelly, E., Heidari, N., & Jamal, B. (2022). Pin-site Infection: A systematic review of prevention strategies. *Strategies in Trauma and Limb Reconstruction, 17*(2), 93–104. https://doi.org/10.5005/jp-journals-10080-1562

U.S. Department of Health and Human Services. (n.d.). *Healthy People 2030*. https://health.gov/healthypeople

U.S. Food and Drug Administration. (2014). *Recommendations for labeling medical products to inform users that the product or product container is not made with natural rubber latex: Guidance for industry and food and drug administration staff.* https://www.fda.gov/media/85473/download

Walker, J. (2018). Assessing and managing pin sites in patients with external fixation. *Nursing Times [online], 114*(1), 18–21. Retrieved May 11, 2023, from https://cdn.ps.emap.com/wp-content/uploads/sites/3/2017/12/171220-Assessing-and-managing-pin-sites-in-patients-with-external-fixation.pdf

Winell, J. J., Baldwin, K. D., & Wells, L. (2020). Torsional and angular deformities of the limb. In R. M. Kleigman, J. W. St. Geme III, N. J. Blum, S. S. Shah, R. C. Tasker, K. M. Wilson, & R. E. Behrman (Eds.), *Nelson textbook of pediatrics* (21st ed., pp. 18838–18871). Elsevier.

Winell, J. J., & Davidson, R. S. (2020). The foot and toes. In R. M. Kleigman, J. W. St. Geme III, N. J. Blum, S. S. Shah, R. C. Tasker, K. M. Wilson, & R. E. Behrman (Eds.), *Nelson textbook of pediatrics* (21st ed., pp. 18787–18837). Elsevier.

DEVELOPING CLINICAL JUDGMENT

PRACTICING FOR NCLEX

1. A child with Duchenne muscular dystrophy is admitted to the pediatric unit. They have an ineffective cough. Lung auscultation reveals diminished breath sounds. What is the priority nursing intervention?
   a. Apply supplemental oxygen.
   b. Notify the respiratory therapist.
   c. Monitor pulse oximetry.
   d. Position for adequate airway clearance.
2. A 7-year-old child with cerebral palsy has been admitted to the hospital. Which information is most important for the nurse to obtain in the history?
   a. Age that the child learned to walk
   b. Parents' expectations of the child's development
   c. Functional status related to eating and mobility
   d. Birth history to identify the cause of cerebral palsy
3. The nurse is caring for a child with cerebral palsy who requires a wheelchair to attain mobility. Which intervention would help the child achieve a sense of normality?
   a. Encourage follow-through with physical therapy exercises.
   b. Restrict the child to a classroom equipped with functional aids.
   c. Encourage afterschool (adj.) activities within the limits of the child's abilities.
   d. Ensure the school is aware of the child's capabilities.
4. The nurse is caring for orthopedic children who are in the postoperative period following spinal fusion. What is the most appropriate activity to delegate to unlicensed assistive personnel?
   a. Ambulate the children twice daily to promote mobility.
   b. Encourage commode use to promote bowel function.
   c. Provide diversionary activities, as the children must stay flat on their backs.
   d. Assist with log-rolling the children every 2 hours.
5. A 2-month-old infant with a history of a repaired myelomeningocele is seen in your clinic for a well-child check. The parents report the child has been irritable. Upon assessment, the nurse notes a _________ and _________ leading the nurse to assess the infant's _______________.
   Blank 1 and 2:
   a. depressed fontanelle
   b. bulging fontanelle
   c. high-pitched cry
   d. heart rate (HR) 148 bpm
   Blank 3:
   a. weight
   b. head circumference
   c. respiratory rate
   d. HR
6. The nurse is teaching a family with a child newly diagnosed with muscular dystrophy. The nurse can determine teaching has been successful when the parents indicate that which symptoms are early symptoms of the condition? Select all that apply.
   a. "Our child did not walk until 20 months old."
   b. "Our child suffers from frequent respiratory infections."
   c. "Our child has obesity."
   d. "Our child has difficulty climbing stairs."
   e. "Our child has increased muscle strength."
   f. "Our child has difficulty getting up from the floor."

DOSAGE CALCULATION QUESTION

The nurse is caring for a child who is experiencing painful spasms. The child is 6 years old and weighs 42 lb. The medication order reads: Baclofen 25 mg per GT (gastrostomy tube) every 8 hours. Baclofen is supplied as 5 mg/mL.

How many milliliters will the nurse administer? Round to the nearest tenth.

CRITICAL THINKING EXERCISES

1. A 5-year-old child, diagnosed with myelomeningocele, is admitted to the hospital for a corrective surgical procedure. Choose four questions from below that the nurse should ask when obtaining the health history that would assist in planning the child's care.
   a. What is the child's current mobility status?
   b. Is there a family history of myelomeningocele?
   c. What is the child's genitourinary and bowel function and regimen?
   d. Does this child have a history of hydrocephalus with the presence of a shunt?
   e. Does the child have known latex sensitivity?
   f. Were there any complications during the pregnancy or birth of this child?
   g. Did the birthing parent take prenatal folic acid supplementation?
2. Based on the case in the above question, develop a nursing plan of care or concept map for the child with myelomeningocele.

3. A 5-year-old child is admitted to the pediatric unit with a history of cerebral palsy sustained at birth. The child is admitted for a scheduled tendon lengthening procedure. Based on your knowledge about the effects of cerebral palsy, list three priorities to focus on when planning their care. Compare this to a child admitted for surgical correction of a broken femur with no significant past medical history.

4. Develop a discharge teaching plan for a 2-year-old who will be in a hip spica cast for 10 more weeks at home.

5. Devise a developmental/education plan for a child who will be confined to traction for 6 weeks. Choose a child in the clinical area whom you have cared for or choose a particular age group and develop the plan.

STUDY ACTIVITIES

- In the clinical setting, compare the growth of a child with muscular dystrophy, SMA, or cerebral palsy to the growth of a similar-age child who has been healthy. What differences or similarities do you find? What are the explanations for your findings?
- Identify the role of the registered nurse in the multidisciplinary care of the child with a debilitating neuromuscular disorder.
- In the clinical setting, interview the parent of a child with Duchenne muscular dystrophy, myelomeningocele, SMA, or severe cerebral palsy. Determine the parent's feelings about the ongoing care that they are responsible for. Reflect upon this interview in your clinical journal.
- In the clinical setting, compare the cognitive abilities of two children with a severe neuromuscular disorder. What are the reasons for the similarities or differences that you find?

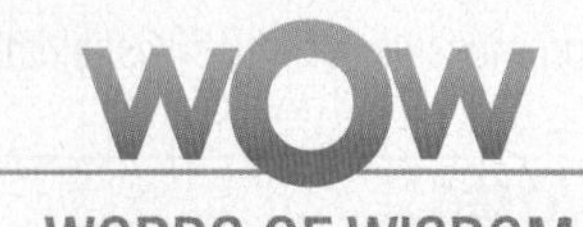

WORDS OF WISDOM

To a nurse the child's skin is life's gift wrapping, but to the child the skin is the space suit for life.

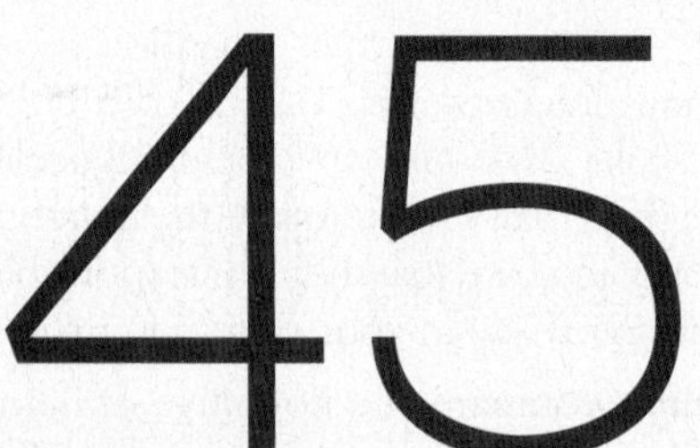

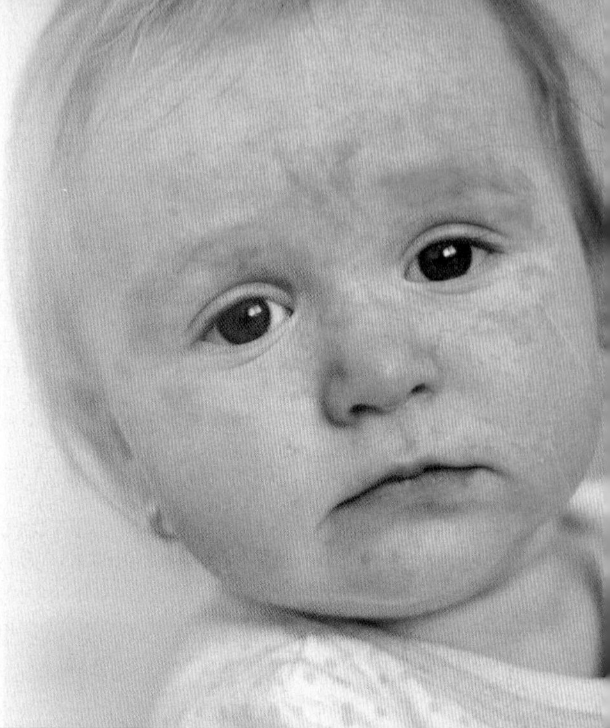

Nursing Care of the Child With an Alteration in Tissue Integrity/ Integumentary Disorder

LEARNING OBJECTIVES

Upon completion of the chapter, you will be able to:

1. Compare the anatomy and physiology of the integumentary system in infants and children to that of adults.
2. Describe nursing care related to common laboratory and diagnostic tests used in the medical diagnosis of integumentary disorders/ alterations in tissue integrity in infants, children, and adolescents.
3. Distinguish alterations in tissue integrity/integumentary disorders common in infants, children, and adolescents.
4. Identify appropriate nursing assessments and interventions related to pediatric integumentary disorders/alterations in tissue integrity.
5. Develop an individualized nursing care plan for the child with an alteration in tissue integrity integumentary disorder.
6. Describe the psychosocial impact of a chronic integumentary disorder on children or adolescents.
7. Develop child and family teaching plans for the child with an integumentary disorder/tissue integrity alteration.

KEY TERMS

annular (an′yŭ-lăr)
dermatitis
erythema (er′i-thē′mă)
macule
papule
pruritus (prū-rī′tŭs)
scaling
vesicle

Eva Lopez, aged 1 year, is brought to the clinic by her parent, who states, "Eva has dry patches of skin, her wrists bleed from her scratching, and she's having trouble sleeping at night."

INTRODUCTION

Tissue integrity refers to the ability of body tissues to maintain normal physiologic processes (Giddens, 2021). Nurses may encounter children with alterations in tissue integrity and should be familiar with various integumentary disorders that children experience. Alterations in tissue integrity or integumentary disorders occur often in children and are caused by exposure to infectious microorganisms, hypersensitivity reactions, hormonal influences, and injuries. Some integumentary disorders are as mild and self-limited as a minor abrasion. Others, such as atopic dermatitis (AD), are chronic and must be managed consistently. Finally, some tissue integrity alterations can be severe and even life-threatening, such as full-thickness burns. If the integumentary disorders are chronic or severe, they can have a major impact on the child's physiologic or psychological status (Teichgräber et al., 2021). Nurses who care for children need to be familiar with common skin disorders of infancy, childhood, and adolescence so they can effectively intervene with children and their families.

VARIATIONS IN PEDIATRIC ANATOMY AND PHYSIOLOGY

The skin is the largest organ of the body and serves to protect the underlying tissues from trauma and invasion by microorganisms. The skin's health reflects the internal well-being of the body. The skin is also important for the perception of pain, heat, and cold and for the regulation of body temperature.

Differences in the Skin Between Children and Adults

The infant's epidermis is thinner than the adult's, and the blood vessels lie closer to the surface because there is a decreased amount of subcutaneous fat. Thus, the infant loses heat more readily through the skin's surface than the older child or adult does. The thinness of the infant's skin also allows substances to be absorbed through the skin more readily than they would be in an adult. Bacteria can gain access via the infant's and younger child's skin more readily than they can through the adult's skin. The infant's skin contains more water than the adult's, and the epidermis is loosely bound to the dermis. This means that friction may easily cause separation of the layers, resulting in blistering or skin breakdown. The infant's skin is also less pigmented than that of the adult (in all races), placing the infant at increased risk of skin damage from ultraviolet (UV) radiation. Over time, the infant's skin toughens and becomes less hydrated and is thus less susceptible to microorganism invasion. The skin thickness and characteristics reach adult levels in the late teenage years.

Differences With Skin Tone

The increased pigmentation in children with darker skin influences the appearance of skin lesions (Armstrong, 2023). Pruritic dermatologic conditions may result in increased lichenification in darker skinned children as compared to lighter skinned children with the same disorders (Sangha, 2021). Dry, darker skin may look whitish or ashy (Armstrong, 2023). Additionally, in darker skin, erythema may be difficult to identify as it may appear as simply a darker area, an ashen gray color, or have a violaceous hue (Armstrong, 2023; Sangha, 2021). Hypopigmentation or hyperpigmentation in the affected area following healing of a dermatologic condition is exaggerated in children with darker skin (Armstrong, 2023). Hypertrophic scarring and keloid formation (Fig. 45.1) occur more often in darker skinned children (Heath et al., 2016).

Sebaceous and Sweat Glands

Sebaceous glands function immaturely at birth. The sebum secreted serves to lubricate the skin and hair. Sebum production increases in the preadolescent and adolescent years, which is why acne develops at that time. The infant's eccrine sweat glands are somewhat functional and will produce sweat as a response to emotional stimuli and heat. They become fully functional in the middle childhood years. Until that time, temperature regulation is less effective compared to older children and adults. The apocrine sweat glands are small and nonfunctional in the infant. They mature during puberty, at which time body odor develops in response to the fluid secreted by these glands.

COMMON MEDICAL TREATMENTS

A variety of medications as well as other medical treatments are used to treat integumentary disorders in children. Most of these treatments will require a health care provider's order when the child is in the hospital. The most common treatments and medications are listed in Common Medical Treatments 45.1 and Drug Guide 45.1. The nurse caring for the child with an integumentary disorder should be familiar with the procedures and medications, how they work, and common nursing implications related to their use.

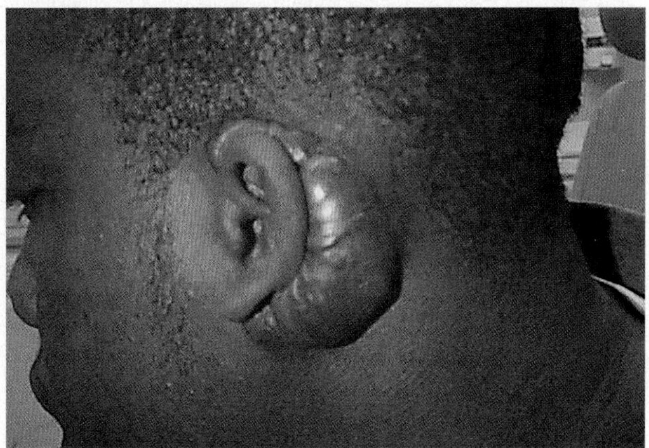

FIGURE 45.1 Keloid formation is more common in dark-skinned than light-skinned children.

COMMON MEDICAL TREATMENTS 45.1

Treatment	Explanation	Indications	Nursing Implications
Wet dressing	Dressing moistened with lukewarm water (sterile water may be required in certain cases.)	In the presence of itching, crusting, or oozing—helps to remove crusts	May use Burow, Domeboro, or saline solutions in certain cases Provide atraumatic care by giving premedication before dressing change.
Sunscreen	Lotion, gel, or cream with a sun-protective factor (SPF)	All children older than 6 months	Use a fragrance-free, para-aminobenzoic acid (PABA)–free preparation with an SPF of 15 or higher. Apply at least 30 minutes prior to sun exposure. Reapply at least every 2 hours while exposed (every 60–80 minutes while in the water). Sweat- and water-resistant preparations are available yet still require reapplication, as noted previously. Use daily in summer and in warm climates, even on overcast and cloudy days.
Bathing	Use of lukewarm water (with or without soap) to bathe	Itchy and irritating skin conditions	Recommend fragrance-free, dye-free soaps such as Dove, Aveeno, Basis, Lubriderm. Colloids (oatmeal baths) are especially helpful. Pat the child dry; do not rub the skin. Leave the child moist before applying medication, dressing, or moisturizer.

DRUG GUIDE 45.1

COMMON DRUGS FOR INTEGUMENTARY DISORDERS

Medication	Actions/Indications	Nursing Implications
Antibiotics (topical)	Decrease skin colonization with bacteria. Indicated for mild acne vulgaris, impetigo, folliculitis	Apply as prescribed to clean skin or a cleansed wound. Be alert for neomycin allergy.
Antibiotics (systemic)	Bactericidal or bacteriostatic against a variety of organisms, depending on the preparation Used for moderate to severe acne vulgaris, extensive impetigo, cellulitis, scalded skin syndrome	Check for medication allergies prior to administration. Teach families to finish entire course of antibiotics.
Corticosteroids (topical)	Antiinflammatory effect in atopic dermatitis and certain kinds of contact dermatitis	Do not use moderate- or high-potency corticosteroid preparations on the face or genitals. Do not cover with an occlusive dressing. Absorption is increased in the young infant.
Antifungals (topical)	Fungicidal used to treat tinea, candidal diaper rash	Apply a thin layer as prescribed. Adhere with length of treatment as prescribed to prevent reemergence of the rash.
Antifungals (systemic): griseofulvin, ketoconazole	Kill fungus; bind to human keratin, making it resistant to fungus Indicated for tinea capitis and severe or widespread fungal skin infections	Griseofulvin: give with fatty food to increase absorption. Requires minimum 4-week course Monitor liver function tests and CBC. May cause photosensitivity Ketoconazole: Administer with food to decrease GI upset.
Benzoyl peroxide	Decreases colonization of *Propionibacterium acnes* in mild acne vulgaris	Available in combination with topical antibiotics Apply sparingly. Shake before application. Avoid contact with eyes and mucous membranes.
Retinoids (topical): tretinoin, adapalene, tazarotene	Anticomedogenic activity in moderate to severe acne vulgaris	Adverse effects: dryness, burning, photosensitivity Instruct child to use SPF 15 or higher sunscreen.
Topical immune modulators (tacrolimus, pimecrolimus)	Inhibit T-lymphocyte action at the skin level. Used for moderate to severe atopic dermatitis, or in conditions resistant to topical steroids	Use only in children older than 2 years. Avoid sunlight exposure. May cause burning, pruritus, flulike symptoms, or headache

DRUG GUIDE 45.1

COMMON DRUGS FOR INTEGUMENTARY DISORDERS

Medication	Actions/Indications	Nursing Implications
Systemic immune modulators (dupilumab)	Inhibit interleukin-4 and interleukin-13 inflammatory processes.	Given by subcutaneous injection every 2 to 4 weeks in children 6 months of age or older
Antihistamines (diphenhydramine, chlorpheniramine, hydroxyzine)	Antihistaminic effect, results in sedation Indicated for hypersensitivity reactions, atopic dermatitis, or contact dermatitis that is severely pruritic	May give three or four times a day unless sedation effect interferes with activities of daily living or school
Systemic corticosteroids (prednisone, dexamethasone, methylprednisolone)	Antiinflammatory and immunosuppressive action Used in severe contact dermatitis	Administer with food to decrease GI upset. May mask signs of infection Monitor blood pressure, urine for glucose. Do not stop treatment abruptly, or acute adrenal insufficiency may occur. Monitor for Cushing syndrome. Doses may be tapered over time.
Isotretinoin	Reduces sebaceous gland size, decreases sebum production, and regulates cell proliferation and differentiation Indicated for cystic acne or severe acne that is resistant to 3 months of treatment with oral antibiotics	Ensure that the adolescent is not pregnant and does not become pregnant. Monitor CBC, lipid profiles, liver function tests, and beta-human chorionic gonadotropin monthly. Monitor for suicide risk.
Coal tar preparations	Antipruritic and antiinflammatory effect Useful in psoriasis, atopic dermatitis	May stain fabrics; strong and unpleasant odor Apply at bedtime and rinse off in the morning to improve adherence.
Silver sulfadiazine 1%	Bactericidal against Gram-positive and Gram-negative bacteria and yeasts Indicated for burns	Cover with occlusive dressing. Apply twice daily. Do not use in children with sulfa allergy. Forms a gel on the burn that is painful to remove May cause transient neutropenia Do not use on the child's face or on an infant younger than 2 months.

CBC, complete blood count; GI, gastrointestinal.

Source: UpToDate, Inc. (2024). *Lexi-comp*® (Version 7.10.0) [Mobile app]. Wolters Kluwer. https://apps.apple.com/us/app/lexicomp/id313401238

COMMON LABORATORY AND DIAGNOSTIC TESTS 45.1

Test	Explanation	Indications	Nursing Implications
Complete blood count (CBC) with differential	Evaluates hemoglobin and hematocrit, white blood cell (WBC) count (particularly the percentage of individual WBCs), and platelet count	Infection or inflammatory process	Normal values vary according to age and sex. WBC differential is helpful in evaluating source of infection. May be affected by myelosuppressive drugs Eosinophils may be elevated in the child with atopic dermatitis.
Erythrocyte sedimentation rate (ESR)	Nonspecific test used to detect presence of infection or inflammation	Infection or inflammatory process	Send sample to laboratory immediately; if allowed to stand for longer than 3 hours, may result in falsely low result.
Potassium hydroxide (KOH) prep	Reveals branching hyphae (fungus) when viewed under microscope	To identify fungal infection	Place skin scrapings on a microscope slide, and add KOH 20% drop.
Culture of wound or skin drainage	Allows for microbial growth and organism identification	Identification of specific organism	Note sensitivities.
Immunoglobulin E (IgE)	Measurement of serum IgE	Atopic dermatitis	Often elevated in allergic or atopic disease, though this is a nonspecific finding; may be increased if the child takes systemic corticosteroids
Patch or skin testing	Needle prick testing with allergens	Atopic or contact dermatitis	Have emergency equipment available in the event of anaphylaxis (rare).

Data from Corbett, J. A., & Banks, A. D. (2019). *Laboratory tests and diagnostic procedures with nursing diagnoses* (9th ed.). Pearson Education Inc.

Clinical Judgment and the Nursing Process for the Child With an Integumentary Disorder

Nursing management of the child with an alteration in tissue integrity or integumentary disorder requires astute assessment skills, development of accurate patient problems and expected outcomes, implementation of appropriate interventions, and evaluation of the entire process. Many skin rashes may be associated with other, often serious illnesses, so the nurse must use comprehensive and excellent assessment skills when evaluating rashes in children. Certain integumentary conditions are chronic and require ongoing care related to health maintenance, education, and psychosocial needs.

Remember Eva, the 1-year-old with the dry patches, itching, and trouble sleeping? What additional health history and physical examination assessment information should the nurse obtain?

Assessment

Nursing assessment of the child with an integumentary disorder or tissue integrity alteration includes obtaining the health history and performing a physical examination. Assisting with or obtaining laboratory tests may also be necessary.

Health History

Determine the child's or parent's chief complaint, which is most often related to **pruritus** (sensation of itching), **scaling** (dry, flaky skin), or a cosmetic disruption. Document the history of the present illness, noting onset, location, duration, characteristics, other symptoms, and relieving factors, particularly as related to a rash or lesion. Also ask about the quantity and quality of any discharge from the rash or lesions. Document accompanying symptoms. Note the child's general state of health, history of chronic medical conditions, recent surgeries, hospitalizations, medications, or immunizations. Has there been a recent change in the child's food intake or environment? Is there a family history of chronic or acute skin conditions? Does anyone in the home have a similar concern at this time? Does the family have pets that go outdoors? Does the child play in the woods or garden? Note usual skin care routines, as well as types of soaps, cosmetics, or other skin care products used. Determine the amount of daily sun exposure and whether the child consistently uses sunscreen.

Physical Examination

Perform a complete physical examination, noting any abnormalities. Perform a focused and thorough examination of the skin. The best lighting for examination of the skin is natural daylight. Look at the skin, in general, noting distribution of any obvious rashes or lesions. Inspect the mucous membranes, noting and describing lesions if present. Examine all surfaces of the skin and scalp carefully. Note temperature, moisture, texture, and fragility of the skin. If a rash or lesions are present, note their location and provide a detailed description of them. Describe whether a rash is macular, papular, pustular, or vesicular.

Provide a description of vascular lesions if present. If lesions are present on the scalp, has hair loss in that region occurred? Describe lesions according to the following criteria:

- Linear: in a line
- Shape: are the lesions round, oval, or **annular** (ring around central clearing)?
- Morbilliform: a rosy, maculopapular rash
- Target lesions: like a bull's eye

If drainage is present, describe it as clear, purulent, honey colored, or otherwise. Note scaling or lichenification of the skin. Palpate for regional lymphadenopathy.

Laboratory and Diagnostic Testing

Common Laboratory and Diagnostic Tests 45.1 details the laboratory and diagnostic tests most commonly used when considering integumentary disorders. The tests can assist the health care provider or nurse practitioner in diagnosing the disorder or can be used as guidelines in determining ongoing treatment. Some of the tests are obtained by laboratory or nonnursing personnel, while others might be obtained by the nurse. In either instance, the nurse should be familiar with how the tests are obtained, what they are used for, and normal versus abnormal results. This knowledge will also be necessary when providing child and family education related to the testing.

Nursing Analysis

After recognizing and analyzing cues from a thorough assessment, the nurse might identify several patient problems, including:

- Impaired skin integrity
- Risk for infection
- Risk for fluid volume deficit
- Altered nutrition
- Disturbed body image
- Pain
- Interrupted family processes
- Risk for caregiver role strain

After completing an assessment of Eva, the nurse noted the following: hypopigmentation of the skin behind her knees, dry patches on her wrists and face, and slight wheezing heard bilaterally on auscultation. Based on these assessment findings, what would your top three patient problems be for Eva?

The foregoing patient problems provide suggestions for nursing care planning or concept mapping. Suggested interventions with rationales are provided further on. Care planning should be individualized, based on the child's and family's needs. Refer to Chapter 36 for the nursing process for pain management and to Chapter 33 for nursing interventions related to interrupted family processes and caregiver role strain risk. Additional information will be included later in the chapter as it relates to nursing management of children with specific disorders, as well as particular nursing interventions for deficient knowledge.

Nursing Analysis

Impaired skin integrity related to infectious process, hypersensitivity reaction, injury, or mechanical factors as evidenced by alteration in skin integrity (rash, inflammation, abrasion, laceration, or disrupted epidermis)

Goal/Outcome

Integrity of skin surface will be restored; rash, abrasion, laceration, or other skin disruption will heal.

Restoring Skin Integrity (interventions with *rationale*)

- Assess site of skin impairment *to determine extent of involvement and plan care.*
- Monitor skin impairment every shift for changes in color, warmth, redness, or other signs of infection *to identify problems early.*
- Determine the child's and family's skin care practices *to establish need for education related to skin care.*
- Individualize the child's skin care regimen depending on the child's particular skin condition *to care for skin most appropriately in light of the child's disorder.*
- In the immobile child, use a risk assessment tool (such as a modified Norton or Braden Q scale) *to identify risk for skin breakdown.*
- Position the child on the opposite side of the skin impairment *to avoid further skin breakdown.*
- Encourage appropriate nutritional intake *as adequate nutrients are necessary for appropriate immune function and skin healing.*
- Consult the wound and ostomy care nurse specialist *to determine the best approach for individualized wound care.*
- Provide dressing change and wound care as prescribed *to promote wound or burn healing.*

Nursing Analysis

Risk for infection related to alteration in skin integrity

Goal/Outcome

Child will remain free from local or systemic infection, will remain afebrile, without additional redness or warmth at skin disruption site.

Preventing Infection (interventions with *rationale*)

- Use appropriate hand hygiene *to decrease transmission of infectious organisms.*
- Assess the skin impairment site for increased warmth, redness, discharge, or new purulence *to identify infection early.*
- Assess temperature every 4 hours or more frequently if needed, *as children develop fever quickly in response to infection.*
- Note white blood cell (WBC) count and culture results, reporting unexpected values to the health care provider or nurse practitioner *so that appropriate treatment may be started.*
- Follow prescribed therapies for skin alteration *to maintain skin moisture and prevent further breakdown, which may lead to infection.*
- Encourage appropriate nutritional intake, *as adequate nutrients are necessary for appropriate immune function and skin healing.*

Nursing Analysis

Risk for deficient fluid volume related to fluid loss through abnormal route (burns)

Goal/Outcome

Fluid volume status will be balanced, child will maintain urine output of 1 to 2 mL/kg/h, oral mucosa will be moist and pink, heart rate will remain within age- and situation-specific parameters.

Promoting Fluid Balance (interventions with *rationale*)

- Assess fluid volume status at least every shift, more frequently if disrupted, *to obtain baseline for comparison.*
- Strictly monitor intake and output *to detect imbalance or need for additional fluid intake.*
- Weigh the child daily on the same scale, at the same time, in the same amount of clothing *as changes in weight are an accurate indicator of fluid volume status in children.*
- Provide intravenous (IV) fluid resuscitation in initial period, followed by encouragement of oral fluid intake in the burned child, *to compensate for fluid loss through burned areas.*

Nursing Analysis

Imbalanced nutrition, less than body requirements, related to insufficient dietary intake in relation to increased metabolic state (burns) as evidenced by poor wound healing, difficulty gaining or maintaining body weight

Goal/Outcome

Child will demonstrate balanced nutritional state, will maintain or gain weight as appropriate for situation, will demonstrate improvement in wound healing.

Promoting Nutrition (interventions with *rationale*)

- Assess the child's food preferences and ability to eat *to provide a baseline for planning nursing care.*
- Consult the nutritionist *because nutritional needs are increased related to altered metabolic state as a result of burns.*
- Collaborate with the nutritionist, child, and parents to plan meals that appeal to the child *to increase the child's intake.*
- Administer vitamin and mineral preparations as prescribed *to supplement nutrients.*
- Provide smaller, more frequent meals and snacks *to promote increased intake.*
- Weigh the child daily *to determine progress.*

Nursing Analysis

Disturbed body image related to injury or alteration in body function (chronic skin changes or burns) as evidenced by child's negative feeling about body or fear of reaction by others

Goal/Outcome

Child will verbalize or demonstrate acceptance of alteration in body, will return to previous level of social involvement.

Promoting Appropriate Body Image (interventions with *rationale*)

- Assess child or adolescent for feelings about alteration in skin *to determine baseline.*
- Acknowledge feelings of anger or depression related to skin changes *to provide an outlet for feelings.*
- Encourage the child or adolescent to participate in skin care *to give some sense of control over what is occurring.*
- Help the child or adolescent to accept self *as the perception of self is tied to knowing oneself and identifying self-values.*

Based on your top three nursing patient problems for Eva, describe appropriate nursing interventions.

INFECTIOUS DISORDERS

Infectious disorders of the skin include those caused by viral, bacterial, or fungal infection. The viral exanthems are discussed in Chapter 37. Bacterial and fungal infections of the skin are discussed in what follows.

Bacterial Infections

Bacterial infections of the skin include bullous and nonbullous impetigo, folliculitis, cellulitis, and staphylococcal scalded skin syndrome. These bacterial skin infections are often caused by *Staphylococcus aureus* and group A beta-hemolytic streptococcus, which are ordinarily normal flora on the skin. Impetigo, folliculitis, and cellulitis are usually self-limited disorders that rarely become severe.

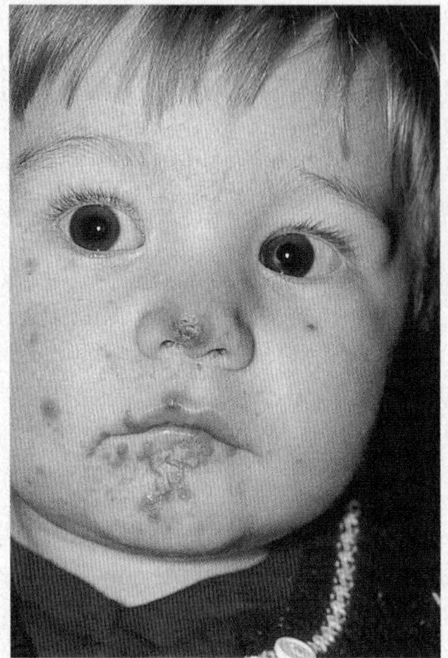

FIGURE 45.2 Note honey-colored crusting with impetigo.

Impetigo is a readily recognizable skin rash (Fig. 45.2). Nonbullous impetigo generally follows some type of skin trauma or may arise as a secondary bacterial infection of another skin disorder, such as AD. Bullous impetigo demonstrates a sporadic occurrence pattern and develops on intact skin, resulting from toxin production by *S. aureus.*

Folliculitis, infection of the hair follicle, most often results from occlusion of the hair follicle. It may occur as a result of poor hygiene, prolonged contact with contaminated water, maceration, a moist environment, or use of occlusive emollient products.

Cellulitis is a localized infection and inflammation of the skin and subcutaneous tissues and is usually preceded by skin trauma of some sort (Fig. 45.3). Periorbital

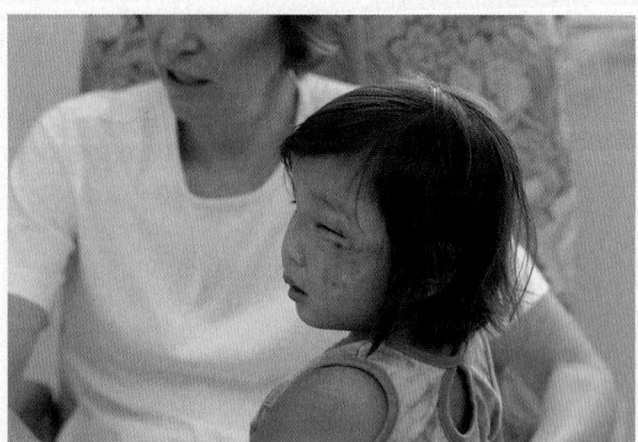

FIGURE 45.3 Note erythema and edema associated with cellulitis.

cellulitis is a bacterial infection of the eyelids and tissue surrounding the eye. The bacteria may gain entry to the skin via an abrasion, laceration, insect bite, foreign body, or impetiginous lesion. Periorbital cellulitis may also result from a nearby bacterial infection, such as sinusitis. *Staphylococcus aureus, Streptococcus pyogenes,* and *Streptococcus pneumoniae* are the most commonly implicated bacteria. The bacteria produce either an enzyme or endotoxins that initiate the inflammatory response. Redness, swelling, and infiltration of the skin by the inflammatory mediators occur.

Staphylococcal scalded skin syndrome results from infection with *S. aureus* that produces a toxin, which then causes exfoliation. It has an abrupt onset and results in diffuse **erythema** (reddening of the skin) and skin tenderness (Fig. 45.4). Scalded skin syndrome is most common in infancy and rare beyond 5 years of age (McMahon, 2022).

Of particular concern are community-acquired bacterial skin infections caused by methicillin-resistant *S. aureus* (CA-MRSA) (Baddour, 2022). CA-MRSA most commonly occurs as a skin or soft tissue infection, such as cellulitis or an abscess. Risk factors for CA-MRSA are turf burns, towel sharing, participation in team sports, or attendance at day care or outdoor camps. If the child presents with a moderate to severe skin infection or with an infection that is not responding as expected to therapy, it is important to culture the infected area for MRSA.

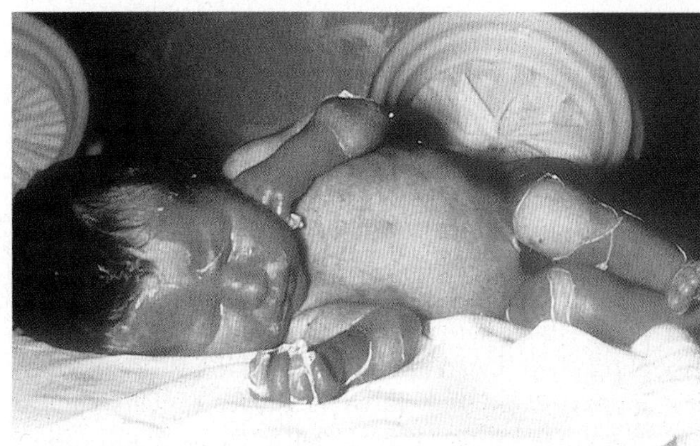

FIGURE 45.4 Staphylococcal scalded skin syndrome (SSSS) with ruptured bullae. (Reprinted with permission from Goodheart, H. P., & Gonzalez, M. E. [2016]. *Goodheart's photoguide to common pediatric and adult skin disorders* [4th ed.]. Wolters Kluwer.)

Therapeutic management of most bacterial skin infections includes topical or systemic antibiotics and appropriate hygiene (Table 45.1). Treatment of periorbital cellulitis focuses on IV antibiotic administration during the acute phase, followed by completion of the course with oral antibiotics. Complications of periorbital cellulitis include bacteremia and progression to orbital cellulitis, which is a more extensive infection involving the orbit of the eye.

TABLE 45.1 • Bacterial Skin Infections

Disorder	Skin Findings	Usual Treatment
Nonbullous impetigo	• Papules progressing to vesicles, then painless pustules with a narrow erythematous border • Honey-colored exudate when the vesicles or pustules rupture, which forms a crust on the ulcer-like base (see Fig. 45.2)	• Limited amount: treat topically with mupirocin ointment. • If numerous lesions, oral first-generation cephalosporin is indicated. • Clindamycin may be needed for MRSA. • Remove honey-colored crust with cool compresses twice daily.
Bullous impetigo	• Red macules and bullous eruptions on an erythematous base • Size may be from a few millimeters to several centimeters.	• Oral first-generation cephalosporin • Good hygiene
Folliculitis	Red, raised hair follicles	• Treat with aggressive hygiene: warm compresses after washing with soap and water several times a day. • Topical mupirocin is indicated; occasionally, oral antibiotics are required.
Cellulitis	Localized reaction: erythema, pain, edema, warmth at site of skin disruption (see Fig. 45.3)	• Mild cases are usually treated with cephalexin or amoxicillin/clavulanic acid. • More severe cases and periorbital or orbital cellulitis require IV cephalosporins.
Staphylococcal scalded skin syndrome	• Flattish bullae that rupture within hours • Red, weeping surface is left, most commonly on face, groin, neck, and axillary region (see Fig. 45.4)	• Mild to moderate cases are treated with oral cephalexin, dicloxacillin, or amoxicillin/clavulanic acid. • Severe cases are managed similar to burns with aggressive fluid management and IV oxacillin or clindamycin.

MRSA, methicillin-resistant *Staphylococcus aureus*

Data from Prok, L. D., & Torres-Zegarra, C. X. (2022). Chapter 15: Skin. In M. Bunik, W. W. Hay, M. J. Levin, & M. J. Abzug (Eds.), *Current diagnosis & treatment: Pediatrics* (26th ed.). McGraw-Hill Education; Baddour, L. M. (2022). Impetigo. *UpToDate*. Retrieved January 29, 2024, from http://www.uptodate.com/contents/impetigo

Nursing Assessment

Obtain the history as noted in the nursing process overview section. Note history of skin disruption such as a cut, scrape, or insect or spider bite (nonbullous impetigo and cellulitis). Note body piercing in the adolescent, which can lead to impetigo or cellulitis. Measure the child's temperature. Fever may occur with bullous impetigo or cellulitis and is common with scalded skin syndrome. Inspect the skin, noting abnormalities, documenting their location and distribution, and describing drainage if present. Table 45.1 gives specific clinical manifestations of the various bacterial skin infections. Assess for pain. In periorbital cellulitis, note marked eyelid edema as well as a purplish or red color of the eyelid (Fig. 45.5) and restricted movement of the eye area.

Palpate for regional lymphadenopathy, which may be present with impetigo or cellulitis. Blood cultures are indicated in the child with cellulitis with lymphangitic streaking and in all cases of periorbital or orbital cellulitis.

CLINICAL REASONING ALERT!

Notify the health care provider or nurse practitioner immediately if any of these signs of progression to orbital cellulitis occur: conjunctival redness, change in vision, pain with eye movement, eye muscle weakness or paralysis, or proptosis.

Nursing Management

Administer antibiotics topically or systemically as prescribed. Teach the family about antibiotic administration and care of the lesions or rash. Soak impetiginous lesions with cool compresses or Burow solution to remove crusts before applying topical antibiotics. Although impetigo is considered a contagious disorder among vulnerable populations, removal from school or day care is not necessary unless the condition is widespread or actively weeping. Prevent transmission of nosocomial MRSA by appropriately isolating children according to the institution's policy when the child is hospitalized. In children with scalded skin syndrome, reduce the risk of scarring by minimal handling, avoiding corticosteroids, and applying soothing ointments as the skin heals.

For periorbital cellulitis, apply warm soaks to the eye area for 20 minutes every 2 to 4 hours. Administer IV antibiotics as prescribed. Instruct parents to call the health care provider or nurse practitioner or have the child evaluated again if the child is not improving or cannot move their eye, if proptosis occurs, or if perceived visual acuity lessens.

Teach families the importance of completing the entire course of oral antibiotic treatment at home. Educate the family about prevention of bacterial skin infections. Stress the importance of cleanliness and hygiene. Teach the family to keep the child's fingernails cut short and to clean the nails with a nail brush at bath time. When a skin disruption such as a cut, scrape, or insect bite occurs, teach the family to clean the area well to prevent the development of cellulitis. Folliculitis may be prevented with diligent hygiene and avoidance of occlusive emollients. Table 45.1 gives additional information about specific treatments for bacterial skin infections. See Dosage Calculation Box 45.1.

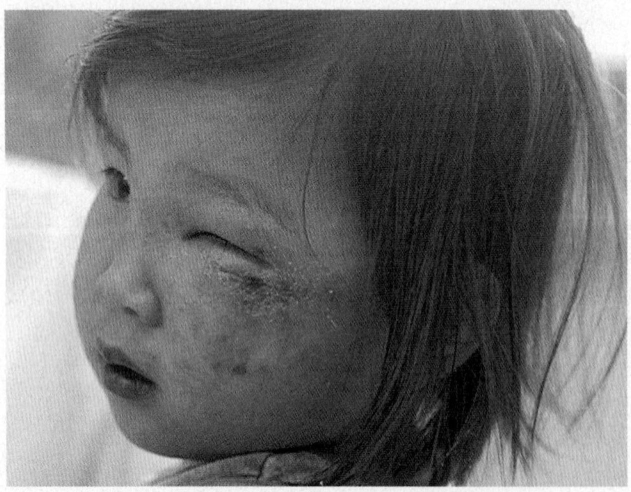

FIGURE 45.5 Periorbital cellulitis.

DOSAGE CALCULATION BOX 45.1

Child's weight: 13 lb 3 oz

Medication order: cephalexin 125 mg/5 mL, 4 mL PO every 6 hours.

Per the Pediatric Dosage Handbook, the recommended dose is 25–50 mg/kg/day divided every 6 to 8 hours daily.

Is the ordered dose safe?

Fungal Infections

Fungi also cause infections on children's skin. *Tinea* is a fungal disease of the skin occurring on any part of the body. The part of the body affected determines the second word in the name. Examples of tinea infections occurring on various parts of the body include:

- Tinea pedis: fungal infection on the feet
- Tinea corporis: fungal infection on the arms or legs
- Tinea versicolor: fungal infection on the trunk and extremities
- Tinea capitis: fungal infection on the scalp, eyebrows, or eyelashes
- Tinea cruris: fungal infection on the groin

The three organisms most often responsible for tinea are *Epidermophyton*, *Microsporum*, and *Trichophyton*,

TABLE 45.2 • Management of Fungal Infections

Disorder	Skin Findings	Usual Treatment
Tinea corporis (ringworm)	Annular lesion with raised peripheral scaling and central clearing (looks like a ring) (see Fig. 45.6)	Topical antifungal cream is required for at least 4 weeks.
Tinea capitis	• Patches of scaling in the scalp with central hair loss • Risk of kerion development (inflamed, boggy mass that is filled with pustules) (see Fig. 45.7)	• Oral griseofulvin for 4–6 weeks • Selenium sulfide shampoo may be used to decrease contagiousness (adjunct only). • No school or day care for 1 week after treatment initiated
Tinea versicolor	• Superficial tan or hypopigmented oval scaly lesions, especially on upper back and chest and proximal arms • More noticeable in the summer with tanning of unaffected areas (see Fig. 45.8)	• Apply selenium sulfide shampoo all over body (from face to knees) and allow to stay on skin overnight, rinsing in the morning, once a week for 4 weeks (this may cause skin irritation). • Topical antifungals in the imidazole family may be used instead.
Tinea pedis (athlete's foot)	Red, scaling rash on soles and between the toes (see Fig. 45.9)	• Topical antifungal cream, powder, or spray • Appropriate foot hygiene
Tinea cruris	Erythema, scaling, maceration in the inguinal creases and inner thighs (penis/scrotum spared)	Topical antifungal preparation for 4–6 weeks
Diaper candidiasis (also called monilial diaper rash)	Fiery red lesions, scaling in the skin folds, and satellite lesions (located further out from the main rash) (see Fig. 45.10)	• Topical nystatin with diaper changes for several days • See section on diaper dermatitis for additional information.

Data from Prok, L. D., & Torres-Zegarra, C. X. (2022). Chapter 15: Skin. In M. Bunik, W. W. Hay, M. J. Levin, & M. J. Abzug (Eds.), *Current diagnosis & treatment: Pediatrics* (26th ed.). McGraw-Hill Education.

although *Malassezia furfur* causes tinea versicolor. *Candida albicans* may cause an infection of the skin, particularly in a warm, moist area such as the diaper area. All fungal skin infections may occur year-round, but tinea versicolor is more common in warm weather.

Therapeutic management of fungal infections involves appropriate hygiene and administration of an antifungal agent. Table 45.2 gives further information about treatment.

Nursing Assessment

Elicit the health history, noting exposure to another person with a fungal infection or exposure to a pet (fungi are often carried by pets). Note onset of the rash and whether it is itchy. Determine if the child has recently visited the barber (tinea capitis). Note contact with damp areas such as locker rooms and swimming pools, use of nylon socks or nonbreathable shoes, or minor trauma to the feet (tinea pedis). Document a history of wearing tight clothing or participating in a contact sport such as wrestling (tinea cruris). Inspect the skin and scalp, noting the location, description, and distribution of the rash or lesions (Figs. 45.6 to 45.10). Table 45.2 describes the clinical findings associated with various types of tinea.

Scraping and KOH preparation show branching hyphae. For tinea capitis, the Wood lamp will fluoresce yellow-green if it is caused by *Microsporum*, but not with *Trichophyton*. A fungal culture of a plucked hair is more reliable for diagnosis of tinea capitis.

Nursing Management

Maintain appropriate hygiene and administer antifungal agents as prescribed (see Table 45.2). Additional specifics related to the individual fungal disorders are as follows:

- Tinea corporis is contagious, but the child may return to day care or school once treatment has begun. Identify and treat family members or other contacts.
- Counsel the child with tinea capitis and parents that hair will usually regrow in 3 to 12 months. Wash sheets

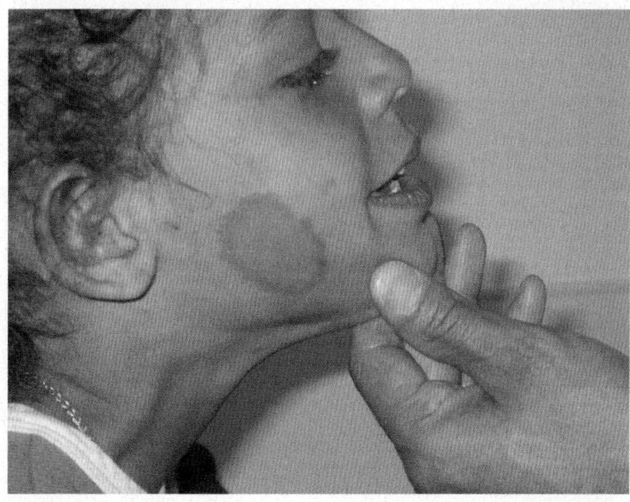

FIGURE 45.6 Tinea corporis: note raised scaly border with clearing in center.

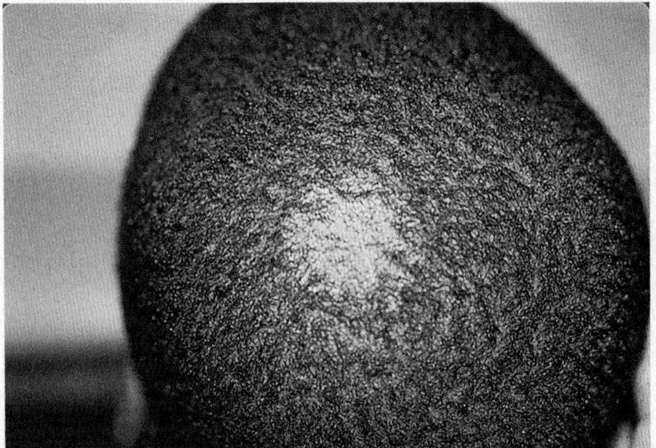

FIGURE 45.7 Note hair breakage and loss with tinea capitis.

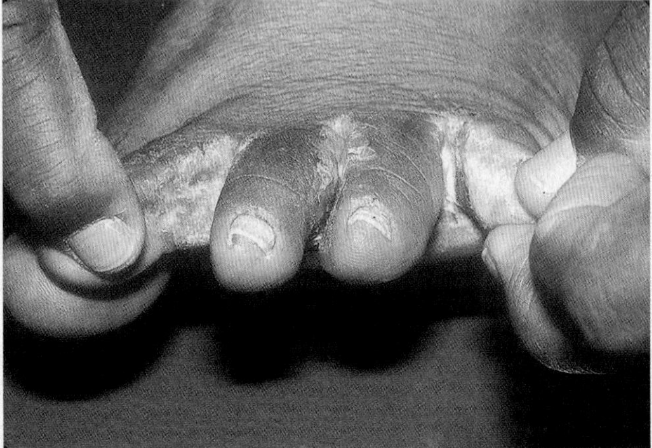

FIGURE 45.9 Tinea pedis. The interdigital pattern of tinea pedis is common. (Reprinted with permission from Goodheart, H. P. [2009]. *Goodheart's photoguide to common skin disorders* [3rd ed.]. Wolters Kluwer.)

and clothes in hot water to decrease the risk of the infection spreading to other family members.

- Instruct the child with tinea pedis to keep the feet clean and dry. Rinse feet with water or a water/vinegar mixture and dry them well, especially between the toes. Encourage the child to wear cotton socks and shoes that allow the feet to breathe. Going barefoot at home is allowed, but flip-flops should be worn around swimming pools and in locker rooms.
- Inform the child with tinea versicolor that return to normal skin pigmentation may take several months.
- Counsel the child or adolescent with tinea cruris to wear cotton underwear and loose clothing. It is important to maintain good hygiene, particularly after sports practice or a sporting event.
- For management of diaper candidiasis, follow the suggestions listed further on in the section on diaper dermatitis.

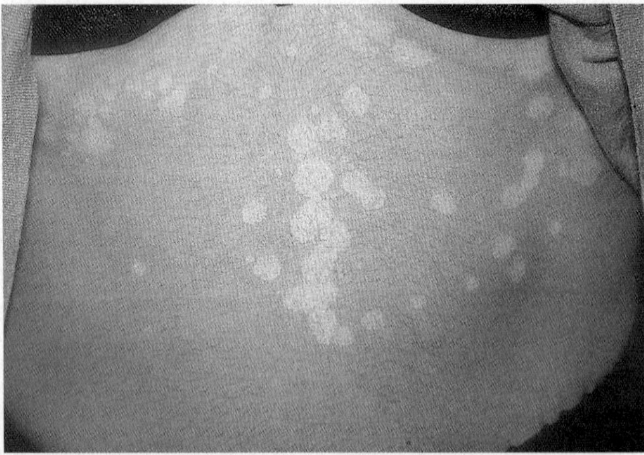

FIGURE 45.8 Tinea versicolor. Hypopigmented scaly lesions on the back of a darkly pigmented adolescent. (Reprinted with permission from Goodheart, H. P., & Gonzalez, M. E. [2016]. *Goodheart's photoguide to common pediatric and adult skin disorders* [4th ed.]. Wolters Kluwer.)

INFLAMMATORY SKIN CONDITIONS

Inflammatory skin conditions (**dermatitis**) may be either acute or chronic. Acute hypersensitivity reactions may cause diaper dermatitis, contact dermatitis, erythema multiforme, and urticaria. AD is a chronic hypersensitivity disorder. Seborrhea and psoriasis are chronic inflammatory skin disorders that do not occur as a result of hypersensitivity.

Diaper Dermatitis

Dermatitis refers to an inflammatory reaction of the skin. Diaper dermatitis refers to an inflammatory reaction of the skin in the area covered by a diaper. It is a nonimmunologic response to a skin irritant that results in skin cell hydration disturbance. Prolonged exposure to urine and feces may lead to skin breakdown (Fig. 45.11). Diaper wearing increases the skin's pH, activating fecal enzymes that further contribute to skin maceration.

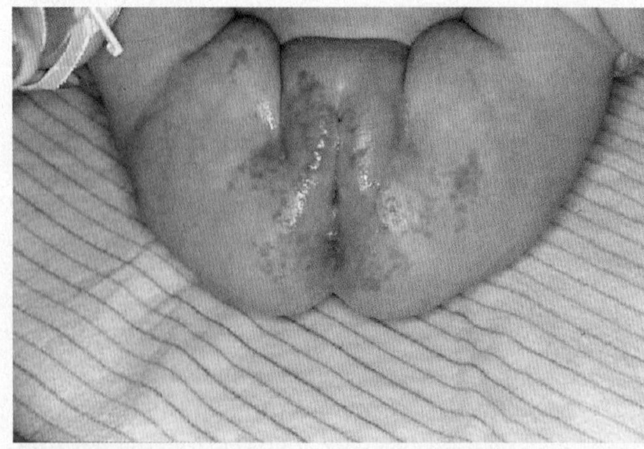

FIGURE 45.10 A bright red rash with satellite lesions occurs with diaper candidiasis.

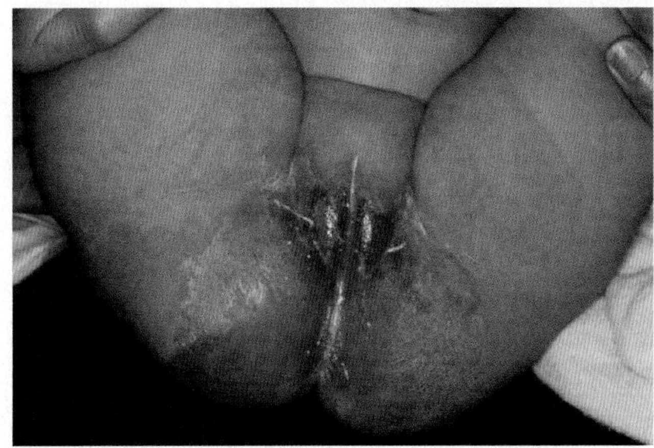

FIGURE 45.11 Diaper dermatitis.

Nursing Assessment

Determine from the history whether the infant or child wears diapers. Ask about the onset and progression of the rash, as well as any treatments and response. Inspect the skin in the diaper area for erythema and maceration (see Fig. 45.11). Ordinary diaper dermatitis does not usually result in a bumpy rash but starts as a flat red rash in the convex skin creases. It may appear red and shiny and may or may not also have **papules** (raised lesion). Untreated, it may become more widespread or severe. Some cases of diaper dermatitis are caused by overgrowth of *C. albicans* (see Fig. 45.9 and the "Fungal Infections" section).

Nursing Management

Prevention is the best management of diaper dermatitis. Topical products such as ointments or creams containing vitamins A, D, and E; zinc oxide; or petrolatum are helpful to provide a barrier to the skin. Teaching Guidelines 45.1 gives further information on prevention and management of diaper dermatitis. See earlier for treatment of diaper rash caused by *C. albicans* infection.

TEACHING GUIDELINES 45.1 Prevention and Management of Diaper Dermatitis

- Change diapers frequently. Change stool-soiled diapers as soon as possible.
- Avoid rubber pants.
- Gently wash the diaper area with a soft cloth, avoiding harsh soaps.
- Use baby wipes in most children, but avoid wipes that contain fragrance or preservatives.
- Once a rash has occurred, follow all the earlier prevention tips and add the following:
  - Allow the infant or child to go diaperless for some time each day to allow the rash to heal.
  - Blow-dry the diaper area/rash area with the dryer set on the warm (not hot) setting for 3 to 5 minutes.

TAKE NOTE!

Discourage parents from using any type of baby powder to avoid the risk of aspiration; inhalation of talcum-containing powders may result in pneumonitis (Hagan et al., 2017).

Atopic Dermatitis

Atopic dermatitis (AD; also called eczema) is one of the disorders in the atopy family (along with asthma and allergic rhinitis). AD affects 16% to 19% of US children (Howe, 2023). Onset of symptoms occurs usually before 2 years of age (Prok & Torres-Zegarra, 2022). AD is often associated with food allergies, allergic rhinitis, and asthma, although not all children with AD will develop one of those other disorders (Howe, 2023).

The chronic itching associated with AD causes a great deal of psychological distress. The child's self-image may be affected, particularly if the rash is extensive. Difficulty sleeping may occur because of the itching. The child is irritable and has difficulty concentrating, and family life is disrupted. Parents' stress related to the child's condition may increase the child's anxiety and lead to an increase in itching and scratching. The child may outgrow AD, its severity may decrease as the child approaches adulthood, or the child may continue to have difficulties into the adult years. Bacterial superinfection may occur as a complication.

Therapeutic management includes good skin hydration, application of topical corticosteroids or immune modulators, oral antihistamines for sedative effects, and antibiotics if secondary infection occurs.

Pathophysiology

AD is a chronic disorder characterized by extreme itching and inflamed, reddened, and swollen skin. It has a relapsing and remitting nature. The skin reaction occurs in response to specific allergens, usually food (especially eggs, wheat, milk, and peanuts) or environmental triggers (e.g., molds, dust mites, and cat dander). Other factors, such as high or low ambient temperatures, perspiring, scratching, skin irritants, or stress, may contribute to flare-ups. When the child encounters a triggering antigen, antigen-presenting cells stimulate interleukins to begin the inflammatory process. The skin begins to feel pruritic, and the child starts to scratch. The sensation of itchiness comes first, and then the rash becomes apparent. The scratching causes the rash to appear. Sweating causes AD to worsen, as does excessively humid or dry environments.

Nursing Assessment

For a full description of the assessment phase of the nursing process, refer to the "Clinical Judgment and the Nursing Process" section earlier in the chapter. Assessment findings pertinent to AD are discussed here.

HEALTH HISTORY

Elicit a description of the present illness and chief complaint. Common signs and symptoms reported during the health history might include:

- Wiggling or scratching
- Dry skin
- Scratch marks noticed by the parents
- Disrupted sleep
- Irritability

Explore the child's current and past medical history for risk factors such as:

- Family history of AD, allergic rhinitis, or asthma
- Child's history of asthma or allergic rhinitis
- Food or environmental allergies

Determine the onset of the rash; its location, progression, and severity; and response to treatments used so far. Note medications used to treat the rash, as well as other medications the child may be taking.

PHYSICAL EXAMINATION

Physical examination consists of inspection and observation and auscultation.

Inspection and Observation

Observe whether the infant is wiggling or the child is actively scratching. Carefully inspect the skin. Document dry, scaly, or flaky skin, as well as hypertrophy and lichenification (Fig. 45.12). If lesions are present, they may be dry lesions or weepy papules or **vesicles** (fluid-filled lesions). In children younger than 2 years, the rash is most likely to occur on the face, scalp, wrists, and extensor surfaces of the arms or legs. In older children, it may occur anywhere on the skin but is found more commonly on the flexor areas. Note erythema or warmth, which may indicate associated secondary bacterial infection. Document areas of hyperpigmentation or hypopigmentation, which may have resulted from a prior exacerbation of AD or its treatment. Inspect the eyes, nose, and throat for symptoms of allergic rhinitis.

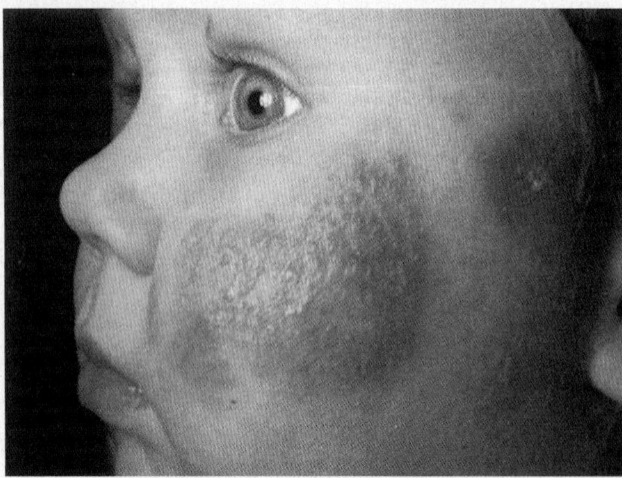

FIGURE 45.12 Atopic dermatitis rash is red, dry, and scaly.

Auscultation

Auscultate the lungs for wheezing (commonly found in the associated condition of asthma).

LABORATORY AND DIAGNOSTIC TESTS

Serum immunoglobulin E (IgE) levels may be elevated in the child with AD. Skin prick allergy testing may determine the food or environmental allergen to which the child is sensitive.

Nursing Management

Nursing management of the child with AD focuses on promoting skin hydration, maintaining skin integrity, and preventing infection.

PROMOTING SKIN HYDRATION

First and foremost, avoid hot water and any skin or hair product containing perfumes, dyes, or fragrance. Bathe the child twice daily in warm (not hot) water. Use a mild soap to clean only the dirty areas. Recommended mild soaps or cleansing agents include:

- Unscented Dove or Dove for sensitive skin
- Tone
- Caress
- Oil of Olay
- Cetaphil
- Aquanil

Slightly pat the child dry after the bath, but do not rub the skin with the towel. Leave the child moist. Apply prescribed topical ointments or creams such as corticosteroids or immune modulators (see Drug Guide 45.1) to the affected area. Apply fragrance-free moisturizer over the prescribed topical medication and all over the child's body. Recommended moisturizers include:

- Eucerin, Moisturel, Curel (cream or lotion)
- Aquaphor
- Vaseline
- Crisco

> ***TAKE NOTE!***
>
> Vaseline or generic petrolatum is an inexpensive, readily available moisturizer.

Apply moisturizer multiple times throughout the day. Avoid clothing made of synthetic fabrics or wool. Avoid triggers known to exacerbate AD.

Herbal supplements and oils (such as evening primrose oil) have demonstrated mixed results for reduction in redness and scaling. If not initially recommended by the health care provider or nurse practitioner, the parent should consult with them first before starting these supplements. Headache and nausea are rare adverse effects of these supplements and, if they occur, are usually mild. Chamomile preparations for topical use help some children and are generally considered safe.

MAINTAINING SKIN INTEGRITY AND PREVENTING INFECTION

Cut the child's fingernails short and keep them clean. Avoid tight clothing and heat. Use 100% cotton bed sheets and pajamas. In addition to keeping the child's skin well moisturized, it is extremely important to prevent the child from scratching. Scratching causes the rash to appear, and further scratching may lead to secondary infection. Antihistamines given at bedtime may sedate the child enough to allow them to sleep without awakening because of itching.

During the waking hours, behavior modification may help to keep the child from scratching. Have the parent keep a diary for 1 week to determine the pattern of scratching. Help the parent to determine specific strategies that may raise the child's awareness of scratching. A handheld clicker or counter may help to identify the scratching episode for the child, thus raising awareness. The use of diversion, imagination, and play may help to distract the child from scratching. The parent and child may create a game together that results in the child participating in a behavior rather than scratching. Pressing the skin or clenching the fist may replace scratching. It is important for the child to stay active to distract their mind from the itching. It is important for the parent to positively reinforce and reward the desired behaviors. See Evidence-Based Practice 45.1.

Contact Dermatitis

Contact dermatitis is a cell-mediated response to an antigenic substance exposure. The first exposure is the sensitization phase. The antigen attaches to cells that migrate to regional lymph nodes and have contact with T lymphocytes, where recognition of antigen is developed. During the second phase, elicitation, contact with the antigen results in T-lymphocyte proliferation and release of inflammatory mediators. An allergic response occurs within 24 to 48 hours after contact with the substance.

Contact dermatitis may occur as a result of allergy to nickel or cobalt found in clothing hardware and dyes, and chemicals found in many hygiene products and cosmetics. One of the more common causes of contact dermatitis in children results from exposure to highly allergenic plants such as *Toxicodendron radicans* (poison ivy), *Toxicodendron quercifolium* (Eastern poison oak), *Toxicodendron diversilobum* (Western poison oak), and *Toxicodendron vernix* (poison sumac).

Direct or indirect contact with the plant's oleoresin found in the leaves, stems, and roots results in an allergic reaction. Even contact with dormant plants or plants perceived to be dead may cause an allergic response. The rash is extremely pruritic and may last for 2 to 4 weeks; lesions continue to appear during the illness. Contact dermatitis is not contagious and does not spread either to other parts of the affected child's skin or to other people. Scratching does not spread the rash, but it may cause skin damage or secondary infection. Complications of contact dermatitis include secondary bacterial skin infections and lichenification or hyperpigmentation, particularly in darker skin tones.

Therapeutic management is directed toward management of itching and the use of topical corticosteroids.

EVIDENCE-BASED PRACTICE 45.1

Phototherapy for Atopic Dermatitis

STUDY

Conventional medications do not always provide the relief children and their parents desire for atopic dermatitis. This review focused on the use of phototherapy (narrow-band ultraviolet B [NB-UVB] therapy) compared to placebo or other treatments for atopic dermatitis. The authors reviewed 32 studies with 1,219 participants aged 5 years and older.

Findings

Overall, the use of NB-UVB did result in modest improvements in signs of eczema as assessed by a health care professional, moderate to significant improvement as reported by the participants, and an increased number of participants reporting less severe itching. Confidence in the findings is limited, as the reviewed studies were quite disparate from each other.

Nursing Implications

The impact of phototherapy on AD has not been well studied. If parents wish to pursue alternative treatments, this study reported on a particular type of phototherapy, NB-UVB. Additional high-quality rigorous studies are needed to establish the benefit of NB-UVB therapy as well as other forms of phototherapy.

Data from Musters, A. H., Mashayekhi, S., Harvey, J., Axon, E., Lax, S. J., Flohr, C., Drucker, A. M, Gerbens, L., Ferguson, J., Ibbotson, S., Dawe, R. S., Garritsen, F., Brouwer, M., Limpens, J., Prescott, L. E., Boyle, R. J., & Spuls, P. I. (2021). Phototherapy for atopic eczema. *Cochrane Database of Systematic Reviews*. https://doi.org/10.1002/14651858.CD013870.pub2

Moderate-potency topical glucocorticoid cream or ointment is used for mild to moderate contact dermatitis, and high-potency preparations are used for more severe cases. Some severe cases of contact dermatitis may require the use of systemic steroids.

Nursing Assessment

Elicit the health history, noting onset, description, location, and progression of the rash, which may be intensely pruritic and vesicular if caused by allergenic plant exposure (Fig. 45.13). Rashes caused by other allergic exposure may be quite variable in their appearance and intensity of pruritus. Document treatment used thus far, and the child's response to it. Examine the skin, noting rash that may vary from maculopapular in nature to an erythematous papulovesicular rash at the site of contact. Some lesions may be weeping; others may erupt and form a crust. The lesions are often distributed in an asymmetric linear pattern on exposed body parts if caused by allergenic plant exposure. If the child's shirt came in contact with the plant and then the shirt was removed by pulling it over the head, widespread lesions might be found over both sides of the face. Lesions near the eyes often cause significant eyelid edema.

> *TAKE NOTE!*
>
> Nickel dermatitis may occur from contact with jewelry, eyeglasses, belts, or clothing snaps. Infants may display a small red circle with scaling at the site of contact with sleeper snaps.

Nursing Management

Contact dermatitis may be prevented by avoiding contact with the allergen. When the condition does occur, nursing management focuses on relieving the discomfort associated with the rash. Administer topical or systemic corticosteroids as prescribed, and teach the family about use of the medications. Teaching Guidelines 45.2 gives more information about the treatment and prevention of contact dermatitis.

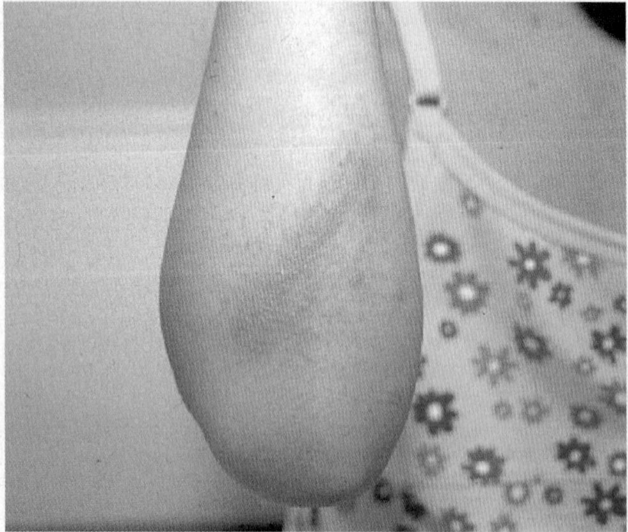

FIGURE 45.13 Note vesicular rash in linear formation characteristic of poison ivy.

Erythema Multiforme

Erythema multiforme, although uncommon in children, is an acute, self-limiting hypersensitivity reaction. It may occur in response to viral infections, such as adenovirus

TEACHING GUIDELINES 45.2 Prevention and Treatment of Contact Dermatitis

Prevention

- Wear long sleeves and long pants on outings in the woods.
- Identify and remove offending plants in the yard by using a commercial weed or underbrush killer.
- Vinyl gloves (not rubber or latex) are an effective barrier.
- The plant's oil residue may be on clothes, pets, garden and sports equipment, and toys; wash those well with soap and water.
- If contact occurs, wash vigorously with soap and water within 10 minutes of contact.
- Zanfel and Tecnu Oak-N-Ivy Outdoor Skin Cleanser (both soap mixtures) may prevent rash if used to wash the skin soon after exposure.
- Ivy Block (an organoclay) is a U.S. Food and Drug Administration–approved preventive treatment for contact dermatitis related to poison ivy, oak, or sumac. It is applied to the skin before possible exposure.

Treatment

- Wash lesions daily with mild soap and water.
- Mildly debride crusted lesions.
- Tepid baths (colloidal oatmeal such as Aveeno) are helpful to decrease itching.
- Avoid hot baths or showers, as they aggravate itching.
- Apply corticosteroid preparations topically as directed (if using high-potency preparations, do not cover with an occlusive dressing).
- Weeping lesions may be wrapped lightly; avoid occlusion.
- Burow or Domeboro solutions with a dressing applied twice daily for 20 minutes may help to dry weepy lesions.
- Over-the-counter preparations such as calamine lotion or Ivy Rest may reduce itching and help the lesions to dry.
- Do not use topical antihistamines, benzocaine, or neomycin because of the potential for sensitization.

BOX 45.1 Stevens–Johnson Syndrome and Toxic Epidermal Necrolysis

- High fever and flulike symptoms for 1 to 3 days prior to rash appearing
- Rash is characteristic of erythema multiforme with the addition of inflammatory bullae on at least two types of mucosa (lips, oral mucosa, bulbar conjunctivae, or anogenital region).
- Stevens–Johnson syndrome results in skin detachment of 10% or less, while toxic epidermal necrolysis involves 30% skin detachment.
- Mortality rate of 23% (Lee, 2024)
- Treatment: hospitalization, isolation, fluid and electrolyte support, treatment of secondary infection of the lesions
- Ophthalmologic consult to determine if corneal ulceration, keratitis, uveitis, or panophthalmitis is present

or Epstein–Barr virus; *Mycoplasma pneumoniae* infection; or a drug (especially sulfa drugs, penicillins, or immunizations) or food reaction. Stevens–Johnson syndrome and toxic epidermal necrolysis are the severest forms of erythema multiforme and most often occur in response to certain medications or to *Mycoplasma* infection (Box 45.1). Therapeutic management of erythema multiforme is generally supportive because it resolves on its own.

Nursing Assessment

Note history of fever, malaise, and achiness (myalgia). Determine onset and progression of rash, as well as presence of pruritus and burning. Document the child's temperature on assessment. Inspect the skin for lesions, which most commonly occur over the hands and feet and extensor surfaces of the extremities, with spread to the trunk. Lesions progress from erythematous **macules** (flat reddened areas) to papules, plaques, vesicles, and target lesions over a period of days (hence the name *multiforme*) (Fig. 45.14).

Nursing Management

Discontinue the medication or food if it is identified as the cause. Ensure that treatment for *Mycoplasma* is instituted if present. Encourage oral hydration. Administer analgesics and antihistamines as needed to promote comfort. If oral lesions are present, encourage soothing mouthwashes or use of topical oral anesthetics in the older child or adolescent. Oral lesions may be debrided with hydrogen peroxide.

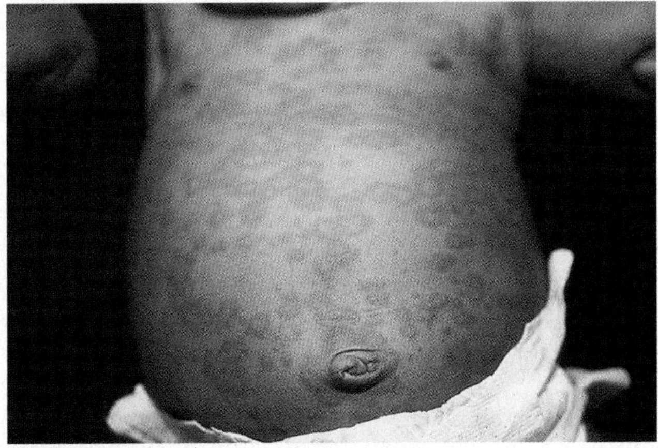

FIGURE 45.14 Erythema multiforme.

Urticaria

Urticaria, commonly called hives, is a type I hypersensitivity reaction caused by an immunologically mediated antigen–antibody response of histamine release from mast cells. Vasodilation and increased vascular permeability result, and erythema and wheals then occur. Urticaria usually begins rapidly and may disappear in a few days or may take up to 6 weeks to resolve. The most common causes of this reaction are foods, drugs, animal stings, infections, environmental stimuli (e.g., heat, cold, sun, tight clothes), and stress. Therapeutic management focuses on identifying and removing the cause as well as providing antihistamines or steroids.

Nursing Assessment

Obtain a detailed history of new foods, medications, symptoms of a recent infection, changes in environment, or unusual stress. Inspect the skin, noting raised, edematous hives anywhere on the body or mucous membranes (Fig. 45.15). The hives are pruritic, blanch when pressed, and may migrate. Angioedema may also be present and is identifiable as subcutaneous edema and warmth, occurring most frequently on the extremities, face, or genitalia. Carefully assess airway and breathing, as hypersensitivity reactions may affect respiratory status.

Nursing Management

Identify and remove the offending trigger. Discontinue antibiotics. Administer antihistamines, corticosteroids,

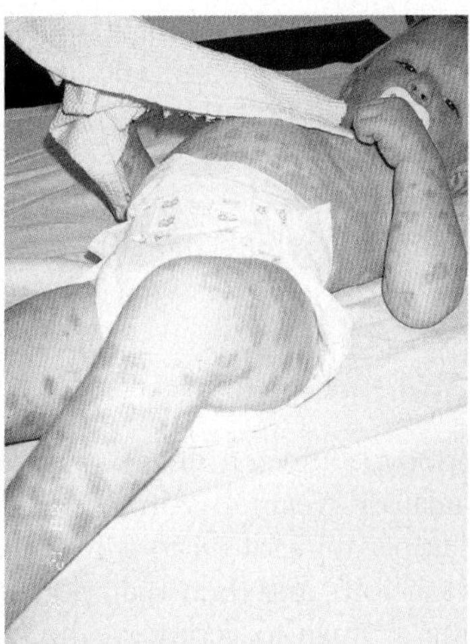

FIGURE 45.15 Ill-appearing child with urticaria. (Reprinted with permission from Fleisher, G. R., Ludwig, S., & Baskin, M. N. [2004]. *Atlas of pediatric emergency medicine* [p. 88]. Lippincott Williams & Wilkins.)

and topical antipruritics as prescribed. Inform the child and family that the episode should resolve within a few days. If it lasts up to 6 weeks, the child should be reevaluated (Covar et al., 2022). Advise the family to obtain a medical alert bracelet for the child if the reaction is severe.

> **TAKE NOTE!**
>
> In an emergency situation when airway and breathing are compromised, subcutaneous epinephrine followed by IV diphenhydramine and corticosteroids is necessary.

Seborrhea

Seborrhea is a chronic inflammatory dermatitis that may occur on the skin or scalp. In infants, it occurs most often on the scalp and is commonly referred to as cradle cap. Infants may also manifest seborrhea on the nose or eyebrows, behind the ears, or in the diaper area. It usually resolves over the course of weeks to months (Sasseville, 2023). Adolescents manifest seborrhea on the scalp (dandruff) and on the eyebrows and eyelashes, behind the ears, and between the shoulder blades.

It is thought that seborrhea is an inflammatory reaction to the fungus *Pityrosporum ovale* and is worsened by sebaceous involvement related to the birthing parent's hormones in the infant and androgens in the adolescent.

Therapeutic management includes treating the skin lesions with corticosteroid creams or lotions. Antidandruff shampoos containing selenium sulfide, ketoconazole, or tar are used to treat the scalp.

Nursing Assessment

Elicit the health history, determining onset and progression of skin and scalp changes. Note response to treatment used so far. In the infant, inspect the scalp and forehead, behind the ears, and the neck, trunk, and diaper area for thick or flaky greasy yellow scales (Fig. 45.16). In the adolescent, note mild flakes in the hair with yellow greasy scales on the scalp, forehead, and eyebrows; behind the ears; or between the scapulae.

Nursing Management

Wash or shampoo the affected areas with a mild soap. Apply antiinflammatory cream to skin lesions if prescribed. In the infant, apply mineral oil to the scalp, massage it well with a washcloth, and then shampoo 10 to 15 minutes later, using a brush to gently lift the crusts; do not forcibly remove the crusts. If needed, selenium sulfide shampoo may safely be used on the infant, following the aforementioned procedure. The adolescent may require daily shampooing with an antidandruff shampoo.

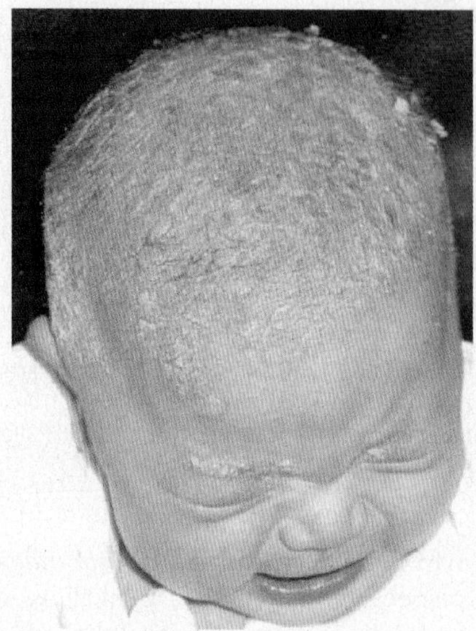

FIGURE 45.16 Severe cradle cap (yellow, greasy-appearing plaques).

Psoriasis

Psoriasis is a chronic inflammatory skin disease with periods of remission and exacerbation; control is possible with conscientious therapy. It is an immune-mediated disorder occurring in people with a genetic predisposition. About 30% of adults with this disorder experienced its onset prior to 2 years of age (Bender & Chiu, 2020).

Hyperproliferation of the epidermis occurs, with a rash developing at sites of mechanical, thermal, or physical trauma. Therapeutic management includes skin hydration with emollient creams, use of tar preparations, topical steroids, and UV light, among others. Narrow-band UV light has been used with some success in children with severe psoriasis.

Nursing Assessment

Note family history of psoriasis. Determine onset and progression of rash, as well as treatments used and the response to treatment. Question the child about pruritus, which is usually absent with psoriasis. Inspect the skin for erythematous papules that coalesce to form plaques, most frequently found on the scalp, elbows, genital area, and knees (Fig. 45.17). Facial plaques may also occur and are more common in children than in adults. The plaques have a silvery or yellow-white scale and sharply demarcated borders. Layers of scale may be present, which, when removed, result in pinpoint bleeding (referred to as the Auspitz sign). Plaques on the scalp may result in alopecia. Examine the palms and soles, noting fissures and scaling. Skin biopsy, although rarely needed for diagnosis, will show hyperplastic epidermis, with thinning of the papillary dermis.

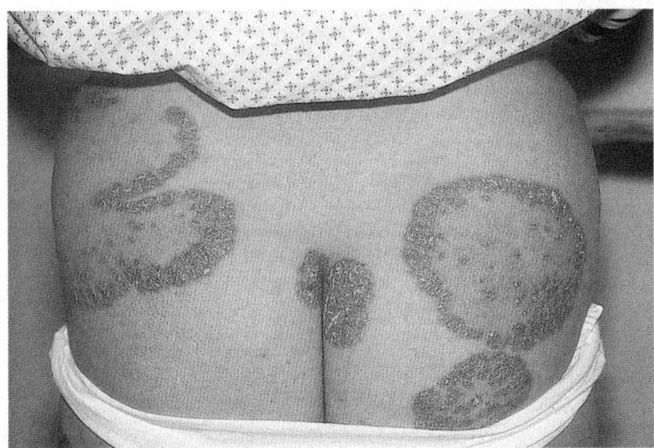

FIGURE 45.17 Psoriasis. (Reprinted with permission from Goodheart, H. P. [2009]. *Goodheart's photoguide to common skin disorders* [3rd ed.]. Wolters Kluwer.)

Nursing Management

Exposure to sunlight may promote healing, but take care not to allow the child to become sunburned. Apply skin moisturizers or emollients daily to prevent dry skin and flare-ups. Apply topical antiinflammatory creams as prescribed during flare-ups. Apply tar shampoos or skin preparations. Use mineral oil and warm towels to soak and remove thick plaques.

THINKING ABOUT **DEVELOPMENT**

Emily Wilson is a 15-year-old girl with a history of moderate psoriasis. She experiences significant scaling along her hairline, forehead, scalp, and arms. Hypopigmentation and striae are beginning to occur on her arms as a result of topical medication use. She is a talented ballerina but expresses increasing concerns about her skin alterations showing while she is performing.

How does Emily's developmental stage affect self-care related to her psoriasis?

What is the most appropriate approach for the nurse to take to educate Emily about control of her psoriasis?

How will the nurse best promote an appropriate body image for Emily?

ACNE

Acne is a disorder that affects the pilosebaceous unit and is common in childhood (Prok & Torres-Zegarra, 2022). Acne that persists past the usual course of time for infantile or adolescent acne may be caused by endocrine abnormalities. It may also occur in response to the use of certain types of drugs such as corticosteroids, androgens, phenytoin, and others. The usual presentation and nursing management of neonatal acne and acne vulgaris are discussed in what follows.

Neonatal Acne

Neonatal acne occurs as a response to the presence of the birthing parent's androgens or to transient androgen production in the newborn. It may be present immediately after birth but often occurs between 2 and 4 weeks of age (Prok & Torres-Zegarra, 2022). Usually, no treatment is necessary, but in severe cases there is a risk of scarring, so a topical preparation may be prescribed.

Nursing Assessment

Note oily face or scalp. Examine the face (especially the cheeks), upper chest, and back for inflammatory papules and pustules. Document absence of fever.

Nursing Management

Instruct parents to avoid picking or squeezing the pimples; to do so places the infant at risk for secondary bacterial infection and cellulitis. Teach parents to wash the affected areas daily with clear water. Avoid using fragranced soaps or lotions on the area with acne. Inform the parents that as the newborn's hormones stabilize over time, the acne usually resolves without additional intervention.

Acne Vulgaris

Beginning as early as 7 to 10 years of age, acne vulgaris affects about 85% of adolescents, and endogenous androgens play a role in its development (Prok & Torres-Zegarra, 2022). It occurs most frequently on the face, chest, and back. Risk factors for the development of acne vulgaris include preadolescent or adolescent age, male sex (due to the presence of androgens), an oily complexion, Cushing syndrome, or another disease process resulting in increased androgen production.

Pathophysiology

The sebaceous gland produces sebum and is connected by a duct to the follicular canal that opens on the skin's surface. Androgens stimulate sebaceous gland proliferation and production of sebum. These hormones exhibit increased activity during the pubertal years. Abnormal shedding of the outermost layer of the skin (the stratum corneum) occurs at the level of the follicular opening, resulting in a keratin plug that fills the follicle. The sebaceous glands increase sebum production. Bacterial overgrowth of *Propionibacterium acnes* occurs because the presence of sebum and keratin in the follicular canal creates an excellent environment for growth. Inflammation occurs as the follicular wall perforates, allowing the contents to leak into nearby tissue.

Therapeutic Management

Therapeutic management focuses on reducing *P. acnes,* decreasing sebum production, normalizing skin shedding, and eliminating inflammation. Teach the adolescent to cleanse the skin gently twice a day. Medication therapy may include a combination of benzoyl peroxide, salicylic acid, retinoids, and topical or oral antibiotics. Isotretinoin may be used in severe cases. Drug Guide 45.1 gives further information on these medications. Oral contraceptives may help lessen acne by decreasing the effects of androgens on the sebaceous glands. Diode laser or blue UV light therapy may also be used. CO_2 lasers and dermabrasion may be used to treat pitted scarring.

Nursing Assessment

Note history of onset of acne lesions, as well as family history of acne. Determine medication use; certain medications may hasten the onset of acne or worsen it when already present. In particular, note use of corticosteroids, androgens, lithium, phenytoin, and isoniazid. Document history of an endocrine disorder, particularly one that results in hyperandrogenism. Note worsening of acne 2 to 7 days before the start of the menstrual period. Inspect the skin for lesions (particularly on the face and upper chest and back, which are the areas of highest sebaceous activity). Note presence, distribution, and extent of noninflammatory lesions, such as open and closed comedones, as well as inflammatory lesions such as papules, pustules, nodules, or cysts (open comedones are commonly referred to as blackheads and closed comedones as whiteheads; Fig. 45.18). Examine the skin for hypertrophic scarring resulting from inflammatory lesions. Table 45.3 explains the acne classification. Note oily skin and oily hair, which result from increased sebum production. Determine remedies that have been used and the extent of success of those treatments. Assess the child's or adolescent's feelings about the disorder.

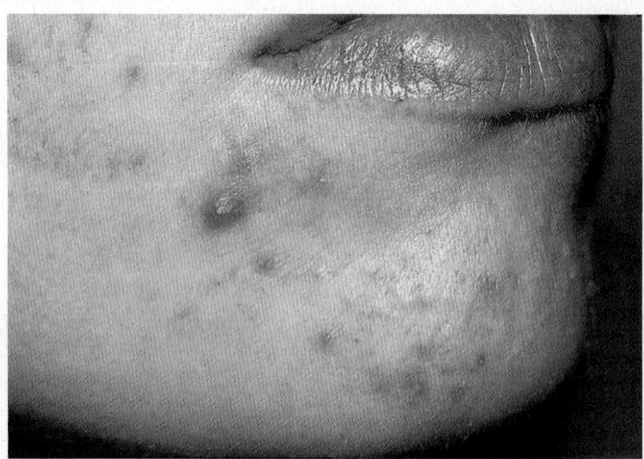

FIGURE 45.18 Acne vulgaris.

TABLE 45.3 • Classification of Acne

Classification	Manifestations
Mild acne	Primarily noninflammatory lesions (comedones)
Moderate acne	Comedones plus inflammatory lesions such as papules or pustules (localized to face or back)
Severe acne	Lesions similar to moderate acne, but more widespread, and/or presence of cysts or nodules; associated more frequently with scarring

Nursing Management

Avoid oil-based cosmetics and hair products, as their use may block pores, contributing to noninflammatory lesions. Look for cosmetic products labeled as noncomedogenic. Headbands, helmets, and hats may exacerbate the lesions by causing friction. Dryness and peeling may occur with acne treatment, so encourage the child to use a humectant moisturizer. Mild cleansing with soap and water twice daily is appropriate. Avoid excessive scrubbing and harsh chemical or alcohol-based cleansers. Avoid picking or squeezing the lesions. Using a noncomedogenic sunscreen with a sun-protective factor (SPF) of 30 or higher is recommended (Kim, 2020).

Teach adolescents that the prescribed topical medications must be used daily and that it may take 4 to 6 weeks to see results. Avoid the use of over-the-counter preparations because they are irritating and aggravate the drying effect of prescription acne treatments. Instruct adolescents who wish to remove facial hair to shave gently and avoid using dull razors, so as not to further irritate the condition. Adolescents taking isotretinoin who could become pregnant must be on a pregnancy prevention program because the drug causes defects in fetal development (Kim, 2020) (Box 45.2).

BOX 45.2 Decreasing Risk of Fetal Exposure to Isotretinoin: iPLEDGE

- As of 2006, health care providers, pharmacists, and patients are required to register in the iPLEDGE program before they prescribe, dispense, or receive isotretinoin.
- The iPLEDGE program is a central registry requiring monthly input as noted following in order to continue isotretinoin treatment.
- Monthly input includes the following:
  - Females of childbearing age are using two forms of contraception.
  - Pregnancy test results are negative.
  - Isotretinoin users do not donate blood during treatment or for 1 month after completion of treatment.
- Additional information available at https://www.ipledgeprogram.com/iPledgeUI/home.u

Data from iPledge. (2021). *iPledge: Committed to pregnancy prevention.* https://www.ipledgeprogram.com/iPledgeUI/home.u

If the acne is severe, depression may occur as a result of body image disturbances. Provide emotional support to adolescents undergoing acne therapy. Refer adolescents for counseling if necessary.

> **CONSIDER THIS!**
>
> Paxton Herman, age 16, comes to the clinic with complaints of acne on his face and back. He states, "I hate the way my face looks." "I'll never get a date looking like this." "I don't even want to take my shirt off at the beach, because there's bumps on my back."
>
> Think back to when you were an adolescent. How would you have felt if you had a skin condition that altered the way your face looked? As the nurse, how can you help Paxton in this situation?

INJURIES

Children, by their inquisitive natures, developmental immaturity, and skin's properties, are prone to experience a variety of skin injuries. Pressure injuries are most likely to occur in hospitalized or otherwise immobile children. Typical healthy, active children are likely to suffer cuts, abrasions, foreign-body penetration, burns and other thermal injuries, bites, and stings.

Pressure Injuries

Skin breakdown involves changes in intact skin, which may range from blanchable erythema to deep pressure injuries. The term pressure injury refers to damage to the skin resulting in skin loss and development of a crater that may range from mild to deep. Pressure injuries develop from a combination of factors, including immobility or decreased activity, decreased sensory perception, increased moisture, impaired nutritional status, inadequate tissue perfusion, and the forces of friction and shear. Common sites of pressure injuries in hospitalized children include the occiput and toes, while children who require wheelchairs for mobility have pressure injuries on the sacral or hip area more frequently.

Nursing Assessment

Note history of immobility (chronic, related to a condition such as paralysis) or lengthy hospitalization, particularly in intensive care. Inspect the skin for areas of erythema or warmth. Note ulceration of the skin. Use the facility's wound assessment scale to document the extent of the injury. Take a photo of the injury if possible.

Nursing Management

Position the child to alleviate pressure on the area of the injury. Use specialized beds or mattresses to prevent further pressure areas from developing. Perform prescribed wound care meticulously, noting the formation of granulation tissue as the injury begins to heal. Prevent pressure injuries in the child who is hospitalized for long periods by turning the child frequently, assessing the entire surface of the child's skin at least every shift, using pressure-alleviating beds and mattresses, and maintaining the child's nutritional status.

Minor Injuries

Children suffer minor injuries frequently. Because of their developmental immaturity and inquisitive nature, children often attempt tasks they are not yet capable of or take risks that an adult would not, often resulting in a fall or other accident. Minor injuries include minor cuts and abrasions, as well as skin penetration of foreign bodies such as splinters or glass fragments. The break in the skin allows an entry point for bacteria, and the complication of cellulitis may occur. Treatment is directed at cleaning the wound and preventing infection.

Nursing Assessment

Obtain the history from the child or caregiver to determine whether dirt or a foreign object may be present in the wound. Inspect the wound, noting depth of injury, a foreign body, and bleeding.

Nursing Management

Cleanse the wound with mild soap and water or with an antibacterial cleanser. Wet gauze helps to scrub away fine and large sand particles. Remove pieces of loose skin with sterile scissors, foreign particles with sterile forceps, and road tar with petrolatum. Small abrasions and minor, well-approximated cuts may be left open to the air. Apply a small amount of antibacterial ointment and cover large abrasions with a loose dressing. Change the dressing 12 hours later and redress after cleaning the wound. Leave it open to air after 23 hours have passed from the time of injury. Assess the wound daily for signs of infection, which include purulence, warmth, edema, increasing pain, and erythema that extends past the margin of the cut or abrasion.

Burns

Burns are a common preventable mechanism of injury among children and adolescents. Young children are at highest risk for burns, and the mortality rate from burns is highest in children younger than 5 years (Joffe, 2023). Most pediatric burn-related injuries do not result in death, but injuries from burns often cause extreme pain, and extensive burns can result in serious disfigurement. In young children, 85% of burns are scald burns, and 18% of pediatric burn injuries result from child abuse (Antoon, 2020). Fires in the home are often related to cooking and cigarette or other smoking materials. Carbon monoxide poisoning often occurs in conjunction with burns as a result of smoke inhalation, and infants and children are at greater risk for carbon monoxide poisoning than adults. Great advances have been made in the care of children with serious burns. As a result of improved burn care, children who in the past would have died as a result of burns over large body surface areas have a much greater chance of survival (Joffe, 2023). Conventional wisdom is that children with severe burns should be transferred to a specialized burn unit. The American Burn Association has developed the following criteria for referral of burned people to a specialized burn unit:

- Partial-thickness burns greater than 10% of total body surface area
- Burns that involve the face, the hands and feet, genitalia, perineum, or major joints
- Full-thickness burns of any size
- Chemical or electrical burns (including lightning injury)
- Inhalation injury
- Burn injury in children who have preexisting conditions that might affect their care
- People with burns and traumatic injuries
- People who will require special social, emotional, or long-term rehabilitative care
- Burned children in a hospital without qualified personnel or equipment for the care of children (Joffe, 2023)

Burns are classified according to the extent of injury, and the terminology used to describe each type includes superficial (formerly first degree), partial thickness (second degree), deep partial thickness (second degree), and full thickness (third and fourth degree) (Antoon, 2020). Superficial burns involve only epidermal injury and usually heal without scarring or other sequelae within 4 to 5 days. In partial-thickness burns, injury occurs not only to the epidermis but also to portions of the dermis. These burns usually heal within about 2 weeks and carry a minimal risk of scar formation. Deep partial-thickness burns take longer to heal, may scar, and result in changes in nail and hair appearance as well as sebaceous gland function in the affected area. They may require surgical intervention. Full-thickness burns result in significant tissue damage as they extend through the epidermis, dermis, and hypodermis. Extensive scarring results, as hair follicles and sweat glands are destroyed. Full-thickness burns require a significant time to heal. If underlying tendons and/or bone are involved, the burn may be termed fourth degree. Contractures and limited function may occur as a complication of full-thickness burns. Skin grafting is usually necessary. Full or partially circumferential burns may result in ischemia from loss of blood flow related to progressive swelling of the area.

Pathophysiology

Burned tissue begins to coagulate after the injury, and direct coagulation and microvascular reactions in the adjacent dermis may extend the burn. The blood vessels demonstrate increased capillary permeability, resulting in vasodilatation. This leads to increased hydrostatic pressure in the capillaries, causing water, electrolytes, and protein to leak out of the vasculature and result in significant edema. Edema forms rapidly in the first 18 hours after the burn, peaking at around 48 hours. Capillary permeability then returns to normal between 48 and 72 hours after the burn, and the lymphatics can reabsorb the edema fluid. Diuresis occurs, ridding the body of the excess fluid. Fluid loss from burned skin occurs at an amount that is five to 10 times greater than that from undamaged skin, and this fluid loss continues until the damaged surface is healed or grafted.

Initially, the severely burned child experiences a decrease in cardiac output, with a subsequent hypermetabolic response during which cardiac output increases dramatically. During this heightened metabolic state, the child is at risk for insulin resistance and increased protein catabolism. Children who are burned during an indoor or chemical fire are at an increased risk of respiratory injury. Children who have aspirated hot liquids are particularly at risk for airway-altering edema.

Therapeutic Management

Therapeutic management of burns focuses on fluid resuscitation, wound care, prevention of infection, and restoration of function. Burn infections are treated with antibiotics specific to the causative organism. If invasive burn damage occurs, surgery may be necessary.

Nursing Assessment

Refer to the "Clinical Judgment and the Nursing Process" section for a full description of the assessment phase of the nursing process. Upon arrival, evaluate the child with burns to determine if they will require intensive management. Remove any smoldering clothing. Obtain a brief history of the burn circumstances while you are assessing the child and providing care.

HEALTH HISTORY

If the burn is severe or there is a potential for respiratory compromise, obtain a brief history while simultaneously evaluating the child and providing emergency care. If the burn does not appear to pose an immediate life-threatening risk, obtain an in-depth history. Elicit a description of how the burn occurred, noting date, time, and cause. Determine if smoke inhalation or an associated fall may have occurred. Document treatment that the parent or caregiver has provided to the child's burn so far. Note the child's recent health status, current medications, recent or chronic illness, and immunization status, noting, in particular, the date of the most recent tetanus vaccination.

Determine whether the history being given sounds consistent with the type of burn injury that has occurred. Inquire about what caused the burn and whether the event was witnessed by anyone. Spatter-type burns resulting from the child pulling a source of hot fluid onto themselves usually yield a nonuniform, asymmetric distribution of injury. In contrast, intentional scald injuries usually yield a uniform "stocking" or "glove" distribution when the child's extremity is held under very hot water as punishment (Ford et al., 2022). It is important for the nurse to pick up on clues in the health history that may indicate that the burn is a result of child abuse rather than an accident (Box 45.3). Children are also burned by curling irons, gasoline, fireworks, room heaters, ovens, and ranges. Obtain a detailed history about the circumstances surrounding these types of burns. Ask the parent what the home hot water heater temperature is.

PHYSICAL EXAMINATION

Emergency examination of the burned child consists of a primary survey followed by a secondary survey. The primary survey includes evaluation of the child's airway, breathing, and circulation. The secondary survey focuses on evaluation of the burns and other injuries. Box 45.4 gives information about emergency assessment of the burned child. Inspect the child's skin, noting erythema, blistering, weeping, or eschar (charred skin).

Classify the burn according to its severity. Superficial burns are painful, red, dry, and possibly edematous (Fig. 45.19). Partial-thickness and deep partial-thickness burns are painful and edematous and have a wet appearance or blisters (Fig. 45.20). Full-thickness burns may be painful or numb or pain-free in some areas. They appear red, edematous, leathery, dry, or waxy and may display peeling or charred skin (Fig. 45.21). Note whether the burn is circumferential (encircling a body part) or partially circumferential.

BOX 45.3 Signs of Child Abuse–Induced Burns

- Inconsistent history given when caregivers are interviewed separately
- Delay in seeking treatment by caregiver
- Uniform appearance of the burn, with clear delineation of burned and nonburned area (as with a hot object applied to the skin)
- In the case of a scald-induced burn, lack of spattering of water but evidence of so-called "porcelain-contact sparing," where the portion of the child's skin that was in contact with the tub or sink is not burned (commonly seen with a forced immersion in extremely hot water used as punishment)
- Flexor-sparing burns or burns that involve the dorsum of the hand
- A stocking/glove pattern on the hands or feet (circumferential ring appearing around the extremity, resulting from a caregiver forcefully holding the child under extremely hot water)

Based on Ford, C. R., Chiesa, A., & Sirotnak, A. P. (2022). Chapter 8: Child abuse & neglect. In M. Bunik, W. W. Hay, M. J. Levin, & M. J. Abzug (Eds.), *Current diagnosis & treatment: Pediatrics* (26th ed.). McGraw-Hill Education.

BOX 45.4 Emergency Assessment of the Burned Child

Primary Survey

- Assess the child's airway, noting whether it is patent, maintainable, or unmaintainable.
- Suspect airway injury from burn or smoke inhalation if any of the following are present: burns around the mouth, nose, or eyes; carbonaceous (black-colored) sputum; hoarseness or stridor.
- Evaluate the child's skin color, respiratory effort, symmetry of breathing, and breath sounds.
- Determine the pulse strength, perfusion status, and heart rate. Note extent and location of edema.

Secondary Survey

- Determine burn depth.
- Estimate burn extent by determining the percentage of body surface area affected. Use a chart for estimation (see Fig. 45.21), or rapidly estimate by using the child's palm size, which is equivalent to about 1.25% of the child's body surface area.
- Inspect the child for other traumatic injuries (children who have jumped or fallen from a house fire may suffer cervical spine or internal injuries).

Based on Joffe, M. D. (2023). Moderate and severe thermal burns in children: Emergency Management. *UpToDate*. Retrieved January 29, 2024, from http://www.uptodate.com/contents/emergency-care-of-moderate-and-severe-thermal-burns-in-children.

TAKE NOTE!

Due to overlying blistering, it is difficult to accurately distinguish between partial- and full-thickness burns. In addition, in the case of third-degree burns, it is difficult to estimate burn depth during the initial evaluation.

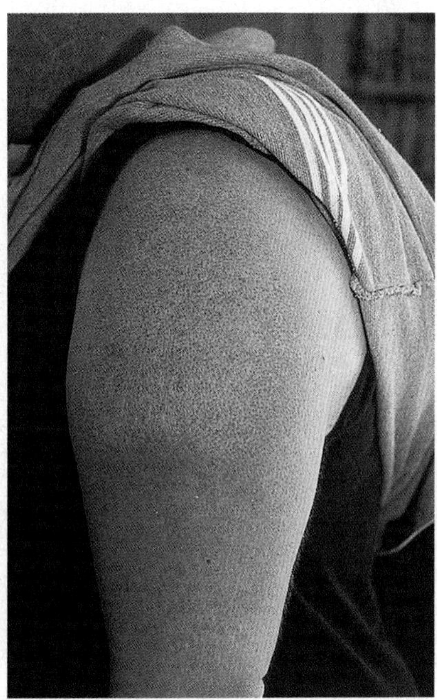

FIGURE 45.19 Superficial burn—painful but without blisters.

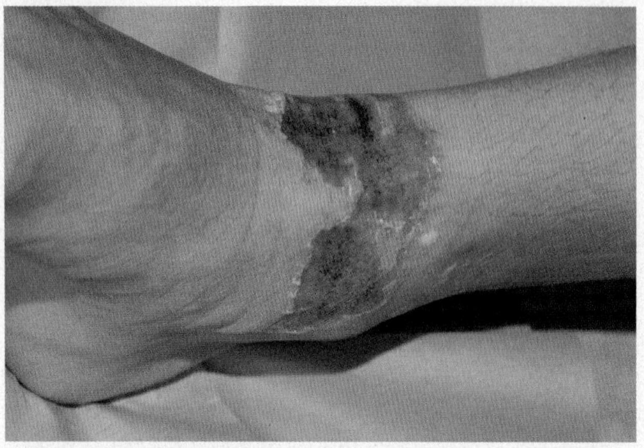

FIGURE 45.20 Partial-thickness burn—very painful, with blistering.

LABORATORY AND DIAGNOSTIC TESTS

In the child with more extensive burns, electrolytes and complete blood count are used to measure fluid and electrolyte balance and to determine the possibility of infection, respectively. If wound infection is suspected, culture of the drainage will determine the particular bacteria. Nutritional indices such as albumin, transferrin, carotene, retinol, copper, cholesterol, calcium, thiamine, riboflavin, pyridoxine, and iron may be evaluated when the child has severe or extensive burns. Pulmonary status may be evaluated via pulse oximetry and end-tidal CO_2 monitoring, arterial blood gases, carboxyhemoglobin levels, and chest radiography. Fiberoptic bronchoscopy and xenon ventilation–perfusion scanning may be used to evaluate inhalation injury. Electrocardiographic monitoring is important for the child who has suffered an electrical burn to identify cardiac dysrhythmias, which can be noted for up to 72 hours after a burn injury.

Nursing Management

Nursing management of the child who has been burned focuses first on stabilizing the child. Place the child on a cardiac/apnea monitor, measure the child with the Broselow tape, monitor pulse oximetry, and apply an end-tidal CO_2 monitor if the child is ventilated. Further management focuses on cleansing the burn, pain management, and prevention and treatment of infection. Fluid status and nutrition are important components of burn care, particularly in the early stages. Rehabilitation of the child with severe burns is also an important nursing function. Providing child and family education about the prevention of burns as well as care of burns at home is critical. The "Clinical Judgment and the Nursing Process" section gives additional interventions related to fluid and nutritional management.

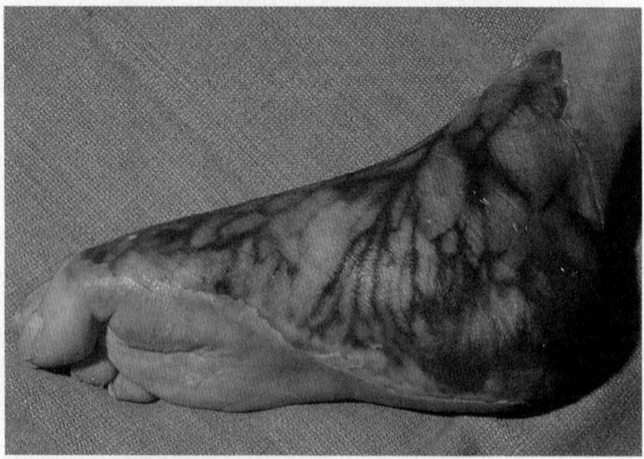

FIGURE 45.21 Full-thickness burn—color ranges from red to charred, or white, minimal pain, marked edema.

PROMOTING OXYGENATION AND VENTILATION

Institute emergency airway management as needed. If the child requires intubation, make sure that the tracheal tube is taped in a secure manner, as reintubation in these children will become increasingly difficult as the edema spreads. The burned child's respiratory status warrants vigilant evaluation and reevaluation, as airway edema that is secondary to a burn may not become evident until 2 days after the injury. Administer 100% oxygen via nonrebreather mask or bag–valve–mask ventilation to all children with severe burns. Continue to reassess the child's pulmonary status, adjusting the interventions as necessary (refer to Chapter 51 for further information about respiratory emergency care).

> **TAKE NOTE!**
>
> High levels of carboxyhemoglobin as a result of smoke inhalation may contribute to falsely high pulse oximetry readings (Mechem, 2024).

RESTORING AND MAINTAINING FLUID VOLUME

Several formulas are available for the calculation of resuscitative fluids in children. Most experts recommend that pediatric burn therapy include:

- Fluid calculation based on the body surface area burned (Fig. 45.22)
- Use of a crystalloid (Ringer's lactate) during the first 24 hours; in smaller children, a small amount of dextrose may be added
- Administration of most of the volume during the first 8 hours (amounts and timing of fluid volume resuscitation will vary from child to child)
- Reassessment of the child and adjustment of the fluid rate accordingly; fluid requirements greatly decrease after 24 hours and should be adjusted to reflect this.
- Administration of a colloid fluid later in therapy once capillary permeability is less of a concern
- Monitoring of the child's urine output as part of ongoing assessment of response to therapy, expecting at least 1 mL/kg/h

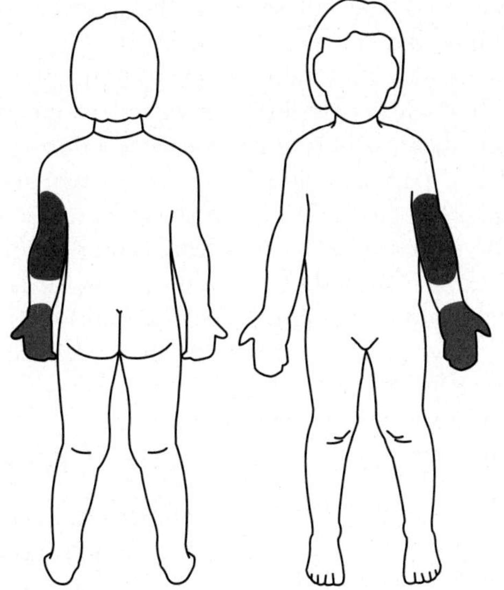

EXAMPLE

Calculating TBSA By Age (Total Body Surface Area)

Color Code
Red - 3° (full thickness)
Blue - 2° (partial thickness)

Area	Birth 1 yr	1–4 yrs	5–9 yrs	10–14 yrs	15 yrs	Adult	2	3	Total
Head	19	17	13	11	9	7	—	8	8.0
Neck	2	2	2	2	2	2	—	1	1.0
Ant. Trunk	13	13	13	13	13	13	1	12	13.0
Post. Trunk	13	13	13	13	13	13	—	—	—
R. Buttock	2 1/2	2 1/2	2 1/2	2 1/2	2 1/2	2 1/2	—	—	—
L. Buttock	2 1/2	2 1/2	2 1/2	2 1/2	2 1/2	2 1/2	—	—	—
Genitalia	1	1	1	1	1	1	—	—	—
R.U. Arm	4	4	4	4	4	4	—	3.5	3.5
L.U. Arm	4	4	4	4	4	4	1	2.5	3.5
R.L. Arm	3	3	3	3	3	3	—	3	3
L.L. Arm	3	3	3	3	3	3	—	3	3
R. Hand	2 1/2	2 1/2	2 1/2	2 1/2	2 1/2	2 1/2	—	2.5	2.5
L. Hand	2 1/2	2 1/2	2 1/2	2 1/2	2 1/2	2 1/2	—	2.5	2.5
R. Thigh	5 1/2	6 1/2	8	8 1/2	9	9 1/2	1	2	3
L. Thigh	5 1/2	6 1/2	8	8 1/2	9	9 1/2	—	2	2
R. Leg	5	5	5 1/2	6	6 1/2	7	—	—	—
L. Leg	5	5	5 1/2	6	6 1/2	7	—	—	—
R. Foot	3 1/2	3 1/2	3 1/2	3 1/2	3 1/2	3 1/2	—	—	—
L. Foot	3 1/2	3 1/2	3 1/2	3 1/2	3 1/2	3 1/2	—	—	—
						Total	3%	42%	45%

FIGURE 45.22 Calculate total body surface area (TBSA) affected by using the child's age and the area affected, as well as whether the burned area is second degree (partial thickness) or third degree (full thickness).

- Daily weights obtained at the same time each day (the best indicator of fluid volume status)
- Monitoring of electrolyte levels (particularly sodium and potassium) for their return to normal levels

PREVENTING HYPOTHERMIA

Due to the loss of the protective dermis, children who are burned are at high risk for hypothermia and secondary infection. Therefore, take care to keep the child warm. Warm intravenous fluids before administration. Maintain a neutral thermal environment, and monitor the child's temperature frequently.

CLEANSING THE BURN

Initially, it is important to stop the burning. Therefore, remove charred clothing. Wash and rinse the burn thoroughly with mild soap and cool water from the tap. Never apply ice. Children who are burned with tar require special care. Remove tar with cool water and mineral oil. Do not routinely remove blisters, because they provide a protective barrier; however, debridement is recommended in certain cases where large blisters impede wound care. Wounds that are open require debridement. Debridement involves the removal of loose skin and eschar (dead, charred skin). This procedure is usually performed with sterile scissors and a pair of forceps or with a gauze sponge. Gently cleanse the burned area; there is no advantage to aggressive scrubbing, and this technique only makes the pain more intense for the child. Wear a gown, mask, head covering, and gloves during dressing changes. Debridement is a necessary, but often excruciatingly painful, procedure. Thus, pain management needs of the child are of utmost importance (refer to the pain management section further on).

When children return for evaluation of a wound that was previously seen in your facility, remove the dressing. Soak the dressing in lukewarm tap water to ease the removal of gauze, which may be stuck to the wound. The nurse plays an important role in ensuring that the dressing change goes smoothly. Be sure to:

- Have all dressing supplies ready.
- Provide pain medication as ordered.
- Promote good infection control technique among your colleagues.
- Assist with restraining young children, using the positions of comfort previously discussed in relation to atraumatic care.
- Encourage participation by the child's parents.
- Talk soothingly to the child, explain what you are going to do, and provide distraction during the procedure.

PREVENTING INFECTION

Prevention of infection is critical to successful outcomes for burned children. If the child's immunization status is unknown or if it has been 5 years or longer since the last tetanus vaccine, administer the tetanus vaccine (Joffe, 2023). If the child has never received tetanus vaccination, also give 250 units tetanus human immunoglobulin intravenously. Apply antibiotic ointment in conjunction with burn dressing changes. Refer to Drug Guide 45.1 for information about topical antibiotics. Membrane dressings such as biosynthetic, hydrocolloid, and antibiotic-impregnated foam dressings are alternatives to topical antibiotics and sterile dressings. Evaluate the child's wound during dressing changes, looking for wound redness, swelling, odor, or drainage. Strictly adhere to infection control procedures and hand hygiene to decrease the risk of burn infection. Maximize the child's nutritional status to decrease their susceptibility to a burn infection. Monitor the child's temperature for the development of fever. Upon discharge, instruct the parents about the signs of a wound infection.

MANAGING PAIN

Pain management is of the utmost importance, and several options are available for the treatment of burn-related pain. Local anesthesia, sedatives, and systemic analgesics are commonly used. Children who have less severe burns that are managed at home can be given oral medications such as acetaminophen with codeine 30 to 45 minutes before dressing changes. In burns that result in more severe pain, the child should be hospitalized and given intravenous pain control with medications such as morphine sulfate. Midazolam (a sedative) may be used in conjunction with pain medication for pain reduction during dressing changes.

Pain may also occur at any time of the day or night, not just in relation to dressing changes. Assess the child's pain status frequently using an age-appropriate pain assessment scale. Administer pain medications as prescribed and/or use nonpharmacologic techniques to alleviate or decrease the child's perception of pain.

• • • ATRAUMATIC CARE • • •

Immersion in virtual reality computer games before and during burn dressing changes provides an exceptionally powerful form of cognitive distraction (Ahmadpour et al., 2019).

TREATING INFECTED BURNS

The potential for burn infection increases if the child has a large, open burn wound and if there are other sources of infection, such as multiple intravenous lines. In addition, children who are immunocompromised have an increased risk of burn infection. In burn wound cellulitis, the area around the burn becomes increasingly red, swollen, and painful early in the course of burn management. With invasive burn cellulitis, the burn develops a dark brown, black, or purplish color, with a discharge and foul odor. Burn impetigo is characterized by multifocal small superficial abscesses. Burn impetigo causes marked destruction of skin-grafted areas. Extensive infected burns may also become infected with a fungus.

When an infection is suspected, antibiotics are usually started, pending wound culture results. Administer antibiotics as prescribed or antifungals if necessary.

PROVIDING BURN REHABILITATION

Children who have suffered a significant burn injury face myriad physical and psychological challenges that extend well beyond the acute injury phase. Burned children may experience higher levels of anxiety than children who have never been burned, and they may display traumatic stress symptoms (Woolard et al., 2021). Skin grafting or special burn dressings are required for some children (Box 45.5). Children who have suffered extensive burns often require multiple skin-grafting surgeries. Figures 45.23 and 45.24 show healed skin grafts. Extensive burns may also result in the need for pressure garments to decrease the risk of extensive scarring. Pressure garments are not comfortable, and they must be worn continuously for at least 1 year, sometimes 2, but they have been shown to be effective in reducing hypertrophic scarring resulting from significant burn injury.

BOX 45.5 Special Burn Care and Skin Grafting

- To prevent infection and promote healing:
  - Biosynthetic skin coverings such as Biobrane (silicone film bonded to flexible nylon fabric and purified collagen peptides) and Mepilex Ag (soft silicone soaked with silver)
  - Kaltostat (calcium alginate dressing) is a brown seaweed extract that is spun into a fiber that is highly absorbent. It reacts with exudate on the wound to form a protective gel.
- Autograft allows for permanent coverage of a deep partial-thickness or full-thickness burn.
  - Consists of child's own skin
  - Split thickness consists of epidermis and superficial layers of dermis. The donor site heals completely.
  - Full thickness consists of full dermal thickness. Cover the donor site with fine-mesh gauze or synthetic wound coverings to allow the site to heal.

Based on Leon-Villapalos, J., & Dziewulski, P. (2022). Skin autografting. *UpToDate*. Retrieved January 29, 2024, from https://www.uptodate.com/contents/skin-autografting; and Tenenhaus, M., & Rennekampff, H.-O. (2023). Topical agents and dressings for local burn wound care. *UpToDate*. Retrieved April 26, 2023, from https://www.uptodate.com/contents/topical-agents-and-dressings-for-local-burn-wound-care

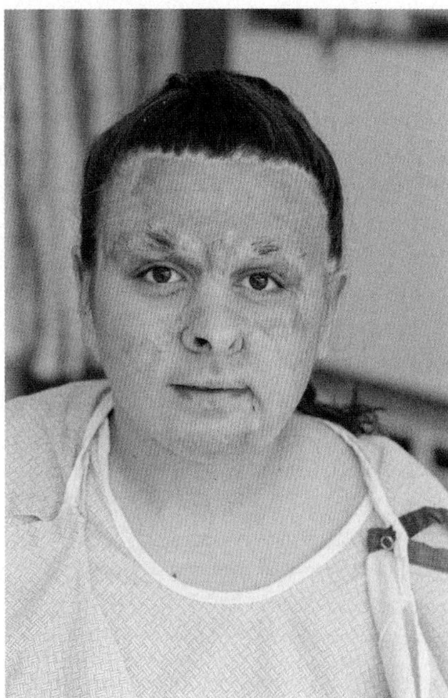

FIGURE 45.24 Extensive grafting to the face.

Physical therapy will usually be initiated in the critical care setting and will continue long after hospital discharge, sometimes throughout life. Positioning, exercise, and range of motion are necessary to maintain joint flexibility.

Nurses play a key role in smoothing the transition from the acute care phase of life-saving interventions and frequent dressing changes to normal activities such as school and play. Body image considerations may have a significant impact on the child when they return to school and should be addressed. Children with altered body image as a result of a burn might benefit from regular counseling and group therapy. Parents often need assistance with the behavioral challenges of caring for a child who is recovering from a burn injury. Various websites are available for support of people who are burned.

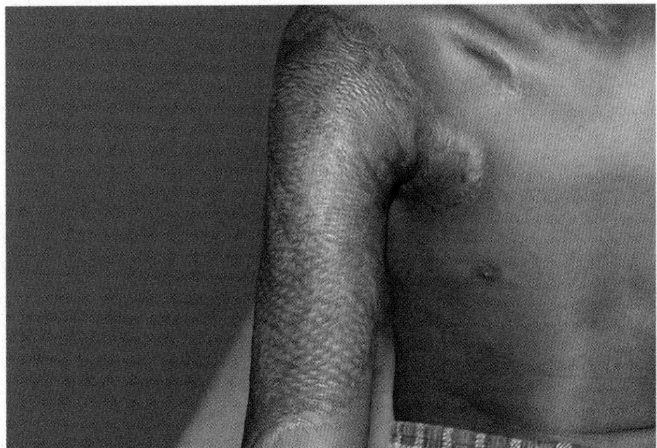

FIGURE 45.23 Healed mesh graft.

Navigating through life after suffering a serious burn injury can be difficult for the child and family, and a skilled nurse can provide valuable assistance to families during the equally important, but less acute, phase of the journey.

PREVENTING BURNS AND CARBON MONOXIDE POISONING

Instruct parents about prevention of burns. Explain that all homes should have working smoke detectors and that batteries should be changed yearly. Instruct families that all homes should be equipped with fire extinguishers and that adults and older teenagers should be taught how to operate them. Explain that children should sleep in fire-retardant sleepwear, parents should not smoke in the house or the car, and parents should keep lighters and matches out of children's reach. Young children are particularly susceptible to burns that occur in the kitchen, such as scalds from hot liquids and foods and burns from contact with hot burners or oven doors. Caution parents about the extreme danger that fireworks present to children. Teaching Guidelines 45.3 gives additional information for parents related to burn prevention. The booklet "Burn Prevention Tips," which includes a coloring book, is available from the Shriners Hospitals for Children.

Children are at significant risk for burns related to hot water. Scald burns can occur when hot water comes into contact with the child's skin, even for a relatively short time. Since hot water presents such a serious risk to children, the temperature on all hot water heaters should be 49°C (120°F) or lower. Figure 45.25 is a graph that

TEACHING GUIDELINES 45.3 Burn Prevention

- Keep hot water heater temperature lower than 49°C (120°F).
- Test bath water temperature before bathing children.
- Keep children away from open flames, stoves, and candles.
- Cook with pots on the inside of the stove with the handles turned in.
- Keep children away from the stove while cooking.
- Place hot liquids out of reach of children.
- Avoid drinking hot beverages while holding a child.
- Keep curling irons out of reach of children.
- Teach older children how to safely get out of the house in case of fire.
- Practice fire drills.
- Teach children to "stop, drop, and roll" if their clothes catch fire.

shows how long a child can be exposed to water of various temperatures before a burn occurs. For example:

- If the water is 66°C (150°F), a child can receive a third-degree burn within 2 seconds.
- If the water is 60°C (140°F), it takes 6 seconds of exposure to cause a significant burn.
- If the water is 54°C (130°F), a child can be burned significantly in only 30 seconds.
- At 49°C (120°F), the recommended maximal home hot water heater temperature, it takes as long as 5 minutes of exposure to burn a person (plenty of time to get out of the tub!) (Accurate Building Inspectors, 2024).

Instruct parents about prevention of carbon monoxide poisoning. All homes should have working carbon monoxide detectors, and batteries should be changed yearly. Teach parents the signs of carbon monoxide poisoning: headaches, dizziness, disorientation, and nausea. If the carbon monoxide detector sounds, turn off any potential sources of combustion, if possible, and evacuate all occupants immediately. Do not attempt to reenter the home until a qualified professional repairs the source of the carbon monoxide leak.

PROVIDING BURN CARE AT HOME

Teach parents about proper burn care in the home. Seek medical attention for burns when:

- The child has a second- or third-degree burn.
- Burns result from a fire, an electrical wire or socket, or chemicals.
- The child has a burn on the face, scalp, hands, feet, or genitals or over the joints.
- The burn appears to be infected.
- The burn is causing prolonged and significant pain.
- Concern exists that the burn was a result of abuse.

If the burn is extensive, even if it appears to be a first-degree burn, seek medical attention immediately. Teaching Guidelines 45.4 gives specific information about burn care at home.

Sunburn

Sunburn occurs as a result of overexposure to the UV rays of the sun. The erythema and eventual blisters occur

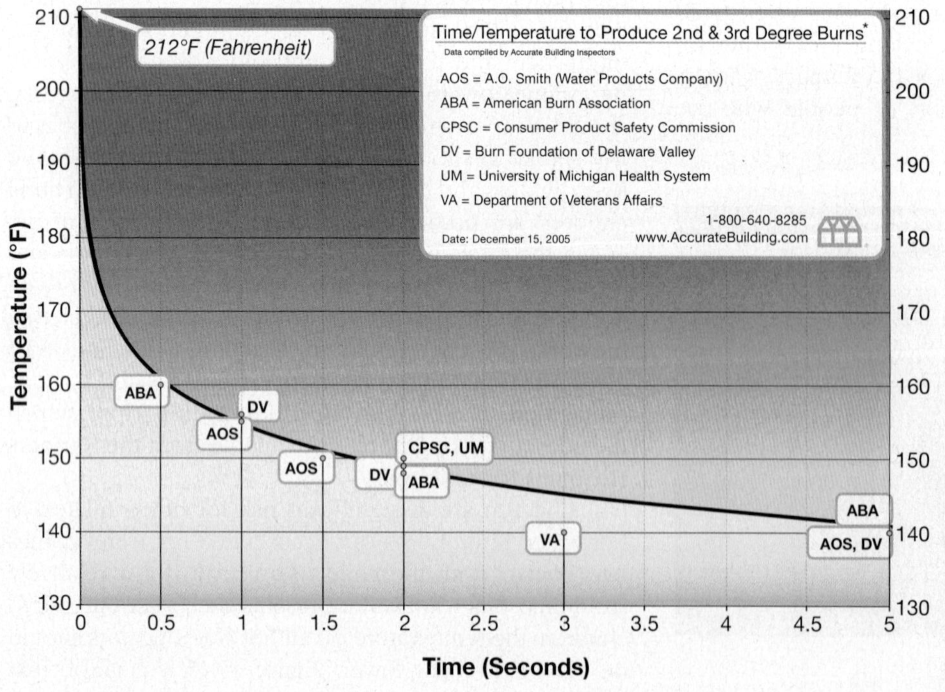

FIGURE 45.25 Length of hot water exposure that results in significant burns based on water temperature. (Used with permission from Accurate Building Inspectors. [2024]. *Water temperature thermometry.* http://www.accuratebuilding.com/services/legal/charts/hot_water_burn_scalding_graph.html)

TEACHING GUIDELINES 45.4 Providing Burn Care at Home

For First-Degree (Superficial) Burns

- Run cool water over the burned area until the pain lessens.
- Do not apply ice to the skin.
- Do not apply butter, ointment, or cream.
- Cover the burn lightly with a clean, nonadhesive bandage.
- Administer acetaminophen or ibuprofen for pain.
- Have the child seen by the health care provider or nurse practitioner within 24 hours.
- Ongoing care: clean in tub or shower with fragrance-free mild soap; pat or air dry.
  - Apply a thin layer of antibiotic ointment.
  - Cover with a nonadherent dressing such as Adaptic, and then cover with dry gauze.

For More Extensive Burns

- Remove clothing only if it comes off easily or if it is still smoldering.
- Check the child's ABCs (airway, breathing, and circulation) and perform cardiopulmonary resuscitation (CPR) if necessary.
- Do not apply butter, ointment, or any other type of cream.
- Cover the burn with a clean, lint-free bandage or sheet.
- Avoid applying large, wet sheets, as this can cause the child to become too cold.
- Do not attempt to break any blisters.
- If the child appears to be in shock, elevate the legs while protecting the burn and call 911.

as a result of the skin's blood flow changes as well as alterations in cell kinetics and pigment products in response to UV exposures. Erythema may occur within 4 hours and blisters within 6 hours. Sunburn is usually treated with cool compresses, cooling lotions, and oral nonsteroidal antiinflammatory agents (Pitone, 2023).

Nursing Assessment

Obtain the health history, noting recent sun exposure. Determine length of exposure and whether any type of sunscreen or sun block product was used. Note redness of the skin on the exposed areas. More severe areas will have a darker red, slightly purple hue. Blisters may be noted with more severe sunburn.

Nursing Management

Cool compresses may help to cool the burn. Aloe vera gel applied topically may provide significant soothing. Rarely are adverse effects reported with the use of aloe vera gel. Administer a nonsteroidal antiinflammatory such as ibuprofen. Discourage hot showers or baths. Instruct the child to wear loose clothing and to ensure that burned areas are covered when going outside (until they are healed). If skin flaking occurs, discourage the child from "peeling" the flaked skin in order to prevent further injury. Refer to Chapter 31 for further information about safe sun exposure.

Cold Injury

The term "frostbite" implies freezing of the tissues. It is described on a continuum from first to fourth degree. When a child is exposed to an extremely cold environment, changes in cutaneous circulation help to maintain the core body temperature. Because circulation is shunted to the core, the most peripheral body parts are those at highest risk for frostbite. Local damage occurs when the tissue temperature drops to 32°F (0°C). Initially, skin sensation is lost, the vasculature constricts, and plasma leakage occurs. Ice crystals develop in the extracellular fluid, and eventually, vascular stasis leads to endothelial cell damage, necrosis, and sloughing of dead tissue (Peters & Buchel, 2023).

Nursing Assessment

Note history of cold exposure. Inquire about pain or numbness. Examine the skin for indications of frostbite. First-degree frostbite results in superficial white plaques with surrounding erythema. Second-degree frostbite demonstrates blistering with erythema and edema. In third-degree frostbite, hemorrhagic blisters occur, progressing to tissue necrosis and sloughing in fourth-degree frostbite.

Nursing Management

Remove wet or tight clothing. Avoid vigorous massage to decrease the chance of damaging the skin further. Immerse the affected part in 40°C (104°F) water for 15 to 30 minutes. Thawing may cause significant pain, so administer analgesics. Keep the thawed part loosely covered, warm, and dry. Splinting may be used to help decrease associated edema. Consult the wound care specialist or plastic surgeon for further management.

Prevent frostbite by:

- Dressing warmly in layers and keeping warm and dry
- Avoiding exertion
- Not playing outside when wind chill advisories are in effect, and locking doors with high locks to prevent toddlers from going outside

Human and Animal Bites

Yearly, significant emergency room visits occur as a result of bites from mammals. In children, dog bites account for the majority of injuries, but human and cat bites account for the most infected bites (Hunstad, 2020). The hand and face are common locations for animal bites. A dog is most often provoked to bite a child when the child is playing with the dog or when the child hits, kicks, hugs, grabs, or chases the dog.

Therapeutic management involves cleansing and irrigating the wound, wound suturing or stapling if necessary, and administering topical and/or systemic antibiotic therapy. Rabies prophylaxis is indicated if the rabies status of the dog is unknown. Secondary bacterial infection of the bite wound with streptococci, staphylococci, or *Pasteurella multocida* may occur.

Nursing Assessment

Determine the history of the attack and whether it was provoked. Determine the child's tetanus vaccination status. Inspect the bite to determine the extent of laceration, avulsion, or crushing injury.

Nursing Management

Provide rabies immunoprophylaxis and a tetanus booster vaccination if indicated. Thoroughly cleanse the wound with soap and water or a povidone–iodine solution. Irrigate the wound well with normal saline after cleansing. If the animal may be rabid, cleanse the wound for at least 10 minutes with a virucidal agent such as povidone–iodine solution. Administer antibiotics as prescribed. Help children who have been bitten by talking about the incident or reading books about this type of event.

Prevention of animal bites is important. Teach children the following:

- Never provoke a dog with teasing or roughhousing.
- Get adult permission before interacting with a dog, cat, or other animal that is not your pet.
- Do not bother an eating, sleeping, or nursing dog.
- Avoid high-pitched talking or screaming around dogs.
- Display a closed fist first for the dog to sniff.
- Keep ferrets away from the face.
- If a cat hisses or lashes out with the paw, leave it alone.

Never leave a child younger than 5 years of age alone with a dog (American Veterinary Medical Association, 2023). Contact the local humane society for a dog bite prevention program that is appropriate for school-age children.

Insect Stings and Spider Bites

Members of the *Hymenoptera* class of insects sting. This class includes bees, wasps, imported fire ants, and yellow jackets. Other insects, such as mosquitos and fleas, bite. Spiders inject their venom when they bite. Stings and bites usually result in a local reaction. A systemic or anaphylactic reaction to a *Hymenoptera* sting may also occur, possibly resulting in airway compromise (refer to Chapter 51 for additional information on anaphylaxis). Serious reactions may occur with brown recluse or black widow spider bites. This discussion will focus on local reactions (Goddard & Steward, 2023).

Local reactions to insect stings and spider bites include pruritus, pain, and edema. A hypersensitivity reaction thought to be mediated by IgE occurs in response to the venom. This may be a physiologic response to the antigens present in the insect's or spider's saliva and other fluids that are transmitted during stinging or biting. Bacterial superinfection may occur as a complication and as a result of scratching. Therapeutic management includes antihistamines to decrease itching and in some cases corticosteroids to decrease inflammation and swelling (Freeman, 2024).

Nursing Assessment

Obtain the history of the bite or sting. Children are usually acutely aware when they have been stung by an insect, but spiders are generally not observed before the bite. Inspect the bite or sting, noting an urticarial wheal or papular reaction. A large local reaction may be mistaken for cellulitis. Note whether a stinger remains present. Assess the child's work of breathing to determine if a systemic reaction or anaphylaxis is occurring (refer to Chapter 51).

Nursing Management

Remove jewelry or constrictive clothing if the sting is on an extremity. Cleanse the wound with mild soap and water. If the stinger is present, scrape it away with your fingernail or a credit card. Apply ice intermittently to decrease pain and edema. Administer diphenhydramine as soon as possible after the sting in an attempt to minimize the reaction.

Prevent insect stings and spider bites by wearing protective clothing and shoes when outdoors. Use insect repellants (with a maximum concentration of 30% *N,N*-diethyl-meta-toluamide [DEET] in infants and children older than 2 months) (American Academy of Pediatrics, 2021). Teach children never to disturb a bee or wasp nest or an anthill.

KEY CONCEPTS

- The infant's epidermis is thinner, loses heat more readily, absorbs substances more easily, and is more accessible to bacterial invasion than the skin of the adult. The increased water content of the infant's skin compared with the adult's places the infant at increased risk of blister development and other skin alterations.
- The child's skin thickness and characteristics reach adult levels in the late teenage years.

- Children with dark skin tend to have more pronounced cutaneous reactions than children with lighter skin.
- Sebum production increases in the preadolescent and adolescent years, contributing to the development of acne at that time.
- Most bacterial skin infections are caused by *S. aureus* and group A beta-hemolytic streptococcus.
- Skin scrapings placed on a slide and prepared with potassium chloride may be evaluated microscopically to determine the presence of fungus.
- Fungal skin infections, referred to collectively as tinea, may require up to several weeks of treatment.
- Contact dermatitis and AD both present as pruritic rashes, whereas psoriasis is generally nonpruritic.
- Hypersensitivity responses may result in erythema multiforme or urticaria.
- Scaling may occur with AD and psoriasis, whereas honey-colored crusting is common with impetigo. Erythema is a common finding with many skin disorders in children.
- Burns may result in significant weeping and fluid loss.
- Keeping the skin well moisturized is a key intervention in the management of AD and psoriasis.
- Appropriate hygiene is of particular importance in integumentary disorders.
- Pain management, prevention of infection, and rehabilitation are the focus of nursing management for the burned child.
- The constant itch–rash–itch cycle of AD may have a considerable impact on the child's sleep, school functioning, and self-esteem.
- Acne vulgaris, particularly if moderate or severe, may have a significant negative effect on the adolescent's self-esteem.
- Teach children with chronic disorders such as AD, psoriasis, and acne (and their parents) to cleanse and moisturize the skin properly, avoid particular skin irritants, and use medications appropriately.
- Many skin disorders are preventable. Teach families how to prevent contact dermatitis, burns, sunburn, frostbite, and bites and stings.
- Educate children and families about the importance of good soap-and-water cleansing of all minor skin injuries.

REFERENCES AND RECOMMENDED READINGS

Accurate Building Inspectors. (2024). *Water temperature thermometry. Ubell Enterprises.* http://www.accuratebuilding.com/services/legal/charts/hot_water_burn_scalding_graph.html

Ahmadpour, N., Randall, H., Choksi, H., Gao, A., Vaughan, C., & Poronnik, P. (2019). Virtual reality interventions for acute and chronic pain management. *The International Journal of Biochemistry & Cell Biology, 114,* 105568. https://doi.org/10.1016/j.biocel.2019.105568

American Academy of Pediatrics. (2021). *American Academy of Pediatrics: Get kids outdoors and use these safety tips to ward off insects and prevent sunburn.* https://www.aap.org/en/news-room/news-releases/health--safety-tips/american-academy-of-pediatrics-get-kids-outdoors-and-use-these-safety-tips-to-ward-off-insects-and-prevent-sunburn/

American Veterinary Medical Association. (2023). *Dog bite prevention.* https://www.avma.org/public/Pages/Dog-Bite-Prevention.aspx

Antoon, A. Y. (2020). Chapter 92: Burn injuries. In R. M. Kliegman, J. W. St Geme, N. J. Blum, S. S. Shah, R. C. Tasker, & K. M. Wilson (Eds.), *Nelson textbook of pediatrics* (21st ed.). Elsevier.

Armstrong, C. A. (2023). Approach to the clinical dermatologic diagnosis. *UpToDate.* Retrieved April 12, 2024, from https://www.uptodate.com/contents/approach-to-the-clinical-dermatologic-diagnosis

Baddour, L. M. (2022). Impetigo. *UpToDate.* Retrieved April 12, 2024, from http://www.uptodate.com/contents/impetigo

Bender, N. R., & Chiu, Y. E. (2020). Chapter 676.1: Psoriasis. In R. M. Kliegman, J. W. St Geme, N. J. Blum, S. S. Shah, R. C. Tasker, & K. M. Wilson (Eds.), *Nelson textbook of pediatrics* (21st ed.). Elsevier.

Corbett, J. A., & Banks, A. D. (2019). *Laboratory tests and diagnostic procedures with nursing diagnoses* (9th ed.). Pearson Education Inc.

Covar, R. A., Fleisher, D. M., Cho, C., & Boguniewicz, M. (2022). Chapter 38: Allergic disorders. In M. Bunik, W. W. Hay, M. J. Levin, & M. J. Abzug (Eds.), *Current diagnosis & treatment: Pediatrics* (26th ed.). McGraw-Hill Education.

Ford, C. R., Chiesa, A., & Sirotnak, A. P. (2022). Chapter 8: Child abuse & neglect. In M. Bunik, W. W. Hay, M. J. Levin, & M. J. Abzug (Eds.), *Current diagnosis & treatment: Pediatrics* (26th ed.). McGraw-Hill Education.

Freeman, T. (2024). Bee, yellow jacket, wasp, and other Hymenoptera stings: Reaction types and acute management. *UpToDate.* Retrieved April 12, 2024, from https://www.uptodate.com/contents/bee-yellow-jacket-wasp-and-other-hymenoptera-stings-reaction-types-and-acute-management

Giddens, J. F. (2021). *Concepts for nursing practice* (3rd ed.). Elsevier.

Goddard, J., & Stewart, P. H. (2023). Insect and other arthropod bites. *UpToDate.* Retrieved April 12, 2024, from https://www.uptodate.com/contents/insect-and-other-arthropod-bites

Hagan, J. F., Shaw, J. S., & Duncan, P. M. (Eds.). (2017). *Bright futures: Guidelines for health supervision of infants, children, and adolescents* (4th ed.). American Academy of Pediatrics.

Heath, C. R., Mazza, J. M., & Silverberg, N. B. (2016). Chapter 84: Pediatrics. In A. P. Kelly, S. C. Taylor, H. W. Lim, & A. M. A. Serrano (Eds.), *Taylor and Kelly's dermatology for skin of color* (2nd ed.). McGraw-Hill Education.

Howe, W. (2023). Atopic dermatitis (eczema): Pathogenesis, clinical manifestations, and diagnosis. *UpToDate.* Retrieved April 12, 2024, from https://www.uptodate.com/contents/atopic-dermatitis-eczema-pathogenesis-clinical-manifestations-and-diagnosis

Hunstad, D. A. (2020). Chapter 743: Animal and human bites. In R. M. Kliegman, J. W. St Geme, N. J. Blum, S. S. Shah, R. C. Tasker, & K. M. Wilson (Eds.), *Nelson textbook of pediatrics* (21st ed.). Elsevier.

iPledge. (2021). *iPledge: Committed to pregnancy prevention.* https://www.ipledgeprogram.com/iPledgeUI/home.u

Joffe, M. D. (2023). Moderate and severe thermal burns in children: Emergency management. *UpToDate.* Retrieved April 12, 2024, from http://www.uptodate.com/contents/emergency-care-of-moderate-and-severe-thermal-burns-in-children

Kim, W. E. (2020). Chapter 689: Acne. In R. M. Kliegman, J. W. St Geme, N. J. Blum, S. S. Shah, R. C. Tasker, & K. M. Wilson (Eds.), *Nelson textbook of pediatrics* (21st ed.). Elsevier.

Lee, H. Y. (2024). Stevens-Johnson syndrome and toxic epidermal necrolysis: Pathogenesis, clinical manifestations, and diagnosis. *UpToDate*. Retrieved April 12, 2024, from http://www.uptodate.com/contents/stevens-johnson-syndrome-and-toxic-epidermal-necrolysis-pathogenesis-clinical-manifestations-and-diagnosis

Leon-Villapalos, J., & Dziewulski, P. (2022). *Skin autografting. UpToDate*. Retrieved April 12, 2024, from https://www.uptodate.com/contents/skin-autografting

McMahon, P. (2022). Staphylococcal scalded skin syndrome. *UpToDate*. Retrieved April 12, 2024, from https://www.uptodate.com/contents/staphylococcal-scalded-skin-syndrome

Mechem, C. C. (2024). Pulse oximetry. *UpToDate*. Retrieved April 12, 2024, from https://www.uptodate.com/contents/pulse-oximetry

Musters, A. H., Mashayekhi, S., Harvey, J., Axon, E., Lax, S. J., Flohr, C., Drucker, A. M, Gerbens, L., Ferguson, J., Ibbotson, S., Dawe, R. S., Garritsen, F., Brouwer, M., Limpens, J., Prescott, L. E., Boyle, R. J., & Spuls, P. I. (2021). Phototherapy for atopic eczema. *Cochrane Database of Systematic Reviews*. *2021*(11). https://doi.org/10.1002/14651858.CD013870.pub2

Peters, B., & Buchel, E. W. (2023). *Cold injuries. Medscape*. https://emedicine.medscape.com/article/1278523-overview

Pitone, M. L. (2023). *How to handle sunburn*. https://kidshealth.org/en/parents/sunburn-sheet.html

Prok, L. D., & Torres-Zegarra, C. X. (2022). Chapter 15: Skin. In M. Bunik, W. W. Hay, M. J. Levin, & M. J. Abzug (Eds.), *Current diagnosis & treatment: Pediatrics* (26th ed.). McGraw-Hill Education.

Sangha, A. M. (2021). Dermatological conditions in skin of color: Managing atopic dermatitis. *Journal of Clinical and Aesthetic Dermatology*, *14*(3 Suppl. 1), S20–S22.

Sasseville, D. (2023). Cradle cap and seborrheic dermatitis in infants. *UpToDate*. Retrieved April 12, 2024, from http://www.uptodate.com/contents/cradle-cap-and-seborrheic-dermatitis-in-infants

Teichgräber, F., Jacob, L., Koyanagi, A., Shin, J. I., Seiringer, P., & Kostev, K. (2021). Association between skin disorders and depression in children and adolescents: A retrospective case-control study. *Journal of Affective Disorders*, *282*, 939–944. https://doi.org/10.1016/j.jad.2021.01.002

Tenenhaus, M., & Rennekampff, H.-O. (2023). *Topical agents and dressings for local burn wound care. UpToDate*. Retrieved April 12, 2024, from https://www.uptodate.com/contents/topical-agents-and-dressings-for-local-burn-wound-care

UpToDate, Inc. (2024). *UpToDate® Lexidrug™* (Version 8.2.0) [Mobile app]. Wolters Kluwer. https://apps.apple.com/us/app/lexicomp/id313401238

Woolard, A., Hill, N. T. M., McQueen, M., Martin, L., Milroy, H., Wood, F. M., Bullman, I., & Lin, A. (2021). The psychological impact of paediatric burn injuries: A systematic review. *BMC Public Health*, *21*(2281). https://doi.org/10.1186/s12889-021-12296-1

DEVELOPING CLINICAL JUDGMENT

PRACTICING FOR NCLEX

1. The nurse is teaching about skin care for AD. Which statement by the parent indicates that further teaching may be necessary?
   a. "I will use Vaseline or Crisco to moisturize my child's skin."
   b. "A hot bath will soothe my child's itching when it is severe."
   c. "I will buy cotton rather than wool or synthetic clothing for my child."
   d. "I will apply a small amount of the prescribed cream after the bath."
2. The nurse is caring for a child who has received significant partial-thickness burns to the lower body. What is the priority assessment in the first 24 hours after injury?
   a. Fluid balance
   b. Wound infection
   c. Respiratory arrest
   d. Separation anxiety
3. The nurse is caring for a child in the emergency department who was bitten by the family dog, who is fully immunized. What is the priority nursing action?
   a. Administer rabies immunoglobulin.
   b. Refer the child to a counselor.
   c. Assess the depth and extent of the wound.
   d. Administer a tetanus booster.
4. The nurse is caring for an infant on the pediatric unit who has a very red rash in the diaper area, with red lesions scattered on the abdomen and thighs. What is the priority nursing intervention?
   a. Administer griseofulvin with a fatty meal.
   b. Institute contact isolation precautions.
   c. Apply topical antibiotic cream.
   d. Apply topical antifungal cream.
5. A varsity high school wrestler presents with a "rug burn" type of rash on their shoulder that is not healing as expected, despite use of triple antibiotic cream. Two other wrestlers on the team have a similar abrasion. What infection should the nurse be most concerned about, based on the history?
   a. Tinea cruris
   b. Methicillin-resistant *Staphylococcus aureus* (MRSA)
   c. Impetigo
   d. Tinea versicolor
6. The nurse has taught the parent of a child with AD how to bathe the child. Which statement by the parent indicates the education was effective?
   a. "I should let my child play in the tub for 40 minutes every night."
   b. "I will be sure to use a moisturizing bubble bath."
   c. "When my child gets out of the tub, I will just pat the skin dry."
   d. "It is important that my child has a bath every night."
7. The nurse is teaching an adolescent about interventions to improve facial acne. What should the nurse include when educating the patient?
   a. Wash the face twice a day with mild soap and water.
   b. Remove whiteheads and blackheads after each face washing.
   c. Apply vitamin E ointment twice daily to each lesion.
   d. Expose the face to the sun after applying tretinoin in the morning.

DOSAGE CALCULATION QUESTION

The nurse is caring for a child who has tinea corporis. The child weighs 18 lb 11 oz. The medication order reads: griseofulvin 85 mg PO every day. Griseofulvin is supplied as 125 mg/5 mL. How many milliliters will the nurse administer? Round to the nearest tenth.

CRITICAL THINKING EXERCISES

1. A 4-year-old presents with their parent for evaluation of a yellowish, runny sore on the head. What questions would be most appropriate to ask the parent when taking the history? Should this child be placed in isolation? If so, why?
2. An 11-month-old comes to the primary care office with the parent for evaluation of a significant flaking red rash on both cheeks. The child is diagnosed with AD. What additional information should be obtained in the health history? What information should be included in the teaching plan for this family?

STUDY ACTIVITIES

1. Plan an educational activity:
   a. For parents of babies about the treatment and prevention of diaper dermatitis
   b. For parents of school-age children about prevention of contact dermatitis (related to poison ivy)
2. During your clinical rotation, spend a day with the wound and ostomy care nurse in a children's hospital. Report to the clinical group about what you learned that day.
3. Talk to adolescents with severe acne, AD, or psoriasis about their feelings about their skin's appearance. Reflect on this information in your clinical journal.

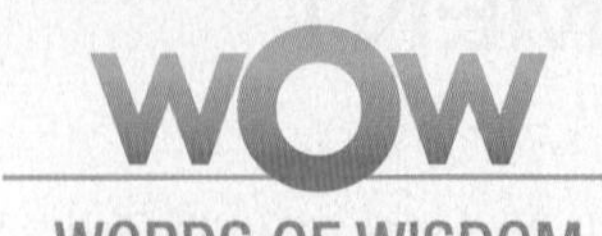

WORDS OF WISDOM

Be inspired by the courage of a child with cancer and reflect it in the care you provide.

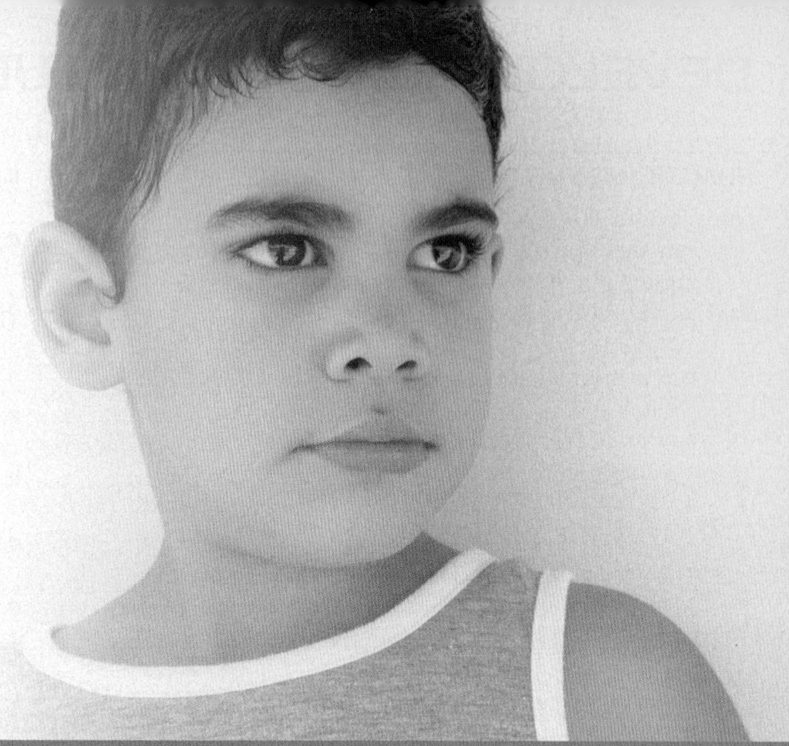

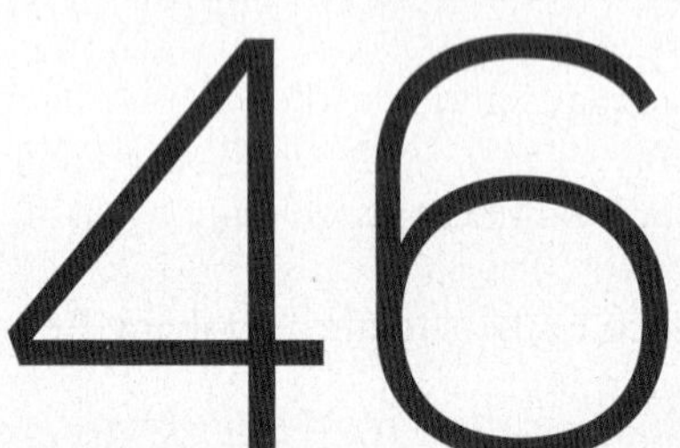

Nursing Care of the Child With an Alteration in Cellular Regulation/ Hematologic or Neoplastic Disorder

KEY TERMS

anisocytosis (an-ī´sō-sī-tō´sis)
chelation therapy (kē-lā´shŭn thăr´ă-pē)
clinical trial
extravasation (eks-trav´ă-sā´shŭn)
hematocrit
hemoglobin
hemosiderosis (hē´mō-sid-ĕr-ō´sis)
hypochromic
macrocytic
malignant
metastasis (mĕ-tas´tă-sis)
microcytic
neoplastic
platelet count
poikilocytosis (poy´ki-lō-sī-tō´sis)
polycythemia
splenomegaly
staging

LEARNING OBJECTIVES

Upon completion of the chapter, you will be able to:

1. Identify major hematologic disorders that affect children.
2. Compare childhood and adult cancers.
3. Identify types of cancer common in infants, children, and adolescents.
4. Determine priority assessment information for children with alterations in cellular regulation/hematologic and neoplastic disorders.
5. Analyze laboratory data and describe nursing care related to common laboratory and diagnostic testing used in alterations in cellular regulation/hematologic and neoplastic disorders.
6. Develop an individualized nursing care plan or concept map for the child with cancer or a hematologic disorder.
7. Identify priority interventions for children with alterations in cellular regulation.
8. Develop a teaching plan for the family of children with hematologic disorders or cancer.
9. Devise a nutrition plan for the child with cancer.
10. Describe the psychosocial impact of cancer on children and their families.
11. Identify resources for children and families with hematologic disorders, or cancer.

Shaun O'Malley, 10 months old, is being admitted to the pediatric unit after being brought to the clinic by his parent for a small laceration that he thought needed stitches. His parent states, "I didn't think the cut was very deep. I was surprised by how long it bled."

INTRODUCTION

Cellular regulation is the process by which cells replicate, proliferate, and grow. The hematologic system is integrally involved in the process of cellular regulation. The hematologic system consists of the blood and blood-forming tissues of the body. These typically function together in a balance that affects the metabolism of the body. The three categories of cells are erythrocytes, or red blood cells (RBCs); thrombocytes, or platelets; and leukocytes, or white blood cells (WBCs). RBCs are responsible for transporting nutrients and oxygen to the body tissues and waste products from the tissues. The platelets are responsible for clotting. WBCs are responsible for fighting infection. WBCs are further divided into granulocytes (neutrophils, eosinophils, and basophils) and agranulocytes (lymphocytes and monocytes).

All blood cells originate from a single type of cell called a multipotent stem cell, which goes on to differentiate into the various types of blood cells. Thrombopoietin (TPO) and interleukin-7 (IL-7) act on the cell and differentiate the cell into either myeloid or lymphoid progenitor cells. The lymphoid cells either, under the influence of IL-6, become B lymphocytes or change directly into T lymphocytes. The myeloid cells are differentiated by the action of either erythropoietin (EPO) or granulocyte–monocyte colony-stimulating factor (GM-CSF). When the cell is acted upon by EPO, which is produced by the kidneys, the cell becomes the megakaryocyte, also known as the erythroid progenitor cell. The megakaryocyte is acted on by either EPO, to become the RBC, or TPO and IL-11, to become a megakaryocyte that goes on to form platelets. GM-CSF influences the cell to become the granulocyte, also known as the macrophage progenitor cell. These cells further differentiate under various influences to become the WBCs (Fig. 46.1).

Certain conditions may cause problems to develop within this system, resulting in an alteration in blood cellular regulation. These problems are related to either the production of the blood cells (too much or too little) or loss and destruction of these cells. Many factors are involved in the development of hematologic disorders, ranging from genetic causes to disorders resulting from injury, infection, or nutritional deficit.

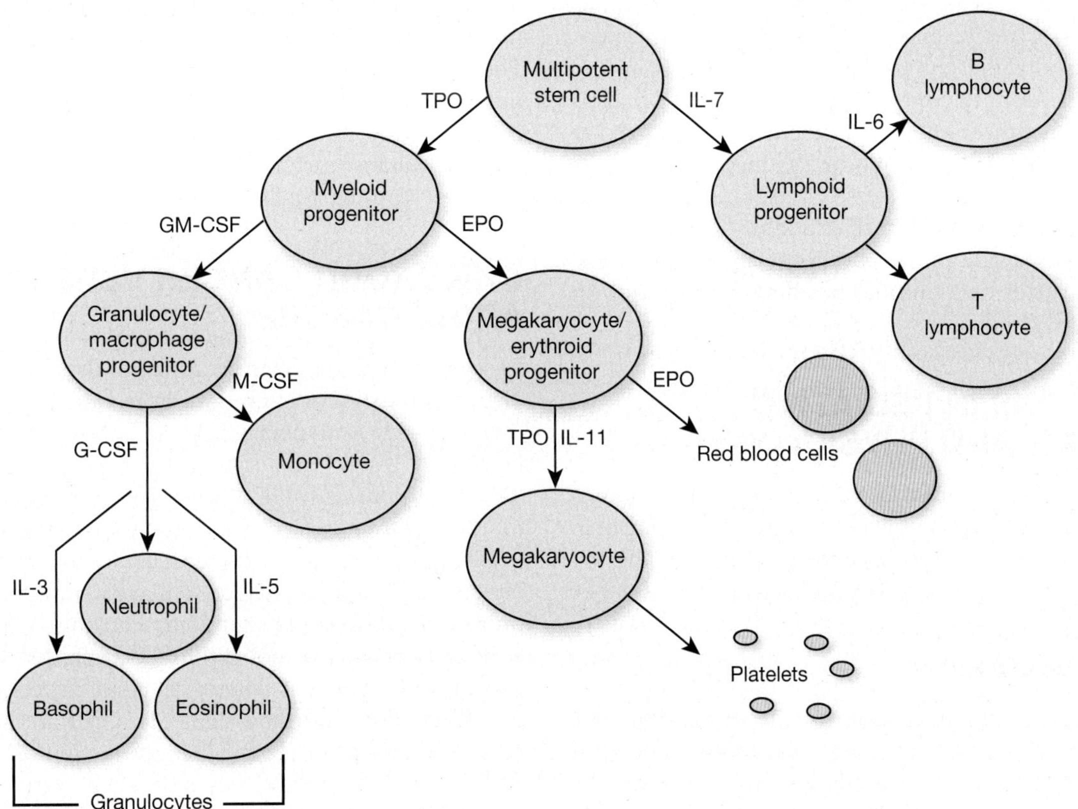

FIGURE 46.1 Process of blood cell formation. EPO, erythropoietin; GM-CSF, granulocyte–monocyte colony-stimulating factor; IL, interleukin; TPO, thrombopoietin.

Neoplastic (referring to cells that abnormally proliferate) disorders are also alterations in cellular regulation. Cancer results from an alteration in cellular regulation resulting in out-of-control cell growth. Cancer accounts for the most deaths from disease in children older than 1 year of age. Cure has been achieved in some children with childhood leukemia and other cancers, but there is no universal long-term cure available for any of the childhood cancers. However, the 5-year survival rate for all cancers in children is 85% (American Cancer Society [ACS], 2024a).

Cancer is a life-threatening illness that involves emotional distress, fear of the unknown, and changes in life priorities for the child and family. Initial and ongoing diagnostic testing and the adverse effects of treatment for cancer, including chemotherapy, radiation, surgery, or other treatments, are often painful as well. Management of cancer also has a significant psychosocial impact on the child or adolescent. Children with cancer are at risk for distress because they have a life-threatening illness and must undergo frequent and stressful tests and treatments (National Cancer Institute [NCI], 2023). In addition, the child often feels isolated from their peers, and the adolescent may have difficulty achieving independence, which is the core developmental task of the adolescent years. Children and adolescents with cancer often demonstrate poorer school performance compared to healthy peers.

Nursing care for the child with a hematologic disorder is often multifaceted. A child who has iron-deficiency anemia requires adequate oxygenation and may require packed red blood cells (PRBCs); a child with hemophilia requires factor replacement and monitoring for safety. Nursing care for the child with cancer is also complex. Nurses caring for children with cellular regulation alterations such as cancer and hematologic disorders need to be not only knowledgeable about the medical treatment of the disease (including adverse effects) but also able to effectively intervene with these children. Nurses need to be particularly aware of the psychosocial and emotional impact of cancer or a chronic hematologic disorder on the child and family.

VARIATIONS IN PEDIATRIC ANATOMY AND PHYSIOLOGY

In the absence of a congenital defect, the hematologic system is intact and functional at birth. RBC and hemoglobin production as well as iron stores undergo changes in the first few months of life; thereafter, hematologic function is stable.

RBC Production

The production of blood cells in the embryo begins by 8 weeks' gestation. In the embryo, blood cells form primarily in the liver; this continues until a few weeks before delivery. Some cell production, lymphoid cells, in particular, takes place in the spleen of the embryo, and the thymus is a site for some transient lymphocyte production. EPO, the hormone that regulates RBC production, is derived primarily from the liver in the fetus, and after birth, the kidneys take over this production.

Hemoglobin

Three types of normal hemoglobin (Hgb) are present at any given time in the blood: Hgb A, Hgb F or fetal hemoglobin, and Hgb A_2. After 6 months of age, Hgb A is the predominant type. In the neonatal period, the largest difference is with the RBCs. Fetal hemoglobin, which has a much shorter cell life, is present in higher quantities, putting the infant at risk for anemia and leading to problems with the oxygen-carrying capacity of the blood. As the production of the cells transfers from the liver to the bone marrow of the long and flat bones, the balance between oxygenation and production is affected.

Iron

The fetus receives iron through the placenta from the pregnant parent. The preterm infant misses out on the final weeks or months of transplacental iron transfer, putting them at increased risk for anemia (Cunningham et al., 2022). In the term infant, a period of physiologic anemia occurs between the ages of 2 and 6 months. This is because the infant demonstrates rapid growth and an increase in blood volume over the first several months of life, and maternally derived iron stores are depleted by 4 to 6 months of age. Sufficient iron intake is critical for the appropriate development of hemoglobin and RBCs. Therefore, the infant must ingest adequate quantities of iron either from breast milk or from iron-fortified formula in early infancy and other food sources in later infancy. Adolescence is also a time of rapid growth, and intake of iron must increase.

CHILDHOOD CANCER VERSUS ADULT CANCER

Cancers in children differ greatly from those in adults. Pediatric cancers most often arise from primitive embryonal (mesodermal) and neuroectodermal tissues, resulting in leukemias, lymphomas, sarcomas, or central nervous system (CNS) tumors (ACS, 2024a). This is in direct contrast to adult cancers, which arise mostly from epithelial cells, resulting in carcinomas. The most common childhood cancers, in order of frequency, are leukemia, CNS tumors, lymphoma, neuroblastoma, rhabdomyosarcoma, Wilms tumor, bone tumors, and retinoblastoma. Comparison Chart 46.1 explains how cancer is different in children versus adults.

In children, warning signs of cancer are most often related to changes in blood cell production or as a result of compression, infiltration, or obstruction caused by the tumor. Changes in blood cell production may result in fatigue, pallor, frequent or severe infection, or easy bruising. Infiltration, obstruction, or compression by a tumor

COMPARISON CHART 46.1 Childhood Cancer Versus Adult Cancer

	Childhood Cancer	Adult Cancer
Cancer usually affects	Tissues	Organs
Histologic type	Embryonal, leukemia, lymphoma	Epithelial in origin
Most common sites	Blood, lymph, brain, bone, kidney, muscle	Breast, lung, prostate, bowel, bladder
Environmental and lifestyle factors	Only a small amount of environmental influence proven	Strong influence on cancer development
Cancer prevention	Little known	80% preventable
Detection	Usually incidental or accidental	Very early detection possible if screening recommendations followed
Latent period	Relatively short	Can be very long (20 years or greater)
Extent of disease	Metastasis often present at diagnosis	Metastasis less often present at diagnosis
Response to treatment	Very responsive	Less responsive

Data from American Cancer Society. (2024a). *Cancer in children.* https://www.cancer.org/cancer/cancer-in-children.html

may result in bone or abdominal pain, pain in other parts of the body, swelling, or unusual discharge.

COMMON MEDICAL TREATMENTS

Various medications as well as other medical treatments are used to treat hematologic and neoplastic disorders in children. Most of these treatments will require a health care provider's or nurse practitioner's order when the child is in the hospital. Deciding on a course of medical treatment for cancer in a developing child is complicated. Some of the treatments can impair the child's growth and development. Many pediatric oncologists and cancer treatment centers are active members of the Children's Oncology Group (COG), an NCI-supported group that approves and administers clinical trials devoted exclusively to childhood and adolescent cancer research. A **clinical trial** is a carefully designed research study that assesses the effectiveness of a treatment as well as its acute and long-term effects on the child. Current cancer care in children is a result of the knowledge gained through clinical trials. A clinical trial may include existing medications or treatments in combination with new drugs or may involve a different approach to sequencing or dosing of medications and treatment (NCI, 2023).

To provide optimal outcomes, the child with cancer should be treated at an institution with multidisciplinary cancer care specialists that can provide the most advanced care available. Each case of pediatric cancer should be considered individually, with the oncology health care team and the family reaching treatment decisions together, whether the treatment plan is standard or involves enrollment in a clinical trial.

In the child with cancer, particularly advanced disease, the decision to provide treatment ("let's do everything we can") or to withhold treatment in the event of an extremely poor prognosis is extraordinarily challenging in an ethical sense. A mature older child or adolescent may have a strong desire to continue or discontinue treatment, and sometimes this desire conflicts with the parents' desires or choices. The American Academy of Pediatrics (AAP) Committee on Bioethics recommends that decision making for older children and adolescents should include the assent of the older child or adolescent (Box 46.1).

Commonly, chemotherapy and radiation therapy are used to treat childhood cancers. In some instances, hematopoietic stem cell transplantation (HSCT) is used. The nurse caring for the child with a hematologic disorder or cancer should be familiar with the procedures used, how the treatments and medications work, and common nursing implications related to use of these modalities. The most common treatments and medications are listed in Common Medical Treatments 46.1 and Drug Guide 46.1.

BOX 46.1 Pediatric Assent

- Give consideration to each child's developmental capacity, rationality, and autonomy.
- Help each child to achieve a developmentally appropriate understanding of the illness.
- Tell the child what they can expect regarding testing procedures and treatments.
- Assess the child's understanding of the situation and how they are responding.
- Note if there is inappropriate pressure to assent to testing or treatment.
- Seriously solicit the child's expression of willingness to accept the proposed plan of care.

Data from Spriggs, M. (2023). Children and bioethics: Clarifying consent and assent in medical and research settings. *British Medical Bulletin, 145*(1), 110. https://doi.org/10.1093/bmb/ldac038

COMMON MEDICAL TREATMENTS 46.1

Treatment	Explanation	Indications	Nursing Implications
Blood product transfusion	Intravenous administration of whole blood, packed red blood cells (PRBCs), platelets, or plasma	PRBCs: severe anemia, thalassemia, sickle cell disease Whole blood: acute hemorrhage or trauma Fresh-frozen plasma: hemophilia Platelets: thrombocytopenia	Follow institution's transfusion protocol. Double check blood type and product label with a second nurse. Use only leukodepleted, CMV-negative blood products in the child with a hemoglobinopathy or cancer. Monitor vital signs and assess child frequently to detect adverse reaction to blood transfusion. If adverse reaction is suspected, immediately discontinue transfusion, run normal saline IV, reassess the child, and notify the health care provider. Some children require premedication with diphenhydramine and/or acetaminophen before receiving blood products.
Leukapheresis	Whole blood is removed from the body, the WBCs are extracted, and then the blood is retransfused into the child.	Hyperviscosity with leukemia (WBC >100,000)	Performed by specially trained personnel Monitor blood pressure and other vital signs.
Hematopoietic stem cell transplantation	Bone marrow transplant: transfer of healthy bone marrow into a child with disease; the transplanted cells can then develop into functional cells. Stem cell transplant: Peripheral stem cells are removed from the donor via apheresis, or stem cells are retrieved from the umbilical cord and placenta. The stem cells are then transplanted into the recipient.	Leukemia, lymphoma, other cancers, sickle cell disease, aplastic anemias, thalassemia	Maintain medical asepsis and protective isolation to prevent infection. Monitor closely for graft-versus-host disease. Provide meticulous oral care. Avoid taking rectal temperatures and inserting suppositories. Encourage appropriate nutrition. Administer immunosuppressive medications as ordered.
Supplemental oxygen	Administration of oxygen via mask, cannula, or blow-by	Hypoxia associated with sickle cell crisis or severe anemia	Frequently monitor work of breathing, oxygen saturation via pulse oximetry, cardiopulmonary status, and level of consciousness.
Biopsy	A small piece of the tumor is removed with a needle or via an open incision.	Solid tumors	Monitor for bleeding at the needle biopsy site. Provide routine incision care for open biopsy site.
Splenectomy	Surgical removal of the spleen	Life-threatening or recurrent splenic sequestration of sickle cell disease; thalassemia	Provide immunization against the following organisms, because they place the child at risk for overwhelming infection: *Streptococcus pneumoniae*, *Neisseria meningitidis*, and *Haemophilus influenzae* type B. Monitor carefully for signs of infection. Administer prophylactic antibiotics. Instruct child or adolescent to wear medical alert bracelet. Teach families to seek medical treatment at first sign of infection or fever.
Surgical removal of tumor	The tumor is completely or partially resected surgically.	Solid tumors	Provide routine postoperative nursing care based on the location of the tumor excision.

COMMON MEDICAL TREATMENTS 46.1

Treatment	Explanation	Indications	Nursing Implications
Radiation therapy	Ionizing radiation (high-energy x-ray) is delivered to the cancerous area. The radiation damages all cells in the locally treated area (normal and cancerous), but the normal cells are able to repair themselves. Usually administered several times a week for several weeks. (A short rest between treatments allows the normal cells time to regenerate.) The lowest possible dose of radiation is used, and it is directed to a specific area.	Solid tumors, before or after surgical resection, leukemia, lymphoma	Do not wash off radiation marking. Keep skin clean and dry. Fatigue is a common side effect. Skin at the site of radiation may become red, dry, or pruritic or may peel; eventually, may become moist and red Mucositis, dry mouth, and loss of taste may occur if head or neck radiated. Radiation may also have adverse effects on the organ irradiated, such as the brain; monitor for changes.
Central venous catheter (see Image A)	IV catheters are inserted into the central circulation for the purpose of administering medications, total parenteral medication, or blood products. A Image A: The central venous access catheter is tunneled under the skin and secured with a cuff.	Any child with cancer who will require long-term IV medications or parenteral nutrition	Complaints of shortness of breath or chest pain may indicate air entry into the central venous catheter. Have child lie on left side and notify health care provider immediately. Keep dressing clean and dry. Perform sterile dressing change per institution policy or health care provider order. Monitor for fever. Monitor insertion site for erythema or drainage. Maintain sterile technique when accessing line, performing dressing change, or administering any fluid through catheter.
Implanted port (see Image B)	A needle-accessible port is implanted under the skin, usually on the chest. The port has a thin catheter exiting it that is tunneled under the skin into the superior vena cava or subclavian vein. 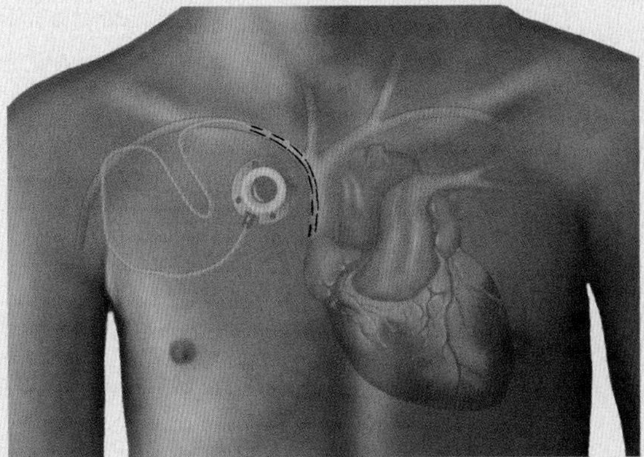 B	Any child with cancer who will require long-term IV medications or parenteral nutrition 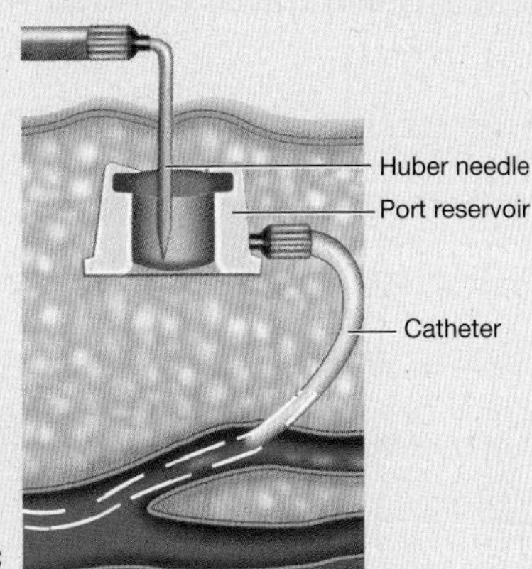 	Flush nonaccessed port with prescribed heparin dose per institution policy. Use sterile technique to access port with Huber needle. Monitor port site for erythema or warmth.

Image B: The implanted port consists of a reservoir under the skin for ready access. The catheter exiting the port is threaded into the subclavian vein or right atrium. Image C: A 90-degree Huber needle is used to access the port.

CMV, cytomegalovirus; WBC, white blood cells.

Based on Anzilotti, A. (2019). *Stem cell transplants.* https://kidshealth.org/en/parents/stem-cells.html; Blaney, S. M., Adamson, P. C., & Helman, L. J. (2021). *Pizzo & Poplack's pediatric oncology* (8th ed.). Wolters Kluwer; and Larson, S. D., Hebra, A., Raju, R., & Lee, S. (2020). Vascular access in children. *Medscape.* Retrieved on April 13, 2023, from https://emedicine.medscape.com/article/1018395-overview#a1

DRUG GUIDE 46.1

COMMON DRUGS FOR HEMATOLOGIC AND NEOPLASTIC DISORDERS

Medication	Actions/Indications	Nursing Implications
Iron supplements (ferrous sulfate, ferrous fumarate)	Supplemental iron in deficient child Iron-deficiency anemia	Dosage is based on milligrams of elemental iron. Give with vitamin C–containing foods to increase absorption. Do not administer with milk or milk products. May color stools and urine black. Liquid can stain the teeth; mix with a small amount of juice; drinking with straw decreases tooth staining. May cause constipation; increase fiber and fluid intake.
Deferasirox	Binds with iron, which is removed in the feces Iron toxicity (as in children chronically transfused)	Oral agent, should be taken at the same time daily, on an empty stomach Do not chew or swallow whole pills; disperse completely in orange juice, apple juice, or water. Monitor iron level, CBC, creatinine, hearing, and vision.
Deferoxamine	Binds with iron, which is removed via the kidneys Iron toxicity (as in children chronically transfused)	Rotate subcutaneous injection sites to decrease local reactions. Apply corticosteroid cream to irritation.
Factor (VIII or IX) replacement	Replaces deficient clotting factors Hemophilia	Use filter needle to draw up medication. Administer IV when bleeding occurs.
Penicillin VK	Kills susceptible bacteria Prophylaxis of infection in asplenia	Determine whether penicillin allergy is present. Monitor kidney and hematologic function during prolonged use.
Folic acid	Replaces the vitamin Folic acid deficiency; questionable use with sickle cell anemia	Administer without regard to meals. Monitor hematologic function.
Hydroxyurea	Stimulates the development of hemoglobin F in sickle cell anemia	Monitor for mild GI discomfort, modest neutropenia, hyperpigmentation of the skin and nails.
L-Glutamine	Conditionally essential amino acid whose production is decreased during times of stress	Decrease frequency of sickle cell disease (SCD) painful vaso-occlusive events.
Intravenous immune globulin (IVIG)	Provides exogenous IgG antibodies Idiopathic thrombocytopenic purpura	Do not mix with IV medications or with other IV fluids. Do not give IM or SQ. Monitor vital signs and watch for adverse reactions frequently during infusion. Child may require antipyretic or antihistamine to prevent chills and fever during infusion. Have epinephrine available during infusion.
Chelating agents: dimercaprol, edetate calcium disodium, succimer	Remove lead from soft tissues and bone, allowing for its excretion via the renal system. Used for blood lead levels >45 mcg/dL	Monitor intake and output closely to ensure adequacy of renal system. Encourage adequate oral hydration or provide IV hydration if required. Follow lead levels as prescribed. Ensure lead is being removed from the child's home.
Allopurinol	Decreases production of uric acid Used to treat secondary hyperuricemia occurring during leukemia or tumor treatment	Give PO after meals with plenty of food. Cardiovascular adverse effects may occur with IV administration. Maintain adequate hydration.
Antibiotics (oral, parenteral)	Treatment of documented bacterial infections Also used as prophylaxis of *Pneumocystis jirovecii* and in the neutropenic child	Check for antibiotic allergies. Should be given as prescribed for the length of time prescribed Start IV antibiotics as soon as possible in the neutropenic child admitted with fever.
Antiemetics: promethazine, metoclopramide, ondansetron	Act on the CNS transmitters to prevent vomiting.	May cause CNS side effects, such as drowsiness or irritability Ondansetron: may cause dry mouth

DRUG GUIDE 46.1

Medication	Actions/Indications	Nursing Implications
Antifungal agents: nystatin, amphotericin B (conventional and lipid complex)	Invade fungal cell wall, enabling its destruction. Indicated for mucositis, or systemic fungal infection	Nystatin: administer after meals Amphotericin B: may cause fever, chills, rigors, cardiovascular adverse effects; monitor child closely throughout infusion; note dose differences between conventional and lipid complex.
Immunosuppressant drugs: cyclosporine A (CyA), mycophenolate, tacrolimus	Inhibition of production and release of interleukin-2 (CyA) Inhibition of T- and B-cell proliferation (mycophenolate). Inhibition of T-cell activation (tacrolimus) Used for treatment of graft-versus-host disease (GVHD) after HSCT	Monitor CBC, serum creatinine, potassium, and magnesium. Monitor blood pressure and for signs of infection. Draw blood levels prior to morning dose. CyA: do not give with grapefruit juice. Mycophenolate: give on empty stomach; do not open capsule or crush tablet. Tacrolimus: give on empty stomach; monitor for anaphylaxis with first IV dose.
Mesna	Binds with and detoxifies cyclophosphamide and ifosfamide metabolites in the urinary bladder to prevent hemorrhagic cystitis	Maintain adequate hydration. Administer concurrently and after cyclophosphamide or ifosfamide. May cause hypotension
Methotrexate antidote: leucovorin	Reduces toxic effects of methotrexate	May cause skin disturbances, wheezing, thrombocytosis Dose depends on methotrexate level. Dose increases with increased creatinine levels.
Biotherapy		
Colony-stimulating factors: darbepoetin alfa, epoetin alfa, filgrastim, sargramostim	Stimulate production of red blood cells (epoetin) or granulocytes (filgrastim, sargramostim) Used to counteract myelosuppressive effects of chemotherapy	Administer SQ or IV. Filgrastim, sargramostim: may cause bone pain Sargramostim may cause hypotension and a first-dose reaction.
Interleukins: aldesleukin	Recombinant DNA interleukin-2 product that recruits T, B, and natural killer cells Indicated for non-Hodgkin lymphoma	Adverse effects are dose-dependent. May cause capillary leak syndrome within 2–12 hours of start of treatment: hypotension and decreased organ perfusion result.
Tumor necrosis factor (protein cytokine)	Increases effectiveness of immune cells, stops cancer cells from dividing, damages tumor blood vessels Used in a variety of cancer protocols	May cause fever, chills, rigors, nausea, vomiting
Monoclonal antibodies: rituximab, gemtuzumab	Bind to CD20 antigen on B lymphocytes Indicated in CD20-positive non-Hodgkin lymphoma, posttransplant lymphoproliferative disorder	Monitor blood pressure for hypotension. Monitor for anaphylaxis and infusion-related reaction. Have epinephrine, antihistamines, and steroids available at bedside for treatment of reaction.
Interferons: alpha, gamma	Alter cancer cell proliferation (alpha), stimulate macrophage production to fight bacteria and fungus (gamma) Indicated in a variety of cancer protocols	May cause flulike symptoms Maintain adequate hydration.
Chemotherapy		
Alkylating agents: busulfan, carboplatin, cisplatin, ifosfamide, temozolomide, thiotepa Nitrosoureas: carmustine, lomustine Nitrogen mustard: chlorambucil, cyclophosphamide, mechlorethamine, melphalan	Interfere with DNA replication and RNA transcription by alkylation (replacing the hydrogen ion with an alkyl group), cross-link DNA Cell cycle nonspecific The nitrosoureas are highly lipid soluble and easily cross the blood–brain barrier. Used in a variety of cancer protocols	Causes myelosuppression, nausea, vomiting, alopecia, mucositis Monitor for signs of infection. Provide adequate hydration. Cyclophosphamide, ifosfamide: Administer in the morning, provide adequate hydration, and have child void frequently during and after infusion to decrease risk of hemorrhagic cystitis. Cisplatin, mechlorethamine, melphalan: Avoid **extravasation** (leakage into surrounding tissues, potentially damaging them). Temozolomide: Avoid opening capsules. Thiotepa: If contact with skin occurs, wash thoroughly with soap and water.

(*continued*)

DRUG GUIDE 46.1 (*continued*)

Medication	Actions/Indications	Nursing Implications
Antitumor antibiotics: bleomycin, dactinomycin, daunorubicin, doxorubicin, idarubicin, mitomycin, mitoxantrone	Interfere with cellular metabolism, causing disruptions in DNA and/or RNA synthesis Cell cycle nonspecific Indicated in a variety of cancer protocols	May cause alopecia, nausea, vomiting, myelosuppression Bleomycin: Fever and chills may occur 20 hours after infusion Dactinomycin, mitomycin: Avoid extravasation. Daunorubicin, doxorubicin, idarubicin: May turn urine red-orange, monitor for arrhythmias, congestive heart failure; avoid extravasation. Mitoxantrone: May color urine, sweat, tears, skin, sclera blue-green; monitor for arrhythmias, congestive heart failure.
Antimetabolites: cladribine, cytarabine, fludarabine, fluorouracil, mercaptopurine, methotrexate, thioguanine	Substitute for a natural metabolite in the molecule, altering the cell's function and ability to replicate. Cell cycle specific (S phase); cladribine is cell cycle nonspecific. Used in a variety of cancer protocols	May cause alopecia, nausea, vomiting, mucositis, and myelosuppression Cladribine: Monitor for fever. Cytarabine: Use corticosteroid eye drops to prevent conjunctivitis with high doses. Fludarabine: Monitor for visual changes and neurotoxicity; maintain adequate hydration. Fluorouracil: Maintain adequate hydration; may cause photosensitivity. Mercaptopurine: Do not give oral doses with meals; may cause drug fever; avoid extravasation. Methotrexate: intensive hydration with high doses; may cause photosensitivity Thioguanine: Maintain hydration; administer on empty stomach.
Antimicrotubulars: paclitaxel	Inhibit mitotic cellular function in late G2 and M phases of cell cycle Indicated for refractory leukemia, recurrent Wilms tumor	May cause alopecia, nausea, vomiting, mucositis, myelosuppression May cause drowsiness Avoid extravasation.
Miscellaneous: asparaginase, pegaspargase	Inhibit protein synthesis by depriving tumor cells of the essential amino acid asparagine Used in acute lymphocytic leukemia, lymphomas	May cause alopecia, nausea, vomiting, and myelosuppression Monitor for vital signs during infusion and for signs of anaphylaxis. Have emergency equipment, oxygen, epinephrine, antihistamines, and steroids available at bedside.
Miscellaneous: dacarbazine, procarbazine	Inhibit DNA and RNA synthesis via cross-linking or suppression of mitosis Indicated in a variety of cancer protocols	May cause alopecia, nausea, vomiting, myelosuppression Monitor for flulike symptoms. Dacarbazine: Photosensitivity may occur; avoid extravasation.
Mitotic inhibitors: etoposide, vinblastine, vincristine	Inhibit mitotic activity by inhibiting DNA topoisomerase (etoposide) Cause metaphase arrest by binding to the mitotic spindle (vinblastine, vincristine) Used in a variety of cancer protocols	May cause alopecia, nausea, vomiting, myelosuppression (only minimal with vincristine) Etoposide: Monitor for anaphylaxis; have emergency equipment, oxygen, epinephrine, antihistamines, and steroids available at bedside. Vinblastine, vincristine: Maintain hydration; administer allopurinol; avoid extravasation.
Topoisomerase inhibitors: irinotecan, topotecan	Bind to DNA complex, preventing religation of single-strand DNA breaks. Indicated for refractory solid tumors	May cause alopecia, nausea, vomiting, myelosuppression, severe diarrhea (irinotecan), hypotension (topotecan) Maintain hydration. Avoid extravasation. Monitor blood pressure during topotecan infusion.
Corticosteroids: prednisone, dexamethasone	Suppress immune system by decreasing lymphatic activity and volume. Also decrease edema caused by tumor or tumor necrosis. Indicated for leukemia and some other cancers	Administer with food to decrease GI upset. May mask signs of infection Monitor blood pressure; monitor urine for glucose. Do not stop treatment abruptly or acute adrenal insufficiency may occur. Monitor for Cushing syndrome. Doses may be tapered over time.

CBC, complete blood count; CNS, central nervous system; GI, gastrointestinal; HSCT, hematopoietic stem cell transplantation; IgG, immunoglobulin G; IM, intramuscularly; IV, intravenous; SQ, subcutaneously.

Data from Blaney, S. M., Adamson, P. C., & Helman, L. J. (2021). *Pizzo & Poplack's pediatric oncology* (8th ed.). Wolters Kluwer; and UpToDate, Inc. (2024). *Lexi-comp®* (Version 8.1.0) [Mobile app]. Wolters Kluwer. https://apps.apple.com/us/app/lexicomp/id313401238

Chemotherapy

To understand how chemotherapy works to destroy cancer cells, it is necessary to review the normal cell cycle, through which all cells progress (Fig. 46.2). The cell cycle consists of five phases:

- G0 phase: the resting phase; lasts from a few hours to a few years; cells have not started to divide
- G1 phase: cell makes more protein in preparation for dividing; lasts 18 to 30 hours
- S phase: chromosomes are copied so that newly formed cells have the appropriate DNA; lasts 18 to 20 hours
- G2 phase: just before the cell splits into two cells; lasts 2 to 10 hours
- M phase: mitosis, the actual splitting of the cell into two new cells; lasts 30 minutes to 1 hour

Chemotherapy drugs work in two different ways in relation to the cell cycle. Cell cycle–specific agents exert their actions during a specific phase of the cell cycle. Cell cycle–nonspecific drugs exert their effect on the cells regardless of which phase the cell is in. Chemotherapy protocols often call for a combination of drugs that act on different phases of the cell cycle, thus maximizing the destruction of cancer cells.

Chemotherapy drugs are divided into classes that exert slightly different actions and have an effect on different portions of the cell cycle. Drug Guide 46.1 gives further explanation about the different classes of chemotherapy drugs.

Unfortunately, chemotherapeutic medications disrupt the cell cycle of not only cancer cells but also normal rapidly dividing cells. This results in a significant number of adverse effects. The cells most likely to be affected by chemotherapy are those in the bone marrow, the digestive tract (especially the mouth), the reproductive system, and hair follicles.

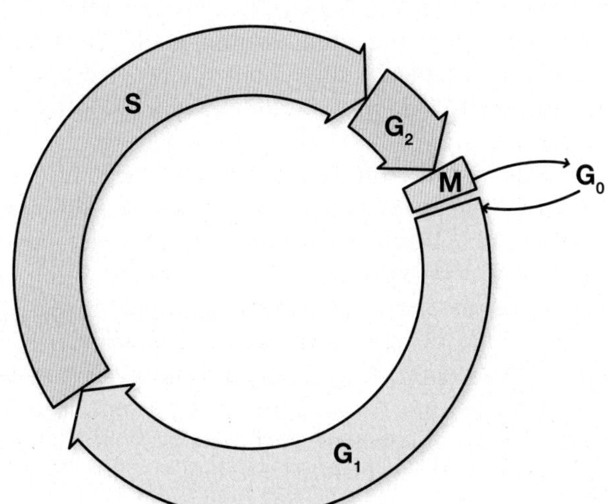

FIGURE 46.2 Phases of the cell cycle.

Adverse effects common to chemotherapeutic drugs include immunosuppression, infection, myelosuppression, nausea, vomiting, constipation, oral mucositis, alopecia, and pain. Long-term complications include microdontia and missing teeth as a result of damage to developing permanent teeth; hearing and vision changes; hematopoietic, immunologic, or gonadal dysfunction; endocrine dysfunction, including altered growth and precocious or delayed puberty; various alterations of the cardiorespiratory, gastrointestinal (GI), and genitourinary systems; and development of a second cancer as an adolescent or adult (ACS, 2024b).

TAKE NOTE!

Acupuncture as an adjunct therapy may help to decrease nausea, vomiting, and aversion to chemotherapy.

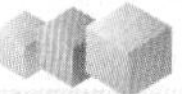 *Concept Mastery Alert*

Chemotherapeutic drugs that act as cell cycle–specific agents are classified as antimetabolites. Alkylating agents are not cell cycle–specific agents.

Radiation Therapy

Radiation therapy uses high-energy radiation to damage or kill cancer cells. Radiant energy in either a gamma or particle form is emitted during the treatment. Radiation affects not only cancer cells but also any rapidly growing cells with which they are in contact. It may be used as a curative, adjuvant, or palliative treatment, either alone or in combination with chemotherapy. Radiation therapy is also used to shrink a tumor prior to surgical resection. The area to be treated is marked carefully to minimize damage to normal cells.

Adverse effects of radiation therapy include fatigue, nausea, vomiting, oral mucositis, myelosuppression, and alterations in skin integrity at the site of irradiation. Long-term complications are related to the area of the body that was irradiated and include alterations in growth; hormone dysfunction; hearing and vision alterations; learning problems; cardiac dysfunction; pulmonary fibrosis; hepatic, sexual, or kidney dysfunction; osteoporosis; and development of secondary cancer (particularly at the site of irradiation) (Mitin, 2023).

Hematopoietic Stem Cell Transplantation

HSCT, also called bone marrow transplantation, is a procedure in which hematopoietic stem cells are infused intravenously into the child. This follows a period of purging of abnormal cells in the child that is accomplished through high-dose chemotherapy or irradiation. The use of high-dose chemotherapy and total body irradiation kills the tumor cells but also destroys the child's bone marrow. The transplanted cells migrate to the empty spaces in the child's bone marrow and reestablish normal hematopoiesis in the child.

HSCT is used for a variety of childhood cancers, including leukemia, lymphoma, brain tumors, neuroblastoma, and other solid tumors. For most pediatric cancers, it is not the first line of treatment but is used for refractory or advanced disease.

Autologous HSCT is achieved through harvest and treatment of the child's own bone marrow, followed by infusion of the treated stem cells. Risk of relapse of the original disease is highest in autologous HSCT. Allogenic HSCT refers to transplantation using stem cells from another individual that are harvested from the bone marrow, peripheral blood, or umbilical cord blood. Allogenic HSCT requires human leukocyte antigen (HLA) matching for antigen-specific sites on the leukocytes. Closely matched HLA donors may be difficult to find from a donor listing, and sibling donors are often the closest match. The degree of match is inversely related to the risk for graft rejection and the development of graft-versus-host disease (GVHD). In other words, the lesser the degree of HLA matching in the donor, the higher the risk of graft rejection and GVHD (Secola, 2022a).

In addition to graft rejection and GVHD, additional initial complications of HSCT are infection; electrolyte imbalance; bleeding; and organ, skin, and mucous membrane toxicities. Long-term complications include impaired growth and fertility related to endocrine dysfunction, developmental delay, cataracts, pulmonary and cardiac disease, avascular necrosis of the bone, and development of secondary cancers.

Palliative Care

Hospice or palliative care may be needed for the child with cancer. Children facing the end of life experience the same symptoms that adults do, including pain, fatigue, nausea, and dyspnea. All dying children have the right to die comfortably and with palliation of symptoms, as has been well established in adult hospice programs. The most recent guidelines for palliative care call for comprehensive assessment and planning by an interdisciplinary team, with care delivered in a culturally sensitive and developmentally appropriate manner (National Hospice and Palliative Care Organization [NHPCO], 2022). For further information related to nursing care of the dying child, refer to Chapter 34.

LABORATORY AND DIAGNOSTIC TESTING

The nurse must understand the main elements of the complete blood count (CBC; hemogram) to recognize critical values and intervene as appropriate. The components of the CBC are:

- RBC count: the actual number of counted RBCs in a certain volume of blood
- **Hemoglobin** (Hgb): measure of the protein made up of heme (iron surrounded by protoporphyrin) and globin, alpha- and beta-polypeptide chains, primarily responsible for the transport of nutrients and oxygen to the tissues
- **Hematocrit** (Hct): an indirect measure of RBCs (number and volume)
- RBC indices:
  - Mean corpuscular volume (MCV): average size of the RBC
  - Mean corpuscular hemoglobin (MCH): a calculated value of the oxygen-carrying capacity of the Hgb in the RBCs
  - Mean corpuscular hemoglobin concentration (MCHC): a calculated value that reflects the concentration of Hgb inside the RBC
  - Red cell distribution width (RDW): a calculated value that is a measure of the width of RBCs
- WBC count: actual count of the number of WBCs in a volume of blood
- **Platelet count:** number of platelets per blood volume
- Mean platelet volume (MPV): a measurement of the size of the platelets

Tables 46.1 and 46.2 provide age-related values for the CBC and leukocyte count. When evaluating the CBC, the nurse must take into account the presenting clinical picture of the child. For instance, the RBC count may be truly elevated (erythrocytosis or **polycythemia**) in certain diseases or in the case of dehydration from diarrhea or burns. When anemia is present, the RBC count is low. When the MCV is elevated, the RBCs are larger than normal (**macrocytic**). When the MCV is decreased, the RBCs are smaller than normal (**microcytic**). A decrease in the MCHC means that the Hgb is diluted in the cell and that less of the red color is present (**hypochromic**). When the Hgb concentration is increased in the RBC, then the pigmentation (red color) is increased (**hyperchromic**). Alterations in these RBC indices assist the health care provider or nurse practitioner with diagnosis.

WBCs are the body's defense against infection or injury. The specific types of WBCs are discussed in Chapter 37. Platelets are necessary for clot formation, and if changes occur, problems may develop. Elevations in platelet levels can indicate an increase in clotting, while decreases can put the child at risk for increased bleeding. Decreases can result if the platelets are being used up when bleeding is present, if an inherited disorder is present, or if the spleen holds them, as in hypersplenism. Platelets are larger when they are new; thus, an elevation in the MPV indicates that an increased number of platelets are being produced in the bone marrow.

TABLE **46.1** • Normal Hemogram Values

Age	WBC ($\times 10^3/mm^3$)	RBC ($\times 10^6/mm^3$)	Hgb (g/dL)	Hct (%)	MCV (fL)	MCH (pg/cell)	MCHC (g/dL)	Platelets ($\times 10^3/mm^3$)	RDW (%)	MPV (fL)
Birth–2 weeks	9.0–30.0	4.1–6.1	14.5–24.5	44–54	98–112	34–40	33–37	150–450	—	—
2–8 weeks	5.0–21.0	4.0–6.0	12.5–20.5	39–59	98–112	30–36	32–36	—	—	—
2–6 months	5.0–19.0	3.8–5.6	10.7–17.3	35–49	83–97	27–33	31–35	—	—	—
6 months–1 year	5.0–19.0	3.8–5.2	9.9–14.5	29–43	73–87	24–30	32–36	—	—	—
1–6 years	5.0–19.0	3.9–5.3	9.5–14.1	30–40	70–84	23–29	31–35	—	—	—
6–16 years	4.8–10.8	4.0–5.2	10.3–14.9	32–42	73–87	24–30	32–36	—	—	—
16–18 years	4.8–10.8	4.2–5.4	11.1–15.7	34–44	75–89	25–31	32–36	—	—	—
>18 years (males)	5.0–10.0	4.5–5.5	14.0–17.4	42–52	84–96	28–34	32–36	140–400	11.5–14.5	7.4–10.4
>18 years (females)	5.0–10.0	4.0–5.0	12.0–16.0	36–48	84–96	28–34	32–36	140–400	11.5–14.5	7.4–10.4

Hct, hematocrit; Hgb, hemoglobin; MCH, mean corpuscular hemoglobin; MCHC, mean corpuscular hemoglobin concentration; MCV, mean corpuscular volume; MPV , mean platelet volume; RBC, red blood cell; RDW, red cell distribution width; WBC, white blood cell.

Data from Fischbach, F. T., Fischbach, M. A., & Stout, K. (2022). *A manual of laboratory and diagnostic tests* (11th ed.). Wolters Kluwer Health.

TABLE 46.2 • Normal Differential for Leukocytes (White Blood Cell Differential)

Age	Bands/Stab (%)	Segs/Polys (%)	Eos (%)	Basos (%)	Lymphs (%)	Monos (%)
Birth–1 week	10–18	32–62	0–2	0–1	26–36	0–6
1–2 weeks	8–16	19–49	0–4	0	38–46	0–9
2–4 weeks	7–15	14–34	0–3	0	43–53	0–9
4–8 weeks	7–13	15–35	0–3	0–1	41–71	0–7
2–6 months	5–11	15–35	0–3	0–1	42–72	0–6
6 months–1 year	6–12	13–33	0–3	0	46–76	0–5
1–6 years	5–11	13–33	0–3	0	46–76	0–5
6–16 years	5–11	32–54	0–3	0–1	27–57	0–5
16–18 years	5–11	34–64	0–3	0–1	25–45	0–5
>18 years	3–6	50–62	0–3	0–1	25–40	3–7

Data from Fischbach, F. T., Fischbach, M. A., & Stout, K. (2022). *A manual of laboratory and diagnostic tests* (11th ed.). Wolters Kluwer Health.

Clinical Judgment and the Nursing Process for the Child With an Alteration in Cellular Regulation/Hematologic or Neoplastic Disorder

Care of the child with a hematologic disorder or cancer includes assessment, nursing analysis, planning, interventions, and evaluation. Development of a plan of care will depend on which component of the blood is altered in the hematologic disorder. A decrease in hemoglobin will necessitate evaluation of oxygen-carrying capacity and effects of hypoxia on the tissues. A reduction in platelet production will lead the nurse to evaluate for prolonged bleeding, hemorrhage, and shock. An elevation in WBCs would require an evaluation for infection.

From a general understanding of the care involved for a child with cancer, the nurse can then individualize the care based on specifics for the particular child. Children with cancer often suffer many physical effects as a result of the disease and its treatment. The nurse must be diligent when assessing for these effects and should involve the parents as a reliable source for reporting the child's physical symptoms.

Assessment

Signs of changes in the hematologic system are often insidious and overlooked. Children with cancer often demonstrate similar signs. Skin color changes such as pallor, bruising, and flushing are often the first signs that a problem is developing. Changes in mental status such as lethargy can indicate a decrease in Hgb and a decreased amount of oxygen being delivered to the brain. Nursing assessment must include a thorough approach.

Health History

Elicit the birth and maternal history, noting low birth weight or gestational diabetes and ascertaining whether vitamin K was given after birth. The past medical history might be significant for recent illnesses that may contribute to a change in blood cell distribution. Determine the child's sleep/wake patterns and bowel elimination patterns, which may be affected by alterations in circulating blood volume or changes in oxygenation. Explore the family history for inherited disorders such as hemophilia, sickle cell disease, thalassemia, or history of cancer. Determine the presence of risk factors such as previous malignancy and treatment; synthetic chemical exposures; parental exposure to radiation, chemicals, or chemotherapeutic agents; and a family history of malignancy (especially childhood), immune disorders, or genetic disorders such as neurofibromatosis or Down syndrome. Evaluate the child's typical diet for nutritional deficits.

Determine risk for lead exposure based on the use of a standard questionnaire. Determine current medical history. When eliciting the history of the present illness, inquire about:

- Fatigue or malaise
- Pallor of the skin
- Unusual bruising or petechiae
- Excessive bleeding or difficulty stopping bleeding

- Pain: location, onset, duration, quality, and relieving factors
- Recurrent fever or frequent infections
- Early-morning headache with nausea or vomiting
- Gait or behavior changes
- Visual disturbances
- History of bone fractures unrelated to trauma

Physical Examination

A child's general appearance gives great insight into their health and can indicate problems such as malnutrition or lead poisoning. A complete physical examination should be performed on any child with, or suspected of having, cancer or a hematologic disorder. Note particular findings as discussed in what follows. Physical examination of the child with a hematologic or neoplastic disorder includes inspection and observation, palpation, and auscultation.

INSPECTION AND OBSERVATION

Observe the child's overall appearance and energy level. Note a thin or frail appearance, fatigue, or altered level of consciousness. Measure weight and height (or length) and plot on standardized growth charts. Examine the oral cavity for bleeding gums or pale mucous membranes. Document visible masses or asymmetry of the face, thorax, abdomen, or extremities. Observe the nail beds, palms, and soles for pallor. Evaluate the fingertips for clubbing, which occurs with chronic hypoxemia. Document the location and extent of bruises, petechiae, or purpura. Count the respiratory rate and observe for work of breathing. Obtain a pulse oximeter reading to determine oxygen saturation of tissues. Note conjunctival color as well as color and moisture of oral mucosa. Determine urinary output, which may be altered with decreases in circulatory blood volume or inadequate oxygenation. Note the child's responsiveness to stimuli and movement of extremities. Observe the child's gait, noting ataxia or limp. Note rectal bleeding or vaginal discharge.

AUSCULTATION

Auscultate breath sounds, noting adequacy of air movement and depth of respiration. Note adventitious sounds or absence of breath sounds (which would occur in an area of the lung filled with blood). Auscultate heart sounds, listening closely for murmurs (which can develop with changes in blood viscosity and volume). Note the rate and rhythm of the heart tones. Auscultate bowel sounds, noting presence and normalcy.

PERCUSSION

Percuss the abdomen, noting dullness over a mass if present.

PALPATION

Measure blood pressure, which may change with alterations in blood volume. Palpate the peripheral pulses for strength and equality. Palpate for lymphadenopathy; in particular, note nontender or firm lymph nodes. Determine capillary refill time, which may be prolonged when the circulating blood volume is decreased. Carefully palpate the abdomen for tenderness, hepatomegaly, **splenomegaly** (increased spleen size), or presence of a mass. Palpate any unusual area of swelling anywhere on the body, noting size and absence of tenderness. Note temperature of the skin. Determine elasticity of skin, noting decreased turgor. Palpate the joints for tenderness and determine if range of motion (ROM) is limited.

Psychosocial Assessment

Assess the child's and family's psychosocial status, using open-ended questions. It is particularly important to determine the child's self-esteem, level of anxiety or stress, and coping mechanisms. Determine the spiritual status of the child and family. Ongoing medical procedures and the fear of dying take a toll on the child and family when cancer is present. Ask the child how things are going at home; how do they get along with brothers, sisters, and parents? If the child is school-age, ask how school is going. Does the child have friends with whom they get to spend time? Ask the child what they do in their spare time; are there any hobbies? These types of queries will provide the nurse with information about how well the child is coping. Assess the parents' status as well. Ask about the parental relationship and how other children in the family are doing. Determine whether certain stressors may need to be addressed.

Laboratory and Diagnostic Testing

Common Laboratory and Diagnostic Tests 46.1 explains the most commonly used laboratory and diagnostic tests for children with hematologic and neoplastic disorders. The tests can assist the health care provider or nurse practitioner in diagnosing the disorder and/or be used as guidelines in determining ongoing treatment. Laboratory or nonnursing personnel obtain some of the tests, while the nurse might obtain others. In either instance, the nurse should be familiar with how the tests are obtained, what they are used for, and normal versus abnormal results. This knowledge will also be necessary when providing child and family education related to the testing.

Remember Shaun, the 10-month-old with the laceration and prolonged bleeding? What additional health history and physical examination assessment information should you obtain?

COMMON LABORATORY AND DIAGNOSTIC TESTS 46.1

Test	Explanation	Indications	Nursing Implications
Alpha-fetoprotein (AFP)	Produced by the fetal liver and yolk sac; normally decreases to very low levels by 1 year of age	May be elevated in Hodgkin disease and other cancers; used to determine tumor burden	No food or fluid restriction required.
Blood type and cross-match	Determines ABO blood type as well as presence of antigens. Cross-match is performed on RBC-containing products to avoid transfusion reaction.	Person who has sustained trauma or any person in whom blood loss is suspected, in preparation for transfusion	Avoid hemolysis of specimen. Appropriately sign and date specimen. Apply "type and cross" or "blood band" to child at the time of blood draw if indicated by the institution. Most type and cross-match specimens expire after 48–72 hours.
Bone marrow aspiration and biopsy	A needle is inserted through the cortex of the bone into the bone marrow (most often the iliac spine), bone marrow is aspirated, and the cells are evaluated.	Evaluation for leukemia or metastasis of other cancers to bone marrow	Use eutectic mixture of local anesthetic (EMLA) or lidocaine to decrease pain with procedure. Often performed under conscious sedation Apply a pressure dressing to arrest bleeding. Assess for tenderness or erythema. May require mild analgesia for postprocedure pain
Bone scan	Administration of IV radionuclide material, which is taken up by the bone and is visible on the scans	Identify metastasis to bone	Requires patent IV for injection Encourage fluid intake after injection to increase uptake of injected radionuclide. Scan will be performed 1–3 hours after injection.
Chest radiography	Radiograph of the chest	Identify tumor or metastasis in the thorax.	Chest must be held stationary for a brief time.
Clotting studies	Prothrombin time (PT), partial thromboplastin time (PTT), activated partial thromboplastin time (aPTT), international normalized ratio (INR)	Evaluation of common pathway in clotting mechanism PT, INR: evaluation of extrinsic system PTT, aPTT: evaluation of intrinsic system	Apply pressure to venipuncture site. Assess for bleeding (gums, bruising, blood in urine or stool).
Coagulating factor concentration	Measures concentration of specific coagulating factors in the blood	Hemophilia, disseminated intravascular coagulation (DIC)	Apply pressure to venipuncture site. Assess for bleeding (gums, bruising, blood in urine or stool). Deliver specimen to laboratory as soon as possible (unstable at room temperature).
Complete blood count (CBC) with differential	Evaluates hemoglobin and hematocrit, WBC count (particularly the percentage of individual WBCs), and platelet count	Anemia, infection, bleeding disorder, clotting disorder, immunosuppression, to determine neutropenia in myelosuppression	Normal values vary according to age and sex. WBC differential is helpful in evaluating source of infection. May be affected by certain medications
Computed tomography (CT) scan	Multiple films taken in successive layers to provide a 3D view of the body part being scanned	Identify tumor location or metastasis.	Some CT scans are done with oral or IV contrast (notify health care provider if child has iodine or shellfish allergy). May require a several-hour period of NPO if contrast is used (contrast may cause nausea). Encourage fluid intake after scan to facilitate excretion of contrast dye.
Hemoglobin electrophoresis	Measures percentage of normal and abnormal hemoglobin in the blood	Sickle cell anemia, thalassemia	Blood transfusions within the previous 12 weeks may alter test results.

COMMON LABORATORY AND DIAGNOSTIC TESTS 46.1

Test	Explanation	Indications	Nursing Implications
Iron	Evaluates iron metabolism	Iron-deficiency anemia, hemosiderosis with chronic transfusion or hemoglobinopathies	Recent blood transfusions increase level. Child should fast for 12 hours before the test. Avoid hemolysis (will falsely elevate result).
Lead	Measures level of lead in blood	Lead poisoning	Normal amount in blood is zero.
Lumbar puncture (LP)	A needle is placed in the subarachnoid space of the spinal column, below the base of the cord, and cerebrospinal fluid is withdrawn for analysis.	Evaluation of tumor or metastasis to brain or spinal cord; also used to administer intrathecal medications	Use EMLA before the procedure to decrease pain. May be performed under conscious sedation. Position child appropriately. Use distraction techniques in the older child or adolescent. Encourage child to recline for up to 12 hours after LP.
Magnetic resonance imaging (MRI)	Based on how hydrogen atoms behave in a magnetic field when disturbed by radiofrequency signals; does not require ionizing radiation; provides a 3D view of the body part being scanned	Identify extent of tumor or metastatic spread.	Remove all metal objects from the child. Child must remain motionless for entire scan; parent can stay in room with child. Younger children will require sedation to keep still. A loud thumping sound occurs inside the machine during the scan procedure; this can be frightening to children.
Reticulocyte count	Measures the number of reticulocytes (immature RBCs) in the blood	Indicates bone marrow's ability to respond to anemia with production of RBCs	Rises quickly in response to iron supplementation in the iron-deficient child
Serum ferritin	Measures the level of ferritin (the major iron storage protein) in the blood	Most sensitive test for determining iron-deficiency anemia	Elevated in hemolytic disease and if transfused recently Iron supplementation increases ferritin levels.
Urine catechol amines (VMA, HVA)	Catabolism of catecholamines causes elevated levels in urine.	Diagnosis of neuroblastoma (produces catecholamines)	24-hour urine collection Levels may be altered with certain foods and drugs or vigorous exercise.
Ultrasound	High-frequency sound waves are directed at internal organs and structures, and an image is made of the waves as they are reflected back through the tissues.	Identify tumor presence, especially in abdomen or on kidney.	Fasting for a few hours may be required when certain organs are to be visualized.

IV, intravenous; HVA, homovanillic acid; NPO, nothing by mouth; VMA, vanillylmandelic acid; RBC, red blood cell; WBC, white blood cell.

Data from Corbett, J. A., & Banks, A. D. (2019). *Laboratory tests and diagnostic procedures with nursing diagnoses* (9th ed.). Pearson Education Inc.

Nursing Analysis

After recognizing and analyzing cues from a thorough assessment, the nurse might identify several patient problems, including:

- Nausea
- Malnutrition risk
- Constipation
- Diarrhea
- Altered oral mucous membrane integrity
- Activity intolerance
- Impaired physical mobility
- Bleeding risk
- Infection risk
- Anxiety
- Altered body image perception
- Coping impairment
- Situational low self-esteem
- Grief
- Pain
- Interrupted family processes
- Caregiver role strain risk

Shaun's health history revealed he bled with all four of the teeth he has cut. Upon physical examination, numerous bruises are noted. Based on these assessment findings, what would your top three patient problems be for Shaun?

The preceding patient problems provide suggestions for nursing care planning or concept mapping. Suggested interventions with rationales are provided further on. Children's responses to alterations in cellular regulation and their treatments will vary; care planning should be individualized, based on the child's and family's needs. Other conditions may contribute to these patient problems and must also be considered when prioritizing care. Refer to Chapter 36 for the nursing process for pain management and to Chapter 33 for nursing interventions related to interrupted family processes and caregiver role strain risk. Additional information will be included later in the chapter as it relates to nursing management of children with specific disorders, as well as particular nursing interventions for deficient knowledge.

Nursing Analysis

Nausea related to exposure to toxin (adverse effects of chemotherapy or radiation therapy) as evidenced by aversion toward food, increase in salivation, increase in swallowing movements, gagging sensation, or sour taste

Goal/Outcome

Child will experience decreased nausea: will verbalize symptom relief and will be free from vomiting.

Alleviating Nausea and Vomiting (interventions with *rationale*)

- Administer antiemetics prior to chemotherapy and as needed thereafter *to decrease frequency of nausea.*
- Assess frequency of vomiting and level of hydration *to provide baseline data and recognize alterations early.*
- Offer frequent, smaller meals or snacks: *smaller amounts are less likely to be vomited.*
- Avoid spicy foods *to avoid stomach upset.*
- Allow bubbles to dissipate from carbonated beverages before they are ingested: *carbonation may contribute to nausea.*
- Remove cover from meal tray before entering child's room: *this will allow the food odor to dissipate outside of the room; food odors may trigger nausea and vomiting.*

Nursing Analysis

Malnutrition risk; risk factors include insufficient dietary intake, and food aversion.

Goal/Outcome

Child will improve nutritional intake, resulting in steady increase in weight and length/height.

Promoting Adequate Nutrition (interventions with *rationale*)

- Determine body weight and length/height norm for age or find out what the child's pretreatment measurements were *to determine goal to work toward.*
- Determine child's food preferences and provide favorite foods as able *to increase the likelihood that the child will consume adequate amounts of foods.*
- Administer antiemetics as ordered *to increase the likelihood that the child will retain the food they ingest.*
- Weigh child daily or weekly (according to health care provider order or institutional standard), and measure length/height weekly *to monitor for growth.*
- Offer highest-calorie meals at the time of day when the child's appetite is the greatest *to increase likelihood of increased caloric intake.*
- Provide increased-calorie shakes or puddings within diet restriction: *high-calorie foods increase weight gain.*
- Administer vitamin and mineral supplements as prescribed *to attain/maintain vitamin and mineral balance in the body.*
- Administer total parenteral nutrition and intravenous lipids as ordered *to provide adequate nutrition for healing.*

Nursing Analysis

Constipation related to decreased gastric motility (effects of vinca alkaloids, opioid use, decreased activity, dietary changes) as evidenced by decrease in stool frequency or volume or inability to defecate

Goal/Outcome

Child's bowel function will return to usual pattern: child will pass a formed, soft stool every day (or modify this criterion according to child's usual pattern).

Preventing or Managing Constipation (interventions with *rationale*)

- Ensure that child increases fluid *intake to provide enough water in the intestines for soft stool formation.*
- Increase fiber in the diet *to provide bulk for stool formation.*
- Administer stool softeners such as mineral oil or docusate sodium; *these help soften the stool, aiding in passage.*
- Provide motivator laxatives such as magnesium hydroxide, lactulose, or sorbitol *to stimulate stool passage.*
- Use stimulant laxatives such as senna or bisacodyl only intermittently rather than on a daily basis *to avoid dependency and diarrhea.*

Nursing Analysis

Diarrhea related to treatment regimen (effects of radiation therapy) as evidenced by bowel urgency, cramping, or loose, liquid stools

Goal/Outcome

Child's bowel function will return to usual pattern: child will pass a formed, soft stool daily (or modify this criterion according to child's usual pattern).

Managing Diarrhea (interventions with *rationale*)

- Assess frequency of diarrhea and level of hydration *to provide data about severity.*
- Obtain weight daily on same scale *to determine extent of fluid loss.*
- Maintain accurate intake and output records *to determine extent of fluid loss.*
- Administer oral rehydration solutions or intravenous fluids as ordered *to maintain or restore adequate hydration.*
- Restrict roughage and residue in diet *to decrease likelihood of diarrhea.*
- Avoid milk products during acute diarrheal phase: *lactose often worsens diarrhea.*
- Provide an elemental diet to relieve symptoms: *absorbed in the upper small bowel.*
- Provide meticulous perineal care *to avoid skin breakdown related to frequent or loose stools.*
- Administer antidiarrheal medications if ordered *to decrease frequency of stools.*
- If severe and related to radiation therapy, a 3- to 4-day rest period from radiation may be required *to begin recovery of normal absorptive capabilities of bowel.*

Nursing Analysis

Altered oral mucous membrane integrity related to chemotherapy, radiation therapy, immunosuppression, decrease in platelets, malnutrition, or dehydration as evidenced by oral discomfort, cheilitis, bleeding, hyperemia, stomatitis, or other oral lesions

Goal/Outcome

Child will maintain intact, moist mucosa free from redness, ulceration, or debris.

Restoring Healthy Oral Mucosa (interventions with *rationale*)

- Frequently assess oral cavity for redness, lesions, ulcers, plaques, or bleeding *to provide baseline for comparison and identify alterations early.*
- Offer ice chips frequently while child is nothing by mouth (NPO) *to maintain hydration of mucosa.*
- Use only a soft toothbrush or toothette for dental care, avoiding excessive pressure with brushing, *to decrease incidence of bleeding with mouth care.*
- Keep lips lubricated with petroleum jelly or fragrance-free lip balm *to maintain moist, hydrated lips.*
- Rinse with salt solution or mouthwash every 1 to 2 hours *to keep oral cavity clean and moist.*
- Administer glutamine and/or beta-carotene supplements, *which have been shown to decrease the incidence and severity of mucositis.*
- Have child swish and spit 1:1 Benadryl/Maalox solution *to decrease pain.*
- Administer antifungal solution *to prevent or treat oral candidiasis.*
- Avoid spicy, acidic, or very hot or very cold foods *to decrease pain.*
- Administer pain medication (usually acetaminophen or codeine) as ordered *to decrease pain.*

Nursing Analysis

Activity intolerance related to imbalance between oxygen supply and demand (treatment adverse effects, anemia) as evidenced by abnormal heart rate response to activity, exertional dyspnea, weakness, or fatigue

Goal/Outcome

Child will display increased activity tolerance: desire to play without developing symptoms of exertion.

Promoting Activity (interventions with *rationale*)

- Encourage activity or ambulation per health care provider's orders: *early mobilization results in better outcomes.*
- Observe child for symptoms of activity intolerance such as pallor, nausea, lightheadedness or dizziness, or changes in vital signs *to determine level of tolerance.*
- If child is on bed rest, perform ROM exercises and frequent position changes: *negative changes to the musculoskeletal system occur quickly with inactivity and immobility.*
- Cluster nursing care activities and plan for periods of rest before and after exertion *to decrease oxygen need and consumption.*
- Refer the child to physical therapy *for exercise prescription to increase skeletal muscle strength.*

Nursing Analysis

Impaired physical mobility related to pain (from sickle cell crisis or acute bleeds), or physical deconditioning as evidenced by discomfort, decreased motor skills, or slowed movement

Goal/Outcome

Child will be able to engage in activities within age parameters and limits of disease: child is able to move extremities, move about environment, and participate in exercise programs within limits of age and disease.

Promoting Physical Mobility (interventions with *rationale*)

- Encourage gross and fine motor activities as able within constraints of pain/bleed *to facilitate motor development.*
- Collaborate with physical therapy to strengthen muscles and promote mobility *to facilitate motor development.*
- Use passive and active ROM exercises, and teach the child and family how to perform them *to prevent*

contractures and facilitate joint mobility and muscle development (active ROM) to help increase mobility.
- Praise accomplishments and emphasize child's abilities *to improve self-esteem and encourage feelings of confidence and competence.*

Nursing Analysis

Bleeding risk; risk factors include decreased platelet count, deficient coagulation factor, treatment regimen effects.

Goal/Outcome

Child will not experience hemorrhage: will experience decreased bruising or episodes of prolonged bleeding.

Preventing Bleeding (interventions with *rationale*)

- Assess for petechiae, purpura, bruising, or bleeding *to provide baseline data for comparison; if present, may warrant intervention.*
- Encourage quiet activities or play *to avoid trauma with active play.*
- Avoid rectal temperatures and examinations. Post sign at head of bed "no rectal temperatures or medications" *to avoid rectal mucosa damage resulting in bleeding.*
- Avoid intramuscular injections and lumbar puncture if possible *to decrease risk of bleeding from a puncture site.*
- If bone marrow aspiration must be performed, apply pressure dressing to site *to prevent bleeding.*
- Teach families about preferred physical activities for the child with immune thrombocytopenia or hemophilia *to provide safe physical activities and decrease risk of injury.*

Nursing Analysis

Infection risk related to immunosuppression or leukopenia

Goal/Outcome

Child will not experience overwhelming infection; child will be free from infection or able to recover if they become infected.

Preventing Infection (interventions with *rationale*)

- Assess for fever, pain, cough, tachypnea, adventitious breath sounds, skin ulceration, stomatitis, and perirectal fissures *to identify potential infection.*
- Administer antibiotics for temperature greater than 38.4°C *to decrease likelihood of overwhelming sepsis.*
- Maintain meticulous hand hygiene (including family, visitors, staff) *to minimize spread of infectious organisms.*
- Maintain isolation as prescribed *to minimize exposure to infectious organisms.*
- Avoid rectal temperatures and examinations, intramuscular injections, and urinary catheterization when child is neutropenic *to decrease possibility of introducing microorganisms.*
- Educate family and visitors that child should be restricted from contact with known infectious exposures (in hospital and at home) *to encourage cooperation with infection control.*
- Strictly observe medical asepsis *to avoid unintentional introduction of microorganisms.*
- Promote nutrition and appropriate rest *to maximize body's potential to heal.*
- Inform family to contact the health care provider or nurse practitioner if child has known exposure to chickenpox or measles *so that preventive measures (e.g., varicella zoster immunoglobulin [VZIG]) can be taken.*
- Administer vaccines (not live) as prescribed (after clearance with oncologist) *to prevent common childhood communicable diseases.*
- Teach family to monitor for fever at home, and report temperature elevations to oncologist immediately *so that antibiotic therapy may be instituted as soon as possible.*

Nursing Analysis

Anxiety related to ineffective coping strategies, or insufficient knowledge to manage a situation, as evidenced by verbalization

Goal/Outcome

Child and/or parents will demonstrate control: child's anxiety/fear will be minimized (verbalization, decreased crying with procedures); parents (and child as developmentally able) will make decisions regarding care as appropriate.

Promoting a Sense of Control (interventions with *rationale*)

- Maintain a quiet and calm environment *to reduce the child's stress.*
- Educate the child, as appropriate, and the family regarding the need for laboratory specimens *to alleviate anxiety related to the unknown.*
- Identify the need for the specific test and explain the procedure before obtaining the specimen *to decrease the anxiety and time required for the procedure.*
- Use topical anesthetic creams or agents for nonemergency laboratory draws to decrease stress related *to needlesticks or venipunctures.*
- Encourage child and family to make decisions regarding care as appropriate, *to increase sense of control.*
- Provide developmentally appropriate activities for the child: *activities can reduce stress and also provide stimulus for children; serves as a model for the family.*

Nursing Analysis

Altered body image perception related to surgery or treatment regimen (amputation or hair loss), as evidenced by negative feeling about body

Goal/Outcome

Child or adolescent will display appropriate body image: will look at self in mirror and participate in social activities.

Promoting Body Image (interventions with *rationale*)

- Acknowledge the child's feelings of anger over body changes and illness: *venting feelings is associated with less body image disturbance.*
- Encourage the child or adolescent to choose a wig or hats and scarves *to involve the child in making decisions about appearance.*
- Support the child's or adolescent's choices of comfortable, fashionable clothing *to disguise weight loss or scarring while promoting self-esteem.*
- Involve the child in the decision-making process, *as a sense of control will improve body image.*
- Encourage the child to spend time with peers who have experienced hair, limb, or weight loss, *as peers' opinions are often better accepted than those of people in authority, such as parents or health care professionals.*

Nursing Analysis

Coping impairment related to prolonged disease (cancer or genetic disorder), or situational crisis as evidenced by protective behaviors incongruent with child's abilities or autonomy, or inadequate understanding/insufficient knowledge interfering with effective behaviors

Goal/Outcome

Child and/or family will demonstrate adequate coping skills: will verbalize feeling supported and demonstrate healthy family interactions.

Promoting Child and Family Coping (interventions with *rationale*)

- Provide emotional support to the child and family *to improve coping abilities.*
- Actively listen to the child's and family's concerns *to validate their feelings and establish trust.*
- Provide open communication with the child and siblings; *children appreciate honesty about their illness, and coping is improved.*
- Refer families to community resources, such as parent support groups and grief counseling, *to improve coping abilities.*
- Give terminally ill children permission to discuss their feelings about their illness, *allowing them to conquer fears and express love for their family and friends.*
- Encourage families to be honest with siblings about the treatment and prognosis of the child with cancer; *children often sense what is going on and cope better when they are prepared and are given an honest explanation of events.*
- Prepare siblings for the death of the child with cancer, using the child life specialist and chaplain as necessary; *the bereavement period is eased when siblings are prepared.*

Nursing Analysis

Situational low self-esteem related to decreased control over environment and developmental transition (inability to progress with quest for independence [adolescents])

Goal/Outcome

Child/adolescent will maintain or increase self-esteem: will display increased coping responses and verbalize control as appropriate as well as discuss plans for future.

Promoting Self-Esteem (interventions with *rationale*)

- Identify the adolescent's positive abilities *to promote self-esteem.*
- Give genuine and honest positive feedback, *as the child or adolescent desires honesty.*
- Explore strengths and weaknesses with the adolescent *to help the adolescent to see similarities and differences with healthy peers of the same age.*
- Encourage the adolescent to perform self-care as possible *to promote independence.*
- Offer emotional support *to reduce psychological distress and increase coping abilities.*
- Encourage participation in a support group *to allow adolescents to discuss body changes and the reactions they perceive in others.*
- When the adolescent is physically able, encourage attendance at camp or an adventure/wilderness event: *these programs have been shown to improve mental health and coping skills.*

Nursing Analysis

Grief related to anticipatory loss of child (diagnosis of cancer), as evidenced by psychological distress, anger, blame, or denial

Goal/Outcome

Family will express feelings of grief: seek help in dealing with feelings, plan for future one day at a time.

Supporting the Grieving Family (interventions with *rationale*)

- Use therapeutic communication with open-ended questions *to encourage an open and trusting relationship for better communication.*

- Actively listen to the family's expression of grief: *just being present and listening conveys support.*
- Encourage the family to cry and express feelings away from the child *to work through feelings while not upsetting the child.*
- Assess for spiritual distress and refer the family to the hospital chaplain or clergy of choice *for support.*
- Educate the family about the child's condition honestly: *knowing what is going on, what is to be expected, and what the treatment plan is gives the family a sense of control.*
- Support the family through discussions with the child about anticipated death when the illness is deemed terminal: *support is needed for this difficult discussion.*

Based on your top three patient problems for Shaun, describe appropriate nursing interventions.

CARING FOR THE CHILD WITH CANCER

Providing Education

Provide education to families of all children with cancer as outlined in Teaching Guidelines 46.1.

TEACHING GUIDELINES 46.1 Education for Families of Children With Cancer

- Obtain a printed or written copy of the child's treatment plan.
- Keep a calendar of all appointment times, blood count lab draw days, and phone numbers of all health care providers and nurse practitioners, home care companies, the laboratory, and the hospital.
- Seek medical care IMMEDIATELY if the child's temperature is 38.3°C (101°F) or higher.
- Call the oncologist or seek medical care if any of the following occur:
    - Cough or rapid breathing
    - Increased bruising, bleeding or petechiae, pallor, or increased levels of fatigue
    - Earache, sore throat, nuchal rigidity
    - Blisters, rashes, ulcers
    - Red, irritated skin on the child's buttocks
    - Abdominal pain, difficulty or pain with eating, drinking, or swallowing
    - Constipation or diarrhea
    - For children with central venous catheters:
        - Pus, redness, or swelling at the site
        - Breakage of the catheter
        - Do not give the child aspirin

Data from Kline, N. E. (2014). *Essentials of pediatric oncology nursing: A core curriculum* (4th ed.). Association of Pediatric Hematology/Oncology Nurses.

Administering Chemotherapy

All chemotherapy medications have the potential to cause toxicities in the child as well as in the people handling or preparing the medication. General guidelines related to the preparation and administration of chemotherapy include:

- Chemotherapy should be prepared and administered only by specially trained personnel.
- Personal protective equipment (PPE) in the form of double gloves and nonpermeable gowns should be worn when preparing or administering chemotherapy. If splashing is possible or a spill occurs, then a face shield and/or mask may also be necessary.
- Dispose of all equipment used in chemotherapy preparation and administration in a puncture-resistant container (Kline, 2014).

It is critical to calculate the chemotherapy dose correctly. Chemotherapy medication doses in children are based on body surface area (BSA). A nomogram is a commonly used device for determining BSA. To use the nomogram, draw a straight line between the child's height on the left and the child's weight on the right. The point at which the straight line crosses the center is the child's BSA expressed in meters squared (Fig. 46.3).

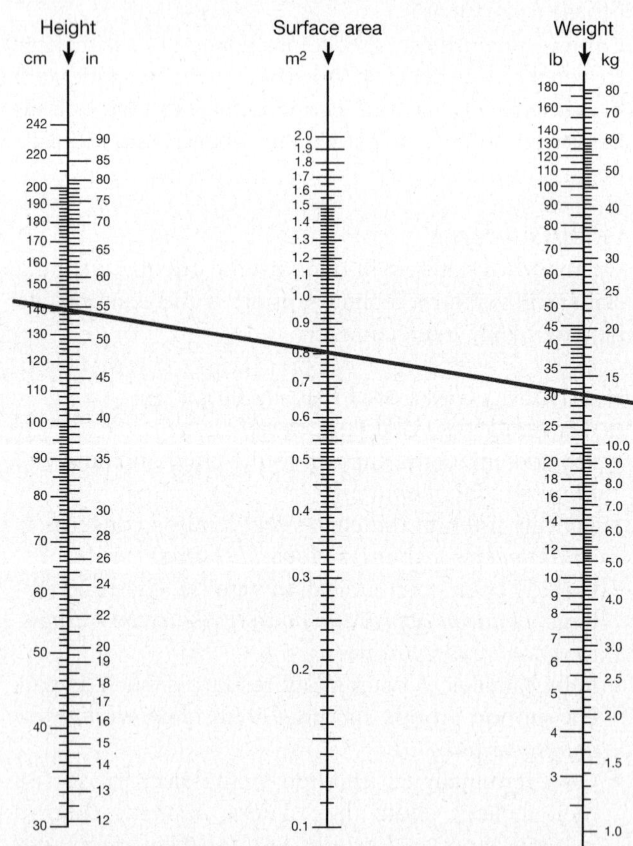

FIGURE 46.3 A child who weighs 13.2 kg and is 140 cm tall has a body surface area (BSA) of 0.80 m^2.

An alternative to using the nomogram is to use the following formula: BSA (m^2) = the square root of (height [in centimeters] × weight [in kilograms] divided by 3,600) (Kline, 2014). For example, for a child 140 cm tall and weighing 30 kg: 140 × 30 = 4,200; 4,200/3,600 = 1.167; and the square root of 1.167 is 1.08. The BSA would be 1.08.

Managing Adverse Effects of Chemotherapy

Chemotherapy can result in multiple adverse effects. Myelosuppression leads to low blood counts in all cell lines, placing the child at risk for infection, hemorrhage, and anemia. Nausea, vomiting, and anorexia may hinder the child's growth. Alopecia and facial changes may affect the child's self-esteem (Fig. 46.4). Nursing interventions related to the effects of myelosuppression, nausea, vomiting, and anorexia are discussed further on. Refer to the "Clinical Judgment and the Nursing Process" section for nursing interventions related to altered body image perception.

> *TAKE NOTE!*
>
> Cooling the scalp during chemotherapy administration with the use of a cooling cap may decrease hair loss (Rugo & van den Hurk, 2023).

PREVENTING INFECTION

Many chemotherapeutic drugs cause significant bone marrow suppression and decreased amounts of circulating mature neutrophils ("segs," or segmented neutrophils). Administer granulocyte colony–stimulating factor (GCSF) as ordered to promote neutrophil growth and maturation (Ahmed & Flynn, 2022). Administer VZIG within 72 hours of exposure to active chickenpox. If the child is actively infected with chickenpox, administer intravenous acyclovir as ordered. Children receiving treatment for acute lymphoblastic leukemia (ALL) are at risk for opportunistic infection with *Pneumocystis jirovecii,* as most children are colonized with this fungus. Administer prophylactic antibiotics as ordered, and teach the parents to administer them at home. Teaching Guidelines 46.2 gives further information about infection prevention at home.

As neutrophils are the primary means of fighting bacterial infection, when the neutrophil count is low, the chance of developing an overwhelming bacterial infection is high. Each drug that causes bone marrow suppression has a point of nadir. *Nadir* is the time after administration of the drug when bone marrow suppression is expected to be at its greatest and the neutrophil count is expected to be at its lowest (neutropenia). Nadir is individual for each drug and ranges from 7 to 28 days after dosing. An absolute neutrophil count (ANC) below 500 places the child at greatest risk (Ahmed & Flynn, 2022). Refer to Box 46.2 for information related to calculating the ANC.

Depending on institutional policy, precautions for neutropenia will be followed if the ANC is depressed. These include the following:

- Place the child in a private room.
- Perform hand hygiene before and after contact with each child.
- Monitor vital signs every 4 hours.
- Assess for signs and symptoms of infection at least every 8 hours.
- Avoid rectal suppositories, enemas, or examinations; urinary catheterization; and invasive procedures.
- Restrict visitors with fever, cough, or other signs/symptoms of infection.
- Do not permit raw fruits or vegetables or fresh flowers or live plants in the room.
- Place a mask on the child when they are being transported outside of the room.
- Perform dental care with a soft toothbrush if the platelet count is adequate.

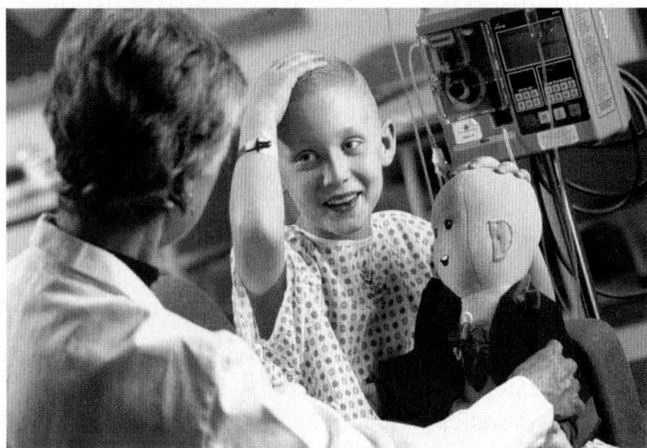

FIGURE 46.4 Chemotherapy often causes alopecia.

TEACHING GUIDELINES 46.2 Preventing Infection in Children Receiving Chemotherapy for Cancer

- Practice meticulous hygiene (oral, body, perianal).
- Avoid known ill contacts, especially people with chickenpox.
- Immediately notify the health care provider or nurse practitioner if exposed to chickenpox.
- Avoid crowded areas.
- Do not let the child receive live vaccines.
- Do not take the child's temperature rectally or give medications by the rectal route.
- Administer twice-daily trimethoprim–sulfamethoxazole for 3 consecutive days each week as ordered for prevention of Pneumocystis pneumonia.

Data from Kline, N. E. (2014). *Essentials of pediatric oncology nursing: A core curriculum* (4th ed.). Association of Pediatric Hematology/Oncology Nurses.

BOX **46.2** **Calculating the ANC**

- Add together the percentage of banded and segmented neutrophils reported on the CBC with differential.
- Multiply the total number of WBCs reported on the CBC by the preceding sum. This yields the ANC (total number of neutrophils present).

Example: Bands 5%, Segs 15%, WBCs 2,500

5% + 15% = 20% (0.20)
2,500 × 0.20 = 500
ANC = 500

ANC, absolute neutrophil count; CBC, complete blood count; WBC, white blood cell.

Data from Children's Oncology Group. (2023). *Low white blood cell count (neutropenia).* https://www.childrensoncologygroup.org/index.php/lowwhitebloodcellcount

Children with neutropenia and fever must be started on intravenous broad-spectrum antibiotics without delay to avoid overwhelming sepsis (Ahmed & Flynn, 2022).

PREVENTING HEMORRHAGE

Assess for petechiae, purpura, bruising, or bleeding. Determine changes from baseline that warrant intervention. Encourage quiet activities or play to avoid trauma. Avoid rectal temperatures and examinations to avoid rectal mucosal damage that results in bleeding. Post a sign at the head of the bed stating, "no rectal temperatures or medications." Avoid intramuscular injections and lumbar puncture, if possible, to decrease the risk of bleeding from a puncture site. If bone marrow aspiration must be performed, apply a pressure dressing to the site to prevent bleeding. For active or uncontrolled bleeding, transfuse platelets as ordered to control bleeding.

TAKE NOTE!

Administer acetaminophen for mild pain; avoid salicylate and NSAIDs due to increased risk for bleeding.

PREVENTING ANEMIA

To maintain blood volume, limit blood draws to the minimum volume required. Encourage the child to eat an appropriate diet that includes adequate iron. Administer EPO injections as ordered. Teach families to give the injections at home if prescribed.

MANAGING NAUSEA, VOMITING, AND ANOREXIA

Many chemotherapeutic drugs produce the adverse effect of nausea and vomiting, which often leads to anorexia. The cycle of nausea, vomiting, and anorexia is difficult to break once it begins. In addition, taste alterations are common in children who have received chemotherapy. During or after chemotherapy, children may develop an aversion to a food that was previously their favorite. Provide foods the child desires or asks for in order to increase the likelihood of eating.

Prevent nausea by administering antiemetic medications prior to the administration of chemotherapy and on a routine schedule around the clock for the first 1 to 2 days rather than on an as-needed (PRN) basis. Herbal or complementary therapies may provide another option for management of nausea.

TAKE NOTE!

Ginger capsules, ginger tea, and candied ginger have been used as a nausea remedy for centuries (ginger ale is usually artificially flavored, so it would not have the same effect). Although ginger is considered safe, instruct families to check with the oncologist before using this remedy.

Bright lights and noise may worsen nausea. Therefore, keep the child's environment dimly lit and calm. Relaxation therapy and guided imagery may also be helpful in preventing or treating nausea and vomiting. Refer to the "Clinical Judgment and the Nursing Process" section for additional interventions.

TAKE NOTE!

Foot massage may decrease the nausea and vomiting associated with chemotherapy (Asha et al., 2020).

Monitoring the Child Receiving Radiation Therapy

Assess the child's skin daily (particularly at the treatment site), as radiation causes damage to the cells in a localized area, which may include normal cells in addition to the cancerous cells. Teach parents not to scrub ink off the marked radiation field, and avoid adhesive tape in that area. Cleanse gently using a mild soap, and pat dry rather than rubbing, so as to avoid skin irritation. Moisturize the skin with aloe vera lotion or other aqueous cream. Administer diphenhydramine or apply hydrocortisone 1% cream to reduce itching and urge to scratch. Apply Silvadene cream once or twice a day to areas of desquamation related to radiation.

Avoid perfumed lotions or soaps, deodorants, heat, cold, or sun, as these will further irritate the skin in the irradiated area. Instruct the child and family that clothing should fit loosely so as not to irritate the site (ACS, 2024c). During the radiation treatment and for 8 weeks thereafter, the skin will be more photosensitive. Explain the importance of protecting the skin with a high-SPF (30 or higher) sunscreen.

Providing Care to the Child Undergoing HSCT

Stem cell transplantation is performed at limited specialty medical centers in the United States. In addition, special training is required for all personnel caring for the child who undergoes a stem cell transplant. The intent of this discussion is to provide only a brief introduction to, and overview of, nursing management related to HSCT.

Care for the child undergoing HSCT may be divided into three phases—the pretransplant phase, the posttransplant phase, and the lengthy supportive care phase. Nursing management of each phase is discussed briefly in what follows.

Nursing Management of the Child During the HSCT Pretransplant Phase

In the pretransplant phase, the child is being prepared to receive the transplant. The child's own bone marrow cells are eradicated through high-dose chemotherapy and total body irradiation. This phase usually occurs over 7 to 10 days. The child will be hospitalized because they are at extreme risk for serious infection. Maintain protective isolation in a positive-pressure room and limit visitors. Administer gamma globulin, acyclovir, or antibiotics as ordered to prevent or treat infection. Lymphohematopoietic rescue occurs with infusion of the donor or autologous cells (Kline, 2014).

Nursing Management of the Child During the HSCT Posttransplant Phase

The posttransplant phase is also a time of high risk for the child. Monitor closely for symptoms of GVHD such as severe diarrhea and maculopapular rash progressing to redness or desquamation of the skin (especially palms or soles) (Fig. 46.5). If GVHD occurs, administer immunosuppressive drugs such as cyclosporine, tacrolimus, or mycophenolate (which place the child at further risk for infection) (Secola, 2022b).

Providing Supportive Care Following the HSCT

During the supportive care phase, which lasts several months after the transplant, continue to monitor for and prevent infection. Administer PRBCs or platelets and GCSF as needed. Families and children who undergo HSCT need prolonged and extensive emotional and psychosocial support.

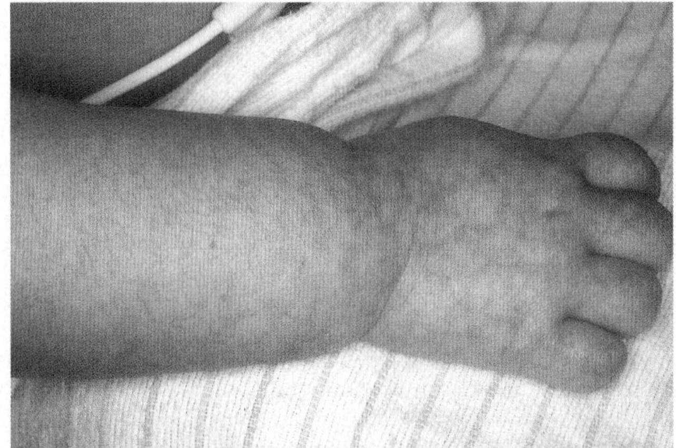

FIGURE 46.5 The first sign of graft-versus-host disease (GVHD) may be a maculopapular rash. (Courtesy of Mary L. Brandt, MD.)

A medical social worker and psychologist or counselor are usually members of the transplant team and are excellent resources for these families' needs (Nuuhiwa, 2022).

Promoting a Normal Life

Children and adolescents want to be normal and to experience the things that other children of their age do. The child should attend school when they are well enough and the WBC counts are not dangerously low. Children, their families, and their teachers should be aware that cancer and its treatment can affect scholastic abilities. Learning disabilities, difficulty with memory, attention disorders, and cognitive deficits can occur (NCI, 2024).

Maintain other activities if the child is able and if platelet counts are within normal limits. Special camps are available for children with cancer. These camps offer an opportunity for children and adolescents to experience a variety of activities safely and to network with other children who are experiencing similar physical and emotional challenges. The Children's Oncology Camping Association and the American Childhood Cancer Foundation provide lists of camps throughout the United States and Canada and internationally for children and adolescents with cancer.

Promoting Growth

Promote growth in children with cancer by encouraging an appropriate diet and preventing nausea and vomiting and also by addressing concerns such as diarrhea and constipation. Chronic diarrhea related to radiation therapy may prevent the child from gaining weight and growing properly (see the "Clinical Judgment and the Nursing Process" section). The use of vinca alkaloids and opioids, as well as the decreased activity level of the child with cancer, may contribute to constipation. Constipation increases the pain experience, contributes to the child's malaise, and decreases quality of life. It directly affects the child's ability to grow by increasing anorexia, nausea, and vomiting (Kline, 2014). Detail for interventions related to preventing and managing constipation is provided in the "Clinical Judgment and the Nursing Process" section earlier in the chapter.

Preventing and Treating Oncologic Emergencies

Oncologic emergencies may occur as an effect of the disease process itself or from cancer treatment. As progress is made in chemotherapy and radiation treatment, children with cancer have an increased survival rate, but they still face the risk of developing an oncologic emergency. Nurses caring for children with cancer need to be familiar with signs and symptoms of oncologic emergencies as well as with their treatment. All of these problems warrant careful, frequent monitoring of respiratory, cardiovascular, neurologic, and kidney status. Table 46.3 provides information about oncologic emergencies.

TABLE 46.3 • Oncologic Emergencies

Emergency	Associated With	Signs and Symptoms	Laboratory or Diagnostic Test Findings	Management
Sepsis	Neutropenia resulting from bone marrow suppression due to chemotherapy	• Fever or low temperature • Respiratory distress • Poor perfusion • Altered level of consciousness	• ANC <500 • Positive blood culture • Increased BUN, creatinine, potassium, clotting times • Decreased platelet count • Metabolic acidosis	• Airway and ventilation maintenance • Fluid volume resuscitation • Inotropic support • Broad-spectrum antibiotics and antifungals • Dialysis if needed
Tumor lysis syndrome	ALL, lymphoma, neuroblastoma	• Nausea, vomiting, diarrhea, anorexia • Lethargy • Increased heart rate and blood pressure • Decreased or absent urine output • Altered level of consciousness	• Hyperuricemia • Hyperkalemia • Hyperphosphatemia • Hypocalcemia • Hypoxia	• Prevent by giving allopurinol for several days prior to chemotherapy (also treat with allopurinol) • Double IV fluid maintenance • Sodium bicarbonate
Typhlitis (neutropenic enterocolitis)	Inflammatory process of GI tract occurring with induction phase of leukemia chemotherapy	• Acute abdominal pain • Nausea, vomiting • Bloody diarrhea and emesis • Fever • Anorexia	• KUB: scarcity of bowel gas, possibly ileus • CT (abdominal): inflammation, bowel wall thickening, peritoneal fluid	• Bowel rest (NPO status) • IV nutrition • Assess for bowel perforation/shock • Broad-spectrum antibiotics and antifungals • Comfort measures
Superior vena cava (SVC) syndrome	Compression on the SVC by NHL or other mediastinal mass, such as neuroblastoma	• Dyspnea and cyanosis • Large cervical lymph nodes • Wheezing, diminished breath sounds	• Chest radiograph or CT shows mediastinal mass • Pleural effusion	• Intubation and ventilation • Comfort measures • Treat cause (usually, surgical removal of mass)
Spinal cord compression	Tumor or metastasis compresses spinal cord	• Back, neck, or leg pain • Sensory or autonomic dysfunction • Extremity weakness or paralysis	• MRI reveals location of tumor or metastasis to epidural space	• Dexamethasone • Careful assessment • Radiation therapy • Comfort measures
Increased intracranial pressure	Brain tumor or metastasis to brain causing compression of brain; may result in herniation	• Headache, visual disturbances • Morning vomiting • Infants: increased head circumference • Altered level of consciousness • Cushing triad • Seizure activity	• Head CT or MRI reveals extent of mass	• Frequent, careful neurologic assessment • Limit fluids • Dexamethasone • Anticonvulsants • Tumor resection, radiation, or chemotherapy • Comfort measures
Massive hepatomegaly	Obstruction caused by neuroblastoma filling a large portion of the abdominal cavity	• Distended, enlarged abdomen • Respiratory distress, hypoxia • Poor perfusion • Tachycardia, hypotension	• Abdominal CT reveals extent of tumor • Coagulopathy	• Tumor resection or debulking • Mechanical ventilation, inotropic support • Nasogastric decompression • Position to minimize abdominal pressure • Blood transfusions • Comfort measures

ANC, absolute neutrophil count; BUN, blood urea nitrogen; CT, computed tomography; GI, gastrointestinal; KUB, kidney, ureters, and bladder scan; MRI, magnetic resonance imaging; NPO, nothing by mouth.

Data from Keating, A. K., Knight-Perry, J., Maloney, K., Levy, J. M. M., Greffe, B. S., Franklin, A. R. K., & Garrington, T. P. (2022). Chapter 31: Neoplastic disease. In M. Bunik, W. W. Hay, M. J. Levin, & M. J. Abzug (Eds.), *Current diagnosis & treatment: Pediatrics* (26th ed, pp. 931–963). McGraw-Hill Education; Hibberd, C., Hibberd, O., Karageorgos, S., & Barnard, G. (2023). Ten oncology emergencies in kids. *Don't Forget the Bubbles*. https://doi.org/10.31440/DFTB.53725

Caring for the Dying Child

Cancer accounts for the most deaths per year from disease for children (CureSearch, 2022). A "do not resuscitate" (DNR) order for the child with progressive cancer is obtained in many situations. This order helps to optimize care in the terminal phase of cancer. Nurses serve as child and family advocates, clarifying terminology and providing support as needed during the discussion of DNR orders and throughout the rest of the terminal phase.

Children with terminal cancer often experience a great deal of pain, particularly when death is imminent. Pain is often accompanied by agitation and dyspnea, which further contribute to the child's discomfort. Whether the child has a DNR order or their status remains that of "full code," pain management is central to the nursing care of the child who is dying from cancer. A primary goal for the child dying of cancer is prevention and alleviation of pain. The health care team partners with the child and parents to manage the child's pain (NHPCO, 2022). Refer to Chapter 36 for further information related to pain assessment and management.

Further discussion related to care of the dying child is found in Chapter 34.

ANEMIA

Anemia is a condition in which the level of RBCs is lower than the age-appropriate normal value. Anemia may develop as a result of decreased production of RBCs or loss and destruction of RBCs. The loss of production can be related to lack of dietary intake of the nutrients needed to produce the cells, alterations in the cell structure, or malfunctioning tissues (e.g., bone marrow). Anemia related to nutritional deficiency includes iron deficiency, folic acid deficiency, and pernicious anemia. Anemia may also result from toxin exposure (lead poisoning) or as an adverse reaction to a medication (aplastic anemia). Blood loss may result from surgery or trauma. Alteration or destruction of cells occurs in certain genetic and cellular development disorders (Nuss et al., 2022).

Anemia caused by the alteration or destruction of the RBCs is termed hemolytic anemia. There are several types of hemolytic anemia, such as sickle cell disease (SCD) and thalassemia; these two disorders are discussed in the section on hemoglobinopathies.

Anemia related to insufficient intake of specific nutrients is the most common type of anemia in children. Nutrient intake may be reduced in children due to food dislikes or conditions that produce malabsorption.

Iron-Deficiency Anemia

Iron-deficiency anemia occurs when the body does not have enough iron to produce Hgb. In the United States, iron-deficiency anemia has a peak prevalence in children between the ages of 12 and 24 months and again during adolescence (Powers, 2023). Cow's milk consumption contributes to iron-deficiency anemia in older infants and young children due to its poor iron availability (Powers, 2023).

The heme portion of Hgb consists of iron surrounded by protoporphyrin. When not enough iron is available to the bone marrow, Hgb production is reduced. Adequate dietary intake of iron is required for the body to make enough Hgb. As Hgb levels decrease, the oxygen-carrying capacity of the blood is decreased, resulting in weakness and fatigue. In addition to delayed growth, iron-deficiency anemia has been associated with cognitive delays and behavioral changes.

> ***TAKE NOTE!***
>
> For appropriate growth to occur in adolescence, increased amounts of iron must be consumed and absorbed.

Therapeutic Management

Iron supplements are usually provided in the form of ferrous sulfate or ferrous fumarate and are available over the counter. The recommended dose is 3 mg/kg of elemental iron daily (Nuss et al., 2022). In more severe cases, blood transfusions may be indicated. Transfusion of PRBCs is reserved for uncompensated anemia. When PRBC administration is warranted, follow specific blood bank guidelines for administration. Monitor subsequent laboratory results for improvement.

Nursing Assessment

For a full description of the assessment phase of the nursing process, refer to the "Clinical Judgment and the Nursing Process" section. Assessment findings pertinent to iron-deficiency anemia are discussed further on.

HEALTH HISTORY

Elicit a description of the current illness and chief complaint. Common signs and symptoms reported during the health history may include irritability, headache, dizziness, weakness, shortness of breath, pallor, and fatigue. Other symptoms may be subtle and difficult for the clinician to identify; these include difficulty feeding, pica, muscle weakness, or unsteady gait.

Explore the health history for risk factors such as:

- Maternal anemia during pregnancy
- Poorly controlled diabetes during pregnancy
- Prematurity, low birth weight, or multiple birth
- Cow's milk consumption before 12 months of age
- Excessive cow's milk consumption (greater than 24 oz a day)
- Infant consumption of low-iron formula

- Lack of iron supplementation after age 6 months in breastfed infants
- Excessive weight gain
- Chronic infection or inflammation
- Chronic or acute blood loss
- Restricted diets
- Use of medication interfering with iron absorption, such as antacids
- Low socioeconomic status
- Recent immigration from a developing country (Powers, 2023)

Evaluate the child's diet for adequate intake of iron-rich foods. Recommended dietary daily intake for iron in children is:

- 0 to 6 months: 0.27 mg
- 7 to 12 months: 11 mg
- 1 to 3 years: 7 mg
- 4 to 8 years: 10 mg
- 9 to 13 years: 8 mg
- Males 14 to 18 years: 11 mg
- Females 14 to 18 years: 15 mg (Diab et al., 2022)

PHYSICAL EXAMINATION

Observe the child for fatigue and lethargy. Inspect the skin, conjunctivae, oral mucosa, palms, and soles for pallor. Note spooning of the nails (concave shape) (Fig. 46.6). Obtain a pulse oximeter reading. Evaluate the heart rate for tachycardia. Auscultate the heart for a flow murmur. Palpate the abdomen for splenomegaly.

LABORATORY AND DIAGNOSTIC TESTS

Laboratory evaluation will reveal decreased Hgb and Hct, decreased reticulocyte count, microcytosis, hypochromia, decreased serum iron and ferritin levels, and an increased free erythrocyte protoporphyrin (FEP) level.

Nursing Management

Nursing management of the child with iron deficiency focuses on promoting safety, ensuring adequate iron intake, and educating the family.

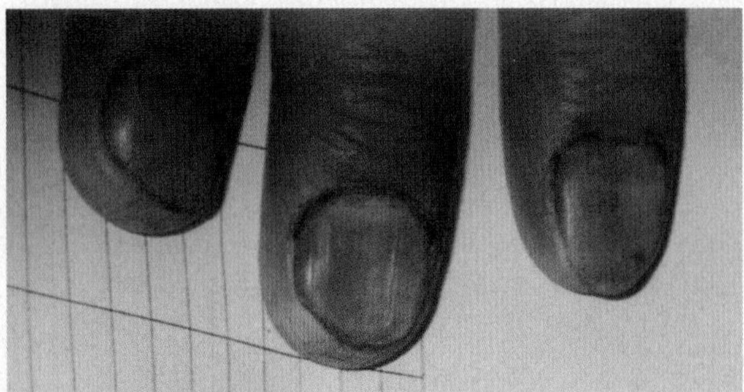

FIGURE 46.6 Note the concave shape of nails ("spooning") that occurs with iron-deficiency anemia.

PROMOTING SAFETY

The child with anemia is at risk for changes in neurologic functioning related to the decreased oxygen supply to the brain. This can lead to fatigue and inability to eat enough. Neurologic effects may be manifested when the child's ability to sit, stand, or walk is impaired. Provide close observation of the anemic child. Assist the older child with ambulation. Educate the parents on how to protect the child from injury due to an unsteady gait or dizziness.

PROVIDING DIETARY INTERVENTIONS

Ensure that iron-deficient infants are fed only formulas fortified with iron. Interventions for breast-fed infants include beginning iron supplementation around the age of 4 or 5 months. Iron supplementation may range from adding iron-fortified cereals to the child's diet to giving iron-containing drops. Encourage breastfeeding parents to increase their dietary intake of iron or take iron supplements when breastfeeding so that the iron may be passed on to the infant. For children over 1 year of age, limit cow's milk intake to 24 oz per day to decrease risk of microscopic GI bleeding and increase appetite for other foods. Limit fast-food consumption and encourage intake of iron-rich foods such as red meats (iron from red meat is the easiest for the body to absorb), tuna, salmon, eggs, tofu, enriched grains, dried beans and peas, dried fruits, leafy green vegetables, and iron-fortified breakfast cereals.

Teach the parents about dietary intake of iron. Encourage parents to provide a variety of foods for iron support and vitamins and other minerals necessary for growth. A big problem for toddlers is their picky eating. This often becomes a means of control for the child, and parents should guard against getting involved in a power struggle with their child. Referring parents to a developmental specialist who can assist them in their approach to diet may prove beneficial. Refer families who meet the financial limits and who have children aged 5 and younger to the Women, Infants, and Children (WIC) program, which provides for supplementation of infants' and children's diets. See the Healthy People 2030 box.

HEALTHY PEOPLE 2030

Objective	Nursing Significance
Reduce iron deficiency among children aged 1–2 years and females aged 12–49 years.	• Encourage use of iron-fortified formulas and infant cereal. • Encourage iron supplementation in the second half of infancy for the breastfed infant. • Educate parents about iron-containing foods. • Encourage adolescent females to consume a diet high in iron-rich foods.

Healthy People Objectives retrieved from http://www.healthypeople.gov

TEACHING ABOUT IRON SUPPLEMENT ADMINISTRATION

The use of iron supplements in infants begins with the use of formula fortified with iron in the formula-fed infant. Oral supplements may also be necessary if the baby's iron levels are extremely low. Oral supplements or multivitamin formulas that contain iron are often dark in color because the iron is pigmented. Teach parents to precisely measure the amount of iron to be administered. Parents should place the liquid behind the teeth, as iron in liquid form can stain the teeth. Iron supplementation can also cause constipation. In some cases, reducing the amount of iron can resolve this problem, but stool softeners may be necessary to control painful or difficult-to-pass stools. Encourage parents to increase their child's fluid intake and include adequate dietary fiber to avoid constipation.

TAKE NOTE!

Teach parents to keep iron-containing supplements out of the reach of young children in order to prevent accidental ingestion leading to overdose or poisoning.

Other Nutritional Causes of Anemia

Other forms of anemia related to nutritional deficit include folic acid deficiency and pernicious anemia. Comparison Chart 46.2 discusses the causes, assessment, and management of these disorders.

Lead Poisoning

Despite concerted efforts in the past few decades to screen for lead poisoning in young children, there are over 500,000 U.S. children between 1 and 5 years of age with elevated lead levels (Halmo & Nappe, 2023). Lead exerts toxic effects on the bone marrow, erythroid cells, nervous system, and kidneys. The presence of lead in the bloodstream interferes with the enzymatic processes of the biosynthesis of heme. The process results in hypochromic, microcytic anemia, and children may exhibit classic signs of anemia. Risk factors for lead poisoning are related to lead exposure in the home, school, or local environment. Sources of lead include:

- Paint in homes built before 1978, at which time lead was banned as an additive to paint used in houses
- Soil where cars that used leaded gas have been in the past (lead was removed from all gasoline in the United States as of 1996)
- Glazed pottery
- Stained glass products
- Lead pipes supplying water to the home
- On the clothing of parents who work in certain manufacturing jobs (battery makers, cable makers)
- Certain folk remedies, such as *greta* or *azarcon*
- Old painted toys or furniture (Centers for Disease Control and Prevention [CDC], 2024)

Complications of lead poisoning include behavioral problems and learning difficulties and, with higher lead levels, encephalopathy, seizures, and brain damage. Therapeutic management for high blood levels of lead involves **chelation therapy** (removal of heavy metals from the body via chelating agents), either orally or intravenously. Drug Guide 46.1 gives further information on chelating agents.

Nursing Assessment

Explore the health history for subtle signs such as anorexia, fatigue, or abdominal pain. Determine whether

COMPARISON CHART 46.2 Folic Acid Deficiency Versus Pernicious Anemia

	Folic Acid Deficiency	Pernicious Anemia
Cause	Low dietary intake of green leafy vegetables, liver, and citrus Malabsorption from medication such as phenytoin (Dilantin) or parasitic infection	Deficiency in vitamin B_{12}
Assessment	Determine risk factors such as prematurity, low socioeconomic status, and history of malabsorption disease. Determine dietary history, noting dislike of fresh vegetables or fruit, ingestion of overcooked foods, or lack of family purchase of fruits and vegetables. Note history of fatigue, headache, poor growth, anorexia, or diarrhea. Inspect the skin for pallor or jaundice, and note presence of a sore on the mouth or tongue.	Note history of anorexia, irritability, or chronic diarrhea. Observe the skin or conjunctivae for pallor and the tongue for smooth texture and bright-red color.
Laboratory analysis	RBC, Hgb, Hct	RBC, Hgb, Hct, low vitamin B_{12} level
Management	Encourage parents to include green leafy vegetables, liver, and citrus in diet. Ensure parents adhere with dietary changes.	Administer monthly injections of vitamin B_{12}. Inform parents that injections will be required throughout the child's life. Provide emotional support related to the chronic nature of this disorder.

Hct, hematocrit; Hgb, hemoglobin; RBC, red blood cell.

behavioral problems, irritability, hyperactivity, or lack of ability to meet developmental milestones have occurred in recent months. Screen children for risk of exposure to lead in the home. Refer to Chapter 31 for a simple screening questionnaire that can be used to determine the need for lead screening in young children. Blood levels of lead greater than 10 mcg/dL require conscientious follow-up. Note pallor of the skin.

Nursing Management

Prevention of elevated lead levels is critical. Screen children for lead exposure risk. The AAP recommends performing a risk assessment at 6, 9, 12, 18, and 24 months, and 3, 4, 5, and 6 years. If positive, the decision may be made to evaluate a blood lead level (Hagan et al., 2017). Table 46.4 gives recommendations for appropriate follow-up depending on lead levels.

Removing old paint is the best way to eliminate the most significant source of lead exposure for a large number of children. If the family rents or lives in public housing, the landlord or owner is responsible for following the guidelines set forth by local and state governmental agencies to correct the problem. Educate families about how to prevent exposure to lead, particularly in young children.

If the child is undergoing chelation therapy, ensure adequate fluid intake and monitor intake and output closely. Refer children with elevated lead levels and developmental or cognitive deficits to developmental centers. These children may need an early intervention program for further evaluation and treatment of developmental delays. See the Healthy People 2030 box.

TABLE 46.4 • Interventions Based on Blood Lead Level

Blood Lead Level (mcg/dL)	Recommended Action
<3.5	May require retesting if determined to be high risk
3.5–14	Repeat test in 1–3 months. Educate parents to decrease lead exposure. Repeat test again in 1–3 months.
15–44	Confirm with repeat test in 1–4 weeks. Educate parents to decrease lead exposure. Report to local health authorities for surveillance.
>44	Retest asymptomatic children with levels 45–69 within 48 hours. Begin chelation therapy and refer to health department as before. Hospitalize child if level ≥70 and begin chelation therapy. Ensure lead is removed from the home.

Data from Sample, J. A. (2024). *Childhood lead poisoning: Management.* Retrieved on February 17, 2024, from http://www.uptodate.com/contents/childhood-lead-poisoning-management

HEALTHY PEOPLE 2030

Objective	Nursing Significance
Reduce blood lead levels in children aged 1–5 years.	Appropriately screen infants and young children for lead exposure at each health care visit.

Healthy People Objectives retrieved from http://www.healthypeople.gov

Aplastic Anemia

Aplastic anemia (failure of the bone marrow to produce cells) is characterized by bone marrow aplasia and pancytopenia (decreased numbers of all blood cells). Most cases are acquired, but there are a few rare types of inherited aplastic anemias (Nuss et al., 2022). The inherited types present as congenital bone marrow failure; the best known is Fanconi anemia, an autosomal recessive disorder. Acquired aplastic anemia is thought to be an immune-mediated response. Most cases are idiopathic, meaning the trigger remains unidentified. Other causes include exposure to environmental toxins, viruses, myelosuppressive drugs, or radiation.

Complications of aplastic anemia include severe overwhelming infection, hemorrhage, and death. Therapeutic management of aplastic anemia in children involves HSCT from an HLA-matched sibling donor; if one is not available, immunosuppressive therapy or high-dose cyclophosphamide can be given.

Nursing Assessment

Determine history of exposure to myelosuppressive medications or radiation therapy. Obtain a detailed family, environmental, and infectious disease history. Note history of epistaxis, gingival oozing, or increased bleeding with menstruation. Anemia may lead to headache and fatigue. On physical examination, note ecchymoses, petechiae or purpura, oral ulcerations, tachycardia, or tachypnea. In addition to suppression of all blood cells, laboratory and diagnostic testing may reveal:

- Guaiac-positive stool
- Blood in the urine
- Severe decrease in or the absence of hematopoietic cells on bone marrow aspiration

Nursing Management

Safety is of the utmost concern in children with aplastic anemia. It is important to prevent injury in order to avoid hemorrhage. Stool softeners may be used to prevent anal fissures associated with constipation. Administer only irradiated and leukocyte-depleted PRBCs or platelet transfusions as necessary. This limits exposure to HLA should the child require bone marrow transplantation in the future. If the child requires HSCT, refer to the section earlier in this chapter for additional nursing management information.

Refer families whose child has only mild or moderate disease to the Aplastic Anemia and Myelodysplastic Syndrome International Foundation.

HEMOGLOBINOPATHIES

Hemoglobinopathy is a condition in which abnormal hemoglobin is present. A large percentage of the newborn's hemoglobin is fetal hemoglobin (Hgb F). Hgb F can exchange oxygen molecules at lower oxygen tensions compared to adult hemoglobin. Over the first several months of life, Hgb F levels fall as it is replaced with Hgb A (adult hemoglobin). The healthy older infant then displays Hgb AA. In hemoglobinopathies, this Hgb configuration is disturbed. Causes of hemoglobinopathies are genetic and include SCD, hemoglobin SC disease, alpha-thalassemia, and beta-thalassemia. This discussion will focus on SCD and beta-thalassemia (Cooley anemia).

Sickle Cell Disease

SCD is a group of inherited hemoglobinopathies in which the RBCs do not carry the normal adult hemoglobin but instead carry a less effective type. In the United States, the most common types of SCD are hemoglobin SS disease (termed sickle cell anemia [SCA]), hemoglobin SC disease, and hemoglobin sickle–beta-thalassemia. SCD is most common in individuals of African, Mediterranean, Middle Eastern, and Indian descent (CDC, 2023a).

The focus of this discussion will be on hemoglobin SS disease. Instead of Hgb AA, individuals with SCA have Hgb SS (Hgb A refers to adult hemoglobin, Hgb S refers to sickle hemoglobin). In hemoglobin S, glutamic acid is replaced with valine in the hemoglobin molecule. This results in an elongated RBC with a shortened lifespan. The elongated cell is more rigid than a normal cell and becomes sickled in shape (Fig. 46.7). One in 325 Black newborns has SCD (CDC, 2023a).

People with heterozygous representation (Hgb AS) are said to have sickle cell trait and are carriers for the disorder; about 1 in 13 Black newborns have sickle cell trait (CDC, 2023a). Generally, individuals with sickle cell trait have only minimal health problems.

SCA is transmitted via an autosomal recessive inheritance pattern. The recessive genes for sickle cell are passed on from both parents who have the gene for Hgb AS (sickle cell trait). Refer to Chapter 49 for further information on autosomal recessive gene transmission.

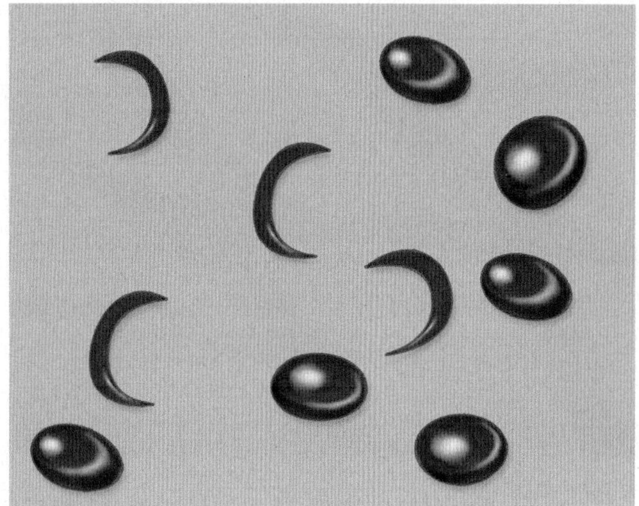

FIGURE 46.7 This peripheral blood smear demonstrates the elongated sickle-shaped red blood cell seen in sickle cell disease.

Figure 46.8 illustrates the inheritance probability with each reproductive event. Infants with SCA are usually asymptomatic until 3 to 4 months of age because Hgb F protects against sickling.

Complications of SCA include recurrent vaso-occlusive pain crises, stroke, sepsis, acute chest syndrome, splenic sequestration, reduced visual acuity related to decreased retinal blood flow, chronic leg ulcers, cholestasis and gallstones, delayed growth and development, delayed puberty, and priapism (the sickled cells prevent blood from flowing out of an erect penis). Children with SCA have an increased incidence of enuresis because the kidneys cannot concentrate urine effectively (Lerma & Vichinsky, 2023). As children reach adulthood, multiple organ dysfunction is common.

Pathophysiology

Significant anemia may occur when the RBCs sickle. Sickling may be triggered by any stress or traumatic

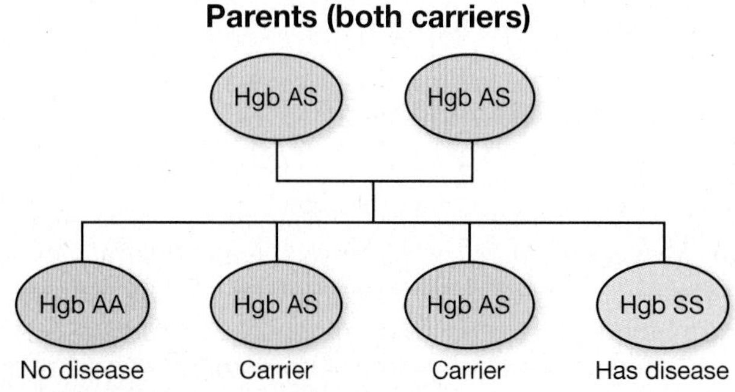

FIGURE 46.8 Simplified genetic scheme for sickle cell disease. *A* denotes adult hemoglobin; *S* denotes sickle hemoglobin. Hemoglobin AA, normal hemoglobin; hemoglobin AS, sickle cell trait; hemoglobin SS, sickle cell disease.

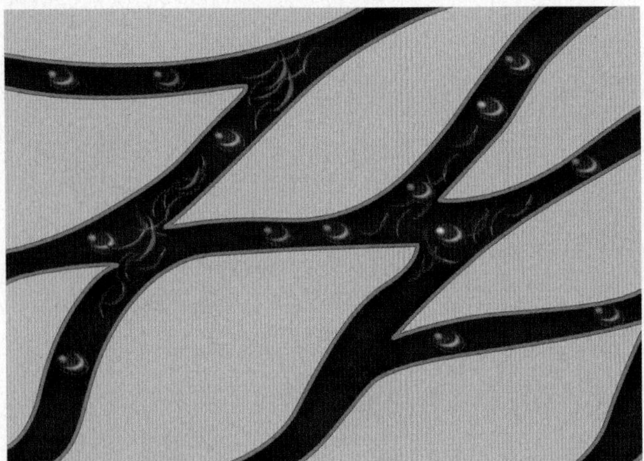

FIGURE 46.9 Clumping of sickle-shaped cells.

event, such as infection, fever, dehydration, physical exertion, excessive cold exposure, or hypoxia (Borhade & Kondamudi, 2022).

As the cells sickle, the blood becomes more viscous because the sickled cells clump together and prevent normal blood flow to the tissues of that area. The sickle-shaped RBCs cannot pass through the smaller capillaries and venules of the circulatory system (Fig. 46.9). This vaso-occlusive process leads to local tissue hypoxia, followed by ischemia and may result in infarction. Pain results as circulation is decreased to the area. Pain can occur in any part of the body but is most common in the joints. Pain causes increased metabolic need by resulting in tachycardia and sometimes tachypnea, which leads to further sickling.

Clumping of cells in the lungs (acute chest syndrome) results in decreased gas exchange, producing hypoxia, which leads to further sickling. Acute chest syndrome and multiorgan failure are the leading common causes of death in children with SCD (Vichinsky, 2023). Sequestration of blood in the spleen leads to splenomegaly and abdominal pain. Hemolysis follows sickling and leads to further anemia. The increased activity of the spleen related to RBC hemolysis leads to splenomegaly, then fibrosis and atrophy. Functional asplenia develops in early childhood (Vichinsky, 2023).

Therapeutic Management

The therapeutic management of children with SCA focuses on preventing vaso-occlusive episodes and infection as well as other complications. Functional asplenia (decrease in the ability of the spleen to function appropriately) places the child at significant risk for serious infection with *Streptococcus pneumoniae* or other encapsulated organisms. Prophylactic antibiotics in the young child and appropriate immunization in all children with SCA can reduce the risk of serious infection (Field & Vichinsky, 2023).

DOSAGE CALCULATION BOX 46.1

Child's weight: 50 lb

Medication order: hydroxyurea 450 mg oral daily

Per the Pediatric Dosage Handbook, the recommended dose is 20 mg/kg/dose, once daily.

Is the ordered dose safe?

Treatment of vaso-occlusive episodes focuses on pain control. Oxygen administration is necessary during episodes of crisis to prevent additional cell sickling. Adequate hydration with intravenous fluids is critical. Close monitoring of Hgb, Hct, and reticulocytes determines the point at which transfusion of PRBCs becomes necessary. Electrolyte analysis is also necessary to ensure that appropriate amounts of electrolytes are present in the serum. When RBCs are administered, there is the potential for hemolysis of the cells, thus increasing the potassium level in the serum. Antibiotic therapy is necessary when infection is present. Box 46.3 describes additional medical treatments that are needed in some children.

Nursing Assessment

Children with SCA experience a significant number of acute and chronic manifestations of the condition (Comparison Chart 46.3). For a full description of the assessment phase of the nursing process, refer to "Clinical Judgment and the Nursing Process" section. Assessment findings pertinent to SCA are discussed in here.

HEALTH HISTORY

Elicit the health history, noting growth and development, frequency and extent of vaso-occlusive crises, past hospitalizations, and treatment for pain crises. Note history of immunizations, including pneumococcal, flu, and meningococcal vaccinations. Determine history

BOX 46.3 Additional Medical Treatments for Some Children With Sickle Cell Anemia

- Cholecystectomy may become necessary if gallstones develop.
- Splenectomy may be performed to prevent recurrence of splenic sequestration if it is life threatening.
- Hydroxyurea increases the percentage of fetal hemoglobin (helping to decrease vaso-occlusive events).
- L-Glutamine in addition to hydroxyurea, or alone, decreases incidence of painful vaso-occlusive episodes.
- Blood transfusions, although not routinely given to children with sickle cell disease, are indicated in children with prolonged or widespread pain, aplastic crisis, or splenic sequestration.
- Partial exchange transfusion may be used to rapidly lower the circulating amount of Hgb SS in the event of stroke or acute chest syndrome.
- HSCT is usually reserved for children with an identical HLA-matched sibling (risk of death and incidence of graft-versus-host disease is high).

Hgb, hemoglobin; HLA, human leukocyte antigen; HSCT, hematopoietic stem cell transplantation.

COMPARISON CHART 46.3 Acute Versus Chronic Manifestations of Sickle Cell Anemia

Acute	Chronic
[a]Acute chest syndrome	Anemia
[a]Aplastic crisis	Avascular necrosis of the hip
[a]Bacterial sepsis or meningitis	Cardiomegaly, functional murmur
Bone infarction	Cholelithiasis
Dactylitis	Delayed growth and development
Hematuria	Delayed puberty
Recurrent pain episodes	Functional asplenia
Pain crisis	Hyposthenuria (low urine specific gravity) and enuresis
[a]Splenic sequestration	Jaundice
[a]Stroke	Leg ulcers
Priapism	Proteinuria [a]Pulmonary hypertension [a]Restrictive lung disease Retinopathy

[a]Often life threatening.

of blood transfusions. Document the current medication regimen. Note history of recurrent infections. Determine history of the present illness that results in a precipitating event, such as hypoxia, infection, or dehydration. Note onset, character, and quality of pain, as well as relieving factors.

PHYSICAL EXAMINATION

Perform a thorough physical examination, because sickling, hypoxia, and tissue ischemia affect most areas of the body (Fig. 46.10). In what follows, note the physical findings discussed that may be detected using inspection, observation, auscultation, and palpation.

Inspection and Observation

Inspect the conjunctivae, palms, and soles for pallor and the skin for pallor, lesions, or ulcers. Note jaundice of the skin or scleral icterus. Document color and moisture of oral mucosa. Measure temperature to evaluate for infection (which can precipitate a sickling crisis). Note blood pressure, which may be decreased with severe anemia or increased with sickle cell nephropathy. Determine baseline mental status. Perform a neurologic assessment frequently, as about 11% of children with SCA will experience an overt stroke (Nuss et al., 2022).

Auscultation

Auscultate heart sounds for a murmur. The heart rate is often elevated with pain, hyperthermia, or dehydration. Listen to breath sounds, noting the rate and depth of respiration as well as the adequacy of aeration. Adventitious breath sounds may be present if a respiratory infection has triggered the sickle cell crisis or in the case of acute chest syndrome. About half of the cases of acute chest syndrome occur in the child already hospitalized for a pain crisis.

Palpation

Palpate the joints for warmth, tenderness, and ROM. Palpate the abdomen for areas of tenderness. Note hepatomegaly or splenomegaly.

CLINICAL REASONING ALERT!

Immediately report symmetric swelling of the hands and feet in the infant or toddler. Termed dactylitis, aseptic infarction occurs in the metacarpals and metatarsals (Fig. 46.11).

LABORATORY AND DIAGNOSTIC TESTING

Newborn screening for SCA is required by law or rule across the United States (CDC, 2023b). Screening by Sickledex or sickle cell prep does not distinguish between SCD and sickle cell trait. If the screening test result indicates the possibility of SCD or sickle cell trait, Hgb electrophoresis is performed promptly to confirm the diagnosis. As the only accurate test for SCD, Hgb electrophoresis will demonstrate the presence of Hgb S and Hgb F only in the young infant; in the older infant or child, the result will be Hgb SS.

Common laboratory and diagnostic studies ordered for the assessment of SCA include:

- Hemoglobin: baseline is usually 7 to 10 mg/dL; will be significantly lower with splenic sequestration, acute chest syndrome, or aplastic crisis
- Reticulocyte count: greatly elevated
- Peripheral blood smear: presence of sickle-shaped cells and target cells
- Platelet count: increased
- Erythrocyte sedimentation rate: elevated
- Abnormal liver function tests with elevated bilirubin

X-ray studies or other scans may be performed to determine the extent of organ or tissue damage resulting from vaso-occlusion.

Nursing Management

Nursing care of the child with SCA focuses on preventing vaso-occlusive crises, providing education to the family and child, managing pain episodes, and providing psychosocial support to the child and family. All children

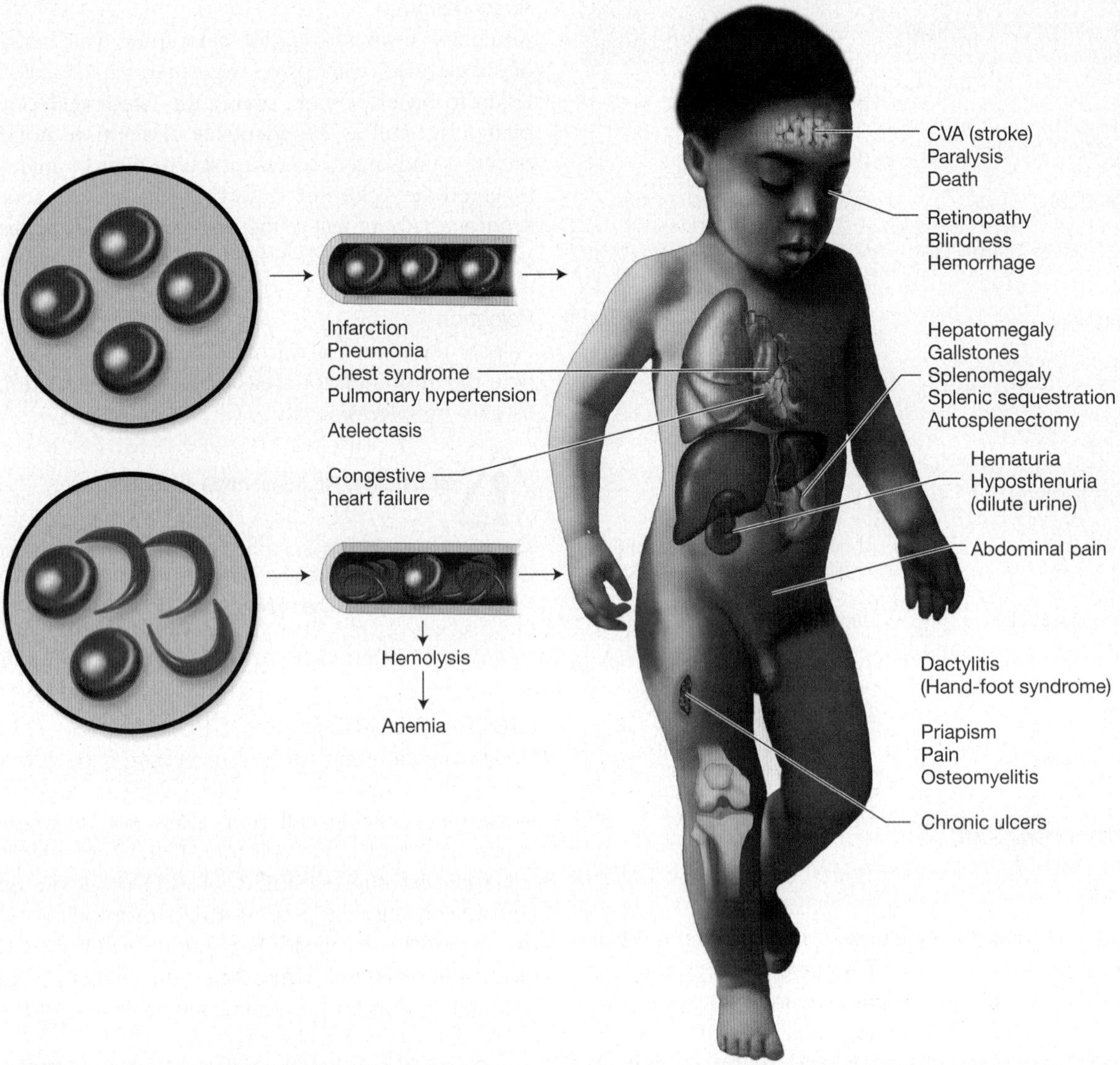

FIGURE 46.10 Effects of sickle cell anemia on various parts of the body. CVA, cerebrovascular accident

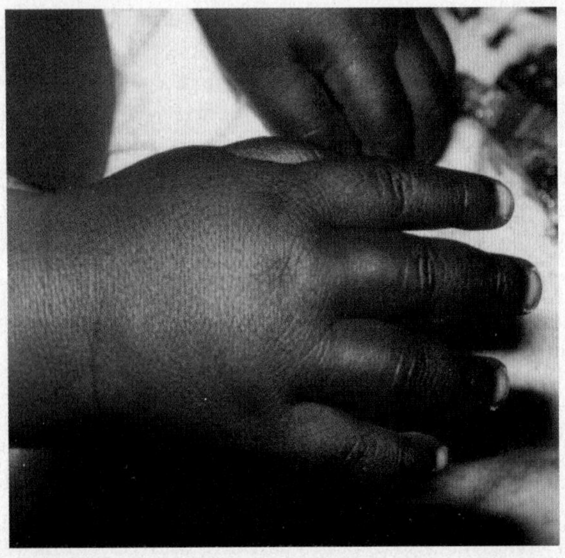

FIGURE 46.11 Swelling of the hands (dactylitis) in a toddler.

with SCA need ongoing evaluation of growth and development to maximize their potential in those areas. Monitor school performance to detect neurodevelopmental problems and seek intervention early. The patient problems and interventions provided in the "Clinical Judgment and the Nursing Process" section should be individualized based on the child's and family's response to the disorder. Specifics related to SCA are discussed further on.

EDUCATING THE FAMILY AND CHILD

Begin child and family education immediately after the diagnosis of SCA is confirmed. Initially, teach the family about the genetics of the disease, and encourage family members to be tested for carrier status. Educate families about the disease process. Emphasize the importance of regularly scheduled health maintenance visits and immunizations. Teach families how to administer prophylactic penicillin for infection prevention and hydroxyurea and/or L-glutamine for prevention of acute pain episodes. Encourage families to seek medical evaluation urgently for any febrile illness. Educate families about how to prevent and recognize vaso-occlusive events (Teaching Guidelines 46.3). Discuss complications such as delayed growth and development, delayed puberty, stroke, cholelithiasis, retinopathy, avascular necrosis, priapism, and leg ulcers.

ATRAUMATIC CARE

Teach the child with SCA age-appropriate distraction and coping skills to assist the child to relieve stress related to their disease and/or recurrent crises.

MANAGING PAIN DURING A VASO-OCCLUSIVE EPISODE

Adequate pain management helps to decrease the child's stress level; elevated stress may contribute to further sickling and additional pain. Initiate pain assessment with a standardized pain scale upon admission. Provide frequent evaluations of pain. Always believe the child's report of pain; only the person suffering the pain knows what it feels like. Moderate to severe pain usually requires opioid medication. To bring the pain under control, initially administer analgesics routinely rather than on an "as needed" (PRN) basis. Once the pain is better managed, medications may be moved to PRN status. Monitor patient-controlled analgesia (PCA) in the child or adolescent. In light of the opioid epidemic concerns, it is important to note that the rate of opioid misuse is lower in individuals with SCD than others with chronic pain syndromes (DeBaun, 2022). Ensure the child is adequately hydrated with hypotonic fluid.

Nonsteroidal antiinflammatory medications and acetaminophen are often used for less severe pain. Use distraction with nonpharmacologic pain management techniques such as relaxation or hypnosis, music, massage, play, guided imagery, therapeutic touch, or behavior modification to augment the pain medication regimen.

TEACHING GUIDELINES 46.3 Prevention or Early Recognition of Vaso-occlusive Events

- Seek immediate attention for ANY febrile illness.
- Obtain vaccinations and penicillin prophylaxis.
- Encourage adequate fluid intake daily.
- Avoid temperatures that are too hot or too cold.
- Avoid overexertion or stress.
- Have 24-hour access to health care provider, nurse practitioner, or facility familiar with sickle cell care.
- Contact medical provider promptly if you suspect a pain crisis is developing.
- Seek medical attention immediately if any of the following develop:
  - Child is pale and listless.
  - Abdominal pain
  - Limp or swollen joints
  - Cough, shortness of breath, chest pain
  - Increasing fatigue
  - Unusual headache, loss of feeling, or sudden weakness
  - Sudden vision change
  - Painful erection that won't go down (priapism)

TAKE NOTE!

Do not use meperidine for pain management during sickle cell crises because multiple dosing has been associated with an increased risk of seizures (DeBaun, 2022).

MANAGING VASO-OCCLUSIVE EPISODES

Treat any underlying conditions such as infection or injury. Deficient fluid volume occurs as a result of decreased intake, increased fluid requirements during vaso-occlusive episode, and the kidney's inability to concentrate urine. Increasing fluid intake will dilute the blood and decrease its viscosity. To promote hemodilution, provide 150 mL/kg of fluids per day or as much as double maintenance, either orally or intravenously. Maintain appropriate electrolyte and pH balance.

Risk of ineffective tissue perfusion related to the effects of RBC sickling and infarction of tissues is another concern. Frequently evaluate respiratory and circulatory status. Encourage incentive spirometry to decrease the incidence of acute chest syndrome. Administer supplemental oxygen if the pulse oximetry reading is 92%; oxygen supplementation in the absence of hypoxia is unnecessary and may inhibit erythropoiesis. Monitor level of consciousness and immediately report changes. See the Healthy People 2030 box.

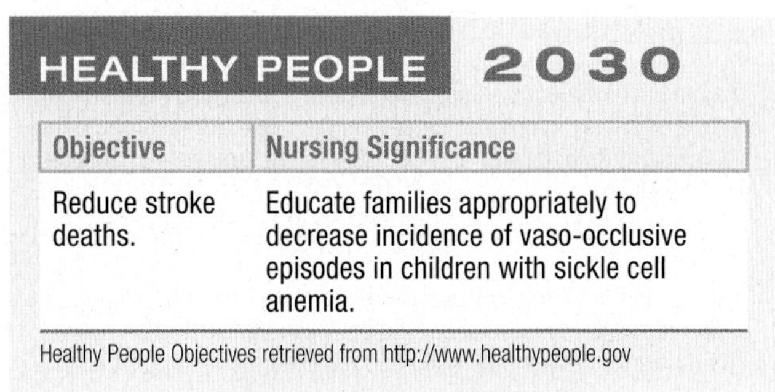

HEALTHY PEOPLE 2030

Objective	Nursing Significance
Reduce stroke deaths.	Educate families appropriately to decrease incidence of vaso-occlusive episodes in children with sickle cell anemia.

Healthy People Objectives retrieved from http://www.healthypeople.gov

PREVENTING INFECTION

To prevent severe infection in the child with SCA, a variety of interventions are necessary. By 2 months of age, begin administration of oral penicillin V potassium as prophylaxis against pneumococcal infection. In the penicillin-allergic child, erythromycin may be used. Continue prophylaxis until at least age 5 years. Administer childhood immunizations according to the currently recommended schedule. To prevent overwhelming sepsis or meningitis as a result of infection with *S. pneumoniae*, the child should receive not only the 7-valent pneumococcal vaccine series in infancy but also the 23-valent pneumococcal conjugate vaccine annually after age 2 years. Meningococcal vaccination is also warranted (refer to Chapter 31 for additional information on these vaccines). Provide influenza immunization annually before the onset of flu season (after 6 months of age) (Field & Vichinsky, 2023).

SUPPORTING THE FAMILY AND CHILD

As with any chronic illness, families of children with SCA need significant support. They often feel guilty or responsible for the disease. Reassure the family and provide education. Refer families to a regional SCD center for multidisciplinary care. See Evidence-Based Practice 46.1.

Thalassemia

Thalassemia is a genetic disorder that most often affects those of African descent, but it also affects individuals of Caribbean, Middle Eastern, South Asian, and Mediterranean descent (Benz & Angelucci, 2022). The genetics of thalassemia are similar to those of SCD in that it is inherited via an autosomal recessive process. Children with thalassemia have reduced production of Hgb.

There are two basic types of thalassemia, alpha and beta. In alpha-thalassemia, synthesis of the alpha chain of the hemoglobin protein is affected. Problems with the beta chain occur more often, and the condition beta-thalassemia can be divided into three subcategories based on severity:

- Thalassemia minor (also called beta-thalassemia trait): leads to mild microcytic anemia; often no treatment is required.
- Thalassemia intermedia: child requires blood transfusions to maintain adequate quality of life.
- Thalassemia major: to survive, the child requires ongoing medical attention, blood transfusions, and iron removal (chelation therapy).

The focus of this discussion will be on beta-thalassemia major (Cooley anemia).

In beta-thalassemia major, the beta-globulin chain in hemoglobin synthesis is reduced or entirely absent. A large number of unstable globulin chains accumulate, causing the RBCs to be rigid and hemolyzed easily. The result is severe hemolytic anemia and chronic hypoxia. In response to the increased rate of RBC destruction, erythroid activity is increased. The increased activity causes massive bone marrow expansion and thinning of the bony cortex. Growth retardation, pathologic fractures, and skeletal deformities (frontal and maxillary bossing) result.

Hemosiderosis (excessive supply of iron) is an additional complication of significant concern. It occurs as a result of rapid hemolysis of RBCs, the decrease in hemoglobin production, and the increased absorption of dietary iron in response to the severely anemic state. The excess iron is deposited in the body's tissues, causing bronze pigmentation of the skin, bony changes, and altered organ function, particularly in the cardiac system. Additional complications include splenomegaly, endocrine abnormalities, osteoporosis, liver and gallbladder

EVIDENCE-BASED PRACTICE 46.1
Comprehensive Clinic for Infants With Sickle Cell Disease

Children with sickle cell disease (SCD) require ongoing comprehensive medical care. Adherence with the medication regimen, infection prevention, and attempts to avoid triggering a vaso-occlusive event are critical to the short- and long-term health of the child. Parents of infants diagnosed with SCD require significant amounts of support and education.

STUDY

In a small convenience sample, parents of 100 children completed a telephone survey in order to determine the impact of the comprehensive clinic for infants with SCD and assess the families' experience with the clinic.

Findings

The results of the survey were mainly positive. One hundred percent of parents reported adherence with penicillin administration, while 78% knew for certain their child had received the meningococcal vaccine. Ninety-eight percent reported knowing to seek care when their child had a fever. A total of 73 of 75 parents participating in group sessions reported feeling comfortable sharing in those sessions, and 95% of parents reported satisfaction with the education received in the clinic.

Nursing Implications

Nurses are in an optimal position to educate and support families of infants with SCD. If high-quality education and support occur early in the child's life, there is potential to decrease the child's morbidity from the disease. Nurses should ensure infants diagnosed with SCD and their families are referred to a comprehensive sickle cell clinic.

Data from Martin, B. M., Thaniel, L. N., Speller-Brown, B. J., & Darbari, D. S. (2018). Comprehensive infant clinic for sickle cell disease: Outcomes and parental perspective. *Journal of Pediatric Health Care, 32*(5), 485–490.

disease, and leg ulcers. Left untreated, beta-thalassemia major is fatal usually by age 5 years, but the use of blood transfusions and chelation therapy has increased the life expectancy of these children (Benz & Angelucci, 2022).

Therapeutic Management

The therapeutic management for children with beta-thalassemia includes monitoring hemoglobin and Hct and transfusing PRBCs at regular intervals. Blood iron levels are also monitored, and iron chelation therapy is provided.

Nursing Assessment

Infants are usually diagnosed by 1 year of age and have a history of pallor, jaundice, failure to thrive, and hepatosplenomegaly (Benz & Angelucci, 2022). Determine the history of the present illness or whether the child is presenting for a routine blood transfusion. Note medications taken at home and any concerns that have arisen since the last visit. Inspect the skin, oral mucosa, conjunctivae, soles, and/or palms for pallor. Note icteric sclerae or jaundice of the skin. Measure weight and height (or length) and plot on an appropriate growth chart. Observe the child for bony deformities and frontal bossing (prominent forehead) (Fig. 46.12). Measure oxygen saturation via pulse oximetry. Evaluate neurologic status, determining level of consciousness and developmental abilities.

Laboratory testing may reveal the following:

- Hemoglobin and Hct are significantly decreased.
- Peripheral blood smear shows prominence of target cells, hypochromia, microcytosis, and extensive **anisocytosis** and **poikilocytosis** (variation in the size and shape of the RBCs, respectively).
- Bilirubin levels are elevated.
- Hgb electrophoresis shows the presence of Hgb F and Hgb A_2 only.
- Iron level is elevated.

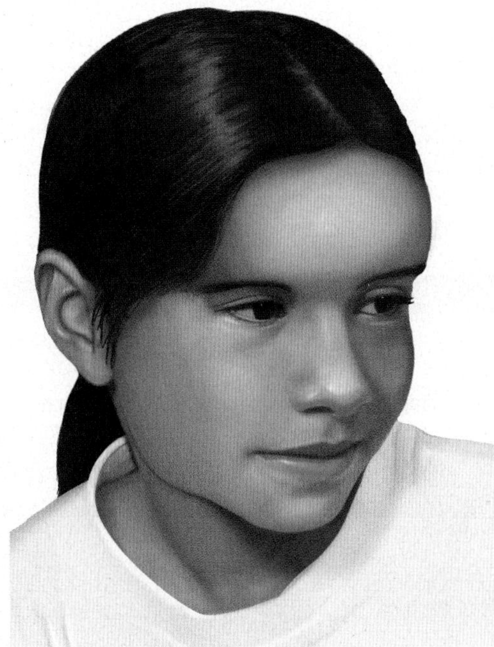

FIGURE 46.12 Iron overload related to thalassemia leads to bony changes such as frontal bossing and maxillary prominence.

Nursing Management

The nursing care of the child with thalassemia is primarily aimed at supporting the family and minimizing the effects of the illness. This includes administering blood transfusions and educating the family.

ADMINISTERING PACKED RBC TRANSFUSIONS

Administer PRBC transfusions as prescribed to maintain an adequate level of hemoglobin for oxygen delivery to the tissues and to suppress erythrocytosis in the bone marrow. Monitor for reactions to the transfusions.

Excess iron is removed by chelation therapy. Administer the chelating agent deferoxamine with the transfusion. Deferoxamine binds to the iron and allows it to be removed through the stool or urine. Oral deferasirox may also be prescribed and is generally well tolerated, with minimal GI side effects.

EDUCATING THE FAMILY

Educate the child and family about the recommended regimen. Ensure that families understand that adhering to the prescribed blood transfusion and chelation therapy schedule is essential to the child's survival. Chelation therapy must be maintained at home to continuously decrease the iron levels in the body. Teach family members to administer deferoxamine subcutaneously with a small battery-powered infusion pump over a period of several hours each night (usually while the child is sleeping). If oral deferasirox is prescribed, instruct the family to dissolve the tablet in juice or water and administer it once daily.

> ***TAKE NOTE!***
>
> Have parents provide return demonstration of subcutaneous infusion of deferoxamine to ensure accuracy and independence in the home environment.

Refer the family for genetic counseling and family support as needed. A good resource for families of children with thalassemia is the Cooley's Anemia Foundation. A group of young adults with Cooley anemia started the Thalassemia Action Group (TAG) (a subgroup of the Cooley's Anemia Foundation) to provide a forum for communication and information, promote a positive outlook on living with the disease, and raise awareness on the importance of continuing therapy for the disease.

TAG is part of the Cooley's Anemia Foundation website, and more information about the group can be found by calling (360) 860–2023.

• • • ATRAUMATIC CARE • • •

When a child is receiving blood transfusion every few weeks, they must experience at least two venipunctures each time, one for the type and cross-match and other relevant laboratory tests on the day before transfusion and another for the intravenous (IV) insertion for the actual transfusion. Minimize trauma by teaching the parent to apply EMLA (eutectic mixture of local anesthetic) cream at home just before leaving for the blood draw or transfusion appointment.

Glucose-6-Phosphate Dehydrogenase Deficiency

Glucose-6-phosphate dehydrogenase (G6PD) is an enzyme that is responsible for maintaining the integrity of RBCs by protecting them from oxidative substances. G6PD deficiency is an X-linked recessive disorder that occurs when the RBCs have insufficient G6PD or the enzyme is abnormal and does not function properly. The RBCs are then affected by oxidative stress more easily. Triggers that may result in oxidative stress and hemolysis include bacterial or viral illness or exposure to certain substances such as medications (e.g., sulfonamides, sulfones, malaria-fighting drugs [such as quinine], or methylene blue [for treating urinary tract infections]), naphthalene (an agent in mothballs), or fava beans.

G6PD deficiency occurs most commonly in children of African, Mediterranean, or Asian descent (Nuss et al., 2022). Complications include prolonged neonatal jaundice and life-threatening acute episodes of hemolysis. Therapeutic management is primarily aimed at avoiding triggers that cause oxidative stress.

Nursing Assessment

Note health history, including fatigue. Determine the parents' understanding of the disorder and the medications and foods to avoid. Inspect the skin for pallor or jaundice. Evaluate neurologic status, which may also be affected. Measure heart rate and respiratory rate, noting elevations. Determine oxygen saturation via pulse oximeter or blood gas analysis. Note tea-colored urine. Palpate the abdomen for splenomegaly. Laboratory studies will reveal anemia.

Nursing Management

Administer oxygen and treat the symptoms. Once the triggering agent is removed or the child recovers from an illness, the child will improve. Provide further education to the child and family about triggers, and advise them that the child should avoid contact with these agents.

CLOTTING DISORDERS

Clotting of blood is a process that occurs after injury. The blood clotting system requires certain factors in the blood and platelets to perform adequately. Individuals with deficiencies of these factors or platelets tend to bleed; they do not bleed more easily than people without these conditions, but it is just more difficult for the clot to form, and bleeding cannot be stopped easily. Factors that are most often involved in problems with clotting include factor VIII, factor IX, and factor XI. Each plays a role in clot formation. Platelets also play a role in the clotting cascade and are necessary for clot formation. Some processes can lead to destruction of the platelets and may lead to a reduction in clotting. Bleeding times are prolonged when a clotting disorder is present. Table 46.5 provides usual values for clotting studies.

Conditions affecting clotting include immune thrombocytopenia (ITP), immunoglobulin A vasculitis, disseminated intravascular coagulation (DIC), and factor deficiencies such as hemophilia A (factor VIII deficiency), von Willebrand disease (vWD), hemophilia B (Christmas disease, factor IX deficiency), and hemophilia C (factor XI deficiency). Table 46.6 reviews the expected levels of proteins involved in coagulation.

Immune Thrombocytopenia

ITP is thought to be an immune response following a viral infection that produces antiplatelet antibodies. These antibodies destroy platelets, which then lead to the development of petechiae, purpura, and excessive bruising. Petechiae are pinpoint hemorrhages that occur anywhere on the body and do not blanch to pressure (Fig. 46.13).

TABLE 46.5 • Clotting Studies

Test	Measure
Prothrombin time (PT)	11.0–13.0 seconds (may vary by laboratory)
Partial thromboplastin time (PTT), activated partial thromboplastin time (aPTT)	21–35 seconds
International normalized ratio (INR) (used to evaluate coagulation)	2.0–3.0 usual target in thromboembolic conditions

Data from Fischbach, F. T., Fischbach, M. A., & Stout, K. (2022). *A manual of laboratory and diagnostic tests* (11th ed.). Wolters Kluwer Health.

TABLE 46.6 • Select Proteins Involved in Coagulation (Factors)

Protein	Synonym	Concentration in Plasma (mg/dL)
Fibrinogen	Factor I	200–400
Factor II	Prothrombin	10–15
Factor V	Proaccelerin; labile factor	0.5–1.0
Factor VII	Stable factor; proconvertin	0.2
Factor VIIIC	Antihemophilic factor; platelet cofactor I	1.0–2.0
Factor IX	Christmas factor; plasma thromboplastin component	0.3–0.4
Factor X	Stuart–Prower factor	0.6–0.8
Factor XI	Plasma thromboplastin antecedent	0.4
Factor XII	Hageman factor	2.9
Factor XIII	Fibrin-stabilizing factor; Laki–Lorand factor	2.5
Von Willebrand factor	Factor VIII–related antigen (VIII: VWD)	1.0

VWD, Von Willebrand disease.

Data from Fischbach, F. T., Fischbach, M. A., & Stout, K. (2022). *A manual of laboratory and diagnostic tests* (11th ed.). Wolters Kluwer Health.

Purpura are larger areas of hemorrhage in which blood collects under the tissues; they are purplish (see Fig. 46.13). ITP may develop within a few weeks after a viral infection. It is most common in young children, and most will recover spontaneously within a few months (Bussell, 2022a). Complications include severe hemorrhage, bleeding into vital organs, and intracranial hemorrhage, although these rarely occur.

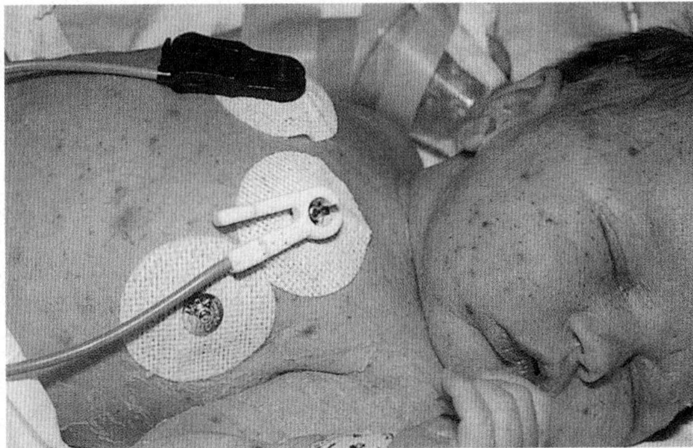

FIGURE 46.13 Pinpoint hemorrhages (petechiae) and large purplish areas of discoloration (purpura) in an infant with idiopathic thrombocytopenia purpura (ITP).

First-line treatment of ITP includes the use of corticosteroids and intravenous immunoglobulin (IVIG) (Bussell, 2022b). Platelet transfusions are not indicated unless life-threatening bleeding is present. ITP is usually self-limiting, but if it persists for a year or longer, splenectomy may be indicated.

Nursing Assessment

Elicit the child's health history (usually a previously healthy child who has recently developed increased bruising, epistaxis, or bleeding of the gums). Note history of blood in the stool. Note risk factors such as recent viral illness, recent measles, mumps, and rubella (MMR) immunization, or ingestion of medications that can cause thrombocytopenia. Inspect for petechiae, purpura, and bruising, which may progress rapidly within the first 24 to 48 hours of the illness. Document the size and location of each lesion. Inspect the lips and buccal mucosa for petechiae. The remainder of the physical examination is usually within normal limits.

Usual laboratory findings include an extremely low platelet count (less than 50,000), normal WBC count and differential, and Hgb and Hct unless hemorrhage has occurred (this is rare). Bone marrow aspiration may be performed to rule out leukemia.

Nursing Management

Many children require no medical treatment except observation and reevaluation of laboratory values. Educate the family about avoiding aspirin, nonsteroidal antiinflammatory drugs (NSAIDs), and antihistamines because these medications may precipitate the development of anemia in these children. The use of acetaminophen for pain control is more appropriate when necessary. Teach the family to prevent trauma by avoiding activities that may cause injury, such as contact sports. Instead, encourage activities, such as swimming, that provide physical activity with less risk of trauma. Explain to parents the signs and symptoms of serious bleeding and whom to call if it is suspected.

Immunoglobulin A Vasculitis (Henoch–Schönlein Purpura)

Immunoglobulin A vasculitis is a condition that affects mostly male young children and develops in association with a viral or bacterial infection (most often respiratory) (Nuss et al., 2022). The classic presentation is vasculitis with immunoglobulin A (IgA)–dominant immune deposits affecting small vessels. These small vessels are generally in the skin, gut, and kidney. In most children, the course of the disease is benign, and the prognosis is good. In a few children, however, ongoing nephrotic syndrome may occur as a result of kidney injury, and those children may have hypertension. Pulmonary, cardiac, and neurologic complications can also occur.

No specific treatment exists for IgA vasculitis since most of the cases resolve without treatment. Treatment with corticosteroids, such as prednisone, may be helpful in children with severe joint or GI manifestations (Nuss et al., 2022). If kidney injury occurs, children may require kidney function testing and evaluation for hypertension and treatment when present.

Nursing Assessment

Note history of viral or bacterial infection. Determine the onset of the complaint and how it has progressed or changed. Note history of joint or abdominal pain. Measure blood pressure. Inspect the skin for a purpuric palpable rash, and document the size and location of lesions. Palpate the rash to determine its extent (Fig. 46.14). Gently palpate the joints for tenderness. Palpate the abdomen for tenderness. Note visible or occult blood in the stool. Note cherry- or tea-colored urine, indicating the presence of blood in the urine; urinalysis can verify the amount of blood present in the urine. Serum IgA levels may be elevated.

Nursing Management

Treatment of the symptoms is the focus. In children with severe joint or abdominal pain, administer analgesics as prescribed, and note the response to pain medications. If the child has normal kidney function, maintaining hydration is the most important intervention. Monitor intake and output. Note the color of urine. Administer corticosteroids and anticoagulants, alone or together, if ordered to reduce kidney impairment. Teach the child and family about the therapy, such as management of hypertension with medications, and sodium restriction. Teach them about signs of kidney injury, such as blood in the urine and changes in weight, as well as frequency and volume of urine output.

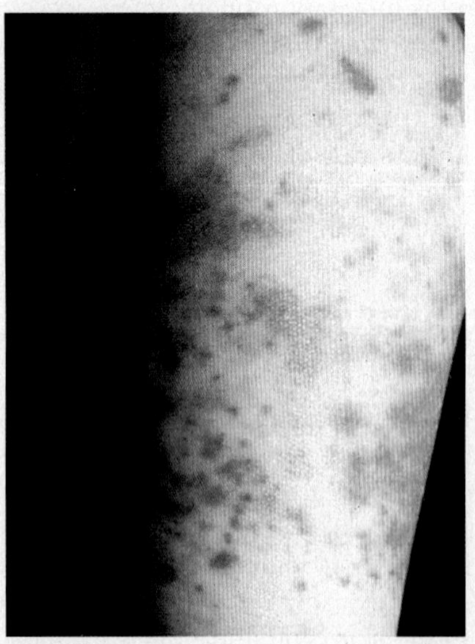

FIGURE 46.14 Palpable purpura on an adolescent's arm.

Disseminated Intravascular Coagulation

DIC is a complex condition that leads to activation of coagulation; it usually occurs in critically ill children. Common triggers of DIC include septic shock, presence of endotoxins and viruses, tissue necrosis or injury, and cancer treatment (Nuss et al., 2022). In DIC, thrombin is generated, fibrin is deposited in the circulation, and platelets are consumed. Deficiencies of coagulation and anticoagulation pathways occur. Hemorrhage and organ tissue damage result and can be irreversible if not recognized and treated immediately.

Therapeutic management of children with DIC requires careful consideration of the etiology. Initial treatment focuses on treating the underlying cause. For example, if DIC occurs secondary to an infection, appropriate antibiotics would be used to treat the infection. Heparin is also used at lower doses to counteract the deficiency in the coagulation/anticoagulation pathway. Heparin reduces consumption of the platelets, resulting in improved platelet counts. Since heparin is an anticoagulant, there is an increased risk of bleeding.

Nursing Assessment

Because DIC occurs as a secondary condition, it may occur in a child hospitalized for any reason. DIC may affect any body system, so a thorough physical examination is warranted. Inspect for signs of bleeding such as petechiae or purpura, blood in the urine or stool, or persistent oozing from venipuncture or from the umbilical cord in the newborn. Evaluate respiratory status, and determine the level of tissue oxygenation via pulse oximetry. Perform a complete circulatory assessment and note signs of circulatory collapse such as poor perfusion, tachycardia, prolonged capillary refill, and weak distal pulses. Note altered level of consciousness and decreased urine output. Careful abdominal palpation may reveal hepatomegaly or splenomegaly.

Laboratory testing may reveal prolonged prothrombin time (PT), partial thromboplastin time (PTT), activated partial thromboplastin time (aPTT), bleeding time, and thrombin time and decreased levels of fibrinogen; platelets; clotting factors II, V, VIII, and X; and antithrombin III. Increases will be noted in levels of fibrinolysin, fibrinopeptide A, positive fibrin split products, and D-dimers.

CLINICAL REASONING ALERT!

Diagnostic tests that indicate the development of DIC include increased fibrinogen/fibrin degradation products, decreased antithrombin III, increased fibrinopeptide A level, and an increased D-dimer assay.

Nursing Management

Continue to provide nursing care related to the triggering event. Assess the child's status frequently. If bleeding is observed, apply pressure to the area along with cold compresses. Elevate the affected body part if this does not affect the child's overall stability. If neurologic deficits are assessed, report the findings immediately so that treatment to prevent permanent damage can be started. Administer anticoagulation therapy (even though hemorrhage is a concern) to interrupt the coagulation process that is present in this condition. Provide ventilatory support as needed and provide continuous cardiac monitoring. Administer clotting factors, platelets, and cryoprecipitate as prescribed to prevent severe hemorrhage. Report changes in laboratory values to the health care provider or nurse practitioner. Changes can occur rapidly, and vigilance is necessary to prevent further tissue damage to the affected system.

Hemophilia

Hemophilia is a group of X-linked recessive disorders that result in deficiency in one of the coagulation factors in the blood. X-linked recessive disorders are transmitted by carrier female parents to their male children, so usually, only males are affected by hemophilia. The coagulation factors in the blood are essential for clot formation either spontaneously or from an injury, and when factors are absent, bleeding will be difficult to stop. There are several types of hemophilia, including factor VIII deficiency (hemophilia A), factor IX deficiency or Christmas disease (hemophilia B), and factor XI deficiency (hemophilia C). The most common, hemophilia A, will be the focus of this discussion (Nuss et al., 2022). Hemophilia A occurs when there is a deficiency of factor VIII in an individual. Factor VIII is essential in the activation of factor X, which is required for the conversion of prothrombin into thrombin, resulting in an inability of the platelets to be used in clot formation.

Hemophilia is classified according to the severity of the disease, ranging from mild to severe. The more severe the disease, the more likely it is that there will be bleeding episodes. When bleeding occurs, the vessels constrict and a platelet plug forms, but because of the deficient factor, the fibrin will not solidify and thus bleeding continues.

Therapeutic Management

The primary goal of managing hemophilia is to prevent bleeding. This is best accomplished by instructing the child to avoid activities with a high potential for injury (e.g., football, riding motorcycles, skateboarding). Instead, encourage the child to participate in activities with the least amount of contact (e.g., swimming, running, tennis). Limiting activities does not mean the child should do nothing; activities that promote health without increased exposure to injury are best.

If bleeding or injury occurs, factor administration is prescribed; this practice has been common in outpatient facilities or the child's home for many years. Once the deficient factor is replaced, clotting factors return to fairly normal levels for a period of time. Factor replacement should be given before any surgeries or other procedures that can lead to bleeding, such as intramuscular injections and dental care.

TAKE NOTE!

The Food and Drug Administration has approved a new long-acting form of factor XIII replacement to be used as routine prophylaxis for bleeding (Antihemophilic Factor (Recombinant), Fc-VWF-XTEN Fusion Protein-ehtl [ALTUVIIIO]) (Sanofi, 2023).

Nursing Assessment

For a full description of the assessment phase of the nursing process, refer to the "Clinical Judgment and the Nursing Process" section. Assessment findings pertinent to hemophilia in children are discussed further on.

HEALTH HISTORY

Elicit the health history, determining the nature of the bleeding episode or bruise. Include in the history any hemorrhagic episodes in other systems, such as the GI tract (e.g., black tarry stools, hematemesis) or caused by injury resulting in joint hemorrhage, or hematuria (Fig. 46.15). Inquire about length of bleeding and amount of blood loss. Because hemophilia A results in difficulty with clotting, the child may bleed for a longer period when injury occurs.

PHYSICAL EXAMINATION

Focus the physical examination on identification of any bleeding. This is of particular concern after injury, but a nosebleed or other spontaneous bleed can occur if factor levels are extremely low. Assess circulation by evaluating pulses and heart sounds if severe or prolonged bleeding is identified. Without intervention, hypovolemia could follow, leading to shock. Note chest pain or abdominal pain, which may indicate internal bleeding. Report these

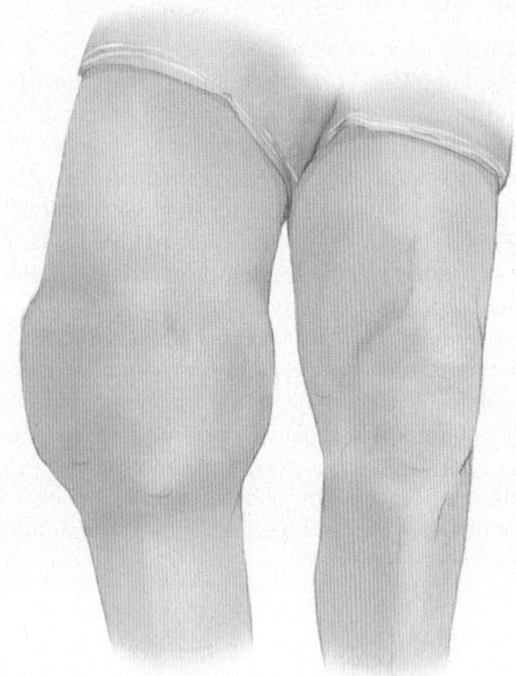

FIGURE 46.15 Significant swelling and discoloration associated with a bleeding episode in the knee of a person with hemophilia.

findings immediately so that the underlying condition can be diagnosed and treated rapidly.

LABORATORY AND DIAGNOSTIC TESTING

Laboratory findings may include decreased hemoglobin and Hct if bleeding is prolonged or severe. Factor levels may be quantified with blood testing.

Nursing Management

Nursing management includes preventing bleeding episodes, managing bleeding episodes, and providing education and support.

PREVENTING BLEEDING EPISODES

All children with hemophilia should attempt to prevent bleeding episodes. Recurrent bleeding into the joints (hemarthroses) may cause joint destruction, thereby limiting ROM and function over the long term (Nuss et al., 2022). Teach children and families that regular physical activity or exercise helps to keep the muscles and joints stronger and that children with stronger joints and muscles have fewer bleeding episodes (see Teaching Guidelines 46.4). Refer the child with moderate to severe hemophilia to a pediatric hematologist and/or a comprehensive hemophilia treatment center.

MANAGING A BLEEDING EPISODE

Administer factor VIII replacement as prescribed. Factor replacement is pooled from multiple blood donors, so families may be concerned about transmission of viruses via the product (specifically, hepatitis and human immunodeficiency virus [HIV]). Several methods of viral inactivation (solvent detergent, dry heat, and monoclonal purification) have been used to treat plasma-derived factors to eliminate the risk of HIV transmission via factor infusion (National Hemophilia Foundation [NHF], 2023).

Administer factor replacement by slow IV push. Document the product name, number of units, lot number, and expiration date. Doses are based on the severity of the bleeding and the weight of the child. Specific dosing guidelines can be obtained from the product insert. In mild cases of hemophilia A, desmopressin may be effective in stopping bleeding (see the nursing management section of VWD for additional information).

If external bleeding develops, apply pressure to the area until bleeding stops. If it is inside a joint, apply ice or cold compresses to the area and elevate any injured extremities, except when contraindicated by further injury. Make sure that all cases of bleeding are followed up to identify whether factor replacement is necessary.

TEACHING GUIDELINES 46.4 Preventing Bleeding in the Child With Hemophilia

- Protect toddlers with soft helmets, padding on the knees, carpets in the home, and softened or covered corners.
- Children should stay active: swimming, baseball, basketball, and bicycling (wearing a helmet) are good physical activities.
- Avoid intense contact sports such as football, wrestling, soccer, and high diving.
- Avoid trampoline use and riding all-terrain vehicles (ATVs).
- Arrange premedication with Amicar if oral surgery is indicated.

PROVIDING EDUCATION

Inform the family that the child should wear a medical alert bracelet. Families should notify the school nurse and teachers of the child's diagnosis and share precautions with them. Instruct all school personnel to call the parent immediately if the child sustains a head, abdominal, or orbit injury at school. Teach parents and caregivers how to administer the intravenous infusion of factor VIII. Administration in the home is the preferred method for factor infusion, as the child will be able to receive treatment in the most timely and efficient manner when a bleeding episode occurs. Alternatives to the parent giving the infusion are to arrange for a home care nursing visit or for the family to keep their own supply of factor VIII that they take to the local emergency room for infusion if bleeding occurs.

Involve children as developmentally appropriate in the infusion process. Young children may hold and apply the Band-Aid; older children may assist with dilution and mixing of the factor. Teach adolescents to administer their own factor infusions. Children with severe hemophilia may need factor infusions so often that implantation of a central venous access port is warranted. Teach the family access, care, and flushing of the implanted port.

TAKE NOTE!

Require a return demonstration of intravenous factor infusion by the parents to ensure independence in the home environment, as well as accuracy of infusion.

THINKING ABOUT **DEVELOPMENT**

Toby Henderson is an 18-month-old male with a history of moderate hemophilia. He is a very active child.

Considering Toby's developmental stage, how will his diagnosis impact his ability to accomplish toddler developmental milestones?

Develop a teaching plan for Toby's parents related to safety for Toby. Incorporate age-appropriate activities that would be safe for Toby in the plan.

How would the safety plan be different if Toby were 13 years old?

PROVIDING SUPPORT

Children with hemophilia may be able to lead a fairly normal life, with the exception of avoiding a few activities. However, accepting the diagnosis of a bleeding disorder in their child is very difficult for parents. They fear the worst (bleeding that won't stop) as well as complications such as infection with bloodborne viruses. Reassure parents that since factor replacement began to be treated, there have been no reports of HIV transmission from factor infusion. Educate and support the parents. Factor replacement is expensive, and bleeding episodes often cause parents to miss work, both of which create financial strains. Refer families to the NHF and NHF Youthworld, which offer support, education, youth leadership, scholarships, and a directory of camps for children with hemophilia and other bleeding disorders.

Von Willebrand Disease

vWD is a genetically transmitted bleeding disorder that may affect any sex or race. The disorder is a deficiency in von Willebrand factor (vWF). Under ordinary circumstances, vWF serves two functions: to bind with factor VIII, protecting it from breakdown, and to serve as the "glue" that attaches platelets to the site of injury. Deficiency in this factor results in a mild bleeding disorder. Children with vWD bruise easily, have frequent nosebleeds (epistaxis), and tend to bleed after oral surgery. Pubescent females often have menorrhagia.

Therapeutic management of vWD is similar to that of hemophilia. Prevention of injury is important. When bleeding or injury does occur, vWF is administered. Desmopressin may also be used to release the factors necessary for clotting. Desmopressin raises the plasma level from stores in the endothelium of blood vessels; this releases factor VIII and vWF from these stores into the bloodstream. These may also be administered before dental work or surgery.

Nursing Assessment

Nursing assessment of the child with vWD is similar to the assessment of the child with hemophilia, although severe bleeding occurs much less frequently.

Nursing Management

Nursing management is also similar to the management of the child with hemophilia. The major difference is the administration of desmopressin. Administer desmopressin nasal spray as prescribed when a bleeding episode occurs. Desmopressin may also be given via an intravenous infusion or subcutaneously (less common). Stimate is the only brand of desmopressin nasal spray that is used for controlling bleeding; the other brands are used for homeostasis and enuresis. Desmopressin is an antidiuretic hormone, so closely monitor fluid balance. Twenty-four hours should elapse between doses, as lessening of the response (tachyphylaxis) occurs with more frequent use (James, 2023). vWD may also be treated with intravenous infusion of vWF, similarly to factor VIII infusion for hemophilia A. Teach children and their families how to avoid or minimize bleeding episodes (see Teaching Guidelines 46.4).

LEUKEMIA

Leukemia is a primary disorder of the bone marrow in which the normal elements are replaced with abnormal WBCs. Normally, lymphoid cells grow and develop into lymphocytes, and myeloid cells grow and develop into RBCs, granulocytes, monocytes, and platelets. Leukemia may develop at any time during the usual stages of normal lymphoid or myeloid development.

Leukemia may be classified as acute or chronic, lymphocytic, or myelogenous. Acute leukemias are rapidly progressive diseases affecting the undifferentiated or immature cells; the result is cells without normal function. Chronic leukemias progress more slowly, permitting maturation and differentiation of cells so that they retain some of their normal function. Acute leukemias, including ALL and acute myelogenous leukemia (AML), occur much more commonly in children and adolescents than do chronic leukemias (Keating et al., 2022). Therefore, they will be the focus of the discussion that follows.

Complications of leukemia include **metastasis** (spread of cancer to other sites) to the blood, bone, CNS, spleen, liver, or other organs and alterations in growth. Late effects include problems with neurocognitive function and ocular, cardiovascular, or thyroid dysfunction. With advances in treatment over the past 50 years, most cases of childhood leukemia are curable. However, children who experience relapse or present with advanced disease have a poorer prognosis (Keating et al., 2022).

Acute Lymphoblastic Leukemia

ALL is the most common form of cancer in children. Eighty-five percent of cases of ALL occur in children between 2 and 10 years of age (Keating et al., 2022). It is more common in White children than in other races. ALL is classified according to the type of cells involved—T cell, B cell, early pre-B cell, or pre-B cell. Most children will achieve initial remission if appropriate treatment is given. The overall cure rate of ALL is over 70% (Keating et al., 2022).

Prognosis is based on the WBC count at diagnosis, the type of cytogenetic factors and immunophenotype, the age at diagnosis, and the extent of extramedullary involvement. Generally, the higher the WBC count at diagnosis, the worse the prognosis. Children between 1 and 9 years of age and with a WBC count of less than 50,000 at diagnosis have the best prognosis. When a child experiences a relapse, the prognosis becomes poorer. Complications include infection, hemorrhage, poor growth, and CNS, bone, or testicular involvement.

Pathophysiology

The exact cause of ALL remains unknown. Genetic factors and chromosome abnormalities may play a role in its development. In ALL, abnormal lymphoblasts abound in the blood-forming tissues. The lymphoblasts are fragile and immature, lacking the infection-fighting capabilities of the normal WBC. The growth of lymphoblasts is excessive, and the abnormal cells replace the normal cells in the bone marrow. The proliferating leukemic cells demonstrate massive metabolic needs, depriving normal body cells of needed nutrients and resulting in fatigue, weight loss or growth arrest, and muscle wasting. The bone marrow becomes unable to maintain normal levels of RBCs, WBCs, and platelets, so anemia, neutropenia, and thrombocytopenia result. As the bone marrow expands or the leukemic cells infiltrate the bone, joint and bone pain may occur. The leukemic cells may permeate the lymph nodes, causing diffuse lymphadenopathy, or the liver and spleen, resulting in hepatosplenomegaly. With spread to the CNS, vomiting, headache, seizures, coma, vision alterations, or cranial nerve palsies may occur (Keating et al., 2022).

CLINICAL REASONING ALERT!

Changes in behavior or personality, headache, irritability, dizziness, persistent nausea or vomiting, seizures, gait changes, lethargy, or altered level of consciousness may indicate CNS infiltration with leukemic cells. Immediately report these findings to the pediatric oncologist.

Therapeutic Management

Therapeutic management of the child with ALL focuses on giving chemotherapy to eradicate the leukemic cells and restore normal bone marrow function. Treatment is divided into three stages. CNS prophylaxis is provided at each stage in order to prevent metastasis to the CNS (Keating et al., 2022). The length of treatment and choice of medications are based on the child's age, risk category, and subtype determined by bone marrow analysis. Table 46.7 discusses the stages of leukemia treatment. For relapsed or less responsive leukemia, HSCT may be necessary.

Nursing Assessment

For a full description of the assessment phase of the nursing process, refer to the "Clinical Judgment and

TABLE 46.7 • Stages of Leukemia Treatment

Stage	Purpose	Length	Usual Medications
Induction	Rapid induction of complete remission	3–4 weeks	Oral steroids, IV vincristine, IM L-asparaginase, daunomycin (high risk)
Consolidation (intensification)	Strengthen remission, reduce leukemic cell burden	Varies	High-dose methotrexate, 6-mercaptopurine; possibly cyclophosphamide, cytarabine, asparaginase, thioguanine, epipodophyllotoxins
Maintenance	Eliminate all residual leukemic cells	2–3 years	Low dose: daily 6-mercaptopurine, weekly methotrexate, intermittent IV vincristine, and oral steroids
CNS prophylaxis	Reduce risk of development of CNS disease	Given periodically in all stages	Intrathecal chemotherapy; cranial radiation is used infrequently.

CNS, central nervous system; IM, intramuscular; IV, intravenous.

Data from Keating, A. K., Knight-Perry, J., Maloney, K., Levy, J. M. M., Greffe, B. S., Franklin, A. R. K., & Garrington, T. P. (2022). Chapter 31: Neoplastic disease. In M. Bunik, W. W. Hay, M. J. Levin, & M. J. Abzug (Eds.), *Current diagnosis & treatment: Pediatrics* (26th ed., pp. 931–963). McGraw-Hill Education; Horton, T. M., & McNeer, J. L. (2022). Treatment of acute lymphoblastic leukemia/lymphoma in children and adolescents. *UpToDate*. Retrieved on April, 26, 2023, from https://www.uptodate.com/contents/overview-of-the-treatment-of-acute-lymphoblastic-leukemia-in-children -and-adolescents

the Nursing Process" section. Assessment findings pertinent to ALL are discussed further on.

HEALTH HISTORY

Elicit a description of the present illness and chief complaint. Common signs and symptoms reported during the health history might include:

- Fever (may be persistent or recurrent, with unknown cause)
- Recurrent infection
- Fatigue, malaise, or listlessness
- Pallor
- Unusual bleeding or bruising
- Abdominal pain
- Nausea or vomiting
- Bone pain
- Headache (Keating et al., 2022)

Explore the child's current and past medical history for risk factors such as:

- Male sex
- Age 2 to 5 years
- White race
- Down syndrome (and many other genetic syndromes)
- Sibling with leukemia
- Radiation exposure
- Previous chemotherapy treatment American Cancer Society, 2024d

Determine the child's history of varicella zoster immunization or disease. Chickenpox infection in the leukemic child may lead to disseminated, overwhelming infection.

PHYSICAL EXAMINATION

Take the child's temperature (fever may be present), and look for petechiae, purpura, or unusual bruising (due to decreased platelet levels). Inspect the skin for signs of infection. Auscultate the lungs, noting adventitious breath sounds, which may indicate pneumonia (present at diagnosis or due to immunosuppression during treatment). Note location and size of enlarged lymph nodes. Palpate the liver and spleen for enlargement. Document tenderness on abdominal palpation.

TAKE NOTE!

Have the child lie flat for 30 minutes after a lumbar puncture, and increase fluid intake for 24 hours after the procedure to decrease incidence of headache.

LABORATORY AND DIAGNOSTIC TESTS

Common laboratory and diagnostic studies ordered for the assessment of ALL include:

- CBC: abnormal findings include low hemoglobin and Hct; decreased RBC count; decreased platelet count; and elevated, normal, or decreased WBC count
- Peripheral blood smear may reveal blasts.
- Bone marrow aspiration: stained smear from bone marrow aspiration will show greater than 25% lymphoblasts. Bone marrow aspirate is also examined for immunophenotyping (lymphoid versus myeloid and level of cancer cell maturity) and cytogenetic analysis (determines abnormalities in chromosome number and structure). Immunophenotyping and cytogenetic analysis are used in the classification of the leukemia, which helps guide treatment.
- Lumbar puncture will reveal whether leukemic cells have infiltrated the CNS.
- Liver function tests and blood urea nitrogen (BUN) and creatinine levels determine liver and kidney function, which, if abnormal, may preclude treatment with certain chemotherapeutic agents.
- Chest radiography may reveal pneumonia or a mediastinal mass.

• • • ATRAUMATIC CARE • • •

The child with leukemia undergoes frequent implantable port accesses for blood draws and chemotherapy, bone marrow aspirations for assessment of blood cell status, and lumbar punctures for laboratory studies and intrathecal medication administration. To decrease trauma produced by these repetitive painful procedures, utilize EMLA (eutectic mixture of local anesthetics) cream appropriately. Teach the child's primary caregiver to apply the cream to the implantable port site 30 minutes to 1 hour prior to the child's clinic appointment time. Apply EMLA cream to the posterior hip or lumbar spine, 1 to 3 hours prior to bone marrow aspiration or lumbar puncture.

Nursing Management

Nursing care of children with ALL focuses on managing disease complications such as infection, pain, anemia, bleeding, and hyperuricemia and the many adverse effects related to treatment. Many children require blood product transfusion for the treatment of severe anemia or low platelet levels with active bleeding.

Individualize nursing care based on the patient problems, interventions, and outcomes presented in the "Clinical Judgment and the Nursing Process" section earlier in the chapter, depending on the child's response to the disease and chemotherapy. Refer to that section for further information related to managing the adverse effects of chemotherapy.

TAKE NOTE!

Blood products administered to children with any type of leukemia should be irradiated, cytomegalovirus (CMV) negative, and leukodepleted. This treatment of blood products before transfusion will decrease the number of antibodies in the blood, an important factor in preventing GVHD if HSCT becomes necessary at a later date (Keating et al., 2022).

REDUCING PAIN

Children and adolescents with leukemia suffer pain related to the disease as well as the treatment. Chemotherapy drugs commonly used in leukemia may cause peripheral neuropathy and headache. Lumbar puncture and bone marrow aspiration, which are periodically performed throughout the course of treatment, also cause pain. The most common areas of pain are the head and neck, legs, and abdomen (probably from protracted vomiting with chemotherapy). Use distraction techniques, such as listening to music, watching TV, or playing games, to help take the child's mind off the pain. Administer mild analgesics such as acetaminophen for acute episodes of pain. Using EMLA cream prior to venipuncture, port access, lumbar puncture, and bone marrow aspiration may decrease procedure-related pain events. In addition, applying heat or cold to the painful area is usually acceptable. Administer narcotic analgesics, as prescribed, for episodes of acute severe pain or for palliation of chronic pain.

> ***TAKE NOTE!***
>
> Administer medications as ordered using the least invasive method possible to avoid pain (intramuscular, subcutaneous, and rectal route should be avoided in the child with thrombocytopenia).

Acute Myeloid Leukemia

AML accounts for about 25% of leukemias in children, yet is responsible for about a third of deaths from leukemia in this age group (Keating et al., 2022). AML affects the myeloid cell progenitors or precursors in the bone marrow, resulting in **malignant** (invasive and fast-growing) cells. The French–American–British (FAB) classification system identifies eight subtypes of AML (M0 to M7), depending on myeloid lineage involved and the degree of cell differentiation. These subtypes are useful for determining treatment. The long-term survival rate for childhood AML is about 50% (Keating et al., 2022). Complications include treatment resistance, infection, hemorrhage, and metastasis. The induction phase of AML requires intense bone marrow suppression and prolonged hospitalization because AML is less responsive to treatment than ALL. Toxicity from treatment is more common in AML and is likely to be more serious than with ALL. Empiric broad-spectrum antibiotics and prophylactic platelet transfusions may be prescribed. After remission is achieved, children require intensive chemotherapy to prolong the duration of remission. HSCT is often required in children with AML, depending on the subtype (Keating et al., 2022).

> ***TAKE NOTE!***
>
> At the time of diagnosis, some children with AML present with a WBC count of above 100,000 (hyperleukocytosis); this results in venous stasis and backup of blast cells in small vessels, causing hypoxia, hemorrhage, and lung or brain infarction. Hyperleukocytosis is a medical emergency. These children require leukapheresis to decrease hyperviscosity by quickly decreasing the number of circulating blasts (Keating et al., 2022).

Nursing Assessment

Explore the health history for common signs and symptoms, including recurrent infections, fever, or fatigue. Explore the medical history for risk factors, such as Hispanic background, previous chemotherapy, and genetic abnormalities, such as Down syndrome, Fanconi anemia, neurofibromatosis, Wiskott–Aldrich syndrome, and Diamond–Blackfan anemia.

Perform a thorough physical examination. Note skin pallor and salmon-colored or blue-gray papular lesions. Palpate the skin for subcutaneous rubbery nodules. Palpate for lymphadenopathy. Note headache, visual disturbance, or signs of increased intracranial pressure, such as vomiting, which may indicate CNS involvement. Upon diagnosis of AML, the child's WBC count is typically extremely elevated (Keating et al., 2022).

Nursing Management

Nursing management of the child with AML is similar to that of the child with ALL. Nursing interventions focus on managing the adverse effects of treatment and preventing infection. Refer to the "Clinical Judgment and the Nursing Process" section earlier in the chapter for appropriate interventions.

LYMPHOMAS

Lymphomas, or tumors of the lymph tissue (lymph nodes, thymus, spleen), account for about 10% to 15% of cases of childhood cancer (Keating et al., 2022). Lymphomas may be divided into two categories—Hodgkin disease (or Hodgkin lymphoma) and non-Hodgkin lymphoma (NHL), which includes more than a dozen types. Hodgkin disease tends to affect lymph nodes located closer to the body's surface, such as those in the cervical, axillary, and inguinal areas, whereas NHL tends to affect lymph nodes located more deeply inside the body.

Hodgkin Disease

In Hodgkin disease, malignant B lymphocytes grow in the lymph tissue, usually starting in one general area of lymph nodes. The presence of Reed–Sternberg cells (giant transformed B lymphocytes with one or two nuclei) differentiates Hodgkin disease from other lymphomas. As the cells multiply, the lymph nodes enlarge, compressing nearby structures, destroying normal cells, and invading other tissues. The cause of Hodgkin disease is still being researched, but there appears to be a link to Epstein–Barr virus infection American Cancer Society, 2024e. Hodgkin disease is rare in children younger than 5 years of age and is most common in adolescents and young adults; in preadolescents, it is more common in males than females (Keating et al., 2022).

In addition to the traditional **staging** (I through IV, depending on the amount of spread of the cancer; Table 46.8), Hodgkin is also classified as A (asymptomatic) or B (presence of symptoms of fever, night sweats, or weight loss of 10% or more). Prognosis depends on the stage of the disease, tumor bulk, and A or B classification (disease classified as A generally carries a better prognosis). Overall, children with Hodgkin disease have a 5- to 10-year survival rate of over 90% (Keating et al., 2022). Complications of Hodgkin disease include liver failure and secondary cancer such as acute nonlymphocytic leukemia and NHL.

Chemotherapy, usually with a combination of drugs, is the treatment of choice for children with Hodgkin disease. Radiation therapy may also be necessary. In the child with disease that does not go into remission or in the child who experiences relapse, HSCT may be an option.

Nursing Assessment

Explore the health history for common signs and symptoms, which may include recent weight loss, fever, drenching night sweats, anorexia, malaise, fatigue, or pruritus. Elicit the health history, determining risk factors such as prior Epstein–Barr virus infection, family history of Hodgkin disease, genetic immune disorder, or HIV infection.

TABLE **46.8** • Staging of Hodgkin Disease

Stage	Clinical Findings
I	Involves a single lymph node region
II	Two or more lymph node regions on the same side of the diaphragm are affected.
III	Lymph node regions or lymphatic structures above and below the diaphragm are affected.
IV	Metastasis to nonlymphatic organs such as the liver, bone, or lungs
A or B suffix	A—Absence of systemic symptoms at diagnosis B—Systemic symptoms present at diagnosis (fever, night sweats, weight loss)

Data from LaCasce, A. S., & Ng, A. K. (2022). Pretreatment evaluation, staging, and treatment stratification of classic Hodgkin lymphoma. *UpToDate*. Retrieved on April 26, 2023, from https://www.uptodate.com/contents/pretreatment-evaluation-staging-and-treatment-stratification-of-classic-hodgkin-lymphoma

Evaluate respiratory status, as the presence of a mediastinal mass may compromise respiration. Palpate for enlarged lymph nodes; they may feel rubbery and tend to occur in clusters (most common sites are cervical and supraclavicular) (Fig. 46.16). Palpate the abdomen for hepatomegaly or splenomegaly, which may be present with advanced disease. The chest radiograph may reveal a mediastinal mass. The CBC may be normal or reflect anemia. Tissue sampling will reveal Reed–Sternberg cells.

> ***TAKE NOTE!***
>
> Pain and pruritus in the affected lymph node region has sometimes been noted after alcohol ingestion (Keating et al., 2022).

Nursing Management

Nursing management of the child with Hodgkin lymphoma focuses on addressing the adverse effects of chemotherapy or radiation. Refer to the "Clinical Judgment and the Nursing Process" section to develop an individualized nursing care plan based on the child's response to treatment.

Non-Hodgkin Lymphoma

NHL results from mutations in the B and T lymphocytes that lead to uncontrolled growth. NHL tends to affect lymph nodes located more deeply within the body. NHL spreads by the bloodstream and in children is a rapidly proliferating, aggressive malignancy that is very responsive to treatment. Prognosis depends on

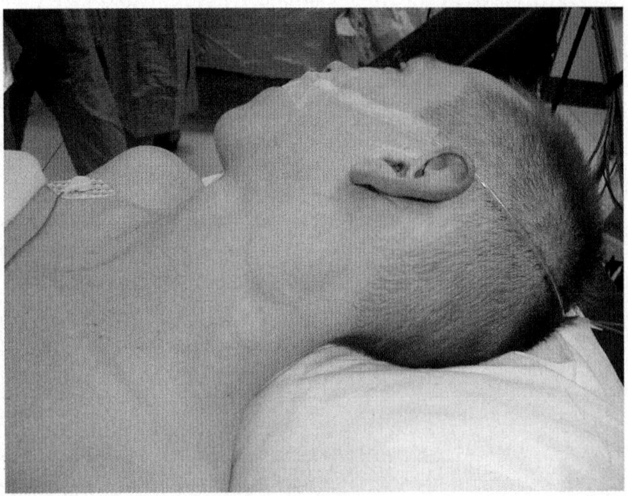

FIGURE 46.16 Hodgkin lymphoma. Large, fixed cervical masses in a 14-year-old with weight loss. (Reprinted with permission from Chung, E. K., Atkinson-McEvoy, L. R., Lai, N. L., & Terry, M. [2014]. *Visual diagnosis and treatment in pediatrics* [3rd ed.]. Wolters Kluwer.)

the cell type involved and the extent of the disease at diagnosis. Ninety percent of children with localized NHL have disease-free long-term survival after treatment (Keating et al., 2022). Complications include metastasis and the development of a secondary malignancy later in life.

Remission is induced with chemotherapy and followed with a maintenance phase of chemotherapy lasting about 2 years. NHL tends to spread easily to the CNS, so CNS prophylaxis similar to that used in leukemia is warranted (Keating et al., 2022). Autologous bone marrow transplantation may be used in some children.

Nursing Assessment

Children with NHL are usually symptomatic for only a few days or a few weeks before diagnosis because the disease progresses so quickly. Note onset and location of pain or lymph node swelling. Document history of abdominal pain, diarrhea, or constipation. Explore the health history for risk factors such as congenital or acquired immune deficiency.

Observe for increased work of breathing, facial edema, or venous engorgement (mediastinal mass). Palpate for the presence of lymphadenopathy, and palpate the abdomen for the presence of a mass. Lymph node biopsy and bone marrow aspiration determine the diagnosis. Computed tomography (CT) scan, chest radiography, and bone marrow results may be used to determine the extent of metastasis.

CLINICAL REASONING ALERT!

Assess for cough, dyspnea, orthopnea, facial edema, or venous engorgement in the child with possible NHL, as mediastinal NHL requires rapid treatment (Keating et al., 2022).

Nursing Management

As with Hodgkin lymphoma, nursing management of NHL is directed toward managing the adverse effects of chemotherapy. Refer to the "Clinical Judgment and the Nursing Process" section to plan nursing care for the child and family based on the responses they exhibit.

BRAIN TUMORS

Brain tumors are the most common form of solid tumor and the second most common type of cancer in children (Keating et al., 2022). Slightly more than half of brain tumors arise in the posterior fossa (infratentorial); the rest are supratentorial in origin. The cause of brain tumors in children is unknown. Some tumors are localized (low grade), while others are of higher grade and more invasive. The prognosis depends on the location of the tumor and extent of tumor. Low-grade tumors and those that are fully resectable have a better prognosis than tumors that are located deeper within the brain or that are more invasive, making them difficult to resect (Keating et al., 2022). There are many different types of childhood brain tumors; Table 46.9 explains the most common ones.

Complications of brain tumors include hydrocephalus, increased intracranial pressure, brain stem herniation, and negative effects of radiation such as neuropsychological, intellectual, and endocrinologic sequelae (Lau & Teo, 2024).

Pathophysiology

Although the cause of brain tumors is generally unknown, the effects of brain tumors are predictable. As the tumor grows within the cranium, it exerts pressure

TABLE 46.9 • Childhood Brain Tumors

Tumor	Location	Characteristics
Medulloblastoma (most common)	Cerebellum	Invasive, highly malignant, grows rapidly. Less favorable outcome with disseminated disease. Progresses quickly to increased intracranial pressure, seeds on CNS pathways. Peak incidence: 5–10 years old
Brain stem glioma	Brain stem	Aggressive, difficult to resect, resistant to chemotherapy. Spreads widely within the brain stem but rarely extends outside of brain stem area. Affects cranial nerve function
Ependymoma	Frequently arises from floor of fourth ventricle	Varying speed of growth. Often causes hydrocephalus. Usually diagnosed before it spreads to other parts of the brain or spinal cord
Astrocytoma	Cerebellum, cerebral hemispheres, thalamus, hypothalamus	Slow course with insidious onset. Responsive to chemotherapy, often resectable. Causes slowly increasing intracranial pressure. Low-grade tumor may be removed completely. High-grade tumors have poor prognosis.

CNS, central nervous system.

Data from Keating, A. K., Knight-Perry, J., Maloney, K., Levy, J. M. M., Greffe, B. S., Franklin, A. R. K., & Garrington, T. P. (2022). Chapter 31: Neoplastic disease. In M. Bunik, W. W. Hay, M. J. Levin, & M. J. Abzug (Eds.), *Current diagnosis & treatment: Pediatrics* (26th ed., pp. 931–963). McGraw-Hill Education.

on the brain tissues surrounding it. The tumor mass may compress vital structures in the brain, block cerebrospinal fluid flow, or cause edema in the brain. The result is an increase in intracranial pressure. Presenting symptoms vary according to location and type of tumor.

Therapeutic Management

The type of tumor may be identified at the time of surgery. The location of the tumor within the brain will determine the extent to which it can safely be resected. Children with hydrocephalus may require a ventriculoperitoneal shunt (see Chapter 38 for further information on hydrocephalus). Radiation is reserved for children older than age 3 years because it can have long-term neurocognitive effects (Lau & Teo, 2024). Chemotherapy is being used increasingly in the treatment of pediatric brain tumors in an attempt to avoid the use of radiation therapy.

Nursing Assessment

For a full description of the assessment phase of the nursing process, refer to "Clinical Judgment and the Nursing Process" section. Assessment findings pertinent to CNS tumors are discussed here.

Health History

Elicit a description of the present illness and chief complaint. Common signs and symptoms reported during the health history might include:

- Nausea or vomiting
- Headache
- Unsteady gait
- Blurred or double vision
- Seizures
- Motor abnormality or hemiparesis
- Weakness, atrophy
- Swallowing difficulties
- Behavior or personality changes
- Irritability, failure to thrive, or developmental delay (in very young children)

Explore the child's current and past medical history for risk factors such as history of neurofibromatosis, tuberous sclerosis, or prior treatment for CNS leukemia.

Physical Examination

Observe for strabismus or nystagmus, 'sunsetting' eyes, head tilt, alterations in coordination, gait disturbance, or alterations in sensation. Note alteration in gag reflex, cranial nerve palsy, lethargy, or irritability. Note the child's posture. Check pupillary reaction, noting size, equality, reaction to light, and accommodation.

Measure blood pressure, which may decrease with increasing intracranial pressure. In the infant, palpate the anterior fontanel for bulging. Assess deep tendon reflexes, noting hyperreflexia.

TAKE NOTE!

A fixed and dilated pupil is a neurosurgical emergency.

Laboratory and Diagnostic Tests

Common laboratory and diagnostic studies ordered for the assessment of CNS tumors are as follows:

- CT, magnetic resonance imaging (MRI), or positron emission tomography (PET) will demonstrate evidence of the tumor and its location within the intracranial cavity.
- Lumbar puncture with cerebrospinal fluid cell evaluation may show tumor markers or the presence of alpha-fetoprotein or human chorionic gonadotropin, which may assist in the diagnosis.

Nursing Management

Nursing management of the child with a brain tumor includes pre- and postoperative care, as well as interventions to manage adverse effects related to chemotherapy and radiation. Refer to the "Clinical Judgment and the Nursing Process" section for a discussion of nursing interventions related to chemotherapy adverse effects and for additional interventions that may be individualized depending on the child's response to the brain tumor and its treatment.

Providing Preoperative Care

Preoperatively, care focuses on monitoring for additional increases in intracranial pressure and avoiding activities that cause transient increases in intracranial pressure. Administer dexamethasone as prescribed to decrease intracranial inflammation. Prevent straining with bowel movements by use of a stool softener. Assess the child's pain level as well as level of consciousness, vital signs, and pupillary reaction to determine subtle changes as soon as possible. Provide a tour of the intensive care unit, which is where the child will wake up after the surgery. Instruct the child and family about the possibility of intubation and ventilation in the postoperative period. If a ventriculoperitoneal shunt will be placed for the treatment of hydrocephalus caused by the tumor, provide education about shunts to the child and family (see Chapter 38).

Shave the portion of the head as determined by the neurosurgeon. Some children may choose to have the entire head shaved. Sometimes, children with long hair may feel better about losing it if they donate it to Locks of Love, an organization that provides hairpieces for financially disadvantaged children who have long-term medical hair loss.

Providing Postoperative Care

Regulate fluid administration, as excess fluid intake may cause or worsen cerebral edema. Administer mannitol or hypertonic dextrose to decrease cerebral edema. Assess vital signs frequently, along with checking pupillary reactions and determining level of consciousness. Extreme lethargy or coma may be present for several days postoperatively. Increases in temperature may indicate infection or may be caused by cerebral edema or disturbance of the hypothalamus. Treat hyperthermia with antipyretics such as acetaminophen and with sponge baths, as increases in temperature increase metabolic need. Reduce the temperature slowly.

Monitor for signs of increased intracranial pressure. Headache is common in the postoperative period. Assess pain level and provide analgesics as prescribed. Minimize environmental stimuli, providing a calm and quiet atmosphere. Check the head dressing for cerebrospinal fluid drainage or bleeding. Assess for and document the extent of head, face, or neck edema. Administer eye lubricant if edema prevents complete closure of the eyelids. Apply cool compresses to the eyes to decrease swelling.

As the child begins to regain consciousness, they may be confused or combative. Restrain the child if needed to keep them in bed and prevent dislodging of tubes and lines.

POSITIONING THE CHILD IN THE POSTOPERATIVE PERIOD

Position the child on the unaffected side with the head of the bed flat or at the level prescribed by the neurosurgeon. Side positioning is usually preferred, as the child may have difficulty handling oral secretions if the level of consciousness is decreased. Do not elevate the foot of the bed, as this may increase intracranial pressure and contribute to bleeding. When changing the child's position, maintain the head in alignment with the remainder of the body. Children with paralyzed or spastic extremities will need additional positioning support.

CLINICAL REASONING ALERT!

Observe pre- and postoperatively for signs of brain stem herniation such as opisthotonos (see Fig. 38.13 in Chapter 38), nuchal rigidity, head tilt, sluggish pupils, increased blood pressure with widening pulse pressure, change in respirations, bradycardia, irregular pulse, and changes in body temperature. Notify the health care provider immediately of these findings.

CONSIDER THIS!

Alice Tice, 8 years old, is scheduled to receive chemotherapy for a brain tumor. Alice states, "I'm scared!" A moment later she cries out, "And I don't want to go bald!" Think about when you were a school-age child—what things were important to you then? As the nurse caring for her, how can you prepare Alice for this?

NEUROBLASTOMA

Neuroblastoma, a tumor that arises from embryonic neural crest cells, is the most common extracranial solid tumor in children (Keating et al., 2022). It most frequently occurs in the abdomen, mainly in the adrenal gland, but it may occur anywhere along the paravertebral sympathetic chain in the chest or retroperitoneum. When diagnosed past infancy or early toddlerhood, by the time of diagnosis, the neuroblastoma has usually already metastasized. Neuroblastoma is the second most frequently occurring solid tumor in children; 90% of cases are diagnosed before the age of 5 years (Keating et al., 2022).

Staging of the tumor at diagnosis determines the course of treatment and prognosis. Table 46.10 discusses the staging of neuroblastomas. The 5-year survival rate for all children with neuroblastoma is about 80% (Shohet et al., 2024). Prognosis depends on the tumor stage, age at diagnosis, location of tumor, and location of metastasis. Metastasis to the bone is a worse prognostic factor than metastasis to the skin, liver, or bone marrow. Children who relapse after initial treatment also tend to have a dismal prognosis. In addition to metastasis, complications may include nerve compression, resulting in neurologic deficits.

The neuroblastoma must be removed surgically. Radiation and chemotherapy are administered to all

TABLE 46.10 • Staging of Neuroblastoma

Stage	Clinical Findings
I	Tumor confined to organ or structure of origin
II	Tumor extends beyond organ or structure, not beyond midline ("A" negative lymph nodes, "B" regional nodes on same side involved)
III	Tumor invasively extends beyond the midline with bilateral lymph node involvement
IV	Metastasis to bone, bone marrow, other organs, distant lymph nodes
IV-S	Tumor would have been considered a stage I or II, but remote metastasis to one or more sites (liver, skin, or bone marrow) has occurred without metastasis to the bone

Data from Keating, A. K., Knight-Perry, J., Maloney, K., Levy, J. M. M., Greffe, B. S., Franklin, A. R. K., & Garrington, T. P. (2022). Chapter 31: Neoplastic disease. In M. Bunik, W. W. Hay, M. J. Levin, & M. J. Abzug (Eds.), *Current diagnosis & treatment: Pediatrics* (26th ed., pp. 931-963). McGraw-Hill Education.

children with neuroblastoma except those with stage I disease, in whom the tumor is completely resected.

Nursing Assessment

For a full description of the assessment phase of the nursing process, refer to the "Clinical Judgment and the Nursing Process" section. Assessment findings pertinent to neuroblastoma are discussed here.

Health History

Presenting signs and symptoms of neuroblastoma depend on the location of the primary tumor and the extent of metastasis. Often, parents are the first to notice a swollen or asymmetric abdomen. Elicit the health history, documenting bowel or bladder dysfunction, especially watery diarrhea, neurologic symptoms (brain metastasis), bone pain (bone metastasis), anorexia, vomiting, or weight loss.

Physical Examination

Note neck or facial swelling, bruising above the eyes, or edema around the eyes (metastasis to skull bones). Inspect the skin for pallor or bruising (bone marrow metastasis) and document cough or difficulty breathing. Auscultate the lungs for wheezing. Palpate for lymphadenopathy, especially cervical. Palpate the abdomen, noting a firm, nontender mass. Palpate for and note hepatomegaly or splenomegaly if present.

Laboratory and Diagnostic Testing

Laboratory and diagnostic testing may reveal the following:

- CT scan or MRI to determine site of tumor and evidence of metastasis
- Chest radiograph, bone scan, and skeletal survey to identify metastasis
- Bone marrow aspiration and biopsy to determine metastasis to the bone marrow
- 24-hour urine collection for homovanillic acid (HVA) and vanillylmandelic acid (VMA); levels will be elevated.

Nursing Management

Postoperative nursing care depends on the site of tumor removal, which is most often the abdomen. Provide routine care after abdominal surgery. Refer to the "Clinical Judgment and the Nursing Process" section for nursing care related to the effects of chemotherapy and radiation. Provide emotional support and possible referrals to help children and families cope with a potentially poor prognosis (due to the fact that the disease has often metastasized significantly by the time of diagnosis).

• • • ATRAUMATIC CARE • • •

The child with cancer often undergoes many painful procedures related to laboratory specimens and treatment protocols. To assist the child to cope with these procedures, provide distraction in the form of reading a favorite book or playing a favorite movie or musical selection.

SARCOMAS

Sarcomas occur in bone and soft tissue in children. Bone tumors are most often diagnosed in adolescence, whereas soft tissue tumors tend to occur in younger children (Keating et al., 2022). This discussion will focus on the most common bone and soft tissue tumors occurring in childhood. The most common bone tumors in children are osteosarcoma and Ewing sarcoma (Keating et al., 2022). These bone tumors often initially go undiagnosed, as adolescents frequently seek care for traumatic events and the pain suffered with a bone tumor may initially be attributed to trauma. Rhabdomyosarcoma is the most common soft tissue tumor in childhood (Keating et al., 2022).

Osteosarcoma

Osteosarcoma accounts for 60% of bone cancer in children, occurring most frequently in adolescents and males (Keating et al., 2022). It presumably arises from the embryonic mesenchymal tissue that forms the bones. The most common sites are in the long bones, particularly the proximal humerus, proximal tibia, and distal femur. Complications include metastasis, particularly to the lungs and other bones, and recurrence of disease within 3 years, primarily affecting the lungs.

Surgical removal of the tumor is necessary. Chemotherapy is often administered before surgery to decrease the size of the tumor; it is usually administered after surgery to treat or prevent metastasis. Radiation is not helpful. The type of surgery performed depends on the tumor size, extent of disease outside of the bone, distant metastasis, and skeletal maturity. Radical amputation may be performed, but often, adolescents undergo a limb-sparing procedure (Keating et al., 2022).

Nursing Assessment

Obtain the health history, ascertaining when pain, limp, or limitation of motion was first noticed. Dull bone pain may be present for several months, eventually progressing to limp or gait changes. Inspect the affected limb for erythema and swelling. Palpate the affected area for warmth and tenderness and to determine the size of the soft tissue mass, if also present. As with other pediatric cancers, a thorough physical examination is warranted to detect other abnormalities that may indicate metastasis.

Laboratory and diagnostic testing may include:

- CT scan or MRI to determine the extent of the lesion and to identify metastasis
- Bone scan to determine the extent of malignancy

Nursing Management

The adolescent will generally be quite anxious about the possibility of amputation and even about the limb salvage procedure. Present preoperative teaching at the adolescent's developmental level, and ensure that they are included in planning treatment. Regardless of the type of surgery performed, provide routine orthopedic postoperative care. Educate the adolescent and parents on the care of the stump, if amputation is necessary, and ensure that the adolescent becomes competent in crutch walking. A prosthesis may be ordered. The adolescent will need time to adjust to these significant body image changes and may benefit from talking with another adolescent who has undergone a similar procedure. Support the adolescent in choosing clothing that may camouflage the prosthesis while still allowing the adolescent to appear fashionable. Provide emotional support, as the adolescent's maturity level allows them to understand the severity of the disease. Peer support groups are often helpful, as adolescents value their peers' opinions and enjoy being part of a group. Examples of comprehensive online support groups are Melissa's Living Legacy Foundation/Helping Teens Live with Cancer and The Wellness Community.

Ewing Sarcoma

Ewing sarcoma is a highly malignant bone tumor. It is rarer than osteosarcoma, accounting for about 30% of childhood bone tumors (Keating et al., 2022). It occurs most frequently in the long bones or pelvis (American Association of Orthopedic Surgeons, 2023). The prognosis for Ewing sarcoma depends on the extent of metastasis. Children with small, localized tumor have a 70% to 75% long-term survival rate, while those with metastasis have a poor survival rate (Keating et al., 2022).

Radiation, chemotherapy, and surgical excision are usually used in combination. Treatment varies depending on the site of the primary tumor and the extent of metastasis at diagnosis. Myeloablative chemotherapy (which destroys the child's marrow) may be used for metastatic disease, followed by a stem cell rescue transplant.

Nursing Assessment

Explore the history for intermittent pain that worsens progressively. Note a possible history of fever. Eventually, the pain becomes constant and severe, sometimes interrupting sleep.

Note the presence of swelling or erythema at the tumor site. CT scan or MRI of the affected area will reveal the extent of the tumor. Biopsy is necessary to establish the diagnosis. CT scan of the chest, bone scan, and bilateral bone marrow aspiration with biopsy determine the extent of metastasis.

Nursing Management

Before treatment begins, discourage active play or weight bearing on the affected extremity to avoid pathologic fracture at the tumor site. Nursing management focuses on addressing the adverse effects of treatment (refer to the "Clinical Judgment and the Nursing Process" section). Give honest and direct answers to adolescents with Ewing sarcoma who ask questions about their disease. These children will undergo intensive therapy and spend a great deal of time in the hospital. Depending on the age of the child, fantasy play, art or pet therapy, drama, writing, humor, and/or music may help the child to work through the psychological impact of this disease. Refer to the nursing process section earlier in the chapter for additional interventions, which should be individualized depending on the child's and family's response to the disease process and treatment.

> **THINKING ABOUT DEVELOPMENT**
>
> Serena Jameson is a 14-year-old cheerleader with newly diagnosed Ewing sarcoma. Her prescribed treatment protocol involves several medications known to cause severe alopecia. Considering Serena's developmental stage, how will this impact her ability and/or willingness to participate in future cheerleading exhibitions? Develop a list of ideas for assisting Serena to cope with the anticipated changes to her body image.

Rhabdomyosarcoma

Rhabdomyosarcoma is a soft tissue tumor that usually arises from the embryonic mesenchymal cells that would ordinarily form striated muscle. The most common locations for the tumor are the head and neck, genitourinary tract, and extremities (Fig. 46.17). The tumor is highly malignant and spreads via local extension or through the venous or lymphatic system, with the lung being the most common site for metastasis. Diagnosis is usually made between 2 and 5 years of age, with 70% of all rhabdomyosarcomas diagnosed by age 10 years (Keating et al., 2022). The prognosis is based on the stage of the disease at diagnosis. Box 46.4 explains the staging of rhabdomyosarcoma. Prognosis is generally favorable for stage I disease (Okcu & Hicks, 2023). Complications of rhabdomyosarcoma include metastasis to lung, bone, or

BOX 46.4 Staging of Rhabdomyosarcoma

- Stage I: completely resectable localized tumor
- Stage II: after local tumor resection, microscopic residual disease remains (or spreads to regional lymph nodes)
- Stage III: after local tumor resection, gross residual disease remains
- Stage IV: distant metastasis present at diagnosis

Data from Okcu, M. F., & Hicks, J. (2023). Rhabdomyosarcoma in childhood and adolescence: Clinical presentation, diagnostic evaluation, and staging. *UpToDate.* Retrieved on April 26, 2023, from https://www.uptodate.com/contents/rhabdomyosarcoma-in-childhood-and-adolescence-clinical-presentation-diagnostic-evaluation-and-staging

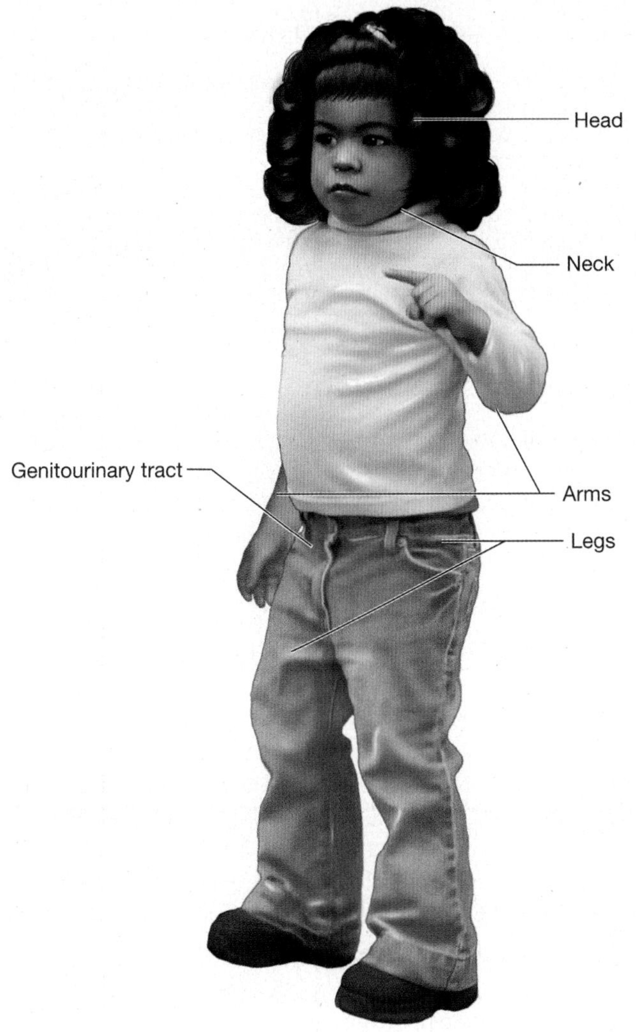

FIGURE 46.17 The most common sites of rhabdomyosarcoma.

bone marrow and direct extension into the CNS, resulting in brain stem compromise or cranial nerve palsy.

Surgical removal of the primary tumor is generally performed. At the time of the surgery, the lesion is biopsied, and the stage of disease determined. Depending on the site (especially head, neck, and pelvis) and size of the tumor, radiation and chemotherapy may be used to shrink the tumor to avoid disability.

Nursing Assessment

The child or parent will often discover an asymptomatic mass and seek medical attention at that time. Obtain a health history, noting recent illness, when the mass was discovered, and whether it has changed since first noted. Examine the history for risk factors such as parental smoking, exposure to environmental chemicals, family history of cancer, or neurofibromatosis. Note respiratory effort and cough, and auscultate the lungs for adventitious sounds. Palpate for lymphadenopathy. Palpate the abdomen for a mass or hepatosplenomegaly. Abnormalities found on physical examination depend on the location of the rhabdomyosarcoma (Table 46.11).

TABLE 46.11 • Presenting Signs and Symptoms Related to Location of Rhabdomyosarcoma

Location of Tumor	Presenting Signs and Symptoms
Orbit	Proptosis
Middle ear	Drainage, pain, facial nerve palsy
Sinuses	Discharge, pain, sinusitis, facial swelling
Nasopharynx	Pain, epistaxis, dysphagia, nasal quality to speech, airway obstruction
Neck	Dysphagia, hoarseness
Thorax, testicle, extremities	Enlarging mass, painless
Retroperitoneum	Gastrointestinal and urinary tract obstruction, pain, weakness, paresthesia
Bladder, prostate	Hematuria, urinary obstruction
Vagina	Mass, vaginal bleeding or chronic discharge

Data from Okcu, M. F., & Hicks, J. (2023). Rhabdomyosarcoma in childhood and adolescence: Clinical presentation, diagnostic evaluation, and staging. *UpToDate*. Retrieved on April 26, 2023, from https://www.uptodate.com/contents/rhabdomyosarcoma-in-childhood-and-adolescence-clinical-presentation-diagnostic-evaluation-and-staging

Laboratory and diagnostic testing may include:

- CT scan or MRI of primary lesion and the chest for metastasis
- Open biopsy of the primary tumor for definitive diagnosis
- Bone marrow aspiration and biopsy, bone scan, and skeletal survey to determine metastasis

CLINICAL REASONING ALERT!

Primary tumors arising in the neck region may compress the child's airway. Assess work of breathing and lung sounds.

Nursing Management

Provide routine postoperative care, depending on the site of surgery. Assess for adverse effects of high-dose radiation, which is generally used to treat the primary tumor as well as metastatic sites. Administer chemotherapy as ordered and assess for adverse effects. Refer to the "Clinical Judgment and the Nursing Process" section to determine an individualized plan of care based on the child's response to the treatment.

WILMS TUMOR

Wilms tumor is the most common kidney tumor and the second most common abdominal solid tumor in children and most commonly occurs between the ages of 2 and 5 years (Keating et al., 2022). It usually affects only one kidney (Fig. 46.18). The etiology is unknown, but some

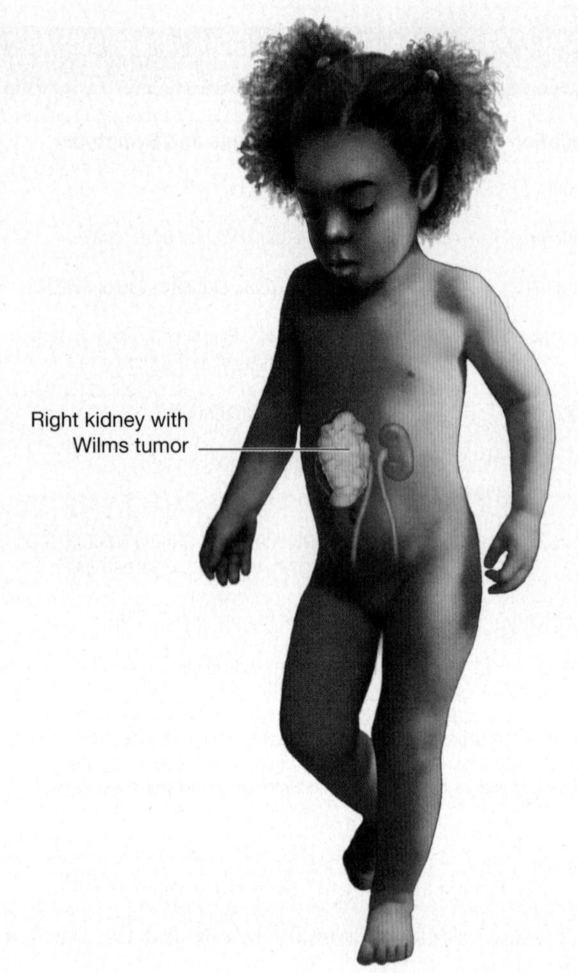

FIGURE 46.18 Wilms tumor is usually unilateral.

cases occur via genetic inheritance. Associated anomalies may occur with Wilms tumor. Wilms tumor demonstrates rapid growth and is usually large at diagnosis. Metastasis occurs via direct extension or through the bloodstream. Wilms tumor most commonly metastasizes to the perirenal tissues, liver, diaphragm, lungs, abdominal muscles, and lymph nodes.

Staging of Wilms tumor is provided in Box 46.5. The tumor is also additionally designated as having favorable histology (FH) or unfavorable histology (UH). UH is noted by the presence of anaplasia (focal or diffuse giant polypoid nuclei). The prognosis depends on staging at diagnosis and the extent of metastasis, with overall survival being more than 90% (Smith & Chintagumpala, 2023). Complications include metastasis or complications from radiation therapy such as liver or kidney damage, female sterility, bowel obstruction, pneumonia, or scoliosis.

Therapeutic Management

Surgical removal of the tumor and affected kidney (nephrectomy) is the treatment of choice and also allows for accurate staging and assessment of tumor spread. Radiation or chemotherapy may be administered either before or after surgery.

BOX 46.5 Staging of Wilms Tumor

- Stage I: unilateral, limited to kidney, completely resectable, renal capsule intact
- Stage II: unilateral, tumor extends beyond kidney but is completely resected
- Stage III: unilateral, tumor has spread outside of kidney, located in abdominal cavity only, not fully removed
- Stage IV: unilateral with metastasis in lung, liver, distant lymph node, bone, or brain
- Stage V: bilateral kidney involvement

Nursing Assessment

For a full description of the assessment phase of the nursing process, refer to "Clinical Judgment and the Nursing Process" section. Assessment findings pertinent to Wilms tumor are discussed further on.

Health History

Parents typically initially observe the abdominal mass associated with Wilms tumor and then seek medical attention. Elicit the health history, noting when the mass was discovered. Note abdominal pain, which may be related to rapid tumor growth. Document history of constipation, vomiting, anorexia, weight loss, or difficulty breathing. Determine risk factors such as hemihypertrophy of the spine, Beckwith–Wiedemann syndrome, genitourinary anomalies, absence of the iris, or family history of cancer.

Physical Examination

Measure blood pressure; hypertension occurs in 25% of children with Wilms tumor (Keating et al., 2022). Inspect the abdomen for asymmetry or a visible mass. Observe for associated anomalies, as noted previously. Auscultate the lungs for adventitious breath sounds associated with tumor metastasis. Palpate for lymphadenopathy.

TAKE NOTE!

Avoid palpating the abdomen after the initial assessment preoperatively. Wilms tumor is highly vascular and soft, so excessive handling of the tumor may result in tumor seeding and metastasis.

Laboratory and Diagnostic Testing

Laboratory and diagnostic testing may include:

- Kidney or abdominal ultrasound to assess the tumor and the contralateral kidney
- CT scan or MRI of the abdomen and chest to determine local spread to lymph nodes or adjacent organs, as well as any distant metastasis

- CBC, BUN, and creatinine: usually within normal limits
- Urinalysis: may reveal hematuria or leukocytes
- 24-hour urine collection for HVA and VMA to distinguish the tumor from neuroblastoma (levels will not be elevated with Wilms tumor)

Nursing Management

Postoperative care of the child with Wilms tumor resection is similar to that of children undergoing other abdominal surgery. Assessment of remaining kidney function is critical. The child may have adverse effects related to chemotherapy or radiation. Refer to the "Clinical Judgment and the Nursing Process" section to individualize care for the child based on the child's response to therapy.

TAKE NOTE!

To avoid injuring the remaining kidney, children with a single kidney should not play contact sports.

RETINOBLASTOMA

Retinoblastoma is a congenital, highly malignant tumor that arises from embryonic retinal cells. It accounts for 5% of cases of blindness in children (Keating et al., 2022). Most children are diagnosed by age 5, and the 5-year survival rate is 95% when the tumor is confined to the retina (Keating et al., 2022). Retinoblastoma may be hereditary or nonhereditary. Nonhereditary retinoblastoma may be associated with advanced paternal age and always presents with unilateral involvement. Hereditary retinoblastoma is inherited via the autosomal dominant mode. These cases may be unilateral or bilateral. The tumor may grow forward into the vitreous cavity of the eye or extend into the subretinal space, causing retinal detachment. The tumor may extend into the choroid, the sclera, and the optic nerve.

Complications include spread to the brain and the opposite eye, as well as metastasis to lymph nodes, bone, bone marrow, and liver. Secondary tumors, most often sarcomas, may also occur in children who have been treated for retinoblastoma. Table 46.12 explains the classification of retinoblastoma.

The goals of treatment are to eradicate the tumor, preserve vision, and provide a good cosmetic outcome. Retinoblastoma may be treated with radiation, chemotherapy, laser surgery, cryotherapy, or a combination of these treatments. Moderate vision may be preserved for most children without advanced disease. In advanced disease or in the case of a massive tumor with retinal detachment, enucleation (removal of the eye) is necessary.

Nursing Assessment

Parents are often the first to notice the "cat's eye reflex" or "whitewash glow" to the child's affected pupil. Obtain the health history, determining when other associated symptoms such as strabismus, orbital inflammation, vomiting, or headache began. Inquire about risk factors such as a family history of retinoblastoma or other cancer, or the presence of chromosomal anomalies. Assess pupils for size and reactivity to light. Note the presence of leukocoria ("cat's eye reflex," a whitish appearance of the pupil) in the affected eye (Fig. 46.19). Assess the eyes for associated signs, which may include erythema, orbital inflammation, or hyphema.

TABLE 46.12 • Classification of Retinoblastoma

Classification	Clinical Findings
A (very low risk)	Small discrete tumor distant from critical structures
B (low risk)	Discrete retinal tumor without subretinal or vitreous seeding
C (moderate risk)	Discrete retinal tumor with only focal subretinal or vitreous seeding
D (high risk)	Large nondiscrete eye tumor(s) and/or diffuse subretinal or vitreous seeding
E (very high risk)	Anatomic or functional destruction of eye by the tumor

Data from Berry, J. L. (2023). Retinoblastoma: Clinical presentation, evaluation, and diagnosis. *UpToDate.* Retrieved on April 26, 2023, from https://www.uptodate.com/contents/retinoblastoma-clinical-presentation-evaluation-and-diagnosis/print

Diagnostic evaluation includes an ophthalmologic examination under anesthesia. CT, MRI, or ultrasound of the head and eyes will help to visualize the tumor. The infant or toddler may also undergo lumbar puncture and bone marrow aspiration to determine the presence and extent of metastasis.

Nursing Management

Provide routine postoperative care to the infant or toddler. If the eye is enucleated, observe the large pressure dressing on

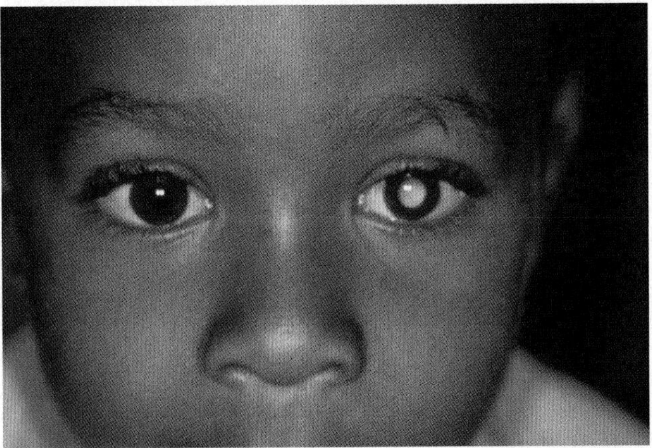

FIGURE 46.19 Note the whitish appearance of this child's pupil (leukocoria). (Reprinted with permission from Strayer, D. E., & Saffitz, J. E. [2019]. *Rubin's pathology: Mechanisms of human disease* [8th ed.]. Wolters Kluwer.)

the eye socket for bleeding. Dressing changes to the socket may include sterile saline rinses and/or antibiotic ointment application. If disease occurs outside of the eye or if metastasis is present, inform the parents that chemotherapy will be necessary. Monitor for side effects of chemotherapy (see the "Clinical Judgment and the Nursing Process" section).

Follow-up will include eye examinations every 3 to 6 months until age 6 and then annually to check for further tumor development. If the eye is enucleated, a prosthetic eye will be fitted several weeks after removal. Teach families use of the prosthetic eye; it does not require daily removal.

Provide parents with support and encouragement. Refer the family for genetic counseling. Children with a family history of retinoblastoma need ophthalmologic examination shortly after birth, at age 1 month, at age 2 months, every 3 months until age 3 years, and then at 4-to-6-month intervals until age 7 years (Berry, 2023).

TAKE NOTE!

Educate parents about protecting vision in the remaining eye: routine eye checkups, protection from accidental injury, use of safety goggles during sports, and prompt treatment of eye infections. Generally, children with one eye should not participate in contact sports.

SCREENING FOR REPRODUCTIVE CANCERS IN ADOLESCENTS

Increasingly, reproductive cancers are being diagnosed in adolescents. Cervical cancer and testicular cancer may be discovered early with appropriate screening, and earlier discovery leads to better outcomes. Starting screening in the adolescent years may also instill a lifelong healthy habit in the adolescent.

Cervical Cancer

Risk factors for cervical cancer include young age at first intercourse, infection with a sexually transmitted disease, and a history of multiple sex partners. More and more adolescents are presenting with these risk factors. Cervical cancer may be prevented through use of the human papillomavirus (HPV) vaccine, which is recommended to be given as a two-dose series to all children between 9 and 11 years of age (Fenton & Perkins, 2022). Despite the availability of the vaccine, not all children will receive it. Counsel all sexually active adolescents to seek reproductive care, which is available without parental consent in most states. The screening Papanicolaou (Pap) smear is efficient and reliable at determining abnormal cervical cells and is a key part of screening for cervical cancer (if cancer is present, the parent will have to be notified). Cervical cancer has a high response to therapy and rate of cure if treated in its early stages. Therefore, encourage adolescents to be responsible for their sexual health by seeking appropriate examination and screening. See the Healthy People 2030 box.

HEALTHY PEOPLE 2030

Objective	Nursing Significance
Increase the proportion of females who receive a cervical cancer screening based on the most recent guidelines.	When an adolescent female makes the decision to become sexually active, counsel them about the importance of getting annual Pap smears, which should begin within 3 years of becoming sexually active.

Healthy People Objectives retrieved from http://www.healthypeople.gov

Testicular Cancer

Although uncommon in adolescents, testicular cancer is most frequently diagnosed in young adult males (NCI, n.d.). It is one of the most curable cancers if diagnosed early. To get into the habit of screening for testicular lumps, encourage adolescents to begin performing testicular self-examinations monthly (Teaching Guidelines 46.5). See the Healthy People 2030 box.

TEACHING GUIDELINES 46.5 Testicular Self-Examination

- Perform the examination once a month, after a shower.
- Be familiar with the size and weight of your testicles.
- Roll the testicle between your fingers. The small rope-like structure is the epididymis; this is normal.
- Report any lump, swelling, or heaviness of one testicle to your health care provider or nurse practitioner.

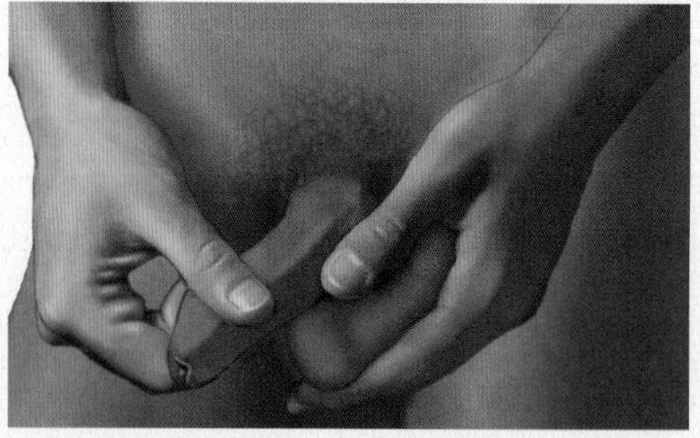

Based on Figueroa, T. E. (2021). *How to do a testicular self-exam.* http://kidshealth.org/teen/sexual_health/guys/tse.html

HEALTHY PEOPLE 2030

Objective	Nursing Significance
Reduce the overall cancer death rate. Increase the proportion of cancer survivors who are living 5 years or longer after diagnosis.	• Teach adolescents testicular self-examination. • Reinforce the importance of this self-screening measure at subsequent visits.

Healthy People Objectives retrieved from http://www.healthypeople.gov

Unfolding Patient Stories: Brittany Long • Part 2

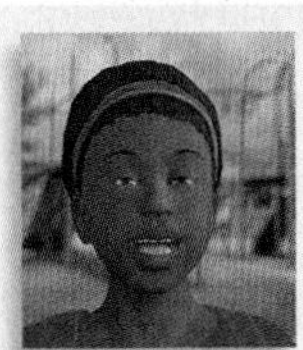

Think back to Brittany Long, whom you met in Chapter 35. Brittany is a 5-year-old Black child diagnosed with sickle cell anemia who lives with her parent, 7-year-old sister, and grandparent. Her pain crises are mostly managed at home, and she has been hospitalized three times. How can the nurse help Brittany and her family cope with a long-term illness and the management of acute crises? How can the reactions of family members influence Brittany's adjustment to sickle cell disease? What effect can a long-term illness have on the sister, and what actions can support her understanding and cooperation?

Care for Brittany and other patients in a realistic virtual environment: ***vSim** for Nursing* (thepoint.lww.com/vSimPediatric). Practice documenting these patients' care in DocuCare (thePoint.lww.com/DocuCareEHR).

KEY CONCEPTS

- The major forms of anemia affecting children are iron-deficiency anemia, lead poisoning, folic acid deficiency, pernicious anemia, sickle cell anemia, thalassemia, and G6PD deficiency.
- The major bleeding disorders affecting children are idiopathic thrombocytopenic purpura, immunoglobulin A vasculitis, DIC, hemophilia, and vWD.
- Childhood cancer tends to develop from embryonal tissue; in general, it is more responsive to therapy than adult cancers, which tend to be derived from epithelial tissue.
- In adults, cancer is influenced to a large extent by environmental factors. Cancer in children is most often not attributed to environmental factors, so generally, there are no routine screening measures or prevention strategies for childhood cancer.
- The pain associated with lumbar puncture or bone marrow aspiration may be minimized with the use of topical anesthetics or conscious sedation.
- CT scans and MRI are used extensively in the diagnosis and follow-up of childhood cancer. The young child may have difficulty holding still for these scans and may need short-term sedation.
- Assess for hypoxia, fatigue, and pallor in the child with anemia.
- Nursing assessment for the child with a bleeding disorder focuses on determining its extent and severity.
- Supplementation with iron is the key intervention for the child with iron-deficiency anemia.
- All young children should be screened for lead exposure.
- Prevention of infection and vaso-occlusive episodes takes priority in children with SCA.
- Multimodal pain management and astute physical assessment for serious complications are critical in the nursing care of the child having a sickle cell crisis.
- The priority intervention for management of thalassemia is chronic transfusion of PRBCs and chelation of iron.
- Idiopathic thrombocytopenic purpura and immunoglobulin A vasculitis are usually self-limiting diseases.
- Administration of factor VIII or desmopressin is the key nursing intervention when a bleeding episode occurs in the child with hemophilia A (desmopressin is also used for vWD).
- Significant anemia may result in hypoxia to the tissues.
- Prolonged bleeding times place the child at risk for hemorrhage.
- Prevention of injury is key for all children with hematologic disorders. Leukemia often presents in children with a history of fever, infection, and fatigue. Bone pain or CNS symptoms may be present if metastasis to the bone or brain has occurred.
- Lymphomas in children present similarly to those in adults, often with an enlarged, nontender lymph node.
- Symptoms of brain tumors depend on the location of the tumor; commonly, they present with signs and symptoms of increased intracranial pressure, such as headache, nausea, and vomiting.
- Neuroblastoma has often significantly metastasized at diagnosis. It most commonly presents as a mass in the abdomen.
- Shortness of breath or chest pain in the child with cancer is a medical emergency; it may indicate superior vena cava syndrome or a tumor in the mediastinal region.
- Retinoblastoma may be identified by the presence of leukocoria in one or both eyes. Retinoblastoma occurs in early infancy up until early childhood.
- Bone cancer does not necessarily require amputation; it may be treated with a combination of limb salvage procedure, radiation, and chemotherapy.
- The symptoms of rhabdomyosarcoma depend on the location of the tumor.

- Avoid abdominal palpation preoperatively in the child with Wilms tumor; palpation may cause seeding of the tumor and metastasis.
- Radiation therapy may result in fatigue, nausea, and vomiting, and long-term cognitive sequelae (if directed to the cranium).
- Nursing care of the child receiving treatment for cancer focuses on preventing or treating adverse effects such as fatigue, nausea, vomiting, alopecia, mucositis, and infection.
- The neutropenic child with fever should receive medical attention as soon as possible so that intravenous antibiotics may be started immediately.
- Cancer is a significant stressor for children and families. Families need support and education throughout the diagnostic process, treatment and cure, or palliative care.
- The child with cancer should lead as near normal a life as possible. When physically able and cleared by the oncologist, the child should resume usual activities such as school. Camps for children with cancer provide an excellent opportunity for children to enjoy everyday activities and meet children experiencing similar alterations in their lives.
- Nutrition may be optimized for children with cancer by managing nausea and vomiting with antiemetics, providing favorite foods, and possibly using total parenteral nutrition.
- Child and family teaching for anemias resulting from nutritional deficiencies focuses on promotion of a diet high in the deficient nutrients.
- Child and family teaching for bleeding disorders focuses on the prevention of injury.
- Numerous nationwide and local resources are available to children with hematologic disorders or nutritional deficits. These organizations offer a wide range of services, including education, support, multidisciplinary care (as appropriate), and financial assistance in caring for the disease.
- Teach adolescents appropriate screening techniques for reproductive cancers.
- Educate the child and family about the adverse effects of cancer treatments.
- Teach parents how to avoid infection in the child receiving chemotherapy, the signs and symptoms of infection, and when to seek medical treatment.

REFERENCES AND RECOMMENDED READINGS

Ahmed, N. M., & Flynn, P. M. (2022). Fever in children with chemotherapy-induced neutropenia. *UpToDate*. Retrieved on February 17, 2024, from https://www.uptodate.com/contents/fever-in-children-with-chemotherapy-induced-neutropenia

American Academy of Orthopedic Surgeons. (2023). *Ewing's sarcoma*. https://orthoinfo.aaos.org/en/diseases--conditions/ewings-sarcoma/

American Cancer Society. (2024a). *Cancer in children*. https://www.cancer.org/cancer/cancer-in-children.html

American Cancer Society. (2024b). *Chemotherapy*. https://www.cancer.org/treatment/treatments-and-side-effects/treatment-types/chemotherapy.html

American Cancer Society. (2024c). *Radiation therapy side effects*. https://www.cancer.org/treatment/treatments-and-side-effects/treatment-types/radiation/coping.html

American Cancer Society. (2024d). Risk factors for acute lymphocytic leukemia (ALL). https://www.cancer.org/cancer/types/acute-lymphocytic-leukemia/causes-risks-prevention/risk-factors.html

American Cancer Society. (2024e). *What causes Hodgkin lymphoma?* https://www.cancer.org/cancer/types/hodgkin-lymphoma/causes-risks-prevention/what-causes.html

Anzilotti, A. (2019). *Stem cell transplants*. https://kidshealth.org/en/parents/stem-cells.html

Asha, C., Manjini, K. J., & Dubashi, B. (2020). Effect of foot massage on patients with chemotherapy induced nausea and vomiting: A randomized clinical trial. *Journal of Caring Sciences, 9*(3), 120–124. https://doi.org/10.34172/jcs.2020.018

Benz, E. J., & Angelucci, E. (2022). Diagnosis of thalassemia (adults and children). *UpToDate*. Retrieved on February 17, 2024, from https://www.uptodate.com/contents/diagnosis-of-thalassemia-adults-and-children

Berry, J. L. (2023). Retinoblastoma: Clinical presentation, evaluation, and diagnosis. *UpToDate*. Retrieved on February 17, 2024, from https://www.uptodate.com/contents/retinoblastoma-clinical-presentation-evaluation-and-diagnosis/print

Blaney, S. M., Adamson, P. C., & Helman, L. J. (2021). *Pizzo & Poplack's pediatric oncology* (8th ed.). Wolters Kluwer.

Borhade, M. B., & Kondamudi, N. P. (2022). Sickle cell crisis. *StatPearls*. https://www.ncbi.nlm.nih.gov/books/NBK526064/

Bussell, J. B. (2022a). Immune thrombocytopenia (ITP) in children: Clinical features and diagnosis. *UpToDate*. Retrieved on February 17, 2024, from https://www.uptodate.com/contents/immune-thrombocytopenia-itp-in-children-clinical-features-and-diagnosis

Bussell, J. B. (2022b). Immune thrombocytopenia (ITP) in children: Initial management. *UpToDate*. Retrieved on February 17, 2024, from https://www.uptodate.com/contents/immune-thrombocytopenia-itp-in-children-initial-management

Centers for Disease Control and Prevention. (2023a). *Data & statistics on sickle cell disease*. https://www.cdc.gov/ncbddd/sicklecell/data.html/

Centers for Disease Control and Prevention. (2023b). *State-based monitoring for selected hemoglobinopathies*. https://www.cdc.gov/ncbddd/hemoglobinopathies/features/keyfinding-state-based.html

Centers for Disease Control and Prevention. (2024). *Childhood lead poisoning prevention program*. https://www.cdc.gov/nceh/lead/

Children's Oncology Group. (2023). *Low white blood cell count (neutropenia)*. https://www.childrensoncologygroup.org/index.php/lowwhitebloodcellcount

Corbett, J. A., & Banks, A. D. (2019). *Laboratory tests and diagnostic procedures with nursing diagnoses* (9th ed.). Pearson Education Inc.

Cunningham, F. G., Leveno, K. J., Bloom, S. L., Dashe, J. S., Hoffman, B. L., Spong, C. Y., & Casey, B. M. (2022). *Williams obstetrics* (26th ed.). McGraw-Hill Education.

CureSearch. (2022). *Childhood cancer statistics*. https://curesearch.org/Childhood-Cancer-Statistics

DeBaun, M. R. (2022). Acute vaso-occlusive pain management in sickle cell disease. *UpToDate*. Retrieved on February 17, 2024, from https://www.uptodate.com/contents/vaso-occlusive-pain-management-in-sickle-cell-disease

Diab, L. K., Haemer, M., Primark, L. E., & Krebs, N. R. (2022). Chapter 11: Normal childhood nutrition & its disorders. In M. Bunik, W. W. Hay, M. J. Levin, & M. J. Abzug (Eds.), *Current diagnosis and treatment: Pediatrics* (26th ed., pp. 269–298). McGraw-Hill Education.

Fenton, R., & Perkins, R. (2022). *Here's why your preteen needs the HPV vaccine*. https://www.healthychildren.org/English/safety-prevention/immunizations/Pages/How-to-Talk-to-Your-Preteen-About-HPV-Vaccine.aspx

Field, J. J., & Vichinsky, E. P. (2023). Overview of the management and prognosis of sickle cell disease. *UpToDate*. Retrieved on February 17, 2024, from https://www.uptodate.com/contents/overview-of-the-management-and-prognosis-of-sickle-cell-disease

Figueroa, T. E. (2021). *How to do a testicular self-exam*. http://kidshealth.org/teen/sexual_health/guys/tse.html

Fischbach, F. T., Fischbach, M. A., & Stout, K. (2022). *A manual of laboratory and diagnostic tests* (11th ed.). Wolters Kluwer Health.

Hagan, J. F., Shaw, J. S., & Duncan, P. M. (Eds.). (2017). *Bright futures: Guidelines for health supervision of infants, children, and adolescents* (4th ed.). American Academy of Pediatrics.

Halmo, L., & Nappe, T. M. (2023). *Lead toxicity*. StatPearls. https://www.ncbi.nlm.nih.gov/books/NBK541097/

Hibberd, C., Hibberd, O., Karageorgos, S., & Barnard, G. (2023). Ten oncology emergencies in kids. *Don't Forget the Bubbles*. https://doi.org/10.31440/DFTB.53725

Horton, T. M., & McNeer, J. L. (2022). Treatment of acute lymphoblastic leukemia/lymphoma in children and adolescents. *UpToDate*. Retrieved on February 17, 2024, from https://www.uptodate.com/contents/overview-of-the-treatment-of-acute-lymphoblastic-leukemia-in-children-and-adolescents

James, P. (2023). Von Willebrand disease (VWD): Treatment of major bleeding and major surgery. *UpToDate*. Retrieved on February 17, 2024, from https://www.uptodate.com/contents/treatment-of-von-willebrand-disease

Keating, A. K., Knight-Perry, J., Maloney, K., Levy, J. M. M., Greffe, B. S., Franklin, A. R. K., & Garrington, T. P. (2022). Chapter 31: Neoplastic disease. In M. Bunik, W. W. Hay, M. J. Levin, & M. J. Abzug (Eds.), *Current diagnosis & treatment: Pediatrics* (26th ed., pp. 931–963). McGraw-Hill Education.

Kline, N. E. (2014). *Essentials of pediatric oncology nursing: A core curriculum* (4th ed.). Association of Pediatric Hematology/Oncology Nurses.

LaCasce, A. S., & Ng, A. K. (2022). Pretreatment evaluation, staging, and treatment stratification of classic Hodgkin lymphoma. *UpToDate*. Retrieved on February 17, 2024, from https://www.uptodate.com/contents/pretreatment-evaluation-staging-and-treatment-stratification-of-classic-hodgkin-lymphoma

Larson, S. D., Hebra, A., Raju, R., & Lee, S. (2020). Vascular access in children. *Medscape*. https://emedicine.medscape.com/article/1018395-overview#a1

Lau, C., & Teo, W-Y. (2024). Overview of the management of central nervous system tumors in children. *UpToDate*. Retrieved on February 17, 2024, from https://www.uptodate.com/contents/overview-of-the-management-of-central-nervous-system-tumors-in-children

Lerma, E. V., & Vichinsky, E. P. (2023). Sickle cell disease effects on the kidney. *UpToDate*. Retrieved April 16, 2024, from https://www.uptodate.com/contents/sickle-cell-disease-effects-on-the-kidney

Martin, B. M., Thaniel, L. N., Speller-Brown, B. J., & Darbari, D. S. (2018). Comprehensive infant clinic for sickle cell disease: Outcomes and parental perspective. *Journal of Pediatric Health Care, 32*(5), 485–490.

Mitin, T. (2023). Radiation therapy techniques in cancer treatment. *UpToDate*. Retrieved on February 17, 2024, from https://www.uptodate.com/contents/radiation-therapy-techniques-in-cancer-treatment

National Cancer Institute. (n.d.). *Cancer stat facts: Testicular cancer*. https://seer.cancer.gov/statfacts/html/testis.html

National Cancer Institute. (2023). *Childhood cancers*. https://www.cancer.gov/types/childhood-cancers

National Cancer Institute. (2024). *Late effects of treatment for childhood cancer (PDQ®)—Health professional version*. https://www.cancer.gov/types/childhood-cancers/late-effects-hp-pdq

National Hemophilia Foundation. (2023). *MASAC document 280—MASAC recommendations concerning products licensed for the treatment of hemophilia and selected disorders of the coagulation system*. https://www.hemophilia.org/healthcare-professionals/guidelines-on-care/masac-documents/masac-document-280-masac-recommendations-concerning-products-licensed-for-the-treatment-of-hemophilia-and-selected-disorders-of-the-coagulation-system

National Hospice and Palliative Care Organization. (2022). *Standards of practice for pediatric palliative care: Quality improvement resource*. https://www.nhpco.org/wp-content/uploads/Pediatric_Standards.pdf

Navin, M. C., & Wasserman, J. A. (2019). Capacity for preferences and pediatric assent implications for pediatric practice. *Hastings Center Report, 49*(1), 43–51.

Nuss, R., McKinney, C. & Wang, M. (2022). Chapter 30: Hematologic disorders. In M. Bunik, W. W. Hay, M. J. Levin, & M. J. Abzug (Eds.), *Current diagnosis and treatment: Pediatrics* (26th ed., pp. 931–963). McGraw-Hill Education.

Nuuhiwa, J. (2022). Module 9: Boundaries and self-care. In M. Evans, J. Nuuhiwa, R. L. Secola, & K. Wolownik, *Foundations of pediatric hematopoietic stem cell transplantation* (3rd ed.). Association of Pediatric Hematology/Oncology Nurses.

Okcu, M. F., & Hicks, J. (2023). Rhabdomyosarcoma in childhood and adolescence: Clinical presentation, diagnostic evaluation, and staging. *UpToDate*. Retrieved on February 17, 2024, from https://www.uptodate.com/contents/rhabdomyosarcoma-in-childhood-and-adolescence-clinical-presentation-diagnostic-evaluation-and-staging

Powers, J. M. (2023). Iron deficiency in infants and children <12 years: Screening, prevention, clinical manifestations, and diagnosis. *UpToDate*. Retrieved on February 17, 2024, from https://www.uptodate.com/contents/iron-deficiency-in-infants-and-children-less-than12-years-screening-prevention-clinical-manifestations-and-diagnosis

Rugo, H. S., & van den Hurk, C. (2023). Alopecia related to systemic cancer therapy. *UpToDate*. Retrieved on February 17, 2024, from https://www.uptodate.com/contents/chemotherapy-induced-alopecia

Sample, J. A. (2024). Childhood lead poisoning: Management. *UpToDate*. Retrieved on February 17, 2024, from http://www.uptodate.com/contents/childhood-lead-poisoning-management

Sanofi. (2023). *FDA approves once-weekly ALTUVIIIO™, a new class of factor VIII therapy for hemophilia A that offers significant bleed protection*. https://ml-eu.globenewswire.com/Resource/Download/23793006-c334-46f9-b225-27df9c8a9285

Secola, R. (2022a). Module 2—HSCT types, selections, stem cell/cellular therapy sources. In M. Evans, J. Nuuhiwa, R. L. Secola, & K. Wolownik, *Foundations of pediatric hematopoietic stem cell transplantation* (3rd ed.). Association of Pediatric Hematology/Oncology Nurses.

Secola, R. (2022b). Module 3—Hematopoietic stem cell transplant (HSCT) conditioning regimens. In M. Evans, J. Nuuhiwa, R. L. Secola, & K. Wolownik, *Foundations of pediatric hematopoietic stem cell transplantation* (3rd ed.). Association of Pediatric Hematology/Oncology Nurses.

Shohet, J. M., Nuchtern, J. G., & Foster, J. H. (2024). Treatment and prognosis of neuroblastoma. *UpToDate*. Retrieved on February 17, 2024, from https://www.uptodate.com/contents/treatment-and-prognosis-of-neuroblastoma

Smith, V., & Chintagumpala, M. (2023). Treatment and prognosis of Wilms tumor. *UpToDate*. Retrieved June 4, 2024, from https://www.uptodate.com/contents/treatment-and-prognosis-of-wilms-tumor

UpToDate, Inc. (2024). *Lexi-comp® (Version 8.1.0) [Mobile app]*. Wolters Kluwer. https://apps.apple.com/us/app/lexicomp/id313401238

U.S. Department of Health and Human Services. (n.d.). *Healthy People 2030*. https://health.gov/healthypeople

Vichinsky, E. P. (2023). Overview of the clinical manifestations of sickle cell disease. *UpToDate*. Retrieved on April 19, 2023, from https://www.uptodate.com/contents/overview-of-the-clinical-manifestations-of-sickle-cell-disease

DEVELOPING CLINICAL JUDGMENT

PRACTICING FOR NCLEX

1. A child on the pediatric unit has morning laboratory results of Hgb 10.0, Hct 30.2, WBC 24,000, and platelets 20,000. What is the priority nursing assessment?

a. Assess for pallor, fatigue, and tachycardia.
b. Monitor for fever.
c. Assess for bruising or bleeding.
d. Determine intake and output.

2. A child with hemophilia A fell while riding his bicycle. He was wearing a helmet and did not lose consciousness. He has a mild abrasion on his knee that is not oozing. He is complaining of abdominal pain. What is the priority nursing assessment?

a. Perform neurologic checks.
b. Assess ability to void frequently.
c. Carefully assess his abdomen.
d. Examine his knee frequently.

3. A 14-year-old with thalassemia asks for your assistance in choosing her afternoon snack. Which choice is the most appropriate?

a. Peanut butter with rice cake
b. Small spinach salad
c. Apple slices with cheddar cheese
d. Small burger on wheat bun

4. The nurse is caring for a child who has just been admitted to the pediatric unit with sickle cell crisis. He is complaining that his right arm and leg hurt. What is the priority nursing intervention?

a. Administer pain medication every 3 hours intravenously until pain is controlled.
b. Perform passive ROM of the arm and leg to maintain function.
c. Try acetaminophen for pain first, moving up to opioids only if needed.
d. Use narcotic analgesics and warm compresses as needed to control the pain.

5. A 5-year-old has been diagnosed with Wilms tumor. What is the priority nursing intervention for this child?

a. Educate the parents about dialysis, as the kidney will be removed.
b. Measure abdominal girth every shift.
c. Avoid palpating the child's abdomen.
d. Monitor BUN and creatinine every 4 hours.

6. A child with leukemia has the following AM laboratory results: Hgb 8.0, Hct 24.2, WBC 8,000, platelets 150,000. What is the priority nursing assessment?

a. Monitor for fever.
b. Assess for bruising or bleeding.
c. Determine intake and output.
d. Assess for pallor, fatigue, and tachycardia.

7. A child with leukemia received chemotherapy about 10 days ago. She presents today with a temperature of 100.4°F, an absolute neutrophil count of 500, and mild bleeding of the gums. What is the priority nursing intervention?

a. Administer IV antibiotics as ordered.
b. Provide vigorous oral care frequently with a firm toothbrush.
c. Monitor pulse and blood pressure for changes.
d. Administer packed RBC transfusion.

8. A child with cancer is receiving chemotherapy, and their parent is concerned that the nausea and vomiting associated with chemotherapy are reducing his ability to eat and gain weight appropriately. Which is the appropriate nursing action?

a. Administer an antiemetic at the first hint of nausea.
b. Offer the child's favorite foods to encourage him to eat.
c. Start antiemetic drugs prior to the chemotherapy infusion.
d. Maintain IV fluid infusion to avoid dehydration.

9. A child is admitted to the hospital with the diagnosis of acute lymphoblastic leukemia (ALL). Which clinical manifestations require the most urgent nursing intervention? Select all that apply.

a. Anorexia
b. Enlarged cervical lymph nodes
c. Fatigue
d. Fever
e. Hepatomegaly
f. Lethargy
g. Petechiae
h. Splenomegaly

10. A child has been newly diagnosed with leukemia, and the nurse has reviewed the child's laboratory report.

Test	Traditional Units	SI Units
Hgb	11.1 g/dL	6.89 mmol/L
Hct	35.6%	0.365
WBC	6,750 mm^3	6.75 * 109/L
Platelets	39,000 mm^3	39 * 109/L

The child is at risk for ________, related to ________.

Blank 1:
a. activity intolerance
b. bleeding
c. impaired tissue perfusion
d. infection

Blank 2:
a. hemoglobin level
b. hematocrit
c. platelet count
d. WBC count

DOSAGE CALCULATION QUESTION

The nurse is caring for a 4-year-old with acute lymphoblastic leukemia. The child weighs 38 lb. The medication order reads: ondansetron 2.6 mg IV every 8 hours for chemotherapy-related nausea/vomiting. Ondansetron is supplied as 4 mg/2 mL. How many milliliters will the nurse administer? Round to the nearest tenth.

CRITICAL THINKING EXERCISES

1. Develop a discharge teaching plan for the parent of a toddler who has just been diagnosed with hemophilia and received factor infusion treatment for a bleeding episode.
2. An 8-year-old has been diagnosed with iron-deficiency anemia. Formulate a nutrition plan for this child.
3. A 5-year-old with beta-thalassemia is resistant to nightly chelation therapy at home. Devise a developmentally appropriate teaching plan for this child.
4. Develop a nursing care plan for a child with sickle cell disease who experiences frequent vaso-occlusive crises.
5. Develop a discharge teaching plan for a child who has just completed the induction phase of chemotherapy for acute lymphocytic leukemia.
6. A 17-year-old female has recently been diagnosed with osteosarcoma. She is worried about how treatment will affect her plans for college, marriage, and children. How will you respond to her concerns?
7. A 3-year-old is going to be starting chemotherapy for rhabdomyosarcoma. Develop an age-appropriate teaching plan for this child.
8. Develop a nursing care plan for an adolescent with cancer who is undergoing radiation and chemotherapy and experiencing a significant number of adverse effects from the treatment.

STUDY ACTIVITIES

1. Visit your local WIC office. Meet with the staff and learn about the services offered for prevention of and nutritional support for anemia. Provide a written report of your learning experience or provide a presentation to your classmates.
2. In the clinical setting, compare the growth and development of a child with sickle cell disease to that of a similarly aged child who has been healthy.
3. Talk to an adolescent with hemophilia about their life experiences and feelings about their disease and their health. Reflect on this conversation in your clinical journal.
4. Visit a public health clinic that provides primary care to children. Spend time with the registered nurse (RN), the advanced practice nurse, and the unlicensed assistive personnel. Write a summary of the roles of the RN in screening for and managing hematologic disorders in children, noting roles that are reserved for the advanced practice nurse and activities that the RN would delegate to unlicensed assistive personnel.
5. While in the clinical area, care for a young child who has undergone therapy for a brain tumor. Compare this child's growth and development to those of a healthy child of similar age whom you know or have cared for.
6. During your clinical rotation, care for a child who has received several chemotherapy treatments. After establishing a therapeutic relationship, talk with the child about their understanding of the disease and the experience the child has had with diagnosis and treatment thus far. If time allows, ask the child to draw a picture describing this experience. Record your observations in your clinical journal, and reflect on the emotions you feel about this experience.
7. Attend the pediatric oncology clinic. Determine the role of the advanced practice nurse (nurse practitioner or clinical nurse specialist) compared to the role of the RN in the outpatient care of children with cancer. Determine which activities the nurse appropriately delegates to unlicensed assistive personnel in that setting.
8. Talk to the hospital chaplain about their experiences with dying children. Reflect on this conversation in your clinical journal.

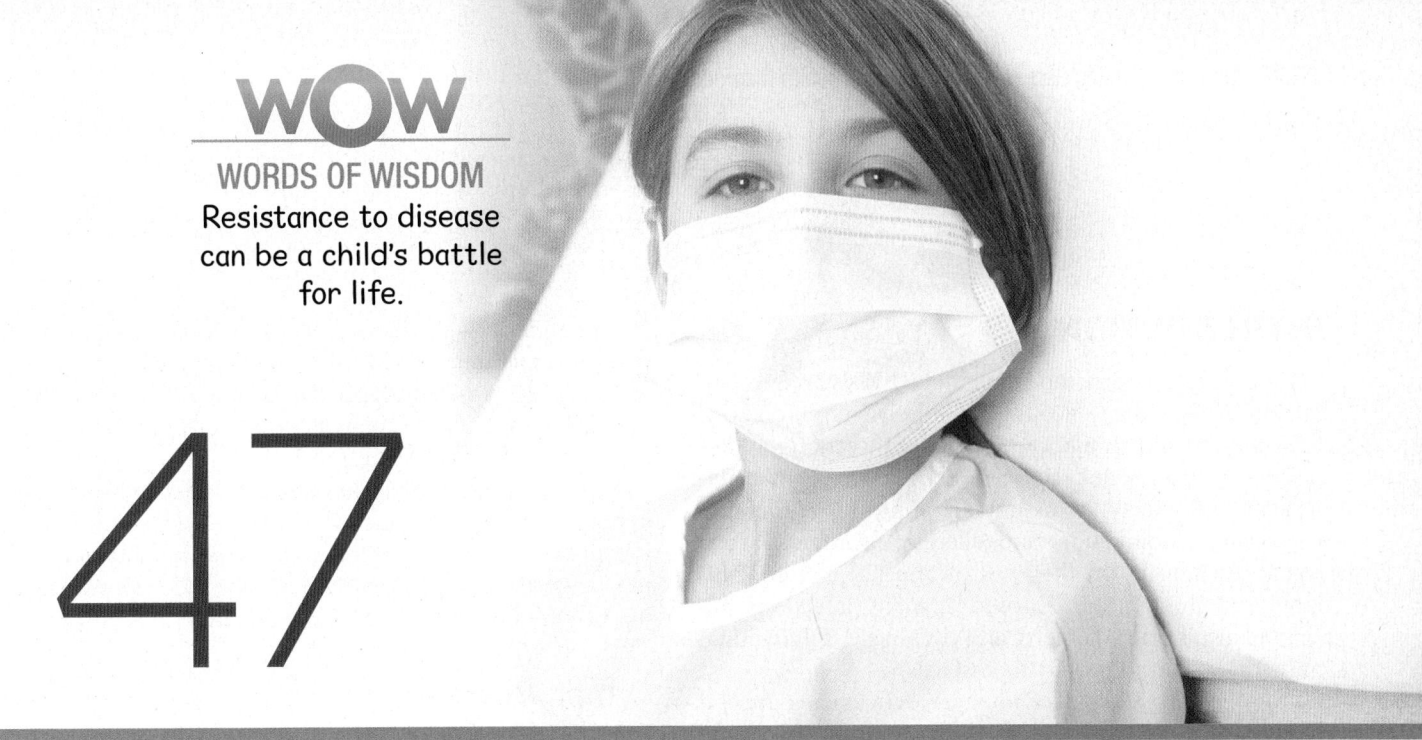

Resistance to disease can be a child's battle for life.

47

Nursing Care of the Child With an Alteration in Immunity or Immunologic Disorder

LEARNING OBJECTIVES

Upon completion of the chapter, you will be able to:

1. Explain the anatomic and physiologic differences of the immune systems of infants and children compared to that of adults.
2. Describe nursing care related to common laboratory and diagnostic testing used in the medical diagnosis of pediatric immune and autoimmune disorders.
3. Distinguish immune, autoimmune, and allergic disorders common in infants, children, and adolescents.
4. Identify appropriate nursing assessments and interventions related to medications and treatments for pediatric immune, autoimmune, and allergic disorders.
5. Develop an individualized nursing care plan or concept map for the child with an immune or autoimmune disorder.
6. Describe the psychosocial impact of chronic immune disorders on children.
7. Devise a nutrition plan for the child with immunodeficiency.
8. Develop child and family teaching plans for the child with an immune or autoimmune disorder.

KEY TERMS

antibodies
antigen
autoantibodies
cellular immunity
chemotaxis (kē′mō-tak′sis)
humoral immunity
immunodeficiency
immunoglobulins
immunosuppressive
opsonization (op′sŏ-nī-zā′shŭn)
phagocytosis (fāg′ō-sī-tō′sis)

Lakeisha Harris, 15 years old, is brought to the clinic by her parent. She presents with complaints of pain and swelling in her joints, weight gain, and fatigue. Lakeisha states, "I'm just very tired all the time, and my knees and ankles ache."

INTRODUCTION

Immunity refers to natural or induced resistance to infection. Nurses may encounter children with alterations in immunity and should be familiar with various immunologic disorders that children experience. **Immunodeficiency** (incapacity to mount an appropriate immune response), autoimmune, and allergic disorders have a significant impact on the lives of affected children. Infants and children are exposed to many infectious microorganisms and allergens and thus need a functional immune system to protect themselves.

Primary or secondary immune deficiencies are the focus of this discussion, along with allergy and anaphylaxis. These immune disorders are chronic, and affected children have more infections compared with healthy children. Recurrent viral or bacterial infections may cause the child to miss significant amounts of school or playtime with other children. Many immunodeficiencies require chronic and frequent clinic visits as well as daily medications. This can be a stress on the family as well. Autoimmune disorders are also chronic, causing significant disruption to the child's and family's life. Allergic disorders in some children may cause significant stress for the child and family. Nurses who care for children need to be familiar with common immunodeficiencies, autoimmune disorders, and allergies to intervene effectively with children and their families.

VARIATIONS IN PEDIATRIC ANATOMY AND PHYSIOLOGY

Normal immune function is a complex process involving **phagocytosis** (process by which phagocytes swallow up and break down microorganisms), **humoral immunity** (immunity mediated by antibodies secreted by B cells), **cellular immunity** (cell-mediated immunity controlled by T cells), and activation of the complement system. The lymphatic system and the white blood cells (WBCs) are the primary players in the immune response. Although these structures and cells are present at birth, the healthy full-term infant's immune system is still immature. The newborn exhibits a decreased inflammatory response to invading organisms, and this increases their susceptibility to infection. Cellular immunity is generally functional at birth, and as the infant is exposed to various substances over time, humoral immunity develops. Comparison Chart 47.1 provides more information on humoral and cellular immunity.

Lymph System

Lymph nodes in the newborn are relatively small, soft, and difficult to palpate. As the infant is exposed to various germs or illnesses, the lymph system passively filters plasma for bacteria or other foreign material before returning it to the bloodstream and back to the heart. As WBCs infiltrate the lymph nodes to attack the foreign substance, the nodes enlarge. Young children have frequent episodes of localized enlarged lymph nodes because of their repeated exposure to viral illnesses (Tosi, 2019). The spleen is functional at birth and also filters the blood for foreign cells. The thymus, responsible for the production of lymphocyte T cells as well as for the development and maturation of peripheral lymphoid tissue, is quite enlarged at birth and remains so until about 10 years of age. It then involutes slowly throughout adulthood. The tonsils are also often enlarged throughout early childhood. The bone marrow is functional at birth, producing stem cells capable of differentiating into various blood cells.

Phagocytosis

Under conditions of stress, the newborn and infant exhibit decreased phagocytic activity. The complement system, which is responsible for **opsonization** (process of making microorganisms more susceptible to phagocytosis) and **chemotaxis** (movement of neutrophils toward microorganisms),

COMPARISON CHART 47.1 Humoral Versus Cellular Immunity

Humoral Immunity (Antibody Protection)	Cellular Immunity (Cell-Mediated Immune Response)
• Lymphocytes: B cells	• Lymphocytes: T cells
• Secrete antibodies to viruses and bacteria; antibodies mark the antigen cell for destruction.	• Direct and regulate immune response (helper T cells).
• Recognize antigens.	• Do not recognize antigens.
• Do not destroy the foreign cell.	• Attack infected or foreign cells (killer T cells and natural killer cells).
• Cross the placenta in the form of IgG.	• Do not cross the placenta.

IgG, immunoglobulin G.

is immature in the newborn but reaches adult levels of activity by 3 to 6 months of age. The infant's phagocytic cells (neutrophils and monocytes) demonstrate decreased chemotaxis, reaching adult levels when the child is several years old. With complement levels being only 50% to 75% of adult levels in the full-term infant, decreased opsonization may be responsible for decreased phagocytic activity compared with adults.

Cellular Immunity

Maternal T cells do not cross the placenta, so the fetal thymus begins production of T cells early in gestation, and the newborn demonstrates a relative lymphocytosis compared with the adult, probably due to increased amounts of T-cell lymphocytes. Although cellular immunity does not cross the placenta, the fetal T cells may become sensitized to antigens that do cross the placenta. Viral infection, hyperbilirubinemia, and drugs taken by the pregnant parent late in pregnancy may contribute to depressed T-cell function in the newborn. Since delayed hypersensitivity reactions are mediated by T cells rather than antibodies, skin test responses (such as purified protein derivative [PPD] for tuberculosis detection) are diminished until about 1 year of age, probably due to the infant's decreased ability to mount an inflammatory response.

Humoral Immunity

The newborn's B cells do not respond as well to infection as do adults'. B cells are responsible for the formation of **antibodies** (specific immunity). The antibodies bind to the **antigen** (substance stimulating an immune response), thus disabling the specific toxin. The fetus is normally in an antigen-free environment and so produces only trace amounts of **immunoglobulins** (Ig; gamma globulin antibody proteins), specifically IgM. Most of the newborn's IgG is acquired transplacentally from the pregnant parent. Hence, the newborn exhibits passive immunity to antigens to which the pregnant parent had developed antibodies. These antibodies wane over the initial months of life as the transplacental IgG is catabolized, having a half-life of only about 25 days.

The newborn begins to make IgG but ordinarily experiences a physiologic hypogammaglobulinemia between 2 and 6 months of age until self-production of IgG reaches higher levels. The breastfed infant will acquire passive transfer of maternal immunity via the breast milk and will be better protected during the physiologic hypogammaglobulinemia phase. By 1 year of age, IgG is 50% of the adult level, and by 7 years of age it reaches the average adult level.

IgA, IgD, IgE, and IgM do not cross the placenta; they require an antigenic challenge for production. IgD and IgE constitute a very small percentage of the immunoglobulins in all ages. IgA increases slowly to about 30% of the adult level at 2 years of age, reaching near-adult levels by age 10 to 13 years. IgM is close to the adult level by 4 years of age (Mayo Foundation for Clinical Education and Research, 2024).

COMMON MEDICAL TREATMENTS

A variety of medications and other medical treatments are used to treat immune deficiencies and autoimmune problems in children. Most of these treatments will require a health care provider's or nurse practitioner's order when the child is in the hospital. The most common treatments and medications are listed in Common Medical Treatments 47.1 and Drug Guide 47.1. The nurse caring for the child with an immune deficiency or autoimmune disorder should be familiar with what the procedures and medications are, how they work, and common nursing implications related to use of these modalities.

COMMON MEDICAL TREATMENTS 47.1

Treatment	Explanation	Indications	Nursing Implications
Immunizations	Killed or modified microorganisms, or components of them, cause the immune system to develop antibodies to the microorganism without developing disease.	Prevention of certain viral and bacterial infections	Do not administer live vaccines to immunosuppressed people. Refer to the individual vaccine for method of administration and contraindications. Report adverse reactions via the vaccine adverse reaction (VAR) reporting system.
Bone marrow or stem cell transplantation	Bone marrow transplant: transfer of healthy bone marrow into the bones of a person with immune malfunction; the transplanted cells can then develop into functional B and T cells Stem cell transplant: Peripheral stem cells are removed from the donor via apheresis or stem cells are retrieved from the umbilical cord and placenta. The stem cells are then transplanted into the recipient	Wiskott–Aldrich syndrome, severe combined immune deficiency (SCID)	Administer immunosuppressive medications as ordered. Maintain medical asepsis and protective isolation to prevent infection. Monitor closely for graft-versus-host disease. Provide meticulous oral care. Avoid rectal temperatures and suppositories. Encourage appropriate nutrition.

DRUG GUIDE 47.1

COMMON DRUGS FOR IMMUNOLOGIC DISORDERS

Medication	Actions/Indications	Nursing Implications
Intravenous immune globulin (IVIG)	Provides exogenous IgG antibodies Indicated for primary immune deficiencies, human immunodeficiency virus (HIV) infection, myasthenia gravis	Do not mix with IV medications or with other IV fluids. Do not give IM or SQ. Monitor vital signs and watch for adverse reactions frequently during infusion. May require antipyretic or antihistamine to prevent chills and fever during infusion Have epinephrine available during infusion.
Nucleoside analog reverse transcriptase inhibitors (NRTIs): abacavir, lamivudine, zidovudine	Inhibit reverse transcription of the viral DNA chain. For treatment of HIV-1 infection as part of a three-drug regimen; zidovudine is also used to prevent perinatal transmission of HIV.	Notify health care provider of muscle weakness, shortness of breath, headache, insomnia, rash, or unusual bleeding. Give IV zidovudine over 1 hour. Fatal hypersensitivity reaction may occur with abacavir.
Nonnucleoside analog reverse transcriptase inhibitors (NNRTIs): efavirenz, nevirapine	Bind to HIV-1 reverse transcriptase, blocking DNA polymerase activity and disrupting the virus life cycle; used for treatment of HIV-1 infection as part of a three-drug regimen	*Nevirapine*: Avoid St. John's wort. Shake suspension gently before administration. Observe for symptoms of Stevens–Johnson syndrome. *Efavirenz*: May cause drowsiness
Protease inhibitors: amprenavir, atazanavir, indinavir, lopinavir, nelfinavir, ritonavir, saquinavir	Inhibit protease activity in the HIV-1 cell, resulting in immature, noninfectious viral particles; used for treatment of HIV-1 infection as part of a three-drug regimen	Multiple drug interactions; review specific medication for adverse effects and administration implications.
Nonsteroidal antiinflammatory drugs (NSAIDs): diclofenac, ibuprofen, naproxen, others	Inhibit prostaglandin synthesis, antiinflammatory action Indicated for juvenile idiopathic arthritis	Administer with food to decrease GI upset. May cause gastric bleeding, increased liver enzymes, decreased kidney function Monitor liver enzymes. Do not crush or chew extended-release or timed-release preparations.
Neuromuscular blocking agent: pyridostigmine	Cholinergic for myasthenia gravis—inhibits destruction of acetylcholine	Note muscle strength, heart rate, and respirations. Overdose may result in a cholinergic crisis. Monitor for sweating, salivation, urinary incontinence.
Corticosteroids	Antiinflammatory and immunosuppressive action; used for juvenile idiopathic arthritis, systemic lupus erythematosus (SLE), myasthenia gravis, and immunosuppression in children with bone marrow or stem cell transplants	Administer with food to decrease GI upset. May mask signs of infection Monitor blood pressure and urine for glucose. Do not stop treatment abruptly, or acute adrenal insufficiency may occur. Monitor for Cushing syndrome. Doses may be tapered over time. *Intravenous pulse:* Monitor for hypertension during infusion.
Cytotoxic drugs (cyclophosphamide)	Interfere with normal function of DNA by alkylation; for treatment of severe SLE	Cause bone marrow suppression; monitor for signs of infection. *Cyclophosphamide*: Administer in the morning. Provide adequate hydration and have child void frequently during and after infusion to decrease risk of hemorrhagic cystitis.
Immunosuppressant drugs (cyclosporine A [CyA], azathioprine)	Inhibition of production and release of interleukin II (CyA) Antagonize purine metabolism (azathioprine); used for severe steroid-resistant autoimmune disease	Monitor CBC, serum creatinine, potassium, and magnesium. Monitor blood pressure and watch for signs of infection. Draw blood levels before morning dose. *CyA*: Do not give with grapefruit juice.

DRUG GUIDE 47.1

COMMON DRUGS FOR IMMUNOLOGIC DISORDERS

Medication	Actions/Indications	Nursing Implications
Antimalarial drugs: hydroxychloroquine sulfate	Impair complement-dependent antigen–antibody reactions to prevent flares in SLE and juvenile arthritis	Funduscopic eye examination and visual field testing every year
Disease-modifying antirheumatic drugs (DMARDs): methotrexate, etanercept	Methotrexate: antimetabolite that depletes DNA precursors, inhibits DNA and urine synthesis Etanercept: binds to tumor necrosis factor (TNF), rendering it ineffective. Used for severe polyarticular juvenile arthritis	*Methotrexate*: Do not give oral form with dairy products. Approximate time to benefit in treatment of arthritis is 3–6 weeks. Salicylates may delay clearance. Protect IV preparation from light. Monitor CBC, kidney and liver function, and symptoms of infection. *Etanercept*: Monitor closely for infection. Do not give live vaccines. Give SQ, twice weekly; effect in 1 week to 3 months

CBC, complete blood count; GI, gastrointestinal; IM, intramuscularly; IV, intravenous; SQ, subcutaneously.

Data from UpToDate, Inc. (2024). *Lexi-comp®* (Version 8.1.0) [Mobile app]. Wolters Kluwer. https://apps.apple.com/us/app/lexicomp/id313401238

COMMON LABORATORY AND DIAGNOSTIC TESTS 47.1

Test	Explanation	Indications	Nursing Implications
Complete blood count (CBC) with differential	Evaluates hemoglobin and hematocrit, WBC count (particularly the percentage of individual WBCs), and platelet count	Infection, inflammatory process, immunosuppression	Normal values vary according to age and sex. WBC count differential is helpful in evaluating source of infection. May be affected by myelosuppressive drugs
Immunoglobulin electrophoresis	Determines level of individual immunoglobulins (IgA, IgD, IgE, IgG, IgM) in the blood	Immune deficiency, autoimmune disorders	Normal levels vary with age. IVIG administration and steroids alter levels.
IgG subclasses	Measure the levels of the four subclasses of IgG (1, 2, 3, and 4)	Determine immune deficiency.	Normal levels vary with age. IVIG administration and steroids alter levels.
Lymphocyte immunophenotyping T-cell quantification	Measures level of T cells (T helper [CD4], T suppressor [CD8]), B cells, and natural killer cells in the blood	Ongoing monitoring of progressive depletion of CD4 T lymphocytes in HIV disease	Do not refrigerate specimen. Steroids may elevate and immunosuppressive drugs may depress lymphocyte levels.
Delayed hypersensitivity skin test	Measures the presence of activated T cells that recognize certain substances	Immune disorders	Administered intradermally Read and document size of reaction at 48–72 hours (tuberculosis, mumps, Candida, tetanus).
Virologic assay (HIV RNA and DNA nucleic acid and polymerase chain reaction tests)	Used to detect HIV RNA and DNA	Diagnosis of HIV infection in children older than 2 weeks of age and ongoing monitoring of viral load	Sensitive and specific for presence of HIV in blood Sequential testing needed to determine perinatal transmission
CD4 count	Measures the number of CD4 T lymphocytes in the blood	Used in people with HIV to determine response to antiretroviral therapy	Normal is $\geq$1,500/mm^3 in the infant, $\geq$1,000/mm^3 in the 1–5-year-old, $\geq$500/mm^3 in children 6 years and older

(continued)

COMMON LABORATORY AND DIAGNOSTIC TESTS **47.1** *(continued)*

Test	Explanation	Indications	Nursing Implications
Complement assay (C3 and C4)	Measures the level of total complement in the blood, as well as levels of C3 and C4	Monitor SLE; determine complement deficiency	Send to laboratory immediately (unstable at room temperature). Usually sent out to a reference laboratory
Erythrocyte sedimentation rate (ESR)	Nonspecific test used to determine presence of infection or inflammation	Immune disorder initial workup, ongoing monitoring of autoimmune disease	Send to laboratory immediately; if allowed to stand >3 hours, falsely low result may occur.
Rheumatoid factor (RF)	Determines the presence of RF in the blood	Juvenile idiopathic arthritis, SLE	Positive RF is also sometimes seen in chronic infectious disorders.
Antinuclear antibody (ANA)	Tests for presence of autoantibodies that react against cellular nuclear material	SLE	Check for signs of infection at venipuncture site. Steroid use can cause false-negative result. May be weakly positive in about 20% of healthy individuals
RAST (radioallergosorbent test)	Measures minute quantities of IgE in the blood Carries no risk of anaphylaxis but is not as sensitive as skin testing	Asthma (food allergies)	Blood test that is usually sent out to a reference laboratory
Allergy skin testing	Suggested allergen is applied to skin via scratch, pin, or prick. A wheal response indicates allergy to the substance. Carries risk of anaphylaxis (Nursing note: Antihistamines must be discontinued before testing, as they inhibit the test.)	Allergic rhinitis, asthma	Close observation for anaphylaxis is necessary. Epinephrine and emergency equipment should be readily available. Some children react to the skin test almost immediately; others take several minutes.
Food-specific IgE antibody testing	Measures IgE antibody to specific food allergens	Accurately determine specific food allergy.	IVIG administration and steroids alter levels.

Ig, immunoglobulin; IVIG, intravenous immune globulin; SLE, systemic lupus erythematosus; WBC, white blood cell.

Data from Corbett, J. A., & Banks, A. D. (2019). *Laboratory tests and diagnostic procedures with nursing diagnoses* (9th ed.). Pearson Education Inc.

• • • ATRAUMATIC CARE • • •

When a child requires repeat injections related to an immune or allergic disorder, use a local anesthetic such as EMLA (eutectic mixture of local anesthetic) cream or a numbing spray to reduce the amount of associated pain.

Clinical Judgment and the Nursing Process for the Child With an Immunologic Disorder

Care of the child with an immunologic or allergic disorder includes assessment, analysis, planning, interventions, and evaluation. There are many general concepts related to the nursing process that may be applied to immunodeficiencies, autoimmune, and allergic disorders. From a general understanding of the care involved for a child with immune dysfunction, the nurse can then individualize the care based on the particular child's specifics.

Assessment

Assessment of children with immunodeficiency, autoimmune disorders, or allergy includes health history, physical examination, and laboratory and diagnostic testing.

Health History

The health history consists of past medical history, including the birthing parent's pregnancy history; family history; and history of present illness (when the symptoms started and how they have progressed), as well as medications and treatments used at home. The past medical history may be significant for:

- Maternal HIV infection
- Frequent, recurrent infections such as otitis media, sinusitis, or pneumonia
- Chronic cough
- Recurrent low-grade fever
- Two or more serious infections in early childhood
- Recurrent deep skin or organ abscesses
- Persistent thrush in the mouth
- Extensive eczema
- Growth failure

Family history may be positive for primary immune deficiency or autoimmune disorder. Document history of known allergy. Note the response that occurs when the child encounters the allergen.

Physical Examination

Physical examination of the child with immunodeficiency or autoimmune disorder includes inspection and observation, auscultation, percussion, and palpation.

INSPECTION AND OBSERVATION

Plot weight and length or height on appropriate growth charts. Inspect the oropharynx for tonsillar size. Note eczematous or other skin lesions, which may occur with allergic diseases or Wiskott–Aldrich syndrome. Document the presence of thrush, which occurs frequently in children with immunodeficiency. Observe gait for unexplained ataxia (neurologic alterations occur with HIV infection).

AUSCULTATION, PERCUSSION, AND PALPATION

Auscultate the lungs for adventitious sounds, which may be present with a concurrent respiratory infection. Note any wheezing that may occur with an allergic reaction. Percuss the abdomen and determine liver span. Palpate for unusually enlarged lymph nodes, particularly in nonadjacent locations. Palpate the abdomen for an enlarged spleen or liver.

Laboratory and Diagnostic Testing

Common Laboratory and Diagnostic Tests 47.1 explains the laboratory and diagnostic tests most commonly used when considering immune disorders. Results of these tests may assist the health care provider or nurse practitioner in diagnosing the disorder and/or be used as guidelines in determining ongoing treatment. Laboratory or nonnursing personnel obtain some of the tests, while the nurse might obtain others. In either instance, it is important for the nurse to be familiar with how the tests are obtained, what they are used for, and normal versus abnormal results. This knowledge will also be necessary when providing child and family education related to the testing.

> Remember Lakeisha, the 15-year-old with joint pain and swelling, fatigue, and weight gain? What additional health history and physical examination assessment information should you obtain?

Nursing Analysis

After recognizing and analyzing cues from a thorough assessment, the nurse might identify several patient problems, including:

- Infection risk
- Malnutrition risk
- Impaired skin integrity risk
- Activity intolerance
- Delayed development risk
- Pain
- Interrupted family processes
- Caregiver role strain risk
- Knowledge deficiency

> After completing an assessment of Lakeisha, you note the following: alopecia, abdominal tenderness, and oral ulcers. Based on these assessment findings, what would your top three patient problems be for Lakeisha?

The foregoing patient problems provide suggestions for nursing care planning or concept mapping for the child with an alteration in immunity. Suggested interventions with rationales for the child with an immunologic disorder, autoimmune disorder, or allergic response are provided next. Care planning should be individualized, based on the child's and family's needs. Refer to Chapter 36 for the nursing process for pain management and to Chapter 33 for nursing interventions related to interrupted family processes and caregiver role strain risk. Additional information will be included later in the chapter as it relates to nursing management of children with specific disorders, as well as particular nursing interventions for deficient knowledge.

Nursing Analysis

Infection risk; immunodeficiency is a risk factor.

Goal/Outcome

Child will not experience overwhelming infection: will be infection-free or able to recover if they become infected

Preventing Infection (interventions with *rationale*)

- Maintain meticulous handwashing procedures (include family, visitors, staff) *to minimize spread of infectious organisms.*
- Maintain isolation as prescribed *to minimize exposure to infectious organisms.*

- Clean frequently touched surfaces with an appropriate cleanser *to minimize spread of infectious organisms.*
- Educate family and visitors that child should be restricted from contact with known infectious exposures (in hospital and at home) *to encourage cooperation with infection control.*
- Strictly observe medical asepsis *to avoid unintentional introduction of microorganisms.*
- Promote nutrition and appropriate rest *to maximize body's potential to heal.*
- Educate family to contact health care provider or nurse practitioner if child has known exposure to chickenpox or measles *so that preventive measures (e.g., varicella zoster immunoglobulin [VZIG]) can be taken.*
- Administer vaccines (not live) as prescribed *to prevent common childhood communicable diseases.*
- Administer prophylactic antibiotics as prescribed *to prevent infection with opportunistic organisms.*

Nursing Analysis

Malnutrition risk; insufficient dietary intake is a risk factor.

Goal/Outcome

Child will consume adequate intake, demonstrating appropriate weight gain and growth of length/height and/or head circumference.

Promoting Adequate Nutritional Intake (interventions with *rationale*)

- Monitor growth (weight and height/length weekly) *to determine progress toward goal.*
- Determine realistic goal for weight gain for age (consulting dietitian if necessary) *to have a specific outcome to work toward.*
- Observe child's physical ability to eat *(if pain from candidiasis or motor impairment is present, will need additional interventions).*
- Provide nutrient-rich meals and snacks *to maximize caloric intake.*
- Supplement milkshakes with protein powder or other additives *to maximize caloric intake.*
- Provide child's favorite foods *to encourage increased intake.*
- Provide smaller, more frequent meals *to reduce sensation of fullness and increase overall intake.*
- If vomiting is an issue, administer antiemetics as ordered prior to meals *to provide optimal state for success at mealtime.*

Nursing Analysis

Impaired skin integrity risk; immunodeficiency is a risk factor.

Goal/Outcome

Skin integrity will be maintained: secondary infection will not occur; rash will not increase.

Preventing Skin Impairment (interventions with *rationale*)

- Assess and monitor extent and location of rash *to provide baseline information and evaluate success of interventions.*
- Keep skin clean and dry *to prevent secondary infection.*
- For the child with limited mobility, turn frequently and use specialty mattress or bed *to prevent pressure injuries.*
- Implement a written plan of care directed toward topical treatment of skin integrity impairment *to provide consistency of care and documentation.*
- Educate child and family to limit direct sun exposure and use sunscreen *to prevent sun damage.*

Nursing Analysis

Activity intolerance related to immobility (from joint pain) or physical deconditioning as evidenced by exertional discomfort, exertional dyspnea, fatigue, or generalized weakness

Goal/Outcome

Child will participate in activities: will demonstrate easy work of breathing and participate in daily routine and play.

Promoting Activity (interventions with *rationale*)

- Cluster care *to decrease disturbances and allow for longer uninterrupted rest periods.*
- Pace activities and encourage regular rest periods *to conserve energy.*
- Administer early morning warm bath *to ease morning stiffness (juvenile arthritis).*
- Use assistive devices such as splints and orthotics *to improve physical function.*
- Plan developmentally appropriate activities that the child can participate in while in bed *to encourage play and continued development.*
- Schedule activities for the time of day the child usually has the most energy *to encourage successful participation.*

Nursing Analysis

Delayed development risk; chronic illness is a risk factor.

Goal/Outcome

Development will be enhanced; child will make continued progress toward expected developmental milestones.

Enhancing Development (interventions with *rationale*)

- Screen for developmental capabilities *to determine child's current level of functioning.*

- Offer age-appropriate toys, play, and activities (including gross motor) *to encourage further development.*
- Encourage peer contact through telephone, e-mail, or letters *to promote/continue socialization.*
- Perform interventions as prescribed by physical or occupational therapist: *repeat participation in those activities helps child improve function and acquire developmental skills.*
- Provide support to families of children with developmental delay: *progress in achieving developmental milestones can be slow, and ongoing motivation is needed.*
- Encourage child to continue school work *so that child will not fall behind.*
- Reinforce positive attributes in the child *to maintain motivation.*

Based on your top three patient problems for Lakeisha, describe appropriate nursing interventions.

PRIMARY IMMUNODEFICIENCIES

Many primary immunodeficiencies have been identified. They are mostly hereditary or congenital. Primary immunodeficiencies may be related to humoral deficiencies, cellular immunity deficiencies, or a combination of the two; phagocytic system defects; or complement deficiencies. This discussion will focus on a few of the more common and/or severe primary immunodeficiencies in children. Box 47.1 lists 10 warning signs that a child may need further evaluation for the possibility of primary immunodeficiency.

BOX 47.1 10 Warning Signs of Primary Immunodeficiency

- Four or more new episodes of acute otitis media in 1 year
- Two or more episodes of severe sinusitis in 1 year
- Treatment with antibiotics for 2 months or longer with little effect
- Two or more episodes of pneumonia in 1 year
- Failure to thrive in the infant
- Recurrent deep skin or organ abscesses
- Persistent oral thrush or skin candidiasis after 1 year of age
- History of infections requiring IV antibiotics to clear
- Two or more serious infections such as sepsis
- Family history of primary immunodeficiency

Data from Abbott, J. K., Dutmer, C. M., & Hauk, P. J. (2022). Immunodeficiency. In M. Bunik, W. W. Hay, M. J. Levin, & M. J. Abzug (Eds.), *Current diagnosis & treatment: Pediatrics* (26th ed.). McGraw-Hill Education.

Hypogammaglobulinemia

Hypogammaglobulinemia refers to a variety of conditions in which the child does not form antibodies appropriately. It results in low or absent levels of one or more of the immunoglobulin classes or subclasses. Table 47.1 provides an overview of several types of hypogammaglobulinemia. Therapeutic management of most types of hypogammaglobulinemia is periodic administration of intravenous immunoglobulin (IVIG).

TABLE 47.1 • Types of Hypogammaglobulinemia

Type	Definition	Characteristics	Treatment
Selective IgA deficiency	Serum IgA <7 mg/dL, normal IgG and IgM	May be asymptomatic Child is more prone to allergies due to lack of the mucosal protection that IgA offers; recurrent infections of respiratory, gastrointestinal, and genitourinary tracts, development of autoimmune disorders	No specific gamma globulin treatment available Treat infections or autoimmune disorders. Severe anaphylactic reaction can occur if child receives transfusion of blood containing IgA and IgA antibodies.
X-linked agammaglobulinemia	Markedly reduced or absent IgG, IgM, and IgA; absence of B cells	Males only Recurrent respiratory and gastrointestinal infections	Routine IVIG infusions Treat infections.
X-linked hyper-IgM syndrome	Defect in protein found on T-cell surface, resulting in decreased IgG and IgA levels with significant increase in IgM levels	Males only Recurrent respiratory infections, diarrhea, malabsorption Neutropenia, autoimmune disorders	Routine administration of IVIG Subcutaneous granulocyte colony-stimulating factor (G-CSF) when neutropenic Bone marrow transplantation Treatment of autoimmune disorders
IgG subclass deficiency	Low levels of one or more of the subclasses of IgG	Recurrent respiratory infections; some children outgrow this condition.	Treatment of respiratory infections Administration of IVIG is helpful in some children.

Ig, immunoglobulin

Nursing Assessment

Note history of recurrent respiratory, gastrointestinal, or genitourinary infections. Palpate for enlarged lymph nodes and spleen in the child with X-linked hyper-IgM syndrome. In children presenting for routine administration of IVIG, determine whether any infections have occurred since the previous infusion.

Nursing Management

Nursing management of hypogammaglobulinemia involves IVIG administration and the provision of education and support to the child and family.

ADMINISTERING INTRAVENOUS IMMUNOGLOBULIN

Determine the amount of IVIG to be given, and reconstitute the product according to the manufacturer's directions (available on the package insert). Some IVIG preparations are provided as a solution, requiring no reconstitution (Fig. 47.1). Others are packaged as two vials, one of IVIG powder and one of sterile diluent. After the diluent is added to the powder, gently roll the vial between your hands to mix. Reconstituted IVIG may be refrigerated overnight but should be brought to room temperature prior to infusion. Assess baseline serum blood urea nitrogen (BUN) and creatinine, as acute renal insufficiency may occur as a serious adverse reaction. Although less common in children than adults, assess for risk factors associated with an increased risk of a thromboembolic event, such as history of atherosclerosis, hyperviscosity or hypercoagulability, stroke, hypertension, hypercholesterolemia, impaired cardiac output, immobility (Lexicomp®, 2024).

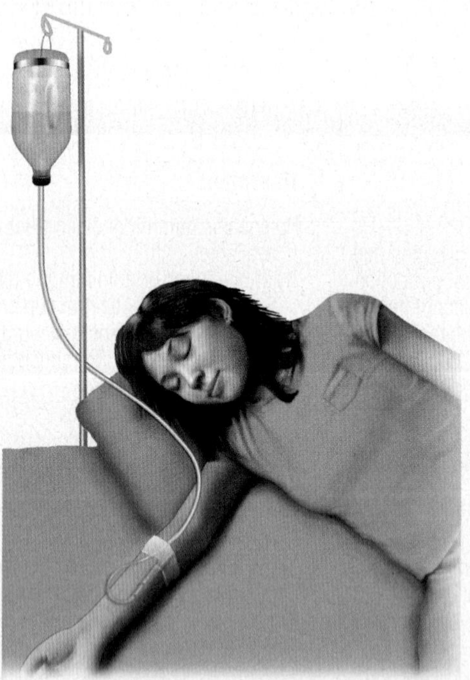

FIGURE 47.1 Intravenous administration of exogenous immunoglobulin every several weeks can decrease the frequency and severity of infections in children with various forms of hypogammaglobulinemia.

TAKE NOTE!

Do not shake the IVIG, as this may lead to foaming and may cause the immunoglobulin protein to degrade (Lexicomp®, 2024).

Ensure the child is well hydrated before the infusion to decrease the risk of rate-related reactions and aseptic meningitis after the infusion. Premedication with diphenhydramine or acetaminophen may be indicated in children who have never received IVIG, have not had an infusion in more than 8 weeks, have had a recent bacterial infection, have a history of serious infusion-related adverse reactions, or are diagnosed with agammaglobulinemia or hypogammaglobulinemia (Lexicomp®, 2024).

The rate for infusion of IVIG is generally prescribed as milligrams of IVIG per kilogram of body weight per minute. Carefully calculate the infusion rate. Obtain a baseline physical assessment and set of vital signs. Begin the infusion slowly, increasing to the prescribed rate as tolerated (see Fig. 47.1). Assess vital signs and check for adverse reactions every 15 minutes for the first hour, then every 30 minutes throughout the remainder of the infusion (the frequency of assessments may vary according to institutional protocol). IVIG is a plasma product, so observe closely for signs of anaphylaxis such as headache, facial flushing, urticaria, dyspnea, shortness of breath, wheezing, chest pain, fever, chills, nausea, vomiting, increased anxiety, or hypotension. If these symptoms occur, discontinue the infusion and notify the health care provider or nurse practitioner. The infusion may be restarted after the symptoms have subsided. Have oxygen and emergency medications such as epinephrine, diphenhydramine, and intravenous corticosteroids available in case of anaphylactic reaction. If the child complains of discomfort at the intravenous site, a cold compress may be helpful.

DOSAGE CALCULATION BOX 47.1

Child's weight: 33 lb

Medication order: intravenous immunoglobulin 6,000 mg IV today.

Per the *Pediatric Dosage Handbook*, the recommended dose is 300 to 600 mg/dose, IV, every 3 to 4 weeks. Infuse at 0.5 mL/kg/h for first 30 minutes, increasing rate every 30 minutes as tolerated, not to exceed 5 mL/kg/h.

Is the ordered dose safe?

IVIG is provided as 100 mg/mL. If the dose is safe, what will the infusion rate be for the first 30 minutes?

TAKE NOTE!

Many children who have had previous reactions to IVIG can tolerate the infusion without reaction if they are premedicated and if the infusion is given at a slower rate (Lexicomp®, 2024).

PROVIDING EDUCATION AND SUPPORT

Provide education and support to the child and family. An excellent book for children with an immune deficiency is *Our Immune System* (1993) by Sara le Bien (available from the Immune Deficiency Foundation).

Wiskott–Aldrich Syndrome

Wiskott–Aldrich syndrome is an X-linked genetic disorder that results in immunodeficiency, eczema, and thrombocytopenia. It affects males only. The defective gene responsible for this disorder is called the Wiskott–Aldrich syndrome protein (WASp). Complications include autoimmune hemolytic anemia, neutropenia, skin or cerebral vasculitis, arthritis, inflammatory bowel disease, and kidney disease (Ochs, 2022).

Autoimmune disease may require high-dose steroids, azathioprine, or cyclophosphamide. Splenectomy may be performed to correct thrombocytopenia. The only cure is hematopoietic cell transplantation, although gene therapy is currently under investigation.

Nursing Assessment

Note history of petechiae, bloody diarrhea, or bleeding episode in the first 6 months of life. Note any history of hematemesis or intracranial or conjunctival hemorrhages. Observe the skin for eczema, which usually worsens with time and tends to become secondarily infected (Fig. 47.2). Laboratory findings include low IgM concentration, elevated IgA and IgE concentrations, and normal IgG concentrations.

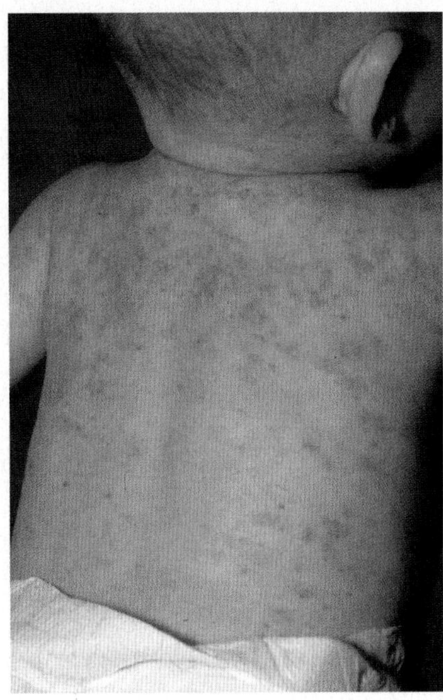

FIGURE 47.2 Children with Wiskott–Aldrich syndrome often have worsening of eczema over time.

TAKE NOTE!

An episode of prolonged bleeding, such as at the umbilical stump or after circumcision, may be the first sign of Wiskott–Aldrich syndrome in the newborn (Ochs, 2022).

Nursing Management

Administer IVIG as ordered to help decrease the frequency of bacterial infections. Perform good skin care and frequently assess eczematous areas to detect secondary infection (refer to Chapter 45 for care of eczema). If the child undergoes splenectomy, in addition to providing routine postoperative care, be aware of the additional risk of development of infection in the asplenic child. Refer to Chapter 46 for information related to hematopoietic cell transplantation.

Severe Combined Immune Deficiency

Severe combined immune deficiency (SCID) is a rare X-linked or autosomal recessive disorder; it can occur in any sex. SCID is characterized by absent T-cell and B-cell function. There are at least five types of SCID, classified according to the exact genetic defect. SCID is a potentially fatal disorder requiring emergency intervention at the time of diagnosis. Gene therapy provides some promise for the future treatment of SCID, but until then, hematopoietic cell transplantation is necessary (Heimall, 2019).

TAKE NOTE!

Use only cytomegalovirus (CMV)-negative, irradiated blood or platelets if transfusion is necessary in the infant with SCID. CMV-positive blood could cause an infection in the infant, and T lymphocytes in blood products may cause fatal graft-versus-host disease (GVHD) to occur (Heimall, 2019).

IVIG infusions may help decrease the number of infections until bone marrow or stem cell transplantation can be done (Heimall, 2019). Certain children with SCID (adenosine deaminase enzyme deficiency) may benefit from lifelong subcutaneous adenosine deaminase enzyme replacement. In addition, long-term antibiotic therapy helps to contain chronic infections in some children with SCID.

Nursing Assessment

Note history of chronic diarrhea and failure to thrive. Note history of severe infections beginning early in infancy. Inspect the mouth for persistent thrush. Auscultate the lungs, noting adventitious sounds related to pneumonia. Laboratory findings include very low levels of all of the immunoglobulins.

Nursing Management

Preventing infection is critical. Teach the family to practice good handwashing. The child must not be exposed to people outside the family, particularly young children. Instruct families to administer prophylactic antibiotics if prescribed. Educate families that the child should not receive live vaccines. Encourage adequate nutrition; supplemental enteral feedings may be necessary in the child with poor appetite. Administer IVIG infusions as prescribed, and monitor for adverse reactions (refer to the nursing management section for hypogammaglobulinemia for further information related to IVIG administration). If the child receives a bone marrow transplant (human leukocyte antigen [HLA]–matched sibling is preferred), provide posttransplant care as outlined in Chapter 46. Teach the family that severe cutaneous human papillomavirus infection may occur after stem cell transplantation (even years later). Refer the family for genetic counseling. Provide ongoing support; this is a difficult disease for families to cope with, and the therapy required is lifelong.

> **TAKE NOTE!**
>
> Monitor the child who had a bone marrow or stem cell transplant closely for a maculopapular rash that usually starts on the palms and soles; this is an indication that GVHD is developing. GVHD is a life-threatening condition in which donor cells attack host cells (Wolownik, 2022).

SECONDARY IMMUNODEFICIENCIES

Secondary immunodeficiency may occur as a result of chronic illness, malignancy, use of **immunosuppressive** (lowering the immune response) medication, malnutrition or protein-losing state, prematurity, or HIV infection. This discussion will focus on HIV infection.

HIV Infection

In the United States, 53 children younger than 13 years old are infected with HIV annually, and 19% of all cases of HIV infection occur in people aged 13 to 24 years (National Institutes of Health [NIH], 2024a, 2024b). Children acquire HIV either vertically or horizontally. Vertical transmission refers to perinatal (in utero or during birth) transmission or via breast milk. Horizontal transmission refers to transmission via nonsterile needles (as in intravenous drug use or tattooing) or via intimate sexual contact. With nationwide screening of blood products, HIV transmission via transfused blood products has become rare (National Hemophilia Foundation, 2023). HIV infection in children may be further classified depending on severity of immune suppression. This classification may serve to guide health care planning.

Infants become infected primarily through their birthing parent, whereas adolescents contract HIV infection primarily through sexual activity or intravenous drug use. In the United States, perinatal transmission of HIV infection has declined dramatically due to improved maternal detection and treatment, as well as newborn treatment (Smith & McFarland, 2022). Currently, there is no cure for HIV infection, although survival has improved since the advent of antiretroviral therapy (ART). In addition to improved survival, improved growth, neurodevelopment, and immune function occur with ART (Panel on Antiretroviral Therapy and Medical Management of Children Living with HIV, 2024).

Pathophysiology

HIV affects immune function via alterations mainly in T-cell function, but it also affects B cells, natural killer cells, and monocyte/macrophage function. HIV infects the CD4 (T-helper) cells. The virus replicates itself via the CD4 cell and renders the cell dysfunctional. Immune deficiency results as the number of normal, functioning CD4 cells drops. Initially, as CD4 counts decrease, the T-suppressor (CD8) counts increase, but as the disease progresses, CD8 counts also fall. The helper T-cell function declines even in asymptomatic infants and children who have not experienced significant decreases in the CD4 cell count. The T cells lose response to recall antigens, and this loss is associated with an increased risk of serious bacterial infection (Smith & McFarland, 2022).

B-cell defects also occur in children with HIV, contributing to high rates of serious bacterial infections. The B cells demonstrate impaired response to mitogens and antigens. They also exhibit defective antibody production in response to antigen exposure or vaccination. Also, infants lack a pool of memory B cells for recall antigens (simply from lack of exposure). Natural killer cells also are affected by HIV infection, as they are dependent on cytokines secreted by the CD4 cells for development of functionality. Functional killer cells play a role in fighting viruses and are critical to immunity in the newborn while the T-cell line develops. Decreased function of the natural killer cells then contributes to increased severity of viral infection in the child or infant with HIV. Although the virus does not destroy monocytes and macrophages, their function is affected. Macrophages in the child with HIV exhibit decreased chemotaxis, and the antigen-presenting capability of the monocytes is defective.

Without appropriate T cell, B cell, natural killer cell, monocyte, and macrophage function, the infant's or child's immune system cannot fight infections it ordinarily could. Recurrent infection with ordinary organisms occurs more frequently in children with HIV infection, and the infections are more severe than in noninfected children. Opportunistic infections also occur in children with HIV, similarly to those in adults with HIV infection. Current guidelines related to prevention of opportunistic infection emphasize ART for prevention as well as ensuring appropriate immunization and antibiotic prophylaxis for certain organisms (Smith & McFarland, 2022).

HIV rapidly invades the central nervous system in infants and children and is responsible for progressive HIV encephalopathy. As a result of encephalopathy, acquired microcephaly, motor deficits, or loss of previously achieved developmental milestones may occur. In children with progressive HIV encephalopathy, neurologic symptoms may present before immune suppression.

Therapeutic Management

Current recommendations for treatment of HIV infection in children include the use of a combination of antiretroviral drugs (Smith & McFarland, 2022). Medication therapy ranges from single-drug therapy in the asymptomatic HIV-exposed newborn to highly active ART, consisting of a combination of antiretroviral drugs. Medications are prescribed based on the severity of the child's illness. One of the goals of ART is to prevent or arrest progressive HIV encephalopathy (Gillespie, 2023).

Nursing Assessment

For a full description of the assessment phase of the nursing process, refer to the "Clinical Judgment and the Nursing Process" section. Assessment findings pertinent to HIV infection in children are discussed further on.

HEALTH HISTORY

Elicit a description of the present illness and chief complaint. Common signs and symptoms reported during the health history might include:

- Failure to thrive
- Recurrent bacterial infections
- Opportunistic infections
- Chronic or recurrent diarrhea
- Recurrent or persistent fever
- Developmental delay
- Prolonged candidiasis

These signs and symptoms may be present in either the child who is undergoing initial diagnosis or the child with known HIV infection. Explore the child's current and past medical history for risk factors such as maternal HIV infection or acquired immunodeficiency syndrome (AIDS), receipt of blood transfusions in a developing country (without adequate screening measures), adolescent or childhood sexual abuse, substance use or misuse (including intravenous drug use), or participation in vaginal or anal sex without the use of a condom. Document who the primary caregiver is, as many children with HIV have lost their parents to the disease. In addition, for the child with known HIV infection, determine the child's medications and dosages as well as the outcome of any recent health care visits or hospitalizations.

PHYSICAL EXAMINATION

Perform a thorough and complete physical examination on the child with suspected or known HIV infection. Note presence of fever. Measure weight, height or length, and head circumference (in children younger than 3 years) and plot this information on standard growth charts, noting whether the measurements fall within the average or below the lower percentiles. Perform a developmental screening test to detect developmental delay. Inspect the oral cavity for candidiasis. Observe work of breathing (may be increased if pneumonitis or pneumonia is present). Determine level of consciousness (may be depressed if HIV encephalopathy is present).

Auscultate the lungs, noting adventitious breath sounds associated with pneumonia or pneumonitis. Palpate for the presence of enlarged lymph nodes (lymphadenopathy) or swollen parotid glands. Palpate the abdomen, noting hepatosplenomegaly.

LABORATORY AND DIAGNOSTIC TESTS

Common laboratory and diagnostic studies ordered for the assessment of HIV infection include:

- RNA or DNA—nucleic acid (NAT) or polymerase chain reaction (PCR) test: positive in infected infants who are not breastfed at 1 month of age and in all infected infants at 6 months of age. Box 47.2 gives information on timing of testing.
- CD4 counts (low in HIV infection)

Nursing Management

Nursing care of the child with HIV infection is directed at avoiding infection, promoting adherence with the

BOX 47.2 Virologic Assay Testing for HIV-Exposed Infants

- 14 to 21 days of age
- 1 to 2 months of age
- 4 to 6 months of age
- In the infant who was not breastfed, two or more negative tests (one at ≥1 month of age and one at ≥4 months of age) determine absence of HIV infection

From Panel on Antiretroviral Therapy and Medical Management of Children Living with HIV. (2024). *Guidelines for the use of antiretroviral agents in pediatric HIV infection.* Department of Health and Human Services. https://clinicalinfo.hiv.gov/en/guidelines/pediatric-arv/whats-new

medication regimen, promoting nutrition, providing pain management and comfort measures, educating the child and caregivers, and providing ongoing psychosocial support. Children with HIV infection may access health services through funding provided by the Ryan White Comprehensive AIDS Resources Emergency Act (Health Resources and Services Administration, the HIV/AIDS Program, 2022). This federal funding provides for primary health care and other services to people with HIV infection. The "Clinical Judgment and the Nursing Process" section lists appropriate patient problems and interventions. In addition, nursing management specific to HIV infection is covered in what follows.

PREVENTING HIV INFECTION IN CHILDREN

It is important to offer all pregnant people routine HIV counseling and voluntary testing. Depending on the stage of pregnancy, the pregnant person should be treated with an antiretroviral drug if they are HIV positive. Children born to HIV-positive birthing parents will receive ART at least until 6 weeks of age, depending on risk (Panel on Antiretroviral Therapy and Medical Management of Children Living with HIV, 2024). Discourage breastfeeding in the parent with HIV, and instruct them about safe alternatives. Early recognition of infection is crucial so that treatment can begin, HIV encephalopathy may be prevented, and progression to AIDS can be prevented. Educate sexually active adolescents about HIV transmission, and urge them to use condoms. Counsel adolescents about the increased risk of HIV transmission with all forms of sexual activity, explaining that vaginal and anal sex are even riskier than oral sex. Urge adolescents to limit the number of sexual partners. Discourage substance use, as the effects of drugs and alcohol often impair the adolescent's ability to make wise choices about sexual conduct. Warn adolescents of the risk of contracting HIV infection via shared needles (as with intravenous drug use or via unclean needles used in tattooing). See the Healthy People 2030 box.

HEALTHY PEOPLE 2030

Objective	Nursing Significance
Reduce the rate of vertically transmitted HIV infection.	• Encourage sexually active adolescents to seek appropriate reproductive health care and screening. • For the pregnant adolescent, encourage HIV testing to determine status. • Encourage the HIV-positive pregnant adolescent to adhere with HIV treatment as prescribed.
Reduce the number of new HIV infections.	• Discourage intravenous illicit drug use. Educate adolescents about the risk of contaminated tattoo needles. • Encourage abstinence in adolescents. • If adolescents are sexually active, educate them about the risks of HIV transmission; encourage condom use with all sexual activity.

Healthy People Objectives retrieved from http://www.healthypeople.gov

PROMOTING ADHERENCE WITH ART

Without treatment, progressive HIV encephalopathy will lead to developmental regression, motor spasticity, and possibly seizures (Gillespie, 2023). To prevent progression of HIV disease and prevent encephalopathy, adherence with the ART regimen is required. Educate the family about the importance of adhering with the medication regimen. Help the caregivers develop a schedule for medication administration that is compatible with the family's home routine. See the Healthy People 2030 box.

HEALTHY PEOPLE 2030

Objective	Nursing Significance
Increase the percentage of people 13 years and older with diagnosed HIV infection who are virally suppressed.	Educate families about the importance of adhering with medication therapy (highly active antiretroviral therapy [HAART]) and receiving regularly scheduled medical evaluations.

Healthy People Objectives retrieved from http://www.healthypeople.gov

REDUCING RISK FOR INFECTION

In the newborn whose birthing parent is infected with tuberculosis, syphilis, toxoplasmosis, CMV, hepatitis B or C, or herpes simplex virus, provide testing and treatment. To prevent infection with *Pneumocystis jirovecii,* administer prophylactic antibiotics as prescribed in any HIV-exposed infant in whom HIV infection has not yet been excluded. Provide tuberculosis screening and childhood immunization in accordance with national guidelines.

THINKING ABOUT DEVELOPMENT

Jasmine Smith is a 5-year-old female with HIV infection. She fights taking her antiretroviral medications because of the nausea and vomiting associated with them. Lucy Panco is a 15-year-old female also with HIV infection. She is noncompliant with her antiretroviral medications, also because of the associated nausea and vomiting.

How will the nurse teach Jasmine about the medications? How will she foster adherence in Jasmine?

What is the most appropriate approach for the nurse to take to educate Lucy about adherence with medications?

How will the approaches to education and encouragement of adherence be different for these two children? How will they be similar?

TAKE NOTE!

Do not administer live vaccines to the immunocompromised child without the express consent of the infectious disease or immunology specialist.

PROMOTING NUTRITION

For the infant, provide increased-calorie formula as tolerated. For the child, provide high-calorie, high-protein meals and snacks. Supplements may be added to milkshakes to increase the protein intake. Ensure that the child is able to choose foods that they prefer from the hospital menu. Document growth through weekly measurements of weight and height/length.

PROMOTING COMFORT

Children with HIV infection experience pain from infections, encephalopathy, adverse effects of medications, and the numerous procedures and treatments that are required, such as venipuncture, biopsy, or lumbar puncture. Refer to Chapter 36 for detailed information about pain assessment and management.

PROVIDING FAMILY EDUCATION AND SUPPORT

Educate caregivers about the medication regimen, the ongoing follow-up that is needed, and when to call the infectious disease provider. Families of children with HIV experience a significant amount of stress from many sources: the diagnosis of an incurable disease, financial difficulties, multiple family members with HIV, HIV-associated stigmas, desire to keep HIV infection confidential, and multiple medical appointments and hospitalizations. Parents of children with HIV often die of AIDS themselves, leaving care of the child to another relative or foster parent. The day care center or school that the child attends will need education about HIV, which can be provided only if the parent or caregiver consents to divulging the child's diagnosis to that agency. Provide education to the school or day care center about how the infection is transmitted (i.e., not through casual contact).

Disclosure of the diagnosis of HIV to the child is another source of stress for the family. The timing of this disclosure will vary considerably depending on the child's and family's situation. Generally, children older than 6 years of age will eventually need to have their diagnosis disclosed to them in an age-appropriate manner. They begin to ask questions and often seem to sense that something is going on other than what they've been told so far. When made aware of the diagnosis and educated about the disease, the child may exhibit a variety of reactions. Anger, depression, or school problems may occur. The child may experience a spiritual dilemma. The nurse should continue to provide emotional support to the child and family. If the disclosure results in significant emotional turmoil, refer the child and caregivers to a counselor, social worker, or psychologist. Anticipatory grieving may also occur. Parents or caregivers may express guilt or anger over the diagnosis of HIV infection. At the other end of the spectrum, families may use denial as their method of coping. Use therapeutic communication with open-ended questions to discover the family's thoughts and fears. Provide emotional support and allow for crying and verbalization. If needed, refer the caregivers to the appropriate professional for additional psychological and emotional intervention.

Many children with HIV have psychosocial, emotional, and cognitive problems. These contribute to a lower quality of life. They are affected by the stigma of their diagnosis and often by the social isolation associated with it. Children and adolescents with HIV infection often exhibit mental health concerns, including mood, anxiety, and substance use disorders (Gillespie, 2023). They may suffer multiple losses within the family related to deaths caused by HIV infection. Children with HIV infection need significant psychosocial support and intervention. Resources for families of children with HIV are listed in Box 47.3.

BOX 47.3 Resources for Children With HIV and Their Families

- www.pedaids.org: Elizabeth Glaser Pediatric AIDS Foundation—resources for children with HIV and their families
- www.avert.org/professionals/hiv-social-issues/key-affected-populations/children: Children page of Avert, Global Information and Education on HIV and AIDS
- www.vachss.com/help_text/hiv_aids_ped.html: Pediatric HIV infection and AIDS resources
- www.thewellproject.org/hiv-information/women-and-hiv: The Well Project: Women and HIV (includes Spanish resources)

AUTOIMMUNE DISORDERS

Autoimmune disorders result from the immune system's malfunction. The body manufactures T cells and antibodies against its own cells and organs (**autoantibodies**). The development of an autoimmune disorder is thought to be multifactorial. Potential influencing factors include heredity, hormones, self-marker molecules, and environmental influences such as viruses and certain drugs.

Systemic Lupus Erythematosus

Systemic lupus erythematosus (SLE) is a multisystem autoimmune disorder that affects both humoral and cellular immunity. SLE can affect any organ system, so the onset and course of the disease are quite variable. The presentation of SLE in childhood most commonly occurs in females 9 to 15 years of age (Soep, 2022). SLE is more common in people who are not White, and young people have a greater relative risk of death from SLE (Klein-Gitelman, 2022).

Pathophysiology

In SLE, autoantibodies react with the child's self-antigens to form immune complexes. The immune complexes accumulate in the tissues and organs, causing an inflammatory response resulting in vasculitis. Injury to the tissues and pain occur. Since SLE may affect any organ system, the potential for alterations or damage to tissues anywhere in the body is significant. In some cases, the autoimmune response may be preceded by a drug reaction, an infection, or excessive sun exposure. In children, the most common initial symptoms are hematologic, cutaneous, and musculoskeletal in origin. The disease is chronic, with periods of remission and exacerbation (flares). Common complications of SLE include ocular or visual changes, cerebrovascular accident (CVA), transverse myelitis, immune complex–mediated glomerulonephritis, pericarditis, valvular heart disease, coronary artery disease, seizures, and psychosis.

Therapeutic Management

Therapeutic management focuses on treating the inflammatory response. Nonsteroidal antiinflammatory drugs (NSAIDs), corticosteroids, and antimalarial agents are often prescribed for the child with mild to moderate SLE. The child with severe SLE or frequent flare-ups of symptoms may require high-dose (pulse) corticosteroid therapy or drugs. When end-stage kidney disease develops as a result of glomerulonephritis, dialysis becomes necessary.

Nursing Assessment

For a full description of the assessment phase of the nursing process, refer to the "Clinical Judgment and the Nursing Process" section. Assessment findings pertinent to SLE in children are discussed here.

HEALTH HISTORY

Elicit a description of the present illness and chief complaint. Common signs and symptoms reported during the health history are history of fatigue, fever, weight changes, pain or swelling in the joints, numbness, tingling or coolness of extremities, or prolonged bleeding. Assess for risk factors, which include female sex; family history; African, Native American, or Asian descent; recent infection; drug reaction; or excessive sun exposure.

PHYSICAL EXAMINATION

Measure temperature and document the presence of fever. Observe the skin for malar rash (a butterfly-shaped rash over the cheeks); discoid lesions on the face, scalp, or neck; changes in skin pigmentation; or scarring (Fig. 47.3). Document alopecia. Inspect the oral cavity for painless ulcerations and the joints for edema.

Measure blood pressure, as hypertension may occur with kidney involvement. Auscultate the lungs; adventitious breath sounds may be present if the pulmonary system is involved. Palpate the joints, noting tenderness. Palpate the abdomen and note areas of tenderness (abdominal involvement is more common in children with SLE than in adults). Box 47.4 lists common clinical findings in SLE.

LABORATORY AND DIAGNOSTIC FINDINGS

Laboratory findings may include decreased hemoglobin and hematocrit, decreased platelet count, and low WBC count. Complement levels, C3 and C4, will also be decreased. Although not specific to SLE, the antinuclear antibody (ANA) is usually positive in children with SLE.

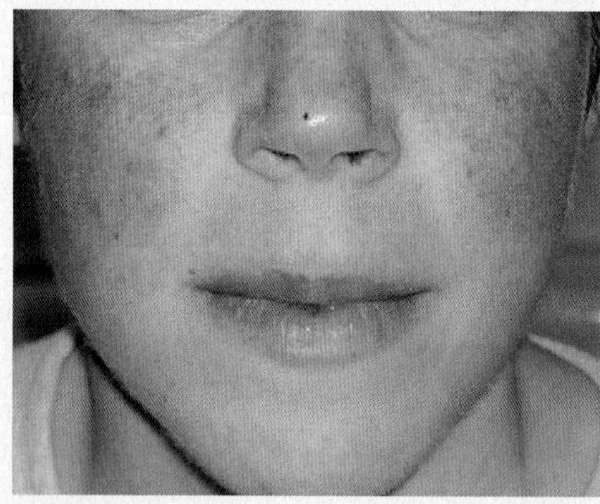

FIGURE 47.3 The malar or butterfly rash (erythema over the cheeks in the shape of a butterfly) is typical in systemic lupus erythematosus (SLE).

BOX **47.4** **Most Common Clinical Manifestations of Systemic Lupus Erythematosus**

- Alopecia
- Anemia
- Arthralgia
- Arthritis
- Fatigue
- Lupus nephritis
- Photosensitivity
- Pleurisy
- Raynaud phenomenon
- Seizures
- Skin rashes, including malar rash
- Stomatitis
- Thrombocytopenia

Nursing Management

Nursing management of the child or adolescent with SLE is long-term and supportive. Management focuses on preventing and monitoring for complications. Educate the child and family about the importance of a healthy diet, regular exercise, and adequate sleep and rest. Administer NSAIDs, corticosteroids, and antimalarial agents as ordered for the child with mild to moderate SLE and pulse corticosteroid therapy or immunomodulators to the child with severe SLE or frequent flare-ups. Assist families to deal with this chronic illness and adolescents with their struggles with body image and independence. Refer families to support services such as the Lupus Alliance of America and the Lupus Foundation of America.

PREVENTING AND MONITORING FOR COMPLICATIONS

Teach families to apply sunscreen (minimum SPF 15) to their child's skin daily to prevent rashes resulting from photosensitivity. Instruct the child and family to protect against cold weather by layering warm socks and wearing gloves when outdoors in the winter. If the child is outside for extended periods during the winter months, inspect the fingers and toes for discoloration. Watch for the development of nephritis by evaluating blood pressure, serum BUN and creatinine levels, and urine output and monitoring for hematuria or proteinuria. Ensure that yearly vision screening and ophthalmic examinations are performed to preserve visual function should changes occur.

TAKE NOTE!

Avascular necrosis (lack of blood supply to a joint, resulting in tissue damage) may occur as an adverse effect of long-term or high-dose corticosteroid use. Teach families to report new onset of joint pain, particularly with weight bearing, or limited range of motion to their health care provider or nurse practitioner (Patel, 2022).

Juvenile Idiopathic Arthritis

Juvenile idiopathic arthritis is an autoimmune disorder in which the autoantibodies target mainly the joints. Inflammatory changes in the joints cause pain, redness, warmth, stiffness, and swelling. Stiffness usually occurs after inactivity (as in the morning, after sleep). Some forms also affect the eyes or other organs. Table 47.2 explains the three types. Juvenile idiopathic arthritis is a chronic disease; the child may experience healthy periods alternating with flare-ups (Soep, 2022). Juvenile idiopathic arthritis was formerly termed "juvenile rheumatoid arthritis," but unlike adult rheumatoid arthritis, few types of juvenile arthritis actually demonstrate a positive RF.

Therapeutic management focuses on inflammation control, pain relief, promotion of remission, and maintenance of mobility. NSAIDs, corticosteroids, and antirheumatic drugs such as methotrexate and etanercept are prescribed, depending on the type and severity of the disease. NSAIDs are helpful with pain relief, but disease-modifying (antirheumatic) drugs are necessary to prevent disease progression (several of which are approved for use in children).

TABLE **47.2** • Types of Juvenile Idiopathic Arthritis

Type	Definition	Nonjoint Manifestations	Complications
Pauciarticular (oligoarticular)	Involvement of four or fewer joints; quite often, the knee is involved. Most common type	Eye inflammation, malaise, poor appetite, poor weight gain	Iritis, uveitis, uneven leg bone growth
Polyarticular	Involvement of five or more joints; frequently involves small joints and often affects the body symmetrically	Malaise, lymphadenopathy, organomegaly, poor growth	Often, a severe form of arthritis; rapidly progressing joint damage, rheumatoid nodules
Systemic	In addition to joint involvement, fever and rash may be present at diagnosis.	Enlarged spleen, liver, and lymph nodes; myalgia; severe anemia	Pericarditis, pericardial effusion, pleuritis, pulmonary fibrosis

Based on Soep, J. B. (2022). Rheumatic diseases. In M. Bunik, W. W. Hay, M. J. Levin, & M. J. Abzug (Eds.), *Current diagnosis & treatment: Pediatrics* (26th ed.). McGraw-Hill Education.

Nursing Assessment

Note history of irritability or fussiness, which may be the first sign of this disease in the infant or very young child. Note complaints of pain, although children do not always communicate this. Document history of withdrawal from play or difficulty getting the child out of bed in the morning (joint stiffness after inactivity). Inquire about history of fever (above 39.5°C for 2 weeks or more in systemic disease).

Measure temperature (fever is present with systemic disease). Inspect skin for evanescent, pale red, nonpruritic macular rash, which may be present at diagnosis of systemic disease. Observe the gait, noting limping or guarding of a joint or extremity. Document growth, which may be delayed. Inspect and palpate each joint for edema, redness, warmth, and tenderness (Fig. 47.4). Note positioning of joints (usually flexed in position of comfort). Mild to moderate anemia and an elevated erythrocyte sedimentation rate are common. Young children with the pauciarticular form may demonstrate a positive ANA, and adolescents with polyarticular disease may have a positive RF.

Nursing Management

Nursing management focuses on managing pain, maintaining mobility, and promoting a normal life. Refer the child to a pediatric rheumatologist to ensure that they receive the most up-to-date treatment. Administer disease-modifying medications and teach children and families how to do so. Refer families to Childhood Arthritis and Rheumatology Research Alliance for clinical research trial information. Encourage regular eye examinations and vision screening to allow for early treatment of visual changes and to prevent blindness.

MANAGING PAIN AND MAINTAINING MOBILITY

Administer medications as prescribed to control inflammation and prevent disease progression. Refer to Drug Guide 47.1 for information related to NSAIDs, corticosteroids, and disease-modifying antirheumatic drugs. Maintain joint range of motion and muscle strength via exercise (physical or occupational therapy). Swimming is a particularly useful exercise to maintain joint mobility without placing pressure on the joints. Teach families appropriate use of splints prescribed to prevent joint contractures. Monitor for pressure areas or skin breakdown with splint or orthotic use.

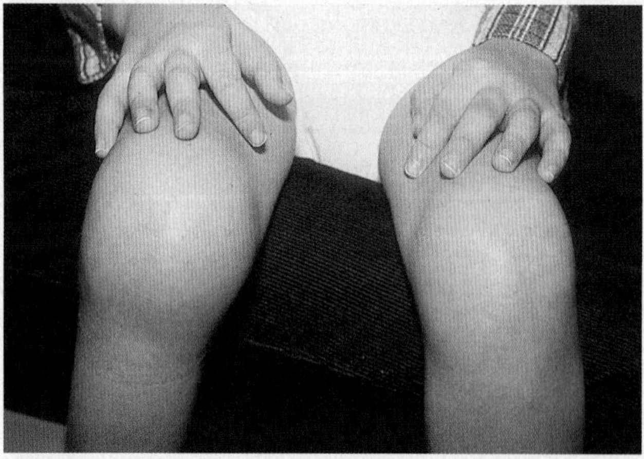

FIGURE 47.4 Note the swollen, reddened joints of this child with juvenile arthritis.

PROMOTING NORMAL LIFE

Chronic pain and decreased mobility may impact the child's psychological and emotional status significantly, during both childhood and adulthood. Providing adequate pain relief and promoting adherence with the disease-modifying medication regimen may allow the child to have a more normal life in the present as well as in the future. In addition to measures described in the previous section, encourage adequate sleep to improve the child's ability to cope with symptoms and with school function. Promote sleep with a warm bath at bedtime and warm compresses to affected joints or massage. To prevent social isolation, encourage the child to attend school and ensure that teachers, the school nurse, and classmates are educated about the child's disease and any limitations on activity. Having two sets of books (one at school and one at home) allows the child to do homework without having to carry heavy books home. Modifications such as allowing the child to leave the classroom early in order to get to the next class on time may seem small but can have a significant impact on the child's life.

Encourage children and families to become involved with local support groups so they can see that they are not alone. Assist children to set and achieve goals to increase their sense of hopefulness. Special summer camps for children with juvenile arthritis allow the child to socialize and belong to a group and have been shown to promote self-esteem in the child with chronic illness. Encourage appropriate family functioning and refer the family to support groups, such as those sponsored by the American Juvenile Arthritis Organization.

Guillain–Barré Syndrome

Guillain–Barré syndrome (GBS) (also called acute immune-mediated polyneuropathies) is a diverse group of syndromes with several forms. In the disorder occurring most often, an immune response within the body attacks the peripheral nervous system but does not usually affect the brain or spinal cord. GBS results in inflammation and demyelinization of the peripheral nerves. Weakness and paralysis occur in a progressive fashion. Progression is usually complete in 2 to 4 weeks, followed by a stable period leading to the recovery phase, which lasts for a few weeks to months in most cases but can take years. Severity of the disorder ranges from mild weakness to total paralysis.

Although not fully understood, it is believed to be an autoimmune condition that is most commonly triggered by a previous viral or bacterial infection, usually described as an upper respiratory tract infection or an acute gastroenteritis with fever. In rare cases, it has occurred after the child has had an immunization or surgery. GBS is more commonly seen in adults than in children (Yiu, 2023).

Therapeutic Management

Treatment of GBS is symptomatic and focuses on lessening the severity and speeding recovery. Management may include plasma exchange and administration of IVIGs, especially in severe cases. The goal of treatment is to keep the body functioning until the nervous system recovers. GBS is a life-threatening condition, and some children will die during the acute phase due to respiratory failure. Most children will make a full recovery, but a few may have residual damage.

Nursing Assessment

Early diagnosis and prompt treatment are essential since the disorder can quickly lead to respiratory failure and death from muscle paralysis. For a full description of the assessment phase of the nursing process, refer to the "Clinical Judgment and the Nursing Process" section. Assessment findings pertinent to GBS are discussed here.

HEALTH HISTORY

Elicit a description of the present illness and chief complaint. The clinical presentation of GBS is fairly similar in children and adults. Note onset of symptoms within a few days or weeks after the causative infection or event. Determine the presence of muscle weakness and paresthesias such as numbness and tingling which have a quick onset. Classically, GBS initially affects the legs and progresses in an ascending manner, but occasionally, it affects the arms or face first and proceeds in a descending manner. Ask about presence of paralysis, ataxia, or sensory disturbances.

PHYSICAL EXAMINATION AND LABORATORY AND DIAGNOSTIC TESTS

Note decreased or absent tendon reflexes, facial weakness, difficulty swallowing, or paralysis. Cerebrospinal fluid (CSF) analysis may reveal an increased level of protein, but this may not be evident until after the first week of the illness. Electrodiagnostic studies, such as electromyogram (EMG) and nerve conduction velocity, can assist in the diagnosis of GBS.

> *TAKE NOTE!*
>
> Tickling may be a successful technique for assessing the level of paralysis in the child with Guillain–Barré syndrome, either initially or in the recovery phase.

Nursing Management

Nursing management is supportive. In severe cases, the child may require intensive nursing care along with mechanical ventilation. Observe the child closely for the extent of paralysis, and monitor for respiratory involvement. Nursing care focuses on the same concerns as in any child with extreme immobility or paralysis.

Prevention of complications associated with immobility is a central concern and involves maintaining skin integrity, preventing respiratory complications and contractures, maintaining adequate nutrition, and managing pain. Turn and/or reposition the child every 2 hours, perform range-of-motion exercises, assess the skin for redness or breakdown, keep the skin clean and dry, encourage fluid intake to maintain hydration status, and encourage coughing and deep breathing every 2 hours and as needed. Provide enteral feeding or parenteral nutrition if swallowing becomes impaired. Perform physical therapy exercises as prescribed to help prevent complications and promote motor skill recovery. Provide support and education to the parent and child. Support the family as the rapid onset and long recovery can be difficult, causing strain on the family and its finances. If residual disability occurs, assist the family to adjust and to care for their child.

> *TAKE NOTE!*
>
> Serial measurement of tidal volumes may reveal respiratory deterioration in the child with Guillain–Barré syndrome.

Myasthenia Gravis

Myasthenia gravis is an autoimmune disease that may be inherited as a rare genetic disease (congenital), may be acquired by infants born to birthing parents with myasthenia gravis (neonatal), or may develop later in childhood (juvenile). The most common form seen is juvenile myasthenia gravis and will be covered here. See Comparison Chart 47.2 for further information on the less common forms, neonatal myasthenia gravis and congenital myasthenia gravis. Juvenile myasthenia gravis is a relatively rare autoimmune disorder (Lin et al., 2023). The child's antibodies attack the acetylcholine receptor (AchR) and other proteins at the neuromuscular junction, inhibiting normal neuromuscular transmission. The result is progressive weakness and fatigue of the skeletal muscles.

There is no cure for myasthenia gravis. Symptoms can be controlled, but it is a lifelong condition, with early detection being the key to managing the disorder successfully. The disease may be aggravated by stress, exposure to extreme temperatures, and infections, resulting in a myasthenic crisis. Myasthenic crisis is a medical

COMPARISON CHART 47.2 Types of Myasthenia Gravis

	Neonatal Myasthenia Gravis	Congenital Myasthenia Gravis
Definition	Transient form resulting from transplacental transfer of maternal antibodies that interfere with neuromuscular junction	A group of disorders resulting from a genetic mutation of components of the neuromuscular junction resulting in neuromuscular junction failure
Characteristics	Present within a few hours after birth; generalized weakness and hypotonia; bulbar and respiratory weakness leads to poor suck and swallow, weak cry, and possible respiratory failure. Neonate will be very ill. Prompt diagnosis and treatment is essential. Recovery usually occurs within a few weeks.	Apparent at birth; frequently have ptosis, ophthalmoplegia, bulbar, and respiratory muscle weakness; Fluctuating generalized weakness and hypotonia, life-threatening apnea; typically improves with age but spontaneous exacerbations seen. Exacerbations are also seen during periods of stress, increased activity, or febrile illness. Management depends on specific type.

emergency with symptoms including sudden respiratory distress, dysphagia, dysarthria, ptosis, diplopia, tachycardia, anxiety, and rapidly increasing weakness.

Therapeutic management generally involves the use of anticholinesterase medications such as pyridostigmine, which blocks the breakdown of acetylcholine at the neuromuscular junction and enhances neuromuscular transmission. If weakness is not controlled, additional medications may include corticosteroids and other immunosuppressants. Other treatments include plasmapheresis to remove antibodies from the blood, IVIG, and thymectomy (however, the role of the thymus gland in the disease process is unclear; therefore, this procedure may or may not improve the child's symptoms).

Nursing Assessment

Note history of fatigue and weakness; difficulty chewing, swallowing, or holding up the head; or pain with muscle fatigue. In the verbal child, note complaints of double vision. Observe the child for ptosis (droopy eyelids) or altered eye movements from partial paralysis. Note increased work of breathing. Laboratory testing may involve the edrophonium (Tensilon) test, in which a short-acting cholinesterase inhibitor is used. AchR antibodies may be present in elevated quantities in the serum.

Nursing Management

The goals of nursing management include prevention of respiratory problems and providing adequate nutrition. Administer anticholinergic or other medications as ordered, teaching children and families about the use of these drugs. Anticholinergic drugs should be given 30 to 45 minutes before meals, on time and exactly as ordered. Encourage families to seek prompt medical treatment for suspected infections. Encourage appropriate stress management and avoidance of extreme temperatures. Teach families that physical activities should be performed during times of peak energy; rest periods are needed for energy conservation. Teach families to call their neurologist immediately if signs and symptoms of myasthenic crisis or cholinergic crisis, which results from overmedication with anticholinergic medications, appear. Myasthenic crisis and cholinergic crisis have a similar presentation: rapidly increasing muscle weakness with resultant respiratory distress. Encourage children to wear a medical alert bracelet.

CLINICAL REASONING ALERT!

Signs and symptoms of myasthenic crisis include severe muscle weakness, respiratory difficulty, tachycardia, and dysphagia. Signs and symptoms of cholinergic crisis include severe muscle weakness, sweating, increased salivation, bradycardia, and hypotension.

Dermatomyositis

Juvenile dermatomyositis is an autoimmune disease that results in inflammation of the muscles or associated tissues. It occurs more often in females and is generally diagnosed between the ages of 5 and 10 years (Hutchinson & Feldman, 2024). The cause remains unclear, but it may be an autoimmune response triggered by exposure to a virus or to certain medications (Hutchinson & Feldman, 2024). As with other autoimmune diseases, a genetic predisposition is present. The inflammatory cells of the immune system cause a vasculitis that affects the skin, muscles, kidneys, retinas, and gastrointestinal tract.

Therapeutic management involving the use of high-dose glucocorticoid or other immunosuppressants is necessary to prevent the complications of painful calcium deposits under the skin, as well as joint contractures. Methotrexate, IVIG, and cyclosporine may also be used. With appropriate treatment, children may recover completely, although some children experience relapses (Hutchinson & Feldman, 2023).

Nursing Assessment

Elicit a health history, which commonly includes fever, fatigue, and rash, usually followed by muscle pain and weakness. Determine onset and progression of muscle weakness. Inspect the skin for the presence of rash involving the upper eyelids and extensor surfaces of the knuckles, elbows, and knees. The rash is initially a reddish-purplish color and then progresses to scaling, with resulting roughness of the skin. Test muscle strength, particularly noting weakness in the pelvic and shoulder girdles. Laboratory and diagnostic testing may include muscle enzyme levels, a positive ANA test, and an EMG to distinguish muscular weakness from other causes.

Nursing Management

Administer medications as ordered and teach families about their use; instruct them to monitor for side effects. Educate the family about the importance of maintaining the medication regimen in order to prevent calcinosis (calcium deposits) and joint deformity in the future. Encourage adherence with physical therapy regimens. Ensure that children are excused from physical education classes while the disease is active.

ALLERGY AND ANAPHYLAXIS

Allergy is an immune-mediated response resulting in an adverse physiologic event or reaction and affects up to 25% of population in developed countries (Covar et al., 2022). The extent of the allergic response is determined by the duration, rate, and amount of exposure to the allergen as well as environmental and host factors. IgE-mediated allergy will be the focus of this discussion. This type of allergic response is mediated by antigen-specific IgE antibodies. When the antibody is exposed to the antigen (allergen), rapid cell activation occurs, and potent mediators and cytokines are released, resulting in changes in the blood vessels, bronchi, and mucus-secreting glands. In addition to the atopic diseases (asthma, allergic rhinitis, and atopic dermatitis), urticaria, digestive allergy, and systemic anaphylaxis are also IgE-mediated. Although any allergen has the potential to trigger an anaphylactic response, food, drug, and insect sting allergies are most common (Campbell & Kelson, 2024).

Food Allergies

A true food hypersensitivity or allergy is defined as an immunologic reaction resulting from the ingestion of a food or food additive. This type of reaction is an IgE-mediated response to a particular food. Food allergy affects approximately 8% of children and can lead to significant medical complications (Covar et al., 2022). The most common food allergies include milk and dairy, eggs, fish and shellfish, peanuts and tree nuts, and wheat, soy, and sesame (American Academy of Allergy, Asthma & Immunology, 2024). Most reactions occur within minutes of exposure, but they may occur up to 2 hours after ingestion. Signs and symptoms of a food allergy reaction include hives, flushing, facial swelling, mouth and throat itching, and runny nose. Many children also have a gastrointestinal reaction, including vomiting, abdominal pain, and diarrhea. In extreme cases, swelling of the tongue, uvula, pharynx, or upper airway may occur. Wheezing can be an ominous sign that the airway is edematous. Rarely, cardiovascular collapse occurs. Although the risk of anaphylaxis is small, parents, caregivers, and health care providers and nurse practitioners should be vigilant when caring for children with food allergies.

Therapeutic Management

Therapeutic management involves verifying the food allergy, avoiding the allergen, and treating the reaction with medications, including antihistamines and epinephrine (in the case of an anaphylactic reaction). To verify the food allergy, a trial elimination diet may be indicated. If symptoms resolve without the food, true allergy may be present. On an elimination diet, the child stops eating all suspicious foods for 1 to 2 weeks and then retries the foods one at a time, over a period of several days, to see whether a similar reaction occurs. Oral challenge testing and retrying of foods after an elimination diet are often done in the health care provider's or nurse practitioner's office or hospital setting if severe reactions have occurred in the past. Food avoidance is recommended for those who have a highly predictive reaction to testing or a history of anaphylactic response. Prevention of food allergies is also important (see Evidence-Based Practice Box 47.1).

Discerning a true food allergy from intolerance to certain foods is an important part of therapeutic management. "Food intolerance" is a general term that describes an abnormal physiologic response to an ingested food or food additive that has not been proven to be immunologic. Often a milk allergy is confused with lactose intolerance. Therefore, a detailed dietary history is important when distinguishing a true allergy versus intolerance.

TAKE NOTE!

To prevent the development of food allergies, infants should be breastfed for at least the first 6 months of life.

Nursing Assessment

It is important to accurately assess children with food allergy reactions. In the initial nursing assessment, immediately assess the child for airway, breathing, or circulation problems (see Chapter 51). If the child's condition is stable, finish the assessment. Make sure that the health history includes a detailed food history and documentation of the reaction, including the food suspected of

EVIDENCE-BASED PRACTICE 47.1

Early Introduction of Peanuts for the Prevention of Allergy

STUDY

Infants with severe eczema and/or egg allergy are at high risk for peanut allergy. Multiple studies over the past couple of decades have indicated that developmentally appropriate food should be introduced at approximately 6 months of age in typical children. These studies have noted a decrease in peanut allergy when peanut exposure occurs during infancy. The researchers conducted a randomized controlled trial involving 640 infants. The infants were divided into two groups: those with positive skin-prick test for peanut allergy and those without. The groups were then further divided. Infants either consumed developmentally appropriate peanut food or they did not.

Findings

The authors noted additional questions remain in relation to the provision of developmentally appropriate peanut food to infants with severe eczema and/or egg allergy. The current recommendation for these infants is to introduce them to peanut food after sensitivity testing is negative.

Nursing Implications

The current recommendation to prevent the development of peanut allergy in typical children is early introduction of developmentally appropriate peanut food for infants once solid foods have been successfully introduced. Children with severe eczema and/or egg allergy may require sensitivity testing prior to the introduction of peanut food. Parents may be fearful of peanut allergy as the recommendation for decades was to avoid peanut foods until after age 12 months. Educate parents that current research demonstrates decreased allergy incidence with earlier introduction. Parents should discuss peanut food introduction with their baby's primary care provider, prior to trying it.

Data from Abrams, E. M., Chan, E. S., & Sicherer, S. (2020). Peanut allergy: New advances and ongoing controversies. *Pediatrics, 145*(5), e20192102. https://doi.org/10.1542/peds.2019-2102

causing the reaction, the quantity of food ingested, the length of time between ingestion and development of symptoms, the symptoms, what treatment has been administered, and the subsequent response. Note gastrointestinal symptoms such as:

- Burning in the mouth or throat
- Bloating
- Nausea
- Diarrhea

Assess for risk factors such as previous exposure to the food, history of poorly controlled asthma, or an increase in atopic dermatitis flare-ups in relation to food intake. Inspect the skin for color, rash, hives, or edema. Auscultate the heart and lungs to determine heart rate and to assess for wheezing.

Allergy skin-prick tests and radioallergosorbent blood tests (RASTs) are used widely by health care providers and nurse practitioners to look for allergic reactions. Food-specific IgE testing is recommended if the child has a history of food allergy. If the child has episodic symptoms, an oral challenge in a controlled setting may be appropriate. For an oral challenge, the child slowly eats a serving of the offending food over the period of 1 hour. Record vital signs and note the presence or absence of allergic symptoms.

Nursing Management

Initial nursing management is aimed at stabilizing the child's condition if an acute reaction to a food allergen is present (see Chapter 51). As stated previously, medications used in the treatment of a food allergy reaction include histamine blockers and, in anaphylactic reactions, epinephrine. Teach the child (if appropriate) and the parents how and when to use these medications during an allergic reaction. The child who has been prescribed an EpiPen should carry the pen with them at all times. Since these reactions can be so sudden (unknown ingestion of allergen) and severe, it is helpful for the family to have a written emergency plan in case of a reaction.

MANAGING THE CHILD'S DIET

Aim dietary teaching at educating the child and family on how to avoid the offending foods. Families should be extremely careful when reading food labels. A dietitian may be helpful in this teaching process. Teaching Guidelines 47.1 gives information about hidden allergens in food. Teach the parents what "safe" foods can be substituted for offensive ones (Box 47.5). Children with peanut allergy should also avoid tree nuts.

Having a child with a food allergy can be anxiety-producing for parents; they often live in fear that the child may accidentally ingest an allergen. Educate the child and family about allergic reactions to help decrease their anxiety. Teach the child and family how to recognize the signs and symptoms of an allergic reaction. It may be necessary to provide information to day

BOX 47.5 Food Substitutions

- Replace milk with water, fruit juice, rice milk, or soymilk.
- Replace each egg with 1.5 tablespoons each of water and oil and 1 teaspoon baking powder; OR 1 packet plain gelatin with 2 tablespoons warm water added at time of use; OR 1 teaspoon yeast and a quarter-cup warm water.
- Replace peanuts or tree nuts with raisins, dates, or crispy cereal.

Data from Winkels, K. (2023). *Allergy-free foods.* http://www.eatingwithfoodallergies.com/allergyfreesubstitutes.html

TEACHING GUIDELINES **47.1** Allergens Hidden in Food

If Child Is Allergic to	Teach Families to Avoid	Unexpected Locations of Common Ingredients
Milk	Artificial butter flavor, casein, lactalbumin, nougat, pudding, whey, yogurt, ghee	Some deli meats and hot dogs, nondairy products, coffee whiteners
Wheat	Cereal extract, couscous, durum, semolina, spelt	Some imitation crab meat and wheat flour shaped to look like shrimp, beef, or pork
Eggs	Albumin, globulin, ovalbumin	Some egg substitutes and foam toppings for drinks, commercially cooked pastas
Peanuts	Fast food cooked in peanut oil, baked goods with nuts, or foods processed on equipment that also processes peanuts	Brown gravy, barbeque sauce, meat sauce, egg rolls, enchilada sauce, hot chocolate

Based on Kids with Food Allergies. (2023). *Recipe substitutions*. https://kidswithfoodallergies.org/recipes-diet/recipe-substitutions/

care providers as well as schoolteachers, staff, and camp counselors. Refer families to the Food Allergy & Anaphylaxis Network.

CONSIDER THIS!

The parent of Mina Stepelman (6 years old) is distraught about the significance of Mina's peanut allergy. She has been prescribed an EpiPen and is comfortable with when and how to use it. Mina's parent says tearfully, "I'm just so scared she'll eat the wrong thing when she's not with me. I'm never letting her go to a party alone or spend the night at someone's house. Even though I've talked to her school nurse, I'm even scared about what she'll eat at school."

Think about if you or your child had this type of significant allergy, how would you feel? How would you deal with this perceived risk?

As a nurse, how should you respond to Mina's parent?

Anaphylaxis

Anaphylaxis is an acute IgE-mediated response to an allergen that involves many organ systems and may be life-threatening. In addition to nuts, shellfish, eggs, and bee or wasp stings, drugs such as beta-lactam antibiotics and NSAIDs, and latex (though rarer) are the leading causes of anaphylaxis (Linzer, 2024). The reaction is severe and usually starts within 5 to 10 minutes of exposure, although delayed reactions are possible. Histamines and secondary mediators are released from the mast cells and eosinophils in response to contact with an allergen. Cutaneous, cardiopulmonary, gastrointestinal, and neurologic symptoms occur. Vasodilation results in a rapid decrease in plasma volume, leading to the risk of circulatory collapse. Prolonged resuscitation may be needed, and death may occur.

Therapeutic management focuses on assessment and support of the airway, breathing, and circulation. Epinephrine is usually required, and intramuscular or intravenous diphenhydramine is used secondarily. Late-onset reactions can be prevented with corticosteroids.

Nursing Assessment

Assess patency of the airway and adequacy of breathing. Determine if circulation is sufficient. Note level of consciousness. Obtain a brief history, inquiring specifically about allergen exposure. Determine whether the child has received any medication (e.g., epinephrine or diphenhydramine) since the onset of the reaction and what effect the medication had on the symptoms. Table 47.3 gives additional signs and symptoms of anaphylaxis.

TABLE **47.3** • Clinical Manifestations of Anaphylaxis

Body Area or System	Manifestation
Oral	• Lip, tongue, or palate pruritus • Lip or tongue edema
Cutaneous	Urticaria (hives), flushing, pruritus, angioedema
Respiratory	• Nasal pruritus, congestion, sneezing, rhinorrhea • Stridor, tightness in the throat, dysphagia, dysphonia, hoarseness • Shortness of breath, dyspnea, tight chest, wheeze
Cardiovascular	Tachycardia, chest pain, arrhythmia, hypotension
Neurologic	Syncope, feeling faint, aura of doom, lethargy, disorientation
Gastrointestinal	Bloating, abdominal pain, diarrhea, vomiting

Based on Covar, R. A., Fleischer, D. M., Cho, C., & Boguniewicz, M. (2022). Allergic disorders. In M. Bunik, W. W. Hay, M. J. Levin, & M. J. Abzug (Eds.), *Current diagnosis & treatment: Pediatrics* (26th ed.). McGraw-Hill Education; Campbell, R. L., & Kelso, J. M. (2024). Anaphylaxis: Acute diagnosis. *UpToDate*. Retrieved April 16, 2024, from https://www.uptodate.com/contents/anaphylaxis-acute-diagnosis

Nursing Management

Nursing management initially focuses on supporting the airway, breathing, and circulation. Provide supplemental oxygen by mask or bag-valve-mask ventilation. Administer epinephrine as ordered to reverse the allergic process. Ensure that bronchodilator inhalation treatment (albuterol) is given if bronchospasm is present. Administer intravenous fluids to provide volume expansion. Observe the child for 4 to 6 hours in case of recurrent attack (Covar et al., 2022).

PREVENTING AND MANAGING FUTURE EPISODES

It is critical to educate the family about preventing and managing future episodes. Teach the family how to use injectable epinephrine in case of subsequent allergen exposure. Intramuscular epinephrine may be given via the EpiPen or EpiPen Jr. Dosage is based on the child's weight. The child should carry the pen with them at all times. Explain to the child and family that the gray safety release on the EpiPen should never be removed until just before use. In addition, teach the child and family that the thumb, fingers, or hand should not be placed over the black tip. Nursing Procedure 47.1 gives further instructions related to EpiPen use. Instruct the child and family to call 911 and seek immediate medical attention after using the EpiPen. Warn the child that the epinephrine may make them feel as if the heart is racing.

Day care providers, school nurses, teachers, and staff who interact with the child must know how to recognize an anaphylactic event. In 2004, Public Law No. 108-377, Asthmatic Schoolchildren's Treatment and Health Management Act, was passed by the U.S. Congress. This law is intended to ensure that students with severe allergies can carry prescribed medications (i.e., EpiPen) with them. All children with allergies should have an action plan in place at the school or day care center. Advise the child to wear a medical ID alert bracelet or necklace at all times.

Teach children and families to avoid known food allergens. Avoid stings from bees and wasps by being alert when eating outdoors, wearing long sleeves and pants when in fields, and having bee and wasp hives or nests removed from areas near the family's home. Immunotherapy (allergy shots) may be indicated in children with a hypersensitivity to stinging insects. Avoid use of cephalosporins in children with severe penicillin allergy. Desensitization is available for children with severe penicillin allergy. Desensitization involves administration of increasingly larger doses of penicillin over a period of hours to days in an intensive care setting.

Latex Allergy

Latex allergy is an IgE-mediated response to exposure to latex, a natural rubber product used in many common

NURSING PROCEDURE 47.1 Using the EpiPen or EpiPen Jr

1. Grasp the EpiPen or EpiPen Jr with the black tip pointing downward, forming a fist (Fig. 1).

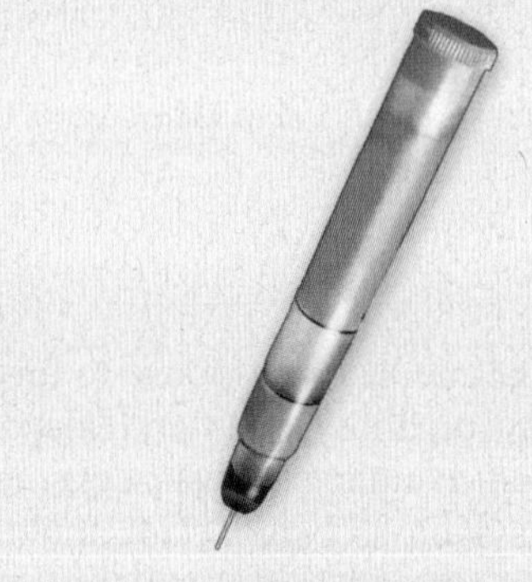

2. With the other hand, pull off the gray safety release.
3. Swing and jab the EpiPen firmly into the outer thigh at a 90-degree angle, and hold firmly there for 10 seconds (Figs. 2 and 3).

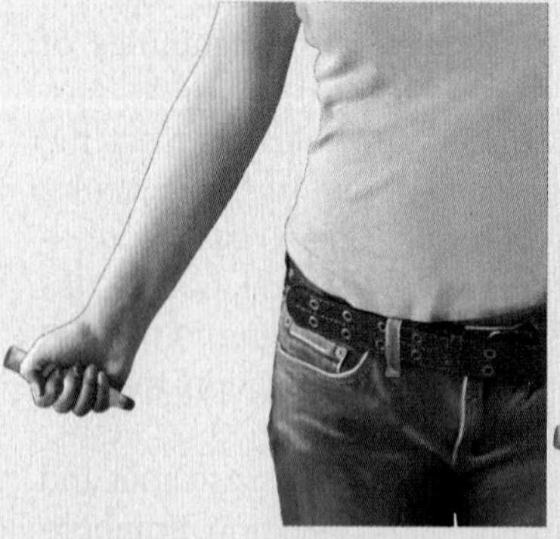

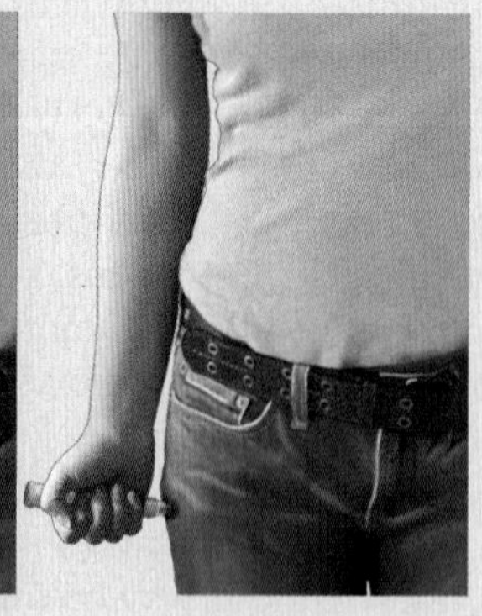

4. Remove the EpiPen and massage the thigh for 10 seconds.

Based on Viatris. (2023). *EpiPen: How to use*. https://www.epipen.com/en/about-epipen-and-generic/how-to-use-epipen

items (especially gloves in the health care setting). The pathophysiology of latex allergy is similar to that of food allergy. Avoidance of latex products is recommended for those who are allergic to it. An immediate allergic reaction may occur if a latex-allergic child comes into contact with latex. Latex allergy can also result in anaphylaxis (refer to previous section on anaphylaxis).

Nursing Assessment

Screen all children who visit a health care facility of any kind for latex allergy. Ask if the child is allergic to rubber gloves or has ever developed hives after exposure to them. Ask the parent if the child has symptoms such as coughing, wheezing, or shortness of breath after glove exposure. Has the child ever had swelling in the mouth or complained that the mouth itched after a dental examination? Determine whether the child has ever had allergic symptoms after eating foods with a known cross-reactivity to latex, such as pear, peach, passion fruit, plum, pineapple, kiwi, fig, grape, cherry, melon, nectarine, papaya, apple, apricot, banana, chestnut, carrot, celery, avocado, tomato, or potato. For the child who has come into contact with latex, assess for symptoms of a reaction such as hives; wheeze; cough; shortness of breath; nasal congestion and rhinorrhea; sneezing; nose, palate, or eye pruritus; or hypotension.

Nursing Management

Nursing management of latex allergy focuses on preventing exposure to latex products. Instruct children and their families to avoid foods with a known cross-reactivity to latex such as those listed earlier. If the child is exposed to latex, remove the irritating substance and cleanse the area with soap and water. Assess for the need for resuscitation and perform it if needed. Become familiar with your institution's latex allergy policy. Know which products contain latex and which do not. Document latex allergy on the chart, the child's identification band, the medication administration record, and the health care provider's order sheet. Refer families to resources for people with latex allergy.

Unfolding Patient Stories: Charlie Snow • Part 2

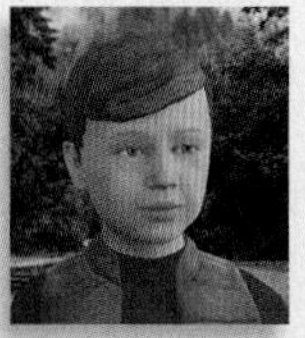

Recall Charlie Snow, a 6-year-old with a known hypersensitivity to dyes, perfumes, and peanuts whom you first met in Chapter 28. Since living with his aunt and uncle while his parents are in the military, he has been treated for a skin reaction and is now hospitalized with an anaphylactic reaction from peanut ingestion. How would the nurse determine if Charlie is at risk for maltreatment or neglect? What measures can the nurse take to ensure his safety at home?

Care for Charlie and other patients in a realistic virtual environment: ***vSim** for Nursing* (thepoint.lww.com/vSimPediatric). Practice documenting these patients' care in DocuCare (thePoint.lww.com/DocuCareEHR).

KEY CONCEPTS

- Waning of maternal antibodies in early infancy while humoral immunity is developing leads to physiologic hypogammaglobulinemia, placing the young infant at risk for overwhelming infection.
- Infants and young children have large lymph nodes, tonsils, and thymus compared with adults.
- Infants have decreased phagocytic activity, placing them at higher risk for serious infection.
- Children with immune disorders often show a decreased or absent response to delayed hypersensitivity skin testing (e.g., the tuberculosis test).
- Primary immune deficiencies such as SCID and Wiskott–Aldrich syndrome are congenital and serious; they can be cured only by bone marrow or stem cell transplantation.
- SLE is a chronic autoimmune disorder that can affect any organ system, primarily causing vasculitis.
- Juvenile idiopathic arthritis results in chronic pain and affects growth and development as well as school performance.
- Nasal, palatal, or throat pruritus and difficulty breathing may indicate an anaphylactic reaction.
- Various forms of hypogammaglobulinemia may be treated with exogenous immunoglobulin administered intravenously every several weeks, allowing children to lead a healthier life with fewer infections.
- Children with severe allergy or previous anaphylactic episodes must avoid contact with allergens.
- Nursing management of lupus focuses on preventing flare-ups and complications.
- Managing pain, maintaining mobility, and administering disease-modifying medications are key nursing interventions in the management of juvenile idiopathic arthritis.
- HIV infection may be prevented in infants by prenatal screening and maternal treatment, as well as postnatal treatment with zidovudine.
- HIV infection in children often results in encephalopathy and developmental delay.
- Spread of HIV infection can be prevented in adolescence by avoiding high-risk behaviors.
- For children with immune deficiency or autoimmune disease, prevention of infection is a primary nursing concern.
- A chronic illness such as immune deficiency, SLE, or juvenile arthritis has a significant impact on the family as well as the child.
- When planning care for the child with an immune deficiency or autoimmune disorder, the nurse should include the child and the family.
- To promote proper growth, encourage the child with an immune or autoimmune disorder to eat a balanced diet.
- Teach families of children with immune deficiencies about infection prevention.
- Teach the family of the child with juvenile arthritis about ways to decrease pain while increasing or maintaining the child's mobility.

- Teach families of children with severe allergy how to avoid allergens and how to use the EpiPen. Make sure that staff at the child's school or day care center are aware of the allergy.
- Explain to the child with severe allergy the importance of wearing a medical ID alert bracelet or necklace.

REFERENCES AND RECOMMENDED READINGS

Abbott, J. K., Dutmer, C. M., & Hauk, P. J. (2022). Chapter 33: Immunodeficiency. In M. Bunik, W. W. Hay, M. J. Levin, & M. J. Abzug (Eds.), *Current diagnosis & treatment: Pediatrics* (26th ed., pp. 976–994). McGraw-Hill Education.

Abrams, E. M., Chan, E. S., & Sicherer, S. (2020) Peanut allergy: New advances and ongoing controversies. *Pediatrics, 145*(5), e20192102. https://doi.org/10.1542/peds.2019-2102

American Academy of Allery, Asthma & Immunology. (2024). Food allergy. https://acaai.org/allergies/allergic-conditions/food/

Campbell, R. L., & Kelso, J. M. (2024). Anaphylaxis: Acute diagnosis. *UpToDate*. Retrieved April 16, 2024, from https://www.uptodate.com/contents/anaphylaxis-acute-diagnosis

Corbett, J. A., & Banks, A. D. (2019). *Laboratory tests and diagnostic procedures with nursing diagnoses* (9th ed.). Pearson Education Inc.

Covar, R. A., Fleischer, D. M., Cho, C., & Boguniewicz, M. (2022). Chapter 38: Allergic disorders. In M. Bunik, W. W. Hay, M. J. Levin, & M. J. Abzug (Eds.), *Current diagnosis & treatment: Pediatrics* (26th ed., pp. 1105–1147). McGraw-Hill Education.

Gillespie, S. L. (2023). Pediatric HIV infection: Classification, clinical manifestations, and outcome. *UpToDate*. Retrieved February 25, 2024, from https://www.uptodate.com/contents/pediatric-hiv-infection-classification-clinical-manifestations-and-outcome

Health Resources and Services Administration, the HIV/AIDS Program. (2022). *About the program*. https://ryanwhite.hrsa.gov/about

Heimall, J. (2019). Severe combined immunodeficiency (SCID): An overview. *UpToDate*. Retrieved February 25, 2024, from http://www.uptodate.com/contents/severe-combined-immunodeficiency-scid-an-overview

Hutchinson, C., & Feldman, B. M. (2023). Juvenile dermatomyositis and polymyositis: Treatment, complications, and prognosis. *UpToDate*. Retrieved February 25, 2024, from http://www.uptodate.com/contents/treatment-and-prognosis-of-juvenile-dermatomyositis-and-polymyositis

Hutchinson, C., & Feldman, B. M. (2024). Juvenile dermatomyositis and other idiopathic inflammatory myopathies: Epidemiology, pathogenesis and clinical manifestations. *UpToDate*. Retrieved February 25, 2024, from http://www.uptodate.com/contents/pathogenesis-and-clinical-manifestations-of-juvenile-dermatomyositis-and-polymyositis

Kids with Food Allergies. (2023). *Recipe substitutions*. https://kidswithfoodallergies.org/recipes-diet/recipe-substitutions/

Klein-Gitelman, M. S. (2022). Pediatric systemic lupus erythematous. *Medscape*. Retrieved April 28, 2023, from https://emedicine.medscape.com/article/1008066-overview#a6

Lexicomp®. (2024). *Lexi-Drugs/immune globulin (Version 8.1.0) [Mobile app]*. Wolters Kluwer. https://apps.apple.com/us/app/lexicomp/id313401238

Lin, Y., Kuang, Q., Li, H., Liang, B., Ly, J., Jiang, Q., & Yang., X. (2023). Outcome and clinical features in juvenile myasthenia gravis: A systematic review and meta-analysis. *Frontiers in Neurology, 14*. https://doi.org/10.3389/fneur.2023.1119294

Linzer, J. F. (2024). *Pediatric anaphylaxis*. Medscape. https://emedicine.medscape.com/article/799744-overview#a1

Mayo Foundation for Clinical Education and Research. (2024). *Pediatric test reference values*. http://www.mayomedicallaboratories.com/test-info/pediatric/refvalues/reference.php

National Hemophilia Foundation. (2023). *MASAC Document 280 - MASAC recommendations concerning products licensed for the treatment of hemophilia and selected disorders of the coagulation system*. https://www.hemophilia.org/healthcare-professionals/guidelines-on-care/masac-documents/masac-document-280-masac-recommendations-concerning-products-licensed-for-the-treatment-of-hemophilia-and-selected-disorders-of-the-coagulation-system

National Institutes of Health. (2024a). *HIV and adolescents and young adults*. https://hivinfo.nih.gov/understanding-hiv/fact-sheets/hiv-and-adolescents-and-young-adults

National Institutes of Health. (2024b). *HIV and children*. https://hivinfo.nih.gov/understanding-hiv/fact-sheets/hiv-and-children

Ochs, H. D. (2022). Wiskott-Aldrich syndrome. *UpToDate*. Retrieved February 25, 2024, from http://www.uptodate.com/contents/wiskott-aldrich-syndrome

Panel on Antiretroviral Therapy and Medical Management of Children Living with HIV. (2024). *Guidelines for the use of antiretroviral agents in pediatric HIV infection*. Department of Health and Human Services. https://clinicalinfo.hiv.gov/en/guidelines/pediatric-arv/whats-new

Patel, S. B. (2022). Avascular necrosis. *Medscape*. Retrieved February 25, 2024, from http://emedicine.medscape.com/article/333364-overview

Smith, C., & McFarland, E. J. (2022). Chapter 41: Human immunodeficiency virus infection. In M. Bunik, W. W. Hay, M. J. Levin, & M. J. Abzug (Eds., pp. 1224–1236), *Current diagnosis & treatment: Pediatrics* (26th ed.). McGraw-Hill Education.

Soep, J. B. (2022). Chapter 29: Rheumatic diseases. In M. Bunik, W. W. Hay, M. J. Levin, & M. J. Abzug (Eds.), *Current diagnosis & treatment: Pediatrics* (26th ed., pp. 865–874). McGraw-Hill Education.

Tosi, M. F. (2019). Chapter 2: Normal and impaired immunologic responses to infection. In J. Cherry, G. J. Harrison, W. J. Steinbach, S. L. Kaplan, & P. Hotez (Eds.), *Feigin & Cherry's textbook of pediatric infectious diseases* (8th ed., pp. 15–40). Elsevier.

U.S. Department of Health and Human Services. (n.d.). *Healthy People 2030*. https://health.gov/healthypeople

U.S. House of Representatives. (2004). *Public law No. 108-377 asthmatic schoolchildren's treatment and health management act of 2004*. Library of Congress.

UpToDate, Inc. (2024). *Lexi-comp® (Version 8.1.0) [Mobile app]*. Wolters Kluwer. https://apps.apple.com/us/app/lexicomp/id313401238

Viatris. (2023). *EpiPen®: How to use*. https://www.epipen.com/en/about-epipen-and-generic/how-to-use-epipen

Winkels, K. (2023). *Allergy-free foods*. http://www.eatingwithfoodallergies.com/allergyfreesubstitutes.html

Wolownik, K. (2022). Common HSCT complications. In M. Evans, J. Nuuhiwa, R. L. Secola, & K. Wolownik (Eds.), *Foundations of pediatric hematopoietic stem cell transplantation* (3rd ed.). Association of Pediatric Hematology/Oncology Nurses.

Yiu, E. (2023). Guillain-Barré syndrome in children: Epidemiology, clinical features, and diagnosis. *UpToDate*. Retrieved February 25, 2024, from http://www.uptodate.com/contents/epidemiology-clinical-features-and-diagnosis-of-guillain-barre-syndrome-in-children

DEVELOPING CLINICAL JUDGMENT

PRACTICING FOR NCLEX

1. The nurse is caring for a 6-year-old with juvenile idiopathic arthritis. The parent states they have trouble getting their child out of bed in the morning and believe the child's behavior is due to a desire to avoid going to school. What is the best advice by the nurse?
- **a.** Refer them to a psychologist for evaluation of school phobia related to chronic illness.
- **b.** Administer a warm bath every morning before school.
- **c.** Give the child prescribed NSAIDs 30 minutes before getting out of bed.
- **d.** Allow the child to stay in bed some mornings if they want.

2. A 14-year-old with SLE wants to know how to care for their skin. What should the nurse teach this adolescent?
- **a.** Careful sun-tanning will give their skin an attractive color.
- **b.** No special skin care is needed.
- **c.** Use sunscreen daily to avoid rashes.
- **d.** Use makeup to camouflage the butterfly rash on their face.

3. The parent of a child with hypogammaglobulinemia reports that their child had a fever and slight chills with an intravenous gamma globulin infusion last month. They want to know what other course of treatment might be available. What is the best response by the nurse?
- **a.** Administration of acetaminophen or diphenhydramine prior to the next infusion may decrease the incidence of fever or chills.
- **b.** Giving the gamma globulin intramuscularly is recommended to prevent a reaction.
- **c.** Talk to the health care provider or nurse practitioner about alternative medications that may be used to boost the gamma globulin level in the blood.
- **d.** If the child is no longer experiencing frequent infections, then the IV infusions may not be necessary.

4. A 4-month-old infant born to a parent with HIV infection is going into foster care because the birthing parent is too ill to care for the child. The foster parent wants to know if the infant is also infected. What is the best response by the nurse?
- **a.** "It's too early to know; we have to wait until the infant has symptoms."
- **b.** "Since the birthing parent is so ill, it's likely the child is also infected with HIV."
- **c.** "The ELISA test is positive, so the child is definitely infected."
- **d.** "The PCR test is positive; this indicates HIV infection, which may or may not progress to AIDS."

5. A parent has received instructions about avoiding wheat and soy allergens. Which response by the parent would indicate that further education is needed?
- **a.** "I will not feed my child any breads made with wheat flour."
- **b.** "I will allow my child to eat semolina pasta, the kind they love."
- **c.** "I will not feed my child shakes made with soy protein."
- **d.** "I will read labels to be sure I am avoiding wheat and soy."

6. The nurse is caring for a child in the acute phase of Guillain–Barré syndrome. What is the priority nursing action?
- **a.** Perform range-of-motion exercises.
- **b.** Take temperature every 4 hours.
- **c.** Monitor respiratory status closely.
- **d.** Assess skin frequently.

7. At a classmate's birthday celebration at school, a child with a known food allergy is coughing and exhibiting retractions when the school nurse assesses them. The child states they "don't feel right" and that they have an itchy throat.
Place the nursing actions in priority order from first to last.
- **a.** Administer the child's prescribed EpiPen.
- **b.** Determine the child's vital signs.
- **c.** Position the child to facilitate breathing.
- **d.** Ask another adult to activate the Emergency Management Systems (EMS).
- **e.** Notify the parents.

8. The charge nurse on the pediatric unit assigns an adolescent with HIV infection and poor growth to the licensed practical nurse (LPN). The LPN states, "I do not want to care for this adolescent." Which is the appropriate response by the charge nurse?
- **a.** "Okay, I will check if the other LPN will care for them."
- **b.** "So you are confident with the adolescent's care, I will help you."
- **c.** "You seem worried about caring for this adolescent."
- **d.** "Let's review blood and body fluid precautions you will using."

DOSAGE CALCULATION QUESTION

The nurse is caring for a term newborn born to a parent with HIV infection. The infant weighs 6 lb 5 oz. The medication order reads: zidovudine 25 mg PO twice daily. Zidovudine is supplied as 50 mg/5 mL. How many milliliters will the nurse administer? Round to the nearest tenth.

CRITICAL THINKING EXERCISES

1. Develop a discharge teaching plan for a 14-year-old with SLE who will be taking corticosteroids long term.
2. Devise a developmental stimulation plan for a 22-month-old with HIV infection and encephalopathy with developmental delay (to the level of a 9-month-old).
3. Determine an appropriate nursing plan of care for an infant who has undergone bone marrow transplantation for SCID.
4. Develop a prioritized list of patient problems for a child with HIV infection, candidiasis, poor growth, and pneumonia requiring oxygen.
5. A child with recurrent infections is being evaluated. Other than information about onset of symptoms and events leading up to this present episode, what other types of information would the nurse ask while obtaining the history?

STUDY ACTIVITIES

1. In the clinical setting, compare the growth and development of two children of the same age, one with HIV infection and one who has been healthy.
2. Attend an outpatient clinic that provides care to children with HIV infection. Observe the health care or nurse practitioner during office visits, and attend a multidisciplinary planning meeting. Identify the role of the registered nurse in providing family education, coordination of care, and referrals.
3. Conduct an internet search to determine the educational material available to children and their families related to immune deficiencies, autoimmune disorders, or allergies.
4. Research your clinical institution's policies related to latex allergy, alternative products available at the institution, and how to obtain them for a child with latex allergy. Provide a presentation to your clinical group about your findings.

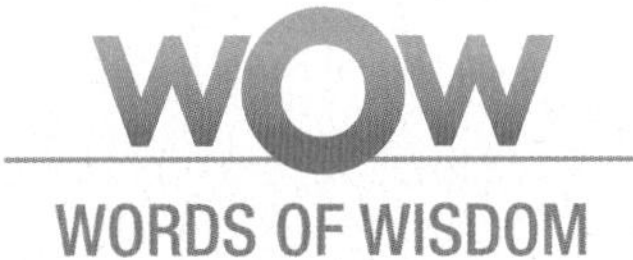

WORDS OF WISDOM

Endocrine disorders in children often elude the medical radar screen.

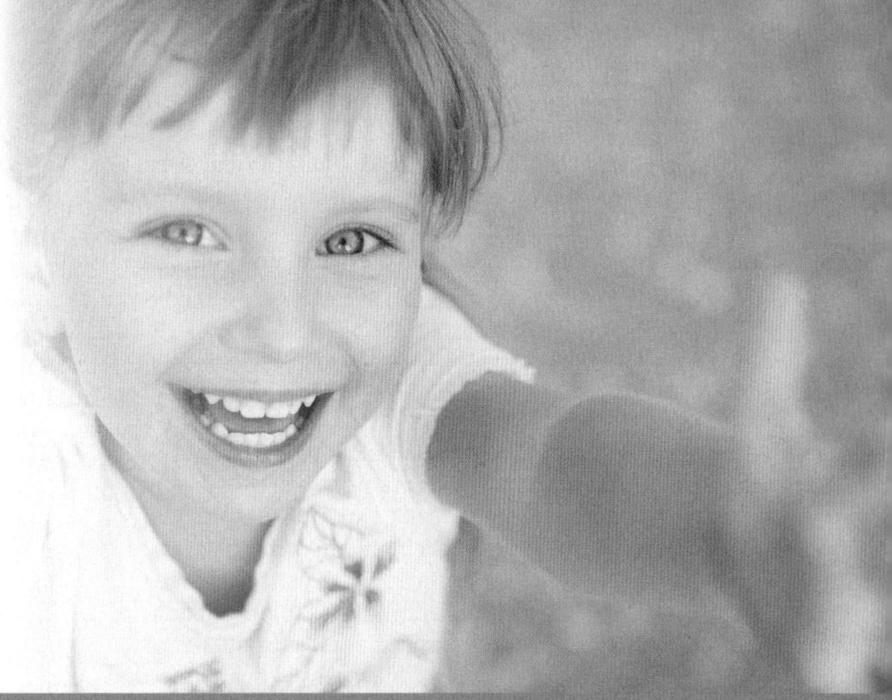

48

Nursing Care of the Child With an Alteration in Metabolism/Endocrine Disorder

LEARNING OBJECTIVES

Upon completion of the chapter, you will be able to:

1. Describe the major components and functions of a child's endocrine system.
2. Differentiate between the anatomic and physiologic differences of the endocrine system in children versus adults.
3. Identify the essential assessment elements, common diagnostic procedures, and laboratory tests associated with the diagnosis of endocrine disorders in children.
4. Identify the common medications and treatment modalities used for palliation of endocrine disorders in children.
5. Distinguish specific disorders of the endocrine system that affect children.
6. Associate the clinical manifestations of specific endocrine disorders with the appropriate patient problems.
7. Establish nursing outcomes, evaluative criteria, and interventions for children with specific disorders in the endocrine system.
8. Develop teaching plans for children and their families regarding endocrine disorders.

KEY TERMS

adrenarche (ad-ren-ahr′kē)
constitutional delay
diabetic ketoacidosis (DKA)
exophthalmos (eks′of-thal′mos)
goiter
hemoglobin A1C
hirsutism (hir′sū-tizm)
hormone
hyperfunction
hypofunction
polydipsia
polyuria

Carlos Rodriguez, a 12-year-old, is seen in the clinic today with complaints of weakness, fatigue, blurred vision, and headaches. His parent states, "Carlos's teacher has noticed mood changes and is concerned about his behavior at school. He's always been a good boy. I'm not sure what's going on."

INTRODUCTION

Metabolism refers to all physical and chemical reactions occurring in the body's cells that are necessary to maintain and sustain life. Nurses encounter potential and actual alterations in metabolism in all types of patients and must detect problems and intervene early to prevent life-threatening or long-term complications. The endocrine system consists of various glands, tissues, or clusters of cells that produce and release hormones. **Hormones** are chemical messengers that stimulate or regulate the actions of other tissues, organs, or other endocrine glands that have specific receptors for the hormone. Along with the nervous system, the endocrine milieu influences all physiologic effects such as growth and development, metabolic processes related to fluid and electrolyte balance and energy production, sexual maturation and reproduction, and the body's response to stress. The release patterns of hormones vary, but the level in the body is maintained within specified limits to preserve health.

Alterations in metabolism develop in the endocrine system when there is a deficiency (**hypofunction**) or excess (**hyperfunction**) of a specific hormone. In children, alterations in metabolism or endocrine conditions often develop insidiously and result from an insufficient production of hormones. If the problem is not diagnosed and treated early, delayed growth and development, cognitive impairments, or death may result. Generally, the treatment plan involves correction of the underlying reason for the dysfunction, such as surgical removal of a tumor, and supplementation of missing hormones or adjustment of specific hormone levels. This allows most children to live normal lives.

VARIATIONS IN ANATOMY AND PHYSIOLOGY

The organs or tissues of the endocrine system include the hypothalamus, pituitary gland, thyroid gland, parathyroid glands, adrenal glands, gonads, and islets of Langerhans located in the pancreas. Figure 48.1 shows the location of these organs or tissues involved in the endocrine system. Typically, most endocrine glands begin to develop during the first trimester of gestation, but their development is incomplete at birth. Thus, complete hormonal control is lacking during the early years of life, and infants cannot appropriately balance fluid concentration, electrolytes, amino acids, glucose, and trace substances.

Hormone Production and Secretion

The hypothalamic–pituitary axis produces a number of releasing and inhibiting hormones that regulate the function of many of the other endocrine glands, including the thyroid gland, the adrenal glands, and the male and female gonads. Some glands regulate their function in connection with the nervous system, such as the islets of Langerhans in the pancreas and the parathyroid glands. Many other cells in the body secrete hormones such as the pineal gland, the scattered epithelial cells in the gastrointestinal (GI) tract, and the thymus. Disorders related to these other cells are discussed in other chapters of this book.

Figure 48.1 shows the major glands, the hormones produced by these glands, and the effects each hormone has on the target cell, tissue, or organ. The process of hormone production and secretion involves the principle of feedback control. One gland produces a hormone that affects another endocrine gland. Once the physiologic effect is achieved, this gland, known as the target organ, inhibits the further release of the original hormone. The reverse occurs when the first gland detects low levels of the target gland hormone. If the original gland does not release enough of the hormone, the inhibition process stops so that the gland increases the production of the hormone. The endocrine system and the nervous system work closely together to maintain an optimal internal environment for the body, a state known as homeostasis.

COMMON MEDICAL TREATMENTS

Primarily, the treatment of endocrine disorders involves decreasing hormone production in cases of hypersecretion or replacing hormones in cases of hypofunction. The first step in treating many of these disorders is to screen for potential problems, especially when familial patterns are present. Since the proper functioning of the endocrine system is critical to growth and development, the child's growth is affected by endocrine dysfunction, and lack of treatment may lead to serious problems such as intellectual disability or even death. Early treatment is often associated with a better prognosis and prevention of long-term problems. The next step in treatment involves identifying underlying causes for the dysfunction (e.g., a tumor or growth that requires surgical removal or irradiation). The use of supplemental hormones in cases of hypofunction is generally successful in children, as is the use of inhibiting substances in cases of hyperfunction.

Common Medical Treatments 48.1 describes the common treatments used in children with endocrine disorders. The table explains and gives indications for each treatment, as well as relevant nursing implications. Advances in technology and our understanding of molecular biology continue to increase our knowledge of these disorders and the modalities needed to prevent them or improve quality of life for affected children. These advances are vital, since the whole body is influenced by the endocrine milieu.

Drug Guide 48.1 lists the medications most commonly used to treat endocrine disorders. The table gives the actions and indications of each drug, as well as pertinent nursing implications. Many of the medications are synthetic preparations of the actual hormones. It is important to maintain specific blood levels of the

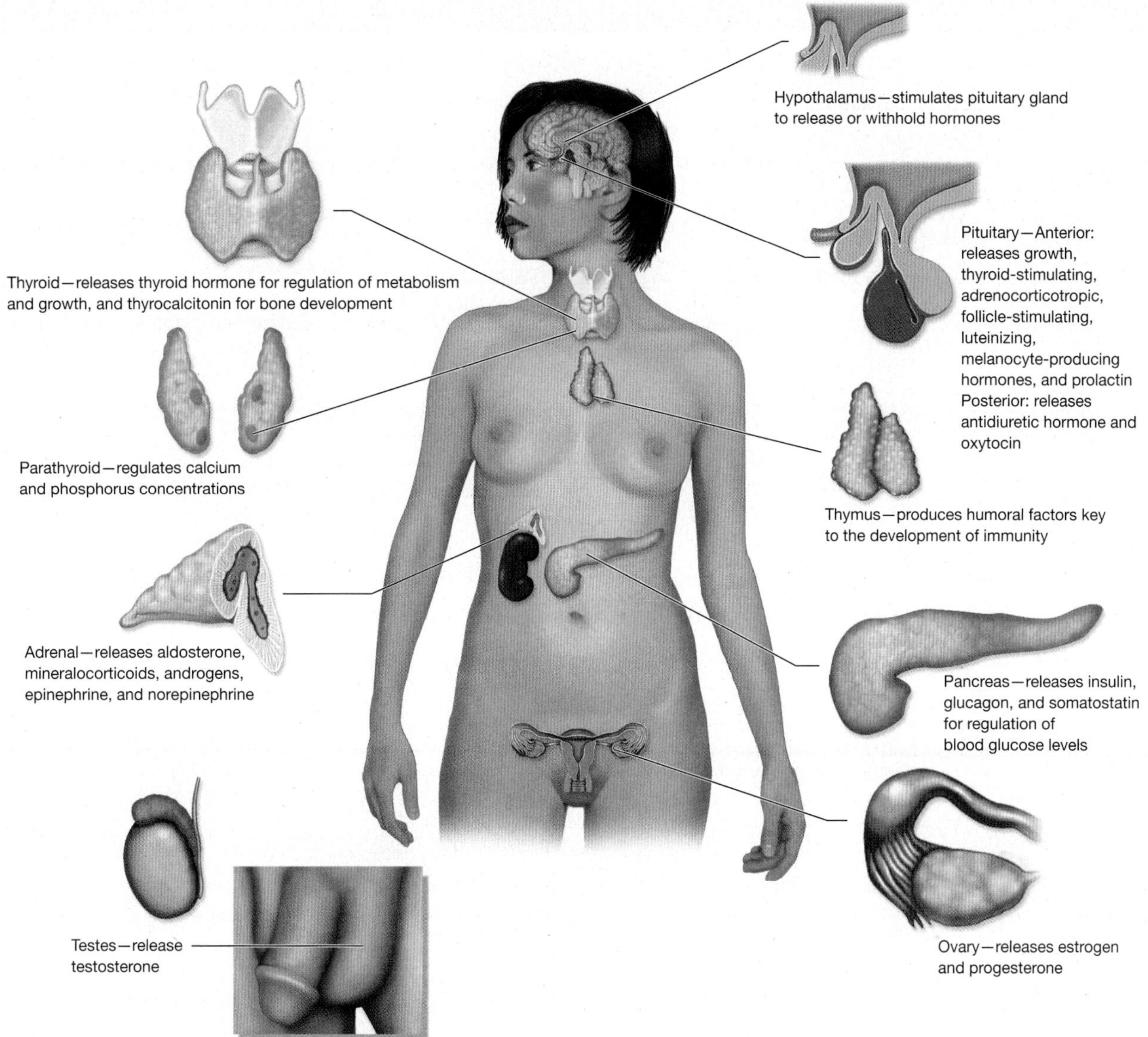
Hypothalamus—stimulates pituitary gland to release or withhold hormones
Pituitary—Anterior: releases growth, thyroid-stimulating, adrenocorticotropic, follicle-stimulating, luteinizing, melanocyte-producing hormones, and prolactin
Posterior: releases antidiuretic hormone and oxytocin
Thyroid—releases thyroid hormone for regulation of metabolism and growth, and thyrocalcitonin for bone development
Parathyroid—regulates calcium and phosphorus concentrations
Thymus—produces humoral factors key to the development of immunity
Adrenal—releases aldosterone, mineralocorticoids, androgens, epinephrine, and norepinephrine
Pancreas—releases insulin, glucagon, and somatostatin for regulation of blood glucose levels
Testes—release testosterone
Ovary—releases estrogen and progesterone

FIGURE 48.1 Location of the endocrine glands in the body, with the major effects of the glands listed.

COMMON MEDICAL TREATMENTS 48.1

Treatment	Explanation	Indications	Nursing Implications
Surgery	Surgical removal of tumors or cysts	Any endocrine malfunction caused by the presence of a mass	• Provide routine preoperative and postoperative care depending on location and extent of surgery. • Keep the family informed of choices.
Irradiation/radioactive iodine	Radiation is used to influence the hormone secretion of a gland; it is less invasive than surgery.	Hyperfunction of an endocrine gland; may be used when surgery is not possible	• Prepare the child for specific procedures following protocols. • Explain the procedure. • Check to ensure the child has no sensitivity to iodine preparations.
Glucose monitoring	Fingerstick blood sample several times per day	Monitoring of glucose control	• Teach the family appropriate procedure. • Refer family to sources for equipment and supplies. • Assist the family with developing a system of record-keeping that works for them.
Dietary interventions (medical nutritional therapy)	Restriction or manipulation of dietary intake	Diabetes mellitus (DM)	• Refer family to a dietitian specializing in pediatric DM. • Reinforce teaching related to special diets.

DRUG GUIDE 48.1

COMMON DRUGS FOR ENDOCRINE DISORDERS

Medication	Actions/Indications	Nursing Implications
Insulin	Used for diabetes mellitus (DM) to replace body's natural insulin, which is necessary for proper glucose use. Indicated for DM type 1 and, sometimes, DM type 2	• Monitor vital signs and blood glucose levels. • Educate the child and the family on proper techniques, actions, and adverse effects. • Rotate site of injections to prevent adipose hypertrophy.
Oral hypoglycemic drugs (glipizide, glyburide, metformin)	Assist the body's production of insulin by stimulating β cells to secrete more insulin. Indicated for type 2 DM	• Monitor vital signs and glucose levels. • Administer with food to minimize gastric upset. • Instruct the child and the family on the use of drug and its adverse effects. • Warn family that some over-the-counter or other drugs may increase hypoglycemic effect.
Growth hormone (GH)/somatropin	Stimulates linear bone, skeletal muscle, and organ growth Used for GH deficiency, growth failure related to inadequate pituitary hormone	• Monitor blood glucose and electrolyte levels. • Administer before epiphyses are fused. • Monitor growth with accurate measurements. • Instruct the child and the family on appropriate route and method of administration. • Periodic thyroid function tests will be needed. • May interact with glucocorticoid therapy • Monitor for limping or complaints in knee or hip related to slipped epiphysis.
Octreotide acetate	Suppresses GH release. Indicated for acromegaly	• Monitor for biliary tract abnormalities, glucose tolerance, and hypothyroidism. • Give subcutaneous injections between meals to decrease gastric effects (may alter absorption of fats). • May switch to intramuscular (IM) depot injection every 1–3 months once stabilized
Corticosteroids (dexamethasone or hydrocortisone)	Cortisol replacement in congenital adrenal hyperplasia, absence of adrenal glands. Also used to close epiphyseal plates in hyperpituitarism	• Give with milk or food. • May need to increase dose if the child is ill or runs fever • Monitor for edema, weight gain, glycosuria, signs of infection, and symptoms of peptic ulcer development. • Do not decrease dose or abruptly stop drug to avoid adrenal crisis.
Desmopressin acetate (DDAVP)	Synthetic antidiuretic hormone that promotes reabsorption of water by action on renal tubules Used to control arginine vasopressin deficiency (AVP-D)	• Monitor for water intoxication, signs and symptoms of hyponatremia, and adverse effects such as nasal irritation, headache, nausea, and increased blood pressure. • Record fluid intake and output and weigh the child daily. • Titrate dose until appropriate fluid output is obtained. • Instruct the child and the family on proper intranasal administration. • May need to be stored in refrigerator
Levothyroxine	Thyroid hormone replacement for hypothyroidism	• Monitor blood pressure and pulse. • Monitor fluid intake and output, daily weights, and thyroid function tests. • Watch for thyroid storm. • Report irritability or anxiety. • Instruct the child and the family to avoid over-the-counter preparations with iodine or foods such as soybeans, iodized salt, tofu, and turnips. If the infant must be on soy formula, administer it between feedings. • Do not administer within 4 hours of antacids (such as simethicone) and iron or calcium supplements. • Administer at same time each day.
Methimazole	Antithyroid drug; blocks synthesis of T_3 and T_4 Indicated for hyperthyroidism	• Monitor pulse and blood pressure. • Monitor input and output, daily weights, serum T_3 and T_4 levels; watch for edema, leukopenia, thrombocytopenia, or agranulocytosis. • Signs of overdose: periorbital edema, cold intolerance, mental depression • Signs of inadequate dose: tachycardia, diarrhea, fever, or irritability
Mineralocorticoid	Promotes reabsorption of Na and K, water from distal renal tubules Used in adrenal insufficiency	• Monitor daily weights, blood pressure, and intake and output. • Observe for potassium depletion. • Titrate dose to lowest effective dose. • Monitor for signs of infection. • Monitor for signs of edema.

T3, triiodothyronine; T4, thyroxine

Source: Lexicomp. (2023). Pediatric drug information. *UpToDate.* Retrieved May 20, 2023, from https://www.uptodate.com/contents/table-of-contents/drug-information

drugs to mimic the actual hormone levels in the body. Nurses must monitor for side effects of both too little and too much of the hormone in the child's system. Most endocrine disorders in children require treatment and follow-up with a pediatric endocrinologist, as well as a multidisciplinary team that includes a registered nurse who specializes in this area.

Clinical Judgment and the Nursing Process for the Child With an Endocrine Disorder

The nursing care of the child with an endocrine disorder requires astute assessment skills, accurate nursing analysis and expected outcomes, skilled interventions, and evaluation of the entire process. Children, especially very young ones, easily develop imbalances such as fluid and electrolyte disturbances that can cause further problems. Most of the endocrine disorders are chronic conditions that require ongoing care related to health maintenance, education, developmental issues, and psychosocial needs. These conditions are sometimes complex and range from mild to profound. Early diagnosis and treatment can improve the long-term outcomes for these children.

Assessment

Nursing assessment of a child with endocrine dysfunction includes obtaining a thorough health history, performing a physical assessment, and assisting with or obtaining laboratory and diagnostic tests. The clinical manifestations of endocrine disorders occur as a result of the altered control of the bodily processes normally regulated by the gland or hormone. These manifestations present in many areas of the body because of the diverse functions associated with the endocrine system.

Health History

The health history should include questions regarding any family history of an endocrine disorder or growth and development difficulties. Use a genogram or family tree to detail the information about the family history in a clear and concise manner.

Discuss prenatal history, including any maternal factors that may affect growth and development, such as substance misuse, use of tobacco or alcohol, and Graves disease; address birth history, including trauma during delivery, birth size, feeding difficulties, and neonatal screening and results. Additionally, consider past medical history, such as any chronic childhood diseases, treatment for endocrine problems, recent gastroenteritis or viral syndromes, or exposures to exogenous steroids or gonadotropins. Finally, evaluate growth and development patterns, including the presence of any delays, learning disabilities, and early or late development of secondary sexual characteristics.

Discuss present complaints or illness. Note the onset of symptoms, whether gradual or sudden. Endocrine disorders often cause problems in normal growth and development, as well as behavioral changes. Question the parent or caregiver about prior growth patterns, achievement of developmental milestones, and the child's behavior. Inquire about recent increases or decreases in weight and height, changes in physical appearance, sleep patterns, muscle weakness, cramps, twitching, or headaches. Have the child and family describe the child's activities on a typical day, including school performance, to identify subtle variations in the child's behavior or moods. For example, a child who is typically quiet might ordinarily be less active than average children of that age, and a child with decreased endocrine function often displays inactivity and fatigue. By having the family and child describe a typical day, the nurse can distinguish between what is appropriate for that child and what may be a change related to endocrine dysfunction.

In addition, obtain a history of dietary and elimination habits. Note any extreme thirst, excessive appetite, vomiting, or frequent voiding. Children with endocrine disorders may exhibit some of these symptoms.

Physical Examination

Physical examination of the child with an endocrine disorder includes inspection and observation, auscultation, percussion, and palpation. Table 48.1 lists key physical examination findings that may be present in children with endocrine dysfunction.

INSPECTION AND OBSERVATION

Note a fatigued appearance, poor muscle tone, sweatiness, faintness, nervousness, or confusion. Inspect the head and face, and note hair texture and growth, a protuberant tongue, drooping eyelids, or **exophthalmos** (protrusion of the eyeballs). Plot the child's height and weight on growth charts to determine abnormal growth velocity, which occurs in many of these disorders.

AUSCULTATION

Auscultate the heart and lungs. Note heart rate and rhythm. During auscultation of the lungs, note labored respiratory effort, such as Kussmaul breathing, which occurs in diabetic ketoacidosis (DKA). Document blood pressure.

PERCUSSION AND PALPATION

Percuss and then palpate the abdomen. Dull (nontympanic) sounds or the presence of masses may indicate constipation or a tumor of the ovaries.

Laboratory and Diagnostic Testing

Common Laboratory and Diagnostic Tests 48.1 describes the diagnostic tests and procedures frequently used in identifying and monitoring endocrine disorders in

TABLE 48.1 • Key Physical Examination Findings Related to Endocrine Problems

Height and weight	Below third percentile or above 90th percentile (pituitary, thyroid, adrenal, or diabetes mellitus)
Hair	Coarse, brittle, excessive (hypothyroidism) Abnormal distribution (adrenal disorders)
Face	Round with hair growth (Cushing syndrome) Deformities or abnormal features (hypoparathyroidism)
Eyes	Blurred or changes in vision (diabetes mellitus, pituitary tumors, precocious puberty)
Mouth	Delayed dentition (hypocalcemia, hypopituitarism) Fruity breath (ketoacidosis)
Neck	Goiter (hyperthyroidism)
Skin	Cool to touch, dry (hypothyroidism) Changes in color or texture (pituitary disorders) Easy bruising, striae (Cushing syndrome)
Chest	Tachycardia (hyperthyroidism) Palpitations, sweating (thyroid disorders) Deep, labored breathing (ketoacidosis) Hypertension (Cushing syndrome)
Abdomen	Extreme weight loss (diabetes mellitus) Extreme fat (Cushing syndrome) Changes in bowel habits (SIADH, AVP-D, diabetes mellitus)
Fingers	Trembling (hyperthyroidism, parathyroid disorders)
Genitals	Excessive growth (adrenogenital syndrome) Early growth (precocious puberty) Delayed growth (hypopituitarism)

AVP-D, arginine vasopressin deficiency; SIADH, syndrome of inappropriate antidiuretic hormone.

COMMON LABORATORY AND DIAGNOSTIC TESTS 48.1

Diagnostic Test or Procedure	Explanation	Indications	Nursing Implications
Newborn metabolic screening programs (refer to Chapter 31 for further information)	Newborn blood testing to identify certain harmful or potentially fatal disorders that are otherwise not apparent at birth. Disorders tested vary by state.	Identify newborns so that treatment can begin early to prevent impact of disorder, such as severe cognitive impairment or death.	• Refer to each state's protocol for fetal or newborn screening for endocrine disorders. • Explain to the family the rationale and procedure. • Collect blood sample accurately. • Collect prior to blood transfusion if possible. • Ensure screening is done for early discharges. • Screening typically between 24 and 48 hours after birth • If collected before 24 hours of age, a repeat test is needed within 14 days. Some states now require a repeat screen at 2 weeks of age.[a]
Random serum hormone levels	Serum levels of various hormones; immunoassay measures levels with very small amounts of blood	High or low levels are used to evaluate the function of specific gland.	• May need to draw specimens at specific times • Keep the child NPO after midnight before test if ordered. • Diurnal variations and episodic secretion of many hormones may require special directions or further testing.
Self-monitoring blood glucose (SMBG)	Fingerstick (monitors that utilize alternative sites, such as the forearm, are available); blood sample several times per day Noninvasive methods available[b]	Monitor glucose level and effectiveness of treatment.	• Teach the family appropriate procedure. • Refer the family to sources for equipment and supplies. • Assist the family with developing a system of record-keeping that works for them. • Refer to Teaching Guidelines 48.2.

COMMON LABORATORY AND DIAGNOSTIC TESTS 48.1

Diagnostic Test or Procedure	Explanation	Indications	Nursing Implications
Fasting plasma glucose	Fasting forces the body to produce glucagon, which causes the release of glucose. In a healthy child, the body will respond by releasing insulin, therefore lowering blood glucose and preventing hyperglycemia.	Detect hyperglycemia related to diabetes or other conditions, such as Cushing syndrome or liver or kidney disease. Can detect prediabetes	• The child should not have had any caloric intake for at least 8 hours. • Draw sample prior to insulin or oral diabetes medications. • Normal value in children 2–18 years of age, 60–100 mg/dL; in children 0–2 years of age, 60–110 mg/dL; impaired fasting glucose or prediabetes is between 100 and 125 mg/dL; diabetes is considered with a result ≥126 mg/dL on two separate occasions.
Two-hour plasma glucose test (2-h PG)	Oral glucose tolerance test Oral glucose is ingested and in a healthy child, insulin will respond and return blood glucose to normal levels.	Usually performed to detect diabetes, often gestational diabetes Can also detect prediabetes	• The child should not have taken any insulin or oral diabetes medication before the test. • Time of oral glucose ingestion needs to be noted. • Specimen to be drawn at specified time interval from ingestion • May have limited value in diagnosing children
Urine or serum ketone testing	Ketones are the result of the metabolism of fat and in a healthy child are present in insignificant amounts.	Screening for ketones in urine is regularly performed in children, people with diabetes, hospitalized patients, preoperatively, and in pregnant people. In children, ketones found in urine during routine urinalysis can detect undiagnosed diabetes. In children with diabetes, the presence of ketones in serum or urine is a sign that their diabetes is not well controlled and can be an early sign of diabetic ketoacidosis (DKA).	• Urine ketone testing can be performed using dipsticks at the bedside and at home (follow manufacturer's directions; time reaction accurately and compare the strip to the control chart on the bottle). • Encourage testing for ketones when blood glucose is elevated, when therapy regimen is changing, or during times of stress or illness.
Hemoglobin A1C (glycated hemoglobin)	Glycated hemoglobin reflects the percentage of hemoglobin to which glucose is attached. In the case of hyperglycemia, an increase in glycohemoglobin leads to an increase in hemoglobin A1C. This test shows the average blood glucose level for the past 2–3 months.	Diagnose diabetes. Indicated for children with diabetes. Provides information regarding long-term glycemic control and effectiveness of therapy.	• Elevated levels seen in newly diagnosed diabetes or poorly controlled diabetes. • Levels can be elevated in children without diabetes with certain conditions such as blood loss, hemolysis, iron-deficiency anemia, sickle cell anemia, and lead toxicity.
Genetic testing	Tests for the presence of the gene for disease or carrier status	Determine genetic involvement of any disorder.	• Explain the procedure and the expense involved. • Refer for genetic counseling if needed.
Serum chemistry levels	Serum blood urea nitrogen (BUN), creatinine, sodium, potassium, glucose, calcium, phosphorus, alkaline phosphatase, etc.	Rule out chronic kidney disease or other chronic illnesses; monitor effects of treatment.	• BUN levels may be elevated with high-protein diet or dehydration and may be decreased with overhydration or malnutrition. • A diet high in meat may cause a transient but not pronounced increase in creatinine. There are also slight diurnal variations in levels. • Avoid hemolysis of specimen, as this may cause elevation in potassium levels. • Calcium and phosphorus: avoid prolonged tourniquet use during blood draw, as this may falsely increase levels. The child should be NPO past midnight prior to the morning of the blood draw.

(continued)

COMMON LABORATORY AND DIAGNOSTIC TESTS 48.1 (*continued*)

Diagnostic Test or Procedure	Explanation	Indications	Nursing Implications
Growth hormone (GH) stimulation	Stimulate release of GH in response to administration of insulin, arginine, clonidine, or glucagon.	Evaluate and diagnose GH deficiency.	• Keep the child NPO for specified time. • Limit stress and physical activity at least 30 minutes before test. • Obtain serial blood samples at specific times. • Monitor blood glucose levels during study. • Observe for signs of hypoglycemia, diaphoresis, and somnolence. • Provide a snack, such as cookies and juice at end of test.
Water deprivation study	The child is deprived of fluids for several hours, and serum sodium and urine osmolality are monitored.	Diagnose AVP-D or AVP-R (previously known as diabetes insipidus [DI]) and distinguish between AVP-D and AVP-R (previously known as central or nephrogenic DI).	• Stop the test if the child exhibits extreme weight loss or changes in vital signs or neurologic status. • Weigh child before, during, and after test. • Rehydrate the child after test. • Monitor for orthostatic hypotension.
Bone age radiograph	Radiographic study of wrist or hand to determine bone maturation compared to national standards	Determine if bone age is consistent with chronologic age to rule out GH deficiency or excess or hypothyroidism.	• Explain the procedure to the child because they need to hold still for the radiograph. • Allow the family to accompany the child. • Enlist the family's help if needed to calm the child during radiography.
Other nuclear medicine studies	Contrast media uptake is assessed with serial radiographs.	Visualize an ectopic, enlarged, absent, or nodular gland.	• Assess the child for allergy to iodine or shellfish. • Explain the procedure to the child.
CT	Noninvasive x-ray study that looks at tissue density and structures. Images a "slice" of tissue	Evaluate the presence of tumors, cysts, or structural abnormalities that may affect specific gland or structure.	• Machine is large and can be frightening to children. • Scan may be lengthy and the child must remain still, so sedation may be necessary. • If contrast medium is to be used, assess for allergy. • Encourage fluids after procedure if not contraindicated.
MRI	Based on how hydrogen atoms behave in a magnetic field when disturbed by radiofrequency signals. Does not require ionizing radiation. Provides a 3D view of the body part being scanned	Evaluate the presence of tumors, cysts, or structural abnormalities that may affect specific gland or structure.	• Remove all metal objects from the child. • The child must remain motionless for entire scan; the parent can stay in room with the child. Younger children will require sedation in order to be still. • A loud thumping sound occurs inside the machine during the procedure, which can be frightening to children.
Ultrasonography	Noninvasive sound waves are used to visualize structures, such as thyroid or pelvic region.	Evaluate the presence of tumors or cysts in a specific gland, such as the adrenal glands or ovaries, to rule out disorders.	• Requires full bladder if in pelvic region. • It is better tolerated by nonsedated children than CT or MRI. • Can be performed with a portable unit at bedside.

AVP-D, arginine vasopressin deficiency; AVP-R, arginine vasopressin resistance; CT, computed tomography; MRI, magnetic resonance imaging; NPO, nothing by mouth.

[a]Kemper, A. R. (2021). Newborn screening. *UpToDate*. Retrieved May 20, 2023 from https://www.uptodate.com/contents/newborn-screening

Data from Fischbach, F. T., Fischbach, M. A., & Stout, K. (2022). *A manual of laboratory and diagnostic tests* (11th ed.). Wolters Kluwer.

children. Serum and urine hormone and other levels are used to determine whether amounts are adequate, deficient, or excessive. Radiographic studies are used to evaluate bone maturation, growth potential, and density or tissue calcification. Genetic studies may be used to determine enzyme deficiencies or chromosome defects. Stimulation studies provide a more accurate or definitive test for identifying the disorder after preliminary serum levels are abnormal. Serial blood sampling identifies peak or trough levels of hormones. Computed tomography (CT) scans, magnetic resonance imaging (MRI), nuclear medicine studies, and ultrasonography are used to look for tumors, cysts, or structural defects. These tests can assist the health care provider or nurse practitioner in diagnosing disorders and guiding ongoing treatment. Laboratory or nonnursing personnel perform some of the tests, while the nurse might perform others. In either instance, the nurse should be familiar with how the tests are performed, what they are used for, and normal versus abnormal results. This knowledge will also be necessary when providing children and family education related to the testing.

Remember Carlos, the 12-year-old, with weakness, fatigue, blurred vision, headaches, and mood changes? What additional health history and physical examination assessment information should the nurse obtain?

Nursing Analysis

After recognizing and analyzing cues from a thorough assessment, the nurse might identify several patient problems, including the following:

- Malnutrition risk
- Dehydration or fluid overload risk
- Delayed development risk
- Altered body image perception
- Knowledge deficiency
- Altered health maintenance
- Interrupted family processes
- Risk for caregiver role strain

After completing an assessment of Carlos, the nurse noted the following: history reveals Carlos has had episodes of bedwetting over the past month and has polydipsia and polyphagia. His weight continues to be above the 95th percentile on the growth chart. Based on these assessment findings, what would be your top three patient problems for Carlos?

The previously listed patient problems or concerns provide suggestions for developing a nursing plan of care or concept mapping. The nurse will then generate solutions by planning interventions (suggested with rationales further on). The plan of care should be individualized, based on the child's and family's needs.

Refer to Chapter 33 for nursing interventions related to interrupted family processes and risk for caregiver role strain. Additional information will be included later in the chapter as it relates to specific disorders. Because of the gradual, insidious onset of many of these disorders, the child may first be seen in an acute situation. It may be easier for the child and family to work with short-term goals until they accept the chronic situation. A major goal will be to achieve adherence to medical management. The goals for the child with a disorder of the endocrine system generally include reestablishing homeostasis, promoting adequate growth and development, establishing appropriate body image, promoting health-seeking behaviors, and providing education so the family can manage the condition.

A key element to include in any plan of care or concept map for a child with an endocrine disorder involves preparing the child, based on their developmental needs, for invasive procedures and tests. Provide an opportunity for the family and child to express their concerns and fears during diagnosis and treatment. Reinforce realistic expectations for treatment and prospects for improvement with the family and child. The plan of care or concept map also needs to address developmental, acute, chronic, and home care issues, as well as child and family education. Families will need assistance with managing the condition from a multidisciplinary team.

Nursing Analysis

Malnutrition risk related to biologic factors, as evidenced by growth parameters less than expected for age

Goal/Outcome

The child's nutritional status is balanced. The child adheres to nutritional guidelines and demonstrates adequate growth (weight and height) patterns within the normal range for age and sex, or shows a progressive increase over time if has growth difficulties.

Maintaining Adequate Nutrition (interventions with *rationale*)

- Determine the body weight and length/height norm for age or what the child's pretreatment measurements were *to determine goal to work toward.*
- Weigh daily or weekly (according to health care provider's order or institutional standard) and measure length/height weekly *to monitor for appropriate growth.*
- Determine the child's food preferences and provide favorite foods when possible *to increase the likelihood of the child consuming appropriate amounts of foods.*

- Instruct the child and family about nutritional requirements *so that they are involved and are prepared for home care.*
- Refer to a dietitian *for more detailed information and assistance.*
- Offer the highest-calorie meals at the time of day when the child's appetite is greatest *to increase the likelihood of increased caloric intake.*
- Provide increased-calorie shakes or puddings within dietary restrictions, *as high-calorie foods increase weight gain.*
- Administer vitamin and mineral supplements as prescribed *to attain/maintain vitamin and mineral balance in the body.*

Nursing Analysis

Dehydration or fluid overload risk related to compromised regulatory function (pathophysiology of endocrine dysfunction), as evidenced by signs and symptoms of dehydration or edema and excessive urine output (fluid overload)

Goal/Outcome

The child will maintain adequate fluid volume, as evidenced by elastic skin turgor, absence of edema, moist and pink oral mucosa, presence of tears, urine output of 1 mL/kg/h or more, vital signs within the normal range for age, and normal electrolyte/hormone serum levels.

Maintaining Adequate Fluid Volume (interventions with *rationale*)

- Assess hydration status (skin turgor, oral mucosa, presence of tears) every 4 to 8 hours *to evaluate the maintenance of adequate fluid volume.*
- Assess the adequacy of urine output *to evaluate end-organ perfusion.*
- Maintain a strict intake and output record *to evaluate the effectiveness of rehydration.*
- Weigh the child daily: *accurate weight is one of the best indicators of fluid volume status in children.*
- Administer specific hormone, fluid, and electrolyte requirements as ordered *to aid in fluid balance.*
- For fluid volume deficit: Maintain the intravenous (IV) line and administer IV fluid as ordered *to maintain fluid volume.*
- For fluid volume excess: Maintain fluid restriction as ordered *to restore homeostasis.*

Nursing Analysis

Delayed development risk (risk factors include chronic illness [endocrine disorder], treatment regimen, and inadequate nutrition)

Goal/Outcome

The child's development will be enhanced. The child will not suffer regression in abilities and will make continued progress toward the attainment of developmental milestones within age parameters and limits of disease. Also, the child expresses interest in the environment and people around them and interacts with the environment appropriately for their developmental level.

Promoting Development (interventions with *rationale*)

- Encourage adherence to hormone supplementation to enhance the ability *to achieve appropriate growth and development.*
- Screen for developmental capabilities *to determine the child's current level of functioning.*
- Offer age-appropriate toys, play, and activities (including gross motor) *to encourage further development.*
- Provide support to families; *due to disability and deficits, the child's progress toward developmental milestones may be slow.*
- Use therapeutic play and adaptive toys *to facilitate developmental functioning.*
- Provide a stimulating environment whenever possible *to maximize the potential for growth and development.*
- Praise accomplishments and emphasize the child's abilities *to improve self-esteem and encourage feeling of confidence and competence.*

Nursing Analysis

Altered body image perception related to an alteration in self-perception (abnormal growth and development or changes in physical appearance due to hormone dysfunction), as evidenced by verbalization of dissatisfaction with the child's or adolescent's looks

Goal/Outcome

The child demonstrates appropriate self-esteem in relation to body image by expressing positive feelings about themselves and participating in social activities.

Promoting Healthy Body Image (interventions with *rationale*)

- Provide opportunities for the child to explore feelings related to appearance; *venting feelings is associated with less body image disturbance.*
- Relate to child on their age level, not appearance level; *"babying" a child who looks younger due to their small size may reduce their self-image.*
- Involve the child, especially the adolescent, in the decision-making process; *a sense of control will improve body image.*
- Encourage the child to spend time with peers who have similar endocrine disorders; *peers' opinions are often better accepted than those of people in authority, such as parents or health care professionals.*
- Refer the child to counseling or support groups *to further support them.*

Nursing Analysis

Knowledge deficiency related to insufficient information (regarding therapeutic regimen), as evidenced by questions about the endocrine disorder and self-management

Goal/Outcome

The child and family will demonstrate sufficient understanding and skills for self-management: verbalize information about disorder, complications/adverse effects, home care regimen, and long-term needs, and provide return demonstrations of medication administration or other procedures.

Promoting Knowledge Required for Self-Management (interventions with *rationale*)

- Assess the child's developmental level and the family's ability to absorb instruction, as well as their willingness to learn, *to determine how to approach teaching sessions; the child and family must be willing to learn for teaching to be effective.*
- Provide the family with time to adjust to the diagnosis *to facilitate their adjustment and ability to learn and participate in the child's care.*
- Establish a teaching plan with the child and family *to gain their cooperation and involvement.*
- Use multiple modes of learning involving many senses (provide written, verbal, demonstration, and videos) when possible; *the child and family are more likely to retain information when it is presented in different ways using multiple senses.*
- Teach and provide printed instructions on disorder, complications, home care, and follow-up requirements *so the family has a reference to use at home.*
- Repeat information *to allow the family and child time to learn and understand.*
- Teach in short sessions: *many short sessions are more helpful than one long session.*
- Gear teaching to the level of understanding of the child and family (depends on age of child, physical condition, memory) *to ensure understanding.*
- Provide reinforcement and rewards *to facilitate the teaching and learning process.*
- Evaluate teaching through return demonstrations *to determine whether the child/family is skilled enough for home management of the disorder.*

For children with diabetes mellitus (DM), include the following:

- First teach "survival skills" (e.g., glucose and urine testing, administering insulin, record-keeping, food guidelines, when to call health care provider) *to provide an initial base of knowledge for self-management.*
- Implement a second-phase home management program with more extensive instruction; *providing additional teaching over time is necessary for managing a significant chronic illness.*
- Monitor the outcomes of teaching with every contact *to ensure progress with child and family education.*

Nursing Analysis

Altered health maintenance related to difficulty managing a complex treatment regimen or insufficient knowledge of the therapeutic regimen, as evidenced by difficulty with the prescribed regimen or failure to include the treatment regimen in daily living

Goal/Outcome

The child and family will adhere to the treatment regimen. They will list treatment expectations, agree to follow through, and keep appointments with providers.

Encouraging Adherence (interventions with *rationale*)

- Listen nonjudgmentally while the child and family describe reasons for nonadherence; *assessment of the problem should begin with a nonthreatening discussion.*
- Help the child and family develop a schedule for medication administration and other home regimens that works best for them; *involving the child and family in planning care will increase adherence by making them feel respected and valued.*
- Work with the child and family to develop a written treatment plan or schedule that best suits their needs *to provide support for the maintenance of the treatment plan.*
- Establish follow-up visits to fit the family's situation *to promote adherence.*
- Encourage monitoring with a pediatric endocrinologist and specialists; *multidisciplinary involvement has been shown to increase adherence.*
- Recognize that behavioral change comes slowly; *allow time for the child and family to adjust to chronic nature of the illness.*

Based on your top three patient problems for Carlos, describe appropriate nursing interventions.

PITUITARY DISORDERS

Because of the close anatomic and functional relationships between the hypothalamus and pituitary gland, we will discuss them together. The hypothalamus affects the pituitary by releasing and inhibiting hormones and may be the cause of pituitary disorders. In general, disorders of the pituitary fall into two major groups: anterior pituitary hormones and posterior pituitary hormones. Anterior pituitary primary disorders in children include growth hormone (GH) deficiency, hyperpituitarism, and precocious puberty. Posterior pituitary disorders include arginine vasopressin deficiency (AVP-D; previously known as diabetes insipidus [DI]) and syndrome of inappropriate antidiuretic hormone (SIADH) secretion.

CLINICAL REASONING ALERT!

Infants with congenital defects of the pituitary gland or hypothalamus may present with symptoms that include apnea, cyanosis, severe hypoglycemia with possible seizures, and prolonged jaundice and should be treated as an emergency (Patterson & Felner, 2020).

GH Deficiency

GH deficiency, also known as hypopituitarism or dwarfism, is characterized by poor growth and short stature. GH is vital for postnatal growth. It is released throughout the day, with most secreted during sleep. GH stimulates linear growth, bone mineral density, and growth in all body tissues.

GH deficiency occurs in approximately one in 4,000 to one in 10,000 children (Patterson & Felner, 2020). Often, this condition is first identified when the health care provider or nurse practitioner assesses growth patterns. Children may start with a normal birth weight and length, but within a few years, their growth falls below the third percentile on the growth chart.

Possible complications related to GH deficiency and its treatment include altered carbohydrate, protein, and fat metabolism; hypoglycemia; glucose intolerance or diabetes; slipped capital femoral epiphysis; pseudotumor cerebri; leukemia; recurrence of central nervous system (CNS) tumors; infection at the injection site; edema; and sodium retention.

Pathophysiology

GH deficiency generally results from the failure of the anterior pituitary or hypothalamic stimulation on the pituitary to produce sufficient GH. This lack of GH impairs the body's ability to metabolize protein, fat, and carbohydrates.

Primary causes of GH deficiency include injury to or destruction of the anterior pituitary gland or hypothalamus. Causes include a tumor (e.g., craniopharyngioma), infection, infarction, CNS irradiation, abnormal formation of these organs in utero, or damage or trauma during birth or afterward. It may also be part of a genetic syndrome, such as Prader–Willi syndrome or Turner syndrome, or the result of a genetic mutation or deletion.

In some cases, the cause of GH deficiency may be idiopathic, such as nutritional deprivation or psychosocial issues, and reversible. Psychosocial dwarfism results from emotional deprivation, which suppresses the production of pituitary hormones, resulting in decreased GH levels. Children with psychosocial dwarfism may exhibit withdrawal, bizarre eating and drinking habits, such as drinking from toilets, and primitive speech. Treatment involves removing the child from the dysfunctional environment and providing normal dietary intake. With normalized eating and behavioral habits, pituitary secretion is restored, and the child experiences dramatic catch-up growth.

Therapeutic Management

Treatment of primary GH deficiency involves the use of supplemental GH and should be started as soon as possible. (See Dosage Calculation Box 48.1.) Secondary GH deficiency requires removal of any tumors that might be the underlying problem, followed by GH therapy. Biosynthetic GH, derived from recombinant DNA, is given by subcutaneous injection. Treatment continues until near-final height is achieved. This can be determined by the child deciding they are tall enough, a growth rate of less than 0.8 to 1 in/year, or bone age greater than 16 years in males and greater than 14 years in females (Patterson & Felner, 2020; Rogol & Richmond Padilla, 2023).

DOSAGE CALCULATION BOX 48.1

Child's weight: 30 lb

Medication order: Somatropin 0.5 mg subcutaneously once a day

Per the *Pediatric Dosage Handbook*, the recommended dose is 0.18–0.3 mg/kg weekly, divided into 6–7 doses.

Is the ordered dose safe?

Nursing Assessment

The focus of the evaluation for GH deficiency is to rule out chronic illnesses such as kidney disease, liver disorders, and thyroid dysfunction. For a full description of the assessment phase of the nursing process, refer to the "Clinical Judgment and the Nursing Process" section earlier in the chapter. Assessment findings pertinent to GH deficiency are discussed further on.

HEALTH HISTORY

The health history may reveal a familial pattern of short stature or a prenatal history of maternal disorders such as malnutrition. The past history may be significant for birth history of intrauterine growth restriction or past history of severe head trauma or a brain tumor such as craniopharyngioma. Evaluate previous and current growth patterns. Note history of chronic illnesses such as cardiac, kidney, or intestinal disorders that may contribute to a decreased growth pattern. Also, assess the child's feelings about their height.

PHYSICAL EXAMINATION

In addition to linear height being at or below the third percentile on standard growth charts, physical assessment findings may show that the child has a higher weight-to-height ratio (Fig. 48.2). Other physical findings may include prominent subcutaneous deposits of abdominal fat; a child-like face with a large, prominent forehead; a high-pitched voice; delayed sexual maturation (e.g., micropenis and undescended testes in males); delayed dentition; delayed skeletal maturation; and decreased muscle mass.

TAKE NOTE!

Growth measurements are often inaccurate and unreliable in children. An important anthropometric measurement is body height, and improved accuracy could yield earlier detection and diagnosis of growth disorders (Warrier et al., 2022). According to the Centers for Disease Control and Prevention (CDC), the stadiometer is the preferred tool for assessing height in children >3 years of age (Warrier et al., 2022) (see Fig. 48.2). To improve and ensure accuracy, the CDC has implemented standardized procedures for measuring body height.

LABORATORY AND DIAGNOSTIC TESTING

The child will undergo laboratory tests to rule out chronic illnesses such as kidney disease, liver dysfunction, and thyroid dysfunction. Laboratory and diagnostic tests used in children with suspected GH deficiency include the following:

- Bone age (as shown by radiographs) will be two or more deviations below normal.
- CT or MRI scans are used to rule out tumors or structural abnormalities.
- Pituitary function testing confirms the diagnosis. This test consists of providing a GH stimulant such as glucagon, clonidine, insulin, arginine, or L-dopa to stimulate the pituitary to release a burst of GH. Peak GH levels below 7 to 10 mcg/mL in at least two tests confirm the diagnosis.

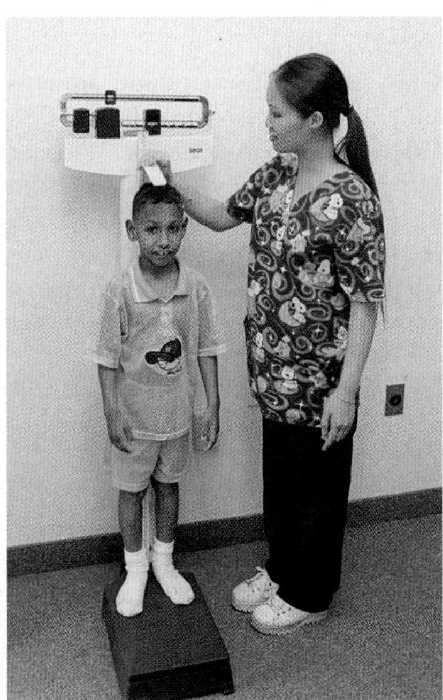

FIGURE 48.2 The child with growth hormone deficiency displays short stature.

Nursing Management

Nursing management for the child with GH deficiency focuses on promoting growth, enhancing the child's self-esteem related to short stature, and providing appropriate education about the disorder.

PROMOTING GROWTH

The goal of growth promotion is for the child to demonstrate an improved growth rate, as evidenced by at least 3 to 5 inches in linear growth in the first year of treatment without complications. With early diagnosis and treatment, the child has a better prognosis for reaching a normal adult height. Growth is usually excellent in the first year of therapy compared to later years (Patterson & Felner, 2020). Treatment stops when the epiphyseal growth plates fuse.

At the beginning of treatment, monitor for height increase and possible side effects related to the medications. Measure the child's height at least every 3 to 6 months and plot growth over time on standardized growth charts. Provide information to the child and family about normal development and growth rates, bone age, and growth potential. Discuss with the family and child their expectations and understanding of what is normal, so they will have realistic expectations of treatment. Consult a dietitian if the child and family need assistance in providing adequate nutrition for growth and development.

ENHANCING THE CHILD'S SELF-ESTEEM

The child with GH deficiency often exhibits younger-looking features and is shorter than their peers. Encourage the child to express positive feelings about their self-image, as shown by comments during health care visits and involvement with peers. Encourage the child to voice any concerns they have. Emphasize the child's strengths and assets. Provide information about community support groups or websites related to GH deficiency. Evaluate for long-term learning problems that may develop if the child had a tumor and underwent surgery or irradiation to remove it. Unidentified learning problems can have a negative impact on the child's self-esteem. Treat and communicate with the child in an age-appropriate manner, even though they may appear younger.

EDUCATING THE FAMILY

GH is available as a powder that is mixed with packaged diluents. Most are available in multidose pen delivery systems, with some systems not requiring reconstitution (Rogol & Richmond Padilla, 2023). Explain how to prepare the medication and give the correct dosage. Encourage rotation of injection sites in the subcutaneous tissue to prevent skin irritation. Have the family provide a return demonstration to make sure they understand the correct dilution and administration of GH. Continue to provide periodic evaluation and ongoing support.

Instruct the family to report any headaches, rapid weight gain, increased thirst or urination, or painful hip or knee joints as possible adverse reactions. Explain to the family that the child will need to visit the pediatric endocrinologist every 3 to 6 months to monitor growth, potential adverse effects, and adherence to therapy. Stress the importance of complying with GH replacement therapy and frequent supervision by a pediatric endocrinologist. Emphasize that the success of the treatment is dependent on adherence to the regimen prescribed. Educate the family about the financial costs of therapy, which may be high, and assist them in obtaining assistance through referral to social services if needed.

Guide the family and child in setting realistic goals and expectations based on age, personal abilities, strengths, and the effectiveness of GH replacement therapy. For example, encourage the family to consider sports that are not dependent on height and to dress the child according to age, not size. Refer the child and family to counseling if indicated. Also, inform families about support groups such as the Human Growth Foundation and the Magic Foundation.

Precocious Puberty

In precocious puberty, the child develops sexual characteristics before the usual age of pubertal onset. Puberty, also known as sexual maturation, occurs when the gonads produce increased amounts of sex hormones. Typically, this occurs around 10 to 12 years of age for females and 11 to 14 years of age for males. In precocious puberty, secondary sex characteristics develop in females before the age of 8 years and in males younger than 9 years (Harrington & Palmert, 2022). The disorder is more common in females, and the majority of the time the cause is unknown in females, while in males, a structural CNS abnormality is often present (Garibaldi & Chemaitilly, 2020). Other causes include benign hypothalamic tumor, brain injury or radiation, a history of infectious encephalitis or meningitis, congenital adrenal hyperplasia (CAH), and tumors of the ovary, adrenal gland, pituitary gland, or testes.

Pathophysiology

Central precocious puberty, the most common form, develops as a result of premature activation of the hypothalamic–pituitary–gonadal axis that results in the production of gonadotropin-releasing hormone (GnRH), which stimulates the pituitary to produce luteinizing hormone (LH) and follicle-stimulating hormone (FSH). These hormones, in turn, stimulate the gonads to secrete the sex hormones (estrogen or testosterone). The child develops sexual characteristics, shows increased growth and skeletal maturation, and has reproductive capability. Peripheral precocious puberty presents with no early secretion of gonadotropin or maturation of gonads but rather early overproduction of sex hormones. The condition results in increased end-organ sensitivity to low levels of circulating sex hormones and leads to premature pubic hair and breast development.

If left untreated, the child may reach fertility. In addition, the hormones stimulate rapid growth. Therefore, the child may appear taller than peers but will reach skeletal maturity and closure of the epiphyseal plates early, which will result in overall short stature.

Therapeutic Management

The clinical treatment for precocious puberty first involves determining the cause. For example, if the etiology is a tumor of the CNS, the child undergoes surgery, radiation, or chemotherapy. The treatment for central precocious puberty involves administering a GnRH analog. This is available as a subcutaneous injection given daily, an intranasal compound administered two or three times daily, a depot injection given every 3 to 4 weeks, a depot injection administered quarterly, or a subcutaneous implant yearly. This analog stimulates gonadotropin release initially, but when given long-term, it suppresses gonadotropin release. With this treatment, the growth rate slows, and secondary sexual development stabilizes or regresses. Medroxyprogesterone injections (Depo-Provera) or tablets (Cycrin) reduce secretion of gonadotropins and prevent menstruation. When treatment is discontinued, puberty resumes according to appropriate developmental stages. The overall aim of treatment is to halt or even reverse sexual development and rapid growth, as well as promote psychosocial well-being.

Nursing Assessment

For a full description of the assessment phase of the nursing process, refer to the "Clinical Judgment and the Nursing Process" section earlier in the chapter. Pertinent assessment findings related to precocious puberty are discussed further on.

HEALTH HISTORY

The health history may reveal complaints of headaches, nausea, vomiting, and visual difficulties due to circulating hormones. Psychosocial development is typical for the child's age, but they may exhibit emotional lability, aggressive behavior, and mood swings. Additional information gathered from the child and family may also reveal risk factors such as exposure to exogenous hormones, a history of CNS trauma or infection, or a family history of early puberty.

PHYSICAL EXAMINATION

The physical examination may reveal acne and an adult-like body odor. The child will present with an accelerated rate of growth. Tanner staging of breasts, pubic hair, and genitalia may indicate advanced maturation for the child's age, although the child typically does not display sexual behavior.

LABORATORY AND DIAGNOSTIC TESTING

Radiologic examinations and pelvic ultrasound can identify advanced bone age, increased uterus size, and development of ovaries consistent with the diagnosis of precocious puberty. Laboratory studies include screening radioimmunoassays for LH, FSH, estradiol, or testosterone. The child's response to GnRH stimulation confirms the diagnosis of central precocious puberty versus gonadotropin-independent puberty. This test involves administering synthetic GnRH intravenously (IV) and drawing serial blood levels, about every 2 hours, of LH, FSH, and estrogen or testosterone. A positive result is defined as pubertal or adult levels of these hormones in response to the GnRH administration. Also, CT, MRI, or skull radiography can reveal any lesions in the CNS or tumors or cysts present in the abdomen, pelvic area, or testes.

Nursing Management

In general, nursing management of a child with precocious puberty focuses on educating both the child and their family about the physical changes the child is experiencing and how to correctly use the prescribed medications and helping the child to deal with self-esteem issues related to the accelerated growth and development of secondary sexual characteristics. Goals of nursing management include appropriate physical development and pubertal progression appropriate for the child's age. Refer to the "Clinical Judgment and the Nursing Process" section earlier in the chapter, and individualize care based on the child's and family's response to this disorder.

PROVIDING EDUCATION

Nursing care involves assessing and documenting the physical changes the child is experiencing, as well as administering medications. Demonstrate correct administration of medication and observe for potential adverse effects (teach this information to the family as well). Encourage families to comply with follow-up appointments, typically scheduled every 6 months, which may include stimulation tests. Inform families that pharmacologic intervention stops when the child reaches the age appropriate for pubertal development. Also, provide appropriate sex education.

DEALING WITH SELF-ESTEEM ISSUES

Due to the body image changes that differ from their peers, these children may develop self-esteem issues. The goal is to foster normal psychosocial development and help the child understand the physical and emotional changes that occur with early onset of puberty. Communicate with the child on an age-appropriate level, even when physical characteristics make the child appear older. Maintain a calm, supportive atmosphere and provide for privacy during examinations. Refer the child and family for counseling as needed. Since the child may have issues with self-image and may be self-conscious, encourage them to express their feelings about the changes, and use role-playing to show the child how to handle teasing from other children. Let the child know that everyone develops sexual characteristics in their own time.

Delayed Puberty

Delayed puberty is a condition of delayed secondary sexual development. In females, it is identified if the breasts have not developed by ages 12 to 13. In males, it is identified when there is no testicular enlargement or scrotal changes by ages 13 to 14 (Crowley & Pitteloud, 2023).

The most common cause for delayed puberty is a hereditary pattern of growth and development known as **constitutional delay** of growth and puberty (or a "late bloomer") (Crowley & Pitteloud, 2023). In these cases, there is a familial pattern of late-onset puberty; affected adolescents typically develop normally, just at a later time than their peers. Hypogonadism may also result when there is decreased stimulation of the gonads due to dysfunction or tumors in the hypothalamus or pituitary gland. Other causes include irradiation, infection, trauma, or genetic syndromes such as Turner or Klinefelter syndrome. Also, chronic conditions, such as anorexia or cystic fibrosis, lead to delayed puberty.

Therapeutic management involves administering testosterone (males) or estradiol-conjugated estrogen (females) in low dosages if there is no underlying medical condition to address. This is usually necessary for only a short time to get puberty started.

Nursing Assessment

Assessment involves obtaining a health history to identify the indications for this condition. Assessment of the growth pattern using correct techniques and standards for comparison is essential. On physical assessment, note the absence of secondary sex characteristics, as noted earlier. Laboratory and diagnostic testing rules out other potential causes for delayed puberty. Blood levels of reproductive hormones may also be evaluated.

Nursing Management

In addition to the general interventions presented in the "Clinical Judgment and the Nursing Process" section earlier in the chapter, instruct the child and family about the medication therapy. Educate them about the different stages of puberty. Help the family develop a home management schedule for the administration of medication. Address any questions the family may have about the condition or potential complications (e.g., infertility), depending on the underlying cause of the condition.

Arginine Vasopressin Resistance (AVP-R) and Arginine Vasopressin Deficiency (AVP-D)

AVP-R (previously referred to as nephrogenic DI) and AVP-D (previously referred to as central DI) are both major causes of polyuria in children (Working Group for Renaming Diabetes Insipidus et al., 2022). AVP-R can be transmitted genetically (e.g., sex-linked, autosomal dominant or recessive forms) or be acquired due to chronic kidney disease, hypercalcemia, hypokalemia, or use of certain drugs such as lithium, amphotericin, methicillin, and rifampin (Breault & Majzoub, 2020a). AVP-R is not associated with the pituitary gland and is related to decreased renal sensitivity to antidiuretic hormone (ADH). Therapeutic management for AVP-R involves diuretics, high fluid intake, restricted sodium intake, and a high-protein diet. Desmopressin acetate (DDAVP) is usually ineffective in the treatment of nephrogenic DI.

AVP-D is a disorder of the posterior pituitary gland and is the most common form of AVP dysfunction (Mutter et al., 2021). Therefore, AVP-D (central DI) will be the focus of the remainder of this discussion. It is characterized by excessive thirst (**polydipsia**) and excessive urination (**polyuria**) that is not affected by decreasing fluid intake. Typically, this disorder occurs in children as a result of complications from head trauma or after cranial surgery to remove hypothalamic–pituitary tumors, such as craniopharyngioma. Some cases can be hereditary; however, 10% of AVP-D cases in children are idiopathic (Breault & Majzoub, 2020a). Other causes include genetic mutations, granulomatous disease, infections such as meningitis or encephalitis, vascular anomalies, congenital malformations, infiltrative disease such as leukemia, or administration of certain drugs that are associated with inhibition of vasopressin release, such as phenytoin (Breault & Majzoub, 2020a). AVP-D is usually permanent and requires treatment throughout life.

Pathophysiology

AVP-D (central DI) results from a deficiency in the secretion of ADH. This hormone, also known as vasopressin, is produced in the hypothalamus and stored in the pituitary gland. ADH is involved in concentrating urine from the kidneys by stimulating the reabsorption of water in the renal collecting tubules through increased membrane permeability. This mechanism conserves water and helps maintains normal osmolality. With a deficiency in ADH, the kidneys lose massive amounts of water and retain sodium in the serum.

Therapeutic Management

Unless a tumor is present (in which case it is removed by surgery), the usual treatment for AVP-D (central DI) involves a low-solute diet (low sodium and low protein), daily replacement of ADH, and possibly the use of a thiazide diuretic (Bichet, 2023). The drug of choice for home treatment is DDAVP, a long-acting vasopressin analog (Breault & Majzoub, 2020a). In children, it is typically given intranasally. However, it can also be administered subcutaneously, orally, or buccally. The dose depends on the child's age, urine output, and urine specific gravity. Treatment of AVP-D and the use of DDAVP in infants and small children can be challenging and complicated due to their inability to access fluids and articulate thirst (Bichet, 2023). In neonates and young infants, treatment often focuses solely on fluid therapy due to their high volume requirements of nutritive fluid (i.e., the drive behind an infant's fluid intake is hunger rather than thirst) (Breault & Majzoub, 2020a). However, some experts suggest that subcutaneously administered DDAVP may be more effective than oral or intranasal therapy in infants and small children due to variable absorption and the challenge of administering accurate doses via these routes (Bichet, 2023).

In the hospital, the child may receive aqueous vasopressin or 8-arginine vasopressin (Pitressin) IV (Breault & Majzoub, 2020a). This is a short-acting drug, so the dosage can be adjusted quickly.

Both the long- and short-acting forms of the medication decrease urinary output and thirst, and the dosages of both forms of these drugs need to be titrated to achieve the desired effect.

TAKE NOTE!

A metered nasal spray form of DDAVP is available, but the prescribed dose must be >10 mcg/0.1 mL for the child to use the spray (Bichet, 2023).

Nursing Assessment

For a full description of the assessment phase, refer to the "Clinical Judgment and the Nursing Process" section earlier in the chapter. Assessment findings pertinent to AVP-D are discussed further on.

HEALTH HISTORY

Nursing assessment involves obtaining a history of any conditions that may have led to the development of the disorder. This review includes information about the neonatal period as well as a current history of infections such as meningitis, diseases such as leukemia, or familial patterns. Although most symptoms of endocrine disorders develop slowly, the onset of this disorder is often abrupt. The health history usually elicits the cardinal symptoms, as well as complaints representing the early signs of dehydration.

The most commonly reported initial symptoms are polyuria and polydipsia (Bichet, 2023; Breault & Majzoub, 2020a). Except for unconscious children, the child typically maintains adequate perfusion by drinking water. Parents or the child may report frequent trips to the bathroom, nocturia, or enuresis. When the child cannot compensate for the excessive loss of water by increasing fluid intake, other symptoms will be reported, such as weight loss or signs of dehydration. For example, irritability may be due to the early signs of dehydration or the frustration the child feels at being unable to quench their thirst. Other signs may include intermittent fever, vomiting, and constipation.

PHYSICAL EXAMINATION

Observation and inspection may reveal weight loss or failure to thrive in young infants. Inspection may also reveal signs of dehydration, such as dry mucous membranes or decreased tears. The child may excrete more than 3 L/m^2 of urine per day. On auscultation, tachycardia or an increased respiratory rate may indicate compensation for the decrease in fluid volume. Palpation may reveal slightly depressed fontanels or decreased skin turgor.

LABORATORY AND DIAGNOSTIC TESTING

Diagnostic tests used to evaluate AVP-D include the following:

- Radiographic studies such as CT scan, MRI, or ultrasound of the skull and kidneys can determine whether a lesion or tumor is present.
- Urinalysis: urine is dilute, osmolality is less than 3,000 mOsm/L, specific gravity is less than 1.005, and sodium level is decreased.
- Serum osmolality is greater than 300 mOsm/L.
- Serum sodium is elevated.
- A fluid deprivation test measures vasopressin release from the pituitary in response to water deprivation. Normal results will show decreased urine output, increased urine specific gravity, and no change in serum sodium levels.

> **TAKE NOTE!**
>
> During a fluid deprivation test, the child may be irritable and frustrated because fluid is being withheld. Don't drink in front of the child.

Nursing Management

Refer to the "Clinical Judgment and the Nursing Process" section earlier in the chapter, and individualize the plan of care based on the child's and family's response to the illness. Specific interventions related to nursing care of the child with AVP-D are discussed further on.

PROMOTING HYDRATION

The goal of treatment is to achieve an hourly urine output of 1 to 2 mL/kg and a urine specific gravity of at least 1.010.

> **CLINICAL REASONING ALERT!**
>
> Notify the health care provider or nurse practitioner if the urine output exceeds 1,000 mL/h for two consecutive voids.

Maintain fluid intake regimens as ordered. Monitor fluid status by measuring vital signs, fluid intake and output, and daily weights (using the same scale at the same time of day). If fluids are stopped too soon, the child may become hypernatremic, which can lead to seizures. Feed infants more frequently, since they excrete more dilute urine, consume larger volumes of free water, and secrete lower amounts of vasopressin than older children. Monitor for signs and symptoms of dehydration during the fluid deprivation test and when starting the treatment regimen.

> **TAKE NOTE!**
>
> Monitor blood pressure closely when initiating vasopressin.

If the child is unconscious or has brain injury, maintain hydration and nutrition by administering nasogastric or gastrostomy feedings.

PROMOTING ACTIVITY

Establish appropriate activity levels for the child, and allow time for them to regain strength and the desire to increase their level of activity. Assess the child's abilities daily, schedule frequent bathroom breaks, and ensure that fluids the child enjoys are available at all times. Tailor the treatment plan to fit the child's daily activities.

EDUCATING THE FAMILY

Involve the family in developing fluid intake regimens. A journal or daily log is essential for maintaining the fluid regimen and identifying problems. Children with intact thirst centers can self-regulate their need for fluids, but if this is not the situation, help the family develop a 24-hour fluid replacement plan. This may require instruction on nasogastric or gastrostomy feedings. Infants will need fluid intake at night. Educate the family about the symptoms of water intoxication (drowsiness, listlessness, headache, confusion, sudden weight gain, and anuria) and dehydration. Help the family develop a plan to inform the school and other people in the child's life about the need for liberal bathroom privileges and extra fluids to prevent accidents or dehydration. Teaching Guidelines 48.1 provides tips on educating the family about the medication regimen. Recommend that the family obtain a medical ID alert bracelet or necklace for the child. Encourage adherence to follow-up appointments, which will probably be every 6 months.

TEACHING GUIDELINES 48.1 DDAVP Intranasal Administration

- Keep desmopressin acetate (DDAVP) in the refrigerator at all times (if directed; some products no longer require refrigeration—refer to product insert).
- Clear the nostrils (medication may be poorly absorbed if the child has nasal congestion).
- Insert the measuring tube into the bottle.
- Fill to the proper dosage and hold the top of the tube closed while inserting the medication-filled end into the nostril.
- Blow the liquid out of the tubing into the nostril.
- When using a metered nasal spray, the spray must be primed before first use.
- If the child sneezes, repeat the dosage.
- Measure urine specific gravity to monitor effectiveness of the drug.
- Monitor for signs and symptoms of overdosage such as confusion, headache, drowsiness, and rapid weight gain due to fluid retention.

Syndrome of Inappropriate Antidiuretic Hormone

SIADH occurs when ADH (vasopressin) is secreted in the presence of low serum osmolality because the feedback mechanism that regulates ADH does not function properly. ADH continues to be released, and this leads to water retention, decreased serum sodium levels due to hemodilution, and extracellular fluid volume expansion. SIADH can be caused by CNS infections such as meningitis, head trauma, brain tumors, intracranial surgery, and certain medications such as analgesics, barbiturates, or chemotherapy. SIADH is rare in children; however, when observed, it is often related to excessive administration of vasopressin during the treatment of AVP-D (central DI) (Breault & Majzoub, 2020b).

The therapeutic management of SIADH includes correcting the underlying disorder, in addition to fluid restriction and intravenous sodium chloride administration to correct hyponatremia and increase serum osmolality.

Nursing Assessment

Obtain a health history, noting a history of CNS infection or tumor, intracranial surgery, head trauma, use of the aforementioned medications, or a history of AVP-D or AVP-R. Note symptoms such as decreased urine output and weight gain, or GI symptoms such as anorexia, nausea, and vomiting. Assess neurologic status, noting lethargy, behavioral changes, headache, altered level of consciousness, seizure, or coma. Neurologic signs develop as the sodium level decreases. Diagnostic tests reveal low serum sodium and osmolality, as well as decreased levels of urea, creatinine, uric acid, and albumin. Urine samples demonstrate elevated osmolality, high sodium concentrations, and specific gravity greater than 1.030. Adrenal, thyroid, and kidney function studies may be used to rule out other causes of hyponatremia.

Comparison Chart 48.1 lists the differences between AVP-D and SIADH.

COMPARISON CHART 48.1 Arginine Vasopressin Deficiency Versus Syndrome of Inappropriate Antidiuretic Hormone

AVP-D (Central DI)	SIADH
• "High and dry" • Increased urination • Hypernatremia • Serum osmolality >300 mOsm/kg • Urine specific gravity <1.005 • Decreased urine osmolality • Dehydration, thirst	• "Low and wet" • Decreased urination • Hyponatremia • Serum osmolality <280 mOsm/kg • Urine specific gravity >1.030 • Increased urine osmolality • Fluid retention, weight gain, and hypertension

Nursing Management

Nursing goals focus on restoring fluid balance and preventing injury. Institute safety precautions if altered levels of consciousness, confusion, or seizures are present. Notify the health care provider or nurse practitioner if headache or irritability is present. Monitor fluid intake and output and weigh the child daily. An indwelling urinary catheter may be needed to allow for hourly monitoring of urine volume and specific gravity. Help the child cope with fluid restriction by offering sugarless candy, a wet washcloth, or, perhaps, ice chips. Administer electrolyte replacement as necessary to correct imbalances.

DISORDERS OF THYROID FUNCTION

Disorders of the thyroid gland are seen in infancy and childhood and are broadly classified as hypothyroidism and hyperthyroidism. These disorders can be serious because thyroid hormones are important for growth and development; they regulate metabolism of nutrients and energy production.

Congenital Hypothyroidism

Congenital hypothyroidism usually results from a defect in the thyroid gland during fetal development or a defect in thyroid hormone synthesis (Connelly & LaFranchi, 2023a). This results in malformation or malfunction of the thyroid gland, which leads to insufficient production of the thyroid hormones that are required to meet the body's metabolic, growth, and development needs. Congenital hypothyroidism leads to low concentrations of circulating thyroid hormones (triiodothyronine [T_3] and thyroxine [T_4]).

Congenital hypothyroidism occurs in one in 2,000 to 4,000 live births (Connelly & LaFranchi, 2023a). It affects a wide range of populations, though less frequently among African Americans, and is more common in females than males (Connelly & LaFranchi, 2023a). Complications include intellectual disability if untreated, short stature, growth failure, and delayed physical maturation and development (Wassner & Smith, 2020). Congenital hypothyroidism is one of the most common preventable causes of intellectual disability. The later it is diagnosed, the greater the disability is (Connelly & LaFranchi, 2023a). Most newborns have few, if any, symptoms, and the occurrence is sporadic, not typically hereditary; therefore, most cases of congenital hypothyroidism are detected via newborn screening programs.

Pathophysiology

Congenital hypothyroidism is due to a defect in the development of the thyroid gland in the fetus, owing to a spontaneous gene mutation, an inborn error of thyroid hormone synthesis resulting from an autosomal recessive trait, pituitary dysfunction, or failure of the CNS–thyroid feedback mechanism to develop. Transient primary hypothyroidism may also occur; it results from transplacental transfer of maternal medications, maternal thyroid-blocking antibodies, iodine deficiency, or fetal or neonatal exposure to excessive iodine (such as the use of iodine antiseptics during delivery or procedures, or excess ingestion of iodine by the birthing parent) (Connelly & Lafranchi, 2023a).

Therapeutic Management

To prevent intellectual disability and restore normal growth and motor development, thyroid hormone replacement with sodium L-thyroxine (Synthroid, synthetic thyroxine, or Levothroid) is given. The recommended starting dosage is 10 to 15 mcg/kg/day (Connelly & LaFranchi, 2023b). There are no adverse effects with physiologic doses, but thyroid function tests are initially performed every 2 weeks to closely monitor for effects and ensure proper dosing. Since thyroid hormone is vital to the infant's developing CNS, the goal is to normalize thyroid function as quickly as possible. This treatment will be needed lifelong to maintain normal metabolism and promote normal physical and mental growth and development.

Nursing Assessment

Nursing assessment of the child with congenital hypothyroidism includes health history, physical examination, and laboratory testing.

HEALTH HISTORY

Inquire whether the neonatal metabolic screening test was performed and if results were obtained. Determine if the test was conducted less than 24 to 48 hours after birth. If so, a repeat test may be warranted (see the "Laboratory and Diagnostic Testing" section). Inquire about maternal history that may indicate a connection to hypothyroidism, such as maternal exposure to iodine. Additional history findings may include sensitivity to cold, constipation, feeding problems, or lethargy. Since parents prefer babies to sleep well, they may not complain that the baby is sleeping too much; rather, they may remark that it is difficult to keep the baby awake.

PHYSICAL EXAMINATION

Most infants do not show symptoms until the first month when they begin to develop clinical signs. Inspection and observation reveal a lethargic baby or a child with hypotonia, hypoactivity, and a dull expression. A combination of lethargy and irritability may exist, with overall delayed mental responsiveness. Measurements of weight and height may reveal delayed growth. Other findings may include a persistent open posterior fontanel, coarse facies with a short neck and limbs, periorbital puffiness, enlarged tongue, and poor sucking response (Fig. 48.3). The skin may appear pale with mottling or yellow from prolonged jaundice, or it may be cool, dry, and scaly to the touch, with sparse hair development on older children. Auscultation of the chest might reveal bradycardia. Signs of respiratory distress and decreased pulse pressure may also be present. On palpation of the abdomen, there may be evidence of an umbilical hernia or a mass due to constipation.

LABORATORY AND DIAGNOSTIC TESTING

Every infant should have a newborn screen for thyroid hormone levels before discharge from the hospital or

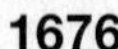

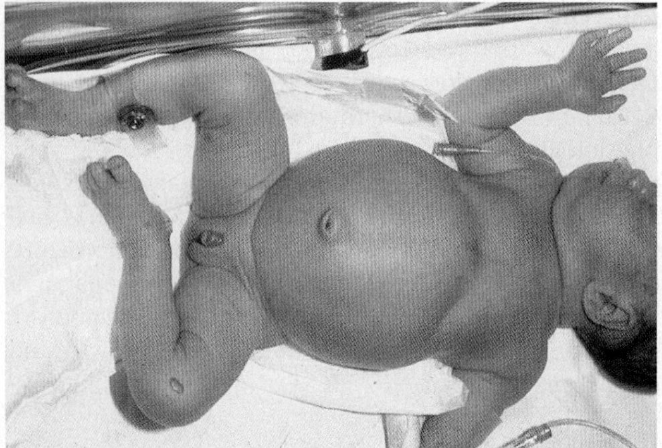

FIGURE 48.3 Newborn with congenital hypothyroidism.

2 to 4 days after birth (Connelly & LaFranchi, 2023a). When the test is performed within the first 24 to 48 hours along with other metabolic screenings, the result may be inaccurate because of the immediate increase in thyroid-stimulating hormone (TSH) shortly after birth (Connelly & LaFranchi, 2023a). Radioimmunoassay is used to measure levels of T_4, which accurately reflect the child's thyroid status. If the T_4 level is low, then a second confirming laboratory test is performed, as well as determining whether the TSH is elevated. A thyroid scan may also be used to check for the absence or ectopic placement of the gland. In addition to serum measurement of T_4, other diagnostic tests include serum T_3, radioiodine uptake, thyroid-bound globulin, and ultrasonography.

Nursing Management

The overall goal of nursing management for infants or children with congenital hypothyroidism is to establish a normal growth pattern without complications such as intellectual disability or failure to thrive. Individualize the nursing care plan based on the infant's responses to the illness.

PROMOTING APPROPRIATE GROWTH

Measure and record growth at regular intervals. Thyroid levels are measured at recommended intervals, such as every 2 weeks until the target range is reached on a stabilized dose of medication, then every 1 to 2 months until the child is 1 year old, every 1 to 3 months until the child is 3 years old, and less frequently as the child gets older (Connelly & LaFranchi, 2023b). A trial off the medication may be performed around the age of 3, under a health care provider's or nurse practitioner's supervision, to confirm the diagnosis (Connelly & LaFranchi, 2023b). Monitor for signs of hypo- or hyperfunction, including changes in vital signs, thermoregulation, and activity level. Provide adequate rest periods and meet thermoregulation needs. If the infant's tongue is unusually large, observe feeding ability, prevent airway obstruction, and position the infant on their side. Fluid restrictions or a low-salt diet may be ordered.

TAKE NOTE!

Observe for signs of thyroid hormone overdose (irritability, rapid pulse, dyspnea, sweating, and fever) or ineffective treatment (fatigue, constipation, and decreased appetite).

EDUCATING THE FAMILY

Since many infants do not show symptoms, the diagnosis may be unexpected, so reassure and convey realistic expectations to the family. Developmental screening may be required if the child showed any symptoms initially or as the child gets older, to ensure that drug therapy is appropriate. Educate the family about the disorder, the medication and method of administration, and adverse effects such as increased pulse rate (which may indicate an overdose of thyroid hormone).

L-Thyroxine is an oral medication. The pill form must be crushed for infants and young children. It can be mixed with a small amount of formula or breast milk and placed in the nipple, but it should not be placed in a full bottle of formula or breast milk because the infant will not ingest all the medication if they do not finish the bottle. The medication can also be mixed with a small amount of liquid and given with a dropper. Medication absorption is affected by soy-based formulas, fiber, and iron preparations (Connelly & LaFranchi, 2023b). Therefore, carefully evaluate the formula the infant is on before administering L-thyroxine.

Inform the family that this medication will be needed throughout the child's life. Explain that missed doses may lead to developmental delays and poor growth. Tell them that frequent blood tests will be needed to evaluate thyroid function and the child's growth rate; genetic counseling may be needed. Clinical examination, including growth and development assessment, should occur every few months until the child is 3 years old. Serum T_4 and TSH should be evaluated often, and more frequent monitoring may be needed if nonadherence occurs, if abnormal values occur, or with any changes in medication dosage or treatment regimen. The nurse may need to help the family to find a nearby laboratory or to handle financial issues related to therapy. Educate the family about infant stimulation programs if the child shows cognitive problems, retarded physical growth, or slow intellectual development. Some information may need to be reinforced during the school-age or adolescent stages of development. Finally, encourage the family to obtain a medical ID bracelet or necklace for the child.

CONSIDER THIS!

Asha Virani, 1 week old, is brought to the clinic. Her newborn screening test was positive for hypothyroidism. Her parents are shocked and upset by the news. Her parent states, "My daughter's been doing so well since she came home from the hospital. She seems to be doing everything she should be. I just can't believe anything's wrong with her. I felt so blessed to have a baby that slept so much but she could have died. What kind of parent will I be?"

Thought: How would you respond to this parent?

Acquired Hypothyroidism

Hypothyroidism also occurs as an acquired condition. This disorder most commonly results from an autoimmune chronic lymphocytic (Hashimoto) thyroiditis (LaFranchi, 2022a). As a genetic condition, antibodies develop against the thyroid gland, causing the gland to become inflamed, infiltrated, and progressively destroyed. It occurs more often in females during childhood and adolescence (LaFranchi, 2022a). Less common etiologies include hypothyroidism associated with pituitary or hypothalamic disease; exposure to drugs or substances such as antithyroid medications, anticonvulsants, lithium, and amiodarone that interfere with thyroid hormone synthesis; thyroid injury such as radiation, thyroidectomy, and hemangiomas; and iodine deficiency or excess (LaFranchi, 2022a).

Therapeutic management is the same as for congenital hypothyroidism. Management involves oral sodium L-thyroxine, which is given at 2 to 6 mcg/kg/day based on age to maintain T_4 in the upper half of the normal range and to suppress TSH (LaFranchi, 2022a).

Nursing Assessment

Interview the family and child to determine activity tolerance and behavior changes. The symptoms may develop over a period of time and may be subtle. Note vague complaints of fatigue, weakness, weight gain, cold intolerance, constipation, and dry skin. The severity of symptoms depends on the length of time that the hormone deficiency has existed and its extent. Reviewing the growth pattern may reveal a slowed or arrested growth rate (height) and increased weight.

Physical examination may reveal a **goiter** (enlargement of the thyroid gland). Deep tendon reflexes may be sluggish, and the face, eyes, and hands may be edematous. Note thinning or coarse hair, muscle hypertrophy with muscle weakness, and signs of delayed or precocious puberty. The diagnostic evaluation involves serum thyroid function studies (TSH, T_3, and T_4), as well as serum thyroid antibodies to confirm autoimmune thyroiditis. MRI and a thyroid uptake test and scan may also be necessary.

Nursing Management

Work with the family to establish a daily schedule for administering L-thyroxine, which should be taken 30 to 60 minutes before a meal for optimal absorption. Explain to the family that growth is related to the child's response to the treatment, and there are no specific strategies to aid in this growth. The family should understand the diagnosis, should be able to recognize signs and symptoms of thyroid hypo- and hyperfunction, and should know when to notify the health care provider or nurse practitioner. The family and child may need assistance in accepting the therapy, as well as the experience of catch-up growth that may occur at the beginning of therapy. The child with chronic or severe hypothyroidism may be at risk for adverse effects such as restlessness, insomnia, or irritability. The child's thyroid levels should be evaluated at recommended intervals, such as every 3 to 6 months, by a pediatric endocrinologist.

Hyperthyroidism

Hyperthyroidism is the result of hyperfunction of the thyroid gland. This leads to excessive levels of circulating thyroid hormones. This condition is uncommon in children, with its peak incidence occurring during adolescence, often due to Graves disease (LaFranchi, 2022b). Graves disease is an autoimmune disorder that causes excessive amounts of thyroid hormone to be released in response to human thyroid stimulator immunoglobulin (TSI). It affects females five times more frequently than males (LaFranchi, 2022b) and a goiter usually develops in this condition. There is a strong genetic factor, with the majority of children having a positive family history of autoimmune thyroid problems (LaFranchi, 2022b). A congenital form of hyperthyroidism, neonatal thyrotoxicosis, occurs in infants of birthing parents with Graves disease. This neonatal condition, which can be life-threatening, is a self-limiting disorder lasting 2 to 4 months. Less common causes of hyperthyroidism are thyroiditis, thyroid hormone–producing tumors, and pituitary adenomas.

Therapeutic management is aimed at decreasing thyroid hormone levels. Current treatment involves antithyroid medication, radioactive iodine therapy, and subtotal thyroidectomy. First-line treatment involves methimazole (MTZ, Tapazole), which blocks the production of T_3 and T_4 (Wassner & LaFranchi, 2021). Adjunct therapy, with beta-adrenergic blockers (such as propranolol or atenolol), may also be used if the child has marked symptoms. Radioactive iodine therapy is restricted to children older than 10 years as a long-term therapy (Wassner & LaFranchi, 2021). This therapy is administered orally and leads to tissue damage and destruction of the thyroid gland within 6 to 18 weeks, but it can result in hypothyroidism. Subtotal thyroidectomy is used when drug therapy is not possible or other treatments have failed. Risks include hypothyroidism, hypoparathyroidism, or laryngeal nerve damage.

Nursing Assessment

Initially, symptoms of hyperthyroidism are mild and can often be overlooked. Many children with hyperthyroidism are first seen in outpatient settings with a history of problems with sleep, school performance, and distractibility. They may become easily frustrated, overheated, and fatigued during physical education classes. Also, the child may complain of diarrhea, excessive perspiration, and muscle weakness. Further, the history may reveal signs of hyperactivity, heat intolerance, emotional lability, and insomnia.

During physical examination, older children may reveal an increased rate of growth, weight loss despite an excellent appetite, hyperactivity, warm and moist skin, tachycardia, fine tremors, an enlarged thyroid gland or goiter, and ophthalmic changes (exophthalmos, which is less pronounced in children; proptosis; lid lag and retraction; staring expression; periorbital edema; and diplopia) (Fig. 48.4). Elevated pulse and blood pressure may also be noted. Laboratory and diagnostic tests reveal that serum T_4 and T_3 levels are markedly elevated, while TSH levels are suppressed.

CLINICAL REASONING ALERT!

The sudden release of high levels of thyroid hormones results in thyroid storm, which progresses to heart failure and shock. Immediately report the signs of thyroid storm, which include the sudden onset of severe restlessness and irritability, fever, diaphoresis, and severe tachycardia (Smith & Wassner, 2020).

Nursing Management

Once the treatment plan is initiated, educate both the family and the child about the medication, its potential adverse effects, the goals of treatment, and possible complications. Monitor for adverse drug effects such as rash, mild leukopenia, loss of taste, sore throat, GI disturbances, and arthralgia. If the medication needs to be taken two or three times a day, teach the family to use a pill dispenser and set alarms. Inform the family of the need for routine blood tests and follow-up visits with the pediatric endocrinologist every 2 to 4 months until normal hormone levels are achieved; then, visits may be decreased to once or twice a year. Instruct the parents to contact the health care provider or nurse practitioner if the child has tachycardia or extreme fatigue.

Help the child and family to cope with symptoms such as heat intolerance, emotional lability, or eye problems. Explain these symptoms to the school or day care personnel and make sure that they understand that the child may require more frequent rest breaks in a cool environment and should refrain from participating in physical education classes until normal hormone levels are attained. Encourage the family to ensure the child maintains a healthy diet with an appropriate level of calories; they may need to eat five or six meals a day. Provide community referrals such as to the Graves Disease and Thyroid Foundation. Also, encourage the family to obtain a medical ID bracelet or necklace for the child.

If surgical intervention is chosen, provide appropriate preoperative teaching and postoperative care. Provide supportive measures such as fluid maintenance, nutritional support, and electrolyte correction. Monitor red blood cell count and liver function tests. Close monitoring for signs and symptoms of hypothyroidism is important.

Comparison Chart 48.2 compares hypothyroidism and hyperthyroidism.

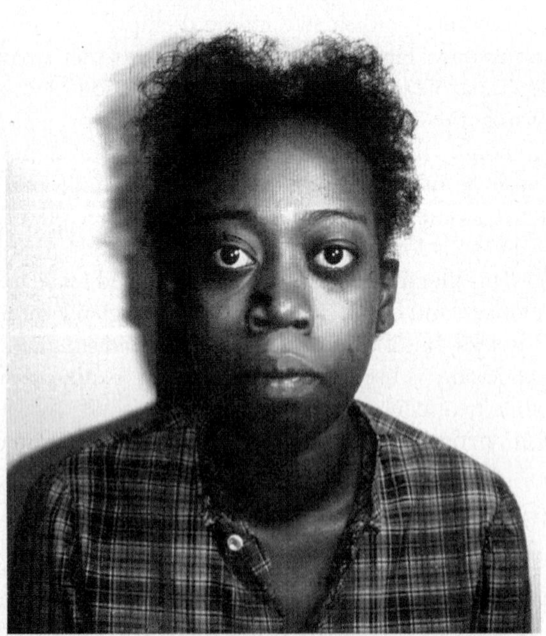

FIGURE 48.4 Adolescent with Graves disease.

DISORDERS RELATED TO PARATHYROID GLAND FUNCTION

The parathyroid glands secrete parathyroid hormone (PTH). This hormone, along with vitamin D and calcitonin, regulates calcium and phosphate homeostasis by increasing osteoclastic activity, promoting calcium absorption in the kidneys, and enhancing calcium absorption in the GI tract while facilitating phosphate excretion

COMPARISON CHART 48.2 Hypothyroidism Versus Hyperthyroidism

Hyperthyroidism	Hypothyroidism
• Nervousness/anxiety • Diarrhea • Heat intolerance • Weight loss • Smooth, velvety skin	• Tiredness/fatigue • Constipation • Cold intolerance • Weight gain • Dry, thick skin; edema of face, eyes, and hands • Decreased growth

by the kidneys. The two primary disorders associated with parathyroid gland dysfunction are hypoparathyroidism and hyperparathyroidism, both of which are rare in children. Refer to Table 48.2, for further information.

DISORDERS RELATED TO ADRENAL GLAND FUNCTION

Disorders of the adrenal gland include both acute and chronic adrenal insufficiency (hypofunction) as well as disorders of hyperfunction like Cushing syndrome (Fig. 48.5). The adrenal cortex is the site of production of glucocorticoids (for blood glucose regulation), mineralocorticoids (for sodium retention), and androgenic and estrogenic steroid compounds (for phallic and secondary sex development). The adrenal medulla is the site of production of the catecholamines (dopamine, norepinephrine, and epinephrine) and is under neuroendocrine control. When production of these compounds is altered, disease results. Pediatric adrenocortical insufficiency is similar to adults, exception for CAH, which will be discussed later. Refer to Table 48.3, for an overview of other disorders of the adrenal gland.

Congenital Adrenal Hyperplasia

CAH is a group of autosomal recessive inherited disorders in which there is an insufficient supply of the enzymes required for the synthesis of cortisol and aldosterone. More than 90% of the CAH cases are caused

TABLE **48.2** • Parathyroid Disorders

Parathyroid Disorder	Cause	Nursing Assessment	Nursing Management
Hypoparathyroidism (deficiency of PTH)	Most common is accidental removal or destruction of the parathyroid gland during thyroidectomy or radial neck dissection; may also be congenital (result of aplasia or hypoplasia of the parathyroid gland)	Hypocalcemia Hyperphosphatemia Hyperexcitability of neuromuscular function, uncontrolled spasms, and hypocalcemic tetany (general muscular hypertonia); positive Chvostek sign (facial muscle spasm elicited by tapping the facial nerve); positive Trousseau sign (carpopedal spasm that results from oxygen deficiency) Laryngeal spasm, stridor Poor eating Lethargy	• Administer intravenous calcium gluconate for acute or severe tetany, then intramuscular or oral calcium as prescribed. • Monitor the child for the development of cardiac arrhythmias. Ensure that the intravenous site is patent; if extravasation occurs, tissue damage or cardiac arrhythmias may result. • Monitor fluid and electrolyte status, weigh the child daily, and measure urinary calcium excretion to prevent nephrocalcinosis. • Institute seizure precautions and reduce environmental stimuli (e.g., loud or sudden noises, bright lights, or stimulating activities). • Observe for signs and symptoms of laryngospasm (e.g., stridor, hoarseness, or a feeling of tightness in the throat). Teach the child and family about the need for continuous daily administration of calcium salts and vitamin D. Have the family observe for vitamin D toxicity by observing for signs such as weakness, fatigue, lassitude, headache, nausea and vomiting, and diarrhea.
Hyperparathyroidism (hypersecretion of PTH)	Parathyroid adenoma is the most common cause; secondary hyperparathyroidism is primarily due to kidney disease.	Hypercalcemia Hypophosphatemia Depression of neuromuscular function, the child may trip and drop objects, general fatigue, failure to thrive, headaches, poor school performance, and irritability, somnolence, stupor, or difficulty concentrating. Irregular heart rate, possibly related to cardiac dysrhythmias. Skeletal pain, fractures, formation of bone tumors, or flank pain related to renal calculi	• Administer IV fluids and diuretics as prescribed to increase urinary excretion of calcium in children without kidney disease. • Administer prescribed medication to treat hypercalcemia, such as oral phosphate (antihypercalcemic agent), pamidronate, calcitonin, or etidronate disodium (by inhibiting bone resorption of calcium). • Increase the child's fluid intake to minimize renal calculi formation. Provide fruit juices to maintain low urinary pH, acidity of body fluids, and calcium absorption. Strain the urine for renal casts. • Dietary calcium is restricted. • Monitor for safety by assessing the child's level of muscular weakness, preventing falls or injury, and checking for fractures. • If the child develops renal rickets (osteodystrophy), long-term braces may be required, so provide family education and encourage adherence. • Surgery may be performed to remove abnormal parathyroid tumor. • Keep the diet low in phosphorus and watch for hypocalcemia and onset of tetany after surgery.

IV, intravenous; PTH, parathyroid hormone.

Doyle, D. A. (2020a). Chapter 589: Hypoparathyroidism. In R. M. Kleigman, J. W. St. Geme III, N. J. Blum, S.S. Shah, R.C. Tasker, K.M. Wilson, & R. E. Behrman (Eds.), *Nelson textbook of pediatrics* (21th ed., pp. 15565-15579). Elsevier;

Doyle, D. A. (2020b). Chapter 591: Hyperparathyroidism. In R. M. Kleigman, J. W. St. Geme III, N. J. Blum, S.S. Shah, R.C. Tasker, K.M. Wilson, & R. E. Behrman (Eds.), *Nelson textbook of pediatrics* (21th ed., pp. 15587-15601). Elsevier.

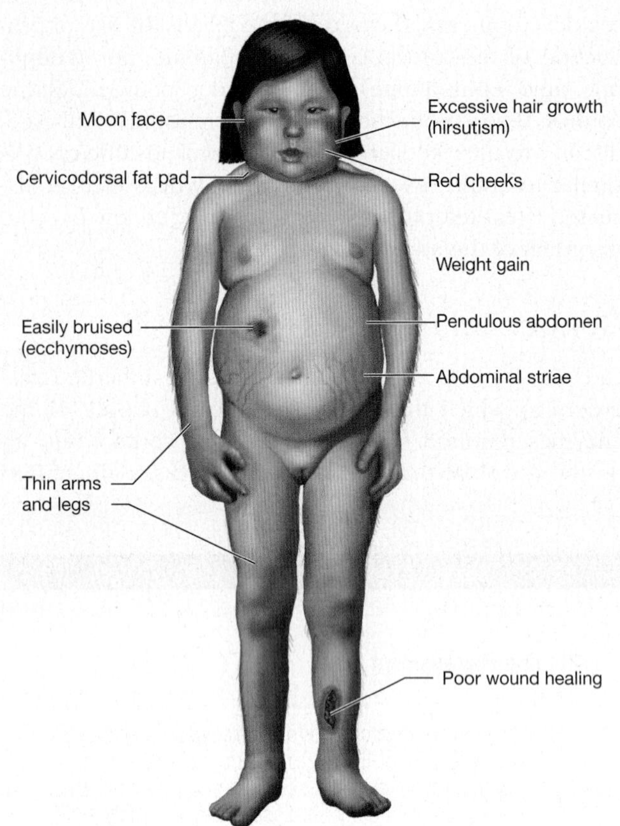

FIGURE 48.5 Cushing syndrome.

by a deficiency of the 21-hydroxylase (21-OH) enzyme (White, 2020b). It is the most common type of adrenocortical insufficiency seen in children with an incidence of about one in 15,000 to 20,000 live births (White, 2020b). Therefore, our discussion will focus on this type. This condition can be life-threatening and requires prompt diagnosis and treatment after birth (White, 2020b). Complications of CAH include hyponatremia, hyperkalemia, hypotension, shock, hypoglycemia, short adult stature, and adult testicular tumor in males.

Pathophysiology

Classic 21-OH enzyme deficiency results in blocking the production of adrenal mineralocorticoids and glucocorticoids. A reduction of cortisol occurs, which leads to increased adrenocorticotropic hormone (ACTH) production by the anterior pituitary to stimulate adrenal gland production. Prolonged oversecretion of ACTH causes enlargement or hyperplasia of the adrenal glands and excess production of androgens, leading to male characteristics appearing early or inappropriately.

In males, the enzyme deficiency of 21-OH with excessive androgen secretion leads to a slightly enlarged penis, which may become adult size by school age, and a hyperpigmented scrotum. Males do not have obvious signs at birth but may enter puberty by 2 to 3 years of age. The female fetus develops male secondary sexual characteristics; thus, CAH causes ambiguous genitalia (Merke & Auchus, 2022; White, 2020b). The clitoris is enlarged and may resemble the penis, the labia have a rugated appearance, and the labial folds are fused, but the internal reproductive organs, including the ovaries, fallopian tubes, and uterus, are typical.

A milder form of 21-OH deficiency becomes evident later (genitals are typical in appearance at birth), in the toddler or preschool years, with premature **adrenarche** (early sexual maturation), pubic hair development, accelerated growth velocity, advanced bone age, early closure of the epiphyseal plates resulting in short stature as an adult, acne, and **hirsutism** (excessive body hair growth). Males usually have typical fertility, while females may have lower fertility.

Aldosterone insufficiency also leads to fluid and electrolyte imbalances, such as hyponatremia, hyperkalemia, and hypotension due to depletion of extracellular fluid. Cortisol insufficiency leads to hypoglycemia.

Therapeutic Management

The goal of treatment is to stop excessive adrenal secretion of androgens while maintaining normal growth and development. Most children with 21-OH deficiency will take a glucocorticoid such as hydrocortisone and the mineralocorticoid fludrocortisone for life. Infants may also require sodium supplementation. When the medications are taken at physiologic doses, there are no adverse effects, but if the drug levels become elevated, hypertension, growth impairment, and acne become a problem. Regular follow-up care and appropriate titration maintain the dose at appropriate levels to allow normal growth and development.

Often when females are born with ambiguous genitalia, standard medical treatment is to correct the external genitalia and establish adequate sexual functioning. Sex can be assigned by karyotyping chromosomes. Typically, a reduction of the clitoris and opening of the labial folds are done within 2 to 6 months of life, with further surgeries at puberty (White, 2020b). Some argue that surgery should be delayed until the child is old enough to decide what kind of correction (if any) should be performed (White, 2020b). The decision to intervene immediately or to delay treatment is a complex one that raises many concerns for the family. The medical team needs to be sensitive to this and provide psychosocial support to the parents and family (Merke, 2022).

Nursing Assessment

Nursing assessment of the child with CAH includes health history, physical examination, and laboratory and diagnostic testing. Specific findings related to CAH are presented further.

TABLE 48.3 • Other Disorders of the Adrenal Gland

Disorder	Cause	Nursing Assessment	Nursing Management
Addison disease (deficiency in the adrenal steroids, glucocorticoids [cortisol], and mineralocorticoids [aldosterone])	It results from damage or destruction of the adrenal glands caused by infections such as tuberculosis, fungal infections, or HIV-related infections; hemorrhage or surgical removal of both glands; or dysfunction of the hypothalamus or pituitary gland. Generally, the etiology in children is an autoimmune process that is familial or sporadic.[a]	Hyponatremia Hyperkalemia Water loss, dehydration, muscular weakness, fatigue, weight loss, anorexia, syncope, nausea, vomiting, and diarrhea Hypoglycemia Hypotension Hyperpigmentation of skin Adrenal crisis, also referred to as Addisonian crisis, can occur (refer to section on CAH for more information)	Similar to that of congenital adrenal insufficiency
Cushing syndrome (excess levels of one or all the hormones [glucocorticoids, mineralocorticoids, and adrenal androgens] but most commonly glucocorticoid excess)	Usually, this condition is due to a small ACTH-producing pituitary adenoma. The most common cause in older children is prolonged or excessive use of corticosteroid therapy.[b]	Note history of rapid weight gain, decreased velocity of linear growth, muscle weakness, fatigue, irritability, sleep disturbance, and hypertension. History of long-term corticosteroid use, water retention, poor wound healing, frequent infections, and missed menstrual periods Refer to Figure 48.5. Skin may be thin and fragile; acne may be present.	• Management varies depending on the cause. • The goal is to restore hormone balance and reverse Cushing syndrome. • If the cause is an adrenal or pituitary tumor, then surgical removal of the tumor alone or the entire adrenal gland is performed. • If the cause is long-term steroid therapy, then the corticosteroid dose is reduced to the lowest dose that is effective in treating the underlying disorder. • Cortisol synthesis–inhibiting medications may be used. • Counsel the family that the cushingoid appearance is reversible with appropriate treatment. • Be alert for signs of adrenal insufficiency if the child has surgery or if corticosteroid withdrawal occurs quickly.

ACTH, adrenocorticotropic hormone; CAH, congenital adrenal hyperplasia; HIV, human immunodeficiency virus.

[a]White, P. C. (2020a). Chapter 593: Adrenocortical insufficiency. In R. M. Kleigman, J. W. St. Geme III, N. J. Blum, S. S. Shah, R. C. Tasker, K. M. Wilson, & R. E. Behrman (Eds.), *Nelson textbook of pediatrics* (21st ed., pp. 15636–15689). Elsevier.

[b]White, P. C. (2020b). Chapter 597: Cushing syndrome. In R. M. Kleigman, J. W. St. Geme III, N. J. Blum, S. S. Shah, R. C. Tasker, K. M. Wilson, & R. E. Behrman (Eds.), *Nelson textbook of pediatrics* (21st ed., pp. 15753–15766). Elsevier.

HEALTH HISTORY AND PHYSICAL EXAMINATION

Obtain the health history, noting any history of atypical genitalia at birth in the infant. For toddlers or preschoolers, take note of any history of accelerated growth velocity and signs of premature adrenarche. During inspection of the infant's genitalia, observe for the presence of a large penis or ambiguous genitalia (Fig. 48.6). When observing toddlers or preschoolers, note pubic hair development, acne, and hirsutism.

LABORATORY AND DIAGNOSTIC TESTING

The most common type of CAH, 21-OH enzyme deficiency, is detected by newborn metabolic screening. If this test has not been done or the results are unavailable, obtain random hormone levels or levels associated with ACTH stimulation. Radiographs reveal advanced bone age and premature closure of epiphyseal plates of the long bones.

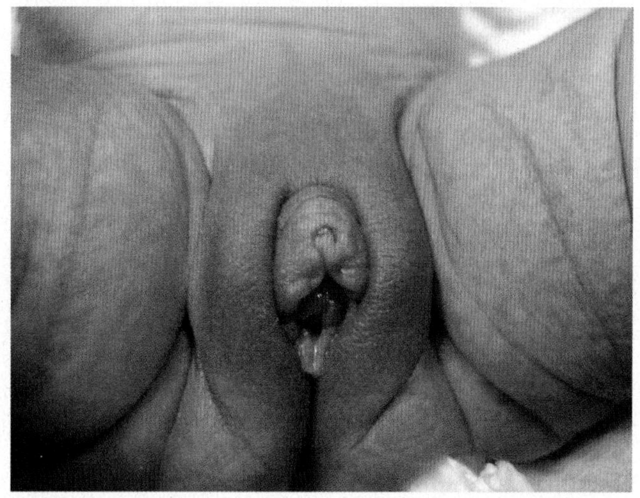

FIGURE 48.6 Newborn with ambiguous genitalia.

Nursing Management

In addition to the common interventions associated with endocrine disorders in childhood (see "Clinical Judgment and the Nursing Process" section earlier in the chapter), nursing management of infants or children with CAH focuses on preventing and monitoring for acute adrenal crisis, helping the family to understand the disease, educating both the child and the family about the importance of maintaining hormone supplementation, and providing emotional support to the family.

PREVENTING AND MONITORING FOR ACUTE ADRENAL CRISIS

Providing continuous assessment of an ill or hospitalized child with a history of CAH is crucial to recognize the development of life-threatening acute adrenal crisis. Signs and symptoms of acute adrenal crisis include persistent vomiting, dehydration, hyponatremia, hyperkalemia, hypotension, tachycardia, and shock. Closely monitor children with CAH and notify the health care provider or nurse practitioner if adrenal crisis is suspected. If signs and symptoms of adrenal crisis develop, the child will receive intravenous steroids, such as hydrocortisone, and aggressive fluid resuscitation, often using 5% dextrose in normal saline (D5NS), to correct electrolyte imbalances.

CLINICAL REASONING ALERT!

Adrenal crisis in newborns is often unrecognized. It presents within the first few days to weeks of life, with vomiting, lethargy, and feeding difficulties.

EDUCATING THE FAMILY ABOUT THE MEDICATION REGIMEN

Medication will be required throughout the child's life because cortisone is necessary for sustaining life. Educate the family on the appropriate oral dosages of hydrocortisone and fludrocortisone. It is critical to maintain tight control over the levels of these medications in the bloodstream. Underdosing or overdosing can lead to short adult stature, while low levels of the hormones may also result in adrenal crisis (as discussed previously). These drugs are usually given orally, but in some instances, will need to be given via intramuscular injections. Teach families how to administer hydrocortisone intramuscularly if the child is vomiting and unable to tolerate oral medication. If the child becomes ill, is under stress, or needs surgery, additional doses of medications may be required. Encourage the family to obtain a medical ID bracelet or necklace for the child.

TAKE NOTE!

Families must keep extra steroids in an injectable form, such as Solu-Cortef or Decadron, at home to administer during emergencies.

PROVIDING FAMILY SUPPORT

Make sure the family of a newborn with ambiguous genitalia feels comfortable asking questions and exploring their feelings. There are many factors to consider, including whether the family will opt to reassign the child's sex, raise the child according to the original assignment at birth, or allow for ambiguity until the child expresses their own gender identification. The birth certificate may pose a problem if the state requires identification of sex. Cultural attitudes, parental expectations, and the extent of family support influence the family's response to the child and the decision-making process related to sex assignment and surgical correction. If corrective surgery is immediately decided upon, then typical surgical concerns for newborns will need to be addressed.

In general, laypeople do not understand adrenal function and what this diagnosis may mean to the family. Provide families with privacy to discuss these issues, and offer emotional support. When referring to infants, use terms such as "your baby" instead of the pronouns "he," "she," or "it," and describe the genitals as "sex organs" instead of "penis" or "clitoris." Refer families to the CARES Foundation (Congenital Adrenal Hyperplasia Research, Education, and Support) and the Magic Foundation, for additional support and resources. Local parent-to-parent support groups are also helpful.

POLYCYSTIC OVARY SYNDROME

Polycystic ovary syndrome (PCOS), also referred to as functional ovarian hyperandrogenism or ovarian androgen excess, is an endocrine disorder that produces a variety of symptoms in adolescent and adult females. The exact cause is unknown. Testosterone production by the ovaries and adrenal cells is excessive, causing hirsutism, balding, topical treatment resistant acne, increased muscle mass, and decreased breast size. Polycystic ovaries may or may not be present.

Complications of excess androgen production in females include infertility, insulin resistance, and hyperinsulinemia, leading to DM, increased risk for endometrial carcinoma, and cardiovascular disease (Shaw & Rosenfield, 2022). Therapeutic management involves the administration of oral contraceptives for their hormonal effects, as well as insulin-sensitizing medications such as metformin (Glucophage).

Nursing Assessment

Explore the health history for oligomenorrhea (irregular, infrequent periods) or amenorrhea. Symptoms typically emerge at or soon after puberty but often go undiagnosed. Note weight in relation to standardized growth charts, and calculate body mass index (BMI) to determine if overweight or higher weight is present. Inspect the skin for acne, acanthosis nigricans (darkened, thickened pigmentation, particularly around the neck or in the axillary region), and hirsutism (excess body hair growth). Assist with collection of timed blood specimens for glucose and insulin levels (which will often show unexpectedly elevated insulin levels in relation to the glucose level). Laboratory tests may show elevated levels of free testosterone and other androgenic hormones.

Nursing Management

One of the most important functions of the nurse in relation to PCOS is to assist with early recognition and treatment. Educate the adolescent about the use of oral contraceptives to normalize hormone levels, which will decrease androgenic effects. Support the adolescent in their efforts to develop nutrition and physical activity habits to maintain a healthy weight. Oral insulin-sensitizing drugs such as metformin (Glucophage) may be prescribed. Encourage the adolescent to comply with the medication regimen. Routinely measure weight to determine progress with weight loss. Monitor blood pressure to screen for hypertension, which may develop as a complication of PCOS. Also, online support groups and education resources are available.

DIABETES MELLITUS

DM is a common chronic disease seen in children and adolescents. In DM, carbohydrate, protein, and lipid metabolism are impaired. The cardinal feature of DM is hyperglycemia. The major forms of diabetes are classified as follows:

- Type 1, which is caused by a deficiency of insulin secretion due to pancreatic beta-cell damage
- Type 2, which is a consequence of insulin resistance that occurs at the level of skeletal muscle, liver, and adipose tissue with different degrees of beta-cell impairment (Weber & Jospe, 2020)
- Other types of diabetes secondary to certain conditions such as cystic fibrosis, glucocorticoid use (as in Cushing syndrome), infections, autoimmune syndromes, and certain genetic syndromes such as Down syndrome, Klinefelter syndrome, and Turner syndrome (Weber & Jospe, 2020)
- Gestational diabetes (diabetes during pregnancy)

The discussion for this chapter will focus on type 1 and type 2 diabetes as these are the most common types seen in children.

Every year, approximately 18,000 children and adolescents are diagnosed with type 1 DM and approximately 5,700 with type 2 DM (CDC, 2020). Historically, diabetes in childhood was assumed to be type 1, and type 2 DM occurred mostly in adults. However, in recent years, type 2 DM has been reported in U.S. children and adolescents at an increasing rate (American Diabetes Association Professional Practice Committee, 2022). This increase in incidence of type 2 DM among children and adolescents can be attributed to factors such as increasing rates of higher weight and decreased physical activity in young people, as well as exposure to diabetes in utero. Many children with type 2 diabetes have a family history of the condition or are overweight. See the Healthy People 2030 box.

HEALTHY PEOPLE 2030

Objective	Nursing Significance
Reduce the annual number of new cases of diagnosed diabetes in the population.	• Screen all children periodically for the development of overweight and higher weight using BMI on the Centers for Disease Control and Prevention growth charts. • Educate families about appropriate diet and exercise beginning in toddlerhood to prevent the development of higher weight.

Healthy People Objectives retrieved from http://www.healthypeople.gov

Care of children with diabetes differs from that of adults due to physiologic and developmental differences. In children, insulin sensitivity varies as the child grows and goes through sexual maturation. Children are dependent on others for their care, and self-management ability varies among children based on factors such as age, developmental level, and unique differences. Care will be needed in a variety of settings, such as schools, daycares, and extracurricular activities. Therefore, teaching and education will need to involve parents and other caregivers throughout childhood and adolescence. Refer to Table 48.4, which discusses developmental issues related to DM.

Pathophysiology

Type 1 DM is an autoimmune disorder that occurs in genetically susceptible people who may also be exposed to one of several environmental or acquired factors, such as chemicals, viruses, or other toxic agents implicated in the development process. As the genetically susceptible person is exposed to environmental factors, the immune system begins a T lymphocyte–mediated process that damages and destroys the beta cells of the pancreas, resulting in inadequate insulin secretion. This deficiency of insulin leads to an inability of cells to take up glucose, resulting in hyperglycemia, glucose accumulation in the blood, and the body's inability to use its main source of fuel efficiently. The kidneys try to lower blood glucose, resulting in glycosuria and polyuria, and protein and fat are broken down for energy. The metabolism of fat leads to a buildup of ketones and acidosis (see discussion of DKA that follows).

TABLE 48.4 • Developmental Issues Related to Diabetes Mellitus

Age Group	Child and Family Implications	Nursing Implications
Infants	Management falls on parents or caregivers. Infant is unable to communicate hypo/hyperglycemic symptoms; signs and symptoms are sometimes difficult to assess. Increased risk of hypoglycemia due to inconsistent feeding times and amounts. Developing brain may experience adverse consequences to severe hypo/hyperglycemia.	Prevent extreme fluctuations in blood glucose. Prevent hypoglycemia and, if present, treat promptly. Attempt to achieve consistent dietary intake. Establish rituals/routines with home management. Provide support for parents and caregivers.
Toddlers	Management falls on parents or caregivers. Increased risk of hypoglycemia due to inconsistent food intake (picky eaters). Developing brain may experience adverse consequences to severe hypo/hyperglycemia. Discipline and temper tantrums common in this age group; may be hard to distinguish between normal toddler behavior and hypoglycemia symptoms. Parents may be overcautious and hinder child's ability to explore and develop normally.	Prevent hypoglycemia and, if present, treat promptly. Assist parents in managing a picky eater. Let toddler choose foods. Get toddler to find a word or phrase to use to describe feelings when hypoglycemic. Help parents provide appropriate discipline and protection while continuing to promote normal development. Establish rituals and routines with home management.
Preschoolers	Increased motor maturity. Widening social circle, so the child will notice that they are "different." Magical thinking presents some issues. Developing brain may experience more adverse consequences to severe hypo/hyperglycemia than older children. Preschooler wants to be an active participant in diabetes care but may lack some of the developmental skills (such as fine motor and cognitive skills). Some children can begin to perform blood glucose testing with the newer devices. Increased risk of hypoglycemia due to varied food intake and activity	Prevent hypoglycemia and if present, treat promptly. Use simple explanations and play therapy when instructing or preparing for a procedure. Encourage the child's participation as appropriate.
School-age children	Can begin to participate in more of the daily diabetes care; may be able to perform self-monitoring blood glucose testing, record glucose levels, choose injection sites and give injections, perform ketone testing, count carbohydrates, recognize need to eat, and treat for hypoglycemia. Begin to rely on others (such as school nurse, child care provider, preschool teacher) to provide diabetes care. Children may feel different from their peers and struggle socially. Must incorporate management into school day and plan for field trips.	Use concise and concrete terms when instructing. Allow the child to proceed at their own rate. Assist the family with incorporating the testing and injections into school day and plan for field trips. Involve the school nurse in helping with the school plan. Encourage the child's participation but emphasize importance of continued adult supervision. Encourage regular attendance at school and participation in extracurricular activities. Assist in the development of a care schedule that is flexible enough to allow for participation in school activities. Assist with education of other care providers as needed.
Adolescents	Undergoing rapid physical, emotional, and cognitive growth. Working toward separate identity from parents and the demands of diabetes care can hinder this. This struggle for independence can lead to nonadherence of diabetes care regimen. Conflicts develop with self-management, body image, and peer group acceptance. They acquire the skills to perform tasks related to diabetes care but may lack decision-making skills needed to adjust treatment plan. Adolescents do not always foresee the consequences of their activity.	Slowly, care is turned over to the adolescent with minor supervision from the family. Encourage parents and adolescent to find the right balance of shared management. Encourage parents to continue to provide guidance and supervision and be actively involved in the plan of care. Assess adherence to diabetes care regimen. Assess for signs and symptoms of depression, eating disorders, or evidence of risky behaviors. In later adolescence, assist the adolescent in transitioning to independent self-management and adult diabetes health care provider or nurse practitioner.

In type 2 DM, the pancreas usually produces insulin, but the body is resistant to the insulin or there is an inadequate insulin secretion response (the body can produce insulin but not enough to meet the body's needs). Eventually, insulin production decreases (resulting from the pancreas working overtime to produce insulin), with a result similar to type 1 DM.

If DM goes unrecognized or is inadequately treated (especially type 1 DM), **diabetic ketoacidosis (DKA)** or fat catabolism develops (a deficiency or ineffectiveness of insulin results in the body using fat instead of glucose for energy), resulting in anorexia, nausea and vomiting, lethargy, stupor, altered level of consciousness, confusion, decreased skin turgor, abdominal pain, Kussmaul respirations and air hunger, fruity (sweet-smelling) or acetone breath odor, presence of ketones in urine and blood, tachycardia, and, if left untreated, coma and death.

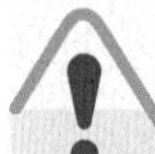

CLINICAL REASONING ALERT!

DKA is a medical emergency. It requires early recognition and prompt intervention. Be alert to the increased chance of DKA during times of stress, such as illness, infection, and surgery, as hormones produced by the body in times of stress result in decreased insulin sensitivity and increased glucose production.

Prolonged exposure to high blood glucose levels results in damage to blood vessels and nerves. Long-term complications of DM include failure to grow, delayed sexual maturation, poor wound healing, recurrent infections (especially of the skin), retinopathy, neuropathy, vascular complications, nephropathy, cerebrovascular disease, peripheral vascular disease, and cardiovascular disease. Consistent, well-controlled blood glucose levels can prevent these complications from developing for many years. On the other hand, poorly controlled DM can lead to complications much earlier.

Therapeutic Management

Treatment for DM must occur as part of a multidisciplinary health care team, with the family and child as a central part of that team. In the past, children would be admitted to the hospital for 3 to 5 days for stabilization and education, but today the trend is toward treating children on an outpatient basis. Established glucose control is essential in reducing the risk of long-term complications associated with DM. Therefore, general goals for therapeutic management include the following:

- Achieving normal growth and development
- Promoting optimal serum glucose control, including fluid and electrolyte levels and near-normal **hemoglobin A1C** (glycosylated hemoglobin, which is hemoglobin that glucose is bound to, a measure of long-term control of blood glucose and diabetes) levels
- Preventing complications
- Promoting positive adjustment to the disease, with ability to self-manage in the home

The key to success is educating the child and family so they can self-manage this chronic condition. Therapeutic management involves blood glucose monitoring, daily insulin injections or administration of oral hypoglycemic medications, following a realistic and well-balanced diet, participating in an exercise program, and developing self-management and decision-making skills.

Research is ongoing to develop alternative medications, including alternative routes for insulin administration and therapies to monitor and treat diabetes.

Monitoring Glycemic Control

Maintain consistent glycemic control leads to fewer long-term diabetes-related complications. Two important methods for monitoring glycemic control include blood glucose monitoring and monitoring hemoglobin A1C (HgbA1C) levels.

BLOOD GLUCOSE MONITORING

Blood glucose monitoring evaluates short-term glycemic control. It allows for tight glucose control because supplemental insulin can be used to correct or prevent hyperglycemia; it also enables children and their parents and their health care providers or nurse practitioners to provide better management of the disease (refer to Common Laboratory and Diagnostic Tests 48.1). The frequency of blood glucose monitoring is based on the individual goals. Children hospitalized for management of their DM or on insulin therapy require blood glucose monitoring before meals and at bedtime, if not more frequently. Additional glucose checks may be necessary if glycemic control has not occurred, during times of illness, during episodes of hypoglycemic or hyperglycemic symptoms, or when there are changes in therapy. Children receiving noninsulin therapy may check their blood glucose levels less frequently, but it can remain a useful guide to their therapy and its effectiveness. The procedure for blood glucose monitoring will vary based on the equipment used but often involves a fingerstick, a reagent strip, and a glucometer.

SMBG at home is essential to improve glycemic control, to provide self-management of this disease, and to help prevent complications such as severe hypoglycemia or hyperglycemia. The child and caregiver need to be aware of the importance of checking blood glucose regularly, and more frequently when needed. Documenting blood glucose values is necessary to provide information on glucose control. This allows their health care provider or nurse practitioner to evaluate the effectiveness of their treatment regimen. Accuracy of SMBG is dependent on proper user technique; therefore, assessment of technique and education reinforcement are important at each visit (see Teaching Guidelines 48.2).

Real-time continuous glucose monitoring should be considered for children with type 1 diabetes. This may be helpful in children with hypoglycemic unawareness or frequent hypoglycemic episodes. A sensor is placed under the skin that measures interstitial glucose. These systems provide valuable information regarding glycemic control. For example, time in range, which is the time in the past 14 days that the child's blood glucose was in the desired range, correlates well with HgbA1C. Additionally, some monitors can provide an estimated HgbA1C (Levitsky & Misra, 2023b).

MONITORING HEMOGLOBIN A1C LEVELS

Hemoglobin A1C (HgbA1C) provides the health care provider or nurse practitioner with information regarding

TEACHING GUIDELINES 48.2 Blood Glucose Monitoring

- Obtain blood glucose levels multiple times daily (up to 6–10 times per day by blood glucose meter or continuous glucose monitoring), including before meals and snacks, at bedtime, and as needed for safety in specific situations such as exercise, driving, or the presence of symptoms of hypoglycemia.
- Perform monitoring more often during prolonged exercise, if you are ill, if you have eaten more food than usual, or if you suspect nighttime hypoglycemia.
- Use the manufacturer's recommendations and perform quality control measures as directed.
- Look for patterns. For example, 3–4 days of a consistent pattern of glucose values above 200 mg/dL before dinner indicates a need to adjust the insulin dose.
- Blood glucose measurements are the best way to determine daily insulin dosages.
- Normal levels are as follows: for children without diabetes: 70–110 mg/dL; target levels should be individualized; time in range is considered 70–180 mg/dL, time below target is <70 mg/dL, time above target is 180 mg/dL.

(American Diabetes Association Professional Practice Committee, 2022).

the long-term control of glucose levels (refer to Common Laboratory and Diagnostic Tests 48.1). In children, especially infants and children younger than 6 years, hypoglycemia poses some unique risks and can be hard to recognize. Therefore, the HgbA1C goals in children need to take into account the risks of severe hypoglycemia, and glycemic control goals need to be individualized (American Diabetes Association Professional Practice Committee, 2022) However, recent data have shown that lower HgbA1C levels lead to reduced long-term complications; therefore, the targets for HgbA1C in children have become lower in recent years. Currently, the American Diabetes Association Professional Practice Committee (2022) recommends that children and adolescents have a target HgbA1C lower than 7.0%.

Insulin Replacement Therapy

Insulin replacement therapy is the cornerstone of management of type 1 DM. Insulin is administered daily by subcutaneous injections into adipose tissue over large muscle masses using a traditional insulin syringe or a subcutaneous injector (Fig. 48.7). U-100 insulin may also be administered using a portable insulin pump (see discussion later). The frequency, dose, and type of insulin are based on how much the child needs to achieve a normal, average blood glucose concentration and to

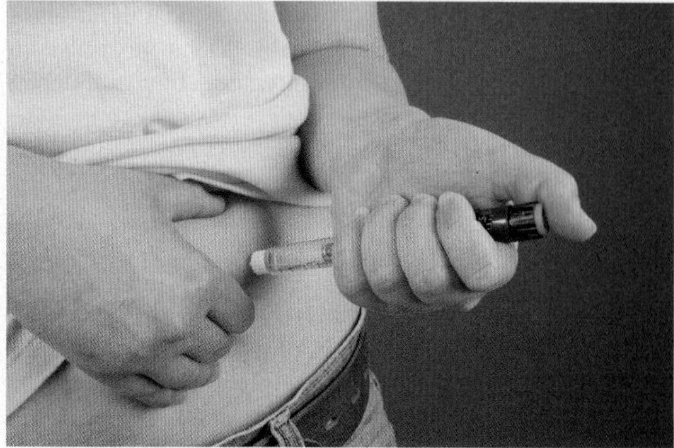

FIGURE 48.7 The subcutaneous injector uses pressure jets to deliver insulin safely and accurately.

prevent hypoglycemia. Typically, two to four daily injections are commonly used, with dosage depending on the needs of the child. The dose may need to be increased during the pubertal growth spurt, as well as during times of illness or stress.

An insulin pump is a device that administers a continuous infusion of rapid-acting insulin. It consists of a computer, a reservoir of rapid-acting insulin, thin tubing through which the insulin is delivered, and a small needle inserted into the abdomen. Insulin pumps attempt to mimic the physiologic insulin release by delivering small continuous infusions of insulin with additional bolus units administered at mealtimes, for planned carbohydrate intake, and if glucose testing results show it is needed. Many insulin pumps have a built-in sensor to monitor blood glucose continuously. Advantages of this kind of therapy include the following:

- There are fewer injections and less trauma.
- Children's food intake can be unpredictable, so insulin delivery can occur after a meal and be adjusted based on actual intake.
- Children can be sensitive to insulin and require only minute doses, which the pump can deliver with precision.
- The pumps can store different basal rates for different times during the day and days of the week. For example, a higher basal rate may be needed in the morning when the child is sitting at their desk and a lower rate may be necessary during the afternoon when the child is more active with recess and physical education classes. In addition, rates can be programmed differently for school days versus weekend days, when the child may sleep later and have differing activity levels.

The use of an insulin pump does require a commitment from the child and caregiver to achieve success and improved glycemic control. The child and caregiver must be able to count carbohydrates, monitor glucose levels frequently, and work closely with the health care provider or nurse practitioner.

TAKE NOTE!

Hybrid closed loop systems (artificial pancreas) will automatically decrease, increase, or stop insulin delivery in response to readings from the continuous glucose monitor. Studies have found these systems to improve glycemic control and decrease hypoglycemic episodes. More advanced closed loop systems are in development (Levitsky & Misra, 2023c).

Types of insulin include ultra rapid-acting, rapid-acting, short-acting, intermediate-acting, and long-acting (Table 48.5). Each type works at a different pace, and most children will use more than one type. Neutral protamine Hagedorn (NPH) and regular insulin are no longer recommended in the routine care of children with type 1 diabetes, but in some cases, premixed combinations of intermediate-acting and short- or rapid-acting, such as 70% NPH and 30% regular, may be used (Levitsky & Misra, 2023c). Again, this depends on the needs of the child. Insulin can be kept at room temperature (insulin that is administered cold may increase discomfort with injection) but should be discarded 1 month after opening even if refrigerated. Any extra, unopened vials should be stored in the refrigerator.

TAKE NOTE!

Do not mix long-acting insulin with other insulins.

TAKE NOTE!

New insulins, including orally absorbed or inhaled insulin, are being developed (Levitsky & Misra, 2023c).

Oral Diabetes Medications

Oral diabetes medications, also referred to as hypoglycemic, antidiabetic, or antihyperglycemic medications, are used in type 2 diabetes if glycemic control cannot be achieved by diet and exercise. The largest clinical trial to date, the Treatment Options for Type 2 Diabetes in Adolescents and Youth (TODAY) study, found that monotherapy with oral diabetes medication did not result in lasting glycemic control in the majority of youth with type 2 diabetes (Laffel & Svoren, 2023). Therefore, children and adolescents with type 2 diabetes need a combination of nonpharmacologic and pharmacologic interventions along with close monitoring and follow-up.

Oral diabetes medications work in a variety of ways. Metformin is the first line of therapy (Laffel & Svoren, 2023). It is an example of a biguanide and is an effective initial therapy unless significant liver or kidney impairment is present. It works by reducing glucose production from the liver and makes the body more sensitive to insulin by increasing insulin-mediated glucose uptake.

Common adverse effects of oral diabetes medications include headache, dizziness, flatulence and GI distress, edema, and liver enzyme elevation. If the oral hypoglycemics fail to maintain a normal glucose level, then insulin injections will be required to manage type 2 diabetes.

Diet and Exercise

Other therapies involve diet and exercise protocols. Medical nutritional therapy (MNT) can be initiated to prevent type 2 diabetes in children showing signs of prediabetes, to help glycemic control in existing diabetes, and to help

TABLE **48.5** Insulin Type, Action, and Duration

Type	Generic (Brand) Name	Onset	Peak	Duration (hours)
Ultra-rapid-acting	Faster aspart Insulin lispro-aabc	6–12 minutes	1–3 hours	3–5
Rapid-acting	Aspart (NovoLog) Lispro (Humalog) Glulisine (Apidra)	Within 15–20 minutes	1–3 hours	3–5
Short-acting	Regular (Humulin R, Novolin R)	0.5–1 hour	2–4 hours	5–8
Intermediate-acting	NPH (Humulin N, Novolin N)	2–4 hours	4–12 hours	12–24
Basal long-acting	Glargine (Lantus) Detemir (Levemir) Glargine 300U Degludec (Tresiba)	2–4 hours 1–2 hours 2–6 hours 0.5–1.5 hours	8–12 hours 4–7 hours None None	22–24 20–24 30–36>42

NPH, neutral protamine Hagedorn

Data from Levitsky, L. L., & Misra, M. (2023c). Insulin therapy for children and adolescents with type 1 diabetes mellitus. *UpToDate*. Retrieved May 23, 2023, from https://www.uptodate.com/contents/insulin-therapy-for-children-and-adolescents-with-type-1-diabetes-mellitus

slow the development of complications associated with diabetes. MNT can be complex and must be individualized to each child, incorporating the child's food preferences, activity level, cultural preferences, and family habits and schedule. Enlisting the help of a registered dietician who has expertise in diabetes management is recommended (American Diabetes Association Professional Practice Committee, 2022).

The appropriate diet for a child or adolescent with diabetes is a balanced, healthy diet that meets the child's growth and development needs. The child and family need to understand the effect that food has on the child's glucose levels. Monitoring carbohydrate intake is an important component of diet management and assists with glycemic control. Nutritional recommendations for a child with diabetes or prediabetes include the following: limit sweets, ensure consistent food intake (eat often and try to avoid skipping meals), monitor carbohydrate intake, eat whole grains and plenty of fruits and vegetables, and limit fat (Gray & Threlkeld, 2019).

It has been shown that regular exercise can improve glycemic control and can prevent the development of type 2 diabetes (American Diabetes Association Professional Practice Committee, 2022). Also, exercise has an important influence on the hypoglycemic effects of insulin (by causing the release of glucagon, which will result in increased blood glucose). Therefore, it is important for the child to maintain or increase their activity levels. Exercise can lead to both hyperglycemia or hypoglycemia; therefore, frequent glucose monitoring before, during, and after exercise is important (American Diabetes Association Professional Practice Committee, 2022). If the child is taking insulin, the family must know how to adjust the medication dosage or add food to maintain blood glucose control. The child needs to have access to rapid-acting carbohydrates, and the child and family should ensure preexercise blood glucose levels of 126 to 180 mg/dL (exact recommendations should be individualized based on the child and the activity) (American Diabetes Association Professional Practice Committee, 2022). Children with type 2 diabetes often are overweight, so the exercise plan is very important in helping the child to lose weight, as well as assisting with the hypoglycemic effects of the medications.

THINKING ABOUT **DEVELOPMENT**

Jayda Jones, a 12-year-old, is recently diagnosed with type 2 diabetes.

Based on her developmental age, how will you instruct her and her caregivers on ways to manage her diabetes at home?

How would your instructions change if she was 16 years old?

Management of Complications

Another important aspect of therapeutic management includes monitoring and managing complications. The American Diabetes Association Professional Practice Committee (2022) has developed recommendations for standards of medical care to help monitor complications and reduce risk. These include the following:

- Retinopathy:
  - Type 1 diabetes: eye examination by ophthalmologist (with expertise in diabetes) once the child is 11 years old or puberty has started (whichever is earlier) and has had diabetes for 3 to 5 years; eye examinations every 2 years unless different recommendation by professional
  - Type 2 diabetes: eye examination by ophthalmologist (with expertise in diabetes) shortly after diagnosis; annual examinations unless different recommendation by professional
- Nephropathy:
  - Type 1 diabetes: annual screening for microalbuminuria (which occurs when the kidneys leak small amounts of albumin into the urine) once the child is 10 years old or puberty has started (whichever is earlier) and has had diabetes for 5 years; if normal then annually
  - Type 2 diabetes: screen at diagnosis and annually thereafter for microalbuminuria
- Neuropathy:
  - Type 1 diabetes: annual foot examination once the child has reached puberty or is 10 years or older (whichever is earlier) and has had diabetes for 5 years, then annually
  - Type 2 diabetes: foot examination at diagnosis and annually
- Dyslipidemia:
  - Type 1 diabetes: Obtain a lipid profile in children above 2 years old at the time of diagnosis (once glucose levels have been stabilized); if normal, repeat at 9 to 11 years of age, and then repeat every 3 years.
  - Type 2 diabetes: Obtain a fasting lipid panel at diagnosis (once glucose levels have been stabilized), then annually.
- Hypertension: blood pressure measured at each routine visit
- In addition, children with type 1 diabetes should be screened for additional autoimmune disorders such as celiac disease (screen after diagnosis and then after 2 years, and again after 5 years, screen more often if symptoms or family history are present) and hypothyroidism (screen after diagnosis, and every 1 to 2 years or sooner if symptoms are present). Children with type 2 diabetes should be screened for nonalcoholic fatty liver disease at diagnosis and annually, and obstructive sleep apnea and PCOS at diagnosis and every visit.

EVIDENCE-BASED PRACTICE **48.1**

What is the Prevalence of Diabetes-Specific Eating Disorder (DSED) in Adolescents With Type 1 Diabetes and Are There Associated Psychopathologies, Such as Anxiety and Depression?

STUDY

Adolescents with type 1 diabetes are at an increased risk for eating disorders and disturbed eating behaviors (DEBs) such as fasting, extreme dieting, binge eating, and omitting or underdosing insulin to cause weight loss (newly referred to as diabulimia). This may be linked to the constant focus on food and its effect on blood glucose and the weight gain related to insulin. This study used cross-sectional data of 92 adolescents aged 12 to 18 years with type 1 diabetes for at least 1 year. It evaluated the frequency of DSED risk and its relationship with metabolic, anthropometric, and socio-demographic parameters and parenting styles, as well as accompanying psychopathologies. The Diabetes Eating Problem Survey-Revised (DEPS-R) was used to determine the risk of DSED along with the Eating Disorder Examination Questionnaire (EDE-Q), Child Anxiety and Depression Scale—Child version, and Parenting Style Scale to help detect if accompanying psychopathologies were present.

In this study, 23.9% of adolescents were found to be at risk for DSED. A weak correlation was found between a higher risk of DSED and higher HgbA1C levels. DEPS-R scores were higher in adolescents with increased BMI. Adolescents with divorced parents were more likely to have DSED, and anxiety and depression scores were higher in adolescents who had a positive DEPS-R.

Nursing Implications

DEBs often are not recognized by clinicians and parents, but the risk of DEBs and eating disorders remains high in children with type 1 diabetes. This study supports the importance of routinely screening people at risk and referring them to child psychiatry services. The American Diabetes Association Professional Practice Committee (2022) recommends screening children with type 1 diabetes for eating disorders beginning between 10 and 12 years of age. The DEPS-R is a reliable, valid, and short screening tool (American Diabetes Association Professional Practice Committee, 2022).

Data from Tarçın, G., Akman, H., Güneş Kaya, D., Serdengeçti, N., İncetahtacı, S., Turan, H., Doğangün, B., & Ercan, O. (2023). Diabetes-specific eating disorder and possible associated psychopathologies in adolescents with type 1 diabetes mellitus. *Eating and Weight Disorders: EWD, 28*(1), 36. https://doi.org/10.1007/s40519-023-01559-y

- Assess for psychosocial and diabetes-related distress generally starting around 7 to 8 years old.
- Screen for eating disorders starting at 10 to 12 years old. Refer to Evidence-Based Practice 48.1.

Nursing Assessment

Assessment involves understanding the everchanging needs of children as they grow and develop. The first phase of assessment involves identifying children who may have diabetes. The second phase involves recognizing problems that may develop in children with diabetes. It is important to always be aware of this when observing for possible complications or management problems. In addition, always be alert for opportunities to provide education that will enhance the understanding and skills related to managing of DM for both the child and the family.

Health History and Physical Examination

During the initial diagnosis of DM, obtain a detailed family history and inquire about any school-related issues that may indicate mental and behavioral changes associated with hyperglycemic state (e.g., weakness, fatigue, mood changes). The child or parent may report unusual or excessive thirst (polydipsia) coupled with frequent urination (polyuria). The child may also complain of blurred vision, headaches, or bedwetting. The child with type 1 diabetes may have a history of poor growth. Comparison Chart 48.3 gives information about common history and physical examination findings in children with type 1 diabetes versus type 2 diabetes.

In a child known to have diabetes, the health history should include any problems related to hyperglycemia or hypoglycemia, dietary habits, activity and exercise patterns, types of medications (insulin or oral diabetes medications) and dose and times of administration, ability to monitor blood glucose levels, and ability to administer insulin. Perform a thorough physical examination, noting any abnormal findings.

Laboratory and Diagnostic Testing

Refer to Common Laboratory and Diagnostic Tests 48.1. A fasting glucose level equal to or greater than 126 mg/dL, a 2-hour plasma glucose level equal to or greater than 200 mg/dL during an oral glucose tolerance test, a random glucose level equal to or greater than 200 mg/dL (accompanied by typical symptoms of diabetes), or a HgbA1C greater than 6.5% are laboratory criteria for the diagnosis of DM (Levitsky & Misra, 2023a). For each of these tests, if hyperglycemia is not explicit, the results should be confirmed with a repeat test on a different day (Levitsky & Misra, 2023a). Other laboratory and diagnostic tests include serum measurements of islet cell antibodies, urea nitrogen, creatinine, calcium, magnesium, phosphate, and electrolytes such as potassium and sodium. Additional tests include a complete blood count, urinalysis, and immunoassay to measure levels of C-peptides after a glucose challenge to verify endogenous insulin secretion.

The American Diabetes Association Professional Practice Committee (2022) recommends screening for type 2 DM if a child presents with overweight or higher

COMPARISON CHART 48.3 Type 1 Versus Type 2 Diabetes Mellitus

History and Physical Findings Usually Present at Diagnosis	Type 1	Type 2
Family history	Less tendency than type 2	Yes
Prone ethnicity	All	Native American, African descent, Hispanic/Latino descents
Polydipsia, polyuria, polyphagia	Yes	Yes, may be mild or absent
Weight	Possibly, weight loss	Usually, higher weight
Age of onset	Usually, younger children	Usually, pubertal children
Incidental finding on screening urinalysis	Rare	Common
Antecedent flulike illness/symptoms	Common	Possible
Autoimmune antibodies	Yes	No
Diabetic ketoacidosis	Common	Possible
Hypertension	No	Common
Acanthosis nigricans	No	Common
Dyslipidemia	No	Common

Data from Weber, D. R., & Jospe, N. (2020). Chapter 607: Diabetes mellitus. In R. M. Kleigman, J. W. St. Geme III, N. J. Blum, S. S. Shah, R. C. Tasker, K. M. Wilson, & R. E. Behrman (Eds.), *Nelson textbook of pediatrics* (21st ed., pp. 15955–16147). Elsevier.

weight after the onset of puberty or at age 10 years or older, along with one of the following risk factors:

- Family history: a parent or relative with type 2 diabetes
- Ethnic background: Native American, African American, Latino, Asian American, or Pacific Islander
- Conditions associated with insulin resistance such as acanthosis nigricans, hypertension, dyslipidemia, or PCOS
- History of maternal diabetes or a birthing parent with gestational diabetes when the child was in utero (Weber & Jospe, 2020).

Nursing Management

Individualize the general nursing care discussed in the "Clinical Judgment and the Nursing Process" section earlier in the chapter, based on the child's and family's response to illness. Additional nursing care topics related to DM are discussed later, including regulating glucose control, monitoring for complications, providing education to the child and family, and offering support to both the child and family.

Regulating Glucose Control

Consistent and established glucose control can reduce the risk of long-term complications associated with diabetes. Therefore, regulating glucose is an important nursing function.

Typically, in children with type 1 diabetes and sometimes in cases of type 2 diabetes, glucose is regulated by subcutaneous insulin via injection or insulin pump. Often, the regimen consists of three injections of intermediate-acting insulin, with the addition of rapid-acting insulin before breakfast and dinner, or three injections of short-acting insulin with a long-acting injection at bedtime. Insulin doses are typically ordered on a sliding scale related to the serum glucose level and how the insulin works. Insulin doses and frequency are based on the needs of the child, utilizing information gained from blood glucose testing. Regulating glucose can be challenging in children due to continual growth, onset of puberty, varying activity levels with unpredictable schedules, unpredictable eating habits, and the inability to always verbalize the way they are feeling. Thus, close monitoring of changing glucose levels through SMBG is essential in determining adjustments needed in insulin therapy, food intake, and activity levels. Adjustment of insulin dosing based on carbohydrate intake is essential for managing blood glucose levels. The use of carbohydrate counting can help children enjoy more freedom to choose their type or amount of food and allow them to vary their mealtime and snack times. It allows them to predict the rise in blood glucose that will occur after eating a specific amount or type of carbohydrate and take into account recent or expected activity levels. It requires knowledge of carbohydrate amounts and calculations with each dose of short-acting insulin. Each scale will vary per child as the insulin per carbohydrate serving is calculated based on the child's specific requirement. See the Dosage Calculation Question under Developing Clinical Judgment at the end of the chapter for an example. Parents will need extensive education and continual follow-up to ensure the successful use of this method.

TAKE NOTE!

Blood glucose level should never be the only factor considered when calculating insulin dosing. Food intake and recent or expected activity/exercise must also be factored.

Teach the child and family to use proper subcutaneous injection techniques to avoid injecting into muscle or vascular spaces. Figure 48.8 shows appropriate sites for subcutaneous injection of insulin. Teach the child and family to rotate sites to avoid adipose hypertrophy (fatty lumps that absorb insulin poorly). If the child is using an insulin pump, additional education will be needed.

• • • ATRAUMATIC CARE • • •

Children with diabetes experience numerous finger pricks and injections. Providing atraumatic care remains important. Allow the child to choose the prick or injection site when possible. Use positioning that is comforting to the child. Encourage participation in care as developmentally appropriate.

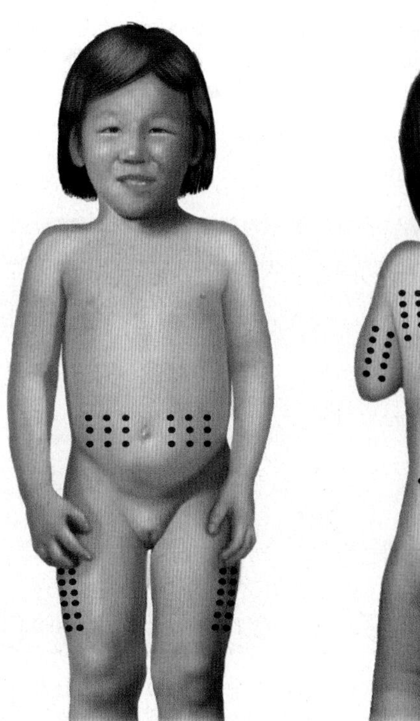

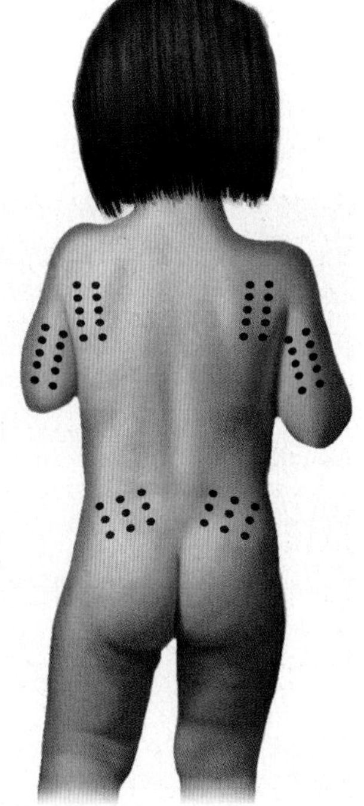

FIGURE 48.8 Insulin injection sites.

COMPARISON CHART 48.4 Hypoglycemia Versus Hyperglycemia

Hypoglycemia	Hyperglycemia
Behavioral changes (tearfulness, irritability, naughtiness), confusion, slurred speech, belligerence	Mental status changes, fatigue, weakness
Diaphoresis	Dry, flushed skin
Tremors	Blurred vision
Palpitations, tachycardia	Abdominal cramping, nausea, vomiting, fruity breath odor

In children with type 2 diabetes, glucose levels can be controlled by diet, exercise, oral diabetes medications, or a combination of all three.

Monitoring for and Managing Complications

While the child is in the hospital, monitor for signs of complications such as acidosis, coma, hyperkalemia, hypokalemia, hypocalcemia, cerebral edema, or hyponatremia. Assess for the development of hypoglycemia or hyperglycemia every 2 hours (Comparison Chart 48.4). Monitor the child's status closely during peak times of insulin action. Perform blood glucose testing as ordered or as needed if the child develops symptoms.

Concept Mastery Alert

Manifestations of hypoglycemia include behavioral changes, confusion, slurred speech, diaphoresis, tremors, palpitations, and tachycardia. In contrast, manifestations of hyperglycemia include blurred vision; dry, flushed skin; and a fruity odor to the breath.

If the child has a severe hypoglycemic reaction, administer glucagon (a hormone produced by the pancreas and stored in the liver) either subcutaneously or intramuscularly. Children under 20 kg receive 0.5 mg; children over 20 kg receive 1 mg (Weber & Jospe, 2020). Dextrose (50%) may be given IV if needed. If the child is not having a severe reaction and is coherent, glucose paste or tablets may be used. Offer 10 to 15 g of a simple carbohydrate, such as orange juice, if the child feels some symptoms of low blood glucose and glucose monitoring indicates a drop in blood glucose level. Follow this with a more complex carbohydrate, such as peanut butter and crackers, to maintain the glucose level.

The child with severe hyperglycemia resulting in DKA is usually treated in the pediatric intensive care unit. In the case of a child presenting with DKA to the hospital, monitor the glucose level hourly to prevent it from falling more than 100 mg/dL/h. A too-rapid decline in blood glucose predisposes the child to cerebral edema. Fluid therapy is given to treat dehydration, correct electrolyte imbalances (sodium and potassium due to osmotic diuresis), and improve peripheral perfusion. Administration of regular insulin, given IV, is preferred during DKA (only regular insulin may be given IV).

Any child exhibiting signs and symptoms of hyperglycemia requires insulin. The dosage is usually based on a sliding scale or determined after consultation with the health care provider or nurse practitioner.

TAKE NOTE!

Double check all insulin doses against the order sheet and with another nurse to ensure accuracy.

Educating the Family

Education is the priority intervention for DM because it will enable the child and family to self-manage this chronic condition. Allow the child and family time to adjust to the diagnosis of a chronic illness that will require self-management. DM is a lifelong condition that requires regular follow-up visits (three or four times a year) to a diabetes specialty clinic. Because approximately 210,000 children and adolescents younger than the age of 20 have diabetes, this becomes a health issue for the community, especially for the schools (CDC, 2020). Daily management of the child with diabetes is complex and dynamic. It will require frequent monitoring of blood glucose levels, medications (including oral diabetes medications and insulin injections), and personalized meal plans, including snacks, while the child is at school. The school nurse will be a principal contact person for both staff and family. With appropriate management, community involvement, and confidence and adherence by the family, the child can maintain a happy, productive life. See the Healthy People 2030 box.

HEALTHY PEOPLE 2030

Objective	Nursing Significance
Increase the proportion of people with diagnosed diabetes who ever receive formal diabetes education.	• Begin diabetes education with the child and family upon knowledge of diagnosis. • Use developmentally appropriate education with children. • Increase the self-management skills taught as the child progresses in age and cognitive development.

Healthy People Objectives retrieved from http://www.healthypeople.gov

Challenges related to educating children with diabetes include the following:

- Children lack the maturity to understand the long-term consequences of this serious chronic illness.
- Children do not want to be different from their peers; having to make lifestyle changes may result in anger or depression.
- Families with limited resources may not be able to afford appropriate food, medication, transportation, and telephone service.
- Families may demonstrate unhealthy behaviors, making it difficult for the child to initiate change because of the lack of supervision or role modeling.
- Family dynamics are affected because management of diabetes must occur all day, every day.

TAKE NOTE!

Children with diabetes have higher rates of depression and may have other comorbid conditions, such as eating disorders, adjustment disorders, or anxiety disorders (American Diabetes Association Professional Practice Committee, 2022; Weber & Jospe, 2020).

The initial goal of education is for the family to develop basic management and decision-making skills. Assess the family's ability to learn the basic concepts and offer psychological support. Teach about specific topics in sessions lasting 15 to 20 minutes for the children and 45 to 60 minutes for the caregivers. Teaching must be geared toward the child's level of development and understanding (see Table 48.4).

Among the topics to include when teaching children and their families about diabetes management are as follows:

- Self-measurement of blood glucose (Fig. 48.9)
- Urine ketone testing

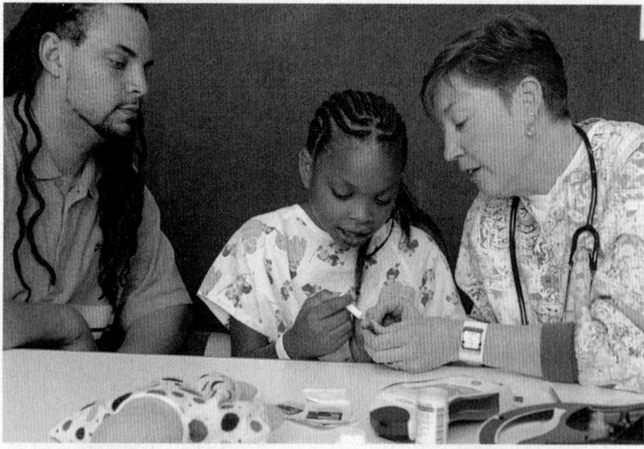

FIGURE 48.9 The school-age child has developed the psychomotor skills needed for blood glucose monitoring and insulin injection.

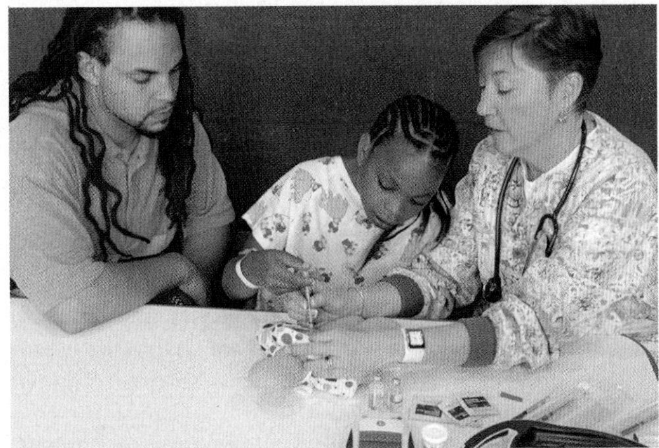

FIGURE 48.10 The school-age child may first practice insulin injections on a doll.

- Medication use (Fig. 48.10)
  - Oral diabetes agents
  - Subcutaneous insulin injection or insulin pump use
  - Subcutaneous site selection and rotation
  - When to alter insulin dosages
  - Use of glucagon to treat severe hypoglycemia
- Signs and symptoms of hypoglycemia and hyperglycemia (refer to Comparison Chart 48.4)
- Treatment for hypoglycemia and hyperglycemia at home or other setting such as school
- Monitoring for and managing complications (see earlier)
- Sick-day instructions
- Laboratory testing and follow-up care
- Diet and exercise as part of DM management (see earlier)

Teaching Guidelines 48.2 presents information to cover when teaching the family about SMBG. Teach families how to give insulin, how to use the insulin pump, and how to rotate injection sites.

Good glucose control is dependent on accurate monitoring and medication administration by the child or caregiver. Assessment of the child's or parent's technique and review of procedure and instructions should occur with each visit. Treatment of hypoglycemia and hyperglycemia may have to occur at home or in another setting such as school. In either case, someone trained to check the child's blood glucose level must be available. In the case of hypoglycemia, early recognition is key. Therefore, all caregivers need to be educated on the causes of hypoglycemia (such as increased physical activity, delayed meals or snacks, insulin, oral diabetes medication, illness, stress, and hormonal fluctuations) along with the signs and symptoms. The child also needs access to glucose tablets or a rapidly absorbing carbohydrate such as orange juice, as well as a snack with complex carbohydrates and protein within 30 to 60 minutes of the hypoglycemic episode. Injectable glucagon should be available in the case that the hypoglycemia is severe and the child is unconscious. In the event of hyperglycemia, the child needs immediate access to rapid-acting insulin injection.

Sick-day instructions may include the following:

- Contact the health care provider or nurse practitioner.
- Perform SMBG more often.
- Check for ketones in the urine, especially if blood glucose is elevated.
- Use a sliding scale to calculate the insulin dosage.

A dietitian can help the family with detailed meal planning and dietary guidelines. Review basic nutritional information with the child and family and provide sample meals. Encourage the child and family to keep a food diary. For the child who needs to lose weight, suggest low-carbohydrate snacks. Encourage all children with diabetes to incorporate physical activity daily (Teaching Guidelines 48.3).

Supporting the Child and Family

Children with diabetes and their families may have difficulty coping if they lack confidence in their self-management skills. Assess the ability of the child and family to handle situations. Role play specific situations

TEACHING GUIDELINES 48.3 Diet and Exercise for Children With Diabetes

- Provide sufficient calories and good nutrition for normal growth and development. The diet should be low in saturated fats and concentrated carbohydrates.
- Learn to identify carbohydrate, protein, and fat foods.
- Make adjustments during periods of rapid growth and for issues such as travel, school parties, and holidays.
- Consult a dietitian with expertise in diabetes education as needed.
- Provide three meals per day and midafternoon and bedtime snacks. Consistency of intake can help prevent complications and maintain near-normal blood glucose levels.
- Encourage the child to exercise routinely to help the body use insulin efficiently, thus reducing the insulin requirement.
- Encourage the child to participate in age-appropriate sports.
- When exercising, monitor insulin dose and nutritional and fluid intake, and observe for hypoglycemic reactions. Add an extra snack containing 15–30 g carbohydrate for each 45–60 minutes of exercise. Avoid exercising excessively when insulin is peaking.

related to symptoms or complications to help them see different ways to solve problems. Work with the child and family to enhance their conflict resolution skills. Provide opportunities for them to express their feelings. Observe for signs of depression, especially in adolescents.

To enhance the child's confidence and promote feelings of mastery and inclusion, refer them to a special camp for children with diabetes. Also refer families to local support groups, parent-to-parent networks, or one of many national support resources and foundations.

KEY CONCEPTS

- The endocrine system consists of cells, tissues, and glands that produce hormones (chemical messengers) and secrete them in response to a negative feedback system involving the hypothalamus and nervous system.
- Hormones (chemical messengers), along with the nervous system, play an intricate role in reproduction, growth and development, energy production and use, and maintenance of the internal homeostasis.
- The pituitary, along with the hypothalamus connection, is considered the "control center," producing hormones that stimulate many glands to produce other hormones or to inhibit the process.
- Hormonal control is immature at birth; this is partly why the infant has trouble maintaining an appropriate balance of fluid concentration, electrolytes, amino acids, glucose, and trace substances.
- Linear growth and cognitive development may be impaired by untreated endocrine dysfunction in the infant or child.
- A thorough health history of the child with a known or potential endocrine disorder often reveals poor growth, school or learning problems, and inactivity or fatigue.
- Serial measurement of growth parameters is a key part of the physical assessment for children with endocrine dysfunction.
- Close monitoring of the child's status is critical during a hormone stimulation test or water deprivation study.
- Hormone supplementation is required lifelong for many of the endocrine disorders.
- The key nursing functions related to hormone supplementation are educating the child and family about medication use and monitoring for therapeutic results and adverse effects.
- Children with adrenocortical dysfunction will require additional hormone supplementation during times of stress such as fever, infection, or surgery.
- GH deficiency is characterized by poor growth and short stature as a result of failure of the anterior pituitary to produce sufficient GH. Early treatment enables the child to reach normal growth.
- Precocious puberty involves early development of secondary sex characteristics as a result of premature activation of the hypothalamic–pituitary–gonadal axis.
- AVP-D is characterized by water intoxication as a result of a deficiency in the ADH that leads to the cardinal signs of polyuria and polydipsia, resulting in hypernatremic dehydration.
- Key findings in congenital hypothyroidism are a thickened protuberant tongue, an enlarged posterior fontanel, feeding difficulties, hypotonia, and lethargy.
- Early diagnosis and treatment of hypothyroidism can prevent impaired growth and severe cognitive impairment.
- CAH results from a genetic defect that causes a breakdown in steroid synthesis and an overproduction of androgens that can lead to ambiguous genitalia in females.
- DM is the most common endocrine disorder now seen in children.
- Type 1 DM is an autoimmune disorder resulting from damage and destruction of the beta cells in the islets of Langerhans in the pancreas; the end result is insulin insufficiency. Peak onset occurs in childhood.
- Type 2 DM results in an insensitivity or resistance to insulin. The incidence of type 2 DM has risen dramatically. It is occurring at an alarming rate in children, especially in those with higher weight and those from certain ethnicity.
- DKA is a medical emergency. The child will usually be admitted to a pediatric intensive care unit.
- The focus of DM management is regulation of glucose control, which is accomplished by medications, diet, and exercise.
- DM education involves instruction in glucose monitoring, administration of insulin or oral hypoglycemics, meal planning, and promotion of a healthy lifestyle.
- Critical areas in the nursing management of children with endocrine dysfunction include maintaining appropriate nutrition and fluid balance and promoting growth and development.
- The nurse provides ongoing assessment and education of the child and family, imparting to them the knowledge and skills required for self-management.
- Encouraging the child to have a healthy body image and working with the family in establishing healthy family processes are also key nursing functions.

REFERENCES AND RECOMMENDED READINGS

American Diabetes Association Professional Practice Committee. (2022). 14. Children and adolescents: Standards of medical care in diabetes—2022. *Diabetes Care, 45*, (Suppl._1), S208–S231. https://doi.org/10.2337/dc22-S014

Bichet, D. G. (2023). Arginine vasopressin deficiency (central diabetes insipidus): Treatment. *UpToDate*. Retrieved May 23, 2023, from https://www.uptodate.com/contents/arginine-vasopressin-deficiency-central-diabetes-insipidus-treatment

Breault, D. T., & Majzoub, J. A. (2020a). Diabetes insipidus. In R. M. Kleigman, J. W. St. Geme III, N. J. Blum, S. S. Shah, R. C. Tasker, K. M. Wilson, & R. E. Behrman (Eds.), *Nelson textbook of pediatrics* (21st ed., pp. 15266–15279). Elsevier.

Breault, D. T., & Majzoub, J. A. (2020b). Other abnormalities of arginine vasopressin metabolism and action. In R. M. Kleigman, J. W. St. Geme III, N. J. Blum, S. S. Shah, R. C. Tasker, K. M. Wilson, & R. E. Behrman (Eds.), *Nelson textbook of pediatrics* (21st ed., pp. 15280–15292). Elsevier.

Centers for Disease Control and Prevention. (2020). *National diabetes statistics report, 2020: Estimates of diabetes and its burden in the United States.* U.S. Department of Health and Human Services. https://www.cdc.gov/diabetes/pdfs/data/statistics/national-diabetes-statistics-report.pdf

Connelly, K., & LaFranchi, S. (2023a). Clinical features and detection of congenital hypothyroidism. In *UpToDate*. Retrieved May 23, 2023, from https://www.uptodate.com/contents/clinical-features-and-detection-of-congenital-hypothyroidism

Connelly, K., & LaFranchi, S. (2023b). Treatment and prognosis of congenital hypothyroidism. *UpToDate*. Retrieved May 23, 2023, from https://www.uptodate.com/contents/treatment-and-prognosis-of-congenital-hypothyroidism

Crowley, W. F., & Pitteloud, N. (2023). Approaches to the patient with delayed puberty. *UpToDate*. Retrieved May 23, 2023, from https://www.uptodate.com/contents/approach-to-the-patient-with-delayed-puberty

Doyle, D. A. (2020a). Hypoparathyroidism. In R. M. Kleigman, J. W. St. Geme III, N. J. Blum, S. S. Shah, R. C. Tasker, K. M. Wilson, & R. E. Behrman (Eds.), *Nelson textbook of pediatrics* (21st ed., pp. 15565–15579). Elsevier.

Doyle, D. A. (2020b). Hyperparathyroidism. In R. M. Kleigman, J. W. St. Geme III, N. J. Blum, S. S. Shah, R. C. Tasker, K. M. Wilson, & R. E. Behrman (Eds.), *Nelson textbook of pediatrics* (21st ed., pp. 15587–15601). Elsevier.

Fischbach, F. T., Fischbach, M. A., & Stout, K. (2022). *A manual of laboratory and diagnostic tests* (11th ed.). Wolters Kluwer.

Garibaldi, L., & Chemaitilly, W. (2020). Disorders of pubertal development. In R. M. Kleigman, J. W. St. Geme III, N. J. Blum, S. S. Shah, R. C. Tasker, K. M. Wilson, & R. E. Behrman (Eds.), *Nelson textbook of pediatrics* (21st ed., pp. 15324–15382). Elsevier.

Gray, A., & Threlkeld, R. J. (2019). Nutritional recommendations for individuals with diabetes. In K. R. Feingold, B. Anawalt, M. R. Blackman, A. Boyce, G. Chrousos, E. Corpas, W. W. de Herder, K. Dhatariya, K. Dungan, J. Hofland, S. Kalra, G. Kaltsas, N. Kapoor, C. Koch, P. Kopp, M. Korbonits, C. S. Kovacs, W. Kuohung, B. Laferrère, . . . , D. P, Wilson (Eds.), *Endotext [Internet]*. https://www.ncbi.nlm.nih.gov/books/NBK279012/

Harrington, J., & Palmert, M. R. (2022). Definition, etiology, and evaluation of precocious puberty. *UpToDate*. Retrieved May 23, 2023, from https://www.uptodate.com/contents/definition-etiology-and-evaluation-of-precocious-puberty

Kemper, A. R. (2021). Newborn screening. *UpToDate*. Retrieved May 20, 2023 from https://www.uptodate.com/contents/newborn-screening

Laffel, L., & Svoren, B. (2023). Management of type 2 diabetes mellitus in children and adolescents. *UpToDate*. Retrieved May 23, 2023, from https://www.uptodate.com/contents/management-of-type-2-diabetes-mellitus-in-children-and-adolescents

LaFranchi, S. (2022a). Acquired hypothyroidism in childhood and adolescence. *UpToDate*. Retrieved May 23, 2023, from https://www.uptodate.com/contents/acquired-hypothyroidism-in-childhood-and-adolescence

LaFranchi, S. (2022b). Clinical manifestations and diagnosis of Graves disease in children and adolescents. *UpToDate*. Retrieved May 23, 2023, from https://www.uptodate.com/contents/clinical-manifestations-and-diagnosis-of-graves-disease-in-children-and-adolescents

Levitsky, L. L., & Misra, M. (2023a). Epidemiology, presentation, and diagnosis of type 1 diabetes mellitus in children and adolescents. *UpToDate*. Retrieved May 23, 2023, from https://www.uptodate.com/contents/epidemiology-presentation-and-diagnosis-of-type-1-diabetes-mellitus-in-children-and-adolescents

Levitsky, L. L., & Misra, M. (2023b). Overview of the management of type 1 diabetes mellitus in children and adolescents. *UpToDate*. Retrieved May 23, 2023, from https://www.uptodate.com/contents/overview-of-the-management-of-type-1-diabetes-mellitus-in-children-and-adolescents

Levitsky, L. L., & Misra, M. (2023c). Insulin therapy for children and adolescents with type 1 diabetes mellitus. *UpToDate*. Retrieved May 23, 2023, from https://www.uptodate.com/contents/insulin-therapy-for-children-and-adolescents-with-type-1-diabetes-mellitus

Lexicomp. (2023). Pediatric drug information. *UpToDate*. Retrieved April 5, 2023, from https://www.uptodate.com/contents/table-of-contents/drug-information

Merke, D. P. (2022). Treatment of classic congenital adrenal hyperplasia due to 21-hydroxylase deficiency in infants and children. *UpToDate*. Retrieved May 23, 2023, from https://www.uptodate.com/contents/treatment-of-classic-congenital-adrenal-hyperplasia-due-to-21-hydroxylase-deficiency-in-infants-and-children

Merke, D. P., & Auchus, R. J. (2022). Clinical manifestations and diagnosis of classic congenital adrenal hyperplasia due to 21-hydroxylase deficiency in infants and children. *UpToDate*. Retrieved May 23, 2023, from https://www.uptodate.com/contents/clinical-manifestations-and-diagnosis-of-classic-congenital-adrenal-hyperplasia-due-to-21-hydroxylase-deficiency-in-infants-and-children?

Mutter, C. M., Smith, T., Menze, O., Zakharia, M., & Nguyen, H. (2021). Diabetes insipidus: Pathogenesis, diagnosis, and clinical management. *Cureus*, *13*(2), e13523. https://doi.org/10.7759/cureus.13523

Patterson, B. C., & Felner, E. I. (2020). Hypopituitarism. In R. M. Kleigman, J. W. St. Geme III, N. J. Blum, S. S. Shah, R. C. Tasker, K. M. Wilson, & R. E. Behrman (Eds.), *Nelson textbook of pediatrics* (21st ed., pp. 15230–15265). Elsevier.

Rogol, A. D., & Richmond Padilla, E. J. (2023). Treatment of growth hormone deficiency in children. *UpToDate*. Retrieved May 22, 2023, from https://www.uptodate.com/contents/treatment-of-growth-hormone-deficiency-in-children

Shaw, N., & Rosenfield, R. L. (2022). Definition, clinical features, and differential diagnosis of polycystic ovary syndrome (PCOS) in adolescents. *UpToDate*. Retrieved May 23, 2023, from https://www.uptodate.com/contents/definition-clinical-features-and-differential-diagnosis-of-polycystic-ovary-syndrome-in-adolescents

Smith, J. R., & Wassner, A. J. (2020). Thyrotoxicosis. In R. M. Kleigman, J. W. St. Geme III, N. J. Blum, S. S. Shah, R. C. Tasker, K. M. Wilson, & R. E. Behrman (Eds.), *Nelson textbook of pediatrics* (21st ed., pp. 15478–15510). Elsevier.

Tarçın, G., Akman, H., Güneş Kaya, D., Serdengeçti, N., İncetahtacı, S., Turan, H., Doğangün, B., & Ercan, O. (2023). Diabetes-specific eating disorder and possible associated psychopathologies in adolescents with type 1 diabetes mellitus. *Eating and Weight Disorders: EWD*, *28*(1), 36. https://doi.org/10.1007/s40519-023-01559-y

U.S. Department of Health and Human Services. (n.d.). *Healthy People 2030*. https://health.gov/healthypeople

Warrier, V., Krishan, K., Shedge, R., & Kanchan, T. (2022). Height assessment. In *StatPearls* [Internet]. StatPearls Publishing. https://www.ncbi.nlm.nih.gov/books/NBK551524/

Wassner, A. J., & LaFranchi, S. (2021). Treatment and prognosis of Graves disease in children and adolescents. *UpToDate*. Retrieved May 23, 2023, from https://www.uptodate.com/contents/treatment-and-prognosis-of-graves-disease-in-children-and-adolescents

Wassner, A. J., & Smith, J. R. (2020). Hypothyroidism. In R. M. Kleigman, J. W. St. Geme III, N. J. Blum, S. S. Shah, R. C. Tasker, K. M. Wilson, & R. E. Behrman (Eds.), *Nelson textbook of pediatrics* (21st ed., pp. 15401–15445). Elsevier.

Weber, D. R., & Jospe, N. (2020). Diabetes mellitus. In R. M. Kleigman, J. W. St. Geme III, N. J. Blum, S. S. Shah, R. C. Tasker, K. M. Wilson, & R. E. Behrman (Eds.), *Nelson textbook of pediatrics* (21st ed., pp. 15955–16147). Elsevier.

White, P. C. (2020a). Adrenocortical insufficiency. In R. M. Kleigman, J. W. St. Geme III, N. J. Blum, S. S. Shah, R. C. Tasker, K. M. Wilson, & R. E. Behrman (Eds.), *Nelson textbook of pediatrics* (21st ed., pp. 15636–15689). Elsevier.

White, P. C. (2020b). Congenital adrenal hyperplasia and related disorders. In R. M. Kleigman, J. W. St. Geme III, N. J. Blum, S. S. Shah, R. C. Tasker, K. M. Wilson, & R. E. Behrman (Eds.), *Nelson textbook of pediatrics* (21st ed., pp. 15690–15735). Elsevier.

White, P. C. (2020c). Cushing syndrome. In R. M. Kleigman, J. W. St. Geme III, N. J. Blum, S. S. Shah, R. C. Tasker, K. M. Wilson, & R. E. Behrman (Eds.), *Nelson textbook of pediatrics* (21st ed., pp. 15753–15766). Elsevier.

Working Group for Renaming Diabetes Insipidus, Arima, H., Cheetham, T., Christ-Crain, M., Cooper, D., Gurnell, M., Drummond, J. B., Levy, M., McCormack, A. I., Verbalis, J., Newell-Price, J., & Wass, J. A. H. (2022). Changing the name of diabetes insipidus: a position statement of The Working Group for Renaming Diabetes Insipidus. *Endocrine Connections*, *11*(11), e220378. https://doi.org/10.1530/EC-22-0378

DEVELOPING CLINICAL JUDGMENT

PRACTICING FOR NCLEX

1. A young parent brings their new baby, diagnosed with congenital hypothyroidism, to the clinic so they can learn how to administer levothyroxine. The nurse should include which of the following instructions?
   a. Crush the medication and place it in a full bottle of formula to disguise the taste.
   b. Administer the medication every other day.
   c. Use an oral dispenser syringe or nipple to give the crushed medication mixed with a small amount of formula.
   d. The medication will not be needed after the age of 7.
2. During a well-child examination, which of the following comments made by the parent would indicate the possibility of a GH deficiency?
   a. "I have to buy my child new clothes every 2 to 3 months."
   b. "I have to buy my child much larger shirts than pants but then the sleeves are too long."
   c. "My child wears out their clothes before they outgrow them."
   d. "I can hand down my child's clothes to their younger brother."
3. The nurse is caring for a 14-year-old child with type 1 diabetes. The child takes Lantus insulin every morning at 7:30 a.m. Which assessment data will the nurse use to evaluate the therapeutic effectiveness of the medication?
   a. Presence of signs and symptoms of hypoglycemia or hyperglycemia during the morning physical assessment
   b. Blood glucose level at 1,630
   c. Appetite and food intake at lunch
   d. Blood glucose level before breakfast
4. When monitoring the blood glucose level of a 12-year-old child with type 2 diabetes, your reading is 50 mg/dL. Which is the most appropriate action?
   a. Encourage the child to get out of bed and increase activity.
   b. Take the child's vital signs.
   c. Ask the child about frequent urine output.
   d. Give the child 4 oz of orange juice.
5. The nurse is caring for a 13-year-old recently diagnosed with Hashimoto disease. Which assessment findings may the nurse find upon examination? Select all that apply.
   a. Fatigue
   b. Weight loss
   c. Constipation
   d. Goiter
   e. Diarrhea
   f. Thinning hair
   g. Nervousness
6. You are the school nurse, and a student recently diagnosed with type 1 diabetes is brought to your office after recess stating they did not eat breakfast and are not feeling well. Which clinical manifestations suggest the student is hypoglycemic? Select all that apply.
   a. Flushed skin
   b. Slurred speech
   c. Diaphoresis
   d. Nausea
   e. Vomiting

DOSAGE CALCULATION QUESTION

The school nurse is caring for a child with type 1 diabetes. The child weighs 56 lb. The sliding scale corrective dose order reads: Insulin aspart before meals: (blood glucose − 120 divided by 70) + (total carbohydrate expected intake divided by 13 carbohydrates per unit). This is the corrective dose + carbohydrate consumption correction. Her blood glucose before lunch is 139 with an expected intake of 47 carbohydrates at lunch and regular activity level the rest of the day. Calculate the insulin dose to be administered. Round to the nearest unit.

CRITICAL THINKING EXERCISES

1. A 12-year-old with type 1 diabetes has the flu. His parent calls the diabetes clinic to report that he stayed home from school and does not have an appetite, so he is not eating. The parent asks the nurse how much insulin the child should take. He is currently taking three injections daily with regular and NPH in the morning before breakfast, regular and NPH in the evening after dinner, and regular before bedtime. What questions should the nurse ask before answering the parent's question? Based on the answers to these questions, how would you instruct the parent?
2. The parent of Robin, a 5-year-old, reports that Robin has a body odor. She is developing breasts and some pubic hair and was teased when she had a sleepover with friends. The review of her growth charts reveals that Robin went from the 50th percentile to the 93rd percentile in the past 6 months. Based on this information, what are the major nursing analyses to begin establishing a plan of care for the child and family? What are the expected outcomes and major interventions associated with the patient problem of knowledge deficit?

3. A parent brings their baby to the clinic after receiving a phone message from the clinic saying there was a problem with the baby's thyroid test. The parent says the trip on the bus took a long time, but the infant slept the entire way, and the baby is sleeping much of the time and does not want to eat very much. The baby was discharged from the hospital 2 weeks ago. The birth was without difficulty and there were no problems during labor. Why is this visit urgent? What would the test show if the disorder was due to a pituitary gland problem and not the thyroid gland?

STUDY ACTIVITIES

1. During your clinical experiences, ask to be on an inpatient unit that provides care for children with alterations in endocrine function. Compare and contrast the health histories, assessments, laboratory tests, diagnostic procedures, and plans of care for these children with those for the care of children on other units. Participate in the teaching plan for these children and their families.
2. Attend an outpatient clinic that provides care to children with endocrine disorders. Identify the role of the registered nurse in providing coordination of care, health teaching, and referrals for these children and their families.
3. Shadow a diabetes nurse educator to observe the teaching methods and strategies they use to provide an education plan for a child with diabetes. Observe how the nurse educator includes the family in the plan. Are there any differences between the teaching plans for type 1 DM and type 2 DM?
4. Conduct a literature review for one of the common endocrine disorders to research current management practices. Are there evidence-based practice guidelines for nursing interventions?
5. Conduct an internet search to research the information that is available to children and their families related to DM.

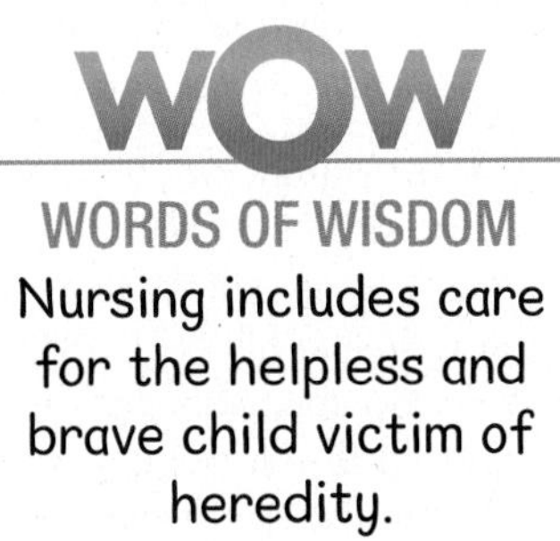
WOW
WORDS OF WISDOM
Nursing includes care for the helpless and brave child victim of heredity.

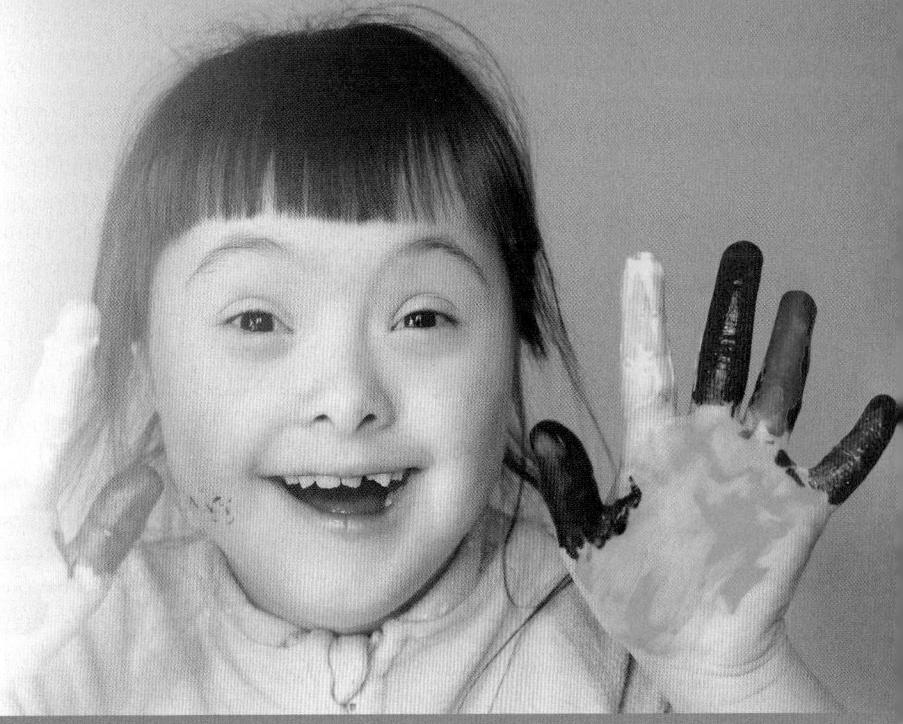

49

Nursing Care of the Child With an Alteration in Genetics

LEARNING OBJECTIVES

Upon completion of the chapter, you will be able to:

1. Discuss the nurse's role and responsibilities when caring for a child diagnosed with a genetic disorder and their family.
2. Identify nursing interventions related to common laboratory and diagnostic tests used in the diagnosis and management of genetic conditions.
3. Distinguish various genetic disorders occurring in childhood.
4. Devise an individualized nursing concept map or plan of care for the child with a genetic disorder.
5. Develop child/family teaching plans for the child with a genetic disorder.

Julie Woods, a 5-year-old, is brought to the clinic for her annual examination. Her parent states, "She's so much smaller than all of the other kindergartners."

KEY TERMS

gene testing
genetics
inborn errors of metabolism
neurocutaneous disorders
newborn screening
trisomy 21

INTRODUCTION

Genetics refers to the study of heredity—its transmission and characteristic variation. Nurses encounter potential or actual alterations in genetics in all types of patients and must detect problems and intervene early to prevent complications. A genetic disorder is a disease caused by an abnormality in a person's genetic material or genome. Some genetic disorders occur in multiple family members (via inheritance of abnormal genes). Other disorders may occur in only a single family member (via spontaneous mutation).

A genetic disorder is caused by completely or partially altered genetic material. In contrast, a familial disorder is more common in relatives of the affected person but may be caused by environmental influences, not genetic alterations.

Many chronic disorders of childhood have a genetic or inherited cause. Common disorders suspected to be caused or influenced by genetic factors include birth defects, chromosomal abnormalities, neurocutaneous disorders, intellectual disability, many types of short stature disorders, connective tissue disorders, and inborn errors of metabolism. Genetic disorders can present at any age, but the most obvious and severe disorders are present in childhood (Scott & Lee, 2020).

Our ability to diagnose genetic conditions is far superior to our ability to cure or treat them. However, accurate diagnosis does lead to improved treatment and outcomes. Nurses should have a basic knowledge of genetics, common genetic disorders in children, genetic testing, and genetic counseling so that they can provide support and information to families and can promote an improved quality of life.

Refer to Chapter 10 for information on advances in genetics, inheritance, and genetic counseling and evaluation.

TAKE NOTE!

Genetic science has the potential to revolutionize health care with regard to national screening programs, predisposition testing, detection of genetic disorders, and pharmacogenetics.

NURSE'S ROLE AND RESPONSIBILITIES

Pediatric nurses will encounter children with genetic disorders in every clinical specialty area. This includes clinics, hospitals, schools, and community-based centers. Talking with families who have recently been diagnosed with a genetic disorder or who have had a child born with congenital anomalies is very difficult. Many times, the nurse is the one who has first contact with these parents and will be the one to provide follow-up care. Genetic disorders are significant, life-changing, and possibly life-threatening situations. The information is highly technical, and the field is still evolving. Therefore, it is important to refer the family to a primary provider or nurse practitioner who specializes in genetics. The nurse should understand who will benefit from genetic counseling and should be able to discuss the role of the genetic counselor with families. Inform families at risk that genetic counseling is available before they attempt to have another baby.

The nurse is in an ideal position to help families review what has been discussed during the genetic counseling sessions and to answer any additional questions they might have. Nurses play an essential role in providing emotional support to the family throughout this challenging time. Nurses should also refer the family to appropriate agencies, support groups, and resources, such as a social worker, a chaplain, or an ethicist.

COMMON MEDICAL TREATMENTS

A variety of medications and other medical treatments are used to treat the symptoms of genetic disorders in children. Genetic disorders do not have specific treatments and there is no cure, so treatment focuses on the specific symptoms of each disorder. Genetic disorders often involve multiple organ systems, and children with these disorders have complex medical needs. Thus, a multidisciplinary approach and good communication are imperative. See "Clinical Judgment and the Nursing Process" section for a discussion on common genetic disorders and their management.

Clinical Judgment and the Nursing Process for the Child With a Genetic Disorder

Care of the child with a genetic disorder includes assessment, analysis, planning, interventions, and evaluation. There are a number of general concepts related to the nursing process that may be applied to the care of children with genetic disorders. From an overall understanding of the care involved for a child with an alteration in genetics, the nurse can then individualize the care based on specifics for the particular child.

Assessment

Assessment of the child with a genetic disorder includes health history, physical examination, and laboratory and diagnostic testing.

HEALTH HISTORY

The health history consists of past medical history, including the birthing parent's pregnancy history; family history; neonatal history; and history of present illness (when the symptoms started and how they have progressed), as well as treatments used at home. Explore the child's current and past medical history for risk factors such as:

- Family history of genetic disorders
- Any complications during the prenatal, perinatal, or postnatal periods
- Changes in developmental status or delays in developmental milestones

The pregnancy history can be extremely relevant when identifying a genetic disorder. The pregnancy history may be significant for maternal age older than 35 years or paternal age older than 40 years, repeated premature births, breech delivery, congenital hip dysplasia, abnormalities found on ultrasound, abnormalities in prenatal blood screening tests (e.g., triple/quadruple screen, alpha-fetoprotein [AFP]), amniotic fluid abnormalities (polyhydramnios, oligohydramnios), multiple births, exposure to medications and known teratogens, and decreased fetal movement.

A focused neonatal history can also help identify a genetic problem. The neonatal history may be significant for symmetric intrauterine growth restriction, large for gestational age without a reason, hearing impaired, persistent hyperbilirubinemia, poor adaptation to the extrauterine environment (demonstrated by temperature and heart rate instability and poor feeding), hypotonia or hypertonia, seizures, and abnormal newborn screening results.

The family history plays a critical role in identifying genetic disorders. Gather data for three generations. If there is a positive family history, the likelihood of a genetic disorder in the child is increased. It is helpful to create a family pedigree (refer to the "Genetic Counseling" section in chapter 10). The family history may be significant for major congenital anomalies, intellectual disability, genetic diseases, metabolic disorders, multiple miscarriages or stillbirths, developmental delays, significant learning disabilities, psychiatric problems, consanguinity, and chronic serious illness (e.g., diabetes, hypertension, kidney disease, hearing impairment, blindness, asthma, seizures, and unexplained death).

When eliciting the history of the present illness, inquire about:

- Developmental delay
- Seizures
- Hypotonia or hypertonia
- Feeding problems
- Lethargy
- Failure to thrive
- Septic appearance
- Vomiting

Children known to have a genetic disorder are often admitted to the hospital for other health-related issues or complications and management of the genetic disorder. The health history should include questions related to:

- Age when the disorder was diagnosed
- Developmental delay
- Complications of the disorder (e.g., thyroid problems, cardiac problems, respiratory problems, leukemia, seizures, cognitive impairment)
- Medications the child takes for complications associated with the disorder
- Dietary restrictions
- Adherence to management regimen

Once complications have been identified, further investigation into their severity, frequency, and management is essential to the care of this child while in the hospital.

PHYSICAL EXAMINATION

Physical examination of the child with a genetic disorder includes inspection and observation, palpation, and auscultation.

INSPECTION AND OBSERVATION

Inspect and observe for congenital anomalies, either major or minor. A major anomaly is an anomaly or malformation that creates significant medical or cosmetic problems and requires surgical or medical management (Bacino, 2023b) (Box 49.1). Minor anomalies are features that vary from those seen in the general population but do not cause an increase in morbidity in and of themselves (Bacino, 2023b) (Box 49.2).

> ***TAKE NOTE!***
>
> Low-set ears are a minor anomaly that is associated with numerous genetic dysmorphisms. If noted, assess thoroughly for other abnormalities.

As the number of minor anomalies present increases, the probability of the presence of a major anomaly increases. In fact, when three or more minor anomalies are present, the risk for a major

BOX 49.1 Examples of Major Congenital Anomalies

- Cleft lip
- Cleft palate
- Congenital heart disease, structural and conduction disorders
- Neural tube defects, such as myelomeningocele
- Chromosomal abnormalities
- Omphalocele; gastroschisis
- Renal agenesis/hypoplasia
- Absent or limb deficiencies
- Generalized dysmorphism
- Ambiguous genitalia

Data obtained from Bacino, C. A. (2023). Congenital anomalies: Epidemiology, types and patterns. *UpToDate.* Retrieved May 26, 2023, from https://www.uptodate.com/contents/birth-defects-epidemiology-types-and-patterns

BOX 49.2 Examples of Minor Congenital Anomalies

- Flat occiput
- Prominent occiput
- Triple hair whorl
- Flat-bridged nose
- Nostrils anteverted
- Ear lobe crease
- Ear lobe notched
- Cup-shaped ears
- Small ears
- Cleft uvula
- Webbed neck
- Short neck
- Extra nipples
- Sacral dimple
- Tapered fingers
- Overlapping digits
- Syndactyly
- Hemangioma
- Nevi

Data obtained from Bacino, C. A. (2023). Congenital anomalies: Epidemiology, types and patterns. *UpToDate*. Retrieved May 26, 2023, from https://www.uptodate.com/contents/birth-defects-epidemiology-types-and-patterns

anomaly or intellectual disability is approximately 19% to 26% (Bacino, 2023b). Assess for a recognized pattern of anomalies that may be associated with certain syndromes.

TAKE NOTE!

Cleft lip and cleft palate are associated with many syndromes. If noted, assess for other anomalies.

Inspect and observe for an abnormal or foul odor of the child's excretions. Certain metabolic disorders or inborn errors of metabolism are associated with specific odors (Table 49.1).

TABLE 49.1 • Inborn Errors of Metabolism and Associated Odor

Inborn Error of Metabolism	Associated Odor
Phenylketonuria	Mousy or musty
Maple syrup urine disease	Maple syrup, burnt sugar, or curry
Tyrosinemia	Cabbagelike, rancid butter
Trimethylaminuria	Rotting fish

Adapted from Shchelochkov, O. A., & Venditti, C. P. (2020). An approach to inborn errors of metabolism. In R. M. Kleigman, J. W. St. Geme III, N. J. Blum, S. S. Shah, R. C. Tasker, K. M. Wilson, & R. E. Behrman (Eds.), *Nelson textbook of pediatrics* (21st ed., pp. 4054–4087). Elsevier.

AUSCULTATION

Physical examination includes auscultation of the heart. Murmurs or dysrhythmias may have a genetic cause. In a child with a congenital heart problem (e.g., ventricular septal defect) and a strong family history of cardiac structural problems, a genetic cause needs to be considered.

PALPATION

Palpation can be used to detect hepatosplenomegaly (an enlarged spleen and liver). However, primary providers or nurse practitioners usually perform this assessment because it requires skill and experience. Hepatosplenomegaly may indicate a metabolic disorder.

LABORATORY AND DIAGNOSTIC TESTING

Common Laboratory and Diagnostic Tests 49.1 explains the laboratory and diagnostic tests used most commonly to detect genetic disorders. The tests can assist the primary provider or nurse practitioner in diagnosing the

COMMON LABORATORY AND DIAGNOSTIC TESTS 49.1

Test	Explanation	Indications	Nursing Implications
Amniocentesis	Ultrasound-guided (to determine placental location) insertion of a needle through the abdomen and into the uterine cavity of a pregnant person to obtain a sample of amniotic fluid. The fluid contains skin cells that have been shed by the fetus and can be isolated and grown in the laboratory to provide enough genetic material for testing.	Test for chromosomal abnormality, neural tube defects, or specific genetic conditions of the fetus. Performed if considered high risk for a genetic disorder or abnormal ultrasound. Most common prenatal test used to diagnose chromosomal and congenital anomalies	Usually not performed until after 15 weeks' gestation Complications include fetal injury, amniotic fluid leakage, infection, spontaneous miscarriage, premature labor, maternal hemorrhage, amniotic fluid embolism, abruptio placentae, and damage to the bladder or intestines. Results are usually not available for 7–10 days or longer, but this varies by laboratory. Monitor the fetus before and after the procedure.

COMMON LABORATORY AND DIAGNOSTIC TESTS 49.1

Test	Explanation	Indications	Nursing Implications
Chorionic villi sampling (CVS)	Involves the removal of a small amount of tissue directly from the chorionic villi (minute vascular projections of the fetal chorion that combine with maternal uterine tissue to form the placenta). In the laboratory, the chromosomes of the fetal cells are analyzed for number and type. Extra chromosomes, such as are present in DS, can be identified. Additional laboratory tests can be performed to look for specific disorders.	Test for chromosomal abnormality, fetal metabolic or blood disorders, or specific genetic conditions of the fetus. Performed if considered high risk for a genetic disorder or abnormal ultrasound. CVS cannot detect alpha-fetoprotein levels; therefore, does not detect neural tube defects	Performed at 7–11 weeks of gestation, so provides early detection of genetic abnormalities Complications include spontaneous miscarriage, infection, bleeding, amniotic fluid leakage, and fetal limb deformities. Results can be available within 24 hours, but this varies depending on the laboratory and location of the procedure (results are usually available sooner than with an amniocentesis). Monitor the fetus before and after the procedure.
Triple/quadruple screen	A maternal serum laboratory screening test that measures the level of three substances made by the developing baby and placenta: alpha-fetoprotein (AFP), human chorionic gonadotropin (hCG), and unconjugated estriol (uE3). Dimeric inhibin A has been added to make the "quadruple test." The addition of dimeric inhibin A increases the detection rate of DS and trisomy 18 in the quadruple screen.	A screening test for low-risk pregnant people to determine pregnancies at an increased risk for open neural tube defects, DS, and trisomy 18	Performed between 15 and 21 weeks of gestation Educate parents that a normal test does not guarantee a healthy baby. Conversely, an abnormal result does not guarantee the baby has a problem. Additional testing will be necessary to confirm or rule out a specific genetic condition.
Fetal nuchal translucency (FNT); may be combined with pregnancy-associated plasma protein (PAPP-A) and beta-hCG to increase the detection rate	Ultrasound prenatal screening to help identify higher risks of DS, trisomy 13, trisomy 18, and Turner syndrome. The ultrasound assesses the amount of fluid behind the neck of a fetus (known as the nuchal fold). Increased fluid increases the risk of a chromosomal abnormality. During this early ultrasound, other markers may be looked at, such as the presence of nasal bones (in DS, hypoplasia or absence of the nasal bones may be noted); short femur or humerus increases the risk of trisomy, echogenic foci (bright spots) in the heart can increase the risk of DS, and echogenic bowel (bowel looks bright and white) can be associated with chromosomal abnormalities. A serum blood test is performed to determine the level of two hormones, PAPP-A and beta-hCG. Using a combination of the results of the ultrasound and the blood test, the risk of having a baby with DS is predicted.	Any pregnant person presenting by 11–13 weeks' gestation can be screened. Particularly for patients with increased risk or desired screening for DS, trisomy 13, trisomy 18, or Turner syndrome	Must be performed between 11 and 13 weeks Genetic counseling before testing may be warranted. Positive tests require follow-up tests and genetic counseling.

(*continued*)

COMMON LABORATORY AND DIAGNOSTIC TESTS 49.1 (*continued*)

Test	Explanation	Indications	Nursing Implications
Ultrasound	Safe, noninvasive, accurate investigation of the fetus. A transducer is placed in contact with the pregnant person's abdomen, and high-frequency sound waves are directed at the fetus. The sound waves are reflected back through the tissues and recorded and displayed in real time on a screen.	Screen for structural malformations	Usually performed at 18–20 weeks of gestation; routinely done Early ultrasound can be performed at 11–14 weeks to evaluate for DS and other chromosomal abnormalities.
Cell-free fetal DNA testing	Fetal circulating cell-free DNA is taken from a sample of maternal blood. It is an advanced screening test that can detect fetal aneuploidies for chromosomes 21, 18, and 13. It can also detect X or Y chromosomes.	Indicated for higher risk pregnancies: • Pregnant people 35 or older at the time of delivery • Prior testing reveals increased risk of trisomy 21, 18, or 13. • History of previous pregnancy with a trisomy • Parental balanced Robertsonian translocation	Can be performed as early as 10 weeks Results usually available in 1 week Not recommended for low-risk pregnancies at this time due to lack of evaluation on this population Positive test results require more invasive testing and genetic counseling. High detection rates with low false positives
Percutaneous umbilical blood sampling	An ultrasound-guided needle is inserted through the abdominal and uterine wall to the umbilical cord, and a sample of blood is retrieved and sent to the laboratory for analysis. Used to detect disorders such as hemophilia, hemoglobinopathies, infections, drug levels, chromosomal abnormalities, and cord blood pH. The procedure is similar to amniocentesis but requires a higher level of expertise and experience. Less risk than fetoscopy	Detect chromosome abnormalities. Usually done when diagnostic information cannot be obtained through amniocentesis, CVS, or ultrasound or the results of these tests were inconclusive.	Performed at or after 18 weeks. Complications include miscarriage, blood loss, infection, and premature rupture of membranes. The risk to the pregnancy is greater than with amniocentesis and CVS. Beginning to replace fetoscopy
Fetoscopy	Endoscopic procedure that allows direct visualization of the fetus through the insertion of a tiny flexible instrument called a fetoscope. It is inserted through the abdominal wall and into the uterine cavity. Ultrasound is used to guide the placement of the scope. Direct visualization can evaluate the fetus for severe congenital anomalies such as neural tube defects. Fetal blood samples from the umbilical cord can be obtained and tested for congenital blood disorders such as hemophilia and sickle cell anemia. Fetal tissue samples (usually skin) can be collected and tested for genetic diseases.	Indicated for any patient at risk for delivering a baby with significant congenital anomalies; can be used to perform corrective surgery (e.g., shunt placement) on the fetus	Performed during or after the 18th week of pregnancy Complications include spontaneous miscarriage, premature delivery, premature rupture of membranes, amniotic fluid leak, intrauterine fetal death, and infection. Monitor the fetus before and after the procedure.

COMMON LABORATORY AND DIAGNOSTIC TESTS 49.1

Test	Explanation	Indications	Nursing Implications
Gene testing	Gene testing is currently available for many inherited diseases. It involves analysis of DNA, RNA, chromosomes, proteins, metabolites, and biochemical agents. Specimens for gene testing can be obtained from numerous sources; leukocytes from blood are the most common and easily obtained site; during pregnancy, amniocentesis, and CVS; and fetal tissue or products of conception after a miscarriage The most common use is DNA or chromosomes isolated from blood. Direct detection of abnormalities in genes and chromosomes is performed using DNA-based test or cytogenetic tests (which look at chromosomes) and other methods. Cytogenetic tests also include fluorescence in situ hybridization (FISH) to assist in detecting chromosomal abnormalities such as duplication, deletion, rearrangements, and translocations; newer testing, known as array comparative genomic hybridization (aCGH), or microarray, analyzes small duplications or deletions across all of the chromosomes.	To detect abnormalities that may indicate actual disease or predict future disease. Indicated in the evaluation of congenital anomalies, intellectual disability, growth retardation, and recurrent miscarriage to determine the reason for the loss of a fetus, and prenatal diagnosis of genetic disease	Provide support, information, and resources to the family. Refer to genetic counseling before and after the test.
Newborn screening (refer to Chapter 31 for further information)	Blood screening performed shortly after birth and is used to identify many life-threatening genetic illnesses that have no immediate visible effects but can lead to physical problems, intellectual disability, and even death. Every U.S. state routinely screens all newborns, but each state dictates which disorders to screen for, so components of the screening vary from state to state.	Identification of newborns so that treatment can begin early to prevent the impact of disorder, such as severe cognitive impairment or death	Refer to each state's protocol for fetal/newborn screening for endocrine disorders. Explain to the family the rationale and procedure. Collect blood sample accurately. Collect prior to blood transfusion if possible. Ideally performed after 24 hours of age; obtain specimen as close to the time of discharge from newborn or labor and delivery unit as possible and no later than 7 days of age Screening typically between 24 and 48 hours after birth The test is less accurate if done before 24 hours of age and should be repeated by 2 weeks of age if the newborn is younger than 24 hours old. Some states now require a repeat screen at 2 weeks of age.[a] Ensure appropriate follow-up with newborn screening results; results are available in 2–3 weeks.

[a]Kemper, A. R. (2021). Overview of newborn screening. *UpToDate*. Retrieved May 25, 2023, from https://www.uptodate.com/contents/newborn-screening

Adapted from Fischbach, F. T., Fischbach, M. A., & Stout, K. (2022). *A manual of laboratory and diagnostic tests* (11th ed.). Wolters Kluwer.

disorder or can be used as guidelines in determining treatment. Laboratory or non-nursing personnel obtain some of the tests, while the nurse might obtain others. In either instance, the nurse should be familiar with how the tests are obtained, what they are used for, and normal versus abnormal results. This knowledge will also be necessary when providing child and family education related to the testing. Due to the nature of the information, a referral to genetic counseling before testing may be appropriate. Advances in genetic technology have led to dramatic increases in the number of diagnostic and screening tests.

Remember Julie, the 5-year-old brought in for her annual examination? What additional health history and physical examination information should you obtain?

Nursing Analysis

Upon completion of an assessment, the nurse might identify several patient problems, including:

- Delayed development risk
- Knowledge deficiency (specify)
- Decisional conflict
- Fear
- Interrupted family processes
- Caregiver role strain

After completing an assessment of Julie, the nurse noted the following: short stature for age and a low posterior hairline. Based on these assessment findings, what would your top three patient problems be for Julie?

The above patient problems or concerns provide suggestions for developing a nursing plan of care or concept mapping. The nurse will then generate solutions by planning interventions (suggested below with rationales). The plan of care should be individualized, based on the child's and family's needs.

Refer to Chapter 33 for nursing interventions related to interrupted family processes and risk for caregiver role strain. Additional information will be included later in the chapter as it relates to specific disorders.

Nursing Analysis

Delayed development risk (risk factors: genetic disorder, treatment regimen)

Goal/Outcome

Child's development will be enhanced: Child will not suffer regression in abilities and will make continued progress toward attainment of developmental milestones within age parameters and limits of the disease. Child expresses interest in the environment and people around them and interacts with the environment appropriately for developmental level.

Promoting Development (interventions with *rationale*)

- Screen for developmental capabilities *to determine the child's current level of functioning.*
- Offer age-appropriate toys, play, and activities (including gross motor) *to encourage further development.*
- Perform exercises or interventions as prescribed by physical or occupational therapist: *these activities promote function and developmental skills.*
- Provide support to families: *due to disability and deficits, the child's progress toward developmental milestones may be slow.*
- Use therapeutic play and adaptive toys *to facilitate developmental functioning.*
- Provide a stimulating environment when possible *to maximize potential for growth and development.*
- Praise accomplishments and emphasize the child's abilities *to improve self-esteem and encourage feeling of confidence and competence.*

Nursing Analysis

Knowledge deficiency related to insufficient information (regarding complex, technical medical condition, prognosis, and medical needs) as evidenced by insufficient knowledge or inaccurate follow-through of instruction

Goal/Outcome

Child and family will verbalize accurate information and understanding about condition, prognosis, and medical needs: Child and family demonstrate knowledge of condition, prognosis, and medical needs, including possible causes, contributing factors, and treatment measures.

Providing Child and Family Teaching (interventions with *rationale*)

- Assess child's and family's willingness to learn: *child and family must be willing to learn for teaching to be effective.*
- Provide family with time to adjust to diagnosis: *will facilitate adjustment and ability to learn and participate in child's care.*
- Repeat information: *allows family and child time to learn and understand.*
- Teach in short sessions: *many short sessions are more helpful than one long session.*
- Gear teaching to the child and family's level of understanding (depends on the age of child, physical condition, and memory) *to ensure understanding.*
- Provide reinforcement and rewards: *facilitates the teaching/learning process.*
- Use multiple modes of learning involving many senses (written, verbal, demonstration, and videos) when possible: *child and family are more likely to retain information when it is presented in different ways using many senses.*
- Refer child and family to a genetics specialist: *genetic information is highly technical; the field is advancing*

at a rapid pace, and information needs to be the most current and accurate. A genetic specialist can provide this along with expertise, support, and resources.

Nursing Analysis

Decisional conflict related to conflict with moral obligation, moral principle, rule, and value supports mutually inconsistent actions (treatment options, conflicting values, and ethical, legal, and social issues surrounding genetic testing) as evidenced by verbalization of uncertainty about choices, or undesired consequences of alternative actions being considered, delay in decision making, physical signs of distress

Goal/Outcome

Family will state they are able to make an informed decision: The family will state the advantages and disadvantages of choices and share fears and concerns regarding choices.

Providing Decision-Making Support (interventions with *rationale*)

- Give family time and encourage them to express their feelings associated with decision making: *the decision-making process becomes more difficult if feelings are not expressed.*
- Encourage the family to list advantages and disadvantages of each alternative: *aids in problem solving and helps family recognize all alternatives.*
- Initiate health teaching and referral to genetic specialist when needed: *genetic testing information is often technical and complex. Families need accurate and up-to-date information to aid in decision making.*
- Maintain a nondirective manner: *this is a difficult decision that the family must make for themselves; the nurse should provide all the necessary information while maintaining an unobtrusive role.*
- Validate the family's feelings regarding the decisional conflict: *validation is a therapeutic communication technique that promotes the nurse–family relationship.*

Nursing Analysis

Fear related to learned response to threat (outcome of genetic testing) as evidenced by apprehensiveness and increased tension

Goal/Outcome

Family will state they can cope with the results of the genetic testing or demonstrate reduced fear: Family accurately discusses chances of offspring having genetic disease, demonstrates positive coping, and asks questions about genetic testing and meaning of results.

Managing Fear (interventions with *rationale*)

- Empathize with the family and avoid false reassurances; be truthful: *allows family to recognize that fear is a reasonable response. Giving false information or reassurance will actually increase fear.*
- Explore coping skills used previously by the family to cope with fear. Reinforce these skills and explore other outlets, such as relaxation, breathing, and physical activity: *encourages the use of coping mechanisms that help control fear.*
- Encourage verbalization of feelings and concerns about genetic testing. Allow time for questions: *provides a safe outlet to express feelings and encourages open communication between the family members.*
- Explain all procedures and review results as available: *knowledge deficit contributes to fear.*
- Refer to appropriate support groups and genetic counseling: *talking with families who have gone through similar situations can help decrease fear and provide methods of coping. Genetic counseling provides information along with support and additional resources.*

No matter what the genetic abnormality is, the news may be shattering to the family. It is difficult for nurses to even begin to understand what the family is going through. When providing support and education to families of children with serious genetic abnormalities, use these guiding principles:

- Build a trusting relationship.
- Stress the authenticity of the parents' feelings.
- Reject your own personal biases.
- Recognize that people cope in various ways; the family's behavior may not be what you would expect.
- Help the family to identify their own strengths and supports, building on those as able.
- Know that the family's emotions may exhaust and disorganize them.
- Assist the family members in maintaining open communication among themselves.
- Provide referrals to local parent groups or other families with a child with a similar disorder.
- Allow the family to verbalize their emotions and ask questions.
- Always ask the parents how *they* are doing (Lashley, 2005).

Based on your top three patient problems for Julie, describe appropriate nursing interventions.

COMMON CHROMOSOMAL ABNORMALITIES

Major chromosomal abnormalities are seen in about one in 140 live births (Giersch, 2022). Many children with chromosomal abnormalities have associated intellectual disabilities, learning disabilities, behavioral problems, and distinct features, including physical birth defects. The most common chromosomal abnormalities will be discussed below. Refer to Table 49.2 for less common chromosomal abnormalities identified in children.

TABLE 49.2 • Less Common Chromosomal Abnormalities

Chromosomal Abnormality	Features
Prader–Willi syndrome (abnormality on chromosome 15)	Affects one in 10,000–30,000 babies[a] Severe hypotonia, obesity, short stature, small hands and feet, hypogonadism, hyperphagia, and intellectual disability (varies from mild to severe)
Angelman syndrome (abnormality on chromosome 15)	Affects one in 12,000–20,000 babies[b] Microcephaly with flatness on the back of the head, fair skin and light hair, large mouth with tongue protrusion, seizures, jerky ataxic movements (resembling a puppet gait), uncontrolled bouts of laughter/smiling, happy demeanor, easily excitable personality, developmental delay and speech impairment, and severe intellectual disability
Cri-du-chat syndrome (abnormality on chromosome 5)	Affects one in 15,000–50,000 babies[c] Hypotonia; short stature; slow growth; low birth weight; failure to thrive; characteristic weak, catlike cry during infancy; microcephaly with protruding metopic suture; moonlike round face; bilateral epicanthal folds (folds of skin over the eyelids); high-arched palate; wide and flat nasal bridge; micrognathia (small receding chin); wide-set eyes (hypertelorism); low-set malformed ears; intellectual disability and developmental delay
Wolf–Hirschhorn syndrome (abnormality on chromosome 4)	Affects one in 50,000 babies[d] Hypotonia, intellectual disability, delayed growth and development, seizures, and characteristic facial features (broad, flat nose bridge; high forehead; widely spaced, protruding eyes; microcephaly)
Williams syndrome (abnormality on chromosome 4)	Affects one in 7,500–75,000 children[e] Affects multiple systems. Cardiovascular disease (supravalvular aortic stenosis most common, hypertension also seen); distinct facial features, such as the broad forehead, flat nasal bridge, short nose with a broad tip, full cheeks, and a wide mouth with full lips; small, wide-spaced teeth with occlusal abnormalities; hypercalcemia; early puberty for both males and females; structural abnormalities of the kidneys, delayed bladder training and urinary frequency, hypotonia, and joint laxity; learning disabilities and intellectual disability, attention deficit disorder, problems with anxiety and phobias such as fears of sounds and tactile issues; unique personality characteristics, such as outgoing and engaging personality; other medical problems involving eyes and vision and digestive tract
Beckwith–Wiedemann syndrome (abnormality on chromosome 11)	Affects one in 10,300–13,700 babies[f] Infants considerably larger than normal and grow at an unusual rate in childhood, growth slows in later childhood with adults not unusually tall, specific parts of the body may grow larger leading to asymmetric appearance; abdominal wall defects such as omphalocele, umbilical hernia; infants present with abnormally large tongue that may interfere with breathing, swallowing, and speaking; abnormally large abdominal organs; crease or pits in skin near ears, hypoglycemia, and kidney abnormalities; increased risk of developing cancerous and noncancerous tumors, such as Wilms tumor, neuroblastoma
22q11 deletion syndrome (DiGeorge syndrome) (abnormality of chromosome 22)	Affects one in 4,000–6,000 babies[g] Hypoplasia or agenesis of the thymus and parathyroid glands, hypocalcemia, hypoplasia of auricle and external auditory canal, cardiac anomalies, immune system abnormalities, cleft palate, short stature, distinctive facial appearance (elongated face, almond-shaped eyes, wide nose, small ears), and developmental delays, learning, speech, feeding, and behavioral problems

Helpful links related to the chromosomal abnormalities and features outlined here are provided on:

[a]Duis, J., & Scheimann, A. O. (2023). Prader–Willi syndrome: Clinical features and diagnosis. *UpToDate.* Retrieved May 29, 2023, from https://www.uptodate.com/contents/prader-willi-syndrome-clinical-features-and-diagnosis

[b]Madaan, M., & Mendez, M. D. (2023). Angelman syndrome. In *StatPearls* [Internet]. StatPearls Publishing. https://www.ncbi.nlm.nih.gov/books/NBK560870/

[c]Ajitkumar, A., Jamil, R. T., & Mathai, J. K. (2023). Cri du chat syndrome. In *StatPearls* [Internet]. StatPearls Publishing. https://www.ncbi.nlm.nih.gov/books/NBK482460/

[d]Genetic and Rare Diseases Information Center. (2023). *Wolf-Hirschhorn syndrome.* https://rarediseases.info.nih.gov/diseases/7896/wolf-hirschhorn-syndrome

[e]Wilson, M., & Carter, I. B. (2022). Williams syndrome. In *StatPearls* [Internet]. StatPearls Publishing. https://www.ncbi.nlm.nih.gov/books/NBK544278/

[f]Hon-Yin, B. C., Shuman, C., Choufani, S., & Weksberg, R. (2022). Beckwith-Wiedemann syndrome. *UpToDate.* Retrieved May 29, 2023, from https://www.uptodate.com/contents/beckwith-wiedemann-syndrome

[g]Lackey, A. E., & Muzio, M. R. (2023). DiGeorge syndrome. In *StatPearls* [Internet]. StatPearls Publishing. https://www.ncbi.nlm.nih.gov/books/NBK549798/

Trisomy 21 (DS)

Trisomy 21 (DS) is a genetic disorder caused by the presence of all or part of an extra 21st chromosome. It is the most common chromosomal abnormality associated with intellectual disability (Ostermaier, 2022b). Trisomy 21 is seen in all ages, races, and socioeconomic levels, but a higher incidence is found with a maternal age older than 35 years (Bacino & Lee, 2020). This is partly explained by the fact that 90% of cases with an extra chromosome 21 originate from the birthing parent (Giersch, 2022). The likelihood of having a baby with DS is around one in 1,000 in females younger than age 30, one in 350 at age 35, one in 85 at age 40, and one in 35 at age 45 (Giersch, 2022).

Trisomy 21 is associated with some degree of intellectual disability, characteristic facial features (e.g., slanted eyes and depressed nasal bridge), and other health problems (e.g., cardiac defects, visual and hearing impairment, intestinal malformations, and an increased susceptibility to infections). The severity of these problems varies.

The prognosis has been improving over the past few decades. Fundamental changes in the care of these children have resulted in longer life expectancy (around 55 to 56 years of age) and an improved quality of life (Ostermaier, 2022b).

Pathophysiology

Trisomy 21 is a disorder caused by nondisjunction or translocation before, at, or after conception.

Each egg and sperm cell normally contain 23 chromosomes. When they join, this results in 23 pairs or 46 chromosomes. Sometimes an extra chromosome originates in the development of either the egg or the sperm, resulting in an embryo with three chromosome 21s in *all* cells (Fig. 49.1). This results in the characteristic features and birth defects of DS. This type and timing of nondisjunction, resulting in the presence of three chromosome 21s in all cells, is responsible for about 96% of the cases of DS (Bull et al., 2022).

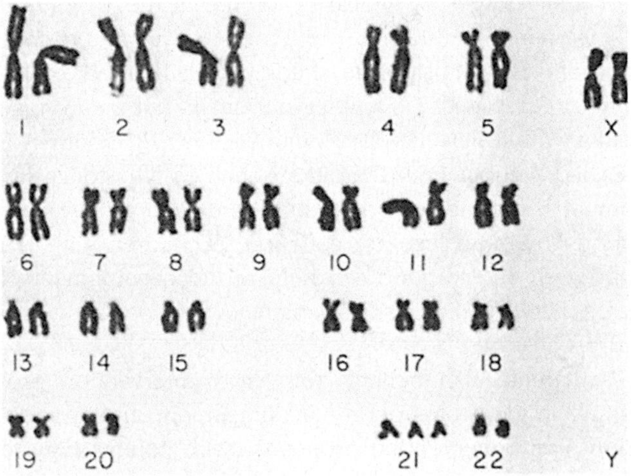

FIGURE 49.1 DS karyotype. Note the third chromosome located at chromosome 21.

In approximately 1% to 2% of cases of DS, the nondisjunction occurs *after* fertilization and a mixture of two cell types is seen (Bull et al., 2022). In these cases, some cells have 47 chromosomes (due to three chromosome 21s), while others have the normal 46 chromosomes (with the normal two chromosome 21s present). This is referred to as the mosaic form of DS. Children with mosaic DS may have a milder form of the disorder, but this is not a general finding.

About 3% to 4% of DS cases involve a translocation, in which part of the number 21 chromosome breaks off during cell division *before or at* conception and attaches (or translocates) to another chromosome (usually chromosome 14) (Bull et al., 2022). The cells will remain with 46 chromosomes, but this extra portion of the number 21 chromosome results in the clinical findings of DS. Cases of translocation are not associated with advanced maternal age, as is the situation with nondisjunction errors (Giersch, 2022).

Therapeutic Management

Management of DS will involve multiple disciplines, including a primary provider; specialty primary providers such as a cardiologist, ophthalmologist, and gastroenterologist; nurses; physical therapists; occupational therapists; speech therapists; dietitians; psychologists; counselors; teachers; and, of course, the parents. There is no standard treatment for all children, and there is no prevention or cure. Treatment is mainly symptomatic and supportive. The overall focus of therapeutic management will be to promote the child's optimal growth and development and function within the limits of the disease.

MANAGING COMPLICATIONS

Children with DS need the usual immunizations, well-child care, and screening recommended by the American Academy of Pediatrics (AAP). In addition, medical management will focus on complications associated with DS.

Congenital heart disease occurs in 40% to 50% of children with DS (Bull et al., 2022). Cardiac problems vary from minor defects that respond to medication therapy to major defects that require surgical intervention. Children with DS also have an increased incidence of gastrointestinal disorders (Bull et al., 2022). These disorders vary from those that can be managed by dietary manipulation, such as celiac disease and constipation, to intestinal malformations such as Hirschsprung disease and imperforate anus, which require surgical intervention.

Hearing and vision impairments also are common. More than 75% of children with DS have hearing loss (Bull et al., 2022). Otitis media is a common problem, affecting 50% to 70% of children with DS and is often the cause of hearing loss (Ostermaier, 2022a). Sixty to 80 percent of children with DS have vision problems (Bull et al., 2022). Therefore, regular evaluation of vision and hearing is essential.

Obstructive sleep apnea is present in 50% to 79% of children with DS (Bull et al., 2022). Often parents are unaware their child is having sleep disturbances, so baseline testing in young children may be warranted.

Children with DS have a higher incidence of thyroid disease, which can affect growth and cognitive function (Bull et al., 2022). Most of these children have hypothyroidism (an underactive thyroid), but sometimes hyperthyroidism (an overactive thyroid) occurs. Periodic thyroid testing may be warranted. Children with DS are also at a higher risk for obesity and delayed dental eruptions or hypodontia (Bull et al., 2022). Some studies have found an increased risk of type 1 diabetes in children with DS (Ostermaier, 2022a).

DOSAGE CALCULATION 49.1

Child's age: 4 years old

Child's weight: 30 lb

Medication order: Levothyroxine (Synthroid) 75 mcg by mouth once a day

Per the *Pediatric Dosage Handbook*, the recommended dose for a child 1 to 5 years of age is 5 to 6 mcg/kg/day.

Is the ordered dose safe?

Children with DS are at an increased risk for atlantoaxial instability (increased mobility of the cervical spine at the first and second vertebrae) (Bull et al., 2022). In most cases, these children are without symptoms, but symptoms may appear if spinal cord compression occurs (Ostermaier, 2022b). Screening for signs and symptoms of atlantoaxial instability is important, especially if the child is involved in sports.

CLINICAL REASONING ALERT!

If neck pain, unusual posturing of the head and neck (torticollis), change in gait, loss of upper body strength, abnormal reflexes, or change in bowel or bladder functioning is noted in the child with DS, immediate attention is required.

Children with DS are at an increased risk for certain hematologic problems, such as anemia, transient leukemia (mostly during the newborn period), leukemia (later onset), and polycythemia during infancy (Bull et al., 2022). Children with DS also have a higher susceptibility to infection and a higher mortality rate from infectious diseases (Ostermaier, 2022b). Precautions to prevent and monitor for infection are needed. Other potential complications include alopecia, communication disorders, and seizures.

Due to their increased risk for certain congenital anomalies and diseases, children with DS will need to be monitored closely, and regular medical care is essential. Children with DS have a higher incidence of autism and other behavioral problems (Bull et al., 2022). Screening for autism spectrum disorder (ASD) may be appropriate. Discuss and assess behavioral and social development and refer children with autism, attention deficit/hyperactivity disorder, or other behavioral or psychiatric issues appropriately. See Evidence-Based Practice 49.1.

EARLY INTERVENTION THERAPY

Early intervention refers to a variety of specialized programs and resources available to young children with developmental delays or other impairments. These programs may involve an array of health care professionals such as physical, occupational, and speech therapists; special educators; and social workers. The programs focus on providing stimulation and encouragement to children with DS. They help encourage and accelerate development and may help to prevent some developmental delays. The earlier the intervention can begin, the more beneficial it will be. The programs are individualized to meet the specific needs of each child.

Children with DS progress through the same developmental stages as typical children, but they do so on their own timetable (refer to Table 49.3 for the average age of skill acquisition in children with DS). For example, children with DS will learn to walk, but the average child with DS walks at 24 months (vs. 12 months for a child without DS). Conditions such as hypotonia, ligament laxity, decreased strength, enlarged tongue, and short arms and legs are common in children with DS, and early intervention can help in the development of gross and fine motor skills, language, and social and self-care skills.

Parents also benefit from early intervention programs in terms of support, encouragement, and information. Early intervention programs teach parents how to interact with their child while meeting the child's specific needs and encouraging development.

EVIDENCE-BASED PRACTICE 49.1

What are the experiences of families of children with a dual diagnosis of DS (DS) and autism spectrum disorder (ASD) (DS-ASD)?

The prevalence rate of ASD is much higher in children with DS compared to the general population. They are often diagnosed later and, in some cases, may go undiagnosed due to the difficulty identifying ASD-associated impairments versus DS-related impairments. Earlier identification of ASD is associated with greater efficacy of interventions. This study aimed to learn about caregiver's perspectives, observations, and experiences when caring for a child with DS-ASD.

STUDY

This was a qualitative study where caregivers, in a closed online community for families who care for a child with DS-ASD, completed a survey, with open-ended questions.

Findings

Data analysis found a 4.65-year gap from when a caregiver first noticed symptoms to the time of diagnosis. Caregivers expressed feelings that their concerns over their child's behaviors were initially dismissed, which contributed to a delay in ASD diagnosis. Caregivers expressed feelings of social isolation, frustration, and increased levels of stress, mainly related to providers' lack of knowledge regarding DS-ASD.

Nursing Implications

It can be challenging to identify children with DS and ASD due to the developmental impairments and behaviors that accompany DS. ASD can contribute to comorbidity of the child with DS, and research has shown children with ASD and DS have lower cognitive, language, and adaptive levels, and increased behavioral problems. Providers and educators need training in recognizing ASD-like symptoms. They need to assess for the presence of multiple signs and symptoms of ASD, listen to parental concerns, and consider referral for evaluation by a specialist. Identification and intervention are imperative. Nurses need to utilize appropriate, valid, and reliable screening tools. Continued research into appropriate screening tools, particularly for children younger than 3 years of age, is warranted. Providers need to provide parental support and resources to minimize feelings of social isolation, frustration, and stress. This study has limitations, including its small sample size. Further research is needed relating to how children with DS-ASD differ from those with DS alone.

Data from Spinazzi, N. A., Velasco, A. B., Wodecki, D. J., & Patel, L. (2023). Autism spectrum disorder in DS: Experiences from caregivers. *Journal of Autism and Developmental Disorders, 54*, 1171–1180. https://doi.org/10.1007/s10803-022-05758-x

Nursing Assessment

For a full description of the assessment phase of the nursing process, refer to the "Clinical Judgment and the Nursing Process" section earlier in the chapter. Assessment findings pertinent to DS are discussed in the following sections.

TABLE 49.3 • Average Age Range of Skill Acquisition in Children With DS

Developmental Milestone	Age Range of Acquisition, Children With DS	Age Range of Acquisition, Typical Children
Smile	1–5 months	1–3 months
Sit alone	6–36 months	5–9 months
Crawl	8–22 months	6–12 months
Stand	1–3.25 years	8–17 months
Walk	1–4 years	8–17 months
First word	1–4 years	1–2 years
Speak in sentences	2–7.5 years	15–32 months
Feed self with fingers	10–24 months	7–15 months
Use spoon	13–39 months	12–20 months
Bowel training	2–7 years	16–42 months
Put on clothes	3.5–8.5 years	3.25–5 years

Data from National DS Society. (2023). *Early intervention.* https://www.ndss.org/resources/early-intervention/

Health History

DS is often diagnosed prenatally using perinatal screening and diagnostic tests. If not diagnosed prenatally, most cases are diagnosed in the first few days of life based on the physical characteristics associated with DS. Identify high-risk deliveries. Explore the pregnancy history and past medical history for risk factors such as:

- Lack of prenatal care or screening
- Abnormal prenatal screening or diagnostic tests for DS (e.g., fetal nuchal translucency, triple/quadruple screen, ultrasound, amniocentesis)
- Maternal age older than 35 years

The older infant or child known to have DS is often admitted to the hospital for corrective surgeries or other complications of the disease, such as infections. Elicit a description of the present illness and chief complaint. In an infant or child returning for a clinic visit or hospitalization, the health history should include questions related to:

- Cardiac defects or disease (treatment regimen, surgical repair)
- Hearing or vision impairment (last hearing and vision evaluation, any corrective measures)
- Developmental delays (speech, gross and fine motor skills)
- Sucking or feeding problems
- Cognitive abilities (degree of intellectual disability)
- Gastrointestinal disorders such as vomiting or absence of stools (special dietary management, surgical interventions)

- Thyroid disease
- Hematologic problems, such as anemia, leukemia
- Atlantoaxial instability
- Seizures
- Infections such as recurrent or chronic respiratory infections, otitis media
- Growth (height and weight changes, feeding problems, unexplained weight gain)
- Signs and symptoms of sleep apnea, such as snoring, restlessness during sleep, daytime sleepiness
- Any other changes in physical state or medication regimen

Physical Examination

The initial assessment after birth may reveal certain physical features characteristic of DS (Box 49.3 and Fig. 49.2).

Observe the child's general appearance. Note the lack of muscle tone and loose joints; this is usually more pronounced in infancy, and the infant has a floppy appearance. Observe growth and development. Plot growth on appropriate growth charts. Because children with DS grow at a slower rate, special growth charts have been developed. Refer to the Centers for Disease Control and Prevention (CDC) website for growth charts for children with DS.

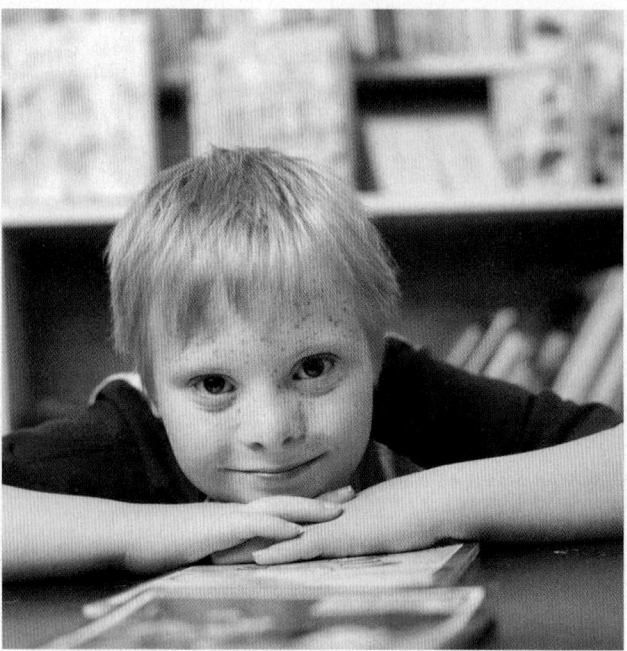

FIGURE 49.2 Child with DS.

BOX 49.3 Common Clinical Manifestations of DS

- Hypotonia
- Short stature
- Flattened occiput
- Small (brachycephalic) head
- Flat facial profile
- Depressed nasal bridge and small nose
- Oblique palpebral fissures (an upward slant to the eyes)
- Brushfield spots (white spots on the iris of the eye)
- Low-set, small ears
- Abnormally shaped ears
- Small mouth
- Protrusion of tongue; tongue is large compared to mouth size.
- Arched, narrow palate
- Hands with broad, short fingers
- A single deep transverse crease on the palm of the hand (simian crease)
- Congenital heart defect
- Short neck, with excessive skin at the nape
- Hyperflexibility and looseness of joints (excessive ability to extend the joints)
- Dysplastic middle phalanx of the fifth finger (one flexion furrow instead of two)
- Epicanthal folds (small skin folds on the inner corner of the eyes)
- Excessive space between the large and second toes

Source: Ostermaier, K. K. (2022). DS: Clinical features and diagnosis. *UpToDate.* Retrieved May 23, 2023, from https://www.uptodate.com/contents/down-syndrome-clinical-features-and-diagnosis; Bull, M. J., Trotter, T., Santoro, S. L., Christensen, C., Grout, R. W., & The Council on Genetics. (2022). Health supervision for children and adolescents with DS. *Pediatrics, 149*(5), e2022057010. https://doi.org/10.1542/peds.2022-057010

When assessing the achievement of developmental milestones in children with DS, it may be more useful to look at the sequence of milestones rather than the age at which they were achieved. Each milestone represents a skill that is needed for the next stage of development.

Perform a subjective assessment of hearing, and refer the child for further evaluation if indicated. Assess vision, especially for cataracts. Assess respiratory status and cardiac status. Auscultate for murmurs and pulmonary changes, which can indicate congenital heart disease. Chronic or recurrent respiratory infections, such as pneumonia and otitis media, may be found.

Laboratory and Diagnostic Tests

A variety of screening tests are available using maternal serum and ultrasound. In recent years, noninvasive cell-free fetal DNA testing has become available and provides a high sensitivity and specificity (Bull et al., 2022). DS risk screening can be calculated incorporating maternal age prenatally between 11 and 14 weeks using ultrasound and blood tests (nuchal translucency and pregnancy-associated plasma protein A [PAPP-A] and human chorionic gonadotropin [hCG]), and around 16 and 18 weeks using triple/quadruple blood tests to detect AFP, hCG, estriol, and/or inhibin A levels (Bull et al., 2022). Ultrasound and amniocentesis or chorionic villi sampling (CVS) to detect chromosomal abnormalities can also occur prenatally. DS can be confirmed after birth using chromosome analysis (see Common Laboratory and Diagnostic Tests 49.1).

Common laboratory and diagnostic studies ordered for the diagnosis and assessment of complications associated with DS include:

- Echocardiogram: to detect cardiac defects
- Vision and hearing screening: to detect vision and hearing impairments
- Thyroid hormone level: to detect thyroid disease
- Cervical radiographs: to assess for atlantoaxial instability
- Ultrasound: to assess for gastrointestinal malformations

These tests will be important in evaluating the severity of the child's physical disabilities.

Nursing Management

Due to the high incidence of DS and the complex medical needs of these children, most pediatric nurses are likely to care for these children in their practice. Nursing management focuses on providing supportive measures such as promoting growth and development, preventing complications, promoting nutrition, and providing support and education to the child and family. In addition to the patient problems and related interventions discussed in the "Clinical Judgment and the Nursing Process" section earlier in the chapter, additional considerations are reviewed in the following sections.

• • • ATRAUMATIC CARE • • •

When planning atraumatic care interventions when caring for a child with DS, be sure to individualize interventions based on the child's developmental level.

Promoting Growth and Development

Children with DS tend to grow more slowly, learn more slowly, have shorter attention spans, and have trouble with reasoning and judgment. Their personality tends to be one of genuine warmth and cheerfulness along with patience, gentleness, and a natural spontaneity. Growth and developmental milestones for children with DS have been developed as a guide for primary providers and nurse practitioners. Table 49.3 gives examples of the average age range at which these children reach selected milestones versus typical children.

THINKING ABOUT DEVELOPMENT

As a nurse in a primary provider's office, how will your education on safety differ when caring for an infant with DS compared to a toddler or adolescent?

Nurses play a key role in connecting families with appropriate resources that can facilitate the child's growth and development. The sooner early intervention programs can begin, the better for the child (see the "Early Intervention Therapy" section). Speech and language therapy, occupational therapy, and physical therapy will be important in promoting the child's growth and development. Special education should fit the child's individual needs, and the child should be integrated into mainstream education whenever possible.

PREVENTING COMPLICATIONS

Children with DS are at risk for certain health problems (see section "Managing Complications"). Even though most nurses will encounter a child with DS in their practice, only a few nurses will become experts in their care. The needs of these children are complex, and the AAP has developed guidelines that can help the nurse care for these children and their families. Refer to the AAP website for health supervision guidelines for children with DS. Nurses play a key role in educating parents and caregivers about how to prevent the complications of DS (see Teaching Guidelines 49.1).

TEACHING GUIDELINES 49.1 Health Guidelines for Children With DS

- Have your child evaluated by a pediatric cardiologist, including an echocardiogram.
- Take your child for routine vision and hearing tests. By 6 months, have your child seen by a pediatric ophthalmologist.
- Make sure your child gets regular medical care, including recommended immunizations and a thyroid test at birth, then every 5 to 7 months until 1 year, then yearly.
- Have your child follow a regular diet and exercise routine.
- Make sure all family members perform proper hand hygiene to prevent infection.
- Monitor for signs and symptoms of respiratory infections, such as pneumonia and otitis media.
- Discuss with your primary provider the use of pneumococcal, respiratory syncytial virus, and influenza vaccines.
- Begin early interventions, therapy, and education as soon as possible.
- Make sure your child brushes their teeth regularly. They should visit the dentist every 6 months.
- Report any changes in gait or use of arms and hands, weakness, changes in bowel or bladder function, complaints of neck pain or stiffness, head tilt, torticollis, or generalized changes in function. Ensure cervical spine positioning precautions (to avoid overextending or flexing of the neck) are utilized during procedures, such as those involving anesthetic, surgery, or radiographs.

Adapted from Bull, M. J., Trotter, T., Santoro, S. L., Christensen, C., Grout, R. W., & The Council on Genetics. (2022). Health supervision for children and adolescents with DS. *Pediatrics*, *149*(5), e2022057010. https://doi.org/10.1542/peds.2022-057010

PROMOTING NUTRITION

Children with DS may have difficulty sucking and feeding due to lack of muscle tone. They tend to have small mouths; a smooth, flat, large tongue; and due to the underdeveloped nasal bone, chronically stuffy noses. This may lead to poor nutritional intake and problems with growth. These problems usually improve as the child gains tongue control. Use of a bulb syringe, humidification, and changing the infant's position can lessen the problem. Breastfeeding a baby with DS is usually possible, and the antibodies in breast milk can help the infant fight infections. The caregiver's hand can be used to provide additional support for the chin and throat. Speech or occupational therapists can work on strengthening muscles and assisting in feeding accommodations. Other feeding problems and failure to thrive can be related to cardiac defects and usually improve after medical management is initiated or corrective surgery is performed.

Children with DS do not need a special diet unless an underlying gastrointestinal disease is present, such as celiac disease. A balanced, high-fiber diet and regular exercise are important. Research has suggested that children with DS have lower basal metabolic rates, which can lead to problems with obesity, so it is important in the early years to develop appropriate eating habits and a regular exercise routine. High fiber intake is important for children with DS because their lack of muscle tone may decrease gastric motility, leading to constipation.

Providing Support and Education for the Child and Family

DS is a lifelong disorder that can result in health problems and cognitive disability. The diagnosis is usually made prenatally or shortly after birth. Parents and caregivers will need support and education during this difficult time. The range of mental impairment varies from mild to moderate; severe deficits occur occasionally. Some families may see having a child with DS as a lifelong tragedy; others may view it as a positive growing experience. Evaluate how the family defines and manages this experience. Base the plan of care on each family's values, beliefs, strengths, and resources.

Family members may have trouble meeting the demands of caring for a child with DS. These children have complex medical needs, which place strain on the family and its finances. From the time of diagnosis, the family should be involved in the child's care. Include parents in planning interventions and care for the child. In most cases, they are the primary caregivers and will provide daily care as well as assisting the child in the development of functioning and skills. They can provide essential information to the health care team and will be advocates for their child throughout their life.

As the child grows, the needs of the family and child will change. Recognize and respect these needs and provide ongoing education and support for the child and family. Children with DS will need meaningful education programs. Many children with DS begin formal education in infancy and continue through high school.

The outlook is brighter than it once was for children with DS. Many go on in adulthood to obtain jobs, to receive secondary education, and to live on their own or in semi-independent housing. Be familiar with local and national resources for families of children with DS so that you can help these children fulfill their potential.

CONSIDER THIS!

"The day after my baby was born I was told they suspected he had DS. Once the diagnosis was confirmed I felt devastated. I grieved the loss of all the dreams I had for him and felt alone and scared. I wonder 'why us.'"

Thoughts: How will you respond to this parent?

Trisomy 18 and Trisomy 13

Trisomy 18 (also known as Edwards syndrome) and trisomy 13 (also known as Patau syndrome) are two other common trisomies. These trisomies are much more severe and debilitating than trisomy 21. The incidence of trisomy 18 (the presence of three number 18 chromosomes) is one in 6,000 births; the incidence of trisomy 13 (the presence of three number 13 chromosomes) is one in 10,000 births (Bacino & Lee, 2020). Like DS, trisomy 13 and trisomy 18 usually result from nondisjunction during cell division. Trisomy 18 and trisomy 13 can be present in all cells or may occur in mosaic forms. Both are associated with a characteristic set of anomalies and severe intellectual disability (Bacino & Lee, 2020).

The prognosis for trisomy 18 and trisomy 13 is usually poor; these children usually do not survive beyond the first year of life. There is no cure for trisomy 18 or trisomy 13. Therapeutic management will focus on managing the various congenital anomalies and health issues associated with the disorders.

Nursing Assessment

Nursing assessment will include a general observation of characteristic anomalies (Table 49.4; Figs. 49.3 and 49.4).

Prenatal screening and diagnostic tests for trisomy 18 and trisomy 13 exist. If not diagnosed during the prenatal period, most cases are diagnosed in the first few days of life based on the physical characteristics associated with the disorders.

TABLE 49.4 • Clinical Manifestations of Trisomy 18 and Trisomy 13

Chromosomal Abnormality	Clinical Manifestations
Trisomy 18	Prominent occiput, low-set ears, short eyelid fissures, severe intellectual disability, severe hypotonia, webbing, clenched fist with index finger over third digit and fifth digit overlapping the fourth, hypoplasia of fingernails, narrow hips with limited abduction, short sternum, congenital cardiac defects
Trisomy 13	Microcephalic head, wide sagittal suture and fontanels, malformed ears, small eyes, extra digits, severe hypotonia, severe intellectual disability, congenital heart defects, cleft lip, cleft palate

Nursing Management

Nursing management will be mainly supportive. This will be a difficult time for the family, so providing support and resources for the family will be an important nursing function. SOFT is a support organization for families who have had a child with a chromosome abnormality.

Turner Syndrome

Turner syndrome is a common abnormality of the sex chromosome. The phenotype is female. It occurs in about one in 2,500 live female births (Bacino, 2023c). The abnormality is due to a loss of all or part of one of the sex chromosomes. About half of the affected people have only one X chromosome; the other half have a variety of abnormalities in one of their sex chromosomes and may present with the mosaic form.

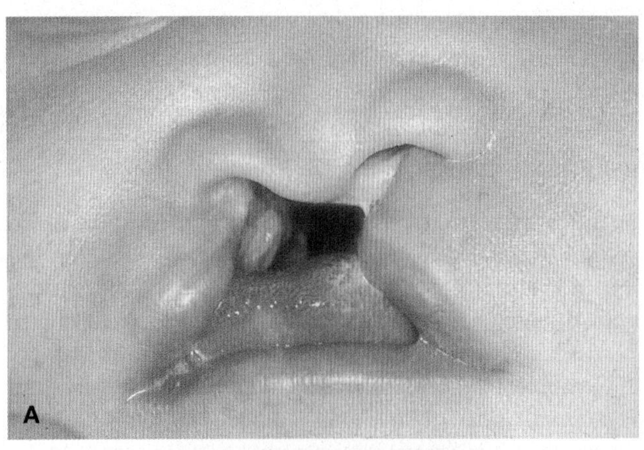

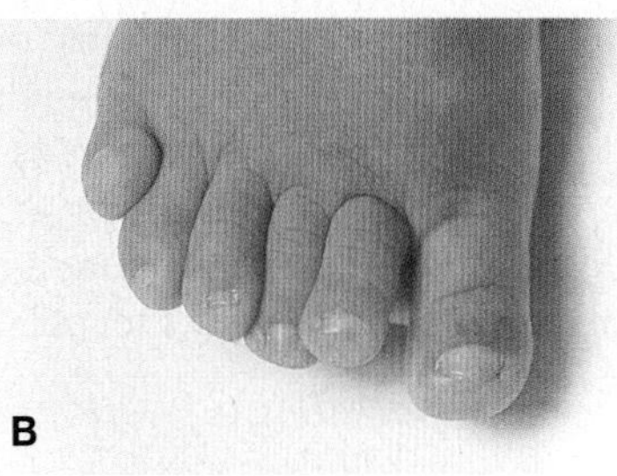

FIGURE 49.4 Trisomy 13.

There is no cure for Turner syndrome. Therapeutic management will focus on managing the health issues associated with the syndrome. Children with Turner syndrome are more prone to cardiovascular problems, kidney and thyroid problems, skeletal disorders such as scoliosis and osteoporosis, hearing and eye disturbances, learning disabilities, and obesity (Bacino & Lee, 2020; Backelijauw, 2022). Infertility is usually present, but a few spontaneous pregnancies have been reported (Backelijauw, 2022). Growth hormone administration is a standard of care and usually begins when the child's height falls below

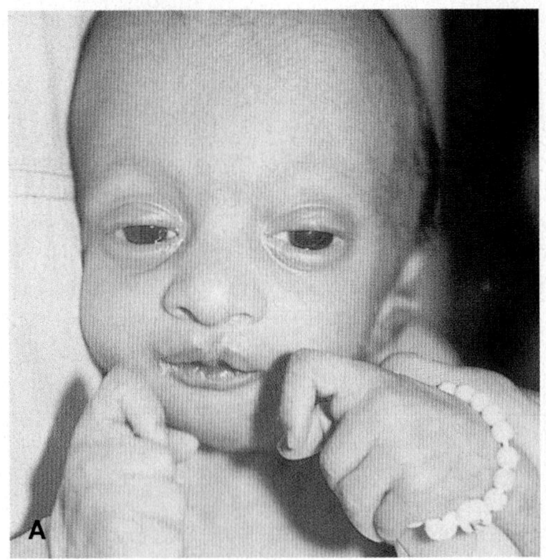

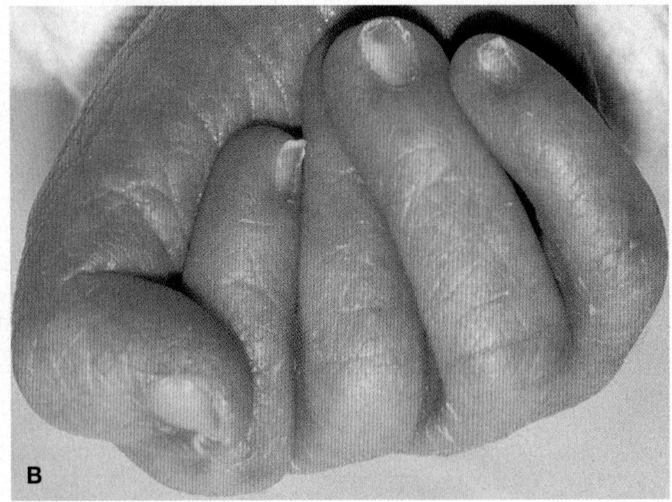

FIGURE 49.3 Trisomy 18. **A.** Note prominent occiput, low set ears and short eyelid fissures. **B.** Note clenched fist with index finger over third digit and fifth digit overlapping the fourth, hypoplasia of the fingernails.

the fifth percentile for healthy females. Hormone replacement therapy may also be given to initiate puberty and complete growth.

Nursing Assessment

On assessment, note patterns of growth; short stature and slow growth will be a characteristic finding and often the first indication. Other physical characteristics include a webbed neck, low posterior hairline, wide-spaced nipples, edema of the hands and feet, amenorrhea, no development of secondary sex characteristics, sterility, and perceptual and social skill difficulties (Fig. 49.5).

Turner syndrome can be suspected prenatally by ultrasound findings such as fetal edema or redundant nuchal skin (Backelijauw, 2022). It can be diagnosed by chromosomal analysis, either prenatally or after birth. Most children are diagnosed at birth or in early childhood when slow growth or growth failure is noted. Some cases will not be diagnosed until the pubertal growth spurt does not occur.

Nursing Management

Nursing management is mainly supportive. Provide education and support to the family; they need to understand that short stature and infertility are likely. Explain that intellectual disability is unlikely, but some learning disabilities may be present. Emphasize that with medical supervision and support, children with Turner syndrome may lead healthy, satisfying lives. Counseling about infertility is important. Parents may be upset that their child will not be able to reproduce, so explain that many alternatives for reproduction, such as in vitro fertilization and adoption, are available.

Providing resources for the family is an important nursing function. The Turner Syndrome Society of the United States provides assistance, support, and education to people with Turner syndrome and their families.

Klinefelter Syndrome

Klinefelter syndrome is the most common sex chromosomal abnormality (Bacino & Lee, 2020). The karyotype and phenotype are male, but one or more extra X chromosomes are present. The abnormality is usually caused by nondisjunction during meiosis, but mosaic forms do present. The incidence of Klinefelter syndrome is one in 500 to 1,000 males (Bacino, 2023c). Males present with some femalelike physical features that are caused by testosterone deficiency. The risk of recurrence in future pregnancies is not increased.

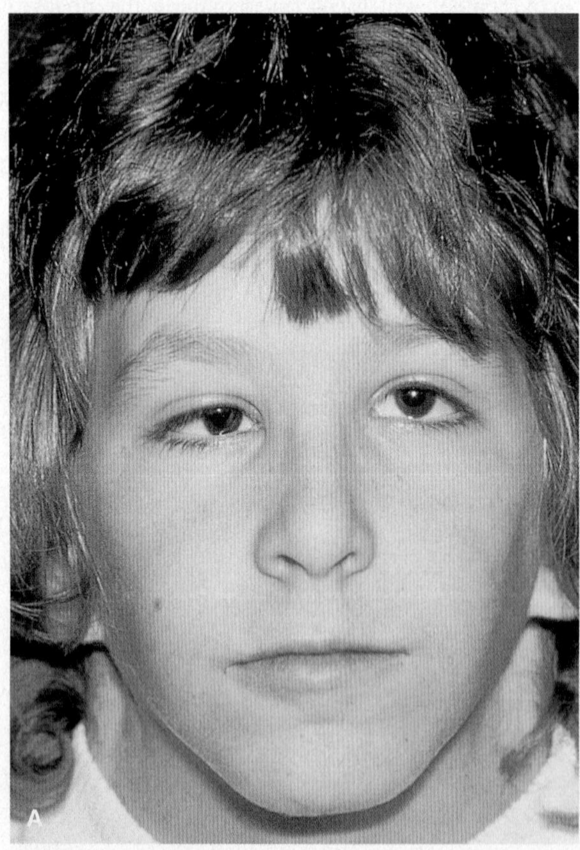

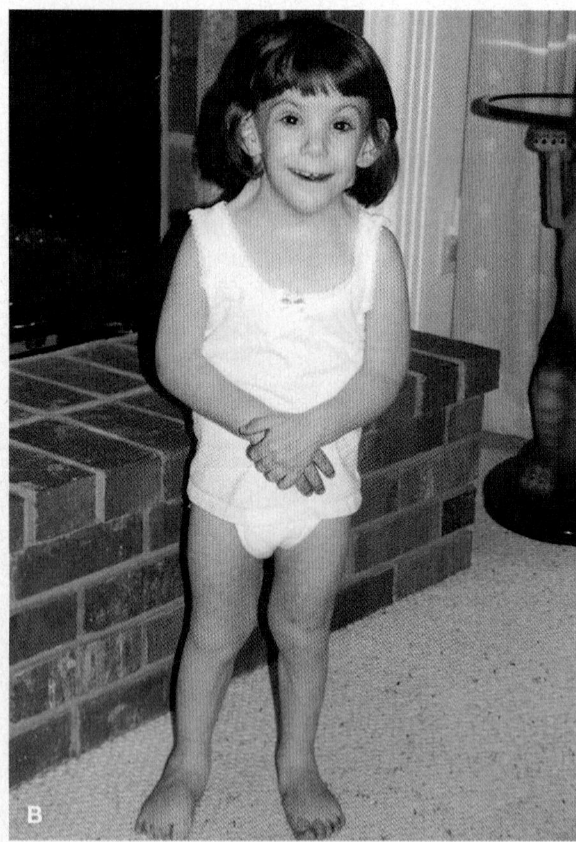

FIGURE 49.5 Note the webbed neck of the child with Turner syndrome. **A.** Note the webbed neck, ocular and ear lobe abnormalities. **B.** Note short stature, webbed neck, genu valgum.

There is no cure for Klinefelter syndrome. Therapeutic management will focus on interventions to enhance masculine characteristics, such as testosterone replacement. Early recognition and hormonal treatment are important to improve quality of life and prevent serious consequences. Cosmetic surgery may be performed to minimize female characteristics such as gynecomastia (increased breast size).

Nursing Assessment

Due to nonspecific findings during childhood, the diagnosis is not usually made until adolescence or adulthood. Prenatal diagnosis is rare unless amniocentesis was performed for genetic testing. Many males with Klinefelter syndrome reach adulthood without being diagnosed (Bacino & Lee, 2020). The diagnosis is confirmed by chromosomal analysis.

On assessment, a lack of development of secondary sex characteristics may be found. The person may have decreased facial hair, gynecomastia, decreased pubic hair, and hypogonadism or underdeveloped testes, which leads to infertility. The person may be taller than average by 5 years of age, with long legs and a short torso (Fig. 49.6). Intellectual disability is not present, but cognitive impairments of varying degrees, such as motor delay, speech or language difficulties, attention deficits, and learning disabilities, may be found.

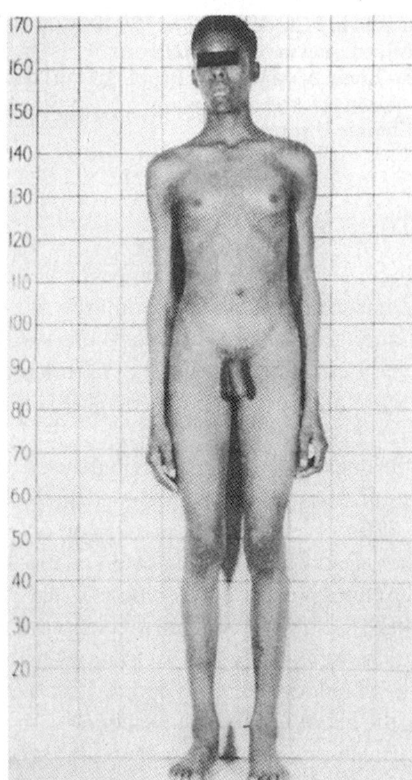

FIGURE 49.6 Klinefelter syndrome.

Nursing Management

Nursing management will be mainly supportive. Provide education and support to the family. The American Association for Klinefelter Syndrome and the Association for X and Y chromosome variations are helpful resources available online.

Counseling about infertility is important. Educate children and families that marriage and sexual relations are possible. Parents may be upset that their child will not be able to reproduce, so explain that many alternatives for reproduction are available and technology is advancing in the field of infertility.

Fragile X Syndrome

Fragile X syndrome is the most common inherited cause of intellectual disability (Van Esch, 2022). It is the outcome of a mutation of a gene (FMR1 [fragile X mental retardation]) on the X chromosome. This mutation essentially "turns off" the gene, triggering fragile X syndrome. Males and females are both affected, but it is more commonly seen in males, and affected females usually have milder symptoms (Van Esch, 2022). The incidence is approximately one in 8,000 females and one in 4,000 males (Stone et al., 2023). The inheritance of fragile X is complex and is less straightforward than single-gene or mendelian inheritance. Some carrier females are affected, and not all males with the gene abnormality show symptoms. Males and females are both fertile and can transmit the disorder to their offspring, so genetic counseling is appropriate. The prognosis for people with fragile X is good, and they tend to live a normal lifespan.

There is no cure for fragile X syndrome. Therapeutic management will be multidisciplinary and aimed at interventions to improve cognitive, emotional, and behavioral impairments.

Nursing Assessment

During childhood, clinical manifestations are subtle, with minor dysmorphic features and developmental delay. Problems with sensation, emotion, and behavior often are the first signs. A delay in attaining developmental milestones will most likely be the first clue found on assessment. Intellectual impairment can range from subtle learning disabilities to severe intellectual disability and autisticlike behaviors. In adolescence, males tend to present with characteristic features such as an elongated face; prominent jaw; large, protruding ears; large size; macroorchidism (large testes); and a range of behavioral abnormalities and cognitive deficits (Fig. 49.7). There is a characteristic pattern to the cognitive deficits, with problems in abstract reasoning, sequential processing, and mathematics. Typical behavior problems include attention deficits, hand flapping and biting, hyperactivity,

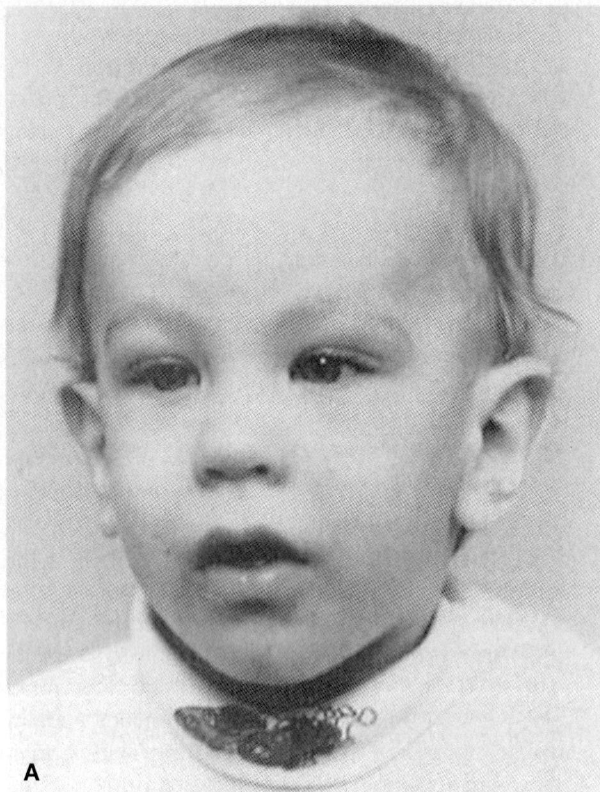

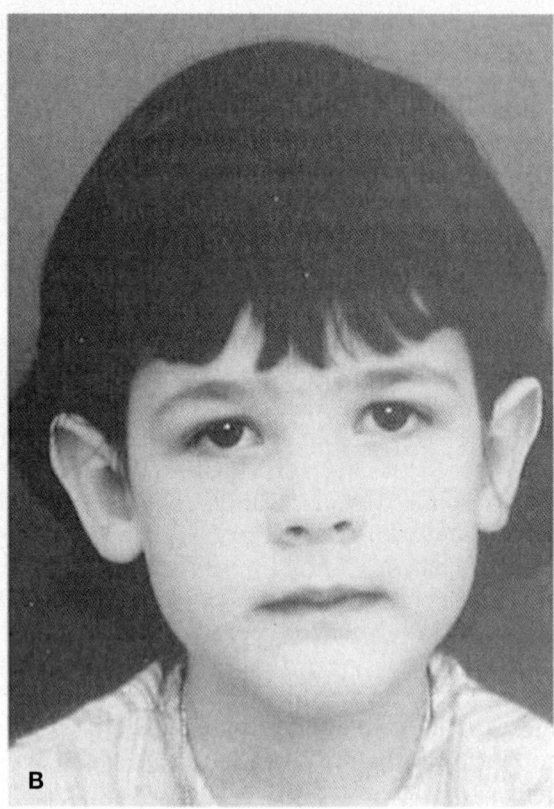

FIGURE 49.7 Fragile X syndrome. **A** and **B.** Note the subtle minor dysmorphic features such as large and protruding ears.

shyness, social isolation, low self-esteem, and gaze aversion. In females, the clinical manifestations are similar but are more varied and often present in a milder form.

Diagnosis is confirmed by molecular genetic testing. Fragile X can be diagnosed prenatally if inheritance is suspected.

Nursing Management

Nursing management will be mainly supportive. Early diagnosis and intervention with developmental therapies and an individualized education plan are ideal. Care of these children will be the same as care of other children with intellectual disability (see Chapter 50 for further information on intellectual disability).

Provide education and support to the family. The National Fragile X Foundation provides education and emotional support and works to increase awareness and advance research for fragile X.

NEUROCUTANEOUS DISORDERS

Neurocutaneous disorders, also referred to as hamartoses, are a group of disorders characterized by abnormalities of both the skin and the central nervous system. Many neurologic conditions are associated with cutaneous manifestations since the skin and the nervous system share a common embryologic origin. They are complex conditions, and most also affect other organ systems such as eyes, bones, heart, and kidneys. Most are hereditary and follow an autosomal dominant inheritance pattern or sporadic occurrence. Neurofibromatosis is a common neurocutaneous syndrome and will be discussed in detail below. Table 49.5 provides information on other neurocutaneous syndromes.

Neurofibromatosis

Neurofibromatoses are neurocutaneous genetic disorders of the nervous system that primarily affect the development and growth of neural cell tissues. There are distinct types: neurofibromatosis 1, *NF2*-related schwannomatosis (NF2, formerly neurofibromatosis type 2), and schwannomatosis (Korf et al., 2023).

Neurofibromatosis 1 (von Recklinghausen disease) is the more common type and is discussed here (Korf et al., 2023). This disorder causes tumors to grow on nerves and produce other abnormalities such as skin changes and bone deformities. Although many affected people inherit the disorder, nearly half of the cases are due to a new mutation (Korf et al., 2023). The inheritance pattern is autosomal dominant; therefore, the offspring of affected people have a 50% chance of inheriting the altered gene and presenting with symptoms. Neurofibromatoses are due to a mutation of the neurofibromin gene on chromosome 17. The estimated prevalence is one in 2,600 to 3,000 live births (Korf et al., 2023).

TABLE 49.5 • Other Neurocutaneous Syndromes

Disorder	Incidence	Clinical Manifestations	Nursing Considerations
Tuberous sclerosis	One in 6,000–10,000[a]	Benign tumors present in the brain and skin. Presents most often as a generalized seizure disorder. Tumors can also involve the heart, kidney, eyes, lung, and bones. Developmental delay and behavioral problems may be noted. Usually evident in early childhood. Wide clinical spectrum from severe intellectual disability with incapacitating seizures to normal intelligence and no seizures	Treatment will be mainly symptomatic with the goal to prevent and treat associated complications. Seizure control will be a primary concern. Provide support and education to the family. Referral for genetic counseling (it follows an autosomal dominant inheritance pattern and half the cases are due to a new mutation) and appropriate resources www.tsalliance.org: Tuberous Sclerosis Alliance
Sturge–Weber syndrome	One in 20,000–50,000[a]	Facial nevus (port wine stain) most often seen on the forehead and on one side of the face, seizures, hemiparesis, intracranial calcifications. In many cases, intellectual disability, behavioral and emotional problems, and learning disabilities are present. Seizures usually begin in infancy and may worsen with age. Convulsions are usually noted on the side of the body opposite the facial nevus. Muscle weakness may be present on the same side. Most affected people have glaucoma at birth or will develop it later in life.	Treatment will be mainly symptomatic. Seizure control will be a primary concern (use of anticonvulsants or surgery). Seizures due to Sturge–Weber syndrome are often difficult to control. Laser treatment may be used to lighten or remove the facial nevus. Surgery may be performed on more serious cases of glaucoma. Physical therapy should be considered for infants and children with muscle weakness. Educational therapy is often prescribed for those with intellectual disability or developmental delays. Provide support and education to the family. Refer to appropriate resources. Genetic counseling may be appropriate (inheritance is unclear and sporadic). www.sturge-weber.org: Sturge–Weber Foundation

[a]Sahin, M., Ullrich, N., Srivastava, S., & Anna Pinto, A. (2020). Neurocutaneous syndromes. In R. M. Kleigman, J. W. St. Geme III, N. J. Blum, S. S. Shah, R. C. Tasker, K. M. Wilson, & R. E. Behrman (Eds.), *Nelson textbook of pediatrics* (21st ed., pp. 16593–16642). Elsevier.

Complications associated with neurofibromatosis include headaches; hydrocephalus; scoliosis; cardiac defects; hypertension; seizures; vision and hearing loss; neurocognitive deficits, including learning disabilities, attention deficit disorder, fine and gross motor delays, ASD, and behavior and psychosocial issues; abnormalities of speech; and a higher risk for neoplasms.

There is no cure for neurofibromatosis. Therapeutic management is aimed at controlling symptoms and managing complications. Surgical intervention can help reduce some of the bone malformations and remove painful or disfiguring tumors. These children should have a yearly physical, including blood pressure and cardiovascular examination, scoliosis screening, ophthalmology examination, developmental screening, and a neurologic examination.

The disease is progressive and symptoms usually worsen over time, but it is difficult to predict the course. Most affected people develop mild to moderate symptoms, with non–life-threatening complications, and live a normal, productive life. Recent studies have shown a decreased life expectancy compared to the general population (Korf et al., 2023).

Nursing Assessment

On assessment, the nurse may find café-au-lait spots (light-brown macules), which are the hallmark of neurofibromatosis (Korf et al., 2023) (Fig. 49.8). These are usually present at birth but can appear during the first year of life and usually increase in size, number, and pigmentation. They are present all over the body, particularly the trunk and extremities, while usually sparing the face. Pigmented nevi, axillary freckling, and slow-growing cutaneous, subcutaneous, or dermal neurofibromas, which are benign tumors, are other signs of neurofibromatosis. Many children with neurofibromatosis have a larger than normal head circumference and are shorter than average. The severity of symptoms varies greatly, but the diagnosis is made if two or more of the clinical signs in Box 49.4 are present.

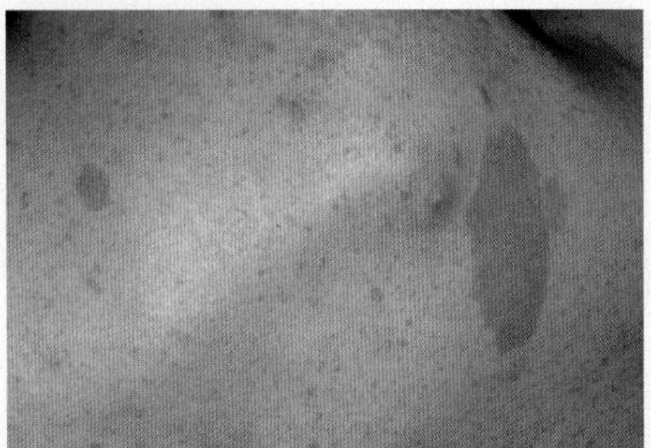

FIGURE 49.8 Café-au-lait spots associated with neurofibromatosis.

TAKE NOTE!

If more than six café-au-lait spots are present, neurofibromatosis should be suspected.

Nursing Management

Nursing management will be mainly supportive. Early detection of treatable conditions and complications is a priority. Provide support and education to the child and family. Discuss genetic counseling with the family. Referral to appropriate resources is essential. The Children's Tumor Foundation is a resource that can be found online.

OTHER GENETIC DISORDERS

Thousands of genetic disorders are known, and new ones are being discovered, but most of them are rare. Table 49.6 lists other genetic disorders that the pediatric nurse may encounter. Nursing management of these disorders will be mainly supportive and will focus on providing support and education to the family and child, with an emphasis on developmental and educational needs. Referral to genetic counseling and appropriate resources is an important nursing function.

BOX 49.4 Clinical Signs of Neurofibromatosis

Diagnosis is made if two or more of the following are present in a child without a parent with a diagnosis of NF1. In a child with a parent with a diagnosis of NF1, a diagnosis is made if one of the following is present:

- Six or more café-au-lait macules (light-brown spots) >5 mm in diameter in children and >15 mm in diameter in adolescents and adults
- Two or more neurofibromas (benign tumors) or one plexiform neurofibroma (a tumor that involves many nerves)
- Freckling in the armpit or groin
- Presence of an optic glioma (a tumor on the optic nerve)
- Two or more growths on the iris of the eye (Lisch nodules or iris hamartomas)
- Presence of a specific osseous lesion such as sphenoid dysplasia, anterolateral bowing of the tibia, or pseudarthrosis of a long bone
- Genetic testing showing NF1 variant

Korf, B. R., Lobbous, M., & Metrock, L. K. (2023). Neurofibromatosis type 1 (NF1): Pathogenesis, clinical features, and diagnosis. *UpToDate*. Retrieved May 29, 2023, from https://www.uptodate.com/contents/neurofibromatosis-type-1-nf1-pathogenesis-clinical-features-and-diagnosis

TAKE NOTE!

Children with VATER syndrome who have only one kidney should not play contact sports.

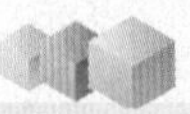

Concept Mastery Alert

Assessment findings in a child with achondroplasia are a trident hand (separation between the middle and ring fingers) and persistent otitis media caused by middle ear dysfunction. In contrast, a child with Marfan syndrome would have slim stature, hypotonia, and a narrow face.

INBORN ERRORS OF METABOLISM

Inborn errors of metabolism are a group of hereditary disorders. They are collectively common, but individually rare with most having an incidence of less than one in 100,000 (Sutton, 2022). Most follow an autosomal recessive inheritance pattern. They are caused by gene mutations that result in abnormalities in the synthesis or catabolism of proteins, carbohydrates, or fats. The body cannot convert food into energy as it normally would. Most inborn errors are due to a defect in an enzyme or transport protein that results in a block in the metabolic pathway. The blocked metabolic pathway allows for the accumulation of the damaging byproduct of the impaired metabolic process or may be responsible for a deficiency or absence of a necessary product. Presentation can occur at any time, even in adulthood, but many affected people exhibit signs in the newborn period or shortly after. Most inborn errors of metabolism presenting in the neonatal period are lethal if specific treatment is not initiated immediately.

Newborn screening is used to detect these disorders before symptoms develop. It began in the early 1960s with screening for phenylketonuria (PKU). Technical advances and developments in screening techniques (such as tandem mass spectrometry) now allow dozens of metabolic disorders to be detected from a single drop of blood (Kemper, 2021). A child who tests positive will require additional testing to confirm the diagnosis (see Chapter 31 for more information on newborn screening for inborn errors of metabolism).

Therapeutic management of these disorders varies depending on the cause of the error of metabolism, but dietary management is often a key component.

TABLE 49.6 • Other Genetic Disorders, Syndromes, and Associations

Disorder	Inheritance/Cause	Signs and Symptoms	Management
CHARGE syndrome (a recognizable pattern of congenital anomalies seen) **C: C**oloboma **H: H**eart disease **A: A**tresia (choanal) **R: R**etarded growth and development and/or central nervous system (CNS) anomalies **G: G**enital anomalies, hypogonadism **E: E**ar anomalies and deafness Incidence is one in 10,000 live births.[a]	Autosomal dominant inheritance possible, but most cases are due to new mutation in the gene *CDH7*. Occurs during fetal development and affects multiple organ systems	Coloboma is a lesion or defect of the eye, usually a fissure or cleft in the iris, ciliary, or choroid; can also see microphthalmos (small eyes) and cryptophthalmos (absent eye). Can lead to vision impairments Heart anomaly can include any type, but the most common are aortic arch anomalies and tetralogy of Fallot. Atresia (choanal) is blocked or narrowed passages from the nose to the throat, which can lead to aspiration. Retarded growth or cognitive development can range from mild to severe. Genital anomaly may include micropenis, undescended testes, and hypoplastic labia. Ear anomalies include short, wide ears with little or no lobe, prominent inner fold, floppy appearance, asymmetry; can have hearing impairment. Each feature occurs in a spectrum from absent to severe; no single feature is present in all people.	Focus is on identifying and treating all defects; early diagnosis is important. www.chargesyndrome.org: CHARGE Syndrome Foundation
Marfan syndrome: disorder of connective tissue Incidence is one in 3,000–5,000.[b]	Autosomal dominant inheritance; in most cases caused by a mutation in the gene fibrillin-1, which results in changes in connective tissue	Primarily involves the skeletal, cardiovascular, and ocular systems. Tall stature with long slim limbs, minimal subcutaneous fat, muscle hypotonia, loose joints, long and narrow face, abnormalities of the skeletal system (e.g., pectus excavatum [funnel chest] or pectus carinatum [pigeon breast]), ocular system (e.g., enlarged cornea or lens subluxation), and cardiovascular system (e.g., dilation of the aorta or mitral valve prolapse) Delayed achievement of gross and fine motor milestones may occur.	Focus is on preventing complications. www.marfan.org: National Marfan Foundation
VATER association (not a diagnosis, but refers to a nonrandom association of defects found to occur together) **V: V**ertebral defects **A: A**nal atresia **TE: T**racheo**E**sophageal fistula with esophageal atresia **R**adial and **R**enal dysplasia May also occur as VACTERL association, with **C: C**ardiac anomalies and **L: L**imb abnormalities added	Sporadic inheritance. Cause is unknown. Can occur with other chromosomal abnormalities such as trisomy 18	One anomaly is present in three body parts (limb, thorax, lower abdomen/pelvis). Anomalies seen include hypoplastic (small) vertebrae or hemivertebra (only half the bones are formed). These anomalies lead to an increased risk of scoliosis. With imperforate anus or anal atresia, the anus does not open to the outside of the body. Tracheoesophageal fistula and/or esophageal atresia leads to increased risk for aspiration, feeding, and swallowing problems. Incomplete formation of one or more kidneys, obstruction of urine flow out of kidneys, or severe reflux back into kidneys can all lead to kidney failure later in life. Cardiac anomalies: most common are ventricular septal defects, atrial septal defects, and tetralogy of Fallot. Absent or displaced thumb, polydactyly (extra digits), syndactyly (fusion of digits) A single umbilical artery at birth is often present. Failure to thrive and slow development in early infancy due to anomalies Usually normal intelligence	Focus is on identifying and treating all defects. http://www.eatef.org: EA/TEF Child and Family Support Connection, Inc.

(*continued*)

TABLE 49.6 • Other Genetic Disorders, Syndromes, and Associations (*continued*)

Disorder	Inheritance/Cause	Signs and Symptoms	Management
Apert syndrome (named for the French physician who described the syndrome) Incidence is 6–15.5 out of 1 million live births.[c]	Autosomal dominant inheritance. Cases are sporadic.	Craniosynostosis and maxillary hypoplasia resulting in a flat recessed forehead and flat midface, bilateral symmetric syndactyly, and craniofacial anomalies such as high-arched palate and associated clefting, short anteroposterior diameter, protruding eyes, down-slanting eyelids, and low-set ears Small nasopharynx can lead to upper airway obstruction and sleep apnea. Acne vulgaris, strabismus, and hearing loss Learning disabilities and mental deficiency	Early surgery for craniosynostosis when increased intracranial pressure is noted. Vigorous early management should occur with a multidisciplinary approach to address multiple anomalies. http://aboutface-usa.org/: About Face USA www.ccakids.com: Children's Craniofacial Association www.faces-cranio.org: National Craniofacial Association
Achondroplasia (most common chondrodysplasia [diseases resulting in disordered growth]) Incidence is one in 20,000.[d]	Autosomal dominant inheritance pattern. Caused by mutations in fibroblast growth factor receptor 3 (FGFR3). 80% new gene mutation[d]	Characterized by abnormal body proportion Small stature (average adult height is 4 ft for all sexes), short limbs with a normal-size torso, low nasal bridge with prominent forehead. Midface hypoplasia, caudal narrowing of the spinal canal, megalocephaly, small foramen magnum; hands are short and stubby with separation between middle and ring fingers ("trident hand"). Delayed motor skills, problems with persistent middle ear dysfunction and infections, and bowing of lower legs Less common complications include hydrocephalus, craniocervical junction compression, upper airway obstruction, and thoracolumbar kyphosis. Usually present with normal intelligence and lead independent, productive lives	Medical management of symptoms Monitor height, weight, and head circumference. Manage and prevent complications (careful and thorough neurologic examination, assessment for sleep apnea). Growth hormone therapy is controversial and currently is not recommended. New treatments such as vosoritide, a recombinant C-type natriuretic peptide analog, may be used. Limb-lengthening surgeries may be performed. http://www.lpaonline.org/: Little People of America

[a]Usman, N., & Sur, M. (2023). CHARGE syndrome. In *StatPearls* [Internet]. StatPearls Publishing. https://www.ncbi.nlm.nih.gov/books/NBK559199/

[b]Wright, M. J., & Connolly, H. M. (2022). Genetics, clinical features, and diagnosis of Marfan syndrome and related disorders. *UpToDate*. Retrieved May 29, 2023, from https://www.uptodate.com/contents/genetics-clinical-features-and-diagnosis-of-marfan-syndrome-and-related-disorders

[c]Firth, H. V. (2023). Craniosynostosis syndromes. *UpToDate*. Retrieved May 29, 2023, from https://www.uptodate.com/contents/craniosynostosis-syndromes

[d]Bacino, C. A. (2023). Achondroplasia. *UpToDate*. Retrieved May 29, 2023, from https://www.uptodate.com/contents/achondroplasia

Nursing Assessment

Clinical signs and symptoms vary with each disorder. Table 49.7 gives information on some common inborn errors of metabolism seen in children.

Because of newborn screening and early identification and management, it is rare to see an untreated newborn with clinical signs and symptoms of disease caused by one of the inborn errors of metabolism disorders. If seen, a newborn who was healthy at birth will often present with lethargy, poor feeding, apnea or tachypnea, recurrent vomiting, altered consciousness, failure to thrive, seizures, septic appearance, or developmental delay. Physical changes that may be seen include dysmorphology, cardiomegaly, rashes, cataracts, retinitis, optic atrophy, corneal opacity, deafness, skeletal dysplasia, macrocephaly, hepatomegaly, jaundice, or cirrhosis.

TAKE NOTE!

When a previously healthy newborn presents with a history of deterioration, suspect an inborn error of metabolism.

The diagnostic workup usually requires a variety of specific laboratory studies and may include:

- Glucose: may be elevated
- Ammonia: may be elevated

TABLE 49.7 • Inborn Errors of Metabolism

Disorder/Explanation	Clinical Manifestations	Management
Phenylketonuria (PKU): deficiency in a liver enzyme leading to inability to process the essential amino acid phenylalanine properly. Phenylalanine accumulation can lead to brain damage unless PKU is detected soon after birth and treated.	No symptoms at birth. Most cases are identified before symptoms are present due to newborn screening (PKU is screened for in all states). If undiagnosed, the most common sign is developmental delay along with vomiting, irritability, eczemalike rash, mousy odor to urine, microcephaly, seizures, and behavioral abnormalities.	Low-phenylalanine diet Can be difficult to follow for entire life so new treatments are being developed such as administrations of large neutral amino acids Phenylalanine is found mostly in protein-containing foods such as meat and milk (including breast milk and formula). www.pkunetwork.org: Children's PKU Network www.pkunews.org: National PKU News
Galactosemia: deficiency in the liver enzyme needed to convert galactose, the breakdown product of lactose, which is commonly found in dairy products, into glucose. Galactose accumulation leads to damage to vital organs.	No symptoms at birth. If undiagnosed, the newborn will have jaundice, feeding intolerance, diarrhea, and vomiting and will not gain weight. Signs and symptoms of sepsis and cataracts are often seen. If untreated, can lead to liver disease, blindness, severe intellectual disability, and death	Ingestion of galactose can produce sepsis in an affected child; therefore, septic workup and antibiotics may be necessary in a child if galactose ingestion has occurred. Elimination of galactose and lactose from the diet is the only treatment. Therefore, milk and dairy products will be eliminated for life. www.galactosemia.org: Parents of Galactosemic Children
Maple sugar urine disease: affects the metabolism of amino acids. A deficiency in the enzyme that metabolizes leucine, isoleucine, and valine, which are components of protein often referred to as the branched-chain amino acids (BCAA). These amino acids then accumulate in the blood and cause damage to the brain.	No symptoms at birth, but if untreated, newborns soon begin to show neurologic signs, vomiting, poor feeding, hypertonicity, increased reflex action, and seizures. Lower intake of protein (as occurs with breastfeeding) may delay the presentation of symptoms. If untreated, can lead to life-threatening neurologic damage	Special low-protein diet; will vary based on the severity of symptoms; limited natural protein requires medical food product supplements such as BCAA free. Thiamine supplements may be given. Diet must be continued throughout life. Liver transplant has been performed with good results (child on normal diet posttransplant). www.msud-support.org: Maple Syrup Urine Disease Family Support Group
Biotinidase deficiency: lack of the enzyme biotinidase results in biotin deficiency.	Typically no symptoms at birth; in the first weeks or months of life, symptoms such as hypotonia, uncoordinated movement, seizures, developmental delay, alopecia, seborrheic dermatitis, hearing loss, optic nerve atrophy, and intellectual disability develop. Metabolic acidosis can lead to death.	Daily oral free biotin
Medium-chain acyl-CoA dehydrogenase deficiency (MCAD): lack of an enzyme required to metabolize fatty acids	Classic presentation is a child 3 months to 5 years with vomiting and lethargy after a period of not eating (fasting typically associated with a viral illness). Recurrent episodes of metabolic acidosis and hypoglycemia, lethargy, seizures, liver failure, brain damage, coma, and cardiac arrest. Can lead to serious and fatal illnesses in children not eating well	Avoid fasting; have frequent meals. Special considerations during illness. If unable to tolerate food, intravenous (IV) dextrose is required. www.fodsupport.org: Fatty Oxidation Disorders (FOD) Family Support Group
Homocystinuria: deficiency in the enzyme needed to digest a component of food called methionine (an amino acid)	Typically, no symptoms at birth. In the first few months of life, symptoms including vomiting, poor feeding, failure to thrive, and hypotonia. If undetected and untreated, can lead to intellectual disability, psychiatric disturbances, developmental delays, displacement of the lens of the eye, abnormal thinning and weakness of bones, and formation of thrombi in veins and arteries that can lead to life-threatening complications such as stroke	Vitamin B_6 and B_{12} supplements and possibly other supplements, such as betaine and folic acid; methionine-restricted diet and cystine supplements; aspirin and dipyridamole to decrease thromboembolic events www.rarediseases.org: National Organization for Rare Disorders

(*continued*)

TABLE 49.7 Inborn Errors of Metabolism (*continued*)

Disorder/Explanation	Clinical Manifestations	Management
Tyrosinemia: deficiency in an enzyme essential in the metabolism of tyrosine; accumulation of the byproducts results in liver and kidney damage.	Symptoms usually appear in the first months of life: fever, failure to thrive, poor weight gain, vomiting, diarrhea, cabbagelike odor, enlarged liver and spleen, increased bleeding tendency, distended abdomen, jaundice, cirrhosis, and liver failure.	The treatment of choice is the administration of nitisinone. Diet low in phenylalanine and tyrosine www.liverfoundation.org: American Liver Foundation
Tay–Sachs (one of GM_2 gangliosidoses) caused by insufficient activity of an enzyme called hexosaminidase A, which is necessary for the breakdown of certain fatty substances in brain and nerve cells	Occurs more frequently among people of Ashkenazi Jewish descent (with one in every 25 being a carrier)[a] Infants appear normal and healthy for the first few months of life. Then, as harmful quantities of the fatty substances (called gangliosides) build up in tissues and nerve cells and cause damage, mental and physical deterioration occur. The child becomes blind, deaf, and unable to swallow; muscles begin to atrophy; and paralysis sets in. Dementia, seizures, and an increased startle reflex may be seen. There is a late-onset type of Tay–Sachs seen in people in their 20s and early 30s, but this is much rarer.	No treatment or cure. Medical management will focus on managing symptoms and maintaining comfort. Anticonvulsants may be given to control seizures. Death usually occurs in early childhood, by age 4 or 5. Carriers can be identified by a blood test, and prenatal testing is available. www.ntsad.org: National Tay-Sachs & Allied Diseases Association

[a]McGovern, M. M., & Desnick, R. J. (2020). Lipidoses (lysosomal storage disorders). In R. M. Kleigman, J. W. St. Geme III, N. J. Blum, S. S. Shah, R. C. Tasker, K. M. Wilson, & R. E. Behrman (Eds.), *Nelson textbook of pediatrics* (21st ed., pp. 4446–4484). Elsevier. Data from Shchelochkov, O. A., & Venditti, C. P. (2020). An approach to inborn errors of metabolism. In R. M. Kleigman, J. W. St. Geme III, N. J. Blum, S. S. Shah, R. C. Tasker, K. M. Wilson, & R. E. Behrman (Eds.), *Nelson textbook of pediatrics* (21st ed., pp. 4054–4087). Elsevier; Shchelochkov, O. A., & Venditti, C. P. (2020). Defects in metabolism of amino acids. In R. M. Kleigman, J. W. St. Geme III, N. J. Blum, S. S. Shah, R. C. Tasker, K. M. Wilson, & R. E. Behrman (Eds.), *Nelson textbook of pediatrics* (21st ed., pp. 4053–4330). Elsevier; Kishnani, P. S., & Chen, Y. T. (2020). Defects in metabolism of carbohydrates. In R. M. Kleigman, J. W. St. Geme III, N. J. Blum, S. S. Shah, R. C. Tasker, K. M. Wilson, & R. E. Behrman (Eds.), *Nelson textbook of pediatrics* (21st ed., pp. 4488–4614). Elsevier; Stanley, C. A., & Bennett, M. J. (2020). Disorders of mitochondrial fatty acid β oxidation. In R. M. Kleigman, J. W. St. Geme III, N. J. Blum, S. S. Shah, R. C. Tasker, K. M. Wilson, & R. E. Behrman (Eds.), *Nelson textbook of pediatrics* (21st ed., pp. 4331–4357). Elsevier; McGovern, M. M., & Desnick, R. J. (2020). Lipidoses (lysosomal storage disorders). In R. M. Kleigman, J. W. St. Geme III, N. J. Blum, S. S. Shah, R. C. Tasker, K. M. Wilson, & R. E. Behrman (Eds.), *Nelson textbook of pediatrics* (21st ed., pp. 4446–4484). Elsevier; McGovern, M., & Desnick, R. J. (2016). Lipidoses (lysosomal storage disorders). In R. M. Kleigman, B. F. Stanton, J. W. St. Geme III, N. F. Schor, & R. E. Behrman (Eds.), *Nelson textbook of pediatrics* (20th ed., pp. 705–714). Saunders.

- Blood gases: may have low bicarbonate and low pH, metabolic acidosis (respiratory alkalosis may also be seen, especially when high ammonia levels are present)

Early diagnosis is the key to saving and improving the lives of these children.

TAKE NOTE!

If an inborn error of metabolism is suspected, feedings will usually be stopped until the test results are received.

When a child who has previously been diagnosed with an inborn error of metabolism is hospitalized, the nurse must determine the prescribed diet and medications so these may be continued while in the hospital setting.

Nursing Management

Ensure that the diet prescribed for the infant or child is followed. For amino acid disorders (e.g., PKU), urea cycle defects (e.g., tyrosinemia type I), and organic acidemia (e.g., maple syrup urine disease), nutritional therapy is the major intervention. Dietary intake of specific amino acids is restricted according to the disorder. Ensure that overall protein and calorie needs are still met, as children need sufficient calories for proper growth. In children with urea cycle defects and organic acidemia, anorexia is common and severe, and the child may need gastrostomy tube feeding supplementation. In fatty acid oxidation disorders (e.g., medium-chain acyl-coenzyme A [CoA] dehydrogenase deficiency), the goal is to avoid prolonged periods of fasting and to provide frequent feeds when the child is sick. Supplementation with specific vitamins may also be important in the treatment of these disorders. Strict adherence to the diet is necessary and will require close supervision by registered dietitians, primary providers, and nurses and the cooperation of both the parent and child.

Nursing management will focus on education and support for the family, who will need thorough knowledge about the child's disease and management. Refer the child and family to a dietitian and appropriate resources, including support groups. In addition, monitor the child's developmental progress and begin therapies as soon as a concern arises.

KEY CONCEPTS

- Nurses play an essential role in providing emotional support and referrals to appropriate agencies, support groups, and resources when caring for families with suspected or diagnosed genetic disorders.
- Referral for genetic counseling prior to genetic testing may be appropriate.
- Many children with chromosomal abnormalities have intellectual disability, learning disabilities, behavioral problems, and distinct features, including birth defects.
- Trisomy 21 (DS) is associated with some degree of intellectual disability, characteristic facial features (e.g., slanted eyes and depressed nasal bridge), and other health problems, such as cardiac defects, visual and hearing impairments, intestinal malformations, and an increased susceptibility to infections.
- In Turner syndrome, short stature and slow growth are characteristic findings.
- Klinefelter syndrome is usually diagnosed in adolescence or adulthood due to a lack of development of secondary sex characteristics.
- Fragile X syndrome's clinical manifestations are subtle during childhood, with minor dysmorphic features and developmental delay. Problems with sensation, emotion, and behavior often are the first signs.
- Café-au-lait spots (light-brown macules) are the hallmark of neurofibromatosis (Korf et al., 2023).
- Inborn errors of metabolism are caused by gene mutations that result in abnormalities in the synthesis or catabolism of proteins, carbohydrates, or fats. Most inborn errors of metabolism presenting in the neonatal period are lethal if specific treatment is not initiated immediately.
- Nurses should have a basic knowledge of genetics, common genetic disorders in children, genetic testing, and genetic counseling so they can provide support and information to families and can help improve their quality of life.
- Genetic disorders usually result in a lifelong complex medical condition. Nurses must provide ongoing education and support for the child and family about the disorder, treatment, and management as well as available resources.

REFERENCES AND RECOMMENDED READINGS

Ajitkumar, A., Jamil, R. T., & Mathai, J. K. (2023). Cri du chat syndrome. In *StatPearls* [Internet]. StatPearls Publishing. https://www.ncbi.nlm.nih.gov/books/NBK482460/

Bacino, C. A. (2023a). Achondroplasia. *UpToDate*. Retrieved May 29, 2023, from https://www.uptodate.com/contents/achondroplasia

Bacino, C. A. (2023b). Congenital anomalies: Epidemiology, types and pattern. *UpToDate*. Retrieved May 26, 2023, from https://www.uptodate.com/contents/birth-defects-epidemiology-types-and-patterns

Bacino, C. A. (2023c). Sex chromosome abnormalities. *UpToDate*. Retrieved May 29, 2023, from https://www.uptodate.com/contents/sex-chromosome-abnormalities

Bacino, C. A., & Lee, B. (2020). Cytogenetics. In R. M. Kleigman, J. W. St. Geme III, N. J. Blum, S. S. Shah, R. C. Tasker, K. M. Wilson, & R. E. Behrman (Eds.), *Nelson textbook of pediatrics* (21st ed., pp. 3903–3999). Elsevier.

Backelijauw, P. (2022). Clinical manifestations and diagnosis of Turner syndrome. *UpToDate*. Retrieved May 29, 2023, from https://www.uptodate.com/contents/clinical-manifestations-and-diagnosis-of-turner-syndrome

Bull, M. J., Trotter, T., Santoro, S. L., Christensen, C., Grout, R.W., & The Council on Genetics. (2022). Health supervision for children and adolescents with DS. *Pediatrics, 149*(5), e2022057010. https://doi.org/10.1542/peds.2022-057010

Duis, J., & Scheimann, A. O. (2023). Prader–Willi syndrome: Clinical features and diagnosis. *UpToDate*. Retrieved May 29, 2023, from https://www.uptodate.com/contents/prader-willi-syndrome-clinical-features-and-diagnosis

Firth, H. V. (2023). Craniosynostosis syndromes. *UpToDate*. Retrieved May 29, 2023, from https://www.uptodate.com/contents/craniosynostosis-syndromes

Fischbach, F. T., Fischbach, M. A., & Stout, K. (2022). *A manual of laboratory and diagnostic tests* (11th ed.). Wolters Kluwer.

Genetic and Rare Diseases Information Center. (2023). *Wolf-Hirschhorn syndrome*. https://rarediseases.info.nih.gov/diseases/7896/wolf-hirschhorn-syndrome

Giersch, A. (2022). Congenital cytogenetic abnormalities. *UpToDate*. Retrieved May 27, 2023, from https://www.uptodate.com/contents/congenital-cytogenetic-abnormalities

Hon-Yin, B. C., Shuman, C., Choufani, S., & Weksberg, R. (2022). Beckwith-Wiedemann syndrome. *UpToDate*. Retrieved May 29, 2023, from https://www.uptodate.com/contents/beckwith-wiedemann-syndrome

Kemper, A. R. (2021). Overview of newborn screening. *UpToDate*. Retrieved May 25, 2023, from https://www.uptodate.com/contents/newborn-screening

Kishnani, P. S., & Chen, Y. T. (2020). Defects in metabolism of carbohydrates. *In* R. M. Kleigman, J. W. St. Geme III, N. J. Blum, S. S. Shah, R. C. Tasker, K. M. Wilson, & R. E. Behrman (Eds.), *Nelson textbook of pediatrics* (21st ed., pp. 4488–4614). Elsevier.

Korf, B. R., Lobbous, M., & Metrock, L. K. (2023). Neurofibromatosis type 1 (NF1): Pathogenesis, clinical features, and diagnosis. *UpToDate*. Retrieved May 29, 2023, from https://www.uptodate.com/contents/neurofibromatosis-type-1-nf1-pathogenesis-clinical-features-and-diagnosis

Lackey, A. E., & Muzio, M. R. (2023). DiGeorge syndrome. In *StatPearls* [Internet]. StatPearls Publishing. https://www.ncbi.nlm.nih.gov/books/NBK549798/

Lashley, F. R. (2005). *Clinical genetics in nursing practice*. Springer Publishing.

Madaan, M., & Mendez, M. D. (2023). Angelman syndrome. In *StatPearls* [Internet]. StatPearls Publishing. https://www.ncbi.nlm.nih.gov/books/NBK560870/

McGovern, M. M., & Desnick, R. J. (2020). Lipidoses (lysosomal storage disorders). In R. M. Kleigman, J. W. St. Geme III, N. J. Blum, S. S. Shah, R. C. Tasker, K. M. Wilson, & R. E. Behrman (Eds.), *Nelson textbook of pediatrics* (21st ed., pp. 4446–4484). Elsevier.

National Down Syndrome Society. (2023). *Early intervention.* https://www.ndss.org/resources/early-intervention/

Ostermaier, K. K. (2022a). Down syndrome: Clinical features and diagnosis. *UpToDate.* Retrieved May 23, 2023, from https://www.uptodate.com/contents/down-syndrome-clinical-features-and-diagnosis

Ostermaier, K. K. (2022b). Down syndrome: Management. *UpToDate.* Retrieved May 27, 2023, from https://www.uptodate.com/contents/down-syndrome-management

Sahin, M., Ullrich, N., Srivastava, S., & Anna Pinto, A. (2020). Neurocutaneous syndromes. In R. M. Kleigman, J. W. St. Geme III, N. J. Blum, S. S. Shah, R. C. Tasker, K. M. Wilson, & R. E. Behrman (Eds.), *Nelson textbook of pediatrics* (21st ed., pp. 16593–16642). Elsevier.

Scott, D. A., & Lee, B. (2020). The genetic approach in pediatric medicine. In R. M. Kleigman, J. W. St. Geme III, N. J. Blum, S. S. Shah, R. C. Tasker, K. M. Wilson, & R. E. Behrman (Eds.), *Nelson textbook of pediatrics* (21st ed., pp. 3821–3837). Elsevier.

Shchelochkov, O. A., & Venditti, C. P. (2020a). An approach to inborn errors of metabolism. In R. M. Kleigman, J. W. St. Geme III, N. J. Blum, S. S. Shah, R. C. Tasker, K. M. Wilson, & R. E. Behrman (Eds.), *Nelson textbook of pediatrics* (21st ed., pp. 4054–4087). Elsevier.

Shchelochkov, O. A., & Venditti, C. P. (2020b). Defects in metabolism of amino acids. In R. M. Kleigman, J. W. St. Geme III, N. J. Blum, S. S. Shah, R. C. Tasker, K. M. Wilson, & R. E. Behrman (Eds.), *Nelson textbook of pediatrics* (21st ed., pp. 4053–4330). Elsevier.

Spinazzi, N. A., Velasco, A. B., Wodecki, D. J., & Patel, L. (2023) Autism spectrum disorder in Down syndrome: Experiences from caregivers. *Journal of Autism and Developmental Disorders, 54*, 1171–1180. https://doi.org/10.1007/s10803-022-05758-x

Stanley, C. A., & Bennett, M. J. (2020). Disorders of mitochondrial fatty acid β oxidation. In R. M. Kleigman, J. W. St. Geme III, N. J. Blum, S. S. Shah, R. C. Tasker, K. M. Wilson, & R. E. Behrman (Eds.), *Nelson textbook of pediatrics* (21st ed., pp. 4331–4357). Elsevier.

Stone, W. L., Basit, H., Shah, M., & Los, E. (2023). Fragile X syndrome. In *StatPearls* [Internet]. StatPearls Publishing. https://www.ncbi.nlm.nih.gov/books/NBK459243/

Sutton, V. R. (2022). Inborn errors of metabolism: Epidemiology, pathogenesis, and clinical features. *UpToDate.* Retrieved May 29, 2023, from https://www.uptodate.com/contents/inborn-errors-of-metabolism-epidemiology-pathogenesis-and-clinical-features

Usman, N., & Sur, M. (2023). CHARGE syndrome. In *StatPearls* [Internet]. StatPearls Publishing. https://www.ncbi.nlm.nih.gov/books/NBK559199/

Van Esch, H. (2022). Fragile X syndrome: Clinical features and diagnosis in children and adolescents. *UpToDate.* Retrieved on May 29, 2023, from https://www.uptodate.com/contents/fragile-x-syndrome-clinical-features-and-diagnosis-in-children-and-adolescents

Wilson, M., & Carter, I. B. (2022). Williams syndrome. In *StatPearls* [Internet]. StatPearls Publishing. https://www.ncbi.nlm.nih.gov/books/NBK544278/

Wright, M. J., & Connolly, H. M. (2022). Genetics, clinical features, and diagnosis of Marfan syndrome and related disorders. *UpToDate.* Retrieved May 29, 2023, from https://www.uptodate.com/contents/genetics-clinical-features-and-diagnosis-of-marfan-syndrome-and-related-disorders

DEVELOPING CLINICAL JUDGMENT

PRACTICING FOR NCLEX

1. You are counseling a couple, one of whom is affected by neurofibromatosis, an autosomal dominant disorder. They want to know the risk of transmitting the disorder. The nurse should tell them that each offspring has a:
   a. one in four (25%) chance of getting the disease.
   b. one in eight (12.5%) chance of getting the disease.
   c. one in one (100%) chance of getting the disease.
   d. one in two (50%) chance of getting the disease.

2. A child born with a single transverse palmar crease, a short neck with excessive skin at the nape, a depressed nasal bridge, and cardiac defects is most likely to have which autosomal abnormality?
   a. Trisomy 21
   b. Trisomy 18
   c. Trisomy 14
   d. Trisomy 13

3. A parent brings their 4-day-old infant to the clinic with vomiting and poor feeding. The newborn was healthy at birth. The nurse should suspect:
   a. Sturge–Weber syndrome.
   b. an inborn error of metabolism.
   c. trisomy 18.
   d. Turner syndrome.

4. The nurse is caring for a child with DS. What should the nurse's focus be?
   a. Teaching hygiene skills to the child in order to increase self-esteem
   b. Screening for anomalies and teaching about the prevention of respiratory infection
   c. Finding opportunities to increase socialization for the child and family
   d. Expecting walking at age 1 year and toilet training completion at age 2 years

5. The nurse is caring for a child with Turner syndrome admitted to the unit for treatment of a kidney infection. What characteristics associated with this syndrome may the nurse expect to find upon assessment? Select all that apply.
   a. Microcephaly
   b. Polydactyly
   c. Short stature
   d. Gynecomastia
   e. Taller than average
   f. Webbed neck
   g. Low posterior hairline
   h. Cleft lip

DOSAGE CALCULATION QUESTION

1. The nurse is caring for a child with DS. The child weighs 26 lb. The primary provider orders intravenous (IV) maintenance fluids. What would be the expected maintenance IV fluid rate? (Round to the nearest mL)

CRITICAL THINKING EXERCISES

1. An 8-month-old is seen in the clinic. On assessment, the nurse finds eight café-au-lait spots on the child's trunk and extremities. What other assessment findings may be pertinent?

2. A child's newborn screen came back positive for PKU. After further testing, the diagnosis is confirmed. What instructions would you give the parents regarding the care of their child?

3. A 6-year-old with DS is admitted to the hospital with pneumonia. Choose three pieces of information that the nurse should seek when obtaining the health history:
   a. Presence of cardiac defects or disease
   b. Last hearing and vision evaluation
   c. Birthing parent's pregnancy history
   d. Presence of thyroid disease
   e. Birthing parent's immunization history

STUDY ACTIVITIES

1. Develop a nursing plan of care for a child with DS.

2. Shadow a genetic counselor. Identify ways they help families understand and cope with genetic disorders.

3. Attend a meeting of an ethics committee at a local hospital. Identify some of the ethical, legal, and social issues in health care that they discuss, particularly related to genetic testing and genetic disorders.

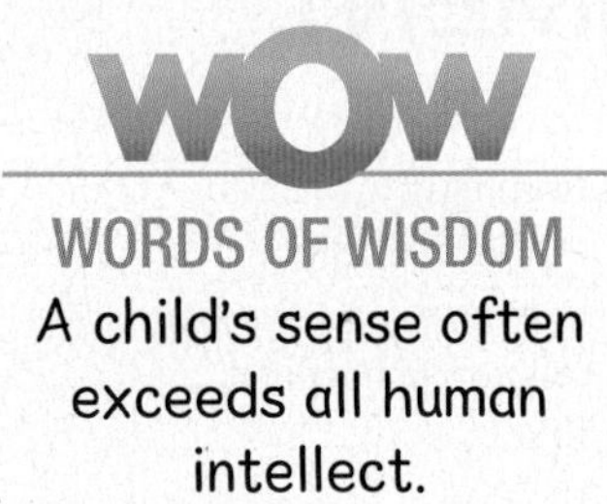

A child's sense often exceeds all human intellect.

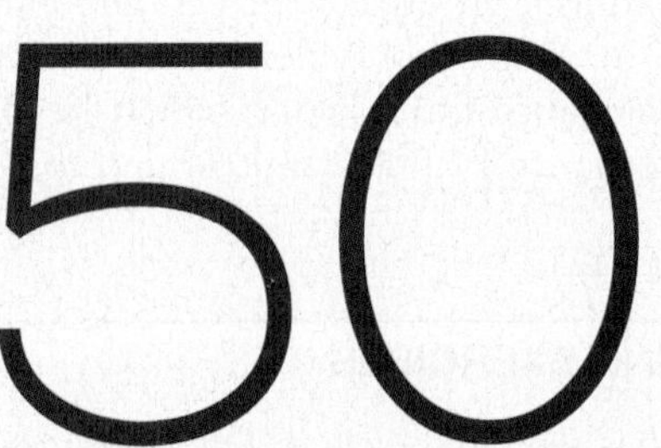

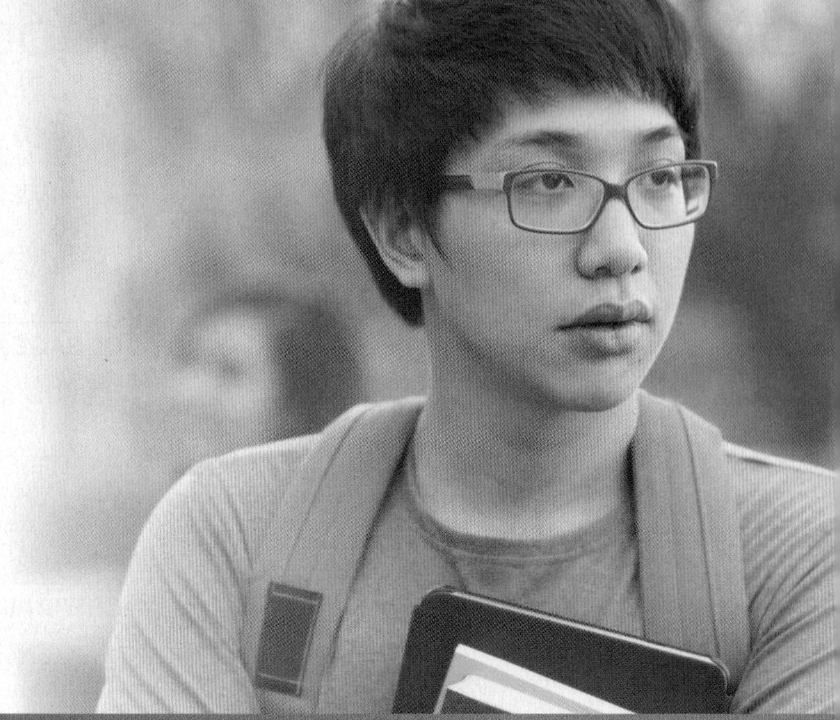

Nursing Care of the Child With an Alteration in Behavior, Cognition, or Development

LEARNING OBJECTIVES

Upon completion of the chapter, you will be able to:

1. Discuss the impact of alterations in mental health on the growth, development, and future health of infants, children, and adolescents.
2. Describe techniques used to evaluate the status of mental health in children.
3. Identify appropriate nursing assessments and interventions related to therapy and medications for the treatment of childhood and adolescent mental health disorders.
4. Distinguish mental health disorders common in infants, children, and adolescents.
5. Devise an individualized nursing care plan or concept map for the child with a mental health disorder.
6. Develop child and family teaching plans for the child with a mental health disorder.

KEY TERMS

affect
bingeing
comorbid
neglect
purging
suicide
violence

John Howard, age 6 years, is brought to the clinic for his annual examination. His parent states, "John has frequent emotional outbursts, and his mood seems to switch from happy to sad rather quickly. His teachers have said his performance at school has been poor."

INTRODUCTION

Mental health issues make up the bulk of the "new morbidity" of children. Such issues include developmental and behavioral disorders, eating disorders, mood disorders, anxiety disorders, and abuse and **violence** (acts of aggression) directed toward children. As many as 14% to 20% of children may be suffering from mental health–related problems (Kelsay et al., 2022). Failure to receive appropriate treatment may lead to further academic and social difficulties. Mental illness manifested in the early years increases the risk of adolescent emotional issues, use of firearms, reckless driving, substance misuse, and risky sexual activity. Some cognitive or neurobehavioral disorders may have a genetic or physiologic cause, whereas others result from family or environmental stressors.

Usually, children with cognitive or mental health disorders are treated in the community or on an outpatient basis, but sometimes, a disorder can have such a significant impact on the child and family that hospitalization is required. Many hospitalized children also experience cognitive or mental health disorders. When a child is diagnosed with a cognitive or mental health disorder, the family may become overwhelmed by the multifaceted services that they require.

Over the past several years, the extensive scope of mental health issues among children, adolescents, and their families has become more apparent, leading the American Academy of Pediatrics (AAP) to create initiatives that address the needs of these children and their families (AAP, 2023). Mental health problems in children are real and painful and can be severe. For affected children to have a chance at a healthy future, nurses must participate in the early identification and referral of children with potential cognitive deficits or other mental health issues.

EFFECTS OF MENTAL HEALTH ISSUES ON DEVELOPMENT AND FUTURE HEALTH

Children's behavior is influenced by biologic or genetic characteristics, nutrition, physical health, developmental ability, environmental and family interactions, the child's individual temperament, and the parents' or caregivers' responses to the child's behavior. The changes that occur with normal growth and development are often a source of stress for children, and in some children, they may lead to dysfunction. Children progress at different rates, so it is often difficult to identify subtle abnormalities. When stress, fatigue, or pain occurs in children, they may quickly regress to earlier patterns of behavior. These regressive behaviors may continue if a mental health concern is present. It is possible that stress placed on developing neurons leads to decreased coping abilities later in life. Children learn through their experiences. Therefore, they may develop maladaptive behaviors through life interactions (Kelsay et al., 2022).

Adverse childhood experiences (ACEs) in childhood are linked to negative long-term adolescent and adult health (Goddard, 2021). ACEs may include abuse, neglect, or other traumatic events experienced by the child. These events trigger the complex stress response humans experience, and when repetitive or chronic, these elevated stress hormones lead to long-term morbidities such as severe obesity, diabetes, and heart disease. Additionally, chronic, toxic stress negatively affects brain development, leading to maladaptive behavioral responses as well as learning difficulties. In order to build resilience during the childhood years, regular screening for ACEs and appropriate referrals may make a difference in the long-term outcome for these children (Goddard, 2021).

COMMON MEDICAL TREATMENTS

A variety of medications and other medical and psychological treatments are used to treat mental health disorders in children. Most of these treatments will require a health care provider's or nurse practitioner's order when the child is in the hospital. The most common medications are listed in Drug Guide 50.1. The nurse caring for the child with a mental health disorder should become familiar with how the treatments and medications work, as well as medication adverse effects for which to monitor. Many mental health disorders are treated with some type of therapy, including behavioral, play, family, and cognitive therapies. Table 50.1 reviews the types of therapies commonly used. These therapies are generally carried out only by specially trained personnel.

Behavior management techniques are also used to help children alter negative behavior patterns. The methods may be used outside of therapy sessions, in the hospital, clinic, classroom, or home. Behavior management techniques include:

- Set limits with the child, holding them responsible for their own behavior.
- Do not argue, bargain, or negotiate about the limits once established.
- Provide consistent caregivers (unlicensed assistive personnel and nurses for the hospitalized child), and establish the child's daily routine.
- Use a low-pitched voice and remain calm.
- Redirect the child's attention when needed.
- Ignore inappropriate behaviors.
- Praise the child's self-control efforts and other accomplishments.
- Use restraints only when necessary.

DRUG GUIDE 50.1

DRUGS USED FOR PEDIATRIC MENTAL HEALTH DISORDERS

Medication	Actions/Indications	Nursing Implications
Psychostimulants: methylphenidate, dextroamphetamine, lisdexamfetamine, pemoline, long-acting methylphenidate, long-acting dextroamphetamine	Increase synaptic levels of dopamine and norepinephrine ADHD	• Methylphenidate has a short half-life; give TID (am, midday at school, at home after school). • Long-acting preparations are given once daily in the morning. • Adverse effects include decreased appetite, headache, abdominal pain, difficulty sleeping, irritability, social withdrawal, and motor tics. If the dose is too high, the child may have a flat affect. • Lisdexamfetamine—If chest pain and fainting occur, notify the provider at once. • Pemoline is only rarely used because of hepatotoxicity.
Antianxiety agent: buspirone	Highly blocks reuptake of dopamine Anxiety, rage, mania, psychosis, depression, Tourette syndrome	• Administer in consistent relation to food (either with or without). • May cause drowsiness • Monitor for disinhibition, agitation, confusion, and depression.
Antimanic agent: lithium	Influences reuptake of serotonin and/or norepinephrine Bipolar disorder, depression, hyperaggression	• Monitor closely. • May cause polyuria, polydipsia, tremor, nausea, weight gain, diarrhea
Selective serotonin reuptake inhibitors: fluoxetine, paroxetine, sertraline	Potentiate serotonin activity in the brain Depression, obsessive-compulsive disorder, anxiety	• Observe for irritability, insomnia, GI distress, nausea, or headache. • Monitor BP for increases.
Atypical antidepressants: trazodone	Inhibit reuptake of serotonin Depression	• Monitor BP for postural hypotension. • Observe for sedation and drowsiness; avoid alcohol use. • Administer after meals or with a snack.
Nonstimulant norepinephrine reuptake inhibitors: atomoxetine	Enhance norepinephrine activity ADHD	• Administer without regard to food once or twice daily. • Monitor weight, height, BP, and heart rate. • May cause dizziness, dry mouth
Alpha-agonist antihypertensive agents: clonidine, guanfacine	Activate inhibitory neurons in the brain stem ADHD, Tourette syndrome, self-harm, aggression	• Clonidine is strongly sedating. • Monitor BP and pulse. • Observe for dry mouth, confusion, depression, urinary retention, and constipation.
Antipsychotic agents: thioridazine, chlorpromazine, haloperidol	Reversibly block type 2 dopamine receptors in the central nervous system Psychosis, mania, self-harm, violent or destructive behavior	• May cause drowsiness • Monitor for anticholinergic effects, drowsiness and dystonia (extrapyramidal effects), and dizziness. • Evaluate for the development of orthostatic hypotension and tachycardia. • Observe closely for the development of tardive dyskinesia, particularly early in treatment.
Atypical antipsychotics: risperidone, clozapine, olanzapine	Reversibly block type 2 dopamine receptors in the central nervous system Psychosis, bipolar disorder, autism spectrum disorder, Tourette syndrome	• Monitor for seizures, agitation, headache, nausea, and sedation. • Olanzapine may cause weight gain. • Note WBC count.
Tricyclic antidepressants: amitriptyline, desipramine, imipramine, nortriptyline	Enhance synaptic concentration of serotonin and/or norepinephrine Depression, ADHD, tics, anxiety	• Monitor for anticholinergic effects or weight loss. • Check blood levels. • Monitor ECG for arrhythmias.

ADHD, attention-deficit/hyperactivity disorder; BP, blood pressure; ECG, electrocardiogram; GI, gastrointestinal; TID, three times a day; WBC, white blood cell.

Data from Halter, M. J., & Fratena, C. A. (2023). *Varcarolis' manual of psychiatric nursing care planning: An interprofessional approach* (7th ed.). Elsevier; UpToDate, Inc. (2024). *UpToDate Lexidrug* (Version 8.2.0) [Mobile app]. Wolters Kluwer. https://apps.apple.com/us/app/lexicomp/id313401238

TABLE **50.1** • Types of Therapy

Treatment	Explanation
Behavioral therapy	Uses stimulus and response conditioning to manage or alter behavior; reinforces desired behaviors, replacing the inappropriate ones; consistency is of utmost importance.
Play therapy	Designed to change emotional status; encourages the child to act out feelings of sadness, fear, hostility, or anger
Cognitive behavioral therapy	Teaches children to change reactions so that automatic negative thought patterns are replaced with alternative ones
Dialectical behavioral therapy	Group and individual sessions to treat chronic suicidal thoughts in borderline personality disorder; individuals learn responsibility for their problems and to better deal with negative emotions.
Family therapy	Exploration of the child's emotional issue and its effect on family members; helps the family focus in more constructive ways
Group therapy	May be conducted in a school, hospital, treatment facility, or neighborhood center; feelings are expressed and participants gain hope, feel a part of something, and benefit from role modeling. Takes advantage of peer relationships as developmental focus in preadolescent and adolescent groups
Milieu therapy	A specially structured setting designed to promote the child's adaptive and social skills; a safe and supportive environment for those at risk for self-harm or those who are very ill or aggressive
Individual therapy	The child and therapist work together to resolve the conflicts, emotions, or behavior problems. Trust is central. Structured based on the child's developmental level (e.g., may use play therapy for a younger child)
Hypnosis	Deep relaxation with suggestibility remarks

Data from American Academy of Child and Adolescent Psychiatry. (2019). *Psychotherapy for children and adolescents: Different types.* https://www.aacap.org/AACAP/Families_and_Youth/Facts_for_Families/FFF-Guide/Psychotherapies-For-Children-And-Adolescents-086.aspx; Halter, M. J., & Fratena, C. A. (2023). *Varcarolis' manual of psychiatric nursing care planning: An interprofessional approach* (7th ed.). Elsevier; and Swick, S. D., & Jellinek, M. S. (2022). Demystifying psychotherapy. *Pediatric News, 56*(10), 18.

Clinical Judgment and the Nursing Process for the Child With a Mental Health Disorder

Care of the child with mental health disorder includes assessment, nursing analysis, planning, interventions, and evaluation. It is important to individualize each step of this process for each child.

Assessment

A careful and thorough health history forms the basis of the nursing assessment of a child with a mental health or cognitive disorder. The physical examination may yield clues to the type of disorder, but the physical examination often yields expected findings (except in cases of physical or sexual abuse).

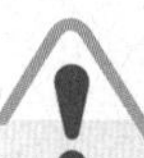

CLINICAL REASONING ALERT!

Observe a child's play or drawings; if the manner or theme of play or nature of the drawings leads you to suspect cognitive or psychological issues, refer the child for further mental health evaluation.

Health History

Elicit the health history, noting the child's prenatal and birth history, past medical history (including previously diagnosed cognitive or mental health disorders), history of neurologic injury or disease, and family history of mental health disorders. Perform a developmental history, noting age of attainment (or loss) of milestones. Question the child and/or parent about behavior changes such as:

- Altered sleep
- Difference in eating patterns, weight loss or gain, change in appetite
- Problems at school
- Participation in risk-taking behaviors
- Alterations in friendships
- Changes in extracurricular activity participation

A number of tools are available for screening for mental health disorders in children and adolescents. Use one of these tools as needed. Note results of any developmental testing performed. Ask the family about progression of the child's skills. Note any unusual deficits or capabilities. Question the family about recent stress, trauma, or change in family structure. Ask if any family members are chronically ill. Note medications the child takes routinely, and ask about any allergies to food, drugs, medications, or environmental agents.

Interview the child at an age-appropriate level to determine their self-perception, future plans, and stressors and how they cope with them. Determine the child's perception of their relationships with parents, siblings, friends, peers, pets, inanimate objects, and transitional or security objects. What is the child's predominant mood? Determine whether the child likes themselves, asking such questions as "What do you like most about yourself?" and "What would you like to change about yourself?" Determine whether the child has a sense of pride in their accomplishments. Has the child developed an appropriate conscience (understanding right and wrong)? Determine the child's gender identity status.

Document whether the child displays any of the following during the health interview:

- Hallucinations
- Aggression
- Impulsivity
- Distractibility
- Intolerance to frustration
- Lack of sense of humor or fun
- Inhibition
- Poor attention span
- Potential cognitive or learning disabilities
- Unusual motor activities

Note history of physical complaints that may be associated with physical abuse such as burns or other injuries or with sexual abuse situations, such as sore throat, difficulty swallowing, or genital burning or itching.

Physical Examination

Observe the child's clothing, noting whether it is appropriate for age, developmental level, and setting. Note the child's facial expression and response to the parent or caregiver and the nurse. Does the child make appropriate eye contact? Determine the child's level of consciousness and extent of interest in and interaction with surroundings. Note the child's posture, **affect** (facial emotional display), and mood. How appropriate to the situation are the child's emotional reactions? Does the child communicate well?

Measure the child's weight and height/length, as well as head circumference if they are younger than 3 years old. Perform a thorough physical examination, noting any physical abnormalities or signs of other physical health disorders. Note abnormal findings that may be associated with particular mental health disorders, such as bruising, burns, contusions, cuts, abrasions, unusual skin marks, soft/sparse body hair, split fingernails, inflamed oropharynx, eroded tooth enamel, reddened gums, or genitourinary discharge or bleeding.

Laboratory and Diagnostic Testing

Mental health disorders are generally diagnosed based on clinical features. However, brain imaging such as computed tomography or magnetic resonance imaging may be used to evaluate for a congenital abnormality or alterations in the brain tissue that may lead to developmental delay. A blood or urine toxicology panel is useful in the diagnosis of substance misuse or overdose, or instances of bizarre behavior.

Remember John, the 6-year-old brought in for his annual examination? What additional health history and physical examination assessment information should the nurse obtain?

Nursing Analysis and Related Interventions

The overall goal of nursing management of cognitive and mental health disorders in children is to help the child and family reach an optimal level of functioning. This may be achieved through interventions designed to decrease the impact of stressors on the child's life. After recognizing and analyzing cues from a thorough assessment, the nurse might identify several patient problems, including:

- Malnutrition risk
- Delayed development risk
- Impulsivity
- Impaired social interaction
- Coping impairment
- Hopelessness
- Caregiver role strain risk
- Knowledge deficiency

These patient problems provide suggestions for nursing care planning or concept mapping for the child with a mental health disorder or an alteration behavior, cognition, or development. Suggested interventions with rationales are provided as follows. Care planning should be individualized, based on the child's and family's needs. Refer to Chapter 36 for the nursing process for pain management and to Chapter 33 for nursing interventions related to caregiver role strain risk. Additional information will be included later in the chapter as it relates to nursing management of children with specific disorders, as well as particular nursing interventions for deficient knowledge.

After completing an assessment of John, the nurse noted difficulty sitting still for the examination, that he was easily distracted and frustrated, and demonstrated a labile mood. Based on the assessment findings, what would your top three patient problems be for John?

See the Healthy People 2030 box.

HEALTHY PEOPLE 2030

Objective	Nursing Significance
Increase the proportion of children with mental health problems who receive treatment and increase the number of children receiving preventive mental health care in school.	• Screen all children and adolescents for mental health problems. • Support families with finding and following up on appropriate treatment. • Assist schools with mental health screenings (either physically or through educating others).

Healthy People Objectives retrieved from http://www.healthypeople.gov

Nursing Analysis

Malnutrition risk; risk factors include insufficient dietary intake, insufficient interest in food, body mass index (BMI) of less than the 5th percentile for age, satiety immediately upon ingesting food, or weight loss with adequate food intake.

Goal/Outcome

The child or adolescent will demonstrate appropriate growth, making gains in weight and stature as appropriate.

Improving Nutritional Intake (interventions with *rationale*)

- Provide favorite foods *to encourage the child with poor appetite to eat more.*
- Assist families with choosing nutrient-rich foods *so that the food the child does eat is most beneficial.*

For the child with an eating disorder:

- Mutually establish a contract related to treatment *to promote the child's sense of control.*
- Provide mealtime structure, *as clear limits let the child know what the expectations are.*
- Encourage the child to choose foods and timing of meals *to develop independence in eating habits.*
- Ensure the eating environment is pleasant and relaxed with minimal distractions *to minimize the child's anxiety and guilt about not eating.*
- Withdraw attention if the child refuses to eat; *secondary gain is minimized if refusal to eat is ignored.*
- Provide continuous supervision during the meal and for 30 minutes following it *so that the child cannot conceal or dispose of food or induce vomiting.*

Nursing Analysis

Delayed development risk; risk factors include inadequate nutrition, presence of abuse, behavioral disorder, chronic (mental) illness.

Goal/Outcome

The child will demonstrate progress toward developmental milestones; the child expresses interest in the environment and people around them and interacts with the environment in an age-appropriate way.

Promoting Development (interventions with *rationale*)

- Use therapeutic play and adaptive toys *to facilitate developmental functioning.*
- Provide stimulating environment when possible *to maximize potential for growth and development.*
- Praise accomplishments and emphasize the child's abilities *to improve self-esteem and encourage feelings of confidence and competence.*
- Follow through with physical, occupational, and speech therapists' recommendations *to maximize exposure to exercises designed to increase the child's skills.*
- Determine parents' expectations of the child's future achievement *to help them work toward these goals.*

Nursing Analysis

Impulsivity related to alteration in cognitive functioning or development, or mood or personality disorder as evidenced by acting without thinking, irritability, sensation seeking, temper outbursts, or violence

Goal/Outcome

Child's impulse control will improve: The child will improve in ability to control impulses, remain free from physical harm, and participate in usual activities as able.

Reducing Impulsivity (interventions with *rationale*)

- Observe for causes of impulsivity *to provide a baseline for assessment and intervention.*
- Perform an age-appropriate mental status examination *to determine the extent of altered thinking.*
- Work together with the child and family to develop a plan for controlling impulses; *individualization will be necessary.*
- Listen carefully and seek clarification *to determine the basis for the child's agitation or other behaviors.*
- Provide validation of the child's thoughts and feelings *to improve trust in the relationship.*
- Establish a daily routine *to provide the child with a sense of security.*

Nursing Analysis

Impaired social interaction related to disturbance in self-concept or thought processes or insufficient skill so as to enhance mutuality as evidenced by dysfunctional interaction or impaired social functioning

(impulsivity, intrusive behavior, feelings of unattractiveness or unworthiness)

Goal/Outcome

The child will demonstrate socially acceptable skills, interacting successfully with peers and in the educational setting, completing tasks as required.

Promoting Appropriate Social Interaction (interventions with *rationale*)

- Identify factors that may aggravate the child's performance *to minimize stimuli that exacerbate the child's undesired behaviors.*
- Modify the environment to decrease distracting stimuli *as the child's ability to deal with external stimuli may be impaired.*
- Ensure that the child hears their name and makes eye contact prior to conversing or receiving instructions *so that the child is engaged and has increased ability to follow through.*
- State expectations for tasks or behaviors clearly *as understanding is necessary to ensure completion.*
- Provide positive feedback for appropriate behaviors or task completion, *encouraging the child to adopt expectations into their behaviors and routine.*

Nursing Analysis

Coping impairment related to inadequate confidence in ability to deal with a situation, insufficient sense of control, or situational crisis as evidenced by alteration in confidence, destructive behavior toward self or others, substance misuse, or ineffective coping strategies

Goal/Outcome

The child will demonstrate improved coping, verbalize feelings, socially engage, and demonstrate problem-solving skills.

Promoting Coping Skills (interventions with *rationale*)

- Encourage discussion of thoughts and feelings, *as this is an initial step toward learning to deal with them appropriately.*
- Provide positive feedback for appropriate discussion, *as this increases the likelihood of continuing performance.*
- Demonstrate unconditional acceptance of the child as a person *to increase self-esteem in the child who has been feeling rejected.*
- Set clear limits on behavior as needed *so the child has a structure to adhere to.*
- Teach the child problem-solving skills *as an alternative to acting-out behaviors.*
- Role model appropriate social and conversational skills *so the child can see what is expected in a nonthreatening manner.*

Nursing Analysis

Hopelessness related to chronic stress (due to mental, behavioral, or developmental disorder), social isolation, or history of abandonment, as evidenced by passivity, decrease in affect, alteration in sleep pattern, or despondent verbal cues

Goal/Outcome

Child will display a sense of hope; they will verbalize feelings, participate in care, and make positive statements.

Promoting Hope (interventions with *rationale*)

- Monitor and document potential for suicide, *as hopelessness often leads to suicidal ideation.*
- Assist the child to identify reasons for hope and for living *so the nurse is aware of the child's values.*
- Help the child set goals that are important to them *to allow the child to see possibilities.*
- Encourage simple decision making on a daily basis, *as hopelessness often occurs as a response to loss of control.*
- Assist the child in identifying positive qualities in themselves and their life *to facilitate the development of hope.*
- Involve parents or others the child loves in the child's care *as social support is critical to the development of hope.*

For each of your top three patient problems for John, choose the top three nursing interventions.

DEVELOPMENTAL AND BEHAVIORAL DISORDERS

Developmental and behavioral disorders make up a large proportion of mental health disorders in children. They include learning disabilities, intellectual disability, autism spectrum disorder (ASD), and attention-deficit/hyperactivity disorder (ADHD).

Learning Disabilities

Up to 15% of children and adolescents have learning disabilities, and in children with chronic illness, learning disabilities are two times more common than in the general population (von Hahn, 2023a). The essential characteristic of learning disability is an innate cognitive difficulty resulting in lower academic achievement than would be expected for the child's intellectual potential (von Hahn, 2023a). Learning disabilities become evident when a child of average intelligence has difficulty mastering basic academic skills. Learning disabilities can affect the child's ability to listen, speak, read, write, and perform mathematics. For example:

- Children with dyslexia have difficulty with reading, writing, and spelling.
- Children with dyscalculia have problems with mathematics and computation.
- Children with dyspraxia have problems with manual dexterity and coordination.
- Children with dysgraphia have difficulty producing the written word (composition, spelling, and writing).

TAKE NOTE!

Sensory processing disorder may be mistaken for a learning disability, but it is not and should be treated differently (Box 50.1).

Therapeutic Management

Therapeutic management may involve remedial or compensatory approaches or may use interventions directed toward social–emotional problems. The focus of the remedial approach is to improve specific skills. The compensatory approach helps the child compensate for the disability, rather than attempting to directly correct it (von Hahn, 2023b). Social–emotional problems may result from frustration or low self-esteem related to capabilities. These may respond to supportive interventions and improvement in coping.

CONSIDER THIS!

Victor Johnson, a third grader with learning disabilities, tells the nurse, "I get made fun of at school." He begins to sniffle and says, "Everybody calls me stupid. It hurts my feelings." Victor's parent adds, "I really just don't know how to help." How should the nurse reply? What would be the most therapeutic response?

BOX 50.1 Sensory Processing Disorder (Also Called Sensory Integration Dysfunction)

- A neurologic disorder in which the child cannot organize sensory input used in daily living
- Hyposensitivity or hypersensitivity to sensory input
- Results in overreaction to different textures, decreasing the child's ability to participate in the world
- Preterm and low-birth-weight infants are at increased risk compared with other infants.
- Occupational and other therapies may increase the child's ability to function.

Data from Star Center Foundation. (2024). *Understanding sensory processing disorder.* https://www.spdstar.org/basic/understanding-sensory-processing-disorder

Nursing Assessment

Elicit the health history, noting risk factors such as a family history of learning disability, problems during pregnancy or birth, prenatal alcohol or drug exposure, low birth weight, premature or prolonged labor, head injury, poor nutritional status or failure to thrive, or lead poisoning. Obtain detailed information about the educational difficulties the child is experiencing (e.g., they seem to do fine in math but always reverse letters when reading). A thorough physical examination may reveal clues to **comorbid** (simultaneously existing) conditions. Ensure the child has undergone a comprehensive education evaluation with assessment testing to diagnose the specific learning disability. Testing may be performed by a school, educational, developmental, or clinical psychologist; occupational therapist; speech and language therapist; or other developmental specialist, depending on the areas of learning with which the child is experiencing difficulty.

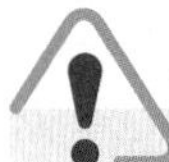

CLINICAL REASONING ALERT!

If a child cannot speak in sentences by 30 months of age; does not have understandable speech 50% of the time by age 3 years; cannot sit still for a short story by 3 to 5 years of age; or cannot tie shoes, cut, button, or hop by 5 to 6 years of age, refer the child to be evaluated for a learning disability.

Nursing Management

Ensure families are aware of their child's rights under the Individuals with Disabilities Education Act (IDEA), which was reapproved in 2004 (108th Congress, 2004). IDEA offers protection from discrimination and the right to assistance in the school or workplace. Each child will need an individualized education plan (IEP) that reflects their particular needs, which must then be provided through the school system. Offer encouragement and support to families as they advocate for their child. Follow up at subsequent health care visits to determine if the child is receiving the services they need to optimize their potential for success. Refer families for additional resources through the National Center for Learning Disabilities, Learning Disabilities Online, or the Center for Learning Differences.

Intellectual Disability

Intellectual disability refers to a functional state in which significant limitations in intellectual status and adaptive behavior (functioning in daily life) develop before the age of 18 to 22 years. Intellectual disability occurs in about 1% to 2% of the population (Pivalizza, 2024). The range of impairments associated with the intellectual disability is variable. Impairments in the adaptive domains of conceptual, social, or practical assist with determining the severity of intellectual disability (from mild to profound) (Pivalizza, 2024).

In the past, people with intellectual disability were confined to institutions and were thought to be harmful to society. In the early 21st century, most children with intellectual disability are receiving their education in public schools with their peers and living at home with their families or elsewhere in the community. Only the most severely affected individuals require separate classrooms or schools.

Pathophysiology

In many instances of intellectual disability, the exact cause remains unknown. Prenatal errors in central nervous system development may be responsible. Other potential causes include an insult or damage to the brain during the prenatal, perinatal, or postnatal period. Prenatal exposure to alcohol or other drugs may impact cognitive development as well. Motor problems such as hypertonia or hypotonia, tremor, ataxia, or clumsiness, or visual motor problems may occur concomitantly with intellectual disability. In addition, functioning at a higher level may be prevented when a learning disability or sensory processing impairment is also present. Intellectual disability may be categorized according to severity of impairment across domains. See Table 50.2.

Therapeutic Management

The primary goal of therapeutic management of children with intellectual disability is to provide appropriate educational experiences that allow the child to achieve a level of functioning and self-sufficiency needed for existence in the home, community, work, and leisure settings. A multidisciplinary approach may be used, and the child's conceptual, social, practical, and intellectual abilities will drive school placement and the focus of the educational experience. The majority of individuals with intellectual disability require only minimal support in the school or home setting, and these individuals are able to achieve some level of self-sufficiency. Only some children and adults with intellectual disability require extensive support and require long-term caregiving.

Nursing Assessment

Perform developmental screening at each health care visit to identify developmental delays early. Elicit the health history, determining the mental and adaptive capacities of the child's parents and other family members. Obtain a detailed pregnancy and birth history. Document sequence and age of attainment of developmental milestones. Note history of motor, visual, or language difficulties. Assess the child's health history for risk factors such as preterm or postterm birth, low birth weight, birth injury, prenatal or neonatal infection, prenatal alcohol or drug exposure, genetic syndrome, chromosomal alteration, metabolic disease, exposure to toxins (e.g., lead), head injury or other trauma, nutritional deficiency, cerebral malformation, and other brain diseases or mental health disorders. Note history of or concomitant seizure disorder, orthopedic problems, speech problems, or vision or hearing deficit.

For the child with known intellectual disability, assess language, sensory, and psychomotor functioning. Determine the child's ability to toilet, dress, and feed themselves. Ask the parents about involvement with school and community services and support.

On physical examination, note dysmorphic features (possibly mild) consistent with certain syndromes (e.g., fetal alcohol syndrome; Box 50.2). Evaluate the newborn or metabolic screening results. Computed tomography

TABLE 50.2 Severity of Intellectual Disability

Severity	Level of Support	Conceptual	Social	Practical
Mild	Intermittent	Requires academic supports	Immature social skills and personal judgment	Usually independent in activities of daily living
Moderate	Limited	Complex tasks require substantial support.	Social cues, judgment, and life decisions need regular support	Independent self-care with moderate supports
Severe	Extensive	Little understanding of written language, time; require extensive supports	Benefit from healthy supportive interactions	Require significant and ongoing supervision for activities of daily living
Profound	Pervasive	May use objects in a goal-directed fashion	May understand gestures and emotional cues; use nonverbal expression	Dependent upon support for all activities of daily living

BOX 50.2 **Fetal Alcohol Syndrome**

- Results from in utero alcohol exposure
- Typical facial features include low nasal bridge with short upturned nose, flattened midface, long philtrum with narrow upper lip.
- Poor coordination, skeletal abnormalities
- Microcephaly
- Failure to thrive
- Hearing loss

Data from Reynolds, A., Angulo, A., Breheney, M., Green, J., & Goldson, E. (2022). Child development and behavior. In M. Bunik, W. W. Hay, M. J. Levin, & M. J. Abzug (Eds.), *Current diagnosis & treatment: Pediatrics* (26th ed.). McGraw-Hill Education.

or magnetic resonance imaging of the head may be performed to evaluate the brain structure. Thyroid function tests may be ordered to rule out thyroid problems leading to developmental delay.

TAKE NOTE!

Due to the extent of cognition required to understand and produce speech, the most sensitive early indicator of intellectual disability is delayed language development.

Nursing Management

When children with intellectual disability are admitted to the hospital (usually for some other physical or medical condition), it is important for the nurse to continue the child's usual home routine. Follow through with feeding and motor supports that the child uses. Ensure that the child is closely supervised and remains free from harm. Allow parents time to verbalize frustrations or fears. For some families, the caregiving burden is extensive and lifelong; arrange for respite care as available. Support the child's strengths, and assist the child and family with following through with therapy or treatment designed to enhance the child's functioning. Assist with the development of the child's IEP as appropriate.

Autism Spectrum Disorder

ASD has its onset in infancy or early childhood and affects one in 68 children (Reynolds et al., 2022). Brain development and function and, ultimately, social behavior and communication are affected (Sohl, 2022). The spectrum ranges from mild to severe. Some children with ASD may be intellectually disabled, requiring lifelong supervision, but the majority will display expected to high intelligence levels (Reynolds et al., 2022). ASD behaviors may be first noticed in infancy as developmental delays or between the ages of 12 and 36 months, when the child exhibits regression or loses previously acquired skills. Parental concerns about development may be sensitive indicators of the development of ASD.

Pathophysiology

Although the exact etiology of ASD continues to be unknown, genetic factors have been well studied in these children, and ASD is considered to be mainly a genetic disorder; however, there may also be issues with brain connectivity (Reynolds et al., 2022). Children with ASD display impaired social interactions and communication as well as perseverative or stereotypic behaviors. They may have difficulty developing interpersonal relationships and experience social isolation.

Therapeutic Management

There are no medications or treatments available to cure ASD. The goal of therapeutic management is for the child to reach optimal functioning within the bounds of the disorder. Each child's treatment is individualized; behavioral and communication therapies are important. Children with ASD respond well to highly structured educational environments, so early, intensive behavioral interventions are necessary. Stimulants may be used to control hyperactivity, and antipsychotic medications are sometimes helpful in children with repetitive and aggressive behaviors.

Some families may be drawn to the use of complementary and alternative medical therapies in attempts to treat a child with ASD. They may use vitamins and nutritional supplements, herbs or restrictive diets, music therapy, art therapy, and sensory integration techniques. The effectiveness of these therapies has not been shown by studies to be beneficial, and herbal and other supplements may interact with prescribed medications (Weissman & Harris, 2022). However, music therapy used within a comprehensive behavioral program has no harmful effects and may improve ASD severity and the child's quality of life (Weissman & Harris, 2022). See Evidence-Based Practice Box 50.1.

Nursing Assessment

Elicit the health history, noting delay or regression in developmental skills, particularly speech and language abilities. Failure to point at objects and to gaze at an object jointly with another by 18 months are concerning signs. The most common early characteristics are a consistent failure to orient to one's name, regard people directly, use gestures, and develop speech (Reynolds et al., 2022). The child may be nonverbal, utter only sounds (not words), or repeat words or phrases over and over. The parent may report that the infant or toddler spends hours in repetitive activity and demonstrates bizarre motor and stereotypic behaviors. The infant may resist cuddling, lack eye contact, be indifferent to touch or affection, and show little change in facial expression. Toddlers may display hyperactivity, aggression, temper

EVIDENCE-BASED PRACTICE 50.1

Early Behavioral Intervention for Autism Spectrum Disorder

STUDY

As the incidence of ASD continues to rise, it is necessary to evaluate the efficacy of interventions for ASD. Early intensive behavioral intervention (delivered at 20 to 40 hours per week) is a commonly used therapy for ASD. The authors reviewed one randomized controlled trial and four clinical control trials with a total of 219 participants under the age of 6 years.

Findings

The Vineland Adaptive Behavioral Scales was used to assess adaptive behavior following treatment. The authors noted that early intensive behavioral intervention resulted in an improvement in adaptive behavior, although it did not change the severity score.

Nursing Implications

Caring for a child with ASD can be challenging for families. If adaptive behaviors can be improved, both the child and the parents will benefit. Assist families with finding schools or centers utilizing early intensive behavioral intervention. Support and encourage parents to encourage interventions in the home setting as prescribed.

Data from Reichow, B., Hume, K., Barton, E. E., & Boyd, B. A. (2018). Early intensive behavioral intervention (EIBI) for young children with autism spectrum disorders (ASD). *Cochrane Database of Systematic Reviews*, (5), CD009260. https://doi.org/10.1002/14651858.CD009260.pub3

tantrums, or self-injurious behaviors, such as head banging or hand biting. The history may also reveal hypersensitivity to touch or hyposensitivity to pain.

Assess the child's functional status, including behavior, nutrition, sleep, speech and language, education needs, and developmental or neurologic limitations. Assist with screening, using an approved ASD screening tool such as the Modified Checklist for Autism in Toddlers-Revised (M-CHAT-R), which is recommended for administration at 18 months of age, and then again at 24 to 30 months of age. Additional screening tools include the Social Communication Questionnaire (SCQ) and the Pervasive Developmental Disorders Screening Test-II (PDDST-II).

Perform a thorough physical examination. Observe the infant or toddler for lack of eye contact, failure to look at objects pointed to by the examiner, failure to point to themselves, failure to let their needs be known, perseverative play activities, and unusual behavior such as hand flapping or spinning. Measure growth parameters, noting, in particular, head circumference (macrocephaly or microcephaly may be associated with ASD). Note the presence of large, prominent, or posteriorly rotated ears. Examine the skin for hypopigmented or hyperpigmented lesions. Note asymmetry of nerve function or palsy, hypertonia, hypotonia, alterations in deep tendon reflexes, toe-walking, loose gait, or poor coordination. Obtain hearing screening results and ascertain that lead screening has been performed.

TAKE NOTE!

Screen all infants and toddlers for warning signs of ASD:

- *Does not imitate*
- *Lack of interest in joint attention*
- *Avoiding eye contact*
- *Delayed language development*
- *Failure to develop symbolic-imaginative play (pretending)*
- *Difficulty with minor changes or transitions* (Augustyn & von Hahn, 2023)

Additional signs at specific ages include:

- At 12 months, does not respond to name
- At 14 months, does not show interest in items by pointing
- At 18 months, does not participate in pretend play (Sohl, 2022)

Nursing Management

When children are initially diagnosed with ASD, provide parents with an extensive amount of emotional support, professional guidance, and education about the disorder while they are attempting to adjust to the diagnosis. Assess the fit between the child's developmental needs and the treatment plan. Help parents overcome barriers to obtaining appropriate education, developmental, and behavioral treatment programs. Ensure that the child younger than 36 months of age receives services via the local early intervention program and that children 3 years and older have an IEP in place if enrolled in the public school system. Stress the importance of rigid, unchanging routines, as children with ASD often have difficulty when their routine changes (which is likely to occur if the child must be hospitalized for another condition). Many specialized schools exist for children with significant developmental disorders, although some are extremely expensive. Assess the parents' need for respite care and make referrals accordingly. Provide positive feedback to parents for supporting their child's unique needs.

ATRAUMATIC CARE

Provide family-centered care, being sure to treat the family and not just the child. Minimize parent–child separation.

Attention-Deficit/Hyperactivity Disorder

ADHD is the most common neurodevelopmental disorder of childhood, estimated to affect 9% to 15% of school-aged children (Krull & Chan, 2023). It is characterized by inattention, impulsivity, distractibility, and hyperactivity. Three subtypes of ADHD exist: hyperactive–impulsive, inattentive, and combined. The child with ADHD has a disruption in learning ability, socialization, and adherence, placing demands on the child, parents, teachers, and community. Children with ADHD often have a comorbidity (disorder accompanying the primary illness) such as oppositional defiant disorder, conduct disorder, an anxiety disorder, depression, a less severe developmental disorder, an auditory processing disorder, or learning or reading disabilities (Krull & Chan, 2023). Comparison Chart 50.1 gives information about oppositional defiant disorder and conduct disorder to distinguish them from ADHD.

Pathophysiology

Although the exact cause of ADHD remains unidentified, an alteration in the catecholamine neurotransmitter system may be responsible, but genetics, environmental exposures, and structural brain abnormalities may play a role (Krull & Chan, 2023). The symptoms of impulsivity, hyperactivity, and inattention begin before 7 years of age and persist longer than 6 months. Symptoms exist in the school and home settings, impairing family and social interactions. Children and adolescents with ADHD may experience frustration, labile moods, emotional outbursts, peer rejection, poor school performance, and low self-esteem. They may also have difficulty with metacognitive skills like organization, time management, and the ability to break a project down into a series of smaller tasks. Box 50.3 provides criteria for the diagnosis of ADHD (Reynolds et al., 2022).

BOX 50.3 Diagnosis of Attention-Deficit/Hyperactivity Disorder

Presence of six or more of the following findings in the child 17 years of age and younger:

- Failure to pay close attention
- Careless mistakes on school work
- Difficulty paying attention to tasks or play
- Doesn't listen
- Doesn't follow through
- Doesn't complete tasks
- Doesn't understand instructions
- Difficulty with organization
- Avoids, dislikes, or fails to engage in activities requiring mental effort
- Loses things needed for task completion
- Easily distracted
- Forgetful
- Fidgety or squirmy
- Often out of seat
- Activity inappropriate to the situation
- Cannot engage in quiet play
- Always on the go
- Talks excessively
- Blurts out answers
- Has difficulty waiting their turn
- Often interrupts or intrudes on others

Additionally, symptoms have been present in two or more settings, and at least two of the symptoms occurred prior to age 12; symptoms have persisted beyond 6 months and to a degree inconsistent with developmental level or negatively interfere with social or academic performance. Symptoms are not associated with purely oppositional behavior or as a component of a psychotic disorder and cannot be explained by the diagnosis of a different mental health disorder.

Data from Reynolds, A., Angulo, A., Breheney, M., Green, J., & Goldson, E. (2022). Child development and behavior. In M. Bunik, W. W. Hay, M. J. Levin, & M. J. Abzug (Eds.), *Current diagnosis & treatment: Pediatrics* (26th ed.). McGraw-Hill Education.

COMPARISON CHART 50.1 Oppositional Defiant Disorder Versus Conduct Disorder

Oppositional Defiant Disorder	Conduct Disorder
• Excessive arguing with adults • Frequent temper tantrums • Active defiance • Revenge-seeking behaviors • Frequent resentment or anger • Touchiness; easily annoyed • Nonadherence with adult requests or limits • Blaming of others for misbehavior or mistakes	• Bullying and threatening of others • Initiation of physical fights • Weapon use to cause others harm • Physical cruelty to animals or people • Destruction of property or arson • Lying and stealing • Serious violation of rules, like staying out past curfew, truancy, running away • Use of force in sexual activity

Based on Kelsay, K., Glaze, K., & Talmi, A. (2022). Child & adolescent psychiatric disorders & psychosocial aspects of pediatrics. In M. Bunik, W. W. Hay, M. J. Levin, & M. J. Abzug (Eds.), *Current pediatric diagnosis and treatment* (26th ed.). McGraw-Hill Education.

Therapeutic Management

Medication management of ADHD includes the use of psychostimulants, nonstimulant norepinephrine reuptake inhibitors, and/or alpha-agonist antihypertensive agents. These medications are not a cure for ADHD but help increase the child's ability to pay attention and decrease the level of impulsive behavior. The child's activity level is not usually affected. Behavior therapy and classroom restructuring may be useful as part of the therapeutic management plan. Concomitant disorders, such as anxiety, should also be treated (see the discussion of anxiety disorders that follows).

Nursing Assessment

For a full description of the assessment phase of the nursing process, refer to the "Clinical Judgment and the Nursing Process" section. Assessment findings pertinent to ADHD are discussed here.

HEALTH HISTORY

Elicit a description of the behavioral issue or school performance problem. Explore the child's history for risk factors such as head trauma, lead exposure, cigarette smoke exposure, prematurity, and low birth weight. The past history may also reveal a larger than usual number of accidents. Determine if there is a family history of ADHD. Question the parent about school behavior. The school-aged child may be unable to stay on task, talk out of turn, leave their desk frequently, and either neglect to complete in-class and homework assignments or forget to turn them in. The adolescent may be inattentive in school, poorly organized, and forgetful.

Several behavioral checklists are available that may assist in the diagnosis of ADHD. They may be completed by the child's teacher and/or parent and focus on behavior patterns related to conduct or learning problems, social competence, anxiety, activity level, and attention. Obtain the completed behavioral checklists (usually one from the parent and one from the teacher) as well as any school records or testing performed.

PHYSICAL EXAMINATION

Perform vision and hearing screening to rule out difficulty with vision or hearing as the cause of poor school performance. Observe the preschool child's behavior, noting quickness, agility, fearlessness, and the desire to touch or explore everything in the room. The older child or adolescent may have difficulty staying on task during the examination or change the subject frequently while conversing.

LABORATORY AND DIAGNOSTIC TESTS

No definitive laboratory or diagnostic test is available for the identification of ADHD. A complete blood count may be performed to rule out anemia, and thyroid hormone levels may be drawn to determine whether they are within the expected range.

Nursing Management

The child's inattention, high activity level, impulsivity, and distractibility can be challenging for caregivers. Parents may doubt their ability to be effective parents or may view their child in a negative light. Children with ADHD may also feel bad about themselves. Provide emotional support, allowing enough time for the family to air their concerns. Work with the child and family to develop goals such as completion of homework, improved communication, and increasing independence in self-care.

Assist the family in advocating for their child's needs through the public school system. The child is entitled to a developmentally appropriate education via an IEP as necessary (refer to Chapter 34 for additional information about special education). The IEP should be updated as needed. Ensure coordination of health and school services. Flag the child's chart and set up a schedule for systematic communication with the family and school. Teach families and school personnel to use behavioral techniques such as time-out, positive reinforcement, reward or privilege withdrawal, or a token system. The token system rewards appropriate behavior with a token and results in a token being taken away if inappropriate behavior occurs. At the end of a specified period of time, the tokens may be exchanged for a prize or privilege. Refer families to local support groups and the national ADHD support group.

Explain that stimulant medications should be taken in the morning to mitigate the risk of the adverse effect of insomnia. Some children may experience decreased appetite, so giving the medication with or after the meal may be beneficial. The child may feel "different" from their peers if they have to visit the school nurse for a lunchtime dose of ADHD medication; this may lead to nonadherence and a subsequent increase in ADHD symptoms with deterioration in school work. In this situation, encourage the family to explore with their provider the option of one of the newer extended-release or once-daily ADHD medications. See Dosage Calculation Box 50.1.

DOSAGE CALCULATION BOX 50.1

Child's weight: 50 lb

Medication order: Start methylphenidate 10 mg PO now.

Per the *Pediatric Dosage Handbook*, for initial dosing, the recommended dose is 0.3 mg/kg/dose.

Is the ordered dose safe?

TOURETTE SYNDROME

Tourette syndrome consists of multiple motor tics and one or more vocal tics occurring either simultaneously or at different times. Children are not tic-free for longer than 3 months. Tics are defined as sudden, rapid, recurrent stereotypical movements and/or sounds over which the child appears to have no control. Tourette syndrome affects about 0.5% of children with onset before 21 years of age (Jankovic, 2023).

Comorbid conditions such as ADHD, obsessive-compulsive disorder (OCD), and others may occur in up to 60% of children with Tourette syndrome (incidence depending upon the comorbid condition) (Jankovic, 2023). The exact pathophysiologic mechanism of Tourette syndrome has yet to be identified, although genetics does seem to play a part. Therapeutic management is highly individualized and involves psychopharmacology and behavioral therapies. Habit reversal training may help in some children.

Nursing Assessment

Evaluate the health history for the occurrence of tics. The child may be embarrassed about or ashamed of the tics, and the parents may feel fearful, angry, or guilty. Determine the presence of symptoms of comorbid conditions. Elicit the child's past health history, noting a family history of tics. Assess the child's psychosocial history to determine the extent to which the tics interfere with friendship, school performance, and self-esteem. Observe the child for simple or complex motor tics. Vocal tics such as sniffling, grunting, clicking, or word utterance may occur. Perform a thorough physical examination, which is usually as expected.

Nursing Management

Inform families that the tics may become more noticeable or severe during times of stress and less pronounced when the child is focused on an activity such as watching TV, reading, or playing a video game. Help the family build on the child's functional behaviors and adaptive skills to improve the child's self-esteem. Encourage the family to pursue classroom accommodations such as allowing for "tic breaks," taking untimed tests or tests in another room, or using note takers or tape recording. Support the family's decisions related to medication use and therapy, and provide appropriate education about the particular drugs and therapies. *Teaching the Tiger* by M. P. Dornbush and S. K. Pruitt (Hope Press) is useful for teachers of children with Tourette syndrome. For additional support, refer families to Tourette Syndrome Association, Tourette Syndrome Foundation of Canada, or Tourette Syndrome Plus.

EATING DISORDERS

Eating disorders include pica, rumination, anorexia nervosa, and bulimia. They affect a significant number of children, especially adolescents. Pica, which occurs most frequently in 2- to 3-year-olds, is an eating disorder in which the child ingests (over at least a 1-month period) a nonnutritive material such as paint, clay, or sand. Rumination is an eating disorder occurring in infants in which the baby regurgitates partially digested food or formula and expels or swallows it. The numbers of children affected by pica and rumination are not known. This discussion will focus on anorexia nervosa and bulimia, as they are more commonly encountered.

Anorexia nervosa and bulimia are common eating disorders affecting primarily adolescents, although younger children may also be affected. In American society, thinness is highly valued, compounding the problem. The lifetime prevalence rate for eating disorders is about 8% for females and 2% for males, and these problems often arise in childhood, particularly adolescence (Guarda, 2023). Anorexia nervosa is characterized by dramatic weight loss as a result of decreased food intake and sharply increased physical exercise. Bulimia refers to a cycle of normal food intake, followed by binge eating and then purging. Typically, the adolescent with bulimia remains around an expected weight. Complications of anorexia and bulimia include fluid and electrolyte imbalance, decreased blood volume, cardiac dysrhythmias, esophagitis, rupture of the esophagus or stomach, tooth loss, and menstrual problems.

Therapeutic management may occur in either the inpatient or outpatient setting. In either case, a multidisciplinary approach including individual and family therapy as well as nutritional therapy is needed for the best chance at successful treatment. Typically, medications are not an initial or primary treatment for eating disorders (Yager, 2022).

Nursing Assessment

Determine the health history, noting risk factors such as family history, female sex, White race, preoccupation with appearance, obsessive traits, and low self-esteem. Adolescents with anorexia may have a history of constipation, syncope, secondary amenorrhea, abdominal pain, and periodic episodes of cold hands and feet. Parents usually note the chief complaint as weight loss. Note history of depression in the child with bulimia. Evaluate the child's self-concept, and pay attention to multiple fears, high need for acceptance, disordered body image, and perfectionism.

Perform a thorough physical examination. The child with anorexia is usually severely underweight, with a BMI of less than 17. Note cachectic appearance, dry sallow skin, thinning scalp hair, soft sparse body hair, and nail pitting. Measure vital signs, noting low temperature, bradycardia, or hypotension. Auscultate the heart, noting murmur as a result of mitral valve prolapse (occurs in about one third of adolescents with anorexia).

The adolescent with bulimia will be of expected weight or slightly overweight. Inspect the hands for calluses on the backs of the knuckles and split fingernails. Inspect the mouth and oropharynx for eroded dental enamel, red gums, and inflamed throat from self-induced vomiting.

Careful laboratory and diagnostic evaluation of serum electrolytes and an electrocardiogram are needed in adolescents with anorexia and bulimia due to severe electrolyte disturbances, and cardiac arrhythmias often occur.

TAKE NOTE!

An adolescent with anorexia nervosa may experience amenorrhea, hypothermia, low blood pressure, and bradycardia. The nurse may also note soft hair on the individual's back and arms.

Nursing Management

Most children with eating disorders can be treated successfully on an outpatient basis, although this treatment may require many months. Those with anorexia who display severe weight loss, unstable vital signs, food refusal, or arrested pubertal development or who require enteral nutrition will need to be hospitalized. Refeeding syndrome (involving cardiovascular, hematologic, and neurologic complications) may occur in the adolescent with severe malnourishment with anorexia if rapid nutritional replacement is given. Therefore, slow refeeding is essential to avoid complications. Give phosphorus supplements as ordered. Assess vital signs frequently for orthostatic hypotension, irregular and decreased pulse, or hypothermia.

Consult the nutritionist for assistance with calculating caloric needs and determining an appropriate diet. Aim for a weight gain goal of 0.5 to 2 lb per week. Instruct the child and family to keep a daily journal of intake, **bingeing** (excessive consumption) and **purging** (forced vomiting) behaviors, mood, and exercise. The journal may be used as an assessment tool as well as to document progress toward recovery. Assist the child and family in planning a suitably structured routine for the child that includes meals, snacks, and appropriate physical activity.

Use the physical findings associated with anorexia to educate the child about the consequences of malnutrition and how they can be remedied with adequate nutrient intake. Refer the adolescent, as appropriate, to behavior or group therapy. Assess the child's need for medical intervention for concomitant depression or anxiety (some also require psychotropic medications). Provide emotional support and positive reinforcement to the child and family. Refer the family to local support groups or online resources such as the Academy for Eating Disorders or the National Eating Disorders Association.

MOOD DISORDERS

Mood disorders in children include depressive disorders and bipolar disorder. It is difficult to quantify the incidence of depression in children under age 5 years due to lack of sophistication of communication skills. In prepubertal children, about 1% to 3% are diagnosed with depression compared to 9% of adolescents (Kelsay et al., 2022). Children may experience major depressive disorder or dysthymic disorder. Females are twice as likely to be affected as males, particularly during adolescence. Bipolar disorder refers to a condition of alternating manic and depressive episodes, and its incidence in children is unknown (Birmaher, 2023). During the manic episode, mood is significantly elevated, and the child displays excess energy.

Depression may cause significant alterations in school performance and social relationships. Anxiety disorders and disruptive behavior may occur together with depression. Substance misuse may also occur concurrently with depression. Divorce and serious family issues may contribute to the development of depression because of the ongoing stress they place on the child and their strong psychological impact.

Children and adolescents experiencing depressive episodes may harm themselves purposefully without intent to kill themselves (**suicide**). They may hit, cut, or burn themselves. Additionally, children with depression are at risk for suicide (Birmaher, 2023). The Centers for Disease Control and Prevention (CDC) Youth Risk Behavior Surveillance 2011-2021 Report revealed that in 2021, the percentage of adolescents who had seriously considered suicide increased to 22%; 18% made a suicide plan, and 10% had attempted suicide (CDC, 2023).

Pathophysiology

Depression in children is likely multifactorial in nature. It may result from neuroendocrine changes (particularly serotonin), genetic transmission, adverse early life events, and/or family factors. Family factors include abuse, parental early-onset mood disorder, parental substance misuse or criminality, or lack of family cohesion and increased incidence of discord (Brent & Maalouf, 2019).

Therapeutic Management

Children with mood disorders usually benefit from psychotherapy, often paired with pharmacologic antidepressants (Brent & Maalouf, 2019). This helps the child deal with the psychosocial consequences of their behavior on their interpersonal relationships with others. Crisis management; parental counseling; and individual, group, or family therapy may be useful. Bipolar disorder may be treated with second-generation antipsychotics for mania and antidepressants for depression, ideally combined with psychotherapy (Axelson, 2022).

CLINICAL REASONING ALERT!

Closely observe children taking antidepressants for the development of suicidal ideation.

Nursing Assessment

Children with untreated depression are at high risk for suicide as well as the development of comorbid disorders such as anxiety disorders, substance misuse, eating disorders, self-harm, and disruptive behavioral disorders (such as conduct disorder or ADHD) (Kelsay et al., 2022). The nurse must screen all children for the development of depression.

Health History

Obtain a health history from the child and separately from the parent. Evaluate the child for history of recent changes in behavior, changes in peer relationships, alterations in school performance, withdrawal from previously enjoyed activities, sleep disturbances, changes in eating behaviors, increase in accidents, or risky sexual behavior. If possible, use a standardized depression screening questionnaire, many of which are available.

Ask about potential stressors such as school concerns, conflicts with parents, dating issues, and abuse (physical or sexual). When bipolar disorder is suspected, the history may reveal rapid, pressured speech; increased energy; decreased sleep; flamboyant behavior; or irritability during manic episodes.

Note history of weight loss, failure to thrive, or increased incidence of infections in the infant. For the toddler, note delay or regression in developmental skills, increase in nightmares, or parental reports of clinginess. The preschooler may have a history of loss of interest in newly acquired skills; manifest encopresis, enuresis, anorexia, or binge eating; or make frequent negative self-statements. The parents of a school-aged child may report that they have a depressed, irritable, or aggressive mood.

Assess for risk factors for suicide, which include:

- Previous suicide attempt
- Change in school performance, sleep, or appetite
- Loss of interest in formerly favorite school or other activities
- Feelings of hopelessness or depression
- Statements about thoughts of suicide

Physical Examination

Observe the infant for weepiness, withdrawn behaviors, or a frozen facial expression. Note a sad or expressionless face in the toddler or preschooler. In any age child, observe for apathy. Inspect the entire body surface for self-inflicted injuries (such as cuts or burns), which may or may not be present. The remainder of the physical examination is generally normal unless the child with depression also has a chronic medical condition.

Nursing Management

Nursing management of children and adolescents with mood disorders focuses on education and support and prevention of depression and suicide.

Educating and Supporting the Child and Family

Teach families that mood disorders are biologic conditions, not personality flaws. They will need to understand how to administer antidepressant medications and to monitor for adverse effects. Encourage and praise the child's and family's efforts at following through with cognitive and behavioral therapies. Support the family throughout the process, as treatment may sometimes be lengthy. Refer parents to local support resources or to the Depression and Bipolar Support Alliance or the Child and Adolescent Bipolar Foundation.

• • • ATRAUMATIC CARE • • •

Promote a family's sense of control through effective communication and teaching and providing the family with appropriate resources and referrals.

Preventing Depression and Suicide

Establish a trusting relationship with the children and adolescents with whom you interact, particularly in the primary care setting, school, or clinic. This trusting relationship may encourage children or adolescents to confide feelings or problems earlier than they may do with their parents. Screen all preadolescents and adolescents for the development of depression (Kelsay et al., 2022). Use standardized screening tools such as those listed in Box 50.4. When a potential problem is identified, immediately refer the child for mental health assessment and intervention. It is important to identify depression early so that treatment can start. When a grief-inducing event is impending (such as the death of

BOX **50.4** **Screening Tools for Depression**

The following tools are used to screen for depression:
- Children's Depression Rating Scale-Revised (CDRS-R)
- Center for Epidemiological Studies Depression Scale Modified for Children (CES-DC)
- Weinberg Depression Scale for Children and Adolescents (WDSCA)
- Children's Depression Inventory (CDI)
- Beck Depression Inventory for Youth (BDI-Y)

a family member), begin preventive intervention to help the child to deal with it. Provide appropriate observation for any child exhibiting suicidal ideation. See the Healthy People 2030 box.

HEALTHY PEOPLE **2030**

Objective	Nursing Significance
Reduce suicide attempts by adolescents.	• Screen all children and adolescents for the development of depression. • When depression or excess stress is present, refer the child to the appropriate support.

Healthy People Objectives retrieved from http://www.healthypeople.gov

ANXIETY DISORDERS

Anxiety disorders are the most commonly diagnosed psychiatric conditions among children and adolescents (Bennett & Walkup, 2022). Anxiety often occurs together with other mental health disorders, especially depression. All children experience fear, worry, and shyness. Infants fear loud noises, being startled, and strangers. Toddlers are afraid of the dark and of separation. Preschoolers fear imaginary creatures and body mutilation. School-aged children worry about injury and natural events, and adolescents are anxious about school and social performance. These normal fears produce a certain level of anxiety that is tolerated by most children, but it is important to distinguish developmentally appropriate anxiety from an anxiety disorder.

Anxiety is considered to be a reaction to a perceived or actual threat. The threat may or may not be distorted by the child, and the emotional distress leads to behavioral responses.

THINKING ABOUT **DEVELOPMENT**

Consider the issue of military deployment of a parent. How might a toddler or preschooler react to the parent's absence and return as contrasted with the response of an adolescent? What types of mental health concerns might be manifested in either group?

Types of Anxiety Disorders

Generalized anxiety disorder (GAD) is characterized by unrealistic concerns over past behavior, future events, and personal competence. Social phobia is a disorder characterized by the child or adolescent demonstrating a persistent fear of speaking or eating in front of others, using public restrooms, or speaking to authorities. Selective mutism refers to a persistent failure to speak. Separation anxiety is more common in children than adolescents. In this disorder, the child may need to remain close to the parents, and the child's worries focus on separation themes. OCD is characterized by compulsions (repetitive behaviors such as cleaning, washing, or checking something), which the child performs to reduce anxiety about obsessions (unwanted and intrusive thoughts). Posttraumatic stress disorder (PTSD) is an anxiety disorder that occurs after a child experiences a traumatic event, later experiencing physiologic arousal when a stimulus triggers memories of the event.

Pathophysiology

Anxiety disorders are thought to occur as a result of disrupted modulation within the central nervous system. Underactivation of the serotonergic system and overactivation of the noradrenergic system are thought to be responsible for dysregulation of physiologic arousal and the resulting emotional experience. Disruption of the gamma-aminobutyric acid (GABA) system may also play a role. Genetic factors may also play a role in the development of anxiety disorders, as may family and environmental influences. Additionally, abnormal thoughts or behaviors may have been learned through observation or conditioning (Bennett & Walkup, 2022).

Therapeutic Management

Therapeutic management of anxiety disorders generally involves the use of pharmacologic agents and psychological therapies. Anxiolytics or antidepressants are the most common pharmacologic approaches. Cognitive behavioral therapy; individual, family, or group psychotherapy; and other behavioral interventions such as relaxation techniques such as yoga may also be useful (Shreve et al., 2021).

Nursing Assessment

Children and adolescents do not always directly express anxiety. Therefore, it is important for the nurse to evaluate somatic complaints and perform a careful health history.

Health History

Explore the child's current and past medical history for risk factors such as depression, anxious temperament, family history of anxiety disorders, certain environmental or life experiences (such as parental dysfunction or significant stressful event or trauma), or unstable parental attachment. Elicit the health history, noting history of social inhibition, panic, or "heart racing." Young children may display overactivity, acting out, sleep difficulties, or separation issues. Older children may describe feelings of nervousness, anger, fear, or tension and may display disruptive behavior. Ask the child to choose a number on a scale from 0 to 10 to describe how much they worry about things. Have the parent rank the child's worry in the same fashion, and ask the parent what the child worries about most. Determine frequency of headaches and stomachaches. Use a standardized screening tool such as the Multidimensional Anxiety Scale for Children (MASC), Spence Children's Anxiety Scale (SACS), Preschool Anxiety Scale, and Beck Anxiety Inventory for Youth.

Physical Examination

Perform a complete physical examination to rule out physiologic causes of the child's symptoms. Note patches of hair loss that occur with repetitive hair twisting or pulling associated with anxiety. Evaluate for evidence of nail biting, sucking blisters, or skin erosion from finger rubbing. Inspect the entire body for signs of self-injury, which may or may not be present.

Nursing Management

Screen children at well-child or other health care visits as well as upon admission to the hospital for anxiety symptoms. If an anxiety disorder is suspected, refer the child to the appropriate mental health provider for further evaluation. When the child is diagnosed with an anxiety disorder and medication is prescribed, teach families about medication administration and any adverse effects. Encourage and praise them for follow-through related to cognitive and behavioral therapy or psychotherapy. Provide emotional support to the child and family. Assess the family for the presence of parental anxiety or insecure attachment. Note parenting style and parent–child interactions. Both the child and the family will benefit from interventions that improve parent–child relationships, decrease parental anxiety, and foster parenting skills that promote autonomy in the child. Thus, refer the child and family to concurrent family therapy if needed.

ABUSE AND VIOLENCE

Abuse and violence contribute significantly to mental illness in children. Children may suffer from child maltreatment, medical child abuse, or substance misuse.

Child Maltreatment

Child maltreatment includes physical abuse, sexual abuse, emotional abuse, and neglect. Physical abuse refers to injuries that are intentionally inflicted on a child and result in morbidity or mortality. Sexual abuse refers to involvement of the child in any activity meant to provide sexual gratification to an adult. Emotional abuse may be verbal denigration of the child or may occur as a result of the child witnessing domestic violence. **Neglect** is defined as failure to provide a child with appropriate food, clothing, shelter, medical care, and schooling (Ford et al., 2022).

Statistics related to family violence as well as child physical and sexual abuse are difficult to determine, as the perpetrator usually forces the victim into silence. Children usually do not want to admit that their parent or relative has hurt them, partly from feelings of guilt and partly because they do not want to lose that person. In 2019, 4.4 million referrals to child protective services were made, alleging child maltreatment in 7.9 million children; however, this may be an underestimate of the prevalence of child abuse (Ford et al., 2022). Abuse and violence occur across all socioeconomic levels but are more prevalent among people with limited resources, and the largest percentage of those affected are under 3 years of age. Despite the lack of complete statistics, it is well known that the problem of abuse and violence is widespread. Parents or caregivers are the most frequent perpetrators of abuse against children (Ford et al., 2022).

A history of childhood abuse is associated with the development of anxiety and depressive disorders, suicidal ideation and attempts, and alcohol and drug misuse. Child maltreatment may result in significant physical injury, poor physical health, and, in some cases, impaired brain development. Abuse places children at risk for developmental and behavioral problems, decreased cognitive functioning, poor academic achievement, and deficits in relationships (Child Welfare Information Gateway, 2019).

Therapeutic management of victims of abuse and violence involves physical treatment of injuries, palliative care in some cases, and intervention to preserve or restore the child's mental well-being as well as family functioning. To protect children, all states legally require health care professionals to report suspected cases of child abuse or neglect (Child Welfare Information Gateway, 2023).

Nursing Assessment

Elicit the health history, noting the chief complaint and timing of onset. Assess for appropriateness of the parent–child attachment (often altered in the case of neglect). Pay particular attention to statements made by the child's parent or caregiver. Is the history given consistent with the child's injury? Identify abuse and violence by screening all children and families using these questions:

- Questions for children:
  - Are you afraid of anyone at home?
  - Whom could you tell if someone hurt you or touched you in a way that made you uncomfortable?
  - Has anyone hurt you or touched you in that way?
- Questions for parents:
  - Are you afraid of anyone at home?
  - Do you ever feel like you may hit or hurt your child when frustrated?

Assess for risk factors in children and parents or caregivers. Risk factors for abuse in children include poverty, prematurity, cerebral palsy, chronic illness, or intellectual disability. Risk factors for parents or caregivers becoming abusive include a history of being abused themselves, alcohol or substance misuse, and extreme stress.

Determine if the child has a history of hurting themselves (e.g., cutting) or others, running away, attempting suicide, or being involved in high-risk behaviors. Note inappropriate sexual behavior for developmental age as this may indicate sexual abuse. Note history of chronic sore throat or difficulty swallowing, which may occur with forced oral sex or sexually transmitted infections. Document history of genital burning or itching (associated with sexual abuse). Note nonspecific symptoms of emotional abuse such as low self-confidence, sleep disturbance, hypervigilance, headaches, or stomachaches.

TAKE NOTE!

A delay in seeking medical treatment, a history that changes over time, or a history of trauma that is inconsistent with the observed injury all suggest child abuse.

Physical Examination

Perform a gentle but thorough physical examination, using a soft touch and calm voice. Observe the parent–child interaction, noting fear or an excessive desire to please. Note the infant's level of consciousness. Vigorous shaking in the infant can lead to intracranial hemorrhage and brain injury. Inspect the skin for bruises, burns, cuts, abrasions, contusions, scars, and any other unusual or suspicious marks. Current or healed scratches or cuts may be found on parts of the body ordinarily covered by clothing in the child who self-mutilates. Burns that occur in a stocking or glove pattern, or only to the soles or palms, are highly suspicious for inflicted burns. Injuries in various stages of healing are also indicative of abuse. Bruises on the chest, head, neck, or abdomen are suspicious for abuse. Nonambulatory children infrequently experience bruises or fractures. Figure 50.1 shows injury sites usually indicative of abuse; Figure 50.2 is a photograph of a child who was beaten with an electric cord. Observe for inflammation of the oropharynx. Inspect the anus and penis or vaginal area for bleeding or discharge.

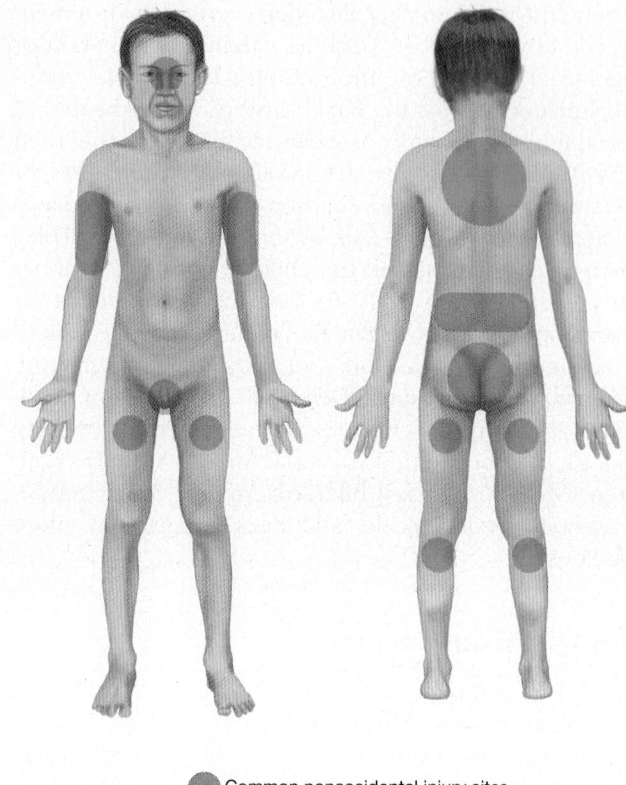

FIGURE 50.1 Injury sites that are suspicious for abuse.

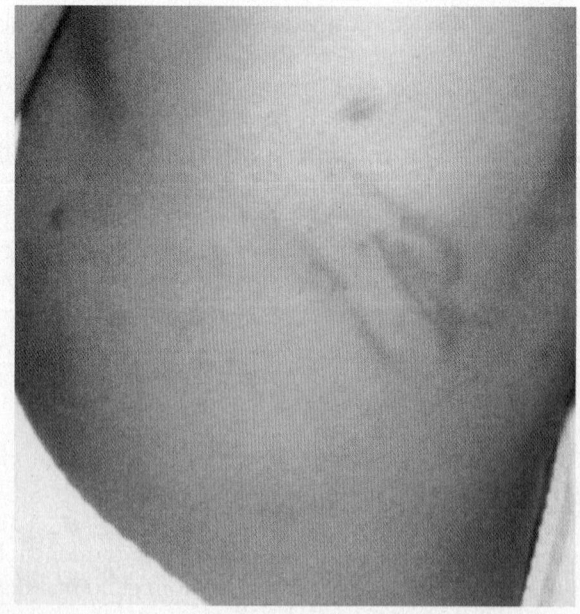

FIGURE 50.2 Note the mark left from a looped electric cord.

Laboratory and Diagnostic Tests

Common laboratory and diagnostic studies ordered for the assessment of abuse include:

- Radiographic skeletal survey or bone scan may reveal current or past fractures.
- Computed tomography scan of the head may reveal intracranial hemorrhage.
- Rectal, oral, vaginal, or urethral specimens may reveal sexually transmitted infections such as gonorrhea or chlamydia.

Nursing Management

Refer suspected cases of neglect or abuse to the local child protection agency. When abusive activity is identified in the hospital, notify the social services and risk management departments. In addition to physical or palliative care needed for the injuries, abused children need to redevelop a sense of trust in adults. Provide consistent care to the abused child by assigning a core group of nurses. Child abuse requires a multidisciplinary approach that will include psychological therapy for the child and the family.

Role model appropriate caregiving activities to the parent or caregiver. Call attention to normal growth and development activities noted in the infant or child, as parents sometimes have expectations of child behavior that may be unrealistic based on the child's age, leading to the abuse. Praise parents and caregivers for taking appropriate steps toward getting help and for providing appropriate care to the child. Refer parents to Parents Anonymous, an organization dedicated to the prevention of child abuse through strengthening of the family (see https://parentsanonymous.org).

When it is determined by the child protective team that the child would be in danger by continuing to live in the current situation, the child may be removed from the home. If the child is removed from the family temporarily or permanently, provide the foster or adoptive family with education necessary to assume the child's care.

Medical Child Abuse

Medical child abuse was historically termed Munchausen syndrome by proxy. It is a type of child abuse in which the parent or caregiver creates physical and/or psychological symptoms of illness or impairment in the child. The adult meets their own psychological needs by having an ill child. Medical child abuse is difficult to detect and may remain hidden for years. In most cases, the birthing parent is the perpetrator (Roesler & Jenny, 2022). Therapeutic management focuses on ensuring the safety and well-being of the child, as well as providing psychotherapy for the perpetrator.

Nursing Assessment

Take a thorough and detailed health history of the child's illness or illnesses. Use quotations to document the parent's responses. Warning signs of medical child abuse include:

- Child with one or more illnesses that do not respond to treatment or that follow a puzzling course; a similar history in siblings
- Symptoms that do not make sense or that disappear when the perpetrator is removed or not present; the symptoms are witnessed only by the caregiver (e.g., cyanosis, apnea, seizure)
- Physical and laboratory findings that do not fit with the reported history
- Repeated hospitalizations failing to produce a medical diagnosis, transfers to other hospitals, discharges against medical advice
- Parent who refuses to accept that the diagnosis is not medical (Roesler & Jenny, 2022)

Observe the parent's behavior with the child, spouse or partner, and staff. Use of covert video surveillance may reveal actions causing illness in the child when the nurse, health care provider, or nurse practitioner is not in the room. Perform a thorough physical examination, noting where the physical examination findings differ from the reported health history.

Nursing Management

Management of medical child abuse is complex. When abusive activity is identified, notify the social services and risk management departments of the hospital. Ensure that the local child protection team and the caregiver's family or support system is present when the caregiver is confronted. Inform the caregiver of the plan of care for the child and of the availability of psychiatric assistance for the caregiver.

Substance Misuse

Substance misuse most often begins before age 20. In 2021, in the United States, 23% of students reported they currently drink alcohol and 16% that they currently use cannabis (CDC, 2023). In addition to alcohol, youths also use cocaine, heroin, methamphetamines, inhalants, ecstasy, nonprescribed steroids, and prescription drugs outside of their intended use (CDC, 2023).

Nursing Assessment

Note risk factors for substance misuse, such as family history of substance use disorder, current parental substance misuse, dysfunctional family relationships, concurrent mental health disorder, aggressive behaviors, low self-esteem or poor academic performance, negative life events, poor social skills, or peers who misuse substances.

Determine the child's history, noting altered school performance or attendance, changes in peer group participation, frequent mood swings, changes in physical appearance, or an altered relationship with or perception of parents. Document history of insomnia, appetite loss, excessive itching, sleepiness or extreme fatigue, dry mouth, or shakiness. Note violent behavior, drunkenness, stupor, blank expression, drowsiness, lack of coordination, confusion, incoherent speech, extremes in emotions, aggressive behavior, silly behavior, or rapid speech. A screening assessment recommended by the AAP is the CRAFFT Screening Tool (Boston Children's Hospital, 2018). Perform a complete physical examination. Observe for an odor of alcohol or cannabis smoke. Assess the eyes, noting wateriness or dilated pupils. Inspect the nares, noting rhinorrhea or absence of nasal hair. Inspect the fingers for glue smears or discoloration and the skin for needle marks or tracks. Palpate the hands and feet for coolness.

Laboratory and diagnostic tests include toxicology studies, such as urine screening, to determine the presence of stimulants, sedative–hypnotics, barbiturates, hallucinogens, opiates, cocaine, and cannabis.

Nursing Management

Help the adolescent acknowledge that they have a problem. Explain the negative consequences of substance misuse, and raise the adolescent's awareness of risks. Remain empathetic while leaving responsibility with the adolescent. Key nursing interventions include promoting participation in treatment programs and preventing substance misuse.

PROMOTING PARTICIPATION IN TREATMENT PROGRAMS

Refer the adolescent to a substance misuse program. Outpatient or day treatment programs are useful in most situations. Family-based programs produce the highest level of recovery. Self-help or 12-step groups are an important element in the recovery process. Serious addiction, the presence of one or more comorbid psychiatric conditions, or suicidal ideation requires residential treatment or hospitalization. See the Healthy People 2030 box.

HEALTHY PEOPLE 2030

Objective	Nursing Significance
Increase the proportion of people with co-occurring substance misuse and mental disorders who receive treatment for both disorders.	• Screen all children and adolescents with mental health disorders for the coexistence of substance misuse (and vice versa). • Refer children and adolescents to appropriate treatment programs and therapy.

Healthy People Objectives retrieved from http://www.healthypeople.gov

PREVENTING SUBSTANCE MISUSE

Establish a trusting relationship with children and adolescents in order to improve acceptance of education about substance misuse and to provide a safe environment for confiding about their problems. Screen all children and adolescents for risk factors. During routine psychosocial screening, be alert to alterations as noted earlier. Teach all children, beginning at the elementary school level (or earlier if appropriate), that all chemicals have the potential to be harmful to the body, including tobacco, alcohol, and illicit drugs. Educate children and adolescents that no matter which administration route is used, the drug still enters the body and affects it negatively. Help children learn problem-solving skills that they can call upon in the future rather than relying on drugs or other substances to avoid their problems. Teach children to "just say no." Reinforce that they are the ones who have control over their bodies and what they expose them to. Encourage children to participate in the local community Drug Abuse Resistance Education (DARE) program, and praise them for completing it. Teach parents that being involved in their child's social life and knowing where they are and with whom when they are outside of the home is an important step toward limiting substance exposure.

KEY CONCEPTS

- Mental health and behavioral disorders account for the bulk of the "new morbidity" among children and adolescents.
- The child with behavioral problems or mental health issues often has difficulty with school, peer relationships, and family, all of which may worsen the child's self-concept, further hindering their emotional health.
- Developmental screening is a key component in the evaluation of a child's mental health.
- Various screening tools are available for depression, ADHD, and anxiety.
- Children with ASD often have impaired social interactions as well as altered communication.
- Learning disabilities and ADHD can have a significant negative impact on the child's education.
- IEPs help children with learning disabilities, intellectual disability, and ADHD receive the educational support they require to optimize their educational capacity.
- Provide support and education to children with mood or anxiety disorders and their families.
- Educating parents about medication administration and any adverse side effects is a critical aspect of nursing management of the child with a mental health disorder.
- Provide nutritional replacement at the appropriate pace in the child with anorexia nervosa. Monitor

the child closely for the development of refeeding syndrome.

- A key nursing function is screening all children and their families for abuse and violence.
- Report suspected cases of child abuse to the appropriate authorities.
- Educate children about the dangers associated with substance misuse. Reward and praise children and adolescents who do not experiment with or use alcohol or illicit drugs.

REFERENCES AND RECOMMENDED READINGS

108th Congress. (2004). *Individuals with Disabilities Education Improvement Act of 2004.* https://www.govinfo.gov/app/details/CRPT-108hrpt779/CRPT-108hrpt779

American Academy of Child and Adolescent Psychiatry. (2019). *Psychotherapy for children and adolescents: Different types.* https://www.aacap.org/AACAP/Families_and_Youth/Facts_for_Families/FFF-Guide/Psychotherapies-For-Children-And-Adolescents-086.aspx

American Academy of Pediatrics. (2023). *Mental health initiatives.* https://www.aap.org/en/patient-care/mental-health-initiatives/

Augustyn, M., & von Hahn, L. E. (2023). Autism spectrum disorder in children and adolescents: Clinical features. *UpToDate.* Retrieved March 22, 2024, from https://www.uptodate.com/contents/autism-spectrum-disorder-in-children-and-adolescents-clinical-features

Axelson, D. (2022). Pediatric bipolar disorder: Overview of choosing treatment. *UpToDate.* Retrieved March 22, 2024, from www.uptodate.com/contents/pediatric-bipolar-disorder-overview-of-choosing-treatment

Bennett, S., & Walkup, J. T. (2022). Anxiety disorders in children and adolescents: Epidemiology, pathogenesis, clinical manifestations, and course. *UpToDate.* Retrieved March 22, 2024, from http://www.uptodate.com/contents/anxiety-disorders-in-children-and-adolescents-epidemiology-pathogenesis-clinical-manifestations-and-course

Birmaher, B. (2023). Pediatric bipolar disorder: Clinical manifestations and course of illness. *UpToDate.* Retrieved March 22, 2024, from https://www.uptodate.com/contents/pediatric-bipolar-disorder-clinical-manifestations-and-course-of-illness#H2995284799

Boston Children's Hospital. (2018). *CRAFFT.* http://crafft.org

Brent, D. A., & Maalouf, F. (2019). Depressive disorders (in childhood and adolescence). In M. H. Ebert, J. F. Leckman, & I. L. Petrakis (Eds.), *Current diagnosis & treatment: Psychiatry* (3rd ed.). McGraw-Hill Education.

Centers for Disease Control and Prevention. (2023). *Youth risk behavior survey: Data summary & trends report 2011-2021.* https://www.cdc.gov/healthyyouth/data/yrbs/pdf/YRBS_Data-Summary-Trends_Report2023_508.pdf

Child Welfare Information Gateway. (2019). *Long-term consequences of child abuse and neglect.* U.S. Department of Health and Human Services. https://www.childwelfare.gov/pubpdfs/long_term_consequences.pdf

Child Welfare Information Gateway. (2023). *Mandatory reporting of child abuse and neglect.* U.S. Department of Health and Human Services. https://www.childwelfare.gov/resources/mandatory-reporting-child-abuse-and-neglect/

Ford, C. R., Chiesa, A., & Sirotnak, A. P. (2022). Child abuse & neglect. In M. Bunik, W. W. Hay, M. J. Levin, & M. J. Abzug (Eds.), *Current diagnosis & treatment: Pediatrics* (26th ed.). McGraw-Hill Education.

Goddard, A. (2021). Adverse childhood experiences and trauma-informed care. *Journal of Pediatric Health Care, 35*(2), 145–155. https://doi.org/10.1016/j.pedhc.2020.09.001

Guarda, A. (2023). Eating disorders: Overview of epidemiology, clinical features, and diagnosis *UpToDate.* https://www.uptodate.com/contents/eating-disorders-overview-of-epidemiology-clinical-features-and-diagnosis

Halter, M. J., & Fratena, C. A. (2023). *Varcarolis' manual of psychiatric nursing care planning: An interprofessional approach* (7th ed.). Elsevier.

Jankovic, J. (2023). Tourette syndrome: Pathogenesis, clinical features, and diagnosis. *UpToDate.* Retrieved March 22, 2024, from https://www.uptodate.com/contents/tourette-syndrome-pathogenesis-clinical-features-and-diagnosis#H5

Kelsay, K., Glaze, K., & Talmi, A. (2022). Child & adolescent psychiatric disorders & psychosocial aspects of pediatrics. In M. Bunik, W. W. Hay, M. J. Levin, R. R. Deterding, & M. J. Abzug (Eds.), *Current pediatric diagnosis and treatment* (26th ed.). McGraw-Hill Education.

Krull, K. R., & Chan, E. (2023). Attention deficit hyperactivity disorder in children and adolescents: Epidemiology and pathogenesis. *UpToDate.* Retrieved March 22, 2024, from http://www.uptodate.com/contents/attention-deficit-hyperactivity-disorder-in-children-and-adolescents-epidemiology-and-pathogenesis

Pivalizza, P. (2024). Intellectual disability (ID) in children: Clinical features, evaluation, and diagnosis. *UpToDate.* Retrieved March 22, 2024, from https://www.uptodate.com/contents/intellectual-disability-id-in-children-clinical-features-evaluation-nd-diagnosis

Reichow, B., Hume, K., Barton, E. E., & Boyd, B. A. (2018). Early intensive behavioral intervention (EIBI) for young children with autism spectrum disorders (ASD*). Cochrane Database of Systematic Reviews,* (5), CD009260. https://doi.org/10.1002/14651858.CD009260.pub3

Reynolds, A., Angulo, A., Breheney, M., Green, J., & Goldson, E. (2022). Child development and behavior. In M. Bunik, W. W. Hay, M. J. Levin, & M. J. Abzug (Eds.), *Current diagnosis & treatment: Pediatrics* (26th ed.). McGraw-Hill Education.

Roesler, T. A., & Jenny, C. (2022). Medical child abuse (Munchausen syndrome by proxy). *UpToDate.* Retrieved March 22, 2024, from http://www.uptodate.com/contents/medical-child-abuse-munchausen-syndrome-by-proxy

Shreve, M., Scott, A., McNeill, C., & Washburn, L. (2021). Using yoga to reduce anxiety in children: Exploring school-based yoga among rural third- and fourth-grade students. *Journal of Pediatric Health Care, 35*(1), 42–52. https://doi.org/10.1016/j.pedhc.2020.07.008

Sohl, K. T. (2022). Understanding physician practice patterns for autism spectrum disorder. *Pediatric News,* 1–8.

Star Center Foundation. (2024). *Understanding sensory processing disorder.* https://www.spdstar.org/basic/understanding-sensory-processing-disorder

Swick, S. D., & Jellinek, M. S. (2022). Demystifying psychotherapy. *Pediatric News, 56*(10), 18.

UpToDate, Inc. (2024). *UpToDate Lexidrug* (Version 8.2.0) [Mobile app]. Wolters Kluwer. https://apps.apple.com/us/app/lexicomp/id313401238

U.S. Department of Health and Human Services. (n.d.). *Healthy People 2030*. https://health.gov/healthypeople

von Hahn, L. E. (2023a). Specific learning disorders in children: Clinical features. *UpToDate*. Retrieved March 22, 2024, from http://www.uptodate.com/contents/specific-learning-disabilities-in-children-clinical-features

von Hahn, L. E. (2023b). Specific learning disorders in children: Role of the primary care provider. *UpToDate*. Retrieved March 22, 2024, from http://www.uptodate.com/contents/specific-learning-disabilities-in-children-role-of-the-primary-care-provider

Weissman, L., & Harris, H. K. (2022). Autism spectrum disorder in children and adolescents: Complementary and alternative therapies. *UpToDate*. Retrieved March 22, 2024, from https://www.uptodate.com/contents/autism-spectrum-disorder-in-children-and-adolescents-complementary-and-alternative-therapies

Yager, J. (2022). Eating disorders: Overview of prevention and treatment. *UpToDate*. Retrieved March 22, 2024, from https://www.uptodate.com/contents/eating-disorders-overview-of-prevention-and-treatment

DEVELOPING CLINICAL JUDGMENT

PRACTICING FOR NCLEX

1. The nurse is caring for a child with ADHD. Which behaviors would the nurse expect the child to display? Select all that apply.
   a. Interruptions
   b. Inability to take turns
   c. Moody, morose behavior
   d. Forgetfulness
   e. Easy distractibility
   f. Pouting
   g. Excessive motor activities
   h. Fidgeting
2. An adolescent who has been receiving treatment for anorexia nervosa has failed to gain weight over the past week despite eating all meals and snacks. What is the priority nursing intervention?
   a. Increase the adolescent's daily caloric intake by at least 500 calories.
   b. Ensure the adolescent's entire fluid intake includes calories.
   c. Supervise the adolescent for 2 hours after all meals and snacks.
   d. Assess the adolescent's anxiety level to determine need for medication.
3. A 15-year-old has been making demands all day, exaggerating every need. They are now crying, saying they have nothing to live for and threatening to kill themselves. What is the priority nursing action?
   a. Ignore the continued exaggerated and melodramatic behavior.
   b. Consult with the health care provider or nurse practitioner to increase the antidepressant dose.
   c. Leave the adolescent alone for a little while until they compose themselves.
   d. Take the suicidal threat seriously and provide close supervision.
4. When trying to manage aggressive or impulsive behaviors in children or adolescents, what is the best nursing intervention?
   a. Train the child to be assertive.
   b. Provide consistency and limit setting.
   c. Allow the child to negotiate the rules.
   d. Encourage the child to express feelings.
5. The nurse is caring for an adolescent who says, "I'm sick of this. I wish I weren't alive anymore." What is the best response by the nurse?
   a. "I often feel sad and sick of things."
   b. "Have you thought about hurting yourself?"
   c. "Are you trying to escape your problems?"
   d. "Do your parents know about this feeling?"
6. The nurse is assessing an adolescent being admitted for an eating disorder. The physical examination reveals temperature 96.7°F oral, heart rate 54 bpm, and blood pressure 88/54 mm Hg. Which eating disorder do these clinical manifestations suggest?
   a. Pica
   b. Bulimia nervosa
   c. Binge eating disorder
   d. Anorexia nervosa
7. The nurse is caring for an adolescent whose physical examination reveals chipped teeth, calluses on the knuckles, and dental enamel erosion. The adolescent is at risk for ____ as related to ______.
   Blank 1:
   a. bradycardia
   b. dysrhythmia
   c. esophagitis
   Blank 2:
   a. decreased oral intake
   b. vomiting
   c. food avoidance

DOSAGE CALCULATION QUESTION

The nurse is caring for a 10-year old diagnosed with depression. The child weighs 72 lb. The medication order reads: fluoxetine 10 mg PO daily. The child refuses to swallow pills. Fluoxetine is supplied as 20 mg/5 mL. How many milliliters will the nurse administer? Round to the nearest tenth.

CRITICAL THINKING EXERCISES

1. A parent tells you that their child's behavior is unmanageable and that they are having difficulty coping with it. The child is argumentative and is bullying others. They are struggling with their school work because they have difficulty staying on task, get out of the chair often, and frequently distract others. What additional assessments should you obtain? What interventions would be helpful in managing the child's behavior?
2. A 14-year-old with moderate intellectual disability is able to feed themselves but is incontinent. Discuss the issues with which the family must deal.

STUDY ACTIVITIES

1. Explore several of the websites related to child abuse prevention. Develop a list of resources for families in your local area.
2. Attend a group therapy session during your pediatric clinical rotation. Observe the children's verbal and nonverbal communication, noting inconsistencies or other interesting observations.
3. Visit a school for children with ASD. Spend time with the various specialists who work with the children, determining their roles and the effect the treatment they are providing has on the children. Report your findings to your classmates.
4. Attend a local Children and Adults with ADHD (CHADD) meeting. Talk to parents about having a child with ADHD.

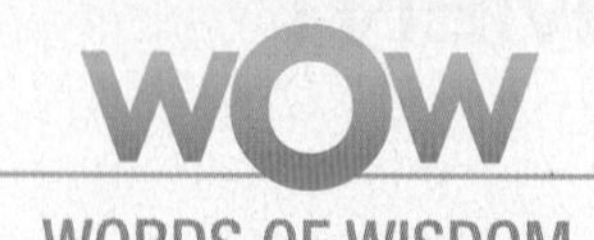

WORDS OF WISDOM

A nurse must possess the knowledge and skills to aid an acutely ill child.

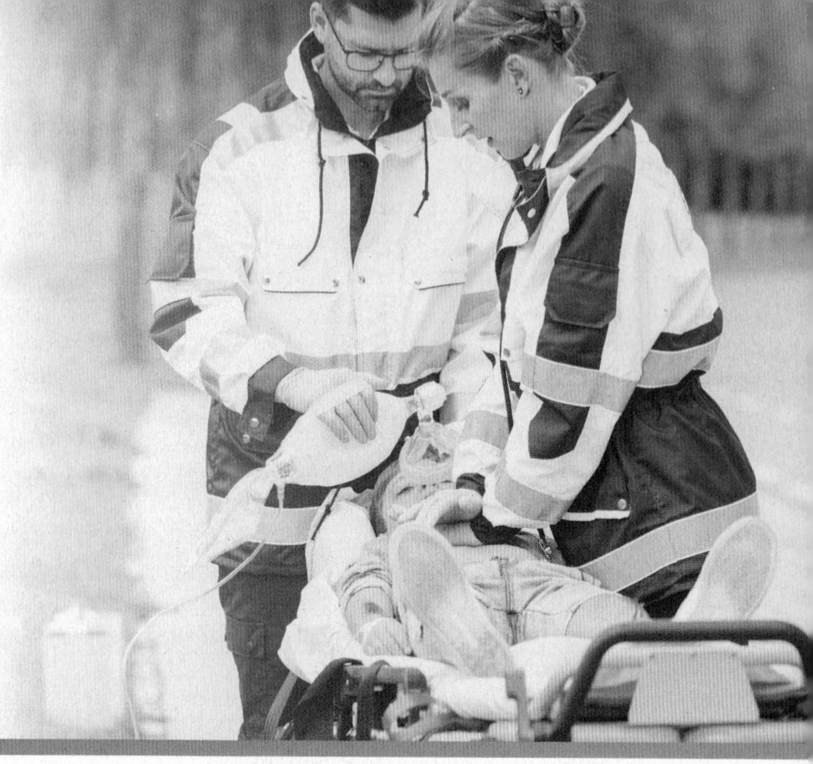

51 Nursing Care During a Pediatric Emergency

LEARNING OBJECTIVES

Upon completion of the chapter, you will be able to:

1. Identify various factors contributing to emergency situations among infants and children.
2. Discuss common treatments and medications used during pediatric emergencies.
3. Conduct a health history of a child in an emergency situation, specific to the emergency.
4. Perform a rapid cardiopulmonary assessment.
5. Discuss common laboratory and other diagnostic tests used during pediatric emergencies.
6. Integrate the principles of the American Heart Association and Pediatric Advanced Life Support in the comprehensive management of pediatric emergencies, such as respiratory arrest, shock, cardiac arrest, near drowning, poisoning, and trauma.
7. Devise an individualized nursing care plan or concept map for the child experiencing a pediatric emergency.

Alma Anderson, age 8 years, has been admitted to the pediatric unit. Her parent calls the nurse into the room, stating, "Alma's having trouble breathing!"

KEY TERMS

asystole (ā-sis′tō-lē)
barotrauma (bar′ō-traw′mă)
bradycardia
cardioversion
defibrillation (dē-fib′ri-lā′shŭn)
hyperventilation
hypocapnia (hī′pō-kap′nē-ă)
hypoventilation
intubation
periodic breathing
tachycardia

INTRODUCTION

Children are uniquely vulnerable to a range of emergency situations. These situations are often life-threatening if not treated quickly and effectively. Because of their developmental level, children are at a greater risk for submersion injury, poisoning, and traumatic injury compared to adults. Most pediatric cardiopulmonary arrests result from respiratory failure or shock. Data suggest that children who have a cardiopulmonary arrest requiring resuscitative measures rarely fare well. For these reasons, the American Heart Association (AHA) has delineated two distinct chains of survival, one for adults and one for children, which should be followed during a life-threatening situation.

The adult chain of survival is:

- Early emergency medical system (EMS) activation
- Early cardiopulmonary resuscitation (CPR)
- Early defibrillation
- Early access to advanced care
- Integrated postcardiac arrest care

In contrast, the pediatric chain of survival is:

- Prevention of cardiac arrest and injuries
- Early CPR
- Early access to emergency response system
- Early advanced care (pediatric advanced life support [PALS])
- Integrated postcardiac arrest care (AHA & American Academy of Pediatrics [AAP], 2020)

Considering the special risks that threaten children, the AHA has also developed specific guidelines for PALS. Courses in PALS are offered for health care professionals so that they can provide expert care for children in emergencies. This chapter emphasizes the principles of PALS in its discussion of the nurse's role in the management of pediatric emergencies.

TAKE NOTE!

The current pediatric basic life support guidelines define an infant as between 0 and 12 months of age, and a child as age 1 year up until puberty. Children in this range should be managed using the PALS guidelines rather than those for adults (AHA & AAP, 2020).

COMMON MEDICAL TREATMENTS

A variety of medications and other medical treatments are used in pediatric emergencies. Most of these treatments will require a health care provider's order when the child is in the hospital, though some emergency departments and pediatric units may have standing orders for pediatric emergencies. The most common medical treatments and medications used in pediatric emergencies are listed in Common Medical Treatments 51.1 and Drug Guide 51.1, respectively. The nurse should be familiar with these procedures and medications, how they work, and nursing implications.

COMMON MEDICAL TREATMENTS 51.1

Treatment	Explanation	Indications	Nursing Implications
Suctioning (oropharyngeal, nasopharyngeal, ET, or tracheostomy)	Removal of secretions via bulb syringe or suction catheter	Excessive airway secretions affecting airway patency	Use caution and suction only as far as recommended for age, ET tube size, or tracheostomy tube size or until coughing or gagging occurs.
Oxygen	Supplementation via mask, nasal cannula, hood, or tent or via ET/nasotracheal tube	Hypoxemia, respiratory distress, shock, trauma	Monitor response via color, work of breathing, respiratory rate, oxygen saturation levels via pulse oximetry, and level of consciousness.
Bag-valve-mask ventilation	Provision of ventilation via a bag-valve-mask device, manual ventilation	Apnea, ineffective ventilation and oxygenation with spontaneous breaths, extremely slow respiratory rate	Ensure adequate chest rise with ventilation. Do not overventilate or bag aggressively to avoid barotrauma. Maintain a seal on the child's face with the appropriate-sized mask. Ensure the oxygen supply tubing is connected to 100% oxygen.
Intubation	Insertion of a tube into the trachea to provide artificial ventilation	Apnea, airway that is not maintainable, need for prolonged assisted ventilation	Determine adequacy of breath sounds with bagging immediately upon insertion of the ET tube. Assess for symmetric chest rise. Tape the tube securely in place and note the number marking on the tube. Connect to ventilator when available.

(continued)

COMMON MEDICAL TREATMENTS 51.1 (*continued*)

Treatment	Explanation	Indications	Nursing Implications
Needle thoracotomy	Insertion of a needle between the ribs into the pleural space to remove air	Tension pneumothorax	There should be a rush of air as the needle reaches the air space. Monitor breath sounds, work of breathing, and pulse oximetry. Ensure patency of IV catheter.
IV fluid therapy	Administration of crystalloid or colloid solutions to provide hydration or improve perfusion	Altered perfusion states such as respiratory distress, shock, trauma, cardiac disturbances	Use intraosseous route if a peripheral IV cannot be obtained quickly in the young child in shock. Reassess respiratory and circulatory status frequently after each IV fluid bolus and during continuous infusion.
Blood product transfusion	Administration of whole blood, packed red blood cells, platelets, or plasma intravenously	Trauma, hemorrhage	Follow the institution's transfusion protocol. Double-check blood type and product label with a second nurse. Monitor vital signs and assess the child frequently to identify adverse reaction to blood transfusion. If adverse reaction is suspected, immediately discontinue transfusion, infuse normal saline solution IV, reassess the child, and notify the health care provider.
Cervical stabilization	Maintenance of the cervical spine in an immobile position	Trauma, near drowning	Use the jaw-thrust maneuver without head tilt to open the airway. Maintain cervical stabilization until the cervical spine radiographs are cleared by the health care provider or radiologist.
Defibrillation and synchronized cardioversion	Provision of electrical current to alter the heart's electrical rhythm	Defibrillation: ventricular fibrillation and pulseless ventricular tachycardia Synchronized cardioversion: supraventricular tachycardia and ventricular tachycardia with a pulse	In the pulseless child, always ensure CPR is ongoing while the defibrillator is being readied. Ensure adequate oxygenation. Provide lidocaine or epinephrine if indicated before defibrillation. Sedate the child if time allows.

CPR, cardiopulmonary resuscitation; ET, endotracheal; IV, intravenous.

DRUG GUIDE 51.1

COMMON MEDICATIONS USED IN PEDIATRIC EMERGENCIES

Medication	Actions/Indications	Nursing Implications
Adenosine (antiarrhythmic)	Slows conduction through AV node, restoring normal sinus rhythm Supraventricular tachycardia (SVT)	• Administer IV at a dose ranging from 0.05 to 0.1 mg/kg for neonates and 0.1 to 0.2 mg/kg. • Administer very rapidly (1–2 seconds) followed by a rapid, generous saline flush. • Repeat every 1–2 minutes, increasing by 0.05–0.1 mg/kg with each dose (maximum dose 0.3 mg/kg). • Monitor for shortness of breath, dyspnea, and worsening of asthma.
Amiodarone (antiarrhythmic)	Prolongs repolarization of action potential, thus slowing the heart rate Ventricular tachycardia, ventricular fibrillation	• Administer IV or IO at a dose of 5 mg/kg over 20–60 minutes. • Avoid use with procainamide.
Atropine (anticholinergic)	Increases cardiac output, dries secretions, inhibits serotonin and histamine Sinus bradycardia, asystole, pulseless electrical activity	• Administer via IV, IO, or ET route at a dose of 0.02 mg/kg (maximum dose 0.5 mg for a child, 1 mg for an adolescent). • Repeat every 5 minutes PRN. • Give undiluted over 30 seconds for IV or IO route. • Dilute with 3–5 mL normal saline for ET route; follow with five positive-pressure ventilations. • Do not mix with sodium bicarbonate (incompatible).

DRUG GUIDE 51.1

COMMON MEDICATIONS USED IN PEDIATRIC EMERGENCIES

Medication	Actions/Indications	Nursing Implications
Dobutamine (adrenergic agent)	Beta-adrenergic agent primarily affecting beta-1 receptors; increases myocardial contractility and heart rate Ongoing short-term management of shock (hypovolemic and cardiogenic)	• Administer via IV or IO route at 2–20 µg/kg/min via a continuous infusion. Monitor for the development of ventricular dysrhythmias • Expect to titrate infusion rate based on cardiac output and BP. • Administer via central line if possible due to the risk of extravasation. • Monitor child closely, preferably in an ICU setting.
Dopamine (inotropic)	Increases cardiac output, BP, and renal perfusion (beta-adrenergic agonist) Bradycardia, hypotension, and poor cardiac output	• Administer via IV or IO route at a dose of 2–20 µg/kg/min via continuous infusion. • Ensure that child has received adequate fluid resuscitation prior to administration. • Due to risk of extravasation, give via central line if possible. • Monitor child closely, preferably in an ICU setting. • Assess for ventricular dysrhythmias
Epinephrine (vasopressor, inotropic)	Stimulates alpha- and beta-adrenergic receptors, increasing heart rate and systemic vascular resistance Bradycardia, anaphylaxis	• Administer via IV or IO route at a dose of 0.01 mg/kg (0.1 mL/kg of 1:10,000 solution) or via ET route at 0.1 mg/kg (0.1 mL/kg of 1:1,000 solution). • During CPR, repeat every 3–5 minutes. • Monitor for ventricular dysrhythmias • High doses may cause tachycardia in newborns. • Due to risk of extravasation and subsequent tissue necrosis, give through a central line if possible. • May also be used as a bronchodilator IV or via inhalation (racemic epinephrine).
Glucose	Increases blood glucose level Hypoglycemia	• Administer via IV or IO route at a dose of 1–2 mL/kg (D50%); maximum dose 2–4 mL/kg. • When administering via a peripheral IV line, dilute 1:1 with sterile water to make D25%. Monitor IV site for infiltration and tissue extravasation. • Monitor blood glucose levels closely.
Lidocaine (anti-dysrhythmic)	Decreases automaticity of conduction tissues of the heart Ventricular dysrhythmias	• Administer via IV or IO route at a dose of 1 mg/kg; administer via ET route at dose two times IV dose diluted with 3–5 mL normal saline, followed by positive-pressure ventilation. Maximum dose 5 mg/kg or 100 mg/dose. • Monitor ECG continuously. • Contraindicated in complete heart block. • With larger than normal doses, monitor for hypotension or seizures.
Naloxone (opioid receptor antagonist)	Antagonizes action of narcotic agents Reversal of respiratory depression related to narcotic effects	• Administer via IV, IO, SQ, or ET route at a dose of 0.01–0.1 mg/kg in children younger than 5 years or $<$20 kg or at a dose of 2 mg in children older than 5 years or $>$20 kg. Onset of action is within 2–5 minutes. • May repeat dose as necessary; narcotic effects outlast therapeutic effects of naloxone.

AV, atrioventricular; BP, blood pressure; ECG, electrocardiogram; ET, endotracheal; ICU, intensive care unit; IO, intraosseous; IV, intravenous; PRN, as needed; SQ, subcutaneous.

Data from American Heart Association & American Academy of Pediatrics. (2020). *Pediatric advanced life support provider manual.* American Heart Association; UpToDate, Inc. (2024). UpToDate Lexidrug (Version 8.2.0) [Mobile app]. Wolters Kluwer. https://apps.apple.com/us/app/lexicomp/id313401238

TAKE NOTE!

Certain emergency drugs for children may be given via an endotracheal tube. Use the mnemonic LEAN (lidocaine, epinephrine, atropine, and naloxone) to remember which drugs may be given via the endotracheal route. These drugs should be followed by sterile normal saline flush and positive-pressure ventilations to ensure that the drugs are delivered (AHA & AAP, 2020).

Clinical Judgment and the Nursing Process for the Child in an Emergency Situation

The nurse may encounter a pediatric emergency in a variety of settings. As a member of a trauma team at a pediatric hospital, the nurse may participate in the stabilization of a child who has suffered a near drowning or trauma. The emergency department nurse may encounter a child who has just been injured, such as from a fall, an accident, or sports. On the hospital unit, a child with asthma may suffer respiratory distress or stop breathing. Regardless of the setting or how the emergency developed, the principles for managing pediatric emergencies are the same.

Care of the child in an emergency includes all components of the nursing process: assessment, analysis, planning, interventions, and evaluation. In an emergency, the nurse must act quickly. It is important to intervene immediately when an abnormality is determined upon assessment. When evaluating a child who presents emergently, always follow the AHA's guidelines for basic life support, which includes evaluating the child's:

- Airway
- Breathing
- Circulation

After evaluating the child's airway, breathing, and circulation, provide care as necessary, including rescue breathing or CPR. Once the child's cardiopulmonary status is stabilized or the child is resuscitated, assessment and management will vary depending on the cause of the emergency.

Assessment

Nursing assessment of the child who presents emergently includes health history, physical examination, and laboratory and diagnostic testing. However, the initial history may be focused and very brief if the child is critically ill; the nurse may need to proceed immediately to rapid cardiopulmonary assessment. Once a child is stabilized, a more comprehensive history is obtained. Laboratory tests, while often important, should never take priority over cardiopulmonary and hemodynamic stabilization.

Health History

Obtain the health history rapidly while simultaneously evaluating the child and providing lifesaving interventions. A brief history is needed initially, followed by a more thorough history after the child is stabilized. The parents or caregiver will provide information about the child's chief complaint. Record the information using the caregiver's own words. For example, the caregiver might say, "He's been having trouble breathing" if the child is presenting in respiratory distress. If the child was injured in a bicycle accident, the caregiver might say, "She was riding her bike down the hill and lost control." This brief statement provides guidance for obtaining more in-depth information about the emergency.

Ask about any significant past history that may affect the care of the child. For example, children who are medically fragile, who were born prematurely, or who have a significant genetically linked disease (e.g., sickle cell anemia) may require special consideration when planning and implementing care.

CLINICAL REASONING ALERT!

When caring for a child injured in an accident, the nurse must always remember that assessment is the first step in the nursing process. So initial questions would relate to how the accident happened. The nurse could then go on to ask other questions such as medication allergies and chronic diseases.

Physical Examination

In an emergency, the nurse must perform a rapid cardiopulmonary assessment and intervene immediately if alterations are noted. The remainder of the physical examination then follows.

RAPID CARDIOPULMONARY ASSESSMENT

As the brief history is being obtained, begin the rapid cardiopulmonary assessment. Most pediatric arrests are related primarily to airway and breathing, and usually only secondarily to the heart. Supported breathing may be all that is needed if the child has a strong, adequate pulse. Always perform the assessment and interventions in that order. In most circumstances, if a child's airway is properly managed and breathing is assisted, the child may not experience a full arrest requiring chest compressions.

Airway Evaluation and Management First, evaluate the airway. Assess its patency. Position the airway in a manner that promotes good airflow. If secretions are obstructing the airway, suction the airway to remove them. If the child is unconscious or has just been injured, open the airway using the head tilt–chin lift maneuver. Place the fingertips on the bony prominence of the child's chin and lift the chin to open the airway. Simultaneously, place one hand on the forehead and tilt the child's head back (Fig. 51.1). If the airway is not maintainable, reposition the airway for appropriate airflow. Place the child immediately on oxygen at 100% and apply a pulse oximeter to monitor oxygen saturation levels.

TAKE NOTE!

If cervical spine injury is a possibility, do not use the head tilt–chin lift maneuver; use only the jaw-thrust technique for opening the airway (see "Trauma" section for explanation and illustration).

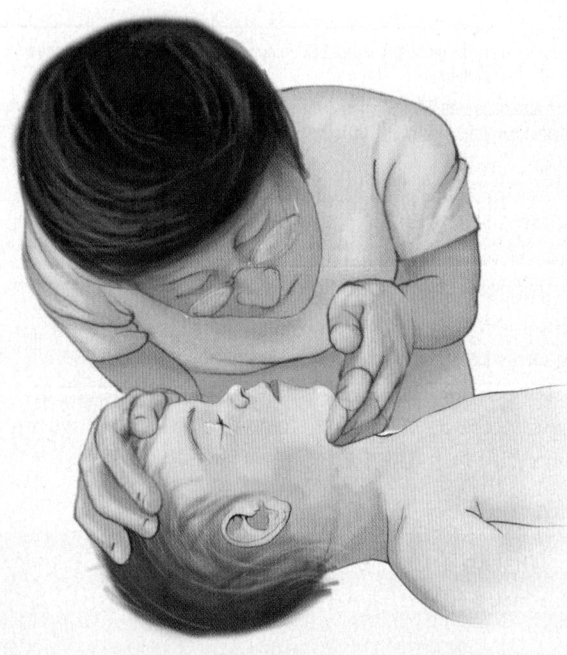

FIGURE 51.1 Head tilt–chin lift maneuver in a child.

Breathing Evaluation and Management After establishing an open airway, look for signs of respiration. Turn your head and place your ear over the child's mouth to "look, listen, and feel" for spontaneous respirations. Look to see if the child's chest is rising, listen for air escaping, and note if you feel any air coming out of the child's nose or mouth. If the child is breathing, evaluate the quality of the respirations: Is ventilation effective, or is the child simply gasping ineffectively for air? Count the respiratory rate. Observe the child's color. Note the depth of respiration, chest rise, adequacy of airflow in all lung fields, and presence of adventitious sounds. Evaluate for increased work of breathing and the use of accessory muscles.

When signs of respiratory distress are noted, immediately place the child on oxygen at 100% and apply a pulse oximeter to monitor oxygen saturation levels. If the child is breathing shallowly and has poor respiratory effort, attempt to reposition the airway to promote better airflow.

For the child receiving 100% oxygen who does not improve with repositioning, begin assisted ventilation with a bag-valve-mask (BVM) device. A need for ongoing BVM ventilation may require airway intubation (process by which an endotracheal [ET] tube is inserted into a child's airway to assist with breathing). See "Respiratory Arrest" section for information on assisting with ventilation using the BVM device and airway intubation.

Circulation Evaluation and Management Next, evaluate circulation. During this phase, evaluate the heart rate (HR), pulse, perfusion, skin color and temperature, blood pressure (BP), cardiac rhythm, and level of consciousness. Determine HR via direct auscultation or palpation of central pulses. Radial and brachial pulses are more difficult to palpate, especially in infants and young children. If perfusion is poor, such as with shock or cardiac arrest, the child may have a weak pulse or no pulse. In the young infant, check the brachial artery for a pulse. In the child and adolescent, evaluate the carotid pulse.

CLINICAL REASONING ALERT!

ALWAYS evaluate the presence of HR by auscultation of the heart or by palpation of central pulses. NEVER use the cardiac monitor to determine if the child has an HR. The presence of a cardiac rhythm is not a reliable method for evaluation of the ability to perfuse the body. In certain circumstances, a rhythm continues but there is no pulse (pulseless electrical activity [PEA]).

If the child has no HR (pulse), begin cardiac compressions. See later for information on performing CPR. High-quality chest compressions of adequate rate and depth are essential (AHA & AAP, 2020). If there is a pulse, note its quality: Is it barely palpable or weak? Is it strong or bounding? Compare the strength and quality of central and peripheral pulses. Assess capillary refill time.

Evaluate the child's perfusion by noting skin temperature and color. Is the skin pink? Is it warm to the touch? The child's skin may be cool to the touch and may appear pale, mottled, or cyanotic. As the child's condition worsens with developing shock and cardiovascular compromise, note a line of demarcation of skin temperature. In this situation, the distal extremities will feel cooler than the proximal regions of the body. Measure the BP and place the child on a cardiac monitor to evaluate the cardiac rhythm. Note the child's sensorium or level of consciousness; if circulation is poor, the child will demonstrate an altered level of consciousness as perfusion to the brain becomes diminished.

If the circulation or perfusion is compromised, then fluid resuscitation is necessary. Establish large-bore intravenous (IV) access immediately and administer isotonic fluid rapidly. Provide 20 mL/kg of normal saline (NS) or lactated Ringer's (LR) as an IV bolus (if the infant is younger than 1 month old, administer 10 mL/kg). If peripheral IV access cannot be obtained in the child with altered perfusion within three attempts or 90 seconds, assist with the insertion of an intraosseous needle for fluid administration (refer to "Shock" section for further information about intraosseous access). Central venous lines or cutdown access may also be used, but these measures take longer to accomplish.

Remember Alma, the 8-year-old with breathing trouble? What additional health history and physical examination assessment information should the nurse obtain?

ADDITIONAL PHYSICAL EXAMINATION COMPONENTS

In addition to assessing and stabilizing the child's airway, breathing, and circulation, perform a thorough physical examination and assess pain.

Neurologic Evaluation Quickly evaluate the sensorium in an older child. Ask the child to state their name. Ask what happened to the child. Does the child know what day it is? Is the child aware of where they are?

If the child is an infant, evaluate their interest in the environment and response to parents. An infant who is not interested in the environment or seems unable to recognize their parents is a cause for concern. In contrast, an infant who enjoys sucking on a finger and making eye contact with the nurse during the assessment is reassuring.

TAKE NOTE!

Use the mnemonic AVPU to quickly determine the level of consciousness:
A–Alert
V–Responsive to voice
P–Responds to pain
U–Unresponsive

Evaluate the child's head. In the infant or young toddler, palpate the anterior fontanel to determine if it is normal (soft and flat), depressed, or full. A sunken fontanel is associated with volume depletion from dehydration or blood loss. If the fontanel is full, note if it is bulging or tense, which may indicate increased intracranial pressure. Next, assess the eyes. Are they open or closed? If closed, do they open spontaneously, to voice, to pain? Does the child focus on and follow the nurse's movements? Evaluate the pupils for equality and reactivity. Sluggish pupillary reaction may occur with increased intracranial pressure.

Evaluate the child's face. Does the child smile or cry? Does the child react to playfulness with a laugh? Does the young infant cry vigorously? Are facial movements equal? In a child, a normal or near-normal neurologic examination can be a reassuring sign. Conversely, obtunded or muted responses to environmental stimuli are a cause for concern.

Next, evaluate for spontaneous movement of the extremities. Young infants cannot walk, so assess their ability to move their arms and legs, and grossly evaluate the tone of their extremities. Does the infant vigorously and equally move the arms and legs? Is the muscle tone normal, or does the infant appear floppy or flaccid? When evaluating the older child, note whether they are ambulatory independently, ambulatory with assistance, or unable to walk. Note whether the child has use of the upper extremities. In the case of trauma, the child may arrive immobilized on a backboard. In this scenario, evaluate the child's motor responsiveness and sensation in each extremity, comparing findings bilaterally while the child is in the supine position. Ask the child if they feel you touching each extremity. Ask the child to squeeze your fingers and to wiggle the toes. This will provide information about cerebral integrity and perfusion, cerebellar health, and spinal cord integrity.

The Pediatric Glasgow Coma Scale may also be used to evaluate the neurologic status in children. Chapter 38 provides a more in-depth discussion of this scale.

TAKE NOTE!

A nonreactive pupil is an ominous sign indicating a need for immediate relief of increased intracranial pressure.

Skin and Extremity Evaluation Remove the child's clothing and thoroughly examine the skin for bruising, lesions, or rashes. If the child has a rash, note the size, shape, color, configuration, and location. Apply pressure to the rash with the fingertips to see whether it blanches. Inspect the trunk, abdomen, and extremities for abrasions or deformities.

CLINICAL REASONING ALERT!

Rashes that do not blanch may be classified as petechiae or purpura. This type of rash may be associated with certain serious conditions, such as meningococcemia. Report this finding to the health care provider or nurse practitioner immediately.

Pain Assessment In emergencies, children may experience pain as a direct result of the injury or disease, and lifesaving interventions such as resuscitation, insertion of IV lines, and administration of medications may cause further pain. The child's pain may also be exaggerated by light, noise, movement of the stretcher or bed, and the sensations of cold or heat. Nurses play a key role in minimizing the child's pain, and this may decrease the child's future distress (Ring et al., 2023). If the child is awake and verbal, use an age-appropriate pain assessment scale to determine the child's pain level. If the child is sedated or unconscious, assess pain with a standardized scale that relies on physiologic measurements as well as behavioral parameters. Refer to Chapter 36 for additional information on pain assessment in children.

Laboratory and Diagnostic Testing

A number of laboratory and diagnostic tests may be ordered in a pediatric emergency. Laboratory tests can help to distinguish the cause of the emergency or additional problems that need to be treated. Standard laboratory tests obtained in most emergency departments include:

- Arterial blood gases (ABGs), obtained initially and then serially to assess for changes
- Electrolytes and glucose levels
- Complete blood count (CBC)
- Blood cultures
- Urinalysis

If ingestion is suspected, then a toxicology panel will be obtained. In suspected sepsis, erythrocyte sedimentation rate (ESR), C-reactive protein (CRP), and urine and spinal fluid cultures may also be obtained. The pediatric trauma victim may have additional laboratory tests performed, including amylase, liver enzymes, and blood type and cross-match.

Diagnostic tests may include radiologic tests, computed tomography (CT) scanning, and magnetic resonance imaging (MRI). One advantage of radiologic diagnostic testing is that the tests are relatively noninvasive. A disadvantage of CT and MRI scans is that before they can be performed, the child must be stabilized. Common Laboratory and Diagnostic Tests 51.1 discusses the tests most commonly used in pediatric emergencies.

COMMON LABORATORY AND DIAGNOSTIC TESTS 51.1

Test	Explanation	Indications	Nursing Implications
Chest radiograph	Radiograph used to evaluate heart and lung structures	To identify: • Infections (e.g., pneumonia) • Foreign body • Injury • Endotracheal tube placement • Central line placement • Pneumothorax • Reevaluation of lungs after chest tube placement	• Radiographs can be obtained quickly during resuscitation, usually available in the emergency department. • Assist the child to lie still if necessary.
Computed tomography (CT)	Use of high radiation (equivalent to about 100–150 chest x-rays) with computer processing targeting specific body areas	Rapid evaluation of tissues and skeletal areas Superior test for the evaluation of internal bleeding	• Expect the child to be transported out of the area for the study. • Accompany the child to provide continued observation and management, especially if child's condition is unstable.
Magnetic resonance imaging (MRI)	Incorporation of responses of hydrogen protons to a dynamic magnetic field	Superior test for the evaluation of the spinal cord and the cerebrospinal fluid spaces; less useful in emergency situations	• Administer sedation as ordered. • Assist child in remaining still; MRI requires child to remain still for a longer period than for a CT. • Assist the conscious child to deal with fear related to loud banging noise of the machine.
Arterial blood gases (ABGs)	Evaluation of blood pH and arterial blood levels of oxygen and carbon dioxide	Evaluation of quality of respiration and evaluation of acid–base balance	• Anticipate serial ABGs to assess for status changes. • Never delay resuscitation efforts pending blood gas results.
Serum electrolytes	Evaluation of electrolyte levels, such as sodium, potassium, and chloride, in the blood	Useful for determining baseline and if dehydration is hypertonic or isotonic	Hemolysis of specimen may lead to falsely elevated potassium levels.
Glucose	Evaluation of glucose level in the blood	Valuable for determining the need for supplementation, as in the case of hypoglycemia	• Use a rapid glucose test at the bedside or obtain serum blood specimen. • Elevated glucose levels can be associated with stress or with the use of corticosteroids.
Toxicology panel (blood and/or urine)	Determination of most commonly misused mood-altering medications, as well as commonly ingested drugs	Drug misuse, overdose, or poisoning	• Standard toxicology panel varies with the agency. • Follow agency protocol; may require special handling or labeling of specimen. • Use a blood specimen that is best for determining overdose or poisoning.
Complete blood count (CBC)	Evaluation of hemoglobin and hematocrit, white blood cell count, and platelet count	Any condition in which anemia, infection, or thrombocytopenia is suspected Trauma if blood loss is suspected	• Be aware of normal values and how they vary with age and sex. • Hemoglobin and hematocrit may be elevated secondary to hemoconcentration in the case of hypovolemia.
Blood type and cross-match	Determination of ABO blood typing as well as the presence of antigens Cross-match is performed on RBC-containing products to avoid transfusion reaction.	Trauma victim or any person with suspected blood loss as preparation for transfusion	• Handle the specimen gently to avoid hemolysis. • Ensure that specimen request and label are appropriately signed and dated. • Apply "type and cross" or "blood band" to child at the time of specimen collection if required by agency. • Most type and cross-match specimens expire after 48–72 hours.

(continued)

COMMON LABORATORY AND DIAGNOSTIC TESTS 51.1 (*continued*)

Test	Explanation	Indications	Nursing Implications
Urinalysis	Evaluation of color, pH, specific gravity, and odor of urine Assessment for protein, glucose, ketones, blood, leukocyte esterase, RBCs, WBCs, bacteria, crystals, and casts	Children with fever, dysuria, flank pain, urgency, or hematuria or those who have experienced trauma to provide information about the urinary tract	• Many drugs can affect urine color; notify the laboratory if the child is taking one. • Notify the laboratory and document on the laboratory form if the child or adolescent is menstruating. • Refrigerate the specimen if it is not processed promptly. • Specimen may be obtained by catheterization, clean-catch voiding sample, or a U-bag.

RBCs, red blood cells; WBCs, white blood cells.

Data from Corbett, J. A., & Banks, A. D. (2019). *Laboratory tests and diagnostic procedures with nursing diagnoses* (9th ed.). Pearson Education Inc.

Nursing Analysis and Related Interventions

After completing a thorough assessment and initial stabilization of the child, the nurse might identify several patient problems, including:

- Ineffective airway clearance
- Altered breathing pattern
- Impaired gas exchange
- Hypovolemia
- Decreased cardiac output (CO)
- Altered tissue perfusion
- Fear
- Interrupted family processes
- Knowledge deficiency

After completing an assessment of Alma, the nurse noted the following: a patent airway, anxious but able to speak in short sentences, and skin temperature cool on the extremities. Based on these assessment findings, what would your top three patient problems be for Alma? Describe appropriate nursing interventions.

Specific nursing goals, interventions, and evaluation for the child in an emergency are based on the patient's problems. Additional information about nursing management will be included later in the chapter as it relates to specific disorders.

Providing Cardiopulmonary Resuscitation

Check for pulse. In the child, the carotid or femoral pulses are easiest to assess. In the infant, check the femoral pulse. Carefully assess for signs of a pulse, but do not spend more than 10 seconds checking the pulse. If there is not a pulse or if the HR is less than 60 beats/min (bpm), begin chest compressions.

Evaluate and manage the airway. Call for help and assign someone to obtain the automatic external defibrillator (AED). Open the airway and assess for adequate breathing. If the child is not breathing, begin rescue breathing.

TAKE NOTE!

When a cardiac arrest occurs in a child out of the hospital and is a witnessed, sudden collapse, initial management is slightly different than that for other arrests. In these sudden, witnessed events, call 9-1-1 or the local emergency number for help first, get the AED, and return to start CPR (AHA & AAP, 2020).

Table 51.1 presents the AHA's most recent recommendations for ratios of breaths and compressions. These recommendations stress the importance of properly performed chest compressions. Therefore, several changes have been made to the guidelines:

- Rescuers must provide compressions of adequate rate and depth.
- Chest recoil should be allowed.
- Minimal interruption of chest compressions should be the goal.
- For infant CPR, two-person infant CPR can be performed by encircling the chest with two thumbs and simultaneously using the hands to provide a thoracic squeeze.
- For two-person CPR, no pauses should occur for ventilation, with the compressing health care provider giving continuous compressions (AHA & AAP, 2020).

Providing Defibrillation or Synchronized Cardioversion

In some cases, the child has an abnormal life-threatening cardiac rhythm or an dysrhythmia that does not respond to pharmacologic therapy or leads to hemodynamic instability. In these cases, electrical therapy, in the form of defibrillation or synchronized cardioversion, may be needed.

Defibrillation is the use of electrical energy to depolarize the cells of the myocardium to terminate an abnormal life-threatening cardiac rhythm, such as ventricular fibrillation (VF). Defibrillation is used in

TABLE 51.1 • Ratios of Breaths to Compressions

Age	One-Person CPR	Two-Person CPR
Infant	• 30 compressions to two breaths • Hand placement: two fingers, placed one fingerbreadth below the nipple line	• 15 compressions to two breaths • Hand placement: two thumbs encircling the chest at the nipple line
Child	• 30 compressions to two breaths • Hand placement: heel of hand or two hands (adult position in larger child), pressing on the sternum at the nipple line	• 15 compressions to two breaths • Hand placement: heel of one hand or two hands (adult position in larger child), pressing on the sternum at the nipple line

Data from American Heart Association & American Academy of Pediatrics. (2020). *Pediatric advanced life support provider manual.* American Heart Association.

conjunction with oxygen, CPR, and medications. The effects of defibrillation are enhanced in an oxygen-rich environment coupled with good artificial circulation (CPR).

Cardioversion, another means of applying electrical current to the heart, is delivered in a synchronized fashion—that is, the electrical current is applied on the R wave of the electrocardiogram (ECG). Cardioversion is used when the child has supraventricular tachycardia (SVT) or ventricular tachycardia with a pulse. Cardioversion may also be enhanced with medications.

The basic defibrillator is equipped with adult- and pediatric-sized paddles. A switch turns the machine on, and controls are used to select the amount of energy (joules). Typically, the initial energy amount is 2 J/kg; it can be increased up to 4 J/kg for defibrillation. Energy for cardioversion is delivered at 0.5 to 1 J/kg.

When the defibrillator is being used in an acute care setting, the leader of the code team will take charge of defibrillator use. The leader is responsible for ensuring that only the child receives the energy from the defibrillator. The code team leader will count to 4 before delivering a shock to the child to ensure that all personnel and other equipment are clear of the bed to avoid accidental shock.

Using Automated External Defibrillation

In cases of sudden, witnessed, out-of-hospital collapse, a dysrhythmia is often the cause. Therefore, the AHA has revised its recommendations about the use of an AED in children (AHA & AAP, 2020). An AED is an alternative to manually defibrillating an individual. The AED device consists of electrodes that are applied to the chest. These electrodes are used to monitor the heart rhythm and deliver the electrical current. AED devices are readily available in a variety of locations, such as airports, sports facilities, and businesses. Traditionally, the AED was designed for use in adults, but newer AEDs with smaller pads and the ability to alter energy delivery are now more readily available. Therefore, the AHA has recommended that an AED be used for children who are older than age 1 year who have no pulse and have suffered a sudden, witnessed collapse (AHA & AAP, 2020).

The AED is designed for people to use it in the prehospital setting. Once the AED is turned on, the machine uses auditory commands to guide laypeople and health care professionals alike through the correct placement of the electrodes and the administration of energy. The AED periodically evaluates the victim's cardiac rhythm and instructs the user about checking the pulse, continuing CPR, and delivering shocks. Nurses who care for children should be able to operate an AED and be prepared to use it in nontraditional settings.

TAKE NOTE!

Currently, the American Academy of Pediatrics (AAP) recommends the placement of AEDs in all secondary schools, in order to improve outcomes should sudden arrest occur in the school (Fuch, 2018).

Determining Medication Doses and Equipment Sizes

Many pediatric acute care facilities prepare code reference sheets when a child is admitted. This sheet uses the child's actual weight to determine medication doses and equipment sizes. The reference sheet is kept on a clipboard at the child's bedside or taped on the wall at the head of the bed. An additional copy is placed in the child's chart.

Ambulatory care providers often use the Broselow tape to estimate the child's weight based on the child's length (Fig. 51.2). The tape is color coded, and emergency equipment for a child of that size is stored in corresponding color-coded packages or in color-coded drawers on the pediatric emergency cart. Medication doses and equipment sizes are also located on the tape. The most accurate calculation for code medications is based on the child's weight, but use of the Broselow tape for estimating the weight has been shown to be successful in children weighing less than 25 kg (Jones, 2023).

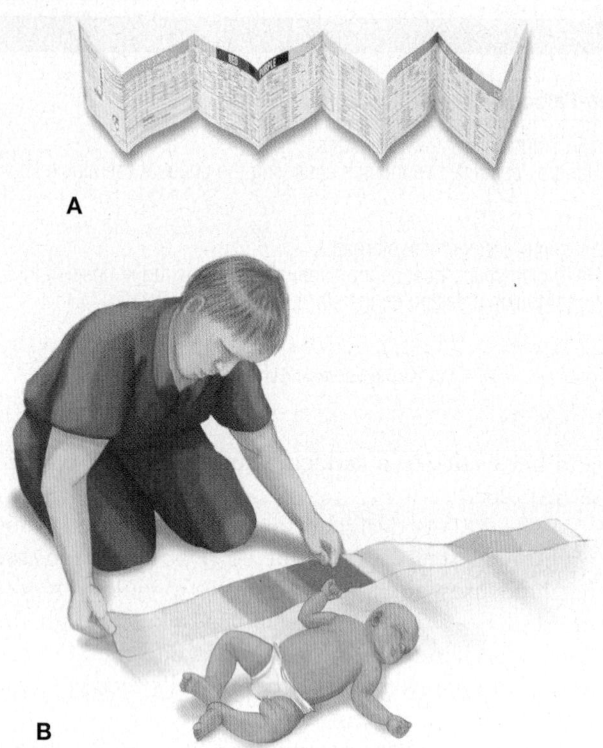

FIGURE 51.2 A. Broselow tape. **B.** Measure the child's length with the Broselow tape to determine medication doses and endotracheal tube size.

Managing Pain

Depending on the child's status and pain level, individualize pain management interventions. For the alert child, nonpharmacologic measures may be used in addition to medications. Provide atraumatic care for procedures and use aggressive pharmacologic treatments to manage pain as the child's condition allows. Refer to Chapter 36 for additional information on pain management strategies.

Ensuring Stabilization

After a child has been resuscitated, the nurse plays a key role in stabilization and transport. Thoroughly document the interventions that were performed as well as the ongoing assessment of the child's response to the interventions. Provide continued monitoring of the child while awaiting transport. Copy and assemble any pertinent documentation, such as the resuscitation record, nurse's notes, and laboratory test results, which will be given to the receiving institution. Ensure that all lines are taped securely and that vascular access sites are dressed and labeled with the date and time of insertion. As soon as possible, bring the child's family in to visit with the child. Provide explanations about the IV lines, monitoring equipment, and other medical equipment and devices. Encourage the family to talk to and touch the child.

Providing Support and Education to the Child and Family

The experience of respiratory distress, oxygen deprivation, and an emergency situation is a frightening one for people of all ages. The lifesaving interventions that take place during an emergency can be especially intimidating and upsetting to children. Infants and young children cannot understand explanations about these interventions, and older children and adolescents may feel frightened and angry about the loss of control. The caregivers may feel fear, anger, guilt, and sadness. They may be concerned about the very real possibility that their child might die.

Resuscitation of a child is often a perplexing and frightening event for laypeople to observe. Therefore, traditionally, family members have been excluded during the resuscitation of children. Recently, however, there has been a trend to allow family members to be present during pediatric resuscitation. Studies have shown that family presence during resuscitation may assist with family coping (Bush & Woodley, 2022).

Considering the highly technical nature of resuscitation, the rapidity with which interventions occur, and the fear associated with a life-threatening event, nurses can play a crucial role in providing understandable explanations to families, coupled with empathic support. During the acute phase, the nurse should give brief explanations as lifesaving interventions are being provided. Examples of these types of explanations include:

- When applying the pulse oximeter sensor: "I need to put this light on your child to check his oxygen level; it won't hurt."
- When connecting the child to the cardiac monitor: "We're going to put these sticky patches on your child and connect them so we can monitor her heart rate on this screen."
- When preparing for intubation and ventilation: "Your child can't breathe on their own right now, so we're going to give them some extra help with this tube. This tube will go through their breathing passage and this machine will help them to breathe" (see Evidence-Based Practice 51.1).

The nurse plays a key role in providing empathy and support. Do not provide false reassurance and say, for example, "Your child is going to be alright." The outcome is never certain. Rather, communicate empathically. For example, say, "This must be very difficult for you. We're doing everything we can to help your child." Provide honest answers in a reassuring manner. Respect each family's diversity and observe their strengths and weaknesses. Be nonjudgmental in all interactions with families, even when the child's emergency situation may have resulted from family neglect.

EVIDENCE-BASED PRACTICE **51.1**

Quality of Pediatric Emergency Care

Children and adolescents comprise a large percentage of the emergency care population, particularly with respect to being seen for injuries and infections. While intervening quickly is often necessary in an emergency situation, it is also important to respect and support children and their parents.

STUDY

Janhunen et al. (2019) conducted a descriptive study of 98 children (ages 7 to 15 years) and their parents from four emergency departments. The authors utilized a survey to compare perceptions of quality of care in the emergency room.

Findings

Overall, parents and children were satisfied with the care received in the emergency room. Interestingly, compared with their parents' scores, children reported the least satisfaction with nursing staff professionalism, ability to talk privately with staff, and ability to participate in planning their own care. Importantly, both parents and children ranked alleviation of the child's pain and fear lowest for all satisfaction items.

Nursing Implications

Though this was a small study, it highlights two important components of care: respect and pain/fear alleviation. When able, nurses should consider speaking with children privately and involve them in care planning, as the situation allows. In all instances, nurses must be vigilant about alleviating fears in children undergoing an emergency situation as well as proactively assessing and managing children's pain.

Data from Janhunen, K., Kankkunen, P., & Kvist, T. (2019). Quality of pediatric emergency care as assessed by children and their parents. *Journal of Nursing Care Quality, 34*(2), 180–184. https://doi.org/10.1097/NCQ.0000000000000346

Parents often feel helpless when their child is in a high-tech environment. Suddenly overwhelmed with the equipment and monitoring devices, they no longer are the people who are the most skilled in caring for their child. Integrate the child's parents into the health care team. Suggest ways the parents can make the hospital experience more normal for their child. For example, simply allowing a parent to read a story to their child or encouraging a parent to hold their child's hand is therapeutic for both the child and the parents. Be aware of this dramatic change and how it affects the parents. Always ensure that they feel like they are a welcome part of their child's care.

Providing the child with familiar comfort objects helps to decrease stress. Once the intubated child is alert and stabilized, assist them with communication. Some children can lift one finger for yes and two fingers for no. If the child is old enough to write, provide paper and pencil. Play is essential to the work of the child, and even if they are immobile, play is still possible. Puppets at the bedside and books help give the child a more normal experience in a scary situation that is far from the norm. Adolescents may enjoy listening to music through headphones. Even children who are comatose should be talked to and allowed to listen to familiar music.

Even if the outcomes are serious, the nurse can provide critical support to children and families. Whether hugging a crying parent or playing "peek-a-boo" with an intubated child, the nurse will be the one who can make a difference during a frightening experience.

• • • ATRAUMATIC CARE • • •

In the conscious child, ensure proximity of the caregiver during the postresuscitation phase to provide security and assist with keeping the child calm.

NURSING MANAGEMENT OF CHILDREN IN EMERGENCIES

Nurses must be adept at identifying the beginning stages of an emergency so they can quickly and appropriately intervene to prevent deterioration to cardiopulmonary arrest. Assessment and management of the most common types of emergencies in children are discussed following. The topics covered include respiratory arrest, shock, cardiac dysrhythmias and arrest, near drowning, poisoning, and traumatic injury.

Respiratory Arrest

Respiratory emergencies may lead to respiratory failure and eventual cardiopulmonary arrest in children. Infants and young children are at greater risk for respiratory emergencies than adolescents and adults because they have smaller airways and underdeveloped immune systems, resulting in a diminished ability to combat serious respiratory illnesses. Young children often lack coordination, making them susceptible to choking on foods and small objects, which may also lead to cardiopulmonary arrest. In addition, sudden unexplained infant death (SUID), also called sudden infant death syndrome (SIDS), is a leading cause of cardiopulmonary arrest in young infants and thus is the leading cause of postneonatal mortality in the United States (Graham & Peoples, 2019). For these reasons, nurses must be skilled at recognizing the signs of pediatric respiratory distress so they can prevent progression to cardiopulmonary arrest. Table 51.2 lists some of the more common causes of pediatric respiratory arrest.

TABLE 51.2 • Causes of Respiratory Arrest in Children

Condition	Cause
Upper airway	Burns Croup Epiglottitis Foreign-body aspiration Reflux Strangulation or near strangulation Tracheomalacia Vascular ring
Lower airway	Asthma Bronchiolitis Burns Foreign-body aspiration Pertussis infection Pneumonia Pneumothorax Reflux
Nonrespiratory origins	Septic shock HIV
Neurologic	CNS infection Guillain–Barré syndrome Poliomyelitis Seizures Sleep apnea Spinal cord trauma Sudden infant death
Chronic illness	Complications of severe prematurity Cystic fibrosis Bone marrow transplant Neutropenia
Metabolic/endocrine disorders	Diabetic ketoacidosis Mitochondrial disorders
Cardiac conditions	Dysrhythmia Congenital cardiac problems Acquired cardiac problems
Traumatic/unintentional/intentional injury	Asphyxia Child abuse/"shaken baby syndrome" Drowning Electrocution Gunshot wound Toxic ingestion Vehicle-related trauma

CNS, central nervous system; HIV, human immunodeficiency virus.

Data from Shaw, K. N., & Bachur, R. G. (Eds.). (2020). *Fleisher and Ludwig's textbook of pediatric emergency medicine* (8th ed.). Wolters Kluwer.

Nursing Assessment

If the child has severe respiratory compromise, obtain a brief history while simultaneously providing respiratory interventions. To obtain the history, use the following questions as a guide:

- When did the symptoms begin and when do they occur?
- Did the symptoms have a sudden onset (as with a foreign-body aspiration)?
- How have the symptoms progressed?
- Is the cough continual, intermittent, or worse at night or with exercise?
- Has there been any stridor? (Stridor is heard upon inhalation and may be associated with swelling of the trachea [as with croup] or with a foreign body in the upper airway.)
- Is there wheezing? If so, is the wheezing on inspiration, on expiration, or both?
- What makes the symptoms better and what makes them worse?
- Does drinking from a bottle induce the symptoms (as with gastroesophageal reflux–induced aspiration)?
- Is the child taking any medication for the symptoms? Does the child or do any members of the immediate family have a history of chronic respiratory disease, such as asthma?
- Are the child's immunizations up to date?
- Was the child born prematurely? If so, did the child require mechanical ventilation? For how long?
- Were there any respiratory problems during the first few days of life?
- When did the child last eat? (This question is important because a recent meal will increase the child's risk of aspiration in the event of a respiratory arrest. In addition, the presence of food in the stomach will increase the risk of aspiration during tracheal intubation.)

If the child can communicate, ask how they are feeling. Are they short of breath? Does their chest hurt? Observe the child while speaking. Children who are in respiratory distress may speak in short sentences with gasping between words.

PHYSICAL EXAMINATION

In an emergency, physical examination is often limited to inspection, observation, and auscultation. First, quickly survey the respiratory status. Determine if the child is breathing.

Inspection and Observation

Establish if the airway is patent, maintainable, or unable to be maintained. The child with a patent airway is breathing without signs of obstruction. The maintainable airway remains patent independently by the child or with interventions such as a towel roll under an infant's neck or the insertion of a nasal trumpet. The airway that cannot be maintained does not remain patent unless a more aggressive intervention, such as the insertion of a tracheal tube, is performed.

Look at the child's posture. Is the child sitting up, leaning forward, and drooling, as with epiglottitis? Observe the child's face: Do they appear anxious or relaxed? Children in respiratory distress often appear anxious. Look at the nose and mouth. Are the nares patent? Is there noticeable nasal congestion or mucus coming from the nose? Note nasal flaring or mouth breathing. Observe for head bobbing. Listen for audible expiratory grunting or inspiratory stridor. Note the child's color. Does the child appear pale, mottled, dusky, or cyanotic? Children may appear mottled in response to poor oxygenation, hypothermia, or stress. Children with severe respiratory compromise may appear dusky. Look for cyanosis around the mouth or on the trunk. Cyanosis is a late and often ominous sign of respiratory distress. Central cyanosis is more likely to be associated with respiratory or cardiac compromise. In contrast, peripheral cyanosis is more likely to be associated with circulatory alteration.

TAKE NOTE!

Closely inspect the color of the area around the mouth. Circumoral pallor is a sign of poor oxygenation.

Evaluate the pattern and quality of respiration, noting the respiratory rate. Tachypnea (increased respiratory rate) is often noted in children in respiratory distress. However, seriously ill children grunt and may have normal or subnormal respiratory rates. **Hypoventilation**, a decrease in the depth and rate of respirations, is noted in very ill children or in children who have central respiratory depression secondary to narcotics. If the child is a young infant (younger than 2 months) or premature, periodic breathing may occur. **Periodic breathing** is regular breathing with occasional short pauses (brief periods of apnea). After the apneic pause, the infant will breathe rapidly (up to 60 breaths/min) for a short period and then will resume a normal respiratory rate. In general, the infant who has periodic breathing looks pink and has a normal HR. Observe for the use of accessory muscles in the neck or retractions in the chest, determining the extent and severity of the retractions.

Auscultation

Auscultate the lungs with the diaphragm of the stethoscope. Breath sounds over the tracheal region are higher pitched and are described as vesicular, while breath sounds over the peripheral lung fields tend to be lower pitched, known as bronchial. Instruct the child to take deep breaths with the mouth open. To encourage the young child to exhale strongly, instruct them to "blow out" the penlight (as with a candle) or to blow on a tissue. Encourage the child not to breathe more rapidly than normal (to prevent **hyperventilation** [increased depth and rate of respirations]) and to avoid making any noises with the mouth.

TAKE NOTE!

Significant upper respiratory congestion often interferes with the assessment of the lower airways because the sound is easily transmitted throughout the chest. Differentiate between the upper and lower airway noises by listening with the stethoscope over the nose. The nurse may be able to determine whether the noise is nasal or bronchial by using this technique.

Auscultate the child's chest systematically. Listen in all anterior, axillary, and posterior regions, comparing the left to the right sides. Note any decreased or absent breath sounds, which may be the result of bronchial obstruction (as with mucous infection) or air trapping (as in children with asthma). Unilateral absent breath sounds are associated with foreign-body aspiration and pneumothorax.

TAKE NOTE!

Sometimes a child's respiratory status is so severely compromised that little or no air movement is noted. This commonly occurs during a severe asthma exacerbation. Minimal or no air movement requires immediate intervention.

Note the presence and location of adventitious breath sounds such as crackles, wheezes, or rhonchi. Document the presence of a pleural friction rub (a low-pitched, grating sound), a sound resulting from inflammation of the pleura.

Palpation

Palpate the chest for any abnormalities. In the older, less severely ill, and cooperative child, assess for tactile fremitus. Using the palm of the hand, palpate over the lung regions in the same manner as for auscultation and percussion while the child says "ninety-nine." Increased vibrations elicited during this maneuver are associated with consolidating conditions, such as pneumonia.

Percussion

Percuss the interspaces of the chest between the ribs in the same systematic fashion as with auscultation. Normally, percussion over an air-filled lung reveals resonant sounds. Note the presence of hyperresonance, which may indicate an acute problem such as a pneumothorax or a chronic disease such as asthma. In contrast, percussion sounds will be dull over a lobe of the lung that is consolidated with fluid, infectious organisms, and blood cells, as in the case of pneumonia.

LABORATORY AND DIAGNOSTIC TESTING

Use continuous pulse oximetry if respiratory status is a concern. Note and report oxygen saturation levels below 95% (see Chapter 40 for additional information about the use of the pulse oximeter).

Additional tests may reveal:

- Arterial or capillary blood gases: hypoxemia, hypercarbia, altered pH
- Chest radiograph: alterations in normal anatomy or lung expansion, or evidence of pneumonia, tumor, or foreign body
- Metal detector: evidence of coins (Gilger & Jain, 2022)

> **TAKE NOTE!**
>
> Children with cardiac conditions resulting in cyanosis often have baseline oxygen saturations that are relatively low because of the mixing of oxygenated with deoxygenated blood.

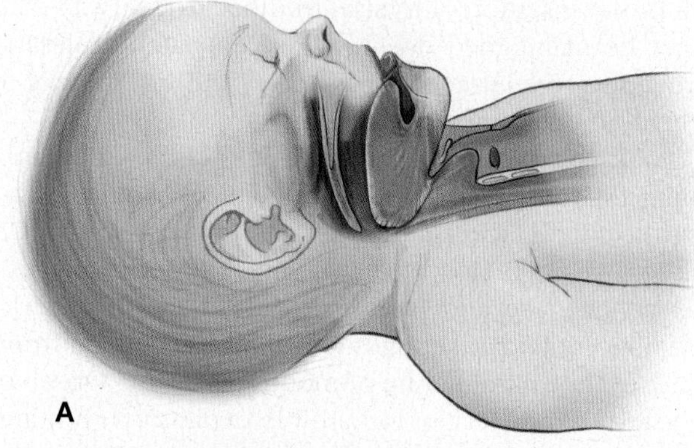

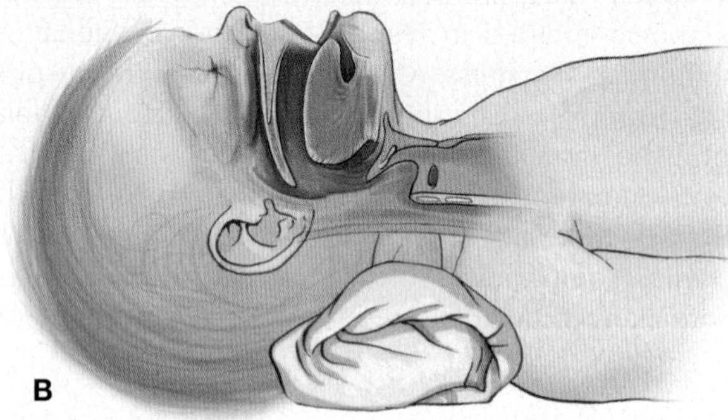

FIGURE 51.3 **A.** The infant and young child's prominent occiput encourages flexion of the neck and may result in airway occlusion. **B.** Putting a towel roll under the shoulders or neck helps to open the infant's or young child's airway by placing it in the neutral or "sniff" position.

Nursing Management

The basic principle of pediatric emergency care and PALS is the prevention of cardiopulmonary arrest (AHA & AAP, 2020). Therefore, the nurse must rapidly assess and appropriately manage children who have signs of respiratory distress. Nursing management of the child in respiratory distress involves maintaining a patent airway, providing supplemental oxygen, monitoring for changes in status, and in some cases assisting ventilation. In addition to providing these lifesaving measures and monitoring the child's progress, offer support and education to the child and family.

MAINTAINING A PATENT AIRWAY

When a child exhibits signs of respiratory distress, make a quick decision about whether it will be safe to allow the child to stay with the parent or whether the child must be placed on the examination table or bed. For example, in the case of croup, the child will often breathe more comfortably and experience less stridor while in the comfort of the parent's lap. Many children in respiratory distress often are most comfortable sitting upright, as this position helps to decrease the work of breathing by allowing appropriate diaphragmatic movement. In contrast, a child with a decreasing level of consciousness may need to be placed in the supine position to facilitate positioning of the airway.

The infant may benefit from a small towel folded under the shoulders or neck (Fig. 51.3). Avoid neck flexion or hyperextension, which may completely occlude the infant's airway. In children older than age 1 year, the optimal method for opening the airway is to hyperextend the neck (AHA & AAP, 2020). If a cervical spine injury is not suspected, use the head tilt–chin lift technique to open the airway. If the child has suffered head or neck trauma and cervical spine instability is a concern, use the jaw-thrust maneuver by placing three fingers under the child's lower jaw and lifting the jaw upward and outward (Fig. 51.4). In either case, never place the hand under the neck to open the airway.

Often the nurse encounters an acutely ill child who cannot maintain an airway independently but may be able to do so with some assistance. For example, sometimes simply opening the airway and moving the tongue

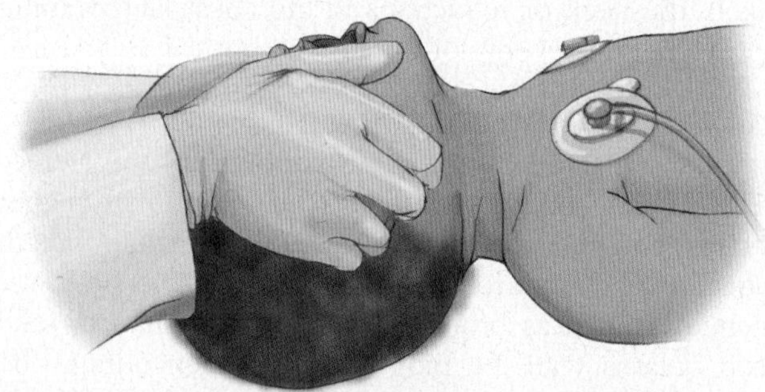

FIGURE 51.4 Jaw-thrust technique for opening the airway.

COMPARISON CHART 51.1 Oropharyngeal Versus Nasopharyngeal Airways

Oropharyngeal airway (used only in unconscious children)	• Consists of a simple plastic curved body that has a central air channel to allow for aeration • Is used when an unconscious child has difficulty maintaining airway patency due to upper airway obstruction, such as from the tongue • Allows for oral suction • Determine the correct size of the airway by placing it next to the child's cheek with the tip pointing down. An airway that is too large will extend past the angle of the child's mandible and can obstruct the glottic opening when inserted. • Choose the airway that best fits the child to decrease the risk of injury to the structures of the mouth.
Nasopharyngeal airway (may be used in conscious children and children who have an intact gag reflex)	• Consists of a flexible curved tube that is inserted nasally • Is used when the child has difficulty maintaining airway patency due to tongue obstruction or palate problems, when neurologic impairment causes poor pharyngeal tone, or in the child with impaired consciousness • Allows for nasopharyngeal suction • When selecting this airway, keep in mind that the diameter of the airway should not be so large that it puts too much pressure on the internal nasal tissue. There are two common methods for measuring this airway: (a) measure the distance from the end of the child's nose to the tragus of the ear; (b) look at the child's fifth digit, which is usually the approximate diameter of the nasopharyngeal airway. • Monitor for mucosal irritation, nasal septum swelling, and laceration of the adenoids. • Do not use this type of airway in children with a history of bleeding disorders and basilar skull fractures. • This airway's small diameter can easily become obstructed with secretions and blood.

away from the tracheal opening is all that is required to regain airway patency. In certain conditions, a nasopharyngeal or oropharyngeal airway may be necessary for airway maintenance. Comparison Chart 51.1 provides additional information about these types of airways.

ASSISTING VENTILATION USING A BVM

The child in respiratory distress may ventilate poorly, hypoventilate, or tire and become apneic. In this case, the child may require assistance with ventilation through BVM ventilation. Refer to Table 51.3 for additional information on BVM ventilation, tracheal **intubation** (the insertion of a tube into the trachea for the purposes of ventilation), the use of an anesthesia bag or flow-inflating ventilation system, and laryngeal mask airways.

BVM ventilation is used in the management of children who cannot ventilate or oxygenate effectively on their own. This technique is a more efficient way of

TABLE 51.3 • Airway and Ventilation Methods

Method	Description	Comments
Anesthesia bag or flow-inflating ventilation systems	A small, collapsible bag that consists of a reservoir bag, an overflow port, and a fresh gas inflow port	• Adjustment of the oxygen flow and of the outlet control valve is necessary. • Useful in providing positive end-expiratory pressure (PEEP) or continuous positive airway pressure (CPAP) • Adequate training and significant skill are needed to properly operate this device. • Hypercapnia and barotrauma may result with improper use. • Used more commonly in the postanesthesia care unit (PACU) and in the neonatal intensive care unit
Bag-valve-mask device or manual resuscitator	A self-inflating oxygen delivery bag that does not require an oxygen source for resuscitation and ventilation. The bag can be connected to oxygen to provide higher oxygen levels than room air. When the child exhales, the nonrebreathing valve closes, allowing exhaled, deoxygenated air to escape.	• Effective in providing oxygen to a child who is in severe respiratory distress or who has suffered a respiratory arrest • A more efficient method of respiratory resuscitation than mouth-to-mouth resuscitation; decreased rescuer exposure to communicable disease • Most medical personnel can be trained to perform resuscitation with this method • Possibly tiring for the rescuer when used to ventilate a child for long periods of time (see discussion on bag-mask ventilation)

(*continued*)

TABLE 51.3 • Airway and Ventilation Methods (*continued*)

Method	Description	Comments
Laryngeal mask airway	An inflatable silicone mask and rubber connecting tube that is inserted blindly into the airway, forming a seal	• The airway is introduced into the pharynx and advanced until it meets resistance; balloon cuff is then inflated. • Easier insertion than an endotracheal tube • Usually used in the unconscious child who benefits from bag-valve-mask ventilation but does not require intubation • Improvement in child comfort
Endotracheal intubation	A plastic tube inserted in the trachea to establish and maintain an airway when the airway cannot be maintained effectively using other measures (e.g., nasal trumpet or bag-valve-mask ventilation)	• Skilled medical professional (health care provider, nurse practitioner, respiratory specialist, emergency medical technician, or health care provider's assistant) necessary for insertion • The nurse acts as a valuable assistant during the intubation procedure.

ensuring ventilation than using only supplemental oxygen. In addition, resuscitating a child in this manner is superior to mouth-to-mouth resuscitation as it provides higher oxygen concentrations and protects the nurse from exposure to oral secretions (AHA & AAP, 2020). However, this technique requires proper training and practice. The proper procedure involves appropriate opening of the airway followed by providing breaths with the BVM.

Ventilation with the BVM may be performed with either one or two rescuers. First, choose an appropriate-sized bag and a corresponding facemask that fits the infant or child. Self-inflating bags are usually available in neonatal, infant, child, and adult sizes. Corresponding masks are available. Choose a facemask that properly fits the child's face and that provides a seal over the nose and mouth and excludes the eyes, thus preventing any pressure on the eyes (Fig. 51.5).

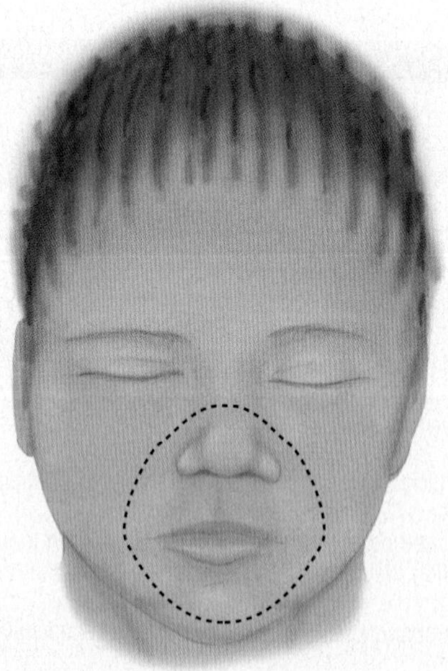

FIGURE 51.5 The mask should form a seal over the nose and mouth, across the chin and nose bridge.

TAKE NOTE!

Facemasks should be clear so that the nurse can see the child's lip color and identify any emesis during resuscitation.

Connect the BVM via the tubing to the oxygen source and turn on the oxygen. When resuscitating infants and children, set the flow rate at approximately 10 L/min. For an adolescent who is adult sized, set the flow rate at 15 L/min or higher to compensate for the larger volume bag. Check to make sure that the oxygen is flowing through the tubing to the bag. Self-inflating bags do not provide free-flow oxygen out of the facemask; manual pumping of the bag is necessary. However, the bags have a corrugated plastic tail that allows oxygen to freely flow. Therefore, check over the tail for oxygen flow through the bag.

After opening the airway appropriately (see earlier), place the mask over the child's face. When one rescuer is providing ventilation (commonly referred to as "bagging"), the person must provide a seal with the mask over the child's face with one hand and use the other hand to manipulate the resuscitator bag. The hand used to provide the mask seal will simultaneously maintain the airway in an open position. Generally, use the left thumb and index finger to hold the mask on the child's face. While maintaining a good seal with the mask, use upward pressure on the jaw angle while pressing downward on the mask below the child's mouth to keep the mouth open (Fig. 51.6). Take care not to put pressure on the neck with the fourth and fifth fingers.

If adequate personnel are available, a more desirable situation involves one person standing behind the child's head to maintain an open airway and to provide a seal of the mask over the face with a hand on each side (usually the thumbs and second fingers). A second rescuer stands on one side of the child and compresses the bag to ventilate the child using both hands. If the child is more difficult to ventilate, the two-rescuer method allows the ventilating nurse to provide better ventilation

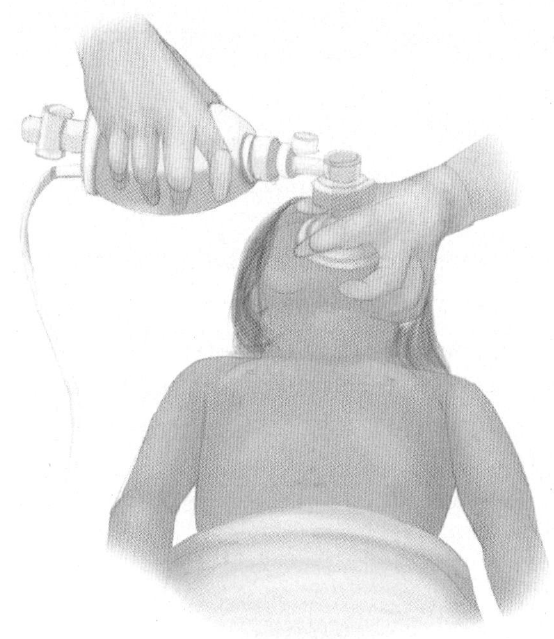

FIGURE 51.6 Proper hand placement for maintaining airway and adequate mask seal using one-rescuer technique.

than with the one-rescuer method. In addition, the two-rescuer method ensures the best possible mask seal, as the rescuer holding the mask can use both hands to maintain the seal.

Regardless of the number of people present, proper placement of the facemask is critical, and a good seal must be maintained throughout the resuscitation. In addition, during ventilation, use only the force and tidal volume necessary to cause a chest rise, no more. If a good chest rise is not observed, attempt to open the airway again. It may be necessary to adjust the position of the airway a few times to achieve a patency conducive to ventilation.

Compress the bag to deliver breaths at the amount recommended in infants and children. Initially, provide two rescue breaths and observe for a chest rise. Rescue breaths should not overinflate the lungs. Breaths should be delivered over 1 second. After the first two rescue ventilations, perform rescue breathing at a rate of one breath every 3 to 5 seconds or about 12 to 20 breaths/min. Delivering each breath should be a steady, one-inhalation-to-one-exhalation ratio. This means that the amount of time delivering the inspiratory ventilation is equal to the amount of time that expiration is allowed. While ventilating the infant or child, work with, not against, any spontaneous respiratory effort; in other words, if the child is breathing out, do not attempt to force air in at the same time.

Monitoring Effectiveness of Ventilation

During the resuscitation, continually reassess the child's response to the resuscitative efforts, noting:

- Adequacy of chest rise
- Absence or minimal presence of abdominal distention
- Improved HR and pulse oximetry readings
- Improved color
- Capillary refill less than 3 seconds with strengthening pulses

If the child's status deteriorates and they become pulseless, then CPR must be started. In addition, periodically and briefly stop ventilating to evaluate for spontaneous respirations.

Preventing Complications Related to BVM Ventilation

During resuscitation, health care personnel usually exhibit high-energy levels, a normal physiologic response that facilitates resuscitative efforts as the rescuers act quickly. However, this heightened state can lead to overzealousness while ventilating an infant or child. Health care providers may inadvertently ventilate the child too rapidly using too much tidal volume, leading to excessive ventilation volume and increased airway pressure. This poor technique can be detrimental to the child, causing:

- Reduced CO (due to increased intrathoracic pressure and increased cardiac afterload)
- Air trapping
- **Barotrauma** (trauma caused by changes in pressure)
- Air leak (thus reducing the oxygen delivered to the child)

Thus, nurses must be mindful of their technique during bagging, not exceeding the recommended respiratory rate or providing too much tidal volume to the child. Ventilate the child in a controlled and uniform manner, providing just enough volume to result in a chest rise.

Assisting With Ventilation Using Tracheal Intubation

ET intubation is needed if the infant or child does not have a maintainable airway or will require artificial ventilation for a prolonged time (see Table 51.3). Intubation of infants and children is a procedure that requires great skill and therefore should be performed by only the most qualified and experienced personnel. Children are most commonly intubated orally, rather than nasally, in acute situations.

Nurses are an essential part of the intubation team, usually assisting a health care provider, nurse practitioner, respiratory therapist, or health care provider's assistant during the intubation procedure (Nursing Procedure 51.1). The nurse may set up the equipment, prepare and administer intubation medications, or assist with suctioning the oral secretions and preparing the tape to secure the ET tube. In a child in full arrest, the nurse might be responsible for performing ongoing chest compressions while other team members manage the child's airway.

NURSING PROCEDURE 51.1 Assisting With Endotracheal Intubation

1. Prepare equipment and supplies.
2. Draw up medications (for rapid sequence intubation).
3. Turn up the volume on the cardiac monitor so that members of the team can easily hear the audible QRS indication of the child's heart rate and note any bradycardia with the procedure.
4. Turn on the suction. Make sure that suction is working by placing your hand over the tubing before you attach the suction catheter.
5. Continue to ventilate the child with the bag-valve-mask (BVM) and 100% oxygen as the team prepares to intubate the child.
6. When there is no suspected cervical spine injury, in the child older than age 2 years, place a small pillow under the child's head to facilitate opening of the airway; this step is unnecessary in children younger than age 2 due to the prominence of their occiput.
7. When assisting with the intubation, stand beside the child's head and prepare to assist with suctioning of oral secretions, providing BVM ventilation as needed, and assisting with securing the tube with tape.
8. Before the initial intubation attempt and after each subsequent attempt to intubate, provide several inhalations of 100% oxygen via the BVM ventilation method (optimally for a few minutes).
9. Administer premedication and medications for sedation.
10. Administer paralyzing medication.
11. Observe as the health care professional who is intubating the child follows the recommended procedure for intubation using the laryngoscope to visualize the vocal cords.

Setting Up Equipment

Appropriate setup and preparation of equipment is essential (Table 51.4). The ET tube size used depends on the child's size. To calculate ET tube size, divide the child's age by 4 and add 4. The resulting number will indicate the size of the ET tube in millimeters. For example, if the child is 2 years old, the proper-sized tube would be 4.5 ([2/4] + 4 = 4.5). Always have one size smaller ready also, so have a 4.0 and a 4.5 ET tube for this child.

TABLE 51.4 • Equipment and Supplies for Endotracheal Intubation

Laryngoscope blades	Straight blades (Miller) are usually used for infants and young children. A curved-blade laryngoscope (Macintosh) may be used for older children and adolescents. The blade has a little light bulb attached to it for visualization of the trachea. The light bulb should be bright and attached securely.
Endotracheal tubes	Three sizes should be readily available: the estimated size, a size smaller, and a size larger. A stylet may be used to guide the tube through the child's vocal cords (it is then removed after the intubation procedure).
Oxygen	100% oxygen is provided using a bag-valve-mask before intubation and after unsuccessful intubation attempts.
Suction	Properly working wall or portable suction with appropriate-sized suction catheters (that fit the endotracheal tube) should be prepared; the package is opened, leaving the sterile-tipped end inside the package, and connecting the other end to the suction tubing. A Yankauer suction catheter (large catheter) should also be available if copious secretions are present in the mouth that interfere with the ability to visualize the airway.
Monitors	Pulse oximeter and cardiac monitor with an audible tone indicating the QRS complex should be in place. Exhaled CO_2 device is needed to detect increased CO_2 levels after the intubation.
Nasogastric (NG) tube	Placing an NG tube will help to mitigate abdominal distention. Children who are manually ventilated typically have some abdominal distention as some air passes into the stomach.
Personal protective equipment	Usually, just gloves, goggles, and a mask are necessary to protect health care workers. In the case of copious bleeding, health care workers should wear gowns also.
Tape, etc.	Tape should be prepared for securing the tube. Benzoin, a sticky substance, is usually applied under the tape for enhanced security of the tape. For children who have had multiple intubations, a protective barrier (as used to protect the skin around an ostomy) may be applied under the tape to protect the skin. Gauze pads should be available to clean up excess secretions that may interfere with taping the endotracheal tube.

Administering Medications

Several medications are often used to facilitate intubation of children. Premedicating a child before passing an ET tube aids in:

- Reducing pain and anxiety (consistent with the concept of atraumatic care)
- Minimizing the effects of passing the ET tube down the airway (vagal stimulation leading to **bradycardia** [decrease in HR])
- Preventing hypoxia
- Reducing intracranial pressure
- Preventing airway trauma and aspiration of stomach contents

The use of medications during the intubation process is known as rapid sequence intubation (Table 51.5). Typically, these medications are used in controlled settings such as the emergency department or the intensive care unit (ICU). Rapid sequence intubation is done only in children who are not experiencing cardiac arrest. If the intubation is expected to be particularly difficult, paralyzing medication should not be used.

The nurse must be aware of the differences in the various medication classes, their advantages, their disadvantages, and adverse effects. The nurse must also be able to distinguish between medications that produce sedation and ones that produce analgesia. Children who are paralyzed and sedated may be suffering severe pain. The pain control needs of children who are acutely ill are of paramount importance and cannot be overstated. Do not mistake a child who is immobilized as a result of sedative and paralytic medications for a child who is pain free.

TABLE **51.5** • Medications for Rapid Sequence Intubation

Medications	Desired Effects	Undesirable Effects
Anticholinergic: atropine	Decreases respiratory secretions and mitigates the vagal effects of intubation, thus decreasing the risk of bradycardia	Doses that are too low (<0.1 mg) can cause a paradoxical bradycardia. Young infants are more prone to the bradycardic effects of atropine, so its use is generally contraindicated in this population.
Sedatives: barbiturates—thiopental (short-acting barbiturate)	Has very rapid onset and short duration of action; reduces intracranial pressure and oxygen demand	Hypotensive effects of this drug are more severe in the dehydrated child. When given in combination with narcotics, respiratory depression is potentiated.
Sedatives: benzodiazepines—midazolam	Has a slightly slower onset than thiopental but is associated with fewer adverse effects Also causes amnesia Can be titrated up or down (at lower doses, it causes conscious sedation; at higher doses, it can induce anesthesia)	When given in combination with narcotics, respiratory depression is potentiated.
Anesthetic agent: ketamine	Has a rapid onset with sedative, amnesic, and analgesic effects. Can be dissociative (child is awake but unaware). May improve BP and cause bronchodilation (helpful for children with status asthmaticus)	Ketamine can cause increased intracranial pressure and increased ocular pressure. Therefore, children who have suffered head trauma or globe injury should not receive this medication. Because of ketamine's sympathetic effects, hypertension can result from its use. Ketamine tends to cause increased secretions, often necessitating the concomitant use of atropine to counteract this adverse effect. May cause hallucinations and is therefore contraindicated in children with psychiatric problems.
Anesthetic agent: lidocaine	Can decrease intracranial pressure at higher doses Has an advantage when used in the management of hypovolemia because it is less likely to cause hypotension	Lidocaine can cause adverse cardiac effects (bradycardia, hypotension, dysrhythmias) in high doses. May be associated with CNS depression and seizures
Narcotic analgesic: fentanyl citrate	A highly concentrated opioid that causes fewer adverse effects (e.g., pruritus) than other opioids Also exerts a less hypotensive effect	Constipation and urinary retention (as is common with opioids) may occur. Increases risk for respiratory depression, increased intracranial pressure, and hypotension Chest wall rigidity is common with this drug and may cause difficulty with ventilation.

(*continued*)

TABLE 51.5 • Medications for Rapid Sequence Intubation (*continued*)

Medications	Desired Effects	Undesirable Effects
Paralyzing or neuromuscular blocking agents: rocuronium, succinylcholine, vecuronium	Used for short-term paralysis during the intubation process. May be used for extended paralysis in the ICU for children in whom movement would be detrimental. For example, a child with epiglottitis has a very precarious airway and must remain intubated until the epiglottis decreases in size. In certain respiratory conditions, spontaneous respiratory effort would interfere with the ventilation of a child, and therefore prolonged paralysis is desirable.	Succinylcholine (a depolarizing agent) has always been the gold standard for paralysis because it has a relatively rapid onset and is short acting. However, it has a greater risk of adverse effects (bradycardia, hyperkalemia, hypertension, increased intracranial, and ocular pressure) and is contraindicated in a variety of clinical conditions. The contemporary approach to paralysis involves the use of longer acting agents, such as rocuronium and vecuronium, because children have fewer adverse effects with these medications. In addition, rocuronium and vecuronium may be used for extended paralysis (not an option with succinylcholine).

BP, blood pressure; CNS, central nervous system; ICU, intensive care unit.

Data from American Heart Association & American Academy of Pediatrics. (2020). *Pediatric advanced life support provider manual.* American Heart Association; UpToDate, Inc. (2024). *UpToDate Lexidrug* (Version 8.2.0) [Mobile app]. Wolters Kluwer. https://apps.apple.com/us/app/lexicomp/id313401238

TAKE NOTE!

Attempts to insert an ET tube should last no longer than 20 to 30 seconds each. After each attempt, the child should receive multiple ventilations by the BVM method using 100% oxygen (AHA & AAP, 2020).

Ensuring and Maintaining Correct Tube Placement

To assess for correct placement once the ET tube is inserted, apply the end-tidal CO_2 monitor to check for placement. Also observe for symmetric chest rise and auscultate over the lung fields for equal breath sounds. Inspect the ET tube for the presence of water vapor on the inside, indicating that the tube is in the trachea. To rule out accidental esophageal intubation, auscultate over the abdomen while the child is being ventilated: There should not be breath sounds in the abdomen. Note improvement in the oxygen saturation level via pulse oximetry.

Once ET tube placement is verified, mark the tube with an indelible pen at the level of the child's lip and secure it with tape. Document the number on the ET tube at the level of the child's mouth. Anticipate a chest radiograph to confirm the correct placement of the ET tube.

After placement is confirmed, the ET tube is connected to the ventilator by respiratory personnel. The ventilator will provide continuous artificial ventilation and oxygenation. Exhaled CO_2 monitoring is recommended as it provides an indication of appropriate ventilation (Box 51.1); the exhaled CO_2 should register yellow.

The nurse plays a key role in ensuring that the ET tube remains taped securely in place by doing the following:

- Using soft wrist restraints if necessary to prevent the child from removing the ET tube
- Providing sedative and/or paralyzing medications
- Using caution when moving the child for radiographs, changing linens, and performing other procedures

Monitoring the Child Who Is Intubated

Provide ongoing and frequent monitoring of the intubated child to determine the adequacy of oxygenation and ventilation as noted earlier. Once the child is intubated, the ventilatory support being provided should result in improvement in oxygen saturation and vital signs. If the child begins to exhibit signs of poor oxygenation, perform a quick assessment. Auscultate the lungs for equal air entry and determine the HR. Are the breath sounds equal? Is the HR normal for age? Perform a quick survey of the equipment and look for any disconnected tubes or kinks in the tubing. Determine oxygen saturation levels via pulse oximeter and evaluate the end-tidal

BOX 51.1 Exhaled CO_2 Monitoring or End-Tidal CO_2 Monitoring

- Device that connects to the child's ventilator circuit to detect CO_2 in the tubing. CO_2 should be noted in the tubing after six ventilations.
- Devices are usually color coded. In the case of endotracheal intubation, observe the color on the device change from purple to tan to yellow.
- Colors on the end-tidal CO_2 device correspond with endotracheal tube placement:
  - Purple = little or no CO_2 detected, <3 mm Hg
  - Tan = 3 to 15 mm Hg exhaled CO_2
  - Yellow = >15 mm Hg exhaled CO_2 (Krauss et al., 2024)
- NOTE: Colorimetric end-tidal CO_2 devices may at times fail to detect the presence of exhaled carbon dioxide, so continue to rely upon visualization of tube placement, symmetric chest rise, and bilateral breath sounds.

(AHA & AAP, 2020)

CO_2 color (see Box 51.1). Use the mnemonic "DOPE" for troubleshooting when the status of a child who is intubated deteriorates:

- D = Displacement. The ET tube is displaced from the trachea.
- O = Obstruction. The ET tube is obstructed (e.g., with a mucous plug).
- P = Pneumothorax. Usually, a pneumothorax results in a sudden change in the child's assessment. The signs of a pneumothorax include decreased breath sounds and decreased chest expansion on the side of the pneumothorax. Subcutaneous emphysema may be noted over the chest. In the case of tension pneumothorax, there may be a sudden drop in HR and BP.
- E = Equipment failure. Relatively simple problems as previously discussed, such as a disconnected oxygen supply, can cause the child to deteriorate. Culprits such as a leak in the ventilator circuit or a loss of power are other types of equipment failure that may be responsible (AHA & AAP, 2020).

Make sure all equipment is appropriately connected and functional. When obstruction with secretions is suspected, suction the ET tube. If the ET tube is displaced from the trachea, remove the tube if it remains in the child's mouth and begin BVM ventilation. In the case of pneumothorax, prepare to assist with needle thoracotomy.

Preparing the Intubated Child for Transport

Once the child is stabilized with a secure ET tube in place, prepare to transport the child. The child will be moved by stretcher to an ICU in the acute care facility or by air or land ambulance to another facility that specializes in the care of acutely ill children. Make sure that all tubes are taped securely. During transport, use portable oxygen and ventilate manually with the BVM. As the sending nurse, ensure that all laboratory results are obtained and provided to the receiving nurse. If the child is going to another facility, complete a detailed summary of the resuscitation or provide a copy of the nurse's and/or progress notes. Complete the appropriate transfer forms as determined by the institution.

If the child is being transported by ambulance, the parents may not be able to accompany their child. In this case, find out as much as possible about the transport and assist the parents by giving directions to the receiving institution.

SHOCK

Shock may be defined as an inability for blood flow and oxygen delivery to meet the metabolic demands of tissue (Herchline & Gaw, 2023). If shock is left untreated, cardiopulmonary arrest will result. Shock, which may be classified as compensated or decompensated, is due to a variety of clinical problems. Compensated shock occurs when poor perfusion exists without a decrease in BP. In decompensated shock, inadequate perfusion is accompanied by a drop in BP. Unchecked decompensated shock leads to cardiac arrest and death. The principles of PALS stress the early evaluation and management of children in compensated shock with the goal of preventing decompensated shock (Herchline & Gaw, 2023). Once the child in shock is hypotensive, organ perfusion is dramatically impaired, and a dire clinical scenario ensues.

Pathophysiology

Shock is the result of dramatic respiratory or hemodynamic compromise. Impaired CO, impaired systemic vascular resistance (SVR), or a combination of both causes shock. CO is equal to HR times ventricular stroke volume (SV) ($CO = HR \times SV$). SV is how much blood is ejected from the heart with each beat. SV is related to left ventricular filling pressure, the impedance to ventricular filling, and myocardial contractility. Left ventricular filling pressure is also known as preload, and the impedance to ventricular filling is commonly called afterload. Young children and infants have relatively small SVs compared to older children and adults. Therefore, infants and young children differ from their adult counterparts in that their CO depends on their HR, not their SV. Clinically, in cases of circulatory compromise and compensated shock in infants and children, HR is increased. The exception to this is a paradoxical phenomenon in neonates, who may have bradycardia rather than tachycardia.

SVR or afterload is the impediment to the heart's ventricular ejection. Increased SVR will result in a decrease in blood flow unless the ventricular pressure increases. Increased vascular resistance is a common problem in shock. In children who have shock-related increased SVR, CO will fall unless the ventricle can compensate by increasing pressure. In cardiac insufficiency, the child's heart will have an impaired ability to compensate for the increased afterload.

Altered microcirculatory status is common in all types of shock. Compensatory mechanisms are activated in response to decreased blood flow. Sympathetic nervous system response results in marked contraction of larger vessel sphincters and arterioles. This compression results in dramatically impaired capillary blood flow. Blood is redirected away from less important body systems, such as the skin and the kidneys, to the vital organs (the heart and brain).

During compensated shock, the body can maintain some level of blood flow to the vital organs. Peripheral vasoconstriction, the body's compensatory response to diminished blood flow, often results in the child's ability to maintain a normal or near-normal BP. As shock continues, capillary beds become obstructed by cellular debris, and platelets and white blood cells aggregate. Endothelial damage occurs as a result of capillary congestion. Poor blood flow to the capillaries results in anaerobic metabolism. Lactic acid accumulates, and this can lead to acidosis. In addition, children with septic shock sustain marked endothelial damage as a result of exposure to bacterial toxins.

The cumulative effect of capillary obstruction and dramatically impaired blood flow is tissue ischemia. As tissue ischemia progresses, the child will show signs of altered perfusion to vital organs. For example, as blood flow to the brain is diminished, the child will demonstrate an altered level of consciousness. Altered blood flow to the kidneys will result in decreased urine output or absence of urine output (oliguria). Commonly, HR will increase in the early stages of shock, but as the heart becomes compromised as a result of poor perfusion, the child will become bradycardic. The child will demonstrate an increased respiratory rate in the initial phase of shock. Tachypnea is seen in septic shock as well. In fact, the child may demonstrate marked hyperventilation in an effort to blow off carbon dioxide in response to the acidosis that is associated with septic shock.

Types of Shock

The most common types of shock are hypovolemic, septic, cardiogenic, and distributive. Hypovolemic shock, the most common type of shock in children, occurs when systemic perfusion decreases as a result of inadequate vascular volume (Peterson & Schuh, 2023). Children commonly have hypovolemic shock that occurs in association with fluid losses. For example, hypovolemic shock may occur with gastroenteritis that results in vomiting and diarrhea, medications such as diuretics, and heat stroke. Other causes of hypovolemia in children include blood loss, such as from a major injury, and third spacing of fluid, such as with burns.

Septic shock is related to a systemic inflammatory response in which there may be increased CO with a low SVR, known as warm shock. More commonly in children, septic shock results in a decrease in CO with an increase in SVR, known as cold shock.

Cardiogenic shock results from an ineffective pump, the heart, with a resultant decrease in SV. Children with structural heart disease and resultant dysrhythmia are at risk for cardiogenic shock (Peterson & Schuh, 2023).

Distributive shock is the result of a loss in the SVR. A relative hypovolemia occurs, most often with neurogenic injury–related shock and anaphylaxis. In relative hypovolemia, the vascular compartment expands due to systemic vasodilation. This results in a relatively larger vasculature requiring more fluid to maintain CO despite no actual loss of fluid.

Finally, toxic drug ingestions may also lead to shock.

Nursing Assessment

Nursing assessment of the child in shock includes the health history and physical examination as well as laboratory and diagnostic testing. The nursing assessment must be performed quickly and accurately so that resuscitation can be expedited.

Health History

In shock, the health history is based on the child's presentation. Children with shock are critically ill and require emergent intervention. Therefore, the history is obtained as lifesaving interventions are provided. Determine when the child first became ill and treatments that have been given thus far. Inquire about sources of volume loss, such as:

- Vomiting
- Diarrhea
- Decreased oral intake
- Blood loss

Ask when the child last urinated. Investigate for other related symptoms such as behavioral changes or lethargy. Has the child had a fever or rash, complained of headache, or been exposed to anyone with similar symptoms? Inquire about day care attendance and whether the family has recently traveled outside of the country. Determine if the child has a history of a congenital heart defect or other heart condition or if the child has severe allergies. Ask the parent about accidental ingestion of medications or other substances and, for the older child or adolescent, about the possibility of illicit substance use.

Physical Examination

The key to successful shock management is early recognition of the signs and symptoms. Obtain vital signs, noting any alterations. Measure BP, although this is not a reliable method of evaluating for shock in children. Children tend to maintain a normal or slightly less than normal BP in compensated shock while sacrificing tissue perfusion until the child suffers a cardiopulmonary arrest. Therefore, other components of the circulatory evaluation will be more valuable when assessing a child.

TAKE NOTE!

Bradycardia is a serious sign in neonates and may occur with respiratory compromise, circulatory compromise, and/or overwhelming sepsis (Aziz et al., 2021).

As with any emergency, determine the presence of a central pulse, if not present begin compressions. Evaluate the airway; is it patent? Then determine if the child is breathing. The child in shock will often demonstrate signs of respiratory distress, such as grunting, gasping, nasal flaring, tachypnea, and increased work of breathing. Auscultate breath sounds to determine the adequacy of air entry and airflow. If the child shows signs of respiratory distress, manage the airway and breathing problem first, as discussed earlier in the chapter.

Assess the skin color. Palpate the skin temperature and determine the quality of pulses. Except in special cases, such as distributive shock, the child in shock will generally have darker and cooler extremities with delayed capillary refill. Note the line of demarcation if present. This refers to the point on the distal extremity where cool temperature begins (the proximal portion of the extremity may continue to be warm). In distributive shock, the initial assessment will reveal full and bounding pulses and warm, erythemic skin. Evaluate the pulse quality. Distal pulses will likely be weaker than central pulses.

Evaluate the child's hydration state and check skin turgor. Decreased elasticity is associated with hypovolemic states, though this is usually a late sign. Observe the child's face; in compensated shock, the child may be awake but obtunded and demonstrate signs of distress. The child in decompensated shock may have their eyes closed and may be responsive only to voice or other stimulation. Evaluate pupillary responses. Determine urinary output, which will be decreased in the child with shock.

After having evaluated and provided initial lifesaving management for airway, breathing, and circulation, evaluate the child's entire body for other disabilities. Injuries warrant vigilant evaluation for ongoing blood loss, although they may also produce internal blood loss (e.g., a femur fracture). Look for signs of malformation, swelling, redness, or pain of the extremities, which may suggest internal blood loss. Also inspect for any open wounds and active sites of bleeding. Children with abdominal injuries also may lose copious amounts of blood internally. Inspect the abdomen for redness, skin discoloration, or distention. Auscultate for bowel sounds in all four quadrants.

Laboratory and Diagnostic Testing

As the child is being resuscitated, laboratory tests and radiographs will be ordered and obtained. However, no diagnostic test should replace the priority of respiratory support, vascular access, and fluid administration. Laboratory results will guide ongoing management. Common laboratory and diagnostic tests used for children with shock include:

- Blood glucose levels: usually performed at the bedside using a glucose meter to obtain a rapid result
- Electrolytes: to evaluate for electrolyte abnormalities
- CBC with differential: to assess for viral or bacterial infection (septic shock) and to evaluate for anemia and platelet abnormalities
- Blood culture: to evaluate for sepsis; preliminary results will not be available for 1 to 2 days
- CRP: to evaluate for infection
- ABGs: to assess oxygen and carbon dioxide levels and to provide information about acid–base balance
- Toxicology panel (if ingestion is suspected)
- Lumbar puncture: to evaluate the cerebrospinal fluid for meningitis
- Urinalysis: to evaluate for glucose, ketones, and protein; concentration (specific gravity) is increased in dehydration states.
- Urine culture: to evaluate for urinary tract or kidney infection
- Radiographs: to evaluate heart size; to evaluate the lungs for pneumonia or pulmonary edema (present with cardiogenic shock)

Nursing Management

Signs of shock in children warrant an emergent response.

Managing the Child's ABCs

Always evaluate and manage the airway and breathing and check for pulses. Initiate CPR if the child is pulseless. All children who have signs and symptoms of shock should receive 100% oxygen via mask. If the child has poor respiratory effort or is apneic, administer 100% oxygen via BVM or ET tube (refer to the "Respiratory Arrest" section for more specific information about the management of airway and breathing). As part of ongoing monitoring, institute cardiac and apnea monitoring and assess oxygen saturation levels via pulse oximetry.

Obtaining Vascular Access

Once the airway and breathing are addressed, nursing management of shock focuses on obtaining vascular access and restoring fluid volume. Children with signs of shock should receive generous amounts of isotonic IV fluids rapidly. However, obtaining vascular access in critically ill children can be challenging. Vascular access must be obtained using the quickest route possible in children whose condition is markedly deteriorated, such as those in decompensated shock.

Various forms of vascular access available for the management of the critically ill child include:

- Peripheral IV route: a large-bore catheter is used to give large amounts of fluid. This route may not be feasible in children with significant vascular compromise.
- Central IV route: central lines can be inserted into the jugular vein and threaded into the superior vena cava.

The femoral route is best for obtaining central venous access while CPR is in progress because the insertion procedure will not interfere with lifesaving interventions involving the airway and cardiac compressions. The subclavian vein, located under the clavicle, is an alternative route for central access.

- Saphenous vein: the saphenous vein (found in the ankle) is an alternative route for venous access that is obtained using a surgical incision.
- Intraosseous access: intraosseous access, obtained by cannulating the bone marrow, is recommended in cases of decompensated shock or cardiac arrest if IV access cannot be attained rapidly. The preferred site is the anterior tibia. Special intraosseous needles are used (generally a 15-gauge needle for older children, 18-gauge for younger children). The needle is inserted using a firm twisting motion slightly away from the growth plate. Any medications or fluids that can be administered using an IV site can be given using this route. Alternative sites include the femur, the iliac crest, the sternum, and the distal tibia.

Restoring Fluid Volume

Administer IV isotonic fluids, such as LR or NS (the isotonic fluids of choice) rapidly. Administer 20 mL/kg of the prescribed fluid as a bolus, infusing the fluid as rapidly as possible. In general, a large-bore syringe, such as a 35- to 60-mL syringe attached to a three-way stopcock, is the preferred method for rapid fluid delivery in children. Infusing the fluid via gravity is too slow. The fluid bolus may be repeated up to two times (for a total of three times) if required.

TAKE NOTE!

Dextrose solutions are contraindicated in shock because of the risk of complications such as osmotic diuresis, hypokalemia, hyperglycemia, and worsening of ischemic brain injury (AHA & AAP, 2020).

Children in septic shock will often require larger volumes of fluid as a result of the increased capillary permeability. Children in shock due to trauma will usually receive a colloid, such as blood, when there is an inadequate response to crystalloid isotonic fluid. After each fluid bolus, reassess the child for signs of positive response to the fluid administration.

Insert an indwelling urinary catheter to allow for accurate and frequent measurement of urine output.

Indicators of improvement include:

- Improved cardiovascular status: The central and peripheral pulses are stronger. The line of demarcation of extremity coolness is diminishing and capillary refill is improved (time is decreased). BP is improved.
- Improved mental status: The child is more alert. For example, the child's eyes are open and watching personnel. If the child is younger, they may be pulling at the IV line.
- Improved urine output: This may not be noted initially but should be noted over the next few hours; the goal is 1 to 2 mL/kg/hour.

The process of fluid resuscitation involves giving the fluid, assessing, and reassessing the child, and documenting findings. Children in shock may require as much as 100 to 200 mL/kg of resuscitative fluid during the initial hours of shock management. Most children in shock need and can tolerate this large volume of fluid. Continued reassessment will determine if the child is beginning to experience fluid overload in the form of pulmonary edema (this is rare but may occur in children with preexisting cardiac conditions or severe chronic pulmonary disease) (AHA & AAP, 2020; Herchline & Gaw, 2023).

CLINICAL REASONING ALERT!

Do not focus solely on the child's circulatory status; you may overlook signs and symptoms of respiratory deterioration.

Administering Medications

In some circumstances, such as septic shock or distributive shock, fluid alone does not adequately improve the child's status and adjunctive medications may be ordered. Vasoactive medications are used either alone or in combination to improve CO and to increase or decrease SVR. The selection of medications is dictated by the child's cardiac and vascular status. For example, dobutamine is a medication with significant beta-adrenergic effects and thus can improve cardiac contractility. Epinephrine, which affects the heart muscle, is also a powerful vasoconstrictor. Dopamine affects the heart at lower doses but increasingly affects the vasculature with increased doses. These medications may be given as a loading dose, followed by a continuous infusion. When vasoactive drugs are administered, monitor for improvement in HR, BP, perfusion, and urine output. Refer to Drug Guide 51.1 for additional information.

CARDIAC DYSRHYTHMIAS AND ARREST

Unlike adults, in whom cardiopulmonary arrest is most often caused by a primary cardiac event, children typically have healthy hearts and thus rarely experience primary cardiac arrest. More commonly, they experience cardiopulmonary arrest from gradual deterioration of respiration and/or circulation (Peterson & Schuh, 2023). In particular, children experiencing a respiratory emergency or shock may deteriorate and eventually demonstrate cardiopulmonary arrest. Thus, the standard of care for managing a child in this situation is vastly different from that for an adult.

Nurses should be skilled in evaluating and managing respiratory alterations and shock in children, as discussed in previous sections. Overwhelming evidence suggests that if primary respiratory compromise or shock is identified and treated in the critically ill child, a secondary cardiac arrest can be prevented.

Rare exceptions do exist, however. For example, electrolyte abnormalities and toxic drug ingestions are primary insults to the cardiovascular system that may lead to a sudden cardiac arrest rather than a gradual progression. Other exceptions in which the child is at risk for a primary and sudden cardiac arrest include:

- History of a serious primary congenital or acquired cardiac defect
- Potentially lethal dysrhythmias such as prolonged QT syndrome
- Hypertrophic cardiomyopathy
- Traumatic cardiac injury or a sharp blow to the chest, known as "commotio cordis" (e.g., when a high-velocity ball hits the chest)

The overwhelming majority of children rarely experience cardiac dysrhythmias so it is beyond the scope of this chapter to discuss the myriad of possible complex rhythm disturbances. Therefore, this discussion will be limited to the management of emergent cardiac conditions that are more typically found in children.

Pathophysiology

The AHA and AAP (2020) have simplified the nomenclature used to describe pediatric cardiac compromise and has established three major categories of cardiac rhythm disturbances:

- Slow: bradydysrhythmia
- Fast: tachydysrhythmia
- Absent: pulseless, cardiovascular collapse

The pathophysiology, causes, and therapeutic management of each of the categories of rhythm disturbances are discussed later.

Bradydysrhythmias

Bradycardia is HR significantly slower than the normal HR for that age. Bradycardia in children is most commonly sinus bradycardia. In other words, there is not a cardiac nodal abnormality associated with the slowed HR. In sinus bradycardia, the P waves and QRS complex remain normal on the ECG. Brief dips in HRs can be normal, such as when the child sleeps. Children are also susceptible to brief drops in HR that are associated with vagal stimulation. For example, passing an orogastric tube down the esophagus of a young infant may induce a temporary bradycardic response. These normal decreases in the child's HR should recover with or without stimulation and are not normally associated with signs of altered perfusion.

Less commonly, children manifest bradycardia as a result of cardiac abnormalities and heart block. Infants with bradycardia related to heart block may exhibit poor feeding and tachypnea, whereas older children may demonstrate fatigue, dizziness, and syncope. Comparison Chart 51.2 compares the causes of sinus bradycardia and heart block in children.

In contrast, the child with a serious and possibly life-threatening bradydysrhythmia will have an HR below 60 bpm, with signs of altered perfusion. The most common causes of profound bradycardia in children are respiratory compromise, hypoxia, and shock. Sustained bradycardia is commonly associated with arrest. It is an ominous sign and should be taken seriously.

Tachydysrhythmias

Children normally have faster HRs than adults, and fever, fear, and pain are common explanations for significant increases in the HR of a child (**tachycardia**). This normal elevation in HR is known as sinus tachycardia. However, once the fever is reduced, the child is comforted, or the pain is managed, the HR should return close to the child's baseline. Hypoxia and hypovolemia are pathologic reasons for tachycardia in the child. If the child has sinus tachycardia that results from any of these causes, the focus is on the underlying cause. It is inappropriate and dangerous to treat sinus tachycardia with medications aimed at decreasing the HR or with a defibrillation device.

Tachydysrhythmias in children that are associated with cardiac compromise have unique characteristics that present differently from sinus tachycardia. Examples of these include SVT and ventricular tachycardia. SVT is a cardiac conduction problem in which the HR is extremely rapid, and the rhythm is very regular, often described as "no beat-to-beat variability." Comparison Chart 51.3 explains the differences between SVT and

COMPARISON CHART 51.2 Causes of Sinus Bradycardia Versus Heart Block

	Sinus Bradycardia	Heart Block
Causes	• Pathologic: medications such as digoxin, hypoxia, hypothermia, head injury • Nonpathologic: well-conditioned athlete	• Congenital: associated with cardiac anomalies • Acquired: endocarditis, rheumatic fever, Kawasaki disease

COMPARISON CHART 51.3 Distinguishing Supraventricular Tachycardia (SVT) From Sinus Tachycardia

	SVT	Sinus Tachycardia
Rate (bpm)	Infants >220, children >180	Infants <220, children <180
Rhythm	Abrupt onset and termination	Beat-to-beat variability
P waves	Flattened	Present and normal
QRS	Narrow (<0.08 seconds)	Normal
History	Usually, no significant history	Fever, fluid loss, hypoxia, pain, fear

sinus tachycardia. The most common cause of SVT is a reentry problem in the cardiac conduction system. Commonly, SVT is the result of a genetic cardiac conduction problem such as Wolff–Parkinson–White syndrome. SVT may also be associated with medications such as caffeine and theophylline. Children often can tolerate the characteristically higher HR that is associated with SVT for short periods of time. However, the increased demand that is placed on the cardiovascular system usually overtaxes the child and results in signs of congestive heart failure if the SVT continues unchecked for a prolonged time.

Ventricular tachycardia is a rhythm involving an elevation of the HR and a wide QRS (greater than 0.08 seconds) that is the result of an abnormal, rapid firing of one or both of the ventricles. Ventricular tachycardia is a rare dysrhythmia in children and usually is associated with a congenital or acquired cardiac abnormality. In addition, prolonged QT syndrome is a conduction abnormality that can result in ventricular tachycardia and sudden death in children. Less commonly, ingestion of medications and toxins, acidosis, hypocalcemia, abnormalities of potassium, and hypoxemia have been associated with the development of ventricular tachycardia in children.

Collapsed Rhythms (Pulseless Rhythms)

A collapsed rhythm, as defined by PALS, is one that produces cardiac arrest with no palpable pulse and no signs of perfusion (cardiac arrest) (AHA & AAP, 2020). Typically, the most common pulseless arrest rhythms in children are asystole and PEA. **Asystole** occurs when there is no cardiac electrical activity, commonly referred to as "a straight line" on the ECG. The child with PEA has some appreciable rhythm on the ECG but no palpable pulses. PEA may be caused by hypoxemia, hypovolemia, hypothermia, electrolyte imbalance, tamponade, toxic ingestion, tension pneumothorax, or thromboembolism. Ventricular tachycardia may also present as pulseless. VF, once thought to be rare in children, occurs in serious cardiac conditions in which the ventricle is not pumping effectively. It may develop from ventricular tachycardia. VF is characterized by variable, high-amplitude waveforms (coarse VF) or a finer, lower-amplitude waveform with no discernible cardiac rhythm (fine VF). In either case, CO is insufficient.

Nursing Assessment

Nursing assessment of the child with a cardiac emergency includes the health history and physical examination as well as laboratory and diagnostic testing. The nursing assessment must be performed quickly and accurately so that resuscitation can be instituted if needed.

Health History

Obtain a brief health history of the child with a cardiac emergency while simultaneously assessing the child and providing lifesaving interventions. Key areas to inquire about include:

- History of cardiac problems, asthma, chromosomal anomaly, delayed growth
- Symptoms such as syncope, dizziness, palpitations or racing heart, chest pain, coughing, wheezing, increased work of breathing
- Activity tolerance with play or feeding: Does the child get out of breath, turn blue, or squat during play? Can the child keep up with playmates? Does the infant tire with feedings?
- Precipitating illness, fever, unexplained joint pains, ingested medications
- Participation in a sport before the cardiac event occurred or injury to the chest
- Family history of cardiac problems, sudden death from a cardiac condition, heart attacks at a young age, chromosomal abnormalities
- Treatment measures performed at the scene: Was CPR initiated? Was an AED used?

Physical Examination

Quickly establish the child's status. A child who is obviously in distress or is arresting must receive emergent lifesaving interventions. Briefly perform the assessment while simultaneously providing lifesaving interventions.

INSPECTION AND OBSERVATION

Assess the child's airway patency and efficiency of breathing. Observe the child's color, noting circumoral pallor or duskiness or central pallor, mottling, duskiness, or cyanosis. Note any increased work of breathing, grunting, head bobbing, or apnea. Inspect the chest for barrel shape, which may be associated with chronic pulmonary or cardiac disease. Observe the pericardium for the presence of lifts or heaves. Note diaphoresis, anxious appearance, or dysmorphic features (almost 50% of children with Down syndrome also have a congenital cardiac defect [Marion & Levy, 2023]). Determine if neck vein distention is present. Inspect the fingertips for clubbing, which is indicative of chronic tissue hypoxemia.

AUSCULTATION

Auscultate the breath sounds, noting any crackles or wheezes. Auscultate the HR. If the child does not have an adequate pulse, initiate CPR. If the child has a strong, perfusing pulse, complete the cardiac assessment. Auscultate with the diaphragm of the stethoscope first and then listen with the bell. Evaluate all of the auscultatory areas, listening first over the second right interspace (aortic valve) and then over the second left interspace (pulmonic valve); next move to the left lower sternal border (tricuspid area); and finally auscultate over the fifth interspace, midclavicular line (mitral area). Evaluate the rate and rhythm of the heart. Listen for any extra sounds or murmurs. Note and describe the quality, intensity, and location of any cardiac murmurs.

> *TAKE NOTE!*
>
> Murmurs are most often systolic and can be benign or associated with pathology.

PERCUSSION AND PALPATION

Percuss between the costal interspaces and note the heart's size. Palpate the heart to find the point of maximal impulse (PMI) and to evaluate for an associated thrill. A thrill feels like a fluttering under the fingers and is associated with cardiac pathology. Palpate and note the quality of the pulses. Evaluate each of the pulses bilaterally and note whether they are absent, faint, normal, or bounding. Compare the quality of pulses on each side of the body and also those of the upper and lower body. Note the skin temperature and evaluate the capillary refill.

Laboratory and Diagnostic Testing

The major diagnostic test used is the ECG. Identify the dysrhythmia according to the ECG reading (Fig. 51.7).

Nursing Management

Provide oxygen at 100%. Institute cardiac monitoring and assess oxygen saturation levels via pulse oximetry. Obtain the child's preprinted code drug sheet or use the Broselow tape to obtain the child's height to estimate the ET tube sizes and medication dosages that are appropriate for the child. Always remember to intervene in this order: first airway, then breathing, then circulation. The remainder of this discussion will assume that the nurse has initiated interventions for airway and breathing as discussed earlier in the chapter.

> *TAKE NOTE!*
>
> Pay attention to the rhythm on the monitor, but continually monitor the child's pulse. If the child does not have a pulse or has a pulse of less than 60 bpm, perform cardiac compressions despite the monitor reading (AHA & AAP, 2020).

MANAGING BRADYDYSRHYTHMIAS

The management of sinus bradycardia is focused on remedying the underlying cause of the slow HR. Since hypoxia is the most common cause of sustained bradycardia, oxygenation and ventilation are necessary. The newborn is particularly susceptible to bradycardia in relation to hypoxemia. Continue to reassess the child to determine if the bradycardia improves with adequate oxygenation and ventilation. If bradycardia persists, administer epinephrine and/or atropine as ordered. Epinephrine is the drug of choice for the treatment of persistent bradycardia.

Other causes of bradycardia such as hypothermia, head injury, and toxic ingestion are managed by addressing the underlying condition. Warming the hypothermic child may restore a normal sinus rhythm. Children with head injury may have bradycardia without any cardiac involvement, and with successful management of the head injury, the bradycardia will resolve. Antidotes to toxins may be necessary in children whose bradycardia is the result of a toxic ingestion.

MANAGING TACHYDYSRHYTHMIAS

The tachydysrhythmias include SVT (stable or unstable) and ventricular tachycardia with a pulse. Examine the ECG to determine if the child is experiencing ventricular tachycardia or SVT. Clinically, determine whether the child in SVT is showing signs that require emergent intervention or if the child is stable. In compensated SVT, the child will appear to be alert, breathing comfortably, and well perfused. The child who is demonstrating signs of compromise, such as a change in consciousness, respiratory status, and perfusion, is considered to be in uncompensated SVT. Uncompensated SVT requires emergent intervention. The child who has ventricular tachycardia with a pulse will have poor perfusion and also require immediate intervention. The evaluation and approaches to the tachydysrhythmias are discussed in Table 51.6.

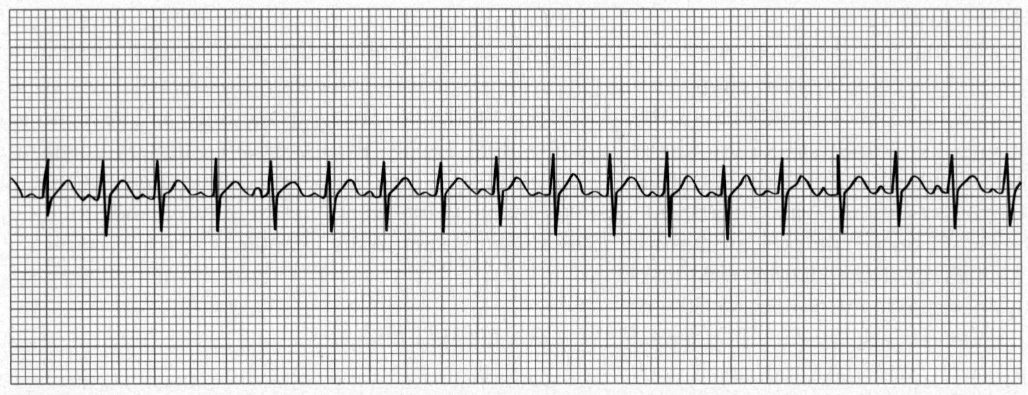

A

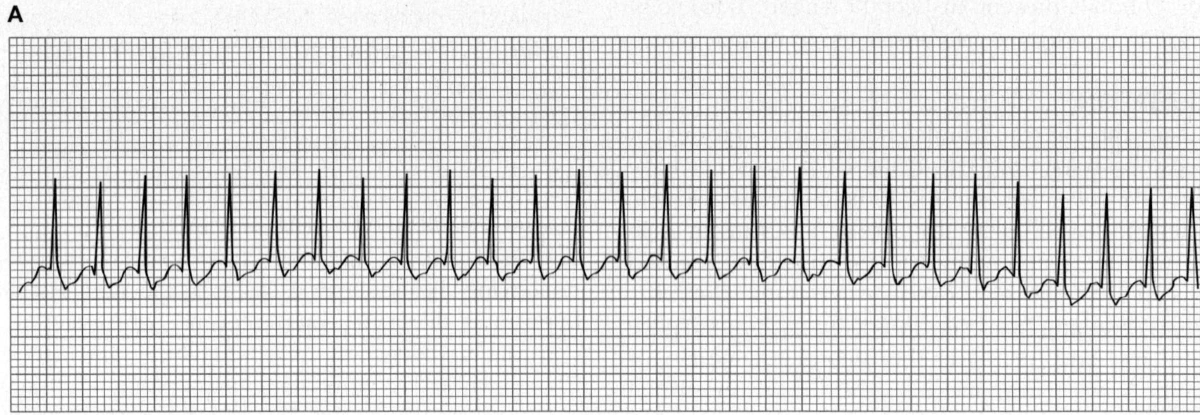

B

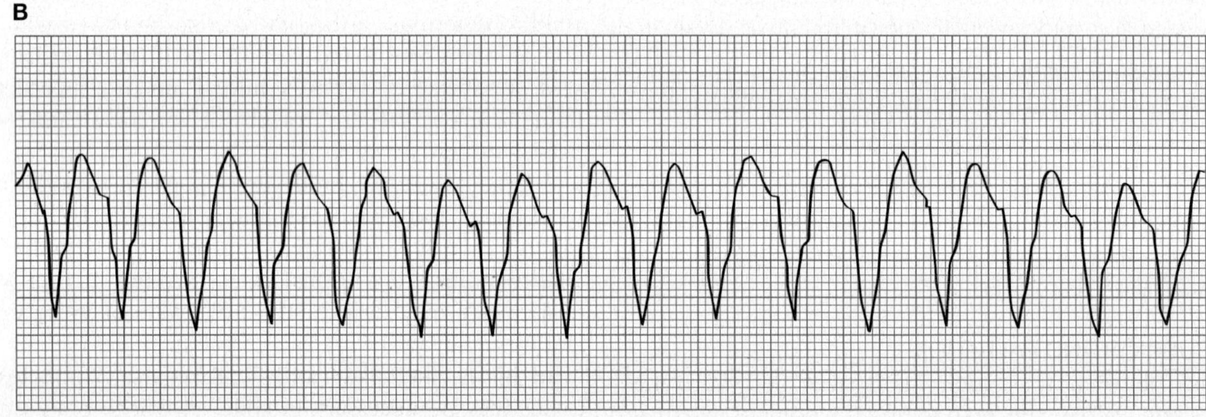

C

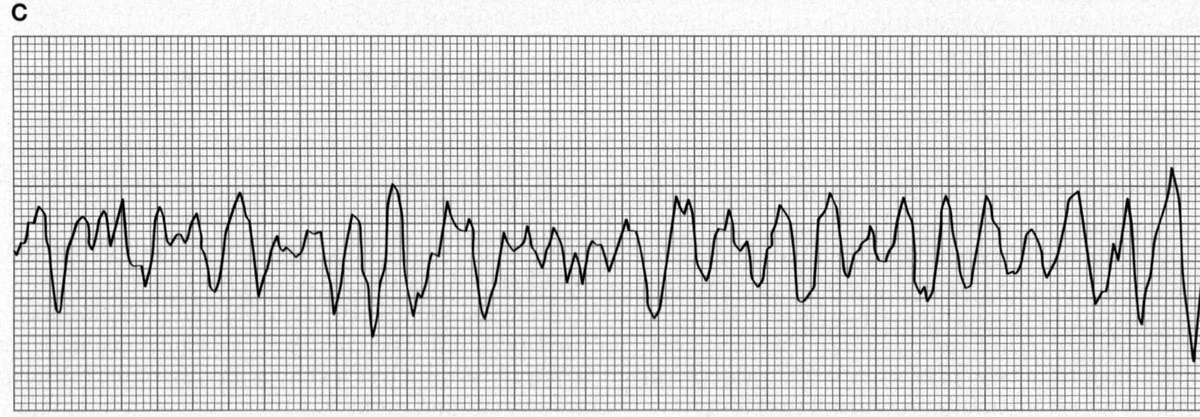

D

FIGURE 51.7 Dysrhythmias **A.** Sinus tachycardia: normal QRS and P waves, mild beat-to-beat variability. **B.** Supraventricular tachycardia: note rate above 220, abnormal P waves, no beat-to-beat variability. **C.** Ventricular tachycardia: rapid and regular rhythm, wide QRS without P waves. **D.** Coarse ventricular fibrillation: chaotic electrical activity.

TABLE 51.6 • Managing tachydysrhythmias

Tachydysrhythmia	Signs and Symptoms	Management
Compensated SVT	• Tachycardia, heart rate >220 • Abnormal P waves • Alert, well-perfused child • Possible complaints of headache and dizziness in older children	• Vagal maneuvers such as ice to face or blowing through a straw that is obstructed • Adenosine if vagal maneuvers fail
Uncompensated SVT	• Tachycardia, heart rate >220 • Abnormal P waves • Signs of shock: altered level of consciousness, poor perfusion, weak pulses	• Adenosine or synchronized cardioversion
Ventricular tachycardia	• Rate may range from normal to 200 bpm. • Wide QRS • No P waves • Pulse present, poor perfusion	• Synchronized cardioversion • IV amiodarone • Treatment of underlying causes

bpm, beats/min; IV, intravenous; SVT, supraventricular tachycardia.

Data from American Heart Association & American Academy of Pediatrics. (2020). *Pediatric advanced life support provider manual.* American Heart Association.

TAKE NOTE!

Adenosine has a rapid onset of action and an extremely short half-life. Administer it extremely rapidly with a generous amount of IV flush; otherwise, it will be ineffective (AHA & AAP, 2020).

MANAGING COLLAPSED RHYTHMS

As in any pediatric emergency, support the ABCs. Manage the airway, provide oxygen, and give fluids. In addition, if the child is pulseless or has HR less than 60 bpm, initiate cardiac compressions (see "Providing Cardiopulmonary Resuscitation" section earlier in the chapter). In addition, some children may require medications and/or defibrillation or synchronized cardioversion. The pulseless rhythms include ventricular tachycardia, VF, asystole, and PEA. ECG characteristics and management of these rhythms are summarized in Table 51.7. Also treat the underlying causes of the dysrhythmia if known.

The AHA emphasizes the importance of cardiac compressions in pulseless individuals with dysrhythmias (AHA & AAP, 2020). Give compressions before and

TABLE 51.7 • ECG Characteristics and Management of Pulseless Rhythms

Pulseless dysrhythmia	ECG Characteristics	Management
Ventricular tachycardia	Wide QRS, no P waves	• CPR • Defibrillation • Epinephrine; also possibly amiodarone, lidocaine, or magnesium • Treat underlying causes
Ventricular fibrillation	• Chaotic ventricular activity • No P waves, no QRS, no T waves	• CPR • Defibrillation • Epinephrine; also possibly amiodarone, lidocaine, or magnesium • Treat underlying causes
Asystole	Flat line	• Check lead placement • CPR if no pulse • Epinephrine
Pulseless electrical activity	Electrical activity that is not consistent with ventricular tachycardia or ventricular fibrillation.	• Check lead placement • CPR if no pulse • Treat underlying cause • Epinephrine

CPR, cardiopulmonary resuscitation; ECG, electrocardiogram.

Data from American Heart Association & American Academy of Pediatrics. (2020). *Pediatric advanced life support provider manual.* American Heart Association.

immediately after defibrillation (see "*Providing Defibrillation or Synchronized Cardioversion*" section earlier in the chapter). Administer medications such as epinephrine, lidocaine, or amiodarone as ordered. In the past, it was recommended that individuals who required defibrillation be given three shocks in a row, but recent research findings have shown that the individual should be defibrillated only once, followed by five cycles of CPR. For defibrillation to be most effective, cardiac compressions must be performed effectively with minimal interruptions (AHA & AAP, 2020).

DOSAGE CALCULATION BOX 51.1

Child's weight: 55 lb

Medication order: epinephrine 100 mg intravenous (IV) STAT

Per the *Pediatric Dosage Handbook*, the recommended dose is 0.01 mg/kg (0.1 mL/kg of 1:10,000 solution) per dose.

Is the ordered dose safe?

SUBMERSION INJURY

Water can be a great source of fun and exercise for children and adolescents, but drowning is the third-leading cause of preventable death in children and adolescents in the United States and worldwide (World Health Organization [WHO], 2023). In warm-weather states where swimming pools are more common, drowning is the primary cause of death in young people. Most drowning deaths are preventable, and the WHO (2023) notes that among younger children, lapse in adult supervision is associated with drowning.

Survival and neurologic outcome of drowning depend on early and appropriate resuscitation. In recent years, with appropriate resuscitation efforts and treatment, children have demonstrated better neurologic outcomes (Chandy & Richards, 2024).

Pathophysiology

Typically, a child who is drowning will struggle to breathe and eventually will aspirate water. Aspiration of relatively small amounts of water leads to poor oxygenation, with retention of carbon dioxide. Alveolar surfactant is depleted during the drowning event and pulmonary edema commonly occurs. Hypoxemia results in increased capillary permeability and resultant hypovolemia. Even small amounts of aspirated water may lead to pulmonary edema within an 8-hour period after the drowning episode (Chandy & Richards, 2024). A drowning survivor is also at risk for renal complications due to altered renal perfusion during the hypoxemic state.

Nursing Assessment

Nursing assessment of the drowning survivor is crucial and must take place quickly and accurately.

Health History

Obtain the history rapidly while providing lifesaving interventions. Ask about the circumstances of the event:

- Where did the incident occur? Was the child in a lake, river, ocean, or swimming pool? Was the child submerged in a toilet, bucket, or bathtub?
- Did someone witness the child's entry into the water?
- Was the water fresh or salty? Cold or warm?
- Is it likely the water was contaminated?
- Were there any extenuating circumstances, such as a diving or automobile accident, associated with the near drowning?
- What was the approximate length of time of the submersion? Was the child conscious or unconscious when rescued?
- What was done at the scene? Was CPR initiated? If so, when?
- If a cervical spine injury was suspected, was the cervical spine immobilized?
- Was an AED used?
- When did the child last eat (to prepare for possible intubation)?

Physical Examination

Evaluate airway patency and breathing. Auscultate all lung fields for signs of pulmonary edema, such as coarseness or crackles. Evaluate the HR, pulse, and perfusion. Note the cardiac rhythm on the monitor and report evidence of dysrhythmias. Evaluate the child's neurologic status. Use a pen light to determine the pupillary reaction. Use the pediatric coma score to further assess the neurologic status. Does the child open the eyes spontaneously, to stimuli, or not at all? Is there any spontaneous movement? Is the younger child crying? Can the older child speak? Measure the child's temperature, as hypothermia often occurs with near drowning.

Laboratory and Diagnostic Testing

While awaiting laboratory and diagnostic testing results, continue resuscitative efforts as addressed following. Laboratory and diagnostic tests typically include the following:

- ABGs: hypoxemia, acidosis
- ECG: cardiac dysrhythmias
- Chest radiography: pulmonary edema, infiltrates
- Serum electrolytes: imbalance related to development of shock

Nursing Management

Because of the potentially devastating effects that drowning-related hypoxia has on the child's brain, airway interventions must be initiated immediately after retrieving a child from the water. Every second counts. Initial interventions for a drowning victim are always focused on the ABCs; commonly, resuscitative efforts have begun before the child arrives at the acute care facility.

If a cervical spine injury is suspected (as in the case of a diving accident), provide stabilization either manually or with a cervical collar. As with any suspected neck injury, do not remove the cervical collar until injury to the cervical spine has been ruled out through a radiograph and clinical evaluation. Suction the airway to ensure airway patency. The child may have aspirated particles from a contaminated water source or emesis, a relatively common complication associated with drowning. A large-bore suction catheter (e.g., Yankauer) is an effective tool for clearing the upper airway. Administer supplemental oxygen at 100%. Children who have poor or absent respiratory effort most likely will require intubation. Insert an orogastric or nasogastric tube to decompress the stomach and prevent aspiration of stomach contents. Initiate chest compressions if a pulse is not present.

Usually, the child exhibits some degree of hypothermia and will require warming. Generally, the core body temperature should be raised slowly, as warming a drowning victim too quickly may have deleterious effects. Remove any wet clothing, dry the child, and cover them with warmed blankets. Warm IV fluids and use other warming methods as prescribed.

CONSIDER THIS!

A parent says to you, "I can't believe my toddler almost drowned. I turned away for a few minutes to check the hamburgers on the grill. I feel terrible. I'll never be able to let her go near a swimming pool again."

Thoughts: What will your response be to this parent? How can you best support them and assist them to work through their emotions?

POISONING

Emergency care of the pediatric poisoning victim consists of rapid nursing assessment and prompt management.

TAKE NOTE!

If a normally healthy child (particularly a young child) suddenly deteriorates without a known cause, suspect a toxic ingestion.

Nursing Assessment

Nursing assessment of the poisoning victim focuses on a thorough health history, followed by physical examination and laboratory and diagnostic testing.

Health History

Obtain the health history from the parents or caregiver or, in the case of an older child or adolescent, from the child. Inquire about the approximate time of poisoning and the nature of the toxin. Was the toxin ingested, inhaled, or applied to the skin? In the case of pill ingestion, does the caregiver have the medication bottle? Did the child experience nausea, vomiting, anorexia, abdominal pain, or neurologic changes such as disorientation, slurred speech, or altered gait? Determine the progression of the symptoms. Did the parent or caregiver call the National Poison Control Center Hotline? Has any treatment been given? In the case of older children and adolescents, inquire about any history of depression or threatened suicide.

TAKE NOTE!

The National Poison Control Center Hotline number is 1-800-222-1222.

Physical Examination

Ingestion of medications or chemicals may result in a wide variety of clinical manifestations. Perform a thorough physical examination, noting alterations that may occur with particular ingestions, such as:

- Hyper- or hypotension
- Hyper- or hypothermia
- Respiratory depression or hyperventilation
- Miosis (pupillary contraction) or mydriasis (pupillary dilatation)

Pay particular attention to the child's mental status, skin moisture and color, and bowel sounds (Velez et al., 2022).

Laboratory and Diagnostic Testing

The suspected poison may direct the laboratory and diagnostic testing. A variety of blood tests may be performed:

- Chemistry panel: to detect hypoglycemia or metabolic acidosis and assess kidney function
- ECG: to identify dysrhythmias or conduction delay
- Liver function tests: to assess for liver injury
- Urine and blood toxicology screens (available for a limited number of medications; may vary per institution)
- Specific drug levels if the substance ingested is known or highly suspected

Nursing Management

When poisoning occurs, give priority to the child's ABCs. Treat alterations as discussed earlier in this chapter. Monitor vital signs frequently and provide supportive care. Few specific antidotes are available for medications or other toxins. Activated charcoal may be administered to bind with the chemical substance in the bowel. Alternatively, whole bowel irrigation with polyethylene glycol electrolyte solutions may be necessary. Occasionally, dialysis is required to lower the level of toxin in the bloodstream. The intervention is based on the source of the ingestion. For example, activated charcoal is an effective method for preventing the absorption of many medications but is not effective in the case of an iron overdose.

If opiate or other narcotic ingestion is suspected, administer naloxone to reverse the respiratory depression or altered level of consciousness. Treatment of seizures and alterations in thermoregulation may also be needed.

Specific treatment of the poisoning will be determined when the toxin is identified, and poison control is queried. Maintain ongoing assessment of the poisoned child because many toxins exhibit very late effects.

TAKE NOTE!

Syrup of ipecac is not recommended for home treatment to induce vomiting after an accidental ingestion (AAP, 2021).

TRAUMA

The leading cause of death in children and adolescents is unintentional injuries (Centers for Disease Control and Prevention [CDC], n.d.). Automobile accidents continue to be a top cause of death in all child age groups (CDC, n.d.). Childhood trauma also results from pedestrian accidents, sporting and bicycling injuries, and firearm use. Children of varying ages are susceptible to various forms of injury due to their developmental level as well as their environmental exposure. Young children rely on their caregivers to promote their safety. Young children also are not developmentally equipped to be able to recognize dangerous situations. Because pediatric injury is so common, nurses must become adept at assessment and intervention in the pediatric trauma victim.

Nursing Assessment

The trauma survey includes a brief health history as the child is being assessed and lifesaving measures are being instituted.

Health History

Begin the health history by asking when the injury happened. If the child sustained a motor vehicle–related injury, ask how fast the vehicle was going. Determine if the child was appropriately restrained in the automobile. If the child was riding a bicycle, was skateboarding, or using in-line skates, were they wearing a helmet, kneepads, and wrist guards? Determine what interventions were performed at the scene. Was the child immobilized on a backboard to protect the cervical spine? If the child is bleeding, ask the person who transported the child to estimate the amount of blood lost.

If the child experienced a fall, ask if the fall was witnessed and the height from which the child fell. Did the child fall onto a hard surface such as concrete? How did the child land: on the head or back, or did the child catch themselves with the hands? Males are at higher risk for injuring their heads (CDC, 2023). Did the child lose consciousness at the scene? What kind of behavior did the child exhibit after the fall? Since the fall, has the child complained of a headache or been vomiting?

While obtaining a detailed history of the fall, think about the child's developmental stage. For example, does it seem plausible that a toddler might fall down the stairs? In contrast, what is the likelihood that a 2-month-old would suffer a fractured femur from a fall? Keep in mind the possibility of child abuse. Critically evaluate the reported circumstances and try to determine if the history, developmental stage of the child, and type of injury sustained match. In addition, evaluate the type of injury that the child sustained, and the history given by the caregiver. For example, children who fall from significant heights often suffer skeletal fractures, but abdominal and chest injuries rarely result from falling from significant heights.

Physical Examination

Physical examination of the child with a traumatic injury should be approached with an evaluation of the ABCs (primary survey) first. Assess the patency of the airway and establish the effectiveness of breathing (as discussed earlier in the chapter). Examine the child's respiratory effort, breath sounds, and color. Next, evaluate the circulation. Note the pulse rate and quality. Observe the color, skin temperature, and perfusion. If bleeding has occurred, the child's circulation may become compromised.

After assessing and intervening for the child's ABCs, proceed to the secondary survey. Assess for disability (D). Rapidly assess critical neurologic function. Determine the level of consciousness, pupillary reaction, and verbal and motor responses to auditory and painful stimuli. If the child is a young infant, palpate the anterior fontanel: A full and bulging fontanel signals increased intracranial pressure. The traumatized child's neurologic status may range from completely normal to comatose.

TAKE NOTE!

Unequal pupils or a fixed and dilated pupil is considered a neurosurgical emergency. Immediately report this finding.

Following the ABCs and D (disability) is E (exposure). Expose the child to observe the entire body for signs of injury, whether blunt or penetrating. Perform a systematic, thorough inspection of the child's body. Note active bleeding and extremity deformity, as well as any lacerations and abrasions. Observe for movement and any complaints of immobility or pain with movement. Inspect the abdomen for redness, skin discoloration, or distention. Auscultate for bowel sounds in all four quadrants. If the child is verbal, ask if they have any pain in the stomach. If the child is younger, ask, "Do you have a tummy ache?" If the child reports abdominal pain, ask the child to point to where it hurts. Note any guarding of the abdomen, which is an indication of abdominal pain. If bowel injury is a possibility, only light palpation is acceptable. Always assess the least tender areas first and palpate the more sensitive areas last.

Laboratory and Diagnostic Testing

As in other pediatric emergencies, never delay lifesaving measures to wait for laboratory or diagnostic test results. In addition to routine laboratory tests, common laboratory and diagnostic tests for the pediatric trauma victim include:

- Type and cross-match: to assess the child's blood type before blood products are given
- Prothrombin time and partial thromboplastin time: to evaluate for clotting dysfunction
- Amylase and lipase: to identify pancreatic injury
- Liver function tests: to assess for liver injury
- Pregnancy test (as appropriate)
- CT scan, ultrasound, or MRI of the head, abdomen, or extremities: to evaluate the extent of the injury

Nursing Management

Nursing management of the pediatric trauma victim focuses initially on the ABCs.

Providing Immediate Care

If head or spinal injury is suspected, open the airway using the jaw-thrust maneuver with cervical spine stabilization (see Fig. 51.4). The guidelines for basic life support recommend that if the airway cannot be opened using the jaw-thrust maneuver, it may be opened using the head tilt–chin lift maneuver since opening the airway is a priority (AHA & AAP, 2020). The head and neck of a trauma victim should be stabilized manually.

TAKE NOTE!

Infants and young children require unique cervical spine management because they have prominent occiputs that result in flexion of the neck in the supine position. To maintain the optimal neutral spinal position in the young child, use a special pediatric backboard with a head indentation, or use a folded towel to elevate the child's torso.

Clear the airway of obstruction using a large-bore suction device such as a Yankauer. If the child is breathing on their own, give oxygen at the highest flow possible (such as with a nonrebreathing mask). If the child is not breathing on their own, intervene with basic life support discussed earlier in this chapter (AHA & AAP, 2020).

If a BVM device is available, connect it to the oxygen source and use the bag to ventilate the child. Observe the chest rise and be careful not to overventilate, as this results in abdominal distention. Deliver breaths at a rate of one breath every 3 seconds (AHA & AAP, 2020). Do not hyperventilate. In the not-too-distant past, head injury in children was managed using hyperventilation. This resulted in **hypocapnia** (decreased amounts of carbon dioxide in the blood). The physiologic effect of hypocapnia is the induction of vasoconstriction, which in turn results in tissue ischemia. Therefore, current management of head injury in children does not use hyperventilation. The only exception to this rule is in an acute situation, if the child is showing signs of a possible brain stem herniation, hyperventilation may be used initially and briefly.

Assess the child for a strong central pulse. If the child has no pulse, initiate CPR immediately. When perfusion is compromised, administer IV fluid resuscitation. Trauma victims are more likely to require colloids or blood products due to blood loss from the injury.

KEY CONCEPTS

- Young children's smaller airways and immature respiratory and immune systems place them at higher risk for respiratory distress than older children and adults. Children generally have healthy hearts and cardiovascular systems and thus rarely present with primary cardiac arrest. Younger children and adolescents are at higher risk for injury due to normal development at those ages.
- Children present with a variety of emergencies and injuries and must be evaluated and treated in an appropriate and timely fashion to achieve a positive outcome. The health history is obtained rapidly while lifesaving measures are performed simultaneously.

- Assess the airway, then breathing, then circulation, providing interventions for alterations before moving on to the next assessment. Provide continuous reassessment, as children respond quickly to interventions and deteriorate quickly as well.
- Pulse oximetry and capnometry can be useful tools for evaluating respiratory status. Never delay intervention pending laboratory results if the child's clinical status warrants immediate action.
- Provide support and education to the child and family involved in an emergency. Teach families why certain procedures are being done, explaining technical medical interventions in simple terms and, for the child, at their developmental level.
- Small amounts of edema or secretions can contribute to significant respiratory effort in infants and young children.
- Children dehydrate more quickly than adults and experience alterations in perfusion related to hypovolemia.
- Children in respiratory distress and shock require supplemental oxygen. Intubation is necessary for the apneic child or the child whose airway is not maintainable.
- Accurate assessment of perfusion status and appropriate fluid resuscitation are critical in the prevention and treatment of shock in children.
- Life-threatening dysrhythmias in children, though uncommon, often must be quickly treated with defibrillation or synchronized cardioversion in addition to CPR.
- In the case of near drowning, maintain ongoing assessment and intervention of pulmonary status.
- Maintain airway, breathing, and circulation in the child who has experienced an accidental ingestion and prepare for gastric lavage or administration of activated charcoal.
- In addition to intervening for airway, breathing, and circulation problems in the pediatric trauma victim, assess for altered neurologic status and extent of bleeding or injury.

REFERENCES AND RECOMMENDED READINGS

American Academy of Pediatrics. (2021). *Using over-the-counter medicines with your child.* https://www.healthychildren.org/English/safety-prevention/at-home/medication-safety/Pages/Using-Over-the-Counter-Medicines-With-Your-Child.aspx

American Heart Association & American Academy of Pediatrics. (2020). *Pediatric advanced life support provider manual.* American Heart Association.

Aziz, K., Lee, H. C., Escobedo, M. B., Hoover, A. V., Kamath-Rayne, B. D., Kapadia, V. S., Magid, D. J., Niermeyer, S., Schmölzer, G. M., Szyld, E., Weiner, G. M., Wyckoff, M. H., Yamada, N. K., & Zaichkin, J. (2021). Part 5: Neonatal resuscitation 2020 American Heart Association guidelines for cardiopulmonary resuscitation and emergency cardiovascular care. *Pediatrics, 147*(Supplement 1), e2020038505E. https://doi.org/10.1542/peds.2020-038505E

Bush, R. N., & Woodley, L. (2022). Increasing nurses' knowledge of and self-confidence with family presence during pediatric resuscitation. *Critical Care Nurse, 42*(4), 27–37. https://doi.org/10.4037/ccn2022898

Centers for Disease Control and Prevention. (2023a). *QuickStats: percentage of children and adolescents aged ≤17 years who had ever received a diagnosis of concussion or brain injury,† by sex and age group—National Health Interview Survey,§ United States, 2022.* https://www.cdc.gov/mmwr/volumes/72/wr/mm7233a5.htm#suggestedcitation

Centers for Disease Control and Prevention. (n.d.). *10 leading causes of death, United States, 2021, both sexes, all ages, all races.* https://wisqars.cdc.gov/pdfs/leading-causes-of-death-by-age-group_2021_508.pdf

Chandy, D., & Richards, D. (2024). Drowning (submersion injuries). *UpToDate*. Retrieved April 10, 2024, from https://www.uptodate.com/contents/drowning-submersion-injuries

Corbett, J. A., & Banks, A. D. (2019). *Laboratory tests and diagnostic procedures with nursing diagnoses* (9th ed.). Pearson Education Inc.

Fuch, S. M. (2018). *AAP policy says more people need access to life support training, AEDs.* https://www.aappublications.org/news/2018/05/23/lifesupport052318

Gilger, M. A., & Jain, A. K. (2022). Foreign bodies of the esophagus and gastrointestinal tract in children. *UpToDate*. Retrieved April 10, 2024, from http://www.uptodate.com/contents/foreign-bodies-of-the-esophagus-and-gastrointestinal-tract-in-children

Graham, J., & Peoples, M. (2019). Nursing student knowledge and compliance with SIDS prevention strategies. *Infant, 15*(1), 29–32. https://www.infantjournal.co.uk/pdf/inf_085_ude.pdf

Herchline, D. J., & Gaw, C. E. (2023). Shock and sepsis. In R. Tenney Soerio & E. P. Devon (Eds.), *Netter's pediatrics* (2nd ed.). Elsevier.

Janhunen, K., Kankkunen, P., & Kvist, T. (2019). Quality of pediatric emergency care as assessed by children and their parents. *Journal of Nursing Care Quality, 34*(2), 180–184. https://doi.org/10.1097/NCQ.0000000000000346

Jones, M. A. (2023). Preparing an office practice for pediatric emergencies. *UpToDate*. Retrieved April 10, 2024, from https://www.uptodate.com/contents/preparing-an-office-practice-for-pediatric-emergencies

Krauss, B., Falk, J. L., & Ladde, J. G. (2024). Carbon dioxide monitoring (capnography). *UpToDate*. Retrieved April 10, 2024, from https://www.uptodate.com/contents/carbon-dioxide-monitoring-capnography

Marion, R. W., & Levy, P. A. (2023). Human genetics and dysmorphology. In K. J. Marcdante, R. M. Kliegman, & A. M Schuh (Eds.), *Nelson's essentials of pediatrics* (9th ed.). Elsevier.

Peterson, T. L., & Schuh, A. M. (2023). The acutely ill or injured child. In K. J. Marcdante, R. M. Kliegman, & A. M. Schuh (Eds.), *Nelson's essentials of pediatrics* (9th ed.). Elsevier.

Ring, L. M., Rana, M. S., & Deutsch, N. (2023). Implementation of a non-sedated procedural pain management practice guideline and order set. *Pediatric Nursing, 49*(1), 12–20.

Shaw, K. N., & Bachur, R. G. (Eds.). (2020). *Fleisher and Ludwig's textbook of pediatric emergency medicine* (8th ed.). Wolters Kluwer.

UpToDate, Inc. (2024). *UpToDate Lexidrug* (Version 8.2.0) [Mobile app]. Wolters Kluwer. https://apps.apple.com/us/app/lexicomp/id313401238

Velez, L. I., Shepherd, J. G., & Goto, C. S. (2022). Approach to the child with occult toxic exposure. *UpToDate*. Retrieved April 10, 2024, from http://www.uptodate.com/contents/approach-to-the-child-with-occult-toxic-exposure

World Health Organization. (2023). *Drowning*. https://www.who.int/en/news-room/fact-sheets/detail/drowning

DEVELOPING CLINICAL JUDGMENT

PRACTICING FOR NCLEX

1. An unresponsive toddler is brought to the emergency department. Assessment reveals mottled skin color, respiratory rate of 10 breaths/min, and a brachial pulse of 52 bpm. What is the priority nursing action?
   a. Prepare the defibrillator and draw up code medications.
   b. Provide 100% oxygen with a bag-valve-mask and start chest compressions.
   c. Start chest compressions and provide 100% oxygen via a nonrebreather mask.
   d. Begin an IV fluid infusion and administer epinephrine IV.
2. A 10-year-old child in respiratory distress requires intubation. Which sizes of endotracheal tubes will the nurse prepare?
   a. 9.5 mm and 10.0 mm
   b. 8.5 mm and 9.0 mm
   c. 6.0 mm and 6.5 mm
   d. 6.5 mm and 7.0 mm
3. A preschooler presents to the emergency department with a history of vomiting, diarrhea, and fever over the past few days. She is receiving 100% oxygen via a nonrebreather mask. Vital signs are temperature 104.5°F, pulse 144 bpm, respiratory rate 22 breaths/min, and BP 70/50 mm Hg. She is listless and difficult to arouse and has weak peripheral pulses and prolonged capillary refill. What nursing intervention takes priority?
   a. Administering acetaminophen rectally for the high fever
   b. Administering IV antibiotics for the infection
   c. Preparing the child for endotracheal intubation
   d. Giving an IV bolus of NS 20 mL/kg
4. Assessment of a 12-year-old who crashed his bicycle without a helmet reveals the following: temperature 99.2°F, pulse 100 bpm, respiratory rate 24 breaths/min with easy work of breathing, and BP 102/70 mm Hg. What is the priority action by the nurse?
   a. Assess neurologic status while observing for obvious injuries.
   b. Administer IV fluid bolus of NS at 20 mL/kg.
   c. Remove the cervical collar if he complains that it bothers him.
   d. Listen for bowel sounds while assessing for pain.
5. An 18-month-old child is brought to the emergency department via ambulance after an accidental ingestion. What is the priority nursing action?
   a. Take the child's vital signs.
   b. Give oral syrup of ipecac.
   c. Insert a nasogastric tube.
   d. Start an IV line.

DOSAGE CALCULATION QUESTION

The nurse is caring for an infant with SVT who is symptomatic and has an IV line in place. The infant weighs 16½ lb. The medication order reads: adenosine 0.01 mg/kg IV STAT followed by rapid flush. Adenosine is supplied as 6 mg/2 mL. How many milliliters will the nurse administer? Round to the nearest hundredth.

CRITICAL THINKING EXERCISES

1. A school-age child presents to the emergency department for evaluation. He had been feeling faint off and on and today fainted at school. On the cardiac monitor, an abnormal cardiac rhythm is noted. At present, the child is stable. What questions would be most appropriate for the nurse to ask when obtaining the child's health history? What objective assessments should the nurse make?
2. A 2-year-old is admitted to the hospital after accidentally ingesting a medication. The parent who brought their child to the hospital is upset and crying. How does this child's age and stage of development affect the child's risk for accidental ingestion? How should the nurse respond to the parent's distress? Develop a discharge teaching plan for this child and family related to poison prevention.
3. A 7-month-old is brought to the acute care facility with a chief complaint of difficulty breathing. The infant's parent says that the cold has gotten worse, and the infant won't eat. What additional questions should the nurse ask about the infant's health history? How would the nurse appropriately manage this infant's airway?

STUDY ACTIVITIES

1. Spend a day in the pediatric emergency department or urgent care center and document the role of the triage nurse.

2. Observe the pediatric emergency medical team at work or observe a pediatric code in the hospital. Compare and contrast the measures performed for the child with those that would be performed for an adult in a similar emergency situation.

3. Develop a teaching project related to injury prevention and present it at a local elementary, middle, or high school. Ensure that the education is geared toward the children's developmental level.

4. Interview the parents of a child who has experienced an emergency situation about how they felt during and after the emergency. Present the information to your classmates.

5. When providing care to a child in an emergency, the nurse performs the following assessments. Place them in the proper sequence.
   a. Pupillary reaction
   b. Presence of cough or sputum
   c. Heart rate and capillary refill
   d. Presence of bruises and abrasions
   e. Work of breathing

APPENDIX A

Clinical Paths

APPENDIX A.1 • Labor and Delivery Clinical Path—Labor: Expected Outcomes

	Active Phase	Expulsion/Pushing	Recovery First Hour Postpartum
PATIENT	Patient coping with labor support Patient utilizing appropriate labor options Patient verbalizes satisfaction with plan. Management interventions	Patient demonstrates effective pushing technique. Patient coping effectively with pushing Support person coping effectively with labor.	Bonding appropriately with baby
PATIENT'S STATUS	Cervix dilated 5 cm—complete Contraction regularly with progressive cervical change Maternal/fetal well-being maintained Hydration maintained If indicated: FSE and/or IUPC placed Pitocin IV started Epidural placed/WE encouraged Medicate with PRN pain meds.	Vaginal birth	Placenta delivered Fundus firm Lochia small–moderate Without clots Perineum intact/repaired Hemodynamically stable EBL $<$ 500 mL
CONTINUUM OF CARE	Prenatal record available after 32 weeks' gestation Prenatal labs WNL Preregistered to hospital Pediatrician identified Support after hospitalization identified. Discharge plan discussed with patient/family Communicates understanding of hospital and community resources		
ASSESSMENT/TREATMENT	Assess: Continuous EFM or auscultation Q15 of 30 minutes as indicated Vital signs hourly/temp Q4 hour if intact membranes/ Q2 hour if membranes ruptured Uterine by monitor or palpation Bladder for distention Hydration status Cervical dilation, effacement, station	Assess: Q15 minutes monitoring of fetal well-being (low risk) and Q5 minutes (high risk) Vital signs hourly/temperature Q2–4 hours depending on membrane status Bladder for distention Hydration status Pushing effectiveness Descent of presenting part Caput	Assess: Uterus–fundus Vital signs Lochia Bladder Perineum Placenta
PATIENT EDUCATION	Reinforce comfort measures. Encourage use of labor options. Inform patient/support person of plan of care.	Teaching of upright pushing positions Discourage prolonged maternal breath holding. Encourage to assume position of choice. Inform patient of progress.	Baby status Breastfeeding
	Interventions		
TESTS/ PROCEDURES	Hgb or Hct (if not done recently) T & S (if ordered) VE as indicated IV therapy AROM by MD or CNM: assess for color, amount, and odor, as appropriate. FSE/IUPC placement if indicated	AROM: assess for color, amount, and odor, as appropriate.	Cord blood or RhoGAM workup if appropriate Cord blood if O+ mother

APPENDIX A.1 • Labor and Delivery Clinical Path—Labor: Expected Outcomes

	Active Phase	Expulsion/Pushing	Recovery First Hour Postpartum
	Interventions		
THERAPIES	Comfort measures/birthing ball/ambulate/telemetry/ shower IV therapy If appropriate, pain management reviewed	Perineal massage Warm soaks to perineal area Allow to rest until feels the urge to push. Frequent position changes Cool cloth to brow	Ice pack to perineum Warm blankets
MEDS	Antibiotics as indicated for +GBS Pitocin if indicated PRN pain medication (encourage WE if requesting this)	Pitocin if indicated	Pitocin IV
ACTIVITY/SAFETY	Labor option usage Position changes	Provide wedge if supine. Promote effective position for pushing: i.e., squatting, side-lying, upright. Breathing technique patient/ support person most comfortable with	Assist with ambulate to bathroom. Infant care Assist with positioning for breastfeeding. Infant ID bands present
NUTRITION	Clear liquids Ice chips Others	Clear liquids Ice chips	Return to previous diet.
UNIQUE PATIENT NEEDS			

APPENDIX A.2 • Integrated Plan of Care for Cesarean Delivery

	Expected Patient Outcomes			
	Phase 1: Preadmission (Cesarean Delivery)	**Phase 2: Surgery/ Immediate Postop/Day of Surgery**	**Phase 3: Postop Day 1**	
USUAL TIME IN PHASE ASSESSMENT/ POTENTIAL COMPLICATIONS	**N/A Date Started**: VS WNL for patient Hgb or Hct/values within normal SLH antepartum range	Up to 23 hours VS WNL for patient Systems assessment: skin warm, dry Clear → Alert and oriented → Breast soft/nipples intact → Lungs clear → Bowel sounds present → Fundus firm u/u or u 1–2 cm below (–/+) Lochia small–moderate Dsg dry and intact No signs infiltration IV site Verbalizes comfort using pain rating scale 0–10	1 day VS WNL for patient Afebrile Voiding without Foley → Passing flatus Incision without redness or drainage Lochia small amount Fundus firm, u/1–2 cm Verbalizes comfort using pain scale 0–10 on oral pain meds	1–2 days Incision well-approximated, without drainage or redness Passing flatus Lochia small–moderate amount Fundus firm, u/1–2 cm Verbalizes comfort using pain medication, as described

(continued)

APPENDIX A.2 • Integrated Plan of Care for Cesarean Delivery (*continued*)

	Expected Patient Outcomes			
	Phase 1: Preadmission (Cesarean Delivery)	**Phase 2: Surgery/ Immediate Postop/Day of Surgery**	**Phase 3: Postop Day 1**	
PATIENT/FAMILY KNOWLEDGE	**Date All Above Met** Verbalizes understanding of condition and need for surgery Verbalizes understanding of all preop teaching	**Date All Above Met** Verbalizes correct use of PCA pain medication pump and when to request pain medication Turn, cough, and deep breathe appropriately.	**Date All Above Met** Can state criteria for when to call doctor for problems post discharge → ↑ Bleeding ↑ Temperature → Incision redness, odor or drainage →	**Date All Above Met** Verbalizes follow-up appointment date and time Verbalizes proper dosing of pain medication
ADLS/ACTIVITY	**Date All Above Met** Verbalizes understanding of NPO status	**Date All Above Met** Able to ambulate with minimal assistance Tolerating clear/full liquid diet Bonding observed with newborn—taking-in phase →	**Date All Above Met** Ambulating without assistance Tolerating soft to regular diet	**Date All Above Met** Ambulating in hall
UNIQUE PATIENT NEEDS	**Date All Above Met** **Entire Phase Outcomes met; progress patient to next phase**	**Date All Above Met** **Entire Phase Outcomes met; progress patient to next phase**	**Date All Above Met** **Entire Phase Outcomes met; progress patient to next phase**	**Date All Above Met** **Entire Phase Outcomes met; progress patient to next phase**
		Plan of Care		
	#1 Preadmission	**#2 Surgery/Immediate Postop/Day of Surgery**	**#3 Postop Day 1**	**#4 Postop Day 2/Discharge**
ASSESSMENTS	Vital signs Fetal status immediately prior to surgery	VS per PACU then Q4 hour Systems assessment: • Skin, LOC, FROM, • Breasts, lungs, fundus, incision • Lochia, bladder, bowel sounds, IV, and site • I & O Q shift • Assess pain control 0–10 scale. • Assess RhoGAM status. • Assess rubella titer status. • ID band on birthing parent	VS Q6 hour Assess pain control 0–10 scale. Incision Foley-voiding Fundus/lochia IV site Breasts ID band on birthing parent Activity	Assess pain control 0–10 scale. Incision Voiding Fundus Lochia IV site as needed ID band on birthing parent Activity
CONSULTS	Anesthesia	Social work as needed, anesthesia, lactation, dietitian as needed	Social work, lactation, dietitian as needed	Social work, lactation, dietitian as needed
PATIENT/FAMILY EDUCATION DISCHARGE PLANNING	Need for surgery Review cesarean delivery. Review procedure, postop expectations. Demonstrate/discuss equipment—PCA, fentanyl pump. Tour of OR area and nursery	Review postop expectations. Review equipment use PRN. Instruct patient on: Hospital/infant security systems Unity orientation Newborn orientation/care/feeding (if breastfeeding problems, see decision trees)	Review dietary needs post-surgery. Review bleeding/lochia. Precautions post–cesarean delivery Review follow-up care and doctor. Appointments Review incision care, pericare. Infant care Infant feeding	Verify follow-up appointment date and time. Activity restrictions Follow-up for staple removal as needed Offer home follow-up care. Discuss birth control.

APPENDIX A.2 • Integrated Plan of Care for Cesarean Delivery

	Expected Patient Outcomes			
	Phase 1: Preadmission (Cesarean Delivery)	**Phase 2: Surgery/ Immediate Postop/Day of Surgery**	**Phase 3: Postop Day 1**	
TESTS AND PROCEDURES	PAT; Hgb, and Hct (if not done recently—within 1 month) T & S (if ordered)			
PHARMACOLOGIC NEEDS		IV fluids as ordered Pain control: PCA, fentanyl pump, IM to PO	IV lock PO pain meds Give RhoGAM if indicated Give rubella if indicated	DC IV lock as ordered
ACTIVITY/ REHABILITATION	Patient's usual	Change position Q2 hour while in bed, OOB stand at bedside postop night/ dangle and transfer to chair Progress to patient endurance. Observe bonding with infant. Observe family support system (if inadequate consult SW).	Progress endurance/begin. Ambulation in hall OOB in AM May shower	Ambulate in halls without assistance.
NUTRITION/ ELIMINATION		NPO then clear liquids to DAT Foley empty Q shift	DAT to regular or previous diet at home Foley discontinued	
MISCELLANEOUS INTERVENTIONS		TCDB Q2 hour while awake	Dressing removed by MD or RN with orders from MD	
UNIQUE PATIENT NEEDS		Assess home preparations for infant arrival and family support system or other available help for postpartum patient. Confirm postpartum and pediatrician appointments made.		

APPENDIX B

Cervical Dilation Chart

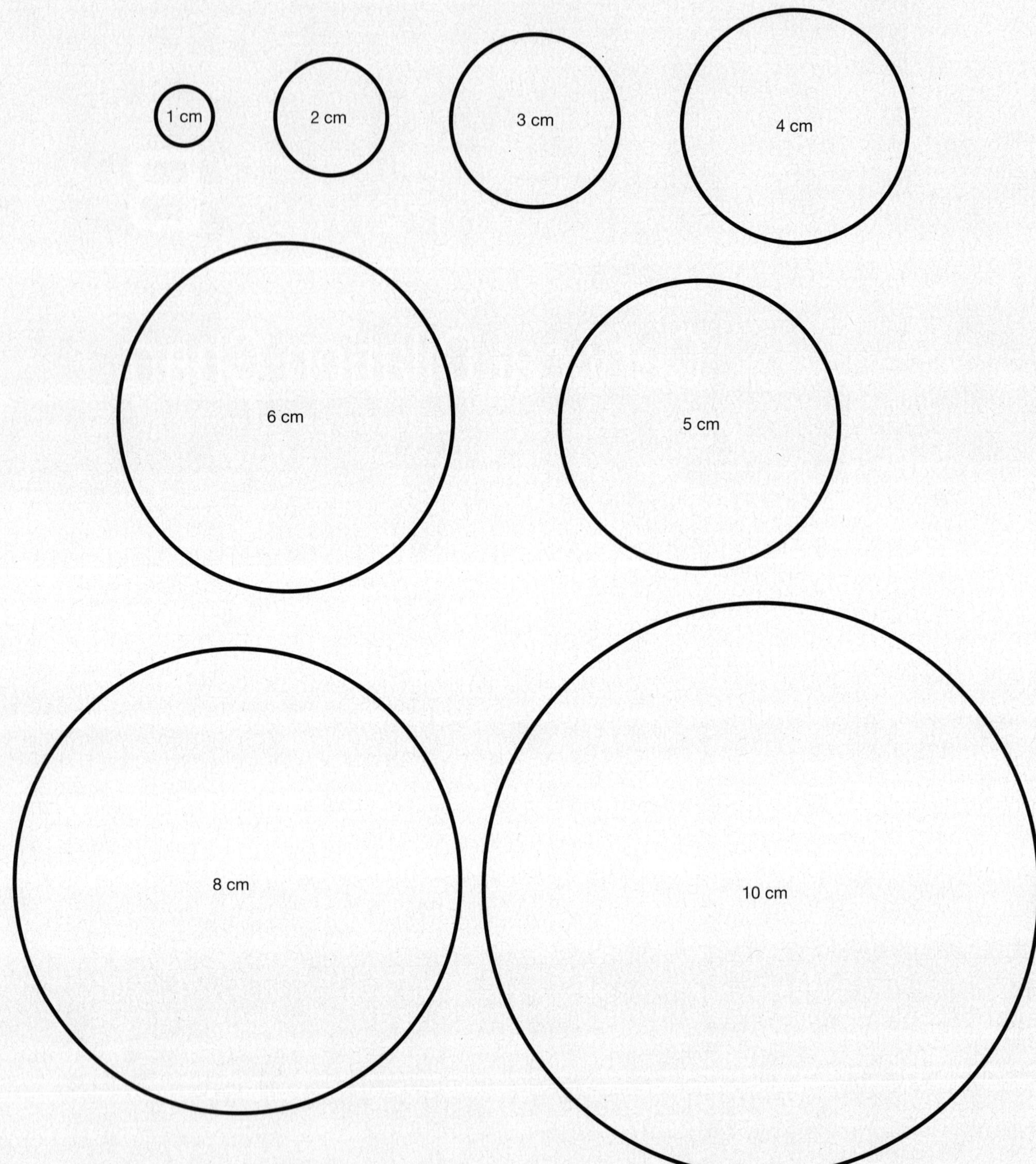
1 cm
2 cm
3 cm
4 cm
6 cm
5 cm
8 cm
10 cm

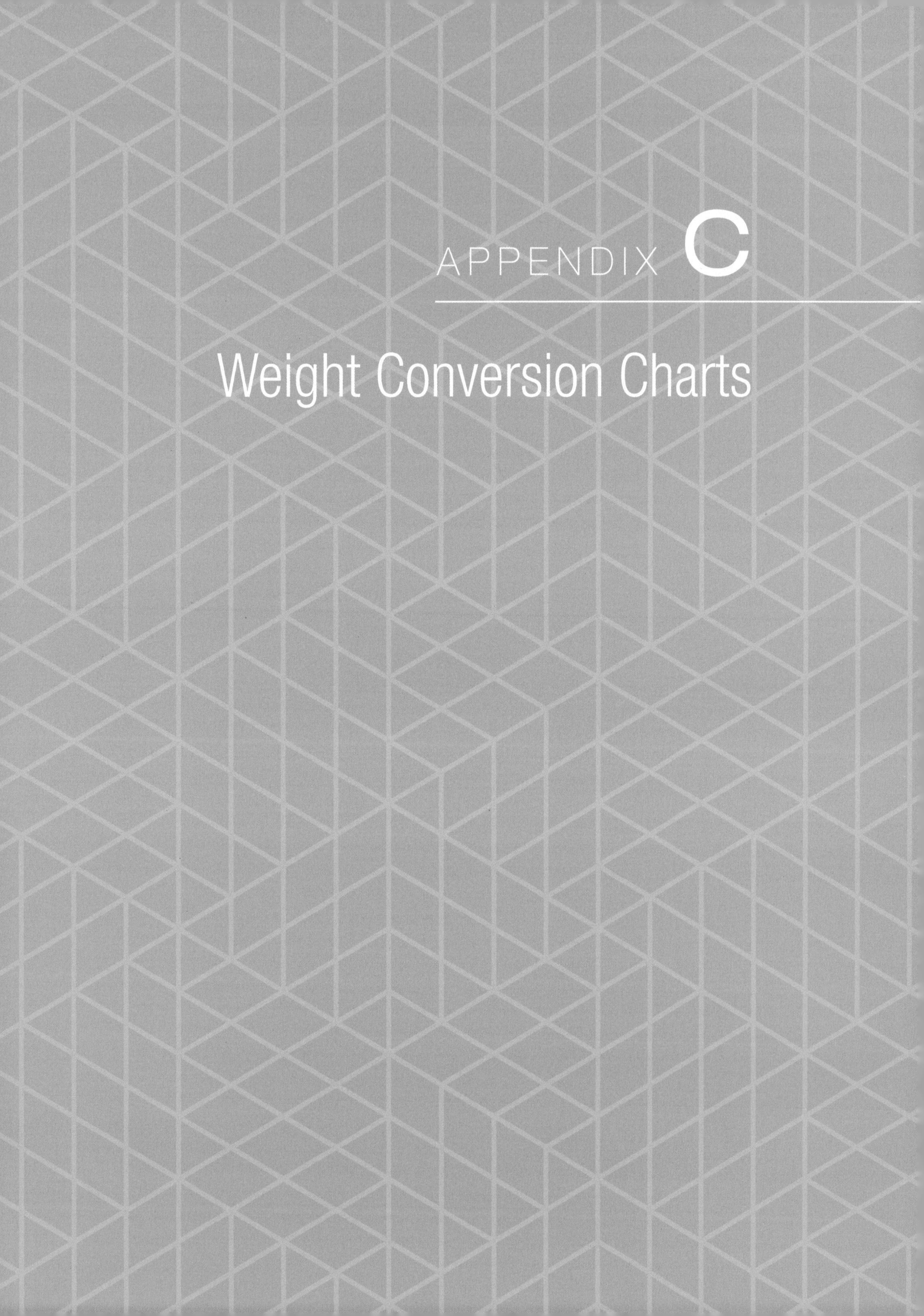

APPENDIX C

Weight Conversion Charts

TABLE C.1 • Conversion of Pounds to Kilograms

Pounds	0	1	2	3	4	5	6	7	8	9
0	—	0.45	0.90	1.36	1.81	2.26	2.72	3.17	3.62	4.08
10	4.53	4.98	5.44	5.89	6.35	6.80	7.25	7.71	8.16	8.61
20	9.07	9.52	9.97	10.43	10.88	11.34	11.79	12.24	12.70	13.15
30	13.60	14.06	14.51	14.96	15.42	15.87	16.32	16.78	17.23	17.69
40	18.14	18.59	19.05	19.50	19.95	20.41	20.86	21.31	21.77	22.22
50	22.68	23.13	23.58	24.04	24.49	24.94	25.40	25.85	26.30	26.76
60	27.21	27.66	28.12	28.57	29.03	29.48	29.93	30.39	30.84	31.29
70	31.75	32.20	32.65	33.11	33.56	34.02	34.47	34.92	35.38	35.83
80	36.28	36.74	37.19	37.64	38.10	38.55	39.00	39.46	39.91	40.37
90	40.82	41.27	41.73	42.18	42.63	43.09	43.54	43.99	44.45	44.90
100	45.36	45.81	46.26	46.72	47.17	47.62	48.08	48.53	48.98	49.44
110	49.89	50.34	50.80	51.25	51.71	52.16	52.61	53.07	53.52	53.97
120	54.43	54.88	55.33	55.79	56.24	56.70	57.15	57.60	58.06	58.51
130	58.96	59.42	59.87	60.32	60.78	61.23	61.68	62.14	62.59	63.05
140	63.50	63.95	64.41	64.86	65.31	65.77	66.22	66.67	67.13	67.58
150	68.04	68.49	68.94	69.40	69.85	70.30	70.76	71.21	71.66	72.12
160	72.57	73.02	73.48	73.93	74.39	74.84	75.29	75.75	76.20	76.65
170	77.11	77.56	78.01	78.47	78.92	79.38	79.83	80.28	80.74	81.19
180	81.64	82.10	82.55	83.00	83.46	83.91	84.36	84.82	85.27	85.73
190	86.18	86.68	87.09	87.54	87.99	88.45	88.90	89.35	89.81	90.26
200	90.72	91.17	91.62	92.08	92.53	92.98	93.44	93.89	94.34	94.80

TABLE C.2 • Conversion of Pounds and Ounces to Grams for Newborn Weights

	Ounces															
Pounds	**0**	**1**	**2**	**3**	**4**	**5**	**6**	**7**	**8**	**9**	**10**	**11**	**12**	**13**	**14**	**15**
0	—	28	57	85	113	142	170	198	227	255	283	312	340	369	397	425
1	454	482	510	539	567	595	624	652	680	709	737	765	794	822	850	879
2	907	936	964	992	1,021	1,049	1,077	1,106	1,134	1,162	1,191	1,219	1,247	1,276	1,304	1,332
3	1,361	1,389	1,417	1,446	1,474	1,503	1,531	1,559	1,588	1,616	1,644	1,673	1,701	1,729	1,758	1,786
4	1,814	1,843	1,871	1,899	1,928	1,956	1,984	2,013	2,041	2,070	2,098	2,126	2,155	2,183	2,211	2,240
5	2,268	2,296	2,325	2,353	2,381	2,410	2,438	2,466	2,495	2,523	2,551	2,580	2,608	2,637	2,665	2,693
6	2,722	2,750	2,778	2,807	2,835	2,863	2,892	2,920	2,948	2,977	3,005	3,033	3,062	3,090	3,118	3,147
7	3,175	3,203	3,232	3,260	3,289	3,317	3,345	3,374	3,402	3,430	3,459	3,487	3,515	3,544	3,572	3,600
8	3,629	3,657	3,685	3,714	3,742	3,770	3,799	3,827	3,856	3,884	3,912	3,941	3,969	3,997	4,026	4,054
9	4,082	4,111	4,139	4,167	4,196	4,224	4,252	4,281	4,309	4,337	4,366	4,394	4,423	4,451	4,479	4,508
10	4,536	4,564	4,593	4,621	4,649	4,678	4,706	4,734	4,763	4,791	4,819	4,848	4,876	4,904	4,933	4,961
11	4,990	5,018	5,046	5,075	5,103	5,131	5,160	5,188	5,216	5,245	5,273	5,301	5,330	5,358	5,386	5,415
12	5,443	5,471	5,500	5,528	5,557	5,585	5,613	5,642	5,670	5,698	5,727	5,755	5,783	5,812	5,840	5,868
13	5,897	5,925	5,953	5,982	6,010	6,038	6,067	6,095	6,123	6,152	6,180	6,209	6,237	6,265	6,294	6,322
14	6,350	6,379	6,407	6,435	6,464	6,492	6,520	6,549	6,577	6,605	6,634	6,662	6,690	6,719	6,747	6,776
15	6,804	6,832	6,860	6,889	6,917	6,945	6,973	7,002	7,030	7,059	7,087	7,115	7,144	7,172	7,201	7,228

APPENDIX D

Growth Charts

Birth to 24 months: Boys
Length-for-age and Weight-for-age percentiles

NAME ______________________

RECORD # ______

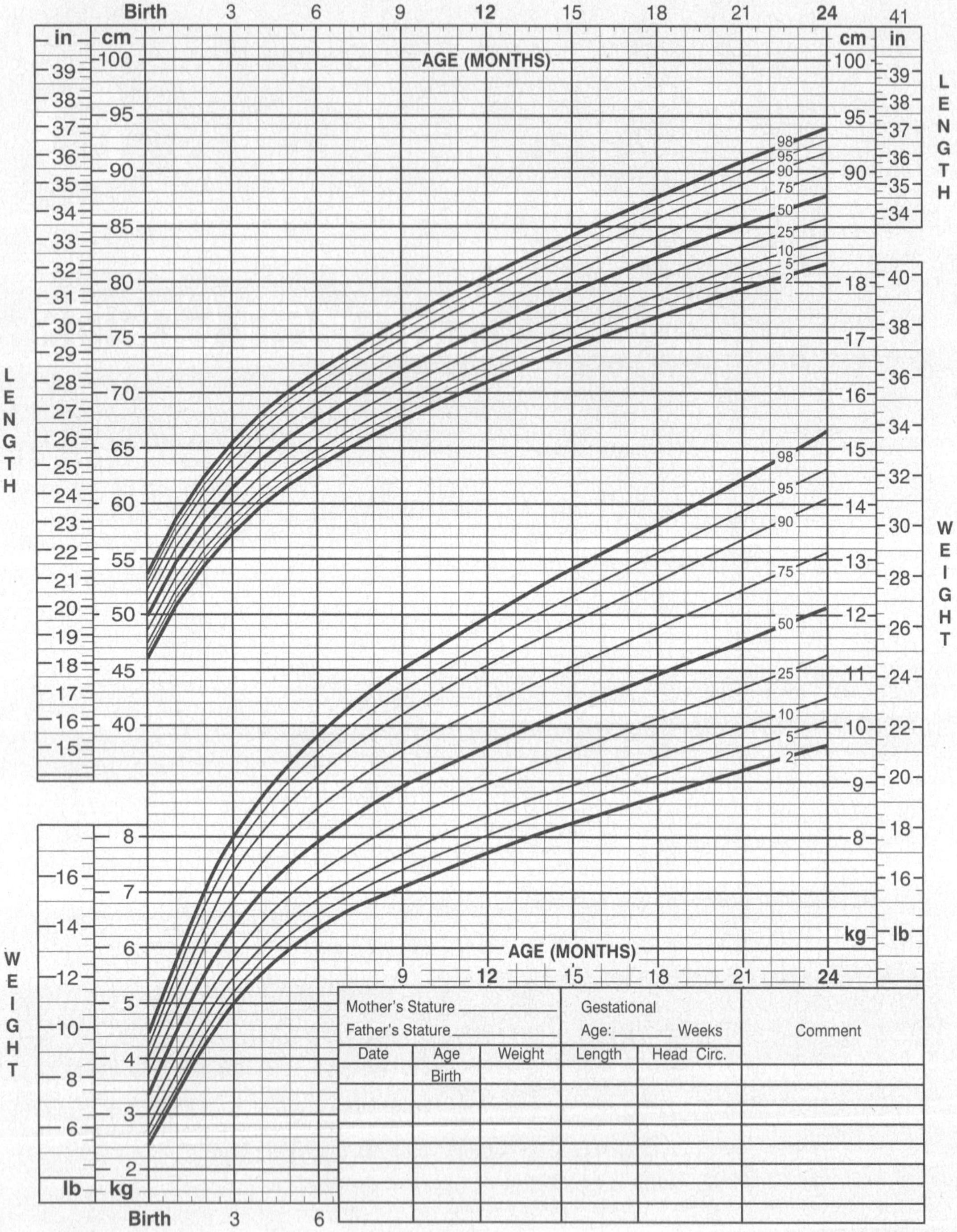

Mother's Stature ______			Gestational		
Father's Stature ______			Age: ______ Weeks		Comment
Date	Age	Weight	Length	Head Circ.	
	Birth				

Published by the Centers for Disease Control and Prevention, November 1, 2009
SOURCE: WHO Child Growth Standards (http://www.who.int/childgrowth/en)

SAFER·HEALTHIER·PEOPLE™

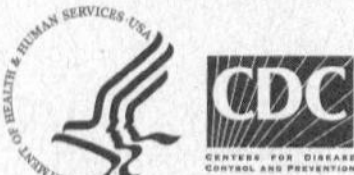

Birth to 24 months: Girls
Length-for-age and Weight-for-age percentiles

NAME ________________

RECORD # ________________

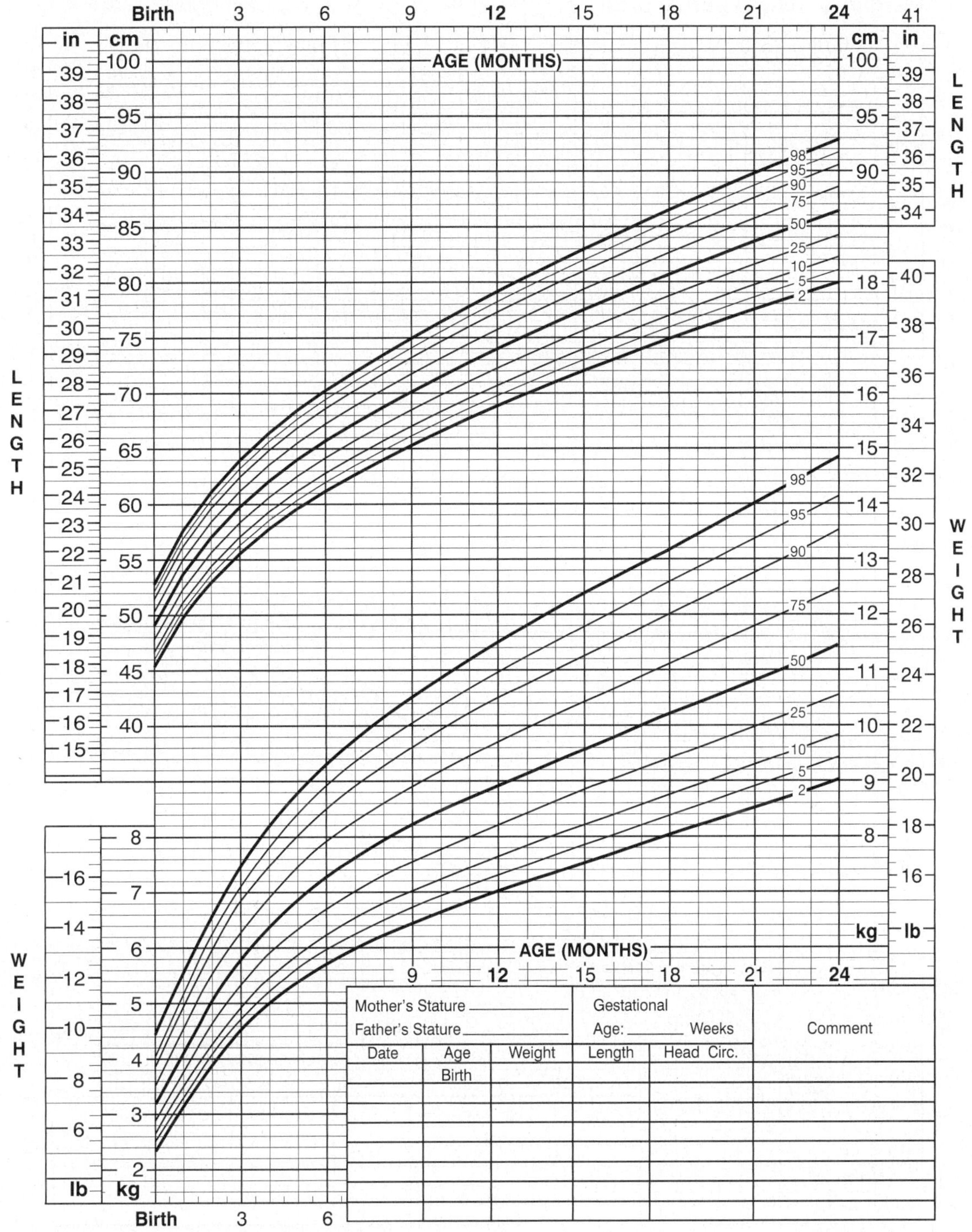

Mother's Stature ______			Gestational Age: ______ Weeks		Comment
Father's Stature ______					
Date	Age	Weight	Length	Head Circ.	
	Birth				

Published by the Centers for Disease Control and Prevention, November 1, 2009
SOURCE: WHO Child Growth Standards (http://www.who.int/childgrowth/en)

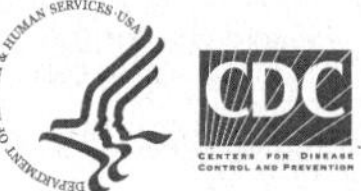

Birth to 24 months: Boys
Head circumference-for-age and Weight-for-length percentiles

NAME ______________________

RECORD # ______________

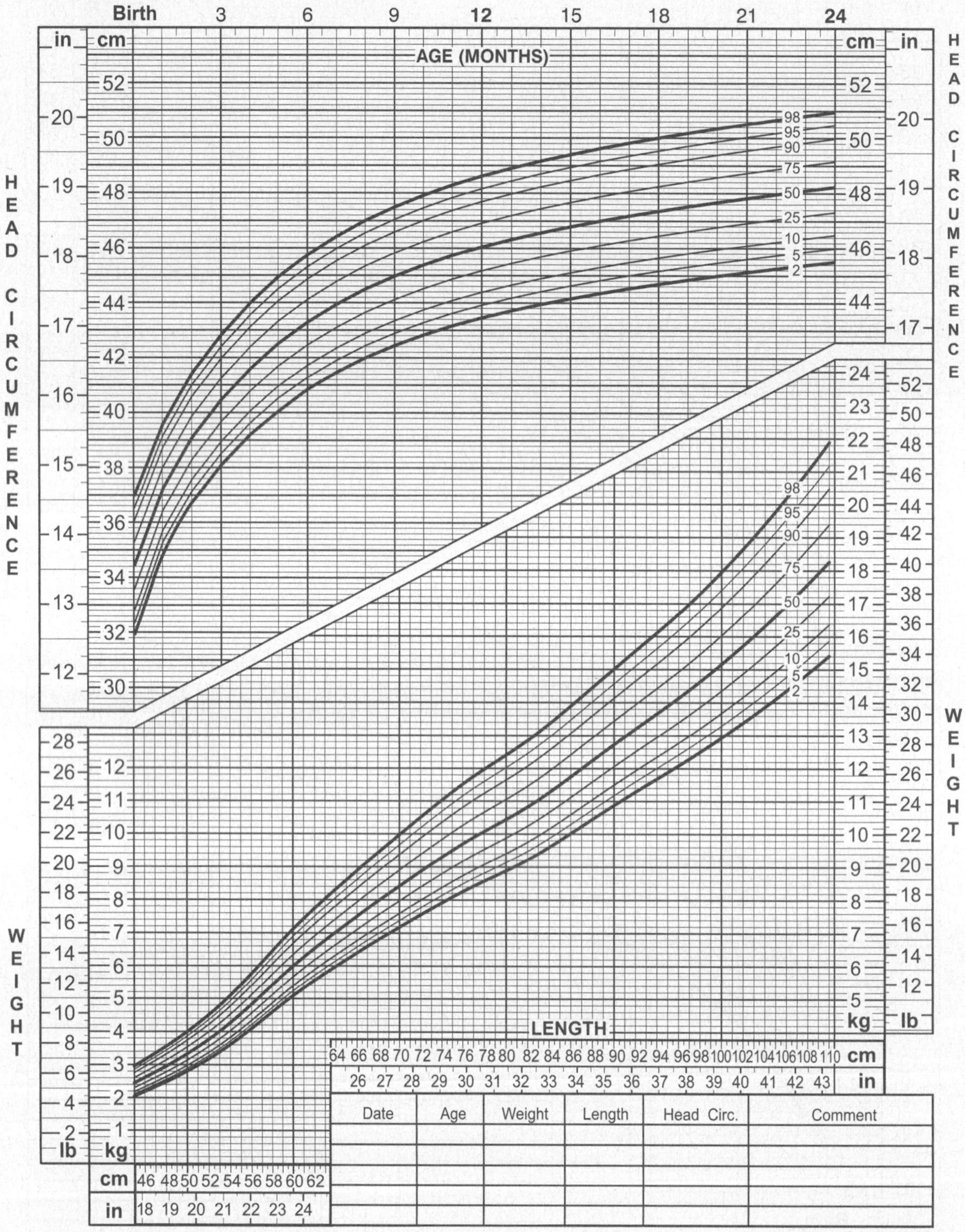

Date	Age	Weight	Length	Head Circ.	Comment

Published by the Centers for Disease Control and Prevention, November 1, 2009
SOURCE: WHO Child Growth Standards (http://www.who.int/childgrowth/en)

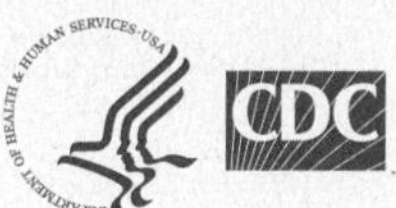

Birth to 24 months: Girls
Head circumference-for-age and
Weight-for-length percentiles

NAME ____________________

RECORD # ____________

Date	Age	Weight	Length	Head Circ.	Comment

Published by the Centers for Disease Control and Prevention, November 1, 2009
SOURCE: WHO Child Growth Standards (http://www.who.int/childgrowth/en)

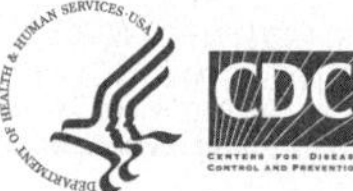

2 to 20 years: Boys
Stature-for-age and Weight-for-age percentiles

NAME ____________

RECORD # ____________

Mother's Stature ________ Father's Stature ________

Date	Age	Weight	Stature	BMI*

***To Calculate BMI**: Weight (kg) ÷ Stature (cm) ÷ Stature (cm) x 10,000
or Weight (lb) ÷ Stature (in) ÷ Stature (in) x 703

Published May 30, 2000 (modified 11/21/00).
SOURCE: Developed by the National Center for Health Statistics in collaboration with the National Center for Chronic Disease Prevention and Health Promotion (2000).
http://www.cdc.gov/growthcharts

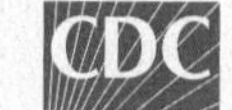

SAFER • HEALTHIER • PEOPLE™

2 to 20 years: Girls
Stature-for-age and Weight-for-age percentiles

NAME ____________________

RECORD # ____________

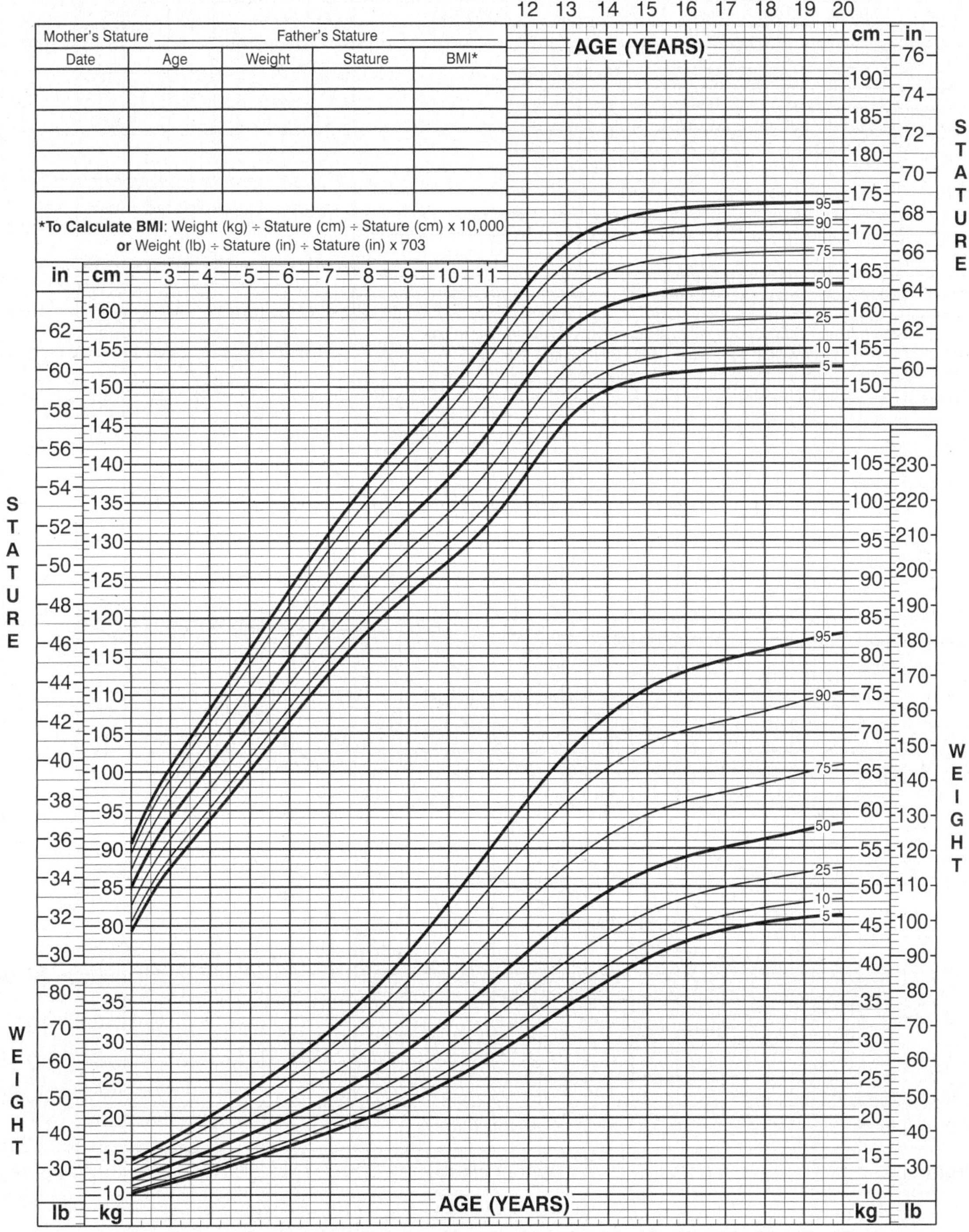

Published May 30, 2000 (modified 11/21/00).
SOURCE: Developed by the National Center for Health Statistics in collaboration with the National Center for Chronic Disease Prevention and Health Promotion (2000).
http://www.cdc.gov/growthcharts

CDC
SAFER • HEALTHIER • PEOPLE™

2 to 20 years: Boys
Body mass index-for-age percentiles

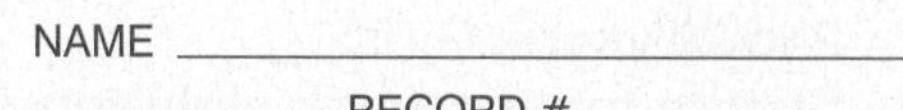

Date	Age	Weight	Stature	BMI*	Comments

***To Calculate BMI**: Weight (kg) ÷ Stature (cm) ÷ Stature (cm) x 10,000
or Weight (lb) ÷ Stature (in) ÷ Stature (in) x 703

BMI

BMI: 12 13 14 15 16 17 18 19 20 21 22 23 24 25 26 27 28 29 30 31 32 33 34 35

Percentiles: 95, 90, 85, 75, 50, 25, 10, 5

kg/m² AGE (YEARS) kg/m²

2 3 4 5 6 7 8 9 10 11 12 13 14 15 16 17 18 19 20

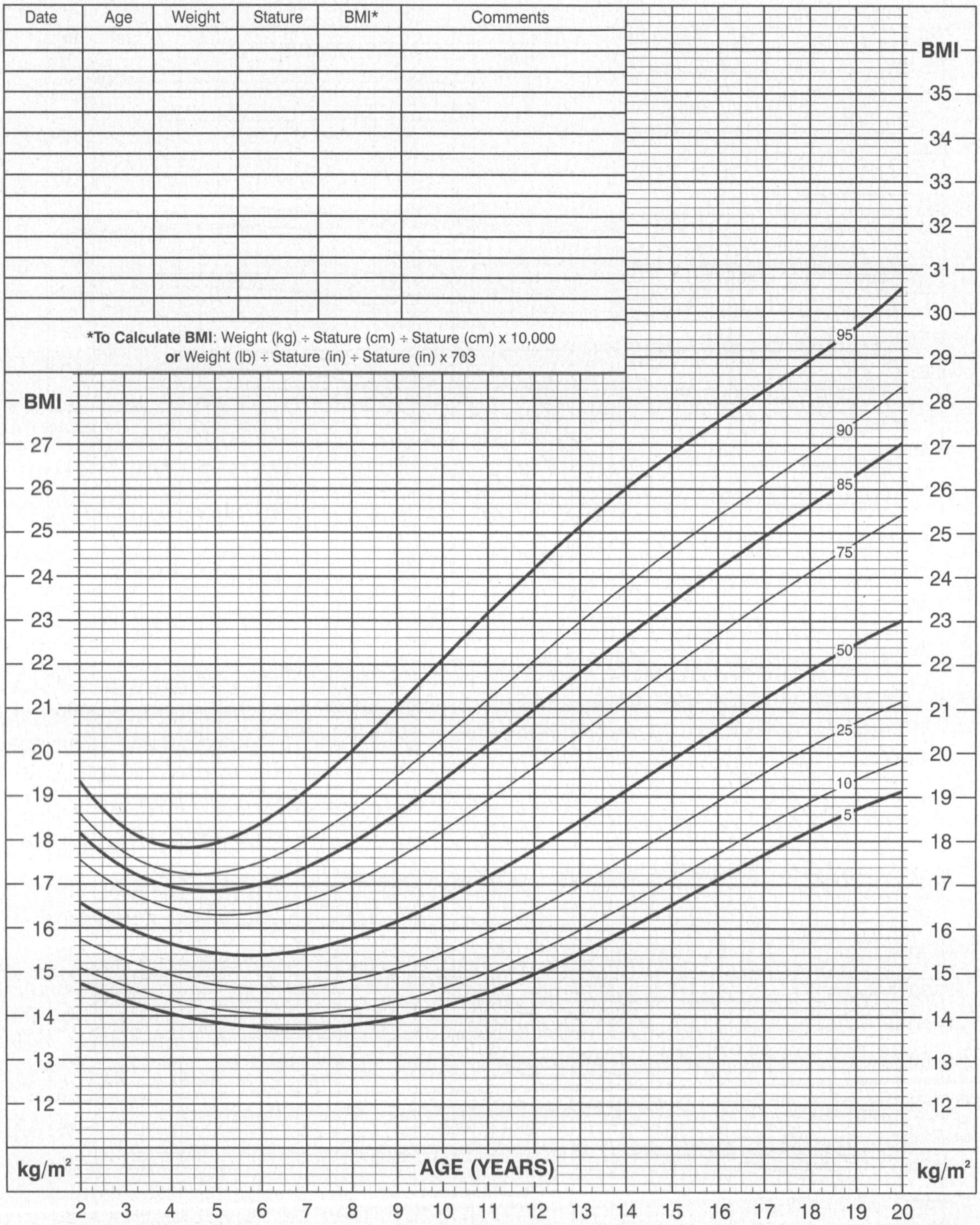

Published May 30, 2000 (modified 10/16/00).
SOURCE: Developed by the National Center for Health Statistics in collaboration with the National Center for Chronic Disease Prevention and Health Promotion (2000).
http://www.cdc.gov/growthcharts

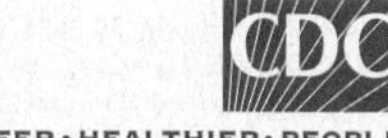

SAFER • HEALTHIER • PEOPLE™

2 to 20 years: Girls
Body mass index-for-age percentiles

NAME ______________________

RECORD # __________

Date	Age	Weight	Stature	BMI*	Comments

***To Calculate BMI**: Weight (kg) ÷ Stature (cm) ÷ Stature (cm) x 10,000
or Weight (lb) ÷ Stature (in) ÷ Stature (in) x 703

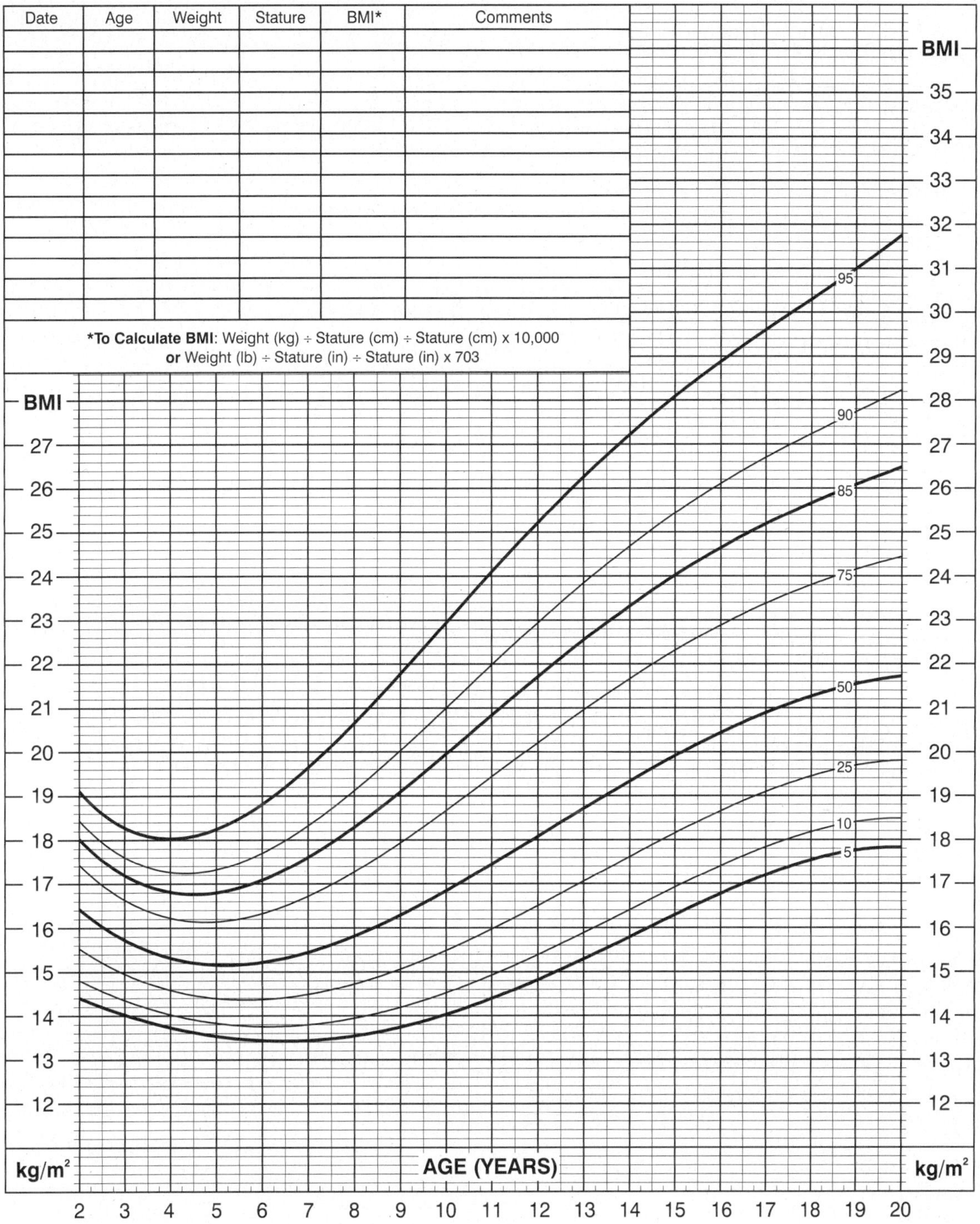

Published May 30, 2000 (modified 10/16/00).
SOURCE: Developed by the National Center for Health Statistics in collaboration with
the National Center for Chronic Disease Prevention and Health Promotion (2000).
http://www.cdc.gov/growthcharts

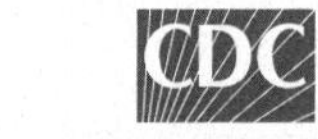

SAFER • HEALTHIER • PEOPLE™

APPENDIX E

Blood Pressure Charts for Children and Adolescents

APPENDIX E.1 • Blood Pressure Levels for Males by Age and Height Percentile

Age (years)	BP Percentile ↓	SBP (mm Hg) ← *Height Percentile or Measured Height* →							DBP (mm Hg) ← *Height Percentile or Measured Height* →						
		5%	***10%***	***25%***	***50%***	***75%***	***90%***	***95%***	***5%***	***10%***	***25%***	***50%***	***75%***	***90%***	***95%***
1	Height (in)	30.4	30.8	31.6	32.4	33.3	34.1	34.6	30.4	30.8	31.6	32.4	33.3	34.1	34.6
	Height (cm)	77.2	78.3	80.2	82.4	84.6	86.7	87.9	77.2	78.3	80.2	82.4	84.6	86.7	87.9
	50th	85	85	86	86	87	88	88	40	40	40	41	41	42	42
	90th	98	99	99	100	100	101	101	52	52	53	53	54	54	54
	95th	102	102	103	103	104	105	105	54	54	55	55	56	57	57
	95th + 12 mm Hg	114	114	115	115	116	117	117	66	66	67	67	68	69	69
2	Height (in)	33.9	34.4	35.3	36.3	37.3	38.2	38.8	33.9	34.4	35.3	36.3	37.3	38.2	38.8
	Height (cm)	86.1	87.4	89.6	92.1	94.7	97.1	98.5	86.1	87.4	89.6	92.1	94.7	97.1	98.5
	50th	87	87	88	89	89	90	91	43	43	44	44	45	46	46
	90th	100	100	101	102	103	103	104	55	55	56	56	57	58	58
	95th	104	105	105	106	107	107	108	57	58	58	59	60	61	61
	95th + 12 mm Hg	116	117	117	118	119	119	120	69	70	70	71	72	73	73
3	Height (in)	36.4	37	37.9	39	40.1	41.1	41.7	36.4	37	37.9	39	40.1	41.1	41.7
	Height (cm)	92.5	93.9	96.3	99	101.8	104.3	105.8	92.5	93.9	96.3	99	101.8	104.3	105.8
	50th	88	89	89	90	91	92	92	45	46	46	47	48	49	49
	90th	101	102	102	103	104	105	105	58	58	59	59	60	61	61
	95th	106	106	107	107	108	109	109	60	61	61	62	63	64	64
	95th + 12 mm Hg	118	118	119	119	120	121	121	72	73	73	74	75	76	76
4	Height (in)	38.8	39.4	40.5	41.7	42.9	43.9	44.5	38.8	39.4	40.5	41.7	42.9	43.9	44.5
	Height (cm)	98.5	100.2	102.9	105.9	108.9	111.5	113.2	98.5	100.2	102.9	105.9	108.9	111.5	113.2
	50th	90	90	91	92	93	94	94	48	49	49	50	51	52	52
	90th	102	103	104	105	105	106	107	60	61	62	62	63	64	64
	95th	107	107	108	108	109	110	110	63	64	65	66	67	67	68
	95th + 12 mm Hg	119	119	120	120	121	122	122	75	76	77	78	79	79	80
5	Height (in)	41.1	41.8	43.0	44.3	45.5	46.7	47.4	41.1	41.8	43.0	44.3	45.5	46.7	47.4
	Height (cm)	104.4	106.2	109.1	112.4	115.7	118.6	120.3	104.4	106.2	109.1	112.4	115.7	118.6	120.3
	50th	91	92	93	94	95	96	96	51	51	52	53	54	55	55
	90th	103	104	105	106	107	108	108	63	64	65	65	66	67	67
	95th	107	108	109	109	110	111	112	66	67	68	69	70	70	71
	95th + 12 mm Hg	119	120	121	121	122	123	124	78	79	80	81	82	82	83
6	Height (in)	43.4	44.2	45.4	46.8	48.2	49.4	50.2	43.4	44.2	45.4	46.8	48.2	49.4	50.2
	Height (cm)	110.3	112.2	115.3	118.9	122.4	125.6	127.5	110.3	112.2	115.3	118.9	122.4	125.6	127.5
	50th	93	93	94	95	96	97	98	54	54	55	56	57	57	58
	90th	105	105	106	107	109	110	110	66	66	67	68	68	69	69
	95th	108	109	110	111	112	113	114	69	70	70	71	72	72	73
	95th + 12 mm Hg	120	121	122	123	124	125	126	81	82	82	83	84	84	85

APPENDIX E.1 • Blood Pressure Levels for Males by Age and Height Percentile

Age (years)	BP Percentile ↓	SBP (mm Hg)							DBP (mm Hg)						
		← Height Percentile or Measured Height →							*← Height Percentile or Measured Height →*						
		5%	*10%*	*25%*	*50%*	*75%*	*90%*	*95%*	*5%*	*10%*	*25%*	*50%*	*75%*	*90%*	*95%*
7	Height (in)	45.7	46.5	47.8	49.3	50.8	52.1	52.9	45.7	46.5	47.8	49.3	50.8	52.1	52.9
	Height (cm)	116.1	118	121.4	125.1	128.9	132.4	134.5	116.1	118	121.4	125.1	128.9	132.4	134.5
	50th	94	94	95	97	98	98	99	56	56	57	58	58	59	59
	90th	106	107	108	109	110	111	111	68	68	69	70	70	71	71
	95th	110	110	111	112	114	115	116	71	71	72	73	73	74	74
	95th + 12 mm Hg	122	122	123	124	126	127	128	83	83	84	85	85	86	86
8	Height (in)	47.8	48.6	50	51.6	53.2	54.6	55.5	47.8	48.6	50	51.6	53.2	54.6	55.5
	Height (cm)	121.4	123.5	127	131	135.1	138.8	141	121.4	123.5	127	131	135.1	138.8	141
	50th	95	96	97	98	99	99	100	57	57	58	59	59	60	60
	90th	107	108	109	110	111	112	112	69	70	70	71	72	72	73
	95th	111	112	112	114	115	116	117	72	73	73	74	75	75	75
	95th + 12 mm Hg	123	124	124	126	127	128	129	84	85	85	86	87	87	87
9	Height (in)	49.6	50.5	52	53.7	55.4	56.9	57.9	49.6	50.5	52	53.7	55.4	56.9	57.9
	Height (cm)	126	128.3	132.1	136.3	140.7	144.7	147.1	126	128.3	132.1	136.3	140.7	144.7	147.1
	50th	96	97	98	99	100	101	101	57	58	59	60	61	62	62
	90th	107	108	109	110	112	113	114	70	71	72	73	74	74	74
	95th	112	112	113	115	116	118	119	74	74	75	76	76	77	77
	95th + 12 mm Hg	124	124	125	127	128	130	131	86	86	87	88	88	89	89
10	Height (in)	51.3	52.2	53.8	55.6	57.4	59.1	60.1	51.3	52.2	53.8	55.6	57.4	59.1	60.1
	Height (cm)	130.2	132.7	136.7	141.3	145.9	150.1	152.7	130.2	132.7	136.7	141.3	145.9	150.1	152.7
	50th	97	98	99	100	101	102	103	59	60	61	62	63	63	64
	90th	108	109	111	112	113	115	116	72	73	74	74	75	75	76
	95th	112	113	114	116	118	120	121	76	76	77	77	78	78	78
	95th + 12 mm Hg	124	125	126	128	130	132	133	88	88	89	89	90	90	90
11	Height (in)	53	54	55.7	57.6	59.6	61.3	62.4	53	54	55.7	57.6	59.6	61.3	62.4
	Height (cm)	134.7	137.3	141.5	146.4	151.3	155.8	158.6	134.7	137.3	141.5	146.4	151.3	155.8	158.6
	50th	99	99	101	102	103	104	106	61	61	62	63	63	63	63
	90th	110	111	112	114	116	117	118	74	74	75	75	75	76	76
	95th	114	114	116	118	120	123	124	77	78	78	78	78	78	78
	95th + 12 mm Hg	126	126	128	130	132	135	136	89	90	90	90	90	90	90
12	Height (in)	55.2	56.3	58.1	60.1	62.2	64	65.2	55.2	56.3	58.1	60.1	62.2	64	65.2
	Height (cm)	140.3	143	147.5	152.7	157.9	162.6	165.5	140.3	143	147.5	152.7	157.9	162.6	165.5
	50th	101	101	102	104	106	108	109	61	62	62	62	62	63	63
	90th	113	114	115	117	119	121	122	75	75	75	75	75	76	76
	95th	116	117	118	121	124	126	128	78	78	78	78	78	79	79
	95th + 12 mm Hg	128	129	130	133	136	138	140	90	90	90	90	90	91	91

(continued)

APPENDIX E.1 • Blood Pressure Levels for Males by Age and Height Percentile (*continued*)

Age (years)	BP Percentile ↓	SBP (mm Hg) ← Height Percentile or Measured Height →							DBP (mm Hg) ← Height Percentile or Measured Height →						
		5%	10%	25%	50%	75%	90%	95%	5%	10%	25%	50%	75%	90%	95%
13	Height (in)	57.9	59.1	61	63.1	65.2	67.1	68.3	57.9	59.1	61	63.1	65.2	67.1	68.3
	Height (cm)	147	150	154.9	160.3	165.7	170.5	173.4	147	150	154.9	160.3	165.7	170.5	173.4
	50th	103	104	105	108	110	111	112	61	60	61	62	63	64	65
	90th	115	116	118	121	124	126	126	74	74	74	75	76	77	77
	95th	119	120	122	125	128	130	131	78	78	78	78	80	81	81
	95th + 12 mm Hg	131	132	134	137	140	142	143	90	90	90	90	92	93	93
14	Height (in)	60.6	61.8	63.8	65.9	68.0	69.8	70.9	60.6	61.8	63.8	65.9	68.0	69.8	70.9
	Height (cm)	153.8	156.9	162	167.5	172.7	177.4	180.1	153.8	156.9	162	167.5	172.7	177.4	180.1
	50th	105	106	109	111	112	113	113	60	60	62	64	65	66	67
	90th	119	120	123	126	127	128	129	74	74	75	77	78	79	80
	95th	123	125	127	130	132	133	134	77	78	79	81	82	83	84
	95th + 12 mm Hg	135	137	139	142	144	145	146	89	90	91	93	94	95	96
15	Height (in)	62.6	63.8	65.7	67.8	69.8	71.5	72.5	62.6	63.8	65.7	67.8	69.8	71.5	72.5
	Height (cm)	159	162	166.9	172.2	177.2	181.6	184.2	159	162	166.9	172.2	177.2	181.6	184.2
	50th	108	110	112	113	114	114	114	61	62	64	65	66	67	68
	90th	123	124	126	128	129	130	130	75	76	78	79	80	81	81
	95th	127	129	131	132	134	135	135	78	79	81	83	84	85	85
	95th + 12 mm Hg	139	141	143	144	146	147	147	90	91	93	95	96	97	97
16	Height (in)	63.8	64.9	66.8	68.8	70.7	72.4	73.4	63.8	64.9	66.8	68.8	70.7	72.4	73.4
	Height (cm)	162.1	165	169.6	174.6	179.5	183.8	186.4	162.1	165	169.6	174.6	179.5	183.8	186.4
	50th	111	112	114	115	115	116	116	63	64	66	67	68	69	69
	90th	126	127	128	129	131	131	132	77	78	79	80	81	82	82
	95th	130	131	133	134	135	136	137	80	81	83	84	85	86	86
	95th + 12 mm Hg	142	143	145	146	147	148	149	92	93	95	96	97	98	98
17	Height (in)	64.5	65.5	67.3	69.2	71.1	72.8	73.8	64.5	65.5	67.3	69.2	71.1	72.8	73.8
	Height (cm)	163.8	166.5	170.9	175.8	180.7	184.9	187.5	163.8	166.5	170.9	175.8	180.7	184.9	187.5
	50th	114	115	116	117	117	118	118	65	66	67	68	69	70	70
	90th	128	129	130	131	132	133	134	78	79	80	81	82	82	83
	95th	132	133	134	135	137	138	138	81	82	84	85	86	86	87
	95th + 12 mm Hg	144	145	146	147	149	150	150	93	94	96	97	98	98	99

BP, blood pressure; DBP, diastolic blood pressure; SBP, systolic blood pressure. ≥90th to ≤95th percentile, or 120/80 or ≤95th percentile (whichever is lower): elevated blood pressure; ≥95th to ≤95th percentile + 12 mm Hg, or 130/80 to 139/89 mm Hg (whichever is lower): stage 1 hypertension; ≥95th percentile + 12 mm Hg, or ≥140/90 mm Hg (whichever is lower): stage 2 hypertension.

Reproduced with permission from Flynn, J. T., Kaelber, D. C., Baker-Smith, C. M., Blowey, D., Carroll, A. E., Daniels, S. R., de Ferranti, S. D., Dionne, J. M., Falkner, B., Flinn, S. K., Gidding, S. S., Goodwin, C., Leu, M. G., Powers, M. E., Rea, C., Samuels, J., Simasek, M., Thaker, V. V., Urbina, E. M., & Subcommittee on Screening and Management of High Blood Pressure in Children. (2017). Clinical practice guideline for screening and management of high blood pressure in children and adolescents. *Pediatrics, 140*(3), e20171904. https://doi.org/10.1542/peds.2017-1904. Copyright © 2017 by American Academy of Pediatrics.

APPENDIX E.2 • Blood Pressure Levels for Females by Age and Height Percentile

Age (years)	BP Percentile ↓	SBP (mm Hg)							DBP (mm Hg)						
		← Height Percentile or Measured Height →							*← Height Percentile or Measured Height →*						
		5%	*10%*	*25%*	*50%*	*75%*	*90%*	*95%*	*5%*	*10%*	*25%*	*50%*	*75%*	*90%*	*95%*
1	Height (in)	29.7	30.2	30.9	31.8	32.7	33.4	33.9	29.7	30.2	30.9	31.8	32.7	33.4	33.9
	Height (cm)	75.4	76.6	78.6	80.8	83	84.9	86.1	75.4	76.6	78.6	80.8	83	84.9	86.1
	50th	84	85	86	86	87	88	88	41	42	42	43	44	45	46
	90th	98	99	99	100	101	102	102	54	55	56	56	57	58	58
	95th	101	102	102	103	104	105	105	59	59	60	60	61	62	62
	95th + 12 mm Hg	113	114	114	115	116	117	117	71	71	72	72	73	74	74
2	Height (in)	33.4	34	34.9	35.9	36.9	37.8	38.4	33.4	34	34.9	35.9	36.9	37.8	38.4
	Height (cm)	84.9	86.3	88.6	91.1	93.7	96	97.4	84.9	86.3	88.6	91.1	93.7	96	97.4
	50th	87	87	88	89	90	91	91	45	46	47	48	49	50	51
	90th	101	101	102	103	104	105	106	58	58	59	60	61	62	62
	95th	104	105	106	106	107	108	109	62	63	63	64	65	66	66
	95th + 12 mm Hg	116	117	118	118	119	120	121	74	75	75	76	77	78	78
3	Height (in)	35.8	36.4	37.3	38.4	39.6	40.6	41.2	35.8	36.4	37.3	38.4	39.6	40.6	41.2
	Height (cm)	91	92.4	94.9	97.6	100.5	103.1	104.6	91	92.4	94.9	97.6	100.5	103.1	104.6
	50th	88	89	89	90	91	92	93	48	48	49	50	51	53	53
	90th	102	103	104	104	105	106	107	60	61	61	62	63	64	65
	95th	106	106	107	108	109	110	110	64	65	65	66	67	68	69
	95th + 12 mm Hg	118	118	119	120	121	122	122	76	77	77	78	79	80	81
4	Height (in)	38.3	38.9	39.9	41.1	42.4	43.5	44.2	38.3	38.9	39.9	41.1	42.4	43.5	44.2
	Height (cm)	97.2	98.8	101.4	104.5	107.6	110.5	112.2	97.2	98.8	101.4	104.5	107.6	110.5	112.2
	50th	89	90	91	92	93	94	94	50	51	51	53	54	55	55
	90th	103	104	105	106	107	108	108	62	63	64	65	66	67	67
	95th	107	108	109	109	110	111	112	66	67	68	69	70	70	71
	95th + 12 mm Hg	119	120	121	121	122	123	124	78	79	80	81	82	82	83
5	Height (in)	40.8	41.5	42.6	43.9	45.2	46.5	47.3	40.8	41.5	42.6	43.9	45.2	46.5	47.3
	Height (cm)	103.6	105.3	108.2	111.5	114.9	118.1	120	103.6	105.3	108.2	111.5	114.9	118.1	120
	50th	90	91	92	93	94	95	96	52	52	53	55	56	57	57
	90th	104	105	106	107	108	109	110	64	65	66	67	68	69	70
	95th	108	109	109	110	111	112	113	68	69	70	71	72	73	73
	95th + 12 mm Hg	120	121	121	122	123	124	125	80	81	82	83	84	85	85
6	Height (in)	43.3	44	45.2	46.6	48.1	49.4	50.3	43.3	44	45.2	46.6	48.1	49.4	50.3
	Height (cm)	110	111.8	114.9	118.4	122.1	125.6	127.7	110	111.8	114.9	118.4	122.1	125.6	127.7
	50th	92	92	93	94	96	97	97	54	54	55	56	57	58	59
	90th	105	106	107	108	109	110	111	67	67	68	69	70	71	71
	95th	109	109	110	111	112	113	114	70	71	72	72	73	74	74
	95th + 12 mm Hg	121	121	122	123	124	125	126	82	83	84	84	85	86	86

(continued)

APPENDIX E.2 • Blood Pressure Levels for Females by Age and Height Percentile (*continued*)

Age (years)	BP Percentile ↓	SBP (mm Hg) ← *Height Percentile or Measured Height* →							DBP (mm Hg) ← *Height Percentile or Measured Height* →						
		5%	*10%*	*25%*	*50%*	*75%*	*90%*	*95%*	*5%*	*10%*	*25%*	*50%*	*75%*	*90%*	*95%*
7	Height (in)	45.6	46.4	47.7	49.2	50.7	52.1	53	45.6	46.4	47.7	49.2	50.7	52.1	53
	Height (cm)	115.9	117.8	121.1	124.9	128.8	132.5	134.7	115.9	117.8	121.1	124.9	128.8	132.5	134.7
	50th	92	93	94	95	97	98	99	55	55	56	57	58	59	60
	90th	106	106	107	109	110	111	112	68	68	69	70	71	72	72
	95th	109	110	111	112	113	114	115	72	72	73	73	74	74	75
	95th + 12 mm Hg	121	122	123	124	125	126	127	84	84	85	85	86	86	87
8	Height (in)	47.6	48.4	49.8	51.4	53	54.5	55.5	47.6	48.4	49.8	51.4	53	54.5	55.5
	Height (cm)	121	123	126.5	130.6	134.7	138.5	140.9	121	123	126.5	130.6	134.7	138.5	140.9
	50th	93	94	95	97	98	99	100	56	56	57	59	60	61	61
	90th	107	107	108	110	111	112	113	69	70	71	72	72	73	73
	95th	110	111	112	113	115	116	117	72	73	74	74	75	75	75
	95th + 12 mm Hg	122	123	124	125	127	128	129	84	85	86	86	87	87	87
9	Height (in)	49.3	50.2	51.7	53.4	55.1	56.7	57.7	49.3	50.2	51.7	53.4	55.1	56.7	57.7
	Height (cm)	125.3	127.6	131.3	135.6	140.1	144.1	146.6	125.3	127.6	131.3	135.6	140.1	144.1	146.6
	50th	95	95	97	98	99	100	101	57	58	59	60	60	61	61
	90th	108	108	109	111	112	113	114	71	71	72	73	73	73	73
	95th	112	112	113	114	116	117	118	74	74	75	75	75	75	75
	95th + 12 mm Hg	124	124	125	126	128	129	130	86	86	87	87	87	87	87
10	Height (in)	51.1	52	53.7	55.5	57.4	59.1	60.2	51.1	52	53.7	55.5	57.4	59.1	60.2
	Height (cm)	129.7	132.2	136.3	141	145.8	150.2	152.8	129.7	132.2	136.3	141	145.8	150.2	152.8
	50th	96	97	98	99	101	102	103	58	59	59	60	61	61	62
	90th	109	110	111	112	113	115	116	72	73	73	73	73	73	73
	95th	113	114	114	116	117	119	120	75	75	76	76	76	76	76
	95th + 12 mm Hg	125	126	126	128	129	131	132	87	87	88	88	88	88	88
11	Height (in)	53.4	54.5	56.2	58.2	60.2	61.9	63	53.4	54.5	56.2	58.2	60.2	61.9	63
	Height (cm)	135.6	138.3	142.8	147.8	152.8	157.3	160	135.6	138.3	142.8	147.8	152.8	157.3	160
	50th	98	99	101	102	104	105	106	60	60	60	61	62	63	64
	90th	111	112	113	114	116	118	120	74	74	74	74	74	75	75
	95th	115	116	117	118	120	123	124	76	77	77	77	77	77	77
	95th + 12 mm Hg	127	128	129	130	132	135	136	88	89	89	89	89	89	89
12	Height (in)	56.2	57.3	59	60.9	62.8	64.5	65.5	56.2	57.3	59	60.9	62.8	64.5	65.5
	Height (cm)	142.8	145.5	149.9	154.8	159.6	163.8	166.4	142.8	145.5	149.9	154.8	159.6	163.8	166.4
	50th	102	102	104	105	107	108	108	61	61	61	62	64	65	65
	90th	114	115	116	118	120	122	122	75	75	75	75	76	76	76
	95th	118	119	120	122	124	125	126	78	78	78	78	79	79	79
	95th + 12 mm Hg	130	131	132	134	136	137	138	90	90	90	90	91	91	91

APPENDIX E.2 • Blood Pressure Levels for Females by Age and Height Percentile

Age (years)	BP Percentile ↓	SBP (mm Hg)							DBP (mm Hg)						
		← *Height Percentile or Measured Height* →							← *Height Percentile or Measured Height* →						
		5%	*10%*	*25%*	*50%*	*75%*	*90%*	*95%*	*5%*	*10%*	*25%*	*50%*	*75%*	*90%*	*95%*
13	Height (in)	58.3	59.3	60.9	62.7	64.5	66.1	67	58.3	59.3	60.9	62.7	64.5	66.1	67
	Height (cm)	148.1	150.6	154.7	159.2	163.7	167.8	170.2	148.1	150.6	154.7	159.2	163.7	167.8	170.2
	50th	104	105	106	107	108	108	109	62	62	63	64	65	65	66
	90th	116	117	119	121	122	123	123	75	75	75	76	76	76	76
	95th	121	122	123	124	126	126	127	79	79	79	79	80	80	81
	95th + 12 mm Hg	133	134	135	136	138	138	139	91	91	91	91	92	92	93
14	Height (in)	59.3	60.2	61.8	63.5	65.2	66.8	67.7	59.3	60.2	61.8	63.5	65.2	66.8	67.7
	Height (cm)	150.6	153	156.9	161.3	165.7	169.7	172.1	150.6	153	156.9	161.3	165.7	169.7	172.1
	50th	105	106	107	108	109	109	109	63	63	64	65	66	66	66
	90th	118	118	120	122	123	123	123	76	76	76	76	77	77	77
	95th	123	123	124	125	126	127	127	80	80	80	80	81	81	82
	95th + 12 mm Hg	135	135	136	137	138	139	139	92	92	92	92	93	93	94
15	Height (in)	59.7	60.6	62.2	63.9	65.6	67.2	68.1	59.7	60.6	62.2	63.9	65.6	67.2	68.1
	Height (cm)	151.7	154	157.9	162.3	166.7	170.6	173	151.7	154	157.9	162.3	166.7	170.6	173
	50th	105	106	107	108	109	109	109	64	64	64	65	66	67	67
	90th	118	119	121	122	123	123	124	76	76	76	77	77	78	78
	95th	124	124	125	126	127	127	128	80	80	80	81	82	82	82
	95th + 12 mm Hg	136	136	137	138	139	139	140	92	92	92	93	94	94	94
16	Height (in)	59.9	60.8	62.4	64.1	65.8	67.3	68.3	59.9	60.8	62.4	64.1	65.8	67.3	68.3
	Height (cm)	152.1	154.5	158.4	162.8	167.1	171.1	173.4	152.1	154.5	158.4	162.8	167.1	171.1	173.4
	50th	106	107	108	109	109	110	110	64	64	65	66	66	67	67
	90th	119	120	122	123	124	124	124	76	76	76	77	78	78	78
	95th	124	125	125	127	127	128	128	80	80	80	81	82	82	82
	95th + 12 mm Hg	136	137	137	139	139	140	140	92	92	92	93	94	94	94
17	Height (in)	60.0	60.9	62.5	64.2	65.9	67.4	68.4	60.0	60.9	62.5	64.2	65.9	67.4	68.4
	Height (cm)	152.4	154.7	158.7	163.0	167.4	171.3	173.7	152.4	154.7	158.7	163.0	167.4	171.3	173.7
	50th	107	108	109	110	110	110	111	64	64	65	66	66	66	67
	90th	120	121	123	124	124	125	125	76	76	77	77	78	78	78
	95th	125	125	126	127	128	128	128	80	80	80	81	82	82	82
	95th + 12 mm Hg	137	137	138	139	140	140	140	92	92	92	93	94	94	94

BP, blood pressure; DBP, diastolic blood pressure; HTN, hypertension; SBP, systolic blood pressure; elevated BP: ≥90th percentile; stage 1 HTN: ≥95th percentile; stage 2 HTN: ≥95th percentile + 12 mm Hg.

Reproduced with permission from Flynn, J. T., Kaelber, D. C., Baker-Smith, C. M., Blowey, D., Carroll, A. E., Daniels, S. R., de Ferranti, S. D., Dionne, J. M., Falkner, B., Flinn, S. K., Gidding, S. S., Goodwin, C., Leu, M. G., Powers, M. E., Rea, C., Samuels, J., Simasek, M., Thaker, V. V., Urbina, E. M., & Subcommittee on Screening and Management of High Blood Pressure in Children. (2017). Clinical practice guideline for screening and management of high blood pressure in children and adolescents. *Pediatrics*, *140*(3), e20171904. https://doi.org/10.1542/peds.2017-1904. Copyright © 2017 by American Academy of Pediatrics.

INDEX

Note: Page numbers followed by *b*, *d*, *f*, and *t* indicates box material, display material, figure, and table, respectively.

B

C

D

E

G

M

N

O

T

U

QUADM0824